Oxford Textbook of

Medicine

Project Administrator Anna McNeil
Project Editor Dr Irene Butcher
Indexer Caroline Sheard
Production Manager Kate Martin
Production Editor Anna Campbell
Design Manager Andrew Meaden
Typographer Jonathan Coleclough
Illustrations Touch Media, Abingdon
Publisher Alison Langton

volume 3

Oxford Textbook of Medicine

Fourth Edition

Volume 3: Sections 18–33

Edited by

David A. Warrell

Professor of Tropical Medicine and Infectious Diseases and Head, Nuffield Department of Clinical Medicine, University of Oxford; Honorary Consultant Physician, Oxford Radcliffe NHS Trust, UK

Timothy M. Cox

Professor of Medicine, University of Cambridge; Honorary Consultant Physician, Addenbrooke's Hospital, Cambridge, UK

and

John D. Firth

Consultant Physician and Nephrologist, Addenbrooke's Hospital, Cambridge, UK

with

Edward J. Benz Jr

President and CEO, Dana Farber Cancer Institute; Richard and Susan Smith Professor of Medicine, Professor of Pediatrics and Professor of Pathology, Harvard Medical School, Boston, USA

OXFORD
UNIVERSITY PRESS

OXFORD
UNIVERSITY PRESS

Great Clarendon Street, Oxford OX2 6DP

Oxford University Press is a department of the University of Oxford.
It furthers the University's objective of excellence in research, scholarship,
and education by publishing worldwide in

Oxford New York

Auckland Bangkok Buenos Aires Cape Town Chennai
Dar es Salaam Delhi Hong Kong Istanbul Karachi Kolkata
Kuala Lumpur Madrid Melbourne Mexico City Mumbai Nairobi
São Paulo Shanghai Singapore Taipei Tokyo Toronto

Oxford is a registered trade mark of Oxford University Press
in the UK and in certain other countries

Published in the United States
by Oxford University Press Inc., New York

First published 1983
Second edition published 1987
Third edition published 1996
Fourth edition published 2003

British Library Cataloguing in Publication Data
Data available

Library of Congress Cataloging in Publication Data
Data available

ISBN 0–19–262922–0 (Three volume set)
0–19–852787–X (volume 1)
0–19–852788–8 (volume 2)
0–19–852789–6 (volume 3)
Available as a three-volume set only

10 9 8 7 6 5 4 3 2 1

Typeset by Interactive Sciences Ltd, Gloucester, England
Printed in Italy
on acid-free paper by LegoPrint

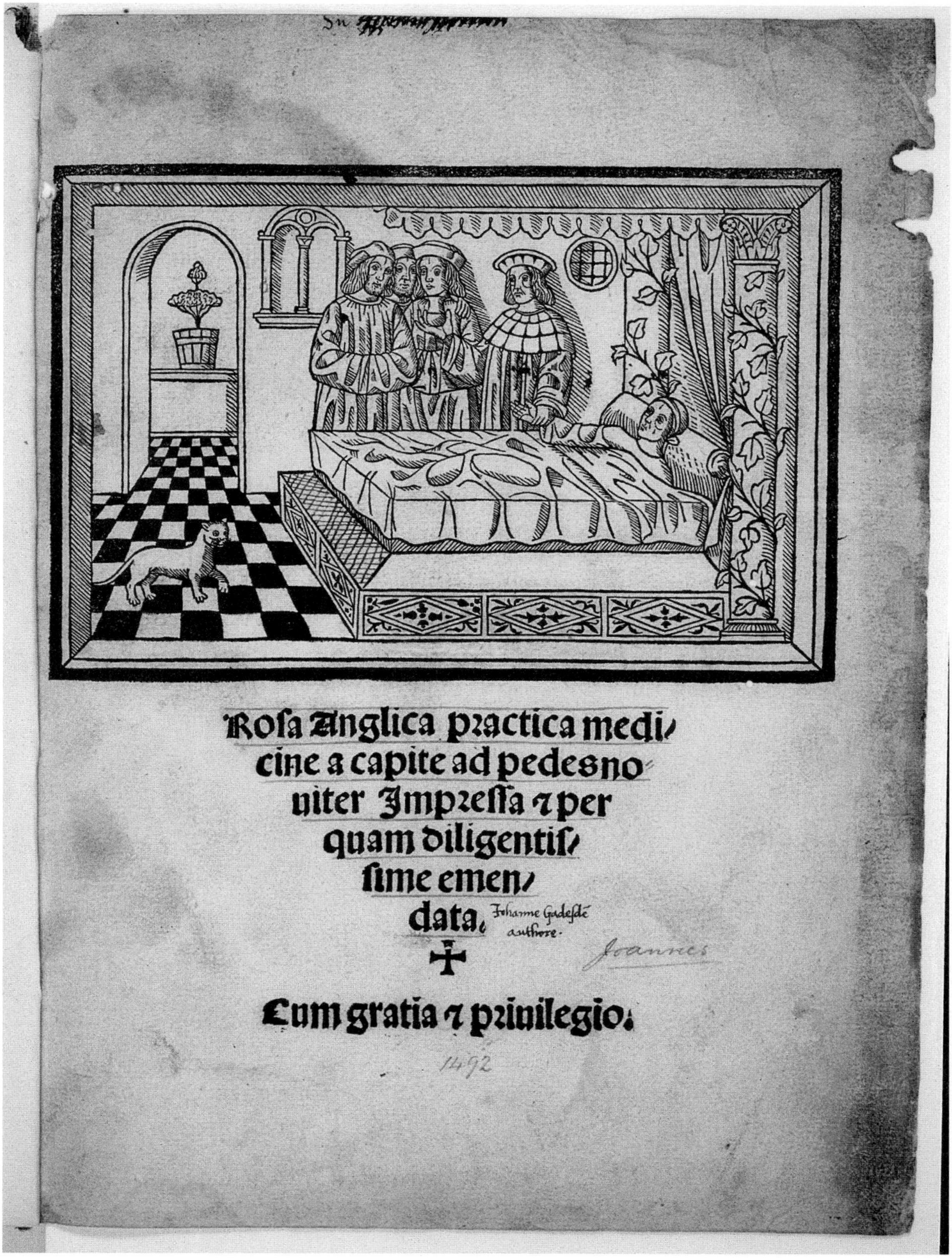

Rosa Anglica practica medicine a capite ad pedes no
uiter Impressa ⁊ per
quam diligentis-
sime emen-
data. Johanne Gadesdē authore.
Joannes

Cum gratia ⁊ priuilegio.

1492

The title page of the 1492 edition of *Rosa Anglica* by John of Gaddesden (1280–1361), which was probably written in 1314. The author was a well known physician attached to Merton College, Oxford in the early part of the 14th century. His famous book was probably the first 'Oxford Textbook of Medicine'. The author was the model for the unsavoury Doctor of Physick in Chaucer's *Canterbury Tales.*

Foreword

by Professor Sir David Weatherall, FRS

It is now 20 years since the first edition of the *Oxford Textbook of Medicine* appeared on the scene, a time when the concept of the all-encompassing textbook of medicine was being questioned. Its predecessor, *Price's Textbook of the Practice of Medicine*, first published in 1922 and by then in its twelfth edition, had come under considerable criticism. One of its most voluble critics, the late J.R.A. Mitchell, had even gone to the trouble of weighing the book, after which he suggested that, because dinosaurs became extinct because of their sheer bulk, medical textbooks would suffer the same fate. In addition, he and many other reviewers suggested that large textbooks are out of date before they are published and hence are of extremely limited value. Notwithstanding Professor Mitchell's outdated views on the extinction of dinosaurs, we thought that he had a point.

After considering these arguments carefully we came to the conclusion that there was still a place for at least one major British work of reference which attempted to cover the whole field of internal medicine.This decision was based largely on the view that, because of the enormous breadth of the subject and the increasing tendency to overspecialization, very few students and practitioners could have immediate access to smaller monographs on every branch of the field; even when they are available they are not always written by those who evaluate their patients in a general medical setting. And if this is true of clinicians in the richer countries, it must apply even more to those in the developing world, where access to libraries and review articles may be limited. Furthermore, although we were well aware that textbooks rapidly become out of date, few advances in medicine lead to major changes in patient care, and those that do often require many years of critical evaluation before they become an integral part of routine clinical practice. For this reason we decided to try to produce a wide-ranging medical textbook which would have a particular emphasis on the global aspects of disease, rather than focus simply on the day-to-day medical problems of the developed world.

Since the *Oxford Textbook of Medicine* first appeared there have been profound changes, both in the practice of medicine and in the problems of the provision of medical care. None of the richer countries has been able to solve the problem of the spiralling costs of health care, which have resulted in part from the introduction of new technology but, even more importantly, from the remarkable increase in the age of their patient populations. If anything, the gap between the quality of the provision of health care between the richer and poorer countries has widened, and although some of the poorer countries have made the epidemiological transition from high death rates due to infection and malnutrition towards a more westernized pattern of illness, particularly in sub-Saharan Africa infectious disease, notably respiratory infection, AIDS, tuberculosis, and malaria, remain the major causes of death; a review of over 11 million childhood deaths in 1998 disclosed, disgracefully, that over 4 million were due to diseases for which adequate vaccines or other forms of prevention already exist. The phenomena of 'globalization', and increasing corporate dominance, are also tending to exacerbate the divide between the rich and poor nations.

Another profound change which has occurred over the last 20 years is the emphasis on the study of disease at the molecular and cellular levels and the increasing role of what is still rather optimistically called 'molecular medicine'. But while this remarkable field promises much for the health of mankind for the future, so far it has had little place in day-to-day clinical practice. Thus, while the fruits of the human genome project offer enormous potential for the better understanding, prevention, and management of the common killers of middle life and old age in richer societies, and the pathogen genome projects offer equal hope for controlling the infectious killers of the developing countries, it is still far from clear when the rich promises of these fields will come to fruition for preventative medicine and clinical care. And there is the danger that when they do, because many of them are likely to be expensive, the gap between the provision of health care in the poorer and richer countries will become even wider. Although many of the solutions to these problems depend on a complete change of attitude of governments and industry in the richer countries, there is no doubt that there will be a rapidly increasing role for their medical schools and doctors to develop collaborative programmes with those of the developing countries and, in general, to take a much more global view of disease, both in medical education and research.

The other major change in the medical field over the last 20 years has been the increasing disquiet about the pattern of medical practice. In many countries doctors have come under increasing criticism for their lack of ability to communicate adequately with patients, for their quality of patient care and, overall, for their lack of humanity. The patient community has become much more sophisticated and demanding, and in most countries there has been a rapid increase in the number of medico-legal actions taken against doctors. This trend has already had wide-ranging repercussions. There has been a major rethink about the pattern of medical education, placing less emphasis on its scientific basis and more on communication skills, ethics, and the social aspects of medicine. The remarkable revolution in the basic biological sciences that underlie medical practice, particularly in the field of genomics, is also raising new ethical issues which would have been undreamed of at the time of the first edition of this book.

In short, medical practice has entered the new millennium in a state of considerable uncertainty. The whole ethos of clinical practice is being questioned, none of the richer countries has got to grips with how to finance the increasing demands of medical care, and many of the poorer countries still have completely dysfunctional health care systems. It is very pleasing therefore to see that the new edition of the *Oxford Textbook of Medicine* reflects so many of these changing issues, as they affect internal medicine. In particular, the textbook has maintained and expanded the aspirations of its original editors towards providing a genuinely global picture of disease, not just as it affects the populations of the richer countries but as it involves the lives of all of those in the poorer countries of the world. As well as continuing to describe the major causes of ill-health and death in the populations of the poorer countries, it includes new sections on screening and the costs of health care, and has greatly increased its coverage of some of the major infectious killers, particularly HIV/AIDS. At the other end of the spectrum it has expanded its sections on the molecular mechanisms of disease and tried to put molecular medicine into perspective by defining its limits. And it has not ignored the remarkable advances in medicine which relate to the richer countries, particularly in its coverage of the problems of the aged. In doing so it has focused on the major killers of Western society, notably cancer, heart disease, and stroke, and has greatly increased the coverage of critical care and emergency medicine. This extensive revision has required the recruitment of many new authors, reflecting a change of over one-third of those from the last edition.

After the publication of the last edition of the *Oxford Textbook of Medicine* my colleague John Ledingham and I decided that it was time to stand aside and pass on our editorial roles to a younger team of editors who are still very active in the fields of medical research and practice. We are delighted to see that our younger colleagues have maintained the tradition of producing a broad-ranging medical textbook which emphasizes the pastoral, scientific, and global aspects of medical care. Despite all its problems medical practice is entering the most exciting and challenging period of its development, and we believe that it still offers the most exciting and enriching of careers for its practitioners. We trust that the 'OTM' will remain their guide and friend for many years to come.

Preface

Textbooks of medicine: *raison d'etre*

Now, in the third millennium, is there any need for a textbook of medicine? Never before has so much information on medical matters been so readily available to so many: physicians are inundated, as are their patients and everyone else. The media seem to carry more and more medical stories in more and more detail every day. The genome has been sequenced. Articulate teenagers speak of stem cells. The internet brings widespread and virtually unlimited access to biomedical information (and misinformation) of a sort: one click of a mouse, and it's all anyone's. A plethora of organizations besieges physicians with guidelines and protocols on every aspect of the practice of medicine. Traditional values are being challenged in all facets of life, including medicine, and there is an unprecedented and entirely appropriate demand for supportive evidence, not just weight of experience, to justify medical interventions.

In these circumstances, some might argue that textbooks of medicine were irrelevant, inappropriate, or even redundant. We strongly refute this. Amidst the maelstrom of 'information' in which physicians now work there is, more than ever, a need for a fixed point of reference, something by which the new, the exciting, and the fashionable can be judged. We make the bold claim that the *Oxford Textbook of Medicine* is just such a fixed point. We argue, unashamedly, that a clinical textbook in the Oslerian tradition is not only required but is essential, to provide expert review, evaluation, and recommendation.

Clinical medicine: changes, challenges, and reconsiderations

This fourth edition of the *Oxford Textbook of Medicine* emerges at a time when discoveries in molecular sciences and advances in technology provide an unprecedented range of diagnostic reagents, drugs, and bioinformatics. Yet, at the same time, there is a widespread recognition that the outcome of treatment for many patients falls short of ideal standards. Microbial resistance to antibiotics, adverse consequences of drugs, and the fallibility of doctors all contribute to failures; and we now realize how dangerous hospitals and clinics can be. Besides this, many contemporary high-tech procedures cannot cure chronic illnesses, and we lack effective weapons to influence the powerful social and behavioural factors that underlie so much illness. The advent of predictive DNA testing also poses complex ethical questions for practitioners, for which few answers are available.

Advances in biomedical science crucially drive innovation and improvement in medical practice. These are not neglected in this book, but the practice of medicine (except in dire emergency) is initiated by a patient talking with a physician and proceeds (as appropriate) through physical examination and investigation to discussion of diagnosis, prognosis, and treatment. These are the core issues of clinical medicine which form the bulk of this textbook.

A culture of public mistrust: the physician–patient relationship

Our political masters in much of the developed world, long tired of being marginalized by old-established networks within the professions, have introduced a new accountability distilled from the concept of audit. This has been exported from the world of finance to embrace the scrutiny of non-financial processes in health care and has created a political climate obsessed with cost effectiveness. The degree of central control often leads to impossible conflicts in the expectations of the public and those entrusted with provision of health care. Baroness O'Neil in her BBC Reith Lectures of 2002* has pointed out that there is often an inconsistency in the demands raised by such control, providing, as it does, perverse incentives for the specious goals and 'output measures' determined by central bodies. While it is true that much better standards of health care delivery are required and careful surveillance of clinical activities is desirable, the *Oxford Textbook of Medicine* presents an affirmation of the physician–patient relationship in the fight against illness, debility, and suffering: for this relationship should remain sacrosanct, based on professional integrity, knowledge, and human feeling.

Aims and emphases: Sir Archibald Garrod's legacy

Garrod first understood the unique interactions between heredity and environment in the genesis of human disease and asked the question: 'Why did this particular person develop this particular illness in this particular environment?' – a question that we are only just beginning to answer in an era of almost naïve enthusiasm for genetics. While the study of the invariant factors in human genetics is almost intoxicating in its simplicity, we now face the formidable challenge of identifying the contribution of the environment, with all its attendant variables, to the generation of the clinical phenotype we define as illness.

This is the background to this edition of the *Oxford Textbook of Medicine*: its remit stretches from disease as it presents to physicians at the bedside, to the attendant disturbances of cellular, tissue, and organ function, all occurring within an individual, inevitably a part of the turmoil of society. To have a complete description of all these aspects of any medical complaint would not be possible, but we recognize that many readers will not have ready access to the latest sources of scientific information. The book is therefore designed to be a proper reference point for both scientific and clinical aspects of medical practice and bears the fingerprints of Osler, Garrod, Doll, and Weatherall, all Regius Professors of Medicine in Oxford.

Limitations and strengths

The bitter practicalities of writing, editing, and producing any book, especially a work of this size, prevent its referring to the last edition of *The*

* *A Question of Trust*. Cambridge University Press 2002.

Lancet, Quarterly Journal of Medicine, New England Journal of Medicine, or any other periodical. But this book can and does provide the medical background against which new information should be assessed and understood. Grounded in the principles that have made the first three editions standard reference textbooks, the new edition has, like medicine itself, evolved to bring all contemporary resources to focus on the teaching and interpretation of medicine. Many new approaches and topics are included and we have incorporated the skill, experience, and perspectives of a truly international complement of highly distinguished authors, including the recently honoured Nobel Laureate in Medicine, Dr Sydney Brenner.

This fourth edition includes, for the first time, an editorial adviser based in the United States (EJB) and a greatly increased and broadened representation of North American authors. By adopting this approach, we hope we have been able to integrate and synthesize in this edition the perspectives on shared medical issues as they confront physicians and medical scientists in different countries.

At a time when there is a tendency for physicians in some parts of the world to be more and more proficient about less and less, this book is a means of their grasping what is happening and what is important in all areas of medical practice. When the movement of people, diseases, and doctors around the world is greater than ever, there is a need for a truly global perspective, which this book provides.

Acknowledgements

This edition contains much that is entirely new, but we wish here to acknowledge that it is built on the firm foundations established by the distinguished co-editors of the previous editions, Professor Sir David Weatherall and Professor John Ledingham. No work of this kind can be produced without the engagement of dedicated professionals who believe in publishing and commit themselves way beyond healthy expectations to see the task through. Mrs Alison Langton has provided guidance and discipline throughout the production and we are enormously grateful to her and her staff at Oxford University Press for their confidence, commitment, and friendship. We are particularly indebted to Dr Irene Butcher who has worked indefatigably to help us realize our aims and at every level has contributed to the organization of the final text and its complex illustrative material. Her experience, knowledge, and uncompromising attention to detail must surely be unique; her forbearance with the editors and, on rare occasions, errant contributors, has been nothing short of miraculous. We thank our contributors for their patience in delivering their sections and review of proofs for which they are responsible. Ultimately, however, the book and any errors it might contain remain the responsibility of the editors.

Finally we thank Mary, Sue, Helen, and Peggy, our constant, supportive, and forgiving wives; Professor Sir David Weatherall, Professor Alastair Compston, Dr Graham Neale, Professor Michael de Swiet, and Dr Michael Sharpe our section advisers; Professor David Lomas, Professor Julian Hopkin, Professor Michael Doherty, Professor David Isenberg, and Dr Christopher Winearls who gave advice and comment for which the editors are very grateful; and our personal secretaries, Eunice Berry (a veteran of four editions), Joan Grantham, Janet Cameron, Naoe Suzuki, and Beverly Comegys for their exceptional dedication.

Oxford, Cambridge, and Boston DAW, TMC, JDF, EJB
January 2003

Contents

12 Endocrine disorders

16 Critical care medicine

17 Respiratory medicine

Volume 3

18 Rheumatology

19 Diseases of the skeleton

20 Nephrology

21 Sexually-transmitted diseases and sexual health

22 Disorders of the blood

23 Diseases of the skin

24 Neurology

Contributors

P. Aaby Research Professor (Novo Nordisk Foundation), Bandim Health Project, Bissau, Guinea-Bissau.
7.10.6 Measles

J. P. Ackers Professor of Postgraduate Education in Public Health, London School of Hygiene and Tropical Medicine, UK.
7.13.13 Trichomoniasis

M. W. Adler Professor of Genitourinary Medicine, Department of Sexually Transmitted Diseases, Royal Free and University College Medical School, London, UK.
21.1 Epidemiology

D. Adu Consultant Nephrologist, Queen Elizabeth Hospital, Birmingham, UK.
20.7.4 Minimal-change nephropathy, focal segmental glomerulosclerosis, and membranous nephtopathy. 20.10.4 The kidney in rheumatological disorders

Graeme J. M. Alexander University Lecturer in Medicine and Honorary Consultant Physician/Hepatologist, University of Cambridge School of Clinical Medicine, Addenbrooke's Hospital, Cambridge, UK.
14.21.4 Liver transplantation

M. Allison Consultant Hepatologist, Hepatobiliary and Transplant Unit, Addenbrooke's Hospital, Cambridge, UK.
5.5 Innate immune system. 14.21.4 Liver transplantation

Chris Andrews Registrar in Anaesthesia, Mater Misericordiae Hospitals, South Brisbane, Queensland, Australia.
8.5.7 Lightning and electrical injuries

Philip Anslow Consultant Neuroradiologist, Radcliffe Infirmary, Oxford, UK.
24.5 Imaging in neurological diseases

Mark J. Arends Senior Lecturer and Honorary Consultant, Pathology Department, University of Cambridge, UK.
4.6 Apoptosis in health and disease

James O. Armitage Dean, College of Medicine, University of Nebraska Medical Center, Omaha, Nebraska, USA.
22.4.3 Lymphoma

J. K. Aronson Reader in Clinical Pharmacology, Radcliffe Infirmary, Oxford, UK.
15.5.1 Pharmacological management of heart failure

Frances M. Ashcroft Royal Society GlaxoSmithKline Research Professor, University Laboratory of Physiology, Oxford, UK.
4.5 Ion channels and disease

T. C. Aw Professor and Head of Division of Occupational Health, Kent Institute of Medicine and Health Sciences, University of Kent at Canterbury, UK.
8.4.1 Occupational and environmental health and safety. 8.5.10 Noise. 8.5.11 Vibration

M. Bagshaw Head of Occupational and Aviation Medicine, British Airways, Harmondsworth, UK.
8.5.5 Aerospace medicine

E. L. Baker Decatur, Georgia, UK.
8.4.1 Occupational and environmental health and safety

L. R. I. Baker Consultant Physician and Nephrologist, London Clinic, London, UK.
20.14 Urinary tract obstruction

C. R. M. Bangham Professor of Immunology, Imperial College Faculty of Medicine, London, UK.
7.10.23 HTLV-I and II and associated diseases

A. P. Banning Consultant Cardiologist, John Radcliffe Hospital, Oxford, UK.
15.3.3 Echocardiography. 15.14.1 Thoracic aortic dissection

D. J. P. Barker Director, MRC Environmental Epidemiology Unit, University of Southampton, UK.
15.4.1.1 Influences acting in utero and early childhood

Roger Barker University Lecturer and Honorary Consultant in Neurology, Department of Neurology, Addenbrooke's Hospital, Cambridge, UK.
24.13.11 Disorders of movement (excluding Parkinson's disease)

D. Barlow Consultant Physician, Department of Genitourinary Medicine, St Thomas's Hospital, London, UK.
7.11.6 Neisseria gonorrhoeae

M. P. Barnes Professor of Neurological Rehabilitation, Hunters Moor Regional Rehabilitation Centre, Newcastle upon Tyne, UK.
24.13.17 Spinal cord injury and its management

John G. Bartlett Chief, Division of Infectious Diseases, Johns Hopkins University School of Medicine, Baltimore, Maryland, USA.
17.5.2.1 Pneumonia—normal host. 17.5.2.2 Nosocomial pneumonia

Christopher Bass Consultant in Liaison Psychiatry, Department of Psychological Medicine, John Radcliffe Hospital, Oxford, UK.
26.5.3 Medically unexplained symptoms in patients attending medical clinics

M. F. Bassendine Professor of Hepatology, Centre for Liver Research, The Medical School, University of Newcastle upon Tyne, UK.
14.20.2.2 Primary biliary cirrhosis

David Bates Professor of Clinical Neurology, Department of Neurology, University of Newcastle upon Tyne, UK.
24.9 Brainstem syndromes. 24.13.1 The unconscious patient

Robert P. Baughman University of Cincinnati Medical Centre, Ohio, USA.
17.11.6 Sarcoidosis

Peter J. Baxter Consultant Physician, Occupational and Environmental Medicine, University of Cambridge, UK.
8.5.12 Disasters: earthquakes, volcanic eruptions, hurricanes, and floods

Peter H. Baylis Provost and Dean of Faculty of Medical Sciences, University of Newcastle upon Tyne, UK.
20.2.1 Water and sodium homeostasis and their disorders

D. Gareth Beevers Professor of Medicine, City Hospital, Birmingham, UK.
15.16.3 Hypertensive emergencies and urgencies

Michael L. Bennish Director, Africa Centre for Health and Population Studies, Mtubatuba, South Africa.
7.11.11 Cholera

M. K. Benson Consultant Physician, Oxford Centre for Respiratory Medicine, Churchill Hospital, Oxford, UK.
17.12 Pleural disease. 17.14.2 Pleural tumours. 17.14.3 Mediastinal tumours and cysts

V. Beral Head, Cancer Research UK Epidemiology Unit, Radcliffe Infirmary, Oxford, UK.
21.6 Cervical cancer and other cancers caused by sexually tramsmitted infections

Anthony R. Berendt Consultant Physician-in-Charge, Bone Infection Unit, Nuffield Orthopaedic Centre, Oxford, UK.
18.7.1 Pyogenic arthritis. 19.3 Osteomyelitis

Nancy Berliner Professor of Medicine and Genetics, Yale School of Medicine, New Haven, Connecticut, USA.
22.4.1 Leucocytes in health and disease. 22.4.2 Introduction to the lymphoproliferative disorders

Michael Besser Professor of Medicine Emeritus, Bart's and The London School of Medicine and Dentistry, Queen Mary College, London, UK.
12.2 Disorders of the anterior pituitary. 12.3 Disorders of the posterior pituitary

Delia B. Bethell Specialist Registrar in Paediatrics, Department of Paediatrics, John Radcliffe Hospital, Oxford, UK.
7.11.1 Diphtheria

Ernest Beutler Chairman, Department of Molecular and Experimental Medicine, The Scripps Research Institute, La Jolla, California, USA.
22.5.11 Erythrocyte enzymopathies

P. C. L. Beverley Professor and Scientific Head, Edward Jenner Institute for Vaccine Research, Compton, Berkshire, UK.
6.5 Tumour immunology

R. W. Bilous Professor of Clinical Medicine, James Cook University Hospital, Middlesbrough, Cleveland, UK.
20.10.1 Diabetes mellitus and the kidney

D. Bilton Consultant in Respiratory Medicine, Papworth Hospital, Cambridge, UK.
17.9 Bronchiectasis

A. E. Bishop Senior Lecturer, Tissue Engineering and Regenerative Medicine Centre, Chelsea and Westminster Hospital, London, UK.
14.8 Hormones and the gastrointestinal tract

Carol M. Black President of the Royal College of Physicians of London and Professor of Rheumatology, Royal Free and University College Medical School, Royal Free Campus, London, UK.
18.10.3 Systemic sclerosis

S. R. Bloom Professor of Medicine and Head, Division of Investigative Science, Imperial College Faculty of Medicine, Hammersmith Campus, London, UK.
12.10 Non-diabetic pancreatic endocrine disorders and multiple endocrine neoplasia. 14.8 Hormones and the gastrointestinal tract

L. D. Blumhardt Emeritus Professor of Clinical Neurology, University of Nottingham, UK.
24.13.5 Syncope. 24.13.16 Diseases of the spinal cord

N. Boon Consultant Cardiologist, Royal Infirmary of Edinburgh, UK.
15.10.4 Cardiac disease in HIV infection

D. R. Booth Senior Hospital Scientist, Institute for Immunology and Allergy Research, Westmead Millennium Institute, Sydney, New South Wales, Australia.
11.12.3 Familial Mediterranean fever and other inherited periodic fever syndromes

Richard T. Booth Professor, Health and Safety Unit, Aston University, Birmingham, UK.
8.4.2 Occupational safety

Leszek K. Borysiewicz Professor and Principal of the Faculty of Medicine, University of Wales, Cardiff, UK.
7.4 The host response to infection

I. C. J. W. Bowler Consultant Microbiologist, Department of Microbiology, John Radcliffe Hospital, Oxford, UK.
7.9 Nosocomial infections

D. J. Bradley Ross Professor of Tropical Hygiene, London School of Hygiene and Tropical Medicine, UK.
7.13.2 Malaria

Thomas Brandt Klinikum Groshadern, Munich, Germany.
24.12.1 Eye movements and balance

P. Brandtzaeg Professor of Paediatrics, Ullevål University Hospital, University of Oslo, Norway.
7.11.5 Meningococcal infections

P. Brasseur Professor and Head of Department of Parasitology, Faculty of Medicine, Rouen, France.
7.13.3 Babesia

J. Braun Professor and Medical Director, Rheumazentrum Ruhrgebiet, Herne, Germany.
18.6 Spondyloarthritides and related arthritides

Sydney Brenner Research Professor, Salk Institute, La Jolla, California, USA, and Honorary Professor of Genetic Medicine, University of Cambridge, UK.
4.2 The human genome sequence

D. P. Brenton Sub Dean (Curriculum), Royal Free and University College Medical School, London, UK.
11.2 Inborn errors of amino acid and organic acid metabolism

Paul H. Brion Rheumatologist in Private Practice, Vista, California, USA.
18.8 Osteoarthritis

Julian Britton Consultant Surgeon, John Radcliffe Hospital, Oxford, UK.
14.3.1 The acute abdomen. 14.18.3.3 Tumours of the pancreas

Anthony F. T. Brown Associate Professor and Senior Staff Specialist, Department of Emergency Medicine, Royal Brisbane Hospital, Queensland, Australia.
16.4 Anaphylaxis

M. J. Brown Professor of Clinical Pharmacology, University of Cambridge and Honorary Consultant Physician, Addenbrooke's Hospital NHS Trust, Cambridge, UK.
15.16.2.3 Primary hyperaldosteronism (Conn's syndrome). 15.16.2.4 Phaeochromocytoma

A. D. M. Bryceson Emeritus Professor of Tropical Medicine, London School of Hygiene and Tropical Medicine, UK.
7.13.12 Leishmaniasis

Philip J. Burke Johns Hopkins Oncology Center, Baltimore, Maryland, USA.
22.3.3 Acute lymphoblastic leukaemia. 22.3.4 Acute myeloblastic leukaemia

G. M. Burnham Associate Professor of International Health, Johns Hopkins Bloomberg School of Public Health, Baltimore, Maryland, USA.
7.14.1 Cutaneous filariasis

Jacky Burrin Professor of Experimental Endocrinology, Bart's and The London School of Medicine and Dentistry, St Bartholomew's Hospital, London, UK.
12.1 Principles of hormone action

Andy Bush Reader in Paediatric Respirology, London, UK.
17.10 Cystic fibrosis

K. Bushby Professor of Neuromuscular Genetics, Institute of Human Genetics, Newcastle upon Tyne, UK.
24.22.2 Muscular dystrophy

Anthony Busuttil Regius Professor of Forensic Medicine, Forensic Medicine Section, Edinburgh University Medical School, UK.
27 Forensic medicine and the practising doctor

T. Butler Professor of Internal Medicine and Chief of Infectious Diseases, Texas Technical University Health Sciences Center, Lubbock, Texas, USA.
7.11.16 Plague

W. F. Bynum Professor of History of Medicine, Wellcome Trust Centre for the History of Medicine at University College London, UK.
2.1 Science in medicine: when, how, and what

I. Byren Consultant in Infectious Diseases and Genito-Urinary Medicine, John Radcliffe Hospital, Oxford, UK.
15.10.3 Cardiovascular syphilis

John Calam* Professor of Medicine, Imperial College London, UK.
14.7 Peptic ulcer diseases

Donald B. Calne Professor Emeritus, University of British Columbia, Vancouver, Canada.
24.13.10 Parkinsonism and other extrapyramidal diseases

P. M. A. Calverley Professor of Medicine (Pulmonary and Rehabilitation), Clinical Science Centre, University Hospital Aintree, Liverpool, UK.
17.7 Chronic respiratory failure

Giovambattista Capasso Professor of Nephrology, Second University of Naples, Italy.
20.13 Urinary stones, nephrocalcinosis, and renal tubular acidosis

* It is with regret that we report the death of Professor John Calam during the preparation of this edition of the textbook.

Jonathan R. Carapetis Senior Lecturer, Research Fellow, and Consultant in Infectious Diseases, Centre for International Child Health, University of Melbourne Department of Paediatrics, Royal Children's Hospital, Melbourne, Australia.
15.10.1 Acute rheumatic fever

Simon Carette Head, Division of Rheumatology, Toronto Western Hospital, Ontario, Canada.
18.4 Back pain and regional disorders

D. J. S. Carmichael Consultant Renal Physician, Southend Hospital, Westcliffe-on-Sea, Essex, UK.
20.16 Drugs and the kidney

D. P. Casemore Senior Research Fellow, CREH, University of Wales, St Asaph, Denbighshire, UK.
7.13.5 Cryptosporidium and cryptosporidiosis. 7.13.6 Cyclospora

D. Catovsky Professor of Haematology, Royal Marsden Hospital and Institute of Cancer Research, London, UK.
22.3.2 The classification of leukaemia. 22.3.5 Chronic lymphocytic leukaemia and other leukaemias of mature B and T cells

Bruce A. Chabner Professor of Medicine, Harvard Medical School and Massachusetts General Hospital, Boston, USA.
6.7 Cancer chemotherapy and radiation therapy

Richard E. Chaisson Professor of Medicine, Epidemiology and International Health, Johns Hopkins University Schools of Medicine and Public Health, Baltimore, Maryland, USA.
7.11.22 Tuberculosis

R. W. Chapman Consultant Gastroenterologist/Hepatologist, John Radcliffe Hospital, Oxford, UK.
14.20.2.3 Primary sclerosing cholangitis

V. Krishna K. Chatterjee Professor of Endocrinology, University of Cambridge, Addenbrooke's Hospital, Cambridge, UK.
12.1 Principles of hormone action

Dominique Chauveau Consultant Nephrologist, Department of Nephrology, Hôpital Necker, Paris, France.
20.9.1 Acute interstitial nephritis

P. F. Chinnery Senior Lecturer in Neurogenetics and Honorary Consultant Neurologist, University of Newcastle upon Tyne and Newcastle upon Tyne Hospitals NHS Trust, UK.
24.22.5 Mitochondrial encephalomyopathies

Seung-Yull Cho Professor, Section of Molecular Parasitology, Sungkyunkwan University School of Medicine, Suwon, Korea.
7.15.4 Pseudophyllidean tapeworms: diphyllobothriasis and sparganosis

Kirpal S. Chugh Professor Emeritus, Department of Nephrology, Postgraduate Institute of Medical Education and Research, Chandigarh, India.
20.7.10 Glomerular disease in the tropics

L. Chwastiak Acting Assistant Professor, Department of Psychiatry, University of Washington, Seattle, USA.
26.5.4 Anxiety and depression

C. M. Clothier Queen's Counsel (retired), London, UK.
1 On being a patient

Andrew J. S. Coats Viscount Royston Professor of Cardiology, Imperial College London and Honorary Consultant Cardiologist, Royal Brompton Hospital, London, UK.
15.2.2 The syndrome of heart failure. 15.5.3 Cardiac rehabilitation

S. M. Cobbe Walton Professor of Medical Cardiology, University of Glasgow, Glasgow Royal Infirmary, UK.
15.2.3 Syncope and palpitation. 15.6 Cardiac arrhythmias

B. J. Cohen Clinical Scientist, Central Public Health Laboratory, London, UK.
7.10.18 Parvovirus B19

J. Cohen Dean and Professor of Infectious Diseases, Brighton and Sussex Medical School, UK.
7.20 Infection in the immunocompromised host

R. D. Cohen Emeritus Professor of Medicine, Bart's and The London School of Medicine and Dentistry, Queen Mary College, University of London, UK.
11.11 Disturbances of acid-base homeostasis

Francis S. Collins Director, National Human Genome Research Institute, Bethesda, Maryland, USA.
4.1 The genomic basis of medicine

R. Collins British Heart Foundation Professor of Medicine and Epidemiology, Clinical Trial Service Unit and Epidemiological Studies Unit, University of Oxford, UK.
2.4.3 Large-scale randomized evidence: trials and overviews

Alastair Compston Professor of Neurology, University of Cambridge, UK.
24.1 Introduction and approach to the patient with neurological disease.
24.16 Demyelinating disorders of the central nervous system

Juliet Compston Reader in Metabolic Bone Diseases and Honorary Consultant Physician, Addenbrooke's Hospital, Cambridge, UK.
19.4 Osteoporosis

C. P. Conlon Consultant Physician in Infectious Diseases, Nuffield Department of Medicine, John Radcliffe Hospital, Oxford, UK.
7.8 Travel and expedition medicine. 7.10.21 HIV and AIDS

Andrew Coop Duke University Medical Center, Durham, North Carolina, USA.
6.2 The nature and development of cancer. 6.3 The genetics of inherited cancers

M. R. Cooper Freelance Science Writer, CAB International, Wallingford, Oxfordshire, UK.
8.3 Poisonous plants and fungi

Susan Copley Consultant Radiologist, Hammersmith Hospital, London, UK.
17.3.1 Thoracic imaging

Fernando F. Costa Professor of Haematology, School of Medical Sciences, Unicamp, Campinas, Brazil.
22.5.10 Disorders of the red cell membrane

J. Couvreur Professeur Associé, Laboratoire de la Toxoplasmose, Institut de Puericulture, Paris, France.
7.13.4 Toxoplasmosis

P. J. Cowen Professor of Psychopharmacology, Warneford Hospital, Oxford, UK.
26.6.1 Psychopharmacology in medical practice

T. M. Cox Professor of Medicine, University of Cambridge, and Honorary Consultant Physician, Addenbrooke's Hospital, Cambridge, UK.
11.3.1 Glycogen storage diseases. 11.3.2 Inborn errors of fructose metabolism. 11.3.3 Disorders of galactose, pentose, and pyruvate metabolism. 11.5 The porphyrias. 11.7.1 Hereditary haemochromatosis. 11.8 Lysosomal storage diseases. 12.13 The pineal gland and melatonin. 14.9.5 Disaccharidase deficiency. 22.5.4 Iron metabolism and its disorders. 33 Emergency medicine

Dorothy H. Crawford Professor of Medical Microbiology, Centre for Infectious Diseases, University of Edinburgh, UK.
7.10.3 The Epstein–Barr virus

Robin A. F. Crawford Consultant Gynaecological Oncologist, Addenbrooke's Hospital, Cambridge, UK.
13.17 Malignant disease in pregnancy

A. J. Crisp Consultant Rheumatologist, Addenbrooke's Hospital, Cambridge, UK.
19.5 Avascular necrosis and related topics

D. W. M. Crook Consultant Microbiologist/Infectious Diseases, John Radcliffe Hospital, Oxford, UK.
24.14.1 Bacterial meningitis

J. Cunningham Professor of Renal and Metabolic Medicine, The Royal London Hospital and Queen Mary's School of Medicine and Dentistry, London, UK.
20.8 Renal tubular disorders

Patrick C. D'Haese Associate Professor, Department of Nephrology and Hypertension, University of Antwerp, Belgium.
20.9.2 Chronic tubulointerstitial nephritis

Tim Dalgleish Research Scientist, MRC Cognitions and Brain Sciences Unit, Cambridge, UK.
26.5.1 Grief, stress, and post-traumatic stress disorder

D. A. B. Dance Director/Consultant Microbiologist, Public Health Laboratory, Derriford Hospital, Plymouth, UK.
7.11.15 Melioidosis and glanders

Chi V. Dang Professor of Medicine and Chief, Hematology Division, Johns Hopkins University School of Medicine, Baltimore, Maryland, USA.
22.3.7 Myelodysplasia

C. J. Danpure Professor of Molecular Cell Biology, Department of Biology, University College London, UK.
11.10 Disorders of oxalate metabolism

John H. Dark Professor of Cardiothoracic Surgery, Freeman Hospital, Newcastle upon Tyne, UK.
15.5.4 Cardiac transplantation and mechanical circulatory support

A. Davenport Consultant Renal Physician/Honorary Senior Lecturer, Centre for Nephrology, Royal Free Hospital, London, UK.
20.3.2 Clinical investigation of renal disease

G. Davey Smith Professor of Clinical Epidemiology, University of Bristol, UK.
15.4.1.2 The epidemiology of ischaemic heart disease

Alun Davies Reader and Honorary Consultant Surgeon, Department of Vascular Surgery, Faculty of Medicine, Imperial College School of Medicine, Charing Cross Hospital, London, UK.
15.14.2 Peripheral arterial disease

P. D. O. Davies Consultant Physician, Fazakerley Hospital, Liverpool, UK.
7.11.23 Disease caused by environmental mycobacteria

Alex M. Davison Professor and Consultant Renal Physician, St James's University Hospital, Leeds, UK.
20.3.1 The clinical presentation of renal disease

Marc E. De Broe Professor in Medicine, Department of Nephrology, University of Antwerp, Belgium.
20.9.2 Chronic tubulointerstitial nephritis

P. de la Motte Hall Professor, Division of Anatomical Pathology, Faculty of Health Sciences, University of Cape Town, South Africa.
14.21.6 Hepatic granulomas

M. de Swiet Professor of Obstetric Medicine, Queeen Charlotte's and Chelsea Hospital, London, UK.
13.7 Thromboembolism in pregnancy. 13.8 Chest diseases in pregnancy

Barbara A. Degar Yale School of Medicine, New Haven, Connecticut, USA.
22.4.2 Introduction to the lymphoproliferative disorders

Eric Demoncheaux Research Associate, Medical School, University of Sheffield, UK.
15.15.1 The pulmonary circulation and its influence on gas exchange

D. M. Denison Emeritus Professor of Clinical Physiology, Royal Brompton Hospital, London, UK.
8.5.5 Aerospace medicine. 8.5.6 Diving medicine

John Dent Director, Department of Gastroenterology, Hepatology and General Medicine and Clinical Professor of Medicine, Royal Adelaide Hospital/ Adelaide University, Australia.
14.6 Diseases of the oesophagus

Christopher P. Denton Senior Lecturer/Consultant Rheumatologist, Centre for Rheumatology, Royal Free Hospital, London, UK.
18.10.3 Systemic sclerosis

Ulrich Desselberger Consultant Virologist and Director, Clinical Microbiology and Public Health Laboratory, Addenbrooke's Hospital, Cambridge, UK.
7.10.7 Enterovirus infections. 7.10.8 Virus infections causing diarrhoea and vomiting

Charles A. Dinarello Professor of Medicine, University of Colorado, Denver, Colorado, USA.
4.4 Cytokines: interleukin-1 and tumour necrosis factor in inflammation

A. K. Dixon Professor of Radiology and Honorary Consultant Radiologist, University of Cambridge and Addenbrooke's Hospital, Cambridge, UK.
14.18.2 Computed tomography and magnetic resonance imaging of the liver and pancreas

Michael Doherty Professor of Rheumatology, University of Nottingham Medical School, UK.
18.3 Clinical investigation. 18.9 Crystal-related arthropathies

R. Doll Emeritus Professor of Medicine and Honorary Member, Cancer Studies Unit, Nuffield Department of Medicine, Radcliffe Infirmary, Oxford, UK.
6.1 Epidemiology of cancer

Michael Donaghy Reader in Clinical Neurology, University of Oxford, Honorary Consultant Neurologist, Radcliffe Infirmary, and Honorary Civilian Consultant in Neurology to the Army, Oxford, UK.
24.13.13 The motor neurone diseases

Dominique Droz Unite de Pathologie Renale, Hôpital Necker, Paris, France.
20.9.1 Acute interstitial nephritis

R. M. du Bois Professor of Respiratory Medicine, National Heart and Lung Institute, University College London and Consultant Physician, Royal Brompton Hospital, London, UK.
17.11.1 Diffuse parenchymal lung disease: an introduction. 17.11.2 Cryptogenic fibrosing alveolitis. 17.11.3 Bronchiolitis obliterans and organizing pneumonia. 17.11.4 The lungs and rheumatological diseases. 17.11.5 The lung in vasculitis

C. R. K. Dudley Consultant Renal Physician, The Richard Bright Renal Unit Southmead Hospital, North Bristol NHS Trust, Bristol, UK.
15.14.3 Cholesterol embolism

D. W. Dunne Reader in Immunoparasitology, Department of Pathology, University of Cambridge, UK.
7.16.1 Schistosomiasis

David T. Durack Consulting Professor of Medicine, Duke University, Durham, North Carolina and Vice-President, Corporate Medical Affairs, Becton Dickinson & Co., Franklin Lakes, New Jersey, USA.
7.2 Fever of unknown origin

S. R. Durham Professor of Allergy and Respiratory Medicine, Imperial College Faculty of Medicine, National Heart and Lung Hospital, and Royal Brompton Hospital, London, UK.
17.4.2 Allergic rhinitis ('hay fever')

P. N. Durrington Professor of Medicine, University of Manchester Department of Medicine, Manchester Royal Infirmary, UK.
11.6 Lipid and lipoprotein disorders

M. Eastwood Post-Retirement Honorary Fellow, Department of Medical Sciences, Western General Hospital, Edinburgh, UK.
10.3 Vitamins and trace elements

Jonathan C. W. Edwards Professor in Connective Tissue Medicine, University College London, UK.
18.1 Joints and connective tissue: introduction

Richard Edwards Emeritus Professor of Medicine, University of Liverpool, UK.
24.22.4 Metabolic and endocrine disorders

M. Elia Professor of Clinical Nutrition and Metabolism, Institute of Human Nutrition, University of Southampton, UK.
10.6 Special nutritional problems and the use of enteral and parenteral nutrition

Matthew J. Ellis Associate Professor of Medicine and Director, Breast Cancer Program, Duke University Medical Center, Durham, North Carolina, USA.
6.2 The nature and development of cancer. 6.3 The genetics of inherited cancers

Monique M. Elseviers Department of Nephrology-Hypertension, University Hospital Antwerp, Belgium.
20.9.2 Chronic tubulointerstitial nephritis

M. A. Epstein Emeritus Professor of Pathology, University of Bristol, UK.
7.10.3 The Epstein–Barr virus

E. Ernst Professor and Director, Department of Complementary Medicine, University of Exeter, UK.
2.5 Complementary and alternative medicine

David Eschenbach Professor, Department of Obstetrics and Gynecology, University of Washington, Seattle, USA.
21.4 Pelvic inflammatory disease

S. M. Evans Specialist Registrar in Gastroenterology, Royal Sussex County Hospital, Brighton, UK.
8.5.8 Podoconiosis

S. J. Eykyn Professor (and Honorary Consultant) in Clinical Microbiology, St Thomas' Hospital, London, UK.
7.11.2 Streptococci and enterococci. 7.11.4 Staphylococci. 7.11.10 Anaerobic bacteria. 15.10.2 Infective endocarditis

C. A. Eynon Director of Neurosciences Intensive Care, Southampton University Hospital NHS Trust, UK.
16.3 Cardiac arrest. 33 Emergency medicine

Christopher G. Fairburn Wellcome Principal Research Fellow and Professor of Psychiatry, Oxford University Department of Psychiatry, Warneford Hospital, Oxford, UK.
26.5.5 Eating disorders

J. J. Farrar Senior Fellow, Wellcome Trust, University of Oxford Clinical Research Unit, The Hospital for Tropical Diseases, Ho Chi Minh, Vietnam.
24.14.1 Bacterial meningitis. 24.14.2 Viral infections of the central nervous system

Ken Farrington Consultant Nephrologist, Lister Hospital, Stevenage, Hertfordshire, UK.
20.6.1 Haemodialysis

D. T. Fearon Wellcome Trust Professor of Medicine, University of Cambridge, UK.
5.5 Innate immune system

John Feehally Professor of Renal Medicine, Leicester General Hospital, UK.
20.7.2 IgA nephropathy and Henoch-Schönlein purpura. 20.7.3 Thin membrane nephropathy

Alvan R. Feinstein* Professor, Yale University School of Medicine, New Haven, Connecticut, USA.
2.4.2 Evidence-based medicine

Eleanor Feldman Consultant Liaison Psychiatrist and Honorary Senior Lecturer, University of Oxford, John Radcliffe Hospital, Oxford, UK.
26.2 Taking a psychiatric history from a medical patient. 26.4 Acute behavioural emergencies

Peter J. Fenner Associate Professor, Schools of Medicine and Health Sciences, James Cook University and National Medical Officer, Surf Life Saving Association of Australia, Mackay, North Queensland, Australia.
8.5.3 Drowning

Robert Ferrari Clinical Assistant Professor, University of Alberta Hospital, Edmonton, Canada.
18.2 Clinical presentation and diagnosis of rheumatic disease

C. ffrench-Constant Professor of Neurological Genetics, University of Cambridge, UK.
24.21 Developmental abnormalities of the central nervous system

R. G. Finch Professor of Infectious Diseases, City Hospital and University of Nottingham, UK.
7.6 Antimicrobial chemotherapy

H. Firth Consultant in Medical Genetics, Department of Medical Genetics, Addenbrooke's Hospital, Cambridge, UK.
24.21 Developmental abnormalities of the central nervous system

J. Firth Consultant Physician and Nephrologist, Addenbrooke's Hospital, Cambridge, UK.
13.5 Renal disease in pregnancy. 15.15.2.2 Pulmonary oedema. 15.15.3.1 Deep venous thrombosis and pulmonary embolism. 15.18 Idiopathic oedema of women. 16.1 The clinical approach to the patient who is very ill. 20.2.2 Disorders of potassium homeostasis. 20.4 Acute renal failure. 33 Emergency medicine

Susan Fisher-Hoch Professor, University of Texas School of Public Health at Brownsville, USA.
7.10.15 Arenaviruses. 7.10.16 Filoviruses

Robert A. Fishman Professor of Neurology Emeritus, University of California San Francisco School of Medicine, USA.
24.7 Lumbar puncture

Edward D. Folland Associate Director of Cardiology and Professor of Medicine, UMass Memorial Medical Center/University of Massachusetts Medical School, Worcester, Maryland, USA.
15.3.6 Cardiac catheterization and angiography. 15.4.2.4 Percutaneous interventional cardiac procedures

J. C. Forfar Consultant Cardiologist, John Radcliffe Hospital, Oxford and Honorary Senior Lecturer, University of Oxford, UK.
13.6 Heart disease in pregnancy

I. S. Foulds Consultant Dermatologist, City Hospital, Birmingham, UK.
8.4.1 Occupational and environmental health and safety

Keith A. A. Fox Professor of Cardiology, Royal Infirmary and University of Edinburgh, UK.
15.4.2.3 Management of acute coronary syndromes: unstable angina and myocardial infarction

Richard Frackowiak Vice Provost (Biomedicine), University College London, Institute of Neurology, London, UK.
24.3 Brain and mind: functional neuroimaging

T. J. R. Francis Consultant in Diving Medicine, Tintagel, Cornwall, UK.
8.5.6 Diving medicine

Keith N. Frayn Professor of Human Metabolism, Oxford Centre for Diabetes, Endocrinology and Metabolism, University of Oxford, UK.
10.2 Nutrition: biochemical background

Alan Freeman Consultant Radiologist, Addenbrooke's Hospital, Cambridge, UK.
14.2.3 Radiology of the gastrointestinal tract

Peggy Frith Consultant Ophthalmic Physician, The Eye Hospital, Radcliffe Infirmary, Oxford and University College London Hospital, UK.
25 The eye in general medicine

Patrick G. Gallagher Associate Professor, Department of Pediatrics, Yale University School of Medicine, New Haven, Connecticut, USA.
22.5.10 Disorders of the red cell membrane

Clare J. Galton Specialist Registrar in Neurology, Neurology Department, Addenbrooke's Hospital, Cambridge, UK.
24.13.8 Alzheimer's disease and other dementias

Hector H. Garcia Associate Professor, Department of Microbiology, Universidad Peruana Cayetano Heredia and Head, Cysticercosis Unit, Department of Transmissible Diseases, Instituto de Ciencias Neurologicas, Lima, Peru.
7.15.1 Cystic hydatid disease (Echinococcus granulosus). 7.15.3 Cysticercosis

K. Gardiner Professor and Managing Director, International Occupational Health Ltd., Birmingham, UK.
8.4.1 Occupational and environmental health and safety

Lawrence B. Gardner Assistant Professor of Medicine, Johns Hopkins University school of Medicine, Baltimore, Maryland, USA.
22.3.7 Myelodysplasia

Christopher S. Garrard Consultant Physician in Intensive Care, John Radcliffe Hospital, Oxford, UK.
16.5.2 The management of respiratory failure

J. S. H. Gaston Professor of Rheumatology, University of Cambridge School of Medicine, Addenbrooke's Hospital, Cambridge, UK.
18.7.2 Reactive arthritis

Duncan Geddes Professor of Respiratory Medicine, Royal Brompton Hospital, London, UK.
17.10 Cystic fibrosis

D. G. Gibson Consultant Cardiologist, Royal Brompton Hospital, London, UK.
15.7 Valve disease. 15.9 Pericardial disease

G. J. Gibson Professor of Respiratory Medicine/Consultant Physician, Freeman Hospital, Newcastle upon Tyne, UK.
17.3.2 Respiratory function tests

A. M. Giles Scientific Officer, Health Systems, Oxford, UK.
32 Reference intervals for biochemical data

I. P. Giles ARC Research Fellow, Bloomsbury Rheumatology Unit, London, UK.
18.10.1 Autoimmune rheumatic disorders and vasculitis

Charles F. Gilks Professor of Tropical Medicine and Senior Adviser on Care, HIV/AIDS Department, World Health Organization, Geneva, Switzerland.
7.10.22 HIV in the developing world

Michael D. J. Gillmer Consultant Obstetrician and Gynaecologist, Women's Centre, John Radcliffe Hospital, Oxford, UK.
13.10 Diabetes in pregnancy

Robert H. Gilman Professor, Department of International Health, Johns Hopkins School of Public Health, Baltimore, Maryland, USA and Research Professor, Universidad Peruana Cayetano Heredia, Lima, Peru.
7.15.3 Cysticercosis

A. E. S. Gimson Consultant Physician and Hepatologist, Cambridge Liver Transplantation Unit, Addenbrooke's Hospital, Cambridge, UK.
13.9 Liver and gastrointestinal diseases during pregnancy. 14.18.1 The structure and function of the liver, biliary tract, and pancreas

P. Glasziou Huntington Centre for Risk Analysis, Boston, Massachusetts, USA.
2.4.1 Bringing the best evidence to the point of care

* It is with regret that we report the death of Professor Alvan R. Feinstein during the preparation of this edition of the textbook.

Peter J. Goadsby Professor of Clinical Neurology, Institute of Neurology, University College and The National Hospital for Neurology and Neurosurgery, London, UK.
24.13.2 Headache

D. Goldblatt Reader in Immunology and Consultant Paediatric Immunologist, Institute of Child Health, Great Ormond Hospital for Children NHS Trust, London, UK.
7.7 Immunization

John M. Goldman Professor of Leukaemia Biology and Chairman, Department of Haematology, Imperial College School of Medicine, London, UK.
22.3.6 Chronic myeloid leukaemia

Irwin Goldstein Director, Institute for Sexual Medicine and Professor of Urology and Gynecology, Boston University School of Medicine, Massachusetts, USA.
12.8.4 Sexual dysfunction

Armando E. Gonzalez Department of Public Health, School of Veterinary Medicine, Universidad Nacional Mayor de San Marcos, Lima, Peru.
7.15.1 Cystic hydatid disease (Echinococcus granulosus)

Timothy H. J. Goodship Reader in Nephrology, University of Newcastle upon Tyne and Consultant Nephrologist, Royal Victoria Infirmary, Newcastle upon Tyne, UK.
20.10.6 Haemolytic uraemic syndrome

Sherwood L. Gorbach Department of Community Health and Medicine, TUFTS University School of Medicine, Boston, Massachusetts, USA.
14.17 Gastrointestinal infections

E. C. Gordon-Smith Professor of Haematology, St George's Hospital Medical School, London, UK.
22.3.11 Aplastic anaemia and other causes of bone marrow failure. 22.8.2 Haemopoietic stem cell transplantation

J. M. Grange Visiting Professor, University College London, Centre for Infectious Diseases and International Health, Royal Free and University College Medical School, London, UK.
7.11.23 Disease caused by environmental mycobacteria

R. Gray Professor of Medical Statistics and Director, University of Birmingham Clinical Trials Unit, UK.
2.4.3 Large-scale randomized evidence: trials and overviews

John R. Graybill Professor, University of Texas Health Science Center, San Antonio, Texas, USA.
7.12.3 Coccidioidomycosis

Jackie Green Director, Centre for Health Promotion Research, Leeds Metropolitan University, Leeds, UK.
3.5 Health promotion

Brian M. Greenwood Professor of Clinical Tropical Medicine, London School of Hygiene and Tropical Medicine, London, UK.
7.11.3 Pneumococcal diseases

Roger Greenwood Consultant Nephrologist and Lead Clinician, Lister Hospital, Stevenage, Hertfordshire, UK.
20.6.1 Haemodialysis

B. Gribbin Honorary Consultant Cardiologist, John Radcliffe Hospital, Oxford, UK.
15.10.3 Cardiovascular syphilis. 15.14.1 Thoracic aortic dissection

John Grimley Evans Professor Emeritus of Clinical Geratology, Green College, Oxford, UK.
30.1 Medicine in old age

Michael L. Grossbard Chief, Hematology/Oncology, St Luke's-Roosevelt Hospital and Beth Israel Medical Center, New York, USA.
6.7 Cancer chemotherapy and radiation therapy

David I. Grove Professor and Director, Clinical Microbiology and Infectious Diseases, The Queen Elizabeth Hospital, Adelaide, Australia.
7.14.5 Nematode infections of lesser importance. 7.16.2 Liver fluke infections. 7.16.4 Intestinal trematode infections

J. P. Grünfeld Professor of Nephrology, Université Paris V - René Descartes and Head of Nephrology, Hôpital Necker, Paris, France.
20.11 Renal involvement in genetic disease

D. J. Gubler Director, Division of Vector-Borne Infectious Diseases, Centers for Disease Control and Prevention, Fort Collins, Colorado, USA.
7.10.11 Alphaviruses. 7.10.13 Flaviviruses

Mark Gurnell Specialist Registrar and Research Fellow, Department of Medicine, Division of Endocrinology and Metabolism, Addenbrooke's Hospital, Cambridge, UK.
12.1 Principles of hormone action

David M. Gustin Section of Hematology–Oncology, University of Chicago, Illinois, USA.
22.3.8 The polycythaemias. 22.3.10 Thrombocytosis

M. R. Haeney Consultant Immunologist, Salford Royal Hospitals NHS Trust, Salford, Manchester, UK.
14.4 Immune disorders of the gastrointestinal tract

Davidson H. Hamer Director, Traveler's Health Service, Tufts-New England Medical Center and Assistant Professor of Medicine and Nutrition, Tufts University, Boston, Massachusetts, USA.
14.17 Gastrointestinal infections

P. J. Hammond Consultant Physician and Endocrinologist, Harrogate District Hospital, Yorkshire, UK.
12.10 Non-diabetic pancreatic endocrine disorders and multiple endocrine neoplasia. 14.8 Hormones and the gastrointestinal tract

J. R. Hampton Professor of Cardiology, Queen's Medical Centre, Nottingham, UK.
15.2.1 Chest pain. 15.2.4 Physical examination of the cardiovascular system

M. Hanna Consultant Neurologist and Reader in Clinical Neurology, National Hospital for Neurology and Neurosurgery and Institute of Neurology, University College London, UK.
24.22.1 Introduction: structure and function

David M. Hansell Professor of Thoracic Imaging, Royal Brompton Hospital, London, UK.
17.3.1 Thoracic imaging

P. Harnden Consultant Urological Pathologist, Cancer Research UK Clinical Centre, St James's University Hospital, Leeds, UK.
20.15 Tumours of the urinary tract

J. M. Harrington Emeritus Professor of Occupational Health, University of Birmingham, UK.
8.4.1 Occupational and environmental health and safety

Anthony Harrison Fellow in Health Systems, King's Fund, London, UK.
3.3 The pattern of care: hospital and community

J. R. Harrison Force Medical Adviser, Sussex Police Authority, Lewes, UK.
8.5.9 Radiation

C. Haslett Professor of Respiratory Medicine, Royal Infirmary, Edinburgh, UK.
16.5.1 Pathophysiology and pathogenesis of acute respiratory distress syndrome. 17.1.3 'First line' defence mechanisms of the lung

Adrian R. W. Hatfield Consultant Gastroenterologist, The Middlesex Hospital, London, UK.
14.2.2 Upper gastrointestinal endoscopy

P. N. Hawkins Professor of Medicine, Royal Free and University College Medical School, London, UK.
11.12.3 Familial Mediterranean fever and other inherited periodic fever syndromes. 11.12.4 Amyloidosis

Keith Hawton Professor of Psychiatry, University Department of Psychiatry and Director and Consultant Psychiatrist, Centre for Suicide Research, Warneford Hospital, Oxford, UK.
26.5.2 The patient who has attempted suicide

R. J. Hay Professor and Dean, Faculty of Medicine and Health Sciences, Queens University, Belfast, UK.
7.11.27 Nocardiosis. 7.12.1 Fungal infections

B. Hazleman Consultant Rheumatologist, Rheumatology Department, Addenbrooke's Hospital, Cambridge, UK.
18.11 Miscellaneous conditions presenting to the rheumatologist

Nick Heather Consultant Clinical Psychologist and Director, Centre for Alcohol and Drug Studies, Newcastle, North Tyneside, and Northumberland Mental Health NHS Trust, Newcastle upon Tyne, UK.
26.7.2 Brief interventions against excessive alcohol consumption

David B. Hellmann Professor, Johns Hopkins University School of Medicine, Baltimore, Maryland, USA.
18.10.7 Polymyositis and dermatomyositis

D. J. Hendrick Consultant Physician and Professor of Occupational Respiratory Medicine, Royal Victoria Infirmary, University of Newcastle upon Tyne, UK.
17.11.8 Pulmonary haemorrhagic disorders. 17.11.9 Eosinophilic pneumonia. 17.11.10 Lymphocytic infiltrations of the lung. 17.11.11 Extrinsic allergic alveolitis. 17.11.12 Eosinophilic granuloma of the lung and pulmonary lymphangiomyomatosis. 17.11.13 Pulmonary alveolar proteinosis. 17.11.14 Pulmonary amyloidosis. 17.11.15 Lipoid (lipid) pneumonia. 17.11.16 Pulmonary alveolar microlithiasis. 17.11.17 Toxic gases and fumes. 17.11.18 Radiation pneumonitis. 17.11.19 Drug-induced lung disease

Mark Herbert Clinical Lecturer in Neonatal Paediatrics, Department of Paediatrics, University of Oxford, UK.
13.15 Infections in pregnancy

Andrew Herxheimer Emeritus Fellow, UK Cochrane Centre, London, UK.
9 Principles of clinical pharmacology and drug therapy

Martin F. Heyworth Chief of Staff and Clinical Professor of Medicine, VA Medical Center and University of Pennsylvania, Philadelphia, USA.
7.13.8 Giardiasis, balantidiasis, isosporiasis, and microsporidiosis

Tim Higenbottam Global Clinical Expert, Astra-Zeneca, Charnwood, Leicestershire and Visiting Professor of Medicine, University of Sheffield, UK.
15.15.1 The pulmonary circulation and its influence on gas exchange. 15.15.2.1 Primary pulmonary hypertension

Katherine A. High William H. Bennett Professor of Pediatrics, University of Pennsylvania School of Medicine and The Children's Hospital of Philadelphia, Pennsylvania, USA.
22.6.4 Genetic disorders of coagulation

S. L. Hillier Research Associate Professor of Obstetrics and Gynecology, University of Washington, Seattle, USA.
21.3 Vaginal discharge

David Hilton-Jones Clinical Director, Oxford MDC Muscle and Nerve Centre, Radcliffe Infirmary, Oxford, UK.
24.17 Disorders of the neuromuscular junction. 24.22.3 Myotonia. 24.22.4 Metabolic and endocrine disorders

John R. Hodges Professor of Behavioural Neurology, MRC Cognition and Brain Sciences Unit and Department of Neurology, Addenbrooke's Hospital, Cambridge, UK.
24.8 Disturbances of higher cerebral function. 24.13.8 Alzheimer's disease and other dementias

H. J. F. Hodgson Sheila Sherlock Professor of Medicine and Director, Centre for Hepatology, Royal Free and University College Medical School, London, UK.
14.9.6 Whipple's disease. 14.20.1 Viral hepatitis—clinical aspects. 14.20.2.1 Autoimmune hepatitis

A. V. Hoffbrand Emeritus Professor of Haematology, Royal Free and University College School of Medicine, London, UK.
22.5.6 Megaloblastic anaemia and miscellaneous deficiency anaemias

Ronald Hoffman Professor, Hematology-Oncology Section University of Illinois College of Medicine, Chicago, USA.
22.3.8 The polycythaemias. 22.3.10 Thrombocytosis

P. A. H. Holloway Consultant Chemical Pathologist in Intensive Care and Honorary Reader in Medicine, John Radcliffe Hospital, Oxford, UK.
32 Reference intervals for biochemical data

Richard H. Holloway Associate Professor of Medicine and Senior Consultant Gastroenterologist, Department of Gastroenterology, Hepatology and General Medicine, Royal Adelaide Hospital, Australia.
14.6 Diseases of the oesophagus

J. M. Hopkin Professor, Experimental Medicine Unit, Swansea Clinical School, University of Wales, Swansea, UK.
17.4.1 Asthma: genetic effects. 17.15 The genetics of lung diseases

Carol Ann Huff Assistant Professor of Oncology, Sidney Kimmel Comprehensive Cancer Care at Johns Hopkins, Baltimore, Maryland, USA.
26.7.3 Problems of alcohol and drug users in the hospital

I. A. Hughes Professor of Paediatrics and Honorary Consultant Paediatric Enterologist, Department of Paediatrics, University of Cambridge, UK.
12.7.2 Congenital adrenal hyperplasia

Lawrence Impey Consultant in Fetal Medicine, The Women's Centre, John Radcliffe Hospital, Oxford, UK.
13.15 Infections in pregnancy

C. W. Imrie Consultant Surgeon and Honorary Professor, Lister Department of Surgery, Royal Infirmary, Glasgow, UK.
14.18.3.1 Acute pancreatitis

H. Irving Consultant Radiologist, St James's University Hospital, Leeds, UK.
20.15 Tumours of the urinary tract

P. G. Isaacson Professor of Histopathology, Royal Free and University College Medical School, London, UK.
14.9.4 Gastrointestinal lymphoma

D. A. Isenberg The Arthritis Research Campaign Professor of Rheumatology at University College London, Centre for Rheumatology, London, UK.
18.10.1 Autoimmune rheumatic disorders and vasculitis. 18.10.2 Systemic lupus erythematosus and related disorders

C. G. Isles Consultant Physician, Medical Unit, Dumfries and Galloway Royal Infirmary, Dumfries, UK.
15.16.1.1 Prevalence, epidemiology, and pathophysiology of hypertension

C. Ison Reader in Medical Microbiology, Department of Infectious Diseases and Microbiology, Faculty of Medicine, Imperial College, St Mary's Campus, London, UK.
7.11.6 Neisseria gonorrhoeae

Alan A. Jackson Professor and Director, Institute of Human Nutrition, University of Southampton, UK.
10.4 Severe malnutrition

H. S. Jacobs Emeritus Professor of Reproductive Endocrinology, University College London Medical School, UK.
12.8.1 Ovarian disorders. 12.8.3 The breast

Robin Jacoby Professor of Old Age Psychiatry, University of Oxford Department of Psychiatry, Warneford Hospital, Oxford, UK.
30.2 Mental disorders of old age

O. F. W. James Head of Clinical Medical Sciences, Medical School, University of Newcastle upon Tyne, UK.
14.21.1 Alcoholic liver disease and non-alcoholic steatosis hepatitis

Paul J. Jenkins Senior Lecturer in Endocrinology, St Bartholomew's Hospital, London, UK.
12.2 Disorders of the anterior pituitary

B. Jennett Emeritus Professor of Neurosurgery, Institute of Neurological Sciences, University of Glasgow, UK.
24.13.6 Brain death and the vegetative state

D. P. Jewell Professor of Gastroenterology, John Radcliffe Hospital, Oxford, UK.
14.9.3 Coeliac disease. 14.10 Crohn's disease. 14.11 Ulcerative colitis. 14.22 Miscellaneous disorders of the gastrointestinal tract and liver

Vivekanand Jha Associate Professor of Nephrology, Postgraduate Institute of Medical Education and Research, Chandigarh, India.
20.7.10 Glomerular disease in the tropics

Anne M. Johnson Professor of Infectious Disease Epidemiology and Head, Department of Primary Care and Population Sciences, University College London, UK.
21.2 Sexual behaviour

A. W. Johnson CAB International, Wallingford, Oxfordshire, UK.
8.3 Poisonous plants and fungi

E. Anthony Jones Chief of Hepatology, Academic Medical Centre, Amsterdam, The Netherlands.
14.21.3 Hepatocellular failure

N. Jones Department of Virology, John Radcliffe Hospital, Oxford, UK.
7.10.25 Orf. 7.10.26 Molluscum contagiosum

S. E. Jones Research Associate, Department of Biology, Imperial College of Science, Technology and Medicine, London, UK.
7.11.33 Syphilis

Kenneth C. Kalunian Professor of Medicine, UCLA School of Medicine, Los Angeles, California, USA.
18.8 Osteoarthritis

Eileen Kaner NHS Primary Care Career Scientist, School of Population and Health Sciences, University of Newcastle upon Tyne, UK.
26.7.2 Brief interventions against excessive alcohol consumption

W. Katon Professor and Vice Chair, Director of Division of Health Services and Psychiatric Epidemiology, University of Washington, Seattle, Washington, USA.
26.5.4 Anxiety and depression

Tomisaku Kawasaki Professor and Director, Japan Kawasaki Disease Research Center, Tokyo, Japan.
18.10.8 Kawasaki syndrome

David Keeling Consultant Haematologist and Director, Oxford Haemophilia Centre and Thrombosis Unit, Churchill Hospital, Oxford, UK.
15.5.2 Therapeutic anticoagulation in atrial fibrillation and heart failure. 15.15.3.2 Therapeutic anticoagulation in deep venous thrombosis and pulmonary embolism

David P. Kelsell Non-Clinical Senior Lecturer, Centre for Cutaneous Research, Barts and The London, Queen Mary's School of Medicine and Dentistry, London, UK.
23.2 Molecular basis of inherited skin disease

John G. Kelton Dean and Vice-President, Faculty of Health Sciences, McMaster University, Hamilton, Ontario, Canada.
22.6.3 Disorders of platelet number and function

Christopher Kennard Professor and Head, Division of Neuroscience and Psychological Medicine, Imperial College London, Charing Cross Campus, London, UK.
24.11 Visual pathways

Rose Anne Kenny Professor of Cardiovascular Research, Institute of Ageing and Health, University of Newcastle upon Tyne, UK.
24.13.5.1 Head-up tilt-table testing in the diagnosis of vasovagal syncope and related disorders

M. G. W. Kettlewell Consultant Surgeon, Oxford Radcliffe Trust, UK.
14.13 Colonic diverticular disease

G. T. Keusch Associate Director for International Research, National Institutes of Health, Bethesda, Maryland, and Professor of Medicine, Tufts-New England Medical Center, Boston, Massachusetts, USA.
7.11.7 Enterobacteria, campylobacter, and miscellaneous food-poisoning bacteria

Munther A. Khamashta Senior Lecturer and Consultant Physician, Lupus Research Unit, The Rayne Institute, St Thomas' Hospital, London, UK.
13.14 Autoimmune rheumatic disorders and vasculitis in pregnancy

Maurice King Honorary Research Fellow, University of Leeds, UK.
3.7.2 Health in a fragile future

Keith P. Klugman Professor of International Health, Rollins School of Public Health and Division of Infectious Diseases, School of Medicine, Emory University, Atlanta, Georgia, USA.
7.11.3 Pneumococcal diseases

R. Knight Associate Specialist in General Medicine, Royal Sussex County Hospital, Brighton, UK.
7.13.1 Amoebic infections. 7.13.9 Blastocystis hominis infection. 7.14.2 Lymphatic filariasis. 7.14.3 Guinea-worm disease: dracunculiasis. 7.14.4 Strongyloidiasis, hookworm, and other gut strongyloid nematodes. 7.14.8 Angiostrongyliasis. 7.15.2 Gut cestodes

Michael D. Kopelman Professor of Clinical Medicine and Deputy Warden, Bart's and The London, Queen Mary's School of Medicine and Dentistry, University of London, UK.
26.3 Neuropsychiatric disorders

Peter G. Kopelman Professor of Clinical Medicine, Bart's and The London Queen Mary's School of Medicine and Dentistry, London, UK.
10.5 Obesity

Christian Krarup Professor, Department of Clinical Neurophysiology, Rigshospitalet, Copenhagen, Denmark.
24.2 Electrophysiology of the central and peripheral nervous systems

J. B. Kurtz Consultant Virologist (retired), Public Health Laboratory, Birmingham Heartlands Hospital, UK.
7.11.35 Legionellosis and legionnaires' disease

Robert A. Kyle Professor of Medicine and Laboratory Medicine, Mayo Clinic, Rochester, Minnesota, USA.
22.4.5 Myeloma and paraproteinaemias

David Lalloo Senior Lecturer in Tropical Medicine, Liverpool School of Tropical Medicine, UK.
7.11.17 Yersinia, Pasteurella, and Francisella

D. J. Lane Consultant Chest Physician (Retired), Oxford Radcliffe Hospital, UK.
17.2 The clinical presentation of chest diseases

Peter Lanyon Consultant Rheumatologist, University Hospital, Queen's Medical Centre, Nottingham, UK.
18.3 Clinical investigation

H. E. Larson Private Practice in Infectious Diseases, Marlborough, Massachusetts, USA.
7.11.21 Botulism, gas gangrene, and clostridial gastrointestinal infections

S. Lawrie Senior Clinical Research Fellow, University Department of Psychiatry, Royal Edinburgh Hospital, UK.
26.5.6 Schizophrenia, bipolar disorder, obsessive–compulsive disorder, and personality disorder

N. F. Lawton Consultant Neurologist, Wessex Neurological Centre, Southampton General Hospital and Honorary Senior Lecturer, University of Southampton, UK.
24.13.19 Benign intracranial hypertension

John H, Lazarus Professor of Clinical Endocrinology, University of Wales College of Medicine, Cardiff, UK.
13.11 Endocrine disease in pregnancy

J. W. LeDuc Director, Division of Viral and Rickettsial Diseases, Centers for Disease Control and Prevention, Atlanta, Georgia, USA.
7.10.14 Bunyaviridae

P. J. Lee Consultant in Metabolic Medicine, Metabolic Unit, National Hospital for Neurology and Neurosurgery, London, UK.
11.2 Inborn errors of amino acid and organic acid metabolism

Tak H. Lee Professor of Allergy and Respiratory Medicine, Guy's, King's and St Thomas' School of Medicine, Guy's Hospital, London, UK.
17.4.3 Basic mechanisms and pathophysiology of asthma

William M. F. Lee Department of Medicine, School of Medicine, University of Pennsylvania, Philadelphia, USA.
4.3 Molecular cell biology

T. Lehner Professor of Basic and Applied Immunology, Department of Immunobiology, Guy's, King's and St Thomas' School of Medicine, London, UK.
14.5 The mouth and salivary glands. 18.10.5 Behçet's disease

Irene M. Leigh Professor of Cellular and Molecular Medicine, Bart's and The London Queen Mary's School of Medicine and Dentistry, University of London, UK.
23.2 Molecular basis of inherited skin disease

G. G. Lennox Consultant Neurologist, Addenbrooke's Hospital, Cambridge, UK.
13.12 Neurological disease in pregnancy

E. A. Letsky Consultant Perinatal Haematologist, Queen Charlotte's and Chelsea Hospital, London, UK.
13.16 Blood disorders in pregnancy

Jeremy Levy Consultant Nephrologist, Imperial College, Hammersmith Hospital, London, UK.
20.7.7 Antiglomerular basement membrane disease

L. M. Lichtenstein Professor of Medicine and Director, Asthma and Allergy Center, Johns Hopkins University School of Medicine, Baltimore, Maryland, USA.
5.2 Allergy

D. C. Linch Professor and Head of Haematology, University College London, UK.
22.2.2 Stem-cell disorders

M. J. Lindop Consultant, Anaesthesia/Intensive Care, Addenbrooke's Hospital, Cambridge, UK.
16.6.3 Brainstem death and organ donation. 16.6.4 The patient without hope

Calvin C. Linnemann, Jr Professor and Director, Infectious Diseases Division, University of Cincinnati Medical Center, Ohio, USA.
7.11.14 Bordetella

Gregory Y. H. Lip Professor of Cardiovascular Medicine, University Department of Medicine, City Hospital, Birmingham, UK.
15.16.3 Hypertensive emergencies and urgencies

P. Little Professor of Primary Care Research, Community Clinical Sciences Division, University of Southampton, UK.
17.5.1 Upper respiratory tract infections

Roderick A. Little Honorary Professor of Surgical Science, University of Manchester, UK.
11.12.2 Metabolic responses to accidental and surgical injury

W. Littler Medical Director, University Hospital NHS Trust, Birmingham, UK.
15.10.2 Infective endocarditis

A. Llanos Cuentas Principal Professor, Facultad de Salud Publica y Administracion, Universidad Peruana Cayetano Heredia, Lima, Peru.
7.11.39.1 Bartonella bacilliformis infection

Diana N. J. Lockwood Consultant Leprologist and Senior Lecturer, Hospital for Tropical Diseases and London School of Hygiene and Tropical Medicine, UK.
7.11.24 Leprosy (Hansen's disease)

S. Logan Senior Lecturer in Paediatric Epidemiology, Institute of Child Health, London, UK.
7.10.12 Rubella

D. J. Lomas Professor of Clinical MRI, University Department of Radiology, Addenbrooke's Hospital, Cambridge, UK.
14.18.2 Computed tomography and magnetic resonance imaging of the liver and pancreas

David A. Lomas Professor of Respiratory Biology and Honorary Consultant Physician, Department of Medicine, University of Cambridge Institute for Medical Research, UK.
11.13 α_1*-Antitrypsin deficiency and the serpinopathies*

Thomas Look Professor of Pediatrics, Harvard Medical School and Vice-Chair for Research, Pediatric Oncology Department, Dana-Farber Institute, Boston, Massachusetts, USA.
22.3.1 Cell and molecular biology of human leukaemias

A. D. Lopez Senior Science Adviser, World Health Organization, Geneva, Switzerland.
3.1 The Global Burden of Disease Study

Elyse E. Lower Professor of Medicine, University of Cincinnati, Ohio, USA.
17.11.6 Sarcoidosis

Linda M. Luxon Professor of Audiological Medicine, University of London, Institute of Child Health, London, UK and Director, National Institute for Cancer Research, Genova, Italy.
24.12.2 Disorders of hearing

Lucio Luzzatto Professor, Department of Human Genetics, Memorial Sloan-Kettering Cancer Center, New York, USA.
22.3.12 Paroxysmal nocturnal haemoglobinuria. 22.5.12 Glucose-6-phosphate dehydrogenase (G6PD) deficiency

G. A. Luzzi Consultant in Genitourinary/HIV Medicine, South Buckinghamshire NHS Trust, Wycombe Hospital, High Wycombe, Buckinghamshire, UK.
7.10.21 HIV and AIDS

D. C. W. Mabey Professor of Communicable Diseases, London School of Hygiene and Tropical Medicine, London, UK.
7.11.40 Chlamydial infections including lymphogranuloma venerum

P. K. MacCallum Senior Lecturer in Haematology, Barts and The London, Queen Mary's School of Medicine and Dentistry, London, UK.
15.1.2.2 The haemostatic system in arterial disease

J. T. Macfarlane Consultant Physician, Nottingham City Hospital, UK.
7.11.35 Legionellosis and legionnaires' disease

K. T. MacLeod Reader in Cardiac Physiology, Cardiac Medicine, NHLI, Faculty of Medicine, Imperial College London, UK.
15.1.3.1 Physical considerations: biochemistry and cellular physiology of heart muscle

William MacNee Professor of Respiratory and Environmental Medicine, University of Edinburgh, and Honorary Consultant Physician, Lothian University NHS Trust, Edinburgh, UK.
17.6 Chronic obstructive pulmonary disease

M. Monir Madkour Consultant Physician, Military Hospital, Riyadh, Saudi Arabia.
7.11.19 Brucellosis

R. N. Maini Professor of Rheumatology in the University of London, Head of the Kennedy Institute of Rheumatology Division, Faculty of Medicine, Imperial College London, and Honorary Consultant Physician, Charing Cross Hospital, London, UK.
18.5 Rheumatoid arthritis

Hadi Manji Consultant Neurologist, National Hospital for Neurology, London and Ipswich Hospital, Suffolk, UK.
24.14.4 Neurosyphilis and neuroAIDS

J. I. Mann Professor in Human Nutrition and Medicine, University of Otago, Dunedin, New Zealand.
10.1 Diseases of overnourished societies and the need for dietary change

D. Mant Professor of General Practice, Department of Primary Health Care, University of Oxford, UK.
3.4 Preventive medicine

Victor J. Marder Orthopedic Hospital/UCLA Vascular Medicine Program, Los Angeles, California, USA.
22.6.2 Evaluation of the patient with a bleeding diathesis

A. F. Markham Professor of Medicine, St James's University Hospital, Leeds, UK.
14.15 Tumours of the gastrointestinal tract

V. Marks Professor of Clinical Biochemistry Emeritus, Post-Graduate Medical School, University of Surrey, Guildford, UK.
12.11.3 Hypoglycaemia

T. J. Marrie Professor and Chair, Department of Medicine, University of Alberta, Edmonton, Canada.
7.11.38 Coxiella burnetii infections (Q fever)

Helen Marriott Research Associate, Department of Respiratory Medicine, University of Shefffield, UK.
15.15.2.1 Primary pulmonary hypertension

C. D. Marsden* Professor of Neurology, National Hospital for Neurology and Neurosurgery, London, UK.
24.15 Metabolic disorders and the nervous system

Jay W. Mason Professor and Chair, Department of Medicine, University of Kentucky College of Medicine, Lexington, USA.
15.8.1 Myocarditis

V. I. Mathan Professor, ICDDR, Dhaka, Bangladesh.
14.9.8 Malabsorption syndromes in the tropics

Christopher J. Mathias Professor of Neurovascular Medicine and Consultant Physician, Imperial College of Science, Technology and Medicine at St Mary's and National Hospital for Neurology and Neurosurgery, Institute of Neurology, University College London, UK.
24.13.14 Diseases of the autonomic nervous system

Peter W. Mathiesen Professor of Renal Medicine, Academic Renal Unit, University of Bristol, Southmead Hospital, Bristol, UK.
20.7.5 Proliferative glomerulonephritis. 20.7.6 Mesangiocapillary glomerulonephritis

R. McCaig Head, Human Factors Unit, Health Directorate, Health and Safety Executive, Bootle, UK.
8.5.10 Noise. 8.5.11 Vibration

Mary E. McCaul Professor, Department of Psychiatry and Behavioral Sciences, Johns Hopkins University School of Medicine, Baltimore, Maryland, USA.
26.7.1 Alcohol and drug dependence

Joseph McCormick Regional Dean, University of Texas School of Public Health at Brownsville, USA.
7.10.15 Arenaviruses. 7.10.16 Filoviruses

William J. McKenna BHF Professor of Molecular Cardiovascular Sciences, Department of Cardiological Sciences, St George's Hospital Medical School, London, UK.
15.8.2 The cardiomyopathies: hypertrophic, dilated, restrictive, and right ventricular. 15.8.3 Specific heart muscle disorders

* It is with regret that we report the death of Professor C. D. Marsden.

A. J. McMichael Professor and Director, Weatherall Institute of Molecular Medicine, John Radcliffe Hospital, Oxford, UK.
5.1 Principles of immunology.

A. J. McMichael Professor and Director, National Centre for Epidemiology and Population Health, Australian National University, Canberra, Australia.
3.2 Human population size, environment, and health

A. McMillan Consultant Physician, Department of Genito-urinary Medicine, Edinburgh Royal Infirmary, UK.
21.5 Infections and other medical problems in homosexual men

Martin McNally Consultant in Limb Reconstruction and Honorary Senior Lecturer in Orthopaedic Surgery, Bone Infection Unit, Nuffield Orthopaedic Centre, Oxford, UK.
19.3 Osteomyelitis

K. McNeil Director of Transplant Services, The Prince Charles Hospital, Brisbane, Australia.
17.16 Lung and heart–lung transplantation

T. W. Meade Emeritus Professor of Epidemiology, London School of Hygiene and Tropical Medicine, UK.
15.1.2.2 The haemostatic system in arterial disease

A. Meheus Professor, University of Antwerp, Belgium.
21.1 Epidemiology

David K. Menon Professor of Anaesthesia, University of Cambridge, Addenbrooke's Hospital, Cambridge, UK.
16.6.2 Management of raised intracranial pressure

Wayne M. Meyers Chief, Mycobacteriology, Armed Forces Institute of Pathology, Washington DC, USA.
7.11.25 Buruli ulcer: Mycobacterium ulcerans infection

Anna Rita Migliaccio Dirigente de Ricerca in Transfusion Medicine, Laboratory of Clinical Biochemistry, Istituto Superiore dei Sanità, Rome, Italy.
22.5.1 Erythropoiesis and the normal red cell

M. A. Miles Professor, London School of Hygiene and Tropical Medicine, UK.
7.13.11 Chagas' disease

G. J. Miller Professor of Epidemiology, Barts and The London, Queen Mary's School of Medicine and Dentistry, London, UK.
15.1.2.2 The haemostatic system in arterial disease

Mary Miller Consultant in Palliative Medicine, Sir Michael Sobell House, Churchill Hospital, Oxford, UK.
31 Palliative care

Robert F. Miller Reader in Clinical Infection and Consultant Physician, Royal Free and University College Medical School, London, UK.
7.12.5 Pneumocystis carinii

K. R. Mills Professor of Clinical Neurophysiology, King's College Hospital, London, UK.
24.4 Investigation of central motor pathways: magnetic brain stimulation

Philip Minor Public Health and Clinical Microbiology Laboratory, Addenbrooke's Hospital, Cambridge, UK.
7.10.7 Enterovirus infections

Raad H. Mohiaddin Consultant and Honorary Senior Lecturer, Royal Brompton and Harefield NHS Trust, London, JK.
15.3.5 Cardiovascular magnetic resonance and computed X-ray tomography

Andrew J. Molyneux Consultant Neuroradiologist, Radcliffe Infirmary, Oxford, UK.
24.5 Imaging in neurological diseases

Kevin Moore Senior Lecturer, Centre for Hepatology, Royal Free Hospital and University College Medical School, London, UK.
14.21.2 Cirrhosis, portal hypertension, and ascites

Pedro L. Moro Fellow, Vaccine Safety Division, National Immunization Program, Centers for Disease Control and Prevention, Baltimore, Maryland, USA.
7.15.1 Cystic hydatid disease (Echinococcus granulosus)

N. J. McC. Mortensen Professor of Colorectal Surgery, Department of Colorectal Surgery, John Radcliffe Hospital, Oxford, UK.
14.13 Colonic diverticular disease

Peter S. Mortimer Professor of Dermatological Medicine and Consultant Skin Physician, St George's Hospital Medical School, Division of Physiological Medicine, London, UK.
15.17 Lymphoedema

Alastair G. Mowat Clinical Lecturer in Rheumatology, Department of Rheumatology, Nuffield Orthopaedic Centre, Oxford, UK.
18.10.4 Polymyalgia rheumatica and giant-cell arteritis

E. R. Moxon Head, Oxford University Department of Paediatrics, John Radcliffe Hospital, Oxford, UK.
7.11.12 Haemophilus influenzae

M. F. Muers Consultant Physician, Respiratory Medicine, The General Infirmary at Leeds, UK.
17.3.4 Diagnostic bronchoscopy, thoracoscopy, and tissue biopsy

Tariq I. Mughal Consultant Haematologist and Medical Oncologist and Senior Lecturer in Oncology, Lancashire Teaching Hospitals NHS Trust and Preston and Christie Hospital NHS Trust, Manchester, UK.
22.3.6 Chronic myeloid leukaemia

J. A. Muir Gray Director of the UK National Screening Committee, Institute of Health Sciences, Oxford, UK.
3.6 Screening

P. A. Murphy Professor of Medicine and Microbiology, Johns Hopkins University and Chief, Infectious Diseases Division, Johns Hopkins Bayview Hospital, Baltimore, Maryland, USA.
7.5 Physiological changes in infected patients

C. J. L. Murray Global Programme on Evidence for Health Policy, World Health Organization, Geneva, Switzerland.
3.1 The Global Burden of Disease Study

Iain M. Murray-Lyon Consultant Physician and Gastroenterologist, Charing Cross Hospital and Chelsea and Westminster Hospital, London, UK.
14.21.5 Primary and secondary liver tumours

Jean Nachega Assistant Scientist, Johns Hopkins University, Baltimore, Maryland, USA.
7.11.22 Tuberculosis

Robert B. Nadelman Professor of Medicine, Division of Infectious Diseases, New York Medical College, USA.
7.11.29 Lyme borreliosis

N. V. Naoumov Reader in Hepatology/Honorary Consultant Physician, Institute of Hepatology, University College London, UK.
7.10.19 Hepatitis viruses (including TTV)

R. P. Naoumova MRC Senior Clinical Scientist/Honorary Consultant Physician, MRC Clinical Sciences Centre, Hammersmith Hospital, London, UK.
15.1.2.1 The pathogenesis of atherosclerosis

D. G. Nathan President, Dana-Farber Cancer Institute, Boston, Massachusetts, USA.
22.2.1 Stem cells and haemopoiesis

Graham Neale Research Fellow, Clinical Risk Unit, University College London, UK.
14.1 Introduction to gastroenterology. 14.1.1.2 Symptomatology of gastrointestinal disease. 14.16 Vascular and collagen disorders

Catherine Nelson-Piercy Consultant Obstetric Physician, Guy's and St Thomas' Hospitals Trust, London, UK.
13.14 Autoimmune rheumatic disorders and vasculitis in pregnancy

A. R. Ness Senior Lecturer in Epidemiology, Department of Social Medicine, University of Bristol, UK.
15.4.1.2 The epidemiology of ischaemic heart disease

Peter Nestor Neurologist, University of Cambridge Neurology Unit, UK.
24.8 Disturbances of higher cerebral function

J. Neuberger Professor of Hepatology and Consultant Physician, Queen Elizabeth Hospital, Birmingham, UK.
14.21.7 Drugs and liver damage. 14.21.8 The liver in systemic disease

John Newell-Price Senior Lecturer in Endocrinology, Division of Clinical Sciences, Sheffield University, Northern General Hospital, Sheffield, UK.
12.3 Disorders of the posterior pituitary

A. J. Newman Taylor Consultant Physician and Head, Department of Occupational and Environmental Medicine, Royal Brompton Harefield NHS Trust, Faculty of Medicine, Imperial College London, UK.
17.4.4 Asthma. 17.4.5 Occupational asthma

C. S. Ng Assistant Professor, Department of Radiology, University of Texas M. D. Anderson Cancer Center, Houston, USA.
14.18.2 Computed tomography and magnetic resonance imaging of the liver and pancreas

S. Nightingale Consultant Neurologist and Honorary Senior Clinical Lecturer, Royal Shrewsbury Hospital and Birmingham University, Shrewsbury, UK.
7.10.23 HTLV-I and II and associated diseases

T. Northfield Professor Emeritus, Department of Biochemical Medicine, St George's Hospital, London, UK.
14.3.2 Gastrointestinal bleeding

John Nowakowski Assistant Professor of Medicine, Department of Medicine, Division of Infectious Diseases, Westchester Medical Center, Valhalla, New York, USA.
7.11.29 Lyme borreliosis

Fujio Numano Director, Tokyo Vascular Disease Institute, Tokyo, Japan.
15.14.4 Takayasu arteritis

D. O'Gradaigh Research Registrar, Department of Medicine, Addenbrooke's Hospital, Cambridge, UK.
18.11 Miscellaneous conditions presenting to the rheumatologist. 19.5 Avascular necrosis and related topics

Stephen O'Rahilly Professor of Clinical Biochemistry, University of Cambridge, and Honorary Consultant Physician, UK.
10.5 Obesity

S. C. O'Reilly Consultant Rheumatologist, Rheumatology Department, Derbyshire Royal Infirmary, Derby, UK.
18.9 Crystal-related arthropathies

P. J. Oldershaw Consultant Cardiologist, Royal Brompton Hospital, London, UK.
15.13 Congenital heart disease in adolescents and adults

James G. Olson Head, Department of Virology, U. S. Navy Medical Research Center Detachment, Lima, Peru.
7.10.6.1 Nipah and Hendra viruses. 7.11.39 Bartonelloses, excluding Bartonella bacilliformis infections

M. Osame Professor, Third Department of Internal Medicine, Faculty of Medicine, Kagoshima University, Japan.
7.10.23 HTLV-I and II and associated diseases

Jackie Palace Consultant Neurologist, Radcliffe Infirmary, Oxford, UK.
24.17 Disorders of the neuromuscular junction

Thalia Papayannopoulou Professor of Medicine (Hematology), University of Washington, Division of Hematology, Seattle, USA.
22.5.1 Erythropoiesis and the normal red cell

S. Parish Senior Research Fellow, Clinical Trial Service Unit, Nuffield Department of Clinical Medicine, University of Oxford, UK.
2.4.3 Large-scale randomized evidence: trials and overviews

G. R. Park Director of Intensive Care Research, John Farman Intensive Care Unit, Addenbrooke's Hospital, Cambridge, UK.
16.6.1 Sedation and analgesia in the critically ill

David Parkes Professor of Clinical Neurology, King's College Hospital, London, UK.
24.13.4 Narcolepsy

C. Parry University of Oxford–Wellcome Trust Clinical Research Unit, Centre for Tropical Diseases, Ho Chi Minh City, Vietnam.
7.11.8 Typhoid and paratyphoid fevers

Steve W. Parry Consultant Physician and Honorary Senior Lecturer, Freeman Hospital and University of Newcastle upon Tyne, UK.
24.13.5.1 Head-up tilt-table testing in the diagnosis of vasovagal syncope and related disorders

J. Paul Consultant Microbiologist and Director, Brighton Public Health Laboratory, Royal Sussex County Hospital, Brighton, UK.
7.11.42 Newly identified and lesser-known bacteria. 7.17 Non-venomous arthropods

Malik Peiris Professor, Department of Microbiology, University of Hong Kong.
7.10.1 Respiratory tract viruses

Edmund D. Pellegrino Emeritus Professor of Medicine and Medical Ethics, Georgetown University Medical Center, Washington DC, USA.
2.3 Medical ethics

T. H. Pennington Professor of Bacteriology, University of Aberdeen Medical School, UK.
7.3 Biology of pathogenic micro-organisms

M. B. Pepys Professor and Head of Medicine, Department of Medicine, Royal Free Campus, Royal Free and University College Medical School, London, UK.
11.12.1 The acute phase response and C reactive protein. 11.12.4 Amyloidosis

P. L. Perine Professor of Epidemiology, School of Public and Community Medicine, University of Washington, Seattle, USA.
7.11.32 Non-venereal treponematoses: yaws, endemic syphilis (bejel), and pinta

G. D. Perkin Consultant Neurologist, Department of Neurology, Charing Cross Hospital, London, UK.
24.13.3 Epilepsy in later childhood and adults

P. L. Perrotta Assistant Professor, Pathology, Stony Brook University Hospital, New York, USA.
22.8.1 Blood transfusion

H. Persson Medical Director and Consultant Physician, Swedish Poisons Information Centre, Stockholm, Sweden.
8.3 Poisonous plants and fungi

M. C. Petch Consultant Cardiologist, Papworth Hospital, Cambridge, UK.
15.4.2.6 The impact of coronary heart disease on life and work

L. R. Petersen Deputy Director for Science, Centers for Disease Control, Division of Vector-borne Infectious Diseases, Fort Collins, Colorado, USA.
7.10.11 Alphaviruses. 7.10.13 Flaviviruses

R. Peto Professor of Epidemiology and Medical Statistics, University of Oxford, UK.
2.4.3 Large-scale randomized evidence: trials and overviews. 6.1 Epidemiology of cancer

T. E. A. Peto Consultant Physician in Infectious Diseases, Nuffield Department of Medicine, John Radcliffe Hospital, Oxford, UK.
7.10.21 HIV and AIDS

A. Phillips Senior Lecturer, Institute of Nephrology, University of Wales College of Medicine, Cardiff, UK.
20.1 Structure and function of the kidney

R. J. Playford Professor, Imperial College School of Medicine, Hammersmith Hospital, London, UK.
14.9.7 Effects of massive small bowel resection

J. M. Polak Professor and Director, Tissue Engineering and Regenerative Medicine Centre, Imperial College School of Medicine, London, UK.
14.8 Hormones and the gastrointestinal tract

Eleanor S. Pollak Associate Director, Clinical Coagulation Laboratory, Hospital of the University of Pennsylvania, University of Pennsylvania Medical Center, Philadelphia, USA.
22.6.4 Genetic disorders of coagulation

P. A. Poole-Wilson Professor of Cardiology and Cardiac Medicine, National Heart and Lung Institute, Faculty of Medicine, Imperial College London, UK.
15.1.3.1 Physical considerations: biochemistry and cellular physiology of heart muscle

F. M. Pope Consultant Dermatologist, West Middlesex University Hospital, London, UK.
19.2 Inherited defects of connective tissue: Ehlers–Danlos syndrome, Marfan's syndrome, and pseudoxanthoma elasticum

Françoise Portaels Professor and Head, Mycobacteriology Unit, Institute of Tropical Medicine, Antwerp, Belgium.
7.11.25 Buruli ulcer: Mycobacterium ulcerans infection

J. S. Porterfield Formerly Reader in Bacteriology, Sir William Dunn School of Pathology, University of Oxford, UK.
7.10.14 Bunyaviridae

Jerome B. Posner Attending Neurologist, Memorial Sloan-Kettering Cancer Center, New York, USA.
24.18 Paraneoplastic syndromes

William G. Powderly Professor of Medicine, Washington University School of Medicine, St Louis, Missouri, USA.
7.12.2 Cryptococcosis

J. J. Powell Senior Lecturer - Nutrition and Medicine, GI Laboratory, Rayne Institute, St Thomas' Hospital, London, UK.
8.5.8 Podoconiosis

Janet Powell Medical Director, University Hospitals, Coventry and Warwickshire NHS Trust, Coventry, Warwickshire, UK.
15.14.2 Peripheral arterial disease

J. W. Powles University Lecturer in Public Health Medicine, Institute of Public Health, Cambridge, UK.
3.2 Human population size, environment, and health

M. A. Preece Professor of Child Health and Growth, Institute of Child Health, University College London, UK.
12.9.2 Normal growth and its disorders

J. S. Prichard* Professor of Medicine, St James's Hospital, Dublin, Eire.
15.15.2.2 Pulmonary oedema

A. T. Proudfoot Consulting Clinical Toxicologist, National Poisons Information Service, City Hospital, Birmingham, UK.
8.1 Poisoning by drugs and chemicals

Charles Pusey Professor of Renal Medicine, Faculty of Medicine, Imperial College, Hammersmith Hospital, London, UK.
20.7.7 Antiglomerular basement membrane disease

N. P. Quinn Professor of Clinical Neurology, Institute of Neurology and Honorary Consultant Neurologist, The National Hospital for Neurology and Neurosurgery, London, UK.
24.10 Subcortical structures—the cerebellum, thalamus, and basal ganglia

Anisur Rahman Senior Lecturer in Rheumatology, Centre for Rheumatology, Department of Medicine, University College London, UK.
18.10.2 Systemic lupus erythematosus and related disorders

Lawrence E. Ramsay Professor of Clinical Pharmacology and Therapeutics, University of Sheffield and Consultant Physician, Royal Hallamshire Hospital, Sheffield, UK.
15.16.2.1 Hypertension—indications for investigation. 15.16.2.2 Renal and renovascular hypertension. 15.16.2.5 Aortic coarctation. 15.16.2.6 Other rare causes of hypertension. 20.10.2 Hypertension and the kidney

M. Ramsay Consultant Epidemiologist, Immunisation Division, PHLS Communicable Disease Surveillance Centre, London, UK.
7.7 Immunization

A. C. Rankin Reader in Cardiology, Glasgow Royal Infirmary, UK.
15.2.3 Syncope and palpitation. 15.6 Cardiac arrhythmias

C. W. G. Redman Professor of Obstetric Medicine, John Radcliffe Hospital, Oxford, UK.
13.4 Hypertension in pregnancy

Laurence John Reed Academic Unit of Psychiatry, St Thomas' Hospital, London, UK.
26.3 Neuropsychiatric disorders

A. J. Rees Regius Professor of Medicine, Institute of Medical Sciences, University of Aberdeen, UK.
20.10.3 Vasculitis and the kidney

Jeremy Rees Clinical Senior Lecturer in Neuro-oncology, National Hospital for Neurology and Neurosurgery, London, UK.
24.13.18.1 Intracranial tumours

D. Rennie Adjunct Professor of Medicine, Institute for Health Policy Studies, University of California, San Francisco, USA.
8.5.4 Diseases of high terrestrial altitudes

J. Richens Clinical Lecturer, Department of Sexually Transmitted Diseases, Royal Free and University College Medical School, London, UK.
7.11.8 Typhoid and paratyphoid fevers. 7.11.9 Intracellular Klebsiella infections

B. K. Rima Professor of Molecular Biology, Medical Biology Centre, Queen's University of Belfast, UK.
7.10.5 Mumps: epidemic parotitis

A. J. Ritchie Consultant Cardiothoracic Surgeon, Papworth NHS Trust, Cambridge, UK.
15.4.2.5 Coronary artery bypass grafting

Eberhard Ritz Professor and Head, Department of Nephrology, University of Heidelberg, Germany.
20.5.2 Bone disease in chronic renal failure

* It is with regret that we report the death of Professor J. S. Prichard.

Harold R. Roberts Sarah Graham Kenan Professor of Medicine and Attending Physician, UNC Hospitals, Chapel Hill, North Carolina, USA.
22.6.1 The biology of haemostasis and thrombosis. 22.6.2 Evaluation of the patient with a bleeding diathesis

William G. Robertson Clinical Scientist, Institute of Urology and Nephrology, University College London, UK.
20.13 Urinary stones, nephrocalcinosis, and renal tubular acidosis

T. A. Rockall Senior Lecturer/Honorary Consultant, St Mary's Hospital, London, UK.
14.3.2 Gastrointestinal bleeding

Allan R. Ronald Professor Emeritus, University of Manitoba, Winnipeg, Canada.
7.11.13 Haemophilus ducreyi and chancroid

P. Ronco Professor of Renal Medicine, Université Pierre et Marie Curie (Paris 6) and Director, Renal Division and INSERM Unit 489, Tenon Hospital (Assistance Publique-Hôpitaux de Paris), Paris, France.
20.10.5 Renal involvement in plasma cell dyscrasias, immunoglobulin-based amyloidoses, and fibrillary glomerulopathies, lymphomas, and leukaemias

Antony Rosen Professor and Director, Division of Rheumatology, Johns Hopkins University School of Medicine, Baltimore, Maryland, USA.
5.3 Autoimmunity

Mark J. Rosen Chief, Division of Pulmonary and Critical Care Medicine, Beth Israel Medical Center, New York, USA.
17.5.2.3 Pulmonary complications of HIV infection

Raymond C. Rosen Professor of Psychiatry, UMDNJ-Robert Wood Johnson Medical School, Department of Psychiatry, Piscataway, New Jersey, USA.
12.8.4 Sexual dysfunction

R. J. M. Ross Professor of Endocrinology, Northern General Hospital, University of Sheffield, UK.
12.9.3 Puberty

D. J. Rowlands Honorary Consultant Cardiologist, Manchester Heart Centre, Manchester Royal Infirmary, UK.
15.3.2 Electrocardiography. 15.3.4 Nuclear techniques

M. B. Rubens Director of Imaging and Consultant Radiologist, Royal Brompton and Harefield NHS Trust, London, UK.
15.3.1 Chest radiography in heart disease. 15.3.5 Cardiovascular magnetic resonance and computed X-ray tomography

David Rubenstein Consultant Physician, Addenbrooke's Hospital, Cambridge, UK.
7.1 The clinical approach to the patient with suspected infection

P. C. Rubin Professor and Dean of Medicine, University of Nottingham, UK.
13.18 Prescribing in pregnancy

Anthony S. Russell Professor of Medicine, University of Alberta, Edmonton, Canada.
18.2 Clinical presentation and diagnosis of rheumatic disease

T. J. Ryan Emeritus Professor of Dermatology, University of Oxford, UK.
23.1 Diseases of the skin

Sara S. T. O. Saad Professor and Haematologist, Department of Internal Medicine, Hematology-Hemotherapy Division, Medical Science Faculty, State University of Campinas, Brazil.
22.5.10 Disorders of the red cell membrane

N. J. Samani Professor of Cardiology, Division of Cardiology, Department of Medicine, University of Leicester, UK.
15.16.1.2 Genetics of hypertension

Brian P. Saunders Senior Lecturer in Endoscopy, St Mark's Hospital, Northwick Park, Harrow, Middlesex, UK.
14.2.1 Colonoscopy and flexible sigmoidoscopy

S. J. Saunders Emeritus Professor, Liver Clinic, Groote Schuur Hospital and Medical Research Council/University of Cape Town Liver Research Centre, Cape Town, South Africa.
14.21.6 Hepatic granulomas

M. O. Savage Professor of Paediatric Endocrinology, St Bartholomew's and The Royal London School of Medicine and Dentistry, London, UK.
12.9.1 Normal and abnormal sexual differentiation. 12.9.3 Puberty

John Savill Professor of Medicine, Royal Infirmary, Edinburgh, UK.
20.7.1 The glomerulus and glomerular injury

K. P. Schaal Professor and Director, Institute for Medical Microbiology and Immunology, Faculty of Medicine, Rheinische Friedrich-Wilhelms-Universität, Bonn, Germany.
7.11.26 Actinomycosis

Michael Schömig Physician in Charge, Division of Nephrology, Ruperto-Carola-University of Heidelberg, Germany.
20.5.2 Bone disease in chronic renal failure

Ruud B. H. Schutgens Head of Department of Clinical Chemistry, Vrije Universiteit Medical Centre (VUMC), Amsterdam, The Netherlands.
11.9 Peroxisomal diseases

J. Schwebke Associate Professor of Medicine, University of Alabama at Birmingham, USA.
21.3 Vaginal discharge

Neil Scolding Burden Professor of Clinical Neurosciences, University of Bristol Institute of Clinical Neurosciences, Frenchay Hospital, Bristol, UK.
24.15 Metabolic disorders and the nervous system. 24.20 Neurological complications of systemic autoimmune and inflammatory diseases

J. Scott Professor of Medicine, Imperial College Faculty of Medicine, Hammersmith Campus, London, UK.
15.1.2.1 The pathogenesis of atherosclerosis

A. Seaton Professor and Head of Department of Environmental and Occupational Medicine, University of Aberdeen, UK.
17.11.7 Pneumoconioses

G. R. Serjeant Professor Emeritus and Chairman, Sickle Cell Trust, Kingston, Jamaica, West Indies.
20.10.7 Sickle-cell disease and the kidney

N. J. Severs Professor of Cell Biology, National Heart and Lung Institute, Faculty of Medicine, Imperial College London, UK.
15.1.3.1 Physical considerations: biochemistry and cellular physiology of heart muscle

C. A. Seymour Professor of Clinical Biochemistry and Metabolic Medicine and Director for Clinical Advice to The Health Service Ombudsman, St George's Hospital Medical School and Office of Health Service Commissioner, London, UK.
11.7.2 Wilson's disease, Menke's disease: inherited disorders of copper metabolism

K. V. Shah Professor, Johns Hopkins Bloomberg School of Public Health, Baltimore, Maryland, USA.
7.10.17 Papovaviruses

L. M. Shapiro Consultant Cardiologist, Papworth Hospital, Cambridge, UK.
15.4.2.2 Management of stable angina. 15.4.2.5 Coronary artery bypass grafting

Michael Sharpe Reader in Psychological Medicine, University of Edinburgh, Royal Edinburgh Hospital, UK.
7.19 Chronic fatigue syndrome (postviral fatigue syndrome,neurasthenia, and myalgic encephalomyelitis). 26.1 General introduction. 26.5.3 Medically unexplained symptoms in patients attending medical clinics. 26.6.2 Psychological treatment in medical practice

J. M. Shneerson Director, Respiratory Support and Sleep Centre, Papworth Hospital, Cambridge, UK.
17.13 Disorders of the thoracic cage and diaphragm

Tom Siddons Clinical Research Assistant, Pfizer Research and Development (UK), Maidstone, Kent, UK.
15.15.1 The pulmonary circulation and its influence on gas exchange

C. A. Sieff Associate Professor in Pediatrics, Dana Farber Cancer Institute, Boston, Massachusetts, USA.
22.2.1 Stem cells and haemopoiesis

J. Sieper Head of Rheumatology, Department of Medicine, University Hospital Benjamin Franklin, Berlin, Germany.
18.6 Spondyloarthritides and related arthritides

Leslie Silberstein Professor, University of Pennsylvania School of Medicine, Philadelphia, Pennsylvania, USA.
22.5.9 Haemolytic anaemia—congenital and acquired

R. Sinclair Senior Lecturer, Department of Dermatology, University of Melbourne, St Vincent's Hospital, Fitzroy, Victoria, Australia.
23.1 Diseases of the skin

Joseph Sinning Yale School of Medicine, New Haven, Connecticut, USA.
22.4.1 Leucocytes in health and disease

Thira Sirisanthana Professor of Medicine and Director, Research Institute for Health Sciences, Chiang Mai University, Thailand.
7.11.18 Anthrax. 7.12.6 Infection due to Penicillium marneffei

J. G. P. Sissons Professor of Medicine, University of Cambridge and Honorary Consultant Physician, Addenbrooke's Hospital, Cambridge, UK.
7.10.2 Herpesviruses (excluding Epstein–Barr virus)

M. B. Skirrow Honorary Emeritus Consultant Microbiologist, Public Health Laboratory, Gloucester Royal Hospital, UK.
7.11.7 Enterobacteria, campylobacter, and miscellaneous food-poisoning bacteria

Geoffrey L. Smith Professor of Virology and Wellcome Trust Principal Research Fellow, The Wright–Fleming Institute, Faculty of Medicine, Imperial College of Science, Technology and Medicine, St Mary's Campus, London, UK.
7.10.4 Poxviruses

P. H. Smith Department of Urology, St James' University Hospital, Leeds, UK.
20.15 Tumours of the urinary tract

R. Smith Consultant Physician, Nuffield Orthopaedic Centre, Oxford, UK.
19.1 Disorders of the skeleton

E. L. Snyder Professor of Laboratory Medicine, Yale University School of Medicine, New Haven, Connecticut, USA.
22.8.1 Blood transfusion

R. L. Souhami Director of Clinical Research, Cancer Research UK and Emeritus Professor of Medicine, University College London, London, UK.
6.6 Cancer: clinical features and management

C. W. N. Spearman Senior Specialist and Co-Head of Liver Clinic, Groote Schuur Hospital, Cape Town, South Africa.
14.21.6 Hepatic granulomas

C. A. Speed Honorary Consultant Rheumatologist, Addenbrooke's Hospital, Cambridge, UK.
19.5 Avascular necrosis and related topics

G. P. Spickett Consultant Clinical Immunologist, Regional Department of Immunology, Royal Victoria Infirmary, Newcastle upon Tyne, UK.
17.11.8 Pulmonary haemorrhagic disorders. 17.11.9 Eosinophilic pneumonia. 17.11.11 Extrinsic allergic alveolitis. 17.11.19 Drug-induced lung disease

S. G. Spiro Professor of Respiratory Medicine and Medical Director, Medicine, University College London Hospitals NHS Trust, Middlesex Hospital, London, UK.
17.14.1.1 Lung cancer. 17.14.1.2 Pulmonary metastases

Jerry L. Spivak Professor of Medicine and Oncology, Johns Hopkins School of Medicine, Baltimore, Maryland, USA.
22.3.9 Idiopathic myelofibrosis

A. Spurgeon Senior Lecturer, Institute of Occupational Health, University of Birmingham, UK.
8.4.1 Occupational and environmental health and safety

Paul D. Stein Director of Research, St Joseph Mercy-Oakland, Pontiac, Michigan, USA.
15.15.3.1 Deep venous thrombosis and pulmonary embolism

Tom Stevens Consultant Psychiatrist, St Thomas' Hospital and Maudsley NHS Trust, London, UK.
26.3 Neuropsychiatric disorders

J. C. Stevenson Reader and Consultant Physician, Endocrinology and Metabolic Medicine, Faculty of Medicine, Imperial College London, UK.
13.20 Benefits and risks of hormone replacement therapy

P. M. Stewart Professor of Medicine, University of Birmingham and Consultant Physician, Queen Elizabeth Hospital, Birmingham, UK.
12.7.1 Disorders of the adrenal cortex

August Stich Consultant in Tropical Medicine, Medical Mission Institute, Unit of Tropical Medicine and Epidemic Control, Wurzburg, Germany.
7.13.10 Human African trypanosomiasis

John H. Stone Associate Professor of Medicine, Johns Hopkins University, Baltimore, Maryland, USA.
18.10.7 Polymyositis and dermatomyositis

J. R. Stradling Consultant Physician and Professor of Respiratory Medicine, Churchill Hospital, Oxford, UK.
17.1.1 The upper respiratory tract. 17.8.1 Upper airways obstruction. 17.8.2 Sleep-related disorders of breathing

Frank J. Strobl Director, Scientific Affairs, Therakos Inc., Exton, Pennsylvania, USA.
22.5.9 Haemolytic anaemia—congenital and acquired

M. A. Stroud Senior Lecturer in Medicine, Southampton University Hospitals Trust, UK.
8.5.1 Environmental extremes—heat. 8.5.2 Environmental extremes—cold

Michael Strupp Associate Professor of Neurology, Department of Neurology, Klinikum Grosshadern, University of Munich, Germany.
24.12.1 Eye movements and balance

P. H. Sugden Professor of Cellular Biochemistry, Imperial College of Science, Technology and Medicine, London, UK.
15.1.3.1 Physical considerations: biochemistry and cellular physiology of heart muscle

Daniel P. Sulmasy Sisters of Charity Chair in Ethics, St Vincent's Manhattan and New York Medical College, New York, USA.
2.3 Medical ethics

J. A. Summerfield Professor of Experimental Medicine, Faculty of Medicine, Imperial College London, UK.
14.19.1 Congenital disorders of the liver, biliary tract, and pancreas. 14.19.2 Diseases of the gallbladder and biliary tree

Pravan Suntharasamai Emeritus Professor of Tropical Medicine, Faculty of Tropical Medicine, Mahidol University, Bangkok, Thailand.
7.14.9 Gnathostomiasis

J. Swales* Professor of Medicine, University of Leicester, UK.
15.16.1.3 Essential hypertension

P. Sweny Consultant Nephrologist, Royal Free Hospital, London, UK.
20.6.3 Renal transplantation

D. Swirsky Consultant Haematologist, Leeds General Infirmary, UK.
22.4.4 The spleen and its disorders

I. C. Talbot Professor of Histopathology, St Mark's Hospital for Colorectal Disorders, London, UK.
14.15 Tumours of the gastrointestinal tract

D. Tarin Director, UCSD Cancer Center, University of California at San Diego, La Jolla, USA.
6.4 Tumour metastasis

D. Taylor-Robinson Emeritus Professor of Genitourinary Microbiology and Medicine, Division of Medicine, Imperial College of Science, Technology and Medicine, St Mary's Hospital, London, UK.
7.11.40 Chlamydial infections including lymphogranuloma venerum. 7.11.41 Mycoplasmas

P. J. Teddy Consultant Neurosurgeon/Clinical Director, Department of Neurological Surgery, Radcliffe Infirmary, Oxford, UK.
24.14.3 Intracranial abscess

H. J. Testa Professor and Consultant (retired), Royal Infirmary, Manchester, UK.
15.3.4 Nuclear techniques

R. V. Thakker May Professor of Medicine, Nuffield Department of Medicine, University of Oxford, UK.
12.6 Parathyroid disorders and diseases altering calcium metabolism

David G. T. Thomas Professor of Neurological Surgery, National Hospital for Neurology and Neurosurgery, London, UK.
24.13.18.2 Traumatic injuries of the head

D. L. Thomas Associate Professor of Medicine, Johns Hopkins School of Medicine, Baltimore, Maryland, USA.
7.10.20 Hepatitis C virus

P. K. Thomas Emeritus Professor of Neurology, Royal Free Hospital School of Medicine and Institute of Neurology, London, UK.
24.6.1 Inherited disorders. 24.13.15 Disorders of cranial nerves. 24.19 Diseases of the peripheral nerves

* It is with regret that we report the death of Professor J. Swales during the preparation of this edition of the textbook.

D. G. Thompson Professor of Gastroenterology, University of Manchester, UK.
14.1.1.1 Structure and function of the gut. 14.12 Functional bowel disorders and irritable bowel syndrome

R. P. H. Thompson Consultant Physician, St Thomas' Hospital, London, UK.
8.5.8 Podoconiosis. 14.19.3 Jaundice

S. A. Thorne Royal Brompton and Harefield NHS Trust, London, UK.
15.13 Congenital heart disease in adolescents and adults

Ph. Thulliez Head, Laboratoire de la Toxoplasmose, Institut de Puericulture, Paris, France.
7.13.4 Toxoplasmosis

Tran Tin Hien Vice Director, Centre for Tropical Diseases (Cho Quan Hospital), Ho Chi Minh City, Vietnam.
7.11.1 Diphtheria

J. A. Todd Professor of Medical Genetics, University of Cambridge, UK.
12.11.2 The genetics of diabetes melllitus

C. Tomson Consultant Nephrologist, Southmead Hospital, Bristol, UK.
20.12 Urinary tract infection

Keith Tones Professor of Health Education (Emeritus), Leeds Metropolitan University, UK.
3.5 Health promotion

P. A. Tookey Lecturer, Centre for Epidemiology and Biostatistics, Institute of Child Health, London, UK.
7.10.12 Rubella

P. P. Toskes Professor of Medicine, Division of Gastroenterology, Hepatology, and Nutrition, Department of Medicine, University of Florida College of Medicine, Gainsville, USA.
14.9.2 Small bowel bacterial overgrowth. 14.18.3.2 Chronic pancreatitis

Thomas A. Traill Professor of Medicine, Johns Hopkins Hospital, Baltimore, Maryland, USA.
15.11.1 Cardiac myxoma. 15.11.2 Other tumours of the heart. 15.12 Cardiac involvement in genetic disease

David F. Treacher Consultant Physician in Intensive Care, St Thomas' Hospital, Guy's and St Thomas' NHS Trust, London, UK.
16.2 The circulation and circulatory support of the critically ill

A. S. Truswell Emeritus Professor of Human Nutrition, University of Sydney, New South Wales, Australia.
10.1 Diseases of overnourished societies and the need for dietary change

D. M. Turnbull Professor of Neurology, The Medical School, University of Newcastle upon Tyne, UK.
24.22.5 Mitochondrial encephalomyopathies

H. E. Turner Consultant Physician, Radcliffe Infirmary, Oxford, UK.
12.12 Hormonal manifestations of non-endocrine disease

A. Neil Turner Professor of Nephrology, Royal Infirmary, Edinburgh, UK.
20.7.8 Infection-associated nephropathies. 20.7.9 Malignancy-associated renal disease

Robert Twycross Emeritus Clinical Reader in Palliative Medicine, Oxford University, Sir Michael Sobell House, Churchill Hospital, Oxford, UK.
31 Palliative care

F. E. Udwadia Emeritus Professor of Medicine, Grant Medical College and J. J. Hospital, Bombay; Consultant Physician and Director-in-charge of ICU, Breach Candy Hospital; Consultant Physician, Parsee General hospital, Bombay, India.
7.11.20 Tetanus

S. Richard Underwood Professor of Cardiac Imaging, Imperial College of Science, Technology and Medicine, National Heart and Lung Institute, and Royal Brompton Hospital, London, UK.
15.3.5 Cardiovascular magnetic resonance and computed X-ray tomography

Robert J. Unwin Professor of Nephrology and Physiology, Centre for Nephrology, The Middlesex Hospital, London, UK.
20.13 Urinary stones, nephrocalcinosis, and renal tubular acidosis

V. Urquidi Assistant Professor, University of California San Diego Cancer Center and Department of Pathology, La Jolla, California, USA.
6.4 Tumour metastasis

J. A. Vale Director, National Poisons Information Service and West Midlands Poisons Unit, City Hospital, Birmingham, UK.
8.1 Poisoning by drugs and chemicals

P. Vallance Professor of Clinical Pharmacology and Therapeutics, Centre for Clinical Pharmacology, University College London, UK.
15.1.1.2 Vascular endothelium, its physiology and pathophysiology

J. van Gijn Professor and Chairman, Department of Neurology, University Medical Centre, Utrecht, The Netherlands.
24.13.7 Stroke: cerebrovascular disease

Sirivan Vanijanonta Emeritus Professor of Tropical Medicine, Faculty of Tropical Medicine, Mahidol University, Bangkok, Thailand.
7.16.3 Lung flukes (paragonimiasis)

Patrick J. W. Venables Professor and Honorary Consultant, Kennedy Institute Division, Imperial College London, UK.
18.10.6 Sjögren's syndrome

B. J. Vennervald Senior Research Scientist, Danish Bilharziasis Laboratory, Charlottenlund, Denmark.
7.16.1 Schistosomiasis

C. M. Verity Consultant Paediatric Neurologist and Associate Lecturer, Faculty of Medicine, University of Cambridge, Addenbrooke's Hospital, Cambridge, UK.
24.21 Developmental abnormalities of the central nervous system

M. P. Vessey Emeritus Professor of Public Health, Unit of Health Care Epidemiology, Department of Public Health, Oxford University, UK.
13.19 Benefits and risks of oral contraceptives

R. Viner Consultant in Adolescent Medicine and Endocrinology, University College London Hospitals and Great Ormond Street Hospital, UK.
29 Adolescent medicine

Peter D. Wagner Professor of Medicine and Bioengineering, University of California, San Diego, USA.
17.1.2 Structure and function of the airways and alveoli

Ann E. Wakefield* Professor of Paediatric Infectious Diseases, Department of Paediatrics, Institute of Molecular Medicine, University of Oxford, UK.
7.12.5 Pneumocystis carinii

D. H. Walker The Carmage and Martha Walls Distinguished Chair in Tropical Diseases, Professor and Chairman, Department of Pathology, and Director, WHO Collaborating Center for Tropical Diseases, Galveston, Texas, USA.
7.11.36 Rickettsial diseases including ehrlichiosis

J. A. Walker-Smith Emeritus Professor of Paediatric Gastroenterology, Royal Free and University College Medical School, London, UK.
14.14 Congenital abnormalities of the gastrointestinal tract

Mark J. Walport Professor of Medicine and Head, Division of Medicine, Faculty of Medicine, Imperial College London, Hammersmith Hospital, London, UK.
5.4 Complement

Julian R. F. Walters Reader in Gastroenterology, Imperial College of Science, Technology and Medicine, Hammersmith Campus, London, UK.
14.2.4 Investigation of gastrointestinal function. 14.9.1 Differential diagnosis and investigation of malabsorption

Gary S. Wand Professor of Medicine, Johns Hopkins University School of Medicine, Baltimore, Maryland, USA.
26.7.1 Alcohol and drug dependence

Ronald J. A. Wanders Professor of Inborn Errors and Metabolism and Deputy Head of the Laboratory for Metabolic Diseases, Academic Medical Centre, Amsterdam, The Netherlands.
11.9 Peroxisomal diseases

B. Ward Anaesthetic Registrar, Coventry School of Anaesthetics, UK.
16.6.1 Sedation and analgesia in the critically ill

T. E. Warkentin Professor, Department of Pathology and Molcular Medicine and Department of Medicine, McMaster University, Hamilton, Ontario, Canada.
22.6.5 Acquired coagulation disorders

D. A. Warrell Professor of Tropical Medicine and Infectious Diseases and Head, Nuffield Department of Clinical Medicine, University of Oxford, UK.
7.8 Travel and expedition medicine. 7.10.9 Rhabdoviruses: rabies and rabies-related viruses. 7.10.10 Colorado tick fever and other arthropod-borne reoviruses. 7.11.28 Rat-bite fevers. 7.11.30 Other borrelia infections. 7.11.32 Non-venereal treponematoses: yaws, endemic syphilis (bejel), and pinta. 7.13.2 Malaria. 7.13.5 Cryptosporidium and cryptosporidiosis. 7.18 Pentostomiasis (porocephalosis). 8.2 Injuries, envenoming, poisoning, and allergic reactions caused by animals. 24.14.1 Bacterial meningitis. 24.14.2 Viral infections of the central nervous system. 24.22.6 Tropical pyomyositis (tropical myositis). 33 Emergency medicine

M. J. Warrell Clinical Virologist, Centre for Tropical Medicine, John Radcliffe Hospital, Oxford, UK.
7.10.9 Rhabdoviruses: rabies and rabies-related viruses. 7.10.10 Colorado tick fever and other arthropod-borne reoviruses

Paul Warwicker Consultant Nephrologist, Renal Unit, Lister Hospital, Stevenage, Hertfordshire, UK.
20.10.6 Haemolytic uraemic syndrome

J. A. H. Wass Professor of Endocrinology and Consultant Physician, Radcliffe Infirmary, Oxford, UK.
12.12 Hormonal manifestations of non-endocrine disease

Laurence Watkins Consultant Neurosurgeon and Senior Lecturer, Institute of Neurology, London, UK.
24.13.18.2 Traumatic injuries of the head

George Watt Department of Medicine, AFRIMS, Bangkok, Thailand.
7.11.31 Leptospirosis. 7.11.37 Scrub typhus

Richard W. E. Watts Visiting Professor and Honorary Consultant Physician, Imperial College School of Medicine, Hammersmith Hospital, London, UK.
11.1 The inborn errors of metabolism: general aspects. 11.4 Disorders of purine and pyrimidine metabolism. 11.10 Disorders of oxalate metabolism

D. J. Weatherall Regius Professor of Medicine Emeritus, University of Oxford, Weatherall Institute of Molecular Medicine, John Radcliffe Hospital, Oxford, UK.
2.2 Scientific method and the art of healing. 22.1 Introduction. 22.5.2 Anaemia: pathophysiology, classification, and clinical features. 22.5.3 Anaemia as a world health problem. 22.5.5 Normochromic, normocytic anaemia. 22.5.7 Disorders of the synthesis or function of haemoglobin. 22.7 The blood in systemic disease

D. K. H. Webb Consultant Paediatric Haematologist, Great Ormond Street Hospital for Children, London, UK.
22.4.7 Histiocytoses

Kathryn E. Webert Clinical Scholar, Hematology and Fellow in Transfusion Medicine, Canadian Blood Services, McMaster University, Hamilton, Ontario, Canada.
22.6.3 Disorders of platelet number and function

A. D. B. Webster Consultant Immunologist, Department of Immunology, Royal Free Hospital, London, UK.
5.6 Immunodeficiency

Anthony P. Weetman Professor of Medicine and Dean, University of Sheffield Medical School, UK.
12.4 The thyroid gland and disorders of thyroid function. 12.5 Thyroid cancer

R. A. Weiss Professor, University College London, UK.
7.10.21 HIV and AIDS. 7.10.24 Viruses and cancer

Peter L. Weissberg BHF Professor of Cardiovascular Medicine, University of Cambridge, UK.
15.1.1.1 Introduction. 15.1.1.3 Vascular smooth muscle cells. 15.4.2.1 The pathophysiology of acute coronary syndromes

Peter F. Weller Professor of Medicine, Harvard Medical School; Chief of Allergy and Inflammation and Co-Chief, Infectious Diseases Division, Beth Israel Deaconess Medical Center, Boston, Massachusetts, USA.
22.4.6 Eosinophilia

A. K. Wells Consultant Respiratory Physician, Royal Brompton Hospital, London, UK.
17.11.4 The lungs and rheumatological diseases

Simon Wessely Professor of Epidemiological Psychiatry, Guy's, King's and St Thomas' School of Medicine and Institute of Psychiatry, London, UK.
26.6.2 Psychological treatment in medical practice

* It is with regret that we report the death of Professor Ann E. Wakefield during the preparation of this edition of the textbook.

Gilbert C. White, II John C. Parker Professor of Medicine and Pharmacology and Director, Center for Thrombosis and Hemostasis, University of North Carolina School of Medicine, Chapel Hill, North Carolina, USA.
22.6.1 The biology of haemostasis and thrombosis. 22.6.2 Evaluation of the patient with a bleeding diathesis

Joseph White SPHTM at TUMC, New Orleans, Louisiana, USA.
3.7.1 The cost of health care in Western countries

H. C. Whittle Visiting Professor, London School of Hygiene and Tropical Medicine and Deputy Director, MRC Laboratories, Banjul, The Gambia.
7.10.6 Measles

D. E. L. Wilcken Professor Emeritus of Medicine and Head, Cardiovascular Research Laboratory, University of New South Wales and Prince of Wales Hospital, Sydney, Australia.
15.1.3.2 Clinical physiology of the normal heart

James S. Wiley Professor and Head of Haematology, Nepean Hospital, Penrith, New South Wales, Australia.
22.5.8 Anaemias resulting from defective red cell maturation

P. J. Wilkinson Consultant Medical Microbiologist, University Hospital, Queen's Medical Centre, Nottingham, UK.
7.11.34 Listeriosis

R. G. Will Professor of Clinical Neurology, Western General Hospital, Edinburgh, UK.
24.13.9 Human prion disease

C. B. Williams Consultant Physician in Endoscopy, St Mark's Hospital for Colorectal Disorders, UK.
14.2.1 Colonoscopy and flexible sigmoidoscopy. 14.15 Tumours of the gastrointestinal tract

D. J. Williams Senior Lecturer/Honorary Consultant in Obstetric Medicine, Division of Paediatrics, Obstetrics and Gynaecology, Imperial College of Science, Technology and Medicine, Chelsea and Westminster Hospital, London, UK.
13.1 Physiological changes of normal pregnancy. 13.2 Nutrition in pregnancy. 13.3 Medical management of normal pregnancy

Gareth Williams Professor of Medicine, Department of Medicine, Clinical Sciences Centre, University Hospital Aintree, Liverpool, UK.
12.11.1 Diabetes

J. D. Williams Professor of Nephrology and Consultant Physician, Institute of Nephrology, University of Wales College of Medicine, Cardiff, UK.
20.1 Structure and function of the kidney

Paul F. Williams Consultant Nephrologist, The Ipswich Hospital NHS Trust, UK.
20.6.2 The treatment of endstage renal disease by peritoneal dialysis

Robert Wilson Consultant Physician and Reader, Royal Brompton Hospital and National Heart and Lung Institute, Imperial College of Science, Technology and Medicine, London, UK.
17.3.3 Microbiological methods in the diagnosis of respiratory infections

C. G. Winearls Consultant Nephrologist, Oxford Kidney Unit, Churchill Hospital, Oxford, UK.
20.5.1 Chronic renal failure

F. Wojnarowska Professor of Dermatology and Consultant Dermatologist, Oxford Radcliffe Hospital, Oxford, UK.
13.13 The skin in pregnancy

R. Wolman Consultant in Rheumatology and Sports Medicine, Royal National Orthopaedic Hospital, Stanmore, Middlesex, UK.
28 Sports and exercise medicine

Kathryn J. Wood Professor of Immunology, Nuffield Department of Surgery, University of Oxford, UK.
5.7 Principles of transplantation immunology

Nicholas Wood Professor of Clinical Neurology, Institute of Neurology, London, UK.
24.6.2 Neurogenetics. 24.13.12 Ataxic disorders

Trevor Woodage Clinical Investigator, Celera Genomics, Rockville, Maryland, USA.
4.1 The genomic basis of medicine

H. F. Woods Professor of Medicine, University of Sheffield, UK.
11.11 Disturbances of acid-base homeostasis

Gary P. Wormser Vice Chairman, Department of Medicine, and Chief, Division of Infectious Diseases, New York Medical College, Valhalla, New York, USA.
7.11.29 Lyme borreliosis

D. J. M. Wright Emeritus Reader in Medical Microbiology, Cell and Molecular Biology Section, Imperial College School of Medicine, London, UK.
7.11.33 Syphilis

V. M. Wright Consultant Paediatric Surgeon, Barts and The London NHS Trust, London, UK.
14.14 Congenital abnormalities of the gastrointestinal tract

F. C. W. Wu Senior Lecturer (Endocrinology), Royal Infirmary and University of Manchester, UK.
12.8.2 Disorders of male reproduction

Andrew H. Wyllie Professor and Head of Department of Pathology, University of Cambridge, UK.
4.6 Apoptosis in health and disease

M. A. S. Yasuda Professor, Department of Infectious and Parasitic Diseases, University of São Paulo Medical School, Brazil.
7.12.4 Paracoccidioidomycosis

Newman M. Yeilding Assistant Professor, University of Pennsylvania, Philadelphia, USA.
4.3 Molecular cell biology

Jenny Yiend Postdoctoral Research Assistant, MRC Cognition and Brain Science Unit, Cambridge, UK.
26.5.1 Grief, stress, and post-traumatic stress disorder

V. Zaman Professor, Department of Microbiology, The Aga Khan University, Karachi, Pakistan.
7.13.7 Sarcocystosis. 7.14.6 Other gut nematodes. 7.14.7 Toxocariasis and visceral larva migrans

18

Rheumatology

18.1 Joints and connective tissue: introduction

Jonathan C. W. Edwards

Modern medicine has moved away from diseases with Latin names towards concepts of disordered physiology. Discussion is increasingly of airflow obstruction, insulin resistance, or reduced ejection fraction. Rheumatology has been behind in this move. Terms such as rheumatoid arthritis and osteoarthritis remain popular and may do so for a few years more. A more physiological approach must come, but old habits die hard.

Five major components of joints are involved in disease: cartilage, bone, tensile tissues (ligament and tendon), and, in diarthrodeal joints, synovium and synovial fluid. Building an understanding of the structure and function of these tissues not only lays down a scientific basis for joint disease, but is also directly relevant to the clinic, providing a framework for explanation and reassurance for patients, which, arguably, is the rheumatologist's main function.

An emerging theme in joint physiology is that biophysics, neurophysiology, and immunoregulation are simply facets of a seamless whole of tissue homeostasis. Disease often arises when interactions between these elements of homeostasis break down.

Cartilage

The primary function of hyaline cartilage is the generation and maintenance of skeletal shape. Most hyaline cartilage ossifies during growth but small amounts are retained in the nose, ribs, and joints. Loss of articular hyaline cartilage reveals two local functions. Spongy bone collapses once cartilage is lost, indicating a force distributing function. The bone margin also remodels progressively in response to changing mechanical stimulation, demonstrating that articular cartilage retains a 'shape memory' function, reflecting its relative resistance to remodelling in response to stress.

Although hyaline cartilage is often seen as adapted to low friction, many human joints (and most avian) function perfectly with fibrocartilaginous surfaces. Fibrocartilage replaces hyaline cartilage following loss, so hyaline cartilage might be considered redundant in this respect.

Cartilage loss

Loss of hyaline articular cartilage is the commonest major joint problem. Loss may occur either by fragmentation, with formation of fissures and the release of debris into the joint, or by resorption. If any central concept survives the debate about what osteoarthritis means, it is cartilage fragmentation under load. Cartilage wear occurs at points of loadbearing. Resorption of cartilage occurs in inflammatory disease and involves replacement of cartilage at the articular margin by fibrovascular 'pannus'. The two processes often coexist.

A major problem with the concept of 'osteoarthritis' is the confusion of events leading up to cartilage fragmentation and the events put in train once fragmentation has started. The events leading to fragmentation are many and affect different joints to differing extents. Dysplasia, heritable biochemical defects, metabolic changes, heritable tendencies to new bone formation, non-physiological usage, obesity, and prior damage from inflammatory disease all contribute. However, it is not clear if all of these factors belong to the concept of osteoarthritis, or whether some represent 'primary' and others 'secondary' disease. In most cases the factors inducing cartilage fragmentation are not understood. The idea that changes in the subchondral bone lead to altered loading on cartilage and subsequent failure is currently popular. This is almost certainly true in Paget's disease, but perhaps more subtle bony changes in middle age underlie many 'primary' cases. It would certainly be the best explanation for the sequential appearance of Heberden's nodes over a period of months in the hands of women who use them rather little.

The events which follow as cartilage fragments are well documented in animal models of non-physiological use, and now in models of excessive bone formation. Changes in glycosaminoglycan composition occur early, with subsequent failure of the collagen framework and disintegration. Disintegration usually starts at the cartilage surface, but there are also examples of cartilage fracturing away from subchondral bone. A major unknown is the role of chondrocyte death in this sequence. Chondrocyte death precedes collagen disruption in at least some cases and could be the critical irreversible event in joints such as the hip.

Resorption of hyaline cartilage is prominent in both septic and aseptic arthritis. Again, several pathways contribute, most involving enzymes. However, chondrocyte death may also play a role here, since most published micrographs of cartilage being resorbed show significant numbers of dead chondrocytes. Toxic factors such as reactive oxygen species and depletion of nutrients may damage cells. Reactive oxygen species and proteolytic enzymes may also attack extracellular matrix. Enzymes may act locally at the surface of cells in pannus activated by cytokines, or indiscriminately, if released into synovial fluid, as may apply to neutrophil elastase.

Chondrocytes also show evidence of degrading their own matrix, both in inflammatory and mechanical disease. Metalloproteinases induced by cytokines such as interleukin 1 and tumour necrosis factor-α are likely mediators. Disruption of collagen by collagenases or gelatinases is likely to be the critical irreversible event. However, depletion of glycosaminoglycan by stromelysin or aggrecanase may make the collagen susceptible to mechanical damage through loss of swelling pressure. Mobilization of aggrecan may also occur through changes in non-covalent interactions involving hyaluronan and binding proteins such as TSG-6 (the product of tumour necrosis factor-senstive gene 6).

Bone

New bone formation commonly occurs in reaction to cartilage fragmentation. However, bone overgrowth has a wider significance. In many joints, subchondral bone remodels gradually over decades, with flaring at the margin and changes in articular congruity. This occurs in the absence of any prior failure of cartilage. In the ninth decade osteophytes are commonplace. One of the major obstacles to effective management of 'hard tissue problems' is the lumping together of new bone formation with loss of (cartilage) joint space as 'degenerative change' in radiographic assessment. The physician cannot reassure the patient with a clear explanation if he or she is not in possession of the facts.

New bone formation

The commonest articular problem attributable to new bone formation is probably pain from impingement of the under surface of the acromion on the rotator cuff tendon of the shoulder. Irritation of the medial collateral ligament of the knee is also common. Compression of other structures occurs, with carpal tunnel syndrome and sciatica being obvious examples.

Very little is known about the factors responsible for the rate of growth of periarticular bone. There is a documented familial element for some sites. A degree of physical stress is probably necessary, in that flaccid limbs may retain a lifelong adolescent bony outline. There is, however, no clear relationship to the degree of use.

A different form of new bone formation occurs at ligament insertion sites. Generalized forms are termed diffuse idiopathic skeletal hyperostosis or Forestier's disease. These patterns of new bone formation may restrict movement, yet may protect against pain.

Tensile tissues—ligament, tendon, and enthesis

Apart from trauma and tenosynovitis (see synovium), tensile tissue problems are focused at entheses—the attachments of ligament, tendon, or aponeurosis to bone. Entheses are variable, containing fibrocartilaginous and hyaline cartilage elements, and undergo structural change at the cessation of growth, which may influence disease onset. Entheses provide routes for vascularization of the tensile tissue.

Enthesopathy is the central lesion of the seronegative spondarthropathies. Two patterns can be separated—axial and peripheral. Axial enthesopathy affects spinal ligaments and the sacroiliac joint. Peripheral enthesopathy affects ligaments around peripheral joints, the plantar ligament origin, and the Achilles tendon insertion.

Axial enthesopathy is strongly associated with the B27 major histocompatability complex class I allotype. This may reflect an unusual immunological microenvironment in tissues under tension. The same sites which overstretch in Marfan's syndrome become inflamed in ankylosing spondylitis: entheses, the lung apices, the aortic root, the ciliary body, and the sacral root sheaths. Several of these sites are favoured by intracellular infections such as tuberculosis and brucellosis, suggesting that major histocompatability complex class I mediated events, such as cytotoxicity, are inhibited there, perhaps to avoid inflammatory resorption of tensile matrix. Inhibition may be mediated by local production of factors such as transforming growth factor-β. Structural differences between B27 and other allotypes are emerging which raise the possibility that local inhibition of class I associated events at sites such as entheses may be defective in the case of B27.

Synovium

Synovium comprises a superficial intimal cell layer and a subintima, which can consist of any type of connective tissue. The intima, unlike epithelium, is an incomplete and loosely arranged layer of modified macrophages and fibroblasts.

Why such a seemingly trivial tissue should be the major target for several autoimmune and inflammatory disorders may appear puzzling. However, tracing the evolution of synovium reveals some clues. Prior to the development of the jaw in cartilaginous fishes the endoskeleton was a semirigid rod of no immunological interest. Primitive immunity and leucocyte activity is likely to have focused on coelomic (serosal) cavities. Splanchnopleura remains the site of lymphocyte origin in mammals. Cartilaginous fish developed cavities within the skeleton, lined by a new tissue—synovium. Synovial intima and serosae share the expression of a complement regulatory protein, decay-accelerating factor and the immunoglobulin IgG receptor FcγRIIIa, suggesting a shared pattern of immunoregulation. Bone marrow and endoskeletal leucocytopoiesis developed later in teleosts, with bone marrow stroma derived from the same perichondrial stock as synovium. Bone and synovial stromal cells therefore share many features, including readiness to express the adhesion molecule VCAM-1. Thus, the cells of the intimal layer show marked immunological specialization. Intimal macrophages may be adapted to an 'early warning' response to immune complexes, in terms of FcγRIIIa expression, and the fibroblasts have an enhanced capacity to support lymphocyte survival via VCAM-1 and decay-accelerating factor. This combination may make the tissue particularly susceptible to autoimmune disease.

Just as tensile stress may regulate the enthesial immunological microenvironment, other stresses may contribute to the synovial environment. Macrophage FcγRIIIa expression appears to be induced at sites of shearing, not only in synovium but also in dermis over bony prominences, matching the distribution of rheumatoid nodules. Hence biophysics and immunology are inseparable.

Functions of synovium

Functions of synovium are not easily defined because removal of synovium causes few problems. It regenerates rapidly. Misconceptions about synovium, such as the existence of 'Haversian glands' have flourished. Largely as a result of the work of J. R. Levick, it has become clear that the dynamics of synovial fluid are unique and quite different from glandular secretion. Other functions have also been reappraised with the general conclusion that synovium has to be understood on its own terms, not by analogy with other tissues.

Functions of synovium are summarized below.

Disconnection

Unlike other connective tissues, synovium maintains a plane of disconnection which allows movement between rather than within solid tissues. This involves the maintenance of a non-adherent tissue surface. The best example of failure of this function is adhesive capsulitis of the shoulder, in which synovium becomes adherent to itself.

Low friction

Synovium contributes to low friction between cartilage surfaces and between synovial surfaces. Three molecules are important: water, hyaluronan, and a glycoprotein, lubricin. Water is a good lubricant, but cannot alone maintain a film between surfaces under load. Hyaluronan is not a lubricant but a film-maintaining agent. It is a carbohydrate polymer which adds viscosity and elasticity to water making it almost impossible to squeeze a film from between two surfaces. Lubricin is a true lubricant, reducing friction to an extremely low level.

Although changes in synovial fluid in disease probably alter lubricating efficiency, this may have little clinical relevance. In the short term joints appear to function well despite dilution of synovial fluid with exudate. The value of the sophisticated lubricating function of normal synovial fluid is that it reduces long-term articular surface wear to zero. The same collagen molecules are present on the surface 50 years after they were put there. Persistent presence of exudate in joints might facilitate wear, but preserved cartilage in reactive arthritis argues against even this. Attempts to modify the properties of synovial fluid are of doubtful value.

Deformable packing

The articular surfaces of most joints are incongruent. The intervening space is packed with synovium. Synovial fluid fills the tiniest crevices, with a film thickness of 40 μm in many places. With joint movement synovium has to deform with minimal resistance. How this is done remains totally unknown. Loss of this deformability is at least as important a source of disability as bone or cartilage damage in inflammatory arthritis, and can be devastating in children. It deserves serious study.

Chondrocyte nutrition

Cartilage is avascular, and chondrocytes must derive nutrition via the subchondral plate or from synovium. The synovial route is most accessible, although there is no proof that cartilage cannot survive without synovium. Synovectomy is not followed by cartilage death. There is also no evidence that synovium is structurally adapted to the nutrition of cartilage since its vasculature is similar when lining tendons, which have their own vascular supply.

It is commonly suggested that synovial fluid is important in transferring nutrients from synovium to cartilage. In fact, synovial fluid impairs nutrient transfer by acting as a diffusion gap. Without it much of the cartilage would be in contact with vascular synovium. During movement synovial fluid may facilitate nutrition of surfaces which do not come in to contact with synovium, but the fluid capacity is small and routes through solid tissue may be effective. The only likely clinical relevance of synovial fluid in nutrition is that large effusions, particularly those containing fibrin, may impair diffusion from synovium to cartilage leading to ischaemia.

Control of synovial fluid volume and composition

The combined action of muscles and lymphatic 'hearts' normally returns free tissue fluid to the circulation. Since synovial surfaces are permeable to water and there is no active pumping of water into synovial cavities, joints might be expected to be dry. The constant presence of a small volume of synovial fluid appears to be due to hyaluronan. Water from plasma transudate can enter the synovial cavity freely, but once in the cavity is mixed with hyaluronan secreted by intimal fibroblasts. If water molecules leave the joint without hyaluronan molecules, the concentration of hyaluronan at the tissue surface rises until it is so great that it obstructs the further flow of water. This curious process, known as solute polarization, means that a given amount of hyaluronan traps a certain amount of water in the synovial space. The volume can increase with inflammatory exudate, but cannot decrease unless the synovium ruptures (well recognized in disease). Chronic leakage through fistulae between synovium and lymphatics is probably also common in rheumatoid joints, and may explain why they often show synovial thickening but are dry on aspiration.

Synovitis and synovial lymphoid metaplasia

Synovial tissue responds to acute stimuli in a similar way to other tissues. Vasodilatation, oedema, hyperalgesia, and granulocyte accumulation occur in response to pyogenic infection or crystals. Synovium may be hyperresponsive: accumulations of crystals cause little inflammation at other sites. Synovial cavities are also reputed to be good sites for induction of an immune response to injected foreign antigen.

A peculiar feature of acute synovitis is that cell migration is polarized and segregated in relation to the cavity. Granulocytes pass rapidly into the fluid compartment and are sparse within the tissue. Mononuclear cells remain largely in the tissue and macrophages accumulate at the tissue surface. This leads to a thickening of the intima, previously misnamed 'hyperplasia'. The differential distribution of cells is partly explained by intimal fibroblast expression of VCAM-1, the ligand for which, $\alpha4\beta1$ integrin, is present on mononuclear but not polymorphonuclear leucocytes. There is also a difference in the behaviour of macrophages and lymphocytes. Macrophages accumulate in the intima but lymphocytes are confined to the subintima. The reasons for this remain unclear.

Prolonged stimulation of synovium leads to a pattern of infiltration peculiar to the tissue. In addition to the features above, both T and B lymphocytes accumulate in the subintima and generate follicles, and the stroma becomes colonized by plasma cells. The tissue effectively becomes a hybrid between bone marrow and lymph node, contributing to the rubbery or 'boggy' feel characteristic of chronic synovitis. The likely reason for this is, again, the readiness with which synovial fibroblasts express VCAM-1. Synovial fibroblasts as a whole show enhanced expression of VCAM-1, and also decay-accelerating factor and complement receptor 2, in response to tumour necrosis factor-α *in vitro*. This suggests that the high-level expression of VCAM-1 and decay-accelerating factor by intimal fibroblasts in normal tissue reflects a combination of a general responsiveness of synovial cells and an unidentified local intimal stimulus. VCAM-1, decay-accelerating factor, and complement receptor 2 are utilized by lymphoid stromal cells to support lymphocyte survival.

It is likely that the formation of lymphoid tissue in synovium is a stereotyped response to the generation of proinflammatory cytokines such as tumour necrosis factor-α. The source of cytokine is likely to be different in different clinical syndromes. In what we call rheumatoid arthritis the characteristic feature of early synovitis is an increase in size, number, and activation of intimal macrophages, suggesting preferential activation of these cells. This is consistent with the initiating stimulus being small immune complexes capable of crossing endothelium and interacting with FcγRIIIa-expressing macrophages. Extra-articular features can be explained in the same way. The most consistent and specific immunological abnormality in rheumatoid arthritis remains the presence of IgG rheumatoid factors, probably formed from IgG oligomers. In systemic lupus other small immune complex species may have a similar effect. However, tissue damage is more limited, perhaps because IgG rheumatoid factor-secreting plasma cells can generate both antibody and antigen locally in synovium, whereas plasma cells secreting the autoantibodies of lupus only produce antibody.

In the seronegative spondarthropathies increasing evidence that the primary lesion is at the enthesis suggests that peripheral synovitis is secondary to cytokines generated at contiguous entheses. This would explain the relatively mild degree of intimal macrophage activation seen. The net result of lymphoid metaplasia may be very similar, although the precise lymphocyte populations involved may be biased by the (unknown) nature of the underlying immune response.

Pain

A structural approach to joints risks overlooking the essence of rheumatic disease—pain. Synovium, tensile tissues, and bone are innervated by pain fibres and there is growing knowledge of their physiology. However, the relationship between pain and events measurable in the terms described above remains about as ineffable as that between the music of Pablo Casals and the motion of a string of catgut. Prostanoids, central nervous system sensitization, depression, hopes and fears, cultural patterns, holidays, and personality interactions are all essential to an effect which can be simultaneously intractable and responsive in an instant to a word or facial expression. A cyclo-oxygenase inhibitor at night may be essential to face the next day, but the best analgesics may remain explanation and trust. Diagnostic terms such as fibromyalgia are often devised to fudge difficult concepts and tend rapidly to lose value. Appropriately, pain is becoming a discipline in its own right.

Applications to therapy

The growing understanding of the biology of joints has contributed to rational therapy in two ways. It has provided rationales for empirically derived current practices, and has generated new therapeutic avenues.

Articular cartilage has little useful capacity for repair. The best treatment for damaged cartilage, as for teeth, may be what we use now—replacement by non-living material. Attempts to induce cartilage regeneration are probably futile and have the disadvantage of needing to maintain a living material. The main remaining problem is osseo-integration of non-living materials. Dentists have achieved a good solution with titanium but optimum materials for joint prostheses are still under review.

Development of rational physical therapies has been slow, owing to our lack of understanding of the relationship between movement and homeostasis in soft connective tissues. Many studies have demonstrated that exercise reduces pain and improves outcome in arthritis, but the reasons are unclear. Physiotherapeutic techniques tend to remain based on pseudophysiological concepts and are rarely validated by well designed trials. The same applies to techniques of 'joint protection' in which specific actions are discouraged to reduce deformity. Pragmatic management of diseased joints by experienced therapists has a major part to play for patient groups whose psychomotor development is limited—especially children and those with central nervous system disease or trauma. For the average adult with arthritis it is less clear that there is justification for more than sympathetic encouragement to exercise.

The discovery of cyclo-oxygenase inhibition confirmed that aspirin and indomethacin were logical agents to use to reduce pain and stiffness due to inflammatory oedema. It explained why these agents have no long-term effect on inflammation, since cyclo-oxygenase products mediate vasodilatation, pain, and oedema rather than cell influx. Cyclo-oxygenase 2 inhibitors follow this path but their place has yet to be evaluated.

Logical treatment of chronic inflammatory disease depends on whether it is the inevitable result of a genetically determined low inflammatory threshold or an acquired immune response. The former is probably important in ankylosing spondylitis and some forms of juvenile arthritis. These conditions may best be treated by long-term modulation of balances in cytokine and growth factor levels but, as yet, we do not know which molecules should be the best targets. In the meantime, suppression of inflammatory cell function by methotrexate remains the main practical, if not very sophisticated, option. This suppressive approach is also currently the mainstay of therapy for disorders such as rheumatoid arthritis which appear to represent an acquired adaptive immune response. Until recently, synovitis has been suppressed by drugs with unknown and probably disparate modes of action. Intramuscular gold and penicillamine appear only to be effective in rheumatoid arthritis. Sulphasalazine is of benefit in inflammatory bowel disease and seronegative spondarthropathies affecting peripheral joints. Methotrexate and azathioprine have a broad spectrum of action. However, none of these agents has a good risk–benefit profile. Rational suppression of synovitis has come with agents which neutralize tumour necrosis factor-α. Antitumour necrosis factor-α antibodies and soluble receptor fusion proteins have been used to mop up tumour necrosis factor-α with very good results. A similar approach has been used for interleukin 1. Anticytokine therapies appear to be broadly safe but are costly, and there is rapid relapse after withdrawal.

There is an increasing view that disorders such as rheumatoid arthritis, based on an acquired immune response, should be amenable to long-term cure if the immune system can be 'reprogrammed' to 'forget' the autoimmune response. Gold is probably the only agent in current use which occasionally induces complete remission that persists indefinitely after drug withdrawal. Rational 'reprogramming' has been attempted with high-dose chemotherapy, followed by stem cell rescue, but the mortality rate for this procedure is significant and long-term results are awaited. Hopes that anti-CD4 therapy might induce a state of tolerance which would abolish the autoimmune response have not been realized, and long-term T-cell depletion has been a problem. B-lymphocyte depletion is currently under study and has shown some promising results, but further information is needed. A combination approach may well be necessary. At least results so far give grounds for optimism that safe definitive therapy may not be a decade away.

Further reading

Archer CW *et al.*, eds (1998). *The biology of the synovial joint.* Harwood Academic Publishers, Reading, MA.

Bird HA, Snaith ML, eds (1999). *Challenges in rheumatoid arthritis.* Blackwell Scientific, Oxford.

Brandt K, Lohmander S, Doherty M, eds (1998). *Osteoarthritis.* Oxford University Press, Oxford.

Edwards JCW, Morris V (1998). Joint physiology: relevant to the rheumatologist? *British Journal of Rheumatology* **37**, 121–5.

Isenberg DA *et al.*, eds (1998). *Oxford textbook of rheumatology*, 2nd edn. Oxford University Press, Oxford.

Isenberg DA, Miller JJ, eds (1998). *Adolescent rheumatology.* Martin Dunitz, London.

Levick JR (1996). Synovial matrix-synovial fluid system of joints. In: Comper WD, ed. *Extracellular matrix*, vol. 1, pp328–77. Harwood Academic Publishers, Amsterdam.

McGonagle D, Gibbon W, Emery P (1998). Classification of inflammatory arthritis by enthesitis. *Lancet*, **352**, 1137–40.

Sokoloff L, ed (1978, 1980). *The joints and synovial fluid.* Academic Press, New York.

18.2 Clinical presentation and diagnosis of rheumatic disease

Anthony S. Russell and Robert Ferrari

'Medicine is a first-rate profession for a second-rate intellect.' Whilst we may not fully agree with that statement from a first-class iconclast (George Bernard Shaw), we do agree that with experience it is possible to discipline the mind to follow routine pathways to arrive at a correct diagnosis and therefore a valid treatment plan. In modern medicine, rheumatologists are almost unique in relying heavily on the patient's history and physical examination before applying a relatively restricted number of valid tests to clarify the diagnosis.

Pitfalls occur at every stage of the diagnostic process. The first trap is the referral note or phone call from the primary care physician, conveying their impression of the case, plus laboratory results which may or may not be of relevance. This information is obviously important but must never be blindly accepted as fact. After all, the patient has been referred for a second opinion, which should be truly unbiased and not merely an automatic repetition of the views of the referring doctor. For example: 'This man has refractory gout which is not responding to treatment and his uric acid level is high. Allopurinol has not helped him and after 5 days he still cannot walk because of pain and swelling in his right foot.' The referring physician's clinical assumption that the patient has gout may be incorrect, and the plasma uric acid level could well be irrelevant. Furthermore, if the clinical assumption is correct, then the treatment is inappropriate. Therefore, whilst at no time hinting to the patient that aspersions are being cast on the referring physician's assumptions, the consultant must start from the very beginning, taking a careful history. This should include any previous or family history of such attacks, a general history for systemic disease, or any cause for secondary gout. There should be a comprehensive physical examination, commencing with inspection of the affected part. The correct diagnostic process can be laid out as in the algorithm (a term which we use for expediency) for monarticular arthritis, but note that algorithms can only be initiated at some distance down the diagnostic pathway (Fig. 1).

General approach

The diagnostic process thus begins with the referral consultation note, followed by observation of the patient as they come in, their gait, demeanour, attire, and whether they are alone or accompanied. These, together with the presenting complaint and the initial features of the history, allow the development of an intuitive approach where the physician attempts to define aspects of the disorder and to arrive at a diagnosis (Table 1). The subsequent interview and examination are used to provide feedback and to support or refute those intuitive diagnoses; some observations necessitating a complete rethink of the process. Sometimes this rethink may relate to results of investigation or the development of new clinical features. Central to this diagnostic process is the classification into systemic rheumatological

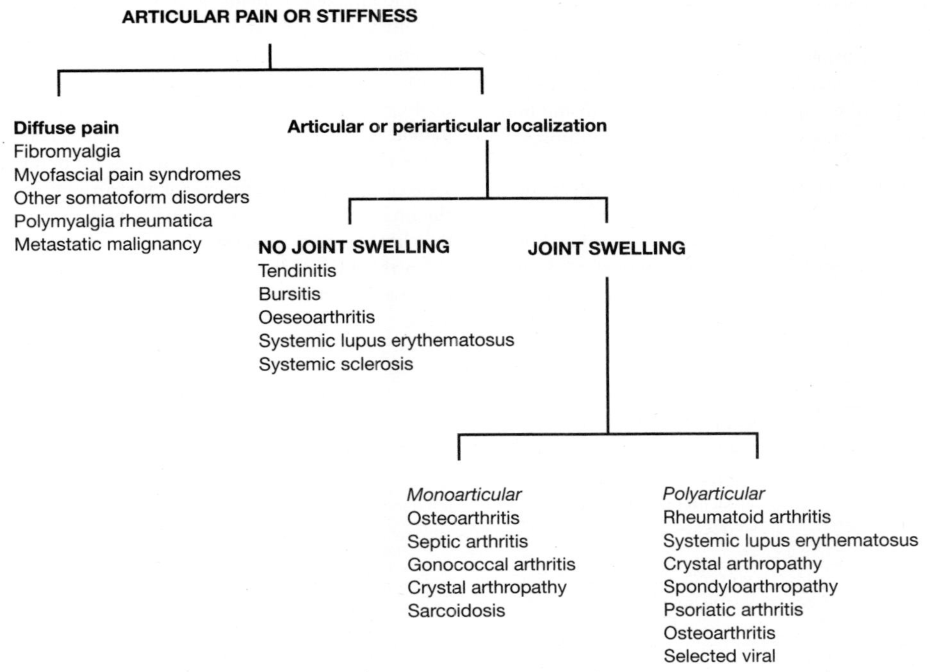

Fig. 1 An algorithm for rheumatology diagnosis.

Table 1 Preconsultation intuitive observations (note that intuitive diagnoses must be constantly subject to reflection and reassessment)

Clinical problem	Possible diagnosis
Painful foot in an elderly lady on diuretics	Gout
Young, sexually active; hot swollen joint	Gonococcal arthritis
Headache with diffuse aches and pains in an elderly person	Polymyalgia rheumatica
Antinuclear antibody-positive, but no symptoms	Referring physician's dilemma, not the patients
On allopurinol with a high uric acid, but no arthritis	Not gout
Postpubertal male with low back pain	Ankylosing spondylitis
Woman, 6 weeks postpartum; small joint arthritis	Rubella vaccination; rheumatoid arthritis
Woman describing excruciating pain (like red hot pokers)	Fibromyalgia/somatoform disorders

problems, localized—usually structural—problems, or functional somatic syndromes—perhaps best thought of as biopsychosocial disorders, an ungainly term, but one which emphasizes that biological, psychiatric, and social factors are all important. While there is obvious overlap between these categories, we believe it provides a useful framework for proceeding, partly because it allows for a positive diagnostic and therapeutic approach to this latter group, rather than simply regarding them as a group of patients where other diagnoses need to be excluded.

Some physicians feel insecure in a rheumatological diagnosis because of a lack of confidence in their rheumatological examination. This is unfortunate, because although the examination will provide important information, we believe that the principal diagnostic pointers come from a good history. The initial interview also provides a useful way of getting to know the patient and their environment. It is important, by open-ended questioning, to find out not only the details of the problem(s), but what the patient's fears and perceptions are, and especially, in a chronic disorder, what led them or their physician to seek a consultation at this time. This format also allows the patient to become at ease, and make them confident that you are truly listening. Specific directed questions are also of importance, both to elicit less frequent complaints, for example photosensitivity, xerophthalmia, recurrent miscarriage, and to elaborate on misleading terms. Thus, patients often describe 'hip pain', meaning pain in the buttocks, rarely due to hip disease; 'weakness' may reflect true neuromuscular disease, but more commonly reflects pain, for example in the shoulders or hip, or simply exhaustion or fatigue. These distinctions are crucial, and will be reviewed below (Table 2).

One of the key questions in rheumatology is 'where is the pain?', but it must be followed up with, 'and do you have pain anywhere else?'. Sometimes the answer to this, eventually, is 'all over', which by itself is very suggestive of a chronic pain syndrome. Instruments such as a pain diagram where the patient is asked to shade in areas that are painful, and also to indicate their intensity, may present a vivid pictorial representation of this. We find these useful, particularly for demonstrating the diagnostic value of this response.

When confronted with the patient who 'hurts all over', the next set of questions will often readily yield the diagnosis. The patient with diffuse pain should be asked to list all their other symptoms: a lengthy list indicates fibromyalgia or another functional somatic syndrome, and hearing extreme descriptions of individual symptoms is the next best clue. Indeed, after this, examination confirming lack of joint swelling and the presence of tender points provides ready and simple confirmation of the diagnosis, avoiding unnecessary consideration of other conditions in most cases. By contrast, when the patient fails to give a lengthy list of other symptoms, the less common causes of diffuse (poorly localized) pain should be sought. Be wary of those who complain of weight loss: this is rarely one of the long list of symptoms of fibromyalgia patients, and its presence in someone suspected of having fibromyalgia mandates a complete history and emphasis on the physical examination to look for another process. Conditions to be carefully considered in this context include polymyalgia rheumatica and metastatic bone disease (see below).

Systemic disorders

These include rheumatoid arthritis, other polyarthritides, systemic lupus erythematosus, polymyalgia, vasculitides, etc. Pointers to this type of disorder are malaise, anorexia, weight loss, rashes, fever, and multifocal symptoms including a description of actual joint swelling or persistent sensory motor deficits. Rheumatoid arthritis may begin as a monarticular problem, and although there are ways, even here, to approach a probable diagnosis, it may require more prolonged observation to establish this with certainty, obviously coupled with empirical management of symptoms. Even though the systemic disorders are typically widespread they are multifocal—that is a widespread focal problem in different joints. By contrast, pain 'all over' or 'from my head to my toes' suggests fibromyalgia, as indicated previously.

Unfortunately, patients' observations and descriptions of joint swelling are often unreliable and are particularly frequent, for example, in fibromyalgia where, by definition, it does not occur (unless there is a second disease process going on). There is little point in going through all the diagnostic questions about rheumatoid arthritis and risk factors for gout in a patient who has never had documented swelling. However, if swelling is present on examination, then a further list of questions is aimed at making a specific diagnosis. This means that in practice it is not uncommon for rheumatologists to immediately examine the hands if the patient says that they hurt, and on seeing swelling, return to diagnostic questions about the polyarthritides to expand on a presumptive diagnosis, for example of rheumatoid arthritis.

Table 2 Misinterpreted physical signs/symptoms

Sign	Misinterpretation	Correct interpretation
Muscle tenderness	Myositis	Muscle tenderness
Tenderness on sacroiliac joint palpation	Sacroiliitis	Probably mechanical back dysfunction
Adson's manoeuvre*	Thoracic outlet root compression	Probably not clinically relevant (as frequently normal)
Positive Tinel's sign†	Carpal tunnel compression	Too non-specific and insensitive to be relied on
'Hip' pain	Hip disease	Buttock pain reflecting a back problem, or lateral hip reflecting trochanteric bursitis
'Weakness'	Neuromuscular disease	Pain and/or fatigue
'Numbness'	Sensory deficit	Paraesthesiae which may be referred
Arm pain	Local lesion	Pain referred to the deltoid from shoulder or cervical spine

*Adson's manoeuvre: the patient inhales, extends the neck fully, and turns the head to the side being examined. A positive test is a reduction in the radial pulse, plus a reproduction of the patient's symptoms.

†Tinel's sign: percussion of the median nerve at the flexor reticanculum produces paraesthesiae in the hand, particularly in the median nerve distribution.

Table 3 Patterns of arthritis

Migratory	Rheumatic fever
	Gonococcal arthritis
Additive	Rheumatoid arthritis
	Psoriatic arthritis
	Chronic polyarticular gout
Intermittent	Palindromic arthritis
	Crystal synovitis
	Familial Mediterranean fever
	Early SLE/rheumatoid arthritis, etc.
	Arthritis of inflammatory bowel disease

SLE, systemic lupus erythematosus.

Inflammatory arthritides are usually associated with morning stiffness of over 30 min, and the patterns of joint involvement (Table 3) and acuteness of presentation may help indicate the likely diagnosis (see Fig. 1). Specific questions directed to associated disorders are important, for example bowel disturbance, rectal bleeding, urethritis, mucosal lesions, conjunctivitis, psoriasis, etc.

Ensure that 'sun sensitivity' is not fatigue, headache, or cholinergic urticaria, but a true photosensitivity. Vague circulatory changes and cold hands are so common in the background population that this is of no help. A diagnosis of Raynaud's requires an extension of this to include at least pallor, usually followed by reactive hyperemia. Even this may occur in 5 per cent of the population without other disease. Always remember to question the validity of previous diagnoses: who made them, and on what grounds?

An important diagnosis in the over-55 age group is polymyalgia rheumatica. Patients may report fatigue and sometimes weight loss. The erythrocyte sedimentation rate is usually very high. Here the problems are located especially around the limb girdles and are associated with marked morning stiffness and sometimes systemic features. The erythrocyte sedimentation rate is virtually always substantially elevated, although this is very non-specific. Commonly the examination may be normal, and muscle tenderness is uncommon. In younger individuals with similar symptoms a somatoform disorder is more likely. Myositis itself is not usually painful, and weakness is the predominant complaint, as it is for myopathies.

Metatastic bone disease is less common. Patients with this condition usually have weight loss and fatigue as well as nocturnal 'bone pain', symptoms which should lead to enquiry about any previous malignancies and risk factors for malignancy.

Although in one sense a focal problem, a patient with a single, hot, swollen joint is best considered as having a systemic disorder. The critical issue here is to decide whether or not the joint is infected. Because of the risk of infection the same initial decision process is involved in a patient with known rheumatoid arthritis who has an acute monarticular 'flare'. If examination confirms an acute synovitis, i.e. not merely tenderness or a periarticular lesion such as cellulitis or erythema nodosum, then joint aspiration and fluid analysis and culture are the most important investigative procedures to be undertaken. Elements of the history are helpful, for example the development 2 to 5 days postoperatively of pain and swelling in the hallux points to gout, and in the knee or wrist to pseudogout. If gonococcus is a possibility then, as culture of joint fluid may be negative, cultures from other sites are equally important. However, the most important point is to remember that even in seemingly classical situations, aspiration remains advisable to achieve a definitive diagnosis.

So-called 'diagnostic criteria' are generally designed not for diagnosis of the individual patient but for classification of groups of patients, for example for studies or reports. They are, however, useful in providing an *aide-mémoire* to direct questions regarding specific features. Thus: the symmetric arthritis of rheumatoid arthritis, the photosensitivity and serositis of systemic lupus erythematosus, the widespread pain above and below the waist of fibromyalgia, the lack of important pain in myositis, the good response of spondylitis to therapy with non-steroidal anti-inflammatory drugs, etc. are all reinforced as important points to record.

Table 4 Clinical pointers in syndromes where pain is poorly localized (other, better localized syndromes, for example calcaneal bursitis, plantar fasciitis, infrapatellar bursitis, should be immediately apparent on examination of the painful area)

Diagnosis	Clinical pointer
Periarticular shoulder pain	Referred to deltoid insertion (e.g. rotator cuff disease)
Tennis and golfer's elbow	Diffuse forearm pain on gripping
Carpal tunnel	Nocturnal paraesthesiae, often diffuse
Digital flexor tenosynovitis	Triggering and/or finger pain on gripping (pulp-pinch sign positive)
DeQuervain's tenosynovitis	Positive Finkelstein test*
Mechanical back pain	Tenderness over gluteals and sacroiliac ligaments frequent
Trochanteric bursitis	Nocturnal pain when lying on that side; focal point tenderness
Hip arthritis	Usually groin and outer thigh pain, occasionally elsewhere
Anserine bursitis	Often nocturnal medial knee pain if knees are touching; localized tenderness

*Finkelstein's test: the thumb is placed in the palm and the fingers flexed over it. Passive ulnar deviation of the wrist stretches the tendons and reproduces pain if positive.

Focal disorders

Here the patient presents with pain or other symptoms in one area, although there may be some radiation or spread. For these it is important to know the relevant anatomy and patterns of referral. Some of these are listed in Table 4 together with diagnostic pointers. To recognize meralgia paraesthetica, for example, one has to know of the existence and supply of the lateral cutaneous nerve of the thigh. A diagnosis of tendonitis should not be made unless it is associated with the name of the specific tendon or, if diffuse, with a systemic disease such as rheumatoid arthritis that can induce this. Too often it is an inappropriate attempt at diagnostic specificity in the presence of vague symptoms; diffuse pain and tenderness are often better considered under the functional section below.

Focal problems can be divided into truly articular and periarticular disorders. It must be remembered that they can be early manifestations of a systemic disease— see Table 5—and this illustrates why an inflammatory lesion is best regarded *ab initio* as a systemic problem.

Diffuse muscle pains are common. In the elderly, where radiological changes of osteoarthritis, particularly of the spine, are frequent, the pains may inappropriately be attributed to 'widespread osteoarthritis'. In general

Table 5 Primarily non-rheumatic illnesses presenting in the rheumatology clinic

Symptom/sign	Illness
Weight loss/bone pain	Multiple myeloma
Carpal tunnel syndrome	Acromegaly, hypothyroidism, amyloid
Bone pain	Secondary tumour
Vasculitis (polyarteritis nodosa)	Hepatitis
Stiffness and difficulty in walking	Parkinson's disease
Chronic synovitis with bowel problems	Inflammatory bowel disease
Stiff fingers, shoulder pain	Diabetic cheiroarthropathy
Ankle swelling/arthritis	Sarcoidosis
Wrist synovitis	CPPD disease/haemochromatosis

CPPD, calcium pyrophosphate deposition.

this is a diagnosis to be avoided. It does occur, for example in haemochromatosis, epiphyseal dysplasias, etc., but should be confirmed by clear-cut joint tenderness and decreased range of movement. However, the elderly may accumulate a number of focal disorders, for example unilateral osteoarthritis of the knee, a frozen shoulder on the right, postural cervical pain, and an osteoporotic fracture of the dorsal spine, the combination of which may simulate a systemic disease.

Functional somatic syndromes

Functional somatic syndromes are common in rheumatological practice, and are often badly managed because physicians tend to focus on organic disease. We are much more likely to be chagrined at missing the rare secondary deposit as a cause of thigh pain than by initially failing to recognize a patient whose somatic symptoms reflect depression or other emotional distress. We are subject to WHIMS (the 'what have I missed syndrome') that encourages repeated and fruitless investigation in this group to eventually arrive at a diagnosis by exclusion.

It is possible and beneficial to make the diagnosis after a good history and examination. Common symptoms are fatigue, weakness, sleep difficulties, headache, muscle aches, joint pains (plus a description of swelling), paraesthesiae, problems with memory and concentration, gastrointestinal symptoms including nausea, and alternating constipation and diarrhoea, and even irritable bladder. Such symptoms have been termed 'idioms of distress' and may be presented with a characteristic hyperbole. Thus, the pain is 'excrutiating' like 'red hot pokers in the back—you know' (as if this were an everyday experience for physicians). Apart from this, excrutiating pain is seen with fractures, septic/crystal arthritis, or nerve involvement. Patients with rheumatoid arthritis or osteoarthritis, however severe, don't normally use this terminology.

Patients with a functional somatic syndrome may also have arrived at a diagnostic label for their illness: repetitive strain injury, chronic whiplash, side-effects of silicone breast implants, candida hypersensitivity, and Gulf War syndrome to name but a few. We would also include fibromyalgia, chronic fatigue, irritable bowel syndrome, and others. It is possible, as has been suggested, that fibromyalgia (for example) may represent a central disorder of pain perception, perhaps associated with altered levels of substance P or nerve growth factor. We are unconvinced, but in any event this could be equally true of individuals with depression, with dysfunctional personalities, etc., and does not affect the overall approach to these disorders, amongst which there is considerable symptomatic overlap. All of these symptoms are common in the healthy population, and it may be more fruitful to ask oneself why the patient has presented to a physician, and at this time, rather than why they have headaches or fatigue in the first place.

Examination

The ability to detect joint swelling is important, but we are referring to obvious changes—if they are merely 'possible' or subtle, then rely more on the history for diagnostic pointers. A distinction between bony swelling and soft tissue/effusion is important and will often be of diagnostic significance.

Contrary to common belief, evident warmth of a joint (or redness) is unusual and would point to infection or crystal synovitis. The knee is normally somewhat cooler than the thigh or foreleg, and a lack of this coolness may actually be a sign that an observed knee swelling is inflammatory.

Careful palpation should allow one to distinguish between joint line tenderness, seen in arthritis, tenderness in between joints, as in an acute flexor tendonitis, periarticular tenderness, for example in lateral epicondylitis, and diffuse muscle tenderness, seen in some patients with local or generalized fibromyalgia (and very, very rarely in myositis).

The tender points found in fibromyalgia and many other somatoform diagnoses reflect a lowered pain threshold, and it has been suggested that they can be thought of as a 'sed(imentation) rate for emotional distress'. Nevertheless, they may provide diagnostic reassurance to the physician as other aspects of the examination are negative. In particular, joint swelling does not occur—although it is frequently referred to and described by the patient. The physician's observations are important here, because if swollen joints are found, then some disease process is going on that may also need assessment, perhaps in addition to fibromyalgia.

With some exceptions, physical signs in rheumatology have not yet been subjected to assessments of their validity or positive predictive value. Thus, the stress tests for sacroiliac inflammation, while often described, are of no value. Tinel and Phalen's (sustained palmar flexion of the wrist for 60 s may induce finger paraesthesiae) signs have become modified and integrated into an approach to improve their use in the diagnosis of carpal tunnel compression. Adson's manoeuvre is also of little value. Palpation of tender muscle bands is subject to great intra- and interobserver error, and the relevance of tender trapezius or gluteal muscles in the diagnosis of postural/mechanical neck and back pain, although clinically probable, remains unproven. Even the classic 'limitation of straight leg raising' has a relatively poor sensitivity and specificity. Crossed straight leg raising appears quite specific, but is relatively insensitive. A great deal still needs to be done here.

Investigations

As physicians we are trained to order tests to help throw light on, and perhaps confirm, a diagnosis. We very commonly use them inappropriately. Thus, the idea of a 'rheumatology screen', so popular with some physicians, is entirely inappropriate. There are far, far more healthy people in the population who have a positive test for rheumatoid factor, antinuclear antibodies, or HLA-B27 than there are those with significant disease. Thus, for any test to be useful diagnostically, a Bayesian approach considering the pretest probability of diagnosis is critical, or to put it simply, the result must be taken in context. If the outcome, positive or negative, cannot affect the diagnostic probability, then the test should not normally be ordered. Otherwise, we subject the patient to unnecessary tests and often, when the results are positive, unreasonable anxiety that may take months and a specialty consultation to assuage. This does not include tests done for reasons other than diagnosis, for example to establish a baseline prior to treatment, or to obtain prognostic information, etc.

Diagnostic tests are sometimes ordered for the false reassurance a negative result provides in the presence of an insecure history and/or physical examination. Unfortunately, a false positive may occur and can be disastrous. Particular caution is therefore advised in ordering tests, or further consultations, to reassure 'the patient', especially those with a somatoform disorder. Negative findings generally fail to reassure, and indeed may heighten anxieties: a negative test is interpreted as puzzling and means that the problem is not yet solved. Similarly, if treatment, such as rest, does not improve the situation, the implication is that the disorder is too bad, not that the treatment was inappropriate. In fibromyalgia, for example, acknowledging and legitimizing the patient's distress and complaints is important. But although the patient may want a diagnostic label, and whilst this seems reasonable, labelling has been shown to increase disability and labels should not be applied that can be used to validate the 'sick role', i.e. they must come with reassurance and explanation. This reassurance will only be perceived as helpful rather than dismissive if the physician has initially taken care to legitimize and accept the validity of the complaints. The goal of treatment becomes the recognition and management of factors increasing symptoms and the focus on coping and improving functional status rather than curing 'the disease'.

Treatment

For many rheumatic diseases therapy has advanced enormously in the past 20 years, but the patient will not benefit if the correct diagnosis is not made. Thus, with allopurinol gout should rarely be an active problem, but patients are frequently still admitted to hospital for antibiotics because the correct diagnostic approach of synovial fluid aspiration has not been performed, or because the fluid has been allowed to clot so that crystals are not seen, or because crystals were not looked for, etc. The therapies for rheumatoid arthritis and ankylosing spondylitis, for example, have all progressed, but not to the stage of a cure. Thus, rheumatologists spend a lot of time informing and 'educating' patients. Many of these educational endeavours, when put to the test, have been shown not merely to convey retained information, but to actually alter behaviour and outcomes. It is always rewarding if we can 'fix' a problem, for example by prescribing antimalarials for palindromic arthritis, but all too often the additional role of the rheumatologist is supportive—to inform, to reassure where possible, and to provide continued advice and encouragement.

Further reading

Barsky AJ, Borus JF (1999). Functional somatic syndromes. *Annals of Internal Medicine* **130**, 910–21.

Deyo RA, Rainville J, Kent DL (1992). What can the history and physical examination tell us about low back pain? *Journal of the American Medical Association* **268**, 760–5.

Goodman SN (1999). Toward evidence based medical statistics. 2: the Bayes factor. *Annals of Internal Medicine* **130**, 1005–13.

Straus SE (1999). Bridging the Gulf War syndrome. *The Lancet* **353**, 162–3.

18.3 Clinical investigation

Michael Doherty and Peter Lanyon

Introduction

Disease 'markers' are pathological or physiological characteristics of an individual that assist in determining the diagnosis, the current activity of disease, or the expected prognosis of the condition in that individual (Fig. 1). Some markers relate to just one of these elements; others may relate to two or occasionally all three.

Clinical markers are derived from enquiry and examination of the patient. For many common rheumatic disorders clinical assessment alone gives sufficient information for patient diagnosis and management. In some situations, however, particularly with inflammatory, metabolic, or multisystem disease, a search for additional investigational markers may be warranted. It is important to emphasize that the requirement for and selection of investigations, as well as their subsequent interpretation, is principally determined by the clinical assessment. Investigations are an adjunct, never a substitute, for competent clinical assessment. There is no place for a battery of 'screening tests'. Investigational markers may include:

- Laboratory markers (biochemical, haematological, microbiological, histological) sought through investigation of body fluids and tissues.
- Structural and physiological markers, mainly assessed by imaging (radiography, scintigraphy, magnetic resonance imaging, ultrasound).
- Genetic disease susceptibility and prognostic markers—these hold promise for the future but at present only have clinical application to rare monogenic disorders.

When considering any investigation the following deliberations are pertinent:

- 'Is this the most appropriate investigation to answer the clinical question?' This may depend on various factors, for example the sensitivity and specificity of the marker being sought, its predictive value (which takes into account disease prevalence as well as the sensitivity and specificity), the cost and availability of the investigation, the pros and cons of invasive versus non-invasive tests.
- 'Will the result of this test alter the diagnosis or clinical management of the patient?' It is easy to initiate more investigations than are really required.
- 'Will I be able to interpret and act on the results of this test?' Tests should only be ordered if the implications of either a normal or abnormal result are understood.

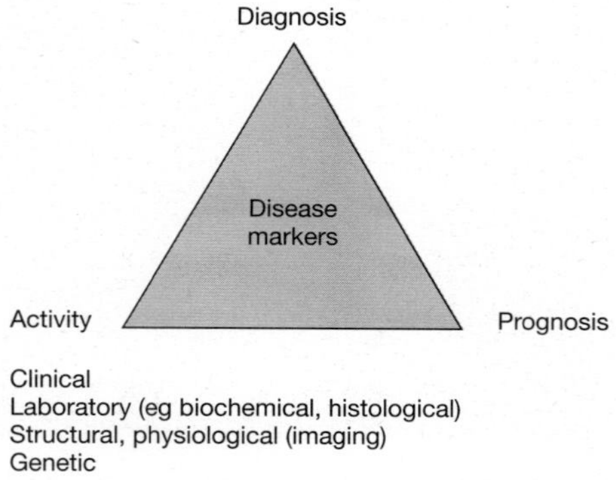

Fig. 1 Markers may be used for diagnosis, assessment of disease activity, or prognosis.

In common rheumatological practice the investigations that are of most use in diagnosis are synovial fluid analysis and the plain radiograph. Confirmation of clinically assessed inflammatory disease activity and its response to treatment is mainly by the full blood count and either direct or indirect measures of the acute phase response. These investigations are therefore given special prominence in this chapter. The usefulness of other investigations will be discussed in the context of specific clinical scenarios.

Synovial fluid analysis

This is the key investigation to confirm the diagnosis of the two curable rheumatic diseases—septic arthritis and gout. Other crystal-associated arthropathies and intra-articular bleeding are also diagnosed in this way. Synovial fluid analysis is thus the pivotal investigation for an acute monoarthritis, especially with overlying erythema.

Synovial fluid can be obtained from almost any peripheral joint and only a small volume is required for diagnostic purposes. Aspiration of large joints should be no more uncomfortable than venepuncture. The patient should be informed of the purpose and nature of the procedure and positioned on a couch in a comfortable and relaxed position with full exposure of the relevant joint. The risk of introducing sepsis is negligible as long as sterile equipment and the same sensible precautions used for venepuncture are employed.

Macroscopic appearance

Normal synovial fluid is present in small volume, contains very few cells, is clear, colourless, to pale yellow, and has high viscosity due to macromolecular hyaluronate (Fig. 2 and Plate 1). In general, with increasing joint inflammation the volume increases, the total cell count and proportion of neutrophils rises (causing turbidity), and the viscosity lowers (due to degradation of hyaluronate by protease). However, there is such overlap between arthropathies that these features are of little diagnostic value. Frank pus or 'pyarthrosis', due to very high neutrophil counts, should always lead to exclusion of sepsis but can occur with any florid synovitis such as acute crystal synovitis or rheumatoid. High concentrations of urate or cholesterol crystals may result in white synovial fluid—joint 'milk'.

Non-uniform bloodstaining of synovial fluid is common and reflects inconsequential needle trauma to synovial vessels. Uniform bloodstaining (haemarthrosis) most commonly occurs in association with florid synovitis

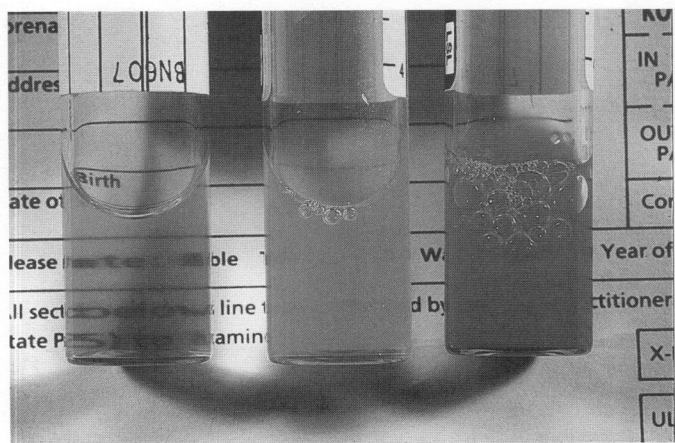

Fig. 2 Different macroscopic appearances of synovial fluids: (a) on the left, clear straw-coloured fluid from an osteoarthritic knee (easy to read writing behind it); (b) less viscous, turbid (high cell count) 'inflammatory' fluid from a rheumatoid knee; and (c) uniform bloodstaining (haemarthrosis) due to acute pseudogout. (See also Plate 1.)

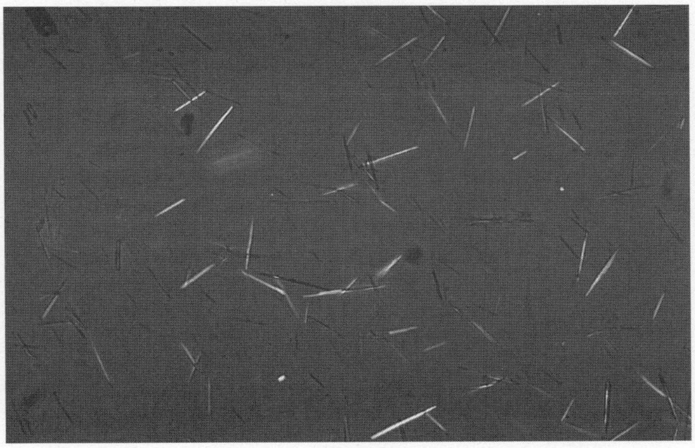

Fig. 3 Monosodium urate crystals viewed by compensated polarized light microscopy (×400) showing bright birefringence (negative sign) and needle-shaped morphology. (See also Plate 2.)

but may also result from a bleeding diathesis, trauma, or pigmented villonodular synovitis. A lipid layer floating above bloodstained fluid is diagnostic of intra-articular fracture.

Gram stain and culture

If sepsis is suspected synovial fluid should be sent for urgent Gram stain and culture. Placement in blood culture bottles in addition to a sterile universal container increases positive yields, especially of anaerobes. If gonococcal sepsis or uncommon organisms are suspected, especially in immunocompromised patients, it is advisable to discuss this with the microbiologist so that the optimal cultures can be established and molecular techniques of antigen detection used if appropriate. Although a positive result on Gram staining is found in over 50 per cent of cases of adult septic arthritis (predominantly *Staphylococcus aureus*), a negative result does not exclude infection. If there is a strong clinical suspicion of sepsis the patient should be given intravenous antibiotics pending the results of the synovial fluid, blood, and other culture results.

Crystal identification

Accurate identification of common synovial fluid crystals requires a compensated polarized light microscope and an experienced observer. Monosodium urate and calcium pyrophosphate crystals may be seen by ordinary light microscopy but confident identification resides in their light characteristics as well as their morphology. Analysis is best performed on fresh unrefrigerated synovial fluid taken into a plain container to avoid problems of crystal dissolution, postaspiration crystallization, and artefacts from tube additives. If only a few drops are obtained these should be placed straight onto a clean microscope slide and a second slide or coverslip placed on top. Even with an apparently 'dry tap' it is worth expelling the contents of the needle onto a slide as a very small amount of fluid is sometimes obtained and may be diagnostic. Urate crystals are long and needle-shaped and show a strong intensity with negative birefringence (Fig. 3 and Plate 2). Pyrophosphate crystals are smaller, rhomboid in shape, usually less numerous than urate, and have weak intensity and positive birefringence (Fig. 4 and Plate 3).

Although usually identified in the setting of acute synovitis, crystals are also often present in fluid aspirated from the joint after the attack has settled. Aspiration of an asymptomatic first metatarsophalangeal joint (gout) or knee (gout, pseudogout) may therefore permit confirmation of a suspected diagnosis. This is particularly important in gout because of the possible implications of life-long hypouricaemic therapy. The diagnosis can also be made by analysis of a tophus aspirate.

Plain radiography

In conjunction with a full history and examination this remains the single most useful imaging technique for assessment of rheumatic disease. Although a radiograph is a static record of predominantly past events, it can demonstrate visually alterations that reflect the underlying pathological processes of rheumatic disease (for example cartilage and bone erosion, bone remodelling, calcification). The abnormalities that may be seen on a plain film include:

- soft tissue swelling—seen as altered skin contours and displaced fat planes and intracapsular fat pads (fat appears dark on a radiograph)
- decreased or increased bone density (localized or generalized; Table 1)
- joint erosion (non-proliferative or proliferative marginal erosion, central erosion)
- joint-space narrowing (osteoarthritis—focal; inflammatory arthritis—generalized)
- new bone formation (osteophyte, enthesophyte, syndesmophyte)

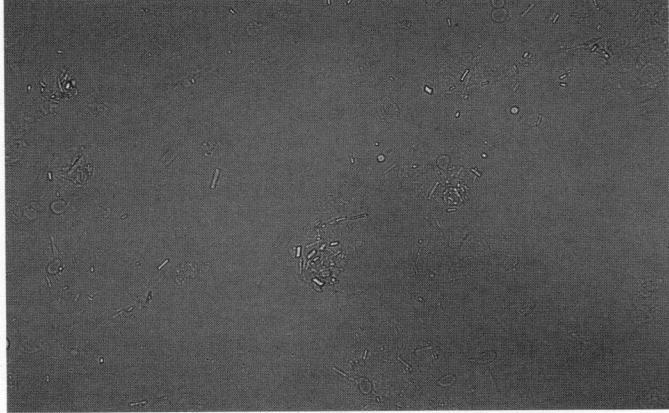

Fig. 4 Calcium pyrophosphate crystals viewed by polarized light microscopy (×400) showing weak birefringence (positive sign), scant numbers, and a predominantly rhomboid morphology. These are clearly more difficult to detect than urate crystals. (See also Plate 3.)

Table 1 Some causes of changes in bone density

Causes of increased bone density	Causes of decreased bone density
Generalized/multiple regional:	
Myelofibrosis	Osteoporosis
Osteopetrosis	Myeloma, leukaemia
	Osteomalacia, rickets
	Hyperparathyroidism
	Vitamin C deficiency
	Osteogenesis imperfecta
Localized:	
Paget's disease (with altered trabecular pattern and radiolucent areas)	Inflammatory arthritis (juxta-articular)
Metastases (especially prostate, breast)	Infection
Osteoid osteoma (sometimes with a central radiolucency)	Algodystrophy (regional)
Bone islands	Extreme disuse

- periosteal reaction (Table 2)
- calcification (cartilage—chondrocalcinosis; synovium, capsule, ligament, tendon, muscle, fat, vascular, skin)
- bone cysts and radiolucent lesions (Table 3)
- intra-articular osteochondral bodies
- deformity.

Although most of these abnormalities taken individually have low specificity, various combinations of some of these features, together with their targeting of certain joint sites (Fig. 5), result in characteristic patterns of abnormality and distribution that have high diagnostic specificity. The distribution of joint involvement, of course, is usually apparent following clinical assessment of the patient, and joints to be investigated by radiography will usually be selected on this basis. An important exception, however, is seronegative spondarthropathy where sacroiliac involvement is often asymptomatic and is difficult to detect clinically. For suspected seronegative spondarthropthy an anteroposterior view of the pelvis and a lateral thoracolumbar spine view (i.e. two films) are usually sufficient to show sacroiliitis and syndesmophytes if these are present.

Radiographs should be selected to answer specific questions. For example, to address the question of whether a patient with chronic inflammatory polyarthritis affecting hands, elbows, neck, knees, and ankles has erosive disease typical of rheumatoid, posteroanterior views of hands and feet (i.e. two films), but not radiographs of all symptomatic joints, are appropriate. This is because rheumatoid erosions appear first in wrists and the small joints of hands and feet, and may first affect the metatarsophalangeal joints, even if they are relatively asymptomatic. However, if the degree of structural damage in one large joint is a principal cause for concern then a radiograph of that particular joint should obviously be taken. For most joints a single (two-dimensional) view is sufficient (for example anteroposterior view of pelvis, posteroanterior view of both hands, posteroanterior view of both feet), although two views are required for some (for example posteroanterior standing view of both knees plus individual lateral or bilateral skyline patellofemoral view). Thus selection of radiographs will often differ for purposes of diagnosis or disease assessment.

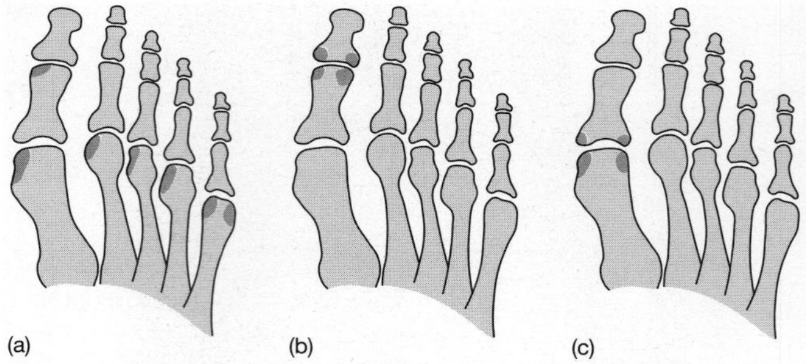

Fig. 5 Diagram to show different target sites of involvement in the forefoot for (a) rheumatoid arthritis, (b) psoriatic arthritis, and (c) osteoarthritis.

Table 2 Some causes of periosteal reaction

Localized:	Infection Trauma Tumour
Multiple sites:	Hypertrophic osteoarthropathy Seronegative spondarthropathy Scurvy

Table 3 Some causes of radiolucent lesions

Bone cysts (isolated or in association with osteoarthritis)
Inflammatory arthritis (erosions)
Infection
Metastases (especially breast, lung, kidney, thyroid)
Myeloma
Osteochondromata
Osteogenic sarcoma
Histiocytosis X

Erosions

An important hallmark of inflammatory arthropathies is cartilage and bone erosion. Intracapsular bone erosion first occurs at the 'bare areas' of the joint margin ('marginal erosion') where bone is exposed directly to inflammatory synovium without the protection of overlying cartilage. Loss of the sharp cortical line, the 'dot-dash' appearance, is the first radiographic sign that precedes more definite scalloping of the bony contour (Fig. 6). Cartilage erosion also commences at the joint margin and slowly works centrally, resulting in relatively late loss of interosseous distance or 'joint space'. Both rheumatoid disease and the seronegative spondarthropathies (especially psoriatic and chronic reactive arthritis) cause marginal erosions. In rheumatoid disease, however, the aggressive synovitis overwhelms any reparative response, presenting a very atrophic appearance ('non-proliferative erosions'; Figs. 6 and 7) with no new bone or periosteal reaction and only juxta-articular osteopenia (a sign of inflammation) and soft tissue swelling as accompanying early radiographic features. By contrast the seronegative spondarthropathies are characterized by a degree of low-grade inflammation that permits some reparative response. Such inflammation results in a tendency to fibrosis, calcification, and ossification. Marginal erosions in these arthropathies are therefore commonly accompanied by

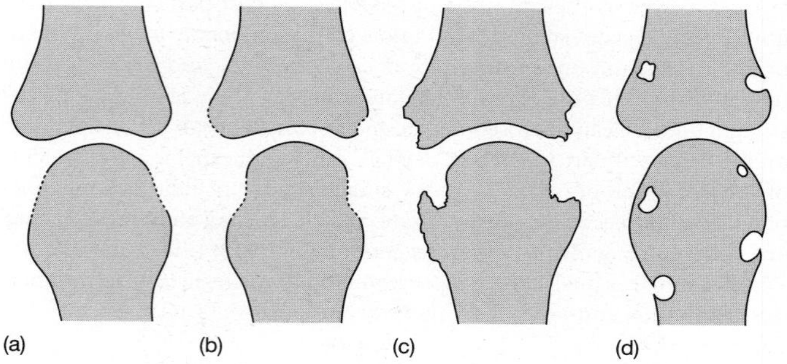

Fig. 6 Diagram of metacarpophalangeal joint showing (a) early dot-dash erosion, (b) the later definite non-proliferative erosion of rheumatoid arthritis, (c) the proliferative erosion of psoriatic arthritis, and (d) the intra- and extracapsular 'pressure erosions' of gout.

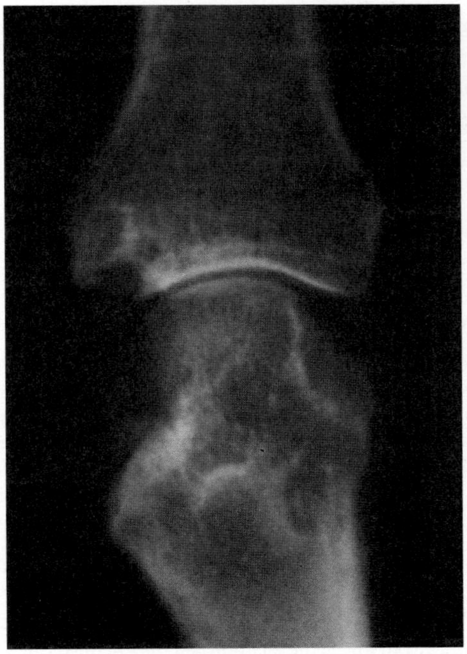

Fig. 7 Radiograph of metacarpophalangeal joint showing late non-proliferative marginal erosions of rheumatoid arthritis, more obvious proximally than distally (reflecting the more proximal than distal distribution of synovium in small finger joints) and eventual global loss of cartilage.

fluffy new bone formation ('proliferative erosions'; Figs. 6 and 8) with normal or increased periosteal and bone density rather than osteopenia. The fact that different joints are targeted in these conditions, and the common accompanying involvement of entheses—fibrous insertions of tendons, ligaments, or capsule into bone—further assists differentiation in most cases.

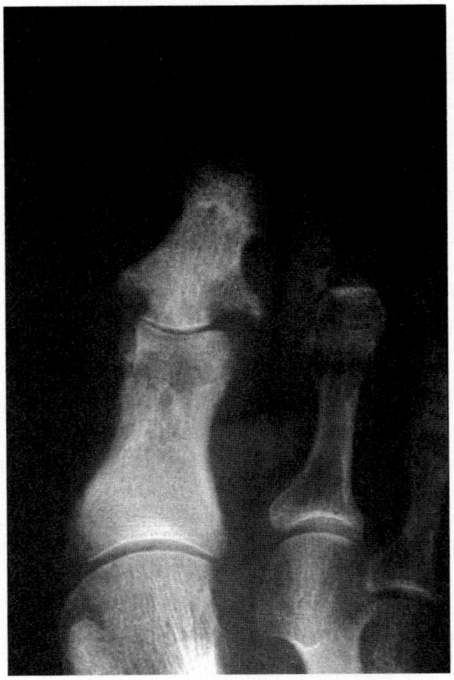

Fig. 8 Radiograph of the hallux showing proliferative erosions and cartilage loss of the interphalangeal joint, and associated increased bone density ('ivory phalanx') typical of psoriatic arthropathy.

In early septic arthritis the radiograph is often normal, apart from osteopenia and soft tissue swelling, for 1 to 2 weeks. However, erosion proceeds rapidly and results in generalized loss of joint space with loss of cortical integrity centrally (central erosion) as well as marginally. In chronic gout bony defects develop slowly as massive crystal concretions ('tophi') causing pressure necrosis to surrounding bone; such 'pressure erosions' (Fig. 6) occur at extracapsular as well as intracapsular sites and are unaccompanied by osteopenia.

Osteoarthritis

The features of osteoarthritis, by far the most common joint disease, are highly characteristic and contrast with those of inflammatory arthropathy. The two cardinal features are narrowing and osteophytes. By contrast to inflammatory arthropathies, joint space narrowing is focal rather than widespread within the joint, mainly targeting the maximum load-bearing region (Fig. 9). Bony osteophyte is most noticeable at the margins of the joint but also occurs centrally and as periosteal osteophyte ('buttressing') at sites such as the femoral neck. Subchondral sclerosis, or increased density of bone is also common, principally below the site of maximal narrowing. Additional features include subchondral 'cysts', osteochondral ('loose') bodies within the synovium, and an increased association with chondrocalcinosis. In contrast to inflammatory arthritis, the bone density is normal or increased and marginal erosions are not a feature.

Calcification

Calcification can affect any locomotor tissue. Calcification of fibro- and hyaline cartilage (chondrocalcinosis) is most commonly due to calcium pyrophosphate crystals, less commonly to apatite or other basic calcium phosphates. This can occur as an isolated phenomenon (mainly age-associated, rarely as a result of metabolic or familial disease predisposition) or in association with structural changes of osteoarthritis (chronic 'pyrophosphate arthropathy'). Less commonly pyrophosphate crystals also cause calcification of the synovium and capsule, and linear tendon calcification (mainly hip adductors, Achilles, triceps).

Periarticular calcification is usually apatite. Isolated periarticular calcification mainly affects central sites such as the shoulder (supraspinatus tendons) or hip (abductor tendons), appearing as single dense concretions with rounded contours, as opposed to the linear calcification of pyrophosphate. Shedding of these crystal deposits can result in severe, self-limiting inflammation (acute calcific periarthritis) with reduction or loss of the radiographic calcification.

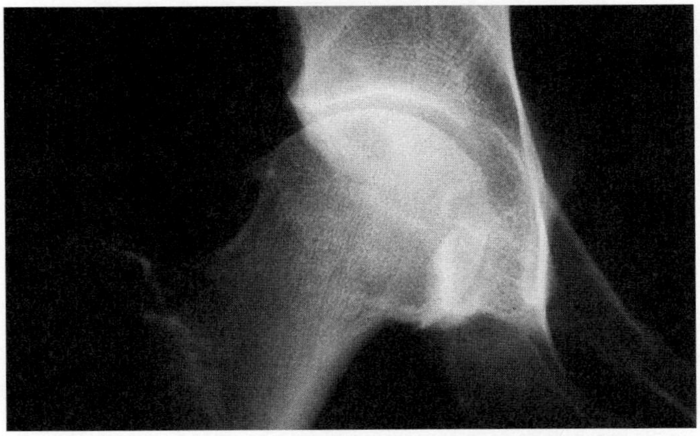

Fig. 9 Radiograph of the hip to show changes of osteoarthritis, specifically superior joint space narrowing, subchondral sclerosis, marginal osteophyte, and cysts.

Spotty, multiple calcification of soft tissues (calcinosis) mainly targets peripheral and intermediate sites such as the finger pulps, wrists, and forearms and is a feature of connective tissue disease, most commonly CREST syndrome (**C**alcinosis, **R**aynaud's, o**E**sophageal dysmotility, **S**clerodactyly, **T**elangiectasia). Calcinosis requires distinction from small blood vessel calcification (increased in diabetes and chronic renal failure) which has a thin, meandering tramline appearance, sesamoids, and solitary dense calcified phleboliths. Myositis ossificans is rare and appears as dense sheets of calcification mainly at proximal sites such as the hip. Fine reticular or linear calcification of subcutaneous fat and muscle may follow young onset dermatomyositis.

Other imaging

Arthrography

Injection of positive (iodinated) or negative (air) contrast, or a combination of both, can help delineate the soft tissue outline of a joint or other tissue space (for example bursa). The main use of plain film arthrography is at the knee to demonstrate a ruptured popliteal ('Baker's') cyst as a cause of calf pain and swelling. It is also commonly used with either computed tomography (**CT**) or magnetic resonance imaging (**MRI**) to provide better anatomical assessment.

Scintigraphy

Scintigraphy is a cheap, readily available technique that delivers only a very small amount of radiation. It involves gamma camera imaging following an intravenous injection of radioisotope, usually $^{99}Tc^{m}$ diphosphonate. Early 'flow' images obtained immediately postinjection, or a little later when the isotope is in the soft tissues ('blood pool' phase), reflect vascularity and will show, for example, the increased perfusion of inflamed synovium, Pagetic bone, or hypervascular primary or secondary bone tumour (Fig. 10). 'Delayed' images, taken a few hours after injection, indicate bone remodelling due to localization of the diphosphonate to sites of active bone turnover. Although non-specific and lacking high spatial resolution, the major advantage of scintigraphy is its high sensitivity for detecting important bone and joint pathology that may not be apparent on plain radiographs. It is particularly useful, following a normal or inconclusive plain radiograph of the presenting painful region, as the second imaging investigation to detect the following:

- bone metastases (at the presenting site and at clinically occult sites)

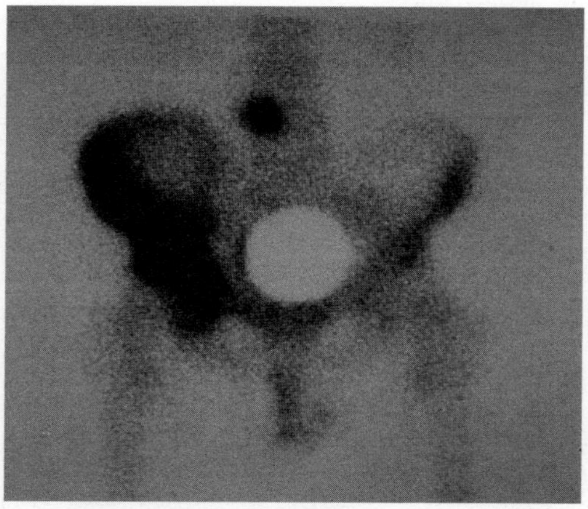

Fig. 10 Bone scan demonstrating secondary deposits of prostate cancer. The presenting painful lesion was in the right hemipelvis and the plain pelvic radiograph was normal. The spinal lesion (and two others not shown on this photograph) were asymptomatic.

- bone or joint sepsis (at the presenting site and at clinically occult sites)
- early osteonecrosis (at the presenting site and at clinically occult sites)
- stress fracture
- reflex sympathetic dystrophy (algodystrophy)
- hypertrophic osteoarthropathy.

Scintigraphy is also useful in delineating the extent and current activity of Paget's disease of bone.

Computed tomography

Computerized reconstruction of multiple radiographic scan sections can give detailed information on anatomy, especially of bone, allowing three-dimensional visualization of structures such as the spinal canal and facet joints. Its principal use is therefore in assessing areas of complex anatomy such as the spine or pelvis where plain radiographs may be inadequate (for example to investigate stenosis of the spinal canal). Drawbacks, however, include limited soft tissue resolution and exposure to a considerable radiation dose; in many situations it is has now been superseded by MRI.

Magnetic resonance imaging

The ability of MRI to image the anatomy and biochemistry of soft tissue as well as bone means that it provides detailed information not only on structure but also on the pathophysiology of all locomotor tissues. Further advantages include its capacity for multiplanar imaging (for example coronal, axial, sagittal, oblique) and its safety, without radiation exposure. The physics of MRI is complex. When a patient is placed in the magnetic field of the scanner the protons in the body align along the central axis of the field. Application of a radiofrequency pulse or 'sequence' causes the protons to spin in phase with each other. When the pulse is stopped the protons return to random spinning and 'dephase'. As they do so they emit a signal that is converted to an image by computer manipulation. In general, T_1-weighted short sequences are useful for defining anatomy, and T_2-weighted long sequences are useful for assessing pathology. Other sequences are selected for special purposes, for example the short tau inversion recovery sequence (**STIR**) is used to image marrow since it suppresses fat and makes the marrow appear dark. MRI, with or without enhancement with gadolinium, is particularly useful in detecting and assessing the following:

- early osteonecrosis (at the presenting site and the contralateral clinically occult site)
- intervertebral disc disease, root entrapment, and spinal cord compression
- osteoarticular and soft tissue sepsis
- osteoarticular and soft tissue malignancy
- internal mechanical derangement of joints (particularly the knee)
- assessment of soft tissue and periarticular pathology (for example early synovitis, rotator cuff tears, bursitis, tenosynovitis).

The choice between three-phase scintigraphy and MRI for detection of conditions such as early osteonecrosis, where both have excellent sensitivity (scintigraphy 90 per cent, MRI 100 per cent), will depend on practical issues such as ease of access, musculoskeletal reporting expertise, and local cost.

Ultrasonography

This is a safe and accessible technique for confirming soft tissue changes such as a hip joint effusion, popliteal cyst, or thickened Achilles tendon. Limited resolution, however, makes it inferior to CT or MRI for defining anatomical abnormality.

Blood tests for inflammation and systemic disease

The full blood count, erythrocyte sedimentation rate, and C-reactive protein may show changes that indicate the presence of inflammation somewhere in the body. These changes are very sensitive but are non-specific. They are mainly used as a semiquantitative measure to complement the clinical assessment of inflammatory disease and its response to treatment.

The systemic response to injury that results in these changes is summarized in Fig. 11. At any site of injury or inflammation macrophages and monocytes release soluble intercellular signalling polypeptides (cytokines) including interleukin 1, interleukin 6, and tumour necrosis factor-α. Some of these cytokines enter the systemic circulation and exert effects on the hypothalamus, bone marrow, and liver. These combined systemic effects are called the acute phase response, even though they accompany chronic as well as acute inflammation. Interleukin 6 is the main cytokine to influence the liver, causing increased production of certain acute phase proteins (including fibrinogen and C-reactive protein) but decreased production of other negative acute phase reactants (such as albumin and transferrin).

Much of the acute phase is beneficial for body defence and adaptation to injury, especially for dealing with the two major complications of injury that threaten life—haemorrhage and sepsis. For example, the thrombocytosis and increased serum levels of clotting factors facilitate haemostasis; neutrophilia and the increased serum levels of complement, immunoglobulin, and C-reactive protein (an opsonin) combat infection; and the anaemia and low serum transferrin levels result in diminished delivery of iron to bacteria and parasites.

Of all the acute phase proteins C-reactive protein shows the greatest shift from very low to very high levels, often representing a several hundred-fold increase in concentration. In addition C-reactive protein closely mirrors the current degree of inflammation, rising rapidly at its onset and falling as inflammation subsides, such that it is therefore the single most useful direct measure of the acute phase response. Interestingly, some rheumatic diseases—specifically lupus, systemic sclerosis, and dermatomyositis—associate with only modest or no elevation of C-reactive protein despite unequivocal pathological evidence of inflammation and tissue damage. The reason for this remains unclear, but patients with such disease are capable of mounting a typical acute phase response, for example in response to infection. In a patient with lupus or scleroderma gross elevation of C-reactive protein should therefore suggest an incidental cause such as sepsis. Some clinical features of active systemic lupus and infection overlap, and in this situation the C-reactive protein can prove a useful test.

The erythrocyte sedimentation rate is an old established indirect measure of the acute phase response. It mainly reflects the degree of rouleaux formation. Normally our circulating erythrocytes do not clump together because of the net balance of three electrical forces (Fig. 12):

- weak attractant van der Waal's forces resulting from red cells being bodies
- a strong repellent net negative surface charge, or zeta potential, due mainly to membrane sialic acid residues, and
- an attractant dielectric constant resulting from the charge characteristics of the plasma constituents.

In health the zeta potential far exceeds the sum of the two attractant forces, so that erythrocytes electrostatically repel each other and remain single. However, during the acute phase response the change in plasma protein concentrations leads to an increase in dielectric constant. Fibrinogen is particularly important in this respect. Although its increase in concentration is relatively modest, fibrinogen is a very asymmetric molecule that exerts a major electrical charge effect. The resulting increase in dielectric constant is sufficient to overcome the zeta potential so that rouleaux form more readily. Rouleaux have a higher ratio of mass per surface area so sediment faster than single red cells. This property is measured in the erythrocyte sedimentation rate. In the Westergren test system a 200 mm capillary tube is filled with the patient's blood. After 1 h the clearance of red cells from the top is measured. If there is little rouleaux formation the discrete red cells sediment only slowly and the clearance is small (less than 5 to 10 mm). However, if there is significant rouleaux formation the clearance is greater and the erythrocyte sedimentation rate in the first hour is elevated. Therefore in a patient with an acute phase response the erythrocyte sedimentation rate and C-reactive protein are both elevated, the erythrocyte sedimentation rate lagging behind the C-reactive protein in terms of speed of change.

The erythrocyte sedimentation rate, however, may be elevated for reasons other than the acute phase response. Immunoglobulins are very

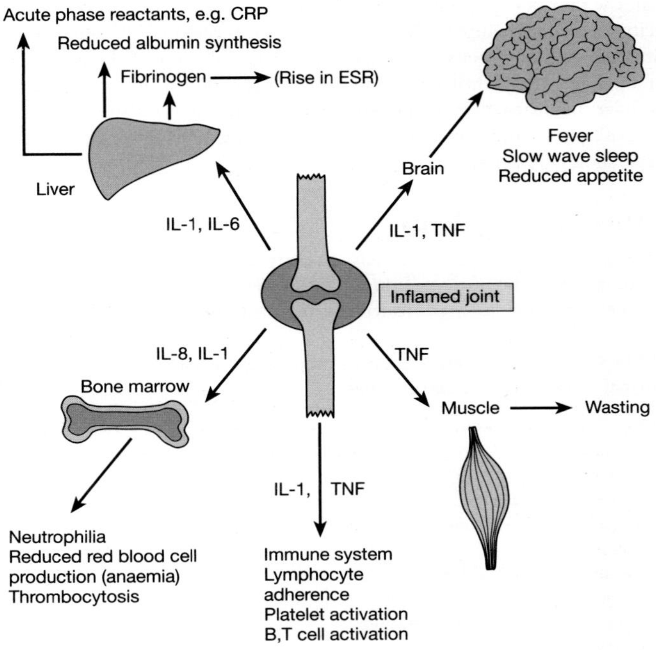

Fig. 11 Diagram to show the important elements of the acute phase response.

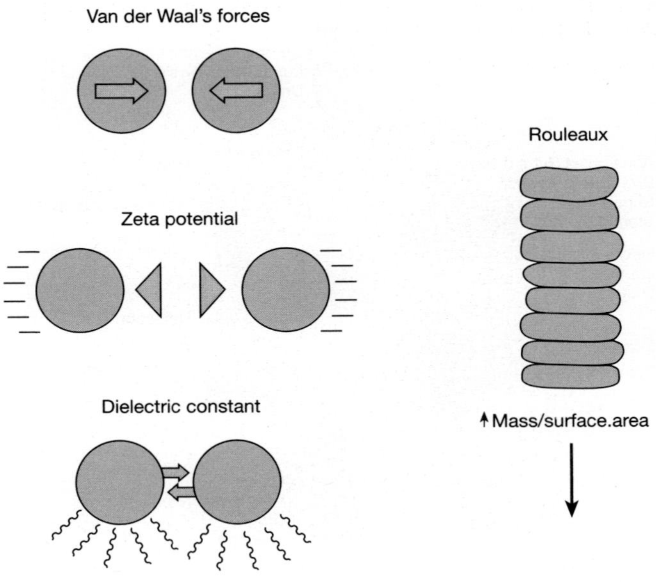

Fig. 12 Diagram showing the balance of three electrical forces that influence clumping of erythrocytes. Rouleaux sediment faster than individual erythrocytes.

symmetrical molecules and their modest increase in concentration during the acute phase response has relatively little effect, compared with fibrinogen, on the dielectric constant. However, large increases in immunoglobulin concentration (for example in multiple myeloma or associated with autoimmune diseases such as Sjögren's syndrome) will increase the dielectric constant and lead to rouleaux formation. In this situation the patient may have a high erythrocyte sedimentation rate but normal or relatively low C-reactive protein. Such discordance between the erythrocyte sedimentation rate and C-reactive protein should lead to consideration of hypergammaglobulinaemia and myeloproliferative disease and to direct measurement of serum immunoglobulins.

In addition to the changes reflecting an acute phase response, the full blood count may show other alterations that are non-specific in themselves but which, taken in the context of the clinical features, may be characteristic of certain rheumatic diseases or their complications (Fig. 13). For example, neutrophilia may be seen in systemic vasculitis, and neutropenia in lupus. Furthermore, many of the slow-acting drugs used to control chronic inflammation have toxicity on the bone marrow so that the full blood count is often included in the routine monitoring of such treatment.

Taken together, therefore, the full blood count, erythrocyte sedimentation rate, and C-reactive protein can be a useful complement of tests in the major rheumatic diseases to:

- assess inflammatory disease activity
- assess response to disease-suppressing treatment
- detect certain disease complications, and
- screen for drug toxicity.

However, it is important to appreciate that although an elevated acute phase response is consistent with inflammatory rheumatic disease, it is non-specific; also that the degree of elevation is often proportional to the amount or 'burden' of inflammatory tissue, for example isolated small joint synovitis in rheumatoid arthritis may not be sufficient to cause a detectable acute phase response, but this does not mean that inflammatory disease is not present.

Immunological tests

There are an increasing number of autoantibodies that can be detected from a serum sample by clinical laboratory services. Production of some of these is a common, age-related phenomenon that may be exaggerated by the presence of chronic inflammation. Their mere presence, therefore, often has low diagnostic specificity and little clinical relevance. If present in high concentrations, however, their disease specificity usually increases, so that it is always important to know how much antibody is present (the titre or concentration in units) rather than just whether it is detectable. For some autoantibodies (for example c-ANCA (antineutrophil cytoplasmic antibody)) their titre, if initially high, may be used to monitor the activity of the associated disease; only a few antibodies (for example anti-dsDNA) have high diagnostic specificity. Again, the correct choice and interpretation of these tests will depend on detailed knowledge of the patient. Different detection and assay systems exist for many of these autoantibodies and close liaison with the local immunology service is required.

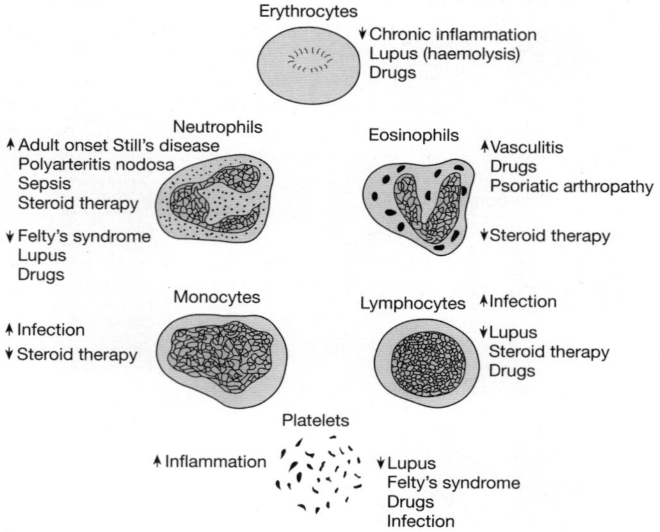

Fig. 13 Diagram showing some of the non-specific changes that may occur in individual elements of the full blood count in patients with systemic rheumatic disease.

Rheumatoid factor

The definition of a rheumatoid factor is an antibody directed against a specific region of the Fc (crystallizable) fragment of human IgG. The antibody itself may be of any immunoglobulin class, although IgM anti-IgG is the rheumatoid factor that is most commonly measured in the first instance. One of the traditional methods used to detect IgM rheumatoid factor is to coat latex beads with human IgG. If the patient's serum is then added to the test system the pentameric IgM antibody binds to the IgG causing the latex particles to flocculate producing a positive 'latex fixation test'. The amount the patient's serum must be diluted before this flocculation is lost is then determined; the higher this 'titre' the higher is the concentration of antibody present. Although 'rheumatoid factor' was so named because it was first detected in the sera of patients with rheumatoid arthritis, it also occurs in association with a variety of other conditions as well as in some normal adults (Table 4). It therefore has low diagnostic specificity, particularly in the elderly, and is not a 'test for rheumatoid arthritis'. In terms of sensitivity, it is present in the majority of patients with erosive rheumatoid disease but may only appear after many months or years of disease, once the diagnosis is beyond dispute. It is therefore of little value in making a diagnosis of rheumatoid arthritis, being neither sufficient nor necessary: rheumatoid arthritis is predominately a clinical diagnosis, based on detecting the presence of synovitis (capsular swelling, joint line tenderness, stress pain). However, if present in high titre at the onset of rheumatoid arthritis it associates with a poorer prognosis. IgG rheumatoid factor has greater specificity for major rheumatic disease, but the above caveats still remain. One situation where a negative rheumatoid factor is of diagnostic significance is in a patient with arthritis and nodules. As a general rule all patients with nodular rheumatoid are seropositive so that in this situation other causes of 'arthritis plus nodules' must be considered, for example tophaceous gout or hypercholesterolaemia.

Antinuclear antibody

An antinuclear antibody is any autoantibody directed against one or more components of the nucleus. Immunofluorescence microscopy after serum has been applied to a nucleated tissue substrate (for example rodent

Table 4 Associations with a positive rheumatoid factor (note that normal subjects can be seropositive)

Rheumatoid arthritis (about 75%)
Lupus, scleroderma, Sjögren's syndrome, dermatomyositis
Chronic infection:
Bacterial endocarditis
Viruses (rubella, cytomegalovirus, infectious mononucleosis)
Parasites
Neoplasms—after irradiation or chemotherapy
Hyperglobulinaemic states:
Hypergammaglobulinaemic purpura
Cryoglobulinaemia
Chronic liver disease

Table 5 Associations with a positive antinuclear antibody (note that normal subjects may be ANA positive)

Systemic lupus erythematosus
Rheumatoid arthritis
Sjögren's syndrome
Polymyositis
Polyarteritis nodosa
Juvenile idiopathic arthritis
Chronic active hepatitis
Autoimmune thyroid disease
Myaesthenia gravis
Extensive burns

organs) or human cell lines (e.g. Hep 2) is the standard method of detection, and four main patterns of staining are reported. As with rheumatoid factor, the higher the titre of antinuclear antibody the greater its significance, but a high titre does not necessarily imply more severe disease. The specificity and sensitivity also vary according to the antigen preparation used in the test system and whether the antinuclear antibody measured is IgG or IgM. However, the tests are not universally standardized, and again, liaison with the laboratory is important in order to determine which cut-off titre is considered to be 'abnormal'. The many causes of a positive antinuclear antibody are outlined in Table 5. The commonest reason to undertake an antinuclear antibody test is in a patient with suspected lupus. For lupus, the antinuclear antibody has high sensitivity (97 to 100 per cent), but because the specificity is very low (10 to 40 per cent) a positive result does not make the diagnosis; by contrast, a negative antinuclear antibody virtually excludes it.

If a screening serum antinuclear antibody test is positive most laboratories will then attempt to determine the specific antigenic determinants. Some of these determinants are soluble and can be extracted from the nucleus, hence 'extractable nuclear antigens' (ENA), although many of the antigen–antibody specificities in human disease remain to be discovered. Compared with the antinuclear antibody, antibodies against specific nuclear antigens may have higher specificity for certain diagnoses or for certain patterns of system involvement within the same disease. For example, antinuclear antibody directed against double-stranded DNA is highly specific for lupus. Unfortunately, it is present in only a minority of patients and those in whom it is positive often have classic severe lupus (for example with renal involvement) and a clear clinical diagnosis.

Antibodies to 'Sm' antigen occur almost exclusively in systemic lupus erythematosus and may imply a poorer disease prognosis. Antitopoisomerase 1 and anticentromere antibodies are found exclusively in diffuse and limited scleroderma respectively. Antibodies to 'Ro' antigen occur predominantly in Sjögren's syndrome and systemic lupus erythematosus and associate with a high frequency of photosensitive rashes and a risk of neonatal heart block. Antibodies to RNP (ribonucleoprotein) are found in systemic lupus erythematosus, but also in a variety of other conditions, including scleroderma, myositis, mixed connective tissue disease, and rheumatoid arthritis. Although these antibodies may associate with disease subsets, there is little evidence that they are involved in disease pathogenesis.

The antiphospholipid syndrome, defined by the occurrence of arterial and venous thromboses, recurrent fetal losses, and thrombocytopenia in the presence of antiphospholipid antibodies, occurs in lupus and other autoimmune diseases and also in subjects with no other underlying disease. Antiphospholipid antibodies can be detected in assays for anticardiolipin antibodies (predominantly directed against $\alpha 2$ glycoprotein 1) and in phospholipid-dependent coagulation studies to detect lupus anticoagulants (prolonged Activated Partial Thromboplastin Time (APTT) which fails to correct with the addition of normal serum). Antiphospholipid antibodies also occur in a wide variety of rheumatic, infectious (bacterial, viral, protozoal) and malignant conditions, although in these situations they are not usually associated with thromboses.

Table 6 Causes of chronic single-site synovitis

Foreign body (e.g. plant thorn)
Infection, including tuberculosis, fungi
Sarcoidosis
Amyloidosis
Pigmented villonodular synovitis
Synovial chondromatosis
Synovial sarcoma

Further information on these tests can be found in Chapters 13.14 and 18.10.2.

Tests for specific clinical situations

Chronic inflammatory disease at a single site

Patients with unexplained inflammatory disease at a single locomotor site (monoarthritis, bursitis, tenosynovitis, osteitis) should be considered for biopsy. The timing for this will vary according to how florid the lesion appears, but in general this should be undertaken for any undiagnosed lesion that has persisted for 6 months. The reason is to determine or exclude specific disease that can only be diagnosed by this means (Table 6). Although these conditions are uncommon or rare they require a specific treatment approach, rather than a continuing empirical symptomatic one. The commonest site for unexplained inflammatory monoarthritis is the knee, followed by the wrist and small hand joints. Arthroscopic biopsy is ideally used for larger joints (for additional information from direct visualization and guided biopsy), open biopsy for smaller joints and periarticular lesions. Tissue should be examined histologically and sent for culture, including mycobacteria. Apart from the specific conditions in Table 6, histopathology has no role in the diagnosis or management of most common rheumatic disease.

Investigation of suspected muscle disease

There are three principal investigations for the diagnosis and monitoring of muscle disease: serum creatine kinase, electromyography, and muscle histology. None are 100 per cent sensitive so that each may be normal despite abnormality detected by one or both of the others. Although creatine kinase is the most indirect measure it is readily available and commonly measured in the first instance. It is important to realize that elevation of the creatine kinase may result from a variety of causes (Table 7) and certain racial groups (e.g. Afro-Caribbean) have higher 'normal range' values. Electromyography or muscle biopsy will usually be undertaken next, the choice depending on local availability and expertise. How much information on diagnosis and disease activity has been gained from the first two tests will then often determine whether the third is also undertaken. The one used for subsequent monitoring of disease activity will be that which was most helpful in confirming the diagnosis.

Electromyography measures the action potentials produced at rest and during voluntary contraction. Normal muscle is electrically silent at rest.

Table 7 Causes of elevation of serum creatine kinase

Inflammatory myositis ± vasculitis
Muscular dystrophy
Motor neurone disease
Alcohol, drugs
Trauma, strenuous exercise
Myocardial infarction
Hypothyroidism, metabolic myopathy

Note: rhabdomyolysis is associated with massive elevation of the serum creatine kinase

On slight contraction motor-unit potentials of 500 to 1000 μV in amplitude and 4 to 8 ms in duration are recorded. On maximal contraction, as many motor units as possible are recruited and an interference pattern develops. With inflammatory polymyositis the electromyography may show a diagnostic triad of:

- spontaneous fibrillation
- short-duration action potentials in a polyphasic disorganized outline, and
- repetitive bouts of high-voltage oscillations produced by contact of diseased muscle with the needle.

Muscle histology can readily be obtained from a needle muscle biopsy sample. This is a relatively simple procedure requiring a local anaesthetic, small skin incision (no stitches required), an appropriate muscle biopsy needle, and no subsequent limitation of activity: it can easily be repeated serially for subsequent monitoring of response to treatment. The quadriceps is usually chosen, although the deltoid or other muscles can also be biopsied this way. The two or more small cores of tissue obtained by the needle need to be transported rapidly to the laboratory to be correctly orientated prior to freezing and sectioning. Immunohistochemical staining in conjunction with plain histology gives considerable information concerning primary and secondary muscle and neuromuscular disease. Although open biopsy will yield more tissue than needle biopsy, only a small amount of muscle is actually required and serial open biopsy is clearly problematic.

For further discussion of the investigation of muscle disease, see Chapter 24.22.4.

Investigation of suspected vasculitis

The clinical features of vasculitis often relate to specific organ involvement (ear, nose, and throat, neurological, renal, respiratory) but may be nonspecific (malaise, weight loss, night sweats). In view of the potential toxicity of appropriate treatment, further investigation is always required. In terms of laboratory tests, simple measures such as a urine dipstick test and microscopy should not be overlooked, as the prognosis of many of these diseases is dictated by renal involvement. Antineutrophil cytoplasmic antibodies (**ANCA**) were initially detected in patients with glomerulonephritis. These antibodies are directed against enzymes present in neutrophil granules. Two main patterns of immunofluorescence are distinguished, cytoplasmic and perinuclear. The majority of c-ANCAs and p-ANCAs are specific for the enzymes proteinase 3 and myeloperoxidase respectively. These two patterns have been correlated with particular disease manifestations, for example c-ANCA with Wegener's granulomatosis and p-ANCA with microscopic polyangiitis. However, positive ANCAs occur in a variety of other settings, including malignancy and infections (bacterial and HIV infection) as well as other autoimmune diseases (inflammatory bowel disease, rheumatoid arthritis, lupus, pulmonary fibrosis). Therefore, the diagnosis of these conditions cannot be made or refuted on the ANCA test alone. Other evidence should be obtained by biopsy of an appropriate organ (nose, kidney, muscle, skin) or angiography.

For further information see Chapter 20.10.3.

Table 8 Investigations to perform in multiple regional pain

Investigation	Condition
ESR/CRP	Systemic inflammation
Creatine kinase	Myositis
Antinuclear antibody	Lupus
Calcium	Parathryoid disease, osteomalacia
Thyroid function tests	Thyroid disease

Investigation of multiple regional pain

In most patients who present with widespread musculoskeletal pain the diagnosis is made from clinical examination alone, for example widespread rheumatoid disease. In some cases, however, there may be little to detect on clinical examination to explain the widespread pain. In most cases the diagnosis will be fibromyalgia. This is confirmed clinically by the appropriate symptoms (for example widespread pain, non-restorative sleep, marked fatigue, 'tension' headache, 'irritable bowel' symptoms, anxiety and depression, poor memory and concentration, urinary frequency) and the presence of widespread hyperalgesic tender sites and negative control sites (see Chapter 18.4). However, a number of other conditions may present similarly with multiple regional symptoms and few, if any, physical findings. In this situation, a limited screen (Table 8) is justified to detect conditions that have a specific treatment approach.

Further reading

Brower A (1997). *Arthritis in black and white*, 2nd edn. WB Saunders.

Gabay C, Kushner L (1999). Acute-phase proteins and other systemic responses to inflammation. *New England Journal of Medicine* **340**, 448–54.

Hoffman GS, Specks U (1998). Antineutrophil cytoplasmic antibodies. *Arthritis and Rheumatism* **41**, 1521–37.

McCarty DJ (1997). Synovial fluid. In: *Arthritis and allied conditions* (Coopman WJ, ed.), 13th edn, pp. 81–102. Williams and Wilkins, Maryland.

18.4 Back pain and regional disorders

Simon Carette

Low back pain

Introduction

Low back pain is one of the commonest symptoms and was the fifth leading reason for all visits to doctors' surgeries in the United States in 1990. Between 60 and 80 per cent of adults will suffer from at least one episode of back pain during their lifetime. Acute back pain is usually self-limiting, and the majority of subjects do not seek medical advice. Of those who do, more than 90 per cent will be back to work within 2 months, independent of the treatment received, including those in whom the acute episode results from a work-related injury for which compensation might be available. The 5 to 10 per cent of patients who remain disabled after this time represent a difficult therapeutic challenge due to the influence of psychological and social factors on the continuation of pain. This small percentage of patients is responsible for more than 75 per cent of the total costs of low back pain to our society, estimated to be between 1 and 2 per cent of the gross national product in most industrialized countries.

Significant risk factors for the occurrence of back pain include older age, heavy labour (in particular jobs requiring lifting in an awkward position), lower education and income, smoking, and obesity. Long-distance driving and whole-body vibration such as experienced by lorry drivers is a well-known risk factor for disc herniation. Prior episodes of back pain are strong predictors of recurrence. A number of psychosocial risk factors, or so-called 'yellow flags', predict poor outcomes. These include beliefs that back pain is harmful or potentially severely disabling, resulting in fear/avoidance behaviour and reduced activity levels, excessive reliance on aids and appliances, depressed mood, withdrawal from social interaction, and job dissatisfaction.

Many structures of the back, including the muscles, ligaments, discs, bones, and zygoapophyseal and sacroiliac joints are innervated and can therefore be a source of pain. However, in more than 90 per cent of patients presenting with low back pain, it is extremely difficult—if not impossible—to identify precisely the anatomical source of the pain on the basis of history and physical examination. These patients should be diagnosed as suffering from 'non-specific low back pain'. A host of clinical entities such as muscle strain, degenerative disc disease, facet syndrome, myofascial pain syndrome, segmental instability, minor intervertebral displacement, ilio-lumbar syndrome, piriformis syndrome, etc. have been described within this broad category based on the localization of pain and tenderness, reproduction of symptoms by specific manoeuvres, radiological features, or pathophysiological hypotheses. Unfortunately, the signs and manoeuvres described for each of these clinical syndromes lack sensitivity and specificity and are not reproducible even by experienced clinicians. Moreover, the claim that any of these entities is responsible for the pain in a given patient can very rarely be validated. For example, it is hazardous to ascribe pain to degenerative disc disease or apophyseal joint osteoarthritis when it has been shown that individuals with similar radiological changes can be completely asymptomatic. The only way to determine if the discs, or zygoapophyseal or sacroiliac joints are the source of pain in a given patient is through injection studies done under stringent, controlled conditions (see below).

Clinical approach to the diagnosis of low back pain

In evaluating a patient presenting with low back pain, the physician should not try to differentiate between the various elusive entities responsible for non-specific back pain but rather should focus on determining if the patient needs emergency surgery, has sciatica with signs of nerve root compression, or has an underlying medical cause of back pain (infectious, inflammatory, metabolic, tumoural, or visceral) (Table 1).

Is this a surgical emergency?

Cauda equina syndrome and an expanding vascular aneurysm are two extremely rare but important conditions to recognize since both are surgical emergencies. In the first instance, the patient will usually present with low back and/or buttock pain, associated with bilateral sciatica, neurological symptoms in the lower extremities, and urinary and/or bowel

Table 1 Causes of back pain

Surgical emergencies		Cauda equina syndrome (disc, tumour mass, abscess)
		Aortic aneurysm (ruptured, dissected)
Sciatica with neurological signs		Ruptured intervertebral disc
		Spinal stenosis (the neurological examination is often normal)
		Spinal cord tumors (extradural, intradural-extramedullary/intramedullary)
Medical conditions		
	Neoplastic	Benign: osteoid osteoma
		Malignant: primary (multiple myeloma); secondary (metastasis)
	Infectious	Acute: pyogenic discitis, osteomyelitis
		Chronic: tuberculosis
	Inflammatory	Ankylosing spondylitis
		Psoriatic arthritis
		Reactive arthritis
		Inflammatory bowel diseases
	Metabolic	Osteoporosis (with fractures)
		Osteomalacia
		Paget's disease of bone
	Visceral	Pelvic organs (endometriosis, prostatitis)
		Renal disease (pyelonephritis, renal colic)
		Gastrointestinal (pancreatitis)
		Aortic aneurysm
Non-specific low back pain		Muscle
		Ligaments
		Discs
		Zygapophyseal joints
		Sacroiliac joints
		Spondylolisthesis

incontinence. Physical examination may show bilateral weakness, sensory losses, saddle anaesthesia, decreased reflexes in the legs, and decreased rectal tone. Diagnostic procedures (magnetic resonance imaging (**MRI**), computed tomography (**CT**) scan, or myelogram) should be performed on an emergency basis if bowel and bladder control are to be preserved. Central disc herniation is the most common cause of the syndrome, followed by tumours and epidural abscesses.

An aortic aneurysm can be responsible for a dull, gnawing back pain due to direct compression of the aneurysm on the lumbar vertebrae. They are typically seen in elderly patients, especially white men, and physical examination may reveal a pulsating abdominal mass and decreased pulses in the lower extremities. Diagnosis is most important because rupture or dissection of the aneurysm can be fatal in 15 to 70 per cent of cases in various series. In this instance, the patient presents with a sudden, excruciating tearing abdominal or back pain radiating to the groin, buttocks, or thighs with haemodynamic compromise (hypotension, tachycardia, and shock). Up to 30 per cent of ruptured aneurysms are initially misdiagnosed. Preventive surgery (before rupture or dissection) is the optimal treatment.

Does the patient have sciatica and/or neurological signs?

Sciatica can be defined as pain radiating below the knee. It is a rare symptom, being reported by only 1 per cent of patients with back pain, but its presence is usually associated with an identifiable aetiology. Typically, sciatica results from compression of the spinal nerve originating between L4 and L5 (L5 nerve root) and/or L5 and S1 (S1 nerve root) by a herniated disc, bone, or a combination of the two (spinal stenosis). Tumours, infections, or epidural haemorrhage can very rarely produce similar symptoms and signs. The pain in a patient with a herniated disc tends to be aggravated by prolonged sitting as well as any manoeuvre that increases intrathecal pressure such as sneezing, coughing, or defaecation. It is often associated with paraesthesiae and weakness in the distribution of the involved nerve.

Patients with spinal stenosis are usually older and typically complain of pain and/or paraesthesiae in one or both buttocks, thighs, and/or legs that develop on standing or walking and are relieved by 15 to 20 min rest ('neurological claudication'). These patients often walk with the trunk flexed since extension aggravates their symptoms by worsening nerve impingement. The neurological examination is most often normal or shows non-specific abnormalities, such as reduced or absent ankle reflexes. Differentiating neurological from vascular claudication can be difficult since both problems occur in the same age category. Typically, pain from vascular claudication is relieved faster with rest than that of neurological claudication.

Does the patient have an underlying medical cause for their back pain?

The history is by far the most important diagnostic step in the search of potential medical aetiologies of low back pain. A number of clues or 'red flags' should be looked for systematically. These include the presence of fever, chills, night sweats, weight loss, and nocturnal pain that should direct the clinician towards the possibility of neoplasia or infection. An insidious onset of back pain accompanied by significant early morning stiffness in a young individual suggests a spondylarthropathy and should prompt the clinician to enquire about the family history and undertake a detailed review of the ocular (conjunctivitis, iritis), cutaneous (psoriasis, mouth ulcers, balanitis, keratoderma blennorrhagica), gastrointestinal (diarrhoea, haematochezia, abdominal pain), genitourinary (urethritis), and musculoskeletal (peripheral arthritis, dactylitis, enthesitis, heel pain) systems. Risk factors for neoplasia (previous or current history of malignancy), infection (history of tuberculosis, AIDS, intravenous drug abuse, or recent genitourinary procedures), and metabolic bone diseases (previous fractures, menopause, corticosteroid intake, history of anorexia nervosa) should also be looked for in patients suspected of having a medical problem underlying their back pain.

Table 2 Physical examination of the patient with back pain

Patient standing	Posture (protuding abdomen, hyperlordosis, loss of lordosis, scoliosis)
	Spinal motion (flexion–extension–lateral flexion)
	Walking on heels (L4–L5) and toes (S1)
	Squatting (L2–L3–L4)
Patient sitting	Straight leg-raising test (tripod sign)
	Knee (L4) and ankle (S1) reflexes
Patient supine	Abdominal examination (mass, bruit)
	Vascular examination
	Sensory examination:
	L4: anteromedial knee and leg
	L5: lateral leg, web space between first and second toes
	S1: lateral aspect of the foot, heel
	Motor examination (if abnormalities are noted in the standing position):
	L4: quadriceps
	L5: dorsiflexion of first toe
	S1: plantar flexion of foot and toes
	Hip examination
Patient prone	Palpation (spinous processes, paraspinal muscles)
	Sensory examination:
	S2–S4: saddle anaesthesia
	Motor examination:
	S1: contraction of gluteus maximus
	Femoral stretch test (L2 to L4)
	Sphincter tone

What are the key signs to look for in the physical examination?

A good examination of the lumbar spine and relevant nerves can be accomplished in less than 5 min if it is done systematically (Table 2). A full physical examination must be completed in patients suspected of having a medical cause for their back pain. The diagnostic utility of the many physical manoeuvres described to identify zygapophyseal and sacroiliac joint pain has been refuted when validated against diagnostic blocks with local anaesthetic. Waddell has described a number of non-organic physical signs (Table 3). When a patient has three or more of these signs, this suggests that psychological factors or secondary gains may be involved.

The classification of non-specific low back pain

In 1987, the Quebec Task Force on Spinal Disorders proposed a classification of activity-related spinal disorders in 11 mutually exclusive categories based on pain localization, neurological examination, paraclinical examinations, and response to treatment. The first four categories are divided according to duration of symptoms and work status as both of these factors can influence management (Table 4).

Who should be investigated and how?

There are now clinical guidelines available from the United States, the United Kingdom, Australia, The Netherlands, Israel, and New Zealand to

Table 3 Waddel's tests for functional low back pain

Tenderness to superficial touch
Simulation tests*
Axial loading
Spinal rotation in one plane
Distraction tests
Inconsistent results on confirmatory testing
Regional disturbances
Abnormalities not following neuroanatomical structures
Over-reaction
Disproportionate verbalization

*A positive test results in aggravation of low back pain.

Table 4 Classification of activity-related spinal disorders.

1*	Back pain without radiation
2*	Back pain plus proximal radiation to extremity (above the knee)
3*	Back pain plus distal radiation to extremity (below the knee)
4*	Back pain plus radiation to extremity plus neurological signs
5	Presumptive compression of a spinal nerve on a simple radiograph (i.e. vertebral instability or fracture)
6	Compression of a spinal nerve root confirmed by: (a) specific imaging (CT, MRI, or myelography) (b) other diagnostic techniques (EMG, venography)
7	Spinal stenosis
8	Postsurgical status, 1 to 6 months after intervention
9	Postsurgical status > 6 months after intervention
10	Chronic pain syndrome
11	Other diagnoses

*Classes 1 to 4 are further divided in three stages: acute, less than 7 days; subacute, between 7 days and 7 weeks; chronic, more than 7 weeks.

Adapted from Spitzer WO *et al.* (1985). Scientific approach to the assessment and management of activity-related spinal disorders: a monograph for clinicians. *Spine* **12**, S1–S59.

help physicians manage patients with acute back pain. No such guidelines exist for chronic back pain. There is a general agreement that the initial assessment should focus on the detection of 'red flags' suggestive of a medical aetiology and that the vast majority of patients with back pain do not need any investigations. Recommendations for ordering a plain radiograph in a patient presenting with back pain include the following: age over 50, fever, weight loss, significant trauma, previous history of neoplasia, use of corticosteroids, drug or alcohol abuse, neurological symptoms and signs, particularly if widespread, night pain, morning stiffness (in which case a pelvic rather than a lumbar radiograph is recommended to detect sacroiliitis), and the persistence of pain after 1 month of conservative therapy.

All other tests should be restricted to patients in whom a medical aetiology is suspected from the history and physical examination, and patients with abnormalities on neurological examination who do not improve with conservative management. Ordering blood tests and imaging in any other situation can hardly be justified since not only are these tests unhelpful but they contribute significantly to medical costs. In addition, as many as 25 to 50 per cent of asymptomatic individuals have been shown to have abnormalities such as disc herniation on CT scans and MRI.

The sedimentation rate is the most useful blood test in patients suspected of having spinal infection since it is elevated in up to 80 per cent of cases. Neutrophilia and anaemia are also commonly seen in patients with neoplasia and infection. Laboratory evaluation of patients with osteoporosis and/or pathological fractures should include serum calcium, phosphorus, alkaline phosphatase as well as serum and urine immunoelectrophoresis (to detect myeloma), particularly if the sedimentation rate is elevated.

Many radiologists consider MRI to be the imaging modality of choice for the diagnosis of lumbar disorders. It provides a unique non-invasive means of studying the spine and is unsurpassed for imaging soft tissues. It is particularly helpful in the evaluation of spinal cord tumours, as well as infections of the spine, including discitis, epidural, and paraspinal abscesses. Computed tomography is superior to MRI for the evaluation of bony structures and therefore is the modality of choice for spinal stenosis, particularly when combined with myelography. Plain myelography is rarely used today except in patients who have contraindications to MRI or CT (claustrophobia in particular). The diagnostic accuracy of MRI, plain CT, and CT myelography is comparable for the assessment of nerve root compression due to disc herniation. While MRI is non-invasive and involves no radiation to the patient, the much lower cost of plain CT makes it an excellent choice in this context. CT-guided percutaneous biopsy is commonly used to obtain histological material from patients with tumour mass or infection.

As mentioned previously, injection studies done under fluoroscopic guidance are the only means of diagnosing back pain of discal, zygoapophyseal, or sacroiliac joint origin. When normal discs are injected with contrast material, the individual does not experience pain. A provocative discography should be considered positive only if the injection reproduces the patient's pain and no pain is experienced during the injection of adjacent discs. In a recent report, 40 per cent of subjects with chronic low back pain attending a large specialist spinal centre satisfied this strict definition and demonstrated a radial fissure on CT. Similarly, between 10 and 15 per cent of subjects report a significant improvement in their pain when their zygoapophyseal joints or their sacroiliac joints are injected with a local anaesthetic but not with isotonic saline. When taken together, these figures suggest that the anatomical source of pain can be established in as many as 70 per cent of patients with non-specific back pain by using these invasive techniques. However, the impact of this approach on patient management is unclear, since no treatment has yet been demonstrated to be effective for these specific entities.

Radionuclide bone scintigraphy with technetium-99m is helpful in conditions characterized by increased bone turnover. These include bone metastases, fracture, Paget's disease, and infections. Gallium-67 binds to polymorphonuclear leucocytes and can he helpful in the evaluation of vertebral osteomyelitis and sacroiliac septic arthritis. Typically, bone scans are negative in patients with multiple myeloma which is characterized by lytic lesions.

Neurophysiological studies are rarely indicated except in patients in whom it is difficult to distinguish between a neuropathy, radiculopathy, or plexopathy. Fibrillations in the paraspinous muscles are the most common and earliest findings seen in radiculopathy. Their presence indicates a lesion proximal to the vertebral foramen and excludes a plexopathy.

How best to manage patients with low back pain?

Surgical emergencies

As mentioned earlier, cauda equina syndrome and a ruptured vascular aneurysm are the only two conditions that must be managed surgically on an emergency basis.

Sciatica and neurological deficits

About 90 per cent of patients with a herniated lumbar disc will improve significantly with limited rest, analgesics, and anti-inflammatory drugs. The role of epidural steroids remains unclear. They may afford short-term improvement in leg pain but they do not reduce the need for surgery. Indications for surgery include persistent disabling buttock and/or leg pain despite 2 to 3 months of conservative management, and/or severe or progressive worsening neurological deficit whilst on treatment. Surgery may also be indicated in patients with neurological claudication due to spinal stenosis, but only after all attempts with conservative management have failed. Patients with spinal stenosis who are more incapacitated by back pain than by neurological claudication probably should not be operated on, since surgery is rarely effective and may even worsen back pain.

Medical back pain

Primary and secondary tumours of the spine can be treated by surgery, radiotherapy, or chemotherapy, while antibiotics with or without surgical drainage are the treatment for discitis and osteomyelitis. Postural exercises and non-steroidal anti-inflammatory drugs remain the cornerstone of treatment for patients with spondylarthropathies. While the efficacy of most non-steroidal anti-inflammatory drugs has been demonstrated, indomethacin and phenylbutazone are the two most effective in resistant cases (because of the risk of agranulocytosis and aplastic anaemia, in the United Kingdom phenylbutazone is only available for the treatment of ankylosing spondylitis when other therapy has failed or is unsuitable). Sulfasalazine and methotrexate are helpful for the peripheral arthritis associated with spondylarthropathies but they have no role in the treatment of the spinal disease. The treatment of metabolic bone diseases is beyond the scope of this chapter.

Non-specific low back pain

A number of systematic reviews of randomized controlled trials of the most common interventions have recently been published and form the basis of the recommendations found in the many guidelines published in the past 10 years. For acute back pain, patients should be advised to stay as active as possible. There is strong evidence for the effectiveness of analgesics, non-steroidal anti-inflammatory drugs, and muscle relaxants. Exercise therapy in the acute phase is ineffective. A very important objective at this stage is to reduce the likelihood of patients progressing to chronicity, not least because there are only a few modalities, including manipulation, back schools (programmes using cognitive, physical, and motivational methods to educate patients on how to manage their back problem), and exercise therapy that have been show to be beneficial in patients with chronic back pain. The early identification of psychosocial risk factors or 'yellow flags' is essential. Screening questionnaires have been developed to help clinicians with this task. Cognitive and behavioural approaches must be used in high-risk patients in an attempt to influence positively some of these factors. Patients with persistent back pain after 6 months represent a very difficult therapeutic challenge, particularly if they have not returned to work. At this stage, their chance of going back to their previous job is only 50 per cent, while after 1 year of absenteeism it decreases to 25 per cent. Health professionals have a major role to play in preventing this unfortunate outcome.

Neck pain

Neck pain is a very common symptom. In a recent large epidemiological survey from Norway, 34.4 per cent of adult respondents reported troublesome neck pain in the previous year, with 13.8 per cent reporting pain lasting more than 6 months. As for low back pain, neck pain can rarely be attributed to a specific anatomical source and the vast majority of patients presenting with this symptom should be diagnosed as suffering from 'non-specific neck pain' or 'cervical spinal pain of unknown origin', rather than applying non-validated diagnostic labels. Trauma, in particular acceleration–deceleration (whiplash) injuries, increasing age, lower education, and psychosocial factors are the most common risk factors associated with the development of neck pain.

The clinical approach to the patient with neck pain should follow the same principles as described for low back pain. Signs of nerve root and/or spinal cord compression should always be looked for, particularly in patients complaining of associated pain, numbness, or weakness in their upper and/or lower extremities. Older patients with cervical spinal stenosis due to severe osteoarthritis may present with wasting and lower motor neurone weakness in the arms or hands and spastic weakness and sensory disturbance in the legs.

A number of diseases from the pharynx (pharyngitis, retropharyngeal abscess), larynx (laryngitis), trachea (tracheitis), thyroid (acute thyroiditis), lymph nodes (lymphadenitis), carotids (carotidynia), lungs (Pancoast tumor), heart (myocardial infarction), pericardium (pericarditis), aorta (dissecting aneurysm), and diaphragm (subphrenic abscess) can refer pain to the neck and should be considered. These conditions will usually have other clinical manifestations to alert the physician to the proper diagnosis. The neoplastic, infectious, inflammatory, and metabolic conditions enumerated in Table 1 can also affect the cervical spine. In addition, rheumatoid arthritis and diffuse idiopathic skeletal hyperostosis should be considered in the differential diagnosis as both can involve the cervical spine and cause spinal cord compression.

A special task force recently proposed a classification of cervical disorders associated with whiplash injuries which takes into account both the severity and duration of symptoms (Table 5). Although the classification was designed to address problems related to whiplash injuries, it can be very useful in classifying and guiding management of patients presenting with non-specific neck pain unrelated to trauma.

Table 5 Classification of whiplash-associated disorders (adapted from Spitzer *et al.* (1995))

Grade	Clinical presentation
I	Neck complaint of pain, stiffness, or tenderness only. No physical signs
II	Neck complaint and musculoskeletal signs*
III	Neck complaint and neurological signs†
IV	Neck complaint and fracture or dislocation

*Musculoskeletal signs include decreased range of motion and point tenderness.

†Neurological signs include decreased or absent deep tendon reflexes, weakness, and sensory deficits.

Symptoms and disorders that can manifest in all grades include deafness, dizziness, tinnitus, headache, memory loss, dysphagia, and temporomandibular joint pain.

Acute, less than 4 days and 4 to 21 days; subacute, 22 to 45 days and 46 to 180 days; chronic, more than 180 days.

Investigation of patients with neck pain—who and how

Guidelines are only available for patients presenting with whiplash injuries. Patients with grade I whiplash-associated disorder do not usually require radiographic evaluation. Those with grade II to IV whiplash-associated disorder need a baseline radiological examination consisting of plain films with anteroposterior, lateral, and open-mouth views. Radiographs are usually unhelpful in patients with non-specific neck pain. Degenerative changes in the discs and zygoapophyseal joints increase with age and do not correlate with symptoms of neck pain. CT is helpful for evaluating the bony structures of the neck but it must be combined with myelography to adequately visualize the neural tissues. Therefore MRI is usually preferred in most cases with spinal cord or nerve root compromise. Fifty per cent of patients with chronic neck pain after motor vehicle accidents respond to diagnostic zygoapophyseal joint injection, suggesting that these joints are responsible for their pain.

Management of patients with neck pain

The majority of treatments recommended for the management of patients with neck pain have not been evaluated in a scientifically rigorous manner. Those that have been have shown very little, if any, evidence of efficacy. These include soft cervical collars, zygoapohyseal joint injections, and acupuncture. Patients with acute neck pain should be encouraged to maintain their usual level of activity. There is evidence that non-narcotic analgesics, non-steroidal anti-inflammatory drugs, mobilization, and manipulation are effective, while the promotion of rest and soft collars tends to prolong disability. Surgery is only indicated for patients with severe radiculopathy not responsive to 2 to 3 months of conservative management. There is no consensus as to how to best manage patients with chronic neck pain.

Regional pain disorders

Regional musculoskeletal pain disorders, defined as painful conditions in a specific region of the body, are extremely common occurrences. A number of clinical entities have been described for the shoulder, elbow, wrist and hand, hip, knee, ankle, and foot regions (Table 6). Most of the regional pain disorders can usually be identified through a careful history and directed physical examination, although recent research indicates that interobserver diagnostic agreement is only moderate for the conditions related to the shoulder region, particularly in patients complaining of severe or chronic pain, and those with bilateral involvement. Paraclinical investigations are not usually required for the diagnosis of most regional pain disorders.

In a patient presenting with regional pain, one should aim to determine whether the pain has its origin in the bones and joints, periarticular soft tissues (tendons, bursa, and fascia), nerve roots and peripheral nerves, or blood vessels or if it is referred from distant musculoskeletal or visceral

Table 6 Regional pain disorders

Diagnosis	Epidemiology	Clinical symptoms	Physical examination	Associations	Investigations	Treatment
Shoulder region						
Rotator cuff tendinitis	Any age	Pain maximum in the deltoid region; increased at night and by specific movements	Painful arc of abduction 60–120 degrees. Full passive movements; pain aggravated by resisted movement of the involved tendon. Positive impingement signs	DM, repetitive movements	Radiograph in chronic cases may show cysts and sclerosis of greater tuberosity	NSAIDs, steroid injection, physio
Calcific tendinitis	Age 20–60	Acute severe pain on the tip of the shoulder	Limitation of both active and passive movements by pain. Occasional swelling when bursa involved		Calcification on radiograph	Rest in sling, NSAIDs, ?steroid injection
Adhesive capsulitis	Age > 40	Diffuse pain in the shoulder area. Progressive restriction of movements	Limitation of both active and passive movements in all directions (external rotation-abduction-internal rotation)	DM, MI stroke, thyroid and pulmonary diseases	Arthrography	NSAIDs, steroid injection, physiotherapy, ?distension
Bicipital tendinitis	Very rare in isolation	Pain anterior aspect of the shoulder and deltoid region	Speed's* and Yerganson's† manoeuvres non-specific	Rotator cuff tendinitis	None	NSAIDs, steroid injection
Rotator cuff rupture	Age > 40	Sudden pain deltoid area	Weakness of abduction if complete tear		US, arthrography, MRI	Surgery if acute and patient <65, NSAIDs physio otherwise
Elbow region						
Lateral epicondylitis	Age 40–60	Pain lateral epicondyle; may spread up and down the arm	Tenderness lateral epicondyle; increased by resisted extension of the wrist	Over use		NSAIDs, physio, steroid injection
Medial epicondyltiis	15 times rarer than lateral epicondylitis	Pain medial epicondyle	Tenderness medial epicondyle; increased by resisted flexion of the wrist	Over use		NSAIDs, physio, steroid injection
Olecranon bursitis		Swelling ± pain olecranon bursa	Swelling ± erythema ± tenderness	Trauma, RA, gout	Bursal aspiration: cell count, Gram stain, culture, crystals	NSAIDs, steroid injection, antibiotics if septic
Wrist and hand region						
DeQuervain tenosynovitis	Women, age 30–50	Pain radial aspect of wrist and thumb base during pinching	Tenderness ± swelling abd.pol.longus. Finkelstein manoeuvre‡ +			NSAIDs, splinting, steroid injection
Trigger finger	Any age	Pain palm of hand; snapping finger	Tenderness ± swelling ± nodule flexor tendon	Diabetes, RA		NSAIDs, steroid injection
Dupuytren's contracture	Males, age 40–80	Flexion contracture of 4th and 5th fingers	Thickening palmar aponeurosis	Alcohol, liver disease, DM		?Steroid injection
Hip region						
Trochanteric bursitis	Women, age 40–70	Pain lateral aspect of hip and thigh; worse at night; increased by lateral decubitus	Tenderness greater trochanter	Hip OA, obesity		NSAIDs, steroid injection
Knee region						
Prepatellar bursitis	Women	Swelling ± pain anterior aspect of knee	Tenderness greater trochanter	Kneeling	Synovial fluid aspiration	NSAIDs, steroid injection
Patello-femoral syndrome	Age 15–40	Pain anterior knee, increased in stairs and by squatting	Tenderness patella ± patellofemoral crepitus			?NSAIDs, exercises
Anserine bursitis	Women, age 40–60	Pain medial aspect upper tibia	Tenderness medial aspect of tibia	Knee OA, obesity		Rest, NSAIDs, steroid injection
Popliteal cyst	Any age	Pain, stiffness, swelling posterior knee	Swelling posterior knee. Leg swelling if rupture	Inflammatory arthritis		Steroid injection

Table 6 Continued

Diagnosis	Epidemiology	Clinical symptoms	Physical examination	Associations	Investigations	Treatment
Ankle and feet						
Achilles tendinitis	Age 20–50	Pain over Achilles tendon	Tenderness ± swelling ± crepitus over Achilles tendon	Spondyl-arthropathies		Rest, NSAIDs
Plantar fasciitis		Pain plantar aspect foot	Tenderness heel, increased by passive flexion of the toes	Spondyl-arthropathies		Orthotics; weight reduction; steroid injection
Morton's neuroma	Women, age 40–60	Burning pain interdigital clefts increased by walking	Tenderness interdigital cleft; rarely sensory alteration, cleft 4th toe	Pes planus, pes cavus, tight shoes		Proper shoes, surgery

*Speed's manoeuvre: the examiner resists shoulder forward flexion while the patient's arm is held in extension and supination. A positive test causes pain in the biccipital groove.

†Yergason's test: the patient's elbow is flexed to 90 degrees and the forearm pronated. The examiner resists the patient's attempts to flex and supinate the forearm. A positive test causes pain in the biccipital groove.

‡Finkelestein's manoeuvre: the patient's thumb is flexed inside the fingers and the wrist is passively deviated in an ulnar direction. A positive test results in pain over the abductor pollicis longus and extensor pollicis brevis tendons at the wrist.

Abbreviations: DM, diabetes mellitus; NSAIDs, non-steroidal anti-inflammatory drugs; physio, physiotherapy; MI, myocardial infarction; US, ultrasonography; MRI, magnetic resonance imaging; RA, rheumatoid arthritis; OA, osteoarthritis.

structures. Lesions of the periarticular soft tissues account for most causes of regional pain disorders. Plain radiographs are helpful in delineating soft tissue calcifications which may or may not be related to the pain presented by the patient. Ultrasonography and MRI are of equal value in confirming a diagnosis of tendon rupture in the shoulder, knee, or ankle regions.

The principles of management include temporary rest, analgesics or non-steroidal anti-inflammatory drugs, local corticosteroid injections, thermal modalities, orthotics, and graded flexibility and strengthening exercises.

Diffuse musculoskeletal pain

Between 8 and 10 per cent of the adult population report suffering from chronic diffuse musculoskeletal pain and about half of these satisfy the classification criteria for fibromyalgia. The aetiology of fibromyalgia is unknown. Patients who seek medical help suffer from more psychological distress than those who don't. Although the pain is felt primarily in the muscles, the muscles show no histological or metabolic abnormalities other than those associated with physical reconditioning. There is evidence that substance P levels are increased in the cerebrospinal fluid of patients with fibromyalgia, thus supporting the hypothesis that the pain may be of central origin. Management which includes patient education, cognitive-behavioural approaches, regular aerobic training, and low-dose tricyclic agents is generally unsatisfactory.

Further reading

Agency for Health Care Policy and Research (1994). Acute low-back pain problems in adults. *Clinical Practice Guideline Number 14.* United States Government Printing Office, Washington, DC.

Boos N, Hodler J (1998). What help and what conclusion can imaging provide? *Ballière's Clinical Rheumatology* **2**, 115–39.

Burton AK, Waddell G (1998). Clinical guidelines in the management of low back pain. *Ballière's Clinical Rheumatology* **12**, 17–35.

Carette S *et al.* (1997) Epidural corticosteroid injections for sciatica due to herniated nucleus pulposus. *New England Journal of Medicine* **336**, 1634–40.

Linton SJ, Halldén K (1998). Can we screen for problematic back pain? A screening questionnaire for predicting outcome in acute and subacute back pain. *Clinical Journal of Pain* **14**, 209–15.

Loney PL, Stratford PW (1999). The prevalence of low back pain in adults: a methodological review of the literature. *Physical Therapy* **79**, 384–96.

Schwarzer AC *et al.* (1994) The relative contribution and clinical features of internal disk disruption in patients with chronic low back pain. *Spine* **19**, 801–6.

Schwarzer AC *et al.* (1995). The prevalence and clinical features of internal disk disruption in patients with chronic low back pain. *Spine* **20**,1878–83.

Schwarzer AC, Aprill CN, Bogduk N. (1995) The sacroiliac joint in chronic low back pain. *Spine* **20**, 31–7.

Spitzer WO (1987). Scientific approach to the assessment and management of activity-related disorders: a monograph for clinicians. Report of the Quebec Task Force on Spinal Disorders. *Spine* **12** (Suppl. 7), 1–59.

Spitzer WO *et al.* (1995). Scientific monograph of the Quebec Task Force on Whiplash-associated Disorders: redefining 'whiplash' and its management. *Spine* **20** (Suppl. 8), S1–73.

Van Tulder MW, Koes BW, Bouter LM (1997). Conservative treatment of acute and chronic nonspecific low back pain. *Spine* **22**, 2128–56.

Wolfe F *et al.* (1990). The American College of Rheumatology 1990 criteria for the classification of fibromyalgia. *Arthritis and Rheumatism* **33**, 160–72.

18.5 Rheumatoid arthritis

R. N. Maini

Historical background

The first clinical description of rheumatoid arthritis in the medical literature is generally accorded to Landry-Beavais (1800), although Garrod was the first to use the term in his book published in 1859. Whether rheumatoid arthritis existed in Western Europe in olden times is debated by scholars of medical history: descriptions of chronic deforming arthritis suggestive of rheumatoid arthritis in classical writings of Galen and others have, for example, been ascribed to chronic polyarticular gout. The suggestion has been made that rheumatoid arthritis was imported to Europe after the discovery of the New World in the fifteenth century, where it pre-existed as evidenced by examination of archaic Amerindian skeletal remains. The possibility that rheumatoid arthritis spread from the New World in recent times is not only of historical interest but has also led to speculation suggesting the importance of environmental factors in its causation.

The concept of rheumatoid arthritis as a disease entity continues to evolve with advances in knowledge of the multiple causes of chronic inflammatory joint diseases. Thus improved microbiological, immunological, and epidemiological methods have led to a reclassification of certain forms of chronic arthritis, which in the past may have been labelled as rheumatoid arthritis. These include arthritis caused by infections, such as rubella, parvovirus, and borrelia (Lyme disease), or due to biological responses to non-viable products of micro-organisms ('reactive' arthritis) such as yersinia, salmonella, and chlamydia. Diseases of uncertain aetiology, for example the spondyloarthropathies, sarcoidosis, and chronic arthritis associated with systemic lupus erythematosus, primary Sjögren's syndrome, and other connective tissue diseases, have all been recognized as distinct from rheumatoid arthritis in the relatively recent past.

Definition

Rheumatoid arthritis has been defined as a chronic systemic inflammatory disorder characterized by deforming symmetrical polyarthritis of varying extent and severity, associated with synovitis of joint and tendon sheaths, articular cartilage loss, erosion of juxta-articular bone, and in most patients, the presence of IgM rheumatoid factor in the blood. In some patients systemic and extra-articular features may be observed during the course of the disease, and rarely prior to joint disease. These include anaemia, weight loss, vasculitis, serositis, mononeuritis multiplex, interstitial inflammation in lungs and exocrine salivary and lacrimal glands, as well as nodules in subcutaneous, pulmonary, and scleral tissues.

The American College of Rheumatology (**ACR**) has developed and revised criteria for the classification of rheumatoid arthritis based on a hospital population of patients with established active disease (Table 1). These combine a constellation of clinical, serological, and radiological features and have become widely accepted for epidemiological and clinical studies. These criteria distinguish active rheumatoid arthritis from other forms of inflammatory arthritis with a diagnostic sensitivity and specificity of about 90 per cent. However, they are of less value in prevalence studies, which should ideally include patients with inactive rheumatoid arthritis.

The classification criteria are too restrictive to diagnose rheumatoid arthritis reliably early in its presentation, since not all the required features may be present at this stage of evolution. Moreover, a minority of patients presenting with polyarthritis who satisfy the classification criteria for rheumatoid arthritis may later differentiate into other disease types or follow a self-limiting course.

Epidemiology

Criteria and methods for diagnosis of rheumatoid arthritis have varied in different epidemiological studies: some have been based on retrospective analysis of hospital records and others on prospective observation of patients attending hospitals where clinical examination, rheumatoid factor tests, and radiography have been employed. Questionnaires and clinical examination, with or without tests for rheumatoid factor and radiography, have also been used in population studies. However, in recent years the more widespread use of ACR criteria, including a version with a modified format for use in population studies, has introduced a measure of standardization. Based on studies carried out in various parts of the world, some generalizations can be made about the occurrence of rheumatoid arthritis amongst different ethnic populations.

Given the inherent variability in the methodology employed it is not surprising that estimates of the incidence of rheumatoid arthritis in the United States and Europe vary. In a recent study the incidence was 54 per 100 000 in women and 24.5 per 100 000 in men. The incidence increased sharply to a maximum in women over the age of 45 and in men continued to rise into the seventh decade (Fig. 1). A declining trend in the incidence of rheumatoid arthritis amongst females has been observed in recent years.

The prevalence of rheumatoid arthritis has been consistently assessed as being between 0.8 and 1.1 per cent of the adult population in cross-sectional studies in United States and Western Europe, and translate into higher prevalence rates in the elderly female population. Lower rates of 0.2 to 0.3 per cent have been reported in China and Japan. The prevalence of rheumatoid arthritis amongst the black population is low in rural South

Table 1 American College of Rheumatology criteria for the classification of rheumatoid arthritis

1. Morning stiffness in and around joints for at least 1 h
2. Soft tissue swelling of three or more joints observed by a physician
3. Swelling (arthritis) of proximal interphalangeal, metacarpophalangeal, or wrist joints
4. Symmetrical swelling of joints
5. Subcutaneous rheumatoid nodules
6. Presence of IgM rheumatoid factor in abnormal amounts
7. Radiographic erosions and/or periarticular osteopenia in hand and/or wrist joints

Criteria 1 to 4 of at least 6 weeks duration. Rheumatoid arthritis is defined by the presence of four or more criteria.

From Arnett FC *et al.* (1988). The American Rheumatism Association 1987 revised criteria for the classification of rheumatoid arthritis. *Arthritis and Rheumatism* **31**, 315–34.

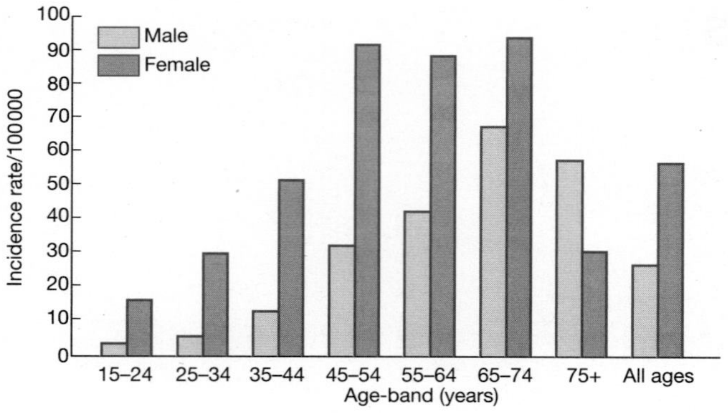

Fig. 1 Age-specific incidence applying modified ACR criteria for rheumatoid arthritis in a United Kingdom population registered in 1990 in whom multiple assessments were made over a 5-year period. Any one of seven criteria may be positive only once during this period. Data from: Wiles N *et al.* (1999). Estimating the incidence of rheumatoid arthritis: Trying to hit a moving target? *Arthritis and Rheumatism* **42**, 1339–46.

Africa (approximately 0.2 per cent) and virtually non-existent in parts of Nigeria. By contrast, prevalence rates of almost 1 per cent have been observed amongst black populations in urban South Africa and in the United States. A strikingly high prevalence rate of over 5 per cent has been noted amongst certain American Indian tribes in the United States, for example the Pima and Chippewa Indians. Differences in both genetic and environmental factors are likely to impact on these variations in incidence and prevalence rates, as are differing access to medical facilities, population age structures, and mortality. Such data are therefore of limited value in providing direct insight into aetiology, but are invaluable in directing research questions and allocating health resources.

Aetiology

Genetic factors

The initiating cause of rheumatoid arthritis remains unknown. A prevalence of 12 to 15 per cent in genetically identical (monozygotic) twins observed in Finland and Great Britain, compared with 4 per cent in non-identical (dizygotic) twins, and between 0.5 to 1 per cent in the general population, strongly favours multigenic influences. It also argues for an environmental trigger.

Advances in molecular genetics have permitted genotyping to confirm an association between the occurrence of rheumatoid arthritis and allelic polymorphisms of genes on the short arm of chromosome 6 that code for a hypervariable region of the β chain of HLA-DR molecules. The critical expressed pentapeptide sequence (glutamine–arginine or lysine–arginine–alanine–alanine) of amino acid residues 70 to 74 has been located to the helical wall of the antigen-binding cleft of the HLA-DRβ chain by molecular structural studies (Fig. 2). This pentapeptide region is also referred to as the 'shared epitope' because of its detection by a specific monoclonal antibody. The sequence is present, for example, on HLA-DR4 subtypes Dw4 and Dw14, and HLA-DR1 subtype Dw1, coded by DRB1*0401,*0404, and 0101 genes, respectively. The shared sequence and corresponding allelic genes have been detected in a frequency of up to 90 per cent in patients with rheumatoid arthritis of Western European descent. Their association with rheumatoid arthritis supports the hypothesis that these particular HLA-DR molecules present antigens to T-cell receptors and activate pathogenic reactions.

By contrast, HLA-DR4 subtypes, of which Dw10 and Dw13 are examples (coded by DRB1*0402 and *0403 genes, respectively), are negatively associated with rheumatoid arthritis. These subtypes are characterized by a substitution of the basic amino acids glutamine and arginine in positions 70 and 71 by acidic amino acids aspartic and glutamic acid. These alterations are sufficient to alter the specificity of binding such that a different set of antigens binds to the HLA cleft. Another possibility is that specific shared epitope sequences influence T-cell receptor interactions with the HLA-DRβ alpha helix independently of peptide. It is proposed that signals delivered to T cells are therefore different and lead to the activation of regulatory pathways that serve a protective function.

It is estimated that major histocompatibility genes confer 30 to 50 per cent of the genetic component of susceptibility to rheumatoid arthritis. However, the presence of DRB1*04 susceptibility genes also correlates with seropositive, erosive, and extra-articular disease. Homozygosity for DRB1*0401 or DRB1*0404, or when they are combined with each other or with DRB1*0101 (as compound homozygotes), appears to correlate with more severe disease, increasing the absolute risk ratio up to 1 in 7 (relative risk of 49). These data have been interpreted as indicating that the shared epitope encoding genes may be more useful as markers of disease severity in established rheumatoid arthritis than as markers of disease susceptibility.

It is intriguing to note that the HLA-DR B1 allele *0405—coding the shared epitope in a different HLA-DR4, Dw15 subtype—is increased in Japanese patients, whilst the DRB1*1402 gene coding HLA-DR6, Dw16 is increased in Yakima American Indians. However, other population studies, for example in black American individuals with rheumatoid arthritis, show no increase in frequency of the gene coding the shared epitope, thus casting some doubt on the hypothesis that it is an essential aetiological factor.

Recent studies have sought positive or negative correlation between disease severity and gene polymorphisms detected by nucleotide sequencing or microsatellite mapping. Using such techniques, associations with polymorphic alleles of candidate genes coding molecules involved in the pathogenesis of rheumatoid arthritis, such as tumour necrosis factor-α (**TNF-α**), a pro-inflammatory cytokine, and interleukin 10 (**IL-10**), an anti-inflammatory cytokine, have been described.

Environmental factors

The similarity of clinical features of rheumatoid arthritis and polyarthritis caused by infectious agents such as rubella, parvovirus B19, and Epstein–Barr virus (**EBV**), and reports of immune hyperactivity to their antigens in rheumatoid arthritis, continues to fuel interest in a potential role for such organisms in initiating rheumatoid disease. In one recent study, for example, the B19 antigen VP-1 was specifically expressed in active lesions in synovium with rheumatoid arthritis but not in osteoarthritis or controls. In

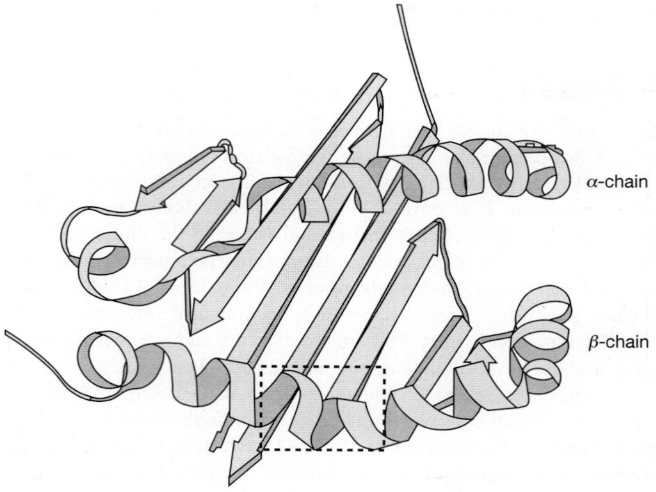

Fig. 2 Ribbon diagram of HLA class II molecule, demonstrating the antigen-binding cleft. The floor consists of a β pleated sheet and the walls are helical structures. The rectangle delineates the hypervariable region of the β chain containing the shared epitope (amino acid residues 70 to 74).

other studies, EBV-specific or rubella-specific lymphocytes have been detected in joints with rheumatoid arthritis. However, the arthritis caused by such known infections is almost always sporadic and self-limiting, and the clustering of new cases that one might expect if rheumatoid arthritis was an infectious disease has not been reported. Moreover, corroboration of claims by independent studies is still lacking, hence these theories of causation remain speculative.

In attempts to define a role for environmental factors in the aetiology of rheumatoid arthritis, epidemiological studies have sought differences in the incidence or prevalence of the disease in genetically similar populations exposed to urbanization, different socio-economic conditions, lifestyles, and known industrial noxious agents. In South Africa, one study found a higher point prevalence of rheumatoid arthritis in Bantu people residing in an urban township area—similar to that recorded for white people in Western countries—compared with Bantu in a rural community. However, in another study, black people living in urban Manchester, United Kingdom, had a lower prevalence of rheumatoid arthritis than white people and the low prevalence of rheumatoid arthritis amongst Chinese people living in urban Hong Kong was no higher than that observed in rural areas. These apparently contradictory data reflect the problems inherent in assessing the relative importance of genetic and environmental factors in heterogeneous populations in a disease with variable expression. The data on correlation with social class are also conflicting. Cigarette smoking, on the other hand, was associated with an increased risk of rheumatoid arthritis in two prospective population studies and in a twin study. Claims of an increased risk have also been made in people exposed to silica dust, organic solvents, and mineral oils.

It is possible that a decline in the incidence of rheumatoid arthritis amongst women noted in Rochester, United States, in the period 1950 to 1975 and in a general practice register in the United Kingdom in the decade following 1976 are indicative of a change in environmental pressures or in lifestyle. Epidemiological studies demonstrating a relationship between the birth weight of babies and future development of cardiovascular disease and premature death have drawn attention to the possibility that the environment of the growing fetus may be as important as environmental factors to which an adult might be exposed.

Host factors

A number of observations implicate sex hormones and prolactin in susceptibility to, or protection from, rheumatoid arthritis. Thus females have a higher incidence of rheumatoid arthritis, which is especially marked before the menopause. Exposure to the oral contraceptive pill confers a level of protection and postpones the onset of rheumatoid arthritis. Pregnancy is associated with suppression of disease, and the incidence of rheumatoid arthritis is increased following parturition and during lactation. Testosterone levels are reported to be low in males with rheumatoid arthritis, and the incidence of disease increases with advancing age when levels of male sex hormones are on the decline. Interconnections between the hypothalmic–pituitary axis, hormones, and cytokines have been described, suggesting possible mechanisms whereby these may influence the evolution of rheumatoid arthritis.

Pathology and pathogenesis

Pathology

Joints

The rheumatoid disease process in the joints is characterized by synovitis, an inflammatory effusion and cellular exudate into the joint space, and by damage to tendons, ligaments, cartilage, and bone in and around articulating surfaces of the joint. Long tendons whose sheaths are lined by synovial membrane, such as in the palms, wrists, ankles, and feet, may also be involved by the inflammatory process and cause malfunction due to damage, rupture, and fibrosis.

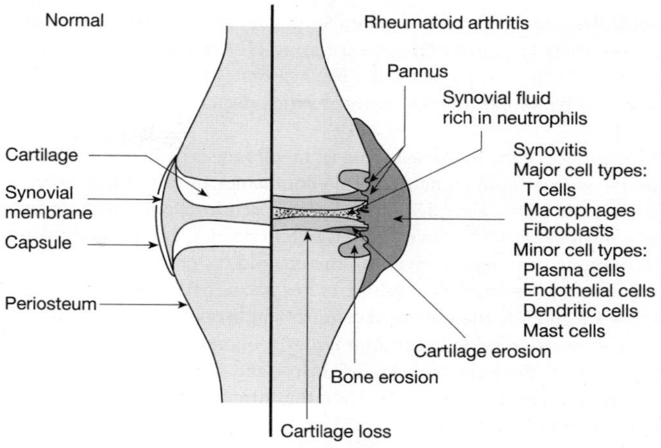

Fig. 3 The pathology of rheumatoid arthritis, normal joint (left) and rheumatoid joint (right).

In health the synovial membrane (the intima) is a film of one or two cells lining the capsule and its circumferential attachment to the periosteum at the cartilage–bone junction of the joint (Fig. 3). The normal synovial membrane consists of type A and B cells, without a basement membrane and lying on a bed of loose connective tissue and a network of small blood vessels (the subintima). Type A cells have morphological and phenotypic features of macrophages. Type B cells are of mesenchymal origin and share many, but not all, of the phenotypic features of typical tissue fibroblasts and are hence referred to as fibroblast-like synoviocytes.

In established rheumatoid arthritis the synovial membrane typically becomes enormously thickened and assumes a villous appearance. The diseased tissue now consists of an intima that is several (2 to 10) cell layers deep and coated by a film of fibrin. Type A cells predominate over type B cells and tend to lie in the more superficial part of the intima. The sublining layer (subintima) is also greatly expanded by newly formed blood vessels and infiltrating mononuclear cells, including T lymphocytes, lymphoblasts, B cells, plasma cells, monocytes, macrophages, dendritic cells, and synoviocytes (Fig. 3). The cellular infiltrate usually has a recognizable architecture, comprising perivascular aggregates of CD4+ T cells (Fig. 4 and Plate 1).

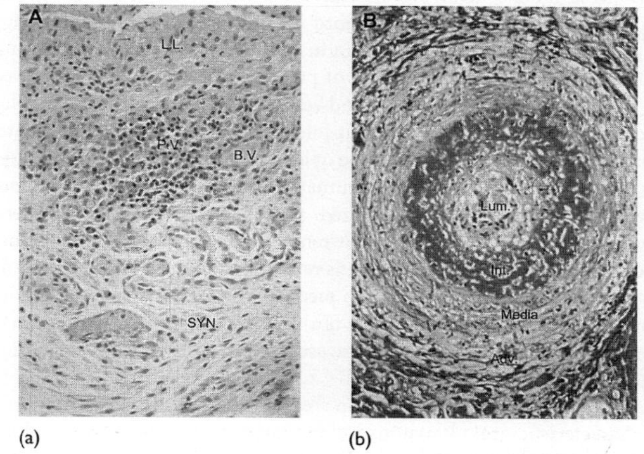

Fig. 4 Histology of rheumatoid arthritis. (a) Rheumatoid arthritis synovitis. L.L., lining layer; P.V., perivascular aggregate of lymphocytes and macrophages; B.V., blood vessel; SYN, synoviocytes; (haematoxylin and eosin staining). (b) Small vessel arteritis. Lum., lumen; Int., Intima; P.V., perivascular inflammation; Adv., adventitial tissue. Arterial wall shows a thrombosed vessel with intimal hyperplasia, destruction of internal elastic lamina, and mononuclear cell infiltration of media and perivascular tissue (methylene blue and safranine staining) (See also Plate 1).

Interaggregate areas show a mixed inflammatory cell population, including dendritic cells and macrophages expressing HLA class II, CD8+ T cells, activated B cells, and plasma cells. The aggregates may be organized into prominent lymphoid follicles, some of which display germinal centre formation.

The surface of the thickened synovial membrane is bathed in an inflammatory synovial fluid containing a predominance of polymorphonuclear cells, but also CD4+ and CD8+ lymphocytes, dendritic cells, macrophages, and synoviocytes. The synovial fluid is rich in pro-inflammatory cytokines and immune complexes containing rheumatoid factor. It is a site of local complement consumption, resulting in low haemolytic complement activity, low C3 and C4, and increased complement breakdown products.

The destructive lesion in the joint typically occurs at the circumferential attachment of the joint capsule, just below and adjacent to the articular cartilage and subchondral bone. Here the intima of the adjacent hypertrophic synovial membrane creeps over the cartilage, and tissue rich in blood vessels, macrophages, and synoviocytes (termed 'pannus') invades and destroys variable parts of articular cartilage and subchondral bone. The cells at the cartilage–pannus junction consist of synoviocytes and macrophages, whereas the pannus invading subchondral bone is enriched in osteoclasts. The connective tissue matrix of cartilage adjacent to pannus tissue becomes depleted of proteoglycans and collagen type II as a result of enzymatic degradation and lack of regeneration. A number of enzymes responsible for degradation of cartilage matrix have been demonstrated in the joint with rheumatoid arthritis, including the collagen-degrading matrix metalloproteinases I, III, and XIII, neutrophil-derived cathepsins L and D, and collagenase, as well as aggrecanase that degrades proteoglycans. The matrix in which chondrocytes are embedded becomes depleted, with loss of chondrocyte numbers, suggesting that matrix degeneration is secondary to degradative effects mediated by both pannus and chondrocyte activity or cell death. There may also be a reparative response in the later stages of disease, as suggested by the presence of fibrous tissue replacing areas of destroyed cartilage and bone in some joints removed at surgery.

Extra-articular disease

Extra-articular features associated with rheumatoid arthritis comprise essentially two types of lesion: the first involves arterial walls and the second leads to extravascular lymphocyte–macrophage granuloma formation.

Of those lesions involving arterial walls, two types of pathology are described. The first type is a bland fibro-intimal hyperplasia, without obvious inflammatory changes, resulting in vascular occlusion. This lesion is typically observed in digital vessels of patients with long-standing disease and is associated with collateral blood vessel formation. It correlates with a history of benign, intermittent nail-fold infarcts that develop in winter months. By contrast, the second type of lesion has a polyarteritic pathology and is observed in patients with rheumatoid systemic vasculitis and a poor prognosis. Medium- and small-sized arteries of the limbs, peripheral nerves, and organs are involved, but renal vessels are spared. Histopathological examination of involved vessels reveals lymphocytic, histiocytic, and inflammatory cell infiltration of the medial and perivascular area, disruption of the internal elastic lamina by fibrinoid necrosis, and proliferation of the vessel wall intima with intravascular thrombosis and occlusion (Fig. 4(b)).

Extravascular nodule formation in areas subject to pressure or friction is the characteristic granulomatous lesion of rheumatoid arthritis. Nodules consist of a central core of fibrinoid eosinophilic material surrounded by a palisade of histiocytes, occasional giant cells, and an outer layer of lymphocytes, fibroblasts, and fibrous tissue. Extravascular granulomatous inflammation, with or without nodule formation, has been documented on the surface of the pleura, pericardium, and endocardial valves. As is the case with systemic vasculitis and Felty's syndrome, the occurrence of nodules correlates with seropositive disease and the carriage of HLA-DRβ1*04 alleles.

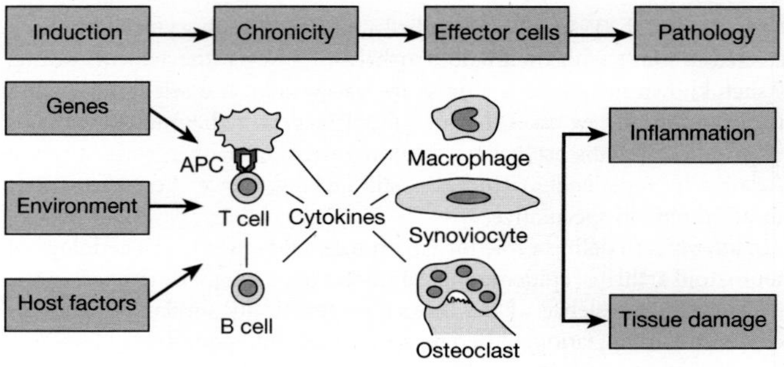

Fig. 5 Aetiopathogenesis of rheumatoid arthritis. In this simplified diagram the four steps in the aetiopathogenesis of rheumatoid arthritis are shown: (a) the induction phase involving interactions among genetic, environmental, and host factors; (b) the chronicity phase dependent upon immunological reactions; and (c) the effector phase of pathology mediated by macrophages, synoviocytes, osteoclasts, and cytokines, which leads to (d) pathology, namely inflammation and tissue damage.

Pathogenesis

Although the initiating cause of rheumatoid arthritis remains uncertain, there has been considerable progress in understanding the cellular and molecular mechanisms involved in chronic inflammation and tissue damage (Fig. 5).

The discovery of rheumatoid factor in the blood of patients with rheumatism over half a century ago led to the immunological hypothesis of disease pathogenesis. Since rheumatoid factor is an autoantibody directed against epitopes on the constant domains of the Fc portion of IgG1, the concept that rheumatoid arthritis is an autoimmune disease gained credibility. However, IgM rheumatoid factor occurs in a variety of other diseases in the absence of joint pathology. In the case of rheumatoid arthritis, rheumatoid factor complexes are present in synovial fluids, and IgG-producing B cells, whose rearranged immunoglobulin gene sequences implicate antigen stimulation, are present in inflamed synovium. B cells in rheumatoid joints also synthesize antibodies to some cartilage components such as collagen type II, although these are not disease specific. By contrast, recent research has shown a highly disease-specific antibody directed against citrullinated peptides in the serum of patients. It seems possible that autoantibodies could interact with complement and Fc receptors expressed on cells in the rheumatoid joint and so contribute to inflammation. Since IgG antibodies are implicated, T-cell help might be required.

The predominance of CD4+ T cells in proximity to antigen-presenting cells in the rheumatoid joint suggests their involvement in perpetuating the immune response. This is also supported by the association of rheumatoid arthritis with HLA class II genes and the beneficial response to T-cell-depleting therapies (lymphophoresis, cyclosporin, and some anti-CD4 monoclonal antibodies). For example, it has been proposed that as a result of molecular mimicry between epitopes on infectious agents and endogenous antigens an immune response is initiated which, by a phenomenon known as 'epitope spreading', overcomes tolerance mechanisms and results in autoimmunity. Alternatively, macromolecules in cells undergoing apoptopic cell death may become modified by oxidative or enzymatic damage and provide neoantigens to which autologous T cells are not tolerant. Candidate autoantigens under current investigation include proteins derived from cartilage, citrullinated peptides, and peptides derived from HLA class II molecules. However, an autoantigen that drives the immune response in rheumatoid arthritis has not yet been identified.

CD4+ T cells in joints appear to be of T_{H1} type, bearing memory and activation markers such as CD45 RO+, CD45B dim+, VLA-4+, CD69+, and HLA class II+. However, whether these T cells are antigen activated is debated since they do not appear to show significant T-cell receptor oligoclonality and do not display the full functional characteristics of such cells,

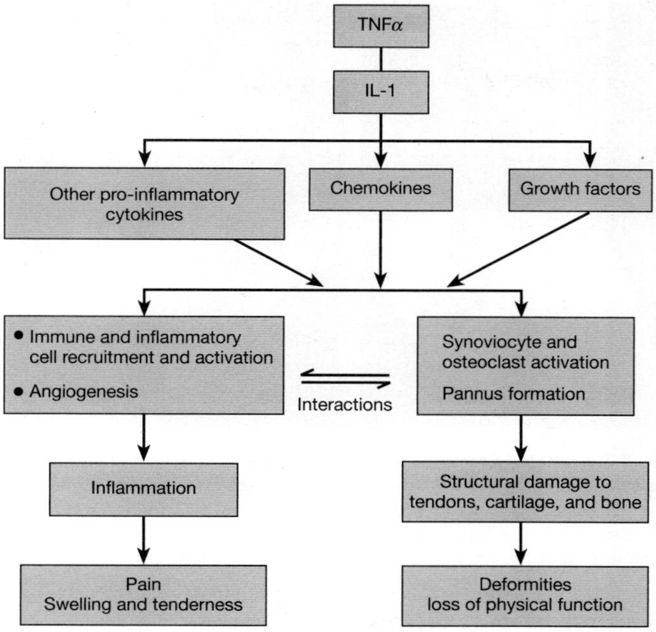

Fig. 6 The role of tumour necrosis factor-α in the pathogenesis of inflammation and structural damage to tendons and bone in rheumatoid arthritis.

for example the production of IL-2 and interferon-γ. Moreover, T cells in joints do not proliferate but increase in number by recruitment and accumulation. It seems possible that T cells are conditioned and activated by cytokines such as IL-15, TNF-α, IL-6, and IL-10 produced by rheumatoid tissues. Cell membrane contact between macrophages and cytokine-activated T cells may also be a key event in driving production of the pivotal cytokine TNF-α (see below).

Cytokines are protein messenger molecules that transmit signals from one cell to another by binding to their specific receptors on the surface of cell membranes. Their activity is usually restricted to adjacent cells in the local milieu. Cytokines are normally produced and exported as soluble molecules into the fluid phase, although some cytokines, such as TNF-α, are also active as molecules displayed on the surface of the producer cells. Expression of mRNA and protein of a large number of cytokines is reported in rheumatoid synovial tissue. These molecules regulate a diverse range of functions relevant to an understanding of the pathogenesis and clinical features of rheumatoid disease. Both pro- and anti-inflammatory cytokines, chemokines, and mitogenic factors are produced, but pro-inflammatory mediators predominate during active phases of disease.

Of the pro-inflammatory cytokines, IL-1 and TNF-α are of key importance in the pathogenesis of rheumatoid arthritis (Fig. 6). They are intimately involved in activation of the cytokine network, leucocyte recruitment and activation, the local immune response, angiogenesis, and fibroblast proliferation. IL-1 and TNF-α also regulate production of a number of mediators of connective tissue damage by synoviocytes, including matrix metalloproteinases and prostaglandins. Furthermore, these cytokines activate osteoclasts that are implicated in bone damage. TNF-α is produced mainly by type A cells of macrophage lineage in the intima, subintima, and the cartilage–pannus junction. The p55- and p75-TNF receptors are coexpressed by cells in the vicinity. The hypothesis that TNF-α is a dominant pro-inflammatory mediator in the cytokine dysequilibrium observed in the rheumatoid synovium has gained considerable support. In particular, TNF-α regulates production of IL-1 and together these two cytokines orchestrate rheumatoid inflammation and damage. The identification of TNF-α as a molecular target for therapy has been validated by clinical trials of biological inhibitors of TNF-α and their recent application in rheumatological practice.

Examples of the importance of TNF-α as a mediator of rheumatoid disease include the following observations after treatment with infliximab, a monoclonal anti-TNF-α antibody.

1. There is a reduction in the cellularity of the rheumatoid synovial membrane associated with a reduction in the number of tissue macrophages and lymphocytes.
2. There is evidence that the reduced cellularity is associated with a reduction of cytokine-induced vascular adhesion molecules—intracellular adhesion molecule-1 (ICAM-1), E-selectin, and vascular cell adhesion molecule-1 (VCAM-1)—as well as chemokines such as IL-8 and monocyte-chemoattractant protein-1 (MCP-1).
3. There is reduction in synovial vascular density and neovascularization (αvβ3 staining of blood vessels), associated with a fall in the concentration of circulating vascular-endothelial growth factor, a major cytokine implicated in new vessel formation.
4. There is direct evidence of reduced retention in joints of autologous ^{111}indium-labelled polymorphonuclear cells (Fig. 7).
5. There is a reduction of serum IL-6 concentrations within 6 h of a single infusion of the anti-TNF-α antibody, followed within 24 h by a reduction in markers of acute-phase response including C-reactive protein, serum amyloid A protein, and erythrocyte sedimentation rate.
6. There is a reduction in the circulating concentrations of pro-matrix metalloproteinase-1 (pro-MMP-1) and pro-MMP-3 in blood. Matrix metalloproteinases are implicated in cartilage and bone degradation and there is clinical trial evidence that anti-TNF-α markedly retards radiographic signs of cartilage loss and bone erosions.

Many other cytokines and chemokines are potential therapeutic targets. Clinical trials have been conducted with anti-TNF-α, anti-IL-1, anti-IL-6, and human recombinant IL-10 and IL-11. So far, anti-TNF-α has been approved for the treatment of rheumatoid arthritis, and in the United States, the IL-1 antagonist, human recombinant IL-1 receptor antagonist (IL-1ra) has been approved.

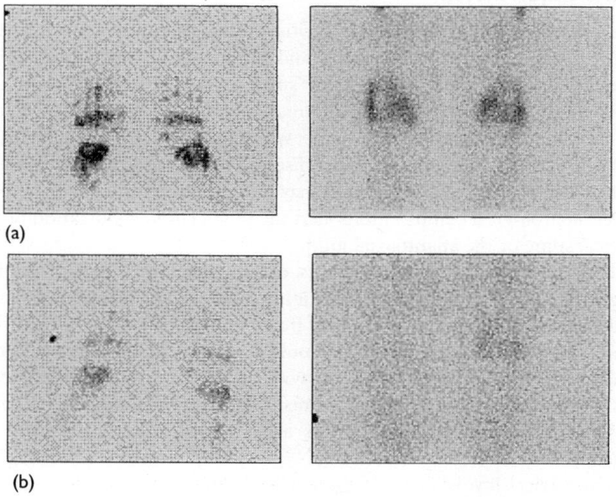

Fig. 7 Gamma camera images of the hands and knees of a patient with rheumatoid arthritis. Images were taken 22 h after a bolus injection of autologous radiolabelled (^{111}indium) granulocytes (a) before and (b) after a single 10 mg/kg intravenous bolus of anti-TNF-α antibody (infliximab). There was a reduction in signal after treatment. (Images kindly provided by P. C. Taylor.)

Clinical features

Presentation

The onset of rheumatoid arthritis is frequently insidious and the principal symptoms are pain and stiffness, mainly of peripheral joints, with associated swelling. Prolonged stiffness of joints on waking and following inactivity is usual and may last an hour or more. There is progressive decline in physical function and ability to perform daily activities. Fatigue and lethargy are common and there may also be low-grade fever and weight loss. Symptoms are persistent in affected joints, although there may be some day to day variation in severity. As the disease evolves, further joints may become involved and some may remit, but ultimately the distribution of arthritis becomes permanently established.

Other patterns of disease presentation are also recognized. Up to one-third of patients present with an explosive or subacute onset of arthritis, leading to severe immobility. In a minority of patients a migratory polyarthritis flitting from joint to joint is observed. This is referred to as 'palindromic rheumatism' and may be a recurring pattern over months before chronic polyarthritis becomes established. About 10 per cent of patients present with features of the syndrome of polymyalgia rheumatica, characterized by prominent limb-girdle pain, stiffness, and painful movement of the neck, shoulders, and hips. Persistent inflammatory arthritis of a single joint such as the knee, wrist, ankle, shoulder, or hip may be the only rheumatological symptom and can antedate the onset of polyarthritis by months or years.

In some patients bilateral diffuse swelling of the fingers and hands may be a presenting complaint, often associated with symptoms of carpal tunnel syndrome. Synovitis of tendon sheaths of the dorsal extensors of the wrist and of flexor tendons in the palm and wrist may be present with concurrent joint signs, but may also occur as a prominent clinical feature in the absence of polyarthritis. Swelling of the ankles with pitting oedema is commonly seen in active rheumatoid arthritis. Lymphoedema of the forearm or lower limb is observed less frequently.

Rarely, the initial manifestations of rheumatoid arthritis are confined to extra-articular disease. Examples include subcutaneous nodules, one or more nodules in the thorax presenting as pulmonary lesions on a chest radiograph, pleurisy with pleural effusion, pericarditis, episcleritis, and vasculitis.

Joint distribution

The expression of rheumatoid arthritis shows interindividual variation with respect to the anatomical sites and numbers of involved joints. For example, some patients have mainly small joints affected, whilst others show simultaneous involvement of small and large joints. The hip and shoulder joints may be spared in some, whilst in others they bear the brunt of the disease. The actual numbers of diseased joints can vary from three or four to over 50. Diseased neck joints may be asymptomatic until, in the late stages, neurological complications alert the physician to subluxation of the cervical spine or the atlantoaxial joint.

In over 80 to 90 per cent of patients, one or more of the metacarpophalangeal and proximal interphalangeal joints of the hand and the metatarsophalangeal joints are involved. Other frequently involved sites include the wrists, glenohumeral joints of the shoulders, knees, and the elbow joints, followed by the mid-tarsal, acromioclavicular, interfacetal, and atlantoaxial joints of the cervical spine and hip joints. The temporomandibular, sternoclavicular, and cricoarytenoid joints are involved in about a third of patients.

Symmetrical involvement of the joints is usual, but joint damage and deformity may be asymmetrical and related to overuse or traumatic injury. Conversely, neurological paralysis of a limb results in joint protection.

In addition to involvement of diarthrodial joints, the rheumatoid process frequently involves tendon sheaths of hands, wrists, shoulders, and ankles.

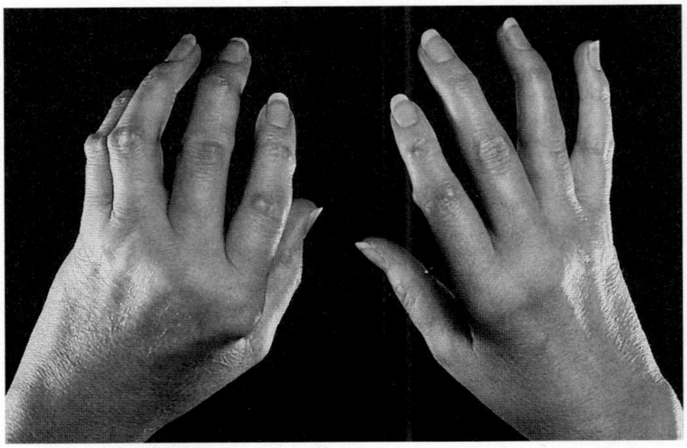

Fig. 8 The hands of a person suffering from rheumatoid arthritis. Features to note include symmetrical soft tissue swelling of the second and third metacarpophalageal joints, early swan-neck deformity of the left ring finger, ulnar deviation at the metacarpophalageal joints, and wasting of the small muscles of the hand. In addition, several small rheumatoid nodules are present. (See also Plate 2.)

Features of joint disease

Hands and wrists

In active rheumatoid disease, soft tissue swelling and tenderness of metacarpophalangeal and proximal interphalangeal joints is observed (Fig. 8 and Plate 2). Thickening and nodularity of flexor tendons in the palms may be palpable and tenosynovitis can be a cause of 'triggering' of the fingers. Wasting of the interossei is prominent and fist closure restricted. Flexor tendonitis and wrist synovitis may be associated with signs and symptoms of median nerve compression (carpal tunnel syndrome).

Ulnar deviation and volar subluxation of the digits and wrists may develop later. Other recognized deformities include Boutonnière (button hole) flexion deformity of the proximal interphalangeal joint and 'swan-neck' deformities of fingers due to hyperextension of the proximal interphalangeal joint and flexion at the distal interphalangeal joint.

Diffuse synovial swelling may be pronounced at the dorsal aspect of the wrist and the ulnar styloid may become dorsally subluxed. The carpus may drift in a volar direction such that supination of the hand is restricted. In this late stage, the extensor tendons appear stretched across a shrunken carpus ('the bowstring' sign). Extensor tendons may occasionally rupture, most commonly affecting the little or ring fingers.

Nail-fold and finger-tip infarcts and splinter haemorrhages indicate digital vascular occlusive disease. Palmar erythema is common but not specific for rheumatoid arthritis.

Elbows and shoulders

Physical signs in early stages include swelling, limitation of movement, and inability to flex or extend the elbow. Later, pronation and supination are restricted, and the head of the proximal radioulnar joint may dislocate. Olecranon bursitis and subcutaneous nodules around the elbow are common. In the shoulder, aside from glenohumeral joint synovitis, there may be accompanying subacromial bursitis and rotator and biceps tendon involvement.

The neck

Rheumatoid involvement of the apophyseal joints of the neck can cause pain, stiffness, and restricted movement. Loss of stability in the spine may occur at several levels and be associated with symptoms and signs of radicular or cord compression. Subluxation of the atlantoaxial joint diagnosed by plain radiography or magnetic resonance imaging occurs in 6 per cent of the rheumatoid population and up to 30 per cent of patients who are admitted to hospital. It may be asymptomatic, but when severe tends to occur in patients who also suffer from severe generalized disease and advanced disability, and is a recognized cause of quadriplegia and sudden death.

The knees

Involvement of the knees is common, and chronically active synovitis is associated with irreversible destruction and rapid deterioration in functional capacity. In early stages especially, high pressure in the knee joint on active flexion, for example during squatting, can lead to joint rupture and leakage of inflammatory fluid into the calf. This complication simulates signs and symptoms of a calf deep vein thrombosis: it can be diagnosed by arthrography using contrast medium, or by ultrasonography of the knee. A chronic effusion in the knee joint may also be associated with a posterior popliteal (Baker's) cyst and occasionally this extends into the medial aspect of the calf.

Ankles and feet

Inflammation of the metatarsophalangeal joints is common and results in subluxation of the metatarsal heads and, ultimately, claw- or hammer-toe deformities. The soft tissue pad that is normally positioned underneath the metatarsal heads becomes displaced such that the heads of the metatarsal bones become painful to walk on. Patients may describe this as feeling as if they were walking on marbles or stones. Involvement of the tarsal and subtalar joints may result in flattening of the arches of the foot and valgus deformity of the hindfoot. These deformities cause difficulties with footwear, and where shoes rub the feet there is a tendency for callosities to form.

Hips

The hips are less often involved, but there may be erosions in severe cases with remodelling of the acetabulum (protrusio acetabuli). There may also be secondary degenerative disease at the hip. Total hip replacement is generally a highly successful treatment for endstage hip disease.

Extra-articular disease

Nodules

Nodules occur in 25 to 30 per cent of patients with rheumatoid arthritis and are associated with seropositive disease. Common sites for subcutaneous nodules include the elbow, ischial tuberosity, heel, and dorsum of fingers. Multiple, small, rapidly evolving nodules can occur in those on methotrexate treatment (Fig. 8). Nodules in the pleura may present as single or multiple round shadows on a routine chest radiograph.

Systemic vasculitis

Rheumatoid vasculitis occurs in patients with seropositive and nodular disease. It presents with a severe systemic illness characterized by fever and weight loss. Associated clinical features are consequent upon occlusion of medium- to small-sized arteries. These include Raynaud's phenomenon, nail-fold and digital infarcts, and gangrene, skin ulceration, mononeuritis multiplex, scleromalacia perforans, and occlusion of arteries to visceral organs. The latter include coronary, pulmonary, coeliac axis, and cerebral vessels. In some patients vasculitis may present as a skin rash associated with necrotizing polyangiitis of small cutaneous blood vessels.

Fibrosing alveolitis and obliterative bronchiolitis

Physiological abnormalities in lung function tests indicative of airways and interstitial disease may be present without symptoms. In a proportion of patients with rheumatoid arthritis, more frequently male than female, dyspnoea of insidious onset, physical signs, characteristic lung function abnormalities, a chest radiograph, and high-resolution computed tomography may reveal characteristic features of chronic fibrosing alveolitis. More rarely, acute pneumonitis may be the presenting feature with rapid deterioration and development of respiratory failure. Patients with fibrosing alveolitis are usually seropositive, have a high frequency of antinuclear antibodies, and may also exhibit evidence of multisystem disease, including vasculitis.

Obliterative bronchiolitis can be associated with rheumatoid arthritis. It is usually rapidly progressive, but some patients follow a chronic protracted course that may respond to corticosteroid and immunosuppressive therapy.

Serositis

Past evidence of pericardial and pleural inflammation is common at autopsy and may be discovered by imaging techniques in asymptomatic patients. Both may present with clinical symptoms, generally following a benign course with resolution associated with disease-modifying antirheumatoid drugs (**DMARDs**) or corticosteroid therapy. Rare cases of constrictive pericarditis have been reported. Typically, pleural effusions are exudates with a high protein content and cellular exudate enriched in lymphocytes, but also containing polymorphonuclear cells and macrophages. A low level of complement activity relative to blood concentrations and a low glucose concentration (usually less than 1.4 mmol/l) is of diagnostic value.

Eye complications

Scleritis, episcleritis, scleromalacia perforans, corneal melt, and keratoconjunctivitis sicca have all been described and need evaluation and treatment by a specialist.

Amyloidosis

Secondary amyloidosis due to deposition of amyloid AA fibrils in blood vessels and parenchyma of kidneys, liver, spleen, and gastrointestinal tract has been described in the tissues of 10 to 15 per cent of patients examined at autopsy, or in the blood vessels in the submucosa of rectal and gingival biopsies. Proteinuria, nephrotic syndrome, or renal failure are less common and have a poor prognosis unless detected and treated before irreversible renal failure has occurred. Effective treatment of rheumatoid arthritis with suppression of the acute-phase response with DMARDs and corticosteroids prevents progression and may reverse the disease. In patients with a continuing acute-phase response despite the standard DMARD therapy, treatment with chlorambucil is reported to be of some benefit. Imaging of radionuclide-labelled serum amyloid P protein in the spleen and kidneys may be used to monitor treatment.

Osteoporosis

Juxta-articular osteoporosis is a common feature of radiographs of affected joints and is related to local disease activity. However, decreased bone mineral density of the spine and pelvis has been described in patients with active severe rheumatoid arthritis. This is likely to reflect the response of bone metabolism to prostaglandins and catabolic cytokines such as IL-6, IL-11, and the receptor for activition of NFκβ (RANK)-ligand, which increase osteoclast activity. This is distinct from immobility-associated or corticosteroid-induced osteoporosis, although these factors may be additive in individual patients. It has been suggested that increased mobility following low-dose prednisolone may be beneficial and reverse, rather than aggravate, corticosteroid-induced osteopenia.

Felty's syndrome

Felty's syndrome is characterized by a combination of seropositive rheumatoid arthritis, neutropenia, and splenomegaly. Lymphadenopathy, leg ulcers, and nodular hyperplasia of the liver have been described. Patients with severe neutropenia are liable to bacterial infections. Some patients also develop anaemia and thrombocytopenia. In a variant of Felty's syndrome, an expansion of large granular lymphocytes is found in the blood: these are cytotoxic CD8+ lymphocytes and may present as clonally expanded cell populations.

Myocardial disease

Myocardial disease due to diffuse fibrosis or granulomatous lesions is recognized in rheumatoid arthritis, although the more frequently recognized association is with coronary artery disease. Systemic vasculitis may also involve coronary vessels. Aortic incompetence due to valvular thickening and nodule formation or dilation of the ascending aorta have been described.

Neurological complications

A number of compression neuropathies may occur in rheumatoid arthritis. These include compression of the median nerve at the wrist, the ulnar nerve and posterior interosseous branch of the radial nerve at the elbow, and posterior tibial nerve at the level of the knee or ankle. It is important to recognize and confirm these neuropathies by nerve conduction studies since surgical decompression usually cures symptoms.

A mild, symmetrical, sensory peripheral neuropathy involving the hands and legs in a 'glove and stocking' distribution also occurs in rheumatoid arthritis. This is distinct from the rarer and more severe sensorimotor mononeuritis multiplex associated with wrist and foot drop and usually due to vasculitis of vasa nervora, when other features of a systemic vasculitis and extra-articular disease may be present. In some patients, however, no vascular pathology is demonstrable and the cause of axonal degeneration is not understood.

Rheumatoid involvement of the transverse ligament and odontoid process of the atlantoaxial joint may lead to posterior subluxation or upward movement of the odontoid and cause cervical cord compression. Cord compression may also occur due to rheumatoid damage at lower levels of the cervical spine. Compression is a recognized cause of tetraparesis and sudden death. Surgical stabilization of the neck can be successful but cannot always be recommended in patients with associated severe disability and poor health status.

Infections

Patients with rheumatoid arthritis are susceptible to local and systemic bacterial and opportunistic infections. Infections of joints and respiratory and urinary tracts, skin ulcers, and septicaemia are all described, and infections are one of the causes of increased mortality in rheumatoid arthritis. Endogenous disease-related immunosuppressive mechanisms are thought to play an important part. In Felty's syndrome, neutropenia compromises host defence. Drugs for treating rheumatoid arthritis such as cytotoxic and immunosuppressive agents may also be contributory factors.

Clinical course, progression, and outcome

Clinical course

Disease activity

The course of the disease activity fluctuates over time, partly due to the endogenous mechanisms of disease and partly as a result of effective therapy. Recurring periods of weeks or months of exacerbation of symptoms, described as 'flares', alternate with periods of relative quiescence of disease. In about 10 to 20 per cent of patients, the disease continues unabated throughout.

The key clinical features of disease activity in rheumatoid arthritis are pain, fatigue, stiffness of joints on waking, swelling, tenderness of joints on palpation, restriction of joint motion, and loss of physical functional capacity. Joint deformities become apparent as the disease progresses. Symptoms are assessed by taking a history in descriptive terms, but also by attempting to quantify their severity. These measurements have been incorporated into various criteria for assessment of disease activity and response to therapy, developed and validated, for example, by the American College of Rheumatology and the European League Against Rheumatism.

Swelling of joints due to synovial thickening may be detected by palpation as a 'spongy' or 'boggy' feel. Concomitant effusion can be demonstrated by fluctuation. In later stages of disease, subluxed surfaces of bones (such as the heads of metacarpals in the hands, the styloid of the ulna, and distal radius at the wrist) can give the appearance of bony swelling. Tenderness is elicited by digital pressure or squeezing of a joint. The classic signs of inflammation, such as redness and increased temperature overlying joints, are not usually prominent, although readily demonstrable by thermography. Active and passive movement of joints through their anatomical range of motion elicits restriction of movement associated with pain.

Functional capacity can be assessed by testing grip strengths using an inflatable bag attached to a sphygmomanometer, walking time over a standard distance, and by standard health assessment questionnaires (such as the Stanford questionnaire). The degree, quantity, and severity of pain is recorded as experienced by the patient, graded on a visual analogue scale of 1 to 10. The duration of morning stiffness is recorded in minutes. A 'global assessment' of disease activity on a visual analogue scale of 1 to 10 as judged by the patient and physician may also be used as a quantitative measurement of disease activity over time.

Structural damage

The rheumatoid disease process leads to structural damage to the cartilage, bone, and associated joint structures. This is cumulative and irreversible and appears to be related to the severity of inflammatory activity over time. In later stages of disease, loss of normal joint architecture and mechanical derangement also contribute to the perpetuation of symptoms and secondary inflammation. Serial radiographs of the hands and feet are employed to assess structural damage to joints.

Prognosis

The longer-term health status of patients presenting to hospital clinics with recent-onset rheumatoid arthritis has been documented in a number of studies. Functional deterioration occurs rapidly. In one study, half the patient population was moderately disabled in 2 years and severely disabled by 10 years. The most marked deterioration occurs in those patients with the most compromised functional capacity in early disease. These data are compatible with the proportion of patients at work whose disease-associated disability prevents continuing employment: around 20 per cent of patients stop work in the first 2 years, increasing to 30 per cent within 5 years, 50 per cent in 10 years, and 90 per cent prior to retirement age. A low level of manual work, job flexibility, and higher educational and psychosocial status are amongst the determinants that correlate best with the ability to continue work.

Patients with rheumatoid arthritis have a higher than expected prevalence of other serious illnesses and an increased mortality compared with the general population. In one study approximately 20 per cent reported concurrent disorders, and iatrogenic disease is not uncommon. In a 35-year follow-up study on 3501 patients, mortality was twice that of a control population, resulting in a shortening of life by 7 to 10 years. Rheumatoid arthritis itself may contribute to premature death in up to 20 per cent of patients as a result of complications such as fibrosing alveolitis, vasculitis, secondary amyloidosis, cardiac disease, or transection of the cord due to cervical spinal subluxation. More frequently, death is the consequence of comorbid conditions or complications of therapy. These include infection, gastrointestinal haemorrhage or perforation, cardiovascular and cerebrovascular disease, renal failure, and lymphoproliferative diseases.

Survival rates of about 50 per cent at 5 years have been recorded in a subset of patients with polyarticular disease, poor functional status, or extra-articular disease (Fig. 9).

Prognostic factors

A number of prognostic factors have been identified in cohorts of patients with rheumatoid arthritis that herald rapid functional deterioration and premature death. These include more than 30 affected joints, a persistently raised level of acute-phase proteins, lower socio-economic status, early development of functional incapacity, a positive rheumatoid factor, cryoglobulinaemia, and in Northern European patients, the presence of the HLA-DRβ*04 genes. However, on an individual patient basis, none of these factors are reliably predictive, either singly or in combination.

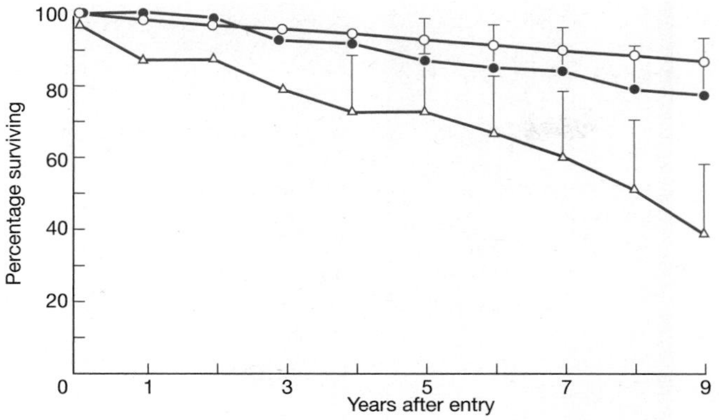

Fig. 9 Survival of female patients with rheumatoid arthritis attending hospital clinics compared with age-adjusted population data for England and Wales. ○—○, survival of whole population; •—• survival of female patients with rheumatoid arthritis and joint disease only (n = 38); △–△ survival of patients with rheumatoid arthritis and extra-articular disease (n = 33). Bars represent 95 per cent confidence limits. (Reproduced from Erhardt CC *et al.* (1989). Factors predicting a poor life prognosis in rheumatoid arthritis: an eight year prospective study. *Annals of the Rheumatic Diseases* **48**, 7 –13, with permission.)

Remission

Remission has been defined by the American College of Rheumatology as an absence of joint symptoms and signs, duration of morning stiffness less than 15 min, freedom from fatigue, and an erythrocyte sedimentation rate less than 30 mm/h for females and 20 mm/h for males, for 2 consecutive months. Remission of disease is seen in a small proportion of patients, especially in the initial stages of disease. More usually, remission follows in approximately 20 per cent of patients treated with a disease- modifying antirheumatoid drug.

Diagnosis and stages of disease

Recent-onset and established disease

A diagnosis of rheumatoid arthritis is likely if three or more symmetrically distributed joints are found to be swollen and tender for more than 6 weeks in a patient with a positive rheumatoid factor test and elevated erythrocyte sedimentation rate or serum concentration of C-reactive protein. However, not all these features are necessarily present at the early stages of disease, at which point arthritis is best termed 'undifferentiated'. The broad spectrum described in the 'presentation' section may cause considerable difficulty in making a definitive diagnosis

With the passage of time, the emergence of other features such as subcutaneous nodules, radiographic evidence of joint space narrowing, juxta-articular osteopenia, and bony erosions add further certainty to the diagnosis.

The ACR criteria (Table 1) may not be fulfilled for 6 to 12 months, by which time the pattern of joint involvement and a chronic disease course are usually evident. Prognostic factors declare themselves and the patient is regarded as having reached the stage of established disease.

Differential diagnosis

In patients with recent onset of symptoms of arthritis, the following disorders should be considered in the differential diagnosis.

Polyarthritis associated with connective tissue disease

Systemic lupus erythematosus may present with chronic non-deforming polyarthritis, but features such as Raynaud's phenomenon, photosensitivity, rashes, alopecia, haemolytic anaemia, leucopenia, thrombocytopenia, and renal or neurological involvement are detectable sooner or later, and diagnostic antinuclear antibodies (anti-ds-DNA, anti-Sm and others) are present. Other connective tissue diseases such as systemic sclerosis, polymyositis, mixed connective tissue disease, 'overlap' syndromes, and primary Sjögren's syndrome may also present with marked polyarthralgia or polyarthritis which mimics rheumatoid arthritis. In many such patients the presence of rheumatoid factor can further confuse the diagnosis. Careful clinical examination and measurement of marker autoantibodies directed against nuclear and cytoplasmic antigens will usually permit recognition of the underlying disorder. In some cases the diagnosis may only unfold after a period of weeks or months of a disorder best labelled 'undifferentiated connective tissue disease'.

Infection-related polyarthritis

The polyarthritis of rubella or other microbial agents, such as parvovirus B19 and *Borrelia burghdorferi*, and reactive arthritis associated with genitourinary or gastrointestinal infections can all cause diagnostic difficulty. A positive diagnosis is made by microbiological tests on relevant body fluids and serological tests for the detection of IgM antibodies or a rising titre of IgG antibodies to the suspected micro-organism in sequential serum samples taken over 2 weeks.

Spondyloarthropathies

Peripheral joint disease can be seen in conjunction with ankylosing spondylitis, psoriasis, and inflammatory bowel disease. Clinical examination of the spine, skin, and nails, radiological examination of the bowel using double-contrast enema or small bowel enema, endoscopy, and biopsy may reveal the underlying diagnosis. A high proportion of patients are HLA B27 positive.

Osteoarthritis

Osteoarthritis may present with inflammatory symptoms and signs but is readily distinguished by its different joint distribution (proximal and distal interphalangeal joints, carpometacarpal joints of the thumb) and radiographs that show joint space narrowing, subchondral new bone formation, osteophytes, and subchondrial cysts. Where there is pre-existing osteoarthritis, the superimposition of rheumatoid arthritis can be difficult to distinguish.

Other conditions

In late middle-aged and elderly patients the clinical presentation of polyarticular chronic pyrophosphate arthropathy may be difficult to distinguish from rheumatoid arthritis. The former diagnosis may be suspected where there is an atypical distribution of synovitis together with periarticular complications. Chronic pyrophosphate arthropathy may be associated with a modest acute-phase response and low-titre rheumatoid factor, but can usually be distinguished from rheumatoid arthritis on the basis of typical radiographic appearances and the finding of calcium pyrophosphate dihydrate (CPPD) crystals in synovial fluid aspirates. Rarely, rheumatoid arthritis and chronic pyrophosphate arthropathy may coexist.

Other diagnoses to be considered include hypermobility syndrome, polyarticular gout, psoriatic arthritis, haemochromatosis, sarcoidosis, sickle-cell disease, primary amyloidosis, and paraneoplastic disease.

Laboratory tests

Laboratory studies are an integral part of the management of patients with rheumatoid arthritis and are employed for diagnosis, evaluation of prognosis, assessment of disease activity, response to therapy, and monitoring toxic effects of drugs. Only routinely used tests are considered here.

The measurement of rheumatoid factors is useful in the early stages of assessment of a patient with suspected rheumatoid arthritis. Tests using sensitized sheep erythrocytes (Rose–Waaler) in an agglutination test give better diagnostic specificity than agglutination of human IgG-coated latex particles. Automated tests using nephelometry or enzyme-linked immunosorbent assays are being increasingly used. All assays have to be standardized against a reference standard and may be expressed in international units. A positive result is one that exceeds concentrations (or titres) observed in less than 5 per cent of normal controls, or the value set by an international reference standard, and is observed in about 70 per cent of patients at some point in their disease course. In a patient with recent-onset polyarthritis, a positive rheumatoid factor is moderately specific for rheumatoid arthritis but can also be observed in patients with other connective tissue diseases such as systemic lupus erythematosus and primary Sjögren's syndrome. A repeat test may be positive after an initial test is negative and is therefore necessary before a patient can be categorized as having seronegative rheumatoid arthritis. A significant titre of rheumatoid factor is associated with a poor prognosis and extra-articular disease.

Measurement of erythrocyte sedimentation rate (Westergren method) and serum C-reactive protein are extensively used. High values correlate with disease severity and a reduction is one criterion of response to therapy. Persistently elevated C-reactive protein concentrations correlate with deforming erosive disease.

Patients with active rheumatoid arthritis show haematological abnormalities as a consequence of disease-related mechanisms, such as the overproduction of cytokines suppressing the bone marrow, immune complexes increasing the clearance of polymorphonuclear cells in Felty's syndrome, and hypersplenism reducing platelet counts. A high level of disease activity is associated with a normocytic normochromic anaemia, polymorphonuclear leucocytosis, and thrombocytosis. These abnormal values tend to return to normal as the inflammatory component of disease responds to therapy.

Active disease may also be associated with a raised serum alkaline phosphatase and a low serum albumin. Serum chemistry is otherwise normal. Serum immunoglobulin and complement C3 and C4 levels may be elevated.

Non-steroidal anti-inflammatory drug (**NSAID**) therapy may cause microcytic iron-deficiency anaemia from blood loss from the gastrointestinal tract. A low serum ferritin level suggests iron deficiency, but this is not a reliable guide in cases of rheumatoid arthritis as serum concentrations may be elevated as part of an acute-phase response. Corticosteroids may be responsible for increased polymorphonuclear cell counts and decreased lymphocyte counts. Many DMARDs show dose-related bone marrow toxicity, and sulphasalazine, D-penicillamine, azathioprine, and gold can cause unexpected agranulocytosis due to hypersensitivity, unrelated to the dose administered.

Of the commonly used drugs, methotrexate, sulphasalazine, azathioprine, and leflunomide are hepatoxic and can cause elevation of liver enzymes and alkaline phosphatase. Repeated monitoring is advisable: persistent or highly raised values should prompt further investigation or discontinuation.

Imaging

Radiographs of hands and feet can be used to assess the presence and progression of cartilage loss and bone erosions (Fig. 10). Standardized measurements (the Larsen or Sharp scoring methods) have been devised to quantify these measures. Changes seen in the hands and feet correlate with radiological changes in other affected joints, showing a linear progression after the initial 1 to 2 years. The erosion count correlates with physical function. Radiographs of affected joints are used for the assessment of integrity and damage. Flexion views of the cervical spine are suitable for demonstration of atlantoaxial subluxation and cervical instability. Arrest or retardation of radiographic change is considered to be a marker of good control of disease.

Magnetic resonance imaging (**MRI**) and computed tomography (CT) are valuable in assessing neck pathology and pressure on the cervical cord. MRI and high-frequency ultrasound examination are sensitive methods to evaluate synovitis and early change in cartilage and bone, but their place in routine management is not yet established. Dual emission x-ray absorptiometry (DEXA) scanning is in routine use for the assessment of bone mineral density.

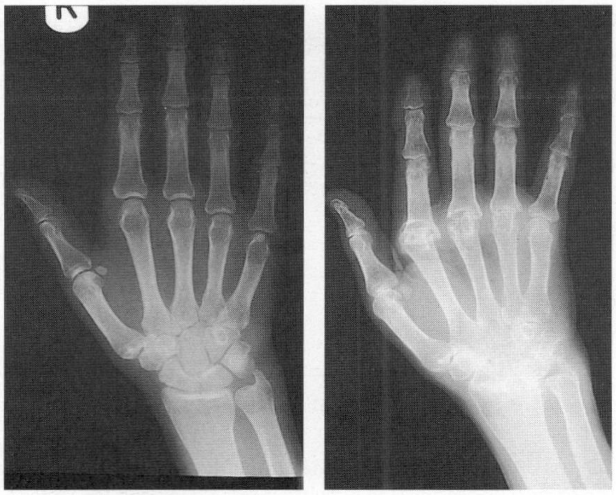

Fig. 10 Hand radiographs taken soon after symptom onset (left panel) and 12 years into established disease (right panel), showing extensive structural damage especially in the metacarpophalangeal, interphalangeal, carpal, and wrist joints.

Management

Aims of treatment

These are:

(1) to relieve symptoms and signs of disease;

(2) maintain physical function;

(3) prevent structural damage to joints and associated structures;

(4) restore and maintain quality of life that permits the pursuit of normal work, domestic, and social life;

(5) reduce the comorbidity and increased mortality associated with the disease and therapies; and

(6) correct abnormal laboratory-based values of haemotopoietic function, acute-phase proteins, and other markers of disease process.

Achievable goals of current therapy

Considerable progress has been made in developing effective therapies for the relief of symptoms and signs of disease. However, despite the best therapies in current use, the goals of halting structural damage and maintaining a normal quality of life have not yet been realized, although significant progress has been made. The realistic aims, therefore, are to maximize gains whilst minimizing toxicity of drugs (an optimum risk:benefit ratio) and to operate within the pharmacoeconomic constraints (cost–benefit and cost–utility) that apply in the setting in which the patient is being treated.

The costs of treatment of rheumatoid arthritis over the lifetime of a patient are considerable. They include direct and indirect costs that are cumulative and incremental as the disease progresses. Direct costs include those in the primary and hospital sectors of medical and allied health professionals, hospital admissions, drugs, surgery, aids, and appliances. Indirect costs include those arising from loss of economic productivity and earnings, unemployment and disability benefits, the cost of maintaining mobility, and domestic help and daily care for the severely disabled. Patients with rheumatoid arthritis become debilitated by pain and fatigue and may experience psychological depression, anxiety, and loss of self-esteem, which require additional medical treatment and psychological support. Iatrogenic diseases caused by anti-inflammatory and other drugs add further socio-economic burdens over the long term. These considerations have been used as an argument for the aggressive use, within safe limits, of drugs and new therapies that offer rapid relief of symptoms and signs, retardation of structural damage, and maintenance of functional capacity.

The physician has to be able to evaluate these factors and, because of the variability of disease expression and progression, individualize and agree the treatment plan with each patient. It is prudent to re-evaluate and revise the goals from time to time as the prognosis and response to therapy unfolds.

General principles

The heterogeneous and variable course of chronic rheumatoid arthritis presents a complex management problem, with each patient requiring an individualized approach for an optimum outcome. Nevertheless, the general principles that may aid the physician's task are summarized below.

Ascertainment of the severity of disease determines the appropriate choice of drugs. Evaluation of the extent of joint and extra-articular involvement, the level of disease activity, and its progression are judged by clinical examination, laboratory tests, and the rate of progression of radiographically determined damage to joints. The full extent may only unfold over months or years of follow-up. Patients with severe and active disease will require more aggressive medical treatment than those with mild disease.

The main aim is to control disease activity as rapidly as possible. Response to therapy should be monitored to ensure efficacy, using quantifiable clinical and laboratory indices of inflammatory activity and impact on the progression of damage to joints. A lack of response to initial therapy should trigger a change in the management plan and consideration of alternative strategies at intervals of 3 to 6 months. A thorough knowledge of the scope and limitations of treatment modalities is essential in the art of management.

In early rheumatoid arthritis the goal should be to achieve disease remission. With aggressive and continuing use of available therapeutic agents there is evidence that it is possible to achieve this in 20 to 40 per cent of patients over a period of 1 to 2 years. Since low or absent disease activity correlates with retardation of joint damage, the benefit of treatment is likely to be most marked in the early phase of disease.

Remission is rare in established rheumatoid arthritis of more than 2 or 3 years duration. Nevertheless, minimizing disease activity by attention to a measurable response to therapy remains at the core of the management plan. Controlled clinical trials support the concept that optimum use of drugs can ameliorate symptoms and signs and retard progression of joint damage and disability even in later stages of disease.

At all stages of disease, irrespective of its severity, drug therapy constitutes only one part of the whole management plan. Other essential elements include measures such as patient education, psychological and employment counselling, setting appropriate levels of rest and exercise, coping with tasks of daily living, and maintaining mobility, access to splints, aids, and appliances for the disabled, and access to social and financial benefits. In addition, successful pharmacological intervention requires the patient's informed consent in instituting therapeutic decisions and involving the patient and other carers in monitoring of drug toxicity. The provision of holistic care thus requires team work and co-ordination between the treating physician and other medical and health-care professionals, including specialist nurses, physiotherapists, occupational therapists, and social workers.

Surgical treatment plays an important role in relieving intractable symptoms and restoring loss of physical function and mobility due to damage to joints, tendons, and associated soft tissues. It is also indicated in the treatment of secondary complications such as entrapment of peripheral nerves at the wrist and elbow and cervical cord compression due to instability of the cervical spine.

Evidence base and profile of drugs used in the treatment of rheumatoid arthritis

Non-steroidal anti-inflammatory drugs (NSAIDs)

NSAIDs are widely used for treating symptoms of rheumatoid arthritis. They act by inhibiting the enzymes cyclo-oxygenase I and/or II, which act on lipid substrates in cells, converting them to prostanoids. Tissues such as the gastric and duodenal mucosa, blood vessels, and platelets constitutively express cyclo-oxygenase I, which in the gastroduodenal mucosa regulates the production of prostaglandins, including prostaglandin E_2, that exert a protective effect on its integrity by reducing acid secretion and increasing the secretion of mucus and bicarbonate. Cyclo-oxygenase I-induced prostaglandin E_2 promotes platelet aggregation and its prothrombotic effects. By contrast, cyclo-oxygenase II is mainly induced in macrophages and polymorphonuclear cells at sites of inflammation by pro-inflammatory cytokines such as IL-1 and TNF-α. NSAIDs that inhibit both cyclo-oxygenase I and II activity therefore compromise the gastroprotective effect of cyclo-oxygenase I, whilst simultaneously exerting a therapeutic effect by inhibiting the production of inflammatory prostanoids. Selective or specific cyclo-oxygenase II inhibitors should in theory block inflammation without gastropathic effects.

The conventional and currently widely used NSAIDs are inhibitors of both cyclo-oxygenase I and II. In the United States they are responsible for admission to hospital of over 1 per cent of patients with rheumatoid arthritis per year for complications such as peptic ulceration, gastric haemorrhage, and perforation, and account for a twofold increase in death over expected rates. It is claimed that the least gastrotoxic are ibuprofen and nabumetone, with naproxen and diclofenac carrying intermediate risk, followed by drugs with a high risk such as fenoprofen, ketoprofen, indomethacin and piroxicam, and azapropazone (see Table 2 for dose ranges).

For patients who develop dyspepsia and/or NSAID-induced gastropathy, or elderly patients who have a high risk of gastroduodenal side–effects, concomitant administration of prostaglandin analogues (such as misoprostol) or proton-pump inhibitors (such as omeprazole or lansoprazole) is recommended, and NSAIDs are best avoided for patients with a history of peptic ulcers. Eradication of *Helicobacter pylori* infection results in long-term healing of pre-existing gastric and duodenal ulcers, but whether it decreases dyspepsia or ulceration caused by NSAIDs is uncertain.

Drugs such as meloxicam and etodolac that act by selective or specific inhibition of cyclo-oxygenase II and thus spare cyclo-oxygenase I have fewer gastropathic effects. Two highly cyclo-oxygenase II selective inhibitors, celecoxib and rofecoxib, possessing no significant cyclo-oxygenase I inhibitory activity at anti-inflammatory therapeutic doses, have been recently introduced. Clinical trials have demonstrated their improved safety profile in respect to endoscopically detectable gastroduodenal ulcers, upper gastrointestinal haemorrhage, and perforation when compared with conventional NSAIDs. Although the inhibition of platelet function by NSAIDs that inhibit cyclo-oxygenase I is associated with serious gastrointestinal haemorrhage in susceptible individuals, certain of these drugs, such as low-dose aspirin, appear to be beneficial in the prevention of strokes and coronary thrombosis, a property not shared by selective cyclo-oxygenase II inhibitors.

NSAIDs are valuable in controlling joint pain and stiffness but have insignificant effect on factors mediating joint damage. There is little difference in the efficacy of available NSAIDs at optimal doses. Preferred NSAIDs have the most favourable risk:benefit ratio at low cost and are administered once or twice daily at doses that achieve 8- to 12-h activity to ensure compliance, alleviation of symptoms during nocturnal sleep, and on waking in the morning.

All NSAIDs can cause fluid retention and oedema by a renin–angiotensin-dependent mechanism that may also aggravate congestive cardiac failure and systemic hypertension. Patients with impaired renal function, cirrhosis of the liver, and decreased plasma volume from any cause are

Table 2 Current non-steroidal anti-inflammatory drugs: dosage for rheumatoid arthritis

Cyclo-oxygenase (Cox) inhibitor	Dose/24 h	Cyclo-oxygenase (Cox) inhibitor	Dose/24 h
Cox I/II (non-selective):		**Cox II selective (Cox II > I):**	
Ibuprofen	400–800 mg, 3 times	Meloxicam	7.5–15 mg, once
Nabumetone	1000 mg at night; to 1000 mg twice	Etodolac	600 mg, slow release once
Naproxen	250–500 mg, twice or slow release 500–1000 mg once		
Diclofenac	25–50 mg, 3 times or slow release 75 mg once or twice	**Cox II specific:**	
Fenoprofen	300–600 mg, 3–4 times	Celecoxib	100–200 mg, twice
Ketoprofen	50 mg, 3–4 times	Rofecoxib	25 mg, once
Indomethacin	(Slow release) 75 mg, once or twice; or 25–50 mg morning and noon, and 50–100 mg at night		
Piroxicam	10–30 mg, once		
Azapropazone	300–600 mg, twice		
Sulindac	200 mg, twice		
Tenoxicam	20 mg, once		
Flurbiprofen	50 mg, 2–4 times Slow release capsule 200 mg once		
Diflunisal	250–500 mg, twice		

at risk from developing NSAID-induced renal toxicity. It is claimed that sulindac may be safer than other NSAIDs in patients with renal failure.

NSAIDs, especially indomethacin, may cause side-effects involving the central nervous system such as headache, dizziness, anxiety, disorientation, and drowsiness. Rarely, use of NSAIDs may be associated with aseptic meningitis. NSAIDs may aggravate asthma and cause hypersensitivity reactions. Blood dycrasias and an increase in serum concentration of liver enzymes and alkaline phosphatase are described. Drug interactions may decrease the efficacy of some concomitantly prescribed therapies, for instance antihypertensives and lithium, and potentiate the effects of others, for instance anticoagulants, anti-epileptics, and oral hypoglycaemics. NSAIDs decrease the excretion of methotrexate but do not appear to increase its toxicity in the dose range used to treat rheumatoid arthritis. They also increase plasma concentrations of cyclosporin and FK-506 and hence may increase the risk of renal toxicity.

Disease-modifying antirheumatoid drugs (DMARDs)

DMARDs, also classified as slow-acting antirheumatoid drugs (SAARDs) because of the lag period of some weeks before their anti-inflammatory effect becomes apparent, are the current cornerstone of drug therapy for rheumatoid arthritis (Table 3). Drugs in this category include: the antimalarials, hydroxychloroquine or chloroquine sulphate; sulphasalazine; weekly low-dose oral or parenterally administered methotrexate; weekly injections of gold aurothiomalate or gold aurothioglucose; leflunomide; cyclosporin; azathioprine; and D-penicillamine. Drugs such as gold, antimalarials, and methotrexate were introduced for use in rheumatoid arthritis by serendipity. Others, such as azathioprine, cyclosporin, and lefluomide, were developed as immunosuppressive agents for preventing transplant rejections and subsequently used to curb the aberrant immunological response in rheumatoid arthritis. The mechanism of action of these drugs in rheumatoid arthritis is complex and still incompletely understood. Inhibitory effects on inflammatory pathways, immune responses, and cell activation have been described in experimental systems and clinical studies.

Clinical trials have demonstrated superior efficacy of all these drugs over placebo in controlling symptoms and signs in patients previously treated with only NSAIDs in early and established rheumatoid arthritis. In addition, compared with placebo, sulphasalazine, methotrexate, and leflunomide appear to retard progression of structural damage as assessed by serial radiographs of the hands and feet in controlled trials lasting 6 to 12 months.

A meta-analysis of clinical trials of commonly used DMARDs has been analysed for efficacy and toxicity relative to each other and to placebo treatment. Methotrexate, sulphasalazine, injectable gold, and D-penicillamine have the best and equal efficacy in the short term compared with placebo. The antimalarials (hydroxychloroquine and chloroquine) and azathioprine appear to be less efficacious in this analysis. The toxicity profile shows a different rank order. Antimalarials are least toxic, followed by methotrexate and sulphasalazine in an intermediate range, and injectable gold, azathioprine, and D-penicillamine at the most toxic end of the spectrum. Methotrexate and sulphasalazine emerge with the best balance between efficacy and toxicity. Since leflunomide was introduced recently it was not included in this meta-analysis, but its efficacy and toxicity profile is similar to methotrexate and sulphasalazine.

Remission of rheumatoid arthritis on DMARD therapy has been described in approximately 20 per cent of those with early disease treated with methotrexate or sulphasalazine as single agents. However, in one example of a follow-up study fewer than 1 in 10 of 18 per cent that achieved remission (i.e. around 2 per cent of the original cohort) sustained it for longer than 3 years. Remissions are rare in patients who have progressed to a stage of physical disability and whose radiographs show bony erosions.

Conclusions from short-term randomized clinical trials do not reflect the effectiveness of DMARDs in controlling disease activity in the longer term. Incomplete responses, relapses, and adverse events are common and account for discontinuation of antimalarials, gold salts, D-penicillamine, sulphasalazine, and azathioprine in the majority of patients in 1 to 3 years. By contrast, responses to methotrexate appear to be more durable in follow-up studies of large cohorts of patients with rheumatoid arthritis, with about 50 per cent continuing therapy at 5 years. Data on long-term effectiveness, tolerability, and toxicity of leflunomide are not yet available.

Combinations of DMARDs have been used in the expectation that their different modes of action might provide added efficacy. However, a meta-analysis showed that there was marginal benefit at the doses and combinations used prior to 1994, especially in the reduction of number of tender joints, with increased toxicity when compared with single agents. Several subsequent randomized controlled trials have demonstrated significantly improved efficacy of combination therapy, without increased toxicity: some examples are given below.

In one trial lasting 2 years, a combination of oral methotrexate (7.5 to 17.5 mg/week), sulphasalazine (0.5 g twice daily), and hydroxychloroquine (200 mg twice daily) showed superior control of symptoms and signs compared with methotrexate alone or a combination of sulphasalazine and hydroxychloroquine. Patients enrolled in this trial with advanced disease had already failed to respond to DMARD monotherapy.

In a further study on patients with disease of less than 2 years duration, the introduction of a combination of methotrexate, sulphasalazine, and hydroxychloquine not only controlled symptoms better but, at the end of 2 years, had induced remission in 37 per cent compared with 21 per cent of patients on sulphasalazine or methotrexate alone.

In another trial lasting 24 weeks, patients with active disease despite methotrexate (mean dose 12.5 mg/week) showed improvement in their signs and symptoms when cyclosporin at 2.5 to 5 mg/kg daily was added, compared with the addition of placebo. Similarly, in an open-label study, the addition of leflunomide at 20 mg daily enhanced the efficacy of ongoing methotrexate treatment in patients whose disease activity was not well controlled, but was associated with greater toxicity.

Corticosteroids

Corticosteroids are potent anti-inflammatory agents and are most efficacious in treating symptoms and signs of rheumatoid arthritis and for amelioration of systemic features, but their use is limited by toxicity related to dose and duration of exposure. The circumstances in which use of corticosteroids has been established and those in which it is debated are described below.

In patients in whom loss of function and disease activity is restricted to a few joints, local corticosteroid therapy can be most effective. This indication may arise in those whose rheumatoid disease is limited to a few joints, or in patients with an incomplete response to NSAID and DMARD therapy. Several alternative corticosteroid preparations are available, the dose being dependent on the size of the joint. Depot methyl prednisolone (dose range 4 to 40 mg) or triamcinolone acetonide (dose range 2.5 to

Table 3 Disease-modifying antirheumatoid drugs

Drug	Dose and comments	Contraindications	Some side-effects*
Methotrexate	Oral 7.5 mg/week initially given as a single dose; usual dose 12.5–15 mg/week; increase up to 20 mg/week orally and try intramuscular route in unresponsive patients or in presence of gastrointestinal intolerance. Folic acid 5 mg daily for 1–5 days/week improves tolerability	Pregnancy and planned conception (teratogenic), alcohol abuse, chronic liver disease, diabetes mellitus, moderate to severe chronic lung disease	Bone marrow suppression, hepatotoxicity, interstital pneumonitis, anorexia, nausea, stomatitis, vomiting, viral and opportunistic infections, possible increased risk of lymphoma
Sulphasalazine	Enteric-coated tablets 0.5 g once a day for initial week; thereafter 0.5 g increment in dose per week to total 2 g/day; maximum dose 3 g/day.	Sulphonamide allergy, glucose-6-phosphate dehydrogenase deficiency	Nausea, anorexia, rashes, blood dyscrasia (especially neutropenia), lupus-like syndrome, oligospermia on taking drug (reversible)
Hydroxychloroquine	200–400 mg in divided doses daily. Maximum dose 6.5 mg/kg (not exceeding 400 mg/day); maintenance dose 200–400 mg daily	Glucose-6-phosphate dehydrogenase deficiency, retinal disease, psoriasis	Maculopathy; test visual acuity and fields, colour vision prior to commencing therapy; if abnormal, full ophthalmology examination required;
Or Chloroquine sulphate	(200 mg, equivalent to chloroquine phosphate 250 mg or chloroquine base 150 mg) Daily dose of chloroquine base 150 mg, daily maximum 2.5 mg/kg	As above	patient to stop drug if any disturbance of vision noted. Annual check-ups advisable; discontinuation after 10 years recommended
Injectable gold aurothiomalate	Deep intramuscular, upper/outer gluteal muscle; 10 mg test dose to check for hypersensitivity; 20–50 mg weekly according to tolerability and severity to a total of 1 g or until response is observed. Maintenance dose 20–50 mg/month	Gold hypersensitivity, chronic liver and renal disease, psoriasis	Blood dyscrasias, aplastic anaemia, nephropathy, dermatitis
Azathioprine	Oral 1.5 to 2.5 mg/kg daily	Up to 1 in 200 of the population have hypersensitivity characterized by severe leucopenia on initial administration	Hepatitis, reversible dose-related bone marrow depression, possible increased risk of lymphoma
Cyclosporin (Neoral)	Oral 2.5–4 mg/kg provided serum creatinine is in normal range and does not increase more than 30 per cent above baseline	Renal disease with compromised function, hypertension	Nephrotoxicity, hirsurtism, hypertension, tremor
D-Penicillamine	Oral 250–1000 mg daily in divided doses	Penicillin hypersensitivity	Taste loss, thrombocytopenia and other dyscrasias, nephropathy, myaesthenia gravis, rashes
Leflunomide	Initial loading dose 100 mg orally, once daily for 3 days. Maintenance dose 20–40 mg daily	Pregnancy (teratogenic), planned conception; long half-life (several months): cholestyramine accelerates clearance	Increases serum concentrations of drugs metabolized by CYPZC9 including NSAIDs; diarrhoea, alopecia, hepatoxicity, and rarely bone marrow suppression

*Refer to *British Society for Rheumatology Drug Monitoring Guidelines*, 2000.

40 mg depending on size of joint) are suitable alternatives. Repeat injections may be necessary, but more than three per joint per year should be avoided.

Corticosteroid administered orally in courses lasting a few weeks to months (such as prednisolone at 7.5 to 10 mg daily), or in the form of 'pulse therapy' (such as depot methyl prednisolone at 80 to 120 mg by intramuscular injection), is a suitable adjunctive therapy in patients in whom the benefit of DMARDs is not yet established. Longer-term, more or less indefinite, treatment with low-dose prednisolone is necessary in patients with moderate to severe disease, especially associated with refractory anaemia that is not controlled with currently used antirheumatoid drugs. Long-term low-dose prednisolone retards the progression of rheumatoid bone erosions in radiographs of hands and feet and, hence it is claimed, deterioration of physical function. Whether this benefit is outweighed by the side-effects and morbidity of corticosteroid therapy is debatable. Higher doses of corticosteroids are indicated in the treatment of severe extra-articular disease.

Prevention of corticosteroid-induced osteoporosis and reduction in risk of fractures requires adequate prophylaxis with calcium and vitamin D intake (for example, daily intake of 1000 mg of calcium and 800 IU of vitamin D). In susceptible patients, or those on doses exceeding the equivalent of 7.5 mg of prednisolone daily, measurement of bone mineral density is used to identify and monitor management. Bisphosphonates may be required in addition to calcium and vitamin D, and hormone replacement therapy is recommended in perimenopausal women.

Biological therapy

The identification of TNF-α as a key mediator of rheumatoid inflammation has led to the development of anti-TNF agents that have been introduced recently into clinical practice. Other targeted therapies are in advanced clinical trials, including recombinant IL-1 receptor antagonist (rIL-ra) that inhibits the activity of IL-1, an important pro-inflammatory cytokine. In clinical trials treatment with rIL-ra has shown significant improvement of signs and symptoms and retardation of radiographic progression of joint damage.

Non-pharmacological measures and support

Specialist physicians co-ordinate the management of patients with rheumatoid arthritis using a team of health professionals. The support provided improves the patient's ability to cope with pain, disability, daily activities, and the prospect of continuing work and retaining independence.

Education and counselling is helpful in preparing patients for the likely consequences of their disease, and its development over time. It also allows the patient to participate fully in making informed decisions about taking and monitoring drugs and retaining control. Studies have demonstrated the benefit of this approach in minimizing costs of medical care and improved outcomes.

Bed rest and the use of resting splints is helpful during the very acute stages of joint disease, but should always be accompanied by daily passive joint movements and appropriate isometric exercises to avoid contractures, muscle atrophy, and osteoporosis, and to retain joint function. Exercise initiated under supervision and maintained by patients on a regular basis does not accelerate joint damage, diminishing pain and promoting a sense of well being in those in whom fatigue is a major feature of active disease.

For patients with disability, aids and appliances can be helpful in undertaking daily tasks and leisure activities such as dressing, turning keys and taps, cooking, lifting, domestic tasks, and gardening. Adjustments in the home are helpful, such as use of cushions and chairs with high seats in the bathroom and toilet. For the very disabled, learning techniques for transfers from bed to chair, chair to the toilet, and the installation of chairlifts and use of wheelchairs need expert help and advice.

Maintenance of mobility requires attention to foot care, podiatry, comfortable shoes, a walking stick or elbow crutches, and specially adapted motor vehicles to get to work and for social purposes.

Disabled people have certain privileges in employment and may qualify for disability allowances. Some may benefit from retraining for suitable work. The health-care team needs to recognize that chronic illness and disability places increased pressure on spouses and family, who generally end up as carers of the patient with rheumatoid arthritis: support and counselling should therefore extend to them.

Dietary manipulation, such as exclusion of certain foods and beverages, has enjoyed popularity and in some patients appears to be beneficial, but there is little evidence that most such diets are of value. Fasting followed by a vegetarian diet was shown to be of benefit in a Norwegian study, but the durability of effect is unknown. Diets rich in fish oils and omega fatty acids appear to be of some benefit. As excessive weight accelerates joint damage and increases the risk of complications when undergoing essential surgery, obese patients should be encouraged to lose weight.

Management strategies

Mild disease

Definition

Mild disease may be defined as rheumatoid arthritis with limited joint involvement, low disease activity, and without markers of poor prognosis. Such patients will typically show most of the following features: involvement of less than six or seven individual joints and sparing of weight-bearing joints; pain readily controlled with NSAIDs; less than 15 min of joint stiffness on waking or following inactivity; lack of extra-articular disease; minimally elevated erythrocyte sedimentation rate or concentration of C-reactive protein; negative rheumatoid factor test; a normal haematological profile; little or no impairment of physical function; and ability to undertake activities of daily living, maintaining employment and enjoying non-strenuous social and leisure activities. Radiographs of hands and feet show a lack of significant osteopenia, joint space narrowing, and bony erosions at baseline and annual follow-up. The disease course may be punctuated by self-limiting exacerbations of symptoms and signs. Patients with mild disease constitute a small proportion of patients referred to specialist clinics but are more numerous in the community and in the primary care setting.

Drug treatment

This consists of a judicious use of non-steroidal anti-inflammatory drugs. Corticosteroid injections into individual affected joints, tendon sheaths, and bursas for persistent swelling, tenderness, or loss of normal range of movement can be very effective. Follow-up assessment is necessary to ensure that the disease has not altered to a more severe pattern. DMARDs are indicated in those with recurrent or persistent symptoms and signs, deformities, or radiographic evidence of structural damage. Hydroxychloroquine or sulphasalazine are used initially. If the decision to embark on the use of DMARDs is made, the aims and management strategy are the same as for patients with moderate or severe disease.

Moderate and severe disease

Definition

This is defined as rheumatoid disease that has evolved into an unremitting pattern of polyarthritis with evidence of significant functional impairment and joint damage. With increasing severity most of the following features are present: 10 to 30 swollen and tender joints; frequent involvement of proximal joints of the upper and lower limbs; moderate to severe pain; inactivity and morning stiffness exceeding 1 h in duration; prominent fatigue; elevated erythrocyte sedimentation rate and/or C-reactive protein concentrations; low haemoglobin concentration; polymorphonuclear leucocytosis and thrombocytosis; and positive rheumatoid factor test. Deformities of joints are apparent early in the course of disease and radiographs of hands, feet, and affected joints already show loss of joint space and subchondral erosions within 2 years of presentation. Such patients show a significant impairment in daily activities and restricted ability to perform domestic and work-related tasks and to enjoy social and leisure activities.

Drug treatment

The aim of drug treatment is to achieve rapid control of disease activity and, if possible, remission of disease. This requires simultaneous or sequential use of drugs belonging to different classes, for instance NSAIDs, DMARDs, corticosteroids, and biological therapies as discussed below.

NSAIDs are used at optimal doses for control of pain and stiffness (Table 2), those most commonly given in practice being naproxen, diclofenac, and indomethacin. Many physicians prefer to administer these drugs in slow-release preparations in the morning and before retiring to bed at night. In the elderly, cyclo-oxygenase II-selective NSAIDs may be preferable, or else the simultaneous use of a gastroprotective agent, most commonly proton pump inhibitors. In addition, simple analgesics such as 0.5 to 1 g of paracetamol every 6 h may be required for relief of pain.

DMARDs should be used in all patients (Table 3), the two most commonly employed being sulphasalazine and methotrexate, provided there are no contraindications. These are given as single drugs in incremental doses over 3 to 4 months to the maximum recommended or tolerated dose. If a clear-cut reduction in disease activity (or remission) is not observed with one of these drugs, then monotherapy with leflunomide, azathioprine, or injectable gold may be attempted. Alternatively, other DMARDs are added at this stage. Commonly used DMARD combinations include: methotrexate and hydroxychloroquine; methotrexate, sulphasalazine, and hydroxychloroquine; and methotrexate and cyclosporin. The choice of therapy is ultimately determined by evaluation of risks of toxicity, efficacy, durability, and direct and indirect costs of treatment. There is no consensus on the most effective combination regimen. Meticulous monitoring of toxic effects is necessary.

In practice over 50 per cent of patients with moderate or severe disease require corticosteroid therapy. If continuing long-term use appears necessary, the aim should be to reduce the dose to the equivalent of 5 to 7.5 mg of prednisolone daily by more aggressive use of DMARDs, or consider anti-TNF therapy.

Despite good initial responses to currently available DMARD treatments, a proportion—probably 10 to 15 per cent of hospital patients—show continuing disease activity and progressive disability. Randomized, placebo-controlled trials of two anti-TNF biological agents have shown these to be efficacious in such cases, and they became available in 2000, although their high cost is likely to restrict widespread use. The two anti-TNF-α drugs licensed for use in rheumatoid arthritis are infliximab (a chimeric monoclonal anti-TNF-α monoclonal antibody) given in combination with methotrexate, and etanercept (a soluble dimeric molecule consisting of a TNF receptor linked to the constant domains of Fc-IgG). Infliximab is given intravenously at a dose of 3 mg/kg over 1 h every 8 weeks to patients already receiving methotrexate therapy once a week. Etanercept given as 25 mg subcutaneously twice weekly is efficacious as monotherapy or when added to methotrexate. Symptoms and signs are rapidly alleviated in approximately 60 to 70 per cent of patients (Fig. 11) in clinical trials. Durable responses are being reported for up to 2 years, with a small increase in upper respiratory infections but without an increase in serious adverse events. Continuing therapy is needed and relapse of disease follows withdrawal.

The combination of infliximab and methotrexate has also been reported to inhibit or even reverse significantly progression of joint damage at the end of 1 year in most patients as assessed by serial radiographs. By contrast, damage continues in the control group of patients with an incomplete response to methotrexate. In another study in rheumatoid arthritis, etanercept was found to be more effective than methotrexate in controlling progression of bone erosions, assessed by radiographs of the hands and feet at baseline and the end of 1 year. These data imply that anti-TNF therapy could preserve physical function and quality of life in the long term and hence prove to be cost-effective.

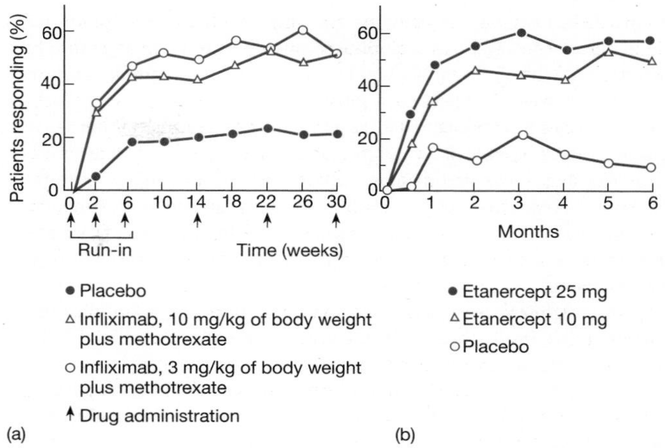

Fig. 11 Anti-TNF therapy. (a) Efficacy of combination of infliximab and methotrexate compared with methotrexate and placebo. Percentage of patients achieving a clinical response of a 20 per cent change from baseline as defined by the American College of Rheumatology 20 (ACR20) criteria. Patients were treated with methotrexate (10 to 35 mg/week) and either placebo, 3, or 10 mg/kg infliximab administered intravenously at time points indicated, in a patient group unresponsive to DMARDs with active disease despite methotrexate therapy (Maini *et al.* 1999). (b) Efficacy of etanercept compared with placebo. ACR 20 results in patients treated with two doses of etanercept or placebo injections administered subcutaneously twice weekly over a 6-month period in a population unresponsive to DMARDs. (Reproduced from Moreland *et al.* (1999), with permission.)

The efficacy of anti-TNF agents represents an important advance in therapy, although their efficacy and safety beyond 2 years of continuous therapy under controlled trial conditions is not yet established. Post-marketing surveillance of adverse events to infliximab and etanercept following exposure of approximately 300 000 patients to date have drawn attention to concerns arising from rare, but significant numbers of cases of sepsis, tuberculosis, fungal, and opportunistic infections. These infections are compatible with the consequences of blockade of the postulated role of TNF in host defence mechanisms. Based on these reports, regulatory authorities in the United States and Europe have advised that anti-TNF therapy is contraindicated in the presence of active serious infections and, in the case of infliximab, latent untreated tuberculosis. Other rare adverse events have included demyelinating syndromes (hence it is advisable not to treat patients with a history of multiple sclerosis), lupus syndrome, and bone marrow depression. Based on reports of an unexpected number of deaths in a phase II clinical trial of infliximab in the treatment of severe congestive cardiac failure, use of infliximab is not advisable for the treatment of patients with rheumatoid arthritis in moderate or severe congestive cardiac failure. Provided suitable screening and monitoring practices are in place, the favourable risk to benefit profile of anti-TNF therapy does not alter the indication for its use in the treatment of moderate to severe rheumatoid arthritis with persistent disease activity despite best available, but also potentially toxic and immunosuppressive, standard therapy. The high cost of anti-TNF drugs has, however, limited access to this treatment in some countries.

Extra-articular disease

Effective treatment of rheumatoid arthritis generally reduces the risk of developing severe extra-articular disease. Systemic rheumatoid vasculitis is potentially a life-threatening complication and may be aggravated by coincidental infection, such as cutaneous ulcers. After due attention to confirming the diagnosis and excluding and treating infections with appropriate antimicrobial drugs, therapy with high-dose corticosteroids and cyclophosphamide is favoured by many specialists, although no randomized placebo-controlled trial data are available. One regimen recommends intravenous methylprednisolone at 1 g daily for 3 days, simultaneously with an initial single pulse of intravenous cyclophosphamide (10 to 15 mg/kg) in a fully hydrated patient to prevent bladder toxicity. Cyclophosphamide is repeated every 3 to 4 weeks, subject to a satisfactory clinical response or lack of toxicity, up to a total dose of 10 to 12 g in a cycle of treatment. Alternatively, oral cyclophosphamide at 2 mg/kg (maximum dose 150 mg daily) may be used. Oral high-dose prednisolone is continued until clinical response is observed or toxic effects occur, when it is rapidly tapered to a maintenance dose, generally about 15 mg daily. Similarly, cyclophosphamide is substituted by the less toxic azathioprine at 1.5 to 2 mg/kg daily or methotrexate at 15 mg/week.

Similar regimens have been used for severe fibrosing alveolitis and for severe scleritis and corneal melt in conjunction with local therapy. Occasional patients with Felty's syndrome and hypersplenism that do not respond to DMARDs benefit from splenectomy, and their neutropenia may respond to recombinant human granulocyte colony-stimulating factor. Keratoconjunctivitis sicca and dry mouth due to secondary Sjögren's syndrome respond to local measures including artificial tears, dental hygiene, and saliva substitute.

Further reading

Arend WP, Dayer JM (1990) Cytokines and cytokine inhibitors or antagonists in rheumatoid arthritis. *Arthritis and Rheumatism* **33**, 305–15.

Arnett FC *et al.* (1988). The American Rheumatism Association 1987 revised criteria for the classification of rheumatoid arthritis. *Arthritis and Rheumatism* **31**, 315–34.

British Society for Rheumatology (2000). *British Society for Rheumatology drug monitoring guidelines.* BSR Headquarters, 41 Eagle Street, London, WC1R 4AR.

Emery P *et al.* (1999). Celecoxib versus diclofenac in long-term management of rheumatoid arthritis: randomised double-blind comparison. *Lancet* **354**, 2106–11.

Erhardt CC *et al.* (1989). Factors predicting a poor life prognosis in rheumatoid arthritis: an eight year prospective study. *Annals of the Rheumatic Diseases* **48**, 7–13.

Feldmann M, Brennan FM, Maini RN (1996). Role of cytokines in rheumatoid arthritis. *Annual Review of Immunology* **14**, 397–440.

Felson DT, Anderson JJ, Meenan RF (1994). The efficacy and toxicity of combination therapy in rheumatoid arthritis: a metaanalysis. *Arthritis and Rheumatism* **37**, 487–91.

Felson DT *et al.* (1995). American College of Rheumatology preliminary definition of improvement in rheumatoid arthritis. *Arthritis and Rheumatism* **38**, 727–35.

Fries JF, Spitz PW, Young DY (1982). The dimensions of health outcomes: the health assessment questionnaire, disability and pain scales. *Journal of Rheumatology* **9**, 789–93.

Furst DE (2000). Aggressive strategies for treating aggressive rheumatoid arthritis: has the case been proven? *Lancet* **356**, 183–4.

Gardner DL (1992). Rheumatoid arthritis: cell and tissue pathology. In: Gardner DL, ed. *Pathological basis of the connective tissue diseases*, pp 444–526. Edward Arnold, London.

Gregersen PK, Silver J, Winchester RJ (1987). The shared epitope hypothesis. An approach to understanding the molecular genetics of susceptibility to rheumatoid arthritis. *Arthritis and Rheumatism* **30**, 1205–13.

Griffiths ID (1998). Extra-articular features of rheumatic diseases. In: Maddison PJ, Isenberg DA, Woo P, Glass DN, eds. *Oxford textbook of rheumatology*, 2nd edn, pp 169–79. Oxford University Press.

Gotzsche PC (2000). Non-steroidal anti-inflammatory drugs. *British Medical Journal* **320**, 1058–61.

Kirwan JR (1995). The effect of glucocorticoids on joint destruction in rheumatoid arthritis. The Arthritis and Rheumatism Council Low-Dose Glucocorticoid Study Group. *New England Journal of Medicine* **333**, 142–6.

Lawrence JS (1970). Rheumatoid arthritis: nature or nurture? *Annals of the Rheumatic Diseases* **29**, 357–69.

Maini RN (1998). The Lumleian lecture: Milestones in the development of anti-tumour necrosis factor α therapy (TNFα) therapy. In: Pusey C, ed. *Horizons in medicine No 11*, pp 131–45. Royal College of Physicians, London.

Maini RN, Feldmann M (1998). Immunopathogenesis of rheumatoid arthritis. In: Maddison PJ, Isenberg DA, Woo P, Glass DN, eds. *Oxford textbook of rheumatology*, 2nd edn, pp 983–1004. Oxford University Press.

Maini RN, Taylor PC (2000). Anti-cytokine therapy for rheumatoid arthritis. *Annual Review of Medicine* **51**, 207–29.

Maini RN *et al.* (1999). Randomised phase III trial of infliximab (Chimeric anti-TNFα monoclonal antibody) versus placebo in rheumatoid arthritis patients receiving concomitant methotrexate. *Lancet* **354**,1932–9.

Mangge H, Hermann J, Schauenstein K (1999). Diet and rheumatoid arthritis—a review. *Scandinavian Journal of Rheumatology* **28**, 201–9.

Moreland LE *et al.* (1999). Etanercept therapy in rheumatoid arthritis. *Annals of Internal Medicine* **130**, 478–86.

O'Dell JR *et al.* (1996). Treatment of rheumatoid arthritis with methotrexate alone, sulfasalazine and hydroxychloroquine, or a combination of all three medications. *New England Journal of Medicine* **334**, 1287–91.

Pinals RS *et al.* (1981). Preliminary criteria for clinical remission in rheumatoid arthritis. *Arthritis and Rheumatism* **24**, 1305–15.

Pincus T (1988). Rheumatoid arthritis: disappointing long-term outcomes despite successful short-term clinical trials. *Journal of Clinical Epidemiology* **41**, 1037–41.

Pincus T, Callahan LF (1993). What is the natural history of rheumatoid arthritis? *Rheumatic Disease Clinics of North America* **19**, 123–51.

Sharp JT *et al.* (2000). Treatment with leflunomide slows radiographic progression of rheumatoid arthritis: results from three randomized controlled trials of leflunomide in patients with active rheumatoid arthritis. Leflunomide Rheumatoid Arthritis Investigators Group. *Arthritis and Rheumatism* **43**, 495–505.

Short CL (1974). The antiquity of rheumatoid arthritis. *Arthritis and Rheumatism* **17**, 193–205.

Silman AJ, Hochberg MC (1993). Rheumatoid arthritis. In: *Epidemiology of the rheumatic diseases*, pp 7–68. Oxford University Press.

Tugwell P *et al.* (1995). Combination therapy with cyclosporine and methotrexate in severe rheumatoid arthritis. The Methotrexate–Cyclosporine Combination Study Group. *New England Journal of Medicine* **333**, 137–41.

Van der Heijde DM *et al.* (1993). Development of a disease activity score based on judgment in clinical practice by rheumatologists. *Journal of Rheumatology* **20**, 579–81.

van Riel PL, Haagsma CJ, Furst DE (1999). Pharmacotherapeutic combination strategies with disease-modifying antirheumatic drugs in established rheumatoid arthritis. *Bailliere's Best Practice and Research: Clinical Rheumatology* **13**, 689–700.

Wiles N *et al.* (1999). Estimating the incidence of rheumatoid arthritis: Trying to hit a moving target? *Arthritis and Rheumatism* **42**, 1339–46.

Wolfe F *et al.* (1994). The mortality of rheumatoid arthritis. *Arthritis and Rheumatism* **37**, 481–94.

Young A *et al.* (2000). How does functional disability in early rheumatoid arthritis (RA) affect patients and their lives? Results of 5 years of follow-up in 732 patients from the early RA study (ERAS). *Rheumatology* **39**, 603–11.

18.6 Spondyloarthritides and related arthritides

J. Braun and J. Sieper

Table 1 First historical descriptions of spondyloarthropathies

Spondarthritis/spondylarthro-pathy	Moll/Wright 1974, ESSG 1991
Ankylosing spondylitis	Connors 1649, Brodie 1888
Reactive arthritis/Reiter's syndrome	Reiter 1916, Ahonen 1973
Psoriatic arthritis	Wright 1959
Arthritis associated with inflammatory bowel diseases	Bargen 1930
Enthesitis	Niepel 1961
HLA B27 association	Brewerton, Schlosstein 1973
Undifferentiated spondyloarthropathy	Khan/van der Linden 1990

ESSG, European Spondylarthropathy Study Group.

Introduction and definitions

The spondyloarthropathies are a heterogenous group of inflammatory rheumatic diseases with predominant involvement of axial and peripheral joints and entheses. In addition to these, the various spondyloarthropathies share other characteristic clinical features, for example anterior uveitis and Crohn-like gut lesions. Symptoms in subsets of spondyloarthropathies can overlap, for example psoriatic skin lesions in Reiter's syndrome, and patients can move from one subset to another, for example from reactive arthritis to ankylosing spondylitis.

The various names which have been and are still used for the spondyloarthropathies include seronegative spondarthropathies, spondarthritis, spondylarthropathy, spondyloarthropathy, and spondyloarthritis. There is no substantial difference between them. The prefix seronegative, referring to the general absence of rheumatoid factors in the spondyloarthropathies, is historical and redundant. The term spondyloarthropathy is preferred in this chapter. The spondyloarthropathies are not modern diseases, with ankylosing spondylitis first having been described in 1649 (Table 1).

Epidemiology

The mean age at onset is 20 to 40 years, with a slight preponderance of males in most subsets of spondyloarthropathy. Next to rheumatoid arthritis, the spondyloarthropathies are the most frequent inflammatory rheumatic diseases (Table 2), with ankylosing spondylitis and undifferentiated spondyloarthropathy being the most common subsets. The overall prevalence of spondyloarthropathies in patients presenting with back pain to general practitioners' surgeries in the United Kingdom has been estimated at 5 per cent.

Table 2 Prevalence of spondyloarthropathies

Disease	Prevalence
Spondyloarthropathy	0.6–2.0%
Ankylosing spondylitis	0.2–1.4%
Undifferentiated spondyloarthropathy	0.2–0.7%
Reactive arthritis	0.01%
Psoriasis	1.0–3.0%
Psoriatic arthritis	0.3%
Arthritis associated with inflammatory bowel disease	0.001%

The spondyloarthropathies are associated with the major histocompatability complex class I antigen HLA B27, and the prevalence of spondyloarthropathies in any population correlates with that of HLA B27. The magnitude of association differs between the subsets (Table 3) and has been mainly shown for ankylosing spondylitis, but in Inuit populations Reiter's syndrome is more frequent.

Pathogenesis

In all forms of spondyloarthropathy there is a strong genetic association with the major histocompatability complex class I antigen HLA B27, as shown in Table 3. The overall influence of genes in the pathogenesis of ankylosing spondylitis has been estimated to be 95 per cent, leaving only 5 per cent to other causative factors such as environmental influences. HLA B27 is responsible for about one-third of the total genetic load: 25 subtypes are now recognized by polymerase chain reaction technology, three of which are not associated with ankylosing spondylitis, or are associated less strongly. There is weaker association of spondyloarthropathies with HLA B60 and HLA DR1, and possibly also tumour necrosis factor-α polymorphisms. Further genes have not yet been identified.

Table 3 HLA B27 association of the spondyloarthropathies. Note that the prevalence of spondyloarthropathies (mainly of the first four listed above) relates to the prevalence of HLA B27 in different populations, which is as shown in the second table

Spondyloarthropathy	HLA B27 prevalence
Ankylosing spondylitis	85–95%
Reactive arthritis	30–80%
Reiter's syndrome	60–90%
Psoriatic arthritis:	
Peripheral arthritis	10–30%
Axial involvement	40–60%
Arthritis associated with inflammatory bowel diseases	
Peripheral arthritis	10–30%
Axial involvement	40–60%
Undifferentiated spondyloarthropathy	50–70%

Population	HLA B27 prevalence
Native Americans	6–50%
Inuit	15–25%
North Europeans	10–25%
Middle Europeans	6–9%
North Americans	6–8%
South Europeans	4–6%
Africans	1–5%

Table 4 Spondyloarthropathy—pathogenetic models

Model	Mechanism
Arthritogenic peptide model	Bacterial protein processed/ presented by B27 to CD8+ T cells
Deficient immune response	Failure of B27+ cells to properly present and eliminate bacteria
Molecular mimicry	Similarity of bacterial and self structures, possibly resulting in autoimmunity
Autoimmunity	Self structures such as B27-derived peptides presented by class I or II molecules

The relevance of HLA B27 to disease pathogenesis is not known: several models have been proposed to explain tissue tropism, the aberrant immune response to certain bacteria, and the HLA B27 association of the spondyloarthropathies (Table 4).

The classical arthritogenic peptide model is backed by the demonstration of HLA B27-restricted CD8+ T-cell clones in the synovial fluid of patients with reactive arthritis. Immunodominant peptide motifs and peptides have been described, but their pathogenetic relevance is not yet clear. Lipopolysaccharide and RNA of bacteria associated with reactive arthritis and a CD4+ T-cell response directed against bacterial antigens have been detected in reactive arthritis, but it is not clear whether this immune response is beneficial or arthritogenic. At the humoral and the cellular level, molecular mimicry (partial sequence homologies at the protein and DNA level) between bacterial antigens and self structures has been described, mainly of the HLA B27 molecule. It also seems possible that patients with HLA B27+ spondyloarthropathies have deficient immune reactivity, for example diminished ability to secrete tumour necrosis factor-α, or a synovial T_{H2} response (secretion of too little interferon-γ, too much IL-4, IL-10) making elimination of bacteria difficult. Presentation of HLA B27-derived peptides themselves by HLA class II molecules, or even by HLA class I molecules, has been proposed as an explanation of the association of HLA B27 with disease.

Clinical features

The characteristic clinical features of the spondyloarthropathies are listed in Table 5.

Table 5 Characteristic clinical features of spondyloarthropathy

Clinical feature	Details
Inflammatory back pain	
Sacroiliitis	
Peripheral arthritis	Affects predominantly but not exclusively the lower limbs; it is often asymmetric but may also involve both knees or ankles
Enthesitis	Inflammation at the insertion sites of tendons and ligaments to bone (Figs 1 and 2 and Plate 1).
Dactylitis	Inflammatory involvement of a whole finger or toe (Fig. 3 and Plate 2) with tendovaginitis and arthritis (sausage digit).
Preceding infection in the urogenital/enteral tract	
Psoriatic skin lesions	
Crohn-like gut lesions	
Anterior uveitis	
Family history of spondyloarthropathy	

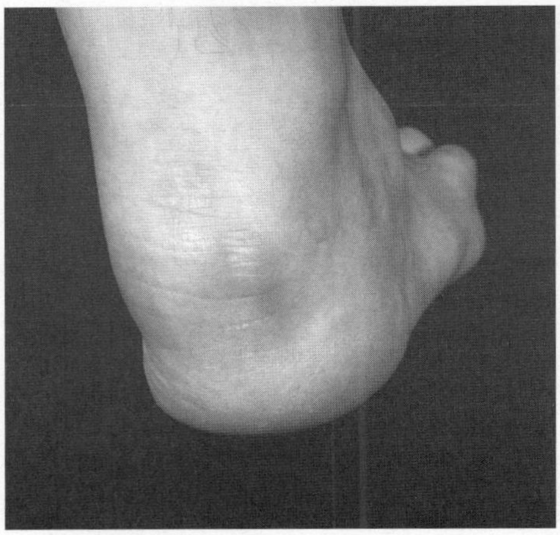

Fig. 1 Enthesitis at the insertion of the Achilles tendon in a patient with reactive arthritis. (See also Plate 1.)

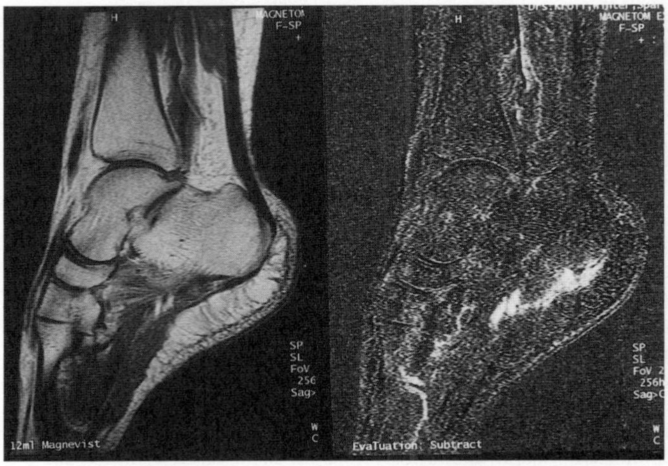

Fig. 2 Magnetic resonance image showing inflammation of the plantar fascia in a patient with undifferentiated spondyloarthropathy.

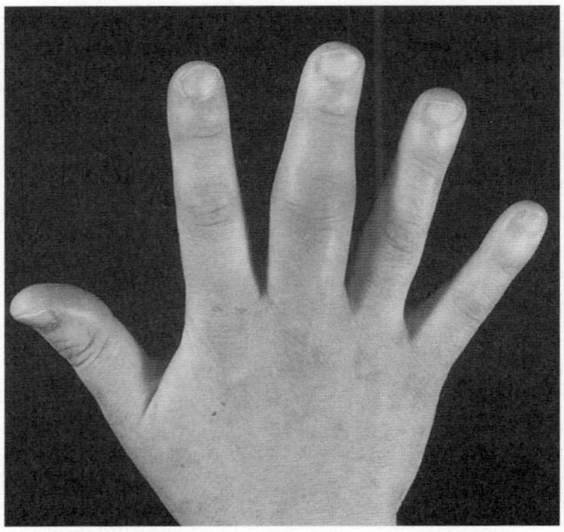

Fig. 3 Dactylitis of the third finger of the right hand in a patient with undifferentiated spondyloarthropathy. (See also Plate 2.)

Diagnosis

Five subsets of spondyloarthropathies can be distinguished on clinical grounds: ankylosing spondylitis, reactive arthritis/Reiter's syndrome, psoriatic arthritis, arthritis associated with inflammatory bowel diseases, and undifferentiated spondyloarthropathy.

Diagnostic criteria for spondyloarthropathies are shown in Table 6. Inflammatory back pain is one of the main clinical criteria used. To diagnose this requires four of the following five to be present: insidious onset, onset before the age of 45 years, duration of more than 3 months, morning stiffness, and relief by exercise but not by rest. Other features of possible relevance include waking up at night, alternating buttock pain, initially deep localization, response to non-steroidal anti-inflammatory drugs (**NSAIDs**), other clinical signs of spondyloarthropathies (enthesitis, arthritis, anterior uveitis, family history), elevated acute phase reactants (C-reactive protein, erythrocyte sedimentation rate), and the presence of HLA B27. Note, however, that HLA B27 can never make a diagnosis but increases the probability of an underlying spondyloarthropathy by about tenfold.

Differential diagnosis

The leading clinical symptom of inflammatory back pain may be pain in the lower back radiating to the thighs. Hence an important initial differential diagnosis is sciatica, particularly if symptoms are not insidious but begin abruptly. In inflammatory back pain radiation is more often bilateral than unilateral, rarely extends below the knees, almost never into the foot, and is not associated with paraesthesia. Cough impulse pain may be present. Diagnostic procedures for the detection of disc herniation by magnetic resonance imaging (**MRI**) or computed tomography (**CT**) can be misleading since disc prolapses are found in as many as 30 per cent of normal individuals.

Diffuse idiopathic skeletal hyperostosis or Forestier's disease, a severe radiographic spondylosis, can be difficult to distinguish from spondyloarthropathy. Scoliosis is not usually a marked feature of anklylosing spondylitis. Sacroiliitis occurs in a number of other rheumatic and infectious diseases, as shown in Table 7. The differential diagnosis of peripheral arthritis of the lower limbs includes Lyme arthritis, sarcoidosis (Löfgren's syndrome), gout, and undifferentiated oligoarthritis. The differential diagnosis of enthesitis includes epicondylitis and fibromyalgia, and that of dactylitis is erysipela and infection.

Prognosis

There are no good studies, but the following seem to be poor prognostic factors: hip arthritis, limitation of lumbar spine movements, dactylitis, oligoarthritis, young age at onset (less than 16 years), poor efficacy of NSAIDs, and an erythrocyte sedimentation rate of more than 30 mm in the first hour.

Table 6 Diagnostic criteria for spondyloarthropathies (1991 European Spondylarthropathy Study Group criteria)

Major criteria
Inflammatory back pain
Oligoarthritis (asymmetric) of the lower limbs
Minor criteria
Enthesitis
Alternating buttock pain
Preceding symptomatic infection
Psoriasis
Crohn-like gut lesions
Family history
Radiographic sacroiliitis

To make the diagnosis requires the presence of one major and one minor criterion. Note that dactylitis, uveitis and HLA B27 are not included in these criteria. The peripheral arthritis does not have to be asymmetric, although it often is; both knees or ankles might well be involved. Inflammatory back pain is mostly due to sacroiliitis but can also be caused by enthesitis.

Table 7 Differential diagnosis of sacroiliitis

Spondyloarthropathies
Reactive arthritis
Psoriatic arthritis
Arthritis associated with inflammatory bowel disease
Undifferentiated spondyloarthropathy
SAPHO syndrome
Other rheumatic diseases
Rheumatoid arthritis
Systemic lupus erythematosus
Sjögren's syndrome
Gout
Osteoarthritis
Paget's disease
Hyper/hypoparathyroidism
Non-rheumatic diseases
Septic sacroiliitis
Acute (staphylococci, steptococci, others)
Chronic (tuberculosis, brucellosis)
Malignancies (lymphoma, metastasis)

Ankylosing spondylitis

Ankylosing spondylitis is a chronic inflammatory rheumatic disease that mainly affects the axial skeleton, starting in the sacroiliac joints and often progressing to the spine, but peripheral joints, enthesial structures, the anterior uvea, and the aorta can also become affected.

The diagnosis is made on the basis of significant radiological changes in the sacroiliac joints, the typical clinical history of inflammatory back pain and stiffness, and evidence of limited spinal movement and/or chest expansion on physical examination.

Epidemiology

The age of onset is commonly in the twenties, but ankylosing spondylitis can begin in childhood, or considerably later (over the age of 50). The male:female ratio is about 2:1 to 3:1. Approximately 90 per cent of Caucasian ankylosing spondylitis patients are HLA B27-positive. The risk of developing ankylosing spondylitis is increased tenfold in HLA B27-positive individuals, rising to 25 to 30 per cent if a first-degree relative or dizygotic twin is affected, and to 50 to 60 per cent in monozygotic twins. Reactive arthritis, psoriasis, and inflammatory bowel disease are additional, partly independent risk factors.

Immunopathology and pathogenesis

The leading features of ankylosing spondylitis are spinal inflammation and ankylosis, but their cause is unknown. The association of ankylosing spondylitis with bacterial infections is less clear than in reactive arthritis. Antibodies to *Klebsiella pneumoniae* are more frequently detected in patients with ankylosing spondylitis than in healthy controls, but similarly often in patients with Crohn's disease and first-degree relatives of those with ankylosing spondylitis. This finding is probably explained by increased gut permeability, and its predominant clinical association is with peripheral (not axial) arthritis.

The sacroiliac joint is the structure most frequently involved in the initial phase of disease. If biopsy is performed, T cells and macrophages are seen to be the predominant infiltrating cells, with CD4+ and CD8+ T cells both present. The reason for this tropism is unclear. The fact that sacroiliac and spinal joints are affected in diseases caused by mycobacteria and other microbes may argue for a pathogen-triggered pathogenesis in ankylosing spondylitis. However, bacteria associated with reactive arthritis have not been detected in the sacroiliac joints.

Clinical features

The most common initial symptom is inflammatory back pain, commonly in the lower back and the buttocks. Early in the course of disease there may be no limitation of spinal movement or chest expansion. As it progresses, there is restriction of lateral flexion, forward flexion, and extension. There is often a flattening of the lumbar lordosis, or an inability to reverse this on forward flexion. With more advanced disease a thoracic kyphosis develops, with concomitant restriction of thoracic rotation and chest expansion due to inflammation and ankylosis of the costovertebral and costotransverse joints. In severe cases movements of the cervical spine are also restricted in all planes, with dramatic limitation of lateral flexion. The combination of cervical stiffness and severe thoracic kyphosis can lead to difficulties with forward vision. An example of a young patient with severe progressive disease is shown in Fig. 4 and Plate 3. Severe spinal disease is more frequent in men than in women. There is no evidence that pregnancy has a significant impact on the course of the disease.

Peripheral joint involvement occurs in 30 to 50 per cent of cases at some time. About 20 to 30 per cent of patients have acute peripheral arthritis of the lower limbs, often with joint effusions as the first symptom, this being especially marked in children. This situation is difficult to differentiate from reactive arthritis. Joint involvement is usually oligoarticular and often asymmetrical. The joints most often involved are the knees, ankles, hips, shoulders, wrists, temporomandibular joints, sternoclavicular joints, manubriosternal joints, costovertebral joints, zygapophyseal joints, and symphysis pubis. Small joints are rarely affected.

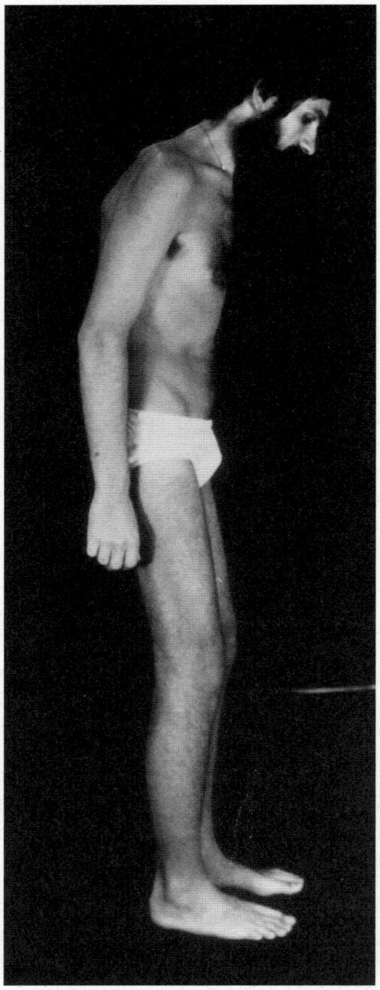

Fig. 4 30-year-old man with rapidly progressive ankylosing spondylitis (disease of 5 years duration). (See also Plate 3.)

Enthesitis occurs at the heel at the insertion of the Achilles tendon (Fig. 1) and the plantar fascia (Fig. 2), and at the iliac crests, the ischial tuberosities, the greater trochanters, and other sites. The diagnosis is often difficult if no swelling is apparent, in which case ultrasound can be revealing. Dactylitis of fingers and toes is uncommon in ankylosing spondylitis, being seen most often in psoriatic arthritis.

Physical examination of the spine and thoracic cage

The physical examination is important in the evaluation of patients with ankylosing spondylitis, in particular to quantitate flexibility of the spine and thoracic cage. The following measurements are useful, but it should be stressed that the values expected of normal individuals are dependent on age and physical training:

1. Schober test (modified):
    - Ventral: with the patient standing upright, a line is drawn across the lumbar spine connecting the two posterior superior iliac spines. Marks are made in the midline over the spine 10 cm cranial and 5 cm caudal to this horizontal line. The patient then bends with legs straight and the distance is measured again. It normally increases by more than 3 cm.
    - Lateral: the distance between the longest finger tip and the floor is measured in the upright position. This is repeated when the patient tries to flex laterally towards the ground as far as possible, normally moving by more than 10 cm.
2. Thoracic excursion. The circumference of the thorax is measured in the fourth intercostal space after maximal inspiration and expiration. It normally alters by more than 3 cm.
3. Occiput/wall distance. In the upright position the patient leans backwards against a wall, and should normally be able to touch the wall with their occiput.
4. Chin/sternum distance. The chin is maximally bent towards the sternum, and should normally be able to touch it.
5. Cervical rotation. The head is rotated to the left and right sides with the angles of rotation measured (normally more than 50°).
6. Intermalleolar distance. The patient tries to stand with their feet together: the malleoli should normally touch.

Physical examination for extra-articular organ involvement

Acute anterior uveitis can occur at any time in the course of disease and is seen in 20 to 30 per cent of patients. It is typically unilateral, but either eye may be affected in separate episodes. Recurrent attacks are common. Aortic regurgitation secondary to aortitis occurs in about 1 per cent of ankylosing spondylitis patients, most frequently in advanced disease, and may be associated with atrioventricular block. Probably on the basis of a restrictive pulmonary defect due to limited chest expansion, apical pulmonary fibrosis occurs in no more than 1 per cent of the patients, especially those with advanced disease. A cauda equina syndrome may complicate severe long-standing disease, with resultant disturbance of the bladder and bowel function. Lumbar diverticulae are seen in myelographic examinations.

Diagnosis

The 1984 modified New York criteria for ankylosing spondylitis are shown in Table 8.

There is a significant diagnostic delay in women (8 years) and in men (5 years). The most probable reason is that back pain is a very frequent

Table 8 Diagnostic criteria for ankylosing spondylitis

Clinical parameters	
Inflammatory back pain	
Limitation of spinal movement in three planes	
Deterioration of chest expansion	
Radiological parameters	
Sacroiliac joint changes of at least:	
Bilateral grade 2	
Unilateral grade 3 or 4	

Note that other spondyloarthropathy-like symptoms and syndesmophytes are not part of these criteria. For a definite diagnosis of ankylosing spondylitis, the radiological criterion is essential and one clinical criterion required. If only clinical symptoms and findings are present, a diagnosis of probable ankylosing spondylitis may be made.

complaint, and that primary care and general physicians are often not trained to distinguish inflammatory back pain from other causes of back pain.

Laboratory features

The erythrocyte sedimentation rate and the C-reactive protein are raised in 30 to 50 per cent of patients, with moderate correlation to overall disease activity. Less commonly, serum IgA levels are raised. Mild to severe normochromic normocytic anaemia occurs.

Radiological features

Sacroiliac radiography

Dependent on stage, severity, and duration of disease, there are sacroiliac joint abnormalities in almost all patients. The radiological changes are graded from 0 (normal), through I (minimal changes), II (sclerosis, some erosions), III (severe erosions, pseudodilatation of joint space, limited ankylosis), to IV (ankylosis) (Fig. 5). They are critical for the diagnosis of ankylosing spondylitis and for the differentiation from undifferentiated spondyloarthropathy, but it must be noted that significant inter- and intra-observer variability has been reported—particularly concerning grades I and II—which creates diagnostic problems and confusion. Sclerosis, joint space narrowing, and even synchondrosis occur in healthy elderly individuals. Oblique and other special views are generally not significantly better than normal anteroposterior pelvic radiographs, but can be helpful in a few cases.

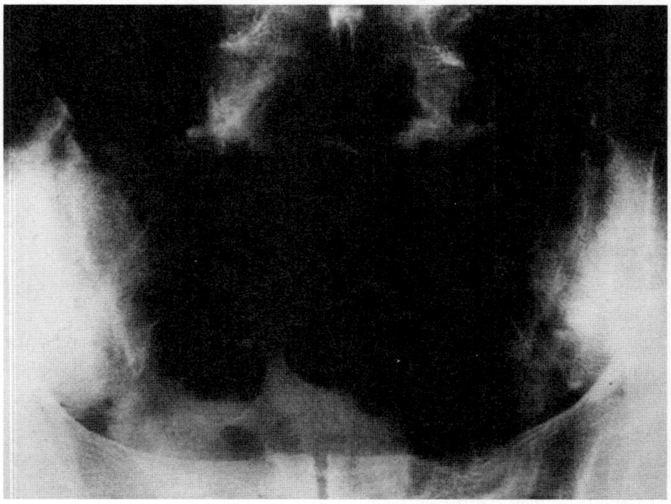

Fig. 5 Radiographic sacroiliitis, stage IV in both joints, in a 28-year-old man with ankylosing spondylitis.

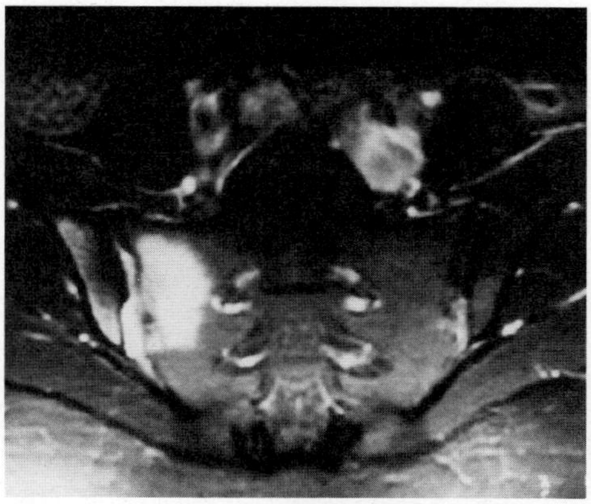

Fig. 6 Dynamic MRI showing right-sided acute sacroiliitis.

Sacroiliac MRI and CT

In early ankylosing spondylitis sacroiliac radiographs may be normal. In clinically suspicious cases dynamic MRI of the sacroiliac joints can be helpful in providing objective evidence of sacroiliitis (see undifferentiated spondyloarthropathy). Active inflammation can be demonstrated by enhancement after application of a contrast agent (gadolinium DTPA) or by special magnetic resonance sequences such as short tau inversion recovery (STIR) or other fat saturation techniques which optimize the visualization of oedematous areas (Fig. 6). Computed tomography of the sacroiliac joints is superior to normal radiographs for documenting bony changes such as erosions and ankylosis. The sacroiliac joint is accessible to biopsy under CT guidance.

Spinal radiography

The characteristic spinal lesion in advanced disease is the syndesmophyte—a bony proliferation originating from an inflammatory area at the ligamentous/discal attachment to the vertebral edge. This early ankylotic structure predominantly grows cranially to fuse with the next vertebral body and has to be distinguished from the spondylophyte, which mainly grows laterally and typically indicates degenerative vertebral disease.

In ankylosing spondylitis the earliest spinal lesions are frequently in the lower thoracic and upper lumbar spine, sometimes preceded by squaring of the vertebrae seen on lateral films. The zygapophyseal joints are frequently involved at all stages. Anterior spondylitis is indicated by lateral spinal radiographs showing hypersclerotic corners (Romanus lesion, Fig. 7).

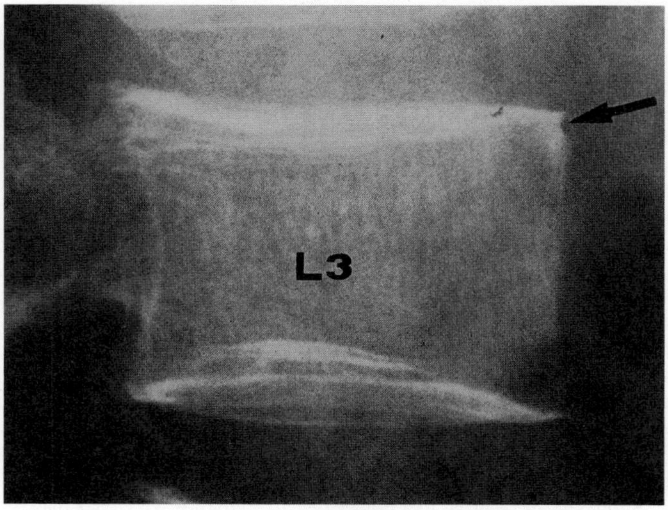

Fig. 7 Radiographic anterior spondylitis (arrow) in a 42-year-old man with ankylosing spondylitis.

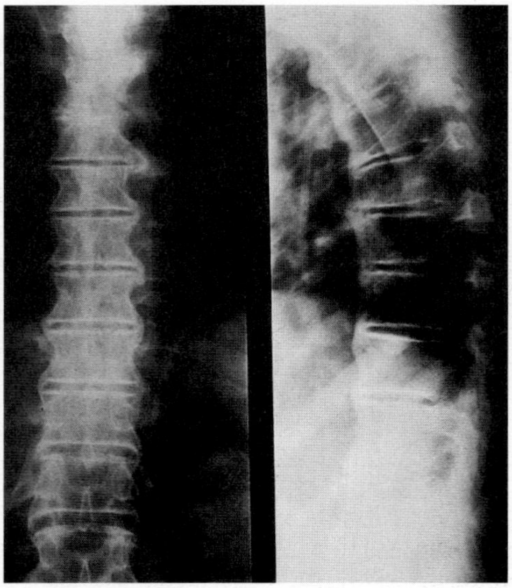

Fig. 8 Spinal radiograph showing classical bamboo spine.

Spondylodiscitis (Anderson lesion) is revealed by erosion of the disc and vertebra with a hypersclerotic lining. In later stages calcification of the anterior and the posterior ligaments occurs, eventually leading to the characteristic 'bamboo spine' (Fig. 8).

Spinal MRI

Early spinal inflammation (spondylitis, spondylodiscitis) can be detected by dynamic MRI, which can be useful for localizing inflammation in the spine in the early stages when plain radiographs are normal.

Treatment

Although there is no cure for ankylosing spondylitis, several treatments are available. The main therapeutic options are as follows:

1. Acute anti-inflammatory therapy: NSAIDs, local corticosteroids, systemic corticosteroids.
2. Disease-modifying therapy: sulphasalazine, methotrexate(?), gold(?), hydroxychloroquine(?).
3. Anti-resorptive therapy: bisphosphonates (pamidronate)

Non-steroidal anti-inflammatory drugs are better than analgesics and can be used in combination with them. Diclofenac (50–150 mg, and higher in extreme cases), meloxicam (7.5–15 mg), and indomethacin (50–150 mg) are commonly given. Thalidomide and phenylbutazone are reserved for severe cases when other agents have failed. The novel Cox-2 specific agents (rofecoxib 12.5–25 mg, celecoxib 100–200 mg) may be useful. The main risk of NSAIDs is gastrointestinal side-effects: 25 per cent of patients suffer these, ranging from dyspepsia to peptic ulceration and (rarely) bleeding, perforation, and death. It is important to provide patients with proper information about possible symptoms, and prophylactic therapy with proton pump inhibitors or misoprostol is indicated in those at particularly high risk (older age, history of ulcer, disability, comorbidity).

Most patients with ankylosing spondylitis do not respond to small doses of corticosteroids. Transient high-dose steroid treatment has been tried in extreme cases with additional symptoms of inflammatory bowel disease. In our experience, mainly female and HLA B27-negative ankylosing spondylitis patients respond to low-dose corticosteroid therapy.

Sulphasalazine is given in a dosage of 2 to 3 g/day, when effects may be seen after 2 to 4 months. The influence on peripheral joint disease is more significant than for axial symptoms, but this may be due to the preferential study of patients with longstanding disease. Sulphasalazine should mainly be given to patients with early, active disease.

The antitumour necrosis factor-α antibody infliximab in a dosage of 5 mg/kg, which has also been found to be effective in Crohn's disease and rheumatoid arthritis, has been used with significant success in open pilot studies in severe ankylosing spondylitis and recently also in a randomized placebo controlled trial.

The aim of physiotherapy is to maintain and enhance function by improving mobility and muscle strength. Patients affected by spinal stiffness should have physiotherapy on a regular daily basis. Hip replacement is indicated for those with severe hip involvement, and osteotomy can be indicated in cases where visual problems are due to severe kyphosis.

Prognosis

The established myth is that 'patients with ankylosing spondylitis generally do well'. However, one-third are severely disabled and experience intense pain and impairment of health to a comparable degree as those with rheumatoid arthritis. Ankylosing spondylitis does not burn out: disease activity and pain are independent of the duration of the disease. Since the disease usually starts in the second or third decade of life, patients with ankylosing spondylitis typically suffer its effects for many years. The mortality of patients with ankylosing spondylitis may be slightly increased: possible causes of premature death are amyloidosis, NSAID gastropathy (ulcers, bleeding), vertebral fractures, and cardiac or respiratory complications.

Reactive arthritis/Reiter's syndrome

For further information see Chapter 18.7.2.

Undifferentiated spondyloarthropathy

Definition

The term undifferentiated spondyloarthropathy (uspondyloarthropathy) was introduced and defined by the European Spondylarthropathy Study Group in 1991. Terms such as incomplete Reiter's syndrome, syndrome of enthesopathy and arthritis, HLA B27-positive oligoarthritis, and others had been used previously. Patients with uspondyloarthropathies have the typical clinical features of spondyloarthropathies but do not fit into any of the other defined categories. The fact that patients with a clinical picture of peripheral oligoarthritis but without spinal symptoms are also classified/diagnosed with uspondyloarthropathies by the European Spondylarthropathy Study Group criteria can be confusing in some cases. It is possible that uspondyloarthropathies may represent an early form of another spondyloarthropathy subset, or be a genuine spondyloarthropathy subset of their own.

Epidemiology

The prevalence of uspondyloarthropathies is not known precisely, but the frequency is not much less than that of ankylosing spondylitis. They are commoner in men. About 70 per cent of patients are HLA B27-positive. In some contrast to other spondyloarthropathies, late onset disease has been reported.

Clinical features

The main clinical features are inflammatory back pain, asymmetric peripheral arthritis, predominantly of the lower limbs, enthesitis, dactylitis, and anterior uveitis.

Diagnosis

The diagnosis of a uspondyloarthropathy requires inflammatory back pain and/or peripheral arthritis of the lower limbs and at least one other characteristic feature in addition—enthesitis, a positive family history for spondyloarthropathy, psoriasis, or inflammatory bowel disease. Dactylitis, anterior uveitis, and HLA B27 are not part of the European Spondylarthropathy Study Group criteria, but are part of Amor's criteria, and may be taken to indicate uspondyloarthropathy in single cases. Radiographs are not essential for a diagnosis, but in clinically suspicious cases MRI of the sacroiliac joints can be helpful in providing objective evidence of sacroiliitis.

The differential diagnosis of asymmetric peripheral arthritis of the lower limbs in spondyloarthropathies comprises Lyme arthritis, sarcoidosis, gout, osteoarthritis, atypical rheumatoid arthritis, and connective tissue diseases and other rarer conditions.

Treatment

Non-specific therapy with NSAIDs, intra-articular steroid injections, transient immobilization, ice packs, and physiotherapy is similar to that of other arthritides. Sulphasalazine may be effective, but no therapeutic trials with disease-modifying agents has been performed in uspondyloarthropathies.

Prognosis

Knowledge of the long-term prognosis in uspondyloarthropathies is limited. In about 30 to 50 per cent of cases a transition to ankylosing spondylitis has been reported over many years.

Psoriatic arthropathy

Definition

All kinds of arthritis occurring in association with psoriasis can be regarded as psoriatic arthritis, but it is clear that there can be considerable variability in arthritic manifestation. Many patients can be classified as having a spondyloarthropathy, but some are affected in a manner more closely resembling rheumatoid arthritis, and there are other unique forms such as arthritis mutilans. Different forms of psoriasis are associated with different forms of arthritis.

Epidemiology

Psoriasis is common, with a prevalence between 1 and 3 per cent of the population. Arthritic symptoms occur in 20 to 40 per cent of these patients, with the axial skeleton affected in 15 to 25 per cent, such that the overall prevalence of psoriatic arthritis is somewhere around 0.1 to 0.3 per cent. The peak age of onset of psoriatic arthritis is between 20 and 40 years: juvenile disease is rare. Both sexes are equally affected, but women more frequently get polyarthritis and men more often have spinal involvement.

Pathogenesis

Familial aggregation and high concordance rates in monozygotic (70 per cent) compared with dizygotic twins (20 per cent) suggest that there is a clear genetic factor in psoriasis and psoriatic arthritis. About 30 per cent of patients give a clear history of affected first-degree relatives. The genetic impact is thought to be multifactorial. Psoriasis is associated with HLA B13, B17, B37, and HLA DR7. The strongest association is with Cw6 (RR = 24). HLA associations of psoriatic arthritis are with HLA B38 and B39 (peripheral arthritis), with HLA DR4 (symmetric polyarthritis) and HLA B27 (spondylitis).

The importance of genetic linkage may lie in determination of the immunological response to particular antigens, and there has been much interest in the possible role of streptococcal infection. A proliferative response of skin and synovial T cells to streptococcal antigens has been detected in psoriatic arthritis, but also in rheumatoid arthritis, and the (immuno)histology is similar in the two conditions, although some differences have been described.

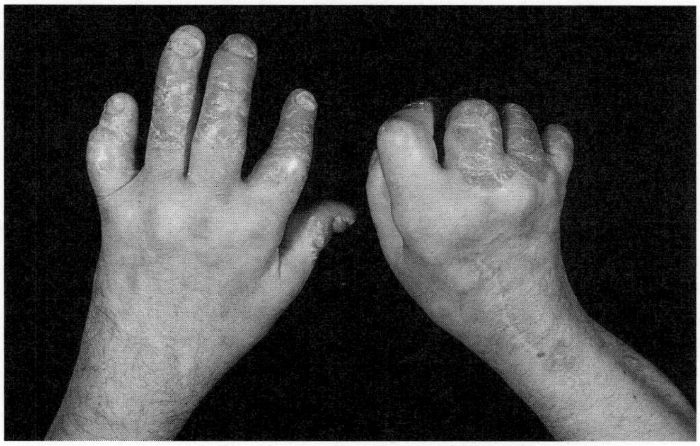

Fig. 9 Severe psoriatic arthritis (arthritis mutilans). (see also Plate 4.)

Koebner's phenomenon is described in psoriasis, when plaques arise at sites of skin injury, scratches, and scars, but the role of trauma in psoriatic arthritis is not clear. Drugs can exacerbate and trigger psoriasis: most well known are β-adrenergic blocking agents, antimalarials, and lithium; and withdrawal of corticosteroids can induce a skin flare; but the relevance of these factors to psoriatic arthritis is uncertain.

Clinical features

Psoriatic arthritis has been divided into five subgroups: distal interphalangeal (overlapping, most common), asymmetrical (spondyloarthropathy-like), symmetrical (rheumatoid arthritis-like), mutilans (unique, rare, Fig. 9 and Plate 4), and spinal (ankylosing spondylitis-like). It must be stressed, however, that these subgroups are not clearcut. In a recent study, when patients were evaluated over a period of 8 years, the initial classification pattern changed significantly over time, and finally only two categories remained: peripheral disease without axial involvement (70 per cent) and axial involvement with or without peripheral arthritis (30 per cent). The latter was correlated with duration of the disease and magnitude of joint involvement. Erosions were found in 70 per cent of the patients.

Psoriasis precedes joint disease in the majority of cases (70–80 per cent), both occur simulataneously in 15 per cent, and in about 10 per cent arthritis comes first. There is poor correlation between onset, severity, and activity of psoriatic skin lesions and arthritis. More than 80 per cent of patients with psoriatic arthritis have nail dystrophy, while this is the case in only 20 per cent of those with uncomplicated skin disease. Nail dystrophy, ranging from some to many nail pits and horizontal (not longitudinal) ridging to onycholysis, occurs most often in those with distal interphalangeal involvement. In some patients the involvement of interphalangeal joints and nails is closely correlated, with both appearing on the same finger(s). Acute anterior uveitis occurs mainly in those with radiological sacroiliitis and ankylosing spondylitis.

Different types of psoriatic skin involvement lead to different types of arthropathy. Most frequent is the common psoriasis vulgaris, but a type of skin disease that frequently affects the palms of the hands and soles of the feet with many psoriatic plaques is also seen: pustolosis palmaris et plantaris. This type is associated with the SAPHO syndrome (see below), which is related to the spondyloarthropathies but has unique features that justify the designation as a separate subset of these disorders.

A severe form of psoriatic arthritis can occur in HIV-infected patients, although is not clear whether HIV increases the overall prevalence of psoriatic arthritis. Severe peripheral enthesitis (predominantly of the heel) and dactylitis are characteristic. Knee arthritis can be rapidly destructive. Axial inflammation is less frequent.

There is a classical overlap between psoriatic arthritis and reactive arthritis in the form of keratoderma blenorrhagicum—a desquamating psoriasis-like lesion mostly occurring on the soles of the feet in patients with Reiter's syndrome.

Psoriatic arthritis often improves during pregnancy. There is no adverse effect of the disease on mother or child.

Diagnosis

Scaling erythematous papules and plaques on the scalp and extensor aspects of the extremities, often surmounted by a silvery white micaceous scale that is easily removed, are suggestive of psoriasis. Elbows and knees are often affected. The diagnosis of psoriatic arthritis is based on the presence of these characteristic skin lesions, which are not always obvious. Less accessible areas such as the navel, perineum, and scalp need to be examined carefully. The patient should be asked whether they have a family history of psoriasis or psoriatic arthritis.

Since psoriasis is a frequent disease, it must be remembered that a patient with psoriasis can have an attack of gout or another form of arthritis. The diagnosis of psoriatic arthritis should be considered in those without skin lesions if there is distal interphalangeal joint involvement, dactylitis, the involvement of a whole finger or toe, tendon sheaths and bone of an affected limb, and/or typical radiographic changes.

Laboratory and radiological features

Acute phase reactants are often raised. HLA determinations including HLA B27 do not provide diagnostic help in those with psoriatic arthritis, but in HLA B27-negative patients who appear to have ankylosing spondylitis, psoriasis should always be searched for. The presence of rheumatoid factor does not formally exclude a diagnosis of psoriatic arthritis, there being a background prevalence of rheumatoid factor positivity, but a positive result should always make the physician consider the diagnosis carefully.

The distribution of radiological changes reflects clinical involvement, with the interphalangeal joints involved earlier than larger joints. A characteristic lesion in advanced cases is the so-called pencil-in-cup deformity (Fig. 10), which evolves by resorption of the distal end of a phalanx or metacarpal with uniform deep erosion of the end of the corresponding distal phalanx. In some cases the joints can be completely destroyed and invisible on the radiograph.

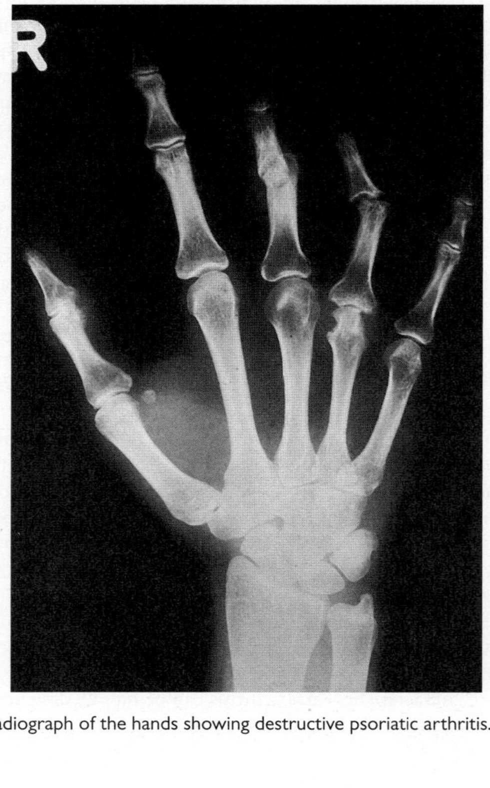

Fig. 10 Radiograph of the hands showing destructive psoriatic arthritis.

Radiological grounds for thinking the diagnosis more likely to be psoriatic arthritis than rheumatoid arthritis are distal interphalangeal joint involvement, asymmetric joint involvement, marginal erosions with adjacent bone proliferation (whiskering), osteolysis, periostitis, proliferative new bone formation, and ankylosis. Radiological sacroiliitis is a finding in 20 to 40 per cent of patients. The axial disease in psoriatic arthritis can be indistinguishable from that in primary ankylosing spondylitis, but in psoriatic arthritis the following are more likely: asymmetrical sacroiliitis, less zygapophyseal joint involvement, fewer, coarser, and asymmetric syndesmophytes, and bony bridging that is more often asymmetrical. Psoriatic arthritis syndesmophytes can be indistinguishable from spondylophytes typical of diffuse idiopathic skeletal hyperostosis (Forestier's disease).

When scintigraphy is used to detect the extent and localization of arthritis, an increased uptake of the isotope ^{99}Tc can frequently be detected in the sternoclavicular and manubriosternal joints—this is not necessarily associated with clinical symptoms.

Treatment

Many patients improve with the use of NSAIDs and intra-articular steroids, especially in the case of large joint involvement or flexor tenosynovitis. However, 20 to 40 per cent of patients will not improve and need to be treated with disease-modifying antirheumatic drugs. Sulphasalazine 2 to 3 g daily is often effective against arthritis. Methotrexate 7.5 to 40 mg daily is also good for arthritis, and even better for the skin. Intramuscular gold and azathioprine can be tried. Antimalarials and penicillamine are not used; the former may exacerbate psoriasis. Cyclosporin A is given in severe cases. There is limited information on the use of combination therapy. Systemic corticosteroids are limited to extreme cases of arthritis: psoriasis usually flares when they are withdrawn.

Local skin therapy has no effect on joint symptoms. Etretinate is not clearly beneficial for arthritis and may cause arthralgias and many other adverse reactions. The role of physiotherapy is similar to that in other spondyloarthropathies, and there are no special considerations for surgical intervention in psoriatic arthritis, apart from the fact that the presence of florid skin lesions close to a joint is a relative contraindication to surgery.

Prognosis

Severe psoriasis can lead to significant disability. There are only limited data from long-term studies in psoriatic arthritis. In cross-sectional studies 10 to 20 per cent of patients with psoriatic arthritis were in a poor functional class; the HLA antigens HLA B27, HLA B39, and DQw3 have been associated with such an outcome.

Arthritis associated with inflammatory bowel disease

Definition

An arthropathy with various clinical symptoms occurring in association with Crohn's disease and ulcerative colitis is termed arthritis associated with inflammatory bowel disease. Other forms of arthropathy occurring in association with enteropathy are Morbus, Whipple's disease, and arthritis after intestinal bypass surgery.

History

A relationship between gut and joint disease was postulated in 1922 when Smith treated arthritis patients with segmental bowel surgery. Bargen and Hench in 1929 and 1935 described arthritis in association with ulcerative colitis and Crohn's disease. Moll and Wright included arthritis associated with inflammatory bowel disease in the concept of spondyloarthropathies in 1973. Mielants and Veys described Crohn-like gut lesions in all subsets of spondyloarthropathy in 1984.

Epidemiology

The prevalence of Crohn's disease and ulcerative colitis is between 0.05 and 0.1 per cent of the population, generally higher in Whites and Jews. The peak occurrence of both diseases is between 15 and 35 years, but it may appear in every decade of life; both sexes are equally involved. Arthritis associated with inflammatory bowel disease occurs in 10 to 30 per cent of patients with inflammatory bowel disease; in general more frequently in Crohn's disease than in ulcerative colitis, and more often in patients with colonic involvement and in those with extended bowel disease.

There is a genetic predisposition for inflammatory bowel disease with documented familial aggregation for both Crohn's disease and ulcerative colitis. The association with HLA B16, HLA B18, and HLA B62 is not strong. The peripheral arthritis of inflammatory bowel disease is not associated with HLA B27, but axial inflammation is (50 per cent). The patient with inflammatory bowel disease who is, by chance, HLA B27-positive, is at high risk of developing spondylitis. The relative frequency of sacroiliitis and ankylosing spondylitis in inflammatory bowel diseases varies between 2 and 20 per cent or more, partly depending on the sensitivity of the diagnostic imaging procedure. Four per cent of patients with ankylosing spondylitis develop overt inflammatory bowel disease, while 60 per cent have microscopically detectable Crohn-like gut lesions.

Pathogenesis

The pathogenesis of inflammatory bowel disease and arthritis associated with inflammatory bowel disease is not known. One hypothesis is of an aberrant immune response to gut bacteria, with gut inflammation leading to increased permeability, allowing bacteria to cross the mucosal border and get access to joints. There is some evidence from the HLA B27 transgenic rat model that gut and joints are closely linked: susceptible rats get both colitis and arthritis once they have left a germfree environment.

Clinical features

Patients with ulcerative colitis and Crohn's disease typically present with bloody diarrhoea and abdominal pain, and in severe cases with fever, weight loss, and fatigue. For further details of gastrointestinal and other non-rheumatological presentations, and criteria for diagnosis, see Section 14.

Similar to the other spondyloarthropathies the arthritis is mostly asymmetric and predominantly affects the lower limbs. The arthritis is migratory, often transient, but tends to recur. It does not frequently become chronic but may be associated with erosive disease in some patients. Flaring of gut symptoms is often associated with arthritis, especially in ulcerative colitis. In Crohn's disease, patients experience significantly fewer joint symptoms after colectomy.

Two types of arthropathy were distinguished in a recent study of almost 1500 patients with inflammatory bowel disease, essentially on the basis of the number of joints involved and importantly without knowledge of spinal radiographs. Pauciarticular disease (type I, fewer than five joints involved) affected 3.6 per cent of patients with ulcerative colitis and 6 per cent of those with Crohn's disease and was acute and self-limiting, with episodes lasting 4 to 5 weeks, in 83 and 79 per cent of the cases. Polyarticular disease (type II, five or more joints) affected 2.5 per cent of patients with ulcerative colitis and 4 per cent of those with Crohn's disease and was associated with persistent symptoms in 87 and 89 per cent of the cases.

The onset of peripheral arthritis is associated with exacerbations of colitis, but there is no link between enteric and spinal symptoms. Acute anterior uveitis occurs in 10 per cent of patients with inflammatory bowel disease. It is associated with axial involvement and with HLA B27. Compared with other spondyloarthropathies, the type of uveitis is somewhat different in inflammatory bowel diseases: posterior uveitis and scleritis may occur. The most common skin lesion in arthritis associated with inflammatory bowel disease is erythema nodosum, occurring in association with exacerbation of enteritis.

Diagnosis

Most arthritic symptoms occurring in patients with inflammatory bowel disease can generally be attributed to spondyloarthropathies. However, as in psoriasis, patients can have more than one disease (osteoarthritis, etc.). As many as 50 to 60 per cent of all patients with ankylosing spondylitis have gut lesions resembling those in Crohn's disease, but the majority are asymptomatic. Clinically apparent ankylosing spondylitis often precedes Crohn-like symptoms. This spectrum of diseases clearly and typically belongs to the spectrum of spondyloarthropathies. The differentiation (if needed) will rarely cause problems since one disease is usually predominant. Along with psoriasis, inflammatory bowel disease should always be looked for in HLA B27-negative patients who appear to have ankylosing spondylitis.

Treatment

Treatment of inflammatory bowel diseases is always the first consideration and will probably influence the peripheral arthritis. Treatment with NSAIDs may be effective for arthritis and spondylitis but can exacerbate the bowel disease. There are few data on the use of disease-modifying antirheumatic drugs. Sulphasalazine is effective in ulcerative colitis and other spondyloarthropathies and may, accordingly, be used in arthritis associated with inflammatory bowel disease. Azathioprine is effective in Crohn's disease and can be tried to treat severe and chronic joint disease. Corticosteroids are the therapy of choice in acute inflammatory bowel disease and will generally help arthritis, but they should not be used for mild and transient joint symptoms.

Prognosis

Patients with inflammatory bowel disease have increased mortality due to peritonitis and sepsis. By contrast, the prognosis of arthritis associated with inflammatory bowel disease is generally good. Joint destruction is a rare event. Patients may have ankylosing spondylitis at presentation of inflammatory bowel disease, or develop this later.

SAPHO syndrome

Definition

The acronym SAPHO stands for **S**ynovitis, **A**cne, **P**ustolosis palmaris et plantaris, **H**yperostosis, and **O**steitis. French workers proposed SAPHO as a unifying diagnosis for several idiopathic bone and skin diseases, thereby combining over 50 different terms published in the literature (including pustulotic arthro-osteitis, chronic multifocal osteomyelitis, Tietze syndrome (German), and acquired hyperostosis syndrome). Their description of the common symptoms and overlapping features of this heterogenous group of rheumatic joint, bone, and skin diseases has led to better recognition of the relatively rare condition.

There is an argument that SAPHO simply represents a subset of psoriatic arthropathy; also that it might not really belong to the spondyloarthropathies at all. Only 43 per cent of patients with SAPHO fulfilled the European Spondylarthropathy Study Group criteria for spondyloarthropathies, and only 1 in 19 was HLA B27-positive in one follow-up study.

Pathogenesis

The pathogenesis is unclear. Some authors think that it is similar to that of reactive arthritis. *Propionibacterium acnes*, which can induce arthritis in animals, has been detected in acne lesions and grown from osteitic lesions

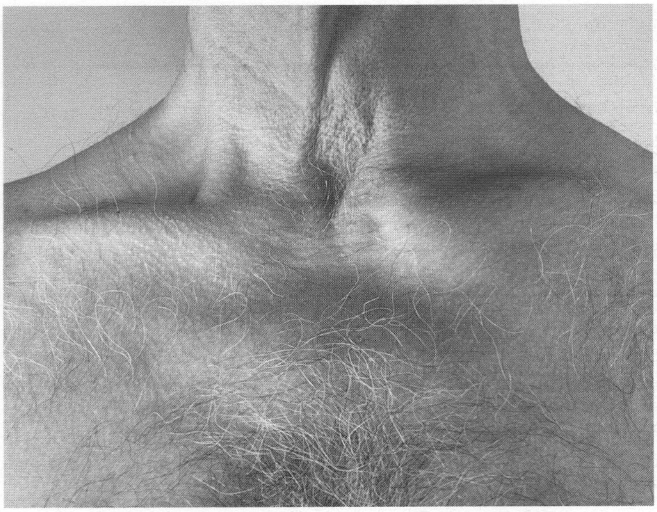

Fig. 11 Arthritis/hyperostosis of the left sternoclavicular joint in a 52-year-old man with SAPHO syndrome. (See also Plate 5.)

in some cases. However, cultures are negative in the vast majority of cases, and antibiotics are ineffective.

Diagnosis

There are no evaluated diagnostic criteria for SAPHO. Most convincing clinically is the combination of a classical skin symptom—such as pustolosis or significant acne (acne conglobata and acne fulminans or hidradenitis suppurativa)—with a characteristic joint or bone lesion such as arthritis of the sternoclavicular joint, osteitis, or hyperostosis in the anterior chest wall.

Diagnosis is important to avoid unnecessary biopsy procedures, but can be very difficult, especially in those without typical skin lesions. The most important differential diagnoses are bacterial osteomyelitis and malignancy. The pattern of joints affected differs from other rheumatic diseases: the sternoclavicular joint (Figs 11 and 12 and Plate 5), the clavicle, the ribs, and the mandible are frequently involved by arthritis, osteitis, and/or hyperostosis. Sacroiliitis, mostly unilateral, occurs in one-third of patients.

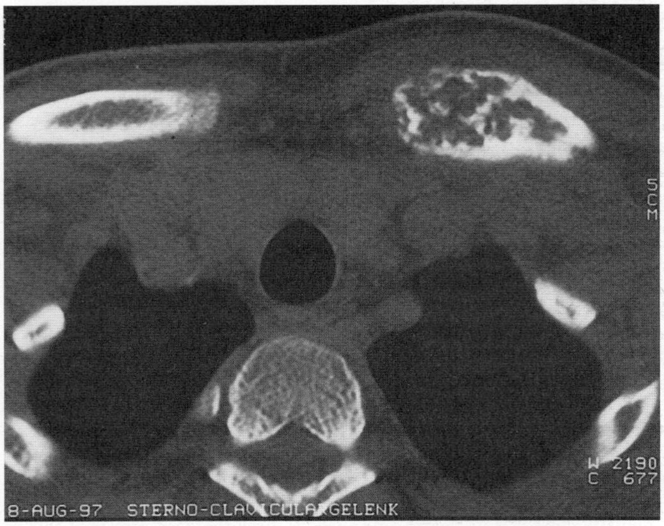

Fig. 12 Radiograph showing severe osteitis of the left sternoclavicular joint in a 35-year-old woman with SAPHO syndrome.

Treatment

Analgesics, NSAIDs, and intra-articular steroids are usually effective. In severe cases systemic corticosteroids should be considered. Immunosuppressive agents can be added if the steroid dose cannot be tapered to less than 10 mg/day. Sulphasalzine, azathioprine, and methotrexate have been tried successfully in some cases. Radiation therapy can also be effective in refractory cases. No controlled studies have been performed.

Prognosis

The course of disease is very variable. Initially, occurrence of several flares per year is common. Further progress is usually favourable, but complications such as axillary vein and C8 compression can occur. Some patients may develop ankylosis and few progress into ankylosing spondylitis.

Other enteric arthropathies

Whipple's disease

Whipple's disease is a rare systemic disease which usually involves the small intestine (see Chapter 14.9.6). The associated arthritis is often symmetric and polyarticular, and may antedate the intestinal complaints by years. It is not usually destructive. Axial involvement occurs but is not typical.

Arthritis associated with coeliac disease

For a description of coeliac disease (gluten-sensitive enteropathy) see Chapter 14.9.3. The joint manifestations show a striking response to a gluten-free diet, which strongly suggests a causal relationship. The pattern of arthritis is very variable and overt bowel symptoms are absent in half of cases, making diagnosis difficult. The lumbar spine, hips, knees, shoulders, elbows, wrists, and ankles are most frequently affected, often symmetrically. The arthritis is not destructive. HLA B8 and DR3 are frequently found in the patients. The pathogenesis is unclear.

Arthropathies associated with collagenous colitis

Collagenous colitis is a chronic diarrhoeal disease characterized by a normal or near-normal mucosa endoscopically and a thick subepithelial collagen layer. More than half of patients with this disorder have some form of arthritis and use NSAIDs regularly.

Arthropathies associated with intestinal bypass surgery

Arthritis has been reported in 5 to 50 per cent of patients in the first 3 years after jejunoileal bypass surgery. A symmetric peripheral polyarthritis involves the knees, wrists, metacarpophalangeal and metatarsophalangeal joints, elbows, proximal interphalangeal joints, and ankles and is usually non-destructive. Almost half of those affected also have vesicopustular skin lesions. No specific HLA association has been found, but two previously healthy HLA B27-positive patients developed spondylitis. Bacterial overgrowth of the blind loop is critical for pathogenesis.

Further reading

Introduction

Amor B *et al.* (1994). Predictive factors for the longterm outcome of spondyloarthropathies. *Journal of Rheumatology* **21**, 1883–7.

Braun J *et al.* (1998). Prevalence of spondylarthropathies in HLA-B27 positive and negative blood donors. *Arthritis and Rheumatism* **41**, 58–67.

Braun J, Bollow M, Sieper J (1998). Radiologic diagnosis and pathology of the spondyloarthropathies. *Rheumatic Disease Clinics of North America* **24**, 697–735.

Calin A *et al.* (1977). Clinical history as a screening test for ankylosing spondylitis. *Journal of the American Medical Association* **237**, 2613–14.

Dougados M *et al.* (1991). The European Spondylarthropathy Study Group preliminary criteria for the classification of spondylarthropathy. *Arthritis and Rheumatism* **34**, 1218–27.

Khan MA, van der Linden SM (1990). A wider spectrum of spondyloarthropathies. *Seminars in Arthritis and Rheumatism* **20**, 107–13.

Moll JM *et al.* (1974). Associations between ankylosing spondylitis, psoriatic arthritis, Reiter's disease, the intestinal arthropathies, and Behcet's syndrome. *Medicine (Baltimore)* **53**, 343–64.

Sieper J, Braun J (1995). Pathogenesis of spondylarthropathies. Persistent bacterial antigen, autoimmunity, or both? *Arthritis and Rheumatism* **38**, 1547–54.

Ankylosing spondylitis

Bollow M *et al.*(2000). Quantitative analysis of sacroiliac biopsies in spondyloarthopathies: T cells and macrophages predominate in early and active sacroiliitis–cellularity correlates with the degree of enhancement detected by magnetic resonance imaging. *Annals of Rheumatic Disease* **59**, 135–40.

Braun J *et al.* (1995). Use of immunohistologic and *in situ* hybridization techniques in the examination of sacroiliac joint biopsy specimens from patients with ankylosing spondylitis. *Arthritis and Rheumatism* **38**, 499–505.

Gran JT, Skomsvoll JF (1997). The outcome of ankylosing spondylitis: a study of 100 patients. *British Journal of Rheumatology* **36**, 766–71.

Kennedy LG, Edmunds L, Calin A (1993). The natural history of ankylosing spondylitis. Does it burn out? *Journal of Rheumatology* **20**, 688–92.

Mau W *et al.* (1988). Clinical features and prognosis of patients with possible ankylosing spondylitis. Results of a 10-year followup. *Journal of Rheumatology* **15**, 1109–14.

McGonagle D *et al.* (1998). Characteristic magnetic resonance imaging entheseal changes of knee synovitis in spondylarthropathy. *Arthritis and Rheumatism* **41**, 694–700.

van der Linden S, Valkenburg HA, Cats A (1984). Evaluation of diagnostic criteria for ankylosing spondylitis. A proposal for modification of the New York criteria. *Arthritis and Rheumatism* **27**, 361–8.

Zink A *et al.*(2000). Disability and handicap in rheumatoid arthritis and ankylosing spondylitis—results from the German rheumatological database. *Journal of Rheumatology* **27**, 613–22.

Uspondyloarthropathies

Olivieri I *et al.* (1995). Late onset undifferentiated seronegative spondyloarthropathy. *Journal of Rheumatology* **22**, 899–903.

Zeidler H, Mau W, Khan A (1992). Undifferentiated spondyloarthropathies.*Rheumatic Disease Clinics of North America* **18**, 187–202.

Psoriatic arthritis

Gladman DD (1998). Psoriatic arthritis. *Rheumatic Disease Clinics of North America* **24**, 829–44.

Helliwell P *et al.* (1991). A re-evaluation of the osteoarticular manifestations of psoriasis. *British Journal of Rheumatology* **30**, 339–45.

Marsal S *et al.* (1999). Clinical, radiographic and HLA associations as markers for different patterns of psoriatic arthritis. *Rheumatology* **38**, 332–7.

Reece RJ *et al.* (1999). Distinct vascular patterns of early synovitis in psoriatic, reactive and rheumatoid arthritis. *Arthritis and Rheumatism* **42**, 1481–4.

Richter Cohen M *et al.* (1999). Baseline relationships between psoriasis and psoriatic arthritis: analysis of 221 patients with active psoriatic arthritis. *Journal of Rheumatology* **26**, 1752–6.

Salvarani C *et al.* (1995). Prevalence of psoriatic arthritis in Italian psoriatic patients. *Journal of Rheumatology* **22**, 1499–503.

Arthritis associated with inflammatory bowel disease

Leirisalo-Repo M *et al.* (1994). High frequency of silent inflammatory bowel disease in spondyloarthropathy. *Arthritis and Rheumatism* **37**, 23–35.

Mielants H *et al.* (1996). Course of gut inflammation in spondylarthropathies and therapeutic consequences. *Baillière's Clinical Rheumatology* **10**, 147–64.

Orchard TR, Jewell DP (1999). The importance of ileocaecal integrity in the arthritic complications of Crohn's disease. *Inflammatory Bowel Disease* **5**, 92–7.

Orchard TR, Wordsworth BP, Jewell DP (1998). Peripheral arthropathies in inflammatory bowel disease: their articular distribution and natural history. *Gut* **42**, 387–91.

Taurog J *et al.* (1994). The germfree state prevents the development of gut and joint inflammatory disease in HLA B27 transgenic rats. *Journal of Experimental Medicine* **180**, 2359–64.

SAPHO syndrome

Boutin RD, Resnick D (1998). The SAPHO syndrome: an evolving concept for unifying several idiopathic disorders of bone and skin. *American Journal of Rheumatology* **170**, 585–91.

Kahn MF, Khan MA (1994). The SAPHO syndrome. *Baillière's Clinical Rheumatology* **8**, 333–62.

Koehler H *et al.* (1975). Sterno-kosto-klavikuläre Hyperostose. *Deutsche Medizinische Wochenschrift* **100**, 1519–23.

Maugars Y *et al.* (1995). SAPHO syndrome: a followup study of 19 cases with special emphasis on enthesis involvement. *Journal of Rheumatology* **22**, 2135–41.

Sonozaki H *et al.* (1981). Clinical features of 39 patients with pustolotic arthroosteitis. *Annals of Rheumatic Diseases* **40**, 547–53.

Other enteric arthropathies

Fleming JL, Wiesner RH, Shorter RG (1988). Whipple's disease: clinical, biochemical and histopathological features and assessment of treatment in 29 patients. *Mayo Clinic Proceedings* **63**, 539–51.

Goff JS *et al.* (1997). Collagenous colitis: histopathology and clinical course. *American Journal of Gastroenterology* **92**, 57–60.

Pinals RS (1986). Arthritis associated with gluten-sensitive arthropathy. *Journal of Rheumatology* **13**, 201–4.

Stein HE *et al.* (1981). The intestinal bypass arthritis-dermatitis syndrome. *Arthritis and Rheumatism* **24**, 684–90.

18.7 Rheumatic disorders associated with infection

18.7.1 Pyogenic arthritis

Anthony R. Berendt

Introduction

Pyogenic arthritis, which may be acute or chronic, describes infection and resulting inflammation in a joint, native or prosthetic. It should not be confused with postinfectious (reactive) arthritis (discussed in Section 18.8). As with other musculoskeletal infections, failings in diagnosis or management may have long-term functional consequences, and clinicians should therefore know when to consider the diagnosis and obtain expert help.

Aetiology

Acute pyogenic arthritis may be primary (by haematogenous spread), or secondary (to trauma, surgery, or arthrocentesis). Organisms that cause primary septic arthritis are usually aggressive pathogens capable of causing a bacteraemia, seeding the joint, and multiplying within it, hence they are also common causes of septicaemia, with *Staphylococcus aureus* dominating in most circumstances. The causes of secondary and chronic septic arthritis are more diverse because they include skin and environmental flora, together with lower-grade pathogens, as well as all the causes of acute infection.

Table 1 in Chapter 19.2 shows the common pathogens involved in both pyogenic arthritis and osteomyelitis.

Epidemiology

The incidence of pyogenic arthritis has been estimated at 7 in 100 000: this is highest in children and the elderly, and more common in males. The increased incidence in the elderly probably reflects a higher prevalence of potential sources of bacteraemia such as urinary tract infection, skin ulceration, pneumonia, and hospitalization with intravenous and/or urinary catheterization. Infection complicates some 0.5 to 2 per cent of total joint replacements, but the true prevalence of prosthetic joint infection is unknown.

Pathogenesis and pathophysiology

In primary septic arthritis, organisms must exit the bloodstream and access the joint. In the case of *S. aureus*, invasion of endothelial cells can occur through interactions between bacterial fibronectin-binding proteins and cell surface-associated fibronectin. This triggers integrin-dependent uptake of bacteria and may be a key first step in bacteraemic seeding.

S. aureus releases a number of toxins and proteases thought to affect host defences. It also expresses numerous cell wall-associated adhesins that mediate attachment to the matrix proteins associated with cell surfaces, cartilage, and bone. Animal models demonstrate that T-cell dependent inflammation plays a central role in damage to articular cartilage following an acute inflammatory response. In these models immunomodulation (for example with corticosteroids) can substantially reduce arthritis, but at the expense of host survival if antibiotic therapy is not also given. Thus the host response appears to reduce the risk of bacteraemia and death, but at the cost of joint damage. If not fatal through septicaemia, untreated septic arthritis generally causes joint destruction or fusion, sometimes with sinus formation and persistent infection (see Fig. 1(a) and (b)).

In a prosthetic joint, the presence of foreign material impairs local antibacterial defences. Bacteria adhere to plastic or metal (in some cases via fibronectin) and in this state become relatively resistant to the action of antibiotics and to phagocytosis. Ineffective but chronic inflammation causes pain and triggers bone loss, with subsequent mechanical loosening.

Clinical features

Patients typically present with fever and an acutely painful joint. The joints involving the long bones are most commonly affected (knee, hip, shoulder, elbow, wrist, and ankle). There may be bacteraemia (in some series up to 70 per cent), giving prostration, vomiting, or hypotension. Infants localize pain poorly and commonly present refusing to use the affected limb. Adults may be unable to localize pain if a sternoclavicular, acromioclavicular, sternocostal, or manubriosternal joint is involved. Infections in these locations often present as chest wall pain. Sacroiliac joint infection presents as buttock or low back pain and may mimic hip or spine pathology.

Clinical examination reveals a joint that is swollen, warm to the touch, tender on palpation, and painful, frequently exquisitely so, on active or passive movement. To minimize pain, the patient will often nurse the joint in a neutral position. A joint effusion is usually present and this may be accompanied by synovitis, depending on the duration of the history. Erythema, not usually prominent, may signal the presence of bursitis.

Septic arthritis must be distinguished from other acute monoarthropathies, notably gout, pyrophosphate arthropathy, and haemarthrosis. Rheumatoid and reactive arthritis can initially present with involvement of only a single joint. Infection is most commonly monoarticular, but multiple joints can be involved. In the patient with known inflammatory arthritis, polyarticular infection may be mistaken for a flare in the underlying disease.

Prosthetic joint infection may present as an acute wound infection, a periarticular abscess, an acute arthritis or with loosening of the implant (as pain). The differential is from superficial wound infection, haemarthrosis, periprosthetic fracture or dislocation, and aseptic loosening. A sinus discharging in or near the operative scar represents infection of the prosthesis until proved otherwise.

Pathology

The synovial fluid contains polymorphs and the synovium shows an acute inflammatory response with a fibrinous exudate on its surface, which may be ulcerated. A chronic synovitis may develop, with a lymphocytic and mononuclear infiltrate. Late changes include chondrolysis and the development of subarticular osteomyelitis. Tissue from infected prosthetic joints shows a polymorph infiltrate accompanied by chronic inflammatory changes representing a reaction to foreign materials.

Laboratory diagnosis

The criterion for diagnosis of pyogenic arthritis is the isolation of a recognized pathogen from samples of synovium or synovial fluid obtained through biopsy or aspiration. Infected synovial fluid is generally turbid or purulent. It should be sent for Gram stain, semiquantitative or quantitative white cell count, examination under polarized light for pyrophosphate or uric acid crystals, and culture. If tuberculosis, brucellosis, or fungi are suspected, the laboratory should be advised so that the sample can be appropriately processed. For suspected *Neisseria gonorrhoeae*, urethral, endocervical, throat, and rectal swabs should also be obtained for microscopy and culture.

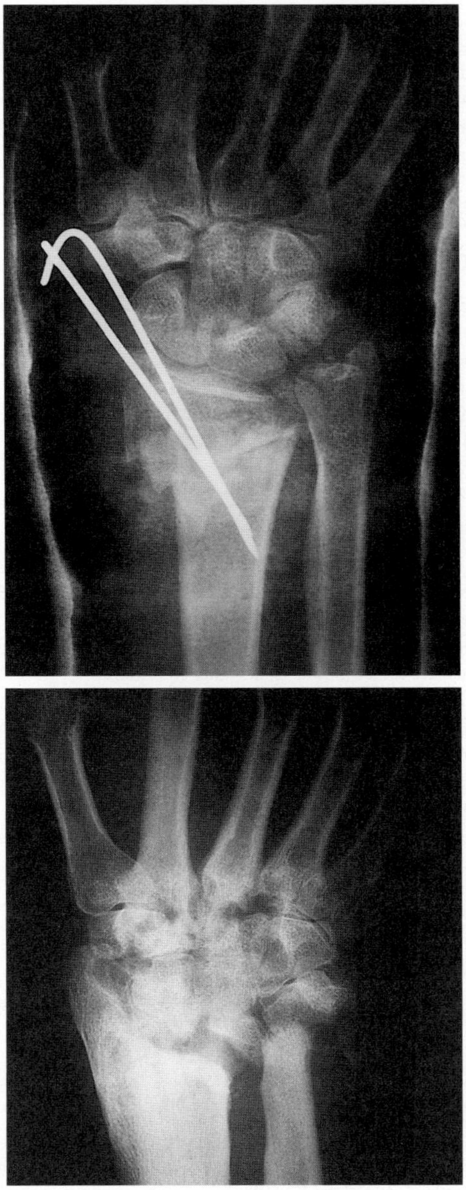

(a)

(b)

Fig. 1 (a) A Colles fracture fixed with percutaneous K wires. (b) A few months later, after *S. aureus* infection associated with the K wires has led to septic arthritis in the wrist, the wrist joint is completely destroyed.

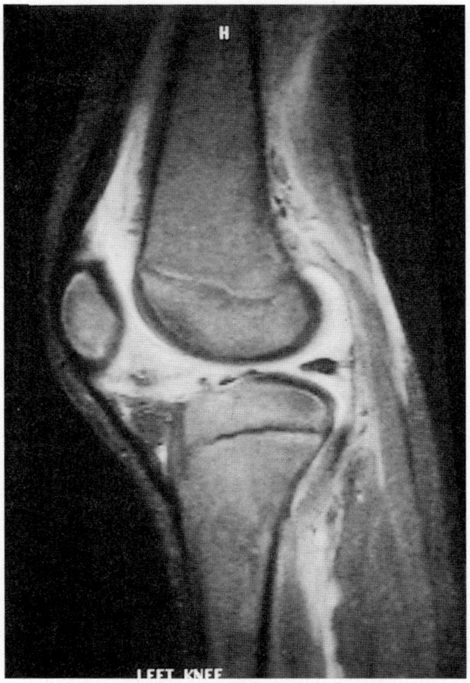

Fig. 2 Marked synovitis, but no osteomyelitis, in a 10-year-old with group A streptococcal infection of the knee.

Blood cultures should always be obtained. The white cell count, C-reactive protein, and erythrocyte sedimentation rate are usually raised, but can also be elevated during flares of inflammatory arthritis or acute crystal arthropathy. Their value is probably greatest in following the response to treatment. Measurement of serum uric acid may be elevated in gout, but cannot be used to establish or refute this diagnosis. Serological tests may be of retrospective value in diagnosing *Borrelia burgdorferi* (Lyme disease) and *Brucella* spp. Detection of bacterial nucleic acid in joints remains a research technique.

Plain radiographs can show fracture, effusion, chondrocalcinosis, bone destruction, or loss of joint space. An effusion may be seen acutely, but bony changes appear slowly. If seen at presentation they either indicate chronic infection or represent underlying arthritis. A radiograph at presentation provides a useful baseline for subsequent comparisons. The role of CT scan or magnetic resonance imaging is to demonstrate or exclude surgical disease in the joint or neighbouring bone (Fig. 2). Ultrasound scanning may assist in this and in distinguishing between effusion and synovitis, allowing diagnostic samples to be obtained more reliably.

Treatment

Acute septic arthritis poses a threat to the joint and is an orthopaedic or rheumatological emergency. Treatment should generally be in an inpatient hospital setting. Patients with suspected chronic septic arthritis may initially be managed as outpatients, but most eventually require surgical intervention.

After obtaining blood cultures and (when possible) synovial fluid, acute pyogenic arthritis should be treated promptly with intravenous antibiotics active against aerobic Gram-positive cocci and Gram-negative organisms. Appropriate regimens would be cefuroxime (or another antistaphylococcal cephalosporin) or a high-dose semisynthetic antistaphylococcal penicillin (flucloxacillin, dicloxacillin, or nafcillin), with or without an aminoglycoside. Patients allergic to β-lactams, or with risk factors for methicillin-resistant *S. aureus*, should receive vancomycin, usually with an aminoglycoside, until culture results are obtained. Treatment can then be modified.

Urgent consultation with an orthopaedic surgeon is advised. Arthroscopic washout has largely replaced arthrotomy, reducing morbidity. Surgery can sometimes be avoided altogether by aspiration once or twice daily until clinical response is evident, but may still be needed if there is clinical deterioration or failure to settle within 5 days. This type of treatment can be applied to children or adults, particularly when anaesthesia is thought to carry high risks. Whether delaying surgery in this way gives worse outcomes than immediate washout is unknown, but there is consensus on the need for prompt surgery on the hip and shoulder joints. The reflection of the capsular vessels up the necks of the humerus and femur makes them vulnerable to thrombosis and subsequent avascular necrosis of the femoral or humeral head. If this occurs, joint destruction, with or without chronic infection of the dead bone, is inevitable.

The optimal duration and mode of administration of antibiotics is unknown. In uncomplicated infection 2 to 3 weeks is adequate, depending on the pathogen (shorter for streptococci, longer for *S. aureus* and aerobic Gram-negative rods). In children it is possible to convert to oral therapy within 48 to 72 h of defervescence, provided that there has been a rapid clinical response. This strategy requires the organism to be sensitive to a reliably bioavailable oral antibiotic, the parents or carers to understand clearly the importance of adhering to the antibiotic regimen, and the clinician to monitor clinical progress carefully. Some authorities treat adults with an oral regimen provided that similar criteria are met, but intravenous antibiotics may be preferred when there has been accompanying bacteraemia or where there are concerns about bony involvement, absorption of antibiotic, or adherence. Many patients are suitable for intravenous therapy at home, provided this is properly organized and supervised.

Chronic septic arthritis has generally led to joint destruction by the time the patient presents. Surgical debridement, arthrodesis, or joint replacement may be necessary, the latter after a considerable interval free of infection. Surgery is commonly required in prosthetic joint infection, although such problems can occasionally be treated successfully with retention of the implant. Antibiotic treatment is usually prolonged in chronic or prosthetic joint infection.

Prognosis

If diagnosed and treated promptly, the prognosis of acute native joint infection is good, with many patients making a complete recovery. Some joint damage is likely when the diagnosis is made late. Infection in young children may lead to disturbance of the growth plate around the infected joint, causing deformity. Mortality is low in uncomplicated septic arthritis, higher when it is complicated by *S. aureus* bacteraemia (up to 20 per cent) and highest in multijoint disease (50 per cent). Recurrence is uncommon and generally indicates a persisting surgical focus in relation to the joint.

Outcomes are less favourable in prosthetic joints, which can be salvaged in 30 to 70 per cent of cases where the prosthesis is retained. Infection can be eradicated in up to 90 per cent of cases with revision surgery, but with very much poorer results when revision surgery for infection is itself complicated by further infection. This and the need for expert surgical and microbiological input, as well as the considerable comorbidity such patients often have, makes the management of infected prosthetic joints a formidable challenge.

Prevention and control

There are no proven means of preventing primary pyogenic arthritis. Secondary cases can be prevented by meticulous attention to infection control measures whenever a joint is aspirated or operated on, and by thorough cleaning and debridement when a joint is contaminated through trauma.

Occupational, quality of life, and psychosocial aspects

The pain of acute pyogenic arthritis generally resolves within the first 1 to 2 weeks of successful treatment, but stiffness and swelling usually persist for very much longer. Chronic infections have significant effects on quality of life through pain and poor function. This is most prolonged and severe in prosthetic joint infection.

Areas of uncertainty needing further research

Further understanding of pathogenesis could potentially offer new targets for therapy or prevention, while diagnostic sensitivity could be improved by robust, well-evaluated molecular methods. Numerous aspects of treatment, including the role of surgery and the duration and route of administration of antibiotics, await clarification in prospective studies, both for native and prosthetic joint infections.

Further reading

Berendt AR (1999). Infections of prosthetic joints and related problems. In: Armstrong D, Cohen J, eds. *Infectious diseases*, pp 2.44.1–2.44.6 Mosby, London. [Review of prosthetic joint infections.]

Dubost J-J *et al.* (1993). Polyarticular septic arthritis. *Medicine* **72**, 296–310. [An extensive review of this challenging condition.]

Girdlestone GR (1943). Acute pyogenic arthritis of the hip: an operation giving free access and effective drainage. *Lancet* **1**, 419. (Reprinted in *Clinical Orthopaedics* **170**, 3–7 (1982).) [Girdlestone's classic description, in the preantibiotic era, of septic arthritis of the hip and the operation that bears his name.]

Howard JB, Highgenboten CL, Nelson JD (1976). Residual effects of septic arthritis in infancy and childhood. *Journal of the American Medical Association* **236**, 932–5. [Outcomes review after infant septic arthritis, emphasizing need for prompt diagnosis and treatment.]

Kaandorp C . *et al.* (1997). The outcome of bacterial arthritis: a prospective community-based study. *Arthritis and Rheumatism* **40**, 884–92.

Le Dantec L *et al.* (1996). Peripheral pyogenic arthritis. A study of one hundred seventy-nine cases. *Reviews in Rheumatology* **63**, 103–10. [Large case series.]

Lowy FD (1998). *Staphylococcus aureus* infections. *New England Journal of Medicine* **339**, 520–9. [Helpful review of this troublesome pathogen.]

Seviour PW, Dieppe PA (1984). Sternoclavicular joint infection as a cause of chest pain. *British Medical Journal* **288**, 133–4. [A catch for the physician.]

Syrogiannopoulos GA, Nelson JD (1988). Duration of antimicrobial therapy for acute suppurative osteoarticular infections. *Lancet* **ii**, 37–40. [Large series that defined oral short course regimens for uncomplicated acute bone and joint infection.]

18.7.2 Reactive arthritis

J. S. H. Gaston

Introduction and historical perspective

The term 'reactive arthritis' was introduced in 1969 by Aho in Finland, where the combination of a high prevalence of HLA B27 and gastrointestinal infection by *Yersinia* afforded opportunities for studying the disease. However, the condition was first recognized in the eighteenth and nineteenth centuries as an arthritis which followed dysentery or venereal disease, and there were descriptions by Hans Reiter and other contemporaries of the disease amongst troops affected by dysentery in the trenches of the First World War. The term 'Reiter's disease' has been used extensively since that time, but is now less favoured for several reasons: Reiter was not the first to describe the disease; he erroneously attributed it to spirochaetal infection; and the triad which makes up Reiter's disease—arthritis, conjunctivitis, and urethritis/cervicitis— is not a clinically meaningful subgroup within reactive arthritis.

Definition

The term reactive arthritis is sometimes used rather loosely to cover any form of arthritis which follows infection, and would then include postviral arthritides, rheumatic fever, Lyme disease, and other forms of arthritis which do not generally have clinical features in common. This usage is not helpful and the term 'postinfectious arthritis' is to be preferred, with this all-embracing term then subdivided into different clinical syndromes, one of which is reactive arthritis (Table 1). Viewed in this way, reactive arthritis is seen as one of the seronegative spondyloarthropathies (ankylosing spondylitis, psoriatic arthritis, arthritis associated with inflammatory bowel disease), sharing clinical and immunogenetic features with those diseases. Other postinfectious arthropathies lack these common features.

In the absence of agreed and validated diagnostic or classification criteria for reactive arthritis, Table 2 presents a useful working classification of those patients who could reasonably be considered to have reactive arthritis. This takes as its starting point the classical pattern of arthritis and typical extra-articular features (Table 3) which are commonly seen after infection by five organisms—*Salmonella, Yersinia, Campylobacter, Shigella flexneri,* and *Chlamydia trachomatis.* The same clinical syndrome (i.e. arthritis and extra-articular signs) is also seen, but more rarely, following many infections, especially of the gastrointestinal tract, for example by *Clostridium difficile,* but genitourinary infections with *Ureaplasma* and respiratory infection with *Chlamydia pneumoniae* can probably also act as triggers of reactive arthritis. The other large group of patients are those who have asymmetric oligoarthritis without extra-articular features, but with definite laboratory evidence of preceding infection by one of the five major reactive arthritis-associated bacteria. Laboratory diagnosis of infection is given priority over symptoms as a classification criterion because infection may be clinically silent. *Chlamydia* is notorious for this, particularly in women, whilst in *Yersinia* infection, arthritis is inversely correlated with the severity of gastrointestinal symptoms. Positively identifying the triggering infection often poses practical problems. Patients in whom arthritis (with or without extra-articular signs) develops after symptomatic episodes of gastrointestinal or genitourinary infection are therefore usually regarded as having reactive arthritis, even when no triggering organism can be identified, although the diagnosis is inevitably less secure in these cases. Improvement in methods for diagnosing preceding infection should decrease the size of this group, and may well show reactive arthritis to be the commonest cause of inflammatory oligo- or monoarthritis in young adults.

Table 1 Postinfectious arthritis

Postviral arthritis, e.g. parvovirus
Poststreptococcal arthritis
Rheumatic fever
Arthritis alone
Post-*Neisseria* arthritis
Lyme disease
Whipple's disease
Reactive arthritis

Table 2 Working definition of reactive arthritis

- Classical clinical features:
  asymmetric oligoarthritis, lower limbs predominate
  enthesitis
  extra-articular signs
  and proven infection by *Salmonella, Campylobacter, Yersinia, Shigella,* or *Chlamydia trachomatis* (whether symptomatic or not)
- Classical clinical features **and** proven infection by other organisms (e.g. *Clostridium difficule, Mycobacterium bovis* BCG)
- Any acute inflammatory arthritis (including monoarthritis) **and** proven infection by reactive arthritis-associated bacteria
- Classical clinical features **and** preceding diarrhoea or urethritis/cervicitis, infection not proven

Table 3 Extra-articular features and their occurrence in other spondyloarthropathies

Eyes
Conjunctivitis
Uveitis (ankylosing spondylitis and inflammatory bowel disease)
Skin and mucous membranes
Oral ulceration
Circinate balanitis
Keratoderma blennorhagica (psoriasis)
Nail dystrophy (psoriasis)
Erythema nodosum (inflammatory bowel disease)
Cardiac
Aortitis (ankylosing spondylitis)
Conduction defects

Epidemiology

This has been best studied in outbreaks of food poisoning where the proportion of infected patients developing arthritis can be accurately assessed. However, in such studies the proportion going on to develop reactive arthritis varies widely (0–21 per cent). The incidence of clinically significant arthritis is generally low in community surveys of infected patients and high in patients whose infection is severe enough to require hospital referral, but careful population studies of *Campylobacter* infection have shown a high incidence (7–16 per cent) of musculoskeletal symptoms not severe enough to need rheumatological attention. As in other forms of spondyloarthropathy, the influence of HLA B27 on incidence is important: 60 to 80 per cent of patients with reactive arthritis presenting to rheumatology clinics will be B27 positive, but amongst those with mild disease the figure drops to 30 per cent, compared with the population prevalence of 7 to 10 per cent. Thus B27 is associated mainly with the severity and persistence of arthritis, rather than its incidence.

Pathogenesis

There is mounting evidence that, following infection of the gut or genitourinary tract, organisms reach the joints. They may arrive intact, when they can be detected by using the polymerase chain reaction, or as antigenic

Table 4 Pattern of joint involvement in reactive arthritis

Oligo- or monoarthritis
Asymmetric
Predominantly lower limbs
Coexisting enthesitis
Sacroiliac joint involvement

material (proteins, lipopolysaccharide) which can be demonstrated by immunofluorescence and immunoblotting techniques in synovial macrophages and polymorphs. This process can continue for months or even years, suggesting that some of the infections, for example *Yersinia*, persist as continuing sources of antigens/organisms. Elevated and persistent titres of IgA antibody to these organisms in reactive arthritis compared with uncomplicated infection also favour the idea of persistence. These findings emphasize that the distinction between septic and postinfectious arthritis has become blurred, since viable organisms can be detected in the joint in various forms of postinfectious arthritis, including Lyme disease and reactive arthritis, although they may be difficult or impossible to culture from synovial fluid or synovium.

Within the joint, cellular immune responses to the bacteria responsible for triggering the reactive arthritis are readily detected, particularly by CD4+ helper T lymphocytes, but also CD8+ T cells. Interestingly, although the association with HLA B27 is often taken to imply that CD8+ T cells are the principal effector cells in the disease, observations on reactive arthritis in HIV-positive patients show that they present with arthritis at stage I infection, when numbers of CD4+ T cells are less depressed. By contrast, arthritis can be relatively quiescent in full-blown AIDS. Both CD4+ and CD8+ lymphocytes produce proinflammatory cytokines such as interferon-γ which could potentially drive joint inflammation by secondary effects on synoviocytes.

There are several hypotheses about how HLA B27 could influence the course of reactive arthritis, particularly its severity and persistence. For instance, infection may generate a B27-restricted response by CD8+ T cells to a bacterial peptide which crossreacts with a component of the joint, i.e. infection triggers autoimmunity by 'molecular mimicry'. No such autoimmune response has yet been demonstrated. Alternatively, B27 may adversely affect the efficiency with which the immune system clears the triggering organism. In this case disease does not require autoimmunity, but is primarily driven by persistent bacterial antigens. Lastly, B27 might affect the immune response to the triggering organism qualitatively, for example by allowing hyper-responsiveness to particular antigens, or biasing the immune response in favour of the production of proinflammatory cytokines.

Clinical features

Preceding illness

A history of urethritis (dysuria or discharge) and diarrhoea must be sought specifically, there being no reason for patients to automatically link these occurrences with their arthritis. The interval between infection and arthritis is variable but is not usually more than 3 weeks. However, by the time a rheumatologist is consulted, many weeks may have passed and the triggering illness be forgotten, particularly if symptoms were mild. Note that urethritis may be triggered by gastrointestinal infection: if this possibility is forgotten minimally symptomatic gastrointestinal infection and prominent urethritis may cause diagnostic confusion.

Arthritis

The clinical picture in reactive arthritis is usually an asymmetric oligoarthritis (generally fewer than six joints), predominantly affecting the lower limbs (Table 4). However, any joint can be affected, and a proportion of patients have monoarthritis only. Affected joints are often hot and markedly swollen, with septic arthritis and crystal-induced arthritis being the most likely differential diagnoses. Dactylitis, similar to that seen in psoriatic arthritis, also occurs. Many patients complain of low back or buttock pain, suggesting involvement of the sacroiliac joint. Arthritis is usually at its worst early in the course of the disease, but new sites can be affected after several months and relapses are not uncommon, even in those in whom disease eventually settles completely. The presence of enthesitis (inflammation of ligamentous and tendinous insertions) in addition to arthritis is helpful diagnostically, with plantar fasciitis and involvement of the Achilles tendon insertion the commonest sites.

Extra-articular features

In acute severe disease patients have constitutional symptoms of malaise, fatigue, and fever. More useful diagnostically are the specific extra-articular signs listed in Table 3 and illustrated in Figs. 1, 2, and 3. The fact that these extra-articular features are common to other forms of spondyloarthropathy greatly strengthens the case for including reactive arthritis in this disease family, and for delineating reactive arthritis as a distinct syndrome within the postinfectious arthritides. Extra-articular features are more common in those with severe joint involvement. Conjunctivitis is often transient and no longer present by the time the patient presents. More persistent eye inflammation or painful eyes should raise the question of an acute anterior uveitis rather than a simple conjunctivitis and prompt full ophthalmological assessment. Circinate balanitis is usually asymptomatic and needs to be looked for specifically in uncircumcized males. Oral ulceration is usually asymptomatic. Keratoderma blennorrhagica is histologically identical to psoriasis; it is most commonly seen on the soles of the feet, but can also involve the hands or trunk. Erythema nodosum is associated with *Yersinia* infection, but is otherwise uncommon in reactive arthritis. Aortitis and cardiac conduction disorders have been described but are rare.

Differential diagnosis

The differential diagnosis of reactive arthritis is summarized in Table 5. The principal concerns in acute disease are septic arthritis, crystal arthropathies, and other forms of postinfectious arthritis such as Lyme disease,

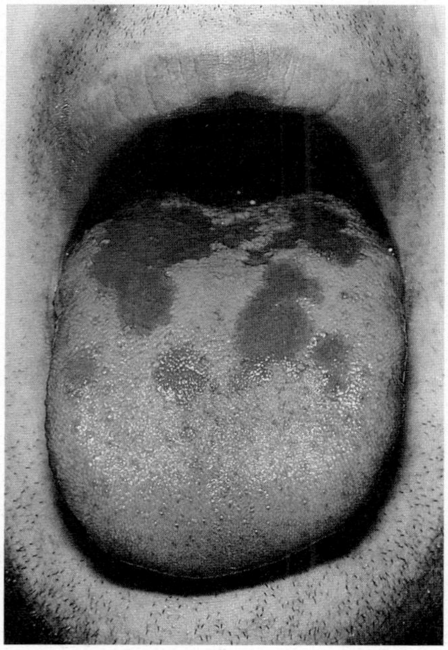

Fig. 1 Ulceration of the tongue in reactive arthritis. (By courtesy of Dr C. J. Eastmond.)

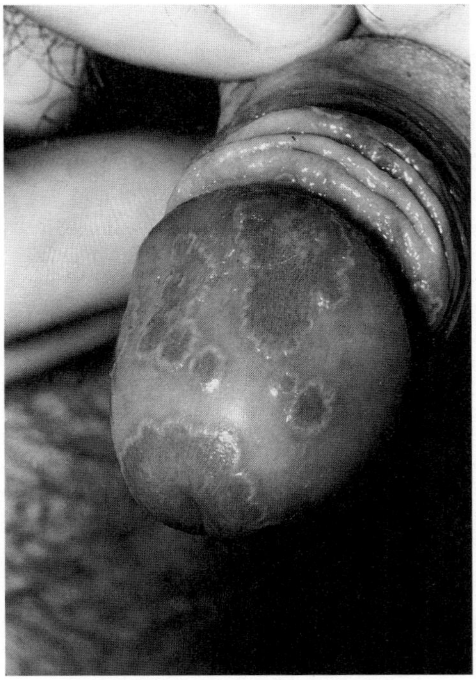

Fig. 2 Circinate balanitis in reactive arthritis. (By courtesy of Dr C. J. Eastmond.)

poststreptococcal arthritis, or gonococcal arthritis. In chronic disease it may be difficult to distinguish reactive arthritis from other forms of spondyloarthropathy, especially in those with inflammatory bowel disease, and many patients in whom no infectious trigger can be implicated are classified as having an 'undifferentiated' spondyloarthropathy.

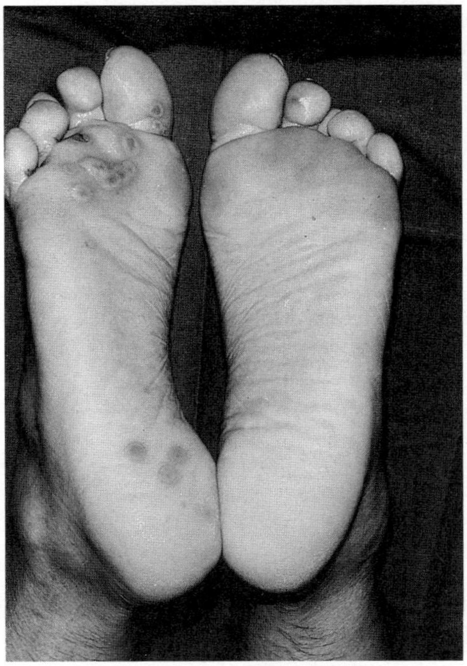

Fig. 3 Keratoderma blennorrhagica in reactive arthritis. (By courtesy of Dr C. J. Eastmond.)

Table 5 Differential diagnosis of reactive arthritis

Septic arthritis
Postinfectious arthritis
Lyme disease
Poststreptococcal or *Neisseria* infection
Viral arthritis
Crystal arthropathies
Other spondyloarthropathies
Behçet's
Sarcoidosis
Trauma, sports injury

Laboratory features

General

The principal aims of investigation are to exclude important differential diagnoses and to identify the triggering organism. Abnormalities in the early stages when arthritis is most active are those of a pronounced acute inflammatory response with elevation of erythrocyte sedimentation rate and C-reactive protein, the latter often very marked (more than 100 mg/litre). Rheumatoid factor and antinuclear antibodies are absent. Positive antineutrophil antiplasmic antibodies have been described, but the antibodies are not directed against proteinase-3 or myeloperoxidase and the test is not useful diagnostically. Septic arthritis and crystal arthropathies are best excluded by aspiration of synovial fluid followed by culture and microscopy. Blood cultures should be performed and serum urate checked. A chest radiograph may reveal hilar lymphadenopathy, suggesting the diagnosis of sarcoidosis, although *Yersinia* can cause both reactive arthritis and a sarcoid-like illness. Throat swab and antibodies to streptococcal antigens may produce evidence of poststreptoccocal arthritis, which does not generally share extra-articular features with reactive arthritis.

Microbiological

Stool should be cultured for pathogens associated with reactive arthritis, although cultures are often negative after gastrointestinal symptoms have settled—despite the recent evidence that persistent infection contributes to pathogenesis. *Chlamydia* infection must be sought in sexually active patients, particularly when there is no clear history of gastroenteritis. Formal referral to a department of genitourinary medicine is often helpful. Patients are not infrequently infected with both *Chlamydia* and *Gonococcus*. This can cause confusion, but gonococcal arthritis differs from reactive arthritis with its characteristic rash and absence of the classical extra-articular features. *Chlamydia* can be cultured from urethral or cervical swabs or from urine, and *Chlamydia* antigens can be demonstrated by enzyme-linked immunosorbent assay techniques or by direct immunofluorescence tests. The latter are highly sensitive, in principle able to detect one organism per smear, but they require highly skilled technicians. Polymerase chain reaction techniques achieve similar sensitivity, and can be used on urine specimens, addressing the natural reluctance of many patients with reactive arthritis (or other conditions) to undergo routine urethral and vaginal instrumentation.

The possibility of spondyloarthropathy in the context of HIV infection also needs to be considered, although this appears rare in developed countries. By contrast, large numbers of reactive arthritis cases, often related to dysentery, have recently emerged amongst the HIV-infected population in Africa, where the disease was previously unknown.. Nevertheless, HIV testing should be considered, particularly in patients with unusually severe disease and with relevant risk factors.

Immunological

When the triggering organism cannot be demonstrated directly, infection can be inferred on the basis of immune responses. However, this evidence needs to be interpreted cautiously, since in many cases the findings simply imply immunological memory for the organism in question and do not demonstrate a clear relationship between infection and arthritis. For enteric pathogens, specific IgM antibodies may be demonstrated and these, along with IgG, form the basis of the agglutination tests which are widely used. Rising IgG titres may also be helpful. However, when patients present several months into their illness, IgM may no longer be evident and IgG titres stable. In these circumstances high and persistent IgA titres to organisms such as *Salmonella* and *Yersinia* may be helpful. The possibility of using antibody responses to particular bacterial antigens diagnostically is currently under investigation. Serological diagnosis of *Chlamydia* infection is particularly difficult because of high levels of infection with *Chlamydia pneumoniae* in the community, an organism which shares several highly conserved antigens with *Chlamydia trachomatis*.

Lastly, cellular immune responses to triggering organisms can be demonstrated, particularly in the synovial fluid. Again, these only demonstrate T-cell memory for the organism and do not demonstrate causality—patients with, for instance, rheumatoid arthritis and incidental *Salmonella* infection, will have *Salmonella*-specific T cells in their synovial fluid. Currently such tests are used in research rather than diagnostically.

Radiology

In the acute stages of disease, radiology is not diagnostically helpful, with soft tissue swelling and occasionally periarticular osteoporosis at affected joints being the only abnormalities. Radionuclide scintigraphy can be useful for demonstrating acute sacroiliitis and may show the full extent of acute synovitis and enthesitis, but is not usually required for clinical management. Radiological changes are confined to the minority of patients with persistent disease (more than 1 year's duration). The principal features are erosion of affected joints, including the sacroiliac, and new bone formation manifested as periostitis of metatarsal and metacarpal bones and 'enthesophytes', such as plantar spurs. In the spine paravertebral ossification can be seen in the lumbar region: this is asymmetric and differs from the classical changes of ankylosing spondylitis. Erosive changes are also seen at sites of enthesitis such as the calaneum.

Treatment

Evidence-based therapies for reactive arthritis are lacking, so that consensus opinion is the current guide. In the acute phase affected joints should be rested until they improve substantially. This often requires emphasizing to young, active patients involved in sports, and alternative forms of exercise should be considered. Synovial effusions should be aspirated and when septic arthritis has been excluded will respond well to injection with long-acting corticosteroids. If *Chlamydia* infection is established or thought likely, patients require conventional treatment with short-term antibiotics, but there is no evidence that this has any effect on the progress of reactive arthritis. Enteric infections do not require antibiotics in their own right. Uveitis requires formal ophthalmological assessment and treatment with local steroids. Physiotherapy and advice on exercise is helpful, with quadriceps function needing particular attention in view of the frequent involvement of the knees.

There are two major unresolved treatment issues in reactive arthritis. Firstly, the place of disease-modifying drugs. Sulphasalazine and methotrexate are useful in spondyloarthropathies generally, and on this basis have been used in reactive arthritis, but without controlled trials confined to this condition alone. The frequency with which the disorder is self-limiting makes controlled trials of second-line agents difficult. The second issue is whether long-term antibiotics confer any benefit. In a controlled trial, a subset of patients with evidence of *Chlamydia* infection benefited from prolonged tetracycline, but subsequent trials using ciprofloxacin, mainly in *Yersinia*-associated reactive arthritis, have been negative. Nevertheless, since persistent infection is implicated in our current understanding of pathogenesis, further work on antibiotics is being undertaken, particularly of agents which might be able to treat quiescent or slow-growing bacteria which are refractory to agents that target bacterial cell division.

Psychological and quality of life issues

Reactive arthritis commonly affects young, fit adults who have not previously experienced any form of prolonged illness or disability. The danger is that the rheumatologist, all too used to the gloomy prognosis of rheumatoid arthritis, may treat reactive arthritis, where there is a high likelihood of complete resolution of disease, too lightly. Patients need to be given a realistic prognosis, i.e. that symptoms are likely to persist at some level for 6 to 12 months, although in the latter stages these are usually very mild compared with those experienced in the first 4 to 8 weeks. Exacerbations during this time are not uncommon and do not imply that the disease will not eventually resolve. The chances of the patient developing chronic arthritis are less than 10 per cent. Patients benefit from continuing psychological and clinical support throughout the course of their illness, with rapid access to joint aspiration and intra-articular steroid injection when there is recurrent joint swelling.

Current areas of uncertainty

Current uncertainties concern classification criteria and management strategies. Both may be resolved by developing more secure diagnostic techniques for identifying the triggering infection. Improved treatment is likely to come from either additional evidence about the importance of persistent infection and how to eliminate it, or from discovery of the immune responses responsible for maintaining joint inflammation, whether these are directed against a bacterial antigen or an autoantigen. If a target antigen can be identified, specific immunomodulation strategies will then be relevant.

Reactive arthritis differs from other forms of human inflammatory arthritis in having a clearly defined onset and being triggered by known infectious agents. Genetic influences that result in a minority of infected individuals developing arthritis are being investigated. These include HLA B27, but it is likely that other genes are also involved. Genome screening now being applied to ankylosing spondylitis may throw up likely candidates.

Further reading

Reviews of pathogenesis

Gaston JSH (1995). Symposium: reactive arthritis. *Rheumatology. in Europe* **24**, 5–22.

Sieper J, Braun J (1995). Pathogenesis of spondylarthropathies: persistent bacterial antigen, autoimmunity, or both? *Arthritis and Rheumatism* **38**, 1547–54.

Incidence following salmonella infection

Mattila L *et al.* (1994). Reactive arthritis following an outbreak of salmonella infection in Finland. *British Journal of Rheumatology* **33**, 1136–41.

Inman RD *et al.* (1988). Postdysenteric reactive arthritis: a clinical and immunologic study following an outbreak of salmonellosis. *Arthritis and Rheumatism* **31**, 1377–83.

Evidence that bacteria or bacterial antigens reach the joint in reactive arthritis

Gaston JSH, Cox C, Granfors K (1999). Clinical and experimental evidence for persistent *Yersinia* infection in reactive arthritis. *Arthritis and Rheumatism* **42**, 2239–42.

Gerard HC *et al.* (1998). Synovial *Chlamydia trachomatis* in patients with reactive arthritis/Reiter's syndrome are viable but show aberrant gene expression. *Journal of Rheumatology* **25**, 734–42.

Granfors K *et al.* (1989). Yersinia antigens in synovial fluid cells from patients with reactive arthritis. *New England Journal of Medicine* **320**, 216–21.

Granfors K *et al.* (1990). Salmonella lipopolysaccharide in synovial cells from patients with reactive arthritis. *The Lancet* **335**, 685–8.

Immune responses in reactive arthritis

Gaston JSH *et al.* (1989). Synovial T lymphocyte recognition of organisms that trigger reactive arthritis. *Clinical and Experimental Immunology* **76**, 348–53.

Granfors K, Toivanen A (1986). IgA-anti-yersinia antibodies in yersinia-triggered reactive arthritis. *Annals of the Rheumatic Diseases* **45**, 561–5.

Hermann E *et al.* (1993). HLA-B27-restricted CD8 T-cells derived from synovial fluids of patients with reactive arthritis and ankylosing spondylitis. *The Lancet* **342**, 646–50.

Reactive arthritis and other spondyloarthropathy in HIV infection

Njobvu P *et al.* (1998). Spondyloarthropathy and human immunodeficiency virus infection in Zambia. *Journal of Rheumatology* **25**, 1553–9.

Treatment in reactive arthritis

Dougados M *et al.* (1995). Sulfasalazine in the treatment of spondylarthropathy: a randomized, multicenter, double-blind, placebo-controlled study. *Arthritis and Rheumatism* **38**, 618–27.

Lauhio A *et al.* (1991). Double-blind, placebo-controlled study of three-month treatment with lymecycline in reactive arthritis with special reference to chlamydia arthritis. *Arthritis and Rheumatism* **34**, 6–14.

Sieper J *et al.* (1999). No benefit of long-term ciprofloxacin treatment in patients with reactive arthritis and undifferentiated oligoarthritis—a three-month, multicenter, double-blind, randomized, placebo-controlled study. *Arthritis and Rheumatism* **42**, 1386–96.

18.8 Osteoarthritis

Paul H. Brion and Kenneth C. Kalunian

Introduction

Osteoarthritis is the commonest form of arthritis, detectable radiographically in 80 per cent of patients over the age of 55. Symptomatic osteoarthritis of the knee (pain with radiographic abnormalities) was noted in 6.1 per cent of adults aged 30 and over in the Framingham Study, and the frequency is comparable in the United Kingdom. Approximately 20.7 million people in the United States have physician-diagnosed osteoarthritis. Whilst some may be asymptomatic, many have significant pain and disability, with one study finding that osteoarthritis accounts for 12.3 per cent of all those with limitation of activity. The prevalence of osteoarthritis is likely to increase, paralleling the increase in the absolute and relative number of people who are over 65 years of age. The social impact of this disease is enormous, accounting for more dependency in walking and stair climbing than any other disease. The estimated annual cost associated with osteoarthritis in the United States is $15.5 billion in 1994 dollars, which approaches 1 per cent of the gross national product, with more than 50 per cent of the costs due to work loss.

Definition

Osteoarthritis was described by Solomon as

> A chronic disorder characterized by softening and disintegration of articular cartilage, with reactive phenomena such as vascular congestion and osteoblastic activity in the subarticular bone, new growth of cartilage and bone (osteophytes) at the joint margins, and capsular fibrosis. Osteoarthritis is not accompanied by any systemic illness, and although there are sometimes signs of inflammation, it is not primarily an inflammatory disorder.

Alternative definitions exist, including those based on symptoms, physical findings, and radiographic and arthroscopic findings. The presence of joint symptoms plus evidence of structural change generally defines clinical osteoarthritis, whereas many studies use radiographic assessment alone as the primary means of identifying the condition. Most clinical investigators use the Kellgren and Lawrence scale for grading osteoarthritis of the knee, which defines osteoarthritis on the basis of osteophytes, the presence of which relates well with the presence of knee symptoms. The American College of Rheumatology has developed classification criteria for the presence of osteoarthritis based on the joint involved (Tables 1, 2, and 3): these are based on clinical criteria alone, clinical and laboratory criteria, and clinical plus radiographic criteria. Initially, only the clinical and radiographic criteria were validated; more recently, Klashman and colleagues have validated the other methods. However, the clinical and radiographic criteria have the best specificity (86 per cent) compared with the clinical and laboratory criteria (75 per cent) and clinical criteria alone (69 per cent). Kawasaki and colleagues have shown that the non-radiographic criteria have adequate interobserver reproducibility for outpatients complaining of knee pain with a wide spectrum of rheumatic diseases; however, sensitivity and specificity are lower than those reported by Klashman and colleagues.

Table 1 American College of Rheumatology clinical criteria for the classification of osteoarthritis of the hand

Hand pain, aching, or stiffness with three of the following four:
Hard tissue enlargement of two or more of ten selected joints
Fewer than three swollen MCP joints
Hard tissue enlargement of two or more DIP joints
Deformity of one or more of ten selected hand joints

- Selected joints are the second and third DIP joints, the second and third proximal interphalangeal joints and the first CMC joint of both hands
- Hand osteoarthritis is readily diagnosed by clinical criteria alone. There are no recommended lab and/or radiographic classification criteria
- Sensitivity = 94%, specificity = 87%

Risk factors and epidemiology

A multitude of risk factors exist for the development of osteoarthritis of the knee. These include being female, increasing age, obesity, family history, increased bone density, trauma, and certain occupational exposures (Table 4).

Age is considered the strongest associated risk factor for the development of osteoarthritis in many studies. The National Health and Nutrition Examination Survey found a prevalence of osteoarthritis of only 0.1 per cent in people aged 25 to 34 years, compared with over 80 per cent in those aged 55 to 64 years. This increased incidence occurs in osteoarthritis of the hands, back, hip, and knees.

Gender differences in osteoarthritis are complicated. There is an overall higher prevalence in women, in whom the disease more often involves multiple joints. However, before the age of 50 years there is a higher prevalence and incidence in men, whereas after 50 years the reverse applies, with increasing female predominance as age increases. There is a plateau or decline in both genders by the age of 80 years. The gender- and age-related differences in prevalence parallel the effect of postmenopausal oestrogen deficiency in increasing the risk of osteoarthritis. Other probable factors

Table 2 American College of Rheumatology clinical, laboratory, and radiographic criteria for the classification of osteoarthritis of the hip

Hip pain for most days in the previous month with two of the following three features:
Femoral and/or acetabular osteophytes on radiograph
Erythrocyte sedimentation rate > 20 mm/h
Joint space narrowing on radiograph

- Clinical and lab criteria alone yield poor results. Only clinical with lab and radiographic criteria are recommended

Sensitivity = 89%, specificity = 91%

Table 3 Criteria for the classification of osteoarthritis of the knee

Clinical criteria*

Knee pain for most days of previous month with three of the following six:

- Age > 50 years
- Morning stiffness < 30 min duration
- Crepitus on active joint motion
- Bony enlargement on examination
- Bony tenderness on examination
- No palpable warmth

Clinical and laboratory criteria†

Knee pain for most days of previous month with five of the following nine:

- Age > 50 years
- Morning stiffness < 30 min duration
- Crepitus on active joint motion
- Bony enlargement on examination
- Bony tenderness
- No palpable warmth
- Westergren ESR < 40 mm/h
- RF titre < 1:40
- Synovial fluid suggestive of osteoarthritis§

Clinical, laboratory, and radiographic criteria‡

Knee pain for most days of the previous month with osteophytes on the radiograph with one of the following three:

- Age > 50 years
- Morning stiffness < 30 min
- Crepitus on active joint motion

* Sensitivity = 95%, specificity = 69%.

† Sensitivity = 92%, specificity = 75%.

‡ Sensitivity = 91%, specificity = 86%.

§ Synovial fluid suggestive of osteoarthritis has a clear colour, viscous fluid, and a white cell count of less than 2000/mm^3.

ESR, erythrocyte sedimentation rate; RF, rheumatoid factor.

that help explain the increase in the incidence and prevalence of osteoarthritis with age include a decreased responsiveness of chondrocytes to growth factors that stimulate repair, an increase in the laxity of ligamentous structures, and a decrease in proprioceptive responses.

Although racial differences in osteoarthritis of the hip are conflicting, the higher relative weight of African-American women may predispose them to higher rates of osteoarthritis of the knee. There are few data available for other racial differences in osteoarthritis of the knee among the population of the United States. Several studies have confirmed that inheritance is a risk factor for osteoarthritis: individuals are at higher risk of developing the condition if their parents had it, especially if the parental disease was polyarticular or had its onset in middle age or earlier. The role of inheritance may be more important among women than men. Numerous extended families with high rates of early onset severe osteoarthritis have been characterized in which the condition has been linked to an autosomal dominant mutation in type 11 procollagen. Although the majority of cases of osteoarthritis of the hand are inherited, the percentage for osteoarthritis of the knee is smaller, perhaps because osteoarthritis of the knee often develops more as a result of repeated mechanical insults.

Table 4 Risk factors and protective factors for osteoarthritis

Risk factors for osteoarthritis

- Age
- Obesity
- Female gender
- Family history
- Prior trauma
- Congenital abnormality
- African-American race
- Increased bone density
- Quadriceps weakness
- Occupation (e.g. farming)
- Competitive level sports

Protective factors for osteoarthritis

- Osteoporosis
- Oestrogen replacement therapy
- Vitamin C
- Vitamin E
- Vitamin D

The incidence of osteoarthritis is lower in the setting of osteoporosis: bone density in osteoarthritis patients is greater than in age-matched controls, even at sites distant from the affected joints. Most studies linking osteoarthritis with high bone density are cross-sectional. Although osteoarthritis and high bone density are both linked to obesity, the association of osteoarthritis with high bone density is independent of body mass index. It has been suggested that osteophyte formation rather than cartilage loss is linked to high bone density, which suggests the presence of a circulating bone growth factor in those with osteophytes; possibilities include insulin-like growth factor type 1, platelet-derived growth factor, fibroblast growth factor, transforming growth factor-β, and colony-stimulating factor.

Oestrogen deficiency has been implicated as a risk factor for the development of osteoarthritis as evidenced by the high incidence of osteoarthritis after the menopause. Several studies suggest that oestrogen replacement therapy reduces the risk of osteoarthritis of the hip and knee. Both the Study of Osteoporotic Fractures and the Framingham Study have reported a strong inverse relationship between oestrogen replacement therapy and osteoarthritis among those undergoing long-term oestrogen replacement therapy.

Reactive oxygen species have been implicated in the development of osteoarthritis, and antioxidants may prevent or delay the onset of osteoarthritis. In the Framingham Study, those in the lowest tertile of vitamin C intake had a threefold greater risk of progression of osteoarthritis of the knee, joint space loss, and onset of knee pain compared with subjects with a higher intake. However, the effects of β-carotene and vitamin E against disease progression were inconsistent. No effect of serum 25-hydroxyvitamin D was seen on incident osteoarthritis; however, among subjects with radiographic osteoarthritis at baseline, those who were in the lowest tertile of serum 25-hydroxyvitamin D had a higher rate of radiographic progression compared with those in the highest tertile.

Local biomechanical factors such as trauma or repetitive joint use are risk factors for osteoarthritis. In animal models, a change in biomechanics that occurs after injury leads to increased shear stress on local areas of cartilage, possibly causing osteoarthritis. In humans, traumatic injury to joints is a common cause of osteoarthritis, and Kellgren and Lawrence found that a history of previous trauma could be elicited in approximately 40 per cent of men and approximately 20 per cent of women aged 55 to 64 years with osteoarthritis of the knee. In the Framingham Study, men with a history of major trauma to the knee had a five-fold increased risk of osteoarthritis of the knee, whilst women with a similar history had a greater than three-fold increased risk. Trauma that causes damage to a cruciate ligament and/or a meniscus has been associated with subsequent development of osteoarthritis of the knee, perhaps through concurrent damage to articular cartilage. With regard to repetitive use, occupations that require kneeling and squatting are associated with a higher prevalence of osteoarthritis of the knee, but heavy physical work is less consistently associated. The level of physical activity increases the risk of developing osteoarthritis. In the Framingham Study, physical activity (generally consisting of walking and gardening in this population) was found to correlate directly with the risk of developing radiographic osteoarthritis of the knee in elderly subjects followed for 8 years. Those with high levels of these activities had a threefold increase in the risk of osteoarthritis compared with sedentary controls. Elite athletes have higher rates of incidence of osteoarthritis of weight-bearing joints compared with controls, probably because athletic activities often involve both increased risk of injury and repetitive use.

Several longitudinal studies suggest that increased weight is a risk factor for the development of osteoarthritis of the knee, and that overweight patients with established osteoarthritis of the knee are at greater risk of developing progressive disease compared with those who are not overweight. The associations between obesity and osteoarthritis of the knee are significantly greater for women than men and are not affected by adjustments for concurrent diseases. Data from the Chingford Study showed that patients in the highest weight tertile had an odds ratio of 6.17 for radiographic osteoarthritis of the knee compared with the lowest weight tertile. For every two-unit increase in body mass index (approximately 5 kg), the odds ratio for radiographic osteoarthritis of the knee increased by 1.36. A follow-up study of incident osteoarthritis of the knee in women with unilateral disease found the tertile with the highest body mass index had a relative risk of 4.69 for developing osteoarthritis in the contralateral knee compared with patients in the lowest body mass index tertile. Similar findings exist for osteoarthritis of the hand and hip, but the association is less robust. The importance of obesity cannot be understated as this may be a modifiable risk factor. A possible mechanism for the effect of obesity on osteoarthritis of the knee is increased force across the weight-bearing joint, which induces cartilage breakdown by altered walking mechanics. However, obesity may also have effects through metabolic intermediaries.

Quadriceps weakness has been associated with radiographic osteoarthritis of the knee. Muscular strength may be required to stabilize the knee, distribute force, or lessen the effect of an impact load, and maintenance of muscular strength may be important in decreasing the incidence of osteoarthritis of the knee and its progression and disability due to established disease. Proprioceptive sensation, which declines with age, is impaired in elderly patients with osteoarthritis of the knee, suggesting that poor proprioception may contribute to functional impairment in these patients.

Pathogenesis and pathological features

The pathogenesis of osteoarthritis remains controversial. Once thought of as a normal consequence of aging, the complex nature of this disease is only now being understood. Current theories suggest that osteoarthritis results from an imbalance in catabolic and anabolic processes that lead to progressive cartilage damage and destruction. Increased catabolism may be the result of acute injuries such as an acute meniscal tear or of chronic microtraumatic events. Initially, anabolic processes such as proteoglycan synthesis maintain balance with catabolic processes and damage to cartilage is repaired. However, with time and age, anabolic processes decline and progressive cartilage damage ensues.

Histological changes in osteoarthritis are complex. Early stages are characterized by increased water content and cartilage swelling. This swollen cartilage is believed to be more susceptible to injury and may lead to fragmentation of the articular surface. Fragmented cartilage is less able to withstand biomechanical insults, resulting in further deterioration. Chondrocytes become activated and proinflammatory cytokines such as interleukin 1 and tumour necrosis factor-α are synthesized. These cytokines increase the synthesis of degradative proteases such as collagenase, gelatinase,and stomelsin. As cartilage destruction progresses, proteoglycan content becomes reduced. Cartilage becomes thinned, fragmented, and proteoglycan depleted.

Reparative processes may initially lead to joint stabilization, but ultimately contribute to progression of the disease. Fibrocartilage may be synthesized in response to loss of the more durable hyaline cartilage. Fibrocartilage may be denuded bone, improving joint mechanics and protecting the subchondral bone. However, fibrocartilage is less able to withstand mechanical loading. The subchondral bone is exposed to increased force relative to that of hyaline cartilage. The synthesis of fibrocartilage, while a temporary improvement, is ultimately less efficient than hyaline cartilage. Subchondral bony changes such as sclerosis and osteophyte formation develop.

The gross pathological findings of osteoarthritis include cartilage loss and reactive bone formation. Cartilage loss occurs primarily in areas of joint loading and may be related to repetitive mechanical insults. Cartilage loss may be best visualized arthroscopially when findings include cartilage softening, fibrillation, and thinning. Areas of complete cartilage loss may be seen. More commonly, the clinician will recognize these findings as radiographic joint space narrowing. Similarly, bony changes may be seen on pathological specimens or arthroscopically. Arthroscopic findings include osteophyte projections and subchondral bone visualized through denuded cartilage. The classic radiographic bony changes include osteophyte formation and subchondral bony sclerosis and cysts.

Clinical features

Precise definition of clinical osteoarthritis has remained elusive since radiographic findings and symptoms may diverge. In addition, osteoarthritis may be categorized by the joint area involved or as being idiopathic or secondary to other disorders. An essential element to diagnosis of osteoarthritis is the correct attribution of symptoms to the affected joint. Initial evaluation of soft tissue abnormalities such as bursitis, tendonitis, and ligamentous strain should be performed. In addition, consideration of neurological or underlying bone abnormalities should be entertained when appropriate.

A thorough history and physical examination should be performed to evaluate for secondary forms of osteoarthritis. These include developmental, mechanical, or biochemical abnormalities known to increase the risk for osteoarthritis. These forms tend to present earlier in life (for example congenital hip abnormality), in atypical joints (for example calcium hydroxyapatite) or as more inflammatory in nature (for example calcium pyrophosphate deposition disease).

Idiopathic osteoarthritis may occur localized to one body area or as a more generalized disease. Common areas of involvement include the hands, hips, knees, and spine. Less commonly, osteoarthritis involves the shoulders, wrists, ankles, feet, and jaw.

Pain is the predominant symptom of osteoarthritis, usually mild to moderate in nature and increasing with joint use and at the end of the day. Pain is generally improved with rest and moderation of activity. Severe disease may cause pain at rest or at night. The source of pain may be the underlying bone, the joint capsule, or surrounding structures. Cartilage is avascular and without nerves and not itself a source of pain.

Stiffness may occur but is generally limited to less than 30 min in duration (gelling phenomenon). It is typical in the morning or after any prolonged rest (theatre sign). Effusions may occur, but warmth and soft tissue swelling is rare and suggests another diagnosis.

Physical examination reveals tenderness to palpation, bony thickening (osteophyte formation), small effusions, and crepitus. Specific joint findings also occur. Typical in the hand are bony enlargement of the proximal interphalangeal joints (Bouchard's nodes) and the distal interphalangeal joints (Heberden's nodes). The first carpometacarpal joint may be involved causing a 'squared appearance' of the lateral aspect of the hand (in anatomical position) (Fig. 1). Involvement of the foot yields bunions, and of the knee pronounced valgus and varus deformities, Baker's cyst or locking suggesting meniscal damage. Early hip findings include limited internal and external rotation. Back findings include pain: true osteoarthritis occurs at the apophyseal joints; degenerative disc disease and diffuse idiopathic skeletal hyperostosis are distinct entities.

In an effort to standardize the diagnosis of osteoarthritis, the American College of Rheumatology formed a subcommittee to define osteoarthritis of the knee, hip, and hand. Clinical, laboratory, and radiographic findings were evaluated by an expert panel and statistical analysis, to yield classification criteria with acceptable sensitivity and specificity values. These instruments should be used with caution in individual patients but provide a framework for analysis (see Tables 1, 2, and 3).

Common clinical mimics of osteoarthritis include rheumatoid arthritis, calcium pyrophosphate deposition disease, and infectious monoarticular arthritis.

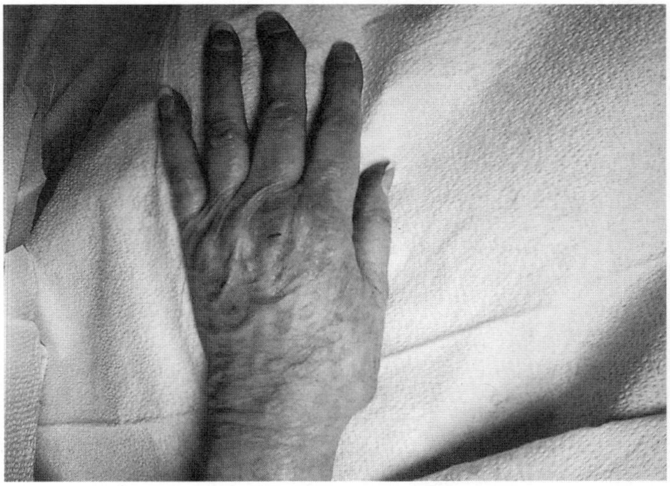

Fig. 1 Osteoarthritis of the hand. Note squaring of first carpometacarpal (CMC) joint and evidence of a Heberden's node on the third distal interphalangeal joint.

Hand osteoarthritis may be confused with rheumatoid arthritis as both cause pain and visible swelling. Less commonly hip or knee arthritis may present as diagnostic challenges. Hand osteoarthritis typically involves the proximal interphalangeal and the distal interphalangeal joints; the 'swelling' is not true swelling but hard, bony thickening due to osteophyte formation; and stiffness is limited. By contrast, rheumatoid arthritis typically involves the proximal interphalangeal, metacarpophalangeal, and carpal joints, sparing the distal interphalangeals. True swelling occurs and is soft with palpation. Multiple joints are involved, symptoms of systemic inflammation occur, and rheumatoid factor is usually positive. In rheumatoid arthritis radiographs demonstrate symmetric joint space narrowing, bony erosions, minimal sclerosis, and minimal osteophyte formation.

Calcium pyrophosphate deposition disease is difficult to differentiate from idiopathic osteoarthritis because the two may coexist. Typical distributions for this disease include the knees, wrist, shoulder, and metacarpophalangeals. Patients may have more prolonged stiffness and pain and swelling may occur. Radiographs with evidence of chondrocalcinosis strongly suggest calcium pyrophosphate deposition disease, but the presence of crystals on arthrocentesis is the gold standard for diagnosis.

Infectious monoarthritis can occasionally mimic osteoarthritis. The distinction is more difficult with subacute infections, such as fungal or mycobacterial. If there is clinical suspicion, radiographs and arthrocentesis should be performed.

Investigation

Laboratory tests, if performed, reveal normal sedimentation rates and non-inflammatory synovial fluid. Radiographic findings include asymmetry, joint space narrowing, subchondral sclerosis, subchondral cysts, and the hallmark osteophyte (Figs. 2, 3, 4, and 5).

Treatment

Traditional treatments

Treatment modalities for all forms of osteoarthritis, listed in Table 5, remain limited. Traditional therapies include analgesics, non-steroidal anti-inflammatory drugs (**NSAIDs**), intra-articular corticosteroid injections, intra-articular hyaluronic acid injections, topical agents, tidal lavage, arthroscopic irrigation, and total joint replacement. With the exception of joint replacement, none of these therapies address the underlying problem of cartilage damage. Newer therapies include weight loss and exercise, both of which have been difficult to maintain over long periods of time. Emerging therapies such as tetracycline, cytokine modulators, and inhibitors of metalloproteinases may potentially alter the progression of osteoarthritis. Nutritional supplements such as glucosamine, chondroitin sulphate, soybean, and avocado products have been reported to provide better long-term analgesia than NSAIDs, and some of these agents may alter the progression of osteoarthritis and repair cartilage damage. However, the efficacy of these emerging therapies and nutritional supplements has not been studied adequately in controlled trials.

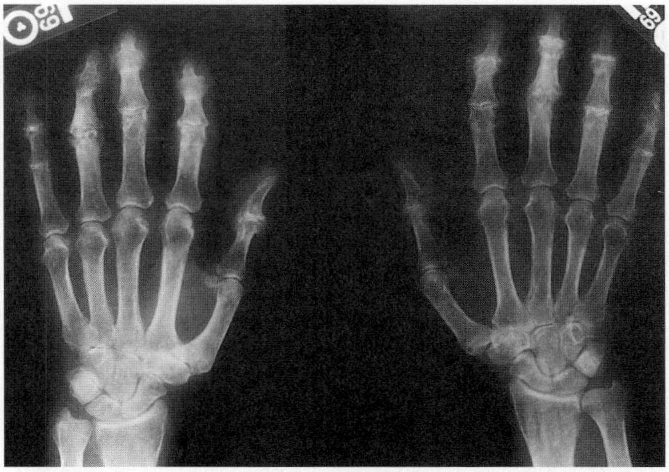

Fig. 2 Osteoarthritis of the hand. Note changes in the distal interphalangeal joints and proximal interphalangeal joints as well as the base of the thumb (carpometacarpal). These changes are typical for osteoarthritis of the hand. Note the loss of joint space, bony sclerosis, and the presence of osteophytes. The bony changes seen in the distal interphalangeal and proximal interphalangeal joints would manifest as Bouchard's and Heberden's nodes on clinical examination.

Weight loss

Weight loss, while effective, is difficult to achieve and maintain. Evidence suggests that a weight loss of 4.5 kg (10 lb) over 10 years may decrease the risk of developing contralateral knee osteoarthritis by 50 per cent. Studies demonstrating improvement in disease outcome are more controversial. However, given potential benefits in osteoarthritis as well as the additional

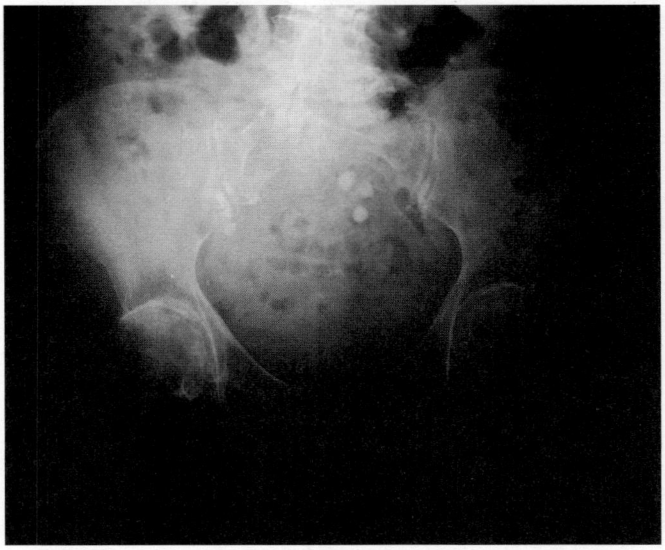

Fig. 3 Hip radiograph demonstrating osteoarthritis. Note joint space narrowing and sclerosis.

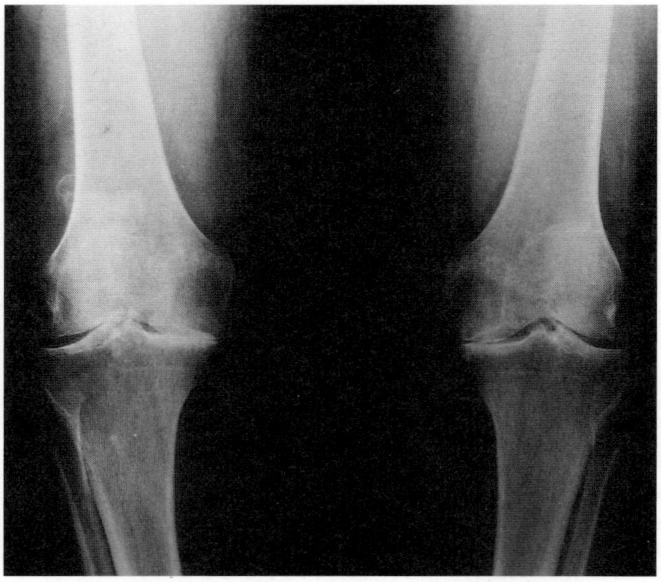

Fig. 4 Bilateral knee osteoarthritis. Note the asymmetric joint space narrowing, bony sclerosis, and the presence of osteophytes.

health benefits of a normal body mass index, obese patients should be encouraged to lose weight.

Exercise and psychosocial support

Physical therapy and exercise are advocated in osteoarthritis for a variety of reasons. Improvements in flexibility and muscle strengthening may decrease joint loading, preventing further damage. They have been demonstrated to improve functional outcome and pain scores in clinical trials. In addition, they provide a sense of self-determination, an adjunct for weight loss, improve depressive symptoms, and decrease patient disability. Obstacles include expense and the lack of motivation to continue exercising after a programme has been completed.

The role of psychosocial support may be significant. Telephone calls providing contact and education have been demonstrated to improve pain and functional status. Education and support improve feelings of frustration, minimize dependency, and improve coping mechanisms.

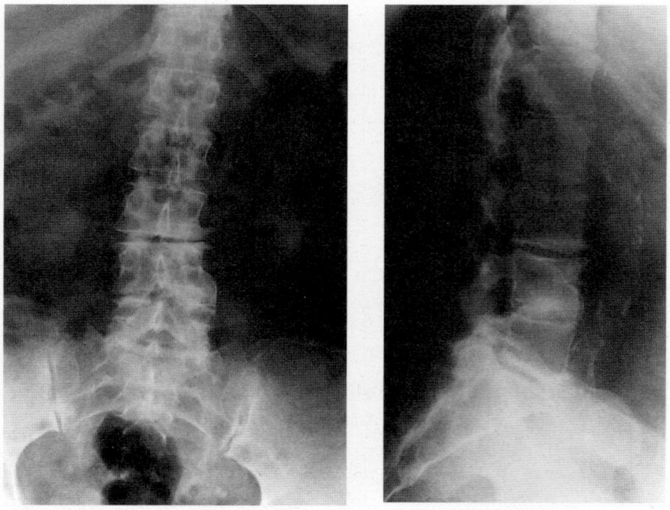

(a) (b)

Fig. 5 (a) and (b) Lumbar spine arthritis. Note the changes of degenerative disc disease as narrowing and large osteophytes. Although often called osteoarthritis these changes are not true osteoarthritis. True osteoarthritis occurs at the facet joints. Sclerosis is seen in the inferior facet joints.

Table 5 Therapies for osteoarthritis

Non-pharmacological
Weight loss
Physical therapy
Exercise
Aids/appliances
Pharmacological
Acetominophen/paracetamol
Non-selective NSAIDs
Cox-2 selective NSAIDs
Narcotic analgesics
Other analgesics
Intra-articular corticosteroids
Intra-articular hyaluronic acid
Surgical
Joint lavage
Meniscectomy
Synovectomy
Realignment osteotomy
Total joint replacement
Potential therapies
Glucosamine salts
Chondroitin sulphate
Tetracyclines
Diacerin
Avocado/soybean
Unsaponifiables

Simple analgesics

Analgesics such as acetaminophen and paracetamol provide analgesic relief comparable with that of NSAIDs. The lower relative risk of complications has favoured their use over that of NSAIDs, especially in older populations. Typical daily doses of acetaminophen are 4 g (3 g in elderly patients). These agents may be associated with liver problems and interactions with other drugs such as warfarin. Narcotic analgesics are generally avoided because of potential complications including constipation, sedation, addiction, and impairment of balance.

Non-steroidal anti-inflammatory agents

NSAIDs remain a cornerstone of osteoarthritis treatment. Availability, dosing schedule, cost and individual side-effect profile influence the choice of a particular agent. The associations of NSAIDs with peptic ulcer disease and renal insufficiency are well established. Less common side-effects include rash, hepatic dysfunction, platelet dysfunction, and central nervous system effects. NSAIDs with specific cyclo-oxygenase-2 (Cox-2) inhibiting activity have become popular because of their decreased dosing frequency, decreased platelet effects, and—most importantly—decreased incidence of gastrointestinal ulceration compared with traditional NSAIDs.

Corticosteroids

Intra-articular corticosteroids may be effective in decreasing joint pain associated with osteoarthritis. Dosage varies depending on patient body size, comorbidity, and the joint involved. They have multiple side-effects, including risk of infection, bleeding, and (possibly) cartilage damage. To minimize the risk of complications, injections should be limited to three to four per year in any given joint.

Hyaluronic acid

The use of hyaluronic acid preparations (Hyalgan™, Synvisc™) has become popular in recent years. These agents are reported to increase viscosity by replacing depleted hyaluronic acid, which occurs in osteoarthritis. Multiple studies demonstrate efficacy similar to NSAIDs, and the risk profile for side-effects is better than that of NSAIDs.

Joint lavage

Irrigation of osteoarthritic joints has been proposed as a method of relieving joint pain by removing debris or inflammatory cytokines, but remains controversial. Livesley compared arthroscopic irrigation with physical therapy and found that the arthroscopic group experienced significant improvement in pain that was sustained over 12 months. Ike and colleagues compared medical management plus joint lavage without arthroscopy with medical management alone in a multicentre, randomized prospective study: significant improvements in pain and stiffness occurred in the group receiving irrigation. Ravaud and colleagues evaluated the efficacy of joint lavage and intra-articular steroid injection in osteoarthritis of the knee. Patients who underwent joint lavage had improved significantly at 6 months; those only given corticosteroids had early improvement but no long-term benefit. Kalunian and colleagues studied the effectiveness of visually guided arthroscopic irrigation in early osteoarthritis of the knee unresponsive to conservative management. Patients received 3 litre or minimal (< 250 ml) arthroscopic irrigation, the former having an effect on pain as measured on two rating scales.

Surgery

Surgical intervention is generally reserved for patients who have failed conservative management including analgesics, physical therapy, and intra-articular injection. Prescribed treatments include synovectomy, repair of meniscal tears, realignment osteotomy, and total joint replacement. Total joint replacement removes the affected structure and is the only known 'cure' for osteoarthritis to date, providing marked pain relief and functional improvement.

Aids and appliances

A joint that is unstable and painful can be made more stable and less painful by appropriate aids. Wheelchairs and other appliances may make it possible for a patient to maintain their independence. Walking sticks can be very effective, and for a painful hip or knee should be held in the contralateral hand to transfer weight from the affected joint. If the main problem is instablility, the stick should be held in the hand that inspires most confidence. Splinting to correct instability, correction of valgus or varus deformity at the knee or ankle, use of a rocker sole to ease hallux rigidus pain, or a heel raise if the legs are of unequal length, can all allow significant reduction of symptoms, as can the simple recommendation of shoes with good shock-absorbing soles. These simple and apparently mundane issues should not be ignored by the physician.

Other therapies

Glucosamine and chondroitin sulphate

Many patients with osteoarthritis feel that glucosamine salts and chondroitin sulphate improve symptoms and there are abundant data to support these claims, but studies generally involve small numbers of subjects. There are, however, few data to suggest that these supplements repair cartilage damage.

Glucosamine, an aminomonosaccharide, is present in almost all human tissues, but particularly in articular cartilage where it is an intermediate substrate in the synthesis of glycosaminoglycan and proteoglycans. Exogenous glucosamine salts significantly enhance chondrocyte synthesis of glycosaminoglycans, collagen, and DNA. Both glucosamine hydrochloride and glucosamine sulphate are rapidly absorbed after oral administration and are not toxic, even at high oral doses.

Several double-blind studies have compared glucosamine to placebo for periods ranging from 5 to 38 weeks in patients with osteoarthritis of the knee, showing that glucosamine produces significant improvements in pain. Vaz found that glucosamine was as effective as ibuprofen in osteoarthritis of the knee: those receiving ibuprofen had greater initial improvement in pain than those randomized to receive glucosamine, but by 4 and 8 weeks the situation had reversed. Qie and colleagues compared glucosamine with ibuprofen in 178 subjects with osteoarthritis of the knee: both significantly reduced knee symptoms, but glucosamine was better tolerated. In a randomized, controlled, double-blind trial involving 329 patients with medial femerotibial osteoarthritis, Rovati and colleagues found that 3 months of glucosamine was more effective than standard NSAID therapy and placebo, and that the safety of glucosamine did not differ from placebo but was significantly better than NSAIDs.

Reginster and colleagues recently presented data regarding the chondroprotective effects of glucosamine sulphate. This randomized, double-blind, placebo-controlled study included 212 patients with osteoarthritis of the knee, who received either oral glucosamine sulphate 1500 mg/day or placebo. Weight-bearing anteroposterior radiographs of each knee were taken at enrolment, year 1, and year 3 and analysed for joint space narrowing: this progressed by 0.24 mm in the placebo-treated group, while the glucosamine-treated group had preservation of the joint space (–0.12 mm progression). The authors concluded that glucosamine sulphate may be a disease-modifying agent. Criticisms of the study include the use of traditional radiographs rather than fluoroscopically guided semiflexed views, which have better reliability in progression studies.

Chondroitin sulphate is a long-chain polymer of a repeating disaccharide. It is the predominant glycosaminoglycan found in articular cartilage and differs from glucosamine in that it stimulates glycosaminoglycan and proteoglycan synthesis by both extracellular and intracellular mechanisms, whereas glucosamine utilizes only intracellular mechanisms. By virtue of its long chains, chondroitin sulphate competitively inhibits enzymes that degrade proteoglycans, and this may be its mechanism of action, with increased availability of substrates for formation of articular matrix another possibility. It is 70 per cent absorbed after oral ingestion, with affinity for synovial fluid and articular cartilage.

In a randomized controlled trial comparing 3 months of treatment with chondroitin sulphate with placebo, the chondroitin sulphate group demonstrated significant reductions in clinical symptoms. Chondroitin sulphate has also been compared with NSAIDs in patients with osteoarthritis of the knee. In one study, patients treated with chondroitin sulphate had statistically significant decreases in pain by 3 months of therapy, with an overall 72 per cent decrease in concomitant usage of NSAIDs. In another study, patients treated with an NSAID showed prompt reduction in clinical symptoms that reappeared after discontinuation of the NSAID, whereas those given chondroitin sulphate had a therapeutic response that appeared later but lasted for up to 3 months after treatment was discontinued.

The combined use of glucosamine and chondroitin sulphate in the treatment of osteoarthritis has become popular: they have been reported to work synergistically in forming glycosaminoglycans, inhibiting degradative enzymes, and stimulating cartilage metabolism and matrix production. In a randomized double-blind placebo-controlled trial of 93 patients with osteoarthritis of the knee, subjects were randomized to receive glucosamine hydrochloride 1000 mg and chondroitin sulphate 800 mg twice daily orally or placebo. There was significantly greater improvement in the glucosamine and chondroitin sulphate treatment group compared with controls, with a significant drop in requirement for pain medication. A National Institutes of Health sponsored multicentre randomized study is under way comparing glucosamine, chondroitin sulphate, the combination of glucosamine and chondroitin sulphate, and placebo in patients with osteoarthritis of the knee: this will involve more than 1000 patients treated for 4 months.

Tetracyclines, interleukin 1 antagonists, and collagenase inhibitors

Tetracyclines have been demonstrated to inactivate matrix metalloproteinases such as collagenase, stromolysin, and gelatinase. Dog models using doxycycline reduce the incidence of osteoarthritis. A National Institutes of

Health sponsored multicentre randomized, placebo-controlled trial of doxycycline is under way.

Other agents demonstrating efficacy in osteoarthritis include use of diacerein and avocado/soybean extracts. Diacerin is an oral agent with analgesic properties, hypothesized to have an effect in osteoarthritis by inhibiting synthesis and activity of interleukin 1 and demonstrating cartilage preservation in an animal model. Human studies have demonstrated improvements in pain and function in hip osteoarthritis, as well as an NSAID-sparing effect. Similarly, avocado and soybean unsaponifiables are believed to exert their effects through interleukin 1. Clinical studies have demonstrated an NSAID-sparing effect and improvement in functional index and pain.

Ro 32–335 (Trocade) is an orally active collagenase inhibitor that has demonstrated chondroprotection by radiographic criteria in a mouse osteoarthritis model. Bay 12–9566 is a stromelysin-1 (MMP-3) inhibitor which demonstrated efficacy both dog and guinea pig meniscetomy models. Further studies of these compounds are needed. Future strategies for chondroprotection include manipulation of tumour necrosis factor, nitrous oxide, and insulin-like growth factor.

Further reading

Altman R *et al.* (1986). Development of criteria in the classification and reporting of osteoarthritis: classification of the knee. *Arthritis and Rheumatism* **29**, 1039–49.

Anderson J, Felson DT (1988). Factors associated with osteoarthritis of the knee in the First National Health and Nutrition Examination Survey (HANES 1). *American Journal of Epidemiology* **128**, 179–89.

Davis MA *et al.* (1988). Sex differences in osteoarthritis of the knee: the role of obesity. *American Journal of Epidemiology* **127**, 1019–30.

Drovanti A, Bignamini AA, Rovati AL (1980). Therapeutic activity of oral glucosamine sulfate in osteoarthritis: a placebo-controlled double-blind investigation. *Clinical Therapy* **3**, 260–72.

Ettinger WH Jr. *et al.* (1997). A randomized trial comparing aerobic exercise and resistance exercise with a health education program in older adults with knee osteoarthritis: the Fitness Arthritis and Seniors Trial (FAST). *Journal of the American Medical Association* **277**, 25–31.

Felson DT *et al.* (1991). Occupational physical demands, knee bending and knee osteoarthritis: results from the Framingham study. *Journal of Rheumatology* **18**, 1587–92.

Felson DT, Zhang Y (1998). An update on the epidemiology of knee and hip osteoarthritis with a view to prevention. *Arthritis and Rheumatism* **41**, 1343–55.

Felson DT *et al.* (1997). Risk factors for incident radiographic knee osteoarthritis in the elderly. *Arthritis and Rheumatism* **40**, 728–33.

Hannan MT *et al.* (1991). Occupational physical demands, knee bending and knee osteoarthritis: results from the Framingham Study. *Journal of Rheumatology* **18**, 1587–92.

Hart DJ, Spector TD (1993). The relationship of obesity, fat distribution and osteoarthritis in women in the general population. The Chingford Study. *Journal of Rheumatology* **20**, 331–5.

Kellgren JH, Lawrence JS (1957). Radiographic assessment of osteoarthritis. *Annals of Rheumatic Disease* **16**, 494–502.

Kelsey JL, Hochberg MC (1988). Epidemiology of chronic musculoskeletal disorders. *Annual Review of Public Health* **9**, 379–401.

Klashman D *et al.* (1996). Validation of nonradiographic ACR knee osteoarthritis classification criteria using arthroscopy damage index as the comparison standard (abstract). *Arthritis and Rheumatism* **39**, S172.

Kujala UM *et al.* (1995). Knee osteoarthritis in former runners, soccer players, weight lifters and shooters. *Arthritis and Rheumatism* **38**, 539–46.

LaPlante MP (1988). *Data on disability from the National Health Interview Survey (1983-5). An InfoUse Report.* National Institute of Disability and Rehabilitation, Washington, DC.

Morreale P *et al.* (1996). Comparison of the antiinflammatory efficacy of chondroitin sulfate and diclofenac sodium in patients with knee osteoarthritis. *Journal of Rheumatology* **23**, 1385–91.

Oliveria SA *et al.* (1995). Incidence of symptomatic hand, hip and knee osteoarthritis among patients in a health maintenance organization, *Arthritis and Rheumatism* **38**, 1134–41.

Setnikar I, Pacinic MA, Revel L (1991). Antiarthritic effects of glucosamine sulfate studied on animal models. *Arzeimitte-Forshung* **41**, 542–5.

18.9 Crystal-related arthropathies

S. C. O'Reilly and M. Doherty

Table 1 Crystalline particles associated with joint disease

Intrinsic
Monosodium urate monohydrate
Calcium pyrophosphate dihydrate (monoclinic, triclinic)
Calcium phosphates
basic: hydroxyapatite, octacalcium phosphate, tricalcium phosphate
acidic: brushite, monetite
Calcium oxalate
Lipids
cholesterol
lipid liquid crystals
Charcot–Leyden (phospholipase) crystals
Cystine
Xanthine, hypoxanthine
Protein precipitates (e.g. cryoglobulins)
Extrinsic
Synthetic corticosteroids
Plant thorns (semicrystalloid cellulose), especially blackthorn, rose, dried palm fronds
Sea-urchin spines (crystalline calcium carbonate)
Methylmethacrylate

Introduction

Diversity and terminology

A large number of crystals have been associated with acute synovitis, chronic arthropathy, or periarticular syndromes (Table 1). In practice only monosodium urate monohydrate, calcium pyrophosphate dihydrate, and basic calcium phosphates (mainly hydroxyapatite) are commonly encountered.

The taxonomy of these conditions is not universally agreed. Difficulties arise from our poor understanding of pathogenesis, historical extrapolation from gout to other crystal-related conditions, and multiple terms for the same clinical syndrome. Possible relationships between crystals and disease are outlined in Fig. 1. A 'crystal deposition disease' is defined as a pathological condition associated with mineral deposits which contribute directly to the pathology. This is probably the situation for all manifestations of gout, for acute syndromes associated with calcium pyrophosphate dihydrate, and for acute apatite periarthritis. However, the role of non-urate crystals in chronic arthropathy is unclear and confounded by the following observations:

1. Most crystals lack disease specificity and occur in a variety of clinical settings, often unaccompanied by symptoms or other abnormality.
2. Crystal deposition may coexist with other rheumatic disease, most commonly osteoarthritis, and often follows rather than precedes articular damage.
3. Combined deposition of several crystal species is common ('mixed crystal deposition').

For descriptive purposes, confusion may be avoided by specifying the crystal, the site of involvement, and the clinical syndrome (for example, chronic urate olecranon bursitis, acute pyrophosphate arthritis of the knee).

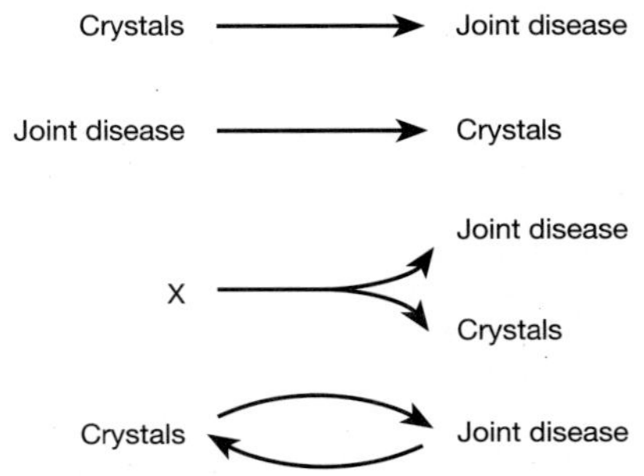

Fig. 1 Possible relationships between crystals and joint disease.

Crystal deposition and clearance

Many factors determine crystal formation and dissolution (Fig. 2). High solute concentrations alone are often insufficient to initiate crystal formation, and the presence of nucleating factors that aid initial particle formation and the balance of growth-promoting and inhibitory factors are probably more important. Little is known of such tissue factors, although they may in part explain:

(1) the characteristic, limited distribution of different crystals;

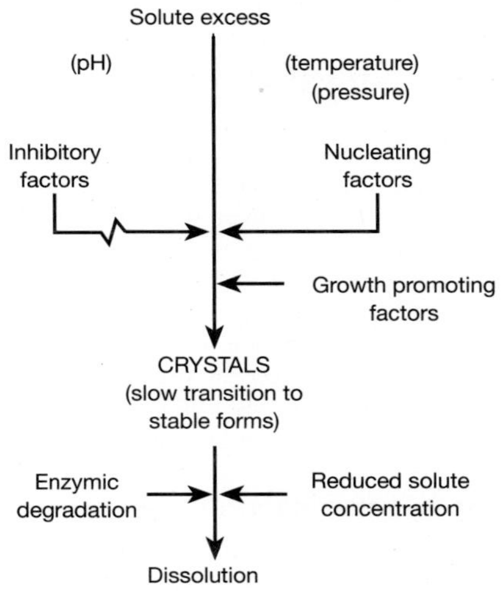

Fig. 2 Factors affecting crystal formation.

(2) the frequency of mixed crystal deposition (via epitaxial nucleation and growth of one crystal on another); and

(3) non-specific predisposition to crystal formation in osteoarthritic tissues (via accompanying alterations in proteoglycan, collagen, and lipid).

Formation of crystals *in vivo* is a dynamic process, although usually slow. At any time the crystal load will depend on the rate of formation, the rate of dissolution, and trafficking of crystals away from their site of formation (via 'shedding' from preformed deposits with secondary uptake by synovial and other cells).

Crystal-induced inflammation and tissue damage

Crystals implicated in joint disease are stable, hard particles that exert biological effects via surface-active and mechanical properties. With respect to acute inflammation, they are all markedly phlogistic agents in a wide range of *in vitro* and *in vivo* systems. Surface-active interaction has been demonstrated with:

(1) humoral mediators: for example complement activation via classical and alternative pathways; activation of Hageman factor;

(2) cell-derived mediators: for example superoxide production and release of lysozymes, chemotactic factor, and lipoxygenase-derived products of arachidonic acid by neutrophils; release of interleukin 1, interleukin 6, and tumour necrosis factor by monocytes and synoviocytes;

(3) cell membranes: for example membranolysis of lysosomes, erythrocytes, and neutrophils; non-lytic platelet and neutrophil secretory responses.

In general, monosodium urate monohydrate is the most inflammatory, followed by calcium pyrophosphate dihydrate, then apatite and the less common crystals. In general, smaller particle size, marked surface irregularity, and high negative surface charge correlate with inflammatory potential. Some surface effects result from direct crystal contact but others are mediated via adsorbed protein, particularly immunoglobulin. Although adsorbed IgG may enhance inflammation, most other protein binding is inhibitory.

Less is known of chronic crystal-induced tissue damage. Postulated effects include persistent synovial inflammation, altered cell metabolism, and deleterious mechanical effects from large deposits. Evidence for activation of inflammatory mediators in chronic crystal-associated synovitis is lacking, although a chronic 'granulomatous' reaction often occurs around large accretions. The physicochemical effects of hard highly charged crystals embedded within cartilage, or occurring as wear particles at the surface, are largely unknown.

Gout (see also Chapter 11.4)

Monosodium urate monohydrate crystals are undoubted causal agents in gout, usually depositing in previously normal tissues and eliciting acute inflammation and eventual tissue damage. Their effective removal halts progression and results in 'cure'. In these respects gout is a true 'crystal deposition disease'.

The incidence of gout varies in populations from 0.2 to 0.35 per 1000, with an overall prevalence of 2.0 to 2.6 per 1000. Prevalence rises with age and increasing serum urate concentration. There is strong predominance in men (about 10:1), particularly under 65 years of age. Untreated gout evolves slowly through four clinical phases: asymptomatic hyperuricaemia, acute gout, intercritical gout, and chronic tophaceous gout.

Asymptomatic hyperuricaemia

Monosodium urate monohydrate crystals preferentially deposit in peripheral connective tissues in and around synovial joints, favouring lower rather than upper limbs. Deposits occur first in articular cartilage, most commonly the first metatarsophalangeal and small joints of the feet. Deposits later develop in synovium, capsule, and periarticular soft tissues, with progressive involvement of more proximal sites. Monosodium urate monohydrate crystals probably take months if not years to grow *in vivo* to detectable size, implying a long asymptomatic phase. Absence of inflammation during this period may relate to low crystal yield, positioning within hypovascular tissues, or inhibitory protein coating. Around 95 per cent of hyperuricaemic subjects remain asymptomatic throughout life, although how many have occult monosodium urate monohydrate deposits is unknown. Of those who develop gout, one in five will have suffered renal colic due to uric acid urolithiasis, sometimes more than a decade earlier. The first presentation of gout is usually acute synovitis, although an insidious onset of chronic arthropathy or nodular deposits ('tophi') occasionally occurs without preceding attacks.

Acute attacks

The classical attack

In almost all initial episodes a single peripheral joint is involved. This is the first metatarsophalangeal joint ('podagra') in 50 per cent of first attacks and 70 per cent of all attacks. Other common sites are the knee, ankle, midtarsal joints, small hand joints, wrist, and elbow. The axial skeleton and large central joints are rarely involved and never as the first site.

Attacks often wake the patient in the early morning with localized irritation and aching. Within a few hours the joint and surrounding tissues are swollen, hot, red, shiny, and extremely painful. The patient cannot bear even bedclothes to touch the joint and it is often described as 'the worst pain ever experienced'. Inflammation is maximal within 24 h and is often associated with pyrexia and malaise. Examination reveals florid synovitis and swelling, extreme tenderness, and overlying erythema. If left untreated, the attack resolves spontaneously over 5 to 15 days, often with pruritus and desquamation of overlying skin.

Although many attacks occur spontaneously, certain situations encourage shedding of preformed monosodium urate monohydrate crystals and triggering of acute attacks. Suggested mechanisms include mechanical loosening (local trauma), partial dissolution and reduction of crystal size (initiation of hypouricaemic treatment), and local increase in cytokines which encourage inflammatory responses to crystals and facilitate crystal escape via alterations in cartilage matrix (intercurrent illness, surgery). Although some triggers (alcohol, dietary excess, diuretics) increase local urate levels, acute crystallization is considered unlikely.

Atypical attacks

Acute attacks may manifest as tenosynovitis, bursitis, or cellulitis. Many patients describe mild episodes of discomfort without swelling lasting a day or so. Ten per cent of all typical attacks involve more than one joint. Sometimes acute gout, by triggering the acute response, provokes migratory attacks in other joints over subsequent days ('cluster attacks'). Polyarticular attacks are rare, usually occurring after a long history of recurrent attacks: marked systemic upset, fever, and confusion may dominate the clinical picture.

Intercritical periods

These are asymptomatic intervals between attacks. Some patients never have a second attack, in others the next episode occurs after many years; in most, however, a second attack occurs within 1 year. Subsequently the frequency of attacks and number of sites involved gradually increase with time. Later attacks are more often pauciarticular or polyarticular and more severe. Eventually, recurrent attacks and continuing monosodium urate monohydrate deposition cause joint damage and chronic pain. The interval between the first attack and development of chronic symptoms is variable, but averages about 10 years. The principal determinant is the serum uric acid—the higher it is, the earlier and more extensive the development of joint damage and tophaceous deposits.

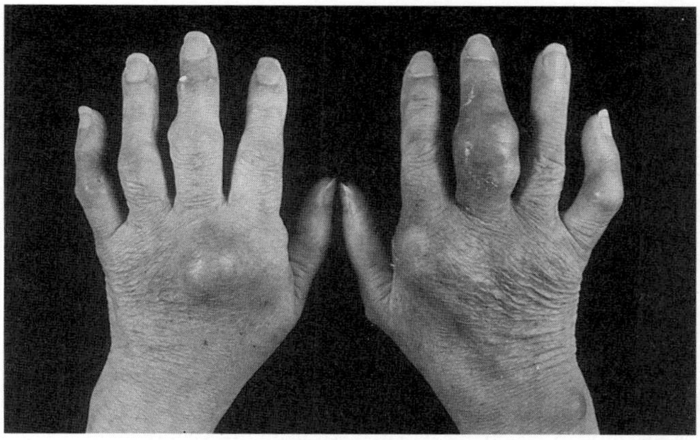

Fig. 3 Chronic tophaceous gout affecting the hands. Note the eccentric nature of the tophi and the asymmetry between sides.

Chronic tophaceous gout

Large crystal deposits ('tophi') produce irregular firm nodules, principally around extensor surfaces of fingers, hands, the ulnar surface of the forearms, olecranon bursae, Achilles tendons, first metatarsophalangeal joints, and the cartilaginous helix of the ear. Marked asymmetry, both locally and between sides, is particularly characteristic (Fig. 3). Monosodium urate monohydrate crystals beneath the skin may give a 'chalky' appearance (Fig. 4). If untreated, tophi can enlarge into gross knobbly swellings that may ulcerate, discharging material which is white and gritty and causes local inflammation (erythema, pus) even in the absence of secondary infection. If extensive, tophi may rarely involve the eyelids, tongue, larynx, or heart (causing conduction defects and valvular dysfunction).

Joints most commonly involved with signs of damage (restricted movement, crepitus, deformity) and varying degrees of synovitis are the first metatarsophalangeal joints, midfoot, small finger joints, and wrists. As with tophi, joint involvement is usually asymmetrical. Occasionally gross destruction may occur in feet and hands, and less commonly other sites. Acute attacks may become less of a feature as chronic symptoms become established. If untreated, the combination of extensive joint destruction and large tophi may cause grotesque deformities, particularly of hands and feet. Ankylosis is a rare late event. Although axial involvement is rare even in late stages, gouty involvement of hips, shoulders, spine and sacroiliac joints, and spinal cord compression by tophi, are all reported.

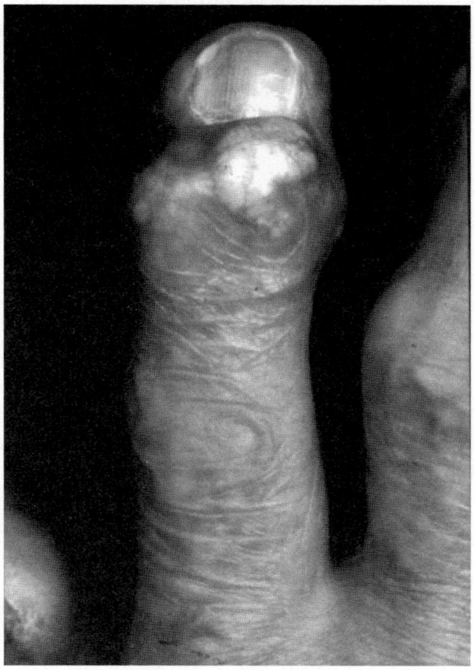

Fig. 4 Diuretic-induced gout in an elderly women, showing tophaceous deposition on pre-existing nodal osteoarthritis; the white monosodium urate monohydrate crystals are clearly visible beneath the skin.

Table 2 Comparison between primary and diuretic-induced gout

	Primary	Diuretic-induced
Sex	Male >> female	Male = female
Age	Middle aged	Elderly
Acute attacks	Common	Uncommon
Tophi	Develop late	Develop early
Associations	Obesity, hypertension, hyperlipidaemia, high alcohol intake	Renal impairment, osteoarthritis

Classification

Traditional classification into primary or secondary gout depends on defining predisposing factors for hyperuricaemia. Most gout is primary, strongly predominating in men, with initial onset between 30 and 60 years of age (Table 2). Presentation is with acute attacks, and untreated disease progresses to chronic tophaceous gout. Such patients often give a family history of gout and are 'undersecretors' of uric acid.

Secondary gout usually results from chronic diuretic therapy and presents in older subjects (over 65 years). This increasingly common form affects women and men and is often associated with osteoarthritis. Upper and lower limb joints are affected equally. Acute attacks are less prominent and presentation is often with painful, sometimes discharging, tophaceous deposits in Heberden's and Bouchard's nodes (Fig. 4).

Associations

Hyperuricaemia

Mechanisms resulting in decreased excretion or increased production of uric acid are fully discussed in Section 11.4. Though hyperuricaemia and gout are strongly linked, they are not synonymous. Most hyperuricaemic subjects never develop gout, emphasizing the importance of local tissue factors in crystal nucleation/growth, and gouty patients may not be hyperuricaemic at presentation. Associations also differ: for example, impaired glucose tolerance, ischaemic heart disease, and hypertension are common in men with gout but do not associate with hyperuricaemia *per se*. The majority (75–90 per cent) of patients with primary gout are 'undersecretors' of uric acid, having inherited an isolated renal lesion that reduces fractional urate clearance; fewer than 10 per cent are 'overproducers' of uric acid. The cause usually remains unclear, although a very few have an inherited purine enzyme defect (see Chapter 11.4). Some patients are both undersecretors and overproducers.

Clinical associations differ according to gender. In men important associations are obesity, excessive alcohol intake, type IV hyperlipoproteinaemia, impaired glucose tolerance, and ischaemic heart disease (Table 3). Obesity and lifestyle, rather than hereditary factors, appear to be central factors linking these 'associations of plenty'. Excessive beer drinking, with its high calorie and alcohol intake, is a common form of alcohol abuse associated with gout. The nineteenth century association with port is partly explained by addition of lead to sweeten the port: lead inhibits uric acid excretion and also promotes nucleation of monosodium urate monohydrate, predisposing to 'the gout, the colic and the palsy' (all features of lead poisoning). However, 'saturnine' gout still occurs in individuals who drink alcohol distilled or stored in lead-contaminated containers ('moonshine'). Alcohol is a less common association in women, usually occurring

Table 3 Clinical associations of gout

Clinical association	Screening test
Obesity (common)	
Alcohol intake (beer) (common)	Liver function test
Diuretic therapy (common)	
Low-dose aspirin, cyclosporin (less common)	
Hypertension (common)	Blood pressure monitoring
Type IV hyperlipidaemia (common)	Fasting lipid
Chronic renal failure	U&Es
Myeloproliferative disorders (rare)	FBC, ESR
Lead poisoning (rare)	

Abbreviations: U&Es, urea and electrolytes; FBC, full blood count; ESR, erythrocyte sedimentation rate.

in young to middle-aged, thin, spirit drinkers. In women the main associations are diuretic therapy, chronic renal impairment, and pre-existing osteoarthritis. Other drugs may predispose to gout, such as aspirin in low doses and cyclosporin.

A strong negative association exists between gout and rheumatoid arthritis. This remains unexplained, but probably reflects impaired nucleation/growth of monosodium urate monohydrate crystals rather than masking of monosodium urate monohydrate crystal-induced inflammation (for example, by crystal coating with rheumatoid factors).

Renal disease

Urolithiasis (see also Chapter 20.13)

Uric acid stones account for 5 to 10 per cent of all stones in the United Kingdom and United States, and up to 40 per cent in Israel. A history of renal colic is seen in 10 to 25 per cent of patients with gout, the important aetiological factors being low urinary pH, low urinary volume, and high urinary uric acid concentration. In particular, high urinary concentrations occur in overproducers of uric acid, if renal urate clearance is increased (uricosuric drugs, defects in tubular reabsorption), and in situations of dehydration with lowering of urinary pH (diarrhoea, ileostomy). Gouty subjects also have an increased incidence of calcium-containing stones, particularly calcium oxalate, with no detectable uric acid nidus.

Acute uric acid nephropathy describes rapid precipitation of uric acid crystals in renal collecting ducts with secondary acute obstructive renal failure. This event correlates with the amount of uric acid excreted rather than the level of hyperuricaemia. Strongly acid urine, which reduces uric acid solubility, potentiates the problem. The condition is most likely in ill, dehydrated patients with lymphoma or malignancy subjected to aggressive chemotherapy without adequate prophylactic treatment with allopurinol. It also occurs in gouty patients with markedly accelerated purine synthesis, for example following excessive exercise or after epileptic seizures. The condition is largely avoidable by appropriate hydration, urine alkalinization, and allopurinol prophylaxis.

Chronic urate nephropathy (see also Section 20.10)

Widespread monosodium urate monohydrate deposition in the interstitium of the medulla and pyramids results in crystal-induced inflammation with surrounding giant-cell reaction and fibrosis, affecting in particular the tubular epithelium of the loop of Henle and juxtaposed interstitial tissues. Subsequent changes include glomerular hyalinization and hypertrophy of the intima and media of arterioles. Hypertensive damage, tubular obstruction, and secondary pyelonephritis may all complicate this picture. Albuminuria and inability to concentrate the urine maximally are early clinical manifestations. Progressive renal disease is an important complication of untreated chronic tophaceous gout, end stage renal failure occurring in up to 25 per cent of cases.

In advanced renal disease of any cause, calcium oxalate or phosphate crystals may deposit in renal parenchyma but are predominantly cortical in location (compare the medullary site of monosodium urate monohydrate).

The association between parenchymal disease and less severe gout remains controversial, being confounded in males by frequent accompanying obesity, hypertension, and drug therapy. The minor progression of renal insufficiency that occurs in most gouty patients, however, is probably largely age-related and life expectancy is not reduced.

Investigations and diagnosis

The history and signs of classical acute or chronic tophaceous gout are highly characteristic, and with a raised serum uric acid a strong presumptive diagnosis is readily made. However, definitive confirmation requires demonstration of monosodium urate monohydrate crystals by compensated polarized light microscopy of fluid from a gouty joint, bursa, or tophus. Synovial fluid in acute attacks is typically turbid with diminished viscosity and greatly elevated cell count (more than 90 per cent neutrophils). Chronic gouty fluid is more variable, but occasionally appears white due to the high crystal load. Only a few drops collected directly on to a slide are required for crystal identification (Chapter 18.3). Monosodium urate monohydrate crystals are seen readily as strongly birefringent (negative sign), needle-shaped crystals, 5 to 20 μm in length, within cells or occurring freely in fluid. In tophaceous material they occur as dense, tightly packed sheets. During intercritical periods, aspiration of an asymptomatic first metatarsophalangeal joint or knee often permits confirmation of the diagnosis by revealing monosodium urate monohydrate crystals.

Hyperuricaemia is confirmed if two or more fasting serum uric acid levels exceed the normal range for the patient's age and sex. Uric acid levels may be lowered during an acute attack of gout and should be remeasured during an intercritical period. In primary gout in a young patient, determination of undersecretion or overproduction of uric acid is best undertaken by measuring total urinary excretion on a low-purine diet, but a quick guide is given by the uric acid/creatinine ratio estimated on a single urine sample (normally less than 0.5). In young overproducers, a purine enzyme defect becomes more likely and should be sought (Chapter 11.4). Assessment of renal function (creatinine, urea, electrolytes, urine testing) should always be undertaken (Table 3). Measurement of fasting lipoprotein concentrations should be made in all patients with primary gout. An intercritical full blood count and measurement of erythrocyte sedimentation rate/viscosity should detect any underlying myeloproliferative disease. During acute attacks a marked acute phase response (high erythrocyte sedimentation rate, neutrophil leucocytosis, thrombocytosis, elevated C-reactive protein) is usual; modest elevations of erythrocyte sedimentation rate also accompany chronic gout.

Radiographs supplement the clinical assessment of structural damage but can also aid diagnosis. In early disease they are usually normal. During acute gout, non-specific soft tissue swelling (rarely juxta-articular osteopenia) may be evident. After repeated attacks, and in chronic disease, joint space narrowing, sclerosis, cysts, and osteophytes (that is, the changes of osteoarthritis) become more frequent in feet and hands. Gouty 'erosions' are a less common but more specific abnormality, occurring as para-articular 'punched-out' bone defects with well-demarcated sclerotic margins, overhanging hooks of bone, and retained bone density (Fig. 5). They are typically asymmetric, eccentric lesions positioned away from the 'bare area' of the joint, contrasting with more symmetrical, ill-defined marginal erosions (with osteopenia) of rheumatoid arthritis. Tophi appear as eccentric soft tissue swellings, occasionally with patchy calcification due to epitaxial growth of apatite. In late disease, severe destructive change with osteopenia may occur and distinction from rheumatoid arthritis or other conditions becomes more difficult.

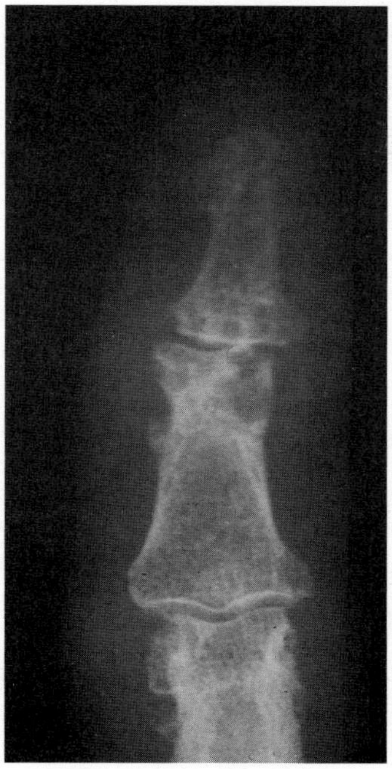

Fig. 5 Characteristic radiographic changes of established gout in a finger: joint space loss and cystic change at the distal interphalangeal joint, 'pressure erosions' with overhanging bony 'hooks' at both interphalangeal joints, and eccentric soft tissue swelling at the proximal joint.

Differential diagnosis

Acute attacks

Sepsis and other crystal-associated synovitis are the main considerations. Gout and sepsis may coexist, as may monosodium urate monohydrate and calcium pyrophosphate dihydrate deposition (particularly in elderly subjects). Examination of aspirated fluid for both crystals and sepsis (Gram stain, culture) is the only sure way of obtaining the correct diagnosis. A wider search for sepsis may be indicated (for example blood and urine cultures), particularly in those who are ill. With less classic attacks, other conditions that may be considered include psoriatic and acute Reiter's arthropathy, acute sarcoid arthropathy, traumatic arthritis, palindromic rheumatism, and exacerbation of osteoarthritis.

Chronic tophaceous gout

Other causes of arthritis and periarticular swellings/nodules that require differentiation are rheumatoid arthritis, generalized nodal osteoarthritis, xanthomatosis with arthropathy, and multicentric reticulohistiocytosis. Gout is usually less symmetrical in distribution than these conditions and, except for xanthomatosis, acute attacks are not a feature. Nodal osteoarthritis, of course, may coexist with gout. Aspiration (joint fluid, nodules) and plain radiographs readily facilitate correct diagnosis.

Treatment

Acute gout

The treatment aim is pain relief by reducing inflammation and intra-articular hypertension. Alteration of uric acid levels is avoided until the attack has resolved, since initiation of hypouricaemic drugs may prolong the attack.

Rapid symptom relief may be obtained with a quick-acting non-steroidal anti-inflammatory drug (**NSAID**), given in full dosage. Although indomethacin has a long tradition in this context, it is preferably avoided in the elderly due to its frequent renal, gut, and nervous system side-effects.

Oral colchicine is rapidly effective within a few hours (1 mg immediately, followed by 0.5 mg every 6 h until symptoms abate). Unfortunately, at the doses necessary, diarrhoea, nausea, and abdominal cramps are common, causing the patient 'to run before he can walk'. Colchicine, however, is a useful alternative if NSAIDs are contraindicated. Intravenous colchicine, however, is particularly toxic and should never be used. Although previously used as a 'diagnostic test' the efficacy of colchicine is not specific to gout: it also ameliorates other crystal-associated syndromes.

Joint aspiration often provides immediate relief by reducing intra-articular hypertension. Intra-articular steroid is useful for large joints such as the knee, or when NSAIDs or colchicine are contraindicated or unsuccessful. In difficult cases, joint lavage may terminate an attack, and for troublesome polyarticular attacks there is support for the use of parenteral steroid.

Long-term management

Once any acute attack has resolved, long-term strategies need consideration. Gout is potentially curable. Treatment may involve:

(1) considering and eliminating modifiable factors that cause hyperuricaemia; and

(2) utilizing hypouricaemic drugs.

Management of gout may require alteration in lifestyle and chronic medication: patient compliance and motivation, which depend on appropriate education and counselling, are essential for success.

Modification of provoking factors

In early primary gout, gradual weight loss, reduction in alcohol consumption, and avoidance of toxins (low-dose aspirin, lead) may alone be sufficient. Similarly, in diuretic-induced gout, stopping the diuretic (plus substitution of alternative therapies) may prove possible and be all that is required.

Hypouricaemic drug therapy

Indications for drug therapy are:

(1) recurrent, troublesome acute attacks;

(2) presence of tophi;

(3) bone or cartilage damage;

(4) coexistent renal disease, uric acid urolithiasis;

(5) very high uric acid levels (particularly with overproduction and hyperexcretion).

The logical approach would be allopurinol for overproducers and uricosurics for undersecretors. In practice, however, allopurinol is the usual drug of choice, permitting flexible tailoring of dose to reduce urate levels below the solubility limit. Allopurinol inhibits xanthine oxidase and often also depresses *de novo* purine synthesis. The starting dose is 100 to 300 mg daily, which is then adjusted within the range 100 to 900 mg daily according to the serum uric acid level (initially checked monthly). In patients with renal insufficiency, particularly the elderly, excretion of the active metabolite oxypurinol is delayed: the starting dose should therefore be 100 mg daily and adjustments made cautiously.

The uricosurics probenecid (0.5–1.0 g twice a day) and sulphinpyrazone (100 mg three or four times daily), which prevent proximal tubular reabsorption of urate, are rarely used. Benzbromarone, a newer uricosuric, is now increasingly used in parts of Europe. Uricosurics are alternatives to allopurinol in patients with normal renal function but are contraindicated in those with renal impairment, urolithiasis, or gross overproduction of uric acid. The therapeutic aim of hypouricaemic therapy is to maintain the serum uric acid well within the normal range (preferably the lower half). Treatment should be lifelong.

Acute attacks may be provoked during the first few months of hypouricaemic treatment. Prophylactic colchicine (0.5 mg twice a day) or a standard dose of NSAID given for the first 2 to 3 months of treatment largely avoids 'breakthrough' attacks. With any uricosuric, high fluid intake and urine alkalinization in the early weeks of treatment are recommended to avoid deposition of uric acid within the kidney.

Serious side-effects are unusual with any hypouricaemic drugs. Rare problems include toxic epidermal necrolysis, interstitial nephritis and vasculitis (allopurinol), nephrotic syndrome (probenecid), and hepatitis and marrow suppression (both drugs). Important interactions with allopurinol occur with coumarin anticoagulants (due to hepatic microsomal enzyme inhibition) and purine analogues (such as azathioprine) which are inactivated by xanthine oxidase. Associated hypertension should be treated, but preferably not with diuretics which elevate serum urate and may provoke acute attacks.

Pyrophosphate arthropathy

Deposition of calcium pyrophosphate dihydrate crystals ($Ca_2P_2O_7.2H_2O$) in articular cartilage is a common age-related phenomenon. Calcium pyrophosphate dihydrate crystals preferentially deposit within fibrocartilage and are the most common cause of cartilage calcification (chondrocalcinosis).

Calcium pyrophosphate dihydrate deposition may occur in otherwise normal cartilage or associate with structural change and clinical arthropathy—'pyrophosphate arthropathy'. A causal role for calcium pyrophosphate dihydrate crystals in acute inflammation is accepted, but their role in chronic arthropathy is unclear. The strong association/overlap with osteoarthritis has led some to consider pyrophosphate arthropathy not as a crystal deposition disease but as a 'subset' of osteoarthritis, with calcium pyrophosphate dihydrate a 'process' marker associating with a hypertrophic articular response.

Radiographic chondrocalcinosis is rare under 50 years of age, but its prevalence rises from 10 to 15 per cent in those aged 65 to 75, to 30 to 60 per cent in those over 85, showing female preponderance (relative risk 1.33) and association with osteoarthritis (relative risk 1.52 at the knee). No epidemiological data exist for pyrophosphate arthropathy, but in patient series the mean age of presentation is around 65 to 75 with female preponderance (about 2:1 to 3:1), particularly in older patients.

Clinical features

Common presentations are acute synovitis, chronic arthritis, or as an incidental finding. Other presentations are rare.

Acute synovitis ('pseudogout')

This is the most common cause of acute monoarthritis in the elderly. Attacks may occur as isolated events or be superimposed upon a background of chronic symptomatic arthropathy. Most attacks occur spontaneously, but provoking factors include intercurrent illness, surgery, and local trauma. Although any joint may be involved, the knee is by far the most common site, followed by the wrist, shoulder, and ankle. Concurrent attacks in several joints are uncommon (fewer than 10 per cent of cases) and polyarticular attacks rare.

The typical attack develops rapidly with severe pain, stiffness, and swelling, becoming maximal within 6 to 24 h of onset. Examination reveals a very tender joint with signs of florid synovitis (increased warmth, tense effusion, restricted movement with stress pain) and often overlying erythema. Fever is common and elderly patients may appear unwell or mildly confused. Attacks are self-limiting, usually resolving within 1 to 3 weeks.

Chronic pyrophosphate arthropathy

This common condition affects mainly elderly women and targets the same large and medium-sized joints as pseudogout. Knees are the usual and most severely affected joint. Presentation is with chronic pain, stiffness, and functional impairment (plus superimposed acute attacks). Symptoms usually relate to just a few joints, although examination often reveals more widespread abnormalities. Affected joints show signs of osteoarthritis (crepitus, bony swelling, restricted movement) with varying degrees of synovitis (often most marked at the knee, radiocarpal, or glenohumeral joint). Knees typically show abnormality of two or three compartments; valgus or varus deformity may occur.

Although symptoms and signs are those of osteoarthritis, chronic pyrophosphate arthropathy may often be distinguished from uncomplicated osteoarthritis by:

(1) the joint distribution: in osteoarthritis wrist, glenohumeral, ankle, elbow, and midtarsal involvement are uncommon;

(2) the often marked inflammatory component; and

(3) superimposition of acute attacks.

The outcome for chronic pyrophosphate arthropathy is generally good, most patients running a relatively benign course, particularly with respect to small and medium-sized joints. If progression occurs, it is usually slow and related to knees, hips, or shoulders. Occasionally severe, rapidly progressive, destructive arthropathy develops at these sites. This is virtually confined to very elderly women and is associated with severe pain, recurrent haemarthrosis (shoulder, knee), and occasional joint leakage.

Incidental finding

As with osteoarthritis, clinical or radiographic evidence of pyrophosphate arthropathy and chondrocalcinosis are not uncommon incidental findings in the elderly, and may confound the cause of regional pain if a through history and examination are not undertaken.

Uncommon presentations

Acute tendinitis (triceps, Achilles), tenosynovitis (hand flexors, extensors), and bursitis (olecranon, infrapatellar, retrocalcaneal) occur uncommonly, usually in patients with widespread calcium pyrophosphate dihydrate crystals. Median and ulnar nerve compression at the wrist may accompany flexor tenosynovitis. Rare tophaceous deposits of calcium pyrophosphate dihydrate usually present as solitary lesions in areas of chondroid metaplasia.

Classification and associations

Calcium pyrophosphate dihydrate deposition is traditionally classified as:

(1) hereditary;

(2) associated with metabolic disease; or

(3) sporadic/idiopathic (by far the commonest, associated with osteoarthritis).

Familial predisposition

This is reported from many countries and different ethnic groups. Two clinical phenotypes occur: early onset (third to fourth decade) florid polyarticular chondrocalcinosis with variable severity of accompanying arthropathy; and late onset (sixth to seventh decade) oligoarticular chondrocalcinosis (mainly knee) with arthritis resembling sporadic disease. The pattern of inheritance varies, although autosomal dominance is usual. Studies on several families have suggested the short arm of chromosome 5 as a potential site for a candidate gene. The mechanism of familial predisposition remains unclear and may differ between families. A primary cartilage abnormality that promotes calcium pyrophosphate dihydrate crystal nucleation and growth (Swedish and Japanese families), and a generalized abnormality of pyrophosphate metabolism resulting in a local increase in cartilage levels (French and American kindreds) have both been reported.

Metabolic disease associations

Inorganic pyrophosphate is a byproduct of many biosynthetic reactions, with a turnover of several kilograms per day. Much extracellular inorganic pyrophosphate derives from ATP via the action of NTP pyrophosphatase, and is rapidly converted to orthophosphate by pyrophosphatases (particularly alkaline phosphatase) (Fig. 6). A number of metabolic diseases associate with deposition of calcium pyrophosphate dihydrate (Table 4), their

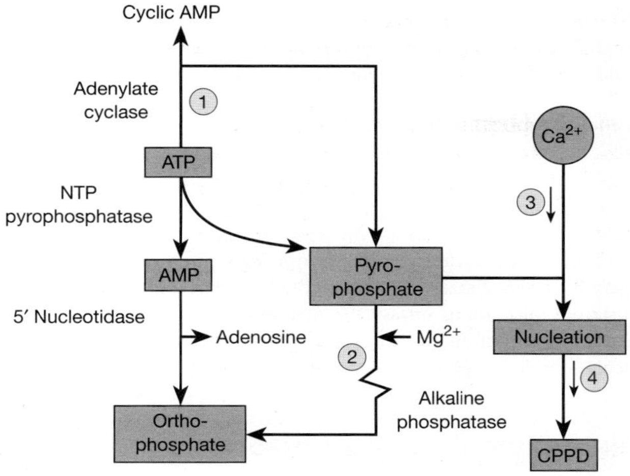

Fig. 6 Simplified scheme of extracellular pyrophosphate metabolism, showing putative sites of interaction by metabolic diseases. Hyperparathyroidism, 1, 2, 3; haemochromatosis, 2, 4; hypophosphatasia, 2; Wilson's disease, 2, 4; and hypomagnesaemia, 2. CPPD, calcium pyrophosphate dihydrate; NTP, nucleotide triphosphate

association being rationalized through putative effects on metabolism of inorganic pyrophosphate. Suggested mechanisms include:

1. Reduced breakdown of inorganic pyrophosphate by alkaline phosphatase, due to (i) reduced levels, (ii) inhibitory ions (calcium, iron, copper), or (iii) impaired complexing with magnesium.
2. Enhanced nucleation by iron or copper.
3. Increased calcium concentration.
4. Increased production of pyrophosphate through stimulation of adenylate cyclase by parathyroid hormone.

Osteoarthritis and joint insult

Several observations support a relationship between osteoarthntis and deposition of calcium pyrophosphate dihydrate, the latter often following rather than preceding joint damage. However, a negative association exists between deposition of calcium pyrophosphate dihydrate and rheumatoid arthritis, with atypical radiographic features in coexistent disease (retained bone density; marked osteophyte, cyst, and bone remodelling) suggesting that the primary association of calcium pyrophosphate dihydrate is with hypertrophic tissue response/osteoarthritis and not joint damage *per se*. The explanation for this association is unknown. Levels of inorganic pyrophosphate in the synovial fluid are increased in pyrophosphate arthropathy and osteoarthritis and are low in rheumatoid arthritis, but the order of change is unlikely to influence formation of calcium pyrophosphate dihydrate significantly. These crystals form in pericellular sites and associate with lipid, proteoglycan depletion, and adjacent hypertrophic chondrocytes containing lipid granules. It is therefore possible that reduction of inhibitors (such as proteoglycan) and increase in promotors (such as lipid) may combine to copromote calcium pyrophosphate dihydrate formation in metabolically active osteoarthritic tissue.

Table 4 Metabolic diseases associated with calcium pyrophosphate dihydrate (CPPD) crystal deposition

	Chondro-calcinosis	Pseudo-gout	Chronic CPPD arthropathy
Definite associations:			
Hyperparathyroidism	+	+	–
Haemochromatosis	+	+	+
Hypophosphatasia	+	+	–
Hypomagnesaemia	+	+	–
Possible associations:			
Hypothyroidism	+	–	–
Gout	+	+	–
X-linked hypophosphataemic rickets	+	+	+
Familial hypocalciuric hypercalcaemia	+	–	–
Wilson's disease	+	–	–
Ochronosis	+	–	–
Acromegaly	+	–	–

Investigations and diagnosis

Critical investigations are synovial fluid analysis and plain radiographs. In pseudogout aspirated fluid is often turbid or bloodstained with an elevated cell count (more than 90 per cent neutrophils). Compensated polarized microscopy reveals calcium pyrophosphate dihydrate crystals as weakly birefringent (positive sign) rhomboids or rods, about 2 to 10 μm long. Calcium pyrophosphate dihydrate crystals are less readily identified and often less numerous than those of monosodium urate monohydrate; examination of a spun deposit may increase detection.

Radiographic aspects relate both to calcification and arthropathy. Chondrocalcinosis signifies extensive deposition and is not always evident: it mainly affects fibrocartilage (particularly knee menisci, wrist triangular cartilage, symphysis pubis), and less commonly hyaline cartilage (Fig. 7). Although occasionally monoarticular, it usually affects several sites. Calcification of capsule, synovium, and tendons is less common. Chondrocalcinosis and calcification may increase or decrease with time, diminishing chondrocalcinosis often accompanying crystal 'shedding' or cartilage loss.

Changes of arthropathy are those of osteoarthritis: cartilage loss, sclerosis, cysts, and osteophyte. However, characteristics which suggest pyrophosphate include:

(1) distribution between and within joints that is atypical of osteoarthritis (for example glenohumeral disease; isolated or predominant patellofemoral or radiocarpal involvement);

(2) prominence of osteophytes and cysts; and

(3) prominent osteochondral bodies.

Such combined features may present a distinctive 'hypertrophic' appearance even in the absence of chondrocalcinosis (Fig. 8). In destructive arthropathy, marked cartilage and bone attrition with fragmentation and loose osseous bodies may resemble a Charcot joint.

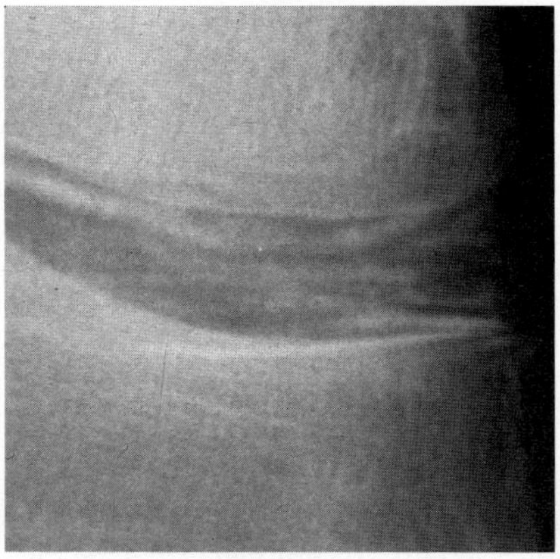

Fig. 7 Radiographic chondrocalcinosis of the knee, affecting meniscal fibrocartilage (central, triangular) and hyaline cartilage (linear, parallel to bone).

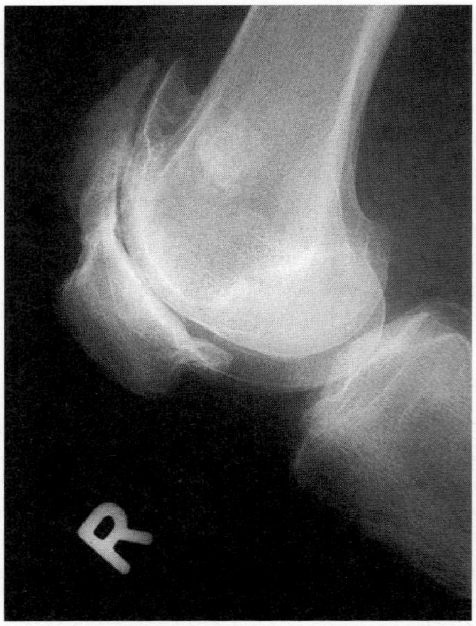

Fig. 8 Lateral knee radiograph showing predominant patellofemoral involvement by 'hypertrophic' osteoarthritis characteristic of pyrophosphate arthropathy.

Metabolic predisposition is rare and routine screening of all patients is unrewarding. Nevertheless, arthritis associated with calcium pyrophosphate dihydrate crystals may be the presenting feature of metabolic disease, and a search is warranted in the following circumstances:

(1) early onset arthritis (under 55 years)

(2) florid polyarticular chondrocalcinosis; or

(3) presence of additional clinical or radiographic clues.

A reasonable screen would include serum calcium, alkaline phosphatase, magnesium, ferritin, and liver function.

Differential diagnosis

The principal differential diagnosis for pseudogout is sepsis or gout, both of which may coexist with calcium pyrophosphate dihydrate deposition. Gram stain and culture of joint fluid should be undertaken even when calcium pyrophosphate dihydrate (and monosodium urate monohydrate) crystals are identified. Marked bloodstaining may lead to consideration of other causes of haemarthrosis, especially a bleeding disorder or subchondral fracture.

Chronic pyrophosphate arthropathy is usually readily distinguished from rheumatoid arthritis by the synovial fluid and radiographic findings, the infrequency of severe systemic upset, absence of extra-articular features, and an acute phase response which is only modest. Proximal stiffness due to glenohumeral involvement may suggest polymyalgia rheumatica, although clinical examination and near normal erythrocyte sedimentation rate should exclude the diagnosis. Destructive pyrophosphate arthropathy may simulate a neuropathic joint, although such joints are severely symptomatic and neurological abnormality is absent.

Treatment

Pseudogout

Since pseudogout usually affects only one or a few joints in elderly patients, local therapy is preferred. Aspiration alone often relieves symptoms, but may be combined with intra-articular steroid in florid cases. Simple analgesics and NSAIDs give additional benefit but should be used cautiously in the elderly. Joint lavage is reserved for troublesome steroid-resistant cases. Colchicine is effective but rarely warranted. Triggering illness (for example chest infection) will require appropriate treatment. Rapid mobilization should be instituted once the synovitis is settling.

Chronic pyrophosphate arthropathy

Unlike gout there is no specific therapy, and treatment of any underlying metabolic disease does not influence outcome. Aims are to reduce symptoms and maintain or improve function. This may include education of the patient in appropriate use of the affected joints, reduction in obesity, improvement of muscle strength, use of a stick or other walking aid, and surgery for severe disease. Chronic synovitis may be improved by intermittent steroid injection or intra-articular radiocolloid (yttrium-90). As with pseudogout, symptomatic drugs are to be used with caution in older patients; simple analgesics are generally preferable to NSAIDs.

Other crystal-related disorders

Apatite-associated syndromes

Hydroxyapatite is the principal bone mineral. Apatites or basic calcium phosphates (partially carbonate-substituted hydroxyapatite, octacalcium phosphate, rarely tricalcium phosphate) are also the usual mineral to deposit in extraskeletal tissues (for example tuberculous lesions, arteries).

The [calcium × phosphate] product must be kept high to maintain skeletal integrity. Specific cellular mechanisms activate calcification where appropriate (for example matrix vesicles in growing cartilage), whilst other mechanisms (such as pyrophosphate and aggregated proteoglycan) inhibit calcification elsewhere. In general, abnormal calcification results from:

(1) elevation of the [calcium × phosphate] product, causing widespread 'metastatic' calcification, or

(2) alteration in the balance between inhibitory and promoting tissue factors, resulting in local 'dystrophic' calcification.

In rheumatic diseases abnormal deposition of basic calcium phosphates may occur in:

(1) periarticular tissues (particularly tendon);

(2) hyaline cartilage, in association with osteoarthritis; or

(3) subcutaneous tissues and muscle, principally in connective tissue diseases.

Apatite crystals are too small (5–500 nm) to be seen by light microscopy. Particles may aggregate, however, to form spherulites visible with the light microscope. Confirmation of basic calcium phosphates requires sophisticated analytical techniques and most clinical diagnoses are presumptive, based on radiographic calcification or non-specific staining of joint fluid or histological material.

Acute calcific periarthritis

Apatite deposition in the supraspinatus tendon (Fig. 9) is a relatively common incidental finding (about 7 per cent of adults). It occasionally results in severe acute inflammation of the subacromial bursa, periarticular tissues, or joint itself. Periarticular sites around the greater hip trochanter, the foot, or the hand are less commonly affected.

Acute episodes may follow local trauma or occur spontaneously. Within a few hours pain and tenderness are often extreme and the area appears swollen, hot, and red. Modest systemic upset and fever are common. Sepsis is usually considered first, but the diagnosis is made following demonstration of radiographic calcification. If the lesion is aspirated, thick white fluid containing many apatite aggregates may be obtained. The condition usually resolves spontaneously over 1 to 3 weeks, often accompanied by radiographic dispersal of modestly sized calcifications (crystal 'shedding'). NSAIDs ameliorate symptoms and the attack can be abbreviated by aspiration and injection of steroid. Large deposits may require surgical removal. Calcific periarthritis rarely results from metabolic abnormality (renal failure, hyperparathyroidism, hypophosphatasia) and measurements of serum

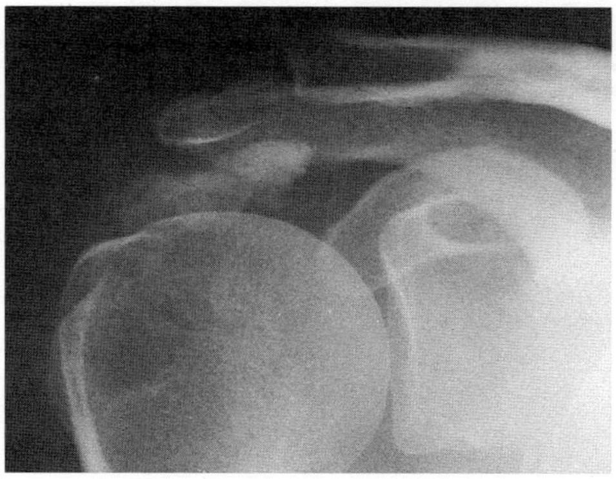

Fig. 9 Shoulder radiograph showing florid supraspinatus tendon calcification (calcific periarthritis).

calcium, alkaline phosphatase, and creatinine are usually normal. Rare families are predisposed to calcific periarthritis at multiple sites with no evidence of altered calcium phosphate product.

Osteoarthritis and apatite-associated destructive arthritis

Modest amounts of basic calcium phosphates are commonly found in synovial fluid from osteoarthritic joints, in isolation or with calcium pyrophosphate dihydrate ('mixed crystal deposition'). Whether apatite plays any part in inflammatory exacerbations or associates with severity or progression of osteoarthritis remains uncertain.

The uncommon condition 'apatite-associated destructive arthritis' is often considered a 'subset' of osteoarthritis. It is virtually confined to elderly women and affects the hip, shoulder ('Milwaukee shoulder'), or knee. It has the general appearance of severe large joint osteoarthritis but is particularly characterized by:

(1) rapid progression, often leading to severe pain and disability within a few months of onset;

(2) development of marked instability;

(3) large, cool effusions;

(4) an atrophic radiographic appearance with marked cartilage and bone attrition and little osteophyte or bone remodelling.

Aspirated fluid has normal viscosity and a low cell count but contains large amounts of apatite aggregates, seen readily on light microscopy following non-specific calcium staining (alizarin red, acidic pH). The differential diagnosis may include sepsis (excluded by synovial fluid culture), late avascular necrosis, or neuropathic joint. The pathogenesis of this condition remains unclear. Although apatite particles could contribute to tissue damage by stimulating release of collagenase and other proteolytic enzymes from synovial cells, it is most likely that the apatite is non-contributory and principally reflects the severity of subchondral bone attrition. The outcome is poor and inevitably requires surgical intervention.

Other apatite syndromes

Deposition of tophaceous periarticular apatite may occur in patients with chronic renal failure managed by dialysis. Apatite has also been incriminated in the occasional erosive interphalangeal arthropathy seen in such patients.

Other crystals

Cholesterol

Cholesterol crystals may induce acute synovitis, acute tenosynovitis, and chronic xanthomatous tendinitis in hypercholesterolaemic subjects. Cholesterol and other lipid crystals may also occur as a non-specific finding in chronic synovitis, most commonly due to rheumatoid arthritis. In this situation the lipid probably derives from cellular debris and its pathogenic significance is uncertain.

Oxalate

Oxalate crystals have been incriminated in acute and chronic articular and periarticular syndromes occurring in association with either primary familial oxalosis (types I and II) or secondary oxalosis (Chapter 11.10). Chronic renal failure managed with dialysis is the commonest cause of secondary oxalosis, particularly if ascorbic acid supplementation has been given. Acute symmetrical interphalangeal and metacarpophalangeal arthritis, with or without tenosynovitis, and digital calcific deposits are the usual manifestation. Large joint involvement, chondrocalcinosis, and tophaceous periarticular masses are less common. Calcium oxalate crystals may also cause life-threatening organ involvement, with peripheral vascular insufficiency and digital necrosis, cardiomyopathy, peripheral neuropathy, and aplastic anaemia. There is no effective treatment.

Extrinsic crystals

These are a rare cause of locomotor problems. Acute flares following intra-articular injection of corticosteroids are uncommon but may represent iatrogenic crystal-induced inflammation. Penetrating injuries involving plant thorns and sea-urchin spines may cause acute and chronic inflammatory synovitis, periostitis, or periarticular lesions which only resolve following surgical removal of the crystalline material.

Further reading

Doherty M and **Dieppe PA** (1986). Crystal deposition disease in the elderly. *Clinics in Rheumatic Diseases* **12**, 97–116.

Emmerson BT (1996). The management of gout. *New England Journal of Medicine* **334**, 445–51.

McCarty DJ, ed (1988). Crystalline deposition diseases. *Rheumatic Disease Clinics of North America* **14**, 2.

Reginato A, Kurnik B (1989). Calcium oxalate and other crystals associated with kidney diseases and arthritis. *Seminars in Arthritis and Rheumatism* **18**, 198–224.

Rosenthal AK (1998). Calcium crystal-associated arthritides. *Current Opinion in Rheumatology* **10**, 273–7.

18.10 Autoimmune rheumatic disorders and vasculitides

18.10.1 Autoimmune rheumatic disorders and vasculitis

I. P. Giles and D. A. Isenberg

Definition and epidemiology

The autoimmune rheumatic diseases are a heterogeneous group of disorders characterized by clinical involvement of the joints, connective tissues, muscles, internal organs, Raynaud's phenomenon, and cutaneous manifestations. Hence the autoimmune rheumatic diseases include a broad clinical spectrum of disease, including systemic lupus erythematosus, rheumatoid arthritis, Sjögren's syndrome, scleroderma, dermatomyositis, polymyositis, antiphospholipid syndrome, and the vasculitides. This latter group of diseases all share inflammation and necrosis of blood vessels as cardinal features, and may be divided into primary (e.g. giant cell arteritis, Wegener's granulomatosis, polyarteritis nodosa, etc.), occurring in the absence of a recognized precipitating cause, or secondary to established disease (e.g. systemic lupus erythematosus or rheumatoid arthritis) or infection (e.g. hepatitis B, C, or HIV) (see Table 1). On the whole these diseases have a predilection for young women and share defects in immune regulation leading to the production of autoantibodies, activation of the complement system, and generation and deposition of immune complex.

Some autoimmune rheumatic diseases are rare, for example systemic sclerosis; others are common, rheumatoid arthritis affecting approximately 1 per cent of the population (see Table 2). Taken as a whole, however, these autoimmune disorders affect as many as 1 in 20 people. Some are severely debilitating or life-threatening illnesses, others produce minor symptoms that require little, if any, medical intervention.

The clinical spectrum

Each of the autoimmune rheumatic diseases is a distinct entity and can be clearly defined clinically, serologically, and in terms of treatment and prognosis. However, many patients with these diseases have non-specific features of malaise, fever, and arthralgia, and there is also much overlap in terms of multisystem involvement, as shown in Table 3. Organ-specific features, for example lung fibrosis, pericarditis, and less frequently glomerulonephritis, can all occur in several of the autoimmune rheumatic diseases and the presence of such a feature is not pathognomonic of an individual disease.

The clinical features of each patient must be considered together with the laboratory investigations, which should include an autoantibody profile. A preliminary 'autoimmune screen' includes a rheumatoid factor and antinuclear antibody test as a bare minimum, the results of which then guide the need for further autoantibody testing. Immunologically rheumatoid factor (especially if the titre is greater than 1 in 320) remains the most important guide to establishing the diagnosis of rheumatoid arthritis, although the American College of Rheumatology classification criteria for rheumatoid arthritis may still be fulfilled in the absence of rheumatoid factor. The antibody is of no value, however, in the monitoring of the disease.

The presence and pattern of staining of antinuclear antibody is a very useful guide to the presence of disease, as shown in Table 4. In the case of the vasculitides the antineutrophil cytoplasmic antibody (**ANCA**) fulfils this role. An important proviso to the antinuclear antibody test is that it is

Table 1 Classification of systemic vasculitis

Dominant vessel involved	Primary	Secondary
Large arteries	Giant cell arteritis	Aortitis associated with RA
	Takayasu's arteritis	Infection (e.g. syphilis)
	Isolated CNS angiitis	
Medium arteries	Classical polyarteritis nodosa	Infection (e.g. hepatitis B)
	Kawasaki disease	
Small vessels and medium arteries	Wegener's granulomatosis*	Vasculitis secondary to RA, SLE, and SS
	Churg–Strauss syndrome*	Drugs
	Microscopic polyangiitis*	Infection (e.g. HIV)
Small vessels (leucocytoclastic)	Henoch–Schönlein purpura	Drugs†
	Essential mixed cryoglobulinaemia	Infection (e.g. hepatitis B,C)
	Cutaneous leucocytoclastic angiitis	

*Diseases most commonly associated with ANCA (antimyeloperoxidase and antiproteinase 3 antibodies), a significant risk of renal involvement, and which are most responsive to immunosuppression with cyclophosphamide.

†For example sulphonamides, penicillins, thiazide diuretics, and many others.

Abbreviations: RA, rheumatoid arthritis; CNS, central nervous sysytem; SLE, systemic lupus erythematosus; SS, Sjögren's syndrome.

Table 2 Occurrence of major autoimmune rheumatic diseases in Western populations aged 15 years and over

Diseases	Annual incidence per 1000	Point prevalence per 1000
Rheumatoid arthritis	0.5	8.0
Systemic lupus erythematosus	0.05	0.4*
Polymyositis	0.005	0.08
Systemic sclerosis	0.01	0.1
Sjögren's syndrome	0.3	0.27

*There is a considerable variation according to ethnic origin, thus Afro-Carribean women are five times as likely to get systemic lupus erythematosus as Caucasian women.

present in a low titre (up to 1 in 80) in about 1 to 2 per cent of the normal population, and more frequently (up to 10 per cent) in healthy people over the age of 75 years. Hence, its presence alone at low titres does not in itself justify the diagnosis of an autoimmune rheumatic disease: the whole clinical picture must be considered. Further confusion may arise because some autoantibodies may be found in more than one disease, such as anti-U1RNP (in systemic lupus erythematosus and undifferentiated autoimmune rheumatic disease), whilst others may be found in other diseases 'beyond' the autoimmune rheumatic diseases, such as perinuclear staining ANCA (p-ANCA) which is well recognized in patients with inflammatory bowel disease, some chronic infections, and malignancies.

Immunopathogenesis

Autoimmune rheumatic disorders

The precise aetiologies of the autoimmune rheumatic diseases remain unknown, but are undoubtedly complex. Inciting agents, such as infection, are involved, as are genetic susceptibility, hormonal factors, and both cellular and immune dysregulation.

Common to all of the autoimmune rheumatic diseases is the phenomenon of production of autoantibodies by activated B cells. Many of the pathogenic autoantibodies are of the IgG class and have undergone somatic mutation in their hypervariable regions leading to a gradual increase in specificity and binding affinity of an antibody produced by a particular clone of cells. This latter finding is particularly true of anti-dsDNA antibodies in systemic lupus erythematosus and antiphospholipid antibodies in the antiphospholipid syndrome.

The origins of autoantibody production remain an enigma. Mechanisms that have been invoked include antigen-driven T helper cell responses, failure of efficient clearance of nuclear antigens which become surface expressed following cellular apoptosis, and epitope spreading. These might act alone, in combination with each other, or together with other factors. Each has been proposed to lead to increased B-cell activation. Impaired tolerance appears to be the central defect and once this has occurred abnormal immunoregulation leads to persistence of the inappropriate self-directed immune response.

Cellular mechanisms also play a role in the development of autoimmunity in the autoimmune rheumatic diseases: T-cell dysfunction, impaired macrophage and natural killer cell cytotoxicity, decreased clearance of immune complexes by the mononuclear phagocytic system, increase in the number of activated B cells, cytokine dysregulation, and upregulation of adhesion molecules have all been reported.

Genetic factors are important, especially in the case of systemic lupus erythematosus, where there is a higher rate of concordance in monozygotic twins (25 per cent) than dizygotic (3 per cent). The best described of the genetic contributions to autoimmune rheumatic disease is the increased risk associated with particular HLA class II molecules. The HLA DR4 (the Dw4 and Dw14 subtypes, notably the DRβ1*0404 allele) and HLA DR1 (Dw1) are particularly associated with rheumatoid arthritis. These subtypes share a similarity of the amino acid sequence in the third hypervariable region of the DRβ1 chain, the shared epitope that has been proposed as the underlying unit of susceptibility to rheumatoid arthritis. There are, however, conflicting data proposing that this epitope is better related to the severity of disease. In systemic lupus erythematosus, among Caucasians, the haplotype A1 B8 DR3 is associated with an approximately tenfold increase in risk, although the primary link may be with the complement C4 null allele with which there is linkage disequilibrium.

HLA associations are not only seen with autoimmune rheumatic disease, but also with certain autoantibodies. Anti-Ro and La are strongly correlated with HLA DR3 and DQ, an association that is stronger than that seen with the disease in which these autoantibodies are most frequently encountered (systemic lupus erythematosus and Sjögren's syndrome).

Vasculitides

HLA class I and class II associations are seen throughout the primary vasculitides, whilst infectious agents and circulating immune complexes are pathogenic in the secondary vasculitides. In the primary vasculitides a pathogenic role has been proposed for antiendothelial cell antibodies and sensitized T cells, but undoubtedly the most important role is that of ANCA. Immunofluoresence studies have localized the antigen to the cytoplasm of granulocytes in the azurophilic granules, and two patterns of staining are seen: cytoplasmic ANCA (c-ANCA), of which 90 per cent of sera recognize proteinase 3; and perinuclear staining ANCA (p-ANCA) which is directed against myeloperoxidase in 70 per cent of p-ANCA vasculitis patients. A positive c-ANCA is strongly associated with Wegener's granulomatosis, although 10 per cent of these patients may be p-ANCA positive, whilst antimyeloperoxidase antibodies occur in necrotizing glomerulonephritis (65 per cent), Churg–Strauss syndrome (60 per cent), and microscopic polyangiitis (45 per cent).

Table 3 The spectrum of the autoimmune rheumatic diseases

Disease	Major organ/system involvement	Principal immunological abnormalities
Rheumatoid arthritis	Joints, skin, eyes, lungs, heart, neurological, renal	Rheumatoid factor, IgM, G, or A, central role for T and B cells
Systemic lupus erythematosus	Skin, joints, kidneys, brain, heart, lungs	AB to polynucleotides, histones, ENA, PL, abnormalities in T and B cells and accessory cells
Poly-/dermatomyositis	Muscle, skin, blood vessels, lungs	Disease-specific AB (e.g. anti-Jo-1) and infiltrates of T cells in muscle
Scleroderma	Skin, gut ,lungs, kidneys, heart, muscle	Disease-specific AB (e.g. anti-Scl-70, anticentromere); T-cell and cytokine abnormalities
Primary antiphospholipid antibody syndrome	Blood vessels any size, skin, fetal loss, thrombocytopenia, neurological	AB to PL, β_2-GP1, and the lupus anticoagulant
Sjögren's syndrome	Exocrine glands, notably lacrimal and parotid	AB to ENA, SS A/Ro, SS B/La; major infiltrate of T cells in glands
Vasculitides (PAN, Wegener's, giant cell arteritis)	Skin, joints, muscles, lungs, central nervous system, kidneys, blood vessels of all sizes	Cellular infiltration of blood vessel walls; disease-related AB, c-ANCA, p-ANCA

AB, antibody; p-ANCA, perinuclear staining antineutrophil cytoplasmic antibody; c-ANCA, cytoplasmic staining antineutrophil cytoplasmic antibody; β_2-GP1, β_2-glycoprotein 1; ENA, extractable nuclear antigen; PAN, polyarteritis nodosa; PL, phospholipid; SS, Sjögren's syndrome

Table 4 Antinuclear antibody use in diagnosis

Antinuclear antibody pattern	Other auto-antibodies	Disease
Homogenous	Histone	Drug-induced lupus
	ds-DNA	Systemic lupus erythematosus
Speckled	Sm, U1RNP	Systemic lupus erythematosus
	Ro, La	Sjögren's syndrome
	High titre U1RNP	Overlap/undifferentiated syndrome
Nucleolar speckled homogenous	Scl-70	Diffuse cutaneous scleroderma
Centromere	Anti-centromere	Localized cutaneous scleroderma

Clinical features

As mentioned previously, the presentation of an autoimmune rheumatic disease may be diffuse and non-specific, with fatigue and arthralgia frequently the major features. In this instance, systemic review should enquire for the presence of alopecia, mouth ulcers, Raynaud's phenomenon, rash, sicca symptoms, and lymphadenopathy. The presence of these would lend an autoimmune flavour to the illness, but not necessarily help to make a precise diagnosis. The history should also seek a possible trigger such as a preceding infection, drugs (for example hydralazine, isoniazid, procainamide in drug-induced lupus), or environmental exposure to chemicals, as may be seen in scleroderma-like illnesses. A family history must pay particular attention to the presence not only of other autoimmune rheumatic diseases but also other autoimmune diseases such as diabetes, pernicious anaemia, and thyroid disease, which are often found in association with the autoimmune rheumatic diseases.

The protean clinical manifestations mean that an autoimmune rheumatic disease may present not only to a rheumatologist but to many other specialists, including those in nephrology, dermatology, and less commonly neurology, cardiology, haematology, or even obstetrics, in the case of recurrent miscarriages in the antiphospholipid syndrome.

In many cases it is not possible to make a precise diagnosis on the first encounter with a patient. In those with mild disease, symptomatic relief can be obtained with a non-steroidal anti-inflammatory drug, whilst the results of baseline investigations and an 'immunological screen' of antinuclear antibody and rheumatoid factor are awaited. It is worth noting, however, that there is increasing emphasis on trying to make the diagnosis of rheumatoid arthritis promptly, so that a disease-modifying drug can be used as early as possible, rather than waiting for the development of erosive, destructive joint disease.

Since the autoimmune rheumatic diseases are systemic disorders, it is always important to search for evidence of involvement of any of the major organ systems. Baseline investigations must therefore include urinalysis, a full blood count, simple blood tests of renal and liver function, measurement of serum inflammatory markers, an ECG, and a chest radiograph. The simple bedside test of urinalysis is particularly important: the finding of proteinuria and haematuria immediately identifies those who require further, often urgent, renal investigation and whose prognosis may be chiefly determined by the extent of renal involvement.

Damage to major organ systems can be part of the presenting illness in a patient with an autoimmune rheumatic disease, but may also occur in a previously diagnosed patient with 'stable' disease. Myocardial infarction can occur as the result of a vasculitic illness, or accelerated atherosclerosis in systemic lupus erythematosus. Pericarditis can lead to tamponade (for example in systemic lupus erythematosus or rheumatoid arthritis), whilst myocarditis may induce complex arrhythmias or even heart failure (for example in systemic lupus erythematosus or polymyositis). Seizures or a disturbed level of consciousness can occur due to cerebral infarction or meningoencephalitis (for example in systemic lupus erythematosus, antiphospholipid syndrome, Wegener's granulomatosis). Rapidly progressive glomerulonephritis (systemic lupus erythematosus, Wegener's granulomatosis, microscopic polyangiitis) may be associated with pulmonary haemorrhage, whilst hypertension requires urgent treatment in scleroderma renal crisis. Pneumonitis or myositis due to systemic lupus erythematosus may be life threatening if not recognized and treated appropriately with adequate immunosuppression. Venous or arterial thromboses are likely to complicate the antiphospholipid syndrome, which in its primary form may be catastrophic and characterized by widespread microvascular disease with adult respiratory distress syndrome, profound thrombocytopenia, and acute renal failure.

Physicians treating patients with autoimmune rheumatic diseases need to be constantly aware of the possibility of organ involvement: prompt diagnosis and treatment being necessary to prevent irreversible end organ damage. The immunosuppressive therapy used will be similar, regardless of the particular diagnosis.

Precise identification of an autoimmune rheumatic disease is reliant upon clinical and laboratory features, of which the presence of antinuclear antibody (and its pattern of staining), antibodies to extractable nuclear antigens, disease-specific antibodies, or ANCA are crucial. There are many instances where the disease may not be precisely labelled, and up to 20 per cent of patients have features of several autoimmune rheumatic diseases, most commonly systemic lupus erythematosus/scleroderma and systemic lupus erythematosus/rheumatoid arthritis, or those who would be considered to have an undifferentiated autoimmune rheumatic disease. In the case of these latter diseases, treatment is guided according to disease features and the pattern of organ/system involvement.

Further reading

Kallenberg CGM, Heeringa P (1998). Pathogenesis of vasculitis. *Lupus* **7**, 280–4.

Mason LJ, Isenberg DA (1998). Immunopathogenesis of SLE. *Baillière's Clinical Rheumatology* **12**, 385–403.

Menon S, Isenberg DA (1996). Small vessel vasculitides. In: Tooke JE, Lowe GDD, eds. *The textbook of vascular medicine*, pp 295–313. Arnold, London.

Morrow J *et al.* (1999). *Autoimmune rheumatic disease,* 2nd edn.Oxford University Press, Oxford.

Scott DGI, Watts RA (1994). Classification and epidemiology of systemic vasculitis. *British Journal of Rheumatology* **33**, 897–900.

18.10.2 Systemic lupus erythematosus and related disorders

Anisur Rahman and David Isenberg

Introduction

Systemic lupus erythematosus is an autoimmune rheumatic disorder that can present with symptoms in almost any organ or system of the body. Classification criteria have been published by the American College of Rheumatology which should universally be used to make the diagnosis. These are shown in Table 1 and demonstrate the wide variety of clinical and serological features that are associated with this condition. They provide a useful guide to the clinical features that should place the suspicion of systemic lupus erythematosus in the mind of a clinician. It is important not to be too dogmatic in searching for 'pathognomonic' features of the disease.

Table 1 Criteria of the American College of Rheumatology for the classification of systemic lupus erytematosus*

1. Malar rash
2. Discoid rash
3. Photosensitivity
4. Oral ulcers
5. Arthritis
6. Serositis
   (a) Pleuritis or
   (b) Pericarditis
7. Renal disorder
   (a) Proteinuria > 0.5 g/24 h or 3+, persistently or
   (b) Cellular casts
8. Neurological disorder
   (a) Seizures or
   (b) Psychosis (having excluded other causes, e.g. drugs)
9. Haematological disorder
   (a) Haemolytic anaemia or
   (b) Leucopenia or $< 4.0 \times 10^9$/litre on two or more occasions
   (c) Lymphopenia or $< 1.5 \times 10^9$/litre on two or more occasions
   (d) Thrombocytopenia $< 100 \times 10^9$/litre
10. Immunological disorders
   (a) Raised antinative DNA antibody binding or
   (b) Anti-Sm antibody or
   (c) Positive finding of antiphospholipid antibodies
11. Antinuclear antibody in raised titre (in the absence of drugs known to be associated with drug-induced lupus)

*'...a person shall be said to have SLE if four or more of the 11 criteria are present, serially or simultaneously, during any interval of observation.' (Tan EM *et al.* (1982). The 1982 revised criteria for the classification of systemic lupus erythematosus. *Arthritis and Rheumatism* **25**, 1271–7.).

For example, although the characteristic butterfly rash over the face is perhaps the best known sign of systemic lupus erythematosus, many patients will never develop such a rash.

Aetiology

The aetiology is multifactorial, incorporating genetic, hormonal, and environmental elements. The best established genetic link is with the presence of null alleles of genes encoding early components of the complement cascade (C1q, C2, and C4). Over 90 per cent of patients homozygous for C1q deficiency and 75 per cent of those with C4 deficiency develop a lupus-like disease (similar clinical features but a relative paucity of antibodies). Major histocompatibility complex genes, particularly HLA A1, B8, and DR3, have also been associated with the presence of lupus in family studies, although part of this association may be due to linkage disequilibrium with the C4 and C2 genes also present in that region of chromosome 6.

Hormones are likely to play a role in pathogenesis, since systemic lupus erythematosus is far commoner in women than men (see below). There is a relatively high incidence of the condition in Klinefelter's syndrome (males with the XXY karyotype) and this is associated with abnormalities in oestrogen metabolism.

Viruses may be important in triggering the autoimmune dysfunction that leads to the production of pathogenic autoantibodies in systemic lupus erythematosus. Reactivation of BK polyomavirus infection, in particular, has been associated with the presence of antibodies to double-stranded DNA (anti-dsDNA) in Norwegian studies. This association has not yet been confirmed in large populations.

Certain drugs induce a form of systemic lupus erythematosus which is generally characterized by the presence of antihistone rather than anti-dsDNA antibodies, a milder course of disease, and total remission when the causative drug is withdrawn. The most common drugs involved are isoniazid, procainamide, hydralazine, minocycline, penicillamine, and anticonvulsants.

Epidemiology

The incidence of systemic lupus erythematosus in the United Kingdom is about four cases per 100 000 people per year. The prevalence varies between the sexes and between different ethnic groups. Systemic lupus erythematosus occurs between 10 and 20 times more frequently in women than in men and is commoner in some ethnic groups. A recent study in Birmingham, United Kingdom gave the prevalence of systemic lupus erythematosus in women as 206 per 100 000 in Afro-Caribbeans, 91 per 100 000 in Asians, and 36 per 100 000 in Caucasians. These gender and racial differences are broadly consistent with those reported from studies in the United States and the Caribbean, although the reported prevalence of systemic lupus erythematosus in Africa is much lower.

Mortality from systemic lupus erythematosus has fallen significantly over the last half century. Whereas systemic lupus erythematosus was reported to have a 50 per cent 5-year survival in the 1950s, 10-year survival rates rose to between 80 and 90 per cent by the 1970s. Since then, survival rates have improved a little, but deaths from renal failure have become less common, whilst those from infection have increased. The latter are generally associated with immunosuppressive therapy, highlighting the need for better and more accurately targeted methods of treating the underlying immunological abnormalities in this disease.

Pathogenesis and immune dysfunction

No single abnormality of the immune system can be considered to be the sole cause of systemic lupus erythematosus. The pathogenesis of the disease depends on the interplay of a number of different factors, the relative importance of which may differ from one patient to another. These include autoantibodies, T lymphocytes, cytokines, the complement system, and apoptosis. Research to unravel this complex system of interrelated factors has been carried out by studying properties of cells and tissue components derived from patients with systemic lupus erythematosus and by studying mouse models of the condition.

B lymphocytes and autoantibodies

Autoantibodies are those which bind to antigens present within the tissues of the body itself. A wide variety of different autoantibodies have been described in systemic lupus erythematosus. Those most frequently reported are listed in Table 2.

Antibodies to double-stranded DNA (anti-dsDNA) have been cited widely as possible causative agents in systemic lupus erythematosus, particularly in lupus glomerulonephritis. Raised titres of anti-dsDNA antibodies are found in 50 to 70 per cent of patients with systemic lupus erythematosus but hardly ever in healthy people or those with other diseases. Levels of these antibodies rise and fall with disease activity in systemic lupus erythematosus, and deposits of anti-dsDNA occur in the glomeruli of patients with lupus nephritis. In experimental murine models of systemic lupus erythematosus, monoclonal anti-dsDNA antibodies can also be shown to deposit in the glomeruli with associated proteinuria.

The titre of anti-dsDNA antibodies present in the bloodstream of patients with systemic lupus erythematosus can be a useful indicator of disease activity. It is increasingly clear, however, that not all anti-dsDNA antibodies are equally likely to be associated with tissue damage. Antibodies of IgG isotype, which show specific, high-affinity binding to dsDNA generally show the closest association with disease activity in patients and the greatest ability to cause renal damage in experimental models.

Why are such antibodies produced in patients with systemic lupus erythematosus? Studies of monoclonal anti-dsDNA antibodies derived from patients or mice indicate that those which show the isotype and binding properties described above often show sequence characteristics suggestive

Table 2 Major autoantibodies associated with systemic lupus erythematosus and their approximate prevalence in patients with the disease

Autoantibodies	Antigen/epitope	Approximate prevalence (%)
Intracellular		
DNA	dsDNA, (ssDNA)	40–90
Histone	H1, 2A, 2B, 3, 4	30–80
Sm	B/B', D, E, F, G	30 (Afro-Caribbean), ~ 10 (Caucasian)
U1RNP	A, C, 70 kDa ribonucleoprotein	20–35
rRNP	Three subunits: 38, 19, 17 kDa	5–15
Ro/SS-A	60, 52 kDa protein bound to cytoplasmic RNA (hY1–hY5)	10–15
La/SS-B	48 kDa protein bound to variety of RNA, U1RNA, hY RNA	10–15
Heat shock protein (hsp)	hsp 90	30
hnRNP	A2 protein (also known as RA-33)	30
Cell membrane		
Cardiolipin	Phospholipids	20–40
Neuronal antigen	Expressed on neuronal cell lines grown *in vitro*	70–90 (+CNS), ~ 10 (–CNS)
Lymphocyte	HLA component	~ 75 (IgM), ~ 45 (IgG)
Red cell	Non-Rh related	< 10
Platelet		< 10
Extracellular		
Rheumatoid factor	Fc region of IgG	~ 25
C1q	Complement component	20–45

of antigen-driven somatic mutation. This is the process whereby mutations accumulate in the expressed immunoglobulin gene sequences of a B lymphocyte under the influence of a particular antigen. The mutations are accumulated non-randomly, such that the end result is an increase in specificity and affinity of binding. This process is dependent on help from T lymphocytes and on the presence of an appropriate antigen. Naked mammalian DNA, however, is a poor immunogen in experimental animals, and the concentration of free DNA in the bloodstream is low even in patients with systemic lupus erythematosus. It is therefore believed that the antigen which stimulates production of high-affinity anti-dsDNA antibodies is probably a complex of DNA and protein. Nucleosomes derived from cell apoptosis may be the most important antigens involved, although a role for viral DNA binding proteins has also been suggested.

How do the autoantibodies exert their pathogenic effects? Deposition of IgG and complement in inflamed tissues such as kidney and skin is a consistent feature of active systemic lupus erythematosus. The pathogenic potential of autoantibodies in systemic lupus erythematosus (particularly IgG anti-dsDNA) may therefore rest upon their ability to deposit in these tissues and to activate complement. However, the role of complement activation has recently been called into question by work showing that knockout mice deficient in both the classical and alternative pathways of the complement cascade still develop a form of glomerulonephritis similar to that seen in systemic lupus erythematosus, but since these mice do not typically produce anti-dsDNA antibodies they may not be an appropriate model of most patients with systemic lupus erythematosus.

Why are anti-dsDNA antibodies deposited in target tissues? Much of the work designed to answer this question has concentrated on autoantibodies in lupus nephritis. Originally, it was felt that DNA–anti-DNA immune complexes would form in the bloodstream and accumulate in glomeruli as the blood was filtered there. It has not been possible to demonstrate large quantities of such complexes in the blood of patients with systemic lupus erythematosus, though their clearance may well be abnormal due to complement deficiency. Anti-dsDNA antibodies may be targeted to the kidney due to cross-reaction with cell surface proteins there, or may deposit due to an interaction with histones and heparan sulphate. According to this latter model, anti-dsDNA antibodies bind to DNA in nucleosomes, and the positively charged histones in these nucleosomes bind to negatively charged heparan sulphate in the renal basement membrane.

Antiphospholipid antibodies

Between 20 and 30 per cent of patients with systemic lupus erythematosus possess serum antiphospholipid antibodies. The origin of these antibodies may be similar to that of anti-dsDNA antibodies since monoclonal antiphospholipid antibodies from patients with systemic lupus erythematosus also show antigen-driven accumulations of somatic mutations. The antigen in this case may be phosphatidylserine on the outer surfaces of blebs derived from apoptotic cells.

The pathological effects of antiphospholipid antibodies are not due to deposition and complement activation but to promotion of thrombus formation. This leads to arterial and venous thromboses that may be particularly harmful in the cerebral and renal circulation. The mechanism by which thrombosis is altered is not fully understood, but it has become clear that antiphospholipid antibodies found in systemic lupus erythematosus and the primary antiphospholipid antibody syndrome recognize a complex of negatively charged phospholipid with the plasma protein β2-glycoprotein 1. Antiphospholipid antibodies found in infectious diseases such as syphilis bind to phospholipids in the absence of this cofactor, and are not associated with increased thrombosis or adverse clinical effects.

T lymphocytes

Since the process of antigen-driven selection of mutations in B lymphocytes is dependent on help from helper T lymphocytes, it would be reasonable to suppose that antigen-specific T cells might also contribute to the pathogenesis of the disease. The isolation of T-cell clones reactive with DNA and/or DNA binding proteins such as histones has been demonstrated from both patients with systemic lupus erythematosus and murine models of the disease. The clones frequently show specificity for histone epitopes that are cryptic (i.e. not exposed) in normal chromatin. These results reinforce the idea that the antigenic stimulus for production of pathogenic T cells and autoantibodies in systemic lupus erythematosus may be a DNA/histone complex rather than DNA alone.

Patients with systemic lupus erythematosus have decreased levels of the subset of T cells carrying the CD4 and CD45Ro surface markers. This population may be involved in stimulation of suppressor T lymphocytes, so that suppression in these patients is insufficient to prevent the production and survival of autoreactive B-lymphocyte and helper T-lymphocyte clones.

Apoptosis and complement

MRL *lpr/lpr* mice are deficient in apoptosis because they lack the Fas protein which plays a major role in promoting this process. These mice develop a disease very similar to systemic lupus erythematosus with death resulting from glomerulonephritis. One possible reason for this might be the failure of the immune system to delete by apoptosis autoreactive clones of T or B lymphocytes which are then able to cause autoimmune disease. By contrast, humans with the equivalent genetic lesion to MRL *lpr/lpr* mice do not develop systemic lupus erythematosus, and other strains of mice show an accumulation of apoptotic debris within nephritic kidneys which resemble those of systemic lupus erythematosus. A simple deficiency in apoptosis is therefore unlikely to be the underlying mechanism in systemic lupus erythematosus.

Apoptosis leads to the production of surface blebs of cellular material. These blebs include a number of the antigens to which autoantibodies develop in systemic lupus erythematosus, notably DNA and associated nuclear proteins and negatively charged phospholipids. A deficiency in the clearance of products of apoptosis has been demonstrated which might allow the production of a wide spectrum of autoantibodies, as found in systemic lupus erythematosus. Removal of immune complexes containing such potentially antigenic material may be compromised in patients with systemic lupus erythematosus. Monocytes derived from such patients show reduced phagocytosis of cell debris *in vitro*. This process may be complement dependent. Humans with homozygous C2 deficiency process immune complexes very differently from normal controls. Administration of fresh frozen plasma to these patients as a source of complement is successful in ameliorating the symptoms of systemic lupus erythematosus and in normalizing (albeit transiently) the processing of immune complexes.

C1q knockout mice develop a form of glomerulonephritis similar to that seen in systemic lupus erythematosus, and their kidneys are characterized by accumulations of apoptotic debris. Similarly, as noted earlier, humans homozygous for C1q deficiency develop a form of systemic lupus erythematosus with the frequent occurrence of nephritis.

The role of cytokines

Cytokines enhance the ability of cells to interact and are therefore critically important in abnormalities in both T- and B-cell functions seen in patients with lupus. Table 3 summarizes the major differences between the different subsets of T helper (T_H) cells in terms of their cytokine profiles and functions. The balance between cytokines from the T_{H1} and T_{H2} cells is essential in determining the outcome of the immune response. Lupus might be expected to be a disease in which T_{H2} cells predominate, resulting in excessive help for B cells and overproduction of antibodies. In support of this notion, increased levels of IL-10 have been found in patients with lupus. This cytokine suppresses T_{H1} cells and thus impairs cell-mediated immunity, a characteristic feature of the disease. Both macrophage and natural killer cell-mediated cytotoxicity are frequently impaired in patients with lupus. γ-interferon-induced enhancement of both types of cytotoxicity is also impaired, despite normal levels of γ-interferon production by lupus T_{H1} cells.

Accessory cells in lupus seem to produce insufficient amounts of IL-1 to provide the necessary activation signals for T cells. Both CD4+ and CD8+ T cells have been described as producing either normal or decreased amounts of IL-2 in response to exogenous antigens. Such a reduction is likely to have a profound effect on T-cell responses.

Table 3 (a) Subsets of CD4+ T cells

	Function	Cytokines
T-helper 1 cell	Cell mediated immunity	IFN-γ, IL-10 (humans only), IL-12, TNF-α
T-helper 2 cell	B cell help	IL-4, IL-10

(b) Cytokine profiles in patients with active systemic lupus erythematosus

Cytokine	Serum level*	Spontaneous	Stimulation *in vitro*
IFN-γ	↑	Low	↓
TNF-α	↑ (or normal)	↓ (DR2, DQw1; ↑ nephritis), ↑ (DR3, 4; ↓ nephritis)	↓
IL-1	n.d.	↑ PBM production	↓ Monocyte production
IL-2	↑	Low	↓
IL-4	n.d.	Low	Low
IL-6	↑	↑	–
IL-10	↑ (or normal)	↑ (or normal)	Normal

*Serum levels of cytokines are difficult to interpret since these may be affected by soluble cytokine receptors which are shed from cells. Among the known shed receptors are those for IL-1, IL-2, IL-6, TNF-α, and IFN-γ. Soluble TNF-αR and IL-2R levels are increased in systemic lupus and correlate with disease activity and lupus nephritis.

Abbreviations: IFN-γ, interferon-γ; n.d. = not detected; PBM = peripheral blood mononuclear cell, TNF-α, tumour necrosis factor-α.

Clinical features of systemic lupus erythematosus

Systemic lupus erythematosus is a chronic condition in which a low level of baseline activity is punctuated by flares of higher activity. The overall severity of the disease in a particular patient depends on the nature and frequency of these flares.

The diverse clinical features of systemic lupus erythematosus mean that the disease may present to any of a number of different specialists, including rheumatologists, dermatologists, nephrologists, and general physicians. It is important to be aware of systemic lupus erythematosus as a possible diagnosis in any patient, especially a woman aged between 15 and 50, in whom a number of different organs are inflamed either simultaneously or sequentially. The frequency of occurrence of symptoms in various organs is shown in Table 4.

According to the diagnostic guidelines published by the American College of Rheumatology (Table 1) systemic lupus erythematosus may be diagnosed where a patient meets at least four of the 11 criteria specified (though not necessarily at a single time). In everyday practice, however, these requirements may be too stringent, and systemic lupus erythematosus is often diagnosed on the basis of typical clinical findings in one organ or tissue combined with the presence of appropriate autoantibodies.

Constitutional symptoms

Patients with systemic lupus erythematosus find fatigue to be the most troublesome feature of the disease. Excessive tiredness is both very common and difficult to treat. Hypothyroidism coexists in 5 to 10 per cent of patients with systemic lupus erythematosus and so thyroid function tests should be performed in the fatigued patient. There is an ongoing debate as to whether fibromyalgia is a significant comorbid condition.

Table 4 Cumulative prevalence of clinical features in patients with systemic lupus erythematosus

Clinical feature	Approximate cumulative prevalence (%)
Musculoskeletal	
Arthralgia/arthritis	90
Tenosynovitis	20
Myalgia	50
Myositis	5
Cardiopulmonary	
Shortness of breath	40
Pleurisy	35
Pleural effusion	25
Lupus pneumonitis	5
Interstitial fibrosis	5
Pulmonary function abnormalities	85
Cardiomegaly	20
Pericarditis	15
Cardiomyopathy	10
Myocardial infarction	5
Gastrointestinal	
Anorexia	40
Nausea	15
Vomiting	< 10
Diarrhoea	< 10
Ascites	< 10
Abdominal pain	30
Hepatomegaly	25
Splenomegaly	10
Renal	
Haematuria	10
Proteinuria	60
Casts	30
Serum albumin < 35 g/l	30
Serum creatinine > 125 μmol/l	30
Reduced 24-h creatinine clearance	35
Cerebral	
Depression	15
Psychosis	15
Seizures	20
Hemiplegia	10
Cranial nerve lesions	10
Cerebellar signs	5
Meningitis	1
Migraine	40
Haematological	
Anaemia (iron deficiency)	30
Anaemia (of chronic disease)	75
Autoimmune haemolytic anaemia	15
Leucopenia	60
Lymphopenia	60
Thrombocytopenia	25
Circulating anticoagulants	15
Dermatological	
Butterfly rash	40
Erythematous maculopapular eruption	35
Discoid lupus	20
Relapsing nodular non-suppurative panniculitis	< 5
Vasculitic skin lesions	40
Livedo reticularis	20
Purpuric lesions	40
Alopecia	70

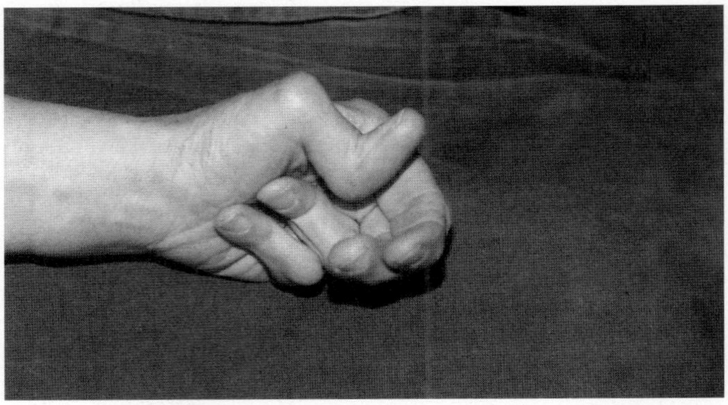

Fig. 1 Deforming Jaccoud's arthropathy. (See also Plate 1.)

Weight loss and low-grade fever may both be indicative of disease activity. Lymphadenopathy is also recognized. The nodes may be markedly enlarged but show no diagnostic features on biopsy, which may nevertheless be necessary to exclude other conditions such as lymphoma.

Musculoskeletal involvement

Arthralgia is the commonest symptom in systemic lupus erythematosus, occurring in 90 per cent of patients. This may be severe but is rarely associated with frank synovitis. Effusions may occur but the fluid shows no diagnostic features.

Erosive arthritis is uncommon, though up to 5 per cent of patients may have an overlap syndrome with features of rheumatoid arthritis as well as systemic lupus erythematosus. These patients tend to have both serum rheumatoid factor and erosions.

When progressive deformity of the hands does occur in systemic lupus erythematosus, it is usually due to an aggressive tenosynovitis and tendon dysfunction rather than to joint damage. This leads to reversible subluxation of the joints, often known as Jaccoud's arthropathy (Fig. 1 and Plate 1).

Development of hip pain in patients who have been treated with corticosteroids should raise the suspicion of avascular necrosis of the femoral head, which may be diagnosed on plain radiograph or, in earlier stages, by magnetic resonance imaging. Corticosteroids also promote osteoporosis, which can be diagnosed in the presymptomatic phase by bone density scanning, but which may present with the acute pain of a vertebral fracture.

Myalgia is common and a true myositis may occur in 5 per cent of cases. Corticosteroid-induced proximal myopathy may also be a problem where these drugs have been used for long periods.

Cutaneous and mucosal involvement

Photosensitivity is very common, particularly in white female patients. Patients should be advised to avoid strong sunlight and to wear protective clothing and/or a high-factor sunblock.

The butterfly rash over the malar area of the face occurs in up to one-third of patients (Fig. 2 and Plate 2). A number of other forms of cutaneous involvement can occur, although these are less specific for systemic lupus erythematosus. These include maculopapular rash, discoid lesions, alopecia, and nailfold infarcts. Scarring alopecia may be particularly distressing and difficult to treat (Fig. 3 and Plate 3).

A variant of systemic lupus erythematosus in which cutaneous manifestations dominate is known as subacute cutaneous lupus. This condition is often associated with anti-Ro antibodies and may be exacerbated by smoking cigarettes.

Antiphospholipid antibodies are associated with a non-raised lattice-like rash concentrated particularly over the thighs and arms. This rash is termed livedo reticularis (Fig. 4 and Plate 4).

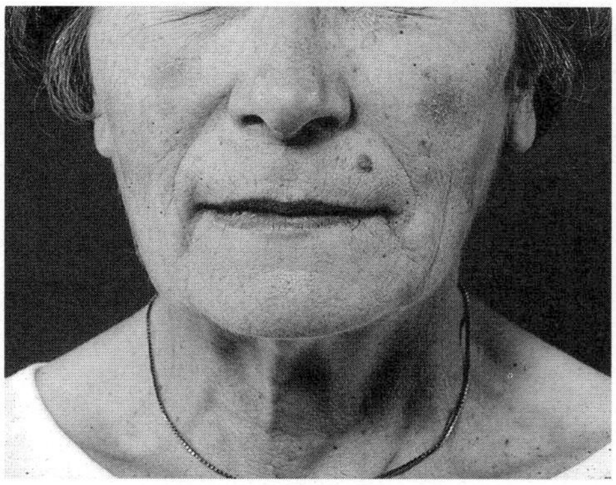

Fig. 2 Malar 'butterfly' rash. (See also Plate 2.)

Painless oral ulcers are common enough to be recognized as one of the diagnostic criteria for systemic lupus erythematosus. However, they are rarely troublesome for the patient. Approximately 20 per cent of patients develop secondary Sjögren's syndrome. The dry eyes and mouth in this condition may respond to artificial tears and saliva.

Renal involvement

Glomerulonephritis is the most serious and potentially lethal manifestation of systemic lupus erythematosus. Its presence may be detected by the finding of haematuria and/or proteinuria on routine stick testing of the urine. It may present as the nephrotic syndrome, or less commonly as a florid nephritis with haematuria, proteinuria, hypertension, and acute renal failure with red cell casts in the urine. The diagnosis and management of glomerulonephritis in systemic lupus erythematosus are more fully discussed in Chapter 20.10.4.

It is important to be aware of the possibility of glomerulonephritis in any patient with systemic lupus erythematosus (Fig. 5 and Plate 5). Measurement of blood pressure and analysis of urine should be carried out at each consultation. Early diagnosis and treatment are invaluable in avoiding deterioration of renal function to the extent that dialysis or renal transplantation become necessary.

Patients with antiphospholipid antibody syndrome may develop a different type of renal lesion characterized by thrombi in small renal vessels rather than by glomerulonephritis. These patients develop hypertension and impairment of renal excretory function, detected as a fall in creatinine clearance, rather than proteinuria and are best managed by anticoagulation rather than immunosuppression.

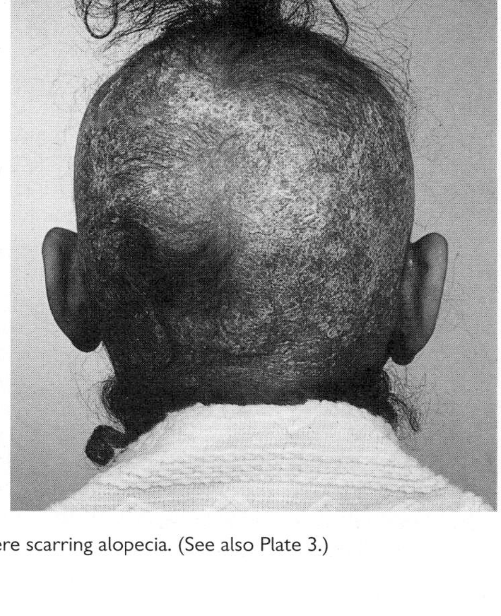

Fig. 3 Severe scarring alopecia. (See also Plate 3.)

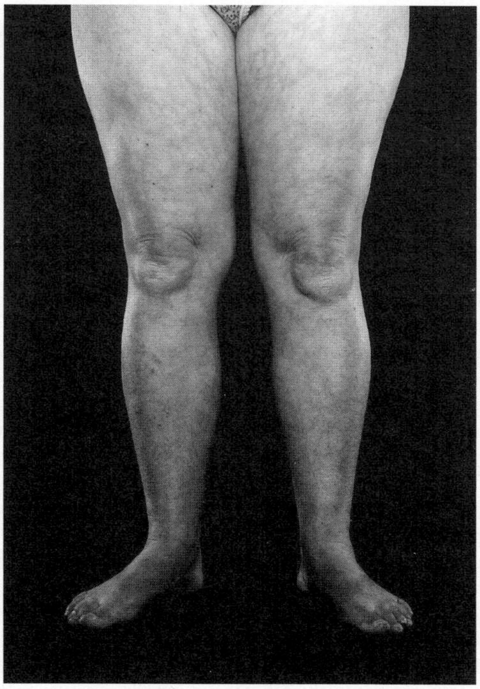

Fig. 4 Livedo reticularis. (See also Plate 4.)

Respiratory involvement

The commonest form of respiratory involvement in systemic lupus erythematosus is pleuritis, manifesting either as pleuritic chest pain or breathlessness caused by pleural effusion. The lung parenchyma is more rarely involved, but fibrosis can occur.

A patient with systemic lupus erythematosus may present with shortness of breath or chest pain for a number of reasons. Pulmonary emboli must be suspected in those with antiphospholipid antibodies. Infections are common in immunosuppressed patients and rib fractures may occur, particularly in those rendered osteoporotic by treatment with corticosteroids.

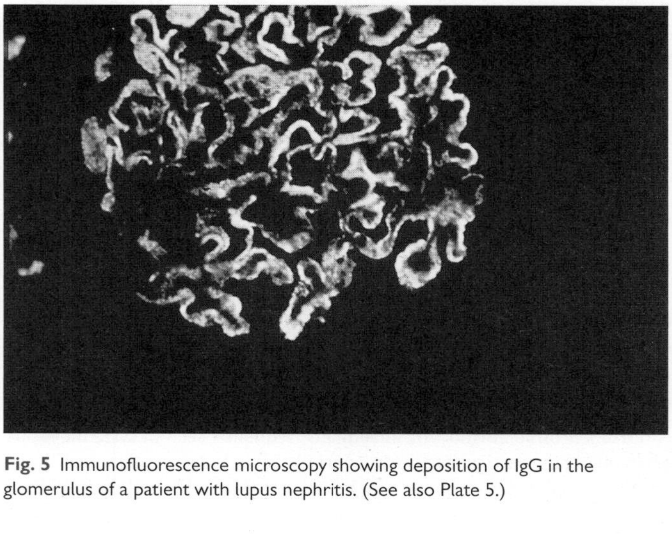

Fig. 5 Immunofluorescence microscopy showing deposition of IgG in the glomerulus of a patient with lupus nephritis. (See also Plate 5.)

The shrinking lung syndrome is characterized by reduced lung volumes and poor respiratory reserve in the face of a normal appearance of the lung parenchyma on computed tomography scanning. It is believed to arise from basal atelectasis in association with diaphragmatic dysfunction.

Cardiovascular involvement

The commonest cardiac manifestation of systemic lupus erythematosus is pericarditis, which occurs in approximately 15 per cent of patients. This generally presents with chest pain or an asymptomatic friction rub. Pericardial effusions may occur but are rarely large enough to cause haemodynamic compromise.

Myocarditis and endocarditis are less common, though post-mortem and echocardiographic studies suggest that both may occur without symptoms in a significant proportion of patients with systemic lupus erythematosus. For example, the classic endocarditis described by Libman and Sacks is characterized by small vegetations that often do not cause murmurs or cardiac compromise, but which have been identified in up to 50 per cent of patients with systemic lupus erythematosus at autopsy.

It is increasingly recognized that atherosclerosis and the attendant deficiencies of cerebral and cardiac circulation are commoner in patients with systemic lupus erythematosus than in the general population. This may be partially due to the use of corticosteroids, which raise serum cholesterol and can promote hypertension. Patients possessing antiphospholipid antibodies are also at a higher risk of stroke or arterial thrombosis.

Raynaud's phenomenon occurs in about one-third of patients with systemic lupus erythematosus, though it is not usually as severe as that seen in systemic sclerosis. Vasculitis presents with a skin rash or ulcers that may be very difficult to heal, but rarely affects the internal organs.

Gastrointestinal involvement

Like pleuritis, peritonitis may occur in patients with systemic lupus erythematosus and must be considered in the event of abdominal pain.

Involvement of the liver and pancreas is recognized but uncommon. The term 'lupoid hepatitis' was previously used for a form of autoimmune hepatitis characterized by the presence of autoantibodies. These patients, however, do not generally have any form of systemic lupus erythematosus and the term is misleading. Minor enlargements of the liver and/or spleen occur in 10 to 25 per cent of cases but these are usually asymptomatic and require no treatment.

Neuropsychiatric involvement

Systemic lupus erythematosus can affect the central nervous system in many ways, so that the true incidence of this type of involvement is difficult to quantify. Symptoms such as poor memory, change of personality, and depression or anxiety occur in many patients. It is difficult, however, to be sure whether these are caused by cerebral systemic lupus erythematosus or represent a reaction to the diagnosis and treatment of the disease.

More florid presentations such as psychotic episodes and convulsions are well recognized. By contrast to the milder symptoms noted above, these manifestations generally call for immunosuppression.

Migraine occurs in up to 40 per cent of patients with systemic lupus erythematosus, particularly in the presence of antiphospholipid antibodies. Peripheral neuropathy can occur, and is usually sensory rather than motor. Cranial nerve palsies are less common, as is transverse myelitis (another feature linked to antiphospholipid antibodies).

Ocular involvement can include episcleritis, conjunctivitis, and the presence of cytoid bodies (white patches on the retina). Patients treated with high-dose steroids may develop cataracts.

Haematological involvement

A normochromic normocytic anaemia is frequently seen in systemic lupus erythematosus, particularly during periods of high disease activity. Microcytic iron-deficiency anaemia may be present due to blood loss from gastritis and ulcers in patients treated with non-steroidal anti-inflammatory drugs. Anaemia may also result from chronic renal failure in lupus nephritis.

A positive Coombs' test, signifying the presence of antibodies to red blood cells, is present in 10 to 15 per cent of patients with systemic lupus erythematosus but does not always indicate haemolytic anaemia.

The presence of lymphopenia (less than 1.5×10^9 per litre) is a common feature, occurring in up to 80 per cent of patients. Neutropenia may occur secondary to the use of cytotoxic drugs such as azathioprine or cyclophosphamide.

Three different types of thrombocytopenia occur in systemic lupus erythematosus. The mildest form is characterized by stable platelet levels of between 50 and 100×10^9 per litre, is rarely symptomatic, and usually requires no treatment. Other patients develop an acute autoimmune thrombocytopenia with levels dropping rapidly below 10×10^9 per litre, but rising when treated with oral steroids. A third group of patients present with thrombocytopenia alone, are treated with steroids, intravenous immunoglobulins, or splenectomy and some years later develop full-blown systemic lupus erythematosus. Thrombocytopenia is also one of the cardinal features of the antiphospholipid antibody syndrome and may be severe enough to necessitate splenectomy in that condition.

Other complicating disorders

Approximately 30 per cent of lupus patients have another autoimmune condition. Sjögren's syndrome is the commonest of these, being present in some 15 to 20 per cent of patients with systemic lupus erythematosus. In the past 15 years it has been recognized that clinical features of the antiphospholipid antibody syndrome, notably venous and arterial thromboses, recurrent miscarriages, thrombocytopenia, and livedo reticularis, may complicate 10 to 15 per cent of patients with systemic lupus erythematosus. When these features, together with the presence of antiphospholipid antibodies (usually cardiolipin, anti-β2-glycoprotein 1 or the lupus anticoagulant) occur in the presence of other more classical lupus features, the condition is known as secondary antiphospholipid syndrome, but they can occur on their own, in which case the patient is said to have primary antiphospholipid syndrome as described elsewhere. Autoimmune thyroid disease (hyper- or hypothyroidism) occurs in 5 to 10 per cent of the patients, and rather less frequently, rheumatoid arthritis, myasthenia gravis, coeliac disease, diabetes, and pernicious anaemia may be found.

Investigations and pathology

Autoantibodies

The most commonly requested test to screen for systemic lupus erythematosus is the antinuclear antibody assay. A positive antinuclear antibody simply indicates that the patient's blood contains antibodies which will bind to the nuclei of a sample of cells used in the test. The test is a sensitive one since over 95 per cent of patients with systemic lupus erythematosus are antinuclear antibody positive. Although a small group of patients do seem to have persistently antinuclear antibody negative systemic lupus erythematosus, the absence of antinuclear antibody in a patient with suspected lupus raises serious doubt about the diagnosis.

The specificity of the antinuclear antibody test for systemic lupus erythematosus is not high. The titre of antibody represents the highest dilution of the patient's serum at which the test is still positive. Low-titre antinuclear antibody (1 in 10) is of little significance and may occur in healthy people. Higher titres (1 in 160 or more) are more worrying and are found in most patients with systemic lupus erythematosus and in a few patients with other autoimmune conditions including rheumatoid arthritis, systemic sclerosis, and Sjögren's syndrome. However, some people with high-titre antinuclear antibody may be followed in rheumatology clinics for years without developing a frank autoimmune disease.

The finding of a positive antinuclear antibody in a patient with symptoms suggestive of systemic lupus erythematosus should lead to a series of other autoantibody tests. These are listed in Table 2 together with the identity of the target antigen and the approximate prevalence of the antibodies.

Anti-dsDNA antibody levels are particularly useful. This test is virtually specific for systemic lupus erythematosus (as is the anti-Sm antibody), especially if the immunoglobulins are of the IgG isotype. The anti-dsDNA result is usually quantified and this value is a measure of the activity of the disease. Indeed, in one study, trial patients were treated with high-dose corticosteroids on the basis of anti-dsDNA levels alone. In comparison with a control group treated only when symptoms or signs also suggested disease activity, the trial group had less disease activity overall and fewer flares. However, frequent large doses of corticosteroids resulted in significant side-effects and a number of subjects dropped out of this arm of the trial. The current evidence therefore suggests that anti-dsDNA should be used only as an adjunct to the clinical impression of disease activity when deciding on a treatment regimen.

Anti-Ro and anti-La antibodies are linked to concurrent Sjögren's syndrome. Mothers who have these antibodies have a higher incidence of neonatal lupus (see below) and should be advised about this before embarking upon a pregnancy. Anti-Ro antibodies are also associated with photosensitivity.

There are no good antibody markers for the presence of disease of the central nervous system. Antibodies to ribosomal protein P were previously thought to have some value in the diagnosis of central nervous system lupus, but this has not been borne out by later results and the test is not available routinely in most laboratories.

Antiphospholipid antibodies can be recognized by one of two assays. The enzyme-linked immunosorbent assay for binding to cardiolipin distinguishes IgM and IgG isotypes. This is helpful because the level of IgG antiphospholipid antibodies is a better predictor of clinical sequelae than that of IgM. Antiphospholipid antibodies can also be diagnosed by testing the clotting properties of the blood *in vitro* in the Russell's viper venom test. An abnormal result in this assay is reported as showing the presence of a lupus anticoagulant. It is quite possible for the anticardiolipin test to be positive while the lupus anticoagulant assay is negative or vice versa. If either is positive, the patient may be at risk of manifestations of the antiphospholipid antibody syndrome. Antibodies to the phospholipid cofactor, known as β2-glycoprotein 1, are now becoming available commercially, offering a third way of detecting antiphospholipid antibodies.

Coombs' test and assays for antithyroid antibodies are often requested in patients with systemic lupus erythematosus, particularly those with coexisting anaemia or hypothyroidism.

Measures of disease activity and end-organ damage

Blood and urine tests

The three most reliable measures of highly active disease are high erythrocyte sedimentation rate, depletion of complement, and high anti-dsDNA levels. The erythrocyte sedimentation rate increases much more than the level of C-reactive protein in active systemic lupus erythematosus. The combination of high erythrocyte sedimentation rate and normal C-reactive protein in a patient with a multisystem disorder should raise the suspicion of systemic lupus erythematosus, leading to appropriate autoantibody tests as described above. The C-reactive protein may, however, be raised in the presence of infection, serositis, or arthritis.

Complement components C3 and C4 are the most commonly measured, and both tend to fall in active systemic lupus erythematosus. A persistently very low level of either C3 or C4 (or a high level of their degradation products C3d or C4d), regardless of immunosuppressive therapy, may signify the presence of a homozygous complement deficiency disorder. Though such disorders are very rare, it is important to diagnose them because they respond better to infusions of fresh frozen plasma than to immunosuppression.

It is important to measure creatinine and electrolyte values regularly and to check the urine for proteinuria and/or haematuria. These measures ensure that renal involvement is diagnosed early. It must be remembered that substantial deterioration in renal function may occur before serum creatinine rises beyond the normal range. It is therefore prudent to note even relatively small rises in creatinine if these are persistent. Renal function may be measured more accurately by creatinine clearance using a 24-h collection of urine or by measuring the clearance of a radio-isotope to obtain the glomerular filtration rate. Persistent proteinuria on bedside testing can be investigated further by measuring the total protein in a 24-h urine sample or the albumin to creatinine ratio in a spot sample.

Liver function tests are not usually abnormal in systemic lupus erythematosus (abnormal in less than 10 per cent of patients), but a baseline value should be measured, particularly in cases where potentially hepatotoxic drugs such as azathioprine may be used. Thyroid function abnormalities, particularly hypothyroidism, are well recognized to coexist with systemic lupus erythematosus.

A full blood count should be measured regularly. Falling haemoglobin, white cell count, and platelet counts may all occur (see under haematological involvement above). Anaemia in the presence of a positive Coombs' test may indicate haemolysis which can be confirmed by requesting a blood film and serum haptoglobins.

Infections occur commonly in patients with systemic lupus erythematosus, particularly in those on high-dose immunosuppressants. Infection may not always be accompanied by high fever or leucocytosis, although C-reactive protein is usually raised. It is wise to carry out blood and urine cultures whenever even mild pyrexia is accompanied by a deterioration in health.

Imaging

Plain radiographs are rarely useful in systemic lupus erythematosus. There is no characteristic appearance in the joints and chest radiographs are unlikely to show abnormalities except in the presence of infection or effusion.

Requests for more specialized imaging studies should be directed by the clinical findings. For example, the presence of dyspnoea and abnormal respiratory function tests often necessitates a computed tomography scan of the thorax, which is the investigation of choice for diagnosis of pulmonary fibrosis. Echocardiography is useful if pericardial effusion, myocarditis, or endocarditis are suspected clinically. Bone density scanning is becoming increasingly important, since patients with systemic lupus erythematosus are often at risk of osteoporosis due to use of corticosteroids and reduced capacity for physical exercise during young adult life.

Histopathology

The two tissues most often subjected to biopsy in systemic lupus erythematosus are the skin and kidneys.

Skin biopsies are chiefly carried out to facilitate the diagnosis of an atypical rash. If systemic lupus erythematosus is suspected, it is important to take a sample of apparently normal skin as well as skin from the rash. Both should show deposition of IgG and complement at the dermoepidermal junction (Fig. 6 and Plate 6).

There are two main indications for renal biopsy in the patient who has, or might have, systemic lupus erythematosus. Firstly, to establish the diagnosis when this is not certain, for example in a patient with poorly characterized multisystem disease with renal involvement. Secondly, to help determine prognosis and decide upon treatment in the patient known to have systemic lupus erythematosus, but with deterioration in renal function, for example development of nephrotic syndrome and/or declining renal excretory function. The activity of glomerular inflammation is graded on a scale of I to V according to World Health Organization criteria. The biopsy can also be used to grade the degree of chronicity of glomerular disease, i.e. how much irreversible damage such as fibrosis and atrophy has occurred. The activity and chronicity scores can both be used to determine

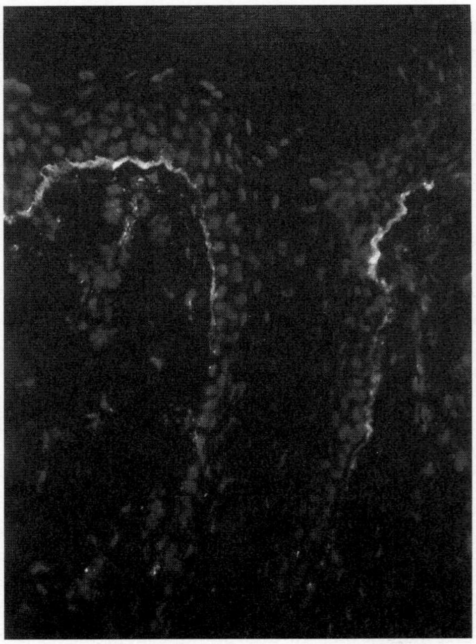

Fig. 6 Immunofluorescence microscopy showing deposition of IgG at the dermoepidermal junction in the skin of a patient with systemic lupus erythematosus (sometimes called the lupus band test). (See also Plate 6.)

appropriate treatment and the risk of a progressive decline in renal function, although the predictive value of such data remains controversial. The subject of renal pathology in systemic lupus erythematosus is considered further in Chapter 20.10.4.

Treatment and prognosis

Systemic lupus erythematosus is a disease that still has the potential to kill young people. In many cases, however, the condition runs a fairly indolent course in which an initial flare is followed by many years of low-grade activity. General measures of value in the treatment of systemic lupus erythematosus are shown in Table 5.

In the pharmacological management of a patient with systemic lupus erythematosus, the clinician will typically seek to answer four questions:

(1) Can the patient be managed without immunosuppression?

(2) If immunosuppression is needed, how should it best be started?

(3) If immunosuppression is being used, is the current level of immunosuppression inadequate or excessive? How should it be increased or reduced?

(4) Is the patient suffering side-effects from the drugs?

Table 5 Treatment of lupus—general measures

1. Rest as appropriate; try to avoid stress
2. Avoid over-exposure to heat and sunlight. Use sun protection factor 15+ (30+ in United States) if in a sunny country; avoid exposing an arm on an open car window
3. Try to adhere to a low-fat diet and consider adding fish oil derivatives
4. Vaccination, for foreign travel etc., apart from 'live' vaccines in patients on immunosuppressives, is not contraindicated though the precise nature of the immune response differs from that in healthy individuals
5. Medium- or high-oestrogen contraceptive pills should be avoided—progesterone only or the lowest possible oestrogen pill (or other methods of contraception) are advised
6. The use of hormone replacement in the menopause remains controversial. Many patients do tolerate it without flaring, but not all

Is immunosuppression required?

Patients whose disease activity is confined to arthralgia, tiredness, and/or mild rash do not usually have greatly raised erythrocyte sedimentation rate or anti-dsDNA antibodies or reduced complement. These patients can often be treated symptomatically, for example with agents such as paracetamol and diclofenac to control joint pain.

Where such symptoms are more severe, the antimalarial agent hydroxychloroquine at a starting dose of 400 mg per day may be useful. This drug has less potential for retinal toxicity than the closely related chloroquine and is therefore preferred in systemic lupus erythematosus. It is often possible to reduce the dose to 200 mg per day after 3 months and gradually withdraw the drug thereafter. Regular blood tests are not required to monitor the effects of hydroxychloroquine, but there is a very small risk of retinopathy such that review by an ophthalmologist every 6 to 12 months is considered advisable in many units.

Where the main symptoms in a patient with systemic lupus erythematosus are those of the antiphospholipid antibody syndrome immunosuppression is rarely useful. Aspirin at a dose of 150 to 300 mg daily is recommended for those with mild symptoms of the disease or who have other risk factors for thrombosis. Patients who have suffered recurrent thromboses or cerebral infarcts and who have serum antiphospholipid antibodies should usually be treated with lifelong anticoagulation. This is a major commitment for a young patient and raises particular problems in pregnancy (discussed below).

Some patients require a low maintenance dose of oral steroids to control their symptoms even though laboratory indices do not indicate high activity of disease. A dose of 5 to 7.5 mg daily is typically used in such cases. Topical steroids may be useful where lupus activity is confined to the skin.

Is the current level of immunosuppression inadequate or excessive?

Corticosteroids and cytotoxic agents are used to treat flares of disease. A mild flare of arthralgia, myalgia, and general fatigue may be alleviated by a single intramuscular dose of a corticosteroid preparation such as prednisolone acetate (usually 50 to 125 mg are given).

More severe flares of arthritis, pleuritis, or pericarditis require oral prednisolone at a dose of 20 to 40 mg daily. This usually leads to a rapid improvement in symptoms and the dose of prednisolone can be reduced by 5 mg every 1 to 2 weeks until it reaches 5 mg per day. It may not be possible to withdraw the drug completely for several months.

Alternatively, a shorter course of corticosteroids can be given intravenously. A typical course would consist of 750 mg to 1 g of methylprednisolone given over 3 to 4 h on each of three successive days. This requires admission to hospital, making it less convenient than oral therapy, and it is generally reserved for those patients who are not responding to oral prednisolone or cannot tolerate that drug in high doses.

Autoimmune haemolytic anaemia requires higher doses (60–80 mg/day) of oral prednisolone, with the dose reduced in 5 to 10 mg increments according to the clinical response. Azathioprine may be required as a steroid-sparing agent and is used at a dose of 2.5 to 3 mg/kg/day.

Renal flares of systemic lupus erythematosus require the most aggressive treatment, generally involving both corticosteroids and cyclophosphamide. A number of regimes have been used and a debate continues as to which is optimal. One of the most common regimes is that recommended by the United States National Institutes of Health, in which the patient is given oral prednisolone at a dose of between 30 and 80 mg/day depending on the severity of the disease. Intravenous boluses of 750 mg to 1 g cyclophosphamide are given at monthly intervals for 6 months, then every 3 months for 2 years. Cyclophosphamide pulses should be accompanied by adequate intravenous hydration and the use of mesna (mercaptoethane sulphonate) to reduce bladder toxicity. It has been suggested that the use of intravenous pulse therapy is preferable to treatment with oral cyclophosphamide on the grounds of improved compliance and less gonadal dysfunction. The latter claim has not been proved beyond doubt and some groups use oral cyclophosphamide (2–4 mg/kg/day) or oral azathioprine (2–3 mg/kg/day) per day as an alternative to intravenous pulses.

In renal systemic lupus erythematosus it is critically important to control the patient's blood pressure. ACE inhibitors, alpha-adrenergic antagonists such as doxazosin, and calcium channel blockers such as nifedipine are the agents most commonly used.

The treatment of central nervous system lupus varies depending on the manifestation of cerebral dysfunction. Mild cases may respond to relatively small doses of oral steroids (up to 30 mg per day). More florid manifestations such as convulsions or major psychosis require treatment with appropriate anticonvulsants or antipsychotic drugs, higher-dose oral steroids (60–80 mg per day), and sometimes azathioprine or intravenous pulses of cyclophosphamide in similar doses to those used in renal systemic lupus erythematosus.

Is the patient suffering side-effects from the drugs?

The side-effects of corticosteroids are well known. The most common early problems are weight gain, hirsutism, easy bruising, and insomnia. It is difficult to prevent them, except by using the lowest dose of steroid that is effective and reducing it as rapidly as possible whilst maintaining control of the disease.

Longer-term sequelae of corticosteroid use include increased susceptibility to infection, osteoporosis, avascular necrosis, and diabetes mellitus. The most rapid loss of bone in steroid-induced osteoporosis occurs within the first year of treatment, though doses of 7.5 mg/day or less of prednisolone are thought to have little effect on bone. At higher doses, it may be advisable to carry out a bone density scan and to give either calcium and vitamin D tablets or a bisphosphonate (either etidronate or alendronate are commonly used) as prophylaxis.

Cyclophosphamide causes alopecia, nausea, bladder toxicity, and gonadal dysfunction that may lead to infertility. The problem of infertility becomes more likely with increasing age. Women over 30 given cyclophosphamide are at particular risk. Again, the best way to prevent such problems is to use as small a cumulative dose of the drug as is feasible. Bone marrow suppression may occur. During a programme of cyclophosphamide pulses, the white blood cell count falls to a nadir 10 days after each pulse and should be measured at that time to decide whether the next pulse can be given safely. Nausea and vomiting during pulses may be so severe that antiemetics such as metoclopramide or granisetron are necessary.

Azathioprine also causes bone marrow suppression and can cause abnormalities of liver enzymes which resolve once the drug is withdrawn.

Systemic lupus erythematosus in pregnancy

Systemic lupus erythematosus itself does not usually reduce the ability to conceive, although as described the drugs used to treat it, notably cyclophosphamide, may induce infertility due to gonadal failure. There is an increased risk of spontaneous abortion, particularly in the presence of high-titre antiphospholipid antibodies. Pregnant mothers with a high antiphospholipid antibody level and a history of previous miscarriage should be considered for anticoagulation until the birth of the baby. Since warfarin is potentially teratogenic, heparin may be used from the second trimester until parturition.

Mothers often ask whether their children are likely to inherit systemic lupus erythematosus. Inheritance of the adult form of the disease is very rare (approximately 1 per cent of all cases), though a transient illness termed neonatal lupus can occur. The characteristics of this condition are rash, hepatitis, anaemia, and thrombocytopenia which usually resolve by 8 months after birth, and inflammation of the cardiac conducting tissues which may lead to heart block in the fetus. The cardiac problem may be diagnosed by ultrasound scans of the fetal heart between 16 and 24 weeks' gestation. Treatment of the mother with 4 mg oral dexamethasone per day may prevent progression from incomplete to complete fetal heart block. If complete heart block occurs, the neonate may require a cardiac pacemaker. Interestingly, children born with neonatal lupus sometimes develop heart block later in life. In one reported case this problem occurred at the age of 35.

The presence of maternal anti-Ro and anti-La antibodies predicts a higher risk of neonatal lupus. Where both are present the risk is approximately 5 per cent. It is believed that the antibodies cross the placenta and bind to some component of the fetal cardiac tissue (laminin is a particular 'suspect'). The mechanism whereby this leads to heart block is mysterious, especially as the mother's heart is never affected.

Although overall the risk of a flare during pregnancy is probably no greater than at other times, systemic lupus erythematosus may exacerbate during the pregnancy. Corticosteroids may be used in moderate doses without affecting the fetus, but higher doses (over 30 mg) given for long periods can potentially cause fetal adrenal suppression. If lupus activity is such that these doses are required, the risk to the fetus of not treating the disease adequately should outweigh any risk from the drug.

Cyclophosphamide, methotrexate, and azathioprine are contraindicated in pregnancy, although there have been many successful pregnancies in transplant patients taking azathioprine without obvious increased risk of adverse effect. Use of hydroxychloroquine is not recommended by the manufacturers, though there is little evidence that it has adverse effects.

It may be difficult to distinguish pre-eclampsia from a flare of renal lupus. Both can cause hypertension and proteinuria. In pre-eclampsia, unlike systemic lupus erythematosus, there are rarely urinary casts and levels of anti-dsDNA and complement are normal. These tests are therefore useful in making the diagnosis.

For further discussion of autoimmune rheumatic disorders in pregnancy see Chapter 13.14.

Occupational and psychological aspects of systemic lupus erythematosus

Systemic lupus erythematosus typically presents in young people, especially women. The onset of a chronic, essentially incurable condition at a time of life when the patient is otherwise healthy and has many plans and responsibilities is an unexpected and unwelcome burden. Many concerns arise, in particular the outlook for fertility and the ability to care for children are major worries. In those cases where the use of high-dose corticosteroids and immunosuppressive agents are essential, detailed explanations of the benefits and risks of these treatments in both the short and long term are necessary. Although a 10-year survival rate of 90 per cent may appear reassuring, it is probably less so to a 25-year-old who recognizes a 10 per cent chance of dying by the age of 35.

In making the diagnosis of systemic lupus erythematosus, therefore, the doctor must consider the effect of this condition on the overall life of the patient as well as his or her individual organs. A sympathetic understanding of the anxieties associated with the diagnosis is vital.

Controversial areas and future prospects

It is clear that we do not yet possess a cure for systemic lupus erythematosus or even a method of controlling the disease without the risk of major side-effects. The main sources of controversy concern attempts to develop new forms of treatment and to establish indices of disease activity that can be used to measure the effects of these treatments.

Plasma exchange and intravenous immunoglobulin therapy have been tried in systemic lupus erythematosus, particularly in renal crises. Overall, the results do not suggest that either form of treatment should be used routinely. New drugs such as tacrolimus and mycophenolate mofetil have been administered to small numbers of patients. Some encouraging results have been reported, but it is too early to decide on the place of these agents in the management of the disease.

There are now many different murine models of systemic lupus erythematosus. These differ in their clinical and serological characteristics and each represents at best a partial approximation to the human disease. This is important because it is now possible to administer agents such as monoclonal anticytokine antibodies to these mice and to assess the effect on the disease process. In deciding which of these agents might be effective in humans it is important to know how far one can extrapolate from the results in mice.

If new drugs or monoclonal antibodies are to be used in human systemic lupus erythematosus, it is necessary, given that mortality is now (thankfully) a rare end point, to have a recognized index by which to judge the response to treatment. Such an index must include a disease activity index, a damage index, a patient health perception index, a record of toxicity, and cost. Several global score disease activity indices, for example the systemic lupus erythematosus disease activity index, SLAM (systemic lupus activity measure), and ECLAM (European Community lupus activity measure) have been developed and provide a 'rough and ready' guide to activity. A more sophisticated approach based on the 'physician's intention to treat principle', has been derived by the British Isles Lupus Activity Group, providing an 'at a glance' review of activity in eight different organs or systems. These indices have all been compared favourably in both paper and real patient exercises. By contrast, a single damage index (the SLICC/ACR damage index) has been developed by a group of investigators and records a wide variety of potential permanent changes (for example avascular necrosis, myocardial infarction) that can occur in patients with lupus as part of the development of the disease. These principally clinical features have to be present for at least 6 months before they count. The medical outcome survey, short form 36 (SF-36), provides a useful health perception index for patients with lupus. Although not designed specifically for this condition, it has been widely used in a number of ongoing drug trials.

It is likely that the treatment of systemic lupus erythematosus in 10 years' time will be different from that given now. Basic science research is starting to identify the various strands of immune dysfunction at the core of this disease. At the same time, drug development is providing agents that are capable of selectively targeting single cell types or cytokines within the immune system. At least some of these agents are likely to be relevant to the dysfunctional mechanisms in systemic lupus erythematosus. In addition, clinicians are becoming more aware that conditions such as atherosclerosis and osteoporosis are common in patients with systemic lupus erythematosus. By increasing efforts to detect and control these associated conditions, as well as seeking to attack the underlying autoimmune disease, it should be possible to improve the lives of patients with systemic lupus erythematosus, even if a cure for the disease remains a distant prospect.

Further reading

Boumpas DT *et al.* (1992). Controlled trial of methyl prednisolone versus two regimens of pulse cyclophosphamide in severe lupus nephritis. *The Lancet* **340**, 741–5.

Casciola-Rosen LA, Anhalt G, Rosen A (1994). Autoantigens targeted in systemic lupus erythematosus are clustered in two populations of surface structures on apoptotic keratinocytes. *Journal of Experimental Medicine* **179**, 1317–30.

Cervera R *et al.* (1993). Systemic lupus erythematosus—clinical and immunologic patterns of disease expression in a cohort of 1000 patients. *Medicine (Baltimore)* **72**, 113–21.

Isenberg DA *et al.* (1997). The role of antibodies to DNA in systemic lupus erythematosus. *Lupus* **6**, 290–304.

Johnson AE *et al.* (1995). The prevalence and incidence of systemic lupus erythematosus in Birmingham, England; relationship to ethnicity and country of birth. *Arthritis and Rheumatism* **38**, 551–8.

Khamashta MA *et al.* (1995). The management of thrombosis in the antiphospholipid antibody syndrome. *New England Journal of Medicine* **332**, 993–7.

Koffler D, Schur PH, Kunkel HG (1967). Immunological studies concerning the nephritis of systemic lupus erythematosus. *Journal of Experimental Medicine* **126**, 607–24.

Morrow J *et al.* (1999) *Autoimmune rheumatic disease*, 2nd edn. Oxford University Press, Oxford.

Okamura M *et al.* (1993). Significance of enzyme linked immunosorbent assay (ELISA) for antibodies to double stranded and single stranded DNA in patients with lupus nephritis: correlation with severity of renal histology. *Annals of the Rheumatic Diseases* **52**, 14–20.

Tan EM *et al.* (1982). The 1982 revised criteria for the classification of systemic lupus erythematosus. *Arthritis and Rheumatism* **25**, 1271–7.

Walport MJ (1993). Inherited complement deficiency—clues to the physiological activity of complement *in vivo*. *Quarterly Journal of Medicine* **86**, 355–8.

18.10.3 Systemic sclerosis

Carol M. Black and Christopher P. Denton

Introduction

The scleroderma-spectrum of disorders includes a number of diseases with similar clinical and pathological features, and which have Raynaud's phenomenon or skin sclerosis in common. They are clinically important because the systemic forms have the highest case-related mortality of any of the rheumatic diseases, and because of the particular difficulties encountered in their management. In the United Kingdom there are approximately 300 new cases of systemic sclerosis per year and the population prevalence has been estimated to be 100 per million. Both these figures are significantly lower than estimates of disease frequency in the United States. Recent epidemiological survival analyses of patients with systemic sclerosis suggest a reduction in mortality compared with earlier studies, but this may partly be accounted for by the greater awareness of the milder forms of the disease. The disease most often develops in the fifth decade of life, and affects women approximately four times as often as men, with this ratio increasing during the childbearing years.

Those disorders included within the scleroderma spectrum are described in Table 1. The term 'prescleroderma' can be applied to the subgroup of patients with autoimmune Raynaud's phenomenon who manifest an abnormal microcirculation and scleroderma-hallmark autoantibodies (anticentromere antibodies, antitopoisomerase, or anti-RNA polymerase I).

Clinical features of localized scleroderma conditions are summarized in Table 2. The importance of distinguishing between these conditions and their subsets lies in the different clinical features, natural history, and patterns of visceral involvement that are characteristic of each subgroup.

There have been important developments in understanding the pathogenesis, clinical diversity, and management of the scleroderma-spectrum disorders over the last few years. This progress has occurred in parallel with improvements in the management of many of the organ-based complications of the condition.

Clinical features

Although thorough baseline and longitudinal investigation of patients with scleroderma-spectrum disorders is central to their management, the diagnosis of scleroderma is essentially clinical. A number of other causes of skin sclerosis or poor peripheral circulation must be considered in the differential diagnosis (summarized in Table 3). Marked differences between the major subsets of systemic sclerosis in the pattern and time-course of clinical features allow most patients to be characterized into the appropriate subset.

Patients with diffuse, cutaneous systemic sclerosis typically present over 1 to 3 years with widespread changes in skin texture, puffy oedematous extremities, generalized pruritis, and profound constitutional and inflammatory symptoms. Vasospastic symptoms are not usually prominent during the early stages, although within 18 months of their onset most patients will describe definite Raynaud's phenomenon. By contrast, the cutaneous and vasospastic symptoms of limited cutaneous systemic sclerosis are very different. The onset of skin changes is more gradual, often preceded by several years of Raynaud's phenomenon, often becoming progressively more severe, with skin sclerosis limited to the face, neck, and hands distal to the wrists. The main differences between the subsets of systemic sclerosis are summarized in Table 4.

Table 1 Scleroderma spectrum of disorders

Localized cutaneous scleroderma	
Morphoea	
– Localized	One or more skin lesions, often on truncal areas
– Generalized	Widespread skin lesions, can be reminiscent of diffuse cutaneous systemic sclerosis, but Raynaud's unusual, no visceral manifestations, and skin changes are less likely to be acral
Linear scleroderma	The most common form occurring in childhood. Skin changes follow a dermatomal distribution, especially on the limbs and lead to important secondary growth defects
En coup de sabre	Midline or parasagittal variant of linear scleroderma, which manifests in childhood and is often associated with defects in underlying fascial and skeletal structures
Systemic sclerosis	
Limited cutaneous systemic sclerosis	Skin sclerosis distal to the wrists(or ankles), over the face and neck Often longstanding Raynaud's phenomenon
Diffuse cutaneous systemic sclerosis	Truncal and acral skin involvement. Presence of tendon friction rubs. Onset of skin changes (puffy or hide-bound) within 1 year of onset of Raynaud's phenomenon
Overlap syndromes	Features of systemic sclerosis together with those of at least one other autoimmune rheumatic disease, e.g. SLE, RA, or polymyositis
Systemic sclerosis sine scleroderma	Vascular or fibrotic visceral features without skin sclerosis (less than 1% cases)
Raynaud's phenomenon	
Autoimmune Raynaud's phenomenon	Raynaud's phenomenon associated with antinuclear antibodies (or other SSc-associated autoimmune serology), usually also abnormal nailfold. capillaroscopy. Some patients later develop systemic sclerosis
Primary Raynaud's phenomenon	Vasospastic symptoms with normal nailfold capillaroscopy and negative autoimmune serology and no other underlying medical/mechanical cause

SLE, systemic lupus erythematosus; RA, rheumatoid arthritis; SSc, systemic sclerosis.

Raynaud's phenomenon

Raynaud's phenomenon is characterized by pallor, cyanosis, suffusion, and/or pain of the fingers in response to cold or stress. The same process can also affect the toes, ears, nose, or jaw. It is present in up to 15 per cent of otherwise healthy individuals. About 1 per cent of those showing the phenomenon develop a connective tissue disease. Other conditions associated with Raynaud's phenomenon include cervical rib, vibration white finger, hypothyroidism, and uraemia. Cold-induced peripheral vasospasm is present in the majority of patients with systemic sclerosis, although generally not in those with localized forms of scleroderma.

It is important to distinguish between the primary and secondary forms of Raynaud's phenomenon. This is most reliably achieved by combining nailfold capillaroscopic assessment with autoantibody testing. Primary Raynaud's phenomenon cases are often familial, typically with onset in the late teens or early adulthood, have normal or only minimally disrupted capillaroscopic architecture, and negative antinuclear antibody tests. Those who present with isolated Raynaud's phenomenon but later develop a connective tissue disease invariably have abnormal autoimmune serology and nailfold capillary studies before they develop associated clinical features. Patients who demonstrate antibodies, including hallmark specificities for lupus or systemic sclerosis, may be designated as having autoimmune Raynaud's phenomenon.

Limited cutaneous systemic sclerosis

This was formerly termed '**CREST**' (calcinosis circumscripta, Raynaud's, (o)esophagus, sclerodactyly, and telangiectasia) and is the most common form of systemic sclerosis, accounting for over 60 per cent of cases. Patients are usually women, between 30- and 50-years old, with longstanding Raynaud's phenomenon.

Early in the disease there is non-pitting oedema of the fingers (sausage-shaped fingers), which, after several weeks or months, is gradually replaced by thickened and shiny skin. This is not usually so closely adherent to underlying structures that mobility is severely impaired, which is in sharp contrast to the findings in those with diffuse disease. Skin involvement does not spread proximally on to the trunk, but the face should be examined carefully for thin, tightly pursed lips, with furrowing and puckering of the surrounding skin, and microstomia. The most striking cutaneous finding is digital and facial telangiectasia caused by dilated capillary loops and venules (Fig. 1). Other evidence of structural vascular change is to be seen in the fingertips, where small areas of ischaemic necrosis or ulceration are common, often leaving pitting scars and pulp atrophy. Loss of the tufts of the terminal phalanges, confirmed on radiography, is also presumed to be due to ischaemia. Patients with limited cutaneous disease often develop intracutaneous and subcutaneous calcification. These deposits frequently occur in the fingers, particularly the digital pads, and in periarticular tissues such as the prepatellar area and olecranon bursa. The calcinotic masses vary in size and are often complicated by ulceration of the overlying skin, extrusion of calcific material, and secondary bacterial infection. Patients may complain of dyspepsia from reflux oesophagitis: this and other visceral complications are discussed in detail below.

Diffuse cutaneous systemic sclerosis

By contrast to limited cutaneous systemic sclerosis, the onset of diffuse disease is often abrupt. It may present with widespread, symmetrical, sometimes itchy, painful swelling of the fingers, arms, feet, legs, and face. Rapid weight loss and constitutional symptoms of fatigue or weakness are frequent. If a patient with early disease presents with headache, blurring of vision, and significant hypertension, then this is a medical emergency, portending hypertensive renal crisis and requiring immediate action (see below).

The clinical findings in diffuse scleroderma depend on the stage of the disease. At onset, examination of the skin will usually reveal cold, painful, swollen hands, with swelling and stiffness already extending to the arms,

Table 2 Localized scleroderma in adults and children

Pattern of disease	Clinical features	Treatment	Prognosis
Localized morphoea	One or a few circumscribed sclerotic plaques with hypo-or hyperpigmentation and an inflamed violaceous border	Often unnecessary Serial measurement to assess progress	Good prognosis, lesions less active within 3 years but pigmentary changes often persist
Generalized morphoea	Widespread pruritic lesions, often symmetrical and following the distribution of superficial veins	Suppress inflammation with oral or IV steroids. Maintenance treatment with D-penicillamine (at least 500 mg/day). Methotrexate and systemic or intralesional interferon may be effective, and ciclosporin has been used in refractory cases	Internal organ pathology very rare. Raynaud's sometimes associated. Generally improves within 5 years of onset, although textural and pigmentary changes can remain
Linear scleroderma	Sclerotic areas occurring in a linear distribution, often on limbs and asymmetrical. In childhood it can lead to serious growth defects of affected limbs. Careful, serial measurement of muscle bulk and limb length is essential	Suppression of inflammation with oral or intravenous steroids. Maintenance treatment with D-penicillamine or methotrexate. Physiotherapy and appropriate regular exercise to minimize growth defects in the childhood-onset form	Long-term effects of childhood-onset form minimized by effective suppression of inflammatory process, and by good physiotherapy. Ultimately the disease tends to resolve, but it can remain active for many years
En coup de sabre	Linear scleroderma affecting the face or scalp, involving underlying subcutaneous tissues, muscles, periosteum, and bone. Underlying cerebral abnormalities have been reported	Therapeutic options as for linear scleroderma; systemic treatment only for active inflammatory lesions	Scarring, growth defects, and alopecia persist, but inflammatory component usually resolves

Table 3 Differential diagnosis of scleroderma

A. Skin sclerosis

Infiltrative disorders
- amyloidosis
- scleromyxoedema
- scleroderma of Buschke
- lichen sclerosis et atrophicus

Metabolic disorders
- myxoedema
- porphyria cutanea tarda
- congenital porphyrias
- acromegaly
- phenylketonuria

Inflammatory disorders
- overlap connective tissue diseases
- eosinophilic fasciitis
- chronic graft-versus-host disease
- sarcoidosis

B. Acral vasospasm

Raynaud's phenomenon
- primary Raynaud's phenomenon
- other autoimmune rheumatic disorders:
  - – systemic lupus erythematosus
  - – rheumatoid disease
  - – dermato/polymyositis

Other vascular disease
- haematological:
  - – cryoglobulinaemia
  - – cold-agglutinin disease
  - – hyperviscosity syndrome
- systemic vasculitis
- macrovascular disease

feet, lower legs, face, and trunk. This oedematous phase is usually replaced within a few months by one of induration, when the skin becomes tight, shiny, and bound to underlying structures. Pigmentary changes (hyperpigmentation or hypopigmentation) accompany skin thickening in many patients. Skin involvement in diffuse scleroderma is quite different from that in the limited form of the disease, and can be mapped semiquantitatively by measuring the degree and extent of cutaneous thickening at multiple sites, from which is derived a skin score. In diffuse scleroderma this score increases rapidly at first, often peaking after 1 to 3 years, and is accompanied by impaired mobility of tendons, joints, and muscles that is clinically all too apparent. Contractures and stretching of the skin over bony points often lead to painful ulcers that are slow to heal, particularly over the proximal interphalangeal joints, elbows, and ankle malleoli.

In its earliest stages, diffuse scleroderma can be confused with an acute inflammatory arthropathy, particularly if Raynaud's phenomenon is absent. The oedematous puffy skin is often accompanied by symmetrically stiff, painful joints (hands, feet, knees, ankles, and wrists), but the classic synovitis of rheumatoid arthritis is usually absent. The clinical sign of tendon friction rubs should carefully be sought in this group of patients: these have a distinctive leathery crepitus and can be elicited during joint movement over elbows, knees, fingers, wrists, and ankles. They frequently antedate a rapid increase in cutaneous involvement, or the onset of visceral disease. Signs of carpal tunnel syndrome may be present, due to flexor tenosynovitis at the wrist.

Mild muscle disease is common and can be detected on examination, but is not usually accompanied by an increase in plasma creatine kinase or inflammatory changes on muscle biopsy. It is generally non-progressive. The few patients with florid changes of polymyositis are usually classified as having an overlap syndrome. As with limited disease, evidence of structural vascular damage—sometimes extensive—may be found in the nailfold capillaries and the digital pads.

Scleroderma sine scleroderma

These patients constitute less than 2 per cent of those with systemic sclerosis, but they are the most difficult group to recognize. They may or may

Table 4 Contrasting clinical features of the two major systemic sclerosis (SSc) subsets

Diffuse cutaneous SSc (dcSSc)

- 33% of patients
- Inflammatory features more prominent at onset
- Raynaud's may develop later
- Skin sclerosis proximal to wrists/elbows and truncal areas
- Prominent pruritis and constitutional symptoms
- Tendon friction rubs associated with progressive disease
- Significant visceral disease more frequent than in lcSSc: renal, pulmonary fibrosis (secondary PHT),cardiac, gut
- Disease activity appears to remain fairly constant over many years, with prominent vasospastic symptoms

Limited cutaneous SSc (lcSSc)

- 66% of patients
- Longstanding Raynaud's phenomenon
- Skin changes: hands, face, neck
- Compared with dcSSc, renal disease less frequent, isolated pulmonary hypertension, severe gut disease, and interstitial lung fibrosis (if antitopoisomerase-1 present)
- Florid telangiectasis and calcinosis (especially anticentromere antibody-positive)
- Disease activity appears to be maximal in first 3 years from onset, then often plateaus and skin involvement may stabilize or improve

Prevalence of organ-based complications in the major systemic sclerosis subsets*

Clinical feature	lcSSc (%)	dcSSc (%)	Overall (%)
Raynaud's phenomenon	99	98	99
Skeletal myopathy	11	23	15
Oesophageal	74	60	69
Other gastrointestinal	7	8	8
Cardiac	9	12	10
Pulmonary fibrosis	26	41	31
Pulmonary hypertension	21	17	20
Renal (overall)	8	18	12
Renal (crisis)	2	10	5

*Data from patients attending The Royal Free Hospital Centre for Rheumatology 1990–99.

not have Raynaud's phenomenon, but by definition they never have the skin changes of scleroderma: common presenting problems include oesophagitis, malabsorption, pseudo-obstruction, renal failure, cardiac arrhythmias, and interstitial lung disease.

Overlap syndromes

There are patients whose disease is not easy to define, having features overlapping with those of other connective tissue diseases. A variety of terms such as 'mixed connective tissue disease', 'undifferentiated connective tissue syndrome', and 'overlap syndromes' have emerged to describe such patients.

Whether or not mixed connective tissue disease is a true entity is controversial. Sharp and colleagues used the term in the 1970s to describe patients with some features of polymyositis, lupus, and scleroderma who ran a benign course with no pulmonary, cerebral, or renal involvement, and no vasculitis. They supposedly responded well to low-dose steroids, and could be identified by the presence of a high-titre antibody with specificity for a nuclear U1 ribonucleoprotein (**RNP**) antigen. However, the clinical features, laboratory tests, and the response to therapy have all proven not to be specific, and these patients do not fulfil the definition of and diagnostic criteria for a single disease. Neither can they be sensibly described as having an 'overlap syndrome', assuming that this definition means the coexistence of two separate diseases. Nevertheless, over time, many do develop major internal organ involvement and evolve into a defined connective tissue disease.

Ribonucleoprotein antibodies can be found in patients with scleroderma or systemic lupus erythematosus. The typical patient with the overlap syndrome presents with Raynaud's phenomenon, puffy hands, arthralgia, myositis, abnormal oesophageal motility, and lymphadenopathy. Over a period of a few years, the skin may become thickened, telangiectasia and calcinosis may appear, signs and symptoms of interstitial lung disease emerge, and the patient has developed scleroderma. Another patient with similar initial findings may develop alopecia, photosensitivity, mouth ulcers, renal disease, antibodies to double-stranded DNA and has developed systemic lupus erythematosus. Other patients may develop a prominent destructive arthropathy reminiscent of rheumatoid disease.

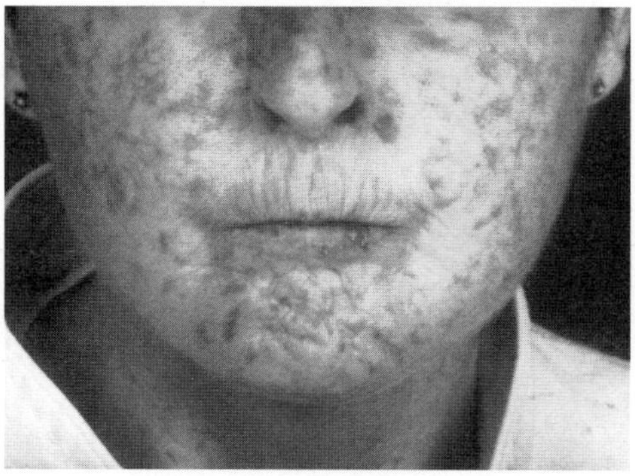

Fig. 1 This patient shows the typical facial features of limited cutaneous systemic sclerosis—microstomia, furrowing, and puckering of the skin around the mouth, beaking of the nose, and telangiectasia on the lips and face.

Autoimmune serology in systemic sclerosis

The majority of patients with scleroderma carry a hallmark autoantibody, and almost all have antinuclear reactivity, often with an antinucleolar pattern on Hep2 cells. Thus either anticentromere, and antitopoisomerase or anti-RNA polymerase III (generally also with anti-RNA polymerase I) are present in most patients and are generally (although not always) mutually exclusive reactivities. Rarer specificities include U3-RNP, PM-Scl, and anti-Th. Each serologically defined group shows somewhat different clinical features, which is of some value in risk stratification for management. There are also well-established class II MHC associations with the various autoantibodies, although some differences in association occur in different racial groups. The reactivities and reported clinical associations of the autoantibodies associated with scleroderma are summarized in Table 5.

Studies using an immunoblotting technique, which is more sensitive than immunofluorescence, have demonstrated that the anticentromere antibody (the antigen actually resides in the kinetochore region of the chromosome) is predictive for the development of limited cutaneous disease (sensitivity 60 per cent, specificity 98 per cent) and Scl-70 (an antibody known to recognize the nuclear enzyme DNA topoisomerase I) for the diffuse subset (sensitivity 38 per cent, specificity 100 per cent). Other serum autoantibodies, notably those to nucleolar antigens, are also relatively specific for scleroderma, and the proportion of patients having one or more antibody is over 80 per cent of the total. Some of these antibodies have been shown to have correlations with class II MHC haplotypes.

Less specific serological abnormalities are also found in scleroderma and include hypergammaglobulinaemia, the presence of immune complexes, low concentrations of complement components, and a weakly positive rheumatoid factor. Antibodies to SSA/Ro and SSB/La are found in 50 per cent of patients with scleroderma who also have Sjögren's syndrome, and are nearly always found in those with glandular lymphocyte infiltration rather than fibrosis.

Organ-based complications of systemic sclerosis

Despite the usefulness of an accurate subset classification of patients with systemic sclerosis, management requires that an organ-based approach be taken once the subset has been assigned. This ensures that important complications, which occur with different frequencies in the different subsets, are not missed. The overall prevalence of the different complications is summarized in Table 4.

Vascular manifestations

Raynaud's phenomenon

Episodic acral vasospasm, precipitated by cold or emotional stress (Raynaud's phenomenon), is almost universally present in patients with systemic sclerosis, although its prominence varies considerably between cases. The pathogenetic mechanism is uncertain, but probably represents an imbalance between vasoconstrictor and vasodilator mechanisms in small blood vessels, or an exaggerated release of vasoconstrictor mediators in response to physiological levels of stimulation by cold or emotion.

Raynaud's phenomenon is common in otherwise healthy individuals, with some series estimating its prevalence to be up to 15 per cent in women, with a much lower frequency in men. It may precede the onset of systemic sclerosis, especially the limited cutaneous subset, by many years, whereas in diffuse cutaneous systemic sclerosis it generally first becomes manifest around the time of the onset of other features of the disorder, or afterwards. Patients who have Raynaud's phenomenon in association with one of the hallmark autoantibodies of systemic sclerosis, such as anticentromere or antitopoisomerase-1, will often develop other features of systemic sclerosis, typically within 3 to 5 years, and so may represent a prescleroderma state—but they can also develop features of other autoimmune rheumatic disorders. Current approaches to the management of patients with Raynaud's phenomenon are summarized in Table 6.

Macrovascular disease

There have been several reports that macrovascular disease is increased in patients with systemic sclerosis. This is plausible, given the number of common aetiopathogenic mechanisms between the processes of atherosclerosis and systemic sclerosis, including endothelial-cell perturbation, activation and damage, and subsequent fibroproliferation. Large-vessel disease has important implications for the organ-based complications of systemic sclerosis such as renal disease, peripheral ischaemia, and bowel involvement. Some non-invasive studies have suggested the presence of flow abnormalities in large vessels in the cerebral and renal circulations in systemic sclerosis. Extrapolating from the results of studies investigating cardiac and pulmonary blood flow variations attributable to vasomotor instability, it is certainly possible that episodic vasospasm is not restricted to the extremities in this disease.

Skin manifestations

Scleroderma means 'hard skin' and is the hallmark of the scleroderma-spectrum disorders. The skin lesions of scleroderma differ between diffuse and limited cutaneous subsets, not only by their extent and distribution,

Table 5 Clinical and laboratory correlates of serum autoantibodies

Antigen	Antinuclear antibody staining pattern	HLA associations	Frequency in patients (%)	Clinical associations	Organ involvement
Scl-70 Topoisomerase 1	Speckled (diffuse fine)	DR5 (DR11) DR3/DR52a DQ7 DQB1	20–25 overall 40 (diffuse) 10–15 (limited)	Diffuse	Lung fibrosis
ACA centromere	Centromere (kinetochore)	DR1 (DQ5) DQB1 DR4 (D13 subtypes)	25–30 70 (limited)	Limited	Pulmonary hypertension, severe gut disease
RNA I and III	Speckled/nucleolar (punctate)	?	20	Diffuse	Renal, skin
U3RNP Fibrillarin	Nucleolar (clumpy)	?	5	Overlap	Pulmonary hypertension, muscle
U1RNP	Speckled nuclear	?	10	Limited overlap, Afro-Caribbeans	Overlap features, muscle
Th (To)	Nucleolar (homogeneous)	?	5	Limited	Pulmonary hypertension, Small bowel
PM-Scl	Nucleolar (homogeneous)	DR3/DR52	3–5	Overlap	Mixed, muscle

but also by the greater tendency for there to be induration and oedema of affected tissues in diffuse cutaneous systemic sclerosis. This may reflect a local release of cytokines or altered endothelial permeability in the diffuse form. The inflammatory phase evolves into established fibrosis, sometimes leading to sheets of thickened skin or a hide-bound texture. The skin sclerosis score (skin-score) is a validated method for assessing the extent of skin involvement, and has been shown to predict survival and to correlate with some other disease features, for example a rapidly increasing skin-score is associated with an increased occurrence of scleroderma renal crisis.

Another common vascular manifestation of scleroderma is the development of local dilated loops of small blood vessels in the skin, termed 'telangiectasias'. These are often distressing for patients and may also cause problems from haemorrhage if they are at sites prone to trauma. Haemorrhage from mucosal telangiectasias is increasingly recognized as a clinical problem that may require local therapy if recurrent: gastrointestinal haemorrhage and epistaxis have both been reported. Men with facial telangiectasia may experience difficulties when shaving. Cosmetic camouflage techniques can be very effective in masking facial telangiectasia, and appropriate advice should be offered to all who might benefit. Recently the pulsed dye laser has also been used with some success.

Pulmonary disease

The most frequent cause of death related to systemic sclerosis is pulmonary disease, which can take the form of interstitial fibrosis or pulmonary vascular disease. These two processes can coexist in patients with secondary pulmonary hypertension, a subgroup that should probably be considered separately from those with isolated pulmonary hypertension.

There has recently been substantial progress in the assessment of pulmonary disease in those patients with systemic sclerosis. This has refined diagnosis and classification, will almost certainly result in different treatment strategies for particular subsets of patients, and illustrates a general theme that the subsetting of organ-based complications is becoming as important as the correct classification of major disease subsets. The investigation and treatment of the pulmonary manifestations of systemic sclerosis are summarized in Table 7.

Fibrosing alveolitis

The initial events in the development of lung disease in patients with systemic sclerosis appear to involve alveolar inflammation and subsequent epithelial and endothelial perturbation. Although all patients should be screened for this complication, it appears to affect only around 25 per cent

Table 6 Treatment of Raynaud's phenomenon

	Treatment	Examples	Comments
1.	*Simple measures:*		
	Non-drug	Hand warmers Protective clothing	Universally helpful; aim to minimize cold exposure and ambient temperature changes in the work environment
	Pharmacological	Evening primrose oil	Evening primrose oil has been shown to be effective in controlled clinical trial
		Fish oil capsules Antioxidant vitamins	Vitamin C, vitamin E are of anecdotal benefit
2.	*Oral vasodilators:*		
	Calcium-channel blockers	Nifedipine retard Nicardipine Felodipine Amlodipine	Responses are often idiosyncratic; therefore best to try several drugs in rotation to find the most effective
	5-HT antagonist	Ketanserin	Only available on named-patient basis, but has shown to be effective in clinical trials
	ACE or angiotensin inhibitors	Captopril Enalapril Losartan	In Raynaud's secondary to dcSSc, may protect from hypertensive renal crisis
3.	*Topical vasodilators*	GTN patches	Shown to be effective in short-term use but often cause headaches
4.	*Parenteral vasodilators*	Carboprostacyclin (iloprost) Prostaglandin E1	Effective and reasonably tolerated; given for severe frequent attacks of Raynaud's phenomenon, digital ulceration, or gangrene and prior to digital surgery
5.	*Antibiotics*	Flucloxacillin Erythromycin	Important in secondary infection in Raynaud's phenomenon; prolonged administration often necessary
6.	*Surgical procedures:*		
	Lumbar sympathectomy Digital sympathectomy Microarteriolysis	Chemical or operative	For severe Raynaud's phenomenon of lower limbs, useful treatment for ischaemia of 1 or 2 digits
	Debridement Amputation	Surgical or auto-	Such surgery should be conservative to allow maximum possibility of spontaneous healing

5-HT, 5-hydroxytryptamine; ACE, angiotensin-converting enzyme; dcSSc, diffuse cutaneous systemic sclerosis; GTN, glyceryl trinitrate.

of those with limited cutaneous disease and up to 40 per cent of those with the diffuse cutaneous form. It is strongly predicted by the presence of anti-topoisomerase-1 autoantibodies and also by the *HLA-Dr52a* genotype. Increased frequency also occurs in patients with anti-RNA polymerase III antibodies, but the presence of anticentromere antibodies (**ACA**) is associated with a reduced risk. These tests are therefore of clinical value in planning the frequency and intensity of lung screening tests.

Technical developments have made the early detection of interstitial lung disease possible. Chest radiography is not sufficiently sensitive. Serial lung function tests including CO diffusing capacity are probably the most sensitive screening tool. A significant reduction from predicted values at baseline with a restrictive pattern, or a worsening of serial tests, warrants further testing with a high-resolution, thin-section (3 mm), computed tomography (**CT**) scan of the lungs and bronchoalveolar lavage. The combined use of these techniques and diethylenetriaminepentaacetic acid (**DTPA**) scans can provide much earlier diagnosis and/or indices of progression.

The earliest detectable abnormality on CT is usually a narrow, often ill-defined, subpleural crescent of increased attenuation in the posterior segment of the lower lobe. Other early CT changes include an amorphous ground-glass pattern of parenchymal opacification, or a more reticular appearance (Fig. 2). The relative extent of each pattern is important because there is good correlation between these appearances and histological findings at open-lung biopsy; an inflammatory biopsy equating to an amorphous pattern and fibrosis to a reticular one. Such information may reduce the need for an invasive biopsy.

Bronchoalveolar lavage often identifies patients with alveolitis before the onset of symptoms or abnormalities on chest radiography or in pulmonary function tests. DTPA scans, particularly serial studies, may become useful predictors of progression or improvement: a persistently abnormal DTPA scan is associated with a higher rate of decline in pulmonary function tests subsequently, whereas a reversion to normal clearance is associated with sustained improvement in pulmonary function.

These tests have obvious value for assessing the progress of the disease and are critically important in evaluating new treatments. Lung biopsy is still the 'gold standard' for establishing the diagnosis of fibrosing alveolitis, although it is required less often than previously. However, it is now recognized that histological and CT scan appearances allow further classification

Table 7 Pulmonary disease in scleroderma

Disorder	Pathology	Frequency	Clinical features	Investigations	Treatment
Pulmonary fibrosis	Alveolitis with mixed cellular infiltrate, predilection for lung bases, progresses to lung fibrosis	More frequent (40%) in dcSSc In both subsets associated with antipoisomerase antibodies	Dry cough, exertional dyspnoea, bibasal crepitations. Finger-clubbing a late sign	Restrictive pattern of lung function tests (proportionate reduction in DLCO and FVC). Leucocytic (especially neutrophilla) BAL sample. Abnormal high-kV chest radiography. Infitrates (ground-glass) or fibroids (reticular) on high-resolution lung CT scan. Biopsy (open or thoracoscopic) remains the 'gold-standard' DTPA clearance accelerated—useful in assessing activity	Prednisolone and cyclophosphamide are widely used. Retrospective studies suggest efficacy. Placebo-controlled trials underway
Pleural disease	Pleurisy, effusion rare	Uncommon	Pleuritic chest pain. Pleural rub	Chest radiography	NSAIDs or low-dose prednisolone
Bronchiectasis	Suppurative inflammation of the airways	Rare	Chest pain, severe acute dysponea.	CT scan	Appropriate antibiotics, postural drainage
Spontaneous pneumothorax	Rupture of cyst into pleural cavity	Rare	Chronic productive cough. Focal, caorse crepitations.	Chest radiography	Intercostal drain—but avoid if possible (?pleuradesis)
Lung carcinoma	Scar-type (especially alveolar-cell carcinoma). All histological types may be increased	Rare	Variable	CT scan, bronchoscopy	Supportive if unresectable
Pulmonary hypertension	Subintimal cell proliferation, endothelial hyperplasia, and microvascular obliteration	10–15% overall. Isolated mainly to lcSSc, secondary to lung fibrosis in both lcSSc and dcSSc	Dyspnoea loud P2 parasternal heave later signs of right ventricular failure	Reduced DLCO (with normal FVC in isolated PHT). Echo-Doppler often diagnostic. ECG. formal exercise assessment (shuttle test). Right heart catheter allows direct measurement, right ventricular functional assessment and vasodilator challenge	Anticoagulation calcium-channel blockers prostacyclin (intermittent or continuous infusion) oxygen Digoxin and spironolactone if evidence of right ventricular dysfunction

Abbreviations: dcSSc, diffuse cutaneous systemic sclerosis; lcSSc, limited cutaneous systemic sclerosis; DLCO, carbon monoxide diffusion in the lung; FVC, forced vital capacity; BAL, bronchoalveolar lavage; DTPA, diethylenetriaminepentaacetic acid; CT, computed tomography; PHT, pulmonary hypertension.

of systemic sclerosis-associated fibrosing alveolitis into 'usual-pattern' (**UIP**) or 'non-specific interstitial pneumonia' (**NSIP**). These have different prognoses and probably require different treatment approaches. In general, the outcome for patients with systemic sclerosis-associated fibrosing alveolitis is better than that for cryptogenic fibrosing alveolitis of equivalent extent. Most patients with active alveolitis receive immunomodulatory therapy and many studies have suggested that this is effective. However, formal prospective controlled trials are still needed to confirm this and to refine therapeutic regimens. The management of interstitial lung disease can be further complicated by the development of secondary pulmonary hypertension.

Pulmonary vascular disease

Pulmonary vascular disease is of substantial clinical importance in patients with scleroderma. The overall prevalence is estimated at between 10 and 20 per cent. This is higher than was previously reported, reflecting the use of non-invasive methods of detection, such as echocardiography with Doppler estimation of the peak pulmonary arterial systolic pressure (from the velocity of retrograde flow into the right atrium in the presence of tricuspid regurgitation).

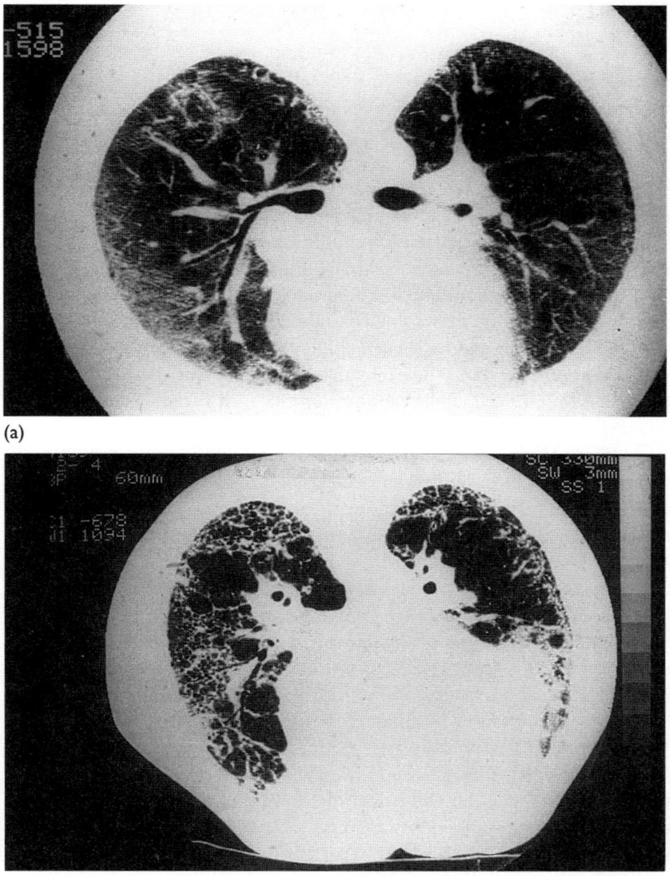

(a)

(b)

Fig. 2 (a) Thin-section CT scan image illustrating the ground-glass appearance of early pulmonary involvement posteriorly. A chest radiograph taken at the same time was normal. (b) Thin-section CT scan image illustrating extensive honeycomb shadowing and cystic air spaces involving both lower lobes. Chest radiographic appearances at the same time were of advanced interstitial lung disease (bibasilar reticulonodular shadowing). (Both images with grateful acknowledgement to Drs A. Wells, R. du Bois, and B. Strickland, Departments of Respiratory Medicine and Radiology, Royal Brompton National Heart and Lung Hospitals.)

Isolated pulmonary hypertension (**PHT**) in scleroderma, occurring without other pulmonary pathology, is characteristic of limited cutaneous systemic sclerosis, especially in the classical CREST form of this subset with florid cutaneous telangiectasias. Some cases of isolated PHT have been seen in the diffuse form of the disease, associated with antibodies to U3-RNP, but pulmonary hypertension in this condition usually occurs in the context of established pulmonary fibrosis and constitutes secondary PHT.

There are considerable similarities between the histological features of isolated PHT in scleroderma and primary pulmonary hypertension. There is evidence of subintimal cell proliferation, endothelial hyperplasia, and the obliteration of small intrapulmonary vessels. It has been suggested that initial proliferative changes lead to the characteristic plexiform pathology of rapidly progressive pulmonary hypertension, with remodelling leading to the concentric obliterative lesions that predominate at necropsy in patients succumbing to severe systemic sclerosis-associated PHT.

Survival analysis suggests that patients with systemic sclerosis-associated PHT may have a better prognosis that those with primary pulmonary hypertension, especially if they have a mild to moderate elevation in pulmonary arterial pressure. Although patients with this condition are being identified more frequently than previously, and probably earlier, treatment remains difficult. The prognosis for those with systemic sclerosis and PHT is still to be fully defined, and haemodynamic predictors of outcome are being sought. Treatment, up to and including continuous ambulatory prostacyclin infusion or heart–lung transplantation, is probably appropriate for the most severe cases.

Cardiac involvement

Autopsy studies have identified at least three patterns of myocardial involvement in systemic sclerosis, when up to 50 per cent of patients show features of myocardial fibrosis. Other histological patterns of cardiac disease include contraction-band necrosis and, less frequently, inflammatory cardiomyopathy, the latter probably occurring most often in those with an inflammatory skeletal myopathy.

Non-invasive imaging techniques such as magnetic resonance imaging (**MRI**) or spiral CT scanning may allow myocardial fibrosis to be detected. Indirect clues of cardiac involvement may be deduced from ECG or echocardiographic studies. The investigation and management of the cardiac manifestations of systemic sclerosis are summarized in Table 8.

Pericarditis is well recognized as a complication of systemic sclerosis. It is seen particularly in the context of severe diffuse cutaneous disease and seems to be most frequently encountered in patients with established or imminent scleroderma renal crisis. Echocardiographic studies often reveal small haemodynamically insignificant effusions in patients with scleroderma: around 17 per cent of those with diffuse cutaneous and 4 per cent of those with limited cutaneous disease. Therapeutic pericardiocentesis is only occasionally required, but pericardial effusion is associated with active progressive diffuse cutaneous disease.

Electrophysiological cardiac abnormalities are commonly seen in patients with scleroderma. Conduction defects are frequent, especially Q–Tc prolongation on 12-lead ECG. Later, conduction tissue fibrosis may lead to varying degrees of heart block, including first- or second-degree block or complete heart block necessitating pacemaker implantation. Bundle-branch blocks may reflect abnormalities in the conducting tissues or be complications of ventricular strain. Thus right bundle-branch block may be seen in association with PHT, and left bundle-branch block may occur when there is left ventricular strain from hypertension or cardiac muscle disease. Paroxysmal arrhythmias are much more difficult to detect than conduction abnormalities, and in those with occult cardiac disease are probably an important cause of unexplained death in patients with systemic sclerosis.

Renal disease

Several patterns of renal pathology are recognized in patients with scleroderma: all involve vascular abnormalities. The most clearly defined is the

Table 8 Investigation and management of cardiac manifestations of systemic sclerosis

Cardiac complication	Pathology	Frequency	Clinical features	Investigation	Treatment
Arrhythmias	Extrasystoles, paroxysmal tachyarrhythmias	30%	Palpitations, syncope	ECG (including 24-h tape or telemetry); exercise stress-test	Treat if haemodynamically significant
Conduction defects	Fibrosis of conduction tissue	15%	Syncope, hypotension	ECG	Pacemaker may be required
Pericardial involvement	Pericarditis	10% clinically	Usually asymptomatic	ECG, Echocardiogram	Often none required.
	Pericardial effusion	35% at autopsy	Haemodynamic effects rare	Echocardiogram	Occasionally pericardiocentesis NSAIDs for pericarditis
Myocardial involvement	Myocarditis	Rare	Congestive cardiac failure, arrhythmias	ECG, echocardiogram, stress-echocardiogram, Cardiac enzymes (CK-MB), troponin levels, MUGA scan, MRI, or spiral CT may be discriminatory.	Myocarditis treated with prednisolone. Cardiac failure managed with digoxin, ACE inhibitors and diuretics, including spironolactone.
	Myocardial fibrosis	30–50% dcSSc	Congestive cardiac failure		

NSAID, non-steroidal anti-inflammatory drug; dcSSc, dcSSc, diffuse cutaneous systemic sclerosis; CK-MB, creatine kinase myocardial-type; MUGA, multigated image acquisition (heart scan); MRI, magnetic resonance imaging; CT, computed tomography.

scleroderma renal crisis, which describes the occurrence of acute renal failure in a patient with scleroderma, usually associated with accelerated hypertension (further compounding the renal pathology), and in whom no other cause for nephropathy is present. Scleroderma renal crisis was almost always fatal prior to the routine use of angiotensin-converting enzyme (**ACE**) inhibitors and the improvement in outcome over the last 20 years represents a considerable therapeutic triumph. However, in addition to scleroderma renal crisis, many patients demonstrate less severe renal complications, probably associated with reduced renal blood flow and the consequent reduction in glomerular filtration rate. The mechanism of this slowly progressive form of chronic renal disease is unclear. A small number of patients develop significant glomerulonephritis.

Acute renal crisis

This generally occurs in patients with diffuse cutaneous systemic sclerosis within 5 years of disease onset. It is often associated with rapidly advancing skin disease and the presence of tendon friction rubs. Patients often carry the antitopoisomerase-1 or anti-RNA polymerase-III autoantibody, and presence of the latter should prompt extra vigilance in monitoring for renal involvement, particularly in those with limited cutaneous disease who otherwise very rarely develop scleroderma renal crisis. The overall incidence of scleroderma renal crisis varies between different systemic sclerosis subsets and disease stages: in high-risk patients it may be as great as 20 per cent, but overall is probably less than 10 per cent.

The following diagnostic criteria for scleroderma renal crisis have been proposed: abrupt onset of arterial hypertension greater than 160/90 mmHg; hypertensive retinopathy of at least grade III severity; rapid deterioration of renal function; and elevated plasma renin activity. Other typical features include hypertensive encephalopathy and the presence of a microangiopathic haemolytic blood film: the presence of fragmented erythrocytes on a blood film is a simple and inexpensive method of identifying early scleroderma renal crisis.

Symptoms of scleroderma renal crisis usually present abruptly and the condition should be regarded as a life-threatening medical emergency requiring prompt intervention. The pulse rate is increased and patients develop headaches, visual phenomena, and convulsions due to accelerated hypertension. Symptoms and signs of left ventricular failure may follow rapidly. Oliguria or anuria lead to a rising serum creatinine level, and death from renal failure can occur within a short time in untreated patients. Proteinuria is almost universal, and although this may be present long before the renal crisis develops, it often increases with the crisis, though not to nephrotic levels. Microscopic haematuria and granular or red cell urinary casts are typically present.

Although renal crisis usually occurs in patients with established systemic sclerosis, it can occasionally be the presenting feature of the disease. For this reason the hands and face of any patient presenting with unexplained severe or accelerated hypertension should be examined for clues that might suggest an underlying connective tissue disorder such as systemic sclerosis. Clinical suspicions should be followed up with appropriate investigations, particularly autoimmune serology and nailfold capillaroscopy.

Hypertension should be treated using ACE inhibitors. It has been suggested that quinapril may be preferable to other agents. Historically, most patients have received either captopril or enalapril together with calcium-channel blockers, aimed at reducing both diastolic and systolic pressure by 10 to 15 mmHg per day until baseline levels of diastolic pressure at 80 to 90 mmHg are achieved. Sublingual nifedipine or subcutaneous hydralazine can be used if the patient is vomiting. Intravenous prostacyclin, which may directly benefit the microvascular lesion, is often administered from diagnosis.

It is generally useful to perform a renal biopsy when hypertension has been adequately controlled. This provides prognostic information, allows histological confirmation of the diagnosis, and permits exclusion of other causes for abrupt-onset renal failure such as glomerulonephritis. Histological examination usually shows fibrinoid necrosis; mucoid or fibromucoid proliferative intimal lesions (when extensive, termed 'onion-skinning') in renal arteries, particularly the arcuate and interlobular vessels; glomerular thrombi; and ultimately glomerulosclerosis. The extent of the glomerular lesion can sometimes be useful in predicting the likely degree of ultimate functional recovery. Occasionally a similar pattern of renal dysfunction occurs without hypertension (normotensive renal crisis), suggesting that the pathological features are not simply the end-organ consequences of raised arterial pressure.

Renal function should be monitored closely with daily measurement of serum creatinine. Regular full blood counts, clotting screens, and fibrin-degradation product estimations are important to detect and monitor microangiopathic haemolytic anaemia, which often reflects activity of the disease process. Short-term haemodialysis should be given if necessary, and peritoneal dialysis often works well if long-term renal replacement therapy is needed. It has been observed that skin sclerosis and other features of systemic sclerosis can improve after a renal crisis, particularly if the patient is undergoing maintenance dialysis. The basis for this is uncertain: it may result from the removal or inactivation of circulating mediators, or simply reflect the natural history of the disease. Considerable recovery in renal function often occurs after an acute crisis, sometimes allowing dialysis to be discontinued, and improvement can continue for up to 2 years. Decisions regarding renal transplantation should not be made before this time.

Chronic nephropathy

Patients who survive scleroderma renal crisis may develop similar but less florid proliferative changes in the interlobular and arcuate arteries. Even those who have never had a renal crisis may show reduplication of elastic fibres, sclerosed glomeruli, tubular atrophy, and interstitial fibrosis, presumably reflecting the chronic changes of scleroderma.

Glomerulonephritis

There are a small number of case reports of glomerulonephritis occurring in systemic sclerosis, including a progressive crescentic glomerulonephritis in association with positive antimyeloperoxidase autoantibodies. More commonly, biopsy reveals coincident pathologies such as drug-induced injury or overlap syndromes with features of other connective tissue disorders such as systemic lupus erythematosus.

Gastrointestinal complications

The majority of patients with systemic sclerosis exhibit at least one gastrointestinal manifestation. Most frequent is oesophageal dysmotility and associated reflux oesophagitis. These symptoms often respond dramatically to treatment with proton-pump inhibitors. Involvement can also occur at other sites: these are described in Table 9, together with current management approaches for each complication.

Gastric involvement typically leads to slow gastric emptying and symptoms of postprandial fullness. This, together with sicca symptoms and difficulty swallowing, encourages poor nutritional intake and is a significant contributor to the weight loss observed in patients with this disease. The earliest feature of small bowel involvement is also dysmotility, leading to increased intestinal transit time, which together with a propensity to form wide-mouthed jejunal diverticulae leads to stagnation of the luminal contents and small intestinal bacterial overgrowth. This may in turn lead to bloating, flatulence, malabsorption, and chronic diarrhoea. Endstage involvement of the small bowel leads to profound malabsorption and malnutrition and is a significant cause of miserable scleroderma-associated death. Large-bowel manifestations include constipation and anorectal incontinence. Alternating constipation and diarrhoea is common and complicates management, which is generally empirical.

Musculoskeletal complications

Musculoskeletal features are almost universal in established systemic sclerosis, although often relatively well tolerated. Most patients with diffuse disease experience muscle weakness, although prominent myositis is unusual. Flexion contractures of the interphalangeal joints are common and can be very debilitating. Surgical intervention can be valuable but should focus on functional rather than cosmetic gain. Arthralgia and stiffness are the most frequent symptoms. Frank arthritis is uncommon and points towards an overlap syndrome. Other musculoskeletal manifestations include carpal tunnel syndrome, tendonitis (with friction rubs—most often in diffuse cutaneous disease), and the consequences of contractures—especially affecting the hands, but also more proximal joints in diffuse disease.

Other organ involvement

Neurological involvement is uncommon, but in the late stages of limited cutaneous disease a small but significant proportion of patients develop unilateral or bilateral trigeminal neuralgia. Impotence is a problem for men, usually occurring 1 to 2 years after disease onset, thought to have an neurovascular cause, and is refractory to treatment. Dryness of the mucous membranes is common, leading to dyspareunia. Hypothyroidism occurs in as many as 50 per cent of patients with systemic sclerosis and is frequently missed. Some patients have antithyroid antibodies, but lymphocytic infiltration in the gland is uncommon, fibrosis being the more typical finding.

Disease course

Since the clinical course of particular subsets of systemic sclerosis can to a great extent be predicted, appropriate classification within the scleroderma-spectrum is valuable in planning disease management.

Patients with limited disease have an 'early phase' that lasts about 10 years, when the picture is usually dominated by vascular problems such as Raynaud's phenomenon, pitting scars, digital ulcers, and telangiectasias. Later there may be worsening of the vascular disease, both cutaneously and in the pulmonary circulation. Pulmonary interstitial disease, usually more indolent than that seen in the diffuse form, can also occur as a late complication. Gut involvement may worsen with time, and oesophageal strictures, malabsorption, pseudo-obstruction, and anal incontinence are all possible late and troublesome events in this subset.

During the early phase of diffuse disease (the first 5 years), the patient is fatigued and loses weight. Hypertensive renal crisis is a real risk, and rapid progression of pulmonary and cardiac disease may occur. Arthritis, myositis, and tendon involvement can be most marked at this time. After 5 years, considered to be the late stage of diffuse disease, the constitutional symptoms settle down, the skin and musculoskeletal problems have usually reached a plateau, and there is progression of existing visceral disease but a reduced risk of new organ involvement. These differences in the pattern and natural history influence evaluation and therapy.

Pathogenesis

Systemic sclerosis involves immunological, vascular, and connective tissue abnormalities. Models of pathogenesis focus upon the importance of an initiating stimulus in a susceptible individual and subsequent amplification of pathogenic processes, leading to one of the different subsets of the disease. There is a complex interplay between a number of factors: some of the mechanisms implicated in pathogenesis of systemic sclerosis are indicated in Table 10.

Current models suggest that initiating events eventually lead to the establishment of a fibrogenic population of interstitial fibroblasts that produce increased amounts of extracellular matrix. Disruption of normal tissue architecture and secondary mechanisms such as ischaemia produce the pathological and clinical features. Determination of the discrete patterns of organ involvement within and between disease subsets is not understood, although associations with class II MHC haplotypes and with particular autoantibodies suggest that genetic or immunological mechanisms may be important. Despite the extreme rarity of familial scleroderma, it seems likely that there is a substantial, if complex, genetic component to the pathogenesis of systemic sclerosis, which is likely to involve both severity and susceptibility loci. Twin data have failed to confirm a substantial inherited component, but some studies—for example, of the Choctaw Native American tribe—have shown a very high incidence of diffuse systemic sclerosis in some populations. A number of candidate genes, including *Fbn-1* (Fibrillin-1), are currently under investigation.

Survival

There have been a number of studies of survival in the past 50 years, and the 5-year cumulative survival rate ranges from 34 to 73 per cent. Even prolonged survival does not protect against an increased mortality risk, which continues for at least 15 years. Factors that adversely affect outcome are increasing age, being male, extent of skin involvement, and heart, lung, and renal disease. Most recent studies point to a substantial improvement in survival over the last 20 years: this is likely to be attributable to the treatment of renal crisis—previously almost invariably fatal—and perhaps to better detection and treatment of other major complications.

Management of systemic sclerosis

There have been significant recent advances in the management of patients with scleroderma, mainly related to improved treatment of organ-based complications and to the appreciation that successful management depends upon accurate diagnosis, subsetting, staging within subset, and screening for specific complications. Many advances have occurred in parallel with the improved treatment of other medical conditions such as hypertension and gastro-oesophageal reflux disease.

One of the most improved areas of clinical understanding of the scleroderma-spectrum of disorders has been the concept of risk stratification. This enables precious resources to be appropriately focused, so that patients at highest risk of particular complications are thoroughly investigated. Subsetting and staging within subsets is the starting point. Associations with particular autoantibodies are helpful, as summarized in Table 5. Additional predictive power is provided by genetic markers, and this is likely to increase considerably over the next few years. In particular, functionally relevant single nucleotide polymorphisms, such as those in cytokine or growth-factor receptors, or other polymorphic markers, including immunogenetic ones, are likely to increase predictive power.

Table 9 Gastrointestinal tract complications of systemic sclerosis

Site	Disorder	Symptom	Investigation	Treatment
Mouth	Tight skin	Cosmetic	None	Facial exercises
	Dental caries	Toothache	Dental radiography	Dental treatment
	Sicca syndrome	Dry mouth	Salivary gland biopsy	Artificial saliva
Oesophagus	Hypomotility	Dysphagia	Barium swallow	Cisapride, avoid NSAIDs and nifedipine
	Reflux oesophagitis	Heartburn	Oesophageal scintiscan	Omeprazole, bed elevation, no late meals, metoclopramide
	Stricture	Dysphagia	Manometry, endoscopy	Dilatation, omeprazole
Stomach	Gastric paresis	Anorexia, nausea, early satiety	Scintigram	Cisapride, metoclopramide
	NSAID-related ulcer	Dyspepsia	Barium meal	Proton-pump inhibitor, H_2 blocker, or misoprostol
Small bowel	Hypomotility, stasis, bacterial overgrowth	Weight loss, postprandial bloating, malabsorption, steatorrhoea	Barium follow-thru' [^{14}C]glycocholate or hydrogen breath test, jejunal aspiration, faecal microscopy	Rotational antibiotics,* cisapride,** metoclopramide,** pancreatic supplements, octreotide (low dose), enteral and parenteral nutritional support
	Pseudo-obstruction NSAID ulceration	Abdominal pain, distension	Plain abdominal radiography	Conservative management *'drip and suck'*
	Pneumatosis intestinalis	Diarrhoea with blood, benign pneumo-peritoneum	Plain abdominal radiography	
Large bowel	Hypomotility	Alternating constipation and diarrhoea	Barium enema	Dietary manipulation, cisapride may help stool expanders, (e.g. ispaghula)
	Colonic pseudo-diverticula perforation	Rare	Barium enema	[resection]
	Pseudo-obstruction	Abdominal pain distension	Plain abdominal radiography	Conservative management 'drip and suck'
Anus	Sphincter involvement	Faecal incontinence	Rectal manometry	Sphincter strengthening exercises ?? Sacral nerve stimulation

*Useful antibiotics: ciprofloxacin, amoxicillin, metronidazole, oral vancomycin, trimethoprim— changing every 4 weeks, with occasional 'antibiotic holiday' that may reduce the development of resistant strains.

**Prokinetic drugs only useful in early neuropathic disease, not later, when smooth muscle is destroyed.

Unfortunately there has been relatively little progress in developing disease-modifying therapies for the most aggressive subset of patients, those with diffuse cutaneous systemic sclerosis, which is probably, in part, a reflection of our relatively limited understanding of the pathogenesis of systemic sclerosis. Effective therapies are likely to be directed against key processes or mediators, and may be different depending upon the subset and stage of disease. In general, it is believed that immunomodulatory strategies are most appropriate in the earlier stages of diffuse disease (1 to 3 years from onset), whereas antifibrotic approaches may be more appropriate in established cases. An induction–maintenance approach has been used in some centres. Current approaches to disease-modifying treatment are summarized in Table 11. Although curative treatments are lacking,

Table 10 Mechanisms implicated in the pathogenesis of systemic sclerosis

	Example	Comments	Potential for therapeutic modulation
Genetic factors	Class II HLA haplotype, Fibrillin-1 (*Fbn-1*)	Linkage studies have shown that autoantibody types associate with particular HLA-D alleles. Recent studies have associated SSc with microsatellites around *Fbn-1* locus	None yet—HLA types may be useful markers of genetic risk, e.g. HLA-DR52a/DR3 associates with lung fibrosis
Chemical exposure	Vinyl chloride, epoxy resin, silica	Epidemiological and anecdotal evidence links various chemical agents to onset of SSc	Avoid exposure to triggering/potentiating factors
Autoimmunity	Hallmark autoantibodies (ACA, anti-topo-1 etc.)	Strong link between autoantibodies and SSc. Mutually exclusive, and some evidence of an antigen-driven production	Specific peptide-based strategies may block antibody production, but antibodies may not be pathogenic. Basis for immunomodulatory therapeutic strategies, including immunoablation and autologous stem-cell reconstitution
Alloimmunity	Fetal microchimerism	Some evidence suggests increased persistence of fetal DNA or cells in mothers who later develop SSc	Benefit of immunosuppression unclear. Could facilitate persistence or amplification of allogeneic cells
Infection	Little direct evidence	Abrupt onset of an immunologically driven disease raises the possibility of an infective trigger	No evidence that anti-infective therapies are useful
Oxidant stress	Increased oxidative metabolites in SSc urine	Body of evidence suggests there is increased oxidant stress in SSc. May fragment autoantigens and trigger autoimmunity or cause vascular damage	Widespread use of antioxidant nutrients
Apoptosis	Conflicting data	Some studies suggest resistance and others increased susceptibility in SSc. Both could facilitate development of populations of fibrogenic cells	None currently
Paracrine interactions	Many examples e.g. IL-6, TGF-β1	Many *in vivo* and *in vitro* studies suggest altered paracrine interactions between endothelial cells, inflammatory/immune cells, and fibroblasts may underlie pathogenesis	Targeted anticytokine strategies proposed. So far, only effective in animal models

ACA, anticentromere antibody; SSc, systemic sclerosis; IL-6, interleukin-6; TGF-β1, transforming growth factor-β1.

Table 11 Disease-modifying therapies for systemic sclerosis

Treatment	Mechanism of action	Comments	Efficacy in clinical trials
Selective immunosuppression			
Ciclosporin-A	Inhibits TH-cell actions by reducing IL-2 release	Reported beneficial effects on skin sclerosis may be confounded by increased incidence of renal crisis	Yes (open study)
Antithymocyte globulin	Temporary suppression of lymphocyte function	Possible benefit for skin sclerosis	Equivocal (open study)
CAMPATH-1H	MAb against activated T cells	Anecdotal benefit in case reports	No formal evaluation
Photopheresis	Extracorporeal photoactivated 8-methoxypsoralen inhibits activated T cells	Benefit has been reported	No (open study)
Oral collagen type I	Induces oral tolerance	Early studies encouraging	Controlled trial underway in USA
Non-selective immunosuppression			
Methotrexate	Folic acid antagonist	Currently under formal evaluation in dcSSc	Yes (open study) Equivocal (controlled trial in Europe). No in American multicentre trial (1999)
Cyclophosphamide chlorambucil, azathioprine	Alkylating agents	Anecdotal benefit reported in open studies, but controlled trial of chlorambucil failed to show superiority over placebo. Cyclophosphamide often combined with corticosteroids	Yes (cyclophosphamide in SSc lung fibrosis—open study). No (chlorambucil, controlled trial 1994)
Stem-cell therapy	Intensive immuno-suppression followed by autologous peripheral stem-cell haemopoietic and immune reconstitution	So far no benefit proven. High treatment-related morbidity/mortality	Formal studies ongoing
Antifibrotic therapies			
D-penicillamine	Inhibits the formation of stable collagen cross-links by forming a complex with hydroxy-lysine aldehyde and lysine groups on collagen precursors	Little used in UK	No (controlled trial) Yes (open study), 1991. Open studies have shown benefit. High dose ineffective in large American trial (1999)
Interferon-α	Inhibits collagen production by dermal SSc fibroblasts *in vitro*, at transcriptional level. May also eliminate high collagen-producing fibroblast subpopulations	Efficacy has been shown in open studies, placebo-controlled trial is negative Must balance benefit with. morbidity connected with interferon	Yes (open study) 1992 Not effective in placebo-controlled trial 1999
Interferon-γ	As above	Considerable support for use from open studies and *in vitro* properties	Yes (open study), 1993 Yes (open study), 1992 Yes (open study), 1998
Recombinant relaxin	Increases collagen breakdown	Initial studies encouraging	Large multicentre USA and European trials under way

TH, T-helper (cell); IL-2, interleukin-2; MAb, monoclonal antibody; SSc, systemic sclerosis; dcSSc, diffuse cutaneous SSc.

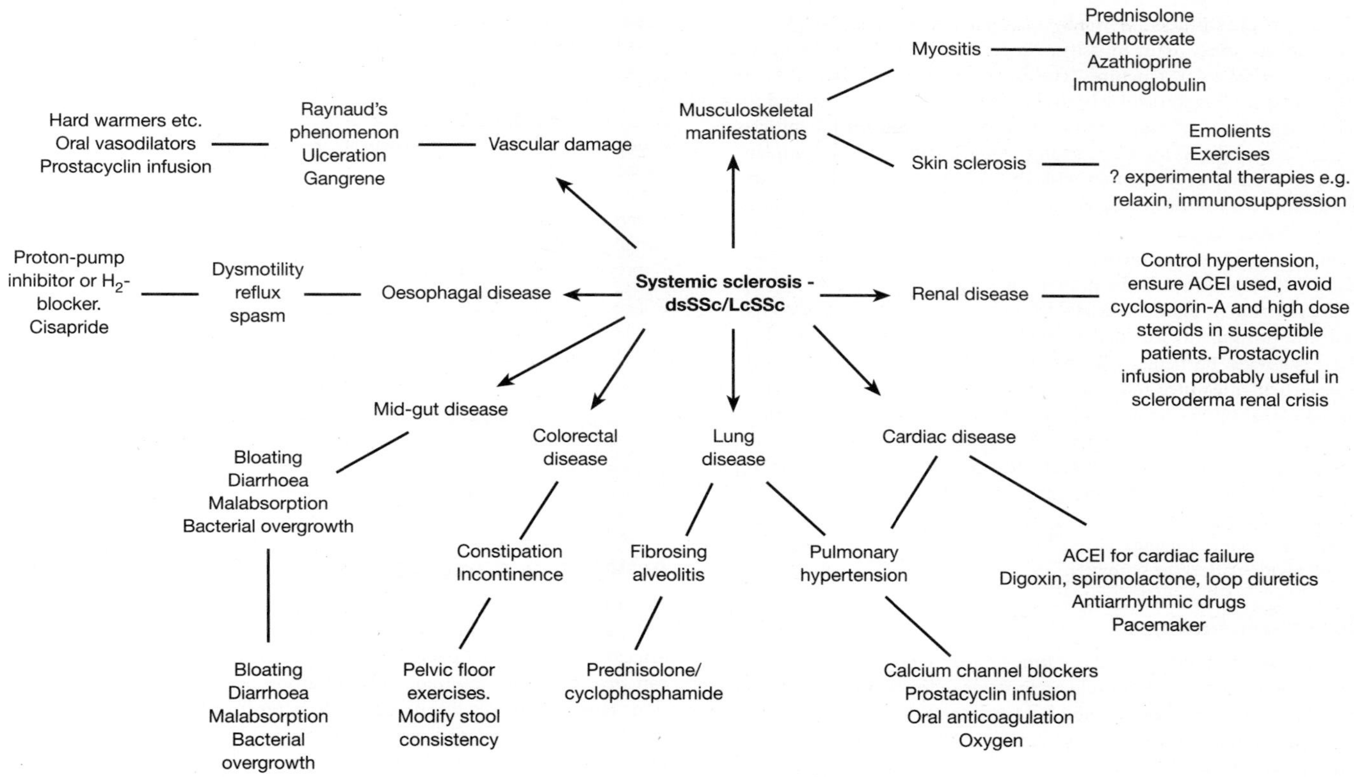

Fig. 3 Overview of the management of organ-based complications of systemic sclerosis.

scleroderma-spectrum disorders, and especially systemic sclerosis, should be considered treatable. Strategies are now available to treat all the diverse manifestations, and an algorithm summarizing current approaches is shown in Fig. 3.

Further reading

Black CM (1995). Measurement of skin involvement in scleroderma. *Journal of Rheumatology* **22**, 1217–19.

Black CM, Denton CP (1998). Scleroderma in adults and children. In: PJ Maddison, DA Isenberg, P Woo, DN Glass, eds. *Oxford textbook of rheumatology*, 2nd edn, pp. 1217–48. Oxford University Press, Oxford.

Bunn CC, Black CM (1999). Systemic sclerosis: an autoantibody mosaic. *Clinical and Experimental Immunology* **117**, 207–8.

Denton CP, *et al.* (1996). Systemic sclerosis: current pathogenetic concepts and future prospects for targeted therapy. *Lancet* **347**, 1453–8.

Denton CP, Black CM (2000). Scleroderma and related disorders: therapeutic aspects. *Ballières Clinical Rheumatology.*

Ho M, Belch JJ (1998). Raynaud's phenomenon: state of the art 1998. *Scandinavian Journal of Rheumatology* **27**, 319–22.

Medsger TA Jr, *et al.* (1999). A disease severity scale for systemic sclerosis: development and testing. *Journal of Rheumatology* **26**, 2159–67.

Silman AJ (1997). Scleroderma—demographics and survival. *Journal of Rheumatology* (Suppl.) **48**, 58–61.

Steen VD, Medsger TA Jr (1997). The palpable tendon friction rub: an important physical examination finding in patients with systemic sclerosis. *Arthritis and Rheumatism* **40**, 1146–51.

White B, *et al.* (1995). Guidelines for clinical trials in systemic sclerosis (scleroderma). I. Disease-modifying interventions. The American College of Rheumatology Committee on Design and Outcomes in Clinical Trials in Systemic Sclerosis. *Arthritis and Rheumatism* **38**, 351–60.

18.10.4 Polymyalgia rheumatica and giant-cell arteritis

Alastair G. Mowat

Polymyalgia rheumatica and giant-cell arteritis are common debilitating conditions that may represent opposite ends of a disease spectrum, but since they appear to present with different clinical symptoms and signs and demand different treatment it is best to describe them separately.

Polymyalgia rheumatica

Polymyalgia rheumatica occurs predominantly in patients over the age of 60 years. There is marked pain and stiffness in the shoulder and pelvic girdles associated with variable systemic symptoms and elevated C-reactive protein and erythrocyte sedimentation rate. While an incidence of some 50 per 100 000 of the population aged 50 years and over has been accepted for hospital referrals on both sides of the Atlantic, careful study of defined elderly populations has shown an incidence of 1.5 per cent which exceeds that of any other inflammatory rheumatic disease in the elderly.

Disease characteristics

Although the most common age group involved is that between 60 and 70 years, a third of patients are under 60 years old. Initial symptoms are seldom seen before 45 years or after 80 years. The male to female ratio is 1:2. The onset is often dramatic, with some patients giving the precise date of their first symptoms, and in most cases it is fully developed within a month. Pain and stiffness are usually localized to muscles, although tenderness is not as severe as in myositis. There may be additional tenderness involving periarticular structures. The onset is most common in the shoulder girdle, spreading to involve both shoulders, the pelvic girdle, and proximal muscles with striking symmetry. Involvement of distal muscles is unusual. Immobility is most severe on waking; a characteristic complaint is a need to roll out of bed, often with the aid of a spouse. Such morning stiffness may persist for hours. Most patients look unwell and complain of general malaise, fatigue, and depression. Anorexia and weight loss can be striking, often suggesting neoplasia, while night sweats and fever are frequent and are occasionally the presenting feature.

The spectrum of musculoskeletal features is broader than is often recognized; the prominent proximal myalgia overshadowing asymmetric peripheral synovitis, particularly of the knee and wrist, while in others there are periarticular features and tenosynovitis. The latter may be the principal cause of carpal tunnel syndrome, found in 10 per cent of cases. Peripheral joint features occur in up to 50 per cent of patients. Radiographs show age-related degenerative change but distinctive erosions may occur in some central joints, for example the sternoclavicular, and provide a basis for the pattern of referred pain. Arthroscopic and isotopic studies and recently magnetic resonance imaging have all supported the existence and importance of a wide pattern of synovitis.

Laboratory findings

An acute phase response (raised erythrocyte sedimentation rate, C-reactive protein) is typical. The elevation in erythrocyte sedimentation rate, often to more than 100 mm/h should not be overinterpreted since polymyalgia rheumatica accounts for only 2 per cent of such high values. Although a normal erythrocyte sedimentation rate may occur in 10 per cent of patients and be associated with the same disease course, 40 mm/h has good diagnostic value. A mild hypochromic normocytic anaemia is common. Rheumatoid factor shows a low incidence of positivity consistent with the patient's age. Serum values of liver enzymes, alkaline phosphatase, and γ-glutamyl transferase are elevated in most patients, and can be correlated with the erythrocyte sedimentation rate and disease severity. Liver biopsy shows only a mild cellular infiltrate and minor changes in the bile canaliculi.

Despite the prominent muscle symptoms, electromyographic studies and serum muscle enzyme values are normal while changes on muscle biopsy, including recent studies of mitochondrial function are non-specific. While several studies have shown changes in the absolute number and percentage of activated CD8 T cells and interleukin receptors these have not provided diagnostic or therapeutic correlation.

Differential diagnosis

Polymyalgia rheumatica remains a clinical diagnosis. It is critical that a careful history is taken and a full examination carried out. This sometimes to leads to claimed disease association, for example connective tissue disease, malignancy, and thyroid disease, but statistically this has not been substantiated. Several diagnostic criteria have been validated over the years but the first remains practical: the seven best discriminatory features are shown in Table 1 of which three or more criteria are required.

Differential diagnosis includes a wide range of conditions (Table 2). Infection may be viral or bacterial, with miliary tuberculosis and infective endocarditis causing confusion. Bone diseases may be difficult to separate as they are common in this elderly group and alkaline phosphatase is raised in polymyalgia rheumatica. This is also the case with neoplastic disease, which may be associated with myalgia even in the absence of secondary spread to bone. Primary muscle disease can be distinguished by electromyography, biopsy, and enzyme values, but joint disease, particularly osteoarthritis, rheumatoid arthritis, and other connective tissue diseases, all of which may start with a polymyalgic pattern lasting for some months in older patients, cause confusion, although appropriate serological tests should help.

Table 1 Validation of diagnostic criteria for polymyalgia rheumatica (after Bird HA *et al.* (1979). *Annals of the Rheumatic Diseases* **38**, 434–9)

Discriminatory feature	Sensitivity* (%)	Relative value†
Shoulder pain and/or stiffness bilaterally	86	155
Onset duration 2 weeks or less	88	151
Initial ESR > 40 mm/h	74	149
Stiffness duration > 1 h	80	141
Age 65+ years	70	139
Depression and/or weight loss	58	139
Upper-arm tenderness bilaterally	36	132

$$\text{*Sensitivity (\%)} = \frac{\text{Individuals with disease with positive test}}{\text{All individuals with disease}}.$$

$$\text{Specificity (\%)} = \frac{\text{Individuals without disease with negative test}}{\text{All individuals without disease}}.$$

†Relative value = sensitivity + specificity (range 0–200).

ESR, erythrocyte sedimentation rate.

Aetiology and pathogenesis

No distinctive pathophysiological mechanisms have been found. Polymyalgia rheumatica may include several different conditions. The distinctive arteritis may occur in up to 15 per cent of cases on biopsy in North American series but much less frequently in Europe, perhaps reflecting case selection. However, newer techniques such as positron emission tomography again suggest that arteritis may be under-recognized. A prodromal malaise and a possible summer/winter peak incidence has promoted a generally unrewarding search for infective causes, although there may be an arteritic subset associated with parainfluenza virus type 1. The evidence for a central arthritis affecting clavicular, shoulder, and sacroiliac joints comes from a study which reproduced the usual pain patterns by injecting hypertonic saline into these joints. In those with proven arteritis, which need not be confined to the temporal and other central vessels but can be found in larger arteries all over the body, a similar pattern of referred pain can be implicated. An immune destruction of the internal elastic lamina is supported by finding circulating immune complexes, together with immunoglobulins, complement deposition, and mononuclear cell infiltrate adjacent to the lamina (Fig. 1).

Table 2 Differential diagnosis of polymyalgia rheumatica

Infection
Viral
Brucellosis
Tuberculosis
Endocarditis
Bone disease
Osteoporosis
Osteomalacia
Paget's disease
Senile hyperostotic spinal ankylosis
Joint disease
Osteoarthritis
Rheumatoid arthritis
Connective tissue diseases
Others
Neoplasia
Muscle disease
Fibromyalgia syndrome
Chronic fatigue syndrome
Parkinsonism
Hypothyroidism

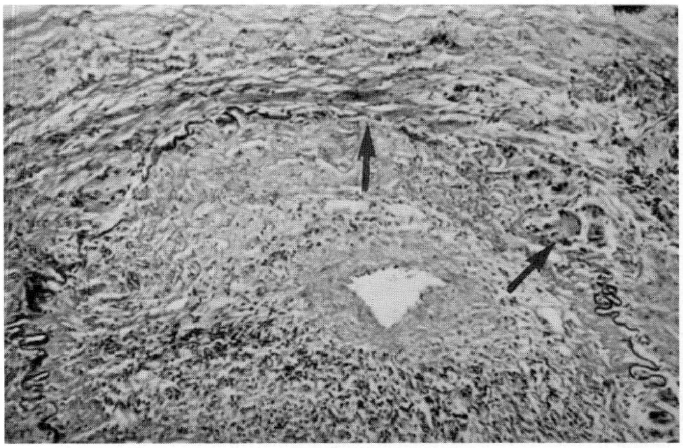

Fig. 1 Photomicrograph of a temporal artery biopsy showing giant cells, mononuclear infiltrate, and disruption of the internal elastic lamina.

Although polymyalgia rheumatica is found worldwide, it is more common in Caucasians, particularly those of Scandinavian extraction. The infrequency of the disease in spouses argues against environmental factors, while familial aggregation and an association with HLA DR4 suggests both genetic and immunological mechanisms, possibly similar to seronegative rheumatoid arthritis. Both polymyalgia rheumatica and giant-cell arteritis are negatively associated with pregnancy, suggesting a vascular protection by the hyperoestrogenic state. No benefit from hormone replacement therapy is documented.

Treatment

A decade ago, the average delay to diagnosis and treatment was 6 months. Now, greater awareness and the fear of the link with giant-cell arteritis and possible blindness has led to overdiagnosis and overtreatment, and the commonness of middle-aged muscle ache has been forgotten. It is a myth that a prompt or dramatic response to corticosteroids confirm a diagnosis; many of the listed differential diagnoses show a similar response. Nevertheless corticosteroids are the drugs of choice.

As the average duration of symptoms is 2 to 3 years, with some persisting for 7 or more years, side-effects of corticosteroids are commonly recorded. Fluid retention, weight gain, diabetes, or osteoporosis are shown by 35 to 75 per cent of patients with polymyalgia rheumatica. Many clinicians now advocate starting therapy appropriate to the patient's age and wishes, to prevent osteoporosis at the outset of corticosteroid therapy. Higher initial erythrocyte sedimentation rates tend to be associated with a longer duration of disease and a greater risk of osteoporosis. Suggested corticosteroid regimes for the first 2 months are shown in Table 3. An intramuscular schedule of 120 mg methylprednisolone every 3 weeks, reducing by 20 mg every 12 weeks appears to be associated with fewer side-effects.

The gradual reduction of corticosteroid treatment over 2 years minimizes the risk of relapse; most clinical problems and associated diagnostic doubts appear to be caused by fluctuating corticosteroid dose. Erythrocyte sedimentation rate and C-reactive protein do not show a sufficiently reliable responce to help in adjusting dosage or in predicting relapse. A few patients can be managed on non-steroidal anti-inflammatory drugs, but the value of poorer and slower symptom control and the risk from different side-effects is debatable. Azathioprine 50 mg twice daily or methotrexate 10 mg per week may be helpful in steroid sparing although the evidence from clinical trials is not striking.

Table 3 Suggested dose of prednisolone (mg/day) for treatment of polymyalgia rheumatica and giant-cell arteritis

	Weeks 1–4 (4 weeks)	Weeks 5–6 (2 weeks)	Weeks 7–8 (2 weeks)
Polymyalgia rheumatica	20	15	10
Giant-cell arteritis	40	30	20

Relationship of polymyalgia rheumatica to giant-cell arteritis

William Bruce, a physician practising in Strathpeffer Spa, Scotland, described polymyalgia rheumatica in 1888 using the term senile rheumatic gout, and Jonathan Hutchison described giant-cell arteritis in 1890. The current names were applied much later. For more than 20 years a common cause has been suggested, emphasized by the term polymyalgia arteritica, and based upon the similar clinical and laboratory features. This has led some to search hard for arterial biopsy evidence lest the patient suffer visual features of giant-cell arteritis. Because the arteritis may be patchy and hence missed, attempts have been made to increase the sensitivity of selection of the biopsy site—angiography, sonography, isotope studies, MRI—without success. However, prospective studies emphasize the difference between the conditions, even if part of a spectrum, and the lack of need for biopsy studies in clear polymyalgia rheumatica. In giant-cell arteritis biopsy proof underpins the need for higher and sustained steroid therapy.

Giant-cell arteritis

Giant-cell (cranial, senile, or temporal) arteritis, which is rare before the age of 50 years, chiefly affects those between 65 and 75 years with a male to female ratio of 1:2. An annual incidence of biopsy-proven disease amongst those aged 50 years or more of 18 per 100 000 (25 per 100 000 for women and 10 per 100 000 for men) has been recorded in the United States and Scandinavia, with the rate for women appearing to rise.

Disease characteristics

The features of giant-cell arteritis are protean, but typical ones are shown in Table 4. The diagnosis depends upon clinical suspicion in less typical cases. As with polymyalgia rheumatica, the onset may be dramatic and the condition always becomes fully developed over a few weeks, although the delay in diagnosis may be months. The malaise, fever, and anaemia are similar to those in polymyalgia rheumatica; the differences are in the vascular symptoms. The majority have temporal features with headache, scalp sensitivity, and tender thickened arteries; the classical nodular red streaks are unusual.

Table 4 Clinical presentation and features of giant-cell arteritis (percentage of cases affected)

Chief presentation	Cases affected
Symptoms of temporal arteritis	30%
Polymyalgia rheumatica	27%
Weight loss, malaise	14%
Fever	13%
Visual disturbance	6%
Headache	4%
Anaemia	4%
Claudication (leg)	2%
Clinical features	**Cases affected**
Signs of temporal arteritis	90%
Polymyalgia rheumatica	55%
Weight loss, malaise	50%
Visual disturbance	40%
Fever	32%
Cranial features	24%
Peripheral neuropathy	12%
Claudication (leg)	7%

Overwhelming generalized headache and the feared complication of irreversible loss of vision are more readily recognized. The clinical features listed emphasize developing arteritis. A wide range of cranial manifestations reflects the involvement of larger arteries with an internal elastic lamina in the face, neck, and brain base but not in the cerebral vessels. They include headache, scalp tenderness, skin necrosis, jaw claudication while talking or chewing, tongue pain and claudication, and face and neck pain with nerve damage. The visual manifestations, which include blurred vision, amaurosis fugax, transient and permanent blindness, diplopia, and visual hallucinations, are due to ischaemic changes in the ciliary arteries causing optic neuritis or infarction, with a smaller number of cases being due to thrombosis of the central retinal artery. Fifteen per cent have evidence of arteritis elsewhere, with intermittent claudication, peripheral neuropathy, widespread vessel tenderness with bruits, myocardial ischaemia and damage, and occasionally an aortic syndrome with valve disease. Stroke due to vascular disease in the brainstem is uncommon, accounting for only 1 to 2 per cent of such cases. In contradistinction to other vasculitides, renal involvement is rare.

Laboratory features

These are the same as in polymyalgia rheumatica. Temporal artery biopsy is the definitive diagnostic test. A 2 cm segment of a tender artery will provide positive histology in 70 per cent of cases. The rate may be enhanced by taking longer segments or by the biopsy of other tender scalp vessels. While biopsy confirmation of the diagnosis is important, it should not be a reason for withholding steroids, since characteristic pathological features persist for at least 2 weeks after treatment has begun, and some argue that scar change never clears.

Differential diagnosis

Since the diagnosis of giant-cell arteritis depends upon a positive biopsy; the differential diagnosis does not include other causes of headache, neck pain, anaemia, and weight loss. The vasculitis of rheumatoid arthritis or systemic lupus erythematosus affects arterioles and is associated with other disease features, particularly arthritis and characteristic immunological tests. Polyarteritis affects small arteries with cutaneous, abdominal, and renal rather than cranial features and the histology is distinctive. Although cranial and central nervous system features occur in Wegener's granulomatosis, involvement usually includes characteristic lesions of the respiratory tract. Takayasu's arteritis, in which the pathological lesions mimic those of giant-cell arteritis, is confined to the aortic arch and its major branches and occurs chiefly in young oriental women.

Treatment

Corticosteroids are mandatory; immunosuppressive therapy has no direct effect and the modest steroid sparing rarely warrants the additional hazard. While doses of prednisolone up to 100 mg per day are often advocated, careful sequential studies indicate that lower doses are quite satisfactory (Table 3). Ophthalmologists, who are likely to see patients with established visual effects or threatening features in the second eye, may use higher doses or methylprednisolone infusions. Dosage reduction must be gradual and should be judged solely on clinical features as acute phase responses are no guide. Most should have achieved a maintenance dose of 10 mg per day after 1 year. Subsequently the known persistence of disease in a significant proportion for 4 years or more and the possible recurrence of symptoms, including blindness, even a year after corticosteroid withdrawal argues for very gradual reduction of dosage. Unfortunately, there are no predictors of these risks. Accordingly, the hazards of therapy are even greater than in polymyalgia rheumatica and require preventive treatment for osteoporosis. Despite all the problems, giant-cell arteritis does not reduce life expectancy.

Further reading

Achkar AA *et al.* (1994). How does previous corticosteroid therapy affect the biopsy findings in giant-cell arteritis? *Annals of Internal Medicine* **120**, 987–92.

Bird HA *et al.* (1979). An evaluation of criteria for polymyalgia rheumatica. *Annals of the Rheumatic Diseases* **38**, 434–9.

Blockmans D *et al.* (1999). New argments for a vasculitic nature of polymyalgia rheumatica using positron emission tomography. *Rheumatology* **38**, 444–7.

Dasgupta B *et al.* (1998). An initially double-blind controlled 96 week trial of depot methylprednisolone against oral prednisolone in the treatment of polymyalgia rheumatica. *British Journal of Rheumatology* **37**, 189–95.

Duhaut P *et al.* (1999). Giant-cell arteritis, polymyalgia rheumatica and viral hypotheses: A multicentre, prospective case-control study. *Journal of Rheumatology* **26**, 361–9.

Duhaut P *et al.* (1999). Giant-cell arteritis and polymyalgia rheumatica: are pregnancies a protective factor ? A prospective, multicentre case-control study. *Rheumatology* **38**, 118–23.

Gonzaley-Gay MA, Garcia-Porrua C, Vazquez-Caruncho M (1998). Polymyalgia rheumatica in biopsy proven giant-cell arteritis does not constitute a different subset but differs from isolated polymyalgia rheumatica. *Journal of Rheumatology* **25**, 1750–5.

Miro O *et al.* (1999). Skeletal muscle mitochondrial function in polymyalgia rheumatica and in giant-cell arteritis. *Rheumatology* **38**, 568–71.

Myklebust G, Gran JT (1996). A prospective stsudy of 287 patients with polymyalgia rheumatica and temporal arteritis: clinical and laboratory manifestations at onset of disease and at time of diagnosis. *British Journal of Rheumatology* **35**, 1161–8.

Pearce G *et al.* (1998). The deleterious effects of low-dose corticosteroids on bone density in patients with polymyalgia rheumatica. *British Journal of Rheumatology* **37**, 292–9.

Proven A *et al.* (1999). Polymyalgia rheumatica with low erythrocyte sedimentation rate at diagnosis. *Journal of Rheumatology* **26**, 1333–7.

Salvarini C *et al.* (1999). Polymyalgia rheumatica: a disorder of extra-articular synovial structures. *Journal of Rheumatology* **26**, 517–21.

18.10.5 Behçet's disease

T. Lehner

Introduction

Behçet's disease is a recurrent, multifocal disorder that persists over many years. It was first described by Hippocrates in ancient Greece and later by Behçet, a Turkish dermatologist. Initial description of the disease comprised oral and genital ulcers and uveitis, but later a number of other clinical features were added, notably skin, joint, neurological, and vascular manifestations. This creates considerable difficulty in diagnosis and a multidisciplinary approach is often required.

An international study group has proposed a set of diagnostic criteria based on data from 914 patients with the disease from 12 centres and seven countries, requiring the presence of recurrent oral ulcers and any two of the following: genital ulcers, defined eye lesions, defined skin lesions, or a positive skin pathergy test. These criteria (Table 1) show better discrimination in sensitivity, specificity, and relative value than the previous criteria. A large number of important clinical manifestations of Behçet's disease have not been included (Table 2) because their lower frequency does not contribute to the accuracy of diagnosis. The same group has proposed that the term 'Behçet's syndrome' be replaced by 'Behçet's disease'.

Table 1 International study group criteria for the diagnosis of Behçet's disease: recurrent oral ulcers plus any two of the four other manifestations

Recurrent oral ulcers	Minor aphthous, major aphthous, or herpetiform ulcers which recurred at least three times a year
Recurrent genital ulcers	Ulcers or scarring
Eye lesions	Anterior uveitis, posterior uveitis, or cells in the vitreous on slit-lamp examination; or retinal vasculitis
Skin lesions	Erythema nodosum, pseudofolliculitis, papulopustular lesions, or acneiform nodules in postadolescent patients not on corticosteroid treatment
Positive pathergy test	Read by physician at 24–48 h

Epidemiology

A striking feature of the disease is the relatively high prevalence in Japan (1 in 10 000), where in 1977 there were an estimated 11 000 patients. The prevalence is also high in countries bordering the Mediterranean: Italy, Greece, Turkey, Israel, Egypt, Lebanon, Syria, Jordan, Saudi Arabia, as well as Algeria, Tunisia, and Morocco. An epidemiological study in the United Kingdom has shown a prevalence of 1 in 170 000, which compares with 1 in 800 000 in a study in the United States.

Although the disease may develop at any age, onset is most commonly in the third decade. However, it can start in childhood with orogenital ulcers, followed by the other manifestations years or decades later. Male predominance is found in most reported series, but this may vary from 2:1 in Japan to 9:1 in the Middle East. Increased familial prevalence of the syndrome has frequently been recorded.

Aetiology

The cause of Behçet's disease is unknown but an immunogenetic basis has been established. HLA B51 is significantly associated with the disease. As with other HLA disease associations, there are at least two interpretations of these findings:

1. The HLA antigen might function as a specific receptor for viruses (or other pathogens).
2. The antigenic determinants of some pathogens might mimic the HLA antigens.

Recently, the *MICA6* allele (*MIC* is the major histocompatability complex class I chain-related gene, thought to be a cell stress response gene), which is in linkage disequilibrium with HLA B51, has been shown to be significantly associated with Behçet's disease.

A viral aetiology for Behçet's disease has often been claimed, but attempts to isolate viruses from patients have failed. Indirect evidence supporting a viral aetiology includes the following. Herpes simplex virus failed to replicate in inactivated cultures of mononuclear cells from patients with Behçet's disease, the interference with viral growth being interpreted as consistent with a viral aetiology of the disease. A more direct approach, using herpes simplex virus DNA probes for complementary DNA obtained from mononuclear cells of patients with Behçet's disease, showed a significant increase in hybridization, suggesting that at least part of the herpes simplex virus genome is transcribed in the circulating mononuclear cells of these patients. However, the role of the virus in the immunopathogenesis has not been elucidated; it may induce some defect in immunoregulation or invoke an autoimmune response.

A variety of streptococci (*Streptococcus sanguis*, *S. pyogenes*, *S. faecalis*, and *S. salivarius*) have been implicated in the aetiology of Behçet's disease, one hypothesis being that heat-shock protein might be a common and perhaps causative agent. Indeed, a significant increase in serum IgA antibodies to the mycobacterial 65 kDa heat-shock protein has been found in patients with Behçet's disease. Earlier reports of autoimmune responses to oral epithelial antigens have been reinvestigated, and a 65 kDa band has been identified with anti-65 kDa heat-shock protein antibodies and mucosal homogenates, as well as streptococci. This evidence, that the 65 kDa heat-shock protein might be involved in the disease is consistent with the finding of a significant increase in circulating T cells with the $\gamma\delta$ T-cell receptor. Furthermore, four peptides derived from the sequence of the mycobacterial 65 kDa heat-shock protein and the corresponding four homologous human heat-shock protein peptides specifically stimulate T cells from patients with Behçet's disease. The potential pathogenicity of some of these peptides has now been established in rats that developed anterior uveitis when the peptides were injected with adjuvant by the subcutaneous route or given orally. Overall, the evidence is growing that Behçet's disease may be closely associated with heat-shock protein peptides of microbial and crossreactive human origin.

Table 2 Clinical manifestations of Behçet's syndrome

Mucocutaneous
- Recurrent oral ulcers: aphthous or herpetiform
- Recurrent genital ulcers: vulval, vaginal, penile, or scrotal
- Skin lesions: pustules, erythema nodosum, perianal ulceration, erythema multiforme

Arthritic
- Polyarthritis of predominantly large joints
- Polyarthralgia of large joints

Neurological
- Brainstem syndrome, resembling minor strokes
- Meningomyelitis or meningoencephalitis
- Organic confusional syndromes
- Multiple sclerosis-like disorder

Ocular
- Uveitis without or with hypopyon
- Iridocyclitis
- Retinal vascular lesions
- Optic atrophy

Vascular
- Venous thrombosis
- Aneurysms

Gastrointestinal
- Abdominal pain, diarrhoea, distension, nausea, and anorexia

Others
- Pulmonary: haemoptysis
- Renal: asymptomatic proteinuria and haematuria

Immunopathology

An early lymphomonocytic infiltration is usually found at the onset of ulceration in the lamina propria, the adjacent epithelium, and around small blood vessels. The latter may show endothelial cell proliferation and some obliteration of the lumen. Although the early stages are suggestive of the type IV cell-mediated immune reaction, this is followed by polymorphonuclear infiltration and fibrinoid necrosis in the blood vessels, consistent with a type III Arthus reaction. The keratinocytes of oral epithelial cells adjacent to an ulcer express HLA class II antigen.

Cell-mediated immune responses can be induced *in vitro* by homogenates of oral mucosa; these elicit lymphoproliferative responses, inhibition of leucocyte migration, and cytotoxicity. The proportion of CD4 cells may be decreased, but that of CD8 cells remains within the normal range.

Circulating immune complexes have been detected in 40 to 60 per cent of patients with Behçet's disease and are associated with disease activity. Although the concentrations of serum C3 and C4 are normal, careful sequential studies have revealed that C3, C4, and C2 are significantly reduced before an attack of uveitis, suggesting consumption of complement by the classical pathway. Electron microscopical examination of centrifuged pellets of serum reveal the presence of small membrane fragments, some of which show complement-dependent holes, suggesting that the soluble immune complex may generate C5b–9 complexes that may bind to the surface of cells and result in lysis.

Acute-phase proteins are increased in Behçet's disease, especially serum C-reactive protein and C9, which is a good marker of disease activity. An increased serum chemotactic activity is found with polymorphonuclear leucocytes and this might be due to IgG complexes releasing chemotactic factors. Serum IgA is often increased in Behçet's disease, but IgG and IgM are variable.

Unlike most autoimmune diseases, nuclear, thyroid, and gastric autoantibodies are not found in greater proportion in Behçet's disease than in the normal population. Rheumatoid factor is also negative, even in patients with joint involvement.

Clinical features

Many patients appear to be generally well and complain only of the localized lesions. However, others present with acute exacerbation of malaise, fever, dysphagia, and loss of weight. Other manifestations are listed in Table 2.

Recurrent oral ulcers

Oral ulcers are the presenting feature in most but not all patients with Behçet's disease. The ulcers can be of the minor or major aphthous or herpetiform type. However, since these ulcers are common in the general population and usually give rise only to local discomfort, they may be missed in the patient's history. Minor aphthous ulcers are found in 67 per cent of the neurological and 76 per cent of the ocular types of Behçet's disease, whereas the more severe major aphthous ulcers are found in 40 and 64 per cent, respectively, of the mucocutaneous and arthritic types. Herpetiform ulcers are found mostly in the mucocutaneous type (45 per cent). An essential feature in relation to the diagnosis of Behçet's disease is that the ulcers recur frequently, at intervals of weeks or months, but this varies from one patient to another. The long-cherished view that oral ulcers in Behçet's disease are rather severe and associated with scarring is no longer tenable. The clinical manifestations can be readily recognized and differentiated from those of similar disorders. The pharynx can also be the site of aphthous ulcers that tend to be rather large, shallow, and covered with a fibrinopurulent exudate (Fig. 1).

Genital ulcers

These are found in most, but not all, patients and can be of the three types described for oral ulcers. They affect women more commonly than men, and scars may follow healing in either sex. Females develop recurrent ulcers of their labia or vagina and they suffer from dysuria and dyspareunia. Males develop recurrent ulcers on the penis or scrotum, again with dysuria and pain on sexual intercourse; occasionally they may develop epididymo-orchitis.

Skin lesions

These vary, but diffuse pustular lesions on the face and (particularly) the back are most common. Erythema nodosum may affect the limbs or other parts of the body. Occasionally, erythema multiforme is found. Both men and women may develop perianal ulcers and, curiously, these may present in the young, well before genital ulcers have appeared.

Ocular lesions

These are the most serious developments in Behçet's disease. Relapsing uveitis, with or without hypopyon, iridocyclitis, retinal vascular lesions, and optic atrophy are common findings. Other manifestations are relapsing conjunctivitis, keratitis, and choroiditis. Gross retinal vascular changes affect both arteries and veins, and fluorescein angiography is particularly helpful in such cases. Both eyes tend to be involved: within 2 years of onset of symptoms in one eye, 90 per cent have involvement of the other eye. There is a painless, bilateral decrease in visual activity, and about 25 per cent of patients with ocular lesions become blind.

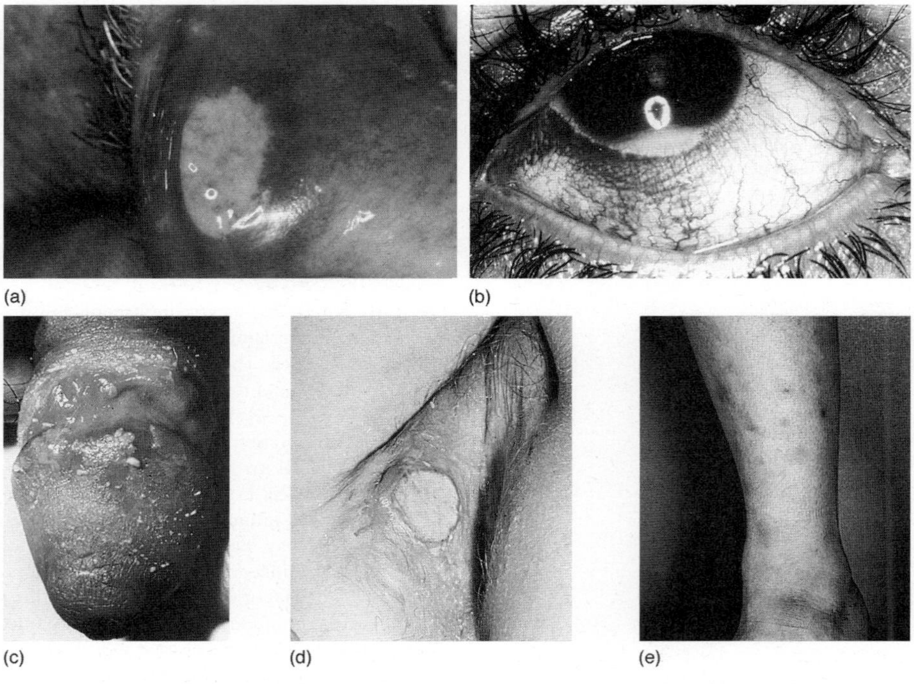

Fig. 1 Behçet's disease: (a) oral ulcer, (b) hypopyon in the eye, (c) ulceration of the head of the penis, (d) vulval ulcers, (e) multiple erythema nodosum lesions of the leg.

Neurological features

These are found in 10 to 25 per cent of patients with Behçet's disease. Patients most commonly develop a transient or persistent brainstem syndrome, resembling a minor stroke, but focal cerebral or spinal cord dysfunction can also occur. Others may present with meningomyelitis or meningoencephalitis, and some with organic confusional syndromes. Multiple sclerosis-like features have also been described. The cerebrospinal fluid sometimes shows pleocytosis, and raised protein and IgG concentrations but more often is normal. Computed tomography scanning does not often reveal abnormalities but the electroencephalogram can show slowing of basic rhythm. Magnetic resonance imaging is the most sensitive and reliable examination, since most patients with neurological involvement may manifest:

(1) atrophy of the cerebral cortex, cerebellum, or brainstem;

(2) the sinuses may be enlarged;

(3) high-intensity focal lesions are found in the brainstem, basal ganglia, or the midbrain;

(4) demyelinating processes may be found in the pons and medulla.

Magnetic resonance imaging can help to differentiate Behçet's disease from multiple sclerosis and other neurological diseases, as well as being useful in assessing the response to treatment.

The prognosis of Behçet's disease with neurological features used to be poor, with mortality of about 40 per cent being recorded in the literature before 1970. However, the prognosis has since been improved with reduced mortality, although whether this can be attributed to steroid and/or cytotoxic agents remains uncertain.

Arthritis or arthralgia

In about half of patients with Behçet's disease the joints are affected, typically at irregular intervals and usually more than one joint. The knees, ankles, and elbows are most commonly involved; less frequently the joints of the hands, feet, shoulders, and hips. Effusions, especially in the knees, cause considerable disability. Radiography of the joints does not usually demonstrate erosive or destructive changes, but a number of exceptions have now been recorded with erosive change in the hips, wrists, and elbows. The test for rheumatoid factor is negative.

Vascular lesions

Recurrent thrombophlebitis of leg veins is a significant feature of Behçet's disease. This has been ascribed to decreased plasma fibrinolytic activity. Less frequently, thrombosis of the superior or inferior vena cava may develop. Arterial aneurysms have also been reported.

Gastrointestinal manifestations

These are ill-defined. The Japanese literature records diarrhoea, distension, nausea, and anorexia in more than half of patients. The ileocaecal region is the most common part of the gut to be affected. However, a British series failed to identify consistent gastrointestinal manifestations, although various transient symptoms were noted in 13 of 70 patients; two of these had rectal ulcers and one each an anal ulcer, a small intestinal ulcer, and perianal fistula. It should be noted that patients with inflammatory bowel disease are excluded from the diagnosis of Behçet's disease by the Mayo Clinic, although they may fulfil current criteria for that diagnosis.

Renal involvement

This has not been established in Behçet's disease. A small number of patients have been reported with Behçet's disease and amyloidosis affecting the kidneys, and a few also with glomerulonephritis. It is doubtful if these renal changes can be considered as primary manifestations of the disease, and they may well be coincidental. Asymptomatic proteinuria and haematuria without evidence either of amyloidosis or nephritis have also been reported in a small number of patients. In a prospective British study, two out of 38 patients with Behçet's disease showed evidence of renal disease: one of these, with biopsy-proven focal proliferative glomerulonephritis, has had no clinical symptoms, and in a 5-year follow-up period the glomerular filtration rate remained normal.

Pulmonary manifestations

These have been reported occasionally, usually with haemoptysis. In some of these patients, pulmonary tuberculosis has been suspected.

Diagnosis

A set of diagnostic criteria is presented in the Introduction (Table 1) that requires recurrent oral ulcers and any two of the following: genital, eye or skin lesions, or a positive pathergy test. However, it is recognized that the wide spectrum of clinical manifestations may not fit the above criteria and the terms incomplete and complete Behçet's disease are often used. The spectrum of the disorder can be divided into four types:

1. Mucocutaneous disease—involving oral and genital ulcers, with or without skin manifestations.
2. Arthritic type—when joint involvement is combined with some or all of the mucocutaneous manifestations.
3. Neurological type—involving the central nervous system and some or all of the features in (1) and (2).
4. Ocular type—affecting the eyes with some or all the features described in (1), (2), and (3).

Thrombosis of blood vessels can be found in any of the types of Behçet's disease, as can some of the other clinical features.

HLA B51 is significantly associated with, but not diagnostic of, the disease. The pathergy test, whereby a sterile subcutaneous puncture (without injection of any material) elicits a pustular reaction within 24 to 48 h, has been used as a diagnostic test in the Middle Eastern countries and in Japan. The presence of immune complexes is consistent with Behçet's disease and so are the raised levels of acute-phase-reacting proteins; C9 is particularly useful in monitoring the course of the disorder.

Patients with rheumatoid arthritis, osteoarthritis, or Reiter's syndrome are excluded from the diagnosis of Behçet's disease, as are patients with a firm diagnosis of ulcerative colitis or Crohn's disease. Stevens–Johnson syndrome may mimic Behçet's disease, but the recurrences are less frequent and tend to be seasonal, the ulcers are large and shallow, the lips are often covered with haemorrhagic crusts, and the skin may show typical lesions of erythema multiforme. Sarcoidosis and viral retinitis should be excluded.

Treatment

The management of patients with Behçet's disease can be difficult, as it requires close liaison between different specialties. Whenever possible, topical treatment of local lesions should be attempted before embarking on systemic anti-inflammatory or immunosuppressive therapy.

Oral and genital ulcers often respond to topical application of steroids or tetracycline or both. Uveitis is initially treated with mydriatic agents and local steroids. However, at some stage systemic prednisolone is usually administered, with a starting dose of 30 to 60 mg/day, which is rapidly brought down to a minimum effective maintenance dose of about 10 mg. There is usually a prompt response, although a small core of patients are resistant to steroid therapy. Azathioprine is often used with prednisolone (2–3 mg/kg body weight daily) and, quite apart from its steroid-sparing function, it may have additional beneficial effects. Colchicine has been advocated by Japanese and Turkish physicians, especially for the treatment of the mucocutaneous type of the disease, with a recommended dose of 0.5 mg twice a day. The rationale is that this drug inhibits the motility of polymorphonuclear leucocytes that is increased in Behçet's disease. There is a general consensus that cyclosporin (2.5–5 mg/kg body weight) should be used in patients with unresponsive uveitis, and is helpful in most patients, though its effect may gradually decline. However, cyclosporin is contraindicated in patients with neurological manifestations, because it may cause or enhance these features. Chlorambucil has also been applied successfully in the treatment of uveitis, but side-effects have limited its application. Recently, interferon-α has been found to be effective in the treatment of ocular manifestations of Behçet's disease. Thalidomide appears to be surprisingly effective in the treatment of orogenital ulcers and pustular lesions, but its teratogenic effect prevents its use in those who are or could become pregnant. Anticoagulant treatment is indicated in deep vein thrombosis.

Further reading

Akman-Demir G *et al.* (1996). Seven-year follow-up of neurologic involvement in Behçet syndrome. *Archives of Neurology* **53**, 691–4.

Benamour S, Zeroual B, Alaoui FZ (1998). Joint manifestations in Behçet's disease: a review of 340 cases. *Review of Rheumatology* **65**, 299–307.

Ehrlich GE (1997). Vasculitis in Behçet's disease. *International Review of Immunology* **14**, 81–8.

Hamuryudan V *et al.* (1997). Azathioprine in Behçet's syndrome: effects on long-term prognosis. *Arthritis and Rheumatology* **40**, 769–74.

Hamuryudan V *et al.* (1998). Thalidomide in the treatment of the mucocutaneous lesions of the Behçet's syndrome: a randomized, double-blind, placebo-controlled trial. *Annales de Medecine Interne* **128**, 443–50.

Hasan A *et al.* (1996). Role of γδ T cells in pathogenesis and diagnosis of Behçet's disease. *Lancet* **347**, 789–94.

International Study Group for Behçet's Disease (1990). Criteria for diagnosis of Behçet's disease. *Lancet* **335,** 1078.

Kaneko S *et al.* (1997). Characterization of T cells specific for an epitope of human 60-kD heat shock protein (hsp) in patients with Behçet's disease (BD) in Japan. *Clinical and Experimental Immunology* **108**, 204–12.

Kotake S *et al.* (1999). Central nervous system symptoms in patients with Behçet's disease receiving cyclosporine therapy. *Ophthalmology* **106**, 586–9.

Lehner T (1999). Immunopathogenesis of Behçet's disease. *Annales de Medecine Interne* **150**, 483–87.

Masuda K *et al.* (1989). Double-masked trial of cyclosporin versus colchicine and long-term open study of cyclosporin in Behçet's disease. *The Lancet* **1**, 1093–5.

Mizuki N *et al.* (1997). Triplet repeat polymorphism in the transmembrane region of MICA gene: A strong association of six GCT repitions with Behçet's disease. *Proceedings of the National Academy of Sciences of the USA* **94**, 1298–303.

Nussenblatt RB (1997). Uveitis in Behçet's disease. *International Review of Immunology* **14,** 67–79.

O'Duffy JD *et al.* (1998). Interferon-alpha treatment of Behçet's disease. *Journal of Rheumatology* **25**, 1938–44.

Pervin K *et al.* (1993). T cell epitope expression of mycobacterial and homologous human 65-kilodalton heat shock protein peptides in short term cell lines from patients with Behçet's disease. *Journal of Immunology* **151,** 2273–82.

Sakane T *et al.* (1999). Behçet's disease. *New England Journal of Medicine* **341**, 1284–91.

Serdaroglu P (1998). Behçet's disease and the nervous system. *Journal of Neurology* **245**, 197–205.

Stanford MR *et al.* (1994). Heat shock protein peptides reactive in patients with Behçet's disease are uveitogenic in Lewis rats. *Clinical and Experimental Immunology* **97**, 226–31.

Yazici H (1981). A controlled trial of azathioprine in Behçet's syndrome. *New England Journal of Medicine* **322**, 281–5.

18.10.6 Sjögren's syndrome

Patrick J. W. Venables

Introduction

Sjögren's syndrome is characterized by inflammation and destruction of exocrine glands. The salivary and lachrymal glands are principally involved, giving rise to dry eyes and mouth. It was originally described by Sjögren in 1933 as the triad of dry eyes, dry mouth, and rheumatoid arthritis. It is now classified as primary Sjögren's syndrome where the disease exists on its own, and secondary Sjögren's syndrome where it is associated with other diseases. Well-recognized secondary associations are rheumatoid arthritis, systemic lupus erythematosus, scleroderma, polymyositis, and primary biliary cirrhosis. The recent descriptions of a Sjögren's syndrome-like illness in patients infected with HTLV-I, HIV-1, and hepatitis C virus infection have drawn attention to the importance of considering these viruses in differential diagnosis, as well intensifying the search for a virus underlying idiopathic disease.

Aetiology and pathology

The aetiology of Sjögren's syndrome is unknown but is often considered to be an interaction between constitutional and environmental factors leading to autoimmunity. Primary Sjögren's syndrome is strongly associated with HLA DR3, and the linked genes *B8*, *DQ2*, and the *C4A* null gene. Aetiological candidates for triggering autoimmunity in Sjögren's syndrome are viruses that infect the salivary gland. Sialotropic herpesviruses including Epstein–Barr virus, cytomegalovirus, and human herpesvirus-6 have been examined with conflicting reports of abnormal responses to infection. Using DNA hybridization techniques, Epstein–Barr virus has been detected in the parotid gland and in labial biopsies, but it remains controversial whether the virus is simply persistent in the glands or whether it is triggering inflammation in Sjögren's syndrome. Retroviruses have also attracted interest recently as they infect and persist in cells of the immune system such as T cells and macrophages, and infect salivary gland epithelium. In spite of increasing circumstantial evidence for their involvement in Sjögren's syndrome, the demonstration of a pathogenic role remains elusive.

The cardinal pathological features of Sjögren's syndrome are inflammation and destruction of salivary gland tissue. The inflammatory infiltrates consist of focal aggregates of lymphocytes, mainly CD4-positive T cells, localized around ducts and acini. Scattered interstitial plasma cells are commonly found, although these are not disease specific and are also found in glands from healthy individuals. The destructive changes are predominantly duct dilation, acinal atrophy, and interstitial fibrosis. These latter findings have also been described in biopsies from people without Sjögren's syndrome, particularly in the elderly, and cannot be regarded as diagnostically specific.

The most striking feature of the systemic autoimmune response in Sjögren's syndrome is the marked activation of B cells which can lead to immunoglobulin levels of over three times the upper limit of the normal range. Rheumatoid factors of all isotypes are observed in blood in about 70 per cent of patients and their detection can lead to some patients with Sjögren's syndrome being misdiagnosed as having rheumatoid arthritis. The typical autoantibodies are those against the cellular ribonucleoprotein antigens Ro and La, named after the patients in whom the antibodies were originally described. Anti-Ro antibodies are more frequently detectable (50–90 per cent of cases) than anti-La antibodies (30–50 per cent of cases), but the latter are more diagnostically specific for primary Sjögren's syndrome. More recently two further potential autoantigens have been described: fodrin, which is a cellular protein involved in apoptosis, and the muscarinic acetylcholine receptor, which is important in mediating parasympathetic stimulation of exocrine glands. An astonishing degree of diagnostic sensitivity and specificity has been claimed for serum antibodies to both antigens in Sjögren's syndrome, but these findings have yet to be confirmed by independent laboratories and must be interpreted with caution.

Clinical features

Sjögren's syndrome is nine times more common in women than men and can develop at any age from 15 to 65. Patients rarely complain of dry eyes, but rather a gritty sensation, soreness, photosensitivity, or intolerance of contact lenses. In early disease excessive watering or deposits of dried mucus in the corner of the eye and recurrent attacks of conjunctivitis may occur. The dry mouth is often manifest as the 'cream cracker' sign, inability to swallow dry food without fluid, or waking up in the night to take sips of water. About half of the patients complain of intermittent parotid swelling, sometimes misdiagnosed as recurrent mumps. When the swelling is excessively painful it is often due to secondary bacterial infection. On examination, xerostomia can be detected as a diminished salivary pool, a dried fissured tongue, often complicated by angular stomatitis, and chronic oral candidiasis. The eyes may be reddened and roughened due to shallow erosions in the conjunctivae. Occasionally the front of the eye is eroded to reveal strands of underlying collagen leading to the appearance of filamentary keratitis.

Other exocrine glands may be affected. Dry nasal passages and upper airways may lead to recurrent bouts of sinusitis, a dry cough, and, possibly, a higher than expected frequency of chest infections. Dry skin and dry hair are symptoms frequently elicited on direct questioning. About 30 per cent of women with Sjögren's syndrome have diminished vaginal secretions and may present with dyspaerunia. Involvement of the gastrointestinal tract leads to reflux oesophagitis or gastritis due to lack of protective mucus secretion, and some patients complain of constipation, which may be attributed to defective mucus in the colon and rectum. Rarely, pancreatic failure leading to malabsorption syndromes may occur.

Recent studies have highlighted yet another complication, namely interstitial cystitis. It has been suggested that this is due to an autoimmune immune response to the muscarinic acetylcholine receptor that is extensively expressed in the bladder wall. There is no doubt about the clinical association, although the serological link awaits confirmation.

There is a higher than expected frequency of thyroid autoimmunity in those with Sjögren's syndrome: whether this is part of the same pathological process is debatable, but it is important to check thyroid function from time to time in patients with this condition.

Systemic manifestations

True Sjögren's syndrome is a systemic disease. Two-thirds of patients complain of fatigue, which, according to a recent epidemiological study, is the single most important cause of disability. Occasionally weight loss and fever mimicking an occult malignancy may be the presenting symptoms, particularly in the elderly. Other features include an arthritis that resembles the Jaccoud-like arthritis of systemic lupus erythematosus (Fig. 1). Raynaud's phenomenon occurs in about 50 per cent of patients, though a true vasculitis is less common. Waldenström's benign hypergammaglobulinaemic purpura affecting the lower legs is found in patients with very high IgG levels. Patients with Sjögren's syndrome may also present with polymyalgia rheumatica or, much less frequently, polymyositis. Pleurisy occurs in about 40 per cent of patients and a high prevalence of abnormalities of pulmonary function has been described, although these are rarely clinically significant. A wide range of neurological diseases has been described: peripheral neuropathies are relatively common, particularly mononeuritis multiplex mediated by vasculitis, and a condition resembling multiple sclerosis has been reported. Interstitial nephritis leading to renal tubular acidosis or nephrogenic diabetes insipidus occurs in about 30 per cent of patients: these are usually subclinical but may lead to hypokalaemia causing muscular weakness or, occasionally, nephrocalcinosis. Lymphoma, almost always of B-cell lineage, is a characteristic but unusual feature. This occurs in about 5 per cent of patients referred to specialist centres and is particularly likely in patients with high levels of immunoglobulins, autoantibodies, and cryoglobulins. As the lymphoma develops, the immunoglobulin levels often fall and the autoantibodies become negative. Women of childbearing age are at increased risk of giving birth to babies with congenital heart block. Although rare, about 1 in 20 000 births, this complication is of great immunopathogenic interest as it is thought to be mediated by transplacental transfer of anti-Ro and anti-La antibodies.

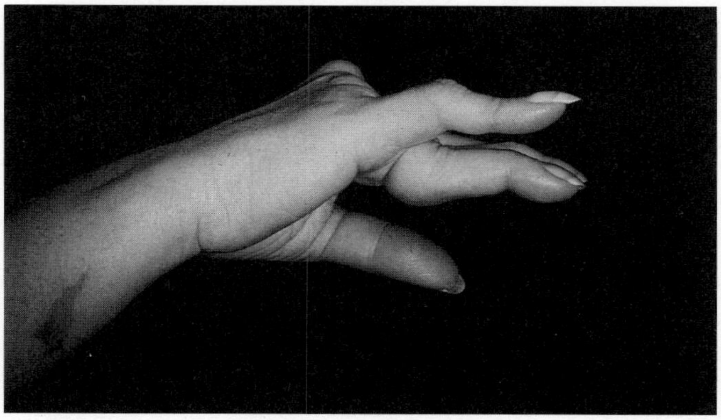

Fig. 1 Hands of a patient with long-standing primary Sjögren's syndrome showing correctable swan-necking deformities similar to the Jaccoud-like arthritis seen in systemic lupus erythematosus.

In secondary Sjögren's syndrome the sicca symptoms are less severe than in primary disease. In rheumatoid arthritis with Sjögren's syndrome the patient tends to have more frequent extra-articular disease manifested as digital infarcts and subcutaneous ulcers. In systemic lupus erythematosus, those with Sjögren's syndrome have a lower frequency of renal disease and a relatively good prognosis.

Diagnosis

Keratoconjunctivitis sicca can be detected by Schirmer's test, tear break-up time, and Rose Bengal staining and xerostomia by a reduced parotid salivary flow rate and by reduced uptake and clearance on isotope scans. It is important to remember that both salivary and lachrymal function decline with age and may be impaired in conditions other than Sjögren's syndrome. One cause of diagnostic confusion arises from treatment with drugs with anticholinergic side-effects, the most frequent being the tricyclic antidepressants.

Biopsy and histology of the labial glands from behind the lower lip provides the most definitive diagnostic test. The area is anaesthetized with lidocaine (lignocaine) containing adrenaline and an incision 1.5 cm long allows access to five to ten glands 2 to 4 mm in diameter that are removed by simple blunt dissection. A diagnosis of Sjögren's syndrome depends on finding foci of periductular infiltrates of at least 50 lymphocytes and/or plasma cells at a density of more than one focus/4 mm^2 (Fig. 2).

The majority of patients have a raised erythrocyte sedimentation rate and a mild normocytic anaemia with leucopenia in about 50 per cent of cases. One of the most remarkable features of primary Sjögren's syndrome is a high level of IgG, which can be up to 50 g/litre. Complement levels are usually normal, although C4 levels can sometimes be reduced because of the link between Sjögren's syndrome and the *C4A* null gene. Anti-La antibodies, although of relatively low sensitivity, are of great diagnostic help when present.

Rheumatoid factors, as measured by routine assays, occur in all forms of Sjögren's syndrome and their detection in primary disease is a common reason for misdiagnosing such patients as having rheumatoid arthritis.

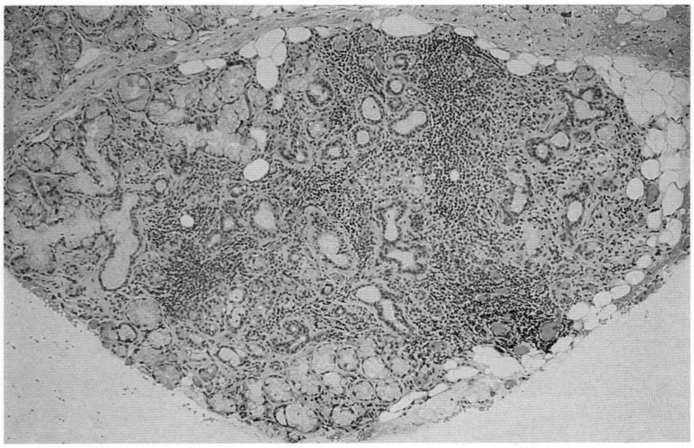

Fig. 2 Biopsy showing a lobule of minor salivary gland from a patient with Sjögren's syndrome. There is a focal inflammatory infiltrate surrounding blood vessels and ducts with the acini being relatively spared.

Similarly, antinuclear antibodies can occur. Both rheumatoid factors and antinuclear antibodies, although not diagnostically specific, can help in distinguishing Sjögren's syndrome from non-autoimmune causes of sicca symptoms. Primary Sjögren's syndrome can be mimicked very closely by infection with HTLV-I, HIV-1, and hepatitis C virus. All three diseases cause dry eyes and mouth, swelling of salivary glands, and biopsy changes very similar to that of primary Sjögren's syndrome. All are associated with hypergammaglobulinaemia, a raised erythrocyte sedimentation rate, and autoantibodies, although anti-Ro and anti-La are unusual. The only way to differentiate them with certainty is by specific serological testing. The Sjögren's-like syndrome associated with HIV infection has been termed diffuse infiltrative lymphocytosis syndrome and occurs in approximately 5 per cent of HIV-positive individuals. Chronic fatigue syndrome is frequently mistaken for Sjögren's syndrome and vice versa (less frequently); a salivary gland biopsy usually clarifies the situation.

Diagnostic criteria

Diagnostic criteria are essential for the standardization of any research involving patient groups, particularly with a disease, or group of diseases, as heterogeneous as Sjögren's syndrome. Currently used criteria depend on the demonstration of keratoconjunctivitis sicca, xerostomia, and a positive labial gland biopsy. The 'European' criteria based on the results of a multicentre European study are probably the most thoroughly evaluated and the simplest to apply. They are based on a short questionnaire (Table 1) about ocular and oral symptoms. Other essential criteria are ocular signs (by Schirmer's test or Rose Bengal staining), lymphocytic infiltrates on lip biopsy, salivary gland involvement (scintigraphy, sialography, or decreased salivary flow rate), and demonstration of serum autoantibodies (rheumatoid factors, antinuclear antibodies, and/or Ro or La antibodies).

Table 1 Questionnaire for eliciting the main ocular and oral symptoms of Sjögren's syndrome.

Ocular symptoms

A positive response to at least one of the three selected questions:

1. Have you had daily, persistent, troublesome dry eyes for more than 3 months?
2. Do you have a recurrent sensation of sand or gravel in the eyes?
3. Do you use tear substitutes more than three times a day?

Oral symptoms

A positive response to at least one of the three selected questions:

1. Have you had a daily feeling of dry mouth for more than 3 months?
2. Have you had recurrently or persistently swollen salivary glands as an adult?
3. Do you frequently drink liquids to aid in swallowing dry food?

From Vitali C *et al.* (1993). Diagnostic criteria for Sjögren's syndrome: results of a European prospective multicentre study. *Arthritis and Rheumatism* **36**, 340–7, with permission.

Treatment

Most treatment in Sjögren's syndrome is topical and symptomatic. Simple measures can help preserve the integrity of the cornea as well as the gums and teeth and are worth pursuing with enthusiasm rather than with the negative attitude that some patients find in their physicians. Tear substitutes, such as hypromellose eye drops, are the mainstay of treatment for dry eyes, and it is generally worth trying several different types before settling on the most suitable preparation. Where thick mucus strands are a particular problem topical acetylcysteine may help. Eye ointments, particularly at night, can help lubricate sticky eyes. Bacterial infection should be treated immediately with chloramphenicol ointment or drops. Some benefit can be achieved by preventing evaporation of tears by fitting side panels to spectacles. Temporary or permanent occlusion of the canaliculi or, rarely, tarsorraphy may help to retain tears within the conjunctival sac.

The dry mouth may be treated with saliva substitutes that are now available as convenient sprays. Pilocarpine tablets have shown promising results in recent controlled trials but patients often seem to stop taking them after a few weeks or months because of cholinergic side-effects such as palpitations, sweating, and abdominal cramps. Candidal infections are extremely common in Sjögren's syndrome and are often missed. They are best treated with prolonged courses of anticandidal drugs such as fluconozole 50 mg daily for ten days. Attention to dental hygiene may help to prevent the premature caries that is a common problem in Sjögren's syndrome.

Attempts to treat the underlying disease with steroids or cytotoxic drugs are generally thought ill-advised unless there are systemic complications. Fever, weight loss, parotid swelling, and interstitial cystitis often respond well to a low dose of steroids. Serious systemic complications such as polymyositis, mononeuritis multiplex, or fibrosing alveolitis are treated with steroids and cytotoxic drugs as in other connective tissue diseases. The arthritis of primary Sjögren's syndrome may be treated with anti-inflammatory drugs, although it also responds to hydroxychloroquine. There is no convincing evidence that methotrexate has a role in Sjögren's syndrome. It is generally agreed that other second-line agents for rheumatoid arthritis such as gold or sulphasalazine are associated with a high frequency of side-effects and this is one of the most important reasons for distinguishing between the arthritis of primary Sjögren's syndrome and rheumatoid arthritis.

There is accumulating evidence that hydroxychloroquine may have a beneficial disease-modifying effect in Sjögren's syndrome. Certainly the drug helps with arthralgia, lowers the erythrocyte sedimentation rate and immunoglobulin levels, and may also prevent bouts of purpura. More importantly there is anecdotal evidence that it may help with fatigue. Properly controlled clinical trials are needed to address this point, but it could be that hydroxychloroquine will emerge as the first disease-modifying drug which can be used in patients with uncomplicated disease.

Further reading

Alexander EL *et al.* (1986). Primary Sjögren's syndrome with central nervous system dysfunction mimicking multiple sclerosis. *Annals of Internal Medicine* **104**, 323–30.

Bacman S *et al.* (1996). Circulating antibodies against rat parotid gland M3 muscarinic receptors in primary Sjögren's syndrome. *Clinical and Experimental Immunology* **104**, 454–9.

Fox RI *et al.* (1986). Sjögren's syndrome: proposed criteria for classification. *Arthritis and Rheumatism* **29**, 577–85.

Fox RI *et al.* (1988). Treatment of primary Sjögren's syndrome with hydroxychloroquine. *American Journal of Medicine* **85**, 62–7.

Fox RI, Tornwall J, Michelson P (1999). Current issues in the diagnosis and treatment of Sjögren's syndrome. *Current Opinion in Rheumatology* **11**, 364–71.

Flescher E, Talal N (1991). Do viruses contribute to the development of Sjögren's syndrome? *American Journal of Medicine* **90**, 283–5.

Haneji N *et al.* (1997). Identification of alpha-fodrin as a candidate autoantigen in primary Sjögren syndrome. *Science* **276**, 604–7.

Harley JB *et al.* (1986). Gene interaction at HLA-DQ enhances autoantibody production in primary Sjögren's syndrome. *Science* **232**, 1145–7.

Price EJ and Venables PJW (1995). Aetiopathogenesis of Sjögren's syndrome. *Seminars in Arthritis and Rheumatism* **25**, 117–33.

Thomas E *et al.* (1998). Sjögren's syndrome: a community-based study of prevalence and impact. *British Journal of Rheumatology* **37**, 1069–76.

Vitali C *et al.* (1993). Diagnostic criteria for Sjögren's syndrome: results of a European prospective multicentre study. *Arthritis and Rheumatism* **36**, 340–7.

18.10.7 Polymyositis and dermatomyositis

John H. Stone and David B. Hellmann

Introduction

Polymyositis and dermatomyositis are the two major types of inflammatory muscle disease. Despite numerous shared features, immunopathological evidence now confirms that they are separate disorders. Polymyositis and dermatomyositis are considered to be autoimmune diseases because of their inflammatory nature and the frequent occurrence of autoantibodies (both antinuclear antibodies and myositis-specific antibodies), but the precise causes of these disorders remain unknown. Both are associated with proximal muscle weakness, and both may affect organs other than skeletal muscle, such as the lungs and heart. In adults, dermatomyositis is so frequently a paraneoplastic disorder that its diagnosis should prompt a search for an underlying malignancy.

Clinical features

Classification and epidemiology

The traditional classification of polymyositis and dermatomyositis distinguishes between five subgroups of patients:

(1) primary idiopathic polymyositis;

(2) primary idiopathic dermatomyositis;

(3) either disorder occurring in association with a malignancy;

(4) childhood dermatomyositis (or, more rarely, polymyositis); and

(5) overlap syndromes, in which polymyositis or dermatomyositis occur along with features of other systemic autoimmune conditions.

This chapter focuses on primary idiopathic polymyositis and dermatomyositis, referring to the other subgroups when appropriate. The principal features of polymyositis and dermatomyositis are displayed in Table 1.

In general, polymyositis and dermatomyositis may afflict individuals of any age and either gender, but female cases outnumber males by a 2:1 ratio. Cases associated with malignancy are clustered among older patients with dermatomyositis, and seldom if ever occur among children.

Polymyositis

Polymyositis is characterized by symmetrical proximal muscle weakness that develops slowly, usually over weeks to months. Routine tasks that require proximal muscle strength, for example rising from a chair or climbing stairs, become increasingly challenging for the patient. In addition to weakness of the extremities, skeletal muscles at many sites, including the upper one-third of the oesophagus, the muscles of neck flexion, the intercostal muscles, and the diaphragm, are also susceptible to muscular inflammation. Dysphagia and nasopharyngeal regurgitation of food may result from oesophageal involvement. Patients with severe neck flexor weakness secondary to polymyositis may be unable to lift their heads from the pillow. Hypercapnoeic respiratory failure sometimes results from weakness of the chest wall muscles and diaphragm. By contrast, polymyositis usually spares the muscles that mediate facial expression and extraocular movements, even in patients with profound weakness elsewhere. Similarly, handgrip strength and the ability to perform fine motor tasks usually remain preserved until advanced stages of the disease.

Prominent muscle pain and tenderness are atypical, and rarely constitute the chief complaint. Deep tendon reflexes and muscle bulk are preserved

Table 1 Principal features of polymyositis and dermatomyositis.

	Polymyositis	Dermatomyositis
Typical patient	Any age Unusual in children Female and African-American predominance	Any age Juvenile form common Female and African-American predominance
Muscle groups affected	Proximal > distal. Symmetrical	Proximal > distal. Symmetrical
CK elevation	40–50 times normal not unusual	40–50 times normal not unusual Weakness sometimes out of proportion to CK level
MSAs	Antisynthetase antibodies, anti-SRP	Antisynthetase antibodies, anti-Mi-2
Histopathology	Endomysial inflammation CD8+ cells invading non-necrotic muscle fibres, which bear HLA class I antigens	Perivascular, interfascicular inflammation CD4+ predominance; complement membrance attack complex present; capillary obliteration; endothelial damage; perifascicular atrophy
Malignancy association	No	Yes
Other features	ILD Cardiac Malignancy	Skin ILD Cardiac Intramuscular calcification Vasculitis Malignancy

Abbreviations: CK, creatine kinase; MSAs, myositis-specific antibodies; ILD, interstitial lung disease; SRP, signal recognition particle.

except in severe, advanced disease. Fasciculations, a manifestation of denervation rather than myopathic injury, are absent in polymyositis. Similarly, sensory function remains normal even as muscle weakness progresses. Endomysial inflammation leads to the release of muscle enzymes into the blood. Thus, polymyositis is characterized by striking elevations of serum creatine kinase, aldolase, aspartate aminotransferase, alanine aminotransferase, and lactate dehydrogenase.

Dermatomyositis

The pattern of muscle involvement in dermatomyositis is clinically indistinguishable from that of polymyositis. In addition to inflammatory muscle disease, however, dermatomyositis has an array of characteristic cutaneous manifestations. Gottron's sign, an erythematous, scaly eruption confined to skin overlying the knuckles, is pathognomonic of this disease (Fig. 1 and Plate 1). Identical lesions known as Gottron's papules also occur over the extensor surfaces of many other joints, particularly the elbows and knees. The heliotrope rash consists of a lilac discoloration of skin over the eyelids, often accompanied by eyelid oedema (Fig. 2 and Plate 2). Cutaneous erythema may involve several sites in dermatomyositis, including the upper back and shoulders (the 'shawl sign'), the upper chest (in a 'V' distribution), and the face and hands. 'Mechanic's hands' (see below) often occur in association with certain types of myositis-specific antibodies.

Patients with dermatomyositis may mimic systemic lupus erythematosus in demonstrating photosensitivity and malar rash. Skin biopsies in these two diseases share the histopathological features of 'interface dermatitis', i.e. immune complex deposition at the dermal–epidermal junction. Acral regions are also affected by characteristic features. Both periungual erythema and capillary loop dilatation underscore the vascular nature of this disorder. Sometimes the classic skin features are apparent for months before muscle weakness becomes evident, in which case the condition is termed amyopathic dermatomyositis (or 'dermatomyositis sine myositis').

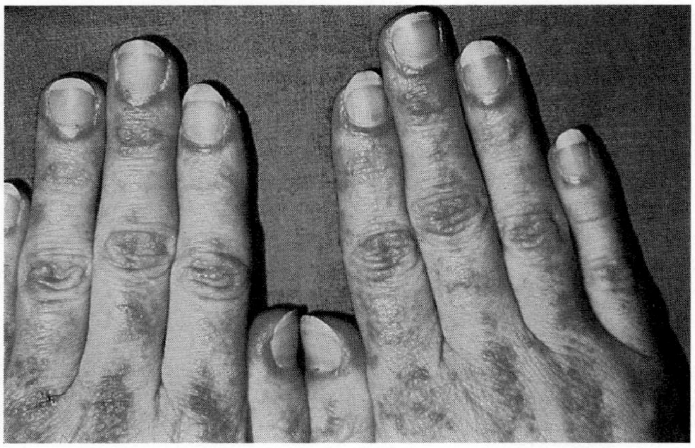

Fig. 1 Gottron's sign. Roughened, violaceous papules over the dorsal surfaces of several metacarpophalangeal and proximal interphalangeal joints. Note also the erythema at the bases of the fingernail, caused by capillary loop dilatation. (See also Plate 1.)

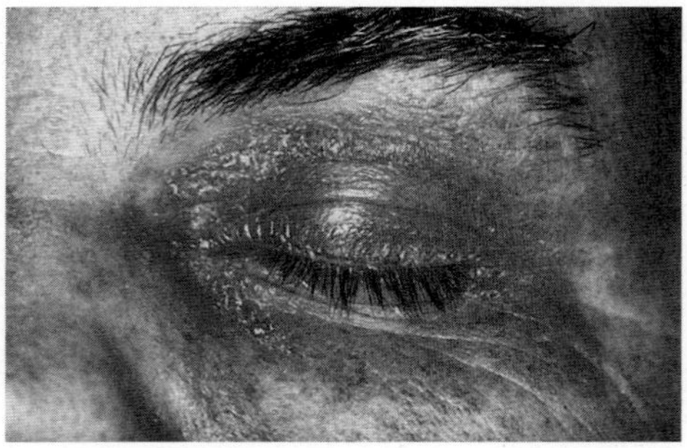

Fig. 2 Heliotrope rash. An erythematous (often lilac-coloured) rash over the eyelids in a patient with dermatomyositis (reproduced from Mousari HC, Wigley FM (2000). *Journal of Rheumatology* **27**,1542-5 with permission). (See also Plate 2.)

Extramuscular features

Lung

Weakness of the intercostal muscles and diaphragm occasionally leads to ventilatory failure in polymyositis or dermatomyositis. More commonly, however, patients suffer pulmonary involvement in the form of interstitial lung disease, a complication that occurs in up to 30 per cent of cases. The pattern of pulmonary involvement in the inflammatory myopathies is typical of that which occurs in connective tissue disorders, namely interstitial fibrosis, predominantly at the lung bases. High-resolution computed tomography is very sensitive for detecting this type of pulmonary change, which in the early stages corresponds to an inflammatory alveolitis. The severity of interstitial lung disease in polymyositis and dermatomyositis ranges from asymptomatic radiological findings to a refractory process indistinguishable from idiopathic pulmonary fibrosis. Lung involvement is often, but not always, associated with antisynthetase antibodies (see below). Restrictive findings on pulmonary function testing are the rule. Another common pulmonary complication of the inflammatory myopathies is aspiration pneumonia, caused by weakness of the hypopharynx and upper oesophagus.

Cardiac

Cardiac involvement in polymyositis or dermatomyositis is usually subclinical, and its prevalence is not known with certainty. When measured, creatine kinase-MB isoenzyme levels are frequently elevated in the absence of overt cardiac symptoms. Electrocardiograms usually demonstrate nonspecific ST-T wave changes. Even so, the occurrence of clinically evident myocarditis in these diseases may lead to cardiac failure or intractable, life-threatening arrythmias.

Gastrointestinal

Involvement of the gastrointestinal tract beyond the pharynx and oesophagus is particularly common in juvenile dermatomyositis (the childhood form). This complication is mediated by vasculitis, and may result in intestinal haemorrhage or perforation.

Malignancy

A significant proportion of adults with polymyositis or dermatomyositis have underlying malignancies, usually carcinomas. The association with malignancy is stronger for adults with dermatomyositis, who die from cancer significantly more often than age-matched controls. The weaker association of polymyositis with malignancy may be attributable to ascertainment bias resulting from more frequent visits to the doctor and cancer surveillance.

Many types of malignancy have been reported in association with dermatomyositis, including lung, oesophageal, breast, colon, and ovarian tumours. Among women with dermatomyositis, the risk of ovarian cancer may be 20 times greater than that of the general population. Most patients diagnosed with primary polymyositis or dermatomyositis (children excepted) should undergo some surveillance for a disease-associated malignancy. This screening should be based upon careful histories, physical examinations, and the performance of a limited number of routine tests (for example chest radiography), in addition to age-appropriate cancer screening such as mammography and flexible sigmoidoscopy. Costly, undirected 'fishing expeditions' rarely benefit the patient.

Differential diagnosis

Polymyositis and dermatomyositis must be distinguished from numerous disorders that cause subacute weakness. These are shown in Table 2.

Table 2 Differential diagnosis of subacute weakness

Neurological	Inclusion body myositis, Guillain Barre syndrome, myasthenia gravis, Eaton–Lambert syndrome, amyotrophic lateral sclerosis, muscular dystrophies (Duchenne's, Becker's, limb-girdle, fascioscapulohumeral)
Endocrine	Hyper- and hypothyroidism, Cushing's syndrome, Addison's disease
Metabolic	Familial periodic paralysis, McArdle's disease, phosphofructokinase deficiency, adult acid maltase deficiency, mitochondrial myopathies
Drugs	Alcohol, chloroquine, hydroxychloroquine, colchicine, penicillamine, corticosteroids, lipid-lowering agents, zidovudine
Infections	Viral (echovirus), retroviral (human immunodeficiency virus, HTLV-1), bacterial (*Staphylococcus*—pyomyositis), parasitic (trichinosis)
Rheumatic	Vasculitis, polymyalgia rheumatica, myositis associated with systemic lupus erythematosus, rheumatoid arthritis, or systemic sclerosis
Other	Rhabdomyolysis, chronic graft versus host disease, rubella vaccinations

Pathology

Polymyositis is characterized by an endomysial infiltrate containing large numbers of CD8+ T cells, combined with foci of cytotoxic T cells and macrophages. The inflammatory infiltrate surrounds and invades non-necrotic muscle fibres. In polymyositis, both uninvolved and involved fibres express increased amounts of HLA class I antigen (normal muscle fibres, by contrast, express neither class I nor class II antigens). Thus, the pathological findings in polymyositis suggest an HLA class I-restricted immune response mediated by cytotoxic T cells. Polymyositis must be distinguished from inclusion body myositis, a more indolent form of inflammatory myopathy associated with asymmetric and distal motor weakness. Inclusion body myositis has distinctive pathological findings: 'rimmed vacuoles' distributed around the myocyte's edge, basophilic 'inclusion bodies' within these vacuoles, and filamentous inclusions within the cytoplasm. Cases of 'refractory polymyositis' are often misdiagnoses of inclusion body myositis.

Muscle biopsies from patients with dermatomyositis contain increased numbers of CD4+ T cells and B lymphocytes. The inflammatory infiltrate in dermatomyositis is localized to perivascular regions. Capillary obliteration, fibrin thrombi, and endothelial cell damage are all hallmarks of dermatomyositis. Evidence of the membrane attack complex, comprising complement components C5 to C9, is present early in dermatomyositis, consistent with the humorally mediated destruction of muscle-associated microvasculature. Focal capillary depletion is one of the earliest pathological changes. In addition to its vascular orientation, the inflammatory infiltrate in dermatomyositis centres on the interfascicular septae and around, rather than within, muscle fascicles. Even in the absence of inflammation, perifascicular atrophy is diagnostic of dermatomyositis.

Myositis-specific antibodies

Approximately 30 per cent of patients with polymyositis/dermatomyositis have myositis-specific antibodies, immune globulins directed against a variety of nuclear or cytoplasmic antigens. Three major types of myositis-specific antibodies have been identified: the antisynthetases; antisignal recognition particle antibodies (**anti-SRP**); and anti-Mi-2 antibodies. Individual patients generally develop only one type of myositis-specific antibody. The antisynthetase antibodies are directed against aminoacyl-tRNA synthetase enzymes, which catalyse the attachment of specific amino acids to their cognate tRNAs. In the case of Jo-1 (the most common type of myositis-specific antibody), the antibody is formed against antihistidyl-tRNA synthetase. Anti-Jo-1 antibodies inhibit the function of their target antigens *in vitro*. In addition to anti-Jo-1 antibodies, antibodies to several other aminoacyl-tRNA synthetase enzymes have been described, including anti-OJ, anti-PL-12, and anti-KJ.

Patients with antisynthetase antibodies often manifest a unique disease phenotype known as 'the antisynthetase syndrome'. This syndrome occurs in 30 per cent of patients with either polymyositis or dermatomyositis. It is characterized by relatively acute disease onset, the presence of constitutional symptoms (for example fever), interstitial lung disease, Raynaud's phenomenon, arthritis, and 'mechanic's hands'. 'Mechanic's hands' consist of roughened, cracked skin on the lateral and palmar surfaces of the fingers and hands, with irregular, dirty-appearing lines, resembling the hands of a manual labourer. The presence of antisynthetase antibodies in a patient denotes a disease phenotype that usually responds to corticosteroid treatment but which is likely to persist. Thus, patients with antisynthetase antibodies may be candidates for early use of immunosuppressive agents in addition to corticosteroids.

Anti-SRP antibodies occur exclusively in polymyositis. They react with the signal recognition particle, a complex of RNA and protein involved in translocating newly synthesized proteins into the endoplasmic reticulum. Anti-SRP antibodies, which occur in approximately 5 per cent of all adult patients with polymyositis, are associated with muscle inflammation of acute onset, severe degree, and refractoriness to therapy.

Finally, anti-Mi-2 antibodies almost always occur in patients with dermatomyositis, often in patients whose cutaneous involvement is prominent. The target of Mi-2 is a complex of nuclear proteins whose function remains unknown. In comparison with patients with antisynthetases and anti-SRP antibodies, those with antibodies to Mi-2 usually have better treatment outcomes.

Diagnosis and treatment

The unequivocal presence of Gottron's sign in association with proximal muscle weakness and elevation of muscle enzymes obviates the need for muscle biopsy because it is pathognomonic. In virtually all other cases of possible polymyositis or dermatomyositis, however, confirmation of the diagnosis by muscle biopsy is essential. Other studies, such electromyography, nerve conduction studies, and magnetic resonance imaging, are adjuncts to diagnosis but do not supplant tissue biopsy.

Corticosteroids, usually beginning with 1 mg/kg/day of prednisone, remain the cornerstone of all initial treatment regimens for polymyositis and dermatomyositis. Decline of the creatine kinase level within 2 weeks of starting treatment may portend a good outcome, but improvement in muscle strength frequently lags and is sometimes not evident for up to 3 months. Patients should be treated with 1 mg/kg/day of prednisone until the creatine kinase is normal (or nearly so), and then undergo a slow taper that does not exceed 10 mg/month. Once the steroid taper has begun, creatine kinase levels are useful in gauging disease activity, but mild creatine kinase elevations do not justify escalations in treatment, particularly if the patient's muscle strength continues to improve. Conversely, once treatment has begun, low creatine kinase levels do not guarantee inactive muscle disease. Dermatomyositis is particularly notorious for the finding of low or normal creatine kinase levels despite active muscle inflammation. Steroid myopathy is a common complication of treatment, and may be difficult to distinguish from active disease.

Many patients with polymyositis or dermatomyositis require additional immunosuppressive agents during their course.

Methotrexate (up to 25 mg/week) or azathioprine (2 mg/kg/day) are the initial second-line agents of choice. Cyclophosphamide may be preferred for patients who have severe interstitial lung disease at presentation or for the rare patient presenting with overt features of necrotizing vasculitis. Intravenous immune globulin is useful in refractory cases of dermatomyositis, but its expense precludes its use in all patients as an initial therapy.

Finally, in addition to pharmacological treatments, physical therapy and rehabilitative medicine play important roles in patient recovery.

Prognosis

Prompter diagnoses, a broader range of therapies, and improved general medical care have improved the 5-year survival rate of patients with polymyositis or dermatomyositis to greater than 80 per cent. However, morbidity from both the diseases themselves and their treatments is high, and few patients emerge from treatment cured and unscathed. Several variables may contribute to worse outcomes or suboptimal therapeutic responses, including delay in diagnosis, the presence of severe myositis, dysphagia, pulmonary or cardiac involvement, the diagnosis of inclusion body myositis, association with malignancy, and the presence of certain myositis-specific antibodies.

Further reading

Bohan A *et al.* (1977). A computer-assisted analysis of 153 patients with polymyositis and dermatomyositis. *Medicine* **56**, 255–86.

Cherin P *et al.* (1993). Dermatomyositis and ovarian cancer: a report of 7 cases and literature review. *Journal of Rheumatology* **20**, 1897–99.

Dalakas MC (1991). Polymyositis, dermatomyositis, and inclusion-body myositis. *New England Journal of Medicine* **325**, 1487–96.

Dalakas MC *et al.* (1993). A controlled trial of high-dose intravenous immune globulin infusions as treatment for dermatomyositis. *New England Journal of Medicine* **329**, 1993–2000.

Kissel JT, Mendell JR, Rammohan KW (1986). Microvascular deposition of complement membrane attack complex in dermatomyositis. *New England Journal of Medicine* **314**, 329–34.

Lie JT (1995). Cardiac manifestations in polymyositis/dermatomyositis: how to get to the heart of the matter. *Journal of Rheumatology* **22**, 809–11.

Plotz PH *et al.* (1995). Myositis: immunologic contributions to understanding cause, pathogenesis, and therapy. *Annals of Internal Medicine* **122**, 715–24.

Schwarz MI (1998). The lung in polymyositis. *Clinical Chest Medicine* **19**, 701–12.

18.10.8 Kawasaki syndrome

Tomisaku Kawasaki

Introduction

Kawasaki disease, first described by Kawasaki in 1967, is an acute febrile, multisystem vasculitic illness of unknown aetiology most commonly affecting children younger than 5 years of age. Originally, the prognosis was believed to be favourable. However, as more studies were carried out, the mortality rate was found to be about 0.3 to 0.5 per cent, but this has subsequently declined to around 0.05 to 0.1 per cent. Autopsy findings revealed exceptional pathological features such as coronary artery aneurysms with thrombosis in many cases. However, since the disease cannot be differentiated histopathologically from infantile periarteritis nodosa (infantile polyarteritis), previously the subject of a few reports in the American and European literature, it is still unclear whether Kawasaki disease is a new entity or a condition that had previously been overlooked. This problem will remain unsolved until the pathogenesis of both diseases is determined.

Although in most cases Kawasaki disease is self-limiting, approximately 25 per cent of untreated patients manifest coronary artery changes such as dilatation and/or aneurysms on echocardiogram. Since 1984, treatment with high-dose intravenous immunoglobulin (**IVIG**) has been used to produce a rapid resolution of the fever and other inflammatory manifestations of Kawasaki disease, in addition to reducing the frequency and severity of coronary artery abnormalities.

Since more than 30 years has elapsed from the first description of Kawasaki disease, some of the earlier patients are now adults. The coronary artery features of the condition may be an important cause of ischaemic heart disease in young adults. Physicians should therefore ask patients with ischaemic heart disease, particularly those under 40 years of age, whether they have a history of childhood Kawasaki disease.

Table 1 The six main features of Kawasaki disease

1.	Fever of unknown aetiology lasting 5 days or more
2.	Bilateral congestion of ocular conjunctiva
3.	Changes in lips and oral cavity
4.	Acute non-purulent swelling of cervical lymph node
5.	Polymorphous exanthema
6.	Changes in the extremities

Clinical manifestations

Kawasaki disease is a clear-cut clinical entity that can be diagnosed after the recognition and analysis of six main symptoms (Table 1). The clinical features can be classified into two categories: principal and subsidiary. At least five of the six main features are required for diagnosis. However, patients with four features can also be diagnosed as having the condition, provided that coronary aneurysms are identified by echocardiography or coronary angiography.

Principal features

Fever of unknown aetiology lasting 5 days or more

In general, the onset of Kawasaki disease is with abrupt high fever but without prodromal symptoms such as coughing, sneezing, or rhinorrhoea. Cervical lymphadenopathy is sometimes felt, particularly if the patient complains of neck pain, and this can precede the fever by a day. Usually the fever is remittent or continuous, ranging from 38 °C to 40 °C, for 1 to 2 weeks. High fever lasting more than 2 weeks is seen in 14 to 20 per cent of untreated cases, but it rarely lasts for more than 30 days. The longer the high fever continues, the greater the possibility of coronary artery aneurysm. Nothing apart from IVIG appears to reduce the fever, which resolves significantly faster when IVIG is administered with aspirin, as compared to therapy with aspirin alone. However, in about 10 per cent of cases, IVIG is not effective in reducing fever.

Bilateral congestion of ocular conjunctiva

Conjunctival infection develops 2 to 4 days after the onset of fever. Each capillary vessel is dilated. There is no purulent discharge, so the term 'conjunctivitis' is inappropriate. In most cases redness of the eyes is obvious, but in some cases it can only be seen upon very close examination. Pseudomembrane formation, iris adhesion, or visual disturbance has not been reported. Anterior uveitis can be observed in 66 per cent of cases upon careful slit-lamp examination early in the course of the disease.

Changes of lips and oral cavity

Dryness, redness, and fissuring of the lips occur 3 to 5 days after the onset of fever. The membranes of the oral cavity and pharyngeal mucosa are diffusely red. There is no vesicle, aphtha, or pseudomembrane formation. Frequently there is prominence of the tongue papillae, referred to as a strawberry tongue and similar to that seen in scarlet fever (Fig. 1 and Plate 1).

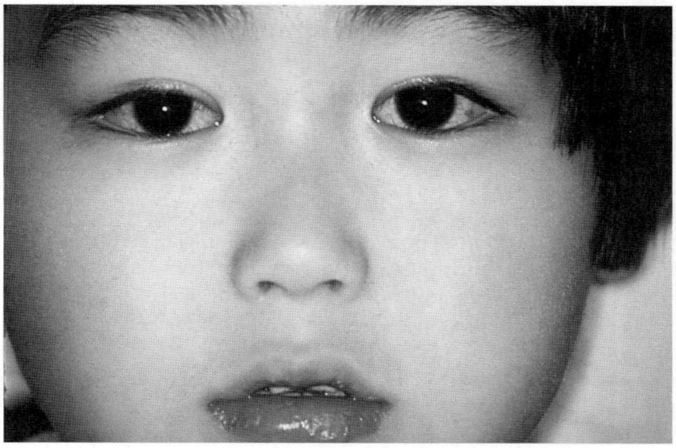

Fig. 1 Typical appearance of a patient with Kawasaki disease, note the red eyes and red lips (picture of a 5-year-old boy, taken on the fourth day of illness). (See also Plate 1).

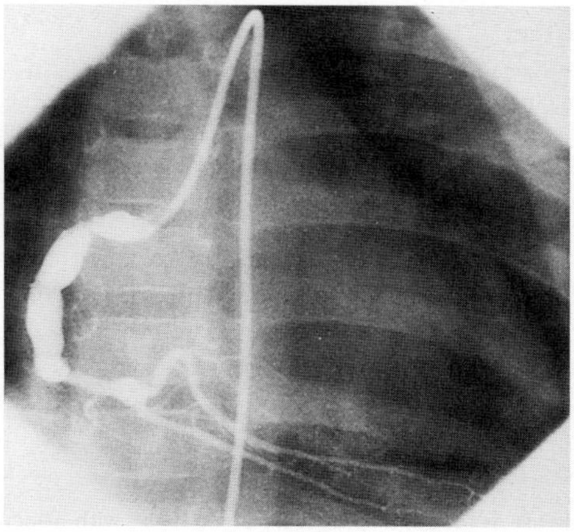

Fig. 2 Right coronary artery aneurysms, seen 1 month after the onset of Kawasaki disease in a boy aged 5 years and 7 months. (By courtesy of Dr T Sonobe of the Japanese Red Cross Medical Center, Tokyo.)

Acute non-purulent swelling of cervical lymph nodes

From the day before the onset of fever, or together with fever, there is swelling of the cervical lymph nodes. The patient complains of pain and often suffers a wry neck. In some cases the swelling occurs several days after the onset of fever. The nodes range from 1.5 to 5 cm in size and form a firm, non-fluctuant mass. Sometimes there is bilateral swelling leading to a misdiagnosis of mumps.

Polymorphous exanthema

From the first to the fifth day after the onset of fever, a polymorphic rash appears on the trunk or extremities. It is variously morbiliform, scarlatiniform, urticariform, or erythema multiform-like. In each case the rash is a different combination of these forms. They are not accompanied by vesicles or crusts, but sometimes there are small aseptic pustules on the knees, buttocks, or other sites. The eruptions usually disappear in less than a week.

Changes in the extremities

Approximately 2 to 5 days after the onset of the disease, when the rash on the trunk has appeared, there is reddening of the palms and soles. Simultaneously, there is an indurative oedema in the hands and feet. From 10 to 15 days after the onset of the illness, desquamation begins from the tips of the fingers and membranous desquamation spreads over the palm up to the wrist. From 45 to 60 days after onset, transverse furrows frequently appear in the nails of both the fingers and toes.

Subsidiary clinical manifestations and complications

Cardiovascular complications

Cardiovascular manifestations can be remarkable in the acute phase of Kawasaki disease and are the leading cause of long-term morbidity and mortality. In this phase, the pericardium, myocardium, endocardium, and coronary arteries may all be involved. Clinically recognizable myocarditis is common, with tachycardia, gallop rhythm, and signs of cardiac failure.

The electrocardiogram is abnormal in one-third of patients, showing low-voltage, ST-segment depression, and T-wave flattening or inversion. Coronary arterial abnormalities develop in approximately 25 per cent of untreated patients (Fig. 2). Aneurysms have been detected within 7 days of illness, but more commonly they occur between 10 days and 3 weeks after the onset of symptoms. The appearance of aneurysms more than 4 weeks after the onset of illness is uncommon. Patients with giant aneurysms (internal diameter of at least 8 mm) have the worst prognosis and are at the greatest risk of developing coronary thrombosis, stenosis, or myocardial infarction. Angiography is sometimes used for diagnosis, particularly in patients with suspected or definite echocardiographic changes or ischaemia. Because of considerable normal variations in the coronary arteries in childhood, only an experienced paediatric cardiologist can properly interpret the angiograms.

Myocardial infarction is the principal cause of death in patients with Kawasaki disease. It may occur within a year; even later in patients who have giant aneurysms. Children with giant aneurysms more likely have other arterial involvement including that of the renal, brachial, and iliac arteries. Valvular involvement, primarily mitral regurgitation, has been described in about 1 per cent of children with Kawasaki disease.

Gastrointestinal tract

Diarrhoea occurs in approximately 35 per cent of patients. Patients with gall bladder involvement (acute acalculous distension: 'hydrops') often suffer severe abdominal pain, especially in the upper right quadrant. Mild jaundice occurs in approximately 5 per cent of cases. The total serum bilirubin level is almost always lower than 10 mg/dl. In the acute phase, serum transaminase levels are often increased. Serum glutamate-oxaloacetate transaminase (**GOT**) and glutamate-pyruvate transaminase (**GPT**) levels increase from 60 to 200 IU, while the lactate dehydrogenase (**LDH**) level increases from 600 to 900 IU. Paralytic ileus has been reported.

Blood

In almost all cases there is leucocytosis with a shift to the left, an increased erythrocyte sedimentation rate (**ESR**), elevated C-reactive protein, and an increased α2-globulin level. The platelet count increases from the second week and may reach 1000 to 1500 $\times 10^9$ per litre. Hypoalbuminaemia and slight anaemia are common.

Urinary tract

Albuminuria is frequently seen in the acute phase, with aseptic microscopic pyuria. These findings disappear in the convalescent phase.

Respiratory system

Preceding or concurrent respiratory symptoms such as cough and rhinorrhoea are occasionally seen. Abnormal infiltrates on the chest radiograph are occasionally observed.

Joints

Arthritis or arthralgia can occur in the initial phase of the illness and are usually polyarticular, involving the knees, ankles, and hands. A pauciarticular arthritis involving the knees, ankles, or hips commonly appears during the second or third week of illness. These symptoms disappear within 30 days after their onset in most cases.

Nervous system

Infants with Kawasaki disease are often more irritable than infants with other febrile illnesses. Signs and symptoms suggestive of aseptic meningitis may be present in some patients, and this is found in 20 to 50 per cent of those with Kawasaki disease who undergo lumbar puncture. Other neurological complications such as facial palsy, hemiplegia, and encephalopathy have been reported.

Other systems

Auditory abnormalities, testicular swelling, and peripheral gangrene have also been reported.

Pathological findings

Kawasaki disease is an acute inflammatory disease with systemic angiitis which is distinguishable from classic periarteritis nodosa of the Kussmaul–Maier type. Coronary aneurysms are usually present at autopsy. The angiitis is characterized by acute inflammation with or without mild fibrinoid necrosis. Middle- or large-sized arteries (such as the main coronary, iliac, axillary, or renal arteries and aorta) are commonly involved. The course of the angiitis can be classified into four stages according to the duration of the illness:

- *Stage 1* (1–2 weeks from onset) shows perivasculitis and vasculitis of the microvessels, small arteries, and veins. There is inflammation of the intima, externa, and perivascular areas in medium- and large-sized arteries. Oedema and infiltration with leucocytes and lymphocytes are also present.
- *Stage 2* (2–4 weeks from onset) shows less inflammation in the vessels than in Stage 1. This stage is characterized by panvasculitis of the main coronary arteries and aneurysm with thrombus in the stems. Myocarditis, coagulation necrosis of heart muscle, lesions of the conduction system, pericarditis and endocarditis with valvulitis are also present.
- *Stage 3* (4–7 weeks from onset) shows subsidence of inflammation in the vessels. Granulation may occur in the medium-sized arteries.
- *Stage 4* (more than 7 weeks from onset) reveals scar formation and intimal thickening with aneurysms, thrombus, and stenosis in the medium-sized arteries.

Other lesions include myocarditis, pericarditis, and inflammation of almost all organs. All these lesions are frequently seen in Stage 1 and 2, but rarely in Stage 4. Ischaemic heart disease usually occurs in Stages 2 to 4. The major cause of death in Stage 1 is myocarditis, including inflammation of conduction systems. In Stage 2 and 3, the causes are ischaemic heart disease, rupture of an aneurysm (rare), and myocarditis. In Stage 4, there may be ischaemic heart disease, and, in rare cases, heart failure due to mitral insufficiency.

Epidemiology

The first nationwide survey was conducted in 1970 by the Japanese Kawasaki disease Research Committee. Since then 15 nationwide surveys have been carried out at 2-year intervals up to December 1998. A total of 153 803 cases (89 272 males and 64 531 females M:F ratio of 1.38:1) has been reported, including 426 (0.28 per cent) deaths. The number of cases reported has been steadily increasing since 1971. There were outbreaks in 1979, 1982, and 1986, when a high incidence of the disease was reported in the early or late spring throughout Japan. A shift of the epidemic wave from warm to cool geographical areas was observed in 1979, but not in 1982 and 1986.

Since 1974, a number of cases have been reported from outside of Japan. Kawasaki disease is now known to have a worldwide distribution, having been observed in all continents and in all ethnic groups. It currently ranks as the leading cause of acquired heart disease in the paediatric population of the United States and Japan.

Aetiology

It is not proven, but the clinical and epidemiological features of Kawasaki disease strongly suggest that it is caused by an infectious agent; one to which the great majority of people become immunized in early life by subclinical infection. The spacing between waves of the disease is determined by the build-up of a new group of susceptible individuals.

The rarity of the illness in the first few months of life and in older children and adults, the low incidence of disease in siblings, and the absence of person-to-person transmission, are all compatible with infection by a ubiquitous agent, to which virtually all adults are immune and from which very young children are protected by passive maternal antibody. The majority of infected individuals probably experience an asymptomatic infection, whilst a select few develop the recognizable clinical features of Kawasaki disease.

Treatment and management

Therapy with the combination of intravenous immunoglobulin (IVIG) and aspirin during the acute phase of Kawasaki disease produces a more marked anti-inflammatory effect and reduction in coronary artery abnormalities than does aspirin alone. It is recommended that patients with acute disease be treated with a single 2 g/kg infusion of IVIG and aspirin (30–50 mg/kg per day) within the first 10 days from onset, and that the aspirin dose be reduced to 3–5 mg/kg per day given as a single daily dose after defervescence. Aspirin is discontinued if no coronary abnormalities have been detected by echocardiography by 6 to 8 weeks after the onset of illness, but continued if coronary artery abnormalities are present. Aspirin should be discontinued if the patient develops an illness suspected to be varicella or influenza, this is to reduce the risk of Reye's syndrome, when the use of an alternative antiplatelet agent should be considered.

Approximately 10 per cent of patients with Kawasaki disease are resistant to IVIG therapy. These patients are at greatest risk for the development of coronary artery aneurysms and long-term sequelae of the disease. As in other vasculitides, blood vessel damage appears to result from an aberrant immune response leading to endothelial cell injury and vessel wall damage. Steroids such as methylprednisolone are the treatment of choice in other forms of vasculitis, yet they have been considered to be unsafe in patients with Kawasaki disease. However, it has been reported that at least some patients with severe disease, resistant to IVIG therapy, may be safely treated with intravenous pulse-steroid therapy and benefit from this treatment.

The management of patients with severe obstructive coronary artery disease, who may develop symptomatic ischaemic heart disease, is an important issue. Patients must be immediately admitted to hospital when myocardial infarction occurs. Management strategies employed are those well defined in the context of atheromatous coronary artery disease. Massive thrombus formation can be visualized by serial echocardiographic studies and is a clear indication for anticoagulation. Recurrence of infarction, which is associated with high mortality, occurs in approximately 20 per cent of patients, and emphasizes the need for the careful management of children with myocardial infarction, even if this is silent.

Patients with cardiac complications or sequelae, such as ventricular dysfunction, heart failure, severe arrhythmias, or postinfarction angina, are managed by conventional medical and/or surgical techniques. As a prelude to surgical treatment, detailed coronary angiography is essential, and viability of the myocardium should be evaluated by thallium scintigraphy. Long-term results and prognosis after surgery remain uncertain. Heart transplantation of patients with Kawasaki disease has been performed in 15 cases.

Further reading

Burns JC, *et al.* (1985). Anterior uveitis associated with Kawasaki syndrome. *Pediatric Infectious Disease* **4**, 258–61.

Checchia P, *et al.* (1995). The worldwide experience with cardiac transplantation for Kawasaki disease. In: Kato H, ed. *Kawasaki disease, Excerpta Medica International Congress Series 1093*, pp 522–6. BV Elsevier Science. Amsterdam.

Dajani AS, *et al.* (1993). Diagnosis and therapy of Kawasaki disease in children. *Circulation* **87**, 1776–80.

Fujiwara H, Hamashima Y (1978). Pathology of the heart in Kawasaki disease. *Pediatrics* **61**, 100–7.

Furusho K, *et al.* (1984). High-dose intravenous gammaglobulin for Kawasaki disease. *Lancet* **2**, 1055–8.

Kato H, Akagi T (1997). Ischemic heart disease in Kawasaki disease. *Progress in Pediatric Cardiology* **6**, 219–26.

Kawasaki T (1967). Acute febrile mucocutaneous syndrome with lymphoid involvement with specific desquamation of the fingers and toes in children. *Japanese Journal of Allergology* **16**, 178–222. [In Japanese.]

Kawasaki T, *et al.* (1974). A new infantile acute febrile mucocutaneous lymph node syndrome (MLNS) prevailing in Japan. *Pediatrics* **54**, 271–6.

Kitamura S, *et al.* (1994). Long-term outcome of myocardial revascularization in patients with Kawasaki coronary artery disease, a multicenter cooperative study. *Journal of Thoracic and Cardiovascular Surgery* **107**, 663–74.

Landing BH, Larson EJ (1987). Pathological features of Kawasaki disease (mucocutaneous lymph node syndrome). *American Journal of Cardiovascular Pathology* **1**, 215–29.

Newburger JW, *et al.* (1991). A single intravenous infusion of gamma globulin as compared with four infusions in the treatment of acute Kawasaki syndrome. *New England Journal of Medicine* **324**, 1633–9.

Shulman ST, Rowley AH (1997). Etiology and pathogenesis of Kawasaki disease. *Progress in Pediatric Cardiology* **6**, 187–92.

Sundel RP, Newburger JW (1997). Management of acute Kawasaki disease. *Progress in Pediatric Cardiology* **6**, 203–9.

Suzuki A, *et al.* (1997). Natural history of coronary artery lesions in Kawasaki disease. *Progress in Pediatric Cardiology* **6**, 211–18.

Tanaka N, Sekimoto K, Naoe S (1976). Kawasaki disease: relationship with infantile periarteritis nodosa. *Archives of Pathology and Laboratory Medicine* **100**, 81–6.

Taubert KA (1997). Epidemiology of Kawasaki disease in the United States and worldwide. *Progress in Pediatric Cardiology* **6**, 181–5.

Yanagawa H, *et al.* (1995). Results of 12 nationwide epidemiological incidence surveys of Kawasaki disease in Japan. *Archives of Pediatrics and Adolescent Medicine*, **149**, 779–83.

Yanagawa H, *et al.* (2000). Results of the 15th nationwide survey on Kawasaki disease in Japan. *Shonika Sinryo* **63**, 121–32. [In Japanese.]

18.11 Miscellaneous conditions presenting to the rheumatologist

D. O'Gradaigh and B. Hazleman

Musculoskeletal symptoms can occur in a wide range of diseases, or as a paraneoplastic manifestation or drug side-effect. Careful assessment of the history, physical signs, and investigation results are required to identify significant underlying conditions that may first present to the rheumatologist. A number of uncommon conditions can present with non-specific musculoskeletal manifestations and are also discussed in this chapter.

Adult Still's disease

In 1971, Bywaters described a series of 14 adults with an illness very similar to the systemic onset-type of juvenile idiopathic arthritis described by Still in 1897. Adult-onset Still's disease is found worldwide with an incidence of 1-3 per million, most commonly in the age range 16 to 35 years and affecting males and females equally in most populations. There is no consistent HLA association.

Features common to both childhood and adult-onset forms are the high, spiking pyrexia, arthralgia or arthritis, and a characteristic rash. The fever typically appears in the evening, and a patient with pyrexia of unknown origin should always be assessed at least once at the end of the day. Spikes in excess of 39°C are typical (and required in diagnostic criteria), though a return to a normal temperature does not occur in 20 per cent. Arthralgia is almost universal and may intensify during the febrile episodes. Distal interphalangeal joint involvement, seen in one in five patients, is useful to distinguish from other inflammatory arthropathies. The classical 'Still's rash' is a maculopapular, salmon-pink rash on the trunk, thighs, and arms or axillae that appears during the temperature spike (termed 'evanescent'). The rash may also appear on the face, palms and soles, and at sites of skin trauma (Koebner phenomenon) in a third of adults. A (culture-negative) severe sore throat is relatively common in adults (though not a feature of the juvenile form).

Other common manifestations are hepatosplenomegaly with or without generalized lymphadenopathy, and polyserositis, of which pericarditis (in a third) and pleuritis are the most common. Rare features include sicca symptoms (dry eyes, mouth), myocarditis, restrictive lung disease, liver or renal failure, panophthalmitis or inflammatory orbital pseudotumour, epilepsy, intravascular coagulopathy or haemophagocytic syndrome, and amyloidosis.

Diagnosis is primarily clinical, it being important to remember that the classical features may only emerge over a period of time, and the possibility of Still's disease may need to be reconsidered as symptoms progress. The differential diagnosis is wide, and while diagnostic criteria have been proposed they have poor sensitivity and specificity until infection (particularly infectious mononucleosis), neoplasia (lymphomas), and connective tissue diseases (such as polyarteritis nodasa and systemic rheumatoid vasculitis) have been excluded.

There are no specific laboratory features, but typical findings include elevated ESR and CRP, thrombocytosis, neutrophil leucocytosis (total leucocytes in excess of 15×10^9/l) and a normochromic normocytic anaemia. Elevated liver enzymes can be found, and may rise further during non-steroidal anti-inflammatory treatment. Both rheumatoid factor and antinuclear antibodies are negative in most cases. A highly elevated (>5 times upper limit) serum ferritin is a useful marker to discriminate from other arthropathies, but is not sufficiently specific to exclude the differentials (especially neoplasia) mentioned above.

Indomethacin (or another non-steroidal anti-inflammatory agent) has largely replaced high-dose (100 mg/kg/day) salicylate as the first line treatment for fever and systemic features. If these agents fail individually, they may be given together, but adequate prophylaxis against peptic ulceration is essential. Corticosteroid is required in two-thirds of cases, and should be initiated without delay in cases of myocarditis, pericardial tamponade, or other severe organ involvement. Doses of prednisolone in the range 0.5–1 mg/kg/day are usually given, and should be continued for 2 to 3 months after remission before gradually tapering the dose.

The role of disease modifying antirheumatic drugs or cytotoxic agents is not established. In refractory cases with systemic features, or as steroid-sparing therapy, methotrexate is particularly useful. Salazopyrin, azothioprine, and intravenous immunoglobulin have also been used. Intramuscular gold is appropriate when arthritis dominates. Most recently, the antitumour necrosis factor-α therapies have been used with some success.

Prognosis is variable. A chronic progressive arthritis is predicted by early arthritis (rather than arthralgia), particularly of the hip and shoulder, and occurs in 30 to 50 per cent of cases, with ankylosis of the carpus and tarsus and involvement of the cervical spine and hips. Equal proportions of the remainder experience either a self-limiting course (lasting up to 1 year), or a polycyclic, relapsing, and remitting course. The rash, fever, and serositis are typically less severe in subsequent relapses, and complete remissions up to 10 years after first presentation have been recorded.

Acne arthralgia

Patients may complain of myalgia, arthralgia, or swelling, typically involving the large joints. Most patients are male adolescents with aggressive acne. *Propionibacterium acnes* has been isolated from joint aspirates; however, effusions are typically sterile and the arthritis is believed to be reactive rather than septic. Hydradenitis suppurativa, producing large abscesses in the axilla and groin, is also associated with a reactive type of large-joint oligoarthropathy. In both conditions, symptoms usually improve with treatment of the skin lesion. A seronegative spondyloarthropathy syndrome of acne, palmoplantar pustulosis, hyperostosis (especially of the clavicles or sternum), and (sterile) osteomyelitis (**SAPHO**) is associated with enthesitis and an inflammatory polyarthritis that often includes the sacroiliac joints.

Neutrophilic dermatoses

The neutrophilic dermatoses include pyoderma gangrenosum and Sweet's syndrome (acute febrile neutrophilic dermatosis). Erythema nodosum is now considered part of this spectrum.

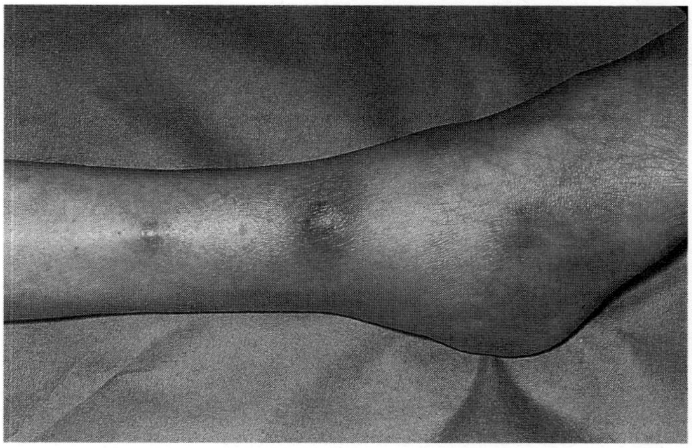

Fig. 1 Pyoderma gangrenosum. (See also Plate 1.)

Pyoderma gangrenosum is a reactive neutrophilic dermatosis associated with ulcerative colitis, rheumatoid arthritis, and monoclonal gammopathies or other haematological malignancies, which produces painful ulcerative skin lesions (Fig. 1 and Plate 1). Approximately 30 per cent of patients describe arthralgia or a seronegative, progressive, erosive polyarthritis. Treatment usually requires corticosteroid therapy in addition to that for the underlying disorder.

Sweet's syndrome presents with tender red or purple raised nodules associated with fever and generalized myalgia and/or arthralgia. Joint effusions may occur, and aspirates reveal high neutrophil counts. Sterile osteomyelitic foci have rarely been described. Skin biopsy is diagnostic. Symptoms typically resolve over 2 to 3 months, requiring symptomatic treatment with a non-steroidal anti-inflammatory drug (**NSAID**) or intra-articular steroid. An association with acute myeloid (particularly premyelocytic) leukaemia is noted in about 15 per cent of cases, and recombinant granulocyte colony-stimulating factor (**rG-CSF**) has also been implicated in a number of cases.

Erythema nodosum presents with discrete nodules on the extensor aspect of the lower leg and less commonly on the upper limbs (Fig. 2 and Plate 2). Joint manifestations (arthralgia in two-thirds) occur in 75 per cent of cases. Arthritis with synovial thickening and joint effusions usually affects the knee and ankle symmetrically. The small joints of the hands, wrists, elbows, and shoulders are less commonly affected. Various underlying conditions, infections, and drugs are associated with erythema nodosum. Whilst their recognition is important, the arthritis is usually self-limiting, responding as it does to treatment with NSAIDs, although corticosteroids are occasionally required, and resolving without sequelae.

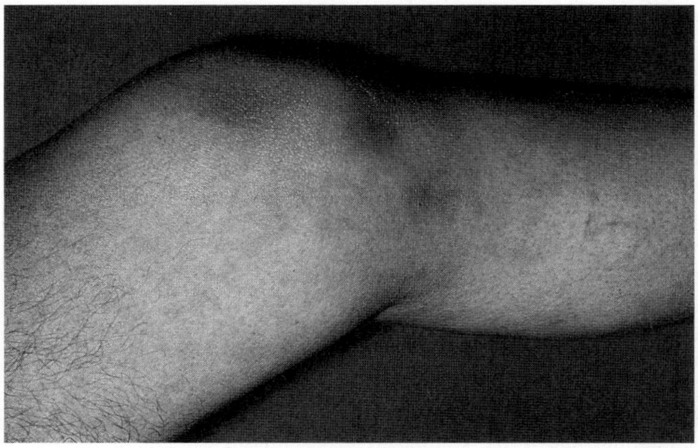

Fig. 2 Erythema nodosum. (See also Plate 2.)

Panniculitis

Also called lupus erythematosus profundus, this is an unusual variation of cutaneous lupus characterized by recurrent inflammation of subcutaneous tissue leading to fibrosis. Asymptomatic, firm, sharply defined subcutaneous nodules or plaques appear on the proximal upper and lower limbs, buttocks, face, and scalp. Histology reveals a non-specific lobular panniculitis with necrobiosis of adipose tissue and fibrotic deposits. Some one in eight patients have systemic lupus erythematosus (**SLE**) at presentation, particularly generalized arthralgia and fatigue. A further 10 to 15 per cent will develop SLE up to 10 years later. Skin and joint features are treated with hydroxychloroquine, though a steroid and dapsone are occasionally required for more florid panniculitis.

Multicentric reticulohistiocytosis

This is a rare systemic disease of unknown aetiology, with infiltration of lipid-laden histiocytes and multinucleate giant cells into various organs. Skin nodules and a rapidly progressive deforming arthritis are the most frequently recognized features. Light copper or red–brown nodules appear on the face and hands, but can appear anywhere, and may number from a few to several hundred. The disease affects middle-aged women who typically present with an insidious onset of polyarthritis in the interphalangeal joints. The spine and other joints may be involved. There is no satisfactory treatment. Underlying malignancy is reported in 20 to 30 per cent of cases.

Sarcoidosis

One-third of patients with sarcoid will have musculoskeletal features, of which an acute symmetrical polyarthritis is the most common. Lofgren's syndrome associates this pattern of arthritis with erythema nodosum and bilateral hilar lymphadenopathy. The ankles and feet are the most commonly affected, followed by the hands, wrists, and elbows. Symptoms develop rapidly and usually respond well to NSAIDs, although corticosteroids are occasionally necessary. Remission without joint destruction occurs after 2 to 4 months. A chronic arthropathy is uncommon, occurring mostly in those with multiorgan involvement and those requiring steroid treatment during the acute phase. Dactylitis, joint space narrowing, and osseous involvement are then the most common features, with superimposed episodes of acute arthritis. Radiographic findings appear late, and include acro-osteolysis, cystic lesions, or a reticulated coarse trabecular pattern in the phalanges. Corticosteroid in doses of 30 to 60 mg are the mainstay of treatment at this stage, but is frequently disappointing, with recurrence of symptoms on cessation of therapy.

Amyloidosis

Musculoskeletal features occur in three main settings. Dialysis-related amyloidosis is due to the accumulation of β_2-microglobulin. Synovitis usually involves large joints such as the hip and shoulder. Magnetic resonance imaging (**MRI**) may show characteristic features, and joint fluid aspiration may identify amyloid deposits, particularly using the more sensitive combination of Congo Red staining and immunocytochemistry. Symptomatic treatment with an NSAID is usually sufficient, considerations of the effect of NSAIDs on renal function only being relevant in those dialysis patients with substantial urine output, but the condition can be disabling and refractory. Significant improvement often follows transplantation. Cystic (lytic) bone lesions are typically painless, and present difficulties in the differential diagnosis. They may be complicated by pathological fracture. Soft tissue amyloid deposits usually present with entrapment neuropathies such as carpal tunnel syndrome.

In primary (AL) amyloidosis, a symmetrical polyarthritis with synovitis and morning stiffness involves large and small joints. Radiographic changes include osteoporosis and, less commonly, joint erosions. Diagnostic confusion can arise, as frequently the erythrocyte sedimentation rate is not significantly elevated. The synovitis is often described as 'pasty', and flexion contractures occur relatively early. The early appearance of carpal tunnel syndrome should also raise the suspicion of underlying amyloidosis. In addition to treatment addressing the underlying paraproteinaemia, joint symptoms may require therapy with a corticosteroid.

Familial amyloidosis and secondary (AA) amyloid due to persistent inflammation are not usually associated with rheumatological symptoms. Exceptions include the Muckle–Wells syndrome of urticaria, deafness, arthritis, and amyloid nephropathy.

Familial Mediterranean fever (FMF)

This is an autosomal recessive disorder appearing in people of Armenian, Arab, and Sephardic Jewish descent. A number of genetic defects have been localized to the *marenostrin* or *pyrin* genes on chromosome 16p. The function of this protein is not known, but the *M694V* mutation is particularly associated with joint involvement. Presenting in childhood with episodes of fever and abdominal pain, synovitis occurs in 75 per cent of cases. Monoarticular involvement of a knee or ankle, or symmetrical involvement of these joints, are the most common of the six patterns of joint involvement described. A symmetrical polyarthritis indistinguishable from juvenile idiopathic arthritis often causes diagnostic confusion, particularly as fever and abdominal pain are not uncommon in this condition. The pattern tends to be similar in subsequent episodes, and despite frequent florid synovitis, residual damage rarely occurs. Episodes typically last for less than 1 week, though more protracted attacks may persist for months. Treatment with colchicine has almost eliminated amyloidosis as a complication of this condition and it also reduces the frequency of symptom relapse. However, it is ineffective once an episode has started, and an NSAID and rest are then the most effective measures. Interferon-α has been used to good effect in resistant cases.

Another two periodic fever syndromes—hyperimmunoglobulin D syndrome (**HIDS**) and familial Hibernian fever (also called autosomal dominant recurrent fever)—occur in The Netherlands and Northern France, and in a few Irish and Scottish families, respectively. To date, neither has been associated with the joint symptoms of FMF. Frequent mouth ulcers resembling Behçet's syndrome appear during attacks of HIDS. However, the markedly elevated levels of IgD and IgA in the latter are diagnostic. The place of colchicine is not yet established in the treatment of these disorders.

Haematological disorders

Leukaemia, lymphoma, and uncommon lymphoproliferative disorders

Between 13 and 60 per cent of patients with acute leukaemia will develop arthralgia or less commonly a frank arthritis. Monoarthritis, symmetrical polyarthritis, and a large joint oligoarthropathy are described. Diagnostic clues include a disproportionate amount of pain, fever, and weight loss, though in children the latter may be mistaken for Still's disease. Arthralgia is an uncommon feature of lymphomas; however, 7 to 25 per cent of patients with non-Hodgkin's lymphoma experience polyarthralgia, secondary gout, or hypertrophic pulmonary osteoarthropathy (see below) during the course of their disease.

Large granular lymphocyte syndrome is a monoclonal expansion of T cells associated with a variety of conditions including rheumatoid arthritis (in one-third of cases). Both neutropenia and splenomegaly can occur, mimicking Felty's syndrome. Some consider it to be indistinguishable in every respect, including its management.

Human T-cell lymphotrophic virus-1 (**HTLV-1**) is associated with the development of leukaemia or lymphoma, and may independently produce a symmetrical polyarthritis closely resembling rheumatoid arthritis.

Haemophilia

Prophylactic, factor replacement between 2 and 18 years of age is cost-effective in preventing disabling joint complications. Without this, acute haemarthroses begin from around 5 years of age, causing recurring episodes of very painful and tender joint swelling, particularly in the hinge joints such as the knee, ankle, and elbow (presumably because these joints are less tolerant of angular or rotational strain). Pain is increased by the additional irritant effect of blood on the synovium. Ultrasonography is useful in the differentiation of haemarthrosis from soft tissue or subperiosteal haemorrhage. Repeated episodes, without appropriate treatment, result in persistent synovitis and joint contracture. Early coagulation factor replacement, ice, joint immobilization, and elevation all reduce further bleeding. Joint aspiration may also be required (after adequate factor replacement). Rehabilitation is required to prevent contraction. Synovectomy by an intra-articular injection of radioactive isotope is a useful treatment in cases of chronic synovitis, but joint replacement continues to be needed where disabling secondary degenerative arthritis has occurred. Acute haemarthrosis due to disseminated intravascular coagulation should be similarly managed.

Cryoglobulinaemia

Cryoglobulins are immune complexes that precipitate spontaneously at low temperatures. Type I (25 per cent) comprises a monoclonal immunoglobulin and is associated with lymphoproliferative disorders including myeloma and Waldenström's macroglobulinaemia. Type II (25 per cent) complexes a monoclonal immunoglobulin, usually of IgM class, with a polyclonal anti-immunoglobulin typically of IgG type (that is, a rheumatoid factor). Previously called mixed essential cryoglobulinaemia, it is now recognized that over 90 per cent of these individuals have serological evidence of hepatitis C virus (HCV) infection. Type III accounts for 50 per cent of cases, and is a complex of two polyclonal immunoglobulins, usually occurring as a paraneoplastic phenomenon.

Precipitation of cryoglobulin leads to complement activation and vasculitis in small vessels. Complete vascular occlusion is less common. A classical triad of a palpable purpuric rash on the extremities, arthralgia, and muscle weakness is described. Joints are involved in 70 per cent of patients in a relapsing and remitting pattern, affecting, in order of frequency, the hands, knees, ankles, and elbows. Inflammatory arthritis is uncommon, and radiological changes do not occur. Other skin presentations include petechiae, urticaria, and acrocyanosis. Other organ involvement is frequently seen in addition to this triad, particularly glomerulonephritis.

Diagnosis requires meticulous attention to phlebotomy and laboratory techniques. A positive rheumatoid factor and raised ESR are supportive features, and urinalysis and microscopy, looking for an 'active sediment' (proteinuria, haematuria, and red cell casts), should always be carried out in patients presenting with purpura and arthralgia. A thorough search is required for underlying malignancy and for associated HCV infection.

Treatment is directed at any underlying cause. NSAIDs, corticosteroids, and steroid-sparing drugs, particularly azathioprine, are used to relieve arthralgia and to prevent the progression of purpura to ulceration. Neurological or renal involvement requires more aggressive therapy, for which cyclophosphamide (oral or intravenous pulses) or chlorambucil are used. Plasmapharesis is sometimes considered for those with rapidly progressive glomerulonephritis, but requires particular care to avoid blood cooling in the extracorporeal circuit.

POEMS

This is an uncommon disorder that may present to any specialty, depending on the dominant feature in the spectrum of **p**olyneuropathy, **o**rganomegaly, **e**ndocrinopathy, **M**-protein (i.e. a monoclonal paraproteinaemia), and **s**kin abnormalities. Skin changes may resemble scleroderma. Radiographs show single or multiple osteosclerotic lesions with unusual patterns of proliferative change, both of which are unexpected in myeloma. The diagnosis of POEMS should therefore be considered in those presenting with osteosclerotic lesions accompanied by paraproteinaemia, particularly when associated with peripheral neuropathy. Treatment must be directed at the principal presenting features—bone lesions are rarely symptomatic unless they result in bone swelling or fracture.

Hypogammaglobulinaemia

Primary hypogammaglobulinaemia is associated in 10 to 30 per cent of patients with a non-erosive polyarthritis resembling rheumatoid arthritis. Features include morning stiffness, pain, and tender swelling in the peripheral joints. Subcutaneous nodules may appear. However, rheumatoid factor is negative, histology reveals the absence of plasma cells, and permanent joint damage is rare. Synovitis may be transient or it may persist for many years, requiring symptomatic treatment. Intra-articular corticosteroid treatment is used, though these patients are somewhat more at risk of septic arthritis. In the absence of any intra-articular procedure, the rate of septic arthritis is approximately 20 per cent over 20 years.

Sickle-cell disease (SCD)

Sickle-cell crises commonly include bone pain. The cause is believed to be intramedullary hypertension due to vascular occlusion resulting in bone ischaemia. Vasodilator drugs have been used with varied results. Avascular necrosis is less commonly associated with other haemoglobinopathies. Synovitis, frequently complicated by haemarthrosis, usually occurs during crises, and is due to synovial infarction. The effusion is non-inflammatory. Osteomyelitis may complicate avascular necrosis due to SCD, *Salmonella* spp. being particularly common. However, septic arthritis is unusual. Hyperuricaemia and gout occur in 40 per cent of adults with SCD, and is treated in the standard way. Less commonly, a hand-and-foot syndrome affects infants aged between 6 months and 2 years, dactylitis and periostitis producing symmetrical tender, diffuse swelling and stiffness lasting several weeks.

Gastroenterological and metabolic conditions

Hepatitis

The common viral hepatitides, hepatitis-A, -B, and -C viruses (**HAV**, **HBV**, and **HCV**, respectively) are associated with a serum-sickness during their prodromal phase. Early morning stiffness and mild arthralgia, or, less commonly, inflammatory arthritis, affect the small joints of the hands, and, in decreasing order of frequency, the knees, ankles, shoulders, wrists, and feet. The spine and hips are not usually affected. Symptoms typically resolve as hepatitis evolves. Less common features include a leucocytoclastic ('hypersensitivity') vasculitis in HAV and an association with polyarteritis nodosa in HBV. HCV is associated with cryoglobulinaemia (in 50 per cent) and with antiphospholipid antibodies and thrombosis.

Enteropathies

Coeliac disease may result in osteoporosis or osteomalacia with bone pain and pathological fracture. Arthritis is uncommon, but can precede overt bowel symptoms by up to 3 years. Symmetrical involvement with swelling and stiffness can affect the lumbar spine, hips, knees, and shoulders. Dermatitis herpetiformis is more common among those with joint involvement. The joint manifestations resolve on changing to a gluten-free diet, and do not reappear on rechallenge with gluten.

Whipple's disease presents with fever and abdominal pain. Acute or subacute migratory polyarthritis may precede bowel symptoms by years, and typically involves the ankles, knees, shoulders, and elbows. Lymphadenopathy is a prominent feature. Duodenal biopsy shows Periodic acid–Schiff (**PAS**) -staining macrophages, and the polymerase chain reaction (**PCR**) detects the causative organism *Tropheryma whippelii*. Its presence within cells implies a mechanism similar to reactive arthritis with a T_H2-dominant response and inability of the T_H1-cellular immune response to clear the microbe from macrophages, which therefore perpetuate the inflammatory reaction.

Surgical procedures that bypass a section of (proximal) small bowel are associated with so-called 'bypass' arthritis. This ranges from a mono- or oligoarthropathy to a diffuse polyarthritis involving large and small joints. Tenosynovitis of the wrist is a particularly common feature. Treatment is symptomatic, though sulfasalazine is occasionally used as a disease-modifying therapy.

Haemochromatosis

An autosomal recessive inherited disorder of iron transportation and storage, this condition may present up to 10 years before the underlying condition is recognized, usually in men between 50 and 60 years of age, with a painful inflammatory synovitis principally affecting the second and third metacarpophalangeal joints. About 80 per cent of those with genetically identified haemochromatosis will develop arthritis at some point. Acute exacerbations may occur due to calcium pyrophosphate dihydrate deposition, particularly in the knee and wrist. The reason for this is unclear, though iron is known to inhibit the clearance of pyrophosphate from the synovial lining layer. Crystals may be identified on polarized light-microscopy of a joint aspirate. Their presence is implied by radiographic evidence of chondrocalcinosis. Radiographs of the hands may also show cyst formation in the affected joints, with erosive changes and characteristically hook-shaped osteophytes. Treatment is symptomatic, intra-articular corticosteroid therapy being of value during acute episodes. Arthritis persists in the majority of cases, and can be relentlessly progressive, despite regular venesection.

Wilson's disease

A disorder of copper metabolism, this condition typically presents in childhood with neurological problems. Some two-thirds of patients with Wilson's disease will develop musculoskeletal manifestations, half of whom being symptomatic by 15 years of age. Features include arthritis (primary, attributed to copper deposition in synovium; or secondary, due to chondrocalcinosis), rhabdomyolysis, hypermobility (due to effects on collagen synthesis), and osteopenia. Radiographic appearances are generally nonspecific, with joint space narrowing, sclerosis, and cyst formation. A fluffy periostitis at the greater trochanter and inferior aspect of the calcaneus, and corticated ossicles near affected joints (particularly the wrist) are characteristic but rare. Diagnosis requires measuring urinary 24-hour copper excretion: caeruloplasmin may be elevated as part of an acute-phase response and therefore is of no diagnostic value in presentations with acute arthritis. Penicillamine is the mainstay of treatment for this condition and alleviates joint symptoms.

Ochronosis

Deficiency of the enzyme homogentisic acid oxidase results in an accumulation of this organic acid. Though a congenital disorder, symptoms rarely appear until the fourth decade. The classical clinical features of pigmentation of the ear and sclera, and urine darkening on standing (giving the alternative name alkaptonuria) allow easy diagnosis. Deposition also occurs in the synovium and may appear in joint fluid aspirate. Pain and swelling affect the large joints, and the thoracolumbar spine is also affected producing pain and stiffness, but the lumbosacral spine is spared. Radiographs show chondrocalcinosis of the intervertebral discs with spondylosis that may progress to ankylosis. In the peripheral joints, radiographic changes of degeneration appear, though osteophytes are often less marked than in other degenerative arthritides. Erosion may occur. Recent treatment efforts are concentrated on early genetic diagnosis, dietary advice, and the possibility in the future of gene therapy.

Hyperlipidaemia

Articular symptoms can occur in a number of the hyperlipidaemias, particularly types II and IV. Joint manifestations typically precede diagnosis of the lipoprotein disorder. Xanthomas of tendons are a useful clue, but the clinical picture is otherwise non-specific. Morning stiffness, pain, and tenderness are noted, but overt joint inflammation is uncommon. A migratory polyarthritis is occasionally described in type II hyperlipoproteinaemia, but oligoarthritis and tendonitis are more common. Tendon xanthomas may result in periarticular bone cyst formation. In two-thirds of patients, symptoms resolve with treatment of the lipid disorder, the remainder requiring symptomatic therapy.

Musculoskeletal manifestations of HIV/AIDS

Rheumatological manifestations include serum-sickness at seroconversion, pyomyositis, and osteomyelitis (particularly in the setting of intravenous drug abuse) and a spectrum of presentations with acute arthropathy. Antiretroviral therapy, particularly zidovudine, may produce a polymyositis with ragged red fibres on muscle biopsy. Very rare manifestations include a vasculitis that appears to be directly induced by the virus, and hypertrophic osteoarthropathy (see below) secondary to *Pneumocystis carinii* pneumonia. Arthritis or arthralgia occur in 1 to 25 per cent of cases. Spondyloarthropathy with dactylitis and enthesitis is the most common. A severe, but self-limiting, large joint oligoarthritis has a predilection for the knees and ankles, resolving over 2 to 6 weeks and responding well to NSAIDs. A generalized articular syndrome is very short-lived though intensely painful, usually lasting only 24 h. Acute symmetrical polyarthritis is relatively uncommon, and septic arthritis is rare.

Reflex sympathetic dystrophy

This is one of a number of terms (including algodystrophy and Sudeck's atrophy) for a condition that has recently been renamed 'chronic regional pain syndrome' (**CRPS**). The dominant feature is pain, with allodynia (pain in response to an innocuous stimuli), hyperalgesia (increased pain perception), and hyperpathia (an exaggerated delayed reaction). Pain usually involves a single limb or body region, typically distal to the site of some traumatic event, but a definite precipitant is recognized in only 50 per cent of patients. Marked joint stiffness and pain on movement cause considerable disability. CRPS may also follow myocardial infarction, stroke, pregnancy, or deep venous thrombosis. There is an association with HLA-DR2. Other cardinal features relate to excessive activity of the sympathetic nervous system, with localized swelling, sweating, and piloerection in the early stages, the skin often appearing stretched and shiny. Hyperaemia is believed to be responsible for osteopenia in the affected part.

Diagnosis is largely clinical, though diffuse osteopenia on plain radiography (comparing the symptomatic and normal limbs on the same film) and the absence of an acute-phase response are supportive. Bone scintigraphy offers the most reliable confirmation of the clinical impression. A three-phase scan is required, comparing the symptomatic and normal sides in the early blood phase (demonstrating hyperaemia in the affected part), the bone pool phase (increased bone turnover), and delayed phase. Physiotherapy is the key element of treatment and must be quite intensive initially. However, pain may limit patient co-operation. Sympathetic nerve blocks (stellate ganglion or lumbar sympathetic chain) with long-acting anaesthetic and/or guanethidine are specialized techniques that are often quite effective. Other pain-relieving modalities include corticosteroid injection to the involved joint, subcutaneous or intranasal calcitonin, intravenous pamidronate, and (oral) gabapentin.

Charcot's arthropathy

This is a disorder of joint destruction associated with neurological injury or damage. Diabetes mellitus, tabes dorsalis, and syringomyelia are the most commonly associated diseases. There are two leading pathogenesis theories. The more widely accepted neurotraumatic theory suggests that loss of sensation allows repeated subclinical trauma, culminating in a destructive arthropathy. The neurovascular theory is proposed to explain how the arthropathy can appear very early in the absence of use of the limb, and the observation, particularly in the tarsus of diabetic patients, that the arthropathy can be quite painful. Here, it is believed that damage to 'trophic centres' results in altered vascular supply and, hence, impaired bone and cartilage nutrition underlying the subsequent joint damage. Radiologically, a gross proliferative osteoarthrosis is most commonly seen, but significant resorption of bone can also feature, and stress fractures occur in up to one-third of patients. Painfree joints rarely require treatment; moreover, orthopaedic procedures are associated with a high failure rate. Management of painful neuropathic joints is very difficult. Orthoses help to prevent stressing of related soft-tissue structures, and a broad range of analgesics, including amitriptyline, should be considered.

Tietze's syndrome/chostochondritis

Both conditions are of unknown aetiology, though a viral trigger has been proposed in Tietze's syndrome (chondropathia tuberosa). A single chostochondral joint (usually the second or third) is involved in 80 per cent of patients. Coughing or deep breathing exacerbates paracentral chest pain. Tietze's syndrome is also associated with firm, tender lumps at the affected sites. Onset may be acute or more gradual, and the subsequent course is similarly variable, ranging from spontaneous remission to prolonged symptoms lasting for years. As these conditions typically affect middle-aged women, a visceral origin for the symptoms must not be overlooked. Local injection with lidocaine (lignocaine) or a corticosteroid may provide symptomatic relief when necessary.

Miscellaneous disorders of synovium, bone, cartilage, and calcification

Synovium

Pigmented villonodular synovitis (PVNS)

This is a benign synovial hyperplasia of unknown aetiology, possibly reactive or neoplastic. To date, three types of PVNS have been described. Giant-cell tumour of the tendon sheath occurs most commonly in extensor tendons of the hand; although painless, large nodules may restrict movement. Treatment is by surgical excision, which allows histological confirmation of the diagnosis. Recurrence is rare. Isolated nodular and true diffuse PVNS are intra-articular lesions occurring most commonly in the knee of adult males aged between 20 and 50 years. Pain, swelling, and a gradual reduction in the range of movement can continue for some years before the diagnosis is made. Aspiration of serosanguinous fluid in the absence of trauma should raise the suspicion. Intra-articular steroid administration gives effective but short-lived relief, and surgical excision is the treatment of choice as it also allows a definitive diagnosis. In the event of a recurrence (uncommon except in the diffuse form), radioisotope synovectomy or radiotherapy may be used. In late stages, haemosiderin deposition and chronic inflammation can lead to destructive changes requiring arthroplasty.

Synovial (osteo-)chondromatosis (Reichel syndrome)

A benign synovial proliferation, this is probably caused by reactive metaplasia secondary to osteoarthrosis, osteochondrosis, or other joint pathology. Most patients are men in their third to fifth decade. Typically monoarticular, usually in the knee, symptoms include joint swelling, locking, and giving way, suggestive of intra-articular loose bodies. Multiple (up to 200) calcified periarticular bodies of hyaline cartilage, 1 mm to 3 cm in size but usually uniform, fill the joint. Surgery is required to remove loose bodies. Rarely, malignant transformation to chondrosarcoma may occur.

Synovial haemangioma

A synovial haemangioma is a benign lesion comprising vascular and non-vascular tissue in an asymptomatic and well-localized intra-articular mass, most commonly in the knee (60 per cent) and elbow (30 per cent). Surgical excision is curative.

Lipomas are most commonly found in the thenar and hypothenar eminences producing compressive symptoms. They may calcify or undergo fibrosis and infarction. Lipoma arborescens occurs particularly in the suprapatellar bursa, producing painless swelling. MRI changes are diagnostic and surgery is curative.

Some two-thirds of 'synovial sarcomas' arise in the thigh. The tissue of origin is mesenchymal, with differentiation to synovium. Prognosis is poor despite surgical excision and radiotherapy.

Bone and cartilage

Bone cysts may be symptomatic or arise as incidental findings, thereby causing diagnostic difficulty. Cysts may be aneurysmal (primary or secondary) or simple (also called unicameral) and can appear in children or adults. Simple cysts are rarely symptomatic or complicated by fracture, and management is expectant. Aneurysmal bone cysts are rare (1 per million), non-neoplastic expansile lesions occurring principally in the metaphysis of long bones (50 per cent), the posterior part of vertebrae (30 per cent), or in the flat bones, particularly the pelvis. Most present with pain, swelling, or pathological fracture at a mean of 13 years of age. Radiological features that suggest the diagnosis include an eccentric location of a cyst containing fluid-fluid levels and trabeculae which remain distinct within it. Management has evolved from the mainstay of curettage with bone grafting or implanting autologous marrow (rich in osteoblasts) to intralesional corticosteroid injection. However, recurrence rates are high (20 to 50 per cent) and other options include embolization and radiotherapy. Secondary aneurysmal cysts complicate giant-cell tumours, chondroblastomas, and osteosarcomas, or they may develop from simple unicameral cysts.

Diffuse idiopathic skeletal hyperostosis (DISH; Forestier's disease)

Presenting in middle age, and more commonly in men (2:1, male:female ratio), this condition of unknown aetiology affects about 10 per cent of men aged 65 years or over, and up to 58 per cent of men with gout. Usually a radiographic diagnosis, the criteria include the presence of new bone forming bridging osteophytes spanning at least four adjacent thoracic vertebrae in the absence of degenerative disc disease or sacroileitis. (The cortex is preserved, unlike the erosive process seen in the Romanus lesion of ankylosing spondylitis.) New bone formation can occur at any site, though entheseal sites are especially common. Phalangeal tufting, and an increase in the cortical thickness of the tubular bones of the hand and in the size of sesamoid bones are recognized. Symptoms include restriction in range of movement, diffuse limb pain, and symptoms of nerve entrapment or myelopathy. Canal stenosis can occur in the lumbar spine. Fracture through bridging osteophytes may also produce pain. Hyperinsulinaemia is frequently associated and related features such as hypertension, type II diabetes, obesity, and hyperlipidaemia are more commonly seen in this group. There is no medical treatment of proven value for established DISH. In the early stages, physical therapy may preserve the range of movement, and weight reduction is of value, both directly and in reducing hyperinsulinaemia. If oral hypoglycaemic agents are required, those that increase serum insulin levels should be avoided. Efforts to reduce heterotopic bone formation at sites of joint replacement have included radiotherapy and perioperative NSAIDs with mixed results. Corticosteroid, given into joints or at entheseal sites may also offer symptomatic relief.

Myositis ossificans (MO)

Calcification of muscle complicates an intramuscular haematoma following direct impact, occurring in 17 to 20 per cent of such injuries. The anterior thigh and upper arm are the most common sites. Predictive signs at onset include local swelling, tenderness, and (particularly) reduced range of stretch in the involved muscle. A sympathetic knee effusion is described in up to half of those with MO in the thigh. Diagnosis may be confirmed radiologically after 3 weeks. Magnetic resonance imaging will detect a haematoma very early, but to date has not identified specific features predictive of MO. Therefore, the classic 'rest, ice, compression, elevation' is appropriate in the acute setting, with NSAIDs where pain and swelling are particularly marked. Physical training should not resume until a full range of passive stretching is restored. Surgical debridement of ectopic calcification should only be undertaken if it interferes with limb function, and then only where bone is matured, as assessed by bone scintigraphy.

Fibrodysplasia (myositis) ossificans progressiva, by contrast, is a rare inherited disorder. It is characterized by abnormally short halluces and ectopic calcification of striated muscle leading to disability as the neck, shoulders, spine, hips, and knees become progressively and relentlessly fixed. Additional variable features include fusion of the lateral masses in the lumbar spine, broad femoral necks, and widened metaphyses, as well as episodes of myositis, principally in the neck and upper paraspinal areas, preceding ossification. Histological misdiagnoses include sarcoma or rhabdomyosarcoma and juvenile fibromatosis. The disease appears to be due to a spontaneous genetic mutation in most cases, and prognosis is extremely variable. It has been difficult to evaluate therapeutic options for this reason, and no single measure is clearly of benefit, though there are theoretical grounds for the use of corticosteroids during episodes of myositis, bisphosphonates, and surgical debridement.

Ectopic calcification in renal disease

This is one aspect of renal osteodystrophy, where painful calcification of soft tissue, particularly at sites of repeated trauma, occurs as a result of serum levels of calcium and phosphate exceeding their combined solubility. Careful monitoring of phosphate and calcium levels, particularly when vitamin D analogues are used, and early treatment of hyperparathyroidism are all important, because established calcification may be intractable. Reversal following renal transplantation has been noted.

Melorheostosis

This is a rare disorder of linear hyperostosis associated with fibrosis of the skin and soft tissue. Thickening of cortical bone appears in a linear fashion (akin to spilling wax on the side of a candle), usually involving one or several bones in the same (more commonly the lower) limb. Many cases are associated with skin changes in the dermatome corresponding to the origin (sclerotome) of the affected bone, resulting in joint contracture. Symptoms include joint pain, intermittent swelling, deformity, and nerve entrapment, usually presenting in the second decade of life. Surgical intervention is most successful.

Paraneoplastic presentations

Rheumatological presentations associated with malignancy include gout, poly- and dermatomyositis, necrotizing vasculitis and cryoglobulinaemia, systemic sclerosis, and the presentations of lymphoproliferative disorders mentioned above. There are two specific conditions: hypertrophic pulmonary osteoarthropathy (**HPOA**) and remitting seronegative symmetric synovitis with pitting (o)edema (**RS3PE**). A seronegative polyarthritis without oedema and otherwise indistinguishable from rheumatoid arthritis may also occur.

HPOA is almost always associated with finger clubbing. Patients complain of pain and stiffness of the wrist and ankles, or of a more diffuse polyarthritis. Radiologically, a proliferative periostitis is noted, particularly at the diaphysis of wrists, ankles, and, less commonly, of knees and elbows. Over 90 per cent of cases have an intrathoracic malignancy, though infections or inflammatory conditions in pulmonary, cardiovascular, or gastrointestinal systems are seen. Primary HPOA (pachydermoperiostitis) also occurs. The cause of the condition is unknown: it has been suggested that cytokines such as platelet-derived growth factor might reach the periphery through pulmonary shunts, thereby producing the clinical proliferative features, but, on the basis of this hypothesis, it is difficult to explain the observation that vagotomy can relieve symptoms and signs in some cases. The arthritis is typically coincident with the malignancy, and will resolve with treatment of the underlying disease. Radiotherapy (to the periostitis sites) and infusion of pamidronate have also been successful in the treatment of resistant cases.

RS3PE was first described in 1985. Mostly affecting older men (mean age 71 years), a symmetrical polyarthritis involves the metacarpophalangeal and interphalangeal joints, wrists, and, less commonly, the elbows and shoulders. Tendon sheath involvement is quite common, and diffuse pitting oedema on the dorsum of the hands is characteristic. This condition has diverse clinical associations, but malignancy is detected in only 10 per cent of cases. Resistance to corticosteroid treatment in this otherwise very responsive condition raises the possibility of malignancy, though in most cases the underlying disease is detected within weeks. In paraneoplastic presentations, symptoms mirror treatment and relapse of the tumour.

Drugs producing rheumatological presentations

Myalgia may occur on withdrawal of steroids, especially in those patients taking 10 mg prednisolone for at least 30 days. This is best managed by reintroducing the steroid with a more gradual reduction in dose (for example, 1-mg steps every few days or weeks, depending on severity). Arthralgia and even arthritis are described as rare adverse effects of steroid therapy. Muscle cramps or aching may also complicate therapy with digoxin, penicillamine, clofibrate, and, more recently, with the statins. Myositis and rhabdomyolysis are also recognized in patients prescribed this latter group of drugs. The oral contraceptive is associated with a syndrome of persisting arthralgia, myalgia, morning stiffness, and even synovitis. Myopathy complicates statin and corticosteroid therapy, and chloroquine may cause neuromyopathy, particularly affecting the lower limbs. Myasthenic weakness is an uncommon complication of penicillamine.

Hypersensitivity reaction is associated with penicillamine, sulphonamides, thiouracils, and allopurinol, to name but a few. Presentations vary, but typically include a small vessel vasculitis and generalized arthralgia or arthritis.

Drug-induced systemic lupus erythematosus is well recognized, though ten times less common than classical SLE. It is characterized by the presence of antihistone antibodies, in distinction to the anti-DNA antibodies of classical SLE. Positive antinuclear antigen (**ANA**) antibodies are considerably more common than any clinical evidence of lupus. Other important distinctions from idiopathic SLE include resolution on withdrawal of the drug—renal and CNS involvement being rare, and rash uncommon—older age of onset (50–60 years compared with a mean age of onset of 29 years in idiopathic SLE). Drug-induced SLE is uncommon among the Black population, though this group accounts for 30 per cent of idiopathic cases. The drugs associated with SLE include hydralazine and procainamide, with minocycline an important recent addition. Most rheumatologists believe that these agents can be used safely by patients with idiopathic SLE, but oestrogen-containing contraceptives are generally regarded as being contraindicated. If a patient develops SLE, any concurrent medication should be withdrawn and the patient observed for a period. However, corticosteroids may be required where there is severe involvement, particularly of the renal, CNS, or cardiorespiratory systems. Antibodies may persist after satisfactory clinical resolution and are not of themselves an indication for continued treatment.

Isoniazid and phenobarbital have been associated with a shoulder–hand syndrome (discussed above as reflex sympathetic dystrophy). The mechanism of this association is unclear, though alteration in serotonin metabolism has been implicated.

Quinolone antibiotics can cause a tendinopathy. This may lead to rupture, most commonly of the Achilles tendon in elderly patients who are also taking corticosteroids.

Retinoids have been associated in recent years with a hyperostosis otherwise indistinguishable from DISH discussed above.

This discussion of the associations between drugs and rheumatological presentations is far from complete, and the physician should always consider drug therapy as a potential cause of new symptoms or signs.

Further reading

Ben-Chetri E, Levy M (1998). Familial Mediterranean fever. *Lancet* **351**, 659–64.

Berman A, *et al.* (1999). Human immunodeficiency virus infection associated arthritis; clinical characteristics. *Journal of Rheumatology* **26**, 1158–62.

Braun J, Sieper J (1999). Rheumatologic manifestations of gastrointestinal disorders. *Current Opinion in Rheumatology* **11**, 68–74.

Brower AC, Allman RM (1981). Pathogenesis of the neuropathic joint: neurotraumatic *vs.* neurovascular. *Radiology* **139**, 349–54.

Bywaters EG (1971). Still's disease in the adult. *Annals of Rheumatic Diseases,* **30**: 121–33.

Cush JJ, *et al.* (1987). Adult-onset Still's disease. Clinical course and outcome. *Arthritis and Rheumatism,* **30**: 186–94.

Cuthbert JA (1998). Wilson's disease. *Gastroenterology Clinics of North America* **27**, 655–81.

Ehrenfeld M, Gur H, Shoenfeld Y (1999). Rheumatologic features of haematologic disorders. *Current Opinion in Rheumatology* **11**, 62–7.

Hamdi N, Cvoke TD, Hassan B (1999). Ochronotic arthropathy: case report and review of the literature. *International Orthopaedics* **23**, 122–5.

Hermaszewski RA, Webster ADB (1993). Primary hypogammaglobulinaemia: a survey of clinical manifestations and complications. *Quarterly Journal of Medicine* **86**, 31–42.

Jones SM, Bhalla AK (1997). Algodystrophy. *Osteoporosis Review* **5**, 1–4.

Kaplan G, Haettich B (1991). Rheumatological symptoms due to retinoids. *Baillière's Clinical Rheumatology* **5**, 77–97.

King JB (1998). Post-traumatic ectopic calcification in the muscle of athletes: a review. *British Journal of Sports Medicine* **32**, 287–90.

Klemp P, *et al.* (1993). Musculoskeletal manifestations of hyperlipidaemia: a controlled study. *Annals of the Rheumatic Diseases* **52**, 44–8.

Kraus A, Alarcon-Segovia D (1991). Fever in adult onset Still's disease. Response to methotrexate. *Journal of Rheumatology,* **18**: 918–20.

Lear JT, Atherton MT, Byrne JP (1997). Neutrophilic dermatoses; pyoderma gangrenosum and Sweet's syndrome. *Postgraduate Medical Journal* **73**, 65–8.

Leclet H, Adamsbaum C (1998). Intraosseous cyst injection. *Radiology Clinics of North America* **36**, 581–7.

Mok CC, *et al.* (1998). Clinical characteristics, treatment, and outcome of adult onset Still's disease in southern Chinese. *Journal of Rheumatology*, **25**: 2345–51

Penrod BJ, Resnik CS (1997). Amyloid arthropathy. *Arthritis and Rheumatism* **40**, 1903–5.

Rodriguez-Merchan EC (1999). Common orthopaedic problems in haemophilia. *Haemophilia* **5**(Suppl. 1), 53–60.

Rydholm U (1998). Pigmented villonodular synovitis. *Acta Orthopaedica Scandinavica* **62**, 203–10.

Sibilia J, *et al.* (1999). Remitting seronegative symmetrical synovitis with pitting oedema (RS3PE): a form of paraneoplastic polyarthritis? *Journal of Rheumatology* **26**, 115–20.

Smith K, Fort JG (1998). Phalangeal osseous sarcoidosis. *Arthritis and Rheumatism* **41**, 176–9.

Smith P, Athanasou NA, Vipond SE (1996). Fibrodysplasia (myositis) ossificans progressiva; clinicopathological features and natural history. *Quarterly Journal of Medicine* **89**, 445–56.

Smythe M, Littlejohn G (1998). Diffuse idiopathic skeletal hyperostosis. In: Klippel JH, Dieppe PA, eds. *Rheumatology*, pp. 8.10.1–8.10.6. Mosby, London.

Trendelenberg M, Schifferli JA (1998). Cryoglobulins are not essential. *Annals of Rheumatic Diseases* **57**, 3–5.

Wong K, *et al.* (1999). Monoarticular synovial lesions; radiologic pictorial essay with pathological illustration. *Clinical Radiology* **54**, 273–84.

19

Diseases of the skeleton

19.1 Disorders of the skeleton

R. Smith

Introduction

Bone is the only tissue, apart from teeth, that is mineralized to allow it to perform its normal function. The presence of mineral should not encourage the belief that bone is inert or that it is metabolically inactive. Many disorders affect the skeleton but only some can be considered here. Fractures, infections, and tumours that are more often dealt with by orthopaedic surgeons, are excluded from this chapter. The descriptions that follow may be divided into:

(1) those disorders generally considered to be metabolic, such as osteoporosis, osteomalacia, Paget's disease of bone, and parathyroid bone disease;

(2) those arising primarily from synthetic defects in the major components of the organic bone matrix and connective tissue, including osteogenesis imperfecta, the skeletal dysplasias, and Marfan's syndrome;

(3) skeletal disorders that are clearly the result of enzyme defects, such as hypophosphatasia, homocystinuria, alkaptonuria, and the storage diseases;

(4) those that appear to be intrinsic disorders of bone cells, such as osteopetrosis, fibrous dysplasia, and inherited ectopic ossification; and

(5) various bone disorders that result from excessive minerals, vitamins, and metallic poisons.

To understand how these disorders arise and how to recognize them, a brief account of relevant aspects of bone physiology and clinical features is given here. More detail can be found in specialized texts (see Further reading list).

Physiology of bone

There is an increasing interest in the cells of bone, their control, activities, and communications, and in the non-collagen as well as the collagen components of the organic bone matrix. Advances in understanding of bone diseases such as osteoporosis, osteopetrosis, osteogenesis imperfecta, and Paget's disease reflect this. The causes of many rare skeletal disorders have been discovered (Table 1). Examples are Marfan's syndrome (mutations in the fibrillin gene); vitamin D-dependent rickets type II (mutations in the 1,25-dihydroxycholecalciferol receptor gene); pseudohypoparathyroidism and fibrous dysplasia (abnormalities in the G-protein signalling system); osteogenesis imperfecta (mutations in the type I collagen genes) and skeletal dysplasias (some with similar mutations in the type II collagen gene). Outstanding recent advances in bone physiology include the identification and elucidation of the functions of the parathyroid hormone-related peptide (**PTHrP**) and the bone morphogenetic proteins, known as **BMPs**. The discovery of the calcium-sensing receptor in the parathyroid and other tissues explains many rare disorders of mineral metabolism (Table 1). Further advances have been made in our understanding of the development of the osteoblast from the stromal-cell precursor and the ways in which the osteoblast controls osteoclast development and function (see below).

The mammalian skeleton serves two main functions, the demands of which often conflict. The first is to provide a rigid structure, the second is to act as an accessible mineral store. Both depend on the activities of specialized bone cells, controlled by genetic, mechanical, nutritional, and hormonal influences, and by a host of short-acting messengers produced by cells, collectively known as cytokines.

Structure

Bone tissue consists of cells and an extracellular mineralized matrix (35 per cent organic and 65 per cent inorganic). Some 90 per cent of the organic component is type I collagen. The remainder includes many non-collagen products of the osteoblast, such as osteocalcin, osteonectin, and proteoglycans. The mineral is present mainly as a complex mixture of calcium and phosphate in the form of hydroxyapatite.

Two anatomical types of bone may be defined, trabecular (cancellous) and cortical. The proportion of these differs from one bone to another; for example, vertebral bodies are predominantly trabecular, and the shafts of the long bones cortical. Such a distribution is related both to the functions of the bones and to the development of disorders of them, such as osteoporosis. Trabecular bone contains more metabolically active surfaces in a given volume than cortical bone. Cellular activities take place on the surfaces of trabecular bone and through resorbing channels (cutting cones) in cortical bone. The fine structure of bone is dealt with in anatomical texts.

Table 1 Molecular basis of some metabolic bone disorders

Disease	Cause
Osteoporosis	Suggestive linkage to many loci
Osteomalacia	Mutations in the *PHEX* gene Mutations in the 1α-hydroxylase gene Mutations in the $1,25(OH)_2D$-receptor gene
Paget's disease	Linkage to chromosome 18 (some families)
Parathyroid disorders	Mutations in *MEN1* Mutations in *Ret* oncogene Loss of function mutations of the G protein gene (pseudohypoparathyroidism) Mutations in the calcium-sensing receptor gene
Osteogenesis imperfecta	Mutations in type I collagen genes
Marfan syndrome	Mutations in the FBN1 gene
Achondroplasia	Mutation in the fibroblast growth-factor receptor-3 gene
Various skeletal dysplasias	See Table 12
Fibrodysplasia ossificans progressiva (FOP)	Overactivity in BMP4 (gene locus not established)

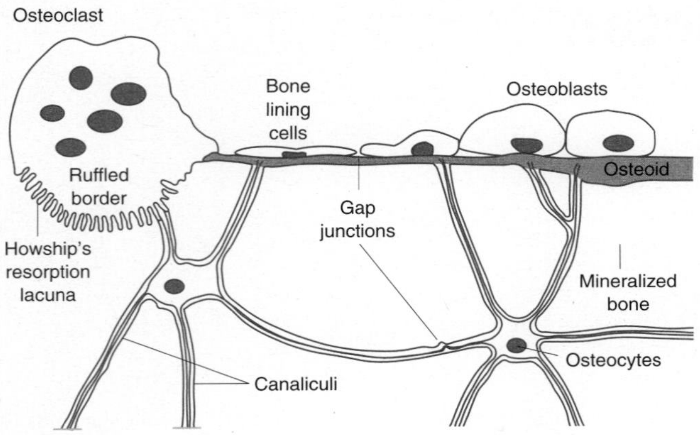

Fig. 1 A diagram showing the structure of bone and the relationship of the different cell types. (From the *Oxford textbook of rheumatology*, with permission.)

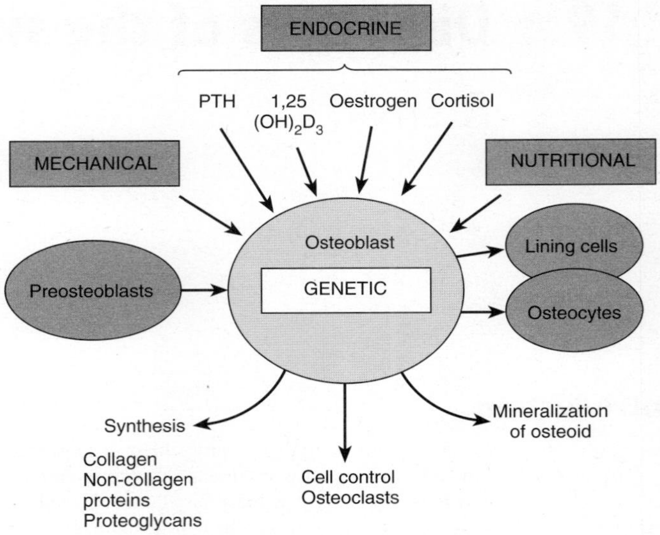

Fig. 2 To show the central position of the osteoblast in bone physiology. (From the *Oxford textbook of rheumatology*, with permission.)

Bone is often assumed to be inert because of its structural rigidity and persistence after death, and to be composed entirely of chalk because it contains 99 per cent of the body's calcium. These assumptions are superficially reasonable: neither is correct.

Bone cells

Conventional histological sections of bone demonstrate three types of bone cells which are clearly different (Fig. 1): osteoblasts, which may be plump and apparently active, or flat and apparently inactive—otherwise called bone-lining cells; multinuclear osteoclasts, which most often occupy areas of resorption; and osteocytes within their lacunae in the mineralized bone, apparently in contact with other osteocytes and bone cells through their extensions in the canaliculi. All these cells are in close contact with the bone marrow, which contains their precursors and brings them into close relationship with the immune system.

Bone cells are at the centre of an information system of astonishing complexity; and it is this complexity of bone that provides both the challenge and the fascination for those interested in its disorders. Histological techniques have been developed to study sequential cellular events in bone tissue; and the techniques of cell biology are used to study the origin and functions of different types of cells and the communications between them. All bone cells communicate with each other to control bone modelling during growth and remodelling throughout life. The constant processes of osteoclastic bone resorption and osteoblastic bone formation which achieve this are closely linked and take place in bone multicellular units (**BMUs**). The cellular cycle of such a unit begins with the activation of multinucleate osteoclasts from their macrophage-like mononuclear precursors, which produce resorption (Howship's) lacunae on the surface of trabecular bone, or cutting cones in cortical bone. These are identical processes; in cancellous (trabecular) bone the BMU may be looked upon as a sagittal section of a cortical BMU. Resorption is followed by a reversal phase, during which a cement line is deposited, and the formation by osteoblasts of new bone matrix which is subsequently mineralized. In the young adult, when the bone mass is constant and there may be several million resorbing sites in the skeleton at any one time, the amount of newly formed bone equals that resorbed. In childhood, more bone is formed than is resorbed; and in later years there is an imbalance between the two processes in favour of resorption, leading to osteoporosis.

The estimated time scale of the remodelling cycle is approximate. In the adult, the replacement of old bone with new occurs at an annual turnover rate of 25 per cent in cancellous bone, and 2 to 3 per cent in cortical bone. In the BMU resorption takes 1 to 2 weeks and new bone formation about 7 weeks. A complete BMU cycle, including reversal and mineralization, takes several months. The turnover of bone at a given site is determined by the frequency with which BMUs are activated and the rates of function of individual cells. Bone loss and gain depend on both factors; and the mechanism of bone loss is different in different disorders. Although the existence of the BMU system is widely accepted, it is far from understood. For instance, what factors lead to activation of the osteoclasts to initiate the resorbing cycle; how do cells talk to each other; and what links osteoblast and osteoclast activity?

It is clear that osteoblasts occupy a central position in bone physiology (Fig. 2). They are derived from the mesenchymal stromal-cell system within the bone marrow. This system is multipotential and the stromal cells can give rise to osteoblasts, fibroblasts, chondrocytes, myocytes, and adipocytes. Under the influence of the differentiation factor identified as CBFA-1 (core-binding factor-a1) the stromal cells develop into osteoblasts. Osteoblasts respond to hormonal factors, both systemic and local (cytokines), and to mechanical stress. They synthesize the organic bone matrix, mainly collagen, and non-collagen proteins, and they control bone mineralization. Importantly, they also appear to direct the activity of other cell types, particularly the osteoclasts. In this respect they may also activate the bone-resorbing cycle. The osteoclast differentiation factor (**ODF**) has now been identified as osteoprotegerin ligand (**OPGL**, also known as **RANKL** and **TRANCE**), a soluble product of the osteoblast, which together with other factors controls the formation and activity of osteoclasts. It is possible that these many functions are divided between different osteoblasts. The bone-lining cells—resting osteoblasts—may not be as inactive as they appear, since they may provide a cellular barrier separating the so-called bone fluid from the general extracellular compartment. The separate existence of bone fluid has yet to be established.

Osteocytes, also derived from osteoblasts, occupy lacunae within the mineralized bone, and communicate with each other through gap junctions via their processes within the canaliculi. They probably have an important function in the detection of mechanical forces and the resultant response of bone.

Osteoclasts have a different origin from osteoblasts, since the former are multinucleated cells derived from the haemopoietic system. The osteoclasts resorb bone by attaching themselves to its surface via integrins and forming a seal to isolate their area of activity. Within this sealed zone they produce a very acid environment, with the aid of a proton pump linked to the enzyme carbonic anhydrase II, to enable digestion of whole bone by lysosomal enzymes. The absence of carbonic anhydrase II is linked to a rare form of osteopetrosis (see below). Osteoclasts have receptors to calcitonin which, when occupied, directly suppress their activity; the existence of any other hormone receptors is controversial. However, they are activated by prostaglandins. The osteoclastic resorptive effects of parathyroid hormone and of 1,25-dihydroxycholecalciferol are probably mediated through the osteoblast.

Bone formation

The factors that control bone formation are complex and not fully understood, but must work largely through the osteoblast. The stromal precursors of osteoblasts are found in the periosteum and the endosteal surfaces close to the bone marrow. The local remodelling stimulus for new bone formation appears to come from some product, or products, of bone resorption, which could, for instance, be a group of polypeptide growth factors or morphogenic proteins liberated from resorbed bone. Such substances are included in the category of cytokines. A cytokine may be defined as 'a peptide produced by a cell which acts as an autocrine, paracrine, or endocrine mediator'. This definition includes a large number of substances with effects on the metabolism of bone and cartilage. Such effects have largely been shown in experimental (and artificial) situations and their physiological role is unknown. Many cytokines have alternative names and multiple actions, featuring both synergism and antagonism. They include interleukins (1 and 6), tumour necrosis factor, γ-interferon, platelet-derived growth factor, fibroblast growth factors, insulin-like growth factors, transforming growth factor-β, and bone morphogenic proteins.

Since bone cells contain, synthesize, and respond to many cytokines, they are part of a complex network. As an example, transforming growth factor-β (**TGF-β**) appears to belong to a family of multifunctional regulatory peptides, and bone is probably its most abundant source. Not only do osteoblasts synthesize TGF-β, but they also have high-affinity receptors for it, and are mitogenically stimulated by it. In addition, most of the bone morphogenic proteins belong to the TGF-β family.

Bone resorption

Osteoclasts are controlled by systemic and local hormones but there is no direct evidence that they are influenced by mechanical stress. Calcitonin directly inhibits the osteoclast, temporarily abolishes the active ruffled border, and suppresses the generation of new osteoclasts. Bone resorption is increased by parathyroid hormone and 1,25-dihydroxycholecalciferol. Since the osteoclast contains no receptors to either of these hormones it is proposed that their resorbing effect is mediated via the osteoblast. It is now realized that the interaction between osteoprotegerin (**OPG**) and its ligand (OPGL) is central to osteoblast/osteoclast interaction. The number and activity of the osteoclasts are also increased by a variety of cytokines produced by lymphocytes and monocytes (lymphokines and monokines, respectively), and by peptide growth factors such as epidermal growth factor. In myeloma the malignant plasma cells release interleukin-1 and -6 and tumour necrosis factor, all of which stimulate osteoclastic destruction of bone.

Bone mass (see also osteoporosis)

The development of the skeleton and its eventual size and density are influenced by important genetic factors modified by mechanical stress, nutrition, the systemic effects of endocrines, and by local factors produced by the bone cells themselves. These determine the balance between resorption and formation, and their relative contribution varies with age.

Recent work re-emphasizes the importance of the genetic contribution to bone mass. Apart from the difference in bone mass between races, this work has confirmed the hereditability of bone mass at all sites, which is greater in monozygotic than dizygotic twins. Clearly, mutations in the structural collagen genes will have a considerable effect on bone mass, as in osteogenesis imperfecta (see below). The contribution of vitamin D receptor-gene polymorphisms and genetic changes in the promoter region of type I collagen has been widely discussed (see osteoporosis).

The main function of the skeleton is mechanical and it has long been known that bone is laid down along its lines of stress. Although the way in which this occurs is obscure, experiments show that osteoblasts *in vitro* may respond to mechanical stress by an increase in levels of cyclic adenosine monophosphate (cAMP) and phosphonositol, partly mediated by prostaglandins. It also seems common sense that the size and density of the skeleton should be related to nutritional intake, particularly of calcium, protein, and energy. This has been difficult to prove, but recent co-twin studies in growing children have demonstrated a significantly greater density of bone (which may be temporary) in those taking calcium supplements, and that the starvation associated with anorexia nervosa reduces bone mineral content. This may also be due to oestrogen deficiency and emphasizes the important effect of reproductive hormones on the skeleton. The sex hormones, testosterone, and oestrogen, encourage new bone formation. It has recently been shown that oestrogen-deficient men have osteoporosis, and thus it is clear that the skeleton depends on a full complement of sex steroids for its integrity. Growth hormone is an important anabolic skeletal agent during the early years of life, partly through the local production of somatomedins (insulin-like growth factors). Several hormones that influence bone resorption may also have anabolic actions mediated by osteoblasts. One is parathyroid hormone, which under certain circumstances increases the proliferation of osteoblast precursors.

Collagen

Collagen is the principal extracellular protein in the body, more than half of which is contained within the skeleton, and is the main product of the osteoblast. There are many different molecular types, with different functions, each encoded by distinct genes (Table 2). Collagen in bone is type I. This heteropolymer is composed of two α-1 chains and one α-2 chain. The general structure of the α-1 chain is $(Gly–X–Y)_{338}$. The α-chains are synthesized as precursors within the osteoblasts and undergo a number of synthetic steps, including post-translational hydroxylation of proline and lysine residues; certain hydroxylysine residues are further modified into aldehydes and are also glycosylated (Fig. 3).

After removal of their extensions, the triple-helical molecules form an exact structure with a quarter-stagger overlap that is subsequently cross-linked. The so-called 'hole zones' within this structure provide a template for early mineralization. Mutations in the collagen genes and defects in post-translational modification cause inherited disorders of connective tissue, of which osteogenesis imperfecta (type I collagen) and type IV Ehlers–Danlos syndrome (type III collagen) are examples (Table 1). Renal excretion of hydroxyproline peptides is an indicator of bone collagen turnover, and excretion of pyridinium compounds is a measure of bone resorption (see below).

Non-collagen proteins

Many such proteins may be extracted from bone, although their abundance differs according to the starting material and the methods used. They include osteocalcin (Gla protein), sialoproteins, various phosphoproteins, such as osteonectin and osteopontin, the bone morphogenetic proteins, and bone-specific proteoglycans.

The nature of non-collagen substances sequestered in bone matrix is complex and most are synthesized by the osteoblasts. Few, if any, are unique to bone, since they can be expressed transiently in other tissues—to date, no unambiguous function has been determined for any of these proteins. Osteonectin is the most abundant non-collagen protein produced by human osteoblasts. It binds strongly to calcium ions, hydroxyapatite, and native collagen, but is not limited to mineralizing tissue, being also found in human platelets. Although osteonectin mRNA is widely distributed in developing tissues, osteonectin is most abundant in bone. Two bone sialoproteins (**BSP**) are now recognized (BSP1 and BSP2). Their relative abundance varies with the species studied: for instance, BSP1 is a minor component of human bone, but a major contributor to total sialoprotein in rat bone. The protein contains an **RGD** (Arg–Gly–Asp) cell-attachment

Table 2 The vertebrate collagens

Type	α-chains	Most common molecular form	Tissue distribution
I	α1(I), α2(I)	$[\alpha1(I)]_2\ \alpha2(I)$	Most connective tissues, e.g. bone, tendon, skin, lung, cornea, sclera, vascular system
II	α1(II)	$[\alpha1(II)]_3$	Cartilage, vitreous humour, embryonic cornea
III	α1(III)	$[\alpha1(III)]_3$	Extensible connective tissues, e.g. lung, vascular system
IV	α1(IV), α2(IV), α3(IV), α4(IV), α5(IV)	$[\alpha1(IV)]_2\ \alpha2(IV)$	Basement membranes
V	α1(V), α2(V), α3(V)	$[\alpha1(V)]_2\ \alpha2(V)$	Tissues containing collagen I, quantitatively minor component
VI	α1(VI), α2(VI), α3(VI)	α1(VI) α2(VI) α3(VI)	Most connective tissues, including cartilage
VII	α1(VII)	$[\alpha1(VII)]_3$	Basement-membrane-associated anchoring fibrils
VIII	α1(VIII), α2(VIII)	$[\alpha1(VIII)]_2\ \alpha2(VII)$?	Product of endothelial and various tumour cell lines
IX	α1(IX), α2(IX), α3(IX)	α1(IX) α2(IX) α3(IX)	Tissues containing collagen II, quantitatively minor component
X	α1(X)	$[\alpha1(X)]_3$	Hypertrophic zone of cartilage
XI	α1(XI), α2(XI), α3(XI)[a]	α1(XI) α2(XI) α3(XI)	Tissues containing collagen III, quantitatively minor component
XII	α1(XII)	$[\alpha1(XII)]_3$	Tissues containing collagen I, quantitatively minor component
XIII	α1(XIII)	$[\alpha1(XIII)]_3$?	Quantitatively minor collagen, found, e.g., in skin, intestine
XIV	α1(XIV)	$[\alpha1(XIV)]_3$?	Tissues containing collagen I, quantitatively minor component

[a] Closely related to α1(II).

Reproduced from Smith R (1998). Bone in health and disease. In: Maddison PJ, *et al.*, eds. *Oxford textbook of rheumatology*, 2nd edn, pp 421–40. Oxford University Press, Oxford.

sequence and is therefore called osteopontin. The major human sialoprotein is BSP2.

There are two bone Gla-containing proteins: osteocalcin—bone Gla protein (**BGP**)—and matrix Gla protein (**MGP**). The term Gla refers to the γ-carboxylated glutamic acid residues, formed by the vitamin K-modulated, post-translational carboxylation of peptide-bound glutamic acid. These proteins have some sequence homology but are products of different genes. MGP is also a cartilage protein and is found at an earlier developmental stage than BGP. The function of BGP is unknown. BGP biosynthesis is regulated by 1,25-dihydroxycholecalciferol ($1,25(OH)_2D_3$) (and no other hormone), which enhances its nuclear transcription and eventual secretion from bone cells. Plasma BGP has been linked to the rate of bone formation or, less specifically, bone turnover.

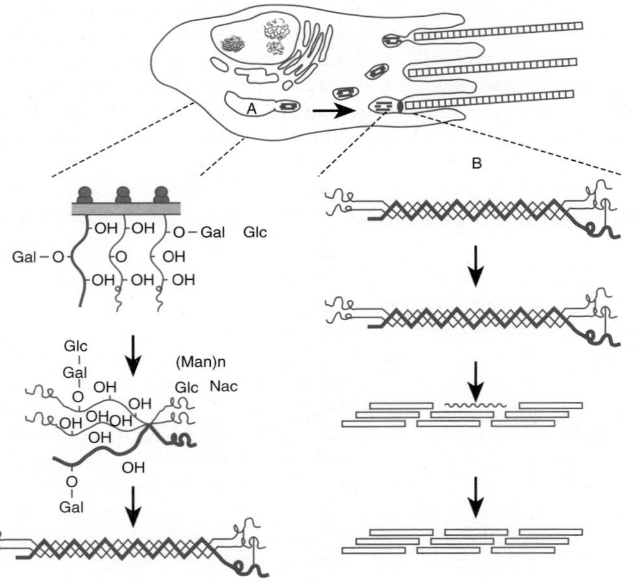

Fig. 3 The synthesis and assembly of collagen molecules. Within the fibroblast (A) the individual pro-α-chains are modified, assembled, and folded into the triple helix. In (B) these chains are exported, shortened, and self-assemble. (From the *Oxford textbook of Rheumatology*, with permission.)

Proteoglycans are proteins with one or more attached glycosaminoglycan chains. They vary widely in form and function. Those of bone, which include decorin and biglycan, have been studied less extensively than those of cartilage, and differ from them in their small overall size and relatively larger amounts of protein. Such small proteoglycans are thought to interact with growing collagen fibrils in a precise manner and to regulate their growth, maturation, and interactions. Type IX collagen, closely associated with type II collagen, bridges the gap between the collagens and proteoglycans since it contains a chondroitin sulphate glycosaminoglycan chain.

It has been known for many years that demineralized bone matrix contains substances capable of inducing ectopic bone formation. Because they are present in such small amounts their extraction and isolation have presented great difficulties, but these bone morphogenic proteins have now been isolated and their genes localized and cloned. Interestingly, most belong to the TGF-β supergene family. Some evidence suggests their overexpression in fibrodysplasia ossificans progressiva (**FOP**).

Bone mineral and mineralization

Mineralization occurs on bone matrix collagen. The way in which it occurs has been long debated, but there is now good evidence that, in most mineralized tissues, calcifying vesicles derived from chondrocytes or osteoblasts provide a focus for mineralization. These vesicles are easily demonstrable in cartilage, but their function in the organized matrix of bone is controversial. The precipitation of calcium within these vesicles may be controlled by the action of a pyrophosphatase that locally destroys pyrophosphate, itself an inhibitor of mineralization. Alkaline phosphatase is one such pyrophosphatase which is readily demonstrable both in osteoblasts and in mineralizing vesicles. It is possible, for the purpose of clarity, to consider two types of mineralization: namely (1) homogeneous nucleation, which occurs in the lumen of the matrix vesicles, from amorphous calcium phosphate to form crystalline hydroxyapatite; and (2) heterogeneous nucleation, which is collagen-mediated and may partly rely on adsorbed non-collagen proteins as nucleators. After this first phase (mediated either by vesicles or collagen) there is a second phase of rapid spread of mineralization initially in the hole zones and later the overlap regions of the collagen matrix.

Calcium and phosphorus balance (see also Section 12)

Much has been written about calcium balance and the main hormones that control it. Phosphate balance is less well understood. The circulating level of plasma calcium is determined by the amount of calcium that is absorbed by the intestine, the amount that is excreted by the kidney, and the exchange of mineral with the skeleton. The relative importance of these exchanges differs during growth and in different disorders. Total plasma calcium concentration is closely maintained between 2.25 and 2.60 mmol/l, of which nearly half is in the ionized form (47 per cent ionized, 46 per cent protein bound, and the remainder complexed). The skeleton contains approximately 1 kg (25 000 mmol) of calcium. The main fluxes of calcium in the young adult are shown in Fig. 4.

Parathyroid hormone (see also Chapter 12.6)

The gene for parathyroid hormone (PTH) is on chromosome 11. PTH is synthesized as a large precursor, in the way of proteins packaged for export, and its secretion is stimulated by a reduction in the plasma ionized-calcium concentration. Changes in plasma calcium are detected by a sensitive calcium-sensing receptor. Mutations in the gene for this receptor can cause hypocalcaemic and hypercalcaemic syndromes (Table 1). Increase in PTH secretion leads to an increase in calcium absorption through the gut, an increase in calcium reabsorption through the kidney, and an increase in bone resorption. Intestinal calcium absorption is mediated by 1,25-dihydroxycholecalciferol, and the 1α-hydroxylation of 25-hydroxycholecalciferol is stimulated by parathyroid hormone, so that the effect of parathyroid hormone in increasing intestinal calcium absorption is indirect. In contrast, the renal effect of parathyroid hormone on calcium reabsorption is direct. The cellular effects of parathyroid hormone on kidney and bone appear to involve two cellular systems, namely cAMP and phosphoinositol. Parathyroid hormone encourages osteoclastic bone resorption by its effects on the osteoblast (as previously described). Peripheral resistance to the effect of PTH due to inherited loss-of-function mutations in the G-protein signalling system occurs in pseudohypoparathyroidism (see below and Chapter 12.6).

Vitamin D

Vitamin D is synthesized either as vitamin D_3 (cholecalciferol) within the skin from its precursor 7-dehydrocholesterol under the influence of ultraviolet light (usually as sunlight), or taken in with food, either as vitamin D_3

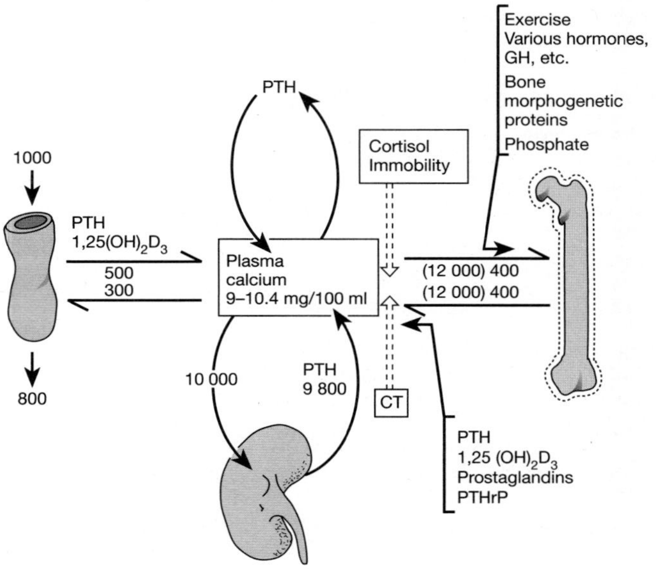

Fig. 4 Factors that control calcium balance. Units are in mg/day (to convert to mmol divide by 40) and refer to an adult. The figures in parentheses are an estimate of exchange through the cellular barrier of bone. CT, calcitonin; GH, growth hormone; PTH, parathyroid hormone; PTHrP, parathyroid hormone-related peptide. (From *Oxford textbook of rheumatology*, with permission.)

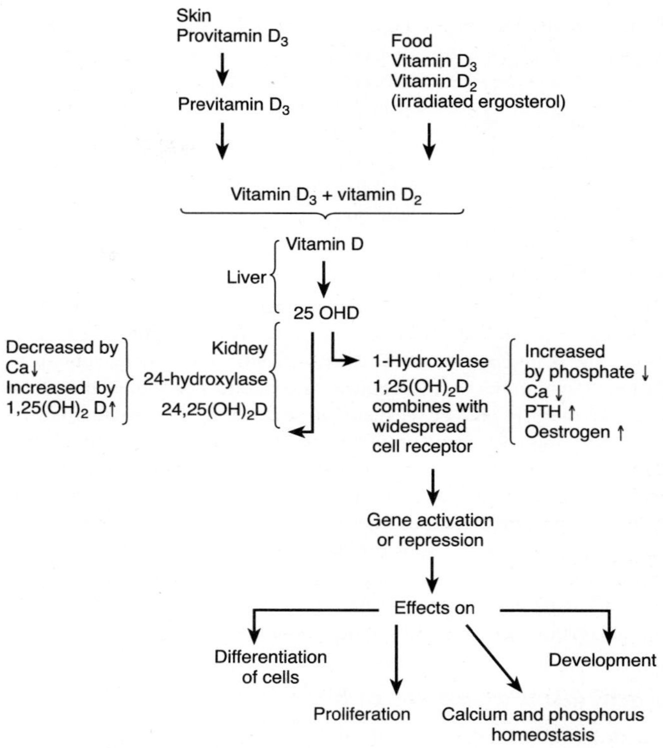

Fig. 5 The synthetic pathways and molecular and cellular effects of $1,25(OH)_2D$. (From *Oxford textbook of rheumatology*, with permission.)

or D_2 (ergocalciferol) (Fig. 5). It is transported to the liver by a binding protein where it undergoes 25-hydroxylation. 25-hydroxy-vitamin D is then hydroxylated in the 1α-position by the renal 1α-hydroxylase. $1,25(OH)_2D$ is the active metabolite of vitamin D and has widespread effects, the extent of which is only just being appreciated. These are mediated through a widely distributed vitamin D receptor which has DNA- and hormone-binding components. In addition to its classic effect on intestinal calcium transport, vitamin D is linked with the immune system and the growth and differentiation of a wide variety of cells. Measurement of the plasma 25-hydroxy-vitamin D concentration has proved to be a useful indicator of vitamin D status, and work on $1,25(OH)_2D$ and its receptors has illuminated the cause of the rarer forms of inherited rickets (see below). The kidney is the main source of $1,25(OH)_2D$ but it is now clear that this metabolite can be synthesized by macrophages in a variety of granulomas, providing an explanation for the hypercalcaemia of sarcoidosis, disseminated tuberculosis, and (occasionally) lymphomas.

Calcitonin

The main effect of administered calcitonin is to reduce bone resorption by the direct and reversible suppression of osteoclasts and by inhibition of their production from precursors. The role of calcitonin is uncertain, although it is thought to protect the skeleton during physiological stresses such as growth and pregnancy. It is produced by alternative splicing of the primary gene transcript also responsible for the production of calcitonin gene-related peptide. Recent work has shown that its receptor is widely distributed.

Parathyroid hormone-related protein (PTHrP)

This hormone was discovered through studies on patients with non-metastatic hypercalcaemia of malignancy. PTHrP has close sequence homology to PTH at the amino-terminal end of the molecule and has very similar effects. Its gene is located on the short arm of chromosome 12, and is thought to have arisen by a duplication of chromosome 11, which carries the human *PTH* gene. It has been detected in a number of tumours, particularly of the lung. There is also evidence that it may have a role in fetal physiology, controlling the calcium gradient across the placenta to maintain the relatively higher concentrations in the fetal circulation. PTH and PTHrP have the same receptor. Mutations of this receptor can cause Jansen's metaphyseal dysplasia and it has become clear that PTHrP is involved in early development of the skeleton.

Other hormones

Apart from the recognized calciotrophic hormones, the skeleton is influenced by corticosteroids, the sex hormones, thyroxine, and growth hormone. The main effect of excess corticosteroids (either therapeutic or in Cushing's syndrome) is to suppress osteoblastic new bone formation, although there is also an element of secondary hyperparathyroidism. Androgens and oestrogens promote and maintain skeletal mass. Osteoblasts have receptors for oestrogens, although they are not abundant. Thyroxine increases bone turnover and increases resorption in excess of formation; thyrotoxicosis thus leads to bone loss. Excess growth hormone leads to gigantism and acromegaly (according to the age of onset) with enlargement of the bones. Absence of growth hormone will lead to proportional short stature; where there is general pituitary failure the reduction in gonadotrophins will also induce bone loss.

Biochemical measures of bone turnover

Knowledge of bone physiology allows one to interpret biochemical measures of bone turnover. These include plasma bone-derived alkaline phosphatase and osteocalcin (BGP), and the urinary total hydroxyproline and crosslinked collagen-derived peptides. The first two are produced by osteoblasts and indicate bone formation, the second two, bone resorption. Since formation and resorption are closely coupled, such measurements are usually closely related to each other and to overall bone turnover.

Total plasma alkaline phosphatase (largely derived from osteoblasts) provides a crude but readily accessible index of bone formation, being increased during periods of rapid growth and particularly when bone turnover is greatly increased, as in Paget's disease. Early measurements of serum BGP gave widely variable results and depended on the origin, sensitivity, and stability of the antibodies used. Total urinary hydroxyproline excretion is influenced by dietary collagen (gelatin) and reflects both resorption and new collagen synthesis. The recent development of methods for the measurement of urinary collagen-derived pyridinium crosslinks promises to give a reliable indication of bone resorption rate, unrelated to new collagen formation, and uninfluenced by diet. There are two forms of crosslinked peptide—pyridinoline and deoxypyridinoline, depending on whether they originate from oxidized hydroxylysine or lysine residues. Early assays were dependent on high-pressure liquid chromatography (**HPLC**) of urinary peptides after hydrolysis with acid. Simple and more direct immunoassays have now been developed.

Correct interpretation of collagen-derived fragments depends on knowledge of collagen's metabolic pathway (Fig. 3). Soon after export from the cell, the amino- and carboxy-propeptide extensions are cleaved from the mainly helical central part of the collagen chain. Measurement of these fragments in the plasma indicates the collagen formation rate. Once the collagen chains are crosslinked, measurement of different crosslinked fragments in the urine indicate (mainly bone) collagen resorption.

The diagnosis of bone disease

The diagnosis of bone disorders increasingly depends on investigation, with the result that important clinical points tend to be forgotten.

History

Deformity, pain, and fracture are common features. To these may be added proximal myopathy (in osteomalacia and rickets) and the symptoms of any underlying disease. The family history is always relevant.

Deformity

Deformity suggests previous skeletal disorder, especially if there is a disturbance of growth. Short stature and disproportion are more frequent than excessive height. In children, a knowledge of growth is essential; in the normal adult, height and span are approximately equal and the crown to pubis measurement is equal to the pubis to heel. Those with short stature can be divided into proportionate and disproportionate, of which the most frequent cause is short limbs. Proportionate short stature may occur in children who appear to be otherwise normal, whereas subjects with disproportionate short stature usually appear abnormal from birth. Some causes of short stature are given in Table 3. Skeletal chondrodysplasias are dealt with further below.

Kyphosis, with loss of trunk height, as in osteoporosis and osteomalacia, is the commonest acquired deformity of adult life. It is often noticed because clothes no longer fit. During childhood vertebral collapse will slow the growth rate. Other deformities are characteristic of the underlying disease; for instance, active childhood rickets produces knock knees, bowed legs, enlarged epiphyses, and bossing of the skull; Paget's disease produces thick limb bones and an enlarged skull vault; and severe osteogenesis imperfecta, very short limbs.

Bone pain and fracture

The cause of bone pain is not well understood. In osteomalacia it may be generalized and associated with tenderness on pressure. It may be due to excessive vascularity, with stretching of the periosteum; certainly it can be rapidly relieved by appropriate treatment, such as calcitonin for Paget's disease, or parathyroidectomy for parathyroid bone disease. Fractures of different sorts occur, examples being: the partial, multiple, and painful microfractures ('fissure' fractures) on the convexity of pagetic bone; the Looser's zones on medial borders of osteomalacic bones; and the multiple vertebral compression fractures of osteoporosis.

Table 3 Some examples of short stature

Proportionate	
Genetic	Familial
Endocrine	Growth-hormone lack
	Hypothyroidism
Metabolic	Lysosomal storage diseases
	Renal glomerular failure
	Cystic fibrosis
Nutritional	Coeliac disease
	Starvation
Chronic disease	Cyanotic heart disease
Intrauterine	Low birth weight dwarfism
Chromosomal	Turner's syndrome
Social	Emotional deprivation
Disproportionate[a]	
Short limbs:	
lethal	Type II osteogenesis imperfecta
	Thanatophoric dwarfism
	Achondrogenesis
non-lethal	Achondroplasia
	Inherited hypophosphataemia
	Metaphyseal dysplasias
Short spine	Spondyloepiphyseal dysplasia

[a] For further details see under Skeletal dysplasias and Osteogenesis imperfecta.

Myopathy

The cause of the proximal muscle weakness in osteomalacia and rickets remains unknown. The symptoms include a waddling gait, and inability to rise from a chair, to lift objects off high shelves, or to climb stairs. Limbs may be described as stiff rather than weak. Myopathy does not occur in subjects with inherited hypophosphataemia.

Underlying disease

It is necessary to be alert for the symptoms of the underlying disease, such as renal failure, steatorrhoea, or myeloma, and to enquire particularly about previous abdominal operations, including hysterectomy and oophorectomy.

Physical signs

It is important to see the patient out of bed so that an abnormal gait or stature is not missed. The appearance may give vital clues; for instance, the large vault of Paget's disease; the coarse features, large nose, big lower jaw, and widely spaced teeth of acromegaly; and the round face, simplicity, and cataracts of pseudohypoparathyroidism. Endocrine disorders affecting the skeleton, such as hypogonadism and hypopituitarism, are readily recognizable. Special facial features should receive attention; these include the eyes for such signs as corneal calcification, arcus juvenilis, and lens dislocation shown by the shimmering of the unsupported iris, iridodinesis. Further examples are corneal clouding (some mucopolysaccharidoses) and cystine crystals (cystinosis). In dentinogenesis imperfecta, often found with osteogenesis imperfecta, the teeth are abnormal in shape, tend to be transparent, and vary in colour from yellow to grey. Enamel defects occur in hypoparathyroidism, teeth are lost early in hypophosphatasia; and dental abscesses are common in hypophosphataemic rickets.

Hands and feet need particular attention. The fingers may be abnormally long and thin, as in Marfan's syndrome, or excessively short and mobile, as in pseudoachondroplasia; alternatively, they may be short, wide, and stiff in some mucopolysaccharidoses; or the hands may have short metacarpals, as in pseudohypoparathyroidism, or additional digits, as in the Ellis–van Creveld syndrome. The monophalangic big toe (and less often short thumbs) is characteristic of fibrodysplasia ossificans progressiva. Abnormal body proportions are common; the spine is relatively short after vertebral collapse. Scoliosis often dates from adolescence; occasionally it may be a clue to an inherited connective tissue disorder. A thoracolumbar gibbus is a particular (though not exclusive) feature of the mucopolysaccharidoses. Spinal deformity produces secondary changes; thus a young patient with severe osteoporosis will develop a prominent sternum with ribs that touch the iliac crest and a transverse crease across the front of the abdomen. Spontaneous tetany is a rare symptom, but there are two recognized bedside tests for latent tetany; of these Chvostek's sign is more convenient, but that of Trousseau more reliable. The first involves tapping the branches of the facial nerves as they spread out from within the parotid gland; a positive sign is twitching of the appropriate facial muscle. In the second the forearm is made ischaemic with a sphygmomanometer cuff for up to 3 min; if positive, carpal spasm will occur.

Investigations

Biochemistry

Many generalized disorders of the skeleton, such as postmenopausal osteoporosis, achondroplasia, osteogenesis imperfecta, and the epiphyseal dysplasias, have normal routine biochemical values; in others changes are diagnostic (Table 3). In normal persons the fasting plasma calcium concentration remains virtually constant through life, the plasma phosphate declines in adolescence to adult values and the plasma alkaline phosphatase level increases temporarily during rapid adolescent growth. Since total plasma calcium includes a protein-bound fraction, it is usual to relate it to the plasma albumin level and, if necessary, correct it to a plasma albumin of 4 g per 100 ml. Acceptable corrections include: corrected calcium (mg per 100 ml) = measured calcium – albumin (g per 100 ml) + 4; or for SI units: 0.02 mmol/l for every 1 g/l change of albumin from 40 g/l. The fasting plasma calcium is normal in osteoporosis and also in Paget's disease unless the patient is immobilized. It is increased in primary hyperparathyroidism, various neoplasms (including humoral hypercalcaemia of malignancy), in sarcoidosis, in vitamin-D overdosage, and in a number of other states, such as acromegaly and thyrotoxicosis (Table 4). It is often low in osteomalacia, but may be restored towards normal by secondary hyperparathyroidism, and is low in parathyroid insufficiency. Normal values are to be expected in inherited hypophosphataemia and in other forms of renal tubular rickets.

Since the main determinant of the fasting plasma phosphate concentration is its renal tubular reabsorption, hypophosphataemia occurs in primary hyperparathyroidism, in the humoral hypercalcaemia of malignancy, and it is also low in inherited hypophosphataemic rickets. Both oral aluminium hydroxide and prolonged intravenous nutrition also lower plasma phosphate levels. Hyperphosphataemia occurs in hypoparathyroidism, in renal glomerular failure, and in the rare, recessively inherited form of tumoral calcinosis.

Total plasma alkaline phosphatase and bone-derived alkaline phosphatase is normally increased in adolescence and in osteomalacia, particularly in the young, but it may be near-normal in renal tubular osteomalacia. Increases occur in primary hyperparathyroidism, but only where there is demonstrable bone disease. The highest values for plasma alkaline phosphatase are found in young patients with active Paget's disease, and in idiopathic hyperphosphatasia; and the lowest in hypophosphatasia.

Other plasma measurements, which have application in particular circumstances and in research, include: tartrate-resistant acid phosphatase (**TRAP**), a product of the osteoclast and therefore an indication of bone resorption; osteocalcin (bone Gla protein), a product of the osteoblast and therefore sometimes useful as an indicator of bone formation; and the N- and C-propeptide extensions of collagen, again an indicator of bone formation rate.

Glucose in the urine of a patient with inherited rickets suggests multiple renal tubular defects, and proteinuria is an important clue to myelomatosis.

The amount of calcium excreted in the urine is related both to the plasma levels and to the percentage of the filtered load reabsorbed through the renal tubules, itself altered by parathyroid hormone. Hypocalcaemia therefore causes hypocalciuria, particularly in osteomalacia and rickets; and hypercalcaemia leads to hypercalciuria, especially when this is due to rapid bone loss as in neoplastic disease of the skeleton, leukaemia, myeloma, and immobilization. Since parathyroid hormone increases the renal tubular reabsorption of calcium, the normal relationship between plasma and urine calcium is disturbed in parathyroid disease; however, most hypercalcaemic hyperparathyroid patients excrete more calcium than normal. Total hydroxyproline in the urine (after acid hydrolysis of the peptides) is a good indicator of bone breakdown and collagen turnover, provided the patient is ingesting a low-gelatin diet. The physiological changes in hydroxyproline excretion are striking, with a particularly sharp peak in adolescence coinciding with the maximum height velocity. The highest values are seen in active Paget's disease, where the excretion may be up to 50-fold the normal value. Hydroxyproline excretion correlates well with plasma alkaline phosphatase, and is therefore increased in some forms of osteomalacia and in hyperparathyroidism with bone disease. Since thyroxine increases collagen turnover, urinary hydroxyproline is also abnormally high in thyrotoxicosis and abnormally low in myxoedema (either primary or secondary).

Hydroxyproline excretion can be most usefully expressed as the amount in a 24-h urine sample in a patient on a gelatin-free diet, or in a fasting urine sample in relation to creatinine. However, hydroxyproline peptide excretion is related both to newly formed and mature collagen, and is not, therefore, a direct measure of bone resorption. The urinary excretion of pyridinium compounds (see above) from the lysyl- and hydroxylysyl-

Table 4 Biochemical and other features in disorders of the skeleton

Disorder	Commonest symptoms	Plasma			Urine		Other biochemical features	Comments
		Ca	P	Alkaline phosphatase	Ca	THP[a]		
Osteoporosis	Fracture	N	N	N	N	N	None	Hypercalcuria if immobilized
Osteomalacia (and rickets)	Bone pain; proximal weakness	N or L	L	N or H	L	N or H	Depends on cause	Plasma P increased in renal glomerular failure
Paget's disease	Pain; deformity	N	N	H	N	H	None	Hypercalcaemia if immobilized
Hyperparathyroidism (with bone disease)	Bone pain; hypercalcaemic symptoms	H	L	H	H	H	Aminoaciduria	Phosphatase and THP normal if clinical bone disease absent
Pseudohypo-parathyroidism	Simple; short metacarpals; cataracts	L	H	N	N	N	None	Mutation in G-protein gene
Osteogenesis imperfecta	Brittle bones	N	N	N	N	N		Many collagen gene mutations
Marfan's syndrome	Tall with scoliosis; dislocated lenses; aortic dissection	N	N	N	N	±H	None	Dominant inheritance; clinically heterogeneous
Homocystinuria	Mentally subnormal; look like Marfan's syndrome	N	N	N	N	N	Homocystine in urine	
Alkaptonuria	Back pain; early arthritis; dark urine	N	N	N	N	N	Homogentisic acid in the urine	Calcified intervertebral discs
Mucopolysaccharidoses	Short stature; thoracolumbar gibbus; mentally subnormal (depends on type)	N	N	N	N	N	Characteristic mucopoly-saccharide in urine	See text
Osteopetrosis (marble bones disease)	Anaemia; blindness, deafness (severe form)	±H	N	N	Low	N	Increase in acid phosphatase in some	Mild form fractures only; rarely carbonic anhydrase lack
Hypophosphatasia	Lethal short-limbed dwarfism; bone disease like rickets	N	N	Low	N	N	Phospho-ethanolamine in urine increased	Fractures in adult
Hyperphosphatasia	Large head, bowing of long bones; occurs in childhood	N	N	Very high	N	Very high	None	Similar to Paget's disease
Fibrous dysplasia	Fracture; sexual precocity in girls; pigmentation	N	N	Slight increase	N	Slight increase	Biochemical changes in polyostotic form only	Mutation in G-protein; occasional hypophosphataemic osteomalacia
Fibrodysplasia (myositis) ossificans progressiva	Pain and swelling in muscles; fixation of joints	N	N	? Increased during myositis	N	N	None	Monophalangic big toe

[a] THP, total hydroxyproline. The same changes occur in pyridinium crosslink collagen-derived peptides. N, normal; L, low; H, high. For changes in other biochemical markers see larger texts (Avioli and Krone 1998).

derived crosslinks of mature collagen is a direct measure of bone resorption, irrespective of dietary collagen.

Radiology

The diagnosis of bone disease often depends on the radiographic appearances, especially where there are no demonstrable biochemical changes. A particular example is in the differential diagnosis of perinatal lethal dwarfism. Conventional radiographs demonstrate well structural changes such as fractures, deformity, areas of resorption, and alteration in size, but are unreliable for the assessment of bone density. As radiographic techniques develop, increasing use is made of isotope bone scans, computed tomographic (**CT**), and magnetic resonance imaging (**MRI**) scans. Bisphosphonate-labelled scanning agents are selectively taken up in areas of increased vascularity or turnover. They are very useful in demonstrating the skeletal extent of Paget's disease of bone, the presence of bony metastases, the pathological fractures of osteoporosis, and Looser's zones in osteomalacia. An isotope scan is preferable to multiple radiographs to assess the distribution (but not the structure) of abnormal bone.

CT scanning can also be very useful in bone disease. Examples include the delineation of ectopic ossification, of spinal cord compression, and of bone tumours. Although magnetic resonance scanning (MRI) finds its most important application in soft-tissue pathology, it is also useful in giving an idea of the composition as well as the structure of bone.

Methods for measuring bone mass are considered under osteoporosis (see below).

Bone biopsy

Direct examination of bone is a valuable but under-used investigation. Bone can be taken by a transiliac trephine (using a local anaesthetic) and sections should be examined with and without decalcification. Ideally the bone should be labelled with tetracycline to allow an estimate of formation rates. In the various metabolic bone diseases the appearances are characteristic, with the: excess osteoid of osteomalacia; the disorganized mosaic pattern, excessive cellular activity, and fibrosis of Paget's disease; and osteitis fibrosa cystica in hyperparathyroid bone disease. In mild osteogenesis imperfecta there is typically an increase in the number of osteocytes, and, in the more severe form, a considerable increase in the amount of woven bone. A normal biopsy will exclude these diseases except where the pathological changes are patchy. Where possible, histological examination should now include transmission and scanning electron microscopy, and the report should include quantitative histomorphometry. More details are given in larger texts (see the Further reading list).

Further investigations

Measurement of the external calcium and phosphorus balance is a classic way of investigating generalized bone disease and the effects of treatment upon it, but it is also tedious. The use of isotopes to measure calcium absorption and apparent bone formation and resorption rates is less direct and also depends on a number of assumptions. This leaves a large number of measurements available for specific problems. Important examples (in the plasma) are intact PTH assays (to investigate hyper- and hypocalcaemia), PTHrP (mainly in research), 25-hydroxy-vitamin D, and 1,25-dihydroxy-vitamin D (for the investigation of rickets and osteomalacia). In inherited disorders, analysis of DNA extracted from whole blood and of collagen synthesized from fibroblast cultures derived from skin samples are used increasingly.

Diagnosis

The diagnosis of a skeletal disorder is not difficult where there are clear biochemical disturbances (Table 4), although, as in osteomalacia, the causes may be many. An exact diagnosis may be impossible when the standard biochemical results are normal, and this is particularly so in some of the rare heritable disorders. Guidance based on the age of the patient and frequency of the disorder is given in Table 5.

Osteomalacia and rickets

Osteomalacia results from a lack of vitamin D or a disturbance of its metabolism; in the growing skeleton it is referred to as rickets, and the terms are often used interchangeably. Very rarely, severe calcium deficiency can lead to rickets. Inherited hypophosphataemia and several other renal tubular disorders may also cause rickets without clear evidence of abnormal vitamin D metabolism. The causal mutations in inherited hypophosphataemia have now been identified.

The main histological feature of osteomalacia is defective mineralization of bone matrix (Fig. 6). Our present understanding of osteomalacia relies on advances in knowledge of vitamin D metabolism (Fig. 7). For clinical purposes two aspects of the physiology of vitamin D require emphasis. The first is the quantitative importance of vitamin D synthesis in the skin in comparison with that in the diet, and the second concerns the relative role of different vitamin D metabolites. The measurement of circulating concentrations of 25-hydroxy-vitamin D (**25(OH)D**) as an index of vitamin D status has identified those groups (Asian immigrants and the elderly) most at risk from vitamin D deficiency; importantly it has also shown the large amounts of vitamin D that can be synthesized in the human skin when exposed to ultraviolet light. The causes of osteomalacia can now be partly understood in terms of its metabolites, and the major importance of **1,25(OH)2D** (1,25-dihydroxy-vitamin D) is established. The effects of giving vitamin D can probably not be ascribed to the actions of $1,25(OH)_2D$ alone, and probably include other biologically active derivatives such as 25(OH)D and possibly 24,25-dihydroxy-vitamin D (**24,25(OH)2D**).

Pathophysiology

The features of osteomalacia can be predicted largely from the known calciotropic effects of vitamin D. Examination of undecalcified bone shows wide osteoid seams with many birefringent lamellae of collagen (Fig. 6) covering more of the bone surface than normal, and absence of the 'calcification front'. The absence of this front is important since excessive osteoid may also be found in conditions other than osteomalacia, such as hypophosphatasia, Paget's disease of bone, and thyrotoxicosis, where the calcification front is normal; in these disorders the increase tends to be in the amount of bone surface covered rather than in the thickness of osteoid. Excess osteoid also occurs when bisphosphonates, such as etidronate, or aluminium accumulate in the skeleton. In rickets the main change is disorganization of the growth plate.

Since there is intestinal malabsorption of calcium in vitamin D deficiency, both the plasma and urine calcium levels are lower than normal; absorption of phosphorus is also defective, with resultant hypophosphataemia. As hypocalcaemia stimulates the secretion of parathyroid hormone, this will correct the low plasma calcium level and exaggerate hypophosphataemia. In osteomalacia, osteoblastic activity is increased and the plasma alkaline phosphatase is therefore also increased. There appears to be no difficulty in laying down bone matrix collagen, but it cannot be properly mineralized. One should recall that the effects of vitamin D are not confined to the skeleton, although they are clinically most obvious in this tissue—thus vitamin D has important effects on cellular differentiation and on the immune system.

Causes

There are many causes of osteomalacia (and rickets), some of which are very rare. They may conveniently be divided into three main groups: nutritional, malabsorptive, and renal (Table 6). Most can be understood in terms of vitamin D metabolism (see Fig. 7). In the elderly and immigrant populations the food intake of vitamin D is often deficient and the requirements may be increased; the absorption of vitamin D is poor in coeliac disease, after partial gastrectomy, intestinal resection or bypass, and in biliary disease. The intestinal absorption of calcium is reduced by phytate and chapatti ingestion, which may also increase vitamin D requirements (see below). Endogenous synthesis of vitamin D in the skin is reduced, especially in towns and city communities in the Northern hemisphere; it is further reduced by skin pigmentation. The 25-hydroxylation of calciferol may be impaired in some chronic liver diseases, and anticonvulsants may induce hepatic enzymes which degrade vitamin D. The 1α-hydroxylation of 25(OH)D is reduced or absent in renal failure, after nephrectomy, in hyperphosphataemia, parathyroid insufficiency, in type-I vitamin D-dependent rickets, and probably in some bone tumours. Many patients have more than one cause for their osteomalacia; in the elderly person vitamin D intake is poor, exposure to sunlight is limited, and renal glomerular failure progressive. Reduced exposure to sunlight is a frequent consequence of physical immobility and may contribute to osteomalacia in rheumatoid arthritis and other chronic diseases.

The effects of renal glomerular failure on the skeleton are complex (Chapter 20.8). Two main events occur: one is an increase in the plasma phosphate level, which leads to a fall in plasma calcium and to secondary hyperparathyroidism with excessive bone resorption; the other is the reduced formation of 1,25$(OH)_2D$, with defective intestinal absorption of calcium and defective bone mineralization. The combination of these events rapidly produces severe deformity, especially in the growing skeleton. In patients receiving dialysis, renal osteodystrophy may be complicated by aluminium intoxication.

Clinical features

The main symptoms of osteomalacia are bone pain and tenderness, skeletal deformity, and proximal muscle weakness, often accompanied by the features of the underlying disorder and by those of hypocalcaemia. In severe osteomalacia all the bones are painful and tender, sometimes sufficiently so to disturb sleep. The tenderness can be particularly marked in the lower ribs and may also be accentuated over Looser's zones. Deformity is most often seen in rickets when the effects of vitamin D deficiency are superimposed on a growing skeleton. The linear growth rate is reduced, there is bowing of the long bones, enlargement of the costochondral junctions (rickety rosary), and bossing of the frontal and parietal bones. Later, osteomalacia may produce a triradiate pelvis, a gross kyphosis, and corresponding deformities of the chest.

Proximal muscle weakness is an important symptom. Its cause is unknown (although myoblasts require 1,25$(OH)_2D$ *in vitro*, and the development of myofibrils in animals without the vitamin D receptor may be abnormal). It is more marked in some forms of osteomalacia than in others. Most commonly there is a waddling gait, a difficulty in getting up and down stairs, out of low chairs, and in and out of small cars. In the

Table 5 Diagnosis of disorders of the skeleton

Age	Main presenting symptom	Most likely diagnosis	Frequency	Exclude
Over 50 years	Pain in the back; loss of height; fracture	Osteoporosis, most common in women	Common	Myeloma (especially in men); secondary deposits; coexistent osteomalacia
	Deformity of long bones; pain in hips; and pelvis fracture	Paget's disease of bone; most common in men	Common	Osteomalacia; hyperparathyroid bone disease skeletal metastases;
	Bone pain and tenderness; difficulty in walking; unable to climb stairs; pathological fracture	Osteomalacia	Uncommon, especially in the adult	Carcinoma; polymyalgia rheumatica
	Bone pain and deformity; thirst; nocturia; depression; vomiting; constipation	Osteitis fibrosa cystica; most common in women	Rare	Carcinoma with hypercalcaemia; myeloma
20–50 years	Loss of height	Probably secondary deposits; or myeloma	Rare	Osteomalacia; accelerated osteoporosis
	Muscle weakness; loss of height; bone pain	Osteomalacia	Rare	Late muscular dystrophy neoplastic; neuromyopathy; Cushing's syndrome
0–20 years	Bowing of bones; deformity; weakness	'Nutritional' rickets	Most common Asian immigrants in in Northern cities	Other causes of rickets; hypophosphatasia
	Multiple fractures; bruising	In infants, inflicted by parents, battered baby'	Not uncommon	Osteogenesis imperfecta
	Bone pain; ill health	Leukaemia	Uncommon	Osteomyelitis; rickets
	Pain in back; difficulty in walking; pain in ankles; less rapid growth	Juvenile osteoporosis	Rare	Leukaemia; osteogenesis imperfecta
	Failure to grow (short stature)	Many causes (Table 3)	Common	Particularly hypothyroidism; Turner's syndrome; and coeliac disease
	Excessive or disproportionate growth	Several causes, often familial	Less common than short stature	Particularly pituitary tumour; Marfan's syndrome; homocystinuria; hypogonadism and chromosomal abnormalities
	Fracture and deformity at birth(often lethal)	Severe osteogenesis imperfecta	Uncommon	Hypophosphatasia; achondrogenesis; thanatophoric dwarfism

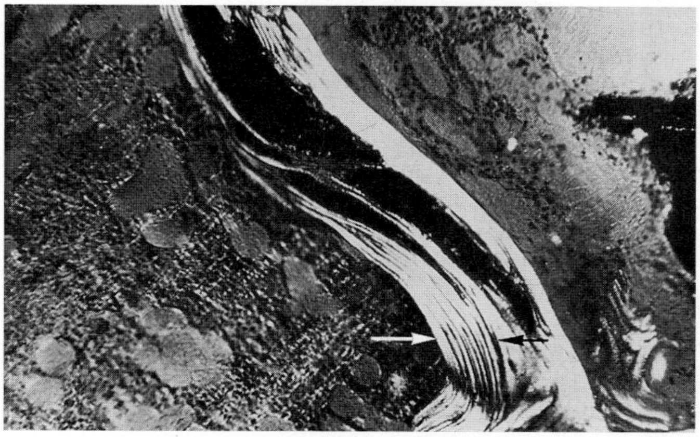

Fig. 6 Bone from a patient with osteomalacia. The birefringent osteoid is abnormally thick (up to 12 lamellae, arrows) and covers all bone surfaces. The bone preparation is undecalcified and viewed under polarized light (von Kossa stain; magnification 300 ×).

elderly, weakness may make walking impossible thereby suggesting paraplegia. In younger subjects even muscular dystrophy may be simulated.

Features of the underlying disorder include anaemia; tiredness and steatorrhoea in coeliac disease; pigmentation, thirst, and nocturia in renal failure. Occasionally hypocalcaemia may cause spontaneous tetany; in children the manifestations of carpopedal spasm, stridor, and fits are more dramatic than in the adult.

Examination of the patient with osteomalacia or rickets confirms the main symptoms. Measurement of the body proportions is useful. Thus patients with inherited hypophosphataemia and rickets have relatively short limbs, whereas those with late-onset osteomalacia will have a relatively short trunk. It is important to look for clues as to the cause of the osteomalacia, such as the scars of previous gastric or intestinal surgery.

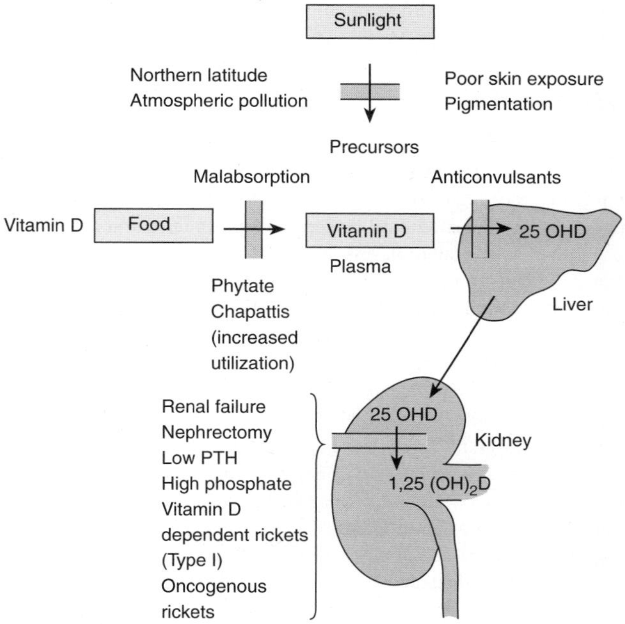

Fig. 7 The causes of rickets and osteomalacia related to the sources and metabolism of vitamin D (From *Oxford textbook of rheumatology*, with permission.)

Table 6 The main causes of rickets and osteomalacia

Lack of vitamin D
Deficient synthesis in the skin
Low intake in the diet
Probably increased requirement
Malabsorption
Gluten-sensitive enteropathy (coeliac disease)
Gastric surgery
Bowel resection
Intestinal bypass surgery
Biliary cirrhosis
Renal disease
Renal-tubular disorders:
inherited hypophosphataemia (vitamin D-resistant rickets)
others[a]
Renal glomerular failure:
renal osteodystrophy
dialysis bone disease
Others
Anticonvulsant osteomalacia
Tumour rickets
Vitamin D-dependent rickets
Phosphate-deficiency rickets

[a] See Table 7.

Investigations

Biochemistry

Since there are many causes of osteomalacia, the detailed biochemical changes differ from one to another. In vitamin D deficiency or malabsorption there are low plasma calcium and phosphate, a low urine calcium, and an increase in the plasma alkaline phosphatase level. However, these may vary with the stage of the disease. Initially, hypocalcaemia may be the only abnormality. Later, with secondary hyperparathyroidism, the plasma calcium level returns towards normal, the plasma phosphate level falls, and the alkaline phosphatase level increases. In inherited hypophosphataemia (vitamin D-resistant rickets) plasma phosphate is low, but the plasma calcium is normal and the alkaline phosphatase may also be normal. Renal glomerular failure causes an increase in plasma phosphate, urea, and creatinine, and hypocalcaemia, and in the rare renal tubular syndromes there may be a marked systemic acidosis. In patients with osteomalacia the urine should always be examined for the presence of glucose and protein. If these are present, it is important to check for the aminoaciduria characteristic of renal tubular disorders.

The measurement of vitamin D metabolites is becoming routine, and a low plasma 25(OH)D level is a good indication of vitamin D deficiency. Estimation of plasma $1,25(OH)_2D$ is important to elucidate the very rare causes of rickets, and particularly to distinguish between type I (low $1,25(OH)_2D$) and type II (high $1,25(OH)_2D$) vitamin D-dependent rickets.

Radiology

The radiological appearances differ according to whether growth has ceased or not. In rickets the main abnormalities are at the ends of the long bones, where the width of the growth plate is increased, and the metaphysis is widened, cupped, and ragged (Fig. 8). Osteomalacia may show the deformities previously described, but the radiological hallmark of active osteomalacia is the Looser's zone (Fig. 9). This is a ribbon-like area of defective mineralization, which may be found in almost any bone but is seen particularly in the long bones, the pelvis, and the ribs, and also around the scapulas. Looser's zones may be bilateral and symmetrical; in bones such as the femur they occur on the medial border of the shaft or neck and

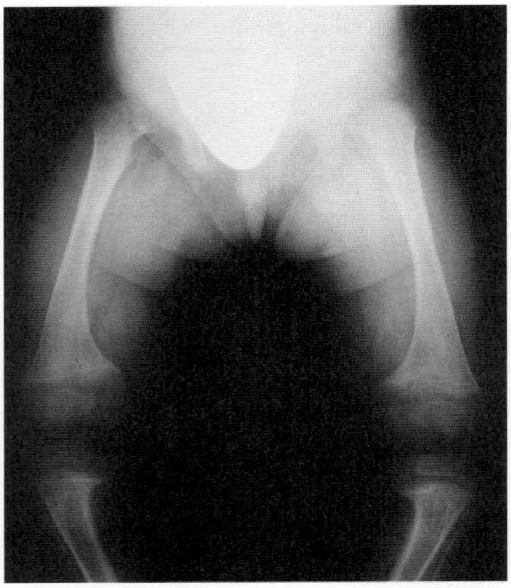

Fig. 8 The radiological appearance of rickets in a child with inherited hypophosphataemia. The growth plates are widened and the metaphyses cupped and ragged.

are usually single, in contrast to the multiple fissure fractures on the lateral convexity of the bone in Paget's disease. In osteomalacia the vertebral bodies are often uniformly biconcave, to produce an appearance likened to a fish spine. Additionally, in renal glomerular osteodystrophy, the endplates may become relatively more dense than the rest of the vertebral body, to produce the so-called 'rugger jersey' spine. In the adult with inherited hypophosphataemia the bones may also become deformed, buttressed, and dense; in this disorder calcification of the tendons and ligaments at their insertions (enthesiopathy) and of the vertebral ligaments can produce an appearance similar to that of ankylosing spondylitis. Ossification of the ligamenta flava narrows the spinal canal and compresses the spinal cord and its roots. This is well shown on CT scans. In patients with osteomalacia and hypocalcaemia the radiological features of secondary hyperparathyroidism appear with subperiosteal bone resorption that affects the phalanges, the pubic symphysis, and the outer ends of the clavicles. In rickets, periostitis of the distal ends of the long bones, such as the radius and ulna, often occur.

The most extreme effects of parathyroid overactivity are seen in the skeleton of the child with renal osteodystrophy, where the region of the growth plate and metaphyses may fracture (an appearance likened to a 'rotting stump'). A bone scintigram may be very useful in cases of osteomalacia, demonstrating multiple pathological fractures often not seen on the plain films. The appearance is similar to that of bony metastases.

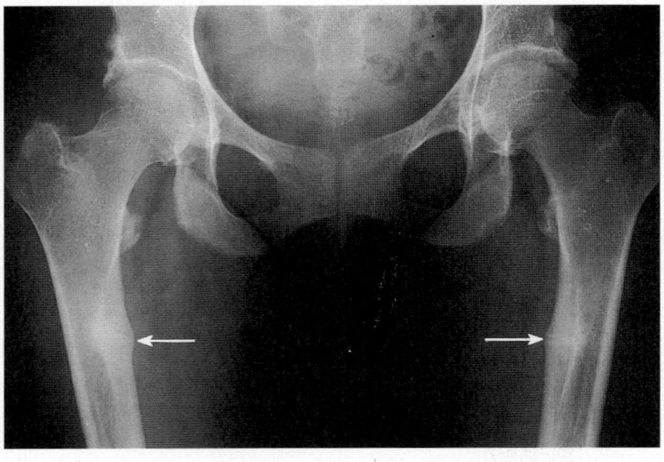

Fig. 9 To demonstrate the bilateral Looser's zones on the medial border of the femora in a woman with osteomalacia due to adult Fanconi's syndrome.

Bone biopsy

The diagnosis of osteomalacia is often clear without examining the bone. Where doubt exists, a transiliac biopsy examined before and after decalcification will demonstrate the failure of mineralization and the wide osteoid seams. It is important to take all surgical opportunities to examine bone, particularly during operations on fractured femurs in the elderly.

Other investigations

Further investigation is not usually needed to diagnose osteomalacia, but may be necessary to identify its cause. Thus patients with vitamin D-deficient rickets and osteomalacia will have a low plasma 25(OH)D, but not all subjects with such low levels have osteomalacia. In the very rare condition of vitamin D-dependent rickets, measurement of circulating $1,25(OH)_2D$ will be necessary to distinguish the absence of 1α-hydroxylase from resistance to $1,25(OH)_2D$. Further, CT scanning may help to identify the presence of a mesenchymal tumour causing hypophosphataemic osteomalacia.

Diagnosis

Osteomalacia is not difficult to diagnose once it is thought of. It should be distinguished from other forms of metabolic bone disease (Table 4), from other causes of proximal muscle weakness, and from other disorders causing bone pain. In patients with proximal muscle weakness, polymyalgia rheumatica, thyrotoxic myopathy, muscular dystrophy, neoplastic neuropathy, dermatomyositis, and polymyositis all need to be considered. Multiple myeloma and leukaemia may need to be excluded as causes of pain. Provided that the plasma calcium, phosphorus, and alkaline phosphatase levels are always measured in patients with these symptoms, those with osteomalacia should be easily identified. Patients with psychological illness may have an abnormal gait and complain of pain and weakness in their limbs, but in such patients the biochemistry will be normal. In practice, symptoms of pain and stiffness often first lead the patient with osteomalacia to a rheumatologist.

Treatment

Rickets and osteomalacia should respond rapidly to vitamin D (or to its metabolites) in an appropriate dose, and the response may be a useful way of confirming the diagnosis. Increased mobility with an increase in muscle strength may be the first clinical response, despite a temporary increase in bone pain. Biochemically, plasma phosphate and urine hydroxyproline levels are the first to increase. The alkaline phosphatase level may show a temporary rise and then fall slowly to normal levels. As the plasma calcium and 25(OH)D concentrations increase towards normal, the parathyroid hormone concentration falls.

The effective dose and the particular vitamin D preparation depends on the cause of the osteomalacia. That due to vitamin D deficiency will respond to microgram doses, but it is often useful to give considerably more than this, such as calciferol 1.25 mg daily for 1 to 2 weeks only. Where there is doubt about compliance, vitamin D may be injected intramuscularly in one large dose (up to 15 mg, 600 000 units). Lack of a response to microgram doses suggest that the osteomalacia is not due to simple vitamin D deficiency but, for instance, to malabsorption or renal failure. It is particularly in the last group that the 1α-hydroxylated metabolites of vitamin D are effective (see Chapter 20.8). Clearly, underlying disorders must be treated at the same time: for example, patients with coeliac disease will need a gluten-free diet.

Particular forms of osteomalacia and rickets

Nutritional osteomalacia

In the United Kingdom and other Northern European countries, so-called nutritional osteomalacia occurs particularly amongst the elderly and in Asian immigrants of all ages. In the elderly, the high incidence of osteomalacia is mainly due to their poor exposure to sunlight and to a low intake of vitamin D; and may be contributed to by the effects of drugs such as anticonvulsants and by increasing renal glomerular failure. Since the elderly are often housebound, they may develop osteomalacia despite a sunny climate. Certainly, the prevalence of osteomalacia in the elderly population is significant. The frequency of osteomalacia in patients with fractures of the femoral neck is also higher than previously suspected, but figures of up to 30 per cent, which continue to be reported (according to the histological definitions used), are probably overestimates. Osteomalacia should always be excluded in elderly people with bone disease, and particularly in those with femoral neck fractures. Where possible this should be done by histological examination of bone taken at operation or by biopsy. When this is not appropriate, a therapeutic trial with vitamin D is often useful. Since it is often difficult to define osteomalacia accurately in elderly people it is important to consider the use of such empirical treatment. In the geriatric population the mean concentration of 25(OH)D is much lower than in non-elderly patients; it shows the usual seasonal variation, with lowest values in the winter and early spring and highest in late summer.

Asian immigrants to the Northern hemisphere develop osteomalacia and rickets more often than the indigenous populations. There are probably several reasons for this. They tend to live in northern cities away from sunlight and, especially in women, do not expose their skin to the limited ultraviolet light. Where dermal synthesis of vitamin D is limited, dietary factors become more important, and it is particularly those on a meat-free diet containing chapattis who develop osteomalacia. The role of chapattis and the phytate they contain is not yet fully understood. Phytates bind to calcium so preventing its absorption, and it can be shown, at least experimentally, that reduced calcium absorption increases the vitamin D requirement by increasing its parathyroid-mediated breakdown. It has been suggested that such a mechanism of reduced calcium absorption may also contribute to the osteomalacia of malabsorptive syndromes, such as that following partial gastrectomy.

Pigmentation of the skin can be shown experimentally, using a standardized dose of ultraviolet light, to reduce vitamin D synthesis, but in practice this is of little significance. Since North European immigrants of Afro-Caribbean descent have a lower incidence of rickets than Asians in the same environment, it is clear that factors other than skin colour are important.

As in the elderly, 25(OH)D levels can be very low, especially in Asian immigrants. They increase in the summer, when there may be spontaneous healing of rickets. Important work in Glasgow has shown that Asian rickets can be prevented by fortifying food such as chapatti flour with vitamin D, although the incidence of osteomalacia in Asian adults remains unaffected. Other local lifestyle changes will also influence the diet of children.

Osteomalacia and malabsorption

Coeliac disease (gluten-sensitive enteropathy) (Chapter 14.9.3) is a relatively common cause of osteomalacia. It should be suspected at any age, and confirmed by the presence of circulating endomysial antibody and, if necessary, by a small intestinal biopsy showing an atrophic mucosa. Other causes of malabsorption vary in their frequency according to surgical practice. Thus it is well established that osteomalacia follows classic partial gastrectomy, but the actual incidence is debated and its cause is probably multifactorial. Postgastrectomy subjects tend to take little vitamin D in their diet and there is defective calcium absorption. Available evidence suggests that clinical osteomalacia is rare after vagotomy and pyloroplasty. Osteomalacia can also follow the removal of long segments of small intestine for conditions such as Crohn's disease, and complicates some intestinal bypass operations used for extreme obesity.

Osteomalacia and liver disease

Osteomalacia is uncommon in those with liver disease; in theory it may be due to a number of factors such as malabsorption of vitamin D and its defective 25-hydroxylation. Most research has concerned the osteomalacia of biliary cirrhosis, and osteomalacia in chronic liver disease appears to be a complication related to prolonged cholestasis.

Osteomalacia and renal disease

It is important to distinguish the osteomalacia and rickets of renal glomerular failure from that attributable to renal tubular disorders. Bone disease in renal glomerular failure (renal glomerular osteodystrophy) is dealt with elsewhere (see Chapter 20.8); this includes bone disease in the dialysed patient and the effects of aluminium. Renal glomerular osteodystrophy is a complex disease with excessive bone resorption, defective bone mineralization, and in some cases osteoporosis. Previously it was treated with large doses of native vitamin D; current therapy now includes 1α-hydroxycholecalciferol or $1{,}25(OH)_2D$.

Many renal tubular disorders lead to osteomalacia (Chapter 20.8) (Table 7). Of these, the most common is inherited hypophosphataemia, so-called vitamin D-resistant rickets, which is normally inherited as an X-linked dominant characteristic; here, the main abnormality is hypophosphataemia due to a reduction in the maximum renal tubular reabsorption rate of phosphate. Some patients in a family will have hypophosphataemia alone, whereas others will have hypophosphataemia with accompanying bone disease. It is now known that inherited hypophosphataemia is caused by mutations in the *PEX* or *PHEX* gene, the cognate protein of which has the features of an endopeptidase. Endopeptidases degrade or activate peptide hormones. It is not yet known how the mutations produce the defect in phosphate homeostasis. Since the $1{,}25(OH)_2D$ levels are normal where the plasma phosphate is low, it is proposed that the sensitivity of the 1α-hydroxylase enzyme is reduced. Children with hypophosphataemic rickets or osteomalacia are unlike patients with other forms of rickets. They present with deformity but are otherwise well, without muscle weakness; however, growth is defective and their eventual height is usually less than 150 cm. Apart from hypophosphataemia there may be no other abnormality in the biochemical values routinely available, and the plasma alkaline phosphatase level can be normal for age. Radiographs show severe rickets, and later the bones are often dense with buttressing and exostoses. The enthesiopathy with ossification of the ligamenta flava can lead to paraplegia. Ligamentous calcification may also contribute to deafness. Finally, abnormal teeth in this disorder cause periapical translucencies and may lead to abscesses.

Table 7 Renal tubular disorders, rickets, and osteomalacia

Inherited hypophosphataemia
Adult-onset hypophosphataemic osteomalacia
Renal tubular acidosis: *Inherited* proximal (bicarbonate wastage) distal (H^+-gradient defect) *Acquired* ureterocolic anastomosis
Multiple renal tubular defects (Fanconi's syndrome) *Inherited* cystinosis oculocerebrorenal syndrome (Lowe's syndrome) Wilson's disease galactosaemia *Acquired* cadmium poisoning multiple myeloma ifosfamide toxicity

The treatment of inherited hypophosphataemia is controversial. For many years its mainstay was large doses of vitamin D; this posed a continuous danger of vitamin D poisoning and did not correct the eventual short stature. There is an improvement in growth rate when oral phosphate is given in addition to vitamin D, but the condition does not appear to respond to phosphate alone. More recently, it has been shown that combined oral phosphate and $1,25(OH)_2D$ produces healing of epiphyseal and trabecular bone and this is now the recommended treatment. This combination produces bone healing and increases eventual stature. However, it is still unusual for affected patients to have an eventual height of more than 1.5 m (5 ft). Accounts of the effects of medical treatment on deformity and height differ; the necessity for corrective osteotomy on the lower limbs is less than previously, but discussion with an orthopaedic surgeon is important.

It is also important that the parents should know the genetics of this condition. Because the defect in phosphate transport is inherited as a dominant on the X chromosome, an affected mother transmits the condition to 50 per cent of her children regardless of their gender. All the daughters of an affected father will have the disease, but none of his sons. In general, affected sons have a more severe disease while some affected daughters may be asymptomatic. Diagnosis can be made from birth, but this demands accurate knowledge of the normal plasma phosphate level at that age. Now that more is known about the exact gene location, prenatal diagnosis may be possible in future. Recently cloned human X-chromosome sequences that reveal restriction fragment length polymorphisms have been used in linkage studies of affected families to map the hypophosphataemic rickets gene. Flanking markers are potentially useful in the identification of mutant gene carriers and in presymptomatic diagnosis, but the distance between these markers and the hypophosphataemic gene is still large, at approximately 10 million base pairs. Hypophosphataemic animal models continue to help in furthering understanding of this disorder. A recently described murine *gy* mutation, in which hypophosphataemia is associated with gyratory activity, has no clear human equivalent. Rare human variants include an autosomal dominant form of hypophosphataemia.

Other renal tubular osteomalacic syndromes include hypophosphataemic osteomalacia presenting in adult life, which may be due to a tumour (see below), inherited and acquired forms of renal tubular acidosis, and rickets associated with multiple renal tubular defects and generalized aminoaciduria (Fanconi's syndrome). Renal tubular acidosis may be proximal or distal, with an inability to reabsorb bicarbonate or to acidify the urine. The osteomalacia may be cured by giving bicarbonate alone or with vitamin D. A persistent acidosis with resultant osteomalacia may also result from ureterosigmoid anastomosis. The commonest cause of Fanconi's syndrome in childhood is nephropathic cystinosis or cystine-storage disease, where there is a widespread deposition of cystine crystals throughout the tissues, and in which thirst, polyuria, dehydration, photophobia, and loss of weight begin at about the age of 1 year. The rickets will heal with the correction of the acidosis, and the administration of phosphate and $1\alpha(OH)D$; renal transplantation corrects the renal failure and prolongs survival, but does not prevent non-renal complications.

Other rare causes of renal tubular rickets and osteomalacia with generalized aminoaciduria are inherited, such as Wilson's disease and the X-linked oculocerebral renal syndrome, or acquired, such as multiple myeloma, cadmium poisoning, and the toxic effects of ifosfamide used in the treatment of childhood malignant disease.

Anticonvulsant osteomalacia

In patients treated with anticonvulsants the incidence of rickets and osteomalacia is higher than normal. This has been attributed to the induction by the anticonvulsants of hepatic enzymes which metabolize vitamin D to biologically inactive derivatives. However, epileptic patients in institutions are often vitamin D-deficient because they are deprived of sunlight, and osteomalacia in such patients probably has several causes.

Tumour rickets

An unusual form of hypophosphataemic rickets or osteomalacia occurs in patients who have mesenchymal tumours, often of a particular histological type, namely sclerosing haemangiopericytomas or non-ossifying fibromas. A tumour should be considered in any adult who develops hypophosphataemic osteomalacia, particularly with prominent myopathy. The disorder is improved by oral phosphate and cured by removal of the tumour. The way in which the tumour induces hypophosphataemia and subsequent osteomalacia is unknown, but current evidence suggests that it interferes with the renal 1α-hydroxylation of 25(OH)D, since the circulating levels of $1,25(OH)_2D$ are abnormally low but rapidly return to normal when the tumour is removed. Rarely, hypophosphataemic osteomalacia may become apparent in adults with neurofibromatosis and polyostotic fibrous dysplasia.

Osteogenic osteomalacia has also been described in cases of prostatic and small-cell carcinoma of the lung.

Vitamin D-dependent rickets

Patients with these very rare, recessively inherited forms of rickets show the features of severe rickets without vitamin D deficiency. There are at least two types of vitamin D-dependent rickets. In type I the activity of the renal 1α-hydroxylase is reduced so that the concentration of $1,25(OH)_2D$ is abnormally low. However, it can be increased by large doses of the native vitamin, which shows that the enzyme block is not complete. In type II there is an end-organ resistance to $1,25(OH)_2D$, which is present in high concentrations. In both forms there is severe rickets and myopathy from infancy; in type II, lifelong total alopecia is a striking feature. Vitamin D-dependent rickets type I responds to very large doses of vitamin D or physiological doses of $1,25(OH)_2D$. Type II may also respond to large doses of vitamin D or its metabolites, or to prolonged intravenous calcium, but some recorded cases suggest that recovery occurs spontaneously with age.

Recent work on type-II, vitamin D-dependent rickets (otherwise known as hereditary $1,25(OH)_2D$-resistant) shows that the $1,25(OH)_2D$-receptor defects, which are responsible for the end-organ resistance in this disease, are due to a variety of point mutations in the gene for the 1,25 receptor, either at its steroid- or DNA-binding domains.

Phosphate-deficiency rickets

If patients ingest large amounts of phosphate-binding drugs, such as aluminium hydroxide, a form of hypophosphataemic osteomalacia may develop. This differs clinically from inherited hypophosphataemic osteomalacia by the presence of severe muscle weakness. Other biochemical features include increased calcium absorption with hypercalcuria, associated with an increase above normal in the concentration of $1,25(OH)_2D$.

Paget's disease of bone

Paget's disease of bone, osteitis deformans, was described more than a century ago, but existed for many years before. It is the most common of the so-called metabolic bone diseases after osteoporosis. Its hallmark is excessive and disorganized resorption and formation of bone. Its cause is unknown, but recent studies on pagetic bone cells, particularly osteoclasts, have provided clues. The new generation of bisphosphonate drugs now provide effective treatment.

Pathophysiology

The natural history of Paget's disease is similar to that of a multicentric neoplasm or a slow virus disease that begins in young adult life. Electron microscopy shows virus-like inclusion bodies in the osteoclasts of patients with Paget's disease. Immunofluorescence studies suggest that these could represent the measles or respiratory syncytial virus. Another candidate has been the canine distemper virus, but the results of polymerase chain reaction amplification of reverse transcribed DNA from Paget's tissue to identify the putative virus remain controversial.

Histology shows multinucleate osteoclasts which appear to be resorbing bone, and busy osteoblasts which appear to be replacing it; these activities are closely linked. There is also excess fibrosis in the marrow. The bone matrix is laid down in all directions and partially loses its birefringence and strength. Mineralization may be defective, probably because of the excessive rate at which the organic bone matrix is laid down. The cement lines and the mosaic appearances of the bone result from the tidemarks of resorption followed by formation. Osteosarcoma which occurs in Paget's disease is presumably the result of the excessive and prolonged activity of the bone cells. Pagetic bone is large, vascular, and deformed. Its physical characteristics depend on the stage of the disorder and it may be hard or soft. In any event, it fractures more readily than normal.

Incidence

Paget's disease occurs in about 3 to 4 per cent of subjects over 40 years of age, is more common in men than in women and its frequency increases with age. It is not unknown in younger people. In Britain, about 750 000 people may have Paget's disease, of whom fewer than 5 per cent have symptoms. It appears to be a peculiarly Anglo-Saxon affliction, being very rare in countries such as Scandinavia and Japan. Within England, early radiological surveys in the 1970s showed that it occurs most often in Lancashire towns and in northern industrial regions (Table 8). It is also more frequent in recent British immigrants to Western Australia than in the Western Australian population, but less frequent than in those relatives who remained in Britain. Such studies do not distinguish between the effect of environment and heredity. In a disorder as common as Paget's disease many striking examples of 'familial' Paget's disease occur by chance. Recent studies suggest a reduction in the prevalence of Paget's disease.

Clinical features

Pain, deformity, fracture

In Paget's disease the bone itself may be painful, or pain may be due to arthritis of a nearby joint, to an associated fracture, or to the development of sarcoma. It has been suggested that there is a specific type of hip joint disorder associated with Paget's disease. Bone pain could be due to stretching of the periosteum, since this part of the bone (and the vessels within bone) contain nerves sensitive to pain. Clinically, the affected bones are enlarged, deformed, and warm. The enlargement is clearly seen in bones such as the tibia and the skull; in the former the bone is typically bowed forwards; the latter shows a characteristic enlargement of the vault that is said to look like a soft beret, or 'tam-o'-shanter', which appears to descend over the ears. Other long bones may become bent and a kyphosis may develop. Although any of the bones can be affected, including the maxilla and the phalanges, the most common sites for Paget's disease are the pelvis and the spine. Fracture may be the first symptom of undiagnosed Paget's disease, for instance at the junction of a resorbing front with normal bone (Fig. 10), or across a fissure fracture (see Fig. 11).

Table 8 Radiological prevalence of Paget's disease

	Prevalence (%) of Paget's disease	
	Men	**Women**
Preston	8.6	6.3
Bolton	7.7	6.4
Blackburn	8.8	3.8
Bradford	7.9	3.6
Hull	7.6	3.1
Southampton	6.6	3.6
Bath	5.3	4.7
Stoke	4.7	4.2
York	5.8	2.5

These data are based on more than 500 patients in each town. The age-standardized incidence is always higher in men than in women. The high incidence in Lancashire towns is not explained. Modified from Barker et *al.* (1977). Recent data (see Further reading list) suggest a decline in radiological prevalence.

Deafness and nerve compression

Deafness in Paget's disease is one of its most disabling symptoms and responds little to treatment. It has many causes, of which nerve compression is only one.

Most nerves can be compressed by enlarging pagetic bone. The spinal cord is particularly at risk, due to the combined effects of increased bone mass, vertebral collapse, and excessive vascularity. Paraplegia or cauda equina lesions may occur. Alterations in the shape of the skull may produce multiple cranial nerve palsies and brainstem lesions, with dysphagia, dysarthria, and ataxia. Basilar invagination with obstruction of cerebrospinal fluid drainage can lead to internal hydrocephalus, raised intracranial pressure, and confusion.

Heart failure

In severe Paget's disease, cardiac output may be increased by the excessive vascularity of the affected bones, but there is no convincing evidence of large arteriovenous shunts within the skeleton. The heart failure which results may be of the high-output variety, but this is excessively rare. Since heart failure and Paget's disease of bone are common in the elderly, their occurrence together is almost always coincidental.

Sarcoma

The incidence of sarcoma in Paget's disease has sometimes been overestimated in the past; it probably occurs in 1 per cent or less of those with symptoms. Paget's sarcoma often occurs in the humerus, although Paget's disease itself is most common in the pelvis and spine. Sarcoma should be

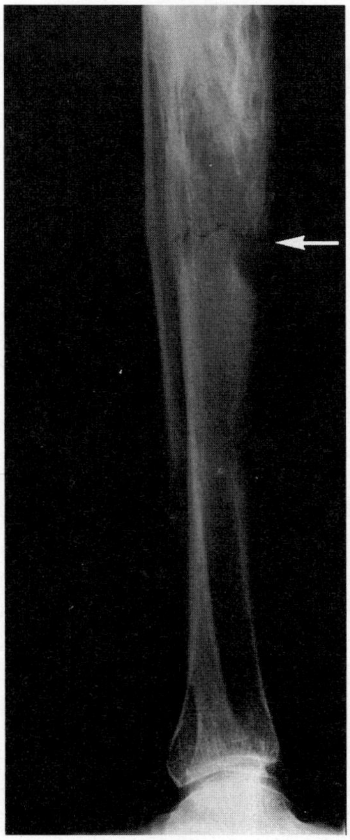

Fig. 10 A fracture in the region of a resorbing front in a pagetic bone (arrowed). Proximal to the area of bone resorption the cortex is thickened and the bone widened by disorganized formation of new bone.

considered in a patient known to have Paget's disease if pain has developed for the first time, or worsened, or if deformity has altered. Radiologically, the appearance of the pagetic bone alters, with evidence of bone destruction (Fig. 12); the tumours occur most often in the medulla. A recent review of 85 bone sarcomas associated with Paget's disease confirmed the humerus as a high-risk site. Rapidly worsening pain was the main symptom; lytic lesions were more common than sclerotic; periosteal reaction was uncommon; and radionuclide bisphosphonate scintigraphy usually showed areas of decreased uptake (contrasting with the underlying pagetic bone).

Associated disorders

Paget's disease is said to be associated with other disorders such as osteoarthritis, gout, vascular calcification, and articular chondrocalcinosis. Since all these occur more often in the elderly the associations have little significance.

Investigations

Biochemistry

There is a marked increase in the level of plasma alkaline phosphatase, derived from the overactive osteoblasts, which is roughly related to the extent of clinical and radiological involvement with Paget's disease. In contrast, the acid phosphatase (derived partly from osteoclasts) level is only slightly increased. The rapid turnover of bone matrix collagen increases urinary hydroxyproline (and hydroxylysine), in proportion to the increase in alkaline phosphatase and also the urinary excretion of crosslinked collagen-derived peptides. Plasma calcium and phosphate levels are normal; hypercalcaemia suggests coexistent hyperparathyroidism, malignant disease, or immobility.

Radiology

The radiological appearances of Paget's disease are legion. The most characteristic is an increase in size of the affected bone. Resorption predominates early in the disease and in the young patient. A resorbing front may be seen in a long bone (as a flame-shaped area) (see Fig. 10) or in the skull (as 'osteoporosis circumscripta'). Excessive resorption is inevitably followed by disordered formation, and at this stage the bone becomes thick and deformed. In elderly subjects the affected bone may be very osteoporotic and liable to fracture. Multiple partial fractures (microfractures, fissure fractures) are common on the deformed convex surface of long bones (see Fig. 11), particularly the femur and tibia.

The use of bone-scintigraphic agents (such as $^{99}Tc^{m}$-labelled disodium etidronate (**EHDP**, [disodium] ethane-1-hydroxy-1,1-diphosphonate) has been particularly informative in Paget's disease. Affected bones take up the isotope avidly, which demonstrates both the extent of the bone lesions and the effects of treatment. In one study, 180 patients with Paget's disease underwent whole-body scintigraphy and 826 lesions were identified—one-third of the patients had only one lesion, and only 10 patients had no symptoms. The increase in plasma alkaline phosphatase and urinary total hydroxyproline was proportional to scintigraphic involvement, and patients with skull involvement had the highest values. Apart from the number of sites involved, any distinction between monostotic and polyostotic disease appeared to be artificial.

Diagnosis

The diagnosis of Paget's disease is usually obvious. Bone biopsy is useful to exclude other generalized bone diseases, such as osteomalacia, as well as to confirm Paget's disease. Paget's disease may initially be confused with osteomalacia because of the high plasma alkaline phosphatase level; rarely,

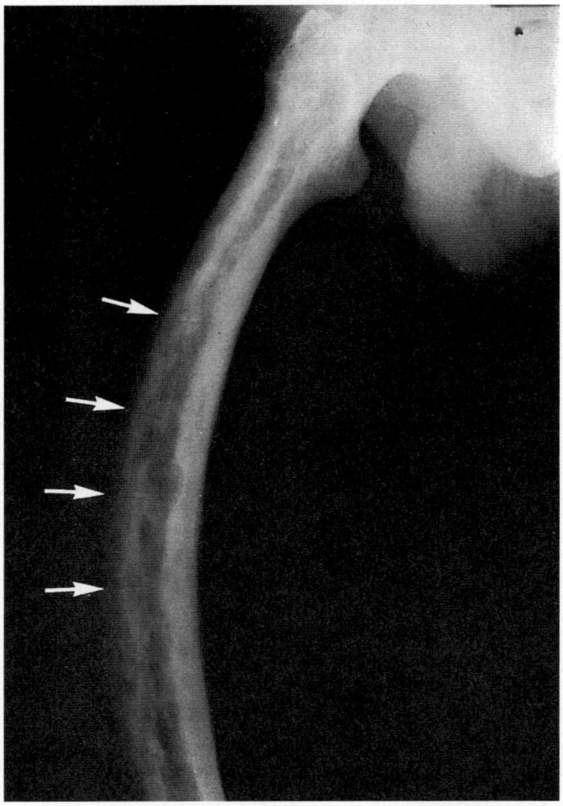

Fig. 11 Multiple microfractures ('fissure fractures' arrowed) on the convex surface of a pagetic femur.

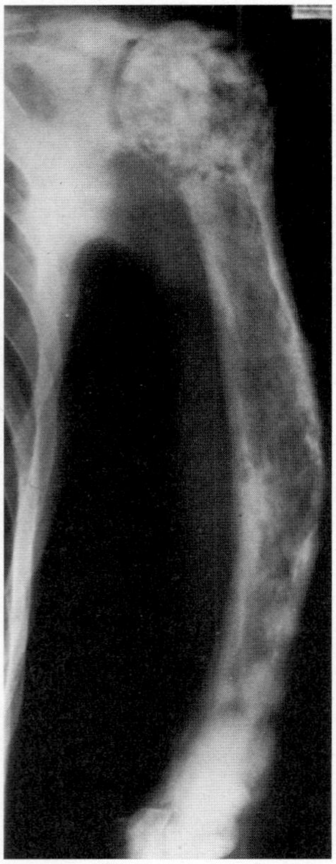

Fig. 12 A sarcoma in the upper end of the left humerus in a 70-year-old man with Paget's disease. The destructive lesion in the proximal humerus has been treated with radiotherapy; there are secondary deposits around the distal end of the bone.

an elevated plasma calcium should suggest additional hyperparathyroidism or malignant disease. In prostatic carcinoma with osteoblastic bone secondaries, the dense bones are not enlarged (as they are in Paget's disease) and the acid phosphatase level is considerably and disproportionately increased in relation to that of alkaline phosphatase. Of many other conditions with similar radiological appearance, fibrous dysplasia (see below), in which the alkaline phosphatase may also be slightly increased, may be difficult to distinguish; in the generalized form the unilateral bone lesions, pigmentation, and sexual precocity (in the female) are characteristic. Another very rare disorder usually mistaken for Paget's disease is fibrogenesis imperfecta ossium (see below), where the bone trabeculae are thickened without bony enlargement and there are multiple abnormal fractures.

Treatment

Many patients with Paget's disease require no treatment, but it may be required for symptoms, to suppress the activity of the disease, and to prevent its further progress. Indications include bone pain, nerve compression, and the suppression of vascularity before elective orthopaedic surgery. Since medical treatment is now so effective, these indications may be widened especially in young people.

Medical treatment

Patients with painful Paget's disease should first be treated with a simple analgesic. Where possible it should be determined whether the pain is directly due to the bone disease or to associated arthritis. Specific treatment aimed at the pagetic bone should be considered for those who have pain due to bone disease despite analgesia, or have the complications of deformity, nerve compression, deafness, or very rarely heart failure. This treatment should also be considered in the young person with Paget's disease to prevent further progression. There is no evidence that the rapid course of pagetic sarcoma is altered by any treatment. Of the many agents previously tried in Paget's disease, such as aspirin, fluoride, and corticosteroids, only three are currently in use, mithramycin, bisphosphonates, and calcitonin. Mithramycin is now rarely used. It is an antimitotic agent given intravenously which is hepatotoxic in high doses. It may rapidly abolish pain in Paget's disease, and rapidly reduce the plasma alkaline phosphatase level, but the effect is usually temporary. Mithramycin has been used on its own and in combination with bisphosphonates or calcitonin.

The bisphosphonates (once called diphosphonates) are a series of compounds with a P–C–P structure resistant to the naturally occurring phosphonates and pyrophosphatases. They are effective both orally and parenterally and reduce excessive bone turnover in Paget's disease. EHDP (Didronel®), one of the early bisphosphonates, also interferes with mineralization if given in high doses (20 mg/kg body weight); subsequent derivatives such as dichloromethylene diphosphonate (**Cl2 MDP**) and 3-amino-hydroxypropylidine-l,l-bisphosphonate (**APD**, pamidronate) do not appear to do this. According to their dose, the bisphosphonates may take up to 6 months to produce their effect on symptoms, histology, and biochemistry. The recommended dose for EHDP is 5 mg/kg per day for up to 6 months. It also has been used in combination with calcitonin, and together these agents suppress Paget's disease more effectively than when given alone. The biochemical effects of EHDP appear to last for a long time (possibly several years) after the drug is stopped. Many new bisphosphonates have now been developed based on side-chain substitutions in the basic P–C–P structure. The aminobisphosphonates are particularly effective. The new bisphosphonates are many times more potent than etidronate. They include pamidronate, tiludronate, alendronate, and risedronate. They may produce almost complete and permanent suppression of Paget's disease without significant side-effects. The dose regimes and expected responses are dealt with in larger reviews (see the Further reading list).

The calcitonins are less widely used for the treatment of Paget's disease, and salmon calcitonin is the most effective commercially available form. Various dose regimens are used, for which 100 IU given three times a week is average. Injected calcitonin may produce nausea and vomiting; if side-effects are troublesome, it is best given in the evening together with an antiemetic. Its main effects are seen during the first 3 months of treatment, and continued treatment is ineffective, especially when the alkaline phosphatase level has ceased to decline.

Antibodies to calcitonin do develop but are not necessarily related to calcitonin 'resistance'. Indications for the bisphosphonates and calcitonins are different. Calcitonin is preferred to treat bone pain, for osteolytic Paget's disease, and for preoperative treatment. Some evidence suggests that calcitonin may halt the progression of deafness. Spinal cord compression is also alleviated. Thus treatment of eight patients with paraparesis due to pagetic vertebrae with either calcitonin or bisphosphonate produced marked clinical improvement, at least comparable to the results of surgical decompression. Calcitonin can also be given preoperatively to reduce excessive bleeding when operations such as total hip replacement have to be performed on pagetic bone. Calcitonin can now be given by the nasal route, which is more acceptable to the patient but less effective.

Surgical treatment

Fractures through pagetic bone require the usual surgical treatment, although union may be delayed. Where fracture occurs through a deformed bone, this deformity should be corrected. In addition, elective osteotomy and intramedullary nailing may be considered for a severe long-bone deformity. Spinal cord compression not responding to medical treatment requires surgery. Rarely, hydrocephalus may require a ventriculojugular shunt. Whatever form of surgery is undertaken, it is important that the period of immobility is as short as possible, to avoid the development of hypercalciuria and hypercalcaemia.

Parathyroids and bone disease

Knowledge of the biochemistry of parathyroid hormone has expanded so rapidly that it now occupies a large and deserved part of any clinical description of parathyroid disorders (see Chapter 12.6). The close relationship between these endocrine glands and the skeleton becomes less obvious with increasing recognition of the many ways in which parathyroid disease presents. However, primary hyperparathyroidism was first identified because of its effects on bone, and only later was it realized that it might more often present with renal stones, with pancreatitis, and with the signs and symptoms of hypercalcaemia—or be a chance discovery as a result of multichannel biochemical analysis.

The subject is discussed further in Chapter 12.6.

Molecular advances

With the discovery of the calcium-sensing receptor (**CaR**) and extensive work on the cause of the multiple endocrine neoplasia syndromes our understanding of the rarer causes of abnormal plasma calcium levels has considerably increased. Thus missense mutations of the *CaR* gene cause both familial benign hypercalcaemia and neonatal hyperparathyroidism, whereas gain-of-function mutations in this receptor can cause familial hypoparathyroidism. Multiple endocrine neoplasia (**MEN**) syndromes have traditionally been divided into two types—type 1 with hyperparathyroidism, pituitary adenomas, insulin- and gastrin-secreting tumours of the pancreas, and gastric hyperacidity (Zollinger–Ellison syndrome); and type 2, also known as Sipple's syndrome, with hyperparathyroidism, medullary carcinoma of the thyroid, and phaeochromocytoma. The molecular elucidation of these differences has identified subgroups. In MEN1 the principal genetic abnormality involves mutations in the *MEN1* gene together with loss of alleles on chromosome 11; in MEN2 (both A and B subgroups) there are mutations in the *RET* proto-oncogene on chromosome 10.

Hypercalcaemia

Of the known causes of hypercalcaemia in hospital inpatients, neoplasm is the most important (Table 9). It should always be considered and excluded

Table 9 Main causes of hypercalcaemia

Diagnosis	Features	Comments
Neoplastic disease[a] Hydrocortisone- sensitive (usually)	Common; with or without secondary deposits; biochemistry often like hyperparathyroidism	Tumours of lung, breast, and others; plasma PTHrP increased, PTH decreased
Multiple myeloma	Bone pain, fractures	High ESR; Bence-Jones (light chain) proteinuria
Hyperparathyroidism	Multiple; does not respond to corticosteroids	Plasma whole-molecule PTH increased
Vitamin D overdosage	May give acute hypercalcaemic symptoms; thirst, vomiting; sore eyes	Most often in patients treated with vitamin D
Sarcoidosis (and other granulomas)	Nephrocalcinosis, splenomegaly, hilar lymphadenopathy; precipitated by sunlight or physiological amounts of vitamin D	May be due to inappropriate formation of $1{,}25(OH)_2D$
Immobility	Especially in young people or in those with Paget's disease	
Thyrotoxicosis	Increased bone turnover. Plasma phosphate increased	Alkaline phosphatase and hydroxyproline increased
Milk alkali syndrome	Associated with milk and alkali ingestion for peptic ulceration; more commonly due to 'indigestion' tablets	Very uncommon in acute forms
Thiazide diuretics		
Hypoadrenalism		
Acute renal failure		

[a] The relative frequency of neoplastic disease and hyperparathyroidism as a cause for hypercalcaemia varies with the population. On screening, more than 85 per cent of healthy outpatients with hypercalcaemia have primary hyperparathyroidism; neoplastic disease is the most common cause in symptomatic inpatients.

clinically. The relative frequency of the causes of hypercalcaemia varies according to the population studied. In apparently healthy outpatients primary hyperparathyroidism is the most frequent cause. In those patients with primary hyperparathyroidism, with hypercalcaemia, hypophosphataemia, hyperphosphatasia, and radiological evidence of osteitis fibrosa, and without clinical evidence of neoplasm, little further investigation is needed. Since only a few patients with hyperparathyroidism have clinical bone disease, further differentiation from other causes of hypercalcaemia is usually necessary. In practice, this means the exclusion of neoplasm, sarcoidosis, thyrotoxicosis, vitamin D overdosage, treatment with thiazide diuretics, or the 'milk alkali' syndrome. The subject is addressed further in Chapter 20. 8.

Secondary (and tertiary) hyperparathyroidism

Where hypocalcaemia is prolonged, as in renal glomerular failure or gluten-sensitive enteropathy, the parathyroid glands increase both their size and activity in an attempt to restore the plasma calcium level to normal. This increases bone resorption and is a particular feature of renal glomerular osteodystrophy. Occasionally hypercalcaemia develops and persists in such patients. It has been proposed that one of the hyperplastic parathyroid glands becomes autonomous and thus the label 'tertiary hyperparathyroidism' has been given. Hypercalcaemia may also occur after renal transplantation (see Chapter 20.8).

Hypoparathyroidism (see also Chapter 20. 8)

Parathyroid insufficiency may occur after surgical removal of the parathyroids, in idiopathic hypoparathyroidism, and in a familial form of hypoparathyroidism which is often associated with manifestations of autoimmune disease, including moniliasis, malabsorption, thyroid and adrenal failure, and pernicious anaemia. In such patients the levels of immunoreactive parathyroid hormone (**PTH**) are undetectably low but the cAMP response to exogenous PTH is maintained. This distinguishes parathyroid insufficiency from pseudohypoparathyroidism, in which the biochemical features of hypoparathyroidism are associated with characteristic skeletal abnormalities (Albright's hereditary osteodystrophy). Pseudohypoparathyroidism is inherited as an autosomal dominant. In the most common form, the cAMP response to exogenous PTH is defective, and the circulating level of immunoreactive PTH is high. Variations of pseudohypoparathyroidism appear to exist, and disorders are described in which the cAMP response is present but there is still end-organ resistance, and also where the cAMP response is restored by giving vitamin D. Patients who have the skeletal manifestations of pseudohypoparathyroidism but with normal biochemistry may be found in families with pseudohypoparathyroidism, and to them the term 'pseudopseudohypoparathyroidism' is applied. Investigation has shown that the loss-of-function end-organ resistance is due to point mutations in the genes controlling one component of the G-protein signalling system.

So far as the skeleton is concerned, the most striking changes are found in pseudohypoparathyroidism. Clinical features include mental simplicity, short stature, round face, short neck, and abnormal metacarpals (or metatarsals), of which the most common change is shortness of the fourth and fifth. The bones may be excessively dense, and widespread ectopic calcification and ossification may also occur, in the basal ganglia and the subcutaneous tissues respectively. Treatment of the hypocalcaemia is the same as for idiopathic hypoparathyroidism, with 1α-hydroxycholecalciferol.

Osteogenesis imperfecta: the brittle bone syndrome

This disorder, which has emerged from the status of an obscure osteopathy to a metabolic bone disease, provides remarkable lessons concerning the effects of mutations in the collagen genes. The correlation between genotype and phenotype is by no means exact and leaves interesting problems.

Osteogenesis imperfecta is said to occur in about 1 in 20 000 births; since the milder forms may never be diagnosed, this could be an underestimate. It is a leading cause of lethal short-limbed dwarfism and crippling skeletal dysplasia. There is no convincing evidence of different racial frequency.

Table 10 Current clinical classification of osteogenesis imperfecta

Type	Clinical features	Inheritance
I	Few fractures; little or no deformity; normal stature; prominent extraskeletal features	Autosomal dominant
II	Multiple fractures; perinatal lethal, short limbs	New dominant mutations
III	Bones deform with age; extreme short stature; dentinogenesis imperfecta common; sclerae less blue with age	Some new mutations; some recessive
IV	Moderate bone deformity and short stature; sclerae normal colour	Autosomal dominant

Many patients with osteogenesis imperfecta do not fit easily into the Sillence classification (Table 10), and in some cases hypermobility and features of the Ehlers–Danlos syndrome (see below) are dominant.

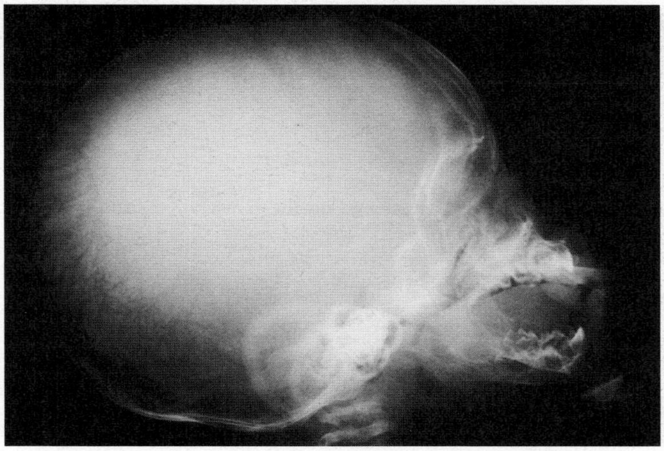

Fig. 13 The innumerable centres of ossification in the occipital region, wormian bones, in an infant with severe (type III) osteogenesis imperfecta.

Pathophysiology

Osteogenesis imperfecta involves those tissues that contain the main fibrillar collagen, type I. These include particularly bone and dentine, but also the sclerae, joints, tendons, heart valves, and skin. The pathology in bone varies with the type and severity of the disease, with age, previous fracture, and surgery. The skeletal effects of osteogenesis imperfecta are most severe in the lethal forms (type II) and at the region of the growth plate. There is faulty conversion of apparently normal mineralized cartilage to defective bone matrix. The collagen fibres are thin but show the normal striated pattern. The endoplasmic reticulum of the osteoblasts is dilated by retained mutant collagen. The bone structure is completely disorganized and structurally useless. In type III osteogenesis imperfecta, which is less severe, there are variable amounts of woven immature bone, with disorganized trabeculae and an apparent excess of osteocytes—as in other forms of the disorder. At the growth plate there are multiple islands of cartilage in the epiphyses and metaphyses. Accounts of the bone pathology in type IV are sparse. Defective mineralization is described in rare forms of osteogenesis imperfecta.

In mild, type I osteogenesis imperfecta there is a reduction in the amount of bone (and hence in measured bone mineral density) and defective bone formation at the cellular level, such that the osteoblasts each make approximately half as much bone collagen as normal. The result is an osteoporotic bone with an apparent excess of osteoblasts and osteocytes. This appearance of 'hyperosteocytosis' suggests (to some) an increase in bone turnover rate. The overall bone structure is otherwise normal, apart from occasional woven bone. In affected dentine, the odontoblasts produce short, branched dentinal tubules and fill in the dental pulp. In the ear, the auditory ossicles may be imperfect or fractured.

The reduction in collagen is repeated in non-skeletal tissues. Thus, the sclerae are thin (leading to their blueness since the pigmented coat of the choroid becomes visible), the tendons are gracile and weak, the thin heart valves may become incompetent, and the aortic root dilated.

Clinical features

Type I is the most frequent and least serious form, and accounts for 60 per cent of all patients with the disorder. Fractures can occur in the perinatal period or even be delayed until the early perimenopause. After the menopause the overall fracture rate has been recorded at seven times more than in the normal population, and the vertebral bone mineral content in adults with type I osteogenesis imperfecta has been found to be 70 per cent of normal.

Childhood fractures in type I osteogenesis imperfecta may be numerous but rarely lead to deformity unless treated inappropriately. Any type of fracture can occur; they become less frequent with age. Overall, fractures are more frequent in the lower limbs. Significant scoliosis is rare. The skull shows interesting changes; in addition to multiple wormian bones (Fig. 13) (which can occur in other disorders, such as pyknodysostosis, cleidocranial dysostosis, Menkes' syndrome, Prader–Willi syndrome, progeria, and, rarely, in normal subjects), the vault may overhang the base, leading to basilar impression requiring surgical correction.

Clinical dentinogenesis imperfecta occurs in only some patients; the appearance varies widely and affects some teeth more than others; the teeth are discoloured and the enamel (which is normal) fractures easily from the dentine, leading to rapid erosion of both the first and second dentition. Blueness of the sclerae is a particularly important physical sign of osteogenesis imperfecta. The cause of the frequently early (juvenile) arcus is unknown: limited investigation excludes hypercholesterolaemia. The cardiac manifestations of osteogenesis imperfecta are also important, not only because of their effects but because tissue fragility makes surgery dangerous. Aortic incompetence, aortic root widening, and mitral valve prolapse all occur. Patients with osteogenesis imperfecta often show hypermobility of joints, with resultant flat feet, hyperextensible large joints, and dislocation.

Type II osteogenesis imperfecta is nearly always lethal, but the severity does differ: some children may be born dismembered, whereas others may (rarely) survive the perinatal period to later merge into the type III form. Not all infants with multiple fractures at birth succumb immediately. It is possible to give a prognosis from the extent of ossification of the skull, the shape of the long bones and ribs, and the number of fractures. In the most frequent form of lethal osteogenesis imperfecta (IIA) the infant is short with disproportionately short and deformed limbs, the skull is deformed and soft, the sclerae are often deep grey-blue. Whole-body radiographs, which distinguish osteogenesis imperfecta from other forms of lethal short-limbed dwarfism, show grossly defective mineralization of the skull, short broad limbs with multiple fractures, and broad ribs with innumerable fractures (Fig. 14). In type IIB, the ribs have some structure; in IIC, the long bones are narrow and beaded at the site of fractures and show some evidence of modelling. Perinatal death results from the mechanical uselessness of the skeleton, which leads to respiratory failure or intracranial haemorrhage.

Type III osteogenesis imperfecta causes most clinical difficulty, since the disability is severe and progressive. During the early years of life, progressive deformity affects the skull, the long bones, the spine, chest, and pelvis; the deformity is associated with fractures but can probably occur without them. The radiological appearance of the bones changes rapidly with age. The face appears triangular, with a large vault, prominent eyes, and small jaw. The sclerae may be blue in infancy but take on a normal colour in childhood. Eventual disability and deformity is considerable. Such patients rarely walk, even after multiple operations, and have a very short stature (–4 to –6 standard deviations (**SD**) below the mean). The changes in the long bones are often bizarre, with long, thin diaphyses and comparatively wide metaphyses. Cartilaginous islands often develop at the end of the long bones in the epiphyses and the metaphyses, spreading into the diaphysis, giving the appearance of 'popcorn' bone. Early death may occur from respiratory infections superimposed on the restrictive reduction in vital capacity associated with severe kyphoscoliosis (Fig. 15). Progressive deformity requires specialized orthopaedic care.

Type IV osteogenesis imperfecta is clinically intermediate between type I and type III and is inherited as a dominant trait. The sclerae are of normal colour after infancy. Overall stature is reduced and disability is variable. The rare complication of hyperplastic callus occurs most often in this form (Fig. 16). This begins with a swollen, painful, and vascular swelling, most often over the long bones, an increase in plasma alkaline phosphatase, and sometimes a systemic illness. Recent investigations of osteogenesis imperfecta-affected families with hyperplastic callus have failed to find collagen mutations in affected children. Some classify this form as type V osteogenesis imperfecta.

Diagnosis

In the perinatal period, the concern is with alternative causes of lethal, short-limbed dwarfism. These include severe hypophosphatasia (see below), achondrogenesis (see below), thanatophoric dwarfism, and the asphyxiating thoracic dystrophies. A perinatal whole-body radiograph is essential.

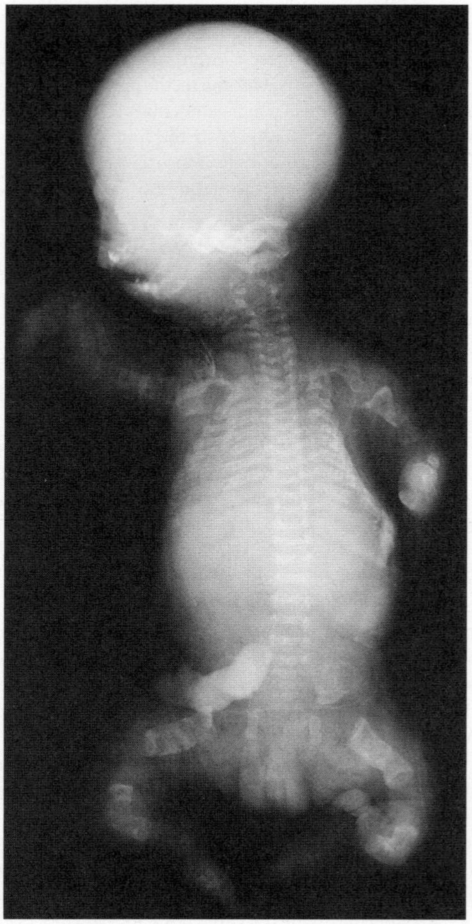

Fig. 14 Whole-body perinatal radiograph (babygram) of lethal (type II) osteogenesis imperfecta. The vault of the skull is not calcified, the ribs and long bones show multiple fractures. There was no family history.

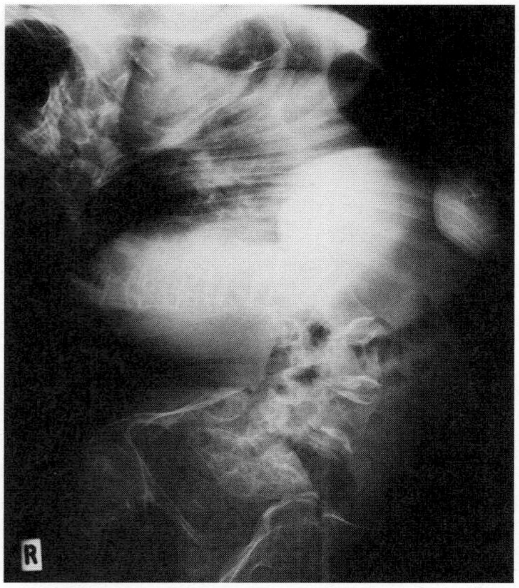

Fig. 15 Severe kyphoscoliosis in type III osteogenesis imperfecta.

In the first few years of life non-accidental injury, 'the battered baby syndrome', is the main differential diagnosis. This is suggested by multiple fractures at different sites and of different ages, especially if associated with clinical signs of neglect. Some fractures, such as metaphyseal 'corner' fractures and posterior rib fractures are more often seen in non-accidental injury, but any type of fracture can occur in osteogenesis imperfecta. The distinction between osteogenesis imperfecta and non-accidental injury is legally important and can be difficult.

Idiopathic juvenile osteoporosis needs to be distinguished during late childhood and adolescence. This begins during growth, with fractures of the long bones, reduction in growth rate (due to vertebral collapse), and metaphyseal compression fractures. In adult life, mild osteogenesis imperfecta may go unrecognized.

Biochemistry

It is impossible to generalize about the clinical effect of a collagen gene mutation but some patterns are emerging. In type I osteogenesis imperfecta there appears to be a null allele for collagen I, so that only 50 per cent of collagen is produced but this is of normal composition. Lethal osteogenesis

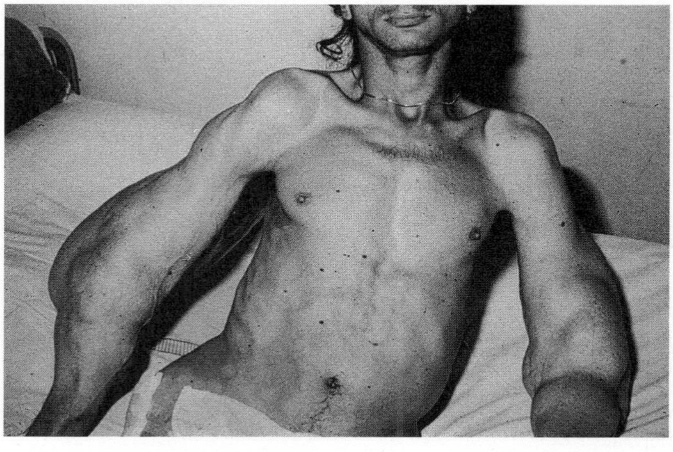

Fig. 16 The appearance of hyperplastic callus in a patient with osteogenesis imperfecta.

imperfecta (type II) may result from large gene deletions but more commonly from single base changes in *COL1A1* or *COL1A2*. Such changes convert a glycine codon to one for another amino acid with a side chain. The effect on the triple helix of incorporating such a mutant chain appears to be most marked when the substitution occurs near the carboxy-terminal end of the chain (the helix winds up from this end), when the substituting amino acid is large; and when it occurs in the α-1 rather than the α-2 chain. Such mutations delay helix formation and render collagen mechanically unsound, and also lead to overhydroxylation and overmodification of the lysine residues, detectable by slowing and widening of the α-chains run on conventional polyacrylamide gels. Such abnormalities are common in type II osteogenesis imperfecta and less well defined in type III, which may rarely result from a failure to synthesize α-2 chains. Type IV osteogenesis imperfecta is most often due to changes in the α-2 chain.

Since the genes for α-1 and α-2 collagen have now been mapped and polymorphic sites identified, the mutant locus for osteogenesis imperfecta can be followed through large, dominantly inherited families. Such information can provide the basis for accurate prenatal diagnosis using fetal DNA derived from a chorionic villus biopsy. Methods are also now becoming available which make it possible to identify the mutation directly in the fetal DNA.

Genetic advice

Parents who have already had an infant with osteogenesis imperfecta need accurate advice about further pregnancies. This can be difficult, because the facts are not clear. Where the mutant gene is dominant (type I and IV) and where one parent is affected, the likelihood of affected children is 50 per cent. Difficulties arise where neither parent is clinically affected, and in the lethal and progressive deforming varieties of the brittle bone syndrome. It is impossible to give a statistically accurate prediction of the likelihood of another affected child, particularly since the strict application of Mendelian principles may be inappropriate because of germline and somatic-cell mosaicism. However, there are some guidelines. Where one offspring of clinically unaffected parents has a form of osteogenesis imperfecta which fits into type I or type IV, this is likely to be a new dominant mutation (50 per cent of whose offspring will be affected) and risk of a further affected sibling is probably no more than normal. It used to be considered that infants with the severe lethal form of osteogenesis imperfect (type II) had inherited a mutant gene from both clinically normal parents and were, therefore, homozygous recessives, so that the risk of a further affected infant was 25 per cent. The evidence is now that the great majority (if not all) result from a new dominant (and lethal) mutation. To allow for the possibility of some recessives, the likelihood of phenotypically normal parents having a second baby with lethal osteogenesis imperfecta is put at approximately 7 per cent (more than normal, but significantly less than 25 per cent).

The recurrence risk in progressively deforming osteogenesis imperfecta (type III) is unknown. If recessive inheritance is included in the definition, it is 25 per cent; if not, it is considerably less.

It is now recognized that germline and somatic-cell mosaicism are important factors in the inheritance and expression of osteogenesis imperfecta, and probably in many other disorders. In brief, germline mosaicism means that the sperm (or ova) of an apparently normal person may contain a proportion of mutant genes for lethal (or other forms) of osteogenesis imperfecta. This accounts for those pedigrees where a phenotypically normal man has two or more babies with lethal osteogenesis imperfecta by separate partners. Somatic mosaicism, with variable proportions of mutant cells in different tissues, likewise provides one (but not the only) explanation for phenotypic variability and differing tissue expression. The many factors that control the regulated expression of the vertebrate collagen genes in different tissues are only partly understood.

Prenatal diagnosis

This may be done from the second trimester by ultrasound and appropriate radiographs, and in the first trimester by analysis of fetal DNA from a chorionic villus biopsy. The appropriateness of such an investigation depends on the information previously available. In a dominantly inherited form of osteogenesis imperfecta, analysis of DNA from affected and unaffected family members can establish linkage to a particular collagen gene polymorphism. In such a situation, analysis of chorionic villus DNA is the most direct approach. Alternatively, the cells from such a biopsy may be cultured and the synthesized collagen examined for abnormalities. Where the collagen mutation is known in a previously affected family member, this method may directly confirm the presence of the mutation in the fetus. Except in well-organized laboratories, culture of cells and analysis of collagen will introduce unacceptable delays. Further, it is usually not possible to exclude an affected fetus merely on the grounds of apparently normal collagen. The rapid direct detection of the mutation in DNA from the chorionic villus is an eventual aim.

Amniocentesis also provides amniocytes for DNA linkage analysis and mutation detection. Amniotic fluid cells tend to produce an α-1(I) homotrimer and are not, therefore, appropriate for collagen analysis.

Diagnosis by ultrasound is possible only in the more severe forms of osteogenesis imperfecta (types II and III). Since the severe forms of osteogenesis imperfecta are sporadic and therefore unsuspected, it is important to be able to detect them early and rapidly by routine scanning. Ultrasound features suggestive of osteogenesis imperfecta are shortness and deformity of the limbs, an abnormal skull shape with lack of mineralization, which makes the intracranial structures abnormally visible, and deformity of the ribs leading to a 'champagne cork' appearance on the anteroposterior projection.

Prognosis and management

For an infant born with manifest osteogenesis imperfecta, important questions are asked: how long will he or she survive; what will be the likelihood of further offspring being affected? The immediate prognosis may already be answered by perinatal death, so that it remains to deal with the prognosis of survivors. Not all born with multiple fractures succumb immediately and radiographic appearances can give a good guide to outcome.

It is in those severely affected survivors classified as type III that management will be a lifelong and specialized problem. Such individuals are of normal intelligence and prolonged admission to hospital, either for repeated surgery or for investigation, should not necessarily take precedence over education. Intramedullary rodding and osteoclasis to correct deformity and improve mobility should be very selective since the bones are often so abnormal as to take no advantage from such procedures. An organized programme of rehabilitation is important. Analysis of life expectancy and cause of death in osteogenesis imperfecta show that survival is normal in type I osteogenesis imperfecta and near-normal in type IV. It is those with type III who have the most disability, of which basilar impression with neurological complications is a newly recognized problem, and the shortest lifespan. There is no convincing evidence that fluoride or calcitonin is beneficial, but cyclic intravenous pamidronate (APD) may alleviate symptoms and increase bone density. In severe osteogenesis imperfecta, attempts to transplant normal stromal cells from bone marrow into severely affected infants with osteogenesis imperfecta have been reported.

The Marfan syndrome (see Chapter 19.2)

The Marfan syndrome (Marfan's syndrome) is most often regarded as an inherited disorder of connective tissue rather than as a metabolic bone disease. Where connective tissue disorders significantly affect the skeleton, this distinction is blurred. For many years, it was thought that the defect underlying the Marfan syndrome involved collagen but recent research excludes this.

Pathophysiology

It is now recognized that Marfan's syndrome is caused by mutations in the epidermal growth factor-like regions of the fibrillin gene on chromosome 15. Fibrillin is the major constituent of the microfibrillar system and of the suspensory ligament of the lens; and it is also associated with elastin-containing tissues such as the aorta. This explains the association between dislocation of the lens and dissection of the aorta. The aorta dilates at its proximal part at the sinuses of Valsalva, and returns to normal diameter below the innominate artery, unless a dissection is present. The cusps of the aortic valve do not close efficiently. Dissection is most often above the aortic valves in the area of greatest dilatation. The dissection may progress forwards or backwards. Retrograde dissection may tear the attachment of the coronary arteries and rupture into the pericardial sac. Histopathology shows a reduction in elastic fibres which are swollen and fragmented. The valve cusps are usually diaphanous and redundant. In the eye, the suspensory ligament of the lens is disorganized.

Clinical features

Marfan's syndrome is dominantly inherited. Its main effects are on the skeleton, cardiovascular, and ocular systems. There is considerable phenotypic variation. In the typical patient with Marfan's syndrome, overall height is increased (relative to unaffected siblings or a matched population) and the limbs are long relative to the trunk (so that the crown to pubis measurement is less than pubis to heel). Long, thin fingers (arachnodactyly) are common. Together with hypermobility, this disproportion forms the basis of clinical signs of variable utility. However, not all patients with Marfan's syndrome are long and thin. The skeletal phenotype differs from one family to another and within families. Asymmetrical anterior chest deformity is associated with either depression or prominence of the sternum. Scoliosis is common, may be severe, and worsens during preadolescent growth as in the idiopathic form. The hard palate is often narrow and high-arched (gothic).

Dislocation of the lens is the main ocular feature of Marfan's syndrome. Typically, this occurs upwards or sideways (in contrast to the downward dislocation in homocystinuria), and this may be present at birth or occur later. Dislocation causes the unsupported iris to wobble on movement (iridodinesis). Less important ocular features are myopia and retinal detachment. The axial length of the globe is increased and the cornea tends to be flattened.

The most severe complication of Marfan's syndrome is dilatation of the ascending aorta leading to aortic incompetence and dissection. Progressive widening of the aorta can be readily measured by serial echocardiography. Less well-known manifestations of Marfan's syndrome include cutaneous striae, hernias, spontaneous pneumothorax, and dural ectasia. The mean life expectancy in those with Marfan's syndrome is reduced by nearly 50 per cent, predominantly due to cardiovascular catastrophe.

Diagnosis

At present, there is no certain biochemical way of excluding or confirming Marfan's syndrome, although this is likely to change. In those with few clinical features and no family history, the diagnosis of Marfan's syndrome can be difficult.

The requirements for the diagnosis of Marfan's syndrome have been revised. Where the family history is not helpful, it is necessary to have major criteria in at least two different organ systems and involvement of a third organ system. Where there is an unequivocally affected relative or a mutation known to cause Marfan's syndrome has been detected, one major criterion in an organ system with involvement of a second organ system is necessary for the diagnosis. Homocystinuria (see below), which has a recessive mode of inheritance, should be excluded. Other important alternative diagnoses include congenital contractural arachnodactyly, familial tall stature, isolated mitral valve prolapse, familial or isolated annuloaortic ectasia, and Stickler's syndrome. The latter is a dominantly inherited connective tissue disorder that affects the eyes, ears, and skeleton with severe myopia in childhood, sensorineural hearing loss from adolescence, and degenerative arthritis from early adult life. The diagnosis can be made at birth if cleft palate and micrognathia are present. There is considerable phenotypic variation. In some families the disorder is linked to the type II collagen gene.

Contractures can occur in Marfan's syndrome but are of a late onset. In congenital contractural arachnodactyly, which is inherited as an autosomal dominant trait, contractures involving the hands, feet, and larger joints are present from birth and tend to improve. Abnormal ears are described. Limited studies suggest that this disorder involves mutations of an additional fibrillin gene on chromosome 5.

Treatment

There is no specific treatment for the underlying defect, but many of the clinical manifestations require attention. Scoliosis may be progressive and severe, particularly in adolescence. Bracing is largely ineffective and operative stabilization may be necessary. Excessive height in girls may be prevented by giving oestrogen together with progestogen in the prepubertal years. Marked sternal deformity may need correction for cosmetic or cardiopulmonary reasons, but opinions on the value of surgery vary widely. In the eyes, it is rarely necessary to remove dislocated lenses unless they prolapse into the anterior chamber, but myopia should be corrected. The main decisions concern the management of the cardiovascular problems: when and if to operate on the dilated ascending aorta or to replace incompetent valves; and whether aortic dilatation can be prevented by reducing the intermittent force on its walls due to left ventricular systole. As far as the second point is concerned, giving a β-blocker such as propranolol probably reduces the rate of aortic dilatation. As regards surgery on the aorta, it is clear that progressive aortic widening (measured regularly by echocardiography), together with progressive aortic incompetence and left ventricular strain, provide strong indications for replacement of the proximal aorta by a prosthesis. Mitral valve replacement may also be necessary.

Since both aortic and mitral valves are susceptible to endocarditis, prophylactic antimicrobials must be given at the time of dentistry.

Genetic advice

Genetic advice is at present based on clinical observations and the knowledge that inheritance is of the autosomal dominant pattern. Numerous mutations in the fibrillin genes have now been described. There is no clear relationship between genotype and phenotype.

Ehlers–Danlos syndrome (see Chapter 19.2)

This syndrome initially included only those conditions with the common clinical features of abnormal velvety hyperelastic skin which healed poorly, hyperextensible joints, and lax ligaments. However, the disorders included in this syndrome have now been increased and have brought with them additional specific features, amongst which is vascular rupture, especially in type IV Ehlers–Danlos syndrome, associated with various mutations in type III collagen. In the currently expanded Ehlers–Danlos syndrome the skeleton is particularly affected in types VI and VII (Table 11).

In type VI (ocular scoliotic) Ehlers–Danlos syndrome) the first disorder in which an inborn error of collagen metabolism was identified, the clinical features are due to lysyl hydroxylase deficiency. Since hydroxylation of peptide-bound lysine is an essential post-translational step in collagen synthesis and a necessary precursor to crosslink formation, this defect weakens collagen structure. The main clinical features are severe scoliosis, microcornea, and ocular fragility.

In type VII (arthrochalasia) there is excessive mobility, perinatal joint dislocations (especially of the hips), and short stature. There is persistence in the tissues of collagen molecules with a retained amino-terminal propeptide which leads to defective fibrillogenesis.

Homocystinuria (see also Chapter 11.3)

Homocystinuria is phenotypically similar to Marfan's syndrome but with a different cause and additional important complications. It is due to a deficiency of cystathionine β-synthase, an enzyme whose gene is located on chromosome 21, and firmly bound pyridoxal phosphate (vitamin B_6) is a feature. Homocystinuria is inherited as an autosomal recessive condition. The amount of residual cystathionine synthase varies from 0 to 10 per cent in patients, and in obligate heterozygotes it is less than 50 per cent of normal.

Pathophysiology

Homocysteine lies at the cross-roads of two metabolic pathways and is converted to cystathionine by the addition of serine. This reaction is controlled by cystathionine β-synthase. The alternative fate of homocysteine is methylation to methionine. Cystathionine β-synthase activity is controlled by pyridoxine, but not all patients with cystathionine-deficient homocystinuria are pyridoxine-sensitive, although this sensitivity or dependency is constant in sibships. In homocystinuria, there is an increase in both homocysteine and homocystine, which accumulate proximal to the metabolic block. Cystathionine, normally present in the brain, is no longer detectable and cysteine (normally made from methionine) becomes an essential amino acid.

The pathological findings include fraying and disruption of the zonular fibres of the lens, defective bone formation, and multiple central nervous system infarcts. It is not known how the biochemical changes lead to the clinical features. The increased thrombotic tendency is not fully explained by changes in platelet function, cellular endothelium, or soluble factors, although abnormalities have been described in all of them. The neurological abnormalities and mental backwardness have not been proven to be due to the biochemical consequences of cystathionine β-synthase deficiency or to repeated vascular thromboses. Homocyst(e)ine may increase the solubility of collagen and interfere with its synthesis; for some, this explains the dislocation of the lens due to failure of the ciliary zonule. Since it is now known that this structure is composed largely of fibrillin, a further explanation is required. There is current interest in the possibility that young adults with premature vascular disease may be heterozygotes for a mutant cystathionine synthase gene. Elevated plasma homocysteine levels are a risk factor for coronary heart disease.

Table 11 Classification and clinical features of the Ehlers–Danlos syndrome

	Type	Inheritance	Skin extensibility and fragility	Bruising	Joint mobility	Other significant features	Biochemical defects
I	Gravis	Dominant	Gross	Severe	Generalized gross	Prematurity; molluscoid pseudotumours; musculoskeletal deformity	Type V collagen
II	Mitis	Dominant	Mild	Mild	Moderate, often limited to hands and feet	None	Type V collagen
III	Benign hypermobile	Dominant	Variable, usually minimal	Mild	Generalized gross	Recurrent joint dislocations; osteoarthritis; skilled contortionists	Not known
IV	Ecchymotic (arterial or Sack–Barabas type; includes acrogeria)	Dominant or recessive	Thin, pale skin with prominent veins	Gross	Minimal, limited to digits	Rupture of great vessels and bowel; elastosis perforans serpiginosa	In synthesis, secretion and structure of type III collagen
V	X-linked	X-linked	Moderate with variable fragility	Variable	Mild	Floppy valve syndrome	Lysyl oxidase deficiency (unconfirmed in other patients)
VI	Ocularscoliotic (hydroxy-lysine deficient disease)	Recessive	Moderate	Moderate	Generalized gross	Scoliosis; microcornea; ocular fragility	Procollagen lysyl hydroxylase deficiency
VII	Arthrochalasis multiplex congenita	Recessive	Moderate	Moderate	Severe	Short stature; congenital dislocations	N-terminal cleavage sites for procollagen peptidase mutated. Different forms described
VIII	Periodontitis	Dominant	Minimal with marked fragility	Mild	Moderate, limited to digits	Advanced generalized periodontitis	Not known
IX	X-linked skeletal	X-linked recessive	Moderate	Moderate	Moderate	Occipital exostoses; deformed clavicles; bowed long bones	Abnormal copper metabolism

Clinical features

The clinical features of cystathionine β-synthase deficiency involve four systems and develop some time after birth; they are ocular, skeletal, central nervous, and vascular. The main ocular manifestation is downward dislocation of the lens. Myopia, glaucoma, retinal degeneration, and detachment also occur, and cataracts, optic atrophy, and corneal abnormalities are described. Some skeletal features suggest Marfan's syndrome. They include a long, thin habitus, pectus excavatum, scoliosis, and genu valgum. There is often radiological osteoporosis and abnormal modelling of the long bones with epimetaphyseal widening. Many subjects with homocystinuria are mentally backward and may also have seizures and strokes. It is unknown how closely these follow the increased tendency to thrombosis or the biochemical changes, especially a lack of cystathionine. Thromboembolism may occur in any vessel and at any age.

Any patient who has the phenotypic features of Marfan's syndrome associated with thrombosis, mental simplicity, and affected siblings should have a cyanide–nitroprusside test performed on their urine, together with an amino acid analysis of the urine and plasma.

The outlook for patients whose biochemical abnormalities are corrected by large amounts of pyridoxine (that is, those with pyridoxine-sensitive homocystinuria) is usually better than those who are pyridoxine-resistant. The main cause of death is thromboembolism.

The management of patients with homocystinuria differs according to the time of diagnosis and whether or not the patient responds to pyridoxine. In pyridoxine-responsive patients diagnosed after the newborn period, giving pyridoxine, in doses that vary from 250 to 1200 mg a day, appears to prevent thromboembolism.

When homocystinuria is detected in the newborn infant (most are discovered by screening and are pyridoxine non-responsive), a diet low in methionine appears to reduce the incidence of low intelligence. After the newborn period, in those who are unresponsive to pyridoxine, methionine restriction and the administration of betaine (as a methyl donor) are also possibly useful lines of approach.

Alkaptonuria (see also Chapter 11.2)

In this rare autosomal recessive disorder, decreased activity of homogentisate oxidase leads to accumulation of homogentistic acid in the urine and increased pigmentation (ochronosis) in cartilage and connective tissues. Darkening of the urine, alkaptonuria, is due to the presence of 2,5-dehydroxyphenylacetic acid derived from the oxidation and polymerization of homogentisic acid. Polymerization increases in alkaline urine and is slowed down by antioxidants such as vitamin C. The structure of the pigment which causes ochronosis is not known. It is granular or homogeneous and may occur within or outside the cell. It is said to be associated with a reduction in lysyl hydroxylase in the tissue concerned, and impairment of the crosslinks of collagen.

Alkaptonuria is more frequent in the former Czechoslovakia and in Germany than elsewhere and occurs equally in the sexes. It is recessively inherited. The mutant gene has now been identified (*HGO*, chromosome 3q2). Abnormal pigmentation is found in the cartilage of the ear (which may be calcified), the nasal cartilage, and the sclerae. The most important effects of this disease are on the spine (Fig. 17) and later on the larger joints. The intervertebral discs lose height and later calcify; they may also herniate acutely. The spine becomes rigid and short and the lumbar lordosis is lost. In the large joints, such as the knees, shoulders, and hips, there are effusions and loose bodies. The symphysis pubis may be affected but not the sacroiliac joints. Ochronotic 'arthritis' is described with episodes of acute inflammation which resemble those of rheumatoid arthritis. Calcification of the aorta is an additional feature.

The diagnosis of alkaptonuria—often made late—should be suspected where there is a premature disc degeneration, even if there is no excessive darkening of the urine. Early degenerative arthritis suggests the disease, confirmed by finding deeply pigmented articular cartilage at the time of operation. In those patients with a lifelong discoloured urine, the differential diagnosis is from other rare causes of urinary pigmentation. The urine of a patient with alkaptonuria contains reducing substances and will therefore give a positive result suggesting glycosuria except where glucose oxidase is used. An increase in homogentisic acid in the urine and plasma confirms the diagnosis.

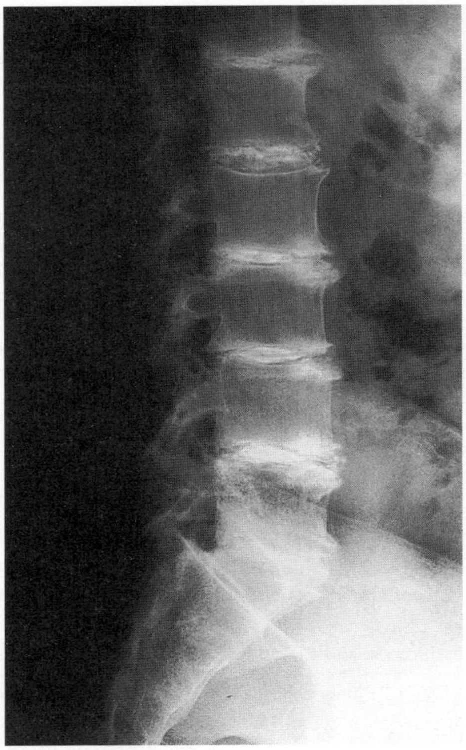

Fig. 17 The appearance of the spine in a man with alkaptonuria. There is universal calcification of the intervertebral discs.

In theory, it should be possible to reduce the amount of homogentisic acid, and presumably the side-effects, by cutting down the protein intake to 30 or 40 g/day, thereby reducing tyrosine intake. There is no evidence that such a procedure alleviates the symptoms of alkaptonuria.

Hypophosphatasia (see also Chapter 12.6.2)

This rare disorder has similarities with rickets and osteomalacia. It is due to a reduction in the tissue non-specific alkaline phosphatase (**TNSAP**), which leads to defective mineralization and a triad of biochemical disturbances: increased urinary phosphoethanolamine, plasma pyrophosphate, and plasma pyridoxal phosphate.

Studies on members of the Mennonite sect in Manitoba, in whom the incidence of hypophosphatasia is high, have linked the defective gene to chromosome 1. Numerous mutations have now been described in the *TNSAP* gene. Although TNASP is widely distributed, its absence leads to lesions only in the bone and teeth.

Pathophysiology

The characteristic biochemical changes result directly from the alkaline phosphatase deficiency. Increased urinary pyrophosphate excretion is more reliable than urinary phosphoethanolamine as a marker for carriers of the hypophosphatasia gene. Often, there is also hypercalcaemia and hypercalciuria in childhood; and up to half of affected children and adults have increased plasma phosphate levels. Hyperphosphataemia is described in carriers of the hypophosphatasia gene. The recorded plasma alkaline phosphatase level must be compared with age-matched control values.

Histological examination of bone shows an excess of osteoid with abnormal tetracycline labelling without evidence of secondary hyperparathyroidism. Matrix vesicles do not contain alkaline phosphatase or hydroxyapatite crystals. The primary dental defect is in the cementum; additionally, the predentine is widened and the dentinal tubules are enlarged and few.

Clinical features

Hypophosphatasia occurs in all races. Since the severe forms are inherited as autosomal recessive traits they are more frequent where there is consanguinity. It has been estimated that hypophosphatasia occurs in 1 in 100 000 live births in Toronto. The four clinical types provide a continuous spectrum, from a lethal perinatal disorder to an asymptomatic disease in adults.

The first is an important cause of lethal, short-limbed dwarfism (see above). Some newborn infants survive for a few days, but fever, failure to thrive, anaemia, seizures, and intracranial haemorrhages occur. Radiographs show grossly defective mineralization, especially in the skull, where only the base may be mineralized, and in diaphyses of the long bones which, rarely, may have bony spurs.

In the infantile form (within the first 6 months), hypotonia, failure to thrive, hypercalcaemia, and hypercalciuria occur. Clinical rickets is noticed and the fontanelle appears wide, but there is a functional synostosis. Craniostenosis can produce optic atrophy, exophthalmos, and raised intracranial pressure requiring surgery.

The most variable expression occurs in childhood. Early loss of deciduous teeth, due to defective cementum, may be the only feature (ondontohypophosphatasia). The pulp chambers are enlarged, the root canals short (shell teeth). If bone disease is present, walking is delayed and deformities occur; for instance, bow legs, knock knees, short stature, and enlargement of the epiphyses at the wrist, knees, and ankles.

In adults, progressive stiffness, pain in the bones, and apparent 'stress' fractures can occur. Approximately 50 per cent of such patients have a childhood history of bone disease resembling rickets, or premature loss of deciduous teeth, or both. There may also be premature shedding of adult teeth, short stature, and abnormal skull shape. Recurrent poorly healing metatarsal fractures occur. Partial fractures of the long bones characteristically occur on the convex outer surface (in contrast to the concave inner position of the Looser's zones in osteomalacia), most often in the upper one-third of the femoral shaft, and are often bilateral; other sites include the ribs, tibias, and ulnas. They may be unaltered for years or increase in size and eventually fracture. Secondary hyperparathyroidism is not seen. Chondrocalcinosis is common and in a proportion is associated with clinical pyrophosphate gout (pseudogout).

Management

In the management of hypophosphatasia, premature synostosis leading to raised intracranial pressure requires surgical relief. Hypercalcaemia may be dealt with by reducing dietary calcium and by giving prednisone. Replacing the defective enzyme by the transfusion of alkaline phosphatase-rich plasma does not produce consistent results. Intramedullary rods may prevent and treat fractures of the long bones. Dental abnormalities, which can occur in biochemically normal members of hypophosphatasia families, may require treatment.

Prenatal diagnosis of a severely affected child can be made by ultrasound. There is also reduced alkaline phosphatase activity in the amniotic fluid cells.

Lysosomal storage diseases (see also Chapter 11.8)

This large group of diseases is due to various inborn errors that affect the function of specific lysosomal enzymes normally responsible for the breakdown of a variety of complex molecules. As a result, these molecules, or their partially degraded derivatives, accumulate in the lysosomes and the tissues that contain them. The effect of this accumulation varies from one tissue to another according to the particular disorder, and the skeleton is significantly involved in only a proportion of them. They include some mucopolysaccharidoses and Gaucher's disease.

Mucopolysaccharidoses

Failure of the normal lysosomal breakdown of complex carbohydrates leads to their accumulation in the tissues, and produces many clinical abnormalities. The disorders may be divided into two main groups according to the chemistry of the accumulated substance, namely the mucopolysaccharidoses and the mucolipidoses. Specific biochemical defects are described elsewhere in this book (see Section 11). Since some of these disorders have a prominent effect on the skeleton, they are briefly mentioned here; they are the Hurler syndrome (mucopolysaccharidosis type IH; **MPS IH**), the Hunter syndrome (MPS II), and the Morquio syndrome (MPS IV). With certain exceptions the bone changes themselves do not permit precise diagnosis of the type of dysplasia present, or distinction from the mucolipidoses.

The Hurler syndrome (MPS IH)

This is the most severe type of mucopolysaccharidosis and causes death at an early age. The enzyme defect is recessively inherited and all patients have the same appearance, to which the term 'gargoylism' was previously applied. Affected infants appear to develop normally in the first few months of life, but then deteriorate mentally and physically. Death often occurs in late childhood, commonly due to pneumonia or to coronary artery disease associated with mucopolysaccharide deposits.

The physical features include proportionate short stature (Table 3), a typical facial appearance, a short neck with a lumbar gibbus and chest deformity, and a protuberant abdomen. The facial features are coarse and ugly, with flattening of the nasal bridge, with large open mouth and tongue, and often with hypertrophied gums over enlarged alveolar ridges. The eyes are prominent with corneal clouding. There is noisy breathing and variable deafness. The vault of the skull may show scaphocephaly or acrocephaly. Other striking features include the stiff, broad trident hands and the large abdomen with hepatosplenomegaly. Radiographs show the abnormal shape of the skull, the slipper-shaped sella turcica, the beaking of the vertebrae with the thoracolumbar kyphosis, and the bullet-shaped phalanges. Similar but less severe features are seen in the Hunter syndrome, which is inherited as an X-linked recessive.

The Morquio syndrome (MPS IV)

In this disorder the orthopaedic manifestations are striking, but intelligence is normal. Although the disorder is probably heterogeneous and only a proportion of cases excrete an excess of keratan sulphate in the urine, the skeletal changes are uniform. In the first years of life the child becomes progressively more deformed and dwarfed. Characteristically the neck is short, the sternum is protuberant, and there may be a flexed stance with knock knees. There is a striking loss of muscle tone in comparison to the stiffness of MPS IH; hypermobility and a loose skin are features. Radiographs in infancy show a spine similar to that seen in those with Hurler syndrome, but later flattening of the vertebrae with anterior beaking lead to relative shortening of the trunk. The small bones of the hands are very different from those of MPS IH and the metacarpals show diaphyseal constriction (Fig. 18).

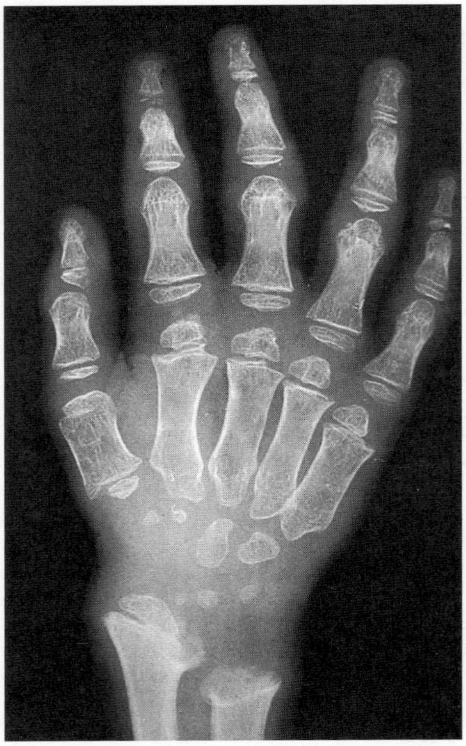

Fig. 18 The appearance of the hands in MPS IV (Morquio syndrome).

Importantly, the odontoid may be hypoplastic, leading to atlantoaxial instability, compression of the long spinal tracts, and paraplegia.

Gaucher's disease (see also Chapter 11.8)

This is a rare lysosomal storage disorder in which glucocerebroside-containing macrophages accumulate within the bone marrow, spleen, liver, and other organs. It is recessively inherited and over-represented in Ashkenazi Jews, where the incidence of the adult form (type I) is about 1 in 2500 births. The skeletal manifestations are often severe and disabling. They vary from a characteristic but clinically insignificant failure of remodelling in the lower femora (Erlenmeyer-flask appearance) to diffuse and localized bone loss and osteosclerotic and osteonecrotic lesions, which cause pain and pathological fracture, often requiring precocious joint replacement surgery.

Skeletal dysplasias

The term 'skeletal dysplasia' has traditionally been used to cover a wide range of generalized disorders of the skeleton, often of unknown cause, affecting both cartilage and bone. With increasing knowledge one can distinguish the chondrodysplasias, which are primarily due to mutations affecting cartilage, from such disorders as diaphyseal dysplasia and assorted dense bone diseases, where the causes are less well known. Since osteopetrosis is a well-defined disorder of osteoclast function, it is dealt with separately below.

The mutations in many of the skeletal dysplasias have been described (Table 1) and the skeletal dysplasias can be classified into biochemical families according to their cause (Table 12). The supposition that many of them could be due to mutations in specific collagens has been partially confirmed with mutations found in type I, IX, X, and XI collagens. Achondroplasia is a striking example of a skeletal dysplasia caused by a non-collagen mutation, that is a mutation in fibroblast growth factor (**FGF**)-receptor 3.

Table 12 Skeletal dysplasias—molecular families

Gene*	Dysplasia
COLIAI	Osteogenesis imperfecta
COLIA2	Osteogenesis imperfecta
COL2A1	Spondyloepiphyseal dysplasia
	Kniest dysplasia
	Achondrogenesis
COL9A2	Multiple epiphyseal dysplasia
COL10A1	Schmid metaphyseal dysplasia
COL11A2	Stickler syndrome
COMP	Pseudoachondroplasia
	Multiple epiphyseal dysplasia
DTDST	Diastrophic dysplasia
	Achondrogenesis
PTP/PTHrP-receptor	Jansen metaphyseal chondrodysplasia
FGFR3	Achondroplasia
	Hypochondroplasia
	Thanatophoric dwarfism
FGFR2	Crouzon syndrome
	Apert syndrome
SOX9	Campomelic dysplasia

* *COL1A1*, etc.; various collagen genes. COMP, cartilage oligomeric protein; DTDST, diastrophic dysplasia sulphate transporter; FGFR; fibroblast growth-factor receptor; *SOX9*, a sex-reversal gene.

Further details can be found in reviews (see the Further reading list) and in Table 12.

Clinical features

The physician confronted by a patient with a skeletal dysplasia is unlikely to make the correct diagnosis without much additional help unless it is clearly one of the most frequent, for instance achondroplasia. However, accurate classification of the dysplasias is important and will make clinical and biochemical advance possible. The most convenient simple classification is a clinical one (Table 13). Most patients with skeletal dysplasias have restricted growth, and most are short-limbed. The bodily proportions of people with skeletal dysplasias will provide a clue about whether the limbs are mainly affected, or the spine, or both. In the short-limbed group, achondroplasia and achondroplasia-like dwarfs are the most typical. Those disorders without conspicuous dwarfing include various inherited epiphyseal dysplasias, diaphyseal dysplasias, and some, but not all, metaphyseal dysplasias. An alternative classification, not based on height, groups the dysplasias according to whether they are predominantly epiphyseal or metaphyseal, whether the spine is predominantly involved, and whether single limbs or segments

Table 13 The main causes of ectopic mineralization

Calcification without bone formation	
Dystrophic:	secondary to tissue damage
Metastatic:	secondary to biochemical abnormalities
Hypocalcaemia	
Hypercalcaemia	
Hyperphosphataemia	
Hypophosphataemia	
Calcification with bone formation (ectopic ossification)	
Acquired	
After injury	
After neurological damage	
In tumours	
Other disorders	
Inherited	
Fibrodysplasia (myositis) ossificans progressiva	
Familial osteoma cutis	

are involved. Radiographs, taken as soon as possible and, where possible, consecutively, are essential to determine whether the metaphyses of the long bones or the epiphyses are primarily affected.

For the purpose of this Section, osteopetrosis (marble bones disease) is dealt with separately as a disorder of bone-cell biology. Other sclerosing disorders of bone, in some of which biochemical abnormalities have been described (Engelmann's disease, van Buchem's disease), receive brief mention.

Achondroplasia

This is the prototype of short-limbed, short stature. It is inherited as an autosomal dominant, with a high mutation rate and the incidence increases with paternal age. It is due to a specific mutation in the gene encoding the FGF-receptor 3. The way in which this produces the skeletal changes is largely unknown. Until recently, any undiagnosed patient with excessively short limbs was given the label of achondroplasia. This explains the apparent high frequency of achondroplasia and its high mortality, since different forms of lethal, short-limbed dwarfism were then included.

As the clinical definition of achondroplasia has not always been exact, its true incidence and natural history are not well defined. There is a failure of the epiphyseal growth cartilage, and bulbous masses of cartilage appear at the ends of the long bones. In contrast, periosteal and membrane bone formation and bone repair are normal. This selective effect on growth cartilage accounts for the skeletal deformity.

Achondroplasia can be diagnosed at birth or within the first year of life, when the disparity between the large skull and short limbs becomes obvious. There is a striking disproportion between the normal length trunk and the short arms and legs. Thus the fingertips may only come down to the iliac crest. The shortness of the limbs particularly affects the proximal segment. The limbs themselves look very broad, with abnormally deep creases, and the hands are trident-like. In contrast to the short limbs is the enlarged bulging vault of the skull, the small face, and flat nasal bridge or 'scooped out' glabella. There is a marked lumbar lordosis and also sometimes some wedging of the upper lumbar vertebrae, which may later lead to a thoracolumbar kyphosis. Radiological features include metaphyseal irregularity and flaring in the long bones, irregular and late-appearing epiphyses, a narrow pelvis in its anteroposterior diameter, with short iliac wings and deep sacroiliac notches, and a spine that shows progressive narrowing of the interpedicular distance from above downwards, which is the reverse of normal.

Children with achondroplasia are of normal intelligence, and the complications of this disease arise particularly from the skeletal disproportion. This may lead to early osteoarthritis, to obstetric difficulties and the need for caesarean section, to hydrocephalus, and to paraplegia. Eventual height can vary between about 80 and 150 cm. Recent reviews emphasize how often narrowing of the spinal canal produces symptoms of spinal stenosis.

Homozygous achondroplasia (the offspring of two affected parents) is severe and lethal. In the condition of hypochondroplasia, which is included in the same *FGFR3* molecular family, the skeletal disproportion and the spinal abnormalities are less and the skull is unaffected.

Achondroplasia-like dwarfism

For details of these and other causes of short-limbed dwarfism the reader should consult more specialized texts). Those that most closely resemble achondroplasia at birth are thanatophoric dwarfism, achondrogenesis, severe hypophosphatasia, and type II osteogenesis imperfecta. All can be distinguished radiologically.

Spondyloepiphyseal dysplasias

This is a heterogeneous group of disorders in which the spine is predominantly affected and the short stature is partly due to shortness of the trunk. The most severe type is spondyloepiphyseal dysplasia (**SED**) congenita; milder forms are referred to as SED tarda. There are various forms of inheritance. Some forms are due to mutations in type II collagen.

SED tarda often has an X-linked mode of inheritance, so that only males are affected and females are carriers. In affected males the disproportionately short trunk becomes obvious at adolescence. Failure of ossification in the anterior part of the so-called ring epiphyses leads to central and posterior humps on the upper and lower parts of the flattened bodies. The condition needs to be distinguished from multiple epiphyseal dysplasia, which involves other major joints more than the spine.

SED congenita can be diagnosed at birth because of the short stature associated with a short trunk. There may be a close resemblance to Morquio's disease (MPS IV, see above). The severe form may be distinguished from the age of about 4 years. The appearance of the capital femoral epiphyses is delayed (in some patients it may never be seen, except by arthrography). Marked lumbar lordosis, waddling gait, back pain, and progressive disproportion may occur. The odontoid is hypoplastic, kyphoscoliosis may develop, and the interpedicular distances of the vertebrae do not increase in the lumbar region. Paraplegia may occur as a result of all these changes. In this disorder there is often myopia and retinal detachment.

There is a form of SED, pseudoachondroplasia, which resembles achondroplasia because of the short limbs, but here the facial appearances are normal. The short stature becomes obvious from about 2 years of age. Lumbar lordosis and scoliosis may develop. The tubular bones are short with irregular metaphyses and small, deformed epiphyses. Hypermobility is marked and early osteoarthritis occurs. The causal mutation is in the gene for the cartilage oligomeric protein (*COMP*, chromosome 19p16).

Proportionate dwarfism

Although it is clinically important to classify short stature into proportionate and disproportionate, there are many conditions in which this distinction is difficult to make. Hypophosphataemic rickets, mucopolysaccharidoses, vitamin D-dependent rickets, and osteogenesis imperfecta may come into both categories.

Bone dysplasias without conspicuous short stature

The height of patients with multiple epiphyseal dysplasia may be only slightly reduced. Although many epiphyses are affected, the spine is virtually normal. There are also variable forms of inheritance. Some are due to mutations in collagen type IX; others to mutations in cartilage oligomeric protein.

In patients with multiple hereditary exostoses (often referred to as diaphyseal aclasis) there is a juxtaepiphyseal disorder of bone growth, limited to bones developed in cartilage, which gives rise to cartilage-capped exostoses that point away from the joint. Inheritance is autosomal dominant and stature is normal. It is likely that there are causal mutations in putative tumour suppressor genes.

The metaphyseal disorders are rare; some, such as the Jansen type of metaphyseal dysostosis (associated with a mutation in the gene for the PTH/PTHrP receptor) do cause severe dwarfing. In others with less severe growth disturbance, such as Type Schmid (due to a mutation in the type X collagen gene), rickets is simulated, and confusion with inherited hypophosphataemia is possible. In progressive diaphyseal dysplasia (see below) the limbs are disproportionately long.

Sclerosing disorders of bone

Apart from marble bones disease (see below) the experience of most physicians of the osteoscleroses is limited by their extreme rarity.

Engelmann's disease (progressive diaphyseal dysplasia: Camurati–Engelmann disease)

This rare condition is autosomal dominantly inherited. It affects endocrine and muscular systems in addition to the skeleton, where the main feature is a variable but progressive endosteal and periosteal thickening of the diaphyses of the long bones. In severely affected subjects the spine, skull, and axial skeleton are all affected. The cause is unknown.

There is a waddling broad-based gait, muscle wasting and weakness, loss of subcutaneous tissues, and pain in the legs during childhood. The appearance is characteristic; the head is large with a prominent forehead and proptosis, the muscle mass is reduced, and the bones are palpably thickened. Cranial nerve palsies, deafness, and blindness with raised intracranial pressure can occur. Puberty is delayed. Bone pain resistant to analgesia is often a presenting and troublesome feature.

Radiographic appearances vary, from limited thickening of the diaphyses (often in the lower extremities) to widespread new bone formation, affecting all bones, including the skull, demonstrated by scintigraphy.

The increased bone turnover causes a moderate increase in plasma alkaline phosphatase and urinary hydroxyproline levels. There may be a markedly positive calcium balance, associated with hypocalcaemia and hypocalciuria. Hyperphosphataemia has been recorded.

Pathological examination confirms gross thickening of the bone with disorganization of internal structure and external shape. The peripheral subperiosteal new bone is woven. The muscles show non-specific, type-II fibre atrophy.

In the differential diagnosis the proximal myopathy and abnormal gait simulate muscular dystrophy. The radiographic appearances are diagnostic, although idiopathic hyperphosphatasia may present some difficulties.

The course of this disorder is unpredictable and remission of symptoms may occur during adolescence or adult life, so it is difficult to assess treatment. Bone pain may respond to corticosteroids in small, alternate-day doses. Etidronate (20 mg/kg daily) has produced hypocalcaemic tetany, but intermittent administration is reported to reduce pain. Limb pain may be relieved by surgical removal of a cortical window in the diaphysis.

Pyknodystosis

In contrast to Engelmann's disease, pyknodystosis has an autosomal recessive mode of inheritance, with parental consanguinity in some 30 per cent of subjects. It has some similarities to osteopetrosis. Since the disease is caused by mutations that lead to deficiency of cathepsin K, an enzyme necessary for osteoclast function, this is not unexpected. Marked reduction in stature with short limbs is a particular clinical feature.

The vault of the skull is large, the face and chin small, the palate high-arched, and the teeth crowded, with retained deciduous teeth. The anterior fontanelle (and other cranial sutures) remain unfused. The painter Toulouse-Lautrec is regarded as a typical example of this disease. The fingers may appear to be clubbed because of associated acro-osteolysis. The chest is deformed with kyphoscoliosis and pectus excavatum. Recurrent fractures of long bones occur, and occasionally rickets. Radiologically, there are similarities to osteopetrosis with generalized osteosclerosis and fractures. However, the osteosclerosis is uniform; there are no defects of modelling and no endobones. In addition to delayed closure of the cranial sutures there are also wormian bones; the bony fragility, wormian bones, and blue sclerae simulate osteogenesis imperfecta.

Idiopathic hyperphosphatasia

This very rare condition is also labelled 'juvenile Paget's disease'. It has autosomal recessive inheritance. The long bones are abnormal, thickened, and bowed from the first year of life, and the skull may be enlarged. Muscular weakness is common and the plasma alkaline phosphatase level is continuously very high.

Sclerosteosis

This condition is due to an autosomal recessive trait. There is progressive overgrowth and sclerosis of the skeleton, including the skull and the mandible. There are similarities to van Buchem's disease (endosteal hyperostosis), but the skeletal problems are more severe and there is often syndactyly. Prophylactic craniectomy may be necessary to reduce the increased intracranial pressure.

van Buchem's disease

In this rare hyperostosis, endosteal thickening of the shafts of the long bones is associated with generalized hyperostosis, including the base of the skull and the mandible. Bilateral facial nerve weakness, deafness, and optic atrophy may ensue. Severe recessive and mild dominant forms are described.

Cleidocranial dysplasia

In this rare condition the clavicles are hypoplastic or absent, the fontanelles remain open, and there are supernumerary teeth. The heterozygous mutation causes a loss of CBFA1, the osteoblast transcription factor (see above).

Osteopetrosis (marble bones disease)

Among those disorders with increased bone density, marble bones disease or osteopetrosis (Albers–Schönberg disease) is the best known. It is a heterogeneous disorder with a widespread increase in bone density. In most cases, the basic defect lies in the osteoclasts which, for various reasons, are unable to resorb mineralized bone. Many animal models of osteopetrosis exist.

Until recently two main forms were distinguished: recessively inherited severe osteopetrosis causing death in childhood; and the dominantly inherited mild form, in which the diagnosis can be made on radiological grounds alone. This distinction is not absolute—two distinct dominantly inherited forms exist, as well as intermediate forms. Deficiency of carbonic anhydrase II can also cause osteopetrosis associated with cerebral calcification, renal tubular acidosis, growth failure, and mental simplicity.

Severe osteopetrosis

In severe recessively inherited osteopetrosis there is widespread increased density of the bones without modelling or remodelling. This produces the Erlenmeyer-flask deformity of the metaphyses. The increase in bone density is often intermittent, producing alternating bands of sclerosis. The failure of resorption leads to a reduction in bone marrow space with a leucoerythroblastic anaemia and hepatosplenomegaly. It also produces nerve compression, with blindness and often deafness. Other clinical features in this severe form can include hydrocephalus, delayed tooth eruption, and osteomyelitis. Fracture of the dense bones is common. The affected infant is short with an apparently large head with frontal bossing, hepatosplenomegaly, and knock knees. The plasma calcium level appears to alter with the dietary intake and may be sufficiently low to contribute to rickets. The acid phosphatase concentration (derived from the defective osteoclasts) is increased. Secondary hyperparathyroidism leads to an increase in calcitriol levels. Apart from transplantation of bone marrow, as a source of normal osteoclasts, from an appropriate donor, other forms of medical treatment deal only with complications; these include surgery for fractures, blood transfusions for anaemia, and antibiotics for frequent infections.

Mild osteopetrosis

The mild forms vary from subjects with an increased number of fractures affecting both the long bones and the small bones of the hands and feet, to those in which the disorder is so mild that the diagnosis is made by radiology alone (accounting for apparently unaffected generations with the dominant form of the disease). There are more severe forms of dominantly inherited osteopetrosis with nerve compression, deafness and blindness, and anaemia at times of increased physiological requirement, such as pregnancy. Other established features include osteomyelitis and facial nerve palsy.

Recent studies of Danish families define two dominantly inherited forms: one with uniformly dense bones with sclerosis of the cranial vault and the spine and no increase in the plasma acid phosphatase level, and another with variable bone density (giving rise to an endobone appearance, Fig. 19) and lack of modelling, with a significant increase in the plasma acid phosphatase level.

Carbonic anhydrase II deficiency

The association of carbonic anhydrase II deficiency with osteopetrosis, renal tubular acidosis, cerebral calcification, some degree of mental retardation, growth failure, and dental malocclusion is of considerable interest because of the clues it provides to the normal function of carbonic anhydrase II in bone resorption. Carbonic anhydrase II is part of the carbonic anhydrase gene family and is widely distributed. It is found in the kidney, brain, red cells, and elsewhere, and its gene is on chromosome 22. Deficiency of carbonic anhydrase II is autosomal recessively inherited, and apparently normal parents of affected offspring have 50 per cent of normal carbonic anhydrase II levels within their red cells. The bone disease is not distinguishable from other forms of osteopetrosis, and fractures occur until adulthood. There is always growth retardation, and height may be more than four standard deviations below the mean. The bone age is also delayed. Radiographic appearances improve in adult life.

The renal tubular acidosis is mixed, both proximal and distal. Cerebral calcification affects the basal ganglia within the first decade. It increases during childhood to include the cortical grey matter and is similar to that occurring in idiopathic or pseudohypoparathyroidism. Bone histology shows unresorbed calcified cartilage and osteoclasts without a ruffled border.

The diagnosis of carbonic anhydrase II deficiency should be considered in any neonate with renal tubular acidosis. Genetic counselling is possible since adult heterozygotes have reduced levels of the enzyme in their red cells. However, the concentration of carbonic anhydrase II is normally very low at birth and cannot be used as a reliable neonatal test for the affected homozygote.

The treatment of carbonic anhydrase II deficiency is symptomatic; it is possible that correction of the renal tubular acidosis temporarily increases the rate of growth.

In the differential diagnosis of osteopetrosis there are many disorders with an excessive amount of bone in various parts of the skeleton; these include other skeletal dysplasias, Caffey's disease (infantile cortical hyperostosis) which causes a temporary increase in bone density from birth, and myelofibrosis, renal glomerular osteodystrophy, inherited hypophosphataemia, and fluorosis in adult life.

Fibrous dysplasia

Fibrous dysplasia of bone is a condition in which areas of immature fibrous tissue, either single or multiple, are found within the skeleton. Recent research has shown a widespread postzygotic activating mutation in the gene for a subunit of the G-protein signalling system. The extent to which this activating mutation affects the bone and other tissues depends on the degree of mosaicism, in other words the proportion and distribution of cells that carry the mutation. It is proposed that such a mutation in the germline would be lethal; certainly the condition is not inherited.

Monostotic fibrous dysplasia

This disorder is relatively common in orthopaedic practice. Although the lesions may occur in any bones, and particularly in the facial bones and ribs, the most frequent presenting symptom at any age is a fracture, often of the upper end of the femur (Fig. 20). The biochemistry is usually normal, and the diagnosis is made from the radiographic and pathological appearances. There is a smooth-walled translucent area within the bone, often with thinning of the cortex and sometimes with associated deformity. Pathologically, areas of disorganized fibrous tissue are are found, associated with woven bone and wide osteoid seams. This represents mosaic tissue with some normal mesenchymal cells and some carrying the mutation. The

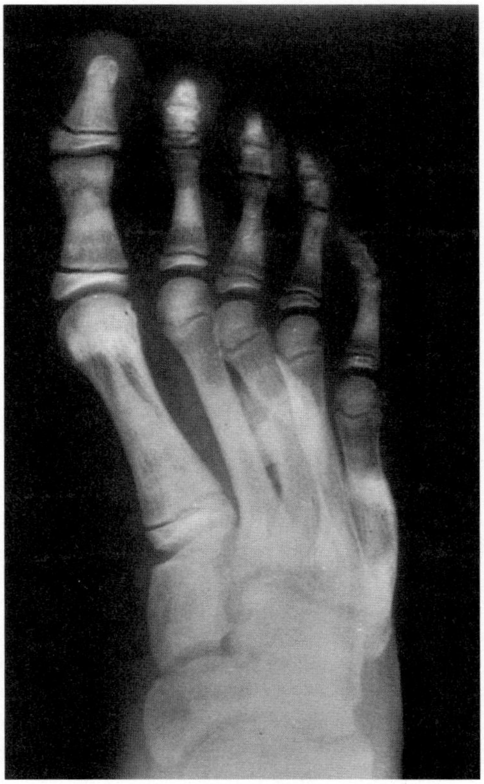

Fig. 19 The appearance of the bones in a boy with dominantly inherited osteopetrosis and a raised plasma acid phosphatase level. There are variations in bone density ('endobones') with recent and old pathological fractures.

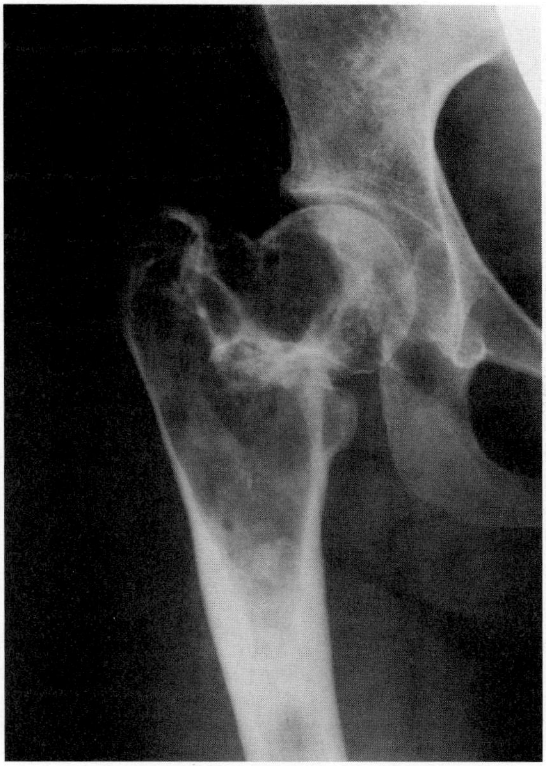

Fig. 20 Polyostotic fibrous dysplasia in a 23-year-old woman. A large cyst in the upper femur led to a spontaneous fracture which subsequently united with conservative treatment. Two ribs on the same side of the body show similar abnormalities. Puberty was precocious but pigmentation absent.

differential diagnosis is from other causes of bone cysts, from Paget's disease, and from hyperparathyroidism with osteitis fibrosa cystica. In the monostotic form treatment is largely orthopaedic. However, the large size of some of the defects in the shafts of the long bones may make conventional stabilization of fractures very difficult. Improvement with intravenous pamidronate (APD) has been reported.

Polyostotic fibrous dysplasia (see Chapter 12.8.6)

Interest in this condition, in which the bone lesions are multiple, arises from its frequent association with pigmentation and sexual precocity, especially in females (McCune–Albright syndrome). The bone lesions and the brown pigmentation are typically associated in position (but not in extent), and may be restricted to one side of the body. Sexual precocity is present in about 50 per cent of females with polyostotic disease, and is then the presenting complaint. It may occur at a very early age, with menstruation and the appearance of secondary sexual characteristics from infancy. Where sexual precocity is not a feature, deformity and fracture are often the first symptoms. Gross deformity of the upper femur and femoral neck produces the 'shepherd's crook' appearance. Asymmetry of the long bones and of the skull are also seen; and in about half of the cases the base of the skull is thickened. The macular pigmentation tends to have smooth borders (in contrast to those of neurofibromatosis) and often does not cross the midline. In a recent long-term follow-up of 15 patients with two or more features of the McCune–Albright triad, the bone lesions tended to increase in size and number, but less rapidly after growth had ceased. Skin lesions were generally bilateral and did not correlate with the site of the bone lesions. There are a number of other features which, like the sexual precocity, are explained by the activating mutation. These include thyrotoxicosis, acromegaly, and Cushing's syndrome. The skeletal lesions may cause complications such as spinal cord compression, and may be associated with hypophosphataemic osteomalacia. Sarcoma formation has been reported, but only after irradiation.

In the polyostotic disease both the plasma alkaline phosphatase and the urinary hydroxyproline levels may be slightly increased and that of plasma phosphate slightly reduced. The pathology is similar to the monostotic form, but it is said that cartilage- and fluid-filled cysts are more common. Microscopically, there is an abundance of woven bone and an increase in osteoblasts and osteoclasts. The cortex and marrow may be virtually replaced by fibrous tissue, so that the bones are fragile. Healing is rapid with abundant callus formation. Radiologically, the bones are deformed, the cortex may be difficult to detect, and the medullary bone takes on a 'ground glass' or 'smoky' appearance.

In polyostotic fibrous dysplasia the main differential diagnosis is from osseous neurofibromatosis; in the former condition there is also pigmentation, bone deformity, and sometimes hypophosphataemic osteomalacia. The borders of the pigmentation are less smooth than in fibrous dysplasia, and there are other cutaneous features of neurofibromatosis; the bone deformity in neurofibromatosis can be quite bizarre, with overgrowth or undergrowth of isolated bones. In neurofibromatosis the characteristic spinal change is a very sharp upper thoracic kyphoscoliosis. Finally, neurofibromatosis often shows clear evidence of dominant inheritance pattern.

The medical treatment of the McCune–Albright syndrome is complex. As for the monostotic from, polyostotic fibrous dysplasia may be improved by pamidronate (APD).

Ectopic mineralization

Deposition of calcium in the soft tissues (ectopic calcification) and on ectopic bone matrix (ossification) has many causes (Table 13). These are nearly always pathological, but often the cause is unknown. In the elderly, calcification in the tissues such as the arteries is so common that it may be regarded as a feature of ageing, in the same way as age-related bone loss. There are some disorders in which calcification and/or ossification are associated with biochemical abnormalities.

Ectopic calcification without bone formation

Calcification can result from previous damage in soft tissues (dystrophic calcification) or from an increase in the circulating concentration of calcium or phosphate (metastatic calcification as, for instance, in advanced renal osteodystrophy).

Dystrophic calcification

This occurs in inherited and acquired disorders involving connective tissue, such as alkaptonuria (intervertebral discs), pseudoxanthoma elasticum (blood vessels), systemic sclerosis, and dermatomyositis, and also after infection, tumours, and trauma. In systemic sclerosis, subcutaneous calcification, often around the phalanges (calcinosis circumscripta), may be part of a syndrome with Raynaud's phenomenon and telangiectases (**CRST**; calcinosis, Raynaud's phenomenon, sclerodactyly, telangiectasia) syndrome; see also Chapter 18.10.3). The calcific deposits can be sufficiently extensive to break through the skin as toothpaste-like material. In dermatomyositis, sheets of subcutaneous calcification can be deposited some time after the initial inflammatory episode characterized by a systemic illness and painful weak muscles; the calcification can be very extensive (calcinosis universalis), but can also disappear rapidly, sometimes in adolescence. Rarely this is associated with hypercalcaemia.

Metastatic calcification

The distribution of the calcification varies inexplicably with its cause; for example, in hypoparathyroidism there is subcutaneous and basal ganglia calcification and in hyperparathyroidism vascular calcification, suggesting that metastatic calcification is not only related to the Ca:P product. Calcification and ossification may also coexist.

Calcification and hypocalcaemia

This occurs in idiopathic and postsurgical hypoparathyroidism, as well as in pseudohypoparathyroidism. There may be extensive ectopic calcification, calcification within the basal ganglia (and outside it), and cataract formation. Pseudohypoparathyroidism is inherited as an autosomal dominant disorder with variable expression; additional clinical features include mental simplicity, round face, short stature, and short third and fourth metacarpals. An important feature is subcutaneous endochondral ossification. End-organ resistance to parathyroid hormone may be due to mutations in the gene responsible for one component ($G_s\alpha$) of the G-protein signalling system (Table 1).

Calcification in hyperphosphataemia

Idiopathic hyperphosphataemia is a rare autosomal recessive disorder, with an increase in the maximal tubular reabsorption of phosphate and an inappropriate increase in the plasma $1,25(OH)_2D$ concentration. Masses of ectopic mineral, which form around the joints from childhood (tumoral calcinosis), may discharge through the skin. Treatment with large oral doses of aluminium hydroxide or other phosphate-binding agents can reduce the plasma phosphate level and the size of the deposits.

Calcification in inherited hypophosphataemia

A particular feature of X-linked inherited hypophosphataemia is the widespread calcification and ossification of ligaments and tendons at their insertions into the periosteum (so-called Sharpey fibres). This is termed an enthesiopathy. Calcification and new bone formation in the ligamenta flava may produce spinal cord compression.

Idiopathic soft-tissue calcification

This includes calcific tendinitis and so-called calcinosis circumscripta.

Ectopic ossification

Acquired ectopic ossification may occur at the site of injury, such as after hip replacement or at a distance from it, for instance, following paraplegia; or in tumours and in a variety of other disorders. Fibrodysplasia (myositis) ossificans progressiva is a very rare disorder inherited as an autosomal dominant (see below).

Acquired ectopic ossification

Post-traumatic ossification

Local ossification can occur after total hip replacement. The quoted incidence varies widely, depending on the method used to detect it. It is said to occur more often in men than in women and in certain individuals; for instance, where ossification follows hip replacement on one side, it is likely to occur if the contralateral hip is also replaced. The reason for this is unknown. The bone mainly forms in the hip abductors and ossification is classified according to its severity. Disodium etidronate may delay mineralization, but only while it is being given, and non-steroidal anti-inflammatory drugs are also useful. A small dose of radiotherapy may also delay ectopic ossification after total hip replacement.

Ossification after neurological injury

Extensive myositis ossificans can also occur 1 to 4 months after injuries to the head or spinal cord, in muscles distant from the injury such as the major muscles of the thigh. Affected muscles become swollen, red, and warm, and, unless the cord lesion is complete, pain and tenderness also occur. At this time the differential diagnosis may include cellulitis, arthritis, and thrombophlebitis. Radiological calcification is initially absent (appearing at about 6 weeks or more after the injury), but an isotope bone scan will show increased uptake before that. Later there is progressive mineralization, with the eventual appearance of organized bone. Because the bone affects the major periarticular muscles, it leads to joint fixation, particularly of the hips. The plasma alkaline phosphatase level may be increased in the early stages.

Attempted surgical removal of ectopic bone is technically difficult and produces little increase in movement. The ectopic bone recurs, especially if it is removed too early. Oral disodium etidronate at full dose (20 mg/kg body weight per day) may delay the onset of mineralization, but only while it is being given. Likewise, the prevention of further ectopic bone formation after its removal may be delayed by non-steroidal anti-inflammatory drugs or radiotherapy, which should be commenced as soon as possible.

Myositis ossificans can also occur after other neurological diseases, such as poliomyelitis and meningitis, and also after prolonged coma. The reason why ectopic ossification occurs after head injury is unknown; interestingly head injury is associated with an increased rate of fracture healing and excessive callus formation. In such patients the serum contains increased mitogenic activity for osteoblast-like cells; the source of this activity is unknown, but there could be an increase in bone morphogenic proteins.

Ossification can coexist with calcification, and, for instance, extensive ossification of the spinal ligaments in hypoparathyroidism can lead to progressive stiffness. The enthesiopathy in inherited hypophosphataemia (vitamin D-resistant rickets) is a form of ectopic ossification. Ossification of the posterior longitudinal ligament and sternoclavicular hyperostosis is particularly described in Japan. Ligamentous ossification has been noted in patients treated with vitamin A analogues, such as etretinate, for dermatological disorders. The term 'osteoma cutis' covers a number of rare conditions of uncertain cause. Finally, ectopic bone may complicate varicose veins, chronic venous insufficiency, and surgical incisions.

Inherited ectopic ossification

The main inherited cause of ectopic ossification is myositis ossificans progressiva. This disorder is currently classified as a 'heritable disorder of connective tissue'.

Histology suggests (to some) that it is the connective tissue within muscles that is primarily involved and therefore the alternative term 'fibrodysplasia ossificans progressiva' is widely used.

Fibrodysplasia ossificans progressiva is rare, with an incidence of between 1 and 2 per million, which increases with paternal age. Since patients rarely reproduce, most instances represent new mutations. The few family histories demonstrate that the mutant gene is inherited as a dominant with full penetrance but variable expression. Diagnosis depends on the combination of progressive myositis, leading to ossification in the major skeletal muscles, and characteristic bony skeletal abnormalities.

Pathophysiology

Initially there is oedema and cellular infiltration throughout the muscle, with myofibrillar breakdown. Later endochondral ossification leads to mature bone, within which is haemopoietic marrow. Information on the earliest histological appearances is scanty because biopsies are often taken after the acute phase of myositis; for this reason there is still doubt about the primary lesion. Ectopic ossification occurs when mesenchymal or stromal cells take on the behaviour of osteoblasts. This form of cell differentiation could result from an increase in bone-inducing substances or (for unknown reasons) a change in stromal-cell expression. Although the timing of myositis differs widely from one affected patient to another, there is a specific order in which they are affected, from the upper paraspinal to the lower, and from the centre to the periphery. Recent work suggests overexpression of the bone morphogenetic proteins (**BMP**-4). Localization of the mutant gene is hampered by the lack of affected families.

Clinical features

Episodes of myositis are the non-skeletal hallmark of this disease. Typically, the affected muscle becomes swollen and hard, sometimes following injury; after a week or two these features subside, but the apparent improvement is followed in a month or so by ossification within the muscle and progressive joint fixation. Myositis usually begins in the upper paraspinal muscles. By late childhood or adolescence ossification will have occurred within the muscles around the shoulders, hips, and knees, to fix these joints and to complete the disability. The large, striated muscles are affected; ossification does not involve the small muscles of the hands and feet, the diaphragm, the cardiac, or the smooth muscles. Ossification in the muscles around the jaw may fix it almost completely. Although the overall sequence of ossification is characteristic from large upper paraspinal to lower limb muscles, it varies considerably in its rate. For instance, neonates may have sufficient ossification to produce torticollis while, in contrast, late and slow ossification producing stiffness may delay the correct diagnosis until adolescence. Likewise, there may be long symptom-free periods.

The diagnostic skeletal abnormalities affect the big toes (Fig. 21) (and to a lesser extent the thumbs), the cervical spine (Fig. 22), and the metaphyses. The big toes are always abnormal; in the infant, bony changes produce bilateral hallux valgus and, in the adult, fusion produces a short fixed monophalangic big toe. In the cervical spine the vertebral bodies are small and the laminae large. Both are variably fused; and this fusion is independent of nearby ossification of the cervical muscles. Finally, the femoral necks are short and wide and there are exostoses from the metaphyses.

Rare clinical features include early onset baldness, difficulty in hearing, and mental retardation.

Differential diagnosis

Bilateral hallux valgus in the neonate should suggest the possibility of fibrodysplasia ossificans progressiva. In childhood, myositis may be mistaken for soft-tissue sarcoma; and a biopsy showing oedema and increased cellularity may support this or suggest an aggressive fibromatosis. Painful swelling of the masticatory muscles simulates mumps; and progressive stiffness with a

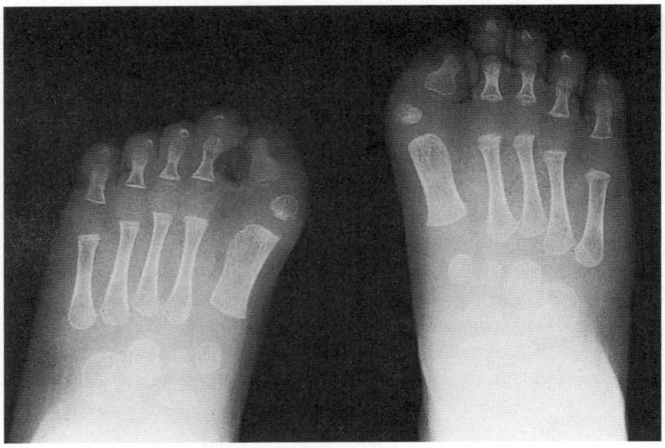

Fig. 21 The abnormal short big toes in an infant with fibrodysplasia ossificans progressiva.

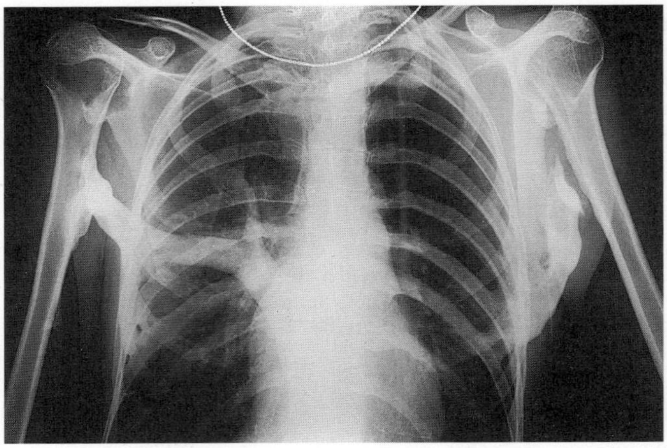

Fig. 23 Extensive ectopic ossification in the paraspinal muscles fixing the shoulders in a patient with fibrodysplasia ossificans progressiva.

fixed abnormal neck suggests the Klippel–Feil syndrome or childhood rheumatoid arthritis.

Management

Once the diagnosis has been made, and this is often delayed, there are four main questions: can the myositis be prevented; if myositis does occur, can subsequent ossification be prevented; what will be the eventual disability; and should ectopic bone be removed?

Since the onset of myositis is quite unpredictable, it is almost impossible to assess the effect of any form of therapy. Corticosteroids have been used, sometimes associated with symptom-free periods. Myositis often follows injury, which should be avoided where possible. It seems likely, but difficult to prove, that myositis is normally followed by ossification. It is to prevent or slow down this ossification that the bisphosphonate EHDP (disodium etidronate) can be given in full doses (20 mg/kg body weight daily by mouth), but there is little evidence that this is effective. In children, continued high-dose etidronate interferes with mineralization, disorganizes the growth plates, and delays fracture healing so that it is not an acceptable long-term treatment. Surgical removal of ectopic bone is technically difficult and recurrence at the site of surgery worsens the disability.

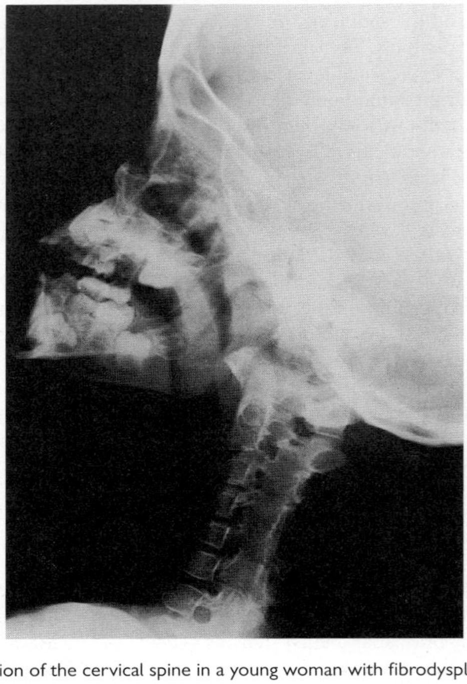

Fig. 22 Fusion of the cervical spine in a young woman with fibrodysplasia ossificans progressiva.

The eventual disability produced by fibrodysplasia ossificans progressiva is severe (Fig. 23). The body moves as in one piece with the legs usually fixed in partial extension. All major joints become completely fixed. The help of a specialized rehabilitation centre is essential.

Familial osteoma cutis

This has been reported as a dominantly inherited disorder in a New Zealand family. The proposita had extensive subcutaneous ossification in one leg; relatives had insignificant multifocal subcutaneous ossification in childhood. Similar patients have been described under the name of progressive osseous heteroplasia.

Miscellaneous bone disorders

The skeleton is affected in many systemic diseases (for example, scurvy and the haemoglobinopathies), by the methods used to treat them (for example, parenteral nutrition), and by excessive ingestion of minerals, vitamins, and metals (for example, fluorosis, overdose of vitamins A and D, and metal poisoning). In some, the skeletal changes are clinically important; in others they are a minor aspect of the general illness. This Section ends with a brief description of the obscure disorder fibrogenesis imperfecta ossium.

Scurvy

Vitamin C (ascorbic acid) is necessary for intracellular hydroxylation of peptide-bound proline. In its absence, formation of the collagen molecule is defective, structurally incompetent precursors accumulate within the cell, and collagen-containing tissues are weak. Scurvy is very rare, occurring most often in neglected infants who do not receive fruit juice or ascorbic acid for several months. Extensive subperiosteal haemorrhage leads to pain and immobility; the legs are held in a 'frog-like' position. In the adult, there is perifollicular haemorrhage, purpura, and bleeding gums. Radiographs in infancy show a widened zone of provisional calcification in the metaphyses, with a proximal disordered area representing the destroyed primary spongiosa and failure of new bone formation. The edges of the metaphyses may show small spurs, and epiphyseolysis may occur. With healing the subperiosteal haematoma calcifies.

The clinical picture of scurvy may suggest non-accidental injury, but scurvy is far less common. Similar radiographic appearances have been described in cases of copper deficiency.

The haemoglobinopathies

In the inherited disorders of haemoglobin (see Section 22) the skeleton is often abnormal. This may result from a hyperplastic bone marrow and overactivity of the osteoblasts, so that the skull, facial bones, and long bones are thickened. Additional features include collapse of the weight-bearing bones and disorganization of the joints following bone infarction. This is especially seen in sickle-cell disease, haemoglobin C disease, and haemoglobin SC compound-heterozygotes. In β-thalassaemia an increase in osteoid thickness has been described which resembles that of osteomalacia.

Parenteral nutrition

Prolonged parenteral nutrition can produce a form of bone disease with similarities to osteomalacia. The main symptom is periarticular bone pain, particularly in the ankles. Histology shows impaired mineralization of bone, and biochemistry an increase in plasma alkaline phosphatase, in urinary calcium, and sometimes in plasma calcium levels. The radiographic appearances suggest osteoporosis. Since patients on total parenteral nutrition are invariably ill to begin with, and many have malabsorption, there are several probable causes for this disorder; aluminium intoxication may contribute.

Fluorosis

Deposition of excess fluoride in the skeleton can result from an excess in the diet (endemic fluorosis), from industrial exposure (during the manufacture of aluminium, steel, and glass, and from exposure to the dust of fluoride-containing rock), and from the administration of sodium fluoride in treatment. The most severe effects are seen in endemic fluorosis, well described from the Punjab.

There is considerable disability, with spinal rigidity, restricted movements of the joints, and flexion deformities of the hips and knees. There is a generalized increase in bone density (with loss of the normal corticomedullary junction), and the tendons, ligaments, and sometimes muscles may be mineralized. This can produce compression of the spinal cord and its roots, with progressive neurological disability. Mineralization of tendon insertions may be seen in other situations, such as inherited hypophosphataemia (see above), retinoid treatment, and fibrogenesis imperfecta ossium (see below).

Increased levels of fluoride can affect the enamel of developing teeth, producing chalky-white patches, yellow-brown discoloration, and other defects.

The diagnosis of fluorosis depends on the radiographic changes and an increased urinary excretion of fluoride (which is an index of current exposure). When a bone biopsy is performed (most often to exclude other causes of increased bone density), histology shows an increase in new bone formation with an increase in the width of osteoid borders. There is also an increase in fibrous tissue and bone resorption. When the biopsy includes an area of tendinous insertion, this may be mineralized.

Sodium fluoride has been given widely to treat osteoporosis and produces increased vertebral density. Current evidence does not suggest that this increases vertebral bone strength and suggests that there is an increase in appendicular bone fracture. The main effect of the fluoride ion is to stimulate new bone formation, while fluoroapatite may also reduce resorption. The new bone appears to be mainly woven in character and imperfectly mineralized. Although there is no doubt about the anabolic effects of fluoride on bone, current controversies about its clinical usefulness depend, in part, on the dose used.

Vitamin A

Retinoic acid and its derivatives have profound effects on osteoblast function. Vitamin A poisoning produces characteristic periostitis in the young skeleton, and therapeutic retinoids (such as etretinate) causes widespread ligamentous calcification. Acute and chronic forms of vitamin A overdosage are described. In infants, it is uncommon under the age of 1 year. There is anorexia and failure to thrive; other features include pruritus, hepatosplenomegaly, jaundice, alopecia, dry skin, and fissures around the lips. Hard, tender masses appear in the limbs, and radiographs show periosteal new bone formation, especially in the diaphyses of the tibias, which later blends into the cortex. A number of other radiological features include shortening of the shafts of the long bones, splaying of the metaphyses, enlargement and premature fusion of the ossification centres, and flexion deformities of the legs.

The prolonged use of retinoids for the treatment of skin disease, such as psoriasis and ichthyosis, leads particularly to calcification of the spinal ligaments, causing stiffness and reduced mobility. There is a resemblance to Forestier's disease (diffuse idiopathic skeletal hyperostosis).

Vitamin D

Vitamin D poisoning can result from inappropriate therapeutic overdosage or accidental overconsumption. This leads to the features of hypercalcaemia (see Chapters 10.3 and 12.6.2) without detectable effects on the skeleton. The main opportunities for overdose exist when potent preparations of vitamin D are used inappropriately (as, for instance, to treat skin conditions and tuberculosis). Chronic vitamin D overdosage leads to soft-tissue calcification, especially in the arteries and kidneys. After several years, progressive stiffness in the spine, major joints, and feet lead to difficulty in walking. Radiographs show ligamentous calcification. Another cause of hypercalcaemia is an excess of $1,25(OH)_2D$ produced by granulomas, especially those of sarcoidosis following exposure of the skin to sunlight. The biochemical effects are the same as those of vitamin D poisoning. The $1,25(OH)_2D$ concentration increases with that of 25(OH)D, and the hypercalcaemia of sarcoidosis often occurs during the spring in persons with outdoor jobs (such as farmers, window cleaners) or after foreign holidays in the sun. Treatment with corticosteroids and removal from sunlight rapidly reduces the hypercalcaemia and the elevated $1,25(OH)_2D$ levels.

Idiopathic hypercalcaemia can occur in infancy. Now named the Williams syndrome, it is associated with an unusual 'elfin face', mental simplicity, and congenital heart disease. Radiographs of the long bones show increased density of the metaphyses. The cause is not fully understood, but the concentration of 25(OH)D may be increased when the patients are hypercalcaemic. Deletion of the elastin locus on chromosome 7 has also been described and may explain the cardiac abnormalities.

Lead (see also Chapter 8.1)

Lead has unique effects on the skeleton, which may be combined with the other manifestations of lead intoxication. Lead deposition in the growing skeleton produces a radiologically dense line near the growth plate. When exposure to lead has been intermittent, or the condition has been treated, this may be a single, relatively narrow line, which is superseded by apparently normal bone. If exposure to lead recurs, a further line will appear.

Lead poisoning due to industrial pollution is thought to be widespread, but the skeleton is affected only when lead exposure has been considerable. In children, one recognized source is lead-containing paint. Other sources include contaminated water from old lead pipes, eye blackener used by Asian women (which contains up to 88 per cent lead sulphide), inhalation of lead fumes from burning old battery cases, and alcoholic drinks stored in vessels of lead glass or coated by lead enamel glaze.

Clinical features involve: the gastrointestinal tract (abdominal pain, colic with constipation, and a blue pigmentation of the gingival margin); the neuromuscular system, with weakness; and encephalopathy, with restlessness, irritability, and lethargy. Renal manifestations are described in Section 20.

Characteristic radiological features include widened skull sutures (due to raised intracranial pressure in infants), dense deposits in the gastrointestinal tract indicating heavy-metal ingestion, and dense lines in the metaphyses (lead lines). Such lines are an important clue to lead poisoning in infants and children up to about the age of 6 years. They occur most commonly around the knees, wrists, and ankles, and appear after about a month of chronic poisoning. The diagnosis of lead poisoning is confirmed by an increase in plasma and urinary lead levels. There are other causes of radiologically dense metaphyses. These include: other heavy metals—bismuth, mercury, or phosphorus; vitamin D intoxication and idiopathic hypercalcaemia of infancy; cretinism; and healing rickets. In practice, there is often difficulty in deciding on the significance of dense metaphyses due to excessive calcium in an otherwise well child, since this appearance can occur in the normal growing skeleton.

Aluminium (See also Chapter 8.1)

Aluminium in water is not significantly absorbed through the intestine, but this barrier was effectively removed in the early days of haemodialysis treatment for endstage renal failure. The resultant accumulation of aluminium in the skeleton in patients in some units where the aluminium content of tap water was high led to the occurrence and recognition of 'dialysis bone disease'. There was a close clinical association with dialysis dementia, also related to aluminium poisoning. The clinical features of this bone disease were proximal myopathy, multiple painful spontaneous fractures with radiographic evidence of osteopenia (osteoporosis), histological evidence of excess osteoid with aluminium deposition near the calcification front, and an absence of response to vitamin D metabolites.

In renal glomerular failure, aluminium may also accumulate in patients given oral aluminium hydroxide to reduce plasma phosphate (in order to lessen hypocalcaemia and subsequent secondary hyperparathyroidism). Aluminium bone disease can also occur in patients on prolonged parenteral nutrition.

The pathology of aluminium bone disease is not fully understood, but it seems likely that in some instances aluminium reduces osteoblast activity. Two different forms are described: in the first, there is excessive osteoid (with an appearance like that of osteomalacia); and in the second, there is little increase in osteoid with reduced osteoblastic activity. It is likely that the different histological features are related to the amount of aluminium in the bones.

Cadmium (See also Chapter 8.1)

Contamination of drinking water by cadmium and its accumulation in the body causes renal tubular damage with multiple biochemical defects. Cadmium intoxication is one of the acquired causes of the Fanconi syndrome which leads to rickets or osteomalacia. Industrial exposure to cadmium fumes can produce hypophosphataemic osteomalacia.

Exceptionally, chronic lead poisoning can also produce osteomalacia by the same mechanism as cadmium; and copper 'poisoning' causes the Fanconi syndrome and bone disease of Wilson's disease.

Fibrogenesis imperfecta ossium

This is a very rare, apparently acquired disorder, characterized by excessive bony fragility due to the replacement of normal bone with a fibre-deficient, poorly mineralized matrix. The cause is unknown. In recorded cases, the main clinical feature has been pathological fractures first presenting in adult life. In most patients, progressive disability has followed, with more fractures that fail to unite. Radiologically, the trabeculae throughout the skeleton appear to be thickened. There is also ectopic mineralization around large joints and tendon insertions. Biochemically, plasma calcium and phosphate levels are normal, but the alkaline phosphatase level is moderately raised. In the urine, monoclonal light chains may be present. The diagnosis is confirmed by the examination of undecalcified bone. This shows defective mineralization and wide osteoid seams suggesting severe osteomalacia, but the osteoid is not birefringent under polarized light and the normal structure of bone collagen under electron microscopy is absent. The differential diagnosis is from those disorders that produce widespread coarse trabeculation throughout the skeleton, and those that produce the histological changes of osteomalacia. In the first category, Paget's disease of bone, renal glomerular osteodystrophy, and fluorosis should be excluded, and in the second, axial osteomalacia has some similarities; in this very rare osteosclerotic disorder, both histology and radiographs suggest that the osteomalacia is limited to the spine, pelvis, and ribs.

Since the cause of fibrogenesis imperfecta ossium is unknown, treatment to date has been largely empirical. The occasional finding of an excess of plasma cells in the bone marrow, or a monoclonal gammopathy, or light-chain proteinuria, has led to apparently successful treatment with melphalan and prednisolone. Where surgery is indicated for fractures, particularly of the femoral neck, this is difficult because of the extreme fragility of the bones.

Although it seems likely that the defect may be related to an acquired disorder of bone collagen, no consistent abnormality has been detected.

Sudeck's atrophy

This is one of many synonyms of what is more often referred to as 'algodystrophy' (painful dystrophy). Its features are pain, swelling, and tenderness, most often of a limb, which is persistent and recurrent. Early oedema and erythema may be replaced by a dystrophic phase that may last for months, with pallor or cyanosis. The skin and subcutaneous tissues may atrophy and there is increased sweating and often worsening of the pain. The main known precipitating cause of algodystrophy is trauma, such as forearm (Colles) fracture. In at least one-quarter of patients there is no identifiable cause. The recorded prevalence of algodystrophy varies widely, depending on its definition and how closely it is looked for; in a specific study made to identify algodystrophy it was found in 25 per cent of patients 9 weeks after Colles fracture, a frequency far higher than normally recorded.

The treatment of algodystrophy is difficult and requires consideration of the whole patient. Adequate pain relief, reassurance, and explanation are essential. Numerous other measures have been proposed; these include courses of corticosteroids and calcitonin, regional sympathetic block, and surgical sympathectomy, none of which is consistently useful. Bisphosphonates, such as pamidronate, may prove to benefit symptoms and outcome, but no controlled trial data are currently available to substantiate their general use where bone loss occurs (see below).

Algodystrophy is often associated with localized bone loss, and some include so-called regional and transient migratory osteoporosis within the algodystrophy syndrome, although the reasons for doing so are tenuous. Characteristically, there is severe localized osteoporosis associated with pain which recurs in different limbs. The increased bone resorptive activity associated with bone loss may be identified by the use of bisphosphonate skeletal scintigraphy, which may assist diagnosis in the early phases of this condition. Further investigation may show that the osteoporosis is more widespread than suspected with, for instance, vertebral compression fractures. Rarely, osteoporosis occurs in pregnancy (see above) predominantly affecting the spine, but also other peripheral bones, leading, for instance, to femoral neck fractures.

Further reading

Bone physiology

Avioli LV, Krane SM (1998). *Metabolic bone disease*, 3rd edn. Academic Press, San Diego.

Bilezikian JP, Raisz LG, Rodan GA (2002). *Principles of bone biology*, 2nd edn. Academic Press, San Diego.

Byers PH (1995). Disorders of collagen biosynthesis and structure. In: Scriver CR, *et al.*, eds. *The metabolic basis of inherited disease*, 7th edn, Volume III, pp 4029–77. McGraw Hill, New York.

Jilka RL (1998). Cytokines, bone modelling and oestrogen deficiency: a 1998 update. *Bone* **23**, 75–81.

Manolagos SC, Jilka RL (1995). Bone marrow, cytokines, and bone remodelling. *New England Journal of Medicine* **332**, 305–11.

Royce PM, Steinmann B (1992). *Connective tissue and its heritable disorders. Molecular, genetic and medical aspects*, 1st edn. Wiley–Liss, New York.

Russell RGG (1997). The assessment of bone metabolism *in vivo* using biochemical approaches. *Hormone and Metabolic Research* **29**, 138–44.

Suda T, *et al.* (1999). Modulation of osteoclast differentiation and function by the new members of the tumour necrosis factor receptor and ligand families. *Endocrine Reviews* **20**, 345–57.

Diagnosis of bone disease

Blumsohn A, Eastell R (1997). The performance and utility of biochemical markers of bone turnover: do we know enough to use them in clinical practice? *Annals of Clinical Biochemistry* **34**, 449–59.

Favus MJ (1999). *Primer on the metabolic bone diseases and disorders of mineral metabolism*, 4th edn. Lippincott, Williams and Wilkins, Philadelphia.

Osteomalacia and rickets

Francis RM, Selby PL (1997). Osteomalacia. *Baillieres Clinical Endocrinology and Metabolism* **II**, 145–63.

O'Riordan JLH (1997). Rickets, from history to molecular biology, from monkeys to YACS. *Journal of Endocrinology* **154**, S3–S13.

Parfitt AM (1998). Osteomalacia and related disorders. In: Avioli LV, Krane SM, eds. *Metabolic bone disease*, 3rd edn, pp 327–86. Academic Press, San Diego.

Paget's disease

Barker DJP *et al.* (1977). Paget's disease of bone in 14 British towns. *British Medical Journal* **1**, 1181–3.

Cooper C, *et al.* (1999). Epidemiology of Paget's disease of bone. *Bone* **24**, 35–55 (Suppl.).

Delmas PD, Meunier PJ (1997). The management of Paget's disease of bone. *New England Journal of Medicine* **336**, 558–66.

Kanis JA (1998). *Pathophysiology and treatment of Paget's disease of bone*, 2nd edn. Martin Dunitz, London.

Parathyroids and bone disease

Bassett JHD, Thakker RV (1995). Molecular genetics of disorders of calcium homeostasis. *Baillieres Clinical Endocrinology and Metabolism* **9**, 581–608.

Osteogenesis imperfecta: the brittle bone syndrome

Glorieux FH, *et al.* (1998). Cyclic administration of pamidronate in children with severe osteogenesis imperfecta. *New England Journal of Medicine* **339**, 947–52.

Pope FM (1998). Molecular abnormalities of collagen and connective tissue. In: Maddison PJ, *et al.*, eds. *Oxford textbook of rheumatology*, 2nd edn, pp 353–404. Oxford University Press, Oxford.

Smith R (1995). Idiopathic juvenile osteoporosis: experience of twenty one patients. *British Journal of Rheumatology* **34**, 68–77.

Smith R (1999). Osteogenesis imperfecta; the brittle syndrome. An update. *Current Orthopaedics* **13**, 218–22.

Marfan's syndrome

De Paepe A, *et al.* (1996). Revised diagnostic criteria for the Marfan syndrome. *American Journal of Medical Genetics* **62**, 417–26.

Pyeritz RE (1993). The Marfan syndrome. In: Royce PM, Steinmann B, eds. *Connective tissue and its heritable disorders*, pp 437–68. Wiley–Liss, New York.

Shores J, *et al.* (1994). Progression of aortic dilatation and the benefit of longterm β adrenergic blockade in Marfan's syndrome. *New England Journal of Medicine* **330**, 1335–41.

Ehlers–Danlos syndrome

Pope FM (1998). Molecular abnormalities of collagen and connective tissue. In: Maddison PJ, *et al.*, eds. *Oxford textbook of rheumatology*, 2nd edn, pp 353–404. Oxford University Press, Oxford.

Steinmann B, Royce PM, Superti-Furga A (1993). The Ehlers–Danlos syndrome. In: Royce PM, Steinmann B, eds. *Connective tissue and its heritable disorders*, pp 351–401. Wiley–Liss, New York.

Homocystinuria

Isherwood DM (1996). Homocystinuria. Early diagnosis and intervention reduces risk of visual impairment and thromboembolism. *British Medical Journal* **313**, 1025–6 [Editorial].

Nygard O, *et al.* (1997). Plasma homocysteine levels and mortality in patients with coronary artery disease. *New England Journal of Medicine* **337**, 230–6.

Skovby F (1993). The homocystinurias. In: Royce PM, Steinmann B, eds. *Connective tissue and its heritable disorders*, pp 469–86. Wiley–Liss, New York.

Alkaptonuria

Hazleman BL, Adebajo AO (1993). Alcaptonuria. In: Royce PM, Steinmann B, eds. *Connective tissue and its heritable disorders*, pp 591–602. Wiley–Liss, New York.

Hypophosphatasia

Whyte MP (1993). Osteopetrosis and the heritable forms of rickets. In Royce PM, Steinmann B, eds. *Connective tissue and its heritable disorders*, pp 563–9. Wiley–Liss, New York.

Whyte MP (1999). Hypophosphatasia. In: Favus MJ, ed. *Primer on the metabolic bone diseases and disorders of mineral metabolism*, 4th edn, pp 337–9. Lippincott, Williams and Wilkins, Baltimore, MD.

Lysosomal storage diseases

Leroy JG, Weismann U (1993). Disorders of lysosomal enzymes. In: Royce PM, Steinmann B, eds. *Connective tissue and its heritable disorders*, pp 613–39. Wiley–Liss, New York.

Mankin HJ, *et al.* (1990). Metabolic bone disease in patients with Gaucher's disease. In: Avioli LV, Krane SM, eds. *Metabolic bone disease*, 2nd edn, pp 730–52. WB Saunders, Philadelphia.

Skeletal dysplasias

Francomano CA, McIntosh I, Wilkins DJ (1996). Bone dysplasias in man: molecular insights. *Current Opinion in Genetics and Development* **6**, 301–8.

Gelb BD, *et al.* (1996). Pycnodysostosis, a lysosomal disease caused by cathepsin K deficiency. *Science* **273**, 1236–8.

Horton WA (1996). Molecular genetic basis of the human chondrodysplasias. *Endocrinology and Metabolism Clinics of North America* **25**, 683–97.

Horton WA, Hecht JT (1993). The chondrodysplasias. In: Royce PM, Steinmann B, eds. *Connective tissue and its heritable disorders*, pp 641–75. Wiley–Liss, New York.

Schipani E, *et al.* (1996). Constitutively activated receptors for parathyroid hormone and parathyroid hormone-related peptide in Jansen's metaphyseal chondrodysplasia. *New England Journal of Medicine* **335**, 708–14.

Osteopetrosis (marble bones disease)

Key LL, Ries WL (1996). Osteopetrosis. In: Bilezikian JP, Raisz LG, Rodan GA, eds. *Principles of bone biology*, 1st edn, pp 941–50 Academic Press, San Diego, CA.

Fibrous dysplasia

Chapurlat RD, *et al.* (1997). Long term effects of intravenous pamidronate on fibrous dysplasia of bone. *Journal of Bone and Mineral Research* **12**, 1746–52.

Ectopic ossification

Connor JM, Evans DAP (1982). Fibrodysplasia ossificans progressiva. The clinical features and natural history of 34 patients. *Journal of Bone and Joint Surgery* **64B**, 76–83.

Kaplan FS (1998). Fibrodysplasia ossificans progressiva. *Clinical orthopaedics and related research* **346**, 1–140 (Symposium).

Smith R, Athanasou N, Vipond SE (1996). Fibrodysplasia (myositis) ossificans progressiva; clinicopathological features and natural history. *Quarterly Journal of Medicine* **89**, 445–56.

Miscellaneous bone disorders

Carr AJ, *et al.* (1995). Fibrogenesis imperfecta ossium. *Journal of Bone and Joint Surgery* **77B**, 820–9.

Smith R (1993). Heritable bone diseases, chondrodysplasias and skeletal poisons. In Nordin BEC, Need AG, Morris HA, eds. *Metabolic bone and stone disease*, 3rd edn, pp 213–48. Churchill Livingstone, Edinburgh.

Sudeck's atrophy

Littlejohn GO (1998). Algodystrophy (reflex sympathetic dystrophy). In: Maddison PJ, *et al.*, eds. *Oxford textbook of rheumatology*, 2nd edn, pp 1679–89. Oxford University Press, Oxford.

19.2 Inherited defects of connective tissue: Ehlers–Danlos syndrome, Marfan's syndrome, and pseudoxanthoma elasticum

F. M. Pope

Introduction

Ehlers–Danlos syndrome, pseudoxanthoma elasticum, and the Marfan syndrome are characterized by the fragility of connective tissues and thus cause diverse clinical disease. These inherited defects disrupt the integrity of structural proteins found in the skin, ligaments, cartilage, and vasculature and share common clinical features (Table 1). Connective tissue is also affected in the pleura, peritoneum, heart valves, gastrointestinal system, muscles, and other tissues with similar scaffolding components. Moreover, defects of connective tissue also disrupt basement membranes present in the eyes, skin, and kidneys.

A notable feature of connective tissues is the existence of molecular interactions between structural proteins and extracellular matrix. These

Table 1 Clinical features shared between inherited disorders of connective tissue

Clinical feature	Disorder	Frequency
Span > height	Marfan's syndrome	Common/consistent
	Ehlers–Danlos syndrome type III	Uncommon
	Ehlers–Danlos syndrome type IV	Rare
	Beals' syndrome	Variable
	Osteogenesis imperfecta	Rare
	Pseudoxanthoma elasticum	Rare
Lens dislocation	Marfan's syndrome	Very common
	Weill–Marchesani syndrome	Variable
	Homocystinuria	Uncommon
Blue sclerae	Osteogenesis imperfecta (I, II, III)	Consistent, very common
	Ehlers–Danlos syndrome type VII	Common
	Ehlers–Danlos syndrome types I, II, and VI	Variable
	Pseudoxanthoma elasticum	Uncommon
Aortic dilatation	Marfan's syndrome	Common/consistent
	Ehlers–Danlos syndrome type IV	Occasional
	Osteogenesis imperfecta (1 and 2 mutants)	Variable
Hypermobility	Ehlers–Danlos syndrome type III	Consistent/common
	Ehlers–Danlos syndrome types VI/VII	Common
	Ehlers–Danlos syndrome types I/II	Variable
	Osteogenesis imperfecta	Variable
	Pseudoxanthoma elasticum	Variable (especially heterozygotes)
Pneumothorax	Marfan's syndrome	Frequent
	Ehlers–Danlos syndrome type IV	Frequent
	Ehlers–Danlos syndrome type III	Variable
	Other Ehlers–Danlos syndromes	Rare
	Osteogenesis imperfecta	Rare
Intestinal perforation	Ehlers–Danlos syndrome type IV	Frequent
	Ehlers–Danlos syndrome type III	Rare to variable
High myopia	Marfan's syndrome	Common
	Stickler syndrome	Common
Low myopia	Marfan's syndrome	Variable
	Ehlers–Danlos syndrome types I/II	Variable
	Pseudoxanthoma elasticum	Variable
Vitreous detachment	Stickler syndrome	Consistent/common
	Ehlers–Danlos syndrome type VI	Variable
	Marfan's syndrome	Rare

interactions are important early in development and involve early embryonic patterning co-ordinated by the expression of homeobox proteins, including those of the hedgehog family. Inherited defects of protein constituents in connective tissues may thus disturb many tissues during development and organogenesis.

For all these reasons, inherited defects of connective tissue impinge widely on the practice of medicine. In the ageing population, increased fragility of the skin, rupture of blood vessels, and laxity of ligaments, as well as defects of cartilage and bone, overlap to form a series of disorders that declare themselves in adult life. Such 'degenerative disorders' include osteoporosis, osteoarthritis, and arterial aneurysms. In the light of spectacular advances in the understanding of the molecular structure and genetics of connective tissue components, it seems likely that many aspects of medicine hitherto ascribed to age-related degeneration, will ultimately prove to have strong genetic components. A valid, molecular understanding of these processes may well emerge. It also appears likely that discrete clinical conditions now recognized as the Marfan syndrome, Ehlers–Danlos syndrome, and pseudoxanthoma elasticum will prove to have diverse and genetically determined counterparts that are responsible for the so-called degenerative disorders in the population at large.

Ehlers–Danlos syndrome (EDS)

Many clinical subtypes of Ehlers–Danlos syndrome have been recognized and increasingly these variants are being associated with distinct abnormalities of collagen structure. Abnormal collagen structure in EDS leads to multisystem disease (Table 2). Common features of this syndrome include fragile skin and laxity of the joints and ligaments (Fig. 1). In certain subtypes there is a particular fragility of tissues including arteries, the wall of the intestine, spinal ligaments, or even teeth; these propensities have led to discrete syndromic recognition (Table 3). The classical form of Ehlers–Danlos syndrome is characterized by excess cutaneous extensibility, bruising, and molluscoid pseudotumours. Careful examination of the skin of patients with EDS may show laxity, pendulousness, and fragility with easy splitting at different stages. In childhood, the skin tends to be hyperelastic but with advancing age, laxity combined with pendulousness, becomes obvious. Other forms of EDS may show hyperelastic and droopy skin in the same or different sites from the outset. The EDS V subtype is now obsolete.

After the original description, it was realized that some patients with EDS were susceptible to spontaneous arterial rupture with its associated lethal consequences. Affected women suffered fetal prematurity, and examination of their skin showed depletion of collagen and an increase in elastin fibres. This particular condition, which is associated with early fatality from vascular rupture, is correlated with defects in a type III collagen, as shown below. There are obstetric, rheumatological, orthopaedic, and abdominal complications of this vascular form of Ehlers–Danlos syndrome (type IV)—as well as an appreciable incidence of bladder-neck obstruction and

Table 2 Clinicopathological correlations in Ehlers–Danlos syndrome

Tissue	Abnormality	Clinical effect
Skin	Increased elasticity; fragility/thinning; abnormal collagen ultrastructure	Atrophy with papyraceous scars; striae, keloid formation; nodules, spherules, tears/splits
Blood vessels	Fragility of veins and arteries	Premature varicose veins; aneurysms of small or medium arteries
Eyes	Visual/refractive errors	Corneal curvature, retinal detachment, scleral rupture
Joints	Hypermobility	Arthralgia, instability/ dislocation
Skeleton (and teeth)	Osteoporosis	Distortion, soft-tissue injury, dysplastic dentine, occasional fractures
Miscellaneous	Hernias Diverticulae Pleuroperitoneal	Pneumothorax Intestinal perforation Peritonitis, strangulation, rectal/pelvic prolapse

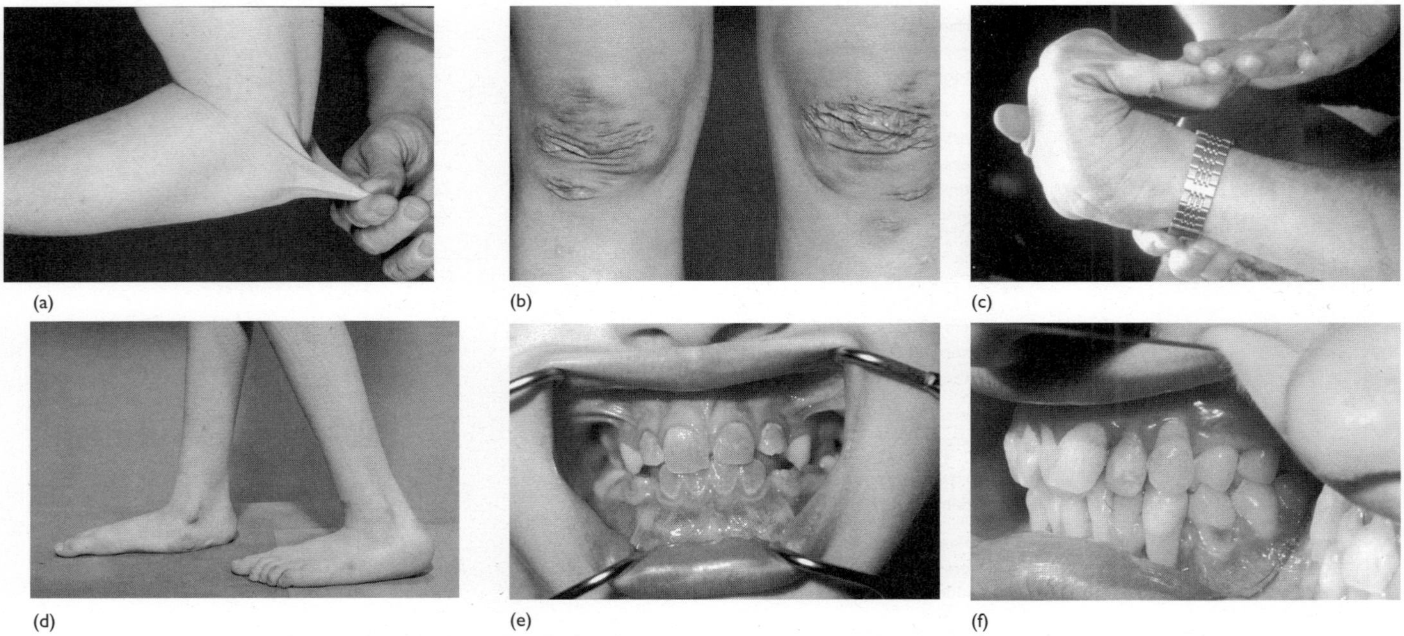

Fig. 1 Ehlers–Danlos syndrome. (a) Hyperelasticity of the skin (EDS II); (b) atrophic and pigmented papyraceous scars (EDS II); (c) joint hypermobility (EDS III); (d) severe pes planus (EDS VI); (e) dentinogenesis imperfecta (EDS VII), this patient had a deletion of exons 3–6 of the *COL1A1* gene; (f) premature periodontitis (EDS VIII).

ureteric reflux. Representative clinical features of EDS subtypes are illustrated in Figs 1 and 2 (and see also Plate 1).

Clinical genetics

Ehlers–Danlos syndrome type VI is caused by a recessively inherited deficiency of lysyl hydroxylase leading to underhydroxylation of collagen molecules (see Fig. 4(b)). Ehlers–Danlos type IV is due to defects and a deficiency of type III collagen in blood vessels, and is inherited as an autosomal dominant disorder. The biochemical defect in autosomal dominant Ehlers–Danlos syndrome type VII results from a failure to remove the N-terminal procollagen extensions of collagen. Defects in type III collagen are now implicated in the cutaneous ligaments and arterial fragility of the three major EDS variants. These defects compromise the assembly of collagen fibrils and provide an important biological model for other EDS subtypes that have now been identified, thus allowing diagnostic criteria to be married to an understanding of the molecular defect in collagen and connective tissue matrix.

Table 3 Diagnostic criteria of Ehlers–Danlos syndrome (EDS)*

Cardinal manifestations in particular tissues	
Skin	Soft, velvety, doughy, and hypoelastic; scars atrophic, papyraceous, especially over bony protuberances; easy bruising—especially on the legs
Connective tissue	Fragile, easily torn ligaments, joint capsules, and skin
Characteristics of EDS subtypes (see text) †	
EDS subtype	**Clinicopathological features**
I	Severe cardinal manifestations
II	Mild cardinal features
Types I and II show cauliflower-like collagen fibrils on transmission electron microscopy. NB Some patients are classified as type I/II to denote intermediate disease severity.	
III	Marked joint hypermobility; moderate skin extensibility no scarring
IV	Thin skin with prominent venous patterns visible; pretibial haemosiderosis; variable hypermobility; colonic perforation; acrogeric facies and extremities; mutated collagen III with variable fibril diameters
VI	Severe cardinal features; early progressive fibrosis; severe motor delay. Underhydroxylated collagen.
VII	Severe cardinal features; short stature; early recurrent hip dislocation; dentinogenesis imperfecta; angulated to hieroglyphic collagen fibres
VIII	Variable cardinal features; aggressive periodontitis and early tooth loss

*Adapted with permission from Beighton *et al.* (1992). † Note EDS V is obsolete.

Ehlers–Danlos syndrome may show classical X-linked, autosomal recessive or autosomal dominant transmission. These patterns reflect the complex assembly of the helical collagen molecule and its susceptibility to protein suicide. Because it is a complex structure, mutations in a single glycine located in the collagen helices disrupt up to seven-eighths of the assembled homocollagen trimers and 75 per cent of collagen heterotrimers, depending on the particular stoichiometry. For these reasons, collagen defects of this type behave as autosomal dominant traits, while the enzymatic deficiencies of collagen formation segregate as autosomal recessive traits with little or no expression in heterozygotes. Convincing autosomal recessive inheritance is common in EDS type VI associated with pronounced cutis laxa, due to gross distortions of the assembly of type I collagen that lead to a hieroglyphic appearance to these fibres under electron microscopy (Fig. 3(a)). In contrast, mutations leading to EDS type IV result from dominant mutations of type III collagen.

Ehlers–Danlos syndrome types I and II

EDS I and II are associated with the classical features outlined in Table 3. Easy skin-splitting, especially over bony prominences on the forehead, elbows, knees, and chin, shows itself in childhood. Notable features of the condition include epicanthic folds, blue sclerae, and fibrous nodules over the knees and ankles. Mitral valve prolapse is common but does not usually result in dilatational rupture of the valve. Unlike Ehlers–Danlos syndrome type IV, fragile blood vessels do not occur, but venous varicosities, premature bilateral hallux valgus, and distortion of the cornea leading to astigmatism, as well as premature osteoarthritis, are common. Most EDS type I or II families show linkage to the collagen V α-1 or V α-2 genes; which are located, respectively, on human chromosomes 9 or 2q34. Mutation analysis usually reveals substitutions of glycines and exon-skipping events. In some instances, null alleles lead to the deficiency of type V collagen domains. It seems likely that defects in the interactive properties of the N-terminus of type V collagen, which normally protrudes from the surface compound fibres comprising types I, III, and V collagen, impair normal interactions with other matrix components. Misdirection of the collagen fibrils leads to the generation of the so-called 'cauliflower' fibrils of EDS types I and II

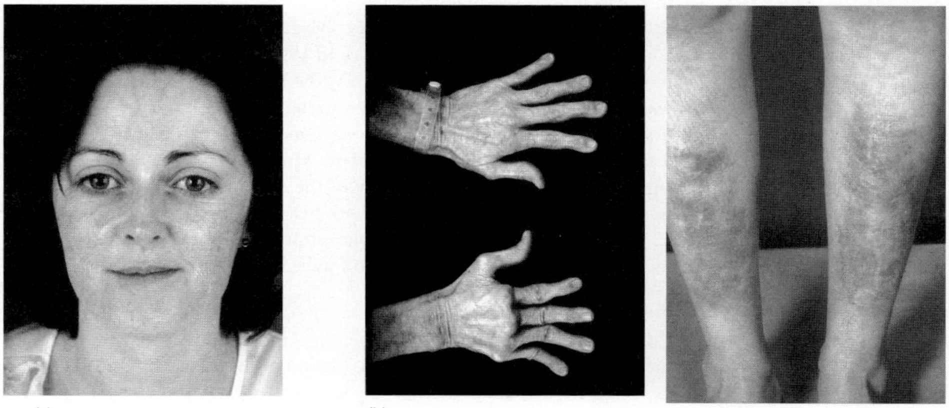

(a) (b) (c)

Fig. 2 EDS type IV (vascular type). (a) Acrogeria—a specific clinical feature of EDS IV. Note the large eyes and thin nose (Madonna facies) with perioral wrinkling. (b) Premature wrinkling of the skin on the dorsum of the hands; note also the joint contractures superficially resembling rheumatoid arthritis. (c) Pretibial bruising and haemosiderosis. (See also Plate 1.)

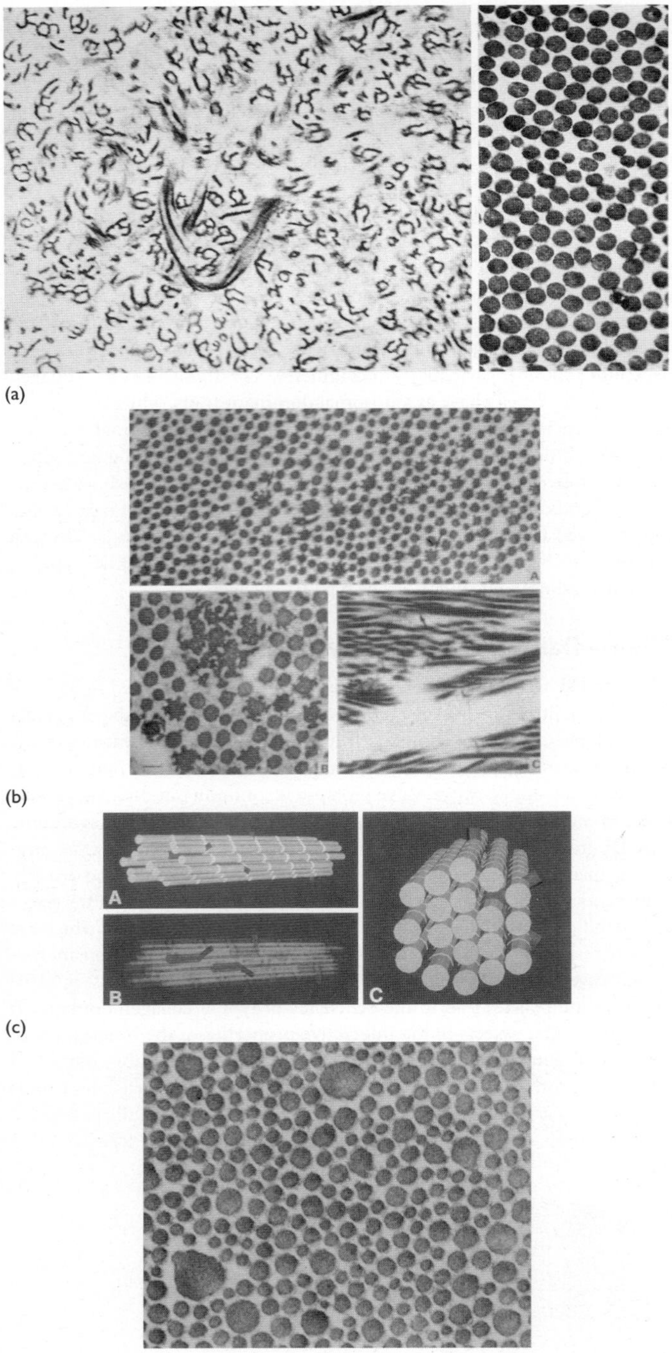

Fig. 3 Ultrastructural abnormalities of collagen in EDS. (a) 'Hieroglyphic' collagen fibres in EDS VII, indicating very severe disruption of fibril packing—compare with healthy collagen shown on the right of the figure. (b) Misassembled 'cauliflower' fibrils of skin and ligaments in EDS II. The left panel shows transversely fused fibres, which in longitudinal sections appear to splay distally. They resemble transversely sectioned cauliflower heads (from Nicholls *et al.* (1996) with permission). (c) Diagrammatic representation (in a) of compound collagen I and III fibres, composed of quarter-staggered individual triple helices. The dark collagen type V molecules (b) regulate fibril diameter; their protruding N-termini (shown in (c)) can interact with other matrix components (from Birk *et al.* (1990) with permission). (d) Dual distribution of collagen fibre size in EDS type IV.

(Fig. 3(b) and (c)). The clinical consequences being of fragile skin, ligaments, tendons, and corneas, as well as defective articular surfaces.

Ehlers–Danlos syndrome type III/benign hypermobile syndrome

This is the most common and least differentiated variant of Ehlers–Danlos syndrome and, for this reason, its diagnosis is frequently overlooked. The disorder is associated with tall stature, ready bruising, blue sclerae, and osteoporosis. Occasionally, more severe defects including osteogenesis imperfecta and Marfan's syndrome occur. Occasionally pseudoxanthoma and other Ehlers–Danlos syndrome variants occur as part of this disorder. As yet uncharacterized defects in collagen, elastin, fibrillin, proteoglycan, and connective tissue-modifying enzymes may all be responsible for the hypermobility of joints and other manifestations in this category of Ehlers–Danlos syndrome (Fig. 1(c)). Patients with Marfan's syndrome may show extensible skin and osteoporosis that complicate Ehlers–Danlos syndrome types III, VI, and VII; Marfan-like stature may be observed in patients with osteogenesis imperfecta.

Ehlers–Danlos syndrome type IV—'vascular form'

This autosomal dominant vascular form of Ehlers–Danlos syndrome is typically accompanied by pretibial ecchymoses over the knees and shins as well as acrogeria (Fig. 2). Acrogeria refers to prematurely aged extremities with thinning of the skin on the dorsum of the hands, feet, and shins. The features are combined with the so-called 'Madonna' facial appearance of large eyes, nasal thinning, and small earlobes. Some patients may have a Marfanic appearance. Rarely there is acro-osteolysis with unexplained androgenic alopecia in females as well as congenital talipes, hip dislocations, and tendon contractures; displacement of the metacarpophalangeal joints in the hands may superficially resemble the changes of rheumatoid arthritis. Fragility of pleuroperitoneal membranes or the colonic wall is a common feature in this vascular subtype but occasionally it may complicate other types of EDS, including types I, II, and III.

The main concern with type IV Ehlers–Danlos syndrome is of spontaneous rupture of medium or large arteries, which may be lethal at any point from mid-adolescence to late-adult life. Aneurysms of small, medium, and large arteries, including the aorta, are common. Angiographic studies reveal a dilatated and tortuous arterial tree, including the carotid bifurcation, and major aortic or iliac disease. Dissections are common especially after ill-advised angiography or surgery; these present with unexplained abdominal pain that proves to be due to intestinal ischaemia. Histological examination of the skin reveals dermal thinning with depletion of dermal collagen and an overproliferation of elastic fibres. Examination of the skin by electron microscopy usually reveals marked variability in collagen fibril size (Fig. 3(d)).

In a recent review by Pepin and colleagues of the medical and surgical complications in 220 index patients and 199 of their affected relatives with biochemically confirmed EDS type IV, the underlying COL 3A1 mutation was identified in 135 propositi. One-quarter of the index patients had had a first complication by the age of 20 years and more than 80 per cent had at least one complication by the age of 40. Most deaths resulted from arterial rupture but bowel rupture, usually of the sigmoid colon was frequent. It was noteworthy that in 81 women with EDS IV who had become pregnant, 12 died as a result of disease complications during pregnancy. Overall the median lifespan of the whole group was reduced to 48 years.

Molecular pathology

Collagen III is the dominant collagen in skin, blood vessels, tendons, ligaments, gastrointestinal tract, and pleuroperitoneal cavity linings. This explains the diverse multisystem phenotype of type IV EDS. Disturbed assembly, as well as haploinsufficiency of type III collagen explains the wide-ranging severity of EDS type IV, although some affected patients suffer a mild clinical phenotype resembling EDS type III (Fig. 4(a)). Numerous mutations in the type III collagen gene have been found in EDS type IV;

most of these mutations are private, although several are associated with 'hot spots' in the complex collagen gene structure that are located in exons 7, 16, and 24. The complications of EDS type IV cannot be predicted from the nature of the specific mutations in COL 3A1.

Ehlers–Danlos syndrome types III, IV, and VI, with overlap to pseudoxanthoma elasticum

Much overlap is seen between these syndromes and others that affect connective tissue, including Stickler syndrome.

A characteristic feature of Ehlers–Danlos syndrome type III is the absence of scarring after skin injury; none the less, the skin is doughy and extensible but without fragility. The benign hypermobile syndrome is associated with joint hypermobility but without extensible skin. While this syndrome may be adapted to extreme sporting skills and gymnastics, it may also indicate heterozygosity for other collagen defects such as Ehlers–Danlos syndrome type VI, or even pseudoxanthoma elasticum.

The syndrome is associated with persistent arthralgia without evidence of inflammatory joint disease and is difficult to treat. Treatment includes physiotherapy, rest, and graded exercise combined with conventional pain relief. Later, joint-stabilizing exercises or supports combine with proprioceptive enhancement, and cognitive therapy may be beneficial. It is unknown whether these patients have defective pain receptors or whether they have acquired or inherited disturbed pain reception as a result of their long-standing collagen abnormality.

Marfan's syndrome

The Marfan syndrome is an archetypal defect of connective tissue with a strong hereditary basis causing characteristic skeletal, cardiovascular, and ocular disease. Patients with Marfan's syndrome are disproportionately tall and thin with abnormally long extremities and, often, a cadaverous physique (Fig. 5). Abraham Lincoln was possibly affected. Marfan's syndrome is caused by mutations in the human fibrillin gene and is an autosomal dominat trait.

Marfan's syndrome is not rare; it affects both sexes and occurs with a frequency of about 1 in 10 000. Marfan's syndrome has been reported in nearly all ethnic groups.

Diagnostic criteria

The Marfan syndrome overlaps with other inherited connective tissue disorders including Ehlers–Danlos syndrome type III, benign hypermobility syndrome, pseudoxanthoma elasticum, osteogenesis imperfecta, and homocystinuria. Typically, there is joint hypermobility, hyperextensibility of the skin with striae, blue sclerae, and tall stature. Combinations of one major and two minor criteria are sufficient to diagnose Marfan's syndrome. Marfan's syndrome also overlaps with ectopia lentis and Beals' syndrome (congenital contractural arachnodactyly)—both of which are unassociated with aortic dilatation and rupture but are caused, respectively, by mutations in the genes encoding fibrillin I or II.

Clinical features

It seems likely, in retrospect, that the patient originally described by Marfan may have suffered from Beals' syndrome with congenital contractural arachnodactyly, elongated feet, and crumpled ears. Classical Marfan's syndrome arises from mutations in fibrillin I. Typically, there are long, elegant (though spidery) fingers and toes with dislocated lenses caused by a rupture of the ciliary zonules early in life. The syndrome is associated with mitral valve prolapse and aortic dilatation. Aortic disease is associated with dissection and rupture; rarely, dissection and rupture of the pulmonary artery occurs in Marfan's syndrome.

Detailed manifestations diagnostic of Marfan's syndrome (Table 4)

Skeletal—anterior chest deformity, including asymmetrical pectus excavatum or carinatum (Fig. 6); dolichostenomelia, arachnodactyly, scoliosis lordosis, tall stature, narrow arched palate and dental crowding, protrusio acetabuli, congenital flexion contractures, hypermobility, ocular ectopia lentis (Fig. 7), flat cornea, elongated globe, retinal detachment, myopia;

Cardiovascular—dilatation of the ascending aorta (Fig. 8), aortic dissection, aortic regurgitation, mitral regurgitation with prolapse, calcification of mitral annulus, abdominal aortic aneurysm, arrhythmia, endocarditis;

Pulmonary—spontaneous pneumothorax, atypical bullae;

Skin—abdominal striae and abdominal hernias, including diaphragmatic and umbilical hernias;

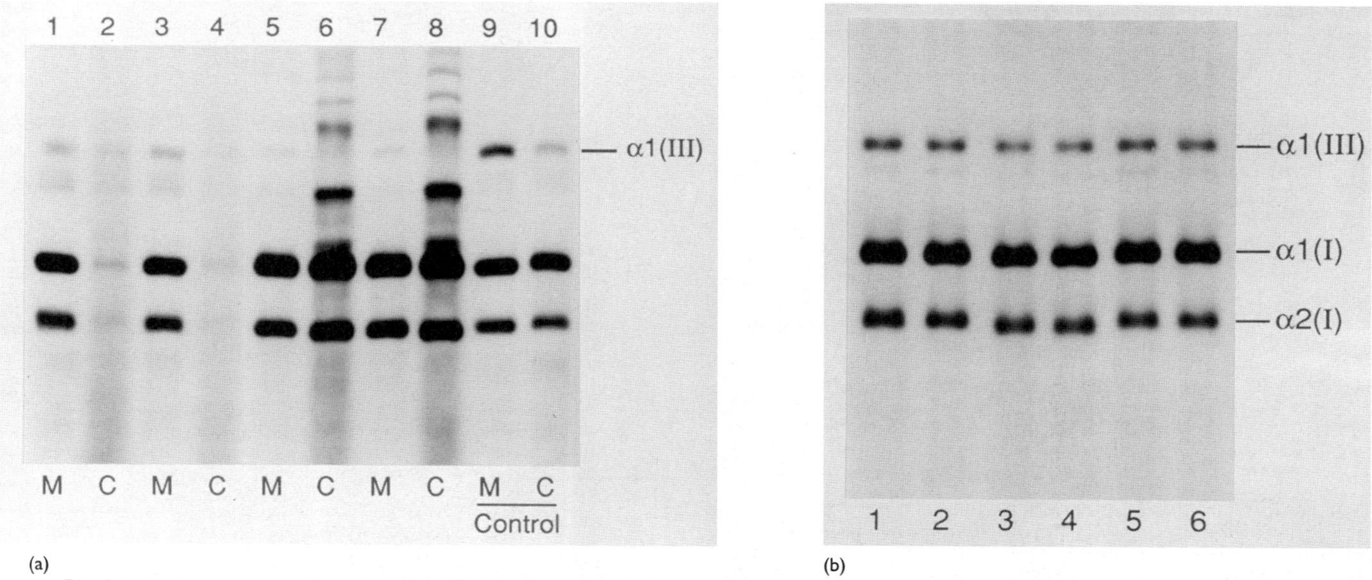

Fig. 4 Molecular analysis of collagen in EDS. (a) Typical collagen type III electrophoretic profile in fibroblasts after biosynthetic labelling in culture. There is virtually complete deficiency (tracks 5–8) or haploinsufficiency (tracks 1–4) compared with the normal pattern (9–10). M, collagen in culture medium; C, collagen recovered from cells. (b) Electrophoresis of radiolabelled collagen proteins in fibroblasts obtained from a patient with severe pes planus due to EDS VI, showing accelerated migration (tracks 3–4) of underhydroxylated, compared with normal, collagen molecules (tracks 1–2; 5–6).

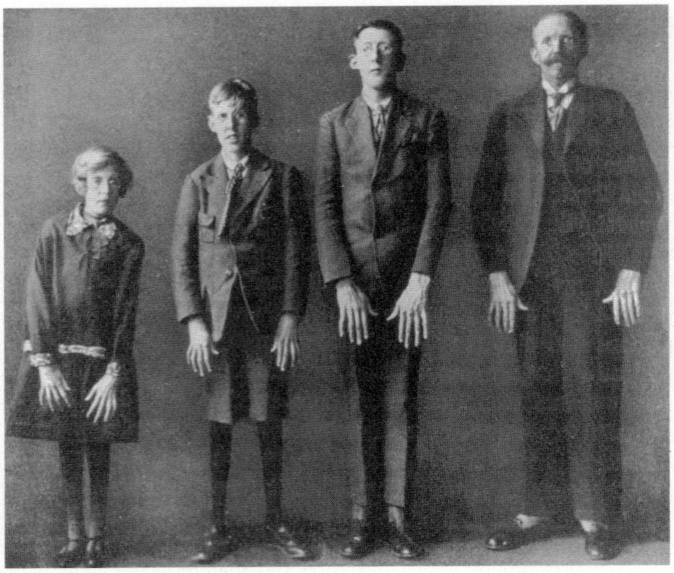

Fig. 5 Marfan's syndrome. Early illustration of a family with skeletal and ophthalmic features transmitted from the affected father to his daughter and two sons.

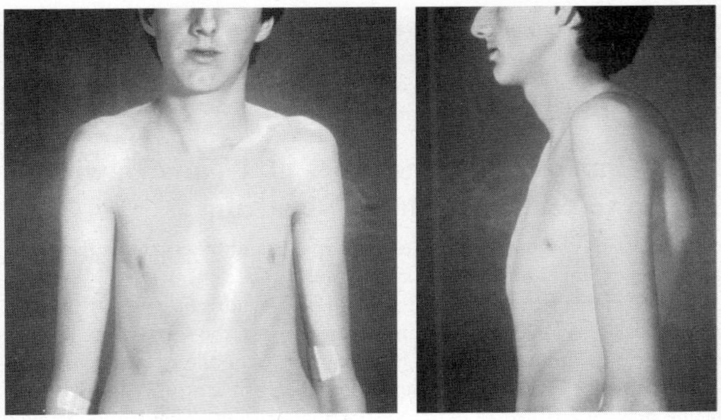

(a) (b)

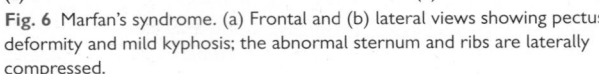

Fig. 6 Marfan's syndrome. (a) Frontal and (b) lateral views showing pectus deformity and mild kyphosis; the abnormal sternum and ribs are laterally compressed.

Central nervous system—dural ectasia, meningocele, dilatation of cisterna magna, learning disability and hyperactivity.

The diagnosis of Marfan's syndrome may be confirmed by the involvement of at least two systems with at least one major manifestation as listed in Table 4; urinalysis (in patients not receiving vitamin B_6 supplements) should confirm the absence of homocystinuria.

The differential diagnosis includes: Stickler syndrome (vitreoretinal changes); osteoarthroses; mid-facial hypoplasia; Shprintzen–Goldberg syndrome (craniocarniosynostosis and retarded neurodevelopment, with Marfanoid features); and homocysteinuria. Since homocystinuria and Marfan's syndrome are distinct disorders—and because many patients with homocystinuria respond to specific therapies, for example pyridoxine supplements—clear distinction is necessary. Confusion between these two conditions is particularly likely in tall young patients with ectopia lentis and, except in unequivocal cases, patients with suspected Marfan's syndrome should always undergo appropriate biochemical testing for homocystinuria due to cystathionine β-synthetase deficiency or other causes.

Table 4 Clinical features of the Marfan syndrome

Tissue	Feature
Skin	Increased elasticity; striae (especially thoracolumbar and sacral) Keloids (rare) EDS-like scarring
Heart and blood vessels	Dilatation—aortic dilatation*/rupture—dissection* Fragility: – aortic and mitral valve prolapse – abdominal aortic aneurysm
Eyes	Lens dislocation* (refractive errors) Corneal/vitreous abnormalities (closed-angle glaucoma) Altered eye length (high myopia)
Joints	Hypermobility, arthralgia, and joint instability
Skeleton	Pectus deformities, misshapen chest Kyphoscoliosis, skeletal deformity Elongated extremities, especially fingers and feet
Miscellaneous	Dural ectasia* hernias (various) Finger contractures, pleural rupture (pneumothorax)

* Major manifestation.

Diagnostic requirements in the absence of an unequivocally affected first-degree relative: involvement of at least two systems; at least one major manifestation preferred, depending on family phenotype. Urine amino acid analysis (in absence of pyridoxine supplementation) must confirm the absence of homocystinuria (see Godfrey M (1993).)

Genetics

Marfan's syndrome is typically inherited as an autosomal dominant trait (see Fig. 5) and belongs to that group of genetic diseases in which a strong paternal-age effect occurs. The mean age of fathers of individuals who appear to harbour 'new' mutations is 5 to 10 years greater than average. Approximately one-third of all patients with Marfan's syndrome appear to be sporadic cases.

The gene responsible for Marfan's syndrome maps to chromosome 15. Mutations in the gene encoding fibrillin, a novel elastin-matrix protein, are responsible for Marfan's syndrome (Fig. 9). A second fibrillin gene maps to chromosome 5, mutations in which are responsible for Beals' syndrome

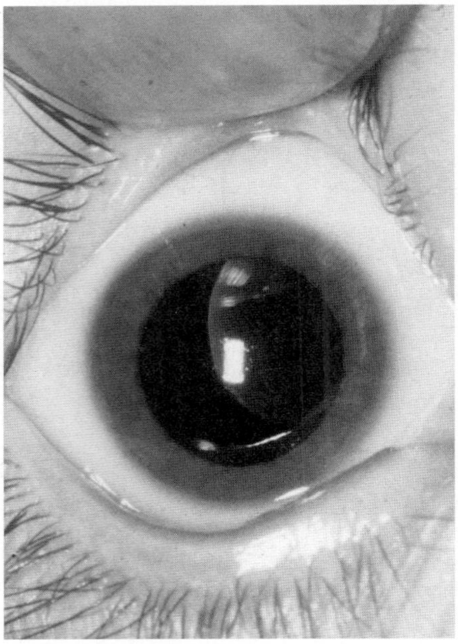

Fig. 7 Ectopia lentis in Marfan's syndrome. The lens is displaced upwards and medially; typically strong concave spectacle (aphakic) lenses are required to correct the high myopia.

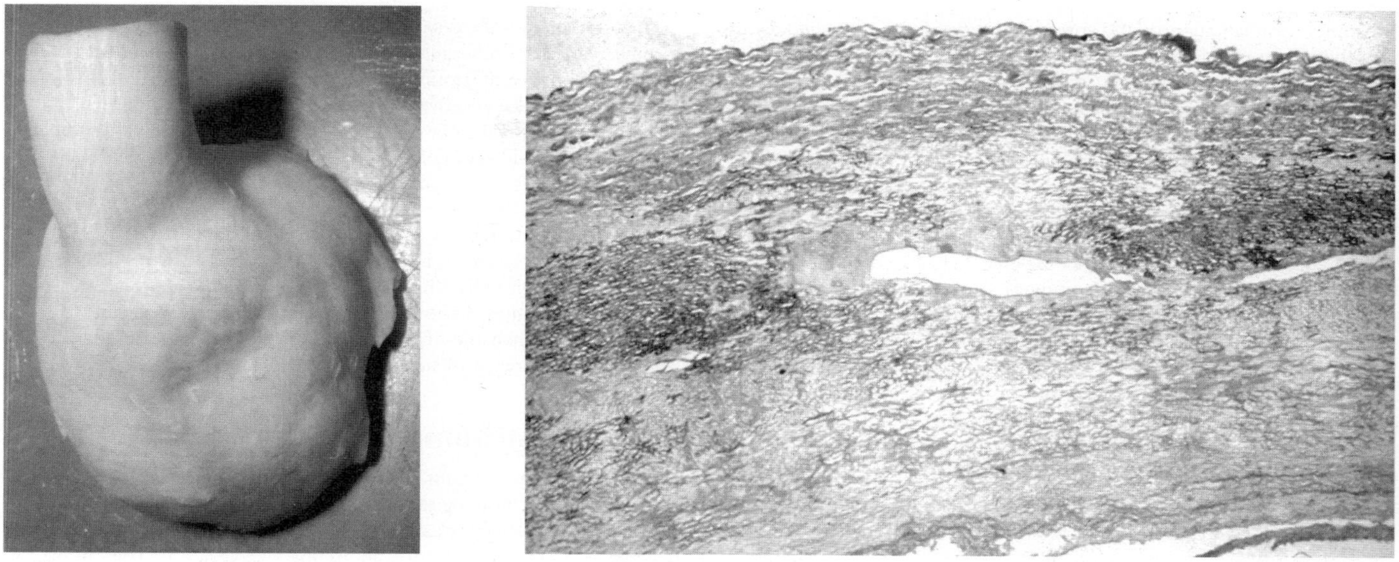

(a) (b)

Fig. 8 Aortic disease in Marfan's syndrome. (a) Excised dilatated aortic root; (b) histological section of the aorta showing elastic degeneration of the aortic media.

(congenital contractural arachnodactyly that is not associated with defects in the ciliary zonules).

The fibrillin I gene has a complex multi-exon organization and encodes calcium-binding, epidermal growth-factor-like and non-calcium binding, epidermal growth-factor regions. The gene encodes 65 exons encoding several conserved cysteines, common mutations of which are responsible for Marfan's syndrome; other fibrillin mutations have also been identified. Mutations in certain cysteines between exons 59 and 65 appear to be responsible for mild Marfan's syndrome that lacks aortic dilatation and is only associated with ectopia lentis. However, substitutions of cysteine codons elsewhere in the fibrillin gene may be responsible for more severe clinical phenotypes. Despite these findings, however, phenotype–genotype correlations in Marfan's syndrome are at present very loose. It is clear, however, that fibrillin mutations responsible for Marfan's syndrome are associated with disruption of the assembly of the fibrillin gene product and that dominant-negative mechanisms operate, as in the collagen defects. It seems likely that mutations of regions encoding epidermal growth-factor domains will disturb important homologous as well as heterologous, protein-matrix interactions of fibrillin.

The fibrillins are elastin-associated microfibrils, which assemble autonomously to form beaded microfilaments with ordered quasi-crystalline structures that can be studied by electron microscopy and other methods. Mutations that lead to the premature termination of the fibrillin I gene also appear to result in a milder phenotype than those mutations that cause small in-frame deletions or insertions. Exon-skipping events lead to the formation of in-frame mutant fibrillins lacking small protein sections which tend to interact normally with their wild-type congeners. In contrast, truncated mutants of fibrillin I typically disrupt the formation of the fibrillar structure. Most mutations in fibrillin I are private, and the presence of 65 exons in this large and complex genetic structure greatly impedes the molecular analysis of the fibrillin gene in patients with suspected Marfan's syndrome.

Treatment

The main causes of death in patients with Marfan's syndrome result from cardiovascular disease and complications elsewhere in the vascular system. Vigorous and regular surveillance is recommended with careful monitoring of aortic-root width and of the function of aortic and mitral valves by transthoracic echocardiography and periodic electrocardiography.

In patients with evidence of progressive aortic disease, including dilatation of the ascending aorta and valve ring, a Dacron graft, with or without an artificial or reconstituted aortic valve (the Bentall procedure), may be considered. There is also a strong case for joint management with experienced cardiac surgical colleagues in special clinics dedicated to the treatment of patients with Marfan's syndrome. Insertion of a Dacron graft to the aortic valvular ring, after excision of a terminally dilated aorta,

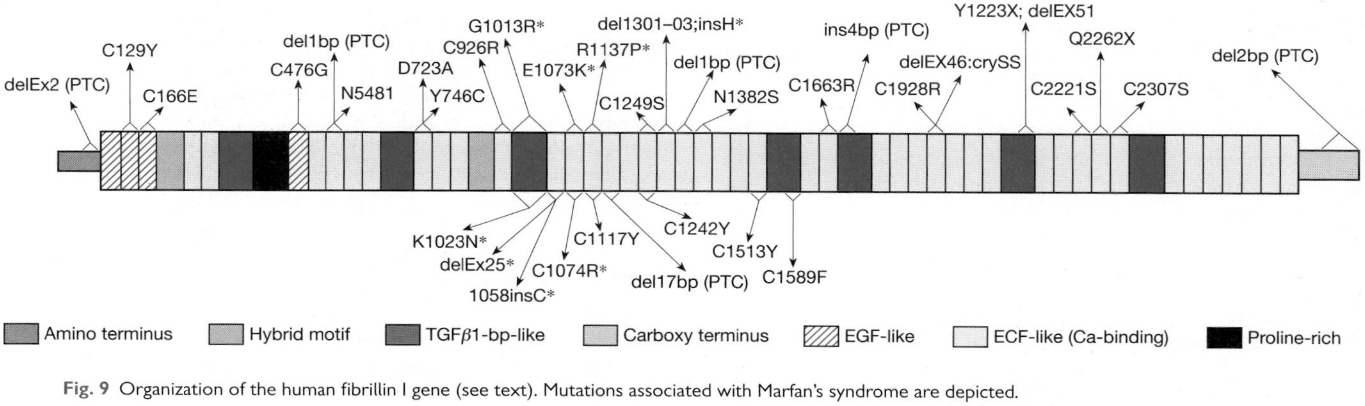

Fig. 9 Organization of the human fibrillin I gene (see text). Mutations associated with Marfan's syndrome are depicted.

requires reimplantation of the coronary arteries; in the best hands, the mortality rate of this procedure is less than 5 per cent, more than three-quarters of patients surviving 5 years. Scrupulous joint cardiac monitoring including echocardiography and magnetic resonance and CT imaging is recommended. A recent report by Gott and colleagues from Johns Hopkins Hospital, in the United States describes the results of aortic root replacement in 271 patients with Marfan's syndrome over the period 1976 to 2000. Most (> 85 per cent) patients underwent the Bentall procedure involving composite graft replacement of the aortic root. There were no 30-day deaths and more than 80 per cent of the operated patients were alive at the time this report was submitted for publication.

Patients with Marfan's syndrome benefit from the early introduction of adrenergic β-blockers to reduce the mean arterial pressure and pulse rate. Serial studies show that the mortality rate for aortic rupture in Marfan's syndrome is significantly reduced by the introduction of prophylactic β-blocking therapy; those so treated have a slower rate of aortic root dilatation. β-Adrenergic blockade should probably be introduced at an early age.

More than half of the patients with Marfan's syndrome suffer from dislocation of the optic lens—often in early childhood. Typically, the lens dislocates upwards. Thus surgical removal is indicated only if cataract or secondary glaucoma, due to the unusual lens position, intervenes. Upward dislocation may also lead to a greatly diminished visual acuity that cannot be corrected with spectacles; extraction of the lens is recommended under these circumstances.

Other complications of Marfan's syndrome including unstable joints, dislocation of the patella, progressive kyphoscoliosis, and recurrent pneumothoraces require surgical intervention. Clearly, many patients with Marfan's syndrome will require support from the psychological aspect and in the light of their diminished life expectancy. Women with Marfan's syndrome require counselling, not only about the genetic risk to their offspring but also because of the intrinsic risks of carrying a pregnancy to term. Re-evaluation of the heart during pregnancy may be recommended as a means of providing reassurance; the introduction of propanolol may be required during the course of labour and delivery to reduce cardiovascular stress.

Patients with Marfan's syndrome are at risk if they participate in competitive athletics. Indeed, the presence of Marfan's syndrome is a common cause of fatal aortic dissection and rupture in young adults. Those individuals with a clear diagnosis of the condition should be advised on an appropriate lifestyle and referred for genetic, as well as cardiological review, upon diagnosis. Several charities exist to support patients with Marfan's syndrome: the National Marfan Foundation in the United States as well as other lay groups in Europe and other countries provide critical information as well as psychological support for these patients and their families. Marfan's syndrome is a complex condition but, as a subject of intensive genetic and clinical study, benefits from active intervention with specific therapy (for instance, β-blockers) as well as rigorous monitoring, counselling, and supportive therapy.

Prognosis

Patients with Marfan's syndrome have a reduced life expectancy, principally as a result of the cardiovascular complications. Indeed, about 80 per cent of all deaths are due to aortic dilatation and its complications; the mean age of death in a series of 257 patients published in 1972 was 32 years. However, with the introduction of β-blocking agents and improvements in vascular and cardiac surgery, the prognosis has improved greatly and the early cohort studies were almost certainly subject to bias, since outcome was better in patients ascertained on the basis of family studies compared with those with sporadic disease.

Men with Marfan's syndrome have a lower survival rate than affected women—a conclusion based on several cohort studies. In a study of patients with Marfan's syndrome in Wales and Scotland between 1970 and 1990, the median survival for men was 53 years and for women, 72 years; the median age at death was 45 ± 16.5 years.

In a trial of 70 adolescent and adult patients with classical Marfan's syndrome, Shores and colleagues reported the results of treatment with propanolol. The treatment group received individualized doses of propanolol sufficient to induce negative inotrophy. When compared with the control group, those treated showed a reduced rate of aortic dilatation and improved survival—fewer of the treated patients reached clinical endpoints as determined by death, congestive cardiac failure, aortic regurgitation, aortic dissection, or the need for cardiac surgery.

Recently, several reports in the surgical literature describe the outcome of aortic root replacement in many hundreds of patients with Marfan disease: about one-third have had aortic dissection and in approximately one-half, aortic dilatation, 6.5 cm or less, was documented. Late operative death occurred in less than one-fifth of patients but subsequent series suggest that the prophylactic repair of smaller aortic aneurysms is preferable.

Pseudoxanthoma elasticum

Pseudoxanthoma elasticum (**PXE**) is an inherited defect of connective tissue with specific histological characteristics that reflect abnormally fragmented and calcified elastic tissue. Fragmented elastin fibres occur principally in the skin, arteries, and retina where they are responsible for the main clinical effects of the disorder. Electron microscopy shows abnormalities of elastic fibres as well as associated collagen fibres. Pseudoxanthoma is now defined principally as a result of examination of the mutational spectrum of the responsible *ABCC6* gene and rigid clinical criteria. The systemic manifestations result principally from premature arterial stiffening and calcification; hypertension, thrombosis, and haemorrhage thus occur with widespread effects. Gastrointestinal bleeding, retinal disease causing visual loss, and stroke phenomena are among the most frequent complications of PXE.

Clinical genetics

The mode of transmission of PXE has been puzzling and controversial. This is reflected in the assignment of several Mendelian inheritance in man (**MIM**) catalogue numbers for autosomal dominant and recessive disease, respectively (MIM 177850, 177860; and 264800). In most (about 85 per cent) affected patients, the disease appears to occur sporadically without an overt family history. A minority of patients with PXE belong to pedigrees in which several siblings are affected in one generation; their parents (and other heterozygotes) often show generalized laxity of the joints, similar to Ehlers–Danlos syndrome type III. Transmission of authentic PXE through two or more generations consistent with an autosomal dominant pattern of inheritance occurs in no more than 5 per cent of cases.

Puzzling segregation patterns are frequent and obligate heterozygotes may show premature atherosclerosis. It is probable that homozygous or doubly heterozygous PXE is relatively common and that the carrier frequency may be as high as 0.5 to 1 per cent. Thus most families exhibiting anomalous inheritance of PXE may prove to be pseudodominant with matings between homozygotes or double heterozygotes and randomly distributed heterozygotes. In practical terms, the sibling recurrence risk for sporadic PXE lies between 1 in 800 and 1 in 4000; for authentic known autosomal recessive disease, this is 1 in 4. The risks of recurrent disease in the offspring of affected or potentially heterozygous children of known heterozygote parents are, providing no matings occur with consanguineous relatives, twice or the same as the odds for the sporadic cases—that is to say, no greater than 1 in 400. In due course, uncertainties about the transmission of PXE and genetic counselling will be clarified by mutation testing of the *ABCC6* gene responsible for this disease (see below).

Clinical features

Until recently there has been a lack of connection between the cutaneous and ophthalmological manifestations of PXE.

Although the typical orange–yellow xanthomatous appearance of flexual skin with underlying fragmentation of elastic had been long known, the association between this syndrome and the development of retinal angioid streaks due to elastic fragmentation of Bruch's membrane was not initially recognized. Pseudoxanthoma elasticum is associated with disease of both large and small arteries, as shown in the retina. Indeed, widespread involvement of the arterial media with attendant thrombotic complications is referable to many organs. Pseudoxanthoma is associated with bleeding from the gastrointestinal tract as well as stroke and, occasionally, lung disease.

Cutaneous

Typical changes of PXE in the skin develop in the face, neck, and flexual regions, including the axillas, antecubital fossas, inguinal folds, as well as the umbilicus. Similar changes may be observed around the mouth and nasolabial creases (Fig. 10 and Plate 2). The first changes are of thickening with a raised yellow discoloration between grooves, leading to plaque formation and an appearance resembling the skin of a plucked chicken, '*peau d'orange*'. With time, the skin becomes inelastic and lax, thus causing considerable cosmetic alarm. In full-blown cases, an unattractive hound-dog appearance to the face and skin folds around the neck and groins develops, 'cutis laxa'. These changes may be aggravated by sun exposure and smoking.

Examination of the palate may show similar changes. Endoscopy of the stomach may reveal nodular submucosal lesions comparable to those present in peripheral skin.

Ophthalmic

The characteristic features of pseudoxanthoma elasticum in the eye are revealed by ophthalmoscopy (Fig. 11 and Plate 3). There may be only minor pigmentary changes, extending to disruption of the fibres in the preretinal membrane of Bruch causing angioid streaks. These retinal streaks vary in colour from dark red or maroon to black. Pressure on the eye, however, may discolour the streaks that underlie the retinal vessels and radiate from the optic disc.

Angioid streaks occur in most patients beyond the age of 50 years but only in about one-third of patients with pseudoxanthoma ascertained in childhood.

In a cross-sectional study of 186 British patients with pseudoxanthoma elasticum conducted by the author in 1973, normal visual acuity was present in two-thirds: central visual loss occurred in 6 per cent; moderate visual impairment in 15 per cent; and mild impairment in 10 per cent. In contrast, fundoscopy was normal in less than 10 per cent of the patients: about one-third had angioid streaks and 13.5 per cent had degenerative maculopathy—a few patients had signs of haemorrhage. Myopia occurred in more than one-third of the patients and appeared to be at least three times more prevalent than in the general population. This implies that PXE may predispose to myopia, perhaps by effects on corneal curvature, lens power, optical length, or vitreous composition.

Cardiovascular

In the cardiovascular system, the most striking abnormality of PXE is hypertension associated with an absence or weakness of peripheral arterial

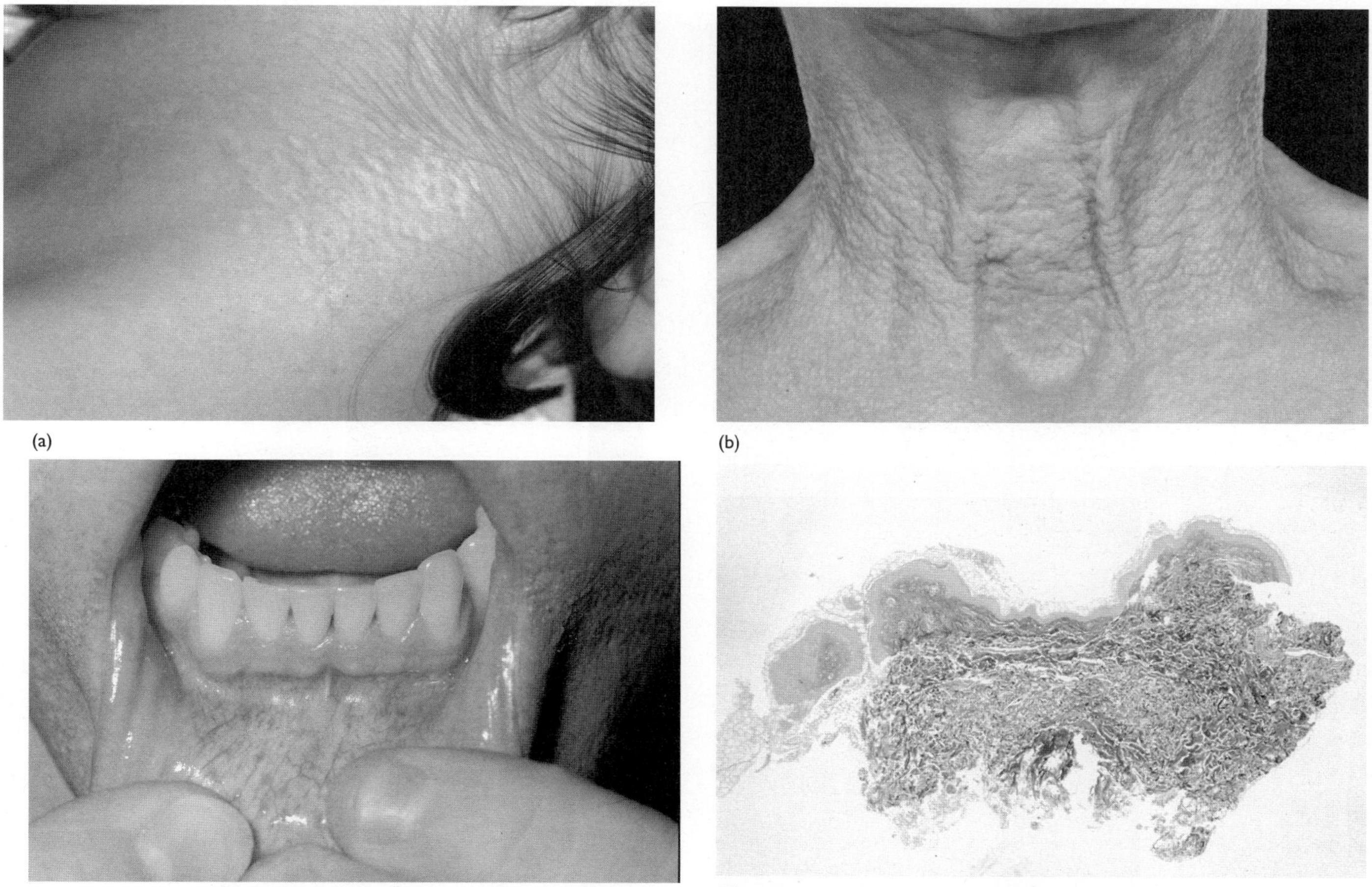

(a) (b) (c) (d)

Fig. 10 Skin lesions in pseudoxanthoma elasticum (PXE). (a) Typical flexural skin lesions of PXE of the lateral neck. (b) Widespread cutis laxa in PXE. (c) Mucosal infiltration of the lower lip in PXE. (d) Elastic van Gieson's stain of skin section showing mid-dermal elastic fragmentation and degeneration. (See also Plate 2).

pulses. The author's cross-sectional survey of 186 British patients with PXE showed that 40 per cent had systemic hypertension: one in five of the patients experienced angina pectoris and one in ten had intermittent claudication; slightly more than 5 per cent had suffered transient ischaemic attacks; and 5 per cent had residual hemipareses following stroke episodes.

Occasionally, ischaemic features develop in the hands associated with resorption of digital tufts; these abnormalities are associated with a diminished Doppler pulse-wave velocity, reflecting a reduced amplitude of the systolic pulse wave. Other features include mitral valve prolapse and episodic and often torrential gastrointestinal haemorrhage usually from the stomach with or without a coincidental hiatal hernia or peptic ulcer. Bleeding may occur at other points including the renal, retinal, uterine, bladder, or subarachnoid spaces.

Many patients with PXE are hypertensive. This appears to increase the risk of bleeding, which may also be associated with premature arterial calcification in peripheral arteries as well as coronary vessels. Women with pseudoxanthoma elasticum often develop severe hypertension during pregnancy and complain of rapid progression of skin changes. Joint manifestations are not a feature of pseudoxanthoma elasticum.

Diagnosis

Several clinical criteria for the diagnosis of PXE have been defined by different authorities. The major and minor criteria preferred by this author are set out in Table 5; any two major, or one major and two minor, criteria are sufficient to diagnose the disease. The most important criteria for establishing the diagnosis are the presence of the appropriate skin eruption with histological evidence of elastic degeneration and calcification as determined by tissue biopsy.

Differential diagnosis

Angioid streaks may be seen in Paget's disease and sickle cell anaemia but are rarely as florid as those occurring in pedigrees affected by pseudoxanthoma elasticum. Rarely, diabetic retinopathy may be associated with angioid streaks. Angioid streaks have also been reported in patients with neurofibromatosis and tuberous sclerosis. Cutaneous manifestations of pseudoxanthoma elasticum may resemble those of extreme solar injury to skin associated with ageing. Characteristically, long-term penicillamine therapy leads to a syndrome that is a close phenocopy of pseudoxanthoma elasticum: elastosis serpingiosa perforans is frequently associated with pseudoxanthoma elasticum-like features. Pseudoxanthoma elasticum may also be considered in patients with Ehlers–Danlos syndrome in which cutis laxa is the sole manifestation.

Pathology

Pseudoxanthoma elasticum is diagnosed principally because of the occurrence of the constellation of clinical features, the family history, and a skin biopsy that reveals a characteristic fragmentation and disruption as well as calcification of the elastic fibres of the middle and deep zones of the corium. The use of von Kossa's stain, which identifies carbonate and phosphate complexes of calcium, together with Van Gieson's stain for elastic fibres is usually diagnostic; electron microscopy usually reveals electron-dense

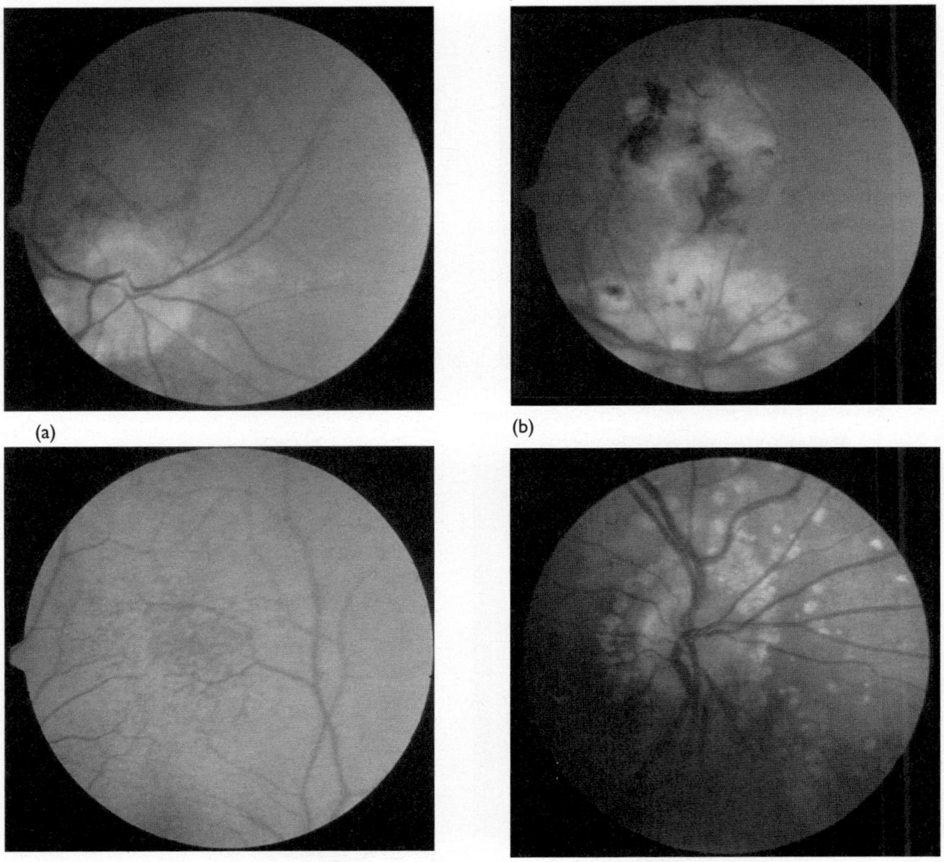

(a) (b) (c) (d)

Fig. 11 Retinal changes in PXE. (a) Angioid streaks caused by fracture of the retroretinal Bruch's membrane—an early feature. (b) Macular haemorrhage with consequential choroideretinitis. (c) Specked *peau d'orange* mottling. (d) Salmon spotting and drusen. (See also Plate 3).

Table 5 Features of pseudoxanthoma elasticum (PXE) in different tissues

Skin
*Classical infiltrative flexural eruption with or without dermal infiltration
*Elastic fragmentation *and* calcification and/or central elastic fibre calcification (by electron microscopy)
Increased cutaneous extensibility (heterozygotes)
†Dermal calcification *without* clinical infiltration
Occasional striae
Blood vessels
Decreased elasticity, hypertension
Arteriosclerosis, claudication
Medial calcification, venous varicosities
Eyes
*Late-onset macular degeneration, macular central visual loss, and/or angioid streaks
†Isolated angioid streaks
Altered corneal geometry, myopia, blue sclerae
†Fundal mottling
Skeleton
Occasional pectus excavatum, osteoporosis (in some heterozygotes)
Scoliosis (rare)
Miscellaneous
†Positive family history of PXE
Mitral valve prolapse
Pleural/parenchymal calcification
Renal stones (questionable)
Hernias

* Major diagnostic criteria; †minor diagnostic criteria.

deposits throughout elastin fibres in the skin with a central core of mineral.

Molecular genetics

The gene responsible for pseudoxanthoma elasticum has been mapped in some affected pedigrees to a single locus on the short arm of chromosome 16 (16p31.1) (Fig. 12). Unexpectedly, the gene proved to be a multidrug-resistance and membrane ion transporter rather than an integral structural matrix protein. It spans 31 exons and encodes at the ATP-binding cassette and is a member of the cystic fibrosis-transmembrane regulator, *CFTR*, gene family.

As discussed above, many patients with pseudoxanthoma elasticum belong to healthy families and are the only member with the condition, thus having no overt family history of the disease. Of the remaining 15 per cent of PXE patients, the most common family pattern is of several affected siblings in one generation showing diverse clinical expression.

Some families appear to show either autosomal recessive or dominant patterns of transmission. The relationship between these defects and mutations in the *ABCC6* gene implicated in pseudoxanthoma is unclear. Most patients appear to be homozygous for a defect in the *PXE* gene and some shared mutations appear to segregate with homozygosity for stop codons. At present, it is unclear what proportion of mutations in the *ABCC6* gene account for pseudoxanthoma elasticum and what proportion of patients are homozygous or compound heterozygotes at this locus. Despite the ambiguities, however, molecular analysis of the *ABCC6* gene provides an opportunity for systematic testing and clarification of the risk of transmission of the disease in affected pedigrees.

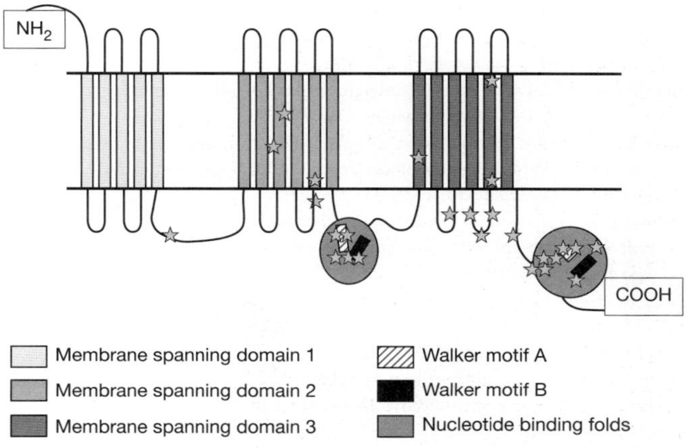

Fig. 12 Organization of the human PXE gene, *ABCC6*, a member of the ABC transmembrane ion transporter family. There are three membrane-spanning domains, each of which contains nucleotide-binding folds.

Disease frequency

At present, the population frequencies of pseudoxanthoma elasticum and mutations in the *ABCC6* gene are unknown, but in the United Kingdom at least 400 families are members of a PXE self-help patient association. Systematic analysis will be needed to provide additional information for diagnosis and genetic counselling in the population affected by PXE at large. So far, no clear correlation between the genotype and phenotype of the complex pseudoxanthoma syndromes has been possible.

Treatment and management

With time, patients with pseudoxanthoma elasticum are prone to premature-ageing phenomena in their skin and cosmetic embarrassment as a result. Patients with PXE are likely to suffer the results of vascular disease with stroke complicating hypertension and subretinal haemorrhages with visual loss; they are at increasing risk from severe gastrointestinal bleeding. Women with pseudoxanthoma elasticum should be advised to limit their family size. Excess exposure to ultraviolet light should be avoided as far as possible and sunscreen lotions used when this is not possible. Regular light exercise and avoidance of cigarette smoking are simple measures that also likely to be beneficial.

Although the skin and vascular lesions of pseudoxanthoma are associated with calcification, there is no evidence that calcium restriction influences the development of the disease. Nonetheless, some authorities recommend restricting calcium intake without evidence that this impedes the progression of the disorder. Because of their severe systemic arterial disease, patients with pseudoxanthoma elasticum are advised to undergo regular monitoring of their vascular integrity and blood pressure. The rapid onset of severe systemic hypertension that is refractory to treatment may be due to unilateral renal artery stenosis—a well-described abnormality in PXE.

Contact sports, including boxing, and arduous exercise such as cross-country running should be avoided. Regular monitoring by a cardiologist and ophthalmologist may be beneficial, in that the occurrence of new vessel formation in relation to angioid streaks can be arrested by ocular laser therapy to prevent or diminish the risk of retinal haemorrhage. Similarly, regular blood pressure monitoring with the prompt use of β-blockers for hypertension where possible may delay the onset of peripheral vascular insufficiency and coronary heart disease.

Prompt treatment of systemic hyperlipidaemia, which may independently complicate the arteriopathy of PXE, is indicated to arrest arterial narrowing and prevent thrombosis. Antiplatelet drugs such as aspirin are contraindicated because of the increased risk of visual loss due to retinal bleeding and of gastrointestinal haemorrhage. Coronary bypass surgery is as successful and no riskier than for the general population; there is little evidence to judge the outcome of vascular surgical procedures that may be indicated for stenoses of carotid or other major peripheral arteries.

Patients with pseudoxanthoma elasticum may benefit from plastic surgery to remove redundant skin around the neck and groins, abdomen and breasts. This is particularly applicable to women who become embarrassed by rapid cutaneous changes after pregnancy or the menopause. Keloid formation may complicate such cosmetic surgery and it is advisable that those who operate are apprised of this risk in PXE.

Special problems in pregnancy

Pregnancy usually proceeds with only minimal difficulties; the theoretical risks of recurrent gastrointestinal haemorrhage and perineal tearing at delivery result only rarely in adverse outcomes in women with pseudoxanthoma elasticum. Maternal PXE does not appear to increase the risk of fetal abnormalities. However, scrupulous monitoring of systemic arterial blood pressure is recommended in pregnant patients with this disorder and during the peripartum period.

Prognosis

In some patients with pseudoxanthoma elasticum, premature death results from vascular disease which may cause critical occlusion of the arterial supply to essential organs or fatal bleeding. Death from a recurrent massive gastrointestinal haemorrhage was recorded in a 13 year-old patient and severe bleeding due to PXE has been reported in many younger children. McKusick has shown that many patients may live beyond 70 years and die of conditions unrelated to their connective tissue disorder; his study of 52 patients with PXE from the case records of the Johns Hopkins Hospital in the early 1970s showed that the median survival of this selected cohort was about 46 years. All the patients in this early group were dead by the age of 76 years.

Further reading

Barabas AP (1967). Heterogeneity of the Ehlers–Danlos syndrome: description of three clinical types and hypothesis to explain the basic defects. *British Medical Journal* **2**, 612–13.

Beighton P (1968). Lethal complications of the Ehlers–Danlos syndrome. *British Medical Journal* **2**, 656–60.

Beighton P (1993). The Ehlers–Danlos syndromes. In: Beighton P, ed. *McKusick's heritable disorders of connective tissue*, 5th edn, pp 189–252. Mosby Year-Book, St. Louis.

Beighton P, *et al.* (1992). Molecular nosology of heritable disorders of connective tissue. *American Journal of Medical Genetics* **42**, 431–48.

Beighton P, *et al.* (1998). International nosology of heritable disorders of connective tissue. *American Journal of Medical Genetics* **29**, 581–94.

Beighton P, *et al.* (1999). Ehlers–Danlos syndrome: revised nosology, Villefrache, 1997. *American Journal of Medical Genetics* **77**, 31–7.

Bergen AAB, *et al.* (2000). Mutations in a gene encoding an ABC transporter cause pseudoxanthoma elasticum. *Nature Genetics* **25**, 223–7.

Birk DE, *et al.* (1990). Collagen fibrillogenesis *in vitro*. Interaction of types I and V collagen regulates fibril diameter. *Journal of Cell Science* **95**, 649–57.

Buntinx IM, *et al.* (1991). Neonatal Marfan syndrome with congenital arachnodactyly flexion contractures and severe cardiac valve insufficiency. *Journal of Medical Genetics* **28**, 267–73.

Burrows NP, *et al.* (1996). The gene encoding collagen alpha 1 type V (COL5A1) to type II Ehlers–Danlos type I/II. *Journal of Investigative Dermatology* **106**, 1273–6.

Byers PH, *et al.* (1979). Clinical and ultrastructural integrity of type IV Ehlers–Danlos syndrome. *Human Genetics* **47**, 141–50.

Carlborg U, *et al.* (1959). Vascular studies in pseudoxanthoma elasticum. *Acta Medica Scandinavica* **350**, 1–17.

Collod-Beraut G, *et al.* (1998). Marfan database (third edition): new mutations and new routines for the software. *Nucleic Acids Research* **26**, 229–33.

De Paepe A, *et al.* (1996). Revised diagnostic criteria for the Marfan syndrome. *American Journal of Medical Genetics* **62**, 417–26.

Elejalde BR, *et al.* (1984). Manifestations of pseudoxanthoma elasticum during pregnancy: a case report and review of the literature. *American Journal of Medical Genetics* **18**, 755–62.

Fattori R, *et al.* (1999). Importance of dural ectasia in phenotypic assessment of Marfan's syndrome. *Lancet* **354**, 910–13.

Godfrey M (1993). The Marfan syndrome. In: Beighton P, ed. *McKusick's heritable disorders of connective tissue*, 5th edn, pp 51–135. Mosby Year Book, St Louis.

Gott VL (2002). Aortic root replacement in 271 Marfan patients: a 24-year experience. *Annals Thoracic Surgery* **73**, 438–43.

Grahame R (2000). Heritable disorders of connective tissue. *Bailliere's Clinical Rheumatology* **14**, 345–61.

Gray JR, *et al.* (1998). Life expectancy in British Marfan syndrome populations. *Clinical Genetics* **54**, 124–8.

James AE, *et al.* (1969). Roentgen findings in pseudoxanthoma elasticum (PXE). *American Journal of Radiology* **106**, 632–47.

Kielty CM and Shuttleworth AC (1994). Abnormal fibril assembly by dermal fibroblasts from two patients with the Marfan syndrome. *Journal of Cell Biology* **124**, 997–1004.

Lee B, Godfrey M, Vitale E (1991). Linkage of the Marfan syndrome and a phenotypically related disorder to two different fibrillin genes. *Nature* **352**, 330–4.

Le Saux O, *et al.* (2001). A spectrum of ABCC6 mutations is responsible for pseudoxanthoma elasticum. *American Journal of Human Genetics* **69**, 749–64.

McKusick VA (1956) and (1972). *Heritable disorders of connective tissue*, 1st and 4th editions. Charles Thomas and Mosby Year Book, St Louis.

Neidner KH (1988). Pseudoxanthoma elasticum. *Clinics in Dermatology* **6**, 1–157.

Nicholls AC, *et al.* (1996). An exon-skipping mutation of the type V collagen gene (COL 5A1) in Ehlers–Danlos syndrome. *Journal of Medical Genetics* **33**, 940–6.

Palz M, *et al.* (2000). Clustering of mutations associated with mild Marfan-like phenotypes in the 3-prime region of FBN1 suggests a potential genotype-phenotype correlation. *American Journal of Medical Genetics* **91**, 212–21.

Pepin M, *et al.* (2000). Clinical and genetic features of Ehlers–Danlos syndrome type IV, the vascular type. *New England Journal of Medicine* **342**, 673–80.

Pope FM (1975). Historical evidence for the genetic heterogeneity of pseudoxanthoma elasticum. Brit. Journal Dermatol. **92**: 493–509.

Pope FM (1997). Molecular abnormalities of collagen. In: Maddison PJ, *et al.*, eds. *Oxford textbook of rheumatology*, 2nd edn, pp. 353–404. Oxford University Press, Oxford.

Pope FM (1998). Components of the dermis in anatomy and organization of skin. In: Champion RH, *et al.*, eds. *Textbook of dermatology*, 6th edn, pp 59–92. Blackwell Science, Oxford.

Pope FM and Burrows NP (1997). Ehlers–Danlos syndrome has varied molecular mechanisms. *Journal of Medical Genetics* **34**, 400–10.

Pope FM, *et al.* (1975). Patients with Ehlers–Danlos syndrome type IV lack type III collagen. *Proceedings National Academy of Sciences, USA* **72**, 1314–16.

Pope FM, *et al.* (1996). CoL3A1 mutations cause variable clinical phenotypes, including acrogeria and vascular rupture. *British Journal of Dermatology* **135**, 1617–20.

Reeve EB, *et al.* (1979). Development and calcification of skin lesions in thirty-nine patients with pseudoxanthoma elasticum. *Clinical and Experimental Dermatology* **4**, 291–301.

Scheie HG and Hogan TT (1957). Angioid streaks and generalized arterial disease. *Archives of Ophthalmology* **56**, 855–68.

Shores J, *et al.* (1994). Progression of aortic dilatation and the benefit of long-term beta-adrenergic blockade in Marfan's syndrome. *New England Journal of Medicine* **330**, 1335–41.

Steinmann B, *et al.* (1979). Evidence for a structural mutation of procollagen type I in a patient with Ehlers–Danlos syndrome type VII. *European Journal of Paediatrics* **130**, 203–5.

Struch B, *et al.* (1997). Mapping of both autosomal recessive and dominant variants of pseudoxanthomata elasticum to chromosome 16p13.1. *Human Molecular Genetics* **6**, 1823–8.

Viljoen DL (1993). Pseudoxanthoma elasticum. In: Beighton P, ed. *McKusick's heritable disorders of connective tissue*, 5th edn, pp 335–65. Mosby Year Book, St Louis.

Viljoen DL, Beatty S, Beighton P (1987). The obstetric and gynaecological implications of pseudoxanthoma elasticum. *British Journal of Obstetrics and Gynaecology* **94**, 884–8.

19.3 Osteomyelitis

Anthony R. Berendt and Martin McNally

Introduction

Osteomyelitis is an ancient disease with a formidable reputation for persistence and relapse. It has been diagnosed in human fossil remains from the late Neolithic and was described by many classical writers including Hippocrates. The term indicates infection of the marrow (the suffix 'myelitis'), but will be used here to indicate any infection of bone, even if confined to the cortex (sometimes called 'osteitis').

Aetiology

The pathogens causing osteomyelitis are dominated by *Staphylococcus aureus*, but there are many other known causes as shown in Fig. 1.

Epidemiology

Classical acute haematogenous osteomyelitis has its peak incidence in childhood. Males are more commonly affected than females. In children, there appears to be a greater incidence in the Southern hemisphere and among certain racial groups (for example, aboriginal Australians), with rates varying from 10 to 100:100 000/year. Socioeconomic factors may contribute to this. Chronic osteomyelitis is such a diverse disease that an overall incidence and prevalence rate is not available, but incidence rises with age due to numerous causes including diabetes, peripheral vascular disease, infirmity, and ulceration.

Pathogenesis and pathophysiology

The critical step in pathogenesis is the access of bacteria to the bone. This may occur from a contiguous focus such as chronic ulceration, surgery, trauma, or soft tissue infection. Alternatively, the route may be haematogenous, with bacteria reaching bone via the circulation. The exact mechanism by which this occurs is uncertain. It is believed that the tortuous capillary loops in the metaphysis of the long bones, a favoured site for haematogenous osteomyelitis, are particularly vulnerable to thrombosis, leading to bacterial seeding. This is supported by a history of recent blunt trauma to the affected part in some 30 per cent of cases, and by observations that in most animal models it is necessary to injure bone to infect it. Even minor bone and soft tissue trauma exposes components of blood clot, extracellular matrix, and bone matrix to the bloodstream. Many pathogens, notably *S. aureus*, can adhere to such host proteins through specific receptors, and hence to tissues and cells, including endothelial cells and osteocytes.

An acute inflammatory response is elicited once bacteria gain access to bone and begin to multiply. This causes oedema within bone and soft tissue, and the procoagulant effect of inflammation may also cause thrombosis in vessels. The result can be bone infarction, possibly contributed to by bacterial toxins.

As infection progresses, it propagates within the bone marrow, and through the cortical bone via the Haversian canals. Pus may form within cancellous bone and beneath the periosteum (see Fig. 2 for a schematic diagram). It may break into the soft tissues and even extend to the surface as a sinus tract. Subperiosteal pus under pressure will strip off the overlying periosteum, tracking along the length of the bone and around its circumference. The vascular consequences of this are critical to the evolution of the disease, since the outer aspect of the cortical bone is vascularized by the periosteum, the inner by the endosteal circulation. If the endosteal blood supply is already compromised, periosteal stripping causes bone death. Thus, large pieces of bone, segments, or even whole long bones can die.

Dead bone can potentially be revascularized and remodelled, but only if it remains in physical continuity with living bone. However, the action of bone-resorbing cells, recruited and activated by inflammation and some bacterial products, is frequently to separate dead from healthy bone. This produces a detached piece of dead bone called a sequestrum. Small sequestra can be extruded from sinuses or wounds and the episode of osteomyelitis may arrest spontaneously; larger sequestra result in continuing infection and inflammation. Over time more bone tends to be involved, sometimes resulting in new sinuses, with extension into soft tissues and contiguous joints. As bone is resorbed and killed, the loss of structure may lead to pathological fracture.

Chronicity and relapse result both from this host response and from features of bacterial physiology. The body cannot mount effective inflammatory responses in dead tissue or chronic abscesses. Bacteria adhere to the inanimate surfaces of dead bone and, as in implant-related infections, form complex structures in which they are enmeshed in an antiphagocytic polysaccharide matrix (the whole known as a biofilm). Their growth state alters within this, rendering them phenotypically resistant to almost all antibiotics. They may even be able to persist as metabolically crippled forms called small-colony variants: these can exist within cells and are also resistant to many antibiotics that would otherwise kill wild-type organisms.

If periosteum has been stripped and remains viable, it produces new bone called the involucrum. This may develop circumferentially, producing a shell of living bone around the dead segment, thus preserving mechanical strength. Defects in the involucrum, through which sinuses communicate with sequestra, are called cloacae.

Variations on this theme occur when flat bones or those of the spine are involved in haematogenous infection. In discitis and vertebral osteomyelitis, infection of the disc space is rapidly followed by involvement of the two adjacent vertebral bodies. The infection may arrest as disc material is replaced by granulation tissue, eventually leading to fusion of the two involved vertebral bodies. In flat bones such as the pelvis or the skull, infection can spread very rapidly in the cancellous bone between the two tables, before exciting a periosteal reaction.

The 'inside-to-out' nature of haematogenous osteomyelitis is in distinction to the 'outside-to-in' nature of contiguous focus osteomyelitis. In this case, periosteum is destroyed as part of the same process that has destroyed the overlying soft tissues. Cortical bone is killed and infection can enter the medullary cavity, thereafter extending as for haematogenous disease.

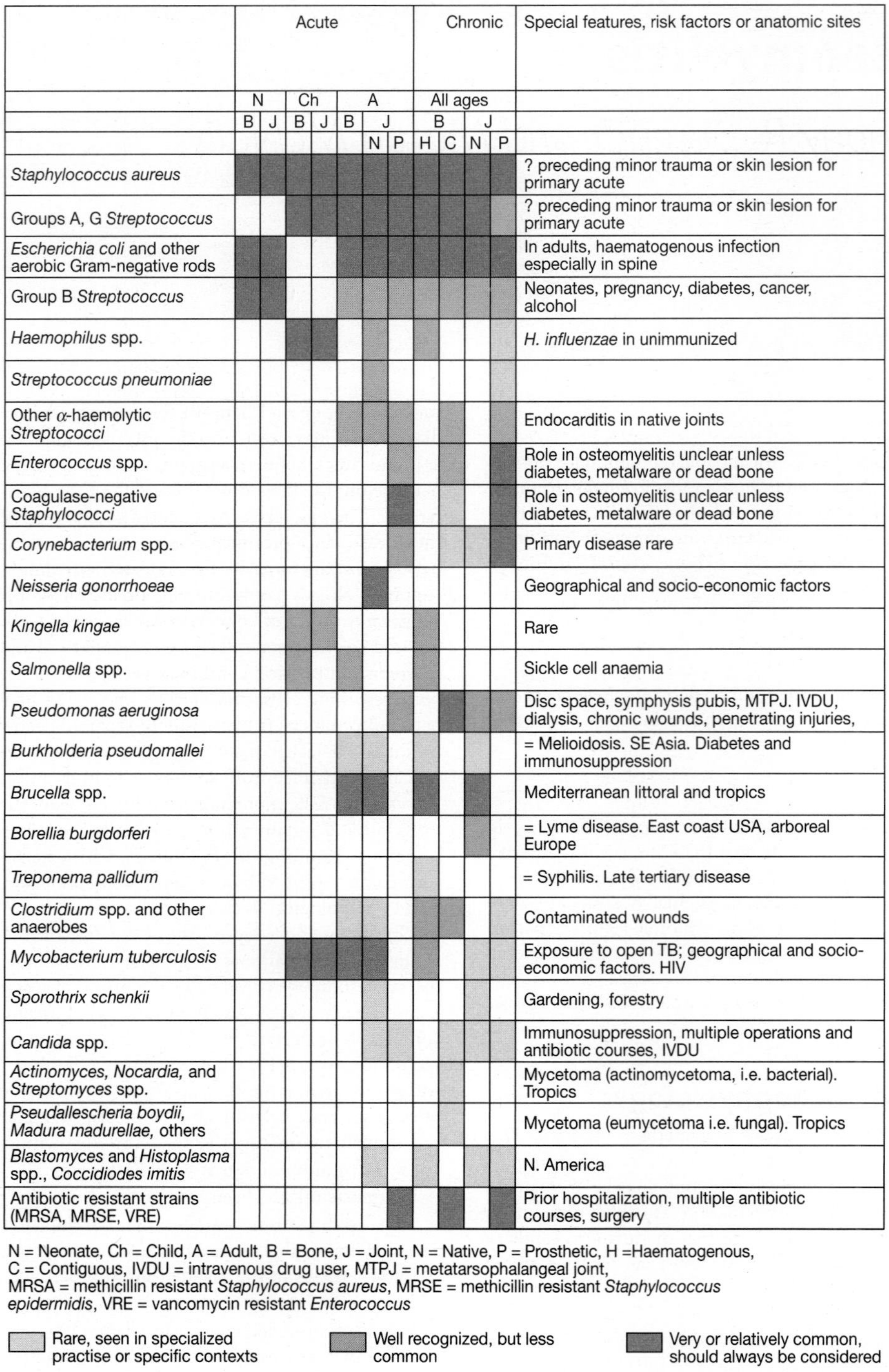
Acute
Chronic
Special features, risk factors or anatomic sites
N
Ch
A
All ages
B J B J B J B J
N P H C N P
Staphylococcus aureus
? preceding minor trauma or skin lesion for primary acute
Groups A, G Streptococcus
? preceding minor trauma or skin lesion for primary acute
Escherichia coli and other aerobic Gram-negative rods
In adults, haematogenous infection especially in spine
Group B Streptococcus
Neonates, pregnancy, diabetes, cancer, alcohol
Haemophilus spp.
H. influenzae in unimmunized
Streptococcus pneumoniae
Other α-haemolytic Streptococci
Endocarditis in native joints
Enterococcus spp.
Role in osteomyelitis unclear unless diabetes, metalware or dead bone
Coagulase-negative Staphylococci
Role in osteomyelitis unclear unless diabetes, metalware or dead bone
Corynebacterium spp.
Primary disease rare
Neisseria gonorrhoeae
Geographical and socio-economic factors
Kingella kingae
Rare
Salmonella spp.
Sickle cell anaemia
Pseudomonas aeruginosa
Disc space, symphysis pubis, MTPJ. IVDU, dialysis, chronic wounds, penetrating injuries,
Burkholderia pseudomallei
= Melioidosis. SE Asia. Diabetes and immunosuppression
Brucella spp.
Mediterranean littoral and tropics
Borellia burgdorferi
= Lyme disease. East coast USA, arboreal Europe
Treponema pallidum
= Syphilis. Late tertiary disease
Clostridium spp. and other anaerobes
Contaminated wounds
Mycobacterium tuberculosis
Exposure to open TB; geographical and socio-economic factors. HIV
Sporothrix schenkii
Gardening, forestry
Candida spp.
Immunosuppression, multiple operations and antibiotic courses, IVDU
Actinomyces, Nocardia, and Streptomyces spp.
Mycetoma (actinomycetoma, i.e. bacterial). Tropics
Pseudallescheria boydii, Madura madurellae, others
Mycetoma (eumycetoma i.e. fungal). Tropics
Blastomyces and Histoplasma spp., Coccidiodes imitis
N. America
Antibiotic resistant strains (MRSA, MRSE, VRE)
Prior hospitalization, multiple antibiotic courses, surgery
N = Neonate, Ch = Child, A = Adult, B = Bone, J = Joint, N = Native, P = Prosthetic, H =Haematogenous,
C = Contiguous, IVDU = intravenous drug user, MTPJ = metatarsophalangeal joint,
MRSA = methicillin resistant Staphylococcus aureus, MRSE = methicillin resistant Staphylococcus epidermidis, VRE = vancomycin resistant Enterococcus
Rare, seen in specialized practise or specific contexts
Well recognized, but less common
Very or relatively common, should always be considered

Fig. 1 Microbiological causes and contexts in pyogenic arthritis and osteomyelitis.

Sequestra may separate and be discharged, but the adverse biological factors that led to the initial soft tissue loss may impair subsequent healing and permit further bone infection to occur.

Clinical features

Acute osteomyelitis presents as a rapid onset of pain and loss of function in the affected limb, usually accompanied by high fever and malaise. It predominantly affects the metaphyses adjacent to the large weight-bearing joints. Prostration, sweating, rigors, and vomiting from accompanying bacteraemia (in 50 per cent of cases) may also be present. In neonates and infants, extension from the medullary cavity of the metaphysis through the cortex leads into the joint space, since the joint capsule extends beyond the growth plate. Thus in this age group an acute septic arthritis can be an early complication, or a presenting feature, of an acute osteomyelitis (see Chapter 18.7.1). In older children, the joint capsule is much tougher and inserts

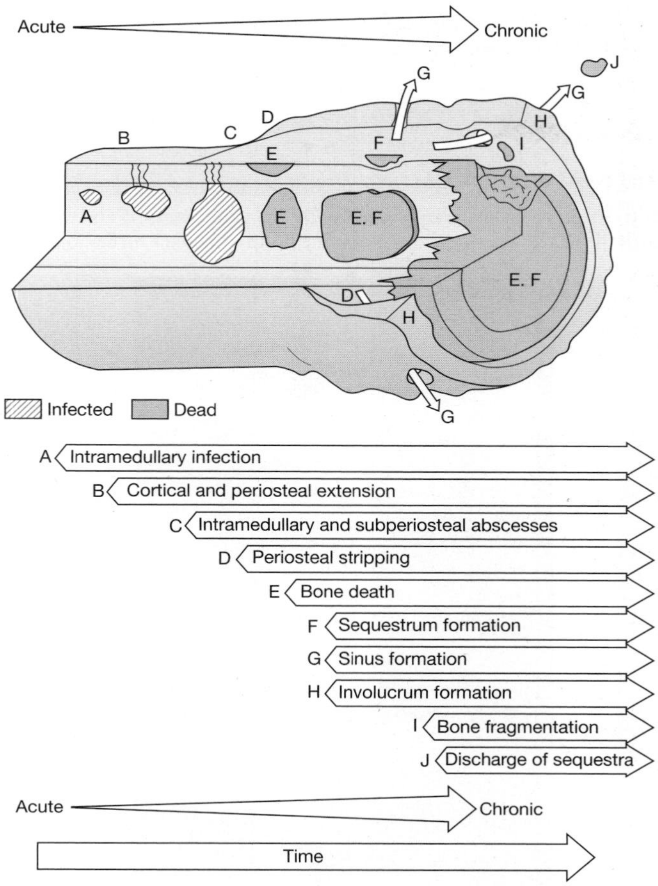

Fig. 2 Schematic diagram showing the evolution from acute to chronic osteomyelitis, with progressive necrosis, sequestration, and sinus formation.

at the growth plate, the cartilage of which forms a barrier to the passage of infection from the metaphysis to the epiphysis and the joint.

Chronic osteomyelitis presents more variably. Pain is the rule, unless there is underlying neuropathy, and there may be severe disability in the context of an ununited fracture or when the spine is involved. Wound or sinus tract drainage is usually present when osteomyelitis complicates ulceration, instrumentation, or other surgery. Bone may be visible, palpable with a gloved finger or located with a sterile metal probe in the base of an ulcer or sinus. There may be evidence of soft tissue swelling or induration, and bony tenderness on palpation or percussion. Some patients experience repeated flares of fever and acute illness due to inadequate drainage of deep pus or rapid extension into previously uninvolved soft tissue or bone. Minor ill health is common, manifesting as weight or appetite loss, general malaise, or poor glycaemic control in diabetics. This is often only noticeable in retrospect, once the infection has been treated.

Patients with vertebral osteomyelitis may present with bacteraemia and acute back pain (raising the possibility of spinal epidural abscess and the need for urgent diagnosis and treatment), but more often they present with chronic back pain and non-specific illness. Differential diagnoses of degenerative back pain, osteoporotic fracture, metastatic disease, and myeloma should be considered. The presence of severe back pain at rest, often of a deep and unremitting character that patients can distinguish from previous back pains, and of night pain, should prompt consideration of the diagnosis. Spinal tenderness is an unreliable sign. Deformity and the development of neurological signs are late features.

Special forms of osteomyelitis include chronic multifocal osteomyelitis (this presents with pain but, despite radiological and histological features of osteomyelitis, is culture-negative), unifocal osteomyelitis with a similar behaviour, and Brodie's abscess (a well-defined chronic abscess in bone with a very indolent presentation). The interested reader is referred to specialist texts for details.

Laboratory diagnosis

The white-cell count, erythrocyte sedimentation rate (**ESR**), and C-reactive protein (**CRP**), though generally elevated in acute infection and flares of chronic disease, are non-specific and occasionally normal in chronic disease. It is helpful to see elevated inflammatory markers fall after treatment, but this may take several weeks. The alkaline phosphatase level is of no value, being neither sensitive nor specific for bone infection. Blood cultures are essential in acute infection, when they may be the only means of obtaining a microbiological diagnosis. Serological tests are useful for the diagnosis of syphilis, yaws, brucellosis, and occasionally bartonellosis.

Plain radiography of chronic osteomyelitis typically shows patchy osteopenia or frank bone destruction, loss of definition of the cortex, areas of sclerosis, or periosteal reaction with new bone formation. These changes take many weeks to develop fully. In acute infection, the earliest changes visible on plain radiography are soft tissue swelling (minimum 2–3 days), followed by periosteal reaction (7 days), and last, bone destruction (10 days). If radiographs are abnormal, the changes need to be distinguished from those of a tumour, trauma, or degenerative bone disease. Repeat imaging at an interval of 2 to 4 weeks can sometimes help as osteomyelitis is usually an aggressive process. For more rapid clarification of diagnosis, however, specialized imaging is needed.

Ultrasound can identify subperiosteal collections and soft tissue abscesses, and demonstrate sinuses. Computed tomography (**CT**) scanning may be able to identify cortical erosion that has been missed on plain films and can demonstrate sequestra within bone. Reformatted images make it possible to produce saggital or coronal images (for example, to view vertebral body endplates) and three-dimensional images for surgical planning. Soft tissue collections are easily identified. Other than a lack of sensitivity early in the disease, the principal pitfalls of CT scanning are the radiation dose, its lack of ability to determine the extent or activity of infection, and its sensitivity to image degradation from orthopaedic metalware.

Isotope scanning is widely used, but there is a lack of consensus on the utility of various tests. Conventional, three-phase, technetium bone scans are sensitive but non-specific. Specificity may be increased by the addition of indium-labelled leucocyte scanning. Other reagents include labelled immunoglobulins, anti-leucocyte monoclonal antibodies, and even radiolabelled antibiotics, but the performance of these tests has not yet been rigorously evaluated.

Magnetic resonance imaging (**MRI**) is the standard and best method for diagnostic imaging of osteomyelitis (Figs 3 and 4). It can detect intra- and extraosseous oedema, abscesses, dead bone, and sinus tracts. It can distinguish active from inactive infection. Other than cost (rapidly falling) and availability (rising), the main problem with MRI is its extreme sensitivity to physiological changes that may persist long after surgery or treatment and to metal artefact from orthopaedic implants (and even to microscopic metallosis when they have been removed).

The microbiological standard for the diagnosis of osteomyelitis is the growth of bacteria from samples of bone, taken with precautions to prevent contamination from superficial flora. Pus or soft tissue associated with infected bone may be acceptable, but sinus tract or wound swab cultures are not. The bacteria isolated from wounds are poorly predictive of the deep flora because of asymptomatic colonization. Cultures of this kind should be reserved for detecting multi-resistant organisms (such as methicillin-resistant *S. aureus* (**MRSA**)) for infection control purposes. Fluid for microscopy and culture can be aspirated from periosteal or subperiosteal abscesses. In infants, needle aspiration of bone itself is safe and well tolerated if performed by someone experienced in the technique. Bone biopsy can be performed surgically or percutaneously (by needle biopsy). In

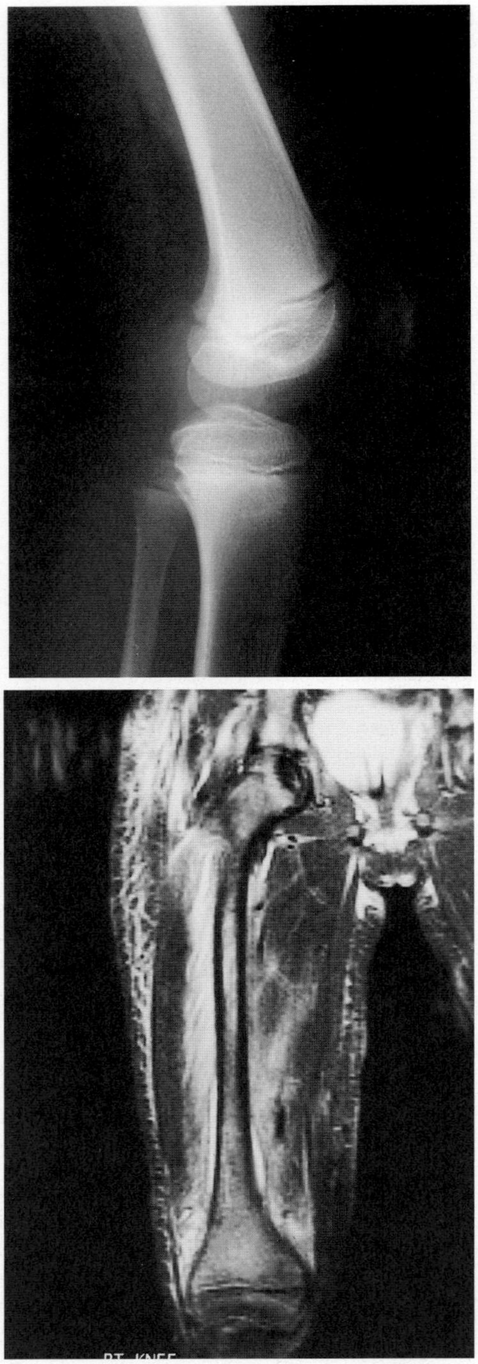

(a)

(b)

Fig. 3 Acute osteomyelitis of the femur in a child. (a) The plain radiograph, after one day of illness, is normal. *S. aureus* was isolated from blood cultures. (b) MRI scan (STIR sequence) of the same patient at day 2. There is marked soft tissue and intraosseous oedema (high signal). Subperiosteal abscesses can clearly be seen as linear areas of high signal just outside the cortex, tracking proximally up the femur from the metaphysis.

neuropathic ulcers, bone can be obtained by curettage. The laboratory must be made aware of the importance and nature of any specimen sent so that it can be appropriately processed and interpreted.

Bone histology is also an important diagnostic test: the presence of inflammatory cells, dead bone, and active bone remodelling are hallmarks of infection. They may provide the only confirmation of infection in cases where the culture results are unhelpful.

Treatment

Acute osteomyelitis

Acute osteomyelitis may respond to antibiotics alone, and with better outcomes, if treated before the onset of bone death or abscess formation. It is

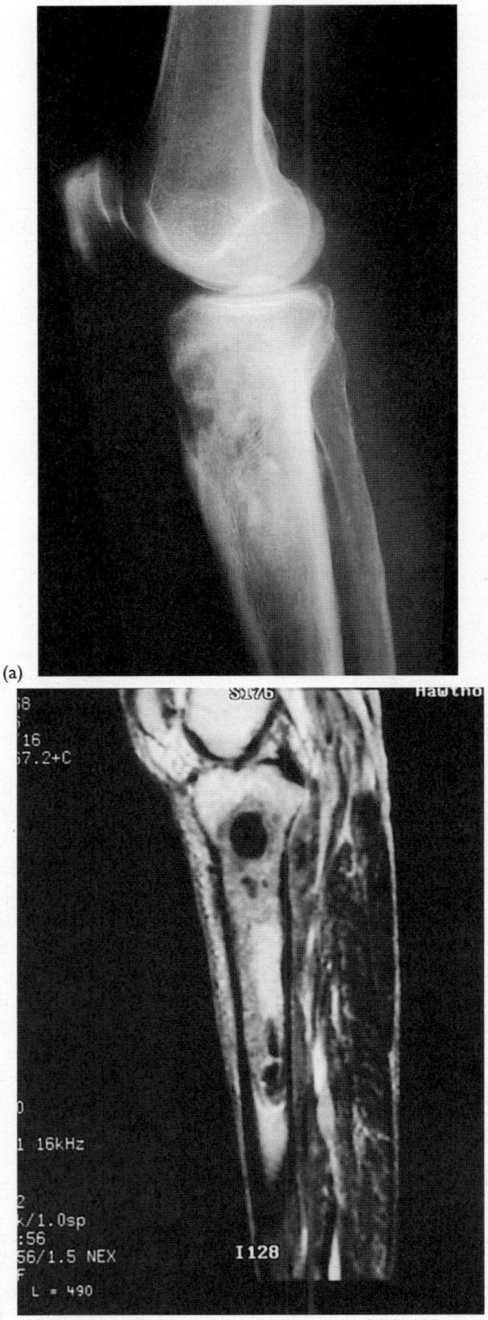

(a)

(b)

Fig. 4 (a) A plain radiograph showing chronic osteomyelitis of the proximal tibia in an adult. There is patchy sclerosis and lysis. (b) MRI of the same patient (*T*1 sequence) showing oedema (low signal) in the area corresponding to plain film changes, but also an additional, distal, intramedullary satellite lesion.

therefore an orthopaedic emergency. Treatment should be initiated on the basis of the clinical diagnosis, with investigations used to confirm the diagnosis once treatment has begun. Following blood cultures, high-dose intravenous antibiotics effective against *S. aureus*, β-haemolytic streptococci, and aerobic Gram-negative rods should be given. Appropriate regimens include a cephalosporin or the combination of an antistaphylococcal penicillin and gentamicin. Vancomycin and gentamicin will be necessary if the patient has risk factors for infection with MRSA. Antibiotics can be modified based on culture results. For patient comfort, the limb should be splinted and elevated, and analgesia given.

Surgery is indicated if abscesses are present: these must be opened, and the bone is usually drilled to allow free drainage of contained pus. The soft tissues are protected to avoid further devascularization and consequent bone death.

The necessary duration of antibiotic therapy is unclear. Treatment for less than 4 weeks is associated with higher rates of relapse.

In children, oral therapy can be considered when:

- the patient is afebrile after an initial 48 to 72 h of intravenous treatment;
- there is no evidence of abscess formation, metastatic infection, or bacteraemia;
- there is no suspicion from the history or imaging that infection has been prolonged or is associated with dead bone;
- the organism is sensitive to reliably bioavailable oral antibiotics; and
- compliance with therapy can be assured.

Less information is available for adults. The greatly lower rates of bone blood flow and turnover make revascularization and absorption of necrotic bone, and delivery of antibiotics and white cells, less certain. For these reasons it is common, but not universal, to treat adult acute osteomyelitis with intravenous therapy for periods of at least 4 weeks. Certain drugs, notably clindamycin and ciprofloxacin, are highly bioavailable and have proved useful in the treatment of osteomyelitis. There are no randomized studies to inform decisions about the requisite total duration or duration of intravenous therapy.

Chronic osteomyelitis

To achieve long-term arrest of infection, the management of chronic osteomyelitis usually requires multiple, co-ordinated inputs. The aims of treatment are to:

- remove dead bone and soft tissue;
- drain abscesses;
- eliminate cavities (which act as surgical 'dead spaces');
- ensure skeletal stability;
- restore soft tissue cover (if necessary using plastic surgery);
- define pathogens from high-quality specimens and administer appropriate antibiotics;
- correct adverse local and systemic host factors;
- support the patient physically and psychologically;
- reconstruct the skeleton if need be; and
- rehabilitate the patient.

Surgery

Detailed consideration of surgical methods is beyond the scope of this book, but major surgical advances include the use of free-tissue transfer and bone transport techniques to close very large bony and soft tissue defects. These permit much more radical approaches to the resection of diseased and dead tissues. In this way, surgery can potentially convert chronic infected wounds with dead bone and soft tissue into contaminated wounds of living bone with healthy soft tissue cover.

Antibiotics

These play an important role in increasing success after surgery, though the 'added value' they confer is uncertain and may depend on the extent of surgical resection. Some conditions often respond well without surgery including:

- discitis and vertebral osteomyelitis, with surgery reserved for abscess formation, progressive pain or deformity, instability, spinal cord compression, or persistent sepsis;
- tuberculous osteomyelitis, reserving surgery for mechanical complications, pain, or persistent infection;
- osteomyelitis of small bones such as the phalanges. In the treatment of a diabetic patient with foot osteomyelitis, accompanied only by limited podiatric debridement of bone, some authorities quote that chronic osteomyelitis can be arrested in 70 to 80 per cent of cases, but recurrences are common.

Antibiotics may also help when the patient refuses surgery, when there is no clearly definable surgical 'target', or when the risks and consequences of surgical resection would be worse than the disease itself.

The choice of antibiotics should be guided by the culture results. Intravenous therapy may need to be prolonged (for up to 6 weeks) where there is thought to be a risk of unreliable compliance, absorption, or efficacy with oral therapy. If properly supervised, many patients can be discharged from hospital while remaining on intravenous therapy. Periods of total antibiotic treatment vary from weeks to many months, but there is a growing trend to shorten the duration of treatment when an expert surgeon has achieved a radical surgical clearance, provided that local and systemic host factors are favourable. Antibiotics can also be delivered locally, by implanting antibiotic-loaded bone cement or collagen fleece at the time of surgery. The relative efficacies of intravenous, oral, or local antibiotics have received little attention and treatment protocols vary widely.

Adjunctive treatment

It is important to correct other host factors that may affect wound and bone healing. These include ischaemia (which may need intervention), anaemia, diabetes, hypoxia from respiratory or cardiac failure, peripheral oedema, poor nutrition, and smoking. Where neuropathy has contributed to ulceration, appropriate pressure relief is essential for healing and for secondary prevention. This must be continued indefinitely through the provision of specialist footwear, cushions, or beds. The patient must be taught about neuropathy and trained in methods to prevent further ulceration. Hyperbaric oxygen therapy has been widely employed with anecdotal success, but its efficacy and precise role are unclear and definitive randomized trials are awaited.

Prognosis

Chronic osteomyelitis can be arrested in 80 to 90 per cent of cases, usually when surgery has been combined with antibiotic treatment. Though most common within the first year, delayed recurrence is well recognized, and relapse can occur up to 50 years after an initial infection has apparently been treated successfully. This poses major difficulties for the design of trials on new treatment, as extended follow-up is needed to make definitive statements about success or failure. Chronic multifocal osteomyelitis has a good prognosis, usually self-arresting, albeit after some years. Long-standing active disease may be associated with the eventual development of squamous metaplasia or carcinoma in a sinus, and rarely with the deposition of amyloid.

Prevention and control

There are no proven means of preventing haematogenous osteomyelitis, but prompt treatment can prevent chronicity. Contiguous osteomyelitis can be prevented by the appropriate management of open fractures, of infective foci close to bone, and of chronic wounds whenever these are close to a bone or joint. Pressure-area care in immobile patients and of a diabetic patient's foot can prevent ulceration and subsequent osteomyelitis.

Occupational, quality of life, and psychosocial aspects

Pain, chronic sepsis, and physical disability have a significant impact on quality of life. Psychological well being is further affected by issues common to all chronic diseases, together with anxiety and depression over:

- risks of death, paralysis (e.g. in spinal infection), and limb loss;
- stigmatizing effects of chronic discharging wounds; and
- feelings of anger or failure where infection has resulted from an accident or surgery.

Areas of uncertainty needing further research

There is a need to define the true health, psychosocial, and economic burden of osteomyelitis. More information is needed on pathogenetic mechanisms and on molecular diagnosis. The optimal duration and route of administration of antibiotics and their place alongside differing forms of surgery needs clarification, as does the role of adjunctive medical treatments such as hyperbaric oxygen.

Further reading

Carr AJ, *et al.* (1993). Chronic multifocal osteomyelitis. *Journal of Bone and Joint Surgery* **75B,** 582–91. [Series of this rare, fascinating, and poorly understood condition.]

Case records of the Massachusetts General Hospital (1993). *New England Journal of Medicine* **328,** 422–8. [Case of late relapsing chronic osteomyelitis with much interesting historical and pathological discussion.]

Cierny, III G, Mader JT (1984). Adult chronic osteomyelitis. *Orthopaedics* **7,** 1557–64. [Classification scheme for chronic osteomyelitis, now widely accepted and used.]

Cremieux A-C, Carbon C (1997). Experimental models of bone and prosthetic joint infection. *Clinical Infectious Diseases* **25,** 1295–302. [Useful review of animal models.]

Gristina A, *et al.* (1985). Adherent bacterial colonisation in the pathogenesis of osteomyelitis. *Science* **228,** 990–3. [Important exposition of the role of bacterial adhesion in disease.]

Jacobs RF, McCarthy RE, Elser JM (1989). Pseudomonas osteocondritis complicating puncture wounds of the foot in children: a 10-year evaluation. *Journal of Infectious Diseases* **160,** 657–61. [Appropriate surgery allowing short-course antibiotic therapy for 'tennis shoe osteomyelitis'.]

Lew DP, Waldvogel RA (1997). Osteomyelitis. *New England Journal of Medicine* **336,** 999–1007. [Review.]

Lipsky BA (1997). Osteomyelitis of the foot in diabetic patients. *Clinical Infectious Diseases* **25,** 1318–26. [Excellent comprehensive review of a common and difficult form of osteomyelitis.]

McNally MA, *et al.* (1993). Two-stage management of chronic osteomyelitis of the long bones. *Journal of Bone and Joint Surgery* **75B,** 375–80. [Combined orthopaedic and plastic surgical management of complex osteomyelitis.]

Mader JT, *et al.* (1990). Hyperbaric oxygen as adjunctive therapy for osteomyelitis. *Infectious Diseases Clinics of North America* **4,** 433–40. [An expert's review of this mode of treatment.]

Norden CW (1996). Bone and joint infection. *Current Opinion in Infectious Diseases* **9,** 109–14. [A still-useful review of advances up to 1996 from an *eminence grise* of bone infection.]

Rissing JP (1997). Antimicrobial therapy for chronic osteomyelitis in adults: role of the quinolones. *Clinical Infectious Diseases* **25,** 1327–33. [Useful review of intravenous and oral therapies.]

Swiontkowski MF, *et al.* (1999). A comparison of short and long course i.v. antibiotic therapy in the post-operative management of adult osteomyelitis. *Journal of Bone and Joint Surgery* **81B,** 1046–50. [Useful paper.]

Syrogiannopoulos GA, Nelson JD (1988). Duration of antimicrobial therapy for acute suppurative osteoarticular infections. *Lancet* **2,** 37–40. [Large series that defined oral short course regimens for uncomplicated acute bone and joint infection.]

Tice AD (1991). Once-daily ceftriaxone outpatient therapy in adults with infections. *Chemotherapy* **37** (Suppl. 3), 7–10. [Description of outpatient intravenous antibiotic therapy.]

Wininger DA, Fass RJ (1996). Antibiotic-impregnated cement and beads for orthopaedic infections. *Antimicrobial Agents and Chemotherapy* **40,** 2675–9. [A review of this mode of treatment.]

19.4 Osteoporosis

Juliet Compston

Introduction

Osteoporosis is characterized by a reduction in bone mass and disruption of bone architecture, resulting in increased bone fragility and an increase in fracture risk. These fractures are widely recognized as a major health problem in the elderly population, resulting in an estimated annual cost to British health services of £1.5 billion. One in three women and one in five men surviving to the age of 80 years will suffer a hip fracture due to osteoporosis; demographic changes over the next 50 years are predicted to lead to at least a doubling in the number of these fractures, largely as a result of increased longevity.

Epidemiology

Osteoporotic fractures are termed fragility fractures (defined as occurring after a fall from standing height or less). They may occur at a number of skeletal sites but fractures of the distal radius (Colles' fracture), spine, and proximal femur are most characteristic. The incidence of osteoporotic fractures increases markedly with age; in women, the median age for Colles' fractures is 65 years and for hip fracture, 80 years. The age at which vertebral fracture incidence reaches a peak has been less well defined but is thought in women to be between 65 and 80 years. In men, no age-related increase in forearm fractures is seen but hip fracture incidence rises exponentially after the age of 75 years. The prevalence of vertebral fractures rises with age in men, although less steeply than in women.

The remaining lifetime risk of osteoporotic fracture in 50-year-old British white women has been estimated at 14 per cent for the hip, 11 per cent for the spine, and 13 per cent for the radius; for any osteoporotic fracture, this risk approaches 40 per cent in women and 13 per cent in men. For women this risk is similar to that of cardiovascular disease and is approximately six times higher than that of breast cancer. In the United Kingdom it is estimated that approximately 60 000 hip fractures and 50 000 Colles' fractures occur annually; for vertebral fractures, the figure of 40 000 reflects only those which are clinically diagnosed and probably represents only about one-third of all fractures. There are marked geographical variations in the incidence of osteoporotic fractures, the reasons for which remain only partially defined. The condition is most common in Asian and Caucasian populations but rare in African and American black populations.

Clinical features

Colles' fractures typically occur after a fall forwards on to the outstretched hand. They cause considerable inconvenience, usually requiring 4 to 6 weeks in plaster and long-term adverse sequelae are seen in up to one-third of patients. These include pain, sympathetic algodystrophy, deformity, and functional impairment.

Spinal fractures are characterized by varying degrees of vertebral deformity (Fig. 1) and may occur spontaneously or as a result of normal activities such as lifting, bending, and coughing. A minority of vertebral fractures (possibly around one-third) present with acute and severe pain at the site of the fracture, often radiating around the thorax or abdomen. The natural history of this pain is variable; in general, there is a tendency for improvement with time but resolution is often incomplete. Multiple vertebral deformities result in spinal deformity (kyphosis), height loss, and corresponding alterations in body shape with protuberance of the abdomen and loss of normal body contours. These changes are commonly associated with loss of self-confidence and self-esteem, difficulty with daily activities, and increased social isolation. The clinical impact of spinal fractures is thus substantial, although often underestimated.

Of all the osteoporotic fractures, hip fractures cause the greatest morbidity and mortality. They almost always follow a fall, either backwards or to the side, and require admission to hospital and surgical treatment. Because hip fractures characteristically affect frail elderly people, postoperative morbidity and mortality are high; at 6 months after fracture, mortality rates of 12 to 20 per cent have been reported. Only a minority of patients regain their former level of independence following a hip fracture and up to one-third require institutionalized care.

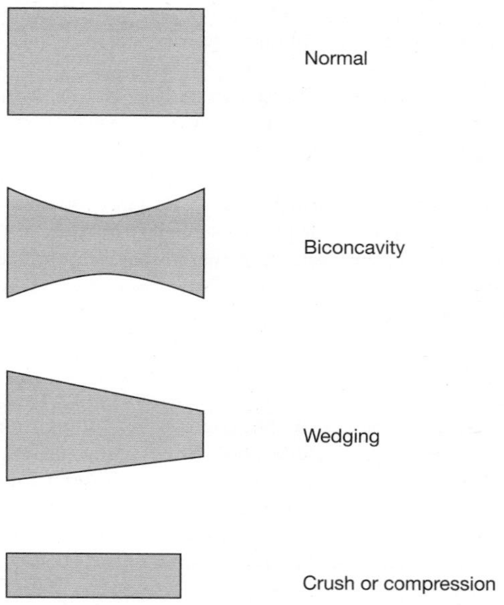

Fig. 1 Vertebral deformities associated with osteoporosis. It should be noted that some degree of biconcavity can be a normal variant and wedge and crush deformities are most commonly associated with symptoms.

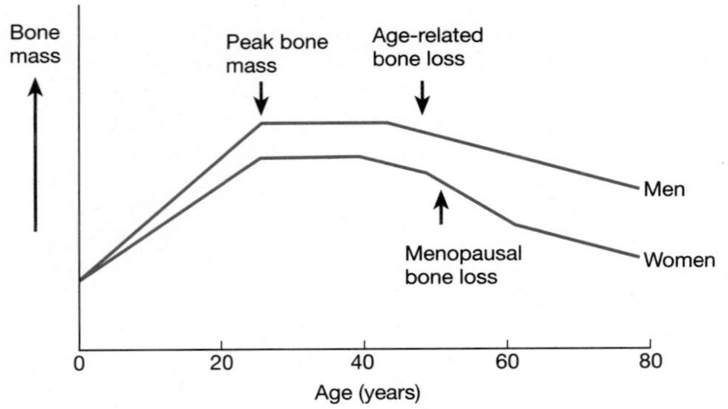

Fig. 2 Schematic representation of lifetime changes in bone mass in men and women. (Reprinted with permission from Compston JE, 1995, Osteoporosis, corticosteroids and inflammatory bowel disease. *Alimentary Pharmacology and Therapeutics* **9**, 237–50.)

Pathogenesis

Lifetime changes in bone mass are shown in Fig. 2. Peak bone mass is attained in the third decade of life and age-related bone loss is believed to start in both men and women around the beginning of the fifth decade; thereafter bone loss continues throughout life. In women, there is an acceleration of the rate of bone loss around the time of the menopause, the duration of which is poorly characterized but may be 5 to 10 years.

Bone mass in later life thus depends both on the peak bone mass achieved in early adulthood and on the rate of age-related bone loss. Genetic factors strongly influence peak bone mass, accounting for up to 70 to 80 per cent of its variance. A number of genes are likely to be involved; a polymorphism of the collagen type IA1 gene has been shown to be associated both with low bone mineral density and fracture and it is likely that other genes will be identified in the near future. Sex hormone status, nutrition, and physical activity also influence peak bone mass.

In women, oestrogen deficiency is a major pathogenetic factor in menopausal bone loss. In men, the relationship between age-related bone loss and declining testosterone levels is less well documented. In the elderly, vitamin D insufficiency and secondary hyperparathyroidism are common and contribute to age-related bone loss. Other potential pathogenetic factors include declining levels of physical activity and intestinal calcium malabsorption.

A number of endogenous and exogenous risk factors for osteoporosis have been identified. In the former category, advancing age, female gender, Caucasian or Asian race, and a family history of osteoporosis (particularly a maternal history of hip fracture) are the most important. Strong exogenous risk factors include hypogonadism in either sex, glucocorticoid therapy, low body weight, and previous or prevalent fragility fracture. Several diseases, including hyperthyroidism, hyperparathyroidism, inflammatory bowel disease, and chronic renal or liver dysfunction are also associated with increased risk of osteoporosis. Finally, low dietary calcium intake, vitamin D deficiency, immobilization, cigarette smoking, and excessive alcohol intake have adverse effects on bone mass.

Risk factors for falling are major determinants of fracture risk, particularly for hip fracture in the elderly. Their recognition is important, since many are modifiable. They include poor visual acuity, neuromuscular weakness or incoordination, reduced mobility, cognitive impairment, and the use of sedatives, tranquillizers, and alcohol. There are also many environmental hazards that increase the risk of falling, such as uneven paving stones, poor lighting, and loose carpets and wires.

Pathophysiology

The mechanical competence of the skeleton is maintained by the process of bone remodelling, in which a quantum of bone is removed by osteoclasts followed by the formation, in the cavity so created, of new bone by osteoblasts. Under normal circumstances resorption always occurs before formation and the amounts of bone resorbed and formed within each bone remodelling unit are similar.

In menopausal bone loss, there is an increase in the number of bone remodelling units on the bone surface (increased bone turnover), resulting in a higher number than normal of remodelling units undergoing resorption at any one time. In addition, within each of these units less bone is formed than resorbed, leading to a negative remodelling imbalance. It is believed that one of the early, and probably transient effects, of oestrogen deficiency is to increase the activity of osteoclasts, probably by suppressing apoptosis. Increased osteoclastic activity causes an increase in the depth of erosion of bone by these cells, contributing to the trabecular penetration and disruption of bone architecture that characterizes postmenopausal osteoporosis.

The pathophysiology of other forms of osteoporosis remains to be fully defined. In glucocorticoid-induced osteoporosis, reduced bone formation and low bone turnover predominate in those treated long term, but there is evidence that in the early stages of treatment there is an increase in bone turnover and osteoclast activity. The alterations in bone remodelling responsible for osteoporosis in men have not been established, but the lesser degree of structural disruption of cancellous bone during ageing suggests that reduced bone formation plays a greater role in age-related bone loss in men than women. Whether this applies to men with osteoporosis, however, is uncertain.

Diagnosis

Several techniques are available for the assessment of bone mass; these include single and dual energy X-ray absorptiometry, quantitative computed tomography, and ultrasound. At present, dual energy X-ray absorptiometry is regarded as the optimal approach in clinical practice because of its ability to measure bone mineral density at axial and appendicular sites, its good reproducibility, and the very low doses of radiation required. However, ultrasonography is currently being evaluated and may become more widely adopted in the future.

The rationale for the use of bone densitometry in clinical practice is the demonstration, in prospective studies, of a continuous and inverse relationship between bone mineral density and fracture risk. For every standard deviation decrease in bone mineral density, there is a two- to threefold increase in fracture risk; this is quantitatively similar to the relationship between blood pressure and stroke and greater than that observed for serum cholesterol and coronary heart disease. Bone mineral density at a wide range of sites, including spine, hip, radius, and os calcis, is able to predict fracture risk, although the best predictive value, at least in the case of hip fracture, is provided by measurement at the potential fracture site.

The relationship between bone mineral density and fracture risk forms the basis for the densitometric classification of osteoporosis. This is based on T scores—standard deviation scores above or below normal peak bone mass—and defines osteoporosis as a bone mineral density T score at the hip and/or spine below –2.5. Osteopenia is defined as a T score between –1 and –2.5 and established osteoporosis as a T score below –2.5 in the presence of one or more fragility fractures. Although these are diagnostic rather than interventional criteria, a T score below –2.5 would generally be considered as an indication for intervention because of the high associated fracture risk.

Since population-based screening cannot be justified at present, patients are selected for bone densitometry in clinical practice on the basis of risk factors and/or symptoms or signs suggestive of osteoporosis. Indications for bone densitometry are shown in Table 1. Bone densitometry should only be performed where the result will influence clinical management; it is not indicated in patients with clear evidence of established osteoporosis and in the very elderly, in whom low bone mass is almost universal, bone densitometry is rarely useful in directing clinical management. In addition, the presence of osteophytes, extraskeletal calcification, and vertebral and/or

Table 1 Indications for bone densitometry

Radiographic osteopenia and/or vertebral deformity
Loss of height and/or thoracic kyphosis
Hypogonadism
Previous fragility fracture
Glucocorticoid therapy
Low body mass index (< 19 kg/m^2)
Maternal history of hip fracture
Diseases associated with an increased risk of osteoporosis, such as inflammatory bowel disease, chronic renal or liver dysfunction, hyperthyroidism, and hyperparathyroidism

spinal deformity in the elderly significantly reduces the accuracy of spinal measurements.

Secondary causes of osteoporosis should be excluded where appropriate. A full blood count, liver function tests, serum calcium and phosphate levels, thyroid function tests, plasma immunoelectrophoresis, and Bence-Jones protein determination should be performed in the first instance with further investigation if indicated. In men, in whom secondary causes are more common, serum testosterone, gonadotrophins and prolactin, and 24-h urinary cortisol should also be performed.

Biochemical markers of bone resorption (such as urinary deoxypyridinoline, pyridinoline, N-terminal and C-terminal cross-linked telopeptides of type I collagen) and formation (such as osteocalcin, bone-specific alkaline phosphatase, C-terminal propeptide of type I procollagen) have been shown to be useful in the prediction of fracture risk, particularly when combined with bone mineral density measurements, and in the monitoring of response to treatment. However, their role in clinical practice has not been firmly established.

Current therapeutic options for osteoporosis

A number of options are now available for the prevention of osteoporotic fractures in postmenopausal women (Table 2). For historical reasons the level of evidence on which the registration of these interventions is based varies widely; thus adequately powered, randomized, controlled trials with fracture as the primary end-point exist only for alendronate, raloxifene, and combined calcium and vitamin D, whereas in the case of hormone replacement therapy, evidence for antifracture efficacy is based almost solely on observational data which are subject to bias and likely to overestimate beneficial effects.

Hormone replacement therapy

Hormone replacement at the menopause, whether unopposed or combined with progestogens, prevents bone loss and there is evidence, mainly from observational studies, for protection against fracture at the hip, spine, and wrist. At least in terms of its effects on bone mineral density, oestrogen replacement is effective both when given at the menopause and if started some years later; however, it is generally less well tolerated in more elderly women and compliance is correspondingly lower.

There is growing evidence for attenuation of the beneficial effects of hormone replacement therapy on the skeleton following cessation of therapy, both in terms of its effects on bone mineral density and protection against fracture. The implications of these findings are first, that lifelong treatment after the menopause is likely to be required to maintain optimal fracture protection, and second, that the most cost-effective treatment strategies will be those which target high-risk women for treatment.

Table 2 Agents used in the prevention of osteoporotic fractures

Hormone replacement therapy
Bisphosphonates (cyclical etidronate, alendronate)
Raloxifene
Calcitonin
Calcitriol
Calcium and vitamin D

Short-term side-effects of hormone replacement therapy include breast tenderness and withdrawal bleeding. Although continuous combined 'no-bleed' preparations are now available, some vaginal bleeding is experienced by up to 30 per cent of women during the first few months of such therapy. The principal concern with long-term use is an increase in the risk of breast cancer; after 5 to 10 years of use, the relative risk increases by around 30 per cent, which is significant in terms of absolute risk for a disease which affects 1 in 12 postmenopausal women. Other adverse extraskeletal side-effects include a two- to threefold increase in risk of venous thromboembolism and there may also be a small increase in the risk of endometrial cancer.

Hormone replacement therapy also has important short-term and long-term benefits. It is effective in alleviating vasomotor and other menopausal symptoms and may also have beneficial effects on postural stability. Observational data indicate a significant reduction in morbidity and mortality attributable to coronary heart disease, although this remains to be confirmed in prospective studies. However, a recent study indicates that combined hormone replacement therapy in older women may not be effective in the secondary prevention of coronary heart disease; in that study, more deaths due to heart disease occurred during the first year in treated women than in controls. Other potential but as yet unproven benefits of long-term hormone replacement therapy include improved cognitive function, protection against Alzheimer's disease, and a reduction in risk of colon cancer.

Accurate evaluation of the risk/benefit ratio of hormone replacement therapy cannot at present be performed because of the lack of prospective data which are required to demonstrate the magnitude of potential risks and benefits. Nevertheless, many women are reluctant to take indefinite hormone replacement therapy because of the increase in breast cancer risk and treatment is thus often limited to a finite period of between 5 and 10 years.

Bisphosphonates

The bisphosphonates are synthetic analogues of the naturally occurring compound pyrophosphate. They inhibit bone resorption by complex and only partially understood mechanisms and may also inhibit mineralization. Three bisphosphonates are currently licensed for use in osteoporosis. Etidronate is administered cyclically and intermittently, the 3-month cycle consisting of 400 mg daily of etidronate for 2 weeks followed by calcium only for 76 days. In contrast, alendronate is given as a single daily dose of 10 mg and calcium is not included in the formulation; once weekly doses of 70 mg of alendronate have an equivalent therapeutic effect. Thirdly, risedronate is given as a single daily dose of 5 mg.

These bisphosphonates have been shown to prevent bone loss in the spine and hip, both in healthy perimenopausal women and in more elderly women with osteoporosis. The magnitude of this effect is similar for both agents; however, unlike the majority of antiresorptive agents, bisphosphonate therapy (at least in the case of alendronate) is associated with a sustained although small increase in bone mineral density, which is believed to be due to hypermineralization of bone. This may occur as a result of the suppression of bone turnover and its consequences for bone strength have not been established.

In a large, randomized controlled trial, treatment with alendronate for nearly 3 years was associated with a reduction of approximately 50 per cent in vertebral and non-vertebral fractures in postmenopausal women with osteoporosis. In the case of cyclic etidronate therapy, the clinical trials did not demonstrate statistically significant fracture reduction, but favourable trends for vertebral fracture were observed after 3 years of treatment and observational data also indicate protective effects against hip and other non-vertebral fractures. Finally, risedronate has been demonstrated to reduce vertebral and non-vertebral fractures, including hip fractures, in postmenopausal women with osteoporosis. A significant reduction in vertebral fractures was observed in the first year of treatment.

Bisphosphonates are generally well tolerated. Gastrointestinal side-effects may occur, especially with aminobisphosphonates, and a small number of cases of erosive oesophagitis have been reported with alendronate. It is therefore important that patients take the drug according to the instructions, namely in the morning with a full glass of water, 30 min before food, drink, or other medications, and remaining upright for 30 min after the dose. Alendronate is contraindicated in patients with oesophageal abnormalities or disease and should be withdrawn immediately if dyspepsia or dysphagia develop during therapy.

The optimum duration of bisphosphonate therapy is unknown. Despite their high skeletal retention, preliminary indications are that bone loss resumes soon after treatment is discontinued, although further studies are required in this area. There are theoretical concerns that prolonged suppression of bone turnover may have adverse effects on bone strength and, at present, treatment is usually given for a period of 5 to 10 years.

Raloxifene

Raloxifene is a selective oestrogen receptor modulator which has oestrogenic effects in the skeleton without the unwanted effects of oestrogen in the breast and endometrium. In randomized controlled trials, raloxifene has been shown to prevent menopausal bone loss in healthy early postmenopausal women; in addition, a 30 per cent reduction in vertebral fracture rate was seen after 3 years of treatment with 60 mg daily in postmenopausal women with osteoporosis. Beneficial effects on bone mineral density are seen both in the spine and proximal femur but no effect of raloxifene therapy on non-vertebral fracture has been demonstrated.

Raloxifene is taken orally as a single daily dose. Minor adverse effects include leg oedema, leg cramps, and hot flushes. As with hormone replacement therapy there is a two- to threefold increase in the relative risk of venous thromboembolism. Raloxifene does not alleviate, and may exacerbate, menopausal vasomotor symptoms; it should therefore be avoided in perimenopausal women with such symptoms.

The extraskeletal effects of raloxifene are of considerable interest. In particular, a highly significant protective effect against breast cancer which is oestrogen receptor positive has emerged in the clinical trials; overall, after 4 years of treatment there was a 75 per cent reduction in new cases of breast cancer, this figure rising to 90 per cent when only cases that were oestrogen receptor positive were considered. Raloxifene use is not associated with vaginal bleeding and does not increase the incidence of endometrial hyperplasia or carcinoma. The effects of raloxifene on cognitive function and cardiovascular disease risk have not been established; in the context of the latter, effects on serum lipid profile similar but not identical to those observed with oestrogen have been reported.

Calcitonin

Calcitonin may be administered parenterally or intranasally; both forms of treatment have been shown to prevent spinal bone loss in postmenopausal women, but treatment benefits at other sites such as the proximal femur and radius have not been clearly demonstrated. The effects of calcitonin on fracture rate are controversial although some randomized controlled trial data indicate beneficial effects on vertebral fracture risk. Adverse effects with intranasal calcitonin are rare. Nausea and flushing may occur shortly after parenteral administration of calcitonin and vomiting and diarrhoea also sometimes occur. These symptoms are usually transient but may persist for some hours after injection.

Vitamin D and calcium

There is increasing evidence that vitamin D and calcium supplementation protects against non-vertebral fractures in elderly subjects. Thus in a randomized controlled trial of vitamin D and calcium in daily doses of 800 IU and 1.2 g, respectively, a significant reduction in hip and other non-vertebral fractures was seen after 12 to 18 months of treatment in a cohort of very elderly women (mean age 84 years) who were living in sheltered accommodation. Subsequently, a significant reduction in non-vertebral fractures was reported in community-dwelling men and women aged over 65 years in a randomized controlled trial of 700 IU of vitamin D and 500 mg of calcium daily. It is not possible from these studies to deduce the relative contribution of vitamin D and calcium to the observed benefits; vitamin D without calcium has been shown in some studies to reduce non-vertebral fracture rate in the elderly, but this finding has not been universal. The important question of whether vitamin D alone reduces hip fracture thus remains unanswered at present.

Calcitriol

Calcitriol (1,25-dihydroxyvitamin D, the active metabolite of vitamin D) preserves bone mineral density in women with postmenopausal osteoporosis and there is evidence that it also reduces vertebral fracture rate, although the latter finding has not been universal. Effects on non-vertebral fracture have not been documented. Calcitriol is given orally in a dose of 0.5 to 1.0 μg daily; hypercalciuria and hypercalcaemia may occur and serum calcium levels should be monitored at regular intervals.

Calcium

Beneficial effects of calcium on bone mineral density have been documented in children and adults, particularly at appendicular skeletal sites. In lumbar spinal bone, these effects are generally less evident and may be transient; the benefits of calcium are also less marked in perimenopausal women, presumably because of the dominant effects of oestrogen deficiency. Although several small studies have reported a reduction in vertebral fracture rate in calcium-supplemented individuals, evidence from adequately powered studies is not available and calcium should be regarded as an adjunct to treatment rather than as definitive therapy.

Non-pharmacological interventions

Hip protectors have been shown to protect against hip fracture in randomized controlled trials in the elderly and should be considered in all those at high risk, including those who have already sustained a hip fracture. Physiotherapy has an important role to play in the management of pain and restricted mobility and measures such as hydrotherapy and TENS (transcutaneous electrical nerve stimulation) are often effective. In elderly patients, occupational therapy is also often helpful and assessment of the risk of falling should be performed with advice on reducing risk where appropriate.

Weight-bearing exercise can produce modest, site-specific increases in bone mineral density in younger adults, but its skeletal effects in postmenopausal women are less certain and it should not be regarded as a definitive treatment. In the elderly, exercise may reduce the risk of falling and, if a fall should occur, improve the neuromuscular protective responses; however, the efficacy of this approach in reducing fracture risk has yet to be proved in randomized controlled trials.

Other aspects of treatment

Pain associated with acute vertebral fracture is often underestimated and can be difficult to manage. Very strong analgesics should be avoided where possible since these may increase the risk of falling and bed rest should be restricted to a minimum to avoid further bone loss associated with immobilization. Calcitonin is often effective in the treatment of pain associated with vertebral fractures; salcatonin is usually given subcutaneously in a dose of 100 IU daily or on alternate days for a period for 3 to 6 weeks.

Treatment of glucocorticoid-induced osteoporosis and osteoporosis in men

Cyclical etidronate, alendronate, and risedronate therapy have all been shown to be effective in the prevention of glucocorticoid-induced osteoporosis and are licensed in the United Kingdom for this indication. In patients receiving high doses of glucocorticoids (such as 15 mg of prednisolone daily or equivalent) for 3 months or more or who have strong risk factors for osteoporosis, bisphosphonate therapy should be started immediately; in those receiving lower doses (more than 7.5 mg) for 6 months or more, bone densitometry should be performed and prophylaxis instituted if the T score is below −1.5.

Alendronate is the only treatment currently licensed for the prevention of osteoporotic fractures in men. Beneficial effects on bone mineral density have been reported after treatment with testosterone or cyclical etidronate, but effects on fracture risk have not been reported for either agent.

Further reading

Adachi JD *et al.* (1997). Intermittent etidronate therapy to prevent corticosteroid-induced osteoporosis. *New England Journal of Medicine* **337**, 382–7.

Barrett-Connor E (1998). Hormone replacement therapy. *British Medical Journal* **317**, 457–61.

Black DM *et al.* (1996). Randomised trial of effect of alendronate on risk of fracture in women with existing vertebral fractures. *Lancet* **348**, 1535–41.

Chapuy MC *et al.* (1992). Vitamin D_3 and calcium to prevent hip fracture in elderly women. *New England Journal of Medicine* **327**, 1637–42.

Cohen S *et al.* (1999). Risedronate therapy prevents corticosteroid-induced bone loss. *Arthritis and Rheumatism*, **42**, 2309–18.

Compston JE (1997). Prevention and management of osteoporosis: current trends and future prospects. *Drugs* **53**, 727–35.

Compston JE, Cooper C, Kanis JA (1995). Bone densitometry in clinical practice. *British Medical Journal* **310**, 1507–10.

Dawson-Hughes B *et al.* (1997). Effect of calcium and vitamin D supplementation on bone density in men and women 65 years of age and older. *New England Journal of Medicine* **337**, 670–6.

Eastell R (1995). Management of corticosteroid-induced osteoporosis. *Journal of Internal Medicine* **237**, 439–47.

Eastell R *et al.* (1998). Management of male osteoporosis: report of the UK Consensus Group. *Quarterly Journal of Medicine* **91**, 71–92.

Ettinger B *et al.* (1999). Reduction of vertebral fracture risk in postmenopausal women with osteoporosis treated with raloxifene: results from a 3-year randomized clinical trial. *Journal of the American Medical Association* **282**, 637–45.

Gluer C-C (1997). Quantitative ultrasound techniques for the assessment of osteoporosis: expert agreement on current status. *Journal of Bone and Mineral Research* **12**, 1280–8.

Harris ST *et al.* (1999). Effects of risedronate treatment on vertebral and non-vertebral fractures in women with postmenpausal osteoporosis. A randomized controlled trial. *Journal of the American Medical Association*, **282**, 1344–52.

Hulley S *et al.* (1998). Randomized trial of estrogen plus progestin for secondary prevention of coronary heart disease in postmenopausal women. *Journal of the American Medical Association* **280**, 605–13.

Kanis JA, McCloskey EV (1999). Effect of calcitonin on vertebral and other fractures. *Quarterly Journal of Medicine* **92**, 143–9.

Lauritzen JB, Petersen MM, Lund B (1993). Effect of external hip protectors on hip fractures. *Lancet* **341**, 11–13.

Marshall D, Johnell O, Wedel H (1996). Meta-analysis of how well measures of bone mineral density predict occurrence of osteoporotic fractures. *Lancet* **312**, 1254–9.

Melton III LJ (1995). How many women have osteoporosis now? *Journal of Bone and Mineral Research* **10**, 175–7.

Michaëlsson K *et al.* (1998). Hormone replacement therapy and risk of hip fracture: population based case–control study. *British Medical Journal* **316**, 1858–63.

Orwell E *et al.* (2000). Alendronate for the treatment of osteoporosis in men. *New England Journal of Medicine*, **343**, 604–10.

Ralston SH (1997). Osteoporosis. *British Medical Journal* **315**, 469–72.

Seibel MJ, Woitge HW (1999). Basic principles and clinical applications of biochemical markers of bone metabolism: biochemical and technical aspects. *Journal of Clinical Densitometry* **2**, 299–322.

Soag KG *et al.* (1998) Alendronate for the prevention and treatment of glucocorticoid-induced osteoporosis. *New England Journal of Medicine*, **339**, 292–9.

Storm T *et al.* (1990). Effect of intermittent cyclical etidronate therapy on bone mass and fracture rate in women with postmenopausal osteoporosis. *New England Journal of Medicine* **322**, 1265–71.

Tilyard MW *et al.* (1992). Treatment of postmenopausal osteoporosis with calcitriol or calcium. *New England Journal of Medicine* **326**, 357–62.

WHO Study Group (1994). Assessment of fracture risk and its application to postmenopausal osteoporosis. *World Health Organization Technical Report Series* **843**.

19.5 Avascular necrosis and related topics

D. O'Gradaigh, C. A. Speed, and A. J. Crisp

Introduction

Osteonecrosis is a non-specific term for the death of bone, which was attributed to suppuration or trauma; Pasteur's study of bacteria in 1860 and the advent of clinical radiography led to recognition that many cases were aseptic. Phemister and others showed the importance of ischaemia in many cases and the collective term avascular necrosis has since been used. Associated disorders are the osteochondroses and osteochondritis dissecans. Although these conditions are separate entities, they are linked by the involvement of ischaemia (Table 1).

Avascular necrosis

There are 15 000 new cases of adult avascular necrosis annually in the United States. Males are more commonly affected (8:1), the majority under 50 years of age, with the exception of knee avascular necrosis, which particularly affects women over the age of 50. Any bone can be affected, the femoral head and condyles, the head of humerus, and the talus being the most commonly involved. The small cuboidal bones of the wrist and foot are less frequently affected. The unifying feature is a relatively poor vascular supply to subchondral bone through end arterioles with a limited collateral network.

Bone comprises osseous tissue and cartilage, with myeloid tissue, fatty marrow, and a sinusoidal network of vessels packing the inexpandable bone compartment. Several local mechanisms may be involved alone or in combination in vascular compromise. These include disruption of the vessel wall, raised intramedullary pressure through intraosseous venous congestion, and intravascular occlusion by atherosclerosis, thrombosis, or embolization. Death and lysis of haemopoietic cells and lymphocytes occurs with a subsequent macrophage and fibroblast response. Revascularization follows with deposition on the dead trabeculae of fibrous tissue (in traumatic

Table 1 Classification of osteochondroses

Type	Site (eponym)	Comments
Articular	Metatarsal head (Frieberg's)	Especially second metatarsal head; uncommon; bilateral in 10 per cent
	Hip (Legg–Calvé–Perthes)	4–10 years; more complications over 8 years; bilateral in 10 per cent
	Navicular (Köhler's)	3–7 years; M:F 5:1; uncommon; may be bilateral
	Talus (Mouchet's)	
	Lunate (Kienböck's)	Rare under 15 years; males, especially trauma; may be associated with short ulna
	Vertebra (Scheuermann's)	13–17 years; M = F; usually lower thoracic more than upper lumbar; often several vertebrae affected (three to five)
Non-articular	Tibial tubercle (Osgood–Schlatter)	10–15 years; M > F; bilateral in 25 per cent
	Lower pole of patella (Sinding–Larsen–Johansson)	10–14 years; 'jumpers knee'
(i) At tendon attachments (apophysitis)	Greater trochanter of hip (Mandl disease)	
	Base of fifth metatarsal (Iselin's apophysitis)	
(ii) At ligament attachments	Ulnar collateral (Panner's disease)	'Little leager's elbow'; 4–16 years, especially males
(iii) At impact sites	Femoral condyles (Ahlback's disease)	
	Calcaneus (Sever's disease)	9–15 years
	Sesamoids (Treve's disease)	
Physeal	Medial/proximal tibia (Blount's disease)	1–3 years; occasionally in adolescents; bowing of the tibia with sharp angulation and metaphyseal beaking; unilateral or asymmetrical

Table 2 Conditions associated with avascular necrosis (incidences where available)

Trauma
Fractures/orthopaedic procedures
Drugs
Corticosteroids (2–5 per cent), alcohol, cocaine, oral contraceptives (rare)
Metabolic and endocrine
Cushing's disease, Gaucher's disease (60 per cent), pancreatitis, hyperlipidaemia (type IV), diabetes mellitus, pregnancy
Systemic lupus erythematosus (16 per cent of those taking steroids)
Transplantation
Sickle-cell disease (5 per cent; 40 per cent on MRI)
Dysbarism (caisson disease) (4 per cent)
Radiotherapy, thermal injury
HIV, AIDS

cases) or of lamellar bone (in non-traumatic cases). Simultaneous formation and resorption occur, with progressive loss of cartilage. Should adequate revascularization and bone deposition not occur, articular collapse ensues.

Numerous conditions have been associated with avascular necrosis (Table 2). Alcoholism and corticosteroids are the most common, where fat embolization precipitating thrombosis is implicated. Higher doses and longer duration of steroid treatment increase the risk of avascular necrosis, though there is considerable variation. Interactions between steroids and the conditions for which they are prescribed may contribute, as some conditions (systemic lupus erythematosus, renal transplantation) appear to confer a particular risk of avascular necrosis.

Avascular necrosis should be considered in anyone presenting with bone pain, particularly those with associated risks. Since dead bone is painless and biomechanically sound, clinical symptoms of activity-related pain and joint dysfunction usually develop insidiously with the onset of repair processes or following articular collapse. Local tenderness, warmth, oedema, synovitis, and reduced range of movement may be evident. Infection must always be excluded.

Low-grade symptoms may precede radiological changes by months or years. In the early stages of avascular necrosis, radiographs are normal. Areas of mottled increase in radiodensity may be seen initially. A radiolucent crescent in subchondral bone (suggestive of fracture), cyst formation, and flattening and fragmentation of the articular surface may be noted in intermediate stages. Joint space narrowing and other degenerative signs occur in advanced stages. Bone scintigraphy is more sensitive in early, potentially reversible, avascular necrosis. A 'cold' area with a surrounding area of increased uptake is characteristic but rare, and non-specific increased uptake is more commonly seen. Magnetic resonance imaging (**MRI**) has become the first choice of investigation for early diagnosis. In addition to its high sensitivity, it is valuable for assessing the extent of the lesion.

Primary prevention is the ideal in 'at risk' groups, where a high index of suspicion must be maintained. Judicious use of corticosteroids, early diagnosis, and treatment of sickle-cell and metabolic syndromes and of alcoholism may reduce risk to bone. Guidelines are available for decompression in divers to reduce dysbaric complications.

Management of avascular necrosis depends on stage classified according to the imaging oulined above. Three main groups can be identified. Early stages (normal radiographs, positive scintigraphy or MRI) may resolve with conservative management. In some centres, raised intramedullary pressure is believed to be a critical factor, and core decompression biopsies (also useful for diagnosis) are therefore advocated; however, fracture is a significant complication. The intermediate group (crescent formation, flattening, etc.) often require surgery, including attempts at reperfusion (with vascularized pedicle grafts or an implanted artery), osteotomy, or arthroplasty. Arthroplasty is recommended in those with advanced degenerative changes. Rare complications of avascular necrosis include osteomyelitis (especially in sickle-cell disease) and malignancy.

Osteochondroses

Osteochondrosis is due to disturbance of endochondral ossification at a previously normal site of growth, involving chondrogenesis and osteogenesis. This can occur through mechanical (macro- or microtrauma) and/or vascular mechanisms which may vary according to the site involved. For example, Legg–Calvé–Perthes disease is considered to be of vascular aetiology. Osteochondrosis can occur at any epiphysis and involve the articular surface, the epiphyseal plate, or apophysis (secondary ossification centre or site of ligament or musculotendinous attachment). These areas are significantly weaker than surrounding soft tissue structures and are particularly vulnerable in growth spurts, where musculotendinous tightness (resulting in poor flexibility) contributes to apophyseal disorders. Growing children and adolescents are most commonly affected, males three times more frequently than females, the onset of symptoms occuring earlier in girls. Osteochondroses are classified into articular, non-articular, and physeal disorders (Table 1). Although they do not continue past the attainment of skeletal maturity, complications may come to light in adulthood.

Specific stages have been identified in the pathogenesis. Arrest of ossification at the affected site occurs, followed by revascularization and bone resorption. Later reossification may result in alteration in shape. It is often difficult to differentiate osteochondroses from normal ossification centres on radiography. Initial reduction in size and fissuring of the ossification centre may appear, followed by sclerosis and alteration in shape. Radiographs of the contralateral side should be obtained for comparison. In early lesions, scintigraphy may show increased uptake, and MRI may show cartilage disruption. While most cases are self-limiting, a poorer prognosis with development of osteoarthrosis is associated with larger lesions and older age at presentation. In apophysitis, radiography is not usually indicated, but may show loose ossicles or bony enlargement at the enthesis. Management is symptomatic, with reassurance, modification of activities, local application of ice, and non-steroidal anti-inflammatory drugs as required combined with a stretching regime.

Osteochondritis dissecans

Osteochondritis dissecans is a distinct form of osteochondral injury through the articular cartilage in a diarthrodial joint. It can affect all ages, but usually presents in teenage males, typically at the distal femur and particularly the lateral aspect of the medial femoral condyle. Other commonly affected sites are the patella, talus, and capitellum of the humerus. Although trauma has been identified in 50 per cent of cases, this is an unlikely aetiological factor in those under 15 years of age. A familial pattern is noted in 10 per cent, and lesions may be multiple and occur at several sites suggestive of multiple epiphyseal dysplasia.

The osteochondral fragment is susceptible to avascular necrosis. It may remain *in situ* or become partially or completely detached, which may precipitate effusion and mechanical symptoms of locking, catching, and giving way. The disorder usually presents with progressive activity-related pain. Local swelling may be evident if trauma has occurred. External tibial rotation when walking is characteristic in medial femoral involvement.

Plain radiographs may be normal and specialized views (such as the notch view of the knee) may be required, showing a typical subchondral crescent sign or loose bodies. Scintigraphic findings resemble those of the osteochondroses, while computed tomography is useful to determine the site and size of the lesion; the overlying cartilage can be evaluated by MRI.

Treatment aims to achieve union of the fragment and restoration of joint surface integrity. In young patients with open epiphyses, healing may be achieved with conservative management, as outlined for osteochondrosis. Joint immobilization may be necessary. Surgery should be considered in skeletally mature patients, those who fail conservative management, or those with detached fragments. This involves debridement and internal fixation of the fragment with drilling or vascular grafting of the base. The prognosis depends on the patient's age, and the stability and location of the fragment. Degenerative joint disease in later life is a major complication.

Further reading

Bohndorf K (1998). Osteochondritis (osteochondrosis) dissecans: a review and new MRI classification. *European Radiology* **8**, 103–12.

Chang CC, Greenspan A, Gershwin ME (1993). Osteonecrosis: current perspectives on pathogenesis and treatment. *Seminars in Arthritis and Rheumatism* **23**, 47–69.

Mitchell DG, Rao VM, Dalinka MK (1987). Femoral head avascular necrosis: correlation of MR imaging, radiographic staging, radionuclide imaging and clinical findings. *Radiology* **162**, 709–15.

Mont MA, Carbone JJ, Fairbank AC (1996). Core decompression versus non-operative management for osteonecrosis of the hip. *Clinical Orthopaedics* **324**, 169–78.

Williams JS Jr, Bush Joseph CA, Bach BR Jr (1998). Osteochondritis dissecans of the knee. *American Journal of Knee Surgery* **11**, 221–32.

20

Nephrology

20.1 Structure and function of the kidney

J. D. Williams and A. Phillips

The organs of the human body were created to perform ten functions, among which is the function of the kidney to furnish the human being with thought.

Leviticus Rabba 3, Talmud Berochoth 61B

Introduction

The human kidney is formed by the fusion of a number of lobes. The structure of a single lobe is best understood by examining the unilobar kidney of a small mammal: in the rat, for example, the medulla is enfolded by the cortex on all sides other than its pelvic aspect, where it projects as a papilla into the renal pelvis. The renal cortex, containing all the glomeruli and the proximal and distal convoluted tubules appears in coronal section to be distinct from the pyramidal-shaped medulla, which contains the loops of Henle. The medulla is divided into an outer and inner medulla, the outer medulla being subdivided into an outer and inner stripe.

The nephron

The functional unit of the kidney is the nephron, which begins at the glomerulus (Fig. 1). The urinary space (the cavity between the glomerulus and its surrounding Bowman's capsule) leads into the proximal tubule, which itself can be subdivided into a convoluted segment and a straight segment. The straight segment of the proximal tubule descends into the medulla and changes abruptly into the descending limb of Henle's loop. This loop penetrates for varying distances into the medulla before returning to the cortex. The longer loops pass all the way into the inner medulla, whilst the short loops only reach the outer medulla. Generally speaking, long loops belong to nephrons of glomeruli lying adjacent to the medullary region, while the shorter loops belong to the more superficial glomeruli. The descending limb of Henle bends sharply back at its lowest point to form the ascending limb, which at another abrupt transition forms the medullary part of the thick ascending limb. This leads up into the cortex where it becomes convoluted and comes into close contact with the vascular pole of its own glomerulus, forming the juxtaglomerular apparatus. Further along the nephron the thick ascending limb becomes the distal convoluted tubule and then the connecting tubule, which joins the cortical collecting duct. Each collecting duct receives connecting tubules from about 12 nephrons and then opens onto the surface of a papilla.

The renal blood supply

Structure

The renal artery divides into the interlobar arteries and enters the renal substance at the columns of Bertin (the area between adjacent lobes). At the junction of the cortex and medulla the arteries divide again and form the arcuate arteries (Fig. 1). Each arcuate artery gives rise to cortical radial arteries that ascend through the cortex: there is no direct arterial supply to the medulla. The afferent glomerular arteries arise from the cortical radial arteries and directly supply the glomeruli. Efferent glomerular arteries drain the glomeruli and then supply the peritubular capillaries of the cortex and medulla, a unique arrangement meaning that the peritubular capillary supply is exclusively postglomerular. Efferent glomerular arteries can be divided into two types: those from the superficial and midcortical glomeruli supply the capillary plexus of the cortex; those from juxtamedullary glomeruli form the blood supply to the renal medulla. Within the outer stripe they divide into the descending vasa recta, which penetrate the inner stripe in vascular bundles. The renal medulla is drained by the ascending vasa recta, which traverse the inner stripe within the vascular bundle and then join the cortical radial veins. The vascular bundles of the medulla represent the vascular component of the countercurrent exchange mechanism between the blood entering and leaving the medulla. Interestingly, the vascular bundles are organized such that the perfusion of the inner medulla is kept totally separate from the perfusion of the outer medulla. The cortical radial veins join the arcuate veins to eventually form the interlobular veins, which run alongside corresponding arteries.

Function

Renal blood flow is influenced by intrarenal and extrarenal factors. Autoregulation within the kidney maintains a relatively stable blood flow to the glomerulus over a range of arterial pressure. This phenomenon seems to be mediated by events intrinsic to the kidney since it has been demonstrated in both denervated and isolated kidney preparations.

The glomerulus

Structure

On entering the glomerulus (Fig. 2(a)) the afferent arteriole divides into primary capillary branches, each of which gives rise to an anastomosing capillary network that forms a glomerular lobule. These capillaries then coalesce into the efferent arteriole within the tuft. The structural organization of the capillaries is unlike that found in any other part of the body. The capillary basement membrane (glomerular basement membrane) forms the barrier across which filtrate is generated. Embryologically, the glomerulus is the interface between the ureteric bud (or hollow nephrogenic vesicle) and the metanephrogenic cap, which develops into the capillary plexus. The result of this is a basement membrane formed by the fusion of the basement membrane of the capillaries and the basement membrane of the nephrogenic vesicle. This glomerular basement membrane (**GBM**) forms the skeletal framework of the glomerular tuft.

Although on electron microscopy the GBM appears as a three-layer structure with a central lamina densa and outer lamina rara interna and externa, this is probably an artefact. Freeze–fracture studies have suggested uniformity in the basement membrane from its outer to inner aspects. The major components of the membrane include a framework of type IV collagen linked by heparan sulphate proteoglycans (**HSPG**) and laminin, the basement membrane charge being provided by the heparan sulphate component (subtypes of which include perlican and agrican). Type IV collagen consists of a triple helix of fibres with a large non-collagenous globular domain at the C-terminal end (called NC1). This NC1 domain of the collagen molecule is the target for Goodpasture's disease, and mutations of the collagen chains are responsible for Alport's syndrome.

The endothelial cells, the basement membrane, and the podocytes form the filtration barrier. The endothelial cells are fenestrated (60 and 100 nm in diameter) and the lack of a diaphragm across the fenestrations exposes the basement membrane directly to the glomerular capillary contents. The luminal surface of the endothelial cells is negatively charged by polyanionic glycoproteins, but these are not present on the fenestrae. The capillary loops are incomplete (a tube of fenestrated endothelial cells surrounded only on its epithelial aspect by a basement membrane) and are held together on their inner aspect by the mesangial cells. Thus the basement membrane has an opening on its mesangial aspect so that the endothelial cells are in direct contact with the mesangium. At the vascular pole of the glomerulus the capillary basement membrane is reflected to form the parietal epithelium of Bowman's capsule.

The outer aspect of the filtration barrier is provided by the epithelial cells (podocytes), which interdigitate on the surface of the glomerular lobules. The foot processes of adjacent podocytes are separated by the filtration slits, which are bridged by the slit diaphragms and are the sites through which the glomerular filtrate passes. The pores have a central proteinaceous core with side arms linking to each adjacent cell, forming a structure with a zipper-like appearance and a width of about 40 nm. The luminal surface of the podocyte and the slit diaphragm are rich in negative charge, being covered in glycoproteins. The podocyte surface adjacent to the basement membrane expresses a number of adhesion proteins that ensure firm anchorage to the membrane.

The mesangium forms the pillar to which the GBM scaffold is attached. The interaction between the mesangial cells and the basement membrane provides the mechanism for the contractility of the glomerular tuft, and the means whereby the surface area of the tuft can be varied. The spaces

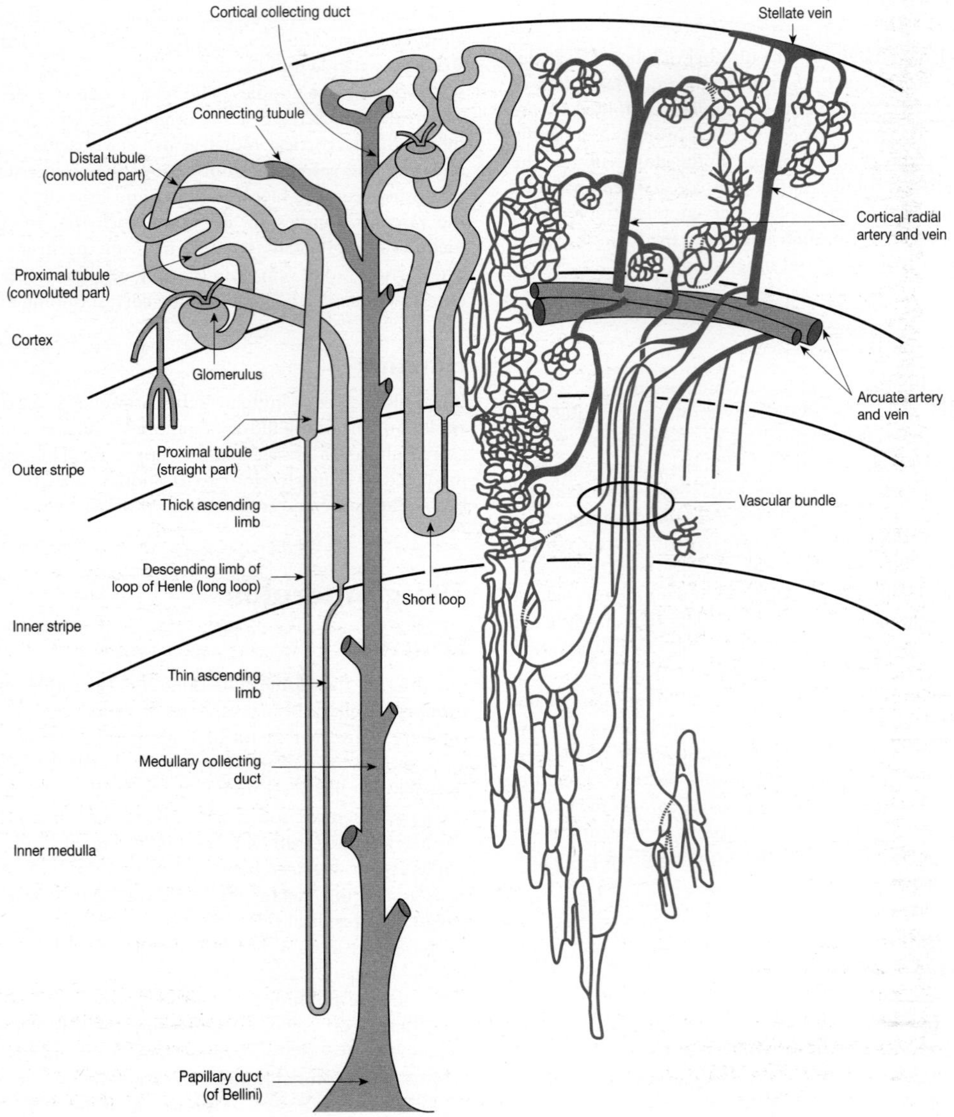

Fig. 1 The nephron and its blood supply. (Reproduced from Williams JD, *et al. Clinical atlas of the kidney.* Gower Publishing, London, with permission.)

between the mesangial cells are filled by the mesangial matrix and consist of a number of different collagens, as well as glycoproteins, fibronectin, and proteoglycans. This mesangial matrix provides a channel for the migration of a variety of molecules from the glomerular capillaries, with trafficking centrally towards the vascular pole of the glomerulus.

Function

The glomerular filtration barrier, consisting of the endothelial pores, the glomerular basement membrane, and slit diaphragms, will exclude molecules on the basis of size, shape, and charge. Size selectivity is imparted by the matrix of the GBM itself, as well as by the integrity of the podocytes. The matrix, formed by the type IV collagen molecules, consists of a series of interlinking pores, the narrowest of which determines the size of molecules that can pass through. Thus any pathological change to the structure of the matrix is likely to result in a greater permeability of the GBM. The resistance to the movement of water and small molecules is provided by the endothelial pores, the basement membrane, and by the available surface area of the slit diaphragms, the last of these probably being the effective barrier. The charge barrier, whose efficiency is disputed, is provided by the negative charge of the basement membrane and to a lesser extent by the surface of the endothelial and epithelial cells.

The effectiveness of the filtration barrier is dependent not only on the integrity of the basement membrane but also on the function of the epithelial cells. Most studies have demonstrated that changes in barrier function are closely correlated with significant alteration to the podocytes. These include changes in the surface area of the slit diaphragm (slit diaphragm frequency) as well as detachment of podocytes from the basement membrane. There is now a large body of evidence to suggest that HSPGs are involved in both the charge- and size-selective properties of the GBM and, furthermore, that alterations in GBM HSPGs may be important in the development of proteinuria.

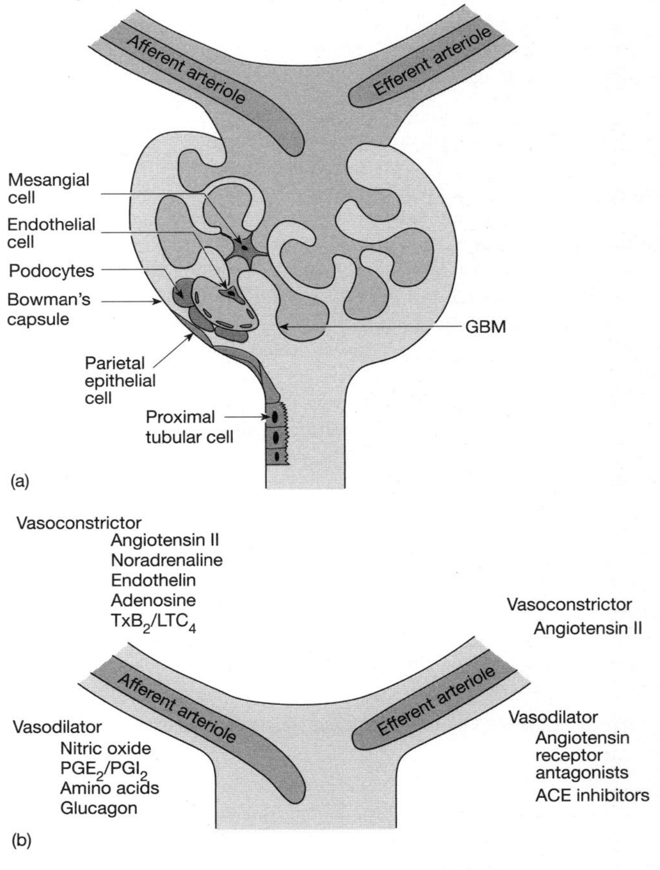

Fig. 2 The glomerulus: (a) structure; (b) regulation of glomerular blood flow by vasoactive agents.

Production of glomerular filtrate

The number of functioning glomeruli and the filtration rate at each single glomerulus determines the GFR. There are approximately a million glomeruli per human kidney, of which 90 per cent are in the outer two-thirds of the cortex and are fairly homogenous in terms of structure and function. The remaining 10 per cent, which are located in the juxtamedullary region, are larger with a higher single-nephron GFR compared with cortical glomeruli.

Single-nephron GFR is determined by a number of factors. First, the pressure of blood in the glomerular capillary and the hydrostatic pressure of the fluid in Bowman's space determine the pressure difference that drives the movement of fluid across the glomerular capillary wall, the transglomerular hydrostatic pressure difference or ΔP. Second, the gradient in colloid osmotic pressure ($\Delta\pi$) across the filtration barrier: this is equal to the colloid osmotic pressure within the glomerular capillary less the colloid osmotic pressure in Bowman's space (which, in effect, is zero). The difference between ΔP and $\Delta\pi$ is the net ultrafiltration pressure. Other determining factors are water permeability (K) and f (the area available for filtration, namely the surface area of the slit pores between podocytes), these two combined forming the glomerular filtration coefficient or Kf. Hence:

$$\text{single-nephron GFR} = (\Delta P - \Delta\pi) \times Kf.$$

SNGFR can be regulated by alterations in the ultrafiltration coefficient Kf, the net ultrafiltration pressure, or both. A change in the net ultrafiltration pressure may arise due to a change in the hydraulic pressure ΔP, the capillary plasma oncotic pressure ($\Delta\pi$), and/or alterations in the initial glomerular capillary plasma flow rate (the latter dictates changes in protein concentration with distance along a capillary network and hence affects colloid osmotic pressure).

Glomeruli contain receptors for a number of hormones that are capable of modifying the filtration rate (see Fig. 2(b)). These include vasoconstrictors such as adenosine, angiotensin II, and endothelin as well as vasodilators including dopamine, bradykinin, prostacyclin, and nitric oxide. Some of these vasoactive molecules are produced within the kidney, whilst others are delivered by the systemic circulation, and many studies have examined the effects of hormones on glomerular ultrafiltration. It is clear from the preceding discussion that, in addition to ΔP (that is, change in hydraulic pressure), the glomerular filtration rate (**GFR**) is dependent on the capillary plasma flow rate and the ultrafiltration coefficient (Kf), all of which may be altered by hormones. Vasoconstrictor substances such as angiotensin II and norepinephrine are capable of producing substantial reductions in renal plasma flow, generally with little change in GFR. Angiotensin II, for example, causes constriction of both afferent and efferent arterioles with a resultant decrease in capillary plasma flow, a reduction in Kf, but little change in the single-nephron GFR (**SNGFR**) due to an increase in ΔP. Increased afferent arterial tone caused by endothelin or adenosine will decrease renal blood flow, decrease ΔP, and therefore decrease GFR. By contrast, dilatation of the afferent arteriole by nitric oxide or prostaglandins will also cause an increase in ΔP, but with an increase in renal blood flow and hence an increase in GFR.

In the normal adult human, water is filtered by the glomerulus at a rate of 80 to 200 ml/min. The glomerular filtration rate is critically related to all functions of the kidney and is closely regulated by mechanisms that maintain a constant high value for GFR. In practical clinical terms, the estimation of GFR is achieved by measuring the renal clearance of a substance that is freely filtered at the glomerulus and not absorbed or secreted by the renal tubules. For discussion of the methods of measuring GFR in clinical practice, see Chapter 20.3.1.

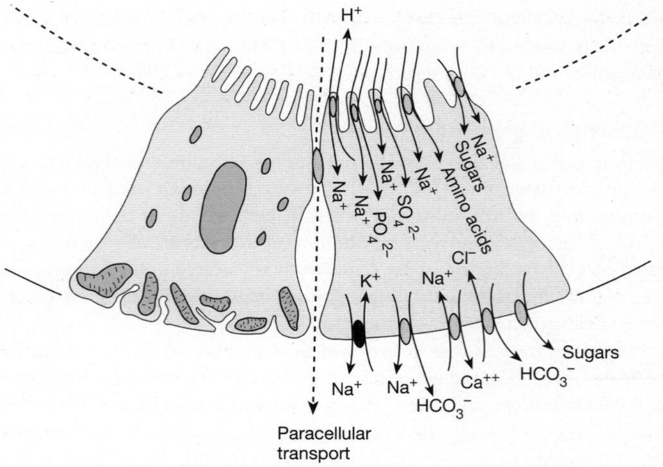

Fig. 3 Proximal tubular cell function. Principal transport processes of the proximal tubular cell.

The proximal convoluted tubule

Structure

The main function of the proximal tubule is to reabsorb the bulk of filtered water and solutes, and its structure shows numerous adaptations for this purpose. Proximal tubular epithelial cells are tall and columnar with a well-developed brush border, resulting in a 40-fold increase in the apical surface area of the cells (Fig. 3). In addition they possess extensive basolateral interdigitation, increasing the basolateral cell surface area. The apices of the cells are held together by junctional complexes: these are called 'tight junctions' (zona occludens), of the leaky variety, with a low electrical resistance that allows some transepithelial transport. The bases of the cells rest on the tubular basement membrane, which separates them from the peritubular capillaries. Another characteristic feature is the presence of large numbers of mitochondria, intimately associated with the basolateral cell membranes where the Na^+/K^+-ATPase is located, and whose function is to provide the energy source for fluid and electrolyte reabsorption.

Function

Sodium and water reabsorption

About seven-eighths of the volume of the glomerular filtrate is reabsorbed in the proximal tubule. Sodium enters the proximal tubular cells passively from the tubular fluid down an electrochemical gradient that is the driving force for fluid and electrolyte reabsorption. This gradient is produced by the action of the Na^+/K^+-ATPase on the basal surface, which transports sodium out of the cell in excess of the potassium transported into the cell, thereby generating a transmembrane potential of −70 mV. Chloride ions follow the same route by cotransport with Na^+, and the resulting increase in osmolality in the intercellular spaces results in the absorption of water by osmosis, such that the volume of the filtrate in the renal tubule is substantially reduced by the time it reaches the beginning of the loop of Henle, although its net osmolality does not change. In addition to this transcellular route for the transport of salt and water, there is also a paracellular route through the 'leaky' tight junctions.

Reabsorption of other substances

The proximal tubule is also responsible for the reabsorption of other substances such as glucose, phosphate, amino acids, and organic anions, including citrate and lactate. These enter the proximal tubular cells across the apical membrane by a series of cotransport systems, each of which binds one or more sodium ions and its specific substrate, and carries them across the cell membrane (Fig. 3). Thus, the rate of sodium entry into the cell is linked by cotransport systems to the reabsorption of these substances.

The energy for secondary active transport or cotransport of substances (glucose, phosphate, etc.) against their concentration gradient is therefore provided indirectly by Na^+/K^+-ATPase, which is responsible for the concentration gradient for sodium across the cell membrane. This is illustrated by the reabsorption of glucose, which involves brush-border, Na^+-coupled glucose transporters, termed **SGLT**, and basolateral facilitated glucose transporters (**GLUT**). In the human, the major site for glucose reabsorption is the early S1 segment of the proximal tubule, where 90 per cent of the filtered glucose is reabsorbed, such that only a small fraction of the filtered load reaches the S2 and S3 segments. Glucose reabsorption in the S1 proximal tubular segment is mediated by the low-affinity, high-capacity, Na^+/glucose cotransporter, SLGT2, whilst reabsorption in the later segments is mediated by the high-affinity, low-capacity SGLT1. Similarly, the high rate of glucose efflux characteristic of the early proximal tubular segment is mediated by the low-affinity, facultative glucose transporter GLUT2 and high-affinity GLUT1, whereas only GLUT1 is expressed in the late proximal tubule where a minor portion of the filtered glucose load is reabsorbed.

The kidneys are also involved in maintenance of the acid–base balance of the body by regulating the serum bicarbonate concentration to approximately 24 mmol/l. The proximal tubule reabsorbs between 80 and 90 per cent of the filtered bicarbonate, largely by the following mechanism. H^+ is secreted by the Na^+/H^+-exchanger on the luminal membrane. It then reacts with the filtered HCO_3– to form H_2CO_3, which is converted to CO_2 and H_2O catalysed by carbonic anhydrase present on the luminal brush-border membrane. CO_2 diffuses passively into the cell where it is split to yield the H^+ that is secreted and OH–, the hydroxyl ion then reacts with CO_2 (catalysed by carbonic anhydrase) to yield HCO_3–, which exits the cell via a Na/HCO_3 synporter thus restoring filtered HCO_3– to the plasma.

Handling of protein

In addition to its role in fluid and electrolyte balance, almost all the protein that is filtered at the glomerulus is reabsorbed by the proximal tubule via a process of endocytosis. To date, four major routes of tubular handling of peptides have been identified: (1) reabsorption of filtered protein/peptides by endocytosis and intracellular lysosomal degradation; (2) luminal hydrolysis and reabsorption of free amino acids; (3) carrier-mediated reabsorption of small intact peptides; and (4) peritubular uptake of peptides. The most important of these is probably the endocytotic route.

In recent years there has been considerable interest in the role of proteinuria in the progression of renal disease. Amongst the hypotheses currently under investigation are those that focus on the effect of excess protein trafficking on the generation of profibrotic factors by proximal tubular cells and the subsequent initiation of interstitial fibrosis. These theories suggest that cells of the proximal tubule play a role in maintaining the normal architecture of the renal interstitium. In support are numerous studies demonstrating that tubular cells are a rich source of many components of the extracellular matrix, which may modify matrix turnover by alterations in the synthesis of both matrix-degrading enzymes and their inhibitors, as well as through the production of cytokines. More recent studies have suggested that cells of the proximal tubule may migrate into the interstitium and transdifferentiate into the cortical fibroblasts during conditions of inflammation.

Interplay between the regulation of GFR and proximal tubular function

One aspect of the control of renal function is the correlation between the volume of filtrate produced by the glomerulus and the reabsorptive capacity of the renal tubule. The movement of sodium and water from the proximal tubular lumen into the capillary network depends on the hydrostatic pressure of the blood in the peritubular capillary complex, as well as the osmotic pressure of the blood within those capillaries. An increased hydrostatic pressure will reduce reabsorption, but an increased oncotic pressure will enhance reabsorption. Thus, increased systemic blood pressure will increase the interstitial pressure within the interstitium and result in the movement of sodium from the interstitial fluid into the lumen (pressure natriuresis).

The loop of Henle

The loop of Henle begins where the straight (S3) part of the proximal tubule changes abruptly in diameter to become the descending thin limb. Long loops pass into the inner medulla, before performing a hairpin bend and returning as the thin ascending limb, when an abrupt transition at the inner stripe of the outer medulla marks the beginning of the thick ascending limb, which is structurally distinct from its thin counterpart. In the case of the short loops the transition to ascending thick limb takes place before the bend, so that the thick part of the tubule forms the loop.

Although there are only minor structural differences between the thin segments of descending and ascending limbs, there are major differences in their permeability properties. The thin descending limb, like the proximal tubule, is highly permeable to water as a result of the presence of aquaporin 1, whereas the thin ascending limb is impermeable to water. By contrast, the descending limb is impermeable to sodium, whilst significant sodium and urea reabsorption occurs in the thin ascending limb. This allows an osmotic gradient to be established in the medulla, which is the basis of the countercurrent multiplier mechanism (Fig. 4).

The juxtaglomerular apparatus

The juxtaglomerular apparatus comprises the macula densa, the extraglomerular mesangium, the terminal portion of the afferent arteriole with its renin-producing granular cells, and the early portions of the efferent arteriole.

The thick ascending limb of the loop of Henle returns to its own glomerulus, where the cells that lie nearest to the glomerulus become taller to form the macula densa, the most obvious structural feature being that these cells are tightly packed and have large nuclei. The basal aspect of the macula densa is firmly attached to the extraglomerular mesangium.

The granular cells (also termed the juxtaglomerular cells) are assembled in clusters within the terminal portion of the afferent arteriole. These are modified smooth muscle cells containing cytoplasmic granules in which renin is stored. This enzyme is responsible for controlling the synthesis of angiotensin II by converting angiotensinogen to angiotensin I. This in turn is converted to angiotensin II by the action of the angiotensin-converting enzyme.

Granular cells appose the extraglomerular mesangial cells, adjacent smooth muscle cells, and endothelial cells, and are densely innervated by sympathetic nerve terminals. The secretion of renin by the granular cells is controlled by signals generated intrarenally (such as perfusion pressure and tubular fluid composition) and extrarenally, due to changes in sympathetic output and by stimuli that decrease the extracellular fluid (**ECF**) volume and blood pressure. Many factors may therefore be involved in the control of renin release, a particularly important one of these being an intrarenal baroreceptor mechanism that causes renin secretion to increase when the intrarenal arteriolar pressure at the granular cells is decreased. A major level of control also lies in the macula densa, where renin secretion is proportionate to the concentration of Cl^- or Na^+ in the tubular fluid. Decreased delivery of Na^+ and Cl^- to the macula densa is associated with increased renin secretion. Angiotensin II, by contrast, inhibits renin secretion by its direct action on the granular cells; it is also a major stimulant of aldosterone secretion, thereby stimulating sodium retention (see below), which closes the renin–angiotensin–aldosterone negative-feedback loop. In addition to these factors, increased activity of the sympathetic nervous system increases renin secretion, both by increased circulating catecholamines and by way of the renal sympathetic nerves.

It has been postulated that the intrarenal renin–angiotensin mechanism is the prime hormonal mediator of the tubuloglomerular feedback system, whereby a stimulus perceived at the macula densa, presumably related to luminal flow or ion concentration, influences filtration rate (Fig. 5). Evidence for this is inconclusive and it is almost certainly not the sole mediator of this feedback mechanism.

The distal tubule and collecting duct

The bulk of sodium and water reabsorption occurs primarily in the proximal tubule, but fine regulation is necessary to maintain a precise sodium and water balance. The distal tubule and the collecting duct are responsible for the necessary final adjustments, which ultimately determine the rate of urinary water and sodium excretion, a mechanism substantially influenced by antidiuretic hormone (vasopressin, **ADH**) and aldosterone, respectively.

Structure

The distal convoluted tubule begins just beyond the macula densa and ends at the cortical collecting duct. Its structure is similar to that of the main part of the thick ascending limb of the loop of Henle. The collecting duct

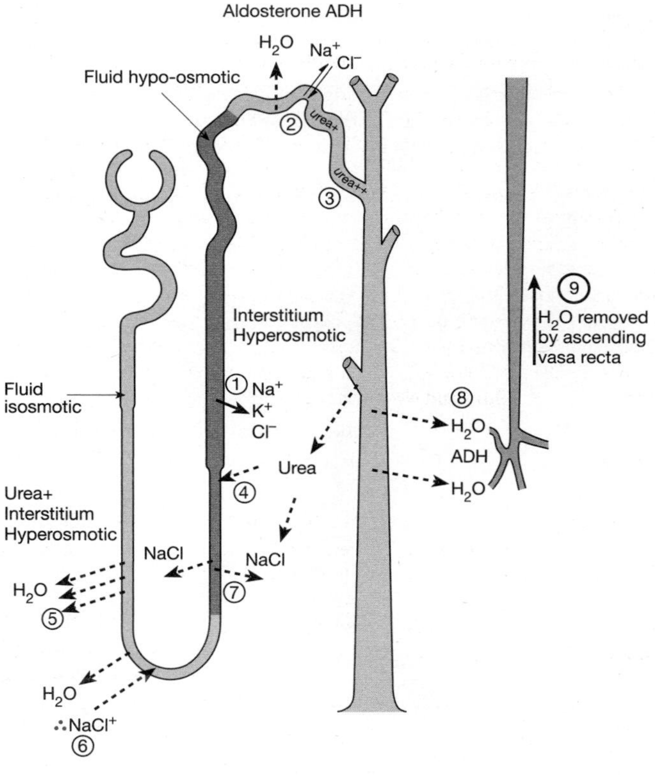

Fig. 4 Diagram to illustrate the mechanism of concentration of the urine. The darkened part of the nephron is impermeable to water. 1, Active transport of Na^+ and Cl^- into the insterstitium. 2, Reabsorption of Na^+ and Cl^-. Passive absorption of water under ADH control. 3, Increased concentration of urea in tubule following reabsorption of water. 4, Urea passes into the interstitium, thereby increasing osmolality. 5, The increased interstitial osmolality results in more water being extracted. 6, This leads to an increased salt concentration in the loop of Henle. 7, In the ascending limb, salt diffuses into the interstitium, further increasing its osmolality. 8, In the presence of ADH the permeability of the distal nephron and collecting ducts is increased and water is reabsorbed. 9, Water is removed from the interstitium by vasa recta. (Reproduced from Williams JD, *et al. Clinical atlas of the kidney*. Gower Publishing, London, with permission.)

system includes the connecting tubule and the cortical and medullary collecting ducts. The connecting tubule and the collecting ducts, unlike the distal tubule, are lined by two cell types: principal cells, with small basal infoldings, some mitochondria, and small microvilli; and intercalated cells with darkly staining cytoplasm that contains mitochondria, smooth endoplasmic reticulum, and prominent Golgi apparatus. There are at least two types of intercalated cells, distinguished on the basis of immunocytochemical and functional characteristics: type A cells express H^+-ATPase at their luminal membrane and secrete protons, whilst type B cells express H^+-ATPase at their basolateral membrane and secrete bicarbonate ions.

Function

Cells of both the connecting tubule and the collecting duct share sensitivity to ADH, but only those of the collecting duct are sensitive to mineralocorticoids. The renal concentrating and diluting processes are ultimately dependent on the ability of ADH to modulate the water permeability of collecting ducts. Regulation of ADH is dependent on osmoreceptors in the hypothalamus, which recognize changes in ECF osmolality, but this can also occur in the absence of changes in plasma osmolality, for example intravascular volume depletion, pain, nausea. Once released from the posterior pituitary, vasopressin exerts its biological action on water excretion by binding to receptors in the basolateral membrane of the collecting duct (Fig. 6). This results in increased adenylate cyclase activity, increased cAMP formation, and ultimately causes the apical (luminal) cell membrane to become more permeable to water through insertion of aquaporin 2 channels.

The principal cells of the collecting duct are responsible for the modulation of sodium reabsorption. Entry of sodium into these cells occurs down a concentration gradient through specific sodium ion channels in the luminal membrane. This creates a negative potential difference in the lumen, which promotes either the secretion of potassium or the reabsorption of chloride via the paracellular route. These processes, which are the final regulators of sodium balance, are under the control of aldosterone, which increases the number of open sodium-ion channels in the luminal membrane (Fig. 7). As previously discussed, angiotensin II is a major stimulant of aldosterone secretion. Hence during periods of volume depletion, activation of the renin–angiotensin system leads to increased aldosterone production and sodium retention; whereas when volume-replete, the system is suppressed and renin release and aldosterone secretion are reduced, resulting in natriuresis. Although the acute production of aldosterone is linked to the renin–angiotensin system, other mechanisms (including that of sodium or potassium balance) can also affect the ability of the adrenal glands to produce aldosterone.

The intercalated cells of the collecting duct are involved in maintenance of the acid–base balance. The method by which they excrete acid by generating ammonium ions is discussed in Chapter 11.11.

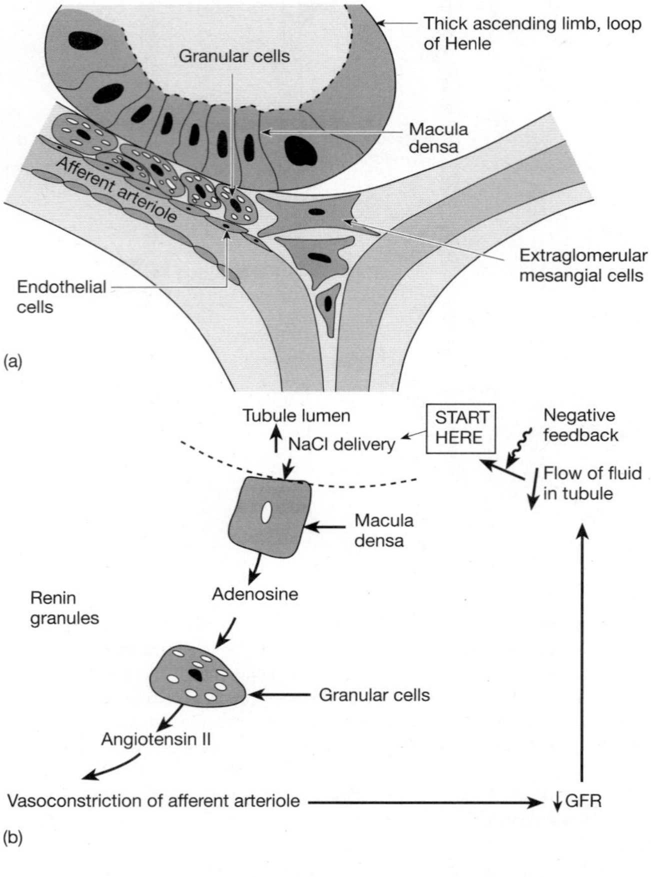

Fig. 5 Tubuloglomerular feedback: (a) anatomical basis; (b) putative mechanism.

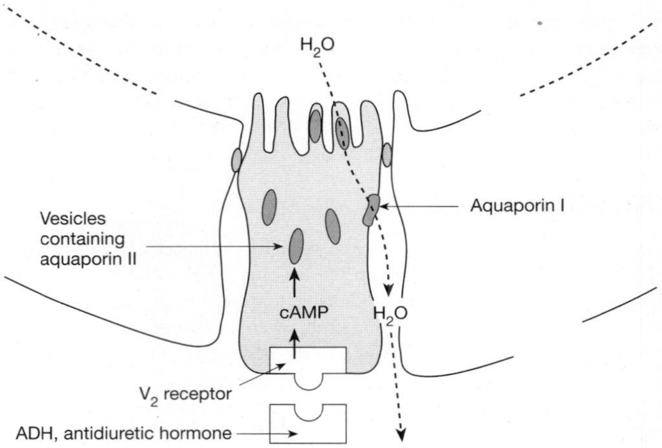

Fig. 6 Action of antidiuretic hormone.

The interstitium

The renal interstitium is the space that is not occupied by the glomeruli or nephrons, and the vasculature of the kidney can be thought of as lying within it. The interstitium amounts to some 5 to 7 per cent of the volume of

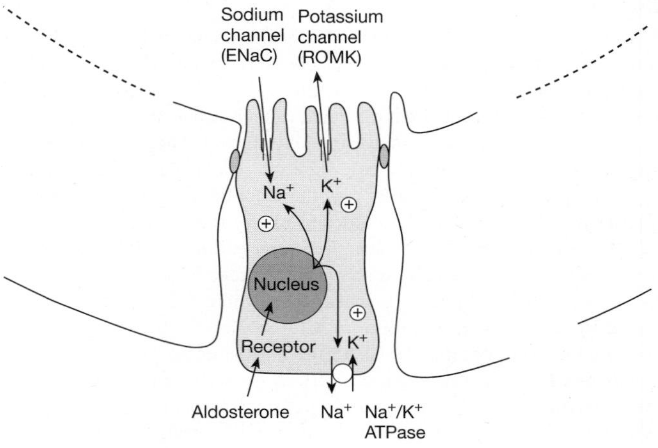

Fig. 7 The action of aldosterone on the collecting duct. Aldosterone stimulates an increase in the numbers and activity of apical ENaC and ROMK, and of basolateral Na^+/K^+-ATPase by direct and indirect effects.

the cortex, 3 to 4 per cent of the outer stripe, 10 per cent of the inner stripe, and up to 30 per cent of the inner medulla. It is involved in virtually all functions of the healthy kidney, as well as in many pathological events. The transit of molecules from the tubules to the blood necessitates a crossing of the interstitial space, and vice versa. Thus, changes to the interstitium have a profound effect on the function of the tubules and indeed of the nephron itself.

The cells of the interstitium are not a homogeneous population but comprise different cell types that vary anatomically within the kidney and between health and disease. The major cellular component is the fibroblast; however, there is evidence to suggest that there is a significant difference between the phenotype of the cortical fibroblast and that of the inner medullary fibroblast. Fibroblasts are important for the integrity of the interstitial matrix and are considered to be the source of matrix component production, as well as being responsible for their turnover. The renal fibroblasts also have endocrine functions: those of the cortex are the source of erythropoietin; the inner medullary fibroblast produces significant amounts of prostaglandins, primarily PGE_2, and has a function in modifying electrolyte transport. Renal fibroblasts may have a pivotal role in renal interstitial fibrosis; it is now well established that the progression of renal disease is intimately linked to the degree of renal interstitial fibrosis, and it is likely that the key cell involved in this may well be the cortical fibroblast.

Dendritic cells are present in small numbers throughout the interstitium and express MHC class II receptors. In addition, there are a few macrophages as well as some large lymphocytes. Dendritic cells, macrophages, and lymphocyte-like cells mostly have immunological and defence-like functions.

Further reading

Davison AM *et al.*, eds (1998). *Oxford textbook of clinical nephrology*, 2nd edn. Oxford University Press, Oxford.

Johnson RJ, Feehally J (2000). *Comprehensive clinical nephrology*. Harcourt Publishers Ltd.

Windhage E, ed. (1992). *Handbook of physiology*, section 8 (renal physiology). Published for the American Physiological Society by Oxford University Press, New York.

20.2 Water and electrolyte metabolism

20.2.1 Water and sodium homeostasis and their disorders

Peter H. Baylis

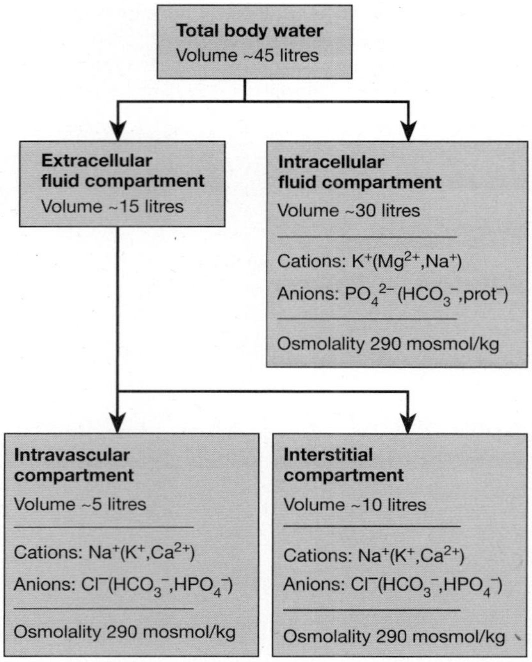

Fig. 1 Composition of body compartments. Body water is distributed uniformly throughout all compartments. Major and some minor (in parentheses) anions and cations are indicated. Osmolality remains the same inside and outside the cell.

Introduction

Total body water accounts for about 60 per cent of the body weight of a healthy adult: two-thirds of this is intracellular and one-third extracellular. The extracellular fluid compartment is divided into the vascular (blood volume) and the interstitial fluid compartments in the ratio 1:2. For a 75 kg adult, the total volume of body water is approximately 45 litres, with intracellular and extracellular volumes of 30 and 15 litres respectively; the latter comprising the blood (5 litres) and interstitial (10 litres) compartments. Sodium is the main extracellular cation, which with its anion, chloride, contributes 95 per cent of the extracellular solute. By contrast, the major intracellular cation is potassium. Many cell membranes are freely permeable to water, but not to most electrolytes, which results in the same total solute but very different electrolyte concentrations in the extracellular and intracellular compartments (Fig. 1).

The maintenance of stable volume and solute concentrations is essential to all complex animals, including humans. In the extracellular fluid compartment, particularly the vascular component, the control of water and sodium balance is inextricably linked. Water is distributed uniformly throughout all compartments, and is clearly a determinant of volume, but is also essential in establishing the concentration of sodium (and other solutes). Sodium, however, contributes not only to its own concentration, but its total quantity in the extracellular fluid is the main factor determining the volume of that compartment. A variety of integrated mechanisms ensure that minimal fluctuations, probably less than 1 per cent, in blood volume and in sodium concentration occur in healthy adults.

Body water and therefore solute concentration is regulated mainly by vasopressin (antidiuretic hormone) mediated alteration of renal water excretion, but also to some extent by thirst as a motivation for drinking. The secretion of vasopressin and thirst are influenced principally by changes in circulating concentration of sodium, but also in part by significant falls in blood volume or pressure, and there are instances where these stimuli can be pulling vasopressin secretion in opposite directions (see later).

The volume of the extracellular compartment is determined by its total sodium content, which is regulated by numerous mechanisms. Sodium intake is poorly controlled in humans, although some animals do demonstrate a specific sodium appetite. The kidney is the major effector organ influencing sodium homeostasis. Complex intrarenal mechanisms contribute to the maintenance of sodium homeostasis, in addition to which are endocrine factors that either tend to reduce excretion of sodium by the kidney (for example the renin–angiotensin–aldosterone system) or which produce a natriuresis (for example atrial natriuretic peptide, ouabain-like substances). The situation is very complex. Blood volume and pressure are also influenced by a variety of vasoactive substances that act locally or systemically (for example catecholamines, prostaglandins, nitric oxide, endothelins), as well as by changes in sympathetic nerve activity. Any change in blood volume and/or pressure will, in turn, have an effect on vasopressin secretion. It can therefore be appreciated that there is an intricate network of homeostatic mechanisms controlling both sodium and water balance.

In clinical practice, the precise measurement of circulating concentrations of electrolytes, specific non-electrolytic solutes (for example glucose), and total solute is relatively simple, and approximates closely to their concentrations in interstitial fluid. Sodium is measured in molar terms (mmol/litre) using flame photometry or an ion-selective electrode. Total solute concentration is assessed by determining the depression of the freezing point of the sample plasma using an osmometer, and is expressed as the number of osmoles of solute per kilogram (osmolality). Thus, a solution of glucose at 1 mmol/litre will provide an osmolality of 1 mosmol/kg but a

1 mmol/litre solution of a salt (for example NaCl), which dissociates completely in the solvent into sodium and chloride ions, will have an osmolality of 2 mosmol/kg. The clinical assessment of volume—whether it be intravascular, interstitial, or extracellular—is extremely important, but difficult and inaccurate.

The physiology of water homeostasis

The maintenance of normal water balance is achieved through the combined action of three main factors: vasopressin, the kidney, and thirst. There needs to be secretion of adequate quantities of osmotically stimulated vasopressin, which must be able to bind to the renal tubule to modulate the flow of solute-free water and produce antidiuresis. Most healthy adults excrete 1 to 2 litres of urine per 24 h, but the normal kidney is capable of wide variation in urine output, ranging from 0.5 to (in very extreme cases) 25 litres per 24 h. Osmotically stimulated thirst must be able to promote drinking and is particularly important when the kidney is concentrating urine maximally but there is still persistent water loss from, for example, excessive sweating or copious watery diarrhoea. Under these circumstances water homeostasis cannot be maintained without adequate fluid intake.

Fine control of water balance ensures that the concentration of solutes, particularly extracellular sodium, remains stable. The extraordinary sensitivity of the function of the three homeostatic mechanisms detailed above allows plasma osmolality to be maintained within the narrow range 285 to 295 mosmol/kg (equivalent to serum sodium, 137 to 142 mmol/litre) in healthy adults.

Thirst and water intake

Drinking behaviour of humans can be divided into two types. The first, primary drinking, occurs as a result of physiological stimulation of thirst. This initiates drinking behaviour to allow ingestion of sufficient fluid to lower blood osmolality. Secondary drinking, which is far more common in our culture, occurs for social reasons (the endless cups of coffee throughout the day, or the ritual visit to the 'pub'), habit, or the need to drink with food. For the majority of adults living in temperate climates, secondary drinking ensures that they remain in a state of mild water excess, and water balance is maintained by regulating renal water excretion.

The mechanism of primary drinking is believed to be as follows: as the body loses water, blood osmolality starts to rise and stimulates thirst osmoreceptors. Studies in animals indicate that these are situated in the anterior hypothalamic structures, probably in the organum vasculosum of the lamina terminalis or the subfornical organ, where there is a defect in the blood–brain barrier. Isolated lesions in this area can occur in humans following haemorrhage from an aneurysm in an anterior communicating artery and result in loss of thirst appreciation, suggesting that human thirst osmoreceptors are located in a similar area to those in animals. The precise mechanism by which blood hyperosmolality stimulates thirst is not known, but it is believed that increase in extracellular osmolality draws water from within the osmoreceptor cells of the organum vasculosum of the lamina terminalis and subfornical organ, resulting in cellular hypovolaemia which is translated into neuronal impulses that migrate to the cortex and allow conscious appreciation of thirst.

With the use of visual analogue scales it is possible to obtain an estimate of the degree of thirst sensation. There is a simple relationship between increasing blood osmolality and the intensity of thirst (Fig. 2(b)). Furthermore, there is also a direct relationship between intensity of thirst and the amount of fluid drunk to quench thirst. The act of drinking quickly reduces thirst, usually within a few minutes and certainly before there are substantial falls in blood osmolality. Drinking is therefore able to override or inhibit osmotically stimulated thirst, probably through an oropharyngeal reflux.

Thirst is not only stimulated by increases in blood osmolality, but also by acute substantial falls in blood volume and/or pressure. A sudden decrease in volume in excess of 15 per cent is required before thirst is influenced. Low-pressure baroreceptors located in the atria of the heart and great veins of the chest mediate the response. In addition, significant extracellular volume depletion is a potent stimulus to the release of renin from the juxtaglomerular apparatus of the nephron: this generates increasing concentrations of circulating angiotensin II, known to be a profound dipsogen in animals. Systemic angiotensin II therefore augments the baroregulatory influence on thirst in acute hypovolaemia. Animal studies have also revealed that intrahypothalamic angiotensin II is the most potent neurotransmitter involved in the generation of the sensation of thirst.

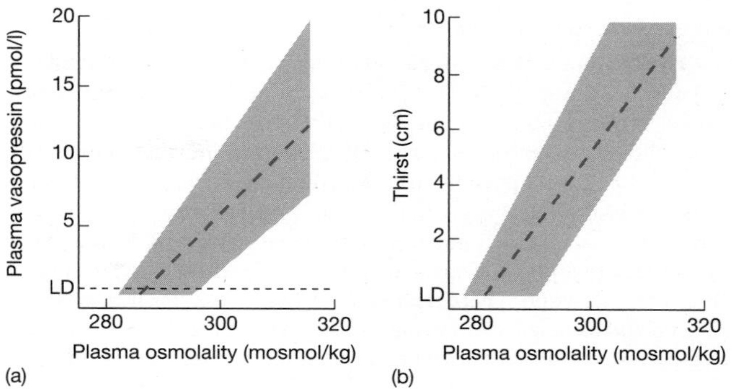

Fig. 2 (a) The relationship between plasma osmolality and plasma vasopressin during infusion of hypertonic (850 mmol/litre) saline in healthy adults. There is a linear relationship between the two variables, represented by the dashed line, termed the mean osmoregulatory line for vasopressin secretion. The abscissal intercept of the line represents the threshold for vasopressin secretion, approximately 283 mosmol/kg. LD is the limit of detection of the assay, and the shaded area is the extent of the normal response. (b) The relationship between plasma osmolality and thirst intensity assessed on a 10 cm visual analogue scale during the same hypertonic infusion. The dashed line is the mean osmoregulatory line for thirst, which has an abscissal intercept (thirst threshold) of 281 mosmol/kg. (Adapted from Thompson CJ *et al.* (1986). The osmotic thresholds for thirst and vasopressin release are similar in healthy man. *Clinical Science* **71**, 651–6, with permission.)

As humans age, so their thirst appreciation becomes blunted, and primary drinking is reduced such that individuals tend to become mildly hyperosmolar and hypernatraemic. Fortunately, most elderly people continue secondary drinking and rely on mechanisms to control renal water excretion, providing protection from significant hypernatraemia.

During human pregnancy there is a fall in plasma osmolality of the order of 10 mosmol/kg, with an appropriate fall in serum sodium. This is due to alteration in the osmoregulatory systems for both thirst and vasopressin secretion. The thirst osmoregulatory line (Fig. 2) is displaced to the left of the normal, non-pregnant position, which runs parallel—but the abscissal intercept, known as the osmotic threshold for thirst, is reset to about 275 mosmol/kg. Similar changes occur with the osmoregulatory line for vasopressin secretion (see below). The precise mechanisms for this 'resetting of the osmostat' are unknown, but they have important implications for the ability of pregnant women to handle a water load.

Vasopressin and renal water excretion

The antidiuretic hormone of humans is arginine vasopressin (in contrast to lysine vasopressin which is specific to the pig family), a nonapeptide, the gene for which is located on chromosome 20. Arginine vasopressin is synthesized from a large precursor molecule in the supraoptic and paraventricular nuclei of the hypothalamus, transported in neurosecretory granules to the posterior pituitary, median eminence of the hypothalamus and to a lesser extent to other areas of the brain and brainstem. It is secreted from the posterior pituitary into the systemic circulation to influence renal function, and into the hypothalamopituitary portal circulation to enhance pituitary ACTH secretion.

Control of vasopressin release

Secretion of vasopressin from the posterior pituitary is regulated mainly by changes in blood osmolality. The vasopressin osmoreceptors, distinct from the thirst osmoreceptors, are located in the same anterior hypothalamic area, i.e. the circumventricular structures, the organum vasculosum of the lamina terminalis, and possibly the subfornical organ. Rising blood osmolality is believed to cause water to flow out of the osmoreceptor cells, with cellular hypovolaemia then initiating a neuronal signal that passes principally to the supraoptic nucleus and stimulates the process of vasopressin synthesis and secretion. There is an exquisitely sensitive linear relationship between blood osmolality and vasopressin secretion (Fig. 2(a)), the slope of the vasopressin osmoregulatory line being a measure of the sensitivity of the system and the abscissal intercept representing the threshold for vasopressin release. At plasma osmolality values below 285 mosmol/kg, on average, vasopressin secretion is inhibited to allow a maximum water diuresis (15–25 litres/24 h) with urine osmolality of 50 to 70 mosmol/kg (Fig. 3). Increase in blood osmolality above this threshold induces progressive vasopressin release, thus increasing urine concentration, so that at plasma vasopressin values of 2 to 4 pmol/litre, maximum antidiuresis occurs. Drinking inhibits osmoregulated vasopressin secretion.

Each individual has a unique threshold and sensitivity for both thirst and vasopressin release. Circulating solutes have varying abilities to stimulate the osmoregulatory system, with sodium chloride being among the most potent and glucose having little or no effect. By contrast to osmoregulated thirst, there is no blunting of the vasopressin response to osmotic stimulation with ageing. Pregnancy is associated with a lowering of the vasopressin threshold similar to the thirst threshold, allowing osmoregulation to occur about a lower set-point of 275 rather than 285 mosmol/kg.

Non-osmotic release of vasopressin is stimulated by a number of factors: acute substantial reductions in blood volume or pressure, of the order of 10 to 15 per cent or more; nausea and/or emesis; hypoglycaemia; and a variety of circulating substances (for example angiotensin II). Low-pressure receptors in the great veins of the chest and cardiac atria mediate the effect of hypovolaemia, while receptors in the arch of the aorta and carotid vessels sense reductions in arterial pressure. The sensory information is carried via the vagus and glossopharyngeal nerves to the brainstem vasomotor centres and then transmitted to the hypothalamus, principally the paraventricular nucleus. There is an exponential relationship between the fall in blood volume/pressure and vasopressin release, such that large reductions (~40 per cent of normal) raise plasma vasopressin to huge concentrations (100 to 500 pmol/litre) that have vasoconstrictor effects. Similarly high vasopressin concentrations can be achieved with nausea/emesis.

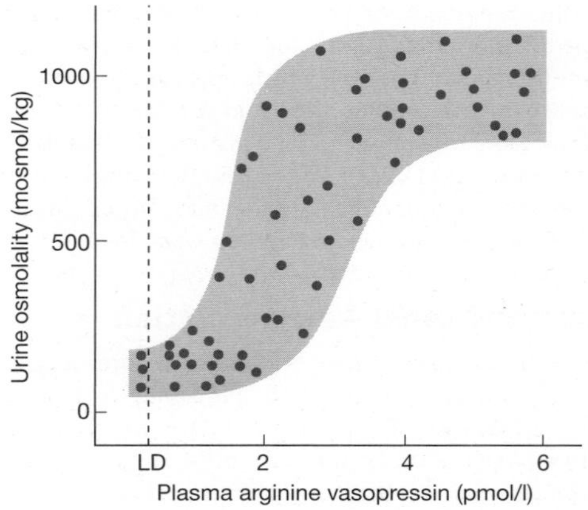

Fig. 3 The effect of vasopressin on urinary concentration during varying states of hydration in humans. Each closed circle represents a single value, and the stippled area the normal range. Values of plasma vasopressin greater than 4 pmol/litre fail to increase urinary concentration further. LD is the limit of the assay.

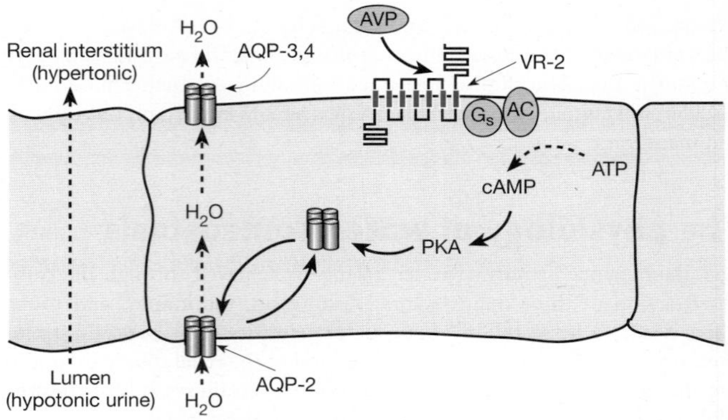

AVP, vasopressin: VR-2, vasopressin receptor-2: Gs, stimulatory G protein: AC, adenylate cyclase: AQP, aquaporin: PKA, protein kinase A.

Fig. 4 A schematic diagram of the distal renal tubule indicating the effect of arginine vasopressin initiating a cascade of intracellular events after binding to the V_2 receptor. Protein kinase A is activated, which mobilizes the arginine vasopressin-sensitive water channel protein, aquaporin 2, for insertion into the luminal tubular membrane. Non-vasopressin-sensitive water channel proteins, aquaporins 3 and 4, are positioned in the contralateral membrane, which allows water to flow through the cell along the osmotic gradient. Loss of arginine vasopressin binding to its receptor promotes re-entry of the luminal aquaporin 2 into the cell, resulting in a shuttling of aquaporin 2.

Actions of vasopressin

The major physiological action of vasopressin is to increase urinary concentration (Fig. 3). Circulating arginine vasopressin binds to a specific renal tubular receptor, designated the V_2 receptor, of the collecting ducts. Adenyl cyclase is stimulated, via the coupled G protein, to produce cyclic 5‘AMP, which activates intracellular protein kinases and accelerates the expression and trafficking of aquaporin 2, the vasopressin-sensitive water channel protein. Aquaporin 2 is organized into a tetramer and inserted into the luminal cellular membrane of the distal tubule, allowing water to flow from the tubular lumen into the cellular compartment. Two other aquaporins (aquaporins 3 and 4) are located on the contraluminal cell membrane: these are not vasopressin responsive but facilitate the flow of water across the distal tubule under the influence of the osmotic gradient between the hypotonic urine within the tubular lumen and the hypertonic renal interstitium. Thus, urine volume is decreased and urine is concentrated (Fig. 4).

Animal studies have indicated that vasopressin also stimulates the transport of urea across the collecting tubule and of sodium chloride across the medullary thick ascending limb of the loop of Henle, both of which enhance the osmotic gradient. As renal prostaglandins reduce the generation of cyclic 5‘AMP, they blunt the effect of vasopressin, and therefore prostaglandin synthetase inhibitors augment the antidiuretic action of arginine vasopressin.

The first action attributed to vasopressin was the elevation of systemic blood pressure by peripheral vasoconstriction. Arginine vasopressin binds to vascular smooth muscle receptors (V_1 receptors) that activate phosphatidyl–inositol pathways, increase intracellular calcium concentration, and cause the contraction of vascular muscles. High circulating concentrations of vasopressin are necessary to achieve this pressor effect: at physiological levels it probably plays little (if any) role in maintaining blood pressure, but it is involved in the pressor response to hypovolaemia or hypotension.

Vasopressin released from the hypothalamic median eminence binds to a modified V_1 receptor on the pituitary corticotroph and acts to enhance the release of ACTH stimulated by corticotrophin-releasing factor. At high concentrations vasopressin increases circulating concentrations of the clotting factors, plasma factor VIII and the von Willebrand factor, by releasing them from vascular endothelium via a V_2 receptor. Hepatic glycogenolysis is also promoted by high concentrations of vasopressin via a V_1 hepatic receptor.

The physiology of sodium homeostasis

The volume of the extracellular compartment is determined by its sodium content, changes in which result in alterations in blood and interstitial volumes (Fig. 1) with little influence on sodium concentration. The reason is that any rise in sodium concentration causes transient stimulation of thirst and increased water intake, as well as increased vasopressin secretion and reduced renal water excretion, both leading to an increase in body water and a return of extracellular sodium concentration to normal. It therefore appears that extracellular osmolality is conserved at the expense of volume in healthy adults, this integration illustrating the close links between sodium and water homeostatic mechanisms.

Sodium intake

There is little regulation of sodium intake in humans, although some animals demonstrate a specific sodium appetite and have sodium receptors in the hypothalamus. Sodium balance is maintained largely by the kidney, which is normally capable of controlling sodium excretion over a very wide range, 1 to 5000 mmol/24 h. In Western countries, including Britain, the usual intake of sodium is grossly in excess of body needs, being about 100 to 200 mmol/24 h. There is little sodium loss from the healthy bowel and in temperate climates sweating is minimal (the sodium concentration in sweat is 40 to 50 mmol/litre). Most people are therefore at continuous risk of sodium excess, which is prevented by the kidney.

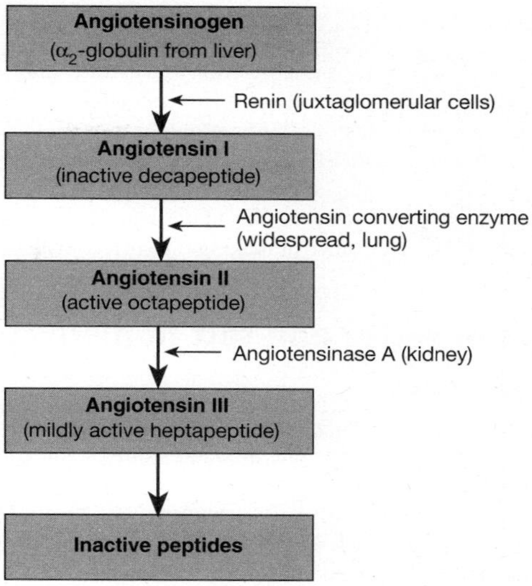

Fig. 5 The renin–angiotensin–aldosterone system. The enzyme, renin, secreted by juxtaglomerular cells of the renal afferent arterioles converts angiotensinogen to angiotensin I (inactive). The active peptides, angiotensin II and III, are potent vasoconstrictors and stimulate aldosterone secretion from the adrenal cortex to expand blood volume and raise blood pressure.

Control of renal sodium excretion

The glomerular filtration rate of normal kidneys is 170 litres per 24 h, the filtrate containing 140 mmol of sodium per litre. Most of the filtered sodium (60–70 per cent) is reabsorbed iso-osmotically by the proximal tubule. Much of the remainder is reabsorbed in the medullary thick ascending limb of the loop of Henle and the distal nephron, such that only a small fraction of the load of sodium filtered at the glomerulus is excreted in the urine (0.1 to a few per cent).

At the single nephron level the glomerulotubular feedback mechanism operates to maintain a balance between the amount of sodium and fluid filtered by the glomerulus and the reabsorptive function of the corresponding nephron. The mechanisms responsible for glomerulotubular feedback are not known precisely, but the macula densa cells of the thick ascending limb detect changes in composition of tubular fluid entering the terminal portion of the thick ascending limb and transmit signals (possibly intrarenal angiotensin II) to modulate glomerular vascular resistance and glomerular pressure. Thus, acute changes in glomerular filtration determine appropriate changes in sodium reabsorption in the proximal tubule, such that if glomerular filtration rate increases, then reabsorption increases proportionally, and vice versa.

Most regulation of sodium balance occurs in the distal nephron, where 'fine tuning' of sodium excretion occurs under the control of a variety of mechanisms.

Renin–angiotensin–aldosterone system

In addition to their role in the glomerulotubular feedback mechanism, the macula densa cells also influence the juxtaglomerular cells of the renal afferent arterioles to synthesize and secrete renin into the systemic circulation if sodium delivery to the distal nephron drops. In addition, reductions of renal perfusion pressure appear to directly increase renin secretion, while baroreceptors within the great veins of the chest influence renin secretion via the sympathetic nerves. Renin catalyses the conversion of angiotensinogen to angiotensin I (Fig. 5), which is then converted into the highly active octapeptide angiotensin II. The activity of angiotensin III is only 30 per cent that of angiotensin II. These peptides influence body sodium content and extracellular fluid volume in a number of ways. Angiotensin II is a potent vasoconstrictor which readily increases systemic blood pressure, stimulates the secretion of aldosterone from the zona glomerulosa of the adrenal cortex to enhance sodium reabsorption in the distal nephron, increases cardiac contractility, stimulates thirst, and is involved in the glomerulotubular feedback mechanism.

Atrial natriuretic peptide

Following the observation that expansion of blood volume caused a rise in renal sodium excretion that could not be accounted for by inhibition of the renin–angiotensin–aldosterone system, specific humoral natriuretic factors were proposed. One that has been well characterized is human alpha atrial natriuretic peptide, which is synthesized and secreted primarily by cardiac atrial myocytes. Moderate increases in blood volume and postural changes cause atrial distension, directly stimulating atrial natriuretic peptide. Its most important actions are on the kidney, where at physiological concentrations it causes a modest natriuresis, minimal diuresis, and reduces plasma renin activity, and plasma aldosterone concentration. In addition, atrial natriuretic peptide acts as a vasodilator agent, reducing systolic blood pressure and cardiac contractility, and is a potent inhibitor of aldosterone synthesis and release. Indeed, many of the effects of atrial natriuretic peptide could be explained by antagonism of the renin–angiotensin–aldosterone system, but this is not its mechanism of action: specific receptors for atrial natriuretic peptide have been identified in the kidney—on cortical glomeruli, the inner medulla, the vasa rectae in the outer medulla, and the collecting duct. Brain natriuretic peptide has similar actions.

Atrial natriuretic peptide and brain natriuretic peptide play minor roles in regulating extracellular sodium content and volume, but do counterbalance to some extent the actions of the renin–angiotensin–aldosterone system. It is likely that there are other natriuretic factors: ouabain-like substances that inhibit renal sodium–potassium ATPase activity have been described, but they have not been characterized fully and their possible significance for sodium homeostasis remains unknown. Furthermore, there are numerous other intrarenal factors that influence renal sodium excretion, including dopamine, prostaglandins (particularly prostaglandin E_2), and the kallikrein–kinin system.

Summary

In health, the control of renal sodium excretion and extracellular volume is multifactorial, complex, and not completely understood: so also in disease. It is not therefore surprising that it can sometimes be difficult to determine precisely why a particular patient has developed a particular disorder of extracellular volume or serum sodium concentration at a particular time. The physician with a good grasp of the underlying pathophysiological mechanisms stands the best chance of making the correct diagnosis.

Disorders of water and salt homeostasis

The polyuric states

Polyuria describes excessive urinary volume, normal being less than 2.5 to 3.0 litres per 24 h. This can occur due to solute diuresis, the commonest cause being hyperglycaemia in poorly controlled diabetes mellitus, but when the urine is hypotonic three basic pathogenetic mechanisms can account for polyuria. First, lack of osmoregulated vasopressin secretion, termed cranial, central, hypothalamic, or neurogenic diabetes insipidus. Second, reduction in responsiveness of the renal tubules to adequate vasopressin, called nephrogenic or vasopressin-resistant diabetes insipidus. Third, persistent excessive intake of fluid due to inappropriate thirst or drinking behaviour, known as primary polydipsia or dipsogenic diabetes insipidus.

Cranial diabetes insipidus

Cranial diabetes insipidus is a disorder of urinary concentration that is due to decreased secretion of osmoregulated vasopressin. At least 80 per cent of vasopressin-synthesizing neurones must be destroyed before overt clinical features become manifest. Cranial diabetes insipidus is rare, with an estimated prevalence of 1 in 25 000 and equal gender distribution.

Aetiology

The causes of cranial diabetes insipidus are given in Table 1.

Familial varieties account for 5 per cent of cases. Autosomal dominant familial cranial diabetes insipidus is caused by mutations of the arginine vasopressin gene located on chromosome 20. Typically the onset is in early childhood (2 to 7 years) and not infancy. A variety of different mis-sense and non-sense mutations and deletions have been identified in numerous kindreds. Mutant arginine vasopressin precursors accumulate in the magnocellular neurones where they are neurotoxic.

Approximately 30 per cent of acquired cases of cranial diabetes insipidus are idiopathic. One-third of these have circulating antibodies to the hypothalamic neurones that produce vasopressin, suggesting an autoimmune aetiology, supported by lymphocytic infiltration of the neurohypophysis that leads to thickening of the pituitary stalk. Trauma to the hypothalamus or pituitary stalk is a frequent cause of cranial diabetes insipidus, but the trans-sphenoidal surgical approach to the pituitary is less traumatic than the transfrontal approach, and rarely causes permanent cranial diabetes insipidus. Head injury may cause cranial diabetes insipidus, with some patients following a triple-phase response to trauma characterized by initial polyuria for a few hours or days, followed by antidiuresis for a variable period, then progressing to permanent polyuria. Primary pituitary tumours rarely cause cranial diabetes insipidus. Germinoma is a common cause of cranial diabetes insipidus in childhood.

Clinical features

The main clinical manifestations of cranial diabetes insipidus are polyuria, nocturia, and excessive thirst and drinking. Children may present with enuresis. Most patients have partial deficiency of vasopressin. Urine volumes range between 3 and 25 litres per 24 h, with random urine osmolalities of 50 to less than 300 mosmol/kg and plasma osmolality within the normal reference range.

Patients with cranial diabetes insipidus maintain normal values of plasma osmolality and serum sodium because they have an intact osmoregulated thirst mechanism. Defective thirst or restricted access to water leads to hypernatraemia and hyperosmolality. With severe polyuria the slightest obstruction to outflow from the urinary tract can lead to hydronephrosis and hydroureter.

Cranial diabetes insipidus may be masked by deficiency of glucocorticoid hormone due either to hypopituitarism or primary adrenal failure because cortisol is necessary for the maximal dilution function of the distal nephron and for normal secretion of arginine vasopressin. The symptoms of partial cranial diabetes insipidus are often worse in pregnancy due to the increase in metabolic clearance of arginine vasopressin caused by cysteine aminopeptidase (vasopressinase), a circulating enzyme of placental origin.

Nephrogenic diabetes insipidus

In nephrogenic diabetes insipidus the renal tubules are partially (most often) or totally resistant to the action of vasopressin.

Aetiology

Table 1 lists the causes of nephrogenic diabetes insipidus.

The X-linked form is rare. Infant males have profound polyuria, dehydration, vomiting, fever, irritability, and fail to thrive. Females, when tested, have slightly impaired urinary concentration. Molecular studies of kindreds with X-linked nephrogenic diabetes insipidus have identified mutations or deletions of the gene that encodes for the V_2 receptor located on Xq28. The V_2 receptor is a classic seven-domain transmembrane protein:

Table 1 Causes of the polyuria–polydipsia syndromes

Cranial diabetes insipidus
Familial
Autosomal dominant inheritance
DIDMOAD* (autosomal recessive)
Acquired
Idiopathic
Inflammatory (lymphocytic infiltration, sarcoidosis, histiocytosis X autoimmunity, Guillain Barré syndrome)
Trauma (neurosurgery, head injury)
Neoplasma (craniopharyngioma, germinoma, pinealoma, hypothalamic metastasis, large pituitary tumour)
Infection (meningitis, encephalitis)
Vascular (sickle cell anaemia, aneurysms of anterior communicating artery, Sheehan's syndrome)
Pregnancy (associated with vasopressinase)
Nephrogenic diabetes insipidus
Familial
X-linked inheritance
Autosomal recessive inheritance
Acquired
Idiopathic
Metabolic (hypercalcaemia, hypokalaemia)
Vascular (sickle cell disease)
Osmotic diuresis (glycosuria, post-obstructive uropathy
Chronic renal disease (renal failure, amyloid, myeloma, sarcoidosis, pyelonephritis)
Drugs (lithium, demeclocycline, amphotericin, glibenclamide, methoxyfluorane)
Primary polydipsia
Unknown aetiology
Psychogenic (compulsive water drinking)
Psychotic (schizophrenia, mania)
Idiopathic
Secondary
Granuloma (sarcoidosis)
Vasculitis
TB meningitis
Multiple sclerosis
Drugs (phenothiazines, tricyclic antidepressants)

*DIDMOAD = diabetes insipidus, diabetes mellitus, optic atrophy, deafness (Wolfram syndrome).

genetic abnormalities have been demonstrated in external and internal segments of the receptor as well as the transmembrane portions.

Approximately 10 per cent of cases of familial nephrogenic diabetes insipidus are due to genetic defects of aquaporin 2, the water-channel protein that is encoded on chromosome 12q13. Mutant aquaporin 2 is misrouted within the distal tubule and fails to be inserted into the cellular membrane. Inheritance is autosomal recessive.

Hypercalcaemia-induced nephrogenic diabetes insipidus is thought to be due to a combination of factors: reduced medullary hyperosmolality and adenyl cyclase activity, dysfunction of aquaporin 2, and calcium deposition with scarring of the kidney. The effect of sustained hypokalaemia on renal function is complex: it inhibits sodium–potassium cotransport in the thick ascending limb, reduces adenyl cyclase activity, increases intrarenal prostaglandin synthesis (which blunts the antidiuretic effect of vasopressin) and may reduce intracellular protein kinase function. Aquaporin 2 trafficking is reduced. Reversal of these metabolic derangements often returns renal function to normal, but does not always do so.

A third of patients taking long-term lithium carbonate develop nephrogenic diabetes insipidus. Lithium blunts the generation and action of cyclic 5′AMP in the distal nephron and may reduce osmoregulated vasopressin secretion and/or stimulate thirst. Demeclocycline also inhibits the generation and function of cyclic 5′AMP.

Clinical features

Adults with nephrogenic diabetes insipidus usually have partial nephrogenic diabetes insipidus with mild symptoms. Similar to patients with cranial diabetes insipidus, these individuals have serum sodium and plasma osmolality within the normal range, but low urine osmolality (< 300 mosmol/kg). The familial forms present soon after birth with profound polyuria, dehydration, and fever (see above). Infants may become hypernatraemic due to inadequate fluid intake.

Primary polydipsia

Some patients drink copious quantities of fluid, well in excess of body requirements, for reasons that are ill understood. This condition is termed primary polydipsia, or dipsogenic diabetes insipidus.

Aetiology

Many patients have a psychological disturbance leading to compulsive drinking, some of whom have a lowered osmotic thirst threshold but a normal threshold for vasopressin release. Up to 20 per cent of patients with chronic schizophrenia have primary polydipsia. Very rarely a structural hypothalamic lesion (for example sarcoidosis) is believed to be the cause of primary polydipsia (Table 1). Some drugs cause a dry mouth, thus stimulating thirst.

Clinical features

Although the clinical manifestations of primary polydipsia are similar to cranial diabetes insipidus and nephrogenic diabetes insipidus, nocturia is less of a feature: patients with primary polydipsia tend to sleep through the night. Individuals with primary polydipsia lower plasma osmolality sufficiently to suppress vasopressin secretion to allow polyuria. Their serum sodium therefore tends to be lower than that of patients with cranial diabetes insipidus and nephrogenic diabetes insipidus, but usually remains within the reference range. The fact that many patients with primary polydipsia can drink up to 20 litres in 24 h and still remain normonatraemic is testament to the remarkable effectiveness of homeostatic mechanisms.

Diagnostic evaluation of the polyuric patient

Before embarking on expensive and time-consuming tests, it is always wise to establish that the urine volume is in excess of 3 litres per 24 h. Urine output less than this with a normal serum sodium and plasma osmolality excludes significant disturbance of water balance. Routine biochemical investigation of glucose, calcium, and potassium may point towards some causes of polyuria (Table 1). Three types of specialized diagnostic tests are available: dehydration tests, measurement of plasma vasopressin after dehydration or osmotic stimulation, and therapeutic trial of desmopressin.

Dehydration tests

These can aid the diagnosis of severe forms of cranial diabetes insipidus and nephrogenic diabetes insipidus. Many protocols have been described: all are based on observing the responses in urine and blood to a period of fluid deprivation, followed by noting the ability to concentrate urine after exposure to exogenous vasopressin (for example desmopressin). A typical commonly used test is (briefly) as follows. The patient is encouraged to drink as usual during the night before the test which is to start in the morning. Basal measurements of urinary volume and osmolality and of plasma osmolality are made, and the patient weighed. All fluid is then withheld for 8 h, with the patient weighed and urine and blood samples taken every 1 to 2 h. The test must be stopped if the patient loses in excess of 5 per cent of their initial body weight. Thereafter 2 μg of desmopressin is injected intramuscularly, the patient being allowed to drink cautiously and eat. Urine samples are collected over the following 16 h.

A guide to interpretation of the results of the water deprivation test is given in Table 2. Substantial difficulty arises in the differentiation of partial diabetes insipidus disorders from each other, and from primary polydipsia. The reason for this is that prolonged polyuria, irrespective of its cause, leads to a reduction in the maximal concentrating ability of the kidney by removing renal medullary interstitial solute and altering aquaporin 2 function, such that exogenously administered vasopressin cannot elicit its maximal renal effect. Direct measurement of plasma vasopressin aids diagnosis of partial nephrogenic diabetes insipidus in these circumstances.

Response of plasma vasopressin to osmotic stimulation and dehydration

Measurement of plasma vasopressin and osmolality during a 2-h hypertonic (850 mmol/litre) saline infusion at a rate of 0.06 ml/kg/min will diagnose partial or complete cranial diabetes insipidus, as the vasopressin response to osmotic stimulation is subnormal (Fig. 6(a)). Patients with nephrogenic diabetes insipidus or primary polydipsia have results that fall within the normal range.

After a period of water deprivation, the measurement of urine osmolality and plasma vasopressin will define nephrogenic diabetes insipidus (Fig. 6(b)), as vasopressin will be inappropriately elevated with respect to the low urine osmolality.

Therapeutic trial of desmopressin

If the water deprivation–desmopressin test gives equivocal results and facilities to measure vasopressin are not available, then a formal therapeutic trial of low-dose desmopressin should be instituted to differentiate the cause of polyuria. The trial must be supervised closely, preferably in hospital, because of the potential hazard of severe water intoxication in those with primary polydipsia. After a basal period of 3 to 4 days, desmopressin (1 μg intramuscularly daily for 10 days) is administered to patients who are weighed and have urine and plasma osmolalities or serum sodium and urine volume measured daily. Patients with cranial diabetes insipidus will

Table 2 Interpretation of results from water deprivation–desmopressin test

Urine osmolality (mosmol/kg)		
After dehydration	**After desmopressin**	**Diagnosis**
> 750	> 750	Normal*
< 300	> 750	CDI
< 300	< 300	NDI
300–750	< 750	Partial CDI or partial NDI or PP

*Assumes that plasma osmolality remains in the normal reference range, 285 to 295 mosmol/kg.

Abbreviations: CDI, cranial diabetes insipidus; NDI, nephrogenic diabetes insipidus; PP, primary polydipsia.

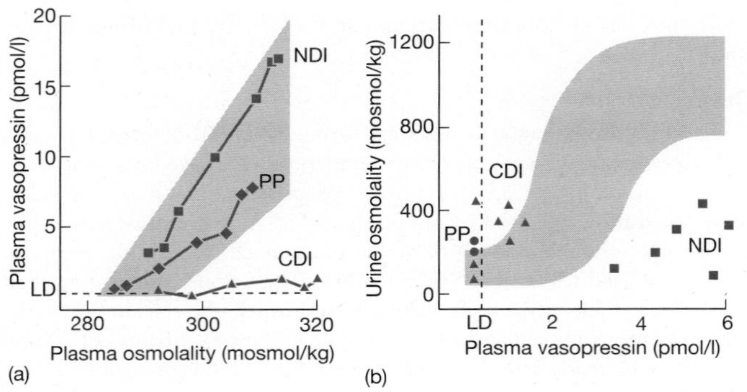

Fig. 6 (a) Relationship between plasma vasopressin and plasma osmolality during hypertonic saline infusion in typical patients with (i) cranial diabetes insipidus (CDI), (ii) nephrogenic diabetes insipidus (NDI), and (iii) primary polydipsia (PP). The shaded area represents the normal response. (b) Relationship between urine osmolality and plasma vasopressin in patients with cranial diabetes insipidus (triangles), nephrogenic diabetes insipidus (squares) and primary polydipsia (circles) after a period of dehydration. The shaded area is the normal relationship under various degrees of hydration. LD represents the limit of detection of the plasma vasopressin assay.

be identified by a reduction of thirst, little or no weight gain, a reduction in urine flow, and normal plasma osmolality. Nephrogenic diabetes insipidus is characterized by a lack of response. Primary polydipsia patients remain thirsty, continue to drink, gain weight, and become progressively hyponatraemic.

Having established the pathogenetic mechanism causing polyuria, it is important to search for a specific underlying cause (Table 1). Magnetic resonance imaging or high-resolution computed tomography scans of the pituitary and surrounding structures are invaluable in those with cranial diabetes insipidus. Patients with cranial diabetes insipidus frequently lose the posterior pituitary bright spot on T_1-weighted MRI.

Treatment

Cranial diabetes insipidus

Mild forms of cranial diabetes insipidus (urine output less than 4 litres/24 h) may not require any specific therapy other than advice to drink sufficient quantities to quench thirst. Such patients can, however, get into difficulty if they are unable to get and retain an adequate fluid intake for any reason. In more severe forms, the drug of choice is desmopressin, a synthetic vasopressin V_2-receptor agonist analogue possessing potent antidiuretic, but no pressor, activity, and with a prolonged duration of action. Desmopressin is administered orally, intranasally by spray or tube, or parenterally. There are wide individual variations in the dose required to control symptoms. Requirements for oral desmopressin range from 50 µg to 1200 µg daily; intranasal from 2.5 µg to 120 µg daily; and parenteral up to 2 µg intramuscularly daily. Dilutional hyponatraemia is a potential hazard if desmopressin is given in excess for a prolonged period: this can be avoided by instructing the patient to forgo the drug for 1 day each week. Other side-effects are minimal. Desmopressin is a safe drug in pregnancy, and is resistant to the circulating placental enzyme, vasopressinase.

Lysine vasopressin, given intranasally, is a shorter-acting alternative but as it possesses pressor activity it can cause intestinal and/or renal colic, increase blood pressure and induce coronary artery vasospasm. Pitressin is rarely used nowadays because of similar pressor side-effects.

Chlorpropamide, clofibrate, carbamazepine, and thiazide diuretics have been used either singly or in combination to reduce urine volume by up to 50 per cent, but they are rarely prescribed these days because of their side-effects and the efficacy of desmopressin.

Nephrogenic diabetes insipidus

Correction of the underlying cause of acquired nephrogenic diabetes insipidus (for example removal of drug or correction of hypercalcaemia) may allow recovery of renal concentrating ability. If matters do resolve, this typically takes a number of weeks.

Severe polyuria of the familial form of nephrogenic diabetes insipidus can be reduced by about 50 per cent using a combination of salt restriction, thiazide and/or amiloride diuretics, and a prostaglandin synthetase inhibitor (indomethacin, 1.5–3.0 mg/kg/day). A promising new therapeutic approach is the combination of a thiazide, indomethacin, and desmopressin, which may reduce urine output by up to 80 per cent.

Primary polydipsia

There is no efficacious drug treatment available for primary polydipsia although propranolol in doses up to 120 mg daily has been recommended to reduce thirst. Therapy directed towards underlying psychiatric problems may prove helpful. Clozapine has reduced polydipsia associated with hyponatraemia in those with chronic schizophrenia.

Hyponatraemic states

Hyponatraemia, defined as a serum sodium less than 130 mmol/litre, is a common electrolyte disturbance, affecting up to 5 per cent of hospital patients. Severe hyponatraemia (serum sodium < 115 mmol/litre) is rare (< 0.5 per cent).

Pseudohyponatraemia

Spuriously low measurements of serum sodium can occur in patients with very high circulating concentrations of lipids or proteins because the volume of these substances contributes substantially to serum volume. The concentration of sodium in the water phase of blood remains normal, hence plasma osmolality is normal and its measurement proves an easy diagnostic test. Pseudohyponatraemia also arises with severe hyperglycaemia, although the mechanism is different: high blood glucose concentration draws intracellular water into the extracellular space, resulting in hyponatraemia. Plasma osmolality will be elevated due to the hyperglycaemia.

Classification and causes of hyponatraemia

In all hyponatraemic states there is an excess of extracellular water relative to the total sodium content of the extracellular compartment. The sodium content, however, can vary markedly, such that patients can be divided into three groups, forming the basis of a classification of hyponatraemia. Total extracellular sodium quantity can be:

- lower than normal, resulting in extracellular hypovolaemia,
- normal, with slightly expanded extracellular volume (not clinically evident), or
- higher than normal causing extracellular hypervolaemia.

Significant extracellular volume changes can be detected clinically:

- hypovolaemia leads to thirst, reduced skin turgor, tachycardia, low jugular venous pressure, and postural hypotension (or supine hypotension in severe cases), and
- hypervolaemia leads to dependent oedema, also possibly to elevation of jugular venous pressure, pulmonary oedema, and ascites.

Minor volume changes are difficult to assess clinically and there are no simple quick diagnostic tests to aid classification.

Table 3 presents the classification and pathogenesis of hyponatraemia. Measurement of urinary sodium helps diagnosis. The majority of hyponatraemic patients have urine osmolalities in excess of 300 mosmol/kg and, of course, plasma is hypo-osmolar (< 280 mosmol/kg).

Table 3 Classification of hyponatraemia

Clinical extracellular volume status	Pathogenesis	Aetiology (examples)	Urinary Na concentration (mmol/litre)
Hypovolaemia	Deficit of TBW, larger deficit of ExNa	**Renal:** mineralocorticoid deficiency, sodium-losing nephritis, diuretic excess, Addison's disease	> 20
		Non-renal: vomiting, diarrhoea, burns, excessive sweating	< 10
Normovolaemia	Normal or slight excess of TBW	Syndrome of inappropriate antidiuresis, glucocorticoid deficiency, hypothyroidism, inappropriate intravenous therapy, 'sick cell' concept	> 20
Hypervolaemia	Excess of ExNa, larger excess of TBW	**Renal:** acute and chronic renal failure, Nephrotic syndrome	> 20
		Non-renal: cardiac failure, cirrhosis, inappropriate intravenous therapy	< 10

Abbreviations: TBW, total body water; ExNa, extracellular sodium.

Large sodium losses and hypovolaemic hyponatraemia commonly occur with persistent vomiting and/or diarrhoea, extensive skin burns, and excessive prolonged sweating. The healthy kidney will conserve sodium and urinary concentration will be less than 10 mmol/litre. Renal sodium loss leading to hyponatraemia can be due to renal diseases, typically those affecting the renal medulla (analgesic nephropathy, chronic pyelonephritis, polycystic kidneys, recovery from acute tubular necrosis, or post bilateral ureteric obstruction), mineralocorticoid deficiency (Addison's disease, hyporeninaemic hypoaldosteronism), or diuretic excess.

Normovolaemic hyponatraemia is usually due to the syndrome of inappropriate antidiuresis (see below) or inappropriate administration of intravenous fluid (for example 5 per cent dextrose solutions) in the postoperative period. Rarely it may be caused by isolated glucocorticoid deficiency (for example partial hypopituitarism) or severe prolonged hypothyroidism. Beer drinker's potomania occurs in some individuals who drink excessive volumes of beer over short periods, for example 10 litres in 6 h, which overwhelms the kidney's capacity to excrete water.

Hypervolaemic hyponatraemia is commonly observed in severe heart failure, decompensated cirrhosis, and nephrotic syndrome. In these disorders glomerular filtration is reduced and proximal tubular sodium reabsorption increased. Renal afferent arteriole perfusion falls leading to increased circulating angiotensin II concentrations, contributing to stimulation of thirst. Furthermore, non-osmotic release of vasopressin also contributes to water retention.

Clinical features

In addition to the features associated with extracellular (and therefore blood) volume reduction or expansion described above, there are clinical manifestations due to hyponatraemia *per se* (Table 4). The severity of hyponatraemic symptoms depends upon both the absolute serum sodium concentration and its rate of fall. Chronic mild hyponatraemia (serum sodium 120–130 mmol/litre) is often totally asymptomatic; but a sudden fall to only 125 mmol/litre from normal values (usually iatrogenic) can cause convulsions.

Table 4 Clinical features of hyponatraemia*

Mild	Anorexia
	Headache
	Nausea
	Vomiting
	Lethargy
Moderate	Personality change
	Muscle cramps
	Muscle weakness
	Confusion
	Ataxia
Severe	Drowsiness
	Diminished reflexes
	Convulsions
	Coma
	Death

*Features depend upon absolute serum sodium concentration and its rate of fall.

General principles of management

Specific therapy for mild hyponatraemia is often not necessary: treatment should be reserved for symptomatic or severe life-threatening hyponatraemia. Treatment of the underlying cause is obviously essential and will frequently correct the serum sodium concentration.

For hypovolaemic hyponatraemia, volume replacement is mandatory. Infusion of isotonic saline is usually sufficient, but occasionally intravascular volume expanders are required to raise blood pressure, particularly in an acute situation. Immediate hydrocortisone and subsequently fludrocortisone are essential to treat Addison's disease.

Treatment of normovolaemic hyponatraemia is described in the section on the syndrome of inappropriate antidiuresis.

Hyponatraemia associated with hypervolaemic disorders responds to single or combined therapy with potent diuretic drugs to remove extracellular sodium, inhibitors of angiotensin-converting enzyme to lower angiotensin II values, and water restriction to less than 1 litre per 24 h.

Irrespective of the cause, chronic severe hyponatraemia (defined as serum sodium < 120 mmol/litre lasting more than 3 days) should be corrected slowly (i.e. at a rate of less than 0.5 mmol/litre/h). Infusion of hypertonic saline should be avoided, but if used the rate of infusion should increase serum sodium by no more than 0.5 mmol/litre/h (10 mmol/litre/24 h) and infusion stopped when serum sodium reaches 120 mmol/litre. A convenient formula determines the likely rate of change of serum sodium concentration following infusion of hypertonic saline and should always be used in patient care:

rate of infusion of 3 per cent NaCl solution (ml/h) = body weight (kg) × desired rate of correction of serum sodium (mmol/litre/h).

Acute symptomatic severe hyponatraemia (developed in less than 3 days; with drowsiness, convulsions, or coma) can be corrected more quickly, with a rate of serum sodium increase of up to 2 mmol/litre/h, but again infusion should stop at a serum sodium concentration of 120 mmol/litre. Regrettably, this condition is almost always iatrogenic, most commonly arising when young women recovering from surgery are ill-advisedly given large quantities of 5 per cent dextrose by intravenous infusion.

Central pontine myelinolysis

The first case of central pontine myelinolysis was described in a young alcoholic. Following many similar cases, it was initially assumed that the condition was due to some form of nutritional deficiency. Association with hyponatraemia was then reported, and the view that this (or its subsequent management) might cause central pontine myelinolysis (also known as osmotic demyelination syndrome) was supported by the finding that dogs made hyponatraemic by repeated injections of vasopressin and intraperitoneal infusions of water, then given hypertonic saline, became quadriparetic with brainstem lesions indistinguishable from those seen in the human condition.

There is undoubtedly a high morbidity and mortality in those with serum sodium concentrations of less than 110 mmol/litre, but debate continues as to whether this is caused by the hyponatraemia itself, or by overzealous treatment of that hyponatraemia. The most feared outcome remains the neurological sequelae of cerebral demyelination, thought to result from large shifts of intracellular water, which occur outside the brainstem as well as in the pons. In most cases reported (if not all), serum sodium has rapidly been corrected to normal levels, hence the recommendation given above that if hypertonic saline is used to correct hyponatraemia, then the infusion must be stopped when serum sodium rises to 120 mmol/litre, allowing more gradual correction from that point onward.

Neurological signs usually develop 2 to 4 days after rapid correction of hyponatraemia. Typical features are quadriplegia and pseudobulbar palsy: these can take the form of a 'locked in' syndrome of mutism with paralysis.

Syndrome of inappropriate antidiuresis

This syndrome is due to inappropriate secretion of vasopressin and is the commonest cause of normovolaemic hyponatraemia. The diagnosis of syndrome of inappropriate antidiuresis is established by ensuring that all the syndrome's criteria are fulfilled (Table 5). This is important: too often the diagnosis is incorrectly claimed on the basis that the first two criteria are met. If they are, this establishes that the level of vasopressin is inappropriate to plasma osmolality, but for the term to be properly applied the level must also be inappropriate to the intravascular volume (it is appropriate to have a high vasopressin level in the context of volume depletion/hypotension). Measurement of urinary sodium is essential: this is persistently elevated in the range 50 to 70 mmol/litre; if it is low, then this suggests that the kidney is attempting to conserve sodium, either due to volume depletion or a sodium-retaining state. The final two criteria specifically exclude those with hypo- and hypervolaemic states, and make the point that the diagnosis can only be confidently made if renal and adrenal function are normal.

Plasma vasopressin estimations are unhelpful in differentiating the syndrome of inappropriate antidiuresis from other causes of hyponatraemia, because the majority of all hyponatraemic states (> 95 per cent) have detectable or elevated values, due to non-osmotic release of the hormone. Persistent circulating vasopressin causes the relative excess of water in all types of hyponatraemia.

Pathophysiology and causes of the syndrome of inappropriate antidiuresis

A very large number of disorders have been associated with the syndrome of inappropriate antidiuresis, some of which are listed in Table 6. In brief, they include a variety of neoplastic conditions, the commonest being small cell carcinoma of the bronchus, non-malignant chest diseases including infections, neurological disorders (infective and vascular), drugs (cytotoxic agents, chlorpropamide, carbamazepine, antidepressants, oxytocin, and thiazide diuretics), recreational agents ('Ecstasy'), and a miscellaneous group (porphyria, cortisol deficiency, idiopathic).

Table 5 Criteria for the diagnosis of the syndrome of antidiuresis

Dilutional hyponatraemia, i.e. plasma hypo-osmolality proportional to hyponatraemia
Urine osmolality greater than plasma osmolality
Persistent renal sodium excretion (~50–70 mmol/litre)
Absence of hypotension, hypovolaemia, and oedema-forming states
Normal renal, thyroid, and adrenal function

The persistent natriuresis, central to the diagnosis of syndrome of inappropriate antidiuresis, can be explained, in part, by the expanded total body water which is not clinically detectable, causing a reduction in aldosterone production, an increase in circulating natriuretic factors, and a decrease in proximal sodium reabsorption.

Treatment of the syndrome of inappropriate antidiuresis

Identification and successful treatment of the underlying cause of the syndrome of inappropriate antidiuresis will usually correct hyponatraemia. If chronic symptomatic or life-threatening hyponatraemia remains, specific measures to remove the excess total body water are required.

Fluid restriction to 500 ml per 24 h to increase serum sodium to about 130 mmol/litre remains the therapy to be tried first. If this approach is unsatisfactory, additional methods to remove water are justified, the most

Table 6 Causes of the syndrome of inappropriate antidiuresis

Neoplastic disease
Carcinoma (bronchus, pancreas, bladder, prostate, duodenum)
Thymoma
Mesothelioma
Lymphoma, leukaemia
Ewing's sarcoma
Carcinoid
Bronchial adenoma
Neurological disorders
Head injury, neurosurgery
Brain abscess
Brain tumour
Meningitis, encephalitis
Guillain Barré syndrome
Cerebral haemorrhage
Cavernous sinus thrombosis
Hydrocephalus
Cerebellar and cerebral atrophy
Shy–Drager syndrome
Peripheral neuropathy
Seizures
Subdural haematoma
Alcohol withdrawal
Chest disorders
Pneumonia
Tuberculosis
Emphyema
Cystic fibrosis
Pneumothorax
Aspergillosis
Drugs
Chlorpropamide
Opiates
Vincristine, cis-platinum
Vinblastine
Thiazides
Dopamine antagonists
Tricyclic antidepressants
MAOIs
SSRIs
'Ecstasy' (3,4-MDMA)
Anticonvulsants
Miscellaneous
Idiopathic
Psychosis
Porphyria
Abdominal surgery

MAOIs = monoamine oxidase inhibitors; SSRIs = selective serotonin reuptake inhibitors; 3,4-MDMA, 3,4-methylenedioxymetamphetamnine.

Table 7 Classification and causes of hypernatraemia

Hypervolaemic (excess extracellular sodium)
Accidental (e.g. salt emetics, infant feeds)
Iatrogenic (e.g. $NaHCO_3$ infusion at cardiac resuscitation)
Hypovolaemic (insufficient total body water)
Decreased water intake:
Hypodipsia or adipsia
neoplasia of the hypothalamopituitary region
vascular (anterior communicating artery aneurysm)
granuloma (sarcoidosis, histiocytosis X)
miscellaneous (trauma, hydrocephalus, ventricular cyst)
Reduced access to water*
travel in desert
limitation of movement (eg. stroke)
Acute excessive fluid loss:
Gastrointestinal
Burns

*Note that dramatic cases of hypernatraemia are seen where polyuria is associated with reduced access to water, e.g. in the patient who is comatose with cranial diabetes insipidus.

successful of which is the induction of partial nephrogenic diabetes insipidus with demeclocycline (600 to 1200 mg daily in divided doses), but the maximal effect may take 2 weeks to achieve. It is preferable to lithium carbonate, which although inducing nephrogenic diabetes insipidus is more nephrotoxic. An alternative approach is the administration of furosemide (frusemide) (40–80 mg daily) in combination with oral sodium chloride supplementation (3 g daily). Phenytoin has occasionally proved helpful by suppressing inappropriate neurohypophyseal vasopressin secretion. Infusion of isotonic or hypertonic solutions of saline are not advised because of the real danger that rapid increase in serum sodium concentration might cause the osmotic demyelination syndrome (see above).

The most logical therapy for the syndrome of inappropriate antidiuresis would be a V_2-receptor antagonist. A recently synthesized, linear non-peptide V_2-receptor antagonist, OPC-31260, increases solute-free water excretion. Clinical trials of the treatment of syndrome of inappropriate antidiuresis with this agent are encouraging. This new class of drugs, called aquaretics, should improve management of the syndrome of inappropriate antidiuresis, and other hyponatraemic states associated with excess arginine vasopressin.

Sick cell concept

This concept was formulated following the observation that hyponatraemia developed quickly in severe trauma or overwhelming infection in humans or animals, and in malnourished very ill patients. It is classified as a cause of normovolaemic hyponatraemia. There is a shift of intracellular water into the extracellular compartment due to reduction of intracellular solute either by leakage across a damaged cell membrane, enhanced intracellular catabolism, or possibly due to movement of sodium into the cell. There is no specific therapy other than treatment of the underlying cause.

Hypernatraemic states and thirst deficiency

Hypernatraemia, defined as a serum sodium concentration greater than 150 mmol/litre, is less common than hyponatraemia.

Aetiology and pathophysiology

Hypernatraemia can be classified into two categories dependent on extracellular volume states (Table 7).

Hypervolaemic hypernatraemia is caused by extracellular sodium excess, usually as a result of accidental iatrogenic overdoses of sodium-containing preparations.

Acute hypovolaemic hypernatraemia occurs when patients lose large quantities of hypotonic fluid (for example gastrointestinal). Chronic hypovolaemic hypernatraemia is the result of prolonged water deficit, usually the result of impaired or absent thirst, hypodipsia, or adipsia, which implies a lesion of the thirst osmoreceptor. It is sometimes associated with abnormal osmoregulated vasopressin secretion. Four patterns of osmoregulatory dysfunction have been described (Fig. 7):

- Type A, shows elevation of osmotic thresholds for both thirst and vasopressin. It has been termed 'essential' hypernatraemia; patients continue to dilute and concentrate urine normally, but do so around a higher serum sodium concentration.
- Type B is characterized by decreased sensitivity (slope) of the vasopressin and thirst osmoregulatory lines.

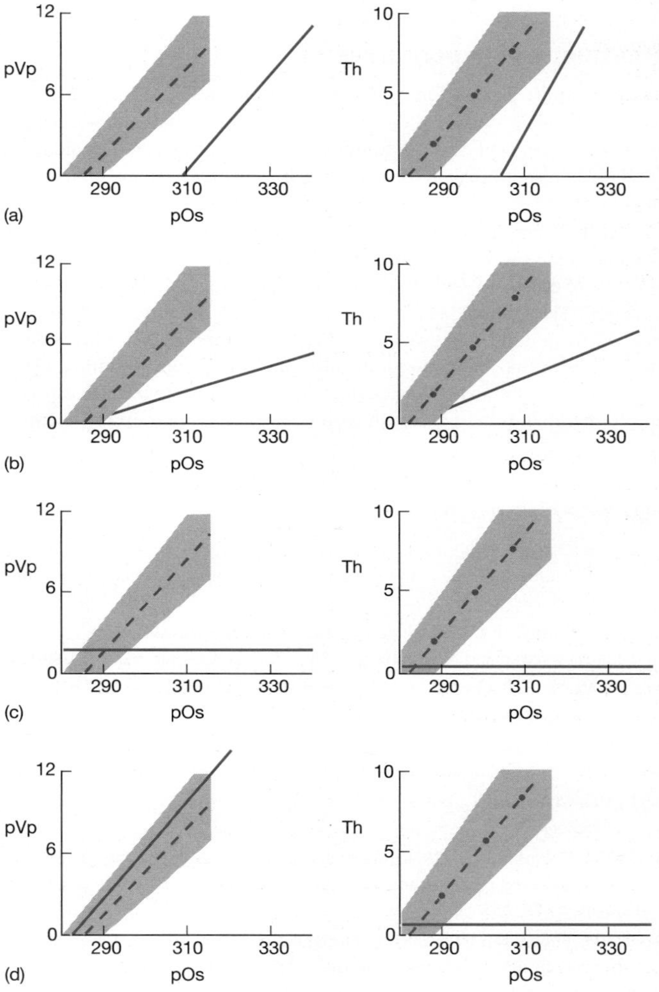

Fig. 7 Patterns of osmoregulated thirst (Th) and plasma vasopressin concentration (pVp) in hypodipsic or adipsic hypernatraemia. The units of pVp are pmol/l and of thirst are 0 to 10 on a visual analogue scale. Stippled areas are the normal responses to increases in plasma osmolality (pOs) and the dashed lines represent mean osmoregulatory lines: (a) reset thirst and vasopressin thresholds or 'essential' hypernatraemia; (b) decreased sensitivity of thirst and vasopressin release; (c) complete destruction of both thirst and vasopressin osmoreceptors; (d) absent thirst osmoregulation with normal osmoregulated vasopressin release. See text for further explanation. (Reproduced from Baylis PH and Thompson CJ (1988). Osmoregulation of vasopressin secretion and thirst in health and disease. *Clinical Endocrinology* **29**, 549–76, with permission.)

- Type C, the most serious defect, termed adipsic hypernatraemia, is due to complete destruction of both thirst and arginine vasopressin osmoreceptors. Patients never experience the desire to drink, even when serum sodium reaches values as high as 190 mmol/litre.
- Type D is very rare, with selective complete loss of thirst but vasopressin osmoregulation remaining normal.

Clinical features

Hypervolaemic hypernatraemia causes severe thirst, irritability, and hypotonia and may lead to convulsions, seizures, and death. Clinical manifestations of hypovolaemic hypernatraemia relate to extracellular and intracellular fluid loss, the striking feature being lack of thirst. The slow development of hypernatraemia is often associated with minimal symptoms of confusion or drowsiness.

Treatment of hypernatraemia

Patients require water to lower serum sodium concentration slowly. The safest route of administration is oral, but unconscious patients will require infusion of 5 per cent dextrose solutions. Care must be taken to avoid rapid falls in serum sodium, with the rate of decline no greater than 10 mmol per 24 h.

'Essential' hypernatraemia (Fig. 7, type A) requires little specific therapy as patients are protected from extremes of hypernatraemia. Patients with total loss of thirst and vasopressin osmoregulation pose major management problems. They should be instructed to drink a daily volume of about 2 litres, which should be adjusted according to changes in daily body weight. Desmopressin may be required. Regular checks of serum sodium concentration are essential to avoid wide fluctuations. Constant vigilance is necessary to maintain water balance in chronic hypodipsic or adipsic patients.

Further reading

Anderson RJ *et al.* (1985). Hyponatremia: a prospective analysis of its epidemiology and the pathogenetic role of vasopressin. *Annals of Internal Medicine* **102**,164–8.

Arieff AL, Guisado R (1976). Effects on the central nervous system of hypernatremic and hyponatremic states. *Kidney International* **10**, 104–16.

Ball SG, Vaidja B, Baylis PH (1997). Hypothalamic adipsic syndrome: diagnosis and management. *Clinical Endocrinology* **47**, 405–9.

Bartter FC, Schwartz WB (1967). The syndrome of inappropriate secretion of antidiuretic hormone. *American Journal of Medicine* **42**, 790–806.

Baylis PH, Cheetham T (1998). Diabetes insipidus. *Archives of Disease in Childhood* **79**, 84–9.

Baylis PH, Robertson GL (1980). Plasma vasopressin response to hypertonic saline to assess posterior pituitary function. *Journal of the Royal Society of Medicine* **73**, 255–60.

Baylis PH, Thompson CJ (1988). Osmoregulation of vasopressin secretion and thirst in health and disease. *Clinical Endocrinology* **29**, 549–76.

Berl T *et al.* (1976). Clinical disorders of water metabolism. *Kidney International* **10**, 117–32.

Bibi D *et al.* (1999). Treatment of central pontine myelinolysis with therapeutic plasmaphoresis. *The Lancet* **353**, 1155.

Bichet DG *et al.* (1994). Nature and recurrence of AVPR2 mutations in X-linked nephrogenic diabetes insipidus. *American Journal of Human Genetics* **55**, 278–86.

Charmondari E, Brook CGD (1999). 20 years of experience of idiopathic central diabetes insipidus. *The Lancet* **353**, 2212–13.

Davison JM *et al.* (1988). Serial evaluation of vasopressin release and thirst in human pregnancy. *Journal of Clinical Investigation* **81**, 798–806.

De Bellis A *et al.* (1999). Longitudinal study of vasopressin cell antibodies, posterior pituitary function and magnetic resonance imaging evaluations in subclinical autoimmune central diabetes insipidus. *Journal of Clinical Endocrinology and Metabolism* **84**, 3047–3051.

Deen PMT *et al.* (1994). Requirement of human renal water channel aquaporin-2 for vasopressin dependent concentration of urine. *Science* **264**, 92–5.

De Zeeuw D, Janssen WMT, de Jong PE (1992). Atrial natriuretic factor: its (patho)physiological significance in humans. *Kidney International* **41**, 1115–33.

Flear CTG, Gill GV, Burn J (1981). Hyponatraemia: mechanisms and management. *The Lancet* **i**, 26–31.

Kenyon CJ, Jardine AG (1989) Atrial natriuretic peptide: water and electrolyte homeostasis. *Baillière's Clinics in Endocrinology and Metabolism* **3**, 431–50.

Martin P-Y, Schrier RW (1998). Role of aquaporin-2 water channels in urinary concentration and dilution defects. *Kidney International* **53** (Supplement 65), 557–62.

McKenna K, Thompson C (1998). Osmoregulation in clinical disorders of thirst and thirst appreciation. *Clinical Endocrinology* **49**, 139–52.

Miller WL (1993). Molecular genetics of familial central diabetes insipidus. *Journal of Clinical Endocrinology and Metabolism* **77**, 592–5.

Mitchell KD, Navar LG (1989). The renin-angiotensin-aldosterone system in volume control. *Baillière's Clinics in Endocrinology and Metabolism* **3**, 393–430.

Robertson GL, Shelton RL, Athar S (1976). The osmoregulation of vasopressin. *Kidney International* **10**, 25–37.

Robertson GL (1995). Diabetes insipidus. *Endocrinology and Metabolism Clinics of North America* **24**, 549–72.

Saito T *et al.* (1997). Acute aquaresis by the non-peptide arginine vasopressin (AVP) antagonist OPC-31260 improves hyponatraemia in patients with the syndrome of inappropriate secretion of antidiuretic hormone. *Journal of Clinical Endocrinology and Metabolism* **82**, 1054–7.

Siggaard C *et al.* (1999). Clinical and molecular evidence of abnormal processing and trafficking of the vasopressin preprohormone in a large kindred with familial neurohypophyseal diabetes insipidus due to a signal peptide mutation. *Journal of Clinical Endocrinology and Metabolism* **84**, 2933–41.

Sterns RH, Riggo J, Schochet SS (1986). Osmotic demyelination syndrome following correction of hyponatremia. *New England Journal of Medicine* **314**, 1535–42.

Strom TM *et al.* (1998). Diabetes insipidus, diabetes mellitus, optic atrophy and deafness (DIDMOAD) caused by mutations in a novel gene (wolframin) coding for a predicted transmembrane protein. *Human Molecular Genetics* **7**, 2021–8.

Thompson CJ *et al.* (1986). The osmotic thresholds for thirst and vasopressin release are similar in healthy man. *Clinical Science* **71**, 651–6.

Thrasher TN, Keil LC, Ramsay DJ (1982). Lesions of the organum vasculosum of the lamina terminalis (OVLT) attenuate osmotically induced drinking and vasopressin secretion in dogs. *Endocrinology* **110**, 1837–41.

Verbalis JG (1989). Hyponatraemia. *Baillière's Clinics in Endocrinology and Metabolism* **3**, 499–530.

Verbalis JG (1998). Adaptation to acute and chronic hyponatraemia: implications for symptomatology, diagnosis and treatment. *Seminars in Nephrology* **18**, 3–19.

Vokes TJ, Robertson GL (1988). Disorders of antidiuretic hormone. *Endocrinology and Metabolism Clinics of North America* **17**, 281–99.

Walker LA, Valtin H (1982). Biological importance of nephron heterogeneity. *Annual Reviews in Physiology* **44**, 203–19.

Yasui M *et al.* (1997). Adenylate cyclase-coupled vasopressin receptor activates AQP-2 promoter via a dual effect on CRE and AP1 elements. *American Journal of Physiology, Renal Fluid and Electrolyte Physiology* **272**, F443–F450.

20.2.2 Disorders of potassium homeostasis

J. Firth

Potassium homeostasis

Introduction

Potassium is the most abundant cation in the body. Total body potassium ranges between 37 and 52 mmol/kg body weight, and of this 98 per cent is found within cells, where its concentration is in the range 150 to 160 mmol/l. By contrast, the normal range of potassium concentration in serum is from 3.5 to 5.0 mmol/l. The ratio of intracellular to extracellular potassium concentration is a critical determinant of cellular resting membrane potential and thereby of the function of excitable tissues, particularly the nerves and muscles. Potassium tends to leak out of cells through a variety of ion-selective potassium channels found in all cell membranes. The maintenance of the intracellular to extracellular gradient is largely dependent on the ubiquitous Na^+,K^+-ATPase enzyme, which pumps two potassium ions into the cell for every three sodium ions extruded.

The mechanisms of potassium homeostasis can be considered in terms of internal balance (the relationship between intracellular and extracellular potassium concentration) and external balance (which determines total body potassium).

Internal balance

A wide variety of factors modulate the distribution of potassium between the intracellular and extracellular fluid compartments. These factors either alter the function of the Na^+,K^+-ATPase or the rate of efflux of potassium from cells, which together dictate intracellular potassium concentration. In view of the importance of the ratio of internal to external potassium concentration for critical neuromuscular functions, some of these mechanisms serve as essential acute defence mechanisms to counteract life-threatening hyperkalaemia. Factors modulating internal potassium balance are shown in Table 1.

External balance

Dietary potassium intake in Western society typically varies between 50 and 150 mmol/day, but balance can be attained with intake of up to 500 mmol/day if homeostatic mechanisms are intact. In normal circumstances potassium excretion in the stool is not regulated, but it amounts to only 5 to 15 mmol/day. When renal function is compromised, the absolute magnitude as well as the proportion of potassium in the faeces is increased, but variation in renal excretion of potassium is usually the only means by which the body achieves external potassium balance by ensuring that excretion equals intake.

With normal intake of potassium, 10 to 20 per cent of the load filtered at the glomerulus is excreted, but fractional excretion of potassium can vary from 1 per cent when intake is restricted to over 100 per cent when intake is excessive. Micropuncture studies have shown that the amount of potassium reaching the distal convoluted tubule does not vary in these circumstances, indicating that modulation of renal potassium excretion is normally a property of the distal nephron. Factors that modify potassium excretion by the distal nephron are shown in Table 2. These factors are clearly interrelated: it is rare that one is modified in isolation and the overall effect on potassium excretion is almost invariably the aggregate result of several complementary or competing stimuli.

Hypokalaemia

A low serum potassium concentration (3.5 mmol/l or less) is the commonest electrolyte abnormality seen in clinical practice, found in up to 20 per cent of patients in hospital. Most have mild hypokalaemia, with serum potassium in the range 3.0 to 3.5 mmol/l, but 5 per cent have a level lower than 3.0 mmol/l, and 0.03 per cent (more in some series) have very severe hypokalaemia with serum potassium concentration less than 2.5 mmol/l.

Clinical features of hypokalaemia

Patients with mild hypokalaemia often have no symptoms attributable to their low serum potassium concentration. A variety of non-specific symptoms develop with more severe hypokalaemia, including lassitude, generalized weakness, and constipation. At a serum potassium level of less than 2.5 mmol/l serious neuromuscular problems sometimes arise. Rhabdomyolysis (see Chapter 20.4) can occur, and increases in serum creatine phosphokinase activity indicative of muscle injury are frequently detectable in those with a serum potassium concentration below 3.0 mmol/l. Hypokalaemia can cause intestinal ileus, and is particularly likely to do so in the postoperative period when other factors also conspire to prevent normal gut motility. Paralysis of skeletal muscle has been reported, most dramatically in cases of hypokalaemic quadraparesis, which appears to be more common in India than elsewhere. Paraesthesias and tetany have rarely been described.

Hypokalaemia can cause polyuria and polydipsia, also a metabolic alkalosis. Severe prolonged potassium depletion is associated with chronic interstitial nephritis, the presence of renal cysts, and with the development of

Table 1 Factors modulating internal potassium balance

Acid–base status	Acidosis (excepting renal tubular acidosis) tends to diminish potassium uptake by cells and to cause hyperkalaemia; alkalosis has the opposite effect. The relationship between pH and serum potassium is not simple: metabolic acidosis produced by mineral acids, such as hyperchloraemic, results in an increment in serum potassium of 0.7 mmol/l for each 0.1 unit fall in blood pH, whereas in acidosis produced by organic acids, such as lactate and β-hydroxybutyrate, the serum potassium may not be altered. Alkalosis reduces serum potassium by 0.3 mmol/l per 0.1 pH unit rise
Pancreatic hormones	Insulin release is stimulated by hyperkalaemia and inhibited by hypokalaemia. It induces cellular uptake of potassium by activating the Na^+,K^+-ATPase directly. Glucagon can increase serum potassium concentration
Catecholamines	β_2-Adrenergic agonists promote cellular potassium uptake by activating the Na^+,K^+-ATPase via a cAMP-dependent mechanism. α-Adrenergic agonists have the opposite effect
Exercise	Exercise results in loss of potassium from muscle cells, which causes local vasodilatation and increases regional blood flow. Serum potassium can increase by as much as 50 per cent after 10 to 15 min of vigorous exercise, falling precipitately in the recovery period
Aldosterone	The most important actions of aldosterone are on external balance, but there is also evidence of effect on internal balance
Osmolality	Hyperosmolality increases the serum potassium concentration
Total body potassium	The distribution of potassium between intracellular and extracellular compartments is influenced by the total amount of potassium in the body. Changes in the extracellular compartment are always proportionately greater than those in the intracellular compartment. The mechanisms are not known

Table 2 Factors that modify potassium excretion by the distal nephron

Aldosterone	Aldosterone is the dominant hormone regulating potassium homeostasis. An increase in plasma potassium directly stimulates aldosterone secretion by the adrenal glands. In the principal cells of the collecting ducts, aldosterone binds to its intracellular mineralocorticoid receptor, is translocated to the nucleus, and induces production of basolateral Na^+,K^+-ATPase and the apical sodium channel. The effect is to increase intracellular potassium concentration and the electrochemical potential favouring potassium secretion into the tubular fluid and hence its excretion from the body. Under normal conditions changes in sodium intake lead to changes in plasma aldosterone (an increase leading to decreased secretion) such that potassium homeostasis is preserved despite alteration in sodium and fluid delivery to the distal nephron
Intravascular volume	Reduction of intravascular volume leads to a 'contraction alkalosis', stimulated largely by aldosterone, and which is associated with hypokalaemia
Dietary potassium intake	Chronic alterations in dietary potassium intake induce profound modifications in the renal capacity to excrete or conserve potassium. A low potassium diet leads to an enhanced renal capacity to conserve potassium and a high potassium diet enhances the ability to excrete a potassium load. The mechanisms involved in these adaptations are poorly understood, although aldosterone is involved
Plasma potassium concentration	The potassium concentration gradient across the basolateral membrane modulates potassium uptake by the cell and/or passive back-leakage, hence hyperkalaemia leads to enhanced potassium excretion
Acid–base status	Systemic pH modulates potassium uptake across the basolateral membrane and conductance of the luminal membrane, with acidosis inhibiting excretion. Chronic metabolic alkalosis is almost invariably associated with potassium depletion
Urine flow rate	Increased flow of tubular fluid lowers potassium concentration in that fluid and favours secretion across the luminal membrane
Sodium	Reduced delivery of sodium ($<$ 30 mmol/l) to the distal nephron impairs potassium secretion by the cortical collecting duct
Other factors	Antidiuretic hormone, poorly reabsorbable anions (such as sulphates), glucocorticoids, and α-adrenergic agonists stimulate potassium secretion

chronic renal failure. It is not always clear, however, whether hypokalaemia is the cause or effect of this condition.

Hypokalaemia may be suspected from the clinical context (for example the patient taking diuretics or vomiting copiously), but there are no specific physical signs. Alterations induced in the ECG include flattening of the T wave, depression of the S–T segment, and the development of prominent U waves, which can give the impression of a prolonged Q–T interval. These changes, typically observed with a serum potassium concentration lower than 3.0 mmol/l, provide a diagnostic clue to the presence of hypokalaemia, but do not have any serious clinical implications in a patient with a normal heart. However, hypokalaemia can cause problems in those whose heart is abnormal. There is a correlation between hypokalaemia and the development of ventricular tachycardia or fibrillation during the acute phase of myocardial infarction; hypokalaemia can provoke life-threatening arrhythmias in those receiving digoxin; and there is controversy as to whether the mild hypokalaemia often produced by diuretic therapy constitutes a risk factor for sudden cardiac death.

Treatment of hypokalaemia

In emergency

Emergency treatment of hypokalaemia is rarely required. In the rare circumstances of life-threatening cardiac arrhythmia or muscular paralysis, intravenous infusion of potassium (usually potassium chloride) should be given immediately. This must be administered into a central vein (internal jugular, subclavian, or femoral) since solutions containing the necessary high concentration of potassium cause pain and phlebitis if given peripherally, and can cause chemical burns if they extravasate. There is no good evidence on which to base a recommendation regarding dose and rate, but the maximum rate of infusion usually employed is 1 mmol/min, which should be controlled with a volumetric pump. The main danger of giving potassium with such rapidity is the development of hyperkalaemia, hence the patient and their ECG should be observed continuously, the serum potassium should be checked frequently, and infusion slowed as soon as the life-threatening problem has resolved (arrhythmia settled, muscular power improved). In one study, administration of 40 mmol of potassium over 1 h was found to increase serum potassium concentration by an average of 1.1 mmol/l in hypokalaemic patients with both normal and impaired renal function.

In cases that are not emergencies

In most circumstances the management of a patient with hypokalaemia requires a methodical approach to establishing the diagnosis, which is often readily apparent (but not always so), rectification (if possible) of the underlying cause, and administration of potassium at a less hurried rate than that described above. In most cases of hypokalaemia, the fall in the serum potassium concentration represents the tip of an iceberg, a reduction of 0.3 mmol/l typically reflecting a 100 mmol deficit in body stores. This relationship is variable, but it is important to remember that patients with even modest hypokalaemia may have a very considerable deficit of total body potassium that needs to be replaced.

Potassium can be given orally or intravenously. Foods with high potassium content are listed in Table 7, but it should be noted that the potassium which they contain is almost entirely coupled with phosphate. In the absence of adequate chloride intake they are therefore ineffective in replenishing body potassium in the many and common causes of hypokalaemia associated with chloride depletion (such as diuretics or vomiting). Potassium chloride can be given in either liquid or tablet form, typically 2 to 4 g (approximately 25 to 50 mmol) daily in divided doses. Both are well absorbed, but the liquid preparations are unpalatable to many patients and slow-release tablets have been associated with gastrointestinal ulceration, bleeding, and stricture, such that they must be taken with fluid whilst sitting or standing and not just before retiring to bed for the night. If intravenous administration of potassium is required, infusions containing a concentration of 20 mmol/l can usually be tolerated through a good peripheral line. If a higher concentration than this is required, central venous access will be necessary. Care must always be taken to monitor serum levels closely.

Common causes of hypokalaemia

There are a very large number of possible causes of hypokalaemia (Table 3), but in most instances the diagnosis is immediately apparent. Whenever this is not so, it is wise to remember that common things are the most likely. In the case of patients with hypokalaemia it is also important to recognize that concealment of the diagnosis is not infrequent, with diuretic abuse or covert vomiting more likely than the more exotic and rare causes of this condition. Hypokalaemia is not a prominent feature of many of the disorders listed in Table 3: discussion in this chapter will be limited to those conditions that are common, or where hypokalaemia is an important manifestation.

Table 3 Causes of hypokalaemia

- **Altered internal balance (redistribution of potassium from extracellular to intracellular compartment)**
- Alkalosis
- Insulin (high doses)
- β_2-Adrenergic stimulants
- B_{12} therapy of deficiency anaemia
- Intoxications
  - Theophylline
  - Toluene (paint/glue sniffing)
  - Barium
- Periodic paralysis
  - Thyrotoxic periodic paralysis
  - Sporadic periodic paralysis
  - Familial hypokalaemic periodic paralysis
- ?Aldosterone
- **Altered external balance (low total body potassium)**
- *Renal losses (urinary potassium > 20 mmol/day)*
- 1. Mineralocorticoid excess
  - Primary hyperaldosteronism (Conn's syndrome)
  - Fludrocortisone
  - Congenital adrenal hyperplasia
  - 11β-Hydroxylase deficiency
  - 17α-Hydroxylase deficiency
  - Renin-secreting tumours
  - Ectopic ACTH production
  - Cushing's syndrome
  - Glucocorticoid-responsive aldosteronism
  - Renovascular hypertension
  - Accelerated (malignant)-phase hypertension
  - Vasculitis
- 2. Apparent mineralocorticoid excess
  - Liddle's syndrome
  - Syndrome of apparent mineralocorticoid excess (hereditary 11β-hydroxysteroid dehydrogenase deficiency)
  - Acquired 11β-hydroxysteroid dehydrogenase deficiency
    - Liquorice
    - Chewing tobacco
    - Carbenoxolone
- 3. Impaired renal tubular ion transport
  - Diuretics
  - Bartter's syndrome
  - Gitelman's syndrome
  - Renal tubular acidosis (distal)
  - High-dose penicillins
  - Magnesium depletion
- *Extrarenal losses (urinary potassium < 20 mmol/day)*
- Gastrointestinal losses
  - Biliary loss
  - Lower gastointestinal loss:
    - Diarrhoea
    - Laxative abuse
    - Villous adenoma
  - Fistula
  - Ureterosigmoidostomy
- Skin losses

A pragmatic approach is first to consider the most frequent causes of hypokalaemia—diuretic ingestion and gastrointestinal fluid loss—and then proceed to a systematic analysis if these are not evidently the cause of the problem.

Treatment with diuretics

The most common cause of hypokalaemia is diuretic therapy. All diuretics other than those acting directly on the collecting duct (amiloride, triamterene, spironolactone) block some form of chloride-associated sodium transport. As a result they increase the delivery of sodium to the collecting duct, where its reabsorption creates a favourable electrochemical gradient for and obligates potassium secretion. Hypokalaemia frequently occurs together with metabolic alkalosis (serum bicarbonate concentration 28 to 36 mmol/l). In general, the hypokalaemia is mild, with serum potassium in the range 3 to 3.5 mmol/l; the average fall after inititation of the usual doses of loop diuretics (frusemide, bumetanide, torasemide) being about 0.3 mmol/l, somewhat more with the usual doses of thiazides (bendrofluazide, chlorothiazide, chlorthalidone) at about 0.6 mmol/l. In one analysis of publications on hypokalaemia and diuretics it was found that the fall in serum potassium was little influenced by the reason for prescription (hypertension or heart failure), or by the dose or duration of treatment.

The question of whether or not patients receiving diuretics prone to induce hypokalaemia should be prescribed potassium supplements or potassium-retaining diuretics has been much debated. There is no strong evidence on which to base recommendations. It seems common sense to monitor for and intervene to prevent hypokalaemia in those considered at particular risk of hypokalaemic complications, including those with a history of cardiac arrhythmia, those on digoxin, and those with liver disease in whom electrolyte imbalance might precipitate encephalopathy. Most patients do not fall into any of these categories, and here the balance is between an attempt to prevent a hypothetical but unproven hazard and the requirement for medication that is unpalatable to many and in rare cases can have significant side-effects. As in many other aspects of medicine, the behaviour of the physician will say as much about them as about the condition that they are dealing with. Those that like all test results to be in the 'normal range' will prescribe, but short of stopping diuretic therapy, correcting diuretic-induced hypokalaemia is not easy. In one study that monitored adverse drug reactions in 5047 consecutive inpatients, 2439 were taking potassium-losing diuretics, in whom serum potassium was less than 3.5 mmol/l in 21 per cent, and below 3.0 mmol/l in 3.8 per cent. If the group taking potassium-losing diuretics was broken down into those taking them without any attempt to prevent hypokalaemia, those taking them in conjunction with potassium supplements, and those taking them together with a potassium-sparing diuretic, then serum potassium below 3.5 mmol/l was found in 24.9, 19.7, and 15.2 per cent, respectively.

Loss of gastrointestinal fluid

In one study of severe hypokalaemia (serum potassium less than 2.5 mmol/l), gastrointestinal fluid loss was the main cause in 22 per cent of cases.

Vomiting

The concentration of potassium in gastric and upper intestinal secretions is between 3 and 12 mmol/l. Reduced intake and direct loss of potassium in vomit are not, therefore, the main causes of hypokalaemia, which arises due to increased renal excretion of potassium. Why does this happen? Circumstances can arise in which the renal response to one pathophysiological abnormality takes precedence over another, and where the attempt to correct one imbalance actually has the effect of worsening another. This is the situation when the kidney responds to prolonged vomiting. Aside from modest quantities of potassium, gastric juices contain sodium ions (30 to 90 mmol/l), protons (90 mmol/l), and chloride (50 to 125 mmol/l). Loss of gastric acid (HCl) pulls the buffer equation $H_2CO_3 + Na^+ + Cl^-$ in equilibrium with $Na^+ + HCO_3^- + H^+ + Cl^-$ to the right, hence the main effect is metabolic alkalosis. Depletion of extracellular fluid volume also occurs, activating the renin–angiotensin–aldosterone system. As the bicarbonate concentration in the blood rises, more is filtered at the glomerulus and some is excreted in the urine, partly in conjunction with potassium, whose distal excretion is stimulated by high levels of aldosterone. Considerations of acid–base balance have taken precedence over those of potassium homeostasis, and hypokalaemia results.

An important point to note is that the combination of direct chloride loss in vomit and contraction of extracellular fluid volume lead to a situation where the kidney avidly retains chloride and the urinary concentration of chloride falls to a very low level (less than 10 mmol/l, sometimes as low as 1 to 2 mmol/l, when the normal range is 30 to 120 mmol/l). This has critical clinical significance in two circumstances. First, since reabsorption of filtered sodium and potassium ions by the renal tubule can only be achieved in combination with an anion, usually chloride, then if urinary chloride concentration is already close to zero there is no way in which sodium and potassium can be reabsorbed efficiently. Hence, sodium and potassium that are administered can only be retained if provided in conjunction with chloride, and not if given as other salts. Second, measurement of urinary chloride concentration can be helpful in making the diagnosis of surreptitious vomiting (see later).

Resuscitation of the patient with hypokalaemia due to vomiting requires the intravenous infusion of 0.9 per cent sodium chloride, together with potassium supplementation as described above. In severe cases the total body deficit of fluid may be in excess of 5 litres, and of potassium of many hundreds of millimoles.

Diarrhoea

The concentration of potassium in stool is 80 to 90 mmol/l. Hence, given normal stool weight of 100 to 200 g/day, faecal loss of potassium is usually in the range 5 to 15 mmol/day. The potassium concentration in the stool decreases as stool volume increases, but volume can increase massively, such that substantial potassium loss and profound hypokalaemia can complicate any severe diarrhoeal illness.

Potassium loss in diarrhoeal states is usually associated with loss of bicarbonate, resulting in a coexisting metabolic acidosis, such that serum levels of potassium may not reflect the true body deficit. In this circumstance the renal excretion of potassium is broadly appropriate, and potassium deficiency is not due to a renal leak. However, in some situations potassium is lost in conjunction with chloride, resulting in a metabolic alkalosis and a picture similar to that seen with vomiting (see above).

A villous adenoma of the colon or rectum can rarely result in profound hypokalaemia. The mechanism seems to involve secretion of cyclic AMP and prostaglandin E_2 by the tumour, leading to disturbance of ion transport in the normal colonic mucosa. Treatment with non-steroidal anti-inflammatory agents can significantly reduce stool volume and help to correct both volume depletion and hypokalaemia. Similar disturbances probably underlie the hypokalaemia of patients with the watery diarrhoea, hypokalaemia, and achlorhydria (WDHA) syndrome, caused by excess vasoactive polypeptide (VIP) secreted by certain tumours. In addition to treatment directed at the tumour itself, somatostatin or somatostatin analogues are effective in controlling symptoms.

Ureteric diversion Diversion of the ureters into the colon (ureterosigmoidostomy) is most commonly performed in children for the treatement of bladder exstrophy, but occasionally for other reasons. If urine remains in contact with the colonic mucosa for a long time there is a tendency for the colon to reabsorb urinary ammonium and secrete bicarbonate, leading to hyperchloraemic acidosis, and also for stimulation of colonic potassium secretion, resulting in hypokalaemia. These can have serious consequences: profound acidosis can occur with concurrent illness, and chronic renal failure can develop. Close metabolic monitoring of patients with ureterosigmoidostomies is essential, and substantial metabolic disturbance is an indication for revision of the procedure, which is performed less frequently following improvement in surgical techniques for ileal conduits and alternative urinary diversions.

Diagnosing the cause of hypokalaemia in difficult cases

The diagnosis of the cause of hypokalaemia is usually straightforward and explained by diuretic therapy or gastrointestinal fluid loss, as described above. In other patients the abnormality is mild, with the occasional serum potassium concentration measured at just below the lower limit of the normal range, such that extensive investigation is almost certainly inappropriate (and likely to be fruitless if pursued). However, some patients present with unexplained severe hypokalaemia, and these represent a considerable challenge for both diagnosis and management. The differential diagnosis in these cases usually lies between concealed ingestion of diuretics, concealed vomiting and/or usage of purgatives, and various abnormalities of tubular potassium transport.

It is important to ask directly for a history of vomiting or diarrhoea, and about present or past use of any medications, particularly diuretics or purgatives. It is also worthwhile to ask about consumption of liquorice or chewing tobacco (see below). Examination is likely to be unremarkable in cases of unexplained hypokalaemia, but pay particular attention to body weight/height/body mass index, and to any other features that might support the diagnosis of an eating disorder such as anorexia nervosa or bulimia nervosa (see Chapter 26.5.5).

One study reported the findings of extensive investigation of 27 adult patients (17 women) who presented with chronic hypokalaemia (serum potassium concentration less than 3.4 mmol/l) that was sustained for over 5 years and which had previously eluded diagnosis. The following diagnoses were established: diuretic abuse (in five patients), surreptitious vomiting (eight), laxative abuse (one), renal tubular acidosis (one), and Gitelman's syndrome (12). Medical work-up that had sought to make the diagnoses by measurement of plasma renin activity, plasma aldosterone concentration, and urinary potassium concentration failed to discriminate between these conditions. Investigations that were diagnostically helpful are given in Table 4, the most useful being the plasma pH and chloride concentration, urinary chloride concentration and screen for diuretics, and (in one case) stool weight.

The finding of a low plasma chloride concentration with the virtual absence of chloride from the urine supports the diagnosis of surreptitious vomiting. Screening the urine for diuretics is appropriate if the urinary chloride concentration is above 20 mmol/l, and if no diuretics are found in samples with a chloride concentration of above 50 mmol/l then Gitelman's syndrome is likely. Vomiting, diuretics, and Gitelman's syndrome all cause alkalosis, whereas laxative abuse is associated with acidosis, as is renal tubular acidosis. The diagnosis of renal tubular acidosis can be established by demonstrating an inability to produce acid urine in the presence of systemic acidosis (see Section 20.8 for further discussion).

The management of cases of surreptitious vomiting, or diuretic or purgative abuse is difficult. Many patients will fulfil diagnostic criteria for anorexia nervosa or bulimia nervosa, and issues other than those simply and directly related to potassium homeostasis will clearly need to be considered. The physician may well need to seek expert psychiatric help. See Chapter 26.5.3 for further discussion.

Rare causes of hypokalaemia

Altered external potassium balance

Mineralocorticoid excess

Hypokalaemia can be caused by a large number of causes of mineralocorticoid excess, as shown in Table 3. Primary aldosteronism is discussed in Chapters 12.7.1 and 15.16.2.3, congenital adrenal hyperplasia in Chapter 12.7.2, and glucocorticoid-remediable aldosteronism in Chapter 15.16.1.2.

Table 4 Diagnostic clues in 26 cases of hypokalaemia that were hard to diagnose

Diagnosis		Diuretic consumption	Vomiting	Laxative consumption	Gitelman's syndrome
Number of cases		5	8	1	12
Plasma	*Normal range*				
Chloride	97–108 mmol/l	Low normal or low	Low	Low	Low normal or low
Bicarbonate	22–28 mmol/l	High normal or high	High	Low	High normal or high
Magnesium	0.8–1.1 mmol/l	NR	NR	NR	Low
Urinary					
Sodium	40–130 mmol/l	Normal	Normal	Low	High normal or high
Potassium	30–110 mmol/l	Normal	Normal	Normal	Normal
Chloride	30–120 mmol/l	Normal	Very low, (less than 10 mmol/l)	Low	High
Calcium	2.5–8.0 mmol per 24 h	NR	NR	NR	Low
Magnesium	2.5–7.5 mmol/l	NR	NR	NR	High
Diuretic screen		Positive	Negative	Negative	Negative
Stool					
Weight	100–200 g/day	Normal	Normal	High	Normal

From Gladziwa *et al.* (1995) *Nephrology, Dialysis, Transplantation* **10**, 1607.
NR, not reported.

Hypokalaemia is rarely a prominent feature of the other conditions of mineralocorticoid excess listed, which are discussed elsewhere in this book.

Apparent mineralocorticoid excess

Activating mutations in the β- or γ-subunits of the epithelial sodium channel in the collecting duct causes Liddle's syndrome. Disabling mutations in the type 2 11β-hydroxysteroid dehydrogenase gene cause a deficiency of the enzyme, allowing cortisol access to the mineralocorticoid receptor and the syndrome of apparent mineralocorticoid excess. Acquired inhibition of the action of 11β-hydroxysteroid dehydrogenase can be caused by liquorice, carbenoxolone, and chewing tobacco. Hypokalaemia with low plasma concentrations of renin and aldosterone are features of all of these conditions, which are discussed in Chapter 15.16.1.2.

Renal transport abnormalities

Patients with renal tubular acidosis type I are prone to hypokalaemia, as discussed in Chapter 20.8.

In 1962 Bartter described 'hyperplasia of the juxtaglomerular complex with hyperaldosteronism and hypokalemic alkalosis: a new syndrome'. Well over a hundred papers were subsequently written to describe features of what was believed to be the same eponymously named condition. The picture became immensely confused, but since 1995 has been clarified by the recognition of distinct phenotypes within the group of patients previously thought to have 'Bartter's syndrome' and the application of powerful molecular genetic methods to their study. These have revealed that most patients previously thought to have Bartter's syndrome do not have this condition, but have Gitelman's syndrome instead.

Bartter's syndrome This is now classified into three types: each is an autosomal recessive disorder caused by mutation of an ion transporter or ion channel that is present in cells of the thick ascending limb of the nephron (Fig. 1).

Bartter's syndrome type I: NKCC2 mutations This was originally described in six consanguineous families. Affected individuals were born prematurely after pregnancies complicated by polyhydramnios and developed severe dehydration in the first few days of life. All affected individuals had severe hypercalciuria in addition to hypokalaemic alkalosis, and most had nephrocalcinosis. In all cases disease was associated with destructive mutations in the gene encoding the Na-K-2Cl cotransporter (NKCC2), which is localized to chromosome 15. Other clinical manifestations can include short stature, mental retardation, rickets, generalized weakness, and muscle cramps. Other reported abnormalities on investigation can include hyperreninism, hyperaldosteronism, increased renal prostaglandin production, erythrocytosis, a platelet aggregation defect, impaired vascular responses to angiotensin II, and hypertrophy or hyperplasia of the juxtaglomerular apparatus. Management is supportive: dehydration must be avoided and potassium supplementation is needed; non-steroidal anti-inflammatory agents may be helpful (although they tend to be more useful in type II disease). There is a high mortality rate before diagnosis, with infants often dying due to volume depletion caused by intercurrent illness, but the prognosis in cases where the diagnosis is made and where care is taken to avoid volume depletion is not known.

Bartter's syndrome type II: ROMK mutations Abnormality of the *NKCC2* gene product was excluded in five families where individuals also presented with severe neonatal dehydration, hypercalciuria, and nephrocalcinosis. The only clinical distinction from Bartter's syndrome type I was that patients often had a transient initial hyperkalaemia, with serum potassium falling rapidly into the hypokalaemic range as soon as they were rehydrated. An obvious explanation was mutation in another gene or genes whose

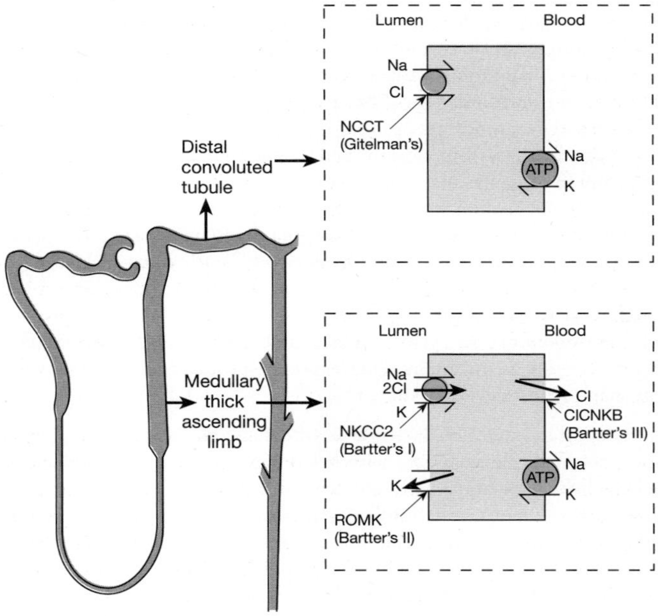

Fig. 1 Some genetic disorders of the renal tubule that cause hypokalaemia. NCCT, Na-Cl cotransporter; NKCC2, Na-K-2Cl cotransporter; ROMK, ATP-regulated potassium channel; CLCNKB, kidney-specific chloride channel.

product interacted with NKCC2 in some way. In 1993 and 1994 a renal potassium channel had been cloned from rat and humans, and this apical ATP-sensitive potassium channel (ROMK) that recycles potassium back into the lumen and is critical for continued activity of the NKCC2 cotransporter was an obvious candidate. Functionally significant mutations of *ROMK* (also known as KCNJ1) were identified in all affected individuals. Management and prognosis is as for Bartter's syndrome type I.

Bartter's syndrome type III: CLCNKB mutations To determine whether mutation of other genes could account for the Bartter's phenotype a large number of patients with inherited hypokalaemic alkalosis, normomagnesaemia, and normocalciuria or hypercalciuria were studied. Most (those in 44 of 66 families) did not have mutations in *NKCC2* or *ROMK*. In 1994 two highly homologous renal chloride channels were cloned, *CLCNKA* and *CLCNKB*, and the latter was shown to be the cause of the Bartter's syndrome in a number of the families. The clinical picture was more varied than that for types I or II Bartter's syndrome, ranging in severity from near fatal volume depletion with hypokalaemic alkalosis and respiratory arrest to mild disease presenting in a teenager with polyuria and weakness. None of the patients had nephrocalcinosis, distinguishing them phenotypically from those with *NKCC2* or *ROMK* mutations. Management is with potassium supplementation and care to avoid dehydration. Long-term prognosis is uncertain.

Gitelman's syndrome Gitelman's syndrome is the commonest genetic cause of hypokalaemia. If it presents clinically, it typically does so in early adulthood with hypotension, alkalosis, and salt wasting, along with hypomagnesaemia, hypocalciuria, and hypermagnesuria (see Table 4). The marked similarity between this picture and that induced by thiazide diuretics, which are potent inhibitors of the Na-Cl cotransporter (NCCT) in the distal convoluted tubule of the nephron, led to a candidate gene approach to the condition as soon as the thiazide-sensitive NCCT gene had been cloned. Mutations in the *NCCT* gene are responsible for Gitelman's syndrome (Fig. 1), which is an autosomal recessive condition.

Since there are no dramatic clinical symptoms or signs, suspicion of the diagnosis of Gitelman's syndrome often arises only when hypokalaemia is found (or in screening of family members of a known case). However, in one recent study it was clearly shown that patients with Gitelman's syndrome are significantly more symptomatic than controls, reporting salt craving, musculoskeletal symptoms (cramps, muscle weakness, and aches), constitutional symptoms (fatigue, generalized weakness, and dizziness), nocturia, and polydipsia. Forty-five per cent of patients considered their symptoms to be a moderate problem or worse.

Management is with potassium and magnesium supplements, it being important to recognize that in the face of magnesium depletion the kidney cannot retain potassium, but these are often poorly tolerated. Diuretics that block sodium reabsorption in the collecting duct (spironolactone, triamterene, and amiloride) can reduce urinary potassium excretion and raise the serum potassium concentration, but they often need to be accompanied by salt-loading to prevent volume depletion and hypotension. Non-steroidal anti-inflammatory agents can sometimes be helpful, but their mechanism of action is uncertain. The long-term prognosis of patients with Gitelman's syndrome is not known.

Heterozygote carriers of Bartter's or Gitelman's mutations The phenotypes that might be associated with heterozygote carriage of the Bartter's and Gitelman's mutations have not been well characterized. Heterozygote carriers of Gitelman's mutations have increased urinary sodium excretion (due to a self-selected higher salt intake), modestly lowered blood pressure (in childhood if not in adulthood), a serum potassium concentration towards the lower limit of the normal range, and increased susceptibility to hypokalaemia induced by diuretics. Similar features would be anticipated in Bartter's heterozygotes. Carriers of Gitelman's mutations have increased bone density; carriers of Bartter's may have a predisposition to osteoporosis or nephrolithiasis caused by hypercalciuria.

Abnormal internal potassium balance

Although there are many causes of hypokalaemia (Table 3), there are relatively few causes of hypokalaemia associated with extreme weakness, the commonest explanation for this rare presentation being hypokalaemic periodic paralysis. In Western countries most cases of hypokalaemic periodic paralysis are familial, termed familial periodic paralysis, whereas in Asian populations the commonest cause is thyrotoxic periodic paralysis. In all forms of hypokalaemic periodic paralysis the hypokalaemia and paralysis result from an acute shift of potassium into cells, the mechanism for which is unknown, although there is speculation that it is due to a transient hyperadrenergic state.

One study reviewed the medical records of 97 patients who presented over a 10-year period to hospital in Taiwan with severe hypokalaemia (plasma potassium less than 3.0 mmol/l, mean 2.2 mmol/l) and acute loss of muscle strength with inability to walk. The final diagnoses established are shown in Table 5.

Treatment of acute attacks of hypokalaemic periodic paralysis traditionally involves the administration of intravenous potassium, some patients recovering with as little as 20 mmol, but others requiring over 200 mmol. In all types of this condition a paradoxical fall in serum potassium concentration can occur at the start of treatment, and rebound hyperkalaemia is also seen.

Thyrotoxic periodic paralysis

The diagnosis of thyrotoxic periodic paralysis is established if hyperthyroidism is present when hypokalaemic paralysis occurs. About 50 per cent of patients give a history of thyrotoxic symptoms, but there is no family history of paralysis. Attacks are often provoked by a large carbohydrate meal (perhaps via the mechanism of an exaggerated response to insulin) or adrenergic stress. Physical findings during an attack include tachycardia (a useful diagnostic discriminator from sporadic periodic paralysis) and high blood pressure; signs of hyperthyroidism are absent in 20 to 40 per cent of cases. In 39 patients reported from Taiwan the mean serum T_3 concentration was 4.5 nmol/l (range 2.3 to 8.4, upper limit of normal being 3.0), the

Table 5 Final diagnoses established in 97 patients initially diagnosed as having hypokalaemic periodic paralysis

	No.	Mean age (years)	Male: female
Patients with hypokalaemic periodic paralysis			
Thyrotoxic periodic paralysis	39	28	39:0
Sporadic periodic paralysis	29	26	23:6
Hypernatraemic hypokalaemic periodic paralysis*	3	18	3:0
Familial periodic paralysis	2	16	2:0
Patients who did not have hypokalaemic periodic paralysis			
Metabolic alkalosis			
Primary aldosteronism	6	39	2:4
Bartter's or Gitelman's syndromes	6	21	4:2
Diuretics	3	40	0:3
Hyperchloraemic acidosis			
Distal renal tubular acidosis	6	47	3:3
Toluene abuse	3	28	1:2

From Lin *et al.* (2001). *Quarterly Journal of Medicine* **94**, 133–9.

*Mean plasma sodium concentration was 167 mmol/l. Two patients had brain tumours and one patient had hypothalamic involvement with tuberculosis. It is possible that diabetes insipidus was the explanation for their presentation and there is insufficient evidence in the paper to justify the naming of a new syndrome.

Patients with hypokalaemic periodic paralysis do not have an acid–base disorder: arterial pH, P_{CO_2}, and bicarbonate are all within the normal range. A key finding is that the urinary potassium concentration is low (mean 8 mmol/l). There is also a low transtubular potassium concentration gradient (TTKG = [urine K/plasma K]/[urine osmolality/plasma osmolality] of < 3: the normal renal response to hypokalaemia of non-renal origin being a TTKG < 2, whereas a renal cause of hypokalaemia is usually associated with TTKG > 5).

mean serum T_4 concentration was 201 nmol/l (range 154 to 299, upper limit of normal 154), and the mean thyroid-stimulating hormone was less than 0.06 mU/l (range less than 0.06 to 0.32; normal 0.5 to 5.0). Hypophosphataemia and hypomagnesaemia are also found, the latter also being low in patients with Gitelman's syndrome.

Although treatment of thyrotoxic periodic paralysis conventionally involves administration of potassium, recent experience suggests that patients with this condition respond rapidly to the β-blocker propanolol (3 mg/kg, given orally). This, rather than potassium, is now the preferred first-line treatment, with the expectation that serum potassium concentration will return to normal and paralysis will resolve within 2 h.

Sporadic periodic paralysis

The cause of sporadic periodic paralysis is not known: patients do not have a family history of hypokalaemic periodic paralysis and do not have hyperthyroidism. There are no obvious precipitating factors. Heart rate at presentation is lower than for those with thyrotoxic periodic paralysis (mean 76 compared with 105 beats/min). Emergency treatment is with intravenous potassium. Propanolol is ineffective. Oral potassium chloride supplements or acetazolamide are used to prevent recurrent attacks. The mechanism of action of acetazolamide is uncertain, but it has been reported in an animal model that it causes activation of the sarcolemmal calcium-activated potassium channel.

Familial hypokalaemic periodic paralysis

The diagnosis is established by finding a family history of attacks of flaccid weakness and hypokalaemia. These can be precipitated by administration of insulin or glucose and aborted by exercise, which induces an exaggerated rise in serum potassium concentration, or by administration of potassium.

Familial hypokalaemic periodic paralysis can be caused by mutations in three genes. First, the *CACNL1A3* gene, which encodes a dihydropyridine receptor that functions as a voltage-gated calcium channel and is also critical for excitation–contraction coupling in a voltage-sensitive and calcium-independent manner. Second, the *SCN4A* gene that encodes for a sodium channel and is also the site of mutations causing hyperkalaemic periodic paralysis. Third, the *KCNE3* gene, which encodes a potassium channel. The conditions are autosomal dominant, with 100 per cent penetrance in males, but much less in females.

Treatment is as for sporadic periodic paralysis. Acetazolamide usually prevents recurrent attacks, but one family has been reported where this made the condition worse (a beneficial response to triamterene was observed).

Sudden unexplained death syndrome

Between 1982 and 1990 there were a total of 235 cases of sudden unexplained death syndrome (**SUDS**) in apparently healthy male Thai migrant workers in Singapore. SUDS, known locally as *laitai*, is a leading cause of death in young men in rural north-eastern Thailand, where one study reported an annual incidence of 38 per 100 000 men aged 20 to 49 years. It is also reported elsewhere in Asia. Women are rarely, if ever, affected. Death occurs at rest and is nocturnal in most (84 per cent) cases. There is a family history of SUDS more often than would be expected by chance. In cases that are observed, witnesses often report that death is preceded by a few minutes of groaning, choking, coughing, and muscular spasticity or paralysis.

The cause of SUDS is not known; hypotheses include stress, genetic factors, dietary deficiency (perhaps of thiamine), potassium deficiency, melioidosis, and sleep disorders. With regard to potassium, survivors of SUDS-like attacks and relatives of victims of SUDS have been reported to have significantly lower activity of erythrocyte Na^+,K^+-ATPase and lower plasma potassium concentration than controls, but the reason for and significance of these findings is not certain.

Hyperkalaemia

Clinical features and treatment of hyperkalaemia

Hyperkalaemia is the most serious of all electrolyte disorders, despite being relatively infrequent, because it typically produces no recognizable symptoms before causing cardiac arrest. Some patients report muscular symptoms such as weakness, stiffness, or simply a 'funny feeling', but the significance of these is rarely appreciated. A high serum potassium concentration leads to membrane depolarization in excitable tissues, making the initation of an action potential more likely, and to increased membrane potassium conductance, which impairs recovery after an action potential. The effect is to cause electrical instability with the risk of life-threatening arrhythmia. The likelihood of such an event increases as the serum potassium concentration rises, but some patients are more resistant to the cardiac effects of hyperkalaemia than others: for instance, those with endstage renal failure on long-term dialysis may be habitually hyperkalaemic (although this is not to be encouraged) and tolerate a plasma potassium concentration that would kill a normal person if imposed acutely.

The best guide to the significance of hyperkalaemia in any particular individual is the impact that it is having on the ECG, and an ECG should be obtained immediately in any patient in whom the question of hyperkalaemia arises. The earliest change is tenting of the T wave, progressing as the plasma potassium concentration rises to P-wave flattening, prolongation of the P–R internal, widening of the QRS complex, and eventually a 'sine wave' pattern as a prelude to ventricular fibrillation and death. All involved in the care of acutely ill patients must be able to recognize this pattern of ECG changes and give effective emergency treatment for severe hyperkalaemia, as described in Chapter 20.5.

Causes of hyperkalaemia

There are many causes of a high serum potassium concentration (Table 6), but a survey of over 400 cases found that renal failure was present in 43 per cent and potassium supplements or potassium-sparing diuretics had been taken by 37 per cent. Life-threatening hyperkalaemia is almost exclusively seen in those with renal failure, often in conjunction with another exacerbating cause. Common scenarios would be the patient with acute renal failure who is hypercatabolic or has extensive tissue destruction, as in rhabdomyolysis, or the patient with endstage renal failure who has missed a dialysis treatment, not adhered to a low potassium diet (see Table 7), or suffered an upper gastrointestinal haemorrhage, thereby inadvertently consuming a high potassium meal.

Hyperkalaemia is not a prominent feature of many of the conditions listed in Table 6: further discussion in this chapter will be limited to disorders other than renal failure that are not discussed elsewhere in this textbook and in which hyperkalaemia is a common or important manifestation.

Pseudohyperkalaemia

Haemolysed samples show hyperkalaemia, which also occurs when there is considerable delay between venepuncture and separation of red cells and plasma or serum in the laboratory, allowing potassium to leak out of red cells after venesection. However, aside from these common and banal explanations, there are other reasons for pseudohyperkalaemia.

Potassium is released from white blood cells and platelets as blood coagulates, causing the serum potassium concentration to exceed, by a few tenths of a millimole per litre, that of plasma estimated in a parallel sample. This process is greatly exaggerated when gross leucocytosis or thrombocytosis is present, such that the serum potassium concentration can be over 2 mmol/l higher than that in plasma. The plasma and not the serum potassium concentration should obviously be measured in this circumstance.

There is also the rare syndrome of familial pseudohyperkalaemia, first described in 16 members of three generations of a kindred from Edinburgh who had elevated plasma potassium if the red cells were not separated

Table 6 Causes of hyperkalaemia

Pseudohyperkalaemia (test tube phenomena where measured potassium concentration does not reflect that in the patient's blood *in vivo*)
- Tight tourniquet with or without limb exercise
- Test tube haemolysis
- Leukaemia with very high white cell count
- Thrombocytosis

Altered internal balance (redistribution of potassium from extracellular to intracellular compartment)
- Exercise
- Acidosis (inorganic)
- Massive tissue destruction:[a]
  - Crush injuries
  - Rhabdomyolysis
  - Burns
  - Tumour lysis
- Drugs/toxins:
  - Digoxin poisoning
  - Succinylcholine
  - Arginine
  - Fluoride intoxication
  - β-Blockade
- Malignant hyperthermia
- Hyperkalaemic periodic paralysis

Altered external balance (high total body potassium)
- *Excessive ingestion*[b]
  - Consumption of high potassium foods (Table 3)
  - Potassium supplements
  - Low salt diet (high in potassium)
  - 'Salt substitutes' (contain potassium)
  - Upper gastrointestinal haemorrhage ('blood meal')
- *Impaired excretion*
  - *General impairment of renal function*
    - Acute renal failure
    - Chronic renal failure
  - *Defects that specifically impair renal potassium excretion*
    - Mineralocorticoid deficiency:
      - Renin deficiency
        - Hyporeninaemic hypoaldosteronism
          - Idiopathic
          - Drug induced
            - Non-steroidal anti-inflammatory drugs
            - Calcineurin inhibitors (tacrolimus, cyclosporin)
      - Angiotensin-converting enzyme inhibition
        - Drug induced (captopril, enalapril, etc.)
      - Angiotensin II receptor blockade
        - Drug induced (losartan, candesartan etc.)
      - Defective aldosterone production
        - Generalized adrenal failure
          - Addison's disease
        - Deficiency of aldosterone synthesis
          - Drug induced (heparin)
          - Enzyme deficiencies
          - Idiopathic
    - Impaired tubular ion transport
      - Drugs
        - Potassium-sparing diuretics[c]
        - Trimethoprim
        - Calcineurin inhibitors (cyclosporin, tacrolimus)
      - Pseudohypoaldosteronism
        - Type I
        - Type II (Gordon's syndrome)

[a]Often associated with acute renal failure.

[b]Note that it is very rare for hyperkalaemia to be caused by excessive ingestion if renal excretory mechanisms for potassium are working normally.

[c]These drugs should be avoided in patients with significant renal impairment.

Table 7 Potassium content of various foodstuffs

High potassium foods (to be avoided in those with hyperkalaemia)	Suitable low potassium alternatives
Dairy products	
Condensed/evaporated milk	Reasonable daily allowance of milk
Food drinks	Various commercial coffee whiteners
Single cream	
Meats	
Ready cooked meals in sauce	All kinds of meat
Fish	
Ready cooked fish pies, fish in sauce, etc	All kinds of fish
Fruit	
All dried fruit	Apple
Apricots	Grapefruit
Avocado pears	Kiwi fruit
Bananas	Passion fruit
Cherries	Pear
Grapes	Satsuma
Melon	Tangerine
Orange	Tinned fruit of all types—but after draining off the juice or syrup, which contains a lot of potassium
Peach	
Pineapple	
Plums	
Raspberries	
Rhubarb	
Strawberries	
Vegetables	
Artichokes	Aubergines
Bamboo shoots	Beans—French, runner
Beans—baked, butter, haricot	Cabbage
Beetroot	Carrots
Cabbage—red	Cauliflower
Corn on the cob	Celery
Mushrooms	Courgettes
Peas—chick, split	Cucumber
Potato— jacket, chips, crisps, sweet	Lettuce
	Marrow
Spinach	Onion
Tomato	Peas
Watercress	Potato—boiled in plenty of water
	Radish
	Spring greens
	Sprouts
	Swede
	Turnips
Cakes	
Any cake containing dried fruit or nuts	Doughnuts
Mince pies	Fruit pies—if fruit not high potassium
Chocolate	Jam tarts
Coffee	Meringue
Flapjack	Scones—plain
Gingerbread	Victoria sandwich—plain
Parkin	
Sweets and biscuits	
Any containing dried fruit or nuts	Barley sugar
Chocolate	Biscuits—plain
Fruit gums	Honey
Fudge	Humbugs
Liquorice	Jam
Marzipan	Marmalade
Toffee	Mints

Table 7 *Continued*

Beverages	
Cocoa	Coca-Cola
Coffee—instant	Coffee—percolated
Drinking chocolate	Fruit squashes—unless with high juice content
Fruit juices—if pure and containing any high potassium fruit	Lemonade and other fizzy drinks
Tea—instant	Soda water
	Tea—infusion
	Tonic water
Cereals	
Muesli and other cereals containing dried fruit or nuts	Bread
	Breakfast cereals—most types
	Pasta
	Rice
Other	
Salt substitutes	

This list is not exhaustive. If a patient with hyperkalaemia seems to be consuming an unusual diet, then obtain dietetic advice.

promptly. Several other families have been described, in each of which there appears to be one of a variety of abnormalities in the temperature sensitivity of the ouabain-plus-bumetanide-resistant potassium flux, which reflects the passive leak. The blood film may show a few target cells, red cell survival is shortened, but there is no frank haemolysis. Other phenotypic abnormalities have been described in some families.

Abnormal external potassium balance

Mineralocorticoid deficiency

Hyporeninaemic hypoaldosteronism It is not uncommon to find patients with chronic renal failure who have hyperkalaemia despite a glomerular filtration rate that should be sufficient to maintain normokalaemia. Two-thirds of these will have the syndrome of hyporeninaemic hypoaldosteronism, which should be suspected in any patient with hyperkalaemia without other obvious explanation. Tubulointerstitial forms of renal disease predominate in this population and diabetes mellitus is common. Hyperkalaemia is usually asymptomatic, but presentation with cardiac arrhythmia and/or muscle weakness has been described.

Characteristics of the syndrome include low levels of plasma renin activity, which are unresponsive to sodium restriction or frusemide, low plasma and urinary aldosterone, hyperkalaemia, and hyperchloraemic metabolic acidosis. Fractional potassium excretion is low for the glomerular filtration rate, and the response to kaliuretic stimuli is blunted. Glucocorticoid metabolism is normal.

The cause of both hyporeninism and hypoaldosteronism is not known. Decreased renin secretion may be the result of pathological involvement of the juxtaglomerular apparatus, but this is not obvious histologically in cases where renal biopsies have been performed. Other hypotheses include defective prostacyclin production and disordered conversion of inactive (prorenin) to active renin, which is a well-documented observation in diabetes mellitus. Chronic expansion of extracellular fluid volume has also been blamed since plasma renin activity may be increased by prolonged sodium restriction or diuretic therapy. By contrast, acute salt restriction can worsen hyperkalaemia in these patients by diminishing the distal delivery of sodium without a concurrent rise in aldosterone secretion, and illnesses causing volume depletion can precipitate presentation with dangerous hyperkalaemia. Hypoaldosteronism is probably related to the low level of plasma renin activity, but the situation is more complicated than this since most patients secrete subnormal amounts of aldosterone in response to infusion of both angiotensin II and ACTH, suggesting a defect in the function of the adrenal gland.

Criteria for establishing the diagnosis of hyporeninaemic hypoaldosteronism are not well defined, and it is uncommon for patients to be intensively investigated in routine clinical practice since treatment is usually straightforward. However, establishing the diagnosis with certainty depends on demonstrating deficient responses of renin and aldosterone to sodium depletion. One study reported plasma renin and aldosterone concentrations in subjects in an upright posture after administration of 60 mg of intravenous frusemide: the renin concentration in those with hyporeninaemic hypoaldosteronism was 6 ± 2 ng/ml per minute (compared with 34 ± 6 in controls matched for degree of renal failure) and aldosterone concentration was 7 ±2 ng/dl (compared with 28 ±2 8 in controls).

Therapy for hyporeninaemic hypoaldosteronism includes dietary potassium restriction and avoidance of drugs that can cause hyperkalaemia. Measures to increase urinary excretion of potassium, such as the use of thiazide or loop diuretics, can be useful. Cation exchange resins can be used to increase elimination of potassium from the gut, but compliance with long-term use of these medications is difficult to achieve. Although mineralocorticoid replacement (fludrocortisone, 0.2 mg/day) effectively treats the hyperkalaemia, sodium retention and worsening hypertension are often unacceptable side-effects.

Effects of drugs on the renin–angiotensin–aldosterone system

Non-steroidal anti-inflammatory agents Prostaglandin synthetase inhibitors produce hyporeninaemic hypoaldosteronism by interfering with prostacyclin-mediated renin secretion, with reduction in glomerular filtration rate and distal sodium delivery as potential contributory factors. These effects, as might be expected, become more important in the context of renal impairment: in one study approximately a quarter of patients with chronic renal failure developed hyperkalaemia after treatment with indomethacin.

Angiotensin-converting enzyme inhibitors and angiotensin II receptor blockers Angiotensin-converting enzyme (**ACE**) inhibitors and angiotensin II receptor blockers produce hyperkalaemia by impairing angiotensin II-mediated secretion of aldosterone. In one study hyperkalaemia was found in 46 of 119 (39 per cent) patients taking ACE inhibitors who were attending a renal clinic. The higher the serum creatinine concentration, the greater the chance of hyperkalaemia. Those with diabetes were also at particular risk. The treatment had to be stopped in 15 patients (13 per cent).

ACE inhibitors and spironolactone have been found to improve prognosis in heart failure, but care is needed when prescribing for those who might be prone to hyperkalaemia. One study reported life-threatening hyperkalaemia (mean serum potassium 7.7 mmol/l) in 25 patients who had received this combination of medications.

Calcineurin inhibitors Hyperkalaemia is a well-documented complication of the immunosuppressive drugs cyclosporin and tacrolimus (FK506). Two mechanisms are possible, both of which may be exacerbated by reduction in glomerular filtration rate caused by nephrotoxicity. First, drug-induced hyporeninaemic hypoaldosteronism, which is well documented with tacrolimus. Second, in association with a distal tubular acidification defect that is caused (mechanism unknown) by both cyclosporin and tacrolimus.

Heparin Hyperkalaemia occurs in about 7 per cent of patients given heparin, which is a potent inhibitor of aldosterone production. It can arise with doses as low as 10 000 units/day, but—as with most other hyperkalaemic stimuli—clinically important elevations in the plasma potassium concentration are found only when more than one homeostatic mechanism for potassium is deranged. Patients with endstage renal failure who receive unfractionated heparin to provide anticoagulation during haemodialysis treatments have a higher predialysis plasma potassium than those given low-molecular-weight heparin.

The most important mechanism of aldosterone inhibition appears to involve reduction in both numbers and affinity of angiotensin II receptors in the zona glomerulosa, which is reduced in width by prolonged use of heparin. Direct inhibition of the enzyme 18-hydroxylase has also been postulated. Production of other corticosteroids is not affected.

Renal transport abnormalities

Tubulointerstitial renal disease A few hyperkalaemic patients with chronic renal failure but a glomerular filtration rate that should be adequate for potassium homeostasis have normal levels of aldosterone and plasma renin activity and seem to have a primary defect in the ability of the distal nephron to excrete potassium. They typically have tubulointerstitial types of renal diseases, the abnormality being documented in patients with obstructive uropathy, renal transplants, sickle-cell disease, systemic lupus erythematosus, amyloidosis, and medullary sponge kidney—all of which can also be associated with hyporeninaemic hypoaldosteronism. In contrast to patients with hyporeninaemic hypoaldosteronism, their hyperkalaemia is unresponsive to mineralocorticoid replacement therapy.

Type IV renal tubular acidosis Hyperkalaemia due to impaired renal excretion of potassium may be a feature of type IV or voltage-dependent renal tubular acidosis. The lumen negative potential difference along the distal nephron normally facilitates the excretion of potassium and hydrogen ions, and hyperkalaemia and metabolic acidosis occur when this is reduced. This condition is discussed in Chapter 20.13.

Drugs Potassium-sparing diuretics are obviously likely to cause hyperkalaemia in those with any predisposition to this condition. They should not be used in those with renal failure, and the serum potassium concentration must be monitored closely in patients taking these agents who become acutely unwell.

Trimethoprim–sulphamethoxazole A review of 80 patients treated with standard-dose trimethoprim (up to 320 mg/day) and sulphamethoxazole (up to 1600 mg/day) showed that this increased the serum potassium concentration by an average of 1.2 mmol/l, whereas there was no change in a control group receiving other antibiotics. Some studies have shown a lesser effect than this, but even larger increases in serum potassium concentration have been reported in those receiving high-dose trimethoprim–sulphamethoxazole to treat pneumocystis, and hyperkalaemia is also reported with use of pentamidine. Both trimethoprim and pentamidine block the apical sodium channel in the distal nephron in a manner similar to amiloride.

Pseudohypoaldosteronism *Pseudohypoaldosteronism type 1* Autosomal recessive pseudohypoaldosteronism type 1 is caused by mutations in the α-, β-, or γ-subunits of the epithelial sodium channel (ENaC). Mutations of the mineralocorticoid receptor gene can cause an autosomal dominant form of this condition.

The recessive form typically presents in infancy with vomiting and feeding difficulty. There are signs of volume depletion and laboratory findings of hyponatraemia, hyperkalaemia, and acidaemia. The plasma renin concentration is usually increased and plasma aldosterone concentration is markedly elevated. The sodium concentration in urine, sweat, saliva, and stool is high. Treatment is with salt supplements that must usually be continued into adulthood. By contrast, the autosomal dominant form has a milder phenotype, with symptoms that remit with age.

Pseudohypoaldosteronism type 2 (Gordon's syndrome) Pseudohypoaldosteronism type 2 (Gordon's syndrome) is a rare autosomal dominant condition in which there is hyperkalaemia despite normal glomerular filtration rate, hypertension, and correction of physiological abnormalities with thiazide diuretics, which may provide effective treatment.

The condition is usually asymptomatic, detected fortuitously if serum potassium concentration is measured for any reason, or in the course of family studies, but can rarely present in late childhood or adulthood with hyperkalaemic periodic paralysis. There is a hyperchloraemic acidosis, a low level of plasma renin activity, and normal or slightly low plasma aldosterone concentration. Giving exogenous aldosterone does not increase urinary potassium excretion or reduce hyperkalaemia.

Loci have been mapped to 1q (PHA2A), 12, and 17q21 (PHA2B), but the gene(s) responsible have not been identified. Because a kaliuresis can be provoked by infusion of sodium sulphate or sodium bicarbonate, but not sodium chloride, it has been suggested that enhanced reabsorption of chloride at a distal nephron site may underlie the abnormality in potassium secretion.

Abnormal internal potassium balance

Exercise

Exercise-related rises in the plasma potassium concentration are a normal phenomenon and usually modest, but increases to 7.0 mmol/l occur during acute, maximal, physical performance and levels as high as 10.0 mmol/l have been reported with prolonged exhaustive exercise such as in marathons. Exercise-induced hyperkalaemia is accentuated by β-adrenergic blockade, α-adrenergic agonists, and in patients with chronic renal failure.

Acidosis

Acidosis diminishes potassium uptake by cells (Table 1) and causes hyperkalaemia. The increase in the plasma potassium concentration is greater with metabolic than respiratory acidosis, and occurs with hyperchloraemic but not with organic acid-induced forms of metabolic acidosis. Stimulation of insulin release by organic acids appears to account for this divergent response, explaining the pathophysiology of disturbed potassium homeostasis in diabetic ketoacidosis. At presentation, when insulin is deficient, potassium is redistributed in a fashion comparable with mineral acid-induced metabolic acidosis and patients are hyperkalaemic. However, the preceding kaliuresis (caused by polyuria) has rendered the body enormously deficient in potassium, and the plasma potassium concentration falls rapidly as soon as insulin is provided, allowing potassium to return to the cells. Indeed, dangerous hypokalaemia can develop if adequate potassium is not given during treatment.

Drugs

Several drugs can produce hyperkalaemia by altering the transcellular distribution of potassium. Digitalis preparations diminish cellular potassium uptake by inhibiting the Na^+,K^+ pump and substantial hyperkalaemia can accompany digitalis intoxication. Succinylcholine and other depolarizing muscle relaxants increase the potassium permeability of muscle: the plasma potassium concentration typically increases by 0.5 to 1.0 mmol/l, but in patients with burns or neuromuscular diseases, hyperkalaemia can be more severe. Infusion of 30 g of the cationic amino acid arginine HCl increases plasma potassium concentration by 0.5 to 1.0 mmol/l and can produce life-threatening hyperkalaemia in individuals with deranged potassium metabolism. Fluoride intoxication appears to increase the plasma potassium concentration by provoking leakage from the intracellular compartment: associated hypocalcaemia enhances the cardiac risks of fluoride-induced hyperkalaemia.

Although β_2-adrenergic stimulants cause hypokalaemia and can be used to treat hyperkalaemia (see section 20.5), the administration of β-blockers typically increases the plasma potassium concentration only modestly (by 0.1 to 0.2 mmol/l). However, the hyperkalaemic effect can be much more prominent when other potassium homeostatic mechanisms are deranged, for example in patients receiving intermittent haemodialysis, the predialysis plasma potassium concentration is increased on average by 1.0 mmol/l.

Hyperkalaemic periodic paralysis

Hyperkalaemic periodic paralysis is a rare autosomal dominant condition in which mutations in the sodium channel gene *SCN4A* are associated with episodes of flaccid generalized weakness (rather than paralysis) and elevation of the serum potassium concentration, typically into the range from 6.0 to 8.0 mmol/l. Mutations in the same gene can cause hypokalaemic periodic paralysis and paramyotonia congenita. Attacks of weakness last from minutes to hours, occurring without any obvious precipitant but sometimes following exercise or administration of potassium.

Treatment with kaliuretic diuretics (not potassium sparing) is used to prevent attacks. β_2-Agonists can be used both to prevent and abort paralytic attacks.

Myotonia of the ocular muscles and tongue is sometimes observed both between and during attacks, the former demonstrable as slow opening of the lids after forced active closure of the eyes, or as myotonic lid lag lasting 15 to 20 s after elevation of the eyes. There can be generalized muscle wasting and progressive myopathy. In some families cardiac arrhythmia, cardiac sudden death, short stature, microcephaly, and clinodactyly (typically a bent little finger) are reported.

Further reading

Brater DC (1998). Diuretic therapy. *New England Journal of Medicine* **339**, 387–95.

Cruz DN *et al.* (2001). Mutations in the Na-Cl cotransporter reduce blood pressure in humans. *Hypertension* **37**, 1458–64.

Cruz DN *et al.* (2001). Gitelman's syndrome revisited: an evaluation of symptoms and health-related quality of life. *Kidney International* **59**, 710–17.

Gennari FJ (1998). Hypokalemia. *New England Journal of Medicine* **339**, 451–8.

Gladziwa U *et al.* (1995). Chronic hypokalaemia of adults: Gitelman's syndrome is frequent but classical Bartter's syndrome is rare. *Nephrology, Dialysis, Transplantation* **10**, 1607–13.

Grier JF (1995). WDHA (watery diarrhea, hypokalemia, achlorhydria) syndrome: clinical features, diagnosis, and treatment. *Southern Medical Journal* **88**, 22–4.

Halevy J *et al.* (1988). Life-threatening hypokalemia in hospitalized patients. *Mineral and Electrolyte Metabolism* **14**, 163–6.

Hamill RJ *et al.* (1991). Efficacy and safety of potassium infusion therapy in hypokalemic critically ill patients. *Critical Care Medicine* **19**, 694–9.

Lin SH, Lin YF (2001). Propranolol rapidly reverses paralysis, hypokalemia, and hypophosphatemia in thyrotoxic periodic paralysis. *American Journal of Kidney Diseases* **37**, 620–3.

Lin SH *et al.* (2001). Hypokalaemia and paralysis. *Quarterly Journal of Medicine* **94**, 133–9.

Morgan DB, Davidson C (1980). Hypokalaemia and diuretics: an analysis of publications. *British Medical Journal* **280**, 905–8.

Nadler JL *et al.* (1986). Evidence of prostacyclin deficiency in the syndrome of hyporeninemic hypoaldosteronism. *New England Journal of Medicine* **314**, 1015–20.

Older J *et al.* (1999). Secretory villous adenomas that cause depletion syndrome. *Archives of Internal Medicine* **159**, 879–80.

Oster JR *et al.* (1995). Heparin-induced aldosterone suppression and hyperkalemia. *American Journal of Medicine* **98**, 575–86.

Paice BJ *et al.* (1986). Record linkage study of hypokalaemia in hospitalized patients. *Postgraduate Medical Journal* **62**, 187–91.

Preston RA *et al.* (1998). University of Miami Division of Clinical Pharmacology therapeutic rounds: drug-induced hyperkalemia. *American Journal of Therapeutics* **5**, 125–32.

Scheinman SJ *et al.* (1999). Genetic disorders of renal electrolyte transport. *New England Journal of Medicine* **340**, 1177–87.

Schepkens H *et al.* (2001). Life-threatening hyperkalemia during combined therapy with angiotensin-converting enzyme inhibitors and spironolactone: an analysis of 25 cases. *American Journal of Medicine* **110**, 438–41.

Simon DB, Lifton RP (1998). Ion transporter mutations in Gitelman's and Bartter's syndromes. *Current Opinion in Nephrology and Hypertension* **7**, 43–7.

Tosukhowong P *et al.* (1996). Hypokalemia, high erythrocyte Na+ and low erythrocyte Na^+,K^+-ATPase in relatives of patients dying from sudden unexplained death syndrome in north-east Thailand and in survivors from near-fatal attacks. *American Journal of Nephrology* **16**, 369–74.

Widmer P *et al.* (1995). Diuretic-related hypokalaemia: the role of diuretics, potassium supplements, glucocorticoids and β_2-adrenoceptor agonists. Results from the comprehensive hospital drug monitoring programme, Berne (CHDM). *European Journal of Clinical Pharmacology* **49**, 31–6.

Wong ML *et al.* (1992). Sudden unexplained death syndrome. A review and update. *Tropical and Geographical Medicine* **44**, S1–19.

20.3 Clinical presentation and investigation of renal disease

20.3.1 The clinical presentation of renal disease

Alex M. Davison

Introduction

Effective diagnosis has four essential requisites: an awareness of the patterns of clinical presentation; obtaining a complete history; undertaking a structured clinical examination; and formulating an appropriate investigative plan. In many instances, the clinical symptoms of renal disease are nonspecific, the underlying condition may not be suspected from the history alone, and the physical examination may be surprisingly unrevealing. It is often routine investigations, such as urine analysis or estimation of renal function, that suggest the presence of renal pathology. Clinicians therefore need to be aware of the symptoms and signs that give a clue to an underlying renal disease, and which act as a prompt for appropriate initial diagnostic investigations.

The presence of renal disease in a patient may be detected because of:

(1) presentation with a symptom or clinical sign that indicates an underlying renal disorder;

(2) the presence of a systemic disease known to involve the kidneys;

(3) a family history of inherited renal disease;

(4) the finding of asymptomatic urinary abnormalities or disordered renal function tests.

Many patients remain asymptomatic, even with advanced renal disease, hence the importance of urine analysis and the estimation of blood urea and serum creatinine in anyone suspected of having renal disease. Unlike most other organ systems, patients with renal failure may remain asymptomatic despite the loss of up to 80 per cent of excretory function. Not surprisingly they may therefore be unaware of the presence of advanced renal disease, and as a consequence find it difficult to come to terms with the severity and seriousness of their illness.

Clinical syndromes

Asymptomatic urinary abnormalities

Asymptomatic proteinuria

Urinary protein excretion can amount to 150 mg daily in normal persons, consisting of albumin, Tamm–Horsfall protein, and secretory IgA. An accurate 24-h urine collection is difficult to obtain, particularly in outpatients, and therefore it is frequently more convenient to estimate the urinary protein/creatinine ratio on a mid-morning sample of urine, a normal value would be less than 130 (as this is a ratio it is without units). Approximately half consists of low molecular weight proteins or protein fragments, with the rest being albumin.

The most common method of detecting proteinuria is by using dipstix. These paper strips are impregnated with tetrabromophenol blue which changes colour from yellow-green to blue-green in the presence of protein. This test is very observer-dependent, and it should be remembered that Bence-Jones protein will not be detected and that false-positive results can occur both in alkaline urine and in urine contaminated with antiseptics (see Section 20.4 for further discussion).

Urinary protein excretion can increase during pyrexial illnesses, with strenuous exercise, congestive cardiac failure, and hypertension. In such patients the proteinuria is commonly mild (generally less than 1.5 g daily) and resolves with remission of the underlying cause. If proteinuria is detected in these circumstances the test should be repeated once the potential cause has resolved. If persistent proteinuria is detected then further investigation to determine the nature of the underlying disease is indicated.

Microalbuminuria

'Microalbuminuria' is the term used for urinary protein excretion greater than normal but still less than that detectable by dipstix testing. The excretion of more than 30 μg/min of albumin in an overnight collection or 70 μg/min in a 24-h collection in a patient with diabetes mellitus is indicative of early diabetic nephropathy. It is, however, not specific for diabetes: microalbuminuria may also be present in hypertension, obesity, systemic lupus erythematosus, and following exercise. Specifically designed stix tests are now available for screening purposes, but these remain only semiquantitative.

Postural (orthostatic) proteinuria

In some patients it has been noted that the proteinuria is present in samples obtained during the day, but absent from samples obtained first thing in the morning after overnight recumbency. This has been termed postural or orthostatic proteinuria. It is most common in children and young adults, and, although the pathogenesis is uncertain, it most likely represents an exaggerated intraglomerular haemodynamic response to a change in posture and/or entrapment of renal veins. Urinary protein excretion in such patients rarely exceeds 1.0 g/24 h. A renal biopsy may be normal or reveal only minor abnormalities.

The long-term prognosis is excellent, hence in patients with minor proteinuria it is important to obtain an early morning sample for testing. If this is found to be negative on stix testing then a diagnosis of postural proteinuria can be made, no biopsy is necessary, and the patient can be reassured that they do not have a sinister renal problem. As the majority of patients with this condition are young adult males this diagnosis may be of value in obtaining employment or insurance.

Investigation of asymptomatic proteinuria

The Scottish Intercollegiate Guidelines Network (**SIGN**) have produced a reasonable guideline for the investigation in primary care and by non-nephrologists of adult patients with asymptomatic proteinuria (Fig. 1). Different nephrologists will take different views regarding further investigation. If there are no symptoms, blood pressure is normal, the glomerular filtration rate (**GFR**) (usually estimated from serum creatinine by the Cockcroft and Gault formula, or from a 24-h creatinine clearance) is within the normal range, and there is no clinical suspicion of a multisystem disorder, then most will adopt a 'watching brief' (reviewing in 6 months and annually thereafter if all parameters remain stable) and perform a renal biopsy only in the event of a change in one or more of these parameters. The justification for this approach is that the chances of a renal biopsy revealing a diagnosis that alters management are extremely small in this context, and that the benefit does not outweigh the risk.

Microscopic haematuria

There is no agreed definition of microscopic haematuria as all urine samples contain some red blood cells. The Scottish Intercollegiate Guideline Network (SIGN) has suggested the presence of a positive result on dipstix

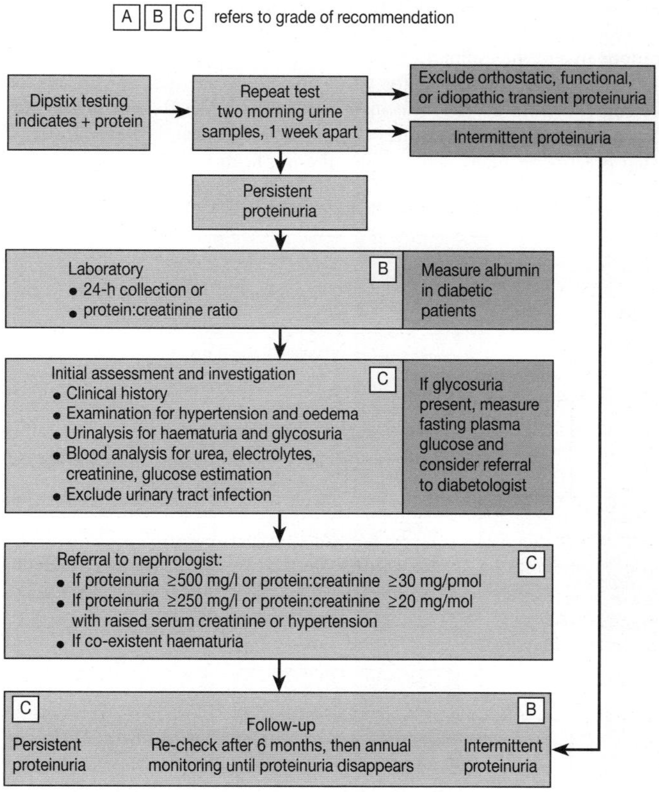

Fig. 1 Summary of the Scottish Intercollegiate Guidelines Network (SIGN) recommendations for the investigation of asymptomatic proteinuria in adults. Evidence required: A, at least one randomized controlled trial as part of the body of literature of overall good quality and consistency, addressing specific recommendations. B, availability of well-conducted clinical studies but no randomized clinical trials on the topic of recommendation. C, expert committee reports or opinions and/or clinical experiences of respected authorities. Note that these recommendations for investigation and referral are made solely on the basis that significant pathology may be detected. It is presently unproven whether there is any effect on patient outcomes. (Reproduced with kind permission from the SIGN Secretariat. Copies of the full text can be obtained from the SIGN Secretariat, Royal College of Physicians, 9 Queen Street, Edinburgh EH2 1JQ, Scotland.)

testing and/or the presence of more than five red blood cells per high-power field on urine microscopy. Asymptomatic microscopic haematuria is occult haematuria, however detected, and excludes haematuria visible to the naked eye or associated with urinary tract pain, infection, or other symptom.

Asymptomatic microscopic haematuria is most commonly detected during routine medical examinations, such as for employment or insurance purposes, in well-person clinics, and when visiting general practitioner or hospital clinics where urine samples are examined by dipstix testing. The dipstix detects the peroxidase activity of haem from its reaction with ortho-toluidine, which shows the presence of haemoglobin, whether in red cells or as 'free' haemoglobin, and myoglobin. False-positive results may be obtained from oxidizing contaminants (for example, from bacteria and from iodine or hypochlorite in antiseptic solutions). In obtaining urine samples for analysis it is important that the labia or prepuce are not first washed with any antiseptic solution. False-negative results may occur in the presence of excess ascorbic acid or the presence of rifampicin or phenolphthalein: if such substances are suspected to be present then a repeat sample should be obtained after appropriate withdrawal of these agents (see Chapter 20.4 for further discussion).

If a positive result is obtained it is important to repeat the test on a different occasion to confirm the result. Tests that are positive in women who are menstruating should be repeated between menses. In many patients stix testing for blood may be positive after exercise, particularly strenuous exercise, and a repeat sample should be obtained after 2 days without exercise. A positive result in the latter situation is probably due to the presence of myoglobinuria—urine microscopy is likely to be negative.

The further investigation of a patient found to have asymptomatic haematuria depends on a number of factors. As haematuria can arise from any part of the urinary tract from the glomerulus to the urethra, the first issue is to determine whether further investigations should be urological or nephrological. In men, particularly those over the age of 50 years, it is most likely that urological investigations will be required because of the increasing incidence of prostatic problems and urothelial malignancy, and in such patients clinical examination must include a rectal examination to determine whether any prostatic abnormality can be detected. By contrast, the presence of significant proteinuria, clinical evidence of renal disease, and/or impaired renal function indicate the need for nephrological investigation.

Urine microscopy can be of value if performed on a fresh sample. Red cell casts are diagnostic of glomerular bleeding and do not arise from bleeding anywhere else in the renal tract. Consideration of the morphology of red cells in the urine can also be useful (Fig. 2): dysmorphic red cells, in particular those appearing as a ring form with bubbles (Fig. 2(d)), are probably the consequence of glomerular bleeding, whereas red cells of normal appearance are more likely to arise from a site in the lower urinary tract. However, discrimination is not always straightforward (Fig. 2(a)), considerable interobserver variability is reported, and the technique is not robust enough to be routinely applied in most centres.

Screening for and investigation of asymptomatic microscopic haematuria

Background

Should patients or the population in general be screened for microscopic haematuria, and what should be done if they test positive and this is confirmed on repeat testing? There is no consensus.

Studies of apparently healthy populations indicate that asymptomatic microscopic haematuria has an incidence of between 2.5 and 13 per cent, the incidence increasing with age, as does the chance of finding an underlying cause. In men over the age of 50 years conditions such as transitional-cell tumours, stones, outflow obstruction, and infections are the most common explanation. However, the chance of a patient with asymptomatic microscopic haematuria detected by population screening having a serious and curable condition is small. A retrospective study using dipstix to screen 10 050 men for asymptomatic haematuria in the United Kingdom found

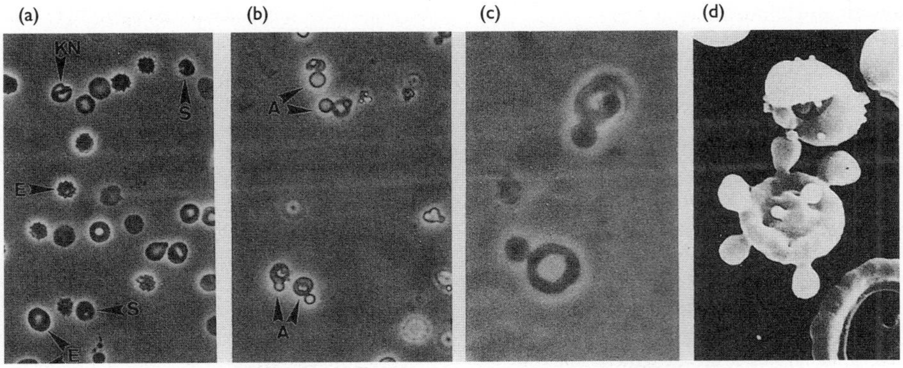

Fig. 2 Appearances of red cells in the urine. (a) phase-contrast microscopy (400 ×) showing a variety of non-specific 'dysmorphic' erythrocytes in acute interstitial nephritis. (b) phase-contrast microscopy (400 ×), (c) phase-contrast microscopy (1000 ×), and (d) scanning electron microscopy (5000 ×), all showing acanthocyturia (ring form and bubbles) in glomerulonephritis. A, acanthocyte; E, echinocyte; KN, knizocyte; S, stomatocyte. (Reproduced with permission from Kohler H, Wandel E (1993). *Nephrology, Dialysis, Transplantation* **8**, 879.)

that 2.5 per cent tested positive. Questionnaires were subsequently sent to the general practitioners of all those who were registered, asking what further investigations had been performed. In 39 per cent (59 of 152 respondents) no further investigations had been undertaken. Abnormalities of some sort were found in 28 per cent of those who had undergone some investigation. This rose to 50 per cent in the few patients (24) who were 'fully investigated' by examination of an midstream urine (**MSU**) specimen, intravenous urography, and cystoscopy: two of whom were found to have bladder cancer. Long-term follow-up of all participants in this study would clearly be of great interest, but is not available. In another study, similar screening was performed in 20 571 men (35 years or older) and women (55 years or older) who were members of a prepaid United States health plan: 867 (4.2 per cent) tested positive, of whom 278 were known to have urological disease to account for this, leaving 589 (2.9 per cent) with newly discovered asymptomatic microscopic haematuria. Over the next 3 years two of these individuals developed prostatic cancer and one bladder cancer. However, the likelihood of developing urological cancer was the same in those whose urine had tested negative for blood on screening. The sensitivity of microhaematuria detected on a single dipstix analysis for urological cancer within 3 years was 2.9 per cent, specificity was 96.7 per cent, and positive predictive value was 0.5 per cent. Multivariate analysis that adjusted for age, gender, and race showed that the relative risk of 2.1 (95 per cent confidence intervals, 0.7 to 6.6) for urological cancer was not significantly increased among patients with asymptomatic microhaematuria compared with patients who had negative test results.

The picture derived from hospital-based studies is rather different. A recent study described the outcomes in 1930 patients referred to a urological clinic because of haematuria, including 982 with microscopic haematuria. Evaluation in all cases consisted of basic demographics, history and examination, routine blood tests, urinalysis and cytology, plain abdominal radiography, renal ultrasound, intravenous urography (**IVU**), and flexible cystoscopy. Of the 982 cases of microscopic haematuria, 53 (5.4 per cent) had cancer, including three with renal and one with urothelial carcinoma.

Recommendations

The report of the American Urological Association Best Practice Policy Panel on Asymptomatic Microhematuria in Adults suggested: 'that the patient's history and physical examination should help the physician decide whether testing is appropriate', and that 'patients with asymptomatic hematuria who are at risk for urological disease or primary renal disease should undergo an appropriate evaluation. In patients at low risk for disease, some components of the evaluation may be deferred'. Risk factors for significant disease are specified as smoking history, occupational exposure to chemicals or dyes, history of gross haematuria, age >40 years, history of urological disorder or disease, history of irritative voiding symptoms, history of urinary tract infection, analgesic abuse, and a history of pelvic irradiation. For patients with any of these risk factors 'complete evaluation' is recommended, comprising upper tract imaging, urinary cytology, and cystoscopy. However, in those with none of these risk factors and thereby at low risk of urological malignancy, the report does not specify clearly which components of the evaluation may be deferred, or for how long.

The Scottish Intercollegiate Guideline Network has also produced recommendations for the investigation of adults detected as having asymptomatic microscopic haematuria (Fig. 3). These do not, however, describe usual practice in many centres, and the implications of employing them

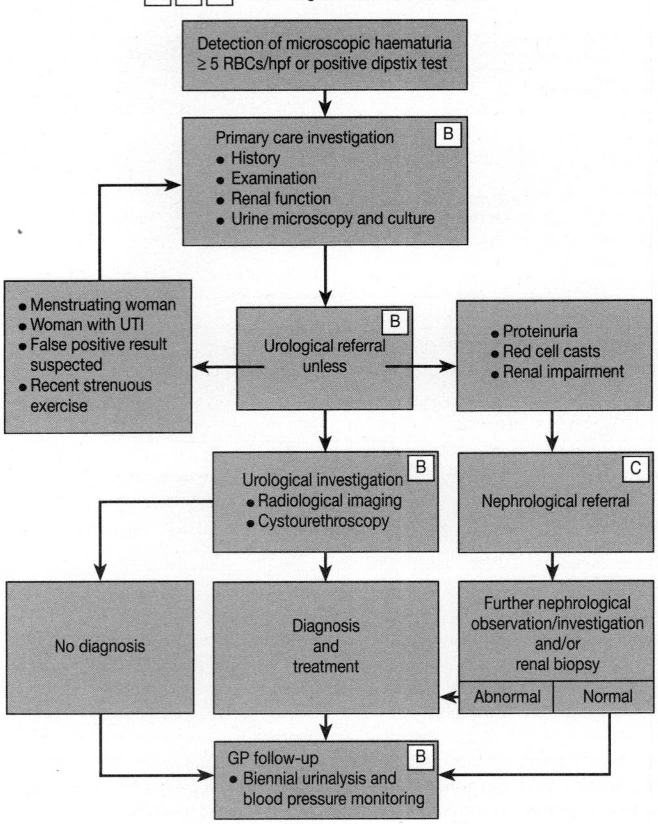

Fig. 3 Summary of the Scottish Intercollegiate Guidelines Network (SIGN) recommendations for the investigation of asymptomatic haematuria in adults. See text for further discussion and caption to Fig.1

would be considerable since they advocate radiological imaging (plain film and ultrasonography of the urinary tract, or intravenous urography) and cystourethroscopy for all those with genuine microscopic haematuria (that is to say, false and known benign positive causes excluded) who do not have clinical suspicion of renal disease. This would mean that (on the figures given above) up to 13 per cent of the population would require cystourethroscopy, which is scarcely sensible and certainly not practicable in most healthcare systems. Given the epidemiology of urothelial malignancy, all would recommend such investigation in patients over the age of 50 years with asymptomatic microscopic haematuria. Some would advocate cystourethroscopy in those over the age of 45, or sometimes 40 years, but many renal physicians and urologists would not do so in their routine practice in those under this age. However, all have seen unfortunate cases of urothelial malignancy in young patients, and prudent instruction to all with microscopic haematuria is that they should report any new symptoms, in particular macroscopic haematuria, immediately. It is also worth noting that knowledge of the length of time for which microscopic haematuria is or has been present is very helpful: malignancies declare themselves eventually, and the patient who is documented retrospectively or prospectively to have microscopic haematuria for more than a few years can almost invariably be reassured with confidence that they do not have urinary tract malignancy.

Symptomatic presentations

Nephrotic syndrome

The nephrotic syndrome is a common mode of presentation of glomerular disease. It is not a diagnosis but rather a term used to describe a clinical syndrome that arises when the urinary protein excretion is sufficient to produce hypoproteinaemic oedema. The correlation between urinary protein excretion, plasma albumin concentration, and the presence of oedema is poor. In adults it is uncommon to develop oedema unless the plasma albumin is less than 30 g/l, but many patients will remain oedema-free with a plasma protein of less than 25 g/l. Similarly, the degree of proteinuria needed to cause hypoprotinaemia is variable: some quote a urinary protein excretion of 3.5 g/day as being 'nephrotic', but it is best to avoid a particular value as some patients develop oedema with an excretion of less than 3.5 g/day, whereas others will excrete greater amounts and remain oedema-free.

Clinically, the presentation is with peripheral oedema. In adults this is commonly of the lower limbs and tends to be progressive throughout the day, in children facial oedema is more common. Ascites and pleural effusions may be present in severe cases. Some patients may mention that they have noticed their urine becoming frothy. Commonly, patients complain of an inexplicable tiredness and lethargy: the cause for which is unknown. Other clinical features include anorexia, muscle wasting, susceptibility to infections, and nail changes (with prolonged severe nephrotic syndrome the nails become white). These latter symptoms and signs are uncommon: they are a feature of prolonged protein loss and the majority of patients present for investigation before they develop. Hypertension and impairment of renal function, if present, will, to a large extent, depend on the underlying cause of the syndrome.

Pathophysiology

Mechanisms of proteinuria

The mechanisms whereby the filtration of protein by the glomerular capillary wall is restricted is poorly understood. The barrier consists of an inner endothelial cell, presenting little in the way of restriction to filtration, a basement membrane consisting of matrix proteins arranged in a complex three-dimensional pattern that allows the passage of small molecules by convection and of larger molecules by diffusion, and an outer cellular layer of epithelial cells producing a complex barrier to filtration. There is also a charge on the surface of the basement membrane due to the presence of negatively charged heparan sulphate that allows the penetration of cationic molecules to the basement membrane but repels anionic (negatively charged) molecules. In addition, the podocytes of the epithelial cells play an important role in controlling glomerular filtration: these adhere to the outer surface of the basement membrane, there being a complex interaction between the podocyte and the basement membrane in maintaining glomerular wall integrity. In patients with proteinuria there is frequently flattening and detachment of the podocyte of the epithelial cell from the basement membrane. The pathogenesis of this is unknown. Proteinuria most likely results from a combination of disruption of the charge barrier, an alteration in the spatial configuration of the basement membrane, and disruption of the normal podocyte–basement membrane interaction. A greater understanding of this may lead to improved methods of controlling proteinuria. (See Chapter 20.1 for further discussion.)

Oedema formation

The mechanisms of oedema formation in the nephrotic syndrome are complex. Initially the loss of protein in the urine will stimulate an increased production of proteins by the liver, but if the proteinuria is sufficient the loss will exceed the capacity to replace them and so the plasma protein concentration will decline. The diminution in plasma protein concentration reduces the plasma oncotic pressure and, as a result, there is accumulation of fluid in the extravascular space, resulting in oedema. Traditional teaching proposes that this is accompanied by a reduction in the intravascular volume and, as a consequence, there is reduced renal perfusion. This results in enhanced renin secretion, and thus through the renin–angiotensin–aldosterone system there is increased sodium retention by the distal tubule. The reduced intravascular volume also stimulates ADH secretion, the net result of these effects being an avid retention of salt and water, which because of the continuing low oncotic pressure increases oedema formation. This proposed mechanism is attractive but does not adequately explain the clinical findings. In the majority of patients with the nephrotic syndrome the plasma volume is not diminished, and in some it is even expanded. In addition, in many patients with the nephrotic syndrome there does not appear to be increased plasma renin, and, furthermore, blocking of the renin–angiotensin system with angiotensin-converting enzyme (**ACE**) inhibitors is not accompanied by a diuresis. It is possible that the retention of sodium and water is due to an intrarenal mechanism involving proximal and distal tubular function, in addition to physical factors such as peritubular oncotic pressure. Hence, oedema formation does not appear to have a uniform mechanism and it is more than likely that it results from a complex of effects within the kidney, the intravascular volume, and possibly the peripheral capillary integrity.

Investigation of patients with the nephrotic syndrome

The presence of the nephrotic syndrome indicates that the patient has at least one of a wide range of glomerular pathologies, which may reflect primary or secondary renal disease. The different conditions have very variable prognoses and responses to treatment, hence making a precise diagnosis is essential to guide management. Aside from the estimation of GFR (usually estimated from serum creatinine by the Cockcroft and Gault formula, or from a 24-h creatinine clearance), quantitation of proteinuria, and measurement of serum albumin, the routine investigation of all patients with the nephrotic syndrome should include a full blood count, tests for systemic lupus erythematosus (**SLE**) (antinuclear antibody tests, anti-double-stranded DNA (-**dsDNA**), estimation of serum complement, hepatitis B and hepatitis C serology, serum immunoglobulins, and protein electrophoresis. Further serological tests may be indicated in some cases. Given the association of membranous glomerulonephritis with malignancy (see Chapter 20.7.9), older patients with the nephrotic syndrome should undergo chest radiography, and there should be a low threshold for the investigation of gastrointestinal symptoms. However, a precise diagnosis of most cases of the nephrotic syndrome can only be made histologically, and renal biopsy should be performed after checking platelets and a coagulation screen, and imaging—usually by ultrasonography—to confirm the presence of two anatomically normal kidneys. Such extensive investigation is not required when a confident diagnosis of the cause of the nephrotic syndrome can be made on clinical grounds, for example in the patient with diabetes and long-standing proteinuria who becomes nephrotic.

Treatment of patients with the nephrotic syndrome

Specific causes of the nephrotic syndrome may require specific treatments: these are discussed in the relevant subsections of Section 20.7, but some general measures are applicable to all nephrotic patients.

Patients with the nephrotic syndrome may feel generally 'washed out' and exhausted, and they may suffer psychologically from uncertainties and fears surrounding their diagnosis and prognosis, but the main concern in all cases is likely to be oedema. This can be massive: over 10 litres of excess fluid is not infrequent, and some have over 20 litres, when the patient is bed-bound with massively swollen and weeping legs, distressing genital oedema, and pitting of the abdominal and sometimes the chest wall.

Patients with the nephrotic syndrome are unable to excrete salt or water normally, hence it is prudent to recommend moderation in the consumption of both. Strict limitation of salt intake renders the diet unpalatable, but patients should be advised not to add salt to food at the table and to avoid foods that are rich in salt. It seems reasonable to suggest a total fluid intake of no more than 1.5 litres per day for those who are very oedematous, and perhaps no more than 1 litre per day in the most severe cases. The mouth can be kept moist using swabs or by sucking boiled sweets, and the daily fluid ration will go much further if the patient is given an ice cube to suck rather than a jug of water if they feel thirsty.

Diuretics are the mainstay of oedema removal, with loop diuretics often the only effective agents. The aim should be to reduce the patient's weight by 0.5 to 1 kg daily. Oral frusemide (furosemide), 40 to 80 mg daily (or other loop diuretic), would be the usual starting dose, but some patients require much higher doses, with up to 250 mg twice daily not uncommon. If oral frusemide proves ineffective, then the addition of oral spironolactone (usually 100 to 200 mg daily, with particularly close monitoring of the serum potassium level) or oral metolazone (usually 2.5 to 20 mg daily, with close monitoring to ensure that it is stopped promptly in the event of massive diuresis) can be helpful. If these fail then admission to hospital for bed rest and intravenous diuretic (usually frusemide 250 to 500 mg) is required, and some would also give daily intravenous infusions of concentrated albumin. There is little evidence that the latter is effective in adult practice, but there is theoretical justification in giving it to those who appear to have intravascular volume depletion (postural hypotension, low jugular venous pressure), and it is reasonable to give it (for example, human albumin solution 20 per cent, 100 ml daily) as a therapeutic trial for a few days to all with severe refractory nephrotic oedema. However, many studies would suggest that the likely effect is simply an increased proteinuria, and if this is indeed the case and no benefit in terms of diuresis/weight loss is seen, then albumin infusion should be abandoned. It is interesting to note that when nephrotic oedema has been removed the patient is often able to sustain a new steady state with a much reduced burden of oedema, with no change in serum albumin or proteinuria.

A number of agents, including ACE inhibitors, non-steroidal anti-inflammatory agents, and ciclosporin, can reduce proteinuria at the expense of some reduction in the glomerular filtration rate. These drugs, most commonly ACE inhibitors, are sometimes used for this purpose (after deliberately inducing volume depletion with diuretics) in managing patients with severe nephrotic syndrome when the difficult judgement has been made that the benefits of reducing proteinuria (and hopefully thereby oedema) more than outweigh the disadvantage of reducing the GFR. This is a step that should never be taken lightly: the reduction in GFR may induce endstage renal failure (so-called 'medical nephrectomy'), and whilst renal replacement therapy may be preferable to intractable massive oedema, this possibility clearly needs to be thoroughly discussed with the patient beforehand.

There is considerable debate about the protein intake that should be recommended for those with the nephrotic syndrome: protein restriction diminishes proteinuria and a high protein diet increases it, but the impact on oedema or long-term prognosis of either manoeuvre is unknown. It is probably reasonable to suggest that patients with the nephrotic syndrome should consume about 1 g/kg per day of mainly first-class protein.

The management of specific complications of the nephrotic syndrome such as infection, thromboembolism, and hyperlipidaemia are discussed below.

Complications of the nephrotic syndrome

A number of complications are recognized in patients with the nephrotic syndrome: these result from the metabolic consequences of prolonged protein loss.

Infections

The incidence of infections, particularly bacterial, is increased in the nephrotic syndrome. Peritonitis is well recognized in children and is an important cause of mortality. Cellulitis, particularly streptococcal, is common and may spread rapidly. The cause of the increased susceptibility to infections is a combination of physical factors such as the accumulation of fluid in the interstitial space, the peritoneal and/or pleural space, and the impairment of defence mechanisms, such as the reduction in immunoglobulin concentration and impaired white cell function. Impairment of the alternative pathway of complement activation through loss in the urine of Factor B, which has a molecular weight of only 55 kDa, is crucial in causing impairment of the phagocytosis of encapsulated organisms. This leads in childhood to the particular vulnerability to *Streptococcus pneumoniae* described above: most adults are protected by virtue of having acquired antibodies against a variety of pneumococcal capsular antigens.

Prompt induction of remission of oedema and proteinuria is the best method of preventing infection. When this cannot be achieved, good skin care is important, and there is a good case for using prophylactic penicillin to prevent pneumococcal infection in oedematous children. Antipneumococcal vaccines against capsular antigens induce an adequate response when given to patients in remission. Any suspicion of infection should be treated aggressively in those with the nephrotic syndrome, with a low threshold for starting a parenteral antibiotic regimen, including benzylpenicillin in children, as soon as necessary cultures have been taken.

Thromboembolism

There is an increase in both arterial and venous thromboses in patients with the nephrotic syndrome, which may be aggravated by the use of excessive diuretic therapy and corticosteroids. There is an increase in the plasma concentration of a number of factors involved in the coagulation cascade, notably fibrinogen, and in addition plasminogen concentration is commonly reduced, thereby increasing the tendency to thrombus formation. Other factors include increased platelet aggregation and alterations in endothelial-cell function.

The increased thrombotic tendency is manifest by an increased risk of deep leg vein thromboses and pulmonary embolism and an increase in arterial thrombotic episodes. Deep leg vein thrombosis is clinically evident in about 6 per cent of nephrotic adults and can be detected in about 25 per cent if Doppler ultrasonography is used. Pulmonary embolism is also clinically evident in around 6 per cent of cases, but if ventilation/perfusion scans are used as a screening test the figure rises to 12 per cent, or even higher in some series. Nevertheless, mortality from thromboembolism appears to be low (only one death in 2100 years of patient follow-up in a series reported by Cameron) and very few nephrologists would routinely anticoagulate all patients with the nephrotic syndrome, although most would have a low threshold for doing so (for instance, during periods of immobility in hospital). Likewise, after any thromboembolic event they would advise anticoagulation for as long as the nephrotic state persisted.

Renal vein thrombosis may occur, presenting acutely with loin pain, haematuria, deterioration in renal function, and with swelling of the kidney detectable on imaging (usually by ultrasonography). It can also present more insidiously with a significant increase in urinary protein excretion and a gradual reduction in renal function. Some one-third of cases are associated with pulmonary embolism. Renal vein thrombosis can be associated with all causes of the nephrotic syndrome but, for reasons that are unknown, is most common in membranous glomerulonephritis, when it is clinically apparent in 6 to 8 per cent of cases and detectable on imaging in 10 to 45 per cent. It is not routine practice to investigate patients with the nephrotic syndrome, even that caused by membranous glomerulonephritis, for renal vein thrombosis: when there is clinical suspicion the diagnosis can be made by magnetic resonance imaging (**MRI**), computed tomographic (**CT**) scanning or renal arteriography (looking at the venous phase). Treatment of symptomatic renal vein thrombosis is by anticoagulation with full-dose therapeutic intravenous heparin or low molecular weight heparin (although there is little experience of using the latter in this condition) followed by warfarinization. Thrombolysis has also been used, although the indications for this are not well defined. The prognosis is usually benign, with recanalization of the veins and recovery of renal function.

Alterations in lipid metabolism

Alterations in lipid metabolism are well recognized in patients with nephrotic syndrome. There is concern that these changes might lead to atheromatous vascular disease and also be an adverse factor with respect to the development of progressive renal function impairment. Moreover, there is some evidence that patients with the nephrotic syndrome have an increased incidence and prevalence of vascular disease, particularly coronary vascular disease leading to ischaemia and infarction, although not all studies have confirmed this.

Patients with the nephrotic syndrome have an increased concentration of both free cholesterol and cholesterol esters, which have an inverse correlation with plasma albumin concentration. There is an increase in phospholipids, although this is not marked, and in severe cases fasting triglycerides are elevated. Plasma free fatty acid concentrations are reduced. The changes are not determined by the nature of the underlying glomerular disease but are closely linked to the degree of hypoproteinaemia. There are alterations in lipoproteins: very low-density lipoproteins (**VLDL**) and low-density lipoproteins (**LDL**) are increased, whilst high-density lipoprotein (**HDL**) concentrations are less predictably affected.

The causes of the alterations in the lipid profile are incompletely understood. There is an increase in the hepatic production of VLDL and LDL, the stimulus for which is unknown but may be related to plasma oncotic pressure. In addition there is evidence for the diminished removal of LDL, possibly due to a reduction in the activity of lipoprotein lipase. The changes in HDL concentrations are probably related to the reduction in lecithin cholesterol acyl transferase (**LCAT**) activity that occurs in nephrotic patients.

Should patients with nephrotic hyperlipidaemia be treated for this? There is no good evidence. It seems reasonable to give dietary advice, although there have been few studies to show how effective (or not) this is in reducing lipid levels, and none looking at cardiovascular outcome. Statins are effective at reducing serum cholesterol, which is virtually always elevated in the nephrotic syndrome, sometimes massively so, but most would not prescribe these as a routine for the following reasons:

1. Given that the aetiology of hyperlipidaemia in the nephrotic syndrome is different from that in the primary hyperlipidaemias, it is not certain that the biological impact is the same, for example it might not be as deleterious from a cardiovascular point of view.
2. Few patients remain nephrotic for years: they either go into remission (spontaneously or after treatment) or develop endstage renal failure.
3. Many patients with the nephrotic syndrome are young and, aside from their hyperlipidaemia, at low absolute risk of vascular events.
4. Many patients will require complex drug therapy, such that there is a reluctance to add further medication, particularly since there is a suspicion that those with the nephrotic syndrome may be more likely to experience side-effects from lipid-lowering medications.

Proteinuria and the progression of renal disease

It is well recognized that prolonged profuse proteinuria is associated with a poor prognosis in patients with glomerulonephritis. In experimental studies proteinuria is associated with interstitial damage, tubular injury, and glomerulosclerosis. Heavy proteinuria is associated with progressive glomerular scarring, and intervention to reduce proteinuria is accompanied by reduction in sclerosis. It is possible that the prolonged and heavy proteinuria has an adverse effect on mesangial cells leading to mesangial sclerosis and eventually global sclerosis, but it is likely that proteinuria is only one of many factors responsible for progressive renal disease.

Acute nephritic syndrome (haematoproteinuria syndrome)

Acute nephritis is a clinical syndrome characterized by the acute onset of haematuria, proteinuria, hypertension, and oliguria. The urine typically appears 'smoky' due to the presence of red blood cell casts, and rarely it will appear frankly red. Proteinuria is variable in amount, but is rarely sufficient to produce a nephrotic syndrome. Hypertension is variable and oliguria depends to a large extent on the degree of glomerular involvement. Not all four clinical features may be present simultaneously. In some patients there is oedema due to salt and water retention in the oliguric phase. Encephalopathy, particularly in children, may occur due to hypertension or electrolyte disorders such as hyponatraemia.

The 'classical' cause of acute nephritis is poststreptococcal glomerulonephritis: this is described in detail in Chapter 20.7.5 and other infective causes in Chapter 20.7.8. However, these diseases are becoming less common, particularly in developed countries, and it is more usual to see patients who have proteinuria and haematuria accompanied by variable hypertension and renal functional impairment in whom no identifiable preceding infection can be identified. The presence of blood and protein in the urine is a sign of glomerular inflammation and is not indicative of any particular glomerular pathology. On investigation such patients have a wide variety of glomerular appearances (Table 1), hence renal biopsy is essential for precise diagnosis. For further discussion of the conditions listed in Table 1 see the relevant subsections of this section.

Recurrent haematuria

'Recurrent haematuria' is the term used to describe patients who have episodic macroscopic haematuria. This most commonly is due to IgA nephropathy, described in Section 20.8.2, where episodes are immediately preceded by mucosal inflammation, usually of the upper respiratory tract but sometimes of the gastrointestinal tract. Some patients with Alport's syndrome may present with episodes of recurrent haematuria but these are

Table 1 Conditions associated with haematoproteinuria

Glomerular diseases
Proliferative glomerulonephritis
Mesangiocapillary glomerulonephritis
Focal segmental glomerulosclerosis
IgA nephropathy
Crescentic glomerulonephritis
Systemic diseases
Henloch–Schönlein syndrome
Polyarteritis (microscopic and nodosa)
Wegener's syndrome
Systemic lupus erythematosus
Other vasculitic diseases

Table 2 Conditions associated with loin pain and haematuria

Loin pain haematuria syndrome
Renal and/or ureteric stones
Urinary tract infections
IgA nephropathy
Thin-membrane nephropathy
Polycystic renal disease
Renal metastases

usually unrelated to mucosal inflammation. It must also be remembered that other causes of repeated episodes of macroscopic haematuria include polycystic renal disease, renal stone disease, sickle-cell disease, and tumours of the renal tract. In such patients there are frequently other clinical indications to allow confident differentiation from IgA nephropathy.

Loin pain haematuria syndrome

This is a relatively uncommon but well-recognized syndrome, which can only be diagnosed by excluding other conditions that can be associated with pain in the loins and microscopic or intermittent macroscopic haematuria (Table 2).

Patients present with intermittent or persistent loin pain accompanied by persistent microscopic haematuria, although on very rare occasions macroscopic haematuria can occur, even to the extent of causing clot colic. Most are young women, many of whom will have undergone numerous investigations. Symptoms are frequently unilateral but usually become bilateral, although one side may predominate. Clinical examination is unremarkable, although there may be some loin tenderness, and blood pressure is normal. The urinary red cells are dysmorphic, suggesting a glomerular origin, but red cell casts are not present. There is no evidence of urinary tract infection, normal urinary protein excretion or only minor proteinuria (occasionally up to 1 g daily), normal GFR (usually estimated from serum creatinine values by the Cockcroft and Gault formula, or from a 24-h creatinine clearance), and no clear structural abnormality on thorough imaging (cystoscopy and at least one of intravenous urography/ultrasound/CT scanning/MRI). Indices of inflammation such as a raised erythrocyte sedimentation rate (**ESR**) or C-reactive protein (**CRP**), or elevated plasma viscosity are notable by their absence.

A radiological abnormality consisting of focal or generalized tortuosity, beading, and occlusion of intrarenal medium-sized arteries leading to cortical infarcts has been described, but these findings are not universal. On renal biopsy the glomeruli appear normal or show only minor changes: a number of reports describe complement deposition (C3 and C4) in arterioles, but the significance of this is uncertain and it may be a non-specific finding.

The syndrome runs a relapsing/remitting course over a number of years, with symptoms gradually subsiding with time. The loin pain can vary greatly in severity, ranging from a mild ache to disabling colic requiring opiate analgesia. There is no effective specific treatment and, not surprisingly, some patients can be difficult to manage as it is difficult for them to accept that there is no 'cure' for their symptoms. Renal denervation and renal autotransplantation have been tried, but pain typically returns over 6 to 12 months, and even after nephrectomy pain can develop in the remaining kidney. These procedures should not be performed, and other methods of pain control (transcutaneous nerve stimulation, amitriptyline, carbamazepine, and similar agents) are usually ineffective. In most cases pain control can be obtained using regular opiate analgesia, after which the dosage can usually be reduced and the patient eventually weaned off medication. Although this can take a long time, it is rare for pain to persist into the patient's forties or fifties.

Disorders of micturition

Frequency

'Frequency' is the term applied when the bladder is emptied more often than normal, hence in obtaining a history it is therefore necessary to determine how often the patient passes urine. This may be associated with a normal or increased 24-hour urine volume. It is important to distinguish between these two situations as frequency in the presence of a normal output indicates a bladder (lower urinary tract) problem, whereas an increase in output is indicative of a disorder of urinary concentration or excessive fluid intake (see 'polyuria').

Frequency in the presence of a normal urine volume is most commonly due to bladder inflammation from a bacterial infection (cystitis), when dysuria is a common accompanying symptom. It can also be produced by chemical irritation (for example, as sometimes occurs during treatment with cyclophosphamide), or from a calculus or tumour involving the bladder wall. A reduction in bladder capacity is uncommon but may result from radiation-induced fibrosis following treatment to a pelvic malignancy. In males, prostatic hypertrophy, benign or malignant, is associated with frequency and a diminution in urinary stream, together with hesitancy (a difficulty in initiating micturition) and dribbling (a difficulty in terminating micturition).

Nocturia

Nocturia may arise from the many conditions that cause frequency. On lying down there is an increase in renal perfusion resulting in increased urine flow, but ADH is secreted during sleep, thereby increasing urinary concentration and meaning that urine volume diminishes during sleep. In patients with sleep disturbance there is less ADH production and thus urine concentration is reduced, with increased urine volume such that nocturia may occur. Enquiry should be made regarding sleep patterns in patients presenting with nocturia, in addition to considering those conditions that cause polyuria and frequency.

Dysuria

Dysuria is pain or discomfort on micturition and one of the most frequent symptoms, accounting for about 2 per cent of consultations in primary care. It is more common in women, and is usually described as a burning, scalding, or tingling sensation in the urethra or at the urethral meatus occurring during or immediately after micturition. Most commonly it is due to urinary infection, but it may also be caused by chemical irritation such as rarely occurs with cyclophosphamide. If associated with frequency and urgency of micturition it indicates bladder irritation such as cystitis. In young women this is usually associated with sexual activity, but in older persons it may indicate a lesion in the bladder or prostate. Prostatic inflammation usually gives rise to perineal or rectal pain. Very young children will be unable to complain of dysuria but urethral irritation may be inferred if the child cries during micturition. (See Chapter 20.12 for further discussion.)

Polyuria

Polyuria is an increase in the daily volume of urine and may arise from a number of different conditions. The normal daily urine volume varies considerably depending on fluid intake and insensible loss, but is normally in the range of 1 to 2 litres. Most patients have no idea of their urine volume and so it is necessary to obtain a 24-h collection to verify urine output. Excessive fluid intake, as occurs in compulsive water drinking, results in an increased volume. An increase in solute load, most commonly due to hyperglycaemia, reduces tubular reabsorption and increases urine production. Inadequate ADH secretion, such as following a head injury or associated with tumours or infection, result in an impaired urinary concentration and increased output (central diabetes insipidus). Conditions that impair the tubular response to ADH, such as potassium depletion, lithium toxicity, and some rare inherited diseases, also increase urine volume (nephrogenic diabetes insipidus), as do renal disorders that impair medullary concentration, such as analgesic nephropathy, papillary necrosis, medullary cystic disease, and nephrocalcinosis.

Oliguria and anuria

Oliguria is a reduction in urine volume to such an extent that there is inability to excrete the residues of normal daily metabolic functions. This normally means to a volume of less than 400 ml daily in an adult, usually indicating acute renal failure of whatever cause (see Chapter 20.4). Anuria is the lack of any urine output and is indicative of obstruction, although it may occur in some forms of severe acute renal failure. If anuria is present it is essential to perform a rectal examination to determine if there is any pelvic malignancy, such as a rectal or cervical carcinoma, to account for the obstruction.

Pain

Renal pain

Stretching of the capsule of the kidney causes renal pain that is felt in the loin ('renal angle'). It can be produced by any condition that distends the kidney, such as inflammation, mass lesions, or an obstruction. The last is the most common cause, particularly obstruction of the pelviureteric junction, when the patient may give a history that anything that causes an acute increase in urine volume (for example, drinking a large quantity of water, beer, or lager or taking a diuretic) precipitates the pain. Inflammatory pain, such as in pyelonephritis and (uncommonly) in glomerulonephritis, develops gradually, is usually constant in nature, and is variable in severity. A perirenal abscess, which may not always be associated with fever or tenderness, can give rise to symptoms and signs of diaphragmatic irritation and/or psoas irritation. In the latter case, the patient usually prefers to rest with the hips flexed, and reports that extension of the hips is accompanied by an increase in pain.

It can be difficult to distinguish renal pain from musculoskeletal pain, hence the history should enquire specifically about the relationship of pain to movement or position, neither of which greatly affects renal pain. Clinical examination of the back and spine should determine any limitation of movement or localized point tenderness, which would suggest a musculoskeletal problem.

Some patients with polycystic renal disease complain of a constant dull loin ache. They may also suffer from the sudden onset of renal pain if there is bleeding into a cyst, or from pain of a more gradual onset if there is cyst infection.

Ureteric colic

Pain arising from an acute obstruction is frequently sudden in onset, severe, colicky, and may radiate to the groin, scrotum, labia, or upper thigh. Many describe it as 'the worst pain that they have ever had', and the patient with ureteric colic typically thrashes about, unable to find comfort, looks pale and sweaty, and often vomits, which can lead to diagnostic confusion. The pain is due to acute distention of the pelvis of the kidney and the upper ureter and the associated increased peristalsis. If the obstruction is ureteric the pain resolves rapidly once the cause is extruded into the bladder, although when in the bladder it may result in bladder irritation with strangury or further obstruction if it becomes impacted at the urethral orifice. The most common differential diagnoses of right-sided renal colic are biliary colic and appendicitis: diagnostic difficulty is less likely on the left side, although colonic pain requires consideration. (See Chapter 20.14 for further discussion.)

Chronic obstruction may be surprisingly asymptomatic. Retroperitoneal fibrosis is accompanied by a dull-aching back discomfort but is not associated with colic in spite of an obstruction.

Disorders of renal function

Acute renal failure

An acute deterioration in renal function may arise in patients with normal renal function or in those with known renal insufficiency, the latter being known as acute on chronic renal failure. The clinical features depend to a large extent on the underlying cause. Patients may be seriously ill with profound hypotension from such causes as multiple trauma or severe sepsis, or they may appear remarkably well, such as with rapidly progressive glomerulonephritis. The diagnosis may be suspected or proven in patients with the following clinical features:

1. *Diminished urine volume.* This is not invariable and some patients have a normal volume but a reduction in urinary concentration to such an extent that there is retention of urea, creatinine, and other substances that are normally excreted. It should be remembered that the quality of urine is as important as the volume.
2. *Increasing blood concentrations of urea and creatinine.* This usually indicates impaired excretion and is the usual way in which the diagnosis of acute renal failure is established. Creatinine is a more accurate reflection of renal function than urea, as its concentration is influenced to a lesser extent by protein catabolism and the state of hydration. An important clinical indicator as to whether a patient has acute or chronic renal failure can be the state of consciousness at a given serum creatinine concentration. If renal function declines rapidly, the patient is often obtunded once the creatinine is in excess of 800 μmol/l, whereas if the creatinine concentration has increased slowly with time the patient is unlikely to have any impairment of consciousness with a creatinine of 1000 μmol/l.
3. *Electrolyte disturbance.* Hyperkalaemia may be the first indication that a patient is developing acute renal failure. In the presence of normal renal function it is difficult to produce hyperkalaemia.
4. *Acidosis.* This is most commonly detected by measurement of a declining serum bicarbonate concentration, reflecting the development of a metabolic acidosis and clinically manifested by tachypnoea.
5. *Pulmonary oedema.* Most patients with acute renal failure are prone to this as their ability to excrete fluid is limited, but it is most commonly iatrogenic, when an oliguric patient is ill-advisedly given inappropriate intravenous fluids.
6. *Appropriate clinical circumstances.* In some instances there is an obvious risk for the development of acute renal failure, such as in septicaemic shock, severe multiple trauma, prolonged hypotension, and indeed any clinical circumstance that impairs normal kidney function.
7. *Consumption of certain medications.* Some medications have the ability to reduce renal function. The most common mechanism is by reduction of effective renal perfusion, such as can be caused by non-steroidal anti-inflammatory agents (**NSAIDs**), ACE inhibitors, and angiotensin II-receptor blockers. Less common mechanisms include the induction of acute interstitial nephritis (for example, caused by NSAIDs, penicillins) or acute toxic tubular dysfunction (for example, aminoglycosides, paracetamol overdose). Rare mechanisms include the precipitation of acute vasculitis (for instance, hydralazine) or stimulation of retroperitoneal fibrosis (for example, methysergide). Commonly it is a combination of medications such as analgesics, antibiotics, and non-steroidal drugs together with radiocontrast agents that result in acute renal failure, because during an illness one agent after another is added without the recognition that renal function is declining.

It must be remembered that to maintain normal renal excretory function there is a need for effective cardiac output and renal perfusion, glomerular filtration, tubular function (reabsorption and excretion), and the drainage of urine from the renal pelvis via the ureters, bladder, and urethra. It is thus possible to acutely disrupt this function in many different ways, and accurate diagnosis is dependent upon obtaining a good history, paying particular attention to detail, followed by a thorough clinical examination supported by a structured investigative protocol. See Section 20.5 for further discussion.

Chronic renal failure

Patients with a slow progressive deterioration in renal function may remain remarkably free from symptoms until renal function is seriously impaired. When symptoms of renal failure do develop, they are non-specific, such that many patients attribute them to increasing age or being less physically active than previously. This can make diagnosis difficult and renal impairment may be unsuspected until the results of some screening investigations, such as haemoglobin and blood urea, are obtained. (See Section 20.5 for further discussion.)

History

Presenting complaint

Obtaining a clear and concise history is about one of the most difficult things to achieve in clinical medicine. It is important to elicit carefully the nature and chronological sequence of all the symptoms experienced by the patient, who should be encouraged to describe each symptom in detail and—if medical terminology is used—the physician needs to determine what exactly the patient understands by the particular word or phrase used. It is not uncommon for a patient to describe their symptoms using words that their friends or previous medical practitioners have used, which may not be appropriate. For each symptom it is necessary to make specific enquiry regarding the mode of onset, whether sudden or gradual, and the nature of any associated features such as precipitating and relieving factors. If the patient describes pain then additional enquiry needs to be made regarding its position, nature, and radiation.

In patients with proteinuria and/or haematuria it is essential to ask about the results of any previous urine testing, even from years previous. It is standard practice to test urine during pregnancy and during employment and insurance medical examinations. It is often profitable to review all available medical notes: frequently urine will have been tested and the results recorded, even if no notice has been taken of an abnormal result.

In most instances the pattern of the symptoms will follow a recognized syndrome; in some an apparently unconnected number of symptoms will suggest the presence of a systemic disease; while in others there will be a condition known to affect the kidneys. In any event, it is important to document carefully all symptomatology and subsequently to record all new or changing symptoms.

Past history

The past medical history of a patient can provide much useful information to aid diagnosis. It is important to obtain as full a history as possible detailing childhood illnesses, all major illnesses, and hospital admissions. A history of unexplained febrile illnesses in childhood or prolonged enuresis suggests the possibility of recurrent urinary infections due to structural urinary abnormalities such as vesicoureteric reflux.

A number of chronic conditions may be associated with renal involvement, either directly as in systemic diseases, or indirectly as in the development of amyloidosis in prolonged inflammatory diseases such as chronic osteomyelitis, bronchiectasis, or rheumatoid arthritis. In addition, certain drugs used to treat chronic conditions may have adverse renal effects such as gold, penicillamine, ciclosporin, NSAIDs and analgesics used in the management of rheumatoid arthritis and similar conditions.

Systemic vasculitides frequently have multisystem manifestations with variable renal involvement. As a general rule the prognosis of any systemic disease is significantly and adversely influenced once there is renal involvement. Diabetes mellitus, either insulin or non-insulin-dependent, may result in glomerulopathy. In the patient with insulin-dependent diabetes the first manifestation of glomerular involvement typically occurs about 10 years after onset. In the non-insulin-dependent patient, however, renal involvement may be detected at or soon after diagnosis, not because of more aggressive glomerular involvement but rather because the condition may well have been present in an undiagnosed form for many years. (See Chapter 20.10.1 for further discussion.)

It is important to obtain details regarding a woman's menstrual, contraception, and pregnancy histories. A delayed menarche may indicate the presence of renal failure, as may the unexplained development of amenorrhoea. Hypertension is more likely in patients taking a combined oestrogen–progesterone oral contraceptive if there is an underlying renal disease. Similarly, hypertension during pregnancy is much more common in patients with renal disease, particularly in the third trimester. Patients with asymptomatic proteinuria will have an increase in proteinuria during pregnancy, which may come to medical attention when the urine is tested for the first time or because it becomes sufficient to produce the nephrotic syndrome. In the latter circumstance it is sometimes difficult to differentiate between a simple nephrotic syndrome and the development of pre-eclampsia. The proteinuria of pre-eclampsia resolves following delivery, usually with 3 months, whereas in patients with glomerular disease, although the proteinuria will diminish, it does not completely resolve (see Chapter 13.5). Recurrent fetal loss may be associated with antiphospholipid antibodies and so prompts appropriate investigations.

It is not uncommon to find that patients are unable to remember significant events in their past medical history. It is important, therefore, to obtain any previous medical notes to obtain the maximum information. It is surprisingly common to find that urinary abnormalities such as proteinuria or haematuria have been documented previously, perhaps during medicals for work or insurance purposes, but not investigated. This can be a reassuring finding, because if it is known that haematuria has been present for many years then it is a safe bet that it is not due to a serious condition (assuming that renal function is normal).

Drug history

It is essential to obtain a detailed history of all medications recently consumed, whether obtained by prescription, over the counter, or from health shops: all have the potential for precipitating adverse renal effects. Many patients do not consider that medications they can buy from their local chemist, such as analgesics, are drugs. In some patients it may be necessary to obtain information from the family practitioner. There may be covert drug use, such as with laxatives and diuretics, which is particularly difficult to detect. The presence of unexplained hypokalaemia may provide the only clue that the patient is abusing diuretics or taking excessive amounts of liquorice (see Chapter 20.2.2). Frequently the patient has some connection to the medical profession and thus access to medications. In addition, some who take diuretics unnecessarily experience oedema on withdrawal of the drug, reinforcing their belief that such medication is necessary and resulting in continued ingestion.

Factors that increase the risk of adverse drug effects include age, impaired renal function, and multiple drug therapy. The elderly are at particular risk as renal function declines with age, and with a diminishing muscle mass this may not be obvious from an estimation of the serum creatinine alone; they may also have multiple pathologies resulting in an increased chance that they are taking many drugs. The pharmacokinetics of drugs are altered in elderly patients and so caution is required when prescribing.

All compartments of the kidney can be involved in adverse drug reactions. In the situation where there is a constraint on renal blood flow there is enhanced secretion of renin from the juxtaglomerular apparatus, activating angiotensin and thereby causing vasoconstriction of the efferent arteriole, resulting in an increase in intraglomerular pressure to maintain filtration. If there is vascular stenosis, whether of the main renal artery or of intrarenal arteries, the introduction of an ACE inhibitor or angiotensin II-receptor blocker may result in a significant reduction in glomerular filtration as a consequence of the abolition of this constrictive effect of angiotensin II. A number of patients, particularly the elderly and those with renovascular disease, are particularly susceptible to this adverse effect of these medications. When the renal circulation is compromised glomerular blood flow is also supported by the action of vasodilator prostaglandins, and in these circumstances NSAIDs can cause substantial decrement in the filtration rate. Much more rarely, the blood vessels may exhibit vasculitis following treatment with hydralazine or propylthiouracil.

Glomerular changes may be induced by gold or D-penicillamine, resulting in proteinuria and, in certain cases, the nephrotic syndrome. The glomerular changes usually revert once the drug is withdrawn.

Tubular function can also be adversely influenced. Lithium is associated with a nephrogenic diabetes insipidus-like syndrome due to inhibition of the action of ADH on the cells of the distal tubule and collecting duct. This may be accompanied by an incomplete distal renal tubular acidosis and, in some patients, with a chronic interstitial nephritis. Acute renal failure due to an acute reversible reduction in glomerular filtration occurs in lithium toxicity.

Interstitial nephritis may occur as an acute allergic reaction occurring shortly after the introduction of a drug, or in a more chronic form after several months of ingestion. In the acute form there may be other manifestations of an allergic reaction such as rash, eosinophilia, and the detection of eosinophils in the urine. In the more chronic form there may be no such indication of an allergic reaction. A wide variety of medications, including antibiotics and analgesics, may give rise to interstitial disease, as can certain herbal remedies, as evidenced by the nephropathy that has been associated with Chinese herbs used as a slimming aid. Analgesic abuse may give rise to papillary necrosis, which may present as polyuria due to impairment of renal concentration or from obstruction if a sloughed papilla occludes the ureter.

Some medications have the ability to elevate blood pressure, and so a drug-induced cause should be considered in any patient presenting with hypertension: this is well recognized in patients receiving oestrogen/progesterone preparations, corticosteroids, ciclosporin, and erythropoietin.

In patients with renal disease there may be a greater propensity for adverse reactions. In the nephrotic syndrome the diminished plasma albumin concentration will result in a lessening of protein binding and thus an increased availability of the 'free' drug. If there is impaired renal function there may be diminished excretion, thus prolonging the half-life of the drug and increasing the risk of toxicity if the dose is not adjusted appropriately. In addition, some treatments given for some renal diseases may have adverse interactions with other drugs, for example high-dose corticosteroids have the ability to displace protein-bound drugs, thereby increasing the concentration of 'free' drug.

Dietary history

A carefully obtained dietary history can, in a few cases, be helpful in reaching a diagnosis. Excessive sodium intake may be associated with hypertension or apparent resistance to antihypertensive medication. Idiopathic, stone-forming patients seem to have a greater than average protein intake, resulting in increased excretion of calcium, oxalate, and uric acid, all of which are risk factors for stone formation. Some patients have a preference for acid-tasting foods that they may consume in excessive amounts: fruit juices and rhubarb, which are high in oxalate, may be the cause of oxalate deposition in the kidney if taken to excess. Other patients consume an excessive amount of liquorice that interferes with the inactivation of cortisol by blocking the enzyme 11β-hydroxysteroid dehydrogenase, and, as a consequence, the cortisol binds to mineralocorticoid receptors mimicking hyperaldosteronism.

There are differences in the composition of some ethnic diets compared to a 'standard' Western diet: Japanese food is high in sodium, whereas Indian food is high in potassium. In addition, some foods may aggravate the effects of renal failure. Unleavened bread, chapattis, with a high phytate content bind intestinal calcium reducing absorption and thereby stimulating parathyroid hormone secretion which, in addition to other effects, increases the metabolism of vitamin D and as a consequence aggravates the osteomalacic or rachitic component of renal osteodystrophy.

Family history

It is important to obtain as full a family history as possible as this can significantly aid diagnosis. If an inherited renal disease is identified, the diagnosis is of value to other members of the family, allowing the identification of affected members and appropriate clinical review to control any associated complications such as hypertension and anaemia. In any patient with suspected renal disease it is advisable to enquire about familial renal disease, deafness (Alport's syndrome), and whether the parents were related (all recessive conditions are much more common with inbreeding). It may be necessary to examine medical notes and obtain death certificates. Sometimes it is possible to infer inherited renal conditions that were unsuspected: a patient with polycystic renal disease may give a history that some relatives have died suddenly from a 'stroke', indicating the possibility of subarachnoid haemorrhage from a ruptured cerebral aneurysm. Similarly, most, if not all, cases of vesicoureteric reflux are familial, when a history of troublesome urinary infections in family members can be informative.

Not all familial conditions seem to have a clear inherited pattern. There is a familial predisposition to systemic lupus erythematosus, other autoimmune diseases, and IgA nephropathy. In some families there is a greater than expected incidence of hypertension or diabetes mellitus, indicating genetic influences as yet undetermined. In some conditions there is considerable genetic heterogeneity: Alport's syndrome is classically an X-linked dominant condition, but an autosomal recessive form has been described, as has a form associated with macrothrombocytopenia (Epstein's syndrome). Furthermore, not all diseases that have similar features are the same condition, for example nerve deafness and urinary abnormalities may be due to Alport's syndrome or to the Muckle–Wells syndrome (heredofamilial amyloidosis), Refsum's syndrome, a rare form of Charcot–Marie–Tooth syndrome, or Cockayne syndrome.

Social history

Socioeconomic factors are important in patients with renal disease. Increasing affluence is associated with an increasing incidence of renal stone disease, possibly related to an increase in protein intake. Low socioeconomic status is associated with an increased incidence of bacteriuria during pregnancy.

Smoking is a risk factor for the development of atherosclerosis, renovascular hypertension, and accelerated hypertension. It is also associated with anti-glomerular basement membrane (**anti-GBM**) nephritis and the risk of developing nephropathy in patients with diabetes mellitus.

Intravenous drug abuse is a risk factor for septicaemia that may lead to bacterial endocarditis with associated glomerulonephritis. In addition, such patients may develop acute renal failure due to septicaemia, rhabdomyolysis or (rarely) vasculitis, or chronic renal failure due to amyloidosis. They are also at risk from needle-transmitted infections such as hepatitis B and C and human immunodeficiency virus (**HIV**) that may lead to vascular and glomerular disease. Many patients will not admit to drug abuse and so obtaining an accurate history may be difficult: on clinical examination particular attention needs to be taken of any skin indication of intravenous needling.

Occupational history

Some renal diseases may be work related, hence specific enquiry should be made with respect to the working environment and, in particular, to exposure to any chemical substances: for example, the use of chemicals, pesticides, exposure to fumes, and the need to wear protective clothing. A full occupational history, proceeding in chronological order from the time of leaving school to the present day, needs to be taken. Aniline dye workers have an increased risk of developing urothelial tumours; exposure to solvents may be causally associated with anti-GBM glomerulonephritis; vaporized lead fumes, as occur in the welding of lead pipes, may cause lead nephropathy and chronic renal failure, which is being associated with exposure to an increasing number of toxic substances. As information becomes available, appropriate health and safety regulations are introduced to lessen the risk to workers, but some workers ignore advice, and in some countries—particularly in the developing world—preventive measures are not enforced or are deliberately ignored.

Acute renal failure may arise from leptospirosis in miners, sewage workers, farm workers, and those recreationally exposed, or from hantavirus infection in laboratory technicians and farmers in endemic areas.

Ethnic and geographical factors

Geographical factors are important in a number of renal diseases. Hantaviruses infect various animal species worldwide, but the incidence of clinical infection is variable. In Asia it is due mainly to the Haantan and Seoul viruses, in China it is known as epidemic haemorrhagic fever, and in Korea as Korean haemorrhagic fever. In Europe infections are mainly caused by the Puumala serotype and result in acute renal failure, whereas in North America, although two serotypes have been identified, no cases of renal disease have been reported. Other infections, such as malaria and schistosomiasis, also have particular geographical prevalence. It is important to obtain a full history of travel abroad, as this will alert the clinician to the potential of diseases not frequently seen in everyday practice but which may have an infective basis. (See Chapter 20.7.10 for further discussion of aspects of renal disease particular to developing countries.)

Patients of African or Asian origin are likely to have been exposed to tuberculosis at some time, which may give rise to clinical disease if they are immunosuppressed for treatment of glomerular disease or following transplantation. It is common practice to treat with prophylactic therapy in such circumstances, generally using isoniazid (with pyridoxine).

Some renal diseases have an ethnic association. The amyloidosis that complicates familial Mediterranean fever occurs in Arabs from the Mediterranean area, Turks and Sephardic Jews, whereas Sephardic Jews from Baghdad, southern Russia, the Balkans, and Ashkenazic Jews are rarely affected. IgA nephropathy is more common in Caucasians and people from some Asian countries (Japan, Singapore, and China) and is apparently less common in Afro-American and African peoples. Systemic lupus erythematosus is more common in those from the Middle East and the Orient than from Europe. Diabetes mellitus has an increased prevalence in Asian communities and in some of the Indian communities of North America.

Tubulointerstitial diseases such as Balkan nephropathy have a particular geographical distribution. Analgesic nephropathy, associated with the regular consumption of compound analgesics, particularly but not exclusively those containing phenacetin (before the use of this drug was restricted or banned), was particularly common in Australia where renal effects may be aggravated by minor dehydration due to increased insensible fluid loss. Less easy to explain is the increased prevalence in Switzerland and certain towns in Belgium.

Further reading

Birch D, *et al.* (1983). Urinary erythrocyte morphology in the diagnosis of glomerular hematuria. *Clinical Nephrology* **20**, 78–84.

Britton JP, *et al.* (1992). A community study of bladder cancer screening by the detection of occult urinary bleeding. *Journal of Urology* **148**, 289–92.

Burden RP, *et al.* (1979). The loin pain/haematuria syndrome. *Lancet* **i**, 897–900.

Castenfors J, Mossfeldt F, Piscator M (1967). Effect of heavy prolonged exercise on renal function and urinary protein excretion. *Acta Physiologica Scandinavica* **70**, 194–206.

Devarajan P (1993). Mechanisms of orthostatic proteinuria: lessons from a transplant donor. *Journal of the American Society of Nephrology* **4**, 36–9.

Dorhout Mees EJ, Geers AB, Koomans HA (1984). Blood volume and sodium retention in the nephrotic syndrome: a controversial pathophysiological concept. *Nephron* **36**, 201–11.

Ginsberg JM, *et al.* (1983). Use of single voided urine samples to estimate quantitative proteinuria. *New England Journal of Medicine* **309**, 1543–6.

Gorensek MJ, Lebel MH, Nelson JD (1988). Peritonitis in children with nephrotic syndrome. *Pediatrics* **8**, 849–56.

Grossfeld GD, *et al.* (2001). Asymptomatic microscopic hematuria in adults: summary of the AUA best practice policy recommendations. *American Family Physician* **63**, 1145–54.

Grossman E, Messerli FH (1995). A side effect of drugs, poisons, and food. *Archives of Internal Medicine* **155**, 450–60.

Hiatt RA, Ordonez JD (1994). Dipstick urinalysis screening, asymptomatic microhematuria, and subsequent urological cancers in a population-based sample. *Cancer Epidemiology, Biomarkers and Prevention* **3**, 439–43.

Khadra MH, *et al.* (2000). A prospective analysis of 1,930 patients with hematuria to evaluate current diagnostic practice. *Journal of Urology* **163**, 524–7.

Little PJ, Sloper JS, deWardener HE (1967). A syndrome of loin pain and haematuria associated with disease of peripheral renal arteries. *Quarterly Journal of Medicine* **36**, 253–9.

MacGregor GA, De Wardener HE (1988). Idiopathic oedema. In: Schrier RW, Gottshalk CW, eds. *Diseases of the kidney*, 4th edn, pp 2743–53. Little, Brown and Co., Boston, MA.

Mallick NP, Short CD (1981). The nephrotic syndrome and ischaemic heart disease. *Nephron* **27**, 54–7.

Messing EM, *et al.* (1992). Home screening for haematuria: results of a multiclinic study. *Journal of Urology* **148**, 289–92.

Mohr DN, *et al.* (1986). Asymptomatic microscopic haematuria and urologic disease: a population based study. *Journal of the American Medical Association* **256**, 224–9.

Naish PF, Aber GM, Boyd WN (1975). C3 deposition in renal arterioles in the loin pain and haematuria syndrome. *British Medical Journal* **3**, 746.

Nuyts GD, *et al.* (1995). New occupational risk factors for chronic renal failure. *Lancet* **346**, 7–11.

Ordoñez JD, *et al.* (1993). The increased risk of coronary heart disease associated with nephrotic syndrome. *Kidney International* **44**, 638–42.

Polenakovic MH, Stefanovic V (1998). Balkan nephropathy. In: Davison AM, *et al.*, eds. *Oxford textbook of clinical nephrology*, pp 1203–10. Oxford University Press, Oxford.

Rabelink TJ, *et al.* (1994). Thrombosis and hemostasis in renal disease. *Kidney International* **46**, 287–96.

Reuben DB, *et al.* (1982). Transient proteinuria in emergency medical admissions. *New England Journal of Medicine* **306**, 1031–3.

Ritchie CD, Bevan EA, Collier StJ (1986). Importance of occult haematuria found at screening. *British Medical Journal* **292**, 681–3.

Robinson RR (1980). Isolated proteinuria in asymptomatic patients. *Kidney International* **18**, 395–406.

Springberg PD, *et al.* (1982). Fixed and reproducible orthostatic proteinuria: results of a 20 year follow-up study. *Annals of Internal Medicine* **97**, 516–19.

van Ypersele de Strihou C (1998). Hantavirus infection. In: Davison AM, *et al.*, eds. *Oxford textbook of clinical nephrology*, 2nd edn, pp 1688–92. Oxford University Press, Oxford.

Wass VJ, Cameron JS (1981). Cardiovascular disease and the nephrotic syndrome. The other side of the coin. *Nephron* **27**, 58–61.

20.3.2 Clinical investigation of renal disease

A. Davenport

Introduction

The key to making any correct diagnosis depends upon a careful history and thorough examination. In patients with renal failure the history and examination should attempt to differentiate acute from chronic renal disease, single-organ system involvement from multisystem disease, and obstruction from intrinsic or prerenal disease. Renal disease may be associated with preceding infections and the ingestion of drugs or herbal remedies. An accurate history and careful examination will determine the sequence and spectrum of clinical investigations required to make a diagnosis.

Examination of the urine

Urine collection

To minimize contamination, standard investigation is of a midstream urine (**MSU**) sample. Voiding from a full bladder containing at least 200 ml of urine should remove urethral organisms before the MSU is collected. Even so, in women, vaginal leucocytes and bacteria may contaminate the urine, and men should retract the foreskin to minimize contamination. Suprapubic aspiration is the technique of choice in babies and infants, and occasionally in adults who can not co-operate to provide an MSU. The second urine of the morning is the best for microscopy as it is still acidic and concentrated, but without the overnight stay in the bladder that results in the degeneration of casts and cells. Cell lysis can occur in both hypotonic and alkaline urine. Only the first 10 ml of the stream are collected in cases of suspected urethritis.

Macroscopic appearance

Fresh urine usually has a yellow colour due to the presence of urochromes. Occasionally urine will have a milky appearance due to pus, spermatozoa, insoluble phosphates in alkaline urine (sometimes seen following heavy meals), or occasionally in cases of chyluria, or urate crystals in acid urine. Foamy or frothy urine is typical of heavy proteinuria.

Certain agents and conditions can discolour urine:

- *Pink to red coloration*—haematuria may result in a range of colours from smoky pink through to port-wine red in cases of frank macroscopic haematuria. Other causes of a pink or red urine include eating sweets containing aniline dyes, beetroot or other foodstuffs containing anthocyanins, haemoglobin, myoglobin, some drugs such as phenindione and phenolphthalein, and (if the urine is left to stand) porphyrins in cases of acute intermittent porphyria.
- *Blue or green coloration*—can be caused by pseudomonas urinary sepsis, methylene blue, biliverdin, triamterene, amitriptyline, chlorophyll-containing breath mints (Clorets®), excessive use of mouthwash and deodorants, magnesium salicylate (Doan's pills®), phenyl salicylate, guanicol (in cough remedies), thymol (in volatile oils and horesemint), iodochlorhydroxyquin, tolonium, Evans blue, methocarbamol, Diagnex blue, indigo blue, resorcinol, azuresin, bromoforium, and occasionally propofol. Phenol and lysol can result in a green or black discoloration.
- *Orange coloration*—can be caused by anthraquinone-containing laxatives, rifampicin, and excess urobilinogen.
- *Yellow urine*—may be found in patients prescribed mepacrine, phenacetin, and those taking excessive amounts of riboflavin, as well as icteric patients with conjugated hyperbilirubinaemia.
- *Black or brown urine*—alkaptonuria results in black or brown urine, whereas myoglobin and melanin only lead to black urine on standing. Other causes of a brown urine include bilirubin, L-dopa, niridazole, furazolidone, and phenazopyridine, and, following standing, haemoglobin and myoglobin. As mentioned above, phenol and lysol can result in a black or green discoloration.

Stick testing

The upper limit of normal for protein excretion in the urine is 128 mg/24 h. Although albumin is the largest single component, more than half of the protein content comprises low molecular weight proteins and protein fragments. Commercial sticks such as Albustix™ are very sensitive, detecting protein in urine starting at concentrations around 100 mg/l. Since these sticks detect protein on a concentration basis, using bromocresol green as an indicator dye, the results they give are affected by urine flow rate and urine dilution or concentration. The sticks are treated with a buffer to keep their pH constant. An elevated urinary protein concentration can erroneously be recorded if the buffer is washed off by leaving the stick in the urine for too long, and with very alkaline urine. Some antiseptics used to clean the skin, including cetrimide and chlorhexidine, may also react and cause a false-positive result.

pH

Normal urine is slightly acidic, but can vary between pH 4.5 and 8.0. If an early morning urine specimen is under pH 5.3, then there is unlikely to be a significant defect in urinary acidification. Alkaline pH is often found in urine infected with urea-splitting bacteria. In some cases of renal calculus disease, particularly in cystinuria and urate nephropathy, crystal solubility is greater in alkaline urine, and patients should regularly check their urine pH. Haemoglobin and myoglobin are also more soluble in alkaline urine. Thus maintaining a forced alkaline diuresis is important in the management of patients following tumour lysis and those with rhabdomyolysis or haemoglobinuria.

Glycosuria

The stick reaction is based on glucose oxidase, which releases hydrogen peroxide from glucose, so producing a graded colour change by oxidizing an indicator. This reaction is specific for glucose, and does not detect other sugars. The reaction can be blocked by large doses of ascorbic acid. A positive stick test for glucose must be interpreted in light of the plasma glucose level, as glycosuria may reflect a defect in renal tubular glucose absorption.

Specific gravity

Specific gravity is a measure of the number of particles dissolved in a litre, whereas osmolality is the number of particles per kilogram. Protein and glucose increase the specific gravity more than the osmolality as they are dense particles. In normal patients the early morning, or concentrated, urine sample should have a specific gravity of 1.024 or more.

Nitrite stick test

Nitrite sticks contain an aromatic amine which reacts with nitrites, produced by bacterial reduction of nitrate, to form a pink-coloured diazonium complex. More than 90 per cent of the common urinary pathogens are nitrite-forming bacteria. However, *Pseudomonas* spp., *Staphylococcus albus*, *Staphylococcus saprophyticus*, and *Streptococcus faecalis* may have minimal or no nitrite producing capacity. Other false-negative results may be obtained in alkaline urine, in patients taking large doses of vitamin C, and with frequent voiding of dilute urine when the urinary nitrite concentration is too low.

Leucocyte esterase stick test

This stick test is based on the presence of a leucocyte esterase, and is very specific for the presence of urinary leucocytes, both intact and lysed. This test may be more accurate than microscopy when the urine is alkaline or hypotonic. However, the test can be inhibited by high concentrations of glucose (≥30 g/l), ketones, and antibiotics including cefalexin, cephalothin, nitrofurantoin, tetracycline, and tobramycin. The sensitivity of this test is also reduced when the specific gravity of the urine is high, for instance in the presence of a heavy proteinuria.

Urine microscopy

To obtain reproducible results urine should be processed in a standard manner and examined under the microscope as soon as possible. In our own institution a few drops of acetic acid (10 per cent v/v) is added to ensure a pH of 6.0 or less; then 10 ml of urine is centrifuged for 5 min at 1500 r.p.m. (750 *g*); following which, 9.5 ml of supernatant is removed and the deposit resuspended. One drop (50 µl) is placed on a microscope slide and covered with a standard coverslip (24 × 32 mm). Although phase-contrast microscopy is an advantage in identifying red cells and casts, a standard microscope will suffice. A semiquantitative assessment of casts is made at low power (160 ×) and other elements at high power (400 ×), expressing the counts as numbers per field. Normal urine contains 1 or 2 leucocytes per high-power field (**HPF**), 1 erythrocyte per 2 or 3 HPF, 1 tubular cell per 10 HPF, and both hyaline casts (1 per low-power field, **LPF**) and granular casts (1 per LPF). Physical exercise can result in haematuria and cylinduria for several hours. Stains such as modified Sternheimer's stain (Sedi-stain™) can be used to help differentiate renal tubular cells from leucocytes. To improve the detection of casts, urine can be filtered through a 5-µm Millipore™ filter, and the retained casts stained with Papanicolaou's stain.

Cellular elements

The morphology of the erythrocytes in the urine can give valuable information as to the source of bleeding. Erythrocytes which have passed through the glomerulus and then along the renal tubule can become distorted or dysmorphic. Those originating from other sources within the urinary tract, such as the bladder, typically show much less signs of damage so that they more closely resemble erythrocytes in the peripheral blood, these are termed isomorphic. To establish a diagnosis of glomerular haematuria there should be a minimum of three different forms of dysmorphic erythrocytes present. One particular type of dysmorphic erythrocyte, the acanthocyte, is reported to have 52 per cent specificity and 98 per cent sensitivity for glomerular haematuria when the acanthocyte count is 5 per cent or more. However, not all workers have found erythrocyte morphology to be useful in discriminating glomerular from non-glomerular bleeding, and the physician who only occasionally examines urine under the microscope is unlikely to obtain clear, reproducible, and useful discrimination between dysmorphic and isomorphic cells.

Some centres use automated haematological cell counters (Coulter Counter™) to assess red cell morphology in both urine and peripheral blood. The red cell size-distribution pattern for lower urinary tract haematuria is similar to that of the peripheral blood, with a relatively narrow size range and a high-frequency distribution curve. Whereas the typical pattern for dysmorphic haematuria is one of a broader range of red cell sizes, with a lower frequency distribution. To have any reliability, urine samples must be processed rapidly by those who do it regularly.

Microscopy may also reveal renal tubular epithelial cells. These cells are shed into the urine in acute tubular necrosis; in response to certain drugs, both nephrotoxic and ischaemic; and also in acute renal allograft rejection. In patients with nephrotic syndrome, these cells are seen as oval fat bodies, laden with lipid droplets. Squamous epithelial cells from the urethra and vagina and transitional cells from the ureter and bladder may also be present in normal urine.

During infection, the urine may contain large numbers of leucocytes and bacteria. When large numbers of leucocytes are present in the absence of bacteria, so called sterile pyuria, then a variety of conditions should be considered: renal calculus disease, analgesic nephropathy, interstitial nephropathy, proliferative glomerulonephritis (rarely), renal tuberculosis, schistosomiasis, and partially treated bacterial urinary tract infection. Phase-contrast microscopy can distinguish lymphocytes from neutrophils, but eosinophils can only be identified with specific stains (Hansel's stain). Classically, urinary eosinophilia occurs in cases of acute interstitial nephritis, typically due to drugs, and also in cholesterol atheroembolic disease.

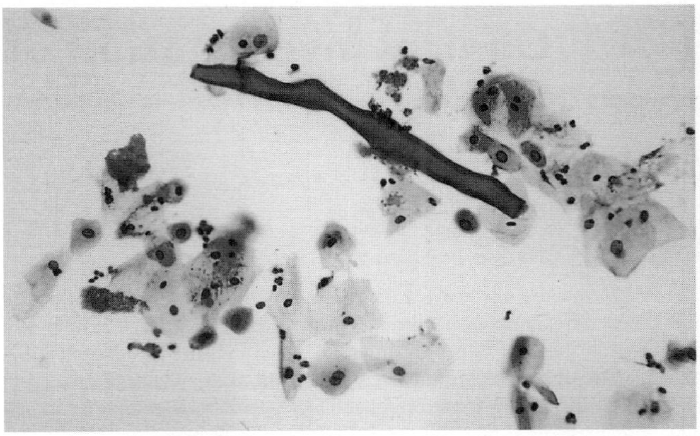

Fig. 1 Papanicolaou-stained urine showing a hyaline cast with both normal transitional and squamous cells and renal tubular cells. (By courtesy of Dr Deery.) (See also Plate 1.)

Urinary casts

Casts form from the transformation of Tamm–Horsfall glycoprotein, secreted by the distal tubular cells, into a gel matrix. They typically assume a tubular structure. Hyaline casts only contain Tamm–Horsfall glycoprotein, and are found in a variable amount in the urine of normal subjects (Fig. 1 and Plate 1). Fever, cardiac failure, strenuous exercise, and some drugs, such as furosemide and ethacrynic acid, increase hyaline cast excretion. During passage through the distal tubule and collecting duct a variety of proteins, pigments, and cells adhere to the Tamm–Horsfall protein, producing a wide variety of casts. Granular casts have deposits of either fine or coarse protein granules (Fig. 2 and Plate 2). Although they may occur in normal subjects, or after exercise, they are typically found in cases of parenchymal renal disease. In patients with proteinuria, the protein deposited comes from the glomerulus, whereas in acute tubular necrosis the protein comes from degenerate tubular cells. Broad waxy casts are much larger than normal casts and have clear-cut edges: they are formed in dilated hypertrophied tubules, as found in patients with chronic renal failure. Casts containing erythrocytes (red cell casts) indicate renal bleeding and are typically found when there is acute glomerular inflammation caused by glomerulonephritis or vasculitis (Fig. 3 and Plate 3). White cell casts (containing

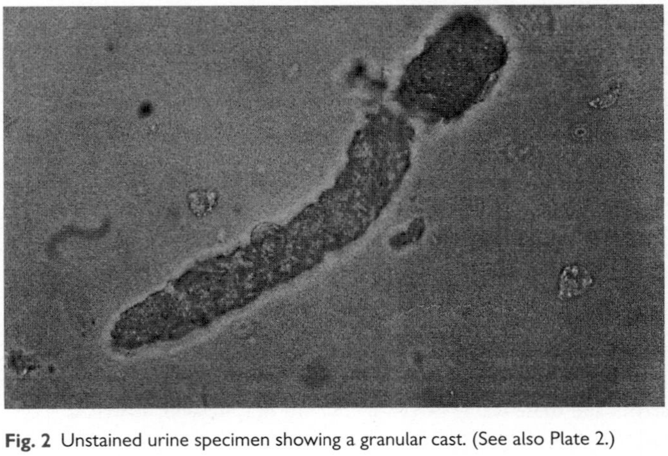

Fig. 2 Unstained urine specimen showing a granular cast. (See also Plate 2.)

leucocytes) can be found in proliferative glomerulonephritis, acute interstitial nephritis, and acute pyelonephritis.

Measurement of proteinuria

Quantification of proteinuria is important as the risk for progression of underlying renal disease to renal failure is related to the amount of protein in the urine. Traditionally, proteinuria has been measured using 24-h urine collections and expressed as grams per day (g/day). This has the advantage that it averages-out protein excretion, and is not therefore affected by the normal diurnal variation in protein excretion (less overnight and first thing in the morning) or urine concentration. Several different methods are used to measure the protein content of 24-h urine collections, ranging from the Biuret method, which uses a copper-based method to precipitate proteins, to dye-binding methods using Coomassie Brilliant Blue as the indicator. These are more accurate than the turbidimetric methods, which use trichloroacetic or sulphosalicylic acid and measure turbidity with a densitometer. Radiocontrast media, and some drugs (including penicillin, sulphonamides, and tolbutamide) may give false-positive results for proteinuria with the sulphosalicylic acid method. The Biuret method measures total proteins, the turbidimetric method provides different readings for albumin and globulins, and the dye-binding methods may do so also.

Testing spot urine samples for protein has been introduced to overcome the inherent problems of patient accuracy and reliability with 24-h urine collections. The urinary albumin concentration is measured by radioimmunoassay. Under resting conditions, urinary creatinine excretion is relatively constant throughout the day. Thus to overcome the problems of timing urinary collections, proteinuria in spot urine samples is expressed as an albumin:creatinine ratio (normal <2.0 mg/mmol creatinine in a daytime urine or 24-h collection, and <1.5 mg/mmol for an overnight or early morning sample). An albumin:creatinine ratio of 100 mg/mmol approximately corresponds to 1.5 g/day, and 350 mg/mmol to nephrotic-range proteinuria. Aside from their use to replace 24-h urine collections, spot urine collections are particularly useful in the diagnosis of orthostatic proteinuria, in other words where the patient has a normal urinary protein excretion when recumbent, or overnight, but has marginally increased proteinuria in the ambulant or daytime sample.

Microalbuminuria

Radioimmunoassays for albumin can detect an increased urinary albumin excretion in patients with normal levels of proteinuria. Normoalbuminuria is defined as an excretion rate of 20 μg/min or less. Proteinuria is usually detectable on dip-stick testing at rates of 200 μg/min or more, and thus microalbuminuria is defined as an excretion rate between 20 and 200 μg/min. The albumin excretion rate (**AER**) is some 25 per cent higher during the day than the night. There is a good correlation between the morning AER and the albumin:creatinine ratio in the first urine sample of the morning. The advantage of spot urines is that all patients can provide a sample when they attend the clinic. Provided the urine samples are taken at the same time, and the patient's dietary intake is relatively constant, then these samples are very useful in assessing patients over time. The advantage of measuring the albumin: creatinine ratio is that it eliminates the timing of urinary samples, which is important in calculating the AER. The albumin-:creatinine ratio can also be used to assess the progress of patients with proteinuria, especially if patients fail to collect 24-h urine samples properly.

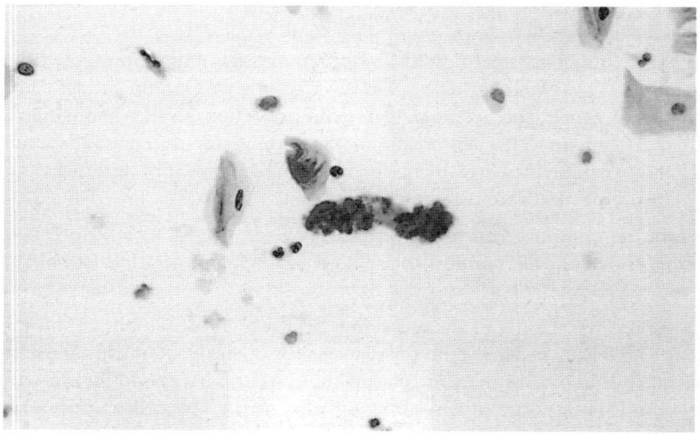

Fig. 3 Papanicolaou-stained urine deposit showing a red cell cast. (See also Plate 3.)

Microalbuminuria is not only an adverse factor for the progression of diabetic renal disease, but is also predictive of cardiovascular events in both the diabetic and non-diabetic population. In addition to diabetic subjects, microalbuminuria may be found in those with hypertension, cardiac failure, and following a pyrexial or viral illness. Similarly, microalbuminuria may be present in healthy subjects after exercise and during normal pregnancy.

Selectivity of proteinuria

Patients with glomerular disease typically have a non-selective proteinuria, with a similar clearance of both high and low molecular weight plasma proteins. However, those with minimal-change disease may have selective proteinuria, with clearance of predominantly small molecular weight proteins. The demonstration of selective proteinuria is useful in paediatric practice, where patients are often treated with steroids without a renal biopsy.

Most laboratories compare the clearance of IgG, as the large molecular weight protein (mol. wt 150 kDa), to that of albumin (or transferrin, mol. wt 88 kDa) as the low molecular weight protein. Both plasma and spot urine samples are required. Protein concentrations are measured either by laser nephelometry or radial immunodiffusion. Non-selective proteinuria is taken as a [IgG]U/[IgG]P × [transferrin]P/[transferrin]U ratio of 0.20 or more, whereas selective proteinuria is taken as a ratio of 0.10 or less (U is the protein concentration in urine, P the protein concentration in plasma).

Spill-over proteinuria

Patients with myeloma, some types of amyloidosis, and those with reticuloendothelial disorders may have a spill-over proteinuria, due to glomerular filtration of complete and incomplete kappa (_) and lambda (λ) chains and immunoglobulin light chains. These small molecular weight proteins are not detected by simple urine stick-testing, or by standard biochemical methods to determine urine protein concentration. Thus, when clinically appropriate, urine should specifically be sent for immunoelectrophoresis to exclude myeloma. However, light chains in particular may still not be detected, hence further investigation with specific antisera may be required if their presence is suspected.

Renal tubular proteinuria

Interstitial renal disease can result in proteinuria, usually less than 2 g/day. Proximal tubular injury leads to increased low molecular weight proteinuria, characterized by an excess of intestinal alkaline phosphatase, *n*-acetylglucosaminidase, retinol binding protein, tissue-specific alkaline phosphatase, α-glutathione *S*-transferase, α_1-macroglobulin, and β_2-microglobulin. By contrast, Tamm–Horsfall glycoprotein and α-glutathione *S*-transferase are increased in distal tubular injury.

β_2-Microglobulin is freely filtered at the glomerulus and then reabsorbed in the proximal tubule, such that less than 1 per cent of the filtered load is excreted in the urine of normal subjects (normal <370 μg/24 h). Thus urinary β_2-microglobulin excretion has been used as a marker of proximal tubular damage. However, β_2-microglobulin is unstable in urine, and its excretion can be affected both by an increased production rate (found in cases of myeloproliferative disease, chronic inflammatory states, and acute liver disease) and by saturation of β_2-microglobulin tubular uptake due to an excess of dibasic amino acids.

More reliable markers of tubular proteinuria are now available. These include α-glutathione *S*-transferase, α_1-macroglobulin, and retinol binding protein. Turbimetric or enzyme assays are now available. Results are expressed as either excretion rates (for example, normal α-glutathione *S*-transferase, <12.5 ng/min or <11.5 μg/l) or as a ratio to urinary creatinine (for example, normal reference range for retinol binding protein:creatinine, <0.019 mg/mmol).

These tests of renal tubular proteinuria are helpful in investigating patients with suspected Chinese herbal nephropathy, Asian subcontinent nephropathy, and Balkan nephropathy. Industrial workers exposed to heavy metals and organic chemicals, such as those used in the dry-cleaning industry, may develop interstitial renal disease characterized by increased urinary low molecular weight proteinuria.

Table 1 Compounds that can affect the measurement of plasma or urinary creatinine concentration

Endogenous compounds	Exogenous compounds
Protein	Acetohexamide
Ketones	Cephalosporins
Ketoacids	5-Fluorocytosine
Glucose	Methanol metabolites
Fatty acids	Phenylacetylurea
Urate	
Urea	
Bilirubin	

Estimation of renal function

Biochemical tests

Measurement of plasma creatinine is the standard biochemical test used to assess renal function. Unfortunately the plasma creatinine concentration is not linearly related to the glomerular filtration rate. Thus some 30 per cent of patients with significantly impaired renal function still have a plasma creatinine value within the normal range (<120 μmol/l).

Creatinine

Creatine, which is endogenously synthesized in the liver or exogenously supplied by meat in the diet, is transported to muscle and converted to creatinine by non-enzymatic dehydration. Muscle mass represents some 98 per cent of the total body creatine pool. Thus gender, racial and age-related differences in body composition, physical training and exercise, muscle-wasting diseases, paralysis, and intercurrent illnesses will all affect the production rate of creatinine, and therefore both the plasma creatinine concentration and urinary creatinine excretion. Hence, in young children there is a steady increase in the plasma creatinine level as their muscle mass increases. Dietary influences will affect plasma creatinine levels, with a reduction in strict vegans and increased values in those with a high meat intake (particularly stewed meat: cooking leads to the conversion of creatine to creatinine) or those taking creatine supplements. For any individual, the plasma creatinine level is relatively constant throughout the day, although there is a tendency for it to increase slightly in the afternoon.

Creatinine is not only freely filtered by the glomerulus, but is also secreted into the renal tubule. Creatinine reabsorption may occur at low urinary flow rates, such as in congestive cardiac failure. The relative proportion of renal tubular creatinine secretion to that filtered increases as renal function declines. In addition, in oedematous states such as nephrotic syndrome, calculated creatinine clearance exceeds inulin clearance, suggesting increased tubular creatinine secretion. Several drugs are known to block the tubular secretion of creatinine, and thus cause an increase in the serum creatinine level: these include the diuretics amiloride, spironolactone, and triamterene; and also cimetidine, aspirin, probenecid, and trimethoprim.

Most laboratories measure plasma creatinine using standard automated analysers, which assess the chromagenic product of creatinine and alkaline picrate (Jaffé reaction). Table 1 lists some substances which in high concentration can act directly or indirectly as chromogens, or affect the background control blanks, and so result in a spurious increase in the plasma creatinine level. In clinical practice these may lead to an overestimation of creatinine in poorly controlled diabetics, and an underestimation in deeply jaundiced patients, such as those with primary biliary cirrhosis. Under these circumstances a more accurate method is to determine the plasma creatinine level enzymatically.

Reciprocal creatinine or logarithm of creatinine values

As the plasma creatinine level roughly doubles for every 50 per cent reduction in glomerular filtration rate (**GFR**), expressing (transforming) the results as the reciprocal or logarithm is useful in assessing serial plasma values—this changes the graph from an exponential to a straight-line plot. The advantage of using a straight-line plot of plasma creatinine is that it allows the rate of renal decline to be calculated, which can then be used to predict the onset of endstage renal failure and the requirement for dialysis treatment in many patients. The reciprocal creatinine plot assumes a constant rate of loss, whereas the logarithm a constant fractional loss of renal function.

Patients with diabetic nephropathy tend to have a faster rate of decline in renal function than those with glomerular disease, who, in turn, have a faster rate than those with tubulointerstitial renal disease. In addition, it is easier to assess the effect of treatment interventions on the progression of renal disease by analysing transformed data, and also to recognize when there has been a sudden and unexpected deterioration in function that requires urgent investigation.

Prediction of creatinine clearance from the plasma creatinine level

Despite the potential inaccuracies in the determination of plasma creatinine, variations in endogenous creatinine production rates, and the relative increase in renal tubular and intestinal creatinine secretion with deteriorating renal function, formulas based on the plasma creatinine level are used in clinical practice to estimate creatinine clearance. The most common equation, validated in adults, is the formula of Cockcroft and Gault, later modified by Gault:

$$\text{GFR ml/min} = 1.2 \times [140 - \text{age (years)}] \times \text{weight (kg)}]/[\text{plasma creatinine concentration}]\ (\mu\text{mol/l}).$$

In the original formula, there was a different equation for women, with a factor of 0.85 (instead of 1.2) to allow for the lower rate of creatinine production in women due to differences in their body composition. Although these formulas may be helpful in clinical practice to provide an estimation of renal function, they are not always accurate, particularly in diabetic subjects and Afro-Americans (due to differences in body composition).

Creatinine clearance

In clinical practice, creatinine clearance remains the most commonly used parameter for assessing the GFR. However, this depends upon patient compliance to provide an accurate 24-h urine collection. Even when patients are in a steady state, urinary creatinine excretion varies from day to day, and reliability can be increased by performing consecutive daily clearances.

Creatinine clearance is calculated thus:

$$\text{creatinine clearance (ml/min)} = [\text{urine volume (ml/24 h)} \times \text{urine creatinine concentration } (\mu\text{mol/l})/\text{plasma creatinine concentration } (\mu\text{mol/l})] \times 24 \times 60.$$

As regards the use of the creatinine clearance measurement as an estimate of GFR, two errors tend to balance each other out. The chromagenic assay tends to overestimate the plasma, but not urinary, creatinine concentration, leading to an underestimation of GFR. By contrast, creatinine is not only excreted by glomerular filtration: some is secreted by the renal tubules, leading to an overestimation of the GFR. However, in patients with impaired renal function these contrasting effects are not balanced, and the relative increase in tubular creatinine secretion results in creatinine clearance exceeding GFR. This problem can be overcome by the administration of 400 mg of cimetidine to block renal tubular creatinine secretion, but this manoeuvre is rarely (if ever) performed in clinical practice solely for this purpose. By convention, creatinine clearance values are commonly corrected for body surface area to adjust for differences in muscle mass, assuming a fixed mathematical relationship between body surface area and the relative proportions of fat to muscle. However, body composition is not only age- and gender-dependent, but also varies from race to race, and other inaccuracies occur in oedematous states.

Cystatin C

Cystatin C is a low molecular weight basic protein (13.26 kDa) produced by all nucleated cells. The cystatin gene is a housekeeping gene and a member of the cystatin superfamily of cysteine proteinase inhibitors. Cystatin C is produced at a constant rate, and is not affected by acute inflammation, nutrition, gender, race, or changes in body mass. The production rate is stable over a wide age range, from infants older than 1 year through to the elderly, although there is a slight increase in the latter age group. As cystatin C is freely filtered by the glomerulus and is unaffected by renal tubular degradation or tubular secretion, it can be used as a marker of GFR. Rapid and fully automated accurate assays are now available, which have a superior analytical specificity and precision to that of serum creatinine.

Carbamylation

Urea accumulates with deteriorating renal function. In plasma, urea can spontaneously dissociate to form a reactive cyanate species which can react with the terminal valine of haemoglobin α and β chains (and also similar valine molecules in other proteins). This reaction is termed 'carbamylation' and the product 'carbamylated haemoglobin' (or other protein). Whereas glycosylated haemoglobin has proved useful in clinical practice for assessing time-averaged diabetic control, carbamylated haemoglobin or carbamyl-lysine adducts have not been shown to be superior to simple serum creatinine measurements in determining stable renal function. However, they are useful in helping to differentiate acute from chronic renal failure, because of the time course of the carbamylation reaction, and also in the assessment of time-averaged urea levels in the dialysis patient with endstage renal failure. However, until the relevant assays are commercially available, their use will remain experimental.

Isotopic methods

The glomerular filtration rate can be determined by the clearance of a compound which is freely filtered by the glomerulus and then passes through the nephron without tubular reabsorption or secretion. Traditionally, inulin—a naturally occurring polyfructose—was given as a constant infusion to achieve a constant plasma concentration, and then clearance determined from timed urinary collections. This was a considerable laborious technique. Furthermore, the biochemical estimation of inulin was initially tedious and difficult, with significant interassay variation, and accurate timed urine collections are unreliable in patients with urinary tract anomalies. To overcome these and other difficulties, compounds other than inulin are generally used to estimate GFR, and methods other than constant infusion.

Following a single bolus injection, depending on the compound used, the fall in plasma concentration follows either a single- or two-compartment model related to renal clearance. Chromium-labelled ethylenediaminetetraacetic acid ([^{51}Cr]EDTA) is the most commonly used isotope. After the single injection, three timed plasma samples are taken to calculate the plasma decay rate, and thereby the GFR. More recently it has been showed that for a GFR over 30 ml/min, only a single blood sample at 4 h is required. At GFRs above 30 ml/min there is a very good correlation between inulin and [^{51}Cr]EDTA clearance, but below 30 ml/min the accuracy of the isotope techniques is reduced, there being some renal tubular reabsorption. Accuracy can be improved in this situation by taking a delayed (24 h) plasma sample.

Other isotopes that have been used to estimate GFR include [^{125}I]iothalamate, which when given as a subcutaneous injection results in a constant plasma concentration equivalent to the infusion technique, and Tc^{99m}-diethylenetriaminepentaacetic acid (**DTPA**), which is less accurate due to its short half-life (6 h) and dissociation of DTPA from the radionuclide.

With all the isotopic methods, it is conventional for the GFR to be corrected for the size of the patient. This correction assumes a fixed relationship between the weight and height of an individual: hence serial estimations to detect a change in renal function are more likely to be accurate than single estimations.

Radiological methods

Iohexol is a non-ionic, low-osmolality, radiocontrast dye. It can be used to estimate glomerular filtration rate following a single bolus injection of between 2 and 5 ml. In patients with a clearance of over 30 ml/min, a single plasma sample taken 3 h after injection provides an accurate estimation, whereas additional later samples are required to improve the accuracy in those with severely impaired renal function.

Summary

When the plasma creatinine concentration is below 150 µmol/l, it cannot be used as an accurate assessment of renal function. When appropriate, an isotopic assessment of GFR is the most accurate method of determining GFR. Otherwise, two 24-h urine collections with corresponding plasma samples should be used to calculate the GFR, although in some centres cystatin C has replaced creatinine for the assessment of renal function. To examine changes in renal function, creatinine concentrations should be transformed to either the reciprocal or the logarithm to assess trends in serial results.

Renal blood flow

Renal blood flow can be estimated non-invasively using Doppler flow probes, provided there is a single renal artery and adequate imaging is possible. This is technically easier for the transplanted kidney than the native kidney. The recent development of contrast agents for ultrasound may increase the reliability of these estimations. Alternatively, renal blood flow can be estimated from the measurement of the renal plasma flow and the haematocrit. However, the haematocrit of peripheral venous blood may not be the same as that entering the renal artery.

Renal plasma flow

Ideally any compound used to assess renal plasma flow should have 100 per cent uptake by the kidney. Thus that fraction not filtered by the glomerulus must be extracted by the tubules and secreted. *p*-Aminohippurate is the most commonly used compound, but is only 85 per cent extracted during a single passage through the kidney, and thus at best only provides an estimate of renal plasma flow. Continuous infusion of *p*-aminohippurate provides a more accurate estimation of renal plasma flow than single injection techniques.

Renal blood flow varies in normal subjects with pain, stress, physical exercise, normal pregnancy, and following a high protein meal. In patients with impaired renal function, the decline in renal plasma flow generally corresponds to the decrease in GFR. However, in some conditions where there may be renal tubular hypoxia or toxicity, such as in patients with severe heart disease or those with ciclosporin nephrotoxicity, the reduction in estimated renal plasma flow is greater than that expected for the change in GFR, due to a reduction in the renal tubular uptake of *p*-aminohippurate. Similarly, *p*-aminohippurate uptake is reduced in small children. [^{125}I]*o*-Iodohippurate has also been used to estimate renal plasma flow, but this has a lower extraction than *p*-aminohippurate (75 per cent), and is less reliable.

Investigation of tubular function

In a normal subject, some 180 litres of glomerular filtrate is produced each day and less 3 per cent of this is excreted, due to reabsorption by the tubules. The proximal and distal tubules have different functions, and traditionally each is considered separately.

Proximal tubular function

Defects in proximal tubular function may be isolated or generalized, as in the Fanconi syndrome. Glucose, amino acids, phosphate, and organic ions are reabsorbed by the apical border of proximal renal tubular cells by sodium-dependent cotransporters, and then cross out from the basolateral membrane by different, sodium-independent, cotransporters.

Glucose

There is a maximum reabsorption rate for glucose (T_MG) in the proximal tubule of 15.1 ± 2.5 mmol/l (T_MG/GFR), above which glycosuria will be present. To determine TMG/GFR, a 20 per cent glucose infusion is administered at increasing rates to produce a slow rise in the plasma glucose up to a maximum of 30 mmol/l, which is maintained for a minimum of 1 h. Plasma and urine samples are collected every 30 min. Renal function is determined by [^{51}Cr]EDTA-GFR. The glucose absorption rate is calculated as the difference between the filtered load in urine (urine volume × $[\text{glucose}]_{\text{urine}}$) and the filtered load in plasma (GFR × $[\text{glucose}]_{\text{plasma}}$). Patients with type A renal glycosuria typically have a reduced threshold of around 5 mmol/l.

Phosphate

Phosphate is normally filtered at the glomerulus and reabsorbed in the proximal tubule, with only 10 to 20 per cent of the filtered load being excreted. The normal tubular reabsorption of phosphate (**TRP**) is above 85 per cent and can be calculated from:

$$\%\text{TRP} = \{1 - (\text{phosphate clearance/GFR or creatinine clearance})\}\times 100.$$

If renal function is normal, then this can be simplified by collecting an early morning specimen of urine, and:

$$\%\text{TRP} = \{1 - ([\text{phosphate}]_{\text{urine}} \times [\text{creatinine}]_{\text{plasma}}/[\text{creatinine}]_{\text{urine}} \times [\text{phosphate}]_{\text{plasma}})\} \times 100.$$

Alternatively, the theoretical maximum tubular threshold of phosphate (T_MP) can be estimated from:

$$T_MP/\text{GFR} = [\text{phosphate}]_{\text{plasma}} - ([\text{phosphate}]_{\text{urine}} \times [\text{creatinine}]_{\text{plasma}}/[\text{creatinine}]_{\text{urine}}),$$

or measured directly as for T_MG, following an infusion of phosphate (1.0 litre of 0.1 M sodium phosphate at pH 7.4) with a corresponding [^{51}Cr]EDTA-GFR.

Excessive urine phosphate losses occur in proximal tubular disorders such as the Fanconi syndrome, primary and secondary hyperparathyroidism. In the various forms of hypophosphataemic rickets, phosphaturia occurs with a characteristically reduced T_MP/GFR of less than 0.56 mmol/l.

Amino acids

Apart from the reabsoption of histidine (90–95 per cent), that of other amino acids is almost complete (97–99 per cent). Although amidoaciduria can occur as a result of overflow when the plasma concentration exceeds the tubular transport maximum, this is very rarely the cause of aminoaciduria in adults. In general, five types of renal aminoaciduria are distinguished: dibasic amino acids, neutral (monoaminomonocarboxylic acids) amino acids, glycine and imino acids, dicarboxylic amino acids, and generalized amino aciduria in the case of the Fanconi syndrome. Generalized and specific amino acidurias can be detected and quantified by thin-layer chromatography. In the Fanconi syndrome amino acids from all four groups are present, whereas there is only excess glycine in glycinuria. Classic cases of cystinuria have increased urinary arginine, ornithine, lysine, and cystine; and patients with Hartnup disease have an excess of neutral amino acids.

For more detailed discussion of other aspects of proximal tubular function and their diseases, see Chapter 20.8.

Distal tubular function

Patients with primary or secondary nephrogenic and/or cranial diabetes insipidus and those with primary polydipsia may present with polyuria. A water-deprivation test can help to differentiate between these conditions, and should be performed as follows. The patient should be admitted to a metabolic ward on the evening prior to the test, be weighed, and have samples taken for baseline plasma osmolality, chemistries, and arginine vasopressin measurement (**AVP**). An osmolality above 295 mosmol/kg and a sodium concentration above 143 mmol/l, excludes a diagnosis of primary polydipsia. After midnight, no oral fluids are allowed until completion of the test. The early morning urine osmolality is measured, and if it is above 800 mosmol/kg (normal response) the test is abandoned. Thereafter the weight, plasma and urine osmolality, and plasma AVP concentration should be recorded regularly. If weight loss exceeds 5 per cent, then the test should be abandoned to prevent dangerous dehydration. Once urine osmolality reaches a plateau (an hourly increase of less than 30 mosmol/kg for 3 consecutive hours), then 5 units of aqueous vasopressin is administered subcutaneously and urine and plasma osmolality measured after a further 30 min, and then at hourly intervals.

Comparison of the last urine osmolality reading prior to the administration of vasopressin with the maximum osmolality following vasopressin helps to categorize patients. Those with nephrogenic diabetes insipidus will produce a urine osmolality under 300 mosmol/kg with no response to exogenous vasopressin and have high AVP levels. Those with severe cranial diabetes insipidus will have dilute urine, again less than 300 mosmol/kg, but they will respond to exogenous vasopressin by increasing urine osmolality by 50 per cent or more, accompanied by low endogenous AVP levels. Both cranial and nephrogenic diabetes insipidus can occur as partial forms, which show some response to dehydration, but they can be discriminated by analysing the relative changes in endogenous AVP and the urinary and plasma osmolalities. Patients with primary polydipsia do not show pituitary suppression, and have little or no response to exogenous vasopressin.

Renally induced electrolyte imbalances

Sodium and water Hyponatraemia may occur both in patients with a reduced effective circulating plasma volume and those with the syndrome of inappropriate ADH secretion (**SIADH**). Patients with reduced renal perfusion, such as those with cardiac failure, chronic liver disease, nephrotic syndrome, and prerenal acute renal failure, will have a reduced fractional excretion of sodium (FE_{Na}) of less than 1 per cent (normal 1–2 per cent), where:

$$\%FE_{Na} = ([\text{Na}]_{\text{urine}}/[\text{Na}]_{\text{plasma}} \times [\text{Cr}]_{\text{plasma}}/[\text{Cr}]_{\text{urine}}) \times 100.$$

Those with SIADH preferentially retain water and have a normal FE_{Na}. However, when interpreting measurements of FE_{Na} it must be remembered that this is increased by diuretic administration and in chronic renal failure.

Both those with a reduced effective circulating plasma volume and those with SIADH have impaired free-water excretion, which can be tested by giving the patient 20 ml of water/kg body weight to drink after voiding. More than 75 per cent of the water load should be excreted within 3 h, and the urine osmolality should fall to under 100 mosmol/kg (specific gravity <1.003). This test can be affected by gastrointestinal disease, smoking, and emotional factors. The free-water clearance (C_{H2O}) can be quantitated from:

$$C_{H2O} = \text{urine volume (ml/min)} - [\text{osmolality}_{\text{urine}}/\text{osmolality}_{\text{plasma}} \times \text{urine volume (ml/min)}].$$

A positive free-water clearance occurs when the urine is more dilute than plasma, and a negative free-water clearance when the urine is more concentrated.

For further discussion of these issues, and the clinical approach to disorders of sodium and water homeostasis, see Chapter 20.2.1.

Potassium To determine whether there is a renal tubular cause for potassium disturbances, the transtubular potassium gradient (**TTKG**) can be calculated. This attempts to estimate the potassium concentration in the cortical collecting duct.

Using TTKG = $[\text{potassium}]_{\text{urine}} \times$ osmolality plasma/urine, a TTKG under 2 suggests a non-renal cause of hypokalaemia, whereas a high TTKG (>10) is associated with mineralocorticoid excess, Liddle's syndrome, or drugs such as acetazolamide, fludrocortisone, and amphotericin. A TTKG above 10 implies a non-renal cause of hyperkalaemia and a low TTKG (<2) would be found in cases of potassium-sparing diuretics, hypoaldosteronism, and pseudohypoaldosteronism. Whilst having theoretical attraction, it is doubtful whether such analysis helps greatly in the diagnosis or management of patients with hypokalaemia or hyperkalaemia. For further discussion of these issues, and the clinical approach to disorders of potassium homeostasis, see Chapter 20.2.2.

For more detailed discussion of other aspects of distal tubular function and their diseases, see Chapters 20.8 and 20.13.

Imaging of the patient with renal disease

Plain radiography

Plain abdominal radiographs may demonstrate opaque renal stones, nephrocalcinosis, and the renal outlines. Ultrafast, non-contrast CT scanning with three-dimensional reconstruction has generally replaced nephrotomograms for detecting low-opacity renal stones.

Chest radiography may be helpful in the diagnosis of pulmonary oedema, and also in demonstrating the cardiac silhouette and lung pathology sometimes associated with renal disease, such as pulmonary haemorrhage and cavitation. Multiple rib fractures may suggest multiple myeloma.

Intravenous urography

Although intravenous urography (**IVU**) is no longer the standard investigation in nephrology, it still has an important place in the investigation of patients with suspected obstruction of the urinary tract, as it does provide imaging of the entire urinary tract. As with all radiographic procedures, potential fetal irradiation should be avoided. Bowel preparation is no longer standard, due to the risks of dehydration in the elderly and of gaseous distension of the bowel obscuring the urinary tract. Even the newer non-ionic contrast media can cause nephrotoxicity in some patients, and care should be taken to ensure that those at risk (elderly and those with diabetes, myeloma, or a pre-existing renal impairment) are adequately hydrated. Normal renal length is between 3 and 4 lumbar vertebrae, with a width approximately half that of the length.

The IVU may provide valuable information about renal size and possible intrarenal masses. It remains the best method for investigating the patient with acute renal colic, and for assessing the level of any obstruction. Other techniques, such as ultrasound and ultrafast computed tomography (**CT**) scanning, can also be used to investigate renal colic—the main advantage of CT scanning being that it can detect other pathologies which mimic this condition.

The calyces and papillae are well demonstrated on the IVU, which may be diagnostic in cases of medullary sponge kidney, papillary necrosis, and sloughed papillae. Similarly, intraluminal radiolucent foreign bodies may be demonstrated surrounded by contrast, typified by radiolucent stones, blood clots, fungal ball, tumour, or sloughed papillae.

Abnormalities of the ureteric wall such as localized thickening are found in cases of transitional-cell carcinoma, oedema, tuberculosis, and parasitic granuloma. The IVU may also demonstrate external compression: this can be due to aberrant blood vessels in the upper tract, retroperitoneal fibrosis affecting the middle ureter, or prostatic pathology in the lower tract.

Other conventional uroradiological techniques

Further information about the site and nature of any obstruction can be obtained by ureteropyelography. This may be performed by an antegrade or a retrograde approach. An antegrade study involves percutaneous puncture of the renal pelvis, with immediate relief of the obstruction by nephrostomy, and allows demonstration of the site of obstruction following an injection of contrast media (antegrade ureteropyelography). A retrograde study requires cystoscopy, allowing direct visualization of the distal ureter, the possibility of removing an obstructing stone, and the passage of double JJ stents from below to relieve the obstruction. Injection of contrast media from below demonstrates the site of any obstruction (retrograde ureteropyelography). Antegrade techniques are usually more successful in relieving obstruction, particularly in those with pelvic malignancy or obstruction of a renal transplant. In cases when renal obstruction is considered, but investigation inconclusive, then a pragmatic trial of antegrade stent insertion should be undertaken. Improvement of renal function confirms obstruction.

Retrograde urethrocystography is performed in female patients to detect lower urinary tract abnormalities, such as fistulas or urethral diverticulae. Sequential films taken during micturition may detect active reflux. In males, urethrocystography can be complicated by trauma and infection to the lower urinary tract, and therefore suprapubic bladder puncture is recommended.

Renal ultrasonography

The normal kidney and chronic renal disease

The normal adult kidney is between 10 and 12 cm long, with a thin, bright capsule surrounded by highly reflective perinephric fat. The healthy cortex returns mid-level grey echoes, the pyramids are darker, and the renal sinus, containing fat and the major vascular pedicle, is bright with high reflectivity. Colour, flow Doppler can be used to visualize the flow of urine from the native ureters into the bladder. In most causes of chronic renal disease the kidneys become smaller, with reduced cortical thickness and increased reflectivity. Diastolic blood flow is reduced on the Doppler scan. The renal ultrasound appearances are characteristic in some conditions: these include focal segmental glomerular sclerosis secondary to HIV infection in which the kidney is reported to be large and the cortex uniformly of a high reflectivity, greater than that of the renal sinus. Scars, either vascular or infective, may often be too small to be detected by ultrasound examination, especially in the neonate.

Renal masses

Ultrasound is useful in the assessment of renal masses. Benign cysts have a smooth outline with well-demarcated borders and an echo-free centre, whereas renal tumours are usually irregular with heterogeneous echo reflectivity. Most tumours are vascular, with high flow during both systole and diastole on colour-Doppler scanning, and adenocarcinomas in particular may be seen to extend into the renal vein. Renal transitional-cell carcinomas are not readily detected unless large, as ultrasound does not visualize individual calyces well. Angiolipomas may have a characteristic appearance due to their fat content which has high reflectivity, but confirmatory CT scanning is required.

In adult polycystic kidney disease, the kidneys are typically enlarged with multiple bilateral cysts. Middle-aged women may also have hepatic cysts. It is important to remember that, if patients are scanned in their teenage years or before, then cysts may not have developed or they may be below the level of resolution for ultrasound detection. Haemorrhage, infection, or malignant change all result in complex echoes within cysts, which cannot be differentiated by ultrasound scanning. Autosomal recessive, polycystic renal disease can be detected *in utero* with antenatal scanning.

There is an increased incidence of cystic change in the kidneys of patients with endstage renal disease, and occasionally these cysts may become malignant. It has been recommended that dialysis patients should be screened by ultrasound every 3 years, and then annually if cystic changes develop.

Urinary obstruction

In most centres, ultrasonography of the urinary tract is the first investigation performed when an obstruction is suspected. When urinary obstruction has been present for some time, the high reflectivity of the central renal sinus becomes replaced by echo-free urine, with distention of the calyces. However, it is important to recognize that in acute obstruction, and in cases where the kidney and ureter are encased (usually the result of tumour), the standard ultrasound examination may appear normal. In these circumstances, a colour-Doppler scan may show reduced diastolic blood flow due to increased intrarenal pressure; also absence of the normal pulsatile jets of urine from the ureter into the bladder on the side with the acute obstruction. Ultrasound is not usually diagnostic of the cause of obstruction, but it may detect para-aortic nodes, a bladder mass, prostatic enlargement, or a ureterocele. Further investigation with transvaginal, transrectal, or transurethral ultrasound may confirm the cause of obstruction, transrectal ultrasound being particularly useful in the detection of local invasion from prostatic carcinoma.

Urinary tract stones

Renal stones appear on ultrasound as a bright echogenic focus with a distal acoustic shadow. Ultrasound can be used to follow up patients with renal calculus disease by assessing the number and size of stones. Nephrocalcinosis may result in an increase in medullary echoreflectivity due to calcium deposition, which usually affects the whole medulla, whereas calcification from papillary necrosis has an appearance more like that of a renal stone.

Renovascular disease

Colour Doppler can be used to investigate renal arterial and venous disease. Thrombosis of major vessels produces absent flow or changes to the intrarenal blood flow pattern. More recently, colour-Doppler scanning has being used as a screening test for renovascular disease, with changes at the site of stenosis characterized by an increase in the peak systolic frequency followed by a diastolic spectral broadening. The sensitivity and specificity of this test has not been determined, and it remains a 'research' rather than a 'standard' clinical investigation.

Renal transplantation

Ultrasound examination is an important investigation in the management of the renal transplant recipient. Early graft dysfunction mandates investigation to exclude a technical problem with either the renal artery or vein, or a urinary leak. Colour-Doppler scanning provides valuable information about the vascular supply of the graft (Fig. 4). Fluid collections (commonly lymphoceles) appear as echo-free or echo-poor areas, and perinephric collections can be drained under ultrasound guidance for diagnostic purposes or to relieve obstruction. As with the native kidney, percutaneous nephrostomy is the emergency treatment of choice for obstruction of the renal transplant. Colour-Doppler scanning can detect the presence of arteriovenous fistulas, not uncommon following transplant biopsy.

Contrast agents for ultrasound

Colour-Doppler ultrasound can detect bubbles present in injected contrast medium. Application of this technique can change the use of ultrasound from simple anatomical visualization of the kidneys to dynamic testing. This will allow ultrasound to determine relative renal function, and improve investigation for obstruction and renovascular disease.

Computed tomography (CT) scanning

Computed tomography has advantages over conventional intravenous urography by imaging the perirenal and retroperitoneal spaces, and differentiating soft tissues within the kidney. Ultrafast CT scanning, without contrast, is being used more frequently to image ureteric renal stones and define the site of ureteric obstruction. In addition, CT provides vital information regarding the cause of ureteric obstruction by imaging the ureter, retroperitoneal space, and pelvis. Spiral, or helical CT scanning allows a three-dimensional reconstruction of the images, overcomes respiratory artefacts, and is useful in the investigation of congenital and anatomical abnormalities of the renal tract, such as renal agenesis. High-resolution CT scanning may detect early nephrocalcinosis, before calcification can be detected on plain films. These imaging techniques can be enhanced by contrast to give additional information: for example, simple renal cysts do not change in density following contrast, but occlusion of vessels may be demonstrated (Fig. 5).

Apart from the investigation of cystic renal disease, CT scanning is used to investigate renal masses. Renal-cell carcinomas vary in appearance: some show calcification both within and surrounding the tumour on non-enhanced scans, some are solid, and others are cystic or have necrotic centres. The majority of tumours are vascular and readily enhance with contrast, but those with heavy calcification may not. CT scanning is important in tumour staging, in determining the extent of perirenal spread, renal vein involvement, and enlargement of local lymph nodes. Occasionally, secondary deposits due to metastatic spread and secondary involvement in lymphomas and leukaemia, can be found on contrast-enhanced scans. These are usually small multiple intrarenal masses, often bilateral, typically homogenous, and solid in lymphomas. Although ultrasound is used to screen and assess Wilms' tumours in children, CT scanning is important in excluding pulmonary metastases.

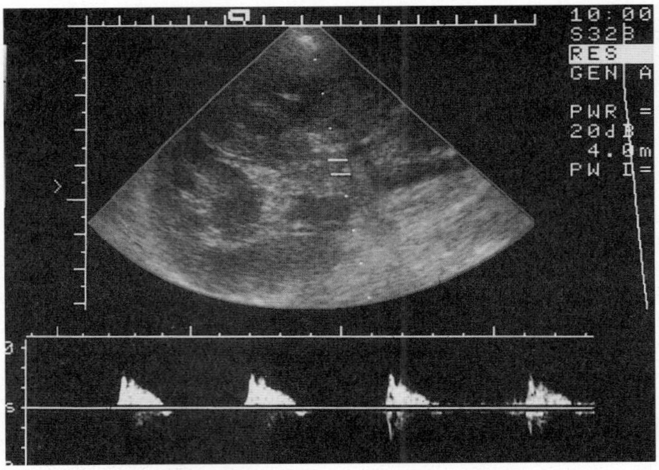

Fig. 4 Doppler ultrasound of a renal transplant showing normal systolic and diastolic wave forms.

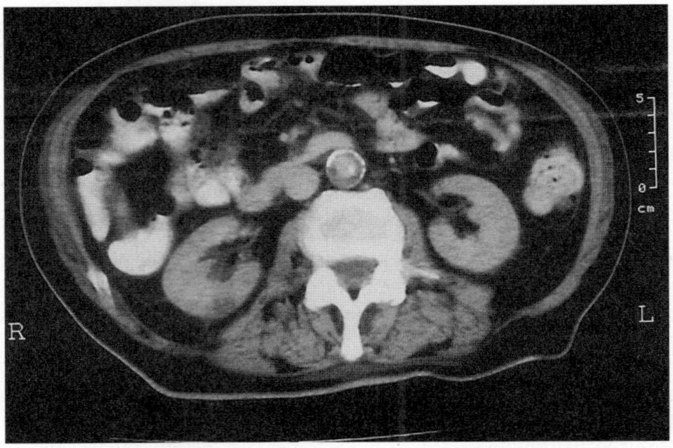

Fig. 5 Contrast-enhanced CT scan showing thrombosed aorta and renal arteries.

Angiolipomas can be recognized with ultrasound, but should be confirmed on CT scanning as some renal-cell carcinomas may contain small amounts of fat. In tuberous sclerosis, angiolipomas may be associated with renal cysts. Although angiolipomas are benign mesenchymal tumours, they can rarely rupture, especially those with intrarenal haematomas and aneurysms. Early detection by CT scanning allows prophylactic embolization of these vascular lesions.

Renal oncocytomas, are another benign renal tumour, and on CT scanning may have a central lucent area due to fibrosis. However, a proportion of oncocytomas may become malignant. Thus any small renal lesion which is not a simple cyst or angiolipoma must be regarded as potentially malignant and therefore surveillance with repeat CT scanning (or ultrasound) should be recommended.

Renal tract imaging in patients with acute pyelonephritis is usually requested to exclude the presence of an obstruction, or when there has been an inadequate response to treatment. CT scanning defines the extent of disease better than ultrasound, detects abscesses, and can also exclude obstruction. Whereas focal acute bacterial pyelonephritis should respond to antibiotics, renal abscesses may require drainage. CT scanning may also detect gas bubbles within the renal parenchyma or perirenal space, characteristic of emphysematous pyelonephritis, typically found in diabetics. Similarly, CT scanning may establish a diagnosis of xanthogranulomatous pyelonephritis, with an enlarged kidney containing areas of scarring, focal loss of renal parenchyma, and multiple low-density masses, often following recurrent infections in patients with staghorn calculi.

In cases where renal trauma is suspected, contrast-enhanced CT scanning provides information not only about renal anatomy and function, but also perirenal collections, differentiating blood from urine. In addition, CT scanning provides valuable information about trauma to other intra-abdominal structures.

Magnetic resonance imaging (MRI)

CT scanning and ultrasound are good reliable techniques for detecting and evaluating renal masses. MRI is an alternative in patients who are allergic to conventional iodine-based radiocontrast media or those at risk of contrast nephropathy. The gadolinium contrast used in MRI is taken up by the proximal tubule, in a similar manner to aluminium, but has not been shown to cause nephropathy. MRI is expensive, but does have some advantages over conventional CT. Tissues surrounded by fat, such as enlarged lymph nodes, or tumour extension into the renal vein, are better demonstrated on MRI than CT. Thus MRI is useful in staging renal-cell carcinoma, and by being able to distinguish blood from tissue can help to differentiate simple cysts complicated by haemorrhage from those that are malignant.

The whole of the urinary tract can be visualized, in a manner similar to an IVU, by using a heavily weighted T_2 fast spin–echo sequence. This rapid acquisition and relaxation enhancement scan can be used to assess potential live donors for renal transplantation, by demonstrating the renal vasculature, renal anatomy, and urinary drainage with one investigation.

The quality of image provided by MRI can be very high (Figs 6 and 7).

Angiography and digital subtraction angiography (DSA)

Formal renal angiography remains the 'gold standard' technique for assessing renovascular disease (Fig. 8). With the advent of expandable renal artery stents, it is important to determine precisely the anatomy of any stenosis, so that appropriate intervention can be planned. Direct pressure measurements can be made either side of any stenosis, so that the degree of stenosis can be assessed both anatomically and functionally. However, renal angiography is not without hazard: it involves an arterial puncture, the use of potentially nephrotoxic contrast agents, and carries the risk of dislodging aortic and renal artery plaques, which can result in intrarenal, intra-abdominal, and peripheral cholesterol embolization.

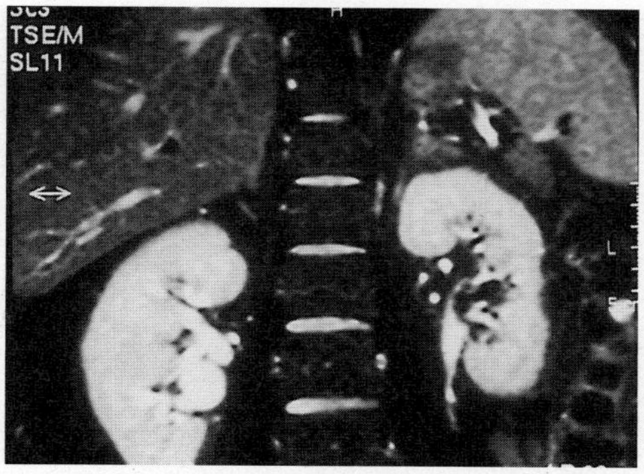

Fig. 6 Gadolinium-enhanced MRI showing left-sided pyelonephritic scarring, with a reduction in cortical thickness and scarring.

Aside from the investigation of suspected chronic renovascular disease, renal arteriography can be indicated in the investigation of sudden renal ischaemia due to renal artery thrombosis or dissection, aortic dissection with extension into the renal arteries, or trauma to the renal artery. In addition, renal and coeliac arteriography can establish a diagnosis of classical macroscopic polyangiitis nodosa. Occasionally renal angiography is helpful in assessing renal tumour vascularity, and in determining whether partial nephrectomy can be performed. In some cases of persistent non-glomerular haematuria, formal renal angiography reveals a vascular abnormality as the underlying cause.

Digital subtraction angiography (DSA) uses a venous injection of contrast and computer-derived images to view the major renal arteries and intrarenal vessels. High doses of contrast media may be required, even so insufficient anatomical definition is obtained in between 5 and 20 per cent of cases. Thus, with appropriate indications, DSA is a good screening test but may need to be followed by formal angiography.

Interventional renal arteriography

Interventional renal arteriography should only be undertaken by experienced interventional radiologists with the support of vascular surgeons, as

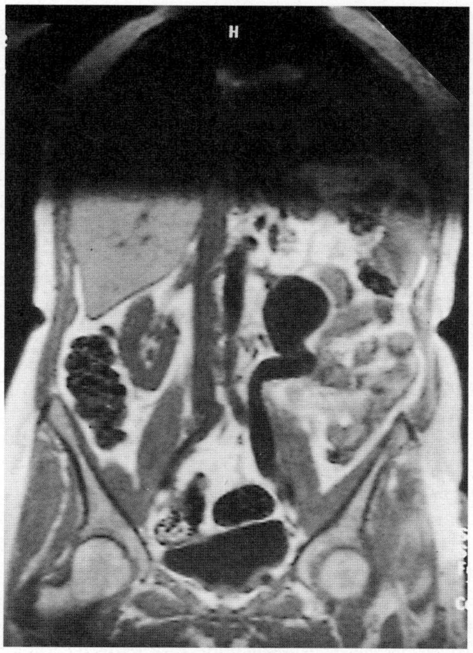

Fig. 7 Gadolinium-enhanced MRI showing a hydronephrotic left kidney and dilated upper two-thirds of the ureter following gynaecological surgery.

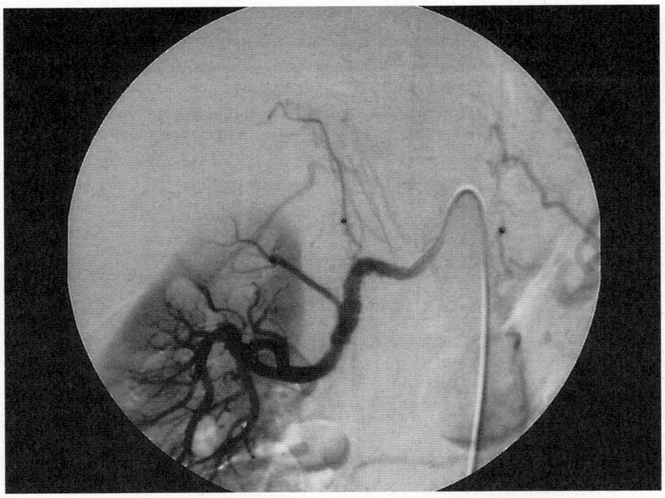

Fig. 8 Renal arteriogram showing fibromuscular hyperplasia of the renal artery.

renal artery dissection or rupture may occur. Embolization with gel foam or metal coils can be used to selectively control renal haemorrhage, which is particularly useful when this follows renal biopsy, and also in cases of arteriovenous malformation or tumour. Occasionally a whole kidney is embolized. Some renovascular stenotic lesions can be usefully treated by transluminal angioplasty or stenting.

Spiral CT angiogram

Spiral CT, by taking pictures which are then reconstructed by computer to provide a three-dimensional picture, can be used to investigate renal vascular disease. Radiocontrast is required, which can be administered by arterial or peripheral venous injection. To reduce the risk of contrast-induced nephropathy, or the possibility of 'flash pulmonary oedema' due to an intravenous volume load, some centres use carbon dioxide gas as the contrast agent. Compared to standard renal angiography, spiral CT renal angiography tends to overestimate any stenosis. The overestimation is greater with carbon dioxide than conventional contrast. However, this is a useful technique for excluding significant renovascular and intrarenal vascular disease.

Magnetic resonance angiography

Magnetic resonance angiography (**MRA**) using gadolinium chelates is indicated when there is a clinical risk of the patient developing contrast-induced nephropathy with standard renal or spiral CT angiography. MRA overemphasizes any stenotic area or other vascular abnormality. Thus MRA is useful in confirming normality, and is used in the preoperative assessment of living related kidney donors. A normal MRA of the renal arteries excludes renal artery stenosis, intrarenal vascular disease, and polyarteritis nodosa.

Magnetic resonance venography

As with MRA, magnetic resonance venography (**MRV**) using gadolinium contrast can be used to assess renal venous patency. Patients with nephrotic syndrome, and those with renal adenocarcinoma, may develop renal venous thrombosis, which can be difficult to positively diagnose with other imaging techniques.

Renal venography

Selective renal venous catheterization for blood sampling is still useful in patients with severe renovascular disease. The relative renal vein renin concentrations may aid the decision-making process in deciding whether to perform a surgical or medical nephrectomy in a patient with a small poorly functioning kidney due to severe renal artery stenosis.

Nuclear medicine

Static imaging

Radiolabelled dimercaptosuccinic acid (DMSA)

Technetium-labelled dimercaptosuccinic acid binds to renal proximal tubular cells, and after an intravenous injection some 70 per cent of the dose is taken up by viable tubules within 3 to 4 h. This can be detected by a gamma camera. DMSA scans provide information about the relative function of each kidney, and show areas of scarring due to renal stone disease, infection, and vascular disease. In children with urinary tract sepsis, suspected of reflux nephropathy, then serial DMSA scans are used to assess progressive cortical scarring. During acute pyelonephritis the DMSA scan may appear to show scars. These photopenic areas are due to inflammation and increased intrarenal pressure and can return to normal following resolution of infection. DMSA scans are also used to confirm the congenital absence of a kidney, to detect ectopic kidneys and other congenital malformations such as horseshoe kidney, and to confirm absence of renal function.

More recently, the introduction of single-photon emission computed tomography (**SPECT**) DMSA scans has improved resolution. These have shown that renal scars occur more frequently than previously thought, both in patients with acute pyelonephritis and also following lower urinary tract infection in renal transplant recipients.

Dynamic imaging

Radiolabelled diethylenetriaminepentaacetic acid and hippuran

Technetium-labelled diethylenetriaminepentaacetic acid (**DTPA**) or ^{131}I-labelled hippuran are both filtered by the glomerulus and then rapidly excreted by the kidney. These renograms have three phases: vascular, accumulation within the kidney, and excretion. Renal artery stenosis and acute tubular necrosis can reduce uptake, flattening the second and third phases of the renogram. Similarly, intrinsic renal disease flattens the second phase, and makes interpretation difficult when renal function is impaired.

Radiolabelled DTPA and hippuran scans are used to assess urological obstruction (Fig. 9). Occasionally patients with polycystic kidney disease

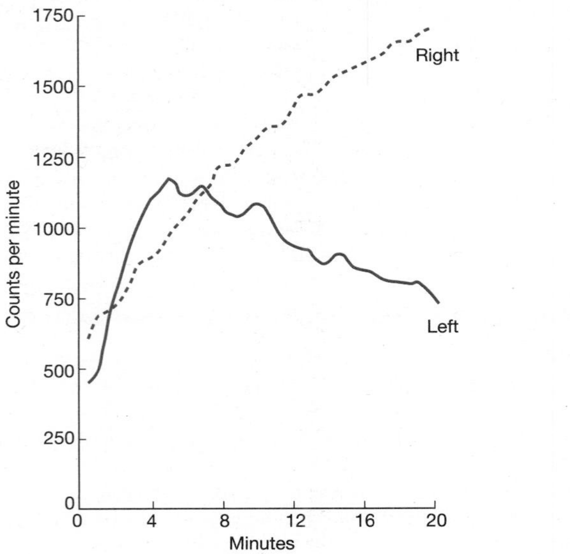

Fig. 9 DTPA renogram showing increasing uptake by the right kidney in a case of right-sided ureteric obstruction.

present with severe pain due to the obstruction of a cyst, and DTPA scanning provides a dynamic test to confirm obstruction. In patients with dilated collecting systems, it is important to a differentiate congenital megaureter from an obstructed system. Excretion may be slow due to pooling in a dilated system, but obstruction is unlikely if there is a brisk wash-out following the administration of intravenous furosemide. Patients with impaired renal function may have a reduced response to furosemide, making interpretation of the renogram less reliable. Thus, in cases with impaired renal function, direct pressure measurement within the renal pelvis following percutaneous puncture may be required to exclude partial obstruction (Stamey test).

DTPA scans are also used to detect reflux in children, as reflux may be demonstrated during the 'emptying' phase of the renogram. If not, then an indirect micturating cystogram can be performed using the radioactivity which has passed into the child's bladder.

Following renal transplantation, DTPA and hippuran isotope scans can be used to monitor graft function. In cases of major arterial or venous thrombosis, and hyperacute rejection, the graft appears to have no perfusion. Acute tubular necrosis, rejection, and immunophylin toxicity may all have similar appearances. Serial scans can help to differentiate these conditions. DTPA scans may also reveal perirenal and urinary leaks before they are clinically manifest. Later isotope scans may detect obstruction due to ureteric stenosis.

Radiolabelled mercaptoacetyltriglycine (**MAG3**)

Technetium-labelled mercaptoacetyltriglycine ([^{99}Tc]MAG3) is protein-bound, and renal excretion is both by glomerular filtration and renal proximal tubular secretion. The excretion pattern is similar to that of hippuran and DTPA. The advantage of MAG3 is that it provides better image definition than DTPA and hippuran, especially in those with impaired renal function. Thus MAG3 can be used to provide both anatomical (as DMSA) and functional (as DTPA and hippuran) information (Fig. 10).

Patients with renal artery stenosis may have a delay in uptake time (the time taken from injection to peak activity) and an increased intensity and duration of MAG3 accumulation (due to increased tubular salt and water reabsorption, not seen in the case depicted in Fig. 10). If there is major stenosis of a major branch artery, then perfusion to one pole may be delayed. To improve the sensitivity and specificity of the MAG3 renogram in the detection of renal artery stenosis, some centres employ a method whereby two scans are performed—one with, and one without, prior administration of captopril. The captopril–MAG3 renogram can also be used as a screening test to determine whether the use of angiotensin-converting enzyme inhibitors or angiotensin II receptor blockers might be detrimental to renal function in patients with an increased risk of atheromatous renovascular disease, including those with severe cardiac failure or diabetes and elderly hypertensive patients.

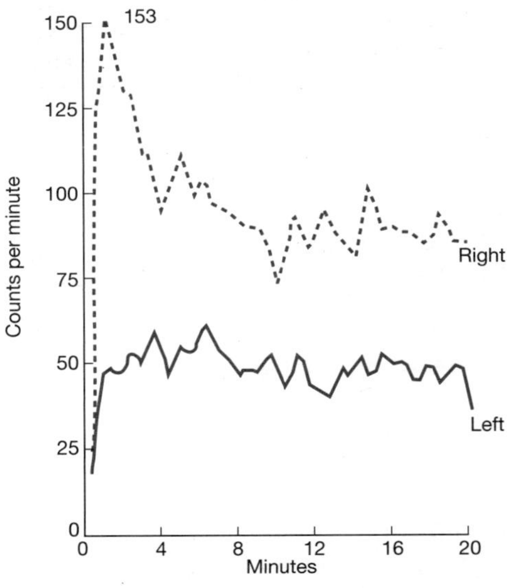

Fig. 10 MAG3 renogram demonstrating reduced uptake by the left kidney in a case of left-sided renal artery stenosis.

Other isotopes

Methyldiphosphonate (**MDP**) is filtered by the glomerulus, providing an immediate dynamic renogram. It is later taken up by inflamed muscles (found in patients with myositis and rhabdomyolysis) and the skeleton (detecting single or multiple bone metastases, and also metabolic bone disease in patients with endstage renal failure).

Renal biopsy

Indications

A renal biopsy should be considered in any patient with disease affecting the kidney when the clinical information and other laboratory investigations have failed to establish a definitive diagnosis or prognosis, or when there is doubt as to the optimal therapy. All renal biopsies have the potential to result in morbidity and (on rare occasions) mortality. The risk of biopsy must therefore be outweighed by the potential advantages of the result to the individual patient. Biopsies which would be 'of interest', but 'not in the patient's interest', should not be performed. Indications for renal biopsy should therefore be considered on an individual basis. Table 2 sets out the clinical presentations that warrant native renal biopsy.

Diabetic patients with proteinuria would not normally be biopsied, unless they had other conditions suggesting there might be an alternative or additional diagnosis to diabetic nephropathy. Most paediatricians would treat small children presenting with nephrotic syndrome with steroids, and only consider renal biopsy if they did not respond to treatment. Some conditions, in particular lupus nephritis and membranous glomerulonephritis, may change histological grading, so requiring repeat biopsy.

Renal biopsy is an important investigation in the management of the renal transplanted patient. Postoperative oliguria requires urgent investigation to differentiate acute ischaemic tubular necrosis from immunophylin (ciclosporin or tacrolimus) or other drug toxicity, acute rejection (vascular and/or cellular), or even frank infarction. Further biopsies may be required to monitor the response to antirejection therapy, and at a later stage to examine for recurrence of the original renal disease, or *de novo* glomerulonephritis in the graft.

Contraindications

Percutaneous renal biopsy should not be undertaken in patients with polycystic kidney disease. Similarly, patients with renal masses, such as tumours or cysts, should only be biopsied under direct vision, either by real-time ultrasound or CT scanning, or by formal open surgical biopsy. Patients with a solitary (or solitary functioning) native kidney are normally considered for open surgical biopsy.

Haemorrhage is more likely to occur in patients with uncontrolled hypertension, hereditary or acquired coagulation disorders, and those taking anticoagulants or antiplatelet agents. Blood pressure should be controlled and coagulation abnormalities treated before biopsy. Patients with renal amyloid also have an increased risk of haemorrhage, as may those with classic polyarteritis nodosa.

Patients with chronic renal failure and bilaterally small kidneys should not undergo biopsy. This would be technically difficult (the kidneys are small and hard) and the biopsy appearances of endstage renal failure are exceedingly unlikely to provide any information that might alter the clinical course or management. Percutaneous renal biopsy should not be performed in patients with untreated acute pyelonephritis due to the risk of developing a perinephric abscess.

Technique

'Blind' biopsy of the native kidney, meaning biopsy without imaging for localization, should not be performed unless there are truly exceptional circumstances. It is possible to visualize the kidney and biopsy under fluoroscopic control after injection of radiocontrast medium as for an IVU, but the most commonly used method for directing biopsy is ultrasound guidance. This can either be used to record the depth of the lower pole from the skin and mark the surface position vertically above it on inspiration, or to provide real-time guidance. The latter technique is described below.

Percutaneous renal biopsy should be carried out using sedation and local anaesthesia. Children may require general anaesthesia. The patient should be placed prone on top of pillows or folded sheets to compress the upper abdomen and lower ribs and fix (to some degree) the position of the kidneys. Under real-time ultrasound the kidneys are visualized, the patient asked to take and hold a deep breath in inspiration, and the kidney which is thought to be technically the most easy to biopsy is targeted. To avoid the major vessels, the aim should be for the lateral border of the lower pole. Either 14- or 18-gauge, trucut-type needles are commonly used, some centres now use an automated spring-loaded biopsy gun. Under direct vision the needle tip is advanced to the renal capsule, and with the kidney fixed in inspiration, biopsy is performed. The advent of colour Doppler means that the operator can deliberately avoid the major intrarenal vessels.

Transjugular biopsy can be performed in patients who have an increased likelihood of bleeding complications. Technical developments have now allowed biopsy needles to be passed reliably from the renal vein into the renal cortex, such that in our own institution all such biopsies in the last 3 years have been diagnostic. Occasionally, open surgical biopsy is required, with the biopsy taken under direct vision and local bleeding controlled.

Renal transplants, usually placed in one or other iliac fossa, are biopsied in the supine position. Pillows can be placed under the side with the transplant to help move bowel and fat pad away from the transplant. Biopsies are taken from the lateral border of the upper pole, avoiding the major vessels and ureter.

The obvious risk of renal biopsy is haemorrhage. All patients should be placed on strict bed rest for at least 6 h after the procedure, and pulse and blood pressure should be checked frequently during this period. Hypotension, tachycardia, abdominal/back pain, and macroscopic haematuria are indications for urgent medical review.

Table 2 Indications for native kidney biopsy

Asymptomatic proteinuria	
≤1.5 g /day	+ controlled hypertension + dysmorphic haematuria + ↓ glomerular filtration rate + any combination of the above
Asymptomatic proteinuria	
>1.5 g/day	
Nephrotic syndrome	
Microscopic haematuria	
dysmorphic haematuria	hereditary condition insurance company requirement patient request + proteinuria + hypertension + ↓ glomerular filtration rate
Acute renal failure	
exclude ischaemic ATN	+ abnormal urinary sediment + proteinuria +ve ANCA/ANA/anti-GBM severe hypertension no obvious cause prolonged history
presumed ischaemic ATN	delayed recovery
Chronic renal failure	
reasonable equal-sized kidneys	+ proteinuria + dysmorphic haematuria
Known renal diagnosis	
reasonable equal-sized kidneys	sudden unexplained ↓ GFR unexplained ↑ proteinuria

Notes: Indications may be clear-cut (e.g. acute renal failure of unknown cause with abnormal urinary sediment; adult with nephrotic syndrome) but they are not always so, and not all nephrologists would recommend biopsy in all of the circumstances listed (e.g. many would elect not to biopsy, but to arrange continued monitoring, for patients with asymptomatic proteinuria and stable renal function).

ATN, acute tubular necrosis; ANCA, antineutrophil cytoplasmic antibody; ANA, antinuclear factor; GBM, glomerular basement membrane; GFR, glomerular filtration rate.

Complications

Postbiopsy scanning has shown that the vast majority of patients develop a perirenal haematoma, which is usually asymptomatic. Arteriovenous fistulas may also develop acutely following biopsy. The majority disappear spontaneously with time, and only the occasional one requires treatment by the interventional radiologist. Macroscopic haematuria occurs in fewer than 10 per cent of patients, and bleeding sufficient to warrant blood transfusion in around 1 per cent. Rarely, severe haemorrhage may require treatment with the insertion of coils or gel foam embolization. Exceptionally, death may occur, usually due to the failure to detect haemorrhage and provide appropriate resuscitation.

Complication rates are increased in patients with both acute and chronic renal failure. Uraemia prolongs the bleeding time, even when the conventional coagulation screening is normal (prothrombin time, activated partial thromboplastin time, and peripheral platelet count). The risk of uraemic haemorrhage can be at least partially reversed prior to biopsy by good dialysis to improve platelet function, correction of the haematocrit and any underlying coagulation defect, and by giving an infusion of deamino-D-arginine vasopressin (**DDAVP**; desmopressin) immediately prior to the procedure (0.3 μg/kg over 30 min).

Further reading

Urine microscopy

Birch DF, *et al.* (1994). *A color atlas of urine microscopy*, 1st edn. Chapman and Hall, London.

Fogazzi GB, *et al.* (1993). *The urinary sediment. An integrated view.* Masson, Milan.

Renal function

Davison AM, *et al.* (1997). *Oxford textbook of nephrology*, 2nd edn. Oxford University Press, Oxford.

Randers E, *et al.* (1998). Serum cystatin C as a marker of the renal function. *Scandinavian Journal of Clinical and Laboratory Investigation* **58**, 585–92.

Seldin DW, Giebisch G (1992). *The kidney physiology and pathology*, 2nd edn. Raven Press, New York.

Valtin H, Schafer JA (1994). *Renal function*, 3rd edn. Little Brown, Boston, MA.

Renal imaging

Allan PL, Dubbins P, Pozniak MA (1997). *Clinical Doppler ultrasound.* Churchill Livingstone, Edinburgh.

Ghantous VE, *et al.* (1999). Evaluating patients with renal failure for renal artery stenosis with gadolinium enhanced magnetic resonance angiography. *American Journal of Kidney Diseases* **33**, 36–42.

Helenon O, *et al.* (1997). Renovascular disease: Doppler ultrasound. *Seminars in Ultrasound* **18**, 136–42.

Testa HJ, Prescott MC (1996). *Nephrourology, British Nuclear Medicine Society*, 1st edn. BPC Wheatons, Exeter.

20.4 Acute renal failure

J. Firth

The clinical approach to the patient with acute renal failure

Introduction

Acute renal failure is defined as a significant decline in renal excretory function occurring over hours or days. This is usually detected clinically by a rise in the plasma concentration of urea or creatinine. Oliguria, defined (arbitrarily) as a urinary volume of less than 400 ml/day, is usually present, but not always. Acute renal failure may arise as an isolated problem, but much more commonly occurs in the setting of circulatory disturbance associated with severe illness, trauma, or surgery; transient renal dysfunction complicates some 5 per cent of medical and surgical admissions. A community-based study conducted during 1993 reported that the incidence of severe acute renal failure in adults (serum creatinine >500 μmol/l) was 172 per million, rising from 17 per million in those under 50 years of age to 949 per million in those aged between 80 and 89 years. A recent (year 2000) study from renal units and intensive care units (ICUs) in a defined geographical area of Scotland found that 131 patients per million per year required renal replacement therapy for acute renal failure. There are many possible causes (Tables 1, 2, and 3), but in any given clinical context few of these are likely to require consideration.

Diagnosis of the presence of acute renal failure

A high index of clinical suspicion is required to diagnose acute renal failure at an early stage of its development. This is because symptoms and signs attributable to the accumulation of fluid, electrolytes, acid or uraemic wastes within the body may not be apparent until the condition is far advanced. Furthermore, the symptoms and signs that may arise are not specific: unsuspected hyperkalaemia is the greatest danger, since this may produce no symptoms whatsoever before causing cardiac arrest.

All patients admitted to hospital with acute illness should be considered at risk of developing acute renal failure. Those who have some pre-existing chronic impairment of renal function are particularly susceptible to acute exacerbations. This group includes all elderly patients, in whom a combination of low muscle mass and low dietary meat consumption may conspire to maintain an apparently 'normal' plasma creatinine level, despite a reduction in glomerular filtration rate to as little as 25 per cent of that expected in a healthy young adult.

To recognize impairment of renal function early, the basic care of all acutely ill patients should include careful monitoring of fluid input and output, daily weighing, lying and standing (or sitting) blood pressure, and regular estimation of plasma creatinine, urea, and electrolytes. Although it might seem to the physician to be a simple matter to monitor fluid input and output, this simplicity is often only present in theory, excepting in patients who are restricted to parenteral fluids and who have a urethral catheter. Drinks may be spilt, extra drinks may be acquired from a variety of sources, urine may be spilt, and vomit and diarrhoea are often found in places where they are difficult to quantitate. These considerations mean that the most likely explanation for fluid balance charts being difficult to interpret is the erroneous recording of input or output. Daily weighing on accurate scales provides a much more reliable picture of net overall fluid

Table 1 Some causes of acute renal failure

Prerenal uraemia
'Acute tubular necrosis':
following haemodynamic compromise, commonly with sepsis
following exposure to nephrotoxins: including drugs, chemicals, rhabdomyolysis, snake bite (see Tables 7 and 8)
Vascular causes:
acute cortical necrosis
large-vessel obstruction
small-vessel obstruction: accelerated-phase hypertension and systemic sclerosis
Glomerulonephritis and vasculitis
Interstitial nephritis
'Haematological' causes:
haemolytic uraemic syndrome/thrombotic thrombocytopenic purpura
myeloma
Hepatorenal syndrome
Urinary obstruction:
intrarenal—crystalluria
postrenal—renal stones, papillary necrosis, retroperitoneal fibrosis, bladder/prostate/cervical lesions

Table 2 Causes of development of acute impairment of renal function in 2216 consecutive medical and surgical admissions

Acute tubular necrosis	
Hypovolaemia	22
Congestive cardiac failure	10
Sepsis	10
Nephrotoxins	25
Postsurgical	23
Other	12
Hepatorenal syndrome	5
Obstruction	3
Vasculitis	2
Other/multifactorial/unknown	17
Total	129 (5.8% of admissions)

Acute impairment of renal function was diagnosed when the serum creatinine concentration rose by a predetermined amount (approximately one-third of the baseline) during the period of hospital admission.

During the period of study, 46 patients were excluded from analysis because they were either admitted specifically for treatment of acute renal failure or were recipients of long-term haemodialysis.

Dialysis was required in 10 cases. (Modified from Hou *et al.* 1983.)

Table 3 Causes of acute renal failure requiring renal replacement therapy at a single centre between 1956 and 1988

	Number of patients (% total)	Diagnoses present (% patients)	
Surgical	638 (47.5)	General surgery	445 (33.1)
		Surgical sepsis	126 (9.4)
		Urinary obstruction	116 (8.6)
		Trauma	94 (7.0)
		Cardiovascular surgery	81 (6.0)
		Malignancy	52 (3.9)
		Pancreatitis	24 (1.8)
		Burns	17 (1.3)
General medical	285 (21.2)	Sepsis	112 (8.3)
		Acute liver disease	44 (3.3)
		Salt and water depletion	43 (3.2)
		Ischaemic heart disease	36 (2.7)
		Diabetes mellitus	30 (2.2)
		Others	53 (3.9)
Renal parenchymal disease	166 (12.4)	Polyarteritis	31 (2.3)
		Crescentic nephritis	25 (1.9)
		Haemolytic uraemic syndrome	21 (1.6)
		Proliferative glomerulonephritis	19 (1.4)
		Histology unknown	19 (1.4)
		Systemic lupus erythematosus	15 (1.1)
		Others	36 (2.7)
Obstetric	142 (10.6)		
Poisoning	112 (8.3)		
Total	1343 (100)		

Modified from Turney JH *et al.* (1990). The evolution of acute renal failure, 1956–1988. *Quarterly Journal of Medicine* **74**, 83–104.
Some patients fell into more than one diagnostic category.
During the period of study there were significant changes in case-mix. Between 1980 and 1988, the following categories were more frequent: general medical (33.2% of all cases) and cardiovascular surgery (15.1%); and the following categories were less frequent: general surgery (26.4%), trauma (2.8%), and obstetric (1.3%).

balance. Patients who are acutely ill invariably lose flesh weight, commonly at a rate of up to a few hundred grams per day. If weight appears to fall at a rate faster than this, then negative fluid balance is likely: the occurrence of greatly increased 'insensible' losses through the skin and lungs during fever being a common explanation. Aside from weight loss, the development of a postural drop in blood pressure is a reliable sign that a patient has become significantly volume-depleted. If weight rises at any time, then this must be due to positive fluid balance, whatever the input/output charts may suggest. It may not be obvious from clinical examination where the fluid has gone: the possibilities of sequestration in the peritoneal cavity or in the tissue interstitium should be recognized.

Plasma urea, creatinine, and electrolytes should be measured on admission in all acutely ill patients, and repeated daily or on alternate days in those who remain so. These measurements will ensure that advanced acute renal failure does not seem to have occurred 'suddenly' in patients already in hospital. However, many patients will be found to have significant renal impairment on admission, and many more will develop some degree of renal impairment whilst on the ward. In all cases the physician must try to make a precise diagnosis of the cause.

Diagnosis of the cause of acute renal failure

In the initial assessment of a patient who appears to have acute renal failure three questions should be asked.

Question 1: is the renal failure really acute?

The only basis for excluding the possibility of pre-existing chronic renal impairment with absolute confidence is the knowledge of a previous normal measurement of renal function. In cases where there is uncertainty, a diligent search for previous notes and biochemical information may save the patient and the doctor the inconvenience (and occasionally hazard) of unnecessary investigation. The finding of two small kidneys on ultrasound examination indicates the presence of chronic renal disease. Other clinical features are poor discriminators between acute and chronic renal impairment. A history of vague ill health of some months' duration, of nocturia, of pruritus, or the findings of skin pigmentation or anaemia would all suggest chronicity (see Section 20.5). However, anaemia is not invariable in chronic renal failure (for example, in polycystic kidney disease the haemoglobin concentration may be normal), and anaemia can develop over a few days in acute renal failure, as may hypocalcaemia and hyperphosphataemia. Radiological evidence of renal osteodystrophy is only found in patients with obviously long-standing renal failure and never aids the clinical distinction between acute and chronic renal failure.

Question 2: is urinary obstruction a possibility?

One of the merits of the traditional division of the causes of acute renal failure into prerenal, renal, and postrenal is that it encourages consideration of the possibility of urinary obstruction, which in community studies accounts for about 25 per cent of severe acute renal failure cases, mostly due to prostatic obstruction.

It is extremely important that obstruction should not be missed, since most cases are readily treatable and delayed diagnosis may lead to permanent renal damage. Obstruction is particularly likely to cause acute renal failure in those with a single functioning kidney, in those with a history of renal stones or of prostatism, and after pelvic or retroperitoneal surgery, but the possibility of obstruction should be seriously considered in all cases where another positive diagnosis cannot be made. The presence of anuria, or of alternating polyuria and oligoanuria, are helpful clues. However, it is not widely appreciated that a patient may pass normal or elevated volumes of urine despite significant obstruction, although this is extremely rare. The mechanism is poorly understood, but three factors present in obstruction tend to impair urinary concentrating ability, thereby leading to the preservation of urinary volume despite obstructive depression of the filtration rate. These factors are structural damage to the inner medulla and papilla, functional changes in the distal nephron resulting from increased intraluminal or interstitial pressure, and loss of medullary hypertonicity at low filtration rates.

Ultrasound examination of the kidneys and bladder is the usual first method of investigation for the presence of obstruction. However, it is important to remember that the quality of the image obtained by renal ultrasonography is highly variable, depending on the patient, the equipment, and the operator. Furthermore, ultrasound detects calyceal dilatation, not obstruction, and the test may be 'negative' (because the calyces fail to dilate, or do so only minimally) in about 5 per cent of cases of acute obstructive renal failure. If doubt as to the diagnosis persists in the clinician's mind, then the examination should be repeated, and other investigations pursued if uncertainty still remains. If renal function is adequate (creatinine concentration less than about 250 μmol/l) then **DTPA** (diethylenetriaminepentaacetic acid) or **MAG3** (mercaptoacetyl triglycine) renography with furosemide (frusemide) injection may be helpful, showing delayed excretion and clearance of radionucleide from the obstructed kidney(s). If renal function is severely impaired then imaging modalities that depend upon renal excretion (including intravenous pyelography) are not useful, and percutaneous antegrade nephrostomy/pyelography or cystoscopy with retrograde ureteric catheterization and pyelography should be undertaken. (See Chapter 20.14 for further discussion.)

Obstruction, once diagnosed, must be relieved urgently by bladder catheterization, percutaneous nephrostomy, or cystoscopic insertion of ureteral stents, as a prelude to definitive treatment (where possible) of the underlying obstructive lesion. The most important causes of urinary obstruction are renal calculi, retroperitoneal fibrosis, and malignant diseases of the uterine cervix, prostate, bladder, and rectum (see Chapter 20.14).

Question 3: are glomerulonephritis, interstitial nephritis, vasculitis, or other rarities possible?

To make these diagnoses, which although rare have critically important management implications, stick testing of the urine and microscopy of the urinary sediment is an essential part of the assessment of any patient with unexplained acute renal failure. If stick testing indicates more than + of protein or more than a trace of blood, then a sample of urine should be examined under the microscope. This should be done by centrifuging 10 to 15 ml of urine at 1500 to 2500 r.p.m. (approximately 400 to 1120 g) for 5 min, carefully discarding all but 1 ml of the supernatant, and then resuspending the pellet. Examination should be made under high power, preferably after staining, which makes the cellular elements of casts more obvious. Red cell casts (Fig. 1) are present in acute glomerulonephritis, renal vasculitis, accelerated-phase hypertension, and (sometimes) in interstitial nephritis, but not in other conditions. Their presence indicates the need for urgent specialist renal referral.

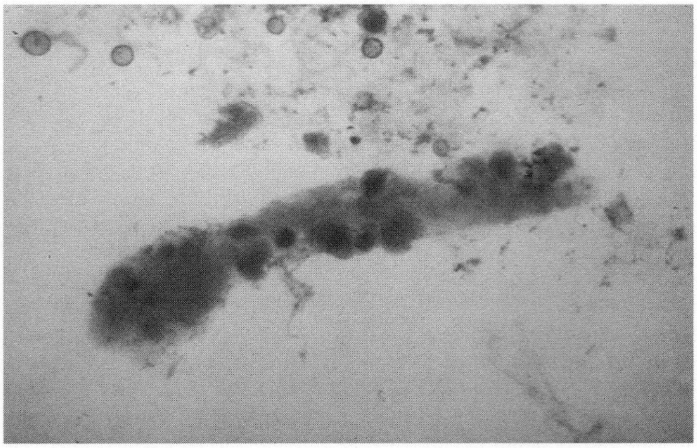

Fig. 1 A red cell cast. The red cells incorporated in the cast, which has a typical cylindrical appearance, look dark in this tone image due to staining with a blue dye.

Clinical features of acute renal failure

In the early stages of acute renal failure there are few warning symptoms. The patient may notice a reduction in urinary volume, but non-oliguric renal failure comprises as many as 50 per cent of cases in some series, and most patients who are unwell do not drink as much as usual and therefore are not concerned if they pass little urine. The clinical picture is likely to be dominated by the primary condition, of which acute renal failure is a complication, and by the effects of intravascular volume depletion, with dizziness caused by postural hypotension a common reason for patients being brought to medical attention.

In the later stages of acute renal failure there are manifestations of uraemia with anorexia, nausea, vomiting (or occasionally diarrhoea), muscular cramps, and signs of encephalopathy—including a 'metabolic' flapping tremor (asterixis), progressing in extreme cases to depressed consciousness and *grand mal* convulsions. Skin bruising and gastrointestinal bleeding may occur. Uraemic haemorrhagic pericarditis is another potentially fatal complication, but this occurs much less frequently in acute renal failure than in (neglected) chronic renal failure.

Biochemical changes

The clinical diagnosis of renal failure, acute or chronic, is made when the plasma urea and creatinine concentrations rise. Other important biochemical changes include the development of hyperkalaemia, metabolic acidosis, hypocalcaemia, and hyperphosphataemia. Hyperkalaemia is due not only to reduced urinary excretion, but also to potassium release from cells—either as a consequence of cell death or as a result of metabolic acidosis. Particularly rapid rises are to be expected when there is extensive tissue damage or hypercatabolism, as in rhabdomyolysis, burns, and sepsis. Transfusion of stored blood is sometimes said to cause dangerous rises in plasma potassium concentration in oliguric patients. However, the transfused blood may not really be to blame, but the circumstances that demand transfusion. Loss of blood into the gastrointestinal tract or body tissues is followed by red cell lysis and the absorption of a considerable potassium load.

Protein catabolism produces sulphuric and phosphoric acids. These are normally buffered by bicarbonate and excreted by the kidney. In acute renal failure these systems fail, leading to the development of acidosis. This is usually modest in degree (plasma pH 7.2–7.35), but can be more severe, manifesting as sighing Kussmaul respiration and/or with circulatory compromise. Acidosis is sometimes the metabolic abnormality most obviously necessitating urgent institution of renal replacement therapy, but overzealous administration of bicarbonate should be avoided (see below).

Calcium malabsorption occurs early in acute renal failure and is probably secondary to disordered vitamin D metabolism. Hypocalcaemia can develop with surprising rapidity. It is usually asymptomatic, but tetany and fits may be provoked by injudicious over-rapid correction of acidosis with resultant depression of ionized calcium. Profound hypocalcaemia and marked hyperphosphataemia, together with hyperuricaemia, is to be expected in rhabdomyolysis. Transient hypercalcaemia is frequently seen during the recovery phase from acute renal failure, and this is particularly common after rhabdomyolysis, probably being caused by secondary hyperparathyroidism related to preceding hypocalcaemia. The hypercalcaemic phase may be prolonged and accompanied by metastatic calcification in patients in whom there has been extensive muscle injury.

The plasma sodium concentration is usually normal in cases of acute renal failure: any deficit of sodium is usually matched by that of water, thus leading to reduction of the extracellular fluid volume but with an unchanged plasma sodium concentration. However, on occasion the intake of water, either drunk in response to thirst or inflicted iatrogenically, may exceed the rate of excretion such that hyponatraemia results.

The retention of uric acid, sulphate, and magnesium occurs in acute renal failure, but these biochemical abnormalities are rarely clinically significant, with the exception of the grossly elevated levels of uric acid that can be seen in rhabdomyolysis and following tumour lysis.

General aspects of medical management

The immediate management of the patient with renal impairment is directed towards three goals. The first is the treatment of any life-threatening complications of acute renal failure. The second is prompt diagnosis and treatment of hypovolaemia. The third is specific treatment of the underlying condition: if this persists untreated then renal function will not improve.

Life-threatening complications

Hyperkalaemia (see also Chapter 20.2.2)

Hyperkalaemia is most commonly dangerous in the context of acute renal failure, and is important because it can cause cardiac arrest. Patients may occasionally notice muscle weakness or paralysis, but the significance of these symptoms is rarely appreciated, and usually there are no symptoms whatsoever. All doctors who work with acutely ill patients should be able to recognize the characteristic electrocardiogram (**ECG**) appearances, which are a better indicator of cardiac toxicity than the serum potassium level. As serum potassium rises, the following changes progressively occur (Fig. 2):

(1) 'tenting' of the T wave;

(2) reduction in size of P waves, increase in the PR interval, widening of the QRS complex;

(3) disappearance of the P wave, further widening of the QRS complex;

(4) irregular 'sinusoidal' ECG;

(5) asystole.

Treatment of hyperkalaemia is described in Table 4.

Pulmonary oedema

The most serious complication of salt and water overload in acute renal failure (usually iatrogenic) is the development of pulmonary oedema. Severe cases are dramatic. The patient is terrified, restless, and confused. Examination reveals cyanosis, tachypnoea, tachycardia, widespread wheeze or crepitations in the chest, and a gallop rhythm (if the heart can be heard). Investigation demonstrates arterial hypoxaemia and widespread interstitial shadowing on the chest radiograph. (See Chapters 15.15.2.2 and 16.1 for further discussion.)

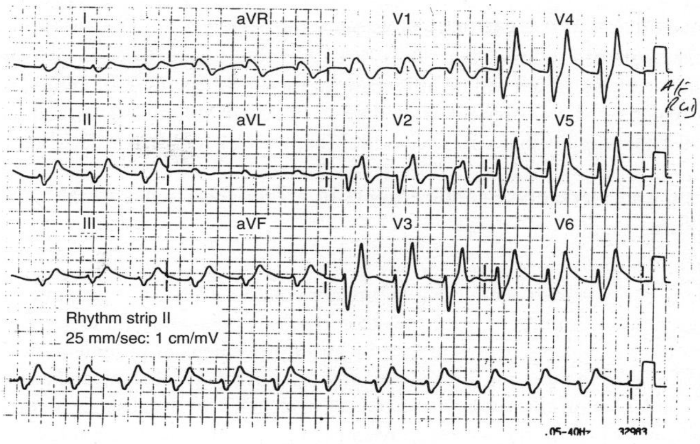

Fig. 2 An electrocardiogram showing severe hyperkalaemic changes in a patient with a serum potassium level of 8.6 mmol/l.

The patient should be sat up and supported, and given oxygen by face-mask in as high a concentration as possible using a reservoir bag. Furosemide (frusemide) may work as a venodilator but is unlikely to provoke a substantial diuresis in a patient with renal failure. Morphine can relieve symptoms rapidly and should be given in small (2.5 to 5 mg) doses, repeated if necessary and if tolerated, and with the opioid antagonist naloxone to hand in the event of deterioration due to toxicity. An intravenous infusion of a venodilator such as isosorbide dinitrate may be helpful.

The definitive treatment for pulmonary oedema caused by renal failure is the removal of fluid by haemodialysis or haemofiltration. Acute peritoneal dialysis is much less effective in this capacity and should only be considered in circumstances where haemodialysis and haemofiltration are not available. The immediate beneficial effects of venesection of 200 to 400 ml of blood from the patient *in extremis* should not be forgotten.

Table 4 Treatment of hyperkalaemia

Treatment		Comment
1.	Intravenous calcium (10 ml of 10% calcium gluconate, over 60 s, repeated until ECG improves)	The treatment to be given immediately if hyperkalaemia is associated with ECG changes more severe than 'tenting' of the T wave. Acts instantly to 'stabilize' cardiac membranes (mechanism unknown). Does not alter serum potassium
2.	Intravenous insulin and glucose (10 units of rapidly acting insulin plus 50 ml of 50% glucose, over 10 min)	Insulin stimulates Na–K-ATPase in muscle and liver, thus driving potassium into cells. Serum potassium falls by 1–2 mmol/l over 30–60 min
3.	Nebulized salbutamol (10–20 mg)	β-Agonists stimulate Na–K-ATPase in muscle and liver, thus driving potassium into cells. Serum potassium falls by 1–2 mmol/l over 30–60 min
4.	Intravenous sodium bicarbonate (50–100 ml of a 4.2% solution, over 10 min)	Traditionally thought to act by increasing blood pH, inducing exchange of intracellular protons for extracellular potassium. May not work in this manner since hypertonic saline has been shown to be effective. Only to be used if there is severe acidosis that merits treatment in its own right (see text for discussion). Glucose/insulin and salbutamol are equally effective and do not have the disadvantages of (1) requiring a large sodium load, and (2) being severe chemical irritants ('burns' requiring surgical debridement and reconstruction can occur if concentrated bicarbonate gets into tissues from peripheral intravenous lines)
5.	Cation exchange resins, e.g. sodium or calcium polystyrene sulphonate (15 g by mouth every 6 h or 15–30 g per rectum every 6 h)	Exchanges sodium or calcium for potassium in the gut lumen and thus induces loss of potassium from body (unlike 1–3 above). Takes 4 h to produce an effect. Precautions against severe constipation are necessary
6.	Haemodialysis/filtration	Except in those rare cases where renal function can be rapidly restored (e.g. relief of obstruction), it is likely that hyperkalaemia will recur and haemodialysis or high-volume haemofiltration will be required

Recognition and treatment of volume depletion

A key part of the immediate assessment and management of any patient who is very ill, which will include many of those with acute renal failure, is to make a correct assessment of the intravascular volume status and to resuscitate rapidly and effectively. (See Chapter 16.1 for further details.)

Fluid and electrolyte requirements in established acute renal failure

Fluid

Many patients with acute renal failure are volume-depleted at the time of presentation. An urgent priority is to correct such depletion rapidly. Once this has been achieved—as judged by an improvement in peripheral perfusion, a fall in pulse rate, loss of postural drop in blood pressure, and a rise in jugular venous pressure—the perspective changes. In the absence of normal renal function the greatest care must be taken to regulate the intake of fluids and electrolytes to match losses in the urine, from the gastrointestinal tract, and from other 'insensible' sources. As a working rule, fluid intake is limited to the volume of the previous day's urine output and gastrointestinal losses, plus 500 ml, but this allocation may need to be substantially increased in the presence of fever or in hot environments, when insensible losses may be much increased. However, as discussed above, fluid-balance charts are frequently inaccurate and unthinking adherence to the 'output plus 500 ml' rule can lead to grief. There is no substitute for careful, twice-daily clinical examination for signs of intravascular volume depletion or excess, supplemented by accurate daily weighing to gauge the overall net fluid balance, and an intelligent flexible response to the findings.

Sodium

In the patient who is not being dialysed, the intake of sodium must also be matched to output. Requirements are usually very small in those who are oliguric, perhaps only 15 to 30 mmol/day, but if the patient is polyuric the requirements can be considerable, with a danger of volume depletion if these are not met. The urine of a patient with polyuric renal failure will usually contain sodium at a concentration of 50 to 70 mmol/l, hence if urine output is 3 litres/day then over 200 mmol of sodium may be required. On occasion, the urine output in polyuric acute renal failure can be massive (even up to 1 litre/hour)—if the response is to administer an even greater quantity of fluid (output plus insensible losses), then it is possible to contrive a vicious cycle whereby an ever-increasing urinary output is rewarded by ever-increasing fluid infusion. To avoid this situation in the patient with polyuria it is best to limit input to urinary output alone, thus allowing other fluid losses to establish a mild overall negative balance, only increasing fluid input if the patient develops significant postural hypotension, which should be checked for twice daily. For unknown reasons, an excess of sodium and water in patients with tubular necrosis leads to peripheral or pulmonary oedema, whereas in those with glomerulonephritis it tends to produce hypertension.

Potassium

Because hyperkalaemia is one of the most important problems in the management of acute renal failure, it is essential to check plasma potassium levels at least daily, and in those with hypercatabolism or gastrointestinal bleeding, or who require surgery, more frequent estimations are advisable. In oliguric cases, dietary consumption should be limited to the minimum compatible with an adequate intake of protein and amino acids (20–30 mmol/day).

Diuretics that work on the distal tubule (for example, spironolactone, amiloride, and triamterene) promote potassium retention: they should never be used in renal failure, and it is important when reviewing the drug chart to remember that these agents are frequent constituents of tablets containing a combination of diuretic/antihypertensive compounds. Intravenous preparations of antimicrobial agents that contain large amounts of potassium should also be avoided whenever possible.

Excretion of potassium can sometimes be enhanced in those who are oliguric by the use of high doses of furosemide (0.5–1 g daily). Oral potassium-exchange resins (e.g. Calcium Resonium), prescribed concurrently with a laxative, can be useful in controlling serum potassium for a few days or weeks, but they are not effective treatments for acute severe hyperkalaemia (see Table 4) and are usually found to be unpalatable for long-term use. By contrast, in polyuric acute renal failure substantial losses of potassium can occur and need to be replaced. Measurement of the urinary potassium concentration can be helpful in estimating how much potassium is required.

Renal replacement therapy

Mandatory indications for immediate instigation of renal replacement therapy are:

(1) refractory hyperkalaemia;

(2) intractable fluid overload;

(3) acidosis producing circulatory compromise;

(4) overt uraemia manifesting as encephalopathy, pericarditis, or uraemic bleeding.

These indications will be present in some patients on their admission to hospital. However, in most cases renal function will be seen to decline over a period of days or a few weeks despite optimal medical therapy. In this situation there is no hard and fast rule as to when renal replacement therapy should be initiated. There is no level of nitrogenous waste at which the patient suddenly becomes susceptible to overt uraemic sequelae. Nevertheless, it is clearly not sensible to wait until an obvious uraemic complication (which might be fatal) arises. Modern practice is (whenever possible) to begin renal replacement therapy when the blood urea reaches 25 to 30 mmol/l and the serum creatinine 500 to 700 μmol/l, unless there is clear evidence that spontaneous recovery is occurring. There are three basic options for renal replacement therapy: peritoneal dialysis, haemodialysis, and haemofiltration.

Peritoneal dialysis

Peritoneal dialysis is technically the simplest form of renal replacement therapy and is commonly used worldwide, although remarkably little has been published recently about its use in those with acute renal failure. The principle is the same as that described for the long-term treatment of patients with chronic renal failure (see Section 20.5), the major differences being: (1) that catheters are used which can be inserted percutaneously using a metal stylet (although some use the same type of catheter as that used for continuous ambulatory treatment); and (2) that smaller volume exchanges with shorter dwell-times are the norm. The technique requires an intact peritoneum and is therefore precluded in the many patients whose renal failure is associated with abdominal surgery. Other problems include difficulties in maintaining dialysate flow, leakage, peritoneal infection, protein losses, and restricted ability to clear fluid and uraemic wastes. These limitations mean that, particularly in the hypercatabolic patient, peritoneal dialysis is frequently unable to provide good dialysis of the patient with acute renal failure as judged by modern standards. It is fair to say that peritoneal dialysis is virtually never the first choice modality for renal replacement therapy in an adult with acute renal failure in those centres that have a range of techniques at their disposal.

Haemodialysis and haemofiltration

Traditional haemodialysis, which is usually performed on alternate days but may be associated with better outcome when applied daily, can provide good control of uraemia in patients with acute renal failure who do not have severe haemodynamic compromise. The major disadvantage and limitation of the technique (apart from cost) arises from the fact that it is intermittent: in each 4-h treatment at least 2 to 3 litres of fluid must typically be removed to make 'space' either for the infusion of drugs/parenteral fluids or for oral fluid intake during the 24- to 48-h period before the next dialysis. This imposes a substantial haemodynamic stress, which often cannot be tolerated by those who are cardiovascularly unstable, and is the main reason why continuous haemofiltration techniques have largely replaced haemodialysis in intensive care units.

The standard haemofiltration technique works as follows: a mechanical pump (but sometimes the patient's own arterial pressure) drives blood through a haemofilter of high hydraulic conductivity. An ultrafiltrate of plasma is removed, usually at a rate of between 1 and 2 litres per hour. This is replaced, minus the volume of other fluid inputs and the amount of 'negative balance' required, using (most commonly) a lactate/acetate-based substitution fluid. The process is tolerated well, even by patients who are very ill, and the continuous nature of the technique permits continuous fine tuning of the intravascular volume. A large number of technical variations are possible—for example, combination of filtration and dialysis elements (haemodiafiltration), use of differing replacement fluids—but there is nothing to suggest that any one of these is better than another, excepting in those who are unable to metabolize lactate, when bicarbonate-based substitution fluid is essential.

In the same way that there is no evidence on which to make firm recommendations as to when to start renal replacement therapy in those with acute renal failure whose chemistry is gradually 'going off', there is also little information on which to base targets for the clearance of metabolic wastes that should be achieved by treatment. One recent study compared the outcome of patients treated with different doses of venovenous haemofiltration: those randomly assigned to ultrafiltration at a rate of 20 ml/h per kg did less well than those receiving 35 ml/h per kg or 45 ml/h per kg, there being no significant difference between the latter two groups.

Other issues in the management of patients with acute renal failure

Indications for renal biopsy

Most cases of acute renal failure are due to prerenal failure or to the clinical syndrome of acute tubular necrosis. They occur in an appropriate clinical setting and follow a typical time course, with recovery of renal function over a few weeks. In such instances renal biopsy should not be performed, since the information gained is exceedingly unlikely to influence management, and the risks of the procedure are therefore not warranted. There are, however, circumstances in which renal biopsy is essential to establish a correct diagnosis, with important implications for both management and prognosis. Biopsy should be considered when:

(1) the history, examination, or laboratory tests suggest a systemic disorder that could cause acute renal failure and could be diagnosed by renal biopsy;

(2) the urine sediment contains red cell casts;

(3) the case history is atypical; and

(4) renal failure is unusually prolonged (say beyond 6 weeks), although in this context cortical necrosis (see below) is better diagnosed by computed tomography (**CT**) scanning or angiography.

Nutrition

Patients with acute renal failure are invariably catabolic and derive a larger fraction of their energy expenditure from protein breakdown than normal. Insulin resistance, metabolic acidosis, the release of proteinases into the circulation, and changes in the metabolism of branched-chain amino acids have all been suggested as possible reasons. If nutrition is neglected, patients with acute renal failure lose weight very rapidly, and those that lose most have the highest mortality. However, it has not been proven in controlled trials that any form of nutritional support can generate a positive nitrogen balance, improve nutritional status, or alter the mortality rate in patients with acute renal failure. Nevertheless, there is a consensus that early institution of nutritional support probably improves prognosis. Despite this, and almost certainly to the patient's detriment, action is frequently delayed or not taken at all, particularly if it is thought that the extra fluid load required will mandate the institution of dialysis or the need for additional dialysis sessions in an already busy unit.

Typical recommended daily adult requirements are total energy 35 kcal/kg body weight, protein 1 g/kg but and nitrogen 0.16 g/kg but there is no good evidence on which to base stipulations and some would advocate more calories and more protein for those who are catabolic. If patients with acute renal failure are oliguric, the nutritional support should be given in a restricted fluid volume, with reduced amounts of sodium, potassium, and phosphate. For practical purposes it is sensible to have enteral and parenteral fluids that satisfy these needs available routinely (a variety of commercial preparations are available): extra water and electrolytes can always be added when required. In the many patients who are too unwell to take adequate food by mouth, commonly those who need it most, tube feeding or parenteral nutrition should be started early. Protein restriction, aimed at moderating the rise of plasma urea, is not appropriate management for the patient with acute renal failure.

Bleeding

In uraemia the bleeding time is prolonged, and in acute renal failure this summates with any abnormality of haemostasis that might be simultaneously induced by the precipitating condition. Better control of uraemia and the routine use of H_2-receptor antagonists have been associated with a greatly reduced risk of upper gastrointestinal bleeding, a previously frequent and grave occurrence. Impairment of haemostasis is not a cause of great clinical concern in most patients, but there are some who bleed—from anywhere and everywhere. Guidelines for the management of such cases are given in Table 5.

Sepsis

Overwhelming septicaemia is a common cause of acute renal failure, and in such instances the diagnosis is often straightforward. However, in many more cases the role of sepsis is insidious and difficult to diagnose with certainty. There is often strong clinical feeling, but little in the way of hard proof, that sepsis underlies the slide towards worsening renal and multi-organ failure in patients who have been apparently successfully resuscitated from major trauma or surgery. Septicaemia is the commonest cause of death in those with acute renal failure. The index of clinical suspicion must therefore be very high: if a patient with acute renal failure appears to be deteriorating in any way, the question must be asked 'is this sepsis?'. Unused intravenous lines and urinary catheters should be removed, and those that are necessary but in any way 'suspicious' should be replaced. The patient should be examined regularly for signs of a septic focus. There should be a low threshold for repeated, thorough microbiological investigation. Proven infection should be treated promptly with appropriate antimicrobial agents (dose modified as required). In many cases, however, it will be necessary to start treatment 'blind', having taken specimens for culture and having made an educated guess as to the likely pathogen, with the possibility of Gram-negative septicaemia high on the list.

In the patient who appears 'obviously septic' or to be 'going off', but in whom no cause can be found, attention should be directed towards the

Table 5 Practical strategies for the management of bleeding in acute renal failure

1	Exclude the possibility of a heparin effect
2.	Blood transfusion to obtain haematocrit >30% (very occasionally erythropoietin is of value)
3.	Cryoprecipitate (10 bags) has its maximal effect between 1 and 2 h after administration. Its effect disappears at 24–36 h
4.	Desmopressin (0.3 µg/kg intravenously) acts by increasing factor VIII coagulant activity. Shown in acute renal failure to shorten prolonged bleeding time. Repeated doses have a lesser effect
5.	Conjugated oestrogen: 0.6 mg/kg per day for 5 days. Shown to reduce bleeding time (for at least 14 days) in patients with chronic renal impairment and haemorrhagic tendency

abdomen, this being the most likely place for hidden mischief, either infective or ischaemic. Radiological investigations, in particular CT scanning, can be very useful in searching for abdominal sepsis or dead bowel, but should not be relied upon too faithfully. However, surgical exploration may be required, both to diagnose and to treat, especially in patients whose renal failure follows previous abdominal surgical procedures.

Prescription of drugs

Many drugs are excreted by glomerular filtration or tubular secretion and must be given in reduced dosage or at longer intervals than normal in patients with renal failure (see Chapter 20.16). For patients with acute renal failure the following should not be given without very good reason: nonsteroidal anti-inflammatory drugs, angiotensin-converting enzyme inhibitors, angiotensin-II receptor antagonists (all of which have adverse effects on renal perfusion and glomerular filtration), and aminoglycoside antibiotics (these are discussed later in this chapter). A note about two other drugs that may be given to patients with acute renal failure is also appropriate here: both aciclovir and penicillins can cause encephalopathy if given in the doses used to treat severe infection in patients with normal renal function. The dose of aciclovir needs to be reduced from between 5 and 10 mg/kg every 8 h to between 2.5 and 5 mg/kg every 24 h in those receiving renal replacement therapy, and physicians should restrain themselves from prescribing the maximum recommended doses of penicillins. If in doubt, consult the manufacturer's data sheet before prescribing any drug to a patient with acute renal failure.

Prognosis

Acute renal failure of sufficient severity to require renal replacement therapy carries a high mortality. In a series of over 1300 cases, the actuarial 1-year survival of all medical and surgical cases rose from 39 per cent to 58 per cent between 1956 and 1988, despite an increase in the median patient age from 41 to 61 years over this period. The prognosis varies according to the cause of acute renal failure: mortality is between 40 and 60 per cent in patients with renal failure as part of the multiple organ failure syndrome, but less than 10 per cent in those who have renal failure alone. Death should rarely be attributable to a primary sequel of renal failure, for example uraemia or hyperkalaemia, and the incidence of life-threatening gastrointestinal haemorrhage is much reduced: sepsis is the major killer. Patients die *with* but not directly *of* renal failure.

Specific causes of acute renal failure

Prerenal failure and acute tubular necrosis

Introduction

Between 80 and 90 per cent of the cases of acute renal failure seen by physicians will fall into the categories of prerenal failure and acute tubular necrosis (those due to prostatic obstruction usually being managed by others). The term 'prerenal failure' is used when renal dysfunction is entirely attributable to hypoperfusion, and where restoration of renal perfusion leads to rapid recovery. The term 'acute tubular necrosis' does not find favour with all; although necrosis of tubular cells can usually be found by diligent examination, the lesion may be inconspicuous and the pathophysiological implications of such necrosis as might be seen remain uncertain. The glomeruli and vessels are usually normal. In common usage (retained here), the term 'acute tubular necrosis' describes a clinical entity comprising acute renal failure with three main characteristics:

(1) it is seen in specific clinical contexts, frequently involving circulatory compromise and/or nephrotoxins;

(2) urinary abnormalities usually suggest tubular dysfunction; and

(3) essentially complete recovery of renal function is expected within days or weeks in most cases if the patient survives the precipitating insult, with a period of polyuria commonly following oliguria (but see the later section on prognosis).

The syndrome can be seen after virtually any episode of severe circulatory compromise, but not all causes of circulatory derangement are equally devastating to renal function. Primary impairment of cardiac performance, for example following myocardial infarction, may cause plasma creatinine to rise somewhat, but rarely causes renal failure of sufficient severity to require renal replacement therapy. By contrast, an apparently similar haemodynamic upset caused by sepsis frequently does, as demonstrated in Tables 2 and 3. Multiple insults are the rule rather than the exception. Circumstances associated with a particularly high risk of acute renal failure include repair of a ruptured aortic aneurysm (20 per cent, as opposed to 3 per cent for elective repair), hepatobiliary surgery (10 per cent), pancreatitis (10 per cent), and burns (2 to 38 per cent, depending on the series).

Pathophysiology

The perfusion of the kidney seems to suffer more than that of any other organ when the circulation is compromised. In the face of modest underperfusion, the glomerular filtration rate is relatively preserved by a compensatory increase in the filtration fraction. This increase has repercussions on tubular function which, along with other factors, leads to the increased tubular reabsorption of sodium, water, and urea—a situation rapidly reversed by restoration of renal perfusion. However, following prolonged circulatory shock, renal function frequently deteriorates in a manner that is not immediately reversible, and it is not at all obvious why this should be so. Lack of a clear pathophysiological understanding has bedevilled all attempts at the development of rational therapy. Under normal conditions the kidney enjoys high blood flow, exceeded on a volume/weight basis only by the carotid body, and oxygen tension in the renal venous effluent is high, suggesting that oxygen supply greatly exceeds demand. Such a situation might be expected to confer protection from the effects of circulatory compromise, but no such benefit is observed: indeed the kidney appears to be more susceptible to damage than other organs. Acute renal failure resembling acute tubular necrosis can be produced in animal models by ischaemia, and the condition often arises clinically in the setting of profound haemodynamic disturbance, leading to the supposition that—despite apparently generous blood flow normally—renal ischaemia is the cause of renal failure in such circumstances. Two main hypotheses, not necessarily mutually exclusive, have been proposed to explain this. The first stresses that arteriovenous shunting of oxygen, resulting from the specialized anatomical arrangement of the vasa rectae that is essential for the countercurrent mechanism involved in urinary concentration and dilution, leads to the presence of areas of profound hypoxia within the normal kidney. These areas might therefore be operating on the verge of anoxia in the normal organ and hence be susceptible to ischaemic damage in response to a modest compromise of whole-organ blood flow. The second hypothesis is based on clinical and experimental evidence of intense constriction of renal vessels during shock, and suggests that very severe reduction in renal blood flow (perhaps only transient) may be responsible for the initiation of ischaemic damage. The justification for many of the interventions proposed in the management of patients at risk of acute renal failure, or with established acute renal failure, is that they might preserve renal blood flow and/or reduce renal oxygen consumption, thus rendering the development of ischaemic injury less likely.

Once damage to the kidney has been sustained, a variety of factors may be responsible for the persistence of excretory failure that is characteristic of the clinical syndrome of acute tubular necrosis. There is evidence from experimental models and in humans that backleak of filtrate can occur from damaged tubules, but reduced renal blood flow and the prevention of fluid flow through tubules by internal blockage or external compression may also contribute to filtration failure. Even in experimental models it is very hard to determine what is happening at any time, and impossible to do so in clinical practice. However, the processes involved are beginning to be dissected, but matters are ferociously complicated and progress is slow. Many of the abnormalities have a structural as well as a functional basis, hence rapid reversal cannot be expected, there being good evidence that recovery from acute tubular necrosis depends upon cellular regeneration.

Diagnosis

The diagnosis of acute tubular necrosis is based on the clinical context, which often involves circulatory compromise, and the exclusion of obstruction or renal inflammatory conditions, usually by ultrasound examination of the kidneys and testing of the urine for blood and protein, respectively.

In prerenal failure the biochemical composition of the urine reflects the response of normal tubules to impaired renal perfusion. There is avid retention of sodium and water, leading to low urinary sodium and high urinary urea and creatinine concentrations, together with a high urinary osmolarity. Restoration of renal perfusion leads to rapid improvement in renal function. By contrast, conventional wisdom holds that in acute tubular necrosis the urinary sodium concentration is elevated and the urinary urea and creatinine concentrations and urinary osmolarity are relatively low, but this is not always so. Biochemical analysis of the urine is rarely useful in clinical practice, as explained in Table 6. From a practical point of view, treatment is begun on exactly the same lines whether the expected diagnosis is of prerenal failure or of acute tubular necrosis. The response to resuscitation retrospectively defines the diagnosis and determines further management.

Circumstances predisposing to prerenal failure are almost invariably associated with raised plasma levels of ADH. This acts on the collecting duct to increase the tubular reabsorption of both water and urea, hence the plasma concentration of urea rises out of proportion to that of creatinine in prerenal failure. Plasma urea may also appear to be disproportionately raised in the presence of sepsis, steroids, tetracycline (catabolic effect), and gastrointestinal haemorrhage (protein meal).

Avoidance

One of the main aims of the basic nursing and medical care provided to all acutely ill patients is to minimize the chances of the development of renal impairment. This can arise despite exemplary treatment, but poor care increases the likelihood. As described above, regular measurement of serum creatinine will permit early recognition of declining renal function, but is not of itself therapeutic. The best way to prevent the development of prerenal failure or acute tubular necrosis is to maintain an optimal intravascular volume (as described above, with further information given in Chapter 16.1), and to avoid or reduce exposure to nephrotoxic agents.

Table 6 Urinary biochemical indices in prerenal failure and acute tubular necrosis

Indices	'Typical' prerenal failure	'Typical' acute tubular necrosis
Urinary sodium (mmol/l)	<20	>40
Urine osmolarity (mosmol/l)	>500	<350
Urine/plasma urea	>8	<3
Urine/plasma creatinine	>40	<20
Fractional sodium excretion (%)	<1	>2

Notes:

1. There are several reasons why urinary biochemical indices are of very limited clinical use:
   - intermediate values are common;
   - 'typical' values do not reliably predict renal prognosis—it is recognized that cases that are otherwise indistinguishable from 'typical' acute tubular necrosis can have a low urinary sodium concentration;
   - diuretics and pre-existing tubular disease will impair the ability of tubules to retain sodium in prerenal failure;
   - treatment is not dictated by urinary indices.
2. Two uncommon circumstances in which measurement of urinary sodium concentration may be helpful are:
   - hepatorenal syndrome, when urinary sodium concentration is low (<10 mmol/l);
   - acute renal artery occlusion (bilateral or of single functioning kidney) when urinary sodium concentration can equal that in plasma.

One common clinical situation worthy of specific note is the patient about to undergo a major elective surgical procedure such as repair of an abdominal aortic aneurysm. In the past the risk of acute renal failure following such an operation was substantial, but this has been considerably reduced by recognition of the importance of careful attention to fluid management—with the aim of avoiding episodes of hypovolaemia—both before, during, and after the procedure. It is good practice to maintain a diuresis, which can often be accomplished simply by infusion of crystalloid at moderate rate, since this appears to render the kidney less susceptible to insult. Although the routine use of diuretic agents is advocated by some, they would appear to have no specific advantages over a simple saline diuresis in protecting the kidney. Modest doses of diuretics (furosemide (frusemide) 40–80 mg, mannitol 25 g) given intravenously to a volume-replete patient undergoing a procedure that might compromise renal blood flow (for example, bile duct surgery, resection of aortic aneurysm, cardiac bypass) will increase urinary volume and may afford protection from acute renal failure. This is not proven, but the treatment should do no harm provided that the patient is not volume-depleted. However, the tendency of some to administer very large doses of diuretic agents should be restrained, since these can provoke massive diuresis (urine output >500 ml/h) and thereby lead to considerable difficulties in the control of electrolytes, especially potassium. A multicentre, randomized, double-blind, placebo-controlled trial of the use of dopamine in critically ill patients with evidence of early renal impairment did not show that this treatment was of any benefit.

For high-risk cases the insertion of a central venous pressure line preoperatively is a sensible precaution: the positioning of the patient for surgery and the presence of drapes may prevent proper intraoperative clinical assessment of cardiovascular status, and the risks of elective insertion of a central venous pressure line in the relative calm of the anaesthetic room are considerably less than those incurred if the attempt is made with the patient 'going off' on the operating table.

Clinical findings

There are no specific clinical features of prerenal failure or acute tubular necrosis. There may be symptoms of acute renal failure, as described previously, but these are also not specific and are rarely prominent, hence the clinical picture at presentation is likely to be dominated by signs of volume depletion and those of the precipitating condition.

If the patient does not die of acute renal failure, either because the degree of uraemia is modest or renal replacement therapy is provided, then renal recovery occurs in the vast majority of those who survive the precipitating insult. This may begin at any time from a few days to a few months (median 10–14 days) after the onset of acute renal failure, with a progressive increase in urinary volume typically preceding improvement in the plasma levels of creatinine and urea. Due to a relatively persistent defect in renal tubular sodium reabsorption and concentrating ability, a period of polyuria may ensue, placing the patient at risk of sodium and water depletion. Young patients can be expected to recover clinically normal renal function, but in those over 70 years of age recovery may be delayed, incomplete, and sometimes does not occur at all—leading to lifelong dependence on renal replacement therapy.

Specific treatment

The importance of effective treatment of the underlying condition and of rapid correction of hypovolaemia are above clinical dispute, although neither has been subject to controlled trial as regards the outcome of prerenal failure and acute tubular necrosis. Diuretic agents, in particular loop diuretics such as furosemide (frusemide), and/or 'renal dose' dopamine are often given to the patient who is thought to have acute tubular necrosis and whose urine output is inadequate. Decent trials are very thin on the ground, but there is no compelling evidence that any of these 'specific' remedies are helpful. In established acute tubular necrosis large doses of furosemide (0.5–2 g/day) may substantially increase urinary volume, and this can ease the management of fluid balance and reduce the degree of hyperkalaemia. However, such treatment is most unlikely to lead to improvement in the renal clearance of metabolic wastes, almost certainly does not alter the requirement for renal replacement therapy, and does not affect mortality. The evidence in favour of 'renal dose' dopamine (1–3 μg/kg per min) is generally weak and, although dopamine receptors certainly exist in the renal vasculature and on the renal tubules, it may well be that the effects that are sometimes observed clinically relate to an improvement in cardiac output rather than to any direct effect on the kidneys. However, many nephrologists have seen cases where the administration of a loop diuretic and dopamine has appeared to a have beneficial effect, hence it is not unreasonable to try such treatment, but not to prolong it if it is ineffective in a particular instance. Practical recommendations are given in Fig. 3.

All other medical treatments should be regarded as experimental and not given except in the context of controlled trials. In experimental models the use of growth factors has been shown to speed renal recovery from acute tubular necrosis, and the possibility that such an approach might be applied clinically has generated the greatest recent excitement. Unfortunately, the only substantial clinical trial published so far showed no evidence of benefit.

Prognosis

Complete recovery of renal function can be anticipated in those with acute tubular necrosis who survive the precipitating insult, excepting in the elderly (over 70 years) in whom there is a substantial chance (10–20 per cent) that dependence on dialysis will be lifelong.

Nephrotoxic causes of acute renal failure

Exogenous nephrotoxins

A wide variety of exogenous agents, including therapeutically prescribed drugs, can cause acute renal failure. Some of these agents are listed in Table 7. The following are worthy of particular note.

Aminoglycosides

Gentamicin, amikacin, kanamycin, and streptomycin are all potentially nephrotoxic, as are tobramycin and netilmicin to a lesser degree. These drugs are usually prescribed for patients thought to be suffering from potentially fatal infections, hence in clinical practice it is frequently impossible to separate with certainty the harmful effects of aminoglycosides from those of the underlying condition, or of other drugs used in treatment. However, evidence from animal models supports the view that these agents are genuinely nephrotoxic, rather than that their prescription is simply a marker for severe infection, which is itself a potent cause of acute renal failure.

The risk of nephrotoxicity is increased by old age, pre-existing renal insufficiency, high dosage, prolonged treatment, combined treatment with other nephrotoxic drugs, renal ischaemia, and volume depletion. It has been stated that acute renal failure complicates up to 25 per cent of therapeutic courses of gentamicin, even when monitoring optimally controls drug levels. Parenteral administration is not required for the development of toxicity: acute renal failure can occur as a result of systemic absorption when aminoglycosides are used in irrigating or bowel-sterilizing solutions. The typical clinical picture is of relatively mild non-oliguric renal failure coming on 1 to 2 weeks after starting treatment. Tubular proteinuria and impaired ability to concentrate the urine precede a loss of glomerular filtration rate. Proximal tubular damage involves the brush border, reflected by increased urinary excretion of γ-glutamyl transferase, alanine aminopeptidase, and of lysosomal enzymes. Recovery may be slow, delayed, or incomplete.

The nephrotoxicity of particular aminoglycosides is related to the strength of their positive charge. They bind to negatively charged membrane phospholipids, particularly in the kidney to parts S1 and S2 of the proximal tubule, where they are delivered to megalin (the Heymann nephritis autoantigen, a member of the low-density lipoprotein (**LDL**) receptor family) in coated pits. The complex is endocytosed and trafficked to the endosome, where gentamicin inhibits fusion *in vivo* and *in vitro*. Polyaspartic acid polymers normalize fusion and ameliorate nephrotoxicity, suggesting that binding of other ligands to megalin may be useful in limiting

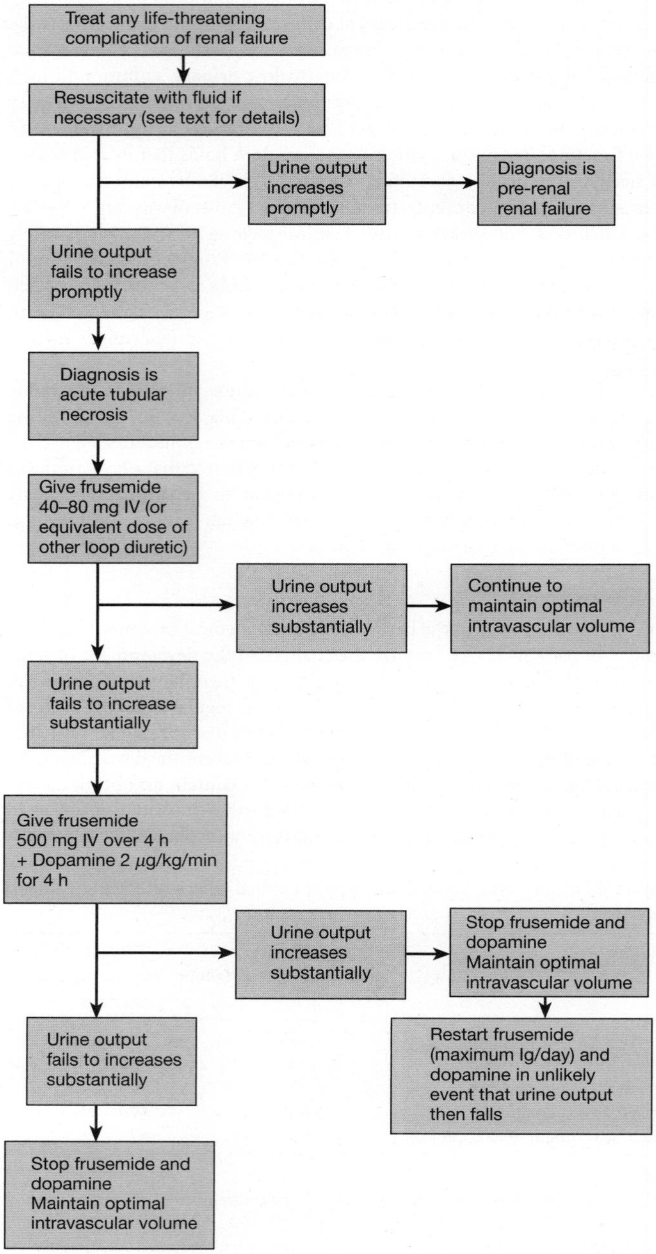

Notes:
(1) Treat precipitating condition vigorously.
(2) Do not forget to exclude urinary obstructions and renal inflammatory causes of acute renal failure if the diagnosis of acute tubular necrosis is not certain, e.g. clinical context not obviously appropriate.
(3) The use of diuretic and dopamine in the way described is commmon practice but not based on controlled trial evidence.

Fig. 3 An algorithm for the practical management of the patient with prerenal failure or acute tubular necrosis.

Table 7 Some nephrotoxins that can cause acute renal failure (excluding causes of interstitial nephritis)

Exogenous	
Antibiotics	Aminoglycosides, tetracyclines, cephaloridine, amphotericin B, sulphonamides, polymyxin/colistin, bacitracin, pentamidine, vancomycin
Radiocontrast media	
Anaesthetic agents	Methoxyflurane[a], enflurane[a]
Chemotherapeutic/immunosuppressive agents	Ciclosporin A, *cis*-platinum, methotrexate
Organic solvents	Glycols (e.g. ethylene glycol[a]), hydrocarbons (e.g. carbon tetrachloride, toluene)
Poisons	Venoms (snake bite, e.g. Russell's viper); stings; insecticides/herbicides/rodenticides (including paraquat, copper sulphate, sodium chlorate); mushrooms (*Amanita* spp.); hemlock; carp bile; herbal medicines
Drugs of abuse	
Heavy metals	
Endogenous	
Pigments	Myoglobin, haemoglobin
Intrarenal crystal deposition	Urate, phosphate (tumour lysis syndrome)
Tumour related	Immunoglobulin light chains

Notes:

In many instances nephrotoxicity arises both from a direct toxic action on renal tissue and from indirect systemic effects.

[a]May be associated with intratubular precipitation of oxalate crystals.

aminoglycoside uptake and nephrotoxicity, but this possibility has not yet been explored clinically.

Aminoglycosides should only be used in the relatively uncommon circumstance that there is no suitable alternative antibiotic that is not nephrotoxic, and careful monitoring of levels is mandatory to avoid toxicity if gentamicin or similar agents must be used.

Radiographic contrast media

The incidence of acute renal failure associated with the use of radiographic contrast media has been reported to vary between 0 and 50 per cent. This extraordinary variability reflects differences in other risk factors in the populations under examination and in the definition of renal failure used. Recent prospective studies, using non-ionic contrast media and in which careful attention has been paid to the maintenance of adequate hydration, have shown a very low incidence of significant renal impairment—even in groups reported to be at high risk (diabetes, myeloma). When renal impairment does occur it is usually mild.

Endogenous nephrotoxins

Myoglobin

Myoglobinuric acute renal failure, the mechanism of which remains uncertain, is typically associated with crush injury to muscle, but there are a large number of causes of non-traumatic rhabdomyolysis (Table 8). A high index of suspicion is required to diagnose cases that are not obviously associated with muscle injury, since muscular pain, swelling, and tenderness may not be prominent features and can even be absent. The key to making the diagnosis is to detect myoglobin in the urine, or a very high level of enzymes released from muscle in the plasma. The former is recognized by the combination of dark-brown ('coca cola') urine that tests positive for 'blood' on a reagent strip, but which does not contain red cells on microscopy. The muscle enzyme usually measured in plasma is creatine kinase: the normal range of this is up to just below 200 U/l; in rhabdomyolysis values above 10 000 U/l are commonly seen, a value of only 1–2000 U/l not being enough to establish the diagnosis of rhabdomyolytic acute renal failure in the absence of other supporting evidence. Extremely high levels of plasma myoglobin, aldolase, and lactic dehydrogenase are also seen, all being released from damaged muscle.

Rhabdomyolysis can be associated with very high plasma levels of urate (>750 μmol/l), phosphate (>2.5 mmol/l), aspartate and alanine transaminase (**AST** in the many hundreds of U/l, exceptionally in the thousands; **ALT** in the few hundreds of U/l; respectively), and with an unusually low plasma calcium concentration (<1.5 mmol/l). Any of these findings should lead to serious consideration of rhabdomyolysis in any patient with unexplained acute renal failure.

If the diagnosis of rhabdomyolysis is made, then the question of whether to initiate an alkaline diuresis arises, since on theoretical grounds it would be anticipated that alkalinization of the urine would lead to enhanced excretion of the putative toxin and protect against acute renal failure. Victims of crush injury have been treated with infusion of very large volumes of fluid (12 litres/day) and high doses of mannitol (160 g/day) and bicarbonate (240 mmol/day). In comparison with historical (almost certainly volume-depleted) controls the incidence of renal failure has been impressively reduced, but the difficulties of controlling potassium balance in the face of such a massive diuresis should not be underestimated. It may well be that avoidance of hypovolaemia using a less aggressive and more easily managed fluid regimen would be equally efficacious.

Haemoglobin

In several situations, acute renal failure is seen in association with massive haemolysis: malaria, glucose-6-phosphate dehydrogenase deficiency, mismatched blood transfusion, arsine poisoning, copper sulphate poisoning, burns, and as a complication of bladder irrigation with hypotonic solutions. In each circumstance it is possible, but not proven, that the development of acute renal failure might be attributable to, or exacerbated by, the presence of large amounts of free haemoglobin within the circulation.

Urate (see also Chapter 20.10.5)

The tumour lysis syndrome is associated with a rapid rise in plasma uric acid concentration (and almost certainly liberation of other nephrotoxins) as a complication of the treatment of lymphoma, leukaemia, myeloma, or other 'high-turnover' tumours. This can result in the deposition of urate crystals in the distal tubule, which can both cause physical obstruction and initiate an inflammatory response, leading to acute renal failure in which

Table 8 Some causes of rhabdomyolysis

Direct muscle injury
Ischaemic muscle injury:
compression
vascular occlusion
Any cause of coma (e.g. opioid overdose, diabetes mellitus, cerebrovascular accident) or of prolonged immobility (e.g. following a fall in the elderly) can be associated with rhabdomyolysis due to a pressure effect
Excessive muscular activity:
seizures
sporting, e.g. marathon running
Inflammatory myositis:
immunological, e.g. dermatomyositis, polymyositis
infection, e.g. viral (influenza, coxsackie)
Metabolic:
hypokalaemia, hypophosphataemia
genetic abnormalities of carbohydrate metabolism, e.g. myophosphorylase deficiency (McArdle's syndrome), phosphofructokinase deficiency
Toxins/drugs:
snake bite, carbon monoxide, alcohol, hemlock, paint/glue sniffing
clofibrate, aminocaproic acid, HMG CoA reductase inhibitors
Others:
malignant hyperpyrexia
neuroleptic malignant syndrome
phaeochromocytoma 'storm'

HMG CoA, 3-hydroxy-3-methylglutaryl coenzyme A.

freshly voided urine is heavily laden with urate crystals. Hyperuricaemia and renal failure have been described on rare occasions after recurrent epileptic seizures.

Hyperuricaemic acute renal failure is predictable and hence potentially avoidable in the context of the treatment of malignancy. The most important issue is that dehydration should be avoided at all costs, and a brisk saline diuresis should be initiated at least 24 h before the initiation of chemotherapy if possible. The use of an alkaline diuresis has been advocated, since uric acid is undoubtedly more soluble in alkaline urine, but this may encourage the precipitation of phosphate within the renal tubules and should not be employed if the serum phosphate is high. It is common practice in many centres to give allopurinol, even at a dosage above the usual 300 mg/day, but others would not do so on the grounds that this may encourage xanthine nephrotoxicity, although the risks of this seem to have been overstated.

If hyperuricaemic acute renal failure does develop, then it is unlikely that any of the treatments described above, or diuretics, will reverse the condition. Prompt improvement usually follows reduction of the plasma uric acid concentration, which is best accomplished by haemodialysis. On very rare occasions the ureters can become obstructed by urate crystals—indicated by colic, pelvicalyceal distension, or persistent oliguria—and ureteral catheterization and washout may be required.

Other endogenous nephrotoxins

More uncommon even than intratubular obstruction by urate crystals is similar obstruction by phosphate, also seen in the context of massive cell destruction in the treatment of malignant disease. Urinary alkalinization should be avoided because it may promote intratubular phosphate precipitation.

The possible role of immunoglobulin light chains in causing acute renal failure related to myeloma is discussed in Chapter 20.10.5.

Vascular causes of acute renal failure

Acute cortical necrosis

Acute cortical necrosis is an uncommon cause of acute renal failure, accounting for around 1 per cent of cases in the developed world, but more (3.8 per cent) in the experience of one large centre in the developing world (North India). However, these figures may be an underestimate, given that investigation is not pursued in many patients who fail to recover from what was presumed to be acute tubular necrosis, on the grounds that test results do not reliably predict prognosis or affect management, which is supportive.

Acute cortical necrosis presents in the same context as acute tubular necrosis, which is almost always the diagnosis made initially on clinical grounds. Suspicion should arise immediately if a patient without obstruction is anuric, as was found in 79 per cent of 113 patients in the largest study reported, but cortical necrosis is often considered only when renal function fails to improve.

Most cases of acute cortical necrosis are the result of obstetric disasters, particularly postpartum haemorrhage, abruptio placentae, eclampsia, or septic abortion. Snake bite, haemolytic uraemic syndrome, acute gastroenteritis, pancreatitis, septicaemia (often with disseminated intravascular coagulation), trauma, and drug-induced intravascular haemolysis are risk factors in the non-obstetric population.

The pathological findings are of microvascular thrombosis, mainly affecting interlobular arteries, arterioles, and glomeruli, with complete infarction of affected areas of cortex. The medulla and a rim of juxtamedullary tissue are spared.

The best investigations to establish the diagnosis of acute cortical necrosis are renal angiography and contrast-enhanced CT scanning. The former reveals attenuation of interlobular arteries, an increase in the subcapsular vessels, and a negative outer cortical nephrogram. The latter shows enhancement of the renal medulla, but no enhancement of the renal cortex and no excretion of contrast. Biopsy necessarily samples only a very small piece of tissue and may mislead because of the patchy nature of renal damage. Radiopharmaceutical investigations that depend upon renal excretion (for example, **DMSA** (dimercaptosuccinic acid) scans) are unhelpful in patients with very poor renal function.

In the months or years after an episode of acute cortical necrosis, the kidneys tend to contract: cortical calcification, producing an eggshell or tramline appearance on the abdominal radiograph, is a characteristic sequel, but this is not useful in making the diagnosis acutely.

Return of renal function in cases of acute cortical necrosis occurs very slowly, if at all, and is attributable to the survival of islands of intact cortical tissue. About 50 per cent of patients recover sufficiently to come off dialysis, but the glomerular filtration rate rarely exceeds 10 to 20 ml/min. Hypertension (including accelerated phase) may be a major problem, and a subsequent decline in renal function with the necessity for a return to dialysis/transplantation is not uncommon.

Large-vessel obstruction

Arterial obstruction

Occlusion of the main renal arteries—or of the artery supplying a solitary functioning kidney—by trauma, dissection, thrombosis, or embolism may rarely be the reason for acute renal failure. Loin pain sometimes occurs, and there is usually a low-grade fever, such that the clinical picture may mimic acute pyelonephritis, but symptoms can be notable by their absence. Proteinuria and haematuria may occur.

Diagnosis is important because thrombolysis and/or renovascular surgery can be surprisingly effective in restoring function, even when undertaken a considerable time after arterial occlusion (up to many weeks), in those with atherosclerotic renovascular disease in whom (prior to occlusion) a collateral blood supply to the renal parenchyma has developed. Suspicion should be aroused by complete, sudden anuria in the absence of urinary obstruction, especially if the clinical setting is appropriate, for example atrial fibrillation in an arteriopath. A useful pointer to the diagnosis is the finding of a urinary sodium concentration similar to that of plasma (see Table 6), but DTPA renography and renal angiography are the appropriate diagnostic tests if the diagnosis of renal artery occlusion is suspected. CT scanning may reveal wedge-shaped infarcts when occlusion is incomplete.

Venous obstruction

Renal vein thrombosis can cause acute renal failure, most commonly in adults as a complication of the nephrotic syndrome, but in infants and children as a result of abdominal sepsis or severe dehydration. Renal pain is common, as is increasing proteinuria and haematuria (which can be macroscopic), but there may be no symptoms. If there is clinical suspicion of the diagnosis, for example unexplained deterioration of renal function in a nephrotic patient, then appropriate investigation includes ultrasound/Doppler examination of the renal veins and inferior vena cava, CT/MRI scanning, or renal arteriography with late films taken specifically to look for filling of the renal veins. Treatment by anticoagulation is the usual practice. (See Section 20.3 for further discussion.)

Small-vessel obstruction

Accelerated-phase hypertension (see also Chapter 15.16.3)

'Accelerated-phase' hypertension (a term preferred to 'malignant' hypertension because the implication of malignancy is terrifying for patients) occurs when the blood pressure is elevated sufficiently to cause fibrinoid necrosis of blood vessels, leading to the development of haemorrhages and exudates in the ocular fundi. It may develop as a consequence of pre-existing renal disease, but does not always do so, and is itself a potent cause of renal damage. Acute renal failure is a common complication in those with previously normal renal function, and is associated with proteinuria, haematuria, and the presence of urinary red cell casts. The higher the creatinine at presentation, the poorer the prognosis for both patient survival and renal outcome: in one study only 9 per cent of those with an initial plasma creatinine below 300 µmol/l progressed to need renal replacement therapy, compared with two-thirds of those with a plasma creatinine above this level. The ability of the kidney to autoregulate perfusion is disturbed in accelerated-phase hypertension, hence the therapeutic lowering of arterial pressure may be associated with reduced renal perfusion and an abrupt decline in renal function. Accelerated-phase hypertension is one of the conditions in which renal function sometimes recovers after a lengthy period on dialysis. Renal failure was the cause of two-thirds of the deaths in patients with accelerated-phase hypertension in the days before dialysis was available.

Systemic sclerosis (see also Chapter 18.10.3)

This disease does not usually involve the kidney, but a syndrome resembling accelerated-phase hypertension and termed 'scleroderma renal crisis' is well recognized in patients with diffuse cutaneous systemic sclerosis. It usually occurs within the first 5 years of the disease, may be the presenting feature, and often appears during the winter months. Rapid worsening of skin manifestations may precede the crisis, but frequently there is no warning. The patient may develop headaches, visual disturbance, and convulsions. Arterial pressure is usually grossly elevated, but the renal syndrome can occur without a rise in arterial pressure. Haemorrhages and exudates are often seen in the ocular fundi. Renal failure, with proteinuria and haematuria, develops rapidly. A microangiopathic haemolytic anaemia may complicate the situation. Plasma levels of renin are grossly elevated. There have been a number of case reports of arrest or reversal of the syndrome after treatment with angiotensin-converting enzyme inhibitors or nifedipine. These agents should be tried, but more in hope than expectation that they will prevent relentless progression to endstage renal failure.

Glomerulonephritic and vasculitic causes of acute renal failure

A large number of glomerulonephritic and vasculitic diseases can cause acute renal failure, sometimes in association with pulmonary haemorrhage (see Table 1 of Chapter 20.10.3). These are discussed in detail in the relevant subsections of Section 20.7, and in Chapters 20.10.3 and 20.10.4. Together they form only 5 to 10 per cent of cases of acute renal failure, but making the correct diagnosis is of extreme importance because of the management implications. Regrettably, most nephrologists have seen cases where the diagnosis has been much delayed because renal impairment has incorrectly been attributed to acute tubular necrosis, and infiltrates on the chest radiograph to oedema or infection. This error, which can be catastrophic, should be avoided in patients in whom the cause of acute renal failure is not obvious, by:

1. A history and examination specifically directed towards determining whether one of the conditions listed in Table 1 of Chapter 20.10.3 might be present.
2. Microscopy of the urine to look for the presence of red cells and red cell casts.
3. The following blood tests:
   (a) measurement of antiglomerular basement membrane (**anti-GBM**) antibodies—positive in Goodpasture's disease (see Chapter 20.7.9);
   (b) measurement of antineutrophil cytoplasmic antigen antibodies (**ANCA**)(screening by indirect immunofluorescence test, specific tests for antiproteinase-3 and antimyeloperoxidase antibodies) —positive in microscopic polyangiitis and Wegener's granulomatosis (see Chapter 20.10.3);
   (c) estimation of serum complement levels (C3 is depressed in postinfectious glomerulonephritis, mesangiocapillary glomerulonephritis, systemic lupus erythematosus) (see Chapters 20.7.7, 20.7.8, and 20.10.4);
   (d) measurement of anti-streptolysin O titre (**ASOT**—elevated in poststreptococcal glomerulonephritis) (see Chapter 20.7.7);
   (e) serological tests for systemic lupus erythematosus (see Chapter 20.10.4);
   (f) cryoglobulins (see Chapter 20.10.5) (tests of serum immunoglobulins and for urinary light chains should also be performed—see below).
4. Considering the possibility that pulmonary infiltrates in a patient with acute renal failure might be due to haemorrhage. The chances of this are increased if there is a history of haemoptysis (associated with several forms of rapidly progressive glomerulonephritis), nasal discharge, or bleeding (associated with Wegener's granulomatosis), or if anaemia is unusually profound and otherwise unexplained. Lung function tests demonstrating an increase in carbon monoxide transfer factor can establish the diagnosis.
5. Performing an urgent renal biopsy. In any patient with acute renal failure and an active urinary sediment, renal biopsy should be performed unless the diagnosis is clear (for example, a classical history of poststreptococcal nephritis, obvious infective endocarditis/shunt nephritis) or there is a strong contraindication, for example a single kidney or serious bleeding disorder.

The possibility of the presence of a rapidly progressive glomerulonephritis/vasculitis constitutes a medical emergency. Anti-GBM disease responds well to immunosuppression with plasma exchange, steroids and cyclophosphamide, but only if treatment is begun before dialysis is required. Immunosuppressive treatment should be given as early as possible in the course of acute renal failure complicating microscopic polyangiitis/idiopathic rapidly progressive (crescentic) glomerulonephritis, Wegener's granulomatosis, and systemic lupus erythematosus. The urgency is such that it may well be appropriate to start these treatments while the results of blood tests and renal biopsy are awaited, and to stop them if the findings do not corroborate the initial clinical diagnosis. The management of these patients is complex and patients benefit from the judgement and expertise of specialists.

Interstitial nephritis as a cause of acute renal failure (see also Chapter 20.9.1)

Drugs

Drugs are the commonest cause of acute interstitial nephritis, the usual culprits being penicillins, non-steroidal anti-inflammatory drugs (**NSAIDs**), and diuretics, but many others have been implicated (see Table 1 of Chapter 20.9.1). The classical clinical picture is that a few days or weeks after taking a drug the patient develops flank pain (sometimes), fever, a skin rash, arthralgias, haematuria, blood eosinophilia and elevated IgE, disturbed liver function (sometimes), interstitial pneumonia (rarely), and renal impairment, but renal failure may be the only manifestation. The urine contains protein and blood, with white and red cell casts. Proteinuria may be in the nephrotic range, particularly in association with NSAIDs. The diagnosis can only be established with certainty by renal biopsy, where typical histological findings are of an interstitial infiltrate of lymphocytes and monocytes/macrophages, together with some eosinophils. Epithelioid granulomas may be seen, strongly supporting the diagnosis of a drug-induced interstitial nephritis, but they are not pathognomonic. When large numbers of cells are present in the renal interstitium the diagnosis is not contentious: more difficult are those cases (not too infrequent) in which the infiltrate is modest—how many cells turn 'acute tubular necrosis' into 'interstitial nephritis'? The importance of making the distinction lies in the belief that, apart from withdrawal of the offending drug, treatment of drug-induced interstitial nephritis with steroids is beneficial. There is some evidence that those given prednisolone (typical dosage 20 to 60 mg/day) have an earlier and more complete recovery of renal function than those left untreated.

Leptospirosis (see also Chapter 7.11.31)

Acute renal failure due to an interstitial nephritis may appear within a few days of the onset of disease, but more commonly in the second week. It occurs in about 10 per cent of cases of leptospirosis and is frequently mild, but may be severe, with the plasma urea level rising rapidly due to hypercatabolism. The diagnosis of leptospirosis should be considered in any patient with unexplained acute renal failure who has myalgias/muscle tenderness, conjunctival infection, and/or haemorrhage or jaundice. Direct enquiry must be made as to whether any such patient has been exposed to rats.

Aside from renal impairment, blood tests commonly reveal a dramatic conjugated hyperbilirubinaemia (often >250 μmol/l) and thrombocytopenia (seen in 40 per cent of cases). There may also be elevation of serum creatine kinase and a slight increase in serum AST. Anaemia may be severe due to intravascular haemolysis. By contrast to most other causes of acute renal failure, serum potassium is often normal or low in cases of leptospirosis. Mild abnormalities of blood clotting tests can be seen, but disseminated intravascular coagulation is not a feature, which is an important point in its distinction from bacterial septicaemia.

The diagnosis is established by culture of *Leptospira* spp. (from blood during the first phase or urine afterwards) or positive serology. Doxycycline prophylaxis is effective at preventing leptospirosis, but antibiotics are not of proven benefit in treating disease. Mild cases are self-limiting; most physicians treat patients who are symptomatic with a 7-day course of oral doxycycline or intravenous benzylpenicillin, on the grounds that this appears to shorten the duration of fever and leptospiruria.

Hantavirus disease (see also Chapter 7.10.15)

In Europe

In Europe the Puumula serotype of hantavirus produces an illness that can have many similarities to that produced by leptospirosis, although serological studies indicate that many patients must have a subclinical infection. In those that are symptomatic, high fever is typically followed within a couple of days by loin/abdominal pain and often by nausea and vomiting; photophobia and signs of meningeal irritation can also occur. Acute renal failure follows when these symptoms have settled and is associated with conjunctival haemorrhage (20 per cent), proteinuria (almost 100 per cent of cases), microscopic haematuria (70 per cent), thrombocytopenia (50 per cent), and a transient mild rise in serum liver enzymes. There may be a small increase in serum bilirubin (maximum 40 μmol/l). Mild abnormalities of blood clotting tests are seen, but disseminated intravascular coagulation is rare.

Renal biopsy, performed for the indication of unexplained acute renal impairment, shows interstitial nephritis. This has no pathognomonic features, leading in this clinical context to the differential diagnosis of leptospirosis and sometimes (depending on exposure) disease induced by NSAIDs. Leptospirosis is much more likely if the serum bilirubin is markedly elevated. NSAID-induced disease does not cause conjunctival haemorrhages or thrombocytopenia. The diagnosis of Puumula hantavirus infection is made on the basis of serological evidence. Prognosis is good: no deaths have been reported and renal function returns to normal.

In some areas of Eastern and Central Europe there is a more severe form of hantavirus infection, which is similar to that seen in Asia.

In Asia

The Hantaan and Seoul viruses cause hantavirus disease in Asia: the former causes more severe illness, but both are considerably more dangerous that the Puumula hantavirus seen in Europe. A total of five phases of disease are recognized, comprising:

(1) high fever and myalgias, followed by headache and severe abdominal/loin pain, often with an erythematous rash that may become petechial, also conjunctival haemorrhages;

(2) severe hypotension;

(3) gradual recovery of blood pressure, but associated with oliguria and renal failure with proteinuria and microscopic haematuria—one-third of patients in this stage have major problems with bleeding: gastrointestinal, intracerebral or massive purpura (hence the terms epidemic or Korean haemorrhagic fever);

(4) presence of polyuria;

(5) convalescence.

Differential diagnosis is from severe leptospirosis and other causes of haemorrhagic fever found in Asia, including dengue and murine typhus. The diagnosis is made serologically. Treatment is supportive. Mortality is between 3 and 7 per cent; survivors recover completely.

'Haematological' causes of acute renal failure

Haemolytic uraemic syndrome and idiopathic postpartum renal failure (see also Chapters 13.5 and 20.10.6)

The haemolytic uraemic syndrome (**HUS**) is a condition, or group of conditions, in which acute renal failure, characterized on biopsy by thrombosis and necrosis of intrarenal vessels, occurs together with thrombocytopenia, haemolytic anaemia, and red cell fragmentation. (See Chapter 20.10.6 for further information.) A similar picture developing immediately (or up to several weeks) after an entirely uneventful pregnancy and delivery is termed 'idiopathic postpartum acute renal failure'.

Myeloma (see also Chapter 20.10.5)

Acute renal failure complicates about 7 per cent of cases of myeloma, often being the presenting feature, and subacute progressive renal failure is even commoner, affecting 14 to 61 per cent of cases. The cause of renal failure is often multifactorial, with varying contribution from the reversible factors of dehydration, infection, hypercalcaemia, and hyperuricaemia, and with renal damage caused by free immunoglobulin light chains. The reason why some patients with myeloma develop renal failure and others do not remains a mystery. There has been much speculation as to whether variation in the isoelectric point of light chains, and hence their capacity for reabsorption by the renal tubules, might be responsible. However, individual patients with light chains of very similar physicochemical properties can present totally different clinical pictures, varying from no perceptible renal involvement to irreversible renal failure.

In a patient with acute renal failure, a history of bone pain, the findings of clumping of erythrocytes on the blood film, or of gross and unexpected elevation of the erythrocyte sedimentation rate, are clues that myeloma might be the underlying diagnosis. Such clues may be absent when excess production of monoclonal light chains is the predominant problem, hence all patients with unexplained acute or subacute renal failure should undergo investigation both of serum for a monoclonal immunoglobulin component (with immunoparesis) and of their urine (if available) for free κ or λ light chains. The renal biopsy appearances are of tubulointerstitial nephritis, with fractured casts in the tubular lumina, tubular atrophy, interstitial oedema/fibrosis, and an interstitial infiltrate that may contain multinucleate giant cells. However, the definitive test for myeloma is a bone marrow biopsy for immunochemical analysis of the plasma-cell population, and this should be performed whenever myeloma is a likely or possible cause of acute renal failure.

The first priority in management is to deal promptly with those factors that can be reversed— dehydration, infection, hypercalcaemia, and hyperuricaemia. Volume resuscitation should be given as described in Chapter 16.1, along with broad-spectrum antimicrobials (after appropriate cultures have been taken) if there is any suspicion of infection. After the intravascular volume has been restored, then (assuming adequate urine output) hypercalcaemia can be treated rapidly and effectively using a two-pronged approach: a diuresis provoked by infusion of 0.9 per cent saline (1 litre every 4–6 h) and furosemide (40 mg as necessary), and intravenous bisphosphonate (for example, disodium pamidronate, 15–60 mg as a single dose, maximum of 90 mg over 2–4 days). It has been suggested that alkalinization of the urine using intravenous sodium bicarbonate may be advantageous in promoting light-chain excretion, but it is unclear whether this is better than adequate rehydration with saline alone.

If there is a clear precipitant for the decline in renal function, then the prospects for renal recovery in patients with myeloma are good; if not, then the renal outlook is less favourable. Although some report that aggressive treatment with cytotoxic agents and/or plasmapheresis can restore renal function in such cases, this is not everyone's experience, and renal recovery seems to be the exception rather than the rule.

The prognosis for patients with myeloma and established renal failure requiring dialysis is poor: 50 per cent 1-year survival, 30 per cent at 2 years. However, many patients will have few symptoms from their myeloma, excepting renal failure, and these patients should certainly be offered the opportunity of renal replacement therapy. In those with considerable extra-renal manifestations the situation is much more difficult, and it may not be appropriate or kind in such circumstances to offer aggressive haematological regimens, producing considerable side-effects, and/or dialysis. The decisions to be made are rarely straightforward: they will substantially depend on an assessment of the overall burden to the patient of their disease and a realistic appraisal of what benefits treatment might produce.

Hepatorenal syndrome

The hepatorenal syndrome consists of the association of severe and usually progressive liver disease with acute renal failure. The renal failure is characterized by:

(1) no evidence of renal parenchymal damage (when kidneys from patients with the hepatorenal syndrome have been transplanted, they function normally in the recipient);

(2) characteristic 'prerenal' urine biochemistry, in particular a very low urinary sodium concentration (<10 mmol/l) (Table 6);

(3) no sustained response to volume expansion; and

(4) exclusion of other causes of acute renal failure.

The mechanism of renal failure is uncertain, but is associated with markedly reduced renal perfusion that may be due to excessive action of the vasoconstrictor endothelin.

One of the aims of the general management of patients with liver disease is prevention of the hepatorenal syndrome, the most important consideration being avoidance of known precipitants (drugs, excessive diuresis, delay in the treatment of sepsis). Nevertheless, the syndrome develops in up to 20 per cent of patients with cirrhosis admitted to hospital. There is no specific treatment and the prognosis is extremely poor. In the presence of potentially reversible liver disease, or with the prospect of liver transplantation, intensive therapy and renal replacement therapy are justified. If these criteria are not met, then aggressive support is almost certainly inappropriate.

Tropical

Acute renal failure in the developing world, as elsewhere, is usually a consequence of acute tubular necrosis. The causes of hospital-acquired acute renal failure are the same as in the developed world, with nephrotoxic drugs, major surgery, and hospital-acquired sepsis the dominant factors. By contrast, the causes of community-acquired acute renal failure are very different.

The Chandigarh study showed that 30 years ago diarrhoeal disease and obstetric complications each accounted for about 25 per cent of cases of acute renal failure in North India, but more recently each has accounted for about 10 per cent. Infections that often cause acute renal failure in the developing world include falciparum malaria, leptospirosis, melioidosis, cholera, salmonellosis, and shigellosis. Intravascular haemolysis is a common feature of many cases, being found in over 20 per cent of 325 patients receiving dialysis for acute renal failure in Chandigarh. This was most frequently seen in those with glucose-6-phosphate dehydrogenase deficiency, with copper sulphate poisoning and snake bite the next commonest causes. Poisoning by deliberate (occasionally accidental) ingestion of paraquat (herbicide) is not uncommon in agricultural communities: aside from renal failure this can lead to inexorably progressive respiratory failure with an extremely high mortality. Treatment with corticosteroids and cyclophosphamide has been used in an attempt to prevent pulmonary fibrosis and may be of benefit. Heatstroke can cause acute renal failure.

Snake bite

Acute renal failure develops in 5 to 30 per cent of the victims of severe viper poisoning and is the cause of between 2 and 3 per cent of cases of acute renal failure, but a very much higher proportion in some centres at some times of the year. It develops from a few hours to 72 h following the bite, and is non-oliguric in 50 per cent of cases. Hyperkalaemia may be prominent in bites associated with myonecrosis, such as those of sea-snakes. The usual renal pathology is acute tubular necrosis, but acute cortical necrosis can occur (see above). Renal management is supportive. (See Chapter 8.2 for further discussion.)

Copper sulphate poisoning

Copper sulphate is extensively used in the leather industry and is a relatively common (although decreasing) cause of poisoning in India. Symptoms include nausea, vomiting, diarrhoea, epigastric pain, gastrointestinal bleeding, and coma. Signs include jaundice, hypotension, and shock. Investigation reveals intravascular haemolysis, methaemoglobinaemia, haemoglobinuria, haematuria, and renal failure, the latter complicating 11 of 29 cases in one series.

Histological examination of the kidneys shows acute tubular necrosis with luminal haemoglobin casts, rupture of tubular basement membranes, and copper in degenerated tubules.

Aside from gastric lavage, management usually involves the administration (urine output permitting) of intravenous 0.9 per cent saline, mannitol, and/or diuretics to encourage copper elimination, intramuscular dimercaprol (but with extreme caution if renal failure has developed), and dialysis.

Further reading

Abassi ZA, *et al.* (1998). Acute renal failure complicating muscle crush injury. *Seminars in Nephrology* **18**, 558–65.

Ash SR (2001). Peritoneal dialysis in acute renal failure of adults: the safe, effective, and low-cost modality. *Contributions to Nephrology* **132**, 210–21.

Barton IK, *et al.* (1993). Acute renal failure treated by haemofiltration: factors affecting outcome. *Quarterly Journal of Medicine* **86**, 81–90.

Bellomo R, *et al.* (2000). Low-dose dopamine in patients with early renal dysfunction: a placebo-controlled randomised trial. Australian and New Zealand Intensive Care Society (ANZICS) Clinical Trials Group. *Lancet* **356**, 2139–43.

Better OS, Stein JH (1990). Early management of shock and prophylaxis of acute renal failure in traumatic rhabdomyolysis. *New England Journal of Medicine* **322**, 825–9.

Bhandari S, Turney JH (1996). Survivors of acute renal failure who do not recover renal function. *Quarterly Journal of Medicine* **89**, 415–21.

Brosius FC, Lau K (1986). Low fractional excretion of sodium in acute renal failure: role of timing of the test and ischemia. *American Journal of Nephrology* **6**, 450–7.

Chugh KS (1989). Snake-bite-induced acute renal failure in India. *Kidney International* **35**, 891–907.

Chugh KS, *et al.* (1977). Acute renal failure following copper sulphate intoxication. *Postgraduate Medical Journal* **53**, 18–23.

Chugh KS, *et al.* (1977). Acute renal failure due to intravascular hemolysis in the North Indian patients. *American Journal of the Medical Sciences* **274**, 139–46.

Chugh KS, *et al.* (1989). Changing trends in acute renal failure in third-world countries—Chandigarh study. *Quarterly Journal of Medicine* **73**, 1117–23.

Chugh KS, *et al.* (1994). Acute renal cortical necrosis—a study of 113 patients. *Renal Failure* **16**, 37–47.

Cramer BC, *et al.* (1985). Renal function following infusion of radiologic contrast material. A prospective controlled study. *Archives of Internal Medicine* **145**, 87–9.

Denton MD, *et al.* (1996). 'Renal-dose' dopamine for the treatment of acute renal failure: scientific rationale, experimental studies and clinical trials. *Kidney International* **50**, 4–14.

Feest TG, *et al.* (1993). Incidence of severe acute renal failure in adults: results of a community based study. *British Medical Journal* **306**, 481–3.

Firth JD (1996). Acute irreversible renal failure. *Quarterly Journal of Medicine* **89**, 397–9.

Gines P, Arroyo V (1999). Hepatorenal syndrome. *Journal of the American Society of Nephrology* **10**, 1833–9.

Hirschberg R, *et al.* (1999). Multicenter clinical trial of recombinant human insulin-like growth factor I in patients with acute renal failure. *Kidney International* **55**, 2423–32.

Holt SG, Moore KP (2001). Pathogenesis and treatment of renal dysfunction in rhabdomyolysis. *Intensive Care Medicine* **27**, 803–11.

Hou SH, *et al.* (1983). Hospital-acquired renal insufficiency: a prospective study. *American Journal of Medicine* **74**, 243–8.

Jha V, *et al.* (1992). Spectrum of hospital-acquired acute renal failure in the developing countries—Chandigarh study. *Quarterly Journal of Medicine* **83**, 497–505.

Kleinknecht D, *et al.* (1973). Diagnostic procedures and long-term prognosis in bilateral renal cortical necrosis. *Kidney International* **4**, 390–400.

Leverve X, Barnoud D (1998). Stress metabolism and nutritional support in acute renal failure. *Kidney International Supplement* **66**, S62–6.

Levy M (1993). Hepatorenal syndrome. *Kidney International* **43**, 737–53.

Liano F, *et al.* (1994). Use of urinary parameters in the diagnosis of total acute renal artery occlusion. *Nephron* **66**, 170–5.

Lieberthal W, Nigam SK (1998). Acute renal failure. I. Relative importance of proximal vs. distal tubular injury. *American Journal of Physiology* **275**, F623–31.

Lieberthal W, Nigam SK (2000). Acute renal failure. II. Experimental models of acute renal failure: imperfect but indispensable. *American Journal of Physiology* **278**, F1–F12.

Lindner A (1983). Synergism of dopamine and furosemide in diuretic-resistant, oliguric acute renal failure. *Nephron* **33**, 121–6.

Maillet PJ, *et al.* (1986). Nondilated obstructive acute renal failure: diagnostic procedures and therapeutic management. *Radiology* **160**, 659–62.

Milligan SL, *et al.* (1978). Intra-abdominal infection and acute renal failure. *Archives of Surgery* **113**, 467–72.

Molitoris BA (1997). Cell biology of aminoglycoside nephrotoxicity: newer aspects. *Current Opinion in Nephrology and Hypertension* **6**, 384–8.

Murphy SW, *et al.* (2000). Contrast nephropathy. *Journal of the American Society of Nephrology* **11**, 177–82.

Nigame S, Lieberthal W (2000). Acute renal failure. III. The role of growth factors in the process of renal regeneration and repair. *American Journal of Physiology* **279**, F3–F11.

Parfrey PS, *et al.* (1989). Contrast material-induced renal failure in patients with diabetes mellitus, renal insufficiency, or both. A prospective controlled study. *New England Journal of Medicine* **320**, 143–9.

Pilmore HL, *et al.* (1995). Acute bilateral renal artery occlusion: successful revascularization with streptokinase. *American Journal of Nephrology* **15**, 90–1.

Ramsay AG, *et al.* (1983). Renal functional recovery 47 days after renal artery occlusion. *American Journal of Nephrology* **3**, 325–8.

Rasmussen HH, Ibels LS (1982). Acute renal failure. Multivariate analysis of causes and risk factors. *American Journal of Medicine* **73**, 211–18.

Remuzzi G (1988). Bleeding in renal failure. *Lancet* **1**, 1205–8.

Ronco C, *et al.* (2000). Effects of different doses in continuous veno-venous haemofiltration on outcomes of acute renal failure: a prospective randomised trial. *Lancet* **356**, 26–30.

Schiffer H, *et al.*(2002). Daily hemodialysis and the outcome of acute renal failure. *New England Journal of Medicine* **346**, 305–10.

Shilliday IR, *et al.* (1997). Loop diuretics in the management of acute renal failure: a prospective, double-blind, placebo-controlled, randomized study. *Nephrology, Dialysis, Transplantation* **12**, 2592–6.

Solez K, Racusen LC (2001). Role of the renal biopsy in acute renal failure. *Contributions to Nephrology* **132**, 68–75.

Solez K, *et al.* (1979). The morphology of 'acute tubular necrosis' in man: analysis of 57 renal biopsies and a comparison with the glycerol model. *Medicine (Baltimore)* **58**, 362–76.

Spital A, *et al.* (1988). Nondilated obstructive uropathy. *Urology* **31**, 478–82.

Sponsel H, Conger JD (1995). Is parenteral nutrition therapy of value in acute renal failure patients? *American Journal of Kidney Diseases* **25**, 96–102.

van Ypersele de Strihou C (1998). Hantavirus infection. In: Davison AM, *et al.*, eds. *Oxford textbook of clinical nephrology*, pp 1688–92. Oxford University Press, Oxford.

van Ypersele de Strihou C, Mery JP (1989). Hantavirus-related acute interstitial nephritis in western Europe. Expansion of a world-wide zoonosis. *Quarterly Journal of Medicine* **73**, 941–50.

Winearls CG, *et al.* (1984). Acute renal failure due to leptospirosis: clinical features and outcome in six cases. *Quarterly Journal of Medicine* **53**, 487–95.

20.5 Chronic renal failure

20.5.1 Chronic renal failure

C. G. Winearls

Introduction

Chronic renal failure is the clinical syndrome of the metabolic and systemic consequences of a gradual, substantial, and irreversible reduction in the excretory and homeostatic functions of the kidneys. It can be difficult to recognize because the symptoms and clinical manifestations are non-specific. However, if suspected, it is easily diagnosed by simple biochemical measurements. Early and specific diagnosis is worthwhile because this allows the application of effective treatments of both cause (in some cases) and consequences (in all cases), and substitution treatments are readily available for complete kidney failure. An understanding of chronic renal failure is important for doctors in both general and specialty practice: they will have to accommodate its consequences in their own work, for example in surgery, obstetrics, and in prescribing, and they will need to refer patients appropriately for specialist investigation and supervision.

For the patients who suffer it, chronic renal failure is an ever-increasing burden that they carry for the rest of their lives. Eventually, when end-stage renal failure (**ESRF**) is reached, they embark on a career of substitution treatments (dialysis and renal transplantation) referred to as renal replacement therapy. The illness and these treatments intrude on every aspect of their lives—physical, social, vocational, and emotional.

Definition

Chronic renal failure is defined as the state resulting from a permanent (and usually progressive) reduction in renal function, sufficient to have adverse consequences on other systems. The threshold at which these develop is at around 40 per cent of normal excretory capacity. A reduction in renal function below the third centile for age and gender (for example, by removing one of a pair of normal kidneys or limited damage to one or both), does not amount to chronic renal failure: although there is a loss of renal reserve, there are no clinical consequences.

The severity of chronic renal failure is graded according to the fraction of kidney function remaining (Table 1). These are useful descriptions because they give an indication of the likely symptoms and complications that

Table 1 Classification of the severity of renal failure

Severity of renal failure	GFR—usually estimated from the creatinine clearance value (ml/min)	Typical creatinine concentration in 65-kg subjects (μmol/l)	Consequences	Action
Reduced renal function	*>50 to <80*	140	None	
Mild	30–50	170	Hypertension, Early secondary hyperparathyroidism	Treat hypertension Start phosphate restriction and vitamin D analogues
Moderate	10–29	350	*As above plus:* Anaemia	Restrict Na and K intake to 60 mmol/day Advise modest protein restriction Plan renal replacement including vascular access (if appropriate)
Severe	<10	700	*As above plus:* Obvious salt and water retention Anorexia and vomiting Higher reduced mental function	Plan elective start of dialysis, or Pre-emptive transplant
Endstage	<5	1500	*As above plus:* Pulmonary oedema Coma/fits Uncompensated acidosis Hyperkalaemia Death	Start dialysis immediately or provide palliative care

should be anticipated, and provide cues to the key steps in both immediate and future management. Accurate measurement of glomerular filtration rate is not necessary to categorize the degree of renal failure: knowledge of the patient's age, gender, and body-weight applied to the Cockcroft–Gault formula:

glomerular filtration rate = [(140 − age in years) × weight (kg)]/plasma creatinine (μmol/l) × 0.82 (subtract 15 per cent for females)

will give an acceptable estimate (see Chapter 20.4 for further discussion). However, this grading of the severity of renal failure has limitations: as ESRF approaches there is a poor correlation between the actual glomerular filtration rate and symptoms which are caused by downstream consequences of that reduction: for example, breathlessness by pulmonary oedema or acidosis, fatigue by anaemia, muscle weakness by abnormalities in calcium and phosphate. The decision when to start dialysis should be made after integrating knowledge of the estimated glomerular filtration rate, symptoms, and recognition of complications. Decisions should not be based on estimates of plasma creatinine or urea.

Incidence and prevalence

The only accurate data on the incidence of chronic renal failure is for ESRF that is treated with renal replacement therapy, that is to say the number of patients starting such treatment. This is available from national and other databases, which also provide data on the prevalence of patients receiving renal replacement treatment (Table 2).

The incidence or prevalence of ESRF that is not treated with renal replacement therapy is unknown, nor is such information available for lesser degrees of chronic renal failure (mild, moderate, and severe): many patients are undiagnosed or not yet referred. This is illustrated by the fact that as many as 30 per cent of new patients starting renal replacement therapy meet a nephrologist for the first time less than 3 months before dialysis is begun. Crude estimates suggest there are about 500 to 1000 patients per million population with significant chronic renal impairment. Many of these patients will never require renal replacement therapy and will die with renal failure and not of it, examples include patients with malignant urinary tract obstruction, diabetes mellitus, renovascular disease with widespread cerebro- and cardiovascular disease.

From a workload point of view there are about 500 to 600 per million patients on renal replacement therapy in the United Kingdom and Australia, and over 1000 per million in the United States and Japan. This means that an average British general practitioner with 2000 registered patients will have only one dialysis or transplant patient on their list, and will see one new ESRF patient every 5 years. They will, however, be involved in the care of one or two patients with chronic renal failure. Renal failure is, when compared to chronic cardiovascular and respiratory diseases, a relatively small part of the general practitioner's workload.

The epidemiological study of renal failure has revealed some stark facts. It is a disease of the elderly: the incidence in a population over 75 years of age is 10 times higher at 400 per million population (**pmp**) than it is in those under 40 years of age; 50 per cent of patients now starting on renal replacement therapy are over 65 years of age. The incidence is higher in males (1.3:1), in areas of social deprivation, and in particular ethnic groups. In the United Kingdom it is 3.5 times higher in citizens of Asian or Afro-Caribbean backgrounds. In 1997 in Australia the incidence in Aboriginals was 435 pmp, which was six to seven times higher than in Caucasoids at 68 patients pmp. In New Zealand the incidence in Maoris is three to four times higher than in Caucasoids. These ethnic variations (which are related to the higher prevalence of diabetes and hypertension) can account only for part of the huge difference in the incidence of ESRF between Europe and the United States. There is still no easy explanation for the higher number of ESRF patients in Caucasian Americans than in the same age groups in Europe. Acceptance criteria for renal replacement therapy are much more stringent in the United Kingdom than in the United States, but although patients with terminal illness, dementia, or severe comorbid conditions are not usually started on dialysis, few patients who would benefit (that is, those who would survive independently for longer than 12 months) are excluded.

The prevalence of treated ESRF, in other words the number of patients receiving dialysis or a life-sustaining renal transplant, varies according to the capacity and availability of renal replacement programmes. In countries such as Germany, the United States, and Japan, where there are no constraints on the acceptance of patients for treatment, the prevalence is higher than elsewhere in the world. There are important health economic implications: renal replacement treatment has proved so successful that it is now accepted as a right in most developed countries. Improvements in patient survival and increases in acceptance rates (these have trebled in the United Kingdom in the last decade) mean that the total numbers of patients, and therefore the aggregate cost of maintenance treatment (already 2 per cent of the National Health Service (**NHS**) budget) is still increasing. A steady state has not yet been reached, and until it does the resources allocated will have to be increased too.

Causes of chronic renal failure

End-stage renal failure databases are the usual sources for descriptions of the causes of chronic renal failure. There are flaws in these because the meaning of terms such as 'pyelonephritis' may vary; diagnoses are allocated as best guesses by clinicians; glomerulonephritis is diagnosed without renal biopsy; and hypertension cited when it may be no more than a consequence of whatever caused the renal failure. The most rigorous database is that of the Australia and New Zealand Data (ANZDATA) Registry. The data in Table 3 should be interpreted with these caveats in mind.

Glomerulonephritis

Primary glomerulonephritis and secondary inflammatory glomerular disease (see Section 20.7, and Chapters 20.10.3 and 20.10.4).

Table 2 Incidence[1] and prevalence[2] of endstage renal failure (pmp)

Country	Year	Incidence	Prevalence	Source
USA	1997	296	1131	USRDS 1999 Annual Report
UK	1998	96	526	UK Renal Registry Report 2001
Australia	1998	85	555	22nd ANZDATA Registry Report 1999
Canada	1997	116	609	Canadian Organ Replacement Register
Japan	1997	229	1397	Japanese Society for Dialysis Therapy
France	1996	123	634	EDTA
Germany	1996	153	683	EDTA
Italy	1996	113	690	EDTA

[1] Incidence, number of new patients starting renal replacement therapy per million population/year.

[2] Prevalence, number of patients with endstage renal failure relying on renal replacement therapy per million population.

USRDS, United States Renal Data System; UK, United Kingdom; ANZDATA, Australian and New Zealand Dialysis and Transplant Registry; EDTA, European Dialysis and Transplantation Association.

Table 3 Given causes of end-stage renal failure

	Percentage of patients starting renal replacement therapy (year)		
	England and Wales (1995)	**Australia (1998)**	**United States (1993–7)**
Glomerulonephritis	12.4	34	12.9
Diabetes mellitus	13.8	21	40.3
Hypertension	7.8	12	24.6
Adult polycystic kidney disease	5.9	6	2.5
Analgesic nephropathy	—	5	0.2
Reflux nephropathy/pyelonephritis	9.1	6	4.2
Miscellaneous	18.3	10	7.8
Uncertain	17.0	6	4.0
Missing	15.7	—	3.5

Glomerulonephritis remains the most common cause of chronic renal failure outside the United States, accounting for 34 per cent of new cases in Australia. The patients usually suffer the common chronic glomerulonephritides, especially IgA disease, but including focal sclerosis, membranous nephropathy, and mesangiocapillary nephritis. These patients, more often males, are identified as marked for ESRF by heavy proteinuria, hypertension, interstitial changes in their renal biopsy specimens, and early and progressive renal dysfunction, in other words they have severe disease. Others have glomerular lesions secondary to systemic diseases such as systemic lupus erythematosis, Henoch–Schönlein purpura, systemic vasculitis, and, rarely, antiglomerular basement membrane antibody disease (**anti-GBM** disease). Progression to ESRF can be rapid or gradual after a severe acute nephritic illness has been halted but leaving substantial residual injury.

Diabetes (see Chapter 20.10.1)

This is now the commonest cause of ESRF in the United States (40 per cent of new patients) but is still behind that for glomerulonephritis in the United Kingdom and Australia (21 per cent). The diagnosis of diabetic nephropathy is usually assumed because of proteinuria, usually with concomitant retinopathy, in patients with a history of diabetes for 10 or more years. About half of the patients have type 2 diabetes, meaning that the onset was in middle life and not immediately requiring insulin.

By 40 years from the onset of diabetes, some 30 to 40 per cent of patients with type 1 diabetes have developed nephropathy and some, but not all, of these will survive long enough to develop ESRF. Between 5 and 10 per cent of type 2 diabetics already have nephropathy at the time their diabetes is diagnosed, and by 20 years from diagnosis 25 per cent of these will have overt nephropathy. It is not possible to predict with certainty which diabetics will develop nephropathy, but it is more likely in Blacks, Asians, and males, and in those with a family history of hypertension. There is now persuasive evidence that good glycaemic control reduces the risk of diabetic nephropathy, and that improving control will reduce the risk of progression of patients with microalbuminuria to overt nephropathy. It has not been shown that glycaemic control affects the prognosis of established diabetic nephropathy. Once overt nephropathy (proteinuria above 0.5 g/day) develops, the median time to ESRF is about 7 years for those with type 1 diabetes but it is more variable in type 2.

Young people with type 1 diabetes present the greatest challenges—they often have many additional complications such as blindness from retinopathy and vitreous haemorrhage, peripheral and autonomic neuropathy, precocious cardiovascular disease, and, unfortunately, some scepticism of conventional medical advice. The older diabetics are usually obese and often have severe peripheral vascular and coronary disease. Both these groups need a multidisciplinary team to care for them—nephrologists, diabetologists, ophthalmologists, vascular surgeons, and podiatrists.

When assessing diabetics with renal problems it should be remembered that they are also susceptible to non-diabetic renal disease such as glomerulonephritis and (particularly) renovascular disease. Their renal failure can be exacerbated by papillary necrosis, usually associated with pyelonephritis. They are more susceptible to renal tuberculosis and fungal infections, especially if autonomic neuropathy has affected bladder function.

There is a general and probably appropriate tendency to start dialysis earlier in those with diabetes. In the younger patient one aims for renal transplantation, ideally with whole pancreas transplantation, as early as possible. Islet-cell transplantation may, in the future, prove to be the best option. Dialysis and diabetes seem to have a synergistically adverse effect on the vasculature. Before embarking on transplantation, a vigorous search for silent coronary artery disease is essential. The prognosis for the survival of all diabetics is much worse than for any other cause of renal failure except malignancy.

Hypertension and renal vascular disease (see Chapters 15.16.2.2 and 20.10.2)

Hypertension is cited as the primary renal disease causing ESRF in 12 per cent of Australian patients and in 25 per cent in the United States. Chronic renal failure is a rare complication of primary essential hypertension, but the large number of patients with hypertension means that it is a relatively common cause. The risk of renal failure is higher in Blacks. Accelerated-phase hypertension was once a frequent cause of ESRF but is now relatively rare, except again in Blacks. Renovascular disease, which is not separately classified, is an increasingly common cause, especially in the elderly. The patients have a history of other vascular diseases—coronary, cerebral, or peripheral—and present with renal impairment, hypertension, and occasionally 'flash' pulmonary oedema. If the arterial stenoses or occlusions are bilateral or the stenosis is in the artery supplying the functionally dominant kidney, angiotensin-converting enzyme (**ACE**) inhibitors or α2-receptor blockers will cause a sharp but usually reversible rise in plasma creatinine. Angioplasty and stenting seldom rescue much renal function but may slow progression or prevent acute occlusion. In atheromatous renal arterial disease, stenting makes relatively little difference to blood pressure control.

Adult polycystic kidney disease (see Chapter 20.11)

The development of renal failure is seldom a surprise in patients with adult polycystic kidney disease whose condition has usually been diagnosed for other reasons (for instance, a family history, hypertension, haematuria, or a loin mass). Once renal impairment is diagnosed, the loss of function is predictable at about 5 to 6 ml/min per year, tending to be more rapid in males than females. Adult polycystic kidney disease accounts for about 6 per cent of those receiving renal replacement therapy in the United Kingdom and Australia, the median age at which ESRF (which is not inevitable) is reached being 55 years, but with a wide range from 25 to 75 years. ESRF occurs 10 to 15 years later in those with type 2 adult polycystic kidney disease than in those with the commoner type 1 disease.

Reflux nephropathy (see Chapter 20.12)

Reflux nephropathy (a congenital and often inherited abnormality of the vesicoureteric junction) and congenital structural abnormalities of the urinary tract are important causes of chronic renal failure in the young, the mean age of entering renal replacement therapy programmes being 30 years. Once a threshold fraction of nephron mass has been lost, perhaps as a consequence of infection-related scarring, the remaining glomeruli develop segmental hyalinosis and eventually sclerosis, manifesting as proteinuria and hypertension, both heralding a steady decline towards end-stage disease. Antireflux procedures make no difference to the prognosis, and management is medical.

Miscellaneous (Table 4)

Many renal conditions, some primary and others secondary to systemic diseases, can cause chronic renal failure.

Drugs

Analgesic nephropathy is declining in incidence but is still common in Australia and parts of Europe (5 per cent). Ciclosporin toxicity can cause chronic renal failure in patients who have received cardiac, liver, and lung allografts. A few patients on long-term lithium medication for bipolar affective disorder develop chronic renal failure. Long-term, non-steroidal anti-inflammatory drugs (**NSAIDs**) use is also associated with chronic renal failure.

Obstructive uropathy (see Chapter 20.14)

Neglected or unrecognized obstruction, associated sometimes with calculi, infection, or malignancy, accounts for a small but significant number of patients requiring dialysis. Any manoeuvre (for example, ureteric stenting) which relieves obstruction, is worthwhile for the preservation of renal function.

Dysproteinaemias (see Chapter 20.10.5)

Primary amyloid, myeloma kidney, and the other immunoglobulin deposition diseases are relatively rare. The patients, usually elderly, generally have a poor prognosis, having to cope with the consequences and treatment not only of the underlying disease, but also the hazards and inconvenience of dialysis. Survival on dialysis is seldom longer than 2 years.

Table 4 Less common causes of chronic renal failure

Metabolic	Cystinosis, cystinuria (stones), oxalosis, nephrocalcinosis, urate nephropathy
Vascular	Ischaemic renal disease, scleroderma, haemolytic uraemic syndrome, postpartum renal failure
Hereditary	Alport's syndrome, Fabry's disease, tuberous sclerosis, sickle-cell disease, medullary cystic disease (and the metabolic conditions listed above)
Vasculitis	Wegener's granulomatosis, microscopic polyangiitis, polyarteritis nodosa, systemic lupus erythematosus, Henoch–Schönlein disease
Malignancy	Renal-cell cancer, von Hippel–Lindau syndrome, lymphoma
Dysproteinaemias	Myeloma, primary (AL) and secondary (AA) amyloid (familial Mediterranean fever), cryoglobulinaemia
Structural/infection/ interstitial	Cystic disease other than ADPKD, congenital and acquired abnormalities of the lower urinary tract, tuberculous and schistosomias, Balkan nephropathy

ADPKD, autosomal dominant polycystic kidney disease.

Pregnancy (see Chapter 13.5)

Irreversible postpartum renal failure is now rare in developed countries but is still a problem in the developing world.

Unknown

In a significant proportion of patients no confident diagnosis of the cause of chronic renal failure can be made. There are no clues in the history, although a renal condition may have been suspected because of long-standing minor urinary abnormalities (such as asymptomatic proteinuria or haematuria). Imaging reveals small echogenic kidneys, which cannot safely be biopsied, and even if tissue does become available it seldom reveals a specific diagnosis. The glomeruli are sclerosed and there is widespread interstitial fibrosis and vascular changes, which are probably secondary. It may be that there are unrecognized renal diseases caused by environmental toxins, but this is speculation. The recent description of the development of renal failure after the consumption of Chinese herbal remedies containing aristocholic acid shows the need to be agnostic on causality. Some patients do probably have unrecognized glomerulonephritis (as shown by the development of IgA nephropathy in subsequent kidney allografts). Others may have silent cholesterol emboli, analgesic nephropathy, or 'burnt out' tuberculosis.

The pattern in developing countries of Asia, Africa, and Latin America is quite different. Chronic glomerulonephritis (especially infection-associated disease, see Chapter 20.7.10) and hypertension are the dominant causes in Africa. In Asia, diabetes mellitus—usually type 2—is almost as common a cause as glomerulonephritis. Obstructive uropathy is a more common cause than in Europe because of the higher incidence of tuberculosis, schistosomiasis, urethral strictures, and renal stone disease. Other diseases more common in these countries, which may cause chronic renal failure, include systemic lupus erythematosus (especially in Asian women), sickle-cell disease, and human immunodeficiency virus (**HIV**) infection.

Pathophysiology of chronic renal failure

In chronic renal failure, compensatory and adaptive mechanisms maintain acceptable health until the glomerular filtration rate is about 10 to 15 ml/min, and life-sustaining renal excretory and homeostatic functions continue until the glomerular filtration rate (**GFR**) is less than 5 ml/min. The favoured explanation for the pathophysiology of this condition centres on the 'intact nephron hypothesis' first proposed by Bricker, which states that despite distortion of renal architecture and a widened range of single nephron GFR in diseased or damaged kidneys, glomerular and tubular function remains closely integrated in all individual nephrons, both normal and damaged. As the GFR of the whole kidney falls, still-functioning nephrons produce an increased volume of filtrate ('hyperfiltration') and their tubules respond appropriately for overall homeostasis by excreting fluid and solutes in amounts that maintain external balance. For sodium and potassium, compensation can occur down to a glomerular filtration rate as low as 5 ml/min and plasma values are commonly normal. For phosphate and urate, adaptation is less precise and plasma concentrations are increased in many patients at a glomerular filtration rate of 20 ml/min and in almost all at 5 to 10 ml/min.

The functional adaptations of individual nephrons that allow homeostasis to be maintained in the face of a substantially reduced GFR do not come without a price, and the 'trade off' hypothesis needs to be considered alongside the intact nephron hypothesis. This describes the concept that adaptations arising in chronic renal failure may control one abnormality, but only in such a way as to produce other changes characteristic of the uraemic syndrome. The best example of 'trade off' is the increase in parathormone secretion essential for the increased fractional excretion of phosphate: as the glomerular filtration rate falls plasma phosphate rises, parathormone secretion increases, and plasma phosphate is lowered by decreased tubular reabsorption. The cost of normal plasma phosphate is then secondary hyperparathyroidism, sometimes leading to metastatic calcification (see Chapter 20.6.1).

Electrolytes and water

Inability to concentrate urine in the presence of dehydration is often the first symptom of chronic renal failure, resulting in polyuria, nocturia, and thirst when GFR is about 30 ml/min, although diseases that predominantly affect the medulla, such as pyelonephritis, interstitial nephritis, and medullary cystic disease, may present with a concentration defect at an earlier stage. Defective urine concentration is due to an increased solute load in surviving nephrons, with minor contributions from decreased tubular function and increased GFR per nephron. Thirst accompanies polyuria and water balance is maintained provided there is free access to fluid. As obligatory water loss is increased, careful attention needs to be paid to fluid balance in the presence of anorexia, fever, surgery, and other sources of extrarenal loss if dehydration, hypotension, and further impairment of renal function are to be avoided.

Diluting capacity is preserved until renal failure is advanced, the asymmetrical narrowing of the range of urinary osmolality eventually producing the fixed (300 mosmol/kg) urinary osmolality of chronic renal failure with its obligatory polyuria (Fig. 1). It should be noted, however, that although urinary dilution is maintained until late in chronic renal failure, large water loads are excreted more slowly than in normal subjects and excessive intake (by drinking or an ill-advised iatrogenic infusion of dextrose-containing solutions) can result in hyponatraemia, mental disturbances, and convulsions.

Sodium excess and hypertension

As renal function decreases, hormonal mechanisms increase the fraction of filtered sodium excreted so that the sodium balance and extracellular fluid volume are maintained until the GFR is less than 10 ml/min. The extent of this adaptation is such that the 1 per cent or less of filtered sodium excreted by normal subjects increases to 30 per cent in those with late chronic renal failure. However, adaptive mechanisms are not unlimited, and in late renal failure increased total body sodium, with water to maintain osmotic equilibrium, presents as fluid overload and hypertension. Initially, excess extracellular fluid does not cause oedema, but in late renal failure an elevated jugular venous pressure, functional incompetence of the mitral valve, and pulmonary and peripheral oedema are often seen. Another major consequence of sodium and fluid excess is hypertension, present in 80 per cent of patients in late chronic renal failure and occasionally presenting in the accelerated phase, although precisely how sodium retention and increased extracellular fluid volume lead to high blood pressure remains uncertain.

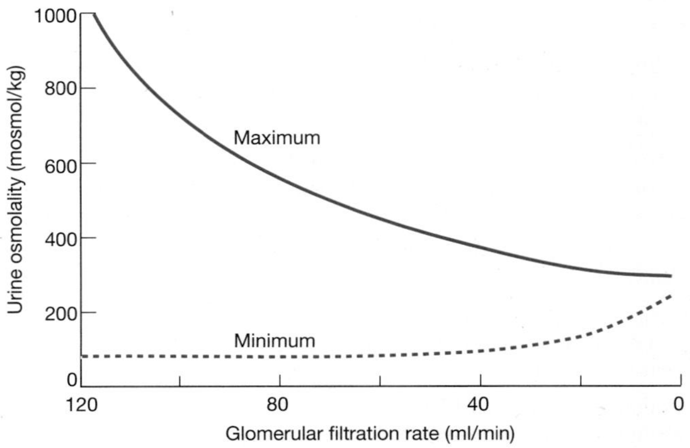

Fig. 1 Progressive loss of flexibility in water handling as renal failure worsens. Concentrating ability is impaired earlier than the ability to excrete a dilute urine.

Sodium depletion

Patients with chronic renal failure can also be vulnerable to sodium depletion. In the presence of dietary sodium restriction or loss of sodium by various routes, functioning nephrons cannot restrict sodium excretion promptly so that the extracellular fluid, plasma volume, and GFR all decrease. Although this sodium and fluid loss has been attributed to an osmotic diuresis, other mechanisms are involved and may dominate; thus, if sodium restriction is induced slowly over months, patients can reduce their urinary sodium concentration to less than 10 mmol/l without significant reduction in GFR. A few patients with early chronic renal failure, usually with diseases affecting the renal medulla (for example, obstructive uropathy and medullary cystic disease), present with a urinary sodium leak and sodium depletion on a normal sodium diet. Blood pressure in these patients is normal or low, often with a postural drop of arterial pressure. Sodium supplements may be needed.

Potassium

Most patients maintain a normal external potassium balance until their GFR is less than 5 ml/min, but their capacity to excrete potassium is limited and severe hyperkalaemia may follow a sudden reduction in residual GFR, excess dietary intake (chocolate, nuts, instant coffee, some fruits and their juices, wine), potassium-sparing diuretics (spironolactone, amiloride, triamterene), medication with a high potassium content, surgery, and hypercatabolic states. Acidosis raises serum potassium by ion transfer out of cells and interference with renal excretion. Hypoxia causes hyperkalaemia by impaired uptake of potassium from extracellular fluid. In some patients, particularly those with diabetes mellitus and/or interstitial nephritis, and sometimes in early chronic renal failure, hyperkalaemia may be due to selective aldosterone deficiency (hyporeninaemic hypoaldosteronism) or the use of angiotensin-converting enzyme (ACE) inhibitors. Tubular resistance to aldosterone is another rare cause of hyperkalaemia. Complications occur at plasma potassium concentrations above 7.0 mmol/l; a weakness in pelvic and shoulder girdle muscles may be the presenting symptom, but in most patients serious electrocardiographic abnormalities and cardiac arrhythmias are the first sign of hyperkalaemia (see Chapter 20.2.2 and Chapter 20.5.2 for further discussion).

Calcium and phosphate and Vitamin D

The role of the kidney in regulating calcium and phosphate in body fluids and tissues is described in Chapter 20.6.1. Magnesium concentrations are usually high and care must be exercised with the use of magnesium-containing drugs.

Acid–base

The kidney is an essential organ for maintenance of the acid–base balance by reabsorption of filtered bicarbonate, acidification of urinary buffers. and excretion of ammonia. As renal failure progresses, at least until GFR is less than 20 ml/min, intact nephrons increase their excretion of hydrogen ions to prevent acidosis. Increasing acidosis, variable between patients, occurs at a GFR of less than 10 ml/min—when normal net acid production exceeds the excretory capacity of remaining nephrons and diminished tubular function impairs ammonia synthesis and bicarbonate regeneration. Renal diseases that principally affect tubules and interstitial tissues are associated with acidosis quite early in the course of chronic renal failure. Acidosis seldom requires treatment unless the bicarbonate concentration is less than 15 mmol/l and the pH less than 7.30, except in children in whom prevention of severe acidosis with bicarbonate supplements may have a beneficial effect on renal osteodystrophy and growth retardation. Delayed excretion of excess base is also a feature of late chronic renal failure so that metabolic alkalosis may occur more easily and resolve more slowly after, for instance, prolonged gastric aspiration.

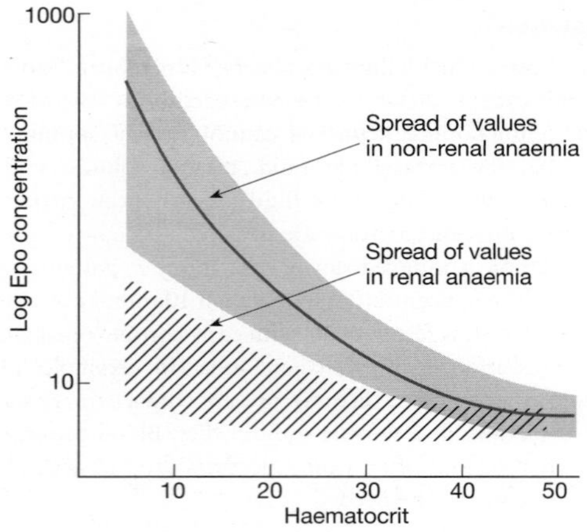

Fig. 2 In renal anaemia the erythropoietin concentration rises in response to anaemia, but to a much lower concentration than in non-renal anaemia. This is a consequence of defective oxygen sensing, reduced synthesis, or both.

Endocrine dysfunction

The endocrine functions of the kidney can be disturbed in kidney disease, for example reduced production of 1,25-dihydroxy vitamin D (see Chapter 20.6.1) and erythropoietin (Fig. 2). There are also diverse abnormalities in the production, control, protein binding, catabolism, and tissue effect of extrarenal hormones in renal failure. Hormone concentrations may be elevated as a result of reduced degradation (insulin) or increased secretion in appropriate response to metabolic alterations (parathormone, **PTH**). Hormone concentrations may be reduced owing to impaired production (oestrogen, testosterone). There may also be disturbances of activation through altered prohormones. Finally, reductions in hormone-binding proteins are most commonly a consequence of protein loss in nephrotic patients or in those on continuous ambulatory peritoneal dialysis.

Thyroid hormones

Total thyroxine (T_4) may be low with increased reverse tri-iodothyronine (T_3) as a result of impaired conversion of T_4 to T_3. Loss of thyroid-binding globulin (**TBG**) may further lower total circulating T_4 concentrations. However, patients are not clinically hypothyroid and measurements of thyroid-stimulating hormone (**TSH**) remain a reliable diagnostic test for hypothyroidism in patients with renal failure.

Growth hormone

Plasma growth-hormone levels are abnormally high in patients in renal failure because of delayed clearance and alterations in the hypothalamic–pituitary control of growth-hormone release. In adults the clinical implications of these changes are not clear. In children with renal failure and growth retardation, production of insulin-like growth factor-1 (**IGF-1**) in response to growth hormone is impaired; this can be overcome by treatment with exogenous recombinant growth hormone in supraphysiological dosage.

Insulin

Decreased clearance of insulin seems to be balanced by increased peripheral resistance to the effects of insulin, hence there are usually no clinical effects and patients are not prone to hypoglycaemia or diabetes, but there is a reduced requirement for insulin in diabetics as renal function declines.

Sex hormones

Males

Prolactin levels are high in renal failure and may contribute to gynaecomastia and sexual dysfunction in men. Testosterone levels are often low to normal in males, but gonadotrophins are raised, implying testicular failure as the cause.

Females

Raised prolactin levels contribute to infertility. In severe renal failure the pituitary–ovary axis is disturbed: luteinizing hormone is raised, but the normal pulsatile release and preovulation surge are absent, hence cycles are often anovulatory, causing oestrogen deficiency.

Middle molecules and the uraemic syndrome

Although many of the manifestations of the uraemic syndrome are attributable to the derangement in electrolyte concentrations, fluid imbalance, and endocrine deficiencies, there are others that are explained by the actions of substances and metabolites retained because of excretory failure. Examples include encephalopathy, glucose intolerance, platelet dysfunction, anaemia, and leucocyte dysfunction. Knowledge of the nature, mode of action, and contribution of those substances referred to as 'uraemic toxins' or 'middle molecules' to the syndrome is incomplete. The best example of a middle molecule is β_2-microglobulin, which is normally excreted by the kidneys, reaches a concentration of 30 times higher than normal in dialysis patients, and accumulates as β_2-microglobulin amyloid in joints and bone. It meets fully the criteria of a 'uraemic toxin'. However, because a substance is retained in uraemia and removed by dialysis does not mean that it can be indicted for a particular element of the uraemic syndrome. To be sure that a substance is relevant to the uraemic syndrome, its concentration should be raised in renal failure, should relate to the severity of the particular effect, and the effect should be reproduced by the substance alone and ameliorated by reducing the concentration. The subject of uraemic toxins has been approached by considering: (1) their existence predicted by abnormalities detected in *in vitro* systems; (2) known chemical effects of urea retention; and (3) identifiable substances.

Urea itself has rather modest effects, but it is used as a marker of accumulation of other metabolites. It inhibits cell-membrane electrolyte transport *in vitro* and is thought to have a direct effect on appetite and protein anabolism. It forms isocyanic acid, which reacts with amino groups on amino acids, carbamoylating them or the proteins of which they are constituents. Similarly, modification of lipoproteins may decrease their binding to receptors, thereby delaying their metabolism.

In a manner analogous to reverse genetics, the existence of certain uraemic toxins can be predicted. Examples include insulin resistance, which in uraemia is improved by dialysis, and a number of factors in uraemic plasma that inhibit glucose metabolism have been found but not identified. Similarly, inhibitors of calcitriol binding to its receptor have been found in ultrafiltrates of uraemic plasma.

Some compounds that accumulate in uraemia are thought to have a direct effect, including:

(1) homocysteine—raised concentrations of which are thought to be atherogenic by an oxidation effect on lipoproteins;

(2) methylguanidine—a neurotoxin that may explain the uraemic peripheral neuropathy;

(3) the aminoguanidine **ADMA** (asymmetric dimethylarginine)— is a potent inhibitor of nitric acid synthesis that may have a bearing on hypertension of renal failure;

(4) β_2-microglobulin—accumulation of which causes β_2-microglobulin amyloid;

(5) drugs such as morphine—which are metabolized to excretable glucuronides that accumulate in renal failure and cause or exacerbate encephalopathy.

Although incomplete, knowledge of the presence of uraemic toxins is what underpins the perceived benefit of early and adequate dialysis for uraemia.

One of the clearest manifestations of the uraemic syndrome is anaemia. The physiological mechanisms controlling red cell mass are shown in Fig. 3.

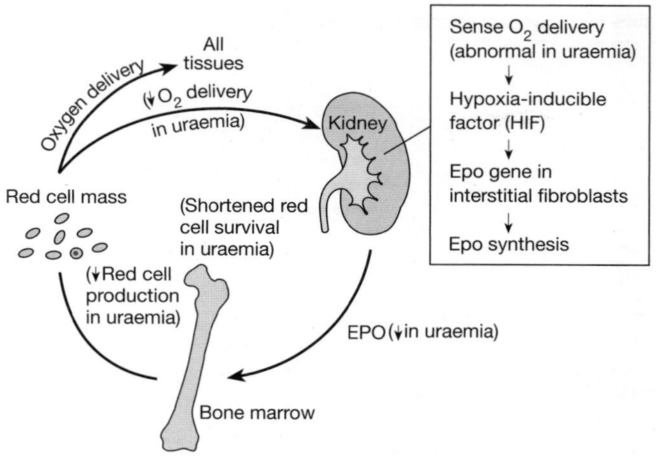

Fig. 3 The relationship between red cell mass, oxygen delivery, anaemia, erythropoietin (Epo) synthesis, and red cell production in the bone marrow. Erythropoietin production is reduced in uraemia, either because of defective sensing or reduced synthesis.

The maintenance of a normal red cell mass requires a rate of red cell production by a healthy bone marrow, with no substrate limitations and under the influence of an adequate amount of erythropoietin, to balance red cell loss and destruction. In uraemia all components are disturbed. Red cell lifespan is shortened by accelerated destruction, possibly caused by substances within uraemic plasma that alter the red cell membrane. To compensate for a shorter lifespan, a higher than normal production of red cells is required, which is dependent on an increase in the erythropoietin secretion rate. Concentrations do indeed rise, but not enough to set erythropoiesis at a sufficient level (Fig. 2). The classic experiment of providing exogenous erythropoietin to treat anaemia shows that: (1) red cell survival is not altered by erythropoietin; (2) red cell mass is restored; (3) marrow activity has to be maintained at a higher than normal level to achieve this. It is a much-argued point whether the marrow is itself normal. *In vitro* experiments reveal that constituents of uraemic plasma can suppress erythropoiesis. However, the fact that the effects of these constituents can obviously be overridden by exogenous erythropoietin does not exclude the possibility of resistance. It is not possible to say whether the doses of erythropoietin required to reverse anaemia are physiological because the modes of delivery—subcutaneous and intravenous injection—are not.

Progression of chronic renal failure

The clinical course of most nephropathies is a progressive decline in renal function. However, the rate of progression varies considerably between patients and diseases, generally being faster in chronic glomerulonephritides than in tubulointerstitial nephritides.

Factors influencing the rate of progression

Proteinuria

The degree of proteinuria correlates with the rate of progression of the underlying nephropathy and is the most reliable prognostic factor in chronic renal failure. In chronic glomerulonephritis, persistent heavy proteinuria (greater than 3 g/24 h) predicts a poor outcome. Conversely, the absence of significant proteinuria or its partial or complete remission indicates a favourable prognosis. In patients with diabetes or tubulointerstitial nephropathy, such as reflux nephropathy, the onset of significant proteinuria (greater than 1 g/24 h) usually predicts a decline in renal function. Proteinuria may be a marker of severe renal disease, but it is possible that the filtration and overloading of the tubules with protein may itself damage the nephron.

Hypertension

The most important factor influencing the rate of progression is systemic hypertension, which appears early in the course of renal diseases and long precedes the onset of ESRF. As with proteinuria, hypertension is a marker of more severe renal disease, but there is good evidence that the raised arterial pressure is itself pathogenetic.

Other factors

Ethnicity and genes

Certain major histocompatibility antigens have been associated with a poor outcome in some forms of glomerulonephritis, for example in membranous nephropathy. In adult polycystic kidney disease, patients with type 1 (abnormal gene on chromosome 16) have an earlier onset and a faster rate of decline compared to those with type 2 (whose abnormal gene is on chromosome 4) (see Chapter 20.11). Afro- and, to a lesser extent, Hispanic Americans suffer a faster rate of progression when compared to Caucasians. Diabetic nephropathy progresses more rapidly in Afro- and native Americans.

Gender

Renal function deteriorates faster in males with adult polycystic kidney disease, mesangial IgA disease, and membranous nephropathy. In Western societies, males tend to have a higher blood pressure than age-matched females, which may explain this difference.

Mechanisms of progression

The loss of filtration rate in chronic renal disorders is a consequence of progressive glomerulosclerosis, tubulointerstitial fibrosis, and vascular sclerosis. Glomerulosclerosis has been attributed to immunological (glomerulonephritis), haemodynamic (hypertension), or metabolic (diabetes mellitus) insults leading to glomerular endothelial injury. In surviving ('remnant') glomeruli, a compensatory increase in intraglomerular capillary pressure (glomerular hypertension) results from a disproportionate afferent arteriolar vasodilatation and the loss of autoregulation, exposing them to systemic hypertension that in turn is associated with endothelial damage. Injury to the glomerular endothelium favours platelet adhesion, aggregation, and the formation of glomerular microthrombi, allowing the transudation of macromolecules, including lipids and growth factors, into the glomerular mesangium. These stimulate mesangial proliferation and the increased synthesis of extracellular collagenous matrix.

Tubulointerstitial scarring

There is a correlation between the severity of tubulointerstitial scarring and GFR. Tubulointerstitial inflammation and widespread interstitial fibrosis are markers of a worse outcome in renal disease: these are characterized by inadequate healing with excessive collagen deposition and involve interactions between renal tubular cells, inflammatory cells, and resident fibroblasts through the release of cytokines and growth promoters.

Vascular sclerosis

The extent and severity of renal vascular changes (arterial and arteriolar) is also relevant to outcome. Although hyalinosis of smaller renal vessels is common in patients of all ages with chronic renal disease, severe arteriolar hyalinosis is often seen in the kidney tissue of patients with chronic nephropathies in the absence of significant systemic hypertension. Moreover, the severity of these vascular changes is greater than that seen in patients with essential hypertension. This arteriolar hyalinosis further jeopardizes the glomerular and tubular blood supply, causing ischaemic injury and further scarring.

Clinical presentation

The presentation of chronic renal failure will depend on the degree of renal dysfunction at the time medical help is sought.

- *Asymptomatic*—At one extreme are asymptomatic patients in whom an abnormal creatinine is noticed on a 'routine' biochemical screen. Such patients may be shocked when it is explained that they have lost what might be a substantial amount of their renal function, and counselling them and persuading them to comply with follow up and medication is sometimes difficult. Patients with illnesses known to cause renal failure, such as adult polycystic kidney disease, are easier to manage because they usually understand the progressive nature of renal failure and the need to introduce various measures in steps.
- *Associated disease*—Much renal failure is picked up in general medical, hypertension, diabetic, cardiac, and urology clinics because clinicians are aware of the effect of other diseases on renal function.
- *Symptomatic presentation*—Relatively few patients are diagnosed because they present with the non-specific symptoms of chronic renal failure, such as lethargy, dyspnoea, and anorexia. Those that are will be relieved that their symptoms have an explanation. At the extreme end of this category are the patients who present with an acute uraemic emergency requiring urgent dialysis, constituting about 5 per cent of patients entering renal replacement treatment programmes. Another 25 per cent are close to end-stage renal failure when they are first seen by a nephrologist and need dialysis within 3 months of the first consultation.

It may at first be difficult to distinguish acute from chronic renal failure, but a systematic history, examination, and appropriate investigations should soon distinguish the two (Table 5). The presentation of ESRF as a uraemic emergency is often the result of missed diagnostic opportunities, but may be the presentation of a rapidly progressive illness such as rapidly progressive nephritis, myeloma, or renal vascular disease.

Assessment

All patients with chronic renal failure should be referred for specialist opinion, although their care can often best be shared with the primary care physician or other specialist, for instance a diabetic physician.

The patient with ESRF

The 5 per cent of patients with chronic renal failure who present as uraemic emergencies may be comatose, may have fitted, and may have asterixis. The skin shows excoriation from pruritus, purpura, and bruising on a sallow yellow-brown background. The blood pressure is raised and examination of the fundi may reveal haemorrhages and exudates. The apex beat is displaced laterally and there is often a pericardial friction rub. There are basal lung crepitations and oedema of the face, sacrum, and ankles. Blood investigations show a urea concentration above 50 mmol/l, a creatinine concentration above 1000 μmol/l, hypocalcaemia, hyperphosphataemia, hyperkalaemia, and a partially compensated metabolic acidosis. There is a normochromic normocytic anaemia, a normal white blood count, and a platelet count in the low normal range.

Table 5 Indications of chronicity of renal failure

History
>6 months' ill health, long-standing hypertension, proteinuria, nocturia for >6 months; sexual dysfunction; abnormalities detected during routine medicals and/or pregnancies; recurrent illness during childhood
Examination
Pallor, pigmentation, and pruritus, brown nails, evidence of long-standing hypertension; the patient often appears 'well' for their very abnormal biochemistry
Investigations
Normochromic anaemia; small kidneys on ultrasound (except: diabetes, amyloid, myeloma, adult polycystic kidney disease); renal osteodystrophy on radiography (this is rarely found but is conclusive evidence if present)

Table 6 Causes of acute deterioration in chronic renal failure

Renal hypoperfusion	Dehydration from diarrhoea, diuretics, surgery Cardiac failure Pericardial tamponade (rare) Renal vascular disease Drugs, especially ACE inhibitors + NSAIDs Systemic infection
Obstruction and infection of the urinary tract	Papillary necrosis and sloughing Stones Bladder cancer Polycystic cysts Clot in the ureter
Metabolic and toxic	Hypercalcaemia Hyperuricaemia Contrast media (especially in diabetes) Drugs, especially aminoglycosides
Progression of underlying diseases	Relapse of nephritis
Development of accelerated-phase hypertension	
Renal vein thrombosis	Usually in chronically nephrotic patients
Pregnancy	At the end of the pregnancy or after delivery, e.g. in patients with reflux nephropathy

ACE, angiotensin-converting enzyme; NSAIDs, non-steroidal anti-inflammatory drugs.

The patient may be too ill to give a history, but family and/or friends report a general deterioration in health over the preceding 6 months with dyspnoea, anorexia, pruritus, and nocturia. Such a patient is easy to diagnose, indeed the ammoniacal smell of the breath often alerts the family practitioner. This medical emergency is now infrequently encountered in societies with developed medical services, but the gradual nature of the deterioration is such that it may take some dramatic event like a fit to provoke referral. The morbidity in such patients is high and it is obvious that the opportunity for halting the underlying pathology or slowing progression will have been lost. Most patients present with a much milder combination of symptoms and signs and are often irritated that their non-specific symptoms had not earlier been attributed to chronic renal failure. They should be told that renal failure is rare and that, in the absence of obvious clues, no doctor should be criticized for missing the diagnosis in the early stages.

Many patients will present to hospitals without dialysis facilities. If so, it needs to be established whether there are any immediately life-threatening complications that mandate urgent transfer to a hospital where dialysis can be provided. These include hyperkalaemia, refractory pulmonary oedema, severe hypertension, metabolic acidosis, and encephalopathy. The specific management of these is described in Section 20.5. After dealing with these issues, the next point is to determine whether there are factors which have caused or are causing an acute reduction in chronically impaired renal function. If so, can they be reversed? (Table 6). Examples include:

- *Hypoperfusion*—This can result from dehydration caused by diarrhoea, vomiting, iatrogenic deprivation of fluid (e.g. following surgery), or the overzealous use of diuretics. An occasional cause is the renal loss of salt and water in conditions such as medullary cystic disease. Significant dehydration is associated with a reduction in weight and postural hypotension. Worsening renal arterial stenosis and cholesterol emboli should be sought in arteriopaths.
- *Drugs*—Many drugs, particularly non-steroidal anti-inflammatory drugs (**NSAIDs**), aminoglycosides, and antihypertensive agents, can cause a reduction in GFR, and many others cause acute interstitial nephritis. Tetracyclines cause nausea and vomiting. Clofibrate causes

rhabdomyolysis and myoglobinuria. Contrast media in the dehydrated patient are another cause of sudden deterioration in function.

- *Infection*—Systemic infection such as pneumonia can reduce the GFR, and renal parenchymal infections in patients with diabetes, analgesic nephropathy, or adult polycystic kidney disease can damage the remaining functioning renal tissue.
- *Obstruction*—Renal function may worsen substantially in a patient with chronic renal failure if one kidney is obstructed by calculi or papillary necrosis, for example. Sloughed papillae should be sought in those with analgesic nephropathy, diabetes, an obstruction, or sickle-cell disease. Retroperitoneal fibrosis may be occult and is not always detected by ultrasound examination (see Chapter 20.14).
- *Relapse* of the underlying disease—Patients with diseases such as systemic lupus erythematosus, IgA nephropathy, or systemic vasculitic syndromes will deteriorate when the underlying disease relapses, causing further damage to glomeruli. Diagnosis can be difficult because the kidneys are too small to biopsy. Serology and examination of the urine deposit can be helpful. Occasionally, membranous nephropathy and membranoproliferative glomerulonephritis can change in character with the development of extracapillary proliferation (crescent formation), and this is associated with a rapid decline in function. Renal vein thrombosis also causes deterioration in function and should be considered in those with chronic nephrotic syndrome, particularly with underlying membranous nephropathy or focal segmental glomerulosclerosis.
- *Hypertension*—The development of accelerated-phase hypertension may cause a sharp and irreversible reduction in residual renal function. This is most likely in patients with glomerulonephritis.
- *Congestive heart failure*—Independent of the salt and water retention of uraemia, congestive heart failure itself can lead to a reduction in GFR. This can be a result of hypertension, myocardial infarction, or arrhythmias.
- *Hypercalcaemia*—The use of vitamin D analogues such as alfa-calcidol (1α-hydroxycholecalciferol) to prevent hyperparathyroidism often leads to hypercalcaemia. When marked (plasma [Ca^{2+}] >3 mmol/l), this causes a reduction in GFR, usually by causing dehydration.
- *Pregnancy*—Early in pregnancy the plasma creatinine concentration tends to fall, but the course of diseases such as reflux nephropathy or glomerulonephritis may accelerate (see Chapter 13.5).

Once the pressure of the emergency situation is resolved, or if the patient has been referred to the outpatient department with apparently stable chronic renal impairment, the clinician will need to make a thorough assessment of the cause and degree of renal failure and its complications, and institute the appropriate treatments, counsel the patient about the prognosis, and (if appropriate) plan for renal replacement treatment.

History and examination

Questions will be directed towards possible causes, duration of illness. and complications (Tables 3, 4, and 5). Patients with advanced chronic renal failure usually admit to a gradual deterioration in health during the previous 6 months, but some are remarkably uncomplaining, claiming to 'feel fine' despite very abnormal blood tests. This is usually an indication of a very gradual decline towards chronic renal failure. Clues as to the cause may come from all past interactions with doctors: for instance, proteinuria during a medical examination for employment and insurance purposes or during pregnancy, or a urological assessment for microscopic haematuria.

The severity of renal failure will be gauged from the uraemic symptoms of anorexia, vomiting, lassitude, breathlessness, and ankle swelling. The clinician will need to know all about the patient's family as well as their social and employment background to allow advice on the future and to plan treatment.

The examination often provides little extra diagnostic help, but it is important to look for evidence of multisystem disorder, generalized vascular disease (which might indicate a renovascular cause for renal failure), and urinary obstruction. The latter cannot be excluded on physical examination, but if the cause of chronic renal failure is not apparent it is essential to palpate carefully for an enlarged bladder and to perform a rectal examination. Examination also allows an assessment of the consequences of chronic renal failure on blood pressure, left ventricular hypertrophy, and salt and water balance.

Investigations

The work-up of a patient newly diagnosed with chronic renal failure (Table 7) is partly diagnostic and partly for staging and preparation for dialysis and/or transplantation.

Radiological

A minimum set of investigations includes: ultrasonography to determine renal size, echogenicity, and calyceal appearance and to ensure complete emptying of the bladder; and a chest radiograph for heart size (cardiothoracic ratio—**CTR**) and lung fields. Some nephrologists would routinely also take radiographs of the hands and pelvis, looking for renal osteodystrophy and vascular calcification.

Biochemical

Creatinine clearance can be estimated using the Cockcroft–Gault formula (see above). The calcium, phosphate, and parathormone levels will give a pointer to the presence of renal osteodystrophy, and hence to the need for dietary advice and to the scope for prescription of vitamin D analogues and calcium-containing phosphate binders. Measurement of cholesterol and triglyceride concentrations will dictate the use of HMG-CoA (3-hydroxy-3-methylglutaryl coenzyme A) reductase inhibitors (statins). There is now a low threshold for statin prescription to patients with hypertensive renal failure because of their very high risk of cardiovascular events.

Haematological

Most patients will have a normochromic normocytic anaemia; although this will be due mainly to erythropoietin deficiency, it can be exacerbated or caused in some by iron deficiency. The iron status (plasma ferritin, percentage hypochromic red cells) should always be measured so that a trial of intravenous iron can be given before the more expensive option of erythropoietin treatment is initiated, the usual threshold for which is a haemoglobin concentration of less than 11 g/dl. Vitamin B_{12} and folate concentrations are rarely abnormal and should not be part of a routine work-up.

Immunological

These tests are mainly of diagnostic use and are performed only when clinically indicated, that is to say when there is diagnostic uncertainty (Table 7).

Cardiac work-up

An ECG is a routine but insensitive marker of left ventricular hypertrophy or ischaemia, except for previous myocardial infarction. Echocardiography is now the preferred investigation to detect left ventricular hypertrophy. In patients being considered for renal transplantation, exercise testing, radionuclide scanning, or angiography are required if there is any suspicion of asymptomatic ischaemic heart disease, for example in juvenile-onset diabetics or a past history of ischaemic events.

Virological

The presence of the hepatitis B surface antigen (**HepBsAg**) and hepatitis C (**Hep C**) antibodies or RNA will need to be established to decide whether a patient needs to be dialysed in isolation (Hep B), or using a dedicated machine (Hep C). HIV testing in many centres is only performed in high-risk groups, or if renal transplantation is contemplated, but in other centres it is done (after appropriate counselling) as a routine. Knowledge of the patient's immune status for cytomegalovirus (**CMV**), Epstein–Barr virus (**EBV**), and herpes zoster virus (**HZV**) will be useful baseline information if the patient is likely to undergo renal transplantation.

Clinical complications of chronic renal failure

The clinical complications of chronic renal failure are widespread (Fig. 4).

The cardiovascular system

The single most important complication of chronic renal failure is raised arterial blood pressure, which accelerates atherosclerosis and is the main cause of the left ventricular hypertrophy that is found in 75 per cent of patients. Left ventricular dilatation, coronary atherosclerosis, ventricular dysfunction, and cardiac failure are common, explaining why cardiac disease is the leading cause of death in patients with ESRF, the relative risk being highest in the young. There is a high risk of acute myocardial infarction, but sudden arrhythmic death is the more common fatal cardiac event. Patients are prone to develop pulmonary oedema with relatively small increases in extracellular fluid and tolerate dialytic removal of fluid poorly.

The factors giving rise to this dangerous combination of left ventricular hypertrophy and coronary atherosclerosis operate early in chronic renal failure and include hypertension, dyslipidaemia, anaemia, hyperparathyroidism, and hyperhomocysteinaemia. The combination of these factors has a synergistic effect on the risk of cardiovascular disease.

Pericarditis is a dreaded complication of chronic renal failure because it may lead to tamponade and death. It was more common in the days when

Table 7 Investigations of a patient newly diagnosed as having chronic renal failure

	Test	Reason
Biochemistry	Plasma creatinine, creatinine clearance	To establish degree of renal impairment and a basline for drawing 1/creatinine plots
	Urea	To give an indication of hypercatabolism, dehydration
	Potassium	Potential cardiotoxicity, response to ACE inhibitors
	Bicarbonate	Metabolic acidosis
	Lipids	Indication for statin or fibrate therapy
	Calcium, phosphates, parathyroid hormone, alkaline phosphatase	Degree of secondary hyperparathyroidism
Haematology	Blood group	In case of need for transfusion; likely need for cadaver renal transplant and/or as a preliminary to arranging a potential live-related donor
	Haemoglobin	To assess need for erythropoietin
	White blood cells	Investigate for sepsis
	Ferritin	Iron deficiency contributing to anaemia
	[Folate + vitamin B12]	[Only if indicated]
Immunology	Serum protein	If myeloma or primary amyloid suspected
	Urine electrophoresis	
	Immunoglobulins	
	ANCA/αGBM/ANF	If diagnostic uncertainty
Urine	Microscopy	For diagnosing underlying GN
	Urine protein excretion	Clue to aetiology: heavy proteinuria suggests glomerular disease
	Culture	Lower UTI, TB if indicated from history or sterile pyuria
Virology	Hepatitis C antibody	Relevant to isolation on dialysis and transplantation
	HBsAg	Relevant to isolation on dialysis and transplantation
	HIV	Relevant to diagnosis of infection, isolation on dialysis and transplantation
	CMV, HSV, HZV, EBV	Relevant to transplantation
Imaging	Ultrasound of kidneys	Size and shape, relevant to diagnosis and chronicity
	Chest radiography	Cardiothoracic ratio, pulmonary oedema, valvular calcification
	Pelvis and hands	Renal osteodystrophy and vascular calcification
Cardiac	ECG	Previous myocardial infarction, left ventricular hypertrophy
	Echocardiogram	Left ventricular hypertrophy or dysfunction Pericardial effusion (rarely)
	Angiography	If transplantation planned in patients at high risk of ischaemic heart disease

ACE, angiotensin-converting enzyme; ANCA, antineutrophil cytoplasmic antibody; ANF, anti-nuclear factor; αGBM, antiglomerular basement membrane antibody; UTI, urinary tract infection; TB, tuberculosis; HBsAg, hepatitis B surface antigen; HIV, human immunodeficiency virus; CMV, cytomegalovirus; HSV, herpes simplex virus; HZV, herpes zoster virus; EBV, Epstein–Barr virus; ECG, electrocardiogram.

dialysis was delayed until the patient was extremely uraemic, but it still occurs in underdialysed, chronically fluid overloaded, and infected patients. Progression to constriction is rare.

Calcific aortic stenosis and mitral valve calcification leading to incompetence occurs in about one-third of patients in dialysis. Endocarditis is not uncommon in haemodialysis patients, but could still be considered as surprisingly rare considering the frequency with which access to the circulation is made. It is usually caused by *Staphylococcus aureus* and leads to destructive valve disease often needing surgery.

Musculoskeletal system

Chronic renal failure causes major problems in the skeleton. Osteitis fibrosa, osteomalacia, and reduced bone turnover are a consequence of hyperparathyroidism, phosphate retention, and deranged vitamin D metabolism. These manifest as bone pain, deformity, pathological fractures, soft tissue and especially vascular calcification, and proximal myopathy. (See Chapter 20.5.2 for further discussion.)

Patients are also prone to develop crystal arthropathy, either from urate or pyrophosphate. Uric acid concentrations are high because of reduced excretion and the effect of diuretics. Long-term dialysis patients develop a specific β_2-microglobulin amyloid, deposits of which cause a large joint and spinal arthropathy, and the carpal tunnel syndrome. Large-joint haemarthroses are seen in anticoagulated renal failure patients, probably because of synergy between the use of heparin and uraemia-associated effects on haemostasis. Gout can be prevented with xanthine oxidase inhibitors such as allopurinol (but note the need for a reduced dosage in patients with renal impairment), or uricosuric agents such as probenecid. Initiation of these agents should be covered by colchicine for they can provoke acute attacks. NSAIDs can be used during acute attacks in chronic renal failure for short periods, provided that the effect on salt retention and GFR is acknowledged. Colchicine or corticosteroids are alternatives. The cyclo-oxygenase-2 inhibitors do not have an advantage over conventional agents.

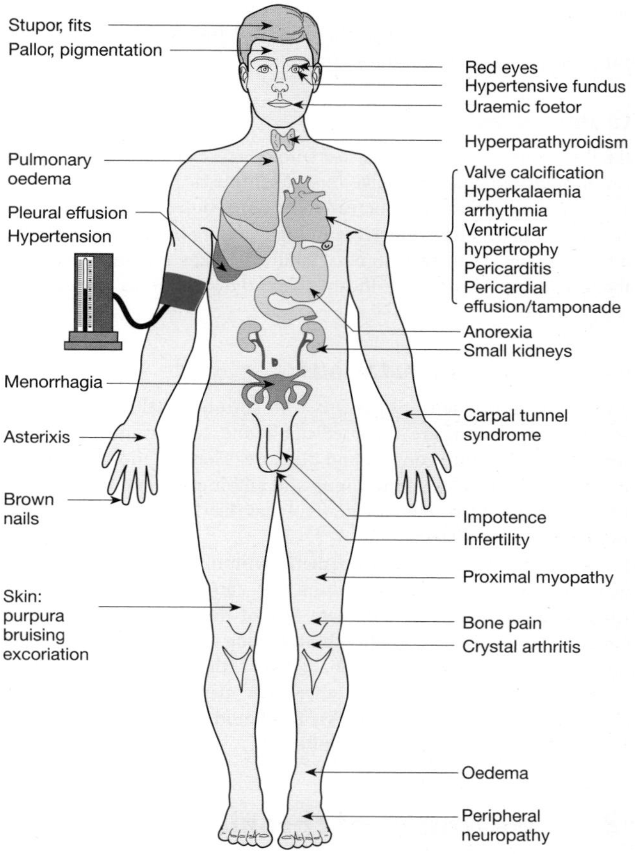

Fig. 4 Symptoms and signs of uraemia.

Gastrointestinal system

Anorexia and nausea are almost universal symptoms in uraemia and are accompanied by a blunting of taste. Both lead to decreased caloric intake and malnutrition. If there is poor oral hygiene, mouth bacteria will break down urea in saliva to ammonia, giving an unpleasant taste in the mouth and uriniferous smell to the breath. Patients often suffer early morning vomiting in the late stages of renal failure. These upper gastrointestinal symptoms are aggravated or even caused by opioid analgesics, the metabolites of which accumulate in renal failure. Diverticular disease is a problem in dialysis patients who may become constipated because of a reduction in the fluid and bulk of their diet. Patients on dialysis with primary amyloid are, for the same reasons, more at risk of perforation of the colon.

Clostridium difficile is endemic in renal units. Elderly patients in particular often develop pseudomembranous colitis after treatment with broad-spectrum antibiotics, especially cephalosporins. Treatment is with oral metronidazole or vancomycin, but if a toxic megacolon develops then colectomy is essential to preserve life.

Gastrin levels are higher in patients with chronic renal failure than in controls, but peptic ulceration is not obviously more common than in the general population. However, gastrointestinal haemorrhage, both acute and chronic, is believed to be more common in renal failure and is attributed to angiodysplasia or non-specific gastric ulceration aggravated by the platelet dysfunction of uraemia. The chronic blood loss is more noticeable because the erythroid bone marrow is already near the limit of compensation for shortened red cell survival.

Pancreatitis is only more common in uraemia because it can be provoked by hypercalcaemia, which is a hazard of vitamin D-analogue treatment. Chronic dialysis patients do have a fibrotic pancreas, but this does not seem to have clinically relevant effects on exocrine secretion.

Hepatitis B infection, if contracted in the presence of renal failure, is likely to become chronic. Patients fail to clear the virus because of their depressed cell-mediated immunity, but they seldom develop severe hepatitis or chronic liver disease. Hepatitis C infections are only more common in renal failure because of exposure to blood transfusions and its transmission in haemodialysis units. The natural history does not seem different in patients in renal failure.

The nervous system

Obvious encephalopathy is a very late manifestation of uraemia, typically leading to confusion, myoclonic twitching of distal muscle groups, and impaired consciousness. Seizures are rare unless there is also accelerated-phase hypertension. Before this preterminal state is reached, higher mental function is impaired and patients will complain of difficulty concentrating and of lethargy. It is important to exclude synergic sedation from drugs such as codeine, dextropropoxyphene, carbamazepine, or benzodiazepines. Electroencephalography (**EEG**), although an unnecessary investigation in these circumstances, shows slowing of the background rhythm. Brain computed tomography (**CT**) scans are unhelpful and magnetic resonance imaging (**MRI**) can be frankly misleading. Treatment is with dialysis—frequent, short, and gentle. The myoclonic jerks can be suppressed by benzodiazepines such as clonazepam, 500 to 2500 μg per day.

A specific encephalopathic ('dialysis disequilibrium') syndrome can occur during or after the institution of dialysis in uraemic individuals. From a normal mental state, the patient develops a headache, confusion, involuntary movements, and seizures, all suggesting the development of cerebral oedema. This is attributed to rapid urea removal leading to changes in the water content of brain cells. It is prevented by slow dialysis, avoiding rapid shifts in urea concentration.

Aluminium-induced encephalopathy—dialysis dementia—has disappeared as a clinical problem since dialysis water is properly purified to exclude aluminium, and aluminium-containing phosphate binders are not given for very long periods. Such patients exhibited a gradual deterioration in intellectual performance, progressing to dementia with involuntary movements.

Sensorimotor peripheral polyneuropathy is a late complication of chronic renal failure. This presents as dysaesthesiae, restless legs, and eventually weakness with foot drop, also loss of power in the small muscles of the hand. Nerve conduction studies do not show specific diagnostic features, there being a delay in the conduction velocity and a reduction in the amplitude of the action potential. The neuropathy is thought to be a result of the effect of an unidentified toxic 'middle' molecule. Dialysis results in a slow improvement, but patients are often left with motor disability. Autonomic neuropathy manifests largely as abnormal cardiovascular reflexes, especially during dialysis.

A specific mononeuropathy of renal failure is the carpal tunnel entrapment syndrome caused by β_2-microglobulin-derived amyloid deposition. Almost all dialysis patients develop this by 10 years of treatment unrelieved by renal transplantation.

One final comment: although renal failure can lead to many neurological problems, as detailed above, it is important that such problems are not automatically attributed to uraemia—drug accumulation and vascular disorders are common differential diagnoses.

The skin

The effects of uraemia on the skin are obvious and cause much distress to the patients. Yellow-brown pigmentation prominent in sun-exposed areas is a feature of prolonged chronic renal failure. It is attributed to an effect of retained melanocyte-stimulating hormone (**MSH**), retention of vegetable-derived lipochrome and carotenoids, and iron.

Pruritus is the most exasperating symptom for both patient and nephrologist because it is so difficult to treat. It is associated with xerosis (dry skin) and is worse when the skin is warm. A number of explanations are advanced including sensitivity to histamines, a raised calcium phosphate product, and uraemia itself. The itch–scratch cycle can lead to infection and nodular prurigo. Treatment includes starting or increasing dialysis, applying skin emollients, controlling the plasma phosphate level, keeping cool, and the prescription of antihistamines, for example chlorphenamine (chlorpheniramine) 4 mg at night (which is also slightly sedative). Naltrexone, an opioid antagonist, and ultraviolet phototherapy are effective in the short-term.

Cutaneous and subcutaneous calcification (calciphylaxis), a result of small-vessel calcification and occlusion, leads to painful livedo reticulosis and ischaemic ulceration. Once established, it is difficult to treat.

Bullous eruptions in sun-exposed areas, mimicking those of porphyria, are seen in dialysis patients. They are attributed to retained uroporphyrins or other photosensitizing chemicals that inhibit porphyrin breakdown. Iron excess is implicated in the pathogenesis, so phlebotomy and erythropoietin are part of the treatment.

Sexual function

Males

A combination of loss of libido and erectile impotence are experienced by about half the men on dialysis. Loss of libido will be a consequence of ill health and depression and is improved when well being is restored. Impotence has many causes, including pelvic vascular disease, venous leakage because of neuropathy, and drugs (for example, thiazides or α-blockers). Treatment of impotence with vacuum devices, intracavernosal injection of phentolamine, or oral sildanefil may be effective. Low sperm counts and motility that are not improved by hormonal treatment account for the lower fertility of uraemic men. *In vitro* fertilization is an option. Priapism is a rare complication of haemodialysis treatment. Gynaecomastia is common.

Females

Most women with severe renal failure develop amenorrhoea or irregular menses due to hypothalamopituitary dysregulation. Oestrogen levels are low, accounting for atrophic vaginitis and contributing to osteoporosis. Women with severe uraemia are usually infertile and the rare pregnancies almost always end in miscarriage. Patients with mild to moderate renal failure do become pregnant, when the risk of an accelerating decline in function and chance of a successful outcome are related to the severity of preconception renal dysfunction, proteinuria, and blood pressure (see Chapter 13.5).

Haematological effects and host defence

Renal anaemia, which is normochromic and normocytic, accounts for many of the symptoms that previously were attributed to uraemia. These include lethargy, cold intolerance, and loss of stamina. Anaemia increases the cardiac output and therefore contributes to the development of left ventricular hypertrophy and dilatation. The low haematocrit itself has an effect on platelet function as measured by prolonged bleeding times.

Platelet numbers are usually normal but function is impaired at the level of endothelial contact. The coagulation system is not affected. The uraemic bleeding diathesis manifests as occult gastrointestinal blood loss, oozing from any injuries or surgical incision, menorrhagia, and epistaxes. It is aggravated by the consumption of aspirin, a regular component of drug regimens in patients with cardiovascular disease.

T-cell immunity is impaired in renal failure, but the mechanism has not been explained. Evidence for this defect is the higher risk of reactivation of tuberculosis and herpes zoster, a failure to clear hepatitis B, and a poor response to immunization with hepatitis B vaccines. Neutrophil function is abnormal in a number of *in vitro* tests and may explain the high incidence and severity of bacterial infections, especially those associated with vascular access. The defect is attributed to the effects of iron, increased cytosolic calcium, and 'granulocyte inhibitory proteins'.

Metabolic effects

Renal failure causes a degree of glucose intolerance explained by resistance to insulin-mediated glucose uptake in skeletal muscle. There are complex effects on lipids resulting in an increased concentration of very low-density lipoproteins (**VLDL**) and an increase in high-density lipoproteins (**HDL**). Protein catabolism is enhanced in renal failure, perhaps as a consequence of metabolic acidosis. This has significant effects during periods of malnutrition and infection.

Psychological manifestations

The psychological problems of patients with chronic renal failure, usually anxiety and depression, are the predictable and understandable consequences of loss of health, control, and pleasure. They are most obvious in those with the most to lose—the young and ambitious—and may be relatively minor in the elderly who are grateful that they have a treatable illness and not an immediately lethal one.

The best treatment is good sympathetic symptomatic care from physicians, nurses, and other staff with whom they can build a relationship. In particular, one should try to eliminate fear of the unknown (caused by ignorance and often by gossip in the clinic waiting room) and encourage an optimistic approach. Psychiatrists usually have little to offer unless there is a specific mental illness, but psychotherapists may be able to help with phobias, guilt, and anger. Antidepressants should be used sparingly, but gentle night sedation is frequently helpful.

Medical treatment of chronic renal failure

Patients with chronic renal failure should be managed by nephrologists (or at least physicians with an interest in renal disease) in 'low clearance clinics' or outpatient departments geared to the three issues—conservation of renal function, compensation for the effects of chronic renal failure, and preparation for eventual renal replacement therapy.

Conservation of function and prevention of progression

Measures to conserve renal function may be specific for the cause of renal disease or general, i.e. applicable to all patients. There are a few treatable causes of chronic renal failure diseases for which the pathology can be modified if not actually arrested.

Specific measures

Urinary obstruction

Relief of obstruction is very rewarding, allowing the patient many years of survival without the need for dialysis because 'natural' progression seems to be relatively slower than for other parenchymal diseases. Proof of a persistent obstruction can be difficult in an already dilated renal tract. Isotope renography with furosemide (frusemide) is unreliable when renal function is poor, so if there is doubt, attempts to improve drainage should be made. This may involve an indwelling bladder catheter for high-pressure bladder outflow obstruction, stenting of ureteric strictures, or even antegrade nephrostomy drainage.

Drug-induced renal disease

If analgesic abusers stop taking the drugs, renal function can stabilize. The same may apply to ciclosporin, NSAIDs, and lithium.

Glomerulonephritis—primary and secondary

The progression of most of the common primary glomerulonephritides is relentless. There are no proven treatments of IgA nephropathy, membranoproliferative glomerulonephritis, or focal segmental glomerulosclerosis. Aggressive membranous nephropathy does respond, but not permanently, to regimens of alkylating agents (chlorambucil or cyclophosphamide) with corticosteroids.

Unsuppressed systemic lupus erythematosus and systemic vasculitis can both accelerate the decline in renal function. Proving 'activity' can be difficult and will require knowledge of serological tests, urinary sediment, and other non-specific markers, such as proteinuria, anaemia, and the concentration of acute-phase reactants. Renal biopsy may help, but is not an option when the kidneys are already small and scarred. A trial of increased immunosuppression is often worthwhile.

Ischaemic renal disease

Angioplasty with or without stenting of atheromatous renal artery stenosis seldom reverses renal failure, but it does seem to stabilize or slow progression. It is now a safe undertaking with a low risk of acute occlusion of the renal arteries.

Myeloma

Chemotherapy, which reduces the paraprotein load, improves renal function in patients with myeloma provided the renal failure is not advanced.

Amyloidosis

Treatment of the underlying cause of amyloid A (AA) disease (for example, familial Mediterranean fever (**FMF**) and Still's disease) improves the renal consequences of the process. Chemotherapy of primary amyloidosis (AL amyloid) has been disappointing. Although prednisone and melphalan regimens improve survival, they do not delay the progression of renal failure. It remains to be seen whether marrow ablation and stem-cell rescue will be an effective and applicable treatment for more than a select minority of patients.

Urinary tract infection

Treatment of renal tuberculosis or infection of polycystic kidneys is effective in reducing renal destruction. In reflux nephropathy, suppressing lower urinary tract infections makes relatively little difference, but true pyelonephritis must be treated with the appropriate antibiotics. Antireflux procedures do not alter the natural history.

Stone disease

Measures to reduce stone formation in cystinuria, hypercalciuria, and hyperuricaemia are effective (see Chapter 20.13). Allopurinol is effective in stabilizing renal function in patients with inherited forms of hyperuricaemia.

Diabetes

Control of blood pressure halts or retards diabetic nephropathy, although there is no evidence that better treatment of diabetes (glycaemic control) has a substantial effect (see Chapter 20.10.1).

General (non-specific) measures

Once there has been a loss of more than 50 per cent of renal function the residual nephrons become vulnerable to injury from glomerular hypertension, quite independent of the primary pathology. The clearest example of this phenomenon is the patient who has 1.5 kidneys removed because of cancer and is left with one-quarter of their normal renal mass. Despite the fact that the remaining kidney tissue has no intrinsic pathology, the patient develops hypertension, proteinuria, and progressive glomerulosclerosis leading to renal failure, the mechanisms involved being described above (see 'mechanisms of progression'). Countering the factors that are thought to favour the vicious cycle of nephron loss and autologous injury could stop or delay the process.

Hypertension

There is good evidence relating the presence of systemic hypertension to progression of chronic renal failure and height of the blood pressure to the rate of decline of renal function. Lowering blood pressure is effective in delaying the rate of progression of renal failure, best exemplified in diabetic nephropathy. The optimum target blood pressure is uncertain, but most nephrologists operate on a 'lower the better' principle. Excepting in diabetic nephropathy, it is still unclear whether ACE inhibitors or α2-receptor blockers are superior to other blood pressure-lowering drugs, but the prejudice of most nephrologists is that they should be the first-line agents. The additional benefit of ACE inhibitors is attributed to their effects on glomerular hypertension and the prevention of angiotensin-induced vascular injury.

Dietary protein

Dietary protein restriction slows the progress of glomerulosclerosis in residual nephrons in animal experimental models of chronic renal failure. Trials in humans have evoked much controversy, but the consensus is that there is a modest effect of a 0.2 g/kg per day reduction in protein consumption (from that consumed in a normal Western diet) in patients with GFRs of 13 to 24 ml/min. In practice, nephrologists do no more than advise against high-protein diets. Promotion of low-protein diets has been abandoned in favour of maintaining good nutrition and starting dialysis earlier.

Other

There is no evidence that antiplatelet drugs, anticoagulants, lipid-lowering measures, and low-phosphate diets delay the progression of chronic renal failure.

Compensation for the effects of chronic renal failure

Although there is usually a remarkable adaptation to the loss of as much as 90 per cent of kidney function, a figure which allows the survival of patients with severe chronic renal failure, there is much that should be done to improve health and prevent complications.

Water and electrolyte balance

Only those with oliguric end-stage renal failure need to restrict their fluid intake precisely, when the usual (but seldom complied with) recommendation is that the patient's daily intake should be 500 ml (for insensible losses) plus a volume equivalent to their daily urine output. Patients with chronic renal failure pass normal volumes of urine. However, they do need to be counselled against binge drinking or ignoring extra fluid losses in hot weather and during episodes of diarrhoea or vomiting, because the free-water clearance is blunted and concentration is impaired in renal failure.

Dietary restriction to 60 mmol/day each of sodium and potassium will not exceed the capacity of the failing kidney to maintain balance. Tolerant and flexible advice to provide a safe and tasty diet is more likely to be adhered to than one with absolute and complete exclusions. Sodium balance and blood pressure will be improved by diuretics, usually of the 'loop' type, and in resistant cases in combination with a thiazide such as metolazone.

If the potassium level rises above 7 mmol/l, haemodialysis should be initiated unless there is an otherwise remediable cause. Occasionally this is an isolated finding in an otherwise stable patient, when the ECG should be checked (with emergency treatment as described in Section 20.5 if there are ominous changes) and the measurement repeated. Causes of hyperkalaemia to be considered in those with chronic renal failure—other than a fruit, chocolate, or coffee binge—include gastrointestinal haemorrhage, acidosis, and tissue necrosis, such as a gut infarction or gangrene. Chronic disproportionate hyperkalaemia (for example, when the GFR is still above 10 ml/min) is encountered in diabetics with hyporeninaemic hypoaldosteronism, hypoadrenalism, and as a response to ACE inhibitors.

Calcium, phosphate, and vitamin D

Secondary hyperparathyroidism—so difficult to suppress or reverse when established—starts early in chronic renal failure, when the GFR falls below 40 ml/min. Prevention requires countering the three key stimuli: hyperphosphataemia by diet and phosphate binders; provision of 1,25-dihydroxycholecalciferol, either as calcitriol or 1α-hydroxycholecalciferol; and maintaining a normal ionized calcium level. To control phosphate, milk products and fish will be limited; the favoured phosphate binder is calcium acetate taken three times a day with meals. A vitamin D analogue should be started in low dose (e.g. 0.25 μg of alfacalcidol three times/week) as soon as the parathormone is found to be above the normal range. It can be quite difficult to persuade patients to adhere to phosphate restriction or to remember to take binders because the immediate benefit is not obvious. (See Chapter 20.5.1 for further discussion.)

Control of blood pressure

A major focus of the follow-up of patients with chronic renal failure is to achieve and maintain a satisfactory blood pressure: the aim is for less than 140/90 mmHg, but in practice this can be difficult to achieve. It is essential that the patients be engaged as partners in the endeavour: it will help if they understand that good blood pressure control will delay the need for dialysis, prevent left ventricular hypertrophy, which will have an adverse effect on survival, and reduce the risk of cardiovascular events. Patients should be encouraged to measure and record their own blood pressures because readings in hurried clinics and general practitioner surgeries are often unreliable. When there is a disparity between clinic and home readings a 24-h ambulatory recording may provide reassurance that increased doses or extra drugs are not needed. Equally, they will justify such a change for a reluctant patient. The choice of drugs will depend on clinician preference and patient tolerance. There is a move towards the use of ACE inhibitors or angiotensin-receptor blockers as first choice because of the potential added benefits, but most patients will require two to four-drug regimens.

Nutrition

Chronic renal failure causes anorexia, acidosis, and insulin resistance. All three contribute to the subtle malnutrition that may develop in the months during which the decision to start dialysis is procrastinated. The dietician's role here is as much to ensure the prevention of malnutrition as to monitor the excess consumption of the problem items. If anorexia causes a reduction in calorie and protein intake, supplements should be prescribed only as a bridge to the starting of dialysis.

Metabolic acidosis

This frequently goes unnoticed as many laboratories do not routinely report plasma bicarbonate levels and it is unusual to take an arterial blood sample in a low-clearance clinic. Acidosis is more common in patients with interstitial renal disease who have an acquired renal tubular acidosis. The usual symptom is effort dyspnoea not explained by pulmonary oedema or anaemia. A chronic acidosis will aggravate hyperkalaemia, inhibit protein anabolism, and accelerate calcium loss from bone where the excess hydrogen ions are buffered. Sodium bicarbonate 1.2 to 1.8 g thrice daily can be prescribed to patients who can bear this sodium load (for example, those with obstructive uropathy who are acidotic salt wasters).

Anaemia

There is no absolute haemoglobin concentration at which the symptoms of anaemia become manifest, so the decision to treat is a matter of judgement: generally the aim is to maintain the haemoglobin level at or above 11 g/dl. Because chronic anaemia leads to left ventricular hypertrophy, which has adverse effects on patient survival and cardiac function, there is a move towards earlier (and even preventive treatment) of anaemia in patients with chronic renal failure. Whether this will improve survival and reduce cardiac complications is a subject of clinical trials.

For patients not yet on dialysis who have a haemoglobin level under 11 g/dl, one can either start erythropoietin, subcutaneously, at 50 U/kg per week (rounded up to reach 1000 units) in two divided doses, or give a trial of intravenous iron first. This can either be a single dose of iron dextran (1 g), taking precautions against the occurrence of anaphylaxis, or intravenous iron saccharate 200 mg weekly for 5 weeks.. A similar regimen is used for dialysis patients. Patients should learn to inject erythropoietin themselves using the prefilled syringe and pens that are available. Longer acting analogues of erythropoietin are now available and will allow once-weekly administration. Doses can be titrated up, the usual maintenance dose being between 25 and 150 U/kg per week. If patients require higher doses or respond poorly they should be investigated for iron deficiency, sepsis, severe hyperparathyroidism (which causes marrow fibrosis), chronic blood loss, or non-compliance. If no cause is found then a bone marrow examination may be helpful. Recently red cell aplasia caused by autoantibodies to erythropoietin has been described. Patients on haemodialysis can receive the erythropoietin intravenously, but the dose required will be about 30 per cent higher and they are especially liable to develop iron deficiency, which can be prevented by the intravenous administration of 100 mg iron saccharate every 2 weeks. The ferritin concentration should be monitored and the iron temporarily stopped if it rises above 500 μg/l. A checklist for the management of renal anaemia is shown in Table 8.

The reversal of anaemia increases blood pressure in about 30 per cent of patients. High/normal haematocrits are associated with an increasing risk of vascular access thrombosis and do not appear to alter cardiac prognosis.

Drugs

It is essential that the appropriateness of the prescription of drugs to patients with renal failure be checked and the doses adjusted according to the estimated GFR (see Chapter 20.16).

Preparation for dialysis and transplantation

Once end-stage renal failure is inevitable, the patient must be prepared physically and psychologically for renal replacement treatment. In many patients it is possible to predict approximately when the end-stage will be reached (Fig. 5). This information is useful for the patient and provides a

Table 8 Checklist for managing patients with renal anaemia

Start	Hb <11 g/dl *and* ferritin <100 μg/l	Give course of intravenous iron	
	Ferritin >100 μg/l	Start Epo, about 50 U/kg per week in two divided doses	
Monitor	Hb <11 g/dl?	Is patient giving injections?	
	Epo dose <50 U/kg	Increase Epo dose	
	Epo dose >150 U/kg	Consider the following:	
		(1) Iron deficiency	Ferritin <100 μg/l, hypochromic red cells >10%
		(2) Blood loss	Gastrointestinal, menses, dialysis
		(3) Inflammation/infection	CRP >12 mg/dl: seek source and treat
		(4) Other haematological conditions	Look for myeloma, thalassaemia, myelofibrosis, vitamin B_{12} or folate deficiency
		(5) Autoantibodies to Epo	This is very rare

Hb, haemoglobin; Epo, erythropoietin; CRP, C-reactive protein

guide for the timing of the creation of vascular access, placement of peritoneal dialysis catheters, or activating the patient on to a transplant waiting list. One should avoid the temptation to delay starting dialysis for as long as possible, for the quality of life and health of a well-dialysed patient is superior to that of a non-dialysed, uraemic malnourished one.

The absolute indications for dialysis are the development of complications that cannot be contained by conservative and pharmacological means. These are hyperkalaemia, fluid overload, severe hypertension, pericarditis, encephalopathy, and neuropathy. To wait for these is bad practice. Nephrologists generally wait until the patient has some uraemic symptoms such as anorexia, lassitude and pruritus, if only because their relief reinforces the need to adjust to regular dialysis. Apart from potassium concentrations and the degree of acidosis, blood tests such as urea and creatinine do not provide a safe guide to when to start. Nevertheless, it is advisable to start dialysis, in the absence of symptoms, at creatinine clearances of less than 10 ml/min. In small patients with little muscle bulk the urea concentration is often between 30 and 40 mmol/l and the creatinine concentration between 650 and 800 μmol/l; in larger subjects the blood urea concentration is typically 45 to 50 mmol/l and that of creatinine above 1000 μmol/l. Initiation of dialysis at lower blood levels of urea and creatinine is recommended in diabetic patients.

The choice of modality—haemodialysis, continuous ambulatory peritoneal dialysis, or renal transplantation—depends on many factors, not least their availability and the patient's preference (see Section 20.6 for further discussion). If transplantation is appropriate, there is no reason not to perform it before dialysis is mandatory. If haemodialysis is chosen, vascular access should be created 4 to 6 months before it is needed. If continuous ambulatory peritoneal dialysis is to be used, the Tenckhoff catheter should be placed 2 to 3 weeks before dialysis needs to be started to allow it to seal.

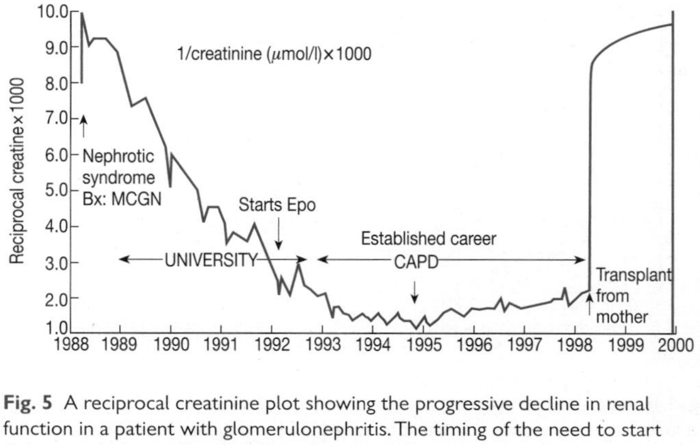

Fig. 5 A reciprocal creatinine plot showing the progressive decline in renal function in a patient with glomerulonephritis. The timing of the need to start dialysis could be predicted sufficiently well to allow planning of treatment.

Management of terminal uraemia

There will be patients for whom dialysis is inappropriate or who either choose not to start or to discontinue treatment. Because, intuitively, one would predict that instituting dialysis in a patient with renal failure and other comorbid conditions should result in some improvement by ameliorating at least one element of their clinical condition, it is very hard not to start. There are those who argue that there is no harm done by starting because treatment can always be stopped or the patient will die despite dialysis. However, withdrawing dialysis or dying while on treatment are traumatic for both the patient's family and staff. If possible, one should discuss the option of not starting before treatment is actually needed. The patient will need to know what the treatment can achieve and at what cost—access, travel to dialysis, restrictions, and complications. If one takes the view that dialysis is a treatment offered to allow the patient to continue living with a reasonable quality of life as opposed to delaying death in the short term, dialysis will not be offered to patients with other life-limiting conditions. Certainly one could argue that it should not be started when survival beyond 3 months outside of hospital is unlikely, indeed at least 10 per cent of deaths in dialysis programmes follow withdrawal of treatment. The ethical and legal issues are complex and require that the patient makes the decision not to start or to discontinue when fully informed and able to do so.

Properly managed death from uraemia is peaceful and free of suffering. It is important to ensure that the patient has peace of mind, in that they are comfortable with the decision, and that their family members are understanding and supportive. They will be comforted to know that their doctor respects their decision. Several distressing symptoms may need to be controlled. The first is breathlessness from pulmonary oedema and acidosis, best controlled with a morphine infusion. The second is nausea and anorexia, which can be helped with regular chlorpromazine 25 mg four times daily: ondansetron 8 mg twice daily can also be effective. Food and fluid should be offered in small palatable helpings and no pressure to eat exerted on the patient. The mouth can become dry and crusted from mouth breathing and will smell foul from the uraemic saliva. Regular mouth washes and gum care will help. Pruritus is managed by keeping the skin cool, and soft with emollients. The patient may not be aware of myoclonic jerks but these will distress the family, so benzodiazepines, such as clonazepam, should be prescribed.

Further reading

Baigent C, Burbury K, Wheeler D (2000). Premature cardiovascular disease in chronic renal failure. *Lancet* **356**, 147–52.

El-Nahas AM, Tamimi N (1999). The progression of chronic renal failure: a harmful quartet. *Quarterly Journal of Medicine* **92**, 421–4.

Hörl W (1999). Neutrophil function and infections in uraemia. *American Journal of Kidney Disease* **33**, xlv–xlviii.

Locatelli F, *et al.* (2000). The management of chronic renal insufficiency in the conservative phase. *Nephrology, Dialysis, Transplantation* **15**, 1529–34.

Luke RG (1999). Hypertensive nephrosclerosis: Pathogenesis and prevalence. *Nephrology, Dialysis, Transplantation* **14**, 2271–8.

McLaughlin K, Jardine AG, Moss JG (2000). Renal artery stenosis. *British Medical Journal* **320**, 1124–7.

Maschio G, *et al.* (1996). Effect of angiotensin-converting enzyme inhibitor benazepril on the progression of chronic renal insufficiency. *New England Journal of Medicine* **334**, 939.

Phillips AO (2000). Diabetic nephropathy—where next? *Quarterly Journal of Medicine* **93**, 643–6.

Ruggenenti P, *et al.* for the GISEN Group (2000). Pretreatment blood pressure reliably predicts progression of chronic nephropathies. *Kidney International* **58**, 2093–101.

Schaefer F, Wiecek A, Ritz E (1998). Endocrine disorders in chronic renal failure. In: Davison AM, *et al.*, eds. *Oxford textbook of clinical nephrology*, 2nd edn, pp 1854–66. Oxford University Press, Oxford.

United States Renal Data System (2000). 2000 Annual Data Report. Atlas of end-stage renal disease in the United States. *American Journal of Kidney Disease* **36**, Suppl. 2.

Working Party (1999). European best practice guidelines for the management of anaemia in patients with chronic renal failure. *Nephrology, Dialysis, Transplantation* 14, Suppl. 5.

20.5.2 Bone disease in chronic renal failure

Michael Schömig and Eberhard Ritz

Introduction

Renal bone disease is a major cause of disability in patients with terminal renal failure. It is mainly, but not exclusively, due to secondary hyperparathyroidism. Previously, aluminium-induced bone disease, secondary to high aluminium concentrations in the dialysate or ingestion of aluminium-containing phosphate binders, played an important role, but this iatrogenic complication has virtually been eliminated. With more efficient prevention and treatment of secondary hyperparathyroidism, patients with uraemia with low bone turnover are encountered with increasing frequency, but whether this condition (so-called adynamic bone disease) has any clinical consequences, other than the propensity to hypercalcaemia, remains unresolved.

It is important to recognize that abnormal calcium/phosphate metabolism impacts not only on parathyroid glands and bone, but also on cardiovascular function; for example, it increases the risk of cardiac death, calcific aortic stenosis, and coronary plaque calcification. This adds a new dimension to the importance of returning calcium/phosphate metabolism to normal in patients with renal failure.

Pathogenesis of renal bone disease

The role of phosphate excess

In early renal failure, plasma phosphate concentration is normal or low, but renal phosphate excretion (more precisely the fractional clearance of phosphate) is increased. Hyperphosphataemia develops when the glomerular filtration rate is approximately 30 ml/min. This causes and aggravates secondary hyperparathyroidism due to indirect mechanisms, such as inhibition of the synthesis of the active vitamin D metabolite 1,25-$(OH)_2$vitamin D_3 (calcitriol) in tubular epithelial cells, and possibly also by inducing a tendency for hypocalcaemia. More recently, it has been shown that phosphate directly stimulates parathyroid hormone (**PTH**) synthesis and secretion as well as causing parathyroid cell proliferation independent of low 1,25-$(OH)_2D_3$ and hypocalcaemia.

The role of 1,25-$(OH)_2$vitamin D_3 (calcitriol) deficiency

The hepatic vitamin D metabolite 25-$(OH)D_3$ is transformed in tubular epithelial cells to the active vitamin D metabolite 1,25-$(OH)_2$vitamin D_3. Synthesis is stimulated by PTH and inhibited by hyperphosphataemia. Even in early renal failure there is a tendency for 1,25-$(OH)_2D_3$ concentration to decrease, although this is very often compensated by increased PTH concentrations. The average concentration of 1,25-$(OH)_2D_3$ falls as renal failure progresses (Fig. 1). One specific problem is that vitamin D metabolites bound to plasma-binding protein (DBP) may be lost in the urine in patients with nephrotic-range proteinuria, so that deficiency of active vitamin D may ensue. The renal 1-α-hydroxylase reaction is normally substrate-independent, but becomes dependent on the availability of the substrate 25-$(OH)D_3$ in some patients with renal failure, hence vitamin D deficiency aggravates the deficit in the synthesis of 1,25-$(OH)_2D_3$.

The role of hypocalcaemia

Plasma (total and ionized) calcium concentrations are maintained until the patient reaches pre-endstage renal failure. Nevertheless, the tendency to hypocalcaemia, which is due to a combination of (1) reduced active calcium resorption in the intestine as a result of insufficient active vitamin D, and (2) resistance of the skeleton to release bone mineral and calcium as a result of (partial) resistance to PTH and active vitamin D, may play a more important role in the genesis of secondary hyperparathyroidism than previously thought. The parathyroid gland senses the calcium concentration in the extracellular space via the calcium receptor (CaR) and there are some observations that argue for abnormal sensing of Ca^{2+} even in early renal failure, which may possibly be reversed by agents that improve calcium sensing (calcimimetics).

Clinical manifestations

Pattern of skeletal involvement

The following bone lesions are found in the skeleton of patients with renal failure, in isolation or in combination (Table 1).

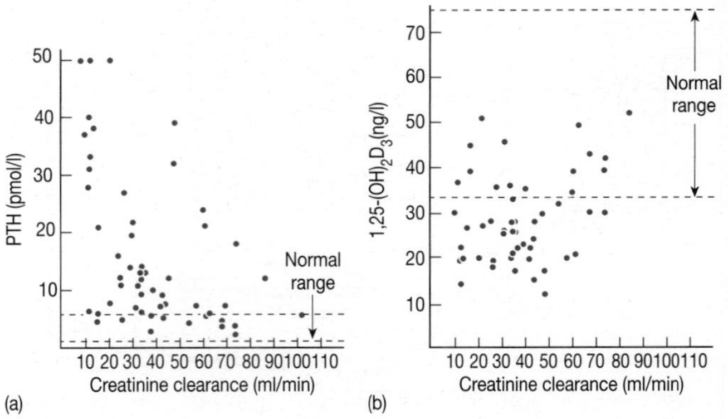

Fig. 1 Intact plasma parathyroid hormone values and serum 1,25-$(OH)_2D_3$ levels as a function of the glomerular filtration rate (GFR) in patients with chronic renal failure.

Table 1 Bone lesions in patients on dialysis

The following bone lesions may be found either in isolation or in combination:
Osteitis fibrosa
Osteomalacia
Mixed lesions
Adynamic bone disease (caused by aluminium or idiopathic)
Further pathologies must to be considered in atypical cases:
β_2-Microglobulin amyloidosis
Sequelae of preceding steroid therapy (fractures, osteonecrosis)
Osteopenia (osteoporosis), particularly in postmenopausal patients
Reflex sympathetic dystrophy
Bony problems caused by primary disease leading to renal failure, e.g. oxalosis

Osteitis fibrosa

This is increased osteoclastic bone resorption and increased osteoblastic bone aposition with (1) consecutive intense remodelling of bone trabeculae in the spongiosa, and (2) rarefaction and tunnelization of cortical bone with or without deposition of fibrous tissue (endosteal fibrosis) (Fig. 2).

Osteomalacia

Osteomalacia is a disparity between the rate of bone matrix synthesis and bone matrix mineralization, leading to widening of the seam of unmineralized bone matrix (osteoid), usually associated with signs of diminished numbers and activities of cells at the bone surface. Pure osteomalacia is rarely seen nowadays. In the past it was mainly due to aluminium toxicity and vitamin D (cholecalciferol) deficiency.

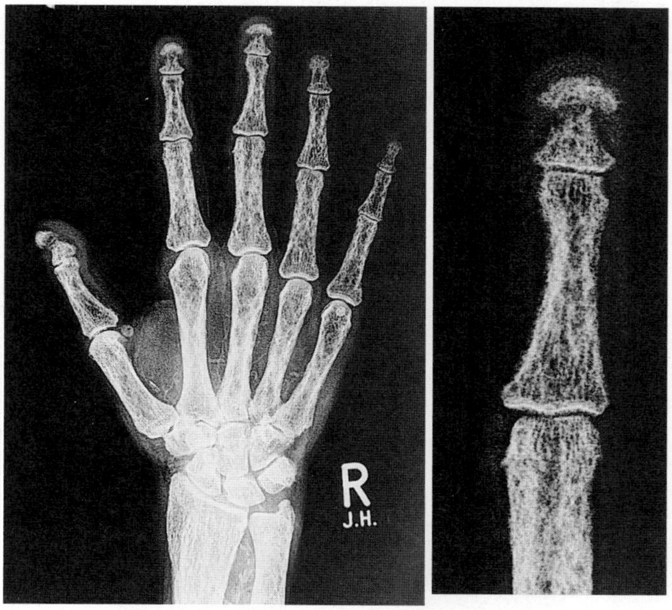

(a) (b)

Fig. 2 The radiograph of the hand (a) shows reduced mineral density as well as fluffy and mottled texture of the bones. Note (i) subperiosteal resorption zones at the radial site of the middle phalanges (see also (b)—erosion cavities with overlying areas of calcification (periosteal neostosis), (ii) longitudinal striation of cortical bone (corresponding to enlarged Haversian channels), (iii) thinning of cortical bone by endosteal bone resorption, and (iv) loss of the terminal lamella of the terminal phalanx. The terminal phalanx of the second digit had collapsed, such that the patient presented with 'pseudo-clubbing'. Vascular calcifications are seen above the first digit and along the exterior side of the radius. A detail of the index finger is shown in (b).

Mixed lesions

In many patients with renal failure a combination of osteitis fibrosa and osteomalacia are present.

Adynamic bone disease

In patients with a low serum PTH concentration the number and activity of cells on the bone surface is strikingly reduced and bone turnover is reduced, as evaluated by isotope- or tetracycline-labelling techniques. This condition is relatively frequent in patients with renal failure treated with active vitamin D. It predisposes to hypercalcaemia because the capacity of the skeleton to sequester calcium is reduced, but whether it has more far reaching clinical implications is currently unknown.

Osteopenia or osteoporosis

The problem of diminished bone mass, superimposed upon uraemia-specific bony abnormalities, is very common in patients with renal failure. The most common causes are a history of treatment with steroids and (premature) menopause. It is currently unresolved whether the risk is aggravated by smoking and low calcium diets and whether it can be prevented by substitution of oestrogens/gestagens or selective oestrogen receptor modulators.

Other pathologies

There are several pathologies unrelated to calcium metabolism that have to be taken into consideration in patients with renal failure (Table 1). A dialysis-specific type of amyloidosis with preferential osteoarticular involvement—β_2-microglobulin-related amyloidosis—must also be considered in the differential diagnosis of bone pain or bone destruction (see Chapter 20.6.1).

The salient differences between osteitis fibrosa and aluminium-related bone disease are summarized in Table 2.

Signs and symptoms

While patients with renal failure left untreated usually have hypocalcaemia and hyperphosphataemia, patients with advanced secondary hyperparathyroidism are characterized by hypercalcaemia and hyperphosphataemia associated with an increase in alkaline phosphatase and its bone isoenzyme.

In the patient with hypercalcaemia it is important to consider causes other than secondary hyperparathyroidism which necessitate specific treatment (Table 3). Similarly, bone pain is not common even in advanced osteitis fibrosa, but bones subjected to mechanical stress (spine, calcaneus, foot) may be painful. Whilst fractures are uncommon, skeletal deformity, leontiasis faciei, and avulsion of the patella may occur. By contrast, osteomalacia, particularly that secondary to aluminium intoxication, may be very painful, especially when Looser zones—fatigue fractures—occur. Again it is important to exclude alternative causes of bone pain (Table 4).

Severe extra-osseous calcifications—periarticular, bursal, or visceral calcifications (see Figs 2, 3, and most dramatically, 4)—are usually the consequence of severe hyperphosphataemia with or without elevated serum PTH concentrations. Tumoral tissue calcification is often triggered by trauma, for instance haematoma. It is favoured by low bone turnover, a situation in which the capacity of the skeleton to sequester calcium phosphate is diminished. Calciphylaxis is a medical emergency where ischaemic skin eschars form secondary to calcification of cutaneous arterial vessels: it usually responds to parathyroidectomy, which may need to be performed as an emergency.

Table 2 The two major forms of renal bone disease—differential diagnosis of serum chemistry findings

	Osteitis fibrosa	Aluminium-related osteopathy
Calcium	Variable, high normal or elevated in advanced hyperparathyroidism	Tendency to hypercalcaemia
Phosphate	Marked increase (dissolution of bone mineral)	Non-specific
Intact PTH	Markedly elevated	Less elevated or normal
Alkaline phosphatase	Usually elevated	Tends to be low
Aluminium	Variable, usually < 60 μg/l	Mostly elevated (> 60 μg/l)
Increase of aluminium after desferrioxamine	Variable	Marked increase, often > 150 μg/dl or threefold above baseline

Prophylaxis of secondary hyperparathyroidism

Rationale

Secondary hyperparathyroidism is the combined result of failing excretory function of the kidney (leading to phosphate excess) and failing endocrine function of the kidney (leading to calcitriol deficiency). Consequently, appropriate management requires that both abnormalities must be treated.

Phosphate control

It is usually recommended that phosphate-lowering interventions should begin once plasma phosphate concentrations exceed the upper limit of the normal range—1.45 mmol/l. This is usually the case when the creatinine clearance is approximately 30 ml/min, but the plasma phosphate concentration depends not only on renal clearance, but also on dietary phosphate intake, protein catabolism, and other confounding factors. The problem of phosphate retention persists when patients are on dialysis: the normal dietary intake of phosphate is 50 to 100 mmol/day, of which 50 to 70 per cent is absorbed in the intestine. This exceeds the amount of phosphate that is eliminated by conventional thrice-weekly haemodialysis (33 mmol per session, i.e. 100 mmol/week), such that an average daily positive phosphate balance of 30 mmol ensues.

The risk of precipitation of calcium phosphate is particularly high if hyperphosphataemia is accompanied by hypercalcaemia, reflected by the calcium × phosphate product (desirable range below 5.6 $mmol^2/l^2$, although the practical value of such calculation is limited).

Phosphate is present in virtually all foods, hence reduction of dietary intake is difficult without incurring the risk of malnutrition. Patients should be advised, however, to avoid items with very high phosphate content, for example dairy products and those to which phosphate is added, such as sausages and phosphate-rich soft drinks. A protein-restricted diet is often recommended to patients with renal insufficiency (although there is controversy regarding this, see Section 20.6) and one desirable consequence is that this diet reduces the dietary intake of phosphate.

However, since dietary restriction of phosphate is usually not feasible or sufficient, patients with uraemia remain in positive phosphate balance unless oral phosphate binders are administered. The agents most commonly used are calcium carbonate and calcium acetate: aluminium-containing substances have been widely used in the past, but because of the risk of aluminium intoxication (encephalopathy, osteopathy, anaemia, etc.) they should generally be avoided. These substances trap phosphate in the intestinal lumen by forming insoluble calcium phosphate complexes, hence it follows that they must be taken together with meals because phosphate in

Table 3 Differential diagnosis of hypercalcaemia in the patient with uraemia

Severe hyperparathyroidism
Vitamin D intoxication (cholecalciferol or active vitamin D)
Immobilization
Inappropriate dialysate calcium concentration
Excessive dose of calcium-containing phosphate binders
Vitamin A intoxication
Granulomatous disease (e.g. sarcoidosis, tuberculosis)
Myeloma
Bone metastases
Pseudohypercalcaemia (elevated total protein concentration)

Table 4 Differential diagnosis of bone pain in the patient with renal failure

Osteitis fibrosa (relatively rare as a cause of pain)
Osteomalacia (secondary to aluminium accumulation)
β_2-Amyloidosis
Skeletal metastases, myeloma
Osteomyelitis, mostly spondylodiscitis (infected vascular access)
Neuromelic pain after arteriovenous fistula
Bone infarction, osteonecrosis (steroid treatment, sickle-cell anaemia)
Osteoporotic fractures

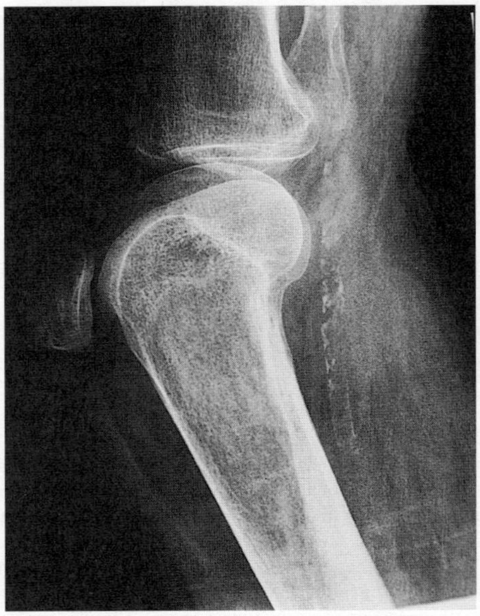

Fig. 3 Calcification of the popliteal artery in a patient with diabetes and severe hyperparathyroidism.

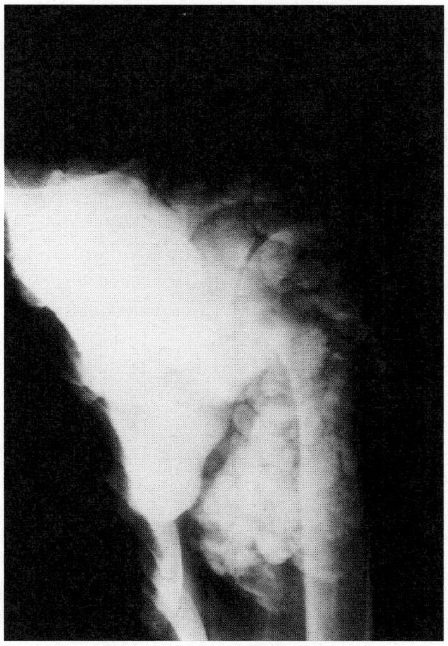

Fig. 4 Tumorous calcification around the left shoulder in a patient on dialysis with aluminium intoxication.

the food can only be precipitated within the intestinal lumen when phosphate binders are present. Furthermore, ingestion of calcium-containing phosphate binders without meals increases the risk of hypercalcaemia. If aluminium-containing phosphate binders are used (in cases where hypercalcaemia develops with calcium-containing phosphate binders), then plasma aluminium concentrations must be monitored at regular intervals (relatively safe range: below 60 µg/l). Phosphate binders without calcium or aluminium are currently under investigation.

If hyperphosphataemia does not respond to intervention, one should consider non-compliance, increased phosphate release from the skeleton (e.g. in marked osteitis fibrosa), or insufficient efficacy of dialysis.

Reversal of cholecalciferol deficiency

Deficiency of the parent compound cholecalciferol (vitamin D_3) is common among patients with renal failure as a result of altered lifestyle with insufficient sun exposure, hyperpigmentation of the skin, and loss of protein-bound vitamin D (metabolites) into proteinuric urine or peritoneal dialysis fluid. Vitamin D deficiency can be diagnosed when plasma 25-$(OH)D_3$ concentrations are low (< 50 nmol/l). In renal failure the synthesis of 1,25-$(OH)_2D_3$ depends on the concentration of the precursor substance 25-$(OH)D_3$, which explains why administration of 1000 U vitamin D per day (which is two to three times the average daily intake) leads to an increase of calcitriol and decrease of intact PTH (**iPTH**) in many patients with renal failure. Note, however, that treatment with pharmacological doses of native vitamin D is never appropriate in renal failure: these are much less effective than hydroxylated metabolites (see below) and, if they do raise the serum calcium concentration, carry a substantial risk of inducing prolonged hypercalcaemia.

Administration of active vitamin D

Although there is not complete consensus, most authorities advise that prophylactic administration of active vitamin D should be considered when 1,84-iPTH concentrations are elevated in early renal failure, or two- to threefold above the normal range in advanced renal failure despite measures to correct plasma phosphate and plasma calcium concentrations. In advanced chronic renal failure, or when patients are on dialysis, complete return of iPTH concentrations to normal is not desirable, because in patients with renal failure a normal bone turnover is found only if PTH concentrations are slightly above the normal range. It is currently unknown whether this reflects PTH resistance of the skeleton or insufficient specificity of the PTH assay, which also measures some inactive fragments of PTH.

It has emerged that relatively low doses of calcitriol or alternative active vitamin D preparations (e.g. 1-α-calcidol) are necessary to prevent the progressive increase of iPTH in patients with renal failure, for instance 0.125 or 0.25 µg 1,25-$(OH)_2D_3$ per day. The rationale for administration of 1,25-$(OH)_2D_3$ is not only the acute reversal of oversecretion of PTH, but also prevention of parathyroid hyperplasia. This is important because hyperplasia is at least partially irreversible. Administration of active vitamin D preparation is fraught with the risks of hypercalciuria, hypercalcaemia, and accelerated loss of renal function. However, monitoring urinary and plasma calcium can prevent this, and the risk is negligible with very low doses, that is, 0.125 µg/day of 1,25-$(OH)_2D_3$. 1-α-Hydroxy-cholecalciferol is a prodrug, which is hydroxylated in the liver *in vivo* to 1,25-$(OH)_2$vitamin D_3. Biotransformation may be abnormal if hepatic disease is present, but otherwise the two compounds yield comparable therapeutic results. Table 5 provides an algorithm for the prophylaxis of secondary hyperparathyroidism.

Selection of dialysate calcium concentration

Active intestinal calcium transport is impaired in uraemia, hence patients with renal failure without additional calcium intake are in negative calcium balance. On dialysis, calcium may be lost into the dialysate, indeed convective calcium loss is obligatory with ultrafiltration and may amount to up to 200 to 400 mg/week. Loss of calcium into the dialysate also occurs by diffusion if the plasma concentration of diffusible calcium is higher than the dialysate calcium concentration. In the past, a high dialysate calcium concentration of 7 mg/100 ml (1.75 mmol/l) was recommended, so that net uptake of calcium occurs during the dialysis session to compensate for convective loss of calcium via ultrafiltration during, and negative intestinal calcium between, dialysis sessions. If calcium-containing phosphate binders or active vitamin D preparations are administered, intestinal uptake of calcium is high and the patients may develop hypercalcaemia. Lowering of dialysate calcium concentration to 6 mg/100 ml (1.5 mmol/l) (temporarily even to 5 mg/100 ml or 1.25 mmol/l) counteracts this tendency. It is important, however, to verify that patients take their medication when low dialysis calcium concentrations have been selected. If calcium carbonate and/or active vitamin D preparations are not taken, there is a definite risk that the calcium balance becomes negative and that secondary hyperparathyroidism is exacerbated.

Table 5 An algorithm for prophylaxis of secondary hyperparathyroidism

Monitoring (plasma chemistry)

Calcium, albumin, phosphate, 25$(OH)D_3$, aluminium, 1,84

Prophylactic measures

If 25-$(OH)D_3$ low, i.e. below 50 nmol/l
→ cholecalciferol 1000 U/day
If plasma calcium decreased and/or plasma phosphate increased
→ calcium carbonate 0.5 to 1.5 g with each meal
If 1,84-iPTH consistently above 12 to 18 nmol/l (two to three times normal) and plasma calcium/phosphate normal (spontaneously or after intervention)
→ calcitriol 0.125 to 0.25 µg/day or equivalent doses of 1-α-calcidol

Treatment of advanced hyperparathyroidism

Administration of active vitamin D

In the patient with advanced hyperparathyroidism (i.e. 1,84-iPTH above approximately 50 pmol/l or eightfold above the normal range), higher doses of active vitamin D are required. However, it is important to stress that active vitamin D must only be administered if hyperphosphataemia and hypercalcaemia are not present (or have been reversed) to prevent extra-osseous calcifications and further stimulation of the parathyroid gland in response to hyperphosphataemia, which is aggravated by administration of active vitamin D. Treatment should start with relatively modest doses, for instance 0.5 μg calcitriol per day. If this dose is tolerated without provoking hyperphosphataemia or hypercalcaemia, then it can be gradually increased until plasma 1,84-iPTH concentrations begin to fall. Several schedules of administration of active vitamin D are currently under discussion, but a complete consensus has not yet emerged.

Continuous compared with pulse administration

In experimental studies, continuous (daily) administration is less effective than intermittent (pulse) administration in lowering PTH concentration and preventing parathyroid hyperplasia. So far, there is no good clinical evidence that this effect is sufficiently marked to be of clinical importance.

Oral compared with intravenous administration

It can be shown that intravenous administration causes rapid lowering of 1,84-iPTH concentrations, but head-on comparisons of intravenous and oral administration have failed to show any superiority of the intravenous route.

Alternative vitamin D analogues

The major side-effects of treatment with active vitamin D are hypercalcaemia and hyperphosphataemia. There has therefore been an intense search for vitamin D analogues that suppress the parathyroid gland while having less hypercalcaemic and hyperphosphataemic potential. Several analogues are available (19-nor-1,25-dihydroxyvitamin D_2, namely Paricalcitol; 19-nor-22-oxa-1α,25-dihydroxyvitamin D_3, namely 22-oxacalcitriol), but so far there is no evidence that they are clinically better.

Calcimimetics

Calcimimetic substances—those that stimulate the calcium sensor—cause substantial acute and sustained decrease in the elevated PTH concentration of patients with moderate and advanced hyperparathyroidism. In experimental studies they also prevent further parathyroid hyperplasia, a finding of great importance because advanced parathyroid hyperplasia is irreversible (see below). There is currently only limited clinical experience, and concerns have been raised because the calcium receptor is expressed on numerous tissues other than the parathyroid gland. Anecdotal observations of long-term administration without side-effects in patients with parathyroid carcinoma raise the hope that these compounds will become an important ingredient in the management of the patient with renal failure.

Parathyroidectomy

It has recently been recognized that marked parathyroid hyperplasia is a process that bears many similarities to tumour growth. In patients whose estimated parathyroid mass exceeds 1 to 1.5 g, nodular hyperplasia is usually found. The nodules frequently exhibit monoclonal growth, with microsatellite analysis showing loss of heterozygosity for many alleles, including putative tumour suppressor genes. These nodules also express few vitamin D and calcium receptors, explaining the frequent lack of response to medical management. It appears that continuous stimulation of the parathyroid gland selectively favours cells with higher proliferative potential, so that the gland progressively escapes from growth inhibitory control mechanisms. This is illustrated by the fact that regrowth, including locally invasive regrowth, occurs in a high proportion (approximately one-third, or even more in studies with longer follow-up) of patients after subtotal parathyroidectomy or autotransplantation of parathyroid tissue.

There has recently been a tendency to consider parathyroidectomy early on if patients with marked elevation of 1,84-iPTH (above approximately 50 pmol/l) fail to respond to medical treatment within 4 to 8 weeks by decreasing their PTH concentration and have massive parathyroid enlargement on imaging procedures, with an estimated mass greater than 1 to 1.5 g.

An absolute indication for parathyroidectomy is calciphylaxis—ischaemic skin necrosis secondary to calcification of skin arteries; a relative indication is intractable pruritus associated with high PTH, or biomechanical problems that require urgent stabilization (e.g. rupture of the patella or epiphyseolysis in children with uraemia).

There is a long-standing debate as to whether total parathyroidectomy or subtotal parathyroidectomy (with a remnant left *in situ* or autotransplanted into the subcutaneous abdominal fat or forearm musculature) is preferable. Leaving parathyroid tissue behind is associated with a relatively high risk of recurrence, presumably because of the higher growth potential of the parathyroid. The risk can be reduced if only non-nodular parts of the gland are autotransplanted. As an alternative to surgery, alcohol injection into the enlarged parathyroids under ultrasonographic guidance has been tried successfully, but this procedure is not completely devoid of risk (paresis of the recurrent nerve).

Table 6 summarizes the approach to the management of patients with advanced renal secondary hyperparathyroidism, and Table 7 gives guidelines on how to interpret the common laboratory values used to diagnose abnormal calcium metabolism or follow therapeutic intervention.

Table 6 Treatment of advanced hyperparathyroidism

If 1,84-iPTH is constantly above 20 pmol/l
→ return plasma calcium and plasma phosphate to normal levels
If plasma phosphate is elevated
→ calcium carbonate (or calcium acetate) with meals
→ reduction of excess intake of dietary phosphate
→ increase of efficacy of dialysis (higher blood flow, longer dialysis sessions, more frequent dialysis sessions)
Note: active vitamin D is contraindicated as long as plasma phosphate elevated
If hypercalcaemia is present
→ reduce dialysate calcium to 6 mg/dl or (transiently) to 5 mg/dl
→ reduce or withdraw calcium-containing oral phosphate binders or active vitamin D
Note: active vitamin D is contraindicated as long as calcium is elevated
If plasma calcium and plasma phosphate have been returned to normal levels
→ increasing doses of calcitriol (0.5 to 3 μg) or alternative active vitamin D preparations daily or one to three times per week; dose and time interval depending on degree of elevation of 1,84-iPTH
→ monitor plasma calcium, plasma phosphate, 1,84-iPTH
If 1,84-iPTH decreases below 12 pmol/l
→ interrupt administration of calcitriol, measure 1,84-iPTH, decide whether low-dose long-term prophylaxis is necessary
If 1,84-iPTH fails to decrease and/or hypercalcaemia/ hyperphosphataemia develop
→ monitor gland size (ultrasonography, MIBI-scan)
→ consider parathyroidectomy

Table 7 Serum biochemistry in the evaluation of renal osteodystrophy

	Comments	Normal range
Calcium	Low, normal, or elevated (elevated in severe HPT, vitamin D excess, therapy with Ca-containing phosphate binders, inappropriate high dialysate Ca, immobilization)	2.2–2.6 mmol/l
Phosphate	Elevated in advanced renal failure (GFR < 30 ml/min)	0.8–1.4 mmol/l
PTH		
Intact 1,84-PTH	Elevated in HPT; can be normal or even low (mostly in cases of Al intoxication, adynamic bone disease, overtreatment with calcitriol, after parathyroidectomy)	1–6 pmol/l or 10–65 pg/ml
25-(OH)D_3 (calcidiol)	Often also low because of reduced sun exposure; seasonal variation, if increased, check for exogenous source	50–200 nmol/l
1,25-$(OH)_2D_3$ (calcitriol)	Usually low (if increased, check for calcitriol ingestion; rarely endogenous overproduction (granulomatous disease))	25–75 pg/ml
Total AP	Normal or increased; elevated in severe HPT (exclude concomitant liver disease by determination of γ-GT)	60–170 IU/l
Osseous AP isoenzyme	Normal or increased; elevated in HPT; measurement by monoclonal antibody technology has better sensitivity and specificity for osteitis fibrosa than total AP	3–22 μg/l
Osteocalcin	Diagnostic information analogous to AP; fragments accumulate in chronic renal failure; probably no extra information in addition to intact PTH and bone isoenzyme of AP	~ 3–8 μg/l* (may depend on assay)
Magnesium	Normal or elevated (decreased renal excretion)	0.8–1.3 mmol/l
Aluminium	Normal; elevated if Al-containing phosphate binders are taken or if dialysate contains Al	< 10 μg/l

Al, aluminium; AP, alkaline phosphatase; Ca, calcium; GFR, glomerular filtration rate; γ-GT, γ-glutamyl transferase; HPT, hyperparathyroidism.

* Range in individual with normal renal function.

Further reading

Arnold A *et al.* (1995). Monoclonality of parathyroid tumors in chronic renal failure and in primary parathyroid hyperplasia. *Journal of Clinical Investigation* **95**, 2047–53. [The first study to document that monoclonal growth occurs in the parathyroid nodules in patients with uraemia with nodular hyperplasia of the parathyroids.]

Couttenye MM *et al.* (1999). Low bone turnover in patients with renal failure. *Kidney International* **56** (Suppl 73), S70–6. [A review summarizing the current information concerning diminished bone turnover in patients with renal disease—so-called adynamic bone disease.]

Drueke TB (1998). Primary and secondary uraemic hyperparathyroidism: from initial clinical observations to recent findings. *Nephrology, Dialysis, Transplantation* **13**, 1384–7. [An up-to-date review of the pathomechanisms of secondary hyperparathyroidism, emphasizing molecular aspects.]

Felsenfeld AJ (1997). Considerations for the treatment of secondary hyperparathyroidism in renal failure. *Journal of the American Society of Nephrology* **8**, 993–1004. [Very complete update on the pathogenesis of secondary hyperparathyroidism and the rationale for therapeutic interventions.]

Fukuda N *et al.* (1993). Decreased 1,25-dihydroxyvitamin D3 receptor density is associated with a more severe form of parathyroid hyperplasia in chronic uremic patients. *Journal of Clinical Investigation* **92**, 1436–43. [A study documenting deficient vitamin D receptor expression in parathyroid glands with nodular hyperplasia. This explains, at least in part, the resistance of advanced hyperparathyroidism to active vitamin D.]

Gagne ER *et al.* (1992). Short- and long-term efficacy of total parathyroidectomy with immediate autografting compared with subtotal parathyroidectomy in hemodialysis patients. *Journal of the American Society of Nephrology* **3**, 1008–17. [A study documenting a high rate of hypoparathyroidism and relapse of hyperparathyroidism in patients with total parathyroidectomy and parathyroid autografts and subtotal parathyroidectomy, respectively.]

Hamdy NA *et al.* (1995). Effect of alfacalcidol on natural course of renal bone disease in mild to moderate renal failure. *British Medical Journal* **310**, 358–63. [A study documenting that early intervention with active vitamin D causes less increase in PTH and interferes with the development of bony lesions.]

Hergesell O, Ritz E (1999). Phosphate binders on iron basis: a new perspective? *Kidney International* **56**(Suppl 73), S42–5. [A review summarizing the rationale for the use of phosphate binders and discussing novel developments in this field.]

Hutchison AJ *et al.* (1993). Correlation of bone histology with parathyroid hormone, vitamin D_3, and radiology in end-stage renal disease. *Kidney International* **44**, 1071–7. [A study documenting marked skeletal abnormalities in patients with renal disease before they are taken into renal replacement therapy programmes.]

Naveh-Many T *et al.* (1995). Parathyroid cell proliferation in normal and chronic renal failure rats. The effects of calcium, phosphate, and vitamin D. *Journal of Clinical Investigation* **96**, 1786–93. [A study showing that phosphate is an important modulator of parathyroid function and involved in the genesis of parathyroid hyperplasia in renal failure.]

Quarles LD *et al.* (1994). Prospective trial of pulse oral versus intravenous calcitriol treatment of hyperparathyroidism in ESRD. *Kidney International* **45**, 1710–21. [A controlled prospective trial documenting the lack of superiority of intermittent intravenous high-dose active vitamin D therapy over oral active vitamin D therapy.]

Ritz E (1994). Early parathyroidectomy should be considered as the first choice. *Nephrology, Dialysis, Transplantation* **9**, 1819–21. [Summarizes the arguments for parathyroidectomy compared with aggressive therapy using active vitamin D in advanced secondary hyperparathyroidism.]

Ritz E *et al.* (1995). Low-dose calcitriol prevents the rise in 1,84 iPTH without affecting serum calcium and phosphate in patients with moderate renal failure (prospective placebo-controlled multicentre trial). *Nephrology, Dialysis, Transplantation* **10**, 2228–34. [A study which documents that very low doses of active vitamin D are effective in preventing the rise of PTH, with no change of serum or urinary calcium, serum phosphate, or creatinine clearance.]

Yalcindag C, Silver J, Naveh-Many T (1999). Mechanism of increased parathyroid hormone mRNA in experimental uremia: roles of protein RNA binding and RNA degradation. *Journal of the American Society of Nephrology* **10**, 2562–8. [A study detailing the molecular mechanism causing increased synthesis of pre-pro-PTH mRNA in experimental uraemia.]

20.6 Renal replacement therapies

20.6.1 Haemodialysis

Ken Farrington and Roger Greenwood

Introduction

The availability of effective renal replacement therapy has transformed the outlook for patients with chronic renal failure over the past 40 years, replacing certain and imminent death with the prospect of long-term survival. Growing numbers of patients worldwide are now dependent on regular dialysis treatment to sustain life, the escalating proportion of older and frailer patients being direct testimony to the durability and flexibility of the treatment. Inevitably this success needs qualification. First, the functions of the kidney are many and diverse and dialysis effects only partial replacement of a few of these, notably the excretion of nitrogenous waste products, and control of water, electrolyte, and acid–base balance. Second, although there is agreement about the general aims of dialysis treatment, to prolong life and prevent or reduce morbidity from the uraemic syndrome, consensus on the way to achieve these aims is still far off. There is still debate about what constitutes adequate dialysis and even about which parameters are appropriate. Third, although dialysis undoubtedly prolongs life in patients with endstage chronic renal failure, mortality still far exceeds that in the general population. This is mainly due to cardiovascular disease, which is endemic and runs an accelerated course in patients on dialysis, whatever the modality employed. This chapter outlines the scope of current practice in haemodialysis stressing those aspects most relevant to clinical management.

The development of haemodialysis

The pioneers

Although dialysis had been known since the mid-nineteenth century as a means of separating dissolved elements by diffusion through a semipermeable membrane, it was not until over 80 years later that haemodialysis was first used clinically to treat acute uraemia. The development of reliable means of vascular access in the 1960s (the Scribner silastic shunt and the Brescia–Cimino arteriovenous fistula) allowed its extension to maintenance treatment for patients with chronic renal failure and Pandora's box was open.

Expanding services

The initial rigid selection criteria for access to dialysis treatment soon bent under the combined strain of ethical concern and patient expectation, eventually giving way to more liberal policies. There were marked geographical variations, largely economically driven, in the rates of the subsequent expansion of dialysis programmes, as well as in the modalities employed and in the patterns of service provision (Figs 1 and 2). Renal transplantation has had a limited impact on this expansion, having hit the ceiling of donor organ availability.

In the United States and most of Europe, haemodialysis was rapidly decentralized from the pioneering units but remained centre-based in hospitals and free-standing facilities in cities, towns, and rural areas. In the United Kingdom little decentralization occurred, with self-supervised home haemodialysis the chosen means of expansion and selection criteria remaining tight. During the 1980s continuous ambulatory peritoneal dialysis (CAPD) was seized upon as the means to liberalize access to treatment in the United Kingdom. It became the dominant dialysis mode, displacing centre-based haemodialysis to a rescue mode for those in whom CAPD was

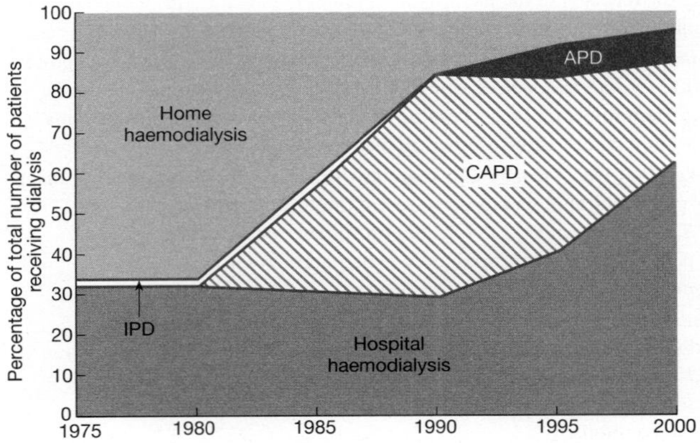

Fig. 1 Dialysis treatment modalities in the United Kingdom. Schematic representation of changes to treatment modality. IPD, intermittent peritoneal dialysis; CAPD, continuous ambulatory peritoneal dialysis; APD, automated peritoneal dialysis.

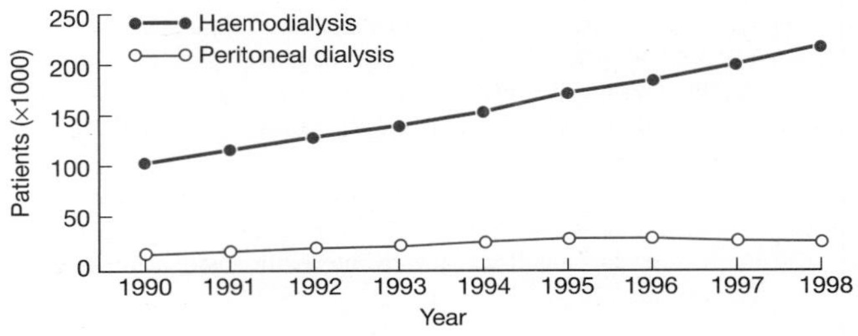

Fig. 2 Dialysis treatment modalities in the United States (United States Renal Data System (USRDS) data).

precluded or had failed. Elsewhere in Europe and in the United States centre-based haemodialysis remained the norm.

The impact of adequacy

Although patients continued to dialyse thrice weekly, there was a general trend to reduce dialysis times below 4 h. This first occurred in the United States as a mechanism to cope with constrained funding. 'Short dialysis' was held responsible for the excess mortality in American patients on haemodialysis during the 1980s, and inadvertently focused attention on the concept of dialysis adequacy, such that most units now prescribe and monitor dialysis dose by urea kinetic methods. Applying the same methods to CAPD, it became apparent that adequacy in this mode was critically dependent on residual renal function. Unless dialysate volumes are increased, adequacy is compromised, sometimes to the point of technique non-viability, when residual renal function has been lost. This has been a major factor in the steady relative decline in the United Kingdom CAPD population during the 1990s (Fig. 1), which has been more than offset by increased centre-based haemodialysis provision. The automated peritoneal dialysis (APD) programme has also grown but remains small. During the last decade, practice in the United Kingdom appears to be converging on United States and European norms.

Changing demographics

The mean age of the dialysis population has increased considerably over the last two decades and is now around 61 years. One-third of all new patients in the United Kingdom are over 70. The elderly, most of whom will not receive transplants, account for most of the increased acceptance and prevalence rates, which now exceed 90 and 300 patients per million population, respectively.

The proportion of patients with non-renal comorbidities, particularly cardiovascular disease, has increased dramatically. Multiple pathologies are common: about 15 per cent of patients on United Kingdom programmes are diabetic, and the United States figure is nearer 50 per cent (see section 20.6). Many such patients have widespread micro- and macrovascular complications at the time of dialysis initiation. These changes have placed increased demands on nephrological and other specialist resources.

Technical aspects

The principles of dialysis

Dialysis is a physicochemical process allowing separation of the components of a complex solution by solute exchange across a semipermeable membrane. Such membranes act as molecular size-selective filters, the size threshold depending on the nature of the membrane. In haemodialysis the membrane is interposed between the patient's bloodstream and a rinsing solution (dialysis fluid). Diffusive and convective mass transfer takes place across the membrane, allowing changes in the composition of body fluid compartments. The rate of diffusive solute transport is dependent on flow rates, concentration gradients, and membrane characteristics. Convection involves the bulk movement of solvent and dissolved solute across the membrane. The driving force is transmembrane hydrostatic pressure, which can be adjusted by application of variable negative pressure to the dialysate side of the membrane. Solute transport (by solvent drag) is independent of diffusion. In general, convection contributes little to the clearance of rapidly diffusible small solutes such as urea (molecular weight 60), but can make a major contribution to the clearance of larger, poorly diffusible molecules such as β_2-microglobulin (molecular weight 11 200), provided the membrane is porous to so-called 'middle' molecules. Convective movement of water from blood across the membrane is known as ultrafiltration.

Membranes and dialysers

The original haemodialysis membranes were fashioned from regenerated cellulose, but technology has since proliferated and there are now three classes of membrane, though there is much overlap (Table 1). Membranes are arranged and supported in devices called dialysers to form separate paths for blood and dialysis fluid flow, usually in a hollow-fibre design. Dialysers are classified by design type, membrane composition, surface area, and permeability characteristics defined in terms of dialyser clearance (K_d) for a range of solutes and ultrafiltration coefficient (K_{uf}), which is the water flux per unit of transmembrane pressure. In contrast to cuprophane, high-flux synthetic membranes are highly permeable (high K_{uf} and high K_d for middle molecules), remove β_2-microglobulin and other potentially toxic middle molecules, and tend to be more 'biocompatible', meaning that they cause less activation of inflammatory cells, the complement cascade, and contact pathways, and less cytokine production. High-flux membranes, when employed in countercurrent mode to maximize diffusion, permit 'back-filtration' of dialysis fluid into blood, hence use of ultrapure water to prepare dialysis fluid is mandatory. Many would argue that this improves biocompatibility and is highly desirable anyway. Synthetic membranes are expensive and dialyser reuse is still an economic necessity in most high-flux programmes.

Dialysis water and fluids

Patients on haemodialysis are intimately exposed to huge quantities of water (300 litres in a single week compared with a standard weekly exposure of 15 litres). The potential for poisoning by waterborne impurities is significant. Aluminium and chloramines are examples of proven toxins, which must be removed. Bacterial and endotoxin contamination can produce acute problems. Ultrapurity is crucial in high-flux modes in which dialysis fluid is passively (back-filtration) or actively (on-line haemodiafiltration) infused directly into the patient. A combination of purification techniques are employed that include filtration, activated carbon adsorption, ion-exchange resin perfusion, reverse osmosis, and ultraviolet irradiation. Regular monitoring ensures chemical and microbiological standards are maintained. Acid and bicarbonate concentrates are then mixed with treated water in a single-patient proportionating system to produce dialysis fluid of the desired composition (Table 2). Regulation of dialysis fluid composition is the main tool to achieve a return to normal of electrolyte and mineral content and acid–base balance in body fluid compartments. Although there is great potential for individualization, a programme-

Table 1 Haemodialysis membranes

Membrane class	Examples	Hydraulic permeability	β_2-Microglobulin clearance	Biocompatibility
Regenerated cellulose	Cuprophane	Low-flux	–	Poor
Modified cellulose	Cellulose acetate Cellulose diacetate Cellulose triacetate	Low/high flux	–/+	Moderate
Synthetic	Polymethylmethacrylate Polyacrylonitrile Polysulphone Polyamide Polycarbonate	High/low flux	+/–	Good

Table 2 Typical dialysis fluid composition

	Concentration (mmol/l)
Sodium	137–144
Potassium	0–3
Calcium	1.25–1.75
Magnesium	0.25–0.75
Chloride	98–112
Acetate	2.5–10
Bicarbonate	27–40
Glucose	0–5.6

standard composition is typically adopted, which may be varied in particular circumstances.

The dialysis machine and the extracorporeal circulation

Dialysis machines control and monitor much of the haemodialysis process and have crucial fail-safe functions. In the standard extracorporeal circuit, arterial blood is withdrawn from the arteriovenous fistula via the 'A' needle by a peristaltic pump (Fig. 3), circulated through the dialyser, through a bubble trap, and returned 'downstream' into the fistula through the 'V' needle. Heparin is infused downstream from the blood pump. The venous pressure monitor (*Pv*) protects against blood loss from the circuit to the environment and detects downstream obstruction to flow. The bubble-trap level detector protects against air embolus. The arterial pressure monitor (*Pa*) protects the fistula by detecting excessive negative pressure. Fail-safe mode activates the venous clamp and switches off the blood pump.

Control of ultrafiltration

Modern dialysis machines utilize volumetric methods that permit precise control of ultrafiltration. A balancing system regulates dialysis fluid flow rates to and from the dialyser allowing for the removal of the required ultrafiltration volume, which is preset by the operator.

Anticoagulation

Routine anticoagulation with heparin, administered by intravenous bolus and subsequent infusion, is monitored by the whole-blood activated clotting time. Heparin-free dialysis, employing regular saline flushes of the circuit, is possible in high-risk patients. Prostacyclin is an expensive alternative.

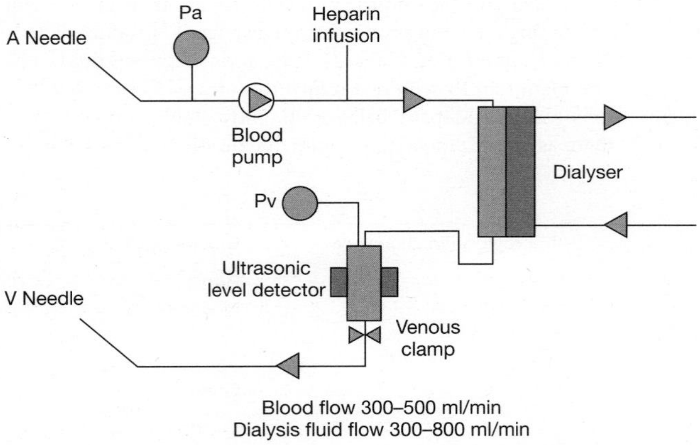

Fig. 3 Standard extracorporeal circuit. *Pa* = arterial pressure detector, *Pv* = venous pressure detector. A needle, arterial needle; V needle, venous needle.

Quantification and adequacy of dialysis

Predialysis blood urea and creatinine concentrations are poor indicators of dialysis adequacy. Low levels have been associated with increased mortality, suggesting that they are as (or more) likely to be due to reduced generation resulting from protein malnutrition and muscle wasting than due to increased clearance indicative of adequate dialysis. This was the lesson of the 1980s.

Urea kinetic modelling

The reanalysed data from the National Cooperative Dialysis Study (**NCDS**), still the only completed randomized study of the effect of haemodialysis dose on outcome, defined a new parameter of adequacy—the normalized urea clearance, Kt/V. This is a dimensionless parameter in which K is the urea clearance of the dialyser, t is the duration of dialysis in minutes, and V is the urea distribution volume, which approximates to total body water volume and is normally estimated from anthropomorphic data. The reanalysis showed that a Kt/V greater than 0.8 per dialysis was associated with good outcomes provided the patients were adequately nourished as defined by a normalized protein catabolic rate (**NPCR**) greater than 0.8 g/kg/day. NPCR can be calculated from urinary urea excretion in an interdialytic urine collection together with blood urea measurements taken at the start and finish of the collection (see equations in Appendix).

It is important to stress that the NCDS findings defined a minimum adequacy standard. The emerging view is that higher delivered Kt/V's produce improved outcomes. It is not yet possible to say whether there is an upper threshold above which no further improvement is obtained. Current guidelines suggest a minimum target Kt/V of 1.2 to 1.3. The dose of dialysis prescribed can be adjusted to achieve the target Kt/V by changing the surface area of the membrane, blood flow rate, dialysis fluid flow rate (these influence urea clearance by the dialyser), and dialysis duration. This logic allows adequate dialysis to be delivered in a shorter time using larger dialysers and high flow rates (high-efficiency dialysis). It is important to have a means of monitoring the effectiveness of delivery of the prescribed dose.

Monitoring dialysis delivery using the urea reduction ratio

The simplest measurement of dialysis dose is the urea reduction ratio (**URR**), which is given by:

$$\mathrm{URR} = 100(1 - C_{\mathrm{post}}/\ C_0)$$

where C_0 is the initial blood urea concentration, and C_{post} is the blood urea concentration in a blood sample taken immediately post-dialysis.

URR is a quality assurance tool, and cannot be used to prescribe dialysis dose. It takes no account of urea generation, ultrafiltration, or residual renal function, but does correlate with outcome testifying to its clinical utility. URR can also be converted to Kt/V (see Appendix).

Monitoring dialysis delivery using urea kinetic modelling

Assuming urea is distributed in a single pool within the body and that the effects of urea generation and ultrafiltration during dialysis are small, the blood urea concentration (C_t) at any time (t) during the dialysis is given by:

$$C_t = C_0 e^{-Kt/V}$$

Hence, the delivered dose of dialysis Kt/V, can be calculated from the expression:

$$Kt/V = \ln(C_0/C_{\mathrm{post}})$$

The expression that corrects for urea generation and ultrafiltration during dialysis is more complex, and the single pool assumption is also an oversimplification. The rapid removal of urea (and other solutes) from the bloodstream during dialysis creates intercompartmental disequilibra. The intracellular concentration of urea exceeds the extracellular, and that in poorly perfused peripheral pools exceeds that in well-perfused body compartments. Urea exchange between these compartments continues after cessation of dialysis and causes a post-dialysis rebound of blood urea concentrations. This rebound can be substantial in high-efficiency treatments and can cause overestimation of Kt/V delivery by as much as 20 per cent, making the single pool assumption untenable in short high-efficiency treatments. There are a number of ways of dealing with this problem: the most straightforward is to delay the post-dialysis sample until rebound is complete (equilibrated post-dialysis sample), but this can be inconvenient (the patients want to leave the dialysis unit as soon as their treatment is completed). Much more complex is to model the system as two pools, requiring the assumption of a number of physiological parameters and iterative solution by computer. There are a number of less complex approximations, which are usually preferred and have been shown to produce equivalent results. The bottom line is that urea kinetic modelling can be used to prescribe the amount of dialysis necessary to attain the target Kt/V. The method has the flexibility to take account of residual renal function, in which case the target Kt/V (total Kt/V) has dialysis (K_dt/V) and residual renal (K_Rt/V) components.

Other approaches to adequacy

Urea clearance is the basis of most current methods of assessment of dialysis adequacy, in spite of the fact that urea transfer is not representative of the kinetics of most uraemic toxins. An alternative, the solute removal index (ratio of mass of solute removed by dialysis to the mass present at the start of dialysis) has a theoretical advantage over Kt/V in that it allows direct comparison of the adequacy of all treatment modalities. Larger molecules such as β_2-microglobulin are certainly toxic in dialysed patients but do not figure in our currently accepted notions of adequacy. Broader definitions are required. Urea kinetic modelling needs to be regarded as an essential component of a more global view of adequacy, which includes clinical as well as other laboratory data.

Initiation of dialysis

Blood urea and creatinine concentrations are poor indicators of dialysis adequacy and are subject to the same misinterpretation in the predialysis phase as endstage chronic renal failure is approached. This may lead to delay in dialysis initiation. The National Kidney Foundation Dialysis Outcomes Quality Initiative (**NKF-DOQI**) guidelines for dialysis initiation are thus based on urea kinetic modelling and suggest that dialysis should be started when weekly renal Kt/V is less than 2.0 unless the patient is asymptomatic, has a stable oedema-free body weight, and a normalized protein equivalent of urea nitrogen appearance (equivalent to NPCR) greater than 0.8. The guidelines have the benefit of aligning the approach to the assessment of severity of uraemia in predialysis and dialysis phases, but still lack a firm evidence base.

Incremental dialysis

This approach recognizes that the target total urea Kt/V has dialysis (K_dt/V) and residual renal (K_Rt/V) components. As residual renal function declines during the first few years of dialysis, the dialysis component is gradually increased to ensure the target continues to be achieved. This allows a gentler initiation and maximizes the use of scarce resources. It does require regular estimates of residual renal function, and also assumes an equivalence of renal and dialyser clearance which holds for urea, but not necessarily for other solutes, or other renal functions. It is relevant that the viability of CAPD as a renal replacement modality also depends on this assumption.

Dry weight

Regulation of salt and water balance is one of the key functions of the kidney. Renal failure results in salt and water retention, which along with activation of the renin–angiotensin–aldosterone system, contributes to hypertension, left ventricular hypertrophy, and dilatation. These are potent causes of morbidity and mortality. 'Dry weight' is an important concept dating back to the early days of maintenance haemodialysis. It assumes that body weight at any time consists of two components: the dry weight or target weight, at which the patient's fluid compartments are normal in volume, and an excess weight consisting of surplus volume, which expands body fluid compartments and elevates blood pressure. The only way of defining dry weight is trial and error. The protocol requires cessation of antihypertensive agents and weight reduction during successive dialyses during the first few weeks or months after initiation. The dry weight is the point at which the patient is oedema free and below which hypotension occurs on further fluid removal. The implicit assumption is that patients on dialysis have normal cardiovascular responses, which may have been reasonable in the highly selected dialysis population of 1970 but is much less tenable in the older, sicker patients on dialysis today. Applying such principles, most of the early patients on dialysis became normotensive without the need for antihypertensive agents. In most current patients the target weight is likely to be the best achievable weight and hypertension is more likely. Shorter treatment times and less rigorous salt restriction have undoubtedly added to these difficulties.

Vascular access

The creation and maintenance of adequate, dependable, and robust vascular access is of vital importance to the continued well-being of patients on haemodialysis, and has rightly been referred to as their 'lifeline'.

Temporary access

For acute haemodialysis, temporary, non-cuffed, dual-lumen catheters can be inserted into femoral, internal jugular, or subclavian veins. The femoral route is simplest and preferred in the very sick patient, but the infection risk is high if femoral catheters are left *in situ* for more than a few days. Temporary catheters in other sites can remain for weeks, though use of the subclavian route risks stenosis of the vein and potentially compromises future permanent access in the ipsilateral arm.

Permanent access

Fashioning an arteriovenous fistula causes arterialization and expansion of the draining vein allowing its repeated puncturing for haemodialysis. A radiocephalic (Brescia–Cimino) fistula at the wrist is preferred, being less likely to produce distal limb ischaemia than proximal fistulas. Forearm vasculature is extremely vulnerable, especially when the patient is in hospital, and needs protecting in those destined for dialysis. Maturation of distal fistulas is slow, so these should be fashioned 3 to 6 months before planned initiation. It may be necessary to resort to other types of access including, in order of preference, an elbow brachiocephalic fistula, an arteriovenous graft composed of synthetic material (e.g. polytetrafluoroethene—PTFE), and cuffed tunnelled internal jugular venous catheters. Many patients still present late for dialysis and require primary central venous access by default. Tunnelled catheters are also required when other access options have been exhausted. Access failure is a significant cause of morbidity and mortality.

Recirculation

If there is a stenosis in the fistula severe enough to limit fistula blood flow to a level less than that demanded by the blood pump in the extracorporeal circulation, then blood returning from the dialyser to the fistula can be drawn directly from the 'V' needle to the 'A' needle and dialysed again. This is known as access recirculation, an effect that can also be produced by misplacement of fistula needles with the 'A' needle downstream to the 'V' needle. Also during dialysis a proportion of the blood returning through the 'V' needle will pass directly to the 'A' needle after passage through the heart and lungs without traversing a capillary bed to be 'replenished' with solute. This is known as cardiopulmonary recirculation and is an inevitable consequence of having a fistula as the access. The higher the blood pump speed the greater the degree of recirculation in all of these circumstances. Access recirculation is a major cause of underdelivery of prescribed dialysis dose, and unexplained reductions of monitored *Kt*/*V* or urea reduction ratios demand further investigation to exclude this. Significant recirculation (greater than 10 per cent), which can be detected and quantified by a variety of sampling and dilution methods (not described here), may require further investigation by Doppler ultrasonography or fistulography to define the lesion before attempting angioplastic or surgical correction.

Haemodialysis and related techniques

Conventional haemodialysis

'Conventional' refers to the use of low-flux cellulosic dialysers in standard circuits (Fig. 3). A decade ago the definition would also have included the use of acetate as buffer, but bicarbonate dialysis is now the norm.

High-flux haemodialysis

Concerns about the biocompatibility of cuprophane, and its poor clearance of middle molecules, especially β_2-microglobulin, have fuelled the increasing use of high-flux membranes, and concomitant investment in the use of ultrapure water for preparation of dialysis fluids.

Haemodiafiltration

Haemofiltration is a purely convective mode of treatment, which involves filtration of uraemic plasma and simultaneous infusion of replacement fluid. This greatly improves middle molecule clearance. However, small molecule clearance is slow (Fig. 4), so the technique is not suitable for routine treatment of patients with chronic renal failure. It has, however, proved highly successful as a continuous treatment for patients with acute renal failure, particularly in the context of multiple organ failure in the intensive care unit (see Section 16). Adding a greater convective component (haemofiltration) to the diffusive and convective clearances offered by high-flux haemodialysis (a technique referred to as haemodiafiltration) allows the benefits of both these modalities to be maximized. The capacity to utilize dialysis fluid as the infusion fluid, made possible by use of ultrapure water in its preparation, means that the technique is economically viable (on-line haemodiafiltration, Fig. 5).

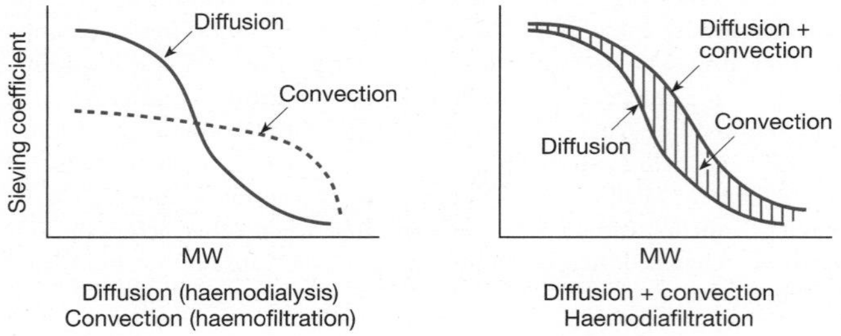

Fig. 4 Comparison of solute removal by diffusion and convection according to molecular weight. Convection has better 'middle molecule' clearance but much poorer clearance of small-molecular-weight solutes than diffusion. Haemodiafiltration combines the strengths of both techniques to broaden the spectrum of solute removal.

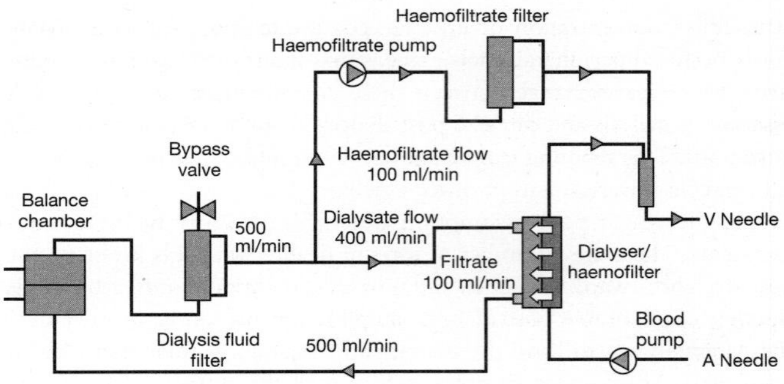

Fig. 5 Circuit for on-line haemodiafiltration. The haemofiltration replacement fluid is haemodialysis fluid pumped through an additional filter before infusion directly into the venous line. HDF, haemodiafiltrate. A needle, arterial needle; V needle, venous needle.

High-efficiency modalities

High-efficiency dialysers have high dialyser urea clearances and large surface areas. Dialysis treatments achieving high urea clearances (usually more than 200 ml/min) are referred to as high-efficiency treatments. Dialysis duration can be shortened by these means, often to below 3 h per session ('short dialysis'). High-efficiency and high-flux relate to different properties of dialysers and dialysis modes, which can be neither, either, or both.

Complications of haemodialysis

Acute complications

Hypotension

Symptomatic hypotension occurs in up to 30 per cent of dialysis sessions. Symptoms include nausea, vomiting, cramps, palpitations, dizziness, and syncope. The major cause is hypovolaemia, resulting from an imbalance between the rate of fluid removal from the circulation by ultrafiltration, and the rate of vascular refilling from the interstitium. Underlying cardiovascular disease, the use of antihypertensive drugs, autonomic dysfunction, and shortened dialysis times, increase the likelihood. The mainstays of management are careful assessment and reassessment of target weight, limited use of antihypertensive agents, reduction of interdialytic weight gain by fluid and sodium restriction, and reduction of ultrafiltration rate. Newer dialysis machines have the capacity to monitor relative blood volume and to profile the sodium concentration of dialysis fluid throughout the dialysis session. These techniques may be useful in particular situations, but neither is yet used routinely. Episodes of hypotension may occasionally have more sinister causes such as primary myocardial events and heparin-induced bleeding.

Disequilibration

The severest forms of disequilibration occur shortly after dialysis initiation (dialysis disequilibrium syndrome). The major predisposing factors are late presentation with severe uraemia and aggressive dialysis initiation with lengthy dialyses and high solute clearance rates. Restlessness, headache, tremors, fits, and coma can result. Dialysis should not be initiated in this way. Cerebral oedema due to fluid shifts induced by intercompartmental differences in urea concentrations and paradoxical cerebrospinal fluid acidosis are among the suggested causes. Post-dialysis headache is a common symptom in patients undergoing regular haemodialysis and may be a minor manifestation of disequilibrium.

Dialyser reactions

Anaphylactic (IgE-mediated) reactions occurring on first use of a dialyser are usually due to ethylene oxide sensitivity, which is used by manufacturers as a sterilizing agent. Reactions with reused dialysers are usually due to disinfectants, such as formaldehyde and peracetic acid, used in reprocessing. Bradykinin-mediated anaphylactoid reactions can occur in patients taking angiotensin-converting enzyme (ACE) inhibitors who are dialysed with polyacrylonitrile synthetic membranes (AN69). All the above occur within the first 20 min of treatment.

Pyrexias

Infected central lines are a potent cause of bacteraemia. Pyrogen reactions due to contaminated water became rare when rebuildable dialysers were replaced by disposable devices in the late 1970s.

Other complications

Use of modern fail-safe dialysis machines and ultrapure water systems has fortunately rendered a number of previously well-described complications exceedingly rare. These include air embolism, severe hypercalcaemia due to dialysis against hard water, and acute haemolysis.

Chronic complications

Hypertension and cardiovascular disease

There are many factors contributing to hypertension in patients on dialysis, including stimulation of the renin–angiotensin–aldosterone system and sympathetic overactivity, but the overriding factor is volume overload. Fluid status varies throughout the dialysis cycle and so does blood pressure. Just what constitutes hypertension in those on dialysis is not well defined, but in most units 60 per cent or more of the patients receive antihypertensive agents, although in other units this is less common. This may be explained by differences in definition and case mix, but other factors are undoubtedly important too, particularly the emphasis placed on the maintenance of optimum sodium balance and adequate ultrafiltration. In some units there may be a tendency to compromise, perhaps too soon, and use drugs, especially in patients with cardiovascular and other comorbidities, making dry weight even more difficult to achieve. Getting this right is crucial since hypertension is an important risk factor for cardiovascular disease, which is the major cause of the excess mortality in the dialysis population.

Volume overload, hypertension, anaemia, hyperparathyroidism, excessive fistula flow rates, and uraemia itself all predispose to left ventricular hypertrophy, which is an independent risk factor for mortality. Correction of anaemia can favourably influence the natural history of left ventricular hypertrophy in patients on dialysis, and early use of erythropoietin in the predialysis period may prevent it. Patients on dialysis also have a variety of lipid abnormalities, hyperhomocysteinaemia, increased oxidative stress, and elevated inflammatory markers, all of which may predispose to cardiovascular disease.

Anaemia

Erythropoietin deficiency is the major cause of anaemia in patients on haemodialysis. The introduction of recombinant erythropoietin in the early 1990s has redefined the uraemic syndrome, in the sense that many debilitating 'uraemic' symptoms can be remedied by successful treatment of anaemia (see Chapter 20.6.2 for further discussion).

A number of additional causes of anaemia may arise from the dialysis process itself. The most common is iron deficiency, which results from the repeated loss of small amounts of blood. Regular iron replacement, preferably given intravenously, is necessary since iron deficiency is a potent cause of resistance to exogenous erythropoietin. Deficiencies of other haematinics can occur, particularly in high-flux treatments and regular supplementation with vitamin B_{12} and folate is recommended. Mechanical and chloramine-induced haemolysis should not occur with modern techniques. There are other causes of erythropoietin resistance, the most potent being infection, often arising from central venous lines in this context, also severe hyperparathyroidism and underlying malignancy.

Bone disease

For discussion of renal bone disease, see Chapter 20.5.2.

Amyloidosis

Dialysis-related amyloidosis is a serious complication of chronic dialysis. The incidence increases with duration of haemodialysis and symptomatic involvement is almost universal after 15 years. Older patients are more susceptible. The syndrome manifests mainly as carpel tunnel syndrome and destructive arthropathy associated with bone cysts, but other organs can be involved. Deposits of amyloid, mainly composed of β_2-microglobulin fibrils, can be found at these and other sites. β_2-Microglobulin is an 11 200-Da protein that is part of the human class 1 major histocompatibility complex. It is 95 per cent eliminated by glomerular filtration, hence levels are elevated in renal failure. Low-flux membranes do not clear β_2-microglobulin but clearance occurs by a combination of convection and adsorption, using high-flux membranes. Elevated plasma levels are the major predisposing factor to amyloid deposition. Other factors may also be important, including modification of β_2-microglobulin by advanced glycation end-products and by oxidative and carbonyl stress. It is also possible that β_2-microglobulin or modified β_2-microglobulin is directly toxic to tissues. Use of high-flux synthetic membranes, especially in haemodiafiltration mode (Fig. 5), reduces plasma levels of β_2-microglobulin, although the level remains about tenfold higher than in those with normal renal function. High-flux dialysis and especially haemodiafiltration may prevent or delay the onset of symptomatic disease. Use of ultrapure water may also be protective. Treatment options are limited for established disease, but renal transplantation may enable slow resorption of deposits.

Patient management

Infection control

Strict adherence to universal precautions is necessary to minimize the risk of cross-infection by bloodborne viruses. Transmission from contaminated external surfaces, rather than through the dialyser membrane, is the major cross-infection threat. Screening of patients about to start dialysis for evidence of prior infection with hepatitis B and C is routine, and should be repeated at least 6 monthly thereafter. Patients negative for hepatitis B surface antigen should be vaccinated: positive patients should be segregated and use a dedicated machine. Patients positive for hepatitis C or HIV should be managed similarly.

Dialysis prescription and monitoring of dialysis delivery

There are a number of elements to the dialysis prescription that should be regularly and systematically reviewed. Target Kt/V is normally 1.2 to 1.3. Patients with intercurrent illness may require more. The value of K is obtained from data sheets from the dialyser manufacturer, taking into account membrane area, and blood and dialyser flow rates. The value of V is obtained empirically from age, sex, weight, and height. If the target Kt/V includes a component for residual renal function then residual urea clearance should be measured monthly and dialysis time readjusted accordingly. Dialysis delivery should be monitored monthly. Prescription and monitoring protocols are now often computer based. Inefficient delivery requires prompt investigation to exclude problems such as access recirculation. Membrane type and flux should be specified. Use of high-flux synthetic membranes is increasingly standard rather than targeted by evidence of amyloid deposition. Setting the dry weight allows the ultrafiltration requirement to be specified for each dialysis. Regular reassessment of dry weight is required, especially during intercurrent illness, when loss of flesh weight predisposes to covert fluid overload. The prescription should also refer to the heparin loading dose and maintenance infusion rate.

Control of hypertension

Predialysis blood pressure measurements may be misleading and cause overdiagnosis and overtreatment of hypertension. Measurements taken 20 min post-dialysis, allowing time for compartmental re-equilibration, are a better reflection of interdialytic ambulatory readings. Target levels have not been defined. We suggest targeting a 20-min post-dialysis reading of 135/85 in patients less than 65 years old. Drug therapy of hypertension is second-line treatment to be deployed after the achievement of optimal fluid status. No class of antihypertensive agent is contraindicated in dialysis patients, although the half-life of renally excreted drugs may be markedly prolonged and care is required with dosing schedules.

Access care and surveillance

Regular clinical examination of fistulas, serial measurement of static and dynamic venous pressures during dialysis, and monitoring of access flow rates by ultrasound dilution may enable access problems to be detected and corrected before the risks of underdialysis supervene.

Diet and nutrition

Malnutrition is common and is usually due to underdialysis. The early signs are subtle and often masked by fluid overload, which can compound the problem. There are no simple, fool-proof laboratory tests. Serum albumin reflects the presence of inflammation as much as it reflects malnutrition. Monitoring of NPCR (normalized protein catabolic rate) may be helpful but cannot replace regular dietetic review. When malnutrition is identified a range of oral nutritional supplements may be deployed. There is a limited role for intradialytic parenteral nutrition. Protein requirements in patients on haemodialysis are not well characterized but have been estimated at 1.2 g/kg ideal body weight/day, which is considerably greater than the non-uraemic requirement. Intakes greatly in excess of this may cause problems unless dialysis dose is correspondingly increased. There is no role for protein restriction. The energy requirement of a moderately active patient on haemodialysis is about 35 kcal/kg body weight/day, which is similar to that of normal subjects.

Attempts should be made to limit interdialytic fluid gains to 1 to 2 litres. This is difficult when residual renal function has been lost. The value of limiting sodium intake (40 to 80 mmol/day) to control thirst is often understated. Potassium restriction (to about 60 mmol/day) is usually required when residual renal function is minimal. The recommended intake of elemental calcium is 1 to 1.5 g/day. Achieving this is seldom difficult given the extensive use of calcium salts as phosphate binders. Phosphate restriction to about 0.8 g/day of elemental phosphorus may reduce the requirement for these agents. There is no consensus on the need to supplement water-soluble vitamins (B and C), but the practice is widespread. Vitamin B_{12} supplements are recommended in high-flux treatments.

Anaemia

Treatment with recombinant erythropoietin has become the mainstay of anaemia management, which is often nurse-led and protocol-driven. Uncertainties remain about the optimal target haemoglobin, recommendations varying between 10 and 12 g/dl. In the dialysis population the use of erythropoietin has unmasked a huge requirement for intravenous iron supplementation. Many patients have a state of absolute or functional iron deficiency, which is difficult to diagnose in those on dialysis. NKF-DOQI recommendations that serum ferritin levels less than 100 ng/ml and transferrin saturation less than 20 per cent are indicative of iron deficiency are reasonably sensitive when taken together, but poorly specific. Other parameters such as the percentage of hypochromic red cells and the reticulocyte haemoglobin content may be useful, but the best test appears to be the pragmatic one of response to intravenous iron. Oral iron is usually ineffective, probably because intestinal iron absorption—already low in endstage chronic renal failure—fails to respond to the stimulus of erythropoiesis, and is further suppressed by high tissue iron stores. Intravenous iron saccharate is used in moderate doses (such as 100 mg on each of 10 successive dialyses) to correct iron deficiency, and as maintenance treatment (such as 50 mg weekly) provided 3-monthly serum ferritin levels remain below about 800 ng/ml. (See Chapter 20.6.2 for further discussion of the use of erythropoietin.)

Bone disease

The goals of treatment are to maintain optimal bone structure and function and prevent metastatic calcification. The short-term surrogate is to maintain biochemical parameters in their target ranges. Serum calcium should be maintained in the normal range. The target range for phosphate is ill-defined and there is confusion about what is desirable and what is achievable. The product of calcium and phosphate (in mmol/l) should be less than 5. Serum parathyroid hormone (**PTH**) levels should be maintained at about two to three times the upper limit of normal. Calcium carbonate and calcium acetate are the phosphate binders in common use. Hypercalcaemia is a real risk. Sevelamer, a new polymeric phosphate binder that does not contan metal ions should be less toxic in this regard. Calcitriol and α-calcidol are used mainly to suppress PTH secretion. When used with calcium salts, the risks of hypercalcaemia are multiplied and careful monitoring is required. Pulsed therapy (usually thrice weekly on dialysis days) may improve the therapeutic ratio, but the benefits of intravenous administration have been overstated. Failure to control hyperparathyroidism still necessitates parathyroidectomy in significant numbers of patients. On the other hand, oversuppression of PTH levels should be avoided, being a risk factor for adynamic bone disease and enhanced metastatic calcification. (See Chapter 20.5.2 for further discussion.)

Other aspects

Selection and preparation of patients on dialysis for transplantation is a crucial aspect of care, which now usually includes rigorous assessment of cardiovascular fitness.

Cardiovascular risk factors such as smoking and lipid disorders should be addressed, and exercise encouraged, both during dialysis sessions and in general. Low-dose aspirin may be beneficial. Folate and vitamin B supplements may reduce elevated homocysteine levels. There is a high incidence of sexual dysfunction, especially in males: some may benefit from androgen replacement, sildenafil may be effective if not contraindicated, skilled counselling may be helpful.

Outcomes

Dialysis undoubtedly prolongs the life of patients with endstage chronic renal failure, but survival remains markedly inferior to that of age-matched peers with normal renal function. Cardiovascular disease is the main cause of death, followed by infection. Comparison of outcome in the different eras of dialysis is fraught with problems, largely because of the dramatic differences in case mix of patients entering programmes. Age, comorbidity, and functional status are independent predictors of morbidity (rate of admission to hospital) and mortality. Late presentation for dialysis has a profound effect on survival; late planned initiation may also have an effect, perhaps mediated through malnutrition; and we have previously alluded to the effects of dialysis adequacy and nutrition on outcome. The relationship between post-dialysis systolic blood pressure and mortality is 'U' shaped, as in the normal population, those with the lowest pressures faring poorly, probably due to coexisting heart failure.

It is difficult to compare the outcome of patients treated with haemodialysis and peritoneal dialysis in any meaningful way. Data from single centres, multicentre studies, and analysis of registry data do not show consistent differences in survival between these modalities. There are a number of confounding factors. Patients initiated on CAPD are younger, have less coexisting non-renal comorbidities, better functional status, and are less likely to have presented late. In addition, technique survival is poor in CAPD, and many patients require transfer to haemodialysis because of peritonitis, inadequate dialysis, or ultrafiltration failure. Haemodialysis can be regarded as the default mode of renal replacement therapy. Quality of life assessments are similar in both groups, but both are inferior to those obtained in patients with successful transplants. It is probably safe to conclude that, in the early years of therapy at least, morbidity and mortality are similar on both modalities if risk-stratified groups are compared.

There are few data to allow comparison of the outcome of conventional haemodialysis and more modern haemodialysis modes. Registry data suggests better survival with more biocompatible membranes, possibly related to enhanced clearance of larger solutes. Evidence is hardening that high-flux modes protect against the development of dialysis-associated amyloidosis.

The future

Haemodialysis is likely to remain centre based for the majority. Technical advances will allow treatments to become more tailored to the specific requirements of the individual. On-line dialysis quantification could guarantee the adequacy of each session. On-line blood volume monitoring coupled with algorithms to control ultrafiltration rate, dialysis fluid temperature, and sodium content, on a minute-to-minute basis, could prevent intradialytic hypotension and allow patients to finish dialysis at their optimal achievable weight. The encouraging results with daily dialysis suggest that this may emerge as a home, self-supervised modality, perhaps for a small proportion of younger, less dependent patients for whom transplantation or retransplantation is not an option. Vascular access will remain the Achilles' heel.

Appendix

$$\mathrm{NPCR} = 148.7(G/V + 0.17),$$

where G is the urea generation rate given by:

$$G/V = [C_{\mathrm{pre2}}(V + w_{\mathrm{g}})/V - C_{\mathrm{post}} + (V_{\mathrm{u}} \times U_{\mathrm{u}})/V]/t_{\mathrm{id}}$$

Where C_{pre2} = predialysis blood urea concentration before succeeding dialysis

w_{g} = interdialytic weight gain

V_{u} = volume of interdialytic urinary collection

U_{u} = urinary urea concentration

t_{id} = duration of intradialytic urine collection

$$Kt/V = -\ln(\mathrm{URR} - 0.008t) + (4 - 3.5\mathrm{URR}) \times (W_2 - W_1)/W_2$$

Where t = duration of dialysis

W_1 = predialysis weight

W_2 = post-dialysis weight

Further reading

Bergstrom J (1993). The nutritional requirements of hemodialysis patients. In: Mitch WE, Klahr S, eds. *Nutrition and the kidney*, 2nd edn, pp 263–89. Little, Brown and Company, Boston.

Block GA, Port FK (2000). Re-evaluation of the risks associated with hyperphosphatemia and hyperparathyroidism in dialysis patients: recommendations for a change in management. *American Journal of Kidney Diseases* **35**, 1226–37.

Chandna SM *et al.* (1999). Factors affecting survival and morbidity on chronic dialysis. Is there a rationale for rationing? *British Medical Journal* **318**, 217–23.

Drucker W (1979). Haemodialysis: a historical review. In: Drucker W, Parsons FM, Maher JF, eds. *Replacement of renal function by dialysis*, pp 3–37. Martinus Nijhoff, The Hague.

Gokal R (1993). Quality of life in patients undergoing renal replacement therapy. *Kidney International* **40**(Suppl 8), S23–7.

Hirsch DH (1989). Death from dialysis termination. *Nephrology, Dialysis, Transplantation* **4**, 41–4.

Keshaviah P, Star RA (1994). A new approach to dialysis quantification: an adequacy index based on solute removal. *Seminars in Dialysis* **7(2)**, 85–9.

Khan IH *et al.* (1993). Influence of coexisting disease on survival on renal replacement therapy. *Lancet* **341**, 415–18.

Lameire N, Van Biesen W (1999). The pattern of referral to the nephrologist: a European survey. *Nephrology, Dialysis, Transplantation* **14**(Suppl.6), 16–23.

Leypoldt JK *et al.* (1999). Effect of dialysis membranes and middle molecule removal on chronic hemodialysis patient survival. *American Journal of Kidney Diseases* **33**, 349–55.

Locatelli F *et al.* (1996). The effects of different membranes and dialysis technologies on patient treatment tolerance and nutritional parameters. The Italian Cooperative Dialysis Study. *Kidney Internationa*l **50**, 1293–302.

Lowrie EG, Lew NL (1990). Death risk in haemodialysis patients: the predictive value of commonly measured variables and an evaluation of death rate differences between facilities. *American Journal of Kidney Diseases* **15**, 458–82.

Mitra SM, Chandna SM, Farrington K (1999). What is hypertension in chronic haemodialysis? The role of interdialytic blood pressure monitoring. *Nephrology, Dialysis, Transplantation* **14**, 2915–21.

National Kidney Foundation (1997). NKF-DOQI clinical practice guidelines for hemodialysis adequacy. *American Journal of Kidney Diseases* **30**(Suppl 2), S15–66.

National Kidney Foundation (1997). NKF-DOQI clinical practice guidelines for vascular access. *American Journal of Kidney Diseases* **30**(Suppl 3), S150–91.

Owen WF *et al.* (1993). The urea reduction ratio and serum albumin concentration as predictors of mortality in patients undergoing haemodialysis. *New England Journal of Medicine* **329**, 1001–6.

Renal Association (1997). *Treatment of adult patients with renal failure. Recommended standards and audit measures.* Royal College of Physicians, London.

Schiffl H *et al.* (2000). Clinical manifestations of AB-amyloidosis: effects of biocompatibility and flux. *Nephrology, Dialysis, Transplantation* **15**, 840–5.

Tattersall JE, Greenwood RN, Farrington K (1995). Urea kinetics and when to commence dialysis. *American Journal of Nephrology* **15**, 283–9.

Tattersall JE, Farrington K, Greenwood RN (1998). Adequacy of dialysis. In: Davison AM, *et al.*, eds. *Oxford textbook of clinical nephrology*, 2nd edn, pp. 2075–87. Oxford University Press, Oxford.

Vonesh EF, Moran J (1999). Mortality in end-stage renal disease. A reassessment of differences between patients treated with hemodialysis and peritoneal dialysis. *Journal of the American Society of Nephrology* **10**, 354–65.

20.6.2 The treatment of endstage renal disease by peritoneal dialysis

Paul F. Williams

Introduction

Peritoneal dialysis has been an established treatment modality for acute and chronic renal failure since the early 1960s, but it was not until 1976 with the description of peritoneal equilibration dialysis (later to become known as 'continuous ambulatory peritoneal dialysis'—**CAPD**) by Popovich and Moncrieff that the technique was popularized. By the end of the twentieth century some 15 to 20 per cent of all chronic dialysis patients worldwide were being treated with either CAPD or automated peritoneal dialysis (**APD**). Peritoneal dialysis plays an important role in the integrated care of the patient with endstage renal disease along with haemodialysis and renal transplantation.

Practical aspects of peritoneal dialysis

The process of peritoneal dialysis involves the instillation of dialysis fluid into the peritoneal cavity via a dialysis catheter, thereby allowing the fluid to come into contact with the uraemic blood in the patient's peritoneal capillaries. Dialysis takes place through the diffusion of uraemic toxins down a concentration gradient from capillary blood to dialysis fluid, with fluid removal from the circulation being achieved by varying the concentrations of osmotic agents (usually glucose) in the dialysis fluid. Once the uraemic toxins in the patient's blood have equilibrated with the dialysis fluid then this can be drained out and replaced manually (CAPD) or by machine (APD).

Peritoneal dialysis solutions

The most commonly used dialysis solutions today contain varying concentrations of glucose as the osmotic agent, along with a balanced electrolyte solution using lactate as a buffer to correct uraemic acidosis. Although these solutions have been in widespread use for many years they are recognized to have a number of disadvantages, including low pH and hyperosmolality, which depends on the glucose concentration. These make the dialysis fluids relatively bioincompatible and may be responsible for long-term membrane damage with mesothelial cell loss and glycation of the membrane. A variety of new peritoneal dialysis solutions have been introduced in recent years in an attempt to improve biocompatibility, membrane viability, fluid removal, and malnutrition. These include: (1) solutions using a bicarbonate/lactate mixture instead of lactate alone as the buffer; (2) a glucose polymer-based fluid that allows reduced membrane exposure to glucose and allows slow prolonged ultrafiltration to take place; and (3) an amino acid-based solution which may help to correct hypoalbuminaemia and malnutrition.

Peritoneal dialysis catheters

Access to the peritoneal cavity can be achieved on a semipermanent basis using a silastic Tenckhoff catheter. A variety of modifications on the basic design exist but none has conclusively been shown to be superior. The intraperitoneal portion of the catheter can be straight or coiled and has side and end holes; the subcutaneous portion provides anchorage and a barrier against infection by means of tissue ingrowth into two Dacron cuffs, one placed preperitoneally in the rectus sheath and one subcutaneously.

Insertion techniques also vary: the catheters may be placed percutaneously via a trochar and cannula, via a laparoscope, or with a formal mini-laparotomy. The success or otherwise of the insertion procedure seems to depend on the skill and experience of the operator rather than any intrinsic advantage for one method of insertion, although a formal surgical procedure is warranted in the presence of significant obesity or suspected adhesions after previous surgical operations. Depending on the urgency of starting dialysis, the insertion technique, and local practice, a variable amount of time is usually allowed to elapse prior to starting peritoneal dialysis to allow satisfactory wound healing to take place. The catheters may remain *in situ* for many years if needed, the main reasons for removal being infection, transfer to haemodialysis, or successful renal transplantation.

Peritoneal membrane function

The transport of small molecular weight uraemic toxins across the peritoneal capillary membrane is governed by its permeability to such solutes. This can be assessed by means of the Peritoneal Equilibration Test (PET) introduced by Twardowski. Instilling a 2.27 per cent glucose-based dialysis solution into the peritoneal cavity and taking samples of blood and dialysate for glucose and creatinine measurements over a 4-h period enables the membrane transport characteristics to be classified as low, low-average, high-average, or high with respect to glucose and creatinine concentrations. A high-transporter status will enable rapid equilibration of urea and creatinine, thus enabling adequate solute removal, but the increased membrane permeability prevents the maintenance of the glucose gradient that is essential for adequate fluid removal. Thus patients will achieve satisfactory small-solute clearance, but may have problems with adequate fluid removal. In a similar fashion, patients with a low-transporter membrane will sustain an adequate glucose gradient and achieve adequate ultrafiltration, but poor equilibration of urea and creatinine will leave them at risk of underdialysis. Knowledge of a patient's membrane function soon after starting dialysis can therefore aid in the rational prescription of peritoneal dialysis and may also have prognostic importance, particularly in large patients with declining residual renal function.

Prescription of peritoneal dialysis

CAPD

In the early years of CAPD many patients received so-called standard peritoneal dialysis prescriptions—4 × 1.5- or 2.0-litre exchanges per day—with little or no regard for body weight, membrane function, or level of residual renal function. With increasing experience worldwide and recognition of the need to attain small-solute clearance targets for maximum patient well being and survival, it has become obligatory to provide an individualized dialysis prescription for each patient.

When patients first begin peritoneal dialysis the great majority will have some degree of residual renal function, which may provide some 25 to 30 per cent of the required small-solute clearance. Under these circumstances most will achieve adequate dialysis with standard CAPD or APD prescriptions. Once residual renal function has been lost after 2 to 3 years on dialysis, then it becomes increasingly important to individualize the patients' prescription to enable adequate dialysis to be delivered. In general, patients who have low-transporter membranes will require high-volume exchanges on CAPD to achieve adequate small-solute clearance. As they still maintain adequate glucose gradients they still have adequate ultrafiltration. Patients with high-transporter membranes will often still achieve adequate small-solute removal, but they will be unable to obtain adequate ultrafiltration to keep them oedema-free unless short frequent exchanges are used. Under these circumstances, if patients do not achieve adequate dialysis in terms of small-solute clearance and ultrafiltration with the above prescription modification, transfer to haemodialysis may be required.

Table 1 summarizes the problems seen with high body-weight anuric patients.

APD

APD makes use of a machine to drain and fill the abdomen with dialysis fluid overnight, usually leaving the patient relatively free from the need to perform any dialysis-related activities during the day. The modality of APD may therefore be particularly suitable for certain groups of patients at the beginning of dialysis, for example the young, or those still at school or work. The increased quality of life achievable with APD is an added benefit in these patient groups, which is partly the reason why APD is the fastest growing renal replacement modality worldwide.

When a patient starts on APD as an initial dialysis modality, the presence of significant residual function may allow the use of relatively low dialysate volumes. However, as the patient's residual renal function declines then the need to reach small-solute and salt and water-removal targets will require the use of larger fill volumes, with the length of overnight dwells matched to peritoneal membrane function. At the other end of the spectrum, APD can also be used to prolong a patient's time on peritoneal dialysis when it is used as a salvage therapy for those no longer adequately dialysed on CAPD.

Table 1 Problems and suggested solutions in anuric patients at the extremes of peritoneal membrane function

Membrane PET status	Small-solute clearance	Fluid removal	Prescription change needed
Low	Poor	Good	Increased volume exchanges or haemodialysis
↓	↓	↓	
			Automated peritoneal dialysis with short cycles and
High	Good	Poor	polyglucose long dwell

PET, peritoneal equilibration test.

But in some patients with membrane failure or some other reason for inadequate dialysis, then elective transfer to haemodialysis is the appropriate course of action.

Outpatient monitoring of the patient on peritoneal dialysis

Once the patient and their family have been trained to perform peritoneal dialysis in the community, then outpatient review need not be that frequent—perhaps monthly initially, and as time passes and confidence increases the intervals between outpatient visits can be increased up to once every 2 to 3 months. At each clinic visit the patient should be assessed by the nephrologist, dialysis nurse, and dietician, with the aim of ensuring that they are compliant with the dialysis regime and adhering to dietary and fluid balance recommendations.

Adequacy of dialysis

As mentioned previously, the need for individualized dialysis prescriptions is paramount. The CANUSA study, and others, have documented the links between adequacy of dialysis, in terms of small-solute clearances, and patient survival, Hence, it is important to monitor the urea and creatinine clearances achieved by the combination of dialysis and residual renal function on a regular basis—at least yearly. If the clearances fall below recommended targets then changes in the dialysis prescription may be needed to keep the patient healthy. Table 2 shows the targets recommended for urea clearance (*Kt*/v urea) and creatinine clearance (Cr Cl) per week.

Nutrition

Malnutrition is a common problem in dialysis patients and may be seen in up to 30 per cent of those on peritoneal dialysis. This may be due to appetite suppression caused by glucose absorption from the dialysate, the presence of dialysis fluid in the abdomen, uraemia secondary to underdialysis, or peritoneal protein losses. If the patient is unable to maintain an adequate protein (1–1.2 g/kg body weight per day) and calorie (30–35 kCal (125–146 joules)/kg body weight per day) intake then malnutrition and hypoproteinaemia will develop with increased risk of death. Dietary advice from an experienced dietician is invaluable under these circumstances.

Table 2 Recommended adequacy targets

Adequacy target	CAPD	APD
Kt/v urea/week	2.0	2.1
CrCl litres/week per $1.73 m^2$	60	63

CAPD, continuous ambulatory peritoneal dialysis; automated peritoneal dialysis; *Kt*/v, urea clearance factored for time and total body water; Cr.Cl, creatinine clearance.

Cardiovascular status

Up to 50 per cent of all deaths in patients on peritoneal dialysis will be from cardiovascular causes, and therefore attention to the control of risk factors may be of benefit. It is important to encourage patients to stop smoking, take exercise, and to control fluid overload and hypertension by a combination of fluid restriction, fluid removal by dialysis, and the use of antihypertensive drugs where appropriate. Control of hyperlipidaemia by diet and drug therapy is also indicated.

Anaemia

The anaemia of renal failure is readily treatable with recombinant erythropoietin and, providing iron stores are kept at adequate levels, it should be possible to keep the majority of patients at or above target haemoglobin levels. This will improve the quality of life, improve exercise tolerance, and may also reduce cardiovascular mortality.

Infective complications

Exit site infections

Bacterial infection around the catheter exit site is a frequent occurrence, which, if neglected or inadequately treated, may lead to peritonitis and/or the need for catheter removal. The majority of these infections are caused by Gram-positive organisms such as *Staphylococcus aureus* and *S. epidermidis*, with occasional episodes being caused by Gram-negative organisms, for example *Pseudomonas* spp.

Meticulous exit site care, with attention to catheter immobilization locally and regular cleaning of the exit site with antiseptics, may diminish the frequency of such infections. Local application of the antibacterial agent mupirocin on a regular basis may also help eradicate *S. aureus* carriage and consequent infections. However, once erythema, purulent discharge, and pain develop, then broad-spectrum antibiotic therapy is indicated. If this is not successful in eradicating catheter sepsis then it may be necessary to replace the catheter.

Peritonitis

Peritonitis remains the major infective complication of peritoneal dialysis, and either acute or repeated episodes of peritonitis are a common cause of transfer from peritoneal dialysis to haemodialysis.

Common causative organisms include *S. aureus*, *S. epidermidis*, coliforms including *Pseudomonas* spp., and, rarely, fungal organisms. The diagnosis of peritonitis is usually straightforward, being based on the presence of cloudy dialysate fluid with or without abdominal pain. Treatment should be initiated on clinical suspicion, before laboratory culture results are available, and should cover both Gram-positive and Gram-negative organisms. Recommended regimes include intraperitoneal cefazolin or vancomycin (to give Gram-positive cover) with an intraperitoneal aminoglycoside or oral quinolone such as ciprofloxacin (to give Gram-negative cover), with subsequent modification of therapy depending on the culture results. The use of vancomycin has declined over recent years because of worries concerning the development of resistant organisms.

The frequency of episodes of peritonitis in patients on peritoneal dialysis has been falling with increasing experience and technological advances, including the use of disconnect systems and APD machines. It should be possible to reduce the frequency of peritonitis to one episode every 2-patient years or better. If peritonitis does develop then the cure rate without removing the dialysis catheter should exceed 85 per cent, and the majority of patients should be able to continue with peritoneal dialysis after the episode has resolved, unless it was caused by bowel perforation or a fungal peritonitis. A successful continuation of peritoneal dialysis is unlikely in both circumstances.

Transplantation

Patients who are established on peritoneal dialysis may be transplanted safely, and there is evidence that they have a lower incidence of delayed graft function and early rejection. The peritoneal dialysis catheter may be used after transplantation if dialysis is required, provided that the peritoneum has not been breached. It is usually removed electively some 2 or 3 months later, when the risk of graft failure has diminished.

Survival data

Studies over the years comparing both technique and survival in patients on haemodialysis and peritoneal dialysis have produced conflicting results. In the absence of a randomized controlled trial the differences in the case mix of patients on the two modalities makes interpretation of the data difficult. It seems likely that providing attention is given to monitoring and adjusting dialysis therapy as residual renal function falls, then the two therapies are equivalent and most patients should be allowed to choose the modality that suits them best. There is some evidence that peritoneal dialysis is the more suitable first modality as residual renal function is better preserved with this technique, but once this advantage is lost after 3 to 5 years then patients are more likely to require haemodialysis as a long-term treatment.

The two techniques should be seen as complementary and both should be available to the patient waiting for renal transplantation. The fact that worldwide peritoneal dialysis varies from less than 5 per cent to more than 60 per cent, with a world average of around 15 per cent, probably reflects factors other than patient selection.

Summary

Peritoneal dialysis has been a well-recognized mode of therapy for endstage renal disease since the mid-1970s. Approximately 15 per cent of the world's dialysis population are currently kept alive and healthy by this technique. Patient survival in the short to medium term with peritoneal dialysis is equivalent to that seen with haemodialysis. In the past, the main complications of peritoneal dialysis have been peritonitis, inadequate dialysis, malnutrition, membrane failure, and patient 'burn-out'. With increasing experience, individualized dialysis prescription, and technological advances including new solutions and improved automated peritoneal dialysis machines, the frequency of these complications is diminishing. Peritoneal dialysis should be seen as part of an integrated care package for patients with endstage renal disease, indeed—there being no significant difference between haemodialysis and peritoneal dialysis—the patient should be encouraged to choose the dialysis technique that fits best with their lifestyle. There may be advantages in starting dialysis with peritoneal dialysis and then, as residual renal function declines, moving to haemodialysis while waiting for a renal transplant to become available.

Further reading

CANUSA Peritoneal Dialysis study group (1996). Adequacy of dialysis and nutrition in continuous peritoneal dialysis: association with clinical outcomes. *Journal of the American Society of Nephrology* **7**, 198–207. [Important trial documenting the link between adequacy of dialysis, nutrition, and patient survival]

Diaz-Buxo JA, Suki WN (1994). Automated peritoneal dialysis. In: Gokal R, Nolph KD, eds. *Textbook of peritoneal dialysis*, pp 399–418. Kluwer Academic, Dordrecht. [Comprehensive review of the history, application, and outcomes of APD]

Fenton SSA, *et al.* (1997). Hemodialysis versus peritoneal dialysis: a comparison of adjusted mortality rates. *American Journal of Kidney Diseases* **30**, 334–42. [Report from Canadian registry showing that peritoneal dialysis and haemodialysis are at least equivalent over the first 5 years of treatment]

Keane WF, *et al.* (1996). Peritoneal dialysis related peritonitis treatment recommendations; 1996 update. *Peritoneal Dialysis International* **16**, 557–73. [Consensus statement by panel of international experts]

Lameire NH (1997). The impact of residual renal function on adequacy of peritoneal dialysis. *Nephron* **77**(1), 13–28. [Important article documenting the importance of residual renal function to adequacy of peritoneal dialysis]

National Kidney Federation (1997). DOQI clinical practice guidelines for peritoneal dialysis adequacy. *American Journal of Kidney Diseases* **30**(Suppl. 2), S67–134. [North American consensus statement on peritoneal dialysis prescription guidelines]

Popovich RP, *et al.* (1978). Continuous ambulatory peritoneal dialysis. *Annals of Internal Medicine* **88**, 449–52. [First description of the technique of CAPD]

Shockley TR, Martis L, Tranaeus AP (1999). New solutions for peritoneal dialysis in adult and paediatric patients. *Peritoneal Dialysis International* **19**(Suppl 2), S429–434. [Review article discussing the role of the new peritoneal dialysis solutions available]

Twardowski ZJ, *et al.* 1987 Peritoneal Equilibration Test. *Peritoneal Dialysis Bulletin* **7**, 128–47. [Important article describing how to perform the PET test and its importance to PD prescription]

Van Biesen W, *et al.* (2000). An evaluation of an integrative care approach for endstage renal disease patients. *Journal of the American Society of Nephrology* **11**(1), 116–25. [Important single-centre report documenting excellent patient survival with integrated PD and HD therapies]

Young G, *et al.* (1991). Nutritional assessment of CAPD: an international study. *American Journal of Kidney Diseases* **17**, 462–71. [International study of the prevalence and causes of malnutrition in CAPD patients]

20.6.3 Renal transplantation

P. Sweny

Introduction

Renal transplantation is the preferred option for the treatment of endstage chronic renal failure in patients for whom there are no major medical contraindications. With improvements in immunosuppression and in the equally important general medical support of the immunocompromised patient, the age ranges and permissible comorbidities continue to be extended. In well-selected recipients, both life expectancy and quality of life are superior to long-term dialysis. The two impediments to the extension of transplantation are the shortage of donor organs and the side-effects of the still crude immunosuppressive agents. Xenotransplantation may remove the first of these hurdles, but is likely to increase our dependence on potent immunosuppressive regimes. In humans, immunological tolerance to the graft with preservation of normal immunoresponsiveness to infections and tumours has not yet been achieved.

Supply, demand, and kidney donation

At the beginning of the year 2000 there were approximately 5000 patients waiting for renal transplantation in the United Kingdom. The annual rate of renal transplantation in the United Kingdom is approximately 1300 per year or 24 per million of the population per year and has not altered greatly over the last 5 years. The dialysis population, however, is increasing by 7 to 10 per cent per annum. In most countries the maximum achievable number of cadaver donors is about 35 per million per year against a need of 50 per million per year. The shortage of cadaver donors has been attributed to three main factors: a decline in deaths from road traffic accidents and cerebral haemorrhage, and inadequate numbers of intensive care unit beds. In the United Kingdom living donation represents only 10 to 15 per cent of all transplants (3 to 5 donors per million of the population), whereas in Scandinavia 10 live donors per million of the population has been achieved.

There are currently three possible sources of donor organs for transplantation: cadaveric, living related, and the living unrelated donor. In most countries the last group is restricted to donors that are closely 'emotionally related', for example spouses and partners. Two factors sustain our continued reliance on living donation as a source of kidneys: the first is the shortfall in available cadaver donors, and the second is the superior survival of a well-matched graft from a living related donor. The continuing need for an adequate supply of cadaver organs for transplantation requires an equally continuing education of both the medical and general population. Acceptance of the brainstem death criteria (see Chapter 16.6.3) in many countries has helped greatly in establishing a secure definition of death for both legal and religious purposes. However, given the continuing shortage of organs, many centres are re-exploring the possibility of the rapid procurement of organs for transplantation from non-heart-beating cadavers.

Living donors

Every care must be taken to protect the interests of the donor. Informed consent is crucial. Potential donors must be aware that giving a kidney carries risks, albeit that the mortality rate is only 0.01 to 0.03 per cent, with most deaths attributable to acute pulmonary embolus. The other risks that are involved in a general anaesthetic and an abdominal operation must also be fully explained. Needless to say, the donor should be in good general physical health and have normal kidney function and surgically acceptable renal anatomy. The assessments required are summarized in Table 1. Apart from exceptional circumstances, donors outside the age limits of 18 to 70 years are not considered. It is usual to wait for a young female potential donor to complete her family.

Most studies have shown an increase in life expectancy of donors when compared with age-matched controls. A small proportion of donors will develop hypertension, but at a risk that is similar to that of the general population. A small number develop proteinuria, but this is usually less than 0.5 g per 24 h and does not affect survival. Renal function usually returns to 75 to 80 per cent of the predonation level.

The superior outcome of living related donor kidney transplantation is partly due to better matching, with donor and recipient sharing one or two extended haplotypes in almost all cases. An additional benefit, shared also by kidneys from living unrelated donors, is the physiological state of the organ when recovered under ideal and planned conditions. Rejection is more likely and more severe with cadaver donors: this may be due to the 'cytokine storm' that accompanies the agonal phase of death and ischaemia reperfusion injury. This is thought to increase the expression of HLA antigens and adhesion molecules in the donor organ, making it more visible to the recipient's immune system.

Cadaver donors

In this situation the prime responsibility is to the potential recipient. The kidney should be in as good a physiological state as possible, and there should be no obvious risk of transfer of infection or malignancy by the donor organ. The major contraindications to organ procurement are listed in Table 2. Marginal donors are increasingly being considered, particularly for older recipients and for those with a limited life expectancy. In some situations it may be appropriate to consider organs from hepatitis C (**HCV**)-positive or hepatitis B (**HBV**)-positive donors for positive recipients. Experience in parts of the world where safe long-term dialysis is not available have shown that an acceptable quality of life can be sustained with substandard kidneys, and—given the shortage of organs—marginal donors should not be discarded out of hand without discussion with the local transplant unit.

Table 1 Assessment of the potential living donor

Medical history
Psychosocial history: at-risk behaviour
Physical examination
Blood group (ABO)
Tissue typing
Lymphocyte crossmatch (donor serum against recipient lymphocytes)
DNA testing to prove family relationship
Urine:
Stick testing—blood, protein, glucose
Culture and microscopy
Quantify protein excretion
Creatinine clearance
Blood:
Glucose—formal glucose tolerance test*
Electrolytes
Urea, creatinine, uric acid
Liver function tests
Full blood count
Glucose-6-phosphate dehydrogenase*
Haemaglobinopathy *
Sickle test *
Procoagulant screen *
Infection screen:
HIV
HIV 1 and 2
Cytomegalovirus
Epstein–Barr virus
Hepatitis B virus
Hepatitis C virus
Kaposi's sarcoma virus (HHV8)
Syphilis
Toxoplasmosis
Schistosomiasis *
Malaria *
Trypanosoma cruzi *
*Strongyloides stercoralis**
Chest radiograph
ECG
Stress cardiac testing *
Formal glomerular filtration rate estimation
Renal imaging:
Ultrasound or intravenous pyelogram
Donor renal arteriogram and late films
Informed consent

* Where clinically indicated, such as specific geographical or other risk.

Recipient assessment

Patients may be transplanted before the need for dialysis (pre-emptive transplantation) or from an established dialysis programme (haemodialysis or peritoneal dialysis). It is essential that all patients are fully assessed by both a transplant surgeon and transplant physician before being placed on the waiting list or offered a kidney, whether it be from a cadaver or a relative. Patients with chronic renal failure develop a multitude of complications that need assessment prior to surgery. Transplantation carries with it the risks of any major surgical procedure together with the added risks of prolonged immunosuppression. An additional consideration is that given the shortage of organs for transplantation, it is important that the best use is made of all organs. Whilst all would agree with this in principle, making decisions in individual cases can be difficult. In some situations the general health and life expectancy of the potential recipient argue strongly against transplantation. In patients with viral hepatitis or cirrhosis there is increasing evidence, particularly for HBV-related disease, that survival will be longer on dialysis. Patients with congenitally abnormal lower urinary tracts can be difficult to transplant and ideally should be managed in centres with urological transplant expertise, some needing complex bladder augmentation or drainage procedures prior to transplantation.

Allocation of kidneys

Fully matched kidneys (zero A, zero B, and zero DR mismatch—denoted 0–0–0 mismatch) and DR identical kidneys do better than less well-matched organs, hence most countries have local or national kidney sharing schemes so that more recipients can receive the benefits of a well-matched organ. Use is increasingly being made of point scoring systems to allocate kidneys fairly, patients accruing points based on the degree of match as well as the length of time they have been waiting for a transplant.

Table 2 Contraindications to cadaver organ procurement

Donor age:
< 3 years
> 70 years*
Cancer not confined to the central nervous system (CNS), but note:
(1) Non-melanoma skin tumours and carcinoma *in situ* of the uterine cervix are permissible
(2) Cancer confined to CNS is acceptable, excepting medulloblastoma and glioblastoma
Risk of transmissable infection:
At-risk behaviour
HCV
HBV
HIV
HTLV 1, 2
Human herpes virus 8
Deep fungal infections
Parenchymal renal infection
Meningoencephalitic syndromes of unknown aetiology
Inadequately treated bacterial infection
Infection with resistant organisms (eg. MRSA, VRE)
Diabetes mellitus *
Acute renal failure *
Hypertension *
Chronic renal impairment
Warm ischaemia > 90 min
Cold ischaemia > 30 h*

* Relative contraindication.

HTLV, human T-cell lymphocytotrophic virus; MRSA, methicillin-resistant *Staphylococcus aureus*;

Surgical technique

The new kidney is placed in one or other iliac fossa, usually in an extraperitoneal position that allows ease of repeated biopsy to detect the cause of graft dysfunction. The renal artery is anastomosed end to side to the common iliac artery or end to end to the internal iliac artery. The renal vein is usually anastomosed to the common iliac vein. The transplant ureter only has a short distance to run before it can be implanted into the bladder, which is usually done through a submucosal tunnel to reduce the chances of reflux of urine from the bladder into the transplant. Some surgeons routinely place a vesicoureteric stent to reduce the risks of urine leakage and to promote healing. A drain is usually placed near the renal hilum. Lymphatics in the perihilar region are tied off. A urethral catheter and/or suprapubic bladder catheter is inserted and left *in situ* for about 5 days. The ureteric stent is removed at cystoscopy after a few weeks. Most units use prophylactic heparin routinely.

Note that in the standard renal transplant operation described above the native kidneys are left *in situ*. In some patients one or both may need to be removed (at a separate operation) before the patient can be listed for transplantation: mandatory indications for this include suspicion of renal tumour (usually in those with cystic disease), chronic renal infection, and massive organomegally, when there is literally no space in which to put a new kidney (in patients with adult polycystic kidney disease). Some would also advocate nephrectomy (Table 3) as a prelude to transplantation in those with gross ureteric reflux, renal stone disease, or analgesic nephropathy.

Retransplantation is increasingly being undertaken as the general medical care of patients with renal failure has improved. Second transplants are now not uncommon, and even third and fourth transplants may be occasionally undertaken. Third and fourth transplants are more surgically demanding as vessels available for anastomosis become limited. Aortic and venocaval anastomoses can be performed.

Ischaemia times

Warm ischaemia is defined as the time between circulatory arrest and renal artery cannulation for ice-cold perfusion, together with the time between the removal of the kidney from ice and release of the vascular clamps at implantation. With the beating heart donor, the first component is zero. The maximum permissible warm ischaemia time before irreversable damage occurs is 60 min.

Cold ischaemia time (preservation time) is defined as the time between ice-cold perfusion of the kidney and removal from the ice at the start of the implantation operation. Cold ischaemia times of up to 96 h have resulted in functioning grafts, but times in excess of 30 h are associated with a less favourable outcome. The permissible cold ischaemia time of 30 h allows for organ sharing and equitable operating times for the surgical team.

Table 3 Indications for native kidney nephrectomy

Intractable hypertension
Multiple cysts
Suspect cyst—risk of malignancy
Analgesic nephropathy
Chronic infection
Stone
Gross reflux
Polycystic kidney
Size—symptoms
Haemorrhage
Risk of malignancy
Uncontrollable nephrotic syndrome

Postoperative management

Excepting for transplants between identical twins, immunosuppression is required to allow transplantation. The first dose of this is often given pre- or intraoperatively. Details are discussed below.

Following implantation, the function of the new kidney is assiduously monitored. Most units give low-dose dopamine, mannitol, or a loop diuretic, singly or in combination, to ensure good urine flow rate on return from theatre. Hourly urine volumes are closely monitored for the first few days. Fluid balance is usually maintained by a prescription that requires 100 per cent replacement of urine volumes and drain losses with crystalloid, and central venous pressure is monitored and maintained in the high normal range (+10 cmH_2O) with blood or colloid.

Serum creatinine is measured daily. A failure to fall rapidly, or a 15 per cent rise once it has fallen to a plateau, is evidence of graft dysfunction and requires prompt investigations. A kidney that fails to function initially, despite good perfusion on the table when the vascular clamps were removed, is usually suffering from acute tubular necrosis, which is expected to recover. A sudden cessation of urine flow usually means a surgical problem, for example clot obstruction, urinary leak, or vascular catastrophe. A slow tailing-off of the urinary volumes is more suggestive of rejection, hypovolaemia, or developing drug nephrotoxicity. Two of the major immunosuppressive agents, cyclosporin A and tacrolimus, are nephrotoxic: doses have to be carefully adjusted to maintain the therapeutic range. Blood pressure should be returned to normal, obstruction excluded, and coagulation checked before a biopsy is undertaken. Close and careful monitoring needs to continue for the first 6 months following transplantation as the risk of rejection is at its greatest during this period.

One of the 'holy grails' of transplant medicine is a method of determining the immunological relationship between the recipient and their transplanted organ, since this would allow tailoring of immunosuppression to immunological need. However, immunological monitoring of transplant recipients is still in its infancy: lympocyte T- and B-cell subsets and activation markers can be of value, particularly when antilymphocyte preparations are being used; serial estimation of post-transplant anti-HLA antibodies can help predict patients at risk of chronic rejection. Much work continues to look for better ways of monitoring patients, such as testing for cytokine gene polymorphisms to predict those at highest risk of rejection, and examination of graft biopsies for expression of adhesion molecules, HLA, cytokines, and enzymes (e.g. granzyme, perforin) to characterize better the rejection process. Protocol biopsies may demonstrate subclinical rejection, and some argue that treatment of these may improve outcome, but most units are not convinced and do not perform 'routine' biopsies.

Complications of renal transplantation

Surgical

Table 4 summarizes the main surgical complications, which include those of any general anaesthetic and laparotomy. Extra risk is added because patients on dialysis are immunosuppressed by uraemia *per se* and transplant patients also require immunosuppressive drugs following surgery. Wound healing is significantly delayed in the early post-transplant period, particularly by steroids. Some patients on dialysis will have a marked bleeding tendency related to defective platelet–endothelial cell interaction. The combination of uraemia, surgical stress, a bleeding tendency, and high-dose steroids produces an increased risk of bleeding peptic ulceration, which the routine use of H_2-blockers has virtually abolished. Many donor organs have small polar arteries that can be lost during or shortly after surgery, in which case the resulting segment of kidney will atrophy. Occasionally a polar infarct can lead to necrosis of a significant segment of renal cortex causing a calyceal fistula and urinary leak. An area of ischaemia around a polar infarct may drive post-transplant hypertension. Perirenal collections of fluid (whether from inadequately tied-off perihilar lymphatics, haemorrhage, or a urinary leak) can become infected: these are best demonstrated by ultrasound, which can guide aspiration for culture and drainage.

Rejection

Rejection can be classified into four main categories (Table 5). These are not mutually exclusive and there is overlap in the pathological processes.

Hyperacute rejection

In the presence of preformed cytotoxic antibodies the new graft infarcts within minutes of insertion. This can occur if transplantation is attempted across ABO incompatibilities. It is a rare event as the lymphocyte crossmatch usually identifies pre-existing anti-HLA antibodies. Transplantation is not undertaken in the presence of a positive lymphocyte crossmatch, but hyperacute rejection can rarely occur in the presence of non-HLA cytotoxic antibodies. There is no treatment save nephrectomy.

Table 4 Complications of renal transplantation

Surgical	Medical
Wound infection	Infections transmitted by graft
Wound haematoma	Opportunistic infections
Perirenal: (collections → infections)	Specific complications of immunosuppression
Lymph	Complex aetiologies:
Haematoma	Accelerated vascular disease
Urine	Hypertension
Vascular catastrophe: (arterial or venous)	Electrolyte disturbances
Haemorrhage	Cosmetic
Thrombosis	Thromboembolism
Segmental artery occlusions:	Erythrocytosis
Ischaemia → hypertension	Marrow suppression
Infarction → calyceal fistula	Liver dysfunction
Devitalization of ureter: (stripping)	Neoplasia
Sloughing	
Ischaemic stricture	
Urinary leaks:	
Cystotomy	
Ureteric–bladder dehiscence	
Venous thromboembolism	
Pancreatitis	
Urinary sepsis	

Table 5 Classification of rejection

	Hyperacute	Accelerated	Acute	Chronic
Timing	Minutes	1–5 days	5 days—3 months	Greater than 3 months
Mediators	Preformed antibodies Complement	Sensitized cells and antibodies	Primary cell-mediated response	Antibodies, complement
Histology	Infarction Platelets Fibrinogen Polymorphs	Tubulitis Endovasculitis (acute)	Tubulitis	Obliterative chronic endovasculitis
Treatment	Nephrectomy	Serotherapy salvage ? Plasma exchange	High-dose intravenous steroids	None proved to be effective, consider: Aspirin/angiotensin II blockers Lipid lowering ↑Azathioprine or add mycophenolate mofetil Fish oils

Accelerated rejection

A fierce, predominantly T-cell mediated rejection crisis may occur within the first few days of transplantation. This is thought to be due to sensitization of the recipient by a previous pregnancy, blood transfusion, or a failed transplant. Patients present clinically with fever, an acutely swollen tender graft, and a rapidly rising serum creatinine. Salvage usually requires the combination of high-dose intravenous pulse methylprednisolone (10 to 15 mg/kg per day infused over 30 min on 3 successive days) and an antilymphocyte antibody such as antithymocyte (ATG) or antilymphocyte globulin (ALG). The murine monoclonal antibody OKT3 may also be used. It is unusual to be able to reverse fully this type of severe rejection and long-term graft survival is compromised

Acute cellular rejection

In most centres about 25 per cent of patients will experience an acute cellular rejection, usually occurring between days 7 to 21 but up to 3 months following transplantation. Acute cellular rejection is often clinically silent as the inflammatory component of the rejection is masked by immunosuppression. Fluid retention, increasing hypertension, and a sharp rise in creatinine are typical. Assessment of renal perfusion (Doppler ultrasound or renography studies) may show a dramatic reduction in graft perfusion, but these tests are not sensitive or specific enough for a confident diagnosis of rejection. Most centres routinely take kidney biopsies for all episodes of graft dysfunction once infection, toxic levels of the calcineurin blocking drugs (cyclosporin and tacrolimus), and mechanical factors causing obstruction have been excluded. Obtaining a histological diagnosis is very important since several processes can mimic rejection, including drug nephrotoxicity, bacterial pyelonephritis, recurrence of original disease, and post-transplant lymphoproliferative disorder. The hallmark of acute cellular rejection is tubulitis in which the invading lymphocytes have penetrated the tubular epithelial cell basement membrane and directly engage tubule epithelial cells. Late acute rejection episodes usually imply inadequate immunosuppression, sometimes due to poor compliance. Treatment is very effective and usually involves a bolus of intravenous steroid therapy as described above. Long-term graft survival is severely jeopardized if the rejection episode is not completely reversed. With some of the newer, very potent induction regimes, the incidence of acute rejection episodes can be reduced to 10 per cent. Whether this will translate into a higher rate of infection and neoplasia awaits further follow-up.

Chronic rejection

Chronic rejection is a complex pathological process that is difficult to define. At its simplest, it represents the breakthrough of humoral immunity with an antibody-mediated attack on the graft endothelium. The result is an insidious and obliterative endovasculitis with progressive graft dysfunction from ischaemia. Clinically, the features of chronic rejection include difficult hypertension, proteinuria, and a slowly rising serum creatinine. (See the subsection on chronic allograft nephropathy for further discussion.) Chronic rejection is associated with the presence of anti-HLA antibodies in the serum and the deposition of C4d complement in the peritubular capillaries.

Immunosuppression

There is no clear consensus on the best immunosuppressive regime for renal transplantation, and for commercial reasons the large multicentre trials that the community of transplant physicians and surgeons would most like to see performed are unlikely ever to be funded. The choice of agents available is summarized in Table 6.

Most centres worldwide use what is now called standard triple therapy, comprising cyclosporin A, prednisolone, and azathioprine. However, in North America in particular, there is widespread use of additional serotherapy given as induction therapy for the first 10 days after grafting, and azathioprine has been replaced by mycophenolate mofetil in many centres, and cyclosporin by tacrolimus in some.

Agents of established efficacy for induction therapy include polyclonal antibodies such as antithymocyte globulin (ATG) or antilymphocyte globulin (ALG), and the murine monoclonal antibody, OKT3. Two anti-CD25 antibodies, daclizumab and basiliximab, which bind to the α-chain of the interleukin 2 (**IL-2**) receptor, have recently been introduced. Both are

Table 6 Choice of immunosuppressive agents in transplantation

Calcineurin-blocking drugs	Purine antagonists	Miscellaneous	Antibodies
Cyclosporin A	Azathioprine	Prednisolone	ALG
Tacrolimus	Mycophenolate mofetil	Rapamicin	ATG
			OKT3
			Anti-CD25: Basiliximab Daclizumab

heavily engineered antibodies, comprising a murine antigen-binding site and human immunoglobulin. Both are very effective and have been shown to reduce acute rejection episodes by about 30 per cent.

Many centres are now exploring the possibility of tailoring immunosuppression to the needs of the individual recipient, but as described above we are not good at assessing immunological risk. In practice this involves giving immunosuppressants that are perceived to be more powerful—for example tacrolimus instead of cyclosporin, mycophenolate mofetil instead of azathioprine, or adding antibody treatments—to recipients who are thought to be at greatest immunological risk, such as those who are highly sensitized, patients who have rejected a previous transplant, or those who have suffered an acute rejection episode.

The best long-term therapy is equally in doubt. This is partly due to the nephrotoxicity of two of the main agents employed for the prevention of rejection: both cyclosporin A and tacrolimus can produce a nodular arterioleopathy resulting in ischaemic renal damage. It is also clear that the morbidity and mortality from long-term steroid therapy is significant, such that many centres are now attempting steroid-free immunosuppression, reducing and even withdrawing steroids at 3 to 6 months despite the associated risk of rejection, which has been reported to be as high as 30 per cent. Unfortunately, it is not possible to predict who is going to reject on withdrawal of steroids, hence one of the main aims of those developing new immunosuppressive drugs and regimens is to devise agents or protocols that allow less dependence on steroids without increased rates of rejection or other unacceptable toxicities.

The side-effects of immunosuppression

It is important to remember that all currently available immunosuppressive regimen are non-specific in the sense that they suppress not only the immune response to the allograft, but also the immune response to infections and tumours. All the agents used have significant side-effects and toxicities, and to a very large extent the long-term complications of renal transplantation are those of the immunosuppressive agents used. Some side-effects are more related to the total burden of immunosuppression rather than to any specific single agent, for example infections and cancer.

Specific side-effects of particular agents

Steroids

Steroids are responsible for many of the complications of transplantation (Table 7). In recent years the dose of steroids used has been safely reduced, thanks in part to the introduction of the calcineurin-blocking drugs, but attempts to produce totally steroid-free transplantation are only successful in about half of cases. One of the most significant side-effects of steroids is that they mask the inflammatory response so that symptoms develop late, which is particularly important in cases of intra-abdominal catastrophy such as a perforated hollow viscus.

Table 7 Side-effects of steroids

Acne
Hypertrichosis
Redistribution of body fat
Obesity
Cushingoid facies
Insulin resistance—diabetes mellitus
Hypertension
Hyperlipidaemia
Proximal myopathy
Osteoporosis—avascular necrosis of bone
Tendon ruptures
Poor wound healing
Skin atrophy/fragility/easy bruising
Scleromalacia
Growth inhibition: premature fusion of the epiphyses
Erythrocytosis
Cataracts
Benign intracranial hypertension
Psychosis
Peptic ulceration
Colonic perforation
Pancreatitis

Calcineurin-blocking drugs

The major drawback of both cyclosporin A and tacrolimus is nephrotoxicity (Table 8), which adds another level of complexity to the differential diagnosis and management of both acute and chronic graft dysfunction. Most consider tacrolimus to be more potent than cyclosporin A, but perhaps more toxic (diabetes mellitus and neurotoxicity). It does, however, have real cosmetic advantages over cyclosporin A, perhaps mediated by lower levels of transforming growth factor-β.

Azathioprine and mycophenolate mofetil

Both agents block purine synthesis. The main side-effects of azathioprine are hepatotoxicity and marrow suppression (Table 9). Mycophenolate mofetil is more potent and more specific than azathioprine, blocking purine synthesis in lymphocytes with a degree of specifity. Its most troublesome side-effect is that of abdominal colic and diarrhoea: about 10 per cent of patients are so badly affected that they are unable to tolerate the drug. A higher incidence of invasive cytomegalovirus disease has been associated with mycophenolate.

Serotherapy

A range of antibodies to lymphocytes is available for clinical use (Table 6). Side-effects vary with the preparation used: it is important to remember that the consequences of augmenting immunosuppression with serological agents may last many months, even though administration is usually limited to 10 to 14 days.

Polyclonal antilymphocyte preparations can cause a marked first-dose effect in which lymphocytes are activated and secrete cytokines. High fever, rigors, and muscle and back pains are common, and hypotension may occur. With successive doses this reaction subsides. The murine anti-CD3 antibody (OKT3) is particularly prone to produce a first-dose effect that can lead to a widespread capillary leak syndrome with non-cardiogenic pulmonary oedema, hypotension, and shock. It should not be given to patients who are fluid overloaded. Aseptic meningitis and encephalitis are also seen occasionally. By contrast, the humanized and chimeric anti-IL2 receptor antibodies that have recently been introduced do not appear to have any short-term side-effects.

General side-effects of immunosuppression

Infectious complications

Introduction

The calcineurin-blocking drugs used for immunosuppression act to inhibit the T-helper cell (CD4) and prevent the elaboration of IL-2 and other cytokines. In some respects this is akin to the effects of HIV infection and it is therefore not surprising that the renal transplant recipient may develop the same range of opportunistic infections and tumours as is seen in patients with AIDS (see Chapter 7.10.21). Clinical features are often dramatic and rapidly evolving, hence prompt and precise microbiological diagnosis is essential. This requires early recourse to invasive techniques, for example biopsy, node aspiration, excision, bronchoalveolar lavage and even lung biopsy. Neurological symptoms and signs may herald central nervous system infection and require urgent CT scanning or MRI and the examination of cerebrospinal fluid whenever possible. Any pyrexial episode in a transplant recipient should prompt a search for infection. Blood and urine cultures should be undertaken routinely.

Table 8 Side-effects of calcineurin-blocking drugs

Side-effect	Cyclosporin A	Tacrolimus
Nephrotoxicity	+ +	+ +
Hypertension/sympathetic overactivity	+ +	+
Hyperuricaemia	+ +	+ +
Hyperkalaemia (type IV renal tubular acidosis)	+	+
Hypomagnesaemia (urine leak)	+	+
Haemolytic uraemic syndrome	+	± ?
Platelet hyperaggregability	+	? ±
Insulin resistance → diabetes mellitus	+	+ /++
Dislipidaemia	+	±
Hepatoxicity	+	+
Breast fibroadenosis	+	–
Coarsening of facial features	+	–
Gum hypertrophy	+	–
Hypertrichosis	+	–
Distal limb pain/periostitis	+	?
Cardiotoxicity	–	+
Neurotoxicity:		
Fits	+	+
Ataxia	+	+
Posterior fossa leucoencephalopathy	+	?
Paraesthesiae	+	+
Tremor	+	+
Neoplasia	+	+
Infection	+	+

Figure 1 summarizes the timetable of infections. In the first month, before immunosuppression is fully established, renal transplant recipients may develop the same sort of infection seen after any general anaesthetic, abdominal operation, or urological procedure. From months 1 to 6, immunosuppression is maximal and the risk of opportunistic infections greatest. Thereafter, the risk of infection declines but remains greater than the general population.

Viral infections

Not all virus infections prove dangerous to the immunosuppressed renal transplant recipient. Those with particularly important clinical sequelae are summarized in Table 10. The most important group are the DNA viruses of the herpes group: infection with these is immunomodulating in its own right and further immunosuppresses the patient, hence they are not infrequently associated with superinfections, for example *Pneumocystis carinii*, listeria, and bacterial sepsis. Several of the viruses have proven oncogenic potential and are considered later.

Table 9 Side-effects of azathioprine and mycophenolate mofetil

Side-effect	Azathioprine	Mycophenolate mofetil
Hepatotoxicity	++	+
Marrow suppression:	++	±
Platelets	±	±
Red cells	±	–
Granulocytes	++	±
Megaloblastic anaemia	+	–
Gut toxicity	±	++
Pancreatitis	+	–
Hypogammaglobulinaemia	±	+
Lung fibrosis	+	±
Alopecia	+	–
Infection	+	+ /++
Cancer	+	?

Cytomegalovirus Cytomegalovirus (**CMV**) is the main infectious complication in solid organ transplantation (Table 11), with a primary infection more likely to produce serious disease than either reinfection or reactivation. Viral load, as indicated by quantitative polymerase chain reaction (**PCR**), and the total burden of immunosuppression, are the main determinants of disease. Use of potent serological agents, either for induction or rescue, is strongly associated with CMV disease. As would be expected, the total number of treated rejection episodes is an important risk factor. Diagnosis is usually via PCR for viral DNA or by an antigen assay (pp65) on peripheral blood leucocytes. Monitoring the serological response for diagnostic purposes is obsolete as it is far too insensitive and routine cultures are too slow. A range of effective prophylactic regimes is available: oral valaciclovir is effective and oral valganciclovir is awaited. Another equally valid approach is careful monitoring combined with pre-emptive treatment of infection, where therapy can be given before clinical disease in vulnerable individuals. Two or three weeks of intravenous ganciclovir is usually effective. Foscarnet is a more toxic alternative.

CMV may play a role in triggering or augmenting both acute and chronic rejection. If this is confirmed then more widespread prophylaxis may be indicated.

Epstein–Barr virus (EBV) EBV-related syndromes (Table 11) are an important cause of morbidity and mortality in renal transplant recipients, the most serious problem being so-called post-transplant lymphoproliferative disorder, which is considered later.

Varicella zoster Reactivation of latent varicella zoster (**VZV**) produces shingles, which is a common and unpleasant complication of transplantation. Immediate treatment with intravenous aciclovir can limit spread and reduce post-herpetic pain. Much more dangerous is a primary VZV infection in an immunocompromised individual: this can cause a fulminating disease with hepatitis, pneumonitis, and disseminated intravascular coagulation occurring within a few days. Mortality is high. All patients who are to receive immunosuppression should have their VZV antibody status established. Those who are seronegative should be counselled about exposure to chicken pox and should report any contact immediately. Vaccination is available, but if exposed, susceptible individuals should be given zoster

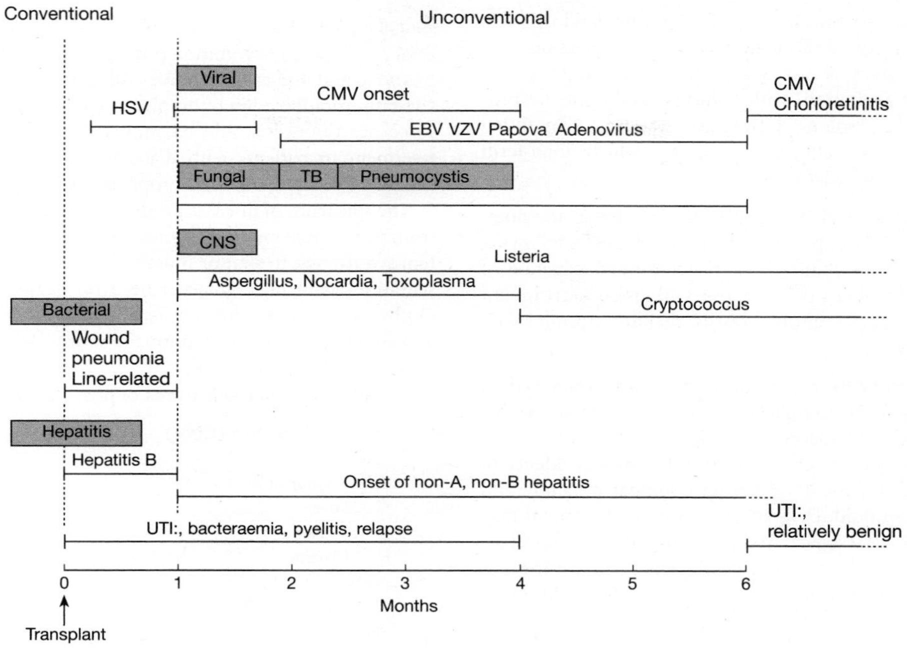

Fig. 1 Timetable of infections (reproduced by permission from Rubin R.H. and Young L.S. (eds) 1994, *Clinical approach to infection in the compromised host*, 3rd edn. Plenum Medical Book Co., New York.)

immune globulin (ZIG) and monitored closely. High-dose intravenous aciclovir should be given at the first suggestion of disease.

Herpes simplex Although the classic herpetic cold sore is common after transplantation, herpes simplex virus (**HSV**) can produce a variety of serious clinical sequelae in the immunocompromised patient (Table 11). Use of prophylactic aciclovir or ganciclovir (primarily for CMV prophylaxis) dramatically reduces the risks of HSV infection. Treatment with aciclovir is very effective.

Human polyomavirus (BK and JC) Most adult recipients are already seropositive for these viruses, indicating childhood infection that is usually asymptomatic. Primary infection can occur from the allograft. In most cases this is also asymptomatic, but rarely these viruses can cause an acute interstitial nephritis and graft dysfunction. The JC virus has been reported to cause a progressive multifocal leucoencephalopathy in renal transplant recipients, although this is very rare.

Papilloma viruses Papilloma viruses cause an extensive range of viral warts in renal transplant recipients. Some types have been implicated in the pathogenisis of anogenital carcinomas and squamous cell carcinomas of the skin (see below). The management of viral warts in the immunocompromised patient is difficult when they are very extensive and consideration should be given to reducing immunosuppression. Localized lesions can be treated conventionally with topical agents such as glutaraldehyde or laser therapy, but widespread surgical excision is sometimes required. Local recurrence in scar tissue is common. A combination of oral etidronate (50 mg daily) and topical tretinoin cream (0.05 per cent) can control the lesions in severe cases.

Human immunodeficiency virus (HIV) Infection with HIV is considered an absolute contraindication to transplantation. The time to AIDS and death is significantly shortened, particularly if HIV is acquired at or shortly after transplantation. However, the recently introduced intensive antiviral therapy for HIV infection may alter this approach. It is important to remember that HIV infection or behaviour considered to be at risk of contracting HIV or other viruses (lifestyle assessment) excludes such individuals from organ donation.

Bacterial infections

There are a limited number of bacterial infections that are significantly more common and more severe in the transplant population (Table 11). However, there is little doubt that bacteraemias are more common in transplant recipients, usually as a result of urinary tract infections. Metastatic abscesses in joints, skin, muscles, and the brain are also more frequent.

Mycobacterial infections Reactivation of mycobacterial infection following transplantation is very common in the 'at risk' population, and most United Kingdom units recommend prophylaxis with isoniazid in these groups, although some debate the need for this. Experience in the Indian Subcontinent suggests that pretransplant BCG vaccination is not effective. Mycobacterial infections (both atypical and tuberculosis) can present in many different guises, for example pneumonia, lymphadenopathy, intracranial space-occupying lesions, discharging sinus, pyrexia of unknown origin, and skin ulcers. Tissue biopsy and cultures and smears employing special stains are essential. PCR, particularly of cerebrospinal fluid, is proving helpful. Gallium scanning may identify nodes that can be aspirated under CT guidance. Skin testing is unreliable in the immunocompromised patient.

Treatment is compromised by serious drug interactions between rifampicin and both the calcineurin-blocking drugs and prednisolone. Rifampicin is such a potent inducer of cytochrome P450 that sub-therapeutic levels of the calcineurin-blocking drugs and steroids can develop within weeks. Graft loss from rejection will occur unless doses are increased: that of prednisolone is usually doubled, and the calcineurin blockers may have to be increased still further and given three times daily. Monitoring of drug levels is essential.

In many units a four-drug antituberculous regimen is recommended, comprising rifampicin, ethambutol, isoniazid, and pyrazinamide. When sensitivities become available, this can be reduced. Treatment should be continued for at least a year, particularly in the case of atypical mycobacterial infections. Therapy may be further complicated by hepatotoxicity, for which the differential diagnosis is complex as many other factors can cause deranged liver function tests in renal transplant recipients (for example virus infections—HBV, HCV, CMV, and other drugs)

Nocardia Nocardia typically produces either a pseudotuberculosis or a pseudostaphylococcal syndrome. Central nervous system infections can occur. Dissemination is common, occurring in 25 to 30 per cent. Diagnosis often requires a biopsy or aspiration, with cultures needing to be prolonged for at least 3 weeks. Prolonged treatment (at least 6 months) with co-trimoxazole is usually effective, following which long-term co-trimoxazole should continue indefinitely.

Non-typhoid salmonella Non-typhoid salmonella infections are noteworthy because of their tendency to produce metastatic abscesses following bacteraemia. With control of the acute illness, the continued excretion of the organism may occur in stool or urine. Relapse is common so treatment needs to be prolonged. Suitable antimicrobials include ciprofloxacin, co-trimoxazole, and ampicillin.

Listeria Listeria has a tendency to localize in the central nervous system following a bacteraemic phase. Neurological syndromes vary from meningitis and meningoencephalitis to space-occupying lesions. It is the commonest cause of post-transplant meningitis. In the absence of evidence of raised intracanial pressure, all patients will require lumbar puncture and examination of cerebrospinal fluid. Delayed or inadequate treatment may result in permanent neurological deficit. Treatment usually includes high-dose ampicillin for at least 6 weeks, combined with gentamicin for the first week. The source of listeria is usually contaminated dairy products, chicken, or uncooked vegetables contaminated by manure.

Table 10 Opportunistic infections in transplant recipients

Viruses	Human herpes viruses (HHV)
	Herpes simplex (HHV1, HHV2)
	Varicella zoster (HHV3)
	Epstein–Barr virus (HHV4)
	Cytomegalovirus (HHV5)
	Kaposi sarcoma virus (HHV8)
	Hepatitis viruses
	Hepatitis B virus (HBV)
	Hepatitis C virus (HCV)
	Papovaviruses:
	Human papilloma virus (HPV)
	Polyoma virus (BK/JC)
	Human immunodeficiency virus (HIV)
Bacteria	Mycobacteria:
	Tuberculosis
	Atypicals
	Nocardia
	Listeria
	Non-typhoid salmonella
	Legionella
Fungi	Hospital acquired:
	Aspergillosis
	Community acquired:
	Candida
	Torulopsis
	Cryptococcus
	Mucormycosis
	Reactivation (geographically restricted):
	Histoplasmosis
	Coccidioidomycosis
Parasites	*Pneumocystis carinii*
	Toxoplasmosis
	Cryptosporidium
	Geographically restricted:
	Strongyloides stercoralis
	Trypanosoma cruzi
	Malaria
	Leishmaniasis
	Schistosomiasis

Fungal infections

Oral candidiasis is a common post-transplant infection. Spread to the oropharynx and lungs may occur. All patients should receive prophylaxis (nystatin mouthwashes or amphotericin lozenges) for at least 6 weeks, but some practitioners would recommend longer courses, or even indefinite treatment in patients with diabetes. Intercurrent courses of antibiotics should be covered with oral prophylaxis against candida.

The spectrum of diseases produced by fungal infections is wide, ranging from mucocutaneous syndromes, severe pneumonias, central nervous system syndromes, to skin or muscle abscesses. This variation in clinical presentation again highlights the need for aggressive invasive investigation. Outbreaks of aspergillus are usually related to hospital building projects and should prompt a search for the source. Deep-seated fungal infections

Table 11 Clinical features of post-transplant viral infections

Cytomegalovirus (CMV)
Asymptomatic
CMV syndrome:
Fever
Wasting
Malaise
Leucopenia
Transaminitis
Hepatitis
Pseudolymphoma
Retinitis
Pneumonitis
Colitis
Gastroduodenitis
Pancreatitis
Myocarditis
Superinfection, e.g. *Pneumocystis carinii* pneumonia
Epstein–Barr virus (EBV)
Asymptomatic
Classic glandular fever
Hairy leucoplakia
Hepatitis
Post-transplant lymphoproliferative disorder
Herpes simplex virus (HSV)
Stomatitis
Oesophagitis
Anogenital ulcers
Corneal ulcers
Kaposi's varicelliform eruption
Haemhorrhagic skin blisters
Paronychia
Pneumonitis
Hepatitis
Pancreatitis
Meningoencephalitis
Varicella zoster virus (VZV)
Reactivation:
Shingles
Primary infection:
Pneumonitis
Hepatitis
Encephalitis
Pancreatitis
Disseminated intravascular coagulation
Human papilloma virus (HPV)
Cutaneous warts
Condyloma acuminatum
Bowen's disease
Squamous cell carcinoma
Anogenital carcinoma (e.g. cervical invasive neoplasia, vulvovaginal invasive neoplasia)

carry a very high mortality. Dissemination is common. Specialist microbiological advice is usually required, but if the fungus is sensitive then liposomal amphotericin is the drug of choice.

Parasitic infections

Some of the parasitic infections listed in Table 10 are geographically restricted and therefore will only be of specific relevance in those areas. Schistosomiasis, for example, can cause ureteric strictures and leaks following transplantation. *Strongyloides stercoralis* is usually found in patients from the West Indies or the Far East: in the immunocompromised it can reactivate, complete its lifecycle in the patient without need for an intermediate host, and produce a hyperinfestation syndrome. A pretransplant eosinophilia is sometimes present. Clinical presentation is with recurrent bouts of Gram-negative septicaemia as the worm penetrates the gut mucosa. Other clinical features include pruritus ani, haemorrhagic enteritis, lava currens, cough, wheeze, and a haemorrhaging bronchopneumonia. Meningitis may also occur. Diagnosis usually requires a duodenal aspirate. Treatment is with thiabendazole, which should be given pretransplant to susceptible patients. Several courses of treatment may be needed to eradicate the infestation.

Scabies may occur in transplant recipients and can produce so-called Norwegian scabies in which there may be many parasitic mites per burrow. In the immunocompromised patient, skin organisms are readily carried into the bloodstream, hence cellulitis and septicaemia are common.

The transplant organ, particularly the heart, can transmit toxoplasmosis. The organism becomes widely disseminated, including the central nervous system. Other clinical features may include low-grade fever, lymphadenopathy, pneumonia, myocarditis, retinopathy, and myositis. It can mimic cytomegalovirus. Treatment is with pyrimethamine and sulphadiazine for at least 4 weeks. Prophylaxis with co-trimoxazole has greatly reduced the incidence of toxoplasmosis following solid organ transplantation.

Pneumocystis carinii Until the widespread introduction of prophylactic low-dose co-trimoxazole, *Pneumocystis carinii* pneumonia was a dreaded complication of solid organ transplantation. Oral co-trimoxazole or inhaled pentamidine (300 mg monthly) is effective prophylaxis. *Pneumocystis carinii* pneumonia is now most commonly seen in the setting of augmented immunosuppression (additional serotherapy) and in patients who already have developed CMV disease. Presentation is with fever, dry cough, and profound shortness of breath, occurring in the context of few added sounds in the chest and a remarkably clear chest radiograph. By the time the chest radiograph has altered, pulmonary fibrosis is occurring. Successful treatment demands an early diagnosis, such that the renal transplant recipient who complains of shortness of breath on exercise and who desaturates on exercise should be admitted and investigated as a medical emergency. Bronchoalveolar lavage is virtually mandatory under these circumstances. Overall immunsuppression should be reduced in patients with *Pneumocystis carinii* pneumonia, but steroids may need to be increased to cover a stress response (e.g. prednisolone at 20 to 25 mg daily). High-dose intravenous co-trimoxazole is given: 15 to 20 mg of trimethoprim and 75 to 100 mg of sulphamethoxazole per kilogram body weight per day, although these doses may need to be reduced in severe renal failure. Treatment should be continued for at least 2 weeks. It is essential to monitor respiratory effort carefully in the renal transplant recipient with an interstitial pneumonitis and intervene with continuous positive airways pressure or full ventilation if the patient tires or cannot protect his airways. Nutrition should be ensured, using total parenteral nutrition if necessary.

Specific infective problems

Pulmonary disease

Recurrent chest infections are common. Many are viral and will be self-limiting, even in the immunosuppressed transplant recipient. An abrupt clinical onset with fever and a lobar pattern of lung infiltrates is likely to be due to a bacterial infection. A more insidious onset with scattered or diffuse pulmonary infiltrates is more likely to be due to an opportunistic infection. Blood and sputum should be cultured urgently. Sputum samples need careful microscopy and cultures should be set up for mycobacteria, fungi, and legionella. PCR is available for *Mycobacterium tuberculosis, Pneumocystis carinii*, and CMV. Antibiotics may be started pending culture results. The regimen that will cover most of the common organisms is penicillin V, clarithromycin (NB drug interactions), and a third-generation cephalosporin.

Failure to respond promptly to therapy or a non-lobar pattern of infiltration is an indication for brochoscopy and bronchoalveolar lavage, the diagnostic accuracy of which is about 80 to 90 per cent. It is essential to examine the fluid thoroughly, which will involve viral and bacterial cultures, special stains, and PCR where available. In clinical practice it is often necessary to start therapy blindly in seriously ill patients. Sometimes this will involve the addition of high-dose co-trimoxazole and ganciclovir to conventional antibiotics. When the results of culture and sensitivity testing become available it may be possible to reduce the antimicrobial regime or change to specific antituberculous or antifungal therapy.

The greatest mimic of a chest infection is pulmonary oedema: measurement of an elevated pulmonary capillary wedge pressure is diagnostic, and a therapeutic test of a potent diuretic sometimes produces a dramatic clearing of the chest radiograph. Other non-infectious causes of acute pulmonary syndromes that may occur in the renal transplant recipient are shown in Table 12.

Urinary tract infection

One-third of renal transplant recipients will develop urinary tract infection. In most this is related to postoperative bladder catheterization and usually resolves with removal of the catheter and a short course of antibiotics. There is an exponential relationship between the incidence of urinary tract infections and the duration of bladder catheterization. Some patients develop numerous recurrent infections, particularly in the first couple of years following transplantation. In some this can be related to a

Table 12 Non-infective differential diagnoses of acute pulmonary syndromes in transplant recipients

- Pneumothorax—central venous lines
- Pulmonary embolus
- Non-cardiogenic pulmonary oedema
    - Cytokine release syndrome
- Left ventricular failure
    - Fluid overload
    - Tacrolimus cardiotoxicity
    - Unrecognized ischaemic heart disease
    - Acute arrhythmias:
        - Hypokalaemia
        - Hypomagnesaemia
    - Uncontrolled hypertension
- Pulmonary fibrosis
    - Mycophenolate mofetil (rare)
    - Azathioprine (rare)
    - Co-trimoxazole
- Bronchospasm
    - Allergic reactions:
        - Antilymphocyte serum
        - X-ray contrast
- Pulmonary vasculitis
    - Recurrence of original disease
- Pulmonary aspiration
    - Diabetic coma
    - Fits
- Impaired ventilation
    - Neuromuscular blockade
- Pulmonary infiltration:
    - Post-transplant lymphoproliferative disorder
    - Kaposi's sarcoma

focus of infection in the native kidneys, when bilateral native nephroureterectomy may be indicated if sepsis is severe. A few patients will develop encrustation or even a stone in the bladder as a result of the surgical implantation of the ureter: a plain abdominal radiograph may reveal such calculi, which should be removed cystoscopically.

More worrying is infection ascending into the transplant kidney itself during the intermediate period of post-transplantation immunosuppression when the patient is most immunocompromised. A severe bacterial pyelonephritis can develop in the transplant, presenting as an acute rejection episode with a swollen kidney, low-grade fever, and deteriorating graft function. Such upper tract infections are frequently complicated by septicaemia, and it is always worth remembering that urinary sepsis is the commonest cause of post-transplant bacteraemia. It is essential that episodes of graft dysfunction due to upper tract infection are clearly diagnosed and aggressively treated with appropriate high-dose parental antibiotics. Misdiagnosis resulting in treatment with high-dose intravenous steroids for a presumed rejection episode can be catastrophic.

The advent of technetium-99m labelled DMSA SPECT isotope scanning (single photon emission computed tomography using dimercaptosuccinic acid labelled with technetium-99m) has enabled three-dimensional reconstructions of the grafted kidney to be produced. Progressive scarring can develop in some patients with recurrent infections and reflux to the graft, hence transplant recipients with recurrent urinary tract infections need full investigation and aggressive treatment. Every effort should be made to establish and maintain sterile urine. Long-term prophylactic low-dose antibiotics may be indicated.

Neurological syndromes

The main concerns are those of post-transplant lymphoproliferative disorder or an opportunistic infection producing progressive neurological deterioration due to an increasing space-occupying lesion. Examples of neurological syndromes seen in the renal transplant recipient and their common causes are given in Table 13. The range of infectious micro-organisms that can cause central nervous system lesions is such that a diagnostic aspirate is usually essential. Tuberculosis is common in at-risk patients. Investigation should include a CT scan with contrast or an MRI so that abscesses are not missed. In the absence of evidence of a raised intracranial pressure, cerebrospinal fluid should be examined. As with the processing of bronchoalveolar lavage fluid, close co-operation between clinician and the cytological and microbiological laboratories is essential.

Fits may occur in the early post-transplant period, when the cause is usually multifactorial, including hyponatraemia, hypertension, hypomagnesaemia, hypocalcaemia, and the toxic effects of the calcineurin-blocking drugs. The rejection process itself can cause a rise in intracranial pressure, so-called rejection encephalopathy. Fits occurring after the first month should prompt a search for a serious intracranial space-occupying lesion.

Renal transplantation in the presence of liver dysfunction

The two main liver conditions encountered in patients on transplant waiting lists that give concern in the post-transplant period are hepatitis B (HBV) and hepatitis C (HCV).

Hepatitis B HBV usually causes persistent infection in patients with chronic renal failure. In many this may be subclinical, but in others a

Table 13 Causes of neurological syndromes in transplant recipients

Syndrome	Causes
Psychosis	Steroids
Space-occupying lesions (focal)	Bacteria:
	Mycobacteria
	Listeria
	Nocardia
	Fungi:
	Aspergillosis
	Mucormycosis
	Parasitic:
	Toxoplasmosis
	Strongyloides
	Other:
	Post-transplant lymphoproliferative disorder
Meningitis: acute/subacute	Listeria
Meningitis: subacute/chronic	Mycobacteria
	Cryptococcus
	Coccidiodomycosis
Meningoencephalitis	Cryptococcus
	OKT3
Encephalitis/multifocal	Herpes simplex and varicella zoster viruses
	Toxoplasmosis
Progressive dementia	Primary measles
	JC polyomavirus
Fits	Hypertension
	Hyponatraemia
	Calcineurin-blocking drugs
	Hypomagnesaemia
	Acute rejection
	Space-occupying lesions
Tremor/ataxia	Calcineurin-blocking drugs
Peripheral neuropoathy	Diabetes mellitus
	Pre-existing uraemic neuropathy
Myopathy	Steroids
	Statins or fibrates

chronic hepatitis and cirrhosis can develop. Serology is of little help in assessing suitability for transplantation, which is contraindicated in the presence of cirrhosis and biopsy evidence of active hepatic inflammation since immunosuppression causes rapid viral replication and progressive liver disease. Death within 5 years of transplantation may occur in up to 50 per cent of patients if wrongly transplanted, usually from extrahepatic sepsis. Long-term therapy with the newer antiviral agents may improve the outlook and allow access to transplantation to those at present denied this.

Hepatitis C Although HCV is now the most common cause of both pre- and post-transplant liver disease, the effects of immunosuppression on HCV seem much less dramatic than the effects on HBV. Occasional patients do develop a fulminating hepatitis post-transplantation, but overall HCV does not appear to have a major impact on the short- to medium-term outcome after renal transplantation.

Post-transplant liver dysfunction

Abnormal liver function tests following transplantation are common: both drugs and infectious agents may be responsible. Full investigation is required, including imaging of the liver, bile ducts, and gallbladder as well as a liver biopsy. In some instances transient elevation of liver transaminases may herald CMV disease. In other situations raised liver enzymes can represent progressive HCV- or HBV- induced liver disease. It is important to remember that the donor organ can transmit most of the hepatotropic viruses. Treatment clearly depends on the cause. Where possible the offending drug (for instance azathioprine) should be withdrawn and antiviral therapy may be appropriate in the case of HBV and HCV. Interferon therapy is contraindicated as it induces expression of HLA antigens and may provoke acute rejection. In the case of HBV it is often possible to reduce the dosage of immunosuppressive agents significantly without precipitating a rejection episode.

Neoplasia

Post-transplant neoplasia is an important cause of morbidity and mortality. There is some debate as to whether some of the conditions often regarded as neoplastic can truly be classed as cancers, since several are clearly viral related and will regress with reduction of immunosuppression. Table 14 summarizes the tumours seen with increased frequency after transplantation. There is a marked geographical variation: for instance in Japan, renal, thyroid, and uterine cancers as well as lymphoma are common; in Saudi Arabia, Kaposi's sarcoma is the most common; in Australia squamous cell carcinoma of the skin is almost ubiquitous 20 years after transplantation (75 per cent). It is also important to remember than the donor organ can transmit cancer.

Table 14 Post-transplant neoplasia

Post-transplant lymphoproliferative disorder (EBV driven)
Lymphadenopathy (33%)
Central nervous system (15–20%)
Graft infiltration
Gut (25%)
Skin masses (1%)
Scar infiltration (1%)
Pulmonary nodules/infiltrates
Widely disseminated (1–3%)
Kaposi's sarcoma (HHV8 driven)
Local (60%): skin infiltrating nodules
Disseminated (40%):
Lymphadenopathy
Upper or lower gastrointestinal tract
Lungs or pleura
Bladder
Oropharynx
Anogenital carcinoma (HPV driven)
Cervical invasive neoplasia
Anal carcinoma
Vulvovaginal invasive neoplasia
Squamous cell carcinoma of the skin (HPV driven)

Post-transplant lymphoproliferative disorder

Post-transplant lymphoproliferative disorder is driven by Epstein–Barr virus (EBV) present in a latent form (episomal or circular DNA) in B lymphocytes. In non-immunosuppressed individuals a normal T-cytotoxic lymphocyte response terminates infected proliferating B cells. In the presence of effective immunosuppression this does not happen and an unrestricted, increasingly monoclonal B-cell proliferation develops. The more potent the immunosuppressive regime, the earlier post-transplant lymphoproliferative disorder occurs. In most centres, the incidence of this disorder is about 2 per cent. The clinical features are summarized in Table 14. In common with many other infections following transplantation, a primary infection (i.e. the recipient is naive or seronegative for EBV antibodies, while the donor is seropositive) leads more frequently to disease.

Early diagnosis is important as the stepwise reduction of immunsuppression with careful monitoring of graft function can lead to regression of the tumour without graft rejection. Stimulating the patient's immune system with interferon-α or IL-2 may be tried. Conventional cytotoxic therapy should be introduced if post-transplant lymphoproliferative disorder progresses despite the withdrawal of immunosuppression, but this further suppresses the patient's immune system and death from overwhelming infection is all too common. Anti-B-cell antibodies (e.g. rituximab) and infusions of EBV-specific cytotoxic T lymphocytes are promising new avenues of therapy.

It remains to be proved, but seems very likely, that the carefully monitored stepwise reduction of immunosuppression may also be appropriate for other virally induced neoplasms in renal transplant recipients, for example Kaposi's sarcoma and squamous cell carcinoma. A few patients who have lost their grafts in the context of post-transplant lymphoproliferative disorder have been successfully retransplanted.

Kaposi's sarcoma

Kaposi's sarcoma is a vascular tumour composed of proliferating spindle cells (latently infected lymphatic endothelial cells) and thin-walled neovascular formations that is driven by the Kaposi's sarcoma virus (KSV), recently designated HHV8. Aetiological factors are very similar to those of post-transplant lymphoproliferative disorder. Lesions may develop at almost any site on the skin and visceral involvement is common. Prompt diagnosis and early reduction of immunosuppression may result in regression. As with post-transplant lymphoproliferative disorder, the use of cytotoxic agents is associated with a greatly increased risk of death from sepsis. Attempts at retransplantation after regression are associated almost universally with recurrence.

Human papilloma virus related carcinoma

Human papilloma virus (HPV) is responsible for skin, vulval, and anogenital warts, and some types are now clearly associated with carcinoma. Renal transplant recipients should therefore receive full dermatological and gynaecological examinations at regular intervals.

Aetiological factors for skin cancer include exposure to ultraviolet light (which may act by depletion of cutaneous Langerhan's cells as well as direct DNA damage), duration and intensity of immunosuppression, and the HPV virus itself. The prevalence increases progressively with time, such that after 20 years most renal transplant recipients will have cutaneous squamous cell carcinoma. Management should involve cautious dose-reduction of immunosuppressive agents. There is great interest in the role of combined oral and topical retinoids, which are associated with repopulation of the skin with Langerhan's cells and augmentation of natural killer cell activity, and may also act by blocking IL-6 pathways. Some cases of squamous cell carcinoma can metastasize, when reduction of immunosuppression dose, interferon-α therapy, and a willingness to abandon the graft should be considered before recourse to systemic cytotoxic chemotherapy.

Hypertension

The aetiology of post-transplant hypertension is complex (Table 15). Over 75 per cent of renal transplant recipients will need drug therapy for hypertension in addition to lifestyle modification. Most units aim for a systolic blood pressure of less than 145 mmHg and a diastolic pressure of less than 85 mmHg, but there is a lack of clear data regarding the ideal blood pressure. Hypertension plays a crucial role in accelerating vascular disease and chronic allograft nephropathy. Care should be taken with the choice of agents. On theoretical grounds, angiotensin-converting enzyme (**ACE**) inhibitors or angiotensin I (**AT-I**) receptor antagonists appear a rational first choice in view of the multiple proinflammatory, profibrotic, and proproliferative actions of angiotensin II. There are overwhelming data showing reduction of proteinuria and a slowing of progression of renal disease in native kidneys treated with ACE inhibitors, and by implication also by AT-I receptor-blocking drugs. However, the risks of using ACE inhibitors in patients with renal artery stenosis should not be forgotten, transplant renal artery stenosis being most likely to develop between 3 and 12 months after transplantation, sometimes (but not always) associated with a bruit over the kidney. Serum creatinine must be carefully monitored, any substantial rise after ACE inhibition leading to immediate cessation of the drug and consideration of angiography of the transplant renal artery. It is preferable to avoid drugs that exacerbate dyslipidaemia, such as β-blockers and thiazides. Poor blood pressure control with short-acting dihydropyridine calcium-channel blockers may increase proteinuria and cardiovascular mortality. In refractory cases, or those where treatment is problematic, estimation of renin levels in the veins draining the native and transplant kidneys may help in the decision to proceed to a native kidney nephrectomy.

Table 15 Aetiological factors for accelerated atherosclerosis in transplant recipients

Factor	Cause
Hypertension	Insulin resistance (sympathetic overactivity)
	Drugs:
	Calcineurin-blocking drugs
	Steroids
	Native kidneys
	Transplant kidneys (ischaemia, rejection)
Hyperlipidaemia	Dialysis and chronic renal failure
	Proteinuria
	Insulin resistance
	Calcineurin-blocking drugs
	Steroids
	β-Blockers
	Thiazides
Proteinuria	Glomerular disease in native/ transplant kidneys
Endothelial cell activation	Oxidized low-density lipoproteins
	Calcineurin-blocking drugs
	Hypertension
	Smoking
Oxidized lipids	Calcineurin-blocking drugs
	Proteinuria
Hyperhomocysteinaemia	Renal failure *per se*
	B_{12} and folate deficiency
Platelet hyperaggregability	Nephrotic syndrome
	Calcineurin-blocking drugs
Hyperfibrinogenaemia	Nephrotic syndrome
	Acute-phase response
Insulin resistance	Steroids, obesity
	Calcineurin-blocking drugs
	Chronic renal failure *per se*
Diabetes mellitus	Primary renal disease
	Acquired post-transplant (e.g. calcineurin-blocking drugs)
Lifestyle	Smoking
	Excessive alcohol
	Diet
	Obesity
Inflammation	Original nephritis
	Haemodialysis *per se*
	Infection and rejection

Accelerated atherosclerosis

In common with patients on dialysis, one of the major causes of death following renal transplantation is cardiovascular disease. Indeed, death with a functioning graft is now the major cause of late graft failure. Much of the cardiovascular disease that shortens life expectancy in renal transplant recipients will have developed and be established pretransplantation. Table 15 summarizes the pre- and post- transplant aetiological factors. Prevention and treatment of established vascular disease is essential. About a third of renal transplant recipients will have hypercholesterolaemia and many will also be hypertensive. Lifestyle modification is important. All renal transplant recipients should be strongly advised not to smoke. Following transplantation, some 10 per cent of transplant recipients become quite grossly obese. It is important to remember that the cardiovascular risk factors multiply rather than summate, hence the long-term management of renal transplant recipients has to address all cardiovascular risk factors.

Electrolyte disorders

Hypophosphataemia

In the presence of inadequately controlled secondary hyperparathyroidism a well functioning transplant will waste phosphate, and in a few cases phosphaturia persists despite resolution of the secondary hyperparathyroidism. In some patients there is steroid-related malabsorption of phosphate. In the first few months following renal transplantation, phosphate wasting can be severe and oral supplements will be required. Untreated chronic hypophosphataemia can lead to bone fractures (hypophosphataemic rickets).

Hyperkalaemia

The calcineurin-blocking drugs cause hyperkalaemia, particularly when levels are toxic. This is thought to be due to type IV renal tubular acidosis in which distal tubular potassium secretion is reduced in response to a fall in renin secretion due to reduced renal prostaglandins. The addition of ACE inhibitors, AT-I receptor-blocking drugs, non-steroidal anti-inflammatory drugs, or potassium-conserving diuretics can produce a brisk rise in serum potassium in renal transplant recipients. Dietary advice and loop diuretics are usually sufficient but a small number of patients may require fludrocortisone (100 to 200 μg daily.)

Hypomagnesaemia

Renal tubular magnesium wasting is a component of the nephrotoxicity of the calcineurin-blocking drugs and can be exacerbated by diuretics and diarrhoea. Hypomagnesaemia may predispose to fits and cardiac arrhythmias in susceptible individuals. Levels should be monitored and oral supplements of magnesium glycerophosphate given if required.

Hypercalcaemia

Hypercalcaemia can develop after grafting if renal osteodystrophy has been poorly controlled and severe secondary hyperparathyroidism is present at the time of transplantation. The transplant kidney produces adequate amounts of 1,25-dihydroxycholecalciferol, which in the presence of high levels of parathyroid hormone will result in hypercalcaemia. Widespread metastatic deposition of calcium can occur if hypercalcaemia is severe. Simple controlling measures include adequate fluids and the use of loop diuretics rather than thiazides. Occasional patients will require regular infusions of pamidronate (15 to 30 mg), which can be combined with intermittent doses of oral α-calcidol to suppress parathyroid hyperplasia. Parathyroidectomy is occasionally required. It may take 12 to 24 months for secondary hyperparathyroidism to resolve following renal transplantation.

Bicarbonate wasting

The transplant kidney may waste bicarbonate as well as phosphate. This may be due to persistent hyperparathyroidism, but can also reflect acute tubule damage from rejection. A chronic metabolic acidosis will contribute to post-transplant osteoporosis and should be treated with bicarbonate supplements.

Hyponatraemia

Hyponatraemia may develop, particularly in the early postoperative period. It is usually due to inappropriate intravenous fluids (excess 5 per cent dextrose or dextrose saline) in the context of deteriorating graft function, and may be an important contributing factor to fits after transplantation.

Musculoskeletal complications

Tendon rupture

Steroids impair collagen synthesis. Tendons and tendon insertions are weakened and avulsions may occur, most commonly in the fingers or Achilles' tendon.

Myopathy

An important complication of steroid therapy is proximal myopathy, which can be incapacitating in some patients. Physiotherapy plus vitamin D supplements and a rapid reduction of steroids (alternate-day prescription or even cessation) can produce improvement. Hypophosphataemia should be corrected. Acute rhabdomyolysis may develop if fibrates or statins are used with the calcineurin-blocking drugs.

Avascular necrosis of bone

Avascular necrosis of bone, particularly of the weight-bearing ends of the long bones, causes an extremely painful joint. When the hips are involved, walking can become impossible and total hip replacement is the only treatment. Prevention may be possible by the careful control of secondary hyperparathyroidism prior to transplantation and the early use of bisphosphonates to minimize post-transplant osteoporosis may be beneficial.

Osteoporosis

Osteoporosis is a common and progressive complication of long-term steroid therapy such that regular bone-density assessment should be part of long-term renal transplant follow-up. The problem is particularly severe in postmenopausal women, in whom hormone replacement therapy is of benefit. Prophylaxis with intravenous pamidronate has been advocated in the first few months after transplantation, but this is not standard practice in most units.

Renal osteodystrophy

In the presence of a poorly functioning graft, control of parathyroid hormone (**PTH**) and the calcium-phosphate product (ideally to be kept at less than 5) is as important as it is in the pretransplant patient with chronic renal failure (see Chapter 20.5.1). PTH levels should be kept at one to two times the upper limit of normal by the careful use of α-calcidol and calcium supplements. Serum phosphate should be kept at 1 to 1.5 mmol/l using calcium carbonate as an oral phosphate binder.

Gout

The calcineurin-blocking drugs impair urate secretion in the proximal tubule, and urate retention is exacerbated by the concomitant use of diuretics, particularly in patients with poorly functioning grafts. Uric acid levels may rise dramatically and be associated with attacks of clinical gout as well as tophi. Management is complicated, both for acute attacks and for prophylaxis. For acute episodes the physician must choose between three treatments, all of which are problematic. Non-steroidal anti-inflammatory drugs are the usual first-line treatment for acute episodes in general medical practice, but in those with renal impairment—including many transplant recipients—they are best avoided, although the recently introduced Cox 2 inhibitors may prove safer. Colchicine can be used for acute attacks, but the transplant recipient tolerates diarrhoea and the attendant hypovolaemia poorly. Oral prednisolone (20 mg daily) can be effective, but will clearly exacerbate steroid side-effects, which are already a problem in many patients. As regards prophylaxis, allopurinol is (relatively) contraindicated if the patient is receiving azathioprine (the dose of azathioprine should be reduced to about 25 per cent of normal) with very careful monitoring for leucopenia. Most uricosuric agents work poorly in the presence of renal impairment, but an important exception to this is benzbromarone (100 to 200 mg daily), which can be safely administered to patients on azathioprine. In some patients it may be helpful to stop azathioprine altogether and use mycophenolate mofetil in its place so that allopurinol can be used safely.

Haematological complications of renal transplantation

Venous thromboembolism is not uncommon following renal transplantation. The local effects of surgery on the pelvic veins together with immediate postoperative bed rest contribute to the risk. The calcineurin-blocking drugs have an activating and procoagulant effect on endothelial cells and platelets. Nephrotic patients have a profound disturbance of many coagulation factors and represent an extremely high-risk group for perioperative venous thromboembolism. Prophylactic subcutaneous low-molecular-weight heparin (e.g. enoxaparin at 20 mg daily) is standard practice, with higher doses (e.g. enoxaparin at 40 mg daily) in those at highest risk.

A direct endothelial effect of the calcineurin-blocking drugs can result in a *de novo* post-transplant haemolytic uraemic syndrome, and it seems likely that both cyclosporin and tacrolimus may increase the risk of recurrent bouts in patients with this as their primary disease.

Bone marrow suppression may occur as a result of intercurrent viral infection and a variety of drugs. In the context of severe CMV infection it is safe to continue with ganciclovir or aciclovir, but the bone marrow should be stimulated with granulocyte colony-stimulating factor. Profound bone marrow suppression may occur when allopurinol is used with azathioprine if the dose of the latter is not appropriately reduced (see above).

An acute haemolytic anaemia can develop at any time following transplantation. Sometimes this is triggered by an intercurrent infection, but in many cases may be due to antibodies to minor blood antigens. Treatment consists of intravenous immunoglobulin and an increase in steroids.

Patients with a poorly functioning graft will become anaemic just as their predialysis counterparts. Haematinics should be prescribed if patients are deficient, using intravenous iron if iron stores cannot be restored by oral supplements. Erythropoietin may be required.

About 20 per cent of renal transplant recipients develop erythrocytosis. The mechanism is probably multifactorial. The transplant kidney may produce an excess of erythropoietin, occasionally stimulated by renal artery stenosis in the donor kidney. The use of diuretics may produce blood volume contraction. Reduction in erythrocytosis following administration of ACE inhibitors or AT-I receptor-blocking drugs suggests that angiotensin II may contribute to pathogenesis. In most cases the condition is self-limiting, but there is a risk of cerebrovascular occlusion if the haematocrit is grossly elevated and most practitioners recommend regular venesection (or ACE inhibitors) to keep the haemoglobin below 15 or 16 g/dl. A high haematocrit will also exacerbate hypertension.

Cosmetic complications

It is important not to underestimate the psychological importance of the cosmetic disfigurement that can be produced by some of the treatment regimes used in transplantation. They are an important contributing factor to non-compliance, particularly in adolescents, and can even lead to agoraphobia and suicide. With the currently available choices of immunosuppressive agents it should be possible to minimize cosmetic complications when these cause great distress, for example steroid withdrawal, substitution of tacrolimus for cyclosporin A, and use of mycophenolate mofetil to reduce reliance on steroids and calcineurin-blocking drugs. The better cosmetic profile of tacrolimus is thought to be due to lower transforming growth factor-β production, but expense may be a limiting factor in some health-care systems.

Outcome

Graft and patient survival

Figures 2 and 3 summarize the graft survival rates for first cadaver and living related transplants. The highest rate of graft loss is within the first few months. Graft losses due to technical factors should be less than 5 per cent. The major cause of early graft loss continues to be acute rejection. However, it is a matter of concern that the attrition of grafts following the first year has not altered, even with the introduction of newer, more potent immunosuppressive agents. Currently some 4 per cent of grafts fail annually for a variety of causes loosely grouped together as chronic allograft nephropathy (see discussion below). Death with a functioning graft is now the most common cause of late graft failure.

Factors affecting graft survival are summarized in Table 16. Even with potent immunosuppressive regimes, HLA matching remains extremely important, forming the rationale for local and national organ sharing schemes to ensure that the best possible matches can be obtained. Figure 2 indicates that beneficially matched cadaver kidneys (1–0–0 or 0–1–0 mismatch) fare significantly better than non-beneficially matched, and well-matched living related transplants do best of all (Fig. 3).

Early studies indicated that an acute rejection episode had a major impact on long-term graft survival, reducing it by almost a half. If an acute

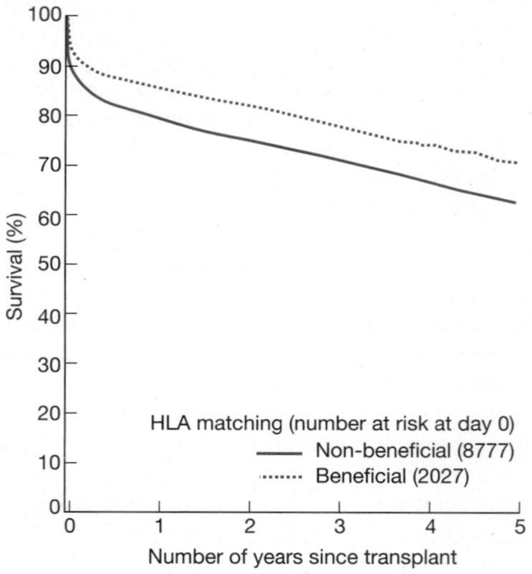

Fig. 2 Graft survival: first cadaver graft (by courtesy of UK Transplant).

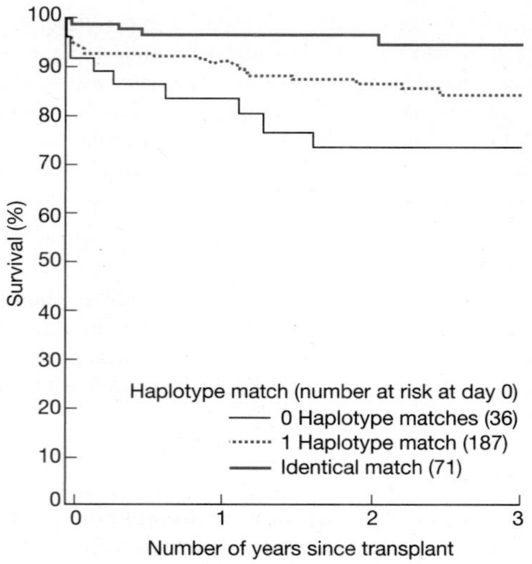

Fig. 3 Graft survival: living related grafts (by courtesy of UK Transplant).

rejection episode is completely reversed the effect on long-term graft survival is markedly reduced. Long-term graft survival can be clearly related to the creatinine level at 1 year. This has led to great emphasis on efforts to reduce the rate of early acute rejection episodes. One crucial observation that predicts those at increased risk is the presence of widely reactive anti-HLA antibodies to potential donors. Those patients who have already rejected a kidney within 6 months of transplantation also do poorly on subsequent transplantation unless immunosuppression is augmented. Increasingly potent induction regimens and combinations of drugs have been introduced, but in the absence of accurate predictors of the risk of rejection this has the effect that a significant number of patients will be grossly over-immunosuppressed, whilst others remain under-immunosuppressed. Poor long-term graft survival is also related to hypertension, proteinuria, hyperlipidaemia, and a high body-mass index (Table 16).

In the early post-transplant period the major causes of death are related to cardiovascular complications of surgery. However, with good patient selection, mortality in the first year should be very low (less than 1 to 2 per cent), despite the fact that increasingly older patients are being offered transplantation, as are those with significant comorbidities, diabetes mellitus in particular. In the first year the major cause of death is infection (Fig. 4). Later on, death from neoplasia and accelerated vascular disease are more common.

Chronic allograft nephropathy

First-year transplant losses from rejection have been dramatically reduced from about 40 per cent in the 1970s to 5 to 10 per cent. Similarly, early rejection rates can be reduced from around 50 per cent to less than 20 per cent. However, as stated above, the rate of chronic graft loss remains at about 4 per cent per year. Some of these graft losses will be due to death with a functioning graft, but many patients present with an insidiously rising creatinine, increasing proteinuria, and worsening hypertension. The causes of this late graft dysfunction are multifactorial and involve many different conditions and several overlapping pathogenic pathways. Histologically, many of these kidneys will show tubular atrophy, interstitial scarring, and an obliterative vasculopathy of the intrarenal arteries and arterioles, but even with a transplant biopsy it may not be possible to define the pathololgical process. Nevertheless, every effort should be made to produce an accurate diagnosis. Obstruction due to ureteric ischaemia must be excluded by renography or ultrasound. A review of past urine cultures and a technetium-99m labelled DMSA SPECT scan may reveal pyelonephritic scarring. Late graft dysfunction due to renal artery stenosis can be demonstrated by angiography. It is possible that the single transplant kidney may

Table 16 Factors affecting graft outcome

Recipient factors	Donor factors
Obesity	Extremes of age (nephron mass)
Compliance	Delayed graft function
Recurrence of original disease	Size mismatch
Hypertension	Ischaemia times
De novo glomerulonephritis	Donor organ quality
Diabetes mellitus/insulin resistance	Source: living or cadaver
Immune responsiveness	Agonal cytokine storm
Race: black individuals	
Infections: CMV	
Creatinine at 1 year	
Proteinuria/hyperlipidaemia	
Smoking	
Hospital factors	
Matching policy	
Choice of immunosuppression	
Surgical and medical expertise	
Nephrotoxicity of calcineurin-blocking drugs	
Adequacy of control of hypertension	
Control of CMV	
Repeated acute rejection episodes	
Poorly reversed acute rejections	
Late acute rejections	
Inadequate long-term immunosuppression	

have insufficient numbers of nephrons to cope with the work demanded of it, particularly if many nephrons have been lost early from acute rejection, manifest as a raised serum creatinine at 1 year. This situation may also arise if there is a very large size mismatch, with a very large recipient being given a kidney from a smaller donor, leading to the self-perpetuating inherently progressive cycle of hyperperfusion and hyperfiltration of the surviving nephrons (Brenner's hypothesis). Treatment is empirical but must involve control of blood pressure, preferably using an ACE inhibitor or an AT-I receptor-blocking drug to reduce intraglomerular blood pressure.

Some pathogenic aspects of insidious graft loss are akin to atherosclerotic changes, and interventions designed to limit vascular damage may prolong the life of poorly functioning kidneys. The early use of ACE inhibitors (especially if there is proteinuria), aspirin, fish oils, and control of cholesterol may help. Chronic allograft nephropathy may also be due in part to the nephrotoxic effects of the calcineurin-blocking drugs. The newer agent, mycophenolate mofetil, may have a particular role to play in that it has been shown to reduce proliferation of smooth muscle cells, which may ameliorate the obliterative vasculopathy typical of the condition, and permit reduced reliance on long-term calcineurin-blocking agents, but this is yet to be proved.

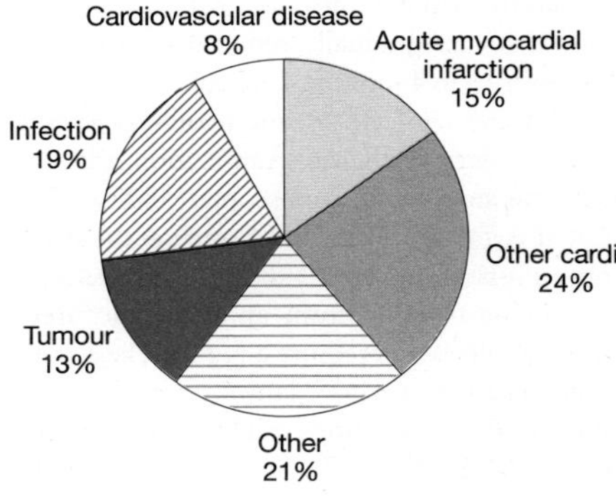

Fig. 4 Causes of death in renal transplant recipients.

Recurrence of original disease and *de novo* glomerulonephritis

Most of the primary glomerular diseases can recur in the transplant, but few are associated with graft loss. Overall, histologically demonstrable recurrence occurs in about 60 per cent of patients, but less than 10 per cent will lose their graft as a result. Accurate recurrence rates are difficult to determine, being roughly 2.5 per cent at 2 years, 10 per cent at 5 years, and perhaps as high as 20 per cent by 8 years. Treatment of recurrent glomerulonephritis is not particularly effective but has usually involved intensive plasma exchange or an increase in immunosuppression.

Oxalosis will recur rapidly in the kidney unless a liver transplant is also done to correct the underlying enzyme defect. Transplantation in the presence of circulating antibody to glomerular basement membrane will result in the immediate recurrence of Goodpasture's disease. The dense deposit variety of mesangiocapillary glomerulonephritis, which is usually associated with hypocomplementaemia, predictably recurs and may destroy the graft. In paediatric practice, the nephrotic syndrome associated with focal segmental glomerulosclerosis may recur in the immediate post-transplant period and can be associated with massive proteinuria, hypovolaemia, and thromboembolism. The risk of recurrence should be taken into account when assessing patients for the possibility of a living related transplant.

Membranous glomerulonephritis can develop *de novo* in patients in whom the original disease was demonstrably different (between 2 and 10 per cent).

Other aspects of medical management of transplant recipients

Drug interactions

Care has to be taken when prescribing drugs for renal transplant recipients. Renal function must be considered, as well as the potential for drug interactions between immunosuppressive agents and other pharmaceuticals. Table 17 summarizes the more common interactions. ACE inhibitors, AT-I receptor antagonists, and non-steroidal anti-inflammatory drugs can compromise the perfusion of a single transplanted kidney, particularly if there is a degree of renal artery stenosis. Great care must be taken with potent

Table 17 Common drug interactions in transplantation

Drugs	Interaction
Cytochrome P450 induction, e.g. Rifampicin Barbiturates Carbamazepam Phenytoin	Subtherapeutic levels of: CNBDs Steroids Oral contraceptives
Cytochrome P450 inhibition, e.g. Macrolides, e.g. erythromycin Imdizoles, e.g. fluconazole Calcium-channel blockers	Toxic levels of CNBDs
Statins (or fibrates) plus CNBDs Colchicine plus CNBDs	Rhabdomyolysis
Allopurinol plus azathioprine	Toxic accumulation of 6-mercaptopurine Marrow suppression
ACE-I (or AT-I receptor antagonists) Calcineurin-blocking drugs NSAIDs Potassium-conserving diuretics	Risk of hyperkalaemia with combinations
Diuretics and CNBDs NSAIDs CNBDs Aminoglycosides Co-trimoxazole	Hyperuricaemia, gout, tophi Nephrotoxins summate—risk of acute renal failure

CNBDs, calcineurin-blocking drugs; NSAIDs, non-steroidal anti-inflammatory drugs.

enzyme inducers such as rifampicin as subtherapeutic levels of steroids and the calcineurin-blocking drugs can occur.

Diet

The help of a renal-trained dietician is essential. Patients may eat voraciously after release from the restrictions of dialysis and, with the euphoric effects of steroids, some gain in excess of 20 kg in the first year. About 5 per cent become grossly obese, which is associated insulin resistance, hyperlipidaemia, sympathetic overactivity, and hypertension. Hypercholesterolaemia is present post-transplant in about 30 per cent of patients and is related to drugs, proteinuria, and diet. Patients should avoid a high intake of saturated fats. Sodium intake—easily gauged from monitoring the 24-h urinary sodium excretion—is often excessive, a desirable intake being less than 100 mmol per day. A high urinary sodium causes urinary calcium wasting and may contribute to post-transplant osteoporosis as well as making hypertension more difficult to control. All patients should spend time with the dietician and be encouraged to adopt healthy eating guidelines. In addition to dietary advice, transplant recipients need education about the risks of contaminated food, for example with listeria, campylobacter, and cryptosporidium.

Additional therapy

The medical complications of renal transplantation are so numerous that many recipients will require many different drugs. The regimen often become intolerable and non-compliance can be a major problem. In the early post-transplant period it is necessary to give prophylaxis with co-trimoxazole, an H_2 antagonist, and possibly a bisphosphonate, as well as an appropriate anti-CMV regime. Patients who are at risk of tuberculosis require isoniazid for the duration of immunosuppression. Hypertension needs aggressive control. In the early post-transplant period there is also the possibility of wasting of magnesium, phosphate, and bicarbonate, each requiring supplements. Uric acid levels may be high and clinical gout may develop requiring either allopurinol or benzbromarone. Long-term management needs to include regular vaccinations (influenza and pneumococcus). To reduce the risks of accelerated vascular disease, aspirins and statins may also be indicated.

In patients with poorly functioning transplants, medical management must include the same measures as would be undertaken in a low clearance clinic for patients expected to start dialysis. Under these circumstances, treatment may include erythropoietin therapy, iron and vitamin supplementation, α-calcidol, and oral phosphate-binders.

Follow-up

With an uncomplicated transplant operation, patients may only be in hospital for about 7 days. Following discharge, patients will need to be seen two or three times a week for the first month, once or twice a week for the second month, and then weekly for the third month. At each visit blood pressure and graft function is checked. Many units undertake weekly CMV surveillance for at least the first 3 months following transplantation. After 3 months, outpatient visits are gradually reduced with patients eventually being reviewed only every 3 to 4 months. Particular attention has to be paid to cardiovascular risk factors, infections, and neoplasia. Ideally, all patients should have an annual dermatological examination and women should have an annual cervical smear and colposcopy if indicated. Bone density should be monitored regularly. Even in an apparently stable transplant, some units perform a renogram every 1 to 2 years to detect deteriorating renal perfusion or an obstruction from an ischaemic ureteric stenosis. Patients at risk of tuberculosis will require a regular chest radiograph. Vaccinations should be kept up to date. Many centres offer an anniversary clinic when these medical complications can be more fully assessed. Accelerated atherosclerosis will lead to early coronary and peripheral vascular disease. Increasingly, renal transplant recipients are being put forward for coronary revascularization procedures, when it is interesting to note that angioplasty alone is less successful in renal patients and should be combined with stenting.

Pregnancy

A successful renal transplant restores fertility and pregnancy with normal vaginal delivery (unless there are obstetric indications for caesarean section) is possible. Most recommend that pregnancy is not embarked upon in the first year or if the serum creatinine is above 150 μmol/l or proteinuria greater than 2 g/day. Many successful pregnancies have been undertaken with renal function worse than this, but the risks are greater.

There is little evidence that immunosuppression with prednisolone, azathioprine, and cyclosporin A has a significant adverse effect on the fetus. Cyclosporin A may be associated with intrauterine growth retardation and prednisolone may produce neonatal adrenal suppression. Experience with tacrolimus is limited but is probably broadly similar to cyclosporin A. Pregnancy with mycophenolate mofetil is contraindicated. There is an increased risk of hypertension and pre-eclampsia in renal transplant recipients. Care has to be taken with the choice of antihypertensive agent. During delivery, intravenous fluid should be given and great care taken to avoid episodes of hypovolaemia and hypotension. It is usual to give an extra dose of steroid during the delivery, for instance 100 mg of intravenous hydrocortisone, and to increase oral prednisolone for a few days afterwards.

Further reading

General

Morris PJ (1994). *Kidney transplantation: principles and practice*, 4th edn. WB Saunders Co., Philadelphia.

Rubin RH, Young LS, eds (1994). *Clinical approach to infection in the compromised host*, 3rd edn. Plenum Medical Book Co., New York.

Suthanthiran M, Strom TB (1994). Renal transplantation. *New England Journal of Medicine* **331**, 365–76.

Infections

Brennan DC, Garlock KA, Lippmann BA (1997). Control of cytomegalovirus-associated morbidity in renal transplant patients using intensive monitoring and either pre-emptive or deferred therapy. *Journal of the American Society of Nephrology* **8**, 118–25.

Jassal SV, Roscoe JM, Zaltzman JS (1998). Clinical practice guidelines: prevention of cytomegalovirus disease after transplantation. *Journal of the American Society of Nephrology* **9**, 1697–708.

Lowance D *et al.* (1999). Valacyclovir for the prevention of cytomegalovirus disease after renal transplantation. *New England Journal of Medicine* **340**, 1462–70.

Lufft V *et al.* (1996). Incidence of *Pneumocystis carinii* pneumonia after renal transplantation: impact of immunosuppression. *Transplantation* **62**, 421–3.

Paya CV (1993). Fungal infections in solid organ transplantation. *Clinical Infectious Diseases* **16**, 677–88.

Sternberg RI *et al.* (1993). Utility of bronchoalveolar lavage in assessing pneumonia in immunosuppressed renal transplant patients. *American Journal of Medicine* **95**, 358–64.

Tumours

Alloub MI *et al.* (1989). Human papillomavirus infection and cervical intraepithelial neoplasia in women with renal allografts. *British Medical Journal* **298**, 153–6.

Barr BBB *et al.* (1989). Human papilloma virus infection and skin cancer in renal allograft recipients. *Lancet* **i**, 124–8.

Bouwes-Bavinck JN *et al.* (1995). Prevention of skin cancer and reduction of keratotic skin lesions during acitretin therapy in renal transplant recipients: a double-blind placebo-controlled study. *Journal of Clinical Oncology* **13**, 1933–8.

Bouwes-Bavinck JN *et al.* (1996). The risk of skin cancer in renal transplant recipients in Queensland, Australia. *Transplantation* **61**, 715–21.

Gotti E, Remuzzi G (1997). Post-transplant Kaposi's sarcoma. *Journal of the American Society of Nephrology* **8**, 130–7.

Opelz G *et al.* (1995). Analysis of non-Hodgkin's lymphomas in organ transplant recipients. *Transplant Reviews* **9**, 231–40.

Penn I (1986). Cancers of the anogenital region in renal transplant recipients. *Cancer* **58**, 611–16.

Penn I (1994). The problems of cancer in organ transplant recipients: an overview. *Transplantation Science* **4**, 23–31.

Rook AH *et al.* (1995). Beneficial effect of low-dose systemic retinoid in combination with topical tretinoin for the treatment and prophylaxis of pre-malignant and malignant skin lesions in renal transplant recipients. *Transplantation* **59**, 179.

Shah KV (1997). Human papillomavirus and anogenital cancers. *New England Journal of Medicine* **337**, 1386–8.

Cardiovascular complications

Arnadottir M, Berg AL (1997). Treatment of hyperlipidaemia in renal transplant recipients. *Transplantation* **63**, 339–45.

Curtis JJ (1991). Distinguishing the causes of post-transplant hypertension. *Pediatric Nephrology* **5**, 108–11.

Fervenza *et al.* (1999). Renal artery stenosis in kidney transplants. *American Journal of Kidney Disease* **31**, 142–8.

Kaisiske BL *et al.* (1996). Cardiovascular disease after renal transplantation. *Journal of the American Society of Nephrology* **7**, 158–65.

Liver disease

Rao KV, Anderson WR (1992). Liver disease after transplantation. *American Journal of Kidney Disease* **19**, 496–501.

Muscoskeletal complications

Julian BA, Quarles LD, Nieman KMW (1992). Musculoskeletal complications after renal transplantation: pathogenesis and treatment. *American Journal of Kidney Disease* **19**, 99–120.

Torregrosa JV, Campistol JM (1999). Reflex sympathetic dystrophy syndrome in renal transplant patients: a mysterious and misdiagnosed entity. *Nephology, Dialysis, Transplantation* **14**, 1364–5.

Haematological complications

Gaston RS, Julian BA, Curtis JJ (1994). Post-transplant erythrocytosis: an enigma revisited. *American Journal of Kidney Disease* **24**, 1–11.

Grupp C *et al.* (1998). Haemolytic uraemic syndrome (HUS) during treatment with cyclosporin A after renal transplantation—is tacrolimus the answer? *Nephrology, Dialysis, Transplantation* **13**, 1629–31.

Diabetes mellitus

Hariharan S *et al.* (1996). Diabetic nephropathy after renal transplantation. *Transplantation* **62**, 632–5.

Vesco L *et al.* (1996). Diabetes mellitus after renal transplantation. *Transplantation* **61**, 1475–8.

Weir MR, Fink JC (1999). Risks for post-transplant diabetes mellitus with current immunosuppressive medications. *American Journal of Kidney Diseases* **34**, 1–13.

Immunosuppression

Denton MD, Magee CC, Sayegh MH (1999). Immunosuppressive strategies in transplantation. *Lancet* **353**, 1083–91.

First MR (1997). An update on new immunosuppressive drugs undergoing preclinical and clinical trials: potential applications in organ transplantations. *American Journal of Kidney Diseases* **29**, 303–17.

Gummert JF, Ikonen T, Morris RE (1999). Newer immunosuppressive drugs: a review. *Journal of the American Society of Nephrology* **10**, 1366–80.

Koene RAP, Hilbrands LB (1998). Choices of long-term immunosuppression in the renal transplantation: balancing the benefits and risks. *Nephology, Dialysis, Transplantation* **13**, 844–6.

Paul LC, Zaltzman J, Cardiella CJ (1995). Prophylactic anti-lymphocyte antibody therapy in kidney transplantation: quo vadis? *Transplant Review* **9**, 200–6.

Chronic allograft nephropathy

Halloran PF, Melk A, Barth C (1999). Rethinking chronic allograft nephropathy: the concept of accelerated senescence. *Journal of the American Society of Nephrology* **10**, 167–81.

Paul LC (1999). Chronic allograft nephropathy. *Kidney International* **56**, 783–93.

Terasaki PI *et al.* (1994). The hyperfiltration hypothesis in human renal transplantation. *Transplantation* **57**, 1450–4.

Pregnancy

Ehrich JHH *et al.* (1996). Repeated successful pregnancies after kidney transplantation in 102 women (report by the EDTA Registry). *Nephrology, Dialysis, Transplantation* **11**, 1314–17.

Recurrance of original disease

Mathew TH (1988). Recurrence of disease following renal transplantation. *American Journal of Kidney Disease* **12**, 85–96.

Outcome

Fischel RJ *et al.* (1991). Long term outlook for renal transplants recipients with 1-year function. *Transplantation* **51**, 118–22.

Hirata M *et al.* (1996). Patient death after renal transplantation: an analysis of its role in graft outcome. *Transplantation* **61**, 1479–83.

Laupacis A *et al.* (1996). A study of the quality of life and cost-utility of renal transplantation. *Kidney International* **50**, 235–42.

Morris PJ *et al.* (1999). Analysis of factors that affect outcome of primary cadaveric renal transplantation in the UK. *Lancet* **354**, 1147–52.

Pratshke J *et al.* (1999). Brain death and its influence on donor organ quality and outcome after transplantation. *Transplantation* **67**, 343–8.

20.7 Glomerular diseases

20.7.1 The glomerulus and glomerular injury

John Savill

Introduction

Patients with glomerular injury consequent upon diverse and often poorly understood stimuli present with remarkably stereotyped clinical features (see Section 20.3). Nevertheless, when investigated by percutaneous renal biopsy, clinically similar patients may exhibit an array of histopathological types of glomerular disease that can bewilder all but the most experienced of clinicians. The patterns of glomerular disease that the skilled histopathologist can recognize will continue to be extremely useful to clinicians. However, recent advances in glomerular cell biology point to a complementary approach toward understanding the pathogenesis and present or future treatment of glomerular disorders. Thus, apparently complex histopathological changes can be viewed as the sum of a small number of pathological alterations in the cell biology of the glomerulus. In this scheme, it is apparent that three potentially reversible cellular processes are active to varying degrees in most forms of glomerulonephritis: (1) leucocyte infiltration; (2) changes in the number, size, or phenotype of resident glomerular cells; and (3) changes in the amount and composition of extracellular matrix, which includes the specialized glomerular basement membrane. Furthermore, although three further processes—(4) crescent formation, (5) glomerular capillary thrombosis, and (6) glomerular sclerosis—may be viewed as irreversible events that are best prevented, there is some hope that resolution of such processes and subsequent repair could be encouraged. Consequently, a basic knowledge of the cellular processes that constitute a threat to long-term function in glomerular disease may not only assist in the understanding of complex glomerular pathologies but will also prepare the contemporary clinician for implementing future therapies targeted at key pathological processes.

Key cellular processes in glomerular disease

Leucocyte infiltration

Accumulation of potentially injurious leucocytes is a hallmark of severe inflammatory glomerular injury (Fig. 1).

Granulocytes (usually neutrophils, but sometimes eosinophils) represent the 'rapid response force' of the inflammatory response and are prominent in severe acute inflammatory conditions such as ANCA-positive vasculitis (**ANCA**, antineutrophil cytoplasmic antibody). Granulocytes threaten to exacerbate injury by generating reactive oxygen species and releasing granules yielding toxic cationic proteins, potent degradative enzymes, and monocyte chemoattractants. However, they are also present in self-limited conditions such as poststreptococcal glomerulonephritis, suggesting that their presence does not *per se* direct progressive glomerular injury. Indeed, this shows that granulocytes can be removed safely from inflamed glomeruli. Neutrophils accumulating in the capillary lumen can return to the circulation, while some extravasated cells reaching Bowman's space are flushed out in the urine. Furthermore, neutrophils 'trapped' in the mesangium or in partially occluded glomerular capillaries are cleared away by undergoing constitutive cell death by apoptosis. In turn this leads to anti-inflammatory engulfment of the intact dying cells by phagocytic cells, including macrophages and mesangial cells, with suppression of the phagocyte synthesis of inflammatory mediators by mechanisms involving local release of the anti-inflammatory cytokine transforming growth factor-β1 (**TGF-β1**).

If granulocytes are the 'storm-troopers' of inflammatory responses to tissue injury, then monocyte/macrophages are the 'regimental officers' controlling the attack. Time-course studies in animal models and in human disease emphasize that blood monocytes are recruited within a few hours of neutrophil sequestration in the injured glomerulus. These monocytes mature, by poorly understood mechanisms, into macrophages, which can be very easily overlooked unless detected by specific immunostaining. This confirms abundant macrophage infiltration in many different types of glomerular injury. There is persuasive evidence that macrophages can, depending on circumstances, either exacerbate injury or promote repair.

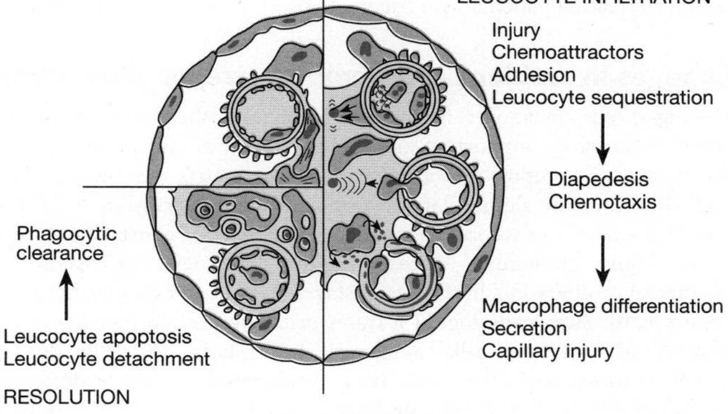

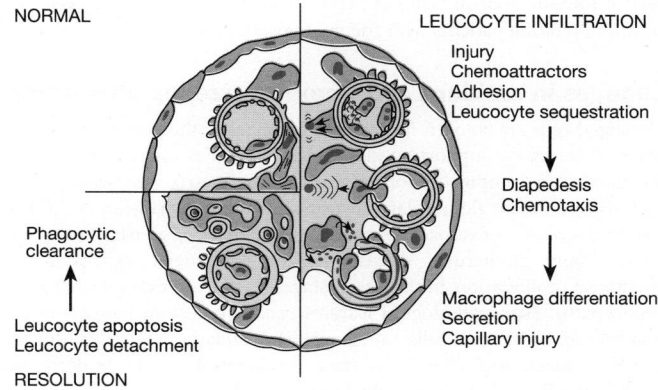

Fig. 1 Leucocyte infiltration in glomerular injury. Generation of chemoattractants and other mediators (consequent upon, for example, immunological injury), causes endothelial cells to express adhesion molecules to which leucocytes bind, these commonly then being sequestered in capillary lumens. However, leucocytes may also migrate towards areas with a high concentration of chemoattractants (chemotaxis), crossing the basement membrane by diapedesis. Monocytes can mature into secretory macrophages, which may further exacerbate capillary injury. Resolution can occur, due to detachment of sequestered leucocytes and apoptosis of leucocytes that have left the bloodstream, the latter leading to anti-inflammatory phagocytic clearance of apoptotic leucocytes.

The microenvironment in which macrophages mature, particularly the cytokines present, can irreversibly 'programme' the cells to adopt particular phenotypes. Thus interferon-gamma (**IFN-γ**) programmes macrophages to adopt an 'activated/inflammatory' phenotype—which, for example, threatens neighbouring cells with injury or death induced by an enhanced macrophage release of nitric oxide, consequent upon IFN-γ-directed induction of the inducible nitric oxide synthase (**iNOS**, also known as **NOS2**). However, if, for example, interleukin-4 (**IL-4**) predominates, macrophages adopt a 'reparative' phenotype in which TGF-β1 secretion will promote extracellular matrix deposition (see below).

T (thymic type) lymphocytes can also infiltrate injured glomeruli, although their presence usually indicates severe damage and a high risk of progression to scarring. T cells have a reciprocal relationship with macrophages—each can tell the other what to do. For example, T cells can summon macrophages to inflamed sites, while macrophage-lineage cells can direct T-cell behaviour by the presentation of antigens on MHC molecules, in the context of other macrophage surface molecules and macrophage-secreted cytokines that help to activate T cells. CD8-positive cytotoxic T cells and their close cousins, the natural killer (**NK**) cells, can injure or kill glomerular cells presenting antigen from infectious or other sources. Helper, CD4-positive T cells are probably important in orchestrating autoimmune glomerular injury, especially where this depends upon autoantibody production by distant B lymphocytes, as in Goodpasture's disease. While T cells may meet their fate by undergoing apoptosis at inflamed sites, these cells are typically 'visitors' circulating through the glomerulus from the blood to the lymphatics, unwanted T cells dying in lymph nodes.

Therapeutic approaches

Glucocorticoids reduce leucocyte infiltration of inflamed tissue by multiple mechanisms, including inhibition of recruitment, promotion of deletion by apoptosis (eosinophils and lymphocytes), and increased phagocyte clearance of dying leucocytes. Immunosuppressive agents such as cyclophosphamide may also reduce leucocyte infiltration, in part by diminishing circulating leucocyte numbers. New therapies in development aim: to inhibit adhesion molecules involved in leucocyte recruitment; to block the action of chemoattractants, such as chemokines or complement fragments; or to inhibit the upregulation of both adhesion molecules and chemoattractants by blocking the action of 'master' proinflammatory cytokines such as tumour necrosis factor-α (**TNF-α**), an approach that has been successful in treating patients with rheumatoid arthritis.

Changes in resident cell number, size, or phenotype

Mesangial cells are smooth muscle-like pericytes of the glomerulus, regulating structure by supporting glomerular capillaries and by modulating the amount or composition of the extracellular matrix (see below). They may also modulate glomerular function, controlling perfusion and filtration by the release of vasoactive mediators and effecting constriction/relaxation. Many glomerular diseases exhibit 'mesangial expansion' or 'mesangial proliferation' in their early stages (Fig. 2), an example being IgA nephropathy. Such pathological features usually reflect an increase in the number of mesangial cells—mesangial hyperplasia, which is due to increased mesangial cell mitosis (true proliferation)—and/or decreased mesangial cell death. Interestingly, however, diabetic nephropathy appears to exhibit a predominant increase in mesangial cell size (hypertrophy) rather than number. Nevertheless, both hyperplasia and hypertrophy involve the activation of intracellular regulatory proteins called cyclin-dependent kinases. In hyperplasia, these cyclin-dependent kinases drive mesangial cells through the cell cycle so that they divide and increase in number, while in hypertrophy such progression does not occur but the cell grows in size. These intracellular controls on mesangial cell number and size are subject to exquisite external controls. Thus, increases in mesangial cell number can be driven by platelet-derived growth factor (**PDGF**) and basic fibroblastic growth factor (**bFGF**). Both mesangial cell hyperplasia

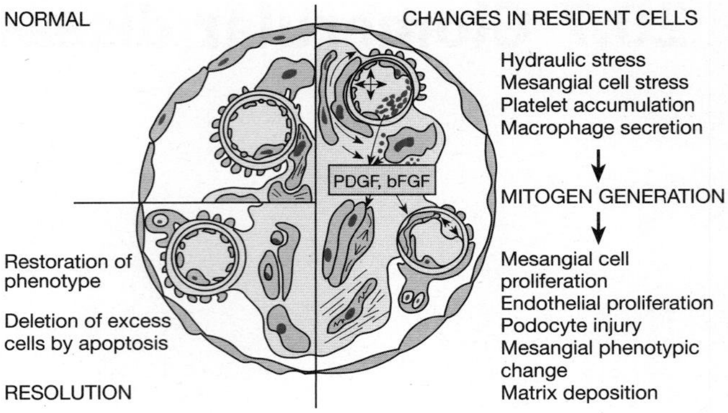

Fig. 2 Resident cell changes in glomerular injury. Hydraulic stress upon mesangial cells (as may occur in glomerular hypertension), secretory macrophages, and recruited blood platelets may all release mitogens such as PDGF (platelet-derived growth factor) or bFGF (basic fibroblastic growth factor). These trigger the proliferation of mesangial and endothelial cells and the phenotypic change seen in these and epithelial cells (podocytes). Such changes are associated with alterations in matrix (see Fig. 3). Resolution involves the deletion of excess resident cells by apoptosis and the restoration of the resident cell phenotype.

and hypertrophy threaten later progression to scarring, this is because these changes in mesangial cell number and size are usually accompanied by the adoption of an abnormal myofibroblast-like phenotype characterized by the expression of α-smooth muscle actin. Such myofibroblast-like mesangial cells are remarkably similar to skin myofibroblasts, which mediate both wound repair and contraction/closure and whose presence is strongly associated with the deposition of excess, abnormal extracellular matrix (see below).

Glomerular endothelial cells seem to obey similar 'rules' as mesangial cells. They undergo true proliferation (i.e. hyperplasia) in poststreptococcal and other forms of glomerular injury, although whether this has the ominous implications of a mesangial cell increase is unclear. By contrast, glomerular epithelial cells or podocytes do not readily undergo proliferation in humans after birth: although they can respond to injury by synthesizing DNA and even becoming binucleate, experimental work in rodents emphasizes that adult podocytes rarely divide. Indeed, it is important to emphasize that the number of glomerular resident cells can also decline undesirably, especially when acute glomerular injury progresses to glomerular sclerosis or scarring (see below).

Therapeutic approaches

It has not been established whether any current therapies specifically modulate changes in the resident cell number, size, or phenotype. However, because such changes may be triggered by mechanical cellular stress resulting from an increased glomerular perfusion pressure, some of the beneficial effects of antihypertensive agents, especially angiotensin-converting enzyme (**ACE**) inhibitors and angiotensin II blockers, may prove to be mediated by effects on resident cells. New therapies in development include drugs that specifically inhibit the cyclin-dependent kinases, which may mediate undesirable glomerular cell hyperplasia and/or hypertrophy.

Increased deposition of abnormal extracellular matrix

The normal glomerular extracellular matrix is a network of proteins and proteoglycans (such as heparan sulphate proteoglycan) of critical importance in regulating the survival and properties of glomerular cells, in addition to supporting the glomerular structure. The accumulation of extracellular matrix (**ECM**) is a prominent feature of most glomerular diseases (Fig. 3) and reflects the combined effects of an increased secretion of matrix components and tissue inhibitors of metalloproteinases (**TIMPs**)

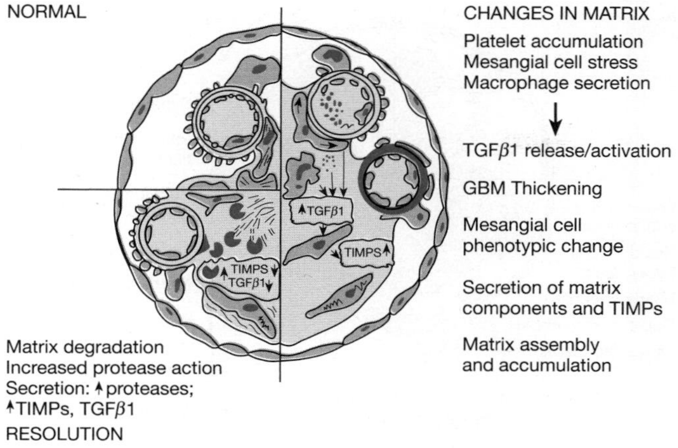

Fig. 3 Extracellular matrix changes in glomerular injury. Mesangial cells (stressed by, for example, hydraulic stimuli), secretory macrophages, and recruited platelets may all release TGF-β1 that is locally activated. In turn, this fibroblastic cytokine causes mesangial cells to adopt a myofibroblastic phenotype, secreting both matrix components and TIMPs, with a net accumulation of abnormal matrix. Similar mechanisms, probably also impinging on endothelial cells, can cause thickening of the glomerular basement membrane (**GBM**). Resolution requires a switch in glomerular cell secretion so that proteases (depicted as 'pacmen') predominate over TIMPs, leading to beneficial matrix degradation.

from glomerular cells. The increased deposition of ECM is thus achieved both by laying down new matrix and preventing the degradation of new or existing ECM. Furthermore, the protein composition of ECM is abnormal in injured glomeruli: there is an accumulation of 'interstitial' type I and type III collagens and of plasma-type fibronectin, alongside an increase in normal constituents such as laminin and type IV collagen. Indeed, there is now a growing body of data to demonstrate that potentially deleterious alterations in glomerular ECM may be dependent upon an excess local secretion (or action) of the cytokine TGF-β1. The propensity of TGF-β1 to promote an undesirable accumulation of ECM is thought to represent the 'dark side' of mechanisms that evolved to promote wound-healing. For example, the accumulation of abnormal ECM is a prominent feature of diabetic nephropathy and may be so exuberant as to form Kimmelstiel–Wilson nodules, constituting a grave threat of progression to scarring. However, in keeping with the dynamic balance between synthesis and degradation that underlies ECM accumulation, abnormal glomerular ECM can be remodelled in self-limited disorders such as some cases of IgA nephropathy.

The general principles of matrix changes in glomerular injury are also evident in the most specialized compartment of the glomerular ECM, the glomerular basement membrane (**GBM**). Thus, thickening of the GBM in cases of diabetic nephropathy largely reflects the accumulation of normal constituents, while grossly similar changes can be caused by the deposition of abnormal proteins, such as amyloid. Examination under polarized light, special stains, immunofluorescence, or electron microscopy may be required to reveal the deposition of abnormal proteins, which can also include immune deposits or fibrils, or intrinsic defects such as those of Alport's syndrome.

Therapeutic approaches

There is no unequivocal evidence that currently available treatments directly and specifically effect changes in the glomerular matrix. New therapies in development include agents to inhibit the profibrotic effects of TGF-β1 (which may be particularly useful in diabetic nephropathy) and drugs that target the control of matrix deposition by antagonizing, for example, TIMPs.

Glomerular crescent formation

Glomerular crescents, abnormal masses of cells filling Bowman's space, are a reflection of severe glomerular injury associated with disorders such as vasculitis, systemic lupus erythematosus (**SLE**), and anti-GBM disease. Indeed, scanning electron microscopy studies of crescentic glomerulonephritis have demonstrated holes in the glomerular basement membrane, consistent with the idea that bleeding into Bowman's space and the deposition of fibrin are crucial pathogenetic factors (Fig. 4). Nevertheless, crescents can be viewed as being a special consequence of the three cellular processes described above. First, monocyte/macrophages and sometimes other leucocytes such as lymphocytes frequently infiltrate them. Second, especially in early crescents, there is prominent evidence of an increase in number and change of phenotype in resident cells, that is to say the 'parietal' epithelial cells of Bowman's capsule, which unlike the 'visceral' glomerular epithelial cells (podocytes) undergo true proliferation in crescentic disease. Third, there is deposition of extracellular matrix, which is obviously abnormal in that it should not be present at all. These cellular processes of glomerular crescent formation are worthy of special consideration because they are widely believed to be incompatible with recovery of function, especially when Bowman's capsule has been breached, potentially allowing ingress of myofibroblasts from the locally injured interstitium.

Therapeutic approaches

In some types of crescentic nephritis there is good anecdotal evidence that glucocorticoids/immunosuppressive agents may retard crescent formation by mechanisms likely to include the downregulation of monocyte/macrophage efflux into Bowman's space. Such drugs might also encourage resolution by promoting apoptosis and safe clearance of cells in crescents. Indeed, most nephrologists will have encountered cases of childhood poststreptococcal glomerulonephritis with 100 per cent crescents, which nevertheless exhibit a large degree of resolution, typically in association with immunosuppressive therapy. The fibrin component may be susceptible to anticoagulants/ancrod but new therapies are urgently required. There is

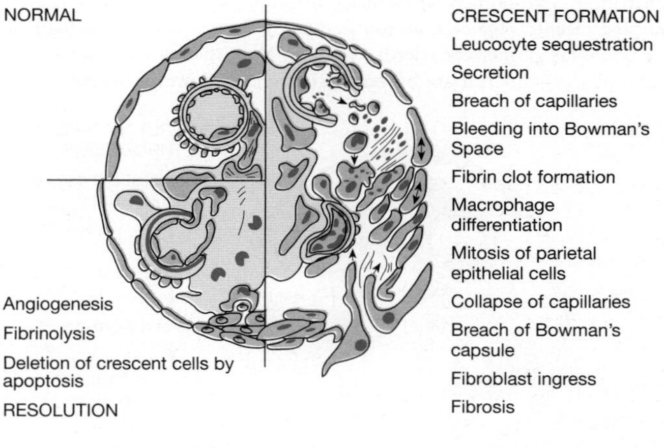

Fig. 4 Crescent formation in severe glomerular injury. Severe glomerular capillary injury, most likely mediated by leucocyte-derived reactive oxygen species and injurious proteins, causes breaches in capillary walls. Bleeding into Bowman's space, with formation of fibrin clot, then ensues. Blood monocytes mature into macrophages and parietal epithelial cells of Bowman's capsule may proliferate. The resultant crescent may compress capillaries, causing their collapse and occlusion, especially when injury is sufficiently severe to allow ingress of fibroblasts from the periglomerular space. It seems that glomerular fibrosis and loss is the rule. However, resolution may occur rarely, for example in poststreptococcal glomerulonephritis. Fibrinolysis, deletion of crescent cells by apoptosis, and repair of damaged capillary networks by angiogenesis may all play a role.

active interest in the antagonism of cytokines/chemokines and in the blockade of leucocyte/endothelial adhesion molecules, but new insights into disease mechanisms are needed.

Glomerular capillary thrombosis

Thrombotic occlusion of glomerular capillaries is another manifestation of severe injury, consequent upon disorders such as systemic vasculitis, SLE, malignant hypertension, and radiation nephritis. Formation of platelet thrombi in glomeruli often reflects loss/retraction of glomerular endothelial cells with exposure to blood elements of the glomerular basement membrane (Fig. 5). Indeed, thrombosis often goes hand in hand with segmental necrosis of glomeruli. In such circumstances there would appear to be little prospect of successful repair and scarring of the affected lobule/glomerulus. However, all may not be lost: the astonishing capacity of mesangial cell precursors to repopulate glomeruli completely denuded of mesangial cells by experimental antibody-mediated injury is a testament to the capacity that the glomerulus may have—under suitable circumstances—to 'rebuild' itself. In keeping with such observations, recent data emphasize that angiogenesis, the growth of new blood vessels, can and does occur in the glomerular response to injury, under the direction of cytokines such as vascular endothelial growth factor (**VEGF**). This raises the possibility that such blood vessel growth could replace occluded, destroyed glomerular capillaries.

Therapeutic approaches

Clinicians dealing with glomerular capillary thrombosis frequently consider using anticoagulants/antiplatelet drugs, and growing experience of using thrombolytic agents in other vascular territories may lead to their increased use in the hope of recanalizing occluded vessels. New therapies under active consideration are likely to concentrate on promoting recovery, but selective stimulation of angiogenesis capable of leading to glomerular repair is a distant prospect.

Glomerular scarring/sclerosis

Leucocyte infiltration, increased glomerular resident cell number/size, increased deposition of abnormal extracellular matrix, glomerular crescent formation, and glomerular capillary thrombosis may all be reversible to varying extents. However, all too frequently these cellular pathologies set the scene for glomerular sclerosis (Fig. 6). Nevertheless, although scarred, functionless glomeruli are beyond resurrection. However, recent insights into the pathogenesis of glomerular sclerosis offer some prospect of prevention and are therefore worthy of consideration.

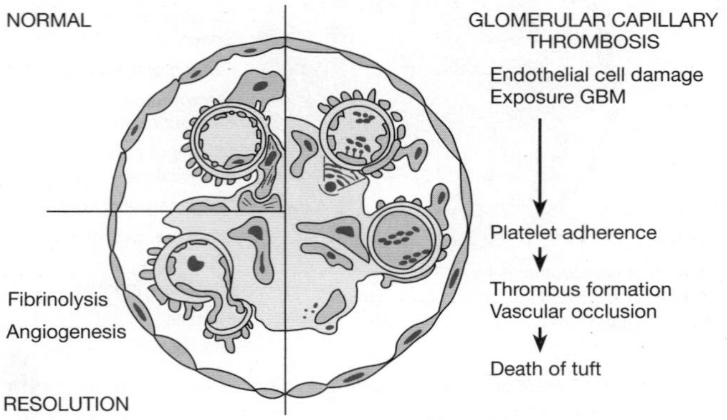

Fig. 5 Glomerular capillary thrombosis. Platelet adherence to the glomerular capillary may reflect mediator generation within the glomerulus, causing endothelial cell activation with adhesion molecule expression, or endothelial cell retraction leading to GBM exposure. Endothelial cells may also be damaged by bloodborne elements or ischaemia–reperfusion injury, as may occur in sickle cell disease. Tufts in which glomerular capillaries are occluded by thrombosis usually die by ischaemic necrosis. However, resolution is possible, since fibrinolysis can result in the recanalization of capillaries, which may be repaired by angiogenesis.

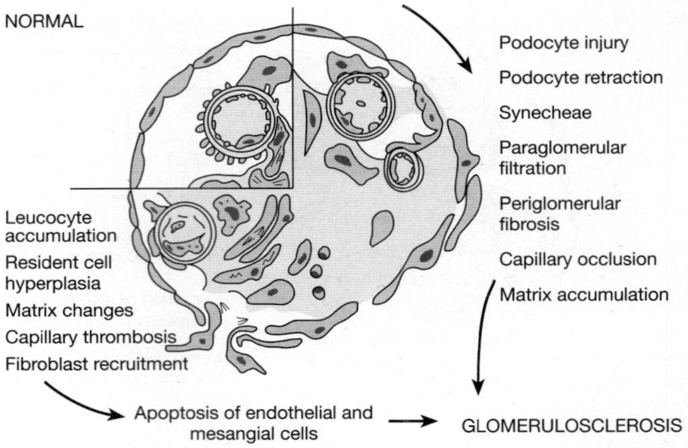

Fig. 6 Two pathways to glomerulosclerosis. At the bottom left, leucocyte accumulation, resident cell hyperplasia, matrix changes, capillary thrombosis, and recruitment of extraglomerular fibroblasts set up a situation in which progressive and unscheduled apoptosis of mesangial and endothelial cells leads to a featureless, non-functioning glomerular scar. This endstage glomerular lesion may also arise because of podocyte injury and retraction (top right), as may occur in HIV infection. 'Naked' GBM then adheres to Bowman's capsule because of local matrix deposition. As the adhesion enlarges, glomerular filtration may occur directly into the paraglomerular space (i.e. 'under' Bowman's capsule) causing gross periglomerular fibrosis and capillary occlusion, with ultimate progression to functionless scarring.

Although an increased number of cells in glomeruli (reflecting leucocyte infiltration and resident cell hyperplasia) characterizes potentially progressive glomerulonephritis, the scarred glomerulus is striking for its lack of cells, being replaced by featureless, acellular matrix. Growing evidence points to the undesirable deletion of resident glomerular cells via unscheduled apoptosis as a final common pathway in glomerular sclerosis. The mechanisms responsible are likely to be complex, since a wide range of possible apoptotic stimuli is likely to occur in injured glomeruli, but the potential consequences of glomerular cell loss are rather easier to appreciate. For example, loss of endothelial cells from glomeruli, as observed in models of progressive glomerular injury, obviously poses a hazard for the disruption of the glomerular blood supply, structure, and function. Such unscheduled loss may be prevented by the antiapoptotic properties of cytokine survival factors. Thus, recent studies suggest that the 165 amino acid isoform of VEGF is of central importance for endothelial cell survival in glomerular injury, while insulin-like growth factor-1 (**IGF-1**) may play a similar role in retarding mesangial cell apoptosis, emphasizing that glomerular cell loss might be preventable.

Recent work, based on elegant morphological studies by Kriz and colleagues, has emphasized the subtle and destabilizing effects of unscheduled glomerular cell loss upon the biomechanics of a delicate multicellular structure, that must contain blood at a much greater pressure than is usual in capillary networks. Loss of supporting mesangial cells is associated with glomerular capillary dilatation, which exerts deleterious mechanical stress upon both glomerular endothelial and epithelial cells, threatening their unscheduled death. Loss of podocytes (see Fig. 6) may be particularly dangerous because of the limited capacity of glomerular epithelial cells for mitosis; rather like precious neurones, if podocytes die they may not be replaced. The consequences of such loss include the formation of tuft adhesions to Bowman's capsule, which may allow abnormal filtration into the interstitium and promote periglomerular fibrosis, the adhesion propagating around an ever-more constricted glomerular tuft. This model may be particularly pertinent to the pathogenesis of focal segmental glomerulosclerosis (**FSGS**). Indeed, the model also predicts the course of the 'collapsing' form of FSGS seen in human immunodeficiency virus (HIV) infection, in which apparent podocyte dedifferentiation seems to deny the glomerulus an essential podocyte-mediated force that counterbalances mesangial cell-mediated constriction of the glomerulus.

Therapeutic approaches

All clinicians employ antihypertensives in the hope of retarding the progression of glomerular scarring, perhaps reducing mechanical stresses that trigger undesirable apoptosis. However, dietary protein restriction has yet to achieve widespread use, despite some encouraging trial evidence and animal data that this reduces potentially harmful glomerular hyperfiltration. New therapies are likely to concentrate on dealing with the cellular pathologies described above in the hope of preventing progression. Nevertheless, the advent of stem-cell therapies and tissue engineering raises the very distant prospect of growing replacement tissue/organs in the laboratory.

Conclusions

When confronted by apparently complex glomerular histopathological changes, it may be helpful to think of the six cellular pathologies described above. Although glomerular histopathology can provide extremely useful prognostic information, considering the cellular pathologies at the root of the problem may help the clinician address the primary concern as to whether the glomerular injury is likely to be amenable to treatment. This will be especially important as new therapies that target pathological cellular processes become available.

Further reading

Kriz W, Lemley KV (1999). The role of the podocyte in glomerulosclerosis. *Current Opinion in Nephrology and Hypertension* **8**, 489–97.

Preisig P (1999). What makes cells grow larger and how do they do it? Renal hypertrophy revisited. *Experimental Nephrology* **7**, 273–83.

Savill J (1999). Regulation of glomerular cell number by apoptosis. *Kidney International* **56**, 1216–22.

Savill J, Rees AJ (1998). Mechanisms of glomerular inflammation. In: Davison AM, *et al*., eds. *Oxford textbook of clinical nephrology*, 2nd edn, pp 403–40. Oxford University Press, Oxford.

Shankland S, Al'Douahji M (1999). Cell cycle regulatory proteins in glomerular disease. *Experimental Nephrology* **7**, 207–11.

20.7.2 IgA nephropathy and Henoch–Schönlein purpura

John Feehally

Introduction and definitions

IgA nephropathy

IgA nephropathy (**IgAN**) is the commonest pattern of glomerulonephritis identified in areas of the world where renal biopsy is frequently performed. It was first described by Berger in 1968 and at one time was known as Berger's disease. It is defined by IgA deposition in the glomerular mesangium, accompanied by a mesangial proliferative glomerulonephritis which may vary greatly in severity. Although recurrent macroscopic haematuria is the hallmark of the disease, the old term 'benign recurrent haematuria' is a discredited misnomer since it is now clear that IgAN is an important cause of endstage renal failure (**ESRF**).

Henoch–Schönlein purpura

Henoch–Schönlein purpura (**HSP**) is a somewhat misleading historical term. The purpuric rash is a cutaneous vasculitis (Plate 1), and HSP is a small-vessel systemic vasculitis characterized by IgA deposition in affected blood vessels. The renal lesion (HSP nephritis) is a mesangial proliferative glomerulonephritis, usually indistinguishable from IgAN.

Aetiology and pathogenesis

Mechanism of mesangial IgA deposition

Mesangial proliferative glomerulonephritis, such as is seen in IgAN and HSP nephritis, may be the consequence of immune complex deposition, either due to trapping of circulating IgA immune complexes or the formation of complexes *in situ* by the reaction of IgA with antigen that has already been deposited. No exogenous antigen has consistently been identified in the mesangial deposits in IgAN, which may indicate that the IgA complexes are a common response to different antigens, or that the initiating antigen has disappeared by the time of the renal biopsy. Alternatively, the IgA may be deposited by some mechanism independent of classical antigen–antibody interactions, such as a physicochemical abnormality of the IgA.

The frequent recurrence of both IgAN and HSP nephritis after renal transplantation strongly suggests that the abnormality resides in the host IgA immune system. The mesangial IgA deposits are polymeric IgA1 (pIgA1). Most pIgA is synthesized in the mucosa, and the clinical association of macroscopic haematuria with mucosal infection originally led to the assumption that an exaggerated mucosal IgA response resulted in mesangial IgA deposition. However, IgA production is downregulated in the mucosal immune system and upregulated in the bone marrow, and exaggerated IgA1 responses to immunization in these patients are marrow rather than mucosally derived.

There is increasing evidence of abnormal glycosylation of both serum and mesangial IgA1 in patients with IgAN and HSP nephritis. The glycosylation abnormality may favour the development of immune complexes or may directly provoke mesangial deposition, but these putative mechanisms have not yet been further defined.

Progression of IgA nephropathy

IgA deposition may occur in many patients with mild disease with little mesangial injury. What decides the prognosis in any individual is the extent to which IgA deposition is followed by mesangial proliferation, inflammation, and scarring. There is nothing to suggest that these subsequent mechanisms of damage and scarring are unique to IgAN, rather they are generic to many forms of glomerulonephritis.

Relationship of IgAN and HSP

There is much indirect evidence to suggest a close relationship between IgAN and HSP. Monozygotic twins have been described, one developing IgAN and the other HSP at the same time. HSP developing on a background of proven IgAN has been described in both adults and children. Many abnormalities of the IgA immune system, including abnormal IgA1 glycosylation, have been described in both conditions. IgAN is increasingly thought of as 'HSP without the rash'. Why some individuals get a renal-limited disease (IgAN) and others a systemic disease (HSP) is not known.

Epidemiology

IgAN is the commonest glomerulonephritis in countries where renal biopsy is widely used, typically found in 30 per cent of biopsies with primary glomerular disease, but the apparent prevalence varies markedly around the world. It is commoner in the Pacific Rim and Mediterranean countries, less so in North America and Northern Europe. At least part of this apparent difference is explained by variations in the use of urine testing in health screening and varying attitudes to the value of renal biopsy in individuals with isolated haematuria or other minor clinical evidence of renal disease. In Japan, for example, where there is routine urine testing of schoolchildren and employed adults, the threshold for renal biopsy is low, and the reported prevalence of IgAN is high.

There are also important racial differences in susceptibility. IgAN is uncommon in Afro-Caribbeans. It is also less common in Polynesians than Caucasians in Australasia—a particularly striking finding given the exaggerated susceptibility of Polynesians to most forms of renal disease. Despite many studies of potential immunogenetic associations, the genetic basis for such variations in susceptibility to IgAN has not yet been identified. IgAN is occasionally familial, one very large kindred having been described in Kentucky, in the United States; but the great majority of cases are sporadic.

Clinical features

IgA nephropathy

Macroscopic haematuria

IgAN can occur at any age, but the peak age of onset is in the second and third decades of life (Fig. 1). IgAN is three times more common in males than females.

The characteristic clinical picture of recurrent macroscopic haematuria occurs in about 40 to 50 per cent of cases. A child or young adult develops episodes of painless macroscopic haematuria occurring within a day or so of the onset of an upper respiratory tract infection, or occasionally infections of other mucosal or IgA-secreting surfaces such as the gastrointestinal tract, bladder, or breast. The urine may be frankly bloody, but more often is brown (like 'Coca-Cola' or tea without milk), there are no clots passed and it is usually painless, although there may be dull loin ache. The episodes settle spontaneously after 1 to 5 days and may be recurrent, but rarely for more than a year or two. Serum IgA is moderately elevated in 30 per cent of cases but serum complement C3 and C4 levels are normal. Between episodes there will be persistent microscopic haematuria. This presentation does not occur beyond the age of 40 years (Fig. 1).

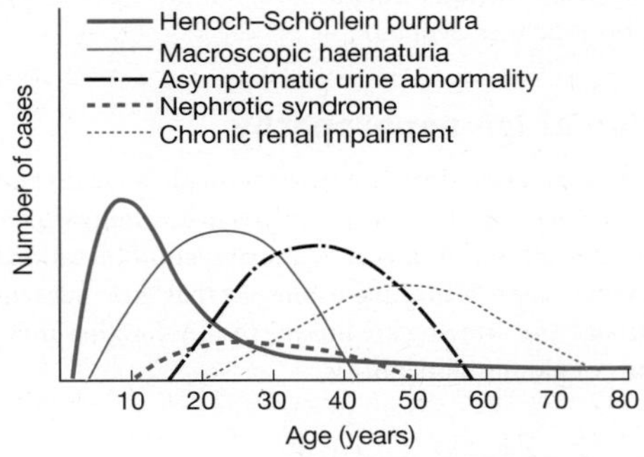

Fig. 1 Clinical presentations of IgA nephropathy (IgAN) and Henoch–Schönlein purpura (HSP) in relation to age at diagnosis. HSP is most common in childhood but may occur at any age. Macroscopic haematuria is very rare in people over the age of 40 years. The importance of an asymptomatic urine abnormality as the presentation of IgAN will depend on attitudes to routine urine testing and renal biopsy. It is uncertain whether those presenting with chronic renal impairment have a disease distinct from that of those presenting at younger ages with macroscopic haematuria. (Reproduced from Johnson RJ, Feehally J. *Comprehensive clinical nephrology.* London: Harcourt Publishers, 1999: 26.3, with permission.)

Asymptomatic haematuria/proteinuria

Some 30 to 40 per cent of cases of IgAN are identified by urine testing—microscopic haematuria may be combined with proteinuria (usually <2 g/24 h). Since this is glomerular haematuria, dysmorphic red cells may be seen on phase-contrast microscopy, but red cell casts are frequently absent in mild disease.

Nephrotic syndrome

Nephrotic syndrome is the presentation in only 5 per cent of patients with IgAN. Very occasionally in children or young adults this appears to be the consequence of coincidental minimal-change nephrotic syndrome: the proteinuria resolves completely with corticosteroid therapy, but haematuria and IgA deposits persist. More commonly, nephrotic syndrome may develop in cases of IgAN with overt mesangial proliferative glomerulonephritis, or it may be a consequence of glomerular scarring in advanced IgAN.

Acute renal failure

Acute renal failure occurs for two reasons in patients with IgAN. Episodes of macroscopic haematuria may produce acute tubular occlusion by red cells in the face of minor glomerular injury. Alternatively, there can be acute severe necrotizing glomerulonephritis with crescent formation—'crescentic IgA nephropathy', which may be the presenting feature or occur on a background of known milder disease.

Chronic renal failure

Patients with IgAN may also present with hypertension and established renal impairment. This often occurs in older patients (Fig. 1). Too little is yet known about the pathogenesis of IgAN to understand whether this is a distinct disease entity, or simply the same disease presenting much later in the absence of macroscopic haematuria or a urine test to bring it to earlier medical attention.

Clinical associations with IgA nephropathy

The commonest secondary cause of IgAN is chronic liver disease, typically alcoholic liver disease, in which it is probable that IgA deposition is a consequence of impaired IgA clearance from the circulation via the liver. Most hepatic IgAN is asymptomatic, and progression to ESRF is unusual. The other best established associations are with coeliac disease and dermatitis herpetiformis; with rheumatoid arthritis, ankylosing spondylitis and Reiter's disease; and with HIV infection. Many other conditions have been reported occasionally with IgAN, but since IgAN is so common it is difficult to know if these are more than chance associations.

Henoch–Schönlein purpura nephritis

HSP can occur at any age but is commonest in the first decade of life (Fig. 1). There is a slight male preponderance. A palpable purpuric rash caused by cutaneous vasculitis is the presenting feature. It has a characteristic extensor surface distribution, with sparing of the trunk and face. Crops of rash, often provoked by intercurrent infection, may continue for some time, but rarely beyond a year from first presentation. Polyarthralgia is common. Abdominal pain, due to gut vasculitis, is usually mild and transient, but severe pain and bloody diarrhoea may develop due to intussusception.

Apart from intussusception the major sequelae of HSP come from renal involvement. Renal disease in HSP is transient in many cases, asymptomatic haematuria or proteinuria disappearing in a few weeks. Of those with persistent evidence of renal disease, asymptomatic haematuria and proteinuria is the commonest clinical state, but 20 per cent will have nephrotic syndrome. Serum IgA is raised in 50 per cent of patients, but complement C3 and C4 levels are normal. Acute renal failure due to crescentic HSP nephritis usually occurs early and is commoner than crescentic IgAN.

Pathology

Immune deposits

IgAN and HSP nephritis are defined by the presence of mesangial IgA detected by immunofluorescence or immunoperoxidase staining (Plate 2). C3 frequently accompanies IgA in the same mesangial distribution, IgG and IgM are less common. Electron microscopy identifies mesangial electron-dense deposits corresponding to the mesangial IgA (Fig. 2).

Light microscopy

Mesangial proliferative glomerulonephritis is the characteristic appearance. Although when haematuria is the only clinical finding, abnormalities seen on light microscopy may be minimal despite florid IgA deposition. Mesangial hypercellularity and matrix expansion are usually global but may be focal and segmental. The hypercellularity is followed by increasing mesangial matrix deposition and eventual sclerosis (Plate 3). In acute renal failure there may be severe glomerular inflammation with crescent formation. In advanced cases there is glomerulosclerosis and corresponding tubular atrophy and interstitial fibrosis, which are entirely non-specific changes of 'endstage kidney'.

Diagnosis and differential diagnosis

IgA nephropathy

By definition, the diagnosis of IgAN requires a renal biopsy: no serological or other laboratory indices provide diagnostic information reliable enough to avoid the need for tissue.

Macroscopic haematuria

Non-glomerular causes of haematuria must always be considered, including renal stones and neoplasia, and excluded where appropriate by urological investigation. While episodic macroscopic haematuria coinciding with an upper respiratory tract infection in children and young adults is the hallmark of IgAN, it is not pathognomonic. Similar episodes can occur with other glomerular diseases, most commonly hereditary nephropathies such as Alport's syndrome and thin membrane nephropathy. The distinction of IgAN from postinfectious (usually post-streptococcal) glomerulonephritis is also important. In post-streptococcal glomerulonephritis there is a 10- to 14-day latency period from the onset of infection and the development of symptomatic renal disease, contrasting with the immediacy of haematuria in IgAN for which the term 'synpharyngitic haematuria' has been coined. The haematuria is usually less heavy in post-streptococcal glomerulonephritis, such that the urine is typically smoky rather than frankly bloody; hypertension, oedema, and other features of the acute nephritic syndrome are usually present. Serological evidence of a recent streptococcal infection (such as antibodies to endostreptosin) and a low C3 level are not found in IgAN.

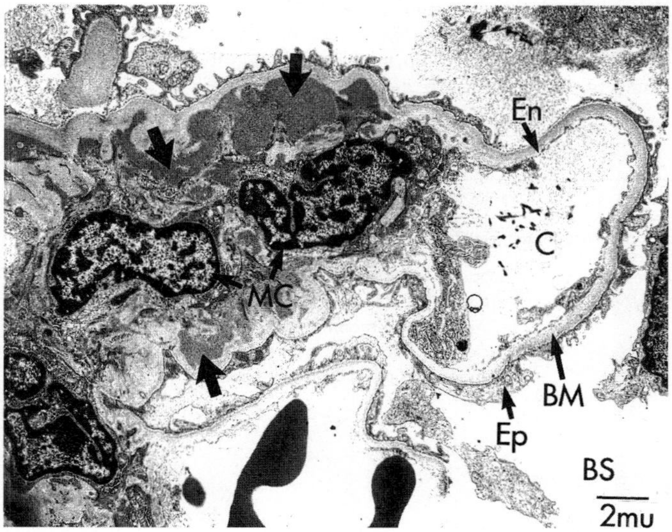

Fig. 2 Electron micrograph of a glomerular capillary loop in IgA nephropathy. Numerous electron-dense deposits representing deposits of IgA (large arrows) are seen within the expanded mesangium (5200 ×). BM, basement membrane; C, capillary lumen; Ep, visceral epithelium; En, fenestrated endothelium; MC, mesangial cell nucleus; BS, Bowman's space.

Nephrotic syndrome

The differential diagnosis when IgAN presents with nephrotic syndrome includes the usual range of glomerular diseases known to cause nephrotic syndrome given the age of the patient.

Chronic renal failure

Advanced IgAN presenting with hypertension, proteinuria, and renal impairment is clinically indistinguishable from many other causes of chronic progressive renal disease. If it is considered important to attempt a precise diagnosis, renal biopsy remains a valuable diagnostic tool since mesangial IgA can often still be identified even when light microscopy shows 'endstage kidney' disease.

Henoch–Schönlein purpura

In children HSP is the commonest form of vasculitis. A clinical diagnosis is often made from the characteristic rash and abdominal pain, but ultimate confirmation requires identification of tissue IgA deposition, which can be found in the vessels of affected skin as well as the kidney. In adults the differential diagnosis is wider, including many other forms of small-vessel vasculitis that must be distinguished on the basis of clinical, serological, and histopathological findings.

Prognosis

IgA nephropathy

Some 30 per cent of children will have a spontaneous clinical remission with complete disappearance of haematuria within 10 years of diagnosis. But IgAN, despite the apparently benign presentation in many cases, is an important cause of endstage renal failure (ESRF). Up to 25 per cent of patients reach ESRF within 20 years of diagnosis. Where a lower risk of ESRF is reported the series will contain larger numbers of patients with mild disease, such as those with isolated microscopic haematuria.

Perhaps unexpectedly, a history of episodic macroscopic haematuria is a favourable prognostic feature. The prognosis for patients who present with microscopic haematuria and minimal proteinuria (<1 g/24 h) is very good, but not perfect. Even in this group up to 5 per cent of patients will develop worsening proteinuria and hypertension during follow-up and are at eventual risk of ESRF. Consequently the long-term follow-up of any patient with biopsy-proven IgAN is mandatory. The risk of progressive renal failure can be predicted by clinical and pathological features at diagnosis (Table 1). These predictive features are not specific to IgAN, but identify the risk of progression in any glomerular disease.

Renal transplantation

Both IgAN and HSP nephritis recur after renal transplantation. Mesangial IgA deposits appear within a few months in 60 per cent of patients with IgAN. Initially this is benign, accompanied by little mesangial injury, but recurrent disease in the long term will contribute to progressive graft loss in a number of patients. However, overall transplant success and graft longevity do not differ in patients with IgAN or HSP from other primary renal disease. The changes in immunosuppressive regimens used to prevent

Table 1 Prognostic markers at presentation in IgA nephropathy

Clinical		
Poor prognosis	*Good prognosis*	*No influence on prognosis*
Increasing age	Recurrent macroscopic haematuria	Gender
Duration of preceding symptoms		Serum IgA level
Severity of proteinuria		
Hypertension		
Renal impairment		
Histopathological		
Poor prognosis		*No influence on prognosis*
Glomerular sclerosis	–	Intensity of IgA deposits
Tubular atrophy		
Interstitial fibrosis		
Vascular wall thickening		
Capillary loop IgA deposits (some reports only)		

rejection over the last two decades have not altered the recurrence rate or its prognosis.

Treatment

IgA nephropathy

Treatment proposals for IgAN are summarized in Table 2. Only in a small minority of patients with IgAN is there any evidence that drug therapy alters the natural history of the disease. Despite being so common among renal diseases, there is still a dearth of well-conducted, prospective, randomized controlled trials in IgAN on which to base therapeutic decisions.

Specific treatment for IgAN would either restrict the formation of relevant pathogenic IgA molecules or prevent their deposition in the mesangium. So little is understood about the pathogenesis of the disease that the prospect for such treatment is still remote.

Haematuria

There is no specific treatment for the great majority of patients with IgAN who have isolated haematuria, with or without low-grade proteinuria (<1 g/24 h).

Microscopic haematuria should merely be observed. Recurrent macroscopic haematuria settles without treatment: there is no role for prophylactic antibiotics, and in any case the majority of precipitating infections are viral. Tonsillectomy may reduce the number of episodes of macroscopic haematuria, but there is no evidence that it reduces the risk of progressive renal failure.

Proteinuria

Those with proteinuria above 1 g/24 h in addition to haematuria have a worse prognosis. Immunosuppressive therapies have been tried, although the frequent recurrence of IgAN in transplanted kidneys when patients are receiving immunosuppressive therapy argues against their value. Short-term, randomized controlled trials of corticosteroids have shown no benefit. However, a 6-month controlled trial of treatment with corticosteroids (prednisolone 0.5 mg/kg per day) showed a significant reduction in proteinuria and a reduced risk of developing renal impairment at 5 years' follow-up. This requires further confirmation: corticosteroid treatment is not presently recommended, except in the rare circumstance where the biopsy suggests coincidental minimal-change nephrotic syndrome which may be fully steroid-responsive. All with proteinuria above 1 g/24 h should receive an ACE inhibitor to minimize protein excretion.

Other immune-modulating drugs have been tried in the treatment of IgAN, including cyclophosphamide, azathioprine, ciclosporin, and pooled human intravenous immunoglobulin. However, there are few properly controlled studies, and for none is there consistent evidence of benefit or an acceptable risk–benefit ratio in the great majority of patients who have indolent slowly progressive disease.

Table 2 Treatment of IgA nephropathy

Microscopic haematuria	No treatment		
Macroscopic haematuria	No treatment	– no indication for prophylactic antibiotics or tonsillectomy	
Macroscopic haematuria + acute renal failure	Biopsy	– *tubular occlusion*	supportive treatment only
		– *crescentic IgAN*	prednisolone 0.5 mg/kg per day reducing to 5–10 mg daily by 3 months cyclophosphamide 2–3 mg/kg per day for 3 months followed by azathioprine 2–3 mg/kg per day
Proteinuria <1 g/24 h	No treatment		
Nephrotic syndrome + minimal change on biopsy	Prednisolone 0.5 mg/kg per day for 8–12 weeks		
All other proteinuria>1 g/24 h	ACE inhibitor		
Hypertension	Control blood pressure to ≤ 130/80 with regimen including ACE inhibitor		
Slowly deteriorating renal function	Consider fish oil (remains unproven)		

Acute renal failure

A renal biopsy is essential when acute renal failure develops in patients with IgAN. If the biopsy shows mild glomerular disease but tubular occlusion with erythrocytes and accompanying acute tubular necrosis, supportive treatment is required while recovery is awaited. If there is crescentic IgAN, a regimen such as that used for renal vasculitis and other forms of crescentic glomerulonephritis should be considered, unless the histological appearances are thought to be advanced and irreversible. Such treatment would typically include oral prednisolone 0.5 mg/kg per day (reducing to a maintenance dose of 5 to 10 mg daily by 3 months), and oral cyclophosphamide 2 to 3 mg/kg per day, the latter being replaced by azathioprine 2 to 3 mg/kg per day after 3 months. There are no randomized controlled trials of these treatments in crescentic IgAN. Although the initial response to treatment is excellent, the medium-term outlook is much less good, and up to 50 per cent of patients may be on long-term dialysis after 12 months.

Progressive renal impairment

Slowly progressive renal impairment due to IgAN requires a management approach common to any form of chronic renal failure. Rigorous control of blood pressure is the one established method of delaying progressive renal failure. Angiotensin-converting enzyme (**ACE**) inhibitors are widely used as first-line therapy for their special role in lessening proteinuria and giving a degree of blood pressure control, although there are no specific prospective studies to prove their additional efficacy in the treatment of IgAN compared to other hypotensive drugs. Fish oil therapy (which provides a supplement of ω-3 fatty acids) has effects likely to impact favourably on mechanisms of progressive renal damage and has been used in randomized controlled trials in IgAN, but there is no reason to expect its effects are specific for IgAN, rather than other progressive disease. One such trial has shown a substantial reduction in the risk of progression to ESRF, but other studies have not shown comparable benefit and at present the use of fish oil is not recommended until confirmatory studies are available.

Henoch–Schönlein purpura nephritis

There is very little information to guide the treatment of patients with HSP nephritis. As there are no published randomized controlled trials, and most therapeutic studies in IgAN exclude patients with HSP, it is unclear whether their conclusions can be extrapolated to HSP.

Transient, early nephritis requires no specific treatment. There is no evidence that corticosteroids or other immunosuppressive regimens alter the natural history of the nephrotic syndrome or slowly progressive glomerular damage in Henoch–Schönlein purpura. Crescentic HSP nephritis is more common than crescentic IgAN. Regimens used in the therapy of renal vasculitis have also been applied to crescentic HSP nephritis with apparent benefit, although there are no controlled trials.

Further reading

Clinical

Galla JH (1995). IgA nephropathy. *Kidney International* **47**, 377–87. [Clinical overview of IgAN]

D'Amico G (2000). Natural history of idiopathic IgA nephropathy: role of clinical and histological prognostic factors. *American Journal of Kidney Disease* **36**, 227–37. [Comprehensive review of the natural history of IgAN]

Pouria S, Feehally J (1999) Glomerular IgA deposition in liver disease. *Nephrology, Dialysis, Transplantation* 14, 2279–82. [Review of hepatic IgAN]

White RHR (1994). Henoch–Schönlein nephritis. *Nephron* **68**, 1–9. [A clinical review of HSP nephritis including long-term outcome]

Pathogenesis

Feehally J (1999). Pathogenesis of IgA nephropathy. *Annales Medicine Interne* **150**, 91–8.

van Es LA, de Fijter JW, Daha MR (1997). Pathogenesis of IgA nephropathy. *Nephrology* **3**, 3–12.

Treatment

Dillon JJ (1997). Fish oil therapy for IgA nephropathy. Efficacy and interstudy variability. *Journal of the American Society of Nephrology* **8**, 1739–44. [Meta-analysis of fish oil studies in IgAN]

Donadio JV *et al.* (1999). The long term outcome of patients with IgA nephropathy treated with fish oil in a controlled trial. *Journal of the American Society of Nephrology* **10**, 1772–7. [Evidence of benefit of fish oil in IgAN]

Feehally J (1999). IgA nephropathy and Henoch–Schönlein purpura. In: Pusey CD, ed. *Treatment of glomerulonephritis*, pp 93–112. Kluwer Academic Publishers, Dordrecht. [Review of all treatment evidence in IgAN and HSP nephritis, except new information on corticosteroids and fish oil cited in the other references here]

Pozzi C *et al.* (1999). Corticosteroids in IgA nephropathy: a randomized controlled trial. *Lancet* **353**, 883–7. [A randomized controlled trial of corticosteroids showing benefit in IgAN]

Roccatello D, *et al.* (1995) Report on intensive treatment of extracapillary glomerulonephritis with focus on crescentic IgA nephropathy. *Nephrology, Dialysis, Transplantation* **10**, 2054–9. [Best available evidence on treatment of crescentic IgAN]

20.7.3 Thin membrane nephropathy

John Feehally

Introduction and definition

Thin membrane nephropathy (**TMN**) must always be considered alongside IgA nephropathy (**IgAN**) in the differential diagnosis of glomerular haematuria. TMN is an autosomal dominant condition diagnosed by examination of a renal biopsy by electron microscopy, which shows thin but otherwise morphologically normal glomerular basement membranes (**GBM**). The term 'benign familial haematuria' was used before the GBM abnormality had been identified.

Aetiology and pathogenesis

The genetic basis for TMN has not been defined, although it seems probable that defects in type IV collagen or other GBM proteins will eventually be identified. The gene defects in the α-3 and α-5 chains seen in Alport's syndrome are not found in TMN. A deletion in the gene for the α-4 chain of type IV collagen has been identified in one kindred, but this is not confirmed in other families and it is likely that TMN is genetically heterogeneous.

Pathology

The GBM is diffusely thin but otherwise morphologically normal (Fig. 1). This contrasts with Alport's syndrome in which the GBM is thickened and lamellated and the normal lamina densa of the GBM is disrupted. The normal range for GBM thickness must be determined in each laboratory

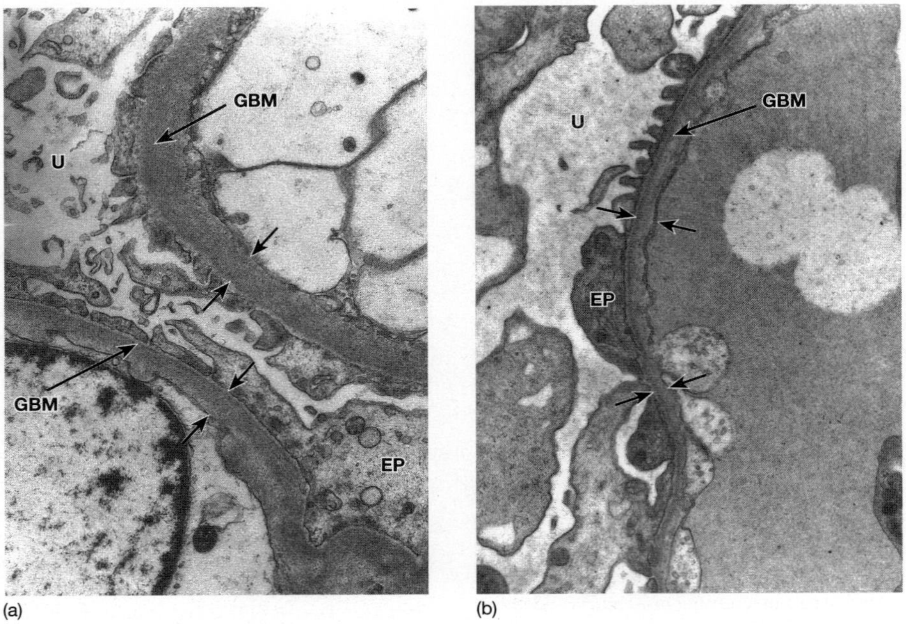

Fig. 1 Thin membrane nephropathy. Electron micrographs contrasting (a) glomerular basement membranes of normal thickness (350–450 nm) with (b) uniform membrane thinning (150–200 nm) in thin membrane nephropathy (both micrographs 20 000 ×). GBM, glomerular basement membrane; Ep, visceral epithelial cells; U, urinary space. (Glutaraldehyde fixation with osmium post-fixation. Ultrathin resin sections stained with uranyl acetate and lead citrate.)

because of the influence of techniques used for tissue fixation, but typically normal GBM thickness is between 350 and 450 nm. A uniform reduction to less than 250 nm is diagnostic of TMN.

Clinical features

TMN is common and is estimated to be the diagnosis in 20 to 25 per cent of patients presenting to a nephrologist with isolated microscopic haematuria. Autopsy studies suggest it may be present in 5 to 9 per cent of the population. It is an autosomal dominant condition but may also be sporadic. Persistent microscopic haematuria is usually lifelong, and episodic macroscopic haematuria may also occur. Proteinuria is uncommon and progressive renal impairment is rare but has been described in a number of families. Deafness and other extrarenal manifestations seen in Alport's syndrome are absent. There is no specific treatment.

Differential diagnosis

TMN can only be distinguished from IgAN by renal biopsy. Although the coexistence of TMN and IgAN is well recorded, it is a matter of debate whether this merely represents the coincidence of two common glomerular diseases. TMN must be distinguished from Alport's syndrome (hereditary nephritis with deafness), of which the commonest form is X-linked. If there is a clear autosomal dominant pattern of haematuria without renal insufficiency or extrarenal problems a clinical diagnosis of TMN may be established with reasonable confidence, but a renal biopsy in at least one family member is still preferable. Once the diagnosis is established in a kindred, biopsy is not required unless there are unexpected clinical findings. The differentiation from the less common autosomal forms of Alport's syndrome may be less straightforward. Subclinical deafness must be excluded by audiography if necessary. The renal biopsy also requires particularly careful assessment: in TMN there is uniform thinning; early in the course of Alport's syndrome, even if the characteristic structural disruption of the GBM has not yet developed, marked variability in GBM width is typical. Staining of GBM for the α-chains of type IV collagen is highly informative since in Alport's syndrome α-3, α-4, and α-5 are absent, whereas normal α-chain distribution is preserved in TMN.

Prognosis

The prognosis is excellent in the great majority of families with TMN, but there is a small but real risk of developing chronic renal failure, identified by the onset of proteinuria and hypertension. Long-term follow up of those with TMN is therefore required: urinalysis and measurement of blood pressure and renal function is recommended every 1 to 2 years.

Further reading

Dische FE, *et al.* (1990). Incidence of thin membrane nephropathy: morphometric investigation of a population sample. *Journal of Clinical Pathology* **43**, 457–60. [Information on the population incidence of TMN]

Kashtan CE (1998). Alport syndrome and thin glomerular basement membrane disease. *Journal of the American Society of Nephrology* **9**, 1736–50. [Review of molecular basis and diagnosis of TMN]

Nieuwhof CM, *et al.* (1997). Thin GBM nephropathy. Premature glomerular obsolescence is associated with hypertension and late onset renal failure. *Kidney International* **51**, 1596–601. [Evidence that TMN may be associated with progressive renal failure]

Tiebosch AT, *et al.* (1989). Thin-basement-membrane nephropathy in adults with persistent hematuria. *New England Journal of Medicine* **320**, 14–18. [The first prospective study of TMN]

20.7.4 Minimal-change nephropathy, focal segmental glomerulosclerosis, and membranous nephropathy

D. Adu

Classification of glomerulonephritis

The most helpful classification of glomerulonephritis is one based on histology. Careful clinical and pathological studies have established the histological patterns of glomerulonephritis in patients with a nephrotic syndrome inhabiting temperate regions of the world (Table 1). The aetiology and patterns of glomerulonephritis in tropical countries differ considerably and are considered elsewhere (see Chapter 20.7.10): discussion in this chapter refers to disease seen in temperate regions. Idiopathic glomerulonephritis accounts for 90 per cent of all childhood cases of the nephrotic syndrome and for approximately 80 per cent in adult patients. Although these histological changes are usually of unknown aetiology, they may also be secondary to well-defined aetiological factors.

General clinical approach

Children

In the original studies of the International Study of Kidney Diseases in Children (**ISKDC**) the diagnosis of minimal-change nephropathy was based on renal biopsies. From these and other studies it was established that for a child aged between 1 and 6 years with nephrotic syndrome and highly selective proteinuria, and who did not have microscopic haematuria, hypertension, or renal impairment, the likely diagnosis was minimal-change nephropathy. When treated with steroids, such children had a greater than 90 per cent chance of going into remission within 4 weeks. Based on these observations, children of this age with the features summarized above are no longer subjected to renal biopsy, but instead are treated with a trial of steroids. This leads to the term 'steroid-responsive nephrotic syndrome of childhood' and most, but not all, of such children will have minimal-change nephropathy. If the proteinuria does not respond to steroids at 1 month then a renal biopsy should be considered to establish the diagnosis. Children over 8 years of age are more likely to have a steroid non-responsive lesion and probably need a renal biopsy. In neonates and in children under 1 year of age there is a high probability of the congenital nephrotic syndrome or diffuse mesangial sclerosis, and therefore renal biopsy should be considered: neither of these lesions respond to steroids.

Table 1 Histology of the nephrotic syndrome

Histology	Children %	Adults %
Minimal-change nephrotic syndrome	76	21
Mesangiocapillary glomerulonephritis	8	4
Focal segmental glomerulosclerosis	7	17
Proliferative (including diffuse mesangial proliferation)	2	0
Membranous	2	28
Other	5	9
Systemic lupus erythematosus	–	7
Amyloid	–	7
Diabetes	–	7

Children: ISKDC study 1978 (excludes secondary causes of nephrotic syndrome, e.g. systemic lupus erythematosus, Henoch–Schönlein purpura—about 10 per cent).
Adults: 469 patients with a nephrotic syndrome. (Howie and Adu 1999 (unpublished).)

Adults

Only 20 per cent of adults with a nephrotic syndrome have minimal-change nephropathy and for that reason a renal biopsy is necessary to establish the type of glomerulonephritis. There have been suggestions that renal biopsy is not essential and that all nephrotic adults should be treated with steroids. However, this approach means unnecessary treatment of a large proportion of patients with a toxic drug, also that no assessment would be available of the type of glomerulonephritis or an estimate of the likelihood of a response to treatment and of the prognosis for long-term renal function. In skilled hands the dangers of renal biopsy are small and outweighed by those of steroid treatment.

General aspects of the management of the nephrotic syndrome

Although steroids and immunosuppressants have been widely used in the treatment of the nephrotic syndrome, general measures remain an important part of the treatment of these disorders. Initial treatment of oedema is with salt restriction and if there is hyponatraemia with fluid restriction. Adults are commonly treated with loop diuretics such as furosemide (frusemide), but this must be used with care, particularly in children, because of the risk of volume depletion and consequent renal impairment. Patients with a nephrotic syndrome are at an increased risk of developing thromboemboli but prophylactic anticoagulation is not normally recommended. There is now good experimental and clinical evidence that angiotensin-converting enzyme (**ACE**) inhibitors reduce proteinuria and slow the progression of renal impairment in patients with glomerulonephritis. These agents are recommended in those who are likely to have a prolonged nephrotic syndrome. Such patients are also likely to benefit from lipid-lowering therapy, although this has not been tested by randomized controlled study.

Minimal-change nephropathy

Aetiology

There is a well-recognized association between Hodgkin's lymphoma and minimal-change nephropathy. Rarely, minimal-change nephropathy has been reported in patients with a carcinoma. There are also case reports of minimal-change nephropathy in individuals, often atopic, exposed to bee stings, poison oak, grass pollen, and cow's milk. Non-steroidal anti-inflammatory drugs can cause an interstitial nephritis, which in some cases is accompanied by a nephrotic syndrome with renal histology showing the changes of minimal-change nephropathy.

Pathogenesis

The responsiveness of the nephrotic syndrome of minimal-change nephropathy to steroids, cyclophosphamide, chlorambucil, and ciclosporin A is strong evidence that this disorder is immune-mediated. The pathogenetic mechanisms remain obscure. The low serum IgG and high IgM levels in these patients appear to be a consequence of the nephrotic syndrome and shed no light on pathogenesis. The hypothesis that proteinuria is caused by a lymphokine produced by an abnormal clone of T lymphocytes has been extensively studied: as yet it has neither been proved nor disproved. In Europe an increased incidence of HLA-DR7 is found in patients with minimal-change nephropathy and in Japan the association is with HLA-DR8, thus suggesting a genetic predisposition.

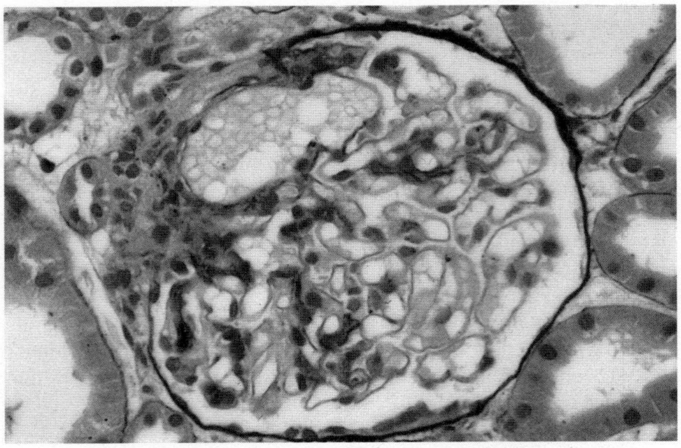

Fig. 1 Minimal-change nephropathy. The glomerulus looks normal on light microscopy. Periodic acid–methenamine silver staining (64 ×). (By courtesy of Dr A. J. Howie.) (See also Plate 1.)

Pathology

The histological features are similar in both children and adults. On light microscopy the glomeruli appear normal or small (Fig. 1 and Plate 1) and on electron microscopy there is effacement of epithelial-cell foot processes over the outer surface of the glomerular basement membrane. Some authors accept a minor degree of mesangial IgM deposition and mesangial proliferation as being consistent with this disorder.

Minimal-change nephropathy in children

Minimal-change nephropathy is found in approximately 76 per cent of children with an idiopathic nephrotic syndrome. Most affected children are under 6 years of age (80 per cent), with a peak age of onset of 2 to 4 years. The condition is responsible for 59 per cent of those aged between 6 and 15 years and about 20 per cent of adults with the nephrotic syndrome. It is more common in boys than in girls, with a male to female childhood ratio of 2:1.

Clinical presentation

The clinical presentation is with a nephrotic syndrome that is characterized by severe hypoalbuminaemia, with a serum albumin level of less than 10 g/l in some 38 per cent of cases. Microscopic haematuria is infrequent (22 per cent), as is hypertension (9 per cent). Renal impairment is infrequent at diagnosis, being found in about 10 per cent of cases, and presentation in acute renal failure is rare. These children are prone to infections, in particular cellulitis and pneumococcal peritonitis.

Diagnosis

The role (or not) of renal biopsy has already been discussed. In 75 per cent of children with minimal-change nephropathy the proteinuria is highly or moderately selective. The concept of protein clearance selectivity was based on the hypothesis that the glomerular basement membrane provided a size-selective barrier to the loss of protein molecules. Although it is now clear that glomerular permselectivity is also based on the charge of molecules, the selectivity test remains useful. A simple version involves dividing the ratio of the urine and plasma concentrations of a large protein (for example, IgG or α_2-macroglobulin) by the ratio of the urine and plasma concentrations of a small molecule (for example, albumin or transferrin).

Treatment of minimal-change nephropathy in children

The first-line treatment of minimal-change nephropathy is prednisolone at an initial dose of 60 mg/m^2 (maximum dose 80 mg) daily for 4 to 6 weeks, reducing the prednisolone to 40 mg/m^2 (maximum dose 60 mg) on alternate days for a further 4 to 6 weeks. With this treatment 93 per cent of children respond with complete loss of proteinuria within 8 weeks. This duration of treatment is more effective in maintaining a remission than a shorter course of steroids. However, once remission is induced, 66 per cent of children have at least one relapse. The major problem is that between 40 and 55 per cent of children who initially respond to steroids develop multiple relapses when steroids are discontinued, or they become steroid-dependent and relapse when the steroid dosage is reduced. Early, frequent relapses (three or more) in the 6 months following an initial response to steroids predict a frequently relapsing course.

Treatment of relapses

Prednisolone 60 mg/m^2 should be given until the urine is free of protein for 3 days (maximum 4 weeks) then prednisolone 40 mg/m^2 on alternate days for 4 weeks. Children's growth should be carefully monitored, using growth curves, during repeated steroid treatment of relapses.

Cyclophosphamide/chlorambucil

Treatment with an immunosuppressant drug should be considered in the following groups of patients: children who are frequent relapsers (two relapses within 6 months of the initial response or four relapses within any 1 year); children who are steroid-dependent (two consecutive relapses occurring during alternate-day treatment for an earlier relapse) or who relapse within 14 days of treatment of an earlier relapse (fast relapse); children in whom two out of four relapses within 6 months were fast relapses; children who are steroid-toxic. There is good evidence that short-term treatment with cyclophosphamide can induce a sustained or even permanent remission in such children. Cyclophosphamide is given in a dose of 2 mg/kg per day (ideally, height for weight) for 8 weeks. Approximately 50 per cent of treated children are in remission at 2 years and 40 per cent at 5 years. One study suggested that the duration of remission was longer with a 12-week course compared with an 8-week course of cyclophosphamide, but this was not subsequently confirmed. Chlorambucil has also been used to treat these patients, but there is no evidence that it is better than cyclophosphamide and it is probably more toxic. Cyclophosphamide has been carefully evaluated in these children and is the drug of choice. Children with the HLA allele HLA-DR7 are less likely to respond to cyclophosphamide.

Toxicity of cyclophosphamide and chlorambucil

The risk of gonadal toxicity is greater in boys than in girls. Gonadal toxicity occurs with chlorambucil at a cumulative dose of 8 to 10 mg/kg. The borderline dose for permanent gonadal toxicity with cyclophosphamide is a cumulative dose of 200 mg/kg. Bone marrow toxicity with both drugs means that the leucocyte count should be regularly measured during treatment. These drugs also increase the long-term risk of developing cancer. Other toxic side-effects of cyclophosphamide include leucopenia, haemorrhagic cystitis, and alopecia. At the doses and duration of treatment outlined above it is relatively safe.

Levamisole

This has been used in children with frequently relapsing or steroid-dependent minimal-change nephropathy and appears to have a steroid-sparing effect. However, the benefits appear marginal and most patients relapse after stopping treatment. Levamisole can cause a reversible neutropenia.

Long-term outcome

The risk of a future relapse is low for those children in whom the nephrotic syndrome goes into remission within 8 weeks of steroid therapy and who do not relapse for 6 months. Early relapse within 6 months is reported to be associated with a risk of relapses for up to 3 years. Some 5.5 per cent of affected children continue to relapse into adult life. All of these children presented with a nephrotic syndrome before the age of 6 years. Children who had persistent proteinuria at 8 weeks had a 21 per cent risk of developing endstage renal failure, and this increased to 35 per cent if they still had proteinuria at 6 months. The long-term mortality rate in children ranges from 2.6 to 7.2 per cent.

Minimal-change nephropathy as part of a spectrum of glomerular disease

In temperate countries, the majority of children with a nephrotic syndrome have minimal-change nephropathy, focal segmental glomerulosclerosis (**FSGS**), or a mesangial proliferative glomerulonephritis (Table 1). Since there is considerable overlap between these conditions, it has been argued that they are all variants of the same disease, termed the 'idiopathic nephrotic syndrome'. In favour of this view is the observation that the histological lesion may evolve with time in a proportion of patients with steroid-responsive nephrotic syndrome. Repeat renal biopsies performed if the character of illness changes—for example, if patients become frequent relapsers, steroid-dependent, or steroid-resistant—sometimes show progression from minimal-change nephropathy or mesangial proliferative glomerulonephritis to focal segmental glomerulonephritis. One study showed that patients with presumed minimal-change nephropathy whose renal biopsies showed large glomeruli were more likely to develop FSGS. In general, those patients with minimal-change nephropathy who develop FSGS but remain steroid-responsive have a good prognosis for renal function, whilst those who are steroid-resistant develop progressive renal failure. The prognosis for renal function is therefore determined by the responsiveness to steroids and not by the histological lesion.

Minimal-change nephropathy in adults

About 20 per cent of adults with a nephrotic syndrome have minimal-change nephropathy. The mean age of onset is 40 years but the condition can occur at any age. The histology is identical to that found in children, with the exception of a higher incidence of globally sclerosed glomeruli that are a feature of ageing.

Clinical presentation

As in children the clinical presentation is with a nephrotic syndrome, although this is not generally as severe. Profound hypoalbuminaemia (serum albumin level under 10 g/l) is rare in adults, being found in only 6 per cent of cases. The disease is slightly more common in men than in women, with a male to female ratio of 1.3:1. More adults than children are hypertensive (30 per cent), have microscopic haematuria (28 per cent), and have renal impairment at diagnosis (60 per cent). These abnormalities are more severe in patients aged over 60 years who are also at particular risk of developing acute renal failure.

Diagnosis

Only 50 per cent of adults with minimal-change nephropathy have highly selective proteinuria, which together with the high incidence of microscopic haematuria and renal impairment makes it impossible to differentiate minimal-change nephropathy from other forms of glomerulonephritis on clinical grounds. A renal biopsy is essential to make the diagnosis in adults with a nephrotic syndrome,.

Treatment of minimal-change nephropathy in adults

Treatment is with prednisolone at an initial dose of 60 mg/day: response occurs slightly less often than in children and also more slowly. Some 80 per cent of adults with minimal-change nephropathy do respond, but remission can take up to 16 weeks to occur. Relapse is less frequent in adults (1.7/patient) than in children, and only 21 per cent of adults develop multiple relapses or are steroid-dependent. In adults as in children, cyclophosphamide is effective in inducing a long-lasting remission. In one study 62.5 per cent of patients treated with cyclophosphamide were in remission at 10 years.

Ciclosporin A

There is now good evidence that ciclosporin A is effective in the treatment of minimal-change nephropathy in both adults and children. Patients who are steroid-responsive or multiple relapsers are more likely to respond with complete or partial remissions (70 to 80 per cent) than patients who are resistant to steroids (40 to 50 per cent). The drug should be considered in those patients who develop steroid toxicity because they have multiple relapses or who are steroid-dependent. Ciclosporin A appears to be effective at blood levels of between 100 and 200 ng/ml, and at these levels significant short-term nephrotoxicity and hypertension are uncommon. However, relapses appear to recur with the same frequency after ciclosporin A has been discontinued as before, and for that reason it is still advisable to use cyclophosphamide as the first-choice treatment in patients with a multiple relapsing or steroid-dependent minimal-change nephropathy in the hope of inducing a sustained remission. In this author's view, ciclosporin A can best be viewed as a steroid-sparing agent in patients with minimal-change nephropathy.

Long-term outcome

Some 6 per cent of adult patients are still nephrotic after a mean follow-up of 7.5 years. The survival in patients over 60 years of age has been reported to be 50 per cent at 10 years, and in those aged 15 to 59 it was 90 per cent.

Focal segmental glomerulosclerosis

Focal segmental glomerulosclerosis (FSGS) was first described by Rich in 1957 at autopsy in children who died from a nephrotic syndrome. Fewer terms have generated more disagreement amongst pathologists and nephrologists: it is not a disease entity but a histological lesion that is often of unknown aetiology.

Secondary FSGS

FSGS may be a sequel of glomerular scarring in patients with previous proliferative glomerulonephritis and is seen in biopsies from patients with Alport's syndrome. It is also seen in patients with reflux nephropathy and other conditions leading to a reduced renal mass, and it is likely that the segmental sclerosing lesions in these circumstances are a consequence of glomerular hypertension and hyperfiltration (Table 2). FSGS has also been

Table 2 Secondary FSGS

Alport's syndrome
Reduced renal mass
- reflux nephropathy
- remnant kidney

Healed glomerulonephritis
- IgA nephropathy
- Vasculitis
- Diffuse proliferative glomerulonephritis

Sickle-cell disease
HIV infection
Intravenous drug abuse (heroin)
Schistosoma mansoni

found late on during the clinical course of patients with a nephrotic syndrome who had an initial renal biopsy showing minimal-change nephropathy.

Pathogenesis

In experimental models, focal segmental sclerosis can develop from different pathogenic mechanisms. These include toxic injury (puromycin nephropathy), immunological injury (anti-GBM nephritis), the lupus-associated nephritis in NZB/NZW F1 mice, and hyperfiltration injury (5/6ths nephrectomy). Some of these models have clinical counterparts, and the diversity of pathogenic mechanisms may explain the variability in the clinical presentation and response to FSGS therapy. As with minimal-change nephropathy there are suggestions that the glomerular injury in FSGS is caused by a lymphokine. The rapid development of heavy proteinuria following renal transplantation in some patients with FSGS indicates that the glomerular injury is caused by a circulating factor.

Primary FSGS

Focal segmental glomerulosclerosis may be apparently idiopathic and found early on during the clinical course of patients with proteinuria or nephrotic syndrome. About 7 per cent of children and 20 per cent of adults with a nephrotic syndrome have FSGS. Even when FSGS is found early on in the course of a nephrotic syndrome there is no evidence to suggest that it represents a homogenous disease.

Pathology

The histological lesions of FSGS comprise segmental areas of glomerular sclerosis with hyalinization of glomerular capillaries, the segmental areas usually being adherent to Bowman's capsule. In childhood FSGS, these lesions predominantly affect juxtamedullary glomeruli. Typically, the areas of segmental sclerosis are randomly distributed within the glomerular tuft with a predilection for the hilar regions, and these patients may be regarded as having classical FSGS (Figs 2 and 3 and Plates 2 and 3). In some biopsies the glomerular lesions are located peripherally at the glomerulotubular junction, the so-called glomerular tip lesion. Focal areas of tubular atrophy and interstitial nephritis are prominent. On immunofluorescent microscopy, deposits of IgM and C3 may be seen in the sclerotic areas. Electron microscopy shows diffuse foot-process effacement in apparently unaffected glomeruli.

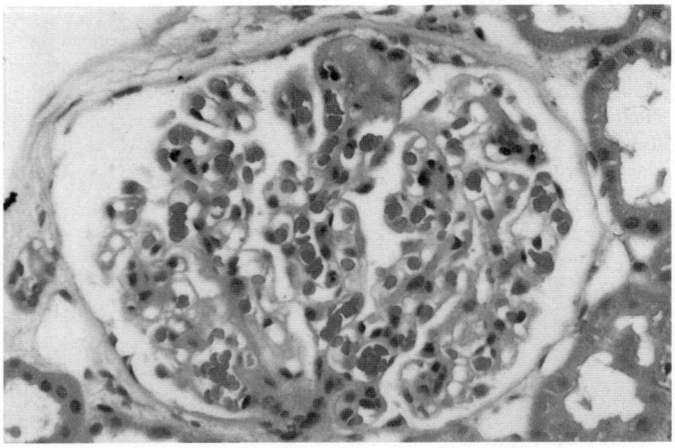

Fig. 2 Classical segmental sclerosing glomerulonephritis at an early stage. The glomerulus shows an erratic increase in mesangium with a segmental area of foamy cells and sclerosis opposite the vascular pole, next to the tubular origin. Haematoxylin and eosin staining (50 ×). (By courtesy of Dr A. J. Howie.) (See also Plate 2.)

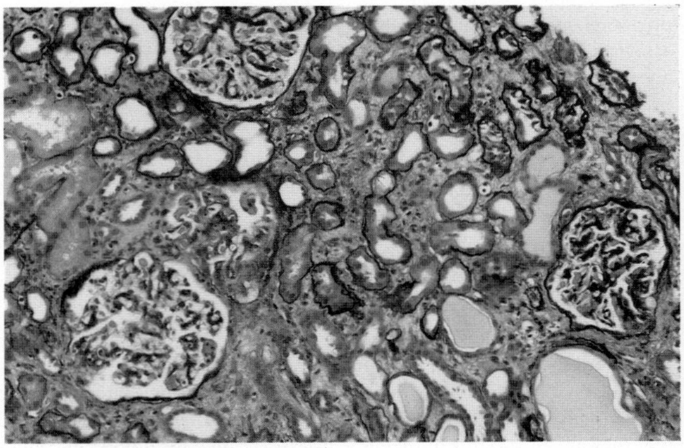

Fig. 3 Classical segmental sclerosing glomerulonephritis at a late stage. Four glomeruli show an erratic increase in mesangium and segmental lesions at various sites. Periodic acid–methenamine silver staining (× 64). (By courtesy of Dr A. J. Howie.) (See also Plate 3.)

Pathogenesis

In approximately 30 per cent of patients with primary FSGS there is a circulating factor that causes an increase in glomerular permeability *in vitro*. This factor appears to be a protein with a molecular weight of between 30 and 50 kDa and is not an immunoglobulin. This factor has also been found in the serum of patients who develop recurrent FSGS postrenal transplantation.

Clinical presentation

Children

Approximately 7 per cent of children presenting with an idiopathic nephrotic syndrome have FSGS. Males and females are equally affected and the peak age at onset is between 6 and 8 years. The majority of patients (75 per cent) present with a nephrotic syndrome, 20 per cent have persistent proteinuria, and 5 per cent haematuria as well as proteinuria. Clinically these patients differ from other children with minimal-change nephropathy, in that two-thirds have microscopic haematuria, half have impaired renal function at diagnosis, and one-third are hypertensive. The proteinuria is usually poorly selective.

Adults

The clinical presentation in adults does not differ in any significant respects from that in children. The mean age at onset is between 20 and 30 years but FSGS has been found in patients aged 70.

Treatment of primary ('classical') FSGS

The prognosis in patients with primary FSGS and proteinuria in the non-nephrotic range is good, and 80 per cent of such patients survive for 10 years without developing endstage renal failure. These patients therefore do not need treatment with either prednisolone or immunosuppressants and should be treated with general measures only.

The main problem is the treatment of patients with FSGS and a nephrotic syndrome. In most studies patients have been given steroids, and approximately 30 per cent of those treated for 8 weeks with prednisolone go into remission. There is now good data from uncontrolled studies that a more prolonged course of steroids, of up to 6 months, is associated with a higher rate of remission. Children are treated with prednisolone at an initial dose of 60 mg/m^2 per day and adults with a dose of 60 mg/day. Patients who go into remission have a good prognosis with fewer than 10 per cent developing endstage renal failure. However, the prognosis in patients who do not respond to steroids is poor, with between 30 and 50 per cent developing endstage renal failure over 5 to 10 years. There is no difference in prognosis between adults and children. Adverse prognostic factors include tubulointerstitial fibrosis and a high serum creatinine level.

Other immunosuppressants

The evidence supporting the addition to prednisolone of cyclophosphamide or chlorambucil in the treatment of FSGS is not convincing. Useful remissions have been reported, but in the absence of controlled trials the value of this is difficult to assess.

Several uncontrolled studies have looked at the effects of ciclosporin A: in general, the responsiveness has been poor and paralleled that of steroids. Recent controlled studies in adults suggest that ciclosporin A when added to prednisolone is more effective in inducing remission of the nephrotic syndrome than steroids alone in patients with steroid-resistant FSGS.

Glomerular tip lesion

Some studies suggest that the site of the segmental sclerosing lesions predicted steroid responsiveness. Adult patients with a peripheral segmental sclerosing lesion at the tubular origin, the glomerular tip lesion, have a steroid- or immunosuppressant-responsive nephrotic syndrome and do not progress to endstage renal failure. Similar observations have been reported in children, although in both children and adults these observations have not been confirmed.

Recurrence after renal transplantation

The nephrotic syndrome recurs in 20 to 40 per cent of patients with primary FSGS, often within days of renal transplantation, and this leads to graft failure in some 50 per cent of cases. After recurrence in a first transplant the rate of recurrence in a subsequent transplant approaches 75 per cent. Plasma exchange and protein immunoadsorption have resulted in a reduction of proteinuria or a remission of the nephrotic syndrome in some patients. These data are not controlled and our experience is that the reduction in proteinuria is transient.

Collapsing glomerulopathy

This is a type of focal segmental sclerosing glomerulonephritis, characterized by segmental or global collapse of glomerular capillaries with basement-membrane wrinkling and crowding of glomerular epithelial cells. These appearances represent a distinct subset of patients with focal segmental glomerulosclerosis, and were initially described in patients with HIV-associated nephropathy in the context of a severe nephrotic syndrome and rapid progression to endstage renal failure. Subsequent reports show that it may also be idiopathic.

Presentation is with a nephrotic syndrome and renal impairment (70 per cent of cases). Treatment with steroids or cytotoxic drugs has been ineffective in inducing remission of the nephrotic syndrome or preventing the development of endstage renal failure. There is a rapid deterioration of renal function and over 70 per cent of patients are in endstage renal failure after a follow up of 5 years.

Membranous nephropathy

Membranous nephropathy accounts for between 20 and 30 per cent of cases of the nephrotic syndrome in adults and about 2 to 5 per cent of those in childhood. Histologically it is defined by the presence of subepithelial immune deposits on the outer surface of the glomerular basement membrane. No cause for this histological lesion is found in most patients living in temperate countries, and it is therefore termed idiopathic membranous nephropathy, but it is unlikely that membranous glomerulonephritis is a homogenous disorder. Its aetiology (where identifiable), genetic basis, frequency as a cause of the nephrotic syndrome, and clinical evolution with or without treatment differ substantially between studies from different countries.

Table 3 Conditions associated with membranous nephropathy

Autoimmune diseases
Systemic lupus erythematosus
Rheumatoid arthritis
Drugs
Gold
Penicillamine
Captopril
Malignancy
Carcinoma (bronchus, colon, stomach, prostate, breast)
Infections
Hepatitis B
Syphilis
Filariasis
Leprosy
Miscellaneous
Autoimmune thyroid disease
Diabetes mellitus

Aetiology

In about 20 to 25 per cent of adults and 35 per cent of children with membranous nephropathy there is an identifiable associated condition (Table 3). The frequency of this varies in different parts of the world. Malignancy, usually a carcinoma and rarely Hodgkin's lymphoma and non-Hodgkin's lymphoma, is found in between 3 and 7 per cent of all cases, rising to 16 per cent in those aged over 60 years. The most common tumours are carcinoma of the bronchus, colon, kidney, breast, stomach, and prostate. Gold and penicillamine are prominent causes of membranous nephropathy and this complication is more common in individuals who carry the *HLA-DR3* gene. There is also some evidence that membranous nephropathy can develop in patients with rheumatoid arthritis who are not taking these drugs. Approximately 3 per cent of all patients with membranous nephropathy have systemic lupus erythematosus; a further 2 per cent of patients have serological features of this disorder or histological changes that are suggestive of it, sometimes predating clinical evidence of the disease by many years. In Northern Europe about 1 per cent of patients with membranous nephropathy have positive hepatitis B serology, but this association is much more common in South-east Asia and in Africa, particularly in children.

Pathogenesis

The immune mechanisms that lead to the development of membranous nephropathy are unknown. In rats, the administration of antibodies against renal tubular epithelial antigen leads to a membranous nephropathy that histologically resembles the human condition. The antibody responsible for this Heymann's nephritis in rats binds to an antigen called gp330, which is found on renal tubular brush border and on glomerular epithelial cells. In glomeruli this leads to the development of subepithelial deposits through the *in situ* formation of immune complexes. Although human renal tubular cells express gp330, this is not found in glomerular epithelial cells, and there is no evidence that a similar mechanism plays a role in human membranous nephropathy. In Europe there is a strong association between membranous nephropathy and the MHC haplotype HLA-A1 B8 DRw3, whilst in Japan the association is with HLA-DR2. By contrast, no such association is seen in the United States.

Pathology

Idiopathic membranous nephropathy is characterized histologically by diffuse thickening of the glomerular basement on light microscopy, usually

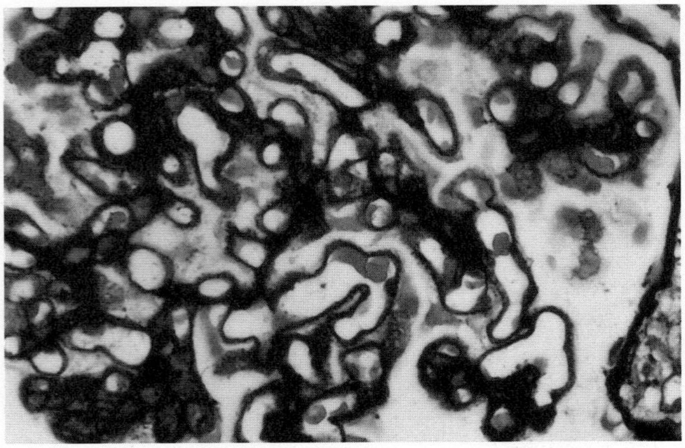

Fig. 4 Membranous nephropathy. There are regular short spikes on the outside of glomerular capillary loops. Periodic acid–methenamine silver staining (80 ×). (See also Plate 4.)

with argyrophyllic subepithelial spikes (Fig. 4 and Plate 4). On immunofluorescent or immunoperoxidase microscopy this thickening is shown to be due to the presence of immune deposits, usually consisting of IgG and C3, on the subepithelial surface of the glomerular basement membrane (Fig. 5 and Plate 5). The size and extent of incorporation of immune deposits into the glomerular basement membrane on electron microscopy forms the basis of histological classification—stage 1: subepithelial deposits without spikes; stage 2: large subendothelial deposits separated by spikes of basement membrane; stage 3: deposits incorporated into a thickened basement membrane with many spikes; stage 4: a very thick irregular basement membrane with no spikes and resorbed deposits. The presence of mesangial proliferation, mesangial immune deposits, and IgA and C1q on immunofluorescent microscopy raises the possibility that membranous nephropathy is secondary to systemic lupus erythematosus.

Clinical presentation

In children, boys are affected three times as often as girls. In adults, most studies report a preponderance of men, with a male to female ratio of 2–3:1. The majority of patients are aged between 30 and 50, although the condition has been described in patients aged up to 80 years. The clinical presentation is with the nephrotic syndrome in about 75 per cent of cases, with the remainder having proteinuria only. Microscopic haematuria is found in 50 per cent of adults and 90 per cent of children. Macroscopic haematuria is found in about 10 to 20 per cent of children but it is rare in adults. About 25 to 40 per cent of adults and 6 per cent of children are hypertensive at diagnosis, and between 10 per cent and 30 per cent of patients have a raised serum creatinine level.

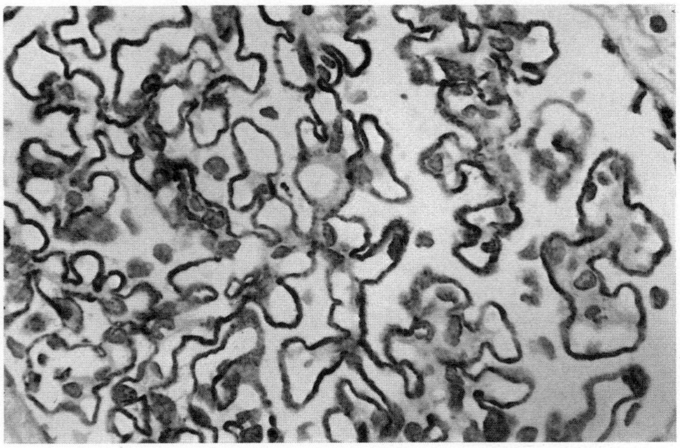

Fig. 5 Membranous nephropathy. Immunoperoxidase staining shows uniform granular deposits of IgG on the epithelial side of glomerular basement membranes (80 ×). (By courtesy of Dr A. J. Howie.) (See also Plate 5.)

Renal vein thrombosis

Patients with membranous nephropathy appear to be at particular risk of developing renal vein thrombosis, although this is not as high as originally suggested. Most such patients are asymptomatic, but they may present with pulmonary emboli. Detection is by Doppler ultrasound of the renal veins, computed tomography (**CT**), magnetic resonance (**MRI**) imaging, or using the venous phase of renal arteriography. In practice, a renal vein thrombosis should be looked for if there is a sudden deterioration of renal function in a patient with membranous nephropathy. It is now known that renal vein thrombosis is a consequence of the hypercoagulable state of the nephrotic syndrome and is not a cause of membranous nephropathy.

Membranous nephropathy with a crescentic glomerulonephritis

About 5 per cent of patients with a membranous nephropathy develop a crescentic glomerulonephritis with rapid deterioration of renal function. Most such patients have antibodies to glomerular basement antigen or to neutrophil cytoplasmic antigens. Treatment has been with prednisolone and cyclophosphamide as for other patients with a crescentic glomerulonephritis.

Clinical evolution of untreated membranous nephropathy

In the long-term, untreated membranous nephropathy evolves either to remission or to the development of chronic renal failure. The rate at which either outcome occurs varies in different studies. After a mean follow-up of 4.5 to 6 years, between 9.5 and 22 per cent of patients are in endstage renal failure, 9.5 to 19 per cent have significantly impaired renal function, and 23 to 50 per cent are in remission. The actuarial survival rate shows that about 75 per cent of patients are alive at 10 years and 60 per cent have functioning kidneys. Examination of the control untreated patients in recent treatment trials shows that, of 205 patients followed for between 2 and 5 years, 15 per cent were in complete remission and 9 per cent in endstage renal failure. Any study of treatment in membranous nephropathy must therefore address the difficulty of treating large numbers of patients with toxic drugs who have little risk of developing endstage renal failure.

Treatment

The twin aims of treating membranous nephropathy are first to induce a remission of the nephrotic syndrome and second to prevent the development of endstage renal failure. Despite several careful studies using steroids and immunosuppressants, there is still no agreement that these aims can be achieved.

Steroid treatment

In the 1979 Collaborative study conducted in the United States, 72 adults with membranous nephropathy were randomized to 8-weeks' treatment with either 125 mg prednisolone on alternate days or placebo. The steroid dose was then tapered and stopped over several weeks. Deterioration of renal function, as measured by the glomerular filtration rate (**GFR**), was significantly more rapid in untreated than in treated patients. Further, a significantly lower proportion of treated patients than untreated patients developed renal failure (serum creatinine level over 440 μmol/l).

In the United Kingdom Medical Research Council (**MRC**) study (1990), 107 adult patients with membranous nephropathy were randomized to treatment with either prednisolone 125 mg on alternate days for 8 weeks or placebo. At 36 months there were no significant differences in the plasma creatinine level, creatinine clearance, and 24-h urine protein between treated and untreated patients. In the Canadian study, 158 patients were treated with either prednisolone 45 mg/m^2 body surface area per day for 6 months or no specific treatment. No benefits were seen in renal function or proteinuria after a mean follow-up of 48 months. These data indicate that short-term steroids are of no benefit in the treatment of membranous nephropathy.

Steroid and chlorambucil treatment

One study reported that chlorambucil was more effective than azathioprine or placebo in the treatment of membranous nephropathy. This provided the rationale for the Italian multicentre study in which patients were randomized to symptomatic treatment only or treatment with the following alternating regime—month 1: intravenous methylprednisolone, 1 g on each of 3 consecutive days, followed by oral methylprednisolone (0.4 mg/kg per day) or prednisolone (0.5 mg/kg per day) for 27 days; month 2: oral chlorambucil (0.2 mg/kg per day) alone for 1 month, the dose was lowered if the leucocyte count fell below 5×10^9/l. Alternating monthly cycles of methylprednisolone and chlorambucil were given for a total of 6 months. After a mean follow-up of 31 to 37 months, significantly more treated than untreated patients were in remission (either total or partial): 23/32 (72 per cent) versus 9/30 (30 per cent). Furthermore, 8 of 30 controls showed a 50 per cent rise in serum creatinine in contrast to none of the treated patients. The side-effects of treatment were minor and consisted of epigastric pain and leucopenia. To answer the question of whether the beneficial effect of this regime was due solely to the steroid component, a further study compared the effect of methylprednisolone alone with methylprednisolone and chlorambucil. Patients treated with the combination were more likely to have an early remission of the nephrotic syndrome, but this benefit was lost after 4 years. There was no difference in the rate of decline of renal function between the two therapies.

Other immunosuppressive regimes

In a recent, randomized controlled study, cyclophosphamide 2.5 mg/kg per day was compared with chlorambucil 0.2 mg/kg per day in the regime described above. The results in terms of remission of the nephrotic syndrome and deterioration of renal function were comparable.

A small, randomized controlled study of 17 patients with a persistent nephrotic syndrome and declining renal function suggested that ciclosporin A slowed the rate of decline of renal function: this requires confirmation in a larger trial.

Meta-analysis of steroid and immunosuppressant treatment of membranous nephropathy

A meta-analysis of four randomized controlled studies comparing treatments of membranous nephropathy showed that regimes comprising chlorambucil or cyclophosphamide, either alone or with steroids, were more effective than symptomatic treatment or treatment with steroids alone in inducing remission of the nephrotic syndrome. These agents increased the relative risk of achieving a complete remission by 4.6 (95 per cent confidence interval of 2.2 to 9.3). The number of patients studied and the design of the clinical trials were such that no conclusion could be drawn on the effects of these treatments on renal function.

Management of the patient with membranous nephropathy and deteriorating renal function

Drug-induced interstitial nephritis, renal vein thrombosis, and crescentic glomerulonephritis should be excluded. In patients with deteriorating renal function due to the progression of membranous nephropathy, several uncontrolled studies have suggested that treatment with intravenous methylprednisolone, or with oral prednisolone and chlorambucil or cyclophosphamide, may reverse the rate of decline in renal function. These studies are difficult to interpret as renal function may stabilize or improve without treatment in some cases.

Prognostic factors

Identifying those patients who at the onset of membranous nephropathy were likely to have a poor outcome for renal function would be helpful in deciding who to treat. Most studies show that adverse risk factors for the development of renal failure include male sex, a nephrotic syndrome, persistent heavy proteinuria, tubulointerstitial fibrosis, renal impairment at diagnosis, and deterioration of renal function in the first 2.5 years after diagnosis. In particular, patients with proteinuria of over 6 g/day for longer than 9 months were found to have a 55 per cent likelihood of progressing to renal failure. Children appear to do better than adults; in one study, 42 per cent of children went into complete remission and only 10 per cent developed endstage renal failure after a mean follow-up of 4 years.

How should membranous nephropathy be treated?

There is still no agreement on how membranous nephropathy should be treated, as up to 40 per cent of patients with this disorder enter spontaneous remission with long-term preservation of renal function. The dilemma is that early treatment of all patients exposes those who were going into remission anyway to the toxicity of drugs, whilst delayed treatment of high-risk patients may be ineffective. The results of current randomized controlled trials into the benefits of treatment with alkylating agents or cyclophosphamide in patients at high risk of progressive renal failure will guide treatment decisions.

Further reading

Minimal-change nephropathy

Arbeitsgemeinschaft fur Padiatrisch Nephrologie (1988). Short versus standard prednisolone for initial treatment of idiopathic nephrotic syndrome in children. *Lancet* **1**, 380–3.

Bargman J (1999). Management of minimal lesion glomerulonephritis: evidence-based recommendations. *Kidney International* **55**(Suppl. 70), 3–16.

British Association for Paediatric Nephrology (1991). Levamisole for corticosteroid dependent nephrotic syndrome in childhood. *Lancet* **337**, 1555–7.

International Study of Kidney Disease in Children (1978). Prediction of histopathology from clinical and laboratory characteristics at time of diagnosis. *Kidney International* **13**, 159–65.

International Study of Kidney Disease in Children (1981). The primary nephrotic syndrome in Children. Identification of patients with minimal change nephrotic syndrome from initial response to prednisolone. *Journal of Pediatrics* **98**, 561–4.

Nolasco F, *et al.* (1986). Adult-onset minimal change nephrotic syndrome: a long term follow-up. *Kidney International* **29**, 1215–23.

Tarshish P *et al.* (1997). Prognostic significance of the early course of minimal changes nephrotic syndrome: report of the International Study of Kidney Disease in Children. *Journal of the American Society of Nephrology* **8**, 769–76.

Ueda N, Kuno K, Ito S (1990). Eight and 12 week courses of cyclophosphamide in nephrotic syndrome. *Archives of Disease in Childhood* **85**, 1147–50.

Focal segmental glomerulosclerosis

Burgess E (1999). Management of focal glomerulosclerosis: evidence based recommendations. *Kidney International* **55**(Suppl. 70), 26–32.

Cattran D, *et al.* (1999). A randomized study of cyclosporine in patients with steroid-resistant focal segmental glomerulosclerosis. *Kidney International* **56**, 2220–6.

D'Agati V (1994). The many masks of focal segmental glomerulosclerosis. *Kidney International* **46**, 1223–41.

Detweiler R, *et al.* (1994). Collapsing glomerulopathy: a clinically and pathologically distinct variant of segmental glomerulosclerosis. *Kidney International* **45**, 1734–46.

Howie A, *et al.* (1993). Different clinicopathological types of segmental sclerosing glomerular lesions in adults. *Nephrology, Dialysis, and Transplantation* **8**, 590–9.

Korbet S, Schwartz M, Lewis E (1994). Primary focal segmental glomerulosclerosis: clinical course and response to therapy. *American Journal of Kidney Disease* **23**, 773–83.

Niaudet P for The French Society of Pediatric Nephrology (1992). Comparison of cyclosporine and chlorambucil in the treatment of idiopathic nephrotic syndrome: a multicenter randomized controlled trial. *Pediatric Nephrology* **6**, 1–3.

Niaudet P for The French Society of Pediatric Nephrology (1994). Treatment of childhood steroid resistant idiopathic nephrosis with a combination of cyclosporine and prednisolone. *Journal of Pediatrics* **125**, 981–6.

Rich A (1957). A hitherto undescribed vulnerability of the juxta-medullary glomeruli in lipoid nephrosis. *Bulletin of John Hopkins Hospital* **100**, 173–86.

Savin V, *et al.* (1996). Circulating factor associated with increased glomerular permeability to albumin in recurrent focal segmental glomerulosclerosis. *New England Journal of Medicine* **334**, 878–83.

Membranous nephropathy

Cameron J, Healy M, Adu D (1990). The Medical Research Council Trial of short-term high-dose alternate day prednisolone in idiopathic membranous nephrotic syndrome in adults. *Quarterly Journal of Medicine* **274**, 133–56.

Cattran D, *et al.* (1989). A randomized controlled trial of prednisolone in patients with idiopathic membranous nephropathy. *New England Journal of Medicine* **320**, 210–15.

Cattran D, *et al.* (1995). A controlled trial of cyclophosphamide in patients with progressive membranous nephropathy: Canadian Glomerulonephritis Study Group. *Kidney International* **47**, 1130–5.

Collaborative Study of the Adult Idiopathic Nephrotic Syndrome (1979). A controlled study of short-term prednisolone treatment in adults with membranous nephropathy. *New England Journal of Medicine* **301**, 1301–6.

Honkanen E, Tornroth T, Gronhagen-Riska C (1992). Natural history, clinical course and morphological evolution of membranous nephropathy. *Nephrology, Dialysis, and Transplantation* **7**(Suppl. 1), 35–41.

Imperiale T, Goldfarb S, Berns J (1995). Are cytotoxic agents beneficial in idiopathic membranous nephropathy? A meta-analysis of the controlled trials. *Journal of the American Society of Nephrology* **5**, 1553–8.

Muirhead N (1999). Management of idiopathic membranous nephropathy: evidence-based recommendations. *Kidney International* **55**(Suppl. 70), S47–55.

Pei Y, Cattran D, Greenwood C (1992). Predicting chronic renal insufficiency in idiopathic membranous nephropathy. *Kidney International* **42**, 960–6.

Ponticelli C, *et al.* (1995). A 10-year follow-up of a randomized study with methylprednisolone and chlorambucil in membranous nephropathy. *Kidney International* **48**, 1600–4.

Ponticelli P, *et al.* (1998). A randomized study comparing methylprednisolone plus chlorambucil versus methylprednisolone plus cyclophosphamide in idiopathic membranous nephropathy. *Journal of the American Society of Nephrology* **9**, 444–50.

Schiepatti A, *et al.* (1993). Prognosis of untreated patients with idiopathic membranous nephropathy. *New England Journal of Medicine* **329**, 85–9.

Books and monographs

Cameron J, Glassock R, eds (1988). *The nephrotic syndrome.* Marcel Dekker, New York.

Cattran DC, ed. (1999). Management of glomerulonephritis. *Kidney International* **55**(Suppl. 70), S1–62.

Kincaid-Smith P, d'Apice A, Atkins R, eds (1978). *Progress in glomerulonephritis.* Wiley, New York.

Pusey CD, ed. (1999). The Treatment of Glomerulonephritis. In: *Developments in nephrology*, Vol. 40. Kluwer Academic, Dordrecht.

20.7.5 Proliferative glomerulonephritis

Peter W. Mathieson

The term proliferative glomerulonephritis covers a variety of conditions (Table 1) where there is increased cellularity of the glomerulus, either due to the proliferation of resident glomerular cells, or infiltration of leucocytes, or both. The proliferative changes may be focal (that is to say, they only affect some glomeruli) and/or segmental (in other words, only affecting parts of each glomerulus). Many of these entities will be considered in other chapters, and only those not covered elsewhere (*) will be described here.

Mesangial proliferative glomerulonephritis

Patients will typically have haematuria and this may be associated with proteinuria and/or impairment of excretory renal function and/or hypertension. The majority of patients whose renal biopsies show only mesangial proliferation will have IgA nephropathy (see Chapter 20.7.2), but a few will have no IgA deposits and their classification is not straightforward: possibilities include IgM nephropathy and so-called 'idiopathic' mesangial proliferative glomerulonephritis (**GN**).

IgM nephropathy

There is continuing controversy about this diagnostic entity. In patients with nephrotic syndrome, if the only abnormalities on the renal biopsy are in the mesangial region, with proliferation of mesangial cells and deposition of IgM, many authorities would assign a diagnosis of minimal-change nephropathy and advocate treatment with corticosteroids; some would consider that these morphological features are markers for a poorer prognosis and a reduced likelihood of a response to corticosteroids. Others would consider the patient to have a completely different disease entity and give a diagnosis of IgM nephropathy. Some of the confusion may be explained by methodological factors: assessment of the degree of mesangial hypercellularity is subjective, and reagents to detect IgM are notoriously unreliable since they may give high background staining. Mesangial IgM has been found in up to 60 per cent of 'normal' kidneys donated for transplantation; the diagnostic significance of IgM is also cast into doubt by its

Table 1 Proliferative GN

(a) Proliferation of mesangial cells
IgA nephropathy ± Henoch-Schönlein disease
IgM nephropathy*
Systemic lupus erythematosus
Idiopathic*
(b) Endocapillary proliferation
Poststreptococcal GN*
Infective endocarditis
Other infections, including leprosy
(c) Extracapillary proliferation (crescent formation)
Small vessel vasculitis (Wegener's/microscopic polyangiitis)
Antiglomerular basement membrane disease
Henoch-Schönlein disease
Systemic lupus erythematosus
Idiopathic (rare)
(d) Diffuse proliferative GN (may include elements of (a), (b), and (c))
Systemic lupus erythematosus
Idiopathic*

presence in over 75 per cent of controls as well as in patients with various other forms of glomerulonephritis. The best support for the existence of IgM nephropathy, as an entity distinct from minimal-change nephropathy, comes from the occurrence of a familial form and from the identification of this pattern of glomerular injury in patients who, after lengthy follow-up, have an appreciable risk of developing impaired excretory kidney function.

Idiopathic mesangial proliferative GN

This term may be applied if there is isolated mesangial proliferation without deposition of IgA or IgM. Again there is overlap with minimal-change nephropathy: if the patient presents with nephrotic syndrome, most nephrologists would not allow the presence of mesangial proliferation to deflect them from treating the patient with corticosteroids, although there is evidence that the presence of this histological finding is associated with a poorer response rate. If, however, the patient has haematuria and/or hypertension and/or impaired kidney function, none of which are typical features of minimal-change nephropathy, it is difficult to resist the need for another separate diagnostic category. Unfortunately there are no informative studies to guide treatment or give information on prognosis.

Endocapillary proliferative GN

Patients will often have impaired excretory function, haematuria, proteinuria, and hypertension, sometimes presenting acutely as a 'nephritic syndrome'. On renal biopsy, the glomerular hypercellularity is confined within the glomerular capillary tuft, which is probably due to the combination of a proliferation of intrinsic (endothelial and mesangial) cells together with an infiltration of inflammatory cells. This can occur in systemic lupus erythematosus and as a complication of a variety of infections (see Chapter 20.7.8). Only poststreptococcal GN will be considered here.

Poststreptococcal GN (Plate 1)

Most infection-related GN occurs concurrently with the infection. By contrast, postinfectious GN (of which poststreptococcal GN is the most frequent and best characterized) occurs, as the name implies, after the infection. In poststreptococcal GN the delay between the inciting infection and the onset of the renal complication may be long enough for the infection to have been forgotten, and this may contribute to diagnostic confusion. The typical case follows infection with streptococci of Lancefield group A (β-haemolytic streptococci, *S. pyogenes*), either causing pharyngitis or skin infections such as cellulitis or impetigo. Children are the most common victims. Around 2 weeks later, sometimes longer after skin infections, the patient develops nephritis which may be sufficiently acute and severe to cause a nephritic syndrome with oliguria, hypertension, and oedema. If a renal biopsy is performed, it will show diffuse proliferative GN, with infiltration by neutrophil polymorphs often particularly prominent (Fig. 1). Immunohistology shows deposition of IgG, IgM, and complement in the mesangial and subepithelial areas, and electron microscopy shows large subepithelial deposits ('humps').

Serological tests

There are typical serological features which give clues to the pathogenesis: these include antibodies to streptococcal antigens and evidence of activation of the complement cascade. The antibodies are IgG; reactivity with numerous streptococcal antigens has been reported including streptolysin O, deoxyribonuclease B, hyaluronidase, and streptokinase. Anti-streptolysin O is the most useful diagnostic test after pharyngitis, anti-DNAse B is best after skin infections. Hypocomplementaemia (low C3 in the majority of cases, also low C4 in a smaller proportion) reflects activation of both the alternative and the classical pathways (the complement system is discussed in more detail in Chapter 20.7.6. In poststreptococcal GN, the alternative complement pathway may be activated by bacterial antigens and/or by IgG

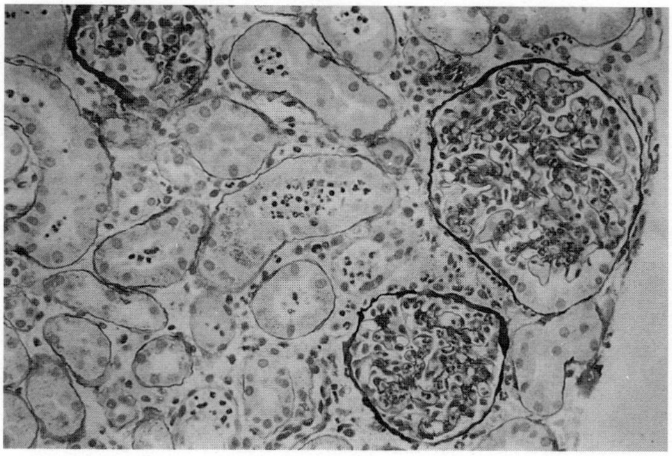

Fig. 1 Poststreptococcal glomerulonephritis.

autoantibodies called nephritic factors which resemble those seen in MCGN; the classical pathway may be activated by circulating immune complexes.

Pathogenesis

It is believed that the pathogenesis of poststreptococcal GN can be explained as follows: streptococcal antigens are deposited in glomeruli, by virtue of some aspect of their charge, size, or other physicochemical characteristics, during the early phase of the infection. After the 10 to 14 days necessary for the host to mount an immune response to the bacterial infection, circulating antibody appears and binds to the 'planted' antigens in the glomeruli. Complement is activated, leucocytes are attracted (by complement-activation products C3a and C5a among other chemoattractants) and an inflammatory reaction is provoked, injuring the glomeruli. The precise nature of the streptococcal antigens that act in this nephritogenic manner remains controversial; only certain serological types of streptococci (referred to as M types and serotyped according to cell-wall protein antigens) are capable of inciting GN, but the M proteins themselves are not believed to be nephritogenic. In addition to the planted antigen mechanism, streptococci may lead to GN by their other complex effects on the immune response. These include the direct activation of T cells by a superantigen effect, whereby M proteins can bind to particular Vβ regions of the T-cell receptor and activate families of T cells sharing receptors of this 'family'. Antigenic crossreactivity ('molecular mimicry') akin to that thought to be responsible for rheumatic fever may also occur, so that anti-streptococcal antibodies crossreact with, and therefore bind to, renal autoantigens such as laminin and collagen.

Management

Poststreptococcal GN is less common in the developed than in the developing world, possibly influenced by socioeconomic factors. Its general importance lies in the fact that early recognition allows appropriate treatment, with the prognosis often being very good, and also that the immunopathological mechanisms outlined above may be instructive in understanding other forms of GN where the inciting stimulus is not so evident. Treatment of patients with poststreptococcal GN should be directed at eradicating the infection (a 10-day course of penicillin or erythromycin is advised even if the original infection appears to have resolved) and providing symptomatic relief of the consequences of the acute nephritis: aggressive treatment of hypertension, salt, and water restriction with or without diuretics for oedema; and dialysis if necessary (which is uncommon). Recovery is the rule, although haematuria and proteinuria may persist and some authors believe that in the long-term there is a risk of chronic renal failure.

Idiopathic diffuse proliferative GN

A few cases will have no preceding history of infection, no evidence of lupus, and/or atypical features on the renal biopsy: these may be assigned the unsatisfactory 'idiopathic' sobriquet, with the implication that the prognosis and the appropriate treatment are uncertain.

Further reading

Bloom PM, Filo RS, Smith EJ (1976). Immunofluorescent deposits in normal kidneys. *Kidney International* **10**, 539. [Report that IgM is present in glomeruli of 60 per cent of kidneys donated for transplantation]

Ji-Yun Y, *et al.* (1984). No evidence for a specific role of IgM in mesangial proliferation of idiopathic nephrotic syndrome. *Kidney International* **25**, 100–6. [High incidence of glomerular IgM deposits in controls as well as in nephritic kidneys]

Kefalides NA, *et al.* (1986). Antibodies to basement membrane collagen and laminin are present in sera from patients with post-streptococcal glomerulonephritis. *Journal of Experimental Medicine* **163**, 585–602. [Suggests 'molecular mimicry' as a pathogenetic mechanism in poststreptococcal glomerulonephritis]

O'Donoghue DJ, *et al.* (1991). IgM-associated primary diffuse mesangial proliferative glomerulonephritis: natural history and prognostic indicators. *Quarterly Journal of Medicine* **79**, 333–50. [Supports a separate diagnostic entity of IgM nephropathy, with implications for prognosis and treatment]

Oliveira DBG (1997). Poststreptococcal glomerulonephritis: getting to know an old enemy. *Clinical and Experimental Immunology* **107**, 8–10. [Editorial review of pathogenetic mechanisms in poststreptococcal glomerulonephritis]

Scolari F, *et al.* (1990). Familial IgM nephropathy: a morphologic and immunogenetic study of three pedigrees. *American Journal of Nephrology* **10**, 261–8. [Suggests familial form of IgM nephropathy]

Watanabe-Ohnishi R, *et al.* (1994). Characterization of unique human TCR V beta specificities for a family of streptococcal superantigens represented by rheumatogenic serotypes of M protein. *Journal of Immunology* **152**, 2066–73. [Evidence of superantigen effects of streptococcal proteins, which may contribute to pathogenesis of poststreptococcal glomerulonephritis]

20.7.6 Mesangiocapillary glomerulonephritis

Peter W. Mathieson

Mesangiocapillary glomerulonephritis (**MCGN**) is synonymous with membranoproliferative glomerulonephritis (**MPGN**). The term describes a morphological pattern of glomerular injury in which there is diffuse thickening of the glomerular basement membrane (**GBM**) associated with increased cellularity, giving a characteristic lobular appearance to the glomeruli (Fig. 1 and Plate 1). As with other forms of glomerulonephritis, such as membranous nephropathy (see Chapter 20.7.4), the appearances on light microscopy are indistinguishable whether the lesion occurs as a primary 'idiopathic' renal disease or secondary to an extrarenal/systemic disorder. Extra information is obtained with the use of immunohistology and electron microscopy, which allow further subdivision into three patterns. In type I MCGN there is typically IgG, IgM, and complement C3 in mesangial areas as well as along the glomerular capillary loops in a subendothelial or intramembranous location, and electron microscopy shows discrete electron-dense deposits in these regions. In type II MCGN there is typically no immunoglobulin deposited, but C3 is detected in a linear distribution along the capillary loops and often also in tubular and vascular basement

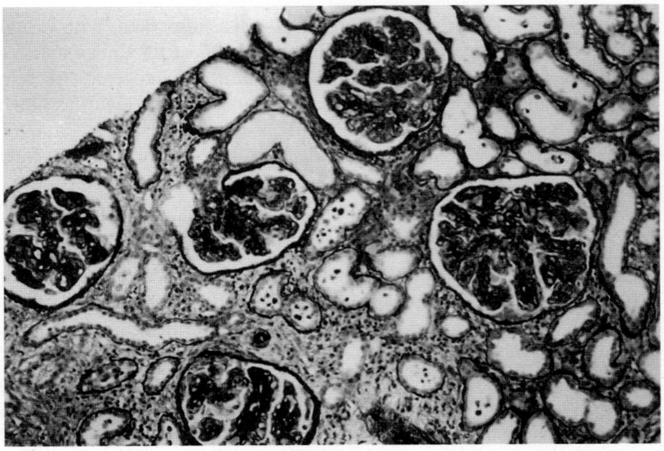

Fig. 1 Mesangiocapillary glomerulonephritis. Note characteristic lobular appearance of expanded glomerulus. (See also Plate 1.)

membranes. Electron microscopy shows typical thick, linear, electron-dense material along these basement membranes, giving rise to the other term for type II MCGN which is '(linear) dense-deposit disease' (Fig. 2). Type III MCGN is similar to type I, except that there are subepithelial as well as subendothelial deposits and there may be disruption of the GBM with accumulation of new basement membrane material in layers. Most 'secondary' forms of MCGN are of the type I pattern.

The complement system

The subdivision of MCGN into types I, II, and III is not just of academic importance. MCGN is the type of glomerulonephritis most closely associated with activation of the complement cascade and there is evidence, at least for some types of MCGN, that complement dysregulation may directly cause the renal lesion. The pattern of complement activation differs between the three subtypes of MCGN. Complement activation can occur via two main pathways, the classical and alternative pathways (Fig. 3). A recently described third pathway, the lectin or mannan-binding pathway, yields similar results to classical pathway activation and is of unknown relevance to nephritis. In general, classical pathway activation leads to depletion of plasma C3 and C4, whereas alternative pathway activation leads to a low C3 with normal C4. This is an oversimplification, since both C3 and C4 are acute-phase reactants whose synthesis is upregulated in inflammation. Thus there may be considerable complement activation without depletion

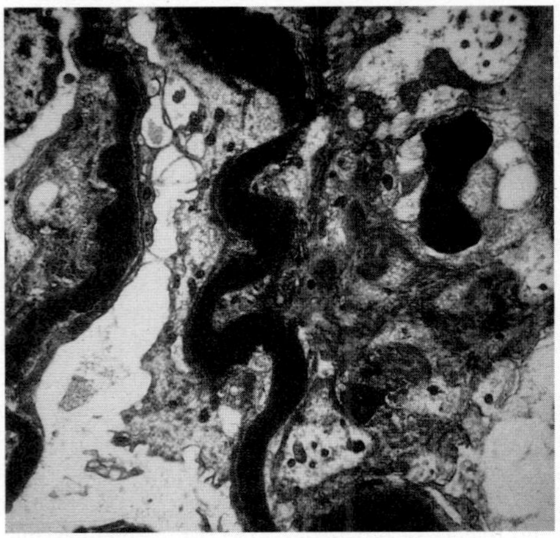

Fig. 2 Electron micrograph of type II MCGN, 'dense deposit disease'. Note linear, electron-dense material along the glomerular basement membrane.

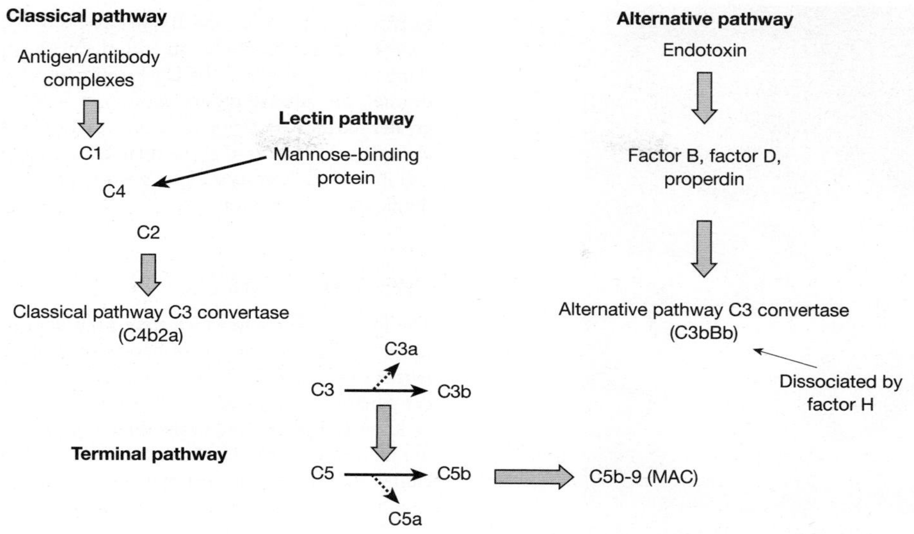

Fig. 3 The complement system.

of circulating levels, due to increased production. Further complexity is introduced by the fact that genetic deficiencies of C4 are common: there are four C4 genes encoded within the major histocompatibility complex (**MHC**) on chromosome 6, and one or more null alleles are commonly present, which result in no C4 protein production. These result in a reduction of circulating C4 concentrations—it is estimated that only 60 per cent of the normal population has all four normal C4 genes. Thus a single low C4 level must be interpreted with caution unless a previous 'normal' result is available for that individual; serial measurements are helpful since they give an indication of the level of C4 consumption.

The classical pathway is activated predominantly by immune complexes: immunoglobulin molecules linked to antigen. The alternative pathway is more concerned with host defence, being activated by bacteria or other foreign surfaces, and existing in a state of constant low-level activity: so-called 'tickover'. This state of constant activity demands tight regulation to avoid excessive activity, and this is achieved by regulatory proteins factor H and factor I. The classical and alternative pathways converge at the point at which C3 is cleaved. The enzyme formed by classical pathway activation is called the classical pathway C3 convertase, and denoted C4b2a. The enzyme formed by alternative pathway activation is the alternative pathway C3 convertase, denoted C3bBb. Each of these enzymes leads to the cleavage of C3, releasing C3a and leading to the formation of a C5 convertase enzyme which cleaves C5, thereby releasing C5a and leading to the formation of C5b–9, the membrane-attack complex (**MAC**).

Pathogenesis of MCGN

In MCGN, the pattern of complement activation (and therefore possibly the pathogenesis) is different in each of the three forms. In type I, the complement activation predominantly affects the classical pathway (causing low levels of both plasma C3 and C4); in type II it is the alternative pathway which is predominantly affected (low C3 with normal C4); and in type III there is activation of the terminal pathway leading to depletion of C5, sometimes associated with mild depletion of C3 and/or C4. 'Secondary' MCGN may occur in systemic lupus erythematosus (**SLE**); cryoglobulinaemia with or without hepatitis C; infections such as infective endocarditis or other chronic bacteraemic states (for example, 'shunt nephritis', originally described with infected ventriculoatrial shunts); or in association with neoplasms. In each of these situations there is activation of the classical pathway which is presumed to be due to circulating immune complexes, and this is associated with a type I MCGN pattern. In idiopathic type I MCGN, a variety of complement-activating factors have been described: there may be circulating immune complexes, some patients have antibodies to Clq which probably directly activate the classical pathway, and some have other autoantibodies which interfere with the normal regulation of the classical pathway. In type II MCGN, the alternative pathway activation is due to the presence of an IgG autoantibody (known as C3 nephritic factor C3NeF, or more simply as nephritic factor, NeF) which binds to a neoantigen formed when the alternative pathway C3 convertase enzyme, C3bBb, is assembled. The antibody stabilizes this enzyme and protects it from degradation by factor H. Thus the half-life of the enzyme is prolonged, and the normal regulatory mechanism is subverted. This type of nephritic factor has also been described in patients with type I and type III MCGN, but its presence is virtually invariable in type II MCGN. In type III MCGN, the presence of a circulating factor which activates complement slowly in a properdin-dependent manner has been postulated; the reasons for the preferential depletion of terminal pathway components, and whether there is a direct relationship of this activation to the renal injury in type III MCGN, remain unanswered questions.

The best evidence for a causative role of complement activation in MCGN comes in type II disease. As mentioned above, most patients with type II MCGN have the IgG autoantibody known as nephritic factor (**NeF**) which allows unregulated alternative pathway activation. Two other situations in which there is similar overactivity of the alternative pathway, and an associated renal lesion with the appearances of type II MCGN, have recently been characterized. First, genetic deficiency of the regulatory protein known as factor H, which normally serves to degrade the alternative pathway C3 convertase, has been reported in a variety of inbred pigs and also in rare human cases. Second, there is a case report of an individual whose serum contained a monoclonal lambda light chain which interacted with factor H *in vitro* and prevented its action, allowing unregulated alternative pathway activation. Therefore, in these three situations (the presence of NeF, genetic deficiency of factor H, or functional blocking of factor H), there is dysregulated alternative pathway activation, but due to completely different mechanisms. In each case, the renal lesion is type II MCGN, strongly suggesting that it is the complement activation *per se* which leads to the renal injury. Importantly, in the factor H-deficient pigs, replacement of factor H leads to prevention of the excessive alternative pathway activation and an improvement in the MCGN. These observations have clear implications for the therapy of human MCGN (discussed further below).

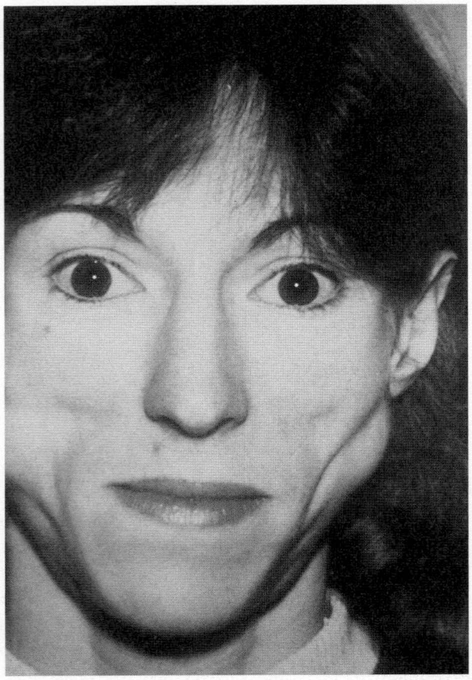

Fig. 4 Facial appearance in partial lipodystrophy. This patient has had silicone pads inserted into her cheeks, accounting for the bulges in the regions where adipose tissue has been completely lost.

The NeF autoantibody, and the resultant unregulated alternative pathway activation, have another striking clinical association: with partial lipodystrophy in which there is permanent loss of adipose tissue from the face and neck and sometimes also from the upper trunk (Fig. 4). Such patients may also have type II MCGN, and as with the renal lesion, there is evidence to suggest that the complement activation directly causes the tissue injury: NeF containing IgG can cause complement-mediated lysis of adipocytes *in vitro*. Furthermore, adipocytes are probably susceptible to this injury because they produce complement components: these observations have contributed to the recent appreciation that the complement system plays a previously unsuspected role in the normal physiological regulation of adipose tissue.

Clinical presentation

This is with proteinuria, which may be sufficiently severe to cause nephrotic syndrome; and/or haematuria, which, especially in children, may be macroscopic. Hypertension and/or impairment of excretory kidney function may be associated. Acute presentation as a nephritic syndrome is recognized in children. As mentioned above, type II MCGN may be associated with partial lipodystrophy; the loss of adipose tissue can precede the onset of nephritis by many years. Abnormalities in the eye are also recognized in type II MCGN, and may rarely be the presenting feature. Drusen-like deposits and mottled pigmentation are visible in the fundi: retinal neovascularization may occasionally threaten sight and require laser therapy.

Natural history of MCGN

Overall, the renal survival in MCGN at 10 years from diagnosis is about 50 per cent. Children tend to have a more acute presentation and a slower decline in renal function, although with lengthy follow-up the overall renal survival is similar to that in adults. The prognosis differs between the three subtypes of MCGN, with type II carrying the greatest risk of the development of endstage renal failure (**ESRF**): in one recent study the median time to ESRF in types I, II, and III was, respectively, 15.3 years, 8.7 years, and 15.9 years. Since presentation with the nephrotic syndrome carries a substantially increased risk of ESRF compared to other milder clinical syndromes, the adverse prognosis of type II MCGN may simply reflect the greater likelihood of nephrotic presentation with this histological type. As in many other forms of glomerular disease the presence of tubular atrophy and interstitial fibrosis indicate a worse prognosis, as does hypertension at the time of presentation.

Treatment of MCGN

The forms of therapy which have been applied to MCGN are similar to those used in other forms of nephritis: antiplatelet drugs, anticoagulants, corticosteroids, and alkylating agents have been used alone or in various combinations. The studies tend to be small, with varying proportions of children and adults, and of the three subtypes of MCGN. There is a dearth of randomized controlled trials and reviews of the subject have usually concluded that there is no treatment of proven efficacy in MCGN. Nevertheless, there are hints from some of the studies that certain drugs may have useful effects. In particular, high doses of prednisone, usually given on alternate days (especially in children) are favoured by some authors, especially the Cincinnati group who have published most extensively on this subject. However, high corticosteroid dosages are required for prolonged periods and the magnitude of benefit obtained may be too small to justify the risks of such treatment. Possibly by refining the dosage schedule and by applying the treatment only to high-risk groups, such as those with severe nephrotic syndrome, the risk:benefit ratio may be more favourable.

Since complement activation is so prominent in MCGN, therapy aimed at the complement system may be rational: promising anticomplement agents are now becoming available. At present, the best strategy is to try to identify any underlying cause of complement activation and remove it if possible. As in other forms of GN, associated hypertension should be aggressively treated. Patients with proteinuria of any cause have their renal prognosis improved if they are treated with angiotensin-converting enzyme (**ACE**) inhibitors. They are at increased cardiovascular risk, and attention should also be paid to other modifiable risk factors, especially cigarette smoking and hyperlipidaemia.

Recurrent MCGN in renal transplants

MCGN is one of the types of nephritis that tends to recur in kidney transplants (see Chapter X): type I recurs in around 25 to 30 per cent of grafts and type II recurs even more frequently, possibly in 85 to 90 per cent of cases. Recurrent MCGN only causes graft failure in a minority of cases, presumably because the antirejection immunosuppressive therapy modulates the damage done by the nephritis.

Further reading

Cameron JS (1982). Glomerulonephritis in renal transplants. *Transplantation* **34,** 237–45. [Review of glomerulonephritis (primary and recurrent) in transplanted kidneys]

Donadio JV, Offord KP (1989). Reassessment of treatment results in membranoproliferative glomerulonephritis, with emphasis on life-table analysis. *American Journal of Kidney Diseases* **14,** 445–51. [Cautionary tale about the assessment of treatment effects in MCGN, refuting earlier claims of effectiveness of antiplatelet therapy]

McEnery PT (1990). Membranoproliferative glomerulonephritis: the Cincinnati experience—cumulative renal survival from 1957 to 1989. *Journal of Pediatrics* **116,** S109–14. [Review of the Cincinnati experience with childhood MCGN, especially supporting the role of corticosteroid therapy]

Mathieson PW (1998). Is complement a target for therapy in renal disease? *Kidney International* **54,** 1429–36. [Review of the role of complement in various forms of renal injury, discussion of currently available anticomplement therapies, and speculation on future possibilities]

Mathieson PW (1999). Mesangiocapillary glomerulonephritis. In: CD Pusey, ed. *Treatment of glomerulonephritis*, pp 81–92. Kluwer Academic, Dordrecht, The Netherlands. [Review of literature on the treatment of MCGN, suggestions for future strategies]

Mathieson PW, Peters DK (1997). Lipodystrophy in MCGN type II: the clue to links between the adipocyte and the complement system. *Nephrology, Dialysis, and Transplantation* **12,** 1804–6. [Review of the evidence for a causative role of complement activation in type II MCGN and partial lipodystrophy, discussion of the complement system's role in the biology of adipose tissue]

Ruggenenti P *et al.* (1998). Renal function and requirement for dialysis in chronic nephropathy patients on long-term ramipril. *Lancet* **352**, 1252–6. [Influential recent trial confirming the benefits of ACE inhibition in patients with proteinuria, irrespective of the underlying cause]

Schena FP, Cameron JS (1988). Treatment of proteinuric idiopathic glomerulonephritides in adults: a retrospective survey. *American Journal of Medicine* **85,** 315–26. [Review of literature on treatment of all forms of glomerulonephritis in adults]

Schwertz R, *et al.* (1996). Outcome of idiopathic membranoproliferative glomerulonephritis in children. *Acta Paediatrica Scandinavica* **85,** 308–12. [Review of natural history of MCGN in children, especially trying to analyse any differences between types I, II, and III]

Sissons JGP, *et al.* (1979). The complement abnormalities of lipodystrophy. *New England Journal of Medicine* **294,** 461–5. [Largest series in which patterns of complement activation have been analysed in patients with different types of lipodystrophy]

Varade WS, Forristal J, West CD (1990). Patterns of complement activation in idiopathic membranoproliferative glomerulonephritis, types I, II, III. *American Journal of Kidney Diseases* **16,** 196–206. [Analysis of patterns of complement activation in subtypes of MCGN, review of reported mechanisms]

20.7.7 Antiglomerular basement membrane disease

Jeremy Levy and Charles Pusey

Introduction

Antiglomerular basement membrane disease is an autoimmune disease in which patients develop pathogenic autoantibodies against the glomerular basement membrane (**GBM**). Patients typically present with renal failure and pulmonary haemorrhage, but isolated renal disease is well recognized. The triad of anti-GBM antibodies, rapidly progressive glomerulonephritis (**RPGN**), and pulmonary haemorrhage is referred to as Goodpasture's disease in the United Kingdom, whilst the term Goodpasture's syndrome describes patients with RPGN and pulmonary haemorrhage of various aetiologies.

The term 'Goodpasture's syndrome' was first used in 1958 by Stanton and Tange in their report of nine patients with pulmonary–renal syndrome, which referred to a patient with fulminant pulmonary haemorrhage and proliferative glomerulonephritis described by Goodpasture during the influenza pandemic of 1919. In retrospect, this original patient may have had systemic vasculitis, not anti-GBM disease. In recent years much has been learnt about the immune response in Goodpasture's disease, but despite huge advances in our understanding of aetiopathogenesis, the therapy has changed little in the last 20 years.

Aetiology and pathogenesis

The Goodpasture antigen

All patients with Goodpasture's disease have circulating antibodies that bind a glomerular basement membrane antigen, the α3 chain of type IV collagen (α3(IV)). Type IV collagen is found in all basement membranes; but the α3, α4, and α5 chains are restricted in their distribution primarily to the GBM and alveolar basement membranes. The epitope for autoantibodies in Goodpasture's disease is carried at the amino terminus of the 230 amino acid, non-collagenous, carboxy-terminal domain of the α3 chain (α3(IV)NC1), which is normally hidden within the collagen network. The α3(IV)NC1 is also found in the basement membranes of the choroid plexus, the cochlea, Bruch's membrane in the eye, retinal capillaries, and the thymus.

Anti-GBM antibodies and the T-cell-mediated immune response

Transfer of antibodies from patients into squirrel monkeys initially confirmed the pathogenicity of the autoantibodies. Clinical studies report a correlation between antibody levels at presentation and disease activity, and the disease recurs immediately in renal transplants when the recipient still has circulating antibodies. All patients have antibodies against α3(IV)NC1, either circulating or bound to the GBM. A small number of patients develop antibodies against other GBM components, particularly the α1 (15 per cent of patients) or α4 (4 per cent of patients) chains of type IV collagen. However, anti-GBM antibodies are unlikely to be the only cause of glomerular injury, and a cell-mediated immune response is also important in inducing renal damage.

Alveolar haemorrhage generally requires a second insult, either local to the lungs (for example, cigarette smoking or pulmonary oedema), or systemic with activation of cytokines and inflammatory mediators (for example, sepsis).

Genetic predisposition

Goodpasture's disease has been reported in four sibling pairs and two sets of identical twins; however, discordant twin pairs are also documented. More striking is the association with the HLA serotype HLA-DR2, which is carried by more than 85 per cent of patients with Goodpasture's disease, compared with 30 per cent of controls. Molecular analysis of HLA alleles has confirmed the association with HLA-DR15 (DRB1*1501 and -1502), and a weaker association with HLA-DR4 (DRB1*04). A negative association with HLA DR7 (DRB1*07) has been demonstrated. Thus, specific characteristics of the HLA molecules on antigen-presenting cells determine susceptibility to Goodpasture's disease.

Environmental factors

No specific pathogens or toxins have been identified that can initiate Goodpasture's disease; but many case reports have documented exposure to hydrocarbons prior to the development of clinical manifestations, and cigarette smoking undoubtedly precipitates pulmonary haemorrhage. It seems more likely that organic solvents trigger overt pulmonary damage (and possibly renal injury) in the presence of circulating autoantibodies than that hydrocarbons are involved in the initiation of autoimmunity. Several clusters of cases have been reported, but no clear associations with influenza virus or other infectious agents have been proved.

Disease associations

Anti-GBM disease is only rarely associated with other autoimmune disorders, apart from systemic vasculitides. Increasing numbers of patients (up to 30 per cent) have been shown to have circulating antineutrophil cytoplasmic antibodies (**ANCA**), generally P-ANCA, in addition to anti-

GBM antibodies. Conversely, only few patients with ANCA-associated vasculitis also have anti-GBM antibodies (2.5–8 per cent). This is an important distinction since the 'double positive' patients tend to behave more like those with 'pure' Goodpasture's disease than systemic vasculitis. Anti-GBM disease has been reported after lithotripsy and urinary tract obstruction, and in some patients with membranous nephropathy. In all these cases it is possible that disruption of the GBM in susceptible individuals can lead to a breakdown in tolerance to the α3 chain of type IV collagen, with the development of autoantibodies and clinical disease.

Epidemiology

Limited epidemiological studies suggest that Goodpasture's disease has an incidence of 0.5 to 1 new case per million of the population per year. It is found in 1 to 2 per cent of renal biopsies. In comparison, systemic vasculitides have an incidence of 15 to 30 new cases per million of the population per year. The disease is less common in Afro-Caribbean and Asian populations. There is a bimodal age distribution, with peak incidence in the third and sixth decades, and a slight excess of males.

Clinical features

Most patients present with RPGN or lung haemorrhage, or both. Some patients have isolated lung haemorrhage and never develop renal failure (although most of these have haematuria and proteinuria), and a few have mild isolated nephritis. General malaise, fatigue, weight loss, and anaemia are the commonest systemic features, whilst other signs and symptoms are much rarer than in patients with systemic vasculitis.

Pulmonary features

Pulmonary haemorrhage occurs in two-thirds of patients, more commonly in young men, it usually precedes presentation with acute renal failure, and is strongly associated with cigarette smoking. Patients often complain of breathlessness and cough, and there is a poor relationship between overt haemoptysis and the degree of alveolar haemorrhage. Haemoptysis can be triggered by cigarettes, inhaled toxins, fluid overload, and intercurrent infection, either local (pneumonia) or systemic (sepsis). Clinical signs are often indistinguishable from those of pulmonary oedema or infection. The most sensitive indicator is an elevated *K*co (diffusing capacity for carbon monoxide), which identifies the presence of haemoglobin in alveolar spaces by increased binding of inhaled carbon monoxide. Radiographic features are not specific, but alveolar shadowing in the central lung fields is typically seen (Fig. 1).

Renal features

Patients can present with isolated haematuria, chronic renal failure, or mild renal insufficiency, but classically present with severe acute renal failure due to rapidly progressive glomerulonephritis. The clinical features of the nephritis are indistinguishable from any other cause of RPGN, with cellular casts in the urine, haematuria, and mild to moderate proteinuria (nephrotic range proteinuria is rare). Hypertension and oliguria are late features. A small number of patients have relatively normal renal function at presentation, but always have abnormal urine findings and evidence of antibody deposition on renal biopsy.

Differential diagnosis

It is crucial to distinguish anti-GBM disease from other cause of RPGN, and especially ANCA-associated vasculitis. There is only a small window of opportunity in which to rescue renal function in patients with anti-GBM disease, by contrast to systemic vasculitis in which renal failure can be reversed at a later stage. All patients with suspected RPGN, acute renal failure of unknown cause, or lung haemorrhage and urinary abnormalities, should have both anti-GBM antibody and ANCA assays performed urgently. Double-positive patients may respond better to therapy at a late stage compared to those with pure anti-GBM disease. Other differential diagnoses to consider include systemic lupus erythematosus (**SLE**), cryoglobulinaemia, haemolytic uraemia syndrome (**HUS**), and other causes of pulmonary renal syndrome (see Table 1).

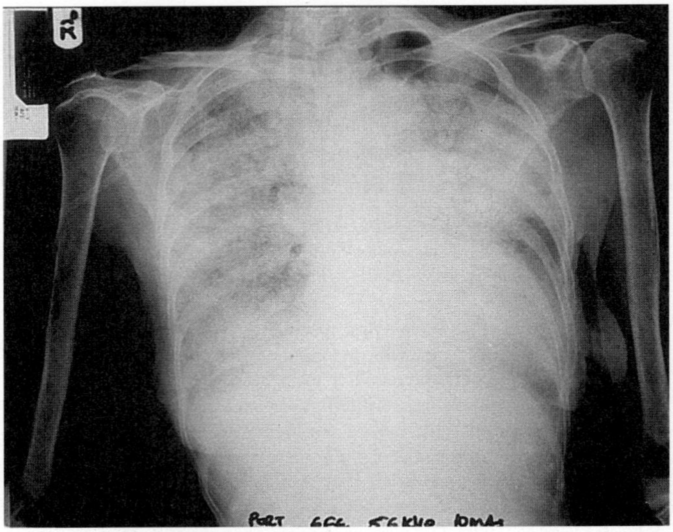

Fig. 1 Chest radiograph from a patient with Goodpasture's disease showing florid pulmonary haemorrhage.

Pathology

Immunohistology is characteristic (Fig. 2 and Plate 1), with linear deposition of IgG (sometimes with IgA or IgM) and complement C3 along the

Table 1 Pulmonary–renal syndromes

(1) Renal and pulmonary failure without alveolar haemorrhage	
Commoner:	Renal failure of any cause with pulmonary oedema (fluid overload)
	Severe pneumonia and renal failure, especially legionella
	Cardiac failure with pulmonary oedema and secondary renal failure
	Infective endocarditis
Less common:	Pulmonary embolism and renal failure (often in nephrotic syndrome)
	Paraquat poisoning
	Organic solvents
	Hantavirus infection
(2) Goodpasture's syndrome (alveolar haemorrhage and nephritis)	
Commoner:	Microscopic polyangiitis
	Wegener's granulomatosis
	Anti-GBM disease (Goodpasture's disease)
	Systemic lupus erythematosus
Less common:	Churg–Strauss syndrome
	Henoch–Schönlein purpura
	Haemolytic uraemic syndrome
	Behçet's disease
	Essential mixed cryoglobulinaemia
	Rheumatoid vasculitis
	Penicillamine therapy

glomerular basement membranes. Rare patients have been reported with IgM or IgA alone. Less intense linear staining with IgG can occasionally be seen in diabetes, SLE, myeloma, and transplanted kidneys. The most characteristic morphological finding is severe crescentic glomerulonephritis, with almost all the glomeruli exhibiting cellular crescents, usually at the same stage of evolution. Segmental necrosis and cellular proliferation may occur. Blood vessels are usually normal, but rarely vasculitis has been reported even in the absence of detectable ANCA. There is often a prominent interstitial cellular infiltrate.

Histological specimens are rarely obtained from lungs, since transbronchial biopsy does not usually penetrate beyond the bronchial mucosa. Open-lung biopsy can reveal alveoli full of red blood cells, macrophages, and fibrin, interspersed between relatively normal alveoli. Immunofluorescence inconsistently reveals linear deposition of antibody.

Laboratory diagnosis

Serological testing for anti-GBM antibodies and ANCA is crucial for confirming the diagnosis, and a renal biopsy is almost always warranted. Some healthy individuals exposed to inhaled oils, hydrocarbons, or solvents may have borderline raised anti-GBM antibody levels, and anti-GBM antibody has also been detected in HIV-negative patients with pneumocystis pneumonia. Other investigations are detailed in Table 2. Alveolar haemorrhage is an important cause of mortality and must be identified early. All patients should have baseline *K*co and chest radiology, repeated as necessary.

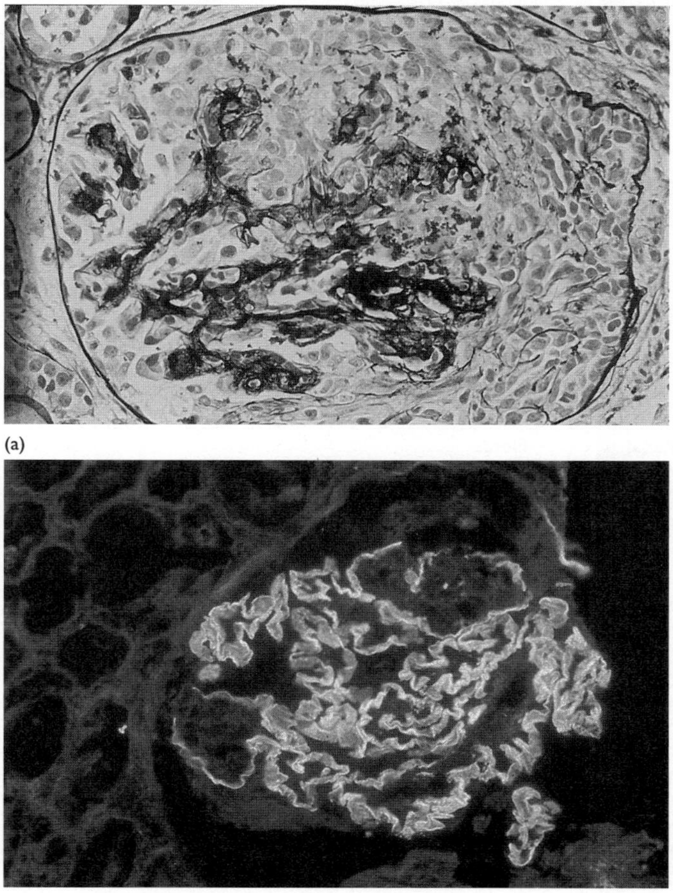

(a)

(b)

Fig. 2 Renal biopsy from a patient with Goodpasture's disease. (a) Light microscopy showing a single glomerulus with cellular crescent and focal necrosis (silver stain). (b) Immunofluorescence of a single glomerulus with linear deposition of IgG along the GBM. (Figure by courtesy of Dr HT Cook.) (See also Plate 1.)

Treatment

Untreated anti-GBM disease is usually fatal, and renal function never recovers. In most centres immunosuppressive treatment is given immediately upon diagnosis to those with a serum creatinine concentration below 600 µmol/l at presentation and/or with active pulmonary haemorrhage. Those with a serum creatinine concentration above 600 µmol/l and without active pulmonary haemorrhage need more careful consideration before being treated since they have a small chance of recovery (see below).

Treatment with plasma exchange, cyclophosphamide, and corticosteroids, together with dialysis when required, can allow up to 90 per cent of patients to survive, but only around 40 per cent of survivors will recover renal function. Daily plasma exchange removes circulating antibodies, whilst cyclophosphamide prevents further antibody synthesis. There has only been one controlled trial of plasma exchange, which utilized a low intensity of exchanges in a small number of patients and showed a non-significant trend towards an improved outcome. However, the dramatic improvement in overall mortality and renal function coincident with the introduction of a treatment regimen of the type described above has led to their widespread use. The regimen we use is shown in Table 3. An alternative to plasma exchange is protein-A immunoadsorption. Ciclosporin has been used in occasional patients unresponsive to other therapies, but is of doubtful benefit. Long-term treatment is unnecessary, and patients can

Table 2 Investigation of patients with anti-GBM disease

Urinalysis	Red cell casts, numerous erythrocytes, mild proteinuria
FBC	Hb often reduced. Monitor WBC count during immunosuppression.
Urea and electrolytes	Severe acute renal failure common
CRP	Moderately elevated (less than in vasculitis)
Immunoglobulins	Normal or mildly raised
Anti-GBM antibodies	Always positive, usually IgG. May be only mildly raised even in typical disease
ANCA	Negative in true anti-GBM disease. If 'double-positive', may have a poor outcome from renal failure
ANA, dsDNA, complement, cryoglobulins, ASOT	Negative or normal
Chest radiography	Usually bilateral airspace shadowing. Difficult to distinguish infection and fluid overload from pulmonary haemorrhage
*K*co	Raised in alveolar haemorrhage. Normal or reduced in pulmonary oedema or infection
Renal biopsy	Crescentic glomerulonephritis and linear IgG deposition along the GBM
Transbronchial biopsy	Not usually diagnostic (difficult to obtain alveoli; open biopsy more useful). Helpful in diagnosis of infection.

GBM, glomerular basement membrane; FBC, full blood count; Hb, haemoglobin; WBC, white blood cells; CRP, C-reactive protein; ANCA, antineutrophil cytoplasmic antibody; ANA, antinuclear antibody; dsDNA, double-stranded DNA; ASOT, antistreptolysin-O titre; *K*co, diffusing capacity for carbon monoxide.

Table 3 Treatment of anti-GBM disease

Initial treatment	
Plasma exchange	Daily, 4-litre exchange for 5% human albumin solution. Use 300–600 ml fresh-frozen plasma within 3 days of any invasive procedure (e.g. biopsy) or in patients with pulmonary haemorrhage. Continue for 14 days, or until antibody levels fully suppressed. Withhold if platelet count <70 × 10^9/ml, or Hb <9 g/dl. Watch for coagulopathy, hypocalcaemia, and hypokalaemia.
Cyclophosphamide	Daily oral dosing at 3 mg/kg per day (round down to nearest 50 mg; reduce to 2 mg/kg per day in patients over 55 years). Stop if white cell count <4 × 10^9/ml, and restart at lower dose when counts >4 × 10^9/ml.
Prednisolone	Daily oral dosing at 1 mg/kg per day (maximum 60 mg). Reduce dose weekly to 20 mg by week 6, and then more slowly. No evidence for benefit of intravenous methylprednisolone and may increase infection risk (possibly use if plasma exchange not available).
Prophylactic treatments	Oral nystatin and amphotericin (or fluconazole) for oropharyngeal fungal infection. Ranitidine or proton-pump inhibitor for steroid-promoted gastric ulceration. Low-dose cotrimoxazole for *Pneumocystis carinii* pneumonia prevention. Consider aciclovir as cytomegalovirus prophylaxis. Consider calcium/ vitamin D for prevention of osteoporosis (but relatively short course of steroids).
Maintenance treatment	
Prednisolone	Reduce dose slowly from 20 mg at 6 weeks, to stop completely by 6 months.
Cyclo-phosphamide	Stop after 2–3 months. No further cytotoxic agents necessary.

stop taking cyclophosphamide after 2 to 3 months, and withdraw prednisolone over approximately 6 months.

Prognosis

The outcome of patients with Goodpasture's disease in published series is shown in Table 4. Most will now survive the acute illness, but pulmonary haemorrhage and infection remain important causes of death. In those with a serum creatinine concentration below 600 μmol/l at presentation, the creatinine should begin to fall within 1 to 2 weeks of treatment, and the majority will recover renal function. However, patients with a creatinine concentration above 600 μmol/l, or with oligoanuria, less commonly recover renal function. For this reason most centres would not give immunosuppressive agents to this group with the sole intention of trying to restore renal function, although they would for concurrent active pulmonary haemorrhage or if the renal biopsy suggests that tubular necrosis may be contributing to the severity of the renal failure (see above). Crescent scores over 50 per cent, high antibody titres, and a delay in diagnosis are also markers of a poor renal prognosis.

The prognosis in anti-GBM disease is in marked contrast to that of patients with a diagnosis of ANCA-associated RPGN. Renal recovery is to be expected in the latter group with immunosuppression, and around 70 per cent of patients presenting with a creatinine concentration above 600 μmol/l will recover renal function.

Relapses of pulmonary haemorrhage and worsening of renal function can occur early during the course of treatment in the presence of circulating autoantibodies, and can be triggered by smoking, infection, or fluid overload. True late recurrence is very unusual. Transplantation is safe once autoantibodies are no longer detectable, and is best delayed until between 6 and 12 months after the disappearance of anti-GBM antibody.

Anti-GBM disease in Alport's syndrome

Patients with X-linked Alport's syndrome have a mutation in the α5 chain of type IV collagen, but also have undetectable Goodpasture antigen in their kidneys despite a normal α3(IV) gene. Transplantation of a normal

Table 4 Outcome of patients with Goodpasture's disease. Data from all published series

Series	Number of patients	1-year patient survival %	1-year renal survival %	Renal recovery[a] (% treated patients)	Notes
Benoit *et al.* (1964)	52	4	4	NA	No treatment. Patients with Goodpasture's syndrome of all causes
Wilson and Dixon (1973)	53	75	23	NA	Immunosuppression only
Beirne *et al.* (1977)	26	46	15	NA	7 patients not treated. Remainder immunosuppression only
Teague *et al.* (1978)	29	62	31	NA	Excluded patients without lung haemorrhage
Briggs *et al.* (1979)	18	83	11	0	7 patients not treated. Remainder immunosuppressed
Peters *et al.* (1982)	41	76	39	4	Hammersmith hospital single centre. All plasma exchanged
Simpson *et al.* (1982)	20	90	59	0	Excluded patients without pulmonary haemorrhage.
Johnson *et al.* (1985)	17	94	45	0	Randomized prospective study of plasma exchange
Walker *et al.* (1985)	22	59	45	18	Australian single centre. All plasma exchanged.
Savage *et al.* (1986)	59	75	8.5	NA	Data from multiple British centres.
	49	84	35	11	Hammersmith hospital single centre.
Williams *et al.* (1988)	10	90	20	NA	Single British unit. Patients presenting over 13 months.
Bouget *et al.* (1990)	14	79	29	0	French single centre.
Herody *et al.* (1993)	29	93	41	0	French single centre. Most plasma exchanged.
Merkel *et al.* (1994)	35	89	40	3	Survival at time of analysis. All plasma exchanged.
Daly *et al.* (1996)	40	—	20	0	All plasma exchanged.
Levy *et al.* (2001)	71	77	53	21	Extended Hammersmith series. All plasma exchanged. Only 8% of patients requiring dialysis recovered renal function

[a] Renal recovery if initial creatinine >600 μmol/l.

kidney into such recipients may allow the development of anti-GBM antibodies as a result of the exposure of the immune system to neoantigens to which tolerance has not developed. These antibodies are usually anti-α5(IV)NC1, but can also be anti-α3(IV)NC1 (classical Goodpasture autoantibodies). Most patients do not develop overt nephritis, but simply deposit antibody along the GBM without recruiting a glomerular inflammatory response. However, a minority develop severe glomerulonephritis. In the absence of lung antigen, pulmonary haemorrhage never occurs.

Further reading

Herody M, *et al.* (1993). Anti-GBM disease: predictive value of clinical, histological and serological data. *Clinical Nephrology* **40**, 249–55. [Detailed description and outcome of French series.]

Johnson JP, *et al.* (1985). Therapy of anti-glomerular basement membrane antibody disease: analysis of prognostic significance of clinical, pathological and treatment factors. *Medicine* **64**, 219–27. [Single controlled trial of plasma exchange in Goodpasture's disease.]

Lerner RA, Glassock RJ, Dixon FJ (1967). The role of anti-glomerular basement membrane antibodies in the pathogenesis of human glomerulonephritis. *Journal of Experimental Medicine* **126**, 989–1004. [Classic paper describing the transfer of disease by anti-GBM antibodies.]

Levy JB, Pusey CD (1997). Anti-glomerular basement membrane disease. In: Wilkinson R, Jamison R, eds. *Nephrology*, pp 599–615. Chapman Hall, London. [Comprehensive review of anti-GBM disease.]

Levy JB *et al.* (2001). Long-term outcome of anti-GBM antibody diseases treated with plasma exchange and immunosuppression. *Annals of Internal Medicine* **134**, 1033–42. [Largest series of patients reported.]

Levy JB, Pusey CD (1999). Plasmapheresis. In: Johnson R, Feehally J, eds. *Comprehensive clinical nephrology*, pp 83.1–8. Mosby, London. [Review of the techniques, use and complications of plasma exchange.]

Lockwood CM, *et al.* (1976). Immunosuppression and plasma exchange in the treatment of Goodpasture's syndrome. *Lancet* **i**, 711–15. [Classic description of treatment of Goodpasture's disease.]

Merkel F, *et al.* (1994). Course and prognosis of anti-basement membrane antibody mediated disease, a report of 35 cases. *Nephrology, Dialysis, Transplantation* **9**, 372–6. [A recent series from Europe documenting prognostic factors.]

Saus J, *et al.* (1988). Identification of the Goodpasture antigen as the α3(IV) chain of collagen IV. *Journal of Biological Chemistry* **263**, 13374–80. [Initial identification of the Goodpasture antigen.]

Savage COS, *et al.* (1986). Anti-GBM antibody mediated disease in the British Isles 1980–1984. *British Medical Journal* **292**, 301–4. [Largest series of patients reported in the United Kingdom.]

Stanton MC, Tange JD (1958). Goodpasture's syndrome, pulmonary haemorrhage associated with glomerulonephritis. *Australasian Annals of Medicine* **7**, 132–44. [Initial description of Goodpasture's syndrome.]

Turner N, *et al.* (1992). Molecular cloning of the human Goodpasture antigen demonstrates it to be the alpha 3 chain of type IV collagen. *Journal of Clinical Investigation* **89**, 592–601. [Molecular characterization of the Goodpasture antigen.]

20.7.8 Infection-associated nephropathies

A. Neil Turner

Introduction

Almost all varieties of renal lesion, particularly glomerular, may be associated with infections. The pathways leading to these are sometimes understood, but sometimes obscure. In the West, infection-associated nephritis was once predominantly recognized during episodes of acute infections in apparently healthy individuals. This is still the pattern in less developed regions; but this could be partly a problem of recognition, as in all populations infections are more common and more severe in malnourished or otherwise debilitated individuals. Improvements in living conditions and healthcare in developed countries have reduced the numbers of healthy people succumbing to complications of infection. By contrast, infections occurring on a background of debilitating illnesses and previous medical interventions have become more common, and are certainly more often diagnosed.

In this chapter, glomerular diseases and interstitial diseases associated with infection are considered in turn. Particular attention is given to those glomerulopathies associated with bacterial endocarditis and other chronic bacterial infections, and to three viral infections of worldwide importance—human immunodeficiency virus (**HIV**), hepatitis B, and hepatitis C.

Pathogenesis

Infection-associated glomerular disease is usually attributed to trapping of circulating antigen–antibody complexes or to immune responses to pathogen-derived antigens that become 'planted' in the glomerulus. The evidence for the deposition of circulating immune complexes is unequivocal for cryoglobulinaemia, and highly plausible for infections occurring within the vascular system such as bacterial endocarditis. In most other infections the evidence is less clear.

Interstitial renal disease is often blamed on direct invasion by microorganisms, and for some, particularly viruses, there is evidence that this is true. The pathogen may cause injury directly, or indirectly by causing cells to express foreign antigens that generate an immune response. More speculatively, an immune response generated to an organism may crossreact with a remote self-antigen, triggering autoimmunity through molecular mimicry, but there are no unequivocal examples of this.

Infection may also involve the kidney by interfering with the circulation either generally (septic shock) or locally (for instance, by causing thrombotic microangiopathy, as for *Escherichia coli* O157), or *Capnocytophaga canimorsus* (previously DF-2). On occasions, toxins may be released that harm the kidney directly (for example, haemoglobin in malaria). Medically administered toxins include antimicrobial agents that impair renal function by crystallization (aciclovir, indinavir, etc.), or by predictable toxicity (e.g. aminoglycosides and amphotericin), or by idiosyncratic reactions such as acute interstitial nephritis (e.g. penicillins).

Glomerulonephritis associated with chronic and acute bacterial infections

Classic, acute postinfectious glomerulonephritis is considered separately elsewhere. This chapter centres on the more subacute or chronic diseases, although other causes of a 'classical' picture are mentioned.

Shunt nephritis was first recognized in the 1960s and remains the archetype of an immune-complex nephritis. The glomerulonephritis occurring in association with infective endocarditis is very similar. Both are caused by subacute infection within the bloodstream, with constant production and shedding of antigen and the formation of antigen–antibody complexes. Other bacterial infections cause similar pictures, or patterns more similar to acute 'postinfectious' glomerulonephritis.

Shunt nephritis

In shunt nephritis a ventriculoatrial shunt implanted for the treatment of hydrocephalus becomes colonized by bacteria, usually of low pathogenicity. More common modern equivalents of this clinical syndrome are due to infected long-term, indwelling, central vein catheters and other intravascular devices. The syndrome does not occur with ventriculoperitoneal shunts, which are therefore now the preferred neurosurgical option. Although *Staphylococcus epidermidis* has been most commonly implicated, *Propionibacterium acnes* or other organisms are sometimes involved. Typically, the diagnosis is only appreciated after weeks to months of symptoms of mild to moderate pyrexia and malaise associated with haematuria, proteinuria, and progressive renal impairment. Fevers have often been attributed to urinary infection in patients with neurogenic bladders. There may be moderate splenomegaly. Investigations show variable renal impairment, complement consumption, and an acute-phase response with a normochromic normocytic anaemia. The renal lesion is characteristically a type-1 mesangioproliferative glomerulonephritis with deposition of multiple immunoglobulins and complement components beneath the endothelium, the classic appearance of a circulating immune-complex nephritis. Sometimes the picture is more severe, showing a diffuse proliferative lesion, occasionally with crescents. In other cases the histological appearances are less pronounced with focal proliferative changes.

Antibiotic treatment alone is almost never adequate to cure these infections, which require removal of the shunt, followed by its replacement after an interval if drainage is still required. Delayed diagnosis and delayed removal may lead to severe and irreversible renal damage and sometimes to endstage renal failure. Substantial recovery often follows successful treatment.

Infective endocarditis

A similar syndrome occurs in patients with subacute bacterial endocarditis (see Chapter 15.10.2), when minor glomerular involvement is probably extremely common. The majority of signs and symptoms in these circumstances are common to shunt nephritis. Typical streptococcal infections are well represented in case series, but there have been many reports involving 'slow' infections such as Q fever (*Coxiella burnetti*) and more unusual causes including chlamydia and fungi. Infection of prosthetic or native heart valves may be implicated. Right-sided endocarditis occurring in intravenous drug abusers may be particularly likely to present as nephritis, perhaps because the diagnosis is often delayed. Depletion of serum complement is again diagnostically useful, but, as for shunt nephritis, most other serological and haematological changes are non-specific. Partial treatment with antibiotics makes diagnosis more difficult, as positive blood cultures are usually a key part of proving the diagnosis and planning appropriate therapy.

The pathological lesion is often similar to that of shunt nephritis. A more acute endocarditis (for instance, that associated with *Staphylococcus aureus*) is more likely to cause glomerulonephritis in a diffuse proliferative pattern, sometimes with crescent formation. A third lesion has been increasingly reported in recent literature – focal changes that are indistinguishable from ANCA-associated vasculitis– indeed, in some cases ANCA have been detected. Cutaneous vasculitis may be seen in association with bacterial infection, and this seems particularly likely in endocarditis (Fig. 1 and Plate 1).

In most cases the outcome depends on the response of the endocarditis to treatment, but renal involvement is a poor prognostic factor for survival, which may be simply because it reflects a long-standing infection. Recovery from dialysis-dependence may occur.

Patients with endocarditis are also prone to two other renal lesions. Interstitial nephritis is frequently due to the prolonged administration of drugs, including high doses of antibiotics. Those with disease on the left side of the heart or with right–left shunts may suffer renal emboli. These are common at autopsies, but glomerulonephritis is probably a more common cause of urinary abnormalities in most patients.

Deep-seated bacterial infections

Amyloidosis is a well-recognized consequence of very chronic bacterial (including mycobacterial) and other infections, and is described in Chapters 11.12.4 and 20.10.4. As in reactive amyloidosis of other aetiologies, progression of the renal lesion may be prevented or even reversed by treatment of the cause.

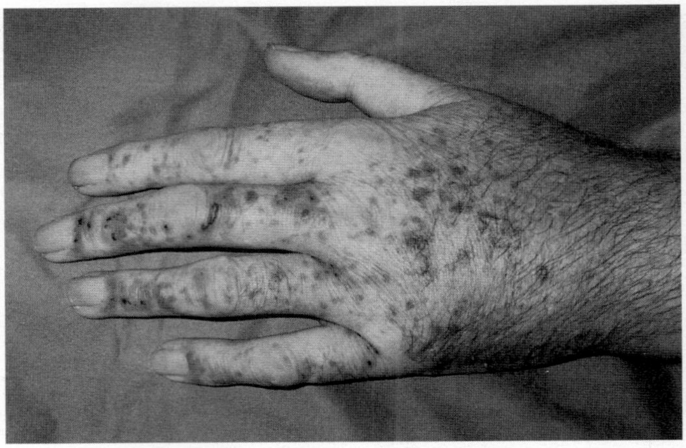

Fig. 1 Cutaneous vasculitis in a patient with *Staphylococcus aureus* endocarditis. (See also Plate 1.)

Deep-seated infections, particularly abscesses, may also be associated with acute renal pathology. Although the mechanisms involved are presumably similar to those of shunt nephritis and nephritis associated with endocarditis, blood cultures have often been negative in reported cases. *Staphylococcus aureus* is the most frequently implicated organism. A specific type of renal disease in association with methicillin-resistant *Staph. aureus* (**MRSA**) infection has been postulated, but without strong support. A wide variety of renal lesions have been described, usually inflammatory/proliferative and with immunoglobulin deposition. Unsuspected abscesses or other deep-seated infections are occasionally found only after the renal biopsy appearances trigger a search. Such hidden abscesses are more likely to occur in the obese, the elderly, and in those prescribed corticosteroids or who are immunosuppressed by other means or by disease.

Acute glomerulonephritis and other infections

Acute glomerulonephritis resembling poststreptococcal nephritis has been reported in association with a large number of other organisms: including current (as opposed to recent) infection with staphylococci, streptococci, and other bacteria, and with acute viral infections that are usually self-limiting. These include Epstein–Barr virus, cytomegalovirus, coxsackieviruses, and the varicella, measles, and mumps viruses. Some may cause a clinical syndrome that is very similar to poststreptococcal nephritis, while others typically cause a less florid 'nephritic' or mixed 'nephritic/nephrotic' picture.

Diagnostic difficulties in bacterial infection-related glomerulonephritis

Infection-related nephritis may present in a very similar manner to nephritis associated with other systemic diseases, notably microscopic polyangiitis and other small-vessel vasculitides. As both types of disease process may be associated with fever, a systemic illness, and an acute-phase response, it is important to consider the possibility of infection in all patients thought to have systemic vasculitis. Blood cultures should be routine. **ANCA** (antineutrophil cytoplasmic antibody) assays are extremely useful, but it is important to note that ANCA positivity has been recorded in many infections, both by fluorescence and by solid-phase assays: ANCA are not diagnostic of small-vessel vasculitides. Renal biopsy is often the most discriminating investigation: infection-associated glomerulonephritis is usually associated with plentiful immunoglobulin deposition, although the pattern is variable, whereas small-vessel vasculitis is characteristically pauci-immune. Non-glomerular causes of renal impairment (interstitial nephritis, acute tubular necrosis) are also distinguished by renal biopsy.

Interstitial nephritis associated with infections

Bacterial infections

Acute bacterial pyelonephritis is usually a florid and painful disorder associated with symptoms of urinary tract infection, as described in Chapter 20.12. Substantial renal impairment is usual only if a single functioning kidney is affected. Occasionally, however, the diagnosis is masked by immunosuppression (for example, in a transplanted kidney), age, or other factors, and the diagnosis is made by the renal biopsy appearances of neutrophils in the interstitium and in tubules, which are rarely found in any other renal lesions.

Acute interstitial nephritis is a key feature of Weil's disease, a severe form of leptospirosis (see Chapter 7.11.31). Jaundice and renal failure follow a febrile illness caused by infection with *Leptospira interrogans*. The renal lesion comprises interstitial oedema with predominantly mononuclear infiltrates and foci of tubular necrosis. Renal failure is usually oliguric but may be polyuric. Dialysis may be required for days to weeks, and renal recovery may sometimes be incomplete.

Other bacterial infections that may cause a similar pathological picture include Rocky Mountain Spotted Fever (*Rickettsia rickettsii*), in which there may be an interstitial nephritis with foci of haemorrhage, and acute *Yersinia pseudotuberculosis* infection, in which an acute lymphocytic interstitial nephritis has been described in several patients. Legionnaire's disease (*Legionella pneumophila*) has been reported to be associated with renal impairment due to an interstitial nephritis, but in some instances may show a picture of acute tubular necrosis. The same is probably true of other severe pneumonias.

Mycobacteria spp. can cause a chronic granulomatous interstitial nephritis that is discussed below.

Viral infections

Hantaviruses

Hantaviruses are carried by small rodents and have been associated with a range of human syndromes that involve the kidneys with varying severity. 'Haemorrhagic fever with renal syndrome' (**HFRS**) was originally described in Eastern Asia. The usual renal syndrome is of oliguric renal failure, associated histologically with lymphocytic interstitial nephritis that may be haemorrhagic in severe cases, reflecting a systemic bleeding diathesis. Some patients have been reported to have persistent renal impairment after recovery.

HFRS was originally associated with Hantaan strains of hantavirus in Korea, while milder disease, usually with less severe or frequent renal impairment and without haemorrhagic diathesis, was associated with the Seoul strain. The milder disease ('nephropathia epidemica') recognized in Northern Europe, and subsequently more widely, was associated with Puumula strain. However, it has become apparent that there are many more subtypes of hantavirus, and that the association of a serotype with a particular clinical picture is not rigid. Severe disease with shock, variable haemorrhage, and (sometimes) pulmonary impairment has been encountered in patients in the Balkans and Greece. Disease with predominantly pulmonary manifestations and shock has been recognized particularly in North America, although these geographical variations in the clinical picture are no more rigid than the strain variations.

Ribavirin was shown to be effective in treating patients with HFRS in China, but in a smaller trial in North American patients with the pulmonary syndrome it was found to be no better than placebo.

Cytomegalovirus and polyomavirus

Cytomegalovirus (**CMV**) may lie dormant in renal tubular cells, and during new or reactivated infection cause characteristic inclusion bodies. This rarely has significant impact on renal function outside the setting of renal transplantation, where CMV infection commonly occurs concurrently with acute rejection. Although there is evidence that CMV infection may precipitate rejection, it is also clear that the risk of CMV infection is greatly increased by most types of antirejection therapy. CMV may also rarely cause a florid glomerular lesion characterized by gross endothelial-cell damage and swelling, resembling pre-eclampsia. This has again been recognized almost exclusively in renal transplant patients, where some believe that the appearances are due to, or complicated by, vascular rejection.

Human polyomaviruses (BK and JC) were previously believed to be benign passenger viruses that replicated without causing damage during immunosuppression. However, BK virus was recently recognized as a cause of impaired renal transplant function, generally months after transplantation. The histological changes of tubulitis had usually suggested acute cellular rejection, leading to further immunosuppression and favouring further infective damage, but inclusion bodies and immunohistochemical or *in situ* hybridization studies provided evidence for active virus replication—one report described an improvement of renal function in several patients after the reduction of immunosuppressive agents. Similar manifestations have not yet been described in other immunosuppressive settings.

Other viruses

A wide range of other viruses and micro-organisms have been less regularly associated with interstitial lesions. HIV may cause an interstitial nephritis and is considered separately below. Another condition that is likely to be infective in origin, Kawasaki disease (see Chapter 18.10.8), is associated with interstitial nephritis, although glomerular lesions have also been described occasionally.

HIV and renal disease

Renal impairment is commonly encountered at some stage of HIV infection, the largest single cause of serious renal disease being the distinct entity of HIV nephropathy. However, this generalization is misleading since this specific diagnosis is largely restricted to Black patients, and there are many other causes of renal disease in patients with HIV infection.

Focal segmental glomerulosclerosis associated with HIV infection (HIV nephropathy)

HIV nephropathy is characterized by heavy proteinuria and renal impairment. It has become the third most frequent cause of endstage renal failure (**ESRF**) in Black adults of working age in the United States. Although it has often been described as the initial manifestation of HIV infection, detailed analyses suggest that even in these cases the infection is advanced and CD4 counts are usually low. The histological appearances are of focal segmental glomerulosclerosis (**FSGS**) of the 'collapsing' form, with injury and hypertrophy of glomerular epithelial cells accompanied by variable interstitial inflammation with oedema and microtubular dilatation. It typically progresses to ESRF very rapidly, over weeks to months. Perhaps because of its association with low CD4 counts, the medium-term prognosis is usually poor despite renal replacement therapy. Highly active antiretroviral therapy is likely to have improved the outlook, and there are isolated reports of responses of nephropathy to such treatment, but at the time of writing no clear picture has emerged. Renal function in some patients has been reported to improve dramatically in response to treatment with corticosteroids, but this is not predictable and carries significant risk. It has been suggested that any improvement may be due to responses of interstitial nephritis rather than the glomerular lesion, as evidenced by the lack of reduction in proteinuria in one study.

Non-FSGS nephropathy in HIV infection

The large proportion of patients with HIV infection and nephropathy of other causes (a majority in most populations) can rarely be reliably distinguished by clinical criteria. Renal biopsies in this group have shown a very wide range of diagnoses encompassing almost all types of glomerular lesion, interstitial nephritis, cryoglobulinaemia, and thrombotic microangiopathy. Some of these lesions may be related to concurrent infections with other micro-organisms. Others may be related to therapy. Aciclovir and indinivar have replaced sulphonamides as common causes of crystal nephropathy. Idiosyncratic reactions to drugs may be more frequent in patients with HIV infection, but they also receive many drugs with predictable nephrotoxicity. The occurrence of autoimmune phenomena in patients with HIV infection may also be accompanied by an increase in immune-mediated primary glomerular diseases.

Nephropathy associated with hepatitis B virus

Chronic infection with hepatitis B virus (**HBV**) is strongly associated with membranous nephropathy and is an important secondary cause of the lesion, with a frequency that depends on the population. A less clear relationship holds with membranoproliferative nephropathy, while for hepatitis C virus (**HCV**) the converse is true.

Chronic HBV infection is much more common in some regions and racial groups, and the distribution of HBV-related nephropathy closely follows this distribution. The clinical picture may be complicated by the concurrence of HBV infection with infection by HCV or other organisms, or by coincidental significant renal and hepatic disease. HBV membranous nephropathy has a close relationship with virus multiplication, so affected individuals are **HBeAg**- and **HBsAg**-positive (hepatitis B e antigen, hepatitis B surface antigen, respectively) and hepatitis usually coexists, although it may be minor and subclinical. Membranous nephropathy is a more common complication of HBV infection in children, but it is also more benign in this group. The lesion may be static or in some cases (particularly in adults) associated with progressive deterioration to ESRF.

The histopathological appearances are typical of membranous nephropathy (see Section 20.8.6), and HBV antigens may be detectable in glomerular deposits. Whether this is relevant to pathogenesis is debatable. Animal models suggest that antibodies to podocyte surface molecules are a more likely way of producing the membranous lesion than trapping of preformed antigen–antibody complexes.

Seroconversion from HBeAg-positive to HBeAb-positive status is associated with remission of the renal lesion, whether the conversion occurs naturally or is induced by treatment. Spontaneous remission of the renal lesion is more likely in children. Antiviral treatment is the appropriate therapy when required, as immunosuppression may increase the viral burden. Unfortunately this is least likely to be successful in those populations in which the problem is greatest.

HBV infection has been associated with classic polyarteritis nodosa (**PAN**) in some populations, such as in France and North America, but even in these areas HBV–PAN is uncommon and apparently decreasing in incidence. Furthermore, the association of the two diseases is rare in some countries with both low (for example, the United Kingdom) and high (for example, Thailand) rates of HBV carriage. Usually the infection has been acquired within months of the onset of arteritic manifestations. Clinically the disease is typical of PAN, affecting medium and somewhat smaller vessels but not capillaries, and therefore not usually associated with focal necrotizing or crescentic nephritis. ANCA are not usually detected. Treatment is difficult as immunosuppression favours viral replication and exacerbation of liver disease, while remission is associated with seroconversion from HBeAg- to HBeAb-positivity.

Nephropathy associated with hepatitis C virus

Chronic hepatitis C virus (**HCV**) infection is the major cause of mixed essential (type II) cryoglobulinaemia in most populations. The mechanism is unknown, but the cryoglobulinaemia associated with HCV infection is entirely typical (see Chapter 20.10.5). The clinical picture includes cutaneous vasculitis, glomerular pathology (membranoproliferative glomerulonephritis), and other manifestations. The cryoglobulins contain quantities of HCV antigens and bound antibody, in addition to monoclonal IgM rheumatoid factors.

HCV may also be associated with mesangioproliferative glomerulonephritis in the absence of detectable cryoglobulins. A relationship with membranous nephropathy has been suggested but is not proven.

As for HBV, reduction of viral replication has been associated with disease remission, but this is harder to achieve for HCV than for HBV with current therapies. Immunosuppression with corticosteroids and sometimes other agents may be required to control disease manifestations caused by vasculitis.

Renal sequelae of other chronic infections

Amyloidosis may be a consequence of all sorts of chronic infection, but of the 'tropical' infections is most frequently associated with schistosomiasis, filariasis, or leishmaniasis.

Mycobacteria

Mycobacterial infections cause a chronic granulomatous interstitial nephritis that is characteristically associated with inflammatory and fibrotic abnormalities in the ureters and lower urinary tract. Symptoms often relate to this lower tract involvement; however, the disease may be asymptomatic and in the earliest stages involvement is presumed to be restricted to the kidneys, with subsequent spread to the lower tract. Sterile pyuria is the rule. Impaired renal function is common at presentation. Intravenous urography will show blunting of the calyces, progressing to changes typical of pyelonephritis or papillary necrosis, along with lower tract abnormalities such as ureteric strictures and scarring and contraction of the bladder. Amyloidosis is a well-recognized secondary complication of mycobacterial infections. Idiosyncratic reactions to antituberculous drugs are the other common cause of late renal dysfunction.

Syphilis

Congenital syphilis may cause severe nephrotic syndrome with the histological pattern of membranous nephropathy. This is also the usual pattern in the rare instances when secondary syphilis causes a nephrotic syndrome. Both respond to antispirochaetal treatment.

Malaria

Plasmodium falciparum infections may cause acute renal disease, but chronic lesions are usually associated with chronic *P. malariae* infection, as described in Chapter 20.7.10.

Schistosomiasis

In renal/urological practice, schistosomiasis is best recognized for causing disease of the lower urinary tract, but chronic infections associated with hepatosplenomegaly may be associated many years later with glomerular disease. In *Schistosoma haematobium* infection this is often due to secondary infections with *Salmonella* species rather than directly associated with schistosomal infection. In *S. mansoni* infection the usual relationship is directly causal, producing a mesangiocapillary or mesangioproliferative picture.

Filariasis

Long-standing filariasis may also be associated with glomerular lesions. An acute syndrome with tubulointerstitial nephritis has also been described in association with the presence of microfilariae in renal capillaries.

Further reading

Bonarek H, *et al.* (1999). Reversal of c-ANCA positive mesangiocapillary glomerulonephritis after removal of an infected cysto-atrial shunt. *Nephrology, Dialysis, Transplantation* **14**, 1771–3. [An example of the association of c-ANCA and proteinase-3 antibodies with infection. Other examples are listed in the discussion.]

Conlon PJ, *et al.* (1998). Predictors of prognosis and risk of acute renal failure in bacterial endocarditis. *Clinical Nephrology* **49**, 96–101.

Daghestani L, Pomeroy C (1999). Renal manifestations of hepatitis C infection. *American Journal of Medicine* **106**, 347–54.

Gee WM, (1993). Causes of death in a hospitalized geriatric population: an autopsy study of 3000 patients. *Virchows Archives A* **423**, 343–9. [Pyelonephritis was commonly clinically unsuspected in this large series of unselected autopsies.]

Guillevin L, *et al.* (1995). Polyarteritis nodosa related to hepatitis B virus. A prospective study with long-term observation of 41 patients. *Medicine (Baltimore)* **74**, 238–53.

Haffner D, *et al.* (1997). The clinical spectrum of shunt nephritis. *Nephrology, Dialysis, Transplantation* **12**, 1143–8. [A report of a condition now rarely seen.]

Johnson RJ, Couser WG (1990). Hepatitis B infection and renal disease: clinical, immunopathogenetic and therapeutic considerations. *Kidney International* **37**, 663–76.

Johnston RJ, *et al.* (1994). Renal manifestations of hepatitis C virus infection. *Kidney International* **46**, 1255–63.

Jones JM, Davison AM (1986). Persistent infection as a cause of renal disease in patients submitted to renal biopsy: a report from the Glomerulonephritis Registry of the United Kingdom MRC. *Quarterly Journal of Medicine* **58**, 123–32. [A rare review of biopsy diagnoses from many centres.]

Klotman PE (1999). HIV-associated nephropathy. *Kidney International* **3**, 1161–76. [A very good general review.]

Koo JW, *et al.* (1996). Acute renal failure associated with *Yersinia pseudotuberculosis* infection in children. *Pediatric Nephrology* **10**, 582–6.

Majumdar A, *et al.*(2000). Renal pathological findings in infective endocarditis. *Nephrology, Dialysis, Transplantation* **15**, 1782–7. [Forty-two of the 62 kidneys studied here were autopsy samples, and of these, half showed localized infarction, whereas this was not identified in biopsies from living patients. Focal changes and crescent formation were the most common glomerular lesions in this group with severe renal and other disease.]

Montseny JJ, *et al.* (1995). The current spectrum of infectious glomerulonephritis: experience with 76 patients and review of the literature. *Medicine (Baltimore)* **74**, 63–73. [Little detail of individual cases but a revealing survey of causes and frequencies in a modern hospital environment.]

Neugarten J, Baldwin DS (1984). Glomerulonephritis in bacterial endocarditis. *American Journal of Medicine* **77**, 297–304. [Although some years old, it describes the current situation.]

Peters CJ, Simpson GL, Levy H (1999). Spectrum of hantavirus infection: hemorrhagic fever with renal syndrome and hantavirus pulmonary syndrome. *Annual Review of Medicine* **50**, 531–45.

Randhawa PS, *et al.* (1999). Human polyoma virus-associated interstitial nephritis in the allograft kidney. *Transplantation* **67**, 103–9.

20.7.9 Malignancy-associated renal disease

A. Neil Turner

Malignant disease may affect the kidneys and urinary tract by five broad mechanisms (Table 1).

Direct involvement of the urinary tract

Solitary kidney tumours in adults are usually caused by renal-cell carcinoma (hypernephroma). Bilateral tumours may occur, but multicentric tumours should lead to the suspicion of an inherited disorder—the least rare of these are von Hippel–Lindau syndrome (see Chapter 20.11; cystic and solid lesions, some malignant), or tuberous sclerosis (see Chapter 20.11; benign lesions), both having an autosomal dominant mode of inheritance. Lymphoma and leukaemia may occasionally invade the renal substance on a sufficient scale to cause renal impairment, but it is rare for other tumours to do so.

A rare and aggressive renal medullary tumour has recently been described in young Blacks with sickle-cell trait or disease: these are easily confused with tumours of the collecting system; all reported cases have been rapidly fatal.

The collecting system and lower urinary tract may be affected by transitional-cell tumours or by invasive malignancies. Transitional-cell tumours affecting the bladder are common, and sometimes cause urinary obstruction if they are extensive or if they block one or both ureters or bladder outflow. Lesions in the ureters and collecting system are less common. They occur multifocally in association with analgesic nephropathy and Balkan nephropathy (see Chapter 20.9.2). Multifocal premalignant or malignant changes have also been described in patients with 'Chinese herb nephropathy', an epidemic of renal interstitial fibrosis associated with the ingestion of a herbal slimming aid in Europe during the early 1990s.

Table 1 Mechanisms by which malignant disease can affect the kidneys and urinary tract

Mode of involvement	Examples
Direct	Tumours of the renal substance Lymphoma, leukaemia deposits Remote metastases from solid tumours Tumours of the urinary tract, prostate gland, etc. Local invasion (cervix, colon)
Metabolic and remote effects	Hypercalcaemia Hypokalaemia Hyperuricaemia Thrombotic microangiopathy (tumour-associated TTP)
Deposition of tumour products	Myeloma kidney (precipitation in tubules) Immunoglobulin deposition diseases
Immune reaction	Minimal-change disease (particularly with lymphomas) Membranous nephropathy (particularly with solid tumours) RPGN (crescentic nephritis) and small-vessel vasculitis
Effect of treatment	Tumour lysis syndrome Direct toxicity of drugs Idiosyncratic (e.g. immune) response

TTP, thrombotic thrombocytopenic purpura; RPGN, rapidly progressing (crescentic) glomerulonephritis.

Metabolic effects

Hypercalcaemia is a feature of many malignancies, both with and without metastasis. Its renal effects are discussed in Chapter 20.10.5. Hypokalaemia may be a consequence of acute leukaemias or rectal tumours, and occasionally may be severe enough to cause renal dysfunction (see Chapter 20.2.2).

Hyperuricaemia and tumour lysis syndrome

Severe hyperuricaemia (>900 μmol/l) is characteristically associated with the occurrence of massive cell death following chemotherapy for haematological or solid tumours (tumour lysis syndrome), when it is usually accompanied by hyperphosphataemia and often hypocalcaemia. High serum lactate dehydrogenase (**LDH**) levels may also be diagnostically useful. Similar gross hyperuricaemia may also be seen following radiotherapy of radiosensitive tumours; sometimes this also occurs in untreated patients who have haematological or other malignancies with a very high rate of cell turnover. Levels this high can lead to precipitation within renal tubules and acute renal failure. Allopurinol should therefore be given prophylactically before commencing any chemotherapeutic regimen where such a response might occur.

Allopurinol therapy is still appropriate once hyperuricaemia has developed, and maintenance of high urinary output, and possibly urinary alkalinization, should theoretically be beneficial. If oliguric renal failure has developed then prolonged haemodialysis treatment may remove enough urate to permit renal recovery. Urate oxidase (uricase) has also been used in these circumstances to convert urate to the more soluble compound allantoin, but the enzyme is not widely available.

Remote effects of malignant tumours on the kidney

Thrombotic microangiopathy

Thrombotic microangiopathy occurring in association with malignant disease (also known as malignancy-associated thrombotic thrombocytopenic purpura, see Section 22). is often attributed to chemotherapy: although this is particularly associated with some agents (for example, bleomycin, mitomycin), isolated reports do implicate other drugs. However, in some instances the classic presentation with thrombocytopenia, microangiopathic haemolytic anaemia, and renal failure occurs in association with primary tumours. This has been particularly reported for malignancies of the stomach, pancreas, and prostate when occasionally it is the presenting sign, but it more often occurs in the setting of a known tumour.

In the absence of specific evidence, tumour-related thrombotic microangiopathy is usually treated in the same way as thrombotic microangiopathy of other types, by plasma exchange with fresh-frozen plasma. Microangiopathy generally subsides if the tumour is responsive to treatment. Renal function may be recoverable if the process is halted rapidly, an outcome most likely to be achieved in patients with prostatic carcinoma.

Other tumour products

The protean effects of the monoclonal overproduction of immunoglobulins, or their component parts, are considered elsewhere in this section. The tubulotoxic effects of light chains may be amplified by hypercalcaemia in patients with myeloma, or by the concurrent administration of other nephrotoxins—notably intravenous contrast media. Although amyloidosis was reported in older series as a consequence of lymphomas, it is now very rarely encountered as a consequence of malignancy.

Immune reactions

Malignant disease is common, so cancer will be associated with nephropathy by chance on occasion. There are therefore many case reports in the literature, but some associations have been reported consistently and are beyond doubt. The best evidence for a linkage between malignancies and intrinsic renal diseases is in minimal-change disease and membranous nephropathy (see Chapter 20.7.4). There is also substantial evidence for an association of malignancy with various types of vasculitis.

Some malignancies are particularly likely to be associated with renal disease. Chronic lymphocytic leukaemia and similar low-grade, B-cell tumours are associated with a variety of types of glomerulopathy. Thymomas have frequently been associated with glomerular lesions, usually causing nephrotic syndrome exhibiting a variety of histological patterns. There is little evidence, by contrast, for a common association of malignancies with primary interstitial renal diseases.

Minimal-change nephrotic syndrome

Lymphomas, usually Hodgkin's disease, are rarely associated with minimal-change nephropathy; this may be the presenting sign of the lymphoma, and it may also herald relapses. More so than with other renal lesions that are putatively associated with malignancy, it has often been possible to show a close temporal relationship between the occurrence of nephrotic syndrome and the presentation of the tumour. However, there is no way of proving the association in an individual patient, or of suspecting an underlying lymphoma in patients who present with nephrotic syndrome without systemic symptoms. As the association is very rare in comparison to the number of young patients with minimal-change disease, screening other than by clinical examination and simple investigations does not seem justified. The renal lesion is typical in its pathological characteristics, and usually also in response to corticosteroid treatment.

Less commonly, minimal-change disease has been associated with solid tumours, and particularly with malignant and benign thymomas.

Membranous nephropathy

Membranous nephropathy is sometimes associated with malignancy, especially in the elderly. Series have reported rates of malignancy ranging from 5 to 11 per cent, with the risk being greatest in those at the upper end of the age range. However, different inclusion criteria have sometimes been used to assess risk: for example, some series have included tumours recognized long after a diagnosis of renal disease has been made, when the association may be coincidental. Most reported tumours have been of solid organs but haematological malignancies are also implicated. Very often the disease is advanced and obvious by the time that nephrotic syndrome or a heavy proteinuria is recognized. In some cases, effective treatment of the malignancy has led to an improvement in the nephrotic syndrome or proteinuria. The use of alkylating agents or corticosteroids to treat membranous nephropathy is not recommended in this setting, unless it would be appropriate for treatment of the malignancy itself.

In patients presenting with membranous nephropathy, controversy surrounds the value of screening for malignancy when this is not apparent from initial investigations. However, palpation of the breasts, faecal occult blood testing, and rectal examination should not be neglected. Routine haematological and biochemical investigations are appropriate for all patients, as is chest radiography and renal ultrasound. In older patients there should be a low threshold for investigating gastrointestinal or other symptoms/signs: for example, with upper gastrointestinal endoscopy, sigmoidoscopy/colonoscopy, or mammography. However, in clinical practice the number of treatable and otherwise subclinical tumours uncovered in this way is low, hence an exhaustive series of investigations is not indicated in the absence of clear and specific clinical indications.

Systemic vasculitis

Focal necrotizing and crescentic nephritis (rapidly progressive glomerulonephritis, RPGN), with or without evidence of small-vessel vasculitis affecting other organs, may occur in association with malignancy. Small-vessel vasculitis is more common in the elderly, so that some of the associations will be chance associations. However, there are sufficient reports of unusual associations to strongly suggest a causal relationship in some cases.

As well as true vasculitis, cancer-related thrombotic microangiopathy and thrombotic events complicating disseminated intravascular coagulation in association with cancer may resemble systemic vasculitis and lead to diagnostic confusion. Recent evidence suggests that thrombotic thrombocytopenic purpura itself may be an autoimmune condition caused by autoantibodies to von Willebrand factor protease, but it is not yet clear whether this association also applies to cases associated with malignancy.

The commonest type of vasculitis to be associated with malignancy is small-vessel cutaneous vasculitis. In other cases, the presence of a small-to-medium vessel systemic vasculitis, not usually associated with autoantibodies to neutrophil granule proteins (**ANCA**, antineutrophil cytoplasmic antibody), has been reported in the bowel and other organs, including the kidney. More typical ANCA-associated vasculitis has also been associated with malignancy, and there may be a particular relationship between Wegener's granulomatosis and renal-cell carcinoma. Usually the kidney is not involved in cancer-associated systemic vasculitis, but when it is the appearances are indistinguishable from those of small-vessel vasculitides of other aetiologies. Immune deposits are not usually found in the glomeruli (pauci-immune). Atrial myomas have been associated with lesions of larger and smaller vessels, and it appears that embolization is not always the explanation for this.

Effects of treatment

These include the tumour-lysis syndrome (discussed above), as well as idiosyncratic or predictable reactions to therapeutic agents. On occasions, minimal-change disease or other lesions have been associated with interferon therapy.

Further reading

Biava CG, *et al.* (1984). Crescentic glomerulonephritis associated with nonrenal malignancies. *American Journal of Nephrology* **4**, 208–14.

Bursteinß DM, Korbet SM, Schwartz MM (1993). Membranous glomerulonephritis and malignancy. *American Journal of Kidney Diseases* **22**, 5–10.

Cosyns JP, *et al.* (1999). Urothelial lesions in Chinese-herb nephropathy. *American Journal of Kidney Diseases* **33**, 1011–17.

Dabbs DJ, *et al.* (1986). Glomerular lesions in lymphomas and leukemias. *American Journal of Medicine* **80**, 63–70.

Gordon LI, *et al.* (1999). Thrombotic microangiopathy manifesting as thrombotic thrombocytopenic purpura/hemolytic uremic syndrome in the cancer patient. *Seminars in Thrombosis and Hemostasis* **25**, 217–21.

Kaplan BS, Klassen J, Gault MH (1976). Glomerular injury in patients with neoplasia. *Annual Review of Medicine* **27**, 117–25.

Kurzrock R, Cohen PR, Markowitz A (1994). Clinical manifestations of vasculitis in patients with solid tumors. A case report and review of the literature. *Archives of Internal Medicine* **154**, 334–40.

Lesesne JB, *et al.* (1989). Cancer-associated hemolytic-uremic syndrome: analysis of 85 cases from a national registry. *Journal of Clinical Oncology* **7**, 781–9.

Ronco PM (1999). Paraneoplastic glomerulopathies: new insights into an old entity. *Kidney International* **56**, 355–77. [Excellent review covering most glomerulopathies, particularly membranous and minimal-change disease, and those associated with haematological malignancy.]

Tatsis E, *et al.* (1999). Wegener's granulomatosis associated with renal cell carcinoma. *Arthritis and Rheumatism* **42**, 751–6. [A retrospective survey of 477 patients showed a specifically increased risk of renal-cell carcinoma, which in five of the seven patients occurred simultaneously with Wegener's granulomatosis.]

Valli G, *et al.* (1998). Glomerulonephritis associated with myasthenia gravis. *American Journal of Kidney Disease* **31**, 350–5. [Of three patients, two had thymomas. Ten previous case reports, including one previous series of three patients (Scadding 1983), are reviewed.]

Warren KE, Gidvani-Diaz V, Duval-Arnould B (1999). Renal medullary carcinoma in an adolescent with sickle cell trait. *Pediatrics* **103**, E22.

20.7.10 Glomerular disease in the tropics

Kirpal S. Chugh and Vivekanand Jha

Introduction

Glomerulonephritis continues to be the commonest cause of endstage renal failure in tropical countries. Reliable statistics on the various types of glomerular diseases encountered in different geographical regions are not available: the published data is mostly based on individual experiences, and suggests a significant difference in the epidemiology, aetiology, and natural history of glomerulonephritis between populations living in countries with tropical and temperate climates. The most important factor that appears to account for this difference is the high prevalence of infection-related glomerulonephritis in tropical regions. Furthermore, the impact of glomerulonephritis on the individual is often more severe: a lower degree of protein loss leads to more severe peripheral oedema and serous effusions in a malnourished individual, and the condition often remains undiagnosed and untreated for long periods due to the lack of uniform access to healthcare, culminating in a higher morbidity and mortality. Because of enormous variation in the prevalence of various endemic infections in different countries, the pattern of glomerulonephritis is different throughout the tropical region.

The overall prevalence of glomerulonephritis appears to be 60 to 100 times higher in tropical countries than in temperate regions. Hospital-based surveys from South Africa, Zimbabwe, Senegal, Uganda, Nigeria, Yemen, and Papua New Guinea show that nephrotic syndrome accounts for between 0.2 and 4 per cent of all hospital admissions. Primary glomerular diseases account for the majority of cases, but secondary causes are responsible for nephrotic syndrome in 40 to 55 per cent of patients in some countries like Zimbabwe and Jamaica.

Primary glomerular diseases

The relative frequencies of the various primary glomerulonephritides in the tropical countries and the rest of the world are shown in Figs 1 and 2. Minimal-change disease is as prevalent in Asian countries as in the developed world, but is seen less frequently in Africa. In a study from South Africa, minimal-change disease was responsible for nephrotic syndrome in 75 per cent of children of Indian ancestry, whereas only 13.5 per cent of Black children showed this lesion. The frequency of membranous nephropathy is high in countries with a high hepatitis B carrier rate. A variant of membranous nephropathy associated with hypocomplementaemia has been described in Senegal.

IgA nephropathy (incorporated under the heading mesangioproliferative nephropathy in Figs 1 and 2) has emerged as the commonest primary

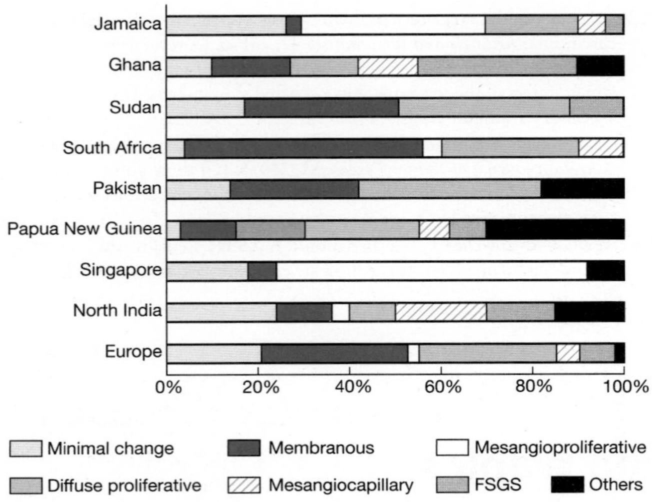

Fig. 1 Prevalence of primary glomerular disease in adults with nephrotic syndrome.

glomerular disease in many parts of the world, including Far Eastern tropical countries where it accounts for between 30 and 50 per cent of all cases of primary glomerulonephritis. By contrast, its frequency is estimated to be 5 to 15 per cent in countries of the Indian subcontinent and South America, and less than 1 per cent amongst the Black population in Africa. However, the reported differences in prevalence may be partly related to the lack of facilities for performing immunofluorescence studies in many centres in the tropical regions. High dietary fibre intake has been suggested to protect Black people from IgA nephropathy.

Postinfectious glomerulonephritis, due to both streptococcal and non-streptococcal organisms, continues to be encountered in a significant proportion of patients in tropical countries.

Glomerular diseases specific to the tropics

In addition to the well-recognized bacterial and viral infections with worldwide distribution that can cause glomerular disease (see Chapter 20.7.8), several other pathogens have been recognized to be associated with glomerular lesions in the kidneys in tropical countries, leading to a significantly different profile of infection-related glomerular disease. Causal relationships are initially suggested by epidemiological studies and then established by demonstrating the resolution of renal lesions following treatment of the infection. More recently, improved diagnostic techniques and well-designed experimental studies have provided more concrete evidence in favour of a cause-and-effect relationship. Direct confirmatory evidence has been obtained by the demonstration of specific antigens (using monoclonal antibodies), immunoglobulins, and complement within the lesions, pointing to the immunological origin of glomerular disease. The infections that cause glomerular lesions specifically in the tropics are listed in Table 1.

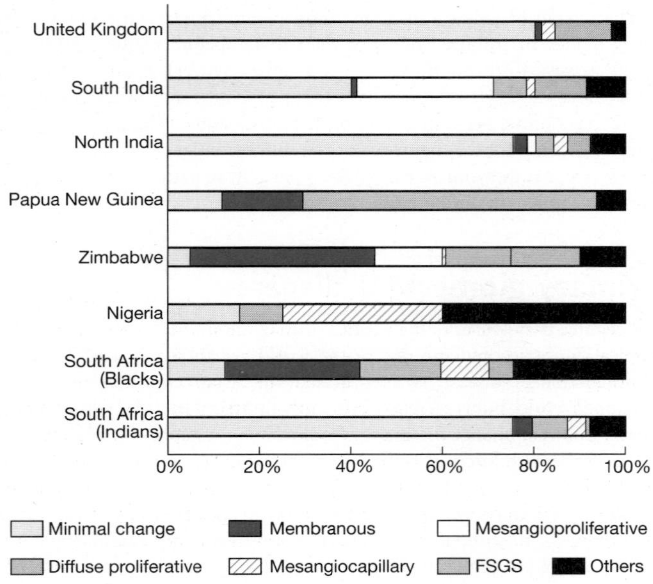

Fig. 2 Prevalence of primary glomerular diseases in nephrotic children.

Table 1 Tropical infections associated with glomerular lesions

Protozoal	*Plasmodium malariae*
	Plasmodium falciparum
	Schistosoma mansoni
	Wuchereria bancrofti
	Loa loa
	Onchocerca volvulus
Bacterial	*Mycobacterium leprae*
	Mycobacterium tuberculosis
	Salmonella typhi
	Brucella abortus
	Leptospira spp.

Malarial nephropathy

Malaria, caused by members of the protozoan *Plasmodium* genus, is endemic in the Indian subcontinent, Middle and Far Eastern Asia, sub-Saharan Africa, and Central America where the hot and humid tropical climate is conducive to multiplication of the disease vector, the Anopheles mosquito. Of the four species that are pathogenic in humans, *P. vivax*, *P. ovale*, *P. malariae*, and *P. falciparum*, only the latter two are associated with clinically significant renal disease. Acute renal failure is the chief complication in falciparum malaria infection. Glomerulonephritis is observed with *P. malariae* infection (quartan malarial nephropathy) and less commonly with *P. falciparum*.

Quartan malaria

Although the first record of quartan malarial nephropathy in the medical literature dates back to 1884, a definite cause-and-effect relationship between *P. malariae* and the nephrotic syndrome was established in 1930 by Giglioli in the surveys carried out in British Guyana. A number of reports subsequently supported his observations, most notable being that by Gilles and Hendrickse who recorded an increased prevalence of *P. malariae* parasitaemia amongst nephrotic children in western Nigeria. The condition has also been reported from Uganda, Kenya, Ivory Coast, Sumatra, New Guinea, and Yemen.

The exact incidence of glomerulonephritis associated with quartan malaria is unknown, but the frequency of nephrotic syndrome in areas endemic for this infection is between 20 and 60 times higher than in non-endemic areas. The prevalence has shown a consistent decline with the eradication of malaria in many areas, most notably in Uganda.

Clinical features

Quartan malarial nephropathy is rare during the first 2 years of life, with the peak incidence being between 5 and 8 years of age. The prevalence declines thereafter, although sporadic cases are reported in adult life. Most patients are poor and malnourished. The most frequent presentation is with a nephrotic syndrome developing several weeks after the onset of quartan fever. Oedema is prominent and accentuated by concomitant protein energy malnutrition. Proteinuria is non-selective in 80 per cent of cases. Gross haematuria is not seen, but microscopic haematuria is noted in some cases. The blood pressure is normal at the onset of disease, but increases once renal failure sets in. Anaemia is a universal feature and enlargement of the liver and/or spleen is noted in over 75 per cent cases. Hypoalbuminaemia is usually profound, with values commonly under 1 g/dl. By contrast with other causes of nephrotic syndrome, the serum cholesterol level tends to be normal or low, reflecting low dietary intake. Serum creatinine is usually normal at presentation. Serum complement (C3) is within the normal range. In the early stages, *P. malariae* parasitaemia is detected in about 75 per cent cases.

Pathology

The predominant light microscopic abnormality is segmental thickening of glomerular capillary walls. This is focal in the early stages, but the number of affected glomeruli increases as the disease progresses. The thickening is due to the subendothelial deposition of Periodic acid–Schiff (**PAS**)- and silver stain-positive fibrils arranged in a plexiform manner. Laying down of new basement membrane material on the opposite side gives rise to the classical 'double contouring'. Eventually the capillary lumina are obliterated and mesangial sclerosis extends to involve all components. Proliferative lesions, including mesangial hypercellularity and small fibroepithelial crescents, have been described in adults.

Immunofluorescence shows deposits of IgG (usually subclass 3), IgM, and C3. Three patterns have been described. The commonest is a coarse, granular deposition along the capillary walls; a minority show diffuse, homogeneously distributed IgG2 deposits; and a mixed pattern is observed in the remaining cases. *P. malariae* antigen is detected in about one-third of patients. Electron microscopy chiefly reveals subendothelial deposits of basement membrane-like material. Intramembranous deposits may also be seen.

Pathogenesis

Demonstration of malarial antigen in the deposits and binding of specific antibody to circulating malarial antigens suggest an immunological basis for the condition. The Rhesus monkey (*Macaca mulatta*) when infected with *P. inui* develops an immune complex glomerulonephritis, and so has been proposed as an experimental model for quartan malarial nephropathy. Subendothelial location of the deposits indicates formation of immune complexes in the circulation rather than *in situ*. The permissive role of environmental factors, such as malnutrition or co-infection with Epstein–Barr virus, has been speculated to explain the development of lesions in some but not all cases of *P. malariae* infection. It has been suggested that the liver may act as a source of continuous antigen supply by harbouring the parasite.

Management

Treatment of quartan malarial nephropathy is highly unsatisfactory. Once established, the disease follows an inexorably progressive course, culminating in renal failure within 2 to 4 years. Antimalarial drugs such as chloroquine and pyrimethamine have been ineffective in controlled trials. Prednisolone is ineffective in inducing remissions and may lead to infections and worsening of hypertension, although some workers have reported a 50 per cent response rate to steroids in those with highly selective proteinuria. Remission of nephrotic syndrome has been reported occasionally with cyclophosphamide in patients with mild histological lesions, but there is no improvement in overall survival. Azathioprine is associated with increased mortality and is contraindicated in this condition.

Falciparum malaria

The incidence of glomerulonephritis associated with falciparum malaria is difficult to estimate as the disease is mild, transient, and overshadowed by other complications. Autopsy studies reveal glomerular lesions in about 18 per cent of cases, but urinary abnormalities including non-selective proteinuria, microhaematuria and casts are noted in 20 to 50 per cent. Full-blown nephrotic and acute nephritic syndromes are seen occasionally. By contrast to quartan malarial nephropathy, glomerulonephritis associated with falciparum malaria resolves within 4 to 6 weeks of eradication of infection.

Pathology

The histological lesions are characterized by mesangial hypercellularity and a modest increase in the mesangial matrix. Basement membrane changes are usually absent. An eosinophilic granular material is present in capillary walls, mesangium, and Bowman's capsule, along with pigment-laden macrophages in the capillary lumina. Immunofluorescence shows finely granular IgG3, IgM, and C3. Malarial antigen can be demonstrated in some cases. Electron microscopy reveals subendothelial and mesangial deposits.

Pathogenesis

Transient glomerular lesions akin to those in falciparum malaria can be induced in BALB/c mice and Sprague–Dawley rats infected with *P. berghei*, also in *P. falciparum*-infected squirrel monkeys, the latter model showing endocapillary proliferation in addition to mesangial hypercellularity. Recent studies have suggested that CD4 cell subpopulations, in particular TH2 cells, may be playing a significant role in the genesis of these glomerular lesions, with renal cytokine expression strongly correlated with the severity of proteinuria in C57BL/6J mice infected with *P. berghei*. The role of concomitant infection, especially with the hepatitis B virus, is under investigation.

Schistosomal nephropathy

Schistosomiasis is a chronic infection caused by trematodes (blood flukes) and affects over 300 million people in Asia, Africa, and South America. Of the seven species pathogenic to man, the most prevalent are *Shistosoma haematobium* (Africa and the Middle East), *S. mansoni* (South America and Africa) and *S. japonicum* (China and the Far East). *S. haematobium* primarily involves the lower urinary tract, whereas *S. mansoni* involves the gastrointestinal tract and portal system, leading to hepatic fibrosis and portal hypertension.

Glomerulonephritis has been described most frequently in association with hepatosplenic schistosomiasis produced by *S. mansoni*. The first reports came from autopsy series in Brazil during 1964. Several clinical observations from endemic areas of Africa, Saudi Arabia, Aden, and Yemen and experimental studies have since confirmed the cause-and-effect relationship of *S. mansoni* infection with glomerulonephritis. *S. japonicum* is known to cause glomerulonephritis only in experimental animals.

In clinical studies, overt proteinuria has been reported in 1 to 20 per cent of patients infected with *S. mansoni* and 2 to 5 per cent with *S. haematobium* infection; microalbuminuria is found in about 22 per cent of patients with hepatosplenic schistosomiasis. Histological studies have documented subclinical glomerular lesions in a much higher proportion of patients, with glomerular abnormalities detected on renal biopsy in 40 per cent of patients who underwent splenectomy in one study, none of whom had clinical evidence of renal disease, hence the true extent of subclinical glomerular involvement remains unknown.

Clinical features

Though described at all ages, glomerulonephritis is seen most commonly in young adults with overt hepatosplenic disease. Males are affected twice as frequently as females. Peripheral oedema and ascites are the hallmarks of clinical glomerular involvement. Hypertension is seen in 50 per cent of cases, appearing late in the disease. Proteinuria is poorly selective and haematuria is uncommon in the absence of lower urinary tract involvement. About 30 per cent of patients exhibit hypergammaglobulinaemia; the serum cholesterol is not elevated in an equal proportion; serum complement (C3) levels are usually low. Non-specific antibody production is demonstrated by false-positive rheumatoid factor or the **VDRL** (Venereal Disease Research Laboratory) test, especially in those with concomitant salmonella infection. Demonstrating viable eggs in the stool or egg-containing granulomas in a rectal or liver biopsy makes the diagnosis of schistosomiasis. It is important to exclude other causes of nephrotic syndrome before attributing the lesions to schistosomiasis. Some patients with schistosomiasis and proteinuria have been shown to have a coexistent salmonella infection.

Pathology

Several patterns of glomerular pathology have been described (Table 2). The Class I lesion is the earliest and most frequent, all three types of mesangioproliferative lesion being seen with equal frequency (see Table 2). It is also the principal lesion in renal allografts with recurrent schistosomal nephropathy. Class II lesions are more frequent in patients with concomitant salmonella infection. The frequency of Class III lesions varies from 20 per cent in asymptomatic patients to over 80 per cent in those with overt renal disease, over 90 per cent of Class III cases belonging to Class III A. Immunofluorescence shows IgG and C3, less commonly IgM and IgA. Schistosomal antigen is detected in a minority of cases. Electron microscopy shows subendothelial and epimembranous deposits in Class IIIA and IIIB, respectively. The Class IV lesion, seen in 15 to 40 per cent of cases, cannot be distinguished from idiopathic focal segmental glomerulosclerosis (**FSGS**) on the basis of light microscopy, but immunofluorescence reveals IgA deposition in most cases. Class III and IV lesions are seen in patients with fibrotic livers. Class V prevalence varies from 15 to 40 per cent, with a higher frequency in African patients. This form is not usually affected by hepatic fibrosis.

Pathogenesis

Schistosomal glomerulopathy is caused by the immunological reaction to specific parasitic antigens. Out of over 100 immunological constituents extracted from adult worms, Cercariae and Schistosomulae, only a few have been identified *in vivo*. The pathogenic antigens originate in the gut of the adult worm, are regurgitated into the host's bloodstream and find their way to the glomeruli. Schistosoma antigens unaccompanied by any immunoglobulin have been demonstrated in the glomeruli of Kenyan baboons infected with *S. mansoni*, suggesting a role for the kidneys in the disposal of circulating antigens. Circulating immune complexes have been documented in humans and experimental animals, with the highest titres in those with hepatosplenic disease. The complexes usually localize in the mesangial region. An additional component of *in situ* immune complex formation is suggested by the extramembranous location of deposits. Interspecies antigenic variation could be responsible for the differential expression of glomerular injury.

Portocaval shunting secondary to hepatic fibrosis is critical in the genesis of an immune reaction to such antigens. Diversion of portal blood carrying the primary load of worm antigen directly into the systemic circulation prevents their normal processing and degradation by hepatic macrophages. This hypothesis is supported by the low frequency of glomerular disease in cases of *S. haematobium* infection that do not show hepatic involvement. Baboons with *S. mansoni* infection develop neither portal fibrosis nor glomerular disease despite heavy infestation. IgA antibodies predominate in the circulation of patients with schistosomal glomerulonephritis, whereas those with hepatosplenic schistosomiasis without glomerular involvement show IgM antibodies. Impaired clearance by the liver and increased production secondary to immunoglobulin isotype 'switching' from IgM- to IgA-producing B cells are postulated to be responsible for this alteration. The number of circulating mononuclear IgA-bearing cells is also increased in these patients.

Elevated immunoglobulin levels and false-positive rheumatoid factor and VDRL tests suggest the presence of an autoimmune disorder. Antinuclear antibodies, specific against the public anti-DNA idiotype 16/6 ID, have been found in the sera and glomerular deposits of humans and experimental animals.

The role of salmonella infection in the genesis of schistosomal nephropathy is unclear. Epidemiological studies have shown that urinary abnormalities disappear following therapy for salmonella alone, suggesting that these abnormalities could be purely due to salmonella infection in some cases.

Management

Treatment of schistosomal glomerulopathy is disappointing. Antischistosomal drugs like oxamniquine, hycanthone, or praziquantel are unsuccessful in altering the clinical course, which is one of inexorable progression to renal failure. Steroids or cytotoxic agents, alone or in combination, are ineffective in inducing remission. Isolated reports of response to these agents have not been evaluated in controlled trials. Salmonella infection should be looked for and treated in all patients.

Table 2 Clinicopathological classification of schistosomal glomerulopathy

Class	I	II	III A	IIIB	IV	V
Light microscopic pattern	Mesangioproliferative (a) 'Minimal lesion' (b) Focal proliferative (c) Diffuse proliferative	Exudative	Mesangio-capillary type I Mesangial IgG and C3, schistosomal gut antigen(early), IgA (late)	Mesangiocapillary type II Mesangial and subepithelial IgG and C3, schistosomal gut antigen (early), IgA(late)	Focal and segmental glomerulosclerosis	Amyloidosis
Immunofluorescence	Mesangial IgM and C3 Schistosomal gut antigens	Endocapillary C3 Schistosomal antigens			Mesangial IgG, IgM, and IgA	Mesangial IgG
Asymptomatic proteinuria	+++	–	+	+	+	+
Nephrotic syndrome	+	+++	++	+++	+++	+++
Hypertension	+/–	–	++	+	+++	+/–
Progression to ESRD	+/–	+/–	++	++	+++	+++
Response to treatment	+/–	+++	–	–	–	–

ESRD, endstage renal disease.

Modified with permission from Barsoum RS (1993). Schistosomal glomerulopathies. *Kidney International* **44**, 1–12.

Filarial nephropathy

Filarial worms are nematodes that dwell in the subcutaneous tissues and lymphatics. These are transmitted to humans through arthropod bites. Clinical manifestations depend upon the location of microfilariae and adult worms in the tissues. Of the eight filarial species that infect humans, *Loa loa*, *Onchocerca volvulus*, *Wuchereria bacrofti*, and *Brugia malayi* are associated with glomerular disease.

Loiasis is prevalent in West and Central Africa and characteristically manifests with localized areas of allergic inflammation and calabar swellings. Onchocerciasis (river blindness) is characterized by subcutaneous nodules, a pruritic skin rash, sclerosing lymphadenitis, and ocular lesions. Bancroftian and brugia infections cause febrile episodes associated with acute lymphangitis and lymphadenitis, leading ultimately to lymphoedema manifesting as hydrocele and elephantiasis. This form of filariasis is endemic in Africa and SE Asia.

The frequency of glomerular involvement in filariasis is difficult to estimate. Urinary abnormalities have been described in 11 to 25 per cent of cases of loiasis and onchocerciasis, with a nephrotic syndrome in 3 to 5 per cent. Nephrotic syndrome is more common in those with polyarthritis and chorioretinitis, and impaired creatinine clearance is more frequent with onchocerciasis than loiasis. Regarding wuchererian and bancroftian filariasis, early studies indicated an increased incidence of proteinuria in patients infected with *B. malayi* compared to controls, but there was no correlation with the severity of filariasis. In a recent survey in an endemic area, proteinuria was detected in over 50 per cent of patients with filariasis, with 25 per cent showing glomerular proteinuria. The frequency of proteinuria, also of microhaematuria and hypertension, is significantly higher in patients with chronic sclerosing filariasis than in those with an acute febrile illness or microfilaraemia. False-positive rheumatoid factor, both of IgG and IgM type, and anti-DNA and antiphospholipid antibodies and autoantibodies against a variety of cytoplasmic proteins may be noted in some cases.

Pathology

Light microscopy reveals a gamut of lesions, including mesangial proliferative, mesangiocapillary, minimal-change disease, chronic sclerosing glomerulonephritis, and the collapsing variant of focal segmental glomerulosclerosis. A diffuse basement membrane thickening with a mild increase in the number of endocapillary cells is the commonest finding. Mononuclear interstitial infiltration and microinfarcts around blood vessels have been demonstrated in patients with loiasis. Microfilariae may be found in the glomerular capillary lumina, tubules, and interstitium. Electron microscopy shows widely spaced subepithelial, subendothelial, and intramembranous deposits and spikes. *O. volvulus* and *B. malayi* antigens along with IgM, IgG, and C3 have been demonstrated in the deposits. Biopsies from patients with loiasis exhibit reactivity with hyperimmune anti-Onchocerca serum, raising the possibility of a shared antigen.

Pathogenesis

Filarial glomerulonephritis appears to be immune complex-mediated. Circulating immune complex levels correlate with the adult worm burden. Dogs infected with *Dirofilaria immitis* develop glomerular lesions similar to human filariasis. Immune complexes can also form *in situ*, as suggested by one experimental study that showed the development of glomerular lesions in kidneys after selective catheterization and infusion of *D. immitis* into the renal arteries. The contralateral kidneys either remained uninvolved or showed very minor lesions. Diethylcarbamazine treatment, by killing the parasite, may lead to antigen release into the circulation, thus exacerbating the immune process. A temporal relationship between the administration of this agent and the development of proteinuria has been noted.

Treatment

A good response to antifilarial therapy with diethylcarbamazine is observed in patients with non-nephrotic proteinuria and/or haematuria. The response is inconsistent in those with nephritic syndrome, and deterioration of renal function may continue despite clearance of microfilariae with treatment.

Mycobacterial infections

Leprosy

Leprosy is a chronic granulomatous disorder caused by the acid-fast bacillus *Mycobacterium leprae*. Nephritis in patients with leprosy was recognized by Hansen and Looft in 1894, and continued to be an important cause of death until the 1950s. The two major glomerular lesions encountered in leprosy include glomerulonephritis and secondary amyloidosis.

Glomerulonephritis

The incidence of glomerulonephritis varies from under 2 per cent on clinical evaluation to over 50 per cent on histology. Interpretation of various studies is confounded by bias in patient selection, with specialized centres reporting high figures. Glomerulonephritis is seen in both lepromatous and non-lepromatous forms of leprosy and is more common during episodes of erythema nodosum leprosum.

Clinical features Most patients present with asymptomatic urinary abnormalities but nephrotic syndrome, acute nephritic syndrome, and rapidly progressive renal failure have all been described in a small number of patients. Hypertension is uncommon. Reduced creatinine clearance is noted in patients with erythema nodosum leprosum, and impaired urinary acidification and concentration may be demonstrated. Hypocomplementaemia is common, and circulating cryoglobulins are present in many cases.

Pathology The histological picture is varied. The most frequent light microscopic lesions are those of mesangial proliferative and diffuse proliferative glomerulonephritis, although other morphological lesions have been reported. Acid-fast bacilli are seen rarely. Electron microscopy reveals electron-dense deposits in the mesangial and subendothelial regions, focal foot-process widening, glomerular capillary basement membrane reduplication with mesangial interposition, and endothelial cytoplasmic vacuolation. Immunofluorescence reveals granular deposits of IgG and C3, and less frequently IgM, IgA, and fibrin in the mesangium and along capillary walls.

Pathogenesis The lesions are manifestations of an immune complex process. Circulating immune complexes can be detected in about one-third of those with lepromatous disease and over 75 per cent of patients with active erythema nodosum leprosum. The antigen is thought to be derived from *M. leprae*, but there is also speculation about the role of a non-mycobacterial antigen derived from co-infecting micro-organisms or dapsone: antidapsone antibodies. Alternate-pathway complement activation by cryoprecipitates can exacerbate the glomerular injury.

Management In general, steroids or antileprosy drugs have no effect on the course of glomerular disease. Prednisolone may hasten the recovery of renal function in patients with renal failure during episodes of erythema nodosum leprosum.

Amyloidosis

The incidence of renal amyloidosis in leprosy ranges from 2 to 55 per cent in different geographical regions. Amyloid was documented in 55 per cent cases in older autopsy and biopsy studies from the United States, but reports from Mexico, Africa, and India found the incidence to be less than 10 per cent. The amyloid is of AA type and is far more frequent in lepromatous compared to non-lepromatous leprosy: erythema nodosum leprosum further increases the risk as each episode is associated with a marked and persistent elevation of serum amyloid A protein. Patients with tuberculoid leprosy who have long-standing and infected trophic ulcers can also develop this complication.

Amyloidosis can be prevented by early and aggressive antileprosy treatment, with particular attention to preventing erythema nodosum leprosum.

Tuberculosis

Renal involvement in patients with tuberculosis takes the form of granuloma formation, interstitial nephritis, and caseous destruction. An association of glomerulonephritis with tuberculosis was postulated in the preantibiotic era, but only stray reports have described immune complex glomerulonephritis and dense-deposit disease in tuberculosis in recent times. The cause-and-effect relationship remains speculative, and a chance association cannot be excluded. A well-known complication, however, is amyloidosis, which is still seen in a significant proportion of patients in poor countries where the disease often remains untreated for long periods. Once established, the course of amyloidosis is unaffected by treatment of the underlying tuberculosis.

Other infections

Variable degrees of glomerular involvement are seen with a variety of infections encountered in the tropical countries. These include: bacterial infections such as typhoid and pneumococcal infection; viral infections including dengue haemorrhagic fever; protozoal infections such as toxoplasmosis, kala-azar, and trypanosomiasis; and parasitic infestations like trichinosis. In most cases, the glomerulonephritis is mild and transient and resolves with treatment of the primary illness. In general, the frequency of glomerular involvement is falling with the reduction in incidence of these infections.

Further reading

Abdurrahman MB, *et al.* (1990). Clinicopathological features of childhood nephrotic syndrome in northern Nigeria. *Quarterly Journal of Medicine* **75**, 563–76.

Aikawa M, *et al.* (1988). Glomerulopathy in squirrel monkeys with acute *Plasmodium falciparum* infection. *American Journal of Tropical Medicine and Hygiene* **38**, 7–14.

Barsoum RS (1993). Schistosomal glomerulopathies. *Kidney International* **44**, 1–12.

Barsoum RS (1999). Tropical parasitic nephropathies. *Nephrology Dialysis Transplantation* **14**, 79–91.

Chugh KS, Jha V (2000). Glomerulonephritis due to other bacterial, viral and parasitic infections. In: Massry SG, Glassock RJ, eds. *Textbook of nephrology*, 4th edn. Williams and Wilkins, Baltimore, MD.

Chugh KS, Sakhuja V (1990). Glomerular diseases in the tropics. *American Journal of Nephrology* **10**, 437–50.

Chugh KS, Sakhuja V (1998). Glomerular disease in the tropics. In: Davison AM, *et al.*, eds. *Oxford textbook of clinical nephrology*, 2nd edn, pp 703–19. Oxford University Press, Oxford.

Eiam-Ong S, Sitprija V (1998). Falciparum malaria and the kidney: a model of inflammation. *American Journal Kidney Diseases* **32**, 361–75.

Gilles HM, Hendrickse RG (1963). Nephrosis in Nigerian children, role of *Plasmodium malariae*, and effect of anti malarial treatment. *British Medical Journal* **1**, 27–31.

Grauer GF, *et al.* (1989). Experimental *Dirofilaria immitis*-associated glomerulonephritis induced in part by *in situ* formation of immune complexes in the glomerular capillary wall. *Journal of Parasitology* **755**, 585–93.

Pakasa NM, Nseka NM, Nyimi LM (1997). Secondary collapsing glomerulopathy associated with Loa loa filariasis. *American Journal of Kidney Diseases* **30**, 836–9.

Sinniah R, Rui-Mei L, Kara L (1999). Up-regulation of cytokines in glomerulonephritis associated with murine malaria infection. *International Journal of Experimental Pathology* **80**, 87–95.

Sitprija V (1988). Nephropathy in falciparum malaria. *Kidney International* **34**, 867–77.

Weiner ID, Northcutt AD (1989). Leprosy and glomerulonephritis. *American Journal of Kidney Diseases* **13**, 424–9.

WHO (1988). *Renal disease, classification and atlas of infectious and tropical diseases*, Sinniah R, *et al.*, eds. ASCP Press, Chicago, IL.

20.8 Renal tubular disorders

J. Cunningham

Renal glycosuria

Definition and pathophysiology

Renal glycosuria occurs when there is failure of tubular mechanisms to reabsorb the entire filtered load of glucose under conditions of normoglycaemia. In health, the volume of the glomerular filtrate is approximately 180 litres/day, containing approximately 800 mmol of glucose. The average daily urinary excretion of glucose is approximately 1 mmol, implying that some 99.9 per cent of the filtered load of glucose is normally reabsorbed, mostly in the proximal tubule. The primary event at this site is the reabsorption of very large amounts of Na+. Glucose reabsorption is a two-step process in which a carrier-mediated Na+-glucose cotransporter moves both sodium and glucose passively across the brush border (apical) membrane and thereby into the proximal tubular cell. The active extrusion of sodium across the basolateral membrane of the cell is subsequently linked with diffusion of glucose facilitated by specific glucose transporters, such that glucose is transported, in a manner tightly linked to sodium transport, from the tubular lumen to the peritubular capillaries. The molecular mechanisms by which cotransported solutes such as glucose are moved across the tubular epithelium are not fully understood, although it is likely that the binding of the cotransported solute (in this case glucose) leads to conformational changes in the transport protein and the opening of a sodium gate. Sodium thus moves down a concentration gradient (from lumen to cell), with secondary active transport linking the movement of glucose to that of Na+. These disturbances can be identified functionally, either as a reduction of the tubular maximum capacity for glucose reabsorption or a reduction of the tubular threshold for glucose.

Clinical features

The isolated form of renal glycosuria is familial with a mixed inheritance pattern, suggesting that the condition results from any one of several mutations affecting the glucose transport processes described above. Isolated renal glycosuria has no clinical sequelae and is easily distinguished from diabetes mellitus by the fact that the patient is normoglycaemic. Isolated renal glycosuria is frequently seen in otherwise normal pregnancies, where it results from the increased glomerular filtration rate (**GFR**) taking the filtered glucose load to a level that exceeds the renal tubular maximum capacity for reabsorption. By contrast with the glycosuria of uncontrolled diabetes mellitus, renal glycosuria is never of sufficient magnitude to drive a clinically significant osmotic diuresis.

Abnormalities of glucose transport may be seen in association with other defects of proximal tubular transport. Collectively these are designated as Fanconi's syndrome, in which renal glycosuria is found as part of a generalized disorder of proximal tubular function with aminoaciduria, renal tubular acidosis, and phosphaturia. It is important to distinguish forms of isolated glycosuria from multiple tubular defects, including the Fanconi syndrome, in which there may be important clinical consequences, albeit not directly in relation to the glycosuria itself.

Many patients with chronic renal insufficiency of mild to moderate degree exhibit renal glycosuria, usually in combination with other disorders of tubular function. These are frequently subtle and of little or no clinical significance. They reflect tubular damage as part of the general renal parenchymal pathology, or the consequences of the high filtered solute load per nephron in patients with reduced numbers and mass of functioning nephrons.

Phosphate-handling disorders

Physiology and pathophysiology

The renal handling of inorganic phosphate is the major determinant of extracellular phosphate concentration. In health, the kidney shows a powerful adaptive capacity that is capable of maintaining a normal phosphate concentration in the face of wide fluctuations in dietary phosphate intake. Between 80 and 95 per cent of the filtered load of phosphate is normally reabsorbed, mostly in the proximal tubule, but up to 20 per cent of phosphate reabsorption occurs at more distal sites, namely the distal convoluted tubule and cortical collecting duct. The initial process is the movement of filtered phosphate into proximal tubular cells via a number of specific Na+–phosphate cotransporters that are located in the luminal membrane and have a $3Na^+:1HPO_4^{2-}$ stoichiometry. This linkage allows the movement of sodium ions down their electrochemical gradient to drive the movement of phosphate up its electrochemical gradient even as the tubular phosphate concentration falls. In the later parts of the proximal tubule other higher affinity phosphate transporters retrieve much of the residual phosphate. The final step, namely the exit of phosphate across the basolateral membrane and into the peritubular capillaries, appears to be passive.

As indicated above, the kidney provides not only the principal means for phosphate excretion, but also acts as the principal regulator of phosphate homeostasis. This regulation takes place over a wide range: the kidneys excrete virtually all the typical dietary phosphate intake of approximately 30 to 40 mmol/day, but phosphate deprivation or hypophosphataemia leads to such effective renal phosphate conservation that renal phosphate excretion virtually ceases. These adjustments are mediated by the cotransporter activity described above.

Parathyroid hormone (**PTH**) is an important hormonal regulator of phosphate excretion, stimulating phosphaturia by acting directly on proximal tubular cells to inhibit sodium-dependent phosphate transport by mechanisms that operate through both the cAMP protein kinase-A and the protein kinase-C phosphoinositide pathways. There are receptors for PTH on both the apical and basolateral membranes of the proximal tubular cells, the functional effect of PTH being to decrease the *V*max of both the more-proximal, high-capacity, low-affinity cotransporter and the more-distal, low-capacity, high-affinity cotransporter systems, both resulting in phosphaturia.

Other hormones influencing proximal phosphate transport include growth hormone, insulin-like growth factor-1 (**IGF-1**), insulin, thyroid hormone, and 1,25-dihydroxyvitamin D, all of which augment phosphate reabsorption. By contrast, in addition to PTH itself, phosphate excretion is augmented by PTH-related peptide, calcitonin, glucocorticoids, and atrial natriuretic peptide (**ANP**).

In addition to the above, it appears that the tubular phosphate transport mechanism can respond to changes in dietary phosphate intake, even when the plasma phosphate level changes little or not at all. The nature of this dietary signal is unclear. In parallel with the antiphosphaturic effect of reduced dietary phosphate, there is an increase in bone resorption leading to mobilization of skeletal phosphate (and calcium). Both the renal and skeletal responses to low dietary phosphate are unimpaired by parathyroidectomy and are therefore not mediated by PTH.

Disorders associated with increased urinary phosphate excretion

There are various types of phosphate transport defect, but all cause hypophosphataemia with inappropriate phosphaturia (Table 1). The fractional excretion of phosphate (the percentage of filtered phosphate that appears in the final urine) is increased and the tubular transport maximum for phosphate (*TmP*/GFR) is decreased. The clinical disturbances that result from such disorders may be very severe, important ones being rickets (in children) and osteomalacia (in adults). The development of these depends on the severity and chronicity of the hypophosphataemia, also on the presence or absence of any associated non-renal abnormalities.

Hereditary hypophosphataemic rickets

The terminology is potentially confusing. Vitamin D-resistant rickets (**VDRR**) originally described a syndrome of hypophosphataemia and metabolic bone disease (rickets or osteomalacia) that in many ways resembled that of vitamin D deficiency but which did not respond to treatment with vitamin D. This condition is now more properly called hereditary hypophosphataemic rickets, a designation more consistent with the phosphate-wasting aetiology. That these patients do not respond to vitamin D is undeniable, but true vitamin D resistance (that is, resistance even to 1,25-dihydroxyvitamin D) appears to exist only in patients with functional defects (usually inherited) of the vitamin D receptor.

Table 1 The kidney and phosphate metabolism

Disturbance	Comments
Hypophosphataemia	
Hereditary hypophosphataemic rickets	
• X-linked hypophosphataemic rickets	The most common
• autosomal dominant and autosomal recessive hypophosphataemic rickets	Rare—variable presentation
• sporadic	Rare
Acquired	
• oncogenous rickets	
• primary hyperparathyroidism	Increased PTH-dependent phosphaturia
• secondary hyperparathyroidism due to vitamin D deficiency	Increased PTH-dependent phosphaturia
Hyperphosphataemia	
Renal failure	Reduced filtered Pi load
Hypoparathyroidism	Reduced PTH-dependent phosphaturia
Pseudohypoparathyroidism	
• type 1	Renal PTH resistance; absent cAMP and phosphaturic responses to PTH
• type 2	Renal PTH resistance; normal cAMP and absent phosphaturic response to PTH

X-linked hypophosphataemic rickets

This is the most important type of renal phosphate-handling disorder. Presentation is generally with poor growth and rickets in early childhood. The inheritance pattern is consistently of X-linked dominant type. There is a defect in proximal tubular phosphate transport that results in persistent hypophosphataemia and inappropriate phosphaturia. Females (heterozygotes) are less severely affected than males (hemizygotes). There also appears to be a subtle disturbance of vitamin D metabolism, such that the plasma 1,25-dihydroxyvitamin D concentration does not show the increase during hypophosphataemia that is seen in otherwise normal subjects.

Understanding of the pathogenesis and molecular biology of X-linked hypophosphataemic rickets has been greatly assisted by the existence of a murine model, the *hyp* mouse. It is clear that the defect of phosphate transport has nothing to do with the normal PTH modulatory control system. Cross-circulation and kidney transplant experiments in *hyp* mice have shown that the defect can be transferred from affected to non-affected animals. This, together with the observation that cultured proximal tubular cells from *hyp* mice exhibit normal phosphate transport, points strongly to mediation by an extrarenal humoral factor termed phosphotonin. The *hyp* gene is called PHEX (Phosphate regulating gene Homologous to Endopeptidases on the X chromosome). It is expressed in bone and not in kidney, a distribution compatible with the extrarenal origin of X-linked hypophosphataemic rickets.

The diagnosis is made on the basis of characteristic clinical features coupled with persistent hypophosphataemia and a reduced *TmP*/GFR, indicating an inappropriate reduction of the tubular reasborptive capacity for phosphate.

Because the bone disease in X-linked hypophosphataemic rickets is at least partly a consequence of the hypophosphataemia, treatment attempts to normalize plasma phosphate—a difficult task in practice. The administration of oral phosphate supplements increases phosphaturia, hence large oral doses have to be taken at frequent intervals, thereby presenting a substantial compliance problem in these patients, many of whom are young children. Additionally, the administration of large doses of phosphate reduces the plasma 1,25-dihydroxyvitamin D concentration, slightly lowers the ionized calcium concentration in plasma, and thereby triggers secondary hyperparathyroidism. This in turn may compound the skeletal disease and also further increase phosphaturia. These troublesome compensations can be attenuated by the addition of calcitriol (1,25-dihydroxyvitamin D) therapy to the phosphate supplement, with substantially improved clinical outcomes. However, treatment must be monitored extremely closely, there being a constant risk of calcitriol-induced hypercalciuria, hypercalcaemia and nephrocalcinosis. If this occurs, the degree of tubular calcium phosphate deposition appears to be largely determined by the oral phosphate dose: the presence of large amounts of phosphate in the gut lumen prevents the normal association of luminal calcium with oxalate, thereby increasing oxalate availability and absorption. Thus the stage is set for enteric hyperoxaluria, another potent risk factor for nephrocalcinosis and stone formation (see Chapter 20.13).

Oncogenic rickets/osteomalacia

A disturbance similar to X-linked hypophosphataemic rickets is rarely acquired in association with certain mesenchymal tumours, especially giant-cell tumours of bone, neurofibromas, and cavernous haemangiomata. Removal of the tumour is followed by complete normalization of renal phosphate handling, an observation that strongly favours the involvement of a tumour-generated humoral factor in the pathogenesis of the hypophosphataemia. Extracts of these tumours have been found to inhibit phosphate transport in renal tubular cells and to initiate phosphaturia in experimental animals. The humoral factor has been named 'phosphatonin' and it is likely that 'phosphatonin' is the same in X-linked hypophosphataemia and in oncogenic rickets/osteomalacia. It affects only phosphate transport and has no direct effects on calcium metabolism, PTH, or the PTH receptor.

Other phosphate-wasting disorders

Autosomal recessive and autosomal dominant phosphaturic disorders have rarely been reported. Common to these disorders is impaired proximal tubular phosphate transport (low *TmP*/GFR) with inappropriate phosphate wasting and variable metabolic bone disease. The clinical presentations are variable: some present during adolescence or even adulthood, while others present in early life, with some cases resolving spontaneously at puberty.

Syndromes of hereditary hypophosphataemia with hypercalciuria are described below in the section on calcium-handling disorders.

Disorders associated with reduced urinary phosphate excretion

Excessive tubular phosphate reabsorption (high *Tm*P/GFR) with resulting hyperphosphataemia is seen in conditions where PTH is lacking or there is renal resistance to PTH (Table 1). In these patients hyperphosphataemia coexists with hypocalcaemia. The hyperphosphataemia is the result of an inappropriately raised *Tm*P/GFR. The hypocalcaemia is largely the result of the failure of adequate 1,25-dihydroxyvitamin D (calcitriol) production by the PTH-deprived kidney, arising because the renal 25-hydroxyvitamin D 1α-hydroxylase is downregulated in the absence of PTH or its receptor.

Hypoparathyroidism

In hypoparathyroidism the renal tubular response to PTH is normal when tested by the administration of exogenous PTH. The metabolic abnormalities merely reflect the lack of PTH. The diagnosis depends on a low or undetectable PTH concentration in plasma, despite a prevailing hypocalcaemia that would normally trigger secondary hyperparathyroidism. For a detailed discussion of hypoparathyroid disorders, see Chapter 12.4.

Pseudohypoparathyroidism

There are two main types of pseudohypoparathyroidism, renal resistance to PTH being a feature of both. In these disorders the resulting hypocalcaemia evokes an appropriate PTH response. Type 1 pseudohypoparathyroidism is associated with a G-protein defect, with failure of coupling between the PTH receptor itself and adenylate cyclase. As a result, PTH (whether endogenous or exogenous) evokes neither a urinary cAMP nor a phosphaturic response. Despite plasma PTH being elevated, the *Tm*P/GFR is high with associated phosphate retention. In the type 2 variant, G-protein activity is normal and PTH induces a cAMP response but no phosphaturia, implying a defect of cAMP-dependent protein kinase C.

Clinically, hypocalcaemia and hyperphosphataemia dominate the metabolic picture. There are also somatic features comprising short stature, short fourth and fifth metacarpals, and a variable degree of mental deficiency.

All types of hypoparathyroidism can be treated effectively using oral calcitriol or alfacalcidol. Pharmacological doses of these agents are needed to bring calcium into the normal range: it is frequently helpful to incorporate a calcium supplement into each meal, principally to reduce the intestinal absorption of dietary phosphate in these hyperphosphataemic individuals.

Calcium-handling disorders

Disorders of urinary calcium output (hypercalciuria and, to a lesser extent, hypocalciuria) are quite common and have important sequelae, particularly in regard to hypercalciuric renal stone disease (see Chapter 20.13). Whilst it is important to recognize that such abnormalities of urinary calcium excretion may reflect intrinsic abnormalities of calcium handling within the kidney, it is also the case that primary disorders remote from the kidneys can also be responsible for disturbances of the calcium excretion rate. For example, hypercalcaemia—as seen in vitamin D intoxication, excessive dietary calcium intake, and osteolytic metastases—is associated with marked hypercalciuria, albeit in circumstances where the kidneys are responding appropriately to the high plasma calcium concentration. Many factors influence the handling of calcium by the renal tubule (Table 2).

Table 2 Tubular calcium reabsorption

Stimulus	Net effect on transport	Excretion
Hypercalcaemia	↓	↑
Volume expansion (sodium loading)	↓	↑
Hypomagnesaemia	↓	↑
Phosphate depletion	↓	↑
Metabolic acidosis	↓	↑
Metabolic alkalosis	↑	↓
PTH (parathyroid hormone)	↑	↓*
PTH-related peptide (PTHrp)	↑	↓*
Vitamin D (calcitriol)	↑	↓*
Loop diuretics (furosemide, bumetanide)	↓	↑
Thiazide diuretics	↑	↓**
Amiloride	↑	↓**

*Unless overwhelmed by an increased filtered load due to hypercalcaemia.
**Thiazide and amiloride effects are additive.

Physiology and pathophysiology

In health, between 200 and 250 mmol of calcium appear in the glomerular filtrate each day, assuming an ultrafiltrable blood calcium concentration of 1.3 mmol/l out of the total blood calcium concentration of 2.5 mmol/l. About 70 per cent of filtered calcium is reabsorbed in the proximal convoluted tubule and the rest in the thick ascending limb of Henle's loop (20 per cent), the distal convoluted tubule (5 to 10 per cent), and the collecting tubule (less than 5 per cent). These reabsorptive processes reclaim nearly all the filtered calcium, such that only about 3 to 5 mmol of calcium appears in the urine each day. Assuming constancy of the total-body calcium content, this urinary calcium loss is equal to the net intestinal calcium absorption.

Calcium reabsorption in the proximal tubule and in the loop of Henle occurs passively down the electrochemical gradient generated by sodium and water reasbsorption at these sites. Regulation of calcium transport occurs at more distal sites where both parathyroid hormone and 1,25-dihydroxyvitamin D augment calcium reabsorption, the former by activation of adenylate cyclase via the PTH receptor and the latter by upregulation of calcium binding proteins – calbindins. Thus, parathyroid hormone itself, and also parathyroid hormone-related peptide (**PTHrp**), acts in an anticalciuric fashion, thereby contributing to the hypercalcaemia of primary hyperparathyroidism and the humoral hypercalcaemia of malignancy, respectively.

The extracellular calcium-sensing receptor (CaR)

It is now clear that the extracellular calcium-sensing receptor plays a central role in regulating the renal handling of calcium. It does this by both indirect and direct mechanisms. Indirectly, the CaR in the parathyroid gland senses extracellular calcium and adjusts the output of parathyroid hormone appropriately. This in turn regulates the renal handling of calcium in the distal nephron, with a fall of plasma calcium concentration triggering PTH secretion and thereby renal calcium retention—an appropriate response. Directly, the CaR in renal epithelial cells (most heavily expressed in the cortical thick ascending limb and also present in the proximal tubule, medullary thick ascending limb of Henle's loop, the distal convoluted tubule, and the collecting duct) regulates the handling of both calcium and water. Binding of calcium to the CaR in Henle's loop is thought to diminish the reabsorption of calcium (and magnesium). Thus, conditions of high calcium delivery to the loop of Henle lead to an appropriate increase in calciuria. In addition, it appears that the CaR in the kidney provides a link between distal tubular calcium delivery and the rate of ADH-stimulated water reabsorption at that site. This mechanism would explain the observed nephrogenic diabetes insipidus that accompanies significant hypercalcaemia and which reduces the likelihood of urinary supersaturation of calcium in circumstances of hypercalciuria.

Action of diuretics

Loop diuretics (furosemide (frusemide) and bumetanide), thiazide diuretics, and amiloride all affect renal tubular calcium transport and, as experimental probes, have been extremely useful in the elucidation of the mechanisms of renal calcium handling, as well as in the therapy of hypercalcaemic and hypercalciuric disorders. Loop diuretics inhibit sodium chloride reabsorption in the thick ascending limb of the loop of Henle and with it the passive reabsorption of various cations, including calcium. The resulting increase in the calcium excretion rate can be beneficial (as in the treatment of hypercalcaemia), or deleterious (increased risk of osteopenia or stone formation in chronic drug-induced hypercalciuria). Conversely, thiazide diuretics substantially reduce the urinary calcium excretion rate. Two mechanisms appear to underlie this effect. First, the mild volume depletion arising from the natriuretic and diuretic actions of the thiazide serves to accelerate proximal sodium and water reabsorption, and with it passive calcium reabsorption in this part of the nephron. Second, thiazides appear to increase distal calcium reabsorption directly, although the mechanism is unclear. These actions of thiazide diuretics are extremely useful in the treatment of hypercalciuric stone disease. In addition, there is evidence that thiazides can reduce the negative calcium balance in elderly people, which may translate to a reduction in the incidence of fractures in this age group. Thiazide diuretics slightly elevate the plasma calcium concentration, although usually to a trivial extent only, but this may become clinically significant in patients who have a tendency to hypercalcaemia, such as those with very mild hyperparathyroidism, Paget's disease, or who are immobilized. Amiloride also exerts a hypocalciuric action, probably at the cortical connecting segment, although the precise mechanism is uncertain. The hypocalciuric effect of thiazides and amiloride are, therefore, exerted at different sites of the renal tubule and in clinical practice are additive. Thus combinations of thiazides and amiloride are useful treatments for patients with hypercalciuric stone disease (see Chapter 20.13).

Disorders associated with increased urinary calcium excretion

Idiopathic hypercalciuria

This is an extremely important metabolic disturbance because of the high associated risk of calcium stone formation. 'Idiopathic' in this context implies hypercalciuria without hypercalcaemia and in the absence of other factors known to accelerate bone resorption (for instance, acromegaly, hyperthyroidism, hyperparathyroidism, osteolytic metastases, immobilization, metabolic acidosis) or reduced tubular calcium reabsorption (such as loop diuretics, chronic metabolic acidosis).

In most cases, the hypercalciuria is driven by calcium hyperabsorption by the intestine, and the hypercalciuria is thus of the 'overspill' type. This usually results from an initial defect of renal phosphate handling (reduction of *Tm*P/GFR and consequent renal phosphate leak), which stimulates the production of 1,25-dihydroxyvitamin D. In a minority of cases the primary defect is of renal tubular calcium reabsorption ('renal leak' hypercalciuria), with a secondary increase of parathyroid hormone, calcitriol, and intestinal calcium absorption.

The assessment and management of these patients has benefited greatly from an increased understanding of the underlying defects. For example, 'absorptive' hypercalciuria is logically managed initially by measures to reduce intestinal calcium absorption, namely avoidance of excessive dietary calcium intake and, in those with evidence of 1,25-dihydroxyvitamin D excess driven by hypophosphataemia, oral phosphate therapy as well. Thiazides and amiloride are added if these initial measures are inadequate. Conversely, the management of 'renal leak' hypercalciuria requires an increase in tubular calcium reabsorption by reducing the dietary sodium and protein intake (acid load) and giving thiazide diuretics and amiloride.

Hereditary hypercalciuric nephrolithiasis

Recent studies have identified four rare disorders, all characterized by low molecular weight proteinuria, hypercalciuria, nephrocalcinosis, renal stone formation, and (in many cases) renal failure. In some, there are also defects of proximal tubular function with aminoaciduria, phosphaturia, renal glycosuria, and uricosuria (Fanconi's syndrome), as well as impairment of urinary acidification (renal tubular acidosis). These four disorders are Dent's disease, X-linked recessive nephrolithiasis, X-linked recessive hypophosphataemic rickets, and idiopathic low molecular weight proteinuria in Japanese children. The underlying defect appears to be the result of a mutation of a chloride-channel gene (*CLCN5*), the functional loss of which results in a widespread defect of proximal tubular transport.

Disorders associated with reduced urinary calcium excretion

Most patients exhibiting hypocalciuria do so in association with hypocalcaemia and a reduced filtered load of calcium. This is seen in patients with secondary hyperparathyroidism as a response to an underlying vitamin D and/or calcium deficiency, when a reduced filtered load of calcium is combined with accelerated tubular calcium reabsorption driven by increased levels of PTH. Most patients with advanced renal failure also exhibit hypocalciuria.

Familial hypocalciuric hypercalcaemia

These conditions reflect functional aberrations of the extracellular calcium-sensing receptor (**CaR**). In familial hypocalciuric hypercalcaemia (**FHH**, also known as familial benign hypercalcaemia) there is an inactivating mutation in the calcium-sensing receptor gene. Several different mutations are known, most appearing to result in receptors that are truncated or have an abnormal amino acid sequence. These render the receptor less sensitive to calcium which, at the level of the parathyroid gland, makes the parathyroid attempt to set calcium at a supraphysiological concentration. At the level of the kidney, the defect leads to increased tubular calcium and magnesium reabsorption. The resulting metabolic disturbance is characterized by hypercalcaemia, hypocalciuria, and hypermagnesaemia. The PTH hormone concentration is within the 'normal range', but this is inappropriately elevated with regard to the serum calcium concentration. The inheritance pattern is autosomal dominant with high penetrance.

Most patients tolerate the hypercalcaemia well and the characteristic symptoms of hypercalcaemia (polyuria, constipation, neuropsychiatric disturbance) are conspicuously absent. The disorder may be distinguished from primary hyperparathyroidism by the presence of a family history, the reduction in urinary calcium excretion rate, and the normal urinary excretion rate of cyclic AMP (increased in conditions of parathyroid hormone excess). It is important to distinguish these patients from those with mild primary hyperparathyroidism: the benign natural history and the poor response to subtotal parathyroidectomy means that parathyroid surgery should not be undertaken in these individuals.

Autosomal dominant hypocalcaemia

By contrast to familial hypocalciuric hypercalcaemia, autosomal dominant hypocalcaemia results from an activating mutation in the calcium-sensing receptor that renders it overly sensitive to extracellular calcium. This leads to a downward setting of the normal parathyroid hormone and calcium relationship with resulting hypocalcaemia. Because the mutation also affects the calcium receptor in the renal tubular cells, urinary calcium excretion is inappropriately high. Principal clinical sequelae are the result of the hypercalciuria that predisposes to stone formation, nephrocalcinosis, and renal insufficiency. The hypocalcaemia is generally well tolerated. Treatment with thiazide–amiloride combinations to reduce hypercalciuria is logical but not of established benefit. Hypocalcaemia is generally asymptomatic and treatment of this with vitamin D or calcitriol is generally inappropriate, serving only to increase the degree of hypercalciuria and the risk of nephrocalcinosis and stone formation.

The Fanconi syndrome and aminoaciduria

Physiology and pathophysiology

Filtered amino acids are subject to very rapid proximal tubular reabsorption, at least 95 per cent having been cleared from the glomerular filtrate by the time it reaches the end of the proximal tubule. The transport of organic solute at this site is a two-step process that is both carrier-mediated and sodium-coupled; amino acids enter the proximal tubular cell via the brush border membrane against an electrochemical gradient, and exit via another transporter at the basolateral membrane. Movement in this fashion is accomplished by secondary active mechanisms, whereby coupling to sodium transport allows the movement of amino acids to be driven indirectly by the basolateral membrane $Na+/K+$-ATPase.

Based on loose structural similarities, the amino acids segregate into four groups, each with a group-specific carrier system (Table 3). Common to many defects of amino acid transport is a reduction of the electrochemical sodium gradient across the proximal tubular cells, leading to the impaired linked transport of glucose, amino acids, phosphate, and a range of other solutes. Some of the amino acid transporters are also expressed in the intestine; in which case defects may be evident at both sites, and clinical disease can result from the intestinal defect, the renal defect, or both.

The Fanconi syndrome

This syndrome comprises a disturbance of proximal tubular functions with generalized aminoaciduria, phosphate wasting (hypophosphataemic rickets and osteomalacia), renal tubular acidosis type-2 (proximal **RTA**), and renal glycosuria. The terms 'juvenile-' and 'adult Fanconi's syndrome' are widely used, but refer only to the age of onset and serve no additional classification purpose. More helpful is to classify, as far as possible, the many causes of the Fanconi syndrome on the basis of aetiology and pathogenesis (Table 4).

Clinical presentations of the Fanconi syndrome usually depend more on the associated underlying abnormality than on the renal tubular defect *per se*. However, the diagnosis ultimately depends on the demonstration of characteristic multiple tubular defects. These may not all be present in all patients and may even fluctuate in an individual patient, hence it is often best to define the specific defects that are present rather than to use the catch-all Fanconi eponym.

Treatment focuses on two issues. First, the cause of the Fanconi syndrome: for example, fructose avoidance in hereditary fructose intolerance, galactose avoidance in galactosaemia, copper chelation therapy in Wilson's disease. Second, the consequences of the Fanconi syndrome: for example, alkali and potassium for RTA type-2, oral phosphate and calcitriol for phosphate wasting.

Specific aminoacidurias

These are classified according to four principal carrier defects (see Table 3).

Neutral aminoacidurias

Hartnup disease

This rare (1:16 000 births), autosomal recessive disorder comprises three features:

(1) intestinal tryptophan malabsorption;

(2) a pellagra-like syndrome with photosensitive skin lesions, ataxia, and neuropsychiatric disturbances; and

(3) neutral aminoaciduria with increased renal clearance of alanine, asparagine, glutamine, histidine, isoleucine, leucine, phenylalanine, serine, threonine, tyrosine, valine, and tryptophan.

The clinical manifestations of Hartnup disease result from the tryptophan malabsorption that leads to nutritional deficiency, which is exacerbated by the accelerated urinary losses of tryptophan. It presents much like pellagra, although is usually less severe and tends to fluctuate in its course. Analysis of the urine distinguishes the two disorders. Hartnup disease responds well to oral nicotinamide therapy (40–200 mg daily).

Dibasic aminoacidurias

These comprise cystinuria, lysinuric protein intolerance, and lysinuria, of which cystinuria is the most common and the most important.

Cystinuria

The group-specific carrier protein for the dibasic amino acids is located on the brush border membrane of the proximal tubular cells and is thought to be the product of a single pair of allelic genes. So far, three potential mutant alleles have been identified that appear to be capable of causing both homozygous and heterozygous forms of cystinuria. When expressed, this transport defect is found in both the kidney and in intestinal epithelium.

Cystinuria occurs in 1 in 7000 births and has serious clinical manifestations. Inheritance is autosomal recessive. Presentation is usually during childhood or adolescence, the syndrome of nephrolithiasis presenting with pain, infection, and, in some cases, renal impairment and hypertension.

Table 3 Aminoacidurias

Type	Diseases	Amino acid	Clinical manifestation of disease
Neutral	Hartnup disease	alanine, asparagine, glutamine, histidine, isoleucine, phenylalanine, serine, threonine, tryptophan, tyrosine, valine	'pellagra' rash, ataxia, mental retardation, diarrhoea (all due to defective gut tryptophan absorption)
	Blue diaper syndrome	tryptophan	no sequelae
Dibasic	Cystinuria	cystine, lysine, arginine, ornithine	cystine stones
Imino acids and glycine	Imminoglycinuria	proline, hydroxyproline, glycine	no sequelae
Acidic	Acidic aminoaciduria	glutamate, aspartate	no sequelae

The stones are radio-opaque (although less so than calcium-containing stones), smooth, and sometimes staghorn-shaped. The diagnosis is confirmed by a positive nitroprusside test, the presence of typical hexagonal crystals in morning urine specimens, and the quantitative measurement of urinary cystine output.

Treatment requires reduction of the cystine concentration in the urine combined with measures to increase its solubility. Typical regimens comprise a high fluid intake, alkalinization of the urine to over pH 7.5 (usually with large quantities of potassium citrate and sodium bicarbonate), and penicillamine. Cystine solubility changes little across the acidic range of pH but increases rapidly above pH 7. At 37 °C and pH 7, the solubility is only 1.66 mmol/l, but this increases to between about 3.3 and 3.5 mmol/l at pH 7.8. However, pushing the pH to even more alkaline levels may be counterproductive since alkalinization decreases the solubility of calcium phosphate, which may be deposited on the cystine stones. Poor compliance is a frequent and unsurprising practical problem with this demanding regimen, particularly in regard to maintenance of a high fluid intake. To be fully effective this requires oral fluids to be taken at least once during the night. Nevertheless, at least 50 per cent of patients respond to these measures if they are rigorously applied and adhered to, and in some cases the stones regress significantly.

Sulphydryl-containing drugs, such as penicillamine, react with cystine to form penicillamine–cysteine, which is much more soluble. In the past this treatment was often reserved for those who failed on the fluid/alkali regimen. However, penicillamine is now used much earlier and often forms part of the initial therapy. Although potentially toxic (cutaneous reactions, marrow suppression, and glomerulopathy), serious reactions are rare, and penicillamine is currently the most effective therapy known. It is given at doses of 1 to 2 g daily, the aim being to reduce the free-cystine concentration in urine to below 1.66 mmol/l, when stone formation is prevented and existing stones can be dissolved.

In cystinuria other basic amino acids (lysine, arginine, and ornithine) are also present in increased amounts in the urine, but only cystine—by virtue of its low solubility—is of clinical importance.

Lysinuric protein intolerance

This is a rare autosomal recessive disorder that results from widespread defects of dibasic amino acid transport, involving particularly the intestine, proximal renal tubule, and liver. Cystine transport is normal. The renal tubular defect plays no part in the pathogenesis of the disease.

Mental retardation, growth failure, and osteopenia are prominent, and are thought to result from reduced activity of the urea cycle with a low plasma urea concentration and hyperammonaemia after food. Treatment with citrulline is sometimes effective, probably by regenerating the deficient urea cycle intermediates, arginine and ornithine.

Imino acids and glycine

Familial iminoglycinuria

This is a relatively common condition, arising in approximately 1 in 15 000 births. Clinically, the inheritance appears to be autosomal recessive, but there are multiple alleles and gene loci for the transport of imino acids and glycine. Proximal tubular transport of proline, hydroxyproline, and glycine is impaired, accompanied in some, but not all, cases with defects in intestinal transport.

Few if any clinical sequelae result from isolated imminoglycinuria, although it was once thought that the abnormality was associated with mental retardation and seizures.

Acidic aminoaciduria

These disturbances are exceedingly rare, involving the dicarboxylic amino acids (aspartic acid and glutamic acid). They are not well understood. The possibility of accelerated renal production and/or failure to transfer these amino acids into the renal circulation is suggested by the observation of renal clearance in excess of the GFR. There are no clinical sequelae.

Table 4 Classification of Fanconi's syndrome

Inherited

Primary idiopathic
- sporadic
- familial

Secondary to inborn error of metabolism
- cystinosis (intralysosomal cystine)
- tyrosinaemia (fumarylacetoacetate)
- Wilson's disease (copper)
- Lowe's syndrome
- galactosaemia (galactose 1-phosphate)
- hereditary fructose intolerance (fructose 1-phosphate)

Acquired

Intrinsic renal disease
- acute tubular necrosis
- hypokalaemic nephropathy
- myeloma
- Sjögren's syndrome
- transplant rejection

Hormonal
- primary hyperparathyroidism
- secondary hyperparathyroidism (vitamin D/calcium deficiency)

Nutritional
- kwashiorkor

Pharmaceuticals
- cisplatin
- ifosfamide
- gentamicin
- sodium valproate/valproic acid

Other exogenous toxins
- glue sniffing
- heavy metals (mercury, lead, cadmium, uranium)
- outdated tetracycline
- 6-mercaptopurine
- maleic acid (in experimental animals)

Further reading

Baron DN, *et al.* (1956). Hereditary pellagra-like skin rash with temporary cerebellar ataxia, constant renal amino-aciduria and other bizarre biochemical features. *Lancet* **ii**, 421–33.

Bergeron M, *et al.* (2001). The renal Fanconi syndrome. In: Scriver CR, *et al.*, eds. *The metabolic and molecular basis of inherited disease*, 8th edn, pp 5023–38. McGraw-Hill, New York.

Brown EM (2000). Familial hypocalciuric hypercalcemia and other disorders with resistance to extracellular calcium. *Endocrinology and Metabolism Clinics of North America* **29**, 503–22.

Brown ME, *et al.* (1995). Calcium-ion-sensing cell-surface receptors. *New England Journal of Medicine* **333**, 234–40

Calcium-sensing receptor. *http://www3.ncbi.nlm.nih.gov/omim/* OMIM Number 601199.

Chesney RW (2001). Iminoglycinuria. In: Scriver CR, *et al.*, eds. *The metabolic and molecular basis of inherited disease*, 8th edn, pp 4971–82. McGraw-Hill, New York.

Coe FL, Parks JH, Moore ES (1979). Familial idiopathic hypercalciuria. *New England Journal of Medicine* **300**, 337–40.

Cystinuria. *http://www3.ncbi.nlm.nih.gov/omim/* OMIM Numbers 220100 (type 1) and 600918 (types 2 and 3).

De Marchi S, *et al.* (1984). Close genetic linkage between HLA and renal glycosuria. *American Journal of Nephrology* **4**, 280–6.

Dent's disease, X-linked recessive nephrolithiasis, X-linked recessive hypophosphataemic rickets, and idiopathic low molecular weight proteinuria of Japanese children. All due to mutations of chloride channel 5; CLCN5. *http://www3.ncbi.nlm.nih.gov/omim/* OMIM Number 300008.

Dicarboxylicaminoaciduria. *http://www3.ncbi.nlm.nih.gov/omim/* OMIM Number 222730.

Familial hypocalciuric hypercalcaemia. *http://www3.ncbi.nlm.nih.gov/omim/* OMIM Number 241530

Familial idiopathic hypercalciuria (hypercalciuria, absorptive, type 1). *http://www3.ncbi.nlm.nih.gov/omim/* OMIM Number 143870

Fitch N (1982). Albright's hereditary osteodystrophy: a review. *American Journal of Medical Genetics* **11**, 11–29.

Gregory MJ, Schwartz GJ (1998). Diagnosis and treatment of renal tubular disorders. *Seminars in Nephrology* **18**, 317.

Hartnup disease. *http://www3.ncbi.nlm.nih.gov/omim/* OMIM Number 234500.

Iminoglycinuria. *http://www3.ncbi.nlm.nih.gov/omim/* OMIM Number 242600.

Kanai Y, *et al.* (1994). The human kidney low affinity Na(+)/glucose cotransporter SGLT2: delineation of the major renal reabsorptive mechanism for D-glucose. *Journal of Clinical Investigation* **93**, 397–404.

Kumar R (2000). Tumor-induced osteomalacia and the regulation of phosphate homeostasis. *Bone* **27**, 333–8.

Levy HL (2001). Hartnup disorder. In: Scriver CR, *et al.*, eds. *The metabolic and molecular basis of inherited disease*, 8th edn, pp 4957–70. McGraw-Hill, New York.

Lloyd SE, *et al.* (1996). A common molecular basis for three inherited kidney stone diseases. *Nature* **370**, 445–9.

Lysinuric protein intolerance. *http://www3.ncbi.nlm.nih.gov/omim/* OMIM Number 222700.

Marx SJ (2000). Hyperparathyroid and hypoparathyroid disorders. *New England Journal of Medicine* **343**, 1863–75.

Nesbitt T, *et al.* (1992). Crosstransplantation of kidneys in normal and Hyp mice: evidence that the Hyp mouse phenotype is unrelated to an intrinsic renal defect. *Journal of Clinical Investigation* **89**, 1453–9.

Palacin M, *et al.* (2001). Cystinuria. In: Scriver CR, *et al.*, eds. *The metabolic and molecular basis of inherited disease*, 8th edn, pp 4909–32. McGraw-Hill, New York.

Pearce SHS, *et al.* (1996). A familial syndrome of hypocalcemia with hypercalciuria due to mutations in the calcium-sensing receptor. *New England Journal of Medicine* **335**, 1115–22.

Pseudohypoparathyroidism type IA. *http://www3.ncbi.nlm.nih.gov/omim/* OMIM Number 103580.

Pseudohypoparathyroidism type IB. *http://www3.ncbi.nlm.nih.gov/omim/* OMIM Number 603233.

Renal glycosuria. *http://www3.ncbi.nlm.nih.gov/omim/* OMIM Number 233100.

Rosenberg LE, Durant JL, Elsas LJ (1968). Familial iminoglycinuria: an inborn error of renal tubular transport. *New England Journal of Medicine* **278**, 1407–13.

Rosenberg LE, *et al.* (1966). Cystinuria: biochemical evidence for three genetically distinct diseases. *Journal of Clinical Investigation* **45**, 365–71.

Rowe PS (2000). The molecular background to hypophosphataemic rickets. *Archives of Disease in Childhood* **83**, 192–4.

Simell O (2001). Lysinuric protein intolerance and other cationic aminoacidurias. In: Scriver CR, *et al.*, eds. *The metabolic and molecular basis of inherited disease*, 8th edn, pp 4933–56. McGraw-Hill, New York.

Strewler GJ (2000). The parathyroid hormone-related protein. *Endocrinology and Metabolism Clinics of North America* **29**, 629–45.

Tenenhouse HS, Econs MJ (2001). Mendelian hypophosphatemias. In: Scriver CR, *et al.*, eds. *The metabolic and molecular basis of inherited disease*, 8th edn, pp 5039–68. McGraw-Hill, New York.

Thakker RV (2000). Pathogenesis of Dent's disease and related syndromes of X-linked nephrolithiasis. *Kidney International* **57**, 787–93.

Tieder M, *et al.* (1985). Hereditary hypophosphatemic rickets with hypercalciuria. *New England Journal of Medicine* **312**, 611–17.

Verge CF, *et al.* (1991). Effects of therapy in X-linked hypophosphatemic rickets. *New England Journal of Medicine* **325**, 1843–8.

Vitamin D resistant rickets with end-organ unresponsiveness to 1,25-dihydoxycholecalciferol. *http://www3.ncbi.nlm.nih.gov/omim/* OMIM Number 277440.

Wright EM, Martin MG, Turk E (2001). Familial glucose–galactose malabsorption and hereditary renal glycosuria. In: Scriver CR, *et al.*, eds. *The metabolic and molecular basis of inherited disease*, 8th edn, pp 4891–908. McGraw-Hill, New York.

X-linked hypophosphataemic rickets. *http://www3.ncbi.nlm.nih.gov/omim/* OMIM Number 307800.

20.9 Tubulointerstitial diseases

20.9.1 Acute interstitial nephritis

Dominique Droz and Dominique Chauveau

Introduction

Acute interstitial nephritis has a clinicopathological definition: acute renal failure with prominent inflammation of the renal interstitium, composed mainly of lymphocytes and more rarely of polymorphonuclear cells or granulomas. Since a variable degree of tubular-cell damage is consistently found, the term 'tubulointerstitial nephritis' is preferred by some authors. Because the clinical presentation of acute renal failure is devoid of specific findings, renal biopsy is required in all cases both to establish the diagnosis of acute interstitial nephritis and to allow appropriate management.

Epidemiology and incidence

Although its precise incidence is difficult to determine, acute interstitial nephritis (**AIN**) is a rare disease, found in 1 to 3 per cent of specimens in unselected series of renal biopsy material. In patients presenting with acute renal failure, the proportion with acute interstitial nephritis varies from 6.5 to 15 per cent. Values at the lower end of this range are found in paediatric series. Higher values are found in studies containing larger numbers of elderly patients, where the increased likelihood of drug ingestion is paralleled by an increase in drug-induced hypersensitivity. Overall, acute interstitial nephritis is the third leading cause of acute drug-induced nephropathy, following haemodynamically mediated and direct tubular injuries.

Pathophysiology of acute interstitial nephritis (AIN)

The pathogenesis of AIN is not completely elucidated, and what we know has been extrapolated from animal models. These include spontaneous T cell-mediated interstitial nephritis in kd/kd mice, interstitial nephritis related to antitubular basement antibodies, interstitial nephritis associated with autoimmune systemic disease, and tubulointerstitial damage associated with glomerular diseases and severe proteinuria. Although in rodents these models induce tubulointerstitial damage, very few reproduce the human picture of AIN.

Experimental evidence implicates both humoral and cell-mediated mechanisms, and both antigen-specific and antigen-nonspecific pathways of T-cell activation, but the relevant antigen responsible for T-cell activation is unknown in the vast majority of cases of human AIN. However, in drug-related acute interstitial nephritis the offending drug or one of its metabolic products could function as a hapten, binding to membrane or cellular proteins and being presented in the context of MHC molecules to T-helper cells. Sensitized activated T-helper cells could then produce cytokines, activate macrophages, induce the differentiation and proliferation of B cells producing specific antibodies, and activate other T cells, either cytotoxic cells or those responsible for the delayed-type hypersensitivity reaction. As a consequence, this cascade of reactions could ultimately result in a variable mixture of specific antibody production, death of the target tubular cells, and development of parenchymal granulomas. This cascade-type response could be modified by a variety of mechanisms such as removal of the antigen (for example, the offending drug) or production of inhibitory cytokines.

Aetiology

The causes of acute interstitial nephritis fall into four main categories: (1) drug hypersensitivity reactions; (2) infections; (3) systemic immune-mediated diseases; and (4) idiopathic (Table 1). A drug hypersensitivity reaction is the most common cause of acute interstitial nephritis, accounting for 40 to 60 per cent of the cases, while infections—of bacterial or viral origin—account for less than 5 per cent of cases today. Table 1 provides a detailed list of drugs and infectious agents repeatedly associated with AIN. Although more than 100 drugs have been implicated in acute interstitial nephritis, only a few are repeatedly incriminated, while most reports remain anecdotal. In the presence of acute interstitial nephritis, this should not distract from considering any drug currently or recently consumed by the patient as a potential culprit.

Clinical and pathological features

Most clinical features are non-specific, but the history may point to AIN when renal failure develops in the context of a systemic infection, typical drug reaction, sarcoidosis, Sjögren's syndrome, or uveitis. Blood pressure remains unchanged. Urinary output is variable with mild or moderate proteinuria (<1–2 g/day). Nephrotic syndrome is only found in cases induced by non-steroidal anti-inflammatory drugs. There is no haematuria except in cases related to β-lactam hypersensitivity. Leucocyte casts are common. Fractional excretion of sodium is often high.

Eosinophilia and eosinophiluria are not always present, but argue in favour of an adverse drug reaction. Eosinophils can be detected in the urine using Wright or Hansel stains, the latter being more sensitive. However, eosinophiluria is not specific for drug-induced acute interstitial nephritis and is therefore of poor predictive value.

Kidney size is typically normal or enlarged. Increased cortical echogenicity shown by ultrasound imaging correlates with the degree of interstitial inflammation. Computed tomography (**CT**) scanning is of limited value in the diagnosis of acute interstitial nephritis and other diffuse renal parenchymal diseases.

Table 1 Main causes of acute interstitial nephritis

1. Drugs	
Antibiotics	
	Methicillin, other penicillin derivatives, cephalosporins, cotrimoxazole and other sulphonamides, rifampicin, ciprofloxacin, erythromycin, vancomycin
Non-steroidal anti-inflammatory drugs	
Diuretics	
	Thiazides, furosemide (frusemide), triamterene
Others	
	Acyclovir, allopurinol, captopril, clofibrate, diphenylhydantoin, fenofibrate, H_2-receptor blockers, indinavir, interferon-α, paracetamol, omeprazole, phenindione, phenobarbital, phenothiazine, salicylate derivatives, streptokinase, valproate, warfarin
2. Infections	
Bacterial	
	Streptococci, including pneumococci, typhoid fever, brucellosis, legionella, mycoplasma, leptospirosis, syphilis, tuberculosis, rickettsia
Viral	
	Hantavirus, cytomegalovirus, Epstein–Barr virus, measles, echovirus, coxsackie virus, parvovirus B19, human immunodeficiency virus
Parasital	
	Toxoplasma, leishmania
3. Systemic diseases	
Sarcoidosis, lupus erythematosus, Sjögren's syndrome	
4. Idiopathic	
Isolated	
Associated with uni- or bilateral uveitis (TINU syndrome)	

Renal biopsy remains the sole means of unequivocally establishing the diagnosis of acute interstitial nephritis. The characteristic lesion is the presence of numerous mononuclear cells in the renal interstitium (Fig. 1 and Plate 1). Tubular changes of focal cell necrosis and tubulitis, together with interstitial oedema, are commonly found. Since a discrete interstitial cell infiltrate may be present in primary acute tubular necrosis (either of ischaemic or toxic origin), the assessment of primary acute interstitial nephritis requires careful evaluation of the abundance of the cell infiltrate in comparison with the degree of tubular damage. In addition, the biopsy must be scrutinized for the presence of glomerular pathology, significant immune complex deposition, and vasculitic lesions. If these coexist with a prominent interstitial-cell infiltrate, then diagnoses such as lupus glomerulonephritis, mixed cryoglobulinaemia, and systemic vasculitis need to be considered. Lymphomas or leukaemias may invade the renal parenchyma and cause acute renal failure. The tumoral (clonal) nature of the infiltrating cells is usually obvious, but needs to be distinguished from acute interstitial nephritis.

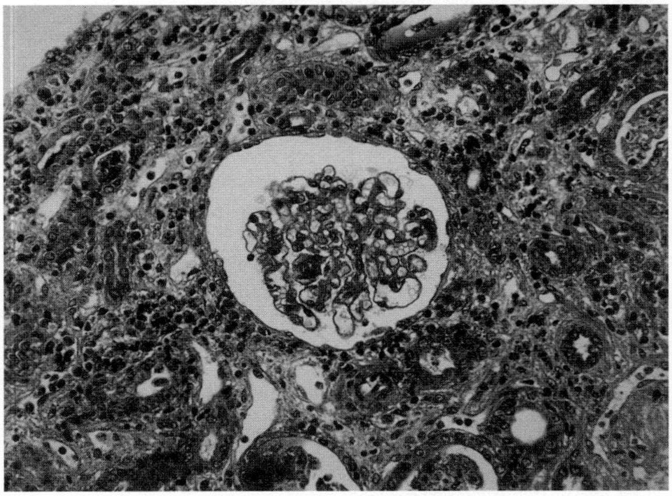

Fig. 1 Acute interstitial nephritis. The renal interstitium is invaded by numerous mononuclear cells. The glomerulus is normal. Mason's trichrome 250 ×. (See also Plate 1.)

In acute interstitial nephritis, the degree of interstitial inflammation is variable and predominates in the cortex. Whatever the cause, T lymphocytes (with an equal proportion of CD4+ and CD8+ cells) and macrophages (CD14+ and CD68+) expressing cell-activation markers, comprise 80 per cent of the infiltrate. Natural killer cells are rare, while polyclonal plasma cells are often observed. Polymorphonuclear cells constitute only a minor part of the cell infiltrate, even in the early phases of the disease, and in cases related to bacterial infection. Eosinophils are rare, even in drug-induced acute interstitial nephritis. Tubular cells express MHC class II antigens. Of note, some interstitial epithelioid and non-caseating granulomas are present in nearly 20 per cent of cases, but they are more common (25 to 45 per cent of cases) in drug-induced acute interstitial nephritis.

In the vast majority of cases (90 per cent), staining for immunofluorescence shows no significant immunoglobulin deposits in the renal parenchyma. However, in rare cases mainly related to systemic lupus erythematosus, granular deposits of immunoglobulin and complement are observed along the tubular basement and in the interstitium. In less than 5 per cent of the cases, linear IgG and C3 deposits are present along the tubular basement membrane, corresponding to the presence of antitubular basement membrane antibodies. Such findings are observed only in cases related to antibiotic use (β-lactams or ciprofloxacin).

Little is known about the long-term histopathological consequences of AIN: most patients recover and serial biopsies have rarely been performed. However, in severe cases, especially those with severe tubule destruction, irreversible lesions with fibrous scars ultimately develop. Late chronic interstitial nephritis is also more frequent when the initial biopsy reveals granulomas, but overall the most reliable histological parameter for prognosis is the extent of interstitial fibrosis on the initial biopsy. The mechanism of fibrogenesis is thought to be that interstitial infiltrating cells and damaged tubular cells release cytokines and growth factors, promoting fibroblast and myofibroblast proliferation and the production of collagen.

Distinctive features of particular causes of acute interstitial nephritis

According to the cause, clinical and laboratory features characterize certain forms of AIN.

Drug-induced acute interstitial nephritis

The most common drugs implicated in acute interstitial nephritis are β-lactam antibiotics and non-steroidal anti-inflammatory drugs (Table 1), but their clinical presentation differs. The β-lactams (and especially methicillin, which is no longer used) give the most characteristic picture of drug-related acute interstitial nephritis. The symptoms occur 2 to 60 days after the beginning of treatment and comprise fever, skin rash (usually maculopapular), arthralgias, liver involvement, abundant haematuria (often macroscopic), blood eosinophilia, and a variable degree of renal failure, requiring dialysis in one-third of the cases. Skin tests or *in vitro* evaluation of hypersensitivity reaction are not valuable for implicating a given drug.

Non-steroidal anti-inflammatory drug-associated acute interstitial nephritis usually affects the elderly, is particularly likely to occur when the drug is taken discontinuously, and evolves with a more progressive course. Renal failure develops several months to years after the initiation of the offending therapy; extrarenal signs of drug sensitization are often lacking. Abundant proteinuria and nephrotic syndrome are found in more than

80 per cent of patients (versus 1 per cent in β-lactam-induced acute interstitial nephritis). In addition to the interstitial lesions, renal biopsy shows minimal glomerular changes with diffuse podocyte foot-process fusion.

How can the physician recognize a drug as being responsible for the onset of acute interstitial nephritis? Given the variability of clinical course, as exemplified for β-lactams and non-steroidal anti-inflammatory drugs, the clinician should first establish an exhaustive list of the drugs used by the patient, including over-the-counter medications, and the date of exposure. This is often a difficult task. In a very few cases, re-challenge with the same drug has mistakenly been performed. When such exposure is elicited and associated with recurrence of the renal and systemic manifestations, then the drug can definitely be regarded as the culprit, but in clinical practice re-challenge should never be recommended. In decreasing order of importance, clues for considering a drug as being responsible for AIN include: (1) appropriate timing, (2) well-documented knowledge of similar nephrotoxicity, and (3) exclusion of other causes (see below).

Infectious acute interstitial nephritis

In children, infections remain the main cause of acute interstitial nephritis. In adults, predisposing factors include old age, diabetes, cytotoxic drug administration, and prolonged corticosteroid therapy. Septicaemia due to various micro-organisms such as *Escherichia coli*, *Proteus* spp., *Staphylococcus* spp., and *Candida albicans* can be associated with direct invasion of the renal parenchyma and acute interstitial nephritis. The clinical picture is that of acute pyelonephritis with a biopsy revealing renal microabscesses.

Haemorrhagic fevers due to Hantaviruses are recognized in Europe with increasing frequency. In these cases, the renal biopsy shows interstitial oedema and medullary haemorrhage, whilst interstitial inflammation remains discrete.

An acute interstitial nephritis with an infiltrate predominantly of CD8+ lymphocytes may be seen in patients with human immunodeficiency viral (HIV) disease, with or without glomerular involvement. Enlargement of the liver and salivary glands with hypergammaglobulinaemia and lymphocytic infiltration of these organs is often found, as well as lymphocytic pneumonitis.

Acute interstitial nephritis in systemic immune-mediated diseases

Lupus erythematosus and Sjögren's syndrome are rare causes of AIN. By contrast, sarcoidosis can present with acute renal failure, with typical sarcoid granulomas found in the renal interstitium. Concomitant hypercalcaemia and/or extrarenal manifestation make the diagnosis of sarcoidosis easy in most cases, but renal involvement can be isolated. In such instances, CT-scanning of the lung may disclose asymptomatic chest involvement. It is conceivable that a localized form of sarcoidosis might be restricted to isolated granulomatous interstitial nephritis, but it is impossible to distinguish between this possibility and that of 'idiopathic' acute interstitial nephritis.

Idiopathic forms of acute interstitial nephritis

Since its description in 1975, an increasing number of cases of acute interstitial nephritis associated with anterior uveitis (or iritis) have been reported. Such an association—referred to as tubulointerstitial nephritis and uveitis, or the **TINU** syndrome—affects mainly young women and adolescent girls. It is characterized by fever, weight loss, blood eosinophilia, hypergammaglobulinaemia, and renal failure. Uveitis may precede the appearance of renal failure by several weeks. An identical clinical picture lacking uveitis has also been described. In the TINU syndrome the biopsy shows diffuse interstitial inflammation, but some granulomas may be present. Whether this association is a manifestation of a limited form of sarcoidosis is still unclear.

Treatment

Treatment of AIN should be first directed against its cause: withdrawal of any drug that might be involved, or prompt treatment of infection. Prednisone improves the renal failure of sarcoidosis and the TINU syndrome, although persistent dysfunction is not uncommon when diagnosis is delayed. Whether or not to use steroids in drug-related AIN remains a matter of debate. Uncontrolled studies suggest that a short course of high-dose prednisone promotes an earlier and more complete decline of serum creatinine toward baseline than in patients left untreated. Some advocate its use when renal failure persists for more than 1 week after withdrawal of the drug or if granulomas are found in the renal biopsy.

In patients with drug-related AIN, the physician should inform the patient that they should not be treated with the presumed culprit or related compounds. More specifically, all β-lactam antibiotics should be avoided in patients who have suffered acute interstitial nephritis attributed to a penicillin compound or a cephalosporin, even though cross-sensitization between the two classes of drugs is not consistent. In those who have recovered from non-steroidal anti-inflammatory-related AIN, acute renal failure may or may not recur after resuming therapy with a non-steroidal anti-inflammatory drug belonging to another family of this class. In some countries, severe drug-induced side-effects, including AIN, should be reported to the health authorities.

Further reading

Buysen JG, *et al.* (1990). Acute interstitial nephritis: a clinical and morphological study in 27 patients. *Nephrology, Dialysis, Transplantation* **5**, 94–9.

Cameron JS (1988). Allergic interstitial nephritis: clinical features and pathogenesis. *Quarterly Journal of Medicine* **66**, 97–115.

Davison AM, Jones CH (1998). Acute interstitial nephritis in the elderly: a report from the UK MRC Glomerulonephritis Register and a review of the literature. *Nephrology, Dialysis, Transplantation,* **13**(Suppl. 7), 12–16.

Dobrin RS, Vernier RL, Fish AL (1975). Acute eosinophilic interstitial nephritis and renal failure with bone marrow-lymph node granulomas and anterior uveitis. A new syndrome. *American Journal of Medicine* **59**, 325–33.

Droz D, Kleinknecht D (1998). Acute interstitial nephritis. In: Davison AM, *et al.* eds. *Oxford textbook of clinical nephrology,* pp 1634–48. Oxford University Press, Oxford.

Ellis D, *et al.* (1981). Acute interstitial nephritis in children: a report of 13 cases and review of the literature. *Pediatrics* **67**, 862–70.

Ivanyi B, *et al.* (1996). Acute tubulointerstitial nephritis: phenotype of infiltrating cells and prognostic impact of tubulitis. *Virchows Archiv* **428**, 5–12.

Kleinknecht D (1995). Interstitial nephritis, the nephrotic syndrome, and chronic renal failure secondary to nonsteroidal anti-inflammatory drugs. *Seminars in Nephrology* **15**, 228–35.

McRae Dell K, Kaplan BS, Meyers CM (1999). Tubulointerstitial nephritis. In: Barratt TM, *et al.* eds. *Pediatric nephrology,* pp 823–4. Lippincott Williams & Wilkins, Baltimore, MD.

Meyers CM, Neilson EG (1995). Immunopathogenesis of tubulointerstitial disease. In: Massry SG, Glassock RJ, eds. *Massry and Glassock's textbook of nephrology,* pp 671–7. Williams & Wilkins, Baltimore, MD.

Michel DM, Kelly CJ (1998). Acute interstitial nephritis. *Journal of the American Society of Nephrology* **9**, 506–15.

Mustonen J, *et al.* (1994). Renal biopsy findings and clinicopathologic correlations in nephropathia epidemica. *Clinical Nephrology* **41**, 121–6.

Nochy D, *et al.* (1993). Renal disease associated with HIV infection: a multicentric study of 60 patients from Paris hospitals. *Nephrology, Dialysis, Transplantation* **8**, 11–19.

Okada H, *et al.* (1993). Steroid-responsive renal insufficiency due to idiopathic granulomatous tubulointerstitial nephritis. *American Journal of Nephrology* **13**, 164–6.

Reddy S, Salant DJ (1998). Treatment of acute interstitial nephritis. *Renal Failure* **20**, 829–38.

Ruffing KA, *et al.* (1994). Eosinophils in urine revisited. *Clinical Nephrology* **41**, 163–6.

20.9.2 Chronic tubulointerstitial nephritis

Marc E. De Broe, Patrick C. D'Haese, and Monique M. Elseviers

Autoimmune

Sarcoidosis

Sarcoidosis is a multisystem disorder of unknown aetiology characterized by the accumulation in many tissues of T lymphocytes, mononuclear phagocytes, and non-caseating granulomas. The pathogenesis and clinical features of the condition are discussed in Chapter 17.11.6.

Clinically important renal involvement is an occasional problem—hypercalciuria and hypercalcaemia are most often responsible, although granulomatous interstitial disease, glomerular disease, obstructive uropathy, and (rarely) endstage renal disease may also occur. The true incidence of renal involvement in sarcoidosis remains unknown, but several small series of renal biopsies suggest that some degree of renal involvement occurs in approximately 35 per cent of patients with sarcoidosis.

Clinical features

Hypercalciuria, hypercalcaemia, nephrolithiasis, granulomatous interstitial nephritis, glomerular disease, and urinary tract disorders can all be observed in patients with sarcoidosis. Macrophages in a sarcoid granulomas contain a 1α-hydroxylase enzyme, but not a 24-hydroxylase enzyme, capable of converting vitamin D to its active form. The resultant increase in the absorption of calcium from the gut, which occurs in up to 50 per cent of those with sarcoidosis, leads to hypercalciuria and, in roughly 2.5 to 20 per cent of cases, to hypercalcaemia. Most patients remain asymptomatic, but nephrolithiasis, nephrocalcinosis, renal insufficiency, and polyuria are potential complications. Nephrolithiasis occurs in approximately 1 to 14 per cent of patients with sarcoidosis and may be the presenting feature. Nephrocalcinosis, observed in over half of those with renal insufficiency, is the most common cause of chronic renal failure in sarcoidosis. The increase in urine output associated with hypercalcaemia and hypercalciuria is due to a reduced responsiveness to antidiuretic hormone.

An interstitial nephritis with granuloma formation is common in sarcoidosis, but the development of clinical disease manifested by renal insufficiency is unusual. A survey of all renal biopsies over a 6-year period at three general hospitals found clinically significant sarcoid granulomatous interstitial nephritis in only four cases. Most affected patients have clear evidence of diffuse active sarcoidosis, although some present with an isolated elevation in the plasma creatinine concentration and no or only minimal renal manifestations. Renal biopsy reveals normal glomeruli, interstitial infiltration mostly with mononuclear cells, non-caseating granulomas in the interstitium, tubular injury, and—with more chronic disease—interstitial fibrosis. Granulomatosis interstitial nephritis is also seen in other diseases, including allergic interstitial nephritis (mainly drug-induced, caused by non-steroidal anti-inflammatory drugs (**NSAIDs**) and 5-aminosalicylic acid), Wegener's granulomatosis, berrylliosis, and tuberculosis. The urinary manifestations of granulomatous interstitial nephritis are relatively non-specific, with urinalysis typical of other chronic tubulointerstitial diseases, being normal or showing only sterile pyuria or mild proteinuria.

Glomerular involvement is rare in sarcoidosis. A variety of different lesions have been described in isolated cases, including membranous nephropathy, a proliferative or crescentic glomerulonephritis, and focal glomerulosclerosis. The presence of heavy proteinuria or red cell casts tends to differentiate these glomerulopathies from interstitial nephritis.

Occasionally, retroperitoneal lymph node involvement, retroperitoneal fibrosis, or renal stones may produce ureteral obstruction.

Diagnosis and treatment

Sarcoid nephropathy should be considered in any patient with unexplained renal failure and hypercalcaemia, nephrocalcinosis, renal tubular defect, or increased immunoglobulins. These patients often have signs and symptoms of pulmonary, ocular, and/or dermal involvement with sarcoidosis. The presence of granulomas on renal biopsy, while not specific to sarcoidosis, should strongly suggest this diagnosis in an appropriate setting. In patients with known sarcoidosis, sarcoid nephropathy should be considered in the presence of renal failure, hypercalcaemia, nephrolithiasis, nephrocalcinosis, or renal tubular defects.

Granulomatous interstitial nephritis can be treated effectively with glucocorticoids, typically prednisolone 1 to 1.5 mg/kg initially, tapered off following signs and symptoms of disease activity. Patients often respond quickly with an improvement in renal function, but this depends greatly on the extent and severity of inflammation and fibrosis before treatment was initiated. There are no controlled trials regarding the dose or length of the treatment.

The hypercalcaemia/hypercalciuric syndrome also responds quickly to corticosteroids: in general the dose needed to treat this complication is significantly lower than that required to treat granulomatous interstitial nephritis, and can be as low as 35 mg of prednisolone daily. Chloroquine, by decreasing the level of 1,25-dihydroxycholecalciferol, is an effective therapy for the hypercalcaemic/hypercalciuric syndrome. Ketoconazole, an inhibitor of steroidogenesis, has been used in a single patient who could not tolerate corticosteroids and was effective in decreasing the level of active vitamin D as well as serum and urinary calcium.

Although uncommon in patients with sarcoidosis, endstage renal failure (**ESRF**) requiring renal replacement therapy is most often due to hypercalcaemic nephropathy rather than granulomatous nephritis. Graft loss due to disease recurrence has not been reported.

Drug-induced nephropathy (Table 1)

Analgesics

Analgesic nephropathy is characterized by renal papillary necrosis and chronic interstitial nephritis caused by the prolonged and excessive consumption of analgesics. It is invariably caused by compound analgesic mixtures containing aspirin or other antipyretic agent in combination with phenacetin, paracetamol, or salicylamide and caffeine or codeine in popular 'over-the-counter' proprietary medicines.

In the recent past, analgesic nephropathy has been one of the commoner causes of chronic renal failure, particularly in Australia and parts of Europe. Estimates made before phenacetin was removed from over-the-counter analgesics and prior to the enactment of legislation making combined analgesic preparations only available by prescription (in Sweden, Canada, and Australia), suggested that analgesic nephropathy was responsible for 1 to 3 per cent of cases of endstage renal disease in the United States as a whole: up to 10 per cent in areas of North Carolina, and 13 to 20 per cent in Australia and some countries in Europe (such as Belgium and Switzerland). During the 1990s, there was a clear decrease in the prevalence and incidence of the condition among patients undergoing dialysis in several European countries and Australia. Some authors have associated this decrease

Table 1 Differential diagnosis of some forms of chronic interstitial nephritis

	Analgesic nephropathy	5-Aminosalicylic acid nephritis	Chinese herb disease	Endemic Balkan nephritis
Course	>10–15 years	>6 months	6 months–2 years	>20 years
Kidney imaging	Shrunken, irregular contours, papillary calcifications	Slightly shrunken, smooth, no calcifications	Shrunken, irregular contours, no calcifications	Shrunken, smooth surface, no calcifications
Histology				
• cellular infiltration	++	+++	+	+
• fibrosis	++	++	++	++
• atrophy	++	+	++	+++
Capillarosclerosis	+	?–	?/+	+
Apoptosis	?	?	?	+
Urothelial malignancies	+ (*)	–	+	+
Familial occurrence	–	–	–	+
Aetiology	Analgesics + addictive substances	5-Aminosalicylic acid +?	Aristolochic acid + vasoconstrictive substances	?

* As long as phenacetin was part of the analgesic mixture.

with the removal of phenacetin from analgesic mixtures. However, it is impossible to draw definitive conclusions from the epidemiological observations since other factors, such as eligibility criteria for dialysis treatment and the availability of analgesic mixtures, may also have had an influence.

Pathogenesis and pathology

The aetiology of analgesic nephropathy remains a controversial issue and the question of which kinds of analgesic are nephrotoxic is still a matter of debate. Since 1955 experimental studies on the nephrotoxicity of analgesics have been performed, mainly using rats fed with large amounts of drugs, sometimes aggravating the renal effects by dehydration or by introducing bacteria into the blood, peritoneum, or bladder. The results have been difficult to interpret, but it could be concluded that renal papillary necrosis was most frequently observed after the administration of aspirin in combination with phenacetin or paracetamol.

In humans, the long-standing excessive use of analgesics observed in patients with analgesic nephropathy is preferentially that of analgesic mixtures rather than single agents, abusers taking these products for their mood-altering effects rather than for the relief of physical complaints. Hence, all these mixtures contain caffeine and/or codeine, substances that can create a psychological dependence. In most of the early analgesic nephropathy reports, nearly all patients had taken large amounts of analgesic mixtures containing phenacetin. There is strong evidence that phenacetin-containing analgesic mixtures showed a high nephrotoxic potency in the past, and several case-control studies, as well as the prospective controlled longitudinal epidemiological study of Dubach *et al.*, demonstrated a high increased risk associated with the regular consumption of analgesic mixtures containing phenacetin.

However, the withdrawal of phenacetin from analgesic mixtures in western Europe, Australia, and the United States gives rise to the question of the nephrotoxic potency of different kinds of products. Clinical observations in countries where analgesics without phenacetin have been on the market for more than 20 years (for example, Australia, Belgium, Germany) have shown that identical renal pathology is observed in patients abusing analgesic mixtures that have never contained phenacetin. We observed a cohort of 226 patients with analgesic nephropathy diagnosed according to objective renal imaging criteria: abuse of analgesic mixtures was documented in all except seven cases, and in 46 patients nephrotoxicity was found in the absence of any previous phenacetin consumption. These patients abused the combinations of: aspirin and paracetamol; aspirin and pyrazolones; paracetamol and pyrazolones; and two pyrazolones.

The mechanisms responsible for the renal injury are incompletely understood. Phenacetin is metabolized to acetaminophen and to reactive intermediates that can injure cells, in part by lipid peroxidation. These metabolites tend to accumulate in the medulla along the medullary osmotic gradient created by the countercurrent system. As a result, the highest concentrations are seen at the papillary tip, the site of the initial vascular lesions. The potentiating effect of aspirin with both phenacetin and acetaminophen may be related to two factors. First, acetaminophen undergoes oxidative metabolism by prostaglandin H synthase to reactive quinoneimine that is conjugated to glutathione. If acetaminophen is present alone, there is sufficient glutathione generated in the papillae to detoxify the reactive intermediate. However, if acetaminophen is ingested with aspirin, the aspirin is converted to salicylate, which becomes highly concentrated and depletes glutathione in both the cortex and papillae of the kidney. With the cellular glutathione depleted, the reactive metabolite of acetaminophen then produces lipid peroxides and arylation of tissue proteins, ultimately resulting in necrosis of the papillae (Fig. 1). Second, aspirin (and other NSAIDs) suppress prostaglandin production by inhibiting cyclooxygenase enzymes. Renal blood flow, particularly within the renal medulla that normally exists on the verge of hypoxia, is highly dependent upon the systemic and local production of vasodilatory prostaglandins. The final injury is therefore due to both the haemodynamic and cytotoxic effects of these drugs resulting in papillary necrosis and interstitial fibrosis.

The renal damage induced by analgesics is most prominent in the medulla. The earliest changes consist of prominent thickening of the vasa recta capillaries (capillary sclerosis) and patchy areas of tubular necrosis; similar vascular lesions can be found in the renal pelvis and ureter, suggesting that the primary effect is damage to the vascular endothelial cells. Later changes include areas of papillary necrosis and secondary cortical injury with focal and segmental glomerulosclerosis and interstitial infiltration and fibrosis.

Clinical features

The renal manifestations of analgesic nephropathy are usually non-specific: normal renal function or slowly progressive chronic renal failure, and urinalysis that may be normal or may reveal sterile pyuria and mild proteinuria (less than 1.5 g/day). Hypertension and anaemia are commonly seen with moderate to advanced disease; more prominent proteinuria that can exceed 3.5 g/day can also occur at this time, a probable reflection of secondary haemodynamically mediated glomerular injury. Most patients have no symptoms referable to the urinary tract, although flank pain or macroscopic/microscopic haematuria from a sloughed or obstructing papilla may occur or as a result of a transitional-cell carcinoma. Urinary tract infection is also somewhat more common in women with this disorder.

Despite the non-specific nature of the renal presentation, there are frequently other findings that point toward the presence of analgesic nephropathy. Most patients are between the ages of 30 and 70 years, and careful questioning often reveals a history of chronic headaches or low back pain that leads to the analgesic use. Also common are other somatic complaints (such as malaise and weakness), and ulcer-like symptoms or a history of peptic ulcer disease due in part of chronic aspirin ingestion.

The decline in renal function can be expected to progress if analgesics are continued, whereas renal function stabilizes or mildly improves in most patients if analgesic consumption is discontinued. However, if the renal disease is already advanced, then progression may occur in the absence of drug intake, presumably due to secondary haemodynamic and metabolic changes associated with nephron loss. The late course of analgesic nephropathy may also be complicated by two additional problems: malignancy and atherosclerotic disease. Urinary tract malignancy will develop in as many as 8 to 10 per cent of patients with analgesic nephropathy, but in well under 1 per cent of phenacetin-containing analgesic users without kidney disease. In women under the age of 50, for example, analgesic abuse is the most common cause of bladder cancer, an otherwise unusual disorder in young women. The potential magnitude of this problem has also been illustrated by histological examination of nephrectomy specimens obtained prior to renal transplantation, when the incidence of urothelial atypia approaches 50 per cent. The tumours generally become apparent after 15 to 25 years of analgesic abuse, usually but not always in patients with clinically evident analgesic nephropathy. Most patients are still taking the drug at the time of diagnosis, but clinically evident disease can first become apparent several years after cessation of analgesic intake and even after renal transplantation. It is presumed that the induction of malignancy results from the intrarenal accumulation of *N*-hydroxylated phenacetin metabolites that have potent alkylating action. The highest concentration of these metabolites will be in the renal medulla, ureters, and bladder (as described above), possibly explaining the predisposition to carcinogenesis at these sites. The pathogenetic importance of phenacetin metabolites is suggested indirectly from the observation that the prolonged ingestion of other analgesics that can cause papillary necrosis, but do not form the same metabolites, such as acetaminophen and the NSAIDs, is not associated with tumour formation. The main presenting symptom of urinary tract malignancy in patients with analgesic nephropathy is microscopic or gross haematuria, hence continued monitoring is essential, and new haematuria should be evaluated by urinary cytology, and—if indicated—cystoscopy with retrograde pyelography. The incidence of urothelial carcinoma after renal transplantation in patients with analgesic nephropathy is comparable to the general incidence, of up to 10 per cent, of urothelial carcinomas in ESRF patients with analgesic nephropathy. Removal of the native kidneys prior to renal transplantation has also been suggested, but the efficacy of this regimen has not been proven.

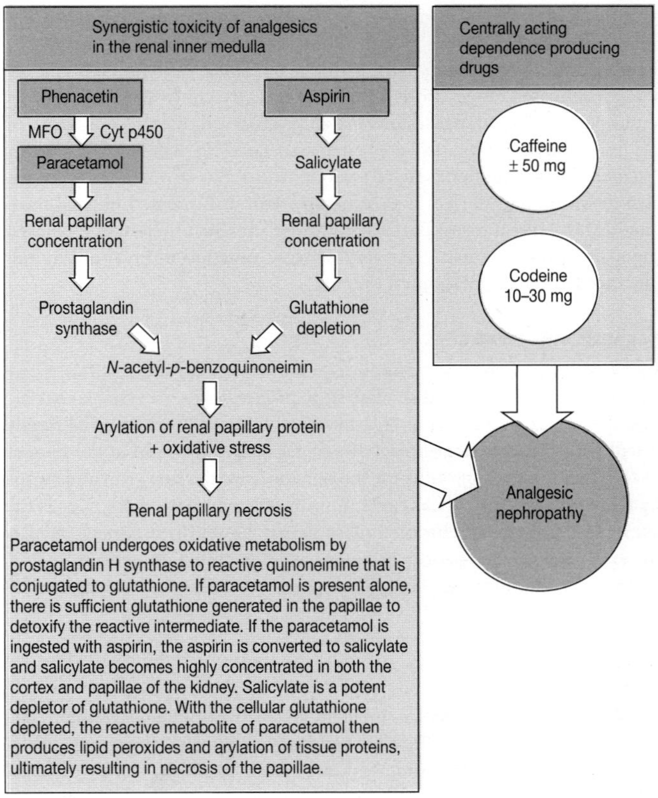

Fig. 1 Synergistic toxicity of analgesics in the renal inner medulla and centrally acting dependence-producing drugs leading to analgesic nephropathy. (Reproduced with permission from Kincaid-Smith P, Nanra RS (1993). In: Schrier RW, Gottschalk CW, eds. *Diseases of the kidney*, pp 1099–129. Little, Brown and Company, Boston, MA, and Duggin G (1996). *American Journal of Kidney Diseases* **28/1** (Suppl. 1), S39–S47.)

Diagnosis and treatment

The lack of reliable criteria and the high prevalence of analgesic nephropathy during the 1980s in Belgium (17.9 per cent in 1984) led us to perform a series of prospective, multicentre, controlled studies to define and validate the diagnostic criteria for this disease. We could provide strong evidence that specific anatomical changes, best seen by non-contrast computed tomography (**CT** scan), have much greater sensitivity and specificity than other clinical signs and symptoms in the diagnosis of endstage renal disease due to analgesic nephropathy. These changes are: (1) decrease in renal volume; (2) bumpy renal contours; and (3) papillary calcifications. In a more recent study, these observations were validated in a representative sample of patients with analgesic abuse with endstage renal disease and extended to patients with moderate renal failure. In patients with ESRF, decreased renal volume had the greatest sensitivity at 95 per cent, whilst papillary calcification had the highest specificity, and contour or papillary necrosis had a sensitivity and specificity of 90 per cent. In patients with moderate renal failure, papillary calcification was most sensitive at 92 per cent and specific at 100 per cent. The combination of papillary necrosis with either a bumpy renal contour or small kidneys did not improve sensitivity or specificity. In clinical practice, however, it is important to remember that the predictive value of this test, like any other diagnostic test, is very much dependent on the prevalence of the disease in the population under study. This test should therefore be utilized in patients with a reasonable risk for analgesic nephropathy and not as a general screening test.

As indicated above, patients with normal or only mildly/moderately impaired renal function should be strongly encouraged to stop taking analgesics, in the hope that further deterioration in renal function can be avoided. Those with severe or endstage renal failure are unlikely to recover renal function, although there may be other valid medical reasons for recommending that they stop ingesting large quantities of analgesics. The medical management of chronic renal failure is along conventional lines, as is provision of renal replacement therapy.

Non-steroidal anti-inflammatory drugs (NSAIDs)

NSAIDs are popular for treating a wide range of clinical conditions, available both over-the-counter and on prescription. Despite their usefulness, there is substantial evidence from experimental and clinical studies that NSAIDs have a variety of effects on the kidney. The most common renal disorder associated with NSAIDs is acute, largely reversible, insufficiency due to the inhibition of renal vasodilatory prostaglandins in the clinical setting of a stimulated renin–angiotensin system. Older age, hypertension, concomitant use of diuretics or aspirin, pre-existing renal failure, diabetes, and plasma-volume contraction are known risk factors for renal failure after the ingestion of NSAIDs. Rarely, NSAIDs may cause acute interstitial nephritis with proteinuria. These effects appear to be common to all NSAIDs, and are likely to be observed with cyclooxygenase-2 inhibitors as well as cyclooxygenase-1 inhibitors because both have been identified in adult and fetal human kidneys, suggesting a role for both enzymes in normal renal physiology.

By contrast to the well-characterized acute effects of NSAIDs on the kidney, the chronic effects are less well documented. However, a recent report demonstrated that NSAIDs are the most frequent cause of permanent renal insufficiency after acute interstitial nephritis. Risk factors for irreversible failure are pre-existing renal damage, long-standing intake of the causative drug, slow oligosymptomatic disease development, and histological signs of chronicity with those of acute interstitial nephritis. Although renal papillary necrosis and chronic renal failure can occur after the prolonged use of NSAIDs, the actual risk of these serious complications is unknown. Furthermore, the frequency of renal papillary necrosis as a primary or contributing cause of endstage renal disease remains unknown.

5-Aminosalicylic acid

Over the past few years an association between the use of 5-aminosalicylic (**5-ASA**) in patients with chronic inflammatory bowel disease and the development of a particular type of chronic tubulointerstitial nephritis has been suggested.

For many years, sulfasalazine, an azo-compound derived from sulphapyridine and 5-ASA, the latter being the pharmacologically active moiety, was the only valuable non-corticosteroid drug in the treatment of inflammatory bowel disease. Since the therapeutically inactive sulphapyridine moiety was largely responsible for the mainly haematological side-effects of sulfasalazine, this stimulated the development of a number of new 5-ASA formulations (mesalazine, olsalazine, balsalazine) for topical and oral use. In the last decade, these new 5-ASA products replaced sulfasalazine as the first-line therapy for mildly to moderately active inflammatory bowel disease. However, a literature search revealed 17 published cases of renal impairment associated with 5-ASA therapy in patients with inflammatory bowel disease, and in several it was shown that this did not recover completely upon stopping the drug, even after a follow-up period of several years. In a retrospective study, nephrologists reported 40 patients with inflammatory bowel disease showing renal impairment, including 15 cases with interstitial nephritis and previous use of 5-ASA. Stimulated by these findings we started a European prospective registration study aiming to register all patients with inflammatory bowel disease and renal impairment and to control for a possible association with 5-ASA therapy. A cohort of 1449 patients with inflammatory bowel disease seen during 1 year in the outpatient clinics of 28 European gastroenterology departments was investigated: preliminary results showed 30 patients (2 per cent) with decreased renal function, and a possible association with 5-ASA therapy was found in half of them.

However, determining the cause of renal disease in those with inflammatory bowel disease is not straightforward. The most frequent renal complications are oxalate stones and their consequences, such as pyelonephritis, hydronephrosis, and (in the long-term) amyloidosis. Chronic inflammatory bowel disease is also associated with glomerulonephritis: minimal-change glomerulonephritis, membranous, membranoproliferative, focal glomerulosclerosis, and proliferative crescentic glomerulonephritis have all been reported. As for many drugs, reversible, acute interstitial nephritis has been described with the use of 5-ASA compounds. In view of this complexity, the association of 5-ASA and chronic interstitial nephritis in patients with inflammatory bowel disease can be difficult to interpret, since renal involvement may be an extraintestinal manifestation of the underlying disease. However, the particular form of chronic tubulointerstitial nephritis in patients with inflammatory bowel disease treated with 5-ASA is characterized by an important cellular infiltration of the interstitium with macrophages, T cells, and also B cells (Fig. 2).

Pathogenesis and pathology

That 5-ASA causes renal disease is supported by the number of case reports appearing in the recent literature of patients with inflammatory bowel disease using 5-ASA as their only medication, the improvement (at least partially) of impaired renal function upon stopping the drug, and a worsening after resuming 5-ASA use. Furthermore, the molecular structure of 5-ASA is very close to that of salicylic acid, phenacetin, and aminophenol, drugs with well-documented nephrotoxic potential (Fig. 1). Calder *et al.* found that necrosis of the proximal convoluted tubules and papillary necrosis developed in rats after a single intravenous injection of 5-ASA at doses of 1.4, 2.8, and 5.7 mmol/kg body weight (high pharmacological doses). The mechanism of renal damage, possibly caused by 5-ASA itself, may be analogous to that of salicylates by inducing hypoxia of renal tissues, either by uncoupling oxidative phosphorylation in renal mitochondria, by inhibiting the synthesis of renal prostaglandins, or by rendering the kidney susceptible to oxidative damage by a reducing renal glutathione concentration after inhibition of the pentose phosphate shunt.

Clinical features

A typical case is shown in Fig. 2. An intriguing aspect of this type of toxic nephropathy is the documented persistence of the renal interstitium inflammation even several months/years after first taking the drug. The disease is more prevalent in men, with a male:female ratio of 15:2. The age of reported cases ranges from 14 to 45 years. By contrast with analgesic nephropathy, where renal lesions are only observed after several years of analgesic abuse, interstitial nephritis associated to 5-ASA was already observed during the first year of treatment in 7 out of 17 reported cases, most of whom had started 5-ASA therapy with documented normal renal function. In several cases, particularly those in which there was a delayed diagnosis of renal damage, recovery of renal function did not occur, and some needed renal replacement therapy.

Diagnosis and treatment

Since this type of chronic tubulointerstitial nephritis produces few if any symptoms, and if diagnosed at a late stage progresses to irreversible chronic endstage renal disease, serum creatinine levels should be measured in any patient with inflammatory bowel disease treated with 5-ASA at the start of the treatment, every 3 months for the remainder of the first year, and annually thereafter. The use of concurrent immunosuppressive therapy, as is the case in severe forms of chronic inflammatory bowel disease, may necessitate extension to the period of intensive renal function monitoring. If serum creatinine increases, a renal biopsy is the only way to demonstrate the cause.

Chinese herbs

In 1992, physicians in Belgium noted an increasing number of women presenting with renal failure, often near end stage, following their exposure to a slimming regimen containing Chinese herbs. An initial survey of seven nephrology centres in Brussels identified 14 women under the age of 50 who had presented with advanced renal failure due to biopsy-proven, chronic tubulointerstitial nephritis over a 3-year period; nine of whom had been exposed to the same slimming regimen. As of early 2000, a total of more than 120 cases had been identified. The epidemiology is unknown, as is the risk for the development of severe renal damage, but the recent publication of case reports from several countries in Europe and Asia would seem to indicate that the incidence of herbal medicine-induced nephrotoxicity is more common than previously thought.

Pathogenesis and pathology

The aetiology of Chinese herbal nephropathy is not fully understood. A plant nephrotoxin, aristolochic acid, was proposed as a possible aetiological agent, but this compound was not part of the herbal preparations used by all the patients. Furthermore, aristolochic acid (0.15 mg/tablet) has been used as an immunomodulatory drug for 20 years in Germany by thousands of patients, sometimes in doses comparable to the Chinese herb slimming regimen; despite this exposure, there is no report relating chronic tubulointerstitial nephritis to aristolochic acid.

In addition to aristolochic acid, patients with Chinese herb nephropathy also received the appetite suppressants fenfluramine and diethylpropion, which have vasoconstrictive properties, and acetazolamide, which alkalinizes the urine, thereby potentially enhancing the nephrotoxic effect of aristolochic acid. Another uncertain factor is why only some patients exposed to the same herbal preparations develop renal disease. Women appear to be at greater risk than men: other factors that might be important include toxin dose, batch-to-batch variability in toxin content, individual differences in toxin metabolism, and a genetically determined predisposition toward nephrotoxicity and/or carcinogenesis.

At one centre in Belgium, 19 native kidneys and ureters were removed in a series of 10 patients during and/or after renal transplantation: multifocal, high-grade, flat, transitional-cell carcinoma (carcinoma *in situ*) was observed in four (40 per cent), whilst all had multifocal moderate atypia. Tissue samples revealed aristolochic acid-related DNA adducts, indicating a possible mechanism underlying the development of malignancy. In another study of 39 patients with Chinese herbal nephropathy and endstage renal disease who underwent prophylactic removal of the native kidneys and ureters, urothelial carcinoma was discovered in 18 and mild-to-moderate urothelial dysplasia in 19. All atypical cells were found to overexpress a p53 protein, suggesting the presence of a mutation in the gene.

The main histological lesion, which is located principally in the cortex, is extensive interstitial fibrosis with atrophy and loss of the tubules (Fig. 3). Cellular infiltration of the interstitium is scarce. Thickening of the walls of the interlobular and afferent arterioles result from endothelial cells swelling. The glomeruli are relatively spared and immune deposits are not observed. These findings suggest that the primary lesions may be centred in the vessel walls, thereby leading to ischaemia and interstitial fibrosis.

Clinical features

Patients present with renal insufficiency and other features indicating a tubulointerstitial disease. Blood pressure is either normal or only mildly elevated, and the urinary sediment reveals only a few red and white cells. The urine contains protein (less than 1.5 g/day), consisting of both albumin and low molecular weight proteins that are normally reabsorbed by the proximal tubules, hence tubular dysfunction—also marked by glycosuria—contributes to the proteinuria. The plasma creatinine concentration at presentation has ranged from 1.4 to 12.7 mg/dl (123 to 1122 μmol/l). Follow-

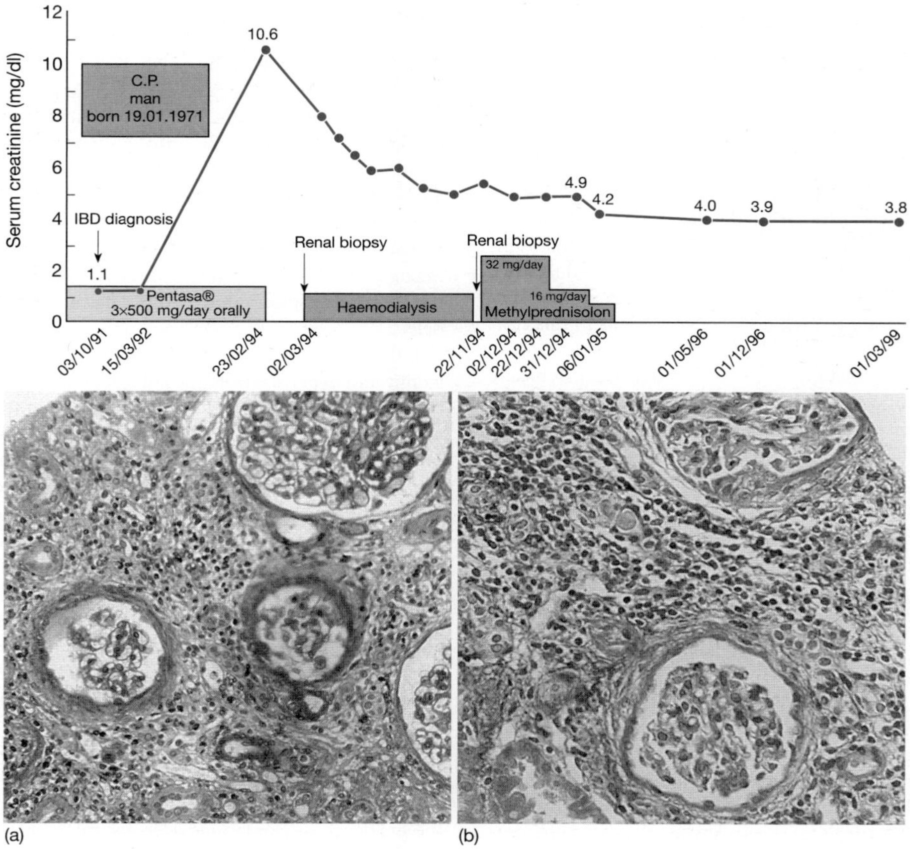

Fig. 2 5-ASA. A 36-year-old male patient suffering from Crohn's disease presented with severe renal failure after 23 months of 5-aminosalicylic acid (Pentasa®) treatment. A first renal biopsy showed widening and massive cellular infiltration of the interstitium, tubular atrophy, and relative spacing of glomeruli. The cellular infiltration was identified using appropriate monoclonal antibodies and consisted not only of T cells and macrophages, but also B cells. A second renal biopsy performed after the drug had been stopped for 8 months, when there was a modest improvement in renal function, again showed a significant cellular infiltration of the interstitium, tubular atrophy, and fibrosis. (a) First renal biopsy, (b) second renal biopsy.

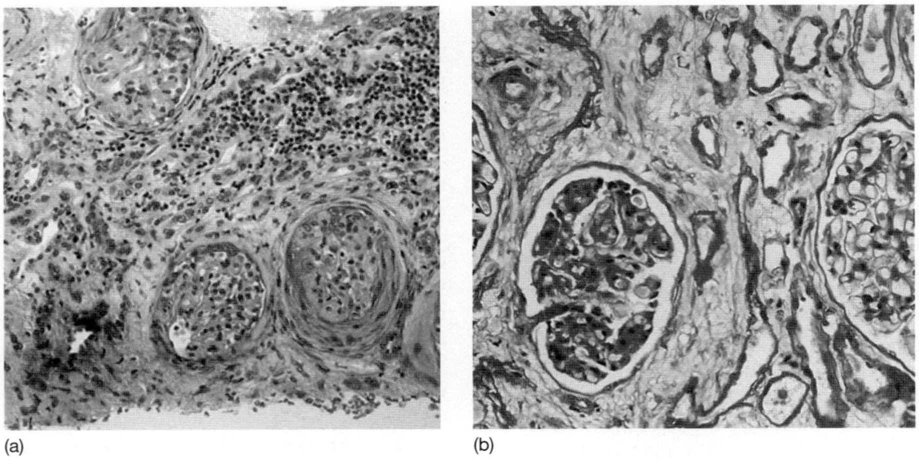

Fig. 3 Renal biopsy showing tubular atrophy, widening of the interstitium, cellular infiltration, and fibrosis, with glomeruli surrounded by a fibrotic ring, in a case of Chinese herb nephropathy. (a) Masson staining, (b) haematoxylin–eosin staining.

up studies have revealed relatively stable renal function in most patients, with an initial plasma creatinine concentration below 2 mg/dl (176 μmol/l). However, progressive renal failure resulting in eventual dialysis or transplantation may ensue in patients with more severe disease, even if further exposure to Chinese herbs is prevented.

An extremely similar clinical and pathological process has been reported in a group of patients from Taiwan who had ingested a selection of uncontrolled traditional Chinese herbs that differed from those of the slimming regimen. Despite discontinuation of these remedies, progressive renal failure was common.

Diagnosis and treatment

There are no specific criteria for the diagnosis of this type of renal disease. The condition should be suspected in any patient with unexplained relatively rapidly progressive renal disease who is using/abusing herbal remedies. The presence of tubular proteinuria may be a clue to the diagnosis, particularly in the early stages. The histological appearances are not specific, but renal biopsy is necessary to exclude other conditions in this clinical context.

There is no proven effective therapy for this disorder, which typically presents with marked interstitial fibrosis without prominent inflammation. An uncontrolled study suggested that corticosteroids may slow the rate of loss of renal function. The high incidence of cellular atypia of the genitourinary tract suggests that, as a minimum, these patients should undergo regular surveillance for abnormal urinary cytology. Whether more aggressive management strategies, such as bilateral native nephrouterectomies (particularly in those undergoing renal transplantation), are required is unclear. Findings from a recent report support the more aggressive option. Renal transplantation is an effective modality for those who progress to endstage renal disease, one report noting no recurrence in five patients.

Lithium

Lithium is used extensively in the treatment of patients with manic-depressive psychosis. Different forms of renal effects/injury have been described: most frequently nephrogenic diabetes insipidus, but also renal tubular acidosis, chronic interstitial nephritis, nephrotic syndrome, and focal segmental glomerular sclerosis/global glomerular sclerosis. Hyperparathyroidism is observed in patients treated with lithium.

Pathogenesis and pathology

Lithium is eliminated from the body almost entirely by the kidney, being filtered at the glomerulus and reabsorbed in the proximal tubule, resulting in a clearance of one-third of the normal creatinine clearance. It moves in and out of cells only slowly and accumulates in the kidney, particularly in the collecting tubule, entering these cells through sodium channels in the luminal membrane. Hence, its principal toxicity relates to distal tubular function, where inhibition of adenylate cyclase and generation of cyclic AMP result in downregulation of aquaporin-2, the collecting tubule water channel, and a decrease in ADH receptor density, leading to resistance to antidiuretic hormone. Further effects compound this. A low intracellular level of cyclic AMP leads to the increased cellular levels of glycogen observed in kidney biopsy specimens from patients taking lithium, as does the fact that lithium also directly inhibits enzymes involved in glycogen breakdown. The ensuing increased glycogen storage may interfere with distal tubular function and be responsible for the observation that polyuria and polydipsia in lithium-treated patients is due to nephrogenic diabetes insipidus.

The tubular defect in the distal nephron can also impair the ability to maximally acidify the urine. A lithium-induced decrease in the activity of the H+-ATPase pump in the collecting tubule may be responsible for this defect.

Lithium treatment has been aetiologically related to parathyroid hypertrophy and hyperfunction, the latter seeming to be due to an upward resetting of the level at which the plasma calcium concentration depresses parathyroid hormone (**PTH**) release. Persistent hypercalcaemia (in 5–10 per cent of the patients) may exacerbate both the concentrating defect and the interstitial nephritis seen in lithium-treated patients.

Renal biopsies from patients taking lithium show a specific histological lesion in the distal tubule and collecting duct. On light microscopy there is swelling and vacuolization in cells associated with a considerable accumulation of Periodic acid–Schiff (**PAS**)-positive glycogen. This is present in all renal biopsies from patients taking lithium, it appears within days after the administration of lithium and disappears when lithium ingestion is ceased.

Hestbech *et al.* were the first to suggest that progressive chronic interstitial lesions occurred in the kidneys of patients receiving lithium. However, a controlled study showed no difference between biopsies from patients taking lithium and those from a group of patients who had affective disorders but were not doing so. Specifically, there was no difference in the incidence of glomerular sclerosis, interstitial fibrosis, tubular atrophy, cast formation, or interstitial volume, but there was a significant increase in the number of microcysts in the lithium-treated patients. One reason why it has been difficult to determine the nature of lithium-induced chronic renal damage has been the lack, until recently, of an animal model in which lesions similar to those noted in human biopsies could be demonstrated. However, a recent study on lithium nephrotoxicity carried out in the rabbit showed clear-cut evidence of progressive histological and functional impairment, with the development of significant interstitial fibrosis, tubular atrophy, glomerular sclerosis, and cystic tubular lesions. A recent publication by Markowitz *et al.* revealed a chronic tubulointerstitial nephropathy in 100 per cent of 24 patients having received lithium for several years, associated with cortical and medullary tubular cysts or dilatation. There was also a surprisingly high prevalence of focal segmental glomerulosclerosis and global glomerulosclerosis, sometimes of equivalent severity to the chronic tubulointerstitial disease. Despite discontinuing lithium treatment, seven of nine patients with initial serum creatinine values above 2.5 mg/dl progressed to endstage renal disease. Nevertheless, an answer to the question as to whether or not chronic lithium therapy causes chronic interstitial nephritis still needs more hard data.

Clinical features

Apart from acute lithium intoxication, chronic poisoning can occur in patients whose lithium dosage has been increased or in those with a decreased effective circulating volume, decreased sodium intake, diabetes mellitus, gastroenteritis, and renal failure, thereby resulting in an increase in serum lithium levels. Symptoms associated with poisoning include lethargy, drowsiness, coarse hand tremor, muscle weakness, nausea, vomiting, weight loss, polyuria, and polydipsia. Severe toxicity is associated with increased deep tendon reflexes, seizures, syncope, renal insufficiency, and coma. The commonest manifestation is altered mental status.

Chronic lithium poisoning is frequently associated with electrocardiogram changes, including ST-segment depression and inverted T waves in the lateral precordial leads. Lithium is concentrated within the thyroid and inhibits the synthesis and release of thyroxine, which can lead to hypothyroidism and hypothermia. It may also cause thyrotoxicosis and hyperthermia. Symptoms of hypercalcaemia may also be present, exacerbating the urinary concentrating defect already present in these patients.

In patients with glomerular lesions such as minimal-change or focal glomerular sclerosis, proteinuria generally begins within 1.5 to 10 months after the onset of therapy, completely or partially resolving in most patients within 4 weeks after lithium is discontinued. Reinstitution of lithium has led to recurrent nephrosis in some cases.

The hyperparathyroidism observed in patients receiving lithium treatment is characterized by elevated parathyroid hormone levels, hypercalcaemia, hypocalciuria, and normal serum phosphate levels, by contrast to primary hyperparathyroidism in which hypophosphataemia and hypercalciuria are seen.

Diagnosis and treatment

The severity of chronic lithium intoxication correlates directly with the serum lithium concentration and may be categorized as mild (1.5–2.0 mEq/l), moderate (2.0–2.5 mEq/l), or severe (>2.5 mEq.l).

Polyuria and polydipsia due to nephrogenic diabetes insipidus and other acute manifestations of the effect of lithium on the kidney usually disappear rapidly if lithium is withdrawn. The decision about management, however, usually revolves around the relative benefit of the lithium in controlling and preventing the manifestation of manic-depressive psychosis, and the disadvantage to the patient of the major side-effect of lithium, namely polyuria. In most cases the lithium is so clearly beneficial that the polyuria is accepted as a side-effect and treatment continued. It is likely that the serum concentration of lithium is important, and that renal damage is more likely to occur if the serum concentration is consistently high or if repeated episodes of lithium toxicity occur. The serum lithium concentration should therefore be monitored carefully (at least every 3 months) and maintained at the lowest level that will provide adequate control of the manic depressive psychosis.

Much more difficult to handle is the situation where a patient on long-term lithium therapy is found to have impaired renal function for which there is no obvious alternative cause. As stated above, renal failure may progress even if lithium therapy is withdrawn, and in some patients the discontinuation of lithium can lead to a devastating deterioration in their psychiatric condition. The decision as to whether or not to discontinue lithium should therefore be made after frank and open discussion, admitting all uncertainties, with the patient, psychiatric colleagues, and (if appropriate) relatives/carers.

Endemic Balkan nephropathy

Endemic Balkan nephropathy (**EBN**) is a chronic, familial, non-inflammatory tubulointerstitial disease of the kidneys. A high frequency of urothelial atypia, occasionally culminating in tumours of the renal pelvis and urethra, is associated with this disorder.

As the name suggests, EBN is most commonly seen in South-Eastern Europe, including the areas traditionally considered to comprise the 'Balkans': Serbia, Bosnia and Herzegovina, Croatia, Romania, and Bulgaria. It is most likely to occur among those living along the confluence of the Danube river, a region in which the plains and low hills generally have a high humidity and rainfall (Fig. 4). There is a very high prevalence in endemic areas, with rates ranging between approximately 0.5 and 4.4 per cent, increasing to as high as 20 per cent if the disorder is suspected and carefully screened for among an at-risk population. A striking observation is that nearly all affected patients are farmers.

Pathogenesis and pathology

Although the aetiology of EBN is unknown, many environmental and genetic factors have been evaluated as possible underlying causes.

Environmental factors

Given that it is endemic to a specific geographic area, toxins and/or environmental exposures that are unique to the Balkans have been investigated. However, no agent and/or general group of compounds or organisms, including trace elements (lead, cadmium, silica, selenium), viruses, fungus, and/or plant toxin, has yet been successfully identified.

One intriguing possibility is that aristolochic acid, a mutagenic and nephrotoxic alkaloid found in the plant *Aristolochia clematis*, may underlie both Chinese herbal nephropathy (see above) and EBN (see Table 1). There are striking pathological and clinical similarities between the progressive interstitial fibrosis observed in young women who have been on a slimming regimen containing Chinese herbs (as well as other agents) and EBN, but this putative association between EBN and aristolochic acid remains speculative.

Genetic factors

Support for a genetic aetiology includes observations that the disease clearly affects particular families, and that some ethnic populations who have lived in endemic areas for generations do not suffer from EBN. The mode of inheritance has not yet been established and possible causative gene(s) have not been identified, but a locus in the region between 3q25 and 3q26 has been incriminated.

By contrast, some observations are inconsistent with a genetic basis. First, EBN is observed in individuals who have immigrated into the 'Balkan' area from regions without the disorder, and in previously unaffected families who have lived for at least 15 years in endemic areas. Second, EBN does not develop in members from previously affected families who have left endemic areas early in life or who spent less than 15 years in these areas.

A unifying hypothesis may be that the disease most likely occurs in genetically predisposed individuals who are chronically exposed to a causative, as yet unidentified agent.

In the early stages of disease, renal histology reveals focal cortical tubular atrophy, interstitial oedema, and peritubuloglomerular sclerosis with limited mononuclear-cell infiltration. Narrowing and endothelial swelling of interstitial capillaries (e.g. capillarosclerosis) is also described. In advanced cases, marked tubular atrophy and interstitial fibrosis develop along with focal segmental glomerular changes and global sclerosis. There

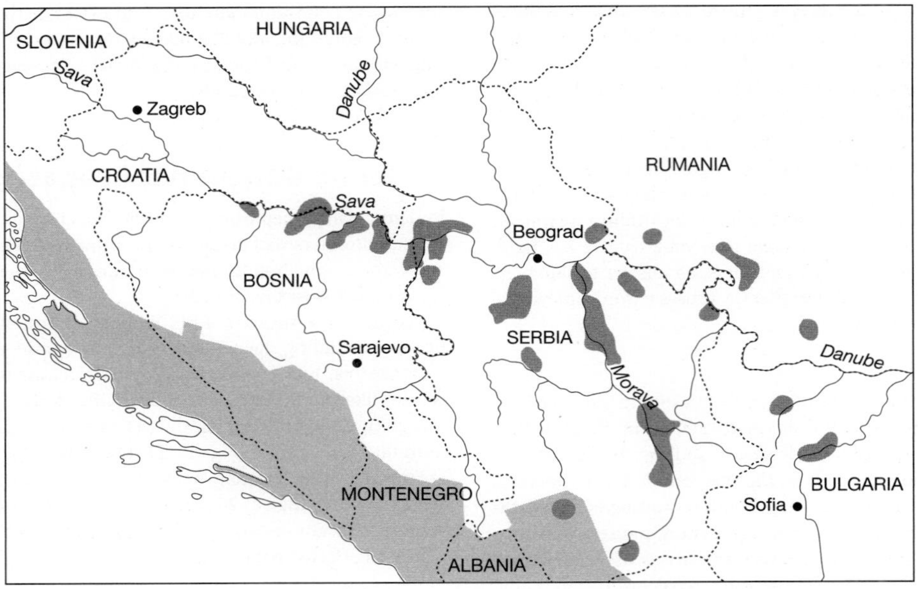

Fig. 4 Foci of endemic Balkan nephropathy.

is an extremely high incidence of cellular atypia and urothelial carcinoma of the genitourinary tract.

Clinical features

EBN is a slowly progressive tubulointerstitial disease that may culminate in endstage renal disease. Clinical manifestations first appear between 30 and 50 years of age, with findings prior to the age of 20 being extremely rare. One of the first signs is tubular dysfunction, which is characterized by an increased excretion of low molecular weight proteins (such as β2-microglobulin). Early tubular injury can also lead to renal glycosuria, aminoaciduria, and diminished ability to handle an acid (NH4Cl) load. Over a period of more than 20 years there is a progressive decrease in concentrating ability (resulting in polyuria) and in the glomerular filtration rate (resulting in endstage renal disease). Patients are usually without oedema and are normotensive, hypertension only developing with endstage disease. A normochromic normocytic anaemia occurs with early disease, which becomes increasingly pronounced as the disorder progresses. Urinary tract infection is rarely observed. Kidneys are of normal size early in the course of the disease. A symmetrical reduction of kidney size with a smooth outline and normal pelvicaliceal system is subsequently observed in patients with late-stage disease. Intrarenal calcifications are not observed.

EBN is also associated with the development of transitional-cell carcinoma of the renal pelvis or ureter, with studies noting a wide range in incidence (2 to nearly 50 per cent). These tumours are generally superficial and slow-growing.

Diagnosis and treatment

The diagnosis of EBN is based upon the presence of some combination of the following findings:

- symmetrically shrunken kidneys with absence of intrarenal calcifications;
- farmers living in the endangered villages;
- familial history positive for endemic Balkan nephropathy;
- mild tubular proteinuria, hyposthenuria; and
- normochromic hypochromic anaemia occurring in patients with only slightly impaired renal function.

As with many other chronic tubulointerstitial diseases of unclear origin, there is no specific prevention or treatment. Therapy is therefore supportive, with renal replacement therapy being initiated in patients with endstage renal disease.

The high incidence of cellular atypia in the genitourinary tract suggests that regular surveillance should be performed for abnormal urinary cytologies. Whether bilateral native nephroureterectomies are required, particularly in those undergoing renal transplantation, is unclear.

Radiation nephropathy

Radiation nephropathy is a renal disorder caused by ionizing radiation. The kidney may be injured by radiation administered to tumours within the kidney or nearby tissues (testis, ovary, retroperitoneum). Clinicians were aware of the potential adverse effects of X-rays on renal function from the beginning of the twentieth century, and between 1940 and 1960 a significant number of cases were reported. In 1953 Luxton established the clinical features of the condition and defined the tolerance of the kidney to irradiation, leading to preventive shielding of the kidneys in patients receiving radiation therapy and to a marked decline in the frequency of radiation nephropathy. In the last decade, however, total-body irradiation preceding bone marrow transplantation has resulted in an increasing incidence of radiation nephropathy, with late chronic renal failure developing in 20 per cent of patients who receive this treatment.

Pathogenesis and pathology

The radiation doses traditionally associated with radiation nephropathy were above 2000 rad (20 Gy) (less in children). By contrast, in patients receiving total-body irradiation preceding bone marrow transplantation, renal impairment was observed after doses of 1000 to 1400 rad (10–14 Gy). Fractionation, time, and effects of cytotoxic chemotherapy can probably explain the differences. In laboratory rodents, fractionation of the total dose into multiple separated doses decreases the risk, probably due to repair of sublethal radiation damage during the time between the fractionated doses. Total-body irradiation before bone marrow transplantation is usually administered over a short period, which does not allow sufficient time for the repair of radiation injury to the kidney. Moreover, the additional cytotoxic chemotherapy given to these patients potentiates the effects of ionizing radiation.

The precise pathogenesis of radiation nephropathy remains to be determined. The initial target of ionizing radiation within the kidney appears to be the endothelial cell. Radiation kills cells by damaging DNA, so that cell death after radiation is delayed until the cell divides. After the initial glomerular endothelial injury, vascular occlusion subsequently develops, leading to tubular atrophy. Because inflammatory cells are not seen in the renal parenchyma, the previously used terminology of 'radiation nephritis' is a misnomer.

The pathological features of radiation nephropathy comprise a continuous spectrum of changes that vary in relation to the dose of irradiation administered and the time elapsed after exposure. Large doses are followed by complete atrophy, thickening of basement membranes, and interstitial fibrosis.

Clinical features

Radiation nephropathy can take several forms. Acute radiation nephropathy occurs between 6 and 12 months after radiation therapy and presents with hypertension, anaemia, and oedema. The severity of hypertension ranges from mild to malignant, and more than half of the patients progress to chronic renal failure. Radiation nephropathy after total-body irradiation before bone marrow transplantation most closely corresponds to this acute form of radiation nephropathy. A more insidious chronic form of radiation nephropathy develops over a period of several years and presents primarily with diminished glomerular filtration rate, hypertension, and (occasionally) proteinuria. Another subset of patients may develop hypertension within a few years of irradiation, evolving in some to malignant hypertension with accelerated loss of renal function. Isolated persistent or intermittent proteinuria may also occur, frequently developing more than a decade after radiation exposure.

Diagnosis and treatment

Radiographic studies may help in the diagnosis of acute radiation nephropathy. CT scans with contrast demonstrate sharply demarcated, dense, persistent nephrograms corresponding to the irradiated areas.

The treatment of radiation nephropathy is supportive. Aggressive treatment of hypertension may slow the progression of renal disease. Hypertension due to unilateral disease may respond to nephrectomy. Additionally, the use of ACE inhibitors may have its classical renoprotective effect independent of antihypertensive action.

Since radiation nephropathy is an irreversible process, preventive measures should be taken during the administration of radiation. This includes selective shielding of the kidneys and the use of fractionated doses. Patients exposed to additional nephrotoxins remain at an increased risk of toxic effects.

Toxins

Lead

Lead toxicity affects many organs, resulting in encephalopathy, anaemia, peripheral neuropathy, gout, and renal failure. It was the epidemic of lead nephropathy in Queensland (Australia) that provided the strongest link between lead and chronic tubulointerstitial nephritis. Henderson noted an excess mortality due to chronic interstitial nephritis in Queensland but not in other parts of Australia, and correlated the incidence of granular contracted kidneys at autopsy with the lead content of the skull in people from Queensland and Sydney, showing that this correlated closely with the incidence of renal failure. Exposure was due to the lead-based paints used between 1890 and 1930, but recently the source of lead is industrial exposure. This type of exposure is often insidious, occurring over a very long period. Two studies have shown an inverse relationship between low-level lead exposure and renal function in the general population. Recent studies have failed to show any effect on renal function 17 to 50 years after an episode of acute childhood plumbism, the difference with Henderson's findings reflecting the greater lead burden in his study compared to the recent ones. Although low-level lead exposure in the general population is associated with mild but significant depression of renal function, its role in the development of endstage renal disease is unclear.

Pathogenesis and pathology

The pathogenesis of renal disease seen in the context of lead exposure may be related to proximal tubule reabsorption of filtered lead, with subsequent accumulation in proximal tubule cells. Aminoaciduria, glycosuria, and phosphaturia representing the Fanconi syndrome are observed after lead exposure, and thought to be related to an effect of lead on mitochondrial respiration and phosphorylation. Since lead is also capable of reducing 1,25-dihydroxyvitamin D synthesis, prolonged hyperphosphaturia and hypophosphataemia caused by lead poisoning in children could result in bone demineralization and rickets. Chronic lead poisoning can affect glomerular function: after an initial period of hyperfiltration the glomerular filtration rate is reduced and nephrosclerosis and chronic renal failure may ensue. Protracted lead exposure also interferes with the distal tubular secretion of urate, leading to hyperuricaemia and gout.

Renal biopsies in patients with subclinical lead nephropathy and a mild to moderate decrease in glomerular filtration rate primarily show focal tubular atrophy and interstitial fibrosis with minimal cellular infiltration. Electron microscopy shows mitochondrial swelling, loss of cristae, loss of basal infoldings, and a lysosomal-like structure containing dense bodies in the proximal tubules. In Australian patients who died as a result of severe lead exposure, their kidneys were fibrotic and shrunken, the interstitium showed variable degree of fibrosis with tubular dilatation, and the vessels had thickened muscular walls with subintimal hyaline deposition in afferent arterioles, but these findings in patients with endstage renal failure were non-specific.

Clinical features

Renal failure becomes apparent years after exposure and is associated with gout in most, if not all, cases. Hypertension is a very common feature of lead nephropathy, and an association between hypertension without renal failure and low-level lead exposure has gained increasing recognition over the past two decades. Although hyperuricaemia is common in renal failure, gout is unusual and its presence should raise the possibility of lead nephropathy.

However, whether chronic lead nephropathy exists as a clinical entity has been questioned. Many studies of occupational lead poisoning have not taken into account the coexposure to other toxins such as cadmium. Additionally, the relationship between early markers of renal tubular dysfunction, such as the urinary excretion of low molecular weight proteins or *N*-acetyl β-D-glucosaminidase, to the subsequent development of renal failure remains to be determined.

Diagnosis and treatment

As the blood lead level only reflects recent lead exposure, and is usually normal in patients with chronic renal failure due to their previously sustained low-level lead exposure, the diagnosis has to be based on measurement of the body lead burden. The test of choice is the **EDTA** (ethylenediaminetetraacetic acid) mobilization test: this involves the administration of 2 g of EDTA intramuscularly in two divided doses 8 to 12 h apart, and collection of three consecutive 24-hour urine samples. A cumulative excretion of more than 600 μg is suggestive for a high lead body burden. Renal failure in itself does not increase body lead load but it does delay the excretion of lead. The diagnosis of lead nephropathy should be considered in any patient with progressive renal failure, mild to moderate proteinuria, significant hypertension, history of gout, and an appropriate history of exposure.

There is very little experience of the therapeutic use of EDTA in patients with chronic renal failure. Wedeen *et al.* treated eight industrially exposed patients with EDTA injections thrice weekly for 6 to 15 months, all having mild renal failure with GFRs of around 50 ml/min before treatment—four patients improved with a 20 per cent increase in their GFR.

Cadmium

Cadmium is a cumulative environmental pollutant and accumulates in the human body after inhalation or gastrointestinal absorption. Due to its various applications and increased industrial production, this element's release into the environment increased considerably from the 1950s onwards, particularly in Belgium and Japan, which are among the most important cadmium-producing countries worldwide. However, the atmospheric emissions of cadmium from zinc smelters have been reduced since the 1970s. At the present, normal cadmium values are set at 0.1 to 0.8 μg/l (non-smokers) in blood and 0.02 to 0.7 μg/g creatinine in urine.

Cadmium is a highly toxic metal. The kidney is the element's most important target organ and it has long been recognized that high-level exposure to cadmium after inhalation or ingestion can give rise to nephrotoxicity in humans, and that this effect is usually considered to be the earliest and most important feature from the point of view of health. Cadmium induces a tubular proteinuria (of low molecular weight plasma proteins). Hence, when exposed to high levels of cadmium (cadmium in renal cortex >100–400 μg/kg wet weight) in the workplace, workers have developed tubular proteinuria, renal glycosuria, aminoaciduria, hypercalciuria, phosphaturia, and polyuria, and in a few severe cases (long-standing high exposure and urinary excretion >20 μg/g creatinine and β_2-microglobulin >1500 μg/g creatinine) renal damage may progress to an irreversible reduction in glomerular filtration. Signs of distal tubular damage such as a cadmium-induced inhibition of ADH-stimulated ion transport have also been reported.

The extent to which chronic low-level environmental exposure to cadmium affects renal function is much less clear. The Cadmibel study, in which a random sample of 1699 subjects was recruited from four areas of Belgium with varying degrees of cadmium pollution, showed that (after standardization for several confounding factors) five markers of renal dysfunction (retinol binding protein, *N*-acetyl-β-glucosaminidase, β_2-microglobulin, amino acids, and calcium) were significantly associated with urinary cadmium excretion. There was a 10 per cent probability of these variables being abnormal when urinary cadmium levels exceeded 2 to 4 μg/24 h. However, in a 5-year follow-up of a subcohort from the Cadmibel study, the so-called Pheecad study, in which 593 individuals with the highest urinary cadmium excretion were re-examined on average 5 years later, it was demonstrated that the subclinical tubular effects previously documented were not associated with a deterioration in glomerular function. Hence, in the environmentally cadmium-exposed population, the renal effects due to cadmium appear to be weak, stable, and even reversible. These findings in environmentally exposed subjects may reasonably be extrapolated to the current, moderately exposed, occupational population, where, in various epidemiological studies, increased cadmium levels/exposure have repeatedly been associated with disturbed levels of markers of early renal dysfunction, but without evidence for accelerated progression towards chronic renal failure.

Metabolic disorders

Chronic hypokalaemia

Several renal abnormalities, most of which are reversible with potassium repletion, can be induced by hypokalaemia. Vasopressin-resistant impairment of the ability to concentrate the urine, increased renal ammonia production, enhanced bicarbonate reabsorption, altered sodium reabsorption, and hyperkalaemic nephropathy have all been described.

Persistent hypokalaemia can induce a variety of changes in renal function, impairing tubular transport, and possibly inducing chronic tubulointerstitial disease and cyst formation. Hypokalaemic nephropathy in humans produces characteristic vacuolar lesions in the epithelial cells of the proximal tubule and (occasionally) the distal tubule. This abnormality probably requires about 1 month to develop. More severe changes, including interstitial fibrosis, tubular atrophy, and cyst formation that is most prominent in the renal medulla, occur if prolonged hypokalaemia is maintained. The pathogenesis of these changes is not well understood.

Renal growth accelerates when rats are placed on a potassium-deficient diet, and within 8 days there is a 25 per cent increase in kidney mass. The changes are most prominent in the outer medulla, especially the inner stripe, where hyperplastic, enlarged, collecting-duct cells form cellular outgrowths that project into the lumen causing partial obstruction. If the potassium-deficient state persists, then cellular infiltrates appear in the renal interstitial compartment and tubulointerstitial fibrosis develops. It has been proposed that some of these pathological changes may be initiated by the high levels of ammonia generated in potassium-deficiency states and may be mediated through the activation of the alternate complement pathway. In support of this hypothesis is the finding that bicarbonate supplementation sufficient to suppress renal ammoniagenesis attenuates the renal enlargement and tubulointerstitial disease: against it are reports that increased renal ammoniagenesis induced by acid loading causes renal enlargement without cellular proliferation or interstitial disease. A recent paper provides results consistent with a sustained role for insulin-like growth factor-1 (**IGF-1**) in promoting the marked tubular epithelial-cell hypertrophy and hyperplasia that occurs in the inner stripe of the outer medulla of the kidney with chronic potassium depletion. The same study also showed that potassium depletion causes a selective increase in the renal expression of transforming growth factor-β (**TGF-β**) in the hypertrophied, non-hyperplastic, thick ascending limb, but—unlike IGF-1—it is absent from the hyperplastic collecting-duct cells. This might be responsible for preventing the conversion of the mitogenic stimulus of IGF-1 into a hypertrophic one. It is possible that TGF-β causes the prominent interstitial infiltrate that develops in chronic hypokalaemia, since this 'growth factor' is a well-known chemoattractant for macrophages.

Hyperoxaluria

Hyperoxaluria may be primary or acquired. The primary form is a rare inherited disorder due to an enzymatic abnormality in the metabolism of glyoxylic acid. The acquired forms of hyperoxaluria are more common and result either from the ingestion of oxalate precursors, such as ethylene glycol and ascorbic acid, and exposure to methoxyflurane anaesthesia, or from increased absorption from the intestinal tract in those with inflammatory bowel disease or who have undergone small-bowel resection.

The microcrystallization of calcium oxalate first occurs in the proximal tubules where oxalate secretion occurs. However, the lesions that develop are more severe in the renal medulla, where the increasing concentration of the tubular fluid and its acidification promote the precipitation of calcium oxalate. If the overload is insidious and chronic, inflammatory-cell infiltration, oedema, interstitial fibrosis, tubular atrophy, and dilatation result in a chronic tubulointerstitial nephritis with progressive renal failure.

Hypercalcaemia

Prolonged elevation of urinary and serum calcium levels may result in the deposition of calcium in the kidney (nephrocalcinosis, see Chapter 20.13). This also occurs in some clinical conditions not associated with hypercalcaemia. Increased intestinal absorption of calcium occurs with vitamin D intoxication, sarcoidosis, and the milk alkali syndrome. Skeletal deossification due to neoplasms, hyperparathyroidism, and multiple myeloma can also produce nephrocalcinosis, stones, and functional abnormalities.

Calcium is most concentrated in the medulla, where degeneration and tubular necrosis begins due to intracellular overload with damage to mitochondria and other critical organelles. Reactive inflammatory changes occur in the adjacent interstitium, and necrotic cells may cause intratubular obstruction and tubular atrophy. The final results of these changes are focal areas of tubular atrophy, interstitial fibrosis, and a mononuclear-cell infiltrate.

Hyperuricaemia/hyperuricosuria

There are three different types of renal disease induced by abnormal uric acid metabolism: acute uric acid nephropathy; chronic urate nephropathy; and uric-acid stone disease—the latter being discussed in Chapter 20.13.

The kidneys are the major organs for the excretion of uric acid and a primary target organ affected in disorders of urate metabolism. Renal lesions result from the crystallization of uric acid either in the urinary outflow tract or in the renal parenchyma. The determinants of uric acid solubility are its concentration and the pH of the medium in which it is dissolved. Hence the supersaturation of fluid within the renal tubules as excreted uric acid becomes concentrated in the medulla, and the acidification of the urine in the distal tubule, are both conducive to the precipitation of uric acid. The major sites of urate deposition are the renal medulla, the collecting tubules, and the urinary tract. The p*Ka* of uric acid is 5.7, and at the acid pH of the fluid in the distal tubule the bulk of filtered urate will be present in its non-ionized form as uric acid, whereas at the more alkaline pH of the blood and interstitium it is in its ionized form as urate salts.

Acute uric acid nephropathy

Acute uric acid nephropathy is an uncommon condition caused by the precipitation of birefringent uric acid crystals in the collecting tubules, with consequent tubular obstruction, dilatation, and inflammation. This can occur in disorders associated with an increased production of uric acid, for example myeloproliferative or lymphoproliferative disorders, tumour lysis syndrome (see Chapter 20.10.5), chronic haemolytic anaemia, psoriasis, or the Lesch–Nyhan syndrome, or when there is increased renal clearance of uric acid, for example inherited or acquired defects of tubular urate transport, uricosuric drugs.

In those prone to acute uric acid nephropathy, management centres on prophylaxis with a plentiful fluid intake, with or without alkalinization of the urine, and pretreatment with allopurinol, although the latter can increase the risk of xanthine nephropathy. Presentation of acute uric acid nephropathy is with acute renal failure, with urine microscopy revealing plentiful birefringent crystals. Management is supportive. If allopurinol is prescribed, then the dose must be substantially reduced in renal failure.

Chronic urate nephropathy

The principal lesion in chronic hyperuricaemia is the deposition of microtophi of amorphous urate crystals in the interstitium, with a surrounding giant-cell reaction. This results in a secondary chronic inflammatory response similar to that seen with microtophus formation elsewhere in the body, potentially leading to interstitial fibrosis and chronic renal failure.

Evidence linking chronic renal failure to gout is weak, and the longstanding notion that chronic renal disease is common in patients with hyperuricaemia has been questioned in the light of prolonged follow-up studies of renal function in people with this condition. Renal dysfunction could be documented only when the serum urate concentration was more than 10 mg/dl (600 μmol/l) in women and more than 13 mg/dl (780 μmol/l) in men for prolonged periods. Furthermore, the deterioration of renal function in those with hyperuricaemia of a lower magnitude has been attributed to the higher-than-expected occurrence of hypertension, diabetes mellitus, abnormal lipid metabolism, and nephrosclerosis. Nonetheless, it seems reasonable to prescribe allopurinol (in a dose appropriate to the level of renal function) to those very rare patients with biopsy evidence of 'gouty nephropathy', and possibly to patients with chronic renal failure who have a grossly elevated serum urate.

There is an association between severe lead intoxication, chronic renal failure, and gout (saturnine gout) (see above). It has also been suggested that there might be an association between renal disease and hyperuricaemia in those with a past history of exposure to lead and consequent subclinical lead toxicity (saturnine nephropathy). Evidence for this association is not clear-cut, nor is the mechanism whereby lead exposure might aggravate hyperuricaemia and renal failure.

Further reading

Bach PH, Hardy TL (1985). Relevance of animal models to analgesic-associated renal papillary necrosis in humans. *Kidney International* **28**(4), 605–13.

Benabe JE, Martinez-Maldonado M (1978). Hypercalcemic nephropathy. *Archives of Internal Medicine* **138**, 777–9.

Bennett WM, De Broe ME (1989). Analgesic nephropathy—a preventable renal disease. *New England Journal of Medicine* **320**, 1269–71.

Bergstein JM (1998). Radiation. In: Davison AM, *et al.*, eds. *Oxford textbook of clinical nephrology*, pp 1190–5. Oxford University Press, Oxford.

Bia MJ, Ansognia K (1991). Treatment of sarcoid-associated hypercalcemia with ketoconazole. *American Journal of Kidney Diseases* **18**, 702–5.

Bjerregaard HF, Faurskov B (1997). Cadmium-induced inhibition of ADH-stimulated ion transport in cultured kidney-derived epithelial cells. *Alternatives to Laboratory Animals* **25**, 271–7.

Blohme I, Johansson S (1981). Renal pelvic neoplasms and atypical urothelium in patients with end-stage analgesic nephropathy. *Kidney International* **20**, 671–5.

Boton R, Gaviria M, Battle CD (1987). Prevalence, pathogenesis, and treatment of renal dysfunction associated with chronic lithium therapy. *American Journal of Kidney Diseases* **10**, 329–45.

Brunner FP, Selwood NH (1994). End-stage renal failure due to analgesic nephropathy, its changing pattern and cardiovascular mortality. *Nephrology, Dialysis, Transplantation* **9**, 1371–6.

Buchet JP, *et al.* (1990). Renal effects of cadmium body burden of the general population. *Lancet* **336**, 699–702.

Calder IC, *et al.* (1972). Nephrotoxic lesions from 5-aminosalicylic acid. *British Medical Journal* **1**, 152–4.

Casella FJ, Allon M (1993). The kidney in sarcoidosis. *Journal of the American Society of Nephrology* **3**, 1555–64.

Ceovic S, Hrabar A, Saric M (1992). Epidemiology of Balkan endemic nephropathy. *Food and Chemical Toxicology* **30**, 183–98.

Cohen EP (2000). Radiation nephropathy after bone marrow transplantation. *Kidney International* **58**, 903–18.

Cosyns JP, *et al.* (1994). Chinese herbs nephropathy: a clue to Balkan endemic nephropathy? *Kidney International* **45**,1680–8.

Cosyns JP, *et al.* (1999). Urothelial lesions in Chinese-herb nephropathy. *American Journal of Kidney Diseases* **33**, 1011–17.

Cremer W, Bock KD (1976). Symptoms and course of chronic hypokalemic nephropathy in man. *Clinical Nephrology* **7**, 112–19.

Dafnis E, Kurtzman NA, Sabatini S (1992). Effects of lithium and amiloride on collecting tubule transport enzymes. *Journal of Pharmacology and Experimental Therapeutics* **261**, 701–6.

De Broe ME (1999). On a nephrotoxic and carcinogenic slimming regimen. *American Journal of Kidney Diseases* **33**, 1171–3. [Editorial]

Depierreux M, *et al.* (1994). Pathologic aspects of a newly described nephropathy related to the prolonged use of Chinese herbs. *American Journal of Kidney Diseases* **24**, 172–80.

Diamond JR, Pallone TL (1994). Acute interstitial nephritis following use of Tung Shueh pills. *American Journal of Kidney Diseases* **24**, 219–21.

Djukanovic L, Velimirovic D, Sindjic M (1998). Balkan nephropathy. In: De Broe ME, *et al.*, eds. *Clinical nephrotoxins—renal injury from drugs and chemicals*, pp 425–36. Kluwer Academic, Dordrecht.

Dubach UC, Rosner B, Pfister E (1983). Epidemiologic study of abuse of analgesics containing phenacetin. Renal morbidity and mortality (1968–1979). *New England Journal of Medicine* **308**, 357–62.

Dubach UC, Rosner B, Sturmer T (1991). An epidemiologic study of abuse of analgesic drugs. Effects of phenacetin and salicylate on mortality and cardiovascular morbidity. *New England Journal of Medicine* **324**, 155–60.

Duffy WB, Senekjian HO, Knight TF (1981). Management of asymptomatic hyperuricemia. *Journal of the American Medical Association* **246**, 2215–16.

Duggin GG (1996). Combination analgesic-induced kidney disease: the Australian experience. *American Journal of Kidney Diseases* **28**(1 Suppl 1), S39–S47.

Elseviers MM, De Broe ME (1996). Combination analgesic involvement in the pathogenesis of analgesic nephropathy: the European perspective. *American Journal of Kidney Diseases* **28**(1-Suppl. 1): S48–S55.

Elseviers MM, *et al.* (1992). Diagnostic criteria of analgesic nephropathy in patients with end-stage renal failure—results of the Belgian study. *Nephrology, Dialysis, Transplantation* **7**, 479–86.

Elseviers MM, *et al.* (1995). Evaluation of diagnostic criteria for analgesic nephropathy in patients with end-stage renal failure: results of the ANNE study. *Nephrology, Dialysis, Transplantation* **10**, 808–14.

Elseviers MM, *et al.* (1995). High diagnostic performance of CT scan for analgesic nephropathy in patients with incipient to severe renal failure. *Kidney International* **48**, 1316–23.

Farkas WR, Stanawitz T, Schneider M (1978). Saturnine gout: lead-induced formation of guanine crystals. *Science* **199**, 786–7.

Ganote CE, *et al.* (1975). Acute calcium nephrotoxicity. An electron microscopical and semiquantitative light microscopical study. *Archives of Pathology* **99**, 650–7.

Henderson DA (1958). The etiology of chronic nephritis in Queensland. *Medical Journal of Australia* **25**, 196–202.

Hensen J, Haenelt M, Gross P (1996). Lithium induced polyuria and renal vasopressin receptor density. *Nephrology, Dialysis, Transplantation* **11**, 622–7.

Hestbech J, *et al.* (1977). Chronic renal lesions following long-term treatment with lithium. *Kidney International* **12**, 205–13.

Hodgkinson A, Wilkinson R (1974). Plasma oxalate concentration and renal excretion of oxalate in man. *Clinical Science and Molecular Medicine* **46**, 61–73.

Hotz P, *et al.* (1999). Renal effects of low-level environmental cadmium exposure: 5-year follow-up of a subcohort from the Cadmibel study. *Lancet* **354**, 1508–13.

Hu H (1991). A 50-year follow-up of childhood plumbism. Hypertension renal function, and hemoglobin levels among survivors. *American Journal of Diseases of Children* **145**, 681–7.

Inglis JA, Henderson DA, Emmerson BT (1978). The pathology and pathogenesis of chronic lead nephropathy occurring in Queensland. *Journal of Pathology* **124**, 65–76.

Ivic M (1970). The problem of etiology of endemic nephropathy. *Acta Facultatis Medicae Naissensis* **1**, 29–38.

Jensen OM, *et al.* (1989). The Copenhagen case-control study of renal pelvis and ureter cancer, role of analgesics. *International Journal of Cancer* **44**, 965–8.

Johnson RJ, *et al.* (1999). Reappraisal of the pathogenesis and consequences of hyperuricemia in hypertension, cardiovascular disease, and renal disease. *American Journal of Kidney Diseases* **33**, 225–34.

Kabanda A, *et al.* (1995). Low molecular weight proteinuria in Chinese herbs nephropathy. *Kidney International* **48**, 1571–6.

Kido T, Nordberg G (1998). Cadmium-induced renal effects in the general environment. In: De Broe ME, *et al.*, eds. *Clinical nephrotoxins*, pp 345–61. Kluwer Academic Press, Dordrecht.

Kim R, *et al.* (1996). A longitudinal study of low-level lead exposure and impairment of renal function. The normative age study. *Journal of the American Medical Association* **275**, 1177–81.

Kömhoff M, *et al.* (1997). Localization of cyclooxygenase-1 and –2 in adult and fetal human kidney: implication for renal function. *American Journal of Physiology* **272**, 460–8.

Korzets Z, *et al.* (1985). Acute renal failure due to sarcoid granulomatous infiltration of the renal parenchyma. *American Journal of Kidney Diseases* **6**, 250–3.

Lakkis FG, Campbell OC, Badr KF (1996). Microvascular diseases of the kidney. In: Barry M. Brenner BM, eds. *The kidney*, pp 1721–2. WB Saunders, Philadelphia.

Luxton RW (1961). Radiation nephritis: a long-term study of fifty-four patients. *Lancet* **2**, 1221.

Markowitz GS, *et al.* (2000). Lithium nephrotoxicity: a progressive combined glomerular and tubulointerstitial nephropathy. *Journal of the American Society of Nephrology* **11**, 1439–48.

Marples D, *et al.* (1995). Lithium-induced downregulation of aquaporin-2 water channel expression in rat kidney medulla. *Journal of Clinical Investigation* **95**, 1838–45.

McCredie M, Stewart JH (1988). Does paracetamol alone cause urothelial cancer or renal papillary necrosis? *Nephron* **49**, 296–300.

McCredie M, *et al.* (1982). Analgesics and cancer of the renal pelvis in New South Wales. *Cancer* **49**, 2617–25.

McCredie M, *et al.* (1986). Phenacetin and papillary necrosis: independent risk factors for renal pelvic cancer. *Kidney International* **30**, 81–4.

McLeary TJ, *et al.* (1986). The effect of chloroquine on serum 1,25-dihydroxyvitamin D and calcium metabolism in sarcoidosis. *New England Journal of Medicine* **315**, 727–30.

Messerli FH, *et al.* (1980). Serum uric acid in essential hypertension: an indicator of renal vascular involvement. *Annals of Internal Medicine* **93**, 817–21.

Mihatsch MJ, *et al.* (1983). Capillary sclerosis of the urinary tract and analgesic nephropathy. *Clinical Nephrology* **20**(6), 285–301

Moel DI, Sachs HK (1992). Renal function 17 to 23 years after chelation therapy for childhood plumbism. *Kidney International* **42**, 1226–31.

Morlans M, *et al.* (1990). End-stage renal disease and non-narcotic analgesics. A case-control study. *British Journal of Clinical Pharmacology* **30**, 717–23.

Murray MD, Brater DC (1993). Renal toxicity of the nonsteroidal anti-inflammatory drugs. *Annual Review of Pharmacology and Toxicology* **33**, 435–65.

Murray MD, Henrich WL, Stoff JS (1996). The renal effects of nonsteroidal anti-inflammatory drugs: summary and recommendations. *American Journal of Kidney Diseases* **28**(Suppl. 1), S56–S62.

Murray TG, Goldberg M (1978). Analgesic-associated nephropathy in the USA: epidemiologic, clinical and pathogenetic features. *Kidney International* **13**, 64–71.

Muther RS, McCarron DA, Bennett VM (1981). Renal manifestations of sarcoidosis. *Archives of Internal Medicine* **141**, 643–5.

Nanra RS (1993). Analgesic nephropathy in the 1990s: an Australian perspective. *Kidney International* **42**(Suppl. 44), 86–92.

Nanra RS, Kincaid-Smith P (1993). Experimental evidence for nephrotoxity of analgesics. In: Stewart JH, ed. *Analgesic and NSAID induced kidney disease*, pp 17–31. Oxford University Press, Oxford.

Nanra RS, *et al.* (1978). Analgesic nephropathy: etiology, clinical syndrome, and clinicopathologic correlations in Australia. *Kidney International* **13**, 79–92.

Nortier JL, *et al.* (2000). Urothelial carcinoma associated with the use of a Chinese herb. *New England Journal of Medicine* **342**, 1686–92.

Petronic VJ, *et al.* (1991). Balkan endemic nephropathy and papillary transitional cell tumors of the renal pelvis and ureters. *Kidney International* **34**, S77–S79.

Piper JM, Tonascia J, Matanoski GM (1985). Heavy phenacetin use and bladder cancer in women aged 20 to 49 years. *New England Journal of Medicine* **313**, 292–5.

Polenakovic MH, Stefanovic V (1998). Balkan nephropathy. In: Davison AM, *et al.*, eds. *Oxford textbook of clinical nephrology*, 2nd edn, pp 1203–9. Oxford Medical Publications, Oxford.

Pommer W, *et al.* (1989). Regular analgesic intake and the risk of end-stage renal failure. *American Journal of Nephrology*, **9**, 403–12.

Reginster F, Jadoul M, van Ypersele de Strihou C (1997). Chinese herbs nephropathy presentation, natural history and fate after transplantation. *Nephrology, Dialysis, Transplantation* **12**, 81–6.

Roels H, *et al.* (1993). Markers of early renal changes induced by industrial pollutants. III Application to workers exposed to cadmium. *British Journal of Industrial Medicine* **50**, 37–48.

Rose BD (1994). *Clinical physiology of acid–base and electrolyte disorders*, 4th edn, pp 802–5. McGraw-Hill, New York.

Sandler DF, *et al.* (1989). Analgesic use and chronic renal disease. *New England Journal of Medicine* **320**, 1238–43.

Schwarz A, *et al.* (2000). The outcome of acute interstitial nephritis: risk factors for the transition from acute to chronic interstitial nephritis. *Clinical Nephrology* **54**, 179–90.

Smilde TJ, *et al.* (1994). Tubulo-interstitiële nefritis door mesalazine (5-ASA)-preparaten. *Nederlands Tijdschrift voor Geneeskunde* **138**, 2557–61.

Staessen JA, *et al.* (1992). Impairment of renal function with increasing blood lead concentrations in the general population. *New England Journal of Medicine* **327**, 151–6.

Staessen JP, *et al.* on behalf of the Working Groups (1996). Public health implications of environmental exposure to cadmium and lead: an overview of epidemiological studies in Belgium. *Journal of Cardiovascular Risk* **3**, 26–41.

Stefanovic V, Polenakovic MH (1991). Balkan nephropathy. *American Journal of Nephrology* **11**, 1–11.

Thompson CS, Weinman EJ (1984). The significance of oxalate in renal failure. *American Journal of Kidney Diseases* **4**, 97–100.

Timmer RT, Sands JM (1999). Lithium intoxication. *Journal of the American Society of Nephrology* **10**, 666–74.

Tollins JP, Hostetter MK, Hostetter TH (1987). Hypokalemic nephropathy in the rat. *Journal of Clinical Investigation* **79**, 1447–58.

Tonceva D, Dimitrov T, Tzoneva M (1988). Cytogenetic studies in Balkan endemic nephropathy. *Nephron* **48**, 18–21.

Torres VE, *et al.* (1990). Association of hypokalemia, aldosteronism, and renal cysts. *New England Journal of Medicine* **322**, 345–51.

Tsao T, *et al.* (2001). Expression of insulin-like growth factor-1 and transforming growth factor-β in hypokalemic nephropathy in the rat. *Kidney International* **59**, 96–105.

Vanherweghem JL (2000). Nephropathy and herbal medicine. *American Journal of Kidney Diseases* **35**, 330–2.

Vanherweghem JL, *et al.* (1993). Rapidly progressive interstitial fibrosis in young women: association with slimming regimen including Chinese herbs. *Lancet* **341**, 387–91.

Vanherweghem JL, *et al.* (1996). Effects of steroids on the progression of renal failure in chronic interstitial renal fibrosis: a pilot study in Chinese herbs nephropathy. *American Journal of Kidney Diseases* **27**, 209–15.

Viero RM, Cavalla T (1995). Granulomatous interstitial nephritis. *Human Pathology* **26**, 1347–53.

Walker RG, *et al.* (1982). Structural and functional effects of long-term lithium therapy. *Kidney International* **21**(Suppl. 11), S13–S19.

Walker RG, *et al.* (1982). A clinicopathological study of lithium nephrotoxicity. *Journal of Chronic Disease*, **35**, 685–95.

Wedeen RP, Batuman V (1983). Tubulointerstitial nephritis induced by heavy metals and metabolic disturbances. *Contemporary Issues in Nephrology* **10**, 211.

Wedeen RP, Mallik DK, Batuman V (1979). Detection and treatment of occupational lead nephropathy. *Archives of Internal Medicine* **139**, 53–7.

Wolf ME, *et al.* (1997). Lithium therapy, hypercalcemia, and hyperparathyroidism. *American Journal of Therapeutics* **4**, 323–5.

World Health Organization (1992). *Cadmium (environment health criteria 134)*, pp 174–88. World Health Organization, Geneva.

World MJ, *et al.* (1996). Mesalazine-associated interstitial nephritis. *Nephrology, Dialysis, Transplantation* **11**, 614–21.

Yang CS, *et al.* (2000). Rapidly progressive fibrosing interstitial nephritis associated with Chinese herbal drugs. *American Journal of Kidney Diseases* **35**, 313–18.

20.10 The kidney in systemic disease

20.10.1 Diabetes mellitus and the kidney

R. W. Bilous

Introduction

Diabetic nephropathy is the commonest single cause of endstage renal failure (**ESRF**) requiring renal replacement therapy in the United States, and the second most common in Europe and Japan. The incidence is increasing, largely because the incidence of diabetes itself is reaching what some have termed epidemic proportions, this growth being greatest in the developing world.

Definition

Nephropathy is a clinical diagnosis based upon the finding of proteinuria in a patient with diabetes and in whom there is no evidence of urinary infection. Conventionally, the level of proteinuria for a diagnosis of 'clinical nephropathy' or 'overt nephropathy' is 0.5 g/day, which is roughly equivalent to a urinary albumin excretion rate (**UAER**) of 300 mg/day. Patients with a UAER between 30 and 300 mg/day are defined as having 'microalbuminuria' or 'incipient nephropathy'. In this chapter, the terms 'incipient' and 'clinical nephropathy' will be used.

Although timed urine collections remain the 'gold standard' for diagnosis, they are cumbersome to use in routine clinical practice and most definitions of clinical or incipient nephropathy depend upon a 'spot' urine sample and thus a test of albumin concentration. Results in excess of 300 mg/l and more than 50 mg/l define clinical and incipient nephropathy, respectively. Sensitivity and specificity can be improved by using an early morning, first-voided specimen and correcting the albumin level for creatinine concentration (albumin:creatinine ratio (**ACR**)). Defining levels are shown in Table 1.

Pathology

Patients with newly diagnosed type 1 disease have large kidneys. Studies in experimental animals suggest that this enlargement is due to tubular hypertrophy and hyperplasia and an expansion of the tubulointerstitium. These changes are probably in response to the increased filtration of glucose and can be reversed in animals, but not man, by glycaemic correction. Otherwise, glomerular and tubular structure is normal at diagnosis in patients with type 1 diabetes.

The pathological hallmarks of diabetic nephropathy are thickening of the glomerular basement membrane (**GBM**) and mesangial expansion with or without nodule formation. GBM thickening can be detected in nearly all patients with diabetes of more than 10 years' duration, irrespective of the UAER. Those with clinical nephropathy almost invariably have GBM widths two to three times the upper limit of normal (350 nm). Mesangial volume remains in the normal range in patients who have a normal UAER. Nodule formation, although virtually pathognomonic, is not invariable. A combination of mesangial expansion and afferent arteriolar hyalinosis with ischaemia leads to eventual total glomerulosclerosis and subsequent loss of filtration capacity, ultimately leading to ESRF.

Patients with type 2 diabetes have been much less well studied, but the pathological appearances of subjects with clinical nephropathy are very

Table 1 Levels of proteinuria, albuminuria, and albumin:creatinine ratio (ACR) that define normal, incipient, and clinical nephropathy. Borderline results should be repeated on early morning samples or confirmed by a time collection

	24-h urine		Timed overnight	'Spot' sample		
	Total protein (g/day)	Albumin (mg/day)	Albumin (μg/min)	Albumin concentration(mg/l)	ACR (mg/mmol)	(mg/g)
Normal	–	<30	<20	<20	<2.5 m <3.5 f	<20 m <30 f
Borderline				20–50	2.5–10 m 3.5–10 f	20–90 m 30–90 f
Incipient nephropathy		30–300	2–2000	50–300	10–30	90–300
Clinical nephropathy	>0.5	>300	>200	>300	>30	>300

m, Male; f, female.

False-positive results with: diurnal variation, exercise, urine infection, other renal disease, haematuria, heart failure

False-negative results with: dilution, diuresis.

Table 2 Natural history of nephropathy

	Normal		Incipient nephropathy		Clinical nephropathy
UAER	<20 μg/min	1–2% p.a →	>20–<200 μg/min (increasing by 20% p.a)	3–4% p.a →	>200 μg/min
GFR	Stable Declines at 1% p.a. >40 years of age		Age-related changes until UAER approaches 200 μg/min or if blood pressure increases		Declines at: 10 ml/min per year (hypertensive), 1–4 ml/min per year (normotensive)
Blood pressure	Stable Significantly higher in those progressing to incipient nephropathy		Initially stable, but higher than in normal UAER controls. Tends to increase with increasing UAER		Most patients hypertensive (>140/80 mmHg)
Pathology	Large kidneys Tubular hypertrophy/ hyperplasia Glomerular enlargement—normal ultrastructure GBM thickening 20 nm p.a.		Kidneys can remain large; GBM thickening by 54 nm p.a. Mesangial expansion 4% p.a.		Increases with declining GFR Kidneys tend to shrink GBM 2–3 times normal, stable. Nodule formation Global glomerulosclerosis Mesangial expansion ~7% p.a.

p.a., per annum; UAER, urinary albumin excretion rate; GFR, glomerular filtration rate; GBM, glomerular basement membrane.

similar to those with type 1. However, the pattern of changes in incipient nephropathy is more heterogeneous and a significant prevalence of non-diabetic pathology (around 10 per cent) has been reported in some biopsy series.

Clinical course

The pathological lesions underpinning nephropathy have been recognized since 1936. However, clinical progression is usually defined in terms of changes in the UAER, glomerular filtration rate (**GFR**), and blood pressure. There are few long-term prospective studies of individual patients, and much of our current understanding is based upon cross-sectional data. Albuminuria is clearly a continuous variable and any separation into stages must be regarded as somewhat artificial. However, the distinction between incipient and clinical nephropathy is a useful one for practical purposes.

Urinary albumin excretion rate (UAER)

UAER may increase at diagnosis of type 1 diabetes and during acute hyperglycaemia, but it rapidly returns to normal with glycaemic correction. Thereafter the majority of patients (>60 per cent) will have a normal UAER throughout their diabetic life. The remainder will develop incipient nephropathy at incidence rates of between 1 and 2 per cent per annum, usually preceded by intermittently positive tests for microalbuminuria. The rate of increase of UAER in patients with incipient nephropathy is around 20 per cent per annum, although these rates will be less in those treated with antihypertensive therapy or intensified insulin regimens (see later).

It is unusual to develop incipient nephropathy within the first 5 years of diabetes onset, but it can develop at any time thereafter, even after 40 years. Most patients with type 1 disease and incipient nephropathy will progress to clinical nephropathy unless treated. The average rate of progression is 20 per cent over 5 years, but those with longer durations of diabetes prior to incipient nephropathy tend to progress more slowly. Once the UAER exceeds 300 mg/day there tends to be a relentless increase, sometimes into the nephrotic range, although the rate of change varies between patients and is very dependent upon systemic blood pressure. Historically, the incidence of clinical nephropathy peaks after diabetes of 15 to 17 years' duration, but these figures were obtained before the availability of effective antihypertensive therapy.

Because the onset of type 2 diabetes is more difficult to define, the precise incidence of incipient nephropathy is difficult to estimate. Up to 7 per cent of patients in the United Kingdom have incipient nephropathy and 1 per cent clinical nephropathy at diagnosis of diabetes. As in type 1 diabetes, the UAER will reduce with glycaemic correction, but usually only in a minority of patients, therefore implying an established nephropathology. The United Kingdom Prospective Diabetes Study (**UKPDS**) in newly diagnosed patients reports rates of transition from normal to incipient nephropathy of 2 per cent per annum and from incipient to clinical nephropathy of 3 per cent per annum, which are very similar to those seen in patients with type 1 diabetes.

Glomerular filtration rate (GFR)

At diagnosis, the GFR is increased in a proportion of patients with type 1 and type 2 diabetes, a phenomenon termed hyperfiltration. The precise prevalence depends upon the definition of 'normal GFR', which varies with methodology and age, but a raised GFR has been described in up to 40 per cent of patients with untreated, non-ketotic type 1 diabetes and in 45 per cent of those newly diagnosed as type 2.

The GFR returns to normal in most patients with treatment, although a significant minority maintain persistent hyperfiltration. In normal people, the GFR declines by 1 per cent per annum beyond 40 years of age, a rate that is no different in normotensive diabetic patients with a normal UAER. Patients with type 1 and type 2 disease with incipient nephropathy also tend to have a stable GFR. However, as the UAER approaches and exceeds the clinical nephropathy threshold there is a steady decline. The rate of loss of GFR is very dependent on systemic blood pressure, and also varies considerably between individuals. In historical series of hypertensive type 1 and type 2 patients, the average decline was 10 ml/min per year, thus leading to ESRF within 7 to 10 years. In patients with well-controlled blood pressure, the rates are around 4 ml/min per year, effectively delaying ESRF by more than 10 years (Table 2).

Blood pressure

In patients with type 1 diabetes, their blood pressure is virtually always normal at diagnosis. In newly diagnosed type 2 patients, over one-third will have hypertension, as conventionally defined (>160/95 mmHg). Type 1 patients who go on to develop incipient nephropathy have significantly higher blood pressures than those who remain with a normal UAER, although the averages remain within the 'normal' range. Patients with newly developed incipient nephropathy show a steady increase thereafter, such that over 45 per cent have a blood pressure of more than 140/90 mmHg within 4 years. Cross-sectional studies also consistently show higher blood pressures with increasing UAER, most type 1 and type 2 patients with clinical nephropathy will be hypertensive.

Clinical concomitants of nephropathy

Most patients with nephropathy will also have retinopathy and neuropathy (the so-called 'triopathy' of microvascular complications), which will also tend to progress along with nephropathy.

However, the most serious comorbid complication of nephropathy is macrovascular disease. The reported relative mortality for European 40-year-old, type 1 patients with clinical nephropathy in Denmark was between 80 and 100 times that of the non-diabetic population, whereas the World Health Organization (**WHO**) study revealed a three- to fourfold excess for patients with type 2 disease. Most of these deaths are due to stroke or myocardial infarction, and in Finland type 1 patients with nephropathy have a 10-fold relative risk for both compared to non-diabetic controls. Similar increases, but of lower magnitude, are seen in type 1 and 2 patients with incipient nephropathy. The reasons are unclear, but increasing blood pressure is certainly a factor, together with the unfavourable blood lipid profile found in patients with an increased UAER.

Non-nephropathic renal disease in diabetes

It is important to remember that not all renal or urinary tract disease in diabetic patients is due to 'diabetic nephropathy'. Urinary tract infection is more common in diabetic women, many of whom are asymptomatic. Urine culture should always be performed in patients with an isolated positive urinalysis for protein. Papillary necrosis is also more common in women with longstanding type 1 diabetes, and is a recognized complication of hyperosmolar coma in patients with type 1 and type 2 disease. Atheromatous vascular disease is common in diabetics and can cause renal artery stenosis, but the prevalence of functionally significant stenosis is not known.

Epidemiology

The incidence of diabetes is increasing worldwide, most rapidly in developing countries. It is estimated that by 2010 there will be a near-doubling of people with the condition to 221 million (5 million with type 1 and 216 million with type 2 disease).

Some of the wide variation in the reported prevalence of incipient and clinical nephropathy can be explained by different selection of the population under study, and by the use of different defining levels of UAER. However, selecting only population-based cohorts with good patient ascertainment, gives prevalence rates for incipient nephropathy of between 5 and 21 per cent for type 1 and 11 to 42 per cent for type 2 disease. Annual incidence rates are similar at around 2 per cent for both type 1 and type 2 patients.

For clinical nephropathy, the prevalence is 6.4 per cent in type 1 patients in the United Kingdom, with a range from 5 to 33 per cent reported worldwide for type 2. A cumulative incidence of approximately 20 per cent after 20 years' duration was found in the type 1 diabetic cohorts of the Steno Hospital in Denmark and Joslin Clinic in the United States, and similar figures have been reported for patients with type 2 diabetes in the United States (25 per cent) and Germany (27 per cent). Although reported annual incidence rates vary from 0.4 to 3.6 per cent, these are highly dependent upon the duration of diabetes in the population under study.

The Steno and Joslin cohorts have shown a 20 to 30 per cent lower incidence of clinical nephropathy in those type 1 patients diagnosed with diabetes in the 1950s and 1960s, compared to those diagnosed 20 years earlier. A single clinic in Sweden reports no patients with clinical nephropathy after 15 years' disease duration in patients diagnosed between 1976 and 1980, compared to 15 per cent and 5 per cent in patients with diabetes onset from 1961 to 1965 and 1966 to 1975, respectively. This reduction has not been seen in other clinics such as the Steno Hospital, for example. There are fewer data in patients with type 2 diabetes, but a recent study from the United States suggests that proteinuria is less common at diagnosis of diabetes, but that its incidence thereafter has not changed in the last 20 years.

Many countries now have registers of patients entering renal replacement therapy and all have shown a dramatic increase in the numbers with diabetic nephropathy. It is not clear, however, whether this is a true increase in the numbers of diabetic patients developing ESRF or a reflection of a change in acceptance policy. Either way, there is going to be a continuing increase in the number of patients with diabetes presenting for renal replacement, particularly from ethnic minorities (Afro-Caribbean and South African), who will make up around 50 per cent of such patients in the United Kingdom by 2001. The reasons for the excess risk of ECRF in these groups is unclear but may be genetic, related to hypertension, or the result of fetal programming. Although patients with type 2 disease have always been thought to develop ESRF less frequently than those with type 1, this may have been because such patients were not referred, or that they died of cardiovascular disease before entering renal failure. In 1997, 71 per cent of all diabetic patients on dialysis in the United States were classified as having type 2 disease.

Pathogenesis

Glycaemia

Observational studies have shown that sustained poor glycaemic control is associated with a greater risk for the development of nephropathy in both type 1 and type 2 diabetes. There are several potential mechanisms by which hyperglycaemia may cause nephropathy. These are common to all the microvascular complications of diabetes and are reviewed in Section 12.11.

Haemodynamic factors

Studies of experimental diabetes in the rat suggested that hyperfiltration alone could cause glomerulosclerosis. The evidence in humans is conflicting, and not helped by differing definitions of an abnormally high GFR. It appears that the rate of decline of GFR in hyperfiltering type 1 patients with a normal UAER is greater than that seen in age- and duration-matched normal GFR controls, but the numbers that go on to develop incipient nephropathy are similar in both groups. In Pima Indians with type 2 diabetes, their baseline GFR is not linked to the subsequent development of incipient or clinical nephropathy.

Growth factors

In experimental animals, the initial increase in kidney size is preceded by an increase in renal production of insulin-like growth-factor 1, and there are reports of increased circulating and urinary levels in diabetic people. However, there is no conclusive link between the initial kidney size or the renal expression of growth factors and the subsequent development of nephropathy in humans.

Hypertension

Systemic blood pressure is higher in patients with type 1 diabetes who subsequently develop incipient nephropathy. In Japanese people and Pima Indians, a prediabetic mean arterial pressure higher than 97 mmHg (>130/80 mmHg) strongly predicts the development of proteinuria. A family history of hypertension has been found in one study of type 1 patients with nephropathy, but not by another.

The situation in Europid type 2 diabetes may be different. In the UKPDS, hypertension (defined as above 160/90 mmHg or above 150/85 on treatment) was present in over 30 per cent of newly diagnosed patients, only a third of whom had increased albuminuria. Cohorts of normotensive (below 140/90 mmHg) type 2 patients with incipient nephropathy from Israel, Japan, and India showed little change in blood pressure over 7, 4, and 5 years, respectively, despite an increase in their UAER over this time.

It is not clear whether the observed changes in blood pressure initiate the nephropathic process or occur as a result of it. What is certain is that progression of nephropathy is much faster in patients with higher systemic blood pressures.

Genetics

There is a greater than 80 per cent concordance for nephropathy and a more than 73 per cent concordance for normal UAER in siblings of patients with type 1 diabetes. In Pima Indians, the prevalence of nephropathy is 14 per cent in the offspring of parents neither of whom have nephropathy, compared to 46 per cent of offspring when both parents have the condition. These observations have led to many studies looking for a possible genetic cause of nephropathy, most of which have used the candidate-gene approach. The most intensively studied genetic abnormality has been the insertion/deletion polymorphism in the angiotensin-converting enzyme (**ACE**) gene, but the results are inconsistent. Other candidate genes that have been studied include polymorphisms of the angiotensinogen, angiotensin-II type 1 receptor, collagen type IV, and aldose reductase genes: results have been variable.

Alterations in cell-membrane ion transporters have been described in patients with nephropathy, notably the red cell sodium–lithium exchanger and the sodium–hydrogen antiporter. Increased activity of the sodium–lithium exchanger is linked to increased blood pressure in non-diabetic subjects, and the sodium–hydrogen antiporter is closely linked to cell responses to growth factors, both of which have a degree of heritability. There is continuing controversy about the importance of these abnormalities in diabetic nephropathy.

Mechanical and structural factors

In experimental diabetes, intraglomerular capillary pressure is closely linked to the development of glomerulosclerosis. It is not possible to measure intraglomerular pressure directly in humans, but mathematical modelling suggests an increase in early nephropathy.

Glomerular volume is increased at diagnosis of type 1 diabetes and is a feature of clinical nephropathy in both type 1 and type 2 disease. A link between baseline glomerular size and subsequent progression to sclerosis has been described in patients with minimal-change disease, but the connection in diabetes is not proven.

Reductions of heparan sulphate proteoglycan in the intercellular matrix of diabetic patients and the GBM of those with incipient and clinical nephropathy have been reported. Workers at the Steno Hospital in Denmark suggested that this might relate to increased tissue damage in the micro- and macrovasculature, but this interesting hypothesis remains unproven.

Fetal programming

The low birth weight-thrifty phenotype hypothesis proposes intrauterine malnutrition as a possible cause of adult hypertension and diabetes, perhaps mediated via reduced numbers of renal glomeruli or islets of Langerhans, respectively. Studies have failed to find lower glomerular numbers in diabetic patients with nephropathy compared to those without, and no consistent correlation between birth weight and adult glomerular number has been found.

Other factors

Smoking rates are higher in diabetic patients with nephropathy, although a plausible mechanism of effect has yet to be defined. A link between raised blood lipids and the causation and progression of renal disease is still hotly debated. Both cross-sectional and prospective studies have shown an association between plasma total cholesterol and triglyceride levels and the UAER, but not between plasma lipids and a change in GFR.

In experimental diabetes, dietary protein restriction can prevent glomerulosclerosis. The cross-sectional EURODIAB study of patients with type 1 diabetes found that the UAER increased in patients with a protein intake of more than 20 per cent of their total food energy, whilst in the Hoorn Study of type 2 diabetic and normal subjects, a 0.1 g/kg body weight per day increase in protein intake was associated with a greater risk of developing microalbuminuria.

Finally, abnormalities of endothelial function, assessed by increases in plasma von Willebrand factor and homocysteine levels, have been described in diabetic patients with initially normal albuminuria who go on to develop incipient nephropathy, as well as in those with a persistently increased UAER at baseline. The EURODIAB investigators suggest that endothelial dysfunction provides a unifying hypothesis of micro- and macrovascular disease in diabetes.

Investigation

The diagnostic criteria for incipient and clinical nephropathy have already been discussed: the choice of urine sample (either timed or spot) and test (either absolute concentration or corrected for creatinine) depend largely upon local factors and patient acceptability. A diagnostic cascade is shown for a single (spot) urine sample in Fig. 1.

Because diabetes is so common, particularly in the elderly, other common nephropathies and uropathies must be excluded if the clinical picture

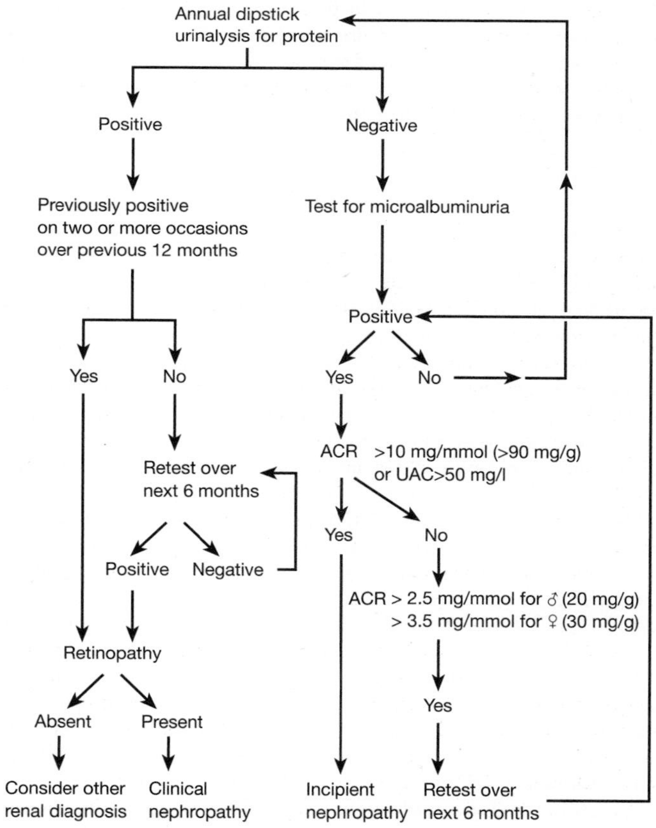

Fig. 1 Flowchart for the diagnosis of incipient and clinical nephropathy. (NB Assumes sterile urine throughout. Exclude infection when proteinuria is first detected and at any time thereafter if there is a history of a urinary tract infection.) ACR, albumin:creatinine ratio; UAC, urine albumin concentration.

Table 3 Comparison of intensive versus conventional therapy in the prevention of incipient nephropathy in type 1 (DCCT) and newly diagnosed type 2 (UKPDS) patients

Study	*n*	Ethnicity (%)	Duration of study (years)	Achieved Hb A_{1c} (%)		Incipient nephropathy (%)	
				Intensive	Conventional	Intensive	Conventional
DCCT		European (96)	9	7.2	9.1	(UAER >40 mg/day)	
No retinopathy	726			(normal <6.05)		15	27
Retinopathy	715					27	42
						(UAC >50 mg/l)	
UKPDS	3867	European (81)	9	7.0	7.9	19.2	25.4
		Indian Asian (10)		(normal 6.2)			
		Afro-Caribbean (8)					

DCCT, Diabetes Control and Complications Trial; UKPDS, UK Prospective Diabetes Study; UAER, urinary albumin excretion rate, annual 4-h collections; UAC, urinary albumin concentration, annual.

is atypical (for example, renal impairment in the absence of significant proteinuria). In addition, non-diabetic glomerular disease should be considered in proteinuric patients without retinopathy, and in those with an unexpectedly rapid deterioration in renal function, or in whom there are features of other systemic disease. Renovascular disease should be considered whenever an acute increase in plasma creatinine follows initiation of ACE inhibitor therapy, or in those with hypertension that is refractory to treatment.

Treatment

Most studies of treatments for diabetic nephropathy have used surrogate endpoints of efficacy such as a reduction in the UAER. Few have had sufficient statistical power to determine whether the therapy under investigation prevents death, reduces the number of patients entering ESRF, slows the rate of decline of GFR, or slows or reverses the progression of the pathological lesions underpinning nephropathy.

Glycaemic control

Up until 1993, there had been several well-planned, but relatively small, studies of the impact of intensified glycaemic control on the development of nephropathy in type 1 diabetes, with meta-analysis confirming significant benefit. Later that year the definitive Diabetes Control and Complications Trial (**DCCT**) showed that 9 years of intensive (mean Hb A_{1c} 7.2 per cent (normal <6.05 per cent)) compared to conventional insulin therapy (Hb A_{1c} 9.1 per cent) produced a 44 per cent reduction of development of incipient nephropathy (UAER >40 mg/day) in patients with no retinopathy, and 35 per cent reduction in patients with early retinopathy at entry (Table 3). However, the cumulative incidence of incipient nephropathy was still 15 and 27 per cent in the intensively treated patients in the two cohorts.

In patients with type 2 diabetes, there has been one small study from Japan ($n = 110$) and the much larger UKPDS cohort of 3867 newly diagnosed patients of mixed ethnicity. The Japanese study used an almost identical protocol to that of the DCCT, and showed a reduction in incipient nephropathy (UAER >30 mg/day) in the intensively treated group from 28.0 to 7.7 per cent ($p = 0.032$) in those without and 32.0 to 11.5 per cent ($p = 0.044$) in those with retinopathy at entry. In the UKPDS, the percentage of patients developing incipient nephropathy (urinary albumin concentration >50 mg/l) was lower at 19.2 versus 25.4 per cent ($p < 0.001$) in the intensively treated cohort after 9 years, representing a risk reduction of 24 per cent (Table 3).

There is continuing controversy as to whether intensive glucose control alone can prevent the progression of incipient to clinical nephropathy. Careful analysis shows that of the 73 patients with a UAER over 40 mg/day at entry into the DCCT, equal numbers developed clinical nephropathy in both the intensive and conventional groups. The UKPDS also found no impact of intensive therapy on the development of a urinary albumin concentration above 300 mg/l (4.4 versus 6.5 per cent at 9 years, relative risk (99 per cent confidence interval (**CI**)) 0.67 (0.42 to 1.07). It therefore seems that once the UAER exceeds 30 to 40 mg/day, other factors (such as blood pressure control) are of more importance for progression.

There are no conclusive data on the impact of improved glycaemic control on the development of endstage renal disease, GFR progression, or death in patients with type 1 diabetes. The UKPDS did show a positive benefit of intensive therapy on the rate of doubling of serum creatinine at 12 years (0.91 versus 3.52 per cent, $p < 0.003$) in patients with type 2 diabetes. Pancreas transplantation in type 1 patients has demonstrated that long-term (10 years) glycaemic normalization can reverse established pathological changes in glomeruli. Thus glomerulopathy may take as long to reverse as it does to develop. Notwithstanding this, it is important to remember that good glycaemic control is of proven benefit for retinopathy and therefore still an important goal of treatment in patients with nephropathy.

Blood pressure control

There have been many more studies of antihypertensive therapy than of improved glycaemic control in diabetic nephropathy. For clarity, these will be dealt with under three headings: primary prevention (of incipient nephropathy); secondary prevention (of clinical nephropathy); and tertiary prevention (of endstage renal disease and death).

Primary prevention

The EUCLID study showed that a UAER between 5 and 20 μg/min could be reduced by 2 years' treatment with the ACE inhibitor lisinopril in normotensive (systolic blood pressure <155, diastolic 75–90 mmHg) type 1 patients. There are no comparable studies in patients with type 2 diabetes, but short-term reductions in the UAER have been demonstrated. In the blood pressure control arm of the UKPDS, the percentage of hypertensive patients developing incipient nephropathy at 6 years was 2.3 per cent in the tight (average blood pressure 144/82 mmHg) and 12.5 per cent in the less tight (average blood pressure 154/87 mmHg) control groups ($p < 0.009$). This benefit was seen whether the main treatment was with ACE inhibitors or β-blockers.

Secondary prevention

All studies falling into this category have shown a short- to medium-term benefit of all antihypertensive therapies on UAER in the incipient nephropathy range, although, as a general rule, ACE inhibitors seem to be more effective.

In an attempt to explore whether ACE inhibitors are uniquely beneficial, investigators have tried to select normotensive patients and compare active treatment to placebo. In mainly European patients with type 1 diabetes with a mean entry blood pressure of 122/77 mmHg, a combined analysis of one European and one American study (total $n = 225$) showed an adjusted risk reduction of 63 per cent (95 per cent CI, 16–84 per cent; $p = 0.017$) for the development of clinical nephropathy comparing captopril 100 mg/day with placebo. Three smaller studies in normotensive (<140/90 mmHg) type 2 patients have reported a similar reduction in the rate of development of clinical nephropathy. In hypertensive type 2 patients, the angiotensin II receptor blocker irbesartan also reduced the rate of progression from incipient to clinical nephropathy by around two-thirds. The much larger Heart Outcomes Prevention Evaluation (**HOPE**) study demonstrated fewer patients progressing from incipient (albumin:creatinine ratio (ACR) >2 mg/mmol) to clinical nephropathy when treated with 10 mg ramipril. Thus blockade of the renin–angiotensin system by any means appears to confer benefit. Accurate data on GFR are not given in these studies, but in type 1 hypertensive patients, long-term ACE inhibitor therapy appears to stabilize renal function. Interpretation of these studies is difficult: actively treated patients have nearly always had significantly lower blood pressures than the placebo groups, and whilst mathematical corrections for these differences can be applied, the magnitude of the biological consequences of blood pressure reduction cannot be precisely determined.

Tertiary prevention

Studies in the early 1980s established that lowering blood pressure in hypertensive (>160/95 mmHg) type 1 patients with clinical nephropathy resulted in a more than 50 per cent reduction in the UAER and a significant slowing down of the rate of decline of the GFR from 10 to 3 ml/min per year. In those with normal blood pressure, the Collaborative Study Group Trial in type 1 diabetes compared the addition of captopril 100 mg per day to placebo in 409 patients with nephropathy and an entry blood pressure of less than 140/90 mmHg. A significant reduction (35 versus 78 per cent, $p < 0.001$) in the numbers of patients doubling their baseline serum creatinine concentration was seen in the captopril-treated patients, although this significance was confined to those with an entry serum creatinine concentration of more than 133 μmol/l (1.5 mg/dl). A similar reduction of 30 versus 70 per cent ($p = 0.002$) in the combined endpoint of death or the need for renal replacement therapy was also seen in the same group.

In patients with type 2 diabetes, the results are less consistent and complicated by the greater frequency of cardiovascular comorbidity. In those studies of more than 2 years' duration, all show sustained reductions in proteinuria but a variable, although usually consistent, slowing of the rate of GFR decline. Two recently reported studies using angiotensin II receptor blocking agents in patients with clinical nephropathy have shown a reduction in the rate of doubling of serum creatinine of between 25 and 33 per cent, less than that seen in type 1 patients but significantly better than that observed in patients randomized to the calcium channel blocker amlodipine. Taken together the studies in type1 and 2 patients support the use of drugs which block the renin–angiotensin system as first-line therapy in both incipient and clinical nephropathy.

Non-renal outcomes

Several large studies of the effect of antihypertensive therapy on cardiovascular mortality and morbidity have been published; many have included sizeable cohorts of diabetic patients, although rarely specifying their nephropathic status. All have shown that low blood pressure is associated with a reduction in overall mortality and stroke incidence, although the effect on myocardial infarction is inconsistent. Diabetic patients on the whole had greater benefit, with no clear-cut advantage from any specific drug.

Treatment targets

There is uncertainty as to what should be the target blood pressure for diabetic patients, irrespective of their nephropathy status. The recommendation of the British Hypertension Society is 140/85 mmHg, and 130/85 mmHg from the American Diabetes Association. Achieving these targets is difficult, particularly in patients with type 2 disease, and especially for systolic hypertension. In the UKPDS by year 9, 27 per cent of 758 patients in the tight blood pressure control arm were on three or more drugs, their average blood pressure was 144/82 mmHg, and 44 per cent had levels above 150/85. However, as with blood glucose levels, it seems that any reduction confers benefit and the lowest achievable (and tolerated) is probably the best target.

Other treatments

Low-protein diets have been shown by meta-analysis to slow the rate of decline of GFR in diabetic patients. Current dietary recommendations are for an intake of between 0.7 and 0.9 g protein/kg body weight per day.

Aspirin in a dose of 325 mg/day reduced myocardial infarction (relative risk (**RR**) 0.72, 99 per cent CI 0.55–0.95) in 3711 type 1 and 2 patients with retinopathy. Although nephropathy status was not determined in this study, aspirin use is advised for all patients with an increased UAER (unless contraindicated) because of their high risk of cardiovascular disease. Similarly, lipid-lowering therapy should also be considered, but there are no data on the impact of such treatment on the progression of nephropathy.

Experimental therapies include agents that inhibit the formation of advanced glycation endproducts (such as aminoguanidine), and third-generation aldose reductase inhibitors. Antagonists of endothelin and neuroendopeptidases are in advanced phase III studies.

Treatment of endstage renal disease

Diabetic patients do less well on all modalities of renal replacement therapy than their non-diabetic counterparts, with higher cardiovascular mortality. The European survival figures for diabetic patients from 1983 to 1992 are dismal: 23 per cent alive at 5 years, compared to 56 per cent of non-diabetic patients. In the United States, the death rate for never-transplanted, 20- to 44-year-old diabetic patients from 1993–1995 was 160.7 per 1000 patient-years, compared to 83.3 for non-diabetic subjects. Overall survival is best in those with a successful kidney transplant, and recent data from the United States estimates an increased survival of 11 years for diabetic patients receiving an allograft compared to those who remain on dialysis.

Management strategy

Because the outcomes of patients with diabetic nephropathy are so poor, many national guidelines now suggest a multiple risk-factor approach to management. These initiatives have been given impetus by the observation that many patients referred to renal units in Europe have: inadequate blood pressure control; low use of therapies of proven benefit in heart and kidney disease (for example β-blockers, ACE inhibitors, lipid-lowering therapy, low-dose aspirin); and poor assessment of comorbidities such as retinopathy and foot care.

The St Vincent Declaration Taskforce recommends that all patients with nephropathy need to be referred to a nephrologist when their plasma creatinine concentration exceeds 200 μmol/l (2.2 mg/dl). However, before this, many are now proposing multiple cardiovascular risk-factor reduction, aiming for:

- a target blood pressure at least below 140/80 mmHg;
- a target total cholesterol concentration below 5 mmol/l;
- ACE inhibitor use as part of, or in addition to, antihypertensive therapy;
- low-dose aspirin; and
- invasive investigation and correction of coexistent cardio-, cerebro-, and peripheral arterial disease.

Screening for nephropathy

Because of the strong associations between an increased UAER and cardiovascular disease, a case for screening for diabetic nephropathy can be made with some confidence, although the evidence base for beneficial intervention at lower levels of albuminuria is less secure. Current recommendations from national diabetes associations recommends at least annual screening based upon the diagnostic flowchart shown in Fig. 1. Extrapolating the known effects of ACE inhibitors on a reduction of UAER to the prevention of clinical nephropathy and thus endstage renal disease, several authors show a potential cost benefit from the early use of these drugs. However, only long-term prospective studies of primary prevention can conclusively answer this question.

Further reading

Useful reference texts

Alberti KGMM, *et al.*, eds (1997). *International textbook of diabetes mellitus*, 2nd edn. Wiley, Chichester.

Mogensen CE, ed. (2000). *The kidney and hypertension in diabetes mellitus*, 5th edn. Kluwer Academic, Boston, MA.

Ritz E, Rychlik I, eds (1999). *Nephropathy in type 2 diabetes*, Oxford University Press, Oxford.

Guidelines for the management of diabetes and its complications

American Diabetes Association: clinical practice recommendations 2001. *Diabetes Care* **24**(Suppl. 1), S1–S133.

European Diabetes Policy Group (1998). A desktop guide to type 1 (insulin-dependent) diabetes mellitus. *Experimental and Clinical Endocrinology and Diabetes* **106**, 240–69.

European Diabetes Policy Group (1999). A desktop guide to type 2 diabetes mellitus. *Diabetic Medicine* **16**, 716–30.

Ramsay LE, *et al.* (1999). British Hypertension Society guidelines for hypertension management 1999: summary. *British Medical Journal* **319**, 630–5.

Epidemiology

Amos AF, *et al.* (1997). The rise in global burden of diabetes and its complications: estimates and projections to the year 2010. *Diabetic Medicine* **14**(Suppl. 5), S7–S85.

Causes of diabetic nephropathy

Cooper ME (1998). Pathogenesis, prevention and treatment of diabetic nephropathy. *Lancet* **252**, 213–9.

Krolewski AS (1999). Genetics of diabetic nephropathy: evidence for major and minor gene effects. *Kidney International* **55**, 1582–96.

Lee HB, Ho H (1997). Experimental approaches to diabetic nephropathy. *Kidney International* **51**(Suppl. 60), S1–S103.

Mogensen CE (1999). Microalbuminuria, blood pressure and diabetic renal disease: origin and development of ideas. *Diabetologia* **42**, 263–85.

Clinical trials

Brenner B *et al.* (2001). Effects of Losartan on renal and cardiovascular outcomes in patients with type 2 diabetes and nephropathy. *New England Journal of Medicine* **345**, 861–9

DCCT (Diabetes Control and Complications Trial) Research Group (1993). The effect of intensive treatment of diabetes on the development and progression of long term complications of insulin dependent diabetes mellitus. *New England Journal of Medicine* **329**, 977–86.

Gaede P *et al.* (1999). Intensified multi-factorial intervention in patients with type 2 diabetes mellitus and microalbuminuria: the Steno type 2 randomised study. *Lancet* **353**, 617–22.

HOPE (Heart Outcomes Prevention Evaluation) study investigators (2000). Effects of ramipril on cardiovascular and microvascular outcomes in people with diabetes mellitus: results of the HOPE Study and micro-HOPE Sub-Study. *Lancet* **355**, 253–9.

Keane WF, Brenner BM, Kurokawa H (1997). Progression of renal disease: clinical patterns, therapeutic options, and lessons from clinical trials. *Kidney International* **52**(Suppl. 63), S32–S53.

Lewis EJ *et al.* (2001). Reno-protective effect of the angiotensin receptor antagonist Irbesartan in patients with nephropathy due to type 2 diabetes. *New England Journal of Medicine* **345**, 851–60.

Parving H-H *et al.* (2001). The effect of Irbesartan of the development of diabetic nephropathy in patients with type 2 diabetes. *New England Journal of Medicine* **345**, 870–8.

The ACE Inhibitors in Diabetic Nephropathy Trialist Group (2001). Should all patients with type 1 diabetes mellitus and microalbuminuria receive angiotensin converting enzyme inhibitors? A meta-analysis of individual patient data. *Annals of Internal Medicine* **134**, 370–9.

UKPDS (UK Prospective Diabetes Study) Group (1998). Intensive blood glucose control with sulphonylureas or insulin compared with conventional treatment and risk of complications in patients with type 2 diabetes (UKPDS 33). *Lancet* **352**, 837–53.

Viberti GC (1994). Outcome variables in the assessment of progression of diabetic kidney disease. *Kidney International* **45**(Suppl. 45), S121–S124.

Wang P-H, Lau J, Chalmers TC (1993). Meta-analysis of effects of intensive blood glucose control on late complications of type 1 diabetes. *Lancet* **34**, 1306–9.

Screening for nephropathy

Bilous RW (1996). Early diagnosis of diabetic nephropathy. *Diabetes and Metabolism Reviews* **12**, 243–53.

20.10.2 Hypertension and the kidney

Lawrence E. Ramsay

This section describes the effects of hypertension on kidney function; renal and renovascular disease causing hypertension are described in Chapter 15.16.2.2. The impact of accelerated hypertension on renal function, and of hypertension and its treatment on the progression of established renal failure, are reasonably clear. There is debate about whether hypertension causes renal failure in the absence of accelerated phase, renovascular disease, or undetected primary renal disease.

Accelerated hypertension and the kidney

Accelerated (or malignant) hypertension is defined by bilateral fundal haemorrhages and exudates. Papilloedema may be present but is not necessary for the diagnosis. The condition is fully described in Chapter 15.16.3. Pathological changes in the kidney include 'onion skin' intimal proliferation in interlobular arteries with narrowing or loss of the lumen, ischaemic atrophy of nephrons, and fibrinoid necrosis of arterioles. These are caused by disruption of the arteriolar wall by severe or rapidly increasing hypertension, allowing insudation of plasma and fibrin deposition. The clinical correlate is moderate to severe renal impairment in one-third of patients with accelerated hypertension, or (uncommonly) oliguric acute renal failure. When blood pressure is controlled there may be slight deterioration of renal function over 1 to 2 days, but renal function then stabilizes and often recovers slightly. Patients with oliguric acute renal failure caused by accelerated hypertension may have excellent recovery of renal function even after prolonged dialysis. However, those who present with serum creatinine of 300 μmol/l or higher (but not oliguric renal failure) often progress to endstage renal disease despite good control of blood pressure and in the absence of a primary renal or renovascular cause. By contrast, in idiopathic accelerated hypertension with serum creatinine less than 300 μmol/l renal function usually remains stable, and deterioration despite good blood pressure control should raise suspicion of a primary renal or renovascular cause.

The 5-year survival of patients with accelerated hypertension has improved dramatically, from 1 per cent without treatment to 75 per cent with modern treatment, but the prognosis is still impaired, with mortality of 25 per cent over 5 years. Renal impairment is a powerful determinant of prognosis, and prevention by urgent treatment of accelerated hypertension is therefore crucial. Bilateral haemorrhages and exudates, even without papilloedema, constitute a medical emergency requiring immediate admission. An underlying cause for hypertension, commonly renal or renovascular disease, is present in about a quarter of patients with accelerated hypertension (see Chapters 15.16.2.1 and 15.16.3).

Hypertension and progression of chronic renal failure

Hypertension is the rule in advanced renal failure of any cause, but occurs earlier in glomerular than interstitial renal disease. The mechanism is inability to excrete a sodium load plus inappropriately high peripheral vascular resistance, i.e. an imbalance between volume and vasoconstriction. Uncontrolled hypertension accelerates the progression of renal failure.

Diabetic nephropathy

As discussed in Chapter 20.10.1, antihypertensive treatment retards the progression of diabetic nephropathy from its earliest stages, slowing progression of microalbuminuria to overt proteinuria, and the decline of glomerular filtration rate in established diabetic nephropathy. Treatment with angiotensin converting enzyme inhibitors confers additional protection, but control of blood pressure probably outweighs any specific effect of angiotensin converting enzyme inhibition. The evidence is stronger for type 1 than type 2 diabetes, but all patients with diabetic nephropathy should have antihypertensive treatment that includes an angiotensin converting enzyme inhibitor. The blood pressure target is (in most cases) as low as is achievable, ideally less than 130/80 mmHg, or less than 125/75 mmHg when there is proteinuria greater than 1 g/24 h.

Non-diabetic nephropathy

There is a relation between the level of blood pressure and the rate of decline of the glomerular filtraton rate in patients with renal impairment, suggesting that uncontrolled hypertension accelerates progression. The putative mechanism is impaired autoregulation in damaged kidneys so that systemic hypertension translates to glomerular hypertension, glomerulosclerosis, and progression of renal failure. Control of blood pressure slows progression, and blood pressure of 140/90 mmHg or more should be treated in any patient with renal disease.

Target blood pressure in renal failure

The Modification of Diet in Renal Disease Study, in addition to looking at the effects of diet, compared antihypertensive treatment titrated to targets equivalent to 140/90 mmHg or 125/75 mmHg in patients with various non-diabetic renal diseases and renal impairment. The overall analysis showed no significant relation between target blood pressure and decline of glomerular filtration rate. However, subgroup analysis showed a substantially slower decline in renal function in patients with proteinuria of 3 g/24 h or more, a similar trend with proteinuria of 1.0 to 2.9 g/24 h, but no benefit when proteinuria was less than 1 g/24 h, or in patients with polycystic kidneys (Fig. 1).

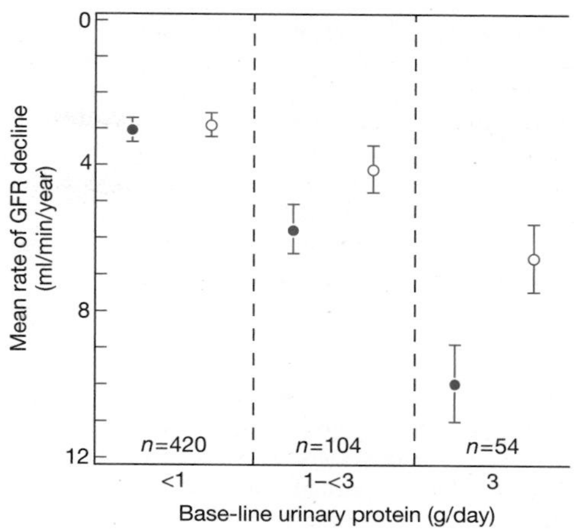

Fig. 1 Decline in glomerular filtration rate related to baseline urinary protein excretion and target blood pressures in patients with non-diabetic chronic renal disease. Solid circles (•) indicate target blood pressure of 140/90 mmHg, open circles (○) a target blood pressure of 125/75 mmHg. More aggressive blood pressure control slowed the rate of progression with proteinuria of 3 g/day or more, with similar trends for proteinuria of 1 to 2.9 g/day. There was no apparent effect with proteinuria of less than 1 g/day. (From the Modification of Diet in Renal Disease Study study (Klahr S *et al.* 1994 *New England Journal of Medicine* **330**, 877–84) with permission.)

Angiotensin converting enzyme inhibitors

Treatment that includes an angiotensin converting enzyme inhibitor slows progression of renal failure in selected patients, and the Ramipril Efficacy in Nephropathy (REIN) study suggests specific benefit from angiotensin converting enzyme inhibition over and above reduction of blood pressure. Benefit is large in those with glomerular disease, and small or absent in interstitial disease, polycystic kidneys, or nephrosclerosis. Rapid progression determines the outcome of treatment with angiotensin converting enzyme inhibitors and is predicted by proteinuria and the severity of renal failure. Treatment with angiotensin converting enzyme inhibitors is indicated in any patient with hypertension (≥ 140/90 mmHg), renal impairment, and proteinuria of 1 g/24 h or more. Angiotensin converting enzyme inhibitors cause renal failure in critical renovascular disease, and there was concern that patients with renal parenchymal disease could be at similar risk because of 'functional' vascular insufficiency. Trials do not support this concern as withdrawals because of renal failure or hyperkalaemia were no more common with angiotensin converting enzyme inhibitor than with placebo.

Conclusions

Blood pressure of 140/90 mmHg or more should be treated in all patients with renal impairment. When proteinuria exceeds 1 g/24 h the regimen should include an angiotensin converting enzyme inhibitor and the target is less than 125/75 mmHg. Angiotensin converting enzyme inhibitors rarely cause serious adverse effects, but renal function and serum potassium should be monitored.

Idiopathic hypertension and renal failure

Introduction

Renal function is altered in early idiopathic hypertension, with reduced renal blood flow, increased efferent arteriolar tone, but maintained glomerular filtration rate. In experimental animals such changes can cause intraglomerular hypertension, hyperfiltration, and glomerulosclerosis. An unresolved question is whether idiopathic non-accelerated hypertension causes similar renal damage in humans, and, if so, whether antihypertensive treatment prevents this. This question is important. If idiopathic hypertension causes endstage renal disease despite conventional antihypertensive treatment, possible responses are to treat even milder hypertension, to lower blood pressure targets, or to prefer antihypertensive drugs that may be renoprotective. If idiopathic hypertension is an innocent bystander when proteinuria or renal failure develops, the response should be to seek the true cause of the renal abnormality which might be undiagnosed glomerular, interstitial, or vascular renal disease.

Pathology

Nephrosclerosis is characterized by hyaline arteriosclerosis in arterioles and intimal fibroelastic reduplication in interlobular arteries. Some view these these changes as confined to vessels, with no encroachment on lumina, glomerular loss, or other important consequences, and consider them entirely benign and not even specific for hypertension. Others believe that preglomerular arteriosclerosis leads to glomerulosclerosis and loss of renal function through narrowing or occlusion causing ischaemia, or by failure of autoregulation causing intraglomerular hypertension.

Outcome trials

The incidence of endstage renal disease or other renal endpoints has been very low in outcome trials and no effect of treatment on renal function has been observed. These trials have included over 50 000 hypertensives, suggesting that renal failure is at most a rare complication of idiopathic hypertension. However, the trials have been short, averaging 2 to 3 years, and have not studied renal function in detail because of the focus on stroke and coronary complications.

Cohort studies

Uncontrolled studies over 5 to 14 years in treated hypertension have shown renal failure or proteinuria developing in 0 to 18 per cent of patients despite adequate control of blood pressure. These studies were in hospital patients with fairly severe hypertension and had inadequate criteria for excluding intrinsic renal disease causing the hypertension. In the MRFIT study (see below) men with serum creatinine of less than 106 μmol/l and proteinuria of less than 1+ at entry were followed for 16 years. The risk of endstage renal disease almost doubled with increased baseline blood pressure of 15/10 mmHg, but the incidence was still very low in absolute terms. Furthermore, undiagnosed primary renal disease could still have caused the endstage renal disease and explained its relation to blood pressure, even in this cohort, because normal serum creatinine and urine protein do not exclude renal causes for hypertension such as renovascular disease, glomerulonephritis, or renal scarring.

Endstage renal disease

Hypertensive nephrosclerosis is said to account for a quarter of entries to endstage renal disease programmes, but this diagnosis is usually presumptive and may often be incorrect. Presumptive diagnoses will include undiagnosed renovascular disease, undiagnosed parenchymal disease, and undiagnosed or forgotten episodes of accelerated hypertension. In one centre 11 per cent of cases having renal replacement were attributed to hypertension. When examined in detail 45 per cent had documented accelerated phase, 15 per cent had scarring or glomerular disease, 4 per cent renovascular disease, and only 2 per cent had documented hypertensive nephrosclerosis. The remaining 34 per cent of patients had hypertension, endstage kidneys, and no definite diagnosis, but had been labelled as having hypertensive nephrosclerosis.

Epidemiological data

The association of endstage renal disease with seven blood pressure strata in the MRFIT cohort of 332 544 men followed for 16 years is shown in Table 1. There is a clear graded association, but the absolute risk in men with mild to moderate hypertension is very small, for example 1/637 over 10 years with blood pressure of (140 to 159)/(90 to 99) mmHg when compared with blood pressure of less than 120/80 mmHg. As discussed above, this association could be explained by undiagnosed intrinsic renal disease or development of renovascular disease. The significant risk factors for developing endstage renal disease were older age, low income, high cholesterol, smoking, diabetes, and hypertension. Note that these are the major risk factors for atherosclerosis, and development of atherosclerotic renovascular disease could cause endstage renal disease in mild to moderate hypertension.

Conclusions

Renal failure and proteinuria in mild to moderate hypertension usually indicate underlying renal or renovascular disease. When renal damage is present, consider whether the hypertension is, or has been, severe enough to cause accelerated phase. If not, assume that intrinsic renal disease or renovascular disease is present and investigate appropriately. If it has, a presumptive diagnosis of renal damage caused by present or past accelerated hypertension should be confirmed by careful follow-up. Deterioration of renal function despite reasonable blood pressure control should prompt investigation for a cause other than the hypertension.

Table 1 Showing risk of endstage renal disease related to initial blood pressure in men followed for 16 years. Note the substantial increase in relative risk, but very small absolute risk, related to mild hypertension—(140 to 159)/(90 to 99) mmHg. Endstage renal disease could be caused by occult primary renal disease, progression to accelerated phase, or development of atherosclerotic renovascular disease, rather than by idiopathic hypertension *per se*. (Adapted from study of MRFIT cohort (Klag MJ *et al.* (1996). *New England Journal of Medicine* **334**, 13–18).)

BP category (mmHg)	Number of men	ESRD (%/10 years)	Relative risk (95% CI)	10-year risk of ESRD attributed to BP*
<120/<80	61 089	0.053	1.0	–
120–129/80–84	81 621	0.066	1.2 (0.8–1.7)	1/7692
130–139/85–89	73 798	0.111	1.9 (1.4–2.7)	1/1724
140–159/90–99	85 684	0.210	3.1 (2.3–4.3)	1/637
160–179/100–109	23 459	0.436	6.0 (4.3—8.4)	1/261
180–209/110–119	5464	0.961	11.2 (7.7–16.2)	1/110
≥210/≥120	1429	1.871	22.1 (14.2–34.3)	1/55

Abbreviations: ESRD, endstage renal disease; CI, confidence interval; BP, blood pressure.

*Attributable to BP when compared with BP stratum of less than 120/80 mmHg.

Further reading

Giatras I, Lau J, Levey AS for the Angiotensin-Converting-Enzyme Inhibition and Progressive Renal Disease Study Group (1997). Effect of angiotensin-converting enzyme inhibitors on the progression of nondiabetic renal disease: a meta-analysis of randomized trials. *Annals of Internal Medicine* **127**, 337–45. [Meta-analysis of trials of angiotensin converting enzyme inhibitors in non-diabetic renal disease.]

Klag MJ *et al.* (1996). Blood pressure and end-stage renal disease in men. *New England Journal of Medicine* **334**, 13–18. [Largest and longest epidemiological study relating endstage renal disease to blood pressure.]

Klahr S (1989). The kidney in hypertension—villain and victim. *New England Journal of Medicine* **320**, 731–2. [Brief review—does idiopathic hypertension cause endstage renal disease?]

Klahr S *et al.* for the Modification of Diet in Renal Disease Study Group (1994). The effects of dietary protein restriction and blood-pressure control on the progression of chronic renal disease. *New England Journal of Medicine* **330**, 877–84. [Modification of diet in renal disease study of different blood pressure targets in non-diabetic renal failure.]

Madhavan S *et al.* (1995). Renal function during antihypertensive treatment. *Lancet* **345**, 749–51. [Cohort study suggesting idiopathic hypertension does not cause endstage renal disease.]

Rostand SG *et al.* (1989). Renal insufficiency in treated essential hypertension. *New England Journal of Medicine* **320**, 684–8. [Cohort study suggesting that idiopathic hypertension may cause endstage renal disease.]

Ruggenenti P *et al.* (1999). Renoprotective properties of ACE-inhibition in non-diabetic nephropathies with non-nephrotic proteinuria. *Lancet* **354**, 359–64. [Second report from REIN trial suggesting that inhibition of angiotensin converting enzyme has a specific renoprotective effect in non-diabetic renal impairment.]

Tomson CRV, Petersen K, Heagerty AM (1991). Does treated essential hypertension result in renal impairment? A cohort study. *Journal of Human Hypertension* **5**, 189–92. [Cohort study and examination of endstage renal disease registry suggesting idiopathic hypertension does not cause endstage renal disease.]

Whitworth JA (1992). Renal parenchymal disease and hypertension. In: Robertson JIS, ed. *Handbook of hypertension, vol 15, Clinical hypertension*, pp 326–56. Elsevier, Amsterdam. [Excellent review of hypertension in renal disease.]

20.10.3 Vasculitis and the kidney

A. J. Rees

Introduction

This chapter is concerned with a heterogeneous group of disorders commonly referred to as the primary systemic vasculitides. These are defined by the presence of inflammation and necrosis of blood vessels, with the individual clinical syndromes defined by the size and distribution of the vessels involved and whether vasculitis is accompanied by granulomas. The diseases include polyarteritis nodosa, Wegener's granulomatosis, microscopic polyangiitis, and Churg–Strauss syndrome, the renal aspects of which are emphasized in this chapter. The aetiology and pathogenesis of these disorders have not been elucidated, but the strong association between some of them and autoantibodies to neutrophil cytoplasmic antigens (antineutrophil cytoplasmic antibodies: **ANCA**) suggests an autoimmune pathogenesis.

Vasculitis is an important treatable cause of renal failure, most commonly when the glomerular capillaries are involved thus causing focal necrotizing glomerulonephritis. This is common in patients with generalized small vessel vasculitis, such as Wegener's granulomatosis and microscopic polyangiitis, both of which are closely associated with ANCA. Some patients presenting with focal necrotizing glomerulonephritis without evidence of involvement of other organs also have positive assays for ANCA. The appearance on renal biopsy is identical to microscopic polyangiitis, as is the response to treatment. Other organs can be involved later in the course of the disease, and autopsies have demonstrated more widespread disease even at the outset. For these reasons, ANCA-associated focal necrotizing glomerulonephritis in the absence of any evidence of generalized disease is usually considered to be a form of microscopic polyangiitis, and will be discussed as such in this chapter.

Focal necrotizing glomerulonephritis usually presents with rapidly deteriorating renal function (rapidly progressive glomerulonephritis) and is caused most frequently by ANCA-associated vasculitis. However, this is not its only cause: focal necrotizing glomerulonephritis can complicate diseases described in other chapters, including hypersensitivity to drugs, systemic infections such as infective endocarditis, systemic immunological diseases (for example systemic lupus erythematosus, Henoch–Schönlein purpura, and rheumatoid arthritis), and as a paraneoplastic syndrome (Table 1). Whilst there are only subtle differences in the morphological appearances of the different types of focal necrotizing glomerulonephritis, there are marked differences in immunohistology, different types usually being separated on the basis of their pattern of glomerular immunoglobulin deposition (Table 1).

Focal necrotizing glomerulonephritis should be regarded as a medical emergency: because different types respond differently to treatment a precise diagnosis must be made promptly on clinical and serological grounds and confirmed by biopsy.

Historical perspective

Vasculitis was first described in autopsy material in the 1840s by Rokitansky but was not recognized as a specific entity until 20 years later. In 1866, Kussmaul and Maier described the case of a young man who presented with fever and muscle, renal, and gastrointestinal disease and at autopsy had widespread inflammation of medium-sized arteries with aneurysms to which the name periarteritis nodosa was applied. The heterogeneity of the disorder was recognized over the next 100 years and various different clinical syndromes were described. In 1923 Wohlwill distinguished a type of vasculitis that affected arterioles, capillaries, and venules as well as muscular arteries. Davson and his colleagues studied this condition in great detail in the 1940s and called it the microscopic form of polyarteritis (now more accurately called polyangiitis). In the 1930s Klinger, and then Wegener, described patients with microscopic polyarteritis in which many of the arthritic lesions were surrounded by granulomas. Disease in these patients had a predilection for the nose, upper airways, and lungs and constituted a distinct clinical syndrome, now called Wegener's granulomatosis. In 1954 Churg and Strauss described another distinct form of primary vasculitis characterized by granulomatous inflammation of medium-sized vessels associated with eosinophilia and asthma: this disease now bears their names. Despite their obvious differences, it should be remembered that Churg in particular regarded Wegener's granulomatosis, microscopic polyangiitis, and Churg–Strauss syndrome as closely related (with macroscopic polyarteritis regarded as being somewhat separate). The subsequent demonstration that ANCA are commonly present in all three of these conditions (but not in macroscopic polyarteritis) supports this suggestion.

Classification

The classic accounts of vasculitis established strict clinical and pathological criteria for diagnosis based on clinical histories and autopsies of patients with endstage disease. They defined the different clinical disorders and remain invaluable descriptions of their evolution. However, the diagnostic criteria they introduced are now far too restrictive because nowadays patients usually present at an early stage, with relatively mild or limited disease that can be controlled by present treatments before it has evolved into a 'classical' syndrome. The current emphasis on early diagnosis and treatment demands a more flexible approach. The finding that most patients with active small vessel vasculitis have circulating ANCA has proved to be especially useful, even though the role of ANCA in pathogenesis is uncertain. Differences in ANCA specificity have also tended to reinforce the idea that different vasculitic syndromes are distinct entities. Thus, most patients with active small vessel vasculitis have positive assays for ANCA, whereas patients whose disease in confined to the arteries do not.

The current more pragmatic approach to diagnosis is exemplified by the criteria developed by Lanham for Churg–Strauss syndrome, but generally the move towards more clinically based definitions has been a source of considerable controversy. New terms were introduced to describe 'incomplete variants', the distinction between classic (large vessel) and microscopic forms of polyangiitis became blurred, and different terms were used for the same entities, not only in different parts of the world but—worse still—by physicians practising in different specialties. In 1990, the American College of Rheumatologists attempted to clarify the situation by establishing standard diagnostic criteria for each of the main vasculitic syndromes, analogous to those that had proved highly successful for systemic lupus erythematosus. These criteria were based on clinical and pathological data collected from patients diagnosed as having the various types of systemic vasculitis, the data being used to derive mutually exclusive sets of criteria for diagnosing each condition. Unfortunately, they have not proved to be robust, especially for patients with extensive renal disease: for example, they do not accurately discriminate between patients with small vessel vasculitis and focal necrotizing glomerulonephritis and those with classical polyarteritis nodosa, or between cutaneous leucocytoclastic vasculitis and Henoch–Schönlein purpura. However, the American College of Rheumatologists project was an important attempt to introduce greater uniformity, although it was flawed because differences in the pattern of disease of patients referred to different physicians was underestimated, and also because the drive for early treatment of patients with vasculitis reversed the injury before patients developed signs that enabled individual conditions to be distinguished from each other with confidence.

In an attempt to overcome these difficulties, the Chapel Hill Consensus Conference in 1994 brought together physicians from all the disciplines to which patients with vasculitis are commonly referred and pathologists with extensive experience of these diseases. The purpose was to establish a classification of vasculitis with a common nomenclature based on set working definitions for the different syndromes. It was recognized that it would not always be possible (or even relevant) to try to distinguish between some of the syndromes before treatment was started, and no attempt was made to establish strict diagnostic criteria although clearly the Chapel Hill classification provided a framework for diagnosis. The definitions of individual clinical syndromes built on previous work that classified vasculitis in terms of the size of vessel involved and the presence or absence of granulomas. Clinical definitions of the different types of vasculitis are shown in Table 2 and illustrated in Fig. 1. The essential feature is that the diagnosis depends on the size of the smallest vessel involved. Thus the term microscopic polyangiitis replaced the term microscopic polyarteritis because capillaries and venules are involved as well as arteries, and the diagnosis depends on their involvement regardless of whether or not small or medium-sized muscular arteries are also affected. By contrast, polyarteritis nodosa was defined as a form of vasculitis in which the vasculitis is confined to muscular arteries and the diagnosis excludes patients with evidence of injury to capillaries or venules. This terminology was justified by differences in the natural history and response to treatment of patients with and without small vessel involvement and is supported by the serological findings. Although not used as a primary diagnostic criterion, ANCA are very frequent in patients with small vessel vasculitis but uncommon in those whose disease is confined to larger vessels.

The Chapel Hill classification has been increasingly widely used since it was first introduced but should not be regarded as definitive. The very high prevalence of ANCA in patients with small vessel vasculitis has lead to the useful generic term ANCA-associated vasculitis, which includes Wegener's granulomatosis and microscopic polyangiitis as well as patients with isolated focal necrotizing glomerulonephritis without clinical evidence of extrarenal disease.

Table 1 Focal necrotizing glomerulonephritis categorized by immunohistology

Linear staining of the GBM*
Anti-GBM nephritis
In membranous nephropathy
In Alport's syndrome and nail-patella syndrome
Following penicillamine (in exceptional cases)
Scanty immune deposits (pauci-immune)
Small vessel vasculitis
Wegener's granulomatosis
Microscopic polyangiitis
Isolated
Drug induced
Penicillamine
Thiouracil
Hydrallazine
Rifampacin
Minocycline
Granular deposits
Postinfectious nephritis
Streptococcal infections
Bacterial endocarditis
Juguloatrial shunt infections
Miscellaneous infections
Deep abscesses
Mycoplasma
Tuberculosis
Legionella
HIV
Syphilis
Leprosy
Complicating systemic disorders
Systemic lupus erythematosus
Henoch–Schönlein purpura
Mixed connective tissue disease
Sarcoidosis
Behçet's syndrome
Cryoglobulinaemia (hepatitis C infection)
Dermatomyositis
Rheumatoid arthritis and juvenile rheumatoid arthritis
Rheumatic fever
Reiter's syndrome
Sjögren's syndrome
Complicating underlying glomerulopathies
Endocapillary/mesangial proliferative glomerulonephritis
Mesangiocapillary glomerulonephritis
IgA nephropathy
Membranous nephropathy

*GBM = glomerular basement membrane.

Antineutrophil cytoplasmic antibodies

ANCA were first identified in patients with small vessel vasculitis thought to be due to Ross River virus and were subsequently reported to be highly specific for Wegener's granulomatosis and microscopic polyangiitis. The antibodies are usually assayed by indirect immunofluorescence using ethanol-fixed normal human neutrophils as the substrate. They are heterogeneous, as reflected in the two distinct patterns of fluorescence that can be seen (Fig. 2 and Plate 1). Some sera display granular staining throughout

Table 2 The Chapel Hill consensus on the nomenclature of systemic vasculitis

Syndromes affecting small vessels (capillaries, venules, and arterioles)	
Wegener's granulomatosis	Granulomatous inflammation in the respiratory tract; necrotizing vasculitis affecting small to medium-sized vessels
Churg–Strauss syndrome	Eosinophil-rich and granulomatous inflammation in the respiratory tract; necrotizing vasculitis affecting small and medium-sized vessels; asthma and eosinophilia
Microscopic polyangiitis	Necrotizing vasculitis, with few or no immune deposits, affecting small vessels
Henoch–Schönlein purpura	Vasculitis, with IgA-dominant immune deposits, affecting small vessels
Essential cryoglobulinaemic vasculitis	Vasculitis, with cryoglobulin deposits, affecting small vessels, and associated with circulating cryoglobulins
Cutaneous leucocytoclastic angiitis	Isolated cutaneous leucocytoclastic angiitis without systemic vasculitis or glomerulonephritis
Syndromes affecting medium-sized vessels	
Polyarteritis nodosa	Necrotizing inflammation of medium-sized or small arteries without glomerulonephritis or vasculitis in arterioles, capillaries, or venules
Kawasaki disease	Necrotizing inflammation involving large, medium-sized, and small arteries: associated with mucocutaneous lymph node syndrome. Coronary arteries are often involved. Aorta and veins may be affected. Usually occurs in children
Syndromes affecting large vessels	
Giant cell arteritis	Granulomatous arteries of the aorta and its major branches, with a predilection for the extracranial branches of the carotid artery
Takayasu arteritis	Granulomatous inflammation of the aorta and its major branches

the cytoplasm (cytoplasmic ANCA or **cANCA**), whereas with others the staining concentrates around the nucleus (perinuclear ANCA or **pANCA**); exceptional patients demonstrate a mixed pattern of staining.

Most ANCA bind to enzymes found in the neutrophil granules, and the commonest antigens in patients with small vessel vasculitis are proteinase-3, which is the principal target of cANCA, and myeloperoxidase, which is the most common target for pANCA. Antiproteinase-3 antibodies are almost invariably present in untreated patients with active systemic Wegener's granulomatosis, as well as a proportion of those with microscopic angiitis. Antimyeloperoxidase antibodies are usually found in the remaining patients with microscopic polyangiitis and in those with isolated focal necrotizing glomerulonephritis. However, it is important to recognize that ANCA are not unique to small vessel vasculitis and there is a growing list of conditions in which they have also been described, including inflammatory bowel disease, systemic lupus erythematosus, and some chronic infections. In these contexts it is rare for the ANCA detected to be directed against proteinase-3 and uncommon that they recognize myeloperoxidase. ANCA that recognize other antigens are found in a minority of patients with small vessel vasculitis (Table 3), and their targets include elastase, cathepsin G, lactoferrin, bacterial-permeability-increasing peptide, and the lysosomal membrane protein h-lamp-2. This last antigen is interesting in that it is also expressed on glomerular endothelium, and antibodies that recognize glomerular endothelium have previously been described in Wegener's granulomatosis.

A critical issue is whether assays for ANCA are specific and sensitive for small vessel vasculitis. Meta-analyses and large-scale multicentre prospective studies have confirmed the original impression that they are, provided that certain safeguards are met. When used alone, ANCA detected by indirect immununoflurescent assays have a sensitivity of 80 to 85 per cent and a specificity of around 75 per cent compared with disease controls. Specificity improves considerably when indirect immunofluorescence assays are used together with specific enzyme-linked immunoabsorbent assays to exclude patients who have ANCA directed against targets other than proteinase-3 and myeloperoxidase, and those with false positive assays caused by antinuclear antibodies. Combining indirect immunofluorescence with specific immunoassays for antibodies to proteinase-3 and myeloperoxidase increases both the sensitivity and the specificity of the assays for Wegener's granulomatosis and microscopic polyangiitis to over 90 per cent. However, the standard enzyme-linked immunoabsorbent assay for proteinase-3 and myeloperoxidase can occasionally give false negative results when circulating ANCA are bound to their natural inhibitors α_1-antitrypsin and caeruloplasmin. There are far fewer data about the use of ANCA for diagnosing

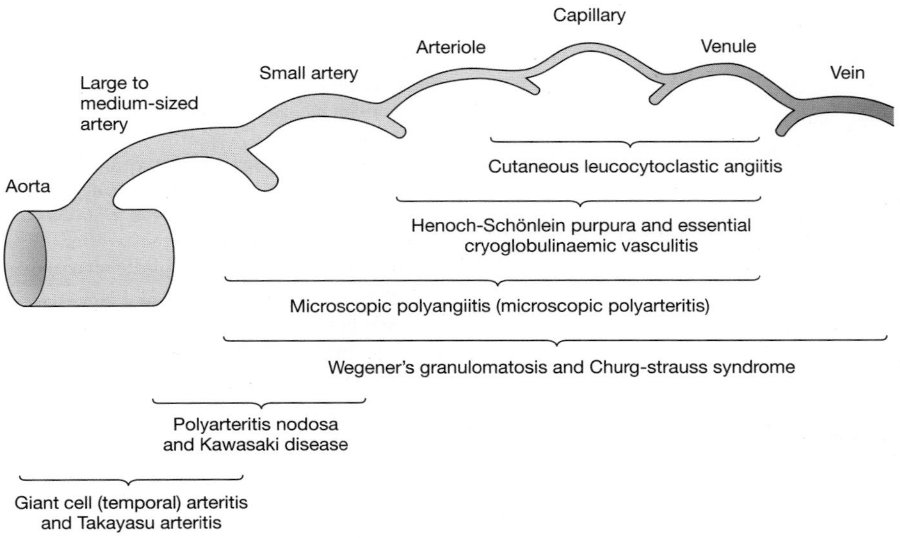

Fig. 1 Summary of the Chapel Hill classification of systemic vasculitis.

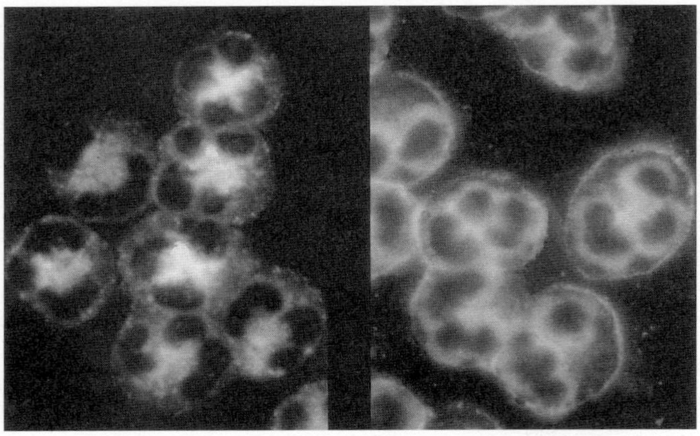

(a) (b)

Fig. 2 Indirect immunofluorescence assay for ANCA. (a) Typical staining of cytoplasmic ANCA that is usually due to antibodies to proteinase 3. (b) Typical staining pattern of perinuclear ANCA most often due to antimyeloperoxidase antibodies. (See also Plate 1.)

Churg–Strauss syndrome: overall about 50 per cent of patients have positive assays for either proteinase-3 or myeloperoxidase, but a sufficiently large cohort of untreated patients has not been studied to establish a true incidence. ANCA are positive in fewer than 10 per cent of patients without evidence of involvement of capillaries or venules.

Incidence and aetiology

Primary systemic vasculitis is relatively uncommon, but the incidence is probably increasing, even allowing for greater awareness and improvements in diagnosis. The overall incidence in southern England is about 20 new patients per million population per year, with a similar incidence reported in Scandinavia. Men are more commonly affected than women, and the incidence rises progressively with age, amounting to 60 per million per year for those aged 65 to 75. The annual incidence of ANCA-associated crescentic nephritis is 6 to 7 per million, accounting for at least 0.5 per cent of patients on dialysis in Europe. However, surveys of the ANCA status of dialysis patients suggest that both figures are underestimates because of underdiagnosis in patients presenting with renal failure and few extrarenal symptoms. The disease appears to be equally common in South Asian caucasoids, but studies from the United States indicate that African Americans are much less susceptible.

Genetic factors

The cause of primary systemic vasculitis is unknown, but heredity undoubtedly influences susceptibility as evidenced by reports of the disease occurring in siblings; however, identical twins discordant for the disease have also been observed. Polymorphisms of the α_1-antitrypsin locus influence susceptibility to Wegener's granulomatosis and cANCA positive vasculitis, case control studies showing that the Z allele, which causes relative antitrypsin deficiency, is much more common in patients than in controls. α_1-antitrypsin is the natural inhibitor of proteinase-3 (but not of myeloperoxidase) and so loss of this inhibition provides an apparent explanation for the findings, although an unconvincing one given the relatively trivial reduction in α_1-antitrypsin activity produced by the Z allele. It should also be noted that nearly 80 per cent of patients have the fully sufficient phenotype. There is a single study describing an association between the complement C3 allele *C3F* and vasculitis, which resulted in a relative risk of 2.6 in heterozygotes and 5.1 in homozygotes. By contrast, studies of the HLA class II complex have produced conflicting results.

Table 3 Target antigens for ANCA

ANCA target antigen on ethanol-fixed PMN	Associated immunofluorescence pattern
Proteinase 3	cANCA; very rarely pANCA
h-lamp-2	cANCA
Myeloperoxidose	pANCA; very rarely cANCA
Elastase	pANCA
Cathepsin G	pANCA
Azurocidin	pANCA
Lactoferrin	pANCA
Lysozyme	pANCA; atypical cytoplasmic
BPI	Atypical cANCA or pANCA

Abbreviations: ANCA, antineutrophil cytoplasmic antibodies; PMN, polymorphonuclear cells; PR3, proteinase-3; cANCA, cytoplasmic ANCA; pANCA, perinuclear ANCA; MPO, myeloperoxidase; BPI, bacterial-permeability-increasing peptide.

Environmental factors

Environmental agents responsible for primary systemic vasculitis have proved even more difficult to identify than genetic factors, but drugs and infections have both been invoked. Hepatitis B carriers have been reported to develop polyarteritis nodosa in some populations (United States and France), but not in others such as the United Kingdom. Infection with parvovirus BIg has also been reported to cause polyateritis nodosa. Hypersensitivity to hydrallazine, rifampicin, and minocycline can cause ANCA-associated vasculitis, and there is convincing evidence that penicillamine causes pANCA-associated crescentic glomerulonephritis with or without pulmonary haemorrhage. Case controlled studies indicate that silica predisposes to ANCA-associated crescentic nephritis and Wegener's granulomatosis. It is difficult to evaluate descriptions of Churg–Strauss syndrome in patients with asthma treated with the leukotriene inhibitor Zafirlukast: asthma could have been the first symptom of the vasculitis, and corticosteroids, which would have been the alternative treatment, would also have been effective treatment for Churg–Strauss.

Pathogenesis

Explanations for the cause of injury in small vessel vasculitis must take account of the close association with ANCA, the extensive infiltration of vessels with neutrophil, endothelial activation, and the near absence of immunoglobulin deposition on immunohistology. Most authorities regard these conditions as autoimmune diseases, but proof is lacking and it is important to remember that 30 years ago they were generally believed to be systemic immune complex diseases.

A direct role for ANCA is suggested by their close association with injury in vasculitis, especially as ANCA titres often, though not invariably, increase before relapses of disease activity. The observation that vasculitis in spontaneous and induced models of autoimmunity in rodents is also associated with ANCA provides further support for the hypothesis. For example, *MRL/lpr* lupus prone mice and Kinjo mice both spontaneously develop vasculitis and focal necrotizing glomerulonephritis in association with ANCA. The real difficulty is to understand how ANCA could cause vasculitis, because neither proteinase-3 nor myeloperoxidase are expressed on endothelium. Three types of explanation have been proposed:

1. They could cause endothelial injury after release from neutrophils and monocytes because they prolong the activity of proteinase-3 and myeloperoxidase by interfering with binding to their natural inhibitors.
2. They activate neutrophils (and possibly endothelium) and so could facilitate endothelial injury.
3. They could bind to endothelium and so facilitate *in situ* immune complex formation between ANCA and their targets.

There has been widespread interest in the effects of ANCA on neutrophil function since the initial reports that they stimulated respiratory burst activity in neutrophils that had been primed with proinflammatory cytokines such as tumour necrosis factor. Proteinase-3 translocates to the plasma membrane when polymorphs are exposed to tumour necrosis factor, and the process is enhanced by the chemokine interleukin 8. *In vivo*, neutrophils from patients with active vasculitis express more proteinase-3 on their surface than neutrophils from controls. Incubation of primed neutrophils with ANCA increases superoxide generation and enzyme release and also interferes with normal control of apoptosis.

Regardless of how ANCA activate neutrophils, there is now a strong body of evidence to show that they facilitate the adherence of neutrophils to endothelium and neutrophil mediated killing of endothelial cells *in vitro*. At one stage it was thought that activated endothelium expressed proteinase-3 but this is now known not to be the case. It seems probable that ANCA aggravate neutrophil-dependent injury once they adhere in the microvasculature.

The question as to whether immune responses to proteinase-3 and myeloperoxidase cause vasculitis and glomerulonephritis directly has also been examined experimentally by infusing neutrophil granule extracts together with hydrogen peroxide (H_2O_2) into the renal arteries of rats that had previously been immunized with myeloperoxidase. This resulted in the development of severe focal necrotizing glomerulonephritis with very transient deposition of immunoglobulin, hence the injury simulated that seen in ANCA-associated vasculitis. Rats in whom the perfusion with H_2O_2 was omitted developed less severe injury and more persistent IgG deposits. In most respects this antimyeloperoxidase model is just another example of '*in situ* complex formation nephritis' similar to models used to examine other types of glomerular injury. The main difference is the transience of the IgG deposits, but even this has been recorded previously in models of chronic serum sickness under conditions of marked excess of antigen. These are exactly the conditions that would be expected in inflamed glomeruli in which neutrophils and monocytes continued to release proteinase-3 and myeloperoxidase in the presence of ANCA. Two additional pieces of evidence support the notion that IgG deposition in ANCA-associated crescentic nephritis might be unusually shortlived: first, proteinase-3 degrades IgG including ANCA, even when complexed to it; secondly, it has been known for many years that IgG deposited in vessels in some forms of cutaneous vasculitis rapidly becomes undetectable. Thus it is entirely plausible that IgG is deposited in glomeruli of patients with crescentic nephritis and is then rapidly removed or destroyed.

In summary, there is no decisive proof that autoimmunity to neutrophil antigens cause injury in human vasculitis, but a number of clear statements can be made:

1. Autoantibodies to ANCA are very closely associated with some types of systemic small vessel vasculitis, both clinically and in experimental models.
2. The autoantibodies modify the function of neutrophil enzymes and promote neutrophil mediated endothelial injury *in vitro*.
3. Injection of antimyeloperoxidase antibodies does not in itself cause glomerular injury, except in rats in which myeloperoxidase has been planted in the kidney, when the result is severe glomerulonephritis with very similar morphological and immunohistological characteristics to human ANCA-associated glomerulonephritis.
4. Injection of antirat myeloperoxidase antibodies into rats with nephrotoxic nephritis markedly aggravates injury.

Thus it reasonable to suggest that the cellular or humoral autoimmune response to neutrophil antigens contributes to the pathogenesis of the glomerular injury in vasculitis.

Clinical features of primary vasculitis

Wegener's granulomatosis and microscopic polyangiitis

Wegener's granulomatosis is characterized by a predominantly small vessel vasculitis associated with granulomas and a predilection for involving the upper and lower airways. Microscopic polyangiitis is characterized by a very similar small vessel vasculitis without granuloma formation or a predilection for the upper airways. These two conditions will be considered together because of the many features they share, and because clinically it can be impossible to distinguish between them. Furthermore, the approach to diagnosis and management of both conditions is identical.

Both Wegener's granulomatosis and microscopic polyangiitis present with non-specific symptoms and signs that can be difficult to distinguish from those of viral infection, except that they are more persistent. These consist of flu-like symptoms with muscle pains, night sweats, and weight loss. Many patients also complain of arthralgia, which is symmetrical, relatively mild, and affects the hands and feet; exceptional patients have frank arthritis. These non-specific symptoms either precede or occur as a background to damage to particular organs, which provides the basis for making a more specific diagnosis.

Features unique to Wegener's granulomatosis

Upper airway involvement

Over 90 per cent of patients with Wegener's granulomatosis have obvious upper airways disease. Nasal discomfort and blockage together with ulceration, crusting, rhinorrhoea, and epistaxis are usually prominent at presentation. Destruction of nasal cartilage with perforation of the nasal septum or the appearance of the characteristic saddle nose deformity rarely occur until much later. Gross destruction of bone is very uncommon and suggests an alternative diagnosis such as malignancy. Disappointingly, nasal biopsies rarely show the characteristic lesions of necrotizing vasculitis with loosely formed granulomas unless special techniques are used to get adequate samples. Nasal disease is frequently accompanied by the involvement of the paranasal sinuses, blockage of the Eustachian tube and otitis media. The larynx is less commonly involved but subglottic stenosis is a characteristic late phenomenon, which may develop insidiously and can be severe.

Pulmonary involvement

Almost all the patients have evidence of granulomatous lung disease at presentation, which is often accompanied by alveolar capillaritis. The bronchi can also be affected and bronchial stenoses occur as late manifestations. Symptoms include cough, dyspnoea, haemoptysis, and chest pain, which can be pleuritic. Signs on chest examination depend on the nature of the pulmonary lesions and include fine crepitations and bronchial breathing or less commonly pleural rubs and signs of pleural effusions. Fixed rhonchi are suggestive of bronchial stenosis and stridor of subglottic stenosis.

Pulmonary granulomas are usually diagnosed from chest radiographs and CT scans. They may appear as single or multiple rounded lesions, which can cavitate (Fig. 3). They are often intermingled with alveolar shadowing to produce composite lesions, which reflect pulmonary capillaritis and haemorrhage as well as granulomas. The radiological findings can be confused with neoplasms, infection, or fluid overload. Results from pulmonary function tests are not specific, but it is important to note that increases in the *K*co are a much less sensitive test for pulmonary haemorrhage in vasculitis than in disease mediated by antiglomerular basement membrane antibodies (see Chapter 20.7.9). Bronchoscopy often reveals granulomatous inflammation and the diagnosis can sometimes be made from bronchial biopsies. By contrast, needle biopsies and transbronchial biopsies of pulmonary lesions are rarely adequate and can delay definitive diagnosis by open or video-endoscopic lung biopsy. Histology of lung biopsies reveals pulmonary necrosis, vasculitis affecting alveolar capillaries and bronchial vessels, and loosely formed granulomas together with a mixed inflammatory infiltrate (Fig. 4 and Plate 2).

Granulomatous inflammation at other sites

Typical Wegener's granulomas have been reported at numerous sites outside the lung, but are much less common in part at least because of the greater difficulty in diagnosing them. Microscopic granulomas are seen in a minority of renal and skin biopsies from patients known to have Wegener's

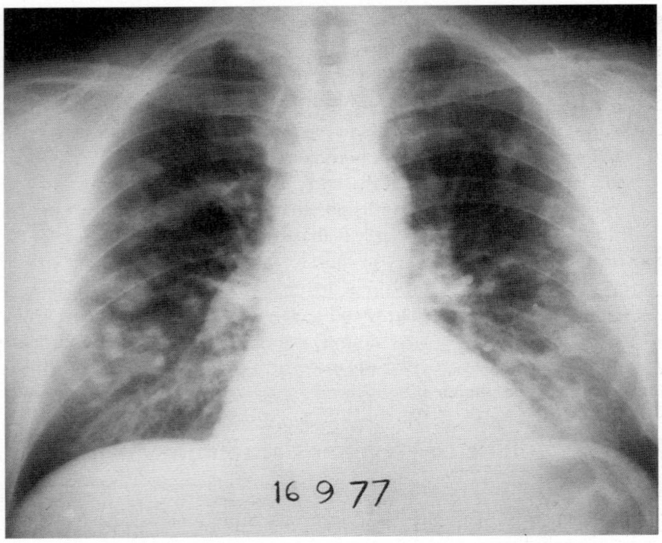

Fig. 3 Chest radiograph from a patient with Wegener's granulomatosis showing the typical appearance of pulmonary granulomas together with alveolar shadowing caused by capillaritis of lung haemorrhage.

granulomatosis, but macroscopically visible granulomas are rare. However, these have been reported in kidney, simulating carcinoma, in the orbit of the eye, causing exophthalmos, and also in the brain, pituitary, salivary glands, prostate, gingiva, and vertebrae. Masses of inflammatory tissue have also been described in the intestine (simulating Crohn's disease) and breast, as well as in the retroperitoneal space and mediastinum.

Features common to microscopic polyangiitis and Wegener's granulomatosis

Renal disease

Focal necrotizing glomerulonephritis is the characteristic renal lesion of generalized Wegener's granulomatosis and microscopic polyangiitis. Typically it presents with deteriorating renal function that progresses to renal failure within 3 months, i.e. as rapidly progressive glomerulonephritis, although a few patients have more indolent disease. Proteinuria (typically 2 to 3 g/24 h, but occasionally in the nephrotic range) and microscopic haematuria provide clinical evidence of glomerulonephritis, as does urine microscopy that reveals granular and red cell casts. Despite the glomerular inflammation hypertension is uncommon, except in patients with pre-existing hypertension or obvious fluid overload. Renal ultrasound examination and CT scans show normal or enlarged kidneys, isotope renograms reflect the renal function, and renal arteriograms only exceptionally demonstrate aneurysms or other evidence of vascular injury in the renal arteries. The diagnosis is made by renal biopsy, the appearances reflecting the extent of the injury and the speed with which it has developed.

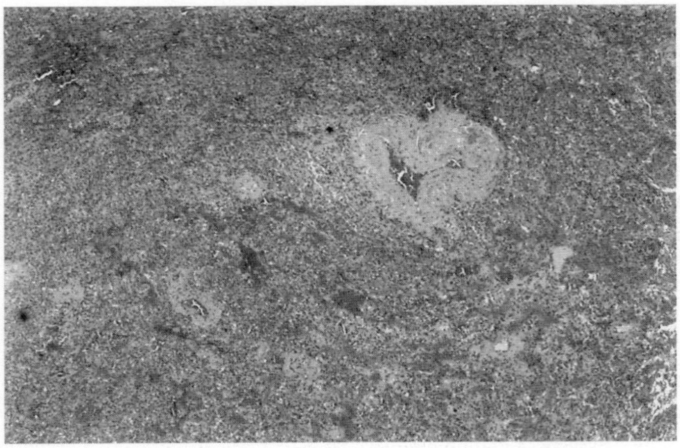

Fig. 4 Morphological appearances of pulmonary granulomas in a specimen obtained by video-endoscopic lung biopsy from a patient with Wegener's granulomatosis. (See also Plate 2.)

Cutaneous vasculitis

Cutaneous vasculitis occurs with equal frequency in Wegener's granulomatosis and microscopic polyangiitis, being present in about half of patients. Typically there is palpable purpura or splinter haemorrhages. Blistering and urcitarial lesions are less common, as are infarcts. Biopsies reveal leucocytoclastic vasculitis without deposition of immunoglobulins.

Vasculitis of the eye

Involvement of the eye occurs in both diseases but is more common in Wegener's granulomatosis. Orbital granulomas and exophthalmos have already been mentioned as features unique to Wegener's granulomatosis, and other manifestations include episcleritis, uveitis, and retinal vasculitis.

Gastrointestinal vasculitis

Vasculitis of the gut can occur in Wegener's granulomatosis and microscopic polyangiitis. Oral ulceration is relatively common. Intestinal vasculitis usually presents as abdominal pain and bloody diarrhoea. Endoscopy reveals purpuric lesions with or without ulceration, and white cell scans show increased uptake and are a useful way of delineating the extent of disease.

Vasculitis of the nervous system

Small vessel vasculitis can affect both central and peripheral nervous systems. Cranial nerve palsies, mononeuritis multiplex, and symmetrical polyneuropathies are straightforward to diagnose but are relatively uncommon in Wegener's granulomatosis and microscopic polyangiitis. Cerebral vasculitis also occurs: this is difficult to diagnose but can cause strokes and convulsions. Computed tomography and magnetic resonance imaging can demonstrate lesions, but appearances are not specific.

Diagnosis

Diagnosis of Wegener's granulomatosis and microscopic polyangiitis depends on an appropriate clinical history together with clinical evidence of vasculitis or focal necrotizing glomerulonephritis and biopsy evidence that is at least consistent with the diagnosis if not pathognomic of it. A positive assay for ANCA with specificity for proteinase-3 or myeloperoxidase provides strong confirmatory evidence, and negative ANCA assays are grounds for reconsidering the diagnosis. However, it is important to remember that 10 per cent of patients with generalized disease have negative ANCA, as do up to 50 per cent of those with Wegener's granulomatosis apparently confined to the respiratory tract. Early diagnosis of the patients with non-specific 'flu-like' symptoms can be very difficult and the value of urinary dipstick testing to search for asymptomatic proteinuria and haematuria cannot be overestimated.

Haematology and biochemistry

Non-specific haematological abnormalities are the rule. The full blood count shows a normocytic normochromic anaemia and often a neutrophil leucocytosis. Thrombocytosis is almost invariably present (typically in the range of 400 to 800 × 10^9/litre) and provides a useful measure of disease activity. Increased values for C-reactive protein and hypoalbuminaemia provide further evidence of the acute phase response. Alkaline phosphatase in often increased, but abnormalities of other liver function tests are much less common. Serum urea and creatinine values reflect the severity of the renal injury.

Serology

The sensitivity and specificity of ANCA for small vessel vasculitis have already been discussed. The results of other serological tests are variable. Up to 50 per cent of patients have detectable antiendothelial cell antibodies, and there is often a polyclonal increase in immunoglobulins. Rheumatoid factors are present in up to a third of patients and positive antinuclear factor without antibodies to double-stranded DNA in at least 10 per cent. Complement concentrations reflect the intensity of the acute phase response and are either normal or increased.

Renal biopsy

Renal biopsies show focal necrotizing glomerulonephritis of varying degrees of severity. Segments of the glomerular tuft are initially infiltrated by leucocytes, individual capillary loops become necrotic, and intravascular contents escape into Bowman's space (Fig. 5(a) and Plate 3(a)). This provokes an intense inflammatory response that is termed extracapillary proliferation, which eventually surrounds the glomerular tuft to form a 'crescent' (Fig. 5(b) and Plate 3(b)). Freshly formed crescents are composed entirely of cells, but gradually these are replaced by fibrosis. Progressively more glomeruli are involved until the disease becomes diffuse, hence it is usual to see crescents in all stages of their evolution, some being entirely cellular whilst others are completely fibrotic. Immunohistology shows that the glomeruli contain scanty deposits of immunoglobulins and complement and for that reason the lesions are often referred to as pauci-immune glomerulonephritis. The glomerular changes are accompanied by interstitial inflammation and progressive tubular atrophy as increasing numbers of nephrons are destroyed. Arteries affected by vasculitis are seen occasionally.

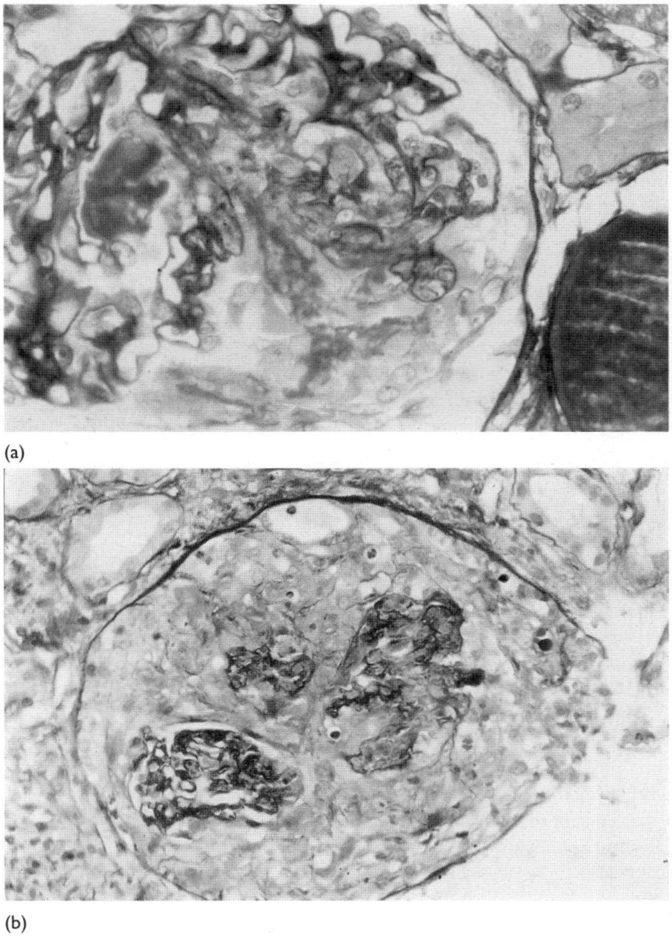

(a)

(b)

Fig. 5 Morphological appearances on a renal biopsy from a patient with pauci-immune focal necrotizing glomerulonephritis. (a) An early lesion with necrosis of one glomerular segment. (b) A much more florid lesion with the whole glomerular tuft surrounded by a crescent. (See also Plate 3.)

Renal morphology on biopsy is critical for diagnosis but has remarkably little prognostic power. In contrast to the situation with Goodpasture's disease (antiglomerular basement membrane antibody disease), even patients whose biopsies show severe glomerular destruction usually respond to treatment with a marked improvement in renal function. Similarly, patients who appear on biopsy to have indolent disease with marked glomerular scarring and tubular atrophy frequently get worthwhile improvements in function with immunosuppressive therapy. The number of normal glomerular capillary loops provides the best, albeit uncertain, guide to prognosis.

Differential diagnosis

Wegener's granulomatosis and microscopic polyangiitis are distinguished from each other on the basis of evidence for granulomatous inflammation and by whether or not the upper airways are involved. They should also be distinguished from other types of vasculitis. Although they often present with similar symptoms, other types of primary vasculitis are distinguished by clinical (for example asthma and eosinophilia in the case of Churg–Strauss syndrome), serological, radiological, and morphological evidence of the size and distribution of the vessels involved. Recognition of secondary forms of small vessel vasculitis (Table 1) depends on making an alternative diagnosis such as rheumatoid arthritis. In some cases this requires a biopsy: for example in adults Henoch–Schönlein purpura can be difficult to distinguish from microscopic polyangiitis without histological demonstration of prominent granular IgA deposits in glomeruli, or in vessels in vasculitic skin. Mixed essential cryoglobulinaemia, rheumatoid vasculitis, and systemic lupus erythematosus can all be diagnosed on the basis of specific serological tests. Infective endocarditis can cause vasculitis that is sometimes associated with positive ANCA assays (usually with specificity for myeloperoxidase) and should therefore be considered in all patients presenting with a vasculitis.

Other causes of rapidly progressive glomerulonephritis should also be considered in patients with few signs of extrarenal disease. Antiglomerular basement membrane disease and crescentic transformation of other types of chronic glomerulonephritis can be excluded on the basis of serology and renal biopsy. Assays for antiglomerular basement membrane antibodies are especially important because 10 to 20 per cent of patients with antiglomerular basement membrane disease also have positive ANCA and 1 to 2 per cent of patients with ANCA also have antiglomerular basement membrane antibodies.

Management of small vessel vasculitis

Before any effective treatments were available, Wegener's granulomatosis was a fatal illness with mean survival of less than 6 months. Corticosteroids extended survival, but the benefits were not prolonged and patients still died with progressive disease. The prognosis was transformed in the 1970s by the introduction of regimens that combined cyclophosphamide and steroids. These proved highly effective at suppressing disease activity and are the basis of treatment today. Cyclophosphamide has become the standard immunosuppressive drug, but prolonged treatment imposes considerable morbidity. The goal is to minimize the long-term use of this drug by developing regimens that control disease activity equally well but with less toxicity.

The prognosis of microscopic polyangiitis in the pretreatment era was little better than that of Wegener's granulomatosis, but a greater proportion of patients were treated successfully with corticosteroids alone, with up to 50 per cent survival at 5 years. Again the combined use of steroids and immunosuppressive drugs has improved the prognosis further. This is especially evident in the prognosis for focal necrotizing glomerulonephritis, which previously almost invariably resulted in endstage renal failure,

Table 4 Treatment of systemic vasculitis

Drug	Dose
Induction regimen (first 3 months):	
Standard	
Prednisolone	60 mg/day for 1 week
reducing to	45 mg, 30 mg, 25 mg and 20 mg at weekly intervals
plus	
cyclophosphamide	2 mg/kg per day orally for 3 months
or cyclophosphamide	0.5–0.75 g intravenously every 2–4 weeks for 3 momths
Fulminant disease	
Standard regimen plus	
plasma exchange	3–4 litre daily for albumin (5–10 days)
or methylprednisolone	0.5 g intravenously daily for 3 days
Limited or mild non-renal disease	
Standard induction regimen	
or methotrexate	10–15 mg weekly increasing to 20 and then 25 mg if needed
Maintenance therapy (after 3 months):	
Prednisolone	5–10 mg daily
plus azathioprine	1–2 mg/kg/day
or methotrexate	10–15 mg weekly
plus or minus	
cotrimoxazole	Applied locally to nares
mupiricin	

whereas nowadays up to 70 per cent of dialysis-dependent patients with ANCA-associated focal necrotizing glomerulonephritis can be expected to regain independent renal function.

Current approaches to management separate immunosuppressive treatment regimens into induction and maintenance phases (Table 4). Effective regimens have evolved empirically without being assessed by well-designed randomized controlled trials. Formal comparisons are increasingly needed to compare newer and potentially less toxic approaches to treatment with the standard protocols.

Induction treatment

The combination of prednisolone and cyclophosphamide is now established as the standard induction therapy for patients with generalized Wegener's granulomatosis or microscopic polyangiitis. There is consensus on how corticosteroids should be used, but less so for cyclophosphamide. Prednisolone is given in doses of around 1 mg/kg/day initially, after which the dose is reduced rapidly, typically at weekly intervals. Controlled trials show that the addition of pulses of methyl prednisolone is unlikely to confer additional benefit.

Traditionally, patients received daily oral cyclophosphamide (2 mg/kg/day), but latterly intravenous boluses have proved increasingly popular, given in doses of 0.5 to 0.75 g/m^2 body surface area at intervals of 2 weeks (at least for short periods) to 2 months. Pulse therapy has three potential advantages: a lower total dose of cyclophosphamide is used, MESNA (2-mercaptoethane sulfonate sodium) can be given with each dose to minimize bladder toxicity, and compliance is assured. Originally it was believed that pulse therapy might also be more effective, but this has not proved to be the case and indeed the opposite may be true. Results of three randomized prospective controlled trials comparing the two regimens have been reported but are not decisive. They show that both regimens are highly effective for most patients, and that pulse therapy has fewer toxic side-effects, including infections. Importantly, however, they suggest that pulse therapy may be less effective for patients with the most aggressive disease, including those with dialysis-dependent renal failure. Thus the available evidence suggests that the daily oral cyclophosphamide regimen should still be employed for patients with very severe disease. The choice of daily versus pulse therapy is open to personal preference for less severely affected patients.

The duration of induction treatment with cyclophosphamide is also controversial. The approach usually employed in North America and Continental Europe has been to use prolonged courses, albeit with progressively smaller doses. The evident toxicity of this approach has forced a re-evaluation and many now switch to weekly methotrexate after an initial course of cyclophosphamide, but there is a problem in that methotrexate is contraindicated in patients with reduced renal function. Management has been different in the United Kingdom, where it has been routine to use a 3-month induction course of cyclophosphamide and then switch to azathioprine as the immunosuppressive drug. There is now controlled trial evidence that this is as effective as prolonged cyclophosphamide. Thus limiting the induction course of cyclophosphamide to 3 months can be recommended and should be used in all patients with evidence of renal involvement.

Induction treatment for less severely affected patients

Another major issue about induction therapy is whether or not drugs which are less toxic than cyclophosphamide should be used for patients with less severe or more localized disease. In the past, azathioprine was used successfully in this situation, it being clear from uncontrolled studies that it was effective in many patients, but not all, and that its substitution by cyclophosphamide was usually effective in the event of treatment failure. Thus azathioprine did not find a regular place in induction therapy, and weekly pulses of methotrexate at an initial dose of 10 to 15 mg/week, increasing to 20 and then 25 mg/week if necessary, is the current most common alternative to cyclophosphamide. This is an effective treatment but is contraindicated in patients with reduced renal function, which limits its use. Controlled trials are now in progress to compare this approach with standard induction therapy for patients without renal disease. Liver function must be monitored carefully in patients receiving methotrexate because of the risk of hepatotoxicity. Other side-effects of methotrexate include infections and pulmonary fibrosis.

The patient with fulminant disease

The management of patients with fulminant or life-threatening disease presents additional problems. It remains controversial whether they benefit from additional treatment. The two regimens most commonly added in this situation are pulse methylprednisolone (typically 0.5 g/day for three doses) or plasma exchange. A prospective randomized controlled clinical trial of plasma exchange (4 litres daily for 7 to 10 days) demonstrated that this had significant benefit for those already on dialysis, but conferred no benefits over conventional treatment for those with less severe renal disease. A second reported trial showed broadly similar results with no overall benefit but a trend in favour of plasma exchange for those on dialysis. There are no controlled trials of methylprednisolone in dialysis-dependent patients but results of uncontrolled studies of dialysis-dependent patients are similar to those achieved using plasma exchange. A formal controlled comparison of the different regimens is being conducted as part of European Multicentre EUVAS trial group.

Antithymocyte and anti-T-cell antibodies have been used with apparent success in small numbers of patients with severe disease, but this approach should be regarded as experimental and restricted to treatment of patients who have failed to respond to conventional therapy in centres with special experience of these disorders. There is not enough experience of the use of newer immunosuppressive drugs to recommend their use outside the clinical trials.

Maintenance therapy

Systemic vasculitis is a chronic disease and so long-term treatment with steroids and immunosuppressive drugs is required both to maintain remission and to preserve renal function. The key to maintenance therapy is to balance the risks of relapse with those of immunosuppression. For this reason the current approach is to minimize the duration of treatment with cyclophosphamide. The evidence from controlled trials already cited has shown that substituting azathioprine (2 mg/kg) for cyclophosphamide after 3 months is as effective as continuing cyclophosphamide. This is continued for at least a year, together with reducing doses of prednisolone. Thereafter the dose of azathioprine is reduced to 1 mg/kg. An alternative approach is to use weekly pulses of methotrexate (10 to 20 mg/week) instead of azathioprine. Further reductions of treatment can be made during the second year provided that the patient's disease remains in remission, and one can consider stopping treatment altogether in patients who are clinically well provided that their assays for ANCA are negative. Even patients with prolonged clinical remissions are at risk of relapse if immunosuppression is stopped when ANCA are still detectable. There are no data that indicate whether it is best to stop the steroids or cytotoxic drugs first, but there is a strong clinical impression that immunosuppressive drugs are better at maintaining remission than are steroids.

Adjunctive therapy

Intravenous immunoglobulin has been widely used to treat autoimmune disease because of its anti-inflammatory properties and possibly because of its proposed effects on idiotypic networks. It appears to have a modest beneficial effect when used to treat vasculitis, but not sufficient to warrant its regular use. Cotrimoxazole has been widely used as adjunctive therapy both during the induction phase of treatment and to prevent relapses. Evidence from controlled trials demonstrates that it confers significant benefit in reducing the incidence of relapses, especially in those with severe upper airway involvement with Wegener's granulomatosis. It is likely that this effect is mediated through better control of infection. Nasal carriage of *Staphylococcus aureus* is associated with an increased risk of relapse and so long-term use of mupirocin cream may be a useful adjunct in affected patients.

Management of relapses

Relapses are common and occur in between a third and a half of patients with small vessel vasculitis, more frequently in those with Wegener's granulomatosis than with microscopic polyangiitis. They may also be more common in patients with microscopic polyangiitis and antiproteinase-3 antibodies. Relapses can occur at any time, even decades after the initial presentation; they may occur spontaneously or be provoked by a reduction of therapy or by the development of an intercurrent infection. As already stated the risk of relapse is significantly greater in chronic nasal carriers of *S. aureus*.

Most relapses occur in patients who are no longer receiving therapy. Clinical evidence of disease activity is the most important determinant of whether to increase therapy. It is usually unwise to increase therapy in the absence of any clinical signs or symptoms, but it is often wise to do so in patients with minimal non-specific symptoms in whom a change in ANCA assays from negative to positive or an increase in titre provide additional evidence of grumbling activity. Minor relapses can usually be managed by minor adjustments to the maintenance dose of steroids, whereas severe ones require more drastic measures. High-dose corticosteroids may need to be introduced, and depending on baseline therapy the dose of azathioprine may need to be increased or cyclophosphamide reintroduced.

Whenever possible overt relapses should be anticipated by prolonged follow-up of patients. This requires careful monitoring, both of clinical symptoms and signs, and also of investigations including full blood count, biochemical profile, urinary protein and sediment, C-reactive protein, and ANCA. Clinical relapses often affect different organs from those of the presenting illness, and the nature of the inflammation can be different, for example granulomas can develop in patients previously thought to have microscopic polyangiitis. The Birmingham vasculitis activity score has been developed to provide an objective assessment of disease activity. Use of such tools is essential for clinical trials and can also be useful in routine practice for monitoring the activity of patients with difficult disease.

Prognosis

Conventional treatments are very effective at suppressing disease activity, with numerous reports in recent literature indicating that more than 90 per cent of patients achieve remission. Resolution of inflammation often leaves patients with long-standing damage to particular organs, including the kidney. None the less, up to 70 per cent of patients with focal necrotizing glomerulonephritis severe enough to require dialysis at presentation regain independent renal function, which is sustained for many years.

One-year survival is around 80 per cent, with 5-year survival in the region of 55 to 75 per cent. About 10 per cent of patients with small vessel vasculitis die early, usually with uncontrolled disease. Opportunist infections contribute to deaths later in the first year, but have become uncommon with increased experience in the use of immunosuppressive drugs in this group of patients. Some units use cotrimoxazole as prophylaxis against *Pneumocystis carinii*. Some late deaths are due to unrelated causes in this elderly population, while others can be attributed to complications of therapy including haematological malignancies and other tumours. Patients with severe renal disease have a worse mortality, as inevitably do the elderly.

Dialysis and transplantation

Patients who develop endstage renal failure due to vasculitis appear to do no worse than other groups when treated by dialysis. Similarly, successful transplantation has been repeatedly reported and recurrence of small vessel vasculitis in renal transplants is exceptional.

Special problems in pregnancy

Vasculitis is uncommon in women of child-bearing age and so pregnancy is rare in these conditions. However, Wegener's granulomatosis has occasionally been reported to present in pregnancy and the puerperium, and there are also reports of a relapse of disease activity in the third trimester. Women of child-bearing age should be warned of the potential teratogenic effects of drugs that they may be taking to control vasculitis, for example cyclophosphamide and cotrimoxazole. Azathioprine does not pose a threat to the fetus but is a contraindication to breast feeding.

Renal involvement in other vasculitic disorders

Churg–Strauss syndrome

Churg–Strauss syndrome (see Chapter 17.11.5) is a small to medium-sized vasculitis frequently associated with ANCA and sometimes with focal necrotizing glomerulonephritis. Characteristic clinical features are those of asthma and transient pulmonary infiltrates, eosinophilia, and a necrotizing vasculitis affecting particularly the peripheral nervous system (mononeuritis multiplex), the bowel, and sometimes the heart and the skin. The full blood count shows normochromic normocytic anaemia and eosinophilia, which may exceed 1.5×10^9/litre, and a raised platelet count. The chest radiograph reveals pulmonary infiltrates and, as with other forms of vasculitis, severe pulmonary haemorrhage can occur. Renal disease is much less common in Churg–Strauss syndrome than in Wegener's granulomatosis or microscopic polyangiitis. When present, it consists of a focal necrotizing glomerulonephritis or, less commonly, a severe interstitial nephritis with large numbers of eosinophils.

Steroids have been the main treatment for many years, but many would advocate the concurrent use of other immunosuppressive drugs in those with severe disease. This should include those with life-threatening pulmonary haemorrhage, rapidly developing mononeuritis multiplex, or focal necrotizing glomerulonephritis. Overall the prognosis of Churg–Strauss

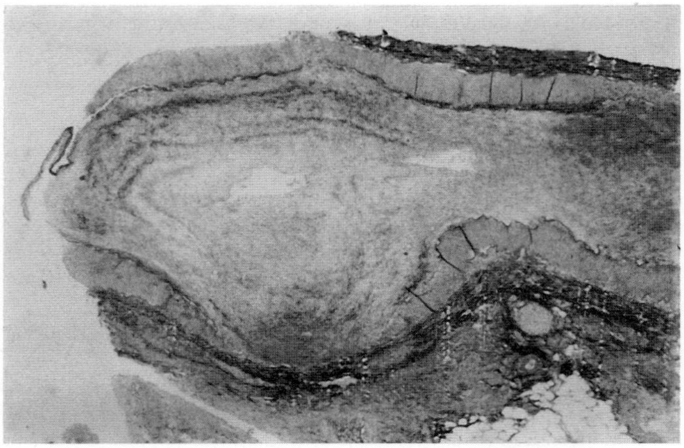

Fig. 6 Morphological appearances of a renal artery from a patient with polyarteritis nodosa. The elastic lamina has been destroyed and the artery has become aneurysmal. (See also Plate 4.)

syndrome is good with initial clinical remission being achieved in over 90 per cent of patients and a 5-year survival of in excess of 75 per cent. However, it should be emphasized that patients with mononeuritis may be left with considerable disability.

Polyarteritis nodosa

Polyarteritis nodosa is an uncommon condition characterized by necrotizing vasculitis affecting small and medium-sized muscular arteries. Affected arteries often develop aneurysmal swellings (Fig. 6 and Plate 4), which can be palpable as nodules when they occur in subcutaneous tissue. By definition the diagnosis excludes patients who also have involvement of capillaries, arterioles, and venules. Typically it is a disease of the middle aged, with males being affected twice as commonly as females. Patients usually present with fever, weight loss, and night sweats. Other symptoms depend on which vessels are involved. Abdominal pain is common and is due to intestinal ischaemia or pressure from aneurysms; some patients present with symptoms of hypertension caused by renal ischaemia.

The aetiology is unknown in most patients, but polyarteritis nodosa has been reported in carriers of hepatitis B virus and also after infection with parvovirus. Further evidence of infective aetiology comes from reports of polyarteritis nodosa in intravenous drug users.

Diagnosis

Polyarteritis nodosa is associated with the usual non-specific signs of inflammation, but in marked contrast to small vessel vasculitis, ANCA are usually negative. The diagnosis depends on the angiographic demonstration of vasculitis in muscular arteries. All patients should be tested to determine whether they are carriers of hepatitis B or infected with hepatitis C.

Treatment

Polyarteritis nodosa is treated with corticosteroids and cytotoxic drugs using the regimen described for small vessel vasculitis (Table 4). This regimen is effective in the short term in those with hepatitis B, but may be deleterious in the longer term, and success has been reported when these patients are treated with antiviral therapy alone, for example interferon-α or lamivudine.

Conclusion

There has been enormous progress in the management of patients with systemic vasculitis over the past decade, in particular for those with severe renal involvement. Common approaches to classification, diagnosis, and treatment have been developed that for the first time provide a basis for prospective randomized controlled trails of treatment methods. There is no doubt that current treatment regimens are highly effective in the short and medium term, but minimizing long-term toxicity of treatment remains a major issue.

The identification of ANCA in patients with vasculitis has been extremely valuable, both for purely practical reasons as an aid to diagnosis, and more generally as a focus for investigation of these disorders. Nevertheless, it is disappointing that despite nearly two decades of research no clear conclusions can be drawn about why ANCA are so closely associated with systemic vasculitis, or about their roll in pathogenesis.

There is an urgent need for better understanding of pathogenesis to rationalize therapy. Controlled clinical trials designed to optimize the use of currently available drugs are certainly needed, but assessing the potential of the large numbers of new immunosuppressive drugs and recombinant molecules presents impossible difficulties. A better understanding of pathogenesis would help in choosing which other new approaches are most likely to be valuable.

Further reading

General

Heeringa P *et al.* (1998). Animal models of anti-neutrophil cytoplasmic antibody associated vasculitis. *Kidney International* **53**, 253–63.

Hoffman GS (1998). Classification of the systemic vasculitides: antineutrophil cytoplasmic antobodies, consensus and controversy. *Clinical and Experimental Rheumatology* **16**, 111–15.

Jennette JC *et al.* (1994). Nomenclature of systemic vasculitides: proposal of an international consensus conference. *Arthritis and Rheumatism* **37**, 187–92.

Pusey CD *et al.* (1991). Plasma exchange in focal necrotising glomerulonephritis without anti-GBM antibodies. *Kidney International* **40**, 757–63.

Watts RA *et al.* (2000). Epidemiology of systemic vasculitis: a ten-year study in the United Kingdom. *Arthritis and Rheumatism* **43**, 414–19.

Antineutrophil cytoplasmic antibodies

Hagen EC *et al.* (1998). Diagnostic value of standardised assays for anti-neutrophil cytoplasmic antibodies in idiopathic vasculitis. *Kidney International* **53**, 743–53.

Hoffman GS, Specks U (1998). Antineutrophil cytoplasmic antibodies. *Arthritis and Rheumatism* **41**, 1521–37.

McLaren JS *et al.* (2001). The diagnostic value of antineutrophil cytoplasmic antibody testing in a routine clinical setting. *Quarterly Journal of Medicine* **94**, 615–21.

Small vessel vasculitis

Adu D *et al.* (1997). Controlled trial of pulse versus continuous prednisolone and cyclophosphamide in the treatment of systemic vasculitis. *Quarterly Journal of Medicine* **90**, 401–9.

Exley AR, Bacon PA (1996). Clinical disease activity in systemic vasculitis. *Current Opinion in Rheumatology* **8**, 12–18.

Gaskin G, Pusey CD (1998). Systemic vasculitis. In: Davison AM *et al.*, eds. *Oxford textbook of clinical nephrology*, vol. 2, pp 877–910. Oxford University Press, Oxford.

Guillevin L *et al.* (1997). A prospective, multicenter, randomised trial comparing steroids and pulse cyclophosphamide in the treatment of generalised Wegener's granulomatosis. *Arthritis and Rheumatism* **40**, 2187–98.

Haubitz M *et al.* (1998). Intravenous pulse administration of cyclophosphamide versus daily oral treatment in patients with antineutrophil cytoplasmic antibody-associated vasculitis and renal involvement: a prospective, randomised study. *Arthritis and Rheumatism* **41**, 1835–44.

Jennette JC, Falk RJ (1997). Small-vessel vasculitis. *New England Journal of Medicine* **337**, 1512–23.

Savage COS *et al.* (1985). Microscopic polyarteritis: presentation, pathology and prognosis. *Quarterly Journal of Medicine* **56**, 467–83.

Westman KWA *et al.* (1997). Relapse rate, renal survival, and cancer morbidity in patients with Wegener's granulomatosis or microscopis polyangiitis with renal involvement. *Journal of the American Society of Nephrology* **9**, 842–52.

Churg–Strauss Syndrome

Eustace JA, Nadasdy T, Choi M (1999). The Churg–Strauss syndrome. *Journal of the American Society of Nephrology* **10**, 2048–55.

Guillevin L *et al.* (1999). Churg–Strauss syndrome: clinical study and long term follow-up of 96 patients. *Medicine* **78**, 26–37

Lanham JG *et al.* (1984). Systemic vasculitis with asthma and eosinophilia: a clinical approach to the Churg–Strauss syndrome. *Medicine* **63**, 65–81.

Polyarteritis nodosa

Gayraud M *et al.* (2001). Long-term followup of polyarteritis nodosa, microscopic polyangiitis, and Churg–Strauss syndrome: analysis of four prospective trials including 278 patients. *Arthritis and Rheumatism* **44**, 666–75.

Guillevin L (1999). The treatment of classic polyarteritis nodosa in 1999. *Nephrology Dialysis Transplantation* **14**, 2077–9.

20.10.4 The kidney in rheumatological disorders

D. Adu

Lupus nephritis

Systemic lupus erythematosus is a multisystem autoimmune disease that is characterized by the presence of antinuclear antibodies (see Chapter 18.10.2). The overall survival of patients with systemic lupus erythematosus and a nephritis has improved considerably over the last few decades; from less than 50 per cent survival at 5 years in the 1960s to over 80 per cent survival at 10 years in the 1990s. This is due the wider use of corticosteroids and immunosuppressants and the availability of more effective antihypertensive drugs, antibiotics, renal dialysis, and transplantation.

Pathogenesis

The pathogenesis of systemic lupus erythematosus in general, and lupus nephritis in particular, is complex and multifactorial. Immunological dysregulation leads to the production of autoantibodies to nuclear (in particular double-stranded DNA) and other cellular antigens. The renal lesions of lupus nephritis show glomerular and (less often) tubular deposits of immunoglobulins and complement in a granular pattern indicating immune aggregation. It now seems likely that this is due to *in situ* assembly of antigen–antibody complexes rather than the deposition of immune complexes from the circulation.

Clinical presentation

Renal disease may rarely be the presenting feature of systemic lupus erythematosus, although at presentation 10 to 20 per cent of patients with the condition have evidence of renal involvement, and this develops in about 40 to 50 per cent of patients, typically during the first 5 years after diagnosis. Whilst renal disease is a major complication of systemic lupus erythematosus it is always important to recognize that lupus is a systemic disease and that nephritis typically occurs in patients with extrarenal symptoms such as a rash, arthralgia, Raynaud's phenomenon, and pleuropericarditis. Other major organ systems may be involved including the central nervous system, heart, and lungs.

Proteinuria is found in all patients with lupus nephritis and in 50 to 60 per cent of cases is heavy enough to lead to a nephrotic syndrome. Microscopic haematuria accompanies the proteinuria in about 80 per cent of patients; hypertension is found at presentation in 20 to 50 per cent; and some 20 to 30 per cent present with rapidly deteriorating renal function that may occasionally be severe enough to lead to acute renal failure.

Diagnosis

Immunology

A fluorescent antinuclear test is positive in more than 95 per cent of patients with systemic lupus erythematosus although it lacks specificity as it is also found in other connective tissue diseases. More specific, but less sensitive, tests include antidouble-stranded DNA and anti-Sm (Smith) autoantibodies. (For discussion of immunological tests for systemic lupus erythematosus see Chapters 18.10.1 and 18.10.2.) In general antidouble-stranded DNA antibody levels reflect disease activity, particularly if accompanied by falling complement levels, but as regards the kidney they are less consistently related to features of active glomerulonephritis. Reduced serum concentrations of the complement proteins C1q and C4 as well as C3 indicate activation of the classical pathway of complement. These are useful in the diagnosis of systemic lupus erythematosus, but although more commonly found in lupus nephritis they are not useful in predicting its onset. Patients with lupus nephritis have antibodies to phospholipids in 30 to 50 per cent of cases, resulting in prolongation of the partial thromboplastin time and leading to the term lupus anticoagulant.

Pathology

A renal biopsy is justified when there is evidence of glomerular disease in the form of proteinuria (more than 200 mg/24 h), microscopic haematuria, a urinary sediment indicative of active nephritis (more than 10 dysmorphic red blood cells per high-power field and/or casts of red and white blood cells), or renal insufficiency. Histology allows an assessment of disease activity and provides a basis for therapy and prognosis.

A distinctive feature of lupus nephritis on light microscopy is the variability of the glomerular changes seen in a single biopsy, and sometimes within the same glomerulus. This makes classification of renal histology difficult, but that most widely used is the modified World Health Organization (**WHO**) classification shown in Table 1. Segmental glomerular thrombosis, necrosis, and extracapillary proliferation (crescents) are frequently found in association with the proliferative type lesions (WHO class III and IV). On immunofluorescent microscopy there is often florid deposition of immunoglobulins IgG, IgA, and IgM as well as complement proteins C3, C4, and C1q.

Patients with minimal changes or mesangial glomerulonephritis (WHO class I and II lesions) (Fig. 1 and Plate 1) usually have an inherently low rate of progressive renal failure. Patients with membranous nephropathy (WHO class V) have an intermediate prognosis for renal function. By contrast, patients with focal or diffuse proliferative glomerulonephritis (WHO class III and IV) (Fig. 2 and Plate 2) have a high risk of progressive renal failure.

Treatment

There are several considerations in the approach to the treatment of patients with lupus nephritis. The first is based on the histological severity of the renal lesion. The second is based on the severity of the clinical presentation. The third consideration is the choice of therapy for inducing remission of acute disease and for maintaining remission and treating relapses. The heterogeneity of the clinical course of lupus nephritis and the relatively few randomized controlled trials means that decision making is

Table 1 The 1995 World Health Organization classification of lupus nephritis

Class I Normal glomeruli (a) Normal (by all techniques) (b) Normal by light microscopy but deposits by electron or immunofluorescence microscopy
Class II Mesangial glomerulonephritis (a) Mesangial widening and or mild hypercellularity (b) Moderate hypercellularity
Class III Focal proliferative glomerulonephritis (associated with mild or moderate mesangial alterations, and/or segmental epimembranous deposits) (a) 'Active' necrotizing lesions (b) 'Active and sclerosing lesions' (c) Sclerosing lesions
Class IV Diffuse proliferative glomerulonephritis (severe mesangial/ mesangiocapillary with extensive subendothelial deposits). Mesangial deposits always present, and frequently subepithelial deposits (a) With segmental lesions (b) With 'active' necrotizing lesions (c) With 'active' and sclerosing lesions (d) With sclerosing lesions
Class V Diffuse membranous glomerulonephritis (a) Pure membranous glomerulonephritis (b) Associated with lesions of category II (a or b)
Class VI Advanced sclerosing glomerulonephritis

difficult and there are still substantial disagreements on the optimum treatment. Steroids and/or immunosuppressants are used—drugs with major toxicities that need to be offset against any benefit.

Treatments for particular classes of lupus nephritis

Mesangial proliferative glomerulonephritis (WHO class II)

Most such patients present with proteinuria and microscopic haematuria, often with little in the way of renal impairment. There are no controlled trials to guide treatment. We treat such patients with corticosteroids in the hope that this will prevent progression to a more severe glomerulonephritis, but this is not certain.

Membranous nephropathy (WHO class V)

In patients with lupus nephritis the frequency of membranous nephropathy is approximately 12 per cent when the definition of the renal histology is confined to pure membranous nephropathy with or without mild

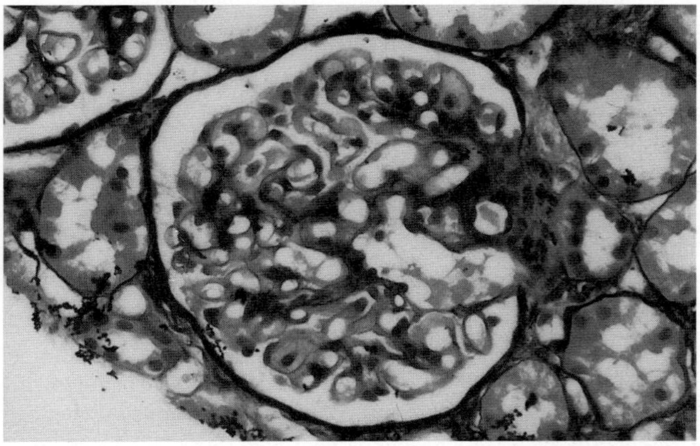

Fig. 1 Lupus nephritis. The glomerulus has mild mesangial increase (WHO class II). Periodic acid-methenamine silver staining (×50). (By courtesy of Dr A. J. Howie.) (See also Plate 1.)

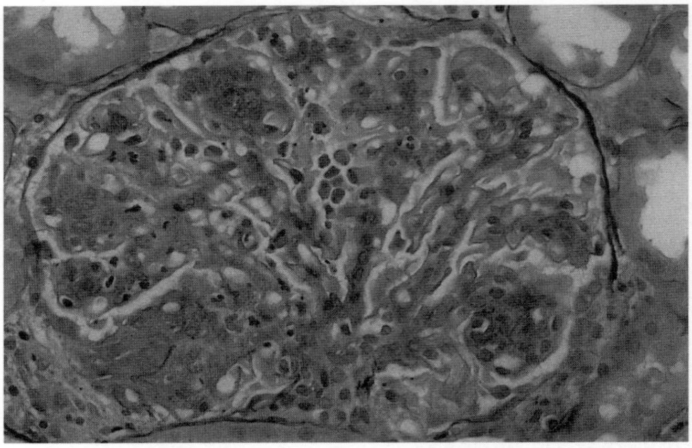

Fig. 2 Lupus nephritis. The glomerulus has marked mesangial increase with wire loops, a few doubled basement membranes and segmental lesions (WHO class IV). Periodic acid-methenamine silver staining (×40). (By courtesy of Dr A. J. Howie. (See also Plate 2.)

mesangial hypercellularity, expansion, and scattered deposits (WHO classes Va and Vb). With the revision of the WHO criteria in 1995, biopsies with focal segmental proliferative or diffuse proliferative glomerulonephritis in addition to membranous changes are now classified as WHO classes III and IV because they behave similarly: this causes some difficulties in interpreting earlier studies where these appearances were classified as Vc and Vd.

The clinical presentation of lupus membranous nephropathy is with proteinuria and in about 50 per cent of cases a nephrotic syndrome. Patients with WHO class Va and Vb lesions have a low rate of progressive renal failure. There are no controlled trials of treatment and thus there is no consensus on treatment. In some studies patients with WHO class Va and Vb disease have been treated with prednisolone, with a smaller proportion also receiving pulses of methylprednisolone or oral cyclophosphamide and azathioprine. By contrast, most patients previously classified as WHO class Vc and Vd have been treated with cyclophosphamide or azathioprine in addition to prednisolone. With these approaches to treatment the 10-year survival free of death and renal failure in WHO class Va and Vb was 72 to 92 per cent and in WHO class Vc and Vd was 35 to 81 per cent.

Most nephrologists treat patients with pure lupus membranous nephropathy with or without minor mesangial proliferation with prednisolone and consider adding in azathioprine as a corticosteroid sparing agent.

Focal and diffuse lupus proliferative glomerulonephritis (WHO class III and IV)

It has been argued that the addition of immunosuppressive drugs to corticosteroids does not improve the prognosis of lupus. Others have concluded that patients treated with prednisolone plus cyclophosphamide or azathioprine have fewer unfavourable outcomes than patients treated with prednisolone alone. Formal meta-analysis has shown that treatment with cyclophosphamide or azathioprine combined with prednisolone reduced the risk of developing endstage renal disease and possibly mortality when compared with prednisolone alone.

A series of clinical trials from the National Institutes of Health provided evidence of the effectiveness of intermittent intravenous cyclophosphamide together with oral prednisolone in preserving renal function in patients with severe lupus nephritis. This regimen is preferable to continuous oral cyclophosphamide as it leads to less bladder toxicity, although the frequency of gonadal toxicity is unaffected and it is not yet known whether pulse cyclophosphamide is less carcinogenic than continuous oral therapy, although this is unlikely. From the National Institutes of Health data, monthly pulse cyclophosphamide (0.5 to 0.75 g/m^2) adjusted for the glomerular filtration rate and leucocyte count at 10 to 14 days is given monthly for the first 6 months, then quarterly for 18 to 24 months, the longer course of cyclophosphamide being associated with fewer relapses than a shorter 6-month course, but at the expense of greater gonadal toxicity. Preliminary data with pulse oral cyclophosphamide have shown encouraging results and, if validated, will minimize the inconvenience associated with intravenous therapy. To reduce the bladder toxicity of intravenous cyclophosphamide patients should be hydrated either with oral or intravenous fluid and mesna given concomitantly. Prednisolone is given in conjunction with the cyclophosphamide at an initial dose of 0.5 to 1 mg/kg/day for 6 to 8 weeks with gradual tapering, preferably to an alternate day regimen to minimize toxicity.

In other uncontrolled but extensive observations, treatment with intravenous methylprednisolone followed by combined prednisolone and azathioprine or oral cyclophosphamide gave long-term results comparable with those of the National Institutes of Health data. It has also been reported that azathioprine may prevent relapse. However, on the basis of the randomized controlled data, we feel that the National Institutes of Health regimen is a reasonable initial treatment for severe lupus nephritis. Much of the toxicity is due to the prolonged maintenance course of pulse cyclophosphamide: whether conversion after 6 months to azathioprine is as effective in maintaining remission as continued pulse cyclophosphamide remains to be established.

A key feature of the care of patients with lupus nephritis is close monitoring of the white cell count and renal function and detailed surveillance and management of infection, extrarenal lupus, and hypertension. A summary of the treatment strategies for lupus nephritis is shown in Table 2.

Notes on particular treatments for lupus nephritis

Toxicity of cyclophosphamide

Intravenous cyclophosphamide often leads to nausea and vomiting: giving serotonin antagonists such as ondansetron together with dexamethasone can control this. The most common toxic effect is depression of normal haematopoiesis, which is dose dependent and reversible on discontinuing therapy. A further major side-effect is an increased risk of infections, worsened by the concomitant use of corticosteroids. In particular, an increased incidence of herpes zoster is seen with cyclophosphamide.

Cyclophosphamide is metabolized to phosphoramide mustard and acrolein that are excreted by the kidneys. Acrolein can lead to a haemorrhagic cystitis, which is particularly common with oral cyclophosphamide. The use of intravenous cyclophosphamide with vigorous hydration and concomitant administration of 2-mercaptoethane sulfonate sodium has essentially eliminated bladder complications. Prolonged oral cyclophosphamide is associated with an increased risk of malignancy and it is likely that intravenous cyclophosphamide also carries this risk.

Cyclophosphamide causes dose- and age-related gonadal toxicity with oligospermia in men and premature ovarian failure in women. Few data on gonadal toxicity in men with lupus are available. In one study of six men treated with oral cyclophosphamide at a daily dose of 50 to 100 mg, germinal aplasia occurred after a cumulative dose of 9 to 18 g. All studies show that the risk of ovarian toxicity rises substantially with age and is correlated with the duration of treatment and the cumulative dose of cyclophosphamide. In patients aged less than 25 the risk of ovarian failure after 6 months of monthly intravenous cyclophosphamide was nil, whilst a further 24 months of quarterly cyclophosphamide increased this risk to 17 per cent.

Table 2 Treatment of lupus glomerulonephritis

Renal histology	Treatment
Mesangial glomerulonephritis (WHO class II)	Prednisolone
Focal and diffuse proliferative glomerulonephritis (WHO classes III and IV)	Oral prednisolone + intermittent intravenous cyclophosphamide (National Institutes of Health regime)
Membranous glomerulonephritis (WHO class V)	Prednisolone ± azathioprine as a steroid sparing agent

Comparable figures for women aged over 31 years were 25 per cent and 100 per cent respectively. By contrast, one out of 20 patients (5 per cent) treated with azathioprine developed ovarian failure. Since lupus nephritis chiefly afflicts women of reproductive age, one must balance this risk of premature ovarian failure, which may be permanent, with the benefits of treatment. Cyclophosphamide, unlike azathioprine, is a potent teratogen and must not be used in pregnancy.

Toxicity of azathioprine

Some patients are intolerant of azathioprine and develop nausea, vomiting, and diarrhoea. It also causes marrow suppression, which can be severe in individuals who have a deficiency of thiopurine methyltransferase. Other toxicities include an increased risk of infection and the development of malignancies with prolonged usage.

Pulse methylprednisolone

Pulse methylprednisolone has been used in at least two different ways. In the first, pulse methylprednisolone has been used in three consecutive daily doses of 0.5 to 1 g at the initiation of treatment of severe proliferative lupus nephritis or for the treatment of renal flares. This has been used together with cyclophosphamide or azathioprine and in conjunction with oral prednisolone. The long-term results of this approach are good, although this approach has not been examined in a randomized controlled study. The second way that methylprednisolone has been used is as monthly pulses together with continuous low-dose prednisolone. However, this is less effective in inducing remission and preventing endstage renal failure than treatments that include cyclophosphamide and it cannot be recommended.

Plasma exchange

Several studies have examined the role of plasmapheresis in the treatment of patients with lupus nephritis: although it was well tolerated with few adverse effects the impact on renal function was disappointing. Controlled trials of plasmapheresis in patients with all types of proliferative or membranous glomerulonephritis showed no benefit over treatment with prednisolone and immunosuppressants alone. We currently use plasmapheresis only in patients with a severe diffuse proliferative glomerulonephritis and pulmonary haemorrhage whose disease does not respond to prednisolone and cyclophosphamide.

Intravenous immunoglobulins

Uncontrolled studies have shown a temporary benefit in patients with systemic lupus erythematosus from the infusion of high doses of intravenous immunoglobulin. Prospective controlled studies are needed to evaluate critically the efficacy of this therapy.

Cyclosporin A

Several studies have examined the effectiveness of cyclosporin A in the treatment of lupus nephritis: none of these were controlled and it is difficult to discern whether cyclosporin was of any benefit. The nephrotoxicity of cyclosporin is a major problem, and pending randomized controlled studies comparing this drug with other immunosuppressive agents we cannot recommend its use in lupus nephritis.

Methotrexate

Methotrexate may be useful as a steroid-sparing agent in lupus with arthritis and serositis, and may have potential benefits in mild nephritis. However, methotrexate is excreted by the kidneys and cannot be used safely in patients with renal impairment.

Mycophenylate mofetil

The active metabolite of mycophenylate mofetil inhibits inosine monophosphate dehydrogenase and thereby the *de novo* pathway of guanosine nucleotide synthesis. Preliminary experimental and clinical studies have indicated a potential role in systemic lupus erythematosus, but this awaits confirmation in controlled trials.

Prognostic factors in lupus nephritis

Patients with proliferative glomerulonephritis (WHO classes III and IV) tend to have a worse outcome for renal function than those with milder lesions, although with treatment this difference is now small. The combination of severe active and chronic histological changes on a renal biopsy adversely affects outcome. Even in the face of active lupus nephritis, patients without chronic histological changes have a lower risk of developing renal failure, 90 per cent or more remaining free of renal failure after 10 years. A number of clinical variables are associated with a greater probability of renal progression in lupus nephritis, including low haematocrit, raised serum creatinine level at diagnosis, 'nephritic flares', hypertension, heavy proteinuria, and poor socio-economic status.

Long-term outcome

Studies reported in the 1990s show a 10-year patient survival in lupus nephritis that ranges from 70 to 90 per cent. Renal failure can now be treated by dialysis and transplantation, the major causes of death now being treatment-related sepsis, which occurs early, and myocardial ischaemia, which occurs late. The other major cause of death is extrarenal lupus.

Between 17 and 30 per cent of patients with lupus nephritis develop endstage renal failure by 10 years. Both haemodialysis and continuous ambulatory peritoneal dialysis are well tolerated and there is a tendency for the activity of lupus disease to diminish after the start of dialysis. We discontinue immunosuppressants in patients on dialysis if there is no overt disease activity, only persisting with a small dose of prednisolone. Overall survival on dialysis is good, being 75 per cent at 10 years. After transplantation, graft survival and function in patients with lupus are comparable to those obtained in patients with other diseases, and recurrence of lupus nephritis is uncommon.

Renal disease in systemic sclerosis

Systemic sclerosis is a systemic disorder characterized by skin thickening due to the deposition of collagen in the dermis (see Chapter 18.10.3). Adverse prognostic features are renal, cardiac, and pulmonary involvement. A major complication is the development of scleroderma renal crisis, which is characterized by the abrupt onset of severe hypertension, usually with retinopathy, together with the rapid deterioration of renal function and heart failure. Scleroderma renal crisis develops in approximately 8 to 15 per cent of patients with diffuse systemic sclerosis, the most important risk factor being the rapid progression of diffuse skin disease. It usually occurs early, within 3 years of the onset of illness, and develops more commonly in the autumn and winter.

Pathogenesis

The pathogenetic mechanisms leading to renal damage in systemic sclerosis are not known. Whilst plasma renin activity is almost always raised in scleroderma renal crisis, there is no evidence that this occurs before the development of this complication and plasma renin activity does not predict the problem. Patients with systemic sclerosis may show cold-induced reduction in renal perfusion and increased plasma renin activity, but this does not correlate with the presence of renal histological vascular abnormalities. There is evidence of endothelial activation in patients who develop renal damage with raised serum levels of circulating endothelial derived adhesion molecules including s-ELAM, s-VCAM, and s-ICAM, but these are likely to reflect the presence of endothelial injury rather than being of pathophysiological significance.

Antecedent hypertension does not increase the risk of development of scleroderma renal crisis, which is as common in men as in women, although systemic sclerosis is more common in the latter, with a female to male ratio between 3:1 and 4:1. In one retrospective case-controlled study the risk of scleroderma renal crisis was increased by prior treatment with steroids (more than 15 mg prednisolone/day) with an odds ratio of 4.37 (95 per cent confidence interval 2.03–9.42) and reduced by treatment with penicillamine (odds ratio 0.41, 95 per cent confidence interval 0.24–0.69). One report suggests that cyclosporin A may predispose to the development of scleroderma renal crisis.

Pathology

The smaller arcuate and interlobular arteries are predominantly involved in scleroderma renal crisis, showing intimal hyperplasia with concentric mucoid intimal degeneration, but the internal and external elastic laminae remain intact. In addition the adventitia of interlobular arteries show an abnormal degree of fibrosis. There is fibrinoid necrosis of afferent arterioles and glomeruli and also glomerular thrombosis. Ischaemia of the glomerular tuft leads to wrinkling and thickening of the glomerular basement membrane and glomerular sclerosis (Fig. 3 and Plate 3). These lesions resemble those seen in accelerated hypertension or the haemolytic uraemic syndrome, although the vessels involved tend to be larger and adventitial fibrosis is not seen in accelerated hypertension.

Clinical presentation

Hypertensive scleroderma renal crisis

The clinical presentation is typically with the symptoms of malignant hypertension with headaches, blurred vision, fits, and heart failure. Renal function is impaired and deteriorates rapidly. The hypertension is almost always severe with a diastolic blood pressure in excess of 100 mmHg in 90 per cent of patients. There is hypertensive retinopathy in about 85 per cent of cases with exudates and haemorrhages and at times papilloedema.

Normotensive scleroderma renal crisis

Scleroderma renal crisis can also develop in individuals with a normal blood pressure. They are more likely to have a microangiopathic haemolytic anaemia (90 per cent versus 38 per cent), thrombocytopenia (83 per cent versus 21 per cent), and pulmonary haemorrhage than patients with hypertensive scleroderma renal crisis.

Diagnosis

The clinical presentation described above in a patient with the typical diffuse skin thickening of systemic sclerosis is diagnostic. Typically the renal impairment is accompanied by a microangiopathic haemolytic anaemia with thrombocytopenia and fragmented red blood cells (schistocytes or burr cells). Once the blood pressure has been well controlled for at least 7 days then, if there is doubt, the diagnosis can be established by renal histology.

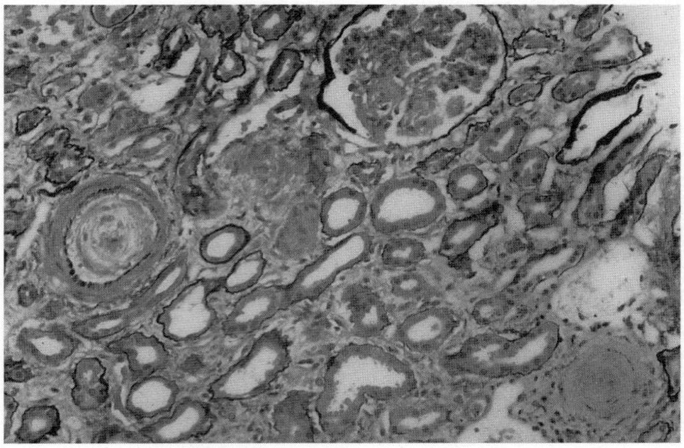

Fig. 3 Scleroderma kidney. A small artery has concentric mucoid intimal thickening, an arteriole has thrombosis and fibrinoid necrosis, and tubules and a glomerulus have ischaemic damage. Periodic acid-methenamine silver staining (×25). (By courtesy of Dr A. J. Howie.) (See also Plate 3.)

Table 3 Renal disease in rheumatoid arthritis

Consequence of rheumatoid arthritis
Amyloid A amyloidosis
Vasculitic glomerulonephritis
Mesangial proliferative glomerulonephritis
Mesangial IgA proliferative glomerulonephritis
Drug nephrotoxicity
Non-steroidal anti-inflammatory drugs—renal impairment, acute tubular necrosis, acute interstitial nephritis with or without a nephrotic syndrome
Gold and penicillamine—proteinuria, nephrotic syndrome. Membranous nephropathy. Rare reports of a crescentic glomerulonephritis

Treatment

Scleroderma renal crisis is a medical emergency. The hypertension should be treated with an angiotensin converting enzyme inhibitor, which can also help with the treatment of the heart failure. The aim should be for a slow and gradual reduction in blood pressure as an abrupt fall can lead to cerebral ischaemia or infarction, as it can in accelerated phase hypertension. Calcium channel blockers may be required in addition to the angiotensin converting enzyme inhibitors. Deterioration of renal function in these patients is often rapid and they can precipitately develop pulmonary oedema, hence they should be treated in a hospital with facilities for dialysis.

Prognosis

Prior to the early 1970s scleroderma renal crisis was almost always a fatal illness with most patients dying within a year. The survival improved slightly with the use of dialysis and better hypotensive agents, but it is only since the introduction of angiotensin converting enzyme inhibitors that prognosis has improved. In one study of 23 patients treated with captopril, 20 responded favourably and in 14 the serum creatinine fell. After a median follow-up of 29 months, six patients had died and four remained dependent on dialysis. Prior to treatment with angiotensin converting enzyme inhibitors, patients with normotensive scleroderma renal crisis had a worse prognosis, with a 1-year survival of 13 per cent as compared with 35 per cent in those who were hypertensive.

Although the renal vascular lesions are acute, recovery of function is unusual once renal failure has developed and most patients require long-term dialysis. However, some patients may recover renal function after a period of dialysis, and there is a tendency for the skin lesions of scleroderma to improve on this treatment.

Renal disease in rheumatoid arthritis

Death certificate and autopsy studies in rheumatoid arthritis show that there is an excess mortality from renal failure, which accounts for between 3 and 20 per cent of deaths. About a half of these are due to amyloid, the remainder being due to nephritis and renal infections. There are no good figures on the prevalence of renal disease during life in rheumatoid arthritis, although this does seem to be lower.

There are three broad categories of renal disease in rheumatoid arthritis (Table 3). The first and the most common is nephrotoxicity from the drugs used in the treatment (see Chapter 18.5). Gold and penicillamine lead to proteinuria and glomerulonephritis in between 10 and 30 per cent of patients, often severe enough to cause a nephrotic syndrome. Non-steroidal anti-inflammatory drugs are widely used for pain relief and are associated with the development of a variety of renal syndromes ranging from a reversible reduction in glomerular filtration rate to acute renal failure, either due to an acute tubular necrosis or an acute interstitial nephritis. The latter may be complicated by nephrotic range proteinuria. The second major but diminishing cause of renal disease in rheumatoid arthritis is amyloidosis. Thirdly, patients with rheumatoid arthritis may develop a renal vasculitis and also a glomerulonephritis.

Secondary amyloidosis in rheumatoid arthritis

Secondary amyloidosis results from deposition of fibrils containing amyloid A protein that is antigenically related to the acute phase reactant serum amyloid A (see Chapters 11.12.1 and 11.12.4 for further discussion). Rheumatoid arthritis is the commonest disease producing secondary amyloidosis in developed countries. At autopsy, prevalence rates of 8 to 17 per cent are found, whilst data from biopsy series show a lower prevalence of around 5 to 10 per cent. There is some evidence for a decline in prevalence of amyloid over the last 20 years, and in the last 5 years the incidence appears to have dropped dramatically (unpublished evidence). The reason for this is likely to be much more aggressive therapy, with fewer patients being left with a persistently elevated acute phase response.

Clinical presentation and diagnosis

The presentation of renal amyloid is with proteinuria that is often severe enough to cause a nephrotic syndrome. Renal vein thrombosis is particularly common. Diagnosis is established by renal biopsy (Fig. 4 and Plate 4), where histological Congo red staining, which is birefringent in polarized light, is characteristic of amyloid. This staining is abolished by potassium permanganate in reactive amyloidosis but not in primary amyloidosis. Monoclonal and polyclonal antibodies that specifically bind amyloid A are now available and are of use for histological diagnosis. The diagnosis of amyloid has also been aided by the availability of scans using radiolabelled serum amyloid P (SAP) protein, utilizing the strong calcium dependent affinity of SAP for amyloid fibrils of any protein type.

Treatment and prognosis

There is no specific therapy for amyloid A amyloidosis, the general principle being suppression of the underlying chronic inflammation. Uncontrolled evidence suggests that aggressive treatment of rheumatoid arthritis may be effective in delaying the deterioration of renal function in patients with renal amyloid. There are some reports that treatment with prednisolone and cyclophosphamide or methotrexate can induce remission of the nephrotic syndrome due to amyloid in patients with rheumatoid arthritis, but in other studies no benefit was seen. Randomized controlled studies are needed to establish the role of aggressive treatment of renal amyloid in this condition.

Renal amyloid leads to progressive renal failure. After 5 years 50 per cent of patients develop endstage renal failure and this rises to 90 per cent at 10 years. Treatment of endstage renal failure from amyloid is by dialysis and renal transplantation.

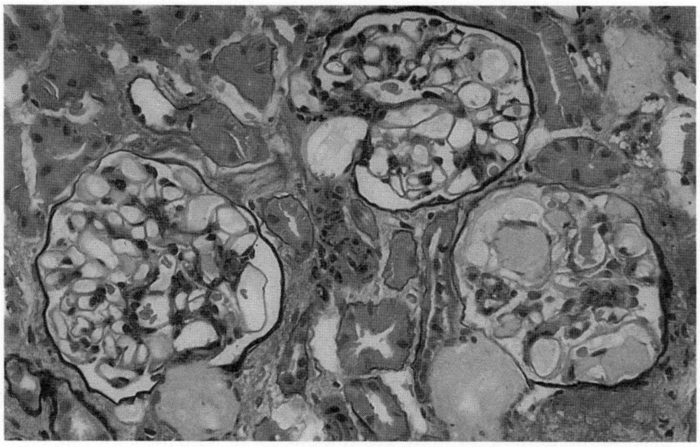

Fig. 4 Amyloidosis in rheumatoid arthritis. Arterioles and glomeruli contain acellular masses of amyloid. Periodic acid-methenamine silver staining (×40). (By courtesy of Dr A. J. Howie.) (See also Plate 4.)

Gold and penicillamine nephropathy

Clinical features

The most frequent presenting feature is proteinuria, which occurs in approximately 10 per cent of patients receiving gold and up to 30 per cent of those taking penicillamine. This progresses to the nephrotic syndrome in 30 and 16 per cent respectively. Haematuria is uncommon, although it is seen more frequently with penicillamine, and still requires the exclusion of other causes when occurring in the context of therapy with these drugs. Renal function is usually normal.

Pathology

About 80 per cent of patients who present with D-penicillamine or gold-induced proteinuria will have a membranous glomerulonephritis. Subepithelial spikes and a mild increase in mesangial cells are usually seen, and the diagnosis can be confirmed with immunofluorescence/immunoperoxidase microscopy that shows granular subepithelial deposits of predominantly IgG. On electron microscopy electron-dense subepithelial deposits are seen.

Other renal lesions are less common and include a mesangial glomerulonephritis, minimal change nephropathy, and tubulointerstitial inflammation. Penicillamine may lead to the development of a rapidly progressive glomerulonephritis with crescents and the clinical picture of Goodpasture's syndrome, also to a renal vasculitis.

Treatment and prognosis

In general gold and penicillamine should be discontinued when significant proteinuria develops (more than 0.5 g/24 h). Renal biopsy should be confined to those patients who have deteriorating renal function, or who fail to improve after withdrawal of the drug. Regular monitoring of proteinuria and the glomerular filtration rate are mandatory. No specific immunosuppression is required although supportive measures for the nephrotic syndrome are given as indicated (see Section 20.3).

After cessation of the drug, proteinuria peaks at around a month then gradually disappears; the majority of patients will have clear urine by 1 year and almost all will achieve this by 2 years. Renal function does not deteriorate in uncomplicated cases.

The susceptibility to gold- or penicillamine-induced nephrotoxicity is linked to the major histocompatibility genes: HLA DR3 confers a relative risk of 14.0 to 32.0 for gold-induced nephropathy and 3.2 to 10.0 for D-penicillamine-induced nephropathy. There also appear to be metabolic factors that determine the toxicity of these drugs: individuals with poor sulphoxidation appear to be at increase risk. Given this basis it is not surprising that rechallenge with the same drug at the same dose usually leads to a recurrence of the renal problem, although a lower dose may be tolerated. The dilemma of whether to restart treatment is now less of a problem because of the increasing number of alternative therapies.

Cyclosporin A nephrotoxicity

The renal toxicity of cyclosporin in rheumatoid arthritis is well documented, hence in these patients cyclosporin should be started at a dose of 2.5 mg/kg/day and not exceeding 5 mg/kg/day, with a reduction of cyclosporin if creatinine rises to 130 per cent of baseline. Indeed, so sensitive is the rise in creatinine in patients with rheumatoid arthritis that other measures of renal function are used only to confirm changes.

Non-steroidal anti-inflammatory drugs increase the nephrotoxicity of cyclosporin A, which can lead to chronic irreversible renal failure: this is more common with doses in excess of 5 mg/kg, in patients with pre-existing renal impairment, in elderly patients, and in those treated for more than 6 months. Renal function should be carefully monitored in patients on cyclosporin therapy.

Non-steroidal anti-inflammatory drugs

Non-steroidal anti-inflammatory drugs are potentially nephrotoxic and in patients with rheumatoid arthritis may lead to a reversible reduction in glomerular filtration rate, acute tubular necrosis, an acute interstitial nephritis often with heavy proteinuria, renal papillary necrosis, and chronic tubulointerstitial nephritis.

Glomerulonephritis

The most commonly described glomerulonephritis in rheumatoid arthritis that is not related to drug use is a mesangial proliferative glomerulonephritis, which in many cases is accompanied by IgA deposits (IgA nephropathy). The other major type of glomerulonephritis reported in rheumatoid arthritis is membranous nephropathy.

Renal vasculitis

The clinical spectrum of rheumatoid arthritis includes a systemic necrotizing vasculitis with involvement of blood vessels ranging in size from capillaries to small and medium-sized arteries. The clinical presentation includes nailfold infarcts, a leucocytoclastic vasculitis, a peripheral neuropathy, pericarditis, gastrointestinal infarcts, and renal vasculitis. Renal abnormalities are found in about 25 per cent of patients with rheumatoid vasculitis, usually microscopic haematuria, proteinuria, and renal impairment. Renal histology shows a large vessel renal arteritis and a segmental necrotizing glomerulonephritis with crescent formation (vasculitic glomerulonephritis) (Fig. 5 and Plate 5). Treatment is with prednisolone and cyclophosphamide, usually leading to improvement of renal function.

Renal disease in juvenile chronic arthritis

Renal failure accounts for 38 per cent of deaths in patients with juvenile chronic arthritis. Proteinuria is found in between 3 and 12 per cent and microscopic haematuria in between 3 and 8 per cent of these patients. Nephrotic range proteinuria is commonly due to renal amyloid, found in between 1.2 and 6.7 per cent of patients with juvenile chronic arthritis, whilst haematuria and proteinuria may be due to amyloid or to gold treatment. Interstitial nephritis is also common and may be due to drug treatment. Amyloid is a major problem, accounting for more than 40 per cent of deaths, the majority due to renal failure.

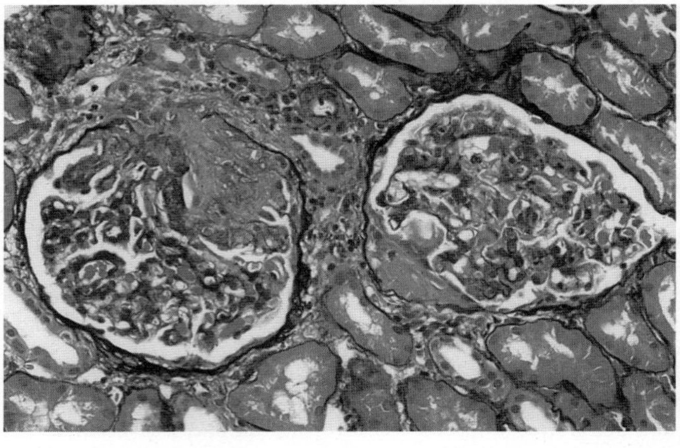

Fig. 5 Vasculitic glomerulonephritis in rheumatoid arthritis. Two glomeruli have sharply defined segmental lesions where there has been disruption of the tuft and partial obliteration of Bowman's space. Periodic acid-methenamine silver staining (×32). (By courtesy of Dr A. J. Howie.) (See also Plate 5.)

Renal disease in primary Sjögren's syndrome

Sjögren's syndrome is characterized by a lymphocytic infiltration of exocrine glands leading to a dry mouth (xerostomia) and dry eyes (keratoconjunctivitis sicca) (see Chapter 18.10.4). It may be primary or secondary to a variety of autoimmune disorders including rheumatoid arthritis, systemic lupus erythematosus, systemic sclerosis, and mixed connective tissue disorder.

Clinically significant renal disease has been reported in about 10 to 25 per cent of patients with Sjögren's syndrome. The most common renal disorder is mild and often subclinical distal renal tubular acidosis, impairment of urinary concentration, and rarely hypokalaemia. Clinical manifestations of these renal tubular disorders include the development of renal calculi, polyuria, and rarely hypokalaemic periodic paralysis. Renal biopsy in these patients shows a tubulointerstitial nephritis with interstitial lymphocytic infiltrates. Glomerulonephritis is rare in primary Sjögren's syndrome, and is most commonly membranoproliferative glomerulonephritis or membranous nephropathy.

Renal disease in mixed connective tissue disease

Some patients with a connective tissue disorder do not fit easily into the accepted definitions of a single disease. In patients with mixed connective tissue disease there is the sequential or concurrent development of the clinical features of systemic lupus erythematosus, systemic sclerosis, polymyositis, and less commonly of rheumatoid arthritis (see Chapter 18.10.2). Renal involvement is found in 10 to 47 per cent of patients with mixed connective tissue disease, the clinical presentation being with asymptomatic proteinuria or haematuria and less commonly with a nephrotic syndrome.

Membranous nephropathy and a mesangial proliferative glomerulonephritis are the most common histological changes, found in 34 and 30 per cent of cases respectively. A focal or diffuse proliferative glomerulonephritis is found in 17 per cent, a mixed lesion with membranous nephropathy in 5 per cent, and in 7 per cent renal histology is normal. Immunofluorescent microscopy of glomeruli in patients with mixed connective tissue disease has shown immunoglobulin and complement deposits; dense deposits are found on electron microscopy.

Treatment of renal disease in mixed connective tissue disease is with steroids, initially in high doses, subsequently tapering to a low maintenance dose over weeks. Treatment of patients with a nephrotic syndrome with high-dose steroids leads to a significant reduction of proteinuria in 62 per cent of cases. Whether those with renal disease resistant to steroids would benefit from the addition of immunosuppressant drugs is not known. Some 14 per cent of patients with mixed connective tissue disease and renal disease develop chronic renal failure.

Further reading

Adu D, *et al.*, eds. (2001). *Rheumatology and the kidney.* Oxford University Press, Oxford.

Lupus nephritis

Austin HA *et al.* (1986). Therapy of lupus nephritis: controlled trial of prednisolone and cytotoxic drugs. *New England Journal of Medicine* **314**, 614–19.

Balow JE *et al.* (1996). Management of lupus nephritis. *Kidney International* **53**, S88–S92.

Bansal VK, Beto JA (1997). Treatment of lupus nephritis: a meta-analysis of clinical trials. *American Journal of Kidney Diseases* **29**, 193–9.

Berden J (1997). Lupus nephritis (nephrology forum). *Kidney International* **52**, 538–58.

Boumpas DT *et al.* (1992). Controlled trial of pulse methylprednisolone versus two regimes of pulse cyclophosphamide in severe lupus nephritis. *The Lancet* **340**, 741–5.

Cameron J (1999). Lupus nephritis. *Journal of the American Society of Nephrology* **10**, 1–17.

Cameron JS (1994). Lupus nephritis in childhood and adolescence. *Pediatric Nephrology* **8**, 230–49.

Donadio JV, Glasscock RJ (1993). Immunosuppressive drug therapy in lupus nephritis. *American Journal of Kidney Diseases* **21**, 239–50.

Fessel WF (1988). Epidemiology of systemic lupus erythematosus. *Rheumatic Disease Clinics of North America* **14**, 15–23.

Lewis EJ *et al.* (1992). A controlled trial of plasmapheresis therapy in severe lupus nephritis. *New England Journal of Medicine* **326**, 1373–9.

Moroni G *et al.* (1996). 'Nephritic flares' are predictors of bad long-term renal outcome in lupus nephritis. *Kidney International* **50**, 2047–53.

Pasquali S *et al.* (1993). Lupus membranous nephropathy: long-term outcome. *Clinical Nephrology* **39**, 175–82.

Tse WY, Adu D (1999). Treatment of glomerulonephritis in systemic disease. In: Pusey CD, ed. *The treatment of glomerulonephritis*, pp 143–76. Kluwer Academic, Dordrecht.

Walport M (1997). The pathogenesis of systemic lupus erythematosus. In: Davison AM *et al.*, eds. *Oxford textbook of clinical nephrology*, vol. 2, pp 917–35. Oxford University Press, Oxford.

Systemic sclerosis

Helfrich D *et al.* (1989). Normotensive renal failure in systemic sclerosis. *Arthritis and Rheumatism* **32**, 1128–34.

Steen V *et al.* (1984). Factors predicting development of renal involvement in progressive systemic sclerosis. *American Journal of Medicine* **76**, 779–86.

Steen V, Medsger TJ (1998). Case-control study of corticosteroids and other drugs that either precipitate or protect from the development of scleroderma renal crisis. *Arthritis and Rheumatism* **41**, 1613–19.

Thurm R, Alexander J (1984). Captopril in the treatment of scleroderma renal crisis. *Archives of Internal Medicine* **144**, 733–5.

Traub Y *et al.* (1983). Hypertension and renal failure (scleroderma renal crisis) in progressive systemic sclerosis: review of a 25-year experience with 68 cases. *Medicine* **62**, 335–52.

Wasner C, Cooke R, Fries J (1978). Successful medical treatment of scleroderma renal crisis. *New England Journal of Medicine* **299**, 873–5.

Rheumatoid arthritis

Adu D *et al.* (1993). Glomerulonephritis in rheumatoid arthritis. *British Journal of Rheumatology* **32**, 1008–11.

Anttila R (1972). Renal involvement in juvenile rheumatoid arthritis. A clinical and histopathological study. *Acta Paediatrica Scandinavica Supplement*, **227**, 1–73.

Boers M *et al.* (1987). Renal findings in rheumatoid arthritis: clinical aspects of 132 necropsies. *Annals of the Rheumatic Diseases* **46**, 658–63.

Boers M (1990). Renal disorders in rheumatoid arthritis. *Seminars in Arthritis and Rheumatism* **20**, 57–68.

Cohen DJ, Appel GB (1992). Cyclosporine: nephrotoxic effects and guidelines for safe use in patients with rheumatoid arthritis. *Seminars in Arthritis and Rheumatism* **21** (suppl. 3), 43–8.

Hall CL *et al.* (1987). The natural course of gold nephropathy: long term study of 21 patients. *British Medical Journal* **295**, 745–84.

Hall CL *et al.* (1988). Natural course of penicillamine nephropathy: a long term study of 33 patients. *British Medical Journal* **296**, 1085–6.

Harper L *et al.* (1997). Focal segmental necrotizing glomerulonephritis in rheumatoid arthritis. *Quarterly Journal of Medicine* **90**, 125–32.

Helin H *et al.* (1986). Mild mesangial glomerulopathy, a frequent finding in rheumatoid arthritis patients with haematuria or proteinuria. *Nephron* **42**, 224–30.

Honkanen E *et al.* (1987). Membranous glomerulonephritis in rheumatoid arthritis not related to gold or D-penicillamine therapy: a report of four cases and review of the literature. *Clinical Nephrology* **27**, 87–93.

Kuznetsky KA *et al.* (1986). Necrotizing glomerulonephritis in rheumatoid arthritis. *Clinical Nephrology* **26**, 257–64.

Table 1 Pathological classification of diseases with tissue deposition or precipitation of monoclonal Ig-related material

Organized			Non-organized (granular)	
Crystals	**Fibrillar**	**Microtubular**	**MIDD (Randall type)**	**Other**
Myeloma cast nephropathy	Light-chain amyloidosis	Cryoglobulinaemia kidney	LCDD	Crescentic GN
Fanconi's syndrome	Non-amyloid fibrillary GN	Immunotactoid GN	LHCDD	Waldenström's macroglobulinaemia
Other			HCDD	

Abbreviations: GN, glomerulonephritis; MIDD, monoclonal immunoglobulin deposition disease; LCDD, LHCDD, HCDD, light-chain, light- and heavy-chain, heavy-chain, deposition disease.

Landewe RB *et al.* (1996). Longterm low dose cyclosporine in patients with rheumatoid arthritis: renal function loss without structural nephropathy. *Journal of Rheumatology* **23**, 61–4.

Maezawa A *et al.* (1994). Combined treatment with cyclophosphamide and prednisolone can induce remission in a patient with nephrotic syndrome with amyloidosis associated with rheumatoid arthritis. *Clinical Nephrology* **42**, 30–2.

Rodriguez F *et al.* (1996) Renal biopsy findings and followup of renal function in rheumatoid arthritis patients treated with cyclosporin A. *Arthritis and Rheumatism* **39**, 1491–8.

Sandler DP *et al.* (1989). Analgesic use and chronic renal disease. *New England Journal of Medicine* **320**, 1238–43.

Scott DGI, Bacon PA, Tribe CR (1981). Systemic rheumatoid vasculitis: a clinical and laboratory study of 50 cases. *Medicine* **60**, 288–97.

Sellars L *et al.* (1983). Renal biopsy appearances in rheumatoid disease. *Clinical Nephrology* **20**, 114–20.

Sjögren's syndrome

Moutsopoulos H *et al.* (1978). Immune complex glomerulonephritis in sicca syndrome. *American Journal of Medicine* **64**, 955–60.

Moutsopoulos H *et al.* (1991). Nephrocalcinosis in Sjögren's syndrome. *Journal of Internal Medicine* **230**, 187–91.

Shearn M, Tu WH (1965). Nephrogenic diabetes insipidus and other disorders of renal tubular function in Sjögren's syndrome. *American Journal of Medicine* **39**, 312–18.

Talal N, Zisman E, Schur P (1968). Renal tubular acidosis, glomerulonephritis and immune complex glomerulonephritis in Sjögren's syndrome. *Arthritis and Rheumatism* **11**, 774.

Mixed connective tissue disease

Kitridou RC *et al.* (1986). Renal involvement in mixed connective tissue disease; a longitudinal clinicopathologic study. *Seminars in Arthritis and Rheumatism* **16**, 135–45.

20.10.5 Renal involvement in plasma cell dyscrasias, immunoglobulin-based amyloidoses, and fibrillary glomerulopathies, lymphomas, and leukaemias

P. Ronco

Introduction

Plasma cell dyscrasias are characterized by uncontrolled proliferation of a single clone of B cells, usually with plasma cell differentiation, that is responsible for the secretion in blood of a monoclonal immunoglobulin (**Ig**) or Ig subunit. This monoclonal component can become deposited in tissues, and the recognized spectrum of renal diseases in which there is deposition or precipitation of Ig-related material has expanded dramatically in recent years.

These conditions can be classified into two categories on the basis of their ultrastructural appearances (Table 1). Those with organized deposits include diseases with crystal formation, mainly myeloma cast nephropathy; diseases with fibril formation, mainly light-chain amyloidosis; and diseases with microtubule formation, including cryoglobulinaemia kidney and immunotactoid glomerulonephritis. A second category of diseases is characterized by the presence of non-organized granular electron-dense deposits made of light and/or heavy chains along the basement membranes of many tissues, most importantly the kidney. First described by Randall and associates, they are named monoclonal immunoglobulin deposition diseases. It is now well established that the spectrum of plasma cell dyscrasia-related renal complications is due to intrinsic properties of the monoclonal component.

Except for myeloma cast nephropathy, diagnosis often relies on careful analysis of a biopsy specimen taken from the kidney, which should systematically include immunohistochemical studies with specific antibodies and also electron microscopy in all ambiguous cases. Since most of these patients will develop renal failure, it is essential to identify the underlying plasma cell dyscrasia because appropriate treatments may halt the extension of visceral deposits, and even induce their regression. Except in patients with myeloma cast nephropathy, who usually present with a high-mass myeloma, 'malignancy' more often results from life-threatening visceral deposits than from the Ig-secreting clone itself.

Renal involvement in Ig light-chain amyloidosis

Definition and epidemiology

Amyloidosis is a general term for a family of diseases defined by morphological criteria and characterized by deposition in extracellular spaces of a proteinaceous material that stains with Congo red and is metachromatic. Amyloid deposits are composed of a felt-like array of 10-nm wide rigid, linear, aggregated fibrils of indefinite length with a β-pleated sheet configuration. They occur in a variety of conditions including Alzheimer's disease and other neurodegenerative disorders, tumoural and inflammatory diseases, and plasma cell dyscrasias. The various types of amyloidosis differ essentially by the nature of the precursor protein that yields the main component of fibrils, and are classified accordingly. (See Chapter 11.12.4 for further discussion.)

Light-chain amyloidosis has become the most frequent form of amyloidosis with renal involvement. Amyloid deposits are found in approximately 10 per cent of myeloma patients, their prevalence reaching 20 per cent in those with pure light-chain myeloma. (Fig. 1 and Plate 1)

Clinical presentation

The main clinical features of light-chain amyloidosis at presentation are fatigue (62 per cent) and weight loss (52 per cent), followed by purpura (15 per cent), pain (5 per cent), and gross bleeding (3 per cent). Hepatomegaly is found in 24 per cent of patients, and macroglossia in 9 per cent. A palpable spleen and lymphadenopathy can also be found.

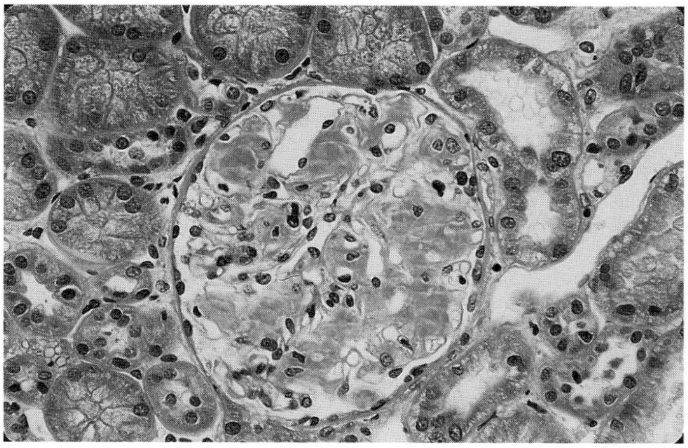

(a)

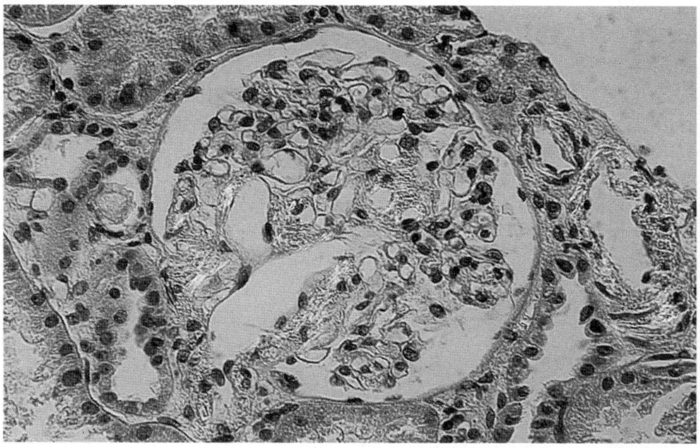

(b)

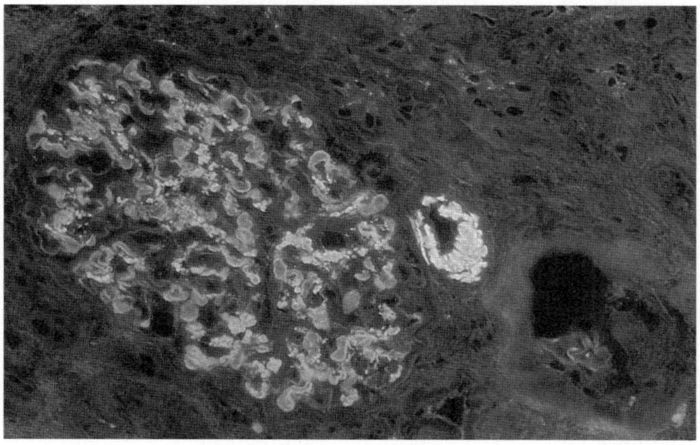

(c)

Fig. 1 Light-chain amyloidosis. (a) Amyloid deposits in a renal glomerulus (Masson's trichrome stain, ×312). (b) Congo red stain. Apple-green/yellow dichroism under polarized light (×312). (c) Immunofluorescence with anti-λ antibody. Note glomerular and arteriolar deposits (×312). (From Béatrice Mougenot's personal collection.) (See also Plate 1.)

Proteinuria is the usual symptom of renal amyloidosis, detected in 55 per cent of patients at presentation and often progressing to a severe nephrotic syndrome, which can be complicated by renal vein thrombosis. Haematuria is uncommon, and when present should prompt examination for a bleeding lesion of the urinary tract. Progressive decline in renal function usually occurs, leading finally to endstage renal failure. In those rare patients in whom renal tubulointerstitial deposits predominate, renal failure may progress without a nephrotic stage, and in some of these cases renal tubular dysfunction may be the presenting problem, including Fanconi syndrome, renal tubular acidosis, or even nephrogenic diabetes insipidus. Hypertension is uncommon but may develop concomitantly with renal failure. The kidneys are generally of normal size or large, even when renal function is impaired.

Light-chain amyloidosis can infiltrate almost any organ and thus be responsible for a wide variety of clinical manifestations. It frequently involves the tongue, gastrointestinal tract, peripheral neural system, carpal tunnel, heart, and skin. Purpuric macules of the superior eyebrow are very typical of light-chain amyloidosis.

Diagnosis

Light-chain amyloidosis should be suspected when the clinical manifestations described above are associated with a monoclonal component. Monoclonal light chains can be detected by immunoelectrophoresis of urine in around 73 per cent of cases, with the λ isotype being twice as frequent as the _. With the use of more sensitive techniques (immunofixation), a monoclonal Ig is found in the serum and/or the urine in nearly 90 per cent of patients, but still not in all of them. Light-chain amyloidosis is, however, always the result of the proliferation of a plasma cell clone. Fifty six per cent of patients with light-chain amyloidosis have an increased number of plasma cells in the bone marrow, and 15 per cent of them have a true myeloma.

In all cases, diagnosis of light-chain amyloidosis should be established by taking a biopsy specimen from a superficial organ including skin, salivary glands, gum, or by aspiration biopsy of abdominal fat. These biopsies should be performed before biopsies of rectal mucosa (which should include vessels of the submucosa where amyloid deposits usually start) and/or of kidney because of the risk of bleeding complications due to factor X deficiency or amyloid infiltration of vascular walls. After Congo red staining, amyloid deposits appear faintly red and show the characteristic apple-green birefringence under polarized light. Metachromasia is also observed with crystal violet, which stains the deposits in red. In the kidney, the earliest lesions are located in the mesangium, along the glomerular basement membrane, and in the blood vessels. Because there are specific diagnostic and therapeutic strategies depending on the type of protein deposited within tissues, immunofluorescence with specific antisera including anti-κ and anti-λ light chains should be performed routinely.

Treatment

Light-chain amyloidosis is a wasting disease with a poor outcome irrespective of the underlying haematological abnormality. Median survival is 18 months in patients treated with chemotherapy (melphalan and prednisolone) and less than 9 months in those given colchicine only. Among patients with the nephrotic syndrome, a normal serum creatinine and no echocardiographic evidence of heart amyloidosis are associated with a higher response rate (39 per cent) to chemotherapy, as defined by a 50 per cent reduction in proteinuria without an increase in serum creatinine.

The results of chemotherapy in amyloidosis are difficult to document because there is no easy way to measure the amount of amyloid present. Resolution of the nephrotic syndrome does not necessarily reflect the disappearance of amyloid deposits, and the progressive deposition of amyloid can occur in the presence of improved clinical and laboratory findings. Scintigraphy after the injection of ^{123}I-labelled SAP may be helpful for monitoring the extent of systemic amyloidosis, but it is available in a rather limited number of centers (see Chapter 11.12.4). The effects of chemotherapy are better evaluated by the level of circulating monoclonal immunoglobulin and by the daily urinary excretion of Ig light chain.

Amyloid nephropathy requires symptomic management of the nephrotic syndrome and of renal failure. Patients in endstage renal disease are candidates for regular dialysis and/or kidney transplantation. Their prognosis is compromised by the risks of extension of extrarenal deposition, especially to the heart, and by recurrence of amyloidosis in the graft, although the latter is uncommon.

Based on promising results in myeloma patients, high-dose melphalan treatment with autologous bone marrow or blood stem cell transplantation is being attempted in light-chain amyloidosis with interesting results. It should be applied in appropriately designed trials in centres with special expertise.

Renal involvement in myeloma

Definition and epidemiology

Renal failure is one of the major complications of myeloma, found at presentation in 20 per cent of patients and occurring in 50 per cent of patients during the course of the disease. It is mostly due to cast nephropathy, although other forms of renal disease can occur as well, including light-chain amyloidosis (10 per cent of myeloma patients), light-chain deposition disease (5 per cent), fanconi syndrome, infiltration of renal interstitium by plasma cells, calcium precipitation, and renal infection. Myeloma cast nephropathy is due both to alterations in tubule cells induced by massive reabsorption of light chains in proximal tubule cells and to cast formation involving light chains and Tamm–Horsfall protein in the distal tubule. The risk of developing renal failure is twice as high in patients with pure light-chain myeloma, and five to six times greater in patients with light-chain proteinuria of more than 2.0 g/day compared with those with proteinuria of less than 0.05 g/day.

Clinical presentation

Myeloma cast nephropathy usually presents as acute or subacute renal failure, often revealing myeloma with a high tumour burden (found in 70 to 80 per cent of myeloma patients with renal failure). Common triggering factors include hypercalcaemia, dehydration, infection, use of toxic compounds including radiocontrast media, non-steroidal anti-inflammatory drugs, and angiotensin converting enzyme inhibitors, all of which reduce renal perfusion, especially in those who are dehydrated.

Renal failure induced by cast nephropathy is remarkably silent. The clinical and urinary syndrome is characterized by non-specific signs including weakness, weight loss, bone pain, and signs of infection, all due to myeloma, and by urinary excretion of a monoclonal light chain. It must be emphasized that urinary dipsticks do not detect the light chain, which is measured by quantitative tests of proteinuria. Light chain accounts for more than 70 per cent of total proteinuria by urine electrophoresis.

Tubular dysfunction is rarely a presenting symptom. fanconi syndrome due to proximal tubule impairment may result from intratubular crystalline inclusions of _ light chains. This can lead to osteomalacia and may precede the diagnosis of myeloma by several years.

Diagnosis

Diagnosis of myeloma cast nephropathy relies on the detection of a urinary monoclonal light chain in patients with subacute or acute renal failure of apparently unknown origin. In those patients with pure light-chain myeloma, diagnosis can be suspected before urinalysis on the basis of dramatic hypogammaglobulinaemia detected by serum electrophoresis.

A renal biopsy should not be performed routinely in patients with a presumed diagnosis of myeloma cast nephropathy. It can, however, be useful for a number of reasons: firstly, to analyse tubulointerstitial lesions and allow diagnosis and treatment of other potential causes of renal impairment in those with multiple possible precipitating factors (infection, drugs, etc.). Secondly, to establish the diagnosis of Fanconi syndrome. Thirdly, to identify glomerular lesions in patients with albuminuria over 1 g/day and no evidence of amyloid deposits in 'peripheral' biopsies. Myeloma casts have unique characteristics, including a 'fractured' appearance due to crystal formation, polychromatism upon staining with Masson's trichrome, and the presence of multinucleated giant cells. They are consistantly associated with dramatic epithelial tubular lesions.

Treatment

The first aim of treatment is to prevent or retard renal impairment in all patients with myeloma, most particularly those with light-chain myeloma, by prevention of dehydration, maintenance of a high urinary output and urine alkalinization, avoidance of nephrotoxic drugs, and control of hypercalcaemia (if present). hypercalcaemia requires correction of salt and water deficit, steroids, and/or bisphosphonates, which are potent inhibitors of osteoclast activity. Renal failure of recent onset should be promptly and vigorously managed. Adequate administration of salt and water and forced alkaline diuresis (which may help to prevent intratubular light-chain precipitation) are required when urine output persists. Plasma exchange has been advocated to remove light chains more rapidly, but its value is unproven. In patients with oliguria, dialysis should be provided early.

Most patients with overt myeloma cast nephropathy should be given chemotherapy to reduce the production of monoclonal light chains, which is justified because partial or complete recovery of renal failure occurs in about half of patients. Only patients with refractory haematological disease should be given purely symptomatic treatment. However, median survival in those with progressive renal failure (about 2 years) remains shorter than that of patients without renal failure (3 to 4 years). Two main options should be discussed. Firstly, conventional chemotherapy regimens can induce remissions, but they have not markedly lengthened median survival. The melphalan–prednisone regimen remains the first choice for chemotherapy, but its drawbacks are slow antitumour action and the necessity of reducing melphalan doses because the drug is renally eliminated. Regimens including vincristine and doxorubicin induce earlier remission and are safer in those with renal failure since the drugs are metabolized in the liver. Secondly, in younger patients (those aged less than 65), high-dose chemotherapy with the support of autologous bone marrow or blood stem cell transplantation should systematically be considered because substantially longer survival can be achieved.

In patients with irreversible renal failure and in those whose renal function deteriorates later, regular dialysis may be indicated if the clinical condition and bone lesions allow it. Recombinant human erythropoietin may be helpful to correct anaemia, although very high doses (and therefore great expense) are likely to be needed.

Light-chain and heavy-chain deposition disease

Definition and epidemiology

It has been known since the late 1950s that non-amyloidotic forms of glomerular disease resembling the lesion of diabetic glomerulosclerosis could occur in multiple myeloma. Randall and associates recognized the presence of monoclonal light chains in these lesions in 1976, defining light-chain deposition disease. Monoclonal heavy chains can also be found in association with light chains (defining light- and heavy-chain deposition disease) or occasionally in the absence of light chains (heavy-chain deposition disease). In clinical and pathological terms light-chain deposition disease, light- and heavy-chain deposition disease, and heavy-chain deposition disease are similar and hence are also collectively referred to as monoclonal immunoglobulin deposition disease. They differ from amyloidosis by the lack of affinity for Congo red and fibrillar organization. Monoclonal immunoglobulin deposition disease occurs in a wide range of ages (31 to 79 years) with a slight male preponderance. Myeloma accounts for only 45 per cent of cases, but as in amyloidosis a monoclonal plasma cell proliferation can be found in virtually all patients by immunofluorescence examination of the bone marrow with specific antiheavy- and antilight-chain antisera.

Clinical presentation

Light-chain deposition disease is a systemic disease with deposition of Ig light chains along basement membranes in most tissues. However, deposition in tissues other than the kidney is often (but not always) totally asymptomatic and renal involvement dominates clinical presentation, mainly in the form of proteinuria and renal failure. In 23 to 67 per cent of patients with light-chain deposition disease, albuminuria is associated with the nephrotic syndrome. In 25 per cent, the urinary albumin output is less than 1 g/day, and these patients mainly exhibit a tubulointerstitial syndrome. Haematuria is more frequent (44 per cent) than one would expect for a nephropathy in which cell proliferation is usually modest. Renal failure is remarkable for its high prevalence (89 per cent), early appearance, and severity, irrespective of urinary albumin output. Hypertension occurs in about half of the patients.

Diagnosis

Diagnosis of monoclonal immunoglobulin deposition disease relies on the association of the clinical features described above with the finding of a monoclonal Ig component in the serum and/or the urine. Since this component cannot be detected even by immunofixation in 15 to 30 per cent of patients, the diagnosis of monoclonal immunoglobulin deposition disease is often made by renal biopsy. In virtually all patients with this condition tubular lesions are characterized by the deposition of a periodic acid-schiff positive ribbon-like material along the basement membrane. This is usually associated with a marked interstitial fibrosis and nodular glomerulosclerosis (found in two-thirds of patients with light-chain deposition disease and in all patients with heavy-chain deposition disease reported so far). Nodules are composed of membrane-like material with nuclei at the periphery (Fig. 2 and Plate 2). A key step in the diagnosis of the various forms of monoclonal immunoglobulin deposition disease is immunofluorescence examination of the biopsy specimen, revealing evidence of monotypic light- and/or heavy-chain deposits along glomerular and tubular basement membranes in all cases. By contrast with light-chain amyloidosis, the κ isotype is two to three times more frequent than the λ one. In those patients with heavy-chain deposition disease, a deletion of the first constant domain of the heavy chain can invariably be demonstrated by immunofluorescence analysis of the kidney specimen with specific antisera. Finally, non-fibrillar granular electron-dense deposits are visible by electron microscopy along tubular basement membranes and in glomerular lesions.

Treatment

The natural history of monoclonal immunoglobulin deposition disease is more uncertain than that of light-chain amyloidosis because extrarenal deposits can be totally asymptomatic or cause severe organ damage, including severe heart failure and occasionally hepatic insufficiency and portal hypertension. The 5-year actuarial rates for patient survival and survival free of endstage renal failure (with chemotherapy) are 70 and 39 per cent respectively.

Patients with monoclonal immunoglobulin deposition disease and myeloma should be treated with conventional chemotherapy if they are over 60 years of age, but intensive therapy with blood stem cell autografting should be discussed in younger patients (see above). As in light-chain amyloidosis, deposited light chains have disappeared in isolated instances after intensive therapy. The correct treatment for those without myeloma is uncertain, the rarity of the disease meaning that there are no controlled trials. A pragmatic approach is to use alkylating agents plus prednisolone in those with moderate but rapidly progressive renal insufficiency in an endeavour to prevent progression to endstage renal failure, but not to treat those with severe renal failure unless there are significant extrarenal complications. Recurrence of the disease has usually been observed in the few patients who have received renal transplants.

Non-amyloid fibrillary and immunotactoid glomerulopathies

Definition and epidemiology

Fibrillary glomerulonephritis and immunotactoid glomerulopathy are recently described entities characterized, respectively, by fibrillar and microtubular deposits in the mesangium and the glomerular capillary loops. These deposits do not have a β-pleated sheet organization and are readily distinguishable from amyloid by the larger thickness of fibrils and the lack of Congo red staining. Whether they are totally distinct entities remains the subject of considerable debate. However, the distinction between the two diseases may be of great clinical and pathophysiological

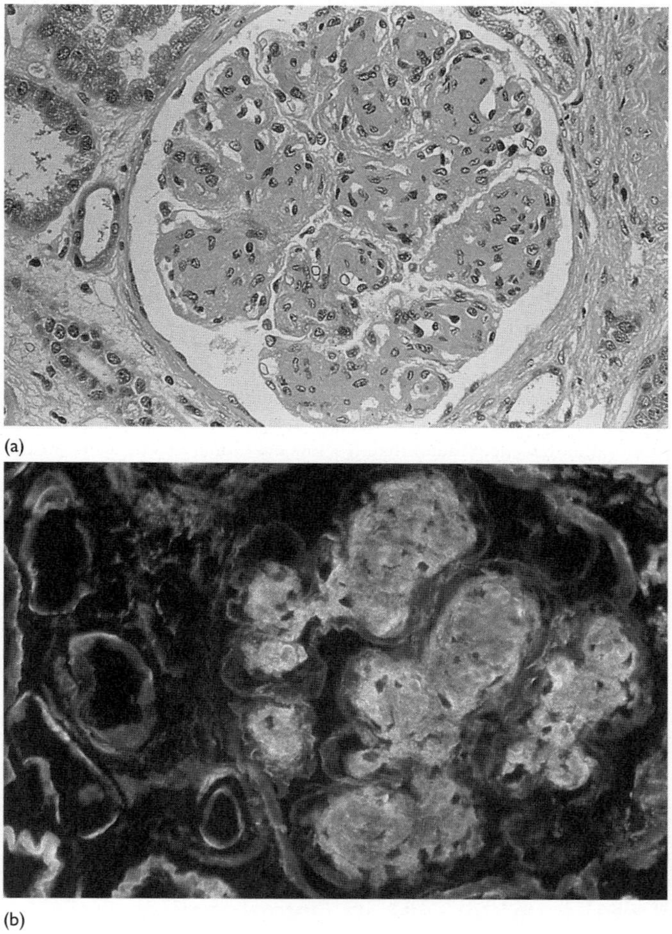

(a) (b)

Fig. 2 Monoclonal immunoglobulin deposition disease. (a) Typical nodular glomerulosclerosis. Note the membrane-like material in the centre of the nodules and nuclei at the periphery. Some glomerular capillaries show double contours. Note also thickening of the basement membrane of atrophic tubules (Masson's trichrome stain, ×312). (b) Bright staining of tubular basement membranes and mesangial nodules and, to a lesser extent, of glomerular basement membrane with anti-κ antibody in a case of κ light-chain deposition disease (immunofluorescence, ×312). (See also Plate 2.)

interest in the context of plasma cell dyscrasias because monotypic deposits are detected in 50 to 80 per cent of immunotactoid glomerulopathies, whilst they are found in fewer than 20 per cent of fibrillary glomerulopathies.

The prevalence of glomerulopathy with non-amyloid deposition of fibrillary or tubular material in a non-transplant adult biopsy population is around 1 per cent, but this is almost certainly an underestimate because insufficient attention is given to atypical reactions with histochemical stains for amyloid and the fact that most specimens are not examined by electron microscopy. The age range extends from 10 to 80 years with a peak incidence between 40 and 60 years.

Clinical presentation

The usual presentation is with the nephrotic syndrome and microscopic haematuria, often in the setting of chronic lymphocytic leukaemia or lymphoma.

Diagnosis

Diagnosis relies entirely on analysis of the renal biopsy specimen by immunofluorescence microscopy with antilight-chain antibodies and by electron microscopy. In immunotactoid glomerulopathy this reveals either membranous glomerulonephritis (often associated with segmental mesangial proliferation) or lobular membranoproliferative glomerulonephritis. Immunofluorescence shows coarse granular deposits of IgG and IgC3 along capillary basement membranes and in mesangial areas. Although monotypic deposits are common, a circulating monoclonal Ig is detected in only a minority of patients. Electron microscopy shows immunotactoid glomerulopathy to be remarkable for the presence of organized deposits of large, thick-walled microtubules, usually greater than 30 nm in diameter, at times arranged in parallel arrays. When immunotactoid glomerulopathy occurs in the setting of chronic lymphocytic leukaemia or related B-cell lymphoma, inclusions showing the same microtubular organization and containing the same IgG subclass and light-chain type as the renal deposits are then often detected in the cytoplasm of leukaemic lymphocytes in the blood (Fig. 4).

Mesangial proliferation and membranoproliferative glomerulonephritis are the commonest lesions observed in fibrillary glomerulonephritis. Immunofluorescence studies mainly show polyclonal IgG deposits (of the $\gamma 4$ isotype in one series). Electron microscopy shows the fibrils to be randomly arranged with a diameter varying between 12 and 22 nm.

Infection wuth hepatitis c virus has recently been reported in patients with non-amyloid fibrillary glomerulonephritis and immunotactoid glomerulopathy.

Treatment

In patients with immunotactoid glomerulopathy and monotypic immunoglobulin deposits, especially in those with chronic lymphocytic leukaemia, corticosteroids and/or chemotherapy are associated with partial or complete remission of the nephrotic syndrome, parallel with improvement of the haemopathy. More variable results are obtained with these treatments in patients with crescentic fibrillary glomerulonephritis. Recurrence of these diseases has been reported in patients receiving a renal allograft.

Renal involvement in cryoglobulinaemia

Definition and epidemiology

Cryoglobulinaemia is a pathological condition in which the blood contains immunoglobulins that precipitate on cooling (4 °C) and resolubilize on warming (37 °C). according to Brouet's classification, there are three types of cryoglobulinaemia defined by their composition. Renal involvement is observed mainly in patients with mixed type II cryoglobulinaemia involving a monoclonal IgM (most often including a κ light chain) with rheumatoid factor activity and a polyclonal IgG. Type II cryoglobulinaemia can be associated with overt lymphoproliferative disorders of the B-cell lineage, although in many cases no underlying haemopathy is found. Therefore, this type of cryoglobulinaemia has long been referred to as essential mixed cryoglobulinaemia (Fig. 3 and Plate 3).

Viral infections may trigger the formation of cryoglobulin. Whereas hepatitis B and Epstein–Barr virus infections have been implicated in the past, the role of hepatitis C virus infection is now recognized to be an important factor in the pathogenesis of type II cryoglobulinaemia. Antibodies to hepatitis C virus and hepatitis C virus RNA are frequently found in the sera of patients with type II cryoglobulinaemia, probably explaining the uneven geographical distribution of mixed cryoglobulinaemias, which predominate in southern Europe where hepatitis C infection is more prevalent.

The condition is commonest in adults in the fifth and the sixth decades of life, with a slight female predominance.

Clinical presentation

Renal disease most often occurs in patients with a long history of cryoglobulinaemia-related vasculitis symptoms including palpable purpura (70 per cent), arthralgias (50 per cent), fatigue, Raynaud's phenomenon, peripheral neuropathy (22 per cent), and hepatic involvement.

The renal disease may present as an acute nephritic syndrome (in 20 to 30 per cent of cases) with gross haematuria, heavy proteinuria, hypertension, and renal failure of sudden onset, sometimes with oliguria (5 per cent of cases). The pathological finding in these patients is membranoproliferative glomerulonephritis with the presence of numerous intraluminal thrombi and/or necrotic vasculitic lesions. Remission may occur spontaneously or during therapy, with relapses following in up to 20 per cent of cases.

Most patients with mixed cryoglobulinaemia (55 per cent) have an indolent and protracted renal course, presenting with proteinuria, haematuria, and hypertension. The usual renal lesion in this context is membranoproliferative glomerulonephritis, with some of the peculiarities described above.

Nephrotic syndrome affects another 20 per cent of patients. Arterial hypertension is observed in more than 80 per cent of patients at the time of onset of renal disease. Endstage uraemia develops in fewer than 10 per cent of patients.

Diagnosis

Mixed type II cryoglobulinaemia should be suspected in patients with the clinical picture described above, an IgM rheumatoid factor, and a very low serum C4 fraction and total haemolytic activity of complement. In this context a careful search for the presence of cryoglobulin must be made, requiring that a blood sample from a fasting patient should be placed in warm water and taken promptly to the laboratory, which needs to be forewarned that such a sample will arrive.

Cryoglobulinaemia-related membranoproliferative glomerulonephritis usually shows several distinctive histological features, including massive subendothelial deposits filling the capillary lumen and forming so-called thrombi, and dramatic infiltration by leucocytes, mainly monocytes. The thrombi are brightly stained with anti-μ and anti-κ antibodies and present a microtubular crystalline structure similar to that of the cryoprecipitate. These glomerular changes may be associated with acute vasculitis of the small and medium-sized arteries (33 per cent) and lymphocytic infiltrates in interstitium. Crescentic extracapillary proliferation is rare and always limited.

Treatment

The best treatment is not firmly established because the course of the disease is unpredictable and acute exacerbations may remit spontaneously. High-dose steroids, cyclophosphamide, and plasma exchanges are used in the more severe cases, particularly those with signs of systemic vasculitis. The place of antihepatitis C virus therapy including interferon-α and vidarabine has still to be evaluated. These antiviral drugs may be useful for controlling virus replication enhanced by steroids and/or immunosuppressive agents. Hypertension needs to be carefully controlled because cardiovascular complications are the major causes of death.

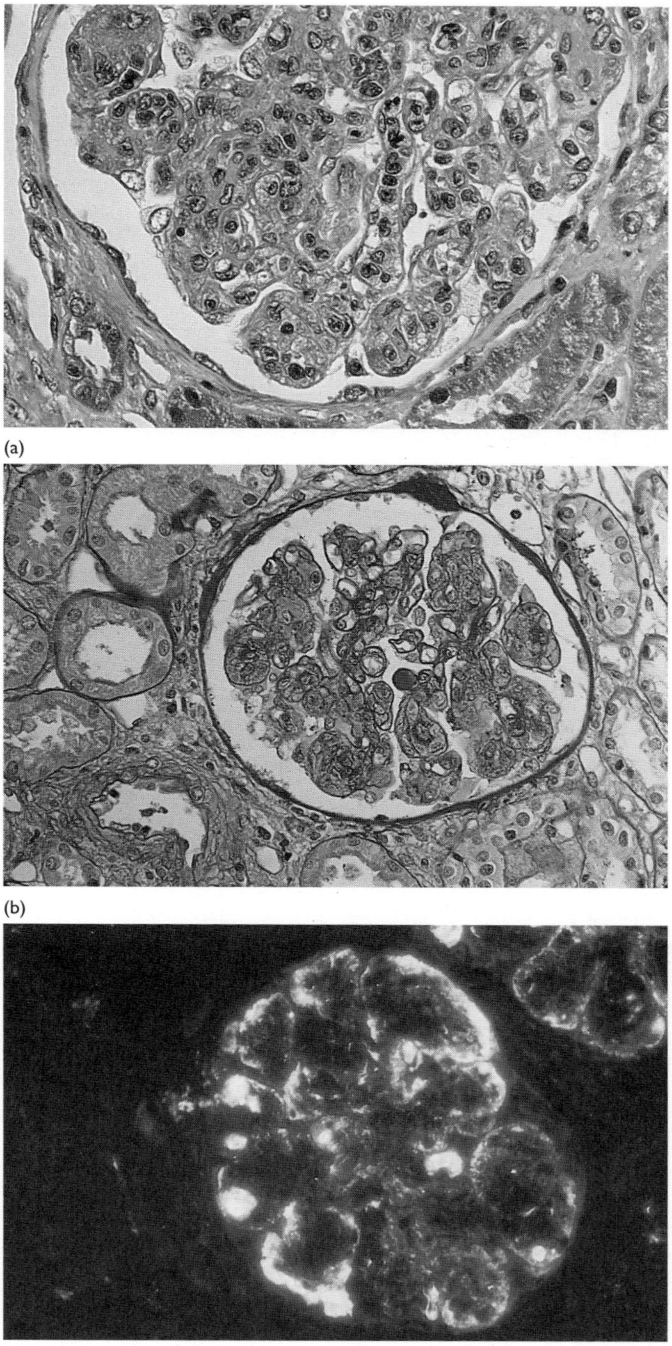

(a) (b) (c)

Fig. 3 Cryoglobulinaemic glomerulonephritis. (a) The glomerulus shows a marked endocapillary hypercellularity with massive infiltration of mononuclear leucocytes (Masson's trichrome stain, ×500). (b) Frequent double-contour aspect, and intraluminal thrombi (periodic acid-Schiff stain, ×312). (c) thrombi and segments of glomerular basement membrane are brightly stained with anti-IgM antibody (immunofluorescence, ×312). (From Béatrice Mougenot's personal collection.) (See also Plate 3.)

Renal involvement in Waldenström's macroglobulinaemia

A glomerulonephritis with intracapillary thrombi of IgM is rare, but is almost specific for Waldenström's macroglobulinaemia. It is characterized by periodic acid-Schiff positive, non-congophilic endomembranous deposits in a variable number of capillary loops, which are sometimes so large as to occlude the capillary lumen either partially or completely, thus forming thrombi. There may also be a B-cell interstitial infiltrate. Renal presentation is with proteinuria or renal impairment. Some patients have a cryoglobulin, in others the amount of circulating IgM seems to be higher than that in patients with Waldenström's without obvious renal involvement, or with amyloidosis, leading to the suggestion that hyperviscosity is important in pathogenesis of the renal lesion. The haemopathy is treated on its own merits (see Section 22). In those with acute renal failure there is anecdotal experience that plasma exchange can be effective in restoring renal function at least temporarily, allowing time for other treatments to be applied.

Renal involvement in lymphomas and leukaemias

Renal complications of lymphomas and leukaemias are summarized in Table 2. Patients with unexplained renal failure should undergo ultrasound examination of the kidney, which should be arranged as a matter of urgency, to identify either enlarged kidneys due to tumour infiltration or hydronephrosis. The presence of heavy albuminuria in this setting is suggestive of paraneoplastic glomerulopathy.

Hodgkin's disease and non-Hodgkin's lymphoma

Glomerulonephritis is a rare complication of lymphoma, most often described in patients with Hodgkin's disease, of whom 0.4 per cent have minimal change disease and 0.1 per cent have AA amyloidosis. This low incidence of amyloidosis in patients with Hodgkin's disease is most likely attributable to modern treatment protocols that induce a rapid remission of the haemopathy. Hodgkin's lymphoma-related minimal change disease shows features of a paraneoplastic glomerulopathy: the nephrotic syndrome usually appears early, revealing the haemopathy in about one-half of the cases; it rapidly disappears after effective treatment of Hodgkin's disease and it usually relapses simultaneously with the haemopathy. Cases of crescentic glomerulonephritis with rapidly progressive renal failure due to anti-glomerular basement antibodies have also been reported.

There are about 50 reports of glomerulonephritis in patients with non-Hodgkin's lymphoma, including both T- and B-cell proliferations. In these

Table 2 Renal complications of lymphomas and leukaemias

Mechanical complications
Infiltration of renal parenchyma
Obstructive uropathy (retroperitoneal fibrosis)
Compression of renal artery or vein
Electrolyte disturbances and disseminated intravascular coagulation
Glomerulopathies (including amyloidosis)
Treatment-induced complications
Tumour lysis syndrome
Lithiasis and urate nephropathy
Radiation nephropathy
Drug-induced toxic nephropathy
Thrombotic microangiopathy and mesangiolysis

conditions, unlike in Hodgkin's lymphoma, minimal change disease is uncommon, and membranoproliferative glomerulonephritis and necrotizing crescentic glomerulonephritis with or without vasculitis are the most frequent lesions. Some cases are associated with type II cryoglobulinaemia or immunotactoid glomerulopathies with monotypic immune deposits. In other cases the association between non-Hodgkin's lymphoma and renal involvement may be coincidental. Presenting renal symptoms are nephrotic syndrome and/or renal impairment. Full remission of these symptoms can be achieved in some patients by aggressive therapy of the lymphoma.

Chronic lymphocytic leukaemia and low-grade B-cell lymphoma

These haemopathies, particularly chronic lymphocytic leukaemia, have been reported in association with glomerular disease in about 50 cases. Most commonly the nephropathy, usually manifesting as nephrotic syndrome with impaired renal function, and the leukaemia are detected simultaneously. The most frequent glomerular disease is membranoproliferative glomerulonephritis with or without cryoglobulinaemia. In the absence of cryoglobulinaemia, a molecular link can be established between the haemopathy and the glomerulopathy when monotypic Ig deposits are found in the glomerulus, which can occur even in the absence of detectable circulating M component. Some of these patients present with typical immunotactoid glomerulopathy or monoclonal immunoglobulin deposition disease (Fig. 4 and Plate 4). Improvement of the nephropathy after treatment for the leukaemia is well described.

Acute leukaemias

Disseminated intravascular coagulation has been associated with acute progranulocytic leukaemia. Other renal complications are commonly due to treatment, most particularly the tumour lysis syndrome (see below).

Tumour lysis syndrome

Tumour lysis syndrome is a life-threatening metabolic emergency. It occurs in patients with haemopathies involving a high cell turnover, mostly at the onset of chemotherapy and/or upon radiation therapy. The ensuing massive cytolysis generates high levels of uric acid, phosphate, potassium, and xanthine (especially in patients treated with allopurinol), with a concomitant decrease in serum calcium concentration. Oliguric or anuric acute renal failure may occur, especially in those who are dehydrated or have preexisting impairment of kidney function. This acute renal failure is mostly the consequence of acute precipitation of urate crystals in the tubular lumen, but in those with a moderate increase in uric acid concentration, the role of severe hyperphosphataemia causing precipitation of calcium/phosphate complexes in renal interstitium and the tubular system has been assumed.

Prevention is better than cure and intensive monitoring is mandatory to prevent the development and the consequences of this syndrome. Patients at risk of the tumour lysis syndrome should be vigorously hydrated with 0.9 per cent saline (assuming normal or near normal baseline renal function, and with care taken to avoid inducing pulmonary oedema) before receiving chemotherapy or radiotherapy. Some physicians would also pretreat with allopurinol, but this does carry the risk of formation of xanthine nephropathy/stones due to accumulation of xanthine and cannot be generally recommended. Urine alkalinization should be avoided because it increases the risk of phosphate precipitation. In those who develop tumour lysis syndrome but are passing urine, vigorous hydration with 0.9 per cent saline to encourage urine output is required, with close clinical monitoring to prevent iatrogenic fluid overload should the urine output drop. Administration of urate oxidase has been advocated as a treatment for acute hyperuricaemia, but experience is very limited and there is no therapeutic formulation that is widely available. Patients with severe acute renal failure should be treated with haemodialysis, which allows recovery of renal function following the reduction of serum phosphate and serum uric acid concentrations.

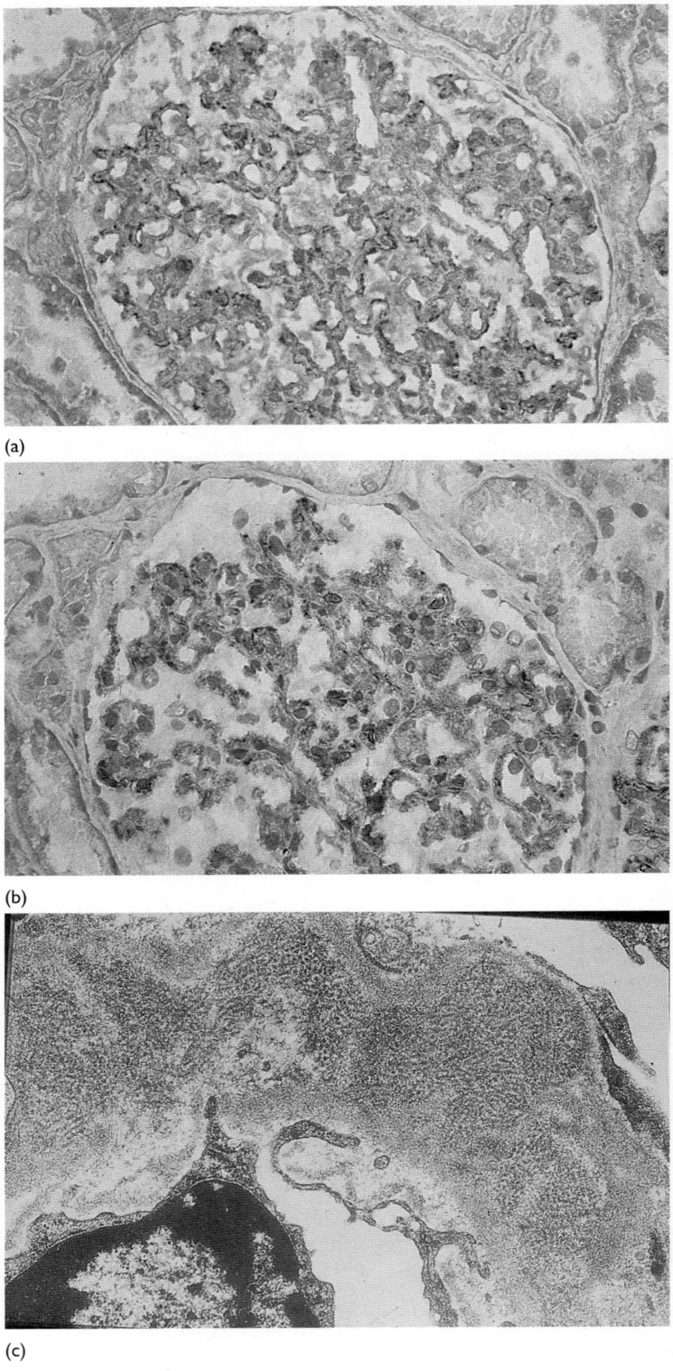

(a) (b) (c)

Fig. 4 Immunotactoid glomerulopathy in a patient with chronic lymphocytic leukaemia. Atypical membranous glomerulonephritis showing exclusive staining of the deposits with anti-γ (a) and anti-κ (b) antibodies (immunohistochemistry, alkaline phosphatase, ×312). (c) Electron micrograph of glomerular basement membrane, showing the microtubular structure of the subepithelial deposits (uranyl acetate and lead citrate, ×12 000). (From Béatrice Mougenot's personal collection.) (See also Plate 4.)

Further reading

Renal involvement in Ig light-chain amyloidosis

Comenzo RL *et al.* (1998). Dose-intensive melphalan with blood stem-cell support for the treatment of AL (amyloid light-chain) amyloidosis: survival and responses in 25 patients. *Blood* **91**, 3662–70.

Kyle RA, Gertz MA (1995). Primary systemic amyloidosis: clinical and laboratory features in 474 cases. *Seminars in Hematology* **32**, 45–59.

Kyle RA *et al.* (1997). A trial of three regimens for primary amyloidosis: colchicine alone, melphalan and prednisone, and melphalan, prednisone, and colchicine. *New England Journal of Medicine* **336**, 1202–7.

Ronco PM, Aucouturier P, Moulin B (1999). Renal amyloidosis and plasma cell dyscrasia-related glomerulopathies. In: Feehally J and Johnson R, eds *Comprehensive nephrology*, section 5, chapter 31, pp 1–14. Mosby, London.

Renal involvement in myeloma

Ronco PM, Aucouturier P, Mougenot B (1997). The kidney in plasma cell dyscrasias. In: Davison AM *et al.*, eds. *Oxford textbook of clinical nephrology*, 2nd edn, vol. 2, pp 811–35. Oxford University Press, Oxford.

Winearls, C.G. (1995). Acute myeloma kidney. *Kidney International* **48**: 1347–61.

Light-chain and heavy-chain deposition disease

Heilman RL *et al.* (1992). Long-term follow-up and response to chemotherapy in patients with light-chain deposition disease. *American Journal of Kidney Diseases* **20**, 34–41.

Moulin B *et al.* (1999). Nodular glomerulosclerosis with deposition of monoclonal immunoglobulin heavy chains lacking C_H1. *Journal of the American Society of Nephrology* **10**, 519–28.

Ronco PM, Aucouturier P, Moulin B (1999). Renal amyloidosis and plasma cell dyscrasia-related glomerulopathies. In: Feehally J and Johnson R, eds *Comprehensive nephrology*, section 5, chapter 31, pp 1–14. Mosby, London.

Non-amyloid fibrillary and immunotactoid glomerulopathies

Brady HR (1998). Fibrillary glomerulopathy. *Kidney International* **53**, 1421–9.

Fogo A, Qureshi N, Horn RG (1993). Morphologic and clinical features of fibrillary glomerulonephritis versus immunotactoid glomerulopathy. *American Journal of Kidney Diseases* **22**, 367–77.

Markowitz GS *et al.* (1998). Hepatitis C viral infection is associated with fibrillary glomerulonephritis and immunotactoid glomerulopathy. *Journal of the American Society of Nephrology* **9**, 2244–52.

Touchard G *et al.* (1994). Glomerulonephritis with organized microtubular monoclonal immunoglobulin deposits. *Advances in Nephrology from the Necker Hospital* **23**, 149–75.

Renal involvement in cryoglobulinaemia

Brouet JC *et al.* (1974). Biologic and clinical significance of cryoglobulins. A report of 86 cases. *American Journal of Medicine* **57**, 775–88.

D'Amico G (1998). Renal involvement in hepatitis C infection: cryoglobulinemic glomerulonephritis. *Kidney International* **54**, 650–71.

Johnson RJ *et al.* (1993). Membranoproliferative glomerulonephritis associated with hepatitis C virus infection. *New England Journal of Medicine* **328**, 465–70.

Renal involvement in Waldenström's macroglobulinaemia

Veltman GA *et al.* (1997). Renal disease in Waldenstrom's macroglobulinaemia. *Nephrology, Dialysis and Transplantation* **12**, 1256–9.

Renal involvement in lymphomas and leukaemias

Moulin B *et al.* (1992). Glomerulonephritis in chronic lymphocytic leukemia and related B-cell lymphomas. *Kidney International* **42**, 127–35.

Ronco PM (1999). Paraneoplastic glomerulopathies: new insights into an old entity. *Kidney International* **56**, 355–77.

Tumour lysis syndrome

Haas M *et al.* (1999). The spectrum of acute renal failure in tumour lysis syndrome. *Nephrology, Dialysis and Transplantation* **14**, 776–9.

Wolf G *et al.* (1999). Hyperuricemia and renal insufficiency associated with malignant disease: urate oxidase as an efficient therapy? *American Journal of Kidney Diseases* **34**, E20.

20.10.6 Haemolytic uraemic syndrome

Paul Warwicker and Timothy H. J. Goodship

Introduction

The haemolytic uraemic syndrome (**HUS**) is characterized by the triad of microangiopathic haemolytic anaemia (Coombs' test negative), thrombocytopenia, and acute renal failure. In thrombotic thrombocytopenic purpura (**TTP**) neurological manifestations and fever occur in addition.

Classification (Table 1)

HUS can be divided into diarrhoeal (D+)- and non-diarrhoeal-associated (D–) disease. Historically, some disorders that present with the characteristic triad of features have been considered separately from HUS. This is illogical, and they too are listed as forms of D– HUS. Because the clinical presentation, prognosis, and treatment differ for each form of HUS they are described separately in this chapter.

Pathogenesis of HUS

The anticoagulant state of normal endothelium is maintained by: (1) a lack of the constitutive expression of tissue factor; (2) the endothelial expression of heparin, tissue-plasminogen activator, and thrombomodulin; and (3) the local secretion of vasoactive substances preventing platelet aggregation, including nitric oxide, prostacyclin, and adenosine.

Table 1 A classification of HUS

D+ HUS
E. coli 0157:H7
Other infective causes
D– HUS
Idiopathic
Familial
Transplantation
Drug-related
Pregnancy-related
Malignancy-related
HIV-related
Other infective causes
Immunological disorders
'HUS-like' syndromes'
• scleroderma renal crisis
• accelerated hypertension
• severe acute vascular rejection of renal allograft

In HUS, several factors can result in endothelial cell activation, these include: antiendothelial antibodies, immune complexes, lipopolysaccharides, toxins, complement, and drugs. Tissue factor and tissue-plasminogen activator inhibitor are expressed. In addition, von Willebrand factor (**vWF**) is synthesized and secreted in increased amounts, promoting platelet aggregation by binding to the $\alpha_{iiib}\beta_3$ integrins on the platelet surface and to the endothelial matrix. Downregulation of this process is usually achieved by endothelial secretion of a metalloproteinase that cleaves vWF, rendering it inactive.

The effect of endothelial activation, a crucial feature of all the conditions listed in Table 1 as causing HUS, is that five core changes occur: loss of vascular integrity, expression of leucocyte-adhesion molecules, cytokine production, upregulation of HLA molecules, and the change in phenotype from an anticoagulant to a procoagulant state. It is the latter that predisposes to the development of a thrombotic microangiopathy.

There have been many descriptions of phenomena associated with HUS, such as complement activation and the secretion of ultra-large vWF, selectins, and tissue plasminogen activator-I. Causal relationships have been proposed. In retrospect many of these observations merely reflect a state of endothelial activation. However, if the mechanisms responsible for downregulating the sequelae of endothelial activation are impaired then it is possible that a procoagulant state will be maintained. This has recently been shown for both HUS (overactivity of the alternative complement pathway) and TTP (abnormalities of the metalloproteinase that cleaves vWF).

Histopathology (Fig. 1 and Plate 1)

In D+ HUS it is predominantly the glomerular endothelium that is affected (hence termed 'thrombotic glomerulopathy'), whilst in D– HUS it is the endothelium of the preglomerular vessels (hence termed 'arterial thrombotic microangiopathy'). Severe intimal proliferation and luminal stenosis also affects arterioles and interlobular arteries in some forms of D– HUS. The subendothelial spaces are widened and these may contain fibrin deposits.

Diagnosis and laboratory features

The diagnosis of HUS is based on demonstrating the aforementioned triad of microangiopathic haemolytic anaemia, thrombocytopenia, and acute renal failure. It should be considered and excluded in all cases of acute renal failure, especially those associated with diarrhoea and/or severe hypertension. Urine output may be reduced, although non-oliguric renal failure is also seen. Urinalysis usually shows microscopic haematuria and proteinuria.

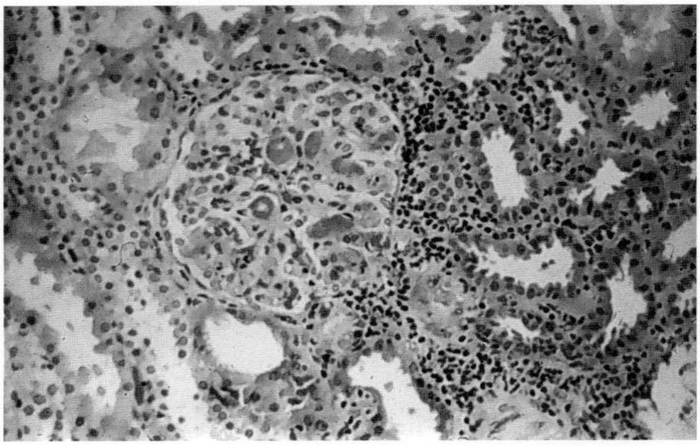

Fig. 1 Typical changes of glomerular thrombotic microangiopathy in a patient with HUS (figure kindly provided by Dr Marie O'Donnell). (See also Plate 1.)

The anaemia of HUS may be severe, with features of haemolysis, including reticulocytosis and increased unconjugated bilirubin, decreased haptoglobin, and raised lactate dehydrogenase (**LDH**) levels, which can be used as a marker of disease. The Coombs' test is negative, and careful examination of the blood film may reveal fragmented and deformed red cells. Thrombocytopenia ranges from severe to mild: 50 per cent of patients will have platelet counts in excess of 100×10^9/l. There may be an associated leucocytosis, the extent of which is correlated with disease severity in D+ HUS. Fibrinogen degradation products may be increased, but clotting tests are characteristically normal. If they are deranged, then septicaemia and disseminated intravascular coagulation should be considered.

Hyponatraemia may complicate D+ HUS, which can then be associated with seizures. Hyperkalaemia is occasionally severe. Complement levels should be measured: C3 is often low in both D+ HUS, where it is associated with a poor prognosis, and D– HUS, where it is associated with recurring or familial types of disease. Human immunodeficiency virus (**HIV**) infection should also be considered in appropriate risk groups.

Diarrhoeal (D+) HUS

Incidence

This is the commonest form of HUS, accounting for over 90 per cent of cases in industrialized countries. It is the commonest cause of renal failure in children and is associated with a diarrhoeal prodrome, hence D+ HUS. The bloody diarrhoea is caused by bacterial infection, predominantly with strains of enterohaemorrhagic *Escherichia coli*, notably *E. coli* O157:H7. This strain has only recently become a significant health hazard—the first descriptions of haemorrhagic colitis and HUS associated with it appeared in 1983. Since then there has been a rapid increase in the number of cases reported. One of the largest and most serious outbreaks was the Central Scotland outbreak of 1996 where 496 individuals were infected, 27 developed HUS, and 18 died. Other diarrhoeal pathogens, particularly *Shigella dysenteriae*-type 1, can also cause D+ HUS.

Clinical features

E. coli is very virulent with as few as 50 organisms causing disease. The bacteria adhere to the large bowel and release a toxin, known as verocytotoxin or Shiga toxin, into the bloodstream. This toxin belongs to the **RIP** (ribosomal inhibitory protein) group of proteins which are amongst the most potent toxins known to man. They include ricin, which gained notoriety in 1978 when an iridium pellet containing trace amounts of the toxin was injected with the aid of an umbrella into the calf of the dissident Bulgarian journalist, Georgi Markov, on Waterloo bridge in London. He subsequently died from multiorgan failure. These toxins consist of five β-subunits and a single α-subunit. The β-subunit binds to Gb3 (a glycolipid found in the membranes of eukaryotic cells), following which the toxin enters the cell by endocytosis and the α-subunit blocks protein synthesis at the ribosome.

The delay between exposure and illness is on average 3 days, typically starting with abdominal cramps and diarrhoea, which becomes bloody over the following 2 days. The majority of patients then recover, although late sequelae such as colonic strictures and chronic pancreatitis are occasionally seen. Between 3 and 20 per cent go on to develop HUS of varying severity. Approximately 50 per cent of patients with D+ HUS require renal replacement therapy, 5 per cent are left with chronic renal failure, and 3 to 5 per cent die of the acute illness. In those who do recover, between 15 and 40 per cent show evidence of persistent renal damage with proteinuria and/or hypertension. Acute neurological complications such as cerebrovascular accident, seizures, and coma develop in approximately 25 per cent of patients with D+ HUS.

Diagnosis

E. coli O157:H7 infection is diagnosed by stool culture and subsequent detection of the O157:H7 antigen. It is also possible to detect antibodies to the O157 lipopolysaccharide in sera from convalescent patients, although this is of limited use in acute illness and is not widely available.

Treatment

Identification of infection and early diagnosis of HUS are important. However, it is unclear whether antibiotics in the early stages of the disease are of benefit, and it is possible that they may increase the risk of developing HUS. Antimotility agents are contraindicated in the early stages as they too may increase the risk of HUS. Treatment of D+ HUS is predominantly supportive, including careful fluid and electrolyte balance, control of hypertension, nutritional support, and renal replacement therapy if necessary. Vigilance should be maintained for complications such as ischaemic colitis, myocardial dysfunction, and pancreatitis. There is limited evidence for a benefit of either plasma exchange or plasma infusion, but plasma exchange continues to be used, particularly in complicated and prolonged cases. Specific treatments such as toxin-binding resins and toxoid vaccines are currently being investigated. Prevention and good public health policy is likely to be of the utmost importance in the future. The recent outbreak in Scotland led to the commissioning of the *Pennington report*, which produced recommendations for disease prevention ranging from the 'farm to the table'.

Non-diarrhoeal (D–) HUS

Different forms of D– HUS

Idiopathic

Idiopathic, also known as sporadic or atypical, HUS accounts for approximately 5 to 10 per cent of cases. It is typically insidious, although it may present following an upper respiratory tract infection. People of all ages can be affected, and there is no seasonal incidence. Severe hypertension is frequent and mortality is higher than with D+ HUS. Renal involvement is usually pronounced with significant proteinuria and uraemia. The disease may recur in both native kidneys and allografts.

As the name suggests, the cause of idiopathic HUS is unknown. Recent research has focused on a dysfunction of complement-pathway modulators; case reports often reveal low levels of C3, indicating overactivity of the alternative complement pathway (see familial HUS below). Other possible aetiological factors implicated include dysfunction of prostacyclin metabolism, abnormalities of von Willebrand factor multimers (see the section on TTP), abnormalities of platelet-activating factor, and tissue plasminogen activator inhibitor-type 1.

Familial HUS

HUS may be inherited as both autosomal recessive and autosomal dominant forms. In autosomal recessive disease the onset is early, with a peak incidence in infancy. Affected children may suffer recurrent episodes. Autosomal dominant disease can affect all ages, and may be precipitated by pregnancy. Phenotypically, familial HUS most closely resembles idiopathic HUS. Severe hypertension is a prominent feature, being found in approximately 80 per cent of autosomal dominant and 40 per cent of autosomal recessive cases. There is usually no diarrhoeal prodrome, prognosis is poor, mortality is high (often over 50 per cent), and recurrence is common. Management includes aggressive control of blood pressure, particularly with angiotensin-converting enzyme (**ACE**) inhibitors, careful fluid balance, and plasma exchange (although it is often unsuccessful in reversing the disease).

Although familial HUS is rare, it affords an opportunity to elucidate underlying mechanisms relevant to the acquired form of D– HUS. Genetic linkage of the familial form of the disease has been established to an area of chromosome 1q32 containing the gene for complement factor H. This is a soluble serum protein that downregulates the spontaneous activity of the alternative complement pathway. Factor H deficiency has now been described in several families with HUS. Mutations in the factor H gene have been identified in both familial and sporadic HUS.

Transplantation

Both *de novo* and recurrent HUS are seen following renal transplantation. HUS is a well-established side-effect of both ciclosporin and tacrolimus (FK506). Other risk factors include acute rejection, cytomegalovirus (**CMV**) infection, and simultaneous pancreas transplantation. Treatment includes discontinuation of the drug, the use of intravenous corticosteroids, and the substitution of other immunosuppressive agents.

HUS is also seen with other forms of transplantation, particularly that of bone marrow, where between 6 and 26 per cent of patients show evidence of a microangiopathy. The aetiology is unclear, but may be related to endothelial damage secondary to total body irradiation, intensive conditioning chemotherapy, ciclosporin treatment, CMV infection, or graft-versus-host disease. Management is supportive, including renal replacement therapy, the aggressive treatment of hypertension with ACE inhibitors, and the withdrawal of ciclosporin. Fresh-frozen plasma replacement may be of benefit, but treatment is usually unsuccessful in the more fulminant forms of the disease and prognosis is poor.

Drug-related

Other drugs besides ciclosporin and tacrolimus are associated with HUS. In particular, several cytotoxic drugs used in chemotherapy are complicated by the syndrome (so-called **C-HUS** or cancer-chemotherapy HUS). They include mitomycin C, 5-fluorouracil, and cisplatin either alone or in combination with daunorubicin, vinblastine, and bleomycin. The disease may be associated with severe hypertension, pulmonary oedema (often after transfusion of blood products), neurological features, and a high mortality (60 to 75 per cent in some series). With mitomycin C the disease is dose-related: it is rarely seen in patients receiving less than 30 mg/m^2, but more frequently at doses above 60 mg/m^2. The incidence is between 2 and 15 per cent, and usually presents weeks or months after the last treatment with mitomycin, often when the patient is in clinical remission. Few treatments have proven effective, although staphylococcal protein-A column perfusion to remove circulating immune complexes seems to be more effective than plasma exchange and may be of benefit in less severe forms of the disease.

Other drugs implicated in HUS include crack cocaine, ticlopidine, and quinine. Use of the oral contraceptive has also been said to be associated with HUS, although with such a commonly prescribed medication it is difficult to be certain whether the association is coincidental. However, it is wise to advise against its use in survivors of D– HUS and in families with the inherited form of HUS.

Pregnancy-related

The incidence of HUS in pregnancy is approximately 1 in 25 000. Presentation is usually peripartum or within a few weeks after delivery, when it is also known as postpartum renal failure. In women presenting in the third trimester, it may be difficult to differentiate HUS from severe forms of pre-eclampsia, such as the **HELLP** syndrome (haemolysis, elevated liver enzymes, and low platelets). Pre-eclamptic syndromes tend to be associated with less severe haemolytic anaemia, the presence of hepatocellular necrosis, and a rapid improvement postdelivery. Features of pregnancy-related HUS include severe hypertension, neurological symptoms, fever, and renal failure requiring renal replacement therapy. Although plasma exchange increases survival rates, maternal mortality remains between 5 and 20 per cent, and preterm delivery and intrauterine fetal death (approximately 30 per cent) are frequent complications. Long-term follow-up is important because of the later development of renal failure and hypertension. HUS will reoccur in approximately 50 per cent of patients, not only during a further pregnancy but also at other times.

Malignancy-related

HUS is associated with malignancy, particularly adenocarcinoma. Patients with a gastric primary and metastatic disease are at increased risk.

HIV-related

There are several forms of nephropathy associated with HIV infection, and a thrombotic microangiopathy with features resembling both idiopathic

HUS and TTP is being increasingly recognized. The incidence of HUS in patients infected with HIV is estimated at approximately 1 per cent; although it usually presents in the later stages of the disease, occasionally it can be the first presentation. HIV infection should be considered in the differential diagnosis of HUS and TTP in high-risk groups and in patients originating from a high-prevalence area. The p24 antigen in endothelial cells may reflect either a direct cytopathic effect of the virus or functional impairment of the endothelium. Concurrent CMV infection has also been associated with HUS. Neurological involvement is common and severe hypertension is a prominent feature. Plasma exchange can lead to renal recovery, but overall the prognosis is poor and few patients survive 1 year from diagnosis. Since ACE inhibitors are used in the therapy of other forms of HIV-associated nephropathy, they would seem a logical choice in the treatment of hypertension.

Other infective causes

Non-diarrhoeal bacterial infections are occasionally associated with HUS. *Pneumococcus* and some *Clostridia* species can produce neuraminidase which strips sialic acid from cell membranes, thereby exposing the cryptic Thomsen–Friedenreich antigen on erythrocytes, platelets, and glomerular cells. An IgM antibody, present in most plasma, causes agglutination, endothelial injury, and HUS. Plasma exchange is therefore contraindicated and treatment consists of washed red cells and antibiotics. Difficulty in red cell typing and a blood film demonstrating both agglutination and red cell fragments may give a clue to diagnosis. Capnocytophagia sepsis from dog bites has recently been associated with cases of HUS.

Immunological disorders

HUS has been reported in association with systemic lupus erythematosus, primary antiphospholipid syndrome, and a variety of glomerulonephritides.

'HUS-like' syndromes

As the renal crisis of systemic sclerosis can be clinically and histologically indistinguishable from idiopathic D– HUS, a diagnosis of systemic sclerosis is often made retrospectively from serological markers or with the development of other features of the disease. Likewise, the thrombotic microangiopathy of accelerated hypertension may be difficult to distinguish from HUS. The most important aspect of treatment in these syndromes is good blood pressure control; ACE inhibitors should be prescribed early, balanced with the requirement to reduce blood pressure gradually. In the renal crisis of systemic sclerosis there may be late recovery of renal function, even when the patient has been established on dialysis for some weeks or months.

Treatment of D– HUS

Few randomized controlled trials have been conducted into the treatment of D– HUS.

Supportive

This consists of careful fluid balance, blood transfusion, and renal replacement therapy. In oliguric patients care should be taken to prevent fluid overload, and central venous monitoring may be required. Platelet transfusions should be avoided, unless there is evidence of bleeding. Patients with deteriorating renal function should always be referred to a renal unit.

Plasma treatment

Previous studies of the efficacy of plasma treatment in HUS are difficult to interpret because of the inclusion of patients with TTP who respond well to plasma exchange. Nevertheless plasma exchange is recommended for most forms of D– HUS.

Corticosteroids

The use of corticosteroids is controversial. Although there is evidence of their efficacy in the treatment of TTP, in small retrospective studies of D– HUS they appear to have no significant effect on survival or the need for renal replacement therapy.

Hypertension

Because of the histological changes in HUS, it is not surprising that hypertension, presumably renin driven, is common. ACE inhibitors are the treatment of choice, with clear parallels existing with their use in the renal crisis of systemic sclerosis. Bilateral nephrectomy has been advocated for severe D– HUS with widespread manifestations unresponsive to plasma exchange. In a series of four patients (three of whom suffered ACE inhibitor-resistant hypertension), bilateral nephrectomy led to complete haematological and clinical remission within 2 weeks.

Renal transplantation

Renal transplantation in patients with renal failure secondary to D+ HUS is safe, with little risk of disease recurrence. In contrast, patients with D– HUS have a 30 to 50 per cent chance of recurrence, usually within the first 2 months, and often within the first 2 weeks. Once recurrent HUS is established, most grafts are lost despite treatment with plasma exchange. This is reflected in the poor 2-year overall graft survival rate of 35 per cent. Graft nephrectomy should not be delayed in this situation. Acute vascular rejection may be difficult to differentiate from recurrent HUS, both clinically and histologically.

Further reading

Reviews of subtypes and treatment of HUS

Kaplan BS, Trompeter RS, Moake JL (1992). *Hemolytic uremic syndrome and thrombotic thrombocytopenic purpura.* Dekker, New York.

Neild GH (1994). Haemolytic-uraemic syndrome in practice. *Lancet* **343**, 398–401.

Neild GH, Barratt TM (1998). Acute renal failure associated with microangiopathy. In: Davison AM, *et al.*, eds. *Oxford textbook of clinical nephrology*, pp 1649–66. Oxford University Press, Oxford.

Remuzzi G, Ruggenenti P (1995). The haemolytic uraemic syndrome. *Kidney International* **48**, 2–19.

Pathophysiology of HUS

Moake JL (1994). Haemolytic-uraemic syndrome: basic science. *Lancet* **343**, 393–7.

Rougier N, *et al.* (1998). Human complement factor H deficiency associated with haemolytic uremic syndrome. *Journal of the American Society of Nephrology* **9**, 2318–26.

Warwicker P, *et al.* (1998). Genetic studies into haemolytic uraemic syndrome. *Kidney International* **53**, 836–44.

Comprehensive review of *E. coli* and D+ HUS

Mead PS, Griffin PM (1998). *Escherichia coli* 0157:H7. *Lancet* **352**, 1207–12.

Editorial summarizing recent studies in TTP and HUS

Moake JL (1998). Moschcowitz, multimers, and metalloprotease. *New England Journal of Medicine* **339**, 1629–31.

Pregnancy-associated HUS

Dashe JS, Ramin SM, Cunningham FG (1998). The long term consequences of thrombotic microangiopathy (thrombotic thrombocytopenic purpura and hemolytic uremic syndrome) in pregnancy. *Obstetrics and Gynecology* **91**, 662–8.

Egerman RS, *et al.* (1996). Thrombotic thrombocytopenic purpura and hemolytic uremic syndrome in pregnancy: review of 11 cases. *American Journal of Obstetrics and Gynecology* **175**, 950–6.

HIV-associated HUS

Badesha PS, Saklayen MG (1996). Hemolytic uremic syndrome as a presenting form of HIV infection. *Nephron* **72**, 472–5.

Sutor GC, Schmidt RE, Albrecht H. (1999). Thrombotic microangiopathies and HIV infection: report of two typical cases, features of HUS and TTP, and review of the literature. *Infection* **27**, 12–15.

Transplantation and HUS

Conlon PJ, *et al.* (1996). Renal transplantation in adults with thrombotic thrombocytopenic purpura/haemolytic uraemic syndrome. *Nephrology, Dialysis and Transplantation* **11**, 1810–14.

Ducloux D, *et al.* (1998). Recurrence of hemolytic-uremic syndrome in renal transplant recipients: a meta-analysis. *Transplantation* **65**, 1405–7.

Verburgh CA, *et al.* (1996). Haemolytic uraemic syndrome following bone marrow transplantation. Case report and review of the literature. *Nephrology, Dialysis and Transplantation* **11**, 1332–7.

20.10.7 Sickle-cell disease and the kidney

G. R. Serjeant

Homozygous sickle-cell (**SS**) disease results in anaemia, a hyperdynamic circulation, less deformable red blood cells, and probably widespread endothelial damage and dysfunction. These processes affect structure and function in the kidney: medullary and glomerular involvement occurs at different ages and with different implications for outcome. Other genotypes of sickle-cell disease such as sickle-cell haemoglobin C (SC) disease, sickle-cell β°-thalassaemia, and sickle-cell β^{+}-thalassaemia manifest similar but less frequent and less severe changes. Even the sickle-cell trait is associated with some abnormalities of renal function.

Medullary involvement

Vascular damage

The vasa rectae system of the renal medulla with its low oxygen tension, high pH, and hypertonicity is uniquely conducive to sickling, causing disruption of the blood vessels and secondary damage to the renal tubules. Microradioangiographic studies have shown almost complete obliteration of the fine-vessel system of the vasa rectae, the remaining vessels being distorted into spirals, dilatations, and appearing to end blindly. These changes have been observed in SS disease in childhood and occur to a lesser extent in the sickle-cell trait in which haemoglobin S levels are only 20 to 45 per cent of total haemoglobin.

Tubular dysfunction

The functional effect of these vascular changes is an inability to concentrate the urine normally, which becomes worse with age but can be improved by transfusion in children under 2 years. Proximal tubular functional abnormalities include an increased secretion of urate and an increased reabsorption of phosphate and of β_2-microglobulin. Distal tubular functional abnormalities include an inability to excrete an acid load, defective maximal potassium excretion, and occasionally evidence of hyporeninaemic hypoaldosteronism.

Clinically, these changes are reflected in hyposthenuria with larger urinary volumes contributing to nocturia, enuresis, and possibly a tendency to dehydration.

Glomerular involvement

Large hypercellular glomeruli are characteristic of SS disease from the age of 2 years, the size continuing to increase with age even over the age of 40 years. The large glomeruli in childhood are associated with supranormal glomerular filtration rates, effective renal blood flows, and effective renal plasma flows. All these indices fall with age and in many patients aged 30 to 40 years are below normal, with particularly rapid decline occurring in some patients who proceed to chronic renal failure. This functional deterioration is assumed to reflect progressive glomerular loss, the mechanism of which is unclear, but there may be contributions from immune complexes derived from renal tubular epithelial antigen and mechanical damage to the nephron from hyperfiltration. The notion that glomerular capillary hypertension might be involved gained support from the observation that angiotensin-converting enzyme inhibitors significantly reduce proteinuria in some proteinuric patients with SS disease.

Clinical syndromes

Nocturnal enuresis

Enuresis is common in SS disease, and in the Jamaican Sickle Cell Cohort study occurred at least 2 nights weekly in 52 per cent of SS males and 38 per cent of SS females aged 8 years compared with values of 22 and 17 per cent in normal control children. Enuretic children with SS disease have slightly higher urine volumes and lower mean maximal functional bladder capacities than those without enuresis, and the ratio of overnight urine volume to bladder capacity was significantly greater in enuretic subjects. Enuresis alarms may therefore be the most appropriate therapy but require testing in controlled studies.

Haematuria

Haematuria occurs in both sickle-cell disease and sickle-cell trait and is believed to result from ischaemic lesions of the renal papilla, varying from minute ulcerations to renal papillary necrosis. Treatment is conservative, although prolonged haematuria may require blood transfusion or rarely limited surgery. Epsilon aminocaproic acid, which inhibits urokinase, has been effective in some cases, but promotes clots that may obstruct the ureters and its use requires assessment in controlled trials.

Urinary tract infections

The frequency of urinary tract infections is increased in subjects with the sickle-cell trait during pregnancy, and may be increased in SS disease, although no reliable data are available. *Escherichia coli*, *Klebsiella*, and *Enterobacter* spp. are most commonly responsible.

Acute glomerular disease

Poststreptococcal glomerulonephritis occurs in SS disease and may affect patients at a later age than the normal population. An association of proteinuria with leg ulceration raised the possibility that leg ulcers acted as a portal of entry for β-haemolytic streptococci, but further analysis did not support this hypothesis.

Nephrotic syndrome

It is unclear whether patients with SS disease are more prone to nephrotic syndrome, but the histological picture of membranoproliferative glomerulonephritis accounts for over half of adult cases. Nephrotic syndrome has been reported following parvovirus B19 infection, and B19-specific DNA demonstrated within renal biopsy tissue 1 year after the onset of nephrotic syndrome. If nephrotic syndrome is due to acute glomerulonephritis, the prognosis is good, but it is not if the cause is otherwise, with a 50 per cent mortality occurring within 16 months in one study.

Chronic renal failure

This is an important contributor to illness and death among adults with SS disease, especially those over 40 years of age. It is usually insidious in onset, manifested initially by a falling haemoglobin level attributable to lowered erythropoietin levels. The renal function of older patients should therefore be monitored regularly. Serum creatinine levels tend to be lower than normal in steady-state SS disease and creatinine levels within the accepted normal range should not be interpreted as indicating normal renal function, indeed in SS disease it is likely that levels of 60 to 70 μmol/l reflect significant renal damage.

Since the early symptoms of chronic renal failure in those with SS disease are principally due to a low haemoglobin level, patients may be maintained in tolerable health for years by regular transfusion. The response to subcutaneous erythropoietin is unpredictable, large doses of erythropoietin being required to induce a response, but some patients showing dramatic increases in haemoglobin that may precipitate painful crises. Endstage renal failure may require long-term renal replacement therapy or renal transplantation, but there are conflicting data on outcome. Successful transplantation can be followed by striking increases in haemoglobin levels sufficient to precipitate painful crises, and recurrent sickle nephropathy may affect the transplanted kidney.

Further reading

Assar R *et al.* (1988). Acute poststreptococcal glomerulonephritis and sickle cell disease. *Child Nephrology and Urology* **9**, 176–9.

Bakir AA *et al.* (1987). Prognosis of the nephrotic syndrome in sickle glomerulopathy. *American Journal of Nephrology* **7**, 110–15.

Barber WH *et al.* (1987). Renal transplantation in sickle cell anemia and sickle disease. *Clinical Transplantation* **1**, 169–75.

Bhathena DB, Sondheimer, JH (1991) The glomerulopathy of homozygous sickle hemoglobin (SS) disease: morphology and pathogenesis. *Journal of the American Society of Nephrology* **1**, 1241–52.

Falk RJ *et al.* (1992). Prevalence and pathologic features of sickle cell nephropathy and response to inhibition of angiotensin-converting enzyme. *New England Journal of Medicine* **326**, 910–15.

Morgan AG, Serjeant GR (1981). Renal function in patients over 40 with homozygous sickle-cell disease. *British Medical Journal* **282**, 1181–3.

Readett DRJ, Morris JS, Serjeant GR (1990). Determinants of nocturnal enuresis in homozygous sickle cell disease. *Archives of Diseases in Childhood* **65**, 615–18.

Statius van Eps LW *et al.* (1970). Nature of concentrating defect in sickle-cell nephropathy. Microradioangiographic studies. *Lancet* **i**, 450–2.

Tejani A *et al.* (1985). Renal lesions in sickle cell nephropathy in children. *Nephron* **39**, 352–5.

Wierenga KJJ *et al.* (1995). Glomerulonephritis after human parvovirus infection in homozygous sickle cell disease. *Lancet* **346**, 475–6.

20.11 Renal involvement in genetic disease

J. P. Grünfeld

Table 1 Main groups of inherited kidney diseases

Cystic kidney diseases (see Table 2)
Alport's syndrome and variants
Inherited metabolic diseases with renal involvement
with glomerular involvement (such as diabetes mellitus, genetic amyloidosis, Fabry's disease)
with non-glomerular involvement (such as cystinosis, primary hyperoxaluria)
Other inherited diseases
with glomerular involvement (such as congenital nephrotic syndrome, nail–patella syndrome)
with non-glomerular involvement (such as nephronophthisis)
Primary immune glomerulonephritis, occasionally familial (such as IgA nephropathy)
Inherited tubular disorders
Various renal diseases with 'genetic influence' (such as reflux nephropathy, haemolytic–uraemic syndrome)

The spectrum of inherited renal disorders (and of inherited diseases with kidney involvement) is summarized in Table 1. Attention will be focused in this section on the commonest inherited kidney diseases leading to renal failure.

Cystic kidney diseases

Autosomal dominant polycystic kidney disease

Autosomal dominant polycystic kidney disease is by far the most frequent inherited kidney disorder, accounting for approximately 7 per cent of cases of endstage renal failure in Western countries. It is one of the most frequent human inherited monogenic diseases (approximately 1 in 1000 individuals). The spectrum of genetic cystic kidney diseases is summarized in Table 2.

Definition

The disease is characterized by the presence of multiple cysts, arising from various segments of the nephrons and involving both kidneys. The mechanisms underlying cyst formation and progression are poorly understood: cysts develop only in a small percentage of nephrons and only focally, whereas all nephron cells carry the mutated gene. This has been explained by a two-hit phenomenon which postulates that renal tubular (or liver biliary) cells which are at the origin of cysts bear first the germinal *PKD* gene mutation, and then acquire a somatic *PKD* gene mutation involving the other allele, this event occurring at random in a limited number of cells. This explanation does not exclude other mechanisms. The link between the genetic event(s) and cystic fluid accumulation is not known.

Table 2 Genetic cystic kidney diseases

Autosomal dominant polycystic kidney disease
Autosomal recessive polycystic kidney disease
Juvenile nephronophthisis–medullary cystic disease complex
Associated with multiple malformation syndrome, such as phacomatoses (autosomal dominant): tuberous sclerosis, von Hippel–Lindau's disease; or other rare syndromes

The disease is also characterized by its autosomal dominant mode of inheritance, so that the risk of any child of either parent carrying the abnormal gene is one in two. New mutations are very rare. The mutant gene responsible for 85 per cent of cases of autosomal dominant polycystic kidney disease has been located to the short arm of chromosome 16 (*PKD1* gene) by linkage analysis, and then identified. A second gene (*PKD2*) has been located to the long arm of chromosome 4 and cloned. The corresponding gene products have been named polycystin 1 and 2. Their normal function is unknown, but the two proteins interact. There is possibly a third locus, so far unidentified.

The diagnosis of autosomal dominant polycystic kidney disease is therefore based on the two following features:

(1) evidence for autosomal dominant inheritance;

(2) demonstration of multiple renal cysts in both kidneys, which are often enlarged, by ultrasonography (Fig. 1).

The latter criterion deserves further comment. Renal cysts are initiated in the fetal kidney and develop progressively in life over the course of years. They may be too small to be detected by ultrasound in childhood, and kidney enlargement also progresses with age. Thus the sensitivity of ultrasonography for detecting autosomal dominant polycystic kidney disease is poor before 20 years of age (but the specificity is high since solitary renal cysts, *a fortiori* bilateral, are very rare at this age). In families with the *PKD1* gene mutation, false-negative ultrasonographic diagnosis is very unlikely at

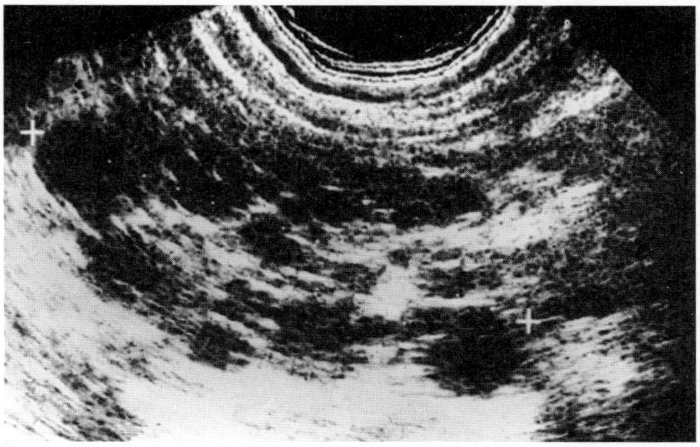

Fig. 1 Typical ultrasonographic findings in a patient with autosomal dominant polycystic kidney disease. The kidney is enlarged and contains multiple cysts of different sizes; the contralateral kidney had similar changes. The concentration of serum creatinine was 120 μmol/l at the time of ultrasonography. (By courtesy of Dr O. Helenon.)

ages above 30 years, and rare at ages 20 to 29 years. Routine screening in asymptomatic members of affected families should not be performed before 20 years of age. By contrast, renal cysts, even bilateral, are relatively common in patients aged 50 years or more, hence strict criteria (multiple cysts in both enlarged kidneys and clear-cut inheritance) are required for diagnosing autosomal dominant polycystic kidney disease in older patients.

Symptoms

Renal manifestations

In some patients, autosomal dominant polycystic kidney disease is asymptomatic and discovered during family investigation or by chance on abdominal ultrasonography. In most cases, however, there are symptoms and patients complain of one or more of the following at some time during their life: renal pain due to cyst development, or stone or blood clot migration; bleeding within a cyst, leading to flank pain, the hyperdense cyst fluid then being visualized by computed tomography; bleeding into the urinary tract, with gross haematuria occurring in approximately 30 per cent of cases; fever due to upper urinary tract infection, which is more frequent in women, or to cyst fluid infection. Renal stones, predominantly uric acid (for unknown reasons), develop in about 20 per cent of the patients.

Hypertension is a common and early finding in autosomal dominant polycystic kidney disease, occurring in about 30 to 50 per cent of patients at a stage when renal function is normal. Subsequently, with the development of renal failure, up to 80 per cent of patients become hypertensive. Why hypertension develops is not known: it has been ascribed to compression and ischaemia of the normal renal parenchyma by cysts.

Renal failure is also a common finding in autosomal dominant polycystic kidney disease. When it occurs, it usually progresses to endstage at between 40 and 60 years of age. However, in 30 per cent of cases it reaches endstage later, and in 5 per cent earlier, including very rare instances when it develops in the first years of life. Recent epidemiological studies have indicated that autosomal dominant polycystic kidney disease may have a much more indolent course in a substantial number of cases: 25 to 50 per cent of affected subjects are not in endstage renal failure by 70 years of age, and some patients may reach 80 or 90 years without the need for renal replacement therapy. This information is crucial for genetic counselling.

Genetic and non-genetic factors determine renal prognosis: the renal disease may progress more slowly in families with *PKD2* disease (mean age at endstage renal disease 55 years in *PKD1* disease compared with 70 years in *PKD2* disease), it progresses more slowly in women than in men, and control of hypertension may reduce the rate of progression.

Extrarenal manifestations

Liver cysts These develop in 70 per cent of patients, usually later in life than renal cysts. Liver cysts are more frequent and more diffuse in women than in men. They are usually asymptomatic, detected by ultrasonography, but may be clinically palpable. Liver function tests are usually normal. Liver cyst infection may occur, particularly in patients on dialysis or transplant recipients. Massive liver involvement can cause severe discomfort in some cases, mostly in women.

Cardiovascular abnormalities These include intracranial aneurysms and mitral valve prolapse. Subarachnoid haemorrhage or intracerebral bleeding due to rupture of intracranial aneurysm are among the most severe complications of autosomal dominant polycystic kidney disease and occur in approximately 1 to 2 per cent of patients. Rapid diagnosis and urgent neurosurgical opinion are required. Diagnosis should be suspected early, before complete rupture, in patients with autosomal dominant polycystic kidney disease with recent and severe headache or with any transient focal neurological deficit.

In cross-sectional studies performed using non-invasive screening methods such as high-resolution computed tomography or magnetic resonance angiography, intracranial aneurysms have been found in 7 to 8 per cent of asymptomatic middle-aged patients with autosomal dominant polycystic kidney disease. The prevalence is higher in those with a family history of intracranial aneurysm. The risk of rupture is largely dependent on aneurysm size. Routine screening by non-invasive methods is not indicated for all asymptomatic patients with autosomal dominant polycystic kidney disease, but it seems reasonable in certain subgroups, in particular those with a family history of intracranial aneurysm or subarachnoid haemorrhage, those who have already bled from an aneurysm (since recurrent aneurysm is possible), and possibly those who are to undergo major elective surgery. In high-risk groups, screening should be repeated every 5 to 10 years since the cerebral vascular disease is progressive.

Mitral valve prolapse is discovered in 20 per cent of patients with autosomal dominant polycystic kidney disease by echocardiography, whereas it is found in only 2 to 3 per cent of the general population. Other cardiac valve abnormalities and occasionally artery dissection or aneurysm may also be detected.

Other extrarenal defects are observed in autosomal dominant polycystic kidney disease: pes excavatum, colonic diverticulas, and abdominal hernias are more prevalent than in the general population.

Treatment

High fluid intake and regular follow-up of blood pressure and renal function are indicated in all patients with autosomal dominant polycystic kidney disease. The control of hypertension is an essential part of management, achieved with standard antihypertensive agents. Haematuria requires conservative management, although bleeding may sometimes be prolonged over several days and even weeks.

The relief of pain or abdominal discomfort can be difficult. In addition to symptomatic treatment, surgical renal cyst decompression should be restricted to very selected cases. Surgery is rarely needed in the management of renal stones. Liver cyst aspirations by needle under CT guidance, fenestration, or resection may be needed when massive involvement gives rise to pain; and in very rare cases such patients have come to liver transplantation.

Kidney infection requires administration of antimicrobials currently used in upper urinary tract infection. In some cases control of infection is not obtained, most probably because agents penetrate some infected cyst fluids poorly and do not achieve adequate concentration. Lipophilic drugs such as trimethoprim–sulphamethoxazole and ciprofloxacin have the best penetration into cyst fluid. Liver cyst infection also requires antimicrobials and drainage if infection is not controlled. Ciprofloxacin penetrates well into liver cyst fluid.

Standard medical management of chronic renal failure is indicated, as are renal replacement therapy and kidney transplantation when the patient reaches endstage, the results being similar to those obtained in other renal diseases.

Genetic counselling

The pattern of inheritance of autosomal dominant polycystic kidney disease means that the offspring of an affected subject have a 50 per cent risk of having the disease. The disease has a highly variable clinical course, even within a given family. Prenatal diagnosis by gene linkage studies using material derived from chorionic villous sampling has been performed and can be considered if required and if adequate family information is available. The demand for such prenatal diagnosis has, however, been very low in Western countries. This is explained by the late onset and the variable clinical course of the disease, often relatively benign, which cannot yet be predicted by DNA analysis.

Ultrasonography may occasionally show renal cysts in the fetus, but late in pregnancy. Obviously, due to the slow and late development of macrocysts, negative ultrasonography in the fetus (as well as in a child) does not rule out the disease.

Autosomal recessive polycystic kidney disease

Autosomal recessive polycystic kidney disease is a rare inherited disease (approximately 1 in 40 000 individuals), the first manifestations of which appear early in childhood.

Three features characterize this disease:

(1) its recessive nature: both heterozygous parents are unaffected, with normal renal ultrasonography; parental consanguinity is found in some families; the mutant gene has been located on chromosome 6;

(2) renal cysts derive from the collecting ducts, accounting for the striations in the dilated collecting system seen on intravenous pyelography; and

(3) the renal disease is invariably associated with congenital hepatic fibrosis: this may be responsible for portal hypertension due to presinusoidal block, or for bacterial angiocholitis due to intrahepatic bile duct dilatation.

In children, autosomal recessive polycystic kidney disease should be differentiated from autosomal dominant polycystic kidney disease, which can be detected in childhood, even in neonates. Family history and renal ultrasonography in parents are decisive for correct diagnosis. In very rare families with *PKD1* disease, renal involvement may be revealed in neonates and may progress to endstage within the first year of life.

The diagnosis of autosomal recessive polycystic kidney disease may be made before birth by antenatal ultrasonography, showing renal enlargement and increased echogenicity (as well as oligohydramnios). However, prenatal diagnosis may be uncertain and, since cystic changes occur in well-developed collecting ducts, these are detected only in the second half of pregnancy. When there is huge renal enlargement, pulmonary hypoplasia and respiratory distress may lead to death within hours after birth. With prolonged survival, liver and renal involvement becomes prominent. Gastrointestinal bleeding due to portal hypertension may be life-threatening and necessitate surgical portocaval shunt. Systemic hypertension is a frequent finding in the first year of life but, surprisingly, it may regress in subsequent years. Urinary tract infection is common. The rate of progression of renal failure is variable. Among patients who survive the neonatal period, approximately 50 per cent reach endstage in childhood, whilst this occurs in adulthood in the remainder.

Other cystic kidney diseases

Renal cysts may be found in von Hippel–Lindau's disease and in tuberous sclerosis (see below). Renal medullary cysts are also found in juvenile nephronophthisis, but not early in the course (see below). By contrast, such cysts—well localized in adults by ultasonography or CT scan—are seen early in autosomal dominant renal medullary cystic disease. This very rare condition progresses to endstage renal failure. Three different genetic loci have so far been localized.

Inherited diseases with glomerular involvement

Alport's syndrome

First described in 1927 by Dr Arthur Cecil Alport, this syndrome is characterized by the association of progressive haematuric hereditary nephritis and bilateral sensorineural hearing loss. Its prevalence is approximately 1 in 5000 individuals. In 85 per cent of kindreds the mode of transmission is compatible with X-linked dominant inheritance. In the remaining families, autosomal dominant or recessive inheritance should be considered.

Symptoms

Renal manifestations

The first clinical manifestation is typically gross haematuria, occurring sometimes in the first year of life, recurring during childhood, and followed by permanent microscopic haematuria. Proteinuria appears later. A nephrotic syndrome, usually moderate, develops in 30 to 40 per cent of patients. In other cases, moderate proteinuria and microscopic haematuria are the presenting symptoms in adulthood. The disease is progressive, leading to renal failure in all affected males, but the rate of progression is heterogeneous from one family to another, although usually homogeneous within a given family. In some endstage is reached at or before 30 years of age, sometimes in childhood; in others renal failure progresses to endstage between the ages of 30 to 60 years.

Carrier females of X-linked Alport's syndrome often have slight or intermittent urinary abnormalities. They may develop mild impairment of renal function late in life but do not usually have progressive renal disease as occurs in males, although this does happen in a few cases. In the autosomal recessive form of Alport's syndrome, renal disease progresses to endstage before 20 to 30 years of age at a similar rate in both affected men and women.

Extrarenal manifestations

The hearing defect may lead to severe perceptive deafness, but it is often moderate or slight, only detected at audiometric testing. The hearing loss labels a given family but is not found in all patients with renal disease. In some kindreds, familial haematuric progressive nephritis without hearing defect is documented: this form belongs to the spectrum of Alport's syndrome.

Other extrarenal manifestations may be found. Eye abnormalities are detected in 30 to 40 per cent of cases. These include bilateral anterior lenticonus detected by slit-lamp examination—a pathognomonic abnormality—and perimacular or macular retinal flecks that are seen by fundoscopic examination and do not alter visual acuity. Recurrent corneal erosions occur in some patients. In some families, macrothrombocytopenia is associated with nephritis and hearing defect. In other rare kindreds the latter features are found in association with diffuse leiomyomatosis, mainly oesophageal, and congenital cataracts.

Pathogenesis

The primary defect in Alport's syndrome involves the glomerular basement membrane. By electron microscopy, this membrane can be abnormally thickened with splitting of the lamina densa, thinned with focal thickening, or diffusely thin in younger children. In some patients, antigenicity of the glomerular basement membrane is abnormal: antiglomerular basement membrane antibodies do not bind linearly along the Alport glomerular basement membrane, whereas they show linear fixation along the glomerular basement membranes of normal and diseased kidneys which contain the corresponding Goodpasture antigen (the Goodpasture syndrome, an autoimmune disorder characterized by the development of antiglomerular basement membrane antibodies directed against this antigen (see Chapter 20.7.7).

In X-linked Alport's syndrome, the molecular defect involves the gene encoding for the α5 chain of the type IV collagen molecule. Type IV collagen is a major component of basement membranes. Six α chains of type IV collagen have been identified so far, with each molecule of type IV collagen being made up of three of these chains, differently associated in various basement membranes. In Alport's syndrome, mutations have been identified in the gene encoding for the α5 chain that maps to the long arm of the X chromosome. The Goodpasture antigen is located in the α3 chain, the gene of which has been mapped on chromosome 2. Absence or severe alteration of the α5 chain possibly prevents normal integration of the α3 chain into the glomerular basement membrane, leading to the defect in antigenicity.

In the autosomal recessive form of Alport's syndrome, the genes encoding for α3 or α4 chains are mutated. Affected subjects are homozygotes in consanguineous families, or compound heterozygotes in other cases. In families with leiomyomatosis, α5 and α6 genes, located contiguously on the X chromosome, are both involved in a large deletion.

Skin biopsy has become valuable for diagnosis of Alport's syndrome. Epidermal basement membrane normally contains α5 but not α3/α4 chains. Thus negative α5 staining by immunofluoresence is highly specific for X-linked Alport's syndrome, but is found in only 75 per cent of cases because α5 chains that are only slightly mutated can be detected. α5 Staining is normal in the autosomal recessive forms of Alport's syndrome.

In the disease with macrothrombocytopenia, mutations involve the *MYH9* gene, encoding the non-muscle myosin heavy chain IIA.

Genetic counselling and treatment

Genetic counselling first requires the correct identification of the mode of inheritance. If X-linked dominant inheritance is documented, affected men will not transmit the disease to their sons, whereas all their daughters will carry the mutant gene; affected women will transmit the mutant gene to 50 per cent of either sons or daughters. DNA analysis may be helpful for genetic counselling in these families.

Treatment of hypertension and supportive management of renal failure are indicated in patients with progressive disease. The results of kidney transplantation are similar to those obtained in other renal diseases. In rare cases, however, antiglomerular basement membrane crescentic glomerulonephritis develops in the graft. It is assumed that this complication is related to alloimmunization to the 'missing antigen' introduced by the transplant.

Benign familial haematuria

This disease is characterized by isolated microhaematuria, without proteinuria and progression to renal failure, in both men and women. Renal biopsy usually shows a thin glomerular basement membrane and immunofluorescence studies are negative. The mode of transmission is compatible with autosomal dominant inheritance. In some families, subjects with microhaematuria are heterozygotes carrying mutations involving the α3 or α4 chain gene.

Congenital nephrotic syndrome of the Finnish type

This disease specifically affects the kidney and is characterized by massive proteinuria, which occurs already *in utero* and then persists in infancy. Intense therapy is needed to afford the children a chance of survival: nutritional support to compensate for protein loss, prevention of infection and thrombosis, bilateral nephrectomy, continuous peritoneal dialysis, and finally kidney transplantation.

It is an autosomal recessive disease. The gene has been located on chromosome 19q and cloned. It encodes for a protein named nephrin, localized at the slit diaphragm between podocyte foot processes, which are both absent in affected subjects. Nephrin probably has a zipper-like structure and plays a key role in the normal glomerular filtration barrier.

Nail–patella syndrome

This syndrome, also known as hereditary osteo-onycho dysplasia, is a rare autosomal dominant disorder, defined by the association of nail hypoplasia or dysplasia, bone abnormalities (including iliac horns), and renal disease. The latter is found in 50 to 60 per cent of cases, progressing to endstage in approximately 15 per cent. The hallmark of renal involvement is the detection by electron microscopy of fibrillar collagen bundles within the glomerular basement membrane. Open angle glaucoma is a feature in rare families.

The mutated gene, *LMX1B* (located on 9q), belongs to a family of transcription factors that are involved in pattern formation during development. *LMX1B* is more specifically involved in the dorsoventral patterning of the limbs, and mice with a deletion in their *lmx1*-homologue exhibit skeletal defects similar to those observed in nail–patella syndrome and abnormal dorsoventral patterning of the extremities of the limbs.

Metabolic diseases with glomerular involvement

Anderson–Fabry disease

This disease is X-linked recessive (prevalence approximately 1 in 40 000 individuals) and due to α-galactosidase A deficiency resulting in glycosphingolipid deposition, mainly in the cardiovascular and renal system. The first manifestations in hemizygotes are painful acroparaesthesias, appearing in childhood, often prevented by continuous administration of carbamazepine or diphenylhydantin. Subsequently, angiokeratomas, anhydrosis, and corneal deposits develop. Ischaemic cerebrovascular complications, cardiac valve abnormalities, myocardial deposition of glycolipids, and coronary accidents are the most severe manifestations, along with renal involvement.

In the kidney, glycolipid deposition involves glomerular epithelial cells, tubular cells, and endothelial and smooth muscle cells of intrarenal arteries. The latter changes are responsible for progressive renal ischaemia. Renal disease is revealed by proteinuria at around 20 years, and then progresses to endstage between 40 and 60 years of age, necessitating regular dialysis and/or kidney transplantation. Glycolipid deposition does not recur in the renal graft that contains normal α-galactosidase activity. Enzyme replacement therapy is available.

Heterozygote female carriers usually have few symptoms. Corneal deposits are found in 70 per cent of them. They can develop cardiac changes and, very rarely, symptomatic renal disease.

Lecithin-cholesterol acyl-transferase (LCAT) deficiency

This is a very rare autosomal recessive disorder. LCAT is a key enzyme in the metabolism of cholesterol, responsible for its esterification. In affected subjects the proportion of cholesteryl ester to total cholesterol is very low. Lipid accumulation occurs in the eyes (causing corneal deposits), erythrocyte membranes (leading to low-grade haemolytic anaemia), arterial walls (contributing to premature atherosclerosis), and kidneys, predominating in glomerular mesangial cells and progressing to endstage renal disease. LCAT is expressed primarily in the liver, hence liver transplantation would theoretically be the treatment of choice, but it has not so far been performed in this disease. Patients have received kidney transplants: lipid deposition recurs slowly in the graft.

Type I glycogen storage disease

Also named von Gierke's disease (see Chapter 11.2), this disease is due to glucose-6-phosphatase deficiency. Affected infants develop hypoglycaemia, growth retardation, and hepatomegaly. Fanconi syndrome may occur as a consequence of glycogen deposition in the proximal tubule. Progressive renal involvement is not due predominantly to glycogen accumulation. It is rather related to the development of focal segmental glomerulosclerosis, the mechanism of which is unclear, usually after 20 years of age. This complication has only been recognized recently since children with severe hypoglycaemia have now survived to adulthood thanks to the progress achieved by paediatricians, dieticians, and families in providing adequate feeding and nutrition.

Familial primary glomerulonephritis

In most types of primary glomerulonephritis, familial cases have been anecdotally reported. The most frequent form, albeit rare, is probably familial IgA nephropathy, either primary (Berger's disease) or associated with Henoch–Schönlein purpura. Familial focal segmental glomerulosclerosis with either autosomal dominant or autosomal recessive inheritance has also been well characterized and several genetic loci have been identified.

Inherited tubulointerstitial disorders

Juvenile nephronophthisis

This complex represents an inherited form of chronic tubulointerstitial disease. Cysts located at the corticomedullary junction or in the medullary region appear late in the course of the disease. Renal pathological examination reveals tubular atrophy and interstitial fibrosis (which are non-specific lesions), and extreme thickening and multilamellation of the tubular basement membrane.

Juvenile nephronophthisis is a major cause of endstage renal disease in children, accounting for 10 to 20 per cent of cases. It is transmitted as an autosomal recessive trait. The gene involved, *NPH1*, has been mapped to the short arm of chromosome 2 and its product has been named nephrocystin. In 80 per cent of cases a homozygous deletion is found. Heterozygotes are asymptomatic.

The clinical manifestations first appear around the age of 4 years and consist of polyuria, secondary enuresis, and polydipsia, reflecting a urinary concentration defect. Renal failure, metabolic acidosis, anaemia, and growth retardation subsequently develop, and endstage renal failure is usually reached at the age of 10 to 13 years. More or less severe renal salt wasting is a common finding. In approximately 10 to 15 per cent of cases renal involvement is associated with retinal changes: tapetoretinal degeneration with or without retinitis pigmentosa, leading to blindness early or later in life (this association is referred to as the Senior–Loken syndrome; in most of these cases, no deletion of the *NPH1* gene has been detected). Other extrarenal features (skeletal changes, cerebellar ataxia, and liver fibrosis) are rare.

Familial nephropathy with juvenile hyperuricaemia and gout (or familial juvenile hyperuricaemic nephropathy)

This disease is characterized by its autosomal dominant inheritance, juvenile onset of gout, hyperuricaemia disproportionate to the age, sex, or degree of renal dysfunction, which is due to low renal fractional excretion of urate, and renal failure often recognized between 20 and 40 years of age. Renal biopsy shows non-specific tubulointerstitial changes. Allopurinol is indicated to prevent gout and perhaps to slow the progression of renal disease.

Genetic disorders with nephrolithiasis

Pertinent clinical data on these disorders are summarized in Table 3. Additional information can be found in Chapters 20.13, 20.8, 11.10, and 11.4.

Other genetic diseases with kidney involvement

Phakomatoses

Two diseases of this group have significant renal involvement: von Hippel–Lindau's disease and tuberous sclerosis.

In von Hippel–Lindau's disease, renal cysts and bilateral multifocal renal cell carcinomas are found in 70 per cent of the patients. Carcinomas are often asymptomatic, should be screened for regularly (Fig. 2), and occur at a mean age of 45 years. Nephron-sparing surgery (tumorectomy) is advocated when technically feasible. The other clinical features of von Hippel–Lindau's disease are described in Chapter 14.8.

The most typical renal lesion encountered in tuberous sclerosis is angiomyolipoma, which is a benign tumour, often multiple and bilateral. By ultrasonography, this tumour is hyperechogenic and by CT is characterized by its fat content (Fig. 3). Bleeding is the main complication of renal angiomyolipoma. Multiple angiomyolipomas may severely reduce renal mass and lead to renal failure, but this is rare. The development of segmental glomerulosclerosis may accelerate the progression to endstage. Renal cysts may also be found in *TSC2* forms (see below). The incidence of renal cell carcinoma is slightly higher than in the general population. The other features of tuberous sclerosis involve the skin and the central nervous system (Chapter 24.8).

The genes mutated in von Hippel–Lindau's disease and tuberous sclerosis are tumour-suppressor genes. Two mutations ('two-hit' phenomenon) are required to trigger tumour formation: the first one germinal, inherited, and the second one somatic. The *VHL* gene has been cloned and located on 3p. Two somatic mutations of the same gene are involved in sporadic renal cell carcinoma. Two genes are identified in tuberous sclerosis: *TSC1* on chromosome 9q encoding for hamartin, and *TSC2* on chromosome 16p, encoding for tuberin.

Cystinosis

Cystinosis results from defective carrier-mediated transport of cystine through the lysosomal membrane. The disease is transmitted as an autosomal recessive trait with an incidence of about 1 in 200 000 live-born babies. The gene has been mapped on chromosome 17, has been identified, mutations have been characterized, and it encodes for a protein named cystinosine. The diagnosis is based on the findings of cystine crystals in tissues, such as the eyes, and on the elevated cystine content in leucocytes. It should be clear that cystinosis is completely different from cystinuria, which is due to a defective reabsorption of cystine in the proximal tubule.

The clinical manifestations are due to progressive intralysosomal accumulation of cystine. In the infantile form, the first symptoms are related to

Table 3 Main inherited disorders with nephrolithiasis

Disease	Mode of transmission	Type of stone	Chronic renal failure	Specific treatment
Cystinuria	AR	Cystine	No	Urine alkalinization D-penicillamine or other chelators
Idiopathic hypercalciuria	Unknown	Calcium	No	Thiazide
Primary hyperoxaluria type I	AR	Monohydrated calcium oxalate	Yes (nephrocalcinosis)	Vitamin B_6 Liver transplantation
Dent's disease	XR	Calcium	Yes (nephrocalcinosis)	
Distal tubular acidosis	AR/AD	Calcium	No	Potassium citrate or bicarbonate
HPRT deficiency (Lesch–Nyhan syndrome)	XR	Uric acid	Yes	Urine alkalinization Allopurinol
APRT deficiency	AR	2,8 dihydroxy adenine	Yes (rarely)	Allopurinol
Xanthinuria	AR	Xanthine	No	

AD, autosomal dominant; APRT, adenine phosphoribosyl transferase; AR, autosomal recessive; HPRT, hypoxanthine-guanine phosphoribosyl transferase; XR, X-linked.

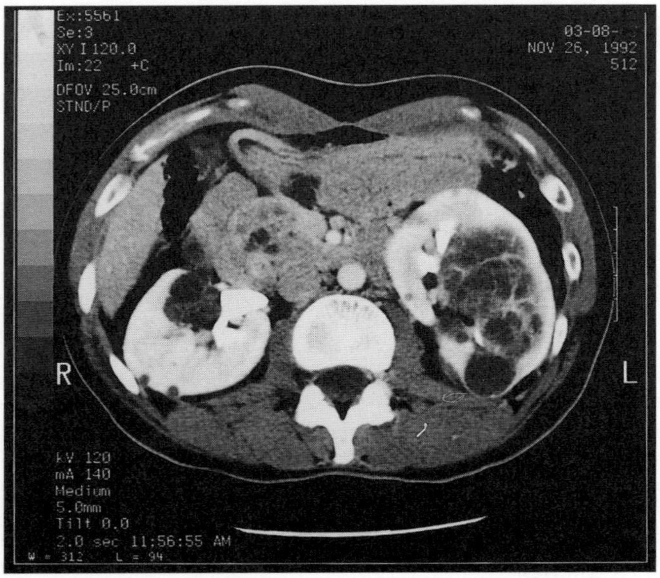

Fig. 2 Computed tomography of the kidneys in a patient with von Hippel–Lindau's disease. In the right kidney, a solid tumour is found as well as cystic changes. In the left kidney, a voluminous multilocular tumour is detected with thick walls, corresponding to renal clear cell carcinoma, associated with other cystic lesions.

the clinical consequences of Fanconi syndrome (salt and water depletion, hypokalaemia, acidosis, rickets) appearing before 6 months of age. Renal failure develops later, reaching endstage generally before 12 years. Cystine accumulates in other tissues, before and after kidney transplantation: eyes (photophobia due to corneal deposits, then retinal depigmentation and visual impairment), thyroid gland (hypothyroidism), liver and spleen (portal hypertension), pancreas (diabetes mellitus), muscles, testis, and central nervous system (encephalopathy) (see Chapter 11.3).

In addition to symptomatic management, cysteamine has proved to be effective in cystinosis. It accumulates within lysosomes, promotes cystine outflow, and thus reduces tissue cystine content. Administration of this drug should be started as soon as the diagnosis is made. It may slow the rate of progression of renal failure and prevent most extrarenal complications. Despite recent progress, tolerance of the drug is not good because of its offensive taste and odour: compliance may therefore be poor. Topical cysteamine prevents corneal crystal deposition.

Juvenile cystinosis presents in late childhood or early adult life. Renal involvement occurs. By contrast, in the adult form only corneal crystals are found. Both forms are very rare.

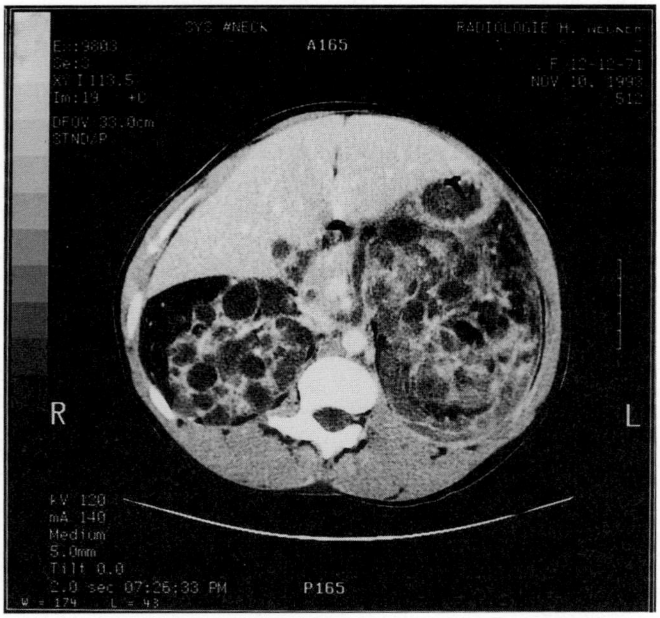

Fig. 3 Multiple bilateral renal angiomyolipomas in a patient with tuberous sclerosis (CT scan). Note the voluminous angiomyolipoma (with high content of fat that is black) at the periphery of the right kidney.

Malformation syndromes with kidney involvement

The most frequent of these rare syndromes is Bardet–Biedl syndrome. This is a heterogeneous autosomal recessive condition for which six different genetic loci have been identified. Clinical features comprise obesity, hypogonadism (in males), polydactyly or dystrophic extremities, retinal dystrophy (leading to blindness), and renal abnormalities. The last have only been recognized recently as a cardinal feature in the syndrome. Renal imaging often shows the following abnormalities: calyceal clubbing and pronounced diverticulas, and lobulated renal outlines of the fetal type. These changes are probably dysplastic in nature, and are characteristic when associated. Renal cortical and medullary cysts have also been found by ultrasonography, but the latter may be difficult to differentiate from calyceal diverticulas. Approximately 25 per cent of patients develop chronic renal failure, progressing to endstage, which is probably the major cause of death. The most important treatment is the provision of specialized education with low-vision aids. Symptomatic management of diabetes mellitus (found in 30 per cent), hypertension, and renal failure is required.

Renal hypoplasia or unilateral renal agenesis is found in other malformation syndromes, such as the following.

1. Kallmann's syndrome—with hypogonadism and hyposmia or anosmia.
2. Branchio-oto-renal syndrome—where laterocervical fistulas or cysts and otic abnormalities, involving the outer, middle, or inner ear are found, and the *EYA1* gene, on the long arm of chromosome 8, is mutated. This gene is the homologue of a gene present in drosophila, the mutation of which leads to eye absence.
3. Renal–coloboma syndrome—with optic nerve coloboma and sometimes hearing defect, and where the *PAX2* gene, located on 10q, is mutated.
4. Alagille's syndrome—characterized by paucity of intrahepatic bile ducts leading to cholestasis, vertebral abnormalities (butterfly vertebra), and heart defects. The gene has been identified.

All these genes implicated in malformation syndromes are involved normally in the control of kidney development.

Further reading

Cystic kidney diseases

Gabow PA (1993). Autosomal dominant polycystic kidney disease. *New England Journal of Medicine* **329**, 332–42.

Pirson Y, Chauveau D (1996). Intracranial aneurysms in ADPKD. In: Watson ML, Torres VE, eds. *Polycystic kidney disease*, pp. 530–47. Oxford University Press, Oxford.

Pirson Y, Chauveau D, Grünfeld JP (1998). Autosomal-dominant polycystic kidney disease. In: Davison AM *et al.*, eds, pp 2393–415. *Oxford textbook of clinical nephrology.* Oxford University Press, Oxford.

Zerres K, Volpel MC, Weiss H (1984). Cystic kidneys: genetics, pathologic anatomy, clinical picture, and prenatal diagnosis. *Human genetics* **68**, 104–35.

Alport's syndrome

Flinter FA *et al.* (1988). Genetics of classic Alport's syndrome. *Lancet* **ii**, 1005–7.

Grünfeld JP, Knebelmann B (1998). Alport's syndrome. In: Davison AM *et al.*, eds. *Oxford textbook of clinical nephrology*, pp 2427–37. Oxford University Press, Oxford.

Kashtan C, Michael AF (1996). Alport syndrome. *Kidney International* **50**, 1145–63.

Pirson Y (1999). Nephrology Forum: making the diagnosis of Alport's syndrome. *Kidney International* **56**, 760–75.

Inherited diseases with glomerular involvement

Morgan SH, Grünfeld JP (1998). *Inherited disorders of the kidney.* Oxford University Press, Oxford.

Inherited tubulointestinal disorders

Cameron JS *et al.* (1998). Inherited disorders of purine metabolism and transport. In: Davison AM *et al.*, eds. *Oxford textbook of clinical nephrology*, pp 2469–84. Oxford University Press, Oxford.

Hildebrandt F, Jungers P, Grünfeld JP (2001). Medullary cystic and medullary sponge renal disorders. In: Schrier RW, ed. *Diseases of the kidney*, pp 521–46. Little, Brown and Company, Boston.

Genetic diseases with kidney involvement

Parfrey PS (1998). Bardet–Biedl syndrome. In: Morgan SH, Grünfeld JP, eds. *Inherited disorders of the kidney*, pp 321–39. Oxford University Press, Oxford.

20.12 Urinary tract infection

C. Tomson

Introduction and definitions

Infection of the urinary tract is important for different reasons in different age groups. In infants and children, ascending infection is thought to be a preventable cause of renal parenchymal scarring and eventual renal failure, although (as discussed below) it is controversial how frequently this occurs. In adult women, recurrent lower urinary tract infection ('cystitis') is a common cause of misery and time off work. In all age groups, persistent or relapsing infection is an important indicator of abnormal host defences, usually due to abnormal anatomy or function of the urinary tract, and may result in irreversible renal damage unless the underlying cause is dealt with. Urinary tract infections are the cause of over 50 per cent of Gram-negative septicaemic episodes. In the elderly, non-specific symptoms including toxic confusional states are often due to occult urinary tract infection, and asymptomatic bacteriuria is associated with increased mortality.

'Urinary tract infection' refers to bacterial or fungal infection of the kidneys, pelvis, ureters, or bladder (viral infections may involve the urinary tract, as in Hantaan virus infection, but viruria more commonly reflects systemic viral infection). Infections primarily involving the urethra are nearly always sexually acquired and are dealt with elsewhere (see Section 21). 'Pyelonephritis' refers to infection primarily involving the kidneys and collecting systems. 'Cystitis' refers to infections localized to the urinary bladder. 'Recurrent' urinary tract infections are due to repeated reinfection, whether by similar organisms on each occasion or by different species; 'relapsing' and 'persistent' infections are due to the continued presence of the same organism, suppressed or not suppressed during antibiotic therapy. 'Uncomplicated' urinary tract infection occurs in an anatomically and functionally normal urinary tract; 'complicated' infection refers to all infections occurring in patients either with impaired host defence (e.g. diabetes) or with abnormal urinary tract anatomy (e.g. urinary tract obstruction).

Epidemiology

Symptomatic bacterial urinary tract infection is one of the commonest bacterial infections. Around 1 per cent of boys and 3 per cent of girls will develop a urinary tract infection during childhood, and 50 per cent of women have a history of at least one episode of urinary tract infection, with recurrent infections in a significant minority. Urinary tract infection is rare in men until after the age of 60, when the rising prevalence of prostatic bladder outflow obstruction leads to an increased risk of infection. Asymptomatic bacteriuria is found in about 10 per cent of elderly men and in 20 per cent of elderly women. Each year in the United Kingdom around 60 women per 1000 population visit their general practitioner with urinary tract infection. Urinary tract infection is responsible for over 25 per cent of all community-acquired bacteraemias, more than any other source of infection, and accounts for over 40 per cent of hospital-acquired infections, often as a result of bladder catheterization.

Causative organisms

The commonest causative organisms in bacterial urinary tract infection are Gram-negative gut organisms, particularly *Escherichia coli* (Table 1). This reflects the fact that most infections reach the urinary tract via the urethra from the perineum. However, as discussed below, only some subtypes of *E. coli* and only some of the other species of gut organisms have the necessary virulence characteristics to enable infection of the normal urinary tract.

Pathophysiology

The great majority of urinary tract infections are acquired by ascent of the infecting organism up the urethra; only a very small minority result from haematogenous spread or—even loss commonly—from vesicoenteric fistulas. The pelvis, ureters, bladder, and urethra possess a highly specialized epithelium, which normally maintains complete impermeability to all components of urine, including toxins and water. This is maintained by tight junctions between the surface layers of epithelial cells, with a very high transepithelial electrical resistance. In the bladder, this impermeability has to be maintained despite repeated large changes in surface area as the bladder fills and empties. This is maintained by unfolding and refolding of the large, highly folded 'umbrella' cells that form the uppermost layer of the epithelium, together with insertion and endocytosis of vesicles, ready-lined with uroplakin, a hexagonal transmembrane protein found only on the surface of umbrella cells. In experimental models, infection is associated with a marked reduction in transepithelial resistance and loss of tight junctions, allowing components of urine to stimulate pain fibres and inflammatory cytokine release.

Ascending infection takes place in a series of steps, at each of which defective host defence increases the chance of successful establishment of infection (Fig. 1).

The ability of a bacterium to colonize the gut and periurethral mucosa, and subsequently to adhere to the uroepithelium, is a major determinant of its ability to cause clinical infection, particularly if other host defences are intact. This ability to adhere is governed by specific interaction between bacterial adhesins, located on the tips of thin filaments ('pili' or 'fimbrias'), with genetically determined glycoproteins on the cell surface of the host cell. Type 1 fimbrias bind to mannose-containing glycoproteins that are

Table 1 Organisms commonly causing uncomplicated urinary tract infection

Escherichia coli
Klebsiella pneumoniae
Proteus spp.
Pseudomonas spp.
Enterococcus spp.
Staphylococcus saprophyticus (in sexually active women and girls)

present on the surface of uroepithelial cells, but also to Tamm–Horsfall protein, which is present in urine and can competitively inhibit binding of bacteria to cell surface glycoproteins. Type P pili bind the α-galactosyl-1,4-β-galactose disaccharide sequence present in some glycoproteins and glycosphingolipids, including the human P blood-group antigen system and also on the cell surface of uroepithelial cells as well as red cells. Some uropathogens are particularly adapted to colonizing foreign surfaces, particularly those coated by biofilm or mucin; for example, *Proteus* spp. are able to transform into a swarming phenotype with massive flagellas, organize into rafts, and move very rapidly against the flow of urine—they are therefore important causes of infection in patients with indwelling urinary catheters and those with ileal conduits.

Following adherence, fimbriae appear to retract, drawing the organism closer to the surface of the uroepithelial cell. Adherence is followed by apoptosis, exfoliation, and excretion of infected superficial cells and replacement by less differentiated cells, a process that may also contribute to host defence.

Bacterial adherence results in the local production of interleukin 8, which results in neutrophil migration through the uroepithelium into the bladder. Inflammatory cytokine release may also be promoted by soluble bacterial stimuli, such as lipopolysaccharide.

Variability in host defence

Frequency and completeness of bladder emptying

For an ascending infection to become established in the bladder, the number of organisms needs to reach a critical mass. The chance of this happening is reduced by increased urine flow rate, causing dilution of organisms within the bladder, and by frequent voiding, which also flushes the urethra and helps to prevent ascent of organisms into the bladder. This is termed 'hydrokinetic' defence. Habitual infrequent voiding is thought to be a risk factor for recurrent urinary tract infection for this reason. Patients with recurrent urinary tract infections are routinely advised to increase fluid intake and frequency of voiding, and some women report that a high fluid intake alone is enough to clear symptomatic infection. Incomplete voiding, which may be present in both sexes and is not necessarily due to outflow obstruction (Table 2) is an important cause of increased susceptibility to urine infection.

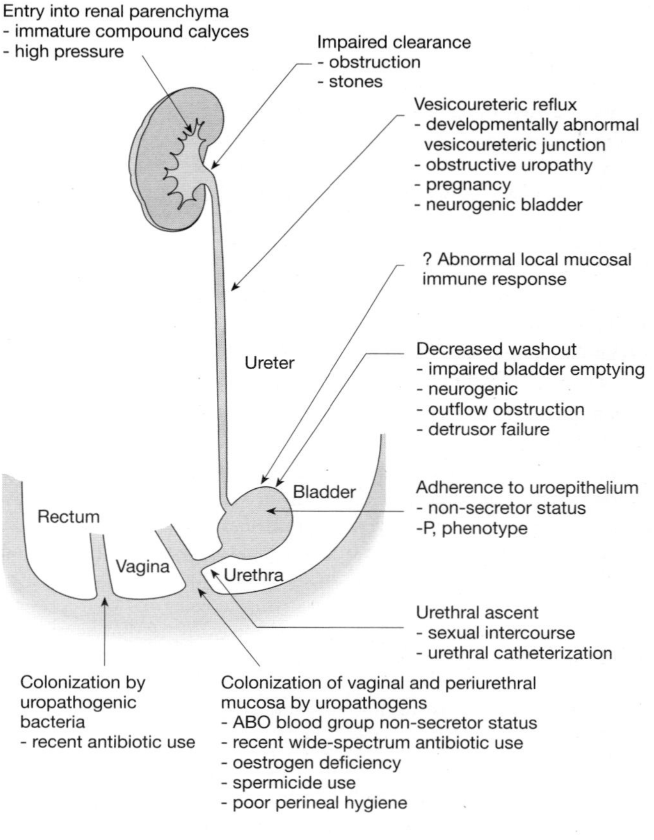

Fig. 1 Mechanisms allowing ascent of infection up the urinary tract.

Table 2 Some of the causes of incomplete bladder emptying

Bladder outflow obstruction	
	Benign prostatic hypertrophy
	Prostate cancer
	Strictures:
	bladder neck
	urethral
	Uterine prolapse
Detrusor underactivity—	
	frequently ill-understood
Abnormal bladder innervation	
	Spinal cord injury
	Autonomic neuropathy, e.g. diabetes

Vesicoureteric reflux

During normal micturition urine is expelled into the urethra, while retrograde flow ('reflux') of urine into the ureters is prevented because muscular contraction of the bladder wall results in closure of the vesicoureteric junctions. Reflux of urine into the ureters can occur if this mechanism is defective, sometimes as far as the renal pelvis, followed by return to the bladder once bladder contraction has finished. The most common cause of reflux is abnormal insertion of the ureters into the bladder: this occurs as a relatively frequent developmental anomaly, the other major cause being abnormally high intravesical pressure, for instance in high-pressure chronic retention of urine due to bladder outflow obstruction, or in neurogenic bladder in patients with partial spinal cord lesions. Whatever the cause, reflux of urine results in failure to expel all bladder urine during micturition, and therefore significantly impairs host defence against infection, as well as being associated with a greatly increased risk of infection ascending to the kidneys and causing acute pyelonephritis. Vesicoureteric reflux is frequently found in children with urinary tract infection. The question of whether ascending infection is a cause of renal damage in children with reflux is discussed later in this chapter.

Foreign bodies, stones, and privileged sites

The presence of a foreign body, such as a urinary catheter or ureteric stent, or of a stone within the urinary tract, creates a protected site where uropathogenic organisms can adhere and multiply, relatively immune to both hydrokinetic and mucosal defence mechanisms. In this situation it is often impossible to eradicate urine infection unless the foreign body or stone is removed completely, and prolonged use of antibiotics often results in the acquisition of resistance by the infecting organism. Urinary infection is nearly inevitable after a few weeks of bladder catheterization, which has led to attempts to develop catheter materials that are less easily colonized by bacteria and might thereby reduce the risk of infection. Meta-analysis shows that silver alloy urinary catheters may be cost-effective in preventing urinary infection in patients catheterized for a short time. Other 'privileged' sites include renal cysts (as in polycystic kidney disease, discussed below) and bladder diverticulas.

Sexual behaviour

Many women first experience acute cystitis shortly after becoming sexually active. Most women have transient bacteriuria after sexual intercourse, which develops into symptomatic cystitis only in a minority. In case–control studies of young women, the risk of urinary tract infection was associated with vaginal intercourse, and increased further by condom use. These findings are explained by the mechanical effect of intercourse encouraging ascent of organisms up the urethra, an effect that may be exacerbated by condom use, particularly without lubricants. The risk of urinary tract infection is also increased by a change in sexual partner, which may reflect male to female transmission of uropathogens. Use of spermicides as an adjunct to barrier contraceptive methods is also associated with an increased rate of periurethral colonization with *E. coli* and other uropathogens and with an increased risk of symptomatic urinary tract infection, probably because the active component in spermicides (nonoxynol-9) is bactericidal against lactobacilli. The protective effect of micturition soon after intercourse, based on the supposition that washout of recently introduced bacteria will prevent establishment of infection, remains unproved.

Vaginal and periurethral flora

Vaginal secretions are normally colonized by lactobacilli that appear to protect against colonization by uropathogenic bacteria such as *E. coli*. The mechanism of this protection is uncertain but may in part be related to the maintenance of an acidic pH, which suppresses growth of some uropathogenic bacteria. Suppression of this normal vaginal colonization by antibiotic treatment or by spermicide use increases the risk of colonization of the periurethral mucosa by uropathogenic bacteria and subsequent ascending urinary tract infection. In addition, atrophic vaginitis caused by oestrogen deficiency is associated with the absence of lactobacillus colonization, which may be part of the reason for the increased risk of urinary tract infection in postmenopausal women. However, attempts to prevent recurrent urinary infection by re-establishing colonization by lactobacilli have so far not yielded convincing results.

Genetic factors

In laboratory studies, adherence of *E. coli* to both vaginal and buccal cells is greater in women with recurrent urinary tract infection than in healthy controls, and women with recurrent urinary tract infection more frequently have gut colonization by uropathogenic strains of *E. coli*, suggesting that they experience more frequent urinary tract infections because they are more susceptible to colonization of the periurethral area by uropathogenic bacteria. It appears that this difference in susceptibility to colonization and infection, especially in patients in whom there is no other defect of host defence (such as vesicoureteric reflux), is due to genetically determined differences in the extracellular antigens to which bacteria adhere, in particular in the expression of blood group antigens. The density of glycosphingolipids is higher in patients with the P1 blood group than those with the P2 blood group, and the P1 blood group is a risk factor for acute pyelonephritis among girls without vesicoureteric reflux. Expression of the large oligosaccharide A, B, H blood group antigens on the cell surface partially or completely obscures the smaller glycosphingolipids, preventing them from being bound by type P pili, which is why women with the secretor phenotype, in which these antigens are both expressed on the cell surface and secreted, are less prone to most *E. coli* infections than non-secretors. Non-secretors also have an increased inflammatory response (fever and acute-phase response) to urinary infection compared with secretors, and non-secretors are over-represented among patients with urographic evidence of reflux nephropathy. However, some *E. coli* strains only bind to cells from subjects who are secretor-positive blood group A.

Local immunity

Another aspect of host defence is the local production of antimicrobial peptides, secreted by uroepithelial cells into the urine, and the secretion of immunoglobulin A into the urine. However, there is little convincing evidence that impaired local IgA secretion is responsible for increased susceptibility to urinary tract infection. Patients with inherited or systemic defects in systemic immunity, whether cellular or humoral, do not appear to be at greatly increased risk of urinary tract infection; the increased risk of urinary tract infection in homosexual men with the acquired immune deficiency syndrome is associated with anal intercourse.

Pathogenicity

A few species of bacteria, collectively known as 'uropathogenic' bacteria, together account for most urinary tract infections (Table 1); the presence of non-uropathogenic species suggests an abnormality of host defence. Within uropathogenic species there are strains that are capable of causing infection and other strains that are far less likely to do so: uropathogenicity is determined by expression of cell surface molecules determining adhesion to receptors on uroepithelial cells, toxin production, factors conferring resistance to the membrane attack complex, and virulence factors. The factors determining pathogenicity of *E. coli* have been studied extensively, but much less is known about the determinants of pathogenicity of other uropathogenic bacteria, although motility may be an important determinant of the ability of *Proteus* spp. to ascend the urinary tract and cause infection; and *Staphylococcus saprophyticus*, an important cause of urinary tract infection in sexually active young women, is probably better able to cause urinary tract infection than *Staphylococcus aureus* or *Staphylococcus epidermidis* because of its possession of a lactosamine adhesin permitting adherence to uroepithelial cells.

Clinical presentation of uncomplicated urinary tract infection

Frequency and dysuria

The commonest presentation of urinary tract infection is with 'cystitis', a symptom complex associated with lower urinary tract infection in which many of the symptoms are directly attributable to increased bladder irritability caused by local infection. Classic symptoms include:

(1) severe dysuria, often described as 'scorching' or 'like peeing barbed wire', worse towards the end or immediately after micturition;

(2) increased urinary frequency, including nocturia—which helps to distinguish cystitis from other causes of daytime frequency;

(3) urgency—the feeling of having to pass urine straight away to avoid incontinence;

(4) urge incontinence—leakage of urine associated with the desire to pass urine;

(5) strangury—the feeling of needing to pass urine despite just having done so;

(6) offensive-smelling urine, often described as 'strong' or 'fishy';

(7) macroscopic haematuria—particularly in women under 50, less commonly in girls or older women;

(8) constant lower abdominal aching, not just in the genital area but also in the back, flanks, and lower abdomen; and

(9) non-specific malaise, aching all over, nausea, tiredness, irritability, and cold sweats.

Not all of these symptoms are specific for lower urinary tract infection. Dysuria may be due to cystitis, urethritis, or vaginitis, but the latter two conditions are usually not associated with urinary frequency, and may be associated with vaginal discharge or itching and with specific findings on vaginal examination. Symptoms of cystitis may be due to causes other than lower urinary tract infection, for instance drug-induced cystitis.

Genuine inflammation of the bladder wall may or may not be present, and it is important to remember that there may be non-infective causes of increased bladder irritability, such as chemical- or drug-induced cystitis. Most patients with cystitis do not have fever, nor is there evidence of an acute-phase response.

Asymptomatic bacteriuria

By definition, this is an incidental finding in patients whose urine is cultured despite the absence of urinary tract symptoms. It is seldom justified to send a urine sample from an asymptomatic patient for culture, so this diagnosis should only rarely be made in clinical practice. An important exception is during pregnancy. Pregnant women with bacteriuria are at increased risk of acute pyelonephritis (occurring in 20 to 30 per cent of untreated women), of delivering low birth-weight babies, and of premature delivery, and antibiotic treatment significantly reduces these risks. Elderly patients with asymptomatic bacteriuria are also at increased risk of death, but this is probably because bacteriuria is a marker of poorer general health, and antibacterial treatment has not been shown to improve survival in this situation.

Acute pyelonephritis

The term acute pyelonephritis denotes infection within the renal pelvis, with or without active infection within the renal parenchyma. The diagnosis is usually made on the basis of the presence of flank pain (usually unilateral), fever, rigors, raised C-reactive protein (or erythrocyte sedimentation rate or plasma viscosity), neutrophilia, and evidence of urine infection on culture of a mid-stream urine sample. However, rigorous tests to localize the site of infection (discussed below) show that the correlation between the presence or absence of bacteriuria in the upper urinary tract and the presence or absence of flank pain, systemic symptoms, and an acute-phase response is dismally poor; many patients with infection confined to the bladder have flank pain and fever, whereas over 60 per cent of elderly women with asymptomatic bacteriuria have upper tract infection. The symptoms and signs of so-called 'acute pyelonephritis' are therefore in reality those of a marked host response to urinary tract infection, irrespective of whether organisms are multiplying in the renal pelvis or in the bladder.

Diagnosis

Inspection and dipstick testing

In a 'classic' case of established urinary tract infection the urine is cloudy, has an offensive smell, and is positive for blood, protein, leucocyte esterase, and nitrite on dipstick urinalysis. In this situation it is reasonable to make a diagnosis of urinary tract infection without further delay, and to institute empirical treatment. Whether a midstream urine sample should also be sent to the laboratory for confirmation and identification of the causative organism depends on the clinical situation, as discussed below. However, in many situations the diagnosis is not so obvious, and the diagnostic accuracy of inspection and dipstick testing less good.

1. Cloudy urine may be caused by bacteria and pyuria, but may also be caused by amorphous phosphate crystals that form in normal urine as it cools. Low concentrations of bacteria and white cells will not cause sufficient turbidity to be detected on visual inspection.
2. An offensive, fishy smell is highly suggestive of urinary tract infection, but relatively infrequent.
3. Macroscopic haematuria can certainly occur as a result of severe cystitis, but is frequently absent in genuine urinary tract infection and is more often due to glomerular bleeding or urothelial bleeding as a result of tumours or stones. Dipstick detection of haematuria is neither sensitive nor specific for the detection of urinary tract infection.
4. Proteinuria can occur in urinary tract infection as a result of the release of proteins from white cells, but is neither specific nor sensitive.
5. Leucocyte esterase is an enzyme released by white cells and a reliable test for pyuria, which is in most situations a major diagnostic criterion for urinary tract infection, as discussed in the next section. A positive test indicates 10 white cells/ml. Transport of urine samples in containers containing boric acid can result in false-negative leucocyte esterase tests, as the boric acid inhibits the enzyme.
6. Nitrite is produced by most uropathogens, which reduce urinary nitrate to nitrite, but not by Gram-positive organisms. A positive test for nitrite is highly suggestive of urinary tract infection. False negative tests can be seen in patients with low dietary nitrate and in those taking high-dose ascorbic acid.

A combination of visual inspection and dipstick testing is therefore a reasonable screening test for patients in whom uncomplicated urinary tract infection is suspected on clinical grounds: in this situation, crystal clear urine and negative dipsticks for nitrite and leucocyte esterase make the diagnosis of urinary tract infection very unlikely (Table 3). The worst that is likely to happen if the diagnosis is missed is that the patient will re-present with more obvious abnormalities due to progression of the urinary tract infection to a more severe stage. However, in situations in which it would be important not to miss the opportunity to start treatment early, for example in patients with known abnormalities of host defence, pregnancy, or previous acute pyelonephritis, or in suspected atypical infections, formal microscopy and culture of the urine is required.

Microscopy and culture of urine

At first sight, the diagnosis of bacterial infection in the urinary tract should be straightforward, relying on culture of freshly voided urine. However, urine samples are very easily contaminated during voiding by bacteria from the perineal skin (or, to a lesser extent, the foreskin in males), resulting in false-positive results. The only certain way to circumvent this problem is to take urine directly from the bladder, either by suprapubic needle aspiration of urine from the bladder, which is invasive and seldom performed in clinical practice, or by urethral catheterization, which carries a 1 to 2 per cent risk of introducing infection into the bladder. In men, contamination of the voided urine sample can largely be avoided by retraction of the foreskin prior to voiding. In women, the reliability of urine culture can be improved by instructing women to part the labia with one hand and ensuring collection of a midstream sample, without either the initial portion or the 'afterdrip', but is not improved further by perineal washing or antiseptic use. These precautions only reduce the risk of contamination, rather than abolishing it altogether.

Microscopy of urine samples allows quantification of pyuria—the presence of white blood cells in the urine. However, the methodology used to report pyuria varies enormously: microscopy of urine that has been centrifuged and resuspended, with reporting of the number of cells per high-power field, gives results which bear little relation to leucocyte excretion rate or to counting cells from unspun urine in a counting chamber, when significant pyuria is usually defined as a urinary white cell count of 10 leucocytes/μl or more.

Bacterial urinary tract infection is by far the commonest cause of pyuria, and symptomatic patients with pyuria whose urine cultures are reported as showing no significant pathogens should be suspected either of having

Table 3 Usefulness of inspection and dipstick testing in the diagnosis of urinary tract infection

Test	Utility	False positive	False negative
Cloudy appearance	Suggestive	Phosphate crystals	Common
Haematuria	Unreliable	Renal disease, stones, tumours	Common
Proteinuria	Unreliable	Renal disease	Common
Leucocyte esterase	Highly suggestive	Some antibiotics	Boric acid
Nitrite	Highly suggestive	Few	Gram +ve

Table 4 Causes of 'sterile pyuria'

Partially treated bacterial urinary tract infection
Bacterial urinary tract infection with a 'fastidious' organism
Chlamydial urethritis
'False-negative' urine cultures due to contamination of midstream urine sample with antiseptic
Contamination by vaginal leucocytes
Chronic interstitial nephritis:
Analgesic nephropathy
Sarcoidosis (urinary white cells may be lymphocytes, not neutrophils)
Urinary tract stones
Acute interstitial nephritis, e.g. allergic interstitial nephritis (urinary white cells may be eosinophils)
Papillary necrosis:
Diabetes
Sickle-cell disease
Renal tract tuberculosis
Fever

'low-count' bacteriuria due to early infection or infection with a slow-growing organism, chlamydial infection, or one of the causes of sterile pyuria (Table 4). However, vaginal leucorrhoea can also result in 'false-positive' pyuria.

Microscopy also gives information on whether the urine sample is contaminated by cells from the periurethral area. Squamous cells are five to seven times larger than red cells and are easily recognized on microscopy: their presence in a midstream urine sample has conventionally been taken to indicate contamination, but they may originate from the urethra as well as from the epithelium of the vulva and vagina, as well as from areas of squamous metaplasia in the bladder, which is a common finding; and squamous cells are frequently seen in urine obtained by bladder catheterization, showing that their presence is not an absolute indicator of contamination.

Once a urine sample is obtained, the conditions under which it is cultured determine whether any organisms present grow. Standard laboratory culture conditions are designed to encourage the growth of recognized urinary pathogens (if present), but may not be optimal for the growth of atypical organisms or of those not usually recognized as urinary pathogens. Because small numbers of organisms are frequently cultured from urine as a result of contamination, growth of an organism is conventionally reported as a 'significant growth' if it meets several criteria:

(1) there is a pure growth, i.e. of a single organism;

(2) the organism grown is a 'recognized' urinary pathogen;

(3) quantitative urine culture results in greater than 10^5 colony-forming units per millilitre (**cfu/ml**); and

(4) there is significant pyuria on urine microscopy, and few if any squamous cells.

However, there are important exceptions to these criteria.

1. Genuine mixed growth of two or more bacteria may occur in complicated urinary tract infection (Table 5), as may the growth of an organism not usually associated with the urinary tract.
2. The spectrum of organisms recognized as capable of causing genuine urinary tract infection is widening. *Staphylococcus saprophyticus* was only fairly recently recognized as a cause of urinary tract infection in sexually active women, and it is possible that other true urinary pathogens are yet to be identified, perhaps accounting for some cases of the so-called urethral syndrome (see below).
3. 'Low-count' bacteriuria may reflect genuine bladder infection, particularly in early urinary tract infections, and may occur in patients who have increased their fluid intake and are 'diluting' their bacterial counts by generating a high urine output; also in patients infected with slow-growing organisms such as *Staph. saprophyticus.* The criterion of 10^5 cfu/ml was originally validated in asymptomatic women, but subsequent studies showed that nearly 50 per cent of women presenting with frequency and dysuria had genuine bladder infection but with counts between 10^2 and 10^5 cfu/ml on culture of a midstream urine sample. If symptomatic women with counts of between 10^2 and 10^4 cfu/ml are left untreated, most have persistent symptoms and counts of more than 10^5 cfu/ml 2 days later.
4. In men, bacterial counts of 10^3 cfu/ml or more are very likely to reflect significant infection, as the potential for significant contamination is lower.
5. The presence of pyuria further increases the likelihood that low counts are significant, although pyuria is not always present in proven bladder infection, particularly if the sample is taken early after the onset. The traditional method of expressing urinary white cell counts as cells per high-power field is very poorly reproducible as the volume in a high-power field is extremely variable. If a counting chamber or equivalent is used, then a criterion of 10 white cells/mm^3 separates patients with genuine bacteriuria from those without.

Table 5 Conditions in which genuine mixed-growth urinary tract infection may occur

Ileal conduits
Neurogenic bladder
Vesicocolic fistula
Urinary tract stones
Renal abscesses
Long-term indwelling urinary catheters or stents

Localization to upper or lower urinary tract

It is sometimes important to discover whether infection is confined to the bladder or whether it has spread to involve one or both kidneys. The 'gold standard' for diagnosis of upper urinary tract infection is culture of urine obtained from each ureter by direct catheterization during cystoscopy, but such an invasive procedure can only be justified in exceptional circumstances, and even then may be difficult to interpret due to contamination of ureteric samples by bladder urine during passage of the catheters. An alternative, the Fairley test, involves a bladder washout using neomycin and fibrinolytic enzymes. Urine is cultured following completion, to confirm eradication of bladder bacteria, and then at 10, 20, and 30 min after completion of the washout. Bacteriuria returns slowly, if at all, in patients with infection confined to the bladder, but because the washout procedure has no effect on bacteria in the upper urinary tracts, rapid reappearance of bacteriuria indicates upper urinary tract infection. Using this test it has been shown that both upper and lower urinary tract infection are frequently asymptomatic and that flank pain and fever are extremely unreliable indicators of the presence of upper urinary tract infection.

Detection by immunofluorescent staining of immunoglobulin-coated bacteria is suggestive of tissue invasion, and has been advocated as a test to distinguish upper from lower urinary tract infection. However, compared with ureteric catheterization or Fairley tests, tests for antibody-coated bacteria are not reliable. This may be partly because tissue invasion can also occur in severe lower urinary tract infection, such as that complicating urethral catheterization. Antibody-coated bacteria may indicate a higher risk of treatment failure after standard antibiotic courses, but this remains uncertain.

Tubular damage due to ascending infection may be detected by measurement of urinary β_2-microglobulin, although this is also raised in patients with chronic renal disease and is therefore not specific for acute pyelonephritis. Renal excretory function usually remains unchanged during acute pyelonephritis unless obstruction is present, but acute renal failure is occasionally seen, often associated with coincident use of non-steroidal anti-inflammatory drugs. Abnormal appearances on contrast CT scanning and/or dimercaptosuccinyl acid (**DMSA**) scanning have been reported, including generalized renal swelling, focal areas of decreased parenchymal enhancement, and perirenal abscess formation, with the development of cortical scars and calyceal diverticulas if imaging is repeated on follow-up. In general, the more severe the infection is clinically (assessed by acute-phase response, duration of fever, etc.), the more marked the scarring. However, significant loss of renal excretory function following acute pyelonephritis in patients without diabetes, obstruction, or pre-existing reflux nephropathy/dysplasia is remarkably uncommon, and the significance of such scars is therefore uncertain.

Culture-negative syndromes

Occasionally patients may present with symptoms and signs highly suggestive of urinary tract infection, with or without pyuria, but with negative urine cultures. These patients may have 'false-negative' urine cultures, for instance a low growth of a genuine pathogen; infection with a 'fastidious' organism, the presence of which is not detected by routine laboratory cultures; or may have a non-infectious cause. It is dangerous to label symptoms in such patients as psychogenic without careful thought and investigation; prolonged symptoms combined with numerous unsuccessful trials of antibacterials or with different explanations from different doctors may result in psychological stress, which in turn may amplify symptoms, whereas there is little evidence that psychological disease is the primary problem even in a subgroup.

'Urethral syndrome'

The term 'urethral syndrome' was used in the past as a synonym for the typical symptoms of cystitis, namely frequency, urgency, and dysuria. More recently it has been applied to the subgroup of women with typical symptoms but in whom a recognized urinary pathogen cannot be cultured from the urine. A significant proportion of these patients, particularly those with pyuria, have chlamydial urethritis, which can be diagnosed by urethral swab or by detection of chlamydial antigens in a first-pass urine sample. Chlamydial infection can be treated with tetracyclines, but as the infection may be sexually transmitted it is also important to treat the patient's sexual partner(s), who may be asymptomatic. Other patients have 'low-count' infection with a true bacterial urinary pathogen. Vaginal infection or atrophy should be excluded, as these can cause similar symptoms.

The pathogenesis and optimal management of the remaining patients with frequency and dysuria with no identifiable bacterial infection remains controversial. There is controversy over the role of 'fastidious bacteria' that are difficult to grow in the laboratory, particularly lactobacilli. Empirical antiobiotic treatment is equally successful in eradicating symptoms in women presenting to primary care whether or not urinary pathogens are found on urine culture, suggesting that the syndrome is frequently due to bacterial infection that is not detected by routine laboratory urine culture. However, a few women with persistent symptoms do not respond to antibiotics, and in these women repeated courses of antibiotics are likely to lead to the emergence of antiobiotic-resistant organisms, which may later cause true infection that is difficult to treat. Psychological distress is common in patients with persistent lower urinary tract symptoms, but the prevalence of emotional or psychiatric disorders is no higher in women presenting to general practitioners with dysuria and frequency whose urine cultures are negative than in those with proven cystitis. Urologists often offer such women urethral dilatation on the assumption that the symptoms are due to urethral spasm or stricture, but there is minimal evidence beyond clinical anecdote that this procedure is of any benefit; one randomized, controlled trial showed no difference in outcome between urethral dilatation and cystoscopy alone. Urethral dilatation may itself cause periurethral fibrosis, resulting in the later formation of genuine urethral strictures.

Women with recurrent episodes of frequency and dysuria, with or without pyuria, whose urine cultures remain sterile should be carefully evaluated for the presence of vaginitis (either infective or atrophic) and for sexually acquired urethritis (where relevant). It is justified in this situation to obtain urine direct from the bladder during an episode, preferably by suprapubic aspiration or alternatively by urethral catheterization, and ensure that this is cultured in conditions permitting the identification of fastidious or low-growing organisms. In urine obtained direct from the bladder, any growth of organisms is clinically significant. Any infection so detected should be treated, preferably with a prolonged course of an appropriate antibiotic to ensure complete eradication. If no infection can be detected, cystoscopy is required to exclude non-infective causes of cystitis. Patients should be treated with compassion and their symptoms believed: attributing the symptoms to psychiatric disease is almost certain to be incorrect and likely to alienate the patient.

Interstitial cystitis

Interstitial cystitis causes chronic suprapubic pain, dysuria, and frequency despite, by definition, sterile urine. Urine microscopy shows pyuria. Cystoscopy shows variable inflammation, sometimes with ulceration. Bladder biopsies show a chronic inflammatory infiltrate; mast cell infiltration is common, but is also seen in infective cystitis. The condition may progress to cause contracture of the bladder. Many of the features would be explained by an acquired defect in the barrier function of the uroepithelium, but the cause of such a defect remains unclear. It remains possible that infection by a fastidious organism is responsible for initiating the disease in some patients. Numerous therapies have been tried, including intravesical instillation of glycosoaminoglycans.

Drug-induced cystitis

This presents similarly, although often more acutely and with macroscopic haematuria. It may be caused by acrolein, a metabolite of cyclophosphamide and ifosfamide, and also by non-steroidal anti-inflammatory drugs, particularly tiaprofenic acid, and by danazol.

Investigation of patients with urinary tract infection

Most women with uncomplicated cystitis do not require investigation other than urine culture, and may even be treated empirically, the choice of antibiotic being based on locally prevalent sensitivity patterns of the most common uropathogens, rather than waiting for the results of culture and sensitivity. The yield in such women of investigation with cystoscopy and/or intravenous urography is low. Because minor abnormalities such as duplex collecting systems are common in the general population, these will often be found in women presenting with cystitis, but detection of such abnormalities does not lead to any change in treatment. Investigation of women should therefore be reserved for those with atypical features (Table 6). In men, urinary tract infection is nearly always associated with an underlying abnormality of host defence, and all men with proven urinary tract infection should therefore be offered investigation. If investigation in either sex is thought necessary, the important abnormalities being looked for are:

- diabetes
- urinary tract stones

Table 6 Indications for further investigation in females with urinary tract infection

Genuine mixed growth
Failure of standard antibiotic treatment to eradicate infection
Relapsing infection (repeated detection of the same organism, as identified by antibiotic sensitivity pattern, or more detailed typing)
Confirmed infection with organisms not usually recognized as uropathogens
Infection with *Proteus* spp.
Marked acute-phase response (or symptoms of 'acute pyelonephritis'), suggesting tissue invasion
Persistent haematuria after treatment of infection
Asymptomatic bacteriuria, for no known cause

- anatomical abnormalities of the upper urinary tract (e.g. papillary necrosis, reflux nephropathy)
- urinary tract obstruction (anywhere from the renal pelvis to the tip of the urethra)
- bladder diverticulas
- impaired bladder emptying.

The choice of investigation of the upper urinary tract depends on local facilities, and usually lies between plain abdominal radiography with ultrasound, on the one hand, and intravenous urography on the other. Both may need to be supplemented by cystoscopy and by bladder voiding studies, using urinary flow rate and measurement of pre- and post-void bladder volumes.

Whether adults should be investigated for vesicoureteric reflux is open to doubt, as there is no good evidence that antireflux surgery (e.g. ureteric reimplantation, injection of Teflon around the ureteric orifice) is of benefit in preventing either ascending infection or renal damage.

Treatment of uncomplicated 'cystitis'

Rational treatment of urinary tract infection requires the physician to balance the costs and dangers of treatment (including cost of the drug, risk of unwanted side-effects, and the induction of resistance) with benefit.

Is treatment necessary at all? Many women with recurrent uncomplicated cystitis report that they can clear their own infections by increased fluid intake and frequent voiding. Many buy alkalinizing agents (e.g. potassium citrate) to ameliorate the symptoms, which work by reducing bladder irritability. Placebo-controlled studies have confirmed that infection may clear spontaneously, although this may take several weeks or even months, and a small percentage of women remain infected until given antibiotics. There is therefore no justification in insisting on antibiotic treatment in those who wish to try to do without.

Choice of antibiotic

It is usually impracticable to await the results of culture and sensitivity testing, if these tests are justified at all. The choice of antibiotic is therefore usually empirical, based on the likelihood that the drug will clear the infection (efficacy), cost, side-effect profile, and the risk of selection of resistant organisms, both in the patient being treated and in the community. The efficacy of antibiotics is not fully predictable from *in vitro* sensitivity testing, which is probably part of the reason why trimethoprim (with or without sulphamethoxazole) remains the first-line choice in many areas, despite resistance rates on *in vitro* testing of up to 20 per cent. This is at least in part because many antibiotics are concentrated in the urine to levels far greater than those found in tissues, and at these concentrations may remain active against organisms that are reported to be resistant to the concentrations found in tissues, which are usually used to define resistance *in vitro.* However, increasing resistance *in vitro* to trimethoprim is sure to lead sooner or later to increased clinical failure rates, as has already been observed for β-lactam antibiotics. Some of the properties of the most commonly used antibiotics are reviewed in Table 7. The most recent recommendations of the Infectious Diseases Society of America are summarized in Table 8.

Duration of treatment

A single high dose of an antibiotic will cure many women and is simple, cheap, and may reduce the risk of side-effects and bacterial resistance. Single-dose treatment is thought to be popular amongst patients, although those paying for prescription medications may feel 'short-changed' by paying a full prescription fee for a single tablet. However, cure rates after single-dose treatment are lower than for longer courses of antibiotics, this difference being more marked for β-lactam antibiotics, which in general need to be given for 7 days, than for trimethoprim (with or without sulphonamide) and for quinolones. Fosfomycin given as a single dose gives higher cure rates than single doses of other antibiotics, but is less effective and more likely to cause adverse effects than 3-day courses of trimethoprim (with or without sulphonamide) or quinolones. The rate of adverse reactions also increases with duration of therapy, particularly for

Table 7 Properties of antibiotics commonly used for urinary tract infections

Antibiotic	Pros	Cons
Trimethoprim	Cheap High concentrations in vaginal and periurethral fluid Low frequency of side-effects	Increasing rates of resistance (20% in some areas)
Trimethoprim–sulphamethoxazole	As for trimethoprim ? Decreased risk of emergence of resistant strains	Increasing rates of resistance Adverse reactions to sulphonamide component
β-Lactams (e.g. amoxycillin, cephalosporins)	Cheap Well tolerated	High rates of resistance (50 per cent in some areas) Less effective than trimethoprim in 3-day or single-dose regimens Allergic reactions High risk of *Clostridium difficile* colitis in hospital or elderly patients with cephalosporins
β-Lactams with β-lactamase inhibitor	As for β-lactams Lower rates of resistance	Cost Risk of emergence of resistance
Quinolones	Low rates of resistance Well tolerated	Cost Risk of selection of resistant strains
Nitrofurantoin	Cheap Does not induce resistance in bowel organisms	Nausea and vomiting (less with macrocrystalline preparations) Less effective in 3-day courses: eradication may require 7-day courses Inactive against *Proteus* spp. Hepatic, neurological, haematological, and pulmonary toxicity (mostly seen with prolonged treatment)

trimethoprim–sulphonamide combinations, which should therefore be given for no more than 3 days. Cure rates of urinary tract infections caused by *Staph. saprophyticus* and in elderly women are low with 3-day regimens, and these infections should be treated with 7-day courses.

Alternatives to antibiotic therapy

Fructose, present in many fruit juices, inhibits binding of type 1 fimbrias of *E. coli* to the uroepithelium. Cranberry juice also contains proanthocyanidin, which inhibits adherence of P-fimbriated *E. coli*. Cranberry juice is popular as an alternative treatment for urinary tract infection, but the evidence for its effectiveness in clinical practice remains uncertain.

Treatment of uncomplicated 'acute pyelonephritis'

Choice of antibiotic

The antibiotic chosen in this situation needs good tissue penetration as well as high urinary excretion, and must be fully active against the infecting organism at typical serum concentrations. It is therefore much more important to identify the infecting organism and its antibiotic sensitivity pattern by sending urine (or blood from patients in hospital) for culture. However, empirical treatment must be started while awaiting culture and sensitivity results, as acute pyelonephritis can evolve rapidly into a life-threatening illness. Oral therapy with a quinolone antibiotic (ciprofloxacin, ofloxacin, norfloxacin) is probably the best choice, although trimethoprim or trimethoprim–sulphamethoxazole are alternatives if local rates of resistance among uropathogens remain low. Treatment with β-lactam antibiotics, even if the infecting organism is fully sensitive *in vitro*, is associated with a high rate of recurrence compared with treatment by other agents. Patients with septicaemia should receive a quinolone (for which oral administration is as effective as intravenous) or a combination of an aminoglycoside with ampicillin plus β-lactamase inhibitor, or an extended-spectrum cephalosporin with or without an aminoglycoside. Once-daily administration of aminoglycosides is as effective as thrice-daily and reduces the risk of toxicity.

Table 8 Recommendations of the Infectious Diseases Society of America for the treatment of uncomplicated acute bacterial cystitis and acute pyelonephritis

Cystitis	
First-line therapy	Trimethoprim–sulphamethoxazole for 3 days
Alternatives	Trimethoprim alone for 3 days
	Ofloxacin*
	Other quinolones* (e.g. ciprofloxacin, norfloxacin)
	β-Lactam antibiotics (less effective when given as 3-day course)
	Nitrofurantoin
	Fosfomycin
Pyelonephritis	
Mild cases	Oral fluroquinolone
	Oral trimethoprim–sulphamethoxazole (if organism known to be susceptible)
	Oral amoxycillin or amoxycillin–clavulanic acid (if causative organism likely to be Gram positive)
Severe cases	Parenteral fluoroquinolone
	Aminoglycoside +/– ampicillin
	Extended-spectrum cephalosporin +/– aminoglycoside
	Ampicillin–sulbactam +/– aminoglycoside (if causative organism likely to be Gram positive)
	Continue treatment for 7 to 14 days depending on severity of initial infection and response to treatment
	All followed by oral treatment to which the organism is susceptible

Full text available at http://www.idsociety.org

*Because of greater cost and the risk of emergence of resistant strains, these drugs should not be used for initial empirical treatment unless the local prevalence of resistance to trimethoprim–sulphamethoxazole is greater than 10 to 20%.

Duration of therapy

It is widely recommended that acute pyelonephritis is treated with a significantly longer course of antibiotics than acute cystitis. Since, as discussed above, the clinical distinction between acute pyelonephritis and cystitis relies on the presence of fever, flank pain, and an acute-phase response, and since all of these may be present in acute cystitis with no involvement of the upper urinary tract and entirely absent in acute pyelonephritis, what these recommendations really mean is that those patients demonstrating a more marked host response should be treated more aggressively and for longer. It is therefore reasonable to suggest that in a patient with systemic symptoms (including flank pain), fever, or leucocytosis, or a raised C-reactive protein, plasma viscosity, or erythrocyte sedimentation rate, antibiotic treatment should be continued until these abnormalities have disappeared. A 14-day course is as effective as a 6-week course in uncomplicated acute pyelonephritis, and a 7-day course may be sufficient for patients with mild illness.

Treatment of asymptomatic bacteriuria

The only situation in which treatment of asymptomatic bacteriuria is mandatory is during pregnancy (see Chapter 13.5). Eradication of asymptomatic infection in children with or without proven vesicoureteric reflux is widely practised in the hope that this will prevent ascending infection and renal damage. However, prophylactic treatment for 2 years of covert bacteriuria in schoolgirls without renal scarring has no effect on glomerular filtration rate at age 18, but is associated with lower fractional reabsorption of glucose and with a smaller increment in glomerular filtration rate and greater degrees of glycosuria during subsequent pregnancy. Screening for asymptomatic bacteriuria with the aim of preventing these minor abnormalities is not currently thought justified. Treatment of asymptomatic bacteriuria in patients with anatomically abnormal urinary tracts or with indwelling urinary catheters is unjustified and is likely only to lead to the emergence of antibiotic-resistance urinary infection. Treatment of asymptomatic bacteriuria in the elderly has been shown to be of no benefit.

Prophylaxis of recurrent urinary tract infection

Some women with recurrent cystitis choose to have antibiotic treatment for each infection as it arises, particularly if they are allowed to self-administer treatment as soon as symptoms start. Others may opt for prophylactic treatment. Long-term low-dose antibiotic treatment has been shown to be effective in reducing the rate of infection in such women, but no regimen offers 100 per cent protection. Prophylactic treatment should be considered in women with at least two symptomatic infections per year and probably works by preventing colonization of periurethral tissues by uropathogens. Trimethoprim (100 mg at night) is widely used for prophylaxis because it achieves very high concentrations in vaginal fluid and may therefore remain active against organisms that are resistant to the concentrations used in *in vitro* sensitivity testing. Nitrofurantoin (100 mg at night) has also been widely used, and may be more effective, but can cause rare but serious adverse effects (pulmonary and hepatic toxicity) with long-term therapy, making regular monitoring of liver enzymes and lung function tests necessary. Because both are well absorbed they do not reach high concentrations in the colon, hence emergence of resistant strains in colonic flora is uncommon, whereas this problem does arise with long-term use of β-lactam antibiotics. Long-term use of quinolones is expensive and associated with a significant risk of selection of resistant strains. There is no proven advantage in 'rotating' antibiotic prophylaxis. A number of dosage regimens have been used, including nightly treatment, thrice-weekly treatment, and postcoital treatment, with no convincing evidence of the superiority of one regimen over another. Treatment should be continued for at least 6 months, because, for reasons that are not clear, this results in a lower relapse rate once treatment is stopped than shorter periods of prophylaxis.

Cranberry juice, as discussed above, contains substances that inhibit adherence of uropathogenic bacteria to the uroepithelium, and has become popular as an alternative treatment to prevent recurrent urinary tract infection. However, the evidence that regular use of cranberry juice reduces the risk of recurrent symptomatic infections remains poor, and there is no consensus on what dosage and regimen, if any, is effective.

Complicated urinary tract infection

'Complicated' urinary tract infections are those occurring in a patient with abnormal host defence, and as a result are often more severe.

Urinary tract infection in men

Cystitis

In the first year of life, urinary tract infection is commoner amongst boys than girls; circumcision reduces the risk. Urinary tract infection in men is uncommon, as the length of the urethra and the fact that the penile mucosa is seldom colonized with faecal organisms including uropathogens confer major protection against ascending infection. The occurrence of urinary tract infection in a man therefore suggests an abnormality of host defence, which may predispose to more severe infection and should be investigated unless the cause is immediately obvious (e.g. the presence of a urinary catheter). Risk factors that may be identified by investigation include:

- bacterial prostatitis and prostatic calcification
- lack of circumcision
- impaired bladder emptying (particularly if this has resulted in bladder catheterization or instrumentation)
- anal intercourse
- urinary tract stones
- reflux nephropathy.

The symptoms of urinary tract infection in men are similar to those in women. The risk of bacterial contamination of voided urine is low apart from in elderly men with foreskins, in whom precautions should be taken to minimize contamination by retraction of the foreskin and collection of a midstream sample. Colony counts of 10^3/ml or higher usually indicate significant infection.

Acute prostatitis

Acute bacterial prostatitis causes fever, rigors, backache, and dysuria, and may result in acute urinary retention. Symptoms and signs of epididymitis may also be present. Rectal examination reveals an enlarged, tender prostate. Untreated, acute prostatitis may culminate in prostatic abscess formation. The causative organism can be identified on urine culture: an antibiotic which has good tissue penetration (e.g. trimethoprim, a tetracycline, or a quinolone) should be used and continued for 4 weeks, as it is thought that this reduces the risk of chronic prostatitis.

Chronic bacterial prostatitis

This is an uncommon syndrome caused by the persistence of a uropathogen within the prostate, with repeated episodes of acute infection caused by the same organism on each occasion, and few if any symptoms between episodes. Obtaining bacteriological proof that the infecting organism is 'hiding' in the prostate gland between acute episodes is difficult. The 'textbook' method described by Stamey and Mears involves culture of four specimens obtained during voiding of the bladder. The first 10 ml voided and a midstream sample are collected. The patient then interrupts the flow of urine, bends forward, and digital prostatic massage is performed, resulting (sometimes) in the collection of a few drops of 'expressed prostatic secretions'. Finally, voiding is completed and a fourth sample collected. Prostatitis is diagnosed when bacterial counts are highest in the expressed prostatic secretions and the final voided urine sample; urethritis, by contrast, results in high counts in the first sample. Due to its complexity and the unpleasantness of performing digital prostatic massage *per rectum* during interrupted micturition, this test is very rarely performed in practice, and many patients are treated with a prolonged course of a quinolone antibiotic. α-Blockers have been shown to reduce recurrence rate, possibly by reducing reflux of urine into prostatic ducts during micturition.

Culture-negative pelvic pain in men

Patients may complain of chronic pelvic pain, dysuria, strangury, urinary frequency, and pain during sexual intercourse but have no evidence of bacterial infection on cultures of prostatic secretions, semen, or post-massage urine specimens. Patients with this symptom complex may be further subclassified as having chronic abacterial prostatitis or non-inflammatory pelvic pain syndrome according to the presence or absence of leucocytes in semen. There is no gold standard for diagnosis, no clear understanding of the pathophysiology, no correlation between symptoms and prostatic histology, and no satisfactory treatment for this ill-understood group of conditions. Occasionally, patients are found to have evidence of prostatic inflammation on biopsy, or to have leucocytes in prostatic fluid in the absence of symptoms. As in the urethral syndrome in women, some cases may be caused by persistent infection by fastidious bacteria, such as *Chlamydia* or *Mycoplasma*; a prolonged trial of a tetracycline is therefore often used. Other treatments include regular prostatic massage, non-steroidal anti-inflammatory drugs, α-blockers, and 5-α reductase inhibitors. α-Blockers have been shown to be of some benefit in all types of symptomatic chronic prostatitis in one randomized study.

Urethral catheterization

Urinary tract infection occurs after 2 per cent of in/out urethral catheterizations, after 10 to 30 per cent of 5-day indwelling catheterization, and is nearly inevitable in patients with long-term indwelling catheters. It is an important cause of hospital-acquired infection, increasing the risk of Gram-negative septicaemia fivefold and carrying a threefold increase in mortality after adjustment for age, severity and type of underlying illness, duration of catheterization, and renal function. Organisms enter the bladder either by migration between the catheter and the urethral mucosa or by ascent up the column of urine in the lumen after entry into the drainage system following contamination at disconnection or drainage points. Although most infections are probably caused by ascent of the patient's own faecal flora, there is evidence from investigation of clusters of infections by highly antibiotic-resistant organisms that inadequate handwashing by hospital staff may also cause some infections. A sample obtained directly from the catheter (not from the drainage bag) represents bladder urine, when any bacterial growth should be considered as evidence of urinary tract infection; low-count infection (e.g. less than 10^2 cfu/ml) usually progresses within days to higher counts. Mixed growths are common in patients with long-term catheterization and may be associated with mixed-growth bacteraemia.

Risk factors for the acquisition of infection include increasing duration of catheterization, increasing age, female sex, renal impairment, diabetes mellitus, and the nature of the underlying illness. Use of prophylactic antibiotics is associated with a delay in the onset of infection and may be justified in high-risk patients requiring catheterization for 3 to 14 days, whereas in those with long-term catheters, antibiotic use simply increases the risk of emergence of antibiotic-resistant pathogens. Use of silver alloy-coated catheters also reduces the risk of infection and may be justified in high-risk patients. Progress is being made in the development of new catheter materials that may provide further resistance against colonization by microorganisms.

Urethral catheters should not be inserted unless absolutely necessary (is knowledge of hourly urine output really going to change your management?) and removed as soon as they are no longer needed. Consideration should always be given to methods of urine collection that may carry lower risks, such as condom drainage in men, intermittent catheterization in patients with abnormal bladder emptying, and suprapubic catheterization.

Abnormal bladder emptying

Incomplete bladder emptying, removing the 'washout' part of host defence, greatly increases the risk of urinary tract infection, as in patients with prostatic bladder outflow obstruction and those with neurogenic bladder due to spinal cord injury. Long-term catheterization only increases these risks. Where possible, the cause of incomplete bladder emptying should be treated. However, patients shown on urodynamic study to have underactive detrusor activity will not benefit from prostatectomy or α-blockade and may require long-term intermittent self-catheterization. Bladder dysfunction in patients with neurogenic bladder, for instance due to spina bifida or spinal cord injury, depends on the level of injury. Patients with lesions above T-11 have hyperreflexic bladder activity, often with sphincter dyssynergia (failure of the sphincter to relax during detrusor contraction), resulting in a high-pressure system, often with high-pressure reflux, combined with impaired emptying. In combination with urinary tract infection, this frequently results in progressive renal damage. Those with lesions below L-1 have decreased detrusor activity with large amounts of residual urine, which also increases the risk of urinary tract infection. Diabetic neuropathy may also cause decreased detrusor activity. The aim of treatment in both situations is to achieve a low-pressure bladder with low residual volumes. This may involve teaching patients to utilize reflexes to induce bladder contraction and sphincter relaxation, condom drainage for incontinence, anticholinergics to reduce detrusor overactivity, sphincterotomy, augmentation cystoplasty, and intermittent self-catheterization. Urethral catheterization should be avoided wherever possible. There is no evidence that regular use of antiseptics to wash the perineum and urethral meatus are of benefit. Bladder washouts with saline or boiled water may be of benefit in eliminating mucus in patients with augmentation cystoplasties: antiseptic bladder washouts are of minimal value in prevention, probably due to the fact that uropathogens become embedded in a biofilm adherent to the bladder wall. Methenamine, a drug that releases formaldehyde into acidic urine, may be of some benefit in preventing infection.

Treatment of urinary tract infection in patients with abnormal bladder emptying should be reserved for those with evidence of invasive infection. The diagnosis is obvious in those with cloudy urine combined with fever, rigors, and flank pain, but it is important to remember that symptoms and signs, particularly flank pain, dysuria, urgency, and frequency may be absent in those with neurological dysfunction.

Urinary diversion

Ileal or colonic conduits have been used for many years in patients requiring cystectomy for malignancy, and occasionally (although increasingly less frequently) for non-malignant conditions such as neurogenic bladder. Such conduits are frequently complicated by urine infection as the bowel mucosa and the mucus it produces readily permits adherence of uropathogens. Upper urinary tract dilatation is common, irrespective of whether the ureteric anastomoses are designed to be non-refluxing or not, and there is a high incidence of recurrent 'acute pyelonephritis' with flank pain, fever, and rigors. Diagnosis of urinary tract infection in patients with a conduit requires insertion of a catheter to the far end of the conduit and collection of urine via the catheter, rather than culture of urine collected from the conduit bag. Preventive measures include ensuring that the ileal segment is as short as possible at the time of surgery and ensuring a high fluid intake. The belief that cranberry juice reduces the incidence of urinary tract infection by reducing bacterial adherence is as yet unproven, although it seems likely that treatments designed to interfere with bacterial adherence or with mucin production are more likely than antibiotic treatment to help prevent symptomatic infection in these patients.

Renal tract stones

Renal tract stones are an important cause of persistent or relapsing urinary tract infection, as they provide a 'hiding place' in which organisms are protected from antibiotics. Management of such patients is complicated, as it may be impossible to eradicate infection without aggressive stone management (which may involve extracorporeal shock-wave lithotripsy, percutaneous and ureteroscopic stone removal). Attempts at stone removal may be complicated by septicaemia unless combined with antibiotic treatment, yet prolonged antibiotic therapy may encourage the emergence of resistance in the infecting organism.

Infection stones are caused by chronic infection with urease-producing organisms, usually *Proteus mirabilis*, and account for around 5 per cent of urinary tract stones. These stones are made of 'struvite' ($MgNH_4PO_4.6H_2O$), which forms as a result of the action of the alkaline pH caused by the production of ammonium and hydroxyl ions from the breakdown of urea by urease. Pure struvite stones may result from *de novo* urinary tract infection by a urease-producing organism, and are commoner in women and, probably, in patients with pre-existing anatomical abnormalities of the upper urinary tract such as reflux nephropathy, pelviureteric junction obstruction, or urinary diversion. Sruvite stones may also form as a secondary complication of metabolic stones. Struvite stones often expand to fill the entire renal pelvis, forming 'staghorn' calculi, but such calculi should not be assumed to be due to infection (rather than a metabolic cause) without demonstration of chronic infection by a urease-producing organism and/or biochemical analysis showing that the stone is made of struvite. The usual presentation is with symptomatic 'acute pyelonephritis' and alkaline urine; renal colic is unusual due to the large size of the stones. Treatment is with a combination of antibiotic and stone removal, which is imperative to prevent stone recurrence, and may require a combination of extracorporeal shock-wave lithotripsy and percutaneous nephrolithotomy, aided by dissolution therapy for larger stones. Urease inhibitors (acetohydroxamic acid, propionhydroxamic acid) may reduce stone recurrence but are too toxic for clinical use. See Chapter 20.13 for further discussion.

Encrusted cystitis and pyelitis occur as a result of chronic infection by urease-producing organisms, including *Corynebacterium* spp., in immunosuppressed patients, causing deposition of struvite in the bladder wall.

Autosomal dominant polycystic kidney disease

Cystitis is common in women with polycystic kidney disease, and in 20 per cent it is the presenting clinical finding, but there is no evidence that host defence in the lower urinary tract is abnormal. However, the risk of upper urinary tract infection is increased, and its diagnosis and treatment complicated. Acute parenchymal infection presents as acute pyelonephritis with flank pain, fever, and infected bladder urine, and usually responds to conventional therapy. Infection of cysts is more difficult to diagnose: the urine may be sterile and there may be no pyuria if the infected cyst does not communicate with the urinary space. Presentation is with fever and a discrete area of tenderness in the affected kidney. Blood cultures are the most reliable way of making a bacteriological diagnosis. Imaging studies, looking for cysts with increased fluid density, septations, and thick walls, are seldom conclusive, as similar appearances may occur normally or after previous cyst haemorrhage. The spectrum of causative organisms suggests that ascending infection rather than haematogenous spread is the usual route of infection. Hydrophilic antibiotics, including aminoglycosides and β-lactam antibiotics, penetrate poorly into those cysts which maintain large ionic gradients, whereas quinolones, trimethoprim–sulphamethoxazole, doxycycline, and clindamycin achieve better penetration. Prolonged courses of antibiotics are usually needed to eradicate infection, with surgical resection a last resort.

Renal transplantation

Urinary tract infection is the commonest bacterial infection after renal transplantation. Risk factors include urethral catheterization in the early postoperative period, the use of ureteric stents, pre-existing abnormalities of bladder emptying (such as diabetic autonomic neuropathy, previous bladder outflow obstruction, small contracted bladders in anuric patients on dialysis), anatomical abnormalities in the upper urinary tract (such as reflux nephropathy), contamination of the transplanted organ during retrieval and storage, abnormal drainage of urine from the transplanted kidney, vesicoureteric reflux into the transplant, areas of renal infarction, and immunosuppression. The commonest causative bacteria are those found in the general population with urinary tract infection, but many organisms not usually considered as urinary tract pathogens may also cause significant infection in these patients. Many infections are asymptomatic. Prophylactic antibiotics may reduce the early postoperative risk and many centres use co-trimoxazole as it also reduces the risk of *Pneumocystis* pneumonia. Antibiotic treatment must be chosen with care because of the risk of interactions with immunosuppressive treatment and of nephrotoxicity.

Infections with the polyomaviruses BK virus and JC virus may cause cystitis, ureteric stenoses, and interstitial nephritis (easily mistaken for acute rejection) in renal transplant recipients. The diagnosis may be suggested by recognition of infected transitional uroepithelial cells on urine cytology or by histological recognition of inclusion bodies on renal biopsy. Treatment is by reduction of immunosuppression, but this is often complicated by further rejection.

Pregnancy

Asymptomatic bacteriuria early in pregnancy is associated with the development of acute pyelonephritis in up to 30 per cent of patients if left untreated. It is commoner in women of lower socio-economic status and is associated with an increased incidence of preterm delivery and low birth weight, particularly if the pregnancy is complicated by acute pyelonephritis towards term. The increased risk of pyelonephritis is attributed to ureteric dilatation caused primarily by progesterone-induced smooth muscle relaxation. Antibiotic treatment of infection reduces the risk of acute pyelonephritis and of preterm delivery and low birth weight. Similar benefit is seen from a short course of treatment and from continued antibiotic prophylaxis. (See Chapter 13.5 for further discussion.)

Reflux nephropathy

As discussed above, vesicoureteric reflux (retrograde flow of urine up into the ureters and, in severe cases, as far as the renal pelvis) is often found in children with recurrent urinary tract infection. At the time of first diagnosis of urinary tract infection or subsequently, a small proportion of such children are found to have a characteristic pattern of renal parenchymal scarring at the upper and lower poles, with underlying clubbing and distortion of calyces. This pattern of scarring has become known by a variety of terms including 'reflux nephropathy' and 'chronic pyelonephritis'. Patients with reflux nephropathy have an increased risk of recurrent urinary tract infection, may develop infection stones, and a proportion develop hypertension, proteinuria, and progressive renal impairment with an inexorable progression to endstage renal failure. Under the age of 1 year, when only relatively severe cases come to clinical attention, slightly more boys than girls are affected; in older children the disease is diagnosed up to 5 times more frequently in girls, possibly because the disease is often discovered during investigation of urinary tract infection, which is commoner in females. Reflux nephropathy is commonly familial, best modelled by an autosomal dominant pattern of inheritance with variable penetrance. Linkage has been demonstrated to an area of chromosome 1 in some large pedigrees.

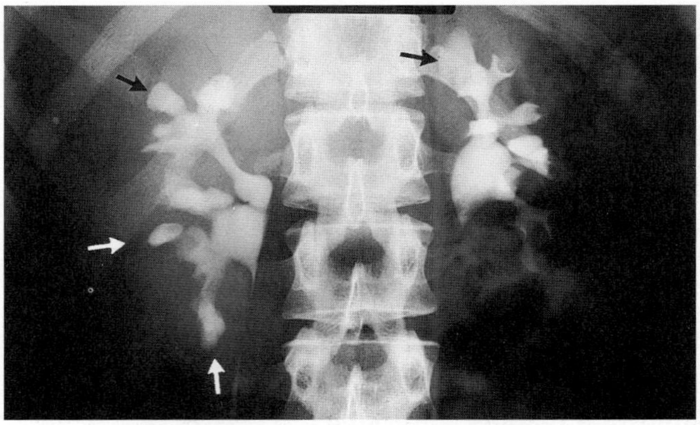

Fig. 2 Reflux nephropathy on intravenous urography, more marked on the right side than the left. Several focal scars (arrowed) involving the full thickness of the renal parenchyma and associated with calyceal clubbing are most obvious in the polar regions (reproduced from Bailey, 1993, with permission).

The diagnosis is conventionally made in adults by intravenous urography, which permits the detection both of focal parenchymal scarring and of the underlying calyceal abnormality (Fig. 2). Ultrasound scanning can show focal scarring but does allow visualization of the calyces. DMSA isotope scanning is the most sensitive test for the detection of parenchymal scars, and is widely used in children, as there are few alternative causes of focal scarring in this age group. Lateral displacement of the ureteric orifices can be demonstrated by Doppler ultrasound in most patients with reflux nephropathy. Demonstration of vesicoureteric reflux by direct or isotopic micturating cystography is commonly used to confirm the diagnosis in children, but is rarely justified in adults, as the absence of reflux could be due to spontaneous resolution of reflux with age (it often resolves in childhood), and its presence seldom justifies a change in clinical management. The histological appearances of 'chronic pyelonephritis' are well described and may occasionally be seen in patients with no scarring on urography or even DMSA scanning, probably because the scars are too small in these patients to be detected radiologically.

The conventional view is that reflux nephropathy is 'postinfectious focal renal scarring' and caused by the ascent of infected urine into the renal pelvis and then into the collecting ducts and renal parenchyma via compound papillas (papillas in which more than one collecting duct opens into the pelvis), which are found at the upper and lower poles but not in the middle calyces—explaining the polar distribution of scars. Sequential radiological imaging studies in children with urinary tract infections appear to support this theory, with the emergence of new scars up until the age of around 5 years, after which it is thought that maturation of the papillas prevents entry of infected urine into the renal parenchyma. Experimental infection in pigs causes a pattern of scarring very similar to that seen in human reflux nephropathy.

An alternative hypothesis is that at least a proportion of children with the radiological diagnosis of reflux nephropathy have congenital renal dysplasia, caused by abnormal nephrogenesis *in utero*, and associated with abnormal embryogenesis of the ureterovesical junction leading to vesicoureteric reflux. Vesicoureteric reflux is often found in the rare genetic syndromes that include renal dysplasia, and in non-syndromic renal dysplasia or aplasia, vesicoureteric reflux in the contralateral ureter is commonly seen. This theory would explain the presence of classic reflux nephropathy in neonates and in children with no documented history of urinary tract infection. Even the emergence of new scars during the first 5 years of life could be due to differential growth around areas of renal dysplasia. The rarity with which acute pyelonephritis in adults results in renal impairment, even in the presence of radiological evidence of scar formation, is perhaps further evidence that progressive loss of renal function is more likely to be due to 'remnant nephropathy' in dysplastic kidneys rather than the result of postinfectious scarring alone.

These two theories have different implications for the prevention of reflux nephropathy. Proponents of the 'postinfectious focal renal scarring' theory believe that diagnosis in infancy and treatment to prevent the ascent of infected urine into the renal pelvis until at least the age of 5 years should prevent the emergence of renal scarring and the later sequelae of hypertension, proteinuria, and progressive renal failure; by contrast, such treatment will not prevent these sequelae if reflux nephropathy is a disease of embryogenesis. Of course, the two theories are not mutually exclusive: in an individual patient reflux nephropathy may be due to the interaction of dysplasia and ascending infection during infancy. Antireflux surgery (ureteric reimplantation) and long-term prophylactic antibiotic treatment have been compared in several large randomized trials. Surgery is more effective at preventing episodes of acute pyelonephritis than medical treatment, but no other major differences in outcome were observed, and potential complications of antireflux surgery include ureteric obstruction, itself a potent cause of renal parenchymal damage.

The confusion over the pathogenesis of reflux nephropathy probably explains the lack of hard clinical evidence to guide the management of children with urinary tract infection. Current United Kingdom guidelines are summarized in Table 9.

Table 9 Summary of guidelines on management of urinary tract infection in childhood

(1) Obtain urine specimen for culture
Clean catch
Aspirate urine from disposable nappies (not applicable with highly absorbent brands)
Bag urine
Suprapubic aspiration
Bladder catheterization
(2) Start antibiotic treatment and continue full dose for at least 5 days
(3) Continue low-dose prophylaxis at least until investigation complete
(4) Investigate for vesicoureteric reflux and renal parenchymal scarring: choice of investigation depends on age of the child, local availability, and expertise:
under age 1 year:
Ultrasound and KUB
Cystourethrogram* once urine is sterile
Repeat ultrasound and DMSA scan (or intravenous urogram if DMSA unavailable) at 3 months
between 1 and 7 years:
Ultrasound and KUB followed by DMSA
Cystourethrogram* only if:
abnormalities on ultrasound, KUB, or DMSA
clinical history suggestive of acute pyelonephritis
family history of reflux nephropathy
recurrent infections
after 7 years:
Renal ultrasound and KUB
IVU and/or DMSA scan if infection recurs or history suggests previous infections

Adapted from Report of a working group of the Research Unit of the Royal College of Physicians (1991). *Journal of the Royal College of Physicians* **25**, 36–42.

*How to image the bladder to look for vesicoureteric reflux depends on local availability and on the age of the child. The choice lies between:

(1) contrast micturating cystourethrogram—requires bladder catheterization and high radiation dose;

(2) direct radionuclide cystogram—requires bladder catheterization and lower radiation dose; and

(3) indirect (intravenous) radionuclide cystogram—does not require bladder catheterization, but only applicable in toilet-trained children.

DMSA, dimercaptosuccinic acid labelled with technetium-99.

KUB, kidneys, ureters, bladder.

Whatever the cause of reflux nephropathy, there is little doubt that women with it are more prone to recurrent acute pyelonephritis than those with anatomically normal upper urinary tracts, particularly during pregnancy.

Invasive/destructive renal parenchymal infection

As discussed above, ascending infection may cause the clinical syndrome of 'acute pyelonephritis' but seldom causes significant renal parenchymal damage. However, this is not the case if there is further impairment of host defence against infection, particularly by diabetes or urinary tract obstruction.

Acute papillary necrosis

This is an unusual complication of acute pyelonephritis, but more likely to occur in the elderly and especially those with diabetes. It should be suspected, as should urinary stones, in the patient with symptoms and signs of acute pyelonephritis who also has pain suggesting renal colic. This situation requires immediate imaging, usually with ultrasonography, to exclude urinary obstruction, and if obstruction is present then it must be relieved urgently, most often by antegrade nephrostomy.

The use of non-steroidal anti-inflammatory drugs is associated with an increased incidence of chronic renal papillary necrosis, perhaps because they compromise the renal medullary circulation. It therefore seems reasonable to say that these agents should be discontinued, at least temporarily, in the presence of acute pyelonephritis.

Renal carbuncle

Renal carbuncle is the formation of renal cortical abscesses, often only in one kidney, caused by bloodborne infection, usually associated with untreated *Staph. aureus* septicaemia. It is most commonly seen in intravenous drug abusers and patients with diabetes. There is usually a significant time delay between the initial infection and presentation with renal carbuncle, typically 6 to 8 weeks. Presenting symptoms include fever, malaise, and abdominal or flank pain, and are often non-specific. Because the infection is limited to the renal cortex and does not communicate with the collecting system, the urine is sterile and acellular. Blood cultures are usually negative. Radiological studies show a semisolid, thick-walled mass, percutaneous aspiration of which yields pus.

Pyonephrosis

Pyonephrosis is bacterial infection within a completely obstructed collecting system, for instance due to an obstructing ureteric stone. Patients usually present with fever, rigors, and flank pain, and have a marked neutrophilia and acute-phase response. Radiological differentiation from hydronephrosis relies on the presence of echogenic material and/or septas in the pelvicalyceal system, and confirmation is by percutaneous aspiration; as with other localized urinary tract infections, the voided bladder urine may be sterile. Untreated pyonephrosis rapidly results in complete destruction of the renal parenchyma, followed by death from complications of sepsis if nephrectomy is not performed; correction of obstruction and aggressive intravenous antibiotic therapy may prevent this if instituted soon enough.

Perinephric abscess

Perinephric abscess may complicate renal carbuncle or, more commonly, acute pyelonephritis—particularly if complicated by an anatomical or functional abnormality of the urinary tract. Typical presenting symptoms are those of acute pyelonephritis, with flank pain, fever, and rigors. If the abscess does not communicate with the collecting system, for instance in abscesses caused by haematogenous spread or complicating obstruction or renal cysts, there may be no lower urinary tract symptoms, no pyuria, and the urine may be sterile. Response to antibiotic treatment is much less rapid than in patients with uncomplicated acute pyelonephritis. Diagnosis is by ultrasound, urography, or CT scanning, followed by percutaneous (or occasionally surgical) aspiration, drainage, and culture of the aspirate. Prolonged antibiotic treatment of the organism identified is needed, stopping only when there is evidence that the infection has resolved, based on defervescence, resolution of the acute-phase response, and repeated radiological studies. This may take as long as 8 weeks.

Xanthogranulomatous pyelonephritis

Xanthogranulomatous pyelonephritis is an atypical form of chronic infection of the renal parenchyma in which bacterial infection, usually in the presence of obstruction or staghorn calculi, results in formation of granulomas with the accumulation of lipid-rich foamy macrophages. The process may be multifocal and can be complicated by extension into the perinephric fat, causing perinephric abscess. Patients are typically febrile and ill, with a history of progressive weight loss, anaemia, and malaise, without lower urinary tract symptoms, and have a mass in the flank on examination. Radiologically, the multifocal mass crossing tissue planes may be indistinguishable from a renal cell carcinoma, which may also cause systemic symptoms such as fever, anaemia, and weight loss. Although both require surgical excision, radical surgery can be avoided if the diagnosis is made preoperatively.

Emphysematous pyelonephritis

Emphysematous pyelonephritis is a rare and life-threatening form of acute pyelonephritis in which there is tissue necrosis together with formation of hydrogen and carbon dioxide, which accumulate in pockets in the renal parenchyma, perinephric space, and collecting systems—'gas gangrene of the kidney' (Fig. 3). The typical patient is an obese, elderly woman with type 2 diabetes; urinary tract obstruction is another important risk factor. Presentation is with fever, vomiting, and abdominal pain. The patient is often extremely ill with hypotension, neutrophilia, and renal impairment. The commonest causative organism is *E. coli*; clostridial infection has not been reported. Even with aggressive medical treatment the mortality is high, and although occasional successes with antibiotics combined with percutaneous drainage have been reported, the standard treatment is nephrectomy.

Malakoplakia

Malakoplakia (Greek: 'soft plaque') is a rare disease characterized by destructive tumour-like granulomatous infiltrates in the urinary bladder, kidneys, and occasionally other organs. Bladder involvement usually presents with haematuria, frequency, and dysuria; renal involvement presents with fever, flank pain, and renal enlargement, and may frequently be bilateral. The diagnosis may be suspected at cystoscopy or on renal imaging, but

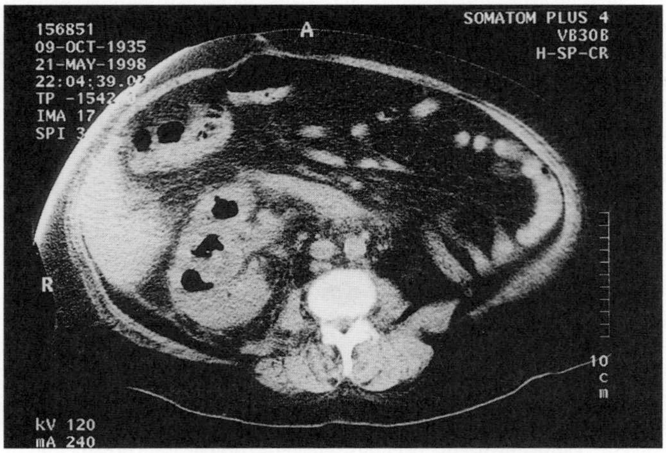

Fig. 3 Gas-forming infection, seen as the three black holes in the single remaining (right) kidney of a patient with diabetes. The left kidney had been removed 2 years earlier for a similar gas-forming infection. This infection was successfully treated by intravenous antibiotics and percutaneous drainage.

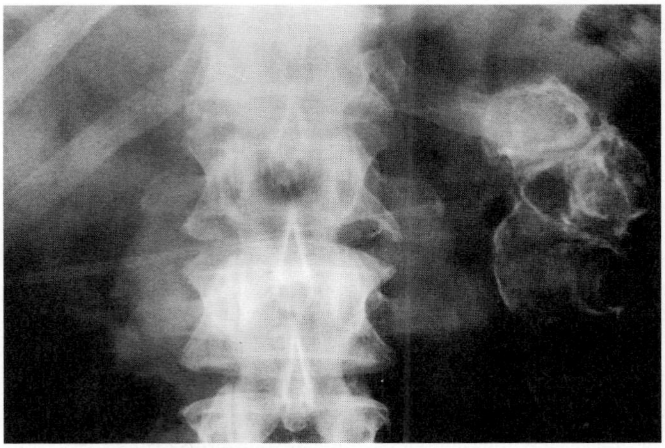

Fig. 4 Calcified 'autonephrectomy' as a result of long-standing tuberculous infection. (Reproduced by permission of Professor P. W. Mathieson.)

is confirmed histologically by detection of large eosinophilic granular macrophages containing characteristic intracellular lamellated 5- to 10-μm inclusion bodies. It is caused by bacterial urinary tract infection, commonly *E. coli*, together with an ill-understood acquired defect of microtubule assembly within phagocytic cells, resulting in the accumulation within the cytoplasm of bacterial remnants that subsequently calcify. Treatment with bethanechol (to stimulate intracellular cGMP and thus microtubule assembly) and ascorbic acid (to stimulate the intracellular hexose monophosphate shunt, which is involved in phagocytosis) have been recommended on theoretical grounds, but seldom arrest the disease. The best chance of avoiding nephrectomy comes from the use of long-term quinolone antibiotics such as ciprofloxacin, which penetrate macrophages well.

Unusual infections

Tuberculosis

Genitourinary tuberculosis is an uncommon late manifestation of tuberculosis, and is often clinically silent, with few if any systemic symptoms. Most cases of renal tuberculosis probably result from haematogenous spread, although unilateral disease is common. Seeding of infection from above leads to ulceration and distortion of the collecting system, pelvis, and ureter, followed by stricture formation and calcification. Obstruction and parenchymal infection may eventually lead to 'autonephrectomy' (Fig. 4). The disease is usually detected either during investigation of asymptomatic sterile pyuria or during investigation of irritative lower urinary tract symptoms or haematuria due to bladder involvement. Reactivation of disease may result from acquired deficiency of 1,25-dihydroxyvitamin D. Occasionally, renal tuberculosis may present with a cold abscess in the flank. Chronic renal failure due to bilateral diffuse interstitial renal tuberculosis may occur, and may account for some of the excess of chronic renal failure in Asian immigrants in the United Kingdom.

Diagnosis of renal tuberculosis is by culture of early morning urine samples. Treatment is with rifampicin, isoniazid, pyrazinamide, and ethambutol for 2 months, followed by rifampicin and isoniazid for a further 4 months, and should be supervised by a physician experienced in the chemotherapy of tuberculosis, and with adjustment of the dose of ethambutol in the presence of renal impairment. Corticosteroids may help to prevent or reverse ureteric obstruction, which may otherwise require stent insertion or surgery to prevent renal destruction. Nephrectomy is seldom necessary.

Schistosomiasis

Schistosoma haematobium infection in the venules of the urinary bladder may cause irritative symptoms and terminal haematuria, starting 2 to 3 months after the initial infection. Eosinophilia may be present. The diagnosis is made by detection of ova in a midday terminal urine specimen or by cystoscopy and biopsy. Treatment is with systemic anthelmintic drugs, currently praziquantel.

Fungal infections

Fungal urinary tract infections typically occur in patients whose host defence is compromised by indwelling urethral catheters or ureteric stents, previous wide-spectrum antibiotic therapy, immunosuppressive drugs, or diabetes. Most infections are caused by *Candida* spp. Many patients with funguria have asymptomatic colonization, but some develop life-threatening ascending disease. Severity of infection does not correlate with pyuria. It is important to differentiate funguria from contamination of voided urine by *Candida* in patients with vaginal candidiasis. Many infections clear spontaneously on removal of the urethral catheter, although this can take many months. Treatment options for patients thought to be at high risk of invasive infection (for instance patients with diabetes with indwelling catheters, renal transplant recipients) include continuous bladder irrigation or antegrade perfusion via a nephrostomy tube with amphotericin B at 50 mg/l, and oral fluconazole. Patients with clinical features of acute pyelonephritis require parenteral antifungal treatment, adjusted to *in vitro* sensitivities.

Fungaemia is often complicated by renal parenchymal infection, possibly because the hypertonic and hypoxic conditions in the renal medulla favour transformation of *Candida* from the yeast to the mycelial phase. Infection starts with multiple cortical abscesses and progresses to invasion of the renal pelvis and ureter, with eventual obstruction by fungus balls.

Prospects for the future

Current methods for prevention and treatment of uncomplicated and complicated urinary tract infection are unsatisfactory, with persisting high morbidity and mortality from complicated infection and increasing rates of antibiotic-resistant organisms. Development of new antibiotics is likely only to remain half a step ahead. We hope to see major advances in the prevention of urinary tract infection, perhaps with the development of substances designed to inhibit bacterial adherence to the uroepithelium, the development of new catheter materials and of alternatives to urethral catheterization, and the possibility of vaccines against the virulence determinants of uropathogenic bacteria.

Further reading

Abrutyn E *et al.* (1993). Does asymptomatic bacteriuria predict mortality and does antimicrobial treatment reduce mortality in elderly ambulatory women? [published erratum appears in *Annals of Internal Medicine* 1994, **121**, 901]. *Annals of Internal Medicine* **120**, 827–33.

Bailey RR (1993). Vesicoureteric reflux and reflux nephropathy. In: Schrier RW, Gottschalk CW, eds. *Diseases of the kidney*, 5th edn, pp 689–727. Little, Brown, Boston.

Cardenas DD, Hooton TM (1995). Urinary tract infection in persons with spinal cord injury. *Archives of Physical Medicine and Rehabilitation* **76**, 272–80.

Cattel WR, ed. (1996). *Infections of the kidney and urinary tract.* Oxford University Press, Oxford.

Chew LD, Fihn SD (1999). Pyelonephritis in non-pregnant women. In: Godlee F *et al.*, eds. *Clinical evidence*, pp. 761–75. BMJ Publishing Group, London.

Franz M, Horl WH (1999). Common errors in diagnosis and management of urinary tract infection. I: pathophysiology and diagnostic techniques. *Nephrology, Dialysis, Transplantation* **14**, 2746–53.

Franz M, Horl WH (1999). Common errors in diagnosis and management of urinary tract infection. II: clinical management. *Nephrology, Dialysis, Transplantation* **14**, 2754–62.

Gordon I (1995). Vesico-ureteric reflux, urinary-tract infection, and renal damage in children. *Lancet* **346**, 489–90.

Gorelick MH, Shaw KN (1999). Screening tests for urinary tract infection in children: a meta-analysis. *Pediatrics* **104**(5). URL: http://www.pediatrics.org/cgi/content/full/104/5/e54

Hooton TM *et al.* (1996). A prospective study of risk factors for symptomatic urinary tract infection in young women. *New England Journal of Medicine* **335**, 468–74.

Hunt GM, Oakeshott P, Whitaker RH (1996). Intermittent catheterisation: simple, safe, and effective but underused. *British Medical Journal* **312**, 103–7.

Kunin CM, White LV, Hua TH (1993). A reassessment of the importance of 'low-count' bacteriuria in young women with acute urinary symptoms. *Annals of Internal Medicine* **119**, 454–60.

Lachs MS *et al.* (1992). Spectrum bias in the evaluation of diagnostic tests: lessons from the rapid dipstick test for urinary tract infection. *Annals of Internal Medicine* **117**, 135–40.

Leibovici L, Wysenbeek AJ (1991). Single-dose antibiotic treatment for symptomatic urinary tract infections in women: a meta-analysis of randomized trials. *Quarterly Journal of Medicine* **78**, 43–57.

Mabeck CE (1972). Treatment of uncomplicated urinary tract infection in non-pregnant women. *Postgraduate Medical Journal* **48**, 69–75.

Platt R *et al.* (1982). Mortality associated with nosocomial urinary-tract infection. *New England Journal of Medicine* **307**, 637–42.

Raz R, Stamm WE (1993). A controlled trial of intravaginal estriol in postmenopausal women with recurrent urinary tract infections. *New England Journal of Medicine* **329**, 753–6.

Saint S, Lipsky BA (1999). Preventing catheter-related bacteriuria: Should we? Can we? How? *Archives of Internal Medicine* **159**, 800–8.

Schaeffer AJ (1994). Urinary tract infection in men—state of the art. *Infection* **22**, S121.

Smaill F (2002). Antibiotics for asymptomatic bacteriuria in pregnancy (Cochrane Review). In: *The Cochrane Library*, Issue 1. Update Software, Oxford. [A substantive amendment to this systematic review was last made on 28 December 2000.]

Stamm WE, Hooton TM (1993). Management of urinary tract infections in adults. *New England Journal of Medicine* **329**, 1328–34.

Stamm WE *et al.* (1982). Diagnosis of coliform infection in acutely dysuric women. *New England Journal of Medicine* **307**, 463–8.

Stapleton A (1999). Prevention of recurrent urinary-tract infections in women. *Lancet* **353**, 7–8.

Svanborg C (1993). Resistance to urinary tract infection. *New England Journal of Medicine* **329**, 802–3.

Warren JW *et al.* (1999). Guidelines for antimicrobial treatment of uncomplicated acute bacterial cystitis and acute pyelonephritis in women. *Clinical Infectious Diseases* **29**, 745–58.

Wong-Beringer A, Jacobs RA, Guglielmo BJ (1992). Treatment of funguria. *Journal of the American Medical Association* **267**, 2780–5.

20.13 Urinary stones, nephrocalcinosis, and renal tubular acidosis

Robert J. Unwin, William G. Robertson, and Giovambattista Capasso

Nephrocalcinosis and urinary stone disease

> 'No stretch of chemical or physical imagination will permit so heterogeneous a group of compounds (as renal stones) to be ascribed to a common origin, or their disposition in the kidney, ureter or bladder to be uniformly charged to an identical cause'
>
> (Howard Kelly)

Nephrocalcinosis and uro-(nephro-)lithiasis frequently coexist and the terms are often loosely combined when describing patients with urinary stone disease. Whether they are aetiologically distinct is unclear, although it is generally believed that nephrocalcinosis represents one end of the spectrum of urinary stone disease. However, although nephrocalcinosis is often associated with urinary stones, most patients with urinary stones do not have macroscopic nephrocalcinosis.

Urolithiasis

Introduction

Urolithiasis has no geographical, demographic, or genetic boundaries: patterns of stone formation have changed in the past and are continuing to change today. The earliest evidence of the disorder is the stones found in mummies entombed in the predynastic Egyptian era, around 4000 BC. In Western countries before 1900, stones occurred commonly in children, particularly boys, and were formed mainly in the bladder. These stones consisted of ammonium urate and/or calcium oxalate and were associated with poor nutrition. Although this form of stone disorder is still found today in rural areas within the so-called 'endemic stone belt' (which stretches from Jordan, through Iraq, Iran, and the Indian subcontinent to the furthest reaches of South-East Asia), it is gradually disappearing with improving standards of nutrition, as it did in most developed countries 100 years ago.

By contrast to the gradual decrease in the occurrence of bladder stones in children, the incidence of upper urinary tract stones (mainly renal) in adults has steadily increased in most countries over the last century. Kidney stones are more common in the industrially developed nations and less so in countries whose economies are more dependent on agriculture. Overall, upper tract stone disease seems to be a disorder associated with affluence, presumably through effects on diet and lifestyle.

Epidemiological factors in the formation of urinary stones

Although stones generally occur more frequently in men than in women (male:female ratio about 2.5:1), recent studies in the United Kingdom and Portugal have shown that, within the past 25 years, there has been a progressive decrease in the age at onset of stone formation in both men and women, particularly women. Within the population of stone formers as a whole, the male:female ratio is now 1.7:1 among patients who formed their first stone before the age of 20 years; but in patients currently aged less than 20 years, the ratio has fallen to 1.1:1. These changes have been attributed to alterations in diet and lifestyle over the last 25 years.

Epidemiological factors important in the formation of urinary stones are summarized in Table 1. Each has been shown to increase the risk of stone formation through effects on the balance between supersaturation and inhibitors and promoters of crystallization in urine (see later).

Calcium oxalate stones

Most (80 per cent) urinary calculi contain calcium oxalate, often on its own, but frequently mixed with calcium phosphate or, occasionally, uric acid. In about 90 per cent of these cases (the so-called idiopathic or primary stone formers), there is no obvious metabolic cause for stone formation. In the remainder, calcium-containing stones form as a result of some disorder of calcium metabolism, oxalate metabolism, or acid–base balance.

For idiopathic calcium stone formation the main epidemiological factors are age, gender, season, climate, stress, occupation, affluence, diet (including fluid intake), and genetic/metabolic factors. The role of diet, in particular, has been studied in detail and appears to explain much of the changing pattern of stone incidence over the past 100 years. As the diet becomes 'richer' in a given population (with an increased consumption of protein, particularly animal protein, refined sugars, and salt), the incidence of stones increases. This often follows periods of economic expansion,

Table 1 The epidemiological factors associated with formation of uric acid and calcium stones and their effects on urinary risk factors

Epidemiological factor	Urinary risk factor(s)
Age (age 20–50 > 60–80 years) Gender (male > female)	↑Calcium, ↑oxalate, ↑uric acid, ↑pH, ↓volume, ↓citrate, ↓magnesium, ↓macromolecular inhibitors, ↑promoters
Climate and season	↓Volume, ↑calcium, ↑oxalate, ↓pH
Stress (unidentified factors)	↑Calcium, ↑oxalate, ↑uric acid, ↓magnesium
Low fluid intake or exercise	↓Volume, ↓pH
Affluence and diet	↑Calcium, ↑oxalate, ↑uric acid, ↓citrate, ↓pH
Metabolic disorders:	
Gout	↑Uric acid
Glycogen storage disease	↑Uric acid
Lesch–Nyhan syndrome	↑Uric acid
Neoplastic disease	↑Uric acid
Ileostomy	↓Volume, ↓pH
Primary hyperparathyroidism	↑↑Calcium, ↑pH
Distal renal tubular acidosis (dRTA)	↑pH, (↑calcium)
Hereditary hyperoxaluria	↑↑Oxalate
Enteric hyperoxaluria	↑Oxalate, ↓pH, ↓citrate, ↓magnesium
Medullary sponge kidney (MSK)	↑Calcium (↑pH)
Cushing's disease	↑Calcium, ↑pH
Vitamin D intoxication	↑↑Calcium
Milk-alkali syndrome	↑Calcium, ↑pH
Immobilization	↑Calcium, ↑pH (from urinary tract infection)

whereas the incidence of stones decreases during periods of recession in parallel with a return to a diet containing more fibre and less energy-rich foods. The recent increase in consumption of soft drinks, especially in the young, is becoming an important 'new' factor in the risk of urinary stone formation. These contain phosphoric acid, providing a small acid load, but one that may become significant if large volumes are drunk. Paradoxically, potential sources of oxalate, such as beer, may be associated with a reduced stone risk, perhaps because a minimum ingestion of oxalate is necessary to bind dietary calcium and limit calciuria. Antacid ingestion (as distinct from 'milk-alkali syndrome') may also reduce stone risk by increasing urine pH, binding oxalate, and providing a source of magnesium.

Infection stones

So-called 'infection stones', composed of magnesium ammonium phosphate, usually in conjunction with calcium phosphate, are more common in women and now constitute between 4 and 15 per cent of stones, depending on the country of origin. They are caused by urinary tract infection with urea-splitting organisms that secrete the enzyme urease. This converts urea to ammonium (NH_4^+) and bicarbonate, making the urine more alkaline (urinary NH_4^+ concentration is normally low in sterile alkaline urine). As a result, phosphate-containing salts, such as calcium phosphate and magnesium ammonium phosphate, precipitate and increase the risk of stone formation. Infection stones can also form secondary to most other types of stone. The relative incidence of infection stones has decreased over the past 25 years in most Western countries, presumably as a result of better clinical diagnosis and earlier treatment of urinary tract infections.

Uric acid stones

Stones consisting of uric acid constitute between 4 and 25 per cent of published series, depending on the relative consumption of animal and vegetable protein in the population studied. There are three factors that promote formation of uric acid stones: (i) low urine volume, (ii) acid urine pH, and (iii) high uric acid excretion. For a given diet, these stones are more common in elderly men, at least in part because of the decline in urine pH with age. Because the pK of uric acid/urate is approximately 5.7, a more acid urine pH favours the less soluble undissociated form of uric acid. 'Pure' uric acid stones are infrequent in most developing countries and are most common in the oil-rich states of the Arabian Gulf, or in countries where there is a cheap local source of meat, fish, or poultry protein. Most uric acid stones are idiopathic; a small number form secondary to some disorder of purine metabolism (such as Lesch–Nyhan syndrome), or to a condition in which there is high tissue turnover (such as tumour necrosis following chemotherapy).

'Rare' stones

In all series of stones analysed, between 1 and 2 per cent consist of a range of 'rare' constituents derived from either some hereditary or congenital inborn error of metabolism, such as cystinuria (not to be confused with cystinosis), xanthinuria, or 2,8-dihydroxyadeninuria, or from a prescribed drug or metabolite, which is relatively insoluble in urine. Examples are silica (from excess ingestion of the antacid magnesium trisilicate, or from the use of pectin and silicium to thicken milk for infant feeding), sulphonamides, indinavir, and triamterene. All stones contain a small percentage by weight of mucoproteinaceous matrix. Some 'stones' consist almost entirely of mucoprotein, and usually result from inflammation of the urinary tract in patients whose urine is not sufficiently supersaturated to mineralize the organic matrix.

Causes of urinary stone formation

Insolubility of mineral components

The overriding factor that is common to all types of stone is the relative insolubility of their respective mineral component(s) in the urine. However, whether or not this is the only factor responsible for the formation of stones is still open to debate. There are two possible models (which are not mutually exclusive) for the initiation of stones. The 'free-particle' model is that stones are initiated when urine becomes so excessively supersaturated with one of the salts or acids occurring in kidney stones that crystals spontaneously precipitate in urine. If this happens frequently, and if the crystals grow or aggregate sufficiently within the transit time of urine through the kidney, then the risk increases that one of these particles will become trapped at some narrow point along the urinary tract and act as a focus around which a stone can form. The other model of stone formation, which is currently favoured, requires chemical 'fixation' of a crystal, or aggregate of crystals, to the renal epithelial cell lining. This fixed particle may result from injury to the cell wall (caused either by the crystals themselves or by viruses or bacteria) and/or from some 'gluing' material—present only in the urine of stone formers—that causes crystals to adhere to these sites and then results in stone formation.

Both models require urine to be supersaturated to some degree with respect to the stone-forming salt or acid concerned, sufficient to cause crystals to be formed by nucleation that is either homogeneous (spontaneous) or heterogeneous (on a pre-existing nucleus of some foreign material). The factors causing urine to become supersaturated with one or more of the various constituents of stones are shown in Table 2.

Modifiers of crystallization

One factor that might affect the kinetics of the processes involved is the presence or absence in urine of so-called modifiers of crystallization, claimed to be of particular importance in the formation of calcium-containing stones. One group of crystallization modifiers is said to retard the rate of growth and/or aggregation of crystals, or the binding of calcium-containing crystals to cell walls. These are known as inhibitors of crystallization and include magnesium, citrate, pyrophosphate, ADP, ATP, at least two phosphopeptides, glycosaminoglycans, Tamm–Horsfall protein, nephrocalcin, calgranulin, fibronectin, various plasma proteins, osteopontin (uropontin), α_1-microglobulin, β_2-microglobulin, urinary prothrombin fragment 1, and inter-α-trypsin inhibitor. Of these, urinary citrate is probably the most important. The second group of modifiers is claimed to promote one or more of the processes involved in crystallization. These are known as promoters of stone formation and include matrix substance A, various uncharacterized urinary proteins and glycoproteins, and the polymerized form of Tamm–Horsfall protein (uromucoid). However, the clinical importance of these compounds in the pathogenesis of stone formation remains unclear.

In the final analysis, stone formation is probably due to an abnormal combination of factors that affect either the thermodynamic (supersaturation driving force) or kinetic (rate-controlling) processes involved in the crystallization of the various stone-forming minerals. For some types of stone formation (cystine, xanthine, 2,8-dihydroxyadenine, uric acid, and probably magnesium phosphate ammonium stones) the thermodynamic factors predominate; in others (calcium oxalate and calcium phosphate) both sets of factors may be involved.

Idiopathic hypercalciuria

This is often familial, accounts for the majority (more than 50 per cent) of patients with renal stones, and can be divided into three types: absorptive, resorptive (or fasting), and renal. The most common is absorptive, due to increased intestinal absorption of calcium, the cause of which remains unknown. Resorptive hypercalciuria is associated with reduced bone mineralization, although primary hyperparathyroidism must be excluded. Renal hypercalciuria is distinct from that seen in tubular disorders such as the Fanconi syndrome (see under renal tubular acidosis). Although the underlying mechanism is not known, there may be a primary defect of renal phosphate reabsorption, suggested in some cases by an increase in plasma calcitriol (1,25-OH vitamin D) levels, which will enhance intestinal absorption of calcium.

Hypocitraturia

This is an important risk factor for renal stone disease. The blood citrate pool is maintained by delivery from bone and the gastrointestinal tract and by removal by hepatic and renal metabolism. High urinary citrate prevents

Table 2 The urinary risk factors for the various types of stones and their effects on the parameters of crystallization

Stone type	Urinary risk factor	Chemical effect
Rare stones	↑Xanthine ↑2,8-dihydroxyadenine ↑Silica ↑Indinavir, etc	↑Supersaturation of relevant stone constituent
Cystine stones	↑Cystine	↑Cystine supersaturation
Uric acid stones	↓pH ↑Uric acid ↓Volume	↑Uric acid supersaturation
Infection stones	↑↑pH ↑NH_4^+ (from urea-splitting) ↑Mucosubstances	↑Magnesium ammonium phosphate and calcium phosphate supersaturation ↑Agglomeration of crystals
Calcium stones	↓Volume ↑Oxalate ↑Calcium ↑pH ↓Citrate ↓Magnesium ↑Uric acid ↓Macromolecular inhibitors ↑Macromolecular promoters	↑Calcium oxalate and/or calcium phosphate supersaturation ↓Crystallization inhibitory activity ↑Crystallization promotive activity

calcium stones by encouraging formation of soluble calcium citrate; it also reduces formation of urate stones by alkalinizing the urine. Hypocitraturia is present in about 40 per cent of calcium stone formers, but in most cases the reason for this is unknown.

Low urinary citrate excretion results from metabolic acidosis in conditions such as chronic diarrhoea, urinary diversion, and distal renal tubular acidosis. The hypocitraturia of distal renal tubular acidosis is due to increased reabsorption of citrate in the proximal tubule as a result of intracellular acidosis (see section on renal tubular acidosis below for more detail). Citrate excretion is also reduced because of acid retention in subjects on a high protein diet. The widely prescribed angiotensin-converting enzyme (**ACE**) inhibitor enalapril has been shown to decrease citrate excretion in rats, although the effect is small in humans. It is not known whether this is true of all ACE inhibitors, or if it is of any significance in patients at risk of renal stones (particularly given the increased prevalence of hypertension in renal stone disease).

Hyperuricosuria

The contribution of increased uric acid excretion to uric acid stone formation occurs mainly in patients on a high protein (purine) diet, which leads to the production of more acid urine and increases the risk of urate precipitation. Hyperuricosuria is less commonly due to a defect of urate metabolism *per se.*

Up to a fifth of patients with gout also have urinary stone disease (urate, calcium oxalate, calcium phosphate, or mixed). Hypertension is commonly associated with both conditions; hence, as already mentioned, it may be important to consider the effect of antihypertensive therapy on the risk of urolithiasis. The angiotensin receptor blocker Losartan lowers plasma urate concentration and increases uric acid excretion by an unknown mechanism, although this does not seem to increase the risk of uric acid stones.

Hyperoxaluria

The excretion of oxalate is often mildly elevated in idiopathic stone formers. Most oxalate is derived from the metabolism of glycine and ascorbic acid, vitamin C intoxication being a rare cause of hyperoxaluria (vitamin C can be non-enzymatically converted to oxalate in urine; this can be prevented by collecting urine in acid or EDTA; up to 4 g/day of vitamin C has no significant effect on urinary oxalate excretion). Intestinal absorption of oxalate is normally low, but rises when dietary calcium content is reduced. It is also increased following small bowel resection and in Crohn's disease (so-called enteric hyperoxaluria), when saponification and the action of bile salts increase the permeability of the large bowel to oxalate. In these conditions diarrhoea and malabsorption can lead to chronic dehydration, low urinary volumes and metabolic acidosis, with the risk of interstitial oxalate deposition causing acute or chronic renal failure.

Recent research suggests that normal bowel colonization with the bacterium *Oxalobacter formigenes* is an important determinant of urinary oxalate excretion, because this organism digests dietary oxalate, thereby reducing its absorption. This might be relevant to the association between renal stones and long-term antibiotic use in patients with cystic fibrosis, although their high protein intake from pancreatic enzyme supplements may also be a factor.

The two genetic types of primary hyperoxaluria are autosomal recessive and cause oxalate overproduction. Type 1 (PH1) is the more severe form, producing widespread tissue deposition of oxalate (oxalosis), early renal failure, and nephrocalcinosis. It is due to a defect of the liver transaminase that converts glyoxylate to glycine, resulting in glyoxylate oxidation to oxalate and reduction to glycollate. The rarer type 2 (PH2) is due to a deficiency of liver D-glycerate dehydrogenase and is characterized by glyceraturia. Since pyridoxine (vitamin B_6) is a cofactor for the defective enzyme in PH1, high doses of this vitamin can sometimes help to reduce oxalate production; more modest doses are sometimes also effective in patients with mild 'idiopathic' hyperoxaluria.

Cystinuria, xanthinuria, and 2,8-dihydroxyadeninuria

A small number of stones are found in patients with cystinuria, xanthinuria and 2,8-dihydroxyadeninuria arising from inherited or congenital errors of metabolism. Cystine is normally excreted in very low concentrations, well below the limit of solubility of cystine in urine (1 to 1.5 mmol/l). In cystinuria, due to a defect in the tubular reabsorption of cystine, the urinary concentrations are 200-fold higher than normal, leading to precipitation of cystine and stone formation. Only homozygotes form stones; the excretion of cystine in heterozygotes is higher than normal, but insufficient to cause crystal formation in most cases. The basic amino acids ornithine, lysine, and arginine share the same amino acid transport mechanism as cystine and their excretion is also increased.

Xanthinuria results from a deficiency of the enzyme xanthine oxidase, such that xanthine is not converted to uric acid. Radiolucent stones form in acid urine. Secondary xanthinuria producing xanthine stones is an unusual complication of allopurinol therapy.

A deficiency of the enzyme adenine phosphoribosyl transferase, inherited as an autosomal recessive trait, is associated with an increased urinary excretion of 2,8-dihydroxyadenine and this sometimes leads to stone formation.

Clinical features

Calculi can occur at any point in the urinary tract, although they are more often located in the kidney and ureter than in the bladder. Upper urinary tract stones can occur on either side and are often bilateral. Over 60 per cent are small enough to be passed spontaneously. Within the kidney itself, concretions may be found in the calyces, in the renal pelvis, or extending from the calyces into the pelvis. They may be attached to the epithelial surfaces of the pelvicalyceal system, be encapsulated within the renal parenchyma, or lie free within the pelvis or lower pole of the kidney. Occasionally, they may occupy the entire pelvicalyceal space to form a so-called 'staghorn' calculus. The clinical presentation of calculi depends primarily upon their position in the urinary tract, and whether or not they cause obstruction to urinary flow.

Pain from urinary stones

The commonest presentation of urinary calculi is with pain. Stones can become lodged at any point in the ureter, but most commonly do so at the upper and lower ends, where there are constrictions at the pelviureteric and vesicoureteric junctions. A stone in the renal pelvis typically causes dull loin pain with occasional colic. The most problematic differential diagnosis is from musculoskeletal pain arising in the back, lower ribs, or their muscular and ligamentous attachments. Such pain is common, and it can be very difficult to decide whether a stone seen on a radiograph is 'incidental' (see later) or the cause of symptoms. Musculoskeletal pain is more likely to be precipitated by bad posture, exercise, or movement, to come on suddenly, to last for a few seconds or minutes only, and to be associated with a localized 'superficial' point of tenderness. Renal pain is less likely to be brought on by exercise or movement and more likely to be felt 'deeper inside', last for hours, and be associated with diffuse loin tenderness and no comfortable position.

Partial or total obstruction of the pelviureteric junction or ureter gives rise to the agonizing pain of renal colic, described by many sufferers as the 'worst pain they have ever had'. The patient can be in absolute agony, rolling around and crying out as the waves of colic strike them. If the stone is at the pelviureteric junction, the pain is felt in the loin. If it moves down the ureter, the pain radiates into the groin and (sometimes) into the scrotum or labia. The patient sweats profusely with the waves of pain and often vomits. Treatment with non-steroidal anti-inflammatory agents may be helpful, but the physician should not refrain from giving prompt and adequate doses of powerful analgesics (pethidine, morphine) and will certainly gain the undying gratitude of their patient if they do so. The diagnosis of renal colic is often straightforward from the history alone, but in some cases differential diagnoses need to be entertained, which include biliary colic, small bowel obstruction, appendicitis, and diverticulitis. Children and pregnant women are less likely to present with characteristic symptoms and a high index of suspicion is sometimes required to make the diagnosis.

The patient with stones in the upper urinary tract may have macroscopic haematuria and frequently will have microscopic haematuria, together with episodes of frequency and dysuria caused by the passage of 'sand' or 'gravel'.

'Staghorn' calculi are associated with infection, as described previously, but urinary infection is probably more common in any individual with urinary stones, and the combination of urinary obstruction with sepsis can be particularly dangerous. Added to symptoms arising from obstruction are those from infection, with high fever (often 39°C or higher), rigors, and (in severe cases) circulatory collapse. These cases are medical emergencies requiring resuscitation, intravenous antimicrobial therapy, and urgent relief of obstruction.

Another circumstance worthy of note is the patient with a single functioning kidney. Obstruction by a stone, or any other cause, will lead to acute obstructive renal failure, demanding urgent relief of obstruction.

Calculi may be found in the bladder, either lying free or lodged in a diverticulum in the vesical wall. Most probably they originate in the upper urinary tract and continue to grow in their new location, although others may be initiated in the bladder. They occur almost exclusively in elderly men and usually consist of uric acid, or are associated with infection due to chronic prostatic obstruction. Stones in the bladder may be asymptomatic, but can cause discomfort in the suprapubic and perineal regions, and also the dramatic symptom of sudden and painful cessation to urine flow.

Imaging

Diagnosis is usually confirmed by a combination of ultrasound, plain abdominal radiography (kidney, ureters, and bladder), and particularly in the case of radiolucent stones (i.e. those composed of uric acid, 2,8-dihydroxyadenine, or xanthine), an intravenous urogram. The place of the intravenous urogram is still hotly debated, although there is really no better means of defining the anatomy of the renal drainage system and at the same time providing some index of renal function, which an ultrasound examination cannot do. Occasionally, a computed tomographic (CT) scan (especially spiral) can provide useful additional information, particularly if there is associated nephrocalcinosis or lucent stones. Magnetic resonance imaging is poor at showing calcium deposits.

Recurrence

If patients are not provided with proper preventative management, the risk of recurrence is high—40 per cent within 3 years, rising to 74 per cent at 10 years, and 98 per cent at 25 years. The rate of recurrence appears to be higher after the use of minimally invasive techniques for the disintegration and/or removal of stones than it was in the days of open kidney surgery. This is particularly noticeable in patients treated with extracorporeal shock-wave lithotripsy, which by the nature of the technique tends to leave behind fragments of stone that may act as foci for subsequent stone formation. Percutaneous nephrolithotomy is slightly less of a problem in this respect, because it is usually easier to ensure that most of the stone fragments are removed during this procedure: it is usually preferred to lithotripsy for treatment of a stone present in the lower pole of the kidney, or greater than 2 cm in diameter. It is important to remember that sole reliance on surgical procedures for the overall management of stone formers is inadequate: stones tend to recur unless dietary and/or medical treatment is also instituted.

Asymptomatic urinary stones

About 3 per cent of patients undergoing abdominal ultrasound or radiographic investigations for other indications are found to have 'silent' kidney stones (Fig. 1(a)). If the stone is greater than 4 mm in diameter and of uncertain location, an intravenous urogram should be performed to determine this in relation to the renal pelvis and ureter and to assess the risk of future obstruction (Fig. 1(b)). A simple metabolic screen (see later) is also required. If the patient remains asymptomatic, no specific abnormality is found, and no intervention deemed necessary, then a follow-up radiograph or ultrasound at 2 years is probably advisable, depending on the size of the stone.

Biochemical screening to determine risk of urinary stones

Once the presence of a stone is confirmed and a decision is reached on the most appropriate urological intervention (if any), the patient should be screened for a biochemical cause. It is usually best to do this when the patient is eating and drinking 'normally', but not when there is haematuria or immediately prior to stone removal or lithotripsy. After such treatment it is sensible to wait for 2 to 3 months, because during this period patients often consume a diet that is very different from their 'normal'one. If they do not form another stone within 3 months of the presenting episode, then

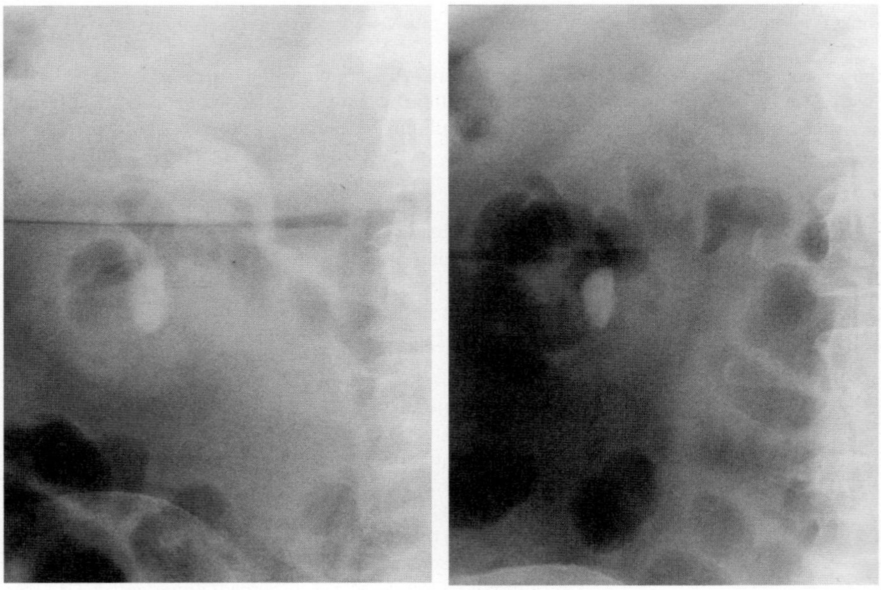

(a) (b)

Fig. 1 A plain radiograph (a) and intravenous urogram (b) of an adult woman showing an incidental right kidney stone. The stone is in a lower pole calyx or calyceal diverticulum and measures 8 by 15 mm.

they will frequently return to former dietary habits and an increased risk of stone formation.

There are several published biochemical screening procedures for assessing the risk of stone formation, most of which require a stone analysis, a metabolic screen, a 24-h urine screen, and in some instances, a dietary history. These should not be carried out when the patient is in hospital, because the diet is usually very different from that consumed at home. In addition to the routine clinical history from the patient, which should include occupation and family history of stones, the screen includes the following.

1. Analysis of a simultaneous blood and spot urine sample. The blood sample should be analysed for urea, creatinine, calcium, magnesium, sodium, potassium, bicarbonate, phosphate, urate, alkaline phosphatase, albumin, and oxalate (where necessary). The urine sample should be analysed for urea, creatinine, pH, calcium, sodium, potassium, phosphate, and urate.
2. Analysis of two 24-h urine samples collected on consecutive days at home: the first in a container with 50 ml of 2.2 mol hydrochloric acid as a preservative and analysed for volume, creatinine, calcium, magnesium, sodium, potassium, phosphate, oxalate, and citrate; the second in a plain container and analysed for volume, creatinine, pH, protein, urate, and a qualitative test for cystine.
3. Dietary assessment carried out using the diet diary system during the week leading up to, and including, the 2 days of the 24-urine collections. The patient is asked to complete a diet diary of everything that he or she consumes each day. This is analysed for fluid intake, calories, calcium, magnesium, sodium, potassium, phosphate, oxalate, purine, protein (and its various fractions, including animal protein, meat plus fish plus poultry protein, dairy protein, and fruit plus vegetable plus cereal protein), fibre, fat, and refined sugars.
4. Quantitative stone analysis (whenever possible). All patients should be encouraged to retain their stones or stone fragments for quantitative analysis by infrared spectroscopy. This is an important tool, often providing the first clue as to the cause of the stone(s) in a given patient.

From the combined analyses, a number of algorithms can be used to assess the overall biochemical risk of forming stones containing uric acid, calcium oxalate, or calcium phosphate, or various mixtures of these constituents (details of several such algorithms that are currently used in various specialist urinary stone clinics can be found in chapter 2 of Coe *et al.*1996). These are used to give an indication of the risk of stone formation in an individual patient. High risk is rarely caused by a single abnormal urinary constituent (except in the case of primary hyperoxaluria), but usually due to a combination of several lesser abnormalities, depending on the stone type. Indeed, it is possible to be at high risk with every single individual risk factor within its 'normal range', but with several lying towards the upper or lower limits of these ranges. This is an important feature of these models because they allow a risk assessment to be made in the patient who would otherwise be described as 'having normal urine', yet has an abnormal combination of the variables that lead to crystalluria and stones. The models can be used both to assess the patient's probability of stones before treatment, and also to follow progress during preventative management.

Prevention of stone recurrence

The main aim in the prevention of stone recurrence is to decrease the likelihood of crystals forming in the urinary tract by reducing the supersaturation of urine with respect to the particular constituent(s) that occurs in a patient's stone.

A summary of the available dietary and medical treatments for the various types of urinary calculi is shown in Table 3. The injunction to 'drink more' is crucially important for all at risk of urinary stones, and patients should aim to maintain a urinary volume of at least 2.5 litres per day. Those with recurrent stones will certainly benefit from maintaining a higher urinary volume than this, and also from making a point of drinking when they get up at night to micturate. This is undoubtedly an inconvenience, but recommended to ensure that the urine is as dilute as possible throughout the 24 h, and does not become concentrated at night. Patients taking treatment to modify their urinary pH should be given appropriate sticks to measure this, instructed how to use them, and how to modify their treatment to achieve the desired effect.

Some patients will benefit from alteration of their diet, in particular those who eat excessive amounts of animal protein and purine from meat, fish, and poultry; those who consume large quantities of oxalate-containing foods; and those who not only consume high amounts of calcium but also hyperabsorb calcium from the intestine. Too low an intake of calcium, on the other hand, may increase the intestinal absorption and hence urinary excretion of oxalate. It is important, therefore, not to advise patients to cut out all dairy produce to correct their hypercalciuria, as they may end up with a higher risk of forming stones than when they started. Other dietary

Table 3 Medical methods for prevention and treatment of urinary stone disease

Stone type	Treatment
2,8-Dihydroxyadenine	Very high fluid intake (> 3 litre/day) + allopurinol (300 mg/day)
Silica	Discontinue magnesium trisilicate antacids
Xanthine	Hereditary form: high fluid intake + oral alkali (urine pH > 7.4) Iatrogenic form: withdraw allopurinol
Cystine	Very high fluid intake (> 3 litre/day) + oral alkali (urine pH > 7.5) or D-penicillamine (2–4 g/day), α-mercaptopropionylglycine, or captopril[a]
Uric acid	High fluid intake (> 2.5 litre/day) + oral alkali (urine pH > 6.2) or reduce purine intake or give allopurinol (up to 300 mg/day)
Infected	High fluid intake + antibiotics + oral acid (pH < 6.2)
Calcium:	
Idiopathic	High fluid intake + relevant dietary advice or thiazide diuretics (bendrofluazide, up to 10 mg/day) or phosphate supplements (1–1.5 g P/day) or magnesium supplements (500 mg Mg/day) or potassium citrate or bicarbonate (20 mEq three times daily)
Hyperparathyroid	Parathyroidectomy or, if contraindicated, high fluids + oral acid
Hereditary hyperoxaluric	High fluid intake (> 3 litre/day) + pyridoxine (400 mg/day) in primary hyperoxaluria type I
Enteric hyperoxaluric	High fluid intake + low oxalate/high calcium diet or potassium citrate
Distal renal tubular acidosis	High fluid intake + sodium bicarbonate or potassium citrate/bicarbonate (thiazide if still hypercalciuric, though may cause significant hypokalaemia)
Medullary sponge kidney	Treat as for idiopathic
Corticosteroid-induced	Discontinue corticosteroids: treat as for idiopathic
Sarcoidosis	High fluid intake
Milk-alkali syndrome	Discontinue alkali and moderate calcium intake + high fluid intake
Vitamin D intoxication	Discontinue high vitamin D intake + high fluid intake
Immobilization	High fluid intake; remobilize as far as possible; treat any urinary tract infection with antibiotics
Drug-related	Discontinue drug concerned as far as possible and replace with alternative therapy + high fluid intake

[a]Cystine is made up of two linked cysteine molecules and drugs like penicillamine and thiola, or the ACE inhibitor captopril, which contain sulphydryl groups, can form soluble disulphides with a cysteine.

excesses that may increase the risk of stones include a high intake of salt, which leads to a renal leak of calcium, and a high intake of refined sugars, which increase the intestinal absorption of calcium. When taken together, gross hypercalciuria often results. A list of foods that should be avoided in excess and taken only in moderation is contained in Table 4.

Although most of the treatments listed in Tables 3 and 4 are effective in reducing the risk of stone recurrence, the main problem in the long-term management of patients with stones is compliance. Stone formers typically feel well for most of the time, except when experiencing an attack of renal colic. It is therefore often difficult to maintain co-operation and motivation to adhere to preventative treatment for long after a first stone episode, particularly since this is socially intrusive, with drinking of large volumes leading to urinary frequency. If patients do not have a recurrent stone within a few months, they will generally return to their original abnormal pattern of urine biochemistry by 3 to 6 months and eventually produce another stone. Once they have had several episodes of renal colic, compliance with treatment is usually better.

Table 4 Foodstuffs that should be avoided in excess and taken only in moderation by patients with a history of forming calcium- and/or uric acid-containing stones

Foodstuff	Constituents that increase the risk of stones	Effect on urinary composition
Rhubarb	↑↑ Oxalate	↑ Oxalate
Spinach	↑↑ Oxalate	↑ Oxalate
Okra	↑↑ Oxalate	↑ Oxalate
Beetroot	↑ Oxalate	↑ Oxalate
Nuts	↑ Oxalate	↑ Oxalate
Chocolate	↑ Oxalate	↑ Oxalate
Meat, fish, poultry	↑ Purine, ↑ acid ash, ↑ amino acid precursors of oxalate	↑↑ Calcium, oxalate, ↑ uric acid, ↓ citrate, ↓ pH
Dairy produce	↑ Calcium	↑ Calcium
Salt	↑ Sodium	↑ Calcium
Refined sugars	↑ Sugar	↑ Calcium

Figure 2 illustrates how the important urinary risk factors for stone formation can be represented visually to encourage understanding, compliance, and motivation. The patient can see immediately how changes in diet and urine composition affect his/her stone risk, which can be an incentive to try and reduce the combined risk by moving it from outside (high risk) toward the central (low risk) 'bull's eye'. It is important to review the patient regularly as an outpatient and to repeat the relevant screening tests, preferably annually but at least biennially, to encourage adherence to the recommended treatment.

Economics of management of urinary stones

The undoubted success of lithotripsy, less invasive surgery (such as percutaneous nephrolithotomy), and ureteroscopy for the disintegration and removal of calculi has lulled some into the belief that urinary stone disease can be managed solely by these interventions. Although these minimally invasive techniques are often the procedures of choice for the removal of stones, they do not prevent their recurrence. Without biochemical screening and appropriate dietary and/or medical management, the patient will often return for further stone removal in the future, which can be uncomfortable for the patient and is expensive to perform. Failure to provide proper prophylactic treatment and follow-up can also result in missed infections and eventually compromised renal function. Financial analysis has shown that the projected costs of treating patients with stones by only removing their stones as they form is much more costly than removing the

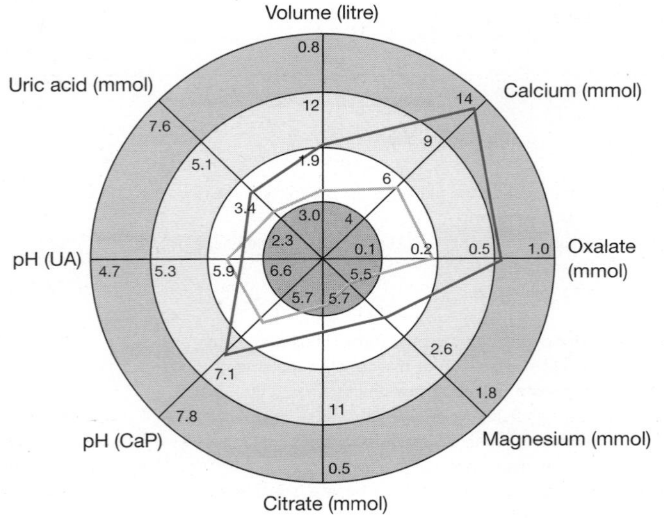

Fig. 2 A radar plot ('target diagram') showing the baseline urinary risk factors for stone formation (purple lines) and the corresponding data during preventative treatment (pink lines) in a patient with 'mixed' calcium oxalate and calcium phosphate stones. The individual urinary risk factors are plotted such that abnormal values fall in the dark pink outer ring and normal values in the grey bull's eye. Intermediate values fall in the white and light pink areas. The objective for the patient is to aim to get his/her risk factors in the 'bull's eye'. Units of axes are urinary volumes or amounts per 24 h. UA, refers to a patient with uric acid stones; CaP, refers to a patient with calcium phosphate-containing stones.

initial stone(s) and then screening to identify risk factors to provide appropriate advice and long-term management.

Nephrocalcinosis

Nephrocalcinosis is the deposition of calcium salts (mainly phosphates and oxalates) within the kidney, but the term is usually reserved for those conditions in which there is a generalized increase in kidney calcium content, rather than any localized intrarenal calcification, as may occur in some tumours, cysts, tuberculous granulomas, and areas of renal infarction.

Microscopic, or mild, nephrocalcinosis is a common incidental finding at autopsy, but macroscopic nephrocalcinosis is uncommon. It is diagnosed by radiography or ultrasound, although there is still some debate amongst radiologists as to whether radiography or ultrasound is more sensitive in detecting early disease. Plain radiographs have the advantage that they can more readily be used to judge progress from one year to the next, and they are better at detecting associated urinary stone disease. It is useful to have both tests, except in children and women of childbearing age.

Cortical nephrocalcinosis is seen following extensive acute cortical infarction, and in chronic glomerulonephritis or pyelonephritis. It can occur in the transplanted kidney and in severe oxalosis, conditions that also produce a medullary distribution. An example of the more common (and clinically more important) medullary form of nephrocalcinosis is shown in Fig. 3. There are many causes of medullary nephrocalcinosis: it is usually associated with disordered calcium homeostasis and can, like urolithiasis, be broadly divided into hypercalcaemic, hypercalciuric/non-hypercalcaemic, and non-hypercalciuric forms. However, the presence of nephrocalcinosis is more likely to signify an underlying metabolic disturbance than is isolated urinary stone disease.

The most important risk factors for nephrocalcinosis are the same as those for urolithiasis:

(1) hypercalcaemia (leading to an increased filtered load of calcium), which is linked to diet;

(2) enhanced intestinal absorption of calcium, increased parathyroid hormone activity, or vitamin D excess;

(3) altered renal tubular handling of calcium resulting in hypercalciuria; and

(4) absence of factors in urine (such as citrate) that help to maintain calcium salts in solution.

Nephrocalcinosis associated with hypercalcaemia

Hyperparathyroidism is a common cause, accounting for approximately a third of cases in the large series of Wrong and Feest. Skeletal breakdown due to neoplasia or bone loss from chronic immobilization and severe osteoporosis can also be associated with nephrocalcinosis, although the latter, especially when the result of steroid therapy, usually only causes hypercalciuria. Vitamin D intoxication is often iatrogenic, a consequence of treating combined hypophosphataemic and hypocalcaemic states with vitamin D, calcium, and phosphate supplements. Sarcoid-induced hypercalcaemia is also related to increased activity of vitamin D, due in this circumstance to increased synthesis in granulomas, and sometimes causing significant hypercalciuria without overt hypercalcaemia. Nephrocalcinosis in association with hypothyroidism has been reported. By contrast, nephrocalcinosis is not seen in thyrotoxicosis, which can cause hypercalcaemia, except when there is an autoimmune basis and may therefore be associated with autoimmune distal renal tubular acidosis (see later in this section). A rare cause is the idiopathic hypercalcaemia of infancy (William's disease).

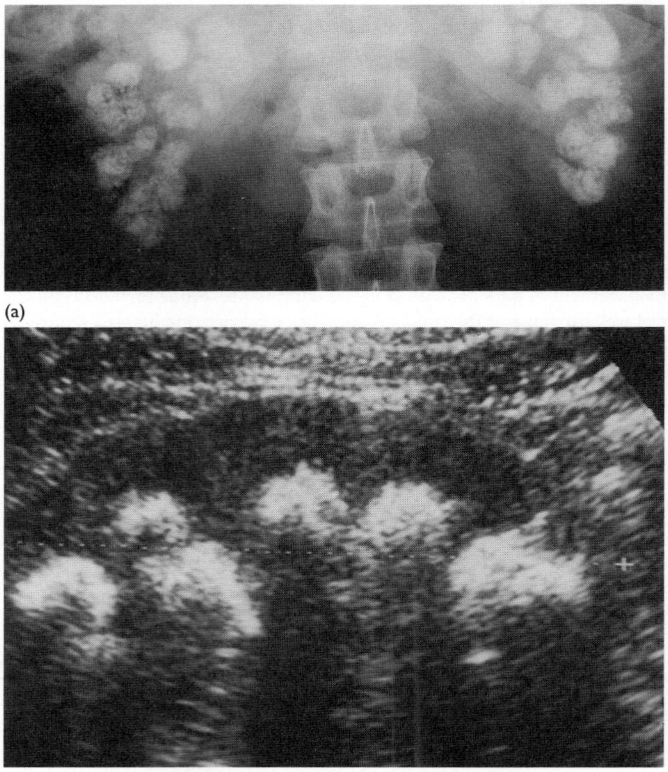

(a) (b)

Fig. 3 A plain radiograph (a) and renal ultrasound scan (b) of a man with familial distal renal tubular acidosis and severe medullary nephrocalcinosis. Note the striking medullary distribution of calcification in the radiographic picture and the increased medullary reflections and acoustic shadows 'behind' in the ultrasound picture.

Nephrocalcinosis associated with hypercalciuria without hypercalcaemia

The commonest cause in this category is distal renal tubular acidosis, which is associated with low urinary excretion of citrate. Hypercalciuria is a consistent finding in patients with the complete form of this disease and systemic acidosis (see under renal tubular acidosis). Although hypercalciuria is also a feature of the Fanconi syndrome and proximal renal tubular acidosis, these conditions are less commonly associated with nephrocalcinosis, presumably because of supranormal excretion of citrate in many cases.

The next most common cause of nephrocalcinosis is medullary sponge kidney. The cause of this condition is unknown. The collecting ducts are dilated and become the site of crystal formation and precipitation, probably related to stasis. The diagnosis can only be made reliably on an intravenous urogram, which shows grape-like clusters of ectatic medullary collecting ducts filled with contrast dye. Medullary sponge kidney can run in families and in some cases is associated with hemihypertrophy affecting the face, an arm, or a leg. Because damage to the collecting ducts can affect acid excretion, medullary sponge kidney can also be associated with a 'secondary' form of distal renal tubular acidosis, as well as mild nephrogenic diabetes insipidus.

Absorptive hypercalciuria is another cause: this may be idiopathic, but is also seen with vitamin D excess and in sarcoidosis. 'Milk-alkali syndrome' as a cause, due to excess calcium ingestion from calcium carbonate, is now rarely seen. Hypercalciuria and nephrocalcinosis can also occur in inherited tubular disorders like Bartter's syndrome and familial magnesium-losing nephropathy, and may follow intensive loop diuretic treatment in premature infants.

Non-hypercalciuric

Hyperoxaluria and oxalosis have been described earlier (see under urolithiasis). Various chronic hypokalaemic states have been associated with nephrocalcinosis. Hypokalaemia causes an intracellular acidosis, which reduces citrate excretion and may cause unspecified tubular damage. Reported examples are the hypertensive syndromes of apparent mineralocorticoid excess, due to a defect in the enzyme 11β-hydroxysteroid dehydrogenase, and Liddle's syndrome, due to an activating mutation of the collecting duct sodium (Na^+) channel (ENaC). Other conditions in which hypokalaemia may be a contributory factor include Bartter's syndrome and loop diuretic use in infancy. These and other causes are listed in Table 5.

Clinical approach to the patient with nephrocalcinosis

In most patients with nephrocalcinosis, a clinical diagnosis can be made and contributory factors identified. However, as with urinary stones, it is still poorly understood why changes in important risk factors (such as urinary calcium or citrate excretion) occur, and why or how calcium is deposited. The impact of nephrocalcinosis on health varies and its presentation can range from incidental, when detected on abdominal radiographs or ultrasounds performed for another reason, to life threatening. It may result in uncontrolled hypertension, renal infection, scarring, renal colic, defects of renal tubular function (impaired urinary concentrating ability and acid excretion—mild diabetes insipidus and secondary distal renal tubular acidosis), and even renal failure, although this is unusual.

Treatment

A metabolic cause must always be sought and treated if found. Treatment and management are otherwise very similar to those for macroscopic renal stone disease, and are mainly symptomatic. Assessment of dietary risk factors may be of some help if the underlying cause, such as distal renal tubular acidosis, cannot be easily corrected. Surgical intervention is only required if significant stones form, are passed frequently, or cause obstruction and infection. There is no place for lithotripsy, which may actually do harm, as the calcium deposition is largely parenchymal.

Renal tubular acidoses

The term 'renal tubular acidosis' is used to describe a group of clinical disorders in which net renal excretion of acid (hydrogen ions, H^+) is impaired as a result of renal tubular dysfunction. Strictly speaking, this definition could also include chronic renal failure, but by convention a reduced glomerular filtration rate as the cause of failure of acid excretion is excluded. Primary abnormalities of urinary acidification, renal tubular acidosis, are responsible for approximately 20 per cent of cases of medullary nephrocalcinosis with stones (see under nephrocalcinosis). To understand the pathogenesis of the renal tubular acidoses, an understanding of the role of the kidney in acid–base balance is required.

Role of the kidney in acid–base balance

Normal H^+ excretion depends on the ability of the renal tubule to reabsorb filtered bicarbonate (HCO_3^-) in the proximal nephron, followed by net H^+ secretion (approximately 50 mmol/day) by excretion of titratable acid and ammonium (NH_4^+) in the distal nephron (distal tubule and collecting duct) (see Fig. 4).

Reclamation of filtered bicarbonate

Normally, almost all filtered HCO_3^- is reabsorbed, the bulk of it in the proximal tubule (about 80 per cent), the remainder in the loop of Henle (about 15 per cent) and distal nephron (about 5 per cent). The mechanism of reabsorption is indirect: H^+ and HCO_3^- are generated in renal tubular cells (with the aid of carbonic anhydrase type II, **CA-II**), and the H^+ are secreted apically into the lumen, while the HCO_3^- enters the plasma via the basolateral cell membrane. In the proximal tubule and loop of Henle, most of the H^+ secretion is via Na^+/H^+ exchange in the apical (luminal) membrane, although there is also a contribution from primary active H^+-ATPase. The secreted H^+ reacts with filtered HCO_3^- to produce carbonic acid (H_2CO_3), which is rapidly converted to CO_2 and H_2O by carbonic anhydrase type IV (**CA-IV**) present on the luminal membrane, and the CO_2 and H_2O diffuse into the cell. The net result is that for every filtered HCO_3^- removed from tubular fluid, another replaces it in plasma.

Addition of 'new' bicarbonate to plasma

The bulk of H^+ generated within tubular cells is involved in reclaiming filtered bicarbonate (more than 4000 mmol/day). However, under normal conditions, because of the excess acid produced from food metabolism (about 50 mmol/day), it is necessary to add 'new' (extra) HCO_3^- to the plasma to replace that which has buffered this acid load. This is achieved by the generation of H^+ (and HCO_3^-) within tubular cells in addition to those needed to effect HCO_3^- reabsorption. The extra HCO_3^- enters the plasma, thus making the bicarbonate content of blood in the renal vein slightly higher than that in the renal artery. What happens to the H^+ produced simultaneously is a little more complicated. It would seem simplest to secrete these H^+ directly and independently into the tubular lumen and excrete them in the urine. However, the excretion of around 50 mmol of free H^+ per day in urine would lower urine pH to approximately 1.5 ($[H^+]$, ≅ 31 mmol/l), which the tubular epithelium cannot do, because it is only able to sustain a maximum pH gradient between plasma (pH ≅ 7.4; $[H^+]$ ≅ 40 nmol/l) and tubular fluid of 3 pH units (minimum urine pH ≅ 4.5; $[H^+]$ ≅ 31 600 nmol/l). The extra H^+ are excreted in two different ways: as titratable acid and as NH_4^+.

Excretion of titratable acid

Some of the extra H^+ are secreted into the lumen, where they can react with buffer anions in the tubular fluid (principally filtered HPO_4^{2-}); any buffer that is not reabsorbed will therefore excrete acid. The total amount of H^+ lost in the urine in this way can be determined by back-titrating the urine with a strong base, such as NaOH, until the urine pH is raised to 7.4 (that of arterial plasma); hence the term 'titratable acid'. It usually amounts to about 20 mmol/day. Approximately half the titratable acid production occurs in the proximal tubule, where tubular fluid pH falls to around 6.8 (equal to the pK of the $HPO_4^{2-}/H_2PO_4^-$ buffer system). The remainder occurs in the collecting duct, where H^+ can be secreted against a higher concentration gradient and consequently, as indicated above, urine pH can fall to approximately 4.5.

Excretion of ammonium

The proximal tubular cells are capable of taking up the amino acid glutamine and deaminating it to form NH_4^+ and α-ketoglutarate. NH_4^+ is secreted into the tubular lumen (substituting for H^+ on the Na^+/H^+ exchanger—Fig. 4) and eventually excreted, whereas α-ketoglutarate is converted to glucose, through reactions that consume H^+. The secreted H^+ (in NH_4^+) is

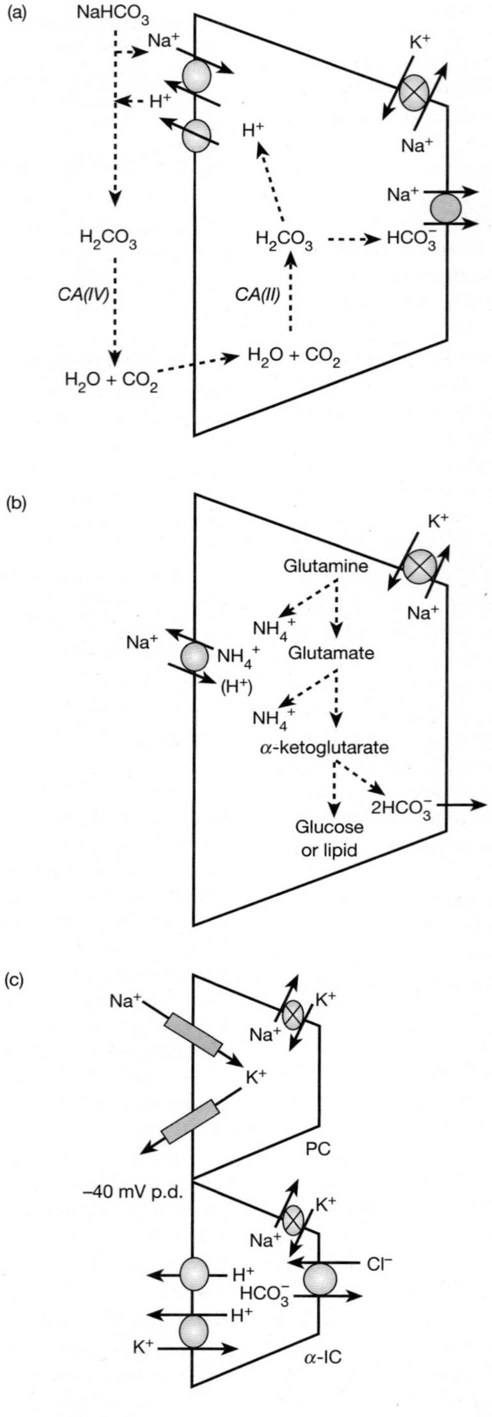

Fig. 4 Diagram showing cellular mechanisms of bicarbonate (HCO_3^-) reabsorption, ammonium (NH_4^+) generation and secretion, and hydrogen ion (H^+) secretion along the nephron. (a) Reclamation of filtered HCO_3^-, also mechanism of titratable acid; (b) generation and secretion of NH_4^+; (c) H^+ secretion. CA, carbonic anhydrase; PC, principal cell; α-IC, α-intercalated cell. See text for further details.

generated from CO_2 and H_2O, and the HCO_3^- that is formed at the same time is added to plasma. It is important that the NH_4^+ produced from glutamine enters the tubular fluid and not the plasma: if it did so it would be taken up by the liver and combined with bicarbonate to produce urea ($CO(NH_2)_2$) and CO_2, effectively neutralizing the bicarbonate generated in the proximal tubule thus: $2NH_4^+ + 2HCO_3^- \rightarrow CO(NH_2)_2 + CO_2 + 3H_2O$. In severe liver disease, metabolic alkalosis occurs because urea synthesis is impaired and bicarbonate consumption in this way is reduced. The converse of this is that when whole kidney NH_4^+ production and 'new' bicarbonate generation are impaired (as in chronic renal failure), continuing synthesis of urea by the liver will generate unneutralized H^+ (from CO_2), which may contribute to the metabolic acidosis of uraemia. This renal NH_4^+ system for the generation of 'new' bicarbonate is adaptable: the activity of the glutaminase enzyme that deaminates glutamine is enhanced during acidosis (including intracellular acidosis due to chronic hypokalaemia).

The elimination of NH_4^+ in the urine occurs only after a complicated process that involves active NH_4^+ secretion in the proximal tubule, NH_4^+ reabsorption in the thick ascending limb of the loop of Henle (which can be blocked by the loop diuretic frusemide—see under urinary acidification and the diagnosis of renal tubular acidosis), and finally, NH_3 secretion by diffusion into the collecting duct. The reabsorption of NH_4^+ in the thick ascending limb leads to accumulation of NH_4^+ in the medullary interstitium, which is increased further by countercurrent multiplication (similar to generation of the corticomedullary osmotic gradient for urinary concentration). At the pH of interstitial fluid, and with a high medullary concentration of NH_4^+, some dissociates and increases the local level of NH_3. This can then diffuse into the collecting duct, where owing to the lower pH it is converted to NH_4^+ again, trapped in the tubular lumen, and excreted. This conversion maintains a concentration gradient for further NH_3 diffusion into the collecting duct ('diffusion trapping'). Anything that interferes with H^+ secretion in the collecting duct, as in distal renal tubular acidosis, would be expected to reduce diffusion trapping and thereby cause not only a higher urine pH (which depends on the presence of free H^+), but also a reduction in NH_4^+ and titratable acid (net acid) excretion; in fact some authorities advocate defining renal tubular acidosis in terms of reduced NH_4^+ excretion. The converse of this is decreased availability of NH_3 (as in hyperkalaemia, which suppresses NH_3 synthesis), but relatively normal tubular H^+ secretion per nephron. In this situation, urine pH will be low (because of less NH_3 to buffer H^+) and net acid excretion reduced. Like distal renal tubular acidosis, in chronic renal failure (uraemic acidosis), urinary excretion of NH_4^+ and titratable acid (mainly phosphate) is decreased; however in contrast to renal tubular acidosis, urine pH is usually low, and when the amounts of excreted phosphate and NH_4^+ are corrected for the reduced glomerular filtration rate (i.e. excretion per nephron), they are both normal or even increased.

What determines the presence of acidosis?

The following factors are important:

(1) H^+ intake and endogenous generation;

(2) Net H^+ excretion in urine = urinary [titratable acid] + [NH_4^+] − [HCO_3^-];

(3) [titratable acid] in urine is dependent on urine pH and the amount of buffer available;

(4) [NH_4^+] in urine is dependent on NH_3/NH_4^+ generation and delivery (proximal tubule secretion, thick ascending loop reabsorption, and diffusion trapping in the collecting duct); and

(5) [HCO_3^-] in urine is dependent on urine pH and pco_2.

Specific transport proteins differentially located on the apical and basolateral membrane of tubular cells mediate the processes described above. They are either responsible for H^+ or HCO_3^- transport. The Na^+/H^+ exchanger and H^+-ATPase, together with a small and uncertain contribution from a renal H^+/K^+-ATPase (similar to that found in the stomach) are responsible for H^+ secretion. Six isoforms of the Na^+/H^+ exchanger have been identified (NHE-1 to NHE-6), but so far none has been linked to a clinical form of renal tubular acidosis. The H^+-ATPase is not a single protein, but composed of at least nine distinct subunits. It is found mainly in the distal nephron, although it is also present in the proximal tubule and loop of Henle. The role of the H^+/K^+-ATPase in normal urinary acidification is still debated, although it seems to be upregulated along the distal nephron in potassium deficiency.

To generalize, it can be said that the main exit pathway for bicarbonate from tubular cells of the proximal tubule and loop of Henle is the Na^+-HCO_3^- cotransporter, while from cells of the distal nephron it is the Cl^-/HCO_3^- exchanger. The latter transporter can also mediate HCO_3^- secretion when present in the luminal cell membrane.

Nomenclature of the renal tubular acidoses

The 'old' numbered classification of renal tubular acidosis is a chronological one and reflects historical description of clinical disease. The numbering is often a source of great confusion to students and doctors alike, since it is not based on any functional understanding of acid excretion by the nephron. It is easier to subdivide renal tubular acidosis into proximal ('old' type II) and distal ('old' type I) nephron types (which may be inherited, or due to a variety of drugs or systemic diseases) and to consider underlying mechanisms. What is now emerging is that we can begin to subclassify these two main types according to the transport defect of acid excretion. The fact that several of the transporters involved in the renal handling of H^+ and HCO_3^- have now been cloned means that our classification of renal tubular acidosis is likely to change in the future, to one based on underlying and specific molecular transport defects.

Tests to diagnose renal tubular acidosis

From the above, it is apparent that in the presence of a normal glomerular filtration rate, renal tubular acidosis can result from (alone or in combination): (1) failure to reclaim filtered bicarbonate in the proximal tubule; (2) failure to generate and excrete NH_4^+; and (3) impaired H^+ secretion along the distal nephron. The finding of a low serum bicarbonate concentration in an appropriate clinical context should raise the possibility of renal tubular acidosis, but to make the diagnosis, specialized tests are usually required. A variety of such tests have been described, some of which we find to be more useful than others, as indicated below.

Measurement of urinary pH and HCO_3– excretion

Dipstix urine pH values are unreliable: pH should be measured in a freshly passed specimen of urine with a glass pH electrode. The pH of a urine sample that has been left to stand, and has not been covered with a film of oil, will rise as CO_2 is lost; this is usually the reason for a measured urine pH of higher than 8, unless it is infected (high NH_4^+ from urea-splitting organisms).

Whilst a high urinary pH might lead one to diagnose renal tubular acidosis in an acidotic patient with normal glomerular filtration rate and uninfected urine, especially if they had nephrocalcinosis and/or urinary stones, the diagnosis of renal tubular acidosis cannot be based on the measurement of urine pH alone. For example, even in the presence of systemic acidosis, and excluding chronic renal failure, a low urine pH may not rule out a diagnosis of renal tubular acidosis, since renal acid excretion can still be impaired if the generation and delivery of NH_3/NH_4^+ are reduced. In addition, in proximal renal tubular acidosis, when bicarbonate reabsorption is impaired, urine pH can be low (rather than high) if previous loss of bicarbonate has lowered plasma [HCO_3^-] to such a level (less than 18 mmol/l) that the filtered load of bicarbonate is then decreased, resulting in low urinary bicarbonate excretion. In this situation, failure of the proximal tubule to reabsorb bicarbonate can only be demonstrated by showing a high fractional (as a proportion of the amount of filtered bicarbonate) excretion (urinary [HCO_3^-]/plasma [HCO_3^-] × plasma [creatinine]/urinary [creatinine]) × 100 per cent), although to do this plasma [HCO_3^-] must be increased to approximately 24 mmol/l by intravenous infusion of bicarbonate. Fractional bicarbonate excretion is normally less than 5 per cent, but in proximal renal tubular acidosis it exceeds 15 per cent. Ammonium generation can also be reduced in proximal renal tubular acidosis (as part of more generalized proximal tubular dysfunction), which may be another reason for the finding of a low urine pH.

Urinary net negative charge and osmolal gap

The difficulty in interpretation of urinary pH in isolation is why some have argued for the calculation of the urinary net charge, or anion gap ($[Na^+] + [K^+] - [Cl^-]$), which is usually negative (because Cl^- is balanced by unmeasured NH_4^+), to estimate urinary NH_4^+ concentration indirectly. Because a non-renal cause of metabolic acidosis will increase NH_4^+ generation and excretion (making the net charge more negative), reduced NH_4^+ excretion is evident as a positive net charge, which would indicate a renal cause for acidosis, including uraemic acidosis (chronic renal failure). However, an increase in the excretion of ketoacid anions (such as in diabetic ketoacidosis) will also make the net charge positive, despite increased NH_4^+ excretion, because excreted NH_4^+ accompanies unmeasured ketoacid anions (A^-), rather than measured Cl^-.

To get around the problem of unmeasured anions, calculation of the urinary osmolal gap (urine osmolality-($2 \times ([Na^+] + [K^+]) + [urea] + [glucose]$)) has been proposed. Assuming that NH_4^+ and its accompanying anion constitute the main unmeasured osmotically active particles in the urine, then urinary $[NH_4^+]$ is approximately half the osmolal gap. A low osmolal gap suggests low NH_4^+ excretion and thus a defect of renal acidification. However, to determine where the defect might lie, urine pH must still be measured: if it is high (more than 6), there may be reduced distal H^+ excretion or increased distal delivery of HCO_3^-, that is, distal or proximal renal tubular acidosis, respectively; if urine pH is low (less than 5), there may be chronic renal failure (low glomerular filtration rate) or hyperkalaemia (inhibiting NH_4^+ generation); an intermediate urine pH of 5 to 6 is said to indicate renal interstitial disease.

However, despite the sound theory, there are too many confounding variables, and both estimation of urinary net negative charge and osmolal gap fail to distinguish reliably between the acidosis of chronic renal failure and renal tubular acidosis. In our opinion these measurements often seem confusing and are of limited practical value in the diagnosis of renal tubular acidosis.

Urinary $p\text{CO}_2$/blood difference

Since the distal nephron H^+ secretory mechanism is intact in proximal renal tubular acidosis, measurement of the urine–blood $p\text{CO}_2$ (U–B $p\text{CO}_2$) difference has been proposed as a means of distinguishing proximal from distal renal tubular acidosis. In the presence of adequate bicarbonaturia and alkaline urine (pH greater than 7.4; intravenous bicarbonate may be necessary to achieve this) this difference is high (around 30 mmHg (4 kPa) or more), whereas it is low (less than 25 mmHg) when distal H^+ secretion is defective. This test is also said to distinguish between reduced distal H^+ secretion due to a primary secretory ('pump') defect and that due to increased cell membrane permeability and backleak of H^+ (see Table 5). Whilst there are theoretical reasons why this may be so, our incomplete understanding of the factors that determine urinary $p\text{CO}_2$ make interpretation difficult; moreover, in practice the test is not easy to perform and results can be variable. Like the urinary anion and osmolal gaps, we do not find it clinically useful.

Acid loading

The most straightforward and reliable means of making the diagnosis of impaired distal nephron acidification is an acid load test. The easiest and best-established method is the short oral ammonium chloride (0.1 g/kg) test of Wrong and Davies. The criterion for a diagnosis of a distal acidification defect is a failure to lower urine pH to less than 5.5, making measurements as urine is passed for at least 6 h (and up to 8 h) after the ingestion of NH_4Cl.

A simpler test, which compares well with the NH_4Cl test in normal subjects, although it has not been formally validated in patients with renal tubular acidosis, is the frusemide/fludrocortisone test. In this much more palatable test, a single dose of fludrocortisone (1 mg) is given orally, followed 1 h later by oral frusemide (40 mg), and urine pH measured for up to 5 h; again the threshold pH is 5.5. Frusemide works by enhancing H^+ secretion through increased delivery of Na^+ (from the thick ascending

Table 5 An anatomical and functional classification of renal tubular acidosis (RTA)

Proximal RTA (pRTA)	Distal RTA (dRTA)
Mutations of carbonic anhydrase type II (CA-II)—deafness and osteopetrosis (because of the widespread distribution of CA-II in tubular cells, it can also manifest as a dRTA and/or mixed type of RTA)	*Autoimmune*—impaired function of both H^+-ATPase and AE1 Cl^-/ HCO_3^- exchanger, and CA-II have all been described, especially in Sjögren's syndrome, in which symptomatic hypokalaemia is often a feature
Fanconi syndrome:	*Inherited*:
Cystinotic	Dominant (mutations of AE1)
Non-cystinotic (inherited metabolic, including X- linked Dent's disease), mitochondrial cytopathies (inherited and drug-related, e.g. zidovudine), drug induced, heavy metal poisoning and myeloma, galactosaemia, hereditary fructose intolerance	Recessive (mutations of AE1)
	Recessive with deafness (mutations of the B1 subunit of the H^+-ATPase)
	Dent's disease (a Cl^- channel—ClC-5—mutation)
After renal transplantation—often a mixture of pRTA and dRTA because of immune-related interstitial inflammation and tubular damage, including reduced NH_3/NH_4^+ generation related to decreased nephron mass	*Real and apparent mineralocorticoid deficiency* ('old'type IV dRTA—reduced transepithelial voltage—with hyperkalaemia):
	Hyporeninaemic hypoaldosteronism (in diabetes mellitus)
	Pseudohypoaldosteronism type 1a (an inactivating mutation of the epithelial Na^+ channel—recessive inheritance)
	Pseudohypoaldosteronism type 1b (a mutation of mineralocorticoid receptor—dominant inheritance)
	Pseudohypoaldosteronism type 2 (Gordon's syndrome, due to a presumed increase in distal Cl^- absorption–dominant inheritance)
Hyperparathyroidism (without nephrocalcinosis)—inhibition of the proximal tubular Na^+/H^+ exchange	*Drug-induced*:
	Amphotericin B (increased permeability)
	Toluene ('glue-sniffing') (increased permeability)
	Lithium (H^+-ATPase dysfunction)
	Trimethoprim (reduced transepithelial voltage)
	Medullary sponge kidney and analgesic abuse—secondary dRTA as a result of medullary (collecting duct) damage
	Obstuctive uropathy—H^+-ATPase dysfunction

limb) to the distal tubule and collecting duct, where increased Na^+ reabsorption facilitates H^+ secretion; fludrocortisone directly stimulates both distal Na^+ reabsorption and H^+ secretion. Frusemide may also promote NH_4^+ excretion by blocking its reabsorption in the thick ascending limb, which could be used to demonstrate that impaired NH_4^+ generation *per se* is not the primary cause of reduced distal acidification. In distal renal tubular acidosis secondary to a defect of H^+ secretion, frusemide should still increase NH_4^+ excretion, although it may be less than normal.

The clinical features of renal tubular acidosis

A hyperchloraemic (normal anion gap) metabolic acidosis is a feature of both proximal and distal forms of renal tubular acidosis.

Proximal renal tubular acidosis

As already mentioned, urine pH in this form of renal tubular acidosis (also known as type 2) is often within the normal range; plasma bicarbonate concentration can range between 10 and 20 mmol/l. This type of renal tubular acidosis is uncommon and an isolated failure to reabsorb bicarbonate is unusual. Most cases are associated with other proximal tubular transport defects, as in the Fanconi syndrome, which may have many causes (see Table 5). Thus, it is likely that other clues to a primary abnormality of proximal tubular function will be present, such as glycosuria, hyperphosphaturia (hypophosphataemia), hyperuricosuria (hypouricaemia), aminoaciduria, and tubular (low molecular weight, e.g. retinol-binding protein) proteinuria. Osteomalacia (rickets and growth retardation in children) is common and due to impaired synthesis of active metabolites of vitamin D and urinary loss of 25-OH vitamin D.

Although hypercalciuria and hyperphosphaturia occur, nephrocalcinosis or urinary stones are rare, probably because of the associated increase in urinary citrate excretion. However, nephrocalcinosis is sometimes seen as a consequence of treatment with vitamin D, calcium, and phosphate supplements, and is often attributable to periods of iatrogenic hypercalcaemia.

Hypokalaemia is common and probably a consequence of osmotic diuresis due to reduced solute reabsorption (mainly bicarbonate) in the proximal tubule, leading to increased flow rate in the distal nephron, the site of potassium secretion. For this reason, bicarbonate supplementation tends to exacerbate hypokalaemia.

The molecular basis of a particular form of inherited non-cystinotic Fanconi syndrome, now known as Dent's disease, has been defined. This condition is X-linked (Xp11.22) and recessive, typically (about 80 per cent) presenting with nephrocalcinosis and urolithiasis, hypercalciuria, and progressive renal failure. A proportion of cases are initially thought to have a proximal or distal type of renal tubular acidosis. The reason for is that the underlying defect is a mutation of an intracellular membrane-associated chloride channel (ClC-5) found in cells of the proximal tubule, thick ascending loop, and collecting duct (α-intercalated cells) (Fig. 5). This channel appears to be involved in normal endosomal function (acidification), which affects both the reabsorption of low-molecular weight-proteins in the proximal tubule and perhaps the normal turnover and recruitment (recycling) to the luminal membrane of transport proteins, like the H^+-ATPase of the α-intercalated cell. Tubular proteinuria is a characteristic feature, distinguishing it from distal renal tubular acidosis proper.

Because the proximal tubule is the dominant site of bicarbonate reabsorption, and this is ultimately dependent on CA-II activity, lack of this enzyme produces a predominantly proximal form of renal tubular acidosis, although it is widely expressed along the nephron. This type of proximal renal tubular acidosis is very rare and associated with increased bone mineralization (osteopetrosis), deafness, and cerebral calcification. Interestingly, a recent publication describing a *CA-II* 'knockout' mouse with renal tubular acidosis (but without bicarbonaturia) demonstrated that the condition could be partially corrected by gene therapy (retrograde injection of

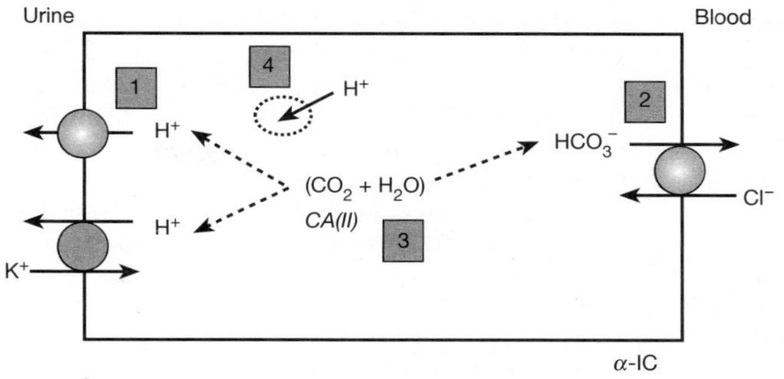

Fig. 5 Diagram of the α-intercalated cell (α-IC) of the collecting duct, showing the sites of ion transport defects that have been linked to distal renal tubular acidosis (dRTA). In boxes: **1**, H^+-ATPase mutations in recessive dRTA with and without deafness; **2**, Cl^-/HCO_3^- exchanger mutation in dominant (and recessive) dRTA; **3**, CA-II (carbonic anhydrase) deficiency in inherited mixed pRTA and dRTA; **4**, Cl^- channel (ClC-5) mutation in Dent's disease (pRTA/Fanconi with some dRTA features).

CA-II cDNA in liposomes), which restored *CA-II* function to the distal nephron.

Distal renal tubular acidosis

The most common form of renal tubular acidosis is 'classic' (or type 1) distal renal tubular acidosis and is due to an underlying defect of H^+ secretion ('pump defect'). The key feature of this form of renal tubular acidosis is an inability to lower urine pH below 5.5. In the absence of systemic acidosis, a patient who cannot reduce their urine pH to less than 5.5 in the face of an acid load is said have the 'incomplete' form. In patients with 'complete' distal renal tubular acidosis, plasma bicarbonate concentration usually ranges between 15 and 20 mmol/l, but can fall to less than 10 mmol/l in severe cases. In patients with 'incomplete' distal renal tubular acidosis, NH_4^+ excretion is normal (in relation to glomerular filtration rate) and this may be why these patients are not acidotic and their plasma bicarbonate concentration stays within the normal range. The causes of distal renal tubular acidosis are listed in Table 5.

Hypokalaemia can occur, especially in the autoimmune form (such as Sjögren's syndrome) and when there is systemic acidosis, but it is not as consistent a feature as it is in proximal renal tubular acidosis. Nephrocalcinosis is common and present in 70 to 80 per cent of adults, whether or not they have a systemic acidosis. Osteomalacia (rickets in children) is seen only in acidotic patients with 'complete' distal renal tubular acidosis. Hypercalciuria is said to be a feature of this form of renal tubular acidosis, but it is not a consistent finding and may depend on the presence of systemic acidosis and resulting calcium loss from bone.

A characteristic of distal renal tubular acidosis, which can be useful in screening for this condition in children, is a low urinary excretion of citrate, which in alkaline urine is normally increased. The probable explanation for reduced citrate excretion in distal renal tubular acidosis is that it is reabsorbed in the proximal tubule by a mechanism dependent on intracellular pH: intracellular acidosis (due to systemic acidosis or chronic hypokalaemia) increases mitochondrial metabolism of citrate and thus its reabsorption. In addition, trivalent citrate buffers H^+ in systemic acidosis and is converted to the more readily reabsorbed divalent form. Because it inhibits the precipitation of calcium salts (mainly phosphate), reduced citrate delivery to the distal nephron is a key factor in the development of nephrocalcinosis and urinary stone disease in distal renal tubular acidosis.

The main site of H^+ secretion along the distal nephron is the H^+-ATPase in the luminal cell membrane of the α-intercalated cell (Fig. 5). As already described, H^+ and HCO_3^- are generated from intracellular hydration of CO_2, the latter exiting the basolateral cell membrane in exchange for Cl^- by an anion exchanger (AE1). This basolateral exchanger is essential for normal apical H^+ secretion in the α-intercalated cell and it has been established that a mutation of the gene encoding this transport protein is the cause of dominantly inherited distal renal tubular acidosis and some cases of the recessive form without deafness. Recessive distal renal tubular acidosis with deafness is due to a mutation of the B1 subunit of the H^+-ATPase (and recently another H^+-ATPase subunit mutation in some cases without deafness) . However, unlike the dominant form, the recessive form appears to be genetically heterogeneous. Expression of both these transport proteins is decreased in the collecting duct α-intercalated cells of patients with autoimmune distal renal tubular acidosis.

A rare drug-related form of distal renal tubular acidosis with hypokalaemia is that due to amphotericin B. This drug accumulates in the kidney and increases the permeability of the tubular cell membrane, resulting in a back-leak of secreted H^+ ('permeability' or 'gradient' defect) and failure to maintain the plasma–urine pH gradient across the tubular epithelium.

Distal renal tubular acidosis with hyperkalaemia is also known as type IV renal tubular acidosis, or voltage-dependent renal tubular acidosis. It occurs in situations in which the lumen negative potential difference along the distal nephron (Fig. 4) is reduced. This normally facilitates potassium and hydrogen ion secretion, depends on sodium reabsorption, and is stimulated by aldosterone. Thus, when sodium reabsorption through the epithelial Na^+ channel is reduced by drugs like amiloride and trimethoprim, or when the Na^+ channel is inactive (autosomal recessive pseudohypoaldosteronism type 1a), there is a decrease in both potassium and hydrogen ion secretion, leading to hyperkalaemia and metabolic acidosis. Because of the stimulatory effect of aldosterone, this form of renal tubular acidosis is also seen in states of hypoaldosteronism.

Another rare and inherited form of hyperkalaemic renal tubular acidosis is autosomal dominant pseudohypoaldosteronism type II, or Gordon's syndrome. The transport defect underlying this condition remains unknown, although it has been proposed that an abnormal increase in collecting duct permeability to Cl^- is responsible, leading to a decrease in the lumen negative potential difference. In contrast to patients with the type 1 variant of pseudohypoaldosteronism, these patients are usually hypertensive, and their blood pressure and hyperkalaemia are particularly responsive to thiazide diuretics.

In all forms of hyperkalaemia, renal NH_3/NH_4^+ generation is reduced, which also impairs acid excretion and exacerbates systemic acidosis.

Treatment

Administration of oral bicarbonate, which can also be given as citrate, is the mainstay of treatment in all forms of renal tubular acidosis, unless the underlying defect can be corrected (for instance drug withdrawal or aldosterone replacement). It can prevent the long-term complications of rickets and growth retardation, and may also limit the progression of nephrocalcinosis and nephrolithiasis in distal renal tubular acidosis by increasing citrate excretion. In both proximal renal tubular acidosis and 'classic' distal renal tubular acidosis, a potassium supplement may also be necessary, since oral sodium bicarbonate tends to increase urinary potassium loss.

Treatment that is more specific to proximal renal tubular acidosis may include vitamin D, calcium, and phosphate supplementation; a thiazide diuretic can also be tried, so as to increase bicarbonate reabsorption (secondary to mild extracellular volume contraction), but this may also exacerbate the tendency to hypokalaemia.

In distal renal tubular acidosis, plasma bicarbonate concentration should be maintained above 20 mmol/l. Morbidity in classic distal renal tubular acidosis is due to calcium phosphate renal stones; endstage renal failure is a rare complication and is usually the result of unrecognized urinary tract obstruction and recurrent infection. In hyperkalaemic distal renal tubular acidosis, a loop diuretic plus fludrocortisone, or an ion exchange resin, can be used to control the hyperkalaemia, and improve NH_3/NH_4^+ generation and thus acid excretion.

A seeming contradiction in the treatment of distal renal tubular acidosis with nephrocalcinosis and urolithiasis is the use of alkali therapy. On the one hand, this treatment will correct acidosis-related hypercalciuria and increase urinary citrate excretion, which should reduce or arrest nephrocalcinosis and stone formation. On the other hand, calcium phosphate precipitation (the main component of nephrocalcinosis and stones related to distal renal tubular acidosis) is favoured by an alkaline urine pH, and if bicarbonate is given as the sodium salt, this will also tend to increase urinary calcium excretion. It is possible that these opposing effects are why amelioration of nephrocalcinosis is often not seen in treated patients followed long-term.

Further reading

Urolithiasis and nephrocalcinosis

Coe FL *et al.*, eds. (1996). *Kidney stones, medical and surgical management.* Lippincott-Raven, Philadelphia.

Lingeman JE *et al.*, eds. (1989). *Urinary calculi.* Lea & Febiger, Philadelphia.

Pak CYC (1998). Kidney stones. *Lancet* **351**, 1797–801.

Robertson WG (1992). Factors involved in stone-formation. In: Cameron S *et al.*, eds. *Oxford textbook of nephrology*, 1st edn, pp 1822–46. Oxford University Press, Oxford.

Robertson WG (1993). Urinary tract calculi. In: Nordin BEC, Need AG, Morris HA, eds. *Metabolic bone and stone disease*, 3rd edn, pp 249–311. Churchill Livingstone, Edinburgh.

Wickham JEA, Buck AC, eds (1990). *Renal tract stone, metabolic basis and practice.* Churchill Livingstone, Edinburgh.

Wrong O (1998). Nephrocalcinsosis. In: Cameron S *et al.*, eds. *Oxford textbook of nephrology*, 2nd edn, pp 1375–96. Oxford University Press, Oxford.

Renal tubular acidosis

Alpern RJ (1990). Cell mechanisms of proximal tubule acidification. *Physiological Reviews* **70**, 79–114.

Bruce LJ *et al.* (1997). Familial distal renal tubular acidosis is associated with mutations in the red cell anion exchanger (band 3, *AE1*) gene. *Journal of Clinical Investigation* **100**, 1693–707.

Capasso G *et al.* (1986). Amphotericin B and amphotericin B methylester: effect on brush border membrane permeability. *Kidney International* **30**, 311–17.

Capasso G *et al.* (1994). Acidification in mammalian cortical distal tubule. *Kidney International* **45**, 1543–54.

Cohen EP *et al.* (1992). Absence of H(+)-ATPase in cortical collecting tubules of a patient with Sjögren's syndrome and distal renal tubular acidosis. *Journal of the American Society of Nephrology* **3**, 264–71.

Halperin ML, Vasuvattakul S, Bayoumi A (1992). A modified classification of metabolic acidosis: a pathophysiologic approach. *Nephron* **60**, 129–33.

Karet FE *et al.* (1999). Mutations in the gene encoding B1 subunit of H+-ATPase cause renal tubular acidosis with sensorineural deafness. *Nature Genetics* **21**, 84–90.

Lai LW *et al.* (1998). Correction of renal tubular acidosis in carbonic anhydrase II-deficient mice with gene therapy. *Journal of Clinical Investigation* **101**, 1320–5.

Lloyd SE *et al.* (1996). A common molecular basis for three inherited kidney stone diseases. *Nature* **379**, 445–9.

Wrong O (1991). Distal renal tubular acidosis: the value of urinary pH, pCO_2 and NH_4^+ measurements. *Pediatric Nephrology* **5**, 249–55.

Wrong O, Davies HEF (1959). The excretion of acid in renal disease. *Quarterly Journal of Medicine* **28**, 259–313.

20.14 Urinary tract obstruction

L. R. I. Baker

Introduction

If the flow of urine is impeded at any point in its course from the renal calices to the exterior, urinary tract obstruction is present. The terms 'obstructive uropathy', 'obstructive nephropathy', and 'hydronephrosis' are frequently used interchangeably and are taken to have the same meaning as the term 'urinary tract obstruction'. A more rigorous approach is preferable: 'obstructive uropathy' should be taken to mean pathological change occurring in the urinary tract and kidney consequent upon urinary tract obstruction. 'Obstructive nephropathy' is present when pathological change in the kidney resulting from urinary tract obstruction is associated with prolongation of the transit time of glomerular filtrate down the nephron. The term 'hydronephrosis' should be taken to denote dilatation of the renal pelvis and calyceal system.

Intraluminal obstruction between the commencement of the proximal tubule and the distal end of the collecting duct, such as occurs in uric acid nephropathy, as a result of sulphonamide crystal deposition, and in multiple myelomatosis, falls outside the definition of urinary tract obstruction employed here and will not be considered further.

Although dilatation of the outflow system proximal to the site of obstruction is a characteristic finding, widening of the ureter and/or pelvicalyceal system does not necessarily indicate the presence of obstruction. Causes of such anatomical abnormality in the absence of obstruction are listed in Table 1.

Obstruction may be partial or complete, unilateral or bilateral. Bilateral obstruction, or obstruction of a single kidney, is a greater threat to the patient than unilateral obstruction. Obstruction associated with infection is a greater threat to kidney function and to life than obstruction in the absence of infection. Since it is common, and often reversible, obstruction of the urinary tract should be considered in every uraemic patient, whether acute or chronic.

Table 1 Causes of non-obstructive dilatation of the collecting system

Anatomical variants
Large major calyx
Extrarenal pelvis
Distensible system after relief of obstruction
Pregnancy
Congenital anomalies
Megacalyces
Vesicoureteric reflux
Children
Abnormality of ureteric insertion into bladder
Adults
Neuropathic bladder, after ileal loop diversion, following vesicoureteric surgery, after renal transplantation
Calyceal pathology
Tuberculosis
Caliceal cyst
Papillary necrosis

Incidence

Urinary tract obstruction occurs most frequently in the young and the old. Hydronephrosis is the most common cause of an abdominal mass in neonates, and obstruction, usually due to congenital abnormalities, is also relatively common in children. Its incidence declines after the age of 10 and is at its lowest in middle age, but begins to rise again after the age of 60, particularly in males, in whom the commonest cause is prostatic enlargement. Although the overall frequency of urinary tract obstruction is the same in both sexes, between 20 and 60 years of age it is more frequent in women, and over the age of 60 years the reverse is true. Urinary tract obstruction has been found in 3.8 per cent of a large series of routine autopsies and 25 per cent of autopsies carried out upon uraemic patients.

Causes

Obstructing lesions may lie within the lumen or the wall of the urinary tract, or may cause obstruction by pressure from outside, the major causes in each group being listed in Table 2.

Calculi and neuromuscular malfunction at the junction of the renal pelvis and ureter are common causes of unilateral obstruction. Prostatic obstruction, stone disease, and bladder tumours account for approximately 75 per cent of cases of bilateral obstruction in developed countries. Wide geographical variations occur in the relative incidence of some causes of obstruction, for example schistosomiasis. To the clinician, the most important questions are whether urinary tract obstruction affects the upper or the lower urinary tract, and whether it is of recent onset (acute obstruction) or is long-standing (chronic obstruction).

Pathophysiology

Acute upper tract obstruction

Urine flows from the kidney to the bladder as a result of ureteric and pelvic peristalsis, the effects of gravity, and the pressure of glomerular filtration. Peristalsis normally generates high pressures within the ureteric lumen, sufficient to propel urine down the ureter without the transmission of the increased pressure to the renal parenchyma. Initially, an upward movement occurs in the ureter: thereafter, proximal contraction of ureteric circular muscle, with eventual complete occlusion of the lumen, forms a bolus of urine. Contraction of longitudinal smooth muscle then propels the bolus along the ureter. Baseline ureteric pressure is similar to that in the renal pelvis, but during this process rises to values between 10 and 25 mmHg. These pressures are not transmitted to the renal pelvis, where pressure seldom rises above 4 mmHg.

Any change in blood flow or glomerular filtration rate resulting from ureteric obstruction would have important effects on tubular pressures and flows. In humans, the time of onset of obstruction is seldom known with

Table 2 Some causes of urinary tract obstruction

Within the lumen
Calculus
Blood clot
Sloughed papillae (diabetes, analgesic abuse, sickle cell disease)
Tumour of renal pelvis or ureter
Bladder tumour
Within the wall
Pelviureteric neuromuscular dysfunction (congenital, 10 per cent bilateral)
Ureteric stricture (tuberculosis, especially after treatment; calculous; following surgery)
Ureterovesical stricture (congenital, ureterocele, calculous, schistosomiasis)
Congenital megaureter
Congenital bladder neck obstruction
Neurogenic bladder
Urethral stricture (calculous, gonococcal, after instrumentation)
Congenital urethral valve
Pinhole meatus
Pressure from outside
Pelviureteric compression (bands, aberrant vessels)
Tumours, for example retroperitoneal growths or glands, carcinoma of colon, diverticulitis, aortic aneurysm
Retroperitoneal fibrosis (peri-aortitis)
Accidental ligation of ureter
Pancreatitis
Retrocaval ureter (right-sided obstruction)
Crohn's disease
Chronic granulomatous disease
Prostatic obstruction
Tumours in pelvis, for example carcinoma of cervix
Phimosis

any precision, and methods of measurement of renal blood flow or filtration rate using clearance techniques are indirect and depend upon tubular function, which is affected by urinary tract obstruction; hence pathophysiological explanations must depend on animal experiments. In the normal dog, pressure within the ureter more than doubles when the ureteric lumen is occluded during peristalsis, and similar changes occur in ureteric wall tension. Baseline and peak pressure and wall tensions are about twice as high as control values 3 min after acute ureteric obstruction; at 5 to 20 min they approximate to peak values; and at 1 h there is a threefold increase. At this point, occlusion of the ureter fails to occur and pressures generated by ureteric wall tension are transmitted to the renal pelvis and parenchyma. Any further increase in pressure results in dilatation of the ureter.

The effect of an increase in pressure within the ureter transmitted to the nephron depends upon the degree of obstruction (whether complete or incomplete), whether obstruction is unilateral or bilateral, and the duration of obstruction. In the dog, renal blood flow falls to 50 per cent of control values 3 or 4 days after induction of complete ureteric obstruction and at 4 weeks it is about one-third that of the contralateral unobstructed kidney. Three phases, which are not well understood, are discernible in the relationship between changes in ureteral pressure and renal blood flow with time (Fig. 1). Phase I occurs during the first hour after induction of obstruction. Renal blood flow increases, presumably owing to a reduction in intrarenal vascular resistance, associated with a gradual increase in ureteric pressure. In phase II, which takes place over the next 2 to 5 h, ureteric pressure continues to rise and renal blood flow begins to fall. Thereafter, in phase III, renal blood flow continues to fall and ureteric pressure returns towards or to normal.

Chronic upper tract obstruction

Three months after the production of experimental obstruction in dogs, baseline ureteric wall tension is increased and there is no difference between baseline and peak values of wall tension, the latter being measured during ureteric occlusion. By contrast, baseline and peak pressures within the ureteric lumen are not significantly different from control values. This is a consequence of the relationship between pressure and wall tension expressed in Laplace's law, which states that $P = K(T/R)$, where P is the transluminal pressure, K is a constant, T is wall tension, and R is the radius of the ureter. In chronic obstruction, therefore, normal intraluminal pressures are maintained as a consequence of ureteric dilatation.

These experimental findings suggest that the major component of damage to the kidney due to obstruction occurs soon after its onset. In humans the highest measured ureteric pressures have been found during acute obstruction (as high as 50 mmHg during passage of a stone) and there appears to be an inverse relationship between pressure within the renal pelvis and time of measurement in patients with complete obstruction. The notion that chronic obstruction with dilatation of the ureter may be relatively benign is supported by the observation that patients with incomplete urinary tract obstruction due to congenital anomalies lose renal function only slowly.

Acute lower tract obstruction

The mechanical efficiency of smooth muscle fibres is reduced when they become overstretched. As obstruction to bladder outflow increases, a point is reached when acute urinary retention will result. Factors which may precipitate acute retention include a sudden diuresis, such as occurs after diuretic therapy (particularly loop agents) for heart failure, urinary infection, and drugs that have pharmacological effects upon the bladder, provoking retention, such as those with antimuscarinic and calcium channel blocking activity.

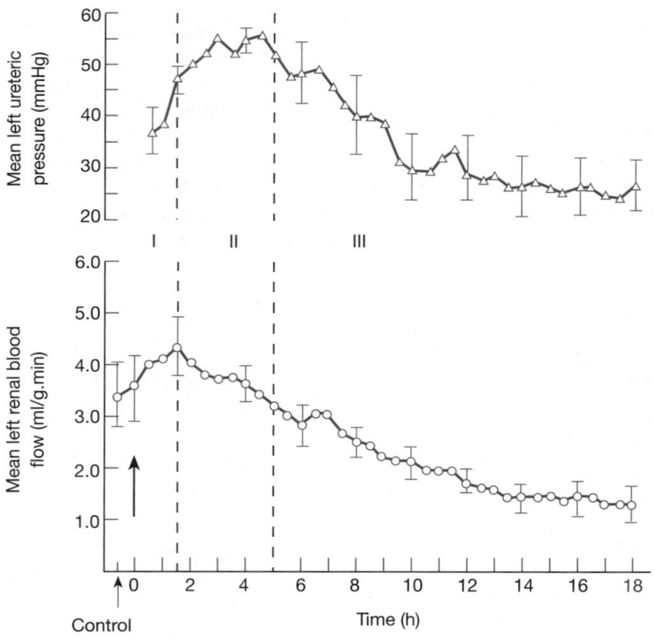

Fig. 1 The relationship between ipsilateral renal blood flow and ureteric pressure during experimental ureteric occlusion in the dog. In phase I, renal blood flow and ureteric pressure rise. In phase II, blood flow declines while ureteric pressure continues to rise. In phase III, both renal blood flow and ureteric pressure decline. The arrow indicates the time of ureteric occlusion. Mean ± standard error; $n = 5$. (Reprinted with permission from Moody *et al.* 1975.)

Chronic lower tract obstruction

In adults, chronic obstruction of the outflow from the bladder is most commonly due to benign prostatic hypertrophy. Prostatic malignancy and urethral strictures may also be responsible. In children, posterior urethral valves and urethral strictures are most often the cause. Such organic causes are easy to understand, but functional obstruction may occur at the bladder neck and at the level of the distal sphincter owing to a failure of co-ordination between bladder contraction and sphincter relaxation. The bladder wall may become increasingly compliant or non-compliant: this is of significance to the urologist, since patients with poorly compliant bladders fare much better after removal of the obstruction than those with highly compliant bladders. The highly compliant bladder tends not to be associated with upper tract dilatation, whereas the high pressure that exists within a bladder of low compliance may be transmitted to the upper tracts and may be the cause of renal impairment, which on occasion will be severe.

Histopathological changes

Acute obstruction results in increased ureteric pressure and decreased renal blood flow, and may be complicated by bacterial infection. The rise in intraluminal pressure and dilatation of the system proximal to the site of obstruction both result in compression of the renal substance. In the early phase of obstruction, the kidney becomes oedematous and haemorrhagic; tubular dilatation initially affects mainly the collecting duct and distal tubular segments; and Bowman's space may be dilated. The ducts of Bellini are first affected by dilatation of the system proximal to the site of obstruction. Subsequently, other papillary structures are affected, and ultimately compression of renal cortical tissue occurs with thinning of the renal parenchyma. Enlargement of the kidney occurs in association with dilatation of the renal pelvis.

Atrophy of the renal parenchyma with reduction in size of the kidney (obstructive atrophy) is believed to result from the effects of compression of the renal parenchyma and from prolonged renal ischaemia. Slowly progressive increasing resistance to outflow tends to result in gross dilatation of the collecting system, dilated calyces, and the renal pelvis being surrounded by only a thin rim of renal parenchyma. In acute complete obstruction dilatation tends to be less marked.

In patients with long-standing obstruction there is flattening of the renal tubular epithelium, periglomerular fibrosis, interstitial fibrosis, and mononuclear cell infiltration. These changes are thought to result in part from renal ischaemia and in part to reflect the effects of bacterial infection (Fig. 2).

Effects of obstruction upon renal function

Little detailed information is available about the effects of urinary tract obstruction on the glomerular filtration rate in humans, but it is clear that ureteric obstruction results in a marked fall in glomerular filtration rate, and that incomplete bilateral obstruction causes progressive renal failure. Glomerular filtration must continue to some extent even after development of complete acute obstruction since a nephrogram (albeit a delayed one) can be obtained after injection of intravenous contrast medium during urography.

Distal tubular function is more strikingly disturbed than proximal tubular function in chronically increased resistance to outflow, as would be expected from the histopathological findings. A characteristic feature of patients with such pathology is an impaired ability to concentrate urine. The concentration defect is resistant to administration of antidiuretic hormone and is thus an example of nephrogenic diabetes insipidus. Such patients may present with polyuria, dehydration, and hypernatraemia secondary to a reduction in free water reabsorption. Animal experiments indicate that production of cyclic AMP in response to vasopressin is reduced in chronic partial obstruction and this may, in part, explain the concentration defect. The extent to which the need to excrete an increased solute load in bilateral ureteric obstruction contributes to the concentration defect is unclear. Chronically increased bilateral resistance to outflow in humans may be associated with a salt-losing state, although the frequency with which this occurs has not been defined.

Since ureteric obstruction preferentially affects distal segments of the nephron, an acidification defect is associated with chronically increased resistance to outflow in humans. In many patients with obstructive nephropathy, urinary pH is inappropriately high for any associated degree of metabolic acidosis. This distal renal tubular acidosis is present in both unilateral and bilateral ureteric obstruction, and may be associated with hyperkalaemia.

Renal function after relief of obstruction

The relationship between duration of obstruction and recovery of function has been defined in experimental animals. In dogs subjected to unilateral ureteric ligation the ipsilateral glomerular filtration rate was 25 per cent of the ipsilateral control value and 16 per cent of that concurrently measured in the contralateral kidney when a ligature causing complete obstruction was removed after 1 week. This discrepancy resulted from a compensatory increase in function of the non-obstructed kidney during the week of complete obstruction of its partner. Improvement in the glomerular filtration rate of the previously obstructed kidney continued up to, but not beyond, 2 months after release of the obstruction, but complete recovery never occurred, maximum improvement being to only 50 per cent of the glomerular filtration rate of the non-obstructed kidney.

In humans, renal blood flow increases after relief of obstruction and the glomerular filtration rate either remains the same or increases, but no large study has been performed in which the duration of obstruction has been correlated with the degree of recovery of glomerular filtration rate. However, there is no reason to doubt that the extent of recovery depends upon whether the resistance to outflow is mild or severe, the duration of obstruction, and whether or not obstruction is complicated by bacterial infection.

After relief of prolonged bilateral obstruction or obstruction of a functionally or anatomically single kidney, there may follow a pronounced salt and water diuresis and kaliuresis, requiring appropriate oral or intravenous

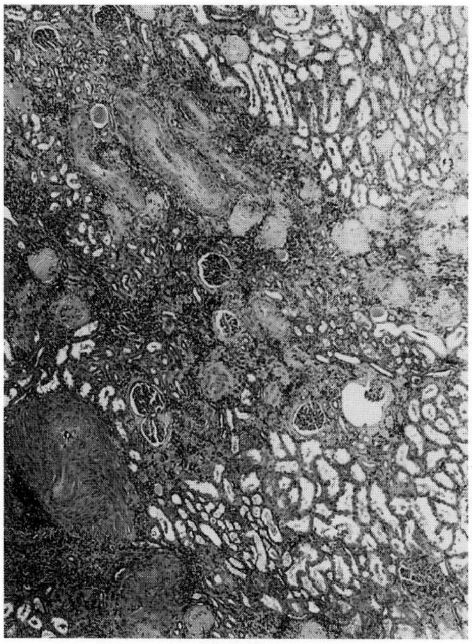

Fig. 2 Histological appearances in long-standing obstruction. Note dilated tubules, interstitial fibrosis, vessel wall thickening, and global sclerosis of some glomeruli.

replacement. This is usually attributed to damage to the renal tubules and collecting ducts induced by the resistance to outflow, resulting in failure of sodium, water, and potassium conservation. However, this cannot be the sole explanation because a salt, water, and potassium diuresis is not seen as a clinical problem in humans following relief of unilateral obstruction. The osmotic diuretic effect of uraemia, hypervolaemia owing to salt and water retention, and perhaps retention in renal failure of natriuretic factors may play a part.

Hormonal changes induced by obstruction

Erythropoietin

Levels of erythropoietin are low in humans with renal failure due to obstructive uropathy, but neither the degree of anaemia nor the degree of depression of erythropoietin concentration is known to differ from that occurring in chronic renal failure of similar severity and different aetiology.

Erythraemia is a recognized association of chronic upper urinary tract obstruction and correction after relief of obstruction has been recorded. Erythropoietin concentrations in such patients have rarely been documented.

Vitamin D metabolism

Anatomical considerations suggest that renal 1α-hydroxylase activity might be particularly severely affected in chronic obstruction, but scant data are available in respect of levels of vitamin D metabolite and vitamin D metabolism in renal failure associated with obstruction, compared with renal failure of similar degree but of different aetiologies. There is an impression that osteomalacia may be more common in patients with chronic renal failure due to obstruction, but the fact that such renal failure is very slowly progressive may account for this. Among patients about to start dialysis, radiological evidence of hyperparathyroid bone disease is most common in those whose renal failure is a consequence of obstruction, even when a correction is applied for duration of renal failure and gender.

Hypertension and the renin–angiotensin system

Hypertension is more common in patients with bilateral urinary tract obstruction than in normal individuals matched for age and sex. The prevalence of hypertension resulting from unilateral obstruction is unknown.

An increase in total exchangeable sodium has been demonstrated in chronic bilateral upper tract obstruction, and blood pressure frequently returns to normal with correction of obstruction. Patients of this sort appear to have a volume-dependent form of hypertension consequent upon salt and water retention. Concentrations of renin in renal and peripheral veins are normal.

Patients with chronic unilateral ureteric obstruction and hypertension have been described in whom renal vein renin concentrations were elevated on the side of obstruction and in whom both blood pressure and renal vein renin concentration returned to normal after the relief of obstruction, but there are no clinical features or preoperative investigations that will predict outcome.

Atrial natriuretic peptide

Release of atrial natriuretic peptide is augmented in patients with bilateral ureteric obstruction and uraemia, probably owing to salt and water overload, and this may contribute to the postobstructive diuresis and natriuresis which occurs after surgical correction of the problem.

Clinical features

Acute upper tract obstruction

Typically, this gives rise to pain in the flank that may radiate to the iliac fossa, inguinal region, testis, or labium. The pain may be dull or sharp, intermittent or persistent, though waxing and waning in intensity. A high fluid intake, alcohol, or diuretics—all measures that increase urinary volume and distend the collecting system—may provoke it, which is particularly noticeable when obstruction occurs at the pelviureteric junction. Loin tenderness may be detected and an enlarged kidney felt. Upper urinary tract infection with malaise, fever, and symptoms and signs of septicaemia may dominate the clinical picture.

Complete anuria is strongly suggestive of complete bilateral obstruction or complete obstruction of a single kidney. The differential diagnosis includes bilateral total renal cortical necrosis, acute anuric glomerulonephritis, and bilateral renal arterial occlusion. Intermittent anuria indicates the presence of intermittent complete obstruction.

Chronic upper tract obstruction

Patients may present with flank or abdominal pain, renal failure, or both, and the symptoms and signs of urinary tract infection and septicaemia may be superimposed. Rarely, presentation is with erythraemia or hypertension and their complications. Some patients are asymptomatic, obstruction being found during investigation of another condition.

Polyuria often occurs when there is chronic resistance to outflow owing to impairment of the concentrating capacity of the renal tubules. Intermittent anuria and polyuria indicate intermittent complete and partial obstruction.

Acute lower tract obstruction

Acute urinary retention is often preceded by a history of symptoms of obstruction of bladder outflow. It is typically associated with severe suprapubic pain, but this may be absent if acute retention is superimposed on chronic retention or if there is an underlying neuropathy. A potential clinical pitfall is failure to recognize that patients who have had an epidural anaesthetic may develop painless acute retention of urine. Most modalities of bladder sensation are mediated via sacral parasympathetic nerves. The pain from overdistension of the bladder is sympathetically mediated and will be abolished by a high epidural reaching to D10. Obstetricians need to be particularly alert to this problem.

Pre-existing obstruction may have provoked changes in the bladder, such as muscle wall hypertrophy, sacculation, and diverticulum formation; these in turn predispose to persistence of lower urinary tract infection once acquired and occasionally to bladder stones. Epididymo-orchitis may occur.

Chronic lower tract obstruction

Symptoms may be minimal or may be accepted by the patient as within normal limits. Hesitancy, narrowing, and diminished force of the urinary stream, terminal dribbling, and a sense of incomplete bladder emptying are typical features. If a large volume of residual urine remains in the bladder after urination, the frequent passage of small volumes of urine may be a prominent symptom even in the absence of infection. Incontinence of such small volumes of urine is termed overflow incontinence or retention with overflow.

There are no pathognomonic clinical features that differentiate high-pressure and low-pressure chronic retention. In each the bladder may be palpably distended if the volume of residual urine is sufficient. The size and consistency of the prostate is variable.

Acute complete retention of urine, usually with severe suprapubic and perineal pain, may complicate chronic retention and is commonly precipitated by lower urinary tract infection. Frequency, urgency, urge incontinence, dysuria, strangury, suprapubic pain, haematuria, and cloudy, smelly urine may be present. Asymptomatic bacteriuria is common.

Examination of the abdomen and genitalia, and rectal and vaginal examination are essential. It should be noted that the apparent size of the prostate is a poor guide to the presence of prostatic obstruction. Median lobe enlargement of a palpably normal prostate may give rise to severe obstruction, whereas an apparently grossly enlarged gland may cause little or no obstruction.

Investigation

Acute upper urinary tract obstruction

The range and specificity of imaging techniques available for the investigation of possible upper urinary tract obstruction is continually expanding. The decision as to which method of investigation to use will be influenced by local expertise and availability, but new developments seem certain to alter the optimum plan of investigation in the future. At present ultrasonography, excretion urography, and computed tomography (**CT**) scanning compete for the role of first-line investigation in this field, each having its advantages and disadvantages. Magnetic resonance urography is an alternative investigation that is currently very little used but shows considerable promise.

Ultrasonography

Ultrasonography appears to be completely safe and is relatively inexpensive. It is non-invasive, no intravenous injection, exposure to radiation, or exposure to contrast medium being involved. It has become the first-line imaging procedure in many centres, but an ultrasound report saying 'normal kidneys and urinary tract' should not be taken as meaning 'obstruction is excluded'. A relative disadvantage is its dependence on the operator: the ultrasonographer sees much more during the course of an examination than the clinician examining the few images produced. Relatively minor degrees of upper tract dilatation may be missed, indicative in some cases of clinically important obstruction. Ultrasound may visualize a few centimetres of dilated upper ureter and can show a dilated distal ureter posterior to the bladder, but it does not visualize most of the mid ureter. Calculi are easily missed: those in a dilated upper or lower ureter may be detected, but since much of the ureter is not visualized, ultrasonography cannot diagnose many ureteric calculi and hence should be accompanied by a full-length plain abdominal radiograph and, if necessary (usually owing to bowel gas overlying the renal areas), plain tomograms. Ultrasonography is less sensitive for detection of opaque renal calculi than either plain films and plain renal tomography or CT. The site and nature of obstruction often cannot be defined by ultrasonography, and upper tract dilatation on ultrasound (Fig. 3) is not synonymous with urinary tract obstruction since ultrasound cannot differentiate a baggy, low-pressure, unobstructed system from a tense, dilated, obstructed one. Ultrasound has advantages compared with intravenous urography, although not with CT, in patients with severe impairment of renal function (see below). In contrast with urography, but again not with CT, it does not exacerbate pain due to obstruction, caused in excretion urography by the diuretic effect of intravenous contrast medium employed.

Intravenous urography

Intravenous urography will usually demonstrate the site, cause, and degree of obstruction and is much less operator dependent than ultrasound since the number of images checked by the clinician is equal to the number of images reported by the radiologist. Its major disadvantage is that the technique carries a mortality owing to contrast hypersensitivity reaction of perhaps 1 in 200 000. It also involves an intravenous injection, exposure to radiation (of particular concern in pregnant women and children), worsening of pain due to the diuretic effect of contrast medium when an upper tract (or tracts) is obstructed, and the potential for contrast nephrotoxicity. Patients with impaired renal function, particularly those with diabetes and perhaps patients with myelomatosis, are at particular risk. Such risk is minimized by employment of low osmolality contrast medium and the avoidance of prior dehydration. As with ultrasound, upper tract dilatation does not necessarily indicate the existence of obstruction, but this is much less often a diagnostic problem in urography than with ultrasonography

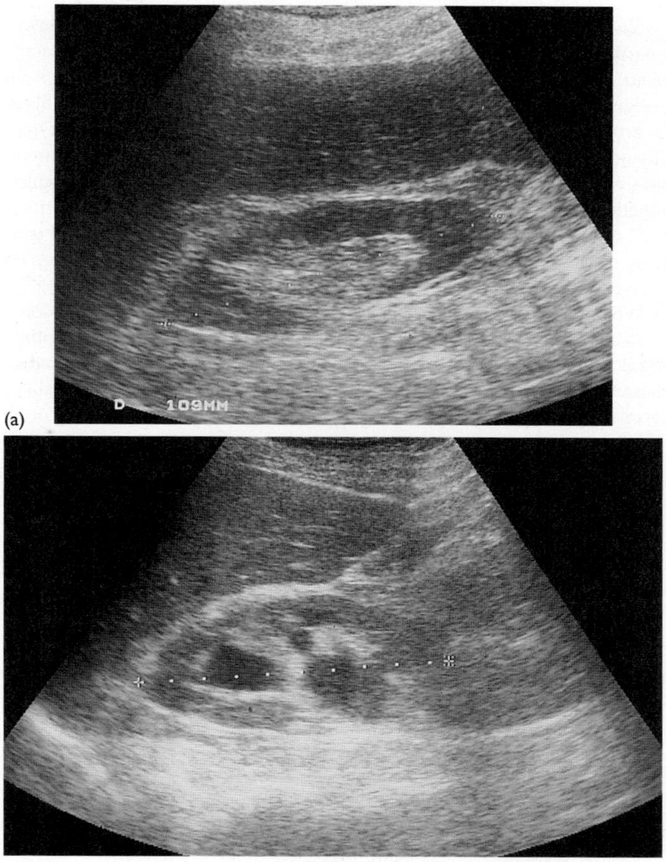

(a)

(b)

Fig. 3 Ultrasound showing (a) a normal kidney, and (b) a kidney with a dilated pelvicalyceal system in urinary obstruction.

because of the better ureteric visualization and the ability to assess drainage of the upper tracts. Ultrasonography has replaced high-dose urography as the first-line method for detecting obstruction in renal failure.

The initial sequence of radiographs must include sufficient films to identify calcifications in the urinary tract, a good combination being a full length and a coned renal area plain film. The plain films must be examined carefully for opaque calculi along the line of the ureter—calculi overlying bone are easily missed (Figs 4 (a and b)). Some obstructing calculi are very small and only faintly calcified or non-opaque. Ureteric calculi within the bony pelvis are often impossible to distinguish from calcified phleboliths on the plain film.

A large dose of contrast, preferably of low osmolality, should be given to those who may have acute obstruction to compensate for the lack of preparation of the patient and the probability of a low glomerular filtration rate. After contrast injection, the recently obstructed kidney is typically enlarged and smooth in outline. There is an immediate nephrogram, but the calyces and pelvis fill with contrast later than normal and the nephrogram becomes increasingly dense over time owing to the prolonged nephron transit time, which allows greater than normal concentration of contrast medium within the tubules (Fig. 5). In time, the site of obstruction may become obvious owing to dilatation of the system to the level of the block (Fig. 6). A full length film should be taken 20 min after contrast injection and after the patient has been asked to empty their bladder, since contrast in a full bladder may cause spurious upper tract dilatation and may obscure the lower end of the ureter and make it impossible to confirm that a ureter is dilated down to an opacity seen in the line of the ureter in the bony pelvis.

Since contrast medium enters the pelvicalyceal system and ureter slowly, opacification of the system and ureter may never be seen in severe acute obstruction. However, in most instances filling of the pelvicalyceal system and ureter to the level of obstruction can be demonstrated on delayed films. In acute ureteric obstruction the pelvicalyceal system and ureter are typically only slightly dilated. Occasionally the only abnormality may be a ureter that remains full throughout its length to the level of the vesicoureteric junction, with this finding persisting on the full length postmicturition film. Acute obstruction is also characterized by increased excretion of contrast medium by the liver, leading to opacification of the gallbladder on delayed films.

When typical obstructive changes are present, with a ureter dilated down to a calcified opacity, diagnosis is simple. If there is an obstructive nephrogram or dilatation of the pelvicalyceal system and/or ureter but no radiodense calculus is seen, diagnosis is more difficult. If the history is of pain of recent onset, the likely diagnostic possibilities are a small low-density stone not detected by urography, recent passage of an opaque stone, a uric acid stone, acute pelviureteric junction obstruction, a blood clot, or sloughed papillae. Ultrasonography can often demonstrate small low-density stones at the vesicoureteric junction not shown by urography. The presence of a uric acid stone may be suggested by a previous history of such stones, a personal or family history of gout, or clinical circumstances associated with uric acid stone formation, such as cytotoxic drug therapy or chronic small bowel disease. Urography shows uric acid stones as lucent filling defects

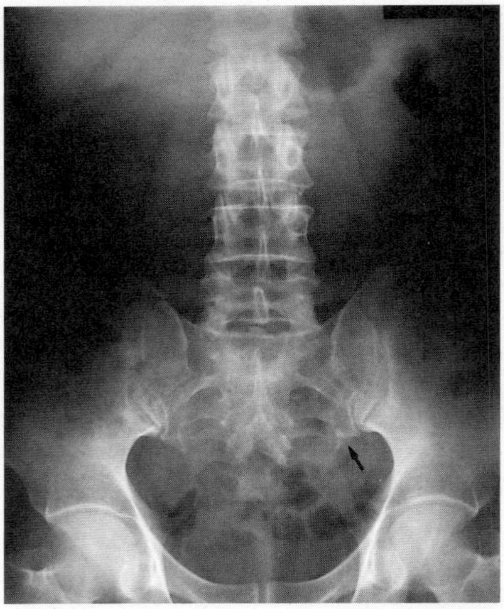

(a)

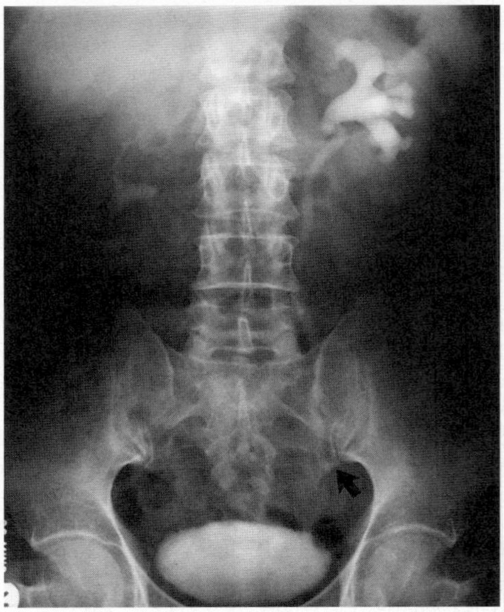

(b)

Fig. 4 (a) Plain abdominal radiograph. Opaque calculus (arrowed) medial to the left lower sacroiliac joint is easy to overlook. (b) Same patient as in (a) after contrast radiograph. Note dilatation of collecting system and ureter to the level of the calculus.

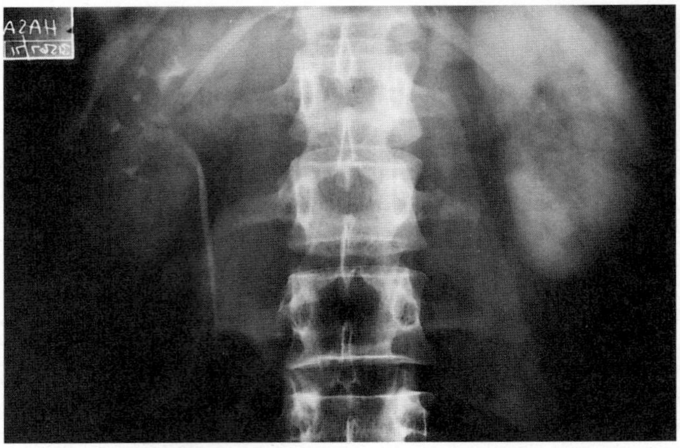

Fig. 5 Acute left ureteric obstruction. Note the increased density of the nephrogram and the absence of a pyelogram on the left side 15 min after injection of contrast.

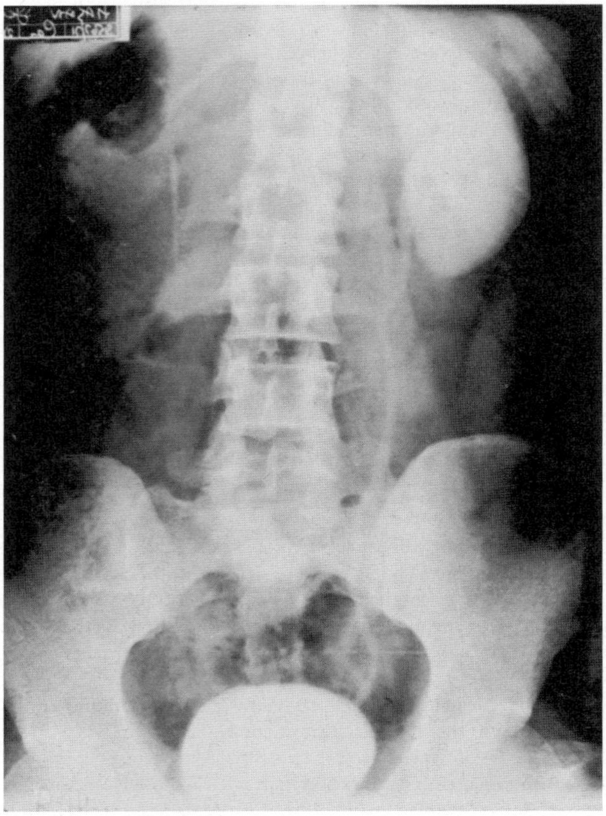

Fig. 6 Same patient as in Fig. 5. A later radiograph showing a persistent dense nephrogram on the left. The pelvicalyceal system and ureter, which have now filled, are only slightly dilated due to the fact that obstruction is of very recent onset. The obstructing calculus at the left ureteric orifice is not visible.

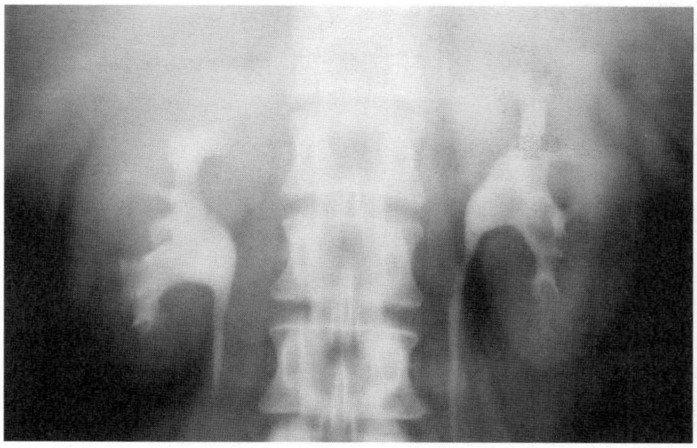

Fig. 7 Uric acid stones seen on intravenous urography as lucent filling defects in the collecting system on the left.

(Fig. 7); similar filling defects may also occur with transitional cell tumours, sloughed papillae, or blood clots. Since most ureteric stones pass spontaneously, investigation of a possible transitional cell tumour or blood clot should be delayed. If a persistent lucency is present, CT scanning may be very helpful (Fig. 8).

Acute idiopathic pelviureteric junction obstruction should be suspected if there is a large, soft tissue density inferomedial to the kidney on the plain film produced by the distended pelvis. This usually fills on delayed films of the urogram, with no filling of the ureter.

Clot colic is always associated with macroscopic haematuria. When it is suspected, the urogram should be repeated after 2 weeks, by which time the clot should have lysed and any underlying lucent filling defect can be seen. Such patients require further investigation to define the cause of bleeding.

Sloughed papillae result from papillary necrosis. Typically, abnormal calyces are seen in both kidneys, but papillary necrosis may occasionally be unilateral, usually as a result of a previous episode of infection associated with unilateral obstruction, especially in diabetics. Occasionally, calcified papillae may mimic stones (Fig. 9).

CT scanning

CT scanning carried out without the use of oral or intravenous contrast medium offers obvious safety advantages compared with intravenous urography, since no intravenous injection is required. The radiation dose is,

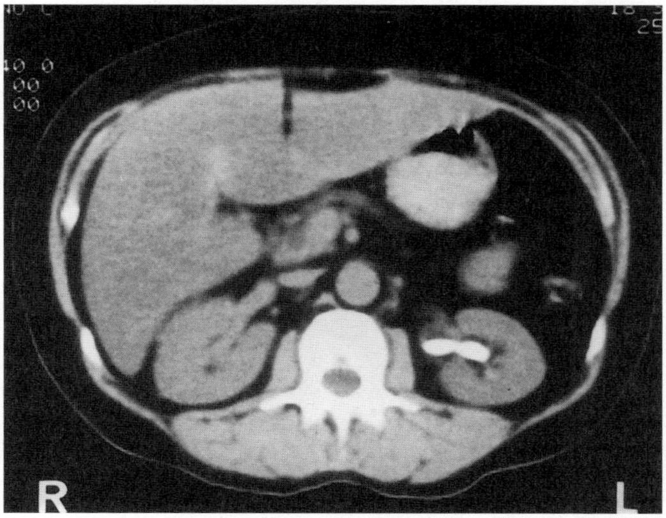

Fig. 8 Same patient as in Fig. 7. The CT scan clearly shows uric acid stones as opacities within the collecting system.

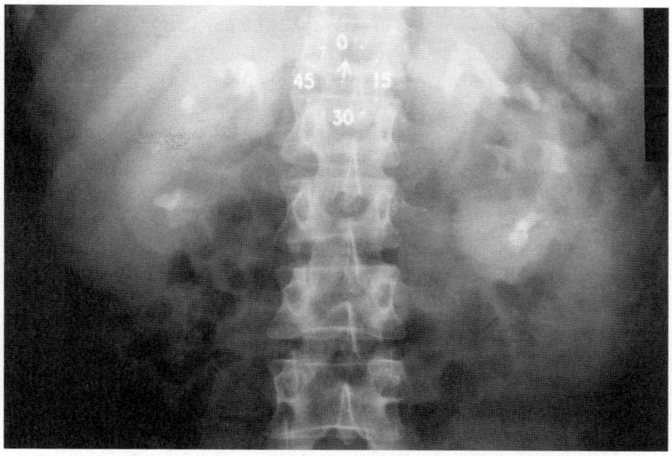

Fig. 9 Bilateral papillary necrosis with papillary calcification mimicking stones.

however, significantly higher (four to 10 times) than with urography. Unenhanced CT is well established as a second-line method for detecting pelvicalyceal and ureteric dilatation when ultrasonography is non-diagnostic in patients with suspected obstruction. CT also has an established role in demonstrating the cause of obstruction when this is not shown by ultrasonography (for example ureteric calculus, retroperitoneal mass). With the advent of helical (spiral) CT, this method is being increasingly widely used, especially in the United States, in patients with suspected ureteric colic where it has a sensitivity and specificity (in expert hands) of over 95 per cent.

A major advantage of helical CT scanning over both ultrasonography and intravenous urography is that it is capable of diagnosing non-urological conditions presenting with flank pain and not associated with urinary tract obstruction, as well as conditions causing obstruction by extrinsic compression of the ureter. These include appendix abscess, diverticular perforation, torsion of an ovarian mass, a leaking abdominal aortic aneurysm, and pancreatitis.

Other techniques

Magnetic resonance imaging

A number of magnetic resonance urography techniques are available. In suspected obstruction when irradiation and/or contrast exposure are contraindicated (for example pregnancy, contrast allergy, impaired renal function) and ultrasonography is inconclusive, heavily T_2-weighted sequences may be used to generate a magnetic resonance urogram. The dilated pelvicalyceal system and ureter show increased signal and can be delineated without using contrast medium. However, since magnetic resonance does not demonstrate calculi, it may be difficult to be sure that the obstructing lesion is a stone.

Antegrade and retrograde pyelography and ureterography

If the site of obstruction is not demonstrated by intravenous urography or other imaging techniques, antegrade or retrograde examination may be helpful. Both have the advantage that they can be initiated as a method of diagnosis and then extended to provide a therapeutic role by providing drainage.

Radionuclide imaging

There is no role for the use of radionuclides in the investigation of acute urinary tract obstruction.

Which imaging technique to use?

The time taken for each of the examinations described above is not a major consideration. With appropriate equipment, unenhanced helical CT is very quick (approximately 5 min), ultrasonography takes approximately 15 min, and standard urography 30 min. If there is an obstruction, delayed films up to 24 h after contrast injection may be necessary with urography. The cost of ultrasound is approximately half that of intravenous urography but neither is expensive by the standards of the developed world. It has been claimed that the cost of helical CT scanning is equivalent to that of urography, although the initial cost of providing the necessary equipment is high.

The plan and sequence of investigation in suspected upper tract obstruction is dictated by the mode of presentation and the presence or absence of uraemia. If there is suspected chronic urinary tract obstruction, ultrasonography is the method of choice. Uraemia, if present due to urinary tract obstruction, must indicate bilateral obstruction or obstruction of a functionally or anatomically single kidney. Renal ultrasonography (plus plain films to screen for the presence of calculi) is the investigation of first choice. The same is true if a palpably enlarged kidney or kidneys are present in the absence of pain or flank tenderness. Where signs of sepsis are present and pyonephrosis (an infected and obstructed system) is suspected, ultrasound is also the investigation of first choice. However, many patients with acute urinary tract obstruction present with pain and without uraemia or signs of sepsis. In this situation, intravenous urography (or unenhanced spiral CT, if available) remains the investigation of first choice for reasons given above. Magnetic resonance urography may be of value in the minority of patients in whom ultrasonography is inconclusive and irradiation and/or contrast exposure are contraindicated.

Chronic upper urinary tract obstruction

Obstruction must be excluded in all patients with unexplained renal failure. In patients with known renal disease, rapid deterioration in renal function unexplained by the primary renal problem also demands investigation. Relapsing urinary tract infections should also raise the possibility of an associated obstructing lesion. The diagnosis of chronic resistance to outflow should not be discounted simply because the volume of urine is normal or even increased.

The history should include questions relating to analgesic abuse (associated with papillary necrosis, transitional cell tumours, and periureteric fibrosis) and vitamin D consumption (associated with calculus formation). Ingestion of methysergide and other drugs may be associated with retroperitoneal fibrosis. A history or family history of gout, diabetes, or renal stone formation should be sought.

Ultrasonography

In suspected chronic upper tract obstruction, including the initial investigation of patients with unexplained impairment of renal function, ultrasonography is usually the imaging method of choice. Plain films should also be obtained, often with plain renal tomography to check for low-density calculi if the bowel overlies the renal area. Ultrasonography has a high sensitivity for the detection of pelvicalyceal dilatation but cannot distinguish between dilatation caused by obstruction and other types of pelvicalyceal abnormality—caused for example by a distensible system, extrarenal pelvis, vesicoureteric reflux, or dilated calyces due to reflux nephropathy (Table 1). To avoid missing the relatively minor dilatation that may occur with some causes of severe functional obstruction (for example in retroperitoneal fibrosis and tumours), all questionable pelvicalyceal visualization on ultrasonography must be evaluated further. This, together with the difficulty in differentiating dilated obstructed from dilated non-obstructed systems, leads to a significant false positive rate when ultrasonography is used to exclude obstruction. Further evaluation with intravenous urography or CT may be necessary depending on renal function. Intravenous urography is the method of choice in patients with loin pain since it best diagnoses the more common causes—calculous obstruction and idiopathic pelviureteric junction obstruction. Scintigraphy is not recommended as the first investigation in suspected obstruction but is useful in defining whether dilatation shown by other methods is obstructive (see below).

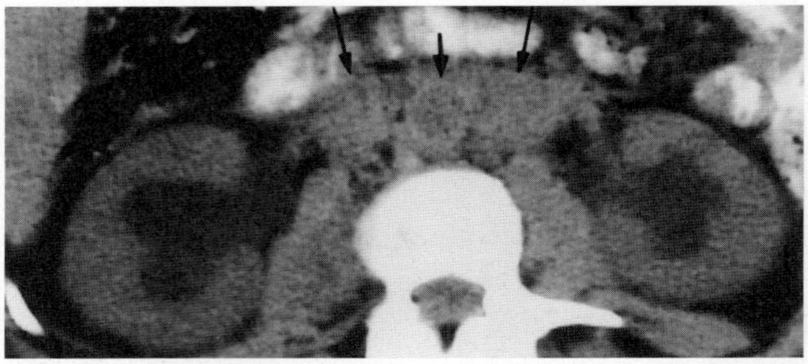

Fig. 10 CT scan in a patient with bilateral urinary tract obstruction due to prostatic cancer. Tumour tissue is clearly delineated on the scan (arrowed).

Intravenous urography and CT scanning

Intravenous urography may be helpful when ultrasonography yields equivocal results in a patient with suspected obstruction, especially when renal function is normal.

Unenhanced CT is used as a secondary method of diagnosing obstruction when the results of ultrasonography are equivocal. On CT the dilated collecting system appears as a multiloculate fluid collection with the density of water in the renal sinus. It is possible to distinguish the intrarenal collecting system from the extrarenal portion of the pelvis; this is important since obstruction can only be diagnosed on CT when there is dilatation of the intrarenal collecting system since a prominent extrarenal pelvis may be a normal variant. The whole dilated ureter is well shown on CT.

The main value of CT in the investigation of chronic upper tract obstruction is in defining the cause (Fig. 10). It is particularly helpful for diagnosing retroperitoneal masses causing obstruction, since the retroperitoneum is often obscured by the bowel at ultrasonography. CT also demonstrates calculi causing obstruction, including 'lucent' calculi such as urate stones that appear with a high density on CT.

Scintigraphy

Renal scintigraphy (also called renography) provides functional evidence of obstruction. A radioactive tracer is injected, its passage through the kidney and pelvis is recorded by serial images, and the data are computerized for further analysis (see section 20.4 for further discussion). A rise in resistance to flow in the pelvis or ureter, sufficient to result in impaired renal function, prolongs the parenchymal transit of tracer and there is usually a delay in emptying the pelvis. On whole-kidney renograms, the activity–time curve fails to fall after an initial peak, or continues to rise (Fig. 11). These activity–time curves alone do not enable a distinction to be made between obstructive nephropathy, in which parenchymal transit time is prolonged, and retention of tracer within a large, baggy, low-pressure unobstructed pelvis, where the parenchymal transit time is normal. Parenchymal transit times must therefore be measured through renographic data analysis to

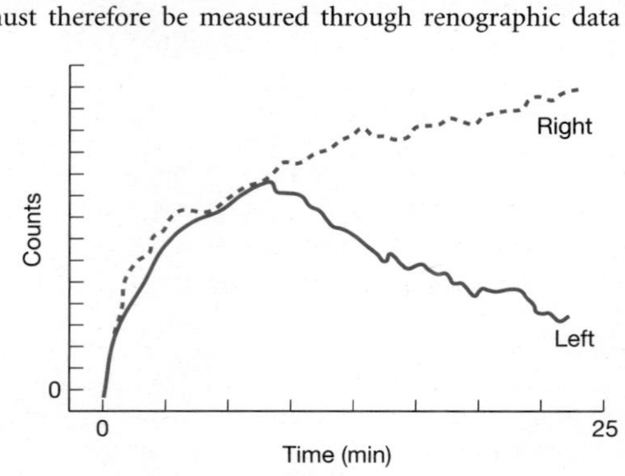

Fig. 11 Dynamic diethylene-triamine penta-aceticacid (DTPA) scintigram. Note the progressive rise of the right kidney curve to a plateau in contrast to the normal left kidney curve.

make this distinction. Whereas obstructive nephropathy is associated with prolonged transit of tracer through the renal parenchyma, a normal parenchymal transit time with delayed outflow indicates a non-obstructed dilated pelvis.When the possibility of obstruction is suspected, a dynamic renal scintigram is performed with diuresis. Frusemide (furosemide) (0.5 mg/kg, adult dose 40 mg) is given intravenously about 18 to 20 min into the study. Activity–time curves show an immediate fall in the normal kidney after the injection of frusemide (furosemide): in the presence of obstructive uropathy activity persists in the pelvis, the activity–time curve fails to fall, or falls to a lesser extent than its previous rate of increase (an 'inappropriate' response). The half-time of the descending part of the activity–time curve is prolonged, meaning that 'outflow efficiency' is impaired, which compares the amount of activity taken up by the kidney with that excreted within 30 min (the normal value is greater than 78 per cent). However, this test is not infallible: a poor response to frusemide (furosemide) may result from poor renal function or blood volume depletion rather than from obstruction and in the presence of massive pelvic or ureteric dilatation washout may not be observed on the images. Under these circumstances this part of the test is uninterpretable. However, the parenchymal transit time index will indicate whether obstructive nephropathy is or is not present.

In conclusion, radionuclide scintigraphy methods are of particular value in differentiating obstructive nephropathy from a baggy, dilated, but unobstructed system and in defining the contribution of each kidney to overall uptake function. A decision as to whether conservative surgery or nephrectomy should be carried out in unilateral obstruction may be much facilitated by the latter assessment.

Antegrade pyelography and ureterography

Percutaneous introduction of contrast medium directly into the renal pelvis or a calyx via a needle, with subsequent radiographic examination of the pelvicalyceal system and ureter (antegrade pyelography and ureterography) is used increasingly to define the site and cause of chronic upper tract obstruction. Diagnostic antegrade examination can be combined with therapeutic drainage of an obstructed system.

Retrograde ureterography

Cystoscopy and catheterization of one or both of the ureters from below, followed by retrograde injection of contrast medium (retrograde ureterography), is indicated if antegrade examination cannot be carried out, or if there is a prospect of dealing with ureteric obstruction from below at the time of retrograde examination. The technique carries the risks of introducing infection into an obstructed urinary tract and of septicaemia, and should be performed only when absolutely necessary. In obstruction due to neuromuscular dysfunction at the pelviureteric junction and in retroperitoneal fibrosis, the collecting system may fill normally from below.

Pressure flow studies

This investigation provides a quantitative assessment of the effect of obstruction on the outflow tract. The technique involves the insertion of a needle transparenchymally into the upper collecting system. Local anaesthetic is sufficient in adults, but general anaesthesia is required in children. The bladder is catheterized and the intravesical pressure measured. The pressure differential between the kidney and the bladder is monitored while the collecting system is perfused with dilute contrast at a rate of 10 ml/min. Perfusion must be maintained for long enough to ensure that the upper urinary tract is filled.

Normal systems can accommodate a flow rate of 10 ml/min without a pressure differential of more than 15 cm of water. If an obstruction is present, there will be a pressure differential of more than 22 cm of water. An equivocal range exists when the differential pressure is between 15 and 22 cm of water, but such a result occurs in only a small proportion of patients.

This diagnostic technique is relatively simple and can readily be extended into a therapeutic one by leaving a catheter *in situ*, to provide drainage of an obstructed system. The disadvantages are that it is an invasive test with a risk (albeit small) of provoking haemorrhage or infection, that the technique investigates the collecting system and gives no information on parenchymal function, and that it is not readily repeatable. Leakage around the needle can invalidate the pressure measurements.

With the advent of more sophisticated renography, pressure flow studies are rarely performed, but they still have a place in the investigation of obstruction in patients with very poor renal function, in whom radioisotope techniques are less reliable, in equivocal obstruction, particularly at the pelviureteric junction, and intraoperatively in patients with retroperitoneal fibrosis undergoing ureterolysis.

Difficult clinical situations

Significant incomplete chronic upper urinary tract obstruction

It may be very difficult to tell whether a given degree of resistance to outflow or intermittent obstruction is impairing, or potentially impairing, renal function or causing symptoms. Symptoms may be present in the absence of deleterious effects upon renal function and the converse may also be true. Different methods of diagnosing obstruction define subtly different pathological features of the condition and a valid correlation between the results of different investigations cannot invariably be made. Incomplete obstruction is clinically important if it causes deterioration in kidney function that can be halted or corrected by intervention, or symptoms that are improved thereby. In patients with one kidney, or in those with bilateral partial obstruction, a decline in serial measurements of glomerular filtration rate attributable to obstruction may define the situation. There may be a similar change in uptake of radionuclides in unilateral obstruction. Other proposed methods of detecting significant incomplete obstruction are given in Table 3. Strict validation of these methods would require them to be carried out in patients with supposed obstruction who would then be allocated randomly to intervention or no intervention. Deterioration in function predicted by each of the methods by comparison with matched controls would provide validation. This study is never likely to be done.

Differential diagnosis of non-obstructive dilatation of the collecting system

A number of non-obstructive conditions may cause dilatation of the collecting system (Table 1).

Extrarenal pelves may mimic pelviureteric junctional obstruction. If intravenous frusemide (furosemide) is administered after the 20-min full length contrast radiograph in this condition, contrast medium will have washed out of the affected side on a full length film 15 min later. In the presence of obstruction of the pelviureteric junction the contrast is retained and the pelvicalyceal system increases in size.

Megacalyces are readily identified on urography. The renal cortex is normal and the calyceal infundibula, pelvis, and ureter are normal with no evidence of obstruction.

Vesicoureteric reflux may be associated with dilatation of the ureters and in severe cases dilatation of the pelvicalyceal system too. The presence of reflux on urography is suggested by the degree of dilatation varying at different times during the examination, by dilatation which is greatest from

Table 3 Detection of significant incomplete obstruction

Introduction of a needle into the renal pelvis with direct measurement of the pressure developing after infusion of fluid at a known flow rate (antegrade pressure flow measurement)
Urographic observation of the degree of distension of the renal pelvis induced by intravenous frusemide (furosemide) (frusemide urography)
Observation of the effect of intravenous frusemide (furosemide) upon the isotope renogram (frusemide renography)
Comparison of activity–time curves after injection of $^{99}Tc^{m}$ DTPA in whole kidney versus renal pelvis (retention function analysis)
Measurement of the nephron transit time of a non-reabsorbable tracer (outflow obstruction may increase the transit time)

the vesicoureteric junction upwards, and by a postmicturition film which shows a large volume of residual urine in the bladder composed of urine that has refluxed into the ureters during voiding and drained back thereafter.

A decision as to whether or not significant obstruction is present at the pelviureteric junction and whether operation is indicated may be facilitated by frusemide (furosemide) urography (Fig. 12) or frusemide (furosemide) scintigraphy. In some patients the urographic findings are unremarkable during asymptomatic periods, while emergency intravenous urography during an episode of pain may define the condition.

In women who have been pregnant, particularly those who have suffered pregnancy bacteriuria, one or both upper ureters (more often the right) may be dilated to the pelvic brim, but the system is seen to empty on a full length postmicturition film and there is no dilatation of the pelvis and calyces (see Chapter 13.5 for further discussion).

Acute lower urinary tract obstruction

Most patients presenting with acute urinary retention require no investigation before treatment. Suprapubic pain coexisting with a bladder that is palpably or percussibly distended above the level of the symphysis pubis is sufficient evidence for immediate catheterization.

If there is doubt about the diagnosis, an ultrasound examination will confirm or refute the presence of a distended bladder. Transrectal ultrasound of the prostrate can demonstrate both the size of the gland and, to some extent, the benign or malignant nature of any enlargement. Such an investigation is not indicated in the acute situation but is of potential benefit after the relief of obstruction.

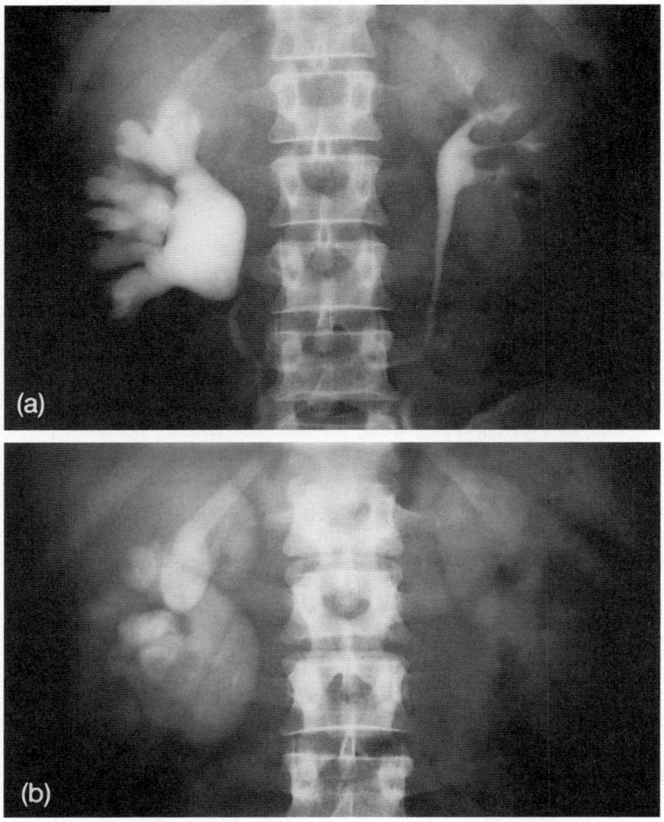

Fig. 12 (a) Right-sided pelviureteric obstruction. (b) Same urogram as in (a) 15 min after intravenous injection of frusemide (furosemide). Note the increase in size of the pelvicalyceal system, indicating significant pelviureteric junction obstruction.

An ascending urethrogram may be indicated if an attempt at urethral catheterization proves unsuccessful. This is done as an elective procedure after bladder drainage has been achieved by suprapubic catheterization.

Chronic lower urinary tract obstruction

In one series of patients presenting with acute retention of urine, approximately half had bladders of low compliance and half of high compliance. Investigation is aimed at demonstrating associated pathology such as urinary tract infection, upper tract dilatation, stones, and renal impairment, and also at defining the severity of obstruction of bladder outflow.

Urine culture is essential. In most centres, ultrasonography of the upper and lower urinary tract, together with a plain abdominal radiograph and measurement of urinary flow rate have replaced the intravenous urogram. Full urodynamic investigations, with combined videopressure cystourethrography may be necessary. Serum biochemistry and routine haematology are also required, as is measurement of the level of prostatic-specific antigen in men.

Management

Acute upper tract obstruction

Stones

Most patients presenting with renal and ureteric colic will have a stone in the lower third of the ureter, often in that portion of the ureter lying within the bladder wall. Such patients can be managed conservatively, since the stone has already passed through two areas of relative ureteric narrowing—the pelviureteric junction and the site at which the ureter crosses the bifurcation of the common iliac artery. A conservative policy is likely to prove successful if the stone is 5 mm or less in its maximum diameter. It is unusual for acute episodes of colic to persist for more than 72 h.

Patients with ureteric colic are usually admitted to hospital, although this is unnecessary in many cases since the only medical requirement is the provision of regular analgesia, which can be given parenterally, orally, or rectally. There is a time-honoured recommendation that patients with colic should be encouraged to maintain a very high fluid intake to induce a diuresis. An antimuscarinic drug such as propantheline is also often prescribed. There is no reason to think that these measures are of benefit, and they may even be harmful since both encourage ureteric dilatation and would be expected to reduce forward peristalsis of the ureter, which is the very effect needed to encourage spontaneous passage of the stone. A diuresis will also tend to increase intratubular pressure and may increase the risk of forniceal rupture. It might be argued that forniceal rupture may, by decompressing the system, encourage the return of peristalsis but few would regard this as an appropriate approach to management.

Although it has long been argued that morphine should be avoided as an analgesic as it may provoke prolonged ureteric constriction, there is no evidence that therapeutic doses of morphine have this adverse effect. Pethidine may provoke nausea and vomiting, particularly when administered parenterally, but since nausea and vomiting frequently accompany colic it is difficult to disentangle the effects of such treatment from the effects of colic alone. Very satisfactory pain relief can often be obtained using non-steroidal anti-inflammatory agents administered orally or rectally.

With the advent of new, less invasive methods of surgical management of ureteric stones, there is a temptation to intervene earlier. Stones in the intramural ureter can be treated readily with most lithotripters, whether imaging is by ultrasound or radiology. Since most stones at that site will pass spontaneously, the extent to which lithotripsy will hasten the process is difficult to establish. Lithotripsy may be worthwhile for stones in the upper third of the ureter since, by disintegrating the stone into small fragments, spontaneous passage will be encouraged. However, the availability of lithotripsy for patients with acute colic varies very markedly between countries and the precise role and benefits of the technique have yet to be established.

Endoscopic manoeuvres, which are usually performed under general anaesthesia, are reserved for those patients with persistent colic.

Drainage of an obstructed system

If there is clinical evidence of infection above an obstruction, drainage must be established as a matter of urgency. The diagnosis is a clinical one, made on the basis that the patient is pyrexial, often with a very high fever and rigors, and the degree of loin tenderness is greater than when obstruction is not associated with infection. Examination of bladder urine may be unhelpful since ureteric obstruction may prevent red and white blood cells and organisms from reaching the lower urinary tract. Leucocytosis may be present but this is not invariably the case, especially in the elderly.

The choice between antegrade and retrograde intervention will depend on the facilities and expertise available. In most specialist centres there is a clear preference for the percutaneous insertion of an antegrade needle to provide a nephrostomy under local anaesthesia. In a dilated high-pressure system the procedure is usually easy, and such a system may be used to provide drainage for weeks or even months if necessary. If excretion of intravenous contrast has outlined renal anatomy, renal puncture may be guided radiographically; if not, the initial puncture may be better directed under ultrasound control using a fine needle. The collecting system is then outlined with contrast and an accurate transparenchymal calyceal puncture can be placed, usually through a lower calyx. By contrast, a retrograde ureteric catheter can be relied on to provide drainage for only for a matter of days at best. Occasionally a retrograde catheter cannot be passed beyond the obstruction and the diagnostic role of retrograde ureterography cannot then be extended to a therapeutic one.

Other causes of acute obstruction

Aside from urinary stone, the two other most common causes of acute obstruction are sloughed papillae and blood clots. The principles of management vary little from those already outlined for ureteric stones, but greater attention must be paid in the acute phase to the underlying cause. In the patient with papillary necrosis, infection is a more common accompaniment of obstruction, and intervention, usually with a percutaneous needle nephrostomy, is required more often. When colic results from a blood clot, treatment of the underlying cause may be necessary at an early stage. Renal parenchymal tumours and transitional cell tumours of the collecting system may both cause persistent bleeding and colic, and ablative open surgery is usually required. More difficulty is encountered when bleeding occurs from a non-malignant cause. An arteriovenous fistula, whether spontaneous or traumatic, may be embolized with every prospect of success. The most difficult case of recurrent bleeding to manage is that associated with papillary necrosis in sickle cell trait or disease. Antifibrinolytic agents may be of value, but administration of such treatment during active bleeding may produce hard, rubbery clots that fill the collecting system and require surgical removal.

Chronic upper tract obstruction

The aim of management is to relieve symptoms, improve or conserve renal function, and avoid complications such as septicaemia. Important surgical advances in the past decade include the increasing use of ureteric stents to provide short-term, or even long-term, relief of obstruction. Recently a means of avoiding problems associated with endoluminal stenting has been described, in which a stent is used to drain urine from the renal pelvis through a subcutaneous tube directly into the bladder, bypassing the ureter.

Obstruction is the most readily reversible cause of chronic renal failure. Acute obstruction caused by ureteric stones commonly resolves spontaneously; but the longer a stone remains in the same position within the ureter the less likely it is that a conservative policy will be successful.

Probably the second most common cause of chronic obstruction in adults is obstruction of the pelviureteric junction. The Anderson–Hynes pyeloplasty gives very satisfactory results and provides the gold standard against which other open and endoscopic techniques (such as endopyelotomy) must be assessed.

Idiopathic obstruction at the pelviureteric junction may present in childhood, when obstructed megaureter and ureteric obstruction secondary to a ureterocele are also more common. Since all three congenital anomalies cause pelvicalyceal dilatation, it is becoming increasingly common for obstruction to be diagnosed *in utero*. Treatment of the obstruction *in utero* by the insertion of a nephrostomy tube has been reported: it is too early to know whether such early intervention will prove to have long-term benefits, but at the moment it seems, on balance, best to wait until immediately after delivery to investigate and relieve the problem.

Ureteric obstruction can occur in a transplanted kidney, most commonly at the site of the ureteroneocystostomy, but sometimes more proximally in the ureter. Vesicoureteric stenosis is caused by ischaemia of the ureter, but it is never possible to define whether this ischaemia is associated with rejection or is a result of poor vascularization following donor dephrectomy. More proximal ureteric obstruction may be due to mechanical kinking of the ureter or, occasionally, to extrinsic compression by a lymphocele. Irrespective of the site and cause of the obstruction, the diagnosis presents special problems. The possibility of obstruction is raised either because of deteriorating renal function or because ultrasound during routine follow-up demonstrates increasing dilataton of the collecting system. The differential diagnosis includes rejection, cyclosporin nephrotoxicity, and arterial insufficiency. An obstruction may be demonstrated by intravenous urography and/or antegrade pyelography. Retrograde studies are usually difficult and not infrequently impossible, and since, in the case of stenosis at a ureteroneocystostomy, they involve passing a catheter across the segment of ureter under suspicion, the investigation is only indicated if intravenous urography and antegrade pyelography prove unsatisfactory.

Minimally invasive stone surgery

The past decade has seen a revolution in the management of urinary tract stones, due to the adoption of minimally invasive techniques including percutaneous surgery and extracorporeal shock wave lithotripsy. Open operation for renal stones can now be avoided in many cases by creating a nephrostomy track to the calculus, dilating the track, and then either removing the calculus endoscopically via the track or causing it to disintegrate by direct application of an ultrasound probe. It is possible to extract ureteric stones endoscopically with the assistance of a ureteroscope, and bladder calculi may be disintegrated by the endoscopic application of electrohydraulically produced shock waves.

Externally delivered shock waves can be used to shatter calculi into many fragments which are then passed spontaneously, hence extracorporeal shock wave lithotripsy offers a solution to the problem of the presence of a calculus or calculi within the kidney without the need for a surgical operation. This carries the promise of a reduction in morbidity and perhaps mortality, a much shorter hospital stay for the patient, a more rapid return to work, and may also be suitable for those who are unfit for conventional surgery. The technique is unsuitable for hard uric acid and cystine stones, for very large stones (which must be debulked percutaneously before lithotripsy), and for some ureteric stones (although a proportion of these can be manoeuvred into the upper collecting system endoscopically and then dealt with by this method). Other disadvantages include the high capital cost of the necessary equipment and the need for further intervention in 10 to 15 per cent of patients in whom stone fragments do not pass. Such fragments can, in general, be removed endoscopically. Despite these difficulties, non-operative dissolution of calculi is being increasingly used. The recurrence rate of stones in the long term seems to be no higher than after open surgery and to date no unforeseen long-term complications have emerged.

Large staghorn calculi are still usually removed by a cutting procedure. Surface cooling of the kidney at the time of operation allows time for more complete clearance of stones with the renal artery clamped, and protects against the development of ischaemic damage to the kidney.

For details of other aspects of diagnosis and management of urinary stones see Chapter 20.13.

Other causes of urinary obstruction

Pelviureteric junction obstruction

This often appears to result from a functional disturbance in peristalsis of the collecting system in the absence of mechanical obstruction. A percutaneous procedure for managing pelviureteric junction obstruction was first described in 1983 (endopyelotomy): this involves a full thickness incision through the stenosed region with a stent left *in situ*; healing occurs by re-epithelialization from either side of the incision and very little new scar tissue is formed. There is no consensus on the indications: patients with secondary pelviureteric junction stenosis in association with stones, infection, or previous surgery tend to be offered the percutaneous operation, whereas those with primary idiopathic obstruction are usually treated by open pyeloplasty.

Malignant obstruction

A wide variety of tumours may cause ureteric obstruction, either by local spread (cervix, prostate, bladder), or secondary to para-aortic nodal enlargement (lymphoma, testicular tumours). The diagnosis rests upon the same investigations as for any other cause of chronic obstruction, but the treatment will vary widely, depending on the cause. An aggressive or radical approach is almost always indicated in a patient who has received no previous treatment for the underlying malignancy. Unilateral or bilateral ureteric stenting or percutaneous nephrostomies may be necessary to cover the period of time during which chemotherapy or radiotherapy is given with the expectation of controlling the tumour. More difficulty arises when ureteric obstruction is due to recurrent tumour, when the potential benefits of chemotherapy and radiotherapy are significantly less and patients may be facing debilitating treatment for an advancing malignant disease, the prognosis of which is poor. To be confined by nephrostomy drainage for what is left of life significantly diminishes its quality, but may be right in certain circumstances. A percutaneously placed pigtail nephrostomy, which can be inserted under local anaesthetic, has a tendency to fall out or to be pulled out. Open surgery can be avoided by the use of a ring nephrostomy inserted percutaneously under general anaesthesia: this provides secure long-term drainage, for years if necessary.

Obstruction in patients with urinary diversion

There are many reasons for diverting the urine into an isolated loop of ileum or colon. One of the recognized complications is stenosis at the site of anastomosis between the bowel and ureter(s).

The thin muscle wall of the ileum means that it is not possible to fashion an antireflux anastomosis between the bowel and the ureter when diverting the urine into an ileal conduit, hence a loopogram (a radiograph carried out after injection of contrast into an ideal loop) will normally show bilateral ureteric reflux, and the absence of such reflux is strong evidence of a stenosis at the ureteroileal junction.

The operation of ureterosigmoidostomy, in which the ureters are anastomosed to sigmoid colon, has fallen into disfavour owing to the associated complications of infection, metabolic acidosis (caused by reabsorption of hydrogen ions from the gut), and osteomalacia.

Idiopathic retroperitoneal fibrosis (peri-aortitis)

In this condition the ureters become embedded in dense fibrous tissue, with resultant unilateral or bilateral obstruction, usually at the junction between the middle and lower thirds of the ureter. The condition is progressive: initially, the fibrous tissue is fairly cellular, later becoming relatively acellular. The mechanism by which obstruction occurs is unclear, not least because of the frequent observation that contrast medium injected into the lower ureter may pass freely up to the pelvicalyceal system despite the presence of clinical, radiological and isotopic evidence of functional urinary tract obstruction.

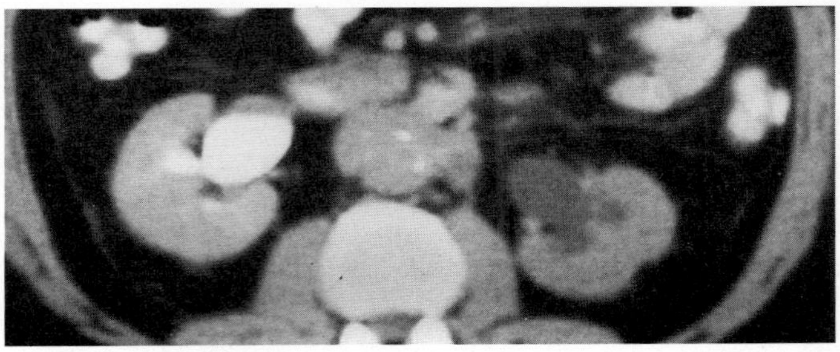

Fig. 13 A CT scan of idiopathic retroperitoneal fibrosis (peri-aortitis) causing urinary tract obstruction. Note the aortic calcification and peri-aortic nature of the mass.

Pathogenesis

'Retroperitoneal fibrosis' is an unfortunate term, since there are many causes of fibrosis in the retroperitoneal area, for example malignant disease of the breast, colon, or prostate, and because it is anatomically misleading and says nothing about pathogenesis.

The location, long known to surgeons and pathologists, and further emphasized by the advent of CT scanning (Fig. 13), is around the aorta, hence the term peri-aortitis is preferable to retroperitoneal fibrosis. The histological appearances are of aortic atheroma, medial thinning, splits in the media, and an increase in the adventitia, which contains an inflammatory infiltrate. These findings are present to some extent in the aortas of some patients with advanced atherosclerosis who have not suffered a clinical illness and may reasonably be classified as having 'subclinical peri-aortitis'. The fibrous tissue itself contains macrophages and plasma cells but not polymorphs, and it now seems likely that this is due to an autoimmune response to leakage of material derived from atheromatous plaques in the diseased aorta.

The substance ceroid, an insoluble polymer of oxidized lipid and lipoprotein, which can be synthesized artificially by oxidizing low-density lipoprotein, may be involved in generating the fibrotic reaction. It is found in atheromatous plaques and is identified by staining with oil red O. Examination of sections of aorta containing such plaques incubated with mouse monoclonal antibody to human IgG localizes the antibody to the region of the plaque where ceroid has been identified by oil red O staining. Identical findings are obtained on incubation with polyclonal rabbit antihuman IgG. Moreover, IgG and some IgM, but not IgA or IgE, can be identified in plasma cells in the fibrotic tissue where there are splits in the adjacent media. Circulating antibodies to oxidized low-density lipoprotein and to ceroid extracted from human atheroma are detected in patients with peri-aortitis in much higher concentrations than in normal individuals and in those with ischaemic heart disease. Stored sera obtained from individuals subsequently shown at autopsy to have had subclinical peri-aortitis also show significantly increased antibody titres compared with controls. It thus seems likely that chronic peri-aortitis has an autoimmune aetiology in which the allergen is a component of ceroid, probably oxidized low-density lipoprotein, produced in human atheroma, and that a specific immune response involves T cells and plasma cells, which secrete IgG. Oxidized low-density lipoprotein is known to be highly immunogenic.

This concept clarifies some issues that were previously difficult to explain. For example, the definite, although uncommon, association between mediastinal fibrosis and idiopathic retroperitoneal fibrosis has always been difficult to understand. If one regards at least some cases of mediastinal fibrosis (see below) as a peri-aortitis, occurring in this instance around the thoracic aorta, the association becomes comprehensible. Surgeons operating on aortic aneurysms quite often see fibrosis around the aneurysm. Sometimes the surgeon encounters technical difficulties in adhesions between the aorta and duodenum, and a dense, fibrotic, chronic inflammatory infiltrate is present around the aorta: the term 'inflammatory aneurysm' is used to describe this condition. The unifying hypothesis of an autoimmune peri-aortitis accounts for this finding. Certainly so-called idiopathic retroperitoneal fibrosis, idiopathic mediastinal fibrosis, perianeurysmal fibrosis, and inflammatory aneurysm have much in common. The hypothesis also accounts for the well-known association between aortic disease, including aneurysm and aortic wall calcification, and retroperitoneal fibrosis. Finally, it may be no coincidence that carcinoid tumours and drugs such as methysergide and ergot derivatives which are sometimes responsible for the condition all have well described effects on the vasculature.

Clinical features

The condition is three times as common in men as in women. Patients' ages range from the third to the ninth decade, but peak incidence occurs in the sixth and seventh decades; in one series of 60 patients the mean age of the group was 56 years. The early clinical manifestations are not distinctive. Most commonly there is pain in a girdle-like distribution from the low back to the lower abdomen, occasionally spreading to the buttocks or thighs. Examination is usually unremarkable apart from hypertension, which is found in over 50 per cent of patients. Oedema of the legs, a palpable kidney, or hydrocele is found in fewer than 10 per cent of patients. There is usually a normochromic, normocytic anaemia and a raised erythrocyte sedimentation rate and plasma C-reactive protein, but a significant minority are normal in one or both of these respects. Proteinuria is uncommon and significant bacteriuria rare.

Diagnosis

Peri-aortic fibrosis is clearly more common than hitherto appreciated, particularly if one takes subclinical forms of the condition into account. Diagnostic delay is the rule: in one series 6 to 12 months, or even longer, elapsed from the onset of symptoms to diagnosis. Perhaps for this reason, bilateral rather than unilateral upper tract obstruction was present in the majority of patients.

When taking the history, enquiry should be made regarding consumption of relevant drugs, including methysergide, β-blockers, methyldopa, and bromocriptine, another ergot-like drug.

Ultrasonography, radionuclide methods, and the intravenous urogram will reveal findings typical of urinary tract obstruction, and the last technique may show medial deviation of the ureters, although this may also be present in normal subjects and is an unreliable guide to diagnosis. CT scanning will show the peri-aortic mass (Fig. 13). The differential diagnosis includes lymphoma (in which case splenomegaly and lymphadenopathy may be seen on CT scanning) and various forms of cancer, including particularly those of the bladder, bowel, and cervix.

A histological diagnosis should be obtained if at all possible, and laparotomy is required in order to obtain a sufficiently large sample to exclude lymphoma and cancer with certainty. Conversely, a CT-guided needle biopsy may be sufficient to make a definitive diagnosis of malignancy.

Management

Management of the idiopathic and probably autoimmune syndrome is empirical and controversial since controlled trials of treatment are lacking. Corticosteroid therapy, with or without temporary relief of obstruction by insertion of ureteric stents, ureterolysis alone, and ureterolysis followed by steroid therapy to shrink the peri-aortic mass and maintain remission are all employed. Corticosteroid therapy alone may correct obstruction, but is not invariably effective. Ureterolysis alone may also correct obstruction in the long term but is sometimes associated with recurrence or the development of a further obstruction in a previously unaffected kidney. Surgical relief of obstruction by ureterolysis followed by corticosteroid therapy (initial dose of prednisolone 20 mg daily, begun when sutures are removed) has proved to be a reliable and successful strategy. Corticosteroid dosage is reduced progressively thereafter according to clinical response. When bilateral obstruction is present, bilateral ureterolysis followed by steroid therapy is preferable to unilateral ureterolysis with reliance upon corticosteroid therapy to free the contralateral side, since this is sometimes unsuccessful. Ureterolysis of kidneys shown to be non-functioning on high-dose excretion urography or by appropriate radionuclide techniques is usually unsuccessful in restoring useful renal function. A reasonable policy for management would seem to be to perform unilateral or bilateral ureterolysis, as appropriate, followed by corticosteroid therapy in patients fit for operation and able to take steroids safely. Surgery alone should be employed in those with a particular contraindication to corticosteroid treatment, such as the presence of a peptic ulcer or severe osteoporosis. Steroid therapy alone (methylprednisolone 500 mg intravenously daily for 3 days, followed by prednisolone 20 mg daily), with or without insertion of ureteric stents, should be reserved for patients unfit for ureterolysis. A dramatic response to parenteral steroid treatment sometimes occurs, a marked diuresis being seen within 24 h of commencing treatment.

In the United Kingdom in recent years there has been an increasing tendency to avoid operation, even in patients fit for ureterolysis, whether unilateral or bilateral. Reliance is placed upon the insertion of a ureteric stent or stents plus corticosteroid therapy. This approach has the advantage of avoiding operative mortality and morbidity, of providing a rapid solution to the problem of urinary tract obstruction, and a much reduced hospital stay. Disadvantages include difficulties in stent insertion, incomplete relief of obstruction by stents, the need for periodic (say 6-monthly) change of stents if steroid therapy is unsuccessful, and the potential for urinary tract sepsis in the presence of a stent, which is a foreign body. To these must be added, in 'real life' clinical practice, the potential for patients to be lost to follow-up and the presence of a stent to be forgotten. No completely reliable method has ever been devised to render this last occurrence impossible. By contrast, when the ureter or ureters are displaced surgically, well away from the periaortic mass, the patient and the patient's urinary tract are secure, and a further advantage of open surgery is the potential it offers to obtain adequate tissue to permit a firm histological diagnosis to be made. Patients judged fit for operation should in general undergo ureterolysis unless or until prospective controlled trials are published showing equivalent or better results from alternative approaches.

Peri-aortitis in the absence of ureteric obstruction

The use of CT scanning in the investigation of abdominal pain has revealed an increasing number of patients to have peri-aortitis before the onset of urinary tract obstruction. Management of these cases is controversial. The development of bilateral ureteric obstruction with severe uraemia within 3 months of diagnosis (at which time renal function was normal and the ureters unobstructed) has occurred in at least one patient. Until more is known of the natural history of the disease in such patients, it would seem prudent to obtain a histological diagnosis at open operation and to consider corticosteroid therapy to shrink the mass. Whether an attempt to reduce the risk of ureteric obstruction by insertion of stents or displacement of the ureters from the mass at the time of the operation should be carried out is not known.

Prognosis

The older and the more uraemic the patient at the time of presentation, the worse is the prognosis. Nevertheless, if treated appropriately, most patients do well.

Follow-up

In some patients long-term remission is achieved by surgery alone. In those receiving maintenance prednisolone, the dose can be reduced progressively, and in some patients long-term remission occurs after complete withdrawal of corticosteroid therapy. In one series of 60 patients, 10 relapsed more than 5 years after the time of diagnosis when steroid therapy had been stopped, in that their erythrocyte sedimentation rates rose to an abnormal level, and obstruction and diminished renal function redeveloped. Five patients relapsed as late as 10 years after the onset of the disease. Lifelong follow-up is therefore mandatory, but the best way to monitor such patients is not certain. Clinical assessment, serial measurement of erythrocyte sedimentation rate and C-reactive protein, and assessment of renal function, together with imaging to detect redevelopment of obstruction, is appropriate. Reduction in size of the peri-aortic mass can be detected on serial CT scanning, but residual peri-aortic tissue is seen frequently, even after steroid therapy, and the usefulness of CT in monitoring disease activity is limited.

Associated fibrotic conditions

Mediastinal fibrosis

The pathological process described in connection with retroperitoneal fibrosis can also develop in the upper mediastinum where it tends to be located around the bronchi, the cardiac atria, the pulmonary arteries and veins, the superior vena cava, and the azygos vein; rarely, it also envelops the oesophagus. Symptoms vary according to the structures principally affected. There may be cardiopulmonary manifestations because of scar tissue about the atria, pulmonary vessels, or bronchi, and dysphagia can result from oesophageal constriction. One of the commonest clinical manifestations results from obstruction of the superior vena cava, with distension of veins in the neck and upper extremities. When mediastinal fibrosis appears without discernible cause, it may be associated with retroperitoneal fibrosis and then probably has the autoimmune origin described above. There are, however, other causes to consider. The condition is encountered most commonly in people who reside in places where histoplasmosis is endemic, notably in the central parts of the United States, and most of the case reports have come from clinics located in the Mississippi river valley (see Chapter 7.13.1 for further information). Studies of some of these patients have revealed the existence of large granulomas due to histoplasmosis, with eventual rupture into the superior mediastinum and subsequent growth of the dense masses of scar tissue characteristic of the fibrosing syndromes. A curious anomaly in this context is that tuberculosis rarely, if ever, causes the syndrome.

The diagnosis is suggested by radiographic demonstration of the fibrous tissue in the affected areas. CT scanning may be of great value in this context, and histological verification of the diagnosis can be made by CT-guided needle biopsy or by mediastinoscopy. Surgical treatment of mediastinal fibrosis is much more hazardous than of retroperitoneal fibrosis and is much less likely to be beneficial. Despite this, some experienced thoracic surgeons recommend that attempts be made to remove large granulomatous masses of histoplasmosis when this is the diagnosis. Chemotherapy for histoplasmosis has not been very effective. In view of the tendency of this fibrosing process to burn out eventually, it may be possible to ameliorate the manifestations by steroid therapy and thus gain time for a collateral circulation to develop. However, there is little experience of the effects of steroid treatment or other forms of immunosuppression, but there is obvious potential for this approach if the origin of the disorder is autoimmune.

Other rarer fibrosing syndromes

In association with retroperitoneal fibrosis and mediastinal fibrosis, other fibrotic processes have been reported to involve the thyroid gland (Riedel's thyroiditis), the pancreas, the salivary glands, and orbital tissue. The last mentioned can cause severe proptosis and damage to the optic nerve leading to loss of vision, some cases of which may be due to undiagnosed Wegener's granulomatosis. Peyronie's disease is characterized by the deposition of fibrous plaques in the corpora cavernosa of the penis. These plaques, which can be detected by palpation, may cause discomfort and angulation during penile erection.

Chronic inflammatory bowel disease

Chronic inflammatory bowel disease is associated with chronic and unsuspected urinary tract obstruction in 10 to 15 per cent of patients. The obstruction is nearly always right-sided in patients with Crohn's disease, and a valuable clue to its existence is pain radiating down from the right iliac fossa into the right leg. The ureter is usually involved in an inflammatory mass. By contrast, in patients with ulcerative colitis the problem may occur on either side and nearly always follows colectomy. There should be a low threshold for ultrasound examination of the urinary tract to detect obstruction in patients with chronic inflammatory bowel disease.

Further reading

Baker LRI *et al.* (1988). Idiopathic retroperitoneal fibrosis. A retrospective analysis of 60 cases. *British Journal of Urology* **60**, 497–503.

Baker LRI *et al.* (1992). Rate of development of ureteric obstruction in idiopathic retroperitoneal fibrosis (periaortitis). *British Journal of Urology* **69**, 102–5.

Better OS *et al.* (1973). Studies on renal function after relief of complete unilateral ureteral obstruction of three months' duration in man. *American Journal of Medicine* **54**, 234–40.

Brooks AP (1990). Computed tomography of idiopathic retroperitoneal fibrosis ('periaortitis'): variants, variations, patterns and pitfalls. *Clinical Radiology* **42**, 75–9.

Dines DE *et al.* (1979). Mediastinal granuloma and fibrosing mediastinitis. *Chest* **75**, 320–4.

Früh D, Jaeger W, Küfer O (1975). Orbital involvement in retroperitoneal fibrosis (morbus ormond). *Modern Problems in Ophthalmology* **14**, 651–6.

Ghose RR (1990). Prolonged recovery of renal function after prostatectomy for prostatic outflow obstruction. *British Medical Journal* **300**, 1376–7.

Gillenwater JY (1986). The pathophysiology of urinary obstruction. In: Walsh PC, ed. *Campbell's Urology*, 5th edn, p 554. WB Saunders, Philadelphia.

Graham JR *et al.* (1966). Fibrotic disorders associated with methysergide therapy for headache. *New England Journal of Medicine* **274**, 359–68.

Higgins PM *et al.* (1988). Non-operative management of retroperitoneal fibrosis. *British Journal of Surgery* **75**, 573–7.

Jaworski ZF, Wolan FT (1963). Hydronephrosis and polycythaemia, a case with erythrocytosis relieved by decompression of unilateral hydronephrosis and cured by nephrectomy. *American Journal of Medicine* **34**, 523.

Keuhnelian JG, Bartone F, Marshall VF (1964). Practical considerations from autopsies in uraemic patients. *Journal of Urology* **91**, 467–73.

McDougal WS, Wright FS (1972). Defect in proximal and distal sodium transport in post-obstructive diuresis. *Kidney International* **2**, 304–17.

Mitchinson MJ (1970). The pathology of retroperitoneal fibrosis. *Journal of Clinical Pathology* **23**, 681–9.

Moody TE, Vaughan ED, Gillenwater JY (1975). Relationship between renal blood flow and ureteral pressure during 18 hours of total unilateral occlusion. *Investigative Urology* **13**, 246–51.

Ormond JK (1948). Bilateral ureteral obstruction due to envelopment and compression by an inflammatory process. *Journal of Urology* **59**, 1072–9.

Parums DV, Brown DL, Mitchinson MJ (1990). Serum antibodies to oxidised LDL and ceroid in chronic periaortitis. *Archives of Pathology and Laboratory Medicine* **114**, 383–7.

Parums DV, Chadwick DR, Mitchinson MJ (1986). The localisation of immunoglobulin in chronic periaortitis. *Atherosclerosis* **61**, 117–23.

Pryor JP *et al.* (1983). Do beta adrenoceptor blocking drugs cause retroperitoneal fibrosis? *British Medical Journal* **287**, 639–42.

Roy C, Saussine C, Jacqmin D (2000). Magnetic resonance urography. *British Journal of Urology* **86** (suppl. 1), 42–7.

Sacks SH *et al.* (1989). Late renal failure due to prostatic outflow obstruction: a preventable disease. *British Medical Journal* **298**, 156–9.

Schowengerdt CG, Suyemoto R, Main FB (1969). Granulomatous and fibrous mediastinitis: a review and analysis of 180 cases. *Journal of Thoracic and Cardiovascular Surgery* **57**, 365–79.

Smith RC, Coll DM (2000). Helical computed tomography in the diagnosis of ureteric colic. *British Journal of Urology* **86** (suppl. 1), 33–41.

Smith RC *et al.* (1996). Diagnosis of acute flank pain: value of unenhanced helical CT. *American Journal of Roentgenology* **166**, 97–101.

Webb JAW *et al.* (1984). Can ultrasound and computed tomography replace high-dose urography in patients with impaired renal function? *Quarterly Journal of Medicine* **xx**, 411–25.

Whelan JS *et al.* (1991). Computed tomography (CT) and ultrasound (US) guided core biopsy in the management of non-Hodgkin's lymphoma. *British Journal of Cancer* **63**, 460–2.

Whitaker RH (1990). The diagnosis of upper urinary tract obstruction. *Postgraduate Medical Journal* **66** (suppl. 1), 25–30.

Whitfield HN *et al.* (1979). Frusemide intravenous urography in the diagnosis of pelvi-ureteric junction obstruction. *British Journal of Urology* **51**, 445–8.

Whitfield HN *et al.* (1981). Renal transit time measurements in the diagnosis of ureteric obstruction. *British Journal of Urology* **53**, 500–3.

Whitfield HN *et al.* (1983). Percutaneous pyelolysis: an alternative to pyeloplasty. *British Journal of Urology* **55**, 93–6.

Wickham JEA, Buck AC, eds (1990). *Renal tract stone.* Churchill Livingstone, London.

20.15 Tumours of the urinary tract

P. H. Smith, H. Irving, and P. Harnden

Introduction

Tumours of the kidney, bladder, prostate, and testis are grouped together only because of their association with the genitourinary tract. Each has, over the years, inspired surgeons to prove that ever more complex operations may be undertaken, but patients have not always benefited from this approach and surgeons now rely increasingly upon physicians working in radiotherapy and medical oncology. Recent emphasis has focused on earlier diagnosis and population screening in the hope that overall mortality will fall as more and more localized tumours are detected. Such an approach carries considerable economic consequences.

Transitional cell carcinoma of the bladder and upper urinary tract

Aetiology and incidence

Risk factors include: tobacco smoking; several chemicals related to the dye, rubber, leather, painting, and organic chemical industries; chronic irritation involving *N*-nitrosamine production; and therapeutic pelvic irradiation in women. Genetic factors modulate individual responses to environmental carcinogens, partially explaining variations in incidences between ethnic groups. The slow *N*-acetylation genotype and inherited defects of the glutathione-*S*-transferase M1 gene are susceptibility factors in occupational and smoking-related bladder cancer. Occupational exposure is thought to account for up to 25 per cent of cases in the United States, but less than 5 per cent of patients with bladder cancer are eligible for prescribed disease benefit in the United Kingdom.

The incidence in males and females is 32.5 and 12.9 per 100 000 population, respectively. The changes in industrial practice (and in supervision of workers) over the last 50 years has reduced the incidence of bladder cancer due to industrial carcinogens and it is now believed that over 40 per cent of all bladder tumours arise primarily as a consequence of cigarette smoking. The recent changes in attitude to smoking, both in the workplace and socially, may well result in a significant fall in the incidence of bladder cancer in the years to come.

The peak age at presentation is 65 to 69 years for men and 75 to 79 years for women, with less than 5 per cent of tumours occurring in patients younger than 60 years.

Clinical features

Though most bladder tumours present because of haematuria, less frequent presentations include bladder irritability, difficulty with micturition, and symptoms of uraemia or backache. Tumours of the renal pelvis and ureter may bleed or may silently obstruct the relevant kidney and ureter.

Investigation and diagnosis

Urinary cytology and high quality ultrasound is usually adequate to make the diagnosis of bladder cancer (Fig. 1). The flexible cystoscope allows the nature and extent of the lesion within the bladder to be seen. Tumours of the upper tract are revealed by intravenous pyelography or by ultrasound.

Patient categories and treatment

The TNM classification of bladder tumours is unique in that it recognizes a category of papillary carcinoma that is non-invasive (invasion through the basement membrane is the hallmark of malignancy in other tumour types, otherwise the lesion is regarded as premalignant or '*in situ*'). This evolved because of the difficulties in using standard microscopical techniques to distinguish urothelial papillomas (implying a benign lesion with no associated cancer risk) from the 70 per cent of tumours which recur and may progress. Understanding the biological behaviour of urothelial tumours has been further hampered by the tendency until recently to group together non-invasive tumours (pTa) and the tumours invading the lamina propria (pT1) under the umbrella of 'superficial disease' for treatment purposes, despite evidence that tumours with lamina propria invasion are at higher risk of progressing further.

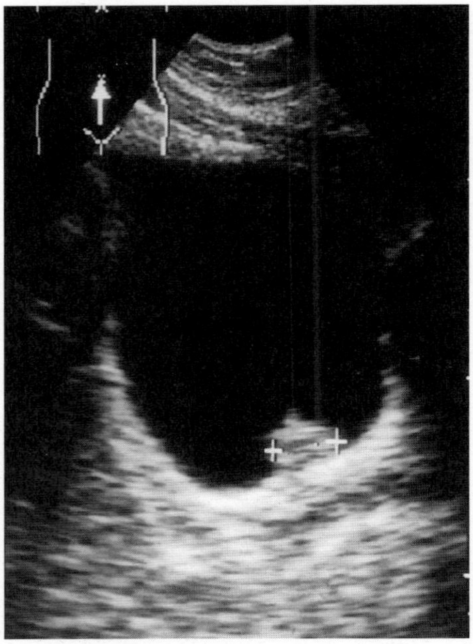

Fig. 1 Bladder ultrasound scan showing small (1 cm diameter) transitional cell carcinoma arising from the posterior wall.

Tumours not invading the lamina propria (pTa)

The now accepted primary treatment of the superficial lesion is by transurethral resection with a single instillation of an intravesical agent. Once the tumour has been resected, continuing supervision by check cystoscopy is mandatory as 70 per cent of lesions recur at some stage, whilst approximately 10 per cent will subsequently show progression of grade or stage requiring additional therapy.

Tumours involving the lamina propria (pT1)

These tumours have already demonstrated their invasive potential and require more intensive treatment. Intravesical BCG is commonly used.

If there is associated carcinoma *in situ*, or if the tumour is poorly differentiated, approximately half of the patients will develop invasive disease within 5 years. Many urologists believe that early cystectomy is better for this small subgroup, comprising perhaps 5 to 6 per cent of the whole.

Muscle invasive disease of the bladder (pT2 and above)

For the patient with disease invading the bladder muscle, cystectomy or radiotherapy will be necessary. Cystectomy is well established, but is a major procedure that still carries a mortality of between 2 and 4 per cent in different institutions and in different trials. In addition, the patient must accept the need for some form of urinary diversion or bladder replacement. Both are inconvenient to a greater or lesser extent, and the large segments of bowel needed for bladder replacement or a continent diversion bring with them the risks of metabolic problems associated with impaired absorption from the bowel, of diarrhoea, and of electrolyte imbalance. Radiotherapy may be thought to be a more attractive option, especially for the elderly patient. It must be accepted, however, that radical radiotherapy causes troublesome proctitis in 10 per cent of patients and, if survival is prolonged, telangiectases within the bladder that lead to haematuria. In addition, bladder contracture due to ischaemic fibrosis can necessitate secondary cystectomy for intractable symptoms.

As the two forms of radical treatment, cystectomy and radiotherapy, have not been adequately compared in randomized trials, comparisons of outcomes are limited as cystectomy may only be offered to fitter, younger patients. However, both treatment types offer similar overall 5-year survival rates related to the depth of invasion (which can only be accurately assessed in surgical series). This ranges from 60 to 70 per cent for tumours involving superficial muscle only, to 0 to 10 per cent for tumours which have spread beyond the bladder.

Adjuvant chemotherapy appeared to be very promising 10 years ago, but randomized trials have shown no survival advantage for single agent therapy or for combinations including cyclophosphamide, methotrexate, and vinblastine (CMV). The addition to this combination of adriamycin (M-VAC) may have marginally greater benefit but is also more toxic.

In the United Kingdom it is increasingly being suggested that patients with muscle invasive bladder cancer be managed in cancer centres in which there is surgical, radiation, and medical oncological expertise to advise the patient of the options and to supervise effectively the treatment that is chosen.

Transitional cell tumours of the upper urinary tract

Radical nephro-ureterectomy excising a cuff of bladder mucosa remains the treatment of choice in most patients whose other kidney is normal, since accurate staging of tumours of the ureter and pelvis is often impossible because of difficulties in obtaining biopsies of adequate depth endoscopically. Similarly, the possibility of regular assessment of the upper tracts for evidence of recurrence or progression is limited. Unifocal small lesions may be treated endoscopically or by local excision. In the patient in whom overall renal function is impaired or in whom there is only one kidney a conservative approach is desirable. Such lesions may be treated endoscopically or by local excision in certain cases.

Other tumours

Squamous and adenocarcinomas may be found in the bladder and, more rarely, in the upper urinary tract in association with long-standing stone disease, schistosomiasis, or spinal cord injury. The management of these tumours is surgical and the prognosis is poor.

Screening for transitional cell tumours of the bladder and upper urinary tract

Routine urinary cytology in workers in the chemical and dye industries is well established. The situation in relation to the general public is more debatable: screening by dipstick for microscopic haematuria in the elderly yields a positive test in up to 20 per cent, but a tumour incidence of only 1 per cent. Whilst a single positive dipstick test may not merit full urological investigation, if the test is repeatedly positive, formal investigation (urinary cytology, ultrasound of the urinary tract, and perhaps flexible cystoscopy) becomes inevitable, even in patients taking aspirin or anticoagulants, to reassure the physician, the patient, (and his lawyer). Unfortunately there is no evidence that 'screening' picks up invasive bladder cancer more effectively than the superficial tumour, nor that—in patients known to have bladder cancer—screening and early diagnosis will prevent invasion in the 10 per cent of patients in whom this subsequently recurs. For further discussion of the approach to microscopic haematuria, see Section 20.7.

Carcinoma of the prostate

Aetiology and incidence

There is some relationship between the number of sexual partners or extent of sexual activity and prostate cancer. The condition is less common in those who are celibate. The tumour does not occur in those who are castrated before puberty. Dietary factors are also of importance. The incidence is high at 50.7 per 100 000 men.

Clinical features

Patients may present themselves with symptoms of bladder outflow obstruction, bladder irritation, or the effect of some secondary deposit. Increasingly, however, the diagnosis is made as a result of a prostate-specific antigen (**PSA**) test. PSA is a glycoprotein of molecular weight 33 000 containing 7 per cent carbohydrate. It is a serine protease and an esterase with chymotrypsin-like and trypsin-like activity. It is found almost exclusively in the epithelial cells of the prostate.

Investigation and diagnosis

The introduction of the PSA test has led to increasing public awareness of prostate cancer, whilst the introduction of the nerve-sparing technique of radical prostatectomy by Walsh in the early 1980s offered the hope of effective cancer surgery with preservation of sexual function for the patients whose disease proves to be localized. As a consequence, diagnosis is increasingly made before metastases in lymph nodes or bone are evident. Bony metastases are very unlikely unless the PSA exceeds 20 ng/ml and a bone scan at diagnosis is probably an unnecessary luxury in patients whose PSA is below 20. Repeated bone scans during the course of treatment are unnecessary in the absence of clinical indications since repeated PSA tests are as effective and much cheaper.

Large numbers of cancers are now diagnosed following a PSA test at a stage before they are palpable (category T1c) by sextant biopsies under transrectal ultrasound control. The usual indication for biopsy is a PSA exceeding 4 ng/ml, but there is logic in taking a biopsy from all patients whose PSA exceeds 3 ng/ml (see below). As a consequence, large numbers of patients without symptoms and with no clinical findings are discovering that they have prostate cancer and are having to consider the form of therapy that they are prepared to accept. The situation is further complicated by the difficulty in staging the disease when it is not advanced. There is no true prostatic capsule. The prostate merges with the muscle of the bladder above and with the fibres of the levator ani below.

Radical therapy is appropriate for patients whose disease is confined to the prostate—a particularly important point with this disease since the surgeon has little opportunity to excise any normal tissue around the prostate because of its close association with the rectum and the base of the bladder. Surgical studies reveal that up to 50 per cent of prostatic tumours are understaged clinically, implying the need for even earlier diagnosis if surgical treatment is to be effective.

Treatment

'Localized disease'

In patients whose PSA is less than 20 ng/ml bone metastases are hardly ever seen and many patients have no involvement of their lymph nodes. Such early diagnosis will be of help only if existing therapy is curative or provides improved survival or quality of life. Unfortunately, 30 to 40 per cent of patients, despite early diagnosis, are found to have tumour extending beyond the prostate at the time of surgical intervention, suggesting that recurrence is likely if not inevitable. This is typically discovered as a rising level of PSA during follow-up ('PSA failure'): following radical prostatectomy or radiotherapy the PSA is expected to fall—to zero after operation or to less than 0.5 after radical radiotherapy since the prostate remains *in situ*. PSA failure is more common in those with higher stage and less well differentiated disease. It is seen in half of patients whose PSA at diagnosis is 10 ng/ml or more and in the vast majority of those with lymph node involvement at the time of treatment. None the less, it is possible that the reduction of tumour bulk by operation or radiotherapy may have affected the natural course of events such that the death rate from prostatic cancer will fall significantly, but this will not be clear for at least another 5 to 10 years.

'Advanced disease'

The dramatic change in outlook following the introduction of oestrogen therapy and orchidectomy in the 1940s was followed 20 years later by a search for agents that were more effective and without cardiotoxicity. Unfortunately, neither the steroidal nor non-steroidal anti-androgens, estramustine phosphate, nor the luteinizing hormone releasing hormone (LHRH) analogues used alone or in combination have been shown to prolong life to any clinically significantly extent, and many have concluded that little progress has been made in hormone therapy in the last 50 years. It is true, however, that sexual function may be preserved somewhat longer if the patient takes a non-steroidal anti-androgen and that the modern compounds have a lower rate of cardiovascular complications than stilboestrol.

Screening for prostate cancer

This topic creates great emotion in urological circles. The debate is polarized between those who believe that screening and radical therapy (prostatectomy) will cure the condition and those who are less certain that screening will identify only those patients whose cancers are likely to be life-threatening during the remaining years of the individual's life.

Post-mortem studies of victims of road accidents reveal that histological changes of prostate cancer can be found at increasing frequency with age from 30 per cent of 40-year olds to 50 per cent of 80-year olds. Of 1000 men in their 50s to 70s approximately 400 will have histological changes of prostate cancer, but only 100 will develop symptoms of the disease in the remaining years of their lives, whilst the 'forces of competing mortality' result in only one-quarter of these dying of the condition. Those anxious to prove that radical prostatectomy will cure the condition are naturally in favour of population screening. Epidemiologists are less convinced of its benefits to society as a whole.

A recent report of a working party of the British Association of Urological Surgeons recommends the following.

1. There is a need for scientifically valid controlled trials. These are currently being undertaken in the United States and Europe by the International Prostate Study for Treatment and Evaluation Group (IPSTEG) and by the European Randomized Study for Screening of Prostate Cancer (ERSPC).
2. Diagnostic tests, particularly prostate-specific antigen (PSA) measurements, should not be used in those for whom they are inappropriate, particularly the very elderly and those with diseases severely limiting their life expectation.
3. No asymptomatic man who requests PSA testing should undergo tests for prostate cancer without adequate counselling as to the possible consequences.
4. The role of PSA as part of a routine protocol for investigating men with lower urinary tract symptoms is controversial.
5. Transurethral ultrasound and biopsy must be carried out by trained operators with appropriate equipment.
6. The diagnosis of early prostate cancer will identify those who need or desire treatment for confined disease.
7. Early prostate cancer should be managed in designated clinics where the patient has access to a urologist and an oncologist.

The approach to a patient who has symptoms or has a genuine fear of having prostate cancer must be different from that adopted towards the population as a whole. Even here, however, it must be remembered that approximately half the men subjected to radical prostatectomy whose PSA at diagnosis is between 4 and 10 ng/ml have disease outside the prostate, and that a PSA limit of 3 ng/ml is probably more effective for population screening since:

(1) 12 per cent of tumours are found in men whose PSA is between 3 and 4 ng/ml;

(2) almost half the patients diagnosed at screening have extraprostatic disease; and

(3) 'PSA failure' (a gradually rising PSA following radical treatment) is found in up to 50 per cent of patients within 5 years of operation.

However, it should be noted that the death rate from prostatic cancer in the United States which rose during the 1990s and peaked in 1996 has since fallen for reasons which are not fully understood, but which may relate to early diagnosis and to radical therapy.

Carcinoma of the kidney

Aetiology and incidence

Though tumours may be produced in animals following irradiation, prolonged administration of oestrogens, exposure to nitrosamines, aromatic agents, and certain alkylating agents, the cause of renal tumours in humans is less well understood. Renal cell cancer is four times as common in males as in females, is linked with smoking, and associated with exposure to cadmium. It is more commonly found in areas with urban or industrial pollution than in rural areas. The incidence in males and females is 10.3 and 5.6 per 100 000 population, respectively.

Rarely, renal cancer appears to run in families, when a defect in the short arm of chromosome 3 is found in many cases (88 per cent in one series). Similar abnormalities are common in non-familial renal cancer and are found uniformly in von Hippel–Lindau disease—an inherited syndrome in which cysts or tumours in the kidney, pancreas, adrenal gland, epididymis, cerebellum, and spinal cord may form. Between one-third and one-half of

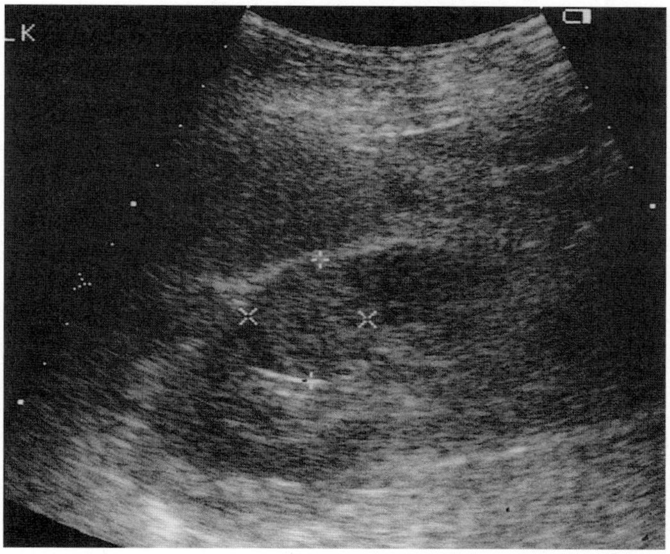

Fig. 2 Renal ultrasound scan showing an incidentally detected, small (2.5 cm diameter) renal cell carcinoma, proved to be stage T1 following nephrectomy. The edge of the tumour is marked by the four crosses.

patients with this condition develop renal cell tumours that are often bilateral and multifocal.

Investigation and diagnosis

Though some tumours are still diagnosed with the classic triad of haematuria, flank pain, and a palpable mass, many tumours are now discovered when completely asymptomatic and at a much earlier stage as a consequence of an incidental upper abdominal ultrasound (Fig. 2). It is also well recognized that renal cancer can present with a variety of apparently unrelated paraneoplastic syndromes. These are a consequence of the production of hormones or cytokines, or perhaps arise from an immune response to the tumour. Relatively common presentations include anaemia, hypertension, pyrexia of unknown origin, fatigue, and an increased plasma viscosity or raised erythrocyte sedimentation rate. Less common presentations include hypercalcaemia, polycythaemia, liver dysfunction, enteropathy, and neuromyopathy.

Until 20 years ago it was necessary to rely upon an intravenous urogram to show evidence of a space-occupying lesion within the kidney and difficult to detect tumours less than 3 cm in diameter. Modern ultrasound and CT can detect and correctly characterize 95 per cent of renal masses greater than 1 cm in diameter. Detection rates for lesions less than 1 cm are 50 per cent.

Survival is crucially dependent upon tumour stage. The free use of upper abdominal ultrasound in the investigation of many patients with upper abdominal symptoms or with symptoms consistent with renal cancer has led to a rapid increase in the diagnosis of early stage tumours that are potentially curable. These small lesions do, however, present diagnostic difficulties to both the pathologist and radiologist whose task it is to separate the renal carcinoma from benign tumours such as oncocytomas, angiomyolipomas, and complex cysts.

The use of ultrasound, CT (Fig. 3), and MRI (Fig. 4), if necessary with image-guided biopsy, can nearly always determine the nature of the tumour and the extent, if any, of lymph node involvement and venous invasion, whilst a bone scan will complete the basic investigations required prior to surgical excision. Tumours diagnosed whilst still small (less than 3 cm) and without extension to lymph nodes or the venous system are likely to have a 10-year survival of 90 per cent if treated effectively.

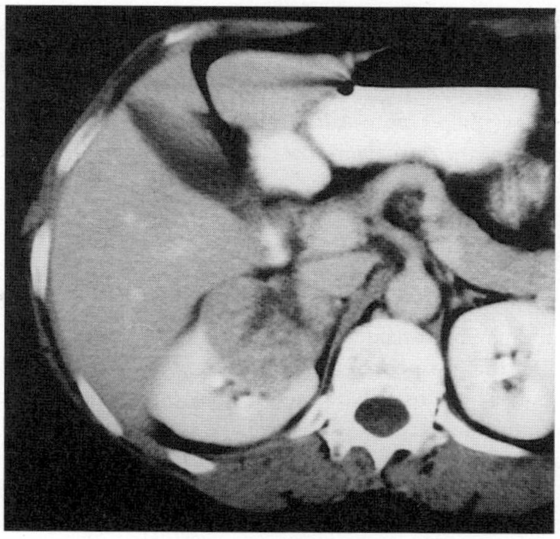

Fig. 3 CT scan showing a renal carcinoma extending into the retrocaval tissues.

Treatment

As yet renal tumours can only be cured by surgical excision. The standard treatment is still that of radical nephrectomy in which the affected kidney is removed with its perinephric fat and fascia. It has not yet been established that routine lymph node dissection is of value, but it is recognized that radiotherapy has little role in the management of the primary tumour or local recurrence, although it can be helpful in 'sterilizing' solitary bone metastases.

The use of nephron-sparing surgery is appropriate for smaller tumours, for the patient with a solitary kidney, for those with bilateral tumours, and in patients with von Hippel–Lindau disease. If the partial nephrectomy which such an excision involves leaves half of one functioning kidney, renal function will be adequate. For patients with very small lesions near the cortex of the kidney a simple wedge excision may be sufficient. If local recurrence occurs following partial nephrectomy, the remaining part of the kidney can be removed. It is often impossible for the surgeon to know exactly what sort of operation will be required until 'they get in there'. If there is any likelihood that the patient may be rendered anephric, this prospect should be fully discussed, and the patient introduced to the local renal unit for discussions regarding long-term dialysis before surgery is undertaken.

As yet neither chemo- nor immunotherapy have proved effective, but the use of interferon and interleukin 2 alone or in combination offers a 10 to 40 per cent chance of a partial or complete response in patients with

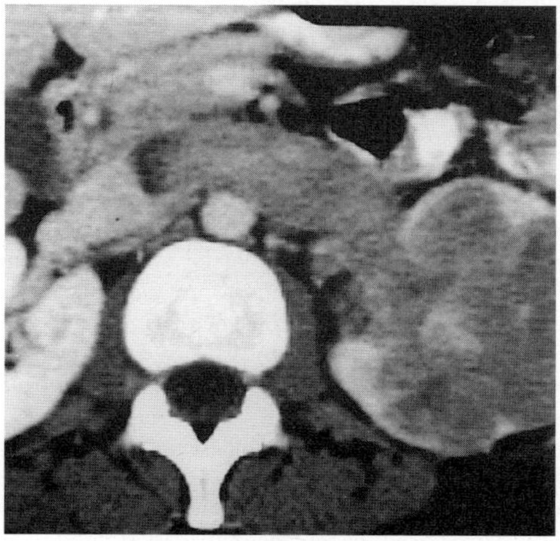

Fig. 4 MR scan showing a renal carcinoma distending and filling the left renal vein and the inferior vena cava.

advanced disease following preliminary nephrectomy and in good general condition. Metastases in the lungs are those which respond most frequently. Patients with a complete response have a two-thirds chance of surviving for longer than 1 year. Adoptive immunotherapy and trials of gene therapy remain at the investigational stage.

Advanced disease

For those in whom the diagnosis of renal carcinoma is not made until the local tumour is advanced, or with invasion of the vena cava, nodal involvement, or distant metastases, the outcome remains poor despite therapy. Nephrectomy may be considered for relief of symptoms but is unlikely to be able to offer the prospect of long-term survival. Spontaneous regression of metastases has been reported in fewer than 1 per cent of patients treated by nephrectomy, the responding lesions usually being in the lungs. The surgeon may also be of help to the patient with an apparently solitary skeletal metastasis, since it may be possible to excise it and provide a prosthetic replacement; also to relieve incipient spinal cord compression. In the management of such metastases adjunctive postoperative radiotherapy also plays a role.

Screening for carcinoma of the kidney

This tumour is relatively uncommon, is known to present with a wide variety of symptoms, and 30 per cent of people have metastases at diagnosis. Though no formal screening programme has been suggested, the increasing use of abdominal ultrasound for investigation of problems arising within the upper abdomen has brought to light many small and asymptomatic space-occupying lesions within the kidneys which present a diagnostic problem to the clinician and radiologist. CT scan or MRI with or without needle biopsy can confirm the diagnosis, but the decision as to the type of treatment to be offered is difficult, especially in the elderly patient in whom so many of these lesions are found.

Testicular tumours

Aetiology and incidence

Maldescent increases the risk of testicular cancer approximately fourfold and a range of other abnormalities in urogenital development, such as testicular atrophy or intersex states, have also been associated with an increased risk. This indicates that there are aetiological events associated with embryonic development, but the nature of these events is not known. Excessive oestrogenic exposure may play a role. The incidence has doubled in the last 20 years for reasons that are not understood, but germ cell tumours of the testis are rare, accounting for no more than 1 to 2 per cent of malignancies in males. The incidence (5.1 per 100 000 men) peaks between the ages of 25 and 34 years.

Clinical features, investigation, and diagnosis

From the clinical perspective it is important for the practising physician to remember that whilst most patients notice a lump, a few have symptoms consistent with epididymo-orchitis and a minority present with symptoms of metastases in nodes or other organs. Any disabling symptoms in a male under 35 years of age, such as malaise, loss of weight, backache, and pulmonary symptoms, including haemoptysis, may arise from a previously unrecognized testicular tumour that has metastasized. In a young adolescent or adult male in whom the diagnosis is in doubt or obscure, blood samples for α-fetoprotein and β-human chorionic gonadotrophin should be taken.

Examination of the abdomen in outpatients or on admission must include examination of the scrotal contents. Unless a completely normal testis can be identified, urgent ultrasound of the scrotum is indicated. This is very accurate in determining whether any mass is intratesticular (probably malignant) or extratesticular (probably benign). Samples of blood for α-fetoprotein and β-human chorionic gonadotrophin are mandatory investigations prior to surgery. Any tumour found must be removed without delay. The urologist should deal with such a patient on their next list by removing the testicle with spermatic cord as far as the internal inguinal ring.

Treatment

Following diagnosis by 'excision biopsy', as outlined above, all further management (staging, treatment, and subsequent follow-up) must be in the hands of a specialist cancer centre where expertise should be available to ensure that appropriate additional care is given without delay. Pathological assessment of the orchidectomy specimen is performed to confirm the germ cell origin of the tumour (other diagnoses to be considered include Sertoli or Leydig cell tumours and lymphoma). Germ cell tumours are divided into two main categories, seminoma and teratoma (non-seminomatous germ cell tumours in the American literature), which differ in terms of their relapse rates, patterns of spread, and treatment. Important clinical distinction is also made between patients who have disease clinically localized to the testis at the time of presentation and those who have evidence of metastatic disease.

Localized tumours

Relapse occurs in 16 per cent of patients with seminomas and twice as many with teratomas. Radiotherapy is the treatment of choice in seminoma because it is radiosensitive, and also because it tends to spread in a contiguous manner, with 80 per cent of relapses occurring in the retroperitoneum. Sites of relapse are less predictable in teratoma, and patients considered to be at high risk (generally because of the presence of vascular invasion in the orchidectomy specimen) are given chemotherapy in the United Kingdom. In North America, standard treatment involves a surgical retroperitoneal lymph node dissection and chemotherapy is reserved for those with evidence of established metastatic disease.

Metastatic disease

The dissemination of testicular cancer beyond the testis was a uniformly fatal illness until the 1960s. During the 1970s the introduction of a series of chemotherapy combinations, particularly those involving cisplatin, resulted in improving cure rates for patients with advanced disease. In modern practice, when treatment is delivered carefully by specialized multidisciplinary teams, 90 per cent of patients with testicular cancer, even if disseminated, can expect to be cured.

The International Germ Cell Consensus Classification, based on multivariate analyses of prognostic factors for progression and survival, determined that the most important factors for patients with a testicular primary were the level of serum markers (α-fetoprotein, β-human chorionic gonadotrophin, and lactate dehydrogenase) and the presence or absence of non-pulmonary metastases. The 5-year survival for patients with non-pulmonary visceral metastases was 18 per cent compared with 80 to 92 per cent for patients without such metastases. For the minority of patients for whom conventional therapy is not curative—identifiable by careful consideration of these prognostic factors—therapy including high-dose treatment, new drugs, and combined modality treatment with surgical resection of residual disease can still result in significant benefit.

Screening for tumours of the testis

Testicular self-examination is to be encouraged. Teenagers and men up to the age of 50 years should examine their testicles on a monthly basis, presenting themselves for consultation, diagnosis, and therapy if any abnormality is detected. Any abnormality not otherwise easily explicable should be investigated urgently by testicular ultrasound together with blood samples for α-fetoprotein and β-human chorionic gonadotrophin. Of the urological tumours, this is the only group for which therapy must rightly be given on an emergency basis.

Further reading

General

Vogelzang NJ *et al.*, eds (1996). *Comprehensive textbook of genito-urinary oncology.* Williams & Wilkins, Baltimore. [A first class and modern reference work on the topic.]

http://www.nice.org.uk/pdf/urologicalcancerimprovingoutcomes.pdf

Bladder

International collaboration of Trialists on behalf of the Medical Research Council Advanced Bladder Cancer Working Party *et al.* (1999). Neoadjuvant cisplatin, methotrexate and vinblastine chemotherapy for muscle invasive bladder cancer: a randomised controlled trial. *Lancet* **354**, 533–40. [A large international randomized trial to investigate the role of neoadjuvant chemotherapy in patients with invasive bladder cancer.]

Mayfield MP, Whelan P (1998). Bladder tumours detected on screening: results at 7 years. *British Journal of Urology* **82**, 825–8. [A good analysis of a screening study.]

Michaud DS *et al.* (1999). Fluid intake and the risk of bladder cancer in men. *New England Journal of Medicine* **340**, 1390–7. [Simple advice for a complex problem.]

Mills RD, Studer UE (1999). Metabolic consequences of continent urinary diversion. *Journal of Urology* **161**, 1057–66. [A detailed analysis of the consequences and complications of urinary diversion.]

Prostate

Auvinen A *et al.* for the International Prostate Screening Trial Evaluation Group (1996). Prospective evaluation plan for randomised trial of prostate cancer screening. *Journal of Medical Screening* **3**, 97–104. [The outline of the two major randomized screening studies.]

Dearnaley DP *et al.* (1999). Diagnosis and management of early prostate cancer. Report of a British Association of Urological Surgeons Working Party. *British Journal of Urology* **83**, 18–33. [A thoughtful analysis of the present situation.]

Prostate Cancer Trialists Collaborative Group (2000). Maximum androgen blockade in advanced prostate cancer: an overview of the randomised trials. *Lancet* **355**, 1491–8. [A meta-analysis showing only a minimal advantage for combination therapy at the time of first treatment.]

Schroder FH (1995). Detection of prostate cancer. *British Medical Journal* **310**, 140–1.

Schroder FH, Bangma CH (1997). The European Randomised Screening Study for Prostate Cancer ERSPC. *British Journal of Urology* **79**(Suppl 1), 68–71. [An analysis of the results of a pilot study leading to the randomized trial.]

Kidney

Avisrror MU (1998). Renal carcinoma and other tumours. In: Davison AM *et al.*, eds. *Oxford textbook of clinical nephrology,* 2nd edn, pp 2573–94. Oxford University Press.

Belldegrun A, deKernion JB (1998). Renal tumours. In: Walsh PC *et al.*, eds. *Campbell's urology,* 7th edn, pp 2283–325. Saunders, Philadelphia.

Davidson AJ *et al.* (1997). Radiologic assessment of renal masses: implications for patient care. *Radiology* **202**, 297–305.

Pavone-Macaluso M, Ingargiola GB, La Martina M (1983). Aetiology of kidney tumours. In: Smith PH, ed. *Cancer of the prostate and kidney,* pp 475–88. NATO ASI series, Plenum Press, New York. [An extensive review of possible aetiological factors.]

Vogelzang NJ *et al.*, eds (1996). *Comprehensive textbook of genito-urinary oncology.* Williams & Wilkins, Baltimore. [A detailed analysis of what is possible and not possible for the patient with renal cell cancer.]

Testis

Bueton SA (1996). Testicular cancer—to screen or not to screen? *Journal of Medical Screening* **3**, 3–7.

Collette L *et al.* (1999). Impact of the treating institution on survival of patients with 'poor prognosis' metastatic non-seminoma. *Journal of the National Cancer Institute* **91**, 839–46. [Emphasizes the importance of treating patients with advanced disease in large centres.]

Colls BM *et al.* (1992). Results of the surveillance policy of stage I non-seminomatous germ cell testicular tumours. *British Journal of Urology* **70**, 423–8.

Donohue JP, Foster RS (1994). Management of retroperitoneal recurrences: seminoma and non-seminoma. *Urological Clinics of North America* **21**, 761–72.

Scheinfeld J, Bajorin D (1993). Management of the post-chemotherapy residual mass. *Urological Clinics of North America* **20**, 133–43.

Sternberg CN (1993). Role of primary chemotherapy in stage I and low volume stage II non-seminomatous germ cell testis tumours. *Urological Clinics of North America* **20**, 93–109.

20.16 Drugs and the kidney

D. J. S. Carmichael

Introduction

The kidney is the major route of elimination for many drugs and their metabolites. This excretion may be by glomerular filtration, tubular secretion, or in some cases both. In practice a minority of drugs need dose adjustment (dosage and/or interval). The major problems occur in those drugs with a narrow therapeutic range or whose adverse effects are related to the concentration of the drug or its metabolites.

Excretion is affected most by reduction in the glomerular filtration rate, but absorption, distribution (including protein binding), metabolism, and pharmacodynamics may be altered in patients with renal impairment. However, the major determinant of alteration in dosage is the change in drug clearance, which can be estimated by measurement of the glomerular filtration rate, and many handbooks provide guidelines for the adjustment of dosage in renal impairment. Many of these data are derived from measurement or estimation of changes in clearance, half-life ($t_{1/2}$), and volume of distribution (V_d). Renal impairment will often be defined as mild (glomerular filtration rate > 50 ml/min), moderate (glomerular filtration rate > 20 to < 50 ml/min) or severe (glomerular filtration rate < 20 ml/min).

Patients with established chronic renal impairment are often on many medications, either for treatment of the primary disease or its consequences (dialysis, transplantation) or concurrent medical problems. Conversely many patients who are prescribed drugs have impaired renal function (often unrecognized) coincidentally or as a result of other medical problems. Although alteration in pharmacokinetics in renal disease is important, problems are more likely to arise for the following reasons:

(i) ignorance of renal impairment before a drug is prescribed;

(ii) ignorance of how a drug is cleared from the body;

(iii) failure to monitor therapeutic and adverse effects.

Pharmacokinetics

Renal excretion

Renal excretion of drugs depends upon:

(i) filtration

(ii) active tubular secretion and reabsorption

(iii) passive diffusion.

Renal clearance of drugs is a function of the glomerular filtration rate, but tubular reabsorption, secretion, and passive diffusion are contributory factors. If renal clearance is less than the glomerular filtration rate, then tubular reabsorption must be taking place; if it is greater than the glomerular filtration rate, then there must be active tubular secretion.

Compounds with a molecular weight below 60 000 Da are filtered through the glomerulus to a variable extent depending on molecular size, unless they are protein bound when only the unbound portion is filtered. Non-polar (lipid soluble) drugs diffuse readily across tubular cells whereas polar (water soluble) compounds do not. Hence polar drugs generally remain in the tubular fluid and are excreted in the urine, whilst non-polar drugs are reabsorbed by passive diffusion down their concentration gradient into plasma. Some polar drugs are eliminated in the urine as a result of active or facilitated transport mechanisms that transport organic acids or bases (see Table 1). Many drugs are metabolized, primarily in the liver, to produce more polar compounds that cannot be passively reabsorbed and so are eliminated in the urine. In renal failure there may be reduced clearance of these metabolites, which could have therapeutic or adverse effects (see Table 2).

Elimination of organic acids (AH) or bases (B) is affected by the H^+ ion concentration of the tubular fluid, with any change of urinary pH that favours ionization leading to more drug excretion:

$$H^+ + B \overset{pK_B}{\rightleftharpoons} BH^+$$

$$AH \underset{pK_A}{\rightleftharpoons} H^+ + A^-$$

The amount of ionized drug at any particular pH is determined by its pK, this being the pH at which 50 per cent of the drug is ionized. If an organic acid has a pK_A of less than 7.5, making the urine alkaline (i.e. increasing its pH) increases the amount of ionized drug (A^-) and therefore its excretion. The converse is true for organic bases with a pK_B of more than 7.5, which are eliminated as the charged (BH^+) form favoured by acid pH. The excretion of salicylates (weak acids) and amphetamines (weak bases) exemplifies these principles.

Although it is an oversimplification to disregard the tubular handling of drugs in renal impairment, both filtration and secretion of drugs appear to fall in parallel and in proportion to the glomerular filtration rate. Hence by far the most important aspect of prescribing in renal disease is awareness of the existence of renal impairment and of changes in renal function: some measure of glomerular filtration rate is needed, serum creatinine measurement usually being sufficient, but more precise measurement is required in some circumstances, for example before the use of known nephrotoxins in chemotherapeutic regimes.

Table 1 Examples of drugs with active tubular secretion

Organic acids	Penicillins
	Cephalosporins
	Sulphanamides
	Furosemide (frusemide)
	Thiazides
	Salicylates
	Probenecid
Organic bases	Amiloride
	Procainamide
	Quinidine

Table 2 Parent drugs, metabolites and possible adverse effects

Drug	Metabolite	Effect of metabolite
Allopurinol	Oxypurinol	?Causes rashes
Clofibrate	Chlorophenoxyiso-butyric acid	Muscle damage, neuropathy
Nitroprusside	Thiocyanate	Toxic symptoms
Primodone	Phenobarbitone	Active drug
Procainamide	*N*-Acetyl procainamide	Antiarrhythmic
Sulphonamides	Acetylsulphon-amides	Rashes
Pethidine	Norpethidine	Causes seizures
Morphine	Morphine-6-glucuronide	Prolongs analgesia and respiratory depression
Codeine	Morphine	Prolongs analgesia and respiratory depression
Propoxyphene	Norpropoxyphene	Cardiotoxicity
Acebutalol	*N*-Acetyl analogue	Confers selectivity
Nitrofurantoin	Nitrofurantoin metabolites	Peripheral neuropathy

Drugs present in tubular fluid may affect the excretion of other compounds; for example, aspirin and paracetamol reduce methotrexate excretion and probenecid reduces tubular secretion of penicillins and cephalosporins.

Drug kinetics

Most drugs that are eliminated by the kidney display first-order kinetics, meaning that the rate of removal is proportional to the concentration of the drug. The elimination rate constant k_e is the proportion of the total amount of drug removed per unit time, producing a simple exponential decline (and therefore a straight line on a semilogarithmic plot) in concentration (Fig. 1). The half-life ($t_{1/2}$) of a drug is the time for its plasma concentration to fall by half after absorption and distribution are complete. It is useful in determining dosage interval, drug accumulation (both extent of accumulation and the time taken to reach steady state), and persistence of drug after dosing is stopped. $t_{1/2}$ is inversely related to k_e:

$$t_{1/2} = 0.693/k_e$$

(note: 0.693 = ln 2). The clearance of a drug depends upon $t_{1/2}$ (k_e) and the volume of distribution (V_d). The latter does not usually correspond to a real (physiological) volume, although for a drug confined exclusively to the plasma it would approximate to the plasma volume: it represents an apparent volume in which the amount of drug administered would have distributed to produce the measured plasma concentration. The volume of distribution itself may be affected by the protein and tissue binding of drugs, changes in intravascular and extravascular fluid volumes, and lean body mass. Digoxin is one of the few drugs in which a smaller loading dose is needed because of changes in V_d in renal impairment.

Clearance can be used to calculate the steady state concentration of a drug (C_{ss}) that can be anticipated in response to any particular dosage regimen. This concentration is proportional to the dose and $t_{1/2}$ of the drug and inversely proportional to the V_d and dosage interval. From these relationships it can be seen that C_{ss} will increase with a longer $t_{1/2}$ and a smaller V_d; it can be reduced either by lowering the dose or by increasing the dose interval.

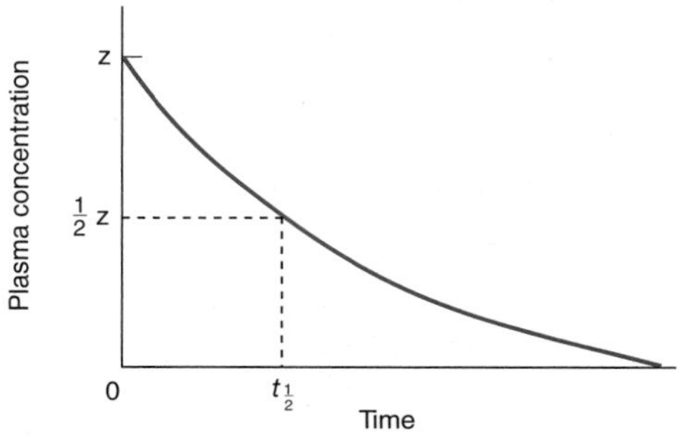

Fig. 1 Plot of log concentration of a drug against time to demonstrate the half-life of a drug.

The relationship between the elimination of a drug in the presence of renal impairment and normal renal function can be estimated and used to gauge the appropriate reduction in dose or increase in dose interval compared with a standard regimen. If non-renal clearance accounts for 50 per cent or more of total drug clearance then no dose adjustment will be needed, provided that non-renal clearance is not affected by renal impairment. If dose reduction is required, then dose, dose interval, or both can be adjusted to reduce dose per unit time. However, in practice the decision whether to reduce dose or prolong dose interval is not always equivalent: for example in the use of aminoglycoside antibiotics, which must achieve a threshold peak concentration in order to kill bacteria effectively, when small but frequent doses may fail to achieve efficacy whereas the same total dose delivered less frequently may achieve the desired therapeutic effect without leading to accumulation and toxicity.

Other pharmacokinetic topics

Gastrointestinal absorption, distribution, metabolism, and renal haemodynamics are other factors that may be altered in the presence of renal impairment. They are less significant than the effects of changes in renal excretion and are dealt with in more specialized pharmacology texts.

Dialysis and haemofiltration

The clearance of drugs by haemodialysis and haemofiltration follows first-order kinetics. Estimates of clearance can be obtained by use of the sieving coefficient, which is the proportion of the drug (or solute) that will cross the membrane and should be constant for a particular drug and membrane (see Table 3). This depends on the drug's molecular weight (and size) and protein binding. Haemofilters have a pore size of 0.01 μm and artificial kidneys for haemodialysis have a pore size of 0.001 μm. In haemofiltration, drugs with a molecular weight below that of inulin (5200 Da) will pass through, whereas in haemodialysis most drugs with a molecular weight

Table 3 Factors influencing the clearance of drugs

Properties of the drug	Molecular weight Protein binding Volume of distribution
Delivery of drug to the filter	Blood flow to filter Blood flow within filter Volume of distribution
Properties of the filter	Pore size Surface area

below 500 Da (which includes most antibiotics) will be cleared, but drugs such as vancomycin (1800 Da), amphotericin (960 Da), and erythromycin (734 Da) behave differentially with respect to haemofiltration/haemodialysis. Heavily protein bound drugs, even those of low molecular weight (propranolol 259 Da), will not be filtered, but drugs that are displaced from binding sites in the presence of renal impairment will become available for filtration. Water soluble drugs pass through filters more readily than those which are fat soluble. The other differences between the different techniques of haemodialysis, haemodiafiltration, and intermittent and continuous haemofiltration are dealt with in Chapter 20.6.1 and other specialized texts.

Digoxin and antidepressants are examples of drugs with a large volume of distribution that will have low plasma concentrations, hence little of the drug is available for filtration.

Peritoneal dialysis clears drugs very much less efficiently than haemodialysis/filtration, some needing careful adjustment of prescription, for example antibiotics in the treatment of continuous ambulatory peritoneal dialysis peritonitis.

Poisoning

Haemodialysis, peritoneal dialysis, haemofiltration, and haemoperfusion have all been used to eliminate poisons and drugs in overdose from the body. Peritoneal dialysis is very slow but can be used to clear alcohols, salicylate, and lithium if haemodialysis or filtration are unavailable. Similar principles apply to those for the handling of drugs in therapeutic dialysis and filtration. A substance that has a low V_d, low protein binding, and is unipolar will be cleared more efficiently. Note, however, that measurements of the amount of any drug in the body almost invariably report the plasma concentration, and simple estimates of the clearance of any substance will reflect the rate at which the plasma is cleared, ignoring the relationship between the plasma and other compartments. This is a gross oversimplification in some instances, when rebound of plasma concentration occurs as drug redistributes from intracellular compartments.

Haemodialysis

All toxins of size 100 to 2000 Da can be removed using conventional filters, preferably by dialysis with bicarbonate buffering as many toxins will cause acidosis. Should rebound of plasma levels of a substance occur after a period of treatment, as described above, then continuous haemofiltration or repeated haemodialysis may be required; for example thallium poisoning may need prolonged treatment over several days. High-flux membranes used in continuous haemofiltration and haemodiafiltration will remove larger sized molecules (up to 10 000 Da).

Haemoperfusion

Haemoperfusion relies on the affinity of an adsorbent for a toxin and can be used preceding filtration or dialysis in series. Activated charcoal or polystyrene exchange resins are usually used in a column arranged like an artificial kidney. The technique is particularly useful for toxins with a low V_d: poisons and drugs that can be removed by these means are listed in (Table 4). Further information should be obtained from the National Poisons Centre (Toxbase http://www.spib.axl.co.uk/toxbaseindex.htm).

Table 4 Poisoning—removal of toxic drugs

Haemodialysis and haemofiltration	Acetic acid
	Boric acid
	Formic acid
	Lactic acid
	Phosphoric acid
	Acetylsalicylic acid
	Acyclovir
	Ethyl alcohol
	Methyl alcohol
	Ethylene glycol
	Bromide
	Lithium
	Thallium
	Barbiturates*
	Paracetamol*
	Paraquat*
Haemoperfusion	Paracetamol
	Paraquat
	Barbiturates

*Less efficient than haemoperfusion.

Prescribing drugs for patients with renal failure

Once the clinician has identified that renal impairment is present, and that a drug to be administered has clinically important renal excretion, the dose can be adjusted in two main ways. Either the size of each dose or the frequency of administration can be reduced. Plasma drug concentrations can be used to confirm that the initial adjustment of dosage is correct in that particular individual. Steady state concentrations of anticonvulsants, digoxin, and theophylline can be measured after the equivalent of five half-lives of the drug. For antibiotics such as gentamicin monitoring is required after the first day's administration and continued if renal function is impaired or changing.

The combination of reduction in dosage and less frequent administration is suitable for most drugs. Dosage reduction alone is more likely to lead to subtherapeutic plasma concentrations. Unfamiliar dosages and administration of drugs at odd times may result in errors, hence adjustments of dose and timing must be kept simple and clear. The physician should use a limited number of drugs and learn about their clearance in renal impairment and changes during renal replacement therapy.

Many of the most complex prescribing problems arise in patients with acute renal failure, particularly if this occurs as part of multisystem failure, perhaps in a patient requiring artificial ventilation and some form of renal replacement therapy.

Acute renal failure on the intensive care unit

Neuromuscular blocking agents

Succinylcholine is rapidly hydrolysed by plasma cholinesterase: no dose adjustment is needed. For more prolonged paralysis atracurium should be used; this is degraded by non-enzymatic Hofmann elimination independent of renal or hepatic function. It is removed by dialysis and haemofiltration: the dose must be titrated to produce a therapeutic effect. Avoid tubocurarine, gallamine, alcuronium, pancuronium, and vercuronium.

Anaesthetic and sedating agents

Propofol, fentanyl, and alfentanyl require no dose adjustment, but the latter two may have prolonged effects if there is concomitant hepatic dysfunction. Metabolites of diazepam accumulate and midazolam is preferable (with dosage reduction) if the glomerular filtration rate falls below 10 ml/min. Phenothiazines, butyrophenones, and chlormethiazole are given in the usual doses.

Treatment of pain or inflammation: analgesics and anti-inflammatories

Narcotic analgesics

Opiates are affected by renal failure, and retention of metabolites can produce adverse effects which may be reduced by intermittent dosing, epidural administration, or low-dose continuous infusions. Diamorphine is metabolized into morphine and then to morphine-3-glucuronide and morphine-6-glucuronide, both of which accumulate to prolong both analgesia and respiratory depression. Morphine and its metabolites are not cleared well by haemofiltration or dialsysis. Pethidine (meperidine) is converted to norpethidine (normeperidine), which accumulates and can cause seizures. Papaveretum is a mixture of alkaloids of opium including morphine, codeine, noscapine, and papaverene: its use is not recommended. Codeine and dihydrocodeine, although weaker analgesics, still have the potential to cause severe respiratory depression in some patients with renal failure, likewise dextropropoxyphene (combined with paracetamol as coproxamol). Its metabolite norproxyphene, which accumulates in renal failure, sometimes causes cardiac toxicity. Buprenorphine is metabolized in the liver and does not appear to have any important toxic metabolites.

If confronted with a patient with renal failure who is inexplicably drowsy or has depressed respiration and who has (or might have) received opiates in the last 72 h, then a trial of intravenous naloxone should be administered: this is sometimes dramatically effective.

Non-narcotic analgesics

Paracetamol (which in overdosage is an important cause of acute renal failure) is excreted in small amounts by glomerular filtration, with some passive tubular reabsorption. Most of the drug is metabolized and the glucuronide and sulphide metabolites, which are subject to active tubular secretion, accumulate in renal impairment, with some regeneration of the parent compound. Despite this, paracetamol is used in the usual doses. Aspirin has the disadvantage of causing gastric damage and increasing the bleeding diathesis of patients with renal failure. Renal elimination of its metabolite salicylate is enhanced in alkaline urine (see above).

Anti-inflammatory agents

Non-steroidal anti-inflammatory drugs including aspirin inhibit the synthesis of prostaglandin by inhibition of cyclo-oxygenase. The principal renal prostaglandins in humans are prostaglandin E_2 and prostaglandin I_2, each of which is vasodilator and natriuretic, having direct effects on both renal blood flow and tubular ion transport. In healthy individuals inhibition of cyclo-oxygenase has no detectable effect on renal function, but in patients with cardiac failure, nephrotic syndrome, liver disease, glomerulonephritis, and other renal disease cyclo-oxygenase inhibitors predictably cause a reversible fall in glomerular filtration rate that can be severe. They can also cause fluid retention and hyperkalaemia. There is evidence that sulindac causes less inhibition of renal cyclo-oxygenase than a dose of ibuprofen that is equieffective on extrarenal tissues and sulindac may cause less renal impairment than other non-steroidal anti-inflammatory drugs. Aspirin may also spare cyclo-oxygenase in the kidney to some extent. The clinical relevance of these observations remains uncertain and caution is needed in severe renal impairment when using any non-steroidal anti-inflammatory drugs.

Indomethacin, azapropazone, and diflunisal have important renal excretion, whereas most other non-steroidal anti-inflammatory drugs are eliminated by metabolism. The non-steroidal anti-inflammatory drugs are highly protein bound and are not removed by dialysis.

Treatment of circulatory disturbance, cardiac disease, or hypertension

Problems can be avoided or minimized by titration of a low starting dose of any drug to produce the required therapeutic effect.

Vasopressors and vasodilators

Adrenaline, dobutamine, dopexamine, dopamine, and noradrenaline should be used in the minimum doses possible to avoid renal vasoconstriction. They all have a short half-life and are not affected by haemo- or haemodiafiltration. Intravenous nitrates are given in the normal dosage. Sodium nitroprusside is metabolized in the liver to sodium thiocyanate, which is eliminated by the kidney and thus may accumulate in renal failure, causing toxicity. It is removed by haemofiltration or haemodiafiltration.

Antiarrhythmics

In patients with abnormal renal function it is advisable to keep treatment simple. Most antiarrhythmic drugs are used without dose modification, for example lidocaine (lignocaine) and verapamil. Digoxin is a notable exception, with a lower loading and maintenance dose than usual. Flecainide and disopyramide require dosage reduction. Amiodarone requires a lower maintenance dose (100 mg daily) when the glomerular filtration rate falls below 20 ml/min.

Diuretics

Spironolactone, triamterene, and amiloride, all potassium sparing diuretics, should be avoided or used with extreme caution in renal impairment because of the danger of hyperkalaemia. The same applies for combination diuretics such as 'Moduretic' (amiloride and hydrochlorothiazide) or 'Dyazide' (triamterene and hydrochlorothiazide). Thiazides, apart from metolazone (a quinolone), become less effective in treatment of both fluid retention and hypertension if the glomerular filtration rate is below 25 ml/min. Higher doses of loop diuretics are needed, but the synergistic effect with metolazone may overcome 'diuretic resistance' in refractory oedema.

Severe sodium and water depletion can occur in diuretic therapy. This may affect renal haemodynamics with secondary effects upon renal function and concomitant drug therapy.

Angiotensin converting enzyme inhibitors

Whether angiotensin converting enzyme inhibitors are being used to treat cardiac failure or hypertension the same precautions apply. Starting doses should be low and increased slowly with careful monitoring of serum creatinine and potassium. Particular caution is necessary if these drugs are used in combination with diuretics or in other high-renin states (for example volume depletion), when marked hypotension ('first-dose effect') may be anticipated. Caution is also necessary when there is (or may be) a possibility of renal artery stenosis, both because of the risk of hypotension and also because of the reduced glomerular filtration rate in the affected kidney(s). Angiotensin converting enzyme inhibitors should not generally be used with potassium sparing diuretics because of the added risk of hyperkalaemia. The kidney eliminates all angiotensin converting enzyme inhibitors, accounting for the reduced dose usually required in the elderly. Exactly the same advice pertains for angiotensin II receptor antagonists.

β-blockers

Atenolol, bisoprolol, pindolol, nadolol, and sotalol are all excreted by the kidney and reduced doses may be needed. The metabolites of acebutolol may accumulate. Other β-blockers are prescribed unchanged.

Vasodilators, calcium channel blockers, and α-blockers

No dose adjustment is needed for any of these drugs. Minoxidil therapy often requires concomitant use of a loop diuretic.

Centrally acting agents

α-Methyldopa, moxonidine, and clonidine are given in the usual doses and titrated for their effect.

Treatment of infection: antimicrobials

Many antimicrobial agents are excreted by the kidney. With the exception of aminoglycosides and vancomycin, most have a wide therapeutic index and little or no dose adjustment is typically made until the glomerular filtration rate is less than 20 ml/min. Antimicrobials that are removed by dialysis should be administered after dialysis, or a supplemental dose given at that time. Adjustments are shown in Table 5.

Penicillins

All penicillins need to be given in reduced dose. Carbenicillin and ticarcillin solutions contain approximately 5 mmol Na^+/g, and caution is needed in the presence of salt and water retention. Mezlocillin (unlike other penicillins) is not removed by dialysis.

Intravenous cephalosporins and other β-lactams

Cephalosporins are excreted in similar fashion to penicillins and need dose reduction in renal impairment (Table 5). The later generation drugs are relatively safe, but caution is still needed with cefuroxime. The carbapenems imipenem and meropenem have a broad spectrum of activity: the former is partially inactivated by a renal dipeptidase and hence administered in combined preparation with cilastatin, an inhibitor of this enzyme. Aztreonam (a monobactam) requires dose adjustment.

Aminoglycosides

Aminoglycosides need dose adjustment in mild renal impairment. Furthermore, they are inherently nephrotoxic and their use may worsen renal impairment as well as causing ototoxicity. Several factors predispose to nephrotoxicity: these include prior or prolonged treatment, hypovolaemia, dehydration, concomitant administration of diuretics, hypokalaemia, and hypomagnesaemia. Obstructive jaundice also increases the risk. The simplest way to prevent aminoglycoside toxicity is to avoid their use altogether in patients with any suspicion of renal impairment and prescribe alternatives.

Nomograms and other guidelines should be used for dose adjustment of aminoglycosides in patients with renal impairment, usually based on conventional multiple dosages. Since the volume of distribution of aminoglycosides is not materially affected by renal impairment, an adequate loading dose is required whatever the method of dose adjustment. Reduction of dose (without alteration in frequency of administration) may lead to an increased likelihood of subtherapeutic peak plasma levels. However, if only the frequency of administration is reduced, then subtherapeutic plasma concentrations are more likely to occur over longer periods. A combination of both methods with frequent peak measurements (taken 1 h after intravenous dosing) and trough measurements (immediately before the next dose) is optimal. An alternative method is to give a single daily dose, there being evidence that gentamicin is less nephrotoxic with an initial dose of 3 to 5 mg/kg body weight, with adjustment made on a daily trough level. Such measurements should be made daily when alterations in renal function are anticipated and two to three times a week under other circumstances. Doses and therapeutic concentrations are shown in (Table 6).

Table 5 Antimicrobial dose adjustment

Drug	Renal function	Dose reduction	Comments
Ampicillin			Seldom needed
Flucloxacillin		Nil	
Amoxicillin + clavulanic acid	GFR < 20 ml/min	By 50%	Half dose postdialysis
Benzyl penicillin	GFR < 20 ml/min		Daily dose should not exceed 20 mU
Piperacillin	GFR 20–50 ml/min	By 50%	Half dose postdialysis
	GFR < 20 ml/min	By 66%	
Cefotaxime	GFR 20–50 ml/min	By 66%	Half dose postdialysis
Ceftazidine	GFR < 20 ml/min	By 75%	Half dose postdialysis
Aztreonam	GFR < 10 ml/min	By 75%	Half dose postdialysis
Imipenem/ cilastatin	GFR < 20 ml/min	By 50%	Half dose postdialysis
Erythromycin		Nil	
Trimethoprim	GFR < 20 ml/min	By half	Half dose postdialysis
Ciprofloxacin	GFR < 10 ml/min		500–750 mg/day maximum
Rifampicin		Nil	Avoid with cyclosporin
Flucytosine	GFR 20–50 ml/min	By half	Half dose postdialysis
	GFR < 20 ml/min	By three-quarters	
Fluconazole	GFR < 50 ml/min	By half	After 2 days
Acyclovir	GFR 50–10 ml/min	Stepwise reduction from 800 mg five times/ day	

GFR = glomerular filtration rate.

Table 6 Doses and therapeutic plasma concentrations of aminoglycosides

Drug	Usual daily dose*	Therapeutic concentration	
		Peak†	Trough‡
Gentamicin	2–5 mg/kg	5–10 mg/l	< 2.5 mg/l
Tobramycin	2–5 mg/kg	5–10 mg/l	< 2.5 mg/l
Netilmicin§	2–5 mg/kg	5–10 mg/l	< 2.5 mg/l
Amikacin	10–30 μg/kg	20–30 mg/l	< 10 mg/l
Kanamycin	10–30 μg/kg	20–30 mg/l	< 10 mg/l

*Usual daily dose is administered 8-hourly.
†Peak concentration measured 1 h postinjection.
‡Trough concentration immediately before next dose.
§Netilmycin dose can be increased to 7.5 mg/kg/day in severe infections but with careful therapeutic monitoring.

Vancomycin and teicoplanin

Vancomycin is excreted by the kidney and is not dialysed (except at extremely high flow rates in haemofiltration, by haemodiafiltration, or by haemodialysis with high-flux dialysers). In patients with endstage renal failure on dialysis, therapeutic concentrations can be maintained for 5 days or more after a single intravenous dose, the target steady state plasma concentration being approximately 15 mg/l. Following a loading dose of 15 mg/kg, further doses are given on the basis of plasma concentration.

Teicoplanin, a glycopeptide related to vancomycin, behaves rather differently. The half-life is prolonged by approximately threefold in renal failure, and after a loading dose of 400 mg the maintenance dose of 200 mg/day is reduced after 3 days, even in mild renal failure. It is not cleared by dialysis.

Ciprofloxacin

Renal excretion exceeds the glomerular filtration rate, and in patients with normal renal function approximately 60 per cent is cleared by passage through the kidneys. It is recommended that the dose should be reduced in renal impairment, but the proportion that is eliminated by the kidney is reduced in renal failure as a result of an increase in hepatic clearance and of secretion through the wall of the bowel. This becomes more problematic if there is combined renal and hepatic or intestinal failure. Ciprofloxacin is not significantly removed by haemodialysis, but is partially removed by haemofiltration.

Tetracyclines

All the tetracyclines, with the exception of minocycline and doxycycline, are renally excreted. Plasma half-lives are markedly prolonged (up to 100 h) in renal impairment. Tetracyclines are antianabolic and cause a concentration-related increase in blood urea, setting up a vicious cycle leading to deterioration in renal function. Doxycycline or minocycline can be used cautiously in patients with renal impairment, but the other tetracyclines are contraindicated. Demeclocycline, peculiar to itself, has an inhibitory effect on the tubular action of antidiuretic hormone.

Sulphonamides and cotrimoxazole and trimethoprim

Sulphonamides are eliminated by acetylation followed by renal excretion, and acetylated metabolites (which have no antibacterial activity) are a cause of crystalluria and tubular damage. High doses of cotrimoxazole are needed in the treatment of *Pneumocystis carinii*, the risk of adverse effects being balanced against the seriousness of the condition. Such patients often have impaired renal function. The dose is trimethoprim 20 mg and sulphamethoxazole 100 mg/kg body weight/day divided into two or more doses. The plasma concentration should be maintained at approximately 5 to 8 μg/l, measured after five doses. Full dosage should be given initially to those with renal impairment and then reduced if necessary.

Pentamidine

The usual dose is 4 mg/kg, given by slow intravenous infusion over 90 min. There is considerable tissue binding and the drug is excreted in the urine over long periods. The dose should be reduced in patients with renal impairment and, since the drug is nephrotoxic, the dose should be reduced by 30 to 50 per cent if the serum creatinine increases by 88 μmol/l (1 mg/dl).

Antituberculous chemotherapy

Rifampicin and isoniazid (given with pyridoxine) are given in the usual doses. Rifampicin is a potent inducer of the cytochrome P-450 system and will therefore affect cyclosporin metabolism. The dosage of ethambutol and pyrazinamide needs to be reduced. Capreomycin is nephrotoxic and, although streptomycin can be used, careful monitoring after each dose is required.

Antiviral agents

Aciclovir and ganciclovir are both eliminated by the kidney and both are dialysed. Similar dose reductions are needed for each (see Table 5). Antiretroviral drugs such as lamivudine, zalcitabine, and zidovudine all need reduced dosage.

Antifungal agents

Amphotericin is nephrotoxic: it should only be used with great caution in patients who already have renal impairment and discontinued if the plasma creatinine concentration exceeds 260 μmol/l. Liposomal amphotericin avoids this toxicity. Amphotericin is cleared by haemodialysis and should therefore be given after treatment. Both flucytosine and fluconazole are excreted in the urine. Fluconazole should be given at a dose of 200 mg/day after an initial dose of 400 mg. Ketoconazole is less well absorbed in renal failure and interferes with cyclosporin metabolism through action on the cytochrome P-450 system (see Table 7).

Table 7 Drugs affecting the cytochrome P-450 system

Inhibitors	Ketoconazole
	Erythromycin
	Oral contraceptives
	Methylprednisolone
	Diltiazem
	Nicardipine
	Verapamil
	Cimetidine
Inducers	Rifampicin
	Phenytoin
	Phenobarbitone
	Carbamazepine
	Sodium valproate

Antiprotozoal agents and malaria

Quinine is given in the usual doses unless acute renal failure develops, in which case the dose is reduced after two to three days. The dose of chloroquine is reduced by half if the glomerular filtration rate is less than 50 ml/min and to a quarter if the glomerular filtration rate is less than 10 ml/min; primaquine is given in the usual doses. For prophylaxis chloroquine (usual dose 300 mg/week) can be given to patients with renal impairment. Proguanil (usual dose 200 mg daily) should be given in half the usual dose if the glomerular filtration rate is less than 10 ml/min. Mefloquine has been used in haemodialysis patients in a dose of 250 mg weekly: it is not cleared by dialysis and no adverse effects were reported.

Drugs acting on the central nervous system

Drugs acting on the central nervous system may have a prolonged effect in renal failure, not only because of changes in pharmacokinetics, but also because of increased sensitivity as a consequence of uraemia.

Antidepressants

The data on antidepressant drugs are conflicting, but all should be used with caution. Tricyclics are given in the usual dosage. Fluoxetine, paroxetine, and other selective serotonin reuptake inhibitors have been used widely in patients on dialysis, although dosage reductions are advised. It is best to avoid citalopram and venaflaxine.

Lithium

Lithium is filtered and then reabsorbed, mainly in the proximal tubule. The dose should be reduced in renal impairment with careful monitoring of plasma concentration. In sodium depletion (for example with chronic use of thiazide diuretics) tubular reabsorption of lithium is increased, leading to higher plasma concentrations and toxicity. Lithium is a cause of chronic tubulointerstitial damage.

Major tranquillizers

No dose change is required when phenothiazines or butyrophenones are used in patients with renal impairment. Newer drugs such as clozapine, rispiridone, and sulpiride should be used with caution.

Minor tranquillizers

Benzodiazepines can be prescribed in the usual dosage. Diazepam and chlordiazepoxide have active metabolites that may accumulate in renal failure: drugs without active metabolites such as nitrazepam and temazepam may avoid hangover the morning after use as night sedation.

Anticonvulsants

Phenytoin, carbamazepine, and valproic acid are given in the usual dosage. Protein binding of phenytoin is reduced in renal impairment with a rise in the free (active) fraction such that plasma or serum levels may need to be adjusted downwards. Vigabatrin and gabapentin need dose reduction.

Antihistamines

Terfenadine should be avoided because of prolongation of the QT interval, perhaps made more likely in renal impairment. Prochlorperazine and chlorpheniramine are used in the usual dosage but may cause drowsiness.

Treatment of hyperlipidaemia and diabetes mellitus

Lipid lowering agents

There is now wide experience in the use of HMG-coenzyme A reductase inhibitors. Simvastatin and pravastatin are given in the usual doses, that of fluvastatin is reduced. All may cause myopathy and myositis, particularly in renal impairment or if used with cyclosporin or gemfibrizol. The fibrates (gemfibrizol, bezafibrate) can be used with dose reduction at a glomerular filtration rate of less than 20 ml/min.

Insulin

Insulin requirements fall with declining renal function, probably as a consequence of the reduced metabolism of insulin by the kidney in both acute and chronic renal failure. In patients on haemodialysis it is often necessary to give supplemental insulin during treatment. The same situation applies in patients on haemofiltration for acute renal failure, particularly if they are being fed parenterally, and in continuous haemodiafiltration when the dialysate is a glucose-based solution. Non-diabetic patients may require insulin temporarily under these circumstances. Patients on continuous ambulatory peritoneal dialysis may need a change in insulin preparation and adjustment in the frequency and route of administration. The intraperitoneal requirement is approximately 50 per cent of that needed intravenously.

Oral hypoglycaemic agents

Glicazide, gliquidone, and glipizide are the safest drugs to use, although dose reduction may be needed if the glomerular filtration rate is below 10 ml/min. Other sulphonylureas, particularly chlopropamide, have a prolonged half-life. The biguanides should not be used if the glomerular filtration rate is below 20 ml/min.

Treatment of asthma

β-Agonists administered by inhalation, oral, or parenteral routes need no adjustment in patients with renal impairment, although tobuterol is an exception. Aminophylline and theophylline can be given in the usual doses but metabolites may accumulate. The leukotrione antagonist zafirlukast (but not montelukast) needs dosage reduction.

Treatment of gastrointestinal disorders

H_2-Antagonists and antiulcer drugs

Cimetidine is cleared by the liver but metabolites accumulate if the glomerular filtration rate is less than 20 ml/min. Ranitidine, which causes less cerebral confusion, is preferable in this situation, but may interfere with creatinine secretion and raises plasma creatinine. It is partly cleared by the kidneys (in common with famotidine) and the dose should be halved when the glomerular filtration rate less than 10 ml/min. It is dialysed, and a supplemental dose is needed after dialysis but not after haemofiltration. Omeprazole and misoprostol are given in the usual doses. Misoprostol may cause reductions in glomerular filtration rate through haemodynamic changes in the kidney.

Antacids

Alginates, magnesium trisilicate mixture (but not magnesium trisilicate powder), and sodium bicarbonate all have high sodium contents. The use of aluminium containing compounds, such as aluminium hydroxide or sulcralfate, in patients with severe renal impairment or those on dialysis is controversial because of the potential risks of aluminium retention with deleterious effects on bone, bone marrow, and the central nervous system. Calcium carbonate should not be used as an antacid but only as a phosphate binder.

Treatment of hyperuricaemia and gout

Allopurinol

Allopurinol is metabolized to oxypurinol, which is retained in renal impairment and may be responsible for some of the adverse effects including rashes, bone marrow depression, and gastrointestinal upset. The dose should be reduced to 100 mg/day when the glomerular filtration rate is less than 20 ml/min. The dose should be given after haemodialysis. Allopurinol interferes with the metabolism of 6-mercaptopurine (an active metabolite of azathioprine) causing accumulation and toxicity (for example leucopenia).

Probenecid

Probenecid inhibits secretion of acids in the proximal tubule and prevents reabsorption of urate from the tubular lumen. It prolongs the effect of penicillins, cephalosporins, naproxen, indomethacin, methotrexate, and sulphonylureas (all of which are weak acids), causing accumulation and the potential for toxicity. It also inhibits tubular secretion (and hence activity) of furosemide (frusemide) and bumetanide.

Colchicine

Colchicine has been largely replaced by non-steroidal anti-inflammatory drugs (see above) for the treatment of acute gout. However, it remains valuable in patients in whom non-steroidal anti-inflammatory drugs are undesirable (for example in those with peptic ulcer disease, cardiac failure, or renal impairment), and can be used without dose adjustment in renal failure.

Treatment or prevention of thrombosis and thromboembolism: anticoagulants and antiplatelet agents

Warfarin is used in the normal dosage and its effect is monitored by measuring prothrombin time in the usual way. It is highly protein bound and there may be slight displacement and consequent reduction in the volume of distribution in uraemia. In nephrotic patients hypoalbuminaemia leads to an increased sensitivity to warfarin, which is not removed by dialysis. Heparin is used in the normal dosage, but dosage reduction is required for tinzaparin. Prophylactic aspirin is given in the usual low dose (75–150 mg/day), but the dosages of clodiprogel and ticlopidine should be reduced.

Treatment of autoimmune rheumatic or vasculitic disorders: corticosteroids and immunosuppressive agents

Prednisone and prednisolone are not eliminated by the kidney. Methylprednisolone is cleared by haemodialysis, and should be given after dialysis. Azathioprine accumulates in renal impairment and the dose should be reduced from a maximum of 3 mg/kg/day to 1 mg/kg/day if the glomerular filtration rate falls below 10 ml/min. The dose of cyclophophamide, if given intravenously for systemic lupus erythematosus or systemic vasculitis, should be at the lower end of the therapeutic range with careful monitoring of the blood count before further doses are given.

Methotrexate is used frequently in rheumatological disorders (rheumatoid arthritis, psoriatic arthropathy), usually as a small (7.5 to 20 mg) weekly dose. It should be noted that the drug is a weak acid and is eliminated by proximal tubular secretion, which can be blocked by salicylates or non-steroidal drugs.

Cyclosporin is a highly lipid soluble drug that is extensively bound to plasma proteins and has a large volume of distribution. It is metabolized in the liver via the cytochrome P-450 system by mono- and dihydroxylation as well as *N*-demethylation. Only minor amounts are excreted as the parent drug or metabolites in the urine. Renal impairment does not affect its metabolism. However, since many other drugs may be prescribed to patients on cyclosporin therapy, several important interactions may occur. These may both increase plasma concentration and therefore increase the risk of nephrotoxicity, or reduce plasma concentrations to increase the risk of transplant organ rejection. Aminoglycosides may have an additive effect upon the nephrotoxicity itself. The common interactions are listed in Table 7.

Miscellaneous drugs

Acetazolamide

Acetazolamide may produce electrolyte disturbance, particularly in renal impairment and in the elderly. Its use should be avoided or carefully monitored.

Bisphosphonates

It is appropriate to use intravenous disodium pamidronate or etidronate in hypercalcaemia caused by malignancy, even if this is causing renal failure. The likely outcome is an improvement in renal function, particularly if other measures such as sodium and water depletion are addressed. Bisphosphonates (with the exception of alendronic acid) can be used to treat post-menopausal or corticosteroid induced osteoporosis and Paget's disease, with dosage reduced in moderate renal impairment. Etidronate may cause hypercalcaemia if combined with calcium supplementation.

Anticancer drugs

The kidney excretes many anticancer drugs or their metabolites, and doses need to be calculated with accurate measurements of glomerular filtration rate (for example cisplatin). It is important to obtain appropriate information before prescribing.

Summary

- Always check the method of elimination of any drug before prescribing in the presence of known or suspected renal impairment.
- Monitor any changes in renal function.
- Look out for any adverse or side-effects.

Further reading

Barclay ML, Kirkpatrick CMJ, Begg EJ (1999). Once daily aminoglycoside therapy. *Clinical Pharmacokinetics* **36**, 89–98.

Bellisant E, Sebilla V, Vaintand G. (1998). Methodological issues in pharmaco-pharmacodynamic modeling. *Clinical Pharmacokinetics* **35**, 151–66.

Benet LZ, Kroetz DL, Sheiner LB (1996). Pharmacokinetics: the dynamics of drug, absorption, distribution, and elimination. In: Hardman JG and Limberd LE, eds. *Goodman and Gilman's the pharmacological basis of therapeutics*, section I, pp 3–28. McGraw-Hill New York.

Benet LZ, Zia-Amirhossaini P (1995). Basic principles of pharmacokinetics. *Toxicology and Pathology* **23**, 115–23.

Bohler J, Donauer J, Keller F (1999). Pharmacokinetic principles during continuous renal replacement therapy: drugs and dosage. *Kidney International* **72**, S24–S28.

Bonate PL, Reith K, Weir S (1998). Drug interactions at a renal level. *Clinical Pharmackinetics* **34**, 375–404.

Carmichael DJS (1998). Handling of drugs in kidney disease. In: Davison AM *et al.*, eds. *Oxford textbook of clinical nephrology*, pp.2659–78. Oxford University Press, Oxford.

Czock D, Keller F (1999). The area under the effect-time curve as a target for dosage adaptation in renal insufficiency. *Nephrology, Dialysis and Transplantation* **14** (suppl. 4), 4.

Davies G, Kingswood C, Street M (1996). Pharmacokinetics of opiods in renal dysfunction. *Clinical Pharmacokinetics* **31**, 410–22.

Golper TA, Marx MA (1998). Drug dosing adjustments during continuous renal replacement therapies. *Kidney International* **66**, S165–S168.

Hammertstein A, Derendorf H, Lowenthal DT (1998). Pharmacokinetic and pharmacodynamic changes in the elderly. *Clinical Pharmacokinetics* **35**, 49–64.

Joos B, Schmidli M, Keusch G (1996). Pharmacokinetics of antimicrobial agents in anuric patients during continous venovenous haemofiltration. *Nephrology, Dialysis and Transplantation* **11**, 1582–5.

Keller F *et al.* (1999). Individualized drug dosage in patients treated with continuous hemofiltration. *Kidney International* **72**, S29–S31.

Keller F, Czock D (1999) Pharmacodynamic half-life and effect-time in renal impairment. *Nephrology, Dialysis and Transplantation* **14** (suppl. 4), 6–8.

Kramer BK, Schweda F, Riegger GAJ (1999). Diuretic treatment and diuretic resistance in heart failure. *American Journal Of Medicine* **106**, 90–6.

Joest M, Ritz E, Mutschler E (1999). Renal handling of drugs in the healthy elderly. *European Journal of Clinical Pharmacology* **55**, 205–11.

Laville M *et al.* (1989). Restrictions on use of creatinine clearance for measurement of renal functional reserve. *Nephron* **51**, 233–6.

Taylor CA *et al.* (1996). Clinical pharmacokinetics during continuous ambulatory peritoneal dialysis. *Clinical Pharmackinetics* **31**, 293–308.

Toxbase http://www.spib.axl.co.uk/toxbaseindex.htm.

21

Sexually-transmitted diseases and sexual health

21.1 Epidemiology

M. W. Adler and A. Meheus

Table 1 Micro-organisms that can be sexually transmitted

Bacteria	**Viruses**
Chlamydia trachomatis	Human immunodeficiency virus 1 and 2
Neisseria gonorrhoeae	Herpes simplex virus types 1 and 2
Treponema pallidum	Wart virus (human papillomavirus)
Haemophilus ducreyi	Hepatitis A, B, and C virus
Calymmatobacterium granulomatis	Molluscum contagiosum virus (poxvirus)
Gardnerella vaginalis	Cytomegalovirus
Shigella spp.	
	Protozoa
Mycoplasmas	*Entamoeba histolytica*
Ureaplasma urealyticum	*Giardia lamblia*
Mycoplasma hominis	*Trichomonas vaginalis*
Arthropods	**Fungi**
Sarcoptes scabiei	*Candida albicans*
Phthirus pubis	

Introduction

The sexually transmitted infections (**STIs**) are mainly spread by sexual intercourse (Table 1). However, some, such as genital candidosis, are only rarely spread in this way; others, like scabies and pediculosis pubis, are spread by close bodily contact without penetrative intercourse. The range of diseases spread by sexual activity continues to increase, with familiar bacterial and treponemal infections now being superseded in developed countries by herpes, warts, and human immunodeficiency virus infection (**HIV**). The detrimental effect of STIs on pregnancy and the newborn (for example, miscarriage, prematurity, congenital and neonatal infections, blindness) are more common and severe than had previously been realized. Furthermore, complications such as pelvic inflammatory disease, ectopic pregnancy, infertility, and cervical cancer are major health problems. The World Bank in 1993 estimated that for women aged 15 to 44 years, STIs, excluding HIV infection, were second only to maternal morbidity and mortality as causes of healthy lives lost.

Their incidence, distribution, and risk of complications is strongly influenced by a wide array of determining factors, including behavioural and sociocultural factors, population composition, susceptibility of individuals, changing characteristics of pathogens, and society's efforts at primary prevention and disease control.

Since the advent of HIV/AIDS, increased attention is being given to the other STIs, because they are important causes of morbidity and mortality in their own right and are important markers of behaviour associated with a high risk of HIV transmission. Some 80 per cent of HIV infection is spread sexually. STIs, especially genital ulcer disease, can enhance the acquisition and transmission of HIV by damaging the mucosa or skin, due to increases in HIV-susceptible macrophages and increased viral shedding.

The global burden of STIs is unknown because of the lack of effective control and notification systems in some countries. The World Health Organization (WHO) has estimated a total of 340 million new cases of curable STDs in adults per annum, mainly in South-East Asia (151 million new cases per year) and Sub-Saharan Africa (69 million). In Eastern Europe and Central Asia, the estimate is 22 million, and 17 million in Western Europe. The prevalence and incidence varies regionally: for instance, between Sub-Saharan Africa and Western Europe, 4.6- and 3.3-fold, respectively (Table 2).

The diseases

The accuracy of European data suffers from the reluctance of private doctors, who may see most of the patients, to notify the appropriate authorities. Notification systems include STD clinics (United Kingdom, France, Italy), laboratory/systems (Denmark, Sweden), and sentinel general practitioner (**GP**) systems (Belgium).

In the United Kingdom, a notification system was established in 1916, which also provided a free and confidential service for people with sexually transmitted infections. This service, mainly run outside hospitals, was integrated into the hospital structure following the creation of the National Health Service in 1948. At that time, syphilis and gonorrhoea made up the majority of the 132 000 cases diagnosed in clinics in England and Wales. Since then, the number of people attending clinics has increased exponentially and the disease profile has changed (Fig. 1). Gonorrhoea and syphilis now represent less than 2 per cent of all cases seen, while the new viral diseases, in particular genital warts and herpes, increased by 236 per cent and 160 per cent, respectively, between 1980 and 2000.

Gonorrhoea

Although rates of gonorrhoea vary between countries, there was a general upward trend over most of the last 40 or so years, with a flattening out in the mid-1970s and a subsequent decrease in the number of cases reported

Table 2 Estimated prevalence and incidence of STIs by region

Region	Prevalence per million	Incidence per million
Sub-Saharan Africa	32	69
South and South-East Asia	48	151
Latin America and Caribbean	18.5	38
Eastern Europe and Central Asia	6	22
North America	3	14
Australasia	0.3	1
Western Europe	4	17
Northern Africa and Middle East	3.5	10
East Asia and Pacific	6	18
Total	116.5	340

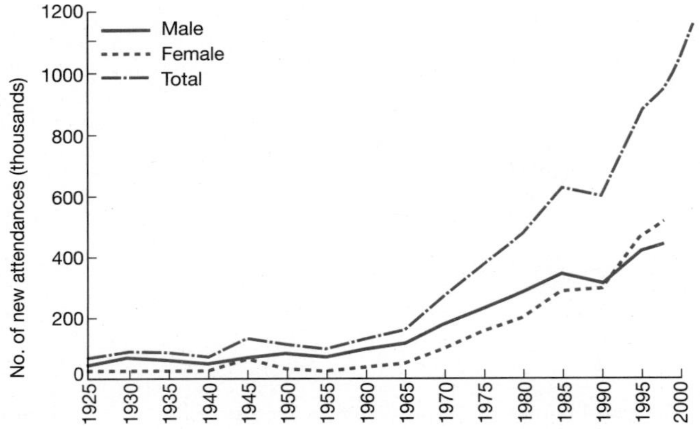

Fig. 1 New attendance at genitourinary medicine (**GUM**) clinics England and Wales 1925–2000.

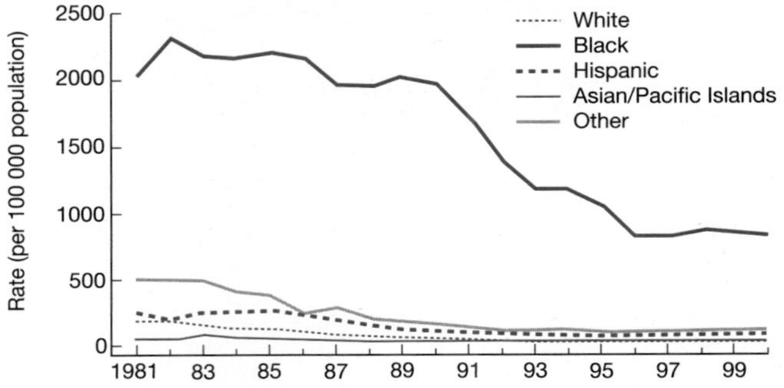

Fig. 3 Gonorrhoea—rates by race and ethnicity: United States, 1981–2000, and the 'Healthy People year 2000 objective'. 'Other' includes Asian/Pacific Islander and Native American/Alaskan populations. Georgia did not report gonorrhoea statistics in 1994.

with recent increases in some countries. It is difficult to interpret differences between countries because of the variation in reporting practices and the provision of facilities.

Data tend to be more complete in developed countries. However, standards vary and countries like the United Kingdom, which has a network of genitourinary medicine/STD clinics and routine notification requirements, produce more accurate figures than some other European and North American countries where most patients are treated by private physicians who do not usually report cases. There was a peak in the number of cases of gonorrhoea during the early to mid-1970s in most European countries. The advent of AIDS/HIV infection in the 1980s led to safer sexual practices and a reduction in the number of cases of gonorrhoea, but this has not been sustained in all countries. Recently, there has been a substantial increase in both male and female cases of gonorrhoea in England and Wales. Between 1995 and 2000 there was a 105 per cent increase in the number of cases in men, from 6759 to 14 231, and in females an 85 per cent increase from 3394 to 6289. In males, this increase was seen in all age groups, particularly in those aged 16 to 19 and 35 to 44 years, but in females, it was mostly in teenagers. The incidence of gonorrhoea has increased since 1993 in homosexual men, particularly in those living in London and its immediate surrounding area.

In Nordic countries, the annual incidence of gonorrhoea declined (Fig. 2) from over 100 per 100 000 population in most countries in the early 1980s to less than 10 per 100 000 population by the late 1990s, but there have been recent slight increases. Although the incidence of gonorrhoea has declined in the United States, there are considerable differences between ethnic groups (Fig. 3). In 2000 there was a total of 358 995 cases.

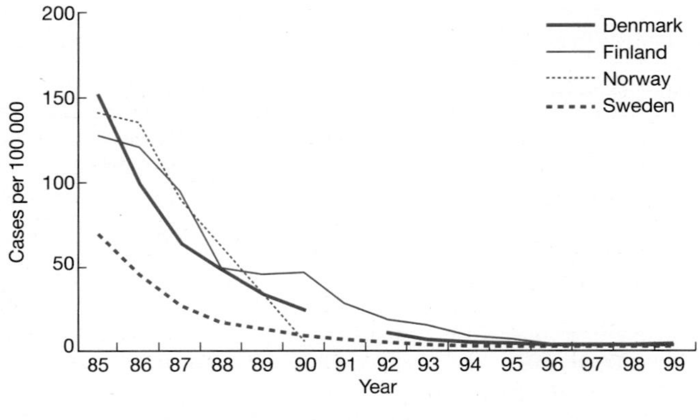

Fig. 2 Annual incidence of gonorrhoea per 100 000 population in Nordic countries.

There is an epidemic of STIs in Eastern Europe, in the newly independent states of the former Soviet Union. The highest rates of gonorrhoea are in Estonia (166), Russia (139), and Belarus (125) per 100 000, compared to France 18.5, Germany 5, The Netherlands 8, and the United Kingdom 22 per 100 000.

Syphilis

The dramatic impact of penicillin on the incidence of early infectious syphilis throughout the world in the 1950s has not been maintained everywhere. The United States has experienced a continuous increase in the total number of cases of primary and secondary syphilis of seven- to ninefold in males and females, respectively, since 1956. These increases were particularly noticeable in the 1990s and are partly explained by the deployment of resources away from traditional STD control programmes to those for AIDS. However, the control of HIV and AIDS will only come through integrated STD/AIDS control programmes.

In most Western European countries, but particularly in Scandinavia, there has been a decline in incidence to below 5 per 100 000. However, in Eastern Europe there is an epidemic of syphilis in all Newly Independent States (**NIS**) of the former Soviet Union. The 1999 incidence of syphilis in these NIS ranged from 55 to 180 per 100 000 (Fig. 4); increases are particularly evident in older adolescents. Between 1986 and 1996, the incidence of syphilis increased in 18- to 19-year-old Russians, from 6 to 607 per 100 000

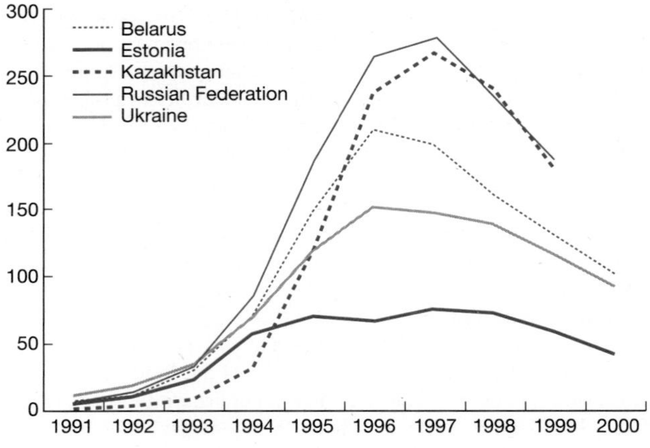

Fig. 4 Annual incidence of syphilis in Belarus, Estonia, Kazakhstan, the Republic of Moldova, the Russian Federation, and Ukraine, 1990–2000 (rate per 100 000 of the population).

in men and from 20 to 1321 per 100 000 in women. The increase in Russia between 1992 and 1996 was 20-fold, Estonia 6-fold, Latvia 12-fold, and Lithuania 14-fold. An HIV/AIDS epidemic can be predicted in Eastern Europe, and already there have been outbreaks of HIV among intravenous drug users, particularly in Belarus, Russia, and Ukraine.

There has been an encouraging fall in the incidence of congenital syphilis in developed countries, largely due to the control of early acquired infectious syphilis in women and the screening of all pregnant women for syphilis. However, congenital syphilis is still a major health problem in the countries of the former Soviet Union and in many developing countries.

Chlamydia

The introduction of antigen detection tests such as direct immunofluorescence techniques and enzyme immunoassays in the 1990s, and, more recently, sensitive nucleic acid detection-based tests such as polymerase or ligase chain reactions, has allowed a more widespread screening for chlamydia in most European countries. After the start of wide-scale screening in Sweden during the 1980s, the number of cases declined from 38 000 in 1987 to 14 000 by 1997, with an associated decrease in ectopic pregnancies.

In England and Wales there has been no such decline, and chlamydia remains a major public health problem; long-term sequelae associated with chlamydial infection include pelvic inflammatory disease, ectopic pregnancy, infertility, and abdominal pain. Genital *Chlamydia trachomatis* infection is now the commonest curable bacterial STI in England and Wales. There has been an increase in the number of cases since 1993, with females outnumbering males; in 2000, 63 037 people attended clinics—27 222 males, 35 815 females. It is commonest in young people: the peak age in men is between 20 and 24 years, and between 16 and 19 in women. Screening surveys carried out in antenatal and gynaecological clinics, general practice, family planning units prior to pregnancy termination, and those attending STD clinics have shown median prevalences ranging from 4.5 to 16.4 per cent. Similar prevalence rates have been seen in the United States. The increased availability of Chlamydia testing and more sensitive detection tests will, to some extent, account for the apparent increase in the number of cases seen.

Genital herpes and warts

The greatest increase in STIs in England and Wales during the 1980s was in the number of reported cases of genital herpes and warts. In 1978, 8406 cases of herpes and 24 136 of warts were seen in STD clinics, increasing to 30 199 and 100 124, respectively, by 2000 (Fig. 5). Compared to Chlamydia and gonorrhoea there has been a slowing down in the increase in the last few years.

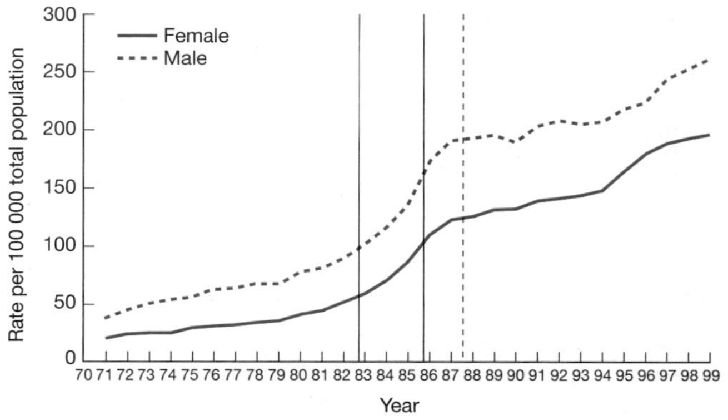

Fig. 5 New cases of genital warts infection seen in GUM clinics, 1970–1999 (England).

Genital herpes

There are between 200 000 and 500 000 new cases of herpes each year in the United States, with a prevalence of approximately 40 million cases. These extrapolations from STD clinic data may not be valid, for most of these patients attending such clinics are of lower socioeconomic status and unrepresentative of the whole population. In a Swedish STD clinic, herpes simplex virus (**HSV**) was isolated from the cervices of 8.4 per cent of all female attenders.

HSV-1 and -2 antibody tests allow prevalence studies to be carried out in different populations. In the United Kingdom, HSV-2 seroprevalence is low in blood donors (3 per cent in men, 12 per cent in women), intermediate in pregnant women (4 per cent in those under 20 years of age, 11 per cent in the 20 to 29 age group, and 16 per cent in those over 29 years), and high in STD clinic attenders (21 per cent in men, 25 per cent in women). In the United States, the pattern is similar but rates are approximately twice as high.

In the United Kingdom, STD clinic attenders showed an increasing proportion of HSV-1 genital infections during the 1980s and early 1990s. HSV-1 now accounts for most first episodes in women. The proportion of HSV-1 in genital specimens was 48 to 68 per cent in women, 25 to 35 per cent in men. In the United States most genital infections are caused by HSV-2.

Genital human papillomavirus (HPV)

Genital warts is now the commonest sexually transmitted disease seen in STD clinics in England and Wales (100 124 cases in 2000). They are difficult and time-consuming to treat. HPV infection is of particular concern because certain types are associated with cervical dysplasia and cervical cancer (see Chapter 7.10.17).

Pelvic inflammatory disease

Pelvic inflammatory disease (**PID**) is the most serious complication following gonococcal, chlamydial, and non-specific infections. Its incidence and prevalence is increasing in most countries. In Western industrialized countries its estimated annual incidence is 10 per 1000 women aged 15 to 39 years, with a peak incidence of 20 per 1000 in the age group 15 to 24 years. Risk factors include STIs, the use of intrauterine devices (**IUDs**), and postabortion and puerperal infections.

STIs cause most cases of PID. In developed countries, 75 per cent of cases in under 25-year-old women are attributable to STIs. In Uppsala, 50 per cent of patients with PID in 1965 had cervical gonorrhoea, but by 1975 this had dropped to approximately 10 to 15 per cent, at which time *Chlamydia trachomatis* was found to be responsible for 60 per cent of cases.

The most serious consequence of PID is infertility (see Chapter 21.4). It is difficult to obtain accurate data on the trends for PID since not all patients are hospitalized or correctly diagnosed.

STD epidemiology in developing countries

The frequency of STIs is much higher in developing countries. They are among the top five causes of consultation at general health services in many African countries. The incidence and prevalence of these infections are very high in specific population groups, such as female prostitutes and their clients. Prostitution is an important factor in the transmission of STIs in developing countries.

Genital ulcers are much more frequent. The so-called 'tropical STIs'—in particular chancroid and, to a lesser degree, lymphogranuloma venereum and granuloma inguinale—are major causes. More genital ulcers in developing countries are caused by syphilis than in industrialized countries; genital herpes accounts for a smaller proportion, but has become the leading cause of genital ulcers in areas of high HIV/AIDS incidence.

The incidence of STI complications and their sequelae is much higher in developing countries due to the lack of resources for adequate diagnosis and treatment. Important STI complications and sequelae include adverse pregnancy outcome for mother and newborn, neonatal and infant infections, infertility in both sexes, ectopic pregnancy, urethral stricture in males, blindness in infants due to gonococcal and chlamydial ophthalmia neonatorum and in adults due to gonococcal keratoconjunctivitis, as well as genital cancers, particularly cancer of the cervix uteri and penis.

The epidemiology of HIV infection and AIDS is very different from that in Western countries: level of sexual activity, not sexual orientation is, apparently, the major risk factor. HIV is predominantly transmitted heterosexually in developing countries. Genital ulceration, and other STIs, facilitate the sexual transmission of HIV. Many governments and international donor agencies have tended to ignore the real magnitude of the problem. It needed a fatal STI to alert decision-makers worldwide and the community to the STI problem and to generate resources for its prevention and control.

Control

Prevention is more effective and cheaper than treatment. The objectives of STI control are to interrupt the transmission of STIs, to prevent their development, complications, and sequelae and to reduce the risk of sexual transmission of HIV. These aims can be achieved by primary and secondary prevention and comprehensive patient care (Table 3).

Primary prevention

Primary prevention is achieved through health promotion (information, education, communication—**IEC**) and counselling activities (see Chapter 3.5). The aim is to educate people about the advantages of discriminative sex and prophylaxis ('safer sex'). Clearly, the best way to avoid STIs is to avoid sexual intercourse. This may not be acceptable to those who are already sexually active, but the dangers of frequent changes of sexual partners and the methods of reducing the risk must be emphasized. It is essential to use a condom to avoid contact with partners who have symptoms or lesions, and to have regular check-ups. This must be taught to children before they become sexually active. The best place for this is at home or school in the context of growing up, understanding one's body, and being responsible for one's own health. Since the arrival of HIV infection and AIDS, sexuality has become less of a taboo in many countries. Health workers and health educators must, therefore, take advantage of this new openness. Through mass media campaigns targeted at the general public, IECs have become part of STD/AIDS control nearly everywhere.

A special target group for health promotion and individual counselling are patients with STIs; such infections prove them to be at risk of contracting STIs, including HIV infection. Their current infection and the awareness of their vulnerability might make STD patients more inclined to change risky sexual behaviour.

Table 3 Structure of a control programme for sexually transmitted infections (STIs)

Intervention strategies		Support components	
1.	Health promotion/counselling: vaccination (HBV) (= primary prevention)	1.	Professional training
		2.	Laboratory service
2.	Early detection of infection (= secondary prevention)	3.	Research
		4.	Information system/ surveillance
3.	Appropriate management of patients with STI: diagnosis and treatment, counselling, contact tracing (= comprehensive care)		

No effective vaccines are as yet available for STIs, apart from that for hepatitis-B virus (**HBV**).

Secondary prevention

Here the aim is to detect STIs early through screening ('check-up') and by education about what to do once disease is suspected (healthcare-seeking behaviour). Sexual intercourse should be stopped until medical care has been sought. Education should indicate how and where such advice can be found, and emphasize the importance of adhering to the treatment and advice.

Screening aims to detect asymptomatic or mildly symptomatic infections, and is carried out in specific populations if the prevalence of STIs is high. Good laboratory support is essential. Pregnant women may be screened for syphilis, HIV, or chlamydial infection. Where prostitution is legal or tolerated, prostitutes can be screened for various STIs. Blood donors are screened for HIV, HBV, and syphilis.

Adequate and comprehensive management of STI patients

The management of infected patients is a cornerstone of STI control. The aims of patient care are: to detect or rule out infection; to give treatment if necessary; to educate and counsel on treatment compliance and on STD/HIV prevention and condom use; to ensure that sexual partner(s) are evaluated and managed (contact tracing); and eventually to test for other STIs, including HIV infection. In a developed country, it is not appropriate to attempt the management of STIs without microbiological facilities, since doctors providing care in these countries usually have specialist knowledge of the diseases. However, in developing countries with limited resources, it is more realistic to use a syndromic approach based on STI signs, symptoms, and simple laboratory tests. To implement major intervention strategies, the following support components need to be developed:

- *Training* should be given to health workers and health educators, for instance in the use of flow-charts to simplify the management of STD patients, or to strengthen their health education and counselling skills.
- *Laboratory services* need to be expanded, depending on the level of healthcare provided. A reference laboratory should be developed in each country to allow the quality control and analysis of referred specimens.
- *Research* should be undertaken to include epidemiological and sociobehavioural baseline studies, assessment of antimicrobial sensitivity, as well as operational research to render the programme more cost-effective.
- *Information systems* or surveillance should be implemented to gather epidemiological data for magnitude and trend assessments, and to provide data for programme planning and monitoring. Various surveillance methods can be used—clinician notification, laboratory notification, sentinel site surveillance (either of syndromes or of aetiological diagnoses), prevalence studies in specific population groups, and aetiological surveys in patients.

Conclusion

A successful STI control programme, by reducing both the incidence and prevalence of STIs, will reduce the morbidity, suffering, and economic cost associated with these diseases. By eliminating STIs as a facilitating factor in HIV transmission, and by contributing to behavioural changes towards safer sex, it will play an important role in the prevention and control of HIV/AIDS.

Further reading

Adler MW (1998). *The ABC of sexually transmitted diseases*, 4th edition. British Medical Association, London.

Adler MW (1980). The terrible peril—a historical perspective on the venereal diseases. *British Medical Journal* **281**, 206–11.

Adler MW (1999). Cinderella and the glass slipper: the growth and modernisation of a specialty. *Sexually Transmitted Infections* **75**, 439–44.

Adler MW, *et al.* (1998). Sexual health and healthcare: sexually transmitted infections—guidelines for prevention and treatment. Department for International Development, London.

Arya OP, Hart CA, eds (1998). *Sexually transmitted infections and AIDS in the tropics.* CABI Publishing, Wallingford, Oxon, UK.

De Schryver A, Meheus A (1990). Epidemiology of sexually transmitted diseases: the global picture. *Bulletin of the World Health Organisation* **68**, 639–54.

Meheus A, Piot P (1986). Provision of services for sexually transmitted diseases in developing countries. In: Oriel, JD and Harris, JRW, eds. *Recent advances in STIs*, 3rd edn. Churchill Livingstone.

World Health Organization (1991). *Management of patients with sexually transmitted diseases.* WHO Technical Report Series 810. WHO, Geneva.

World Health Organization (1995). *An overview of selected curable sexually transmitted diseases.*

World Health Organization/United Nations Programme on HIV/AIDS (1997). *Sexually transmitted diseases: policies and principles for prevention and care*, pp 1–47. WHO/UNAIDS, Geneva.

21.2 Sexual behaviour

Anne M. Johnson

Most men and women are sexually active for a large part of their adult lives and sexual fulfilment is an important part of the quality of life. Patterns of sexual behaviour in populations are a key determinant of fertility and transmission of sexually transmitted infections (**STIs**).

Discussion of sexual lifestyle and the ability to take a sexual history is relevant to a wide range of clinical consultations. A few common examples include management of genitourinary symptoms, contraceptive advice, sexual dysfunction, and resumption of sexual activity following childbirth, major illnesses, and surgery.

Sexual orientation

Sexual behaviour studies in representative population samples show that the majority of men and women are predominantly attracted to, and have experience with, members of the opposite sex throughout their lives. However, sexual orientation is not a simple dichotomy between 'homosexual' and 'heterosexual', but varies between individuals from exclusively heterosexual experience through various shades of attraction and experience with both genders, to exclusively homosexual experience.

In a large-scale British study of adults aged between 16 and 44, 8.5 per cent of men and 9.7 per cent of women reported having had any sexual experience with someone of the same gender. For some this may be a fleeting experience in adolescence, with subsequent exclusively heterosexual partnerships. A smaller proportion of the British population report homosexual partnerships involving genital contact (5.4 per cent of men and 4.9 per cent of women). Similar findings are reported from surveys in France and the United States. Most of those with same-gender partners have also experienced heterosexual intercourse at some time in their lives. Exclusively homosexual experience throughout life is thus a relatively unusual phenomenon.

Homosexual experience is more common among men in large metropolitan areas. For example, 10.5 per cent of men sampled in Greater London reported ever having a homosexual partner. Capital cities typically provide a more tolerant atmosphere and better social facilities for those with a homosexual lifestyle. This is reflected in the high proportion of homosexually acquired STIs which are reported from clinics in London, and the higher rates of homosexually acquired HIV and AIDS reported in many metropolitan areas in Europe and the United States.

Age of first heterosexual intercourse

The age of first heterosexual intercourse has been gradually declining over recent decades. The proportion of people having sexual intercourse before marriage has rapidly increased so that sex before marriage has become almost universal in Britain. For men born in between 1930 and 1935, the median age of first intercourse was 20 and for women 21. For men and women born between 1965 and 1975, the median age at first intercourse was 17. Similar trends have been observed in France and the United States.

English law gives the age of consent for heterosexual intercourse as 16 and it is illegal for a man to have sex with a women under 16 in England. The proportion of men and women reporting first intercourse before the age of 16 has risen rapidly over recent decades to 30 per cent of men and 26 per cent of women aged between 16 and 19 in 2000 in Britain. This has important implications for the provision of sex education. Those who are embarking on their sexual careers may be most susceptible to the unwanted consequences of unprotected sexual intercourse. The incidence of sexually transmitted diseases and termination of pregnancy is higher among 16- to 24-year-olds than in older men and women.

Heterosexual partners

There is great variability between individuals in the number of reported heterosexual partners. While many people have few partners, a small proportion have many. Among 16- to 44-year-old men in Britain, 51 per cent reported having none or one partner in the last 5 years; 8 per cent reported more than 10; and a small proportion reported hundreds or even thousands of partners in the course of their lives.

The risk of acquiring or transmitting an STI increases with the number of sexual partners. Those with high numbers of partners may account for a relatively high proportion of STI transmission in a society, and for sustaining endemic STI transmission. They are sometimes referred to as a 'core group for STI transmission'. The choice of partner also influences STI transmission in populations. Age, gender, and ethnic mixing are important, as well as the extent to which people choose partners with similar lifestyles to their own (assortative mixing) or different from their own (disassortative); and whether they have serially monogamous or concurrent partnerships.

Prostitutes and their clients remain at high risk of contracting HIV and STI in some parts of the developing world where condoms are rarely used. In some countries, such as Thailand, public health campaigns have recently led to considerable success in increasing the use of condoms during client and prostitute contacts. In many developed countries, although prostitutes are at increased risk of STIs, they use condoms frequently to protect both themselves and their clients.

The proportion of men who use prostitutes varies widely between countries. In the British survey, 4 per cent of men reported having paid money for sex with a woman in the last 5 years but considerably more frequent exposure is reported in other countries.

Multiple heterosexual partnerships are most common among the young, and among those who are neither married nor cohabiting. Close to one in seven men between the ages of 16 and 24 in Britain reported more than 10 partners in the last 5 years, even though in this group a high proportion are not yet sexually active. Age *per se* is not the only influence on sexual behaviour. Whatever their age, those who are separated, divorced, or widowed are more likely than married people of a similar age to have multiple partners, illustrating the effects of the lifecourse on patterns of partnership formation. Since the emergence of the HIV epidemic, public health campaigns have emphasized the need for a change in sexual behaviour. STI incidence fell in the 1980s but rose again in the late 1990s. In Britain since there has been an increase in number of partners as well as an increase in condom use. In some parts of the developing world, such as Uganda and Thailand, there is evidence of a reduction in the incidence of HIV infection attributable to a recent change in behaviour.

Heterosexual practices

There is variability in the repertoire and frequency of sexual practices between individuals. In heterosexual relationships, vaginal intercourse is the most common practice, but most couples include other practices in their repertoire, particularly mutual masturbation and orogenital contact.

The frequency of sexual contact varies with age, lifestage, and the availability of a sexual partner. For married couples, the median frequency of sexual intercourse is in the order of four times per month, but this is highly variable. The frequency of intercourse appears to decline with age in married and cohabiting couples, although this is partly a function of the increasing length of their relationship.

Among 16- to 44-year-old men and women in Britain, close to 80 per cent reported experience of orogenital contact in the last year, with the majority of couples who experience any orogenital contact practising both cunnilingus and fellatio. There is evidence of an increasing practice of orogenital stimulation in recent decades. Mutual masturbation is also a common practice and has become more frequent in recent decades.

Anal intercourse is a relatively infrequent activity in heterosexual couples. In the British survey, 26 per cent of men and 24 per cent of women had experienced anal intercourse, but only around 12 per cent had experienced it in the last year. Anal intercourse can result in transmission of STIs. The practice of anal intercourse in addition to vaginal intercourse may increase the risk of heterosexual transmission of HIV. Since anal intercourse is a relatively infrequent practice in all parts of the world, most heterosexual HIV transmission worldwide is attributable to vaginal intercourse.

Homosexual behaviour

Male homosexual lifestyles have been rather more intensively studied than female homosexual lifestyles. Research in the 1970s of volunteer samples of homosexual men in the United States identified a particular lifestyle characterized by multiple casual sexual partners, often encountered at gay meeting places such as bars, clubs, and 'bath-houses'. These men were at high risk of contracting STIs and were among the first to suffer high rates of HIV infection. Research in Britain identified a group of homosexual men with similar lifestyles. However, studies of homosexual men recruited from sites other than STD clinics and gay meeting places show lower rates of sexual partner change and a lower prevalence of sexually acquired pathogens.

Men with multiple homosexual partnerships are at increased risk of HIV infection as well as other STIs, including hepatitis B and syphilis. Women with homosexual partnerships tend to be at low risk of STI and HIV as a result of their different sexual lifestyles and sexual practices, such as non-penetrative sex and orogenital contact.

Many male homosexual partnerships do not involve penetrative anal intercourse, but are restricted to mutual masturbation or orogenital contact. Anal intercourse, however, is the most important mode of transmission of sexually acquired organisms between homosexual men. Many men practise both anal receptive and insertive intercourse. Receptive anal intercourse is the highest risk behaviour for HIV transmission. Since the emergence of the HIV epidemic, there is evidence of a reduction in high-risk behaviour among gay men, characterized by increased condom use and reduced exposure to unprotected anal intercourse. However, there have been recent concerns of a resurgence in high-risk behaviour.

Risk-reduction strategies and sexual health

Increasing attention is being paid to promoting sexual health and reducing the adverse consequences of sexual behaviour. Extensive discussion of population strategies is outside the scope of this chapter. However, people can reduce their risk of STI and unwanted pregnancy by reducing the numbers of partners with whom they have unprotected intercourse, by using condoms, by using effective contraception, and by enjoying sexual practices that may reduce transmission risks. Negotiating sexual fulfilment is a more difficult matter, but greater focus on communication between partners, and sexual technique, is also important. Health professionals have an important role to play, not only by being well informed but by including tactful sexual history-taking among their clinical skills and by being concerned about sexual health and health promotion.

Further reading

ACSF investigators (1992). AIDS and sexual behaviour in France. *Nature* **360**, 407–9.

Cleland J, Ferry B (1995). *Sexual behaviour and AIDS in the developing world.* Taylor and Frances, London.

Johnson AM, *et al.* (1994). *Sexual attitudes and lifestyles.* Blackwell Scientific, Oxford.

Johnson AM, *et al.* (2001). Sexual behaviour in Britain: partnerships, practices, and HIV risk behaviours. *Lancet* **358**, 1835–42.

21.3 Vaginal discharge

J. Schwebke and S. L. Hillier

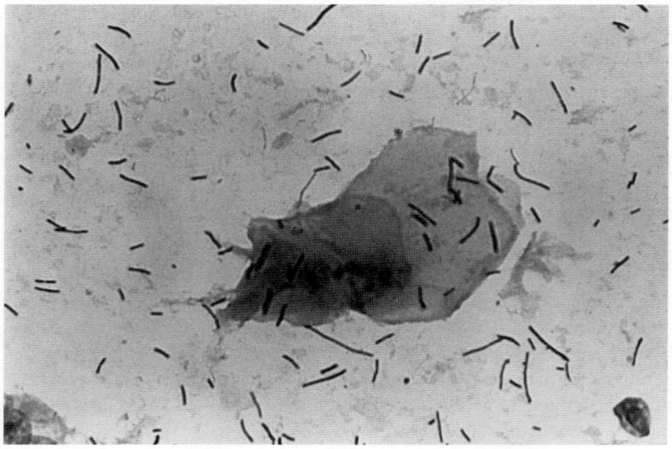

Fig. 1 Gram stain of normal vaginal fluid (copyright Dr Sharon Hillier).

Vaginal discharge is an extremely common reason for women to seek medical care, but its causes, treatment, and potential complications are poorly understood by patients and medical personnel. In the past, it has often been regarded as simply a nuisance. Only recently have accurate diagnosis and treatment of vaginal discharge been recognized as means of preventing future costly morbidity.

The healthy vagina

It is important to understand the normal vaginal ecosystem. At puberty the vagina becomes colonized predominantly with lactobacilli (Fig. 1). These Gram-positive facultative bacilli convert glucose to lactic acid, which helps maintain the normal vaginal pH at less than 4.5. This acidic environment helps to stabilize the ecosystem, as many pathogens, with the exception of *Candida* spp., are inhibited at this pH. Vaginal lactobacilli produce other antibacterial compounds, most notably hydrogen peroxide, which can inhibit the growth of bacterial vaginosis-associated pathogens *in vitro*. Women with peroxide-producing lactobacilli in the vagina are less likely to have gonorrhoea, chlamydial infection, trichomoniasis, or bacterial vaginosis.

Factors that alter the normal vaginal milieu and predispose the vagina to infection are poorly understood. They probably include hormonal and immunological factors as well as exogenous influences such as antimicrobial therapy, multiple sexual partners, and the use of vaginal douches.

Vaginitis and vaginosis

There are three main types of vaginal infections: trichomoniasis, bacterial vaginosis, and vulvovaginal candidiasis. Trichomoniasis is the only one known to be sexually transmitted, although bacterial vaginosis is most commonly seen in sexually active women and frequently coexists with sexually transmitted infections.

Trichomoniasis (see also Chapter 7.13.13)

Trichomoniasis is one of the few sexually transmitted infections that is more easily diagnosed in the female than in the male. In males, infection is usually asymptomatic and so they may be an important reservoir of infection. Annual worldwide incidence is estimated at 180 million cases. Prevalence varies with the population being studied. It is high among women attending sexually transmitted disease clinics. *Trichomonas* spp. and *Neisseria gonorrhoeae* are frequent coinfections. Symptomatic patients with trichomoniasis most frequently complain of discharge and vaginal pruritus. Intermenstrual or postcoital spotting may occur because the ectocervix is involved. Occasionally the urethra and Skene's glands may be infected, resulting in dysuria. Some 50 per cent of all infected women are probably asymptomatic.

Signs of trichomoniasis are vaginal discharge (42 per cent), odour (50 per cent), oedema or erythema (22–37 per cent). The often copious discharge is described as frothy and yellowish-green, but varies in consistency and colour and is actually frothy in only 8 to 12 per cent of women. Colpitis macularis ('strawberry cervix'), detected by colposcopy, is reported in almost half the patients and is the most specific clinical sign for trichomoniasis, but is rarely seen during routine examination.

Because the clinical signs and symptoms are not diagnostic, the organism should be sought either by direct wet-mount preparation or culture. Trichomonads are motile by means of flagella that can be seen beating even when the organism is at rest; the organism is about the size of a white blood cell (10–20 μm wide). The vaginal fluid contains numerous polymorphonuclear neutrophils because this disease is a true vaginitis, causing a local inflammatory response. The vaginal pH is usually elevated to above 4.5 and can be as high as 6.5 to 7.5. The background bacterial flora is often abnormal as bacterial vaginosis may also be present. The sensitivity of microscopical examination of the vaginal fluid for the diagnosis of trichomoniasis ranges from 40 to 80 per cent. Culture is the current diagnostic 'gold standard' but requires 2 to 5 days before a result can be obtained. As trichomoniasis can occur with other sexually transmitted diseases, screening should be carried out for gonococcal and chlamydial infections.

Treatment is with nitroimidazoles; metronidazole is most frequently used. A single oral dose of 2.0 g is preferred to 250 mg orally three times daily for 7 days because of better compliance and reduced total dosage. The use of nitroimidazoles is often complicated by gastrointestinal side-effects. Some strains of *T. vaginalis* are resistant to metronidazole, but treatment fails most often because the sexual partner has not been treated. For strains of *T. vaginalis* with decreased susceptibility to metronidazole, higher doses are given orally (up to 1 g three times daily), often in combination with intravaginal metronidazole.

New data link trichomoniasis with preterm labour, and no adverse outcomes of pregnancy have been associated with the use of metronidazole, therefore treatment during pregnancy is recommended.

Women in whom *T. vaginalis* is detected, but who are asymptomatic, should be treated as above. If left untreated they may later become symptomatic and, without treatment, they serve as an important reservoir for continued transmission of the disease. Furthermore, there is data which suggests that trichomoniasis may facilitate the transmission of the human immunodeficiency virus (**HIV**). Because *T. vaginalis* is sexually transmitted it is imperative that the male partners of women with trichomoniasis be treated empirically for *T. vaginalis* and screened for other sexually transmitted diseases.

Bacterial vaginosis

Bacterial vaginosis is the most common diagnosis made in women complaining of abnormal vaginal discharge. The microbiology of bacterial vaginosis is now much better understood, but not its pathogenesis. Recently, complications associated with bacterial vaginosis have been recognized, such as preterm birth, low birth weight, and infectious complications of pregnancy including postabortive endometritis, intra-amniotic infection, and postpartum endometritis. Among non-pregnant women, bacterial vaginosis has been linked to infection of the vaginal cuff following hysterectomy, and possibly pelvic inflammatory disease.

Despite the fact that bacterial vaginosis is most often diagnosed in sexually active women and is frequently seen together with other sexually transmitted infections, there remains no direct proof that it is exclusively sexually transmitted.

Unlike trichomoniasis and candidiasis, bacterial vaginosis does not appear to be caused by a single organism. Instead there is a change in the entire vaginal flora, resulting in the loss of normal hydrogen peroxide-producing lactobacilli and the appearance of increased numbers of mycoplasmas, *Gardnerella* spp., and anaerobic bacteria. Included among the anaerobes are the black-pigmented *Bacteroides (Prevotella)* spp., *B. (Prevotella) biviens*, *Peptostreptococcus* spp., and *Mobiluncus* spp. There is no inflammation of the vaginal epithelium, unlike in trichomoniasis and candidiasis, hence use of the term 'vaginosis' instead of 'vaginitis'. However, one-third of women with bacterial vaginosis and without other infections have more than 30 white blood cells per high-power field in the vaginal fluid. The predominant cell type is the squamous epithelial cell, many of which are covered by adherent bacteria ('clue cells') (Fig. 2).

The symptoms of bacterial vaginosis are vaginal discharge (90 per cent) and an unpleasant odour (90 per cent). The odour is often first noticed after intercourse as the alkaline semen mixes with the vaginal fluid releasing volatile amines. Many women complain of increased odour during menses,

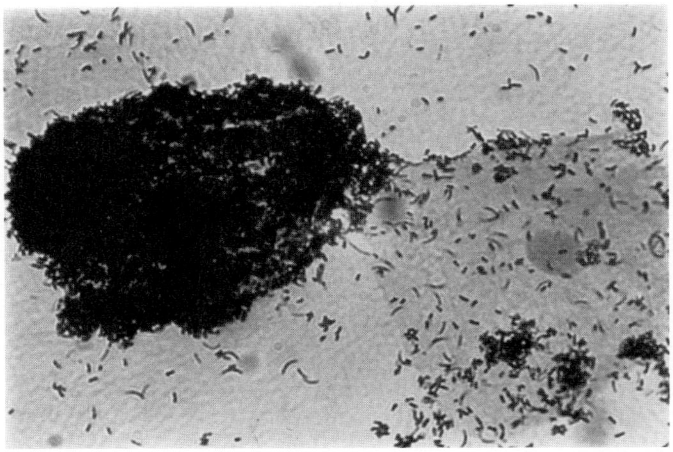

Fig. 2 Gram stain from a patient with bacterial vaginosis (copyright Dr Sharon Hillier).

at which time vaginal pH increases due to the presence of menstrual blood. As with sexually transmitted infections there is a wide range of symptoms, and many women with bacterial vaginosis are asymptomatic or unaware of their symptoms. Thus, it is of great importance to make a careful evaluation of the following clinical signs:

(1) homogeneous-looking, white to grey vaginal discharge;

(2) vaginal pH greater than 4.5;

(3) positive amine odour when vaginal secretions are mixed with 10 per cent potassium hydroxide ('whiff' test);

(4) the presence of 'clue cells'.

It is important to note the type of bacteria present in the vaginal fluid. Careful observation will alert the microscopist to the absence of characteristic lactobacilli and the presence of large numbers of coccobacilli and curved, motile rods (*Mobiluncus* spp.). Culture techniques are not helpful in the diagnosis of this infection, as many of the offending organisms are present in the normal vagina but in low numbers.

Antimicrobial therapy directed at anaerobic organisms is the mainstay of treatment. The most commonly used antibiotic is metronidazole (500 mg orally twice a day for 1 week). Clindamycin is also effective. Intravaginal therapy in the form of clindamycin 2 per cent cream or ovules and metronidazole 0.75 per cent gel is associated with fewer side-effects than oral metronidazole and are of equivalent efficacy.

Although antimicrobial therapy alleviates symptoms in up to 80 per cent of women, recurrences are common. There is no proven regimen for the management of recurrences; however, retreatment with an identical regimen is generally successful in four out of five women. Recurrences may occur because therapy is directed towards eliminating organisms rather than re-establishing the normal vaginal flora. Microbiological studies have shown that the return to normal is slow, often taking several weeks. During this time the vagina is vulnerable to regrowth of the organisms associated with bacterial vaginosis and to clinical relapse. Future directions in treatment may involve some means of reintroducing healthy lactobacilli into the vaginal ecosystem.

Treatment of women with asymptomatic bacterial vaginosis remains controversial. Further studies are needed to define the natural history of bacterial vaginosis in these women. However, because of the association of bacterial vaginosis with infectious complications of gynaecological surgery, treatment is justified in this setting. Although bacterial vaginosis has been associated with complications of pregnancy, routine screening and treatment of pregnant women with asymptomatic bacterial vaginosis is not yet recommended. There is some data to support screening and treatment of women at high risk for preterm delivery, namely those who have had a prior preterm delivery. However, published studies have yielded different results, suggesting that simple treatment of bacterial vaginosis is inadequate to prevent preterm birth. A clearer understanding of the mechanisms by which bacterial vaginosis could cause preterm birth are needed before devising appropriate intervention trials. Because bacterial vaginosis has now been associated with an increased risk for acquisition of HIV, there is interest in promoting widespread screening and treatment in areas with high incidences of HIV. However, the current suboptimal cure rates and high recurrence rates associated with current therapies may make these initiatives untenable.

Candidiasis (see also Chapter 7.12.1)

Vaginal candidiasis or 'yeast' infections are perhaps the best known of vaginal infections to patients and physicians alike. Any type of vaginal discharge is likely to be self-diagnosed as a yeast infection by the patient, yet these represent only 20 to 30 per cent of all vaginal infections. Therefore, many women who have identified themselves as having yeast infections actually have other types of infections, or sometimes no infection at all.

Risk factors for candidiasis include the use of oral contraceptives, containing a high dose of oestrogen, recent use of broad-spectrum antimicrobials, pregnancy, diabetes mellitus, and immunosuppression.

Table 1 Diagnosis and treatment of vaginal infections

	Bacterial vaginosis	Trichomoniasis	Candidiasis
Symptoms[1]	Odour (fishy), discharge	Pruritus, discharge	Pruritus, discharge
Signs[2]	White-grey, homogeneous discharge	Thick, yellow discharge	Cottage-cheese discharge, erythema, fissures
Laboratory tests			
pH[3]	>4.5	>4.5	<4.5
'Whiff'[3]	Positive	Positive	Negative
Saline wet-slide preparation	'Clue cells', abnormal vaginal flora	Motile trichomonads, leucocytes	Pseudohyphae and budding yeasts leucocytes,
Treatment	Metronidazole (oral or topical), clindamycin (oral or topical)	Metronidazole	Imidazole (oral or creams/suppositories, triazoles (oral)[4]

[1]Patients may be asymptomatic.

[2]Characteristics of the discharge are quite variable; these are the classical descriptions.

[3]Not reliable during menses or after recent intercourse; pH may be normal in trichomoniasis.

[4]Fluconazole should not be used during pregnancy.

Vaginal candidiasis is not thought to be a sexually transmitted infection but an overgrowth of vaginal yeasts with the development of local symptoms. The most common species causing vaginitis is *Candida albicans*, although other candidal species account for 10 per cent of genital yeast infections.

The symptoms of vaginal candidiasis are a thick, white discharge and pruritis. Frequently, there is extensive inflammation, which may involve the vulva. Examination may reveal a discharge, erythema, and often excoriations. The discharge is classically described as resembling cottage cheese but it can be variable.

Diagnosis is confirmed microscopically by the presence of pseudohyphae and budding yeasts in the vaginal fluid. Addition of 10 per cent potassium hydroxide may help to clarify these appearances by dissolving epithelial cells and bacteria. Typically the pH is below 4.5 and there are many neutrophils present, although candidiasis can occur simultaneously with trichomoniasis or bacterial vaginosis. Culture is not useful because low numbers of yeasts may be present in the vagina without causing disease. Culture may be of use when characteristic signs and symptoms are present, but pseudohyphae are not identified in the wet-mount examination.

Treatment of vaginal candidiasis relies heavily upon intravaginal imidazole preparations such as clotrimazole, terconazole, miconazole, and butoconazole for 3 to 7 days. Fluconazole is an attractive, single-dose, oral alternative to the topical preparations in women with uncomplicated vaginal candidiasis.

Diagnostic approach to the patient with vaginal discharge

As with any problem in medicine, the history is of great importance. This should include a detailed sexual history to help assess the patient's level of risk for sexually transmitted infections. During the examination the pH of the vaginal fluid should be determined and a sample of the fluid placed in small amounts of both saline and 10 per cent potassium hydroxide for microscopy. The presence or absence of an amine odour when the potassium hydroxide preparation is made should be noted ('whiff test'). The presence of blood, semen, or exogenous vaginal preparations (douches, creams) will interfere with the determination of pH and with the 'whiff test'. Microscopical examination of the saline preparation should be done at 400 × to look for pseudohyphae, 'clue cells', motile trichomonads, and polymorphonuclear leucocytes. The predominant type of bacteria should also be noted.

Vaginal Gram stains may also be useful to determine if 'clue cells' and bacterial morphotypes suggestive of bacterial vaginosis are present. Table 1 reviews the bedside diagnosis and treatment of vaginal infections.

Conclusion

The aetiology of vaginal discharge can be easily determined by taking a careful history, by physical examination, and simple laboratory techniques. Timely and appropriate treatment will prevent recurrent illness and costly complications to the patient and, perhaps, to neonates.

Further reading

Eschenbach DA, *et al.* (1988). Diagnosis and clinical manifestations of bacterial vaginosis. *American Journal of Obstetrics and Gynecology* **158**, 819–28.

Holmes KK, *et al.* (1999). *Sexually transmitted diseases*, 3rd edn. McGraw-Hill, New York

Joesoef MR, Schmid GP, Hillier SL (1999). Bacterial vaginosis: review of treatment options and potential clinical indications for therapy. *Clinical Infectious Diseases* **28**, 57–65.

Lossick JG (1990). Treatment of sexually transmitted vaginosis/vaginitis. *Reviews of Infectious Diseases* **12,** S665–81.

Mårdh P (1991). The vaginal ecosystem. *American Journal of Obstetrics and Gynecology* **165**, 1163–8.

Wolner-Hanssen P, *et al.* (1989). Clinical manifestations of vaginal trichomoniasis. *Journal of the American Medical Association* **261**, 571–6.

21.4 Pelvic inflammatory disease

David Eschenbach

Pelvic inflammatory disease (**PID**) comprises a spectrum of female upper genital tract infections that includes any combination of endometritis, salpingitis, tubo-ovarian abscess, and pelvic peritonitis. Salpingitis, or infection of the fallopian tubes, is the most important feature of PID. This is one of the most common and serious infections of the female genital tract because of the long-term effects after PID including infertility, ectopic pregnancy, and pelvic pain.

PID is caused by the canalicular spread of micro-organisms along the mucosal surfaces from the cervix, and to a lesser extent from the vagina, into the upper genital tract. Cervical mucus provides a relative barrier to this spread, but virulent microbes can traverse cervical mucus, which, in any case, is lost during menses. Little is known of local defence mechanisms to prevent this spread of micro-organisms. Certain HLA types appear to be important in chlamydial PID. Factors that appear to influence the ascent of microbes from the cervix into the upper genital tract include surgical procedures such as dilatation and curettage, induced abortion, intrauterine device (**IUD**)-insertion, and hysterosalpingograms. Vaginal douching with medicated products disrupts the vaginal flora and appears to increase the incidence of PID. Furthermore, contraceptive use influences PID rates. Barrier contraception reduces the risk of PID by preventing the acquisition of *Gonorrhoea* and *Chlamydia* spp. Oral contraceptives also appear to decrease the incidence of PID, perhaps by reducing the inflammatory response to chlamydia infection. The IUD appears to increase the risk of PID by allowing the attachment of bacteria.

Most initial episodes of PID are attributable to *Neisseria gonorrhoeae* and *Chlamydia trachomatis.* While one or both bacteria can be isolated from the cervix in up to 75 per cent of patients with PID, there is a wide variation in the prevalence of these bacteria. In populations where gonorrhoea is highly endemic, there is a 50 to 80 per cent prevalence of *N. gonorrhoeae* in women with PID. A study conducted across eight countries of 1900 patients with PID found that the prevalence of *N. gonorrhoeae* varied from 5 to 80 per cent, with a mean of 26 per cent. In the same 1900 patients, *C. trachomatis* was isolated from 5 to 50 per cent of these women (mean prevalence of 29 per cent). In Europe, there was a 30 to 50 per cent prevalence of *C. trachomatis* in women with PID, and a 5 to 15 per cent prevalence of *N. gonorrhoeae.* Between 10 and 20 per cent of patients with PID harbour both bacteria. However, the use of DNA amplification techniques may reveal even higher numbers of infections with these bacteria.

Mycoplasma hominis and *M. genitalium* cause tubal infection in primates, but their role in human PID is unclear. *Ureaplasma urealyticum* has been isolated from the fallopian tubes but appears to play little role in the development of PID.

Facultative and anaerobic bacteria common to the vagina are also isolated from the fallopian tubes of women with PID. In the initial episode of PID, these bacteria appear less frequent than *N. gonorrhoeae* and *C. trachomatis,* but they can become secondary invaders and are important among women with prolonged symptoms. Anaerobic bacteria are virtually always present in pelvic abscesses associated with initial or recurrent episodes of PID. These bacteria are important in recurrent PID, where *N. gonorrhoeae* and *C. trachomatis* are infrequent.

Women with PID have a vast array of clinical symptoms, ranging from virtually no symptoms to ones that are severe. No symptom, clinical sign, or laboratory result is pathognomonic of PID. In women with mild or uncharacteristic manifestations, the diagnosis of PID is usually missed. Perhaps two-thirds of cases of PID go unrecognized. Some patients' symptoms are too mild or are suggestive of common, less serious conditions. The diagnostic threshold of PID must be sufficiently low to include women with mild PID, but as the threshold is lowered, specificity decreases. However, it is better to overdiagnose than to fail to treat mild PID. Most recognized cases of PID present with moderate symptoms and signs such as lower abdominal pain. Symptoms such as abnormal vaginal discharge or bleeding, dysuria, or vomiting do not distinguish women with PID from those with apparently normal fallopian tubes at laparoscopy. Among women with PID diagnosed by laparoscopy, a temperature over 38 °C is present in only 40 per cent of cases, 60 per cent have a leucocytosis, and 75 per cent an elevated erythrocyte sedimentation rate. Women with severe symptoms and signs usually have peritonitis, often from *N. gonorrhoeae* infection, or they have an abscess. These patients can be very ill. Laparoscopy should be considered both for those with florid peritonitis, to exclude other causes such as appendicitis, and for those with abscesses greater than 6 cm in diameter to allow percutaneous drainage.

Perihepatitis occurs in about 10 per cent of women with PID. Often there is moderate to severe pleuritic pain and tenderness, usually in the right upper quadrant. These symptoms are often so severe that lower abdominal pain, suggesting PID, may not be noticed. Perihepatitis must therefore be distinguished from other causes of upper quadrant pain and tenderness by careful pelvic examination. Perihepatitis is associated with *N. gonorrhoeae, C. trachomatis,* and other aetiologies.

Cervical samples should be obtained to identify *N. gonorrhoeae* by culture or DNA technology and to identify *C. trachomatis* by DNA technology. Patients with severe manifestations should have peripheral white blood cell counts. Other laboratory tests are usually of little benefit. Ultrasound is helpful for identifying the presence, and particularly the size, of an abscess. Dilated or thickened tubes or fluid within tubes are found in 80 to 90 per cent of women with severe to moderate PID, but in only two-thirds of those with mild PID. Most sonographers have little experience with these findings. Laparoscopy provides an accurate diagnosis and is particularly useful for excluding serious surgical conditions such as ectopic pregnancy, appendicitis, bleeding ruptured ovarian cyst, or a ruptured abscess. Laparoscopy is also useful for difficult cases, such as those unresponsive to antibiotics in which the only objective finding is pelvic tenderness.

Differential diagnosis of PID

Among 814 women who underwent laparoscopy because of a clinical diagnosis of PID, 12 per cent had intra-abdominal conditions other than PID: ectopic pregnancy, appendicitis, ruptured ovarian cysts, and endometriosis. In older women, pyelonephritis, gastroenteritis, and diverticulitis can masquerade as PID. A patient with severe signs of peritonitis should be admitted to hospital for ultrasound examination and/or exploratory laparoscopy. A pregnancy test is needed. If positive, an ectopic pregnancy or other pregnancy complications must be considered. If the pregnancy test is negative and a wet mount of vaginal/cervical secretions reveals no neutrophils or bacterial vaginosis, an ultrasound is needed to diagnose gynaecological diseases other than PID or a gastrointestinal or urinary disorder. If the wet mount shows more neutrophils than vaginal epithelial cells, PID is probable, but other pelvic conditions are not completely excluded. Ultrasound or an endometrial biopsy examined for plasma cells is useful to increase the accuracy of diagnosis.

Treatment is aimed at eradicating *N. gonorrhoeae* and *C. trachomatis*, and, especially for those with moderate to severe disease, anaerobic bacteria (Table 1). Women with PID who are HIV-seropositive appear less likely to be infected with *N. gonorrhoeae* and *C. trachomatis*, but they are more likely to develop abscesses. These patients respond to treatment as promptly as those who are HIV-seronegative, unless they are severely immunosuppressed.

Table 1 Inpatient and outpatient PID treatment regimens

Inpatient
Regimen A
Cefoxitin 2 g IV every 6 h, or cefotetan 2 g IV every 12 h,
+
Doxycycline 100 mg IV or orally every 12 h
Regimen B
Clindamycin 900 mg IV every 8 h,
+
Gentamicin loading dose IV, or intramuscular (2 mg/kg of body weight) followed by a maintenance dose(1.5 mg/kg) every 8 h. The intravenous regimens should be continued for at least 48 h after substantial clinical improvement (but beware of gentamicin toxicity!), then followed by 100 mg doxycycline twice daily or 450 mg clindamycin 4 times daily (both orally) for a total of 14 days of therapy.
Outpatient
Regimen A
Cefoxitin 2 g intramuscular plus probenecid, 1 g orally in a single dose concurrently, or ceftriaxone250 mg intramuscular or other parenteral third-generation cephalosporin (e.g., ceftizoxime or cefotaxime)
+
Doxycycline 100 mg orally 2 times daily for 14 days.
Regimen B
Ofloxacin 400 mg orally 2 times daily for 14 days,
+
Either clindamycin 450 mg orally 4 times a day, or metronidazole 500 mg orally 2 times daily for 14 days.

IV, intravenous.

Despite prompt treatment, sequelae are common. Tubal infertility is the most common and disturbing complication. About 10 per cent of women develop tubal infertility after a single episode of PID. Tubal infertility is increased by delaying the treatment of abdominal pain by more than 3 days in chlamydial PID, in women aged over 25 years at the time of PID, and particularly by the number of episodes of PID. Tubal infertility occurs in about 20 per cent of women after two episodes and 40 per cent after three episodes of PID. Tubal infertility occurs in about two-thirds of those with a pelvic abscess or severely damaged tubes observed laparoscopically. There is no correlation between clinical manifestations and the degree of tubal damage observed laparoscopically. Thus, women with mild symptoms but severe tubal damage may become infertile from a single episode of PID. About 7 to 10 per cent of women who become pregnant following PID develop an ectopic pregnancy. Chronic pelvic pain of over 6 months' duration occurs in about 15 per cent of patients following PID.

Attempts should be made to prevent PID. Ideally *N. gonorrhoeae* and *C. trachomatis* infection should be diagnosed and treated before PID can develop. Reduction of *C. trachomatis* infection has lowered the incidence of PID. This should be the aim of primary care providers, especially since *C. trachomatis* can now be diagnosed more readily using new sensitive DNA detection methods.

Further reading

Centers for Disease Control and Prevention (1998). 1998 Guidelines for treatment of sexually transmitted diseases. *Morbidity and Mortality Weekly Report* **47**(No. RR-1), 79–86.

Cohen CR, *et al.* (1998). Effect of human immunodeficiency virus type 1 infection upon acute salpingitis: a laparoscopic study. *Journal of Infectious Disease* **178**, 1352–8.

Eschenbach DA, *et al.* (1975). Polymicrobial etiology of acute pelvic inflammatory disease. *New England Journal Medicine* **293**, 166–71.

Jacobsen L, Westrom L (1969). Objectivized diagnosis of pelvic inflammatory disease. Diagnostic and prognostic value of routine laparoscopy. *American Journal of Obstetrics and Gynecology* **105**, 1088–98.

Scholes D, *et al.* (1996). Prevention of pelvic inflammatory disease by screening for cervical chlamydial infection. *New England Journal of Medicine* **334**, 1362–6.

Spirtos NJ, *et al.* (1982). Sonography in acute pelvic inflammatory disease. *Journal of Reproductive Medicine* **27**, 312–20.

Westrom L (1980). Incidence, prevalence, and trends of acute pelvic inflammatory disease and its consequences in industrialized countries. *American Journal of Obstetrics and Gynecology* **138**, 880–92.

Westrom L, Eschenbach D (1999). Pelvic inflammatory disease. In: Holmes KK, *et al.*, eds. *Sexually transmitted diseases*, pp 783–809. McGraw-Hill, New York.

21.5 Infections and other medical problems in homosexual men

A. McMillan

Many homosexual men have adopted safer sexual practices to prevent the acquisition or transmission of the human immunodeficiency virus (**HIV**). However, condom use is often inconsistent and these men may be at risk of contracting sexually transmissible infections (**STIs**), spread by unprotected receptive/insertive genitoanal and orogenital sex, and faecal–oral infections.

An approach to patients with a suspected sexually transmitted infection that has been acquired homosexually

History

Symptomless, sexually transmissible infections in homosexual men are common, particularly when the pharynx or rectum is affected. A history of a sore throat developing within a few days of receptive orogenital contact is common, and often is not associated with a detectable infection. However, pharyngeal gonorrhoea sometimes produces a sore throat. In HIV-infected men, oral discomfort may be a feature of candidiasis or of oral hairy leucoplakia. A rash may be a feature of several STIs, including primary HIV infection. The patient with various viral STIs, including HIV infection, may notice the presence of enlarged lymph nodes. There may be symptoms of viral hepatitis. Constipation, a mucopurulent anal discharge, anal bleeding, perianal discomfort or pruritus ani, and, in severe cases, pain and tenesmus are symptoms of proctitis caused, for example, by *Neisseria gonorrhoeae*. Many men with proctocolitis, such as results from campylobacter infection, have similar symptoms, but diarrhoea with abdominal cramping, bloating, and fever are the principal features in some people. Diarrhoea, epigastric fullness, abdominal cramps, increased flatulence, and nausea may be features of enteritis caused by *Giardia intestinalis*. All patients, but particularly those with a diarrhoeal disease, should be asked about recent travel to tropical or subtropical areas and sexual contacts there. Perianal pain may be a feature of proctitis, but it is also a symptom of localized disease such as traumatic anal fissure and perianal haematoma. A common cause of pruritus ani is threadworm infestation.

Urethral discharge and dysuria are symptoms of urethritis, caused, for example, by *N. gonorrhoeae*.

The proper interpretation of serological tests for syphilis requires information about previous infection. Similarly, a history of vaccination against hepatitis B should be noted.

Since many homosexual men have psychological problems, careful enquiry should be made about, for example, problems with sexual identity.

Physical examination and investigations

The following should be examined:

- *The skin*: for example, a macular rash may indicate early secondary syphilis, acute HIV, or primary Epstein–Barr virus infections. There may be other dermatological features of HIV (see Chapter 7.11.23). Patients with acute hepatitis may be jaundiced.
- *The mouth and pharynx:* tender superficial ulceration may be caused by herpes simplex virus infection but can also occur during acute HIV infection. Other oral manifestations of HIV infection may be seen (Chapter 7.10.21). Painless superficial ulceration may be a manifestation of secondary syphilis.
- *The superficial lymph nodes*: generalized lymphadenopathy (each node being at least 1 cm in diameter) may be associated with some STIs, including HIV infection. Tender enlargement of the inguinal or femoral nodes may be found in, for example, herpes simplex virus infection of the external genitalia or of the perianal region, respectively.
- *The abdomen*: tender hepatic enlargement is a feature of viral hepatitis and splenomegaly may be found in acute viral infections.
- *The external genitalia:* see Chapter 7.10.21.
- *The anal region*: erythema without specific features may be found in patients who have pruritus ani secondary to an anal discharge. Threadworms may be seen. Multiple tender ulcers are most commonly caused by herpes simplex virus (**HSV**) infection. A solitary ulcer at the anal margin may be traumatic in origin, but primary syphilis must always be excluded. Papillomatous lesions of the perianal region are usually caused by human papillomavirus infection, although the condylomata lata of secondary syphilis should always be considered in the differential diagnosis.
- *The rectum*: the distal rectal mucosa should be inspected in those who give a history of receptive anal intercourse or who have anorectal symptoms. In primary perianal and anal HSV infection, however, proctoscopy should be postponed until the lesions have healed. Signs of proctitis are: loss of the normal vascular pattern of the mucosa (although sometimes this may be a normal finding in the distal rectum), mucosal oedema, friability with contact bleeding, and the presence of mucopus in the lumen (Plate 1). Table 1 lists the sexually transmissible causes of proctitis. Ulceration may be noted in HSV infection, and rarely in primary syphilis or lymphogranuloma venereum. As the proctoscope is withdrawn, the anal canal should be examined for ulceration and condylomata (Plate 2).

In patients with anorectal symptoms and in whom microbiological tests yield negative results for the more common pathogens, sigmoidoscopy may define the extent of proctitis and may identify any lesions beyond the reach of the proctoscope. Rectal biopsy is only occasionally helpful in the diagnosis of rectal sexually transmitted diseases (for example, in lymphogranuloma venereum), but may help to exclude other causes of proctocolitis such as Crohn's disease.

Table 2 indicates the routine microbiological investigations that should be undertaken in the management of a symptomless homosexual man who requests a sexual health screen.

Table 1 Association of sexually transmissible organisms with the clinical features of intestinal disease in immunocompetent individuals

Organisms associated with: Proctitis	Proctocolitis	Enteritis
Neisseria gonorrhoeae	*Campylobacter* spp.	*Cryptosporidium* spp.
N. meningitidis[a]	*Salmonella* spp.	*Giardia intestinalis*
Chlamydia trachomatis:	*Shigella* spp.	
– oculogenital serovars	*Entamoeba histolytica*[b]	
– lymphogranuloma venereum serovars		
Treponema pallidum ssp. *pallidum*		
Herpes simplex virus		
Cytomegalovirus[a]		

[a]Rare.
[b]Rare in temperate climates.

Homosexually transmissible infections

The clinical features, diagnosis, and treatment of these conditions are detailed elsewhere and only those aspects that particularly concern homosexual men are discussed here.

Bacterial infections

Gonorrhoea

In homosexual men the urethra is the most frequently infected site, but infection at multiple sites occurs in about 10 per cent of men.

Although pharyngeal gonorrhoea is usually symptomless, occasionally the patient complains of a sore throat, the pain sometimes radiating to the ear. The physical signs are non-specific but include pharyngeal erythema and sometimes tender enlargement of the anterior cervical lymph nodes. Systemic spread of the gonococcus from the site is extremely rare.

At least 40 per cent of homosexual men with rectal gonorrhoea are symptomless and the rectal mucosa appears normal. When present, symptoms and signs are those of a distal proctitis; the histological findings are non-specific. Perianal abscess is an uncommon complication and disseminated infection is rare.

Neisseria meningitidis infection

N. meningitidis is the most common *Neisseria* species to colonize the oropharynx, and is isolated more frequently from this site in homosexual than in heterosexual men. Urethral carriage of the organism occurs in fewer than 1 per cent of homosexuals and rarely causes urethritis. The rectum is colonized in about 2 per cent of homosexually active men, but this organism is a rare cause of proctitis.

Syphilis

The primary lesion may occur on the penis and have the classical features. A chancre may be found at the anal margin or, rarely, in the distal rectum or in the oropharynx. The clinical presentation of extragenital lesions is often atypical. For example, an anal chancre often resembles a traumatic anal fissure—it is often painful, tender, bleeds easily, and often lacks induration; there is usually femoral lymph-node enlargement. The most common symptoms of primary syphilis of the rectum are rectal pain, an alteration of bowel habit, a mucoid anal discharge, and bleeding; the lesion is usually ulcerative but can be polypoidal, resembling a carcinoma. Biopsy can cause profuse haemorrhage.

Table 2 Microbiological tests that should be undertaken in the routine management of a symptomless homosexual man seeking a sexual health screen

Pharynx	Culture for *Neisseria gonorrhoeae* in all cases
Urethra[a]	• Gram-smear microscopy for diagnosis of symptomless gonococcal or non-gonococcal urethritis • Culture for *N. gonorrhoeae* • EIA for chlamydial antigen *or* culture for *Chlamydia* spp. *or* PCR or LCR for chlamydial DNA
Distal rectum	• If signs of proctitis, Gram-smear microscopy for diagnosis of symptomless gonococcal infection • Culture for *N. gonorrhoeae* in all cases • If signs of proctitis, culture for *Chlamydia* spp. *or* PCR or LCR for chlamydial DNA *and* culture for herpes simplex virus
Blood	Serological tests for: – syphilis – hepatitis B virus infection (if not known to be immune)b – hepatitis A virus infection (if not known to be immune)b – HIV infection[c]

[a]A first-voided specimen of urine is a less invasive test for chlamydial infection (Chapter 7.11.40)
[b]Vaccination should be offered to those who are not immune.
[c]Only after appropriate counselling.
EIA, enzyme immunoassay; PCR, polymerase chain reaction; LCR, ligase chain reaction.

Chlamydia infection

Although non-gonococcal urethritis is common in homosexual men attending sexually transmitted disease (**STD**) clinics, *C. trachomatis* is isolated much less frequently from homosexual than heterosexual men with non-gonococcal urethritis. The aetiology of non-chlamydial, non-gonococcal urethritis is uncertain. Rectal chlamydial infection is found in about 6 per cent of STD clinic attenders who have had unprotected, receptive anal intercourse. Pharyngeal chlamydial infection, diagnosed either by culture or by the detection of chlamydial DNA, is uncommon. In temperate climates, infection with the lymphogranuloma venereum serovars of *C. trachomatis* is rare.

The clinical features of non-gonococcal urethritis associated with infection by the oculogenital serovars (D–K) of *C. trachomatis* are described in Chapter 7.11.40. Pharyngeal infections are often symptomless but can be associated with pharyngitis lacking specific features. Most men with rectal infection are symptomless with normal proctoscopic findings, but there may be features of a distal proctitis. Histologically, there is a non-specific proctitis consisting of a mild increase in the number of chronic inflammatory cells and polymorphonuclear leucocytes within the lamina propria.

Infection with lymphogranuloma venereum serovars is associated with a more severe proctitis with systemic features. Although the sigmoidoscopic findings are those of a severe proctitis, the inflammatory changes seldom extend more proximally than 12 cm from the dentate line. Occasionally, the inflammation is more localized, with an irregular ulcerated mass that may be polypoidal and extend circumferentially to produce stenosis. Inguinal lymph-node involvement may be a feature of lesions of the anal canal and distal rectum. Untreated, lymphogranuloma venereum can be complicated by perianal abscess formation, strictures, and fistulas in the anus. Histologically, there is a dense infiltration of the lamina propria and submucosa by lymphocytes, plasma cells, histiocytes, and sometimes eosinophils. Occasionally, granulomas with giant cells are found with focal areas of acute inflammation with crypt abscesses.

Chancroid

Chancroid, caused by *Haemophilus ducreyi*, is common in tropical countries. Although there are few reports on the features of perianal chancroid, it is likely that the ulceration is similar to that occurring on the genitalia (Chapter 7.11.13).

Donovanosis (granuloma inguinale)

Klebsiella granulomatis infection is regarded as a sexually transmitted disease. Perianal donovanosis usually occurs in homosexual men, presenting as ulceration. Extensive fibrosis with anal stenosis may occur and, rarely, extensive areas of skin and subcutaneous tissue undergo necrosis. Basal-cell or squamous-cell carcinomas may complicate the infection.

Shigellosis

The sexual transmission of *Shigella* spp. among homosexual men was first recognized in 1974 in San Francisco. Subsequent reports have confirmed the spread of this organism through oroanal sexual contact.

Salmonellosis

Cases of typhoid fever acquired from anilingus with symptomless carriers of *Salmonella typhi* have been described.

Campylobacter infection

In some areas of the United States, *Campylobacter* spp. (particularly *C. jejuni* and, to a lesser extent, *C. fetus, C. fennelliae*, and *C. cinaedi*) can be isolated from over 20 per cent of homosexual men with diarrhoea. The source of infection is often uncertain but symptomless carriers are known to exist.

Corynebacterium diphtheriae infection

An increased pharyngeal carriage rate of non-toxigenic *C. diphtheriae* has been reported, but, although these organisms may be associated with pharyngitis, the significance of the finding is uncertain.

Viral infections

Human papillomavirus (**HPV**)

Condyloma is the most common clinical presentation of HPV infection, a lesion that is almost always associated with HPV type 6/11. In homosexual men, condylomas are found on the genitalia and in the perianal region and within the anal canal, where they may cause pruritus ani and bleeding during defaecation. Rarely, condyloma acuminata may develop in the oropharynx. Although condylomas may be very extensive and persistent in immunocompetent individuals, this is particularly so in immunocompromised patients, including those with HIV infection.

Non-condylomatous HPV lesions of the anal canal may be associated with squamous intraepithelial lesions (SIL). The lesions can be identified through an operating microscope after the application of acetic acid (5 per cent v/v), they are white, well-demarcated from the surrounding mucosa, and have a punctate appearance similar to that seen in HPV infection of the uterine cervix. Definitive diagnosis is by biopsy.

Herpes simplex virus (HSV)

Both HSV-1 and -2 can affect the anogenital region. In Edinburgh, between 1989 and mid-1999, 65 per cent of 65 primary or initial episodes of anogenital disease in homosexual men were associated with HSV-1. These had probably been acquired during orogenital or oroanal sexual contact. Inapparent infection with either type is common.

Primary perianal herpes causes anal pain, constipation, tenesmus, anal discharge, and bleeding on defaecation; systemic symptoms are often prominent. Sacral nerve-root involvement may result in paraesthesia in the affected nerves, urinary hesitancy or acute retention, and impotence. There are often multiple tender ulcers in the perianal region and within the anal canal. Distal proctitis associated with HSV may have no specific features but discrete vesicular or pustular lesions or ulcers may be seen. HSV is an uncommon cause of proctitis. It can occur in the absence of perianal or anal ulceration. Rectal biopsies show a marked infiltration of the lamina propria with neutrophils (sometimes with the formation of crypt abscesses), perivascular infiltration of the submucosal vessels with lymphocytes, and multinucleated cells occasionally with intranuclear inclusions.

HSV-2 is more likely to recur than in HSV-1, but the symptoms and signs are generally much less severe and there are no systemic features.

Cytomegalovirus (**CMV**)

CMV infection is more prevalent among homosexual than heterosexual men and women. A study in San Francisco during 1981 reported that 94 per cent of sexually active, homosexual men were seropositive for CMV compared with only 54 per cent of heterosexuals. Receptive anal intercourse is the most likely means of acquisition. The virus is present in semen. Restriction enzyme analysis of serial isolates from homosexuals has shown that infection with multiple strains of CMV is common and that multiple strains can be shed simultaneously. CMV is a rare cause of anorectal ulceration.

Hepatitis A virus (**HAV**)

HAV is transmitted by the faecal–oral route and, although there are conflicting data, homosexual men may be at increased risk of infection. Epidemic outbreaks of homosexually acquired, acute hepatitis A are reported occasionally. Inactivated HAV vaccine may be indicated in sexually active homosexual men to prevent the spread of this infection.

Hepatitis B virus (**HBV**)

The homosexual transmission of HBV was first recognized more than 20 years ago when it was shown that the prevalence of hepatitis B surface antigen (**HBsAg**) was significantly higher in sera of Caucasian homosexuals than in the sera of Caucasian heterosexual men attending an STD clinic in London. HBV-seropositivity has been related to the duration of regular homosexual activity and to the numbers of different sexual partners. As hepatitis B e antigenaemia is closely associated with infectivity, and as the sera of some 70 per cent of homosexual men who are persistent carriers of HBsAg contain e antigen, their sexual contacts are at particular risk of infection. The means of transmission of HBV between homosexual men is uncertain. In some areas there has been a recent decline in HB prevalence, presumably as a result of the adoption of safer sexual practices to avoid HIV infection and to the more widespread use of hepatitis B vaccine. Vaccination of sexually active homosexual and bisexual men who are antiHBs-negative, is a cost-effective method of preventing spread. However, in HIV-infected homosexual men, the humoral response to vaccination is frequently impaired.

*Hepatitis C virus (**HCV**)*

HCV can be transmitted sexually, but the risk of infection to homosexual men who do not inject drugs is low.

*Hepatitis D virus (**HDV**)*

In the United States, sera from 7.7 per cent of 298 homosexual men who were HBsAg-positive contained anti-HDV antibodies. There was an association with the number of sexual partners and the occurrence of anorectal trauma in the 2 years before testing. These data, and the finding of HDV markers in the serum and viral RNA in liver tissue from HBV-infected homosexuals who had never injected intravenous drugs, suggests that sexual transmission of this virus occurs within this population.

Hepatitis G virus/GB virus C

The prevalence of serum antibodies against this virus is significantly higher among homosexual than heterosexual men, suggesting that it is sexually transmissible. The pathogenic significance of the virus, however, remains uncertain.

Human immunodeficiency virus (HIV)

The epidemiology, pathogenesis, and manifestations of this viral infection are discussed in Chapter 7.10.21.

*Human T-cell leukaemia viruses (**HTLV**) types 1 and 2*

Although HTLV-1 and HTLV-2 can be transmitted sexually, the prevalence of infection among homosexual men is low.

*Human herpesvirus 8 (**HHV-8**)*

Kaposi's sarcoma is more common among homosexual men than other groups affected by the HIV. The association with HHV-8 is now well established, but its epidemiology is not fully understood. The prevalence of antibodies against HHV-8 in the sera of homosexual men is significantly higher than that of the general population and correlates with the number of male sexual partners. Orogenital insertive and orogenital receptive sex have been implicated in the transmission of HHV-8 amongst homosexual men.

Protozoal infections

Amoebiasis

Entamoeba histolytica can be transmitted sexually, but the incidence of infection among homosexual men in industrialized countries is low. Previous reports on the apparent high prevalence of infection were erroneous because the organism that was reported as *E. histolytica* was almost invariably *E. dispar*, a non-pathogenic protozoan that is morphologically indistinguishable from *E. histolytica*.

Giardiasis

The prevalence of *Giardia intestinalis* in homosexual men attending STD clinics in temperate climates varies between 2 and 12 per cent. Most infections are symptomless, but a diarrhoeal illness may result.

Cryptosporidiosis

Cryptosporidium parvum can cause diarrhoeal illness. Person-to-person spread has probably been responsible for infection in household contacts. It is a cause of diarrhoea in some homosexual men, but the importance of sexual transmission in the epidemiology of cryptosporidium is uncertain.

Nematode infection

Enterobius vermicularis

Sexual spread by oroanal contact is the most likely route of infection in homosexual men.

Strongyloides stercoralis

Non-infective rhabditaform larvae may develop into infective filariform larvae before leaving the colon. During oroanal contact, these larvae may be transmitted by ingestion of faeces. Penetration of the skin or mucous membrane of the penis by these larvae cause infection during or after anal intercourse.

Other medical conditions in homosexual men

Urinary-tract infection and epididymitis

Bacteriuria may be more prevalent among homosexual men. Acute epididymitis in homosexuals under 35 years of age is more likely to be caused by enterobacteria than *N. gonorrhoeae* or *C. trachomatis*, the most common aetiological agents in heterosexual men under the age of 35 years.

Anorectal trauma

Violent anal intercourse can cause anal fissure or a perianal haematoma. Profuse rectal haemorrhage from mucosal laceration or rupture of the colon at the rectosigmoid junction may result from the insertion of a closed fist into the rectum. Extraperitoneal microperforation of the rectum during 'fisting' may result in pelvic cellulitis: within a few days, lower abdominal and rectal pain develops and the temperature rises. Abdominal examination is usually normal but there may be tenderness in the left iliac fossa. There is marked proctitis and induration of the pararectal tissues. Treatment is with broad-spectrum antimicrobial agents.

Rectal spirochaetosis

In this condition, spirochaetes lie parallel to the microvilli of the epithelial cells of the rectum and superficial portions of the crypts. The condition is indicated by the presence in a haematoxylin and eosin-stained section as a haematoxyphil zone, 3 μm wide, on the luminal surface of the cells. At least one species of spirochaete, *Brachyspira aalborgi*, has been associated with this condition.

Rectal spirochaetosis is found in at least one-third of homosexual men who attend STD clinics but in only 2 to 7 per cent of patients attending general outpatient departments, suggesting sexual transmission. The pathogenicity of the spirochaetes is uncertain.

Carcinoma of the anal canal

In men, receptive anal intercourse may be a risk factor for squamous- and transitional-cell carcinomas of the anal canal. HPV types, particularly HPV-16, have been detected in anal squamous-cell carcinomas. The development of squamous-cell carcinomas in HIV-infected individuals is now well recognized. The immune deficiency associated with HIV infection may permit reactivation of latent HPV resulting in epithelial abnormalities. The situation may be analogous to the development of cancers at other sites in iatrogenically immunosuppressed patients.

Anal squamous intraepithelial lesions (**SIL**) were first described in 1986 and are most commonly found at the junction of the squamous epithelium of the anal canal and the columnar epithelium of the rectum. SILs have been found in tissue removed from the anal canal of homosexual men, and with the operating microscope, after the application of acetic acid, high-grade SILs may be seen as irregular white areas with cobblestoning and mosaicism, and corkscrew vessels.

Low-grade SILs tend to be associated with HPV types 6 and 11 and high-grade SILs with types 16 and 18. Abnormal anal cytology is common in homosexual men with late-stage HIV disease (Centers for Disease Control group IV) and is significantly associated with infection with multiple types of HPV, including those with oncogenic potential. The natural history of SILs, particularly progression to invasive cancer and whether treatment is necessary, is as yet unknown.

Further reading

Doll LS, Ostrow DG (1999). Homosexual behaviour and bisexual behaviour. In: Holmes KK, *et al.*, eds. *Sexually transmitted diseases*, pp 151–62. McGraw-Hill, New York. [Well-referenced review in specialist textbook]

Friedman RC, Downey JI (1994). Homosexuality. *New England Journal of Medicine* **331**, 923–30. [Useful review of psychosocial aspects of homosexuality]

Frisch M *et al.* (1997). Sexually transmitted infection as a cause of anal cancer. *New England Journal of Medicine* **337**, 1350–8.

Katz MH *et al.* (1997). Seroprevalence of and risk factors for hepatitis A infection among young homosexual and bisexual men. *Journal of Infectious Diseases* **175**, 1225–9. [Study that identified risk factors for the acquisition of hepatitis A in young men in the United States]

Martin JN *et al.* (1998). Sexual transmission and the natural history of human herpesvirus 8 infection. *New England Journal of Medicine* **338**, 948–54. [Epidemiological study]

Palefsky JM *et al.* (1998). High incidence of anal high-grade squamous intraepithelial lesions among HIV-positive and HIV-negative homosexual and bisexual men. *AIDS* **12**, 495–503.

Scallan MF *et al.* (1998). Sexual transmission of GB virus C/hepatitis G. *Journal of Medical Virology* **55**, 203–8. [Epidemiological study]

21.6 Cervical cancer and other cancers caused by sexually transmitted infections

V. Beral

Occurrence

Worldwide, cervical cancer is the second most common cancer in women. It is far more frequent in Third World countries than in the West (Fig. 1). About 1 per cent of women in Britain have invasive cervical cancer diagnosed during their lifetime, and 0.4 per cent die from it. Mortality rates have been falling throughout the twentieth century, except among recent generations of women who became sexually active during the 1960s, a time when exposure to sexually transmitted diseases increased rapidly: 0.2 per cent develop vulval cancer and 0.2 per cent anal cancer.

The role of human papillomaviruses and other factors

There is now overwhelming evidence that the vast majority of cervical, vulval, anal, and penile cancers are caused by specific types of the human papillomavirus (see Chapter 7.10.2). DNA from human papillomavirus types 16, 18, 31, 33, and 35 (mostly type 16) has been found in as many as 99 per cent of cervical and other anogenital cancers. Fewer than 10 per cent of people without such cancers have detectable evidence of these types of papillomaviruses in their anogenital cells.

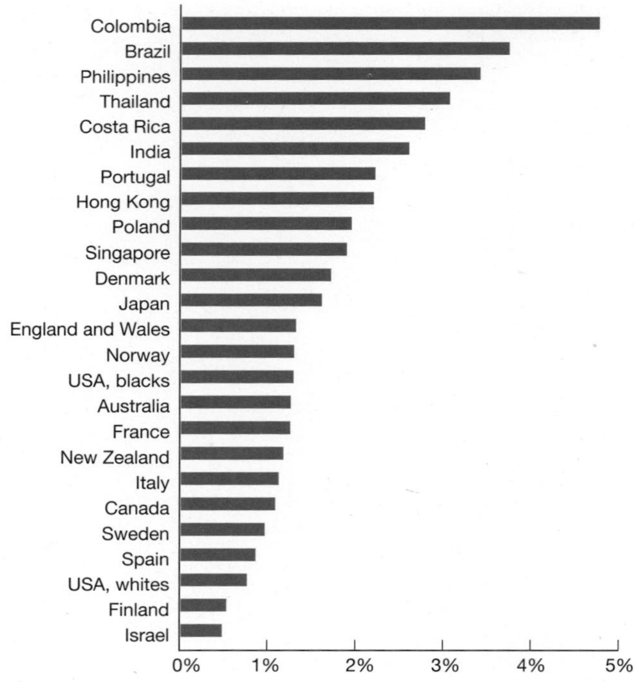

Fig. 1 Percentage of women who develop cervical cancer before the age of 75 years, by country.

The risk of cervical cancer is increased in women who are poor, have little education, were young when they first had sexual intercourse, had many sexual partners and multiple sexually transmitted infections, had many children, especially when they were young, and who smoked cigarettes and used oral contraceptives. Recent evidence suggests that hormonal and reproductive factors and cigarette smoking may independently influence the development of cervical cancer in papillomavirus-infected women, whereas other sexually transmitted infections may be of no direct aetiological significance.

The natural history of infection with the human papillomavirus and associated changes in the cervical epithelium

Some cervical papillomavirus infections cause no obvious epithelial changes—cervical colposcopy, cytology, and biopsy are normal—and the only way infection can be identified is by virological study. Other papillomavirus infections cause 'cervical warts', which are asymptomatic but can be seen as white patches at colposcopy after acetic acid has been applied to the cervix. Cervical smears from women with cervical warts may show various degrees of dysplasia or dyskaryosis, and cervical biopsy may show various grades of cervical intraepithelial neoplasia (**CIN**) (or squamous intraepithelial lesions (**SIL**) according to a new classification known as the 'Bethesda system'). The most extreme change in the epithelium is the development of invasive cervical cancer, which seems to be associated with persistent viral infection and long-standing epithelial abnormalities.

Very little is known about why some lesions progress or regress. Most changes (up to the development of invasive cancer) seem to be reversible. Moreover, lesions of different severity often coexist in the same woman. The more severe lesions tend to be rarer and found in older women: estimates of the proportion of women in Britain likely to develop various types of lesions are given in Table 1, and the age-specific prevalences of some of these lesions are shown in Fig. 2. At least 1 woman in 10 is likely to be infected with human papillomavirus types 16 or 18; 1 in 20 is likely to develop persistent infection or some abnormality of her cervical epithelium; 1 in 50 is diagnosed with *in situ* cervical cancer; and 1 in 100 develops invasive cervical cancer. Papillomavirus infection is most prevalent in women in their twenties, corresponding to the age when they acquire other sexually transmitted infections; the peak prevalence of *in situ* cancer tends to be about 10 years later (in women in their thirties), whereas invasive cancer is rare before 30 years of age.

Clinical implications

Most premalignant cervical changes are caused by papillomaviruses, although most infections resolve spontaneously. Cervical infection with

Table 1 Estimated proportion of women in Britain likely to be infected by the papillomavirus and to develop abnormalities of the cervical epithelium, including cancer

Outcome	%*
Acquire cervical papillomavirus infection	20–50
Develop persistent infection with papillomavirus	5–10
Develop abnormalities of the cervical epithelium such as dyskaryosis or cervical intraepithelial neoplasia (CIN)	5–10
Have carcinoma *in situ* of the cervix diagnosed	2–5
Have invasive carcinoma of the cervix diagnosed	1.0–1.5
Die from cervical cancer	0.3–0.5

*Ranges are given because exposure to the papillomavirus and the risk of associated abnormalities of the cervical epithelium are not the same for different generations of women, definitions and diagnostic criteria for cervical lesions vary, screening programmes are leading to a reduction in the incidence of invasive cervical cancer and mortality from it, and the magnitude of this reduction cannot be estimated with precision.

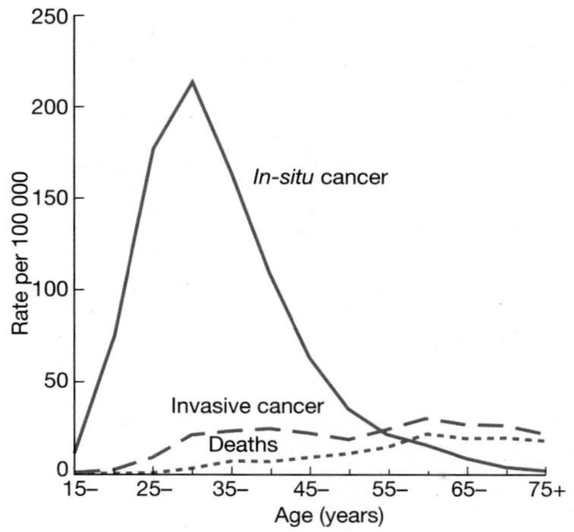

Fig. 2 Age-specific incidence of *in situ* and invasive cervical cancer and of death from cervical cancer in England and Wales.

papillomaviruses is especially common in young women, but invasive cervical cancer is rare before the age of 30 years and seems to be associated with persistent infection and long-standing epithelial abnormalities.

We do not know why infection persists in some women and what determines who goes on to develop cervical cancer. Although intensity of infection, age at exposure, immune response, genital hygiene, reproductive history, and the use of oral contraceptives could be relevant, further research is needed to clarify the role of these possible risk factors. In the meantime, it seems sensible not to resort to active treatment for women in their twenties with papillomavirus infection and related mild cervical lesions, but to reassure them that most lesions will resolve spontaneously and encourage them to have regular cervical smears. Only in young women with severe lesions and older women with persistent epithelial abnormalities is there an appreciable risk of progression to invasive cervical cancer, and active treatment is required.

Prevention

Well-organized screening programmes, based on exfoliative cervical cytology, are known to be effective in reducing the incidence and mortality of cervical cancer. Testing for papillomaviruses should not replace cervical cytology as a first-line approach in screening, since this would result in unnecessary treatment in many young women and because not all cervical cancers are associated with papillomavirus infection. Testing for papillomaviruses may be useful, however, in deciding how to manage the large number of women who have equivocal cervical cytology. Its efficacy must be evaluated before it is adopted on a large scale.

Effective vaccines have already been produced for bovine tumours caused by papillomavirus. Vaccines against the human papillomaviruses have been developed in the last few years and are now being tested in clinical trials.

Further reading

Schiffman MH (1992). Recent progress in defining the epidemiology of human papillomavirus infection and cervical neoplasia. *Journal of the National Cancer Institute* **84**, 394–8.

22

Disorders of the blood

22.1 Introduction

D. J. Weatherall

The study of blood is one of the most fascinating branches of clinical medicine. Almost all diseases produce changes in the blood at some time during the course of the illness. Furthermore, the primary disorders of the blood and blood-forming tissues can give rise to extremely diverse clinical manifestations, which may involve any of the organ systems. Textbooks often give their readers an unbalanced picture of haematology in the real world. Primary disorders of the blood and blood-forming organs account for only a small percentage of a haematologist's practice. Most patients who are referred with haematological abnormalities have diseases in other systems. Anaemia is a good example. Most anaemias are due to blood loss, infection, renal failure, malignant disease, and malnutrition or parasitic infestation. Anaemia may be the first indication of a chronic urinary tract infection, hypothyroidism, pituitary failure, bacterial endocarditis, polymyalgia rheumatica, or even that endemic disease of 'medical grand rounds', atrial myxoma.

This section emphasizes primary diseases of the blood and blood-forming organs, but the reader should be aware that many of these conditions are relatively uncommon. The summary of the haematological manifestations of non-haematological diseases that appears later in this section should leave the reader with a more balanced view of the scope of this absorbing subject.

An approach to patients with haematological disorders

The diagnosis of blood diseases follows the same process as any other condition; expertise in the laboratory will never make up for an inadequate history and clinical examination. It should be remembered that many patients who are referred to hospital for a specialist opinion on their blood are worried about the possibility of leukaemia, although they will rarely say so. It is important to reassure them as soon as possible if this is not the diagnosis. Where leukaemia is suspected, no time should be lost in determining an accurate diagnosis and a well-worked out plan of management. The situation can then be discussed frankly with the patient and his or her family; knowledge of what they face and precisely what form of treatment is to be instituted often engenders a great sense of relief after weeks or months of fearing the worst.

History

In taking a history from a patient who is suspected of having a haematological disorder, certain factors are of particular importance. The symptoms of anaemia are described in detail later in this section. However, a slowly developing anaemia may be completely asymptomatic, even when the haemoglobin level is extremely low. Individuals who are otherwise healthy should be able to compensate for a relatively mild anaemia; a young individual with a haemoglobin level of 10.5 g/dl who complains of tiredness and an inability to cope with life is more likely to have these symptoms because of chronic anxiety rather than the anaemia. Other general symptoms are of great importance, particularly weight loss, night sweats, bone pain, and pruritis. Moderate nocturnal sweating is common in anxiety states; drenching sweats requiring several changes of nightclothes and sheets are a more ominous symptom, often associated with infection or lymphoproliferative disease. Pruritus occurs in conjunction with many disorders of the blood. When associated with lymphoma it is non-specific, but when it accompanies the myeloproliferative disorders it is often precipitated by warmth such as getting into bed or a hot bath. A detailed drug history is essential; many drugs produce haematological side-effects.

Although a complete systematic history must be taken, gastrointestinal and haemostatic functions are particularly relevant to diseases of the blood. A detailed dietetic history is essential when investigating anaemia, and it is important to ask specifically about symptoms such as a sore tongue, bleeding gums, dysphagia, dyspepsia, disturbance of bowel habit suggestive of malabsorption, and rectal bleeding. Patients are often referred to haematological departments for investigation of easy bruising. Many people, particularly women, bruise easily and the key question is whether the bruising is unusual for them. Is it spontaneous or related to only mild trauma? It is also extremely helpful to enquire into certain key episodes in a patient's life that may provide a clue as to whether there is an inborn bleeding tendency. These include circumcision, dental extraction (was a return to the dentist for stitching or packing ever required?), menstruation, surgical procedures, and so on.

Assessment of menstrual blood loss is an important part of the history in women with iron deficiency, as well as for assessing haemostatic function. It is not enough to ask a woman whether she considers that her periods are normal. If she only uses internal tampons, she probably does not have menorrhagia. However, the use of one or more packets of the more absorbent brands of external pads, or the need to get up at night to change pads or to stay at home during the menstrual period, suggests a heavy loss.

Family histories are particularly important for the diagnosis of blood diseases. It is not only essential to ask for a family history of anaemia or bleeding disorders, the racial origin of the patient's ancestors may also give valuable clues to the cause of anaemia. The long-forgotten, Italian great-grandparent may have been the source of the thalassaemia gene that is responsible for a refractory hypochromic anaemia or the red-cell enzyme deficiency that leads to a haemolytic drug reaction. A detailed personal history is also essential. Cigarette- or cigar-smoking is probably the most common cause of mild polycythaemia. Alcohol can produce remarkably diverse haematological changes. A detailed occupational history may reveal exposure to industrial solvents or other agents responsible for bone marrow depression; unusual hobbies may also result in contact with toxic agents.

Physical examination

The examination of a patient with a haematological disorder follows the same pattern as any physical examination, but there are certain aspects of particular importance. On general inspection it is essential to examine the skin carefully for evidence of bruising, purpura, infiltration, or ulceration. The distribution and pattern of bruising or petechiae may be diagnostic, particularly in disorders such as Henoch–Schönlein purpura, senile purpura, scurvy, purpura due to venous obstruction, and the painful bruising syndrome. Thrombocytopenic purpura is often seen most easily over pressure areas; a few lesions in these regions are easily overlooked. Cutaneous lymphoma may mimic a variety of skin diseases. Chronic leg ulceration is a common finding in sickle-cell anaemia; it occurs occasionally with other genetic haemolytic anaemias. The perianal region and perineum should be carefully inspected. There may be perianal infiltration, particularly in the monocytic leukaemias, and it is very important to recognize perianal infection early in neutropenic patients. Digital examination of the rectum should be avoided in neutropenia for fear of disseminating an infection. Potential sites of infection in compromised patients must be examined daily. They include the skin, intravenous infusion sites, the mouth and throat, and the perineum. The mucous membranes, nailbeds, and palmar creases should be examined carefully for pallor, always remembering that the clinical assessment of anaemia is very inaccurate. Pigmentation of the face is sometimes a feature of folic acid deficiency. Mild jaundice may be a useful indicator of haemolysis, while a greyish pigmentation of the skin is common in patients with iron overload, both primary and secondary to repeated transfusion. There is an association between vitiligo and pernicious anaemia. In patients with polycythaemia there may be suffusion of the conjunctivae, a high colour, and prominence of the vessels over the face, neck, and upper part of the chest. The nails should be examined for unusual fragility; flattened, spoon-shaped nails, koilonychia, which are supposed to be diagnostic of chronic iron deficiency, are now rarely seen.

An assessment of the size of the lymph nodes and an inspection of other lymphatic tissue are a major part of the examination of patients with haematological disorders. It is most important to develop a systematic approach to lymph-node examination. Each group of nodes in the head and neck, axillae and groins, together with the epitrochlear nodes, must be examined in detail. In the head and neck it is useful to start with the occipital nodes, then move to the preauricular and postauricular nodes, and, finally, to examine systematically the anterior and posterior triangles and supraclavicular regions. In patients with enlarged occipital or posterior cervical nodes, the scalp should be inspected for signs of infestation and secondary infection due to scratching. A simple way of describing enlarged lymph nodes should be used, without the use of too many adjectives. Nodes should be labelled as hard, firm, or soft, and tender or non-tender. Ambiguous terms such as 'rubbery' should be avoided. Soft, tender nodes usually indicate infection. Large, firm nodes are characteristic of lymphoma. Hard nodes occur in secondary carcinoma, although calcified nodes, matted together and attached to skin, are still encountered in patients with tuberculous adenitis. The approximate size of the nodes should be recorded, together with whether they are mobile, attached deep or superficially, and discrete or matted together. It is also very important to examine the tonsils and adenoids, particularly in a patient suspected of having a lymphoproliferative disease.

A detailed examination of the mouth should include the state of the tongue, mucous membranes, gums, teeth, and fauces. Glossitis, as evidenced by a smooth, depapillated tongue, occurs in iron-deficiency and megaloblastic anaemia. Small, black bullae (blood blisters) on the tongue or mucous membranes, which burst and leave superficial ulcers, are characteristic of thrombocytopenic purpura. Gingival hypertrophy is sometimes found in patients with acute leukaemia, particularly the monocytic type, and in some individuals with megaloblastic anaemia due to phenytoin therapy. Ulcers of the mouth and fauces occur in all forms of acute leukaemia. Oral infection, often associated with ulceration, is very common in neutropenic patients. Candidosis may be seen on the fauces, tongue, or mucous membranes. Candidal infection of the throat, associated with dysphagia, should raise the suspicion of oesophageal candidosis (-iasis). The teeth may be badly formed and the bite may be abnormal in patients with severe forms of thalassaemia. Dental abscesses are common in patients with neutropenia; suspect teeth should be gently percussed for evidence of apical infection. Telangiectases may be found on the lips and oral mucous membranes of patients with hereditary telangiectasia.

On abdominal examination the most important questions are the size of the liver, whether there is splenomegaly, and if there are any palpable para-aortic lymph nodes. It is not possible to learn how to examine the spleen from a textbook, but a few hints may be helpful. Large spleens can often be seen to move up and down on respiration if the abdomen is well illuminated and the observer stands at the end of the bed. Very large spleens tend to move downwards and medially towards the right iliac fossa and can be missed if the examiner does not start palpating from this region, moving upwards and medially towards the left subcostal region. A sure way to miss a moderately enlarged spleen is to go digging in with the fingers without eliciting the patient's help. With the left-hand hooked round the region above the left costal margin, and the right hand resting lightly on the abdomen, the patient should be asked to gently breathe in and out through the mouth. The secret of success is to persuade the patient to breathe just deeply enough to move the spleen down without contracting the abdominal muscles. The examiner should wait for the spleen tip to meet their fingers rather than to try to find it by deep palpation. Once defined, the position of the lower border of the spleen should be recorded in centimetres, vertically below the costal margin. Manoeuvres designed to facilitate the palpation of a slightly enlarged spleen, such as turning the patient on their right side, while useful for impressing clinical examiners, are rarely of much help in practice. Be gentle! The author has seen enlarged spleens ruptured by overenthusiastic medical students. If there is pain over the spleen or referred to the left shoulder, don't forget to listen for a rub. Finally, remember that spleens come in all sizes and shapes, and often lie more laterally than expected. Do not be disappointed not to feel the much publicized notch; it happens once or twice in a clinical lifetime! The differential diagnosis of palpable masses in the region of the spleen is considered later in this section.

The eyes are a mine of information in patients with haematological disorders. Periorbital oedema is sometimes seen in infectious mononucleosis. The conjunctivae may show mild icterus not obvious in the skin, and there may be haemorrhages in bleeding disorders. Pingueculae of the conjunctivae are seen in Gaucher's disease. Retinal haemorrhages are common in patients who have had a sudden fall in haemoglobin level. They are less frequent in severely thrombocytopenic patients with normal haemoglobin levels; the combination of anaemia and thrombocytopenia is particularly likely to lead to severe retinal bleeding. Papilloedema occurs commonly in patients with leukaemia involving the central nervous system. Proliferative abnormalities of the retinal vessels are often seen in patients with sickling disorders, particularly haemoglobin SC disease. The hyperviscosity syndrome associated with macroglobulinaemia and some forms of myeloma is characterized by fullness of the retinal veins, which are sometimes broken up into segments like a string of sausages. These changes are often associated with widespread retinal haemorrhages. Optic atrophy may occur in patients with severe vitamin B_{12} deficiency. Unilateral exophthalmos occurs occasionally in patients with myeloma deposits or lymphoma involving the orbit.

Examination of the musculoskeletal system may be particularly rewarding in patients suspected of having genetic blood disorders. In patients with coagulation defects such as haemophilia or Christmas disease, recurrent bleeding into joints may produce a chronic deforming arthritis. Muscle haematomas are also common and are easily missed. For example, bleeding into the psoas sheath may produce a discrete swelling above the inguinal ligament, which may later be associated with nerve compression leading to weakness of the quadriceps and anaesthesia over the anterior aspect of the thigh. If muscle pain is the presenting symptom, it is very important to palpate the muscle groups carefully for the cystic swellings that may occur in haemophiliacs after bleeding into muscles. The joints have other important associations with blood disorders. A mild refractory anaemia is a very common accompaniment of rheumatoid arthritis. Painful arthritis of the large joints may be the presenting symptom of primary haemochromatosis. Gout is a common complication of all the myeloproliferative diseases; the ears should be examined carefully for tophi, in addition to a full assessment of the joints. The value of bone tenderness in the diagnosis of acute leukaemia has been overemphasized. When present it is best elicited by carefully palpating the sternum or tibias, or by rib compression. Be gentle, because sometimes the tenderness is quite exquisite. Bone tenderness or local swelling are also found in patients with myeloma or sickle-cell anaemia. In children with thalassaemia or other hereditary haemolytic anaemias there may be reduced growth, bossing of the skull, and facial deformities. A wide variety of skeletal changes may occur with congenital hypoplastic anaemia.

The use of the laboratory

The diagnosis and management of blood disease requires an examination of the blood and, if appropriate, the bone marrow. Clinicians will obtain the maximum information from their colleagues in the laboratory if they ask the right questions. Scribbling down 'full blood count' on a laboratory request form is useless. It is essential to ask for an examination of the blood film in any patient who is suspected of having a haematological disorder. More can be learned from the help of an experienced morphologist than any other investigation in clinical haematology. Some haematological investigations are underused; others are requested far too often. For example, the often forgotten reticulocyte count is an invaluable guide to the response of the bone marrow to anaemia and for the recognition of bleeding or mild haemolysis. On the other hand, bone marrow examination is an unpleasant investigation and should only be requested with very clear indications. For example, clinicians should stop and think why they are ordering a bone marrow examination in an elderly patient with a peripheral blood lymphocyte count of 80×10^9/l. This can only be chronic lymphatic leukaemia; the bone marrow will be infiltrated with lymphocytes. Why put the patient through this traumatic investigation? The result is predictable and will not help in their management.

It cannot be emphasized too strongly that the most useful information is obtained by very close liaison between the laboratory and the ward. Clinicians should visit the haematology laboratory regularly, review films and haematological data with their laboratory colleagues, and be very precise in setting out the reasons for the investigations they order. Much valuable information is lost because of the lack of good liaison between the bedside and laboratory.

Examination of the blood

Constituents of normal blood

Blood consists of several different types of cells suspended in plasma. The classification and morphological analysis of blood cells was made possible by the studies of Ehrlich, who, in 1877, described the use of aniline dyes for staining dried blood films. This approach has been refined over the years. The fine structure of the blood cells has been analysed in greater detail with the electron microscope and, more recently, with the scanning electron microscope (Fig. 1).

The formed elements of the blood, or blood cells, consist of the red cells, white cells, and platelets. The red cells are biconcave discs approximately 7 to 8 μm in diameter (Fig. 1). They consist of a membrane that contains a concentrated solution of haemoglobin and a variety of other proteins, salts, and vitamins. Normally they are of a uniform shape and size, and contain similar amounts of haemoglobin. On supravital staining, approximately 1 per cent of the red cells show a reticular appearance. These are newly released cells and because of their staining characteristics are called reticulocytes.

The white cells are classified according to their morphological appearances into granulocytes (polymorphonuclear leucocytes (PMNs)), monocytes, and lymphocytes. The granulocytes and monocytes are phagocytic cells, while the lymphocytes are involved in a variety of immune mechanisms. The granulocytes can be further classified according to their maturity. In the newly produced forms, band cells or juvenile polymorphonuclear leucocytes, the nucleus is horseshoe-shaped but single. In a normal blood film the majority of the granulocytes have matured beyond this stage

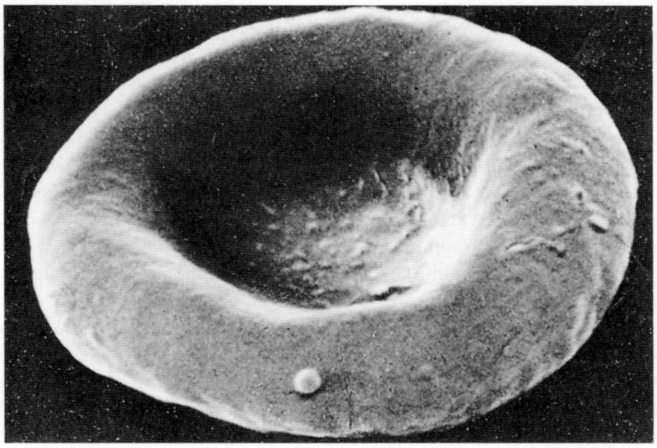

Fig. 1 A human erythrocyte as viewed through the scanning electron microscope. (By kind permission of Dr S. M. Lewis.)

and their nuclei consist of two or more lobes separated by thin, filamentous chromatin strands. These cells are about 12 to 15 μm in diameter. The granulocyte series is further classified according to the staining characteristics of the granules into neutrophils, eosinophils, and basophils. The monocytes are of similar size to the granulocytes but have oval nuclei with a slate-coloured cytoplasm, which may contain some fine granules.

There are two morphologically distinct forms of lymphocyte: a large cell with a diameter of 8 to 16 μm and a smaller one measuring 7 to 9 μm. Both forms are round and have a light blue cytoplasm. In the large lymphocytes the nucleus fills about half of the cell whereas in the small lymphocytes it almost completely fills the cell.

The platelets are disc-shaped cells measuring approximately 2 to 3 μm in diameter. In normal blood they are relatively homogeneous in structure; their fine structure cannot be distinguished by conventional light microscopy.

A more detailed description of the structure and function of these different blood cells and their precursors appears later in this chapter.

Investigation of the blood—the normal blood count

A full blood count can be carried out on a 5-ml anticoagulated blood sample. A stained blood film is prepared for examination of the morphology of the different cells. Using either chemical and physical methods, or the more accurate electronic cell counters, the relative volume of packed red cells and white cells, the haemoglobin level, and the red-cell, white-cell, and platelet counts can be determined. From a series of calculations relating the volume of packed cells, haemoglobin level, and red-cell count, it is possible to derive a series of absolute indices that provide useful information about the size and degree of haemoglobinization of the red cells. Finally, the relative numbers of reticulocytes and the erythrocyte sedimentation rate can be determined.

The stained blood film

An examination of the stained blood film is the most important investigation in haematology. Each of the cell types is studied separately.

The red cells are examined to assess their degree of haemoglobinization and their shape; if both are normal, they are described as normochromic and normocytic. Disorders of the red cell are frequently associated with changes in their morphology or staining properties. These include variation in size or anisocytosis; an increase in size or macrocytosis; a reduction in size or microcytosis; variability in shape or poikilocytosis; pale staining or hypochromia, which suggests underhaemoglobinization; and variation in the degree of staining from cell to cell, which is called anisochromia. In addition to these changes there may be more specific alterations in the morphology of the red cells. Some of these, together with the different clinical disorders with which they are associated, are summarized in Table 1 and illustrated in Fig. 2.

The white cells may be abnormal in number or morphology. An increased white-cell count is called a leucocytosis. If this involves the polymorphonuclear series, it is called a polymorphonuclear leucocytosis or granulocytosis. An elevated eosinophil, basophil, monocyte, or lymphocyte count is called an eosinophilia, basophilia, monocytosis, or lymphocytosis, respectively. A reduced white count is called a neutropenia or lymphopenia, depending on the cell type involved. An absence of granulocytes in the blood is called agranulocytosis. Much can be learned by morphological examination of the white cells. A blood film is said to show a 'shift to the left' if there are relatively more 'young' polymorphonuclear leucocytes present than normal. This is reflected by an increased proportion of band forms and, in more extreme cases, by a variable number of myelocytes or metamyelocytes. In acute bacterial infections, vacuoles may appear in the cytoplasm of polymorphonuclear leucocytes. In addition, the granules may become morphologically abnormal; heavy granulation of this type is called toxic granulation. This change is sometimes associated with the presence of small (1–2 μm) oval bodies called Döhle bodies. A variety of genetic changes of nuclear configuration or of the granules of the polymorphonuclear leucocytes has been described; these are discussed later in this section.

Table 1 Significance of morphological and staining variations of the red cells

Change	Clinical significance
Hypochromia	Defective haemoglobinization; usually iron deficiency or defective haemoglobin synthesis
Microcytosis	As above
Macrocytosis	Dyserythropoiesis or premature release; may indicate megaloblastic erythropoiesis or haemolysis
Anisochromia	Variability of haemoglobinization or presence of young red-cell populations, e.g. in haemolysis
Spherocytosis	Usually indicates damage to membrane; may result from a genetic disorder of the membrane or an acquired defect often due to antibody or other damage to the cell
Target cells	Large 'floppy' cells that occur with deficient haemoglobinization or in liver disease; also occur in hyposplenism
Elliptocytes	May result from a genetic defect in the red-cell membrane but also occur in a variety of acquired conditions including iron deficiency
Poikilocytes: include burr cells, helmet cells, schistocytes, fragmented forms etc.	Usually indicates trauma to red cells in microcirculation or severe oxidant damage
Sickle cells	Occur in sickling disorders
Acanthocytes	Occur in genetic disorders of lipid metabolism
Inclusions: iron granules(siderocytes), Howell–Jolly bodies and Cabot's rings (nuclear remnants), basophilic stippling, and Heinz bodies	Iron granules and nuclear remnants are often seen after splenectomy. Basophilic stippling indicates accelerated erythropoiesis or defective haemoglobin synthesis. It also occurs in some hereditary haemolytic anaemias Heinz bodies are precipitated haemoglobin or globin subunits

The packed-cell volume, haemoglobin level, and red-cell indices

A great deal can be learned about the character of an anaemia from a few simple haematological tests. The volume of packed red cells (**PCV** or haematocrit) can be estimated either by centrifugation of a blood sample, or by a conductivity method in which it is derived from measurement of the red-cell volume and the number of red cells using an electronic counting system. The haemoglobin concentration is usually determined spectrophotometrically by comparing a test sample with a stable standard, usually of the cyanmethaemoglobin derivative. Red-cell counting has become part of a standard blood count because of the accuracy of electronic cell counters.

Normal values for the PCV, haemoglobin level, and red-cell count are shown in Table 2. It is important to become familiar with the variability of these figures between the sexes and at different stages of development (Table 3). Furthermore, it should be emphasized that the accuracy of these measurements relies very much on the method used for their determination. An electronic cell counter gives extremely reproducible results for all three measurements, whereas a red-cell count made with a counting chamber is of little value. The red-cell indices can be estimated by combining information obtained from these measurements. The mean cell haemoglobin (**MCH**), which is derived from the haemoglobin value and the red-

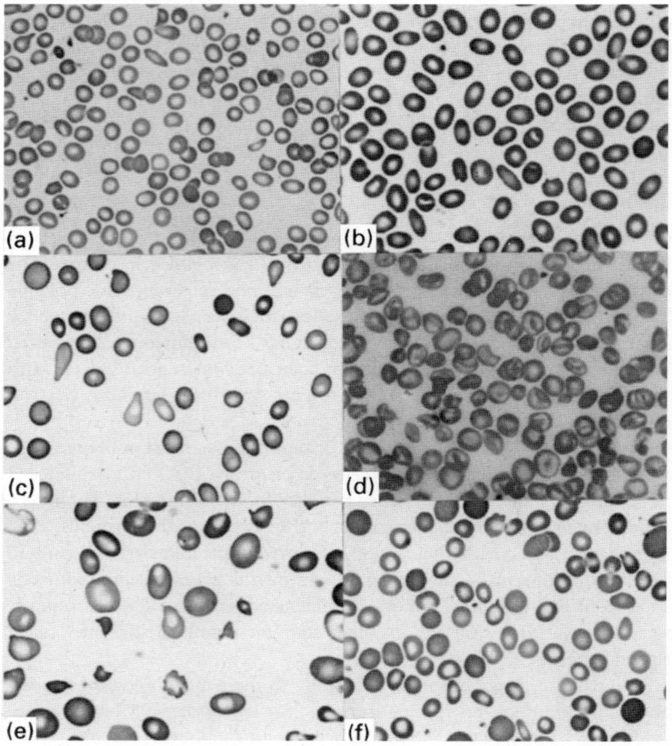

Fig. 2 Morphological changes of the red cells (600–800 ×). (a) Hypochromia and microcytosis. (b) Elliptocytosis. (c) Poikilocytosis (myelosclerosis). (d) Target cells and intracellular crystals (haemoglobin C disease). (e) Macrocytosis and anisocytosis (pernicious anaemia). (f) Dimorphic picture—normochromic and hypochromic (sideroblastic anaemia).

cell count and is expressed in picograms (pg), gives a reliable indication of the amount of haemoglobin per cell. The mean cell haemoglobin concentration (**MCHC**) represents the concentration of haemoglobin in g/dl (g/100 ml) of erythrocytes. The mean cell volume (**MCV**), calculated in femtolitres (fl), gives an indication of the size of the erythrocytes. Hence it is elevated in patients with macrocytic disorders and reduced in the presence of microcytic red cells. The normal values at different stages of development are summarized in Table 3.

It should be emphasized that the red-cell indices give an indication of the average size and degree of haemoglobinization of the red cells. They are only of value if combined with an examination of a blood film to provide information about the relative uniformity of any changes in size or haemoglobin concentration.

The total and differential leucocyte count

The leucocyte count can be determined either by using a counting chamber or electronically. The differential count is obtained from analysing the different types of white cells in a total of 200 to 300 cells, or more if the total white-cell count is unusually low. It should be remembered that the total white-cell count shows remarkable variability even in the same individual at different times. There are variations during the menstrual cycle and a

Table 2 Haematological values for normal adults

Red-cell count		*β-Thromboglobulin*	<50 ng/ml
Men	5.0 ± 0.5 × 10^{12}/l	*Platelet factor 4*	<10 ng/ml
Women	4.3 ± 0.5 × 10^{12}/l	Protein C	<10 ng/ml
Haemoglobin		Function	0.70–1.40 u/ml
Men	150 ± 20 g/l	Antigen	0.61–1.32 u/ml
Women	140 ± 20 g/l	*Protein S*	
Packed-cell volume (PCV; haematocrit value)		Total	0.78–1.37 u/ml
Men	0.45 ± 0.05 (l/l)	Free	0.68–1.52 u/ml
Women	0.41 ± 0.04 (l/l)	*Heparin cofactor II*	55–145%
Mean cell volume (MCV)		*Autohaemolysis (37 °C)*	
Men and women	92 ± 10 fl	48 h without added glucose	0.2–2.0
Mean cell haemoglobin (MCH)		48 h, with added glucose	0–0.9%
Men and women	29.5 ± 2.5 pg	*Cold agglutinin titre (4 °C)*	<64
Mean cell haemoglobin concentration (MCHC)		*Serum iron*	13–32 μmol/l (0.7–1.8 mg/l)
Men and women	330 ± 15 g/l	*Total iron-binding capacity*	45–70 μmol/l (2.5–4.0 mg/l)
Red-cell diameter (mean values)		*Transferrin*	1.2–2.0 g/l
Dry films	6.7–7.7 μm	*Ferritin*	
Red-cell density	1092–1100 g/l	Men	20–300 median 100 μg/l
Reticulocyte count	0.5–2.0% (25–85 × 10^9/l)	Women	15–150 median 30 μg/l
Blood volume		*Serum vitamin B_{12}*	160–760 ng/l
Red-cell volume		*Serum folate*	3–20 μg/l
Men	30 ± 5 ml/kg	*Red-cell folate*	160–640 μg/l
Women	25 ± 5 ml/kg	*Plasma haemoglobin*	10–40 mg/l
Plasma volume	45 ± 5 ml/kg	*Serum haptoglobin*	0.6–2.7 mg/l
Total blood volume	70 ± 10 ml/kg	*HbA2*	2.2–3.5%
Real cell lifespan	120 ± 30 days	*HbF*	<1.0%
Leucocyte count	7.0 ± 3.0 × 10^9/l	*Methaemoglobin*	<2.0%
Differential leucocyte count		*Sedimentation rate* (1 h at 20 ± 3 °C)	
Neutrophils	2.0–7.0 × 10^9/l (40–80%)	(upper limits)	
Lymphocytes	1.0–3.0 × 10^9/l (20–40%)	Men:	10 mm
Monocytes	0.2–1.0 × 10^9/l (2–10%)	17–50 years	12 mm
Eosinophils	0.04–0.4 × 10^9/l (1–6%)	50–60 years	14 mm
Basophils	0.02–0.1 × 10^9/l (<1–2%)	61–70 years	30 mm
Platelet count	130–400 × 10^9/l	>70 years	
Bleeding time		Women:	19 mm
(Ivy's method)	2–7 min	17–50 years	19 mm
(Template method)	2.5–9.5 min	50–60 years	20 mm
Prothrombin time	12–16 s	61–70 years	35 mm
Partial thromboplastin time (PTT)	30–46 s	>70 years	
Thrombin time	15–19 s	*Plasma viscosity*	1.50–1.72 mPa/s
Plasma fibrinogen	2.0–4.0 g/l	25 °C	1.16–1.33 mPa/s
Fibrinogen titre	≥128	37 °C	<80
Plasminogen		*cell) agglutinin titre*	
Function	0.75–1.35 u/ml	*Heterophile (anti-sheep red*	<10
Antigen	0.76–1.36 u/ml	After absorption with	
Euglobulin lysis time	90–240 min	guinea-pig kidney	
Antithrombin III			
Function	0.86–13.2 u/ml		
Antigen	0.79–1.11 u/ml		

Expressed as mean ± SD (95% range).

After Dacie and Lewis (1994).

Table 3 Haematological values for normal infants and children

	At birth (full term)	Day 3	1 month	2–6 months	2–6 years	6–12 years
Red-cell count (× 10^{12}/l)	6.0 ± 1.0	5.3 ± 1.3	4.2 ± 1.2	3.8 ± 0.8	4.6 ± 0.7	4.6 ± 0.6
Haemoglobin (g/l)	165 ± 30	185 ± 40	140 ± 30	115 ± 20	125 ± 15	135 ± 20
Packed-cell volume/haematocrit	0.54 ± 0.10	0.56 ± 0.11	0.43 ± 0.12	0.35 ± 0.07	0.37 ± 0.03	0.40 ± 0.05
Mean cell volume (MCV) (fl)	110 ± 10	108 ± 13	104 ± 19	91 ± 17	81 ± 6	86 ± 8
Mean cell haemoglobin (MCH) (pg)	34 ± 3	34 ± 3	34 ± 6	30 ± 5	27 ± 3	29 ± 4
Mean cell haemoglobin concentration (MCHC) (g/l)	330 ± 30	330 ± 40	330 ± 40	330 ± 30	340 ± 30	340 ± 30
Reticulocytes (%)	2–5	1–4.5	0.3–1	0.4–1	0.2–2	0.2–2
Leucocyte count (× 10^9/l)	18 ± 8	15 ± 8	12 ± 7	12 ± 6	10 ± 5	9 ± 4
Neutrophils (× 10^9/l)	5–13	3–5	3–9	1.5–9	1.5–8	2–8
Lymphocytes (× 10^9/l)	3–10	2–8	3–16	4–10	6–9	1–5
Monocytes (× 10^9/l)	0.7–1.5	0.5–1	0.3–1	0.1–1	0.1–1	0.1–1
Eosinophils (× 10^9/l)	0.2–1	0.1–2.5	0.2–1	0.2–1	0.2–1	0.1–1

Expressed as mean ± 2 SD or 95% range.
After Dacie and Lewis (1994).

marked diurnal rhythm with minimum counts in the morning with subjects at rest. Activity may increase the white-cell count slightly, as may emotional stress and eating. Furthermore, the differential white-cell count varies considerably during normal human development. There is a preponderance of lymphocytes during the first few years of life and of polymorphonuclear leucocytes during later development and in adult life. These normal variations are shown in Table 3.

The platelet count

This is most accurately determined with an electronic cell counter, although a rough approximation can be obtained by using a counting chamber. There is marked variation in the normal platelet count and the range in health is approximately 150 to 400×10^9/l. A slight drop in the count occurs before menstruation but on the whole it varies less within an individual than the white-cell count.

Blood volume, red-cell mass, and plasma volume

Because the haemoglobin level or PCV may vary due to expansion or contraction of the plasma volume, it is sometimes necessary to measure the red-cell mass and plasma volume directly. This is usually done by radioisotope dilution. The red-cell volume (**RCV**) is measured by labelling the red cells with ^{51}Cr and the plasma volume (**PV**) by the use of isotope-labelled albumin. These measurements are fraught with difficulties because of the variation of vascularity and PCV between different organs, and because fat is a relatively avascular tissue. There is still considerable controversy about how best to express the results. A variety of correction factors has been derived, which attempt to relate the measured RCV or PV to an ideal body weight. In practice it is usual to simply calculate the RCV or PV in ml/kg. The wide range of normal values is summarized in Table 2.

The erythrocyte sedimentation rate (ESR)

The ESR is a measure of the suspension stability of red cells in blood. It is usually expressed in millimetres (mm) and is obtained by measuring the distance from the surface meniscus to the upper limit of the red-cell layer in a column of blood after 60 min. The ESR depends on the difference in specific gravity between the red cells and plasma but is influenced by many other factors, particularly the rate at which the red cells clump or form rouleaux. The increased sedimentation rate of clusters of cells reflects reduced fluid friction resulting from a decreased surface:volume ratio. Rouleaux formation is related to the concentration of fibrinogen and, to a lesser extent, of α_2- and γ-globulins in the plasma. Unfortunately, the ESR is also subject to many technical difficulties including the dimensions of the tube, the nature of the anticoagulant used, and any degree of tilt of the tube from the horizontal.

The ESR is still widely used as a non-specific index of organic disease. It is elevated in many acute or chronic infections, neoplastic diseases, collagen diseases, renal insufficiency, and any disorder associated with a significant change in the plasma proteins. Anaemia may cause an increased rate of sedimentation. Although many attempts have been made to develop correction factors to allow for this variable, none is satisfactory. Like all haematological measurements, the ESR changes in certain physiological states, particularly in pregnancy and with increasing age. In men and women over the age of 60 a slightly elevated ESR is often found without an obvious cause (Table 2).

Other haematological investigations

The simple tests that have been outlined in this section form the general screening investigations for all haematological disorders. In later sections we will describe the more specialized investigations that are often required to diagnose specific disorders of the red cells, white cells, and platelets, or of haemostasis and coagulation. Normal values for some of these investigations are given in Table 2.

Examination of the marrow

Bone marrow can be examined by needle aspiration, closed needle biopsy, or open surgical biopsy. In adults the sites most easily available are the sternum and the anterior or posterior iliac crests, although the marrow at the iliac crests tends to become rather fatty in elderly subjects. In under 1-year-old children the anterior surface of the tibia is the site of choice, but in older children the iliac crest or the lumbar vertebral spines are suitable. After aspiration of the marrow, films are made and stained with a Romanowsky stain. Needle or surgical biopsy samples are fixed and sectioned by standard methods.

The marrow films are initially examined under low power to assess the overall cellularity and for the presence of abnormal cells. It is sometimes useful to obtain a differential count and from this to determine the myeloid/erythroid (**M/E**) ratio. This is approximately 3:1 in health, although, if there is increased erythroid activity, it may fall to unity or less. It should be remembered that differential counts may be quite inaccurate because the precursors may not be distributed homogeneously. This is a particular problem in disorders in which there are abnormal cells in the marrow. Having determined the overall cellularity, the morphology of the individual cells is examined. The degree of maturation of the red cells, white cells, and megakaryocyte series is assessed and the marrow examined carefully for the presence of any abnormal cells.

A biopsy specimen is particularly useful for looking at overall cellularity and relating the amount of haemopoiesis to the amount of fatty tissue. It is of particular value if an aspiration yields a 'dry tap' when it may show replacement by fibrous or tumour tissue, which may not aspirate readily. Using appropriate stains it is possible to estimate the amount of iron and reticulin in the marrow.

Assessment of bone marrow activity and distribution

Some indication of marrow function is obtained from its morphological appearances and from the M/E ratio. It is also possible to measure the rates of production and turnover of the red-cell series using radioactive iron. It is sometimes necessary to attempt to estimate the distribution of the haemopoietic marrow, and this is usually done by using isotopes to produce scintograms that show the distribution of erythropoietic or reticuloendothelial marrow throughout the body. Erythropoietic marrow can be visualized using the short-lived, positron-emitting isotope ^{52}Fe with a scintillation camera. In health this shows erythropoietic marrow in the ribs, spine, pelvis, scapula, and clavicle, with a variable amount in the skull. The reticuloendothelial portion of the marrow can be labelled with a radiocolloid with an appropriate particle size; the most effective and commonly used is $^{99}Tc^{m}$-sulphur colloid.

Further reading

Beutler E, *et al.*, eds (2001). *Williams hematology*, 6th edn. McGraw-Hill, New York.

Dacie JV, Lewis SM (1994). *Practical haematology*, 8th edn. Churchill Livingstone, Edinburgh.

Hoffman R, *et al.* (2000). *Hematology. Basic principles and practice*, 3rd edn. Churchill Livingstone, New York.

Nathan DG, Orkin SH (1998). *Hematology of infancy and childhood*, 5th edn. WB Saunders, Philadelphia.

22.2 Disorders of the blood

22.2.1 Stem cells and haemopoiesis

C. A. Sieff and D. G. Nathan

Introduction

Normal haemopoiesis in the adult depends on the production of blood cells from their recognizable precursors in the bone marrow, their survival in the vasculature, and their demise in the reticuloendothelial system, predominantly in the spleen, liver, lung, and the marrow itself. Though the concentration of cells in the blood varies widely, the values observed in normal individuals are remarkably consistent, particularly considering the vast differences in the lifespans of these cells. For example, the mean lifespan of granulocytes in the peripheral blood may be measured in hours. In contrast, platelets survive for 7 to 10 days. Though platelets are removed from the blood in part by random forces, most of their lifespan is dictated by metabolic changes within them that lead to predetermined death. Normally, red cells are lost by a process of metabolic decay that begins after the erythrocyte has attained an age of approximately 100 days. Lymphocytes have very dramatic differences in lifespan. Some are removed from the circulation in 2 or 3 weeks by a process that is not understood. Others, particularly certain T lymphocytes, appear to survive for the entire lifespan of the individual, carrying within them the programmes embossed upon them by the thymus.

The steady-state concentrations of blood cells vary from one another by three logs or more, but the marrow production rates that maintain them are very similar. Approximately 5×10^4 red cells, 2×10^4 platelets, and 2×10^4 granulocytes are produced per microlitre of blood per day to maintain a normal blood count. Lymphocyte production must be considerably lower because the bulk of lymphocytes in the peripheral blood are long-lived T lymphocytes.

The relatively constant production rates of blood cells are regulated by a highly complex marrow tissue characterized morphologically by recognizable, differentiating precursor cells. These are partially renewed by a variable population of invisible progenitor cells, some of which have the characteristics of stem cells. Precursor cells and their progenitors are packed together into fronds surrounded by endothelial cells that separate marrow cells from the venous sinuses. The completed blood cells find apertures through the endothelial cells and migrate between them to fall into the sinuses, the currents of which carry them into the peripheral blood.

In this chapter, we shall describe critical aspects of the physiology of haemopoiesis in the marrow. To understand this process, we must first review its ontogeny and comparative development.

Phylogeny and ontogeny

In the developing human being, haemopoiesis moves through several overlapping anatomical and functional stages, beginning in the yolk sac, entering the hepatic phase at 6 weeks', and the marrow phase at 20 weeks' gestation. Transfer to the bone marrow phase is generally complete at birth. These anatomical shifts are associated with marked alterations in functional properties, particularly with respect to the pattern of globin synthesis in the red cell. These changes are referred to as the 'fetal switch'. This transition is not a single event involving only the γ-chains of fetal haemoglobin, it is instead polygenic involving a series of changes regulated in a programmed fashion. The mechanism of this co-ordinated series of changes is as yet undetermined. It appears to be mediated at the level of the progenitors of haemopoietic cells and is strongly influenced by site-specific regulatory factors.

Marrow anatomy

The relative red (active) marrow space of a child is much greater than that of an adult, presumably because the high requirements for red-cell production during neonatal life demand the resources of the entire production potential of the marrow. During postnatal life the demands for red-cell production ebb. Much of the marrow space is progressively filled with fat (Fig. 1). In certain diseases that are usually associated with anaemia, such as myeloid metaplasia, haemopoiesis may return to its former sites in the liver, spleen, and lymph nodes and may also be found in the adrenals, cartilage, adipose tissue, thoracic paravertebral gutters, and even in the kidneys.

The microenvironment of the marrow cavity is a vast network of endothelial cell-lined vascular channels or sinusoids that separate clumps of haemopoietic cells, including fat cells, that reside in the intrasinusoidal spaces. These two compartments are separated by reticular cells (derived from fibroblasts) that form the adventitial surfaces of the sinuses and extend cytoplasmic processes to create a lattice on which blood cells are found. The lattice is demonstrated by reticulin stains of marrow sections (Fig. 2). The conformation of the meshwork of cytoplasmic extensions and the placement of haemopoietic cells in the network of sinuses are best illustrated by scanning electron microscopy. The fibroblast–endothelial cell network provides two major functions: (i) an adhesive framework on to which the developing cells are bound by fibronectin and other integrins, and (ii) the production of haemopoietic growth factors by these cells. Cell–cell adhesion may be mediated by binding of the haemopoietic VLA-4 integrin to stromal fibronectin or VCAM-1.

The central and radial arteries ramify in the cortical capillaries, which in turn join the marrow sinusoids and drain into the central sinus. Cells that egress from the marrow sinusoids then join the venous circulation through concomitant veins. The inner, or luminal, surface of the vascular sinusoids is lined with endothelial cells, the cytoplasmic extensions of which overlap, or interdigitate, with one another. The escape of developing haemopoietic cells into the sinus for transport to the circulation occurs through gaps that develop in this endothelial lining and even through endothelial-cell cytoplasmic pores.

The haemopoietic growth factors comprise a family of small glycoproteins that not only affect immature cells but also influence the survival and

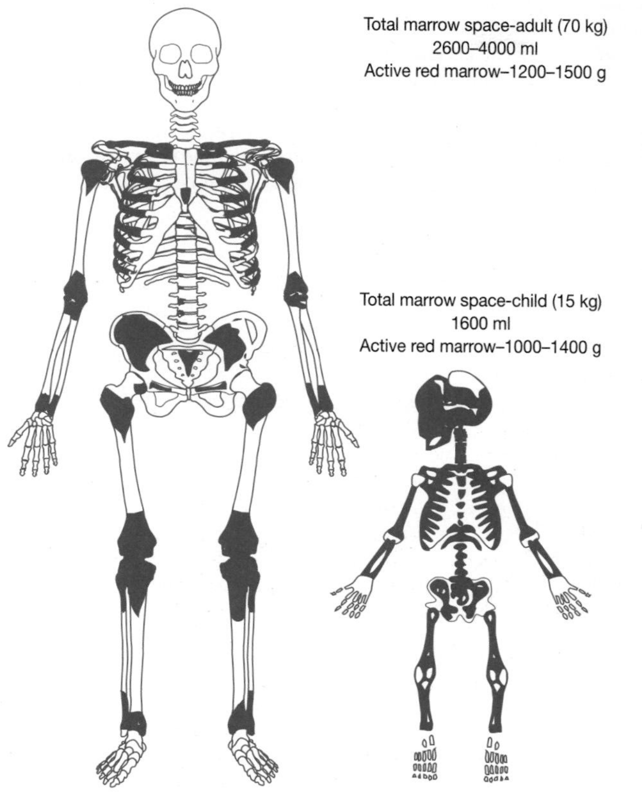

Fig. 1 A comparison of active red marrow-bearing areas in a child and adult. Note the almost identical amount of active red marrow in the child and adult despite a fivefold discrepancy in body weight. (Reproduced from MacFarlane RG and Robb-Smith AHT, eds, 1961. *Functions of the blood*, p 357. Blackwell Scientific, Oxford, with permission.)

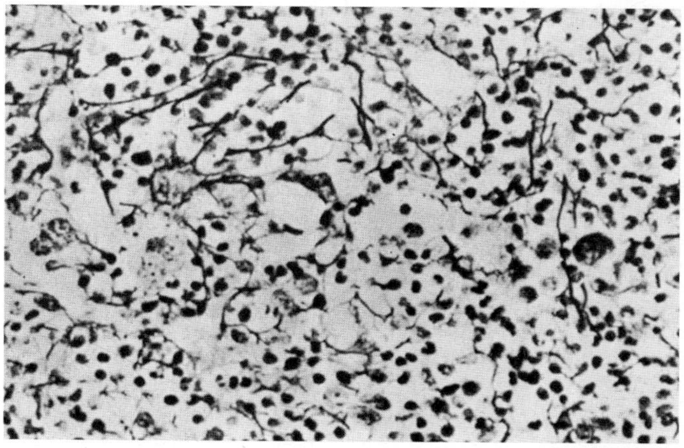

Fig. 2 Bone marrow biopsy of a patient with mild myelofibrosis. A slight increase in the number of reticulin fibres in a delicate discontinuous fibre network is present. Gomori stain, ×350. (Reproduced from Lennert K *et al.*, 1975, *Clinical Haematology* **4**, 335, with permission.)

function of mature cells. They do so by binding to specific cell-surface receptors. The genes for many of the growth factors and their receptors have been isolated. The cellular origin and the major sites of action of important members of the haemopoietic growth-factor family are shown in Fig. 3. Three of the receptors, c-*kit*, the receptor for Steel factor, Flt-3, the receptor for Flt-3 ligand, and c-*fms*, the monocyte colony-stimulating factor (**M-CSF**) receptor, are members of the transmembrane tyrosine kinase family. In contrast, the receptors for the other haemopoietic growth factors such as interleukin 3(**IL-3**), granulocyte–macrophage colony-stimulating factor (**GM-CSF**), granulocyte-CSF (**G-CSF**), IL-5, IL-6, erythropoietin, and thrombopoietin are members of the haemopoietic growth-factor receptor family. They share several structural features; lacking cytoplasmic tyrosine kinase domains, they activate cells by dimerizing after binding their cognate ligands. This promotes the recruitment and activation of cytoplasmic tyrosine kinases such as members of the Janus kinase (**JAK**) family. The JAK proteins in turn activate members of the signal transducer and activator of transcription (STAT) family and phosphorylate tyrosines of the cytoplasmic domains of the receptor itself. This stimulates recruitment of other signalling or adaptor proteins that activate pathways, such as that involving the RAS protein.

The location of the different haemopoietic cells is not random. Clumps of megakaryocytes are found adjacent to marrow sinuses. They shed platelets, the fragments of their cytoplasm, directly into the lumen. This reduces the requirement for movement of bulky mature megakaryocytes, a mobility characteristic of the granuloid- and erythroid-differentiated precursors as they approach the point at which they egress from the marrow.

The formed elements of blood in vertebrates, including humans, continuously undergo replacement to maintain a constant number of red cells, white cells, and platelets. The number of cells of each type is maintained in a very narrow range in normal adults—approximately 5000 granulocytes, 5 $\times 10^6$ red blood cells, and 150 000 to 300 000 platelets per microlitre of whole blood. In the following section we shall review the nature of the signals that affect the proliferation of the stem and progenitor cells, and the normal regulatory mechanisms that maintain balanced production of new blood cells.

Function of stem cells and progenitors

The progenitors of recognizable precursor cells are mononuclear 'blast' cells with large nuclei, prominent nucleoli, and basophilic cytoplasm devoid of granules. These primitive progenitors are present at extremely low frequencies, approximately 1 in 10^4 to 10^5 marrow cells for the stem cell population and 1 in 10^3 for their committed progenitor progeny. A single pluripotent stem cell is capable of giving rise, in a stochastic fashion, to increasingly committed progenitor cells according to the schema outlined in Fig. 3. These committed progenitors are destined to form differentiated recognizable precursors of the specific types of blood cells.

Pluripotent stem cells are defined as cells capable of both self-renewal and multilineage differentiation under the influence of certain non-lineage-specific growth factors such as Flt-3 ligand, Steel factor, IL-6, and thrombopoietin. Their differentiation programme is random and leads to a broad array of more mature lineage-committed progenitors that are themselves responsive to broadly active factors such as IL-3, GM-CSF, IL-11, and subsequently to the more lineage-restricted growth factors, including erythropoietin, thrombopoietin, G-CSF, IL-5, and M-CSF. Some of the lineage-restricted growth factors, particularly erythropoietin, are produced in response to the circulating levels of differentiated blood cells.

Lineage-committed progenitors are characterized by limited proliferative potential that depends upon the presence of specific growth factors that interact with specific receptors on progenitor surfaces. Progenitors are not capable of indefinite self-renewal. In fact, they 'die by differentiation' to mature precursors of the blood cells. The maintenance of their numbers ultimately depends upon the presence of lineage-specific growth factors and on random influx into their pool from the pluripotent stem-cell pool. Therefore, amplification of blood-cell production occurs at the level of the committed progenitor pool, while maintenance of the progenitors depends upon the capacity of members of the pluripotent stem-cell pool to differentiate into the committed progenitor pool.

Haemopoietic differentiation requires an appropriate microenvironment. In normal adults, this is confined to the bone marrow, whereas in the mouse it includes both the spleen and bone marrow. The existence of certain strains of mice that exhibit a deficiency in the haemopoietic microenvironment suggests that the interactions between haemopoietic cells and the bone marrow microenvironment involve very specific molecular mechanisms. Insight into the nature of one of these interactions has come from isolation of the genes that determine the *White Spotting (W)* and *Steel (Sl)* mutations in mice. Animals affected by mutations at both of these loci have a severe macrocytic anaemia associated with defects in skin pigmentation and fertility. The mutations, however, map to different chromosome loci (*W* to chromosome 5, *Sl* to chromosome 10). This is consistent with the results of transplant experiments, which demonstrate that the *W* mutation is one of stem cells whereas the *Sl* defect is one of the bone marrow microenvironment. The *W* gene has now been shown to be allelic with the c-*kit*

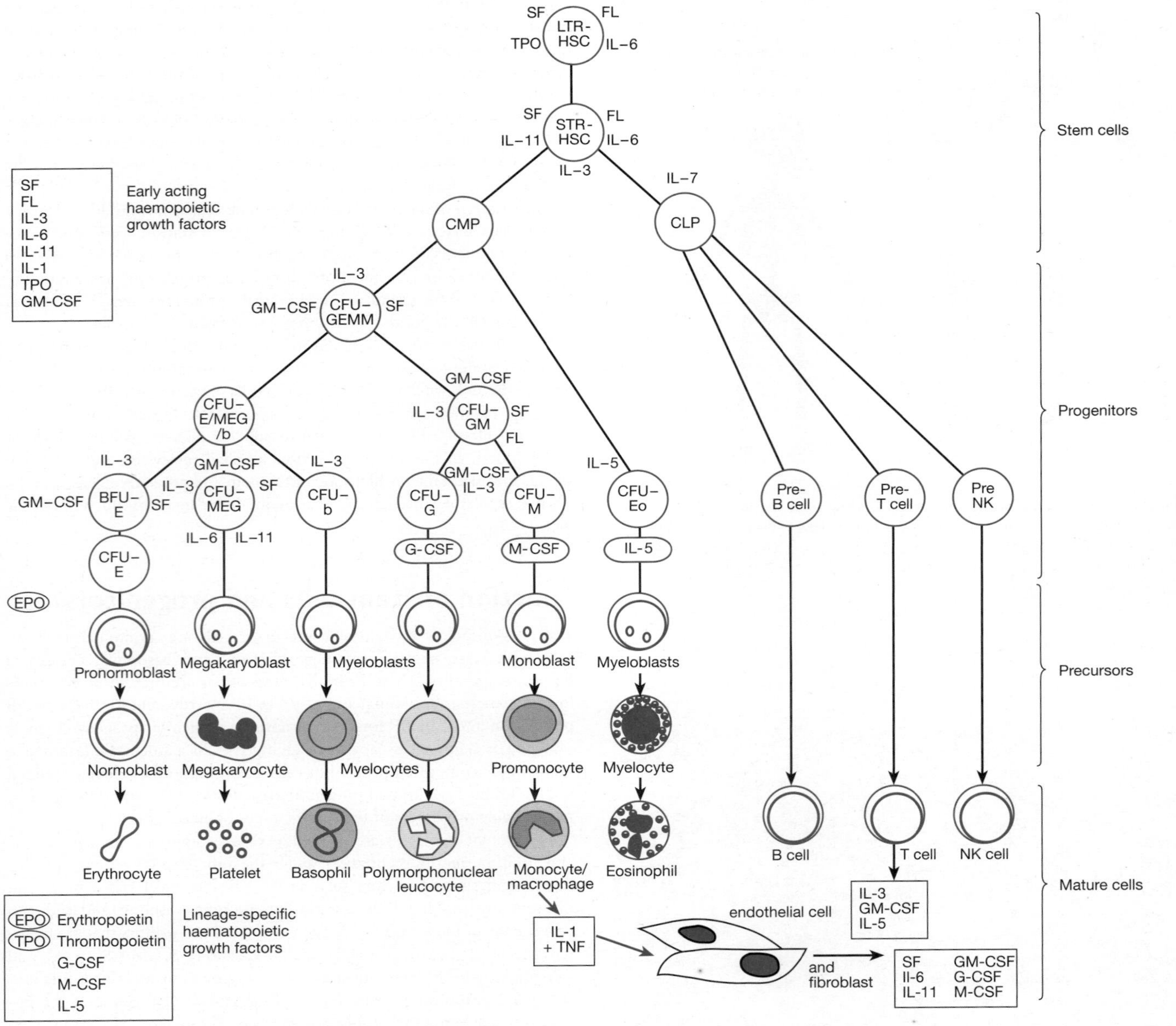

Fig. 3 Maturation of haemopoietic cells and sources and actions of haemopoietic growth factors (HGFs). The predominant actions of several major HGFs are indicated diagrammatically. Steel factor (SF), Flt-3 ligand (FL), IL-11, IL-3, IL-6, and thrombopoietin (TPO) act early during haemopoiesis on haemopoietic stem cells (HSC), while GM-CSF probably act slightly later. The lineage-specific factors erythropoietic (EPO), granulocyte colony-stimulating factor (G-CSF), monocyte-CSF (M-CSF), IL-5, and thrombopoietin act on single lineage-committed progenitors and precursors. Monocytes and macrophages also produce IL-1 and tumour necrosis factor (TNF), potent inducers of HGF production by microenvironmental endothelial and reticular fibroblastoid cells. In addition, macrophages can produce these factors after induction with endotoxin (not shown) and T cells produce IL-3, GM-CSF, and IL-5 in response to IL-1 plus antigenic stimulation.

proto-oncogene, a member of the tyrosine kinase cell-surface receptor family; in contrast, the *Sl* mutation results in defective production of the ligand for this receptor (Steel factor, also known as kit ligand, stem-cell factor, or mast-cell growth factor). Interestingly, Steel factor is produced in both a secreted and membrane-bound form by fibroblasts and other cells. The latter form may thus provide one molecular explanation for interactions between the stem cells and their microenvironment.

Progenitors can exist outside the marrow. Early haemopoietic cells, including the pluripotent stem cells and certain committed progenitor cells, have been demonstrated in the circulation of normal individuals and experimental animals. The capacity of haemopoietic stem cells to negotiate the circulation is especially significant in relation to stem cell transplantation. While this procedure is still often carried out by infusion of bone marrow from the donor into the circulation of the recipient, mobilized blood stem and progenitors cells are now frequently being used.

The relatively limited production of lymphocyte progenitors has made it difficult to demonstrate that the lymphocyte is derived from the same population of stem cells as the other cellular elements of blood. Recent evidence indicates, however, that both T and B lymphocytes and natural killer cells are derived from a common lymphoid progenitor, while a common myeloid progenitor cell matures to form the committed progenitors of red blood cells, phagocytes, and megakaryocytes (Fig. 3).

The pluripotent stem cell

The concept that sustained haemopoiesis comes from pluripotent stem cells derives from the observation that mice can be protected from the lethal effects of whole-body irradiation by exteriorization and shielding of the spleen. This protective effect was shown to be cell mediated as the injection of spleen cells could initiate recovery and re-establish haemopoiesis in irradiated animals. Till and McCulloch demonstrated that colonies of haemopoietic cells could be observed in the spleen in bone-marrow transplanted, irradiated recipient mice within 10 days after the transplant. These spleen colony-forming units (**CFU-S**) produce colonies that contain precursors of erythrocytes, granulocytes, macrophages, and megakaryocytes. Subsequent experiments using karyotypically marked donor cells confirmed the clonal origin of the differentiated cells. Recent experiments in which foreign genes have been inserted into spleen colony-forming cells have further substantiated this finding. Each colony contains a variable number of stem cells that could again form spleen colonies of differentiated progeny in a second irradiated recipient, indicating the self-renewal property of stem cells. The demonstration of a stem cell that can differentiate to form progenitor cells for erythropoiesis, granulopoiesis, and megakaryopoiesis is completely consistent with subsequent observations in diseases such as chronic myeloid leukaemia and polycythaemia vera in which a clonal origin of abnormal erythroid, granulocytic, and megakaryocytic precursor cells can be demonstrated (see Chapter 22.3.5). In addition, these studies of chronic myeloid leukaemia have demonstrated a pluripotent stem cell that gives rise to B cells as well as to the aforementioned blood cells.

Recent studies provide a model in which the CFU-S is viewed as part of a continuum of cells with a decreasing capacity for self-renewal, increasing likelihood for differentiation, and increasing proliferative activity. The cells progress in a unidirectional fashion in this continuum. CFU-S can be distinguished from a more primitive precursor that has the capacity for long-term haemopoietic reconstitution after bone marrow transplantation (**LTR-HSC**, Fig. 3). In the mouse, as few as 30 cells of a highly purified marrow population that lacks lineage-specific antigens but expresses Ly-6 (Sca-1) and low levels of Thy-1 (that is, lin^- $Sca\text{-}1^+$ $Thy\text{-}1^{lo}$) can reconstitute haemopoiesis in 50 per cent of lethally irradiated mice. This fraction appears to comprise virtually 100 per cent CFU-S, but single-cell transfer experiments have shown that it is still heterogeneous. Indeed, cell elutriation studies have shown that most of the CFU-S population is contained within a cell fraction that confers short-term radioprotective capacity (STR-HSC, Fig. 3). It can be separated from a cell fraction with the capacity for long-term haemopoietic reconstitution.

Differences in physical properties and expression of the antigens CD34 and CD33/CD38 have been used to enrich for human stem cells. Most colony-forming cells express all three cell-surface molecules. Cells that give rise to colony-forming cells in long-term bone marrow cultures (that is, long-term culture-initiating cells; LTC-IC) can be separated by their expression of CD34, lack of expression of CD33, CD38, and other lineage-specific markers, and intermediate forward light scattering properties. The importance of $CD34^+$ marrow cells is emphasized by *in vivo* simian studies. Like human bone marrow, the CD34 antigen is expressed by a minority of baboon cells. Infusion of these purified cells can reconstitute lymphohaemopoiesis in lethally irradiated baboons. The recent cloning of the murine CD34 cDNA has cast some doubt on expression of CD34 by LTR-HSC. A monoclonal antibody raised to a murine CD34–GST fusion protein was use to separate marrow cells into $CD34^{lo/-}$, $CD34^{lo}$, and $CD34^+$ fractions. Interestingly, long-term multilineage reconstitution was observed after transplantation of the $CD34^{lo/-}$ cells, whereas the $CD34^+$ fraction gave early but unsustained multilineage reconstitution. These data are supported by experiments demonstrating that a tiny subset of murine bone marrow cells that exclude the Hoechst 33342 dye at blue and red wavelengths (called the side population) contains all the LTR-HSC activity, but is $CD34^-$. Recent human studies have also raised the possibility that LTR-HSC do not express CD34. When primitive human lin^- cells are separated into $CD34^+$ and $CD34^-$ fractions, the capacity to reconstitute haemopoiesis in immunodeficient mice (called SCID repopulating cells or SRC) is found in both cell fractions. A resolution to this controversy may come from the recent demonstration that resting murine haemopoietic stem cells are $CD34^-$, while activated haemopoietic stem cells express the CD34 antigen.

Studies with purified populations of stem cells have shown that combinations of specific haemopoietic growth factors such as Steel factor, Flt-3 ligand , IL-6, and surprisingly, thrombopoietin can act at the stem cell level to induce cell cycling and proliferation. IL-3, produced by T cells and natural killer cells, and GM-CSF, a product of both stromal cells and T cells, appear to be factors essential for the survival *in vitro* of a class of stem cells that forms blast colonies in methylcellulose culture. These 'blast' colonies contain multilineage and unilineage progenitors. They are probably at the myeloid stem-cell stage of differentiation (Fig. 3). When isolated from bone marrow, these stem cells are mostly in a non-cycling, quiescent state. The addition of IL-3, GM-CSF, or Steel factor or other stromally produced haemopoietic growth factors such as IL-6, IL-11, or G-CSF shortens the G_0 phase in these cultures, thus hastening the onset of blast colony formation.

The factors that control the fate of stem cells to undergo either self-renewal or commitment to differentiate down a lineage pathway are poorly understood. However, nuclear transcription factors have been shown to play a role in haemopoietic cell proliferation and lineage commitment. The tal-1/SCL, Rbtn2/LMO2, and GATA family of transcription factors are important in this regard. In particular, tal-1/SCL, a basic helix–loop–helix (bHLH) transcription factor, is expressed in biphenotypic (lymphoid/myeloid) and T-cell leukaemias, and in both early haemopoietic progenitors and more mature erythroid, mast, megakaryocyte, and endothelial cells. Targeted disruption of the *tal-1/SCL* gene in murine embryonic stem cells leads to death *in utero* from absence of blood formation; a lack of *in vitro* myeloid colony formation suggests a role for this factor very early during haemopoiesis.

Another transcription factor implicated in T-cell ALL is the LIM domain nuclear protein rhombotin 2 (rbtn2/LMO2). Mice that lack this factor die *in utero* and have the same bloodless phenotype as the $tal\text{-}1/SCL^{-/-}$ animals. GATA-2 is expressed in the regions of the *Xenopus* and zebrafish embryos that are fated to become haemopoietic, and is highly expressed in progenitor cells. Overexpression of GATA-2 in chicken erythroid progenitors leads to proliferation at the expense of differentiation. Targeted disruption of the *GATA-2* gene by homologous recombination in embryonic stem cells leads to reduced primitive haemopoiesis in the yolk sac and embryonic death by day 10 to 11. Definitive haemopoiesis in liver and bone marrow is profoundly reduced with loss of virtually all lineages. *In vitro* differentiation data show a marked deficiency of Steel factor-responsive definitive erythroid and mast cell colonies and reduced macrophage colonies, suggesting that GATA-2 serves as a regulator of genes that control haemopoietic growth factor responsiveness or proliferation of stem and/or early progenitor cells. These data contrast with the later time of embryonic death from anaemia (day 15) in mice with targeted disruption of the c-*myb* or retinoblastoma (*Rb*) genes, or with severe forms of *W* and *Sl* mutations. Similarly, loss of function of the AML-1 gene, which encodes one of the α subunits of the heterodimeric core-binding factor (**CBF**), results in fetal death by day 12.5 due to failure of production of all definitive haemopoietic lineages. CBF recognition sequences are present in the IL-3, GM-CSF, M-CSFR, and T-cell antigen receptor promoters. The *AML-1* gene is frequently rearranged in acute myeloid leukaemia (AML) and childhood acute lymphoblastic leukaemia (ALL), and is expressed in myeloid and lymphoid cells.

The survival of a particular stem cell in the marrow requires a 'niche'; thus isogeneic marrow infusions are not successful unless the recipient is irradiated or treated with sufficient doses of cytotoxic drugs to create an adequate number of niches. Therefore, reports of failure of engraftment in aplastic anaemia using identical twin donors do not necessarily implicate an immunological basis for the disease. Equally likely is persistence of nonfunctional pluripotent progenitors in the aplastic marrow niches. These abnormal cells must be destroyed in order to allow implantation of transfused normal progenitors.

The stem cell model of haemopoiesis has parallels in other organ systems. That rapidly self-renewing epithelial tissues like skin and intestine have stem cells that continually replenish the cells lost by differentiation is well described. It is likely that most epithelial tissues, for example liver and pancreas, also contain stem cells that are brought to bear after organ damage. The demonstration of the existence of neural stem cells in the adult brain has raised the possibility that many organ systems might retain a population of self-renewing stem cells. Muscle satellite cells also appear to fulfil this role.

Much more surprising are recent demonstrations of stem cell plasticity. Transplantation of genetically marked bone marrow showed that the donor cells can migrate into areas of damaged muscle, differentiate into myogenic cells, and participate in tissue regeneration. Similarly, transplanted haemopoietic cells can differentiate into glial cells in adult mouse brain, into endothelial cells, and into hepatocytes in damaged liver. Mesenchymal stem cells, derived from an adherent bone marrow cell population, express neither CD34 nor CD45, markers of primitive haemopoietic cells. Mesenchymal stem cells are capable of marked expansion in culture, and can then be induced to differentiate into osteoblasts and osteocytes, chondrocytes, adipocytes, and myotubules.

That stem cell plasticity may be therapeutically useful is suggested by bone marrow transplant studies in three patients with ostegenesis imperfecta, in which low-level osteoblast engraftment was demonstrated 3 months post-transplantation, with histological changes indicating new dense bone formation. These studies do not address the question of the identity of the engrafting cell, since whole unfractionated marrow was used. Further studies with purified cell populations and longer follow-up will be required. The relationship of the mesenchymal stem cells to the haemopoietic stem cells is not clearly defined, especially in view of the recent demonstration that the highly purified CD34– side population of murine marrow can reconstitute not only haemopoietic activity, but also contribute nuclei to muscle fibres, partially restoring expression of dystrophin in the *mdx* mouse, a model of Duchenne muscular dystrophy. Finally, it is now apparent that the plasticity of primitive cells is not confined to the haemopoietic system, with the demonstration that blood cells can be derived from both neural and myogenic satellite cells.

Erythropoiesis

The rate of erythropoiesis is driven by anaemia or hypoxia. Both stimulate a class of peritubular kidney cells, through a haem-containing oxygen sensor, to transcribe the erythropoietin gene and release the hormone into the blood. The hormone binds to the erythropoietin receptor in erythroblasts and erythroid progenitors to stimulate their division and differentiation. The least mature committed erythroid progenitor is known as an erythroid burst-forming unit (**BFU-E**), because when it differentiates *in vitro* it forms large colonies of erythroblasts and reticulocytes that may contain as many as 50 000 cells. The colonies, derived from single cells, have a burst-like appearance because they may be composed of multiple subcolonies. Thus one BFU-E may first divide in culture to form subcolony-forming cells, which then differentiate into colonies of erythroblasts and reticulocytes. BFU-E progressively mature during their sojourn in the marrow. In doing so they lose their capacity to divide and migrate *in vitro*, but gain in sensitivity to erythropoietin until they reach the stage at which they are known as erythroid colony-forming units (**CFU-E**).

The regulated proliferation and maturation of erythroid progenitors depends on interaction with a number of growth factors. Erythropoietin is essential for the terminal maturation of erythroid cells. Its major effect appears to be at the level of the CFU-E during adult erythropoiesis. Recombinant preparations are as effective as the natural hormone. These very mature progenitors and proerythroblasts do not require 'burst-promoting activity' in the form of IL-3, GM-CSF, or Steel factor. Their dependence on erythropoietin is emphasized by the observation that they will not survive *in vitro* in its absence.

Steel factor has also been shown to have marked synergistic effects on BFU-E cultured in the presence of erythropoietin. Alone, it has no colony-forming ability. The majority of CFU-E are in cycle; their survival in the presence of erythropoietin is probably tightly linked to their proliferation and differentiation to proerythroblasts and mature erythrocytes. Erythropoietin also acts on a subset of presumptive mature BFU-E that require it for survival and terminal differentiation. A second subset of BFU-E, presumably less mature, survive deprivation of erythropoietin if 'burst-promoting activity' is present, either as Steel factor, IL-3, or GM-CSF. Under serum-deprived culture conditions, the combination of erythropoietin and IL-3 or GM-CSF results in more BFU-E-derived colonies than when erythropoietin is added alone.

Factors distinct from the classic colony-stimulating factors may positively regulate erythropoiesis, either directly or indirectly. Limiting dilution studies of highly purified CFU-E in serum-free culture show that insulin and insulin-like growth factor I act directly on these cells. The presence of erythropoietin is also essential. CFU-E and mature BFU-E are highly responsive to the mitogenic effect of erythropoietin as well as to its differentiating role. Therefore, in haemorrhagic or haemolytic anaemias with elevated levels of erythropoietin, the numbers of CFU-E and mature BFU-E may rise remarkably in the marrow. Immature BFU-E are less responsive to the mitogenic effect of erythropoietin, and therefore, the frequency of this subset of BFU-E changes little in anaemia.

Negative regulation of erythropoiesis

Subsets of lymphocytes with an immunological suppressor phenotype isolated from normal subjects can inhibit erythroid activity *in vitro*. Similarly, some patients with anaemia or granulocytopenia have an associated expansion of certain T-lymphocyte populations. In the rare disorder 'T lymphocytosis with cytopenia', *in vitro* suppression of erythropoiesis (or granulocytopoiesis) has been correlated with the expansion of a T-lymphocyte population that may be the counterpart of the haemopoietic suppressor cells isolated from normal peripheral blood. The phenotype of these cells has been described in detail. The cell is a large, granular lymphocyte that is both CD2 and CD8 (classic suppressor phenotype) positive. Suppressor T cells may also be involved in some cases of aplastic anaemia or neutropenia without any underlying immunological disorder or an overt T-cell proliferation.

Exactly how suppressor T cells interact with haemopoietic progenitors, and what surface antigens are 'seen' by the suppressors is not known. There is evidence to support the concept that suppression of erythroid colony expression *in vitro* can be regulated by T cells and may be genetically restricted. Certain phenotypes of T cells 'recognize' distinct classes of histocompatibility antigens on immunological cell surfaces. Thus, the observation that haemopoietic progenitors have a unique distribution of class II histocompatibility antigens on their cell surface suggests a role for these antigens in the cell–cell interactions that regulate haemopoietic differentiation.

T cells may also inhibit erythropoiesis in a non-HLA restricted fashion by the production of inhibitory cytokines. Some lymphokines may inhibit erythropoiesis *in vitro* by a complex lymphokine cascade. Activation of T cells by the T-cell antigen receptor CD3 results in cell-surface expression of the IL-2 α-chain (p55) and the acquisition of IL-2 responsiveness. IL-2 inhibits BFU-E in the presence of these IL-2R positive cells, possibly by inducing their release of interferon-γ. CD2 can serve as an alternative pathway of T-cell activation, and may do so through binding to its ligand LFA-3 on antigen-presenting cells. Blockade of CD2 with monoclonal antibody leads to abrogation of IL-2/ interferon-γ-mediated BFU-E suppression. These data are difficult to reconcile with the observation that IL-2 incubation of activated CD4+ T cells leads to marked expansion of IL-3 and GM-CSF mRNA-positive cells by *in situ* hybridization. Most, but not all, CD4+ T cells express CD28 as well, and there is evidence to suggest that IL-3 production is restricted to CD28+ T cells. It thus appears paradoxical that potent stimulating and inhibitory lymphokines can be produced by activation of T cells through the same pathway.

Tumour necrosis factor also suppresses erythropoiesis *in vitro*. The injection of peritoneal macrophages into animals infected with Friend murine leukaemia virus results in rapid but transient resolution of the massive erythroid hyperplasia associated with this disease. This may be due to elaboration by macrophages of IL-1α, which does not suppress erythropoiesis itself, but acts by the induction of tumour necrosis factor. This effect is reversed by erythropoietin.

Proerythroblasts represent the ultimate stage of differentiation of committed erythroid progenitors. In contrast to the progenitors, which comprise less than 0.1 per cent of the marrow cell population, proerythroblasts are present at 3 to 5 per cent, and their daughters, the recognizable erythroid precursors, comprise 30 per cent of the population.

Estimates of reticulocyte production and erythroblast content of marrows, together with measurements of the rate at which the proerythroblast compartment is renewed from the progenitor pool, suggest that approximately 10 per cent of the daily reticulocyte production is derived from the terminal differentiation of proerythroblasts newly developed from the progenitor department. During anaemic stress the rate at which progenitors differentiate to proerythroblasts may increase 10-fold or more. This increase in the rate of proerythroblast formation from progenitors is associated with an increase in the production of fetal haemoglobin in a large fraction of the erythroid cells derived from them. The basis of this reactivation of fetal haemoglobin synthesis is not understood. The extent to which fetal haemoglobin may be increased in such settings could be genetically controlled. It is an important phenomenon because those with the capacity to develop large increases in fetal haemoglobin who are also homozygous for major β-chain haemoglobinopathies may have a remarkably mild course. Fetal haemoglobin elevation occurs in many forms of accelerated erythropoiesis and is a marker of such a condition.

Phagocytopoiesis

The development of a clonal assay for granulocyte and macrophage progenitors preceded the development of erythroid progenitor assays by nearly a decade, yet a clear understanding of the regulation of myeloid differentiation remains elusive. Figure 3 describes the development and regulation of granulocyte, monocyte, and macrophage production from the pluripotent stem cell. The colony-forming unit-granulocyte-macrophage (**CFU-GM**) is derived from the pluripotent progenitor. It gives rise to separate granulocyte and monocyte progenitors (CFU-G and CFU-M), which, under the influence of unique colony-stimulating factors, differentiate to mature granulocytes and/or monocytes, respectively. Both IL-3 and GM-CSF affect a similar broad spectrum of human myeloid progenitor cells. This includes colonies that contain granulocytes, erythrocytes, monocytes, and megakaryocytes (**CFU-GEMM**), eosinophils (**CFU-Eo**), CFU-GM, CFU-G, and CFU-M. Data from serum-free cultures suggest that in the presence of IL-3 or GM-CSF alone, myeloid colony formation is much reduced. Optimal CFU-G or CFU-M proliferation requires the addition of G-CSF or M-CSF, respectively, to the cultures. Even in serum-replete conditions, IL-3 acts additively or synergistically with G-CSF to induce more granulocyte colony formation than is observed with either factor alone.

Serum-free studies may have important implications for the use of combinations of colony-stimulating factors *in vivo*. The use of such culture conditions should provide further insight into the *in vitro* activities of the different factors.

Colony-stimulating factors also induce a variety of functional changes in mature cells. GM-CSF inhibits polymorphonuclear neutrophil migration, induces antibody-dependent cellular cytotoxicity (**ADCC**) for human target cells, and increases neutrophil phagocytic activity. Some of these changes may be related to GM-CSF-induced increase in the cell-surface expression of a family of antigens that function as cell adhesion molecules. The increase in antigen expression is rapid and is associated with increased aggregation of neutrophils. Granulocyte–granulocyte adhesion can be inhibited by an antigen-specific monoclonal antibody. GM-CSF also acts as a potent stimulus of eosinophil ADCC, superoxide production, and phagocytosis. G-CSF acts as a potent stimulus of neutrophil superoxide production, ADCC, and phagocytosis, while M-CSF activates mature macrophages and enhances macrophage cytotoxicity.

Monocytes leave the circulation and differentiate further to become fixed tissue macrophages. These tissue macrophages include alveolar macrophages and hepatic Kupffer cells, dermal Langerhans cells, osteoclasts, peritoneal macrophages, pleural macrophages, and possibly brain microglial cells, though the origin of these is still uncertain. The wide variety of cells with diverse functions that must be supplied from the granulocyte–macrophage progenitor requires that this system be highly regulated at many levels of differentiation.

The granulocyte compartment itself is more complex than either the erythroid or megakaryocyte compartments. The circulating half-life of the newly rapidly deployed granulocyte is only 6.5 h. In order to meet sudden demands, an additional non-circulating granulocyte pool exists in the spleen, marginated around blood vessels, and in a readily releasable bone-marrow pool. The rate at which new myeloblasts or monoblasts are produced by progenitors *in vivo* is not known, but exhaustion of progenitors in infection, particularly in the neonatal period, is associated with a fatal outcome due to a failure of granulocyte production.

Suppression of phagocyte production

An elaborate system exists for suppression of granulocyte and macrophage production. It involves T lymphocytes and their products, particularly interferon-γ, monocytes, and perhaps acidic isoferritins. In some circumstances, clones of T cells that suppress granulocyte production *in vitro* and *in vivo* have caused profound granulocytopenia. Clearly, a twin regulatory system exists that contributes to the fine control of phagocyte production by close control between progenitors and adventitial cells that secrete inducer and suppressor molecules. It is well established that T lymphocytes capable of the suppression of phagocyte colony formation may be present in human marrow and induce neutropenia.

Megakaryocytopoiesis

The cloning of thrombopoietin has greatly clarified our understanding of the regulation of megakaryocytopoiesis. Prior to the discovery of thrombopoietin, several factors including IL-3, IL-6, IL-11, Steel factor, and even erythropoietin were shown to stimulate megakaryocytopoiesis and thrombopoiesis *in vitro* and *in vivo*. IL-11 has even entered clinical trials. Hence, all of the above mentioned haemopoietic growth factors, except erythropoietin, can contribute collectively to 'megakaryocyte colony-stimulating activity' (**Meg-CSA**). Meg-CSA is therefore a 'soup' of growth factors that transduce three of the four classes of receptors that drive haemopoietic differentiation; these comprise the β common, tyrosine kinase, and gp130 families. All of these receptors, when engaged, drive early progenitor proliferation and partial differentiation to more mature progenitors. The final steps of lineage-committed mature progenitor development into recognizable marrow precursors require a lineage-specific growth factor—G-CSF for the granulocyte, M-CSF for the macrophage, IL-5 for the eosinophil, and erythropoietin for the erythrocyte.

The discovery of thrombopoietin provides the final step of understanding of megakaryocytopoiesis because this factor, and probably none other, actually induces lineage-restricted megakaryocyte progenitor proliferation, differentiation of those committed progenitors to megakaryoblasts, and finally, differentiation of megakaryoblasts to the megakaryocytes that in turn produce platelets. However, this in no way implies that other Meg-CSA components may not be useful in the therapy of hypoplastic thrombocytopenias. Circulating thrombopoietin levels are high in those conditions, just as erythropoietin levels are elevated in the erythroid hypoplasias. Administration of high doses of erythropoietin is usually of little benefit in the latter conditions. Thrombopoietin may be just as unsuccessful in certain megakaryocyte hypoplasias because those conditions are often associated with severe depletion of lineage-specific or multipotent progenitors. One or more of the growth factors that comprise Meg-CSA, such as IL-11, may be more useful in such circumstances. Clinical trials now in progress will decide this issue.

Thrombopoietin

Identification of the proto-oncogene c-*mpl* revealed an orphan haemopoietic growth factor receptor that proved to be crucial for megakaryocytopoiesis. In 1993, Methia and coworkers performed a critically important experiment, when they demonstrated that exposure of CD34+ progenitor cells in culture to oligonucleotides that were antisense to c-mpl inhibited the ability of these cells to form megakaryocyte, but not other haemopoietic colonies. In 1994 several laboratories cloned the all-important ligand for this receptor, the growth factor thrombopoietin, and important physiological studies of thrombopoietin were launched.

The thrombopoietin gene is localized on the long arm of chromosome 3. It contains five exons, the boundaries of which line up precisely with those of the erythropoietin gene. The gene is widely expressed in liver, kidney, smooth muscle, endothelial cells, and fibroblasts. Thus thrombopoietin is produced at the site of stoma supporting haemopoiesis. Though its activity is increased in the blood during episodes of thrombocytopenia, it does not necessarily function as a hormone because it is produced directly at the site of thrombopoiesis. In this sense, it differs from erythropoietin, which is not produced at all in marrow stroma. It is likely that the level of production of thrombopoietin is quite constant in all tissues. The blood levels may increase in thrombocytopenic states merely because circulating platelets and tissue megakaryocytes sop up the growth factor and carry it out of the circulation. This theory has received support from observations in mice with disruption of the murine transcription factor gene called *NF-E2*; although these animals are thrombocytopenic they have an increase in megakaryocyte mass and no increase in serum thrombopoietin levels.

The thrombopoietin molecule is considerably longer than the other haemopoietic growth factor polypeptides. Its 5' half bears 23 per cent sequence homology to erythropoietin, while the 3' half bears no structural homology to any cytokine and may be removed by a proteolytic mechanism. Indeed, removal of this half does not ablate physiological function. The resemblance of the 5' domain of the molecule to erythropoietin may explain the synergy of thrombopoietin and erythropoietin in megakaryocyte colony formation and platelet production. It is well recognized that splenectomized individuals with persistent anaemia usually have significant thrombocytosis and many individuals with red cell aplasia and high erythropoietin levels also have thrombocytosis and megakaryocytosis.

Circulating platelets

The differential diagnosis of thrombocytopenia rests first on evaluation of platelet morphology. In conditions in which megakaryocytopoiesis is accelerated, circulating platelet volume (and usually diameter) is increased. The reasons for this shift in volume are disputed. Some claim that young platelets are larger than old platelets, while others suggest that large megakaryocytes give rise to large platelets. Neither explanation satisfies all experimental and clinical conditions, but in general, thrombocytopenia secondary to increased destruction of platelets is associated with platelets of large volume. Thrombocytopenia related to decreased production of platelets is associated with platelets of normal size.

There are major exceptions to this rule. Patients with hyposplenism tend to have large platelets in their blood, whether thrombopoiesis is increased or not, and patients with primary abnormalities of platelet function, such as Wiskott–Aldrich syndrome or Bernard–Soulier syndrome, have small and large platelets, respectively, that bear no relationship to platelet production. Thrombopoietin increases platelet production by increasing both the number and size of individual megakaryocytes. Though thrombopoietin is probably solely responsible for the later stages of recognizable megakaryocyte differentiation and proliferation of megakaryocyte progenitors, its function depends, at least in part, on the additional stimulation of earlier megakaryocyte progenitors with other growth factors, including IL-3, IL-11, and Steel factor.

Down-regulation of megakaryocytes

There is great uncertainty about possible down-regulation of megakaryocytes. Platelet factor 4 seems to down-regulate colony formation *in vitro*. If active *in vivo*, this would provide an interesting feedback loop. Transforming growth factor-β is also a potent inhibitor *in vitro*. Natural killer cells, which are thought by some to be general suppressors of haemopoiesis *in vitro*, actually enhance megakaryocyte colony formation *in vitro*. In addition, an antibody to natural killer cells, when it is given intraperitoneally in massive doses to mice, abolishes the formation of colonies of megakaryocytes that can be grown in culture from murine marrow. Natural killer cells may thus actually play a stimulating role *in vivo*.

Megakaryocyte progenitors in disease

A number of attempts have been made to relate diseases associated with elevated or depressed platelet counts to the number or the growth characteristics of megakaryocyte progenitors. Megakaryocyte progenitors in essential thrombocythaemia are similar in their growth characteristics to the expanded numbers of erythroid progenitors in polycythaemia vera. The latter develop into erythroid colonies without additions of erythropoietin to the culture medium. The trace of erythropoietin in the serum is sufficient to drive the sensitive receptor system in these progenitors. In a similar fashion, the numerous CFU-Meg in essential thrombocythaemia develop into megakaryocyte colonies in the absence of stimulation by aplastic anaemia serum. They are 'thrombopoietin independent' and many produce endogenous thrombopoietin.

Clinical studies with haemopoietic growth factors

Several recombinant haemopoietic growth factors are currently in use and under evaluation in a variety of clinical settings. Initial studies focused on erythropoietin in the anaemia of chronic renal failure, and GM-CSF and G-CSF in both transient and long-standing bone marrow-failure syndromes. These three factors are now commercially available for clinical use. More recently, other haemopoietic growth factors such as M-CSF, IL-3, and Steel factor are coming under scrutiny.

Anaemia is a major complication of endstage renal failure, and is due primarily to a reduction in erythropoietin production. Several phase I, II, and III studies have documented that recombinant human erythropoietin can induce a dose-dependent increase in effective erythropoiesis. The extension of this treatment to patients who do not yet require dialysis has met with similar success. Erythropoietin may also be useful in the anaemia of chronic disease and in the anaemia that complicates azidothymidine treatment of patients with acquired immune deficiency disease (**AIDS**).

G-CSF has proven to be useful for shortening the period of neutropenia following myelosuppressive anticancer chemotherapy, and has been approved in the United States and Europe for reduction of infection in patients with non-myeloid malignancies. GM-CSF and G-CSF can accelerate haemopoietic reconstitution after bone marrow transplantation, and GM-CSF has been approved for use in the United States in autologous transplantation. In the context of bone marrow failure, GM-CSF is a useful palliative treatment as it can increase the neutrophil count, particularly in the majority of children with acquired aplastic anaemia. GM-CSF can also increase neutrophils, eosinophils, and monocytes in AIDS. Most patients with Kostmann syndrome, a rare inherited severe failure of neutrophil production, respond dramatically to G-CSF treatment. Patients with other defects of neutrophil production such as cyclic neutropenia and chronic idiopathic neutropenia have also responded to this factor.

Recombinant human thrombopoietin or its polyethylene glycol (**PEG**)-derivatized 163 residue aminoterminus (PEG-MGDF) stimulates megakaryocyte proliferation and endoreduplication *in vitro* and is a potent inducer of megakaryocytopoiesis and platelet production *in vivo* in mice and non-human primates. Both recombinant human thrombopoietin and PEG-MGDF are safe and show no organ toxicity. In normal volunteers a single bolus of 3 μg/kg per day of PEG-MGDF doubles the blood platelet concentration by day 12, with a return to baseline by day 28. A stimulatory effect on platelet production was observed when thrombopoietin or PEG-MGDF was administered after chemotherapy to more than 100 patients with cancer, with a decrease in the time for platelet counts to return to normal and elevated platelet nadirs. Antibodies to thrombopoietin have been reported in one patient with cancer and in volunteers given subcutaneous PEG-MGDF. Further clinical development of this thrombopoietin formulation has been stopped, since transient decreases in platelet count were noted. It is possible that the factor is more antigenic when given by the subcutaneous route.

Summary

Haemopoiesis is the process of terminal differentiation of recognizable immature precursors of the formed elements of the blood. Renewal of the precursor pool is accompanied by the differentiation of committed progenitor cells that are themselves renewed by a process of stochastic maturation of stem cells. A group of haemopoietins derived from T cells, monocytes, and fibroblasts governs the differentiation of committed progenitor cells by mechanisms yet to be defined.

The *mélange* of marrow cells described above exists in delicate fronds thrust into the venous sinuses. Cells are packed in close proximity within the fronds, held together by extensions of fibroblast cytoplasm and fibronectin. Such a delicate anatomy is subject to a myriad of abnormalities that can disturb the orderly progress of cell–cell interactions that govern the system. The multiple symptoms of bone marrow failure are the results of these disturbances.

Further reading

Clark S, Nathan DG, Sieff CA (1997). The anatomy and physiology of hematopoiesis. In: Nathan DG, Orkin SH, eds. *Hematology of infancy and childhood.* W.B. Saunders, Philadelphia. [Comprehensive chapter that discusses haemopoiesis in more detail.]

Cosman D *et al.* (1990). A new cytokine receptor superfamily. *Trends in Biochemical Sciences* **15**, 265–70. [Review of the haemopoietic growth factor receptors.]

Drachman JG (2000). Role of thrombopoietin in hematopoietic stem cell and progenitor regulation. *Current Opinion in Hematology* **7**, 183–90.

Gerson SL (1999). Mesenchymal stem cells: no longer second class marrow citizens. *Nature Medicine* **5**, 262–4.

Goodell MA *et al.* (1997). Dye efflux studies suggest that hematopoietic stem cells expressing low or undetectable levels of CD34 antigen exist in multiple species. *Nature Medicine* **3**, 1337–45. [Demonstration that purified murine and rhesus 'side population' cells do not express CD34 and have stem cell properties.]

Gussoni E *et al.* (1999). Dystrophin expression in the mdx mouse restored by stem cell transplantation. *Nature* **401**, 390–4. [Example of the plasticity of both haemopoietic and muscle stem cells.]

Horwitz EM *et al.* (1999). Transplantability and therapeutic effects of bone marrow-derived mesenchymal cells in children with osteogenesis imperfecta. *Nature Medicine* **5**, 309–13.

Kaushansky K (1995). Thrombopoietin: the primary regulator of megakaryocyte and platelet production. *Thrombosis and Haemostasis* **74**, 521–5.

Metcalf D (1984). *The hemopoietic growth factors.* Elsevier, Amsterdam.

Metcalf D, Moore MAS (1971). *Haematopoietic cells.* North-Holland Publishing Company, Amsterdam.

Miyajima A *et al.* (1992). Cytokine receptors and signal transduction. *Annual Review of Immunology* **10**, 295–331. [Review of haemopoietic growth factor signal transduction pathways.]

Nicola NA (1989). Hemopoietic cell growth factors and their receptors. *Annual Review of Biochemistry* **58**, 45–77.

Osawa M *et al.* (1996). Long-term lymphohematopoietic reconstitution by a single CD34– low/negative hematopoietic stem cell. *Science* **273**, 242–5. [Original paper showing that murine long-term reconstituting stem cells do not express CD34.]

Shivdasani RA, Orkin SH (1996). The transcriptional control of hematopoiesis. *Blood* **87**, 4025–39.

Weissman IL (2000). Translating stem and progenitor cell biology to the clinic: barriers and opportunities. *Science* **287**, 1442–6. [Review of current research and clinical potential of haemopoietic stem cells.]

22.2.2 Stem-cell disorders

D. C. Linch

Concept of the haemopoietic stem cell and its disorders

The haemopoietic stem cell is a poorly defined entity with an undifferentiated phenotype, which resides within the haemopoietic tissue. It has the ability to self-renew, and the capacity to generate large numbers of mature progeny of multiple haemopoietic lineages. It was considered that such cells were irreversibly committed to haemopoiesis. More recent data suggest that stem cells have far greater plasticity than previously appreciated. Within the adult marrow, stem cells have been found that can give rise not only to blood cells, but also to other mesodermally derived tissues such as endothelium and muscle and to hepatic and neuronal cells traditionally thought to be derived from the endoderm and ectoderm, respectively. In some instances the extensive repertoire is due to the presence of non-haemopoietic mesenchymal stem cells within the bone marrow, but there is also evidence that stem cells with haemopoietic potential can give rise to other tissue-types. In addition, stem cells within the brain have been shown to be capable of generating cells that are embryologically derived from all three germ layers, and this includes the generation of haemopoietic cells. Either very undifferentiated multipotent stem cells persist in many adult tissues or, under appropriate conditions, some stem cells can undergo dedifferentiation and reprogramming. The most dramatic evidence for the possibility of dedifferentiation comes from 'Dolly the sheep', generated by the transfer of a mature cell nucleus into an enucleated egg. Clearly, the environment within the egg cytoplasm can reprogramme the genetic material within the nucleus. It is conceivable that similar processes could be induced by an appropriate extracellular milieu. It is not yet clear whether these new insights into the potential of the stem cell will alter the way in which we consider the haemopoietic stem cell disorders, but some of the fundamental assumptions of recent decades may be challenged.

Quantitative and qualitative abnormalities of haemopoietic stem cells can be envisaged. The stem-cell population might become depleted and fail to produce adequate mature progeny. Similarly, a normal number of abnormal stem cells could fail to proliferate normally and thus generate the same deficiency of end-cells. Abnormal stem cells could also produce normal numbers of defective end-cells, or the stem cells could undergo malignant transformation. These possibilities are not mutually exclusive and transitional forms can be envisaged.

In practice, the definition of a stem-cell disorder is often extremely difficult. Self-renewal, one of the hallmarks of a stem cell, cannot be considered in the context of malignant disorders, as any malignant clone, arising in any tissue, at any stage of differentiation, must have undergone immortalization and be capable of self-renewal. The term 'stem-cell disorder' is usually used, therefore, to imply that the target cell for the disease process has occurred in a cell with the potential to develop into cells of different lineages. Such a cell could be a relatively 'late' or 'lineage-restricted, stem-cell' capable, for example, of giving rise to phagocytes and erythrocytes, or it could be a very primitive stem cell capable of giving rise to all myeloid and lymphoid lineages. There are, however, a number of difficulties with such a definition. First, malignant change in a very primitive cell does not necessarily lead to the production of mature cells of multiple lineages. It is a feature of the acute leukaemias that there is a block in differentiation; in some cases of acute myeloid leukaemia (**AML**), no mature progeny are produced by the malignant clone. In other cases of AML, neutrophils alone are produced. However, it cannot be assumed that the target cell of the original oncogenic event was not a cell with the potential to form all the myeloid elements, including the red cell series. Second, whereas an immature phenotype of a malignant cells was always considered to be indicative of the transformation of a very early cell, we must now consider the possibility that transformation could arise in a later cell with subsequent dedifferentiation.

The concept of a haemopoietic stem-cell disorder is, therefore, imprecise. Pragmatically a stem-cell disorder is most easily considered as a disease with multilineage involvement.

Detection of multilineage involvement

In the bone marrow hypoplastic states, stem-cell involvement is obvious because of the pancytopenia that occurs. In the myeloproliferative disorders examination of the blood count and blood film also reveals the involvement of multiple lineages; neutrophil leucocytosis may coexist with eosinophilia, basophilia, and thrombocytosis. A number of more sophisticated techniques have also been used to demonstrate that a particular cell lineage is involved in a clonal process (Table 1).

Analysis of non-random cytogenetic abnormalities represents one of the most longstanding techniques for examining cell-lineage involvement in the haematological malignancies. This approach was used in the investigation of acute myeloid leukaemia to show that the large majority of T cells in the peripheral blood were not part of the malignant clone. The combination of this technique with immunophenotyping for lineage-specific markers provides a powerful addition to this approach. Conventional cytogenetic studies suffer the disadvantage that only cells in metaphase can be analysed, but techniques such as fluorescent *in situ* hybridization (**FISH**) (with or without immunophenotyping) allow cells in interphase to be examined.

Somatic mutations, from major chromosomal alterations to point mutations, can also be detected using non-microscopic methods employing recombinant DNA technology. Polymerase chain reaction (**PCR**) methods are particularly sensitive and make it possible to study small samples of cells, but it is difficult to make the techniques fully quantitative. Errors in interpretation can readily arise from minor contaminating cells in supposedly purified cell populations. Analysis of somatic mutations is subject to a further potential problem if the mutation is a secondary event in the disease process. Under these circumstances the mutation observed could have arisen in a subclone and not be present in all the malignant cells. In acute myeloid leukaemia mutations in *N-ras* may be present in all or just a few cells; sometimes a mutation detected at presentation cannot be found

Table 1 Assessment of clonality in haematological disorders

1.	*Chromosome analysis by microscopy*	
	Conventional cytogenetic analysis	
	Dual cytogenetic analysis with surface immunophenotyping	
	Fluorescent *in situ* hybridization (FISH) for specific chromosome translocations, and changes in chromosome number, e.g. trisomy 8	
	Dual FISH and immunophenotyping	
2.	*Detection of somatic mutations by non-microscopic means*	
	Detection of chromosome loss	) RFLP analysis
	Detection of translocations	) and
	Detection of point mutations	) PCR
	DNA fingerprinting	) methodology
3.	*Lymphocyte gene rearrangements*[*]	
	Expression of surface light chains on B cells	
	Rearrangement of immunoglobulin heavy- and light-chain genes	
	Rearrangement of T-cell receptor genes (β, γ, δ)	
4.	*X- chromosome inactivation*	
	Protein expression, e.g. isoforms of G6PD	
	DNA expression:	
	PGK	
	HPRT	
	M27B	
	HUMARA	
	MOA	
	Fragile X (FMR1)	
	mRNA expression:	
	HUMARA	
	G6PD	
	IDS	
	P55	

[*] Detection of lymphocyte gene rearrangements is not usually applicable to the stem-cell disorders, but a small proportion of cases of acute myeloid leukaemia do have rearrangements of the immunoglobulin heavy chains or T-cell receptor genes.

RFLP, restriction fragment length polymorphism; PCR, polymerase chain reaction; G6PD, glucose-6-phosphate dehydrogenase; PGK, phosphoglycerate kinase; HPRT, hypoxanthine phosphoribosyl transferase; HUMARA, human androgen receptor; MOA, monoamine oxidase-A.

in relapse, indicative of the process of clonal evolution and the fact that the *ras* mutation was not an early event in the leukaemogenic process.

The use of polymorphic X-linked markers has been a very useful tool for examining clonality in informative females, and is not subject to the problems of clonal evolution. The original studies used the enzyme glucose-6-phosphate dehydrogenase (**G6PD**). However, there are many structural variants of this enzyme, the most common normally active variant being designated as B type. In populations of African descent a common normal variant exists which is designated as A type. Although this variant only differs by one amino acid it can be readily separated from the B type on starch-gel electrophoresis. Because the gene which codes for G6PD is on the X-chromosome, individual cells of a heterozygous female (AB) express only one enzyme type, with approximately half the cells expressing type A and half type B (in other words, the individual is a mosaic). This restricted pattern of gene expression arises because of the process of random X-inactivation, known as lyonization, which occurs in early embryonic life and is passed on to the progeny of those cells in a stable manner. (Fig. 1). Malignant disorders nearly always arise in a single cell, and thus all the malignant cells in a particular patient will have the same X-chromosome inactivated. In an informative G6PD female all the tumour cells will express either type A or type B enzyme. Analysis of the G6PD levels in blood cells of different lineages will help to determine whether they are involved in a haematological malignancy. This technique is limited by the low frequency of informative polymorphisms in populations other than those of African descent.

Clonality can also be investigated using X-linked DNA polymorphisms which do not result in different protein products. This is based on the fact that the active and inactive genes are differentially methylated at specific cytosine residues. DNA samples are first digested with an appropriate restriction endonuclease to distinguish maternal and paternal copies of the gene, and subsequently with a restriction endonuclease sensitive to cytosine methylation in its recognition sequence to distinguish active from inactive copies of the gene. Useful genes to study include the hypoxanthine phosphoribosyl transferase (*HPRT*) gene and the phosphoglycerate kinase (*PGK*) gene (Fig. 2). The X-linked, multiple tandem repeat recognized by the probe M27B is highly informative (approximately 80 per cent of females are heterozygous), but as this is not a gene it is not really correct to talk about active and inactive copies. None the less, it acts as a useful marker of the inactivated X-chromosome, and results with this probe are concordant with those obtained with HPRT or PGK. PCR-based assays have also been developed to examine the methylation status of a number of genes, including the monoamine oxidase A gene (*MOA*), the human androgen-receptor gene (*HUMARA*), and the Fragile X gene. These assays require far fewer cells than are required for techniques based on Southern blotting and hence are now more frequently used. The *HUMARA* gene is the most informative, with heterozygosity rates in Caucasian populations of about 90 per cent. More recently a number of reverse transcriptase, polymerase chain reaction (**RT-PCR**) assays have been introduced that enable direct analysis of the relative expression of the two alleles at the transcript level, which may circumvent the problem of complex DNA methylation patterns. Informative genes must contain polymorphisms in the coding sequence, although these do not necessarily have to lead to changes in the amino acid sequence. It is also essential that the gene to be analysed is expressed by the cell type being investigated.

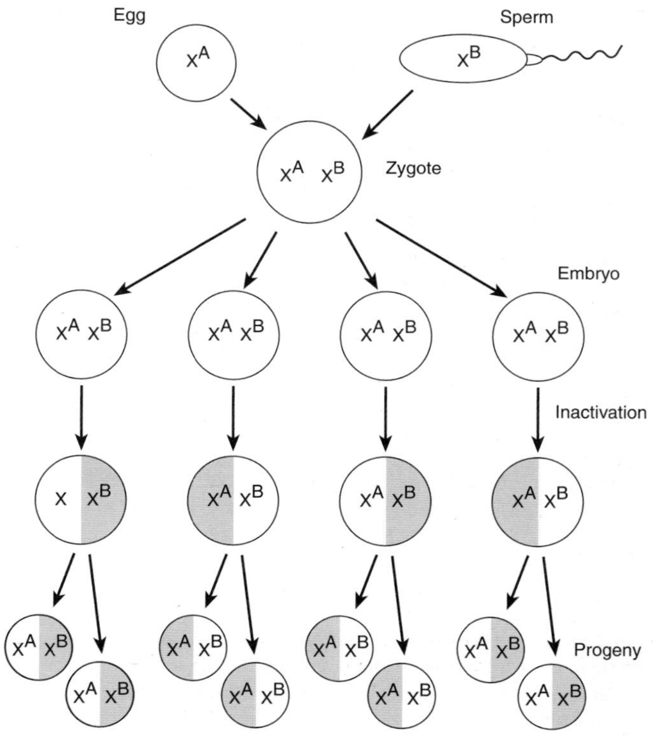

Fig. 1 X-chromosome inactivation.

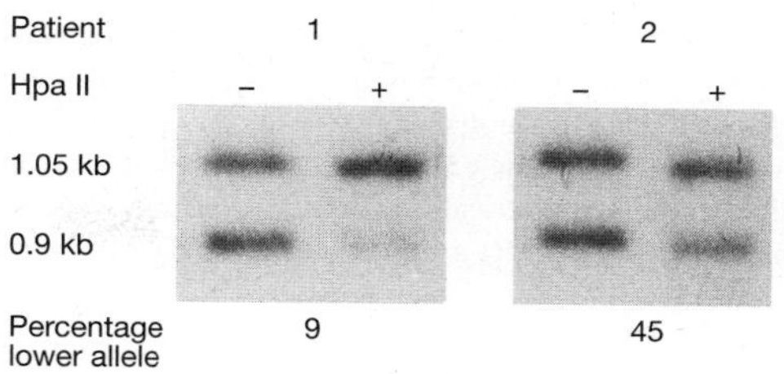

Fig. 2 Clonal analysis of PCK heterozygotes.

The *HUMARA* gene is again the most informative gene as the polymorphic variable number tandem repeat (**VNTR**) is contained within the coding sequence. The two alleles can be readily distinguished on electrophoresis of the RT-PCR product, but unfortunately this gene is not expressed in all haemopoietic tissues. The transcripts most commonly studied in haematological samples include G6PD, iduronate-2-sulfatase (**IDS**), and the palmitoylated membrane protein p55 (p55). Together these three RNA transcripts are informative in about 70 per cent of females. Once the mRNA has been reverse-transcribed into cDNA the different alleles, which differ only by single base changes, are then be detected by allele-specific PCR or allele-specific restriction analysis. Even with these genes expression is not constant between different haemopoietic cell-types. In one study IDS expression was shown to be sixfold higher in T cells than in neutrophils. High sample purity is thus essential when using this methodology.

Clonality studies based on X-chromosome inactivation patterns have three main drawbacks. First, it must be appreciated that lyonization occurs early in embryogenesis when there are few stem cells destined to give rise to the different tissues. As a consequence of this and the random nature of X-inactivation, considerable constitutive skewing away from the expected 50:50 expression of maternal and paternal alleles occurs in some individuals. An ill-defined inherited component may also contribute to this random process. In approximately one-quarter of females more than 75 per cent of the expressed genes derive from the same allele, and in 3 per cent of normal individuals more than 90 per cent. It is therefore essential that X-chromosome inactivation patterns are interpreted with reference to normal tissue. This has frequently been omitted and many of the reports in the literature are thus suspect. Furthermore, in the case of the haematological malignancies it is not always easy to obtain appropriate control samples. Non-haemopoietic tissues can be misleading controls, as X-inactivation patterns can vary between tissues. T cells are probably a good control in most myeloid malignancies as they derive from the same stem-cell pool as the myeloid cells, and it is unlikely that the majority of T lymphocytes will be involved in the malignant clone. Second, it has been clearly demonstrated that skewing of the myeloid lineages is acquired in a significant proportion of elderly females, so clonal analysis of haemopoietic lineages must be limited to females under the 65 years of age. Third, it must be remembered that the study of X-inactivation patterns is an insensitive technique which can not be used to detect a minor clone within a polyclonal population.

Myeloproliferative disorders

The term 'myeloproliferative disorders' was invented by Dameshek and others in the 1950s in an attempt to explain the variability of the haematological findings in polycythaemia rubra vera, chronic myeloid leukaemia, and myelofibrosis, and the existence of intermediate and transitional forms. The myeloproliferative disorders are characterized by the predominant cell type produced by the malignant clone, but they all involve a primitive stem cell (Fig. 3). Acute myeloid leukaemia frequently arises at the stem-cell level and diseases such as chronic myeloid leukaemia and polycythaemia rubra vera not infrequently terminate in 'blastic transformation'. By convention, however, the term 'myeloproliferative disorders' is usually reserved for the chronic malignancies where mature myeloid cells predominate.

Lineage involvement was first studied in chronic myeloid leukaemia because of the presence of the characteristic Philadelphia chromosome [t(9;22)(q34;q11)]. Not only were all cells of the phagocytic- and red-cell series found to be involved, but Epstein–Barr virus (**EBV**)-transformed B lymphocytes were also shown to contain the Ph1 chromosome, thus indicating that the target cell for malignant transformation was a primitive stem cell with both myeloid and lymphoid potential. This is confirmed by the fact that about one-third of blastic transformations are due to the accumulation of primitive B cells.

A similarly primitive stem cell is thought to be the cell of origin of polycythaemia rubra vera (**PRV**), and at least some cases of essential thrombocythaemia (**ET**). Clonality studies have revealed, however, that a significant proportion of cases of ET are polyclonal and not malignant disorders, despite fulfilling the usual diagnostic criteria. The cause of the dysregulated blood cell production in such cases is unknown. An important observation made by several groups is that people with the polyclonal forms of ET have a lower incidence of thrombosis.

Dameshek had considered that idiopathic myelofibrosis was part of the myeloproliferative disease spectrum, and indeed this is the case. The fibroblasts are not part of the malignant clone, however, but are a reaction to an underlying myeloid malignancy. Where studied, the myeloid cells have been shown to be clonal. Fibrosis is particularly common when cells of the megakaryocytic series predominate, and may be due to the excessive local production of platelet growth factors such as platelet-derived growth factor (**PDGF**) and transforming growth factor-β (**TGF-β**).

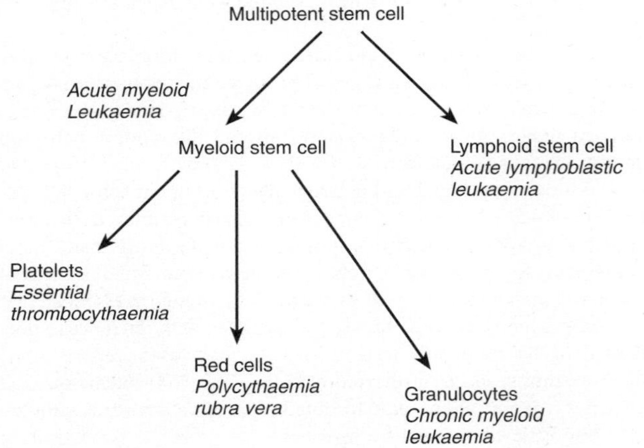

Fig. 3 The myeloproliferative disorders.

Acute leukaemias

In children with acute myeloid leukaemia (**AML**) the red cells and platelets do not appear to be part of the malignant clone, whereas such tri-lineage involvement is frequent in adults. There is no convincing evidence of lymphoid involvement. Considerable attention has been focused on the notion that remission in AML may represent persistence of the malignant clone with full differentiation to give a normal blood count. This view is based on studies that did not pay adequate attention to the skewing of X-inactivation patterns that can occur in normal individuals; true 'clonal remission' is rare.

Myelodysplasia, which frequently precedes AML, often involves all myeloid lineages, as is evident from examination of the blood and bone marrow films. There is considerable controversy within the literature, but the majority of studies do not demonstrate involvement of the lymphoid series.

Acute lymphoid leukaemia (**ALL**) is usually restricted to the B-cell or T-cell lineage. An exception occurs in cases of Ph1-positive ALL where the myeloid lineages are often involved. This entity is akin to chronic myeloid leukaemia (**CML**) presenting in lymphoid blast crisis.

Aplastic anaemia

Aplastic anaemia by definition refers to involvement of multiple myeloid lineages (pancytopenia). In severe cases the lymphocyte count is also reduced, suggesting that the defect is at the level of stem cells with the potential to give rise to both myeloid and lymphoid elements. Although T-cell numbers tend to be relatively well preserved, it must be appreciated that many T cells are long-lived cells and their numbers would not be expected to fall rapidly if their production from stem cells ceased. Furthermore, the basis of immunological memory, and a characteristic difference between myeloid and lymphoid cells, is that the mature progeny of the lymphoid stem cells can undergo amplification-division and self-renewal.

In those patients who respond (at least partially) to immunosuppression, with long-term follow-up there is a very high incidence of the development of clonal disorders such as paroxysmal nocturnal haemoglobinuria (**PNH**), myelodysplasia, and AML. In some patients at presentation, the few remaining granulocytes are clonal, although it is not clear how a clonal disorder can give rise to a hypoplastic bone marrow.

Paroxysmal nocturnal haemoglobinuria

PNH is a clonal disorder, due to a somatic mutation in the haemopoietic stem cell in the X-linked phosphatidylinositol glycan-A (**PIG-A**) responsible for the assembly of glycosyl phosphatidylinositol (**GPI**)-linked proteins on the cell surface of that cell and its progeny. This results in complement hypersensitivity and low-level expression of a number of antigens which are useful for defining lineage involvement. These include CD59 for red cells, platelets and T cells, CD67 for granulocytes, CD14 for monocytes, and CD24 for B cells. Flow cytometric studies have revealed variable lineage involvement: red cells, granulocytes, and monocytes and natural killer (**NK**) cells are involved in most cases; B cells are involved in a proportion of cases, and there is one report of a subpopulation of T cells involved in the PNH clone. It is possible that the variable lineage involvement represents differences in the target cell for the initiating mutation. The immunophenotypic studies have also confirmed that there is variable persistence of normal haemopoiesis, and some patients have more than one PNH clone with different levels of expression of GPI-linked molecules. One of the major unresolved questions in PNH is how does the PNH clone, which is not usually considered to be a malignancy, acquire a growth advantage over the normal haemopoietic tissue.

Further reading

Abrahamson G, *et al.* (1991). Clonality of cell populations in refractory anaemia using combined approach of gene loss and X-linked restriction fragment length polymorphism-methylation analyses. *British Journal of Haematology* **79**, 550–5.

Adamson JW, *et al.* (1976). Polycythaemia vera: stem cell and probable clonal origin of the disease. *New England Journal of Medicine* **295**, 913–16.

Beutler E, Collins Z, Irwin LE (1967). Value of genetic variants of glucose-6-phosphate dehydrogenase in tracing the origin of malignant tumours. *New England Journal of Medicine* **276**, 389–91.

Bjornson CR, *et al.* (1999). Turning brain into blood: a haemopoietic fate adopted by adult neural stem cells *in vivo*. *Science* **283**, 534–7.

Busque L, *et al.* (1996). Nonrandom X-inactivation patterns in normal females: lyonization ratios vary with age. *Blood* **88**, 59–65.

Dameshek W (1951). Some speculations on the myeloproliferative syndromes. *Blood* **6**, 392–5.

Fialkow PJ (1972). Use of genetic markers to study cellular origin of development of tumours in human females. *Advances in Cancer Research* **15**, 191–226.

Fialkow PJ, Jacobson RJ, Papayanopoulou T (1977). Chronic myeloid leukaemia: clonal origin in a stem cell common to the granulocytic, erythrocyte, platelet and monocyte/macrophage. *American Journal of Medicine* **63**, 125–31.

Fialkow PJ, *et al.* (1987). Clonal development, stem cell differentiation and clinical remissions in acute non-lymphocytic leukaemia. *New England Journal of Medicine* **317**, 468–73.

Gale RE, Wheadon H, Linch DC (1991). X-chromosome inactivation patterns using HPRT and PGK polymorphisms in haematologically normal and post-chemotherapy females. *British Journal of Haematology* **79**, 193–7.

Gale RE, *et al.* (1993). Frequency of clonal remission in acute myeloid leukaemia. *Lancet* **341**, 138–42.

Gale RE, *et al.* (1994). Tissue specificity of X-chromosome inactivation patterns. *Blood* **83**, 2899–905.

Gale RE, *et al.* (1997). Acquired skewing of X chromosome inactivation patterns in myeloid cells of the elderly suggests stochastic clonal loss with age. *British Journal of Haematology* **98**, 512–19.

Harrison C, *et al.* (1999). A large proportion of patients with a diagnosis of essential thrombocythaemia do not have a clonal disorder and may be at lower risk of thrombotic complications. *Blood* **93**, 417–25.

Hillmen P, Richards SJ (2000). Implications of recent insights into the pathophysiology of paroxysmal nocturnal haemoglobinuria. *British Journal of Haematology* **108**, 470–9.

Kurzrock R, Gutterman JU, Talpaz M (1988). The molecular genetics of Philadelphia chromosome-positive leukaemias. *New England Journal of Medicine* **319**, 990–8.

Lyon MF (1961). Gene action in the X-chromosome of the mouse (*Mus musculus* L). *Nature* **190**, 372–3.

Naumova AK, *et al.* (1996). Heritability of X-chromosome inactivation phenotype in a large family. *American Journal of Human Genetics* **58**, 1111–19.

Nissen C, *et al.* (1986). Acquired aplastic anaemia: a PNH-like disease? *British Journal of Haematology* **64**, 355–62.

Rowley JD (1973). A new consistent chromosomal abnormality in chronic myeloid leukaemia identified by quinacrine fluorescence and Giemsa staining. *Nature* **243**, 290–3.

Turhan AG, *et al.* (1988). Molecular analysis of clonality and *bcr* rearrangements in Philadelphia chromosome positive acute lymphoblastic leukaemia. *Blood* **71**, 1495–500.

van Kamp H, *et al.* (1991). Clonal haematopoiesis in patients with acquired aplastic anaemia. *Blood* **78**, 3209–14.

Vogelstein B, *et al.* (1987). Clonal analysis using recombinant DNA probes from the X-chromosome. *Cancer Research* **47**, 4806–13.

Weissman I (2000). Translating stem and progenitor cell biology to the clinic: barriers and opportunities. *Science* **287**, 1442.

22.3 The leukaemias and other disorders of haematopoietic stem cells

22.3.1 Cell and molecular biology of human leukaemias

*Thomas Look**

Introduction

The human leukaemias arise from haemopoietic stem and progenitor cells, and exhibit differentiation arrest in any lineage and in any stage of maturation. Attempts to understand the pathobiology of these diseases have focused on clinical presentation, cell morphology, histochemistry, cell immunophenotype, cytogenetics, and, in recent years, molecular genetics. Although useful in diagnosis and risk assessment, clinical and cell-biological findings ultimately fail to reveal underlying mechanisms of leukaemic transformation and, therefore, cannot account for treatment failures among groups of patients with ostensibly similar features. The emerging picture of leucocyte transformation indicates that most cases of leukaemia involve chromosomal translocations that result in aberrantly expressed transcription factors or activated tyrosine kinases, which drive malignant conversion and maintain the leukaemic phenotype. Some of these genetic changes affect cell proliferation or survival, while others exert their primary effects on cell differentiation. Almost always, the critical lesion involves a 'master' transcriptional regulatory gene or tyrosine kinase signalling molecule that stands near the top of a hierarchy of gene control, so that leukaemia is efficiently instigated by a limited number of alterations rather than by multiple changes affecting tens of responder genes in the biochemical cascade.

This chapter describes the human leukaemias in terms of their characteristic molecular genetic and developmental features. A recurring theme is that the genes most frequently altered in these diseases are those with evolutionarily conserved roles in the embryological development of various cell lineages and organ systems, including, but not limited to, genes that control normal blood cell production (haemopoiesis). Whenever possible, I have attempted to link advances in the molecular biology of a particular leukaemia to any unique implications for treatment and prognosis.

Oncogenic transcription factors and activated tyrosine kinases

Transcriptional control genes are common mutational targets in the human leukaemias because their protein products (transcription factors) bind to regulatory elements in DNA, such as promoters and enhancers, and stimulate or inhibit gene expression. These proto-oncogenes are frequently activated by chromosomal translocations, either by fusion of disparate gene fragments or by mobilization of the gene into the vicinity of transcriptionally active T-cell receptor (*TCR*) or immunoglobulin (*IG*) genes. More than 80 per cent of the oncogenic transcription factors identified to date can be classified according to the structural motifs within their DNA- and protein-binding domains: **bHLH** (basic region/helix–loop–helix), **bZIP** (basic region/leucine zipper), **HTH** or homeodomain (helix–turn–helix), A–T hook, Ets-like, Runt homology, zinc finger, and LIM (cysteine-rich). Each of these motifs has functional significance, in that it defines the downstream responder genes that determine the altered patterns of gene expression during normal development and malignant transformation.

Current observations indicate that oncogenic transcription factors act positively to aberrantly upregulate critical target genes that coordinate the production of proteins needed for normal cell proliferation, differentiation, or survival (gain of function), or negatively to interfere with normal regulatory cascades controlling apoptosis and the growth that normally accompanies differentiation (loss of function). Similarly, activated tyrosine kinases act through signal-transduction cascades that ultimately dysregulate the transcriptional control of gene expression. The oncogenic transcription factors or activated tyrosine kinases involved in the human leukaemias have unique transforming properties, which tend to be specific for different types of progenitor cells developing in the lymphoid or myeloid pathways. In most cases of acute lymphoblastic leukaemia and acute promyelocytic leukaemia, the initial lesion appears to affect progenitors at the same stage of differentiation as the predominate phenotype in the malignant clone. However, most types of acute myeloid leukaemia appear to arise in a primitive haemopoietic stem cell rather than a committed myeloid progenitor, with subsequent blockade of differentiation that determines the morphological (FAB) subtypes of myeloid leukaemia apparent at diagnosis. Primitive normal stem cells are also thought to be the targets of leukaemic transformation in chronic myeloid leukaemia and in some cases of acute lymphoblastic leukaemia, at least those expressing the *BCR–ABL* and *MLL* fusion oncogenes.

Acute lymphoblastic leukaemia

Approximately 3000 to 4000 people in the United States, two-thirds of them children, develop acute lymphoblastic leukaemia (**ALL**) each year. Only 20 to 25 per cent of the childhood cases are resistant to modern multiagent therapy, attesting to the remarkable treatment advances that have been made over the past three decades. Unfortunately, the prognosis for adults with ALL remains poor. Fewer than 50 per cent of the patients treated solely with chemotherapy become long-term survivors, and many patients are ineligible for or fail in spite of bone marrow transplantation. The difference in curability between acute leukaemias in children and adults can be attributed partly to the much larger proportion of adult cases with the *BCR–ABL* chimeric tyrosine kinase oncogene, resulting from the

* I would like to thank Markus Seidel and Adolfo Ferrando for assistance and helpful discussions, and John Gilbert for editorial review and critical comments. Supported in part by NIH grants CA-59571,

Philadelphia chromosome, and to the poor tolerance of intensive chemotherapy by patients over 50 years of age. There is also the possibility that ostensibly similar cases of ALL in children and adults differ in, as yet undefined, genetic ways that influence the outcome of therapy.

B-Lineage ALL

Normal B-lymphoid cell populations undergo diverse, clonal rearrangements of their *IG* genes, followed by highly regulated proliferation of cells that successfully complete the process and produce immunoglobulin. When this developmental process is altered, the developing B lymphocytes may undergo transforming events that eventually lead to overt ALL. In most instances, the pathobiology of transformed lymphoid cells mirrors the altered expression of genes that contribute to the normal functioning of pro-B (immunoglobulin undetectable) or pre-B (cytoplasmic immunoglobulin-positive) lymphocytes or occasionally mature virgin B cells (surface immunoglobulin-positive), although it may involve the aberrant expression of normally quiescent genes. Approximately 80 per cent of patients with ALL have lymphoblasts whose phenotypes correspond to those of B-cell precursors. Only 2 to 3 per cent of these patients have mature B-cell leukaemia, which is thought to represent a disseminated form of Burkitt lymphoma. The prevailing concept is that lymphoid leukaemic cells are classified immunophenotypically according to their 'normal' developmental stage, as this convention provides a firm basis for the study of cell type-specific genetic alterations.

BCR–ABL

The first constitutively activated tyrosine kinase described in ALL results from fusion of 5′ sequences of the *BCR* proto-oncogene to 3′ sequences of *ABL* due to action of the t(9;22) translocation, leading to creation of the so-called Philadelphia (**Ph**) chromosome. Most investigators agree that the t(9;22) translocation occurs in haemopoietic stem cells possessing both lymphoid and myeloid differentiative potential. Differences between *BCR–ABL*$^+$ leukaemias in children and adults are striking. Found in only 3 to 5 per cent of newly diagnosed paediatric ALL cases, they represent at least 25 per cent of adult cases. Also, the *BCR* breakpoints on chromosome 22 in paediatric cases cluster mainly in the *m-bcr* (minor breakpoint cluster region), whereas in adults they can occur in either the *m-bcr* or the *M-bcr* (major breakpoint cluster region). Breaks in the former region lead to fusion genes encoding a 190-kDa protein (p190), while those in the latter generate a 210-kDa protein (p120).

Very little is known about the normal function of ABL, although as a nuclear protein with tyrosine kinase activity, it may stimulate p53-dependent growth arrest, suggesting a role as a cell-cycle checkpoint after damage to the cellular genome. Both the p190 and p210 forms of BCR–ABL are localized in the cytoplasm and have increased tyrosine kinase activity. Their enforced expression can transform haemopoietic cells *in vitro* and can induce a syndrome similar to chronic myeloid leukaemia in mice. The precise mechanism by which BCR–ABL transforms human haemopoietic cells is unclear, but this process almost certainly involves activation of the *CRKL* gene, whose product stimulates JUN kinase and ultimately JUN through the RAS signalling pathway, as well as STATs, MYC, and cyclin D1.

Patients with *BCR–ABL*$^+$ ALL respond poorly to conventional therapy but are excellent candidates for bone marrow transplantation. A new drug, STI-571, has been identified that selectively inhibits the ABL tyrosine kinase and appears to be highly active in BCR–ABL$^+$ CML (see below). Trials are currently underway to test the activity of this drug in BCR–ABL$^+$ leukaemias that present initially as ALL.

TEL–AML1

One of the exciting recent developments in molecular genetics research of ALL was the identification of *TEL–AML1* (also termed *ETV6–CBFA2*) as the most common genetic alteration in leukaemic pro-B lymphoblasts. This chimeric oncogene is generated by the t(12;21), a translocation that is difficult to detect by standard Giemsa-banding, but which is identified in 25 per cent of cases by molecular assays. The resultant TEL–AML1 oncoprotein consists of the HLH domain of TEL, an ETS family transcription factor, fused to the DNA-binding and transactivation domains of AML1. AML1 is the DNA-binding component of the core-binding factor (**CBF**) transcription-factor complex, which is also the most frequent target of myeloid cell-associated translocations, including the t(8;21), t(3;21), and inv(16), and a critical participant in normal haemopoiesis.

The relative contributions of TEL and AML1 to leukaemia induction are only beginning to be understood. One attractive model suggests that the crucial pathogenic event is interference with AML1-mediated expression of *HOX* or other master control genes, which have pivotal roles in normal lymphopoiesis. Thus, the leukaemogenic role of TEL–AML1 may well depend on the DNA-binding and transactivating domains of AML1, although a definitive explanation will probably not be found until better *in vitro* transformation assays become available.

The prognostic impact of *TEL–AML1* expression is controversial. Some treatment centres claim long-term, event-free survival rates of approximately 90 per cent in patients with this genetic abnormality, while others report a lack of a favourable prognostic significance. Evaluation of the components of the treatment regimens suggest that TEL–AML1$^+$ cases respond better to drug combinations that rely on the intensive use of L-asparaginase and increased dosages of methotrexate with leucovorin (calcium folinate) rescue. Thus, the *TEL–AML1* fusion gene may identify a large, previously unrecognized subset of pro-B ALL cases that can be treated with regimens that rely on antimetabolites and an enzyme that depletes an essential amino acid in lymphoid cells, rather than genotoxic agents (for example, epipodophyllotoxins) that are associated with secondary AML.

E2A fusion genes

The *E2A* gene, which encodes a bHLH transcription factor on chromosome 19, is targeted by two reciprocal translocations in patients with ALL—the t(1;19) in 5 per cent of children and 3 per cent of adults, and the t(17;19) in approximately 0.5 per cent of children. The former generates one of the best-characterized fusion oncogenes in ALL, in which the two transcriptional transactivation domains of *E2A* are linked to the homeodomain of *PBX1*. *PBX1* is an orphan *HOX* gene that shares homology with the *exd* gene of *Drosophila*, which regulates in segment identity through direct interaction of its product with specific HOM proteins of the *Bithorax* and *Antennapedia* complexes.

E2A–PBX1, which binds to DNA in a site-specific manner, is clearly oncogenic in fibroblast transformation assays and in mice, and appears to induce programmed cell death (apoptosis) in lymphoid cells. Like its exd homologue, PBX1 is directed to its consensus DNA-binding site by a subset of interacting HOX proteins, whether or not it is fused to E2A. Surprisingly, these site-specific recognition sequences of PBX1 are not required for the transforming activity of E2A–PBX1. How, then, would the chimeric oncoprotein induce leukaemia, if not by disruption of gene expression normally regulated by HOX proteins? The answer appears to lie in a short peptide sequence that regulates the HOX-specific protein–protein interaction, and which is essential for leukaemogenic activity.

In about 0.5 per cent of childhood ALL cases, the t(17;19) translocation generates the *E2A–HLF* fusion gene, consisting of the amino-terminal transactivation regions of *E2A* and the C-terminal DNA-binding and dimerization domains of *HLF*, a member of the bZIP transcription factor gene family. E2A–HLF mediates leukaemic transformation by inhibiting a normal apoptotic pathway in pro-B lymphocytes, one that closely resembles the pathway responsible for eliminating extraneous neuronal cells in the nematode *Caenorhabditis elegans*. Of seven reported patients with ALL whose blast cells expressed *E2A–HLF*, each has died of leukaemia during or after aggressive treatment, suggesting a profound resistance to chemotherapy, which may arise from E2A–HLF-induced inhibition of drug-induced apoptosis.

MLL fusion genes

Structural abnormalities of chromosome 11, band q23, are found in 80 per cent of infants with ALL, but only 7 per cent of older children and adults with this disease. Recent findings of Greaves and co-workers in the United Kingdom, indicate that translocations affecting the 11q23 region can arise *in utero*, predisposing the child to the very early development of leukaemia. The vast majority of 11q23 translocations affect the *MLL* gene, which encodes a protein of 3968 amino acids with a predicted molecular mass of 431 kDa and with three regions of homology with the *Drosophila* trithorax protein (two central zinc-finger domains and a C-terminal segment of 210 amino acids). The N-terminal region, which is uniformly retained in reciprocal translocations, contains three A–T hook motifs that apparently bind A–T-rich sequences in the minor groove of DNA. The A–T hook motifs are separated from the zinc-finger regions by a 47-amino-acid sequence with homology to the non-catalytic domains of human DNA-methyltransferase, an enzyme that produces fully methylated double-stranded DNA from a hemimethylated substrate. The structural features of MLL indicate that its normal physiological function, as well as its role in leukaemogenesis, is mediated through direct interactions with DNA and other DNA-binding and signal-transduction proteins.

As with PBX1, the MLL protein appears to play a role in *HOX* gene regulation. Homozygous inactivation of the *Mll* gene in mice is lethal during embryogenesis, with homeotic transformations of the skeleton reminiscent of the phenotype associated with *trithorax* mutation in flies. Knockout mice heterozygous for *Mll* are small at birth, have retarded growth, and develop both anaemia and thrombocytopenia. Thus, loss of function of one *MLL* allele through chromosome breakage and translocation of the resultant fragment to a new site, together with a gain of function due to gene fusion, would be expected to interfere with the normal haemopoietic role of HOX proteins, thereby contributing to leukaemogenesis.

More than 30 discrete chromosomal sites participate in 11q23 translocations, most commonly 4q21, 9p22, and 19p13, resulting in fusion of the *AF4*, *AF9*, and *ENL* genes to *MLL*,. A recurring question has been whether the partner DNA fragments in *MLL* gene fusions are needed to induce leukaemia. In the case of *MLL–ENL*, created by the t(11;19), neither the *MLL* fragment alone nor a fusion gene lacking the *ENL* C-terminal region is sufficient to transform retrovirally transduced haemopoietic cells, suggesting that a gain of function due to the *ENL* C-terminus is required for *MLL–ENL*-induced leukaemia. Similar results have been obtained for *AF9*, in regions of the molecules required for transcriptional activation, which occurs through recruitment of co-activators like **CBP** to the transcriptional machinery. In fact, CBP itself has recently been identified as a fusion partner with MLL in rare leukaemia cases. Taken together, recent findings suggest a model in which CBP or related histone acetylases like p300 contribute in a highly regulated fashion to normal MLL function. MLL fusion proteins apparently result in aberrant gene regulation through the constitutive association of this enzymatic activity with the MLL DNA-binding domain.

The *MLL–AF4*, *MLL–AF9*, and other *MLL* fusion genes predict a dismal outcome in infants and adults treated exclusively with chemotherapy. Trials testing the efficacy of high-dose chemotherapy and radiation with stem cell replacement are currently underway.

MYC

Chromosomal translocations in B-lineage cells can also mobilize proto-oncogenes to sites adjacent to normally active enhancer or promoter elements of *IG* genes. The prototype for this mechanism in B-lineage ALL is the t(8;14), which arises in mature B cells and places the *MYC* proto-oncogene on chromosome 8 under the control of *IG* heavy-chain gene regulatory sequences on chromosome 14. Similar repositioning of *MYC* adjacent to the light-chain regulatory sequences results from the t(2;8) or the t(8;22), although in much smaller percentages of cases. Through one of these translocations, *MYC* expression becomes dysregulated, leading to abnormally increased amounts of the MYC protein, a transcription factor that forms a DNA-binding complex with another cellular protein (MAX), and eventually leads to disruption of gene expression involved in the control of cell proliferation.

Dysregulated *MYC* genes confer an exceptionally poor prognosis in children and adults with mature B-cell ALL who are treated with conventional regimens used for other types of ALL. Recent studies, however, indicate that at least 80 per cent of these patients can be cured with intensive short-term chemotherapy including high-doses of cyclophosphamide, methotrexate, and cytarabine. Thus, B-cell ALL provides the first example of a subtype of ALL requiring tailored therapy with a vastly different drug regimen for effective disease control.

T-Lineage ALL

Cell biology

First recognized as a distinct clinical entity in the early 1970s, T-cell ALL accounts for 10 to 15 per cent of acute lymphoid leukaemias in children and 20 to 25 per cent of cases in adults. The disease can arise in thymocytes at any stage of maturation, defined on the basis of reactivity with monoclonal antibodies (CD4/CD8 double-negative immature thymocytes, cytoplasmic CD3+ CD7+ CD2+ CD5+; CD4/CD8 double-positive common thymocytes, cytoplasmic CD3+ CD1+ CD2+ CD5+ CD7+ CD10+ CD4+ and CD8+; and CD4/CD8 single-positive late thymocytes, cytoplasmic CD3+ CD2+ CD5+ CD7+, CD4+ or CD8+).

Molecular oncogenesis

In contrast to the fusion oncogenes that drive the development of B-cell precursor ALL, oncogene activation in T-cell ALL reflects the mobilization of genes encoding structurally intact T-cell proto-oncogenes into the vicinity of transcriptionally active sites of the beta or alpha/delta loci of the T-cell receptor genes (TCRβ or TCRα/δ). Among the genes that are aberrantly expressed in thymocytes and cause leukaemic transformation through this mechanism are those representing the bHLH family of transcription factors (TAL1/SCL1, TAL2/SCL2, LYL1, and BHLHB1), the bHLH/ZIP family (MYC), other nuclear regulatory proteins (LMO1 and LMO2), homeotic proteins (HOX11), and a truncated and constitutively activated form of the human homologue of the *Drosophila* Notch 1 receptor (TAN1). The relationship of these genes to the pathogenesis of T-cell ALL has been established by their recurrent involvement in translocations that affect thymocytes or their precursors. Surprisingly, most of the T-cell oncogenes identified to date are not usually expressed in T cells; hence, their ability to induce leukaemia most likely reflects the misexpression of master transcriptional control genes with the disruption of normal T-cell developmental pathways. This is illustrated by *HOX11*, which is not normally expressed in lymphoid cells, but has been shown to be absolutely essential for normal development of the spleen.

Despite intensive cytogenetic research, chromosomal translocations have been identified in only about 25 per cent of T-cell ALL cases, suggesting that additional pathogenetic mechanisms remain to be identified. One intriguing possibility is that such cases harbour mutations (not attributable to translocations) that disrupt key transcriptional control networks in thymocyte development, leading to overt ALL. Support for this hypothesis comes from the existence of mechanisms that can induce misexpression of bHLH transcription factor genes, including *TAL1/SCL*, without a requirement for rearrangement to a site near the *TCR*α/δ locus. Thus, *TAL1/SCL* may be abnormally expressed in as many as 60 per cent of T-cell leukaemias, in contrast to the 3 per cent accounted for by chromosomal translocations. Even so, it is unlikely that dysregulation of *TAL1/SCL* by itself would be sufficient to generate a fully malignant phenotype; rather, consistent misexpression of two or more T-cell oncogenes and their cooperative interaction, both among themselves and through a lack of other regulatory proteins encoded by tumour suppressor genes, is probably needed to induce clinically apparent leukaemia.

Therapeutic implications

With the availability of effective multidrug regimens, the prognostic importance of T-lineage leukaemia has disappeared in children. In adults, the addition of cyclophosphamide and cytarabine to first-line treatments boosted complete remission rates from 72 per cent to 85 per cent and improved the probability of continuous complete remission from less than 10 per cent to 46 per cent or more. The best prospect for accelerated therapeutic progress in this disease appears to lie in a fuller understanding of the molecular aspects of T-cell pathogenesis and how they relate to available modes of treatment. Ongoing studies to clarify these interactions should greatly enhance the value of molecular genetics in predicting the clinical responses of patients with T-cell ALL and, ultimately, could provide lucrative targets for novel drug therapies.

Acute myeloid leukaemia

The estimated number of new cases of acute myeloid leukaemia (**AML**) occurring annually in the United States is vastly higher in adults than in children (22 500 versus 500). Prognosis is poor in both age groups, especially in older patients with AML, although recent improvements in allogeneic bone marrow transplantation may boost cure rates above 50 per cent in those patients under 50 years of age with histocompatible donors. AML can develop from transformed cells within the granulocyte/monocyte lineage or from haemopoietic stem cells capable of differentiating into erythrocytes and megakaryocytes, as well as granulocytes and monocytes. Regardless of the cell of origin, AML pathogenesis is a multistep process, involving alterations of both proto-oncogenes and tumour suppressor genes. Although important tumour suppressors are thought to exist in regions of non-random loss of heterozygosity in this disease (for example, monosomy 7, 5q$^-$, 20q$^-$), current knowledge focuses on chromosomal translocations which activate transcription factor genes, reminiscent of those giving rise to ALL.

Differentiation stage in AML is best described in the context of the French–American–British (**FAB**) cell-classification system, which distinguishes among eight morphological subtypes of myeloid leukaemia, allowing useful cell type-specific comparisons of molecular genetic findings.

Acute promyelocytic leukaemia

Characterized by the clonal expansion of transformed myeloid cells blocked at the promyelocyte stage of development, the FAB M3 subtype of AML harbours a t(15;17) translocation that generates the *PML–RARα* fusion gene. *RARα* is a member of the nuclear hormone-receptor superfamily, functioning as a ligand-dependent, zinc-finger transcription factor with a critical role in normal myeloid cell differentiation. Much less is known about the normal biological function of PML, although it is a nuclear protein thought to function with p53 in cellular senescence induced by oncogene expression. The fusion protein contains nearly all the key functional domains of each molecule, including the protein–protein interaction motifs of PML and the DNA-binding, dimerization, ligand-binding, and transcriptional activation domains of RARα. The PML–RARα oncoprotein induces leukaemia by inhibiting, in a dominant fashion, the normal biological activities of both RARα and PML. The net effect is a blockade of differentiation with immortality and sustained proliferation among promyelocytes, the hallmark of acute promyelocytic leukaemia (M3 AML).

Treatment of *PML–RARα+* AML with pharmacological dosages of the RARα ligand all-*trans*-retinoic acid (**ATRA**) results in the release of co-repressor complexes from the PML–RARα fusion protein, reversing the protein's inhibitory activity and enabling the leukaemic promyelocytes to proceed to terminal differentiation. The unique specificity of ATRA for the underlying molecular lesion in M3 AML affords a paradigm for molecularly targeted cancer chemotherapy.

Acute myeloblastic leukaemia

AML1–ETO

The *AML1–ETO* fusion gene results from the t(8;21) translocation in approximately 40 per cent of cases involving myeloblastic leukaemic cells with some evidence of differentiation (FAB M2 subtype). The oncogene product consists of the N-terminal portion of AML1, including its entire Runt homology domain (RHD), and the C-terminal portion of ETO, the mammalian homologue of the *Drosophila* protein, nervy. The AML1–ETO chimeric oncoprotein exerts its leukaemic activity by dominantly repressing the DNA-binding sites normally recognized by the AML1/CBFβ core-binding factor transcriptional complex, whose function is essential for the development of all haemopoietic lineages.

Patients with *AML1–ETO+* leukaemia respond more readily to chemotherapy than most other patients with AML, so that most experts advise reserving stem-cell transplantation for patients in first relapse. Multiple groups have documented the persistence of *AML1–ETO* fusion transcripts in patients with long-term remissions, suggesting that additional mutations within the leukaemic clone are essential for manifestation of the malignant phenotype. Since AML–ETO is a dominant-negative chimeric transcription factor that relies on co-repressor complexes, novel treatments that disrupt the formation, stability, or activity of such complexes, such as histone deacetylase inhibitors, might reverse the leukaemic phenotype, as seen with the use of ATRA in patients with acute promyelocytic leukaemia carrying the *PML–RARα* oncogene.

CBFβ–MYH11

The *CBFβ–MYH11* fusion product, due to inv(16) or t(16;16), is another frequent genetic lesion in newly diagnosed cases of AML. Once thought to be pathognomonic of cases with dysplastic eosinophilic precursors among myeloblasts and monoblasts (M4Eo subtype), this finding has since been made in acute myeloblastic leukaemia (M1 and M2 subtypes). These genetic rearrangements fuse the N-terminal portion of CBFβ to a variable amount of the C-terminal α-helical rod domain of MYH11, a smooth-muscle, myosin heavy-chain protein that possesses both actin binding and ATPase activity. *CBFβ–MYH11* also inhibits the normal activity of the AML1/CBFβ transcription factor complex, depriving the cell of requisite developmental signals. There are also suggestions that the oncoprotein generates positive signals resulting in abnormalities of cell growth. As with *AML1–ETO*, the *CBFβ–MYH11* oncogene confers a better-than-average probability of achieving a sustained remission with chemotherapy.

Chronic myeloid leukaemia

Several forms of leukaemia are included under the generic term 'chronic myeloid leukaemia' (**CML**). About 90 per cent of patients with CML, both children and adults, harbour the classic t(9;22) translocation in myeloid cells, giving rise to the Ph chromosome and the *BCR–ABL* oncogene. In most patients the resulting disease is biphasic, with an initial (chronic) phase that lasts 3 years on average, and a terminal (blast) phase that is refractory to all treatment and is generally fatal within a median of 2 to 4 months. Children also can develop a juvenile form of CML (**JCML**) that often involves loss of the NF1 tumour suppressor.

Allogeneic bone marrow transplantation is the main curative treatment for CML. Patients with either the adult or juvenile form of the disease, who lack histocompatible sibling donors, may benefit from long-term treatment with interferon-α, which improves karyotypic responses, delays progression of the disease, and prolongs overall survival in randomized clinical trials. An exciting new development is the experimental agent STI-571, which targets the tyrosine kinase activity of BCR–ABL. STI-571 has produced striking improvements in each of 31 patients who were resistant to interferon and who then received STI-571 in cumulative doses of at least 300 mg per day. In three cases, the drug eradicated all cells with the t(9;22) chromosomal marker, and the malignant clone has remained undetectable in these patients for the relatively short duration of this trial.

Table 1 Clinical applications of common oncogenic transcription factors in the human leukaemias

Altered gene	Leukaemia subtype*	Risk of treatment failure†	Recommended treatment‡
ALL			
TEL–AML1 (ETV6–EBFA2)	Pro-B cell	Low	Well-tolerated chemotherapy (antimetabolites primarily)
E2A–PBX1	Pre-B cell	Intermediate	Intensive chemotherapy (genotoxic drugs and antimetabolites)
MYC	B cell	High	Intensive chemotherapy (rotation of genotoxic drugs)
MLL–AF4	CD10– pro-B cell	Very high	Allogeneic stem-cell transplantation
BCR–ABL	Pro-B cell(predominantly)	Very high	Allogeneic stem-cell transplantation
AML			
AML1–ETO	Acute myeloblastic leukaemia with maturation (M2 morphology)	Intermediate	Intensive chemotherapy (including high-dose cytarabine)
CBFβ–MYHII	Acute myelomonocytic leukaemia with eosinophils (M4Eo morphology)	Intermediate	Intensive chemotherapy (including high-dose cytarabine)
PML–RARα	Acute promyelocytic leukaemia (M3 morphology)	Intermediate	Intensive chemotherapy (including all-*trans*-retinoic acid and an anthracycline)

ALL, acute lymphoblastic leukaemia; AML, acute myeloid leukaemia.

* Subclassifications of AML are those of the French–American–British (FAB) cooperative group.

† As determined in standard programmes of chemotherapy (without haemopoietic stem-cell rescue). Treatment failure refers to either remission induction or remission maintenance, or both. The average rates of long-term, leukaemia-free survival in children and adolescents with ALL or AML range from 65–70 per cent and from 30–40 per cent, respectively.

‡ The choice of therapy is based on detection of the indicated fusion gene at diagnosis by cytogenetic analysis, Southern blotting, or RNA-polymerase chain reaction assays for chimeric mRNAs.

Clinical summary

Molecular genetic changes at diagnosis are sensitive markers of potential leukaemia aggressiveness and therefore can be used as guides to treatment. Table 1 summarizes the clinical utility of recognized oncogenic transcription factors in the human leukaemias. Thus far, only two specific lesions, the *PML–RARα* fusion gene in acute promyelocytic leukaemia and the BCR–ABL kinase in CML and ALL, have been productive targets for molecular-oriented therapy, but this number will likely increase as we learn more about the genetic mechanisms that transform normal blood cells and maintain leukaemic phenotypes.

Further reading

Bash RO, *et al.* (1995). Does activation of the *TAL1* gene occur in a majority of patients with T-cell acute lymphoblastic leukemia? A pediatric oncology group study. *Blood* **86,** 666–676.

Blackwood EM, Eisenman RN (1991). Max: a helix–loop–helix zipper protein that forms a sequence- specific DNA-binding complex with Myc. *Science* **251,** 1211–1217.

Bonnet D, Dick JE (1997). Human acute myeloid leukemia is organized as a hierarchy that originates from a primitive hematopoietic cell. *Nature Medicine* **3,** 730–737.

Clark SS, *et al.* (1987). Unique forms of the abl tyrosine kinase distinguish Ph[1]-positive CML from Ph[1]-positive ALL. *Science* **235,** 85–88.

de The H, *et al.* (1990). The t(15;17) translocation of acute promyelocytic leukaemia fuses the retinoic acid receptor alpha gene to a novel transcribed locus. *Nature* **347,** 558–561.

Fletcher JA, *et al.* (1991). Translocation (9;22) is associated with extremely poor prognosis in intensively treated children with acute lymphoblastic leukemia. *Blood* **77,** 435–9.

Ford AM, *et al.* (1993). In utero rearrangements in the trithorax-related oncogene in infant leukaemias. *Nature* **363,** 358–60.

Golub TR, *et al.* (1995). Fusion of the TEL gene on 12p13 to the AML1 gene on 21q22 in acute lymphoblastic leukemia. *Proceedings of the National Academy of Science, USA* **92,** 4917–21.

Head DR, Pui CH (1999). Leukemia diagnosis and classification. In: Pui CH, ed. *Childhood leukemias,* pp 19–37. Cambridge University Press, New York.

Hughes TP, Goldman JM (1995). Chronic myeloid leukemia. In: Hoffman R, *et al.*, eds. *Hematology,* pp 1142–59. Churchill Livingstone, New York.

Hunger SP (1996). Chromosomal translocations involving the *E2A* gene in acute lymphoblastic leukemia: clinical features and molecular pathogenesis. *Blood* **87,** 1211–24.

Inaba T, *et al.* (1996). Reversal of apoptosis by the leukaemia-associated E2A-HLF chimaeric transcription factor. *Nature* **382,** 541–4.

Look AT (1997). Oncogenic transcription factors in the human acute leukemias. *Science* **278,** 1059–2064.

Look AT, Kirsch IR (1997). Molecular basis of childhood cancer. In: Pizzo PA, Poplack DG, eds. *Pediatric oncology,* pp 37–74. Lippincott-Raven, Philadelphia.

Meyers S, Downing JR, Hiebert SW (1993). Identification of AML-1 and the (8;21) translocation protein (AML-1/ETO) as sequence specific DNA binding proteins: the runt homology domain is required for DNA binding and protein-protein interactions. *Molecular and Cellular Biology* **13,** 6336–45.

Okuda T (1996). AML1, the target of multiple chromosomal translocations in human leukemia, is essential for normal fetal liver hematopoiesis. *Cell* **84,** 321–30.

Pui CH, Evans WE (1998). Acute lymphoblastic leukemia. *New England Journal of Medicine* **339,** 605–15.

Rabbitts TH (1994). Chromosomal translocations in human cancer. *Nature* **372,** 143–9.

Rubnitz JE, *et al.* (1997). *TEL* gene rearrangement in acute lymphoblastic leukemia: a new genetic marker with prognostic significance. *Journal of Clinical Oncology* **15,** 1150–7.

Shtivelman E, *et al.* (1985). Fused transcript of *abl* and *bcr* genes in chronic myelogenous leukemia. *Nature* **315,** 550–4.

Thirman MJ, *et al.* (1993). Rearrangement of the MLL gene in acute lymphoblastic and acute myeloid leukemias with 11q23 chromosomal translocations. *New England Journal of Medicine* **329,** 909–14.

Wang Q, *et al.* (1996). The CBFβ subunit is essential for CBFα2 (AML1) function *in vivo. Cell* **87,** 697–708.

Warrell RP, Jr, *et al.* (1991). Differentiation therapy of acute promyelocytic leukemia with tretinoin (all-trans-retinoic acid). *New England Journal of Medicine* **324,** 1385–93.

22.3.2 The classification of leukaemia

D. Catovsky

Introduction

The classification of leukaemia has evolved from a purely morphological approach, based on the appearances of the leukaemic cells in peripheral blood and bone marrow films, through cytochemical techniques and, more recently, with the use of monoclonal antibodies (**MAbs**) against cellular antigens. There has also been a major input from cytogenetic and molecular methods. The new methodologies are introducing greater precision and objectivity to the diagnostic criteria and in the assessment of prognosis in the well-defined disease entities. A new WHO classification on haemopoietic malignancies is a positive step forward and represents the consensus of most pathologists and clinicians in the field.

A broad classification of acute leukaemia includes two large groups, historically designated 'acute' and 'chronic'. Acute leukaemias represent malignancies with little evidence of differentiation; the characteristic cells are immature precursors or blasts. It is for this group where techniques other than morphology are essential for classification. The chronic leukaemias (lymphoid and myeloid) show maturation that is easily recognized morphologically, although in the diseases of lymphocytes the various subtypes can only be accurately defined by means of immunological methodology using panels of MAbs (Chapter 22.3.5).

Acute leukaemia

There are two major groups of acute leukaemia, lymphoblastic (**ALL**) and myeloid (**AML**) (Table 1). Both affect children and adults but with different frequency: 80 per cent of patients with AML are adults (over the age of 15 years) and 20 per cent children, including infants; in contrast, 85 per cent of those with ALL are children (under 15 years) and 15 per cent are adults. There are few differences in most disease features in AML between children and adults; conversely, the biological and clinical differences between childhood ALL and adult ALL are substantial.

For a diagnosis of acute leukaemia it is necessary to identify blasts as the major cellular component. With a few cytochemical reactions, namely myeloperoxidase (**MPO**), Sudan Black B, and α-naphthyl acetate esterase (**ANAE**), it is possible to distinguish the two main forms, ALL and AML. However, because cytochemistry is largely negative in ALL, it is essential to apply a battery of MAbs which can be used as markers for the two ALL cell lineages, B and T, and which can also characterize the AML blasts (Table 2). These MAbs define the immunophenotype of the disease. In immature cells some antigens are first expressed in the cytoplasm then in the cell membrane. This must be taken into account when testing blasts in suspension by flow cytometry as this method needs to be adapted for the detection of cytoplasmic antigens. Some of the markers that are specific for the T, B, and myeloid lineages, CD3, CD22, CD79a, and MPO (Table 2), are localized in the cytoplasm and not in the membrane.

Table 1 The classification of acute leukaemia

Acute myeloid leukaemia (AML)
AML with recurrent cytogenetic abnormalities
AML not otherwise categorized (including FAB subtypes M0 to M7)
AML with multilineage dysplasias
AML therapy-related
Acute lymphoblastic leukaemia (ALL)
Precursor B-ALL
Precursor T-ALL
Burkitt leukaemia/lymphoma

Table 2 Differential diagnosis of the acute leukaemias by immunological methods and MAbs

Marker	Precursor B-ALL	Precursor T-ALL	AML
CD10	+	–	–
CD19	+	–	–
CD22(c)	+	–	–
CD79a(c)	+	–	–
TdT	+	+	–
CD2	–	+	–
CD3(c)	–	+	–
CD7	–	+	–
CD1a	–	–/+	–
CD13	–	–	+
CD33	–	–	+
CD117	–	–/+	+
MPO(c)	–	–	+*

(c) cytoplasmic expression; all other markers are usually detected in the cell membrane.

* Anti-MPO is negative in erythroid precursors (M6) and megakaryoblasts (M7). M6 cells react with antibodies to glycophorin A and Hb A; M7 cells react with antibodies to platelet glycoproteins CD41(gpIIb/IIIa) and CD61(gpIIIa).

Bone marrow trephine biopsies may be useful for the diagnosis of those rare cases that yield a dry tap or a hypocellular specimen in aspirates. This is the case in two uncommon forms of acute leukaemia: megakaryoblastic, or AML-M7, and hypocellular acute leukaemia, the blasts of which may be myeloid or lymphoid.

In the last decade it has become apparent that some of the acute leukaemias, both AML and ALL, can be defined by distinct chromosome translocations. These translocations often result in a fusion gene that encodes a new chimeric protein. The leukaemias so classified correlate with their response to therapy and their prognosis. For this reason, the new WHO classification has defined several types of AML and ALL by the molecular events crucial in their pathogenesis. It is therefore essential that, whenever possible, cytogenetic analysis and/or molecular methods—such as fluorescent *in-situ* hybridization (**FISH**), polymerase chain reaction (**PCR**), or Southern blots—should be part of the diagnostic procedures performed in all these cases.

Acute myeloid leukaemia (Table 3)

AML with cytogenetic abnormalities

There is now good evidence that four types of AML defined by reciprocal chromosomal translocations represent distinct disease entities: these are listed in Table 3.

The translocation t(8;21)(q22;q22) is seen in 10 per cent of cases of AML, most of which have the M2 morphology (myeloblastic with maturation). This form of AML is relatively more common in children than adults. In rare cases the percentage of blasts in the bone marrow is less than 20 per cent, which is currently the recommended threshold for the diagnosis of AML. The immunophenotype of this type of AML is similar to others (Table 2), except for the frequent expression of the B-lineage antigen CD19, in 70 per cent of cases. AML with t(8;21) is associated with a high

Table 3 The classification of acute myeloid leukaemia

AML with recurrent cytogenetic abnormalities
AML with t(8;21)(q22;q22) [*ETO/AML1*]*
AML with t(15;17)(q22;q21) [*PML/RARα*]* or acute promyelocytic leukaemia [FAB M3]
AML with abnormal eosinophils and inv(16)(p13;q22), del(16)(q22), or t(16;16)(p13;q22) [*CBFB/MYH11*]*
AML with 11q23 [*MLL*]* abnormalities
AML not otherwise categorized (see Table 4) [Includes all FAB subtypes M0–M7 and others]
AML with multilineage dysplasia
AML (or MDS) therapy-related

* Genes involved in the molecular rearrangement.

Table 4 AML not otherwise categorized*

Myeloblastic	
M0	minimal differentiation
M1	without maturation
M2	with maturation
Promyelocytic	
M3	hypergranular
M3V	microgranular variant
Myelomonocytic/monocytic	
M4	granulocytic/monocytic
M5	monoblastic/monocytic
M6	**Erythroleukaemia**
M7	**Megakaryoblastic**
Acute basophilic leukaemia	
Acute panmyelosis with myelofibrosis	
Myeloid sarcoma	

* Does not include cases with the recurrent abnormalities defined in Table 3 but they may have other cytogenetic changes.

complete remission rate and a long-term disease-free survival. In a proportion of cases, mainly children, t(8;21) presents as a chloroma (myeloid sarcoma), sometimes with little bone marrow involvement.

The translocation t(15;17)(q22;q21) is consistently associated with acute promyelocytic leukaemia (FAB M3). The chromosome abnormality is seen in both the typical or hypergranular form and the less common microgranular type or M3V. The translocation involves the *PML* and *RARα* (retinoic acid receptor) genes, resulting in a *PML/RARα* fusion gene. M3 represents 7 to 8 per cent of all AMLs. Typical cases can be recognized morphologically: the blasts are bilobed, heavily granular, and show bundles of Auer rods or 'faggots'. MPO and Sudan Black B are strongly positive, myeloid antigens are expressed but HLA-DR and CD34, a feature of myeloblasts, are negative. AML M3 affects young adults who present with low white blood counts (**WBC**) and a bleeding tendency. M3 variant cases have high WBC, and the blasts are deceptively hypogranular and may resemble monocytes but the nucleus is bilobed rather than reniform. Cytochemistry helps to exclude monocytic leukaemia by a strong MPO and weak or negative ANAE reaction. Patients with the rare variant translocations such as t(11;17)(q23;q21) also involving *RARa* usually lack typical M3 morphology and do not respond to treatment with all-*trans* retinoic acid (**ATRA**).

AML with myelomonocytic features and abnormal eosinophils (FAB M4Eo) is associated with abnormalities of chromosome 16, inv16, del(16) or t(16;16) (Table 3). The cytogenetic changes result in the fusion of the *CBFb* and *MYH11* genes and often require analysis by FISH or PCR as they may be missed by conventional karyotype analysis. The granules of the bone marrow eosinophils are often large and react with chloracetate esterase.

Analysis of more than 4000 AML cases entered into MRC AML trials (MRC AML 10, 11, and 12) showed that patients with t(8;21), t(15;17), or inv(16) represent 23 per cent of all cases, and have a significantly better prognosis and treatment outcome than those with normal karyotypes or other abnormalities. In contrast, a particularly unfavourable prognosis is seen in AML with abnormalities of chromosomes 3, 5, and 7.

Translocations involving the *MLL* gene at 11q23 take place with close to 20 other partner chromosomes. These abnormalities are more common in childhood AML and include the t(9;11)(p21;q23) and t(11;19)(q23;p13). The demonstration of *MLL* rearrangement, which is also affected in childhood ALL, is better shown by Southern blot and FISH than by conventional karyotyping. Abnormalities of the *MLL* gene are seen mainly in infants (<1 year) with AML and therapy-related AML (see below). Morphologically, these cases often have monocytic/monoblastic features and a strong ANAE reaction sensitive to inhibition by sodium fluoride.

AML not otherwise categorized

These represent more than two-thirds of cases of AML not included in the above group. Some have distinct chromosome abnormalities, but because they are uncommon they have not yet been considered as specific entities. The WHO classification has retained the FAB categories (M0 to M7) with some additions for this large group of AML (Table 4).

AML M0 represents the most immature form of myeloblastic leukaemia. The blasts are negative with MPO and ANAE cytochemistry, negative with B- and T-lymphoid markers, as distinct from ALL, and positive with one or more of the AML markers (Table 2), including anti-MPO which is more sensitive than the cytochemical method for MPO. The incidence of M0 is around 3 per cent of all AML. There is evidence that this disease has a poor prognosis with a lower remission rate and shorter survival than other forms of AML.

AML M1 is also poorly differentiated; it differs from M0 in the demonstration of myeloid features by the cytochemical reactions with MPO and Sudan Black B. The majority of cases have more than 25 per cent positive blasts and often show Auer rods. It is advisable, in cases with less than 10 per cent MPO-positive blasts, to confirm the diagnosis of AML with myeloid markers (Table 2; Fig. 1).

Some one-third of cases with AML M2 will show t(8;21) and will therefore be included in the group defined by cytogenetic abnormalities. Other cases may have other changes, for example the rare variants of M2 and basophilia involving abnormalities at 12p or the translocation t(6;9)(p23;q34) with the chimeric fusion of the *DEK* and *CAN* genes.

The majority of cases of M3 and M3V recognized morphologically will have the t(15;17) described above. It has been retained here only for cases in which cytogenetic or molecular studies are not possible.

The myelomonocytic (M4) and pure monocytic (M5) leukaemias can be defined by morphology and cytochemistry. The variant M4Eo is associated with inv(16) and is included in the group with cytogenetic abnormalities.

There are two forms of M5 AML identified by morphology. M5a is immature, common in infants, and is recognized by a strong ANAE cytochemical reaction. In M5b the cells are more mature and lysozyme levels are raised. M5 is associated with high WBC, lymphadenopathy, gum hypertrophy, skin deposits, and central nervous system involvement. A rare form of M4 or M5 has heavily granular blasts, prominent haemophagocytosis, and a bleeding diathesis and is characterized by the translocation t(8;16)(p11;p13).

M6 (erythroleukaemia) may show features of trilineage dysplasia. The WHO recommends that the 20 per cent blasts required for the diagnosis of AML could be reached in M6 by excluding erythroblasts in the bone marrow differential count. The blasts in M6 are often myeloblasts. A rare pure form of AML M6 with erythroid precursors could be identified with MAbs against glycophorin A and Hb A.

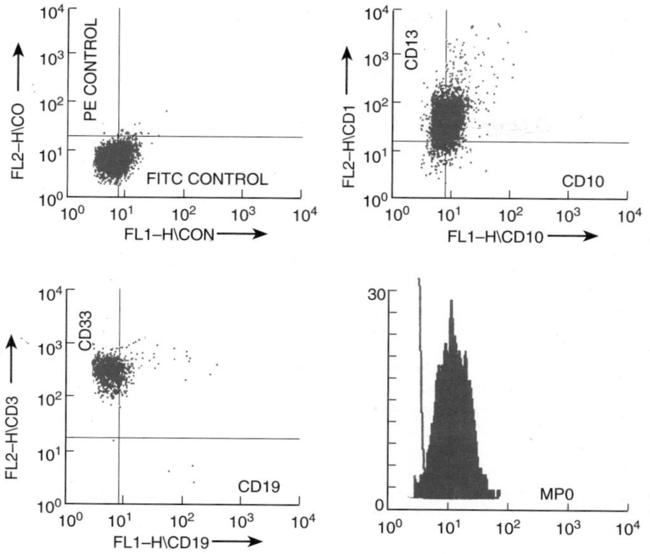

Fig. 1 Flow cytometry analysis of a case of AML using double MAbs conjugated with two different fluorescent dyes (phycoerythrin (**PE**) and fluorescein-isothiocyanate (**FITC**)) shown in the control panel (top left). The blast cells are CD13+ and CD10– (top right), CD33+ and CD19– (bottom left) and anti-MPO+ (bottom right). (See Table 2 and Farahat *et al.* (1994) for technical details).

AML M7 has a fibrotic bone marrow with more than 20 per cent blasts, abnormal megakaryocytes, and circulating blasts shown to be megakaryoblasts by their reactivity with MAbs against platelet glycoproteins, for example CD41/42/61. Bone marrow trephines are essential for diagnosis if there are insufficient blasts to examine with MAbs. Electron microscopy shows that the megakaryoblasts contain peroxidase activity in their nuclear membranes and endoplasmic reticulum. Both M6 and M7 are associated with a poor prognosis.

A subtype of AML seen in children with Down's syndrome has been described as a transient myeloproliferative disorder. If they develop acute leukaemia this is often megakaryoblastic in type.

Other rare forms of AML, acute basophilic leukaemia, acute panmyelosis with myelofibrosis (which may be indistinguishable from AML M7), and myeloid sarcoma (a myeloid tumour developing in an extramedullary site) are now incorporated in the WHO classification (Table 4).

AML with multilineage dysplasia

This form of AML is seen mainly in elderly patients and is defined by the presence of dysplasia in the three bone marrow lineages: granulocytic, erythroid, and megakaryocytic. Chromosome abnormalities, gains or losses, involving chromosomes 7 (–7,7q–) and 5 (–5,5q–), are common. These cases include those evolving from a myelodysplastic syndrome (**MDS**) or arising apparently *de novo*. The key element to distinguish from MDS is the presence of more than 20 per cent blasts in the bone marrow.

Therapy-related AML and MDS

This new category recognized in the WHO classification results from the increased number of patients developing AML and MDS following therapy for other malignancies. Two major types are recognized:

1. *Related to therapy with alkylating agents.* These cases occur late, 5 to 6 years following exposure. A phase of MDS often precedes AML. Morphologically, these cases have trilineage dysplasia and are difficult to classify in the types listed in Table 4. Abnormalities of chromosomes 5 and 7 are also common.
2. *Related to therapy with topoisomerase II inhibitors.* This form of AML is seen in patients treated with drugs targeting topoisomerase II, such as etoposide and teniposide, and also with anthracyclines. It has a short period of latency, usually from 12 to 50 months (median 33 months) and is rarely associated with MDS changes. Chromosome abnormalities often involve the *MLL* gene, e.g. t(9;11) and t(11;19), and also t(8;21), inv(16), and t(6;9).

Acute lymphoblastic leukaemia

ALL represents the clonal proliferation of immature lymphoid precursors. The characteristic cell is the lymphoblast, which has a high nuclear to cytoplasmic ratio and usually lacks cytoplasmic granules. Staining reactions with MPO, Sudan Black B, and ANAE are negative. Evidence of lymphoid differentiation towards a B or T lineage is provided by immunological markers (Table 2), including a positive terminal deoxynucleotidyl transferase (**TdT**) response.

In the morphological groups described by the FAB group, L1 is seen in 80 per cent of childhood cases, L2 in 20 per cent, and L3 (or Burkitt type) in 1 to 3 per cent. However, only the latter—which corresponds to membrane Ig-positive B-lineage ALL and has the same chromosome translocation, t(8;14), as Burkitt lymphoma—remains as a morphological/pathological entity described as Burkitt leukaemia/lymphoma (Table 5). The L1 and L2 types are no longer taken into consideration for classification purposes.

The current classification of ALL takes into account the cell lineage, B or T, which is based on the sequential appearance of B- and T-cell antigens during differentiation (Table 2), and distinct and consistent abnormalities that define discrete forms of the disease (Table 5). The immunophenotype of ALL correlates at the DNA level with the rearrangement of the immunoglobulin heavy-chain genes and T-cell receptor (**TCR**) genes in the B and T lineages, respectively. This type of analysis is not necessary for diagnosis or classification purposes, but it is important for monitoring minimal residual disease. Molecular techniques, such as PCR and FISH analysis, on the other hand, are also becoming more informative for the detection of rearranged genes and chimeric mRNA involved in the specific chromosome abnormalities of ALL.

Precursor B-lineage ALL

This is more frequent in children and the elderly. In infants with precursor B-ALL, there is a strong association with translocations of the *MLL* gene, which confers a poor prognosis.

An important marker of the B lineage is the common-ALL antigen recognized by MAbs of the CD10 cluster. CD10 is expressed in the blasts of 75 per cent of childhood ALL cases. Less mature lymphoblasts (early or pro-B ALL) do not express CD10, and this is seen in 10 per cent of childhood cases and in 30 per cent of adult patients. Pre-B ALL blasts express cytoplasmic μ chains (without light chains).

The various forms of B-lineage ALL have distinct prognostic features that are best characterized by the associated chromosome abnormalities (Table 5). The best two prognostic groups of precursor B-ALL defined by

Table 5 The classification of acute lymphoblastic leukaemia

Precursor B-lineage ALL
ALL with t(9;22)(q34;q11) [*ABL/BCR*]*
ALL with *MLL** translocations t(v;11)(v;q23)
ALL with t(12;21)(p21;q22) [*TEL/AML1*]*
ALL with t(1;19)(q23;p13) [*PBX/E2A*]*
ALL with hyperdiploidy (51–65 chromosomes)
Precursor T-lineage ALL
Burkitt leukaemia/lymphoma (FAB L3)

* Genes involved in the molecular rearrangements.

cytogenetic/molecular rearrangements are t(12;21)(q21;q22) and hyperdiploidy (51–65 chromosomes). The t(12;21) translocation is the most common, found in 25 per cent of cases, but it is difficult to detect by conventional cytogenetics and needs FISH analysis or Southern blotting to identify rearrangements of the *TEL* gene. Recent data show that at 5 years' follow-up the event-free survival of children with *TEL* rearrangements is 91 per cent. Similarly, 85 per cent of children with ALL and 51 to 65 chromosomes can be cured with current protocols. One of the possible explanations for this high cure rate is the propensity of lymphoblasts from hyperdiploid cases to undergo apoptosis.

The translocation t(1;19) is associated with the expression of cytoplasmic μ chain and immunologically it corresponds to a pre-B precursor. Although formerly associated with a poor prognosis, this has improved with newer modalities.

Poor prognosis in patients with ALL is associated with two molecular events: *MLL* rearrangement and the *BCR/ABL* fusion gene (Table 5). The *MLL* gene is rearranged in several translocations. The most common in infants is t(4;11)(q21;q23); this event is now known to occur before birth. The t(4;11) translocation is seen in 4 to 8 per cent of adult cases of ALL, 3 to 5 per cent of childhood ALL, and in up to 70 per cent of infants with ALL.

The t(9;22), which results in a short chromosome 22, the Philadelphia (**Ph**) chromosome, and the associated *BCR/ABL* fusion gene, increases in frequency with age. In childhood ALL up to 5 per cent of cases have been reported, but 25 to 30 per cent of adult patients with ALL have the translocation. There are important subtle differences between children and adults. In the latter, 50 per cent of the *BCR/ABL* fusion results in a p210 chimeric protein (as in all cases of Ph-positive CML), whilst in childhood ALL the common product is p190. In addition to the higher incidence of t(9;22) in adult ALL, their poor prognosis is compounded by the rarity of hyperdiploidy and of the t(12;21) translocation.

Precursor T-lineage ALL

T-lymphoblasts are defined by several T-cell markers (Table 2). In about one-third of cases, chromosome translocations involving the *TCRα/d* loci at 14q11 and the *TCRβ/γ* loci at 7q34. Examples are t(1;14)(p32;q11) involving the *TAL1* gene, t(10;14)(q24;q11) with the *HOX11* gene, and t(11;14)(p13;q11) involving the *RBTN2* gene. In 25 per cent of cases of T-ALL the *TAL1* locus (1p32) is dysregulated by submicroscopic deletion.

Precursor T-ALL comprises 15 per cent of childhood ALL and is more common in adolescents and males. In adult ALL it comprises 25 per cent of cases. Disease characteristics are a high WBC, large mediastinal mass, and less involvement of the bone marrow than precursor B cases.

Burkitt leukaemia/lymphoma

This leukaemia represents the leukaemic presentation of Burkitt lymphoma and is defined by evidence of membrane immunoglobulin (heavy and light chains); it is associated with L3 morphology and the translocation t(8;14)(q24;q32). In adults it may also represent the transformation of a pre-existing follicular lymphoma; in such cases t(8;14) coexists with t(14;18), but this is rare. The lymphoblasts have a deep basophilic cytoplasm and prominent nucleolus. L3 blasts are TdT- and CD34-negative and CD19-, CD20-, and CD22-positive; CD10 may be expressed, although it is more frequently absent.

Patients present with bulky disease and, biochemically, a high lactate dehydrogenase (**LDH**) level. Prognosis has now improved with very intensive protocols of short duration.

Biphenotypic acute leukaemia or acute leukaemia of ambiguous lineage

The wider use of MAbs has brought to light the existence of cases in which markers of different cell lineages (usually B and myeloid) are coexpressed on the same blast cells. Many of the markers used for defining the immunophenotype of acute leukaemia are not always lineage-specific. Hence, it is necessary to use restrictive criteria to define as 'biphenotypic' those cases that coexpress two markers of which at least one is lineage specific, for example: CD22, CD79a, and μ chain for the B lineage; CD3 for the T lineage; and MPO or CD117 for the myeloid lineage.

Some cases of biphenotypic leukaemia have all the features of ALL but coexpress two or more myeloid markers. Others present as typical AML and, in addition to myeloid antigens (Table 2), they express TdT and two or more B (or rarely T) antigens. Biphenotypic leukaemias may represent up to 5 per cent of all acute leukaemias and frequently show rearrangement of immunoglobulin and/or *TCR* genes, even in cases presenting as AML. Because of the distinct biological and molecular changes and current poor prognosis associated with these cases, it is relevant to recognize biphenotypic leukaemia as a distinct type using well-defined criteria. Cytogenetic changes include t(4;11) and other 11q23 abnormalities as well as t(9;22), which may explain the overall poor prognosis.

Chronic leukaemias

These are malignancies in which mature leucocytes are the predominant cells. As in the acute leukaemias, there are two main groups: myeloid and lymphoid, with two representative disorders, chronic myelogenous (**CML**) and chronic lymphocytic (**CLL**) leukaemia. The latter, as well as the less common forms of leukaemias of mature B and T lymphocytes, are described in Chapter 22.3.5. The chronic myeloid leukaemias reflect granulocytic or monocytic differentiation, or a combination of both: myelomonocytic (Table 6).

CML (Ph-positive)

CML (or CGL) has a distinct chromosome marker, the Ph chromosome, resulting from the reciprocal translocation t(9;22), found in 95 per cent of cases. Cases with similar haematological features, but which are cytogenetically Ph-negative, often have the same molecular rearrangement that results from the juxtaposition of the *BCR* and *ABL* genes to form a hybrid *BCR/ABL* gene. Understanding of the molecular biology of CML leads to significant advances in treatment (see Further reading list).

The diagnosis of Ph-positive CML can be established by the morphological appearance of peripheral blood and bone marrow films, and confirmed by cytogenetic and/or molecular analysis. The leucocyte differential count in CML shows the full spectrum of granulocytic cells but with a predominance of myelocytes (about 30 per cent) and mature neutrophils (about 50 per cent), as well as almost invariably basophilia (approximately 5 per cent) and frequent eosinophilia; the percentage of monocytes is low, usually less than 3 per cent. Blasts represent 1 or 2 per cent of the circulating cells unless the disease is in accelerated phase or in transformation; myelodysplastic changes are minimal. The bone marrow aspirate is hypercellular with granulocytic hyperplasia and numerous megakaryocytes, and is less useful than the peripheral blood for a differential diagnosis between CGL and the other chronic myeloid leukaemias. The myeloid:erythroid ratio is greater than 10:1 with few erythroblasts. The bone marrow trephine is necessary to assess the degree of fibrosis and, occasionally, to distinguish from idiopathic myelofibrosis.

Table 6 Chronic myeloid leukaemias

Chronic myelogenous (CML), Ph-positive t(9;22)(q34;q11) *BCR/ABL*
Chronic neutrophilic (CNL)
Atypical CML (Ph-negative)
Chronic eosinophilic/hypereosinophilic syndrome
Chronic myelomonocytic (CMML)
Juvenile CMML

Atypical chronic myeloid leukaemia (Ph-negative)

Patients with high leucocyte counts who are Ph chromosome-negative (and *BCR/ABL*-negative) represent a slightly heterogeneous group. Most cases have atypical morphological features compared with those with Ph-positive CML: namely, slight monocytosis, absence of basophilia and eosinophilia, granulocytic dysplasia (Pelger and hypogranular neutrophils), and 2 to 3 per cent circulating blasts.

Chronic myelomonocytic leukaemia (CMML)

CMML has features of MDS and myeloproliferative disorders. The two main differences with atypical CML and Ph-positive CML are the proportion of monocytes, which ranges from 25 to 50 per cent in CMML, and the lower percentage of immature granulocytes (5–10 per cent) in the bone marrow. The erythroid cells in the bone marrow are also more prominent in CMML, with a lower myeloid:erythroid ratio than in the other conditions. CMML cases are always Ph-negative and *BCR/ABL*-negative, and show moderate to high levels of serum and urinary lysozyme and myelodysplastic changes in the bone marrow. The WHO includes CML in an MDS/myeloproliferative grouping and no longer purely as MDS.

Rare forms of chronic myeloid leukaemia

Chronic neutrophilia

This occurs in adults over 50 years of age. Haemoglobin and platelet counts are normal. The blood film shows predominantly neutrophils without immature forms. The neutrophil alkaline phosphatase score is high, in contrast with the very low levels in classic Ph-positive CML. Most cases were thought to be Ph-negative. Recent evidence suggests that some cases have the t(9;22), but, in contrast to CML, the *BCR/ABL* rearrangement results in a p230, rather than a p210, protein product.

Juvenile CMML

Juvenile chronic myelomonocytic leukaemia represents 2 per cent of the childhood leukaemias. Patients are under 5 years of age and have systemic symptoms. In contrast to CML, there is monocytosis without basophilia or eosinophilia. Characteristically, the levels of fetal haemoglobin are high. Cytogenetic analysis is important to distinguish juvenile CMML from Ph-positive CML in childhood and from the myelodysplastic syndrome with monosomy 7 seen in young children.

Chronic eosinophilic leukaemia (CES)

CES is now included together with the hypereosinophilic syndrome because a clear distinction between these conditions is currently not possible. A comprehensive review of the topic has recently been published (see Further reading list).

Further reading

Bain BJ (2000). Hypereosinophilia. *Current Opinion in Hematology* **7**, 21–5.

Bennett JM, *et al.* (1976). Proposals for the classification of the acute leukaemias. *British Journal of Haematology* **33**, 451–8.

Bennett JM, *et al.* (1985). Criteria for the diagnosis of acute leukemia of megakaryocyte lineage (M7). *Annals of Internal Medicine* **103**, 460–2.

Bennett JM, *et al.* (1991). Proposal for the recognition of minimally differentiated acute myeloid leukaemia (AML-M0). *British Journal of Haematology* **78**, 325–9.

Bennett JM, *et al.* (1994). The chronic myeloid leukaemias: guidelines for distinguishing chronic granulocytic, atypical chronic myeloid, and chronic myelomonocytic leukaemia. Proposals by the French–American–British Cooperative Leukaemia Group. *British Journal of Haematology* **87**, 746–54.

Farahat N, *et al.* (1994). Demonstration of cytoplasmic and nuclear antigens in acute leukaemia using flow cytometry. *Journal of Clinical Pathology* **47**, 843–9.

Harris NL, *et al.* (1999). World Health Organization classification of neoplastic diseases of the hematopoietic and lymphoid tissues: report of the Clinical Advisory Committee meeting—Airlie House, Virginia, November 1997. *Journal of Clinical Oncology* **17**, 3835–49.

Jaffe ES, *et al.* (2001). *World Health Organization classification of tumours – pathology and genetics of tumours of haematopoietic and lymphoid tissues.* IARC Press, Dijon.

Löwenberg B, Downing JR, Burnett A (1999). Acute myeloid leukemia. *New England Journal of Medicine* **341**, 1051–62.

Melo JV (1996). The diversity of BCR–ABL fusion proteins and their relationship to leukemia phenotype. *Blood* **88**, 2375–84.

Rowley JD (2000). Molecular genetics in acute leukemia. *Leukemia* **14**, 513–17.

Savage DG, Antman KH (2002). Imatinib mesylate–a new oral targeted therapy. *New England Journal of Medicine*, **346**, 683–93.

Wheatley K, *et al.* (1999). A simple, robust, validated and highly predictive index for the determination of risk-directed therapy in acute myeloid leukaemia derived from the MRC AML 10 trial. United Kingdom Medical Research Council's Adult and Childhood Leukaemia Working Parties. *British Journal of Haematology* **107**, 69–79.

22.3.3 Acute lymphoblastic leukaemia

Philip J. Burke

Acute lymphoblastic leukaemia (ALL)

Some 40 years ago prednisone and vincristine were found to be effective in reducing visible leukaemia in children with ALL. The concepts of remission, consolidation, and maintenance therapies for all leukaemias evolved from trials in this disease, and until now have been the mainstay of tumour control strategies. Although the outcome in children has been excellent, outcomes in adults have so far been discouraging. However, with improved support, thereby permitting more intensive treatment modalities, the survival rate in patients at obvious poor risk has improved. Unfortunately, a significant increase in the cure rate without untoward early and late toxicity is unlikely using currently available drugs.

It is unclear how best to increase the cure rate in older patients. Real improvement may lie in applied molecular biology aimed at specific genetic targets. Subset identification will help to resolve the question of risk versus benefit in individual patients. The next step will be to obtain evidence supporting biological intervention with specific novel agents. The most appropriate candidates for study are patients with minimal leukaemia after initial tumour reduction and bone marrow homeostasis.

Diagnosis

Classically, acute lymphoblastic leukaemia has been categorized by morphology. There are three groups in the French–American–British (**FAB**) carcinoma staging classification, with L1 being defined by small monomorphic cells, L2 by large heterogeneous cells, and L3 by a Burkitt's cell-type with vacuoles. These distinctions are not as definitive as for acute myeloblastic leukaemia (**AML**), but flow cytometry has relieved some of the confusion with identification by phenotype. A prognosis in ALL can now be more accurately assigned with the addition of both immunophenotyping and cytogenetics (Table 1). Some 20 per cent of ALL are T cell, 75 per cent are precursor B cell, and 5 per cent are mature B cell in origin. In adults, 35 per cent of cases express both lymphoid and myeloid antigens. These more immature subtypes, early-pre-B-ALL and pre-T-ALL occur more frequently in adults than in children. Classification by immunological

Table 1 Characteristics of subgroups of AML and ALL

Cytogenetic determinant		FAB	Proto-oncogene	Reciprocal gene	Product
Myeloid					
t(8;21)—X;Y	M2	Abnormal maturation granulocytes	*AML-1* runt homologene	*ETO*	Protein DER(8)
t(9;22)—5, -7	M2	Trilineage proliferation/maturation	*ABL* tyrosine kinase	*M-BCR*	Fusion protein (210 kDa)
t(6;9)	M2 baso	with basophils	*DEK-7*	*CAN*	Fusion protein
t(15;17)	M3	Hypergranular progranulocytes	*PML* zinc finger	*RAR*-(alpha)	Fusion protein
	M4V	Microgranular progranulocytes			
Inv(16)	M4eo	Trilineage dyspoiesis with eosinophils	*CBF-B*	*MVH-11*	Fusion protein
t(3;v)	M7	Blocked terminal differentiation	*EVI-1* zinc finger		Hypermethylated GATA-1
t(3;21)			*EVI-1*	*MDS-1*	
(9;11)	M4, M5	Mixed hypercellularity	*MLL/HRX/ALL-1 AT-HOOK*		Fusion protein
Lymphoid					
t(1;19)	L2	Pre-B lymphocytes	*E2A*	*PBX-1*	Fusion protein
t(1;14)	L2	T lymphocytes	*TAL-1*	*TRC*	
t(8;14)	L2	Burkitt's-vacuolated lymphoblasts	*MYC*	*IqG*	Fusion protein
t(9;22)	L2	B-mixed myeloid/lymphoid	*ABL*	*mBCR*	Fusion protein (190 kDa)
t(11;14)	L2	B lymphocytes	*MLL/HRX*	*IqG*	
t(4;11)	L2	T lymphocytes	*MLL*	*AF4*	
t(12;21)			*AML-1*	*TEL*	

subtype is reviewed in Chapter 22.3.2. In brief, early pre-B-ALL expressing HLA-DR, terminal deoxynucleotidyl transferase (**TdT**), and CD19 occur in 10 per cent of adults and 5 per cent of children. Common ALL, found in 50 per cent of adults, is characterized by CD10 and CD19. Some 15 per cent of ALL are pre-B with expression of a cytoplasmic immunoglobulin absent in common ALL.

The T-cell phenotype is present in 25 per cent of adult ALL, with CD7, CD2, and/or CD1. In most, the T-cell receptor gene is rearranged. Bilineage or biphenotypic hybrid leukaemias which express both lymphoid and myeloid antigens account for 35 per cent of adult cases.

Cytogenetic analyses of lymphoblasts reveal clonal chromosomal aberrations in 50 to 75 per cent of ALL. Most are structural abnormalities with a balanced translocation. Other more random aberrations are classed by chromosomal number—hypo- or hyperploidy. This syndrome identification confers prognosis for outcome with standard therapy.

Pathophysiology

Clinical manifestations

The pathophysiology of ALL is the consequence of bone marrow failure caused by tumour-related suppression of normal haemopoiesis and the clinical expression of the malignant clone. The growth of lymphocytic precursors arrested at an immature stage of differentiation suppresses production of the normal bone marrow elements, resulting in anaemia, infection, and bleeding. Circulating leukaemic cells infiltrate the central nervous system, liver, spleen, testes, ovary, lymph nodes, skin, and gastrointestinal tract. Diffuse lymphadenopathy and hepatosplenomegaly occur in half the cases. Varied degrees of failure of each organ, and the metabolic effects of increased cell turnover, contribute to the overall symptom complex at presentation. Centripetal joint swelling and bone pain with rheumatic symptoms in the adult contrast with the distal bone involvement seen in children. Punched out bony lesions may be present on the radiograph.

In children, the history of a recent severe upper respiratory infection is frequently elicited. Although evidence for a viral aetiology is sketchy, immune stimulation may lead to proliferation of B-cell precursors. There are models in the lymphomas with similar theoretical pathogenesis.

Failure to obtain disease remission late in therapy involves either failure of support or tumour resistance, while early mortality relates to the pathophysiology of the tumour and its immediate management.

Infection

As seen with AML, clinical signs and symptoms are those of bone marrow failure and tumour mass, but because of a lack of normal lymphocytes there is an associated immunosuppression in addition to neutropenia. This loss of immune surveillance places the patient at risk for infections unique to the immunocompromised host. In addition to the infectious agents encountered in the myeloid malignancies with granulocytopenia, nosocomial and parasitic infections, such as *Pneumocystis carinii* and atypical fungal organisms, must be suspected with each new fever. Since therapy is prolonged in ALL, consistent monitoring for pathogenic organisms is necessary even during remission (Chapter 22.3.4).

Lymphoblastosis

The immediate challenge at presentation is the diagnosis of the leukaemia presenting with a high white blood cell (**WBC**) count. Acute causes of an increased WBC count which may be mistaken for lymphoid leukaemia include the FAB classifications M0 and M7 of acute myelocytic leukaemia, chronic myelocytic leukaemia, and chronic lymphocytic leukaemia.

The WBC can range from zero to more than 100×10^9/l, with a count of less than 5×10^9/l in 25 per cent of patients. The need for immediate intervention is less urgent with lymphoblasts because they are relatively small and deformable compared with young myeloid cells, lessening the probability of hyperviscosity. Their rupture with chemotherapy, however, releases high levels of phosphates and urates which can cause tumour-lysis syndrome unless precautions are taken. An approach to hydration, leukapheresis, and possible early dialysis is reviewed in Chapter 22.3.4. If the diagnosis remains in doubt after slide review, flow cytometry will quickly distinguish between myeloid and lymphoid cells. The untoward effects of inappropriate chemotherapy prior to leukapheresis and fluid balance must be avoided in ALL.

Occasionally (less than 5 per cent of patients) the differential count shows reactive myelopoiesis with pseudo Pelger–Huët cells, but without circulating lymphoblasts. Normal lymphocytes may be absent. A bone marrow aspirate will provide the diagnosis in these cases of subleukaemic leukaemia.

Prognostic factors

Although statistics indicate considerable improvement in the treatment of adult ALL over the past decade, the majority of patients relapse and die of their disease. Certain subsets of patients are predicted to respond poorly with current therapies. For example, those with leukaemia characterized by the Philadelphia chromosome (Ph_1) or its molecular equivalent, the fusion gene *BCR–ABL*, have essentially no chance of cure without allogeneic bone marrow transplantation. Even then, only 40 per cent of patients who achieve remission will be cured.

Other adverse prognostic factors include over 60 years of age, WBC in excess of 30×10^9/l, absence of a mediastinal mass, L3 morphology, myeloid phenotype, and lack of expression of CD10. Combinations of these markers decrease the predicted survival. In one trial, the presence of three high-risk factors in B-lineage ALL decreased the 1-year survival rate from 75 per cent (one risk factor present) to 25 per cent. There were no long-term survivors among patients with four risk factors.

The strongest variable, genetic identification, now provides a reliable basis for assigning risk and selecting therapies (see cytogenetic and phenotypic classification, Chapters 22.3.1 and 22.3.2). Patients known to do poorly with childhood-type strategies, usually those with the chromosomal anomalies t(9;22), t(4;11), t(8;14), or 14q 11–13 (T-ALL), now respond to intensive initial treatment schedules.

Management

Therapy

The highly successful treatment of ALL in young children combines numerous drugs known to be active against malignant lymphoblasts. Therapy consists of a three-phase treatment induction, CNS prophylaxis, and maintenance. Induction therapy with prednisone, vincristine, L-asparaginase, and daunorubicin produces remission rates of 85 per cent. Maintenance therapy with 6-mercaptopurine, methotrexate, cyclophosphamide, and prednisone is given in a cyclical fashion for 2 or more years.

In contrast, complete remission (**CR**) rates in adults with ALL range from 65 per cent to 85 per cent, the time to remission is longer, the relapse rate is higher, and cure rates are between 20 per cent and 40 per cent. Multiple factors related to both the biology of leukaemic cells and ability of the host to tolerate treatment contribute to the inferior prognosis in adults as compared with childhood ALL.

A variety of strategies are designed to decrease the relapse rates in adults. Early intensive therapy to rapidly destroy more leukaemic cells that have not yet developed drug resistance is a logical approach. Increasing induction intensity with sequential high-dose cytotoxic agents results in an improved long-term outcome in poor-risk groups. In recent studies, the addition of early intensification therapy, particularly a timed sequence of daunorubicin and cytarabine, effectively prolongs remissions and prevents relapse. This approach in children results in a CR rate of 95 per cent, with 70 per cent of children remaining in CR beyond 5 years.

Intense therapy derived from AML models, given early in remission (consolidation) using drugs not previously employed and at high doses, effectively destroys residual leukaemic cells. Cyclophosphamide and cytarabine are examples of AML drugs of obvious value which are now better tolerated, and with a greater therapeutic advantage provided by effective support measures. The role of colony-stimulating factors remains unclear.

The present investigative approach focuses on intensification of therapy in all subgroups with ALL. Repeatedly given high-dose drugs rapidly reduce tumour mass, reduce the possibility of drug-resistance, and invade sanctuary sites to eliminate sequestered cells. With these more aggressive therapies, CNS relapse in adults is less than 5 per cent.

However, in contrast to the experience with two short, intensive courses in AML, long-term success in ALL requires prolonged chemotherapy with multiple courses similar to present lymphoma regimens. Long-term maintenance therapy remains standard in most group trials but long-term value is not proven (Table 2).

The model of high-dose chemotherapy is intense induction followed by bone marrow transplantation (**BMT**). The optimal indications for BMT in adult ALL remain to be determined. While a definitive role of allogeneic BMT during first remission in patients with high-risk features has been established, significant controversy exists regarding the indications for BMT in patients with standard-risk adult ALL. Autologous BMT has a failure rate similar to that of high-dose chemotherapy.

High-dose treatment in poor-risk patients with ALL

Below are examples of cytogenetically poor-risk groups of ALL which respond to aggressive therapies:

1. ALL-L3 (B-ALL) treated with intensive therapies with high doses of five drugs (vincristine, doxorubicin, cytarabine, methotrexate, cyclophosphamide) given in short repeated cycles now achieve CR rates of 70 per cent with 50 per cent long-term survival rates in patients with this rare (5 per cent) leukaemia. CNS prophylaxis with high-dose systemic therapy or intrathecal drugs is essential.
2. t(4;11) ALL with a pro-B-cell phenotype occurs in 5 per cent of adults and infants. Intensive therapy with high-dose cytarabine and mitoxantrone has improved the dismal outcome, with a predicted 50 per cent disease-free survival. Bone marrow transplantation is a reasonable alternative therapy.
3. t(9;22) ALL with *BCR–ABL* fusion gene occurs in 30 per cent of adults; 50 per cent of adults with B-lineage surface antigens have this fusion protein p190, in contrast to the p210 subtype of CML. Although remission rates of 75 per cent can be achieved with intensive therapy, even with BMT the relapse rate is between 40 and 80 per cent.
4. t(1;19), 11q23, t(12;21) are specific syndromes which have also demonstrated a significantly improved outcome with aggressive treatment.

Allogeneic bone marrow transplantation in poor-risk patients is a reasonable choice, since the median age in adults is 33 years. Relapse after BMT is 30 per cent, with a 15 to 20 per cent mortality from immediate and late toxicities.

With present support and intensive treatment, most patients can achieve a stable and durable remission. Most will relapse with resistant disease. A

Table 2 Multiagent remission-induction regimens and postremission therapy for adult acute lymphoblastic leukaemia

	No. of patients	Median age	No. of drugs used			Complete remission (%)	Median survival (months)
			Induction	Consolidation	Maintenance		
Germany	368	25	7	5	2	74	28
SWOG	168	28	4	7	8	68	18
UCSF	109	25	4	7	2	88	28
Italy	541	30	4	8	4	80	NR
France	511	33	4	5	6	76	18
CALGB	197	32	5	8	4	85	36
MDA	128	39	4	2	4	91	36

NR, not reported.

continued search for new approaches to the treatment of such patients with these non-random subsets of ALL is critical.

Proto-oncogene leukaemogenesis (see Table 1)

Most of the lymphoid malignancies appear to be related to oncogene rather than tumour-suppressor malfunction. Oncogenes direct the synthesis of products that contribute to the malignant transformation of a cell. When a genetic alteration activates a particular proto-oncogene, it is implicated in malignant transformation. The mechanisms may also involve either a point mutation or insertional mutagenesis. The most mechanistically defined are those syndromes related to visible translocation of proto-oncogenes to active promoter sites, a coupling that results in production of a unique protein or overproduction of the normal product. The diseases may also be associated with a single-point mutation in cells committed to specific lineage. A number of the leukaemias have been fully characterized. Minimal numbers of leukaemia cells are quantifiable by detection of the residual fusion gene with the polymerase chain reaction.

Measuring cause and change in these specific and cytotoxic drug-responsive leukaemias may determine and remedy the oncogenic mechanism, and establish models for treatment strategies in similar, but less definable, tumours.

Regulation of lymphoid-cell growth

Biological modifiers of lymphoid-cell proliferation are being sought for therapy. These are best understood by reviewing the normal regulation of cell growth and survival. The proliferation and maturation of lymphocytes is ultimately determined by peptide growth factors that bind and activate specific receptors. These activated receptors propagate the signal through a series of protein interactions to the cell nucleus where the signals are converted into predetermined responses. Proto-oncogenes encode growth factors and growth-factor receptors, transcription factors, and cell-cycle proteins that determine the level of gene expression. Abnormalities of these functions are produced by genetic change in haematological malignancies.

The rate of proliferation versus its maturation and normal programmed cell death by growth factors is determined by the cell. In the nucleus, low levels of MYC cause apoptosis (cell death) in response to cytokines. MYC is an intracellular protein ordinarily sequestered in the cytoplasm by the retinoblastoma suppressor protein (**Rb**). MYC protein, functioning in the nucleus as a heterodimer with another molecule, MAX, regulates transcription and therefore gene expression and cell survival. BCL-2 allows MYC to drive the cells to proliferation by blocking the pathway to cell death, determining the ultimate expansion of the cell population. This activity of BCL-2 is balanced by an opposing protein, BAX, whose activity as a dominant regulator of BCL-2 is increased by expression of P53. P53 overcomes the BCL-2 block of cell death and inhibits cell-cycle traverse of mutated or damaged DNA. It blocks cyclin-dependent phosphorylation, forcing DNA repair, or apoptosis if repair is faulty. For example, elimination of excess lymphoid cells activated by antigenic stimuli via the programmed cell-death mechanism is a physiological event involved in normal immune responses.

The initial aim of intervention in the lymphoid tumours is to down-regulate the overexpressed gene *BCL2*, and to force apoptosis in patients with leukaemias defined by this *BCL2* abnormality. In those without specific abnormalities in gene translocation and protein production, the transfer of lymphocytes to upregulate cytoplasmic antigens for tumour-specific attack is a testable thesis.

Novel agents

A few of many targets for investigation in patients with senescent leukaemia in remission are listed below. See Table 5 of Chapter 22.3.4 for a wider list of potential agents.

Drug resistance

Although most leukaemias are responsive to initial therapies, most patients relapse and die of drug-resistant disease. The refractory clone, either acquired or selected with chemotherapy, contains the multidrug resistance gene and its encoded 170-kDa P-glycoprotein. This mechanism may also protect normal bone marrow stem cells from cytotoxicity. Drugs that modulate the effect of this gene—the rapid pumping out of drug from the cell—are calcium-channel blocking agents such as verapamil and ciclosporin-A.

Telomerase

Telomeres are structures at the ends of chromosome which in normal cells progressively shorten with each cell division. Without telomerase action terminally short telomeres cause cell-growth arrest. Suppression of telomerase is a tumour-suppressor and ageing mechanism. In contrast, most cancer cells activate telomerase, resulting in stable telomeres and immortalization. Normal stem cells may express telomerase in the adult, allowing perpetuation, while tumours arising from stem cells may have a similar prolongation of survival. Telomerase inhibition is a therapeutic target to force cell senescence. Since telomerase levels reflect the persistent growth of AML, measurable suppression of telomerase activity in patients with minimal residual disease in remission may force tumour senescence and cell death.

Methylation

An imbalance of DNA methylation, involving widespread hypomethylation, regional hypermethylation, and increased cellular capacity for methylation is characteristic of human neoplasia. Beginning in preneoplastic cells, it becomes extensive in subsequent stages of tumour progression. This aberrant methylation, particularly of cytosine, may mark abnormalities of chromatin reorganization and mediate progressive losses of gene expression associated with tumour development.

Abnormal methylation sites have been detected in both myeloid and lymphoid malignancies. Drugs presently in trial to prevent leukaemic transformation or suppress relapse are the butyrates and cytidine analogues.

Angiogenesis

Leukaemia-cell growth requires the aggressive infiltration of capillaries into nests of tumour in excess of that seen in normal bone marrow. Relative selectivity of this neovascularization results in selective tumour regression on administration of antiangiogenic agents. These include angiostatin, endostatin, vasostatin, and other endogenous inhibitors of angiogenesis that block the effects of vascular endothelial cell-growth factor (**VEGF**). Other drugs act to block oncoprotein function by inhibiting signal transduction, for example Ras farnesyltransferase inhibitors. Such factors will prevent blood supply to new tumour growth when given at the time of maximal leukaemia-cell reduction.

Monoclonal antibodies

Cell-surface directed approaches are now in large clinical trials with encouraging responses. Constructs aimed directly at receptors include monoclonal antibodies (MAbs) specific for the cell-surface receptors CD20, CD19, and CD33 linked with a radionuclide, an endotoxin, or an antibiotic. All have achieved early success in relatively resistant leukaemias.

Unequal expression of surface receptors in the leukaemic clone may require upregulation for sensitivity.

Monoclonal antibodies have achieved utility in the treatment on lymphoma and hold promise in ALL.

Further reading

Cassileth PA, *et al.* (1992). Adult acute lymphocytic leukemia: the Eastern Cooperative Oncology Group experience. *Leukemia* **6**,178–81.

Chao NJ, *et al.* (1991). Allogeneic bone marrow transplantation for high-risk acute lymphoblastic leukemia during first complete remission. *Blood* **78**,1923–7.

Copelan EA, *et al.* (1995). The biology and treatment of acute lymphoblastic leukemia in adults. *Blood* **85**,1151–68.

Hoelzer D, *et al.* (1988). Prognostic factors in a multicenter study for treatment of acute lymphoblastic leukemia in adults. *Blood* **71**,123–31.

Hoelzer DF (1993). Therapy of the newly diagnosed adult with acute lymphoblastic leukemia. *Hematology/Oncology Clinics of North America* **7**,139–60.

Kantarjian HM (1994). Adult acute lymphocytic leukemia: critical review of current knowledge. *American Journal of Medicine* **97**,176–84.

Larson RA, *et al.* (1995). A five-drug remission induction regimen with intensive consolidation for adults with acute lymphoblastic leukemia: cancer and leukemia group B study 8811. *Blood* **85**, 2025–37.

Linker Ca, *et al.* (1991). Treatment of adult acute lymphoblastic leukemia with intensive cyclical chemotherapy: a follow-up report. *Blood* **78**, 2814–22.

Mandelli F (1992). GIMEMA ALL 0288: a multicentric study on adult acute lymphoblastic leukemia. Preliminary results. *Leukemia* **6**,182–5.

Rivera GK (1993). Treatment of acute lymphoblastic leukemia. 30 years' experience at St. Jude Children's Research Hospital. *New England Journal of Medicine* **329**,1289–95. [See comments.]

Rohatiner AZ, *et al.* (1990). High dose cytosine arabinoside in the initial treatment of adults with acute lymphoblastic leukemia. *British Journal of Cancer* **62**, 454–8.

Woods WG, *et al.* (1996). Timed-sequential induction therapy improves postremission outcome in acute myeloid leukemia: a report from the Children's Cancer Group. *Blood* **87**, 4979–89.

Yeager AM, *et al.* (1986). Autologous bone marrow transplantation in patients with acute nonlymphocytic leukemia, using *ex vivo* marrow treatment with 4-hydroperoxycyclophosphamide. *New England Journal of Medicine* **315**,141–7.

22.3.4 Acute myeloblastic leukaemia

Philip J. Burke

Introduction

Efforts in leukaemia research over the last 30 years or so have been rewarded with much success. Moreover, the principles of clinical research and their application to patient care are now defined.

With the availability of effective extrinsic haemopoietic support, leukaemia-induced bone marrow failure no longer restricts the intensity of therapy necessary to achieve maximal tumour kill. Pharmacologically determined drugs and schedules combined with rational concepts of maximal therapy have improved the survival rates of patients with leukaemia. The identification of tools and specific targets heralds a new era of therapy in patients with small amounts of residual leukaemia.

Many new technologies—DNA hybridization, purified specific probes, monoclonal antibodies marking lineage specificity, genetic array, and rapid measures of hybrid proteins—permit the genetic classification and identification of the origin and activity of a tumour. For some types of leukaemias, a combination of these methods provides an accurate prognosis for tumour eradication with the utilization of enhanced chemotherapy regimens and the application of new biological modalities. Single-site genetic mutations, translocations or deletions on chromosomes, loss of suppression or overexpression of genes, and transcription of an abnormal product that induces a malignant phenotype are all obvious targets for unique approaches to tumour control. Future success depends on understanding genetic multistep pathogenesis and its control, ultimately with specific interdiction of the premalignant clone.

Pathogenesis of myeloid leukaemia

There is evidence for a multistep pathogenesis of solid tumours. Similarly, many of the acute myeloid leukaemias are the final stages of clonal homeopathies initially transformed by exposure to ionizing radiation, certain chemicals, some chemotherapeutic drugs—especially alkylating agents and topoisomerase inhibitors—or by progression (for example, in certain genetic disorders).

Leukaemogenesis proceeds after the deleterious effect of a chemical or environmental agent on chromosomes. In some cases amplification or modification of the gene product then perpetuates the process. These events can be subclinical and of long duration in the prodromal stage. Progression occurs, for instance, when DNA damage is not repaired in proliferating cells which then escape programmed cell death.

The prima-facie evidence of induced genetic instability comes from the leukaemias that developed in people exposed to high-dose radiation from the Hiroshima and Nagasaki atomic bombs. A similar leukaemogenic effect of alkylating agents was manifested in 10 per cent of patients treated with **MOPP** (mechlorethamine, Oncovin (vincristine), procarbazine, prednisone) for Hodgkin's disease. These therapy-related leukaemias (**tAML**; secondary AML, **sAML**) usually have non-random genetic deletions of -5, -7, 5q, and/or 7q, while those related to topoisomerase II inhibitors (etoposides and anthracyclines) have consistent abnormalities of chromosome 11 (11q,23), and FAB 4 to 5 morphology of the French–American–British carcinoma staging classification. Many evolve from trilineage bone marrow failure (myelodysplastic syndrome, **MDS**), suggesting a genetic instability of multistep origin. These syndromes of long duration culminate in an aggressive phase with a clonal cohort that escaped DNA repair. The increasing numbers of patients with MDS reflect the cumulative effects of a series of sporadic incidents having their ultimate expression in an ageing population.

Some 30 per cent of patients have leukaemic syndromes associated with a non-random loss or gain of DNA on chromosomes 5, 7, and 8. These are stem-cell derived, trilineage tumours classified by FAB as either M_6, M_7, transformed MDS, or secondary acute myelocytic leukaemia (**sAML**). As in colon cancer, sequential genetic alterations ultimately result in metastatic malignancy. Secondary leukaemia may take years to evolve (Fig. 1). This class of haematological malignancy—the loss of a tumour-suppressor gene(s)—only transiently responds to current therapeutic modalities. However, remissions of predictable duration are achievable with intensive therapy in 40 per cent of such patients. Once stable, these genetic carcinoma-like tumours are targets for specific novel agents.

In contrast, myeloid leukaemias which occur spontaneously or with only brief incubation periods are probably clonal progeny with a single proto-oncogene, non-random genetic mutation. In these, chromosomal malfunction at the gene level follows transposition of genetic material to promoter areas and activation. These leukaemias, representing 20 per cent of all cases of AML, have either a chromosomal balanced translocation or an inversion. Some 50 per cent of patients with a normal karyotype have submicroscopic genetic mutations and overexpression. These alter nuclear oncogenes, many yet to be defined, which affect signal transduction, transcription, gene splicing, protein kinase C, and many other cellular activities.

Pretreatment management of acute leukaemia

Initial evaluation

The clinical signs and symptoms of acute leukaemia result from the suppression of normal haemopoiesis and the extramedullary expression of the malignant clone.

Bone marrow failure

Tumour suppression of the trilineage elements of the bone marrow produces pancytopenia. The signs and symptoms of anaemia result from the non-production of red blood cells, and may be associated with overt blood loss and with petechia and purpura at pressure sites in the skin. Variations in the dominance of loss of function of any the trilineage products relate to the specific type of AML (see FAB classification). Neutropenia is not commonly associated with infection in the rapid-onset subsets of AML. With a lymphoid-sparing pathogenesis, immunosuppression and its associated opportunistic infections are not frequently encountered in patients with AML. The incidence of compounding medical diseases is no greater that in the general population. Most signs and symptoms of acute multiorgan impairment disappear with adequate tumour control and homeostasis. The performance factor score is not a reliable indicator for making treatment decisions.

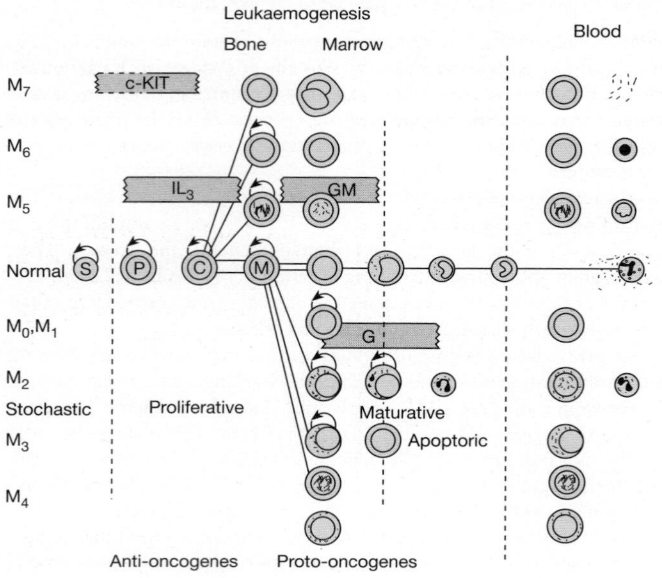

Fig. 1 Myeloid leukaemogenesis. Normal proliferation and maturation of granulopoiesis is contrasted to those leukaemias of proto-oncogene and antioncogene derivation. This is a conceptual model loosely relating FAB with a cytogenetic classification. The activities of growth factors relative to proliferation, maturation, and apoptosis are shown. The figure depicts the progression of leukaemia according to the FAB classification and ligand stimulation. During the stochastic kinetic period the stem cell reproduces itself, with some cells distributed to the committed pool in a random manner. While in this proliferative pool they are influenced by normal regulatory factors. The first legend, *c-kit*, affects the stem cell directly, with the subsequent committed cells filling various compartments. In the M7 through M5 leukaemias, this compartment consists of trilineage-derived cells. The disease reflects the activities of the cell type most prominently involved, i.e. megakaryocyte, erythrocyte, or monocyte. Leukaemias of FAB classification M1 through M3 are specifically derived from cells committed to the granulocytic pathway, while M4, a combination of monocytic and granulocytic phenotypes, is probably derived from one or more earlier cells. Normal growth factors, which modify proliferation and maturation, are c-kit, IL-3 (active early), and GM-CSF (active late) in the proliferation period; and G-CSF specifically affecting the more mature granulocytic precursors (GM-CSF, granulocyte–macrophage colony-stimulating factor; G-CSF, granulocyte colony-stimulating factor). The resultant forms commonly released to the peripheral blood are blasts, some showing signs of maturation. The leukaemias with balanced translocations represent a loss of oncogene control, while those derived from earlier progenitors, more likely to be involved with a loss of DNA, relate to a loss of suppressor gene activity. Patients with balanced translocations or inversions comprise 20 per cent of the total AML population, while 50 per cent have grossly normal cytogenetics. Most of these are found within FAB classifications M0–5, while those antioncogene tumours with DNA loss occur in the FAB M5–7, secondary AMLs, and transformed MDS. This distribution is not absolute, and prognosis cannot be determined by FAB classification alone.

Extramedullary disease

A minority of patients present with a subleukaemia without circulating blast cells and require a bone marrow aspirate for diagnosis. The white blood cell (**WBC**) count may reach levels in excess of 100 000 × 10^9/l in 5 per cent of patients, although in the majority it is between 5 and 20 × 10^9/l. However, even in those patients with low WBC counts at presentation the initial decisions are urgent. Disseminated intravascular coagulation (**DIC**) can occur in promyelocytic leukaemia (M3) in young patients with pancytopenia. Emergency approaches have been designed to manage patients who will suffer the morbidity of leucostasis and tumour-lysis syndrome before and during treatment.

Diagnosis and supportive care

The advent of HLA typing, recognition of the risks of neutropenia, evidence of stem-cell resilience, availability of blood products, the acceptance of new aggressive chemotherapy regimens, recognition of genetic subsets, and identification of special training needs of staff now provide the basis for maximal levels of support for the patient presenting with acute leukaemia. These concepts of oncology care are essential for patients' survival throughout the intensive therapy required to reduce their leukaemic state to a minimum.

Support at presentation

Although the combination of bone marrow failure and tumour invasion determine the presenting clinical features of acute leukaemia, the aspects of clonal expression based on tumour mass, specific leukaemia-cell characteristics, and the rate of cell turnover determine the need for prompt intervention. Paradoxically, rapid cell killing with intensive drug treatment results in severe metabolic imbalances that are sometimes difficult to ameliorate. Survival depends on the prevention of both disease and treatment-related complications. The rational use of supportive measures combined with treatment permits both disease eradication and survival with treatment.

Immediate intervention is required in some cases. Efforts to decrease tumour mass both rapidly and safely entail awareness, rapid intervention, and aggressive treatment. Intense and appropriate critical-care management in emergency situations in patients with hyperleucocytosis, tumour-lysis syndrome, and DIC has now markedly reduced the historical early death rate of 50 per cent.

Hyperleucocytosis

Early mortality is related to the sheer mass of tumour cells. Patients with hyperleucocytic leukaemia (WBC count of more than 75 000 × 10^9/l), can suffer early death with central nervous system (**CNS**) haemorrhage and pulmonary capillary leakage sometimes due to a delay in treatment. These patients are at grave risk of vessel rupture. Clinically, high leukaemia blast-cell counts in AML and chronic myelocytic leukaemia (CML) are associated with fever and evidence of functional impairment of the lungs and brain. The most predictive sign of ongoing vascular rupture is a target purpura with a single, deep central nodule. The rigidity of the myeloblast causes stasis with expanding aggregates, arteriole infarction, and bleeding (Fig. 2

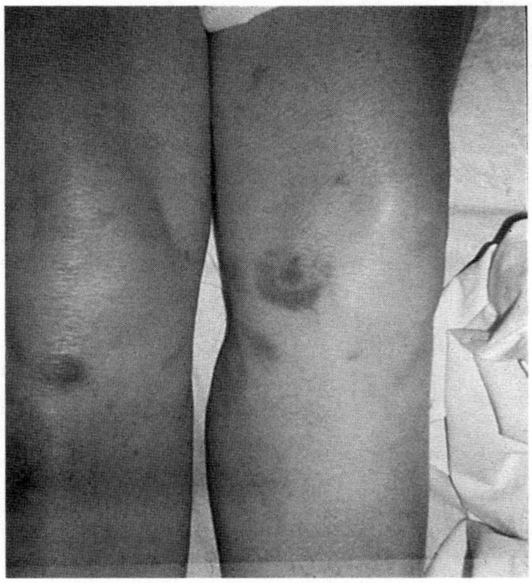

Fig. 2 Target purpura. Classic target appearance of purpura formed by infarction of an arteriole by a dividing cluster of leukaemic myeloblasts. Typically, a deep, firm nodule can be felt in the pale centre of the lesion. (See also Plate 1.)

and Plate 1). Increased viscosity is offset by a concurrent anaemia. The combined haematocrit and leucocrit at presentation is usually no more than 45 per cent. Because this critical level is not exceeded unless iatrogenically increased by red blood cell transfusions, the incidence of clinical leucostasis in patients with WBC counts less than 75×10^9/l is low.

Not all patients with an elevated WBC count are at risk of leucostasis. Those with acute lymphocytic leukaemia (**ALL**) and chronic lymphocytic leukaemia (**CLL**) are less likely to be affected, as are those with CML. Those in jeopardy are patients with myeloblasts having a high proliferative rate and short cell-cycle time. These patients form thrombi in the slow-flow microcirculation, with haemorrhage and necrosis of lung and brain tissue.

In a high percentage of patients CNS damage can be prevented with the rapid institution of a continuous infusion of high-dose cytarabine. Hydroxycarbamide (hydroxyurea) (6 g/m^2) and cyclophosphamide (3 g/m^2) are also of value in rapidly reducing the WBC count (Table 1).

Tumour lysis

An indwelling, triple-lumen catheter provides access for all necessary parenteral support throughout the treatment and recovery period. Initial platelet support and subsequent prophylactic antibiotics prevent the complications of bleeding and infection at the puncture site. Measures to allay the complications of rapid tumour kill and chemotherapy toxicity include hydration and diuresis. Allopurinol offsets the metabolic consequences of hyperuricaemia, particularly in lymphoid leukaemias, and aluminium hydroxide counters the opposing phosphataemia. The addition of bicarbonate is unnecessary. Furosemide (frusemide) given every 6 h is the critical component affecting the morbidity associated with the tumour-lysis syndrome and fluid overload. Low-dose dopamine helps to maintain renal blood flow and the essential high urinary output. The toxicity of cytarabine when given by continuous infusion—namely, pulmonary vascular permeability—is prevented by rigorous control of the fluid balance. If major renal insufficiency does occur, then early dialysis effectively maintains the metabolic balance for the short at-risk period.

Disseminated intravascular coagulation (DIC)

An aggressive attack on ongoing or anticipated DIC has changed the dire prognosis of patients presenting with FAB M3, M3V, and occasionally M2 to M4 and M_5 myeloid leukaemias. Prophylactic infusion of heparin at 10 units/kg per hour in patients with M_3 and M_3V disease, together with close monitoring of changes in the prothrombin and partial thromboplastin times, fibrinogen, fibrin degradation products, and the platelet count, will prevent haemorrhage in these ultimately long-term survivors. Ongoing platelet consumption is countered with platelet infusions to maintain counts in excess of 50×10^9/l, and heparin to prevent the fibrinogen level from falling below 100 mg/ml. Some centres depend more heavily on the use of cryoprecipitate infusions.

Bleeding as a result of low-dose anticoagulation is seldom encountered; the risk of fatal haemorrhage is far greater without its use. This syndrome of DIC is driven by tumour-cell destruction, and should be monitored and treated throughout the initial days of chemotherapy. The WBC count will fall to 10 per cent of the presenting count within 72 h. The major cause of morbidity is any delay in the institution of leukaemic treatment.

Fever

At initial presentation, fever is related either to disease progression (B signs) or caused by a sensitive Gram-positive organism. Opportunistic and Gram-negative organisms and parasites are uncommon in patients with AML prior to their initial therapy. However, if a patient has been previously treated, the manifestations and organisms previously encountered must be anticipated.

Prophylactic antibiotics

If the patient is afebrile, prophylaxis is begun with an oral antiviral agent and vancomycin to prevent the first fever, most frequently caused by *Staphylococcus epidermitis* and/or *Corynebacterium* spp. This approach prohibits the use of empirical Gram-negative antibiotics for up to 5 days. The guidelines for antibiotic use at the Johns Hopkins' Oncology Center (**JHOC**) are outlined in (Table 2).

Laboratory monitoring

Laboratory data for tumour lysis, DIC, and chemotherapy-induced organ toxicity are determined daily until after tumour clearance, then twice a week.

Table 1 Management of hyperleucocytosis and tumour-lysis syndrome

All patients with leukaemia

- Institute oral allopurinol at an initial dose of 600 mg; followed by 300 mg, once a day, for 5 days
- Institute aluminium hydroxide 30 ml orally, immediately, and every 4 h for 5 days
- Hydrate with 0.45 M NaCl without bicarbonate 150 ml/h for 5 days
- Maintain urine output equal to hydration:
  - furosemide (frusemide) IV as needed and effective
  - dopamine ≤3 μg/kg per min infusion
- Monitor K^+, PO_4, Cr, SUN, blood gases, every 12 h until stable
- Monitor PT, PTT, fibrinogen, FDP every 12 h until stable
- If positive tests develop, add heparin
- Dialyse early for increasing uric acid and/or renal failure
- Maintain platelet count >20×10^9/l

Hyperleucocytosis

- Begin cell-cycle-specific antileukaemic therapy within 2 h of admission
- Transfuse RBC only when WBC <50×10^9/l, or when clinically imperative
- Maintain platelet count >50×10^9/l
- Monitor PT, PTT, fibrinogen, FDP every 12 h during drug infusion and until stable

Coagulopathy-M3, ongoing DIC

- Heparin 10 U/kg per h by continuous infusion 6 h prior to treatment or with treatment if hyperleucocytic
- Maintain platelet count >50×10^9/l
- Monitor PT, PTT, fibrinogen, FDP every 12 h during drug infusion and until stable

IV, intravenous; Cr, creatine; SUN, serum urea nitrogen; PT, prothrombin; PTT, partial thromboplastin; FDP, fibrin degradation product.

Blood products

Once the WBC count is less than 50×10^9/l the haematocrit is maintained above 24 per cent. If evidence of bleeding and platelet deficiency is present on admission, and to anticipate DIC in all patients with AML, the platelet count is maintained at 50×10^9/l until measurements are reviewed and the leukaemia stabilized.

Hyperalimentation

Nausea and vomiting associated with intensive induction therapy limits a patient's oral intake to less than 500 calories/day. Parenteral feeding provides nourishment for normal bone marrow stem-cell regrowth and decreases the mitotic activity of the villus crypt cells of the gut, thereby eliminating them as a target for DNA synthesis-dependent drugs.

Three-step treatment

The immediate goal of therapy is to alter disease progression and stabilize the biology in favour of the patient by eradicating leukaemia and restoring bone marrow homeostasis. Currently, the use of potent chemotherapeutic agents is the first-choice therapy at diagnosis. Early and aggressive therapy, in contrast to the so-called 'standard' regimens, greatly improves survival.

Reviews of large randomized studies confirm that early intensive therapy with the few available drugs used at full dose cures a growing percentage of patients with myeloid malignancies, while providing a period of meaningful survival for many others (Table 3). This approach calls for an initial aggressive reduction of a large tumour mass with cautious management of tumour and therapy-related physiological instabilities, as well as chronic biological infirmities (stroke, myocardial infarction, DU, emphysema, etc.). When followed by greater intensification in remission this two-course sequence of rapid high-dose cytotoxicity results in a 40 per cent long-term survival in definable, selected populations. The key second course eliminates leukaemia in some, or substantially reduces it to small amounts in others, resulting in measurable and anticipated stable periods prior to relapse. These subgroups of patients with predicted outcomes furnishes the model for studies of novel therapeutic agents. Once homeostasis has been re-established and the patient is in remission, further interventions with novel agents are warranted in all groups, since there is a risk of relapse in all such patients. Many varied approaches now exist, or soon will, which are non-cytotoxic innovative modalities based in new biology.

Table 2 Antibiotic guidelines

Prophylactic antibiotics at presentation	
• Norfloxacin 400 mg, orally, twice daily	Day 0 until ANC >0.5×10^9/l
• Valtrex 500 mg, orally, three-times daily	Day 0 until ANC >0.5×10^9/l
• Vancomycin 1g, IV, per day	Day 0 until first fever
Empirical	
First fever >38.3 °C	
• Piperacillin 18 g, IV, per day by continuous infusion	
• Tobramycin 5 mg/kg, IV, per day	
• If *Stenotrophomonas maltophilia* is suspected, add bactrim 5.0 mg/kg IV load then 3.3 mg/kg IV every 8 h	
Second fever (or unremitting fever of 72-h duration)	
• Add amphotericin B 0.5 mg/kg per day IV	
Third fever (or unremitting fever of 144-h duration)	
• Increase amphotericin B to 1.25 mg/kg per day	
• Flucytosine 25 mg/kg every 6 h orally	
Fever progression	
• Option 1:	Add vancomycin only if documented Gram-positive infection is only sensitive to vancomycin
• Option 2:	Discontinue piperacillin/tobramycin Start: imipenem 500 mg IV every 8 h and amikacin 8 mg/kg IV every 8 h
Laboratory	
• Surveillance cultures (throat, urine, stool) are done twice a week	
• Antibiotic coverage must treat any positive bacterial and non-*Candida albicans* surveillance cultures	

ANC, absolute neutrophil count; IV, intravenous.

Management of induction therapy—step 1

Drugs and dose

Variables predicting early failure must be taken into account when clinical instability is identified in patients presenting with leukaemia. However, since a delay in intervention is frequently not a valid option, it is important to select a dose schedule that provides stability and some therapeutic advantage based on the anticipated duration of bone marrow failure. The use of a moderately intense induction regimen (compared to the aggressive second course in remission) has reduced the clinical failure rate in successive studies. Examples of some two-step therapies are given in Table 4.

Support in remission

The interval between remission and the second course of therapy should be long enough to allow the patient to fully recover from all untoward consequences of the induction treatment. Those with FAB 1 to 5 disease usually recover without sequelae within a month, whereas those patients with FAB 6 to 7, SAML, and transformed MDS may be slower to recover. Any infections, but most importantly previous fungal infections, require treatment with appropriate antibiotics/antifungal agents prior to the patient receiving further chemotherapy: the use of amphotericin B will prevent the recurrence of fungal infections during the second course of therapy. On admission to hospital, patients should be treated with prophylactic antibiotics, since past infections in the patient will recur (Table 2).

Management of augmentation therapy—step 2

Intensive chemotherapy

Until recently it was assumed that cures could only be achieved in AML with therapy that destroyed both leukaemic and normal host bone marrow tissues. Requiring bone marrow transplanted from a suitable donor, this strategy is the ultimate aggressive single-course therapy. Although a high cure rate is apparent in those patients surviving allogeneic bone marrow transplantation, its application is limited by the age and availability of a suitable donor.

Another approach considers the infinite character of the bone marrow stem cell. With the development of four drugs effective in the treatment of AML, and the exploration of more intensive therapy, evidence accumulates that cures can be attained. Central to the success of these intensive regimens is the relative resistance of the host progenitor haemopoietic cell to tumoricidal doses of drugs. Such aggressive therapies contrast with those based on some of the principles developed in rodent lymphoid models and

Table 3 Response and long-term results achieved with intensive therapies in ***de novo*** leukaemia

Study	Year study terminated	Chemotherapy Induction	Chemotherapy Postremission	Age (years)	CR %	DFS %	Percentage survival All patients
JHOC	1988	INT TST	INT TST × 1	18–83	71	40	25
Canadian	1991	INT TST	INT × 1	15–60	90	30	–
AMLCG	1992	INT	STD + MAINT	16–83	62	33	24
ECOG	1992	STD	INT + MAINT	15–65	68	27	7
UCLA	1992	STD versus INT	INT	16–68	67	13	33
AMLEG	1992	INT	STD/MAINT	16–83	62	18	30
EORTC	1995	STD × 2	INT	16–83	62	29	24
CALGB	1995	STD × 2	INT HDAC × 4	16–86	64	21	31
			+ MAINT			25	35
SEOG	1995	STD × 2	STD + AMSA	15–50	63	38	–
CCG	1996	TST	INT TST	0–21	75	60	63
ALSG	1996	INT TST (1–3)	INT + MAINT	15–60	71	41	31
ECOG	1998	STD	INT HDAC × 1	Young	70	39	52

CR, complete remission; DFS, disease-free survival; INT, intensive; STD, standard; TST, timed sequential therapy; MAINT, maintenance; HDAC, high-dose cytarabine; AMSA, amsacrine.

extrapolated to trials in children with lymphocytic leukaemia. These regimens initially reduce the tumour bulk to levels allowing the recovery of normal haemopoiesis, but they require continued long-term treatment to suppress tumour regrowth. These approaches using low-dose drugs are generally effective for only short periods in patients with AML. Conceptual change, using intensive high-dose therapy to eradicate residual leukaemia after its initial reduction, has prompted a number of successful innovative studies that have matured sufficiently to allow comparison of the two approaches.

Patients with good-risk prognostic factors—normal genetics or balanced translocations with core-binding transcripts—are candidates for intensive non-ablative chemotherapy in remission. The data strongly support the use of a brief exposure to an intense regimen, high-dose cytarabine (**HDAC**) or timed sequential therapy (**TST**), which, with one or two courses, produce significant improvements over lesser therapies. There is no role for 'maintenance' therapy with similar cytotoxic drugs after the recovery of normal bone marrow function.

Alternately, patients with poor-risk prognostic factors (that is to say, genetic loss of a tumour suppressor) or with negative prognostic factors are candidates for bone marrow transplantation with stem-cell ablation.

Bone marrow transplantation (BMT)

The outcome, availability, and technology for BMT have all improved, and the indications for its use have increased in recent years. The number of bone marrow transplants performed annually has increased 10-fold since 1985, when essentially all transplants were allogeneic; 60 per cent are now autologous and 50 per cent use sources of stem cells other than from bone marrow.

Non-myeloablative BMT regimens are now used to produce mixed donor chimerism instead of full donor engraftment. This approach

Table 4 Chemotherapy plans

Treatment type	Drug	Dose	Timing and route of administration
Induction			
• 'Standard' 3 and 7	Cytarabine	200 mg/m^2	days 1–7, continuous infusion
	Daunorubicin	45 mg/m^2	days 8–10, IV infusion
• More intense	'AC_2–D–VP16' (TST)		
	Cytarabine	667 mg/m$_2$	days 1–3, continuous infusion
	Daunorubicin	45 mg/m^2	days 1–3, IV infusion
	Etoposide	200 mg/m^2	days 8–10, IV infusion
Augmentation (consolidation)			
• 'Standard' 3 and 7	Cytarabine	200 mg/m^2	days 1–7, continuous infusion
	Daunorubicin	45 mg/m^2	days 8–10, IV infusion
	(No role in good-risk patients)		
• Intensive TST	'AC_4–D–AC_2'		
	Cytarabine	1.33 g/m^2	days 1–3, continuous infusion
	Daunorubicin	45 mg/m^2	days 1–30, IV infusion
	Cytarabine	667 mg/m^2	days 10–12, continuous infusion
	(All patients—rigid fluid balance on days 8–14)		
• Intensive 'HDAC'	Cytarabine	1.5 g/m^2	every 12 h on days 1, 3, 5
	(Age restricted ≤60—cerebellar toxicity)		
Maintenance	Any		
	(No role in in AML in remission)		

TST, timed sequential therapy; HDAC, high-dose cytarabine.

(referred to as 'minitransplants' or 'transplant-lite') can serve as a foundation for adoptive immunotherapy with donor lymphocyte infusions against leukaemias.

T-cell depletion and intensive immunosuppression can successfully prevent graft-versus-host disease, but these approaches are associated with an increased frequency of Epstein–Barr virus-associated lymphoproliferative disease.

High-dose cytotoxic therapy followed by BMT produces high response rates, prolongation of survival, and cures in some patients. It is indicated in patients with AML who are at risk of a poor response to non-ablative intensive chemotherapy. Autologous transplantation procedures are not as successful as intensive non-ablative chemotherapy.

Limitations of two-step treatment

Currently available drugs allow the most aggressive therapy to be rationally applied, and meaningful survival achieved. These brief intensive treatments aimed at leukaemia cure include doses of active drugs given to host tolerance levels, although some patients will require bone marrow rescue. Initial tumour reduction with a less intense regimen is followed by a more aggressive tumour-ablative treatment in a medically stable patient with normal bone marrow function. In an attempt to further reduce the amount of leukaemia while preserving host recovery capability, this approach, as in the ablative therapy for BMT, produces a large tumour kill while sparing host stem cells.

However, much more needs to be done for treating patients with all subsets of leukaemia. Only 70 per cent of adults with AML achieve complete remission (**CR**) following cytotoxic therapy. Further intensive chemotherapy or BMT during a patient's early first complete remission results in a longer than 5-year disease-free survival (**DFS**) in 35 to 50 per cent of adults treated in this manner. However, 30 per cent of all newly diagnosed AMLs are primarily refractory to induction therapy, in particular those evolving from myelodysplastic syndrome (**MDS**), an antecedent haematological disorder, and those linked to environmental/occupational exposures, including the secondary AMLs. The myelodysplastic syndrome-associated AMLs occur in older adults (over 60 years of age). Current treatment approaches to these AML variants yield CR rates of 40 per cent or less (however, the CR is brief, at less than 12 months), and low cure rates even with BMT.

At present, the cure rate for all adult acute leukaemias is only between 25 and 30 per cent. New approaches are needed to improve the clinical outcome of those adult leukaemias which are refractory to current therapeutic modalities.

Elimination of senescent leukaemia—step 3

New strategies with biological agents will test current approaches in all patients with minimal residual leukaemia. These new agents will probably be most effective after two courses of intensive timed sequential therapy, which reduces the tumour mass to minimal amounts, frequently to levels only detectable using PCR or fluorescent *in situ* hybridization (**FISH**) techniques.

Therapeutic strategies (novel agents)

Genetically engineered, human biological agents having minimal host toxicity and possessing activity at multiple levels of gene function are expanding the scope of applied medicine.

Brief, two-course, tumour-reduction therapy in all patients with AML provides a biologically stable array of genetically determined subgroups with predictable cell mass. These residual cells are vulnerable to designer agents. Coupled with the immunologically intact host, novel agents with a wide therapeutic advantage could annihilate the remaining 100 cells.

Examples of possible novel genetic agents of use in the treatment of varied leukaemias with minimal residual disease are outlined in (Table 5).

The ability to detect probable subtle differences in early outcome induced by the new biological agents is critical to expanding their trials, and hence rapidly moving to alternate treatments. These methods vary with the disease syndrome. In some good-risk patients, such as those with balanced chromosomal translocations, fluctuation of hybrid proteins may reflect and quantify any modifying effects of new agents. A prime example is the signal transduction inhibitor (STI571). Designed by flow-through and configuration technologies, this selected blocker of a tyrosine kinase specific for bcr-able has demonstrated significant antitumour effect and apoptosis in patients with CML in all stages. Persistent bone marrow depression and activity of STI571 against the rare gastrointestinal stromal tumours may relate to interaction with platelet derived growth factor and C-KIT as well as abl. Less effect in CML blast crisis may relate to the second-step genetic changes in that disease, with progressive proto-oncogenes characteristic of carcinoma.

In other groups of patients, the persistence of molecular abnormalities detectable in leukaemic cells (such as *RAS* mutations), kinetic responses to recruiting agents, or maturation effects may all be of specific value, but are as yet not clinically relevant to the study design. The duration of complete remission will be a valuable tool for measuring effect, particularly in that group of patients with leukaemic syndromes mirroring one-step carcinogenesis. Those with a loss or gain of DNA are predicted for relapse within a defined period. These genetic abnormalities promote biological instability and a tumour growth advantage. When minimal residual disease after induction therapy is achieved, any effective intervention that alters the time of relapse may be transferable to the management of patients with cancer, since the genetics of these leukaemias mimic those of carcinoma. Thus, the paradigm for the leukaemic model of cure of carcinoma is in those patients

Table 5 Therapeutic strategies (according to the Johns Hopkins' Oncology Center)

Steps 1 and 2	
Cytoreduce	
TST × 2 or BMT	Minimal residual disease
or TST+ BMT	Stable clone
Step 3	
Oncogene tumours	
– Lymphoid	
Downregulate BCL2	
Upregulate BAX	
Tumour antigen recognition	
Vaccines	
– Myeloid—defined syndromes with gene translocations	
Block specific fusion proteins	
Block signal transduction	
Anticytokines	
Cytokine vaccines	
Antisense oligonucleotides	
– Myeloid—genetic cause undefined	
Specific antidote	
Farnesyltransferase inhibitors	
Apoptotics, wild p53, Rb, BAX, BCLX	
Vaccines	
Antioncogene tumours	
Maturation agents	
Cytokine inhibitors	
Stem-cell transfer	
Antisense oligonucleotides	
Cytotoxic antibodies	
Soluble receptors	
Demethylators	
Ribozymes	
Antitelomerases	
Antiangiogenesis factors	
Vaccines	

TST, timed sequential therapy; BMT, bone marrow transplantation.

with an anti-oncogene with significant tumour reduction, but an anticipated short remission. Lengthening of this duration, or cure with genetically targeted novel biologies, will be of great significance.

Further reading

Bishop JF, *et al.* (1996). A randomized study of high-dose cytarabine in induction in acute myeloid leukemia. *Blood* **87**, 1710–17.

Bloomfield CD, *et al.* (1998). Frequency of prolonged remission duration after high-dose cytarabine intensification in acute leukemia varies by cytogenetic subtype. *Cancer Research* **58**, 4173–9.

Burke PJ (1993). Leukemia and the new biology. In: Niederbeuber JE, ed. *Current therapy in oncology*, pp 575–91. Mosby, New York.

Cassileth PA, *et al.* (1998). Chemotherapy compared with autologous or allogeneic bone marrow transplantation in the management of acute myeloid leukemia in first remission. *New England Journal of Medicine* **23**, 1649–56.

Fearon ER, *et al.* (1986). Differentiation of leukemia cells to polymorphonuclear leukocytes in patients with acute nonlymphocytic leukemia. *New England Journal of Medicine* **315**, 15–24.

Geller RB, *et al.* (1989). A two-step timed sequential treatment for acute myelocytic leukemia. *Blood* **74**, 1499–506.

Jaffee EM, *et al.* (1995). Use of murine models of cytokine-secreting tumor vaccines to study feasibility and toxicity issues critical to designing clinical trials. *Journal of Immunotherapy with Emphasis on Tumor Immunology* **18**, 1–9.

Mayer R J, *et al.* (1994). Intensive postremission chemotherapy in adults with acute myeloid leukemia. *New England Journal of Medicine* **231**, 896–903.

Phillips GL, *et al.* (1991). High-dose cytarabine and daunorubicin induction and postremission chemotherapy for the treatment of acute myelogenous leukemia in adults. *Blood* **77**, 1429–35.

Woods WG, *et al.* (1996). Timed-sequential induction therapy improves postremission outcome in acute myeloid leukemia: a report from the Children's Cancer Group. *Blood* **87**, 4979–89.

22.3.5 Chronic lymphocytic leukaemia and other leukaemias of mature B and T cells

D. Catovsky

Advances in the last decade have revealed a greater recognition of the heterogeneity in leukaemias arising from immunologically mature B and T cells. These advances resulted mainly from the systematic use of monoclonal antibodies against lymphocyte differentiation antigens, greater attention to morphological detail, and a more consistent evaluation of the patterns of lymphocytic infiltration in the bone marrow, lymph nodes, and spleen. Precise diagnosis is critical because there are new treatment modalities for these disorders and the related low-grade non-Hodgkin's lymphomas.

The principal methods used for diagnosis and classification include: films of peripheral blood and bone marrow aspirates, bone marrow trephine biopsies, monoclonal antibodies against lymphocyte differentiation antigens and antibodies specific to immunoglobulin (**Ig**) heavy and light chains, histology of involved organs such as lymph nodes and spleen, and cytogenetic analysis, chiefly by means of fluorescence *in situ* hybridization (**FISH**), which allows the study of cells in interphase. DNA analysis may help to elucidate pathogenesis and demonstrate clonality in cases of uncertain diagnosis. Other investigations which may provide information are protein electrophoresis, tests for free light chains in the urine, and imaging techniques. Physical examination should include palpation of lymph nodes, liver, and spleen, and detection of any skin infiltration.

There are two broad disease categories to be considered: primary lymphoid leukaemias and leukaemia/lymphoma syndromes, which as a rule correspond to non-Hodgkin's lymphomas manifesting with peripheral blood and/or bone marrow involvement. Both groups can be subdivided, according to their cell derivation, into B- and T-cell types (Table 1).

Table 1 Disease categories in leukaemia

Primary lymphoid leukaemias
B-cell type:
Chronic lymphocytic leukaemia
B-cell prolymphocytic leukaemia
Hairy cell leukaemia and the variant form
T-cell type:
T-cell large granular lymphocyte leukaemia
T-cell prolymphocytic leukaemia
*Leukaemic phase of non-Hodgkin's lymphomas**
B-cell type:
Follicular lymphoma
Mantle cell lymphoma
Splenic marginal zone lymphoma with villous lymphocytes
Lymphoplasmacytic lymphoma
T-cell type:
Adult T-cell leukaemia/lymphoma
Sézary syndrome
Peripheral T-cell lymphoma

* With small or medium-size lymphoid cells.

Chronic lymphocytic leukaemia

This is the most common form of lymphocytic leukaemia, accounting for at least 50 per cent of cases presenting with a lymphocyte count of 5×10^9/l or higher. In Western countries chronic lymphocytic leukaemia accounts for 25 per cent of all cases of leukaemia. It is less common in the Far East, comprising 2 per cent of cases. It is estimated that 1000 new cases are diagnosed in the United Kingdom each year.

Chronic lymphocytic leukaemia affects adults over the age of 50 years, with only 5 per cent of patients aged between 30 and 50, and it is rare below the age of 30. The peak incidence is between 60 and 80 years. The male to female ratio is 2:1. This ratio is greater in younger patients and lower in older patients.

Diagnostic criteria include lymphocytosis greater than 10×10^9/l and more than 30 per cent lymphocytes in the bone marrow aspirates. With the use of membrane markers it is possible to make a diagnosis with lymphocyte counts of at least 5×10^9/l. The lymphocytes in chronic lymphocytic leukaemia have distinct morphology (Plate 1): small size, round nucleus, clumped nuclear chromatin, and scanty cytoplasm; smear cells are common. A minority of cells are larger with a prominent nucleolus and have been designated prolymphocytes. Cases with more than 10 per cent prolymphocytes have a progressive clinical course, a higher proliferation rate than stable cases, and a correspondingly shorter lymphocyte doubling time. This variant form of chronic lymphocytic leukaemia has been described as chronic lymphocytic leukaemia/prolymphocytic.

Clinical features

Almost one-third of patients are diagnosed by chance with lymphocytosis and no specific symptoms or physical signs. Others present with lymphadenopathy or symptoms of anaemia. The lymphadenopathy is usually symmetrical and of moderate size, involving the neck, axillas, and inguinal regions. Other nodal areas can be ascertained by chest radiography and abdominal CT scan. Splenomegaly of variable size is found in 50 per cent of cases; hepatomegaly is less common and more difficult to document as being of clinical relevance.

Systemic symptoms such as weight loss or night sweating are not common but, when present, they correlate with bulky abdominal disease. Fever in chronic lymphocytic leukaemia usually indicates infection, but if the latter is excluded it may suggest transformation (see below).

Membrane markers

Chronic lymphocytic leukaemia lymphocytes are clonal B cells with weak kappa or lambda light-chain expression (**SmIg**) in the membrane. The immunophenotype of chronic lymphocytic leukaemia is unique within the B-cell disorders: CD5 and CD23 positive, FMC7 negative, and weak or negative expression of CD22 and CD79b. These markers, including the weak SmIg expression, represent the typical immunophenotype of chronic lymphocytic leukaemia. In a majority of cases (about 90 per cent) chronic lymphocytic leukaemia lymphocytes will show the expected findings with four or five of the above reagents. The most consistent markers are CD5 and CD23, positive in 92 and 94 per cent of cases, respectively. This contrasts with observations in other B-cell leukaemias and non-Hodgkin's lymphoma in leukaemic phase (Table 2). Chronic lymphocytic leukaemia/prolymphocytic has the same membrane markers as typical chronic lymphocytic leukaemia although in 20 to 30 per cent of cases it departs from the expected phenotype by expressing strong SmIg or CD79b or FMC7. As CD5 is a marker of both B and T cells, it may be necessary to establish in cases with a low white blood cell count that another B-cell antigen, such as CD19, is coexpressed in the CD5+ lymphocytes by simultaneous double labelling.

The expression of CD38 on chronic lymphocytic leukaemia lymphocytes seems to provide a strong new marker of prognosis. To be accurate, the assessment of CD38 needs to be done simultaneously with CD5 and CD19 to identify chronic lymphocytic leukaemia cells. CD38 appears also to be a surrogate marker for two forms of chronic lymphocytic leukaemia: (i) a benign one, CD38 negative, which arises from post-follicular (memory) B cells as shown by somatic mutations of the IgVH genes; and (ii) a more active and progressive form of chronic lymphocytic leukaemia, CD38 positive, which usually requires treatment and is associated with unmutated IgVH genes (naive B cells). The proportion of cases with one or other form of chronic lymphocytic leukaemia appears to be similar.

Bone marrow findings

A bone marrow trephine biopsy should always be performed in chronic lymphocytic leukaemia to complement the clinical staging (see below), to exclude other B-cell leukaemias and non-Hodgkin's lymphoma, and as a baseline to assess disease progression and/or response to therapy. Immunohistochemistry with CD20 and CD79a is useful to highlight the areas of leukaemic infiltration.

Table 2 Membrane immunophenotype in leukaemias of mature B cells[a]

Marker	CLL	CLL score[b]	B-PLL	HCL	NHL[c]
SmIg	Weak	1	Strong	Strong	Strong
CD22/CD79b	Weak	1	Strong	Strong	Strong
CD5	+	1	–/+	–	–/+
CD23	+	1	–	–	–
FMC7	–	1	+	+	+

[a] The B-cell antigens CD19 and CD20 are positive in all cases; CD20 expression in chronic lymphocytic leukaemia is weaker than in the other disorders.

[b] Chronic lymphocytic leukaemia cases score 4 or 5; all other B-cell leukaemias score 0, 1, or 2.

[c] Follicular, mantle cell, and splenic marginal zone lymphoma as tested in peripheral blood lymphocytes. Mantle cell lymphoma is, as a rule, CD5+/CD23– and scores 2 or 3.

B-PLL, B-cell prolymphocytic leukaemia; CLL, chronic lymphocytic leukaemia; HCL, hairy cell leukaemia; NHL, non-Hodgkin's lymphoma.

The patterns of bone marrow infiltration in chronic lymphocytic leukaemia are variable and correlate with clinical stages. Early chronic lymphocytic leukaemia shows minimal interstitial or nodular involvement; with disease progression the normal bone marrow fat spaces are gradually replaced by lymphocytes. There is a mixed interstitial and nodular pattern and in advanced disease, the involvement is diffuse or 'packed'. The latter correlates with the presence of anaemia and/or thrombocytopenia. A paratrabecular pattern characteristic of non-Hodgkin's lymphoma, follicular lymphoma in particular, is not seen in chronic lymphocytic leukaemia. A nodular pattern, on the other hand, is common in lymphoplasmacytic, mantle cell, and splenic lymphoma with villous lymphocytes.

Bone marrow aspirates are necessary to confirm lymphocyte morphology and to evaluate infiltration. A minimum of 30 per cent lymphocytes is required for a diagnosis of chronic lymphocytic leukaemia, but this needs to be confirmed by cell marker studies.

Examination of the bone marrow is important in chronic lymphocytic leukaemia for three reasons: (i) to assess the degree of infiltration, which is an independent prognostic factor; (ii) to establish the possible mechanism of anaemia or thrombocytopenia by assessing the normal haemopoietic reserves; and (iii) to distinguish chronic lymphocytic leukaemia from cases of low-grade non-Hodgkin's lymphoma by the pattern of involvement in trephine biopsy sections. In patients with cytopenias and a large spleen, assessment of the bone marrow is critical to decide whether splenectomy may be beneficial.

Staging

The course of chronic lymphocytic leukaemia is very variable. Some patients may never require treatment and others have a progressive course with short survival. A major advance in the management of chronic lymphocytic leukaemia was the development of staging systems which can predict prognosis. The first system, used in the United States, was described by Rai *et al.* (1975). A new, simplified proposal by Binet *et al.* (1981) was subsequently adopted by the International Workshop on Chronic Lymphocytic Leukaemia (1981) whilst retaining some aspects of Rai's staging.

Both systems use simple information: blood counts and physical signs, namely lymphadenopathy and hepatosplenomegaly. Findings by imaging techniques are not taken into account for staging but are useful for assessing accurately disease bulk and measuring response to treatment.

Binet's system is currently used in chronic lymphocytic leukaemia trials in the United Kingdom. Stages A and B have no anaemia (haemoglobin, **Hb** > 10 g/dl) or thrombocytopenia (platelets > 100×10^9/l) and have a different degree of organ enlargement. Patients with stage A disease have either no palpable nodes (including liver and spleen as nodal areas) or have one or two involved areas. Patients with stage B disease have three, four, or all five nodal areas involved, which include nodes in cervical, axillary, and inguinal regions, spleen, and liver. Patients with stage C disease have anaemia (Hb < 10 g/dl) and/or thrombocytopenia (platelets < 100×10^9/l) and correspond to stages III and IV of the Rai system. The relative distribution of stages at presentation in chronic lymphocytic leukaemia is as follows: stage A, 45 to 50 per cent; stage B, 25 to 30 per cent; and stage C, 20 to 25 per cent. The proportion of patients in stages A, B, and C varies between the sexes. More women are likely to present with stage A and more men with stages B and C. Stage A is also more common over the age of 70 years in both sexes. Stage is the single most important prognostic factor of the disease (see below).

Attempts have been made to identify, within the large stage A group, further prognostic substages. One is to retain Rai stage 0 (lymphocytosis with no physical signs) as stage A(0). The other, proposed by the French Cooperative Group on Chronic Lymphocytic Leukaemia (1990), is to separate stage A into patients with (i) haemoglobin greater than 12 g/dl and a lymphocyte count less than 30×10^9/l (stage A′) or (ii) haemoglobin less than 12 g/dl and a lymphocyte count greater than 30×10^9/l (stage A″). The 5-year survival of the first group was 87 per cent and of the latter 60 per cent. This difference was confirmed in the analysis of the United Kingdom Medical Research Council (**MRC**) Chronic Lymphocytic Leukaemia 3A study, which also confirmed the survival advantage of patients with stage A disease with lymphocyte doubling times greater than 12 months.

Chromosome abnormalities

Progress in this area has resulted from the routine use of fluorescence *in situ* hybridization (FISH), which helps detect the abnormalities in chronic lymphocytic leukaemia with a higher frequency (80 per cent of cases) than conventional cytogenetic methods (30 per cent). The most common abnormality is the interstitial deletion of 13q14 (50 to 60 per cent of cases), followed by trisomy 12 (20 per cent), 11q23 deletion (20 per cent), 17p13 (p53 locus) deletion (10 per cent), and 6q21 deletion (5 per cent of cases). Chromosome translocations have been described in chronic lymphocytic leukaemia but with low frequency. None of the above abnormalities are unique to chronic lymphocytic leukaemia as they may also be seen in other low-grade non-Hodgkin's lymphomas. On the other hand, translocations seen in non-Hodgkin's lymphomas such as t(11;14)(q13;q32), a feature of mantle cell lymphoma, and t(14;18)(q32;q21) are not a feature of chronic lymphocytic leukaemia.

Some of the changes detected by FISH in chronic lymphocytic leukaemia have been associated with distinct disease characteristics, namely: trisomy 12 with high proliferative rate and increased number of prolymphocytes; p53 deletion, which correlates with p53 overexpression and gene mutation, is associated with chronic lymphocytic leukaemia/prolymphocytic and poor response to therapy; 11q23 with younger age, massive lymphadenopathy, and poor prognosis; and 6q21 with high lymphocyte counts and bulky disease. It is likely that most of the abnormalities described in chronic lymphocytic leukaemia are relatively late events in the evolution of the disease. The nature of the early genetic event triggering naive (unmutated IgVH genes) or memory (mutated IgVH genes) B cells to become neoplastic is unknown.

Prognostic factors

The main features of poor prognosis in chronic lymphocytic leukaemia are listed in Table 3. The most important one for predicting survival is clinical stage, assessed by either the Binet or Rai systems, followed by age, sex, and response to therapy. The median survival of patients with stage A disease is more than 10 years, with stage B disease it is 6 years, and stage C disease 4 to 5 years.

For patients with stage A disease, both the French substaging (A′, A″) and the lymphocyte doubling time are important independent prognostic variables (see above). A period of close observation with blood counts every 2 or 3 months for the first year is recommended in newly diagnosed patients with stage A disease in order to assess the pace of the disease and calculate the lymphocyte doubling time. The degree of bone marrow infiltration is also an independent prognostic variable, particularly in patients with stage B disease. A packed bone marrow pattern is associated with worse prognosis. In contrast to the anaemia caused by bone marrow infiltration, autoimmune haemolytic anaemia is not necessarily considered to indicate poor prognosis. Because chronic lymphocytic leukaemia affects elderly people, it is essential to investigate thoroughly other causes of anaemia and exclude, as not related to chronic lymphocytic leukaemia, those caused by iron, folate, or vitamin B_{12} deficiency, before deciding that the patient has stage C disease and requires chemotherapy.

The prospective value of new prognostic factors such as CD38 expression, IgVH mutations, and cytogenetic changes as detected by FISH analysis is still being evaluated. However, they are likely to define or to be associated with distinct clinical behaviour and to explain in large part the contrasting evolution of chronic lymphocytic leukaemia seen in patients.

Table 3 Features of poor prognosis in chronic lymphocytic leukaemia

Advanced clinical stage[a]
Age (> 70 years); Sex (male)
No response to therapy
Lymphocyte count > 30 × 10^9/l and Hb <12 g/l (substage A')
Lymphocyte doubling time (< 12 months)
Diffuse bone marrow histology[b]
More than 10 per cent prolymphocytes (CLL/PL)
Membrane antigens: CD38+, FMC7+ (for stage A)
Chromosome abnormalities by FISH analysis:
11q23 deletion, trisomy 12, p53 deletion

[a] Rai III–IV or Binet C staging consider haemoglobin (Hb) < 10 g/l and platelets < 100 × 10^9/l as advanced; Binet stage B includes patients with three or more nodal disease sites.

[b] Or packed bone marrow, worse than the other patterns (interstitial, nodular, and mixed).

CLL/PL, chronic lymphocytic leukaemia/prolymphocytic.

Complications

Infections, particularly of the upper respiratory tract, are the main cause of morbidity in chronic lymphocytic leukaemia. Pneumonia is the main cause of death in 30 per cent of cases, usually in patients with advanced disease. The major predisposing factor for infections is hypogammaglobulinaemia.

Autoimmune phenomena, commonly haemolytic anaemia with a positive direct antiglobulin test due to warm autoantibodies, is a feature in 5 to 7 per cent of cases at presentation. However, the proportion of cases with a positive Coombs' test is higher than the number with frank haemolysis. Not infrequently, the haemolytic anaemia is precipitated by the initiation of therapy, particularly the nucleoside analogue fludarabine, which causes a drop in CD4+ T cells, or following a viral illness. Immune thrombocytopenia is seen in 2 per cent of cases.

Other malignancies are not uncommon in chronic lymphocytic leukaemia and it is not clear whether this relatively high incidence correlates with age or with a greater predisposition of the disease itself or its associated immunodeficiency. Up to 30 per cent of patients may die of causes unrelated to chronic lymphocytic leukaemia and in half of them the cause is another cancer. In patients with early chronic lymphocytic leukaemia (stage A), half of the causes of death are not due to the disease itself and are often age related, such as cardiovascular events. In contrast, in advanced stages (stages B and C) 80 to 90 per cent of deaths are a direct consequence of chronic lymphocytic leukaemia and its complications.

Treatment

Because of the variable outlook of patients, which relates to stage and other disease features, it is important to consider the treatment separately for patients with early and stable disease and for those with progressive, symptomatic, and/or advanced disease. For this purpose staging is the first criterion to take into account.

The majority of patients with stage A disease have no symptoms and may be observed for a while to determine, by the lymphocyte doubling time or other features, whether the disease has a stable pattern, before deciding whether treatment is necessary. A number of randomized trials have considered whether patients having stage A disease should be treated early with chlorambucil, with or without prednisolone, and these have been summarized in an overview (Chronic Lymphocytic Leukaemia trialists, 1999) which showed conclusively that patients treated early did not fare better and, if anything, show a trend towards shorter survival.

Treatment is indicated for patients with stage B and C disease or stage A with evidence of progression. Disease progression is defined as a downward trend in haemoglobin or platelets, rising lymphocyte counts, development of lymphadenopathy, and systemic symptoms, among other parameters. Most of the treatments listed in Table 4 have been, or still are, subject to clinical trials. It is accepted that the addition of prednisolone to an alkylating agent, chlorambucil or cyclophosphamide as in **COP** (cyclophosphamide/oncovin/prednisolone) does not confer a survival advantage. There is good evidence, on the other hand, that the use of prednisolone alone for the first 4 weeks in patients who present with stage C disease facilitates the

Table 4 Treatment modalities used in chronic lymphocytic leukaemia

Alkylating agents	
	Chlorambucil intermittently (10 mg/m^2.day × 7 days, monthly) or continuously (5–10 mg/day)
Combinations	
	COP: cyclophosphamide, oncovin, prednisolone (5-day monthly courses)
	Chlorambucil plus epirubicin(chlorambucil intermittently as above; epirubicin: 60 mg/m^2 day 1; both monthly)
	CHOP: COP plus doxorubicin(doxorubicin: 50 mg/m^2 intravenously day 1, or 25 mg/m^2 'mini' CHOP; monthly)
Corticosteroids	
	Prednisolone: 30 mg/m^2 for 3 weeks plus 1 week tailing off for initial treatment of patients with stage C disease
	High-dose methylprednisolone intravenously (or oral) at 1 g/m^2 (5-day monthly courses)
Nucleoside analogues	
	Fludarabine: intravenous push at 25 mg/m^2 daily or oral daily at 40 mg/m^2 (5-day monthly courses; usually six)
	Fludarabine (25 mg/m^2) plus cyclophosphamide (250 mg/m^2) intravenous push (3-day monthly courses)
	Pentostatin intravenous push 4 mg/m^2 (once a week or every 2 weeks)
	Cladribine intravenous infusion (0.1 or 0.15 mg/kg.day × 5 days every 4 weeks)

subsequent introduction of other drugs and corrects more rapidly the cytopenias. One needs to be aware that the use of corticosteroids results in a significant rise in the lymphocyte count whilst lymph nodes and spleen are reducing in size.

The role of anthracyclines, as in the combination **CHOP** (cyclophosphamide/oncovin/ prednisolone/doxorubicin) or by adding epirubicin to chlorambucil (Table 4), has been tested in several trials, including recently MRC CLL 3, but no survival advantage has been shown in a large meta-analysis of randomized trials. Although the response rates are slightly higher with anthracycline-containing combinations in previously untreated patients, for example 80 per cent for partial plus complete remissions, against 70 per cent with chlorambucil or COP, this has not translated into a survival advantage. The 5-year survival in the MRC CLL 3 trial was 44 per cent with chlorambucil and 45 per cent with chlorambucil plus epirubicin.

One of the difficulties in assessing survival as the only end point in clinical trials of chronic lymphocytic leukaemia is that patients who do not respond to a first-line therapy may respond to another and whenever there is a response (partial or complete) the outlook improves. Only patients who do not respond to any modality, such as those with p53 deletion/mutation or 11q23 deletion, fare really badly with respect to survival.

A new generation of drugs, the nucleoside analogues (Table 4), have shown promise for the treatment of chronic lymphocytic leukaemia and other low-grade lymphoid malignancies. The agent with greater activity in chronic lymphocytic leukaemia is fludarabine. The encouraging findings with fludarabine result from higher complete remission rates, for example 33 per cent in previously untreated patients, which compares favourably with the 15 per cent rate of complete remission that is observed with other agents. Furthermore, there is no evidence for cross-resistance between fludarabine and chlorambucil or anthracyclines. This makes fludarabine the agent of choice for second-line therapy in chronic lymphocytic leukaemia. It is not yet clear whether using fludarabine as first-line treatment provides any survival advantage.

Trials carried out in previously untreated patients by American and French co-operative groups have shown a higher rate of complete remission with fludarabine over chlorambucil or the combination CHOP and a prolonged disease-free interval, but no survival advantage. The reason for the latter, as stated above, may be that crossover design allowed good responses to fludarabine in the non-responders to chlorambucil or CHOP.

Data from the MD Anderson group in Texas suggest that fludarabine inhibits DNA and RNA synthesis as well as DNA repair, thus being potentially beneficial in combination with DNA-damaging agents. The combination of fludarabine with cyclophosphamide is currently being tested as first-line therapy in the Chronic Lymphocytic Leukaemia 4 trial in the United Kingdom. The potential benefit of the monoclonal antibodies, anti-CD20 and CD52 (Table 4), is currently being explored in chronic lymphocytic leukaemia with promising results. High-dose methylprednisolone is an effective salvage therapy for highly resistant patients, including those with p53 abnormalities. Although complete remissions are rare, partial responses, including some reverting to a bone marrow nodular pattern, have been observed. We have used high-dose methylprednisolone alone or in combination with other agents, such as vinca alkaloids, depending on results of an *in vitro* cytotoxicity assay (Bosanquet *et al.* 1999).

Stem cell transplantation

Efforts to improve treatment results in younger individuals with chronic lymphocytic leukaemia led to protocols using allogeneic and autologous stem cell transplantation. Allogeneic transplants may be curative in a minority, but this procedure is limited to those with an HLA-identical donor and has been associated in chronic lymphocytic leukaemia with a high (about 35 per cent) treatment-related mortality. To improve treatment-related mortality, less intensive conditioning regimens ('mini' transplants) have been devised in an attempt to exploit the host versus leukaemia effect. Currently, the use of the patient's own stem cells harvested after a good remission has been achieved is the preferred method of transplant for chronic lymphocytic leukaemia. The treatment-related mortality of autografts worldwide is less than 10 per cent and is more likely to be less than 5 per cent with improvements in supportive care and the ability to mobilize peripheral stem cells using haemopoietic growth factors such as granulocyte colony-stimulating factor (**G-CSF**). Due to its low toxicity, the 3- to 5-year survival after autografts is in the order of 75 to 80 per cent. However, the event-free survival is shorter due to 40 per cent relapses in the first 3 years. Thus, autologous transplants seem to increase survival in chronic lymphocytic leukaemia but may not be considered a curative procedure. The MRC Chronic Lymphocytic Leukaemia Working Group has conducted a pilot study since 1996 in which 102 patients have been entered so far. Remissions were induced with fludarabine and stem cells were harvested after cyclophosphamide priming followed by G-CSF. A harvest was not possible in a minority (about 15 per cent). The projected 5-year survival of the 50 patients who received transplants is 80 per cent, with a high proportion of bone marrow samples after autograft showing no sign of chronic lymphocytic leukaemia by polymerase chain reaction (PCR) for IgH gene rearrangement. A European randomized trial is planned, to assess further the value of autografts in younger patients with chronic lymphocytic leukaemia.

Splenectomy in chronic lymphocytic leukaemia

There are three indications for splenectomy in chronic lymphocytic leukaemia. First, for therapy-resistant disease with significant residual splenomegaly. Second, in patients with evidence of hypersplenism, that is cytopenia(s) and active bone marrow haemopoiesis. Third, for autoimmune complications, haemolytic anaemia, or thrombocytopenia that do not respond to therapy with corticosteroids and immunosuppressive drugs. In our experience, splenectomy is always beneficial in any of the above indications. In patients in whom the spleen is the dominant organ, with little or no lymphadenopathy, splenectomy could revert the clinical staging from C to A with the corresponding improvement in survival.

Because of the poor humoral immunity in chronic lymphocytic leukaemia, the prophylaxis after splenectomy should rely on oral penicillin as well as on antipneumococcal vaccines. The latter should also be used in all patients with chronic lymphocytic leukaemia.

Supportive care

The recurrent infections in patients with chronic lymphocytic leukaemia, particularly with advanced disease, makes supportive care an important component of management. This includes long-term antibiotics and their availability as soon as signs or symptoms of infections appear, and intravenous gammaglobulin replacement therapy to prevent serious upper respiratory tract infections in selected patients. Co-trimoxazole should be used in all patients treated with fludarabine or other nucleoside analogues that cause lymphopenia. Blood products should always be irradiated after fludarabine. Annual influenza vaccinations are strongly recommended. Other measures include blood transfusions and vitamin supplements such as folic acid to correct deficiencies. Anaemia in chronic lymphocytic leukaemia should always be thoroughly investigated and it should not be assumed that it is caused by bone marrow infiltration. The treatment of autoimmune complications includes corticosteroids, splenectomy, danazol, azathioprine, cyclophosphamide, and cyclosporin A.

Transformation

There are two forms of transformation in chronic lymphocytic leukaemia: a subtle one with increased proportion (usually more than 10 per cent) of prolymphocytes, known as chronic lymphocytic leukaemia/prolymphocytic, and a more dramatic change to a high-grade non-Hodgkin's lymphoma with diffuse large B-cell/immunoblastic histology, known as Richter's syndrome. Chronic lymphocytic leukaemia/prolymphocytic may be seen in 10 per cent of patients and Richter's syndrome in at least 5 per cent. The former has a progressive course and is associated with trisomy 12 and p53 abnormalities in about 50 per cent of cases. The immunophenotype of chronic lymphocytic leukaemia/prolymphocytic is identical to typical chronic lymphocytic leukaemia with occasional cases scoring 3 instead of the usual 4 or 5. Chronic lymphocytic leukaemia/prolymphocytic should not be confused with B-cell prolymphocytic leukaemia (see below), which is a distinct entity and in which the immunophenotype usually scores less than 2 (Table 2).

The large cell transformation may be localized or generalized; very rarely, it may resemble an acute leukaemia with circulating large blasts. Richter's syndrome is associated with deteriorating clinical status and the systemic symptoms of fever, weight loss, and sweating, particularly when large para-aortic nodes are involved. Systemic symptoms or rapidly enlarging asymmetric nodes should always raise the question of transformation and be properly documented. Hypercalcaemia, a rare feature of chronic lymphocytic leukaemia, has been documented in patients developing Richter's syndrome.

One question which has generated interest is whether Richter's transformation represents a new malignancy or a new change within the chronic lymphocytic leukaemia B-cell clone. Studies with anti-light-chain antibodies and DNA analysis with probes for heavy- and light-chain genes seem to indicate that in 50 per cent of cases the transformation occurs within the pre-existing chronic lymphocytic leukaemia cells; in the rest it represents a new B-cell clone. In cases arising from a separate clone, it has been suggested that the new malignancy may be mediated by the Epstein–Barr virus (**EBV**) as shown by the expression of the EBV latent membrane protein (LMP-1) and EBV mRNA in tissue sections. Severe immunosuppression, usually through CD4 lymphopenia such as caused by fludarabine, may be involved in the development of the new malignancy, which, in the strict sense, is not truly a transformation event. Cases which histologically resemble Hodgkin's disease have been documented with an incidence of 0.5 per cent. These may also relate to treatment with nucleoside analogues.

Richter's syndrome has been associated with poor prognosis with a median survival of less than 6 months following presentation. Alkylating agents are no longer effective at this stage and neither is fludarabine. Combinations of the type used in high-grade non-Hodgkin's lymphoma, such as CHOP, may induce remissions in some patients. If complete remission is obtained, the outlook may be favourable. Patients with localized transformation seem to respond better than those with generalized lymphadenopathy.

B-cell prolymphocytic leukaemia

B-cell prolymphocytic leukaemia was originally described by Galton in 1974 as a variant form of chronic lymphocytic leukaemia but is now recognized as a distinct clinicopathological entity. The main disease features are splenomegaly without peripheral lymphadenopathy, anaemia, and thrombocytopenia and a high white blood cell count, usually over 100×10^9/l. The diagnosis is made by examination of peripheral blood films in which the predominant cells are prolymphocytes (Plate 2); small lymphocytes, as in chronic lymphocytic leukaemia, are rarely seen. B-cell prolymphocytic leukaemia is rare, representing 1 per cent of cases of lymphocytic leukaemia. Most patients are over the age of 60, with a median age of 70 years.

The immunophenotype of B-cell prolymphocytic leukaemia (Table 2) is different from that of chronic lymphocytic leukaemia: most cases express strongly SmIg, FMC7, CD22, and CD79b; two-thirds of cases are CD5 negative and CD23 is also often negative. The differential diagnosis should be considered with chronic lymphocytic leukaemia/prolymphocytic, mantle cell non-Hodgkin's lymphoma, and a rare variant form of hairy cell leukaemia. In chronic lymphocytic leukaemia/prolymphocytic the proportion of prolymphocytes is less than 50 per cent, there are many small lymphocytes in the blood films, and the immunophenotype is similar to that of chronic lymphocytic leukaemia. The circulating cells in the leukaemic phase of mantle cell lymphoma have a pleomorphic appearance, the nucleolus is not prominent, and they often have stippled nuclear chromatin and an indented nuclear outline. The membrane phenotype may be similar to B-cell prolymphocytic leukaemia except for CD5 which is positive in most cases. The cells in variant hairy cell leukaemia have a prominent nucleolus resembling prolymphocytes but their cytoplasm is abundant and has distinct 'hairy' projections. Their immunological profile may be similar to that of B-cell prolymphocytic leukaemia.

Many cases of B-cell prolymphocytic leukaemia have been reported with break points at chromosome 14q32 including the translocation t(11;14)(q13;q32) in 20 per cent. Such cases need to be distinguished from blastoid forms of mantle cell lymphoma presenting with leukaemia, but this may not be easy; cases with t(11;14) in both conditions overexpress cyclin D1. Abnormalities of the p53 gene (loss of heterozygosity, overexpression, and mutations) have been reported in more than 50 per cent of cases of B-cell prolymphocytic leukaemia, the highest incidence reported in lymphoid malignancies. Deletions at 11q23 and 13q14 have also been shown by FISH.

Treatment and prognosis

In contrast to chronic lymphocytic leukaemia, the evolution of B-cell prolymphocytic leukaemia is always progressive with a median survival of 3 to 4 years. Several treatment modalities have been used with moderate success: splenic irradiation, the combination CHOP, and splenectomy. Recently the nucleoside analogues fludarabine and cladribine have been shown to induce remissions in 50 per cent of patients. Chlorambucil and other alkylating agents are largely ineffective. The high incidence of p53 abnormalities may underlie the resistance of B-cell prolymphocytic leukaemia to chemotherapy.

Hairy cell leukaemia

Hairy cell leukaemia is a rare disorder comprising 2 per cent of lymphoid leukaemias characterized by pancytopenia and splenomegaly in two-thirds of cases; monocytopenia is a consistent finding. Most patients have circulating hairy cells but leucocyte counts rarely exceed 10×10^9/l. Hairy cells are larger than lymphocytes, their nuclei show a homogeneous loose chromatin pattern without a visible nucleolus (except in variant hairy cell leukaemia) and have an abundant cytoplasm with broad-based projections or villi. The nuclear outline is often kidney shaped.

The bone marrow trephine biopsy is the main diagnostic test and shows a unique pattern of infiltration with characteristic clear zones in between the cells. This infiltration is usually interstitial but may be also be focal. Bone marrow aspirates are, as a rule, unsuccessful (dry tap) due to the heavy deposition of reticulin fibres.

Hairy cells are B cells positive with CD19, CD20, and SmIg with light-chain restriction. When tested with the five markers listed in Table 2, the immunophenotype is different from chronic lymphocytic leukaemia but similar to other B-cell disorders. Four other monoclonal antibodies, CD103, CD11c, CD25, and HC2, which have shown specificity for hairy cells, are positive in most cases. Cases of variant hairy cell leukaemia have high white blood cell counts and no monocytopenia. Histologically they resemble typical hairy cell leukaemia. The cells are CD11c+, CD103+ (in 50 per cent of cases), but always HC2 and CD25 negative.

A cytochemical property of hairy cells is the presence of tartaric acid-resistant acid phosphatase, which is still used for diagnosis. In paraffin-embedded sections of bone marrow, hairy cells are positive with the monoclonal antibodies CD20 and DBA44. These reagents can help monitor residual disease after treatment as recognition of clusters of hairy cells in histological sections may be difficult.

Treatment and prognosis

The prognosis of patients with hairy cell leukaemia has improved dramatically with the advent of three treatment modalities: interferon-α, pentostatin, and cladribine. Splenectomy is reserved for patients presenting with very large spleens that are disproportionate to the degree of bone marrow involvement. Interferon-α improves the blood counts and the bone marrow but does not induce prolonged remissions when treatment is discontinued. Pentostatin induces complete remissions in 85 to 90 per cent of patients with few (less than 5 per cent) non-responders. Once treatment is discontinued the majority of responders remain in remission for more than 5 years; 40 to 50 per cent of patients are still in remission after 10 years. The response to these agents in variant hairy cell leukaemia is usually poor and the survival significantly shorter than in the typical form.

Transformation

A subtle transformation takes place in patients with hairy cell leukaemia in the form of massive abdominal lymphadenopathy with few systemic symptoms. The overall incidence of abdominal nodes in hairy cell leukaemia is about 25 per cent and is documented by performing routine CT scan investigations. The proportion with lymphadenopathy is higher in patients who relapse after previously successful treatments and/or who had long-standing disease. Abdominal lymphadenopathy may be associated with resistance to further therapy and with the presence of large hairy cells in both the bone marrow and the enlarged lymph nodes, supporting the concept of transformation suggested by clinical findings.

B-cell lymphomas in leukaemic phase

Several types of low- or intermediate-grade non-Hodgkin's lymphoma of B-cell type present or evolve with a leukaemic blood picture, for example more than 5×10^9/l circulating lymphoid cells (Table 1). The types of non-Hodgkin's lymphoma that most commonly develop a leukaemic phase are follicular lymphoma (Plate 4), mantle cell lymphoma (Plate 3), and splenic marginal zone lymphoma with villous lymphocytes (**SLVL**) (Plate 5). The main differential diagnosis is with chronic lymphocytic leukaemia, other non-Hodgkin's lymphoma, and in the case of SLVL, with hairy cell leukaemia.

The circulating cells in follicular lymphoma are small, have no visible cytoplasm, the nuclear chromatin has a smooth pattern and shows regularly deep nuclear clefts or indentations and an angular or irregular nuclear shape. Leukaemia in follicular lymphoma is associated with widespread disease, such as hepatosplenomegaly and lymphadenopathy. The membrane phenotype is different from chronic lymphocytic leukaemia (Table 2) and the cells often express CD10. Lymph node biopsy is essential for a definitive diagnosis. Cytogenetic analysis will show the translocation t(14;18)(q32;q21) and rearrangement of the BCL-2 gene by molecular techniques. Cases with leukaemia tend to run a more aggressive course and require a more intensive treatment approach than those without leukaemia.

SLVL is a distinct low-grade non-Hodgkin's lymphoma characterized by splenomegaly, moderate lymphocytosis (10 to 30×10^9/l), a small monoclonal band, and/or free light chains in the urine in 50 per cent of cases. The circulating lymphocytes have a small nucleolus and a cytoplasm with conspicuous villous projections that are often seen polarized in one end of the cell (Plate 5). A minority of cells show plasma cell differentiation. The bone marrow is minimally involved early in the disease and the biopsies show a nodular pattern and intrasinusoidal infiltration highlighted in trephine biopsies by CD20 staining. The immunophenotype of SLVL cells can be distinguished from that of chronic lymphocytic leukaemia (Table 2) and hairy cell leukaemia, both diseases with which it can be confused. SLVL lymphocytes do not express HC2 and CD25 as typical hairy cells. The distinction with variant hairy cell leukaemia is difficult unless there is tissue histology.

Splenectomy is a useful treatment modality for SLVL and fludarabine has recently been shown to induce complete remissions. The spleen histology shows predominant white pulp involvement with a prominent marginal zone, which contrasts with the predominantly red pulp infiltration pattern in typical and variant hairy cell leukaemia. Most cases have somatic mutations of the IgVH genes, suggesting a disease derivation from late B cells. Chromosome abnormalities are not consistent but chromosome 7q21–32 deletion has been found in 40 per cent of cases with abnormalities of the CDK6 gene at 7q21. Trisomy 3, a feature of marginal zone lymphoma of MALT type, has been found in 17 per cent of SLVL cases. The disease course is indolent. Transformation to a high-grade diffuse large B-cell lymphoma has been observed in 5 per cent of cases.

Leukaemia is common in mantle cell lymphoma presenting with splenomegaly and lymphocytosis. The circulating cells in mantle cell lymphoma (Plate 3) are of medium to large size with an irregular nuclear outline. The bone marrow biopsy shows nodular or paratrabecular involvement (Plate 6). In addition to histology, mantle cell lymphoma is characterized by the translocation t(11;14)(q13;q32) in 80 per cent of cases, involving the BCL-1/PRAD-1 gene at 11q13. This chromosome translocation, which can be shown in interphase cells by FISH, results in the overexpression of cyclin D1 in the nucleus, which can be demonstrated by immunohistochemistry in tissue sections and by flow cytometry in cell suspensions.

Large granular lymphocytic leukaemia

Most cases with persistent T-cell lymphocytosis greater than 2×10^9/l lasting for more than 6 months without an identifiable cause are likely to represent clonal proliferations of large granular lymphocytes. Clonality can be demonstrated by the rearrangement of T-cell receptor genes and sometimes, also, by chromosome translocations, which are not consistent in every case. Large granular lymphocytes have abundant cytoplasm with prominent azurophil granules and an excentric nucleus without a visible nucleolus. Half of the patients have splenomegaly without lymphadenopathy and are neutropenic or, less frequently, suffer from other cytopenias, in particular red cell hypoplasia. Rheumatoid arthritis and the presence of autoantibodies are a feature of 25 to 30 per cent of cases. The membrane phenotype shows mature T cells which are CD4–, CD8+ and, characteristically, express one or more antigens associated with natural killer cells, such as CD11b, CD16, CD56, and CD57. Bone marrow involvement is variable but is usually present in true large granular lymphocyte leukaemia. The spleen involvement is in the red pulp with reactive normal follicles (white pulp) and frequent granuloma formation. The bone marrow involvement is variable, often with an interstitial pattern, but representing less than 50 per cent of the bone marrow cells. Although many patients do not require active treatment, a significant number (about 60 per cent) present a therapeutic problem related to the associated cytopenia. Treatments that have been effective in some patients are cyclosporin A, prednisolone plus an alkylating agent, and pentostatin.

T-cell prolymphocytic leukaemia

This aggressive form of T-cell leukaemia is characterized by hepatosplenomegaly, lymphadenopathy, and high leucocyte counts, usually rising fairly rapidly above 100×10^9/l, but cases with an initial indolent course have been recognized. There is skin infiltration in the dermis around the blood vessels and appendages in 20 per cent of cases and pleural effusions are often seen. The blood picture (Plate 7) may resemble B-cell prolymphocytic leukaemia but typical T prolymphocytes are smaller than B prolymphocytes and have some distinct features: irregular nuclear outline and a deep basophilic cytoplasm with protrusions or blebs. The nucleolus is often prominent, but it may be hidden in 20 per cent of cases when small cells predominate (small cell variant). In 5 per cent of cases the cells have a cerebriform configuration (Sézary cell variant), but erythroderma is not a feature in these patients. Serology for HTLV-I is always negative.

The membrane phenotype corresponds to that of mature (post-thymic) T lymphocytes, CD2+, CD3+, CD7+, with CD4+, CD8– markers. One-third of cases coexpress CD4 and CD8 or are CD4–, CD8+. The diagnosis is made by examination of peripheral blood and bone marrow films and confirmed by the appropriate markers. Ultrastructural examination has been used to define the morphology in cases with small cells.

Cytogenetic abnormalities

There are consistent non-random chromosome abnormalities in T-cell prolymphocytic leukaemia affecting 90 per cent of cases. The most commonly involved inversion is of chromosome 14 with break points at 14q11, the T-cell receptor (**TCR**) a/b locus, and 14q32.1, locus of the proto-oncogenes TCL1 and TCL1b, which are activated through the translocation. Other karyotypic changes include: idic(8)(p11), t(8;8)(p11–12;q12) and trisomy 8q, and deletions at 12p13. The translocation t(X;14)(q28;q11) is less common but also involves the TCR a/b locus and the MTCP1 gene, which has 70 per cent homology with TCL1. Both TCL1 and MTCP1 can induce a T-cell leukaemia with a CD4–, CD8+ immunophenotype in a transgenic mouse model. Deletions and missense mutations involving the ataxia telangiectasia mutated (ATM) gene at 11q23 have been documented in a high proportion of cases. It is of interest that patients with ataxia telangiectasia have circulating T-cell clones with inv(14)(q11;q32) and that some develop a T-cell leukaemia indistinguishable from T-cell prolymphocytic leukaemia.

Treatment and prognosis

The median survival of T-cell prolymphocytic leukaemia in our historical series has been 7 months. Responses can be obtained in 50 per cent of cases with pentostatin, but the majority of these are partial. Complete responses can now be obtained with the humanized monoclonal antibodies CAMPATH-1H in two-thirds of patients who are resistant and only partially responsive to other agents. Currently CAMPATH-1H should be considered the best first-line therapy for T-cell prolymphocytic leukaemia. Autologous stem cell transplantation has been used in patients achieving a complete remission, with some success.

T-cell lymphomas in leukaemic phase

T-cell non-Hodgkin's lymphomas develop leukaemia with higher frequency that B-cell lymphomas. Two diseases in particular regularly evolve with circulating lymphoma cells in the peripheral blood: adult T-cell leukaemia/lymphoma and Sézary syndrome.

Adult T-cell leukaemia/lymphoma has a distinct geographical distribution affecting mainly the south-west islands of Japan, the Caribbean basin, and some parts of South America—Brazil and Chile. The serological demonstration of antibodies to HTLV-I, the causative agent of adult T-cell leukaemia/lymphoma, is one of the tests necessary for diagnosis. At genomic level there is evidence of clonal integration of HTLV-I in the malignant T cells. Diagnosis is further suggested by the demonstration of adult T-cell leukaemia/lymphoma cells in peripheral blood films (Plate 8). These cells have an irregular nucleus with polylobed configuration and many atypical forms including large transformed ones. These cells have been described as 'flower' cells. Patients with adult T-cell leukaemia/lymphoma have generalized lymphadenopathy, splenomegaly, and skin rashes. Leucocyte counts are variable but often less than 50×10^9/l. Hypercalcaemia is present in two-thirds of patients and tends to be difficult to control.

The pathogenesis of the T-cell malignancy by HTLV-I involves multiple steps. Infection with HTLV-I is essential but only 1 out of 2000 infected patients may develop full-blown adult T-cell leukaemia/lymphoma. Cases with non-specific symptoms and signs and minimal lymphocytosis are considered as smouldering disease. Lymphoma forms without blood or bone marrow involvement have been recognized in 20 per cent of cases.

Adult T-cell leukaemia/lymphoma cells may resemble Sézary cells. The latter have more uniform features and a cerebriform rather than a hyperlobulated nucleus. Lymph node histology in adult T-cell leukaemia/lymphoma shows diffuse infiltration with pleomorphic T cells of small, medium, and large size (Plate 10). The median survival of acute forms of adult T-cell leukaemia/lymphoma is less than 12 months. Patients are treated as those with high-grade non-Hodgkin's lymphoma, but remissions are transient and opportunistic infections are common. Some benefit has been reported using the combination of interferon-α and zidovudine.

Sézary syndrome is a distinct form of cutaneous T-cell lymphoma characterized by erythroderma and circulating Sézary cells, usually of small size (also known as Lutzner cells) (Plate 9). The skin infiltration is epidermotrophic with the formation of Pautrier microabcesses. Sézary cells, as well as adult T-cell leukaemia/lymphoma cells, are mature T cells with a CD4+, CD8– immunophenotype. The main difference is strong expression of the interleukin-2 receptor, demonstrated by the monoclonal antibodies CD25, in adult T-cell leukaemia/lymphoma but not in Sézary cells. Cases of T-cell leukaemia without skin involvement and with cells that resemble Sézary cells morphologically but lack skin involvement are now considered as part of the spectrum of T-cell prolymphocytic leukaemia (see above).

Further reading

Bennett JM *et al.* (1989). Proposals for the classification of chronic (mature) B and T lymphoid leukaemias. *Journal of Clinical Pathology* **42**, 567–84.

Bolam S, Orchard J, Oscier D (1997). Fludarabine is effective in the treatment of splenic lymphoma with villous lymphocytes. *British Journal of Haematology* **99**, 158–61.

Bosanquet AG, Johnson SA, Richards SM (1999). Prognosis for fludarabine therapy of chronic lymphocytic leukaemia based on *ex vivo* drug response by DiSC assay. *British Journal of Haematology* **106**, 71–7.

Brito-Babapulle V *et al.* (1997). The impact of molecular cytogenetics on chronic lymphoid leukaemia. *Acta Haematologica* **98**, 175–86.

Catovsky D, Foa R (1990). *The lymphoid leukaemias.* Butterworths, London. [A description of the clinical and laboratory features of chronic lymphocytic leukaemia and other B- and T-cell leukaemias and lymphomas evolving with leukaemia.]

Catovsky D, Matutes E (1999). Splenic lymphoma with circulating villous lymphocytes/splenic marginal zone lymphoma. *Seminars in Hematology* **36**, 148–54.

Chronic Lymphocytic Leukaemia Trialists' Collaborative Group (1999). Chemotherapeutic options in chronic lymphocytic leukemia: a meta-analysis of the randomized trials. *Journal of the National Cancer Institute* **91**, 861–8.

Damle RN *et al.* (1999). Ig V gene mutation status and CD38 expression as novel prognostic indicators in chronic lymphocytic leukemia. *Blood* **94**, 1840–7.

Dearden CE *et al.* (1999). Long-term follow-up of patients with hairy cell leukaemia after treatment with pentostatin or cladribine. *British Journal of Haematology* **106**, 515–19.

Dearden CE *et al.* (2001). High remission rate in T-cell prolymphocytic leukaemia. *Blood* **98**, 1271–6.

Döhner H *et al.* (1997). 11q deletions identify a new subset of B-cell chronic lymphocytic leukemia characterized by extensive nodal involvement and inferior prognosis. *Blood* **89**, 2516–22.

Döhner H *et al.* (1999). Chromosome aberrations in B-cell chronic lymphocytic leukemia: reassessment based on molecular cytogenetic analysis. *Journal of Molecular Medicine* **77**, 266–81.

Dreger P *et al.* (1998). Early stem cell transplantation for chronic lymphocytic leukaemia: a chance for cure? *British Journal of Cancer* **7**, 2291–7.

Dyer MJ *et al.* (1997). *In vivo* 'purging' of residual disease in CLL with Campath-1H. *British Journal of Haematology* **97**, 669–72.

Grever M *et al.* (1995). Randomized comparison of pentostatin versus interferon-α_{2a} in previously untreated patients with hairy cell leukemia: an intergroup study. *Journal of Clinical Oncology* **13**, 974–82.

Hamblin TJ *et al.* (1999). Unmutated Ig VH genes are associated with a more aggressive form of chronic lymphocytic leukemia. *Blood* **94**, 1848–54.

Jaffe ES *et al.*, eds. (2001). *World Health Organization classification of tumours–pathology and genetics of tumours of haematopoietic and lymphoid tissues.* IARC Press, Lyon.

Keating *et al.* (1998). Long-term follow-up of patients with chronic lymphocytic leukemia (CLL) receiving fludarabine regimens as initial therapy. *Blood* **92**, 1165–71.

Lamy T, Loughran TP Jr (1999). Current concepts: large granular lymphocyte leukemia. *Blood Reviews* **13**, 230–40.

Lens D *et al.* (1997). p53 abnormalities in B-cell prolymphocytic leukemia. *Blood* **89**, 2015–23.

Lens D *et al.* (1997). p53 abnormalities in CLL are associated with excess of prolymphocytes and poor prognosis. *British Journal of Haematology* **99**, 848–57.

Maljaei SH *et al.* (1998). Abnormalities of chromosomes 8, 11, 14, and X in T-prolymphocytic leukemia studied by fluorescence *in situ* hybridization. *Cancer, Genetics and Cytogenetics* **103**, 110–16.

Matutes E (1999). *T-cell lymphoproliferative disorders—classification, clinical and laboratory aspects.* Harwood Academic Publishers, Australia.

Matutes E *et al.* (1991). Clinical and laboratory features of 78 cases of T-prolymphocytic leukemia. *Blood* **78**, 3269–74.

Matutes E *et al.* (1996). Trisomy 12 defines a group of CLL with atypical morphology: correlation between cytogenetic, clinical and laboratory features in 544 patients. *British Journal of Haematology* **92**, 382–8.

Matutes E *et al.* (1999). FISH analysis for BCL-1 rearrangements and trisomy 12 helps the diagnosis of atypical B cell leukaemias. *Leukemia* **13**, 1721–6.

Mercieca J *et al.* (1992). Massive abdominal lymphadenopathy in hairy cell leukaemia: a report of 12 cases. *British Journal of Haematology* **82**, 547–54.

Mercieca J *et al.* (1994). The role of pentostatin in the treatment of T-cell malignancies: analysis of response rate in 145 patients according to disease subtype. *Journal of Clinical Oncology* **12**, 2588–93.

Montserrat E *et al.* (1996). Bone marrow assessment in chronic lymphocytic leukaemia: aspirate or biopsy? A comparative study in 258 patients. *British Journal of Haematology* **93**, 111–16.

Moreau EJ *et al.* (1997). Improvement of the chronic lymphocytic leukemia scoring system with the monoclonal antibody SN8 (CD79b). *American Journal of Clinical Pathology* **108**, 378–82.

Österborg A *et al.* (1996). Humanized CD52 monoclonal antibody Campath-1H as first-line treatment in chronic lymphocytic leukaemia. *British Journal of Haematology* **93**, 151–3.

Pawson R *et al.* (1997). Treatment of T-cell prolymphocytic leukemia with human CD52 antibody. *Journal of Clinical Oncology* **15**, 2667–72.

Pawson R *et al.* (1997). Sézary cell leukemia: a distinct T-cell disorder or a variant form of T prolymphocytic leukaemia? *Leukemia* **11**, 1009–13.

Pekarsky Y *et al.* (1999). Abnormalities at 14q32.1 in T cell malignancies involve two oncogenes. *Proceedings of the National Academy of Sciences (USA)* **96**, 2949–51.

Sainati L *et al.* (1990). A variant form of hairy cell leukemia resistant to α-interferon: clinical and phenotypic characteristics of 17 patients. *Blood* **76**, 157–62.

Sood R *et al.* (1998). Neutropenia associated with T-cell large granular lymphocyte leukemia: long-term response to cyclosporine therapy despite persistence of abnormal cells. *Blood* **91**, 3372–8.

Vorechovský I *et al.* (1997). Clustering of missense mutations in the ataxia-telangiectasia gene in a sporadic T-cell leukaemia. *Nature Genetics* **17**, 96–9.

22.3.6 Chronic myeloid leukaemia

Tariq I. Mughal and John M. Goldman

Introduction

Chronic myeloid leukaemia (**CML**)—a term historically used interchangeably with chronic granulocytic leukaemia, chronic myelogenous leukaemia, and chronic myelocytic leukaemia—is a clonal malignant myeloproliferative disorder believed to originate in a single abnormal haemopoietic stem cell. It involves myeloid, monocytic, erythyroid, megakaryocytic, B-lymphoid, and sometimes T-lymphoid lineages. The first cases were described in the 1840s. A major landmark in the study of CML was the discovery of the Philadelphia (**Ph**) chromosome in 1960. Later it was established that the Ph chromosome was linked to the genetic events that cause CML. CML became the first human cancer in which a specific cytogenetic abnormality could be linked to its pathogenesis.

The past two decades have witnessed an enormous increase in our understanding of the molecular biology of CML. Such knowledge has enabled specialists to define precisely some of the molecular events and relate them to the prognostic factors of the individual patients with CML. During this period the prognosis of patients with CML has evolved from incurable to potentially curable by treatment with allogeneic haemopoietic stem-cell transplantation (allo-**SCT**). However, only a relatively small proportion of all patients with CML are eligible for allo-SCT, which still carries an appreciable risk of mortality and morbidity. For the majority of patients, interferon-alpha (IFN-á) have been found to suppress the CML cells and prolong survival in comparison to hydroxyurea. Adoptive immunotherapy using donor-lymphocyte infusions have proven valuable in treating selected patients with mini-SCT, and for rescuing those who relapse following a conventional allogeneic SCT. A new Abl-specific tyrosine kinase inhibitor, designated STI571 or imatinib mesylate, has recently been introduced and early clinical results are extremely encouraging.

Epidemiology

The annual incidence of CML is about 1 to 1.5 per 100 000 of the population. It accounts for approximately 15 per cent of all leukaemias in adults but less than 5 per cent of all childhood leukaemias. In the United Kingdom there are about 700 new cases each year. The median age of onset is 60 years and there is a slight male excess. With the possible exception of China there appears to be no clear geographical variation in the incidence.

Aetiology

Most cases of CML occur sporadically. No aetiological factor can be incriminated in the great majority of cases. A marginally increased risk of developing CML has been reported following exposure to high doses of irradiation, as occurred in survivors of the Hiroshima and Nagasaki atomic bombs in 1945. No familial predisposition or specific HLA genotypes have been recognized, but a small number of families with a high incidence of the disease have been reported.

Natural history

Characteristically CML is a biphasic or triphasic disease. Most patients present in the initial stable 'chronic' phase which typically lasts for 4 to 7 years. The natural history involves a spontaneous but largely predictable progression to an 'advanced phase', a term that covers the 'accelerated' phase and also 'blast crisis' or 'blastic transformation' (Table 1). About half of all patients in chronic phase transform directly into blast crisis, and the remainder do so following an intervening period of accelerated phase. In blastic transformation the CML cells fail to mature, and the blast cells resemble either the myeloblasts (myeloid blastic transformation) or lymphoblasts (lymphoid blastic transformation) found in patients with *de novo* acute myeloid or acute lymphoblastic leukaemia respectively.

Clinical features

Most patients typically present with lethargy and anorexia or abdominal discomfort due to splenomegaly, but 30 to 40 per cent of patients are asymptomatic and the diagnosis is made following a routine blood test. The principal physical finding is a palpable spleen, which is found in up to three-quarters of patients. Hepatomegaly and lymphadenopathy are uncommon. The clinical features of 430 patients referred to the Hammersmith Hospital in London are shown in Table 2. Occasional patients have 'chloromas' or 'granulocytic sarcomas' with subcutaneous deposits of extramedullary leukaemia.

In contrast to patients in the chronic phase, patients in the advanced phase are often symptomatic with fever, bone pain, bleeding, and/or excessive sweating. Splenic pain due to splenic infarct is not uncommon. During the accelerated phase patients often require increasing doses of hydroxycarbamide (hydroxyurea) to control the neutrophil counts.

Table 1 Different phases of chronic myeloid leukaemia

Chronic phase

Ability to reduce spleen size and restore and maintain 'normal' blood count with appropriate therapy

Accelerated phase

Presence of any one of the following:

- Anaemia (<8.0 g/dl)[a]
- Leucocytosis (>100 × 10^9/l)[a]
- Thrombocytopenia (<100 × 10^9/l)[a]
- Thrombocytosis (>1000 × 10^9/l)[a]

Splenomegaly[a]

- >10 per cent blasts in blood or marrow
- >20 per cent blasts plus promyelocytes in blood or marrow
- >20 per cent basophils plus eosinophils in blood
- New cytogenetic changes (in addition to Ph)

Blastic phase

More than 30 per cent blasts plus promyelocytes in blood or marrow

Note: Classification of disease phase must take account of the treatment the patient is receiving. Thus (a) indicates features that are indications of accelerated-phase disease only if a patient is already receiving therapy that would be considered adequate for the control of chronic-phase disease.

Table 2 Clinical features of 430 patients with CML referred to Hammersmith Hospital in London between 1979 and 1995

	n	%
Symptoms		
Fatigue	140	34
Bleeding	89	21
Weight loss	84	20
Splenic discomfort	76	18
Abdominal mass	62	14
Sweats	61	14
Bone pain	31	7
Infections	26	6
Priapism	8	2
Others	65	15
Incidental finding	85	20
Signs		
Spleen palpable	314	76
1–10 cm	153	37
>10 cm	161	39
Spleen not palpable	100	24
Purpura	66	16
Palpable liver	9	2
No signs	85	20

Molecular biology

The Ph chromosome is an acquired cytogenetic abnormality present in all CML cells (Fig. 1). It is formed as a result of a reciprocal translocation of genetic material from the long arm of one of the two no. 9 chromosomes with material from the long arm of one of the no. 22 chromosomes, referred to as t(9;22)(q34;q11). This translocation involves transections of the *BCR* (breakpoint cluster region) gene normally on chromosome 22 and the *ABL* (Abelson) gene normally on chromosome 9 and so results in the juxtaposition of 5′ sequences from the *BCR* gene with the 3′ sequences from

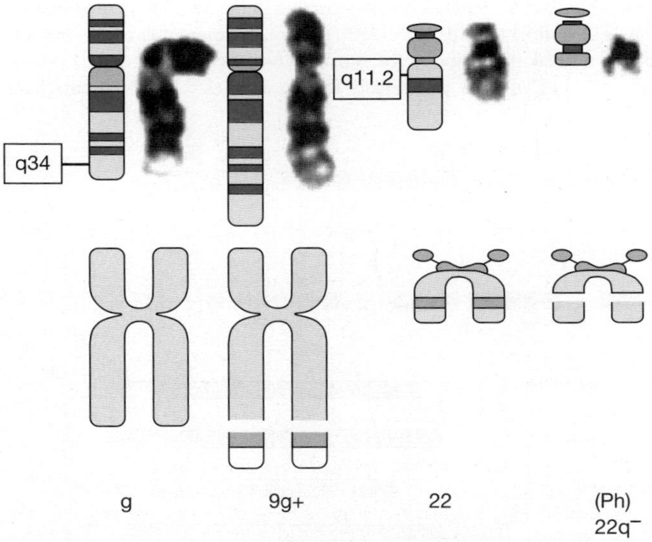

Fig. 1 Partial karyotype showing the Philadelphia chromosome translocation t(9;22)(q34;q11) with the positions of the breakpoints on chromosomes 9 and 22.

the *ABL* gene. The end results is the creation of a chimeric or 'fusion' *BCR–ABL* gene.

The classical Ph chromosome is easily identified in 80 per cent of patients with CML. Variant translocations are seen in a further 10 per cent of patients; these variants may be 'simple' involving chromosome 22 and a chromosome other than chromosome 9, or 'complex', where chromosomes 9, 22, and other additional chromosomes are involved. About 8 per cent of patients with classical clinical and haematological features of CML lack the Ph chromosome and are referred to as cases of Ph-negative CML. About half of such patients have a *BCR–ABL* chimeric gene and are referred to as Ph-negative, BCR-ABL-positive cases; the remainder are BCR-ABL-negative, and some of these have mutations in other genes. It is probable that these latter patients have a more aggressive clinical course than those with Ph-negative, BCR-ABL-positive disease. As the disease progresses patients may acquire additional cytogenetic abnormalities, including duplication of the Ph chromosome, trisomy 8, and isochromosome 17q. Mutations or deletions of tumour-suppressor genes such as *p16* and *p53* may contribute to the disease progression.

The *BCR–ABL* fusion gene transcribes an mRNA which encodes a protein that has a greater tyrosine kinase activity than the normal ABL protein. Depending on the site of the breakpoint in the *BCR* gene, the fusion protein can vary in size from 185 kDa to 230 kDa (Fig. 2). To date, three separate breakpoint locations on the *BCR* gene have been identified. When the break occurs in *major breakpoint cluster region* (**M-BCR**) it is nearly always in the intron between exons e13 and e14 or in the intron between exons e14 and e15 (toward the telomere). By contrast, the position of the breakpoint in the *ABL* gene is highly variable and may occur at almost any position upstream of exon a2 (toward the centromere). Most patients with the classical Ph chromosome have express transcripts with e13a2 or e14a2 junctions which translate as 210-kDa oncoproteins ($p210^{BCR-ABL}$) (Table 3). A break in the first intron of the *BCR* gene, between exons e1 and e2, in an area designated the *minor breakpoint cluster region* (m-bcr) results in the transcription of an e1a2 mRNA which encodes a 190-kDa protein ($p190^{BCR-ABL}$). This is found in about two-thirds of patients with Ph-positive acute lymphoblastic leukaemia. The third position for a break in the *BCR* gene is between exons e19 and e20, in an area designated *micro breakpoint cluster region* (**μ-bcr**). The associated mRNA product, e19a2, encodes a larger protein of 230 kDa ($p230^{BCR-ABL}$), which is found in the very rare cases of chronic neutrophilic leukaemia associated with a Ph chromosome.

The different breakpoints in the M-BCR result in two slightly different chimeric *BCR–ABL* genes. A break occurring in the M-BCR intron between exons e13 and e14 yields an e13a2 (previously known as b2a2) mRNA, whereas a break occurring in the intron between exons e14 and e15) produces an e14a2 mRNA (previously known as b3a2). Most patients have

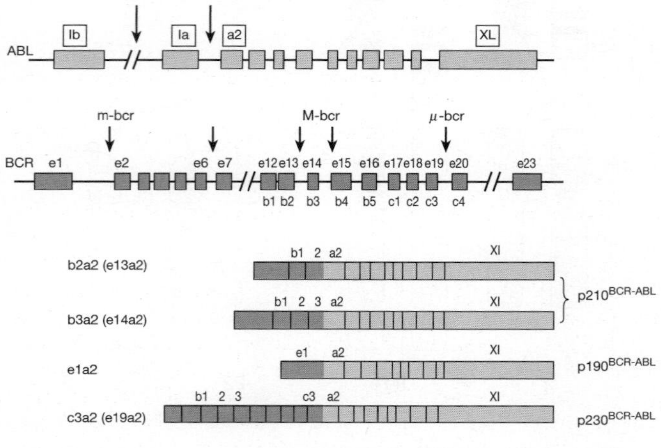

Fig. 2 Schematic representation of the various breakpoints in the *ABL* and *BCR* genes and the encoded proteins in the BCR–ABL-positive leukaemias

Table 3 The BCR-ABL-positive leukaemias

p190 disease	– Usually ALL phenotype
	– Very rarely CML with monocytosis and dysplasia
p210 disease	– Classical Ph-positive CML
	– About 5 per cent of cases are Ph-negative
	– Includes 3–20 per cent of cases of Ph-positive ALL
p230 disease	– Chronic neutrophilic leukaemia (Ph-positive)
	– Absence of immature cells from peripheral blood

ALL, acute lymphoblastic leukaemia; CML, chronic myeloid leukaemia.

either e13a2 or e14a2 transcripts, although both transcripts are present in about 10 per cent of cases. The type of BCR-ABL transcript has no important prognostic significance, altough patients with the e14a2 transcripts may have higher platelet counts.

It is believed that the various BCR–ABL transcripts play a central role in the pathogenesis of CML, though the precise details are still not fully understood. Various efforts to determine the function of the BCR–ABL proteins have established that, as a consequence of increased tyrosine kinase activity, the BCR–ABL protein can phosphorylate several substrate molecules, such as CRKL, p62Dok, paxillin, CBL, and RIN, thereby activating multiple signal-transduction pathways affecting cell growth and differentiation. The details of the pathways are incomplete, but a popular hypothesis is that the BCR–ABL protein activates the same pathways as are activated by cytokines that control the growth and differentiation of haemopoietic cells, thereby allowing CML cells to circumvent normal cellular growth and differentiation and become malignant. This would not, however, explain the mechanism by which the preferential proliferation and differentiation of myeloid progenitors occur. The molecular basis for transformation of CML from chronic phase to more advanced phases remains poorly understood, although several molecular changes, in particular mutations or deletions of p53, p16, retinoblastoma protein, and mutations or overexpression of Ras and EVI-1, have been identified.

Normal haemopoietic stem cells may be maintained in a resting state (designated G_o) as a result of the proliferation of CML cells. Under certain circumstances, however, these normal cells can be induced to proliferate, and this provides the rationale for autografting as a treatment of CML. There may also be a subpopulation of deeply quiescent Ph-positive CML cells, that might be relatively resistant to eradication by cycle-active cytotoxic drugs even when administered in high doses.

Diagnosis

The diagnosis of CML is commonly based on the characteristic appearances of the peripheral blood film and bone marrow aspirate and trephine biopsy. Cytogenetic analysis for the presence of the Ph chromosome is confirmatory. Molecular studies for the evidence of the BCR–ABL product provide additional confirmation.

The peripheral blood usually shows a leucocytosis which involves cells at all stages of differentiation within the myeloid lineage (Fig. 3 and Plate 1). Basophilia is an important diagnostic feature as its absence suggests other myeloproliferative disorders, particularly if the Ph chromosome and *BCR–ABL* gene are also absent. Eosinophilia may also be present but has no diagnostic relevance. There is a relative monocytopenia, although absolute numbers may be increased corresponding with the leucocytosis. This differentiates CML from chronic myelomonocytic leukaemia. Thrombocytosis with platelet anisocytosis and nucleated red cells are common.

The bone marrow is markedly hypercellular with an increased myeloid to erythroid ratio due to the predominance of myeloid cells, particularly

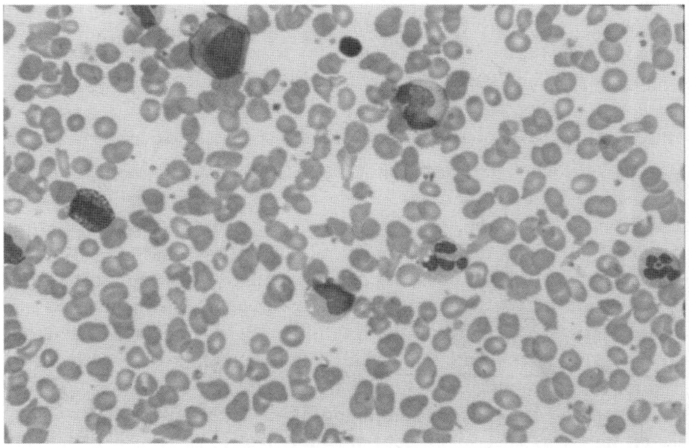

Fig. 3 Peripheral blood film from a patient with CML in chronic phase. (Photograph kindly provided by Professor Barbara Bain, Imperial College London.) (See also Plate 1.)

neutrophils and myelocytes. There may be no features of abnormal maturation in the precursors. Megakaryocytes are increased and may form clusters, which are less striking than those seen in essential thrombocythaemia. Reticulin fibrosis is usually absent or mildly increased at diagnosis.

Blastic transformation is often abrupt and striking with blast cells comprising up to 100 per cent of nucleated cells seen in the blood and marrow; it thus resembles an acute leukaemia arising *de novo*. These blast cells are of myeloid lineage in about 70 per cent of the patients, while in about 20 per cent the express lymphoid surface markers, have rearrangement of immunoglobulin genes and are presumably lymhoid in origin. The remaining patients in blast crisis have a blast population with a mixed or indeterminate morphology and immunophenotype.

Prognostic factors

Various efforts have been made to establish criteria definable at diagnosis that may help to predict survival for individual patients. Historically the most frequently used method was that proposed by Sokal, whereby patients can be divided into various risk categories based on a mathematical formula that takes account of the patient's age, blast-cell count, spleen size, and platelet count at diagnosis. The Sokal index has recently been updated by a retrospective study of patients treated with IFN-α in Germany — the new Euro or Hasford system is similar to the Sokal index but includes consideration of basophil and eosinophil numbers. Currently the best prognostic indicator may be the response to initial treatment with **IFN-α**; patients who achieve a degree of cytogenetic response have the best survival. These approaches help to predict survival with a non-transplant strategy. Other methods, such as the risk assessment proposals by Gratwohl *et al.* and Lee *et al.*, are designed to calculate the risk of transplant-related mortality after an allo-SCT. Other possible prognostic factors are the presence or absence of deletions in the derivative 9q+ chromosome and the rate of shortening of telomeres in the leukaemia clone.

Management

The substantial recent developments in treating CML, including the introduction of IFN-α and allogeneic SCT in the 1980s and of STI571 very recently, have made management decisions for individual patients in chronic phase fairly complex. Thus some patients with CML can be cured by an allogeneic SCT, but the risks associated with it need to be carefully assessed. In contrast, IFN-α induces haematological control in a significant proportion of patients and confers some improvement in survival in comparison with hydroxyurea, especially for those patients who achieve a degree of cytogenetic response. It is rare, however, to achieve a molecular remission with IFN-α. STI571 induces haematological remission in almost all patients and is associated with a high incidence of cytogenetic response, but there is not yet information on its ability to confer molecular remission; neither is there any evidence as yet that it prolongs survival in comparison to the other treatments of CML. It is therefore prudent to discuss the relative merits of the various treatments with the patient at the time of diagnosis and to explain some aspects of the disease and the proposed management strategy.

Non-transplant treatment options

IFN-α is a member of a large family of glycoproteins of biological origin with antiviral and antiproliferative properties. It is active in reducing the leucocyte count and reversing the clinical features in 70 to 80 per cent of patients with CML. Five to 15 per cent of patients achieve a major reduction in the proportion of Ph-positive marrow metaphases. A number of prospective studies comparing IFN-α to hydroxycarbamide (hydroxyurea) and busulfan have been reported. The standard treatment for most patients with CML in the 1980s was hydroxycarbamide which had largely replaced busulfan. By the mid-1990s it was suggested that IFN-α was probably superior to both hydroxycarbamide and busulfan, and, more importantly, it appeared that IFN-α treatment resulted in prolongation of survival, in particular for patients achieving substantial cytogenetic responses. A meta-analysis of seven prospective randomized trials has confirmed the superiority of IFN-α over both busulfan and hydroxycarbamide. The meta-analysis involved over 1500 patients and found a 5-year survival of 57 per cent for the IFN-α treated patients compared to 42 per cent for the chemotherapy treated cohort. A major cytogenetic response (>66 per cent Ph-chromosome negativity in the marrow) was seen in 10 to 38 per cent of all patients and occurred usually within 12 to 18 months of starting IFN-α therapy.

There are several key issues still unresolved with regard to IFN-α. The optimal dose remains a matter of some controversy although the recent study conducted by the UK Medical Research Council found no difference between 'high' and 'low' doses. Moreover, the optimal duration of IFN-α treatment remains undefined. Toxicity is common but is generally mild and reversible. Most patients suffer from influenza-like symptoms on starting treatment. Later they may experience lethargy and weight loss. Less common effects include autoimmune-mediated complications, such as thrombocytopenia and hypothyroidism. In an effort to improve the treatment results, several trials focused on combining IFN-α with cytotoxic drugs. Encouraging cytogenetic results have been obtained with the addition of cytarabine to IFN-α in French trial and a survival advantage in comparison to IFN-α was observed; this has not however been confirmed in a comparable Italian study. In an attempt to reduce the toxicity of IFN-α therapy, a pegylated form of IFN-α has also been investigated and preliminary experience is encouraging.

The precise mode of action of IFN-α remains uncertain. *In vitro* studies, mainly from long-term cultures of CML cells, suggest a prominent antiproliferative effect of IFN-α in CML. Some of this activity against CML cells may be mediated through the dendritic cells. IFN-α may also indirectly influence the survival of CML cells by restoring the defective cytoadhesion of the CML cells or by recruiting accessory cells of the immune surveillance system, by inhibiting other cytokines or by augmenting the action of natural killer cells.

Clinical trials designed to assess the efficacy and safety of STI571 in patients in all phases of CML began in 1998. In patients with CML in chronic phase refractory to or intolerant of IFN-α who receive at least 300mg of STI571 daily the incidence of complete haematological response is 98 per cent of the patients; about 40 to 45 per cent achieve cytogenetic responses. STI571 was administered orally and so far no important side-effects have been noted. The drug also demonstrated significant activity in CML in accelerated phase and in blast crisis. The follow-up is still relatively short, but if the responses are sustainable, this novel drug will become the preferred non-transplant treatment option. The drug is now licensed for these indications on both sides of the Atlantic and studies to compare STI571 alone with STI571 plus IFN-á and STI571 plus cytarabine are being designed. The combination of STI571 with pegylated IFN-á is also being tested.

Stem-cell transplantation

Allogeneic SCT, using blood- or marrow-derived stem cells derived from an HLA-matched sibling donor, performed in the chronic phase can cure a substantial proportion of patients with CML. International Bone Marrow Transplant Registry (**IBMTR**) showed that the leukaemia-free survival (**LFS**) at 5 years is 55 to 60 per cent. The probability of relapse at 5 years was 15 per cent. In contrast, the results of allogeneic SCT performed in the advanced phase of CML were generally poor. The probabilities of LFS at 5 years for those transplanted in the accelerated phase and blast crisis were 28 per cent and 10 per cent, respectively. The clinical results of transplantation using HLA-matched sibling donors appear to be relatively consistent worldwide.

The major determinants for survival, other than the phase of the disease, include the patient's age at transplant and the cytomegalovirus (**CMV**) status of the patient, and the age and sex of the donor. Survival appears to be best for patients who are transplanted within 1 year of diagnosis, are less than 40 years of age, have a young male donor, and both patient and donor are CMV-negative. For such a cohort, the 5-year LFS is probably 70 to 80 per cent; the relapse rate would be 10 to 20 per cent. It is possible that the precise details of the transplant procedure also influence the outcome. The cytoreductive regimens used prior to the transplant and the preventive measures for graft-versus-host disease (**GvHD**) appear especially important. The source of stem cells may also influence the result; following a peripheral-blood SCT patients achieve rapid engraftment, but there is a slight excess of chronic GvHD, perhaps due to the increased T-cell numbers in the peripheral blood compared to the bone marrow. There has also been some concern with regard to the effect of prior IFN-α therapy following an initial report suggesting a possible detrimental effect, further careful monitoring is therefore necessary.

Although allogeneic SCT using an HLA-matched sibling donor appears to cure some patients with CML, this treatment is only available to about 15 to 20 per cent of all patients with CML. This is largely due to a lack of suitable family donors and to age limitations. The rigors associated with SCT mean that most patients over the age of 60 years have a substantial incidence of transplant-related mortality (**TRM**). For these reasons, efforts have been made to identify suitable volunteer unrelated donors (**VUD**) and better conditioning regimens to reduce the toxicity. Historically, the results of VUD-SCT are inferior to those of HLA-matched sibling SCT due to an increased rate of graft failure, GvHD, and TRM. The presence of GvHD greatly increases the risk of TRM and morbidity post-SCT from infections. GvHD prophylaxis with a combination of ciclosporin and methotrexate is superior to ciclosporin alone. T-cell depletion of the allograft effectively abrogates GvHD, in particular in the VUD-SCT setting, but it is accompanied by a relapse rate of over 60 per cent. The observation that removal of donor T cells greatly increased the incidence of relapse was the unequivocal proof of the existence of a graft-versus-leukaemia (**GvL**) effect.

Current results of VUD-SCT from the Seattle group suggest an LFS of 74 per cent at 5 years in CML patients who are under the age of 50 years and are transplanted within a year of diagnosis. These and other similar results have led to further refinements toward the search for suitable VUDs to make SCT more available. Newer molecular techniques for subtyping the HLA class I genes should improve the chances of finding optimally matched or acceptably mismatched donors. Syngeneic SCT has comparable overall survival, but, due to the lack of a GvL effect, there is a higher relapse rate resulting in a lower LFS.

Efforts to minimize the toxicity of conditioning regimens have been benefited by the use of the purine analogues (for example, fludarabine) which are potent immunosuppressive drugs. These regimens are non-myeloablative but ensure engraftment and are designed to exploit maximally the GvL effect. These procedures have been termed reduced intensity conditioning SCTs (also mini-SCTs or non-myeloablative SCTs) and reflect the exciting advances in our understanding of how SCT actually works.

Treatment of relapse of CML post-transplantation

Most patients who relapse after allogeneic SCT (allo-SCT) do so within the first 3 years. This relapse tends to follow an orderly progression, with the patient initially demonstrating evidence of a molecular relapse with increasing positivity of BCR–ABL transcripts assayed by the polymerase chain reaction (**PCR**), followed by a cytogenetic relapse (finding of the Ph chromosome in marrow metaphases), and then by haematological and clinical relapse. Molecular monitoring of allo-SCT recipients is therefore valuable. For patients with molecular relapse, remission can be induced by withdrawing immunosuppression or by the infusion of lymphocytes collected from the original transplant donor (**DLI**) without any other antileukaemic measures. DLI can induce remissions in 60 to 80 per cent of patients with molecular or cytogenetic relapse. These important results lend further support to the concept that a GvL effect plays an important role in the cure of CML after allografting. Patients who fail to enter remission with DLI may be candidates for treatment with STI571 or a second allo-SCT but the risk of TRM is relatively high. The 4-year LFS for a second allo-SCT is around 28 per cent. The potential benefit of using STI571 initially instead of DLI is now being assessed.

The mechanisms by which T lymphocytes exert a GvL effect remain highly speculative. It is possible that they release cytokines, such as interleukin-2, IFN-α, or transforming growth factor-α, that selectively suppress the proliferation of Ph-positive cells. It is possible that T cells or natural killer cells act directly against leukaemia cells. A third possibility is that CML cells express leukaemia-specific antigens, possibly coded by the *BCR–ABL* chimeric gene, that provoke a true leukaemia-specific, T-cell response.

Autologous stem-cell transplantation

Despite the qualified success of allo-SCT, the majority of CML patients are not eligible for this therapy and a substantial number have a marginal survival benefit from IFN-α treatment. Autologous SCT following high-dose chemotherapy has a lower TRM and is available to more patients. Retrospective analyses suggest that autografting with blood- or marrow-derived stem cells can prolong survival. The fact that some Ph-negative stem cells survive at the time of diagnosis in most patients provides the rationale for developing techniques that favour reconstitution with Ph-negative haemopoiesis. The Genoa group has pioneered procedures where Ph-negative stem cells are harvested during the recovery phase after chemotherapy; they demonstrated successful engraftment resulting in Ph-negative haemopoiesis. In most cases, however, the Ph-positive haemopoiesis recurs. This recurrence may be due in some cases to residual Ph-positive cells in the autografted material and this provides the rationale for 'purging' techniques. Various *in vitro* and *in vivo* methods have been developed with variable degrees of success. The new generation of *in vitro* purging studies using tyrosine kinase inhibitors targeted against the *BCR–ABL* oncoprotein, such as STI571, may be informative. Although the clinical feasibility and safety of these differing autografting strategies have been demonstrated, the precise therapeutic role of autografting remains unclear.

Conclusions and a suggested therapeutic algorithm

The choice of therapy for the younger CML patient newly diagnosed in chronic phase now requires the benefits and risks of SCT to be balanced against the predicted results of non-transplant therapy. The decision to offer an allogeneic SCT early after diagnosis to a patient under the age of 40 years, in particular if an HLA-matched sibling donor is available, is probably straightforward. For most other patients it is useful to assess all

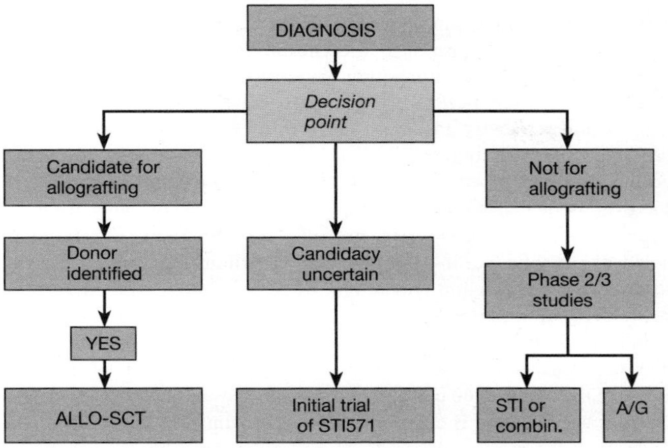

Fig. 4 A suggested therapeutic algorithm for the management of patients with CML.

the treatment options carefully. For the present, patients over the age of 60 years cannot safely be treated by SCT, but this may change in the near future following further experience with non-myeloablative SCT. For patients aged between 40 and 60 years who have a suitable molecularly matched unrelated donor and wish to be transplanted, the risk of TRM is such that a trial of STI571 in the first instance is reasonable. We suggest this form of an integrated approach in the therapeutic algorithm shown in Fig. 4. It is likely that some of the other new treatment strategies currently being investigated, such as immunotherapy to activate a leukaemia-specific immune response, will also be integrated in the treatment plans of patients with CML in the near future.

Further reading

Ahuja H, *et al.* (1991). The spectrum of molecular alterations in the evolution of chronic myeloid leukemia. *Journal of Clinical Investigation* **87**, 2042–6.

Allan NC, Richards SM, Shepherd PCA (1995). UK Medical Research Council randomised multicentre trial of interferon-αn1 for chronic myeloid leukaemia: improved survival irrespective of cytogenetic response. *Lancet* **345**, 1392–7.

Barrett AJ, Malkovska V (1996). Graft-versus-leukaemia: understanding and using the allo-immune response to treat haematological malignancies. *British Journal of Haematology* **93**, 754–61.

Barrett AJ, van Rhee F (1997). Graft-versus-leukemia. *Baillière's Clinical Haematology* **10**, 337–56.

Bolin RW, *et al.* (1982). Busulfan versus hydroxyurea in the long-term therapy of chronic myelogenous leukemia. *Cancer* 50, 1683–7.

Carella AM, *et al.* (1997). Mobilization and transplantation of Philadelphia-negative peripheral blood progenitor cells early in chronic myelogenous leukemia. *Journal of Clinical Oncology* **15**, 1575.

Collins RH, *et al.* (1997). Donor leukocyte infusions in 140 patients with relapse malignancy after allogeneic bone marrow transplantation. *Journal of Clinical Oncology* **15**, 433.

Devergie A, *et al.* (1995). Allogeneic bone marrow transplantation for chronic myeloid leukemia in first chronic phase: a randomized trial of busulfan–cytoxan versus cytoxan–total body irradiation as preparative regimen: a report from the French Society of Bone Marrow Graft (SFGM). *Blood* **85**, 2263.

Druker BJ, *et al.* (2001). Efficacy and safety of a specific inhibitor of the Bcr-Abl tyrosine kinase in chronic myeloid leukemia. *New England Journal of Medicine* 344, 1031-1037

Druker BJ, *et al.* (1996). Effects of a selective inhibitor of the Abl tyrosine kinase on the growth of BCR–ABL positive cells. *Nature Medicine* **2**, 561.

Faderl S, *et al.* (1999). The biology of chronic myeloid leukemia. *New England Journal of Medicine* **341**, 164–72.

Fialkow PJ (1981). Evidence for a multistep origin of chronic myeloid leukemia. *Blood* **58**, 158–63.

Goldman JM, *et al.* (1986). Bone marrow transplantation for patients with chronic myeloid leukemia. *New England Journal of Medicine* **314**, 202.

Goldman JM (1998). Cost effectiveness of interferon-α for chronic myeloid leukaemia. *Annals of Oncology* **9**, 351–2.

Goldman JM (1999). Donor lymphocyte infusion for chronic myelogenous leukemia. *Blood* **94** (Suppl. 1), 60.

Goldman JM (2000). Tyrosine-kinase inhibition in treatment of chronic myeloid leukaemia. *Lancet* **355**, 1031–2.

Gratwohl A, *et al.* (1998). Risk assessment for patients with chronic myeloid leukaemia before allogeneic blood or marrow transplantation. *Lancet* **352**, 1078–92.

Gratwohl A, *et al.* (1986). Bone marrow transplantation for chronic myeloid leukemia: long-term results. *Bone Marrow Transplantation* **12**, 509.

Groffen J, Heisterkamp N (1997). The chimeric *BCR–ABL* gene. *Baillière's Clinical Haematology* **10**, 187.

Guilhot F, *et al.* (1997). Interferon alpha-2b combined with cytarabine versus interferon alone in chronic myelogenous leukemia. *New England Journal of Medicine* **337**, 223.

Hansen JA, *et al.* (1998). Bone marrow transplantation from unrelated donors for patients with chronic myeloid leukemia. *New England Journal of Medicine* **338**, 962.

Hasford J, *et al.* (1998). A new prognostic score for survival of patients with chronic myeloid leukemia treated with interferon alfa. *Journal of the National Cancer Institute* **90**, 850–8.

Holyoake T, *et al.* (1999). Isolation of a highly quiescent subpopulation of primitive leukemic cells in chronic myeloid leukemia. *Blood* **94**, 2056–64.

Horowitz MM, *et al.* (1996). Effect of prior interferon therapy on outcome of HLA-identical sibling bone marrow transplants for chronic myelogenous leukemia (CML) in first chronic phase. *Experimental Hematology* **24**, 1143.

Horowitz MM, Rowlings PA, Passweg JR (1996). Allogeneic bone marrow transplantation for CML: a report from the International Bone Marrow Transplant Registry. *Bone Marrow Transplantation* **17**(Suppl. 3), S5–6.

Huntly BJ, *et al.* (2001) Deletions of the derivative chromosome 9 occur at the time of the Philadelphia translocation and provide a powerful and independent prognostic indicator in chronic myeloid leukemia. *Blood* **98**, 1732–38.

Ichimaru M, Ishimaru T, Belsky JL (1978). Incidence of leukemia in atomic bomb survivors belonging to a fixed cohort in Hiroshima and Nagasaki, 1950–1971: radiation dose, years after exposure, age at exposure, and type of leukaemia. *Journal of Radiation Research* **19**, 262.

Kantarjian HM, *et al.* (1995). Prolonged survival in chronic myelogenous leukemia after cytogenetic response to interferon-a therapy. *Annals of Internal Medicine* **122**, 254–61.

Lee S, *et al.* (1998). Initial therapy for chronic myelogenous leukemia: playing the odds. *Journal of Clinical Oncology* **16**, 2897–903.

Lee SJ, *et al.* (1997). Unrelated donor bone marrow transplantation for chronic myelogenous leukemia: a decision analysis. *Annals of Internal Medicine* **127**, 1080–8.

Lin F, *et al.* (1996). Kinetics of increasing BCR–ABL transcript numbers in chronic myeloid leukemia patients who relapse after allogeneic bone barrow transplantation. *Blood* 87, 4473.

McGlave P, *et al.* (1994). Autologous transplant therapy for chronic myelogenous leukaemia prolongs survival: results from eight transplant groups. *Lancet* **343**, 1486.

Marmont A, *et al.* (1984). Recurrence of Ph'-leukemia in donor cells after marrow transplantation for chronic myelogenous leukemia. *New England Journal of Medicine* **310**, 903.

Melo JV (1996). The diversity of the BCR–ABL fusion proteins and their relationship to leukemia phenotype. *Blood* **88**, 2375.

Mughal TI, Goldman JM (1995). Chronic myeloid leukaemia: a therapeutic challenge. *Annals of Oncology* **6**, 637–44.

Mughal TI, Hoyle C, Goldman JM (1993). Autografting for patients with chronic myeloid leukemia—The Hammersmith experience. *Stem Cells* **11**, 20–2.

Mughal TI, *et al.* (2001). Molecular studies in patients with chronic myeloid leukaemia in remission 5 years after allogeneic stem cell transplant define the risk of subsequent relapse. *British Journal of Haematology* **115**, 569–74.

Nowell PC, Hungerford DA (1960). A minute chromosome in human chronic granulocytic leukemia. *Science* **132**, 1497.

Pane F, *et al.* (1996). Neutrophilic-chronic myeloid leukemia: a distinct disease with a specific molecular marker. *Blood* **88**, 2410–14

Sawyers CL (1999). Chronic myeloid leukemia *New England Journal of Medicine* **340**, 1330–8.

Schofield JR, *et al.* (1994). Low doses of interferon-α are as effective as higher doses in inducing remissions and prolonging survival in chronic myeloid leukemia. *Annals of Internal Medicine* **121**, 736.

Shepherd P, *et al.* (1995). Analysis of molecular breakpoint and mRNA transcripts in a prospective randomized trial of interferon in chronic myeloid leukaemia: no correlation with clinical features, cytogenetic response, duration of chronic phase, or survival. *British Journal of Haematology* **89**, 546–54.

Silver RT, *et al.* (1999). An evidence-based analysis of the effect of busulfan, hydroxyurea, interferon, and allogeneic bone marrow transplantation in treating the chronic phase of chronic myeloid leukemia: Development for the American Society of Hematology. *Blood* **94**, 1517–36

Slavin S, *et al.* (1998). Nonmyeloablative stem cell transplantation with cell therapy as an alternative to conventional bone marrow transplantation with lethal cytoreduction for the treatment of malignant and non-malignant hematologic diseases. *Blood* **91**, 756.

Sokal JE, *et al.* (1984). Prognostic discrimination in 'good-risk' chronic granulocytic leukemia. *Blood* **63**, 789.

Spencer A, *et al.* (1995). Cytotoxic T-lymphocyte precursor frequency analysis in bone marrow transplantation with volunteer unrelated donors: value in donor selection. *Transplantation* **59**, 1303.

Spencer A, *et al.* (1995). Bone marrow transplantation for chronic myeloid leukemia with volunteer unrelated donors using '*ex vivo*' or '*in vivo*' T-cell depletion: a major prognostic impact of HLA class I identity between donor and recipient. *Blood* **86**, 3590.

Szydlo R, *et al.* (1997). Results of allogeneic bone marrow transplants using donors other than HLA-identical siblings. *Journal of Clinical Oncology* **15**, 1767.

Talpaz M, *et al.* (1998). The MD Anderson Cancer Center experience with interferon-a therapy in chronic myelogenous leukemia. *Baillière's Clinical Haematology* **10**, 291.

The Chronic Myeloid Leukemia Trialists' Collaborative Group (1997). Interferon versus chemotherapy for chronic myeloid leukemia: a meta-analysis of seven randomized trials. *Journal of the National Cancer Institute* **89**, 1616–20.

Tura S (1998). Cytarabine increases karyotypic response in alpha-IFN treated chronic myeloid leukemia patients: results of a national prospective randomized trial. *Blood* **92**, 317a.

van Rhee F, *et al.* (1994). Detection of residual leukemia more than 10 years after allogeneic bone marrow transplantation. *Bone Marrow Transplantation* **14**, 609.

22.3.7 Myelodysplasia

Lawrence B. Gardner and Chi V. Dang

Definition

The myelodysplastic syndromes are a collection of acquired, clonal, haemopoietic disorders characterized by cytopenias and abnormal cellular morphologies. The vast majority of myelodysplastic syndromes (**MDS**) are marked by progressive, multilineage cytopenias, ineffective maturation of cells with dysplastic appearances and chromosomal abnormalities, and a tendency to degenerate into poorly responsive leukaemias. Historically, these syndromes have been referred to as preleukaemias, smouldering leukaemias, and refractory anaemias. In 1976 the French–American–British (**FAB**) Cooperative Group proposed a classification system of these heterogeneous disorders based on the histological appearance of the peripheral blood and bone marrow, with primary emphasis placed on the percentage of immature cells, or myeloblasts, present. This artificial classification has provided a helpful outline for physician communication and research. However, the presentation and prognosis of individuals with MDS vary greatly, depending on the biological impact of the genetic mutation(s) present in an individual's clone. MDS is more common in adults than any acute or chronic leukaemia. While MDS can occur at any age, it is primarily a disease of the old; over 80 per cent of those affected are older than 60 years, and after age 70 there is a prevalence of approximately 33/100 000. The incidence of the disease appears to be increasing, probably in part due to more common screening with complete blood counts, and an increase in secondary, treatment-related MDS. There is currently no effective cure for MDS, except for allogeneic bone marrow transplantation, which is often not an option for the older patient with MDS. Treatment therefore remains supportive, consisting of transfusion and antibiotic treatment for documented infections. Patients often die as a result of their cytopenias (for example, from bleeding or infection) or transformation to leukaemia.

Pathogenesis and pathophysiology

The biology of MDS is difficult to study, since disorders grouped under MDS probably include diagnoses of disparate aetiologies. It is clear from karyotypic analysis, including chromosomal studies, and X-linked inactivation of genetic markers, that MDS is a clonal disorder involving a defect in an early haemopoietic progenitor cell. Thus erythrocytes, platelets, neutrophils, and monocytes may all be affected in MDS. The ability of progenitor cells from patients with MDS to form colonies *in vitro* is markedly diminished. Haemopoietic growth-factor production by lymphocytes from these patients is often decreased, and growth-inhibitory cytokines may be increased. In addition to the abnormal growth characteristics found in MDS progenitor cells in culture, there appears to be a higher rate of programmed cell death, or apoptosis, in such cells, which may contribute to the peripheral cytopenias and ineffective haemopoiesis noted on bone marrow examination.

Chromosomes are often abnormal in MDS. In both therapy-related and *de novo*-acquired MDS, specific chromosomal abnormalities (including deletions of chromosomes 5 and 7, and trisomy 8) are relatively common. A specific chromosomal translocation resulting in an oncogenic fusion protein is often found in a subtype of chronic myelomonocytic leukaemia (**CMMoL**). While the regions of chromosome 5 and 7 often deleted in MDS contain several genes important for haemopoiesis, including granulocyte–macrophage colony-stimulating factor (**GM-CSF**), erythropoietin, interleukin-6 (**IL-6**), and the receptors for several haemopoietic growth factors, no single gene, or group of genes, has been found to be consistently mutated in MDS. In addition, the pathogenic importance of specific deletions has not been well established. A number of genes important for proliferation and apoptosis have been described to be abnormally expressed in MDS, including the mutated *ras* oncogene which is present in up to 30 per cent of cases, but the importance of these abnormalities in the causation of MDS is unclear. Progression of MDS is often associated with the accumulation of additional chromosomal abnormalities. This stepwise accumulation of mutations, often found in many types of cancers, suggests the dominance of new clones with a proliferation and/or survival advantage.

Primary acquired sideroblastic anaemia is a unique subset of MDS. Other causes of an anaemia with the morphological appearance of ringed sideroblasts include an X-linked inherited form, and a secondary toxic form. Inherited and secondary sideroblastic anaemias are believed to result from a disruption in haem synthesis, producing ineffective haemopoiesis and iron overload. Alcohol, isoniazid, and pyrazinamide are among the common medications that can cause acquired sideroblastic anaemia.

Clinical features

While MDS has been described in children, it is uncommon and other congenital haemopoietic diseases should be strongly considered. And while secondary MDS may occur in younger adults, MDS is primarily a disease of the older adult. The clinical presentation of a patient with MDS depends on the specific cytopenias present, and the extent to which a lineage is depressed. Most commonly, patients present due to a symptomatic anaemia. Because the onset of MDS is gradual and progressive, patients typically present with signs and symptoms of chronic, not acute, anaemia, including fatigue and exertional dyspnoea. If the platelet count is are low, petechiae or other forms of bleeding, typically mucosal or gastrointestinal, may be present. Infections occur with suppressed numbers of white cells, particularly when the absolute neutrophil count is below 500/ml. One form of MDS, CMMoL, shares many characteristics with myeloproliferative diseases. In CMMoL the monocyte count can be quite high, resulting in pleural, pericardial, and peritoneal effusions, as well as splenomegaly. Rheumatological and autoimmune processes have been noted to occur with MDS.

Laboratory diagnosis

Because MDS is a chronic disease, obtaining old laboratory data documenting a progressive, often macrocytic anaemia, thrombocytopenia, and leucopenia, can be invaluable in making the diagnosis. All patients diagnosed with MDS have an anaemia, which is typically either normocytic or macrocytic, although extreme macrocytosis (mean corpuscular volume (**MCV**) >120 fl) is not common. Anaemia and leucopenia in the setting of a normal or elevated platelet count should lead one to consider a subtype of MDS, the 5q-syndrome. The hallmark of MDS is dysplasia, which is often noted on a peripheral blood smear (Fig. 1(a)). Erythrocytes may show anisocytosis (varying sizes), poikilocytosis (abnormal morphology) with bizarre shapes, and basophilic stippling. Polymorphonuclear neutrophils may be hyperlobulated or, more commonly, hypolobulated, sometimes showing the characteristic bilobed appearance of pseudo-Pelger–Huët cells. Hypogranulation may be present, and chromatin may be abnormally clumped. Myeloblasts may be seen in the periphery, and are a poor prognostic sign.

A bone marrow aspirate and biopsy, along with cytogenetics, are crucial for the diagnosis of MDS (Fig. 1(b)). Although the bone marrow biopsy may reveal a hypocellular bone marrow, this is rare, and should lead one to question the diagnosis and consider aplastic anaemia as the cause of a cytopenia. Typically, the bone marrow biopsy reveals a hypercellular marrow, consistent with the ineffective haemopoiesis common in MDS. The morphology of early progenitor cells shows a lack of maturation, with abnormal forms. Dyserythropoiesis, with multilobed erythroid progenitors, may be present. Megaloblastoid erythropoiesis is common; this is evidenced by an asynchrony of nuclear/cytoplasmic maturation, so that haemoglobin synthesis occurs while the erythroid nucleus is large and young. Megakaryocytes may be diminished, and/or be small and hypolobulated The bone marrow biopsy may show an abnormal localization of immature myeloid precursors (**ALIP**); typically, granulopoiesis occurs in a paratrabecular location, but in MDS there may be a shift to a central intratrabecular site. Depending on the stage of MDS, the number of blasts may be elevated. According to the FAB classification scheme, more than 30 per cent blasts in the marrow defines acute leukaemia, while less than 30 per cent are consistent with MDS. Staining the bone marrow biopsy for CD34+ cells may be helpful in the diagnosis.

Chromosomal abnormalities (deletions, additions, translocations) are very common in MDS. In MDS as a whole, chromosomal abnormalities are found 40 per cent of the time. While MDS may be associated with a normal karyotype, especially in an early stage with few blasts, some chromosomal abnormalities are so typical that their presence strongly suggests the diagnosis. Similarly, multiple complex chromosomal abnormalities leads one to strongly consider a diagnosis of MDS. Typically, the longer a patient has MDS, the more chromosomal abnormalities may occur, leading to a more aggressive clone. The most common abnormalities include monosomy 7, 7q-, monosomy 5, 5q-, trisomy 8, and 20q-. 11q23 is commonly found in secondary MDS due to treatment with topoisomerase II inhibitors, such as the epipodophyllotoxin, VP16 (etoposide). As discussed below, chromosomal abnormalities are important not only in suggesting the diagnosis of MDS, but also in its prognosis. Other diagnostic tests, such as abnormal growth of progenitor colonies in *in vitro* assays, are not widely utilized.

Differential diagnosis

When working up the possible aetiologies of a mild asymptomatic anaemia or pancytopenia in the older patient, where making a diagnosis may not change management, the extent of the work-up should depend on the patient's wishes. However, certain reversible diseases, several of which may be significant to the patient's overall health, must be ruled out. Aplastic anaemia also presents with pancytopenia; however, in contrast to MDS, the bone marrow is hypocellular, CD34+ early progenitor stem cells in the bone marrow are relatively diminished, and there is little evidence of dysplasia. In paroxysmal nocturnal haemoglobinuria the absence of the marker CD59 on the surface of cells, a lack of dysplasia, and low iron stores should differentiate this disease from MDS. Macrocytic, megaloblastoid anaemias as well as pancytopenias are common in patients with vitamin

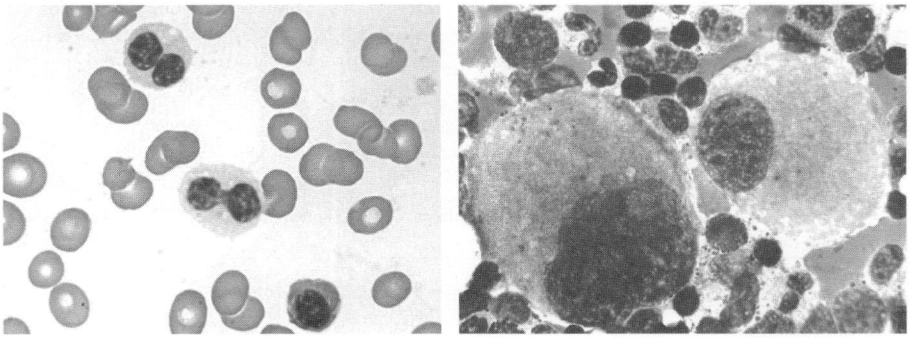

(a) (b)

Fig. 1 (a) Peripheral blood smear and (b) bone marrow appearance in MDS. (a) Several dysplastic neutrophils, including a pseudo-Pelger–Huët neutrophil with a bilobed nucleus. The chromatin in the neutrophils is clumped, and the red cells show a range of sizes and appearances. (b) A bone marrow aspirate with a small, monolobed megakaryocyte, typical in MDS.

B12 and folate deficiency. These may be ruled out with serum and red cell measurements, respectively. Additionally, these defects should respond rapidly to replacement therapy. The anaemia of chronic disease is primarily a clinical diagnosis, but little dysplasia should be present. Alcoholism and/or hypersplenism can result in a mild pancytopenia, and an abnormal physical examination and normal bone marrow biopsy will rule these out. Bone marrow infiltration by a tumour or fibrosis usually presents with a myelophthisic blood smear consisting of nucleated red cells, teardrop red-cell forms, and a left-shifted myeloid series. Although both MDS and myeloproliferative diseases may present with a hypercellular marrow, it should not be difficult to delineate these two. Myeloproliferative disorders are not marked by dysplasia and bone marrow failure, but by increased proliferation and usually elevated cell counts.

Classification

The 1976 FAB classification divided MDS into five subgroups based on the morphological appearance of the peripheral blood and bone marrow (Table 1). While newer prognostic systems, including a modification of the FAB classification recently proposed by the World Health Organization, are becoming more popular, and aspects of the FAB MDS classification, especially the inclusion of CMMoL, have been criticized, this classification system remains helpful clinically and is the basis of patient stratification in most recent MDS research. In many patients, there is a gradual progression through the subgroups, eventually leading to acute leukaemia.

Refractory anaemia

Refractory anaemia accounts for approximately 25 per cent of all cases of MDS. By definition, less than 5 per cent blasts are present in the bone marrow, and less than 15 per cent ringed sideroblasts are seen with iron staining. Typically, dysplasia in the peripheral blood and bone marrow are minimal, and there are few chromosomal abnormalities. These patients have a relatively low risk of progressing to leukaemia, and may do well for prolonged periods of time.

Refractory anaemia with ringed sideroblasts (RARS)

Ringed sideroblasts are erythroblasts with iron-laden mitochondria encircling more than one-third of the nucleus. More than six Prussian Blue-stained iron granules must be noted, in more than 15 per cent of the cells to make the diagnosis of RARS. In addition, fewer than 5 per cent blasts must be found in the bone marrow. As alluded to above, several drug-induced and hereditary syndromes may also present with ringed sideroblasts: for example, alcohol- and isoniazid-induced and X-linked disease, respectively. It is important to differentiate these states, as their prognosis and treatment may be different than for RARS. For example, inherited RARS may sometimes be successfully treated with pyridoxine, and the most common complication is usually iron overload. RARS, like refractory anaemia, has a relatively low risk of progression to acute leukaemia (approximately 10 per cent), especially when only the erythroid series is suppressed. Median survival is 50 months.

Refractory anaemia with excess blasts (RAEB)

RAEB accounts for approximately 25 per cent of cases of MDS. While ringed sideroblasts may be present, a diagnosis of RAEB is made when the bone marrow contains 5 to 20 per cent blasts. Multiple lineages of cells are usually affected, and chromosomal abnormalities are often found. RAEB has a high rate of progression to acute leukaemia and of bone marrow failure.

Refractory anaemia with excess blasts in transformation (RAEBt)

A diagnosis of RAEBt is made when there are more than 5 per cent blasts in the peripheral blood, or 21 to 30 per cent blasts in the bone marrow. Auer rods (that is, abnormal, oblong lysosomes) may be present in these blasts. These patients have multiple chromosomal abnormalities and a dismal prognosis, with most progressing to acute leukaemia. Obviously the decision that 29 per cent blasts in the marrow confers a diagnosis of MDS, while 31 per cent blasts meet the criteria of leukaemia is artefactual and arbitrary. Even some cases of RAEB, where the bone marrow blasts are less than 20 per cent, clinically behave as—and might be better considered—an evolving acute leukaemia. Thus a proportion of RAEBt cases may be acute leukaemia diagnosed relatively early. The classification of RAEBt is most helpful in those with documented long-term cytopenias and MDS, and characteristic chromosomal abnormalities. Mortality of patients with RAEBt is not dramatically different than those with acute leukaemia, and in fact survivors whose acute leukaemia has evolved from RAEBt have a higher rate of relapse after aggressive chemotherapy.

Chronic myelomonocytic leukaemia (CMMoL)

CMMoL, characterized by fewer than 20 per cent bone marrow blasts and a peripheral monocytosis of more than 1000 monocytes/μl, has many similarities to myeloproliferative diseases such as chronic myelogenous leukaemia. The white blood cell count is typically very elevated, marrow fibrosis can occur, and extramedullary diseases (hepatosplenomegaly, skin) and serositis are common. Splenomegaly is found in approximately 20 per cent of the cases. However, similar to other MDS types, trilineage dysplasia is typically evident. Prognosis best correlates with the percentage of bone marrow blasts, not with the degree of peripheral monocytosis. Approximately 25 per cent of patients progress to acute leukaemia, and death due to cytopenia is common.

Other subtypes of MDS- 5q- and secondary MDS

The 5q- syndrome is a unique subtype of MDS with specific morphological, laboratory, and clinical characteristics. Platelet counts are typically normal, or even elevated. Megakaryocytes are small and hypolobulated. When the only chromosomal abnormality is a deletion of 5, patients have

Table 1 General characteristics of MDS subtypes

MDS type	Peripheral blood blasts (%)	Bone marrow blasts (%)	Monocytosis (>1000/ml)	Ringed sideroblasts (%)	Chromosomal abnormality	AML progression (%)	Median survival (months)
RA	<5	<5	No	–	–	10–15	50
RARS	<5	<5	No	>15	+	10	51
RAEB	<5	5–20	No	± >15	++	30	12
RAEBt	>5	21–30	No/Yes	± >15	+++	60	6
CMMoL	<5	5–20	Yes	± >15	+	20–30	16

RA, refractory anaemia; RARS, refractory anaemia with ringed sideroblasts, RAEB, refractory anaemia with excess blasts; RAEBt, refractory anaemia with excess blasts in transformation; CMMoL, chronic myelomonocytic leukaemia.

an excellent prognosis with a low risk of transforming to a leukaemic state.

Secondary, or treatment-related MDS, is becoming more prevalent. This is probably due to several factors. Patients with solid malignancies are being treated with more aggressive chemotherapeutic regimens, and they are living longer after these treatments. In addition, it has been postulated that haemopoietic growth-factor support during intensive chemotherapy may be a contributing factor to the development of MDS. Most cases of secondary MDS present within the first decade after treatment. Chromosomal abnormalities are common, occurring more than 90 per cent of the time. Chromosomes 5 or 7, are typically involved, with monosomy 7 occurring in 60 per cent of the cases. Alkylating agents and topoisomerase II inhibitors are the most commonly implicated in causing secondary MDS.

Treatment

With the exception of allogeneic transplant there is no curative treatment for MDS. In addition, once acute leukaemia has evolved from MDS, treatment with aggressive chemotherapy does not usually result in long-term, curative, remission. Although there are several treatments for MDS, there are little data to suggest that drug treatment of MDS prolongs survival over that of standard, supportive care. However, treatment can improve quality of life, and new treatments are being explored.

Because of the limits of therapy, there is no need to treat asymptomatic patients, except when an allogeneic bone marrow transplant is clinically possible and the patient wishes to undergo such a procedure. Thus, mild anaemia and thrombocytopenia without bleeding do not necessitate transfusion. There is no evidence that prophylactic antibiotics are beneficial. However, for symptomatic anaemia, or anaemia in the older patient with cardiovascular disease, and for severely thrombocytopenic patients with episodes of bleeding or who are at high risk for significant bleeds, supportive transfusions are the mainstay of care. Patients may need regular transfusions. It is important to recognize patients who will live for long periods with red cell transfusion; such patients should have their iron status followed, and be initiated on iron chelation therapy to avoid the side-effects of haemosiderosis.

A wide range of myeloablative chemotherapeutic regimens have been explored; for instance, regimens commonly used to treat acute myelogenous leukaemia (**AML**), including aplasia-inducing doses of cytosine arabinoside (**Ara-C**), anthracyclines, cytoxan, and topotecan. A few studies have suggested that selected patients with good-risk characteristics may do as well with such regimens as patients with AML, but the results have usually been disappointing. Complete responses have ranged from 10 to 50 per cent, but these are generally of short duration and accompanied by significant morbidity and mortality. This is probably due to several factors, including the relatively older age of most patients with MDS, the drug resistance of MDS due to the increased expression of multidrug resistance proteins, and limited reserves of normal, healthy marrow for recovery. Low-dose chemotherapy has also been used. While initially explored because these dosing regimens are better tolerated in the older MDS population, many of these agents may have differentiating as well as cytotoxic effects. Low-dose Ara-C, 5-azacytidine, and topotecan have been used. These have resulted in complete responses from 10 to 40 per cent, but again these responses are not durable. Trials with low-dose Ara-C or 5-azacytidine showed no improvement in survival over supportive care. There is still significant scientific enthusiasm for exploring other dosing regimens, other differentiating agents, alone or in combination with growth factors and cytotoxic agents, in the treatment of MDS. For CMMoL, hydroxycarbamide (hydroxyurea) and the control of peripheral monocytosis has been shown to be as effective as aggressive chemotherapy.

Although most patients with MDS are ineligible for an allogeneic stem-cell transplant (either because of their age, comorbid disease, or lack of suitable donor), for some this remains a viable option and hope for cure. Bone marrow transplantation has been successively carried out in highly selected 55- to 66-year-old patients with MDS. The 5-year survival rate for all patients undergoing transplantation ranges from 30 to 70 per cent, but early mortality is common. Patients with refractory anaemia and RARS and younger patients have the best outcomes with transplantation. Normal or good chromosomal abnormalities are also predictive of a better response with a transplant. All high-risk (see next section) young patients should be considered for allogeneic bone marrow transplantation.

Multiple trials have utilized haemopoietic growth factors, such as erythropoietin and granulocyte colony-stimulating factor (**G-CSF**) (or granulocyte–macrophage colony-stimulating factor, **GM-CSF**), sometimes in combination. Short-term (1–2 weeks) and prolonged treatment with erythropoietin and G-CSF or GM-CSF do not appear to increase the progression to acute leukaemia. In a majority of patients, neutrophil counts increase, sometimes with a documented decrease in infection, and there are often improvements in red cell and platelet counts with decreased transfusion requirements. Some patients may actually respond with a decreased platelet count, and some patients may not tolerate some of the side-effects of the injections. Current evidence suggests that overall survival does not appear to be improved. Generally higher doses of erythropoietin (>200 U/kg per day) may be necessary, and patients with lower serum erythropoietin levels (<500 mU/ml) tend to have better responses. Laboratory data has suggested that the combination of erythropoietin and G-CSF may be synergistic in promoting the growth of haemopoietic progenitor colonies. Several clinical studies have suggested that the combination of erythropoietin and G-CSF is more effective than either alone, especially in patients with low serum erythropoietin levels and in those with ringed sideroblasts. Ciclosporin, an immunosuppressant, has also recently been reported as effective in MDS, especially when the marrow is hypocellular. In general, treatment choices should be based on the patient's performance status and age, the prognosis of the disease, and, whenever possible, in the setting of a clinical research protocol.

Prognosis

The median survival of all those with MDS has been reported to be between 12 and 28 months. However, since MDS consists of a variety of diseases, prognosis varies widely. A number of prognostic factors have been studied. Many of the factors which have proven to be predictive in prospective and retrospective studies are intuitive. Because the most common causes of death in patients with MDS are transformation to leukaemia or symptomatic cytopenias, a poorer prognosis is seen in those with increased bone marrow blasts and with more severe cytopenias. Other important prognostic factors include age and specific karyotypic abnormalities.

Because the FAB classification is for the most part dependent on the percentage of bone marrow blasts, the FAB subtypes closely correlate with both overall survival and evolution to acute leukaemia (Fig. 2). Those with refractory anaemia (**RA**) and RARS have a low incidence of leukaemia, both within the first 2 years and overall, and an improved survival rate. Patients with increased blasts, seen in RAEB and RAEBt do worse, and the overall survival in RAEBt is not significantly different than AML. Virtually all patients with RAEBt evolve to acute leukaemia within 30 months. Univariate analysis has also indicated that those with two or three cytopenias do worse than those with none or just one cytopenia, probably because those with more cytopenias have increased blasts, and are more prone to bleeding and infection. Marrow cytogenetics have also been found to be important. A relatively good prognosis is found in deletions of 5q, 20q, -Y in men, or normal cytogenetics. Of note, when these deletions are accompanied with other chromosomal abnormalities, they do not connote a good prognosis. Those with complex chromosomal abnormalities, or deletions of 7 do particularly poorly, with a high progression to acute leukaemia.

Several of these prognostic indicators have been combined in various scoring systems to predict the survival of patients with MDS. One of the most accurate, and most widely used, is the International Prognostic Scoring System (**IPSS**) (Table 2). The IPSS assigns points for unfavourable characteristics, such as unbalanced chromosomal translocations, percentage of blasts in the bone marrow, and lineages affected by the MDS. Although the IPSS is somewhat cumbersome to use for clinicians, and no scoring system is perfect for individual patients, the IPSS is useful for investigators and for making general decisions regarding the aggressiveness of treatment.

Further research

Increasing information on normal stem-cell biology and haemopoiesis will clearly lead to increased understanding of the abnormal haemopoietic development seen in MDS. Particular areas of research being explored include the role of apoptosis in MDS, and specific genetic mutations (or

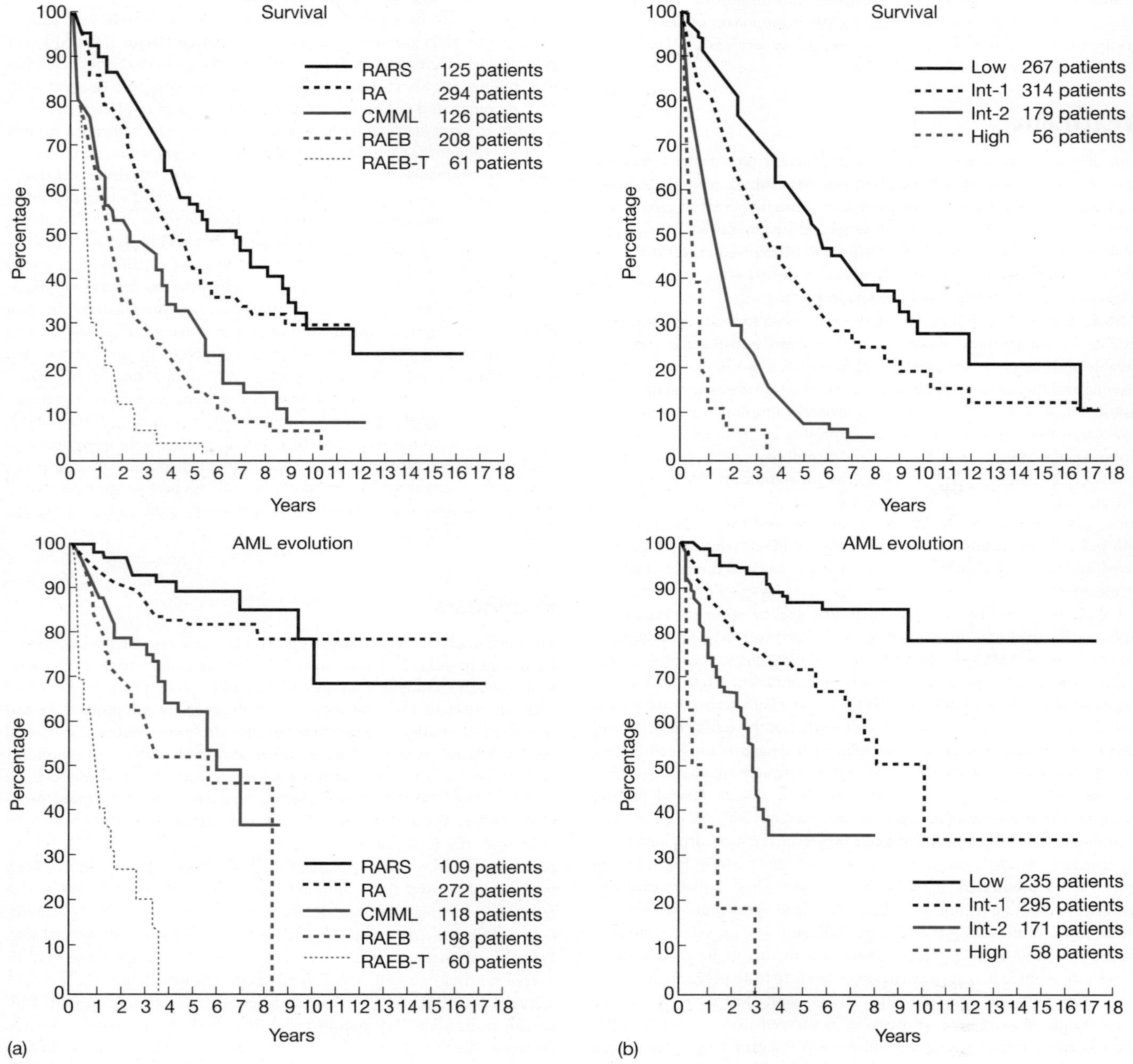

Fig. 2 Survival and evolution to leukaemia in MDS in groups defined by FAB classification (a) and IPSS (b). RA, refractory anaemia; RARS, refractory anaemia with ringed sideroblasts; RAEB, refractory anaemia with excess blasts; RAEBt, refractory anaemia with excess blasts in transformation; CMMoL, chronic myelomonocytic leukaemia. IPSS as defined in Table 2. (Figures taken from Greenberg P, *et al.* (1997). International scoring system for evaluating prognosis in myelodysplastic syndromes. *Blood* **89**, 2079–88, with permission from the publisher.)

Table 2 The International Prognostic Scoring System (IPSS)

Prognostic variable	Score 0	0.5	1.0	1.5	2
Marrow blasts (%)	<5	5–10	–	11–20	21–30
Cytogenetics	Good	Intermediate	Poor		
Cytopenias	0–1	2–3			

Risk category	Combined score
Low	0
Intermediate-1	0.5–1.0
Intermediate-2	1.5–2.0
High	≥ 2.5

Cytogenetics: 'good', normal, -Y, del(5q), del(20q); 'poor', complex, chromosome 7 abnormalities; 'intermediate', all others.

Cytopenias: neutrophils <1.8 × 103/μl; platelets <105/μl; haemoglobin <10 g/dl.

groups of mutations) that are necessary for the development of MDS. The importance of individual mutations or chromosomal abnormalities for prognosis is still being explored. A major emphasis in the stem-cell transplantation field is on increasing the availability of transplants. This includes making transplantation less toxic through non-myeloablative induction strategies, capitalizing on the graft-versus-tumour phenomena, and increasing the number of potential donors with international registries and by minimizing the importance of HLA barriers. Clearly these improvements will aid in the treatment of MDS. The most active area of research in specific treatment of MDS, is in the role of non-toxic differentiating agents.

Further reading

Bennett JM, *et al.* (1982). FAB Cooperative Group L Proposal for the classification of the myelodysplastic syndromes. *British Journal of Haematology* **51**, 189–99.

Cheson BD (1998). Standard and low-dose chemotherapy for the treatment of myelodysplastic syndromes. *Leukemia Research* **22**(Suppl 1), S17–21.

Deeg HJ, Appelbaum FR (2000). Hematopoietic stem cell transplantation for myelodysplastic syndrome. *Current Opinion in Oncology* **12**, 116–20.

Deeg HJ *et al.* (2000). Allogeneic and syngeneic marrow transplantation for myelodysplastic syndrome in patients 55–66 years of age. *Blood* **15**, 1188–94.

Eillman CL (1998). Molecular genetic features of myelodysplastic syndromes. *Leukaemia* **12**(Suppl 1), S2–6.

Estey EH (1998). Prognosis and therapy of secondary myelodysplastic syndromes. *Haematologica* **83**, 543–9.

Greenberg P (2000). Myelodysplastic syndrome. In: Hoffman R, *et al.*, eds. *Hematology: basic principles and practice*, pp 1106–29. Churchill Livingstone, New York.

Greenberg P, *et al.* (1997). International scoring system for evaluating prognosis in myelodysplastic syndromes. *Blood* **89**, 2079–88.

Hellstrom-Lindberg E, *et al.* (1997). Erythroid responses to treatment with G-CSF plus erythropoietin for the anaemia of patients with myelodysplastic syndromes: proposal for a predictive model. *British Journal of Haematology* **99**, 344–51.

Sole F, *et al.* (2000). Incidence, characterization and prognostic significance of chromosomal abnormalities in 640 patients with primary myelodysplastic syndromes. Grups Cooperativo Espanol de Citogenetica Hematologica. *British Journal of Haematology* **108**, 346–56.

Yoshida Y, Mufti GJ (1999). Apoptosis and its significance in MDS: controversies revisited. *Leukemia Research* **23**, 777–85.

22.3.8 The polycythaemias

David M. Gustin and Ronald Hoffman

Introduction

Polycythaemia or erythrocytosis is associated with an aetiologically distinct group of disorders characterized by an abnormal increase in the numbers of red blood cells, leading to an elevation in the haemoglobin concentration and haematocrit. Absolute polycythaemias (increased red cell mass) can be attributed to either an intrinsic defect of haemopoietic stem cells (primary) or to the stimulation of progenitor cells by excessive levels of circulating growth factors (secondary). A pathophysiological classification of polycythaemia is offered in Table 1. Patients with absolute polycythaemias should be distinguished from individuals in whom a minimally elevated haematocrit is not accompanied by a corresponding absolute increase in the red cell mass (spurious polycythaemia, stress erythrocytosis, Gaisbock's syndrome), but rather by a contraction of plasma volume.

Erythropoiesis

Erythropoietin (EPO), a 34.4-kDa glycoprotein hormone, is the primary humoral regulator of red blood cell production. Erythropoiesis occurs at a low baseline level to replace normal, senescent red blood cells. Decreased tissue oxygen tension increases erythropoietin levels by enhancing expression of the *EPO* gene. The circulating, secreted erythropoietin binds to receptors present on erythroid progenitor cells, promoting the proliferation and differentiation of erythroid precursors, ultimately resulting in an increased red cell mass. This complex process enhances the oxygen-carrying capacity of blood, leading to elevated tissue oxygen tension and down-modulating erythropoietin production. A peritubular interstitial cell is the primary site of erythropoietin production in the kidney. An oxygen-sensing haem protein present in these cells is essential for the control of erythropoietin production. It induces the transcription of EPO mRNA, a phenomenon mediated by hypoxia-inducible factors (**HIF**), a group of nucleoproteins that interact with the enhancer element of the *EPO* gene. The kidney has no preformed stores of erythropoietin. Increases in plasma levels are primarily due to new hormone synthesis. Since anaemia or hypoxia does not seem to influence, to any significant degree, the plasma clearance of erythropoietin, the control appears to occur mainly at the level of gene expression. Erythropoietin production also occurs in the liver to a lesser degree. The severity of hypoxia required to induce its production is much greater than that required in the kidney.

Table 1 Classification of polycythaemia

Relative polycythaemias	
Associated with volume loss or contraction:	
	Gastrointestinal losses: diarrhoea, vomiting, ileostomy
	Renal losses: osmotic diuresis, therapeutic diuresis, Addison's syndrome, hypercalcaemia
	Insensible losses: profuse sweating, fever
	Stress or Gaisbok's polycythaemia
Absolute polycythaemias	
Primary polycythaemias	
	Primary familial and congenital polycythaemia (PFCP)
	Polycythaemia vera
Secondary polycythaemias associated with appropriate secretion of EPO	
	Smokers' polycythaemia
	Hypobaric hypoxia
	Chronic pulmonary disease
	Alveolar hypoventilation
	Congenital heart diseases associated with right-to-left shunts
	High-affinity haemoglobins
	2,3-DPG deficiency
	Methaemoglobinaemias
	Chuvash polycythaemia
Secondary polycythaemias associated with inappropriate secretion of EPO	
	Polycythaemia of renal disease
	Tumour-associated polycythaemia
	Endocrine disorders: phaeochromocytomas, aldosterone-producing adenomas, Cushing's syndrome[1]

EPO, erythropoietin; 2,3-DPG, 2,3-diphosphoglycerate.

[1] Probably related to marrow stimulation by steroid hormones.

Oxygen transport is a complex process dependent on a number of variables, such as ambient oxygen levels, minute ventilation, lung diffusion capacity, cardiac output, red cell mass, regional blood flow, tissue capillary density, and haemoglobin–oxygen affinity. Acute changes in tissue oxygen demands or in environmental oxygen levels are compensated not only by increased erythropoietin production but also in minute ventilation, cardiac output, blood flow distribution, and haemoglobin–oxygen affinity (through the modulation of 2,3-diphosphoglycerate (**2,3-DPG**) production). Sustained hypoxia is required for polycythaemia to occur as a compensatory mechanism.

Relative polycythaemias

A common group of disorders is marked by an elevated haemoglobin or haematocrit as the result of the contraction in plasma volume. The red cell mass remains normal. There are two major groups of patients with relative polycythaemias. The first includes patients with more acute conditions associated with significant degrees of dehydration with a consequent decrease in extracellular volume: for example, gastrointestinal fluid losses, therapeutic diuresis, endocrine disorders such as Addison's disease, and hypercalcaemia. In most cases, the presence of volume contraction is clinically obvious. The aetiology of the increase in haematocrit does not usually present a diagnostic challenge.

The second group is associated with a chronic low-level increase in the haematocrit. These patients are frequently active, hard-working, middle-aged, mildly hypertensive, obese males subjected to considerable stress who present with persistent polycythaemia. Characteristically, they appear plethoric but without any of the other typical features of polycythaemia vera. The cause for the contraction in the plasma volume is poorly understood, but autonomic dysregulation with changes in venous capacitance have been suggested.

The usual range of haemoglobin in these individuals is between 18 and 20 g/dl with haematocrits ranging from 49 to 55 per cent. Most of these patients seek medical evaluation for an unrelated condition, and are incidentally found to have increased haemoglobin and haematocrit values.

Suitable advice regarding weight reduction, control of hypertension, and smoking cessation is usually given to these patients. Evidence associating the mild elevations in viscosity encountered in this condition with episodes of thrombosis is incomplete. It seems sensible to recommend phlebotomy for those patients who have already experienced thrombotic episodes and who have persistent elevations of their haematocrits. It is more difficult to justify phlebotomy in asymptomatic individuals with mild elevations in haematocrit.

Absolute polycythaemia

Absolute polycythaemias may be classified as being primary, due to autonomous cell growth or to an enhanced response to growth factors that promote the proliferation of developing erythroid cells, or secondary, due to excessive production of erythropoietin in response to a variety of stimuli. Primary polycythaemia caused by defects in haemopoietic stem cells, is accompanied by low levels of circulating erythropoietin. Germline mutations that lead to enhanced erythropoiesis cause primary familial congenital polycythaemias. Polycythaemia vera, the most common primary polycythaemia, is caused by an acquired defect in haemopoietic stem cells resulting in an excessive proliferation of myeloid cells. By contrast, secondary polycythaemia is generally associated with elevated erythropoietin production. Raised levels of plasma erythropoietin can accompany systemic hypoxaemia, certain neoplasms, and disorders that impair oxygen delivery to tissues.

Absolute polycythaemias are accompanied by an elevated red cell mass. Documentation of such a mass to confirm the presence of an absolute polycythaemia usually requires a blood volume study with direct quantitation of both the red cell mass and plasma volume. An haematocrit greater than 60 per cent in men and greater than 55 per cent in women, however, are almost always associated with absolute erythrocytosis. In such cases it is frequently unnecessary to perform blood volume studies to be assured that the patient has an absolute polycythaemia.

Secondary polycythaemias associated with appropriate erythropoietin secretion

This group of polycythaemias encompasses a number of conditions that are ultimately the result of tissue hypoxia and subsequent excessive erythropoietin production leading to erythrocytosis. These disorders are collectively regarded as hypoxic erythrocytoses.

Hypobaric hypoxia

At high altitudes the barometric pressure and, consequently, the ambient oxygen tension are reduced, resulting in alveolar and arterial hypoxia. Natives of the Andes mountains who live above 4200 metres have been reported to have haematocrits 30 per cent higher than individuals who live at sea level. Acutely, changes in minute ventilation, heart rate, blood flow, and haemoglobin–oxygen affinity occur as an individual reaches a high altitude. Serum erythropoietin is elevated initially, but eventually returns to the normal range in the absence of extreme hypoxia. This decline will not prevent the increase in red cell mass, which will be sustained, because early unsustained elevations of erythropoietin promote expansion of the erythroid progenitor pool. Only very small quantities of the hormone are subsequently required to sustain the red cell mass under normal circumstances.

A decrease in the plasma volume frequently accompanies hypoxic erythrocytoses resulting in further elevation of the haematocrit. Some individuals who live at high altitudes for prolonged periods develop chronic mountain sickness. They suffer from headaches, fatigue, impaired exercise tolerance, cyanosis, clubbing, right heart failure, and absolute polycythaemia. These symptoms frequently resolve with therapeutic phlebotomy.

Chronic pulmonary disease

Pulmonary diseases are a common cause of secondary polycythaemias. Defects in gas exchange result in hypoxia, with consequent increases in erythropoietin and red cell mass. Not every patient with hypoxia secondary to respiratory disease develops polycythaemia. The presence of concurrent inflammation or infection may blunt the marrow response to hypoxia. It is important to be aware that smoking itself may also contribute significantly to the polycythaemia associated with chronic respiratory disease. Phlebotomy may be indicated in patients with relatively high haematocrits (55–60 per cent), given the known deleterious effects of increased viscosity on tissue perfusion.

Alveolar hypoventilation

Hypoventilation may lead to hypoxia and an erythropoietin-mediated increase in red cell mass. These disorders include the sleep apnoea syndrome and supine hypoventilation. In these conditions, significant degrees of hypoxia may occur without evident parenchymal pulmonary disease. Decreases in blood oxygen content may occur intermittently, consequently erythropoietin levels and arterial blood gas values may be normal. Diseases affecting the central nervous system may impair respiratory centre function and trigger hypoventilation. These defects have been described in association with encephalitis, cerebrovascular accidents, and drug intoxication (that is, barbiturates). Impaired skeletal muscle function of the chest wall or diaphragm may also sufficiently compromise alveolar ventilation to trigger polycythaemia. In these cases, correction of hypoxia is warranted. The role of phlebotomy is unclear, but not unreasonable in patients with significant elevations in haematocrit and associated cardiovascular or cerebrovascular disease.

Cardiovascular disease

Cyanotic congenital heart diseases with associated right-to-left shunt result in oxygen desaturation and an elevation of erythropoietin, causing secondary polycythaemia. After compensatory erythrocytosis in response to oxygen desaturation occurs, serum erythropoietin levels may return to normal levels. Characteristically, therapeutic phlebotomy is associated with marked increases in erythropoietin levels. Some children with congenital heart disease may develop extreme haematocrit values (80 per cent or higher), which lead to a clear risk of a thrombotic event, especially during periods of dehydration. Phlebotomy may be indicated in some instances: for example, in preparation for elective surgery. Further clinical information is required to establish the precise target haematocrit value for therapeutic phlebotomy in the management of these disorders.

Carbon monoxide intoxication

Chronic carbon monoxide intoxication most commonly occurs as a consequence of smoking. Elevated haematocrits have been reported in 3 per cent of all smokers. Other less common causes include work-related exposures such as those seen in caisson workers or tunnel toll-collectors. Carbon monoxide has a much higher affinity for haemoglobin than oxygen, thereby reducing the amount of oxygen that can be bound and transported by haemoglobin. It also shifts the oxygen–haemoglobin dissociation curve to the left, decreasing the ability of haemoglobin to release oxygen to peripheral tissues. Furthermore, carbon monoxide impairs normal compensatory mechanisms; carboxyhaemoglobin is known to decrease 2,3-DPG production by red cells and to reduce the affinity of haemoglobin for 2,3-DPG. Polycythaemia due to chronic carbon monoxide intoxication may be associated with an increased risk of thromboembolic phenomena. Phlebotomy may be indicated in patients with very high haematocrits (>55–60 per cent).

The decreased oxygen-carrying capacity associated with carbon monoxide intoxication is not detected by standard blood gas measurements, therefore a direct measure of carboxyhaemoglobin levels is required. Morning carboxyhaemoglobin levels ranging from 4 per cent to 20 per cent have been reported. Individuals with chronic carbon monoxide poisoning may experience neuropsychiatric and cardiac abnormalities. The treatment is smoking cessation or removal of the patient from the alternative source of carbon monoxide.

High-affinity haemoglobins

At least 50 haemoglobin variants exhibit increased avidity for oxygen. Oxygen transport by haemoglobin occurs as a function of the oxygen–haemoglobin affinity curve. This function is represented by a sigmoid-shaped curve and is a reflection of the initial binding of oxygen by deoxygenated haemoglobin occurring with significant difficulty. As oxygen molecules are bound to normal haemoglobin, further binding is facilitated by structural changes that occur to the haemoglobin molecule. High-affinity haemoglobin variants arise when mutations alter key amino acid residues in regions of haemoglobin that affect these rearrangements, or at the interface between α- and β-chains. Another group of mutations induces changes in oxygen affinity indirectly, by causing structural changes in haemoglobin regions that are critical for the binding of 2,3-DPG.

Increases in oxygen affinity result in a shift of the oxygen dissociation curve to the left. Consequently haemoglobin binds oxygen more readily and retains more oxygen at lower P_{O2} (partial pressure of O2) levels. This ultimately results in decreased delivery of oxygen to tissues where capillary P_{O2} is low (35–45 mmHg). Mild tissue hypoxia then triggers an increase in the production of erythropoietin with consequent polycythaemia.

Oxygen affinity by a variant haemoglobin is usually measured as the $P_{50}O_2$, which represents the partial oxygen pressure at which 50 per cent of haemoglobin is saturated with oxygen. This analysis is necessary for the identification of patients with high-affinity haemoglobins. High-affinity haemoglobins are associated with lower than normal values of $P_{50}O_2$. Haemoglobin electrophoresis may, on occasion, aid in the recognition of an abnormal haemoglobin, but many high-affinity haemoglobins display normal electrophoretic mobility. Conversely, the presence of an abnormal band *per se* does not provide information regarding oxygen affinity. A study of family members is important, but a negative family history does not negate the diagnosis since there is a high rate of spontaneous mutations.

Most patients with high-affinity haemoglobins have mild polycythaemia and are asymptomatic since the compensatory polycythaemia results in normal oxygen delivery to tissues. On rare occasions, very high haematocrits (>55–60 per cent) associated with elevated blood viscosity may be sufficient to warrant therapeutic phlebotomy.

Methaemoglobinaemias

Hereditary methaemoglobinaemia may be associated with a mild polycythaemia. Methaemoglobin results from the oxidation of ferrous ions (Fe^{2+}) to the ferric state (Fe^{3+}). Oxygen does not bind reversibly to methaemoglobin, so resulting in a left shift of the oxygen dissociation curve, impaired oxygen delivery, and chronic tissue hypoxia.

2,3-Diphosphoglycerate (2,3-DPG) deficiency

This rare familial form of polycythaemia is due to a deficiency of the enzyme diphosphoglyceromutase. Deficiency leads to a decrease in 2,3-DPG, resulting in the increased affinity of oxygen to haemoglobin, peripheral tissue hypoxia, and hypoxic erythrocytosis. This disorder should be suspected in patients with familial polycythaemia with a low $P_{50}O_2$ in the absence of a mutant haemoglobin. Measurements of 2,3-DPG in fresh red cells reveals reduced levels.

Chuvash polycythaemia

Chuvash polycythaemia is a recently recognized form of congenital and familial polycythaemia that is endemic to the Chuvash population of the Russian Federation. The extreme elevations of haemoglobin in this autosomal recessive disorder are accompanied by increased erythropoietin levels.

Excessive elaboration of erythropoietin is thought to be due to an abnormality of the oxygen-sensing mechanism. These patients present with isolated erythrocytosis without elevations of white cells or platelets. Death frequently occurs before the age of 40 due to thrombotic and haemorrhagic complications.

Secondary polycythaemias associated with the inappropriate secretion of erythropoietin

Enhanced erythropoietin levels and secretion occur in the absence of tissue hypoxia in this group of disorders. The erythropoietin response is therefore inappropriate to systemic oxygen requirements.

Polycythaemia of renal disease

As the kidney is the major site of erythropoietin production, it is not surprising that renal disorders may be associated with erythrocytosis or anaemia. Patients with hypertension and renal artery stenosis have a higher incidence of erythrocytosis than similarly hypertensive patients without renal artery disease. Other benign kidney diseases associated with an increase in erythropoietin production and erythrocytosis include polycystic kidney disease (acquired or familial) and renal cysts. Unusual patients with glomerulonephritis may also occasionally present with an elevated haematocrit. An uncommon cause of polycythaemia is Bartter's syndrome, an hereditary tubular disorder characterized by hypokalaemia secondary to renal potassium loss in association with elevated plasma renin activity and aldosterone secretion. Between 5 and 13 per cent of patients have been reported to develop erythrocytosis following renal transplantation. It has been postulated that the excessive erythropoietin response originates from the patient's own kidneys and not from the transplanted one. Angiotensin-converting enzyme inhibitors may prove useful in controlling post-transplantation polycythaemia. Phlebotomy may be required in patients with haematocrit levels over 55 to 60 per cent.

Tumour-associated polycythaemia

A number of tumours are associated with an inappropriately increased production of erythropoietin, including benign and malignant tumours of the kidney, hepatomas, cerebellar haemangioblastomas, and phaeochromocytomas. Polycythaemia occurs in 1 per cent of patients with renal carcinomas, 9 to 20 per cent of patients with cerebellar haemangioblastomas, and 10 per cent of patients with hepatomas. Resection of the tumour, if feasible, may be associated with regression of the polycythaemia. Therapeutic phlebotomy is recommended in patients with extreme increases in the haematocrit.

Endocrine disorders

Phaeochromocytomas and aldosterone-producing adenomas have been associated with increased levels of erythropoietin. Mild forms of polycythaemia have also been observed in some patients with Cushing's syndrome, probably related to marrow stimulation by steroid hormone.

Primary polycythaemia

Primary familial and congenital polycythaemia (PFCP)

PFCP is an inherited form of polycythaemia caused by mutations in the erythropoietin receptor, thereby resulting in the hypersensitivity of erythroid progenitor cells to erythropoietin and low serum erythropoietin levels. In the autosomal dominant form of the disease, family members have plethora, headaches, dizziness, nose bleeds, and exertional dyspnoea. These symptoms resolve with phlebotomy and reduction of the haematocrit. Not all cases of PFPC can be attributed to the mutations of the erythropoietin receptor, suggesting that other genetic defects can lead to a similar phenotype.

Polycythaemia vera

Polycythaemia vera is a malignancy characterized by excessive proliferation of erythroid, myeloid, and megakaryocytic elements in the bone marrow. Its hallmark is an absolute increase in the red cell mass usually associated with leucocytosis, thrombocytosis, and splenomegaly. In contrast to other haematological malignancies, patients suffering from polycythaemia vera may enjoy prolonged survival, provided that the excessive production of red cells and platelets is controlled. This survival is occasionally punctuated by the development of myelofibrosis and/or acute leukaemia.

Epidemiology

Polycythaemia vera is a rare disorder, the estimated yearly incidence in the Western world is between 5 and 17 cases per 1 million of the population. Its true prevalence is unknown but it seems to be more common in Ashkenazi Jews and rarer in Afro-Americans. A very low incidence of 2 cases per year per million population has been reported in Japan. These differences suggest that environmental as well as genetic factors might be important.

Polycythaemia vera is slightly more common in males than in females, with a male to female ratio of 1.2:1. The average age at diagnosis is 60 years, it is very rare in individuals younger than 30 years of age. Only a handful of cases have being reported during childhood.

Biological and molecular aspects

The exaggerated production of red cells, granulocytes, and platelets in polycythaemia vera suggests that the fundamental defect occurs at the level of the pluripotent haemopoietic stem cell. The clonal, and thereby malignant, nature of polycythaemia vera was first established by the cellular analysis of blood cell production, in heterozygous Afro-American women, of X-linked glucose-6-phosphate dehydrogenase (**G6PD**) isoenzymes. These results have recently been confirmed using restriction fragment length polymorphisms (**RFLPs**) of the active X-chromosomes.

In patients with polycythaemia vera, erythropoietin levels often fall below the 95 per cent confidence interval for normal individuals. These low levels persist even after repeated phlebotomies, suggesting that excessive production of erythropoietin is not a critical component in the pathogenesis of this disorder. Using *in vitro* cell-culture systems, polycythaemia-vera bone marrow can form erythroid colonies in the absence of erythropoietin (endogenous colonies). Erythroid progenitor cells derived from normal individuals are incapable of forming such colonies in the absence of exogenous erythropoietin. In addition to the erythroid colonies, mixed-lineage colonies are frequently formed in the absence of exogenous erythropoietin, suggesting the involvement by not just erythroid precursors but also of more primitive haemopoietic progenitor cells. Both malignant and normal cells are present in the bone marrow of patients with polycythaemia vera, but the malignant cells have a growth advantage. Most peripheral blood elements are thus derived from the neoplastic clone. We now know that the clonal assay systems that were first used to produce endogenous erythroid colonies contained trace quantities of erythropoietin. In newer systems that are absolutely devoided of erythropoietin, the progenitor cells in polycythaemia vera require erythropoietin, but clearly demonstrate increased sensitivity to this growth factor.

Polycythaemia vera progenitor cells are also hypersensitive to other cytokines such as steel factor, interleukin-3 (**IL-3**), and granulocyte–macrophage colony-stimulating factor (**GM-CSF**). These responses require the presence of insulin-like growth factor-1 (**IGF-1**) or of its binding protein (**IGFBP-1**). At present, the primary signalling protein defect that underlies the characteristic hypersensitivity to this broad group of cytokines remains unknown.

Pathobiology

Patients with polycythaemia vera have an increased thrombotic tendency resulting from the expansion of the red cell mass. There is a direct relationship between the risk of thrombosis and age, suggesting that the presence of vascular disease might be important. Younger individuals are also at risk for thrombotic episodes, many of them life-threatening. The main rheological abnormality is elevated total blood viscosity. Cerebral blood flow is reduced in patients with polycythaemia vera and a haematocrit of 53 to 62 per cent. Reductions in blood flow are correctable by phlebotomy. Even small reductions in the haematocrit result in significant reduction in blood viscosity and cerebral blood flow. An increased haematocrit may facilitate the transport of platelets to the vessel wall, an event that may lead to thrombus formation. Elevation in blood viscosity also results in greater peripheral vascular resistance and a consequent reduction in organ blood flow, thereby increasing the likelihood of thrombus development. Thrombocytosis and functional platelet abnormalities are frequently present, and may play a role in the development of thrombosis. This relationship is still highly controversial.

Patients with polycythaemia vera are also at an increased risk of developing life-threatening haemorrhagic complications. Abnormalities in platelet function and number have been implicated. Qualitative platelet abnormalities include defective platelet aggregation *in vitro*, acquired storage pool disease, and dysregulated thromboxane A_2 metabolism. Patients with acquired von Willebrand syndromes have been described who have very high platelet counts ($>1000 \times 10^6/\mu l$), in association with life-threatening bleeding episodes. Leucocytosis, found in 50 per cent of patients, may impact negatively on the rheology of the microcirculation. No laboratory test has proven useful for the *a priori* identification of patients at an increased risk of developing haemorrhagic or thrombotic events.

The progression to the so-called 'spent phase' is a common cause of morbidity. This stage, also known as postpolycythaemic myeloid metaplasia (**PPMM**), is characterized by cytopenias, myelofibrosis, and extramedullary haemopoiesis. The fibroblastic component represents a reactive event, and may be due to the local release of growth factors, particularly platelet-derived growth factor. The association between the treatment modality and the development of myeloid metaplasia is as yet unclear. Clearer is the association between treatment type (alkylating agents and ^{32}P; see below), and the development of acute leukaemia. It must be emphasized, however, that even those patients treated with phlebotomy alone have a leukaemogenic risk significantly higher than that expected in the general population.

Clinical manifestations

The clinical manifestations of polycythaemia vera are the direct consequence of the excessive proliferation of cellular elements of the various haemopoietic cell lineages.

The routine and widespread use of laboratory screening tests during medical evaluations has led to an increased detection of asymptomatic patients. In contrast, symptomatic patients may present to their physician with a large array of non-specific complaints including headache, weakness, pruritus, dizziness, excessive sweating, visual disturbances, paraesthesias, joint symptoms, and epigastric distress. Some one-third of patients will have lost 10 per cent of their body weight by the time they present, presumably due to the associated hypermetabolism. Joint disease is usually the manifestation of gout, due to the increased production of uric acid. The most important signs on physical examination include ruddy cyanosis, conjunctival plethora, hepatomegaly, splenomegaly, and hypertension.

Patients left without appropriate treatment are at a particularly high risk of developing thrombotic or haemorrhagic events. In fact, thrombosis may be the cause of death in up to 30 to 40 per cent of patients. Thrombosis may occur in the deep venous system of the lower extremities, or present as a pulmonary embolism. Cerebrovascular, coronary, and peripheral vascular occlusions are not rare.

Thromboses at unusual sites are characteristic of polycythaemia vera. They include occlusion of the splenic, portal, hepatic, and mesenteric veins. Cardiac valve abnormalities affecting the aortic or the mitral valves are commonly seen, frequently in the form of leaflet thickening or frank vegetations. These lesions are associated with the occurrence of arterial thromboembolism. Hepatic venous or inferior vena caval thrombosis is known as Budd–Chiari syndrome. It is characterized by hepatosplenomegaly, ascites, oedema of the peripheral extremities, jaundice, abdominal pain, and distension of superficial abdominal veins due to portal hypertension. Some ten per cent of patients who present with Budd–Chiari syndrome have polycythaemia vera. At times, these patients will present with normal haemoglobin and haematocrit levels as a consequence of blood loss and expansion of the plasma volume. This phenomenon is regarded as 'inapparent polycythaemia vera' and requires direct quantification of the red cell mass for confirmation. Iron deficiency may also mask the expected erythrocytosis in some patients with polycythaemia vera. Leucocytosis, thrombocytosis, and splenomegaly are usually present. The definitive diagnosis of polycythaemia vera in this patient population requires the documentation of an elevated red cell mass.

Neurological abnormalities are also common and occur in up to 60 to 80 per cent of patients. They include transient ischaemic attacks, cerebral infarction, cerebral haemorrhage, confusional states, fluctuating dementia, and involuntary movement syndromes. Dizziness, paraesthesias, tinnitus, visual problems, and headaches are common symptoms attributed to the hyperviscosity state. Small infarcts in the basal ganglia region, also known as lacunae, might be related to some of the transient neurological manifestations. Symptoms of carotid or vertebral and basilar artery insufficiency occur frequently. Peripheral vascular insufficiency may be manifested by intense redness or cyanosis of the digits, burning, classical erythromelalgia, digital ischaemia with palpable pulses, or thrombophlebitis. Erythromelalgia consists of a burning pain in the digits of either the lower and/or upper extremities, an objective sensation of increased temperature, and relief by cooling. If left untreated it may evolve into gangrene. Antiplatelet aggregation therapy rapidly reverses the symptoms. Peripheral pulses are usually normal in these patients, as this phenomenon is due to changes in the microcirculation related to arteriolar activation and aggregation of platelets *in vivo*.

Haemorrhagic complications are the cause of death in 2 to 10 per cent of patients with polycythaemia vera: 30 to 40 per cent of patients will experience a haemorrhagic event sometime during the course of their disease. Peptic ulcer disease occurs frequently and contributes to the gastrointestinal tract being the most common source of bleeding. The bleeding diathesis may relate to abnormalities in platelet function, and thus occurs frequently after the ingestion of anti-inflammatory agents. Spontaneous bleeding is rare. Recent data suggests that low-dose aspirin might not increase the frequency of life-threatening haemorrhages.

The risk of postoperative complications is high in patients with polycythaemia vera. Bleeding, thrombosis, or a combination of both can occur. The risk is higher for those patients who undergo surgery with uncontrolled erythrocytosis. Generalized pruritus affects 50 per cent of all patients, but its aetiology is unknown. Increased blood and urine histamine levels have been implicated by some. Pruritus triggered by water contact is characteristic and tolerated very poorly. There is no relationship between the severity of the disease and the intensity of the pruritus. Up to 20 per cent of patients experience persistent pruritus in even after normalization of their counts.

Polycythaemia vera evolves to PPMM in up to 50 per cent of the patients 10 years, on average, after the initial diagnosis. It is characterized by increased splenomegaly, tear-drop red cells, a leucoerythroblastic blood picture, marrow fibrosis, and a normal or decreasing red cell mass. Fatigue, dizziness, weight loss, anorexia, progressive anaemia, and thrombocytopenia associated with bleeding are common. Patients with progressive anaemia should be evaluated for folate and iron deficiency. Occasional patients will respond to iron supplementation with resurgence of erythropoiesis. Severe hyperuricaemia may induce gout or uric acid nephropathy. PPMM portends a very grave prognosis with over two-thirds of patients dying within 3 years.

The evolution to acute leukaemia is probably the natural consequence of the malignant nature of polycythaemia vera, which can be accentuated by the therapeutic interventions commonly used for its treatment, such as alkylating agent use or radioactive phosphorus (^{32}P) administration. A randomized study conducted under the auspices of the Polycythaemia Vera Study Group (**PVSG**) comparing chlorambucil, ^{32}P, and phlebotomy is instructive. After 15 years of follow-up, 17.5 per cent of patients treated with chlorambucil and 10.9 per cent of those who received ^{32}P had developed acute leukaemia. Only 1.5 per cent of patients treated with phlebotomy alone developed acute leukaemia. This still represents a much higher incidence than the one expected in a normal age-matched population. Between 30 and 50 per cent of patients who develop leukaemia have previously entered the spent phase, whereas 50 per cent progress directly from the erythrocytotic phase. A significant number of patients experience a myelodysplastic interval before transforming. Large-cell lymphomas have been observed in roughly 3.5 per cent of patients treated with chlorambucil.

Laboratory evaluation

Polycythaemia vera is a panmyelosis. Some two-thirds of the patients present with leucocytosis and approximately 50 per cent with thrombocytosis. Red cell morphology usually reflects an underlying iron deficiency state: microcytosis, hypochromia, polychromatophilia, poikilocytosis, and anisocytosis are frequently seen. White blood cell morphology is usually normal. Increased numbers of basophils, eosinophils, and immature myeloid cells are observed. Megathrombocytes are often seen in the peripheral blood smear. Platelet counts are usually under $1 \times 10^6/\mu l$, but higher counts may be seen. The PPMM phase is characterized by a leucoerythroblastic response with the presence in the peripheral blood of tear-drop red cells (dacrocytes), immature myeloid cells, and nucleated red blood cells. Bleeding time and platelet aggregation studies are frequently, but not always, abnormal. Prolongation of prothrombin and partial thromboplastin times are frequently encountered, usually reflecting a laboratory artefact due to erythrocytosis (the volume of plasma in the collection tube might be too small relative to the amount of anticoagulant (citrate) present in these tubes).

Acquired von Willebrand factor (**vWF**) defects are frequently characterized by a significant decrease in large vWF multimers. This acquired defect resembles type II vWF disease. It occurs mainly in patients with very high platelet counts ($>1 \times 10^6/\mu l$), implicating the adsorption of larger forms of vWF multimers on to platelet membranes. The defect is corrected by normalization of the thrombocytosis. Elevations in leucocyte alkaline phosphatase (70 per cent), serum vitamin B12 levels (40 per cent), and serum vitamin B12 binding proteins (70 per cent) are common, as are hyperuricaemia and increased histamine levels.

Bone marrow examination reveals a hypercellular marrow with an increased number of megakaryocytes. The cellular elements are morphologically normal. Iron stores are usually absent prior to treatment. Reticulin is often seen, but is not predictive of evolution into the spent phase. At diagnosis, erythropoietin levels are either reduced or within the lower limits of normal. Low levels persist in two-thirds of patients after normalization of their haematocrit. Cytogenetic abnormalities have been described, but none are characteristic. Abnormalities in chromosomes 1, 5, 7, 8, 9, 12, 13, and 20 have been detected. The frequency and complexity of these chromosomal abnormalities are a function of the disease longevity and duration of treatment.

Diagnostic criteria of polycythaemia vera

Clinical criteria for the diagnosis of polycythaemia vera have been developed. These criteria have proven useful in defining a homogeneous study population for incorporation into clinical studies, but, in our opinion, the previously utilized criteria have a number of shortcomings that are of clinical relevance. In Table 2 we offer what we believe to be a more flexible and useful criteria utilizing modern diagnostic tools for the diagnosis of polycythaemia vera.

Table 2 Diagnostic criteria of polycythaemia vera[1]

1.	Elevated red blood cell mass of >25 per cent above the mean predicted value
2.	Normal arterial oxygen saturation (≥92 per cent) in the presence of erythrocytosis as defined in criterion 1
3.	Splenomegaly
4.	Thrombocytosis (platelet count ≥400 000/μl) and leucocytosis (white blood cell count of ≥12 000/μl)
5.	Bone marrow hypercellularity associated with clustered mature megakaryocytes with hyperlobulated nuclei and absent iron stores
6.	Low serum EPO levels (<3.0 U/L) in the presence of an increased red blood cell mass as defined in criterion 1
7.	Abnormal marrow proliferative capacity as manifested by the formation of erythroid colonies in the absence of exogenous EPO

EPO, erythropoietin.

[1] The presence of criterion 1 and any three additional criteria are diagnostic of polycythaemia vera.

With permission from Hoffman R (2000). Polycythemia vera. In: Hoffman R, Benz EJ Jr, Shattil SJ, Furie B, Cohen HJ, Silberstein LE, McGlave P, eds. *Hematology basic principles and practice*, pp 1130–55. Churchill Livingstone, Philadelphia, PA.

Approach to the patient with polycythaemia

It is wise to avoid the temptation of diagnosing polycythaemia on the basis of a single blood count determination unless extremely high levels are identified. A rational diagnostic approach is required to avoid unnecessary emotional distress to the patient as well as expensive and unnecessary evaluations (see Fig. 1).

Dehydration from any cause can produce a spurious elevation in the blood counts. Heavy smokers with mild polycythaemias should be asked to stop smoking and their counts repeated after a few weeks. Once a genuine elevation of haemoglobin or haematocrit has been established, the next step is to decide whether this represents an absolute increase in total red cell mass, or just a relative phenomenon. A blood volume study with direct quantitation of both red cell mass and plasma volume is helpful in making this distinction. If absolute polycythaemia is confirmed, it is essential to elucidate whether it is the consequence of a primary myeloproliferative disorder such as polycythaemia vera or a secondary condition.

The determination of erythropoietin levels may prove to be of diagnostic utility. An elevated serum erythropoietin level is indicative of the presence of a secondary polycythaemia and a low level supports the diagnosis of polycythaemia vera, but a normal erythropoietin value excludes neither hypoxia nor the autonomous production of erythropoietin as the cause. Normal values may also be encountered in some cases of polycythaemia vera.

The presence of leucocytosis, thrombocytosis, or splenomegaly is suggestive of polycythaemia vera as the cause for the elevated red cell mass. Arterial blood gases and the direct determination of oxygen saturation in arterial blood, if decreased they may aid in the recognition of a chronic pulmonary or congenital cardiovascular abnormality. If blood oxygen saturation is normal, the quantification of haemoglobin's oxygen affinity ($P_{50}O_2$) may indicate the presence of a high-affinity haemoglobin variant. Otherwise, causes for a physiologically inappropriate polycythaemia should be sought.

There is a small but definite group of patients in whom a specific cause for polycythaemia remains elusive, despite appropriate diagnostic testing. Examining close relatives might disclose the presence of a hereditary polycythaemia, a rare condition caused by an abnormality in erythropoietin control. Regular, continued surveillance is recommended for all non-categorized patients, as some of them develop polycythaemia vera in the future.

Management of polycythaemia

The two major tasks in the management of polycythaemia involve the identification of a correctable cause and the reduction of the red cell mass. The untoward effects of an increased red cell mass on tissue blood flow occur independently from the specific cause of the polycythaemia. It is thus reasonable to recommend that all patients with uncorrectable erythrocytosis be offered phlebotomy. A haematocrit under 45 per cent represents a reasonable target.

Polycythaemia vera is an incurable disorder. The main therapeutic goals are the maintenance of well being and the prevention of complications for as long as possible. Several therapeutic strategies have resulted in dramatic increases in the survival of patients. Historical evidence suggests a median survival of approximately 18 months in untreated patients, whereas with appropriate management survival of over 10 years is now common. The main therapeutic objective is the reduction of the haematocrit to a safe level. This is usually accomplished by the implementation of repeated phlebotomies. Every possible effort should be made to discourage patients with polycythaemia vera from smoking. A regimen of phlebotomies should be prescribed as soon as the diagnosis has been clearly established. It is often feasible to remove between 350 and 500 ml of blood every other day until the desired haematocrit level is attained. Haematocrit levels of less than 50 per cent and preferably below 45 per cent are desirable. The removal of smaller aliquots might be necessary in older patients.

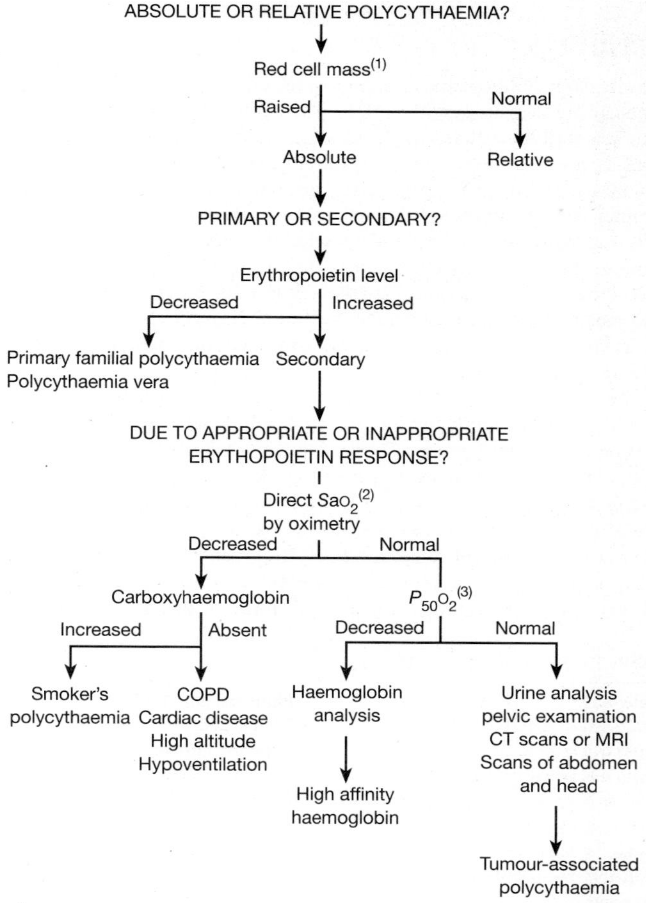

(1)Unnecessary if haematocrit is greater that 60% in men or greater than 55% in women
(2)Oxygen saturation in arterial blood
(3)Partial oxygen pressure at which 50% of haemoglobin is saturated with oxygen

Fig. 1 Diagnostic approach to the patient with polycythaemia.

Once the target haematocrit level is achieved, a maintenance regimen should be instituted. Venesection is preferred in those younger individuals without critical elevations in their platelet counts. Myelosuppressive therapy should be considered in elderly patients who are intolerant of phlebotomies, and in younger individuals with repeated thrombotic episodes and extremely high platelet counts. There is controversy regarding what represents the optimal myelosuppressive agent. A major concern has been the growing evidence that supports the association between exposure to some of these agents and the development of leukaemia. A number of clinical studies have been conducted in order to clarify the risk/benefit ratios of some of these approaches.

The Polycythemia Vera Study Group conducted a randomized comparison of three interventions: (1) phlebotomy only; (2) chlorambucil supplemented by phlebotomy; and (3) ^{32}P supplemented by phlebotomy. Median survival was shorter for the chlorambucil group (9.1 years) and statistically similar for ^{32}P (10.9 years) and for the phlebotomy-only group (12.6 years). Chlorambucil treatment was clearly associated with an unacceptably large number of acute leukaemias. Thrombosis as a cause of death was much more common in the phlebotomy-only group, whereas the use of ^{32}P led to a higher incidence of leukaemias, lymphoma, and non-haematological malignancies. In a subsequent study, high-dose platelet antiaggregating agents (aspirin and dipyridamole) were added to phlebotomy and compared with ^{32}P. Surprisingly, a higher number of thrombotic and serious bleeding episodes were seen in the former group. In a recent study, however, 40 mg/day of aspirin was administered to patients with polycythaemia vera in order to prevent thrombosis and minimize the bleeding risk. This regimen was shown to be well tolerated, safe, and appeared to reduce the thrombotic risk. Hydroxycarbamide (hydroxyurea) is useful for the management of a number of patients with polycythaemia vera, despite emerging evidence suggesting a mild leukaemogenic potential. At present, hydroxyurea is the chemotherapeutic drug of choice in those patients who can not be treated with phlebotomy alone.

In younger patients, given their potential long-term survival, strong consideration should be given to the use of phlebotomy therapy in combination with low-dose aspirin, as well as with other apparently non-leukaemogenic interventions such as interferon-α and anagrelide. In patients where uncontrolled thrombocytosis is a problem, anagrelide, an inhibitor of megakaryocytic maturation, has proven effective.

Elective surgery should only be undertaken after adequate and sustained control of the blood count has been achieved. When emergency surgery is required the patient should be phlebotomized rapidly until a normal haematocrit is achieved, and platelets should be available in case excessive operative bleeding occurs. Patients should be mobilized promptly, and the use of prophylactic doses of low molecular weight heparin should be considered unless contraindicated. Dental extractions are associated with an increased bleeding risk and should only be pursued in patients with good haematological control.

In the later spent phases of the disease the management is quite similar to that for primary myelofibrosis. It mainly consists of blood product replacement, folate and iron replacement, and splenectomy if there is significant hypersplenism. The prognosis of patients with acute leukaemia that has evolved from pre-existing polycythaemia vera is very poor, with very few long-term survivors after aggressive combination chemotherapy.

Pregnant patients with polycythaemia vera experience an increased incidence of fetal wastage, with 30 per cent of pregnancies culminating in spontaneous abortions. Interestingly, pregnancy in patients with polycythaemia vera is frequently associated with a gradual normalization of blood values, and it is not unusual for a woman who has required extensive therapy for control of her disease to no longer require phlebotomies during pregnancy.

Delivery appears not to be complicated by excessive haemorrhage or by an increased risk of venous thrombosis.

Prognosis

The outcome of patients with secondary polycythaemia is usually related to the prognosis of the underlying disorder. In polycythaemia vera, the nature and severity of the complications during the clinical course of the disease are the most important determinants of outcome. Disease duration is also important, as long-term survival is strongly associated with progression into the spent phase or acute leukaemia. As was previously emphasized, prompt and appropriate therapy results in dramatic improvements in survival. Young patients should be initially managed with phlebotomy and low doses of aspirin. Supplemental therapy with interferon, anagrelide, or hydroxyurea might be required in patients with serious haemorrhagic or thrombotic episodes. The use of either hydroxyurea or ^{32}P appears warranted in the treatment of elderly patients who, because of their age, have a limited survival.

Further reading

Copelan EA, Balcerzak SP (1995). Secondary polycythemia. In: Wasserman LR, Berk PD, Berlin NI, eds. *Polycythemia vera and the myeloproliferative disorders*, pp 195–221. WB Saunders, Philadelphia.

Fruchtman SM, *et al.* (1997). From efficacy to safety: a Polycythemia Vera Study Group report on hydroxyurea in patients with polycythemia vera. *Seminars in Hematology* **34**, 17–23.

Gruppo Italiano Studio Policitemia (1995). Polycythemia vera: the natural history of 1213 patients followed for 20 years. *Annals of Internal Medicine* **123**, 656–64.

Gruppo Italiano Studio Policitemia (GISP) (1997). Low dose aspirin in polycythaemia vera: a pilot study. *British Journal of Haematology* **77**, 453–6.

Hoffman R (2000). Polycythemia vera. In: Hoffman R, *et al.*, eds. *Hematology basic principles and practice*, pp 1130–55. Churchill Livingstone, Philadelphia, PA.

Messinezy M, *et al.* (1995). Low serum erythropoietin—a strong diagnostic criteria of primary polycythaemia even at normal haemoglobin levels. *Clinical and Laboratory Haematology* **17**, 217–20.

Michiels JJ (1996). The myeloproliferative disorders, a historical appraisal and personal experiences. *Leukemia and Lymphoma* **22**(Suppl. 1), 1–14.

Michiels JJ, *et al.* (1985). Erythromelalgia caused by platelet mediated arteriolar inflammation and thrombosis in thrombocythemia. *Annals of Internal Medicine* **102**, 466–71.

Michiels JJ, *et al.* (1996). Erythromelalgic thrombotic and hemorrhagic manifestations in 50 cases of thrombocythemia. *Leukemia and Lymphoma* **22**(Suppl. 1), 47–56.

Pearson TC, Messinezy M (1996). The diagnostic criteria of polycythemia rubra vera. *Leukemia and Lymphoma* **22**(Suppl. 1), 87–93.

Pearson TC, Wetherley-Mein G (1978). Vascular occlusive episodes and venous haematocrit in primary proliferative polycythemia. *Lancet* **2**, 1219–22.

Petitt RM, Silverstein MK (1997). Anagrelide for control of thrombocythemia in polycythemia and other myeloproliferative disorders. *Seminars in Hematology* **34**, 51–4.

Prchal JF, Prchal JT (1999). Molecular basis for polycythemia. *Current Opinion in Hematology* **6**, 100–9.

Silver RT (1997). Interferon alpha: effects of long term treatment for polycythemia vera. *Seminars in Hematology* **34**, 40–50.

Spivak JL (2000). Erythrocytosis. In: Hoffman R, *et al.*, eds. *Hematology basic principles and practice*, pp 388–96. Churchill Livingstone, Philadelphia, PA.

22.3.9 Idiopathic myelofibrosis

Jerry L. Spivak

Introduction

Idiopathic myelofibrosis (also called myelofibrosis with myeloid metaplasia, agnogenic myeloid metaplasia, primary myelofibrosis, or primary myelosclerosis) is a chronic clonal disorder of unknown aetiology, involving a multipotent haemopoietic progenitor cell that results in abnormalities in red cell, white cell, and platelet production in association with marrow fibrosis and extramedullary haemopoiesis. Although myelofibrosis in association with leucoerythroblastosis and splenomegaly are the clinical hallmarks of idiopathic myelofibrosis, these abnormalities can also be seen in other chronic myeloproliferative disorders such as polycythaemia vera and chronic myelogenous leukaemia as well as in a variety of benign and malignant disorders that involve the bone marrow (Table 1). Since there is no specific clonal marker for idiopathic myelofibrosis and since many of the disorders listed in Table 1 are responsive to specific therapies not effective in idiopathic myelofibrosis, the diagnosis of this disorder is one of exclusion.

Aetiology

The aetiology of idiopathic myelofibrosis is unknown. Analysis of glucose-6-phosphate dehydrogenase (**G6DP**) isoenzyme expression and X-linked gene inactivation patterns in informative women, as well as N-*ras* mutations, have established the clonality of idiopathic myelofibrosis and its origin in a multipotent haemopoietic progenitor cell. In some patients, T lymphocytes express the same clonal marker as B lymphocytes and myeloid cells, suggesting involvement at the level of the pluripotent stem cell. Nonrandom chromosome abnormalities primarily involving chromosomes 13 (del. 13q), 20 (del. 20q), and 1 (partial trisomy 1q) occur, but are found in fewer than 40 per cent of patients at the time of diagnosis. No abnormalities of the known tumour suppressor genes associated with these chromosomes have yet been identified.

The basis for the myelofibrosis has proved equally problematic. Marrow fibroblasts in idiopathic myelofibrosis are polyclonal, suggesting that the fibrosis is a reactive process initiated by expansion of the monoclonal malignant clone. Marrow collagen is argyrophilic, so that changes in its distribution and content can be analysed histochemically by silver staining. Under normal circumstances, the connective tissue stroma of the bone marrow is composed of collagen types I, III, IV, and V together with non-collagen proteins such as fibronectin, laminin, vitronectin, and the proteoglycans. Collagen types I, III, and V form a delicate and usually

Table 1 Causes of marrow fibrosis

Malignant	Non-malignant
Acute lymphocytic leukaemia	HIV infection
Acute myelogenous leukaemia	Hyperparathyroidism
Acute megakaryocytic leukaemia	Renal osteodystrophy
Chronic myelogenous leukaemia	Systemic lupus erythematosus
Hairy-cell leukaemia	Thorium dioxide exposure
Hodgkin's disease	Tuberculosis
Idiopathic myelofibrosis	Vitamin D deficiency
Lymphoma	
Multiple myeloma	
Metastatic carcinoma	
Polycythaemia vera	
Systemic mastocytosis	

non-continuous supporting network for haemopoietic cells, while type IV collagen, laminin, and fibronectin are localized in the basement membranes of arteries in a continuous fashion and along marrow sinusoids in a discontinuous fashion. With increasing marrow cellularity, the collagenous supporting network also increases. In myelofibrosis, however, there is both an increase in the collagen network and a change in its physical characteristics. Condensation of the interstitial fibres results in the formation of thick, continuous and often wavy bundles in association with an increase in reticular or fibroblastic cells. Sinusoidal basement membrane collagen becomes continuous, leading to sinusoidal dilatation and obliteration with an associated capillary neovascularization. The content of basement membrane fibronectin as well as stromal fibronectin and vitronectin also increases. While best studied in idiopathic myelofibrosis, the types of collagen involved in marrow fibrosis in this condition do not appear to differ from those involved in the marrow fibrosis associated with the other disorders listed in Table 1.

Neither the stimulus nor the molecular basis for the increase in marrow collagen and non-collagenous extracellular matrix proteins in idiopathic myelofibrosis is understood. The commonality of the types of collagen involved and the similarity of the histological process, regardless of disease association, implies that marrow fibrosis *per se* represents a final common pathway involved in the response to diverse immunological, metabolic, toxic, or infectious stimuli (Table 1). Megakaryocytic hyperplasia, dysplasia, and clustering is characteristic of idiopathic myelofibrosis. These cells produce proteins such as platelet-derived growth factor (**PDGF**) and transforming growth factor-β (**TGF-β**) that promote fibroblast proliferation, and platelet factor 4, which, like TGF-β, inhibits collagenase. These findings suggest that inappropriate release of these fibrogenic proteins by dysfunctional megakaryocytes is the stimulus for myelofibrosis. In support of this contention, elevated levels of PDGF and TGF-β as well as basic fibroblast growth factor have been observed in platelets and megakaryocytes from patients with idiopathic myelofibrosis. Circulating levels of TGF-β are also increased in idiopathic myelofibrosis, as is the urinary excretion of basic fibroblast growth factor and calmodulin, another potential fibroblast stimulant present in platelets.

However, these findings must be reconciled with the observations that neither overexpression of PDGF nor high levels of circulating TGF-β alone are associated with marrow fibrosis, presumably because PDGF in the circulation is inactivated by α2-macroglobulin and TGF-β usually circulates in an inactive from. Furthermore, in some studies the appropriate control populations were not examined, while in others there was significant overlap in the overexpression of these proteins when they were examined. Importantly, there was no correlation between marrow TGF-β content and megakaryocyte number, nor was there a correlation between marrow fibrosis and platelet number, although such a correlation existed between the extent of fibrosis and granulocyte number. Nevertheless, given what is known about the process of tissue fibrosis in other organs, it is likely that a combination of cytokines and growth factors such as TGF-β, PDGF, basic fibroblast growth factor, interleukin-1, and tumour necrosis factor (**TNF**) acting in synergy are required to initiate and perpetuate collagen deposition. In addition, thrombopoietin may also have a role, since overexpression of this hormone can cause myelofibrosis in animal models. Neither the cells responsible for the elaboration of these cytokines nor their targets, whether reticulum cells or fibroblasts, have been defined but recent evidence suggests that monocytes may be an important source of cytokine production. What has been learned, however, is that myelofibrosis is reversible by chemotherapy or bone marrow transplantation and occasionally spontaneously resolves.

Clinical features

Although considered to be an uncommon disorder with an incidence of approximately 1/100 000 person-years, clinical studies of more than 1000 patients have been reported over the last 40 years. In contrast to the other chronic myeloproliferative disorders, the median age at diagnosis of myelofibrosis, 61 years (range 15–94), is much older. No gender differences exist and familial clustering is sufficiently unusual that another myeloproliferative disorder such as polycythaemia vera should be considered when this occurs. The presenting manifestations depend on the state of the illness but are often bland. Many patients are asymptomatic at the time of discovery. Fatigue is the commonest presenting complaint followed by weight loss, night sweats, fever, dyspnoea, and abdominal discomfort due to splenomegaly. Hearing loss due to otosclerosis is an interesting but often non-elicited symptom. Easy bruising or bleeding and acute gout or renal stones are other presenting manifestations that are reasonably common and directly related to the underlying disease process. Rarely, periostitis may occur.

Splenomegaly is present in virtually every patient with idiopathic myelofibrosis at diagnosis. When absent, one should consider other causes for the clinical abnormalities. The degree of splenomegaly varies but is frequently substantial. Moreover, the rate of splenic enlargement is also variable; spleen size cannot be used as an indication of disease duration. Hepatomegaly, invariably of a lesser extent than the splenomegaly, is present initially in approximately 50 per cent of patients and is usually proportional to the degree of splenomegaly. Lymphadenopathy is uncommon. With substantial splenomegaly, wasting may be prominent.

Laboratory studies

Because of its origin in a multipotent haemopoietic progenitor cell, idiopathic myelofibrosis affects all cell lines but not in a predictable manner. Anaemia, usually mild, is the most consistent abnormality. Indeed, a normal haemoglobin or haematocrit in the presence of substantial splenomegaly should lead to immediate consideration of polycythaemia vera, since the expanded plasma volume associated with splenomegaly can mask a substantial increase of the red cell mass. The leucocyte and platelets counts can be low, normal, or high without reference to spleen size. Inevitably, due to extramedullary haemopoiesis, metamyelocytes, myelocytes, promyelocytes, myeloblasts, and nucleated red cells will be present in the circulation together with the tear drop-shaped red cells characteristic of this situation (Fig. 1). While this so-called leucoerythroblastic reaction is not specific for idiopathic myelofibrosis, its absence should challenge the clinical impression. Abnormalities in liver function tests are not uncommon, usually mild

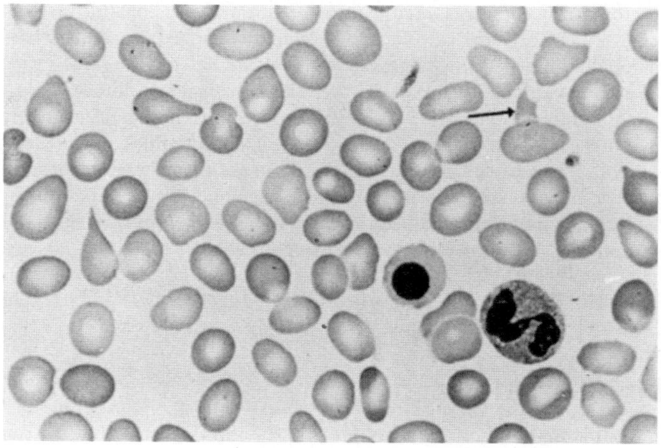

Fig. 1 Haematological changes in myelosclerosis. (a) A peripheral blood film showing tear-drop cells, a nucleated red cell, and a grossly distorted cell marked by the arrow. (From Liebold PF, Weed RI (1975). *Clinical Haematology*, **4**, 353, reproduced with permission.) (b) A scanning electron-microscope study showing characteristic poikilocytes. (From Liebold PF, Weed RI (1975). *Clinical Haematology*, **4**, 353, reproduced with permission.) (c) A leucoerythroblastic reaction in myelosclerosis showing young red-cell precursors. Note, in addition, the abnormal platelet morphology and platelet clumps.

and most often involve a reduction in serum albumin and an elevation of the alkaline phosphatase, an abnormality that is magnified by splenectomy. The lactate dehydrogenase (**LDH**) level is usually mildly increased and correlates best with the leucocyte count. Hyperuricaemia is not infrequent. The leucocyte alkaline phosphatase concentration can be low, normal, or high and so cannot be recommended as a diagnostic test.

Perhaps the most intriguing laboratory abnormalities in idiopathic myelofibrosis are those linked to autoreactivity, such as circulating immune complexes, complement activation, elevations in antinuclear antibody (**ANA**) and rheumatoid factor titres, and a positive Coombs' test in the absence of an overt connective tissue disorder. Although marrow fibrosis has been documented in patients with systemic lupus erythematosis, the linkage between autoimmune abnormalities and marrow fibrosis is unclear. It does, however, provide another therapeutic option as discussed below.

The presence of marrow fibrosis is essential for a diagnosis of idiopathic myelofibrosis and usually results in a 'dry tap' or the inability to aspirate marrow from a properly placed needle. A prefibrotic phase of idiopathic myelofibrosis has been described retrospectively. However, given the similarity of the histopathology of polycythaemia vera, essential thrombocytosis, and premyelofibrotic myelofibrosis, prospective substantiation of the latter disorder is not possible in the absence of marrow fibrosis and/or a specific clonal marker. Even the presence of myelofibrosis, while mandatory, is not in itself sufficient for diagnosis. This is because polycythaemia vera and chronic myelogenous leukaemia and other disorders such as hairy-cell leukaemia, myelodysplasia, and acute leukaemia can present with myelofibrosis. Thus, it is essential to employ the appropriate diagnostic tests (cytogenetics, *BCR–ABL* polymerase chain reaction (**PCR**), flow cytometry, and immunohistochemistry) to exclude these and the other disorders listed in Table 1 that can cause myelofibrosis.

Marrow cellularity in idiopathic myelofibrosis may be increased with trilineage hyperplasia and erythroblastic and megakaryocytic islands, decreased with scattered areas of hyperplastic marrow embedded in a collagenous matrix, or hypoplastic with intense osteomyelosclerosis and residual megakaryocytic islands (Fig. 2). While there is a correlation between the degree of fibrosis and osteosclerosis, there is no correlation between bone marrow histology and disease duration, platelet count, or splenomegaly; marrow fibrosis does, however, appear to correlate with the leucocyte count. In general, marrow fibrosis and extramedullary haemopoiesis with myeloid metaplasia appear unrelated, and the latter abnormalities cannot be considered as compensation for the former. Increased marrow angiogenesis is a recently recognized feature of idiopathic myelofibrosis which correlates with increased cellularity and extramedullary haematopoiesis independently of marrow fibrosis.

In conjunction with the most severe form of marrow fibrosis, osteosclerosis, radiographic abnormalities become apparent. These primarily involve the axial skeleton but can include the skull, with thickening of bony trabeculae and patchy or coalescent sclerosis. With obliteration of axial marrow, extension of the marrow into the long bones occurs. Interestingly, the increase in trabecula bone formation in idiopathic myelofibrosis is not accompanied by an increase in either osteoblastic or osteoclastic activity. This feature distinguishes the osteosclerosis of idiopathic myelofibrosis from that associated with metabolic causes of osteosclerosis.

Course and prognosis

Idiopathic myelofibrosis is a chronic progressive disorder with a median lifespan (5.5 years) that is much shorter than for polycythaemia vera and essential thrombocytosis. However, the heterogeneity characterizing the initial clinical presentation is also evident with respect to survival, which can range from less than a year to more than 30 years. Death is usually a consequence of bone marrow failure (haemorrhage, anaemia, or infection), transformation to acute leukaemia, portal hypertension, heart failure, cachexia, or myeloid metaplasia with organ failure. Retrospective analysis of the adverse prognostic value of presenting manifestations has identified a number of factors that may be useful for both prognostic and therapeutic purposes. These include age at onset (>64 years), anaemia (haemoglobin <10 g/dl), constitutional symptoms, white cell count abnormalities (<4000/μl or >12 000/μl), thrombocytopenia, circulating blast cells (>1 per cent), and cytogenetic abnormalities. A number of scoring systems have been devised for identifying long- and short-term survivors based on the presence of more than one adverse presenting manifestation. Two such scoring systems that are useful in separating patients of any age with myelofibrosis into low- and high-risk groups with respect to survival are shown in Table 2.

Complications

The major complications of idiopathic myelofibrosis are the consequences of bone marrow failure and extramedullary haemopoiesis.

Anaemia may be the result of ineffective erythropoiesis, but haemodilution due to the expanded plasma volume associated with splenomegaly, iron deficiency due to gastrointestinal blood loss, folic acid deficiency due to the increased demands of haemopoiesis, haemolysis due to autoimmune phenomena or hypersplenism, and, rarely, pyridoxine deficiency are also considerations. In some patients, erythropoietin production may be inappropriately low for the degree of anaemia but in this instance haemodilution needs to be excluded. Red cell survival and splenic sequestration studies can be useful in determining the splenic contribution to anaemia. Ferrokinetic studies, although no longer easily obtained, provide a means of assessing effective marrow erythropoiesis.

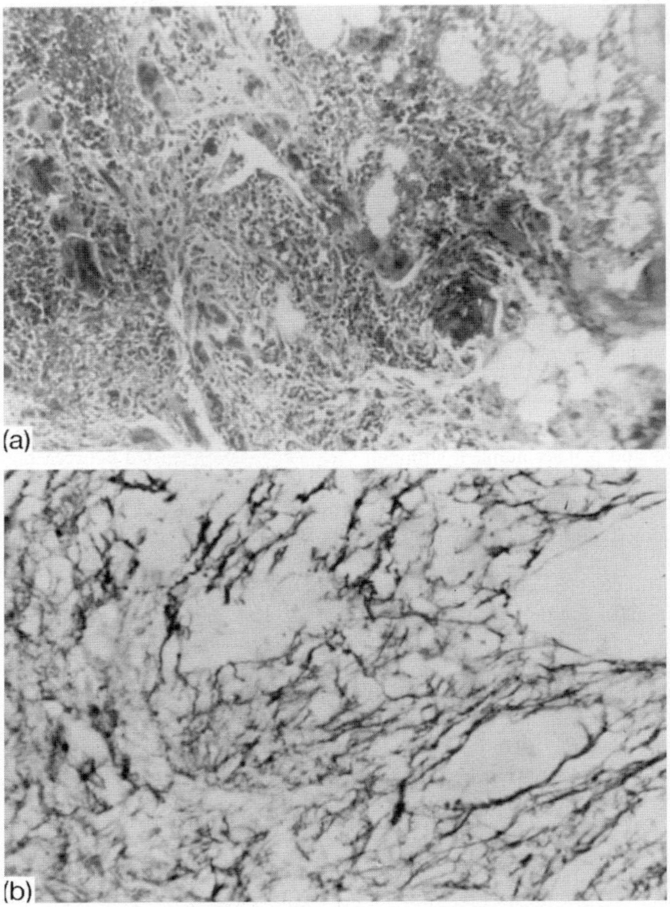

Fig. 2 Bone marrow appearances in myelosclerosis. (a) A biopsy showing a hyperplastic fragment with marked megakaryocytic hyperplasia; (b) silver stain showing the marked increase in reticulin.

Table 2 Two scoring systems for predicting survival in patients with idiopathic myelofibrosis

(a) Prognostic factors:		
HgB <10 g/dl		
WBC <4 or <30 × 10^9/μl		
Number of prognostic factors	*Risk group*	*Median survival (months)*
0	Low	93
1–2	High	17
(b) Prognostic factors:		
HgB <10 g/dl		
Constitutional symptoms		
Blast cells ≥1%		
Number of prognostic factors	*Risk group*	*Median survival (months)*
0–1	Low	99
2–3	High	21

(a) Taken with permission from Dupriez B, *et al.* (1996). Prognostic factors in agnogenic myeloid metaplasia: a report on 195 cases with a new scoring system. *Blood* **88**, 1013–18.

(b) Taken with permission from Cervantes F, *et al.* (1997). Identification of 'short-lived' and 'long-lived' patients at presentation of idiopathic myelofibrosis. *British Journal of Haematology* **97**, 635–40.

Hyperuricaemia is a consequence of increased cell turnover and can provoke acute gout or renal stone formation if left untreated.

Splenic enlargement is inevitable and can lead to splenic infarction, malnutrition due to early satiety, plasma volume expansion, hypersplenism, portal hypertension, extreme discomfort due to its mass, and eventually cachexia (Fig. 3). Hepatomegaly is associated with splenomegaly. Impaired hepatic function is a consequence of extramedullary haemopoiesis, which can lead to hepatic fibrosis and portal hypertension.

Although myeloid metaplasia due to exuberant extramedullary haemopoiesis is most common in the spleen and liver, it can occur at any site and compromise organ or tissue function. For example: peritoneal involvement can lead to ascites; epidural involvement to spinal cord compression; retroperitoneal involvement to obstructive uropathy or portal hypertension; and intravascular haemopoiesis to pulmonary thrombosis. The reason why myeloid metaplasia is more aggressive in some patients than in others is unclear.

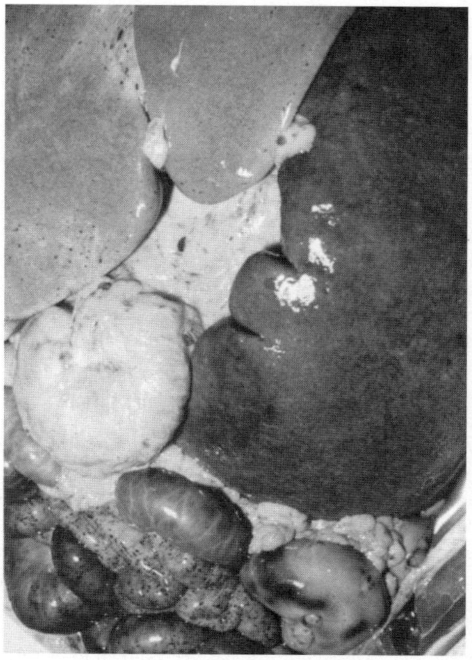

Fig. 3 Autopsy showing massive splenomegaly together with a splenic infarct on the medial surface of the spleen in a patient with advanced myelosclerosis.

Approximately 20 per cent of patients with idiopathic myelofibrosis develop acute leukaemia as a terminal event. Although some clinicians do not distinguish acute leukaemia presenting with myelofibrosis (malignant myelosclerosis) from idiopathic myelofibrosis, they are clinically distinct entities. The extent to which therapeutic intervention with mutagenic drugs such as hydroxycarbamide (hydroxyurea), alkylating agents, or irradiation predisposes patients with idiopathic myelofibrosis to progress to acute leukaemia (as it does in patients with polycythaemia vera or essential thrombocytosis) is unknown. Again for unknown reasons, splenectomy also appears to be a predisposing factor for the development of acute leukaemia.

Platelet dysfunction is a common feature of the chronic myeloproliferative disorders and can lead to spontaneous haemorrhage as well as increased bleeding during surgical procedures. Although abnormalities in platelet morphology, prolongation of the bleeding time, and abnormal platelet aggregation are frequently observed in patients with idiopathic myelofibrosis, no consistent biochemical abnormality has been identified and no platelet function test is predictive for the risk of haemorrhage.

Therapy

There is no specific therapy for idiopathic myelofibrosis. Treatment should be individualized based on the patient's risk group and age. Asymptomatic, low-risk patients without hyperuricaemia or a remedial cause of anaemia require no therapy, although the oral administration of folic acid (1 mg per day) and a trial of oral pyridoxine (250 mg per day for 3 months) appears reasonable. Anaemia associated with an inappropriately low endogenous erythropoietin level may respond to recombinant erythropoietin therapy but the hormone can cause an increase in splenomegaly or hepatomegaly. Hyperuricaemia should be treated with allopurinol. Asymptomatic leucocytosis or thrombocytosis requires no therapy. Patients of appropriate age, who are in a high-risk category and who have a matched, related donor should be considered for allogeneic bone marrow transplantation. In the absence of a suitable donor, therapy with recombinant α-interferon should be employed. This can alleviate splenomegaly and reduce myeloid metaplasia but may not reverse marrow fibrosis. Interferon therapy can be limited by the induction of leucopenia or thrombocytopenia and by its side-effects in elderly patients, in whom interferon therapy should be initiated at a low dose.

Given the known sensitivity of patients with polycythaemia vera to chemotherapeutic agents and irradiation, these forms of therapy should be used judiciously in the treatment of idiopathic myelofibrosis. Hydroxycarbamide, while easy to use and with a low incidence of acute toxicity, is leukaemogenic and should not be employed before a trial of interferon.

Busulfan is another effective agent that has been demonstrated to reduce organomegaly, reverse marrow fibrosis, and improve blood counts, occasionally in a durable fashion. However, busulfan has significant toxicities, not least of which is prolonged marrow aplasia. Its influence on the development of acute leukaemia in patients with idiopathic myelofibrosis is unknown.

Splenomegaly is the most distressing complication of idiopathic myelofibrosis, leading to mechanical discomfort, inanition, splenic infarction, portal hypertension, and blood cell sequestration. Reduction in splenic size can be achieved with interferon, alkylating agents, hydroxcarbamide, splenectomy, and splenic irradiation. Interferon is the treatment of choice followed by chemotherapy with either busulfan or hydroxycarbamide. Splenic irradiation can be effective at alleviating splenic pain and temporarily reducing spleen size. However, its use should be restricted to inoperable patients since there is an unpredictable risk of severe cytopenias as well as an increased risk of haemorrhage if the irradiation precedes splenectomy. Local irradiation is, of course, appropriate for the management of patients with symptomatic extramedullary haemopoiesis.

Splenectomy in idiopathic myelofibrosis is a prodigious procedure, given the large size of the spleen and its vessels, the inevitable presence of adhesions, the haemorrhagic tendency of patients with idiopathic myelofibrosis, and their often poor nutritional status. Evaluation for portal hypertension should precede surgery and, if necessary, parental hyperalimentation should be employed to avoid postoperative complications. Epsilon-aminocaproic acid should be used if bleeding is a problem.

Leucocytosis, thrombocytosis, and postoperative hepatic enlargement are the usual consequences of splenectomy, as is elevation of the alkaline phosphatase. Postoperative splenic and portal vein thrombosis occur in approximately 10 per cent of patients, most often in the first few weeks after surgery and presumably due to the size of the splenic vein remnant. However, there is no correlation between splenic or portal vein thrombosis and the platelet count. Surveillance by sonography or computed tomography may useful in identifying this complication with the intent of administering anticoagulants or thrombolytic agents. Although most patients tolerate splenectomy well, the incidence of the transformation of idiopathic myelofibrosis to acute leukaemia is increased postsplenectomy, for unknown reasons.

Finally, as mentioned earlier, both autoimmune phenomena and capillary neovascularization are features of idiopathic myelofibrosis. The use of antiangiogenetic and immunosuppressive agents such as thalidomide are currently undergoing clinical trials. Corticosteroids may also be beneficial if autoimmune phenomena are clinically significant. Finally, tuberculosis was a frequent complication of idiopathic myelofibrosis early in the nineteenth century. Thus, constitutional symptoms in these patients should not be attributed to the myeloproliferative disease without first excluding an infectious process.

Further reading

Barosi G (1999). Myelofibrosis with myeloid metaplasia: diagnostic definition and prognostic classification for clinical studies and treatment guidelines. *Journal of Clinical Oncology* **17,** 2954–70.

Cervantes F, *et al.* (1997). Identification of 'short-lived' and 'long-lived' patients at presentation of idiopathic myelofibrosis. *British Journal of Haematology* **97**, 635–40.

Dupriez B, *et al.* (1996). Prognostic factors in agnogenic myeloid metaplasia: a report on 195 cases with a new scoring system. *Blood* **88**, 1013–18.

Elliott MA, *et al.* (1998). Splenic irradiation for symptomatic splenomegaly associated with myelofibrosis with myeloid metaplasia. *British Journal of Haematology* **103**, 505–11.

Frey BM *et al.* (1998). Adenovector-mediated expression of human thrombopoietin cDNA in immune compromised mice. *Journal of Immunology* **160**, 691–9.

Glew RH, Wolfgang HH, McIntrye PA (1973). Myeloid metaplasia with myelofibrosis. The clinical spectrum of extramedullary hematopoiesis and tumor formation. *Johns Hopkins Medical Journal* **132**, 253–70.

Mesa RA *et al.* (2000). Evaluation and clinical correlations of bone marrow angiogenesis in myelofibrosis and myeloid metaplasia. *Blood* **96**, 3374–80.

Reilly JT (1997). Idiopathic myelofibrosis: pathogenesis, natural history and management. *Blood* **11**, 233–42.

Reilly JT, *et al.* (1997). Cytogenetic abnormalities and their prognostic significance in idiopathic myelofibrosis: a study of 106 case. *British Journal of Haematology* **98**, 96–102.

Sterkers Y, *et al.* (1998). Acute myeloid leukemia and myelodysplastic syndromes following essential thrombocythemia treated with hydroxyurea: high proportion of cases with 17p deletion. *Blood* **91**, 616–22.

Tefferi A *et al.* (2000). Splenectomy in myelofibrosis with myeloid metaplasia: a single-institution experience with 223 patients. *Blood* **95**, 226–33.

Truong LD, Saleem A, Schwartz MR (1984). Acute myelofibrosis. a report of four cases and review of the literature. *Medicine* **63**, 182–7.

Varki A, *et al.* (1974). The syndrome of idiopathic myelofibrosis. A clinicopathologic review with emphasis on the prognostic variables predicting survival. *Medicine* **62**, 353–71.

22.3.10 Thrombocytosis

David M. Gustin and Ronald Hoffman

Thrombocytosis refers to a platelet count elevated above the accepted normal range (more than 500×10^9/l). The widespread use of automated cell counters has made the identification of platelet count abnormalities a relatively common event requiring further evaluation. The clinical consequences are usually determined by the cause of the thrombocytosis, ranging from the uneventful recognition of a laboratory abnormality, to medical emergencies such as life threatening thrombosis or haemorrhage.

Pathophysiology and classification

An understanding of the disorders of platelet production requires knowledge of the regulatory events that occur during normal megakaryocytopoiesis. Megakaryocyte development is a complex process in which a wide variety of regulatory signals work in concert to direct a highly specific response to thrombopoietic demand. A large number of cytokines including interleukins (IL-3, IL-6, IL-9 and IL-11), c-kit ligand, granulocyte–macrophage colony stimulating factor (GM-CSF), thrombopoietin (TPO) and, possibly, erythropoietin have been shown to stimulate megakaryocyte development, but TPO and its receptor, c-mpl, are the primary physiological regulators of *in vivo* magakaryocytopoiesis. The liver and the kidney contribute most of the basal, constitutive production of TPO. Levels are regulated by the total mass of platelets and megakaryocytes. TPO binding to its receptor on these cells, and its subsequent degradation, represents its main pathway of clearance. During times of thrombopoietic stress, there is increased TPO production by the spleen and bone marrow. Inappropriately elevated levels of TPO may be observed in primary thrombocythaemia. This is probably not due to excessive production but rather impaired TPO clearance associated with decreased expression of the TPO receptor by megakaryocytes and platelets. Molecular abnormalities in the TPO gene, however, have been recently identified in several families with an autosomal dominant form of hereditary thrombocytosis where serum TPO levels are significantly elevated. This syndrome has been shown to be due to a mutation in a portion of the TPO gene which plays a crucial role in regulating its expression.

Table 1 Classification of the causes of thrombocytosis

Autosomal dominant thrombocytosis
Secondary thrombocytosis (reactive)
Infection
Post-splenectomy (or hyposplenism)
Malignancy
Trauma
Inflammation (non-infectious)
Blood loss
Major surgery
Exercise
Rebound from myelosupression
Primary thrombocytosis (non-reactive)
Chronic myelogenous leukaemia
Primary or essential thrombocythaemia
Polycythaemia vera
Agnogenic myeloid metaplasia with myelofibrosis
Unclassified myeloproliferative disorders
Myelodysplastic syndromes
Uncertain aetiology

Modified from Buss DH *et al.* (1994). Occurrence, etiology and clinical significance of extreme thrombocytosis: a study of 280 cases. *American Journal of Medicine* **96**, 247–53.

Thrombocytosis can occur in response to many underlying clinical conditions (secondary or reactive), or as an expression of a primary abnormality in bone marrow function (primary). A classification of the causes of thrombocytosis is offered in Table 1. Reactive or secondary thrombocytosis account for over 80 per cent of all recognized cases of thrombocytosis (platelet count more than 500 $\times 10^9$/l). Short-lived, secondary thrombocytosis may be observed in situations such as trauma, acute bleeding, major surgery, or after strenuous physical exercise. Longer-term thrombocytosis is associated with the presence of chronic disorders such as malignancy, inflammation, chronic infections, and iron deficiency anaemia. The pathophysiology of reactive thrombocytosis is not fully understood but probably involves the increased generation of inflammatory cytokines such as IL-1, IL-6, GM-CSF and, possibly, TPO. Primary thrombocytosis by contrast is associated with a group of bone marrow disorders including chronic myeloid leukaemia, primary thrombocythaemia, polycythaemia vera, myeloid metaplasia with myelofibrosis, and the myelodysplastic syndromes. The level of elevated platelet numbers is not helpful in differentiating a reactive from a primary process.

For the most part, the presence of an underlying cause for reactive thrombocytosis can be identified by clinical criteria. A number of laboratory tests can be useful in distinguishing primary from secondary thrombocytosis. C-reactive protein synthesis in the liver is mediated by IL-6, with C-reactive protein levels being high in those patients with elevated IL-6 levels. Elevated levels of both IL-6 and C-reactive protein are strongly indicative of the elevated platelet count being reactive. The presence of 'endogenous erythroid colonies' (erythroid progenitor cells that proliferate *in vitro* without the addition of erythropoietin) and of megakaryocyte progenitor cells that are hypersensitive to certain stimulatory cytokines *in vitro* may be helpful in the identification of myeloproliferative disorders. Assays using probes for genes located on the X chromosome might help identify clonal haemopoiesis. In a number of female patients with a primary thrombocytosis, this can indicate the malignant origin of these underlying disorders.

The natural history and prognosis of reactive thrombocytosis is defined by its underlying cause. The thrombocytosis per se is probably inconsequential and does not require specific therapy. The thrombocytosis usually resolves after the treatment of the underlying cause. In contrast, the thrombocytosis due to underlying myeloproliferative disorders can cause life-threatening thromboembolic phenomena and bleeding episodes, and frequently requires specific cytoreductive therapy, emphasizing the need for accurate recognition. Primary or essential thrombocythaemia is the most important cause of primary thrombocytosis.

Primary thrombocythaemia

Primary thrombocythaemia, also known as essential thrombocythaemia or essential thrombocytosis, is a chronic myeloproliferative disorder characterized by marked megakaryocytic hyperplasia. The clinical course is punctuated by episodes of thrombosis and/or bleeding. In 1951, Dameshek suggested that primary thrombocythaemia represented a myeloproliferative disorder and hypothesized its clonal nature. The myeloproliferative disorders are currently thought to represent primary stem cell disorders.

Aetiology and pathogenesis

The causative factors of primary thrombocythaemia are poorly understood. Its pathogenesis involves the abnormal proliferation of a blood cell precursor that differentiates mainly towards the megakaryocytic/platelet compartment. Current evidence suggests that hypersensitivity to stimulatory cytokines such as IL-3, IL-6, TPO, and GM-CSF, coupled with relative insensitivity to inhibitory soluble factors such as transforming growth factor-β (TGF-β), might provoke the expansion of the megakaryocytic progenitor pool. Its clonal origin was initially established through biochemical isoenzyme characterization of the blood cells of affected women who were heterozygous for glucose-phosphate dehydrogenase (G-6PD). More recently, analysis of X-linked restriction fragment length polymorphisms in affected women has confirmed a clonal pattern in some cases. Recent evidence, however, suggests that a significant number of patients have polyclonal myelopoiesis and that these non-clonal cases may have a decreased risk for thrombosis. This information therefore suggests that primary thrombocythaemia, as diagnosed by the currently accepted clinical and laboratory criteria, is a heterogeneous disorder in terms of clonality. The pathogenesis of such sustained non-reactive polyclonal thrombocytosis is as yet unclear.

Epidemiology

The true incidence of primary thrombocythaemia is unknown. Approximately 6000 new cases are identified each year in the United States. There seems to be a slight female predominance and the usual age at onset is between 50 and 60 years. Approximately 20 per cent of all cases occur in individuals younger than 40, but it is very rarely seen during childhood.

Pathobiology

The characteristic clinical features are dominated by the thrombocytosis and abnormalities in platelet function. The association between increased numbers of circulating platelets and ischaemic episodes remains unclear, but duration of thrombocytosis may play a role. Microvascular thrombosis results in a variety of clinical syndromes associated with digital and cerebrovascular ischaemia. Abnormalities in platelet aggregation occur in 35 per cent to 100 per cent of patients, and prolongation of the bleeding time in 7 per cent to 19 per cent. Despite being common, these abnormalities are poor predictors of bleeding and/or thrombotic risk. This is in contrast to the acquired von Willebrand syndrome and erythromelalgia, clinical entities not infrequently seen in association with primary thrombocythaemia. In acquired von Willebrand syndrome, extreme thrombocytosis (more than 1000 $\times 10^9$/l) induces the adsorption of larger von Willebrand multimers on to platelet membranes and their subsequent degradation, triggering a haemostatic defect that induces a bleeding diathesis quite similar to that observed in Type II von Willebrand disease. Erythromelalgia refers to redness and burning pain in the extremities which results from platelet-mediated thrombosis of the arterial microvasculature. If left untreated it may progress to frank gangrene. Its exquisite response to cyclo-oxygenase inhibitors such as aspirin and indomethacin suggests that prostaglandin endoperoxides produced by the metabolism of arachidonic acid play a major role in the generation of platelet-associated thrombosis.

Clinical features

As many as two-thirds of patients are asymptomatic when diagnosed. Most symptomatic patients present with either a thrombotic episode or a minor bleeding episode. Bleeding can occur spontaneously but is frequently associated with the recent use of a non-steroidal anti-inflammatory drug. Common sites of haemorrhage include the gastrointestinal and the genito-urinary tracts as well as easy bruisability of the skin. Thrombosis leads to the most common presenting symptoms and can occur in arteries and veins, large or small. Occlusion of the splenic vessels and of the superficial and deep veins of the lower extremities is common. Pulmonary emboli may also occur. An occasional patient presents with thrombosis of the hepatic veins causing the Budd–Chiari syndrome or with occlusion of the renal veins manifesting clinically as nephrotic syndrome.

When the microcirculation is involved, a number of clinical syndromes may occur. Palpable lesions with small areas of gangrene indistinguishable from vasculitic lesions of rheumatoid arthritis or systemic lupus erythematosus may be observed. Erythromelalgia may occur in association with transient ischaemic attacks or acute episodes of cardiac angina. Peripheral pulses are usually preserved; this helps differentiate erythromelalgia from atherosclerotic-related ischaemia. Neurological symptoms are common and include headaches and paresthesias of the extremities. Transient ischaemic attacks may present with symptoms of unsteadiness, dysarthria, dysphoria, motor hemiparesis, scintillating scotomas, amaurosis fugax, vertigo, dizziness, migraine headaches, and seizures. On occasion, transient ischaemic attacks may progress to established infarcts. Myocardial ischaemia with normal angiograms occurs occasionally. Thrombotic non-bacterial endocarditis, usually affecting the mitral or aortic valves, may manifest with findings of distal emboli. Splenic enlargement is often seen. Patients unaware of their diagnosis who have undergone splenectomy as part of the diagnostic work-up for splenomegaly will predictably develop extreme increases in their platelet counts with a consequent increased risk for bleeding and/or thrombosis.

Laboratory diagnosis

Elevated platelet counts, often above 600 to 1000 × 10^9/l are characteristic. The absolute number of platelets, even if higher than 1 million/μl, is not diagnostic of primary thrombocythaemia. Extreme increments have been observed in reactive thrombocytosis. Marked changes in platelet morphology, which include large and bizarre-looking platelets sometimes forming aggregates, are also characteristic and may be more useful in helping distinguishing primary from reactive thrombocytosis. The bone marrow is hypercellular with megakaryocytic hyperplasia. Clusters of megakaryocytes are often observed. Absent or diminished iron stores are seen frequently. This may be an epiphenomenon of an underlying myeloproliferative disorder or a true expression of iron depletion in patients with chronic bleeding. Reticulin is present in one-quarter of bone marrow specimens but collagen is usually absent. Mild leucocytosis is common.

Platelet function abnormalities are commonly found and include defective platelet aggregation in response to adrenaline, ADP, and collagen. Aggregation in response to arachidonic acid and ristocetin is often normal. An acquired platelet storage pool disease also occurs due to abnormalities in the content and release of α granules associated with a state of increased platelet activation. The bleeding time is occasionally prolonged but does not predict bleeding risk. Cytogenetic evidence for a Philadelphia chromosome and/or the molecular identification of the *brc/abl* fusion gene aids in distinguishing primary thrombocythaemia from chronic myeloid leukaemia. The presence of dyspoietic changes in bone marrow precursor cells and of characteristic chromosomal abnormalities suggests the diagnosis of myelodysplasia. The diagnostic criteria and management of the other myeloproliferative disorders associated with thrombocytosis are outlined in other chapters. Cytogenetic abnormalities occur in approximately 5 per cent of patients with primary thrombocythaemia. The most common chromosomal alterations include 1q–, 20q–, 21q–, and 1q+. Elevated vitamin B-12 levels occurs in 25 per cent of patients.

Diagnostic criteria and differential diagnosis

Diagnostic criteria are listed in Table 2. The exclusion of an identifiable cause of reactive thrombocytosis is a necessary condition. Primary thrombocythaemia is mainly a diagnosis of exclusion. Any condition associated with elevations in circulating platelets is part of the differential diagnosis. Thrombocytosis may be the consequence of primary bone marrow disorders associated with increases in platelet production (non-reactive thrombocytosis), or a secondary response to an underlying disorder (reactive thrombocytosis). Table 1 summarizes the most important. Clearly, secondary causes of thrombocytosis occur more frequently (more than 80 per cent). Infection, hyposplenism, malignancy, trauma, and non-infectious inflammation are the most commonly encountered disorders. Chronic myelogenous leukaemia and primary thrombocythaemia are the most frequent causes of primary thrombocytosis.

Risk assessment

Primary thrombocythaemia is associated with a very low risk of life-threatening complications. Most patients enjoy survival fairly similar to that of their unaffected peers. Exposure of every patient with primary thrombocythaemia to myelosuppresive therapy is unwarranted. A risk-based decision approach to therapy is outlined in Table 3. Advanced age (60 years or older) and previous history of thrombosis clearly define a group at high risk for

Table 2 Criteria for the diagnosis of primary thrombocythaemia

1. Platelet count > 600 000/mm^3 on two different occasions separated by a 1 month interval
2. Absence of identifiable cause of reactive thrombocytosis
3. Normal red cell mass (measured red cell mass < 25 per cent above the predicted normal value)
4. Absence of significant fibrosis of the marrow (> 1/3 cross-sectional area of the bone marrow biopsy)
5. Absence of the Philadelphia chromosome and the fusion *bcr/abl* gene by PCR; absence of clonal cytogenetic abnormalities associated with myelodysplastic disorders
6. Presence of splenomegaly by physical examination, ultrasonography, or other scans
7. Bone marrow hypercellularity, as shown by a bone marrow biopsy and the presence of megakaryocytic hyperplasia with clusters of multilobulated large megakaryocytes
8. Absence of iron deficiency, as documented by the presence of stainable marrow iron and/or normal serum ferritin
9. In females, the demonstration of clonal haematopoiesis by means of restriction fragment length polymorphism analysis of genes present on the X-chromosome is suggestive of the diagnosis; however, non-clonal haematopoiesis may also be seen.
10. Presence of abnormal marrow haematopoietic progenitor cells as determined by the formation of endogenous erythroid and/or megakaryocytic colonies with increased sensitivity to IL-3
11. No elevation of plasma C-reactive protein and IL-6 levels

Patients who meet criteria 1–5 and 3 or more of criteria 6–11 should be considered to have primary thrombocythaemia.

Modified from Hoffman R. Primary thrombocythemia. In: Hoffman R, Benz EJ, Shattil SJ, Furie B, Cohen HJ, Silberstein LE, Mc Glave P, eds. *Hematology: basic principles and practice*, pp. 1188–204. Churchill Livingston, Philadelphia.

Table 3 Risk stratification-based treatment of primary thrombocythaemia

Risk category	Treatment
Low risk	Observation
age < 60 years, and	
no history of thrombosis, and	
platelet count < 1.0 million/mm^3, and	
no cardiovascular risk factors (smoking, obesity)	
High risk	Hydroxyurea[1]
age ≥ 60 years, or	Anagrelide[2]
a previous history of thrombosis	Interferon[3]
Intermediate risk[4]	Anagrelide[2]
platelet count > 1.0 million/mm^3, or	Interferon[3]
cardiovascular risk factors (smoking, obesity)	Hydroxyurea[1]

[1] Hydroxyurea is the drug of choice in patients whose age is 60 or more. It can be used in younger patients if anagrelide and interferon prove ineffective or are not tolerated.

[2] Anagrelide is the drug of choice in young patients. It should be used with caution in patients with pre-existing heart disease.

[3] Interferon is a reasonable choice for young patients (less than 60) who are either intolerant or do not respond to anagrelide. It is the drug of choice during pregnancy.

[4] The decision to treat is at the discretion of the clinician. We offer treatment to most of our patients with platelets more than 1.0 million. Behavioural risk modification only, might be appropriate for patients at intermediate risk on the basis of the presence of cardiovascular risk factors. All patients in the intermediate risk category are younger than 60 years of age, as age 60 or more defines high risk.

the development of life-threatening complications. The degree of thrombocytosis and the presence of associated cardiovascular risk factors, particularly smoking and obesity, is also taken into consideration when making treatment decisions.

Treatment

A number of agents can lower the platelet count of patients with primary thrombocythaemia. There is now firm evidence that cytoreduction using hydroxyurea, at least in high-risk patients, results in a significant reduction in the number of thrombotic episodes. However, only a handful of randomized clinical trials have been conducted given the relatively small number of patients diagnosed with this disease each year. Alkylating agents have been extensively used in the past to treat primary thrombocythaemia. Within this group of agents, busulfan has been shown to be quite effective and relatively non-toxic, with predictable cytopenias as its major untoward effect. It is usually prescribed at 4 mg/day until a platelet count of 400 000/μl is reached. Additional 2-week courses are given if and when the platelet count rises over 400 000/μl. Extensive experience has also accumulated with radioactive phosphorus (^{32}P). Its advantages include ease of administration and the relative absence of significant, acute side-effects. It is usually given as a single dose of 2.3 mCi/m^2 that may be repeated in 3 to 6 month. Its effects are seen 4 to 8 weeks after administration. Excessive doses of ^{32}P can be associated with cytopenias. Alkylating agents and ^{32}P have been associated with significant increases in the risk of leukaemic transformation.

The use of hydroxyurea, an antimetabolite that interferes with DNA repair, decreased the number of thrombotic events in a randomized study of high risk patients when given at 15 mg/kg initially with subsequent adjustments based on initial response. In this study, the target was a platelet count of less than 600 000/μl, but it is possible that tighter control (less than 350 000) may be more effective. Onset of action is usually 3 to 5 days. Frequent side-effects include dose-related neutropenia, nausea, stomatitis, hyperpigmentation, rash, nail changes, leg ulcers, and hair loss. Its leukaemogenic potential when given as a single agent is still a subject of major controversy although it is clearly less leukaemogenic than alkylating agents or ^{32}P.

Interferon-α, a biological response modifier, also is useful in treating patients with primary thrombocytosis. Ninety per cent response rates with median times to response of approximately 3 months are seen when 3 to 5 million units are administered subcutaneously 3 to 5 days per week. It is non-mutagenic and does not cross the placenta. Frequent side-effects include flu-like symptoms, fatigue, lethargy, and depression. Its long-term use is associated with mild weight loss, alopecia, autoimmune thyroiditis, and autoimmune haemolytic anaemia. Interferon's extensive toxicity profile and the need for parenteral administration limit its use as initial therapy, particularly in elderly patients.

Anagrelide is at present the treatment of choice for younger patients and acts by selectively inhibiting megakaryocytic maturation. Responses have been documented in over 90 per cent of treated patients with a median time to response of 2.5 to 4 weeks and an onset of action of 6 to 10 days. It is non-mutagenic and its use has not been associated with the development of acute leukaemia. The usual initial dose is 0.5 mg, two to four times per day, which is increased at 0.5-mg increments per week according to response. Excessive dosing predictably causes thrombocytopenia. The current recommendation is not to exceed a total of 10 mg/day or 2 mg (single) doses. The average daily maintenance dose is 2 mg in divided doses. The most common side-effects include headaches, dizziness, fluid retention, palpitations, nausea, abdominal pain, and diarrhoea. They develop within 2 weeks of use and usually improve within 2 weeks of continued treatment. It may also, on occasion, trigger episodes of tachyarrhythmias and heart failure. For this reason, it should be used carefully in the elderly and avoided in patients with known heart disease.

Recent evidence suggests that the administration of low doses of aspirin (250 mg daily, or less) is safe, and may decrease the recurrence of microcirculatory events (erythromelalgia/ transient ischaemic attacks) and prevent the development of other thrombotic phenomena, especially in combination with myelosuppressive agents. These data are still preliminary and require further study in large, randomized trials. In order to minimize the risk of iatrogenic bleeding, only patients with platelet counts less than 1 000 000/μl and without evidence of an acquired von Willebrand syndrome should be considered for low-dose aspirin administration.

Given the number of available therapeutic options and their different toxicity profiles, the choice of the appropriate cytoreductive drug for a given individual requires the consideration of a number of variables. These include age, childbearing potential, projected life expectancy, co-morbidities, and cost of treatment. Furthermore, the overall low risk for the development of life-threatening complications that affects patients with primary thrombocythaemia highlights the need for systematic, risk-based approaches to therapeutic decision making (see Table 3). The optimal therapy for patients with primary thrombocythaemia remains unclear. All patients should stop smoking. Indiscriminant use of high doses of non-steroidal anti-inflammatory agents should be avoided. Their excessive use is clearly associated with bleeding episodes.

Low-risk patients have a risk of thrombosis similar to that of the age and sex-matched population and a very low risk of life-threatening bleeding, supporting close observation without cytoreductive therapy as the most sensible approach. Hydroxyurea is an adequate choice for patients 60 years of age or older who are otherwise in good health. For elderly patients with limited projected survival (less than 10 years) and who have problems with either drug compliance or are too ill to comply with the minimum follow-up requirements during cytoreductive therapy, ^{32}P administration might be appropriate. Anagrelide should be offered to younger patients (less than 60) who are at high risk by virtue of a prior history of thrombosis or to patients at intermediate risk who the physician feels the necessity to treat. This drug should be used with extreme caution in elderly individuals and should be avoided in patients with cardiac disease. α-Interferon may be an acceptable option in the younger population of patients but is usually not used initially given the need for parenteral administration and its prominent side-effect profile. Alkylating agents, ^{32}P, and hydroxyurea are usually avoided in younger patients given their known (alkylators and ^{32}P) and possible (hydroxyurea) leukaemogenic potential. If a young patient, however, is resistant or intolerant to α-interferon and/or anagrelide, and requires treatment, we feel comfortable prescribing hydroxyurea at this point. In patients at intermediate risk based on platelet numbers at or more than 1 000 000/μl and who have the acquired von Willebrand syndrome, platelet reduction therapy is indicated to avoid the high risk of haemorrhage.

Smokers and obese individuals, unless symptomatic, should be managed by risk modification. In patients who suffer from thrombotic episodes, especially episodes involving the microcirculation or large vessels, we usually administer low-dose aspirin (100 mg/day). This dose appears safe and is effective in the treatment of thrombotic events, and is usually given in addition to cytoreductive therapy. In severe, life-threatening episodes, rapid cytoreduction may be achieved by plateletpheresis or by the administration of a single dose of 0.4 mg/kg of nitrogen mustard. In patients who present with a life-threatening, acute bleeding episode, the site of bleeding should be promptly identified and any antiplatelet agent should be stopped. Those suffering from an acquired von Willebrand's syndrome, can be treated with desmopressin (DDAVP) and factor VIII concentrates that contain high concentrations of von Willebrand factor. Cytoreductive therapy with hydroxyurea must be promptly initiated. In bleeding patients who fail to respond to DDAVP and factor VIII administration, the bleeding frequently resolves following platelet transfusions.

The management of patients who are or want to become pregnant requires special consideration. The risk of fetal loss is quite high (approximately 40 per cent). No clinical features other than the previous history of a miscarriage are predictive. Patients at low or intermediate risk should be managed by observation. Specific treatment should be considered during subsequent pregnancies if fetal loss were to occur. Uncontrolled studies have suggested that the careful use of heparin, aspirin, or α-interferon may decrease the chance for miscarriages. These data require further confirmation. Patients at high risk (for maternal thrombosis) are candidates for cytoreduction. Despite the lack of endorsement by the manufacturers of α-interferon, it may be the drug of choice during pregnancy given its lack of mutagenic potential and its inability to cross the placenta. Hydroxyurea, given its mechanism of action, could theoretically cause fetal malformations and anagrelide, due to its small molecular size, probably crosses the placenta and may cause life-threatening thrombocytopenia and haemorrhage in the fetus. Despite these concerns, recent case reports have described first trimester exposures to these two drugs resulting in the delivery of normal newborns. We therefore do not consider unintended exposures to hydroxyurea or anagrelide as absolute indications for the termination of pregnancy.

Prognosis

The probability that a patient with primary thrombocythaemia will survive 10 years is within the range of 64 to 80 per cent and is not substantially different from that of a control age- and sex-matched population. The actual risk for the development of a catastrophic thrombotic or haemorrhagic event in an asymptomatic patient is quite low. The majority of deaths come from thrombotic complications. Transformation to myelofibrosis and/or acute leukaemia has been reported with increasing frequency at a rate of transformation of 3 to 10 per cent. Prior administration of cytotoxic therapy is the strongest predictor of evolution to leukaemia but spontaneous transformations also occur, as in other myeloproliferative disorders. In rare instances, primary thrombocythaemia may also evolve into a clinical picture that resembles one of the other chronic myeloproliferative disorders.

Future directions

Better means to establish thrombotic and/or bleeding risk are required, and will help to improve the individualized risk-based selection of therapy. It is now clear that high-risk patients do benefit from cytoreductive therapy. Randomized comparisons to establish the efficacy of α-interferon and anagrelide in younger individuals at high risk is still needed. Although there is clear evidence that low-dose aspirin is safe and useful for the treatment of microcirculatory events such as erythromelalgia and transient ischaemic attacks, its additional therapeutic contribution when used in combination with anagrelide, hydroxyurea, or α-interferon requires further confirmation. The ideal therapeutic target in terms of the most desirable platelet number also requires better definition. A better understanding of the mechanisms involved in the regulation of platelet production and of the molecular abnormalities specifically associated with primary thrombocythaemia will offer rational targets against which to develop new and more specific therapies.

Further reading

Barbui T *et al.* (1996). Treatment strategies in essential thrombocythemia: a critical appraisal of various experiences in different centers. *Leukemia and Lymphoma* **22** (Suppl.1), 149–60.

Buss DH *et al.* (1994). Occurrence, etiology and clinical significance of extreme thrombocytosis: a study of 280 cases. *American Journal of Medicine* **96**, 247–53.

Cortelazzo S *et al.* (1995). Hydroxyurea for patients with essential thrombocythemia and a high risk of thrombosis. *New England Journal of Medicine* **332**, 1132–9.

Greisshamer M, Heimpel H, Pearson TC (1996). Essential thrombocythemia and pregnancy. *Leukemia and Lymphoma* **22** (Suppl.1), 57–63.

Harrison CN *et al.* (1999). A large proportion of patients with a diagnosis of essential thrombocythemia does not have a clonal disorder and may be at lower risk of thrombotic complications. *Blood* **93**, 417–24.

Hoffman R. Primary thrombocythemia. In: Hoffman R, Benz EJ, Shattil SJ, Furie B, Cohen HJ, Silberstein LE, Mc Glave P, eds. *Hematology: basic principles and practice*, pp. 1188–204. Churchill Livingston, Philadelphia.

Kaushansky K (1995). Thrombopoietin: the primary regulator of platelet production. *Blood* **86**, 419–31.

Kondo T *et al.* (1998). Familial essential thrombocythemia associated with one-base deletion in the 5'-untranslated region of the thrombopoietin gene. *Blood* **92**, 1091–6.

McIntyre CJ *et al.* (1991). Essential thrombocythaemia in young adults. *Mayo Clinic Proceedings* **66**, 149–54.

Murphy S *et al.* (1997). Experience of the Polycythemia Vera Study Group with essential thrombocythemia: a final report on diagnostic criteria, survival and leukemic transition by treatment. *Seminars in Hematology* **34**, 29–39.

Ruggeri M *et al.* (1998). No treatment for low-risk thrombocythaemia: results from a prospective study. *British Journal of Haematology* **103**, 772–7.

Silverman MN and Tefferi A (1999). Treatment of essential thrombocythemia with anagrelide. *Seminars in Hematology* **36** (Suppl. 2), 23–5.

Tefferi A *et al.* (1994). Plasma interleukin-6 and C-reactive protein levels in reactive versus clonal thrombocytosis. *American Journal of Medicine* **97**, 374–8.

Tefferi A *et al.* (1997). New drugs in essential thrombocythemia and polycythemia vera. *Blood Reviews* **11**, 1–7.

Tefferi A, Hoagland HC (1994). Issues in the diagnosis and management of primary thrombocythemia. *Mayo Clinic Proceedings* **69**, 651–5.

Van Genderen PJJ *et al.* (1996). The reduction of large von Willebrand factor multimers in plasma in essential thrombocythemia is related to the platelet count. *British Journal of Haematology* **93**, 962–5.

Van Genderen PJJ *et al.* (1996). Acquired von Willebrand disease in myeloproliferative disorders. *Leukemia and Lymphoma* **22** (Suppl.1), 79–82.

Van Genderen PJJ *et al.* (1997) Prevention and treatment of thrombotic complications in essential thrombocythemia: efficacy and safety of aspirin. *British Journal of Haematology* **97**, 179–84.

22.3.11 Aplastic anaemia and other causes of bone marrow failure

E. C. Gordon-Smith

Introduction

The concept of bone marrow failure as a cause of peripheral blood cytopenias is imprecise but convenient. Broadly, it indicates that the cause of the peripheral blood disturbance lies within the dividing pool of cells in the marrow itself. Fundamental to the classification of disorders within this group is the idea that normal development of cells within the bone marrow and release of cells into the peripheral blood depend upon an interaction between haematopoietic cells and the environment in which they proliferate and differentiate (see Chapter 22.2.1). The pathogenesis of most of these disorders is unknown and their separation depends mainly upon morphological criteria. The classification shown in Table 1 attempts to group the syndromes where there is a failure of circulating cell production according to the presumed cell stage involved and indicates inherited or congenital syndromes which mimic the acquired disorders.

Aplastic anaemias

Aplastic anaemia is defined by peripheral blood pancytopenia associated with a hypocellular marrow in which the normal haematopoietic tissue is replaced to a greater or lesser extent by fat cells. Remaining cells, both in the peripheral blood and bone marrow, appear morphologically normal and there is neither fibrosis nor infiltration by malignant cells in the marrow. Vitamin B_{12} and folate levels are normal and the disorder is not associated with other dietary deficiencies.

Classification

As defined above, aplastic anaemia may occur in a number of ways. There is no universally acceptable classification but a number of more or less well-defined entities may be identified (Table 2). In each of these, the pathogenesis seems to involve damage to the early haemopoietic progenitor cells, either stem cells or early lineage-committed progenitor cells.

Inevitable aplastic anaemia

Myelosuppression occurs following exposure to cytotoxic drugs or irradiation. The severity and duration of aplasia depends upon the nature of the cytotoxic agent and is dose related. Recovery usually occurs 1 to 6 weeks after the cytotoxic agent is discontinued. With very-high-dose radiation and certain cytotoxic agents, which do not depend on cell cycling for their action, stem cell killing may be complete and recovery does not occur.

Acquired aplastic anaemia

Incidence and epidemiology

Aplastic anaemia is a rare disease. In Europe and the United States, the incidence is probably between 2 and 4 per million of the population per year. All age groups may be affected, possibly with peaks between 20 and 30 and again in older patients. There is a slight preponderance of males, possibly reflecting the greater risk of exposure to toxic substances at work amongst men. In the Far East, the incidence of aplastic anaemia is two to three times higher and the male preponderance much more obvious. The risk factors seem to be environmental rather than genetic since people of the same ethnic groups in the West have a lower incidence.

Aetiology

In about two-thirds of cases of aplastic anaemia it is not possible to identify any likely cause. Amongst the rest, drugs, viruses, and environmental toxins may be identified as probable causes. There is no test to pinpoint the cause of the aplastic anaemia. The implication of any particular agent depends upon temporal associations and previous reports. Drugs have been implicated in the aetiology for 50 years or more and the list of drugs is long. In many cases, the association is weak and often confounded by the patient having received other drugs at the same time. The agents most commonly implicated are some antibiotics, of which chloramphenicol is the best known, and drugs used in the treatment of rheumatoid arthritis including non-steroidal anti-inflammatory agents (NSAIDS) and disease modifying agents in rheumatoid disorders (DMARDs). Table 3 includes a list of the more frequently reported drugs.

Table 1 Classification of bone marrow failure

Pathogenesis	Diseases	
	Acquired	**Congenital**
Haematopoietic stem cell failure	Acquired aplastic anaemia	Fanconi anaemia Dyskeratosis congenita Pearson's syndrome Shwachman–Diamond syndrome Reticular dysgenesis
Proliferative dysplasias with abnormal differentiation	Myelodysplastic syndromes Hypoplastic myelodysplastic syndromes	Congenital dyserythropoietic anaemias
Abnormal environment	Proliferative dysplasias with fibrosis Severe vitamin D deficiency Myelofibrosis	Osteopetrosis
Haematopoietic failure during differentiation	Pure red cell aplasia Parvovirus B19 Amegakaryocytic thrombocytopenia Chronic acquired neutropenia Cyclic neutropenia	Diamond–Blackfan anaemia Thrombocytopenia with absent radii (TAR) Kostmann's syndrome Cyclic neutropenia
Infiltrations	Amyloid (leukaemias/lymphomas)	Lipid storage disease (e.g. Gaucher's disease)
Infections	HIV Dengue fever	
Bone marrow necrosis		

Table 2 Classification of aplastic anaemia (AA)

Disease	Causes	Characterization
Inevitable AA	Cytotoxic drugs Radiation	Dose dependent, predictable recovery
Idiosyncratic AA	Drugs/chemicals Viruses (e.g. hepatitis)	Not dose dependent, prolonged course, recovery unpredictable
	Idiopathic	Most cases
Immune AA	Autoimmune disease Viruses (e.g. Epstein–Barr)	Usually short duration, antibodies may be detectable
Inherited AA	Autosomal recessive inheritance	Fanconi anaemia Pearson's syndrome Shwachman–Diamond syndrome
	Sex linked (usually)	Dyskeratosis congenita
Malignant AA	Acute leukaemias (usually acute lymphoblastic leukaemia)	Transient, leukaemia develops later
	Myelodysplastic aplasia	Prolonged or preleukaemic, cytogenetic abnormalities common

Viruses are also implicated. Up to 10 per cent of patients in Western and Japanese series of aplastic anaemia, particularly in the younger age group, give a history of jaundice and/or hepatitic symptoms some 6 weeks before the pancytopenia develops. In many instances, disturbances of hepatocellular function consistent with viral hepatitis have been demonstrated. However, a specific hepatitis virus is not usually identifiable. Aplastic anaemia has occurred following liver transplantation for fulminant infectious hepatitis but not other causes of liver failure. Occasional reports of aplastic anaemia following Epstein–Barr or other viruses have been published.

Table 3 Drugs which are strongly associated with an increased risk of aplastic anaemia

Class of drug	Examples
Antibiotics	Chloramphenicol Sulfonamides Salazopyrine Co-trimoxazole
Anti-inflammatory agents	Phenylbutazone Oxyphenbutazone Indomethacin Sulindac Diclofenac Piroxicam Penicillamine Gold salts
Thyrostatic	Carbimazole Thiouracils Potassium perchlorate
Anticonvulsant	Hydantoins Phenytoin Mephenytoin Carbamazepine Ethosuximide
Psychotropic	Phenothiazines
Antimalarial	Quinacrine (Mepacrine) Maloprim
Antidiabetic	Chlorpropamide Carbutamide Tolbutamide

Many of these drugs have also been associated with a variety of other blood dyscrasias, particularly neutropenia or agranulocytosis.

Various domestic and recreational drugs and chemicals have been implicated, though the evidence against any particular agent is not always very convincing. Wood preservatives, pesticides, and various organic solvents have been associated with the disease. Benzene is known to produce proliferative dysplasias, including acute leukaemias, when exposure is high. Its part in causing aplasia is not so certain.

Pathogenesis

The way in which the various agents bring about aplastic anaemia is unknown. The main defect is a failure of the pluripotent haematopoietic stem cells in the bone marrow to proliferate and differentiate into mature blood cells. *In vitro* experiments with long-term bone marrow culture show that aplastic marrow stroma cells are able to support haemopoiesis from normal stem cells but aplastic stem cells continue to grow abnormally on normal stroma. There is indirect evidence that cellular immune reactions play a role in the pathogenesis or at least the perpetuation of stem cell damage. The strongest evidence for this is the response of aplastic anaemia to immunosuppressive treatment.

Diagnosis and pathology

The diagnosis of aplastic anaemia is made on the basis of the peripheral blood and bone marrow findings and by excluding other causes for pancytopenia. In the peripheral blood there is pancytopenia with no abnormal cells present. The anaemia is usually normocytic at presentation but becomes macrocytic, even strikingly so, in chronic cases. The reticulocyte count is low. Neutrophils are invariably reduced and the count may be very low. Circulating neutrophils may have rather heavy granulation, so-called 'toxic' granulation, and have a high alkaline phosphatase content. The eosinophils, basophils, and monocytes are usually also depleted. The reduction in the lymphocyte count is more variable; in children particularly it may be relatively high so that the total white cell count may be normal. The platelet count is reduced.

Aspiration of bone marrow is usually easy, fragments are obtained which are fatty, and there is a reduction of haematopoietic cells in the trails. The cellularity of the marrow may be judged to some extent from the marrow aspirate, but a so-called 'dry-tap' (no material obtained from an aspirate) or 'blood-tap' (no fragments obtained) does not allow an assessment of bone marrow activity. In aplastic anaemia, there may be a patchy loss of cellularity throughout the marrow so that an aspirate may yield relatively normal-looking marrow. The diagnosis cannot therefore be made on a bone marrow aspirate alone. Assessment of cellularity is made on a trephine biopsy, which shows replacement of the normal cellular marrow by fatty marrow (Fig. 1). The reticulin network of the marrow is reduced commensurate with the reduction in the general overall cellularity. Focal areas of preserved cellularity may be seen in the bone marrow trephine, so called 'hot pockets' (Fig. 1). The morphology of remaining haematopoietic progenitor cells is broadly normal though there may be some changes in the erythroid precursors which constitute mild dyserythropoiesis. Erythrophagocytosis by macrophages may be prominent, especially early in the disease. Megakaryocytes are often absent but when present have normal maturation and morphology.

Clinical features

The clinical features of aplastic anaemia arise from the deficiencies of the cellular elements of the blood. There are no specific physical signs. Haemorrhagic manifestations are common at presentation. The development of thrombocytopenia takes place over a matter of weeks or months so that catastrophic haemorrhage as a presenting feature is unusual; minor signs of the bleeding tendency, easy bruising, gum bleeding, or purpuric rash, are more usual. Haemorrhages in the buccal mucosa may occur; retinal haemorrhages may be a portent of serious bleeding. The anaemia also develops slowly and the patient may complain only of mild fatigue or shortness of breath on marked exertion. Infections, particularly of the oropharynx or upper respiratory pathways, may be a presenting feature. Infections anywhere aggravate the effect of thrombocytopenia, particularly in the mouth. If the aplastic anaemia has followed an episode of apparent hepatitis, there may be some residual jaundice with enzyme abnormalities consistent with post-hepatitic cholestasis.

The progression of the disease is variable and depends upon the severity and completeness of the marrow damage. In earlier series of patients with aplastic anaemia where only support in the form of transfusions and available antibiotics was given, about half the patients died within 3 to 6 months as a result of infection or haemorrhage. Patients alive at a year, however, had a better chance of surviving, at least for the next 2 or 3 years. This suggested that there was a group of patients with severe disease with a very poor chance of recovery and another group with a milder disorder. This lead to the establishment of criteria for severe aplastic anaemia (Table 4) which have proven to be useful in stratifying patients when different treatments have been compared. The designations severe aplastic anaemia (neutrophils less than 0.5 but more than 0.2×10^{9}/l) and very severe aplastic anaemia (neutrophils less than 0.2×10^{9}/l) are useful in planning therapy.

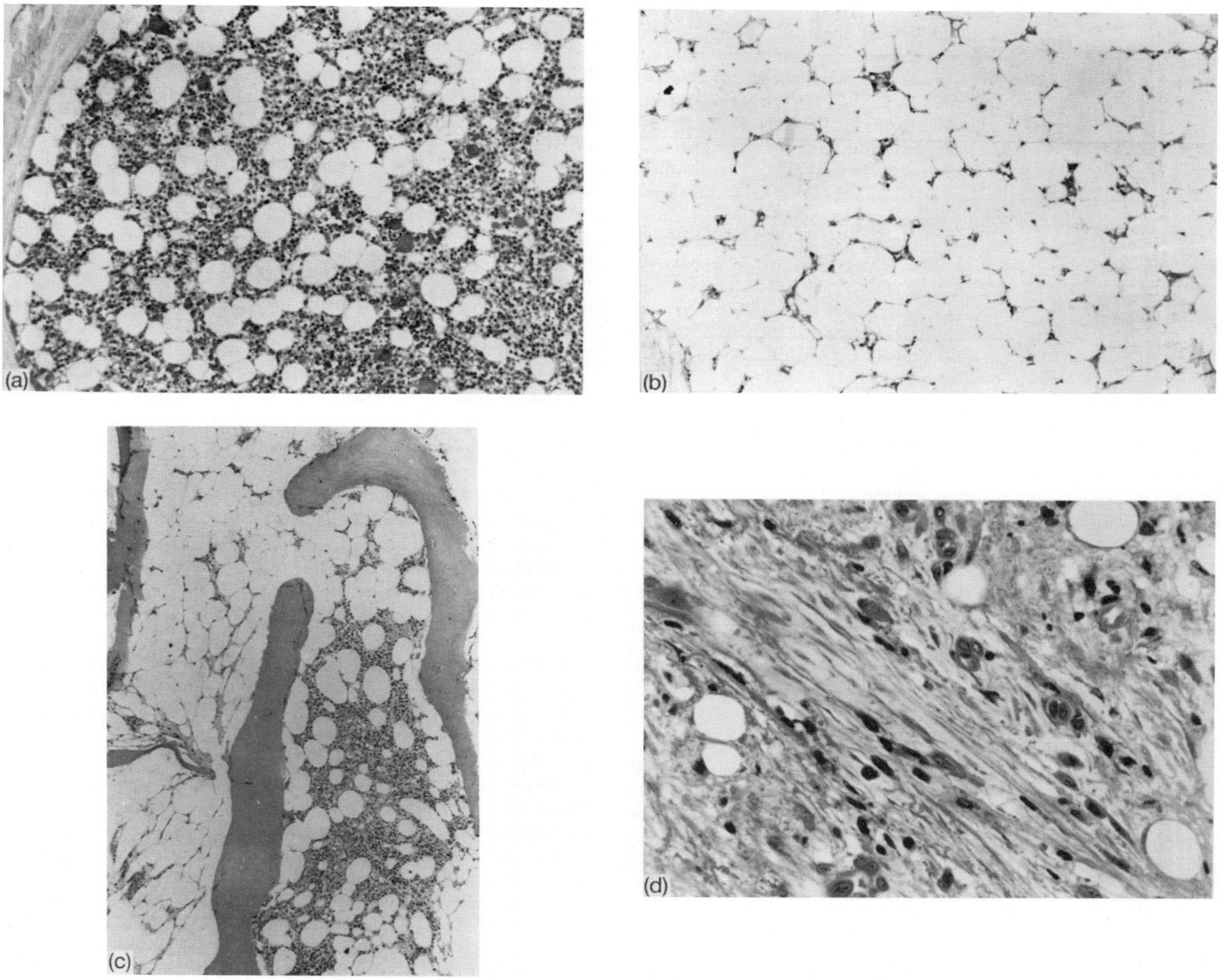

Fig. 1 Trephine biopsies of adult posterior iliac crest: (a) normal marrow; (b) severe aplastic anaemia; (c) cellular focus in severe aplastic anaemia; (d) proliferative dysplasia with fibrosis.

Table 4 Criteria for classifying the severity of aplastic anaemia

Designation	Criteria
Severe aplastic anaemia	Peripheral blood: 2 of 3 Neutrophils $<0.5 \times 10^9$/l Platelets $<20 \times 10^9$/l Reticulocytes <1% (corrected for haematocrit) Bone marrow trephine Markedly hypocellular, <25% cellularity Moderately hypocellular, 25–50% cellularity <30% remaining cells haematopoietic
Very severe aplastic anaemia	As above but neutrophils $<0.2 \times 10^9$/l
Non-severe aplastic anaemia	Remaining cases with pancytopenia and hypocellular marrow

The natural history of the disease has been so modified by improvement in transfusion support and infection control that it is difficult to decide, in some cases, whether subsequent events are part of the disease or the consequences of treatment. Spontaneous recovery, apparently to complete normality, may occur even after several years of pancytopenia. Other patients may remain stable for many years before haematopoietic activity decreases further. The emergence of abnormal clones, both benign and malignant, transient or progressive, is common. Paroxysmal nocturnal haemoglobinuria (PNH) is the most frequent. PNH arises from a somatic mutation involving a gene on the X chromosome which codes for a protein involved in the assembly of phosphatidyl inositol glycan (PIG), which anchors many proteins to the surface of cell membranes. Two enzymes which inactivate complement complexes, decay accelerating factor (DAF; CD59) and membrane inhibitor of reactive lysis (MIRL; CD55) are absent in PNH red cells, which then become sensitive to lysis by complement. PNH may be recognized by the Ham's test or directly by using fluorescence-activated cell scanning to identify populations which lack the PIG anchored proteins. Myelodysplastic syndromes and acute myeloid leukaemia may also develop following aplastic anaemia and the relationship between these blood diseases is discussed below.

Until platelet transfusions became readily available, the usual cause of death in these patients was haemorrhage. Most patients who fail to respond to treatment now succumb to infection or a mixture of infection and haemorrhage, often after many months of treatment with antibiotics. It is virtually impossible to eradicate infection in the severely neutropenic patient until such time as neutrophil production returns.

Treatment

The treatment of aplastic anaemia has two main components. The first is to protect and support patients from the consequences of pancytopenia. The second is to try to accelerate the recovery of the bone marrow by whatever means without eradicating the chance of spontaneous recovery.

Support and protection

For the aplastic patient this depends upon reducing potential sources of infection to a minimum and replacing deficient cells by transfusion (see Section 7). Infections may arise from the environment or from sources of bacteria and other agents with the patient. As with all immunosuppressed patients, significant and lethal infections may arise from contamination with organisms which are not normally pathogenic. Exogenous infections are more likely in a hospital environment than at home, so any patient with aplastic anaemia admitted to hospital must be nursed in a clean, and preferably sterile, area. Measures to prevent nosocomial infections should be of the highest standards. Virus infections are not in themselves especially likely in the neutropenic host, but if they occur they produce an environment in which secondary bacterial infections may flourish. When the neutropenic patient is also immunosuppressed in other ways, virus infections assume a very important role in causing morbidity. Patients with non-severe aplastic anaemia are not at greatly increased risk of opportunistic infection.

Endogenous infections arise from organisms carried within the patient, particularly the upper respiratory passages and the gastrointestinal tract. Scrupulous attention to oral hygiene minimizes the risk of infection from this source and diminishes gum bleeding. The extent to which potential pathogens should be removed from the gastrointestinal tract is debatable. Mostly these are aerobic organisms which are easily eliminated by antibiotics. Some would argue that removal of anaerobic bacteria may actually be harmful. So-called complete decontamination of the gut is achieved by giving a variety of non-absorbable antibiotics together with antifungal agents such as nystatin or amphotericin. Co-trimoxazole or ciprofloxacin, together with an antifungal agent, may be equally effective in eliminating most aerobic pathogens although it has yet to be demonstrated conclusively that this prevents infections. Recolonization of the bowel by potential pathogens can be avoided by using freshly cooked, low bacterial food. It should be remembered that patients with aplastic anaemia may require months of protective isolation and therefore measures must be practical as well as effective.

Once an infection is established, it is essential to treat it as soon as possible. Systemic antibiotics, particularly to treat Gram-negative organisms, must be given as soon as fever or signs of infection occur and appropriate samples have been sent to the laboratory. Delay in the severely neutropenic patient may be fatal. Gram-positive infections, mainly with coagulase-negative staphylococci, are now common because of the extensive use of indwelling central venous lines, but rarely lead to rapidly progressive endotoxic shock. Since the most common exogenous infections arise from *Pseudomonas* or *Klebsiella* spp. and the endogenous ones from aerobic organisms of the gastrointestinal tract, the antibiotics used in the first instance must be appropriate to those organisms. Most centres use a combination of aminoglycoside with a second antibiotic likely to have activity against *Pseudomonas* or a third-generation cephalosporin (suitable regimens are described in Section 7). A difficulty in aplastic anaemia is to decide when to discontinue the antibiotics. The patient may become afebrile and apparently well, but when the antibiotics are stopped, infection by the original organism is all too likely to return unless the neutropenia recovers. Granulocyte stimulating cytokines, filgrastim or lenograstim, or granulocyte–macrophage stimulating cytokine, rhGM-CSF, may stimulate the remaining bone marrow sufficiently to raise the neutrophil count enough to eradicate the infection. Granulocyte transfusions do not seem to be helpful (see Section 7).

Transfusion of red cells and platelets is the other main standby in the management of aplasia. Red cell transfusions usually present few problems, but it must be remembered that the platelet count will fall and haemorrhage may occur during such transfusions. Platelets should always be given with red cell transfusion in the severely pancytopenic patient. Repeated platelet transfusion leads to the development of antibodies and resistance to platelet concentrates in about 40 per cent of patients. This complication is reduced by using white-cell-depleted products. The antibodies may be anti-HLA or antiplatelet-specific antigens. Resistance is indicated by an inability to raise the platelet count by platelet transfusion. Conventionally, platelets are only transfused when there is a clinical indication for their use. Indications include the rapid development of purpura, extensive bleeding from the gums and in the buccal mucosa, retinal haemorrhages, and headache. In aplastic anaemia, particularly when the patient is being managed on an outpatient basis, catastrophic and fatal haemorrhage may be the first indication of severe bleeding, particularly so if the patient develops an infection. For this reason centres manage their outpatients with regular platelet transfusions to maintain a count above 15×10^9/l.

Further details of the management of patients with marrow failure are given elsewhere.

Specific measures

There are two main approaches to the treatment of aplastic anaemia. Haematopoietic stem cell transplantation is curative but carries a high risk of treatment-related mortality and morbidity and is only available to patients with a suitable HLA-matched allogeneic donor. Immunosuppressive treatment, with antilymphocyte or antithymocyte globulin (ALG, ATG) and/or cyclosporin, is the other treatment option. The choice of treatment for any individual with aplastic anaemia depends on the age of the patient, the severity of the disease, and the availability of a suitable donor.

Haematopoietic stem cell transplantation

Recolonization of the aplastic bone marrow with normal stem cells from a suitable donor has long been considered the most rational treatment for aplastic anaemia. The first successful transplants from HLA-matched siblings for severe aplastic anaemia were carried out in Seattle in 1969 by E. Donall Thomas and colleagues. Subsequent, world-wide experience has shown that such transplants are the most effective treatment for very severe aplastic anaemia and severe aplastic anaemia in patients of suitable age. Patients up to the age of 55 years and, in certain instances, older, with very severe aplastic anaemia should be considered for stem cell transplantation. Children and young adults with severe aplastic anaemia should be offered transplantation as the first choice. The problems of stem cell transplantation for aplastic anaemia are the same as for other conditions, namely graft rejection and graft-versus-host disease. Graft rejection may be increased by sensitization to multiple blood transfusions, so transplants are best carried out early, once the diagnosis has been confirmed, the severity established, and a suitable donor identified. Stem cells for transplantation may be obtained from the bone marrow or from the peripheral blood following mobilization of the stem cells from the marrow by granulocyte colony stimulating factor (G-CSF). Peripheral blood stem cell transplants lead to quicker recovery of peripheral blood counts (at about 14 days compared with 20) but may cause more chronic graft-versus-host disease. On-going trials may establish the superior outcome for one or other source in the future. Conditioning of the patient for sibling transplant is relatively mild in that irradiation is not required. Various regimen have been used, the most wide experience being with intravenous cyclophosphamide 50 mg/kg per day for 4 days before the transplant. Commonly this is combined with ALG given for 4 or 5 days before the cyclophosphomide and continuing up to the transplant. The cell dose given is important. Graft rejection is uncommon after transfusion with greater than 3.0×10^6 nucleated cells per kg recipient body weight. Cyclosporin is given for graft-versus-host disease prophylaxis, initially intravenously and subsequently orally, and continued for up to 1 year to prevent late graft rejection. Successful outcome is achieved in about 70 to 80 per cent of cases overall with an incidence of chronic graft-versus-host disease of about 10 to 15 per cent. Children have a success rate of 90 per cent or better. Growth rate, endocrine development, and fertility appear to be normal following this type of transplant and the recovered marrow behaves normally without an increased risk of leukaemia or other clonal disorder.

Problems of bone marrow transplantation are considered further elsewhere.

Immunosuppression

Immunosuppressive treatment for aplastic anaemia was introduced in Europe in 1977, following observations by Georges Mathé in Paris and experimental work by Bruno Speck in Basel. Subsequent controlled trials confirmed that 5 days treatment with ALG was an effective way of achieving remission in all degrees of severity of aplastic anaemia and for all ages. Immunosuppression is the treatment of choice for all patients who are not suitable for transplantation. Recovery following treatment is usually slow with little response before about 3 months and often up to 6 months. Many patients treated in this way still require some transfusion support for this time and may continue with neutropenia and/or thrombocytopenia for many years, though independent of transfusion or hospital care. If the patient fails to respond to the first course of ALG, a second course using an alternative ATG may be given. Some 60 per cent of patients respond to the first course with partial or complete remission and about 40 per cent of non-responders will achieve some improvement with a second. The optimum timing of a second course still has to be determined but most groups wait about 4 to 6 months before a second course. Further courses may be tried in non-responders if they have not been sensitized to the animal protein. There are several preparations of ALG/ATG which are not necessarily bioequivalent so treatment schedules may vary. Reactions during infusion of ALG or ATG are common and may be severe. Serum sickness occurs in some 75 per cent of patients, requiring treatment with corticosteroids. The routine addition of high-dose methylprednisolone (5 mg/kg per day) has no obvious therapeutic advantage and produces a high incidence of avascular necrosis of the hip.

Cyclosporin, 5 mg/kg per day, the dose then adjusted to individual requirement, appears to increase the speed of remission when given after ALG and may also be used alone as an alternative to ALG, though the proportion of responders is less. Recovery, as with ALG, is slow and may be incomplete.

Relapse, or the emergence of PNH or myelodysplastic syndrome clones, leading to a requirement for transfusion, occurs in about 25 per cent of remitting patients over a 10-year period, though some patients respond to further course of immunosuppression. Relapse may follow virus infections, immunizations, or in pregnancy. Some patients seem to be dependent on a continuing dose of cyclosporin post ALG.

Anabolic steroids

Anabolic steroids may be useful in non-severe aplastic anaemia when immunosuppressive therapy fails. The virilizing side-effects make their use unpopular and hepatotoxicity is a problem. A trial of oxymethalone, 2.5 mg/kg per day, or other anabolic steroid in equivalent dose, may be warranted.

Congenital aplastic anaemias

There are a number of inherited disorders which may be associated with bone marrow failure. Table 5 lists the better characterized disorders; familial pancytopenias, which do not fit these diagnoses, sometimes occur.

Fanconi anaemia

The commonest of the inherited disorders which produce aplastic anaemia is that described by Fanconi in 1927. The disorder is inherited as an autosomal recessive and is associated with multiple developmental abnormalities, particularly of the skin and skeleton (Table 6). There is wide genetic and phenotypic heterogeneity. Cases have been described in all populations.

Genetic basis of Fanconi anaemia

Somatic cell fusion studies have shown that there are at least seven distinct genes identifiable, *FANC(A–G)*. Four of these genes have been cloned, *FANCA* (16q24.3), *FANCC* (9q22.3), *FANCF* (11p15), *FANCG* (9p13). For

Table 5 Inherited and congenital causes of bone marrow failure

Disorder	Inheritance	Genetics
Fanconi anaemia	Autosomal recessive	Eight different genes *FANC(A–H)* (see text)
Dyskeratosis congenita	X linked (most cases)	Xq28, *DKC1* (dyskerin)
Pearson syndrome[1,2]	Congenital	Mitochondrial DNA deletion
Shwachman–Diamond syndrome[1]	Autosomal recessive	Unknown

[1] Also have exocrine pancreatic insufficiency.

[2] Ringed sideroblasts.

Table 6 Abnormalities associated with Fanconi anaemia

Condition	Patients affected (%)[1]
Hyperpigmentation of the skin	75
Malformation of the skeleton	
all patients	66
aplasia or hypoplasia of the thumb	50
aplasia or hypoplasia of the radii	17
syndactyly	15
reduced number of carpal bones	30
microsomy/microphthalmia	60
microcephaly	40
malformation of the kidneys	28
strabismus	30
Cryptorchidism	20
Mental retardation	17
Deafness	7
Short stature	80
Growth hormone deficiency[2]	Rare

[1] Percentages are approximate. Data derived mainly from Fanconi (1967).
[2] Many patients have normal levels despite short stature.

each of these genes, multiple mutations have been described. *FANCG* is identical to a gene, *XRCC9*, which is thought to be involved in cell cycle regulation or postreplication repair but the function of the other genes is unknown and the products of the cloned genes have no homology to each other or to other known proteins. It is presumed that the various gene products are part of a pathway involved in chromosome protection, probably through the formation of a functional complex. The genetic heterogeneity accounts for much of the phenotypic heterogeneity.

Cytogenetic findings

The diagnostic test for Fanconi anaemia is the appearance in metaphase of multiple chromosome breaks in phytohaemagglutinin-stimulated peripheral blood lymphocytes. Breakage rate is increased in baseline cultures but is markedly enhanced when cultures are exposed to clastogens such as diepoxybutane or mitomycin C (Fig. 2). Other inherited disorders which are thought to have underlying chromosome instability and a defect in DNA repair also have an increased tendency to develop acute leukaemia, though not usually with an aplastic phase (see Table 7).

Haematological features

Patients with Fanconi anaemia usually have a normal or nearly normal blood count at birth and during infancy. Bone marrow failure develops slowly. The age at which it is manifest clinically depends in part on the underlying genetic cause. In many cases the failure appears between 5 and 10 years, in other families the defect becomes apparent in adolescence whilst in some cases it presents in adult life. A severe form caused by a mutation in *FANCC*, the IVS-4 mutation found in Ashkenazi Jews, has a particularly rapid development of aplasia and a very high transformation to acute leukaemia. In all cases the bone marrow becomes progressively hypocellular, eventually being indistinguishable from acquired aplastic anaemia. Early on, macrophages showing active phagocytosis are prominent, perhaps indicating the removal of cells in apoptosis. Granulopoiesis may be relatively well-preserved. Dyserythropoiesis may be prominent. Evolution to acute leukaemia is common, particularly in some gene types. Patients may present with acute leukaemia, usually myeloid, without a prior period of aplasia. Red cells are macrocytic but there are no specific features in the peripheral blood to suggest the diagnosis.

Clinical features

The features of the full-blown Fanconi anaemia are characteristic (Table 6). There is marked phenotypic variation between patients in different families but considerable similarities within families, which reflects the genetic variation. In some cases, diagnosis may be difficult because of absence of the characteristic skeletal and skin features. Infants are of low birth weight and most remain small-for-age after birth. The skin is often mildly pigmented with areas of deeper pigmentation producing café-au-lait spots, sometimes

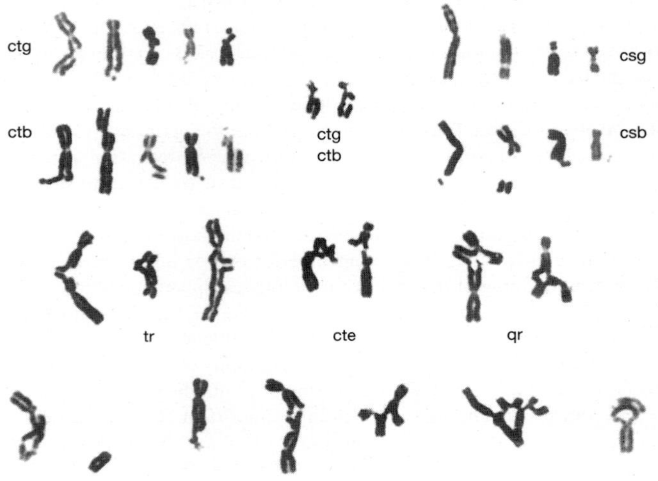

Fig. 2 Chromosomes from a metaphase preparation of peripheral blood lymphocytes from a patient with Fanconi anaemia incubated in the presence of diepoxybutane (DEB) show multiple breaks and rearrangements. ctg, chromatid gap; csg, chromosome gap; ctb, chromatid break; csb, chromosome break. Rearrangements: cte, chromatid exchange; tr, triradial; qr, quadriradial.

Table 7 Disorders with possible defective DNA repair mechanisms associated with increased risk of leukaemia and other malignancies

Disease	Clinical features	Evidence for DNA repair defect	Malignancy
Fanconi anaemia	Aplastic anaemia Skeletal disorders Skin disorders	Chromatid breaks	Acute leukaemia ?Hepatocellular carcinoma
Xeroderma pigmentosa	Keratosis of the skin Neurological disease Mental deficiency Bone marrow failure	Excessive chromatid fragility to ultraviolet light Excision repair defect	Skin cancers
Bloom's syndrome	Growth disorder Sun-sensitive eruptions Disturbed immune function	Chromatid breaks Sister chromatid exchanges	Acute leukaemia
Ataxia telangiectasia	Cerebellar ataxia Oculocutaneous telangiectasia Combined immune deficiency	Defective excision	Acute leukaemia and other lymphoreticular malignancies

with areas of depigmentation. Skeletal abnormalities involve particularly the bones of the forearm and thumbs. Abnormalities in the anatomy of the kidneys are also common. Intellectual development is usually normal.

Prognosis and treatment

The outlook in Fanconi anaemia is poor. Untreated, the disease is usually relentless. Despite support with transfusions over many years most patients die of haemorrhage, infection, or of acute leukaemia. Fanconi anaemia should also be suspected in all children and adolescents presenting with acute myeloid leukaemia. Identification of the familial nature of the disease is important for genetic counselling. The median interval between presentation and death is about 2 to 4 years. Patients who survive to adult life have an increased risk of solid tumours of squamous origin, particularly of the tongue, oesophagus, vulva, cervix, and breast. Most adult females are fertile whilst most males are infertile.

Treatment with anabolic steroids may bring about a remission of variable duration. Several years free from transfusion requirements may be obtained, but at the price of virilization and liver toxicity. Hepatocellular carcinoma, often accompanying peliosis hepatis, seems to be particularly common in children treated for years with 17α-alkylated anabolic agents (Fig. 3).

Bone marrow transplantation is the only curative form of treatment but carries special risks. The Fanconi anaemia cells are very sensitive to cyclophosphamide and irradiation used to immunosuppress patients prior to transplant and the doses given to these patients have to be greatly reduced. With these modifications, the success of bone marrow transplantation from HLA-matched sibling donors is similar to that for acquired aplastic anaemia. Transplantation from unrelated, HLA-matched donors is less successful but given that no other treatment is effective, should be offered whenever possible.

Dyskeratosis congenita

Dyskeratosis congenita is an inherited disorder involving the mucocutaneous system with the development of bone marrow failure in about 50 per cent of cases. The inheritance is X linked in the majority of cases with the defective gene located at Xq28.The gene mutated in these cases is designated *DKC1*, the protein dyskerin. Dyskerin may take part in the assembly of ribosomes and their export from the nucleus to the cytoplasm. Some families show recessive inheritance with female members also being affected.

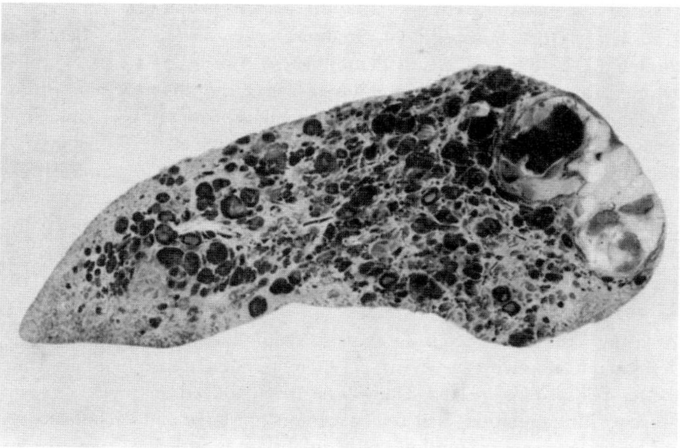

Fig. 3 Hepatocellular carcinoma in the liver of a patient with Fanconi anaemia treated for 4 years with anabolic steroids; the liver also shows multiple venous lakes (peliosis hepatis), another side-effect of anabolic steroids.

Patients have reticular skin pigmentation of the upper body; leukoplakia and nail dystrophy usually appearing in childhood. There is a high incidence of squamous carcinoma of the oropharynx and gastrointestinal tract but not an increased risk of leukaemia. Marrow aplasia develops in the second or third decade. Treatment with anabolic steroids may be temporally effective in some patients as with Fanconi anaemia but most patients become refractory. Stem cell transplantation should be considered as the only possible cure for the haematological problems but results are poor. Late complications post-transplantation include renal failure, pulmonary fibrosis, and diffuse vasculitis.

Aplastic presentation of malignant disease

Aplastic anaemia is one response to bone marrow damage and acute leukaemia is another. At presentation, the distinction between the two may not always be clear, at least on histological and morphological criteria.

Acute lymphoblastic leukaemia (ALL)

ALL may present in a form indistinguishable from aplastic anaemia, usually, but not exclusively, in children. Blasts are not seen in the peripheral blood, and the bone marrow aspirate and trephine are hypocellular without any obvious infiltration by malignant cells. Presentation with severe infection, often of the pharynx, is more common than in acquired aplastic anaemia. The aplasia usually recovers spontaneously, sometimes in response to steroids. Some 6 to 8 weeks later there is the emergence of leukaemic cells in the peripheral blood. Whilst ALL in childhood is the commonest association, aplasia preceding acute myeloid leukaemia in this way has been described, and adults are occasionally affected.

Hypoplastic myelodysplasia

Hypoplastic myelodysplastic syndrome is a disease characterized by a hypocellular marrow in which a small proportion of blasts may be seen, sometimes with occasional blasts in the peripheral blood. The proportion of blasts in the marrow is less than 5 per cent but there may be abnormal aggregations of primitive precursors. Circulating granulocytes, reduced in number, are hypogranular in contrast to the toxic granulation of aplastic anaemia. The condition differs in a number of ways from aplastic anaemia, but the differences may be subtle and there is considerable overlap. The distinction by morphological criteria is subjective. The presence of cytogentically abnormal metaphases has been used to distinguish hypoplastic myelodysplastic syndrome from aplastic anaemia but transient clones may appear in the latter. The condition may remain stable for months or years during which the patient requires transfusions but is otherwise well. The prognosis is in the low-risk group of the international prognostic scoring system. If a suitable bone marrow donor is available, transplantation is indicated. Recent trials have shown that as many as two-thirds of patients may achieve meaningful remissions with ALG, indicating another link with aplastic anaemia.

Proliferative dysplasia with fibrosis

Occasionally, fibrosis of the bone marrow appears without evident underlying cause and in the absence of hepatosplenomegaly or extramedullary haemopoiesis. The condition is characterized by pancytopenia sometimes with the presence of red cell and white cell precursors in the peripheral blood, a leucoerythroblastic picture. Bone marrow aspirate is usually unsuccessful, and a trephine biopsy shows a variable degree of reduction in haemopoietic cells with the marrow replaced by reticulin and fibroblasts. Primitive cells are not seen at this stage of the illness. Some of these patients probably have an unusual form of myelofibrosis, particularly those who

Table 8 Bone marrow failure affecting surface cell lines

Deficiency	Inherited	Acquired
Pure red cell aplasia	Diamond–Blackfan anaemia	Pure red cell aplasia ± thymoma Drug-induced Parvovirus 19 infection Transient erythroblastopenia of childhood
Neutropenia	Kostmann's syndrome Shwachman–Diamond syndrome	Cyclical neutropenia Drug-induced
Thrombocytopenia	With total absence of radii (TAR)	Amegakaryocytic thrombocytopenia

present in childhood. Others may have hypoplastic failure in which abnormal megakaryocyte development leads to the fibrosis.

Bone marrow failure affecting single cell lines

There are a number of conditions in which anaemia, neutropenia, or thrombocytopenia develop in isolation as a result of the failure of production by the marrow. The conditions may be inherited or acquired and the main disorders are listed in Table 8. The majority of acquired cytopenias are immune in origin with peripheral destruction so do not represent examples of bone marrow failure.

Amegakaryocytic thrombocytopenia

Thrombocytopenia caused by deficiency of megakaryocytes may be acquired or inherited. Inherited syndromes include amegakaryocytic thrombocytopenia with total absence of radii (TAR syndrome) and other congenital cases with normal skeleton. If children with TAR survive the first year of life, when cerebral haemorrhage is most likely, the platelet count usually increases spontaneously to safe levels and the outlook is good. Acquired amegakaryocytic thrombocytopenia is probably a variant of aplastic anaemia or myelodysplastic syndrome. The condition is rare. About one-third of patients remain thrombocytopenic, another third progress slowly to aplasia, and the remainder develop myelodysplastic syndrome. Immunosuppressive therapy may produce remission and stem cell transplantation may be curative for appropriate patients.

Pure red cell aplasia (PRCA)

PRCA is defined by anaemia with a marked reduction or absence of reticulocytes in which the neutrophil and platelet count are normal. The bone marrow is cellular with normal granulopoiesis and megakaryocytes. There may be a complete absence of red cell precursors or there may be red cell precursors present up to a certain stage of development but not beyond, so-called 'maturation arrest'. Apart from the changes in the red cell series, there are no other abnormalities in the peripheral blood and there is no evidence of peripheral destruction of red cells. The patients are in other respects normal. Both congenital and acquired forms exist.

Congenital pure red cell aplasia—Diamond–Blackfan anaemia

This has also been called rather confusingly 'congenital hypoplastic anaemia' but is better known by its eponym, the Diamond–Blackfan syndrome. In most instances, anaemia is present at birth or is detected shortly afterwards. There is a profound reticulocytopenia often with no reticulocytes present in the peripheral blood. There is macrocytosis and raised HbF. Red cell adenosine deaminase is increased. There is no hepatosplenomegaly. The white count and platelet counts are normal. Skeletal abnormalities may be present, particularly of the head and upper limb. About 50 per cent have no dysmorphic features. There may be disturbances of growth, either inherent in the disease or brought about by anaemia, iron overload, or steroid therapy. There are no abnormalities of the skin or other organs as seen in Fanconi anaemia.

Pathogenesis

There seem to be a number of genetic abnormalities underlying the disorder. About 20 per cent of patients have a family history, usually in earlier generations, suggesting dominant inheritance. The remainder has no such history but adenosine deaminase may be elevated in first degree relatives and sporadic cases may go on to have affected children. One gene in which mutations are associated with Diamond–Blackfan anaemia is located on chromosome 19 and codes for RPS19, a ribosomal protein. The function of the protein in the pathogenesis of Diamond–Blackfan anaemia is unknown. About a quarter of Diamond–Blackfan anaemia families have this defect. At least two other unrelated defects produce the phenotype.

Treatment

Treatment presents many problems. Most of these children, if treated early enough with corticosteroids, will respond. However, if the condition is steroid-dependent, major problems may result from the continued use of corticosteroids in the doses necessary to maintain remission. Patients may become steroid resistant. Some patients fail to respond to corticosteroids, and this seems to be particularly true if the corticosteroids are instituted late in the illness. These patients rely on blood transfusions for survival. Transfusion will permit normal growth but produces all the problems of iron overload, including delayed or absent puberty. Chelation therapy is required from an early stage. Stem cell transplantation should be considered if there is a matched family donor but the potential donor should be checked for raised adenosine deaminase levels as well as anaemia before being accepted.

During the course of the disease, the spleen may enlarge and transfusion requirements increase. In these patients, splenectomy may reduce transfusion requirements and occasionally is associated with a marked increase in steroid responsiveness or even complete remission. This only seems to apply to those patients whose spleen is enlarged, and relapse may occur after a few years.

Transient erythroblastopenic anaemia in childhood (TEC)

Transient erythroblastopenia of childhood may have a viral aetiology though this is not always clearly demonstrated. The anaemia with reticulocytopenia most often occurs in children from 6 months to 5 years with a peak incidence around 2 years. There is usually a history of preceding viral illness. More than one member of the family may be affected making distinction from Diamond–Blackfan anaemia difficult. The anaemia is normocytic and adenosine deaminase levels are normal. Neutropenia is common. Recovery occurs within a few weeks of diagnosis though the patient may need transfusion in the meantime.

Parvovirus infection

'Aplastic crises' may occur in patients with haemolytic anaemia who develop infection with Parvovirus B 19. The term is confusing because only the red cell series is affected. The virus is tropic for red cell precursors and prevents differentiation. Red cell precursors are large and vacuolated. As antibodies to the virus develop, so the inhibition is removed. The reticulocytopenia lasts for up to 7 days so that the effect is trivial or unnoticed in people with red cell survival of 120 days. In patients with short red cell survival, such as patients with sickle cell disease and other congenital haemolytic anaemias, the effect may be devastating. Anaemia develops rapidly and transfusion may be required urgently. Antibodies to the virus are lacking in the serum initially, followed by an IgM response. The presence of IgG antibodies precludes the diagnosis.

Acquired pure red cell aplasia

This may occur *de novo*, following administration of various drugs, or in association with lymphoma, and about one-third are associated with a thymoma. PRCA may precede, accompany, or follow the development of the thymoma and excision of the tumour has variable effect with no guarantee of recovery of the anaemia. The haematological features of the disorder are similar to that seen in the congenital red cell aplasia, with anaemia and reticulocytopenia associated with absence of red cell precursors or maturation arrest of the red cell series in the bone marrow. There is an unpredictable responsiveness to corticosteroids. Immunosuppression with azathioprine or cyclophosphamide may be effective. Autoantibodies are thought to play a role in the pathogenesis and occasionally immunoglobulins have been identified which inhibit haem synthesis or prevent the development of red cell colonies *in vitro*. Very rarely antierythropoietin antibodies have been found.

Acquired PRCA may occur in association with common variable hypogammaglobulinaemia and in association with other autoimmune diseases. The presence of such autoimmune phenomena suggests that the patient has a better chance of responding to corticosteroids than in their absence. PRCA may be associated with lymphomas and evidence of an underlying lymphoma may be obtained by finding evidence of immunoglobulin or T-cell receptor gene rearrangement in the marrow even when histological proof is lacking. Occasionally, splenectomy may increase responsiveness to corticosteroids or immunosuppression. An enlarging spleen, which increases transfusion requirements, is an indication for splenectomy. A chronic transfusion regimen with iron chelation may be required for non-responding patients.

Isolated defects in white cell or platelet production

These conditions are described elsewhere and are summarized in Table 7.

Further reading

Barrett J, Sauntharajah Y, Molldrem J (2000). Myelodysplastic syndrome and aplastic anemia: distinct entities or diseases linked by a common pathophysiology? *Seminars in Hematology* **37**, 15–29.

Fanconi G (1967). Familial constitutional panmyelopathy, Fanconi's anaemia (FA). I. Clinical aspects. *Seminars in Hematology* **4**, 233–40.

Gluckman E (1998). Fanconi anaemia. In: Barrett J, Treleaven J, eds. *The clinical practice of stem cell transplantation,* pp. 259–65. Isis Medical Media, Oxford.

Gordon-Smith EC, Issaragrisil S (1992). Epidemiology of aplastic anaemia. *Clinics in Haematology* **5:2**, 475–91.

Marsh J, Gordon-Smith T (1998). Aplastic anaemia. In: Barrett J, Treleaven J, eds. *The clinical practice of stem cell transplantaion,* pp. 238–58. Isis Medical Media, Oxford.

Marsh JC, Gordon-Smith EC (1998). Treatment options in severe aplastic anaemia. *Lancet* **351**, 1830–1.

Schrezenmeier H, Bacigalupo A, eds (2000). *Aplastic anemia. Pathophysiology and treatment.* Cambridge University Press, Cambridge.

Schroeder-Kurth TH, Auerbach AD, Obe G, eds (1989). *Fanconi anemia.* Springer-Verlag, Heidelberg.

Schwartz RS (1994). PIG-A—the target gene in paroxysmal nocturnal hemoglobinuria. *New England Journal of Medicine* **330**, 283–4.

Sieff CA, Nisbet-Brown E, Nathan DG (2000). Review. Congenital bone marrow failure syndromes. *British Journal of Haematology* **111**, 30–42.

Wagner JL, Storb R (1999). Allogeneic transplantation for aplastic anemia. In: Thomas ED, Blume KG, Forman SJ, eds. *Hematopoietic cell transplantation*, 2nd edn, pp. 791–806. Blackwell Science, Oxford.

Wright EG (1999). Inherited and inducible chromosomal instability: a fragile bridge between genome integrity mechanisms and tumourigenesis. Review. *Journal of Pathology* **187**, 19–27.

Young NS, Alter BP (1994). *Aplastic anemia acquired and inherited.* W.B. Saunders, Philadelphia.

22.3.12 Paroxysmal nocturnal haemoglobinuria

Lucio Luzzatto

Definition

Paroxysmal nocturnal haemoglobinuria (**PNH**) is an acquired chronic disorder characterized by persistent intravascular haemolysis, subject to recurrent exacerbations, often associated with pancytopenia, and with a distinct tendency to venous thrombosis. The triad of haemolytic anaemia, pancytopenia, and thrombosis makes PNH a truly unique clinical condition: however, even in the absence of one or more of these manifestations a conclusive diagnosis can be made by appropriate laboratory investigations (see below).

Epidemiology

PNH is encountered in all populations throughout the world, and it can affect people of all socioeconomic groups. The prevalence of PNH is not accurately known: however, it is more rare than the related disorder, acquired aplastic anaemia (**AAA**). A rough estimate of the frequency of PNH is between 1 in 100 000 and 1 in 1 million. It has been suggested that, like AAA, PNH may be somewhat less rare in South East Asia and in the Far East. Most patients present as young adults, but we have seen PNH in a 2-year-old child and in people in their seventies. PNH has never been reported as a congenital disease, and there is no reported evidence of inherited susceptibility. The sex ratio is not far from even.

Clinical features

The patient may seek medical attention because, one morning, she or he has 'passed blood instead of urine'. This distressing or frightening event—the direct evidence of haemoglobinuria—may be regarded as the classical presentation; however, not infrequently the haemoglobinuria may be initially less spectacular, or it is suppressed. Indeed, the patient often presents simply as a problem in the differential diagnosis of anaemia, whether symptomatic or discovered incidentally; this may be associated with jaundice, immediately suggesting it may be a haemolytic anaemia. Sometimes the anaemia is associated from the outset with neutropenia, or thrombocytopenia, or both. Venous thrombosis may be the first clinical manifestation in other patients. Although any vein may be affected, the most common localization is intra-abdominal: indeed, recurrent attacks of severe abdominal pain defying a specific diagnosis, and eventually found to be related to thrombosis, have given to PNH the attribute of being a great impostor. On the other hand, when thrombosis affects the hepatic veins it may produce acute hepatomegaly and ascites—that is to say, a fully fledged Budd–Chiari syndrome.

The natural history of PNH can extend over decades. Without treatment the median survival is estimated to be about 8 to 10 years (see Fig. 1); in the past—but unfortunately even today—the most common causes of death have been thrombosis, or infection associated with severe neutropenia, or haemorrhage associated with severe thrombocytopenia. PNH may evolve

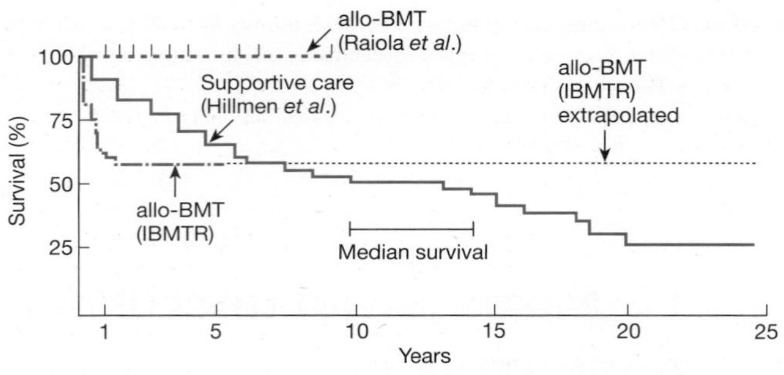

Fig. 1 PNH is a chronic disorder, the time course of which is often measured in decades. From a series of 80 patients who received only minimal supportive treatment we estimate a median survival of about 10 years. Allogeneic BMT has still been associated with significant mortality, and therefore may have reduced the survival of some patients; but recently more encouraging data have been reported on a small series from a single centre.

into AAA, and PNH may manifest itself in patients who previously had AAA. Rarely (estimated 1–2 per cent of all cases), PNH may terminate in acute myeloid leukaemia. On the other hand, full spontaneous recovery from PNH has been also well documented.

Laboratory investigations and diagnosis

The most consistent blood finding is anaemia, which may range from mild to moderate to very severe. The anaemia is usually normomacrocytic; if the mean cell volume (**MCV**) is high it is usually largely accounted for by reticulocytosis, which may be quite marked—up to 20 per cent. The anaemia may become microcytic if the patient is allowed to become iron-deficient as a result of chronic urinary blood loss through haemoglobinuria. The red cell morphology is otherwise usually normal. Neutropenia and/or thrombocytopenia may or may not be present from the outset, or may develop subsequently. Unconjugated bilirubin is mildly or moderately elevated; lactate dehydrogenase (**LDH**) is typically markedly elevated; haptoglobin is usually undetectable. All these findings make the diagnosis of haemolytic anaemia compelling. Haemoglobinuria may be overt in a random urine sample: if it is not, it may be helpful to obtain serial urine samples, since haemoglobinuria can vary dramatically from day to day, and even from hour to hour (it is more common, but not always, in the early morning: hence the adjective 'nocturnal'). Obviously, haemoglobinuria must be distinguished from haematuria. Surprisingly, even today a patient may undergo extensive urological investigations before it is realized that the patient has PNH. There may be free haemoglobin in the serum, and sometimes this is so high as to interfere with clinical chemistry. These findings clearly indicate intravascular haemolysis, thus increasing, by an order of magnitude, the likelihood that the haemolytic anaemia is in fact PNH (see Table 1). The bone marrow is usually cellular, with marked to massive erythroid hyperplasia, often with mild to moderate dyserythropoietic features. However, at some stage of the disease the marrow may become hypocellular or even frankly aplastic (see below).

The definitive diagnosis of PNH must be based on the demonstration that a substantial proportion of the patient's red cells have an increased susceptibility to complement, due to the deficiency on their surface of proteins that normally protect the red cells from activated complement. Classically, this is proven by the Ham test (acidified serum test): if appropriately carried out with all the necessary controls this test is still valid. By contrast, the sucrose haemolysis test can give both 'false-negatives' and 'false-positives', and therefore must be regarded as obsolete. Nowadays, the presence of a PNH red blood cell population can be easily demonstrated and quantified by flow cytometry, using anti-CD59 or anti-CD48. This analysis can also be carried out on granulocytes with a higher sensitivity (see Fig. 2).

Pathophysiology

Haemolysis

Haemolysis in PNH is due to an intrinsic abnormality of the red cell, which makes it exquisitely sensitive to activated complement, whether it is activated through the alternative pathway or through an antigen–antibody reaction. The former mechanism is probably the reason why there is chronic intravascular haemolysis in PNH. The latter mechanism explains why the haemolysis can be dramatically exacerbated in the course of a viral or bacterial infection. Hypersusceptibility to complement is due to the deficiency of several protective membrane proteins, of which CD59 is the most important, because it hinders the insertion into the membrane of C9 polymers.

The molecular basis for the deficiency of these proteins has been pinpointed not to a defect in any of the respective genes, but rather to the shortage of a unique glycolipid molecule, glycosyl phosphatidyl inositol (**GPI**), which, through a peptide bond, anchors these proteins to the surface membrane of cells. The shortage of GPI is due in turn to a mutation in an X-linked gene, called *PIG-A*, required for an early step in GPI biosynthesis. In virtually each patient the *PIG-A* mutation is different. This is not surprising, since these mutations are not inherited: rather, each one takes place *de novo* in a haemopoietic stem cell (in other words, they are somatic mutations). As a result, the patient's bone marrow is a mosaic of mutant and non-mutant cells, and the peripheral blood always contains both PNH cells and normal (non-PNH) cells (see Fig. 2).

Thrombosis

This is one of the most immediately life-threatening complications of PNH, and yet one of the least understood pathogenetically. It could be due to impaired fibrinolysis, because the urokinase plasminogen activator receptor (**uPAR**) is a GPI-linked protein; alternatively, complement activation could cause hypercoagulability, or hyperactivity of platelets, or both. For instance, it could be speculated that deficiency of CD59 on the PNH platelet could lead to abnormal insertion of the C5b–9 complex in the platelet membrane, as is the case with the red cell.

Table 1 Differential diagnosis of dark urine

Different sorts of dark urine	Causes	Additional tests	Possible diagnosis
Haematuria	Many	Clears on centrifugation	Mostly urinary tract pathology
Myoglobinuria	Rhabdomyolysis	Ultrafiltration; spectroscopy	March myoglobinuria
Haemoglobinuria	Intravascular haemolysis	Serology after blood transfusion	Incompatible blood transfusion
		Donath–Landsteiner antibody	Paroxysmal cold haemoglobinuria
		G6PD activity	G6PD deficiency
		Blood film for malaria parasites	'Blackwater fever'
		Ham; flow cytometry for CD59	PNH

G6PD, glucose-6-phosphate dehydrogenase; PNH, paroxysmal nocturnal haemoglobinuria.

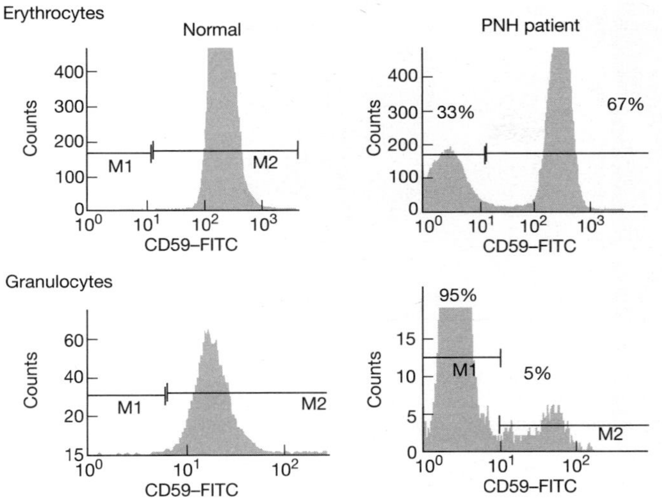

Fig. 2 Flow cytometry analysis of blood cells in a patient with PNH. On the left, red cells and granulocytes from a normal person display a unimodal distribution of surface expression of the GPI-linked protein CD59, which protects red cells against complement-mediated lysis. On the right, a similar analysis reveals, in a patient with PNH, a clearly bimodal distribution: from this analysis the size of the PNH cell population can be quantitated. (Figure by courtesy of Dr David Araten.)

Bone marrow failure and the relationship between PNH and AAA

PNH has an intimate link with AAA, for several reasons. (1) As stated above, sometimes a patient with PNH becomes 'less haemolytic' and 'more pancytopenic' and ultimately evolves to frank AAA. (2) In terms of pathogenesis, it is believed that AAA is essentially an organ-specific autoimmune disease mediated by 'activated' cytotoxic (CD8+) T lymphocytes, which are able to inhibit haemopoietic stem cells. Recently, skewing of the T-cell repertoire, indicating the presence of abnormally expanded T-cell clones, has also been observed in cases of PNH. (3) Most important, intensive immunosuppressive treatment is the standard of care in those with AAA, and a beneficial response to the same treatment can also be obtained in patients with PNH (see below).

In view of these facts, it seems that an element of bone marrow failure in PNH is the rule rather than the exception: an extreme view is that PNH is a form of AAA, in which bone marrow failure is masked by the enormous expansion of the PNH clone that populates the patient's bone marrow. In other words, it appears that two different mechanisms co-operate in producing PNH (see Fig. 3): autoimmune damage to stem cells, and a somatic mutation in the *PIG-A* gene. This notion is supported by two further lines of evidence. (1) By targeted inactivation of the *pig-A* gene in mouse embryonic stem cells one can produce mice with a PNH cell population. However, this population does not grow further, as it does in patients with PNH. (2) By using refined flow cytometry technology, PNH cells harbouring *PIG-A* mutations can be demonstrated in normal people at a frequency in the order of 10 per million. Both these findings indicate that some other factor is required, in addition to a somatic mutation in the *PIG-A* gene, in order to cause PNH. Most likely, the same cytotoxic damage to stem cells that would otherwise cause AAA spares the PNH stem cells, thus allowing the PNH clone to grow to the size when it gives clinical PNH. The mechanism whereby the PNH cells escape damage is not yet known.

Complications

Given the chronic course and the complex nature of PNH, many events can cause concern and sometimes threaten life. The most important complication is certainly thrombosis, which is nearly always venous, and mostly affects the abdominal veins (see Fig. 4). The Budd–Chiari syndrome has already been mentioned: because of its characteristic clinical picture it is usually easy to recognize. However, in PNH it is sometimes associated with portal vein thrombosis, and this may limit the extent of liver enlargement. Thrombosis of the splenic vein should be suspected whenever a patient with PNH has, or develops, splenomegaly. Thrombosis of one of the mesenteric veins is much more difficult to diagnose clinically. Appropriate investigations include Doppler ultrasound, contrast-enhanced computer tomography (**CT**), and magnetic resonance imaging (**MRI**): in our experience, the most sensitive methodology is MR venography. Another life-threatening site of thrombosis is in the cranial veins, particularly the sagittal and transverse sinuses. Assessment of the location and extent of these complications is of great practical importance, because thrombolytic therapy with tissue plasminogen activator (Fig. 4) has been carried out successfully even after 3 weeks from the onset of signs and symptoms.

Treatment (see Fig. 5)

In the management of patients with PNH it is important to keep in mind two cardinal points: (1) unlike other acquired haemolytic anaemias, PNH may be lifelong; and (2) in view of the unique pathophysiological features reviewed in the section above, we may have to deal with any or all of three components: haemolysis, thrombosis, bone marrow failure. At the moment, the only form of treatment that can provide a cure for PNH is allogeneic bone marrow transplantation (**BMT**): when an HLA-identical sibling is available, BMT should be offered to any young patient with PNH, especially if there is severe pancytopenia. Results similar to those for AAA can be expected, with long-term disease-free survival ranging from 60 to 100 per cent in the few series that have been published (see Fig. 1: by contrast, the past record of BMT from unrelated donors in PNH is poor). The majority of patients will not have a potential sibling donor, and some of those who do may not wish to undergo BMT. Given the common pathogenesis of PNH and AAA, a logical alternative is immunosuppressive treatment with antilymphocyte globulin (or antithymocyte globulin) and ciclosporin A. Although no formal trial has ever been conducted, this approach has particularly helped to relieve severe thrombocytopenia and/or neutropenia in patients in whom these were the main problem(s): by

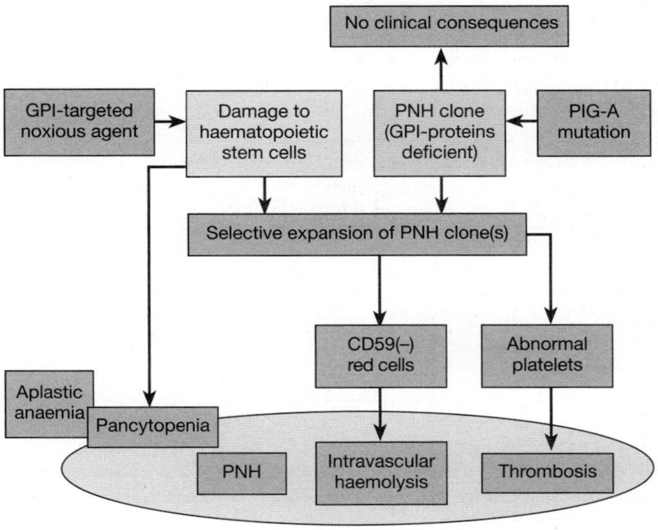

Fig. 3 The role of somatic mutation and bone marrow failure in causing PNH. This cartoon aims to emphasize that two separate factors are required to bring about PNH as a clinical disease. On the one hand, a *PIG-A* mutation on its own will produce a PNH clone, but there will be no basis for it to expand; on the other hand, damage to haemopoietic stem cells (HSC) can cause aplastic anaemia without PNH. When both factors co-operate, and if the damage to HSC is GPI-mediated, then there will be selective expansion of the PNH clone.

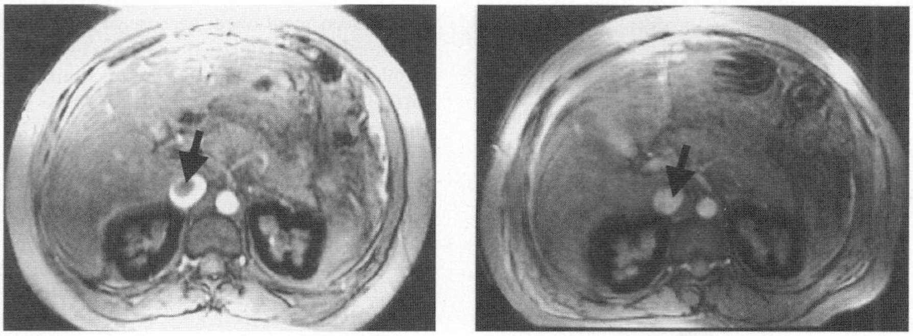

(a) (b)

Fig. 4 Abdominal vein thrombosis in PNH can resolve with thrombolytic therapy. (a) shows extensive thrombus in the inferior vena cava in a patient with known PNH who had developed Budd–Chiari syndrome a few days earlier: it is not infrequent in PNH for thrombosis to involve multiple veins in the abdomen all at once. (b) shows a thrombus-free vena cava 2 days after an intravenous infusion of tissue plasminogen activator.(Figure by courtesy of Dr Raymond Thertulien.)

contrast, there is often little beneficial effect on the haemolysis itself. For all patients, supportive management supervised by somebody who has previous experience of PNH can help the patient to 'live with PNH' for years, sometimes for decades, and sometimes with a good quality of life. The mainstay of support is the transfusion of filtered red cells whenever necessary. Folic acid supplements (at least 3 mg/day) are mandatory; the serum iron concentration should be checked periodically and iron supplements added as indicated. Prednisone (often administered at a dose of 15–30 mg on alternate days) is still quite popular; however, there is no evidence that prednisone decreases the rate of haemolysis, and long-term administration of prednisone, even at a low dosage, is **contraindicated**, in view of the serious potential side-effects. By contrast, a short course of prednisone may sometimes appear helpful during the course of an episode of massive haemoglobinuria associated with intercurrent infection. Any patient who has had a deep vein thrombosis at any one site in the abdomen or in a limb should be given anticoagulant prophylaxis.

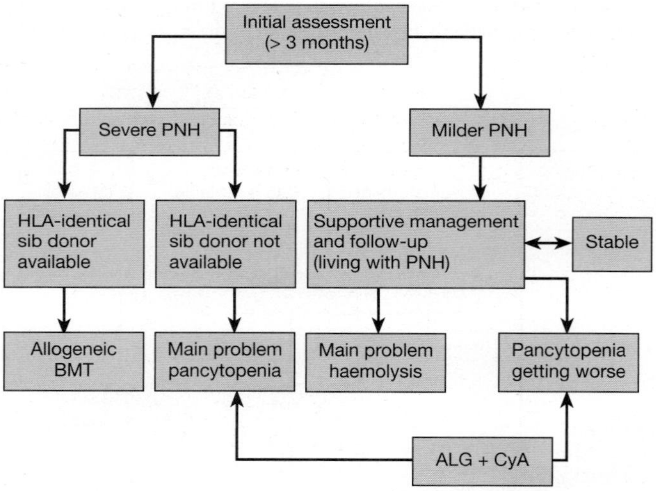

Fig. 5 An algorithm for the management of PNH. This algorithm is based on the consideration that patients with this condition vary considerably (1) in terms of clinical severity, and (2) in terms of the contributions of the PNH clone and of bone marrow failure, respectively, to determining the overall clinical picture. Some patients have been cured by bone marrow transplantation (BMT); other patients who for a long time have been 'living with PNH' have eventually experienced spontaneous recovery (see Hillmen *et al.*, 1995).

Further reading

Araten D, *et al.* (1999). Clonal populations of hematopoietic cells with paroxysmal nocturnal hemoglobinuria genotype and phenotype are present in normal individuals. *Proceedings of the National Academy of Sciences USA* **96**, 5209–14.

Dacie JV (1999). *The haemolytic anaemias*, 3rd edn, Vol. 5. Churchill-Livingstone, London.

Hillmen P, *et al.* (1993). Specific defect in *N*-acetylglucosamine incorporation in the biosynthesis of the glycosylphosphatidylinositol anchor in cloned cell lines from patients with paroxysmal nocturnal hemoglobinuria. *Proceedings of the National Academy of Sciences USA* **90**, 5272–6.

Hillmen P, *et al.* (1995). Natural history of paroxysmal nocturnal hemoglobinuria. *New England Journal of Medicine* **333**, 1253–8.

Karadimitris A, *et al.* (2000). Abnormal T-cell repertoire is consistent with immune process underlying the pathogenesis of paroxysmal nocturnal hemoglobinuria. *Blood* **96**, 2613–20.

Luzzatto L (1999). Paroxysmal murine hemoglobinuria (?): a model for human PNH. *Blood* **94**, 2941–4.

Luzzatto L, Bessler M, Rotoli B (1997). Somatic mutations in paroxysmal nocturnal hemoglobinuria: a blessing in disguise? *Cell* **88**, 1–4.

Oni SB, Osunkoya BO, Luzzatto L (1970). Paroxysmal nocturnal hemoglobinuria: evidence for monoclonal origin of abnormal red cells. *Blood* **36**, 145–52.

Raiola AM, *et al.* (2000). Bone marrow transplantation for paroxysmal nocturnal hemoglobinuria. *Haematologica* **85**, 59–62. [See comments]

Rosse W (1995). Paroxysmal nocturnal hemoglobinuria. In: Handin RI LS, Stossel TP, eds. *Blood—principles and practice of hematology*, pp 367–76. Lippincott, Philadelphia.

Rosse WF (1997). Paroxysmal nocturnal hemoglobinuria as a molecular disease. *Medicine (Baltimore)* **76**, 63–93.

Rotoli B, Luzzatto L (1989). Paroxysmal nocturnal hemoglobinuria. *Seminars in Haematology* **26**, 201–7.

Saso R, *et al.* (1999). Bone marrow transplants for paroxysmal nocturnal haemoglobinuria. *British Journal of Haematology* **104**, 392–6.

Takeda J, *et al.* (1993). Deficiency of the GPI anchor caused by a somatic mutation of the PIG-A gene in paroxysmal nocturnal hemoglobinuria. *Cell* **73**, 703–11.

Young NS, Moss J, eds (2000). *Paroxysmal nocturnal hemoglobinuria and the GPI-linked proteins.* Academic Press, New York.

22.4 The white cells and lyphomproliferative disorders

22.4.1 Leucocytes in health and disease

Joseph Sinning and Nancy Berliner

Introduction

Leucocytes perform a critical role in the host defence against pathogens. They mediate inflammation and modulate the immune response. Leucocytes can be divided into granulocytes (neutrophils, eosinophils, and basophils) (Plate 1), monocytes, and lymphocytes. This chapter will focus on the role of granulocytes and monocytes in the normal host response and pathological manifestations of abnormalities of their number and/or function. Lymphocytes are discussed elsewhere.

Neutrophils

Morphology

Under normal conditions neutrophils make up over half of the leucocytes in the peripheral blood. The morphological hallmarks of these cells include heterogeneous granules and a multilobated or segmented nucleus. The two predominant types of granules in the neutrophil's cytoplasm are the azurophilic (or primary) granules and the specific (or secondary) granules. Azurophilic granules arise at the promyelocytic stage of differentiation. They contain myeloperoxidase, proteases, acid hydrolases, and microbicidal proteins. Specific granules and their content proteins are synthesized at the myelocytic stage of differentiation. Their contents include lactoferrin, lysozyme, vitamin B_{12} -binding protein, gelatinase, and neutrophil collagenase. The specific granules are not a uniform population, and vary by their content with the time of their formation. Those formed early in the myelocyte stage contain abundant lactoferrin, while those formed later are enriched for gelatinase, and are often referred to as 'tertiary' granules or gelatinase granules. The specific granule membrane contains the cytochrome b-558 component of the respiratory burst oxidase, as well as chemotactic and opsonic receptors, which are transferred to the plasma membrane upon activation of the neutrophil. Finally, the neutrophil cytoplasm also contains secretory vesicles that are endocytic vesicles containing primarily plasma proteins, and are the most rapidly mobilized fraction of cytoplasmic granules in the neutrophil. The membrane of secretory vesicles is rich in receptors and cytochrome b, and the vesicles contribute these proteins to the plasma membrane upon neutrophil activation.

Common variants of neutrophil morphology include the Pelger–Huet anomaly, hypersegmentation of the nucleus Dohle bodies, and toxic granulations. The Pelger–Huet anomaly is a dominantly inherited defect in nuclear segmentation that results in a dumb-bell- or rod-shaped nucleus. Neutrophils with nuclei similar to this ('pseudo-Pelger–Huet anomaly') may be seen in acquired myelodysplastic syndromes. Hypersegmented nuclei (containing five or more segments) are characteristic of megaloblastic haematopoiesis due to folic acid or vitamin B_{12} deficiency. Dohle bodies are large basophilic inclusions that may be seen in sepsis, pregnancy, and following cytotoxic chemotherapy. Toxic granulations are abnormally staining primary granules that arise when neutrophils are released prematurely from the marrow, as in severe bacterial infections.

Maturation

There are three cellular compartments that contain myeloid cells: the marrow, the intravascular compartment, and the extravascular space. Maturation from the haematopoietic stem cell occurs in the bone marrow and takes from 10 to 14 days. The marrow compartment can be subdivided into the mitotic compartment and the post-mitotic and storage compartment. In the marrow mitotic compartment neutrophils arise through serial division of myeloid precursors. The mitotic compartment contains myeloid cells with the ability to replicate: myeloblasts, promyelocytes, and myelocytes. The marrow post-mitotic and storage compartment contains myeloid elements that have lost the ability to divide, including metamyelocytes, bands, and segmented neutrophils. Neutrophils are released from the storage pool into the intravascular space, where they remain for 4 to 12 h. Within this space approximately half of the neutrophils circulate freely in the peripheral blood while half remain 'marginated' along the vascular endothelium. The marginated and circulating cells are in dynamic equilibrium with one another. Neutrophils then migrate through the vascular endothelium into the extravascular space, where they survive for 1 to 3 days. At any given time approximately 90 per cent of neutrophils are in the marrow compartment and 2 to 3 per cent are in the intravascular space, with the remainder in the extravascular space.

Neutrophilia

Neutrophilia is defined as an elevation of the circulating neutrophil count (greater than $7.5 \times 10^6/\mu l$). Although it may reflect a primary haematological process, it usually occurs as a secondary manifestation of an underlying disease process or drug. The causes of an elevated neutrophil count are summarized in Table 1.

Hereditary neutrophilias

Hereditary neutrophilia

This is a dominantly inherited syndrome manifested by leucocytosis, splenomegaly, and widened diploë of the skull. Laboratory evaluation reveals a white blood count of 20 000 to 70 000/μl with a neutrophilic predominance, and an elevated leucocyte alkaline phosphatase. Its clinical course is benign.

Chronic idiopathic neutrophilia

This is a sporadically occurring condition manifest as a white blood count of 11 000 to 40 000/μl with a neutrophilic predominance. Patients are

Table 1 Differential diagnosis of neutrophilia

Primary haematological disease	
Chronic idiopathic neutrophilia	
Hereditary neutrophilia	
Leucocyte adhesion deficiency	
Myeloproliferative disorders:	
	Chronic myelogenous leukaemia
	Polycythaemia vera
	Agnogenic myeloid metaplasia
Secondary to other disease processes or drugs	
Infection:	
	Acute
	Chronic
Acute stress:	
	Exercise
	Surgery
	Seizure
	Myocardial infarction
Drugs:	
	Steroids
	Lithium
	β-Agonists
	Cytokines (G-CSF, GM-CSF)
Chronic inflammation	
Myelophthysis	
Marrow hyperstimulation:	
	Chronic haemolysis
	Immune thrombocytopenia
	Recovery from marrow suppression
Post-splenectomy/hyposplenism	
Non-haematological neoplasms	

G-CSF, granulocyte colony-stimulating factor; GM-CSF, granulocyte–macrophage colony-stimulating factor.

otherwise well and have been followed for up to 20 years without the development of significant pathology.

Leucocyte adhesion deficiency

This is a rare inherited disorder characterized by recurrent life-threatening bacterial and fungal infections, cutaneous abscesses, gingivitis, or periodontal infections. Expression of the CD11b/CD18 integrin is deficient, resulting in the inability of neutrophils to migrate to sites of infection (see below under disorders of neutrophil function for further discussion).

Acquired neutrophilias

Infection

The most common cause of an elevated leucocyte count is infection. Acute infection often causes a modest rise in the white blood count, which may be accompanied by an increase in circulating immature precursors ('left shift'). This occurs more commonly with bacterial infection but can also occur with viral processes. Along with a left shift, morphological changes in the neutrophil may be seen with bacterial infection, including toxic granulation, Dohle bodies, and cytoplasmic vacuoles. Neutrophilia resolves with treatment or resolution of the infectious process. In chronic inflammation, marrow granulocyte production is stimulated, resulting in moderate neutrophilia, sometimes with monocytosis. Chronic infections such as osteomyelitis, empyema, and tuberculosis can also give rise to a leukaemoid reaction with white blood counts markedly elevated (greater than $50\ 000/\mu l$), usually associated with a marked left shift.

Drugs

Drugs can cause leucocytosis by several different mechanisms. Steroids increase the release of mature neutrophils from the marrow and should not cause a left shift. β-Agonists acutely raise the neutrophil count by inducing the demargination of neutrophils adherent to the vascular endothelium, and may result in a neutrophil count twice that of baseline. Acute stress also results in demargination of neutrophils, which is probably mediated by adrenergic stimulation. Stresses that can cause this include exercise, surgery, seizure, and myocardial infarction. The cytokines granulocyte colony-stimulating factor (**G-CSF**) and granulocyte–macrophage colony-stimulating factor (**GM-CSF**) stimulate marrow production of neutrophils and can cause dramatic elevations in the white blood count. The majority of white cells formed are neutrophils and a left shift is often seen. The use of these cytokines therefore requires careful monitoring.

Primary haematological conditions

In other situations, neutrophilia may reflect a primary haematological condition. Marrow hyperstimulation in the setting of autoimmune haemolytic anaemia, immune thrombocytopenia, or recovery following chemotherapy or toxic insult to the marrow may result in a reactive leucocytosis. In autoimmune haemolytic anaemia and immune thrombocytopenia, neutrophilia may reflect disease activity, but steroid therapy or splenectomy may contribute. Splenectomy or hyposplenic states (for instance sickle-cell disease) may also result in modest neutrophilia at baseline with more marked neutrophilia at times of stress or infection, reflective of the loss of the spleen as a site of margination and sequestration of leucocytes.

Myeloproliferative disorders

Neutrophilia is a common feature of the myeloproliferative disorders chronic myelogenous leukaemia, polycythaemia vera, and agnogenic myeloid metaplasia, as well as familial myeloproliferative disorders. Elevated eosinophil and basophil counts are also often seen in these disorders. Leucocyte alkaline phosphatase may be low or undetectable in chronic myelogenous leukaemia. The myeloproliferative disorders are discussed in further detail elsewhere.

Non-haematological malignancies

Various non-haematological malignancies including lung and breast tumours may also cause neutrophilia. Tumours may secrete colony-stimulating factors or may cause a leukaemoid reaction. Tumour metastatic to the bone marrow may cause leucoerythroblastic changes, characterized by fragmented erythrocytes, teardrops, and nucleated red cells (myelophthysic changes), as well as leucocytosis with a left shift.

Evaluation of neutrophilia

The evaluation of neutrophilia should take account of the fact that leucocytosis is usually reactive, and that primary haematological aetiologies are relatively rare. The abnormal laboratory value should be verified to rule out laboratory error or a transient unexplained leucocytosis that resolves spontaneously. A careful history and physical examination are essential to evaluate for potential infectious processes, and to obtain a history of medication use. Examination of the bone marrow is usually not necessary for the evaluation of neutrophilia, but examination of a peripheral smear may be very helpful. Evidence of leucoerythroblastic changes warrants examination of the bone marrow to rule out granulomatous disease or tumour infiltration of the marrow. If a bone marrow biopsy is performed, evaluation should include culture of the marrow for fungus or mycobacteria.

Features that raise the question of myeloproliferative disease include concomitant elevation of platelets and haematocrit, basophilia and/or eosinophilia, and splenomegaly. In that setting, evaluation should include stem cell culture of the peripheral blood or bone marrow to assay for cytokine-independent colony growth. Evaluation for myeloproliferative disease is discussed in detail elsewhere.

Neutropenia

Neutropenia is defined as an absolute neutrophil count (**ANC**) of less than $1.5 \times 10^6/\mu l$. In some populations, such as Africans and Yemenite Jews, normal absolute neutrophil counts are lower, with a lower limit of normal of $1.2 \times 10^6/\mu l$. Neutropenia may pose a risk of serious bacterial infection, and this risk is directly related to the degree of neutropenia. In mild neutropenia (ANC 1000 to $1500 \times 10^6/\mu l$) the risk of life-threatening infection is not increased, and in moderate neutropenia (ANC 500 to $1000 \times 10^6/\mu l$) the risk of severe infection is only mildly elevated. Severe neutropenia (ANC $< 500 \times 10^6/\mu l$) markedly increases the risk of life-threatening infection. The duration and acuity of neutropenia may also be important, as the acute onset of severe neutropenia is associated with a higher risk of serious infection than is chronic neutropenia of similar severity. Neutropenia in the setting of marrow failure is more threatening than neutropenia with an intact marrow, as the marrow reserve pool may afford protection. Fever of new onset in the setting of severe neutropenia is a medical emergency requiring immediate evaluation and treatment. Common causes of infection in these patients include Gram-negative enteric pathogens such as *Escherichia coli*, *Pseudomonas* spp., and *Klebsiella pneumoniae*, as well as *Staphylococcus aureus*. The causes of neutropenia are summarized in Table 2.

Congenital neutropenia

Congenital agranulocytosis (Kostmann's syndrome)

This is characterized by severe persistent neutropenia, and the early onset of frequent, life-threatening infections. Bone marrow aspirate reveals a maturation arrest at the promyelocyte stage. This syndrome was originally described as an autosomal recessive disorder, but recent evidence suggests that most cases are autosomal dominant or sporadic. These patients respond to G-CSF with increases in their absolute neutrophil count and decreased incidence of infection. Haematopoietic cell transplantation is another viable treatment option.

With the prolongation of life offered by G-CSF therapy, it has become apparent that patients with Kostmann's syndrome have an increased incidence of acute myeloblastic leukaemia (AML) and myelodysplastic syndrome (MDS). These malignancies develop in association with an acquired mutation in the G-CSF receptor. A relationship has been speculated to exist between G-CSF therapy and the development of these mutations in the G-CSF receptor, but this connection remains unproven, as has the pathogenetic role of the mutations in the subsequent development of acute myeloblastic leukaemia (AML) and myelodysplastic syndrome (MDS). Recent studies have established that Kostmann's syndrome is linked to mutations in the gene encoding neutrophil elastase, a neutrophil primary granule protein. How mutations in the elastase gene give rise to agranulocytosis remains to be elucidated.

Table 2 Differential diagnosis of neutropenia

Decreased production of neutrophils
Constitutional neutropenia
Congenital neutropenia (Kostmann's syndrome)
Cyclic neutropenia
Postinfectious
Nutritional deficieny:
Vitamin B_{12}
Folic acid
Copper
Anorexia nervosa
Drug or toxin induced
Primary marrow failure:
Aplastic anaemia
Myelodysplastic syndromes
Acute leukaemia
Paroxysmal nocturnal haemoglobinuria
Pure white-cell aplasis
Schwachman–Diamond–Oski syndrome
Chediak–Higashi syndrome
Reticular dysgenesis
Dyskeratosis congenita
Large granular lymphocytosis
Increased peripheral destruction of neutrophils
Overwhelming infection
Immune destruction:
Drug-related
Collagen vascular disease-associated
Felty's syndrome
Isoimmune
Hypersplenism/sequestration

Cyclic neutropenia (cyclic haematopoiesis)

This is a rare, dominantly inherited, marrow disorder characterized by cyclic fluctuations in neutrophil counts approximately every 21 days and lasting 3 to 7 days. Along with the neutropenia, cyclic drops in the reticulocyte and monocyte counts are also observed. This suggests that the entire pattern of haematopoiesis is cyclic in these patients, although because of the short half-life of the neutrophil, only neutropenia is clinically significant. Episodes of neutropenia may be severe, often with an absolute neutrophil count less than $200 \times 10^6/\mu l$, and may be accompanied by fevers, pharyngitis, stomatitis, and other bacterial infections. Cyclic neutropenia has also been linked to mutations in the neutrophil elastase gene, although why some mutations give rise to cyclic haematopoiesis and others to agranulocytosis is still a matter of speculation. Cyclic neutropenia can be treated safely and effectively with G-CSF. Unlike Kostmann' s syndrome, cyclic haematopoiesis is not associated with an increased incidence of AML and MDS.

Acquired neutropenias

Postinfectious neutropenia

This is commonly seen following viral infections. It usually occurs several days after the onset of infection and may last several weeks. Varicella zoster, measles, Epstein–Barr, cytomegalovirus, influenza A and B, and hepatitis A and B are some of the viruses most commonly associated with postinfectious neutropenia. The neutropenia resolves spontaneously. Transient neutropenia may also be seen with parvovirus infection. Neutropenia occurs commonly in patients with HIV. The causes are multifactorial and may be related directly to the viral infection, to opportunistic infections or associated conditions, or to the treatment of the virus or its complications.

Several bacterial infections can cause neutropenia, including rickettsial infections, typhoid fever, brucellosis, and tularaemia. Bacterial sepsis of any cause can result in acute neutropenia. This occurs both as a result of marrow suppression and increased destruction of neutrophils. Acute severe neutropenia in bacterial infections suggest that egress to tissue exceeds the capacity of the marrow reserve pool. The neutropenia may be severe and it portends a poor prognosis. Fungal infections, such as disseminated histoplasmosis, and mycobacterial diseases may also cause neutropenia.

Nutritional deficiencies

Nutritional deficiencies of vitamins B_{12} and folic acid result in megaloblastic haematopoiesis with ineffective myelopoiesis. Deficiency of copper is a rare nutritional cause of neutropenia seen in the setting of severe malnutrition or long-term parenteral alimentation. Mild neutropenia may also be seen with anorexia nervosa.

Drugs and toxins

Numerous drugs and toxins are known to cause neutropenia. Mechanisms of drug-induced neutropenia include: (i) direct marrow suppression, (ii) immune destruction with antibody- or complement-mediated damage of myeloid precursors, and (iii) peripheral destruction of neutrophils. In most cases direct marrow suppression is dose dependent. Common offending drugs that cause dose-dependent neutropenia include cancer chemotherapeutic agents, phenothiazines, anticonvulsants, and ganciclovir. Alcohol can also cause neutropenia by marrow suppression. If a drug is suspected of causing dose-dependent neutropenia, it is best to stop the suspected offending agent when possible. However, if it is not possible to stop the drug and the neutropenia is not severe, the drug may be continued with careful monitoring. Neutropenia is often related to the dose and duration of therapy. In contrast, those drugs that cause immune neutropenia usually cause profound agranulocytosis, resulting from both intramedullary destruction of myeloid precursors and peripheral destruction of mature neutrophils. Such drugs include antithyroid medications, sulphonamides, and semisynthetic penicillins. Examination of the bone marrow shows a maturation arrest of the myeloid lineage, reflecting immune destruction of myeloid precursors. The offending agent must be stopped. Recovery of the neutrophil count can be accelerated by the administration of G-CSF.

Autoimmune neutropenia

This may occur in association with collagen vascular disorders such as systemic lupus erythematosis and rheumatoid arthritis, as well as with immune thrombocytopenia and autoimmune haemolytic anaemia. Destruction may be mediated by IgG or IgM antibodies. The neutropenia may be severe but the degree of neutropenia frequently does not correlate as well with the risk of infection as in other conditions. The marrow typically is hypercellular with a late myeloid maturation arrest. Treatment is indicated in the setting of severe, recurrent infections.

Treatment options include intravenous immunoglobulin, splenectomy, and other therapies directed at the underlying collagen vascular disorder. In Felty's syndrome, neutropenia accompanies rheumatoid arthritis and splenomegaly and neutropenia probably reflects both immune destruction and splenic sequestration. Granulopoiesis is inhibited by either antibodies or T cells. This can lead to severe and recurrent infections. It may be managed with G-CSF. Splenectomy relieves the neutropenia in the majority of cases.

Large granular lymphocytosis

This may cause profound neutropenia accompanied by severe infections. It occurs in an older population, and is frequently seen in association with rheumatological diseases such as rheumatoid arthritis. Because of the association with systemic inflammatory disease, large granular lymphocytosis was originally hypothesized to be a polyclonal abnormal immune response. However, gene rearrangement studies have confirmed that large granular lymphocytosis is frequently a clonal disease representing a form of T-cell lymphoma. There are two distinct subtypes, with cells expressing either an unusual Tγ phenotype (CD3+,CD8+, CD56–) or an natural killer phenotype (CD56+). When seen in association with rheumatoid arthritis, the disease may be confused with Felty's syndrome. Neutropenia related to large granular lymphocytosis is associated with a myeloid maturation arrest in the marrow, consistent with immune-mediated neturophil destruction. Surprisingly, however, the neutrophil count will often respond to G-CSF. The course of lymphoma in large granular lymphocytosis varies from indolent to rapidly progressive.

Other causes

Aplastic anaemia reflects a primary failure of haematopoiesis with neutropenia, anaemia, and thrombocytopenia. In the myelodysplastic syndromes and acute leukaemias the marrow does not produce adequate numbers of neutrophils.

Isoimmune neutropenia occurs in 1 in 500 babies born alive. It is caused by placental transfer of maternal IgG directed against fetal neutrophils, and it presents in the first days of life.

Hypersplenism usually causes mild or moderate neutropenia along with anaemia and thrombocytopenia. Normal myeloid maturation is seen in the marrow. The neutropenia is rarely severe.

Evaluation of neutropenia

In contrast to the evaluation of neutrophilia, most patients with confirmed neutropenia require bone marrow examination. A comprehensive history and physical examination may identify the occasional patient with mild neutropenia and no other evidence of disease that may warrant close observation only. However, recurrent infections, including oral and mucosal infections, abnormalities observed in a peripheral blood smear, or severe neutropenia increase the likelihood of significant marrow pathology and marrow aspiration and biopsy is indicated. If neutropenia is accompanied by anaemia or thrombocytopenia, marrow examination is required to rule out aplasia, leukaemia, myelodysplasia, or other primary marrow malignancy. A marrow that shows hyperplastic myeloid precursors and a maturation arrest supports a diagnosis of peripheral neutrophil destruction and/or immune neutropenia, which should lead to a search for an underlying collagen vascular disorder or drug-induced neutropenia.

Management of neutropenia

Fever of new onset in the setting of severe neutropenia (ANC $< 500 \times 10^6/\mu l$) is a medical emergency. A careful history and physical examination should be performed in a timely fashion. Because of the lack of neutrophils, sites of infection may be difficult to find as significant inflammation or tissue infiltration by neutrophils may not occur. Blood and bodily fluids should be cultured. Empirical broad-spectrum antibiotics should be initiated without delay. In patients with fever in the setting of neutropenia that is expected to resolve (usually neutropenia induced by chemotherapy or drug reaction), antibiotics should be continued until the neutrophil count recovers to over 500/μl. In patients with chronic neutropenia that is expected to persist indefinitely, antibiotics should be continued for several days past the resolution of fever. If fever persists for more than 1 week despite antibiotic therapy, empirical antifungal therapy should be given. Granulocyte transfusion should be considered in culture-positive Gram-negative sepsis not responsive to antibiotics in the setting of continued neutropenia.

Granulocyte colony-stimulating factor (G-CSF)

G-CSF (Filgrastim) is a haematopoietic growth factor that has effects primarily on the neutrophilic myeloid lineage. G-CSF reduces the time of maturation of committed neutrophil precursors, prolongs the lifespan of mature neutrophils, and primes them for enhanced function of the respiratory burst, phagocytosis, and chemotaxis. Clinically, G-CSF is used in the treatment and prevention of neutropenia. When used in conjunction with myelosuppressive chemotherapy, G-CSF has been shown to reduce the severity of neutropenia, shorten the duration of neutropenia, reduce the risk of developing neutropenic fever, and reduce the length of stay in hospital. G-CSF has also been utilized successfully in the treatment of severe neutropenia secondary to congenital disorders such as cyclic neutropenia and Kostmann's syndrome, and may be useful in the treatment of autoimmune neutropenia as seen in Felty's syndrome and systemic lupus erythematosis. The neutropenia of marrow failure states, such as the myelodysplastic syndromes, may respond to G-CSF.

Neutropenia secondary to the treatment of HIV infection can also be controlled with G-CSF. The other major use of G-CSF is in the mobilization of haematopoietic progenitor cells from the bone marrow to the peripheral blood. While in the peripheral blood, these cells can be collected by cytopheresis for use in haematopoietic cell transplantation.

Disorders of neutrophil function

Chronic granulomatous disease

Chronic granulomatous disease is a heterogeneous group of rare disorders characterized by defective production of superoxide (O_2^-) by neutrophils, monocytes, and eosinophils. The majority of cases are inherited in an X-linked fashion, but autosomal recessive inheritance also occurs. The genetic lesions causing chronic granulomatous disease have been characterized, and involve mutations in any of four genes encoding the proteins of the respiratory burst oxidase. These include the 91-kDa (X-linked) and 22-kDa (autosomal) components of the membrane cytochrome b-558 complex, and the 47- and 67-kDa soluble components (autosomal) of the oxidase complex. Patients usually present in childhood with severe infections, often with catalase-negative pathogens. The most common infection in patients with chronic granulomatous disease is pneumonia, with *Staphylococcus aureus*, *Burkholderia cepacia*, *Aspergillus* spp., and enteric Gram-negative bacteria often implicated. Other common infections in chronic granulomatous disease include lymphadenitis, cutaneous infections, hepatic abscesses, and osteomyelitis. Aphthous ulceration of the oral mucosa is common, as are chronic mucosal inflammation, perirectal abscesses or fissures, and granulomas of the gastrointestinal and genitourinary tract. The diagnosis of chronic granulomatous disease should be considered in an individual with a history of multiple severe bacterial and fungal infections or a family history of the disorder. The diagnosis is established by confirming abnormal neutrophil oxidative metabolism with tests such as the nitroblue tetrazolium (NBT) slide test or measurements of superoxide or peroxide production. The management of chronic granulomatous disease is based on aggressive prophylaxis and prompt treatment of infection. Prophylactic trimethoprim–sulphamethoxazole or dicloxacillin can significantly decrease the number of bacterial infections in patients with chronic granulomatous disease. Potentially serious infections require the prompt initiation of parenteral antibiotics. Surgical interventions including drainage of abscesses and resection of infected tissue are in important adjunct to antimicrobial chemotherapy. Prophylaxis with recombinant human interferon-γ has been shown in a phase III trial to decrease substantially the number of serious infections in patients with chronic granulomatous disease.

Leucocyte adhesion deficiency

Leucocyte adhesion deficiency is an inherited disorder of neutrophil function. Two types of leucocyte adhesion deficiency have been characterized. Type 1 deficiency is a rare autosomal recessive disorder resulting from mutations in CD18, the gene encoding for the β-chain of leucocyte function antigen-1 (LFA-1, CD11a/CD18), Mac-1 (CD 11b/CD18, CR3, the receptor for the opsonin C3Bi), and gp150,95 (CD11c/CD18). Deficient expression of these three integrin complexes on the neutrophil cell surface results in decreased neutrophil adhesion to the endothelium, impaired chemotaxis, and defective C3Bi-mediated pathogen ingestion, degranulation, and respiratory burst activation. Patients with leucocyte adhesion deficiency typically present in early childhood with recurrent pyogenic infections of the skin, respiratory and digestive tracts, and mucosal membranes. A history of delayed umbilical cord separation is also often noted. Common pathogens in patients with type 1 leucocyte adhesion deficiency include *Staphylococcus aureus* and Gram-negative enterics. Foci of infection notably lack neutrophil infiltration. A mild leucocytosis persists due to impaired margination. The diagnosis is confirmed by flow cytometric measurement of neutrophil CD11b/CD18 expression. The treatment of type 1 leucocyte adhesion deficiency includes aggressive use of parenteral antibiotics for pyogenic infections. Prophylactic trimethoprim–sulphamethoxazole may benefit some patients. Patients with a severe phenotype often die in the first 2 years of life, but patients with mild disease may survive to early adulthood. Type 2 leucocyte adhesion deficiency is caused by a deficiency of Sialyl–Lewis X moieties on neutrophil selectins. In addition to neutrophil function abnormalities, this extremely rare syndrome also is characterized by mental retardation, short stature, and the rare Bombay erythrocyte phenotype.

Myeloperoxidase deficiency

Myeloperoxidase deficiency is a relatively common, autosomal recessively inherited, disorder of neutrophil function. Complete deficiency occurs in 1 in 2000 individuals and partial deficiency occurs twice as frequently. Myeloperoxidase catalyses the production of hypochlorous acid, which is an antimicrobial agent. Myeloperoxidase deficiency is often of no clinical consequence because other host defence mechanisms can adequately compensate for the defective myeloperoxidase; however, when myeloperoxidase deficiency coexists with another defect in host defence, such as diabetes mellitus, disseminated candidal or fungal infections may occur. The diagnosis of myeloperoxidase deficiency is made by histochemical staining of neutrophils and monocytes. Therapy consists of aggressive treatment of fungal infections as well as careful control of glucose levels in patients with diabetes. An acquired form of myeloperoxidase deficiency occurs in some myeloid leukaemia.

Chediak–Higashi syndrome

Chediak–Higashi syndrome is a rare disorder of neutrophil function. Neutrophils and monocytes contain giant primary granules and demonstrate impaired degranulation and fusion with phagosomes. Chemotaxis is also defective. Neutropenia results from defective granulopoiesis. Chediak–Higashi syndrome is inherited in an autosomal recessive manner. The gene responsible has been cloned, and is homologous to a murine lysosomal trafficking protein. Chediak–Higashi syndrome manifests in childhood or infancy with infections of the skin, lungs, and mucous membranes. *S. aureus*, Gram-negative enterics, *Candida*, and *Aspergillus* species are responsible for most infections in this syndrome. Non-haematological manifestations of Chediak–Higashi syndrome include partial oculocutaneous albinism, progressive peripheral and cranial neuropathies, and in some cases, mental retardation. The majority of patients will develop an accelerated phase of the syndrome, manifested by lymphohistiocytic proliferation in the liver, spleen, bone marrow, and lymphatics. The diagnosis of Chediak–Higashi syndrome is made by the demonstration of giant peroxidase-containing granules in peripheral blood or bone marrow myeloid cells, outside of the setting of myelogenous leukaemia. Chediak–Higashi syndrome is treated in the early or stable phase with prophylactic antibiotics and aggressive parenteral antibiotics for infections. Ascorbic acid may also be of benefit. The accelerated phase is treated with vinca alkaloids and glucocorticoids, but often responds poorly to these measures. Allogeneic haematopoietic cell transplantation from HLA-compatible donors is the only potentially curative therapy for Chediak–Higashi syndrome.

Specific granule deficiency

An extremely rare disorder, neutrophil specific granule deficiency is characterized by absent or empty neutrophil specific granules. Specific granule deficiency is manifested clinically as recurrent skin and pulmonary infections resulting from the absence of antimicrobial neutrophil granule proteins such as lactoferrin and defensins. An inability to upregulate the expression of integrins stored on the specific granule membrane may also be responsible for the impairment of host defence. The diagnosis of specific granule deficiency is made by microscopic examination of neutrophils. With appropriate antibiotic prophylaxis and aggressive treatment of infections, patients may live to adulthood. A truncation mutation in the transcription factor C/EBPε has recently been demonstrated to be responsible for some, but not all, cases of specific granule deficiency.

Monocytes

Monocytes are large circulating cells with a non-segmented nucleus and cytoplasmic granules. They function as phagocytes both in antimicrobial defence and in clearing cellular debris. Their granules are essentially identical to neutrophil azurophilic granules, and contain acid hydrolases and myeloperoxidase. Monocytes are also capable of producing reactive oxygen and nitrogen compounds with microbicidal activity. Monocytes play a critical role in the immune response as they present antigens in the context of MHC to T cells. They also produce a variety of immunomodulatory cytokines including interleukins 1 and 6, tumour necrosis factor-α, and β-interferon.

Monocytes arise from bone marrow stem cells. They share a common myeloid precursor with granulocytes. The differentiation to the monocyte is modulated by several cytokines, most importantly monocyte colony-stimulating factor and granulocyte–monocyte colony-stimulating factor. The majority of monocytes are marginated to the vascular endothelium. Upon stimulation, they migrate to the tissue where they develop into macrophages. In the tissue they kill bacteria, mycobacteria, fungi, and protozoa. They are especially important in defence against intracellular pathogens. Specialized resident tissue macrophages include the Langerhans cells of the skin, dendritic cells of lymph nodes, Kupffer cells of the liver, and alveolar macrophages.

Monocytosis is defined as a monocyte count of greater than $0.9 \times 10^6/\mu l$. Disorders causing monocytosis are heterogeneous. Recovery of the marrow following chemotherapy or agranulocytosis is heralded by monocytosis prior to the return of neutrophils. Monocytosis is also seen in syndromes such as cyclic neutropenia, Kostmann's syndrome, and idiopathic neutropenia.

The most common causes of monocytosis include chronic infection, inflammation, or tumour, as well as some primary haematological disorders (Table 3). Chronic infections leading to monocytosis include subacute bacterial endocarditis and mycobacterial diseases. Monocytosis is typically moderate and resolves with treatment of the infection. Autoimmune processes such as systemic lupus erythematosis, rheumatoid arthritis, and vasculitis also cause moderate monocytosis. Monocytosis may arise from primary malignancies of the marrow or in the setting of marrow infiltration with solid tumours (myelophthysis).

Primary marrow disorders causing monocytosis include acute monocytic leukaemia, chronic myelogenous leukaemia and other myeloproliferative disorders, and chronic myelomonocytic leukaemia, which has features of both myelodysplastic and myeloproliferative disorders. Juvenile chronic myelogenous leukaemia is a rare disorder occurring in children less than 4 years of age. Lymphadenopathy and splenomegaly are also prominent features.

Monocytopenia in isolation is uncommon. Monocytopenia is sometimes seen following steroid administration, endotoxaemia, or in marrow failure syndromes such as aplastic anaemia.

Eosinophils

Morphology

Eosinophils have a bilobate nucleus and contain characteristic elliptical granules that stain with eosin. There are three types of eosinophil granules. Primary granules are round in shape. Secondary granules are abundant and contain crystalloid material, and account for the eosinophil's staining properties. The third type of granule is small and contains lysosomal enzymes. Granules contain high concentrations of eosinophil major basic protein, histaminase, eosinophil cationic protein, hydrolases, and peroxidase. Eosinophils are capable of phagocytic function but more commonly release their granule contents to the environment. Eosinophils are also capable of producing reactive oxygen species, and produce prostaglandins, thromboxane A_2, and leukotriene C_4. Eosinophils play a prominent role in defence against helminths and parasites. They arise in the marrow from a common myeloid precursor, and their production is dependent on GM-CSF, IL-3, and IL-5.

Table 3 Causes of monocytosis

Inflammatory diseases
Infectious diseases:
Tuberculosis
Syphilis
Subacute bacterial endocarditis
Fungal infections
Kala-azar
Brucellosis
Autoimmune processes
Systemic lupus erythromatosis
Rheumatoid arthritis
Polyarteritis
Inflammatory bowel disease
Sarcoidosis
Malignancy
Acute myelogenous leukaemia
Chronic myelogenous leukaemia
Chronic myelomonocytic leukaemia
Juvenile chronic myelogenous leukaemia
Hodgkins disease
Non-Hodgkins lymphoma
Histiocytoses
Solid tumours
Miscellaneous
Chronic neutropenia
Post-splenectomy
Marrow recovery

Congenital eosinophilia

Job's syndrome is an inherited disorder characterized by recurrent cold abscesses, eczema, and coarse facies. Patients typically have eosinophilia and significantly elevated levels of IgE.

Acquired eosinophilia

Allergic reactions

These are the most common cause of eosinophilia, including allergies to drugs and environmental agents (Table 4). Moderate eosinophilia is common in collagen vascular diseases including rheumatoid arthritis, vasculitis, and eosinophilic fasciitis. Malignancies such as Hodgkin's disease, non-Hodgkin's lymphoma, and various solid tumours may present with eosinophilia. Moderate eosinophilia is commonly seen in chronic myelogenous leukaemia.

Eosinophilic leukaemia

This is an extremely rare disorder. It presents with extreme eosinophilia, and may be difficult to differentiate from the hypereosinophilic syndrome. However, in eosinophilic leukaemia, the eosinophils are clonal and may contain clonal cytogenetic abnormalities. Furthermore, eosinophilic leukaemia is often associated with cytopenias, infections, and an increase in marrow blasts.

Idiopathic hypereosinophilic syndrome

This is characterized by prolonged eosinophilia and end-organ damage secondary to tissue infiltration by eosinophils. Organs commonly involved include the heart, lungs, central nervous syndrome, kidneys, gastrointestinal tract, and skin. Eosinophilia may be severe ($> 50–100 \times 10^6/\mu l$). Eosinophils deposit toxic proteins in the infiltrated tissues which lead to thrombosis and fibrosis. In the heart the fibrosis results in restrictive cardiomyopathy. The diagnosis of an idiopathic hypereosinophilic syndrome requires eosinophil counts greater than $1.5 \times 10^6/\mu l$ for 6 months, organ

Table 4 Causes of eosinophilia

Allergies
Atopy
Inflammation
Collagen vascular diseases:
Rheumatoid arthritis
Polyarteritis nodosa
Eosinophilic fasciitis
Infection:
Helminths
Parasites
Neoplasms
Hodgkin's disease, non-Hodgkin's lymphoma
Chronic myelogenous leukaemia
Eosinophilic leukaemia
Job's syndrome
Idiopathic hypereosinophilic syndromes
Addison's disease

dysfuncton secondary to eosinophilic infiltration, and no other cause to explain the eosinophilia.

Churg–Strauss syndrome

Primary hypereosinophilic syndrome may be difficult to distinguish from Churg–Strauss syndrome, an eosinophilic vasculitis associated with eosinophilia, pulmonary infiltrates, asthma, and neuropathy. The presence of Churg–Strauss syndrome is suggested by the presence of asthma, which is not characteristic of hypereosinophilic syndrome, and the diagnosis can be confirmed by the finding of necrotizing vasculitis of small vessels, often in association with extravascular granulomas.

Eosinophilia–myalgia syndrome

This is a disorder associated with the ingestion of L-tryptophan supplements from a single source. Affected individuals have eosinphilia and severe myositis. Tissues are infiltrated with eosinophils. In many cases the syndrome responds to steroids, but in some cases it is fatal.

Eosinopenia

Eosinopenia is seen in the setting of steroid use, stress, and acute infection. It typically is clinically benign.

Basophils

Basophils are rare circulating cells, accounting for less than 0.1 per cent of white blood cells. They are non-phagocytic granulocytes. Their large heterogeneous granules account for their purple-black staining. Their granules contain histamine, heparin, tryptase, chemotactic factors for neutrophils and eosinophils, leukotrienes, prostaglandins, and platelet-activating factor. They arise in the marrow from the same myeloid precursor as eosinophils. Basophils function in immediate-type hypersensitivity. They are structurally similar to mast cells but the exact relationship between these cell types is not clear. Basophilia ($> 0.2 \times 10^6/\mu l$) is seen in myeloproliferative disorders such as chronic myelogenous leukaemia and polycythaemia vera, hypersensitivity reactions, and with some viral infections including varicella and influenza. Mast cell leukaemia is a rare disorder with a poor prognosis.

Further reading

Baehner RL (2000). Normal neutrophil structure and function. In: Hoffman R *et al.*, eds. *Hematology: basic principles and practice*, pp 667–86. Churchill Livingstone, Philadelphia.

Curnutte IT, Coates TD (2000). Disorders of phagocyte function and number. In: Hoffman R *et al.*, eds. *Hematology: basic principles and practice*, pp 720–62. Churchill Livingstone, Philadelphia.

Dale DC *et al.* (2000). Mutations in the gene encoding neutrophil elastase in congenital and cyclic neutropenia. *Blood* **96**, 2317.

Malech HL, Gallin JI (1987). Current concepts: immunology. Neutrophils in human disease. *New England Journal of Medicine* **317**, 687.

Pizzo PA (1993). Drug therapy: management of fever in patients with cancer and treatment-induced neutropenia. *New England Journal of Medicine* **328**, 1323.

Rothberg ME (1998). Mechanisms of disease: eosinophilia. *New England Journal of Medicine* **338**, 1592.

Stock W, Hoffman R (2000). White blood cells 1: non-malignant disorders. *Lancet* **355**, 1351.

Winkelstein JA *et al.* (2000). Chronic granulomatous disease: report on a national registry of 368 patients. *Medicine (Baltimore)* **79**, 155.

22.4.2 Introduction to the lymphoproliferative disorders

Barbara A. Degar and Nancy Berliner

The human immune system has the capacity to identify and respond specifically to invading pathogens. It can also 'remember' the exposure, such that subsequent exposure to the same pathogen results in a more rapid and potent immune response. Lymphocytes play the key role in the adaptive immune response, mediating both specificity and memory.

Lymphocytes

The lymphocytes can be divided into two morphologically indistinguishable types, which play different and complementary roles in the immune system. Both are derived from lymphohaemopoietic stem cells that reside in fetal liver and in adult bone marrow. B cells develop in the marrow (the human equivalent of the avian bursa of Fabricius) and their principal role is to generate immunoglobulin (antibodies). B cells represent about 20 per cent of the lymphocyte population in peripheral blood. T cells mature within the thymus. T cells orchestrate the immune response: they are capable of cell-mediated cytotoxicity, they generate inflammatory cytokines, and they provide help for B-cell function. T cells account for approximately 80 per cent of the lymphocytes in the peripheral circulation. A much smaller population of lymphoid-appearing cells express neither B-cell nor T-cell markers. These null cells, also known as natural killer (**NK**) cells and large granular lymphocytes (**LGLs**), are capable of cell-mediated cytotoxicity, especially against tumour cells and virally infected cells. NK cells are a component of the innate immune response, as they do not demonstrate immunological memory.

Lymph nodes

In their role in infection surveillance, lymphocytes circulate through the body via a network of lymphatic and blood vessels. At strategic locations, lymphoid cells are organized to allow direct interaction among lymphocytes and other specialized cells of the immune system.

These interactions permit the production of specific, functional effector cells. The network includes approximately 500 to 600 discrete lymph nodes, lymphoid populations in the oropharynx (Waldeyer's ring), bronchial tree and gut, as well as in the thymus, the bone marrow, and the spleen.

Within lymph nodes, lymphocytes are arranged in a central medulla surrounded by an outer cortex contained within a connective tissue capsule (Fig. 1) Afferent lymphatics penetrate the cortex and lymphocyte-rich fluid filters toward the medullary sinusoids and the efferent lymphatics at the hilum of the node. The vascular supply to the lymph node includes specialized postcapillary venules that allow the passage of peripheral blood lymphocytes into the node. Lymphocytes are ultimately returned to the bloodstream via the thoracic duct.

Roughly spherical follicles are found in the lymph node cortex and predominantly comprise B cells. Primary follicles contain clusters of naïve, unstimulated B cells. Secondary follicles, with pale 'germinal centres' surrounded by a darker 'mantle' zone, represent foci of B cells proliferating and differentiating in the presence of antigen-bearing dendritic cells and activated 'helper' T cells (T_H cells). The interfollicular and paracortical zones of the lymph node are densely populated by T cells. Macrophages, follicular dendritic cells, and interdigitating reticulum cells all process and present antigen to the lymphocytes within the node.

The design of the lymph node facilitates the process whereby the subpopulation of lymphocytes capable of responding to a specific antigen is expanded. Antigens are delivered to the subcapsular sinus of the node via

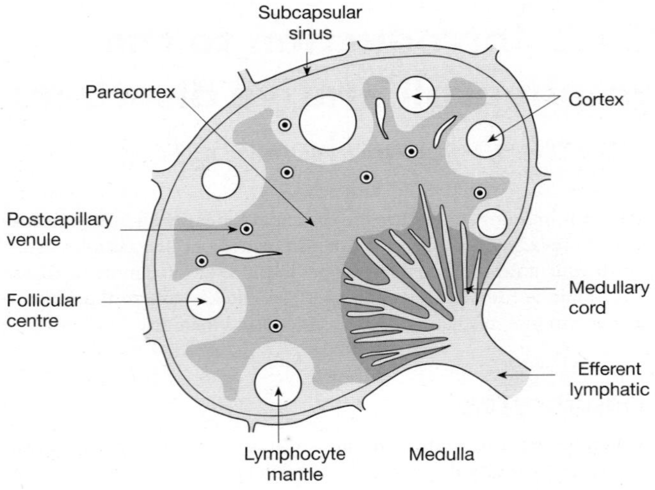

Fig. 1 Functional architecture of a normal lymph node. (Reproduced from Arno J (1980). *Atlas of lymph node pathology*, with permission.)

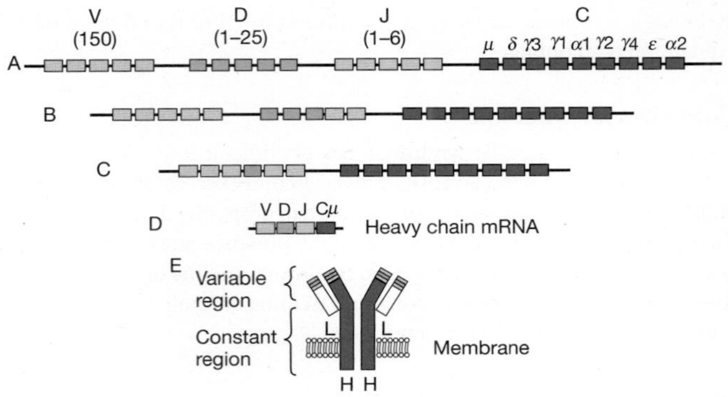

Fig. 2 Immunoglobulin gene rearrangement. The top line (A) represents the germline pattern of the immunoglobulin heavy chain locus found on human chromosome 14. B-cell progenitors express recombination activating genes which mediate the random, sequential rearrangement of gene modules (lines B and C) such that only one of several variable (V)₁ diversity (D), and joining (J) segments is expressed by a B-cell clone (line D). As the gene components are spliced, terminal deoxynucleotidyl transferase (TdT) randomly inserts additional nucleotides at splice junctures. Diverse antigenic specificity is thus somatically generated from a relatively small amount of genetic material. The immunoglobulin molecule (line E) is a tetramer of two heavy and two light chains which may be cell-associated (as shown) or secreted. The region of the molecule which interacts specifically with antigen is the variable region. The constant region of the light chain are of either the κ or λ types. The constant region of the heavy chain determines the isotype of the antibody (IgM, IgD, IgG, IgA, IgE).

afferent lymphatics, and are taken up by reticulum cells and presented on their surface in the context of the major histocompatibility complex (**MHC**) proteins. Specific T-lymphocyte responses require that peptide antigens, which are derived from 'foreign' proteins, appear on the surface of antigen-presenting cells in close association with a 'self' MHC molecule. B cells, on the other hand, are capable of responding to some antigens in solution. Optimal B-cell responses require the 'help' of T cells both via direct cell–cell contact and in response to cytokines secreted by T cells. Only those T cells and B cells that have been genetically preprogrammed to interact with a specific antigen will proliferate and differentiate in response to it.

Antigen receptors

Both B and T cells express transmembrane proteins on their cell surfaces, these proteins bind antigen and define the antigenic specificity of the cell. In the case of B cells, the immunoglobulin molecule represents the B-cell receptor (Fig. 2) Each immunoglobulin molecule is a bivalent tetramer comprising a pair of heavy chains bound to two light chains (of either kappa or lambda type). Genetic recombination of approximately 400 immunoglobulin gene segments (located on chromosomes 2, 14, and 22), generates about 10^{15} distinct antibody specificities. The expression of recombination activating genes (*RAG1* and *RAG2*) early in B-cell development mediates the random rearrangement of variable (**V**), diversity (**D**), and joining (**J**) gene segments. Terminal deoxyribonucleotidyl transferase (**TdT**) contributes to the diversity of immunoglobulin molecules by inserting additional nucleotides during the splicing of gene segments. This process gives rise to a vast repertoire of antibody molecules, each with a unique antigen-binding cleft. All of the progeny cells of a B cell that has rearranged its immunoglobulin genes have the same antigenic specificity and are referred to as a clone. Most protein antigens are complex and contain many different epitopes (structures capable of binding an antigen receptor). Therefore, most pathogens stimulate many lymphocyte clones to proliferate: that is to say, they result in polyclonal responses. As B-cell clones mature, the isotype of the antibodies they produce 'switches' from IgM/IgD to IgG, IgA, or IgE.

In an analogous fashion, T-cell precursors rearrange the T-cell receptor (**TCR**) genes. The TCR consists of a heterodimer of α and β chains, or γ and δ chains in a minority of T cells. The α and β genes are encoded on chromosomes 14 and 7, respectively, while the γ and δ chains are on chromosomes 7 and 14, respectively. T-cell precursors randomly assemble variable, joining, and diversity gene segments to generate a vastly diverse array of antigen-specific T-cell clones. When the T cell encounters antigen to which it can productively bind, the cell undergoes clonal expansion, and generates both activated effector cells and long-lived memory cells.

Lymphocyte ontogeny

As lymphocytes develop and mature from multipotent progenitors to terminally differentiated effector cells, they express a sequential pattern of surface proteins. Some of these cell-surface molecules subserve known, critical functions in the cells that bear them. Others are of less clear biological significance, but are useful markers of cell type and status of differentiation and activation. Malignant lymphomas and lymphoid leukaemias are frequently classified and understood on the basis of their expression of cell-surface markers (Fig. 3) In some cases, the stage of differentiation at which malignant transformation occurred can be inferred from the pattern of the surface antigens expressed by the malignant cells.

Lymphocytes develop from haemopoietic stem cells. Although the surface characteristics of these elusive cells are not well understood, it is likely that human stem cells express the cell-surface glycoprotein CD34. The first recognizable sign of commitment to the B-lymphoid lineage is the expression of TdT and the rearrangement of the immunoglobulin heavy chain. As differentiation progresses, B-cell progenitors turn on the expression of class II MHC molecules (HLA-DR) as well as CD19 and then CD10 (the latter is also known as 'common acute lymphoblastic leukaemia antigen', **CALLA**). The immunoglobulin light chain is rearranged and the cells (now termed pre-B cells) express the μ heavy chain within their cytoplasm. As the cells progress to the early B-cell stage, CD34, TdT, and CD10 expression are extinguished, and CD19, CD20, and CD21, as well as IgM are expressed on the cells' surface. Mature B cells express surface IgM and/or IgD, in addition to CD19 and CD20. Plasma cells, the end result of B-cell differentiation, produce cytoplasmic as well as secreted immunoglobulin, but do not express surface immunoglobulin. They lack CD19 and CD20 expression.

Similarly, as T cells mature they progress through an orderly cascade of genetic and cell-surface events. CD34-positive progenitors that are destined for a T-lymphoid fate migrate from the marrow to the thymus and express

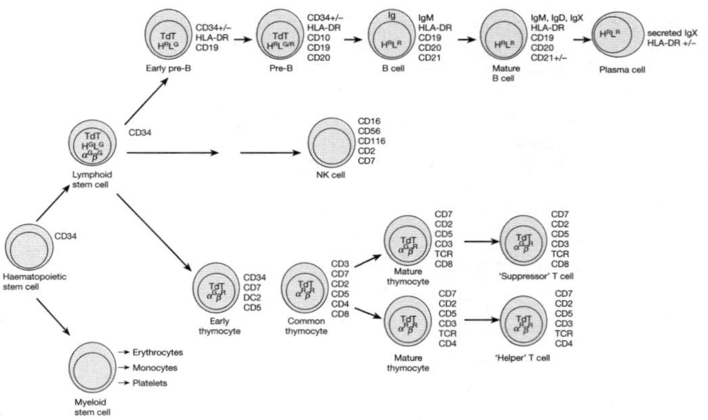

Fig. 3 Simplified depiction of lymphocyte ontogeny. Lymphocytes derive from lymphoid progenitors in the bone marrow, which in turn are derived from multipotent haemopoietic stem cells. B-lymphoid progenitors are recognized by their expression of terminal deoxynucleotidyl transferase (TdT) and the rearrangement of the immunoglobulin heavy chain locus. As B cells mature, the light chain is rearranged and immunoglobulin is expressed first within the cell cytoplasm, then on the cell surface, and is ultimately secreted. T-lymphoid progenitors migrate to the thymus where they express TdT and rearrange the β-subunit followed by the α-subunit of the T-cell receptor (TCR). An overlapping sequence of cell-surface proteins are expressed as the cells differentiate, these have been numerically classified using cluster of differentiation (**CD**) designations. The status of the immunoglobulin and *TCR* genes are represented as follows: H, immunoglobulin heavy chain; L, light chain; α, TCR-α; β, TCR-β; G, germline; R, rearranged.

TdT as well as CD7. Next, the cells express the CD2 molecule, which, among other things, mediates the binding of T cells to sheep erythrocytes. The T-cell receptor genes are then rearranged and subsequently expressed on the surface of the thymocyte in association with the CD3 molecule. Distinct populations of mature thymocytes emerge: those that express CD4 and function as cytokine-secreting 'helper' cells and those that express CD8 and function as cytotoxic 'killer' cells. Rare 'double-positives' (CD4+CD8+) and 'double-negatives' (CD4–CD8–) also exist. The CD4 molecule mediates the binding of T cells to MHC class II molecules, whereas CD8 binds MHC class I proteins.

The third descendant of the lymphoid stem cell, the NK cell, is characterized by its expression of CD7, CD2, CD16, and CD56, in addition to other surface proteins. NK cells are distinguished from T cells by the fact they do not express CD3 (and therefore the T-cell receptor).

Lymphoproliferative disorders

A variety of conditions that span the spectrum of benign, reactive processes to frank malignant transformation result in the expansion of lymphocyte populations. Lymphoproliferative diseases are typically manifested by lymphocytosis and/or lymphadenopathy. Distinguishing these processes clinically and pathologically is not always easy. The lymphoproliferative disorders are a loosely defined group of malignant and non-malignant entities characterized by the autonomous, poorly controlled proliferation of lymphoid cells. Malignant tumours are clonal in nature; they result from the uncontrolled proliferation of a single transformed cell. In contrast, non-malignant lymphoproliferation contains polyclonal lymphocyte populations. Lymphoproliferative disorders may result from chronic antigenic stimulation, certain viral infections, or from an imbalance among interacting lymphocyte populations, as may occur in congenital or acquired immunodeficiency syndromes. In addition, lymphocytes are prone to the acquisition of chromosomal translocations, particularly involving the immunoglobulin and T-cell receptor genes, and such changes may contribute to malignant transformation (see Table 1).

Lymphocytosis

Normal peripheral blood usually contains approximately 1000 to 5000 lymphocytes/μl, accounting for approximately 40 per cent of the circulating leucocytes. Infants and young children typically have higher absolute lymphocyte values. Increased numbers of circulating lymphocytes (lymphocytosis) and/or the appearance of abnormal (or atypical) lymphocytes in the blood are usually caused by either viral infection or lymphoid malignancy. The appearance of the circulating lymphocytes on a peripheral blood smear may provide clues to the pathogenesis of the elevated lymphocyte count. For example, infectious mononucleosis results from primary infection with the Epstein–Barr virus (**EBV**), and gives rise to large numbers of 'atypical' lymphocytes with abundant cytoplasm in the peripheral blood. Chronic lymphocytic leukaemia (**CLL**) leads to an increase in circulating normal-appearing 'mature' lymphocytes. CLL is also frequently associated with the appearance of 'smudge' cells in the peripheral smear, a preparation artefact caused by the destruction of the fragile CLL cells. Follicular lymphoma may be associated with the circulation of characteristic cells with a cleaved nucleus.

Lymphadenopathy

Enlargement of one or more lymph nodes (lymphadenopathy) is an extremely common clinical finding. With the exception of inguinal nodes, normal lymph nodes are non-palpable. Nodes that are palpable and/or exceed approximately 1 × 1 cm on imaging studies are considered pathological. Lymph node enlargement often results from the body's normal and adaptive response to an immunological challenge; however, it may signify a pathological inflammatory or malignant disease. The causes of lymphadenopathy fall into three main categories: infectious, inflammatory (reactive), and neoplastic (Table 1) Younger patients, especially children, are more likely to develop adenopathy as a result of infection, while the likelihood of haematological or metastatic malignancy increases with age.

Approach to the patient with lymphadenopathy

The history of the patient with lymphadenopathy should take into account the age and general health of the patient, the duration of the adenopathy, the coexistence of fever, weight loss, night sweats, pruritis, and cough, and any recent infections, medications, travel, and animal exposures. The physical examination should make note of the location (generalized versus regional), the texture (hard versus rubbery), and the mobility of the nodes (fixed versus mobile), and the presence or absence of signs of inflammation (warmth, tenderness, erythema). The skin and oropharynx should be examined and the size of the liver and spleen should be assessed. Additional screening studies may include a complete blood count, and measurement of the erythrocyte sedimentation rate (**ESR**). Serological studies for certain viral pathogens and for rheumatological diseases can be diagnostically helpful. Radiographs of the chest should be obtained if mediastinal adenopathy is suspected. Ultrasound may demonstrate central suppuration, which is characteristic of acute lymphadenitis. A computed tomography (**CT**) scan is required to diagnose intra-abdominal adenopathy.

Lymph node biopsy

In the absence of an obvious infection or underlying illness associated with lymphadenopathy, or when malignancy is suspected, a lymph node biopsy is recommended. Depending on the clinician's level of concern, a trial of observation with or without empirical antibiotics (usually an antistaphylococcal agent) is sometimes chosen. Empirical treatment with steroids should be avoided because it may undermine the diagnosis and proper therapy of lymphoid malignancy. If there is no resolution within 2 weeks, then a lymph node biopsy should be strongly considered. The largest accessible node is most often selected for biopsy. A fine-needle aspiration of lymph nodes is adequate for diagnosis in a restricted set of clinical circumstances: for example, diagnosis of recurrent disease or metastatic carcinoma or melanoma. Culture of a lymph node aspirate may yield a microbiological diagnosis in infective lymphadenitis. Most pathologists prefer an

Table 1 Causes of lymphadenopathy

	Clinical features	Histological characteristics
Infectious		
Bacterial	Regional, often tender	Suppurative
Mycobacterial (tuberculosis, leprosy)	Regional or generalized	Suppurative granulomas
Viral (EBV, CMV, HIV)	Often generalized	Follicular hyperplasia
Fungal (*Histoplasma, Coccidioides* spp.)	Often hilar	Suppurative granulomas
Parasitic (*Toxoplasma, Chlamydia* spp.)	Usually regional(cervical, inguinal)	Suppurative granulomas
Reactive		
Rheumatological conditions (SLE, RA)	Often generalized	Follicular hyperplasia
Sarcoidosis	Especially hilar	Epithelioid granulomas
Drugs (e.g. phenytoin)	Generalized	Paracortical expansion
Castleman's disease	Localized/multicentric	Follicular hyperplasia (hyaline vascular or plasma cell)
Rosai–Dorfman disease	Usually cervical	Sinus hyperplasia
Neoplastic		
Leukaemia/lymphoma	Often generalized, 'rubbery'	Effacement of nodal architecture
Metastatic(carcinoma, melanoma)	Regional, rock hard	Subcapsular expansion, effacement of nodal architecture
Other		
Storage diseases(e.g. Gaucher's)	Generalized	Paracortical or sinusoidal lipogranulomas

EBV, Epstein–Barr virus; CMV, cytomegalovirus; HIV, human immunodeficiency virus; SLE, systemic lupus erythematosus; RA, rheumatoid arthritis.

excisional biopsy, when possible, because nodal architecture is preserved. A portion of the sample should be reserved fresh (that is, not fixed in formalin) for flow cytometry and cytogenetic studies, if indicated.

Histopathology Histological examination of lymph nodes is the mainstay of diagnostic studies, however non-diagnostic or non-specific inflammatory findings are frequently encountered. Reactive lymph nodes demonstrate characteristic, but by no means specific, histological patterns which involve the three functional domains of the lymph node: the follicles, the paracortex, and the medullary sinuses.

An increase in the size and/or number of lymphoid follicles (which contain proliferating B cells,) is termed 'follicular hyperplasia'. The specific cause is rarely identified. This pattern of lymph node reactivity is characteristic of rheumatological conditions and of HIV infection and Castleman's disease. Castleman's disease is a rare and poorly understood non-neoplastic cause of lymphadenopathy that occurs in localized and multicentric forms. The multicentric form is a systemic illness without defined therapy that is associated with infection with human herpesvirus-8 (HHV-8, also known as Kaposi's sarcoma herpesvirus).

Paracortical expansion accompanies T-cell proliferation and is characteristic of certain viral causes of lymphadenopathy, such as EBV infection. Paracortical expansion with granuloma formation is typical of mycobacterial infections and sarcoidosis. In Kikuchi's disease and Kawasaki's disease (mucocutaneous lymph node syndrome), paracortical necrosis is seen in involved lymph nodes.

Sinus hyperplasia is caused by an increased number of histiocytes in the medullary sinuses. This pattern of lymph node reactivity is seen in the histiocytic syndromes and in the storage diseases. A rare condition known as sinus histiocytosis with massive lymphadenopathy or Rosai–Dorfman disease is characterized by an extreme polyclonal proliferation of macrophages. This entity often involves the cervical lymph nodes, but may occur in virtually any nodal or extranodal site and is usually, but not always, self-limited.

Involvement by a malignant lymphoma leads to effacement of the lymph node structure to a greater or lesser degree. Histology correlates with clinical behaviour and will be described in subsequent sections focused on the classification of lymphoma.

Immunohistochemistry and flow cytometry

Histology alone may be inadequate to distinguish the malignant from the non-malignant lymphoproliferative disorders. Supplemental information from flow cytometry, cytogenetics, and immunoglobulin/TCR gene rearrangement studies demonstrate the clonal nature of malignant disease and provide data with prognostic and therapeutic significance. Immunohistochemistry is used to characterize the pattern of surface marker expression in fixed or frozen tissue samples. Flow cytometry is performed on cells in suspension, such as peripheral blood or bone marrow, or on cell suspensions prepared from a lymph node or other solid tumour. For flow cytometry, solid specimens should not be fixed or frozen but kept refrigerated until processing. Both techniques detect the binding of monoclonal antibodies of known specificity to the clinical sample. Using a panel of antibodies, these studies demonstrate the types of cells present in the sample. Non-haemopoietic metastatic tumours can be identified. The lineage of lymphoid malignancies can be revealed, for example B cell versus T cell versus NK cell. In the case of B-cell lymphoproliferation, the relative expression of kappa and lambda light chains can be measured. As described above, B cells express either the kappa or the lambda light chain, but not both. Predominant expression of either the kappa or lambda light chain by a population of B cells, a phenomenon known as light-chain restriction, suggests a clonal process. Using flow cytometry, lymphoid neoplasms can be placed within the hierarchy of normal lymphocyte ontogeny, and clinical behaviour, such as response to cytotoxic therapy, can often be predicted. These studies may be used to demonstrate the presence of a surface antigen to which monoclonal antibody-based therapy has been developed (for example, CD20 and rituxumab). Sometimes, malignant cells demonstrate lineage infidelity, with expression of a pattern of surface markers that does not correspond to a normal cellular counterpart. This may fortuitously provide an immunophenotypical fingerprint to detect small amounts of disease, early relapse, or minimal residual disease after therapy.

Genetic studies

The high proliferative rate of lymphocytes and the genetic events that occur within them, sets the stage for the development of chromosomal translocations which are aetiologically linked to malignant transformation. Increasingly, haemopoietic cancers are being defined genetically by the presence of specific, non-random chromosomal translocations. The detection and study of these translocations has increased diagnostic precision, has provided insights into the molecular mechanisms of oncogenesis, and has revealed molecular targets for rational therapeutic design. Chromosomal translocations can be demonstrated using classical cytogenetic techniques. When cytogenetics is technically unsuccessful, specific translocations may also be detected using the polymerase chain reaction (**PCR**) and fluorescence *in situ* hybridization (**FISH**). In addition, these methods may be used to identify the presence of specific viral sequences, such as those encoded by EBV and HHV-8. These highly sensitive and specific techniques are increasingly being applied to the detection of minimal residual disease.

As described above, the hallmark of lymphocyte differentiation is the somatic rearrangement of the antigen-receptor genes, immunoglobulin in the case of B cells and the TCR in the case of T cells. Each lymphocyte clone has a unique arrangement of the components of the antigen-receptor genes, while cells of non-lymphocyte lineage preserve the germline structure of these genes. Lymphoproliferative malignancies are composed of clonal proliferations arising from a single cell with a rearranged antigen-receptor locus. The pattern of gene rearrangement helps to characterize the lineage and stage of differentiation of the tumour. For example, pre-B-cell acute lymphoblastic leukaemia cells usually contain rearranged heavy-chain genes with germline light-chain genes, whereas B-CLL cells usually have a rearrangement of both heavy- and light-chain genes and express surface immunoglobulin. Furthermore, since clonal populations of lymphocytes all contain the same antigen-receptor rearrangement, these cells possess a 'molecular signature' that is unique to the malignant clone.

Consequently, antigen-receptor rearrangements have become the target of DNA diagnostic techniques for diagnosing and following lymphoproliferative malignancies. Antigen-receptor rearrangements can be detected by several methods including Southern blot and PCR-based techniques. The genetic detection of clonal B-cell populations was first achieved using Southern blotting. For Southern analysis, DNA is digested with restriction endonucleases, blotted on nitrocellulose membranes, and hybridized with probes specific for the immunoglobulin loci. Somatic rearrangement of the immunoglobulin loci, with concomitant excision of the intervening DNA, results in loss of the normal restriction endonuclease sites that lie within the immunoglobulin locus. Clonal populations of B cells then give rise to restriction fragments of altered size when probed with immunoglobulin gene sequences. This technique is still the 'gold standard' for determining B-lymphoid clonality of confusing lymphoproliferations. It has also been used for the detection of minimal residual disease (**MRD**). However, PCR-based techniques have largely supplanted Southern analysis for the detection of MRD. For these studies, PCR is performed using oligonucleotide primers based on conserved sequences within the immunoglobulin heavy-chain locus; approximately 70 to 90 per cent of rearrangements can be detected by this approach. To detect MRD with maximal sensitivity, such rearrangements are then subjected to sequence analysis to determine the antigen-specific sequences unique to the tumour rearrangement. An allele-specific oligonucleotide can then be synthesized and used in a PCR analysis that can detect residual clonal populations representing as few as $1:10^5$ cells.

Further reading

Berliner N, Smith B (1991). The pathobiology of lymphoproliferative disease. In: Hoffman R, *et al.*, ed. *Hematology basic principles and practice*, pp 897–911. Churchill Livingstone, New York.

Delves P, Roitt I (2000). Advances in immunology 1. *New England Journal of Medicine* **343**, 37–49.

Delves P, Roitt I (2000). Advances in immunology 2. *New England Journal of Medicine* **343**, 108–17.

Foon KA, Todd RF 3rd (1986). Immunologic classification of leukemia and lymphoma. *Blood* **68**, 1–31.

Look A (1997). Oncogenic transcription factors in human acute leukemias. *Science* **278**, 1059–64.

Macintyre EA, Delabesse E (1999). Molecular approaches to the diagnosis and evaluation of lymphoid malignancies. *Seminars in Hematology*, **36**, 373–89.

Sell S (1996). *Immunology, immunopathology, and immunity.* Appleton and Lange, Stamford, CT.

Strauchen J (1998). *Diagnostic histopathology of the lymph node.* Oxford University Press, New York.

Wickremasinghe R, Hoftbrand A (1999). Biochemical and genetic control of apoptosis: relevance to normal hematopoiesis and hematological malignancies. *Blood* **93**, 3587–600.

22.4.3 Lymphoma

James O. Armitage

Introduction

Lymphomas represent malignancies of lymphoid cells and almost always present as solid tumours, ranging from among the least to among the most aggressive of the human malignancies. They have in common a frequent response to available therapies, and a significant subset of patients who develop lymphomas can be cured.

Lymphomas are usually divided into Hodgkin's disease and non-Hodgkin's lymphomas. The non-Hodgkin's lymphomas are much more frequent, with almost 60 000 new cases being diagnosed in the United States annually and approximately 8000 new cases diagnosed each year in the United Kingdom. Non-Hodgkin's lymphomas are increasing in incidence at a higher rate than almost all other malignancies; for instance, in the United States the incidence has increased at a rate of approximately 4 per cent per year since 1950. In contrast, Hodgkin's lymphomas occur approximately 7500 times per year in the United States and 1200 times per year in the United Kingdom. The incidence of Hodgkin's disease appears to be stable.

Presenting manifestation

Patients with lymphoma most commonly present with lymphadenopathy. However, a variety of presentations are possible. These include systemic symptoms such as fevers, night sweats, weight loss, and pruritus, which are believed to be the result of the release of cytokines by normal or malignant cells. Patients can present with symptoms secondary to a mediastinal or retroperitoneal mass such as superior vena cava obstruction, pleural effusion, pericardial tamponade, abdominal or back pain, intestinal obstruction or perforation, gastrointestinal bleeding, or renal failure from urethral obstruction. Central nervous system presentations include primary brain tumours and signs of meningeal involvement and spinal cord compression. Patients might present with cytopenia secondary to either bone marrow involvement or autoimmune destruction of the formed elements of the blood. Symptoms secondary to the overproduction of a monoclonal immunoglobulin or hypogammaglobulinaemia can be seen. In short, the possible presentations of lymphomas are so varied that the diagnosis should be considered in almost all patients and not just restricted to those presenting with lymphadenopathy or splenomegaly.

Establishing a diagnosis

The diagnosis of lymphoma should always be based on evaluation by an expert haematopathologist of, preferably, an adequate lymph node biopsy, or an extranodal tumour mass if lymph nodes are unavailable. Needle aspirates or small biopsies should be avoided as the basis for diagnosing lymphoma whenever possible. As one of the major challenges that pathologists face is the diagnosis of lymphoma, it is important not to handicap the haematopathologist by providing inadequate material. The differential diagnosis that the pathologist considers when diagnosing a lymphoma includes benign proliferations of lymphoid tissue, malignancies of myeloid cells, non-haemopoietic malignancies, viral infections, and unusual disorders such as Castleman's disease and giant lymph node hyperplasia. Having tissue available for immunological studies and/or genetic studies will frequently help to confirm the diagnosis.

Table 1 The Ann Arbor Staging system

Stage	Characteristics
I	1 nodal site involved
IE	1 site of localized extranodal involvement
II	2 or more nodal sites involved, but only on 1 side of the diaphragm
IIE	1 site of localized extranodal involvement plus regional nodes involved—all on 1 side of the diaphragm
III	Nodal involvement (i.e. spleen counts as a nodal site) on both sides of the diaphragm
IV	Bone marrow, liver, or other extensive extranodal involvement (e.g. multiple pulmonary nodules)
A	Absence of unexplained fever (i.e. >38 °C), drenching night sweats, or weight loss (i.e. ≥10% in 6 months)
B	Presence of unexplained fever (i.e. >38 °C), drenching night sweats, or weight loss (i.e. ≥10% in 6 months)

Table 2 Staging evaluation for a new patient with lymphoma

- Complete history and physical examination
- Haematological studies:
  complete blood count, sedimentation rate (for Hodgkin's disease)
- Chemistry studies to predict prognosis:
  serum lactate dehydrogenase (LDH) and β_2-microglobulin (both for non-Hodgkin's lymphoma (NHL))
- Chemistry studies to measure normal organ function:
  serum creatinine, liver function studies
- Miscellaneous chemistry studies:
  serum protein electrophoresis
- Imaging studies:
  chest radiograph, computed tomograms of the chest, abdomen, and pelvis
  gallium scan (Hodgkin's disease and aggressive NHL)
- Bone marrow biopsy
- Other studies as appropriate to evaluate specific complaints and to follow-up abnormal results found from the studies listed above

Patient evaluation

Once the diagnosis of a type of lymphoma has been established, a series of studies should be carried out to determine the extent of disease. The anatomical spread of disease is usually expressed as an Ann Arbor Stage (Table 1). This staging system was originally developed for Hodgkin's disease and divides patients into those with disease confined to one lymphatic site, multiple lymphatic sites on one side of the diaphragm, lymphatic involvement on both sides of the diaphragm, and those with bone marrow involvement, liver involvement, or other extensive extranodal disease. The Ann Arbor Stage also includes a suffix A or B indicating the absence (A) or presence (B) of unexplained fevers above 38 °C, weight loss of more than 10 per cent of the body weight in the preceding 6 months, or drenching night sweats. Additional factors can also have an impact on a patient's response to therapy and survival. For non-Hodgkin's lymphomas, these factors are incorporated into the International Prognostic Index. In this system, the Ann Arbor Stage represents one factor with an adverse risk associated with stage III or IV. Other adverse risk factors include an elevated serum lactate dehydrogenase (**LDH**) level, age of 60 years or greater, multiple sites of extranodal disease, and a reduced performance status. The International Prognostic Index Score is determined by adding the adverse risk factors.

The laboratory and radiological evaluation of patients with lymphoma typically involves a standardized series of tests, such as a complete blood count, erythrocyte sedimentation rate determination, chemistry studies reflecting major organ function, computed tomography scans of the chest, abdomen, and pelvis, and a bone marrow biopsy (Table 2). In patients with non-Hodgkin's lymphoma, serum LDH, serum β_2-macroglobulin, and serum protein electrophoresis are often useful adjuncts. A gallium scan performed before therapy can identify sites of involvement in the majority of patients with Hodgkin's disease and those with aggressive non-Hodgkin's lymphoma. In addition to potentially altering the diagnostic stage, this technique allows a more accurate restaging of disease at the completion of therapy than can be obtained simply with computed tomography (**CT**) scans. However, CT scans only show anatomical findings, and some patients with lymphomas in the mediastinum and retroperitoneum do not have complete regression of their initial masses because of a sclerotic reaction to the tumour. Moreover, in patients who have actually achieved a complete remission, the gallium scan (that is to say, a functional as opposed to an anatomical study) will typically have reverted to normal. Other studies can be useful in particular situations. Most patients will be given a chest radiograph. This offers an easy way to follow mediastinal or pulmonary involvement. Magnetic resonance imaging (**MRI**) studies are particularly useful in evaluating suspected bone or central nervous system sites of involvement by a lymphoma. Technetium scans of bone or the liver and spleen are occasionally valuable in detecting occult sites of involvement by a lymphoma. In some patients, abdominal ultrasonography will provide a more economical way to follow intra-abdominal disease.

Bilateral, lower limb lymphangiography was formerly used to evaluate pubic and retroperitoneal node involvement in most patients with lymphoma. However, this study is difficult to perform and is used only occasionally today. Patients with Hodgkin's disease and many patients with non-Hodgkin's lymphoma once routinely underwent staging laparotomy before the initiation of therapy to search for occult intra-abdominal disease. This approach is rarely used today because of the quality of available non-invasive staging procedures and the effectiveness of therapy. The one remaining place for staging laparotomy is for a patient with supradiaphragmatic disease who wants to be treated with limited radiotherapy alone. A laparotomy provides the surest evidence of the absence of intra-abdominal disease in this patient.

The studies necessary to evaluate a new patient with lymphoma and provide prognostic information and a therapy plan are presented in Table 2.

Pathobiology of lymphoma

Introduction

Increased understanding of the biology of the immune system has allowed the various lymphomas to be subclassified, and provided new prognostic information and new potential targets for therapy. Since lymphomas are malignancies of lymphocytes, the surface proteins involved in cell recognition and intercellular signalling can be expected to be important. Although the genetics of lymphomas are complicated, they too are beginning to be unravelled. Information gleaned from all these studies is likely to further change both the classification and therapy of the lymphomas.

Immunology

The recognition of new surface antigens has improved the ability to recognize specific subtypes of lymphoma. For example, discovery of the Ki-1 (CD30) antigen by investigators in Germany provided a marker for the Reed–Sternberg cells in classical Hodgkin's disease. However, it was soon discovered that this antigen was found on the surface of cancers that were previously felt to be undifferentiated carcinomas and malignant histiocytosis. This observation allowed the description of anaplastic large T/null-cell lymphoma as a diagnostic entity and, more importantly, allowed some patients with lymphoma to receive appropriate therapy.

The recognition of specific antigens by standardized antibodies has improved the accuracy of diagnosis. Some of the more commonly recognized antigens are presented in Table 3. A characteristic pattern of occurrence can be a key factor in making an accurate diagnosis. Some types of lymphoma, such as follicular lymphoma and nodular sclerosing Hodgkin's disease, can be diagnosed accurately without immunological studies. Others such as all T-cell lymphomas, diffuse large B-cell lymphoma, and

Table 3 Immunological markers useful in the diagnosis of lymphomas

Marker	Target	Characteristically positive lymphomas
CD3	T cells	T-cell lymphomas
CD4	Helper/inducer T cells	Some T-cell lymphomas
CD5	T cells, early B cells	T-cell lymphomas, small lymphocytic lymphoma, mantle-cell lymphoma
CD8	Cytotoxic/suppressor T cells and NK cells	Some T-cell lymphomas
CD10	CALLA	B-lymphoblastic lymphoma
CD15	Lewis-X	Classical Hodgkin's disease
CD20	B cells	B-cell lymphomas and nodular lymphocyte-predominance Hodgkin's disease
CD23	IgE receptor	Small lymphocytic lymphoma
CD25	IL-2 receptor	Peripheral T-cell lymphomas
CD30	Ki-1	Classical Hodgkin's disease and anaplastic large T/null-cell lymphoma
CD57	HNK-1	NK-cell lymphomas

NK, natural killer; CALLA, common acute lymphoblastic leukaemia antigen; IL-2, interleukin-2.

mantle-cell lymphoma can only be accurately diagnosed with immune markers.

Genetics

A theme common to malignant disorders is the abnormal expression of specific genes. The search for these genes was facilitated by the frequent occurrence of chromosomal abnormalities detectable by cytogenetic studies. These abnormalities include chromosomal deletions or deletions of parts of a chromosome, chromosomal duplications, and translocation of genetic material from one chromosome to another. Chromosomal translocations, through studying the sites of chromosome breakage, led to the discovery of a number of genes that appear to be important in lymphomagenesis or in determining the character of a particular lymphoma. The best documented chromosomal translocations associated with lymphomas along with the involved oncogenes are presented in Table 4.

Genetic abnormalities determine the nature of the lymphoma by leading to the overexpression, underexpression, or abnormal expression of specific genes. The genes involved, termed 'oncogenes', are typically those that regulate the cell cycle or differentiation. Since the work of genes is done by the proteins for which they code, the underexpression, overexpression, or abnormal expression of specific proteins is an increasing source for study. In some cases, protein expression might be abnormal despite no obvious translocation. For example, diffuse large B-cell lymphoma displays the t(14;18) in approximately 30 per cent of patients. This translocation involves the *BCL-2* gene on chromosome 18, whose protein product is involved in suppressing apoptosis (that is, the mechanism of cell death usually triggered by chemotherapeutic agents). Tumours can overexpress the BCL-2 protein with or without the t(14;18). Overexpression of BCL-2 protein might be expected to lead to the increased survival of lymphoma cells when they are exposed to therapeutic agents. In patients with diffuse large-cell lymphoma, an increased relapse rate has been associated with overexpression of the BCL-2 protein, rather than with the t(14;18).

Table 4 Recurring chromosomal translocations in non-Hodgkin's lymphoma

Translocation	Associated oncogene	Type of lymphoma
t(8;14) (q24;q32)	*c-myc*	Burkitt's
t(14;18) (q32;q21)	*BCL-2*	Follicular, diffuse large B-cell
t(3;14) (q27;q32)	*BCL-6*	Diffuse large B-cell
t(11;14) (q13;q32)	*BCL-1*	Mantle-cell
t(2;5) (q23;q35)	*NPM/ALK*	Anaplastic large T/null-cell
t(9;14) (p13;q32)	*PAX5*	Lymphoplasmacytoid
t(11;18) (q21;q21)	–	MALT

MALT, mucosa-associated lymphoid tissue.

Specific chromosomal translocations are highly associated with certain subtypes of lymphoma and thus are useful in diagnosis. These include the t(2;5) and anaplastic large T/null-cell lymphoma, the t(14;18) in follicular lymphoma, the t(8;14), t(2;8), and t(8;22) in Burkitt's lymphoma, and the t(11;14) in mantle-cell lymphoma. Cytogenetic studies in most patients with non-Hodgkin's lymphoma display a large number of chromosomal abnormalities. However, only a few have been shown to be of diagnostic or prognostic significance. No such abnormalities have been consistently identified in patient's with Hodgkin's disease.

Future genetic studies in lymphomas are likely to focus on specific gene expression. The new 'lympho chip' technology will allow the several thousand genes typically expressed in lymphoid cells to be studied simultaneously. Patterns of gene expression may well provide new methods of classifying lymphomas, provide new prognostic information, and direct therapy or provide new targets for therapy.

The general principles of therapy of lymphoma

Those treatments effective in the management of patients with cancer include surgery, radiotherapy, cytotoxic chemotherapy, and a variety of new approaches developed through increasing understanding of the biology of the immune system. The latter include cytokines, antibodies, and attempts to direct an immune reaction against cancer. Because few patients with lymphoma have truly localized disease, surgery has not been a major treatment modality. Radiotherapy, since its utilization in medicine in the first part of the twentieth century, has been a major treatment modality for patients with lymphoma. Radiotherapy is limited in its application by toxicity. Its curative potential depends upon being able to achieve a tumoricidal dose (typically 3000–4000 cGy) without irreversibly injuring normal organs. Thus, the site of involvement by a lymphoma, as well as the number of sites involved, can limit the effectiveness of this treatment, since toxicity increases with the volume of tissue radiated. If a lymphoma is truly localized, radiotherapy is often a curative. Two approaches have been utilized to make radiotherapy a 'systemic' treatment. One involves radiation of the total body. When this is part of a bone marrow transplant regimen, a total dose of 1000–1500 cGy can be administered. More recently, it has been demonstrated that it is possible to give higher doses of radiotherapy to multiple areas by attaching radioactive molecules to antibodies that home to sites of involvement by lymphoma.

Cytotoxic chemotherapeutic agents were first discovered in the 1940s when mechlorethamine (that is, the nitrogen mustard gas used in warfare) and, subsequently, methotrexate were found to cause regressions in immune system malignancies. A wide variety of agents have since been shown to be able to cause regressions in a significant proportion of patients with lymphomas (Table 5). Unfortunately, early studies showed that regressions induced by single agents were almost invariably followed by regrowth of the tumour and eventual death of the patient. In an attempt to circumvent this, combinations of chemotherapeutic agents were first utilized in the 1960s and early 1970s. The drugs were combined by attempting to choose agents with different mechanisms of action and non-overlapping toxicities to allow the administration of doses that were near to the maximum tolerated dose with an individual agent. In both childhood acute leukaemia and Hodgkin's disease this approach was validated by the cure of a significant number of patients. Today, several combination-chemotherapy regimens with acceptable toxicity have been shown to be effective and are widely used worldwide (Table 6). All regimens are not equally good for treating all types of lymphoma.

Increasing knowledge of the immune system has further led to the recognition that a number of biologically active molecules can cause regression

Table 5 Active drugs used in treating patients with lymphoma

Alkylating agents:	*Nitrosoureas:*
mechlorethamine (H)	carmustine (H)
chlorambucil (B)	lomustine (H)
cyclophosphamide (N)	
ifosfamide (N)	*Other cytotoxics:*
	dacarbazine (H)
Antimetabolites:	procarbazine (H)
methotrexate (N)	cisplatin (N)
cytarabine (N)	
pentostatin (N)	*Hormones:*
fludarabine (N)	corticosteroids (B)
Antitumour antibiotics:	*Biologics:*
doxorubicin (B)	interferon-alpha (N)
mitoxantrone (N)	rituximab (N)
bleomycin (B)	tositumomab (N)
	bagiliximab (N)
Alkaloids:	daclizumab (N)
vincristine (B)	
vinblastine (B)	
vindesine (N)	
etoposide (N)	

H, primarily used in Hodgkin's disease; N, primarily used in non-Hodgkin's lymphoma; B, used in both.

of lymphomas and, in some cases, impact on survival. The first such agent to be widely used was interferon-alpha, which has some activity in both non-Hodgkin's lymphoma and Hodgkin's disease. When administered at an adequate dose (at least 36 units per month), it has been shown to prolong survival in patients with poor-prognosis follicular lymphoma who received an anthracycline-containing chemotherapy regimen as their initial treatment. The ability to produce monoclonal antibodies has provided new therapeutic molecules. In B-cell non-Hodgkin's lymphomas, antibodies directed against the CD20 molecule have been incorporated into clinical practice. Rituximab has been shown to be active in a variety of B-cell lymphomas, and the new radiolabelled antibodies such as tositumomab will soon become available. An antibody directed against CD25 has been introduced into therapy for patients with cutaneous T-cell lymphoma.

Very high doses of cytotoxic chemotherapeutic agents with or without radiotherapy and biologically active molecules have been utilized in the treatment of patients with lymphomas as part of the bone marrow transplantation procedure. This involves the administration of very high doses of antilymphoma therapy in an attempt to overcome presumed treatment resistance. Patients are rescued from the toxicity of treatment by the reinfusion of haemopoietic stem cells. The patient's own haemopoietic stem cells (an autologous transplant) or those from another individual with identical HLA genes (an allogeneic transplant) can be utilized. Cells for this procedure can be obtained from either bone marrow or peripheral blood. Autologous transplantation has been widely used for patients with lymphoma and shown to be able to cure patients with relapsed Hodgkin's disease and aggressive non-Hodgkin's lymphoma. In aggressive non-Hodgkin's lymphomas, a probable increased cure rate has been demonstrated by utilizing adjuvant transplantation following initially effective standard chemotherapy in patients with a poor prognosis. Transplantation is being widely utilized in patients with follicular lymphoma, but the curability of autologous transplantation in this setting remains a point of controversy, and allogeneic transplantation, while apparently curative, has a high mortality rate.

Various new treatments are being studied for patients with lymphoma. These include attempts to stimulate the patient's endogenous immune system to develop antibodies against lymphomas; such 'tumour vaccines' are now in clinical trials. Another approach has been called 'antisense therapy', which involves the use of antisense oligonucleotides aimed at interrupting the transcription and expression of key genes.

A number of factors need to be taken into account when formulating a treatment recommendation for a patient with lymphoma (Table 7). These include the patient's age, general health, extent of disease, likelihood of cure, coexisting illnesses, long-term goals, and concerns about treatment toxicity. This decision should be made in conjunction with the patient, and requires good judgement in addition to technical knowledge. The aggressiveness of the treatment that is finally chosen will often depend upon the physician's interpretation of the chances for cure. It is obvious that more toxicity would be acceptable if the goal was cure rather than palliation. For this reason, patients with definitely curable lymphomas, such as diffuse large B-cell lymphoma and Burkitt's lymphoma, are almost always treated promptly with intensive regimens. In contrast, the best treatment for patients with follicular lymphoma remains a point for intense debate. Since the curability of this disease is in question, many physicians would favour no initial therapy in an asymptomatic patient. However, as discussed below, this is not a simple decision.

For most patients, the goal of therapy is to achieve a complete remission. This implies the disappearance of all symptoms and objective evidence of lymphoma. In practice, a complete remission is documented by repeating all abnormal staging studies after several cycles of therapy or at the completion of the planned therapy. Sometimes, persisting masses visualized on CT scans represent residual fibrosis rather than persisting tumour. In certain patients, a previously abnormal gallium scan reverting to normal would resolve this dilemma, but, on rare occasions, a biopsy might be required. Documentation of complete remission is important. Patients who achieve a complete remission have a chance for cure; those who do not achieve a complete remission with initial therapy will often go directly to second-line treatments.

Patients who fail to be cured with initial therapy, either because they do not achieve an initial remission or they relapse from remission, are candidates for what has been termed 'salvage therapy.' These second-line regimens can regularly cause tumour regression in most patients with lymphoma and can occasionally produce long-term, disease-free survival. However, for most patients, the only curative approach in this setting is bone marrow transplantation. The toxicity of bone marrow transplantation limits its use to patients under certain ages (under 70 years of age for autologous transplantation and under 55 years for allogeneic transplantation), who have a good performance status, without serious compromise of major organ function, and to patients who do not have bulky/chemotherapy-refractory disease.

Hodgkin's disease

In 1832, Thomas Hodgkin of Guy's Hospital, London, reported seven patients who died from a disorder involving lymph node and spleen enlargement. Then, early in the twentieth century, Sternberg and Reed independently described the characteristic giant cells that now bear their name. This made it possible for pathologists to separate the disorder we now know as Hodgkin's disease from other lymphomas.

Incidence and epidemiology

Unlike non-Hodgkin's lymphomas, the incidence of Hodgkin's disease appears to be stable with approximately three new cases per 100 000 per year in western countries. As demonstrated in Fig. 1, this illness displays a peculiar bimodal distribution of occurrence with peaks in young adulthood and older age. This dual peak has led some to propose that Hodgkin's disease actually represents two illnesses, with the earlier peak being related to an infectious aetiology and the latter representing a true malignancy. However, there is little evidence to support this distinction.

A strong association has been demonstrated between the occurrence of Hodgkin's disease and infection by the Epstein–Barr virus (**EBV**). Monoclonal or oligoclonal proliferation of EBV-infected cells is found in 20 to 40 per cent of patients with Hodgkin's disease. Patients infected by the human immunodeficiency virus (**HIV**) are at an increased risk for Hodgkin's disease in addition to non-Hodgkin's lymphomas.

The subtypes of Hodgkin's disease vary geographically and by age group. Patients in western countries who develop Hodgkin's disease in young adulthood usually have the nodular sclerosis subtype. Patients from Third-World countries, elderly patients, and those infected with HIV usually have mixed-cellularity or lymphocyte-depletion Hodgkin's disease.

Hodgkin's disease is approximately 100 times more likely in an identical twin of an infected patient. Numerous instances of case-clustering have been described. While these might be taken as evidence of a genetic or infectious aetiology, the cause of Hodgkin's disease remains unknown.

Pathology

The diagnosis of Hodgkin's disease requires the identification of Reed–Sternberg cells in a characteristic cellular background; however, the cell of origin for the Reed–Sternberg cell remains unknown. The subtypes of Hodgkin's disease are presented in Table 8. Nodular sclerosing Hodgkin's disease is characterized by bands of fibrosis that are often visible to the naked eye when a slide is held to the light. Mixed-cellularity Hodgkin's disease typically displays a larger number of Reed–Sternberg cells in a mixed-cellular background including lymphocytes, macrophages, and eosinophils. Lymphocyte-depletion Hodgkin's disease can present with a very large number of Reed–Sternberg cells and atypical mononuclear cells, or a background of diffuse fibrosis with occasional Reed–Sternberg cells. Lymphocyte-predominance Hodgkin's disease is characterized by large numbers of small lymphocytes and histiocytes with occasional Reed–Sternberg cells. The growth pattern can be nodular or diffuse.

It is now clear that patients with nodular lymphocyte-predominance Hodgkin's disease have a different illness that is, in many ways, more like a B-cell non-Hodgkin's lymphoma. The Reed–Sternberg cells in nodular lymphocyte-predominance Hodgkin's disease express the leucocyte common antigen and other B-cell markers including CD20. Typical Reed–Sternberg cells do not express the leucocyte common antigen, but are CD15- and CD30-positive. Staining for CD15 and CD30 can resolve difficult diagnostic problems in some cases.

Clinical features and evaluation

Patients with classical Hodgkin's disease usually present with palpable non-tender lymphadenopathy. In most patients, lymph nodes are discovered in the cervical, supraclavicular, and axillary regions. More than half the patients have mediastinal lymphadenopathy at diagnosis, and symptoms

Table 6 Popular combination chemotherapy regimens used in treating patients with lymphoma

Regimen	Drug	Dose in mg/m²	Route	Schedule
Hodgkin's disease				
ABVD	Doxorubicin	25	IV	D1 and 15
	Bleomycin	10	IV	D1 and 15
	Vinblastine	6	IV	D1 and 15
	Dacarbazine	375	IV	D1 and 15
	28-day cycles			
BEACOPP	Bleomycin	10	IV	D8
	Etoposide	100	IV	D1 thru 3
	Doxorubicin	25	IV	D1
	Cyclophosphamide	650	IV	D1
	Vincristine	1.4 (max. 2)	IV	D1
	Procarbazine	100	PO	D1 thru 7
	Prednisone	40	PO	D1 thru 14
	Requires filgrastim			
	21-day cycles			
Non-Hodgkin's lymphoma				
CVP	Cyclophosphamide	400	PO	D1 thru 5
		or		
		1200	IV	D1 thru 5
	Vincristine	1.4 (max. 2)	IV	D1
	Prednisone	100 total dose (not by m²)	PO	D1 thru 5
	21-day cycles			
CHOP	Cyclophosphamide	750	IV	D1
	Doxorubicin	50	IV	D1
	Vincristine	1.4 (max. 2)	IV	D1
	Prednisone	100 total (not by m²)	PO	D1 thru 5
	21-day cycles			
ACVBP	Doxorubicin	75	IV	D1
	Cyclophosphamide	2200	IV	D1 thru 5
	Vindesine	2	IV	D1
	Bleomycin	5	IV	D1
	Methylprednisolone	60	IV	D1 thru 5
	14-day cycles			

Table 7 Factors to consider in therapy for a patient with lymphoma

- Specific type of lymphoma
- Age
- Performance status
- Presence of other diseases
- Stage
- Systemic symptoms
- Pace of disease
- Potential side-effects
- Is there a chance of cure?
- Patient's concerns about specific treatments
- Convenience
- Patient's immediate and long-term goals
- Quality of life

from a large mediastinal mass are often the initial presentation. Subdiaphragmatic presentation of Hodgkin's disease is unusual and more common in older males. Approximately one-third of patients with classical Hodgkin's disease present with fevers, night sweats, and/or weight loss.

Hodgkin's disease can present as a fever of unknown origin. Presentation as a 'fever of unknown origin' is more common in older patients who have mixed-cellularity or lymphocyte-depletion Hodgkin's disease and who present with disease in abdominal nodes. Fevers associated with Hodgkin's disease occasionally persist for days to weeks, followed by afebrile intervals, and then reoccurrence of the fever. This pattern is known as Pel–Ebstein fever. Unusual presentations of Hodgkin's disease include severe and unexplained pyloritis, paraneoplastic cerebellar degeneration, nephrotic syndrome, immune haemolytic anaemia and thrombocytopenia, hypercalcaemia, and pain in lymph nodes on alcohol ingestion.

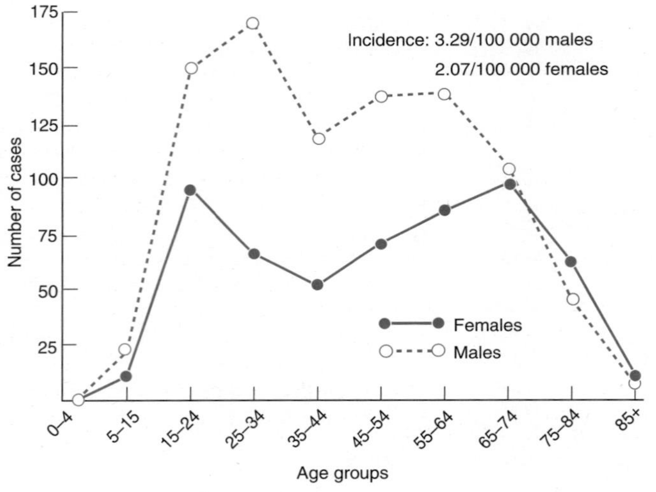

Fig. 1 Age distribution of Hodgkin's disease expressed as new cases registered in England and Wales in 1973.

Table 8 Histological subtypes of Hodgkin's disease

- Nodular sclerosis
- Mixed cellularity
- Lymphocyte-predominance:
  - nodular
  - diffuse
- Lymphocyte-depleted
  - reticular
  - diffuse fibrosis

The diagnosis of Hodgkin's disease is based on a review of an adequate biopsy by an expert haematopathologist. Subsequent evaluation should include a careful history and examination, complete blood count, erythrocyte sedimentation rate determination, serum chemistry studies including serum lactate dehydrogenase, chest radiograph, computer demography of the chest, abdomen, and pelvis, and bone marrow biopsy. Gallium scans can be performed to document radioisotope uptake by the tumour, which can then be repeated at the completion of therapy to document remission. Bipedal lymphangiograms can be useful if radiologists expert in carrying out the procedure are available. Staging laparotomies are now rarely indicated.

Nodular lymphocyte-predominance Hodgkin's disease, as noted above, is a different clinical entity from classical Hodgkin's disease. These patients represent less than 5 per cent of all patients found to have Hodgkin's disease. The evaluation of such patients is carried out in a similar way to that for classical Hodgkin's disease. However, nodular lymphocyte-predominance Hodgkin's disease tends to follow a chronic, relapsing course and sometimes transforms to diffuse large B-cell lymphoma.

Prognostic factors

The major factors determining treatment outcome for patients with Hodgkin's disease include the Ann Arbor stage, the presence or absence of systemic symptoms, age, and gender. Patients with asymptomatic, localized disease who are young and female have the best outlook. Histological subtypes do not appear to have major independent prognostic significance. Patients with nodular sclerosing Hodgkin's disease have a better outcome than those with mixed-cellularity or lymphocyte-depleted Hodgkin's disease. However, adverse prognostic factors are more commonly found in patients with the latter histological subtypes. The results of several laboratory studies can predict outcome in patients with Hodgkin's disease. These include anaemia, an elevated erythrocyte sedimentation rate, and a low albumin level. The erythrocyte sedimentation rate is sometimes used to follow the course of patients with Hodgkin's disease since it tends to normalize with successful treatment.

The most important factor in predicting outcome for patients with Hodgkin's disease is their response to therapy. Patients who have a prompt, complete response to chemotherapy and/or radiotherapy have the best outlook and are most likely to be cured. It is important to note that residual masses do not always represent persisting disease. This is particularly true for residual mediastinal and retroperitoneal masses. These sites tend to be associated with a considerable amount of fibrosis that can persist after effective therapy. Normalization of a gallium scan can be used to document remission. Patients who relapse after initial successful treatment for Hodgkin's disease can sometimes be effectively treated with further chemotherapy or radiotherapy. The chances for successful treatment, in part, depend upon the duration of initial remission in addition to other prognostic factors present at relapse. Patients with a longer initial remission are more likely to be successfully retreated.

Primary therapy

Patients with localized Hodgkin's disease (stage I or non-bulky stage II) can be cured with extended-field radiotherapy. Patients with supradiaphragmatic disease are typically treated with a radiotherapy port that is often referred to as a mantle. This involves treatment of the cervical, supraclavicular, axillary, and mediastinal lymph nodes. In the absence of a staging laparotomy before therapy, upper abdominal nodes and spleen are also often treated. A dose of 3500 to 4400 cGY is usually administered in fractions of 175 to 200 cGy daily, 5 days per week for approximately 4 weeks.

Patients with otherwise localized Hodgkin's disease who present with a large mediastinal mass pose special therapeutic problems. A large mediastinal mass is often defined as one whose maximum diameter is greater than one-third of the maximum thoracic diameter. Treatment with radiotherapy alone, or chemotherapy alone, is associated with a high relapse rate. Large mediastinal masses are one definite indication for combined modality therapy.

Patients who present with B-symptoms or stage III or IV disease are best treated initially with a combination-chemotherapy regimen. If complete remission is documented after completing a course of chemotherapy, the majority of patients will be cured. Patients who have large masses often receive adjuvant radiotherapy to the sites of previous bulky disease after completing the chemotherapy regimen. While the original **MOPP** (mechlorethamine, Oncovin (i.e. vincristine), procarbazine, prednisone) regimen was effective in the treatment of Hodgkin's disease, it has now been shown that regimens which include **ABVD** (doxorubicin (Adriamycin), bleomycin, vinblastine, dacarbazine) are associated with a better outcome (Table 6).

Elderly and pregnant patients pose special therapeutic problems. In Hodgkin's disease, the elderly have a much worse prognosis than younger patients: patients over 60 years of age at the time of diagnosis have a survival rate less than half that of younger patients. Elderly patients with localized disease seem to benefit from radiotherapy in a manner comparable to younger patients. However, older patients tolerate aggressive chemotherapy regimens much less well and, even if the drugs can be administered, have a higher relapse rate.

Hodgkin's disease, since it occurs frequently in young adults, is not rarely diagnosed in pregnant women. It is now clear that Hodgkin's disease can be treated with chemotherapy at any point during pregnancy with a chance of a good treatment outcome and a surviving infant. However, the risks are higher in the first trimester. Most physicians would favour delaying therapy past the first trimester, if possible, and would discuss the possibility of a therapeutic abortion with the patient. If the decision is made to treat a pregnant patient with chemotherapy, it must be remembered that the fetus will be myelosuppressed in a manner similar to the mother. This must be taken into account when planning delivery of the baby. Radiotherapy is generally not used in pregnant patients because of its teratogenic potential.

The optimal treatment for lymphocyte-predominance Hodgkin's disease is unclear. Some clinicians favour no initial therapy in asymptomatic patients. However, potentially curative radiotherapy to localized disease seems wise. The clinician must be alert for transformation to diffuse, large B-cell lymphoma.

Treatment of relapse

Approximately 25 to 35 per cent of patients treated with chemotherapy for stage III or IV Hodgkin's disease will suffer relapse after achieving a remission. A small proportion of patients will fail to enter initial complete remission. Patients who fail to enter complete remission or relapse within 1 year of completing therapy have a poor prognosis with further standard chemotherapy. Autologous bone marrow transplantation can be curative in 25 to 50 per cent of such patients, and is the treatment of choice. Patients who have an initial remission of longer than 1 year pose a more complicated therapeutic problem. These patients are likely to achieve a second remission with a standard chemotherapy regimen. However, long-term follow-up has demonstrated that the majority of these remissions are not durable, and many physicians would recommend autologous transplantation to such patients. The occasional patient with a localized relapse after chemotherapy can sometimes be cured with radiotherapy. Patients who relapse after treatment with initial radiotherapy have an excellent result with standard chemotherapy regimens and a high likelihood of cure.

Treatment complications

The treatment of Hodgkin's disease is associated with both short-term and long-term complications. Prominent short-term complications include hair loss, emesis, fatigue, anaemia, and infection due to chemotherapy-induced neutropenia. Hair loss is usually transient. Emesis can be prevented in almost all patients by 5-hydroxytryptamine antagonists such as ondansetron and granisetron. Anaemia and fatigue do not usually limit the administration of therapy. Chemotherapy-induced neutropenia is a major problem and neutropenic fever needs to be managed aggressively with intravenous antibiotics after cultures are obtained. Even so, treatment for Hodgkin's disease is administered entirely on an outpatient basis.

Delayed toxicity from the treatment of Hodgkin's disease has become a major problem for young patients who are cured of Hodgkin's disease and have been followed for extended periods. In fact, for patients with good-prognosis Hodgkin's disease, long-term complications might lead to a higher mortality rate than the Hodgkin's disease itself.

Most of the serious complications of radiotherapy appear after long follow-up. In the first few months after treatment, some patients will develop an electric shock sensation down the spine and into the legs on flexion of the neck. This represents Lhermitte's syndrome and needs to be recognized so that further evaluation is not carried out. It is usually transient. In some patients, delayed pulmonary fibrosis or cardiac injuries are associated with thoracic radiotherapy. Modern radiotherapy techniques have minimized the risk of these problems, but accelerated coronary artery disease is a significant problem and leads to a number of treatment-related deaths. The major delayed problem with radiotherapy is the development of secondary cancers. This risk begins to appear beyond 10 years post-therapy, and by 20 years after therapy leads to a significant number of deaths. Patients treated with thoracic radiotherapy for Hodgkin's disease should be strongly encouraged not to smoke to reduce the risk of lung cancer. Young women should have screening mammography instituted 5 to 10 years earlier than for women not irradiated, or by 10 years after completing treatment.

Patients who receive radiotherapy to the neck have a high risk of developing subsequent hypothyroidism. Follow-up in such patients should include periodic quantitation of their thyrotropin levels to anticipate this problem. Some patients treated with either radiotherapy or chemotherapy will develop herpes zoster. This diagnosis does not necessarily signify a relapse of Hodgkin's disease.

Long-term problems associated with chemotherapy include treatment-related leukaemia, infertility, and aseptic necrosis of bone. Infertility is most likely in patients who receive alkylating agent-containing regimens. Most young males who received MOPP become infertile. In women, the risks of infertility are age-related. Women over 30 years of age are much more likely to be permanently infertile than those under 30 years. However, in any patient, resumption of fertility is possible and the patient should be aware of this. Infertility is less of a problem in patients who receive the ABVD regimen. Males very anxious to retain fertility can be offered semen storage and women, in extraordinary cases, can be offered egg storage.

Treatment-related leukaemia is most frequent in patients who receive chemotherapy regimens containing alkylating agents and who are treated on more than one occasion. Young patients treated with only one chemotherapy sequence are unlikely to develop leukaemia. The incidence of leukaemia rises dramatically in patients over 40 years of age, and in those who receive alkylating agents on more than one occasion. Leukaemia is unusual in patients treated with ABVD. The combination of chemotherapy and radiotherapy seems to increase the risk of leukaemia. The leukaemias that occur in this setting usually present with myelodysplasia and typically have genetic abnormalities involving chromosomes 5, 7, and 8. Etoposide can lead to the development of acute leukaemia without a preceding myelodysplasia that involves abnormalities on chromosome 11.

Patients who receive corticosteroid treatment as part of a combination therapy are at risk for aseptic necrosis of the femoral heads. Those who develop hip pain on follow-up should be evaluated for this possibility.

Non-Hodgkin's lymphoma

Incidence

In much of the world, it appears that the incidence of non-Hodgkin's lymphoma is increasing, but the incidence still varies widely between countries. The incidence appears to be approximately 2 cases per 100 000 per year in the Orient, 10 per 100 000 per year in the United Kingdom, and more than 15 per 100 000 per year in the United States. In the United States, the disease increased in frequency by approximately 4 per cent per year between 1950 and the mid-1990s. This increased incidence is seen in patients of all ages but more striking in the elderly. However, recent data suggest that the rate of increase may be slowing.

A recent study showed that the specific types of non-Hodgkin's lymphomas vary in occurrence between countries. For example, follicular lymphoma is more common in North America than in Europe or Asia. T-cell lymphomas have been seen more frequently in Asia, and certain types of T/NK-cell lymphomas (**NK**, natural killer) such as angiocentric nasal lymphomas seem restricted to only a few countries in Asia and Latin America. The explanation for this difference in different geographical settings is unclear.

Aetiology

Various aetiological factors, either proven or suggested to be associated with the development of non-Hodgkin's lymphoma, are listed in Table 9. It is now clear that exposure to certain agriculture chemicals does increase the risk of this disease. A variety of immune deficiencies, such as those associated with immunosuppression following organ transplantation and various inherited immune deficiencies, are also associated with an increased risk of developing non-Hodgkin's lymphoma. Patients with rheumatoid arthritis and systemic lupus erythematosus appear to be at increased risk.

A variety of infectious agents have been shown to be associated with the development of non-Hodgkin's lymphoma. Gastric *Helicobacter pylori* infection is associated with the development of gastric **MALT** (mucosa-associated lymphoid tissue) lymphoma. In the case of MALT lymphomas, eradication of the *Helicobacter pylori* infection by antibiotics can lead to regression of the lymphoma in a significant number of patients. **HTLV**-1 (human T-cell lymphoma/leukaemia virus-1) appears to be the cause of a specific type of non-Hodgkin's lymphoma, seen predominantly in southern Japan and the Caribbean, called adult T-cell lymphoma/leukaemia. The Epstein–Barr virus has been associated with Burkitt's lymphoma in Africa, the development of aggressive B-cell lymphomas in immunosuppressed patients, Hodgkin's disease, and certain aggressive T-cell lymphomas. HHV-8 (human herpesvirus-8) has been closely associated with a rare, diffuse, large B-cell lymphoma called effusion lymphoma. HIV (human immunodeficiency virus) infection can lead to the development of aggressive B-cell lymphoma. It is likely that the future will see more associations between lymphomas and specific infectious agents.

Table 9 Factors predisposing to the development of non-Hodgkin's lymphoma

• Immune deficiencies: organ transplantation inherited immune deficiencies AIDS
• Agricultural chemicals
• Autoimmune disorders: rheumatoid arthritis lupus erythematosus
• Treated Hodgkin's disease
• Infectious agents: *Helicobacter pylori* vEBV HTLV-1 HIV HHV-8 HCV

AIDS, acquired immune deficiency syndrome; EBV, Epstein–Barr virus; HTLV-1, human T-cell leukaemia virus-1; HIV, human immunodeficiency virus; HHV-8, human herpesvirus-8, HCV, hepatitis C virus.

REAL/WHO classification

The classification of non-Hodgkin's lymphomas has changed several times during the twentieth century. The first popular classification proposed by Gall and Mallory divided lymphomas into giant follicular lymphoma, reticulum-cell sarcoma, and lymphosarcoma. Both the lack of adequate clinical correlation and clear definitions of the entities led to further proposals. Henry Rappaport recognized the importance of growth pattern in the prognosis of non-Hodgkin's lymphomas, and put forward his system that divided patients into those with nodular (i.e. follicular) or diffuse lymphomas and those with large- or small-cell lymphomas. However, this system was proposed before the recognition that lymphomas were all malignancies of lymphocytes and before the discovery of the existence of subtypes of lymphocytes. The advent of modern immunology led to new classification systems proposed by Carl Lennert and colleagues in Europe and Lukes and Collins in the United States. The Kiel classification proposed by Lennert and colleagues became the most widely used system in Europe. An attempt to unify the classifications of lymphomas led to the development of the Working Formulation. This is a compromise system taking major elements from the Rappaport classification, Kiel classification, and the Lukes/Collins classification. It became widely used in the United States but less so in Europe.

In the 1990s a group of haematopathologists from Europe, North America, and other parts of the world proposed a new system based on not just morphology and immunophenotyping, but taking into account other genetic and biological information that had become available. In the 1990s, a number of 'new' lymphomas were discovered that did not fit into previous classification systems. These included mantle-cell lymphoma, anaplastic large T/null-cell lymphoma, and MALT lymphomas. The Revised European/American Lymphoma classification (**REAL**) classified lymphomas based on clinical pathological syndromes (in other words, real diseases) rather than simply morphology. This system was tested in a large international study and shown to be more accurate than previous systems and to have high clinical relevance. Leaders in the fields of both haematopathology and clinical haematology/oncology agreed on a modified REAL classification to be endorsed by the World Health Organization and published as the WHO classification (Table 10). This, with modifications, is likely to be the major lymphoma classification for at least the next decade. The incidence of major lymphoma subtypes according to the WHO classification are listed in Table 11. Knowledge of 10 to 12 specific subtypes of non-Hodgkin's lymphoma will allow a clinician to care for almost all patients.

International Prognostic Index

Knowledge of the specific subtype of non-Hodgkin's lymphoma is only one of two pieces of information necessary to plan the intelligent management of patients with these disorders. The other that must be available involves the delineation of the prognostic characteristics of the individual patient. While it is true that follicular lymphoma has a higher median overall survival than diffuse large B-cell lymphoma, individual patients with follicular lymphoma might have a much worse survival because of adverse prognostic characteristics than an individual patient with diffuse large B-cell lymphoma who has good prognostic characteristics. Codification of these prognostic characteristics into a practical clinical tool was accomplished by a large international study that yielded the International Prognostic Index (**IPI**) (Table 12). The IPI is a summation of a number of specific adverse

Table 10 WHO classification of non-Hodgkin's lymphoma*

Precursor B-cell	*Precursor T-cell*
B lymphoblastic	T lymphoblastic
Mature (peripheral) B-cell	**Mature (peripheral) T-cell**
B-cell CLL/small lymphocytic lymphoma	Mycosis fungoides/Sezary syndrome
	Adult T-cell lymphoma/leukaemia
Lymphoplasmacytic lymphoma	**Anaplastic large T/null-cell lymphoma**
Extranodal marginal-zone B-cell lymphoma of MALT type	**Peripheral T-cell lymphoma**
	Not otherwise specified
Nodal marginal-zone B-cell lymphoma	Angioimmunoblastic T-cell lymphoma
	Entranodal nasal NK/T-cell lymphoma
Splenic marginal-zone B-cell lymphoma	Exteropathy type T-cell lymphoma
	Hepatosplenic γδ T-cell lymphoma
Mantle-cell lymphoma	Subcutaneous panniculitis-like T-cell lymphoma
Follicular lymphoma	
Diffuse large B-cell lymphoma	
Burkitt's lymphoma	

* Lymphomas representing 5 per cent or more of all non-Hodgkin's lymphomas are presented in **bold** print.

prognostic factors in an individual patient. The important factors include age greater than 60 years, Ann Arbor Stage III/IV, serum lactate dehydrogenase level greater than normal, reduced performance status, and multiple extranodal sites of involvement by lymphoma. The impact of the IPI score on the survival of patients with follicular lymphoma and diffuse large B-cell lymphoma are presented in Fig. 2. As mentioned above, the treatment plan for a patient with lymphoma must always include knowledge of the specific subtype of lymphoma and the patient's prognostic characteristics.

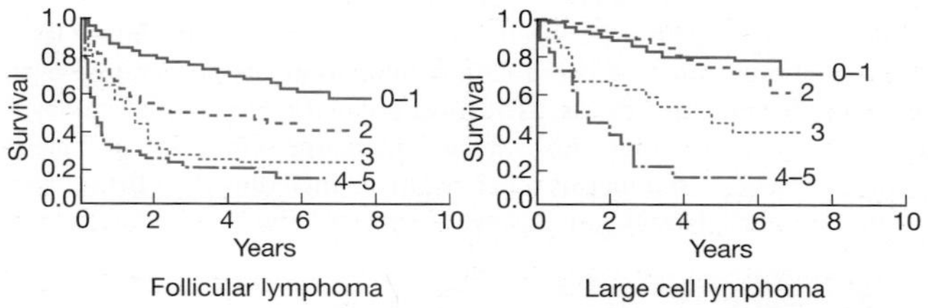

Fig. 2 The survival of 275 patients with follicular lymphoma and 388 patients with diffuse large B-cell lymphoma are shown by International Prognostic Index score.

Lymphoblastic lymphoma of B-cell and T-cell origin

Lymphoblastic lymphoma is a tumour of the precursor cells of T- and B-lymphocytes. It is intimately related to the acute lymphoid leukaemias, with the difference being the method of presentation. Sometimes it is difficult to determine when a patient should be said to have acute lymphoid leukaemia or lymphoblastic lymphoma, since bone marrow involvement is frequent with a lymphomatous presentation and lymphadenopathy and mediastinal mass are common in patients who present with leukaemia.

Table 11 The relative frequency of occurrence of major subtypes of non-Hodgkin's disease

Type of NHL	Percentage of All NHL
Diffuse large B-cell	31
Follicular	22
Small lymphocytic/LLL	6
Mantle-cell	6
Peripheral T-cell	6
MALT	5
Anaplastic large T/null-cell	2
Lymphoblastic	2
Burkitt's	<1

LLL, large lymphocytic leukaemia; MALT, mucosa-associated lymphoid tissue.

Table 12 International Prognostic Index (IPI)

Adverse risk factor	Score
Age >60 years	1
Ann Arbor Stage III or IV	1
Serum LDH >normal	1
Reduced performance status	1
Multiple extranodal sites involved	1

- IPI score = sum of adverse risk factors (i.e. 0–5)
- Age-adjusted IPI used in patients <60 years of age considers only stage, LDH, and performance status—i.e. maximum score is 3.

LDH, lactate dehydrogenase.

Most patients with lymphoblastic lymphoma have tumours derived from T-lymphoblasts, but approximately 10 per cent are B-cell in origin. The differential diagnosis of lymphoblastic lymphoma includes a blastic variant of mantle-cell lymphoma, acute myeloid leukaemia, and small round-cell lymphoma in children and young adults.

The median age of patients with lymphoblastic lymphoma is the late twenties and the majority of patients are male. Most patients have widely disseminated disease and an elevated serum LDH level. Approximately 50 per cent of patients will have bone marrow involvement. The IPI predicts outcome in lymphoblastic lymphoma. However, it has been suggested that patients can be divided into two prognostic groups. One group includes patients who have stage IV disease, elevated LDH levels, and bone marrow or central nervous system involvement; adults with these characteristics have a poor outlook. The second group comprises patients without these adverse characteristics, and these patients have a high cure rate.

Most patients with lymphoblastic lymphoma will be treated with a leukaemia-like regimen. This includes an intensive induction therapy along with central nervous system prophylaxis, and an ongoing maintenance or consolidation phase of treatment. The majority of children and young adults can be cured with this treatment approach. Patients who present with adverse risk characteristics or who relapse after initial therapy are candidates for bone marrow transplantation.

Diffuse large B-cell lymphoma

Diffuse large B-cell lymphoma is the most common non-Hodgkin's lymphoma, representing approximately one-third of all patients. It most commonly presents *de novo*, but also can develop after histological transformation of a small-cell lymphoma such as follicular, small lymphocytic, and MALT lymphoma. This tumour can arise in lymph nodes or essentially on any extranodal site including the central nervous system. Rare presentations include pleural effusions from involvement of serosal surfaces (effusion lymphoma) and multiple organ system dysfunction secondary to endothelial involvement (intravascular lymphomatosis).

B-cell lymphomas will display the CD20 antigen. Several cytogenetic abnormalities are frequently associated with diffuse large B-cell lymphoma including t(14;18) t(3;14) and t(8;14). The differential diagnosis includes undifferentiated carcinoma, acute myeloid leukaemia, and Hodgkin's disease. Occasional patients with diffuse large B-cell lymphoma have a large number of infiltrating T cells, and so can be confused with a peripheral T-cell lymphoma.

The clinical characteristics of patients with diffuse large B-cell lymphoma are presented in Box 1. The median age at presentation is 64 years and there is a slight male predominance. Approximately 50 per cent of patients will have stage I or II disease and approximately 50 per cent will have a more widely disseminated lymphoma. Approximately two-thirds of patients will have some sign of extranodal involvement. B-symptoms are seen at presentation in approximately one-third of patients and approximately half of the patients have an elevated LDH. Bone marrow involvement is seen in approximately 15 per cent of patients.

Since the early 1970s it has been known that patients with diffuse large B-cell lymphoma could be cured with combination chemotherapy—even those with disseminated disease. The most popular regimen in use today is **CHOP** (cyclophosphamide, doxorubicin, vincristine (Oncovin), and prednisone), although a number of other regimens including **ACVBP** (doxorubicin, cyclophosphamide, vindesine, bleomycin, and prednisone) are at least as active. A recent randomized trial in older patients found that adding rituximab to CHOP improved both the failure-free and overall survival. When a staging evaluation shows disease confined to one site (that is, stage I) or two nearby sites (minimal stage II) a brief course of chemotherapy followed by radiotherapy gives the highest cure rate. In patients with more disseminated disease, a complete course of one of the combination-chemotherapy regimens mentioned earlier is appropriate. In patients who present with the multiple adverse risk factors listed in the IPI, adjuvant autologous haemopoietic stem-cell transplantation after achieving an initial remission seems to yield a higher cure rate.

Approximately 75 per cent of patients with localized disease can be cured with abbreviated chemotherapy and radiotherapy, and approximately 35 to 40 per cent of patients with more disseminated disease can be cured with combination chemotherapy. Patients who relapse from complete remission can be cured with autologous transplantation. Patients who remain chemotherapy-sensitive after relapse have an approximately 40 per cent cure rate with autologous transplantation, while chemotherapy-resistant patients are cured only approximately 10 per cent of the time.

Follicular lymphoma

The second most common type of non-Hodgkin's lymphoma is follicular lymphoma. The clinical characteristics of patients with this disease are presented in Box 2. The differential diagnosis of follicular lymphoma includes benign follicular hyperplasia and the follicular variant of mantle-cell lymphoma. Patients with follicular lymphoma are subdivided based on the

Box 1 Diffuse large B-cell lymphoma

Median age	64 years
Percentage male	55%
Stage: I	12%
IE	13%
II	13%
IIE	16%
III	13%
IV	33%
B-symptoms	33%
Elevated LDH	53%
Reduced performance status	24%
Tumour mass >10 cm	30%
Bone marrow involvement	16%
Gastrointestinal tract involvement	18%
International prognostic index score	
0–1	35%
2–3	46%
4–5	19%

Survival and disease-free survival

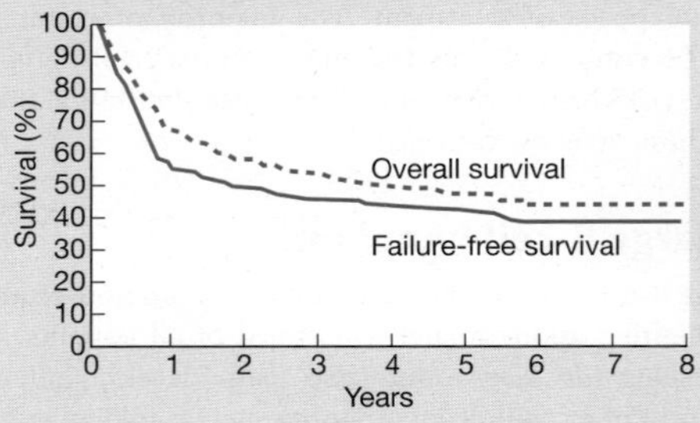

Box 2 Follicular lymphoma

Median age	59 years
Percentage male	42%
Stage: I	16%
IE	2%
II	11%
IIE	4%
III	16%
IV	51%
B-symptoms	28%
Elevated LDH	30%
Reduced performance status	9%
Tumour mass >10 cm	28%
Bone marrow involvement	47%
Gastrointestinal tract involvement	4%
International prognostic index score	
0–1	45%
2–3	48%
4–5	7%

Survival and disease-free survival

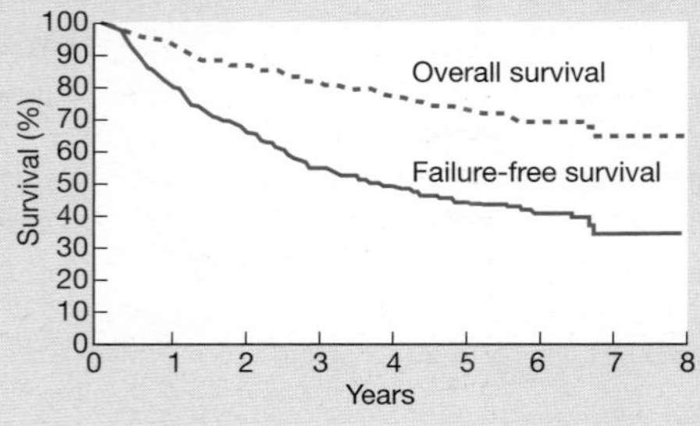

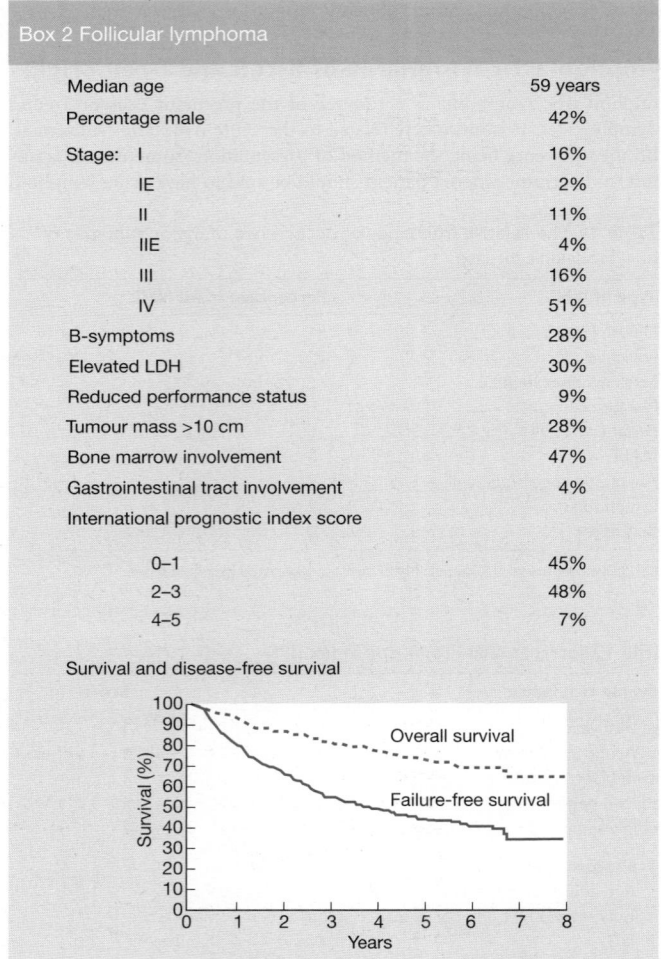

Table 13 Treatment regimens used for patients with follicular lymphoma

- Close observation and no initial therapy
- Radiotherapy: involved field, total nodal, low-dose total body
- Single-agent chemotherapy: chlorambucil, cyclophosphamide, fludarabine
- Combination chemotherapy: CVP, CHOP, FND
- Interferon-alpha
- Antibodies: rituximab, tositumomab
- Tumour vaccines
- Haemopoietic stem-cell transplantation: autologous, allogeneic

CVP: cyclophosphamide, vincristine, prednisone; CHOP: cyclophosphamide, doxorubicin, vincristine, prednisone; FND: fludarabine, mitoxantrone, dexamethasone.

number of large cells in the tumour. In general, a higher proportion of large cells is associated with a higher proliferative rate, more rapid tumour progression, and, perhaps, a better response to anthracycline-containing combination-chemotherapy regimens. The natural history of follicular lymphoma involves a reduction in the degree of follicularity in the tumour over time and an increase in the proportion of large cells. At autopsy, the majority of tumours will be found to have undergone transformation to diffuse large B-cell lymphoma. This is recognized during life in approximately 50 per cent of patients. Histological transformation to diffuse large B-cell lymphoma is associated with a poor prognosis in most patients.

Follicular lymphomas are B-cell lymphomas that display the CD20 antigen. Most patients' tumours will display the translocation t(14;18) and overexpress the *BCL-2* oncogene. Transformation to diffuse large B-cell lymphoma is frequently associated with additional cytogenetic abnormalities and the expression of other oncogenes such as *p53*.

Treatments commonly utilized in the management of patients with follicular lymphoma are presented in Table 13. Asymptomatic patients are often managed with no initial therapy—a strategy that is sometimes called 'watchful waiting'. When followed in this manner, approximately 25 per cent of patients will undergo at least a partial spontaneous regression, although these regressions are not durable. The most popular treatment worldwide for follicular lymphoma is probably single-agent oral chlorambucil. This is particularly true in elderly or infirm patients requiring therapy. Combination chemotherapy with **CVP** (cyclophosphamide, vincristine, and prednisone) or **CHOP** (cyclophosphamide, doxorubicin, vincristine, and prednisone) causes a more rapid response and a higher proportion of complete remissions. Approximately 20 per cent of completely responding patients have remissions that last more than 10 years. Recently, a meta-analysis was conducted of all available trials of interferon incorporated into primary therapy in follicular lymphoma, which demonstrated an improved survival of patients who received adjuvant interferon if they presented with poor risk characteristics and received an anthracycline, such as doxorubicin, as part of their primary therapy. Using **PCR** (polymerase chain reaction) technology, bone marrow specimens from patients with follicular lymphoma frequently test positive for the *BCL-2* gene rearrangement. The goal of some treatment regimens is to eradicate any evidence of *BCL-2* gene rearrangement in the bone marrow, but what the ultimate effect of this will be on survival has not been proven.

Patients with localized follicular lymphoma are often treated with radiotherapy alone. These patients have an excellent outlook with a 10-year survival of 70 to 90 per cent in most series.

Most patients with follicular lymphoma will eventually fail their initial treatment regimen. There is a high response rate to retreatment utilizing single-agent chemotherapeutic agents such as chlorambucil or fludarabine, many combination-chemotherapy regimens, antibodies such as rituximab, and bone marrow transplantation. Both autologous and allogeneic bone marrow transplantation have been demonstrated to produce long-term, disease-free survival in a proportion of patients with follicular lymphoma. Allogeneic transplantation is associated with a higher mortality rate, but there is more convincing evidence that the procedure might be curative.

The median survival in series of patients treated for follicular lymphoma is approximately 10 years, although the median time to relapse is only 3 years. Prolonged survival after relapse is a characteristic of this disease, as are late relapses. This has made study of the treatment of patients with follicular lymphoma difficult and led to controversy of the curability of this illness.

MALT (mucosa-associated lymphoid tissue) lymphoma

This lymphoma, also known as the extranodal marginal-zone B-cell lymphoma of MALT-type, always presents in extranodal sites. A nodal presentation of a similar lymphoma is referred to as nodal marginal-zone lymphoma or monocytoid B-cell lymphoma (see below). Before the recognition of the existence of MALT lymphomas, orbital, pulmonary, and gastric presentations were sometimes referred to by pathologists as pseudolymphoma. The differential diagnosis of MALT lymphoma includes benign lymphocytic infiltration of extranodal organs and other small-cell B-cell lymphomas.

MALT lymphomas are tumours of CD5– and CD23– B cells that express CD20. The commonly seen cytogenetic abnormalities include trisomy 3 and t(11;18). Gastric MALT lymphomas are associated with infection by *Helicobacter pylori.* Thyroid MALT lymphomas are frequently associated with Hashimoto's thyroiditis, and orbital MALT lymphomas are sometimes associated with Sjögren's syndrome. MALT lymphomas can undergo histological transformation to diffuse large B-cell lymphomas. After this transformation, the patient should be treated for diffuse large B-cell lymphoma.

MALT lymphomas have a slight female predominance with a median age at presentation of approximately 60 years. The symptoms of the disorder are those associated with involvement of the extranodal site. The disease is usually localized and the presence of systemic symptoms or elevated LDH is unusual. The characteristics of patients with this lymphoma are presented in Box 3.

Gastric MALT lymphomas are the first example of a lymphoma that can be treated by eliminating a chronic infection. If the tumour does not transform to a large-cell lymphoma, and has not deeply invaded the stomach, the majority of patients will have their tumour regress with the eradication of *Helicobacter pylori* using antibiotics, proton-pump inhibitors, and bismuth. It appears that in some patients this treatment might be curative. Other local therapies are also effective, and patients with MALT lymphomas can be treated with local radiotherapy or, in some cases, surgery if radiotherapy would be contraindicated. These lymphomas also respond to single-agent chemotherapy or combination chemotherapy. Patients with disseminated MALT lymphoma regularly respond to therapy, but are rarely curable.

The majority of patients with localized MALT lymphoma can be cured, and the 5-year survival in such patients is approximately 90 per cent. However, patients with disseminated disease have a more serious illness and those with a high International Prognostic Index score have a 5-year survival of only 40 per cent.

Small lymphocytic lymphoma/chronic lymphocytic leukaemia

Small lymphocytic lymphoma is the tissue manifestation of chronic lymphocytic leukaemia. Patients who present predominantly with blood and bone marrow involvement will have chronic lymphocytic leukaemia and those who present with lymphadenopathy will have small lymphocytic lymphoma. These are CD5+ B-cell lymphomas. Patients with plasmacytoid differentiation and monoclonal IgM protein in the serum can present the syndrome of Waldenström's macroglobulinaemia. Small lymphocytic lymphoma makes up approximately 7 per cent of non-Hodgkin's lymphomas worldwide, although it is more often seen in western countries.

The differential diagnosis of small lymphocytic lymphoma includes other small B-cell lymphomas. Patients with small lymphocytic lymphoma can undergo histological transformation to diffuse large B-cell lymphoma. This syndrome is seen in approximately 3 per cent of patients and is called Richter's syndrome. It is associated with a poor prognosis.

Chronic lymphocytic leukaemia/small lymphocytic lymphoma is a B-cell neoplasm that typically expresses CD20 and CD23. Approximately 30 per cent of cases have trisomy 12, but there is no specific chromosomal translocation associated with small lymphocytic lymphoma.

The clinical characteristics of patients with small lymphocytic lymphoma are presented in Box 4. Unusual immunological manifestations are sometimes seen, including hypogammaglobulinaemia, autoimmune thrombocytopenia, and autoimmune haemolytic anaemia. When present, these immune abnormalities should be specifically treated, in addition to any treatment given for the lymphoma. Hypogammaglobulinaemia should be treated with intermittent immunoglobulin interfusions and autoimmune cytopenias should be treated with prednisone and/or splenectomy.

Patients with small lymphocytic lymphoma can be followed with no initial therapy if they are symptomatic, but most patients will require treatment within the first few years. The two most popular treatments for small lymphocytic lymphoma/small lymphocytic leukaemia are single-agent oral chlorambucil and single-agent fludarabine. Fludarabine is associated with a higher complete response rate, but is somewhat more difficult to administer. Neither treatment is curative. Patients frequently respond to further treatment after relapse. Only a small proportion of patients are candidates for bone marrow transplantation. However, occasional patients seem to have a long-term, disease-free survival following allogeneic bone marrow transplantation.

Mantle-cell lymphoma

The clinical characteristics of patients with mantle-cell lymphoma are presented in Box 5. This lymphoma was recognized as a specific entity because of its characteristic cytogenetic abnormality. These tumours regularly express the t(11;14) that involves the *BCL-1* gene on chromosome 11 and the tumour cells overexpress the BCL-1 protein. This can be useful in diagnosis. Before the recognition of mantle-cell lymphoma, patients with this disorder were placed in many other histological categories. In the Kiel classification, mantle-cell lymphoma was usually called centrocytic lymphoma. An expert haematopathologist is important in making the diagnosis, since this lymphoma can be confused with small lymphocytic lymphoma, follicular lymphoma, and lymphoblastic lymphoma.

Extranodal sites of involvement by mantle-cell lymphoma are not unusual. Large bowel involvement with mantle-cell lymphoma presents as the syndrome of lymphomatous polyposis. Patients with distal gastrointestinal tract lymphoma often have Waldeyer's ring, and the converse is also true.

Mantle-cell lymphoma responds poorly to available therapies. Combination therapy regimens lead to a complete remission in less than 50 per cent of patients, and most complete responders relapse quickly. The median survival is 3 to 4 years and the 5-year survival for all patients is approximately 25 per cent. Patients who present with a high International Prognostic

Box 3 MALT lymphoma

Median age	60 years
Percentage male	48%
Stage: I	0%
IE	39%
II	0%
IIE	28%
III	2%
IV	31%
B-symptoms	19%
Elevated LDH	27%
Reduced performance status	15%
Tumour mass >10 cm	8%
Bone marrow involvement	14%
Gastrointestinal tract involvement	50%
International prognostic index score	
0–1	44%
2–3	48%
4–5	8%

Survival and disease-free survival

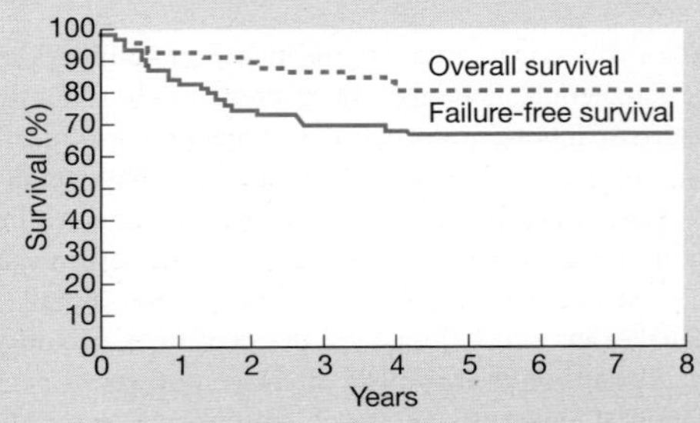

Box 4 Small lymphocytic lymphoma

Median age	65 years
Percentage male	53%
Stage: I	4%
IE	0%
II	2%
IIE	3%
III	8%
IV	83%
B-symptoms	33%
Elevated LDH	41%
Reduced performance status	11%
Tumour mass >10 cm	13%
Bone marrow involvement	72%
Gastrointestinal tract involvement	3%
International prognostic index score	
0–1	23%
2–3	64%
4–5	13%

Survival and disease-free survival

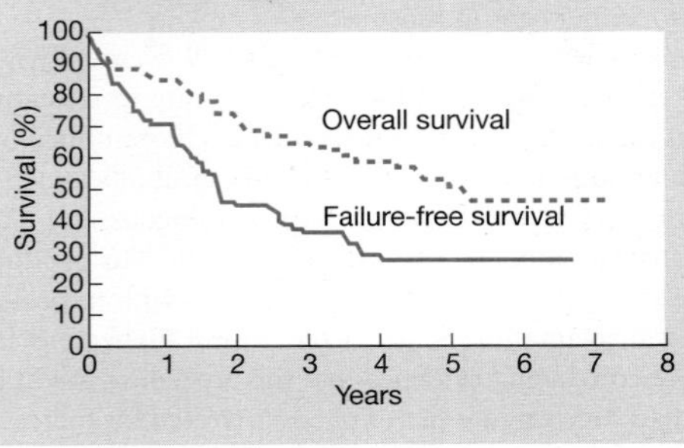

Index score rarely survive 5 years. Because of the poor outlook, autologous and allogeneic bone marrow transplantation have been increasingly utilized in younger patients.

Less common B-cell lymphomas

Burkitt's lymphoma was originally described by Dennis Burkitt while studying an aggressive lymphoma that occurred in the jaw of children in Central Africa. An association has been demonstrated between infection by the Epstein–Barr virus and this lymphoma. It is much more frequent in children than in adults and in patients infected by HIV. This very rapidly progressive lymphoma is associated with specific chromosomal translocations involving the heavy chain immunoglobulin gene on chromosome 14 or the light chain immunoglobulin genes on chromosomes 2 and 22. In each case, the associated oncogene is the *c-myc* gene on chromosome 8 (namely, t(8;14), t(2;8), and t(8;22)). Burkitt's lymphoma can present as acute leukaemia. This lymphoma can frequently be cured utilizing short courses of very intensive regimens that incorporate high doses of cyclophosphamide.

Nodal marginal-zone lymphoma or monocytoid B-cell lymphoma is immunologically related to MALT lymphoma (see above), but presents in a manner similar to follicular lymphoma. These patients respond to therapy and have an overall survival similar to those with follicular lymphoma. Splenic marginal-zone lymphoma is a rare disorder also known as splenic lymphoma with villous lymphocytes. This rare and indolent lymphoma often responds to splenectomy.

Primary, mediastinal, diffuse large B-cell lymphoma varies from other diffuse large B-cell lymphomas in that it occurs at a younger age and has a striking female predominance. However, the treatment and response to therapy are similar to other diffuse large B-cell lymphomas.

Lymphoplasmacytic lymphoma is a subtype of small lymphocytic lymphoma, which is a tissue manifestation of Waldenström's macroglobulinaemia.

Box 5 Mantle cell lymphoma

Median age		63 years
Percentage male		74%
Stage:	I	10%
	IE	3%
	II	6%
	IIE	1%
	III	9%
	IV	71%
B-symptoms		28%
Elevated LDH		40%
Reduced performance status		21%
Tumour mass >10 cm		81%
Bone marrow involvement		64%
Gastrointestinal tract involvement		9%
International prognostic index score		
	0–1	23%
	2–3	54%
	4–5	23%

Survival and disease-free survival

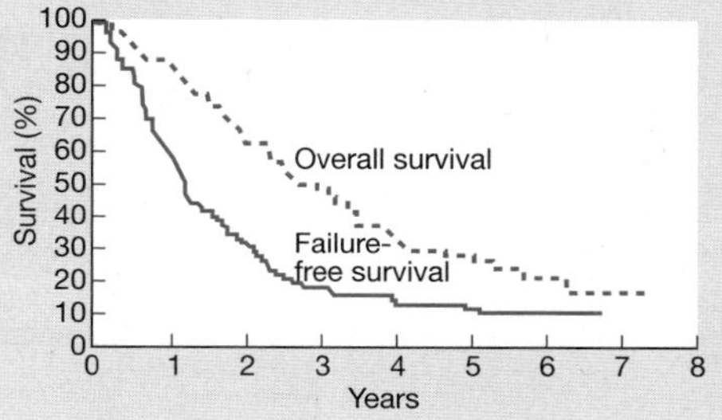

Peripheral T-cell lymphoma

The illnesses classified together as 'peripheral T-cell lymphoma, unspecified type', are a heterogeneous group of non-Hodgkin's lymphomas. The accurate diagnosis of peripheral T-cell lymphoma involves the review of adequate histological material by an expert haematopathologist who has tissue available for immunophenotyping. The diagnosis cannot be made accurately in the absence of immunophenotyping. These tumours are generally CD3- and CD4-positive, although a few will be CD8-positive. Some display CD57 and an NK-cell immunophenotype. Cytogenetic abnormalities are frequent, but there is no consistent genetic abnormality. In occasional cases, demonstrating a T-cell receptor gene rearrangement will help to resolve a difficult diagnostic dilemma and confirm the diagnosis. The differential diagnosis of peripheral T-cell lymphoma includes diffuse large B-cell lymphoma and T-cell hyperplasia as seen in viral infection and drug reactions.

The clinical characteristics of patients with peripheral T-cell lymphoma are presented in Box 6. There are a number of distinctive clinical syndromes grouped together in the category of peripheral T-cell lymphoma. These include the angiocentric nasal NK-cell lymphoma that typically presents with necrotic nasal or facial lesions. Angioimmunoblastic T-cell lymphoma includes most patients who before would have been classed as having angioimmunoblastic lymphadenopathy with dysproteinaemia. These patients present with widespread disease, systemic system disease, skin rash, and polyclonal hypergammaglobulinaemia. Enteropathy-type intestinal T-cell lymphoma is a rare disorder that occurs in patients with gluten-sensitive enteropathy. Patients are frequently wasted and sometimes present with intestinal perforation. Hepatosplenic γ,δ T-cell lymphoma presents as a systemic illness with sinusoidal infiltration of the liver, spleen, and bone marrow by malignant T cells. Subcutaneous panniculitis-like T-cell lymphoma is a rare disorder that presents with subcutaneous nodules, which are often confused with panniculitis on biopsy. All subtypes of peripheral T-cell lymphoma have a poor prognosis.

The treatment for patients with peripheral T-cell lymphoma involves the same regimens utilized for diffuse large B-cell lymphoma. Unfortunately, the overall 5-year survival is only 25 per cent and patients with a high International Prognostic Index score have a particularly poor outlook. Bone marrow transplantation can cure some patients who fail primary therapy, and this has been included in the initial treatment of patients with poor prognosis.

Anaplastic large T/null-cell lymphoma

Patients with this lymphoma were previously often diagnosed as having undifferentiated carcinoma, undifferentiated malignant neoplasm, or malignant histiocytosis. Discovery of the Ki-1 antigen (i.e. CD30) led to the recognition that some patients with anaplastic malignancies actually had non-Hodgkin's lymphoma. Subsequent discovery of the t(2;5) and the resultant overexpression of the ALK protein led to the confirmation of anaplastic large T/null-cell lymphoma as a specific entity. In some patients, the B-cell lymphoma has an anaplastic appearance, but these patients have the same outcome as others with diffuse large B-cell lymphoma.

The clinical characteristics of patients with anaplastic large T/null-cell lymphoma are presented in Box 7. The diagnosis can be made confidently by an expert haematopathologist when facilities for immunophenotyping and staining for the ALK protein are available. The median age of patients with anaplastic T/null-cell lymphoma is approximately 30 years, and 70 per cent of the patients are male. Half the patients have localized (stage I/II) and half have disseminated (stage III/IV) disease. Systemic symptoms are present in 50 per cent of patients and a similar proportion have an elevated LDH level. Occasional patients present with localized disease in the skin and probably have a different and somewhat more indolent disorder.

Despite the anaplastic appearance of the lymphoma and frequent poor prognostic characteristics, patients with anaplastic large T/null-cell lymphoma respond well to therapy. The 5-year survival is approximately 75 per cent, and this lymphoma has one of the highest cure rates from combination chemotherapy of any non-Hodgkin's lymphoma. Patients relapsing can respond favourably to bone marrow transplantation.

Mycosis fungoides/Sezary syndrome

Mycosis fungoides or cutaneous T-cell lymphoma is an indolent lymphoma of mature T cells predominantly involving the skin. Patients who present with circulating, atypical (that is, Sezary) cells and erythroderma are said to have Sezary syndrome. The median age is approximately 50 years and the disease is more common in males and Blacks.

Mycosis fungoides often presents with eczematous or dermatitic skin lesions for many years before the diagnosis is firmly established. Frequently, patients will have several biopsies before the diagnosis is confirmed. Lymphoma first manifests itself as superficial lesions in the skin that thicken and eventually ulcerate. In the late stages of the illness, lymphoma can metastasize to lymph nodes and visceral organs.

Treatments utilized for mycosis fungoides include topical corticosteroids, topical nitrogen mustard, phototherapy, **PUVA** (psoralen ultraviolet A-range) therapy, electron-beam radiation, interferon, and systemic cytotoxic therapy. Some patients with localized mycosis fungoides can be cured with radiotherapy. However, the majority of patients will progress. In the end stages of this disease, management is difficult and the ulcerating cutaneous lesions present unpleasant problems for both the patient and the physician. The median survival from diagnosis averages over 10 years.

Adult T-cell lymphoma/leukaemia

The two major manifestations of infection by the human T-cell lymphoma/leukaemia virus-1 (HTLV-1) are tropical spastic paraparesis and adult T-cell lymphoma/leukaemia. Patients can be infected with HTLV-1 through sexual transmission, blood transmission, and transplacentally. The risk of developing lymphoma in a patient infected with HTLV-1 is between 1 and 7 per cent according to various studies. The latency between infection and the development of lymphoma averages approximately 20 years. The diagnosis is established by review of an adequate biopsy by an expert haematopathologist, demonstration of a T-cell immunophenotype, and demonstration of antibodies to HTLV-1. Most patients will have circulating tumour cells with a characteristic pleomorphic histology.

Adult T-cell lymphoma/leukaemia is most frequently seen in the southern islands of Japan and the Caribbean. Most patients seen in Europe and North America will be immigrants from those regions. Blood transfusion

Box 6 Peripheral T-cell lymphoma

Median age	63 years
Percentage male	55%
Stage: I	10%
IE	7%
II	6%
IIE	6%
III	15%
IV	65%
B-symptoms	50%
Elevated LDH	64%
Reduced performance status	32%
Tumour mass >10 cm	12%
Bone marrow involvement	36%
Gastrointestinal tract involvement	15%
International prognostic index score	
0–1	17%
2–3	52%
4–5	31%

Survival and disease-free survival

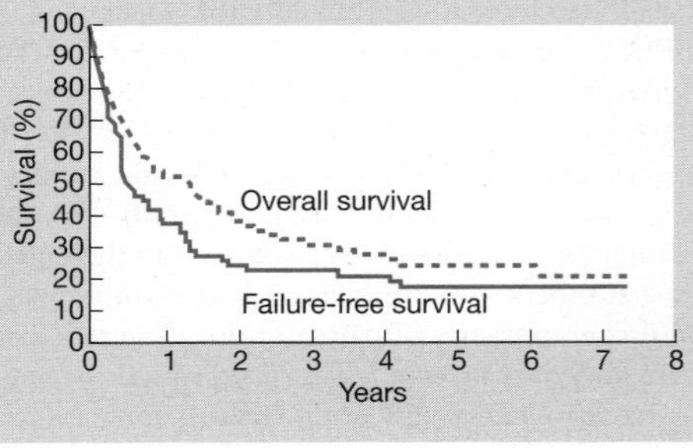

Box 7 Anaplastic large T/null cell lymphoma

Median age	34 years
Percentage male	69%
Stage: I	16%
IE	3%
II	22%
IIE	10%
III	10%
IV	39%
B-symptoms	53%
Elevated LDH	45%
Reduced performance status	26%
Tumour mass >10 cm	17%
Bone marrow involvement	13%
Gastrointestinal tract involvement	9%
International prognostic index score	
0–1	61%
2–3	18%
4–5	21%

Survival and disease-free survival

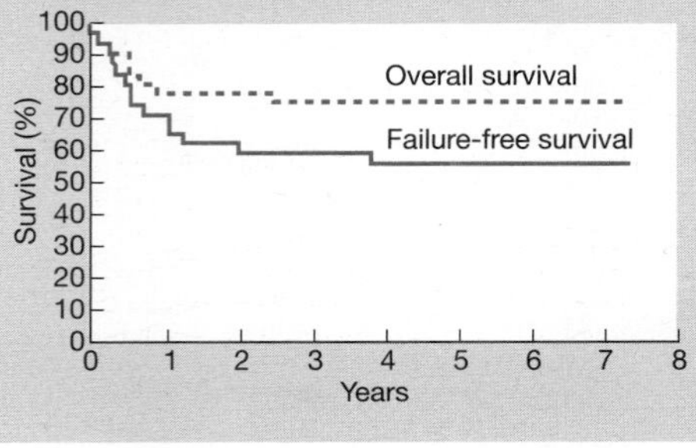

provides a possible source for infection, but screening for HTLV-1 has reduced the risk.

The clinical characteristics of patients with adult T-cell lymphoma/leukaemia vary considerably. Some patients present with an indolent disease manifested by lymphadenopathy and skin lesions and survive for extended times without specific therapy. Others present with progressive lymphadenopathy, hepatosplenomegaly, skin infiltration, hypercalcaemia, lytic bone lesions, and elevated LDH levels. Although patients sometimes respond to combination-chemotherapy regimens, complete remissions are unusual and survival is poor.

Lymphoma-like disorders (see Chapter 22.4.2)

Lymphadenopathy caused by infectious mononucleosis, drug reactions to diphenylhydantoin or carbamazepine, autoimmune disorders such as rheumatoid arthritis and lupus erythematosus, and bacterial infections such as cat-scratch disease can all be confused on biopsy with lymphoma. Castleman's disease is a specific condition that can present with localized or disseminated lymphadenopathy and systemic symptoms. The disease appears to be related to an overproduction of interleukin-6. The disseminated form of Castleman's disease is frequently accompanied by anaemia and polyclonal hypergammaglobulinaemia. Patients with localized disease can frequently be treated with local therapy, while systemic disease sometimes responds to systemic glucocorticoids. Sinus histiocytosis with massive lymphadenopathy (Rosai–Dorfman's disease) typically presents with bulky lymphadenopathy in children or young adults. The disease is usually non-progressive and self-limited. Lymphomatoid papulosis is a cutaneous lymphoproliferative disorder that can be confused with T-cell lymphoma in the skin. The cells in lymphomatoid papulosis stain for CD30 and sometimes have a monoclonal T-cell receptor gene rearrangement. The condition is characterized by waxing and waning skin lesions that usually heal leaving small scars. Although these patients have an increased risk of developing lymphoma, aggressive therapy is inappropriate.

Further reading

Armitage JO, Weisenburg ER for the Non-Hodgkin's Lymphoma Classification Project (1998). New approach to classifying non-Hodgkin's lymphomas: clinical features of the major histologic subtypes. *Journal of Clinical Oncology* **16**, 2780–95.

Cheson BD, *et al.* (1999). Report of an. International Workshop to Standardize Response Criteria for non-Hodgkin's lymphomas. *Journal of Clinical Oncology* **17**, 1244–53.

Diehl V, Josting A (2000). Hodgkin's disease. *Cancer Journal* **6** (suppl.2), S150–S158.

Foon KA (2000). Monoclonal antibodies in the treatment of lymphomas for the year 2000. *Principles and Practice of Oncology Updates* **14**, 1.

Godwin JE, Fisher KC (2001). Diffuse large-cell lymphomas; a review of therapy. *Clinical Lymphoma* **2**,155–63.

Jaffe ES *et al.*, eds (2001). *World Health Organization classification of tumours, pathology and genetics of tumours of haematopoietic and lymphoid tissues.* IARC Press, Lyon.

Mauch P *et al.*, eds (1999). *Hodgkin's disease.* Lippincott Williams & Wilkins, Philadelphia, PA.

Ruzich J, Fisher RJ (2000). MALT lymphoma. *Clinical Oncology Updates* **3**, 1–7.

The International Non-Hodgkin's Lymphoma Prognostic Factors Project (1993). A predictive model for aggressive non-Hodgkin's lymphoma. *New England Journal of Medicine* **329**, 987–94.

Winter JN (1999). High-dose therapy with stem-cell transplantation in the malignant lymphomas. *Oncology,* 1635.

22.4.4 The spleen and its disorders

D. Swirsky

Since Hippocratic times the role of the spleen has been controversial. Galen called it an organ of mystery. Its structure was described during the seventeenth and early eighteenth centuries by Harvey, Glisson, Wharton, Malpighi, and van Leeuwenhoek. In 1777 William Hewson recognized an association with the lymphatic system, and in 1846 Virchow demonstrated that the Malpighian follicles are associated with the formation of white blood cells. In 1885 Ponfick showed that the spleen can remove particles from the blood and might be involved in the destruction of blood cells. Two years later Spencer Wells performed a laparotomy on a 27-year-old woman with a lifelong history of passing dark urine with attacks of jaundice and who had an abdominal tumour thought to be a fibroid. This turned out to be a large spleen and its removal was followed by a complete remission. The retrospective diagnosis of hereditary spherocytosis was made by Lord Dawson of Penn some 40 years later, by which time splenectomy was being performed quite frequently for the treatment of leukaemia, Hodgkin's disease, Banti's haemolytic jaundice, Gaucher's disease, polycythaemia, and thrombocytopenic purpura. The frequent success of the operation led Doan and Dameshek to engage in a lively argument on the mechanisms by which the spleen might destroy blood cells or suppress their formation, a process which Chauffard had earlier called 'hypersplenism'.

There is now a greater understanding of the splenic function in health and of the spleen's involvement in disease. Methods have been developed by which the various functions of the spleen can be defined and measured, sometimes with important clinical application.

Structure of the spleen

At birth the spleen has a mean weight of 11 g. By the age of 1 year the weight is 15 to 25 g; by 5 years it is 40 to 70 g, and by 10 years it is 80 to 100 g. It reaches a maximum weight of 200 to 300 g soon after puberty, and is slightly lighter throughout adult life until the age of about 65 years, when it decreases to 100 to 150 g or less. These figures have been derived from autopsy studies and are probably underestimates. This is mainly due to the splenic red cell pool which will be described later. Ultrasound, computed tomography (**CT**), magnetic resonance imaging (**MRI**) scans and scintigraphic radionuclide scans have shown that, *in vivo,* the normal adult spleen has a length of 8 to 13 cm, a width of 4.5 to 7 cm, a surface area of the order of 45 to 80 cm^2, and a volume less than 275 cm^3. A spleen greater than 14 cm long is usually palpable.

The spleen has a complicated structure (Fig. 1). It consists of a connective tissue framework, vascular channels, lymphatic tissue, lymph drainage channels, and cellular components of the haemopoietic and mononuclear phagocyte systems. There are two main components: (1) the red pulp; and (2) the white pulp. The red pulp consists of sinuses and pulp cords. The sinuses, 20 to 40 μm in diameter, are lined by endothelial macrophages. The white pulp consists of a periarteriolar lymphoid sheath and the adjoining lymphoid follicles (Malpighian bodies), which contain a germinal centre and are structurally similar to lymphoid follicles. From the capsule many lace-like trabeculae extend into the pulp, carrying blood vessels and autonomic nerve fibres. Within the spleen the trabeculae are in direct continuity with a mesh of reticular fibres that supports the pulp vessels and forms the basement membranes of arterial capillaries and the splenic sinuses. Along the reticular fibres lie adventitial reticular cells. These cells have an important role in regulating blood flow through the interendothelial slits of the vascular sinuses.

Blood is supplied by the splenic artery and passes through the trabecular arteries, into the central arteries, which are sited in the white pulp. The

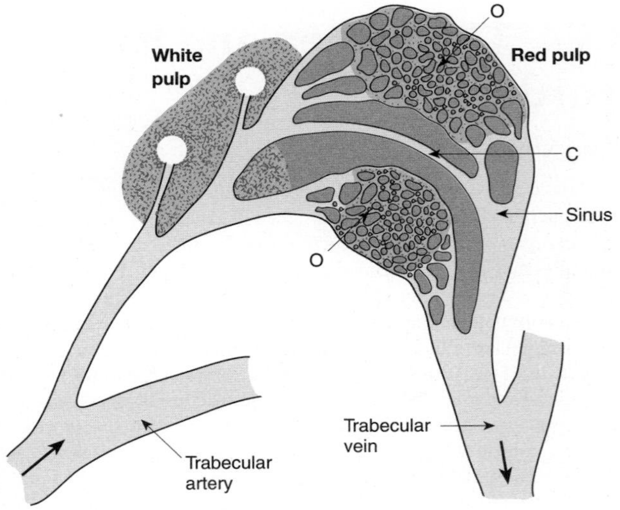

Fig. 1 Diagrammatic illustration of the spleen. The blood passes either directly into a sinus (C, closed system) or first into the cord space in the red pulp (O, open system).

central arteries run into the central axis of the periarteriolar lymphatic sheaths; they give off many arterioles and capillaries, some of which terminate in the white pulp whilst others go on to the red pulp. There they either connect directly with the sinuses and thence, via the collecting vein, to the trabecular vein (closed system), or they first pass into the cord spaces before joining up with the sinuses (open system).

Thus, as blood flows through the spleen it will come into contact with the reticular fibres, and also with endothelial macrophages, which line the interstices of the reticular mesh.

Blood flow in the spleen

Because the spleen has two vascular systems (open and closed) as described above, there are both rapid- and slow-transit components in the splenic circulation. The rapid transit (closed system) is of the order of 1 to 2 min and the slow transit (open system) about 30 to 60 min. In normal subjects the open system has a minor role and the blood flows through the spleen as rapidly as through organs possessing a conventional vasculature, at a rate of 5 to 10 per cent of the blood volume per minute, so that each day the circulating blood has repeated passages through the spleen. When the spleen is enlarged, blood flow increases up to 20 per cent or more of the blood volume per minute. At the same time, a proportion of the blood may be pooled in the cord spaces (see below). As blood traverses the spleen, the plasma and leucocytes pass preferentially to the white pulp by a process of plasma skimming, and the plasma rapidly reaches the venous system, whilst blood with a relatively high packed-cell volume remains in the axial stream of the central artery. Some of this blood flows directly through the sinusoids to the venous system, while the remainder passes into the cords of the red pulp. The normally flexible red cells squeeze through the endothelial slits into the sinuses, whilst inflexible cells with fixed membranes or with inclusions remain in the cords where they either become conditioned for later transit or are destroyed.

Functions of the spleen

Haemopoiesis

In the fetus and compared with the liver, the spleen is a minor haemopoietic organ. There is, however, some erythropoiesis and granulopoiesis in the spleen from the 12th week of gestation; this continues until birth, after which there is normally no demonstrable haemopoiesis. However, the potential remains, and under severe haematological stress, in thalassaemia and in chronic haemolytic anaemias for example, extramedullary haemopoiesis may occur together with intense erythroid hyperplasia of the bone marrow. This must be distinguished from myeloid metaplasia occurring in myelofibrosis, chronic myeloid leukaemia, and occasionally other leukaemias and secondary carcinomas. In these conditions, foci of haemopoietic tissue become established in the spleen and elsewhere outside the bone marrow. They represent an abnormal proliferation which is distinct from compensatory haemopoiesis.

Cell sequestration, phagocytosis, and pooling

The spleen has a remarkable ability to 'cleanse' or 'recondition' red cells for recirculation and also to remove from the circulation effete or damaged cells as well as foreign matter. Of particular importance is the trapping of encapsulated bloodborne bacteria. It is important to distinguish between the three mechanisms involved. Sequestration is a temporary (reversible) process whereby cells are held in the spleen before returning to the circulation; phagocytosis represents the irreversible uptake of non-viable cells by macrophages, or the destruction of viable cells that have been damaged; pooling is the presence in the spleen of an increased amount of blood (or some of its component parts). In contrast to sequestration, pooled cells are in continuous exchange with the circulation.

As blood flows through the sinuses and cords, effete and damaged cells, and particulate foreign matter, are promptly phagocytosed by the endothelial macrophages. Intact red cells are held up temporarily, during which time siderotic granules, Howell–Jolly bodies, and Heinz bodies are removed. After the inclusions have been removed the red cells return to the circulation. Sequestration of reticulocytes also occurs, and they are retained in the splenic cords for part of their last 2 or 3 days of maturation while they lose their intracellular inclusions, alter their surface membrane composition, and become smaller. The spleen normally sequesters 30 to 45 per cent of the total circulating platelet content of the blood. This platelet pool is rapidly mobilized under conditions of stress, and normally there is a constant transit between the spleen and vascular pools.

As the blood becomes more viscous in the spleen, red cells are subjected to a further hazard. Because they are packed together in the presence of metabolically active macrophages, they are depleted of glucose and oxygen. This increases their membrane rigidity and reduces their deformability. Cells may become inflexible if: (1) they are metabolically abnormal (as in some congenital haemolytic anaemias) and thus unduly sensitive to the unfavourable environment of the spleen; (2) if they are held up in the spleen for a prolonged period and are thus rendered metabolically abnormal; and (3) if they are already spherical (as in hereditary spherocytosis), fragmented (as in microangiopathic haemolytic anaemia), or misshapen in some other way. This results in their being trapped in the cord spaces where they subsequently undergo phagocytosis.

Immune function

The spleen contains the largest single accumulation of lymphoid tissue in the body; about 25 per cent of the total T-lymphocyte pool and 10 to 15 per cent of the B-lymphocyte pool, with very marked exchange between circulating and splenic lymphocytes. Splenic macrophages are instrumental in antigen presentation to lymphocytes. The spleen is a major, but not unique, site for the conversion of naive circulating B cells into plasma cells which migrate to the bone marrow and into long-lived memory cells.

Micro-organisms or other antigens that find their way to the spleen are taken up and processed by cord macrophages and are presented to immunocompetent cells in the lymphoid tissue. This stimulates antibody production and an increase in size of the lymphoid germinal centres of the spleen. Secondary stimulation with the antigen enhances antibody production, usually IgG.

Antibody-coated red cells lose pieces of their membrane as they come in contact with the Fc receptors on macrophages, and become spherical and less flexible each time they pass through the sinus vasculature, until finally they become too rigid to traverse the endothelial pores and are trapped and destroyed. Red cells sensitized by IgG do not, as a rule, agglutinate in the peripheral blood, but the environment in the spleen promotes local agglutination with consequent sequestration and destruction (autoimmune haemolysis). Antibody-coated neutrophils and platelets are similarly destroyed by splenic macrophages.

Blood pool

The normal red cell content of the spleen is less than 80 ml of red cells, and always less than 5 per cent of the total red cell mass. There is no significant red cell pool in human spleens. However, enlarged spleens are capable of developing remarkably large pools with a relatively slow exchange of red cells with the general circulation. In the myeloproliferative disorders, as much as 40 per cent of the blood volume may be present in the spleen. Increased pools also occur in lymphoproliferative disorders, especially hairy-cell leukaemia and prolymphocytic leukaemia.

In health there is a good correlation between the amount of blood in the spleen and its size. In lymphomas, however, the splenomegaly is greater than can be accounted for by the pool alone; in such cases the increase in spleen size is due primarily to an expansion of the lymphoid components with replacement of splenic sinuses by tumour. In myelofibrosis there is an increase in the reticular element with expansion of the closed system in the red pulp. A similar effect occurs in hairy-cell leukaemia.

Not unexpectedly, the red cell content of the spleen increases with increasing body haematocrit. There is a disproportionately increased pool in primary proliferative polycythaemia compared with secondary polycythaemia, where the pool remains small irrespective of the haematocrit level. Increased pools are also found in patients with hepatic cirrhosis. Here it is the increased portal pressure that leads to an increased splenic blood flow: the splenic arteries are dilated and the splenic pulp becomes expanded with prominent dilated sinuses. Portal hypertension may result from myeloproliferative disorders associated with splenomegaly.

In myeloproliferative disorders and some other conditions an enlarged splenic blood pool may contribute significantly to anaemia. A low venous haematocrit can be present despite a normal red cell mass (pseudoanaemia). Direct measurement of the splenic red cell volume makes it possible to predict the extent to which splenectomy will improve anaemia and reduce transfusion requirements.

There is also a significant reservoir of platelets in the spleen, which is rapidly interchangeable with the circulation. In some cases of thrombocytopenia, destruction occurs mainly in the spleen and it is essential to distinguish this from pooling. As far as granulocytes are concerned, no pool is demonstrable in the normal spleen, but an abnormally large marginal pool has been found in cases of splenomegaly associated with neutropenia.

Plasma volume

Splenomegaly is frequently associated with an increased plasma volume, which may lead to an apparent anaemia (pseudoanaemia or dilutional anaemia), when a reduced venous haematocrit is the result of an expanded plasma volume in the presence of a normal or slightly reduced red cell mass.

Splenomegaly

A palpable spleen is usually enlarged. Occasionally a normal spleen is palpable if it is displaced downwards, by a pleural effusion for example. The spleen has to be 1.5 to 2 times its normal size to be palpable. Ultrasound, CT, and MRI provide reliable methods for measuring the actual spleen size.

Investigation of splenomegaly

The clinical history should include a relevant travel history (for example, to tropical areas) and family history (for example, Gaucher's disease, hereditary spherocytosis). Physical examination should specifically include assessment for hepatomegaly and lymphadenopathy. Laboratory investigations should include a full blood count, liver function tests and hepatitis serology, serum protein electrophoresis, total cholesterol, triglyceride and lipoprotein determinations, as well as immunoglobulin measurements. A bone marrow aspirate and trephine biopsy, and/or lymph node biopsy, with appropriate cytogenetic and immunophenotyping studies, should be done as indicated. These investigations will reveal the diagnosis in most haematological disorders and many chronic infections. CT or ultrasound scanning, with liver biopsy as required, will reveal hepatic or thrombotic causes of portal hypertension. HIV serology should always be done in puzzling cases of splenomegaly; in patients of Ashkenazi Jewish ancestry, Gaucher's disease or Niemann–Pick disease may be reasonably excluded by determining lysosomal hydrolase activity in leucocytes. If all investigations are negative, diagnostic splenectomy may be necessary, and in non-tropical areas the diagnosis will usually be non-Hodgkin's lymphoma or Hodgkin's disease.

Causes of splenomegaly

So many conditions are associated with splenomegaly that it is impossible to give a comprehensive list. It is even more difficult to list the 'common' causes as these depend on geographical pathology. In Western Europe and the United States viral infections and portal hypertension are the most common causes of splenomegaly, and these together with leukaemias, malignant lymphomas, myeloproliferative disorders, haemolytic anaemias, and other infections account for most cases. Isolated splenomegaly is a common manifestation of type I Gaucher's disease. Globally, however, the incidence of these haematological causes of splenomegaly is swamped by the great preponderance of splenic enlargement caused by parasitic infections, particularly malaria, leishmaniasis, and schistosomiasis. Human immunodeficiency virus (**HIV**) infection, particularly in the later stages of the disease, is an increasing cause of mild to moderate splenomegaly. Haemoglobinopathies head the list in some countries. Portal hypertension is an important cause of splenomegaly in most tropical countries but it is especially prevalent in north-eastern India and southern China. The 'tropical splenomegaly syndrome' associated with malaria is seen commonly in New Guinea and Central Africa.

Some of the causes of splenomegaly are listed in Table 1. The conditions which commonly give rise to massive splenomegaly are marked with an asterisk. The spleen sizes indicated are only a rough guide. Most of the conditions listed are described in other chapters.

Hypersplenism

Hypersplenism is a clinical syndrome of varied aetiology. It is characterized by:

1. Splenomegaly, although this may only be moderate.
2. Cytopenias: pancytopenia, single cytopenias, or any combination of anaemia, neutropenia, and thrombocytopenia.
3. A cellular or hypercellular bone marrow, sometimes showing a paucity of mature granulocytes.
4. A premature release of cells into the peripheral blood, resulting in a mild reticulocytosis with nucleated red cells and occasional immature granulocytes.

Other features are:

(1) decreased red cell survival;

(2) decreased platelet survival;

(3) hypervolaemia (that is, increased plasma volume) if splenomegaly is marked.

The haematological features may be obscured or dominated by the primary disease, especially if it involves the marrow. The diagnosis of hypersplenism is ultimately confirmed by the response to treatment of the underlying cause or of splenectomy, although an immediate remission may be followed in the longer term by relapse with a return of cytopenia.

Tropical splenomegaly syndrome 'big spleen disease'

In areas where malaria is endemic, adults may present with moderate to massive splenomegaly, no obvious signs of active malaria, but all the features of hypersplenism including pancytopenia, expanded plasma volume, and haemolysis. The serum IgM level is usually high, and malarial antibody titres are raised. The spleen shows diffuse proliferation of macrophages. The relationship to malaria is evident by the response to long-term antimalarial treatment, which produces a sustained reduction in spleen size and reversal of the cytopenias. It is unclear why this effect is only seen in a proportion of individuals in areas of the world where malaria is endemic.

A similar degree of splenomegaly occurs in schistosomiasis (see Chapter 7.16.1). However, in this condition there is the further complication that the eggs (especially of *Schistosoma mansoni*) have a direct effect on the liver, resulting in hepatic fibrosis and leading to portal hypertension, which may be further exacerbated by splenic vein thrombosis.

Table 1 Some causes of enlargement of the spleen

Acute viral and bacterial infections
Chronic bacterial infections: mycobacterial and brucellosis
Chronic parasitic infections: malaria, kala azar, schistosomiasis*
Histoplasmosis
Idiopathic non-tropical splenomegaly*
Tropical splenomegaly*
'Congestive': portal and biliary cirrhosis, portal vein obstruction, splenic vein obstruction, Budd–Chiari syndrome, cardiac failure
Inherited haemolytic anaemias
Hereditary spherocytosis
Haemolytic hereditary elliptocytosis
Structural haemoglobinopathies
Thalassaemia major and intermedia
Red-cell enzyme defects
Acquired haemolytic anaemias
Warm-antibody immune haemolytic anaemia
Cold-agglutinin disease
Primary blood disorders
Chronic myeloid leukaemia*
Chronic lymphocytic leukaemia*
Prolymphocytic leukaemia*
Hairy-cell leukaemia*
Acute leukaemia
Myelofibrosis*
Polycythaemia vera
Megaloblastic anaemia
Malignant lymphoma
Hodgkin's disease
Non-Hodgkin's lymphoma
HIV infection
Acute seroconversion
Advancing disease, pre-AIDS
AIDS
AIDS-related lymphoma
AIDS-related opportunistic infection
Connective tissue disorders
Systemic lupus erythematosis
Felty's syndrome
Miscellaneous
Amyloid
Sarcoidosis
Castleman's disease
Storage diseases*
Cysts
Haemangiomas
Littoral-cell angioma

* May be associated with massive splenomegaly.

Non-tropical idiopathic splenomegaly

Rare patients present with marked splenomegaly and the haematological features of hypersplenism but without exposure to malaria or other parasitic disorders. There may be a positive antiglobulin test and other evidence of autoantibody production. Some of these patients have a malignant lymphoma at the time of presentation, but in others the essential feature is non-neoplastic lymphoid hyperplasia, which probably represents an immunological reaction to as yet unidentified stimuli. The chances of long-term cure after splenectomy appear to be good. However, a lymphoma may appear from months to years after splenectomy. The disorder is diagnosed by the finding of massive splenomegaly in the absence of any other cause and by the non-specific histological appearances in the spleen.

Storage disease

The storage diseases are described in detail in Section 11.7. Some of them, notably Gaucher's disease and Niemann–Pick disease, may be complicated by marked splenomegaly. This may lead to hypersplenism, particularly in Gaucher's disease. The advent of specific enzyme therapy for Gaucher's disease has largely removed the need to consider splenectomy. The clinical picture of Niemann–Pick disease is dominated by hepatosplenomegaly and mental retardation. The disorder presents in infancy, and death often occurs between the second and third years of age, but, as with Gaucher's disease, it may present later in life. Hypersplenism becomes a feature in the older age groups, but anaemia and thrombocytopenia are uncommon in the childhood cases, and, if present, are mild. Several other lipid storage diseases may cause hypersplenism. They include Tangier's disease, in which cholesterol esters fill the histiocytes, and Wolman's disease, which is associated with an accumulation of triglycerides and cholesterol esters. Sea-blue histiocytosis is characterized by splenomegaly, hepatomegaly, thrombocytopenia, and, occasionally, neurological damage. The bone marrow and spleen contain cells that have an accumulation of glycosphingolipids, phospholipids, and mucopolysaccharides.

Rarely, Histiocytosis X (including Hand–Schuller–Christian disease, eosinophilic granuloma, Letterer–Siwe disease, and Langerhans' cell histiocytosis) cause splenomegaly. This is usually moderate, but occasionally it is more marked and may be associated with hypersplenism.

Space-occupying lesions and injury of the spleen

The most common causes of splenic masses are trauma leading to haematoma or rupture, abscesses, tumours, and cysts.

Splenic injury

The spleen is relatively unprotected and easily injured. Spontaneous rupture has been reported in a number of conditions in which the spleen is enlarged: these include typhoid, malaria, Epstein–Barr virus infection, leukaemia, Gaucher's disease, and polycythaemia. This may be restricted to a subcapsular haematoma or there may be rupture into the peritoneal cavity.

The diagnosis is suggested by the symptoms of shock, left upper quadrant tenderness, guarding, pain referred to the left shoulder, and clinical and laboratory evidence of bleeding. Plain abdominal radiography is not, as a rule, helpful in diagnosis but CT scanning, ultrasound examination, and splenic arteriography are more useful.

Abscess

Although the spleen is frequently enlarged in association with systemic infection, splenic abscesses are rare. They result from direct or haematogenous spread, or when a haematoma becomes infected. Conditions associated with splenic infarction, such as sickle-cell disease, are particularly likely to give rise to splenic abscesses. Almost any organism can be involved.

Tumours

The spleen may be affected by benign tumours such as hamartomas. The very rare littoral-cell angioma is the only tumour confined to the spleen. Metastases in the spleen are uncommon by comparison to other organs, possibly because the spleen, unlike lymph nodes, lacks an afferent lymphatic system. They occur late in the course of carcinoma and are not found in the absence of metastases elsewhere. Metastases in the spleen are most frequently derived from malignant lymphomas, especially Hodgkin's disease. Lung, breast, prostate, colon, and stomach are the primary sites from which carcinoma is most likely to disseminate to the spleen. Melanoma is also a relatively frequent primary source.

Cysts

Splenic cysts are rare. The most frequent cause is *Echinococcus granulosum* (hydatid); other causes include haemangiomas, lymphangiomas, and dermoids. Cysts may also develop in areas of haemorrhage or infarction.

Loss of spleen function and splenic infarction

Splenic hypoplasia or atrophy

Congenital hypoplasia is rare; in some cases it is associated with extensive developmental abnormalities of the heart and gut. Splenic atrophy may occur in a number of conditions—sickle-cell disease, coeliac disease, dermatitis herpetiformis, ulcerative colitis, Crohn's disease, amyloidosis, selective IgA deficiency, and Fanconi's anaemia. There is evidence of reduced splenic reticuloendothelial function in alcoholics. The spleen shrinks in size in old age. Vascular blockade and repeated infarction is the basis for splenic atrophy in sickle-cell disease, and occurs in early childhood. The peripheral blood changes of hyposplenism, when present, are proportional to disease activity in gut diseases. In coeliac disease, withdrawal of gluten from the diet reverses the changes unless splenic atrophy has occurred. The mechanism of the splenic atrophy is unknown.

Splenic hypofunction and atrophy are characterized by changes in the blood film appearances; the main features are the presence of Howell–Jolly bodies and siderotic granules in some of the red cells. This is due to the loss of the spleen's macrophage 'pitting' function. Reduced sequestration (pooling) of red cells also occurs.

Splenic infarction

Splenic infarction occurs quite frequently in patients who have very large spleens from any cause. It is particularly common in association with myelosclerosis and chronic myeloid leukaemia. It also occurs in most patients with sickle-cell anaemia. In this disorder, splenic infarction occurs early in life and repeated episodes result in an autosplenectomy. Occasionally, when there is rapid growth of the spleen in association with an aggressive form of non-Hodgkin's lymphoma there may be multiple infarctions and spontaneous rupture of the spleen. Splenic infarcts are one of the presenting features of chronic myeloid leukaemia.

Splenic infarction causes pain in the left upper quadrant. If the diaphragmatic surface of the spleen is involved, the pain may be referred to the left shoulder tip. The physical signs include tenderness over the spleen, and sometimes a loud splenic rub is heard. Treatment is by rest and analgesia. The occurrence of repeated splenic infarction may be an indication for splenectomy, which may be complicated by adhesions between the spleen and the overlying peritoneum.

Specialized investigation of splenic function

Assessment of splenic function may be helpful, particularly in assessing the likely effect of splenectomy in haematological disorders. In many conditions it is sufficient to assess the spleen size, examine the peripheral blood for evidence of pancytopenia or a reduction in the number of neutrophils and platelets, and to examine the bone marrow to determine whether haemopoiesis is normal. Often this simple approach, combined with a knowledge of the likely effects of splenectomy for a particular haematological disorder, will be all that is necessary to make a decision about whether to proceed to surgery.

Studies with radionuclides provide information about the extent of splenic involvement in a disease process, the role of the spleen in producing anaemia, and the likely benefits of splenectomy. Details of the methods used and analysis of the results obtained in various conditions are to be found in specialized textbooks.

The following list summarizes the various *in vivo* tests useful for investigating splenic function:

- *Delineation of functional splenic tissue.* The spleen can be visualized and its size estimated by scintillation scanning following injection of isotope-labelled, autologous, heat-damaged red cells, which are selectively removed by functional splenic tissue. A gamma camera or rectilinear scanner visualizes splenic tissue (Fig. 2). The technique is most useful for identifying accessory spleens (splenunculi) associated with a post-splenectomy relapse of immune thrombocytopenia. The rate at which heat-damaged red cells are cleared from the circulation provides a rough guide to the competence of splenic function. A slow clearance may identify splenic hypofunction before the blood film shows Howell–Jolly bodies and other morphological changes.
- *Measurement of splenic red cell pool.* Quantitative scanning of the spleen after injection of undamaged, isotope-labelled, autologous red cells allows measurement of the splenic red cell pool. The size of the splenic red cell pool should be taken into account when assessing the significance of anaemia in the presence of splenomegaly. Measuring the pool is particularly useful for distinguishing polycythaemia vera (increased pool) from secondary polycythaemia (normal pool) and assessing the (useless) spleen pool in massive splenomegaly (Fig. 3).
- *Identification of sites of red cell destruction and quantification of splenic red cell destruction.* Surface counting over the spleen, heart, and liver following injection of autologous ^{51}Cr-labelled erythrocytes provides a qualitative indication of splenic red cell destruction in various haemolytic anaemias; quantitative scanning provides a more accurate measurement of the actual proportion of the cells that are destroyed in the spleen and elsewhere. These studies are moderately predictive of the outcome of splenectomy.
- *Identification and quantification of splenic extramedullary erythropoiesis.* Normally, transferrin-bound iron passes to the bone marrow, where the iron is released and enters erythroblasts for incorporation into the haemoglobin of developing erythrocytes. In the normal spleen, iron does not dissociate from transferrin. Hence, the uptake of iron demonstrable by surface counts shortly after administration of radioactive iron (^{59}Fe or ^{52}Fe), indicates that there is erythropoiesis in the spleen. Extramedullary erythropoiesis in the spleen occurs in the majority of patients with myelofibrosis (Fig. 4), and some patients with essential thrombocythaemia, but not in patients with polycythaemia vera. ^{52}Fe studies are useful for detecting early stages of transition from polycythaemia vera to myelofibrosis and for diagnosing the syndrome of

transitional myeloproliferative disorder. Extramedullary haemopoiesis can be accurately identified in thalassaemia major or intermedia and sickle-cell disease by positron emission tomography (**PET**) after ^{52}Fe administration, for example paraspinal, mediastinal, or in lymph nodes.

- *Role of the spleen in platelet destruction.* About one-third of an injection of ^{51}Cr-labelled platelets disappears from the circulation during their lifespan, mainly in the spleen pool. Splenomegaly is associated with a marked increase in pooling: by contrast, in asplenia, nearly 100 per cent of the labelled platelets are recovered in the circulating blood. Surface counting and quantitative scanning have been used to assess the role of the spleen in thrombocytopenia, but are less reliable in predicting the response to splenectomy than in autoimmune haemolytic anaemia.

The combinations of investigations used depends on the particular clinical problem. In many conditions associated with splenomegaly, it is important to distinguish increased macrophage activity causing cell destruction from increased red cell accumulation in a large pool, and to determine to what extent enlargement of the spleen is due to tumour infiltration. In myelofibrosis and hypersplenism, it may be helpful to ascertain the relative importance of the splenic red cell pool, red cell destruction, and extramedullary erythropoiesis, if present.

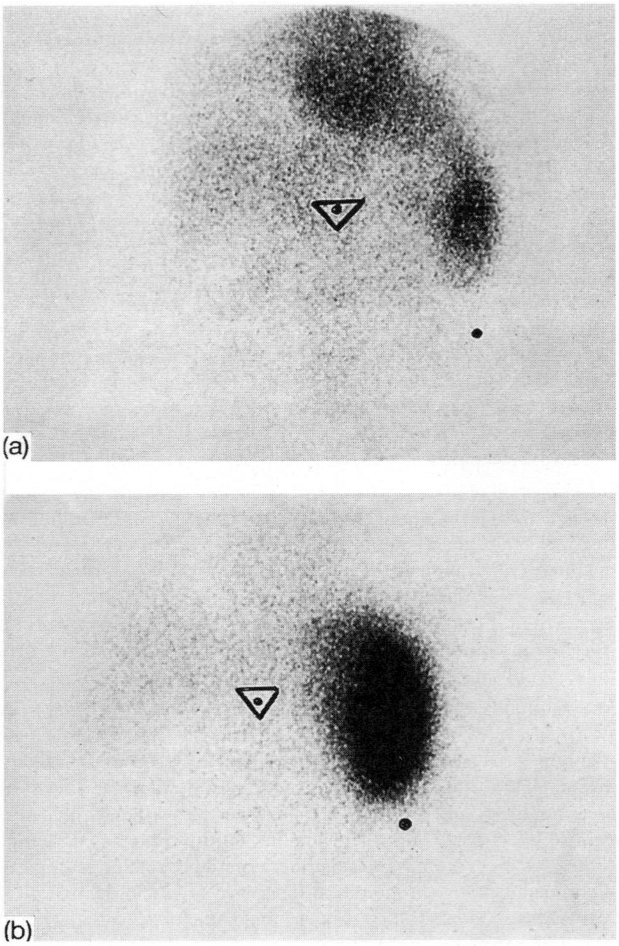

Fig. 2 Images obtained by scintillation camera following administration of (a) ^{99}Tc-labelled red cells and (b) ^{111}In-labelled, heat-damaged red cells.

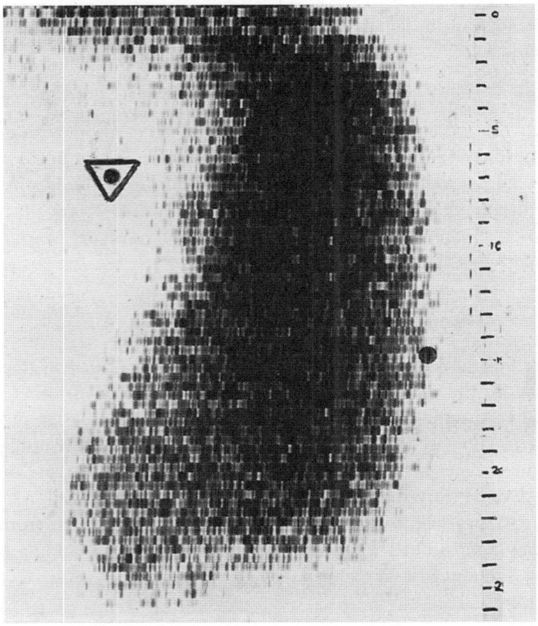

Fig. 3 Splenic enlargement and increased red cell pool in a patient with myelofibrosis. Demonstrated by scanning after the administration of ^{113}In^{m}-labelled red cells. The markings indicate the costal margin. The upper pole of the spleen merges with the image produced by labelled blood in the heart.

Indications for splenectomy

The main indications for splenectomy are summarized in (Table 2). Splenectomy should not be undertaken lightly. Where traumatic damage, usually from a blunt injury, has occurred, every effort should be made to preserve the spleen in whole or in part. Ultrasound and CT imaging are vital in assessing the damage as rupture and haematoma can be confused clinically. Surgical techniques for repairing or partially preserving the spleen have

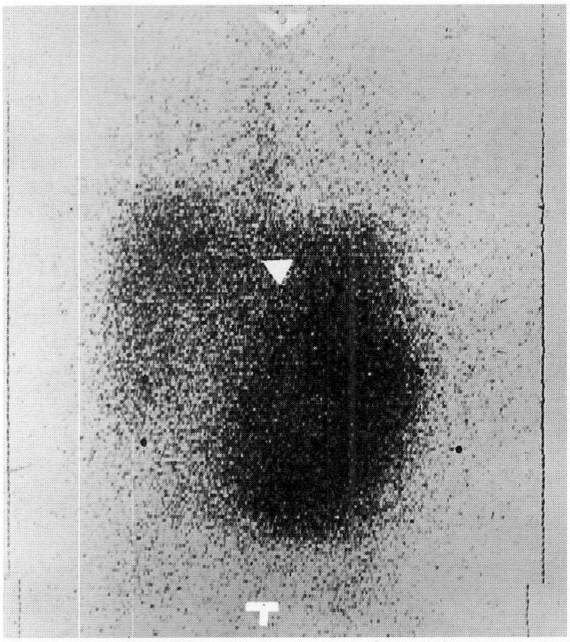

Fig. 4 ^{52}Fe scan in a patient with myelofibrosis showing the extent of splenic erythropoiesis. Vertebral erythropoiesis is markedly reduced.

Table 2 Indications for splenectomy

Definite
Irreparable damage
Severe haemolytic hereditary spherocytosis
Refractory idiopathic immune thrombocytopenia
Occasional
Repeated infarction or chronic discomfort in massive splenomegaly
Severe hypersplenism
Excessive transfusion requirements in massive spleen red-cell pooling
Carcinoma of the colon, pancreas, etc. involving the spleen
Diagnostic splenectomy

improved and should be encouraged. The use of diagnostic laparotomy and splenectomy in Hodgkin's disease has fallen into disuse, partly as a result of improved imaging in the CT and MRI scans, and partly because of the absence of therapeutic advantage, combined with the long-term dangers of splenectomy. In primary haematological disorders, splenectomy is indicated to alleviate complications—repeated infarction, massive red cell pooling, and hypersplenism for example. The decision is usually based on clinical assessment, but radioisotope studies to measure the splenic red cell pool, splenic erythropoiesis, and red cell survival may be helpful in difficult cases. Diagnostic splenectomy may still be required for splenic lymphomas where no other organ is affected. Increasingly, diagnostic splenectomy may be required in HIV-related diseases, particularly for a suspected lymphoma or opportunistic infection. The course of HIV disease is not influenced by splenectomy.

Clinical and haematological effects of splenectomy

Removal of the spleen is associated with certain immediate and delayed clinical complications, and with the presence of permanent changes in the peripheral blood picture.

Clinical complications

Early

In some splenectomies, particularly when the spleen is bound down by adhesions following a previous splenic infarction, there may be difficulty in achieving haemostasis, particularly if the preoperative platelet count is less than 50×10^9/l. Platelets should be infused as soon as the splenic pedicle has been ligated. Subphrenic abscess is a significant complication and may occasionally be fatal. Because the platelet count tends to rise immediately after the operation, there is an increased risk of thromboembolic disease in the first 2 or 3 weeks after splenectomy.

Subcutaneous heparin can be used if the preoperative platelet count is 50 $\times 10^9$/l or greater. After wound healing, aspirin 75 mg daily should be given if the platelet count is elevated above 500×10^9/l, and continued until this normalizes. There is a small, long-term increase in myocardial infarction in splenectomized patients with persistently raised platelet counts, and in these patients aspirin should be given indefinitely.

Mortality depends on the clinical condition of the patient and the size of the spleen. Laparoscopic techniques for splenectomy are safer and reduce morbidity for small or moderately enlarged spleens. In patients with massive splenomegaly, usually myeloproliferative disorders, the mortality rate is up to 15 per cent in those patients thought fit for surgery.

Long term

All patients, whatever the reason for splenectomy, are at risk of overwhelming postsplenectomy infection (**OPSI**). Classically, OPSI presents with a vague general prodrome, followed by prostration, bacteraemic shock, and frequently disseminated intravascular coagulation. Death may occur within 6 h of the onset. The mortality rate in patients reaching hospital alive is in excess of 30 per cent. By far the most important causative organism is the pneumococcus (*Streptococcus pneumoniae*), but *Haemophilus influenzae*, *Neisseria meningitidis*, *Escherichia coli*, and *Pseudomonas* spp. have all been implicated. In endemic areas, plasmodium and babesia infections are of increased severity in non-immune individuals. Special warnings should be given to splenectomized patients travelling to malarial areas. Viral illnesses may also be of increased severity postsplenectomy.

The risk of OPSI does not decline significantly in the years after splenectomy. Children are at the greatest risk, followed by adults splenectomized for an underlying disorder that itself is immunosuppressive, or who require immunosuppressive treatment. Adults splenectomized for trauma are at least risk, but they still carry a lifelong susceptibility. OPSI has been recorded more than 40 years after splenectomy. The relative risk of severe infection compared with the non-splenectomized population is about 10-fold for traumatic splenectomy and as much as 100-fold for small children and patients with Hodgkin's disease.

Infections indistinguishable from OPSI also occur in non-splenectomized individuals who have hypofunctional spleens. It is well recognized as a cause of death in patients sickle-cell disease, particularly in children. Fatal overwhelming pneumococcal sepsis has been reported in patients with coeliac disease and primary amyloidosis affecting the spleen. Dermatitis herpetiformis and inflammatory bowel disease are also associated with splenic hypofunction. Bone marrow transplant recipients, particularly in the presence of chronic graft-versus-host disease are hyposplenic and have an increased risk of pneumococcal disease. Patients with lymphoproliferative disorders, particularly myeloma, are at increased risk of sepsis with encapsulated bacteria and should be considered for prophylaxis.

Strategies for preventing OPSI

All patients undergoing elective splenectomy should be immunized with polyvalent pneumococcal vaccine ('Pneumovax'), which currently gives variable protection against 23 strains of *S. pneumoniae*. Where possible, it should be given at least 1 month prior to splenectomy to allow IgG antibody production. Antibody responses may be suboptimal in patients with immunosuppressive diseases or in those receiving immunosuppressive treatment, or when it the vaccine is given perioperatively in an emergency. Patients should also be immunized against *H. influenzae* type b. Protection against *N. menigitidis* is of relatively short duration, and vaccination should be reserved for patients travelling to high incidence areas. Pneumovax is not fully protective, and a small proportion of patients fail to make detectable antibodies after vaccination. There are reports of OPSI occurring with strains of *S. pneumoniae* covered by the type of vaccine given, and therefore it should always be combined with life-long prophylactic antibiotics. Revaccination with Pneumovax every 5 to 10 years is recommended. Splenectomized individuals should always carry a card or wear a bracelet stating they have no spleen. At the onset of any febrile illness, particularly upper and lower respiratory infections, penicillin V should be stopped and therapeutic doses of a broad-spectrum antibiotic started. The penicillin V is resumed at the end of the course of antibiotics.

Prophylactic penicillin V, 250 mg twice daily, should be started postoperatively. Erythromycin can be substituted in penicillin-sensitive patients. The lifesaving value of prophylactic penicillin V in children with sickle-cell disease (that is to say, functional asplenia) has been proven beyond doubt, and there are only rare reports of OPSI in splenectomized patients regularly taking penicillin V. Surveys of patients dying of OPSI have identified the failure to follow the above guidelines as the greatest risk factor. While the penicillin does not prevent infection, it prevents the rapid onset of the OPSI syndrome. There is controversy as to the effectiveness of penicillin V in areas where resistant strains of pneumococci are common.

Following spleen rupture, splenic tissue may seed into the peritoneum, giving rise to nodules of recognizable splenic tissue (splenosis). These nodules have been shown to have some phagocytic function. This has led to the deliberate autotransplantation of splenic tissue at the time of splenectomy where partial splenic preservation has not been possible. Although such nodules of splenic tissue can phagocytose damaged red cells and reduce hyposplenic changes on the blood film, their protective capacity from infection is not established. The presence of demonstrable splenosis should not be relied upon to replace vaccination and penicillin prophylaxis.

The safest course is to immunize all patients, counsel them carefully about the dangers of infection, and impress upon them the need for lifelong penicillin prophylaxis. This should be reinforced at outpatient follow-up visits, and every effort should be made to maintain good compliance.

Further reading

Anon (1996). Guidelines for the prevention and treatment of infection in patients with an absent or dysfunctional spleen. *British Medical Journal,* **312,** 430–4.

Berman RS, *et al.* (1999). Laparoscopic splenectomy in patients with hematologic malignancies. *American Journal of Surgery,* **178,** 530–6.

Bowdler AJ (ed.) (1990) *The spleen. Structure, function and clinical significance.* Chapman and Hall Medical, London.

Crane CG (1981). Tropical splenomegaly. Part 2: Oceanian. *Clinics in Haematology,* **10,** 976–82.

Dacie JV, Lewis SM (1995). *Practical haematology,* 8th edn. Churchill Livingstone, Edinburgh.

Fakunle YM (1981). Tropical splenomegaly. Part 1: Tropical Africa. *Clinics in Haematology,* **10,** 963–75.

Frank JM, Palomino NJ (1987). Primary amyloidosis with diffuse splenic infiltration presenting as fulminant pneumococcal sepsis. *American Journal of Clinical Pathology,* **87,** 405–7.

Gaston M, *et al.* (1986). Prophylaxis with oral penicillin in children with sickle cell anemia. *New England Journal of Medicine,* **314,** 1593–9.

Lucas CE (1991). Splenic trauma. Choice of management. *Annals of Surgery,* **213,** 98–112.

O'Donoghue DJ (1986). Fatal pneumococcal septicaemia in coeliac disease. *Postgraduate Medical Journal,* **62,** 229–30.

Oksenhendler E, *et al.* (1993). Splenectomy is safe and effective in human immunodeficiency virus-related immune thrombocytopenia. *Blood,* **82,** 29–32.

Spickett GP, *et al.*(1999). Northern region asplenia register—analysis of first two years. *Journal of Clinical Pathology,* **52,** 424–9.

Tefferi A, *et al.* (2000). Splenectomy in myelofibrosis with myeloid metaplasia: a single-institution experience with 223 patients. *Blood,* **95,** 2226–33.

Traub A, *et al.* (1987). Splenic reticuloendothelial function after splenectomy; spleen repair and spleen autotransplantation. *New England Journal of Medicine,* **317,** 1559–64.

Waghorn DJ, Mayon-White RT (1997). A study of 42 episodes of overwhelming post-splenectomy infection: is current guidance for asplenic individuals being followed? *Journal of Infection,* **35,** 289–94.

22.4.5 Myeloma and paraproteinaemias

Robert A. Kyle

The paraproteinaemias are a group of neoplastic, or potentially neoplastic, diseases associated with the proliferation of a single clone of immunoglobulin-secreting plasma cells. They include: multiple myeloma (**MM**); smouldering multiple myeloma (**SMM**); Waldenström's macroglobulinaemia (**WM**); heavy-chain diseases (**HCD**); solitary plasmacytoma of bone, extramedullary plasmacytoma, plasma-cell leukaemia, osteosclerotic myeloma (**POEMS** syndrome); monoclonal gammopathy of undetermined significance (**MGUS**); and primary systemic amyloidosis (**AL**).

The paraproteinaemias are characterized by the secretion of electrophoretically and immunologically homogeneous (monoclonal) (M) proteins (Table 1). Each M-protein consists of two heavy (H) polypeptide chains of the same class and subclass and two light (L) polypeptide chains of the same type. The heavy polypeptide chains are designated by Greek letters: γ in IgG, α in IgA, μ in IgM, δ in IgD, and ε in IgE. The light-chain types are κ (kappa) and λ (lambda).

Recognition of M-proteins

Agarose gel electrophoresis is preferred for the detection of M-proteins. Immunofixation should be used to confirm the presence of an M-protein and distinguish the immunoglobulin class and its light-chain type.

Serum protein electrophoresis should be done when MM, WM, or AL amyloidosis is suspected. A paraprotein is characterized by a narrow peak or spike in the densitometer tracing, or as a dense, discrete band on agarose gel (Fig. 1). In contrast, an excess of polyclonal immunoglobulins (having one or more heavy-chain types and both κ and λ light chains) produces a broad-based peak or broad band. It is important to differentiate an M-protein from a polyclonal increase because the former is associated with a malignant process or a potentially neoplastic condition, whereas a polyclonal increase in immunoglobulins is associated with a reactive or inflammatory process. Immunofixation is the preferred technique for identifying an M-protein. Diseases associated with a paraprotein, as found in our practice in 2000, are shown in Fig. 2. Immunofixation of an adequately concentrated 24-hour urine specimen is best for detection of a monoclonal light chain (Bence Jones protein). The presence of a monoclonal light chain in nephrotic urine is strongly suggestive of AL or light-chain deposition disease.

Table 1 Classification of plasma-cell proliferative disorders

I.	*Monoclonal gammopathies of undetermined significance (MGUS)*		
	A.	Benign (IgG, IgA, IgD, IgM, and, rarely, free light chains)	
	B.	Associated neoplasms or other diseases not known to produce monoclonal proteins	
	C.	Biclonal gammopathies	
	D.	Idiopathic Bence Jones proteinuria	
II.	*Malignant monoclonal gammopathies*		
	A.	Multiple myeloma (IgG, IgA, IgD, IgE, and free light chains)	
		1.	Overt multiple myeloma
		2.	Smouldering multiple myeloma
		3.	Plasma-cell leukaemia
		4.	Non-secretory myeloma
		5.	IgD myeloma
		6.	Osteosclerotic myeloma (POEMS syndrome)
		7.	Solitary plasmacytoma of bone
		8.	Extramedullary plasmacytoma
	B.	Waldenström's macroglobulinaemia	
		1.	Other lymphoproliferative diseases
III.	*Heavy-chain diseases (HCDs)*		
	A.	γ-HCD	
	B.	α-HCD	
	C.	μ-HCD	
IV.	*Cryoglobulinaemia*		
V.	*Primary amyloidosis (AL)*		

Modified from Kyle RA (1986). Classification and diagnosis of monoclonal gammopathies. In: Rose NR, Friedman H, Fahey JL, eds. *Manual of clinical laboratory immunology,* 3rd edn, pp 152–67. American Society for Microbiology, Washington, DC. By permission of the publisher.

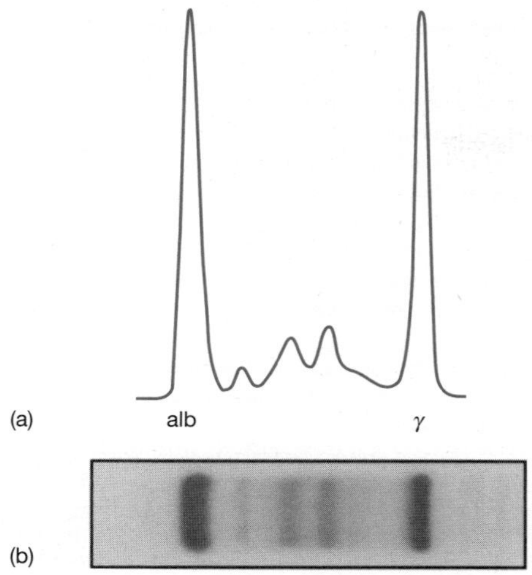

Fig. 1 (a) Monoclonal pattern of serum protein as traced by a densitometer after electrophoresis on agarose gel; tall, narrow-based peak of γ mobility.
(b) Monoclonal pattern from electrophoresis of serum on agarose gel (anode on left); dense, localized band representing monoclonal protein of γ mobility. (From Kyle RA and Katzmann JA (1997). Immunochemical characterization of immunoglobulins. In: Rose NR, *et al.*, eds. *Manual of clinical laboratory immunology*, 5th edn, pp 156–76. ASM Press, Washington, DC. By permission of the American Society for Microbiology.)

Monoclonal gammopathy of undetermined significance (MGUS)

The term 'monoclonal gammopathy of undetermined significance' (MGUS) (benign monoclonal gammopathy) denotes the presence of a paraprotein in persons without evidence of MM, WM, AL, or related disorders. MGUS is characterized by a serum paraprotein concentration of less than 30 g/l; fewer than 5 per cent plasma cells in the bone marrow; no or only small amounts of paraprotein in the urine; absence of lytic bone lesions, anaemia, hypercalcaemia, and renal insufficiency; and, most important, the stability of the paraprotein and the failure of other abnormalities to develop. The prevalence of MGUS is 1 per cent in patients 50 years or older and 3 per cent in those over 70 years of age.

In a series of 241 patients with MGUS followed for 24 to 39 years, 26 per cent developed MM, WM, or AL. The median age at diagnosis was 64 years. Laboratory abnormalities such as anaemia or renal insufficiency were the result of unrelated disorders. The paraprotein concentration ranged from 3 to 30 g/l (median, 17 g/l). The paraproteins consisted of IgG (73 per cent), IgA (11 per cent), IgM (14 per cent), or biclonal (2 per cent). The bone marrow plasma cells ranged from 1 per cent to 10 per cent (median, 3.0 per cent).

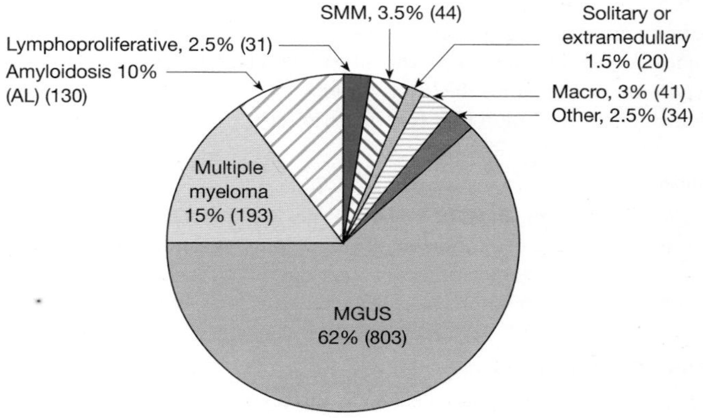

Fig. 2 Types of monoclonal gammopathies in 1296 Mayo Clinic cases in 2000.

Table 2 Course of 241 patients with monoclonal gammopathy of undetermined significance

Group	Description	Follow-up No.	(25–39 years) %
1	No substantial increase of monoclonal protein (benign)	24	10
2	Increase in monoclonal protein to ≥30 g/l	25	10
3	Died of unrelated causes	129	54
4	Development of myeloma, macroglobulinaemia, amyloidosis, etc.	63	26
	Total	241	100

Modified from Kyle RA (1984). 'Benign' monoclonal gammopathy: a misnomer? *Journal of the American Medical Association* **251**, 1849–54. By permission of the American Medical Association.

After 24 to 39 years of follow-up, the 241 patients were classified into four groups (Table 2). Of these patients, 10 per cent have remained stable and could be classified as having 'benign' monoclonal gammopathy, but they must continue to be observed because serious disease may still develop. More than half of the patients died of unrelated causes without developing MM or a related disorder. In 26 per cent, MM (18 per cent), WM (3 per cent), AL (3 per cent), or related disorders (2 per cent) developed; the actuarial rate was 16 per cent at 10 years, 33 per cent at 20 years, and 40 per cent at 25 years. The interval from the time of recognition of the paraprotein to the diagnosis of serious disease ranged from 2 to 29 years (median, 10 years). In seven patients, MM was diagnosed more than 20 years after detection of the paraprotein.

Differential diagnosis of MGUS from MM and WM

The size of the paraprotein in the serum or urine is of some help. SMM is characterized by the presence of a paraprotein concentration of more than 30 g/l, more than 10 per cent plasma cells in the bone marrow, but no anaemia, renal insufficiency, or skeletal lesions. Affected patients must be recognized because they may remain stable for years and not require therapy. The presence of a urinary paraprotein suggests MM, but small amounts of κ or λ paraprotein may persist in the urine and remain stable for years. Large numbers of plasma cells in the bone marrow suggest MM, but some patients may have a plasmacytosis of more than 10 per cent and remain stable. The presence of osteolytic lesions strongly suggests MM, but metastatic carcinoma must be excluded. The plasma-cell labelling index measures the synthesis of DNA, and when increased it is good evidence that the patient has MM. The presence of circulating plasma cells in the peripheral blood usually indicates MM rather than MGUS. No single test will distinguish the patient with MGUS who remains stable from those who develop MM or related disorders. The paraprotein level in the serum and urine should be serially measured, along with periodic re-evaluation of clinical and other features to determine whether MM or a similar disorder is present.

Multiple myeloma (MM)

MM (myelomatosis, Kahler's disease) is characterized by the neoplastic proliferation of a single clone of plasma cells producing a paraprotein. Proliferation of the plasma cells in the bone marrow produces skeletal destruction that leads to bone pain and pathological fractures. The paraprotein can lead to renal failure, recurrent bacterial infections, or hyperviscosity syndrome.

Epidemiology and aetiology

MM accounts for 1 per cent of all malignant diseases and slightly more than 10 per cent of haematological malignancies in the United States. The annual incidence is 4 to 5 per 100 000. The apparent increase during the past few decades is probably related to the increased availability and use of medical facilities, especially in older persons. The incidence in African–Americans is twice that in Caucasians, whereas rates are lower in Asian populations. The median age at diagnosis is about 65 years. Only 18 per cent of patients are younger than 50 years, and 3 per cent are younger than 40 years. The cause of multiple myeloma is unknown, but herbicides, insecticides, and organic solvents may play a role. Human herpesvirus-8 (HHV-8) has been reported in dendritic cells and may play a role in the pathogenesis of MM.

Biological aspects

The plasma cells are phenotypically CIg^+, $CD38^+$, $PCA\text{-}1^+$, $CD56^+$, with only a minority expressing CD10, CD20, and HLA-DR. Although still unknown, the clonogenic cell in MM appears to arise from the germinal centre, circulates in the peripheral blood, and may home to the bone marrow by means of adhesion molecules. Interleukin-6 (**IL-6**) is a potent plasma-cell growth factor and may be increased in MM, in contrast to MGUS. Overproduction of interleukin-1 (IL-1) and tumour necrosis factor, which have bone-resorbing activity, have been found in MM. Approximately 15 per cent of patients have point mutations of *p53*, a tumour suppressor gene.

Conventional cytogenetic studies reveal an abnormal karyotype in only 40 per cent of patients because of the low proliferative rate of plasma cells. Fluorescence *in situ* hybridization using chromosome-specific probes identifies abnormalities in more than 90 per cent of patients with MM, but no specific pattern has been identified.

Clinical manifestations

Bone pain, frequently in the back or chest, is present at diagnosis in more than two-thirds of patients. Loss of height from multiple vertebral collapses may occur. The most common symptoms are weakness and fatigue, which are often due to anaemia. Fever is rare and, when present, is usually due to an infection. An acute infection, renal failure, hypercalcaemia, or amyloidosis may be the presenting feature. The liver is palpable in about 20 per cent of patients, and the spleen in 5 per cent. Extramedullary plasmacytomas are uncommon and are usually observed late in the course of the disease as large, purplish, subcutaneous masses.

Laboratory findings

If MM is suspected, the laboratory tests listed in Table 3 should be performed. Anaemia is initially present in two-thirds of patients but eventually is found in almost all. The serum protein electrophoretic pattern shows a spike or localized band in 80 per cent of cases, hypogammaglobulinaemia is present in 10 per cent, and no apparent abnormality is found in the remainder. The paraprotein is IgG in about 50 per cent of patients, IgA in 20 per cent, and Bence Jones proteinaemia in almost 20 per cent. IgD occurs in 2 per cent, and biclonal paraproteinaemias are found in 1 per cent, whereas the remainder of the patients have no serum M-protein at diagnosis. Immunofixation of the urine shows a paraprotein in approximately 75 per cent of cases. The κ/λ ratio is 2:1. A paraprotein is found in the serum or urine at diagnosis in 98 per cent of cases. Hypercalcaemia is initially present in 15 per cent, about one-fifth of whom have a serum creatinine value of 20 mg/l or more.

The bone marrow usually contains more than 10 per cent plasma cells, but involvement may be focal, and repeat bone marrow examination may be necessary for diagnosis. The presence of monoclonal κ or λ in the cytoplasm of plasma cells, identified by immunoperoxidase staining, is useful for differentiating monoclonal from reactive plasmacytosis (polyclonal) due to connective tissue disorders, metastatic carcinoma, liver disease, or chronic infections.

Table 3 Suggested tests for patients in whom multiple myeloma is suspected

Complete history and physical examination
Complete blood cell count and differential; peripheral blood smear
Chemistry screen (including calcium and creatinine determinations)
Serum protein electrophoresis, immunofixation, quantitation of immunoglobulins
Serum viscosity if IgG value >60 g/l, or IgA value >50 g/l, or if symptoms of hyperviscosity are present
Routine urinalysis, 24-hour urine collection for electrophoresis and immunofixation
Bone marrow aspiration, biopsy, plasma-cell labelling index, and cytogenetics
Metastatic bone survey, including single views of humeri and femurs
Peripheral blood labelling index
β_2-Microglobulin, C-reactive protein, and lactate dehydrogenase determinations

From Kyle RA (1996). Multiple myeloma, macroglobulinemia, and the monoclonal gammopathies. In: Bone RC, ed. *Current practice of medicine*, Vol. 3, pp XI:19-1–19-6. Churchill Livingstone, New York. By permission of *Current Medicine*.

Conventional radiographs show abnormalities consisting of lytic lesions, osteoporosis, or fractures in almost 80 per cent of patients at diagnosis. The vertebrae, skull, thoracic cage, pelvis, and humeri and femurs are the most commonly involved sites. Osteoblastic lesions are rare. Technetium-99m bone scanning is inferior to conventional radiography and should not be used. Magnetic resonance imaging reveals abnormalities in 90 per cent of patients with MM. It is particularly helpful in patients who have back pain but no abnormalities on radiography, in whom spinal cord compression must be considered.

Organ involvement

Renal

The serum creatinine value is 20 mg/l or more in 20 per cent of patients at diagnosis. Bence Jones proteinuria is present in 75 per cent. The two major causes of renal failure are myeloma kidney and hypercalcaemia. Myeloma kidney is characterized by the presence of dense, waxy, laminated casts in the distal and collecting tubules. The casts consist mainly of monoclonal light chains. Dilatation and atrophy of the tubules occur, and the entire nephron becomes non-functional. Dehydration contributes to acute renal failure and must be avoided. Hypercalcaemia, present in 15 per cent of patients initially, is a major and treatable cause of renal insufficiency. Amyloidosis occurs in about 10 per cent of patients and may produce nephrotic syndrome and renal insufficiency. Hyperuricaemia, contrast media, antibiotics, and dehydration may contribute to renal failure.

Neurological

Radiculopathy is the most frequent neurological complication and usually involves the thoracic or lumbosacral areas. Compression of the spinal cord from extradural myeloma occurs in 5 per cent of patients. Leptomeningeal involvement is uncommon but is being recognized more frequently.

Other organ systems

The incidence of bacterial infection is increased in MM. Impairment of antibody response, neutropenia, treatment with glucocorticoids, and reduction of normal immunoglobulins increase the likelihood of infection.

Coating of platelets by paraprotein may cause bleeding. Occasionally, a tendency to thrombosis is present.

Diagnosis

The diagnosis of MM depends on the presence of an increased number of plasma cells in the bone marrow (usually more than 10 per cent), a paraprotein in the serum (usually more than 30 g/l), Bence Jones proteinuria, and osteolytic lesions. The clinical features of MM must also be present for diagnosis. Metastatic carcinoma, connective tissue disorders, lymphoma, or chronic infections must be considered in the differential diagnosis.

Monoclonal gammopathy of undetermined significance (MGUS), smouldering multiple myeloma (SMM), primary systemic amyloidosis (AL), and metastatic carcinoma are the main conditions considered in the differential diagnosis. In MGUS, the paraprotein value is less than 30 g/l, and the bone marrow contains fewer than 10 per cent plasma cells. There are no osteolytic lesions, anaemia, hypercalcaemia, or renal insufficiency. SMM is characterized by the presence of a paraprotein value of 30 g/l or more and more than 10 per cent plasma cells in the bone marrow but no other findings or symptoms of MM. An increased plasma-cell labelling index strongly suggests that the patient has or soon will have symptomatic MM. However, it must be kept in mind that this value is normal in one-third of patients with symptomatic MM. Monoclonal plasma cells of the same isotype are present in the peripheral blood in 75 per cent of patients with active MM, but patients with MGUS or SMM have few or no circulating plasma cells.

The differentiation of AL and MM is arbitrary because both diseases are plasma-cell proliferative disorders with different manifestations. In AL, the bone marrow plasma-cell content is usually less than 20 per cent, there are no osteolytic lesions, and the amount of Bence Jones proteinuria is modest. Obviously, there is considerable overlap between AL and MM.

Prognostic features

The median duration of survival in MM is approximately 3 years, but there is a great deal of variability from one patient to another. In our experience, the plasma-cell labelling index and the β_2-microglobulin level are the two most powerful prognostic factors. The presence of a low index and a low β_2-microglobulin level is associated with a median survival of almost 6 years when treated with conventional chemotherapy. Cytogenetic abnormalities are an important prognostic factor. The deletion of chromosome 13 and the presence of translocations are predictors of poor outcome. The level of C-reactive protein correlates with the serum IL-6 level and is a useful prognostic factor. Plasmablastic morphology, circulating myeloma cells in the peripheral blood, and increased levels of IL-6 are all associated with more aggressive disease. The Durie–Salmon clinical staging system, in use for almost 25 years, has been superseded by these newer parameters.

Treatment

Although most patients with MM have symptomatic disease at diagnosis and require therapy, some are asymptomatic and should not be treated. All symptoms, physical findings, and laboratory data must be considered in making the decision to begin therapy. An increasing level of the paraprotein in the serum or urine, development of anaemia, hypercalcaemia, or renal insufficiency, and the occurrence of lytic lesions or extramedullary plasmacytomas are all indications for therapy. If there is doubt about beginning treatment, the most reasonable approach is to re-evaluate the patient in 2 months and to delay therapy until progressive disease is evident.

If the patient is younger than 70 years, the physician should discuss the possibility of autologous peripheral blood stem-cell transplantation. Haemopoietic stem cells should be collected before the patient is exposed to alkylating agents.

Chemotherapy is the preferred initial treatment for overt symptomatic MM in persons older than 70 years or in younger patients in whom transplantation is not feasible. Oral administration of melphalan and prednisone produces an objective response in 50 to 60 per cent of patients. A reasonable schedule is melphalan orally in a dosage of 8 to 10 mg/day for 7 days and prednisone 20 mg three times a day orally for the same 7 days. The melphalan should be given when the patient is fasting, because absorption is reduced after food is eaten. Leucocyte and platelet counts must be determined at 3-week intervals after the start of therapy, and the melphalan dosage should be altered until mid-cycle neutropenia or thrombocytopenia occurs. Melphalan and prednisone therapy should be repeated every 6 weeks and the dosage altered depending on the blood counts. Unless the disease progresses rapidly, at least three courses of melphalan and prednisone should be given before therapy is discontinued. An objective response may not be achieved for 6 to 12 months, or even longer in some patients.

Because of the obvious shortcomings of melphalan and prednisone, various combinations of therapeutic agents have been tried. In an overview of individual data in 4930 patients from 20 randomized trials comparing melphalan and prednisone with various combinations of therapeutic agents, the response rates were significantly higher with combination chemotherapy (60 per cent) than with melphalan and prednisone (53 per cent) ($p < 0.00001$). There was no evidence that any subset of patients benefited from receiving combination therapy.

Chemotherapy should be continued until the patient is in a plateau state, or for at least 1 year. A plateau state is defined as stable serum and urine paraprotein levels and no other evidence of progression. Chemotherapy should be discontinued when a plateau state occurs, because continued therapy may lead to the development of a myelodysplastic syndrome or acute leukaemia.

Autologous transplantation

Autologous peripheral stem-cell transplantation has virtually replaced autologous bone marrow transplantation, because engraftment is more rapid and there is less contamination by myeloma cells. Autologous, peripheral stem-cell transplantation is applicable for more than half the patients with MM. The two major shortcomings are that: (1) the myeloma is not eradicated even with large doses of chemotherapy and total body radiation; and (2) autologous, peripheral stem cells are contaminated by myeloma cells and their precursors. Fortunately, the mortality from autologous transplantation is currently 1 per cent if patients are appropriately selected.

Most physicians initially treat the patient with vincristine (Oncovin), doxorubicin (Adriamycin), and dexamethasone (**VAD**) for 3 to 4 months to reduce the number of tumour cells in the bone marrow and peripheral blood. The peripheral stem cells are then collected after treatment of the patient with high-dose cyclophosphamide and granulocyte colony-stimulating factor (**G-CSF**). One can then proceed with the transplant, in which the patient is given high-dose chemotherapy followed by infusion of the peripheral blood stem cells. The other choice is to treat the patient with alkylating agents after stem-cell collection until a plateau state is reached, and then treat with α_2-interferon (**IFN-α_2**) or no therapy until early relapse. At that time the patient is given high-dose melphalan or total-body radiation, and the previously collected peripheral blood stem cells are infused. In a French study, 185 patients with primary resistant or relapsed disease were treated with three or four courses of VAD and then randomized to high-dose chemotherapy and autologous stem-cell transplantation or to conventional therapy with high-dose chemotherapy and autologous transplantation given at relapse (early versus late transplantation); the two groups showed no difference in median overall survival (65 versus 64 months).

The largest single-institution experience with autologous transplantation in myeloma included 496 patients enrolled in a tandem transplant programme. Complete response was obtained in 36 per cent and the transplant-related mortality was 7 per cent. The overall survival from the time of the first transplant was 41 months. This series was heterogeneous and included patients with resistant disease and those with disease sensitive to conventional chemotherapy. In a recent report of 231 patients receiving tandem transplants, the overall median survival was 68 months.

A randomized trial performed by the French Myeloma Group compared high-dose chemotherapy and autologous bone marrow transplantation with conventional chemotherapy in 200 previously untreated patients under 65 years of age. The rates of response (81 per cent versus 57 per cent) and complete responses (20 per cent versus 5 per cent) were superior in the transplant group. The transplant group had a higher rate of 5-year, event-free survival (28 per cent versus 10 per cent) and overall survival (52 per cent versus 12 per cent).

It has been suggested that better results could be obtained with two (tandem) autologous peripheral stem-cell transplants. In a randomized trial of 400 patients from France, there was no difference in event-free or overall survival between double and single autologous stem-cell transplantation at 2 years. Longer follow-up analysis is necessary.

A major hurdle is improvement of the preparative regimen because residual myeloma is the likely source of relapse in most patients. In a comparison (non-randomized) of melphalan (140 mg/m^2) plus total-body radiation or melphalan (200 mg/m^2), no difference was found in remission status, event-free survival, or overall survival. The other major shortcoming of autologous stem-cell transplantation is the presence of myeloma cells and their precursors in the blood. Collection of CD34$^+$ cells produces a lower number of tumour cells, but it remains to be seen whether this results in better responses and survival. Because relapse occurs in nearly all patients, the use of dendritic cells and vaccines after autologous transplantation shows some promise.

Allogeneic bone marrow transplantation

This is advantageous because the graft contains no tumour cells that can lead to relapse. Unfortunately, the mortality rate is approximately 25 per cent within 3 months. Furthermore, more than 90 per cent of patients with MM are ineligible for an allogeneic transplant because of their age, lack of an HLA-matched sibling donor, or inadequate renal, pulmonary, or cardiac function.

The mortality rate for allogeneic transplantation must be reduced before it can assume a major role in the treatment of MM. A preparative regimen using fludarabine and melphalan ('mini-allotransplant') may result in a lower mortality. The use of T-cell-depleted peripheral allogeneic stem cells decreases the incidence of graft-versus-host disease and transplant mortality. The use of donor leucocyte infusions for relapses after allogeneic transplantation produces benefit in about half of patients. However, allogeneic transplantation is currently associated with a high mortality and cannot be recommended as a routine procedure.

Maintenance therapy

It would be desirable to keep the patient in a plateau state indefinitely, but this is not possible. An overview by the Myeloma Trialists' Group revealed relapse-free survival at 5 years in 23 per cent of patients receiving IFN-α_2 and 16 per cent without IFN-α_2 (p <0.001). The overall survival at 5 years was only modestly prolonged. Consequently, IFN-α_2 cannot be strongly recommended for maintenance therapy. Patients should be monitored closely during the plateau state, and the same therapy should be reinstituted if relapse occurs more than 6 months after the plateau state has begun.

Refractory multiple myeloma

The highest response rates have been reported with VAD given by continuous infusion for 4 days and dexamethasone (40 mg daily on days 1–4, 9–12, and 17–20). The response rate is approximately 60 per cent for patients who relapse while not receiving chemotherapy, but only 40 per cent for those who relapse while receiving alkylating agent therapy. Dexamethasone can be used as a single agent in the same dosage and schedule as VAD because the steroids probably account for 80 per cent of the benefit of VAD. Methylprednisolone (2 g three times weekly intravenously for 4 weeks) is helpful for refractory disease with pancytopenia. **VBAP** (vincristine (Oncovin), carmustine [BCNU], and doxorubicin [Adriamycin] on day 1 and prednisone daily for 5 days every 3 to 4 weeks) produces benefit in 30 per cent of patients and is easily administered. If the leucocyte and platelet levels are satisfactory, cyclophosphamide (600 mg/m^2 daily, intravenously, for 4 days) plus prednisone (50 mg twice daily for the same 4-day period) followed by G-CSF has been helpful for patients with refractory, advanced disease. The use of IFN-α_2 as a single agent benefits some patients, but the results have been disappointing.

Thalidomide has shown to be of benefit in approximately 30 per cent of patients with refractory disease. Resistance to chemotherapeutic agents is a major problem.

Supportive care

Skeletal complications

Skeletal involvement often leads to pathological fractures, spinal cord compression, pain, or hypercalcaemia. These complications result from increased osteoclastic bone resorption, which is inhibited by bisphosphonates. In a prospective placebo-controlled study, patients receiving pamidronate had fewer skeletal complications and experienced a reduction in bone pain as well as improved quality of life. Pamidronate in a dosage of 90 mg intravenously every 4 weeks is recommended for patients with MM who have lytic lesions or osteopenia. Its use should be continued indefinitely. Clodronate, an orally administered bisphosphonate, has also been reported to be beneficial.

Patients should be encouraged to be as active as possible, but they must avoid undue trauma. Fixation of fractures or pending fractures with an intramedullary rod and methyl methacrylate has produced good results. Bone pain should be treated with analgesics or narcotics as necessary.

Hypercalcaemia

This is present in 15 per cent of patients at diagnosis and should be suspected in the presence of anorexia, nausea, vomiting, polyuria, polydipsia, increased constipation, weakness, confusion, or stupor. If untreated, renal insufficiency develops. Hydration plus prednisone (25 mg four times a day until the serum calcium level decreases) is effective in most cases. If these measures fail, pamidronate or etidronate is effective.

Renal failure

Two major causes of renal insufficiency are 'myeloma kidney' and hypercalcaemia. Maintenance of a high urine output (3 litres/day) is important for preventing renal failure in patients with Bence Jones proteinuria. Haemodialysis or peritoneal dialysis is necessary in the event of symptomatic azotaemia. Plasmapheresis may be useful in acute renal failure, but patients with severe myeloma cast formation or other irreversible changes are unlikely to benefit. Allopurinol should be administered if hyperuricaemia is present. Patients with acute renal failure should be treated with VAD or dexamethasone to reduce the tumour mass as quickly as possible.

Infection

Appropriate therapy for bacterial infections is essential. Patients should receive pneumococcal and influenza vaccination despite their suboptimal antibody response. Prophylactic daily oral penicillin (500 mg daily indefinitely) often benefits patients with recurrent pneumococcal infections. Because many infections occur in the first 2 months after instituting therapy, trimethoprim–sulfamethoxazole is useful. Intravenously administered gammaglobulin can be used for recurrent infections, but it is very expensive.

Neurological

Spinal cord compression should be suspected in patients with severe back pain who develop weakness or paraesthesias of the lower extremities or bladder or bowel dysfunction. Magnetic resonance imaging (**MRI**) or CT scans must be done immediately. Radiation therapy and dexamethasone are usually effective, and surgical decompression is rarely necessary.

Hyperviscosity

This is characterized by oral or nasal bleeding, blurred vision, paraesthesias, headache, reduced cerebration, or congestive heart failure. Serum viscosity levels do not correlate well with the symptoms or clinical findings. A decision to perform plasmapheresis depends on the symptoms and changes in the ocular fundus. Plasmapheresis promptly relieves the symptoms and should be done regardless of the viscosity level if the patient has signs or symptoms of hyperviscosity.

Anaemia

Anaemia occurs in almost all patients during the course of MM. Erythropoietin (150 U/kg 3 times weekly or 40 000-U weekly) will increase haemoglobin in 50 to 60 per cent of patients.

Emotional support

All patients with MM need substantial and continuing emotional support. The physician's approach must be positive and emphasize the potential benefits of therapy. It is reassuring for patients to know that some survive for 10 years or more. It is vital that the physician caring for patients with MM has the interest and capacity to deal with an incurable disease over the space of years with assurance, sympathy, and resourcefulness.

Variant forms of multiple myeloma

Smouldering multiple myeloma (SMM)

See above.

Plasma-cell leukaemia

Plasma-cell leukaemia is defined as the presence of more than 20 per cent plasma cells in the peripheral blood and an absolute plasma-cell count of more than 2×10^9/l. It is classified as primary when it presents *de novo* (60 per cent of cases) and as secondary when it is a leukaemia transformation of a previously recognized myeloma (40 per cent). Patients with primary plasma-cell leukaemia are younger and have a higher platelet count, fewer bone lesions, a smaller serum paraprotein, a greater incidence of hepatosplenomegaly and lymphadenopathy, and a longer duration of survival than patients with secondary plasma-cell leukaemia. Cytogenetic abnormalities are more common than in patients with MM. Autologous stem-cell transplantation after high-dose chemotherapy is beneficial for some patients. Those with secondary plasma-cell leukaemia rarely respond to chemotherapy because they already received treatment and are resistant.

Non-secretory myeloma

These patients have no paraprotein in either the serum or the urine and account for only 2 per cent of patients with myeloma at diagnosis. The diagnosis is established by identification of an M-protein in the cytoplasm of the plasma cells by immunoperoxidase or immunofluorescence staining.

Osteosclerotic myeloma (POEMS syndrome)

This is characterized by polyneuropathy (P), organomegaly (O), endocrinopathy (E), M-protein (M), and skin changes (S). The major clinical finding is a chronic inflammatory-demyelinating neuropathy with predominantly motor disability. Sclerotic bone lesions are found in most patients. The cranial nerves are not involved except for the presence of papilloedema. Hepatomegaly occurs in almost half of patients, but splenomegaly and lymphadenopathy occur in a minority. Hyperpigmentation and hypertrichosis are frequent but may be easily overlooked. Gynaecomastia and atrophic testes as well as clubbing of the fingers and toes may be present. Angiomatous lesions of the trunk are often prominent. Pulmonary hypertension has been recognized in several instances. Ascites, pleural effusion, and peripheral oedema may be present. In contrast to MM, the haemoglobin level is usually normal or increased, and thrombocytosis is common. The bone marrow usually contains fewer than 5 per cent plasma cells, and hypercalcaemia and renal insufficiency rarely occur. Most patients have a λ light chain, and IgA is the most common heavy-chain type. Castleman's disease may be present. The diagnosis is confirmed by the identification of monoclonal plasma cells obtained from an osteosclerotic lesion. If the skeletal lesions are in a limited area, radiation almost always produces a substantial improvement of the neuropathy. If widespread osteosclerotic lesions exist, chemotherapy or an autologous stem cell transplant should be used for therapy.

Solitary plasmacytoma (solitary myeloma) of bone

The diagnosis depends on histological evidence of a plasma-cell tumour but no evidence of MM. Complete skeletal radiographs, bone marrow aspiration and biopsy, and immunofixation of the serum and urine should reveal no evidence of MM. Occasionally, a small paraprotein may be found in the serum or urine, but it usually disappears after radiation of a solitary lesion. Treatment consists of tumoricidal radiation (40–50 Gy). Overt MM develops in approximately 55 per cent of patients, and new solitary lesions or local recurrence develops in about 10 per cent. MRI scans may be helpful for identifying patients in whom MM will develop in the near future.

Extramedullary plasmacytoma

This is a plasma-cell tumour that arises outside the bone marrow. It is located in the upper respiratory tract in approximately 80 per cent of cases, and the nasal cavity and sinuses, nasopharynx, and larynx are most often involved. The gastrointestinal tract, central nervous system, urinary bladder, thyroid, breast, testes, parotid gland, and lymph nodes have all been reported as the initial site of an extramedullary plasmacytoma. There is a predominance of IgA M-protein in extramedullary plasmacytomas. The diagnosis depends on the finding of a plasma-cell tumour in an extramedullary location and the absence of MM on bone marrow examination, radiography, and appropriate studies of serum and urine. Treatment consists of tumoricidal radiation (40–50 Gy). Regional occurrences develop in approximately 25 per cent of patients, but the development of typical MM is uncommon.

Waldenström's macroglobulinaemia (WM)

This malignant plasma-cell proliferative disorder produces a high concentration of immunoglobulin M (IgM) paraprotein. It bears similarities to MM, lymphoma, and chronic lymphocytic leukaemia. The incidence rate is 0.5/100 000, and in our practice it is one-seventh as common as MM. The median age is approximately 65 years, and 60 per cent of patients are male.

Clinical findings

Weakness and fatigue are the most common features. Chronic nasal bleeding or oozing from the gums is characteristic, but postsurgical or gastrointestinal bleeding may occur. Blurring or loss of vision may be prominent. Dyspnoea and congestive heart failure may develop. Dizziness, headaches, vertigo, nystagmus, ataxia, and diplopia have been seen. Constitutional symptoms including fever, night sweats, and loss of weight may be present. Bone pain is rare. Hepatomegaly occurs in about 25 per cent of patients at diagnosis, and splenomegaly and lymphadenopathy are slightly less common. Retinal vein engorgement and flame-shaped haemorrhages are common and are a better measure of symptomatic hyperviscosity syndrome than is the measurement of serum viscosity.

Pulmonary involvement may be manifested by diffuse pulmonary infiltrates, isolated masses, or pleural effusion. Retroperitoneal and mesenteric lymphadenopathy are common, but they are usually asymptomatic. The most common neurological manifestation is sensorimotor peripheral neuropathy. It is often related to amyloid deposition.

Laboratory findings

Anaemia is found in most patients with symptomatic WM. Spuriously low haemoglobin and haematocrit levels may result from an increased plasma volume due to the large amount of paraprotein.

Serum protein electrophoresis reveals a tall, narrow spike or dense band usually migrating in the γ area. About 75 per cent of the IgM paraproteins are κ. The IgM level obtained by nephelometry is often 1000 to 3000 mg/l more than that found with serum protein electrophoresis. A reduction of uninvolved IgG and IgA immunoglobulins is less striking than in MM. About 10 per cent of macroglobulins precipitate in the cold (cryoglobulin). A monoclonal light chain detected by immunofixation is present in the urine in 75 per cent of patients.

Fewer than 5 per cent of patients with WM have lytic bone lesions. The bone marrow aspirate is often hypocellular, but the biopsy specimen is usually hypercellular and extensively infiltrated with lymphoid or plasmacytoid cells.

Diagnosis

The diagnosis of WM depends on the presence of an IgM paraprotein and a lymphocyte–plasma cell infiltration of the bone marrow producing symptoms and physical findings consistent with WM. The differential diagnosis includes MM, MGUS of the IgM type, chronic lymphocytic leukaemia, lymphoma, and undifferentiated lymphoplasma-cell proliferative processes.

Treatment

Patients with WM should not be treated unless they are symptomatic. Symptoms and findings of hyperviscosity are quickly controlled by plasmapheresis with a cell separator. Therapy must be directed against the proliferating lymphocytes and plasma cells because symptoms will recur quickly.

Chlorambucil (Leukeran) is usually given orally in an initial dosage of 6 to 8 mg daily and is reduced when the leucocytes or platelets decrease. It also may be given intermittently at monthly intervals. Patients should be treated until the disease has reached a plateau state, which occurs in about 70 per cent of patients. Patients should be treated for at least 6 months before chlorambucil therapy is abandoned because of a slow response. Cyclophosphamide or combinations of alkylating agents such as the M2 protocol (vincristine, BCNU, melphalan, cyclophosphamide, and prednisone) have also been beneficial. Patients must be followed closely, and chemotherapy of the same type should be reinstituted when the disease relapses. Fludarabine and cladribine (2-chlorodeoxyadenosine) have been reported to produce responses in 80 per cent of patients. However, in a recent report, only one-third of patients with symptomatic WM responded to fludarabine. Rituximab (Rituxan) produces a response in approximately half of patients with refractory disease.

Packed red cells should be transfused into patients with symptomatic anaemia. Erythropoietin may be of help. The median duration of survival for patients with macroglobulinaemia is approximately 5 years.

Heavy-chain diseases

Gamma heavy-chain disease (γ-HCD)

The paraprotein consists of a monoclonal γ chain with significant amino-acid deletions. The median age of patients is approximately 60 years, but the disease has been recognized in persons under 20 years of age. The initial presentation is often a lymphoma-like illness, but the symptoms and clinical findings are diverse and range from an aggressive lymphoproliferative process to an asymptomatic state. Weakness, fatigue, and fever are the most common presenting symptoms. Hepatosplenomegaly and lymphadenopathy are found in about 60 per cent of patients. Anaemia is present in 80 per cent. The serum protein electrophoretic pattern usually shows a broad-based band more suggestive of a polyclonal than an M-protein. The urinary heavy-chain protein value is usually less than 1 g/24 h. Bence Jones proteinuria is not found. The bone marrow and lymph nodes contain an increased number of plasma cells, lymphocytes, and lymphoplasmacytoid cells.

Only symptomatic patients should be treated. Therapy with cyclophosphamide, vincristine, and prednisone is a reasonable choice. If there is no response, a doxorubicin-containing regimen should be used. The median duration of survival is approximately 1 year.

Alpha heavy-chain disease (α-HCD)

α-HCD is the most common type of heavy-chain disease, with more than 200 reported patients since its recognition. It usually occurs in the second or third decade of life, and about 60 per cent of patients are male. Most patients have been from the Mediterranean region and Middle East. Gastrointestinal tract involvement is most common and is manifested by malabsorption with loss of weight, diarrhoea, and steatorrhoea. It is similar to 'immunoproliferative small intestinal disease' (**IPSID**), but patients with IPSID do not synthesize α heavy chains. The serum protein electrophoretic pattern shows no spike. The diagnosis depends on recognition of a monoclonal α heavy chain in the serum or jejunal fluid. Bence-Jones proteinuria never appears. The bone marrow is not infiltrated with lymphocytes. α-HCD is progressive and fatal without therapy. Surprisingly, antibiotics may produce remission, particularly if given early in the course of the disease. Patients who have advanced disease or who do not respond to antibiotics should be treated with a combination of chemotherapy consisting of cyclophosphamide, doxorubicin (Adriamycin), vincristine, and prednisone.

Mu heavy-chain disease (μ-HCD)

μ-HCD is characterized by the presence of a monoclonal μ-chain fragment in the serum. Most patients have a chronic lymphoproliferative process resembling chronic lymphocytic leukaemia or lymphoma. The serum protein electrophoretic pattern contains a spike or localized band in about 40 per cent of patients. Bence Jones proteinuria, which is usually κ, has been recognized in two-thirds of cases. Vacuolization of the plasma cells in the marrow is an important clue for the diagnosis of μ-HCD. There is an increase in lymphocytes, plasma cells, and lymphocytoid cells in the marrow. The course of μ-HCD is variable, with a median survival of approximately 2 years. Treatment with corticosteroids and alkylating agents has produced benefit.

Primary amyloidosis (AL)

Amyloid is a substance consisting of fibrils that appear homogeneous and amorphous under the light microscope and stain pink with haematoxylin–eosin. With polarized light, amyloid stained with Congo red produces an apple-green birefringence. Linear, non-branching, aggregated fibrils 7.5- to 10-nm wide and of indefinite length are seen with electron microscopy. These fibrils consist of various proteins such as monoclonal κ or λ light chains in AL, protein A in secondary amyloidosis, transthyretin (prealbumin) in familial or senile systemic amyloidosis, and β_2-microglobulin in dialysis-associated amyloidosis. Because paraproteins are associated only with primary amyloidosis, the other types are not discussed here.

Aetiology and epidemiology

The annual incidence of AL is 0.9/100 000. The median age at diagnosis is 64 years, and only 1 per cent of patients are younger than 40 years. The cause of AL is unknown.

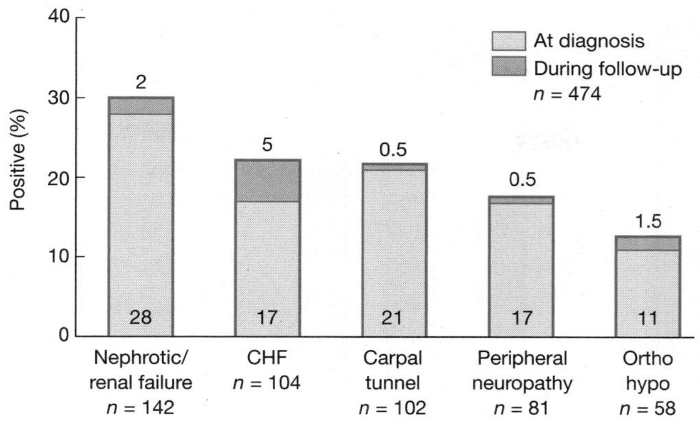

Fig. 3 Frequency of amyloid syndromes at diagnosis of primary systemic amyloidosis. CHF, congestive heart failure; Ortho hypo, orthostatic hypotension. (From Kyle RA and Gertz MA (1995). Primary systemic amyloidosis: clinical and laboratory features in 474 cases. *Seminars in Hematology* **32,** 45–59. By permission of WB Saunders Company.)

Clinical features

Weakness, fatigue, and weight loss are the most common initial symptoms. Light-headedness, syncope, change in the tongue or voice, jaw or hip claudication, paraesthesias, dyspnoea, and oedema are the most frequent symptoms. Macroglossia is present in 10 per cent of patients, and purpura, particularly in the periorbital and facial areas, is found in 15 per cent. The liver is palpable in 25 per cent of patients, but splenomegaly occurs in only 5 per cent. Nephrotic syndrome or renal failure is found in more than 25 per cent of patients at diagnosis (Fig. 3). Congestive heart failure, carpal tunnel syndrome, sensorimotor peripheral neuropathy, and orthostatic hypotension are other important features. The presence of one of these syndromes and a paraprotein in the serum or urine are strong indications of AL, for which appropriate biopsy specimens must be taken for diagnosis.

Laboratory findings

Anaemia is not a prominent feature of AL and, when present, is usually the result of MM, renal insufficiency, or gastrointestinal bleeding. Thrombocytosis (platelets $>500 \times 10^9$/l) is present in about 10 per cent of cases. Renal insufficiency is present in almost half of patients at diagnosis; 20 per cent have a serum creatinine value of 20 mg/l or more. The serum protein electrophoretic pattern shows a modest localized band or spike in about half of the patients (median, 14 g/l). A paraprotein is found in the serum or urine in 90 per cent of patients, and λ light chains are twice as common as κ. The bone marrow contains 5 per cent or less plasma cells in almost half of patients. Only one-fifth of patients have more than 20 per cent plasma cells in the bone marrow, but they usually do not have the other features of MM.

An increased serum alkaline phosphatase level is not uncommon. Hyperbilirubinaemia is infrequent, but when present it is an ominous sign. The factor X level is decreased in more than 10 per cent of patients but is rarely the cause of bleeding.

Congestive heart failure is present in about 20 per cent of patients at diagnosis. Electrocardiography frequently reveals low voltage in the limb leads or characteristics consistent with anteroseptal infarction (loss of anterior forces). Arrhythmias, including atrial fibrillation or heart block, are common. Almost two-thirds of patients have an abnormal echocardiogram at diagnosis. Early cardiac involvement is characterized by abnormal relaxation followed by the features of constrictive cardiomyopathy. Amyloid heart disease may closely resemble constrictive pericarditis or hypertrophic obstructive cardiomyopathy. A sensorimotor peripheral neuropathy is present in about 15 per cent of patients at diagnosis. Autonomic dysfunction may be a prominent feature and is often manifested by orthostatic hypotension, diarrhoea, and impotence.

Diagnosis

The diagnosis depends on the demonstration of amyloid deposits. The possibility of AL must be considered in every patient who has a paraprotein in the serum or urine and who has a nephrotic syndrome, congestive heart failure, sensorimotor peripheral neuropathy, carpal tunnel syndrome, giant hepatomegaly, or idiopathic malabsorption syndrome. A paraprotein in the serum or urine or a monoclonal proliferation of plasma cells in the bone marrow occurs in 98 per cent of patients with AL.

The initial diagnostic procedure should be an abdominal fat aspiration, which is positive in about 80 per cent of patients (Fig. 4). A bone marrow aspiration and biopsy should be done to determine the degree of plasmacytosis, and amyloid stains will be positive in more than half of patients. The abdominal fat or bone marrow biopsy is positive in 90 per cent of cases; if negative, a rectal biopsy (including submucosa) or biopsy of a suspected involved organ such as the kidney, liver, heart, or sural nerve is indicated. Specific antisera to κ, λ, protein A, transthyretin, and β_2-microglobulin are useful for identifying the type of systemic amyloidosis. ^{123}I-labelled human serum amyloid-P component is helpful for detecting amyloid deposition.

Prognosis

The median duration of survival for patients with AL is approximately 13 months. Survival varies greatly depending on the associated syndrome. It is 6 months after the onset of congestive heart failure but more than 2 years in patients presenting with peripheral neuropathy. Almost half of the deaths are due to cardiac involvement.

Treatment

Because amyloid fibrils consist of a monoclonal light chain, treatment with alkylating agents has been a common approach. In a randomized trial, survival of patients receiving the two melphalan–prednisone-containing regimens (17–18 months) was superior to that of patients receiving colchicine (8.5 months). Patients have had substantial clinical improvement after the administration of 4′-iodo-4′-deoxyrubicin (**I-DOX**). This agent appears to bind to the amyloid fibrils and contributes to the resolution of amyloid deposits. Encouraging results have been reported with high-dose intravenous melphalan (100 mg/m^2 for 2 days) followed by autologous peripheral blood stem-cell rescue. The impact of this treatment approach needs to be determined because of the short follow-up to date.

Further reading

Attal M, *et al.*, for the Intergroupe Français du Myélome (1996). A prospective, randomized trial of autologous bone marrow transplantation and chemotherapy in multiple myeloma. *New England Journal of Medicine* **335**, 91–7. [A landmark comparison of bone marrow transplantation versus standard chemotherapy.]

Barlogie B, *et al.* (1999). Total therapy with tandem transplants for newly diagnosed multiple myeloma. *Blood* **93,** 55–65.

Berenson JR, *et al.*, for the Myeloma Aredia Study Group (1998). Long-term pamidronate treatment of advanced multiple myeloma patients reduces skeletal events. *Journal of Clinical Oncology* **16,** 593–602. [This randomized trial proves the value of pamidronate for multiple myeloma bone disease.]

Bladé J, *et al.* (1998). Renal failure in multiple myeloma: presenting features and predictors of outcome in 94 patients from a single institution. *Archives of Internal Medicine* **158,** 1889–93.

Falk RH, Comenzo RL, Skinner M (1997). The systemic amyloidoses. *New England Journal of Medicine* **337,** 898–909. [A comprehensive review of amyloidosis.]

Fermand JP, *et al.* (1998). High-dose therapy and autologous peripheral blood stem cell transplantation in multiple myeloma: up-front or rescue

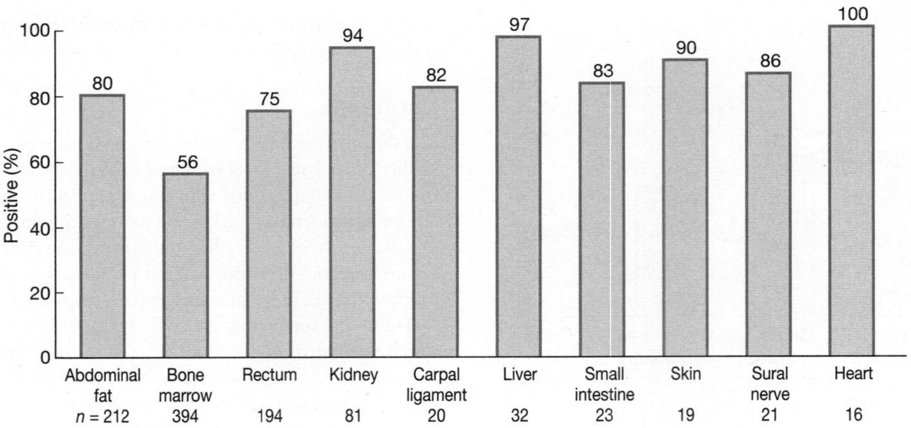

Fig. 4 Diagnosis of amyloidosis on the basis of deposits in tissues. (From Kyle RA and Gertz MA (1995). Primary systemic amyloidosis: clinical and laboratory features in 474 cases. *Seminars in Hematology* **32,** 45–59. By permission of WB Saunders Company.)

treatment? Results of a multicenter sequential randomized clinical trial. *Blood* **92,** 3131–6.

Gahrton G, *et al.* (1995). Prognostic factors in allogeneic bone marrow transplantation for multiple myeloma. *Journal of Clinical Oncology* **13,** 1312–22.

Garcia-Sanz R, *et al.* (1999). Primary plasma cell leukemia: clinical, immunophenotypic, DNA ploidy, and cytogenetic characteristics. *Blood* **93,** 1032–7. [A current review of plasma-cell leukaemia.]

Gertz MA, Kyle RA (1995). Hyperviscosity syndrome. *Journal of Intensive Care Medicine* **10,** 128–41. [A comprehensive review of the hyperviscosity syndrome.]

Hallek M, Leif Bergsagel P, Anderson KC (1998). Multiple myeloma: increasing evidence for a multistep transformation process. *Blood* **91,** 3–21. [An excellent review of the biological aspects of multiple myeloma.]

Kyle RA (1975). Multiple myeloma: review of 869 cases. *Mayo Clinic Proceedings* **50,** 29–40. [A good review of the clinical features of a large series of patients with multiple myeloma.]

Kyle RA (1993). 'Benign' monoclonal gammopathy—after 20 to 35 years of follow-up. *Mayo Clinic Proceedings* **68,** 26–36.

Kyle RA (1999). High-dose therapy in multiple myeloma and primary amyloidosis: an overview. *Seminars in Oncology* **26,** 74–83. [A discussion of the advantages and disadvantages of high-dose therapy.]

Kyle RA, Garton JP (1987). The spectrum of IgM monoclonal gammopathy in 430 cases. *Mayo Clinic Proceedings* **62,** 719–31.

Kyle RA, Gertz MA (1995). Primary systemic amyloidosis: clinical and laboratory features in 474 cases. *Seminars in Hematology* **32,** 45–59. [A detailed description of the features of primary amyloidosis.]

Kyle RA, Katzmann JA (1997). Immunochemical characterization of immunoglobulins. In: Rose NR, *et al.*, eds. *Manual of clinical laboratory immunology,* 5th edn, pp 156–76. ASM Press, Washington, DC.

Kyle RA, *et al.* (1997). A trial of three regimens for primary amyloidosis: colchicine alone, melphalan and prednisone, and melphalan, prednisone, and colchicine. *New England Journal of Medicine* **336,** 1202–7.

Liebross RH, *et al.* (1998). Solitary bone plasmacytoma: outcome and prognostic factors following radiotherapy. *International Journal of Radiation Oncology, Biology, Physics* **41,** 1063–7.

Myeloma Trialists' Collaborative Group (1998). Combination chemotherapy versus melphalan plus prednisone as treatment for multiple myeloma: an overview of 6,633 patients from 27 randomized trials. *Journal of Clinical Oncology* **16,** 3832–42. [This large meta-analysis fails to show a survival advantage for combination chemotherapy compared with single-agent chemotherapy.]

Susnerwala SS, *et al.* (1997). Extramedullary plasmacytoma of the head and neck region: clinicopathological correlation in 25 cases. *British Journal of Cancer* **75,** 921–7. [A helpful recent review of extramedullary plasmacytoma.]

Waldenström JG (1992). POEMS: a multifactorial syndrome. *Haematologica* **77,** 197–203. [Editorial]

22.4.6 Eosinophilia

Peter F. Weller

Eosinophilia is associated with distinct diseases that include helminth parasitic infections, allergic diseases, and varied diseases of often ill-defined aetiologies. This chapter considers the clinical disorders associated with eosinophilia, with additional information on these diseases available in other chapters and then discusses the idiopathic hypereosinophilic syndrome.

In comparison with other leucocytes, eosinophils are distinguished by their morphologies, constituents, products, and associations with specific diseases. The cytokine interleukin 5 (**IL-5**), specific in promoting the development, differentiation, and release of bone marrow-derived eosinophils, is principally responsible for increases in eosinophilopoiesis. Eosinophils are normally tissue-dwelling cells primarily distributed in those tissues with an epithelial interface with the environment, including the respiratory, gastrointestinal, and lower genitourinary tracts. Eosinophils are distinguished morphologically from neutrophils by their cytoplasmic granules which uniquely contain crystalloid cores visible by electron microscopy. Within these granules are four specific cationic proteins, major basic protein, eosinophil peroxidase, eosinophil cationic protein, and eosinophil-derived neurotoxin. The heavy content of these cationic granule proteins, which bind acidic dyes like eosin, are responsible both for the identifying tinctorial properties of eosinophils and for many of the functional properties of eosinophils. As recently established, eosinophils are sources of over two dozen cytokines; and many, if not all, of these are stored preformed within eosinophil granules. In addition to their content of preformed granule cationic and cytokine proteins, eosinophils also synthesize lipid mediators, including the 5-lipoxygenase pathway-derived eicosanoid, leukotriene C_4. The potential functional roles of eosinophils in parasite–host defence, in the pathogenesis of allergic diseases, and in other immunological responses remain uncertain, due to varied and at times conflicting experimental findings, but are subjects of active ongoing investigations.

Eosinophils normally number less than 450/µl in the blood with a mild diurnal variation, being higher in the morning and falling as endogenous glucocorticosteroid levels rise. Blood eosinophil numbers, however, do not always reflect the extent of eosinophil involvement in affected tissues in various diseases; and at times, as in eosinophilic pneumonias, eosinophils may be recruited into involved tissues without a concomitant increase in enumerable blood eosinophils. Eosinopenia, diminished blood eosinophil levels, occurs with corticosteroid administration and is frequent with active bacterial and viral infections. Thus, even normal blood eosinophil numbers in a febrile patient suggest that an illness is not simply due to a bacterial or viral infection.

Some, but not necessarily all, patients with sustained blood eosinophilia can develop organ damage, especially cardiac, as found in the idiopathic hypereosinophilic syndrome, and patients with sustained eosinophilia should be monitored for evidence of cardiac disease.

Diseases associated with eosinophilia (Table 1)

Infectious diseases

Parasitic diseases

Eosinophilia is not elicited by infections with protozoan parasites (with the sole exceptions of the intestinal parasites, *Isospora belli* and *Dientamoeba fragilis*), but rather characteristically by multicellular helminth parasites. Magnitudes of eosinophilia tend to parallel the extent of tissue invasion, especially by helminth larvae. Eosinophilia may be absent in established infections which are well-contained within tissues or are solely intraluminal within the gastrointestinal tract (e.g. *Ascaris*, tapeworms). Even with helminth diseases, superimposed bacterial infections (e.g. in disseminated strongyloidiasis) can suppress expected eosinophilia. In patients with eosinophilia, geographical and dietary histories are pertinent in suggesting potential exposures to helminth parasites. Stool examinations for diagnostic ova and larvae should be obtained. In addition, for several helminth parasites that cause eosinophilia, diagnostic parasite stages are never present in faeces. Hence, negative stool specimens do not necessarily exclude a helminth aetiology for eosinophilia; and examination of appropriate blood or tissue biopsies, as guided by clinical findings and exposure histories, may be needed to diagnose specific tissue- or blood-dwelling infections, including trichinellosis and filarial infections.

Other infectious diseases

The characteristic response in acute bacterial and viral infections is eosinopenia. One fungal disease, coccidioidomycosis, either following primary infection, at times with progressive disseminated disease, or with central nervous system infection (with cerebrospinal fluid eosinophilia), may be associated with eosinophilia.

HIV and retroviral infections

Eosinophilia may be associated with HIV infections: (i) leukopenia may elevate the percentages, but not true numbers, of eosinophils; (ii) adverse reactions to medications may elicit eosinophilia; and (iii) eosinophilia may be due to adrenal insufficiency in patients with AIDS from cytomegalovirus and other infections. In addition, eosinophilia, often modest, is observed in some HIV-infected patients and may accompany eosinophilic folliculitis in HIV infection. Uncommonly, marked hypereosinophilia has developed with HIV infections, including those with a hyperimmunoglobulin E syndrome or exfoliative dermatitis. Eosinophilia frequently develops with HTLV-1 infections.

Allergic and immunological disorders

Common allergic diseases, including allergic rhinitis, asthma, and atopic dermatitis, are accompanied by tissue eosinophil infiltration and usually modest blood eosinophilia. The occurrence of marked blood eosinophilia suggests the presence of other diseases, such as Churg–Strauss vasculitis.

Table 1 Diseases and disorders associated with eosinophilia

Infectious diseases
- Helminth parasites
- Coccidioidomycosis
- Other infections—infrequent, but includes HIV-1 and HTLV-1

Allergic and immunological disorders
- Allergic rhinitis, asthma
- Medication-related eosinophilias
- Immunodeficiency diseases: Job's syndrome and Ommen's syndrome
- Transplant rejections

Myeloproliferative and neoplastic disorders
- Hypereosinophilic syndromes
- Leukaemia, notably M4Eo subtype of acute myelogenous leukaemia
- Lymphoma- and tumour-associated, notably with nodular sclerosing Hodgkin's disease
- Mastocytosis

Pulmonary syndromes
- Parasite-induced eosinophilic lung diseases:
  - Transpulmonary passage of developing larvae (Löffler's syndrome): patchy migratory infiltrates, especially *Ascaris*
  - Tropical pulmonary eosinophilia: miliary lesions and fibrosis; heightened immune responses to lymphatic filariae with increased IgE and antifilarial antibodies
  - Pulmonary parenchymal invasion: paragonimiasis
  - Heavy haematogenous seeding with helminths: disseminated strongyloidiasis, trichinellosis, schistosomiasis, larva migrans
- Allergic bronchopulmonary aspergillosis
- Chronic eosinophilic pneumonia: dense peripheral infiltrates, fever; blood eosinophilia may be absent; steroid responsive
- Acute eosinophilic pneumonia—acute presentation, often without blood eosinophilia; diagnosed by bronchoalveolar lavage or biopsy
- Churg–Strauss vasculitis: small and medium-sized arteries; perivascular eosinophilia early and granulomas and necrosis later; asthma often antecedent; extrapulmonary, e.g. neurological, cutaneous, cardiac, or gastrointestinal, vasculitic involvement likely
- Drug- and toxin-induced eosinophilic lung diseases
- Other: neoplasia, idiopathic hypereosinophilic syndrome, bronchocentric granulomatosis

Skin and subcutaneous diseases
- Skin diseases: atopic dermatitis, blistering diseases, including bullous pemphigoid, urticarias, drug reactions
- Diseases of pregnancy: pruritic urticarial papules and plaques syndrome, herpes gestationis
- Eosinophilic pustular folliculitis
- Eosinophilic cellulitis (Well's syndrome)
- Kimura's disease and angiolymphoid hyperplasia with eosinophilia
- Shulman's syndrome (eosinophilic fasciitis)
- Episodic angio-oedema with eosinophilia: recurrent periodic episodes with fever, angio-oedema, and secondary weight gain; may be long-standing without untoward cardiac dysfunction

Gastrointestinal diseases
- Eosinophilic gastroenteritis: (i) blood eosinophilia; (ii) eosinophil cell infiltrates in the mucosa, muscularis, or serosa; (iii) oedema of stomach or intestines; and (iv) absence of extraintestinal involvement
- Inflammatory bowel disease and collagenous colitis: eosinophils in tissue lesions

Rheumatological diseases
- Churg–Strauss vasculitis
- Cutaneous necrotizing eosinophilic vasculitis

Endocrine disease
- Hypoadrenalism: Addison's disease, adrenal haemorrhage, hypopituitarism

Other causes of eosinophilia
- Atheromatous cholesterol embolization
- Hereditary
- Serosal surface irritation, including peritoneal dialysis and pleural eosinophilia

Medication-related eosinophilias

Therapeutic agents, including herbal or 'natural' therapies, can elicit eosinophilia. Eosinophilia may develop without other manifestations of adverse drug reactions, such as rashes or drug fevers. In the absence of organ involvement, blood eosinophilia by itself need not mandate cessation of drug therapy, if such is medically indicated. Drug-induced blood eosinophilia, however, should prompt an evaluation of whether organs, including the lungs, kidneys, and heart, are involved in the eosinophil-associated drug reaction. If organ involvement develops, cessation of drug administration is necessary.

Some cytokines are potential causes of eosinophilia. Granulocyte–macrophage colony-stimulating factor (GM-CSF), but not granulocyte colony-stimulating factor (G-CSF), stimulates eosinophilopoiesis and can cause prominent blood and tissue eosinophilia and, less commonly, eosinophil-associated diseases, including eosinophilic pneumonia and eosinophilic endomyocardial fibrosis. Administration of IL-2 or IL-2-stimulated lymphocytes frequently elicits eosinophilia, most likely due to production of IL-5. Eosinophilic myocarditis and endocardial thrombosis may complicate high-dose IL-2 therapy.

Diverse agents, including many antimicrobial agents and non-steroidal anti-inflammatory agents (**NSAIDs**), may elicit pulmonary eosinophilia. Blood eosinophilia is usually, but not always, present; and if blood eosinophilia is absent, sputum or bronchoalveolar lavage eosinophilia is necessary to help make the diagnosis.

In drug-induced acute interstitial nephritis, eosinophilia is common in the involved kidneys, urine, and at times, the blood. In addition to eosinophilia, fever, rash, and arthralgia support the diagnosis, but these are commonly absent in cases of drug-induced acute interstital nephritis. Agents that elicit acute interstitial nephritis include semisynthetic penicillins, NSAIDs, cimetidine, sulphonamides, ciprofloxacin, and aztreonam. Eosinophiluria is not uniformly present in all with drug-induced interstitial nephritis.

Acute necrotizing eosinophilic myocarditis is a serious but uncommon type of hypersensitivity myocarditis, with reactions to medications, such as ranitidine or penicillin, responsible in some cases. A syndrome of hepatitis with eosinophilia can be a manifestation of drug reactions, including to minocycline, ranitidine, sulpha antibiotics, and trovafloxicin. Other medication-related eosinophilic responses include drug-induced hypersensitivity vasculitis and forms of gastroenterocolitis elicited by medications, including clozapine and NSAIDs. Adverse reactions to contaminated L-tryptophan in 'natural' medications has previously caused a widespread development of the eosinophilia–myalgia syndrome.

Immunological disorders

The hyper-IgE syndrome is characterized by recurrent staphylococcal abscesses of the skin, lungs, and other sites, pruritic dermatitis, hyperimmunoglobulinaemia E, and blood, sputum, and tissue eosinophilia. Eosinophilia is characteristic of Omenn's syndrome, combined immunodeficiency with hypereosinophilia.

Eosinophil infiltration accompanies rejection of lung, kidney, and liver allografts. Tissue and blood eosinophilia occur early in the rejection process, and eosinophil counts and granule protein levels have correlated with prognosis, severity, and response to rejection therapy.

Myeloproliferative and neoplastic diseases

The hypereosinophilic syndrome is considered below. Eosinophilia may accompany chronic myelogenous leukaemia and the M4Eo subtype of acute myelogenous leukaemia. Blood eosinophils may be elevated in the nodular sclerosing form of Hodgkin's disease. Some patients with carcinomas, especially of mucin-producing epithelial cell origins, have blood eosinophilia. Eosinophilia may accompany angio-immunoblastic lymphadenopathy, mycosis fungoides, Sézary's syndrome, lymphomatoid papulosis, and systemic mastocytosis.

Pulmonary syndromes

Diverse eosinophilic pulmonary syndromes are noted in Table 1.

Skin and subcutaneous diseases

Various cutaneous diseases can be associated with a heightened level of blood eosinophils (Table 1). In episodic angio-oedema with eosinophilia, recurrences are marked by prominent blood eosinophilia, significant angio-oedema, at times with excessive weight gain due to fluid retention, and less frequently by fever.

Gastrointestinal diseases

Eosinophilia is common with eosinophilic gastroenteritis, and tissue eosinophils are found in inflammatory bowel diseases and collagenous colitis.

Rheumatological diseases

The principal eosinophil-related vasculitis is the Churg–Strauss syndrome. Cutaneous necrotizing eosinophilic vasculitis with hypocomplementaemia and eosinophilia, a distinct vasculitis of small dermal vessels which are extensively infiltrated with eosinophils, may occur in patients with connective tissue diseases. Eosinophilia may uncommonly accompany rheumatoid arthritis itself but is more commonly due to adverse reactions to medications or concomitant vasculitis.

Endocrine diseases

Loss of normal adrenoglucocorticosteroid production causes increased blood eosinophilia.

Other disorders

The syndrome of atheromatous cholesterol embolization can be associated with eosinophilia and eosinophiluria. Uncommonly, kindreds with hereditary eosinophilia have been recognized. Irritation of serosal surfaces, as in eosinophilic pleural effusions and peritoneal, and at times blood, eosinophilia developing during chronic peritoneal dialysis, can be associated with eosinophilia.

Idiopathic hypereosinophilic syndrome

Eosinophilia may be associated with a variety of clinical disorders, including common allergic diseases, infections with helminthic parasites, and obvious neoplastic disease. However, in other patients eosinophilia that is pronounced, prolonged, and not associated with identifiable aetiologies has been classified as the idiopathic hypereosinophilic syndrome (HES), in which the heart is the most commonly affected organ due to the development of endomyocardial damage. With time, however, it has become clear that HES includes a clinically heterogeneous and aetiologically diverse group of eosinophilic disorders, with clonal abnormalities in T lymphocyte subsets or eosinophils themselves recognized in some HES patients. Thus, there is a range of syndromes that present with hypereosinophilia and may share some clinical features: as yet these are not fully delineated or differentiated.

Definition

HES is increasingly recognized not to be a single entity but rather a constellation of leucoproliferative disorders, each characterized by sustained overproduction of eosinophils. The three original defining criteria for this syndrome, identified by Chusid and colleagues, need to be expanded to encompass increasing clinical experience with varied eosinophilic syndromes. Contemporary criteria include:

(1) Eosinophilia in excess of 1500/μl of blood, persisting for longer than 6 months.

(2) Lack of an identifiable parasitic, allergic, or other aetiology for eosinophilia. Thus, varied eosinophil-associated diseases need to be sought and excluded. Amongst the potential parasitic aetiologies of eosinophilia it is especially important to exclude *Strongyloides stercoralis*, which may persist for decades and be difficult to diagnose solely by stool examinations, not only because of its capacity to cause marked eosinophilia mimicking HES, but also because it, unlike other helminthic causes of marked eosinophilia, can develop into a disseminated, often fatal, disease (hyperinfection syndrome) in patients given immunosuppressive corticosteroids.

(3) Absence of other idiopathic eosinophilic syndromes clinically distinct from HES. This criterion was not included in the initial analysis of HES, but is needed to help exclude several other defined eosinophilic syndromes whose aetiologies remain unknown. These would include Churg-Strauss vasculitis (see Chapter 17.11.5) as well as syndromes that involve only limited organ systems (e.g., eosinophilic gastroenteritis, eosinophilic pneumonias) and do not have a propensity to cause eosinophil-associated damage to tissues outside their primary target organs. By this criterion, the syndrome of episodic angioedema with eosinophilia would be distinguished from HES.

(4) Evidence by symptoms and signs of organ involvement. Not all patients with prolonged eosinophilia develop organ involvement and many have benign courses. These patients are often not reported or subjected to evaluation at referral centres due to the absence of eosinophil-associated disease. Blood eosinophilia *per se* does not warrant therapy in the absence of evidence of concomitant organ involvement.

Aetiology

The current diagnostic criteria for HES encompass a diversity of eosinophilic disorders of varying, and as yet often unknown aetiologies. Clonal abnormalities in the eosinophil lineage have been detected uncommonly: these are based on analyses of X-linked polymorphisms and hence applicable only to the minority of women with HES, but they do indicate that in some patients HES may be a manifestation of chronic eosinophilic leukaemia. Some patients with HES develop blast crises similar to those of chronic myelogenous leukaemia, or they evolve into chronic myelogenous leukaemia-like diseases. Included in the differential diagnosis of neoplastic causes of eosinophilia are chronic myelogenous leukemia with eosinophilia, the M4EO variant of acute myelogenous leukaemia, and acute lymphocytic leukaemia with eosinophilia. Some patients with the typical clinical and haematological features of HES have subsequently developed T cell lymphomas or acute lymphoblastic leukaemia. However, chromosome studies are normal in most patients with HES, with abnormal findings in only 1 of 18 in a British series and 8 of 33 patients at the National Institutes of Health.

Other potential aetiologies for HES might include dysregulated production of eosinophilopoietic cytokines, such as interleukin 5 (IL-5), IL-3, or granulocyte-macrophage colony stimulating factor (GM-CSF). In some patients with HES the disorder has been correlated with either clonal expansions of $CD3^-CD4^-$ or $CD4^-CD3^+CD8^+$ Th2-like lymphocytes, or other aberrant T cells or NK cells elaborating IL-5. A case with eosinophilia associated with polyclonal expansion of activated $CD3^+$ T cells expressing NK cell markers (CD16 and CD56), associated with IL-2 and IL-15 overproduction, has been reported. In other eosinophilic patients, however, it appears that overproduction of IL-5 is not solely responsible for the eosinophilia. In a kindred with autosomal dominant inheritance of eosinophilia, studies mapped the gene close to, but not involving the IL-3, IL-5, and GM-CSF genes, on chromosome 5q31-q33, suggesting an unidentified gene may regulate eosinophil production. However, for most patients with HES the aetiology of the eosinophilia is not currently understood.

Clinical features

HES is more common in men than women (9:1) and tends to occur between the ages of 20 and 50, although cases have developed in children. The initial manifestations may be due to sudden cardiac or neurological complications, but tend to be more insidious and present over months or longer. Eosinophilia may be detected only incidentally. Other frequent presenting symptoms include tiredness, cough, breathlessness, muscle pains, angioedema, rash, sweating, pruritus, or retinal lesions. Patients with HES do not exhibit a propensity to bacterial or other infections. Weight loss and cachexia are not usually seen. Some patients experience alcohol intolerance with abdominal pain, flushing, nausea, or diarrhoea.

Haematological manifestations

The defining haematological abnormality is sustained eosinophilia. Total leucocyte counts are usually less than 25 000/μl, with between 30 and 70 per cent eosinophils, but extremely high leucocyte counts (>90 000/μl) develop in some patients and are associated with a poor prognosis. Eosinophils in the blood may be mature or less commonly can include numbers of eosinophilic myeloid precursors. Eosinophils often exhibit morphological abnormalities including diminished granule numbers, cytoplasmic vacuolization, and nuclear hypersegmentation. At the ultrastructural level there may be loss of granule contents, either of the crystalline core or matrix of specific granules, fewer and smaller specific granules, increased tubulovesicular structures, and increases in cytoplasmic lipid bodies.

Although not often emphasized, many patients with HES will have an absolute neutrophilia along with their eosinophilia, further contributing to elevations in the white blood cell count. Band forms and less mature neutrophilic precursors may be present in the peripheral blood. Leucocyte alkaline phosphatase levels may be abnormally elevated or decreased. Serum vitamin B_{12} and vitamin B_{12} binding proteins may be normal or elevated. Anaemia is present in about 50 per cent of patients.

Bone marrow findings demonstrate increased numbers of eosinophils, often 30 to 60 per cent, with a shift to the left in eosinophil maturation. Increased numbers of myeloblasts are not usually seen. Myelofibrosis is encountered in a minority of patients. Splenomegaly is found in about 40 per cent of cases.

Cardiac manifestations

In HES, the heart is the most commonly affected organ due to the development of endomyocardial damage leading to a restrictive cardiomyopathy. This distinct form of cardiac involvement may also complicate other varied diseases marked by sustained eosinophilia, including Churg-Strauss vasculitis, eosinophilic leukaemia, eosinophilia with carcinomas or lymphomas, eosinophilia from GM-CSF or IL-2 administration or drug-reactions, and eosinophilia from helminthic infections such as trichinosis, visceral larva migrans, and filariasis. However, many patients with eosinophilia do not develop any evidence of endomyocardial damage; hence in addition to increased numbers of eosinophils, the pathogenesis of eosinophil-mediated cardiac damage probably involves some, as yet ill-defined, activating events that promote eosinophil-mediated endomyocardial damage. Patients with sustained eosinophilia should be monitored by echocardiography for evidence of cardiac disease.

Cardiac damage progresses through three stages, the first involving acute necrosis in the early weeks, the second involving the development of endocardial thrombi over many months, the final stage being the fibrotic stage after a couple of years of disease.

The risks of developing cardiac disease in two series of patients with HES were not related to the extent of eosinophilia or duration of disease. Those who developed evident cardiac disease were more likely to be male and to have splenomegaly, thrombocytopenia, elevated levels of vitamin B_{12}, hypogranular or vacuolated eosinophils, and abnormal early myeloid precursors in their blood. HES patients free of cardiac disease tended to be female and have angio-oedema, hypergammaglobulinaemia, and elevated serum levels of IgE.

Neurological manifestations

Neurological complications may be of three types. The first type is due to thromboemboli originating from the left ventricle, which may occur before cardiac disease is demonstrable by echocardiography and can be the presenting manifestation of HES. The second type of neurological disease is primary central nervous system dysfunction, presenting as an encephalopathy including changes in behaviour, confusion, ataxia, and memory loss, and exhibiting upper motor neurone signs with increased muscle tone, deep tendon reflexes, and a positive Babinski. Impaired cognitive abilities may persist for months. The pathological basis for this form of diffuse central nervous system disease remains unknown. Peripheral neuropathies constitute the third type of neurological dysfunction. Symmetric or asymmetric polyneuropathies manifest by sensory deficits, painful paraesthesiae, or mixed sensory and motor deficits are most common, but mononeuritis multiplex occurs with HES, as do radiculopathies and muscle atrophy due to denervation. Biopsies of affected nerves generally show an axonal neuropathy with varying degrees of axonal loss and no evidence of vasculitis or contiguous eosinophil infiltration.

Cutaneous manifestations

The skin is one of the most frequently involved organs, with cutaneous manifestations occurring in more than 50 per cent of patients. The most common skin manifestations are of two types, either angio-oedematous and urticarial lesions, or erythematous, pruritic papules and nodules. Patients who experience angio-oedema and urticaria are likely to have benign courses without cardiac or neurological complications and either do not require systemic therapy or respond to prednisone alone. Some patients with angio-oedema and eosinophilia are now recognized to have a syndrome, episodic angio-oedema and eosinophilia, that is distinct from HES. Particularly incapacitating mucocutaneous manifestations of HES are mucosal ulcers that may occur in the mouth, nose, pharynx, penis, oesophagus, stomach, and anus. Biopsies demonstrate only a non-specific mixed cellular infiltrate without a prominence of eosinophils and no evidence of vasculitis or microthrombi.

Pulmonary manifestations

Pulmonary involvement is reported in about 40 per cent of HES patients, the commonest respiratory symptom being a chronic, persistent, generally non-productive cough. The basis for this may be sequestration of eosinophils in pulmonary tissues, although most symptomatic individuals have clear chest radiographs. As noted by Spry, asthma is rare in patients with HES.

Pulmonary involvement in HES may be secondary to congestive heart failure, pulmonary emboli originating from right ventricular thrombi, or primary infiltration of the lungs by eosinophils. Infiltrates may be diffuse or focal without a predilection for any region of the lungs, in contrast to the often peripheral infiltrates in chronic eosinophilic pneumonia (see Chapter 17.11.9). Pulmonary fibrosis may develop over time, especially in those with cardiac fibrosis.

Ocular manifestations

Patients with HES can experience visual symptoms, most commonly blurring. Even in those without visual symptoms, fluorescein angiography demonstrates that over 50 per cent of HES patients have choroidal abnormalities, including patchy and delayed filling, and retinal vessel abnormalities.

Rheumatological manifestations

Arthralgias, large joint effusions, cold-induced Raynaud's phenomenon, and digital necrosis of fingers or toes can occur with HES. Although myalgias are frequent, focal myositis or polymyositis occur only uncommonly.

Digestive system involvement

Gastrointestinal tract involvement can accompany HES, and 20 per cent of patients at some time may have diarrhoea. Eosinophilic gastritis, enterocolitis, or colitis may be present. Pancreatitis and sclerosing cholangitis occur rarely. Hepatic involvement with HES includes chronic active hepatitis and the Budd-Chiari syndrome from hepatic vein obstruction.

Diagnosis

There are no specific diagnostic tests for HES. Other diseases associated with eosinophilia need to be excluded. Bone marrow and chromosomal analyses should be performed, and phenotypic studies of blood lymphocyte subsets should be considered. IgE levels should be ascertained. Echocardiography is indicated to search for evidence of endocardial thrombi or fibrosis.

Treatment

For those eosinophilic patients without organ damage, no therapy need be administered. There is no clear threshold value of blood eosinophilia that predicts organ involvement or damage. For those requiring therapy, prednisolone is the initial agent, administered at 60 mg/day in adults. Those more likely to respond to this treatment alone are patients with angio-oedema, urticaria, or elevated serum IgE levels, and also those who experience prolonged eosinopenic responses to single doses of prednisolone. Patients less likely to respond include those with splenomegaly and those with cardiac or neurological dysfunction at the time of presentation. For those not responsive to prednisolone, daily hydroxyurea is one option, but increasing the currently preferred therapy for HES is interferon-α (1–10 million units/day or 3 times a week).

Medical management of cardiac complications, including arrhythmias and congestive heart failure, are important and effective measures in the longer-term management of HES, as is surgical replacement of damaged valves. Although early reports emphasized the mortality due to this disorder, many of the deaths were due to congestive heart failure and complications of endomyocardial damage. If the sequelae of organ damage, especially to the heart, can be managed, the hypereosinophilic syndrome can have a prolonged course in many patients.

Further reading

Bain BJ (2000). Hypereosinophilia. *Current Opinions in Hematology* **7**, 21–5. [A contemporary discussion of eosinophilic syndromes, especially as they relate to leukaemias.]

Chusid MJ, *et al.* (1975). The hypereosinophilic syndrome: analysis of fourteen cases with review of the literature. *Medicine (Baltimore)* **54**, 1–27. [An early analysis of this syndrome.]

Davies J, *et al.* (1983). Cardiovascular features of 11 patients with eosinophilic endomyocardial disease. *Quarterly Journal of Medicine* **52**, 23–39.

Gleich GJ, *et al.* (1984). Episodic angioedema associated with eosinophilia. *New England Journal of Medicine* **310**, 1621–6. [Delineation of a syndrome clinically distinct from HES.]

Guillevin L *et al.* (1999). Churg–Strauss syndrome. Clinical study and long-term follow-up of 96 patients. *Medicine (Baltimore)* **78**, 26–37. [A compromise review of the major eosinophil-associated vasculitis.]

Lim K, Weller PF (1998). Eosinophilia and eosinophil-related disorders. In: Adkinson NF, Jr *et al.*, eds. *Allergy: principles and practice*, 5th edn, pp 783–98. Mosby, St. Louis. [A thorough review of the clinical disorders associated with eosinophilia.]

Lin AY, *et al.* (1998). Familial eosinophilia: clinical and laboratory results on a U.S. kindred. *American Journal of Medical Genetics* **76**, 229–37. [An analysis of a kindred with autosomal dominant inheritance of hypereosinophilia.]

Ommen SR, Seward JB, Tajik AJ (2000). Clinical and echocardiographic features of hypereosinophilic syndromes. *American Journal of Cardiology* **86**, 110–3. [A contemporary update on the value of echocardiographic evaluations of potential eosinophil-mediated endomyocardial damage.]

Roufosse F, *et al.* (2000). Clonal Th2 lymphocytes in patients with the idiopathic hypereosinophilic syndrome. *British Journal of Haematology* **109**, 540–8.

Spry CJF, Davies J, Tai PC, Olsen EG, Oakley CM, Goodwin JF (1983). Clinical features of 15 patients with the hypereosinophilic syndrome. *Quarterly Journal of Medicine* **52**, 1–22.

Spry CJF (1988). *Eosinophils. A comprehensive review and guide to the scientific and medical literature.* Oxford Medical Publications, Oxford.

Weller PF, Bubley GJ (1994). The idiopathic hypereosinophilic syndrome. *Blood* **83**, 2759–79. [A thorough review of HES.]

Wilson ME, Weller PF (1999). Approach to the patient with eosinophilia. In: Guerrant RL, Walker DH, Weller PF, eds. *Tropical infectious diseases: principles, pathogens and practice*, pp 1400–19. Churchill Livingstone, New York. [Considerations of the aetiologies of eosinophilia with special emphasis on helminth infections.]

22.4.7 Histiocytoses

D. K. H. Webb

Introduction

The histiocytoses are characterized by the infiltration of affected tissues with cells of monocyte/macrophage lineage. A classification subdividing the disorders into three classes has been proposed (Table 1). However, the boundaries between classes I and II may be blurred, and more than one class of disorder may be present in the same child.

Aetiology and epidemiology

Histiocytes are of bone marrow origin, derived by the migration and differentiation of blood monocytes, although local proliferation in the tissues may occur following contact with antigen, and in disease states. Growth and differentiation are controlled by haemopoietic growth factors produced by bone marrow stromal cells, fibroblasts, macrophages, and lymphocytes.

Normal histiocytes are divided into two subgroups: (1) dendritic cells (Langerhans' cells, dendritic reticulum cells, and interdigitating reticulum cells); and (2) macrophages. Langerhans' cells are normally found in the epidermis, the mucosa of the bronchial tree, in lymph nodes, and in thymus. Characteristic features include the expression of the CD1a surface antigen, and the presence of specific cytoplasmic organelles (Birbeck granules). These arise either by invagination of the surface membrane during endocytosis of antigen, or as secretory organelles derived from the Golgi apparatus. CD1a has considerable homology with HLA class I molecules and may have a role in antigen presentation to T cells. Following stimulation by antigen, Langerhans' cells migrate to lymph nodes, where they present antigen to T cells. Dendritic and interdigitating reticulum cells are localized to lymph nodes, where they present antigen to B and T cells, respectively.

Macrophages occur widely throughout the tissues where they have multiple functions in the immune response, wound healing, bone remodelling, haemopoiesis, haemostasis, the secretion of inflammatory cytokines, phagocytosis of particulate matter/antigens, and the release of proteases, antiproteases, and arachidonate metabolites.

Table 1 Classification of the histiocytosis syndromes

Class I *Disorders of dendritic cells*			
	(a)	Langerhans' cell histiocytosis (formerly histiocytosis X)	
	(b)	Juvenile xanthogranuloma	
	(c)	Solitary dendritic-cell histiocytomas	
Class II *Disorders of macrophages*			
	(a)	Haemophagocytic lymphohistiocytosis	
		(i)	primary (genetic)
		(ii)	sporadic
	(b)	Sinus histiocytosis with massive lymphadenopathy	
	(c)	Solitary macrophage histiocytomas	
Class III *Malignant histiocyte disorders*			
	(a)	(i)	Acute monocytic leukaemias (AML FAB types M4/M5)
		(ii)	Extramedullary monocytic tumours
	(b)	Malignant histiocytosis	
	(c)	Disseminated or localized malignancies with dendritic-cell phenotype	
	(d)	Disseminated or localized malignancies with macrophage phenotype	

Classification

Class I disorders

Langerhans' cell histiocytosis (LCH)

The term 'Langerhans' cell histiocytosis' has been widely adopted to replace the diagnosis 'histiocytosis X', following the recognition that the presence of Langerhans' cells is characteristic of lesions in the disorder. LCH is rare and can occur at any age, although there is a paucity of epidemiological data regarding the disease in adults. It affects 4 per million children each year, with a peak incidence between 1 and 3 years of age, and is considered to be a reactive disorder resulting from immune activation. Searches for potential triggers have been unsuccessful. There is no evidence for a viral aetiology. High levels of cytokines have been demonstrated both in lesions and in the serum of children with multisystem disease. Two studies of X-linked DNA polymorphisms have demonstrated clonality in lesional Langerhans' cells, but these data do not define LCH as a neoplastic disorder. Clonality has been demonstrated in a variety of non-neoplastic disorders. There is a recognized association between LCH and malignancy. A literature review revealed details of 87 LCH-associated malignancies—39 lymphomas, 22 acute leukaemias, and the remainder solid tumours, including secondary tumours arising within fields of previous irradiation. Amongst 341 children registered in two large international treatment trials, the incidence of secondary malignancy was 1 per cent.

Juvenile xanthogranuloma

Juvenile xanthogranuloma usually presents with single or multiple yellow–red skin lesions in newborns and infants—in one series, the median age at presentation in 36 children was 0.3 years (range from birth to 12 years). Histology shows a cutaneous accumulation of lipid-filled macrophages, Touton giant cells, and fibroblasts. Extracutaneous disease may occur in about 10 per cent of patients involving the CNS, liver, spleen, lung, eye, oropharynx, and muscles.

Class II disorders

Haemophagocytic lymphohistiocytosis (HLH)

This is a rare disorder with typical histology showing tissue infiltration by lymphocytes and macrophages, some manifesting haemophagocytosis (Fig. 1 and Plate 1). It appears likely that HLH is due to the abnormal function of T lymphocytes. Tissue infiltrates and haemophagocytosis is probably due to the dysregulated secretion of cytokines, rather than by a primary disorder of macrophages. The disorder occurs in primary and secondary forms. Primary HLH is an autosomal recessive disorder with an incidence of between 1 and 2 cases per million children each year in the United Kingdom and Sweden. Linkage studies indicate the involvement of at least three genes. In about 20 per cent of cases there is a history of previously affected siblings (familial HLH). Parental consanguinity or onset in early infancy are further supportive features.

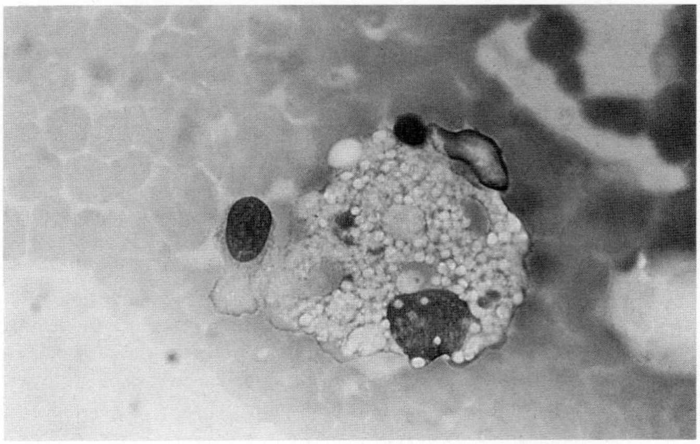

Fig. 1 Macrophage exhibiting haemophagocytosis in the bone marrow of a child with haemophagocytic lymphohistiocytosis. (See also Plate 1.)

Secondary HLH is at least as common as primary disease. Precipitants include viral, bacterial, fungal, or protozoan infections, often in an immunocompromised host. Other precipitants include malignancy, particularly T-cell lymphoproliferative states, autoimmune diseases, and lipid infusions.

Criteria for the diagnosis of HLH are shown in Table 2, although not all features are present in every case. The tissues which are most frequently sampled to substantiate the diagnosis are bone marrow, lymph node, and liver, although fine-needle aspiration of the spleen is reported to have a high diagnostic yield. Diagnostic changes may be difficult to demonstrate, and the bone marrow in particular is hypercellular and reactive in the early stages of the disease. Haemophagocytosis may not be a feature on liver biopsy, but there may be prominent sinusoidal Kupffer cells and lymphoid portal infiltrates similar to those seen in chronic persistent hepatitis.

Sinus histiocytosis with massive lymphadenopathy

This disease was described in 1969 by Rosai and Dorfman as a syndrome of cervical lymphadenopathy with typical histology showing preserved lymph node structure, dilated lymph node sinuses containing mixed inflammatory cells, with vacuolated macrophages manifesting haemophagocytosis and emperipolesis of lymphocytes (that is, a process whereby lymphocytes move straight through the cytoplasm of cells). Fibrosis may be marked. Although most cases are isolated, it has occurred in individuals with malignancy, autoimmune diseases, or other histiocyte disorders, especially LCH.

Table 2 Diagnostic guidelines for haemophagocytic lymphohistiocytosis

Clinical criteria
Fever
Splenomegaly
Laboratory criteria
Cytopenias (affecting >2 of 3 lineages in the peripheral blood)
Haemoglobin (<9g/dl)
Platelets (<100 × 10^9/1)
Neutrophils (<1.0 × 10^9/1)
Hypertriglyceridaemia and/or hypofibrinogenaemia fasting triglycerides >2 mmol/l, fibrinogen <1.5g/1
Histopathological criteria
Haemophagocytosis in bone marrow, spleen, or lymph nodes
No evidence of malignancy
All criteria are required for the diagnosis of HLH. In addition, the diagnosis of familial HLH is justified by a positive family history, and parental consanguinity is suggestive.
The following findings may provide strong supportive evidence for the diagnosis:
(a) spinal fluid pleocytosis (mononuclear cells);
(b) histological picture in the liver resembling chronic persistent hepatitis;
(c) low natural killer-cell activity;
(d) high serum ferritin.

Class III disorders

Acute myelomonocytic and acute monocytic leukaemia account for 30 per cent of cases of acute myeloid leukaemia. Considerable controversy exists regarding other malignancies of the monocyte/macrophage system, due to difficulties in nosology. Malignant histiocytosis was described as a clinical picture of lymphadenopathy, hepatosplenomegaly, fever, wasting, and pancytopenia, with histology showing tissue infiltration by large cells with copious cytoplasm and irregular nuclei. However, recent studies of cell lineage in such cases indicate that the majority of these tumours are in fact of lymphoid origin, and reclassifiable as anaplastic large-cell (Ki 1-positive) lymphomas. Accordingly, true 'malignant histiocytosis' is an extremely rare entity, requiring careful pathological assessment to substantiate the diagnosis. Both localized and disseminated malignancies of dendritic cells occur, although these are extremely rare.

Clinical features

LCH

Some 60 per cent of children with LCH have single-system disease of skin or bone. The remaining 40 per cent have multisystem disease affecting two or more organ systems. There are inadequate data regarding the patterns of disease in adults, although lung involvement appears common, perhaps due to the association with smoking (see below). However, it is clear that adults may manifest a similar pattern of disease to that seen in childhood.

Skin

The skin rash comprises red or yellow-brown papules to the trunk, erythema in skin folds and behind the ears, and scaling, particularly affecting the scalp. Rarely, young infants manifest a vesicular rash, similar to varicella, which may be present at birth.

Ears

Ear discharge is a classic sign, and may be due either to skin involvement in the external auditory canal, or bone destruction around and in the middle ear, with polyp formation. Such destructive lesions may result in hearing loss, and formal ENT assessment is essential.

Bone

Bone lesions may be occult, but present clinically with pain and soft tissue swelling. They are best seen on plain radiographs as irregular lytic areas sometimes with marked periosteal reaction, most commonly affecting the skull and long bones (Fig. 2). There may be pathological fractures. Involvement of the axial skeleton may result in vertebral collapse and vertebral plana, although spinal cord compression is rare. Orbital disease may cause proptosis, a classical feature, but visual impairment is unusual.

Diabetes insipidus

Diabetes insipidus due to involvement of the hypothalamus and pituitary stalk is most common in multisystem disease, reaching 40 per cent in some series. Other risk factors include skull lesions, especially of the orbits or parietal bones. Magnetic resonance imaging (**MRI**) may demonstrate thickening of the pituitary stalk, a suprasellar mass, and/or loss of the posterior pituitary bright signal on *T*2-weighted images due to the absence of vasopressin. Once true diabetes insipidus is established it is irreversible.

Lungs

Lung disease occurs in one-third of children with multisystem disease but is very rare as a single site, it is characterized by cough, chest pain, and tachypnoea, with diffuse micronodular shadowing on chest radiograph. Progression to cyst formation and a honeycomb lung appearance occurs, and hypoxia, pleural effusions, and pneumothorax may occur in advanced disease. Amongst adults, tobacco smoking is a risk factor for pulmonary disease. There may be doubt as to the cause of pulmonary signs, but the diagnosis can be confirmed, and infection excluded, by bronchoalveolar lavage or lung biopsy. As Langerhans' cells are normally present in the bronchial tree, over 5 per cent CD1a-positive cells should be present in lavage fluid to support the diagnosis.

Liver

Hepatomegaly and elevated transaminases may occur without evidence of liver infiltration on biopsy. Jaundice may result from obstruction of the biliary tract by enlarged portal nodes, and therefore is not necessarily diagnostic of liver dysfunction. These provisos emphasize the need for careful assessment of the methods used for clinical findings and of the investigation results in the initial evaluation. Severe liver disease may result in fibrosis, sclerosing cholangitis, and hepatic failure.

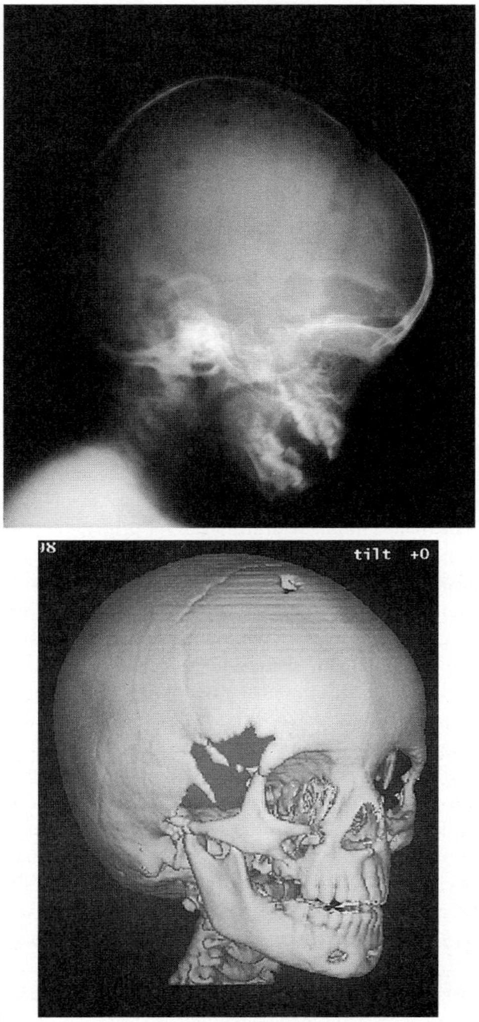

(a)

(b)

Fig. 2 Plain radiograph and 3D computed tomography scan showing bone lesions of Langerhans' cell histiocytosis in the skull.

Bone marrow and blood

A low haemoglobin due to anaemia of chronic disease is a common finding in active disease. Iron deficiency should be excluded in children with microcytosis and hypochromia. Pancytopenia due to secondary bone marrow infiltration by macrophages and haemophagocytosis may occur. CD1a-positive cells may be demonstrated with monoclonal antibodies by flow cytometry or by the alkaline phosphatase/antialkaline phosphatase technique on slides, but their significance is unclear. Pancytopenia associated with liver disease and splenomegaly carries a poor prognosis.

Gut

Gut involvement with vomiting, diarrhoea, malabsorption, and protein-losing enteropathy occurs in under 5 per cent of children, and requires full investigation, including adequate biopsy. Although infiltrates may be seen in the mucosa and submucosa, biopsy of the muscle wall may be required. Barium studies may reveal alternate dilated and stenotic segments throughout the intestine. Mandibular and maxillary disease may result in floating teeth, and there may be gingivitis and buccal ulceration.

Central nervous system

Disease in the central nervous system, excluding diabetes insipidus, occurs in around 4 per cent of cases, and typically affects the cerebellar and cerebral white matter, with ataxia, dysarthria, nystagmus, and cranial nerve palsies. CNS disease usually develops around 5 years from the original presentation. The mechanism of CNS disease is unknown. Most cases occur in individuals with multisystem disease, but also in the setting of single-system bone disease especially of the skull, and in children with diabetes insipidus. On imaging, several patterns are seen:

- poorly defined changes in the white matter of the cerebellum, cerebrum, and basal ganglia—biopsy in these cases shows perivascular and parenchymal infiltrates of macrophages and lymphocytes associated with oedema and demyelination;
- well-defined lesions in the white and grey matter;
- hypothalamic–pituitary involvement including suprasellar masses;
- extraparenchymal masses, generally not in continuity with skull lesions, which on biopsy comprise xanthomatous histiocytes, lymphocytes and Touton giant cells similar to those found in juvenile xanthogranuloma.

Lymph nodes

Lymphadenopathy occurs in both single- and multisystem disease, and may be gross. Local pressure effects may cause obstruction of the airways, vasculature, or biliary tree, and discharging sinuses may form to the overlying skin. Involvement of the thymus may be detected on chest radiography, and may be present on tissue examination even without enlargement of the organ.

HLH

Clinical manifestations include fever, splenomegaly, hepatomegaly, lymphadenopathy, pancytopenia, abnormal liver function, coagulopathy, and signs and symptoms referable to the central nervous system. Occasionally CNS involvement has been the only evidence of disease at presentation. Initial blood changes may show anaemia or thrombocytopenia, with the development of pancytopenia as the disease progresses. Other features include high fasting triglyceride levels, low fibrinogen, mononuclear pleocytosis and increased protein in the cerebrospinal fluid, high serum ferritin, and reduced or absent natural killer-cell function. Many of these changes result from immune activation with cytokine production. Involvement of the central nervous system varies from asymptomatic cerebrospinal fluid pleocytosis (usually to moderate levels comprising lymphocytes and macrophages) to symptomatic disease with encephalitis, abnormal head movements, fits, cranial nerve palsies, ataxia, regression of developmental milestones, and coma. In children who have died with CNS disease, histology of the brain shows oedema, softening and destruction of tissue, perivascular, parenchymal, and leptomeningeal infiltrates, with necrosis and destruction, especially of white matter.

Sinus histiocytosis with massive lymphadenopathy (SHML)

The lymphadenopathy may be gross. It is often painless, and may wax and wane with time. Involvement of cervical lymph nodes is present in most cases, but other groups are affected, either jointly or alone. Extranodal disease of the head and neck or a variety of other sites is present in almost half of cases, either alone or in association with lymphoid masses. Other features of SHML include: systemic ill health with fever and weight loss; destructive infiltrates in skin, bone, and other extranodal sites; hypergammaglobulinaemia; an elevated erythrocyte sedimentation rate; reactive leucocytosis; and immune dysfunction including autoimmune anaemia and neutropenia.

Management of histiocyte disorders

LCH

Initial work-up requires confirmatory biopsy and an accurate assessment of the extent of disease. Identification of Langerhans' cells within the lesional inflammatory cell infiltrate, with demonstration of either the CD1a surface antigen on immunohistochemistry or the presence of Birbeck granules on electron microscopy, is recommended. Thorough physical examination and investigations are required to determine the extent of disease, and investigations must include a full blood count, liver function tests, serum albumin, a coagulation screen, paired urine and plasma osmolalities, and skeletal survey by plain radiographs. Further investigations should be guided by the need to explain specific symptoms and signs. It is important to carefully assess the function of affected organs, as dysfunction carries prognostic significance (see below).

The majority of cases of LCH eventually resolve spontaneously. No therapy is uniformly effective. Approaches to treatment have varied, with particular controversy regarding the role of chemotherapy for children with multisystem disease. Deaths occur in 10 to 15 per cent of cases, and are largely restricted to children with organ dysfunction. For most cases the primary objectives are control of symptoms, and limitation of long-term disability, which affects 50 per cent of those with extensive disease. For children with skin disease requiring therapy, topical application of corticosteroids may prove beneficial. For those with more severe skin involvement, topical mustine has proved highly effective—in one study rapid improvement within 10 days occurred in each of 16 children, with complete healing in 14. Some children require systemic therapy. Oral corticosteroids result in improvement in over half of cases. Bone lesions may resolve following biopsy, but further local therapies include curettage or injected steroids. Radiotherapy is now uncommon due to concerns over late effects—in particular, secondary malignancies have been described within the radiation field. Systemic therapy is indicated for children with multifocal bone disease (30 per cent of all children with bone disease), or single, symptomatic lesions unsuitable for local therapy. Indomethacin may be effective, but it is unclear whether the drug provides more than symptomatic relief. Further lesions and reactivations of initially responding lesions develop in up to one-third of patients.

Children with multisystem disease may be managed conservatively with systemic therapy reserved for those who have organ dysfunction, pain, systemic upset, or failure to thrive. This issue is controversial. There are claims for better results if initial treatment employs relatively intensive chemotherapy, especially in regard to response rates and late effects. There is no evidence that a more-intensive therapy reduces the 40 per cent mortality rate in children with organ dysfunction. For children who require systemic treatment, the accepted agents are prednisolone, vinblastine, and etoposide in varying combinations. The uncertainty regarding the most effective and least toxic approach to treatment, together with the rarity of LCH, emphasizes the need for international collaborative randomized studies. Hepatic failure due to LCH has been successfully treated by orthoptic liver transplantation—80 per cent of children reported in the literature were alive at a median follow-up of 3 years. For children who fail first-line treatment, further options are limited. There is little evidence that immune modulation with cyclosporin or antilymphocyte globulin, or bone marrow transplantation are effective. Responses have been obtained with cladribine (2-chlorodeoxyadenosine). Further studies are underway.

LCH is associated with a wide range of potential late effects, particularly skeletal deformity and dysfunction, diabetes insipidus, growth hormone deficiency, ataxia, intellectual impairment, and lung and liver fibrosis. These data stress the need for therapeutic trials to include standardized assessments for late effects which can be compared between treatments.

Juvenile xanthogranuloma

Spontaneous resolution is usual, and no treatment has been proven to be undoubtedly beneficial. Excision may be indicated for lesions resulting in complications.

Class II disorders

HLH

It can be difficult to determine whether a patient has primary or secondary disease, particularly in children with evidence of recent viral infection. Amongst 93 children with HLH reported to the Histiocyte Society registry, there was no difference in outcome between 40 children with and 53 children without evidence of viral infection. These data emphasize the overlap between these disorders, and the need for circumspection in determining the best approach to therapy in each case.

There are two standard approaches to treatment for primary HLH, one using etoposide and corticosteroids, and the other antithymocyte globulin, corticosteroids, and cyclosporin. Around 80 per cent of patients respond, but eventual disease recurrence is usual in primary HLH unless the child receives an allogeneic bone marrow transplant. Inadequate disease control, or reactivation, may also occur in some secondary cases. These children should then be treated in line with strategies for primary disease. Adequate control of CNS involvement is very important, but the role of routine intrathecal methotrexate in the control of CNS disease is controversial. Cranial radiation is no longer recommended. Experience with bone marrow transplantation is greatest using matched sibling donors, with around 80 per cent of children remaining disease-free. Increasing use of alternative donors, including matched and mismatched unrelated donors has demonstrated that similar results may be achieved by this approach. Full engraftment following transplantation is not a prerequisite for cure, as low levels of donor T cells may provide adequate disease control. A particular worry regarding the use of a sibling donor is that in familial disease there is a 25 per cent risk that the donor will also develop HLH. Continued improvement in the results of alternative donor procedures may make these the treatment of choice. It must also be remembered that some children, usually sporadic cases aged over 2 years at diagnosis, remain well following initial therapy. Bone marrow transplantation is not indicated for this group.

Case reports regarding the prognosis for secondary HLH are conflicting. The appropriate approach for these patients is treatment of the associated condition or removal of immunosuppression, with specific HLH therapy for individuals who fail to improve.

Sinus histiocytosis with massive lymphadenopathy

The natural history of the disorder is chronic with spontaneous resolution over months or years in many cases, although approximately 5 per cent of patients have died due to immune-mediated organ dysfunction, amyloidosis, or infection. Few individuals have died directly due to lymphohistiocytic infiltrates. Therapy with steroids, cytotoxic drugs, particularly vincristine and alkylating agents, or radiotherapy has been variably effective, and is unnecessary in most cases.

Class III disorders

The outlook for monocytic variants of AML has improved considerably over recent years, with around a 50 per cent survival at 5 years from diagnosis in children and young adults following standard chemotherapy regimens. The uncertainty over the pathology of reported cases of malignant histiocytosis clouds the issues regarding therapy. It appears appropriate to treat malignancies of macrophages with AML chemotherapy. Due to the rarity of dendritic-cell malignancies, treatment recommendations are anecdotal, but based on excision with or without adjuvant therapy.

Further reading

Egeler RM, D'Angio G (1998). The histiocytoses. *Hematology and Oncology Clinics of North America* **12**, 2. [Editorial]

Favara BE, *et al.* (1997). Contemporary classification of histiocytic disorders. The WHO committee on histiocytic/reticulum cell proliferations. Reclassification working group of the Histiocyte Society. *Medical Pediatric Oncology* **29**, 157–66.

Henter J-I, *et al.* (1991). Incidence and clinical features of familial hemophagocytic lymphohistiocytosis. *Acta Paediatrica Scandinavica* **80**, 428–35.

Henter J-I, Elinder G, Ost A (1991). Diagnostic guidelines for haemophagocytic lymphohistiocytosis. *Seminars in Oncology* **18**, 29–33.

Ladisch S, Gadner H (1994). Treatment of Langerhans' cell histiocytosis—evolution and current approaches. *British Journal of Cancer* **70**(Suppl xxiii), S41–S46.

Schmidt D (1994). Monocyte/macrophage system and malignancies. *Medical and Pediatric Oncology* **23**, 444–51.

22.5 The red cell

22.5.1 Erythropoiesis and the normal red cell

Anna Rita Migliaccio and Thalia Papayannopoulou

Introduction

Mature circulating red cells are specialized cellular elements of the blood responsible for both the delivery of oxygen to and for the removal of carbon dioxide from all tissues of the body. In the adult, their number is constantly maintained by the balance of two ongoing processes: the destruction of old red cells, mainly in the spleen; and the generation of new red cells within the bone marrow by a process referred to as erythropoiesis.

The generation of new red cells, like other cellular elements, is accomplished through a complex interplay between haemopoietic cells, stromal cells, and the extracellular matrix within the bone marrow microenvironment. Unique to the erythropoietic process is its regulation not only by growth factors produced *in situ* in the bone marrow, but also by circulating erythropoietin (**EPO**), a true 'hormone' produced by the kidneys in the adult. Positive or negative alterations of erythropoietin production, whether acquired or congenital, and/or of its signalling pathway, result in quantitative changes in red cell production—that is to say, anaemia or erythrocytosis.

This chapter will summarize key biological features of normal human erythropoiesis, both in the adult and during embryonic/fetal life, and highlight pathogenetic mechanisms that can lead to perturbations of erythropoiesis.

The erythroid compartment

Erythropoiesis is a highly regulated, multistep process through which 10^{11} functional red cells are generated daily from very few haemopoietic stem cells ($1{:}10^4$–10^5 marrow cells). Stem cells, after a series of amplification divisions, generate multipotential progenitor cells, then oligo- and finally unilineage erythroid progenitors, which give rise to morphologically recognizable erythroid precursors and mature red cells (Fig. 1).

Erythroid progenitors

Progenitor cells committed to a specific lineage are defined by their ability to generate colonies of differentiated cells *in vitro*. In these assays, multipotential progenitors generate colonies consisting of cells of several lineages, whereas unilineage cells give rise to colonies of only one lineage. The earliest erythroid progenitor is the burst-forming unit-erythroid (**BFU-e**), which generates colonies containing several thousand erythroid cells. The colony-forming unit-erythroid (**CFU-e**) generates smaller colonies that mature early in culture. Between these two extremes, there exist intermediate classes of BFU-e with less proliferative potential and shorter maturation time in culture. BFU-e tend to have an antigenic profile similar to progenitor cells of other lineages with few exceptions (that is, they are negative for CD45 RA, CD33, and AC133, but express higher levels, or possibly specific isoforms, of the transferrin receptor). CFU-e, in contrast, begin to express more of the markers found specifically in mature erythroid cells (that is, glycophorin A and blood group antigens). The first blood group antigen to be expressed at the BFU-e level is the glycoprotein (**gp**) Kell, followed by the orderly activation of the expression of Rh gp, Landersteiner–Wiener (**LW**) gp, glycophorin A, Band 3, Lutheran gp, and finally, at the erythroblast level, Duffy gp.

Progression of progenitor cells to terminal differentiation is marked not only by the acquisition of phenotypic markers, but also by the acquisition of specific responses to growth factors. The most active of these on early

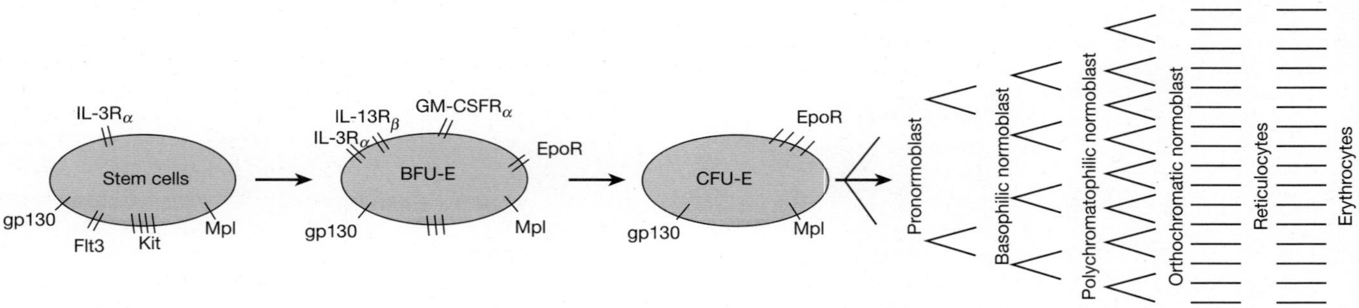

Fig. 1 Adult erythroid progenitor- and precursor-cell compartments. The number of bars on the cell surface is an estimate of the growth factor-receptor concentration/cell responsiveness during erythroid differentiation. A complex of interleukin-6 (**IL-6**) and its soluble receptor (or a fusion molecule called hyper IL-6) may induce growth of burst-forming units-erythroid (**BFU-e**) and erythroid maturation in the absence of exogenously added erythropoietin through activation of an autocrine erythropoietin loop.

progenitors are stem-cell factor (**SCF**, or Steel factor, or kit ligand), interleukin-3 (**IL-3**), granulocyte/macrophage colony-stimulating factor (**GM-CSF**), and erythropoietin and thrombopoietin (**TPO**) on later progenitors.

The special importance of SCF in erythropoiesis is shown by genetic mutations of SCF (such as Sl/Sl^d), or of its receptor, kit (such as W/W^v), that result in mice with anaemia, the severity of which correlates with impairment in kit kinase activity. In humans, heterozygotes with c-*kit* mutations have been reported in individuals with piebaldism, but no homozygotes have been described. Furthermore, mice treated with anti-kit antibodies became anaemic, whereas human kit-antisense containing cultures did not expand the BFU-e compartment.

Erythroid precursors

Erythroid precursors, in contrast to progenitor cells, are morphologically recognizable and include cells at different maturation stages (Fig. 1). The earlier cell is the proerythroblast which, after around 7 days of proliferation and further maturation, gives rise to mature red cells. The maturation process includes haemoglobin synthesis, chromatin condensation (orthochromatic normoblast), and, finally, extrusion of the nucleus and a reduction in cell size (reticulocytes). These morphological changes are paralleled by the accumulation of haemoglobin and by several biochemical changes in the cytoskeleton, which guarantee maximum resistance to stress and flexibility during capillary passage. It has been estimated that about 64 reticulocytes are generated from each pronormoblast, 90 to 95 per cent of which egress into the bloodstream. Within a day or two in the peripheral circulation, the reticulocytes mature further into red cells.

Ontogeny of erythropoiesis

The ontogenetic development of the erythroid system encompasses a series of well co-ordinated events during embryonic and early fetal life, the timing of which is distinct for each mammal. Erythroid cells are the first differentiated haemopoietic cells to appear during ontogeny, initially in the blood islands of the yolk sac, and later in the fetal liver. The recruitment of new erythropoietic sites during ontogeny (from yolk sac to fetal liver to bone marrow) is accompanied by profound differences in the stem-cell differentiation programme and the phenotypic/functional properties of the erythroid cells being developed in each site. Haemopoietic cytokines, specifically expressed and/or sequestered by each microenvironment, may probably mediate these changes in concert with cell intrinsic transcriptional factors. Furthermore, adhesion receptors on haemopoietic cells and their counter-receptors in the microenvironment ensure patterns of firm adherence, migration, and colonization of the successive haemopoietic sites.

Yolk sac erythropoiesis

In humans, the first erythroid cells (the primitive nucleated erythroblasts) are detected in the yolk sac at 3 to 4 weeks and are the only red cells circulating until week 8 of gestation. They synthesize mainly embryonic haemoglobins, such as Gower I ($\zeta_2\varepsilon_2$), Gower II ($\alpha_2\varepsilon_2$), and Portland ($\zeta_2\gamma_2$).

In addition to differentiated primitive erythroid cells, the yolk sac contains progenitor cells of definitive lineage that do not differentiate in the yolk sac but generate BFU-e-like colonies *in vitro*, which are composed of definitive erythroblasts. It is currently undecided whether primitive and definitive progenitor cells derive from the same stem cell.

Gene ablation studies indicate that yolk sac and fetal liver/bone marrow erythropoiesis have clearly distinct growth factor and molecular requirements. Primitive erythropoiesis is not affected by the ablation of several transcription factors (GATA1, AML-1, Rb, Myb, etc.) that affect definitive cells. Also, primitive erythropoiesis *in vivo* is SCF- and erythropoietin-independent, whereas thrombopoietin, but not erythropoietin, is produced *in situ* and may be important for cell survival and partial differentiation. Within the yolk sac, erythroid cells are found in close proximity to endothelial cells and macrophages. Therefore, they are most probably exposed to growth factors produced by these cells, including vascular endothelial growth factor (**VEGF**) and M-CSF. In this regard, yolk sac-derived endothelial cell lines *in vitro* produce leucocyte inhibiting factor (**LIF**), IL-6, flt-3 ligand, SCF, and M-CSF, but not G-CSF, GM-CSF, IL-3, IL-1, erythropoietin, and thrombopoietin. The exchange of trophic signals between endothelial and haemopoietic cells is also mutual at these early stages.

Fetal liver haemopoiesis

The major anatomical site of erythropoiesis in fetal life is the liver, in which newly formed definitive erythroblasts appear at 7 to 8 weeks' gestation within the sinusoidal walls of its parenchyma. Definitive erythroblasts are released into the blood after week 8 and remain the main circulating erythroid cells until birth.

The haemoglobin (Hb) patterns expressed by erythroid cells during ontogeny represent one of the best-studied developmental differences in gene expression. In contrast to primitive erythroblasts, the definitive cells synthesize mainly fetal haemoglobin (Hb F, $\alpha_2\gamma_2$), together with a small component (10–15 per cent) of adult haemoglobin (Hb A, $\alpha_2\beta_2$). The fetal pattern of haemoglobin expression remains stable until 30 weeks' gestation, when a progressive increase in Hb A and a parallel slow decline in Hb F begins. At birth, approximately equal amounts of Hb A and Hb F are synthesized, with the final adult erythroid pattern (adult Hb with <1 per cent fetal Hb) being reached a few months after birth. The fetal to adult Hb switch is strictly related to gestational age and occurs within the same population of cells that undergo an intrinsic modification of its gene expression programme. Its molecular mechanism involves the formation and activation of specific transcriptional complexes within cells at specific stages of ontogeny, but details remain elusive.

Fetal erythroid progenitor cells display a unique phenotypic and functional profile, including higher cell-cycling rates (>30 per cent versus the adult rate of 10 per cent), a lower doubling time (20 h versus the 32 h for the adult cells), and faster kinetics of *in vitro* differentiation (10 days versus 16 days). The average telomeric length is also different (12.8 ± 0.35 kb versus 8.4 ± 0.3 kb). Human fetal BFU-e are exquisitely sensitive to erythropoietin, which is sufficient to sustain their maximal differentiation, whereas SCF complemented by IL-6 alone is sufficient for their maximal *ex vivo* expansion. Whether fetal progenitors do not truly require any other factors, or whether they, unlike adult cells, do not produce autocrine growth inhibitors (transforming growth factor-β (TGF-β)) or are insensitive to them, is unclear.

Unique to the fetal liver stage of haemopoiesis is its almost exclusive erythroid output, whereas its microenvironment is less conducive to myelomonocytic cell differentiation despite the abundant presence of their progenitors.

At the end of fetal development, liver erythropoiesis is suppressed and the organ enters the adult hepatic phase. Oncostatin-M, produced in the liver by haemopoietic CD45+ cells, may facilitate this transition by inhibiting the growth of haemopoietic progenitors while promoting the growth of the hepatocytes expressing its receptor. Increasing glucocorticoid concentrations in fetal liver near term may also contribute to the suppression of liver erythropoiesis.

Bone marrow erythropoiesis

The final site of erythroid cell production maintained throughout life is the bone marrow. Haemopoiesis in the marrow appears between 6.6 and 8.5 weeks after the establishment of a rudimental stroma of cartilagenous and endothelial cells, and is accomplished in four separate phases. Within the bone marrow, granulopoiesis predominates during all the stages of development (fetal and adult).

Erythropoietin and the regulation of erythropoiesis

Erythropoietin was the first haemopoietic growth factor to be identified. Its existence was hypothesized in 1906 by Carnot and Deflandre, but formal proof was obtained by Reissman in 1950 and by Stohlman *et al.* in 1954. Human erythropoietin, a 33- to 38-kDa sialoglycoprotein, was purified to homogeneity in 1977 and its gene, localized on chromosome 7q11, was cloned in 1984. Erythropoietin was also the first growth factor to be used in the treatment of patients because of the clear-cut relationship between its concentration in the blood and the numbers of red cells in the circulation.

Erythropoietin production

Erythropoietin has a short half-life (<5 h; 90 per cent of erythropoietin is rapidly degraded by the liver and 10 per cent secreted in urine), but its blood concentration (0.02 units/ml) is kept constant by continuous production. Erythropoietin levels are exquisitely regulated by changes in O_2 tension, and the kidney is in the ideal anatomical position for sensing these changes (Fig. 2). The kidney is the major producer of erythropoietin, although the liver, which is the main source of erythropoietin in the fetus, retains some capacity of low hypoxia-sensitivity in the adult. Low levels of erythropoietin are also produced in the marrow by the erythroid progenitors themselves.

As the kidney is the primary site of erythropoietin production, it is not surprising that irreversible damage to this organ results in low or no erythropoietin production and consequently results in anaemia. Anaemia in chronic inflammatory states, such as rheumatoid arthritis, is due instead to the fact that proinflammatory cytokines, such as IL-1 and tumour necrosis factor (**TNF**), inhibit erythropoiesis both directly (by inhibiting the proliferation of the progenitor cells) and indirectly (by inhibiting erythropoietin synthesis by the kidney). At the other extreme, some kidney cancers, by increasing the number of erythropoietin-producing cells, also increase erythropoietin production and then lead to secondary erythrocytosis. Furthermore, disorders that impair O_2 delivery to the tissue are sensed as hypoxia and are also associated with secondary erythrocytosis, such as in chronic lung diseases and congenital heart anomalies. In haemoglobin mutations, because there is inefficient O_2 delivery to the tissues due to altered Hb/O_2 affinity, hypoxia is sensed and causes increased erythropoietin serum levels and secondary erythrocytosis. There are more than 50 different mutations in which changes in either the α- or β-globin gene result in increased Hb/O_2 affinity. Secondary autosomal recessive erythrocytosis (polycythaemias) can also be caused by abnormalities in enzymes such as 2,3-diphosphoglycerate (**2,3DPG**) mutase, involved in the regulation of tissue O_2 delivery (familial 2,3-bisphosphoglycerate deficiency). Secondary asymptomatic polycythaemias are also seen in methaemoglobinaemias. Methaemoglobin is a derivative of haemoglobin in which Fe^{2+}, which binds O_2 reversibly, is replaced by its oxidized form (Fe^{3+}), which binds O_2 irreversibly.

Genetic abnormalities in the O_2-sensing system (summarized briefly in Fig. 2) have not yet been described. Mice lacking hypoxia-inducible factor (HIF)-1α are viable, but are unable to increase their hematocrit levels in response to hypoxia, suggesting that mutations may eventually be found which are not likely to be lethal. In this regard, a congenital polycythaemia common in the Chuvashia region of Russia is characterized both by increased erythropoietin responsiveness of the erythroid cells and by increased erythropoietin concentration in serum. This polycythaemia is not associated with mutations in either *EPO* or *EPO-R* and represents a good candidate for a defective O_2-sensing apparatus such as mutations in the *HIF-1α* gene. Examples of acquired polycythaemias due to defects of the hypoxia-sensing mechanism are renal and neuronal cancers associated with mutations in the von Hippel-Lindau (*VHL*) gene. The product of this gene is a member of the protein complex responsible for the stabilization/degradation of HIF-1α. *VHL* mutations result in overexpression of VEGF and of other O_2-regulated genes.

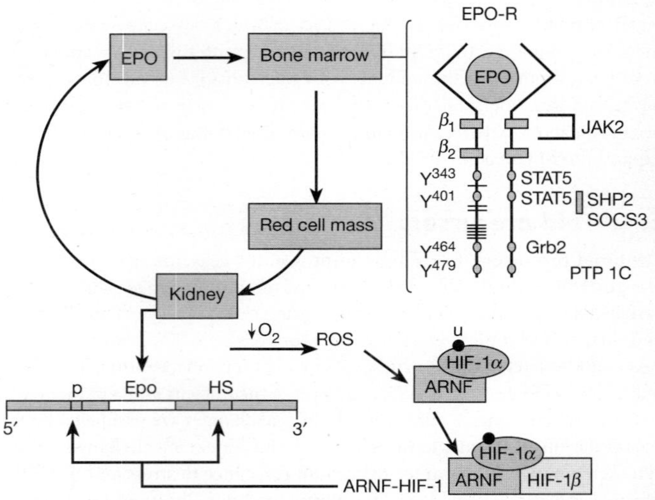

Fig. 2 The regulation of erythroid cell mass. The number of circulating red cells is regulated by the levels of erythropoietin (**EPO**) produced by the kidney under the exquisite control of the hypoxia-sensing machinery. Several pathways are involved in hypoxic recognition and respond by producing reactive O_2 species (**ROS**). The purpose is to rescue (by ubiquitination) hypoxia-induced factor-1α (**HIF-1α**) from degradation, to facilitate its complex formation with aryl-hydrocarbon nuclear translocator (**ARNF**) and with the ubiquitously expressed β subunit of HIF-1. ARNF–HIF-1 activates the expression of several hypoxia-responsive genes such as *EPO*, glucose transporters, glycolytic enzymes, platelet-derived growth factor (**PDGF**), and vascular endothelial factor (VEFG). (ARNF ablation results in embryonic lethality attributed to the loss of induction of VEGF). ARNF–HIF-1 activates the expression of hypoxia-inducible genes by binding to specific cognate sequences, that, in the case of *EPO*, are present both in its promoter (indicated as p, a typical TATA less promoter) and in its DNA-hypersensitive site (**HS**), which has the function of a hypoxia-inducible enhancer. The enhancer is activated by the binding of a protein complex formed by HIF-1 itself, by the constitutively expressed hepatic nuclear factor-4 (**HNF-4**), and by the general transcriptional activator p300. Of note, the EPO promoter and enhancer also contain binding sites for the steroid hormone receptor, closing the bridge between activation of these receptors and control of the haematocrit level. Another link between a response to stress and EPO expression is provided by p38α, a member of the mitogen-activated protein (**MAP**) family that may be involved in cobalt-induced stabilization of HIF-1α and induction of EPO expression, at least in the fetal liver. EPO induces its effects in the marrow by binding to a specific receptor (**EPO-R**) present on erythroid cells. EPO/EPO-R binding induces tyrosine autophosphorylation and the activation of JAK2 (Janus kinase-2) which is physically associated to its cytoplasmic Box 1 (β1) domain. The activation of the JAK2 catalytic domain is responsible for the phosphorylation of several other proteins, including the EPO-R itself (phosphotyrosine residues involved in docking EPO-R with its transducer proteins are indicated as filled circle, not to scale), STAT5 (signal transducer and activator of transcription-5), and proteins involved in the Ras and PKC (protein kinase C) signal-transduction pathways. On the other hand, at least three other pathways are involved in bringing the receptor complex back to its resting configuration after activation: the phosphatase PTP-1C (protein tyrosine phosphatase-1C) /SHP2 (Src-homology-phosphatase 2), SOCS3 (suppressor of cytokine signalling-3) (overexpression of SOCS3 in transgenic mice results in embryonically lethal anaemia), and the proteasomes, which downregulate the number of activated receptors on the cell surface. PTP-1C becomes physically associated through its SH2 domains with Y479 after EPO stimulation, and SOCS3 becomes associated with the Y401 of EPO-R and with JAK2. The narrow bars on the left side of the EPO-R diagram indicate mutations identified in humans that result in familial erythrocytosis.

Erythropoietin signalling pathway

Erythropoietin triggers its biological effect by binding to a specific 64- to 78-kDa (depending on its glycosylation degree) receptor, EPO-R, encoded by a gene on human chromosome 19p. This gene is expressed in erythroid, megakaryocytic, and endothelial cells. Also, marrow cells express high levels of soluble EPO-R species. These may be involved in the fine tuning of erythropoietin concentrations in specific marrow niches, thus allowing erythroid versus myeloid development. In addition to the full-length EPO-R (EPO-RF), immature erythroid cells express a truncated form of the receptor (EPO-RT) that acts as a dominant negative regulator of the EPO-RF mediated signals in mice.

The concentration of EPO-R on the surface of erythroid cells is roughly proportional to their erythropoietin responsiveness *in vitro* (Fig. 1). EPO-R is first detected on BFU-e (around 300 high-affinity erythropoietin binding sites per cell). Its expression increases as the cells progress to CFU-e and proerythroblasts (about 1100 high-affinity sites), but is virtually absent on late normoblasts and reticulocytes. The increase in EPO-R expression observed during erythroid differentiation is also accompanied by a decreased expression of receptors for early-acting growth factors, such as SCF and IL-3 (Fig. 1).

The rapid dimerization induced by erythropoietin binding to its receptor triggers a conformational change that results in autophosphorylation and activation of the kinase catalytic domain of JAK2, a member of the Janus kinase family (Fig. 2). JAK2 phosphorylates and activates several proteins, some of which are responsible for further transmitting the signal to the nucleus, while others, such as the protein tyrosine phosphatases (PTP)-1C (also called HCP or SHP) and -1D (or Syp), dephosphorylate the receptor complex, bringing it back to its resting configuration (Fig. 2). PTP-1C is physically associated with the carboxyterminal domain of EPO-R, a region that is deleted in all of the eight different mutations of *EPO-R* found to be associated with congenital erythrocytosis. 32D cells transfected with one such mutant receptor required erythropoietin to activate the JAK2/STAT5 pathway, but in these cells the activation lasted longer than in cells transfected with the normal receptor. This may explain why congenital polycythaemia/erythrocytosis is characterized by hyper-responsive, erythropoietin-dependent, CFU-e growth. Not all mutations of *EPO-R* cause polycythaemia, however. Two additionally described single-point *EPO-R* mutations are not accompanied by functional consequences or changes in hematocrit.

Signalling through EPO-R triggers several cellular responses, including inhibition of apoptosis, stimulation of cell proliferation, and the induction of expression of erythroid specific genes—that is, the globin genes. The best-studied effect of erythropoietin on erythroid cells is suppression of apoptosis. In fact, mice with targeted deletions of either *Epo*, of its receptor, or of its immediate signal-transduction protein JAK2, die prenatally because of profound anaemia. The livers of these fetuses contain normal numbers of BFU-e and CFU-e, but very few erythroblasts, all of which display signs of apoptosis. These results suggest that these defects impair the final stages of erythroid differentiation by interfering with the erythroblast's ability to survive. Erythropoietin/EPO-R signalling inhibits apoptosis through suppression of caspases (cysteine proteases with aspartate specificity). In erythroid cells, these degrade the erythroid-specific transcription factor GATA1, which is responsible not only for the activation of all the erythroid-specific genes analysed so far, but also of the antiapoptotic protein Bcl-xL. An indirect confirmation of the role of GATA1 in preventing apoptosis of erythroid cells is provided by a recent mutation described in the DNA-binding domain of *GATA1* causing anaemia and thrombocytopenia. As *GATA1* is on the X chromosome, it is possible that other X-linked anaemias or thalassaemia may be due to *GATA1* mutations yet to be identified.

Since survival is a cellular function which is dominant over proliferation, the phenotype of the deletion *Epo*/*Epo-R* mutant mice cannot exclude that erythropoietin may also play a role in the control of proliferation (or differentiation) at later stages of the erythroid differentiation. BFU-e are at least partially dependent on erythropoietin for proliferation and differentiation *in vitro*, but are insensitive to endogenous erythropoietin levels, and neither sustained anaemia nor hypertransfusion alters their frequency and cell-cycle characteristics. In contrast, both the number and cycling characteristics of CFU-e are increased three- to sixfold over the control value. Furthermore, fetal murine CFU-e which constitutively express either Bcl-2 or Bcl-xL survive but do not form colonies in the absence of erythropoietin.

Although the effects of erythropoietin on cell proliferation are not as well characterized as its effects on apoptosis, it can be expected that defects in the proliferation pathway may also result in altered red cell output. In this regard, polycythaemia vera is a human myeloproliferative disorder caused by an acquired presumed mutation at the stem-cell level that results in the formation of CFU-e-derived colonies in the absence of erythropoietin. A familiar autosomal dominant predisposition towards acquiring polycythaemia vera between the ages of 50 and 60 years of age has been described. Since, polycythaemia vera, in contrast to familial polycythaemia, may evolve into leukaemia, it is possible that its defect involves alterations in the proliferative control of erythroid cells.

Red cell homeostasis

Normal red cells have a finite lifespan of 120 ± 20 days. With red cell ageing, metabolic changes decrease their flexibility as they traverse through the microvasculature and promote their lysis or phagocytosis. Thus, the red cell's longevity and ability to carry out its proper function is critically dependent on cell-membrane structure and metabolism. The red cell membrane consists of a lipid bilayer and structural and integral membrane proteins which provide a lattice network under the bilayer and create the red cell cytoskeleton. Inherited defects in protein structure (hereditary spherocytosis, **HS**; hereditary elliptocytosis, **HE**; hereditary pyropoikilocytosis, **HPP**; etc.) lead to haemolytic anaemias. A number of specific receptors and enzymes are also associated with membrane proteins, several of which are important for the maintenance of its structural integrity or for nutrient and ion transport. Enzyme defects in metabolic pathways (pyruvate kinase, **PK**; hexokinase, **G6PD**), or haemoglobin defects (sickle-cell anaemia) can also increase the haemolytic potential of the red cell.

The character of the external red cell surface is defined by its antigenic structure. Over 300 antigens have been identified and many of these contribute to 15 genetic blood group systems. The latter are composed of oligosaccharide prosthetic groups of the integral membrane proteins and complex glycolipids. Nearly all (the Lewis system is an exception) are intrinsic components of the membrane and appear early in the differentiation process. Coating of red cell surface antigens with antibodies in cases of acquired autoimmunity interferes with the membrane functional integrity and allows rapid phagocytosis.

The transport of O_2 by red cells is dependent on their number, their haemoglobin content, and the ability to release O_2 or to increase 2,3DPG, according to tissue needs. However, O_2 transport by red cells is but one of the elements in a multicomponent highly integrated process that is responsible for appropriate O_2 supply to the tissues. A number of other physiological parameters, such as pulmonary function (sufficient O_2 loading in lungs), and haemodynamic factors (cardiac output, blood volume, and viscosity) must be incorporated in an integrated fashion. When anaemia is present, restoration of red cell number is dependent on the degree of erythropoietin stimulation, the ability to increase erythroid proliferation (adequate folic acid, vitamin B_{12} levels, etc.) within the bone marrow, and on the circulating levels and a normal erythroid cell response to iron. Several of these issues are addressed in more details in other chapters.

Finally, several hormones involved in the control of the cellular metabolism, such as corticosteroids, androgens, growth hormone, thyroxine, β-adrenergic agonists, and certain prostaglandins, stimulate erythroid differentiation *in vitro* in synergy with erythropoietin, or can alter hematocrit levels *in vivo*. A direct involvement of glucocorticoids in the control of the red cell mass has recently been provided by the observation that mice lacking the glucocorticoid receptor recover very poorly from haemolytic anaemia caused by phenylhydrazine treatment.

Further reading

Adamson JW (1968). The erythropoietin–hematocrit relationship in normal and polycythemic man: implications of marrow regulation. *Blood* **32**, 597–609.

Arcasoy MO, Harris KW, Forget BG (1999). A human erythropoietin receptor gene mutant causing familial erythrocytosis is associated with deregulation of the rates of Jak2 and Stat5 inactivation. *Experimental Hematology* **27**, 63–74.

Bauer A, *et al.* (1999). The glucocorticoid receptor is required for stress erythropoiesis. *Genes and Development* **13**, 2996.

Broudy VC, *et al.* (1996). Interaction of stem cell factor and its receptor c-kit mediates lodgment and acute expansion of hematopoietic cells in the murine spleen. *Blood* **88**, 75–81.

Carnot P, Deflandre C (1906). Sur l'activitéhématopoietique des serum au cours de la régénération du sang. *Academie des Sciences Medicale* **3**, 384.

Charbord P, *et al.* (1996). Early ontogeny of the human marrow from long bones: an immunohistochemical study of hematopoiesis and its microenvironment. *Blood* **87**, 4109–19.

Dybedal I, Jacobsen SE (1995). Transforming growth factor beta (TGF-beta), a potent inhibitor of erythropoiesis: neutralizing TGF-beta antibodies show erythropoietin as a potent stimulator of murine burst-forming unit erythroid colony formation in the absence of a burst-promoting activity. *Blood* **86**, 949–57.

Ebert BL, Bunn HF (1999). Regulation of the erythropoietin gene. *Blood* **94** 1864–77.

Era T, *et al.* (1997). Thrombopoietin enhances proliferation and differentiation of murine yolk sac erythroid progenitors. *Blood* **89**, 1207–13.

Eschbach J, *et al.* (1987). Correction of the anemia of endstage renal disease with recombinant human erythropoietin. *New England Journal of Medicine* **316**, 73.

Fennie C, *et al.* (1995). CD34+ endothelial cell lines derived from murine yolk sac induce the proliferation and differentiation of yolk sac CD34+ hematopoietic progenitors. *Blood* **86**, 4454–67.

Fleischman RA, Gallardo T, Mi X (1996). Mutations in the ligand-binding domain of the kit receptor: an uncommon site in human piebaldism. *Journal of Investigative Dermatology* **107**, 703–6.

Gallagher PG, Benz EJ, Jr (2001). The erythrocyte membrane and cytoskeleton: structure, function and disorders. In: Stamatoyannopoulos G, *et al.*, eds. *The molecular basis of blood diseases*, 3rd edn, pp. 275–305. WB Saunders, Philadelphia.

Hiyake T, Kung CK-H, Goldwasser E (1977). Purification of human erythropoietin. *Journal of Biological Chemistry* **252**, 5558.

Huehns ER, *et al.* (1964). Human embryonic haemoglobins. *Nature* **201**, 1095.

Ihle JN (2001). Signal transduction in the regulation of hematopoiesis. In: Stamatoyannopoulos G, *et al.*, eds. *The molecular basis of blood diseases*, 3rd edn, pp. 103–125. WB Saunders, Philadelphia.

Iliopoulos O, *et al.* (1996). Negative regulation of hypoxia-inducible genes by the von Hippel-Lindau protein. *Proceedings of the National Academy of Sciences, USA* **93**, 10595.

Jacobs K, *et al.* (1985). Isolation and characterization of genomic and cDNA clones of human erythropoietin. *Nature* **313**, 806.

Kelemen E, Calvo W, Fliedner TM (1979). *Atlas of human hemopoietic development.* Springer, Berlin.

Koury MJ, Bondurant MC (1990). Erythropoietin retards DNA breakdown and prevents programmed death in erythroid progenitor cells. *Science* **248**, 378–81.

Kralovics R, Prchal JT (2000). Congenital and inherited polycythemia. *Current Opinion in Pediatrics* **12**, 29–34.

Lin CS, *et al.* (1996). Differential effects of an erythropoietin receptor gene disruption on primitive and definitive erythropoiesis. *Genes and Development* **10**, 154–64.

Maltepe E, *et al.* (1997). Abnormal angiogenesis and responses to glucose and oxygen deprivation in mice lacking the protein ARNT. *Nature* **386**, 403–7.

Marcus D, ed. (1981). Blood group immunochemistry and genetics. *Seminars in Hematology* **18** 1.

Marine JC, *et al.* (1999). SOCS3 is essential in the regulation of fetal liver erythropoiesis. *Cell* **98**, 617–27.

Migliaccio AR, Papayannopoulou Th (2001). Erythropoiesis. In: Steinberg MH, *et al.*, eds. *Disorders of hemoglobin, genetics, pathophysiology, clinical management.* pp. 52–71.

Moore MA, Metcalf D (1970). Ontogeny of the haemopoietic system: yolk sac origin of *in vivo* and *in vitro* colony forming cells in the developing mouse embryo. *British Journal of Haematology* **18**, 279–96.

Moritz KM, Lim GB, Wintour EM (1997). Developmental regulation of erythropoietin and erythropoiesis. *American Journal of Physiology* **273**, 1829–44.

Nakamura Y, *et al.* (1998). Impaired erythropoiesis in transgenic mice overexpressing a truncated erythropoietin receptor. *Experimental Hematology* **26**, 1105–10.

Nichols KE, *et al.* (2000). Familial dyserythropoietic anaemia and thrombocytopenia due to an inherited mutation in GATA1. *Nature Genetics* **24**, 266–70.

Orkin SH, Weiss MJ (1999). Cutting red-cell production. *Nature* **401**, 433–6.

Orkin SH (2001). Transcription factors that regulate lineage decisions. In: Stamatoyannopoulos G, *et al.*, eds. *The molecular basis of blood diseases*, 3rd edn, pp.80–94. WB Saunders, Philadelphia.

Papayannopoulou T, Abkowitz J, D'Andrea AD (2000). Biology of erythropoiesis, erythroid differentiation, and maturation. In: Hoffman R, *et al.*, eds. *Hematology. Basic principles and practice*, pp 202–19. Churchill Livingstone, New York.

Ponka P (1997). Tissue-specific regulation of iron metabolism and heme synthesis: distinct control mechanisms in erythroid cells. *Blood* **89**, 1–25.

Raskind WH, *et al.* (2000). Mapping of a syndrome of X-linked thrombocytopenia and thalassemia to band Xp11–12: further evidence of genetic heterogeneity of X-linked thrombocytopenia. *Blood* **95**, 2262.

Reissmann KR (1950). Studies on the mechanism of erythropoietic stimulation in parabiotic rats during hypoxia. *Blood* **5**, 372.

Rico-Vargas SA, *et al.* (1994). c-kit expression by B cell precursors in mouse bone marrow. Stimulation of B cell genesis by *in vivo* treatment with anti-c-kit antibody. *Journal of Immunology* **152**, 2845–52.

Russell ES (1979). Hereditary anemias of the mouse: a review for geneticists. *Advances in Genetics* **20**, 357–459.

Sasaki A, *et al.* (2000). CIS3/SOCS3 suppresses erythropoietin signalling by binding the EPO receptor and JAK2. *Journal of Biological Chemistry* July 5, on-line.

Sato T, *et al.* (2000). Erythroid progenitors differentiate and mature in response to endogenous erythropoietin. *Journal of Clinical Investigation* **106**, 263–270.

Semenza GL (1999). Perspectives on oxygen sensing. *Cell* 98, 281–4.

Shimizu R, Komatsu N, Miura Y (1999). Dominant negative effect of a truncated erythropoietin receptor (EPOR- T) on erythropoietin-induced erythroid differentiation: possible involvement of EPOR-T in ineffective erythropoiesis of myelodysplastic syndrome. *Experimental Hematology* **27**, 229–33.

Southcott MJ, Tanner MJ, Anstee DJ (1999). The expression of human blood group antigens during erythropoiesis in a cell culture system. *Blood* **93**, 4425–35.

Spivak JL (2000). The blood in systemic disorders. *Lancet* **355**, 1707–12.

Spritz RA, Beighton P (1998). Piebaldism with deafness: molecular evidence for an expanded syndrome. *American Journal of Medical Genetics* **75**, 101–3.

Stamatoyannopoulos G, Grosveld F (2001). Hemoglobin switching. In: Stamatoyannopoulos G, *et al.*, eds. *The molecular basis of blood diseases*, 3rd edn, 135–65. WB Saunders, Philadelphia.

Stohlman K Jr, Rath CE, Rose JC (1954). Evidence for a humoral regulation of erythropoiesis: studies on a patient with polycythemia secondary to regional exposure to hypoxia. *Blood* **9**, 721.

Stopka T, *et al.* (1998). Human hematopoietic progenitors express erythropoietin. *Blood* **91**, 3766–72.

Takakura N, *et al.* (2000). A role for hematopoietic stem cells in promoting angiogenesis. *Cell* **102**, 199–209.

Tamura K, *et al.* (2000). Requirement for p38α in erythropoietin expression: a role for stress kinases in erythropoiesis. *Cell* **102**, 221–31.

Vaziri H, *et al.* (1994). Evidence for a mitotic clock in human hematopoietic stem cells: loss of telomeric DNA with age. *Proceedings of the National Academy of Sciences, USA* **91**, 9857–60.

Verdier F, *et al.* (2000). Proteasomes regulate the duration of erythropoietin receptor activation by controlling down-regulation of cell surface receptors. *Journal of Biological Chemistry* **275**, 18375–81.

Verfaillie CM (2000). Anatomy and physiology of hematopoiesis. In: Hoffman R, *et al.*, eds. *Hematology. Basic principles and practice*, pp 139–54. Churchill Livingstone, New York.

Winearls C, *et al.* (1986). Effects of human erythropoietin derived from recombinant DNA on the anemia of patients maintained on chronic hemodialysis. *Lancet* **2**, 1175.

Wu H, *et al.* (1995). Generation of committed erythroid BFU-E and CFU-E progenitors does not require erythropoietin or the erythropoietin receptor. *Cell* **83**, 59–67.

Yu AY, *et al.* (1999). Impaired physiological responses to chronic hypoxia in mice partially deficient for hypoxia-inducible factor 1α. *Journal of Clinical Investigation* **103**, 691–6.

Zucali JR, Stevens V, Mirand EA (1975). *In vitro* production of erythropoietin by mouse fetal liver. *Blood* **46**, 85–90.

22.5.2 Anaemia: pathophysiology, classification, and clinical features

D. J. Weatherall

The main function of the red blood cells is oxygen transport. Hence a functional definition of anaemia is 'a state in which the circulating red-cell mass is insufficient to meet the oxygen requirements of the tissues'. However, many compensatory mechanisms can be brought into play to restore the oxygen supply to the vital centres, and therefore in clinical practice this definition is of limited value. For this reason anaemia is usually defined as 'a reduction of the haemoglobin concentration, red-cell count, or packed cell volume (**PCV**) to below normal levels'.

The definition of anaemia

It has been extremely difficult to establish a normal range of haematological values, and hence the definition of anaemia usually involves the adoption of rather arbitrary criteria. For example, the World Health Organization recommends that anaemia should be considered to exist in adults whose haemoglobin levels are lower than 13 g/dl (males) or 12 g/dl (females). Children aged 6 months to 6 years are considered anaemic at haemoglobin levels below 11 g/dl, and those aged 6 to 14 years below 12 g/dl. The disadvantage of such arbitrary criteria for defining anaemia is that there may be many apparently normal individuals whose haemoglobin concentration is below their optimal level. Furthermore, the published 'normal values' for adults (see Chapter 22.1) indicate that there is such a large standard deviation that many adult females must be considered 'normal' even though they have haemoglobin levels below 12 g/dl.

Prevalence of anaemia

Anaemia is a major world health problem and its distribution and prevalence in the developing world are considered in detail in the next chapter.

The prevalence of anaemia has been studied in many populations, but it is difficult to compare data from different sources because of variations in methodology and criteria. Certain patterns emerge, however. An early survey carried out in Great Britain established that haemoglobin levels were low in a significant proportion of the population, particularly susceptible groups being children under the age of 5 years, pregnant women, and those in social classes IV and V. A later random population study in the United Kingdom reported a prevalence of anaemia of 14 per cent for women aged 55 to 64 years and 3 per cent for men aged 35 to 64 years. These and similar studies have shown that anaemia is most common in women between the ages of 15 and 44 years and that it then becomes relatively less frequent, although the prevalence increases again in the 75-and-over age group. Interestingly, it is only in the last group that the prevalence in males and females is almost the same. Where the cause of the anaemia has been analysed in these surveys, the majority of cases have been due to iron deficiency. No doubt these prevalence data vary considerably between the developed countries, but it is clear that nutritional anaemia is relatively common in most populations at certain periods during development and late in life.

Adaptation to anaemia

The function of the red cell is to carry oxygen between the lungs and the tissues. However, tissue oxygenation is the result of a complex series of interactions of different organ systems, of which the red cell is only one (Table 1). Obviously the cardiac output, ventilatory function, and state of the capillaries are of great importance as well. Each of these oxygen supply systems is regulated differently. Ventilation responds to changes in pH, CO_2, and hypoxia. Cardiac output responds to the amount of blood entering the heart, and this is regulated mainly by the effects of tissue metabolism as it modifies the resistance to blood flow in the microvasculature. The erythron itself responds to changes in haemoglobin concentration, arterial oxygen saturation, and to the oxygen affinity of the circulating haemoglobin. Thus a decreased capacity of any of these components may be compensated for by increased activity of the others in an attempt to maintain tissue oxygenation.

Oxygen diffuses across the alveolar membrane and into the blood, which equilibrates with the alveolar gas; the approximate oxygen tension is 100 mmHg, at which the blood is fully saturated with an oxygen content of 20 vol per cent. As blood is pumped through the tissue capillaries oxygen diffuses out. Although the venous oxygen tension varies between organs, the oxygen tension of the pooled venous blood in the pulmonary artery, the 'mixed venous oxygen tension', is remarkably constant at 40 mmHg. At this oxygen tension the oxygen content is 15 vol per cent. Hence, oxygen delivery, as measured by the arteriovenous oxygen difference, is normally 5 vol per cent. By reducing the oxygen-carrying capacity of blood, anaemia tends

Table 1 The steps involved in the transport of oxygen to the tissues

Steps	Factors involved
Ambient O_2 tension ↓	Altitude
Ventilation ↓	Alveolar ventilation Gas-to-blood diffusion Ventilation/perfusion ratio Anatomical shunt
Circulation ↓	Cardiac output Blood: haemoglobin concentration oxygen-dissociation curve
Tissue diffusion	Intercapillary distance

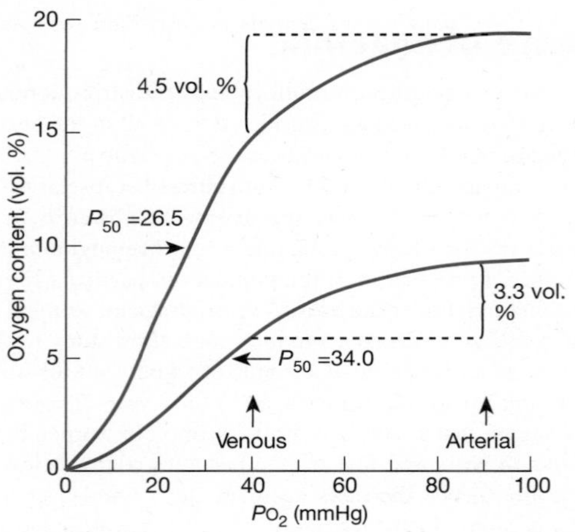

Fig. 1 Enhancement of oxygen loading by decreased red-cell oxygen affinity in a patient with anaemia. An anaemic patient with a 50 per cent reduction in haemoglobin concentration has only a 27 per cent reduction in oxygen unloading. (Based on Klocke RA (1972). *Chest*, **69**, 795.)

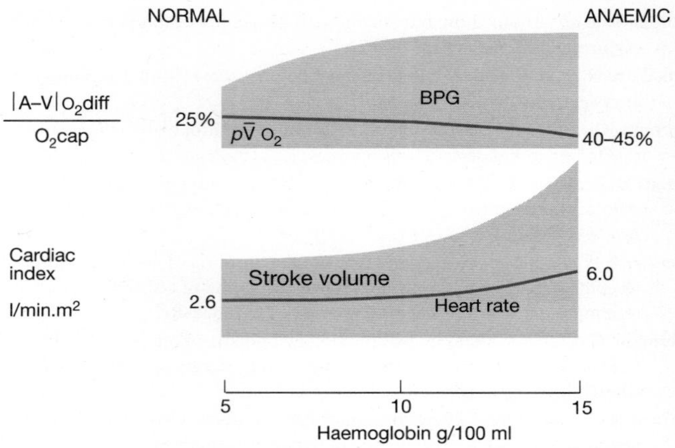

Fig. 2 The changes in factors involved in oxygen delivery with progressive anaemia. As anaemia becomes more severe, cardiac compensation becomes more significant ($P(V)O_2$, mixed venous oxygen tension). (From Bellingham, 1974.)

to reduce the arteriovenous oxygen difference, and this may be compensated for by the following mechanisms: (1) modulation of oxygen affinity; (2) redistribution of flow between different organs; (3) increase in cardiac output; and (4) reduction of mixed venous oxygen tension to increase the arteriovenous oxygen difference.

Intrinsic red-cell adaptation

The consequences of anaemia on the normal oxygen-binding curve of blood are shown in Fig. 1. Anaemia, by lowering the haemoglobin concentration, proportionately reduces the oxygen-carrying capacity of the blood. As a response to this there is an increase in the 2,3-biphosphoglycerate (**2,3-BPG**) concentration in the red cell, shifting the dissociation curve to the right, so significantly enhancing tissue oxygen delivery (Fig. 1).

With increasing severity of anaemia there is a progressive increase in 2,3-DPG, which may increase oxygen delivery by as much as 40 per cent for the same haemoglobin concentration. It should be noted, however, that a consequence of this adaptation is a lower venous oxygen content and hence a lower reserve of oxygen available for a further increase in oxygen demand, as might occur on exercise for example. Hence the increase in 2,3-BPG in anaemia tends to ameliorate the effects of the diminished oxygen-carrying capacity of the blood, so reducing the adaptation required by other steps involved in tissue oxygen delivery (Fig. 2). 2,3-BPG levels vary in a variety of other clinical conditions, some of which are summarized in Table 2.

Local changes in tissue perfusion

The total blood volume does not change greatly in anaemia and therefore increased tissue perfusion has to be achieved by shunting blood from less to more vital organs. There is vasoconstriction of the vessels of the skin and kidney; this mechanism has little effect on renal function. The organs that gain from the redistribution seem to be mainly the myocardium, brain, and muscle.

Cardiovascular changes

It seems likely that mild anaemia is compensated for by shifts in the oxygen dissociation curve. Overall, oxygen consumption is unchanged in anaemia. However, when the haemoglobin level falls below 7 to 8 g/dl, there is an increase in cardiac output, both at rest and after exercise (Fig. 2). The stroke rate increases and a hyperkinetic circulation develops, characterized by tachycardia, arterial and capillary pulsation, a wide pulse pressure, and haemic murmurs. The circulation time is shortened, left ventricular stroke work is increased, and coronary flow increased in proportion to the increased cardiac output. It has been found that there is an acute reversal of the high-output state of chronic anaemia in response to orthostatic stress or pressor amines. This suggests that redistribution of blood volume and vasodilatation with reduced afterload play a dominant role in the hyperkinetic circulatory responses to chronic anaemia. The mechanism of the vasodilatation is not known; it may be a direct result of tissue hypoxia. An additional factor that may be of some importance in increasing cardiac output is the reduction in blood viscosity produced by a relatively low red-cell mass.

While the normal myocardium may tolerate sustained hyperactivity of this type indefinitely, patients with coronary artery disease or those with extreme anaemia may have impaired oxygenation of the myocardium. In such cases, cardiomegaly, pulmonary oedema, ascites, and peripheral oedema may occur, and a state of high-output cardiac failure is established. At this stage the plasma volume is almost always increased.

Pulmonary function

As blood, regardless of its oxygen-carrying capacity, is almost completely oxygenated in the lungs, the oxygen pressure of arterial blood in an anaemic patient should be the same as that in a normal individual, and hence an increase in respiratory rate should not improve the oxygenation of

Table 2 Some conditions in which there is a change in red-cell 2,3-diphosphoglycerate (DPG) levels leading to modification of oxygen transport

Increased 2,3-BPG; increased p50, reduced whole-blood oxygen affinity
Anaemia
Alkalosis
Hyperphosphataemia
Renal failure
Hypoxia
Pregnancy
Cyanotic congenital heart disease
Thyrotoxicosis
Some red-cell enzyme deficiencies
Decreased 2,3-BPG; decreased p50, increased whole-blood oxygen affinity
Acidosis
Cardiogenic or septicaemic shock
Hypophosphataemia
Hypothyroidism
Hypopituitarism
Following replacement with stored blood

the tissues. Curiously, however, severe anaemia is associated with dyspnoea. Although in some patients this may be related to incipient cardiac failure, in most cases it appears to be an inappropriate response to hypoxia which is centrally mediated.

Clinical manifestations and classification of anaemia

Clinical effects of anaemia

Because anaemia reduces tissue oxygenation it is not surprising that it is associated with widespread organ dysfunction and hence an extremely varied clinical picture. The picture depends, of course, on whether the anaemia is of rapid or more insidious onset.

After acute blood loss the red-cell mass and plasma volume are reduced proportionately and the symptoms are mainly of volume depletion. Depending on the amount of fluid replacement there may be a small fall in the PCV during the first 10 h; volume replacement by the influx of albumin from the extravascular compartment takes between 60 and 90 h. Hence the picture of rapid blood loss is characterized by the typical syndrome of shock, with collapse, dyspnoea, tachycardia, a poor volume pulse, reduced blood pressure, and marked peripheral vasoconstriction.

With anaemia of a more insidious onset, the compensatory mechanisms outlined above have time to come into play. In mild anaemia there may be no symptoms or simply increased fatigue and a slight pallor. As the anaemia becomes more marked the symptoms and signs gradually appear. Pallor is best discerned in the mucous membranes; the nailbeds and palmar creases, although often said to be useful sites for detecting anaemia, are relatively insensitive for this purpose. Cardiorespiratory symptoms and signs include exertional dyspnoea, tachycardia, palpitations, angina or claudication, night cramps, increased arterial pulsation, capillary pulsation, a variety of cardiac bruits, reversible cardiac enlargement, and, if cardiac failure occurs, basal crepitations, peripheral oedema, and ascites. Neuromuscular involvement is reflected by headache, vertigo, light-headedness, faintness, tinnitus, roaring in the ears, cramps, increased cold sensitivity, and haemorrhages in the retina. Acute anaemia may occasionally give rise to papilloedema. Gastrointestinal symptoms include loss of appetite, nausea, constipation, and diarrhoea. Genitourinary involvement causes menstrual irregularities, urinary frequency, and loss of libido. There may be a low-grade fever.

In the elderly, in whom associated degenerative arterial disease is common, anaemia may present with the onset of cardiac failure. Alternatively, previously undiagnosed coronary narrowing may be unmasked by the onset of angina. Other symptoms of arterial degenerative disease may be also exacerbated or unmasked; intermittent claudication and a variety of neurological pictures associated with cerebral arteriosclerosis for example. It is important that anaemia is recognized as a contributing factor to the symptoms of these degenerative diseases as its correction may frequently bring about considerable symptomatic improvement.

Causes and classification of anaemia

A reduction in the red-cell mass can result from either the defective production of red cells or an increased rate of loss of cells, either by premature destruction or bleeding. Decreased production of red cells may result from a reduced rate of proliferation of precursors in the bone marrow or from failure of maturation leading to their intramedullary destruction: that is to say, ineffective erythropoiesis. Based on this approach we can derive a very simple pathophysiological classification of anaemia, as shown in Table 3, in which the causes are divided into failure of red-cell proliferation, defective maturation, haemolysis, and blood loss.

Table 3 The main groups of anaemias classified according to the underlying cause

Reduced red-cell production:
Defective precursor proliferation
Defective precursor maturation
Defective proliferation and maturation
Increased rate of red-cell destruction:
Haemolysis
Loss of red cells from the circulation:
Bleeding

Anaemia due to defective proliferation of red-cell precursors

The major causes of this group of anaemias are an inadequate supply of iron, primary diseases of the bone marrow that involve stem cells or later erythroid precursors, and a reduction in the amount of erythropoietin reaching the red-cell precursors (Table 4).

Iron deficiency results in defective erythroid proliferation and also in abnormal maturation of the red-cell precursors due to defective haemoglobin synthesis. Red-cell precursors require adequate iron supplies for normal proliferation, and the anaemia of iron deficiency tends to be hypoproliferative as well as dyserythropoietic. Chronic inflammatory disorders and related conditions also interfere with the iron supply to precursors, probably by blocking the release of catabolized red-cell iron from reticuloendothelial cells. The basic defect in iron-deficiency anaemia and that due to inflammation is similar, therefore, in that the supply of iron is inadequate to meet the requirements for erythropoiesis.

Defective proliferation of red-cell precursors can result from any of the causes of bone marrow failure, including infiltration with leukaemic or

Table 4 Main causes of anaemia due to defective production of red cells

Reduced proliferation of precursors
Iron deficiency anaemia
Anaemia of chronic disorders:
Infections, malignancy, collagen disease, etc.
Reduced erythropoietin production:
Renal disease
Reduced oxygen requirements:
Hypothyroidism
Hypopituitarism
Reduced O_2 affinity of haemoglobin
Primary disease of the bone marrow:
Aplastic anaemia:
primary
secondary to drugs, irradiation, chemicals, toxins, etc.
Pure red-cell hypoplasia
Infiltrative disorders:
leukaemia
lymphoma
secondary carcinoma
myelofibrosis
Defective maturation of precursors
Nuclear maturation:
Vitamin B_{12} deficiency
Folate deficiency
Erythroleukaemia
Cytoplasmic maturation:
Iron deficiency
Disorders of globin synthesis
Disorders of haem and/or iron metabolism
Disorders of porphyrin metabolism
Unknown mechanism:
Congenital dyserythropoietic anaemias
Myelodysplastic syndrome
Infection
Toxins and chemicals

other neoplastic cells, damage due to ionizing radiation, drugs, or infection, and various intrinsic lesions of the stem cells or red-cell precursors. The intrinsic disorders include the congenital hypoplastic anaemias, involving either all the formed elements or the red-cell precursors alone.

Finally, decreased proliferation of the red-cell precursors may result from erythropoietin deficiency. The most common cause is chronic renal failure. A similar mechanism may be involved in conditions in which the tissue requirement for oxygen is reduced. These include various endocrine disorders such as hypothyroidism and hypopituitarism. It may also explain the mild anaemia associated with haemoglobin variants with decreased oxygen affinity.

As a group, the hypoproliferative anaemias are associated with a low reticulocyte count and defective proliferation of the bone marrow precursors. The red cells are usually normochromic and normocytic, although there may be a mild macrocytosis. If the anaemia is due to iron deficiency, the cells are hypochromic. If granulopoiesis is normal, the defect in red-cell proliferation is reflected by an increase in the myeloid:erythroid (**M/E**) ratio.

Defective red-cell maturation

Defects of red-cell maturation may involve primarily nuclear or cytoplasmic maturation (Table 4). Those involving nuclear maturation include vitamin B_{12} and folic acid deficiency and other causes of megaloblastic anaemia, and some of the primary marrow disorders including erythroleukaemia. The important causes of defective cytoplasmic maturation include the inherited disorders of globin synthesis, the thalassaemia syndromes, and the genetic and acquired defects of iron metabolism that characterize the sideroblastic anaemias. There are other genetic defects of red-cell maturation, the congenital dyserythropoietic anaemias, in which the aetiology is unknown. Furthermore, agents such as drugs, chemicals, and infections may interfere with erythroid maturation.

The main pathological mechanism common to all the anaemias that result from maturation abnormalities is ineffective erythropoiesis. In other words, there is marked erythroid proliferation but many of the precursors are destroyed in the bone marrow before they enter the circulation. Hence, the characteristic finding is marked erythroid hyperplasia with a reduction in the M/E ratio, associated with a low reticulocyte count. Because of the significant intramedullary destruction of precursors there is usually an elevated level of bilirubin and lactate dehydrogenase. Furthermore, there are nearly always morphological abnormalities of the red-cell precursors. The anaemias that are associated with abnormal nuclear maturation, such as those due to vitamin B_{12} and folic acid deficiency, are characterized by megaloblastic erythropoiesis and macrocytic red cells, while those caused by abnormal cytoplasmic maturation are characterized by normoblastic hyperplasia and hypochromic and microcytic red cells. However, even in the last conditions, there is marked anisocytosis and there may be a proportion of macrocytes in the peripheral circulation.

Blood loss

As mentioned earlier, the clinical picture associated with an acute loss of a large volume of blood is that of hypovolaemic shock.

Anaemias due to chronic blood loss may develop very insidiously and cause considerable diagnostic problems. Chronic blood loss from the gastrointestinal tract or uterus of more than 15 to 20 ml per day produces a state of negative iron balance. Assuming that the patient starts with a normal body store of iron, which is usually in the region of 1 g, the bone marrow will be able to maintain a normal haemoglobin level until the iron stores are totally depleted. At this stage there is no demonstrable iron in the bone marrow and the plasma iron level starts to fall but the patient is not anaemic. With a further fall in the plasma iron level, the haemoglobin level starts to fall, although at this stage the erythrocyte morphology may be relatively normal, as are the red-cell indices. It is only when iron-deficiency anaemia is well established that the typical morphological appearances of the red cells develop, and only after extreme periods of iron depletion that the tissue changes of iron deficiency become manifest.

Table 5 General classification of haemolytic anaemia. A more detailed classification is shown in Chapter 22.4.9

Genetically determined
Defects involving the structure and/or metabolism of the membrane
Haemoglobin disorders
Enzyme deficiencies involving the main metabolic pathways
Acquired
Immune (iso- or auto-)
Non-immune:
Trauma
Membrane defects
Drugs, chemicals, toxins
Bacteria, parasites
Hypersplenism

From these considerations it is apparent that there may be prolonged blood loss before a patient presents with the symptoms and signs of anaemia. During the earlier stages the peripheral blood film may not be helpful in diagnosis, even though the serum iron level may be extremely low. Indeed, sometimes a dimorphic blood picture with normochromic and hypochromic cell populations may be seen. With chronic blood loss there is quite often a persistent thrombocytosis, and a hypochromic blood picture with thrombocytosis should always raise the possibility of chronic bleeding. In practice, the most common sites of such bleeding are a hiatus hernia, peptic ulcer, and tumour of the large bowel or the uterus.

Haemolytic anaemia (Table 5)

When the lifespan of red cells is shortened there is a reduction in the circulating red-cell mass, which leads to relative tissue hypoxia. This causes an increased output of erythropoietin with stimulation of the bone marrow and an increased rate of red-cell production. This is reflected by a raised reticulocyte count and a macrocytosis due to the presence of young cells in the peripheral circulation. Because of the increased rate of red-cell destruction, there is an increased production of bilirubin, which leads to mild icterus and the presence of increased amounts of urobilinogen in the urine and stool. Thus the haemolytic anaemias are characterized by a variable degree of anaemia, a reticulocytosis, and hyperbilirubinaemia. Their pathophysiology is considered in detail elsewhere.

Red cells are prematurely destroyed either because of an intrinsic lesion or as a result of the action of an extrinsic agent. The intrinsic abnormalities of the red cells that lead to their premature removal are nearly all genetic defects of either the membrane, haemoglobin, or metabolic pathways. The extrinsic agents that may cause premature destruction of the cells include a variety of antibodies, chemicals, drugs, and toxins, or bacteria and parasites. In addition, red cells may be damaged by direct trauma in the microcirculation or on body surfaces.

Premature destruction of red cells may take place either intravascularly or extravascularly, or, as occurs more commonly, in both sites. The site of destruction depends on the type and degree of damage to the red cell. For example, complement-damaged cells develop large holes in the membrane and are destroyed in the circulation, whereas IgG-coated cells are removed mainly in the reticuloendothelial system.

Clearly, there are numerous causes of premature destruction of red cells. These will be considered in detail later in this section. Usually it is easy to recognize that a particular anaemia has a haemolytic basis, by virtue of the reticulocytosis and macrocytosis associated with erythroid hyperplasia of the bone marrow, hyperbilirubinaemia, and increased urinary urobilinogen. However, it should be remembered that many anaemias associated with the abnormal proliferation or maturation of red cells have a haemolytic component. For example, there may be a slightly shortened red-cell survival in patients with pernicious anaemia or thalassaemia and yet there may be a very poor reticulocyte response. Similarly, there is a haemolytic component in the anaemia due to inflammation or malignancy but again the marrow response is poor. In such cases it may be necessary to measure the lifespan of the red cells directly in order to determine the magnitude of the haemolytic component as compared with defective proliferation or maturation.

General approach to the anaemic patient

Clinical assessment

The clinical assessment of patients with anaemia has two main objectives. First, it is essential to determine the degree of disability caused by the anaemia and hence how quickly treatment must be started. Second, as much information as possible about the likely cause of the anaemia must be obtained from a detailed clinical history and physical examination. There is no place for the 'blind' treatment of anaemia without first establishing the cause.

In assessing the severity of the anaemia and how urgently treatment should be instituted, a detailed history of the patient's exercise tolerance must be obtained. This should include a specific enquiry of symptoms suggestive of cardiac complications including angina, dysrhythmias, positional dyspnoea, cough, or ankle swelling. The clinical examination should include a careful assessment of the degree of pallor, the position of the neck veins, whether there are warm extremities and a bounding pulse with a large pulse pressure, the presence of ankle or sacral oedema, and whether there are basal crepitations. The finding of profound anaemia with signs of cardiac failure indicates that urgent treatment is required. If the anaemia is associated with marked splenomegaly there will almost certainly be an increased blood volume and, particularly if there are already signs of cardiac failure, the patient may well go into acute left ventricular failure if transfused. Severely ill patients with profound anaemia require immediate treatment in an environment where they can be under constant observation, have regular measurements of their central venous pressure, and where they can be managed by experienced clinical and nursing staff.

An account of history taking and clinical examination in patients with haematological disorders was given earlier in this section (Chapter 22.1). It cannot be emphasized too strongly that in many cases the anaemia is a symptom of a non-haematological disorder. A detailed history and clinical examination will often provide a clue as to the likely cause of the anaemia, and which laboratory investigations are likely to be most productive for confirming the diagnosis.

Haematological investigation

A preliminary blood count and blood film examination should classify anaemia into hypochromic-microcytic, and macrocytic or normochromic, normocytic varieties (Table 6). In middle-aged women with a history of several pregnancies or heavy menstrual loss it is reasonable to assume that a hypochromic anaemia is due to iron deficiency, and to treat them with iron without further investigation. However, hypochromic anaemia in males or young or postmenopausal women always suggests blood loss and should be investigated accordingly. If there is any doubt about a hypochromic anaemia being due to iron deficiency, the serum iron level and total iron-binding capacity should be established. Hypochromic anaemia with a normal serum iron suggests a genetic or acquired defect in haemoglobin synthesis, common causes being thalassaemia and sideroblastic anaemia. The diagnosis of a macrocytic anaemia always requires further investigation and should be followed up with a bone marrow examination. A macrocytosis with a normoblastic bone marrow may result from alcohol abuse, haemolysis, or, occasionally, one of the refractory anaemias with hyperplastic bone marrow (see Chapter 22.5.8). Macrocytic anaemias with megaloblastic bone marrows are usually due to vitamin B_{12} or folate deficiency and should be investigated accordingly. If there is macrocytosis with a reticulocytosis, hyperbilirubinaemia, and a normoblastic marrow, a haemolytic anaemia is likely; an approach to the further investigation of haemolysis is described in Chapter 22.5.9.

The normochromic, normocytic anaemias often cause more diagnostic difficulty. Some help can be gained from a determination of whether the white-cell and platelet counts are normal. If there is associated neutropenia and thrombocytopenia, a primary disease of the bone marrow is likely; hence, bone marrow examination should be made to determine whether there is hypoplasia of the various precursor forms, hypoplastic or aplastic anaemia, or whether the pancytopenia results from infiltration of the bone marrow as occurs in the various forms of leukaemia. If there are nucleated red cells or young white cells on the peripheral film (that is, a leucoerythroblastic picture), a bone marrow examination is essential, as this type of reaction usually indicates infiltration of the bone marrow with abnormal cells, either as part of a primary marrow disease such as leukaemia, or metastatic carcinoma. In the normochromic, normocytic anaemias in which the white-cell count and platelet count are normal, it is also helpful to make a bone marrow analysis. The most common cause is anaemia of chronic disorders, the diagnosis of which is described in detail below. Another particularly common cause is chronic renal failure. After these conditions have been excluded, there remain the chronic anaemias associated with endocrine deficiencies (see Chapter 22.7) or the primary red-cell hypoplasias (Chapter 22.3.11).

The management of anaemia

The management of specific forms of anaemia is described in detail in subsequent chapters. However, a few principles can be outlined here. In general, a cause should always be sought before treatment is instituted. There is no place whatever for treating anaemia 'blind' with multihaematinic preparations. As mentioned above, most cases of iron-deficiency anaemia require further investigation for a source of blood loss. If there is a clear-cut history of poor diet, multiple pregnancies, or obvious uterine bleeding, it is reasonable to start iron therapy and observe the haemoglobin level both during the period of treatment and for some months after iron therapy has

Table 6 The main causes of anaemia classified according to the associated red-cell changes

Hypochromic–microcytic (reduced MCV, MCH, and MCHC)
Genetic:
Thalassaemia
Sideroblastic anaemia
Acquired:
Iron deficiency
Sideroblastic anaemia
Chronic disorders (mildly hypochromic, occasionally)
Normochromic–macrocytic (increased MCV)
With megaloblastic marrow:
Vitamin B_{12} or folate deficiency
With normoblastic marrow:
Alcohol, myelodysplasia
Polychromatophilic–macrocytic (increased MCV)
Haemolysis
Normochromic–normocytic (normal indices)
Chronic disorders:
Infection, malignancy, collagen disease, rheumatoid arthritis
Renal failure
Hypothyroidism, hypopituitarism
Aplastic anaemia or primary red-cell hypoplasia
Primary disease of bone marrow, leukaemia, myelosclerosis, infiltration with other tumours
Leucoerythroblastic (indices usually normal)
Myelosclerosis
Leukaemia
Metastatic carcinoma

MCV, mean cell volume; MCH, mean corpuscular haemoglobin; MCHC, mean corpuscular haemoglobin concentration.

been stopped. A rise in the haemoglobin level of approximately 1 g/dl per week indicates a full haematological response. For the megaloblastic anaemias it is quite reasonable to start treatment with vitamin B_{12} and folic acid once a diagnosis has been established and blood samples have been obtained for serum folate and vitamin B_{12} levels. The precise cause of the megaloblastic anaemia can be established at leisure once these samples have been obtained. A brisk reticulocyte response 5 to 7 days after initiating therapy suggests that there will be a full restoration of the haemoglobin level to normal. Failure of response of a hypochromic anaemia to adequate iron therapy should be managed by first finding out whether the iron is being taken by the patient and, if so, by determining the serum iron level. If it is normal, causes of hypochromic anaemia that are not associated with iron deficiency—thalassaemia and sideroblastic anaemia for example—should be sought. Similarly, refractory macrocytic anaemias require detailed analysis of the bone marrow morphology as there may be an underlying preleukaemic state.

Blood transfusion should always be avoided unless the haemoglobin level is dangerously low, in which case it is reasonable to transfuse the patient up to a safe level and then allow the haemoglobin to return to normal following appropriate treatment of the underlying cause. The decision whether to transfuse an anaemic patient depends mainly on the severity of the anaemia and its cause. For example, a young patient with a haemoglobin of 5 g/dl who is shown to have an active duodenal ulcer should probably be transfused because they would be at severe risk from a further brisk bleed from the ulcer. On the other hand, a patient of similar age with a similar haemoglobin level due to chronic nutritional iron deficiency might well be allowed to restore their haemoglobin level by oral iron therapy.

Occasionally, patients present in gross congestive cardiac failure with profound anaemia. This picture is usually seen in elderly patients with long-standing pernicious anaemia or iron deficiency. This type of condition still carries a high mortality and requires urgent treatment. Such profoundly anaemic patients require transfusing up to a safe level, that is a haemoglobin value of 6 to 8 g/dl. This can usually be achieved by the slow transfusion of two or three units of red cells with the intravenous administration of a potent diuretic such as furosemide (frusemide) with each unit; the diuretic should never be mixed directly with the blood. A very careful check on the neck veins and lung bases should be made throughout the period of transfusion. Ideally, a central venous-pressure line should be inserted before the transfusion is started. Occasionally, patients are encountered in such gross heart failure that the administration of packed cells and diuretics worsens the failure. In this situation it is possible to raise the circulating red-cell mass by infusing packed cells or whole blood through one arm while removing an equal volume of blood from the other. By carrying out a two-to-three unit exchange transfusion of this type it may be possible to tide the patient over while treating the heart failure by conventional means.

Further reading

Adamson JW, Finch CA (1975). Haemoglobin function, oxygen affinity and erythropoietin. *Annual Review of Physiology* **37,** 351–69.

Bellingham AJ (1974). The red cell in adaptation to anaemic hypoxia. *Clinics in Haematology* **3,** 577–94.

Bunn HF, Forget BG (1986). *Hemoglobin: molecular, genetic and clinical aspects.* Saunders, Philadelphia.

Hjelm M, Wadman B (1974). Clinical symptoms, haemoglobin concentration and erythrocyte biochemistry. *Clinics in Haematology* **3,** 689–704.

Oski FA (1993). Differential diagnosis of anemia. In: Nathan DG, Oski FA, eds. *Hematology of infancy and childhood,* pp 346–53. Saunders, Philadelphia.

Varat MA, Adolph RJ, Fowler NO (1972). Cardiovascular effects of anemia. *American Heart Journal* **83,** 415–26.

Viteri FE, Torun B (1974). Anaemia and physical work capacity. *Clinics in Haematology* **3,** 609–26.

Weatherall DJ, Bunch C (1985). The blood and blood forming organs. In: Smith LH, Their SO, eds. *Pathophysiology,* 2nd edn, pp 173–320. Saunders, Philadelphia.

Woodson RD (1974). Red cell adaptation in cardiorespiratory disease. *Clinics in Haematology* **3,** 627–48.

22.5.3 Anaemia as a world health problem

D. J. Weatherall

Despite improvements in nutrition and hygiene, which have reduced childhood mortality in many emerging countries, anaemia continues to be a major world health problem. It is not, of course, a disease in its own right but simply a by-product of a wide variety of different disorders, most of which are described in detail elsewhere in this book. However, because of its importance as a source of chronic ill health in many populations, the global aspects of the aetiology and manifestations of anaemia are summarized briefly in this chapter. Readers who wish to learn more of the complex literature on this important topic are referred to the extensive reviews cited at the end of the chapter.

Definition and prevalence

It has been very difficult to produce an adequate definition of anaemia. 'Normal' haematological values vary with age, between sexes, at different altitudes, and, possibly, between races. On the other hand, it is helpful to have a standard set of haemoglobin levels at different ages below which 'anaemia' is defined. The World Health Organization (WHO) have attempted to set out criteria of these kind, summarized in Table 1. Despite their many shortcomings, including methodological vagaries, they at least provide a way of obtaining an approximate comparison of the distribution and frequency of anaemia among the different countries of the world.

The global prevalence of anaemia, based on WHO criteria, was estimated in the 1980s. A review of the epidemiological data available at this time suggested that about 1.3 billion people were affected by anaemia, particularly in the developing countries. Infants, young children, menstruating, and, especially, pregnant women were the most severely affected groups (Table 2). The highest prevalence of anaemia was found in southern Asia and Africa. More recent work suggests that while there has been some improvement, anaemia is still a major public health problem in many developing countries. Though found most frequently in poorer countries, anaemia is still an important problem in richer societies, particularly in infancy, pregnancy, and old age.

Table 1 Definition of haemoglobin levels below which anaemia is said to exist in populations at sea level (WHO, 1968)

	Haemoglobin (g/dl) below
Children, 6 months–6 years	11.0
Children, 6–14 years	12.0
Adult males	13.0
Adult females (non-pregnant)	12.0
Adult females (pregnant)	11.0

Table 2 Estimated prevalence of anaemia by region and sex

Region	Percentage anaemic				
	Children		Women 15–49 years		Men
	0–4 years	5–12 years	Pregnant	All	15–59 years
Developing	51	46	59	47	26
Developed	12	7	14	11	3
World	43	37	51	35	18

Data from DeMaeyer and Adiels-Tegman (1985).

The complex and multiple aetiology of anaemia in the Third World

The major causes of anaemia in the developing countries are summarized in Table 3. It is very difficult to determine their relative importance, particularly in tropical countries. Most surveys have focused on one particular mechanism, iron or folate deficiency for example. To obtain a true picture of the cause of anaemia in a particular population it is essential to obtain consecutive data over a long period. For example work in the Gambia has shown that the haemoglobin levels in children vary significantly at different times of the year; anaemia is much more common in the wet season when malaria transmission is at its highest. To complicate matters, this is also the time when diarrhoea and malnutrition are most common. Heavy rains after many dry months have profound effects on the community; sanitation measures are disrupted and food stores are at the lowest level in the annual cycle (Fig. 1).

These observations underline the multifactorial aetiology of anaemia in the developing world. Nonetheless it is clear that iron deficiency, which probably affects at least 20 per cent of the world's population, is the most important factor; the many other diseases that can exacerbate anaemia are often operating in the background of low body-iron stores.

Iron deficiency

It was estimated in the 1980s that some 600 to 700 million individuals suffer from anaemia due to iron deficiency. Surveys using more sensitive indicators of iron status showed that iron depletion is even more prevalent than frank anaemia. The causes of iron deficiency anaemia are extremely complex and vary widely among different populations. The absorption of non-haem iron, except from breast milk, is comparatively restricted, and the content of iron in breast milk is very low. Iron deficiency is particularly common in communities in which food is predominantly of vegetable origin. The three great staples in these populations are rice, wheat, and maize. Sorghum and millet are also important in parts of Africa and Asia. Soy and similar legumes are a major source of protein in many countries. The iron content of these diets is generally low, and, furthermore, absorption is inhibited by fibre, phytates, phosphates, and polyphenols, all of which occur in high levels in vegetarian diets. Populations who have remained as hunter-gatherers, and pastoralists who eat blood and meat, appear to have a lower frequency of iron deficiency anaemia.

Against this background of deficient or borderline dietary iron intake, there are a number of other factors which may exacerbate iron deficiency. Iron requirements are greatly increased during pregnancy because of the expansion of the maternal red cell mass (approximately 500 mg), iron transport to the fetus (approximately 300 mg), and the constitution of the placenta (approximately 25 mg), together with any blood loss at birth. Although there is some compensation by the cessation of iron loss due to menstruation (approximately 200 mg), the total requirements for a single pregnancy are greater than 1000 mg. Iron is also excreted in breast milk and although the concentration is low this loss, particularly with prolonged breast feeding, places a further burden on maternal iron stores.

In many tropical countries, there are important sources of pathological iron loss due to parasitic infection. Hookworm infestation affects millions of people world-wide. These parasites attach themselves to the mucosa of the intestinal tract. With a worm-load of 1000 eggs per gram of faeces, the intestinal blood loss averages about 2.5 ml/day, representing 1 mg of iron. Although some of this is reabsorbed, perhaps up to 40 percent, hookworm infestation is an important source of iron imbalance. Infection with *Schistosoma mansoni* results in intestinal blood loss, while *S. haematobium* results in chronic haematuria. In Kenyan children, for example, mean iron losses in those infected with *S. haematobium* varied from 149 to 652 μg/day, according to the magnitude of the egg counts.

Finally, it should be remembered that chronic ill health due to protein–calorie malnutrition or chronic infection may, by its effect on a patient's appetite, result in further depletion of iron intake.

It must be emphasized that many surveys for assessing body iron stores have used methods which are confounded by associated inflammatory disease or other disorders. These problems are particularly germane to surveys

Table 3 Important causes of anaemia in the developing countries

Acquired
Nutritional
iron, folate, vitamin B_{12}
Chronic infection
malaria, leishmaniasis, schistosomiasis, tuberculosis, AIDS
Blood loss
hookworm
schistosomiasis
Protein–energy malnutrition
Malabsorption
tropical sprue and related disorders
Hereditary
Thalassaemias
Haemoglobin variants
Glucose-6-phosphate dehydrogenase deficiency
Ovalocytosis

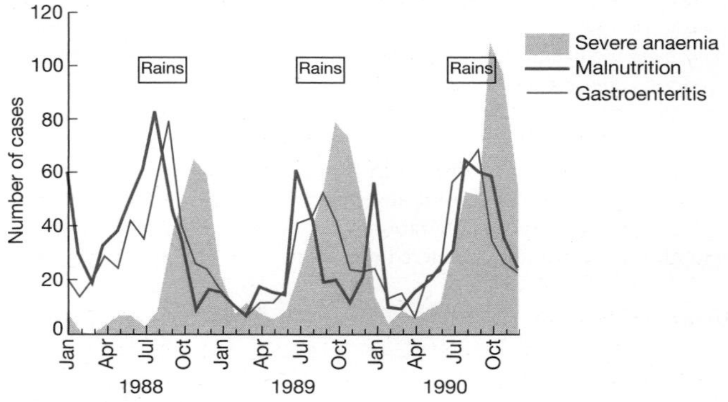

Fig. 1 Admissions to the children's ward in a hospital in The Gambia over dry and rainy seasons. (Data from Brewster DR and Greenwood BM (1993). Season variation of paediatric disease in The Gambia, West Africa. *Annals of Tropical Paediatrics* **13**, 133.)

which have been based on serum iron or ferritin levels. More recently, screening methods based on estimation of transferrin receptor levels have been developed but their application to large populations is, as yet, limited.

Folate deficiency

Folate deficiency is thought to be the second commonest cause of nutritional anaemia in the world population. The mechanisms are complex and differ widely between different populations depending in the way in which food is prepared, in particular the temperature at which it is cooked. It is also clear that dietary folate deficiency is not the whole story. Research in Africa suggests that the continuous anorexia which accompanied recurrent infections, such as malaria or tuberculosis, is a major cause of folate deficiency in children. Postinfective malabsorption and the tropical sprue syndrome are also important causes of folate deficiency, particularly in the Indian subcontinent. Folate requirements may be increased in patients with erythroid hyperplasia secondary to chronic haemolytic anaemia, sickle cell anaemia for example, or chronic malarial infection. They also increase markedly during pregnancy. In women with low baseline folate stores, megaloblastic anaemia in pregnancy or the puerperium is particularly common.

Vitamin B_{12} deficiency

Nutritional vitamin B_{12} deficiency is uncommon, although it is observed in true vegans, particularly in the Indian subcontinent. Infants born of mothers with sprue or postinfective malabsorption who are fed on breast or goats milk containing insufficient vitamin B_{12} may develop megaloblastic anaemia with locomotor complications during the early months of life.

Infection

Almost any chronic infection may produce anaemia. Globally, the most important are the parasitic disorders, malaria, visceral leishmaniasis (kala-azar), schistosomiasis, and some forms of trypanosomiasis. The anaemias due to chronic hookworm infestation were considered in Chapter 22.5.2

Malaria is still the most important parasitic illness of humans. Currently it is estimated that it has a global incidence of about 200 million cases per year, with over one million deaths. Its transmission and clinical manifestations are considered in Section 7. Profound anaemia is a major cause of mortality and morbidity during acute attacks of *P. falciparum* malaria in non-immune persons but, from the perspective of health in the developing world, chronic infection with this organism in childhood is an extremely common cause of anaemia. This is most commonly seen in areas of high malarial transmission and is a growing problem in regions of lower transmission because the rise in antimalarial drug resistance prolongs the average duration of infection. The anaemia of chronic malaria has a complex basis involving haemolysis, hypersplenism, and a suboptimal bone marrow response, often set against a background of iron or folate deficiency. In some populations, notably those of Africa, India, and parts of Southeast Asia, chronic malarial infection may be complicated by the hyper-reactive malarial splenomegaly syndrome, in which hypersplenism plays a major role in the generation of chronic anaemia.

The haematological manifestations of the other common parasitic illnesses in the tropics are considered elsewhere.

Malabsorption

A large proportion of people in tropical climates, both indigenous populations and expatriates who have worked in rural areas, have abnormalities of the intestinal mucosa, often associated with impairment of absorption. These structural and functional alterations of the gut have been called 'tropical enteropathies'. It is likely that they result from adaptation to life in the contaminated environment of the tropics, with frequent gastrointestinal infections and differences of diet.

More severe malabsorption syndromes, called sprue and postinfective malabsorption, are associated with chronic diarrhoea, wasting, and a variable degree of anaemia. The pathophysiology and world distribution of these syndromes are considered in Section 14. They are nearly all associated with anaemia which has a complex aetiology including folate deficiency and, in some cases, iron deficiency.

It should also be remembered that in a tropical setting malabsorption can also result from colonization of the small bowel by specific parasites, including *Giardia lamblia*, *Strongyloides stercralais*, *Cryptosporidium*, and others. Abdominal tuberculosis with malabsorption is also common. In Africa, HIV infection is now an important cause of malabsorption.

Inherited anaemias

The inherited haemoglobin disorders are becoming an increasingly common cause of anaemia, particularly in tropical countries. They are described in detail elsewhere.

Because of heterozygote advantage against *P. falciparum* malaria, the important inherited haemoglobin disorders, notably sickle cell anaemia and the thalassaemias, have a high frequency throughout tropical populations of the Old World. Sickle cell anaemia and its variants are particularly common in Africa, some Mediterranean populations, and throughout the Middle East and parts of India. They also occur at a high frequency in the Caribbean and in other regions with large African populations. The thalassaemias occur at a high frequency in parts of Africa, the Mediterranean, the Middle East, the Indian subcontinent, and throughout Southeast Asia. There is now clear evidence that these conditions will produce a major public health problem in these countries in the future. As poorer countries go through the demographic transition, resulting from better hygiene and control of infectious illness, infants with these genetic anaemias are now surviving long enough to present for diagnosis and treatment. Some estimated figures for the annual numbers of new births of babies with sickle cell anaemia or β thalassaemia are shown in Fig. 2.

The effect that a high frequency of a disease such as thalassaemia can have on the health economy of an emerging country was shown graphically in the case of Cyprus after is passed through the demographic transition in the 1950s. It was estimated that if every patient with this disease was treated with regular blood transfusion and appropriate medication, within 15 years the management of this one condition would consume up to

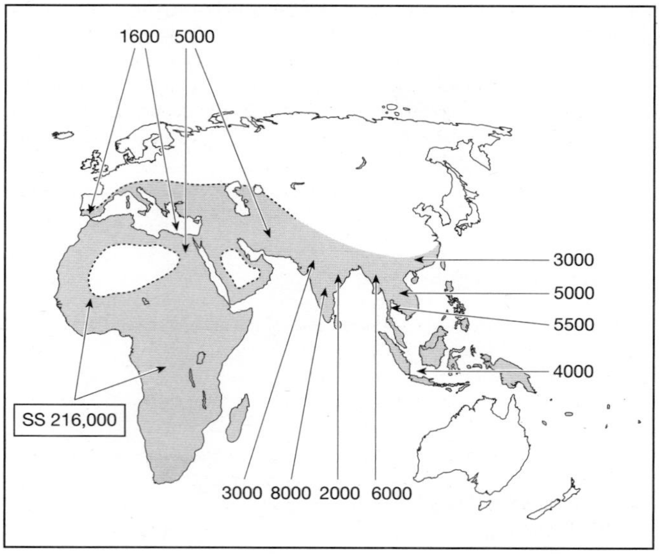

Fig. 2 Estimated annual numbers of births of babies with β thalassaemia and sickle cell anaemia (SS). (Original data in Weatherall and Clegg (2001). *The thalassaemic syndromes*, 4th edn, p.599. Blackwell, Oxford.)

40 per cent of the island's health budget. Recent studies in Indonesia indicate that, at a minimum estimate, approximately 1.25 million units of blood will be required each year to treat a proportion of the thalassaemic population in future years.

In many populations, there are hundreds of thousands of carriers for β thalassaemia or the more common severe forms of α thalassaemia. Although they are asymptomatic they have haemoglobin values which, on average, are 1 to 1.5 g/dl below normal. During pregnancy they retain this difference so that in the midtrimester they have haemoglobin values of approximately 8 g/dl or less. They have increased folate requirements and, in some populations, there appears to be an increased frequency of folate deficiency in pregnancy.

It should be remembered that the inherited anaemias may be exacerbated by other illnesses which are widespread in tropical countries. Folate requirements are increased in all these conditions and secondary folate deficiency is extremely common. They may also be exacerbated by malaria; children may develop malarial infection from infected blood donors. There is also a high frequency of other blood-borne infections, particularly hepatitis C and, in some populations, HIV. Furthermore, there is clear evidence that sickle cell anaemia and thalassaemia can render children more prone to infection. In short, like all forms of anaemia in the tropical world, the inherited disorders of haemoglobin may present with a complex series of complications due to a background of nutritional deficiency and a wide variety of infections.

These complex interactions have a major effect on the prognosis for the important inherited haemoglobin disorders. Early studies in Africa reported a marked paucity of patients with sickle cell anaemia despite a very high carrier frequency, indicating that very few patients with this disorder were surviving beyond early childhood. This may still be the case in parts of rural Africa. On the other hand, in more advanced countries, and with a high quality of medical care, patients with this disease are regularly surviving into adult life; the mean survival time in the United States is now approximately 42 years, with many patients surviving to old age. A similar situation exists for β thalassaemia. In poorer countries, supplies of blood may be limited, there may be difficulties in screening blood for agents such as hepatitis C and HIV, and the prohibitive cost of iron chelating agents means that even children who do receive transfusion die from iron loading before they reach the age of 20 years.

There are other inherited anaemias which are particularly common on tropical countries due to heterozygote advantage against malaria. Glucose-6-phosphate dehydrogenase deficiency is estimated to occur in some 100 million individuals world-wide. Its clinical and haematological manifestations are discussed in Chapter 22.5.12. They include haemolytic reactions to a wide variety of drugs, and, of particular public health significance, to certain foods (favism). There is a form of ovalocytosis which is particularly common in Melanesia which is associated with a mild and well compensated haemolytic anaemia. Recent studies have shown that carriers of Melanesian ovalocytosis are completely protected against cerebral malaria.

Consequences of anaemia

The results of many studies directed at determining the functional consequences of anaemia are still controversial. It is often difficult to distinguish between the effects of anaemia *per se* and the consequences of iron or folate deficiency on other physiological functions. Whatever the mechanism, chronic anaemia is associated with diminished function.

Many studies have suggested that even mild anaemia may reduce near-maximal work capacity. There is some evidence that both in iron-deficient animals and children it reduces mental performance and immune function. There is no doubt that anaemia increases maternal mortality and morbidity. There is a very large literature on the effect of iron deficiency on resistance to infection, as mediated through either immune function or the bacteriostatic and bacteriocidal roles of iron-containing proteins such as transferrin and lactoferrin. The entire complex relationship between iron status and susceptibility of infection requires further work. It is clear that folate deficiency is associated with an increased prevalence of obstetric complications and fetal malformation, although its effect on intellectual and immune function is less clear.

In short, because of the remarkable ability of otherwise healthy individuals to adapt to moderate anaemia it seems likely that many of the associated manifestations which have been observed result from the effects of different deficiency states on other physiological functions rather than the anaemia *per se*. On the other hand, chronic severe anaemia, particularly in childhood, results in a wide variety of complications including failure of growth and development and, possibly, proneness to infection.

Prevention

It is beyond the scope of this brief review to discuss the protean aspects of the prevention of anaemia, particularly in poorer countries. Its high prevalence is a reflection of gross poverty, particularly as manifested by nutritional deficiency, infection, and malabsorption. Its control requires action on many different fronts, including improvements in diet, fortification of commonly eaten foods with iron, the use of modified milk formulae for infants, malaria and hookworm control, iron and folate supplementation in pregnancy, and all round improvements in hygiene. The problem of the population control of sickle cell anaemia and thalassaemia is discussed in Chapter 22.5.7. Good antenatal care helps to prevent anaemia in childhood by reducing prematurity, increasing average birth weight, and improving the nutritional status of the newborn.

Summary

The extremely high prevalence of anaemia in the poorer countries is a reflection of the abject poverty of many of their populations. The anaemia of the developing world, particularly in childhood, seems to reflect a series of vicious circles. Maternal anaemia due to iron or folate deficiency and chronic malaria is associated with the birth of underweight infants who frequently have low iron stores and may also be folate depleted. Anaemia is usually present from about 6 months of age. Such infants are prone to infection, particularly gastrointestinal, and may be further depleted of iron or folate by inappropriately prolonged breast feeding or weaning onto an inadequate diet. They are exposed to hookworm infection as soon as they start to crawl, malaria becomes a major problem after 6 months, and in many populations the increasingly common haemoglobinopathies are a further cause of anaemia after the first few months of life.

Further reading

Beales PF (1997). Anaemia in malaria control: a practical approach. *Annals of Tropical Medicine and Parasitology* **91**, 713–18.

DeMaeyer EM, Adiels-Tegman M (1985). The prevalence of anemia in the world. *World Health Statistics Quarterly* **38**, 302–16.

DeMaeyer EM, Dallman P, Gurney JM, Hallberg L, Sood SK, Srikantia SG (1989). *Preventing and controlling iron deficiency anaemia through primary health care.* World Health Organization, Geneva.

Eskeland B, Hunskaar S (1999). Anaemia and iron deficiency screening in adolescence: a pilot study of iron stores and haemoglobin response to iron treatment in a population of 14–15-year-olds in Norway. *Acta Paediatrica* **88**, 815–21.

Fleming AF (1989). Tropical obstetrics and gynaecology. 1. Anaemia in pregnancy in tropical Africa. *Transaction of the Royal Society of Tropical Medicine and Hygiene* **83**, 441–8.

Flowers CH, Cook JD (1999). Dried plasma spot measurements of ferritin and transferrin receptor for assessing iron status. *Clinical Chemistry* **45**, 1826–32.

Gallacher PG, Ehrenkranz RA (1995). Nutritional anaemias in infancy. *Clinical Perinatology* **22**, 671–92.

Hercberg S, Galan P (1992). Nutritional anaemias. *Clinical Haematology* **5**, 143–68.

Khusun H, Yip R, Schultink W, Dillon DH (1999). World Health Organization hemoglobin cut-off points for the detection of anemia are valid for an Indonesian population. *Journal of Nutrition* **129**, 1669–74.

Morris SS, Ruel MT, Cohen RJ, Dewey KG, de la Briere B, Hassan MN (1999). Precision, accuracy and reliability of hemoglobin assessment with use of capillary blood. *American Journal of Clinical Nutrition* **69**, 1243–8.

Viteri FE, Torun B (1974). Anaemia and physical work capacity. *Clinical Haematology* **3**, 609–26.

Weatherall DJ, Kwiatkowski D (1997). Hematologic manifestations of systemic diseases in children of the developing world. In: Nathan DG, Orkin SH, eds. *Hematology of infancy and childhood*, 5th edn, pp. 1893–914. WB Saunders, Philadelphia.

Wharton BA (1999). Iron deficiency in children: detection and prevention. *British Journal of Haematology* **106**, 270–80.

World Health Organization (1968). *Nutritional anaemias.* Technical Report Series No. 405. WHO, Geneva.

22.5.4 Iron metabolism and its disorders

T. M. Cox

Homeostasis, transport, and storage of iron

Iron is a critically important micronutrient. As a component of metalloenzymes and complexed to form haem, it participates in the transport of oxygen by haemoglobin and myoglobin and in the harnessing of metabolic energy by cytochromes of the electron transport chain.

Iron is abundant in the environment and is the fourth most common element in the earth's crust but iron chemistry poses exceptional problems for living organisms. The metal exists in two readily interconvertible redox states (divalent ferrous and trivalent ferric iron) which are very reactive. In the environment, most iron is oxidized to the trivalent state which, under neutral conditions, is then rapidly hydrolysed to insoluble polyhydroxide complexes that are metabolically inaccessible. High-affinity iron-binding proteins that complex ferric iron have evolved to ensure its transport in the body and delivery to sites of utilization and haem biosynthesis. In bacteria and archaebacteria, a family of compounds termed siderophores have evolved that are secreted into the environment to complex ferric iron competitively for uptake. The availability of iron is limiting for growth for many microbes and for algal growth in the oceans.

In humans, iron deficiency is probably the most frequent organic illness. It affects infants, children, young adults, and the elderly in many populations. Iron deficiency is associated with anaemia and non-haematopoietic disturbances that impair work efficiency and contribute to chronic ill health as well as loss of mucosal integrity; iron-deficiency anaemia is frequently associated with pica, which has important environmental and behavioural associations with hookworm infection. In any event, the prevalence of iron deficiency worldwide provides strong evidence of the critical availability of iron in available nutrients.

Iron may be toxic and excess iron in the tissues is associated with structural injury and functional impairment. The harmful effects of iron are a consequence of its electrochemical properties and potential for the formation of reactive oxygen and nitrogen species which injure cell structures including DNA. There are many causes of excess iron in the tissues but all represent disturbances of iron homeostasis that overwhelm the mechanisms which the body uses to acquire, transport, and store iron safely.

Body iron composition

The total amount of iron in the adult body is between 3 and 4 g—most of which is co-ordinated in protoporphyrin IX as haem (Fig. 1). Haem is found principally as haemoglobin and myoglobin, although appreciable quantities are found in the viscera, especially the liver, kidney, and intestine. Cytochromes of the electron transport chain and of the P-450 system for the metabolism of xenobiotics are abundant in these organs and remarkably selective regions of the brain. In an adult, about 2.5 g of iron is complexed in haemoglobin with an additional 0.5 g as myoglobin in the muscles. In the plasma compartment, very small amounts of iron circulate, bound in the ferric form to the glycoprotein transferrin—this protein is normally only one-third saturated with iron, so that with a mean concentration of 3 g/l for a protein of molecular weight 80 000, it represents less than 2 mg of elemental iron. The normal level of serum ferritin is up to about 250 μg/l, which does not represent an appreciable amount of iron; however, the concentration of ferritin in the serum faithfully reflects the stores of iron in the body. Iron is stored in the mononuclear phagocyte (previously reticuloendothelial) system principally as intracellular ferritin and its proteolytic degradation product, haemosiderin. Body iron stores do not exceed 1.5 g in men and are usually 0.5 g or less in adult women. Non-haem deposits of iron that serve as stores in the iron-rich tissues may be visualized by staining with Perls's reagent (acid potassium ferrocyanide) with which they give a strong Prussian-blue reaction. Faint staining with Perls's reagent may be observed in normal parenchymal liver cells, but in health the principal deposits of storage iron are observed in bone marrow and spleen macrophages as well as in Kupffer cells of the liver.

Erythropoiesis and iron balance

The mean lifespan of the red cell is 120 days and thus approximately 1 per cent of the steady-state haemoglobin pool is resynthesized each day—this requires *de novo* synthesis of approximately 6 g of haemoglobin into which 20 mg of iron is incorporated. The principal fraction of the iron required

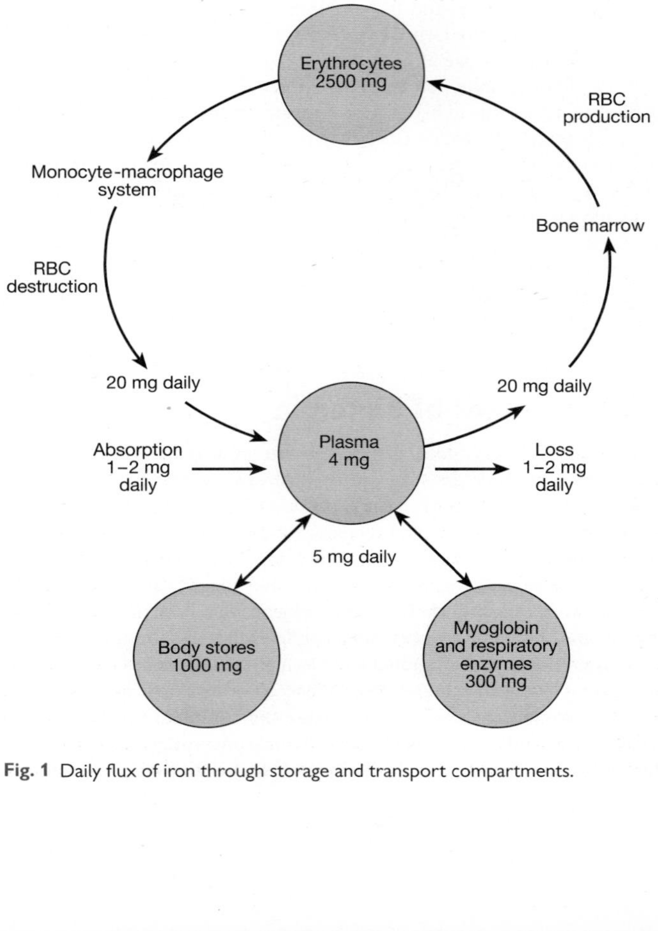

Fig. 1 Daily flux of iron through storage and transport compartments.

for daily haemoglobin production in the basal state is recycled from senescent red cells after their destruction by macrophages; the iron is delivered to the erythron in the plasma by transferrin that binds to cell surface receptors and erythroid precursors (Fig. 1). The transferrin–receptor complex is internalized and, after acidification in endosomes, the iron is released leaving the apotransferrin to be recycled to the surface and re-utilized. Transferrin is the normal mediator of iron delivery and transport in the body.

Under circumstances in which erythropoiesis is stimulated, for example under conditions of reduced oxygen saturation, after bleeding and haemolysis, as well as in dyserythropoietic conditions (including thalassaemia and megaloblastic anaemia), uptake and delivery of iron are greatly increased. Increased delivery of iron occurs in association with an expansion in the number of erythroid precursors that express cell surface transferrin receptors under the influence of the hepatorenal hormone, erythropoietin.

Iron homeostasis

Iron, an essential nutrient, is fastidiously conserved by the body and only a fraction of that which is utilized in the bone marrow is subject to obligatory daily losses through the exfoliation of epithelia and intercurrent blood loss, such as that incurred in trauma or menstruation. The requirements for iron are met from the diet by the specific absorption of iron in the upper small intestine. The amount of iron available in the diet varies greatly and even under optimal circumstances only a fraction is normally absorbed: in adult men the daily requirement is on average 0.8 mg, whereas in adult women of the reproductive age group, the requirement is usually more than 2 mg daily—the recommended daily allowance in the diet is 10 to 20 mg depending on the bioavailability of food iron components. Inorganic and haem iron complexes are released by digestion; there is a belief that haem iron may be more readily absorbed than inorganic iron in the human intestine and, depending principally on the content in meat, may constitute an important source of iron. Dietary phytates and medication including antacids and tetracyclines, as well as proton pump inhibitors, H_2 antagonists, and prior upper gastrointestinal surgery, all greatly influence the absorption of food iron. The requirement for iron is clearly increased in patients with recurrent bleeding, or in those who are blood donors; iron requirements are also increased during periods of growth in childhood and adolescence. In pregnancy, the daily requirement may be as much as 5 mg and the maternal investment of iron, depending in part on peripartum blood losses, may be as much as 1.5 g—this greatly exceeds the savings due to the cessation of menstruation. Given its iron content, the exsanguination of 1 ml of blood constitutes a loss of approximately 0.5 mg of iron; this relationship facilitates estimates of iron requirements as a result of blood losses, for example those incurred by menorrhagia (more than 80 ml/month) or from other sources.

Iron absorption

In health, iron absorption in the duodenum and upper jejunum is a scrupulously regulated process that matches the acquisition of iron from the diet to body requirements for erythropoiesis and to meet obligatory losses. Under conditions of iron deficiency or on depletion of body iron stores, a greater proportion of bioavailable iron is taken up by the intestine. For reasons that are not fully understood, certain anaemias, particularly those associated with ineffective erythropoiesis and dyserythropoiesis, are also associated with enhanced absorption of iron in the intestine. Where the anaemia is longstanding, for example congenital or acquired sideroblastic anaemia, or in haemoglobinopathies such as β-thalassaemia, intestinal absorption of iron may be such as to cause iron overload leading to tissue injury—secondary haemochromatosis.

The regulation of iron balance by the intestine normally protects the body from iron-rich diets; only under exceptional circumstances, such as the ingestion of alcoholic beverages containing abundant iron as a result of toxic manufacturing processes (for example the kaffir beers that are fermented in iron pots by the South African Bantu), does excess dietary iron lead to iron storage disease. It seems probable that those individuals who develop iron storage disease because of longstanding excessive oral intake do so as a result of the operation of genetic cofactors such as mutant alleles of the adult haemochromatosis gene product, *HFE*, or because of an underlying haematological disorder such as α- or β-thalassaemia trait.

Evaluation of body iron status

Clinical features

The most useful clinical measures of iron status include the detection of pallor and non-erythropoietic manifestations of disease including angular cheilosis, atrophic glossitis, and dystrophy of the nails with longitudinal ridging and koilionychia. Iron deficiency has been associated with behavioural changes in experimental animals. In humans, unusual syndromes of food craving (pica) have been recorded and appear to respond to iron supplementation: this includes craving for soils and the ingestion of silica-rich earths as a cult practice in black populations of the Southern United States—geophagia. Pagophagia (ice-craving) combined with the abnormal taste preferences of pregnancy may account for the bizarre food craving that constitutes part of the folklore of pregnancy. Severe iron deficiency may occasionally be associated with splenomegaly and the signs of underlying disease include peripheral oedema (hypoalbuminaemia associated with massive hookworm infection) and oronasal telangiectasia associated with Osler–Rendu–Weber disease (hereditary haemorrhagic telangiectasia).

Laboratory findings

The most useful measurements apart from those identifying the hypochromic microcytic anaemia associated with abnormal blood cell indices and confirmed by microscopy of the blood film involve surrogate measures of body iron stores. A raised platelet count would suggest a haemorrhagic component associated with iron deficiency anaemia. Iron-deficient erythropoiesis is associated with an elevation of free protoporphyrin in red cell precursors which is reflected in a raised free erythrocyte protoporphyrin in the peripheral blood; this may be easily identified in small samples of blood, taken for example as part of population screening, by the use of portable fluorimeters.

In iron-deficiency anaemia, the absolute concentration of transferrin is raised, with an increase in transferrin iron-binding capacity (**TIBC**). This is reflected by a decrease in serum iron and serum iron transferrin saturation. Such measurements may often serve to discriminate the hypochromic microcytic anaemias of thalassaemia and sideroblastic anaemia from true iron-deficiency anaemia. Such discrimination is necessary before a commitment to iron therapy is ever undertaken.

Measurement of the serum ferritin is often helpful in iron deficiency; serum ferritin concentrations are low, reflecting reduced or absent body iron stores. Neither the serum transferrin saturation nor serum ferritin, however, are absolutely infallible measures of iron deficiency: serum transferrin iron saturation may be artificially elevated with a low transferrin and low serum iron in chronic inflammatory states associated with the anaemias of chronic disorders. Likewise, serum ferritin serves as an acute-phase reactant and may be elevated in malignant disease (especially lymphomas including Hodgkin's disease), or released from the liver in hepatitis and in chronic inflammatory states. Recently there are advocates for the measurement of free circulating transferrin receptors which may be determined by immunoassay. Expression of soluble transferrin receptor protein is enhanced under conditions of iron deficiency and plasma concentrations are elevated in the presence of functionally iron-deficient erythropoiesis; however, greatly increased serum transferrin receptor concentrations are found under conditions of erythroid hyperplasia in the bone marrow and especially when ineffective erythropoiesis occurs (megaloblastic anaemia, haemoglobinopathies, sideroblastic anaemia).

Staining of iron stores in the bone marrow with Perls's reagent is a robust and relatively simple method for resolving difficulties that arise in the investigation of patients with suspected iron-deficiency anaemia. Although an examination of the amount of iron (usually graded semiquantitatively on a scale from 0 to 4, reflecting the strength of Prussian-blue staining) does not provide any information as to the availability of the iron for haemoglobin formation, it does provide useful information as to the appropriateness of iron therapy for hypochromic anaemia. Bone marrow examination, moreover, may be diagnostic in patients suffering from hypochromic anaemias due to primary or sideroblastic change in the marrow, since the characteristic ring sideroblasts with or without other myeloblastic changes will be apparent.

In summary, the laboratory evaluation of patients with suspected iron deficiency should include a full examination of haematological parameters including microscopy of the blood film. Quantification of serum iron, serum transferrin, and transferrin saturation (TIBC) may be valuable in establishing the cause of the hypochromic or microcytic anaemia. Serum ferritin measurements are often confirmatory in the absence of malignant, hepatitic, or other inflammatory diseases—as may fluorimetric red-cell protoporphyrin assays. Determinations of serum transferrin receptor concentration may provide evidence of increased demands for iron by the marrow or indeed expansion of the erythron but this test is not readily available. Microscopic examination of a bone marrow aspirate, including staining with Perls's reagent, may provide valuable information about iron stores in macrophages and the need for iron supplementation.

Disturbances of iron metabolism

Disorders of iron metabolism are common contributory factors in disease: iron deficiency is rife, particularly amongst the poor and others whose access to meat is limited and those in whom hookworm infestation occurs. At the same time, the prevalence of haemoglobinopathies and other anaemias such as myelodysplasia and sideroblastic syndromes that require transfusion and cause hyperabsorption of iron associated with ineffective erythropoiesis mean that iron storage disease also represents a major world health problem. In addition, as discussed in Chapter 11.7.1, hereditary haemochromatosis occurs at a high gene frequency in certain populations: this includes peoples of North European descent (adult haemochromatosis, due to mutations in *HFE*) and those of sub-Saharan African origin (African iron overload), in whom the nature of the predisposing gene is unknown.

Iron deficiency

About 30 per cent of the world's population, nearly two billion individuals, are anaemic and at least half of this group are believed to have iron-deficiency anaemia. Up to 20 per cent of menstruating females even in rich countries, such as the United States and in Europe, have signs of iron deficiency. In children and young adults, there is a frequency of between 5 and 10 per cent of iron-deficiency anaemia—particularly in deprived socioeconomic groups.

Many population studies have in the past been based on erroneous attribution of anaemia solely to iron deficiency: there are many conditions, including the anaemia of chronic disorders and haemoglobinopathies such as β-thalassaemia trait, that lead to hypochromic or microcytic red-cell indices. Population surveys based on the detection of iron-deficient erythropoiesis, especially those using determination of free red-cell zinc protoporphyrin concentrations by fluorimetry, may enhance the detection of true iron-deficiency anaemia; determinations of serum ferritin concentrations also facilitate discrimination between the anaemia of chronic disease and true iron deficiency.

Causative factors

Iron-deficiency anaemia in populations is often attributed solely to an iron-poor diet, but in the absence of significant blood loss or intestinal parasites including hookworm, even the most iron-poor diets rarely cause iron-deficiency anaemia, except in growing children. The amount of iron required to repair obligatory losses is very small so that at least 90 per cent of the iron required for *de novo* haemoglobin formation in erythropoiesis is retrieved from senescent erythrocytes broken down by the mononuclear phagocyte system. Furthermore, once iron deficiency develops, striking adaptive changes occur in the absorptive mechanism for iron in the upper small intestine. In experimental animals with iron deficiency, mucosal expression of the divalent metal transporter 1 (**DMT 1**), on the brush border membrane of the intestinal epithelium, is induced. Iron-deficiency anaemia is also associated with enhanced intestinal expression of mucosal ferrireductase activity.

These changes may not represent the portfolio of adaptive changes that occur. There is evidence that iron deficiency is associated with the recruitment of a greater length of mucosal surface in the upper small intestine for participation in the absorption of luminal iron. Iron deficiency, and the response to the removal of a unit of blood, may increase the overall absorptive efficiency of the intestine for iron up to 10-fold—thus greatly enhancing the bioavailability of dietary iron.

Alcoholic beverages may provide a source of iron and the absorption of haem iron present in red meat, poultry, and fish is usually between 15 and 35 per cent. Between 2 and 20 per cent of non-haem iron present in fruit and vegetable sources is absorbed. Natural enhancers of iron absorption such as ascorbic acid, which maintains ferrous iron in its reduced form in the intestinal lumen, promote direct uptake by DMT 1. Fructose and other organic compounds of low molecular weight also form soluble and reduced complexes with iron released from non-haem sources in food. In the West, normal individuals ingest between about 10 and 15 mg of iron daily. Adult men with normal iron stores absorb approximately 2 per cent of the non-haem iron ingested, whereas men with iron deficiency absorb more than 20 per cent of iron from this source in the diet; the comparable figures for haem iron are 26 and 47 per cent, respectively.

Many compounds present in the diet also inhibit or impede the absorption of iron released by digestion in the lumen. These compounds include tannin, especially present in tea, phytates present in bran and nuts, dietary fibre, and other inhibitory factors such as drugs, including tetracycline and alkalis. Some vegetarians of Asian origin ingest large amounts of phosphate and phytates which inhibit the absorption of iron provided in diets that may contain up to 30 mg of assayable total iron each day. A typical example is spinach which, although rich in iron, leads to the appearance of black stools when consumed in small or moderate amounts; these stools are black because of the passage of iron through the small intestine and its delivery to the colon where it forms insoluble ferrous sulphide complexes through the action of colonic sulphur-reducing bacteria.

Malabsorption of iron

The inability to release and absorb adequate amounts of iron from the diet is an important but unusual cause of iron deficiency. Disease of the stomach, duodenum, and upper jejunum may be responsible for the malabsorption of food iron, which may not be readily detected by studies involving the use of simple radioactive tracer measurements. On the other hand, properly conducted radioactive food labelling studies show that after gastric bypass surgery and after intestinal resection, malabsorption of non-haem and haem food iron sources is the rule. Rarely, iron deficiency may result from inflammatory disease of the upper intestine that causes malabsorption: coeliac disease in infants and adults may be responsible, and the iron deficiency may be combined with deficiency of folic acid. Sometimes large pharmacological doses of iron with or without folic acid may overcome the anaemia caused by coeliac disease but unless a strict gluten-free diet is instituted, the anaemia recurs rapidly after iron therapy is stopped. Although malabsorption of food iron is an important aspect of the iron deficiency associated with coeliac disease, loss of iron exacerbates the effects of malabsorption. In coeliac disease this results from increased exfoliation of the epithelium in association with crypt hyperplasia and bleeding due to ulceration. The abnormal motility and maldigestion associated with upper gastrointestinal surgery compounded by anacidity caused by gastritis or acid-suppressing drugs, also impair the absorption of food iron.

Loss of iron

Women in the reproductive age group lose iron regularly at menstruation. An increased recommended daily allowance for women is higher than in all other groups: the average requirement for healthy menstruating women is approximately 1.4 mg of iron daily to replace losses, compared with normal men who lose about 0.8 to 0.9 mg of iron per day. Pregnancy is often associated with iron deficiency when growth of the fetus is rapid. Twin pregnancies and frequent childbirth, especially in women of low socio-economic groups, are associated with iron-deficiency anaemia. Although anaemia is important, a very large study has been conducted that shows no reliable association between maternal anaemia and the complications of pregnancy, including preterm labour. Pregnancy itself is associated with the development of adaptive responses in the intestine and iron transport proteins that enhance the avidity of the gastrointestinal tract for bioavailable food iron. Clearly socio-economic and sociopolitical considerations are likely to influence the population occurrence of iron deficiency in women of the reproductive age group, particularly since the investment of about 1 to 1.5 g of iron occurs with each pregnancy carried to term. This estimate includes blood loss associated with the birth and the investment of iron placed in human milk, which contains up to 0.5 mg/l of iron bound to the whey protein, lactoferrin.

Other sources of iron loss

Intestinal parasites

Several hundred million people are heavily infested with hookworms. The two common hookworms of humans are *Anclyostoma duodenale* and *Necator americanus.* These helminths attach themselves to the lining of the small intestine by their buccal capsules and cause chronic blood loss by sucking blood from the intestinal villi. Hookworm infestation may be light, so that iron loss is not sufficient to cause iron deficiency. In hookworm disease, involving Old World and New World hookworms, heavy infestation occurs as a result of repeated exposure of the skin to contaminated soil. Mucosal immunity may also be reduced in the susceptible host. Although it is not known exactly what hookworms abstract from human blood, microscopic preparations show red cells expelled from the worm: each *Anclyostoma* induces the loss of up to 300 μl of blood daily, whereas each *Necator* causes the loss of up to 50 μl of blood. Clearly the occurrence of anaemia is dependent on the iron content of the diet, the extent of tissue iron stores, and the duration and intensity of the mucosal helminth infestation itself.

Since up to two-thirds of the haemoglobin iron released by the worms can be reabsorbed in the intestine, significant anaemia requires a very heavy parasite load; none the less, extremely severe anaemia may develop in patients with hookworm disease with all the attendant symptoms of fatigue, dyspnoea, palpitations, and mental changes—including pica. Non-specific abdominal pain may occur and radiographic examination of the intestine or endosccopy may reveal duodenitis with a punctate inflammation associated with partial villus atrophy of the duodenojejunal mucosa. Oedema may result from cardiac failure in severe cases and also in association with hypoalbuminaemia, since heavy infestation may lead to significant protein-losing enteropathy. Hookworm disease may be associated with other helminth infections such as strongyloidiasis and ascariasis and itself may contribute to poor socio-economic circumstances as a result of incapacity for work due to illness.

Major hookworm parasites are widely distributed in Southern Europe, Africa, the Middle and Far East, and the New World, including the Southern United States. The heaviest infections usually affect rural workers in agricultural communities where repeated exposure occurs in isolated locations and where crops are harvested under conditions of poor sanitation. The iron-deficiency anaemia of hookworm disease may present difficulties for diagnosis when the mucosal inflammation that accompanies heavy infestation is associated with reduction in serum proteins such as albumin and transferrin; this, combined with an acute-phase response, may at first lead to a mistaken diagnosis of the anaemia of chronic disorders.

Other sources of blood loss

The gastrointestinal tract represents an important source of blood loss which should always be considered in patients with iron-deficiency anaemia. Ulcerating lesions of the small and large intestine, including cancers, are frequent causes of iron-deficiency anaemia. However, chronic intermittent bleeding can arise from unusual sources such as Meckel's diverticula, angiodysplastic lesions, hamartomas, and other benign ulcerating tumours such as leiomyomas. Gastric ulcers may be associated with chronic intermittent bleeding, but duodenal ulcers rarely cause chronic gastrointestinal blood loss.

Oesophageal ulceration and inflammatory lesions can cause iron-deficiency anaemia, but precaution is needed in attributing blood loss sufficient to cause iron deficiency to such a source unless other potential sites of bleeding have been excluded. Other unusual sources of gastrointestinal bleeding include multiple telangiectatic lesions of Osler–Rendu–Weber disease (hereditary haemorrhagic telangiectasia)—in which bleeding may occur anywhere from the nasal or oropharynx down to the stomach and upper intestine. The blue bleb naevus syndrome, the Peutz–Jeghers syndrome, and other hereditary gut polyposes are rare causes of chronic gastrointestinal bleeding. Inflammatory disease of the lower small intestine and colon such as Crohn's disease and ulcerative colitis, usually associated with chronic intestinal blood loss, may present with an abdominal history in which iron-deficiency anaemia is prominent. Very occasionally, artefactual iron-deficiency anaemia due to self-bleeding may occur; blood may be removed from any source but bizarre methods may be adopted to conceal it, thus requiring considerable ingenuity, and often detective work, to identify the cause. Because of the striking appearance of expectorated blood, iron-deficiency anaemia associated with frank haemoptosis requires little diagnostic skill, but occasionally recurrent intra-alveolar lung haemorrhage causes unexplained illness and anaemia. Occasionally, iron may be lost in the urine through the kidney in conditions where chronic intravascular haemolysis occurs. Losses may be sufficient to induce iron deficiency in the absence of marked changes in urine colour. Patients with haemolysis due to prosthetic or paraprosthetic cardiac valve malfunction may be revealed by the presence of characteristic red-cell changes; likewise in paroxysmal nocturnal haemoglobinuria, chronic intravascular haemolysis causes chronic urinary iron loss with or without visible haemoglobinuria. In these circumstances, free haemoglobin is released which quickly saturates the capacity of the plasma protein, haemopexin to bind it; free haemoglobin spills into the glomerular filtrate where it is taken up by the proximal tubular cells and degraded. After degradation to haemosiderin, iron is lost in the urine when the iron-loaded epithelial cells are exfoliated.

Clinical and laboratory features of iron deficiency

Symptoms of iron deficiency include fatigue, pallor, palpitations, irritability, and little-recognized mental changes, such as pica. The patient may complain of a sore tongue, deleterious changes in the appearance of hair or hair loss, and angular cheilosis. Examination of the nails may reveal longitudinal ridging and, most often in elderly women with chronic iron deficiency for many years, koilionychia. There may be a complaint of dysphagia associated with the development of an oesophageal web (Patterson–Brown–Kelly or Plummer–Vinson syndrome). This again usually occurs in elderly or middle-aged women with chronic iron deficiency. A small proportion of patients with iron-deficiency anaemia have detectable but modest splenomegaly.

Diagnosis

Blood parameters will reveal microcytic anaemia usually in association with an unequivocal reduction in serum transferrin saturation (below 16 per cent) and a reduced serum ferritin concentration (below 12 μg/l). The absence of these features and of an acute-phase reactive response may suggest dyserythropoietic or sideroblastic anaemia or β-thalassaemia trait. Lead poisoning may be associated with iron deficient indices with or without full-blown sideroblastic changes. A bone marrow aspirate stained with Perls's reagent for iron in marrow macrophages will rapidly confirm reduced or absent stainable iron in the storage compartment and may also be revealing about other aspects of the anaemia, such as the presence of ring sideroblasts, dyserythropoietic features, and/or megaloblastic change.

The presence of immunoreactive serum transferrin receptors may provide additional evidence in favour of iron-deficiency anaemia but because increased serum concentration of these receptors may be observed in several disorders of the bone marrow and the ELISA tests are relatively expensive, the role of this determination in the routine diagnosis of iron deficiency is as yet unestablished. Red-cell zinc protoporphyrin concentrations greater than 35 μg/dl of whole blood are usually observed in patients with iron deficiency; values in excess of 100 μg/dl are generally associated with lead toxicity. Extremely high levels may indicate the presence of erythropoietic protoporphyria or lead poisoning. Modest elevations in erythrocyte protoporphyrin can be observed in patients with haemolytic anaemias, sideroblastic anaemia, and occasionally, the anaemia of chronic disorders.

Investigations and management

The identification of iron-deficiency anaemia should be regarded in a sense as a symptom rather than a diagnosis of a patient's malady: the management of those affected should always include an attempt to determine the cause. Common errors occur when, in elderly patients, iron deficiency is cynically ascribed to the presence of mild oesophagitis or gastritis observed at endoscopy, when the underlying cause is bleeding due to a coincidental but sinister gastrointestinal cancer elsewhere—and for which a diligent search is often required.

A full evaluation of the patient with iron deficiency should include an adequate dietary history including the consumption of drugs, such as aspirin and non-steroidal anti-inflammatory drugs, that may be responsible for gastrointestinal bleeding. An enquiry should be made about additional gastrointestinal symptoms and other signs of blood loss; reasonable attempts should be made to evaluate the extent of menstrual loss, if the bleeding is to be ascribed to menorrhagia in women of the reproductive age group. Attention should be placed on the family and a travel history to exclude causes such as hereditary haemorrhagic telangiectasia or hookworm disease.

Clinical examination should extend from an enquiry about previous gastrointestinal disease or surgery to an examination for visceral enlargement, abdominal lymphadenopathy, splenomegaly, and other features suggestive of intra-abdominal pathology such as portal hypertension and abdominal cancer. Hereditary haemorrhagic telangiectasia may be detected by the presence of the most subtle oronasal lesions.

In patients in which the cause of the iron deficiency is not apparent, further studies may be needed to search for gastrointestinal bleeding, including detection of occult faecal blood on several samples taken consecutively. Endoscopic and radiographic studies of the gastrointestinal tract, and serological studies for the presence of coeliac disease may be required and occasionally there is a need to quantify the amount of blood loss daily in the faeces or during menstrual flow by using radiolabelled chromium red-cell studies. In difficult cases, percutaneous visceral angiography of the coeliac and mesenteric arteries has proved invaluable for detecting sites of active gastrointestinal bleeding that are beyond the reach of conventional endoscopic procedures. In those patients who are actively bleeding, such a procedure can identify local sites of blood loss greater than 0.5 to 1.0 ml/min. Meckel's diverticulum is a potential cause of obscure gastrointestinal bleeding in young adults and children. Some Meckel's diverticula can be diagnosed by scintigraphic studies using technetium-99m labelled pertechnetate which may be concentrated in the ectopic gastric mucosa. Meckel's diverticulum and intestinal strictures, particularly in the ileum, may be occasionally revealed by retrograde colonic contrast radiographic studies. Other diagnostic tests include searching for endomysial antibodies, with confirmatory duodenojejunal biopsy to detect coeliac disease. Examination of the urine and sometimes sputum may be required to detect occult iron loss in exfoliated macrophages or proximal tubular cells, respectively, where intrapulmonary haemorrhage or renal iron loss is suspected.

Sometimes extensive diagnostic procedures fail to identify the cause of iron deficiency when occult gastrointestinal bleeding is responsible. Under these circumstances, it remains appropriate to conduct a diagnostic laparotomy, after consultation with an experienced surgeon, to identify the bleeding lesion. In adults of any age, an appreciable number of obscure gastrointestinal malignancies or treatable benign tumours can be identified by such a procedure which, when combined with angiography with or without enteroscopy, may permit identification of angiodysplastic lesions at remote sites. In younger adults and children, diagnostic laparotomy may be indicated to identify Meckel's diverticula, intestinal stricture, and congenital abnormalities such as duplications that serve as occult sources of blood loss.

It is not unusual for the patient with recurrent chronic iron-deficiency anaemia to present a challenge for diagnosis. Even the most experienced physician would be well advised to consult widely with colleagues with expertise in radiology, nuclear medicine, and surgery before either prematurely abandoning the search of the causal lesion or requesting an ill-considered laparotomy without a thorough appreciation of the further difficulties it may pose.

Replenishing iron stores is but one aspect of the treatment of iron-deficiency anaemia. Iron should be replaced not only to restore the normal haemoglobin concentration but to replenish body iron stores. It is necessary to replace iron depleted in systemic tissues such as the muscles, where it is an essential component of cytochromes and other enzymes critical for optimal aerobic metabolism. Occasionally a therapeutic trial of oral iron for a defined period may be used to verify the suspected diagnosis of iron-deficiency anaemia. Adequate replacement of iron should be monitored for its effects: a reticulocyte response should be observed in peripheral blood maximally between the 7th and 10th days after initiating treatment and significant increases in blood haemoglobin concentration should be apparent within 2 to 4 weeks. If there is no evidence of continued blood loss, the haemoglobin concentration should come within the normal range within 2 months. Failure to meet these expectations suggests either that the anaemia is not caused by iron deficiency or that there is continued depression of bone marrow function—or that there is bleeding for which further investigation is needed.

Therapeutic preparations of iron

Iron salts should be administered by mouth unless there are overwhelming reasons for using the parenteral route—parenteral preparations of iron are associated with a greatly increased risk of toxicity and hypersensitivity reactions including anaphylaxis. Ferrous salts are better absorbed than ferric salts and show little difference amongst preparations in terms of rate of repair of anaemia at a given dosage of elemental iron.

It is usual to treat iron-deficiency anaemia with at least 100 to 200 mg of elemental iron daily. For full-blown iron-deficiency anaemia, ferrous sulphate is administered three times daily (equivalent to 3×65 mg of elemental iron). Some patients are unable to tolerate such a dose of iron because of constipation, diarrhoea, or abdominal pain; the presence of tarry, black stools may interfere with personal hygiene and thus lead to ultimate rejection of iron therapy by the patient. Under these circumstances the dose of iron may be reduced and this, rather than a change of iron salt preparation, usually improves tolerability. The frequency of unwanted effects with ferrous sulphate is the same as that of other iron salts when compared with the amount of elemental iron ingested. Once established, the optimal therapeutic response to oral iron increases the blood haemoglobin concentration by 0.1 to 0.2 g/dl per day. Replenishment of iron has a slow effect on the epithelial changes of iron deficiency and the atrophic glossitis may take several months to improve as iron stores are replenished.

Slow-release oral preparations of iron are available, which the manufacturers often claim release sufficient iron over a 24-h period for optimal haematological responses after once daily dosages. However, these preparations are likely to distribute the iron beyond the upper jejunum and thereby bypass those regions of the intestine in which iron absorption is most avid. Compound preparations of iron including B vitamins and folic acid are available but there is little justification for prescribing these except for prophylactic use in pregnancy (see below). In infants and children, sugar-free preparations of iron complexes are available in the form of polysaccharide iron or iron–sodium EDTA (sodium ironedetate) complexes, which can be used as recommended by the manufacturer. In premature infants, up to 2.5 ml of a syrup containing approximately 5 mg/ml may be used twice daily; up to 5 ml three times daily may be given to children aged 6 to 12 years.

Pregnancy

Prophylactic iron preparations are recommended in pregnant women who have risk factors for iron deficiency such as poor diet, prior menorrhagia, or those in whom gastric surgery has been carried out. Prophylactic iron may also be used in the management of infants of low birth weight including premature babies, twins, and infants delivered by caesarian section. Compound preparations of iron with folic acid may be used for the treatment of iron and folic acid deficiencies in pregnancy. For the prevention of neural tube defects in women planning a pregnancy, the United Kingdom Department of Health advises that a medicinal or food supplement of 400 µg of folic acid daily be taken before conception and during the first 12 weeks of pregnancy. Lone or combined iron compound preparations are not routinely indicated for prophylaxis in patients with chronic haemolysis or in renal dialysis since they may lead, in the circumstances of dyserythropoiesis, to chronic iron overload and secondary haemochromatosis.

Parenteral preparations of therapeutic iron

Given its potential toxicity, the only justification for the use of parenteral iron is in patients who are unable to co-operate with or tolerate oral iron therapy, or those with severe gastrointestinal disease that causes malabsorption or continuing severe blood loss. Provision of iron by the parenteral route does not normally lead to more rapid repair of anaemia than when adequate oral iron preparations are administered. Some patients with renal failure who receive haemodialysis have obligatory blood losses which cannot be treated adequately with oral iron preparations. These patients, and occasional patients receiving peritoneal dialysis, may require intravenous iron regularly. Two parenteral preparations of iron are now available in the United Kingdom: a ferric hydroxide–sucrose complex containing 20 mg/ml of iron (2 per cent) and iron sorbitol citrate that consists of a colloidal stabilized preparation of iron containing 50 mg/ml. Severe sensitivity reactions to these agents may occur and facilities for cardiopulmonary resuscitation should be at hand with the use of iron–sucrose complex. Moreover, administration of these preparations should not be followed by oral iron therapy until at least 5 days after the last injection.

Unwanted and toxic effects of parenteral iron preparations

A history of allergic disorders including asthma, eczema, and prior anaphylaxis are regarded as contraindications to the use of parenteral iron, as is liver disease and concurrent infection. Moreover, these drugs are not recommended for children. Side-effects include nausea, vomiting, taste disturbances, hypotension, parasthesias, abdominal disorders, fever, flushing, anaphylactoid reactions, and the reactivation of inflammatory arthropathies. Injection site reactions, including phlebitis, have been reported. Iron sorbitol is contraindicated in patients with untreated urinary tract infections and early pregnancy as well as liver disease and kidney disease. Parenteral iron should probably be avoided in patients with pre-existing cardiac disease including arrythmias or angina.

Administration

Iron sorbitol is given only by deep intramuscular injection, whereas iron–sucrose complex may be given slowly intravenously or by intravenous infusion. In both instances the total dose is calculated according to body weight and the presumed iron deficit set out in the manufacturer's product literature.

General aspects of iron therapy

Treatment of causes of anaemia, including bleeding, is clearly a critical aspect of the management of iron-deficiency anaemia and its diagnosis. Coeliac disease should be treated with a gluten-free diet; bleeding lesions in the gastrointestinal tract may require definitive surgery directed to their healing. Occasionally, patients with a chronic bleeding disorder for which surgery is not indicated, such as hereditary haemorrhagic telangiectasia, may require long-term iron supplementation at doses less than that required to treat the acute iron-deficiency state. Periodic monitoring is required to ensure that the level of iron replacement is adequate to meet the demands of the bone marrow for *de novo* haem synthesis and that iron overload is not occurring. It should be recognized that relief of iron deficiency will improve many symptoms suffered by a patient even though they may suffer from an incurable underlying disease.

Treatment with iron should be continued until iron stores are replenished: there is no excuse for inadequate therapy—especially in those patients who are likely to suffer recurrent bleeding. Particular attention is needed for iron-deficient patients who have had episodes of acute bleeding treated by blood transfusion and who at the time of therapy are not anaemic. These patients require appropriate iron replacement to replenish iron stores for their long-term restitution of health. Because iron therapy leads to a reduction in the avidity of the transport system of the intestine for iron, it should be continued for several months after the anaemia has been corrected to re-establish appropriate iron stores, ideally as reflected by a serum ferritin determination within the normal range.

Unusual syndromes with iron-deficient erythropoiesis

Congenital deficiency of serum transferrin

There are a few reports of deficiency or virtual absence of serum transferrin in infants with disturbed growth, marked hypochromic anaemia, and disordered iron metabolism associated with systemic iron storage leading to tissue injury. This disease is extremely rare but holds great fascination for those investigators with an interest in the pathophysiology of iron metabolism. Profound deficiency of serum transferrin disturbs the normal ligand–receptor signalling mechanisms indicated in the overall control of body iron balance and absorption in the intestine. Hypo- or atransferrinaemia in humans appears to be inherited as an autosomal recessive trait; the gene encoding human serum transferrin maps to chromosome 3.

Studies of a naturally occurring mutant mouse, the *hpx* mouse, that also has deficiency of serum transferrin associated with runting and hypochromic anaemia due to iron-deficient erythropoiesis indicate that the disorder responds to infusions of serum transferrin or plasma. These infusions restore normal growth and improve the abnormalities of iron homeostasis; iron-deficient erythropoiesis is also corrected, with resolution of the anaemia. The half-life of transferrin in the plasma is 5 to 10 days and so infusions of plasma or purified preparations enriched with transferrin can be administered at intervals. Since most individuals with transferrin deficiency do express limited amounts of the protein antigen, immune reactions to exogenous human transferrin appear to be either mild or rare. Absolute deficiency of transferrin receptors, for example as occurs in mouse embryos generated as a result of gene disruption technology in embryonic stem cells, is incompatible with normal development beyond the late embryo stage.

Other causes of refractory iron-deficient erythropoiesis

There are sporadic reports of iron deficiency occurring in children and adults for which no cause can be established after intensive investigation. In some instances the expected parameters of iron deficiency associated with iron-deficient erythropoiesis can be demonstrated in individuals who fail to respond to generous oral supplementation with iron salts; administration of parenteral iron, however, leads to an improvement in reticulocytosis with resolution of iron-deficient red-cell indices. Although at the time of writing no molecular lesions have been identified in any of the implicated iron and transport proteins, it is not impossible that disturbed function of DMT 1, ferroportin, haephastin, or as yet uncharacterized moieties involved in the transport of iron across the intestine will be found in these disorders.

Occurrence of iron-deficient erythropoiesis in both females and males that responds only to parenteral iron supplementation is unlikely to be caused by hephastin mutations since this gene maps to the long arm of the X chromosome in humans. It is possible that acquired defects of the intestinal mucosa other than inflammatory disorders may contribute to malabsorption of therapeutic iron. Several young children have been reported with iron-deficiency anaemia refractory to oral therapy but which was corrected by parenteral supplementation. Careful investigation revealed an absorptive defect for iron which was corrected itself by systemic iron supplementation and raises the possibility that severe iron deficiency itself prejudices the ability of the mucosal epithelium in the upper small intestine to carry out its normal absorptive function. However, no further investigations to identify the nature of this acquired metabolic defect have been provided. There is at least one well-documented instance of an acquired defect of iron delivery associated with signs of iron-deficient erythropoiesis caused by loss of human transferrin receptor function. This condition was associated with the development of antinuclear factor and other autoantibodies as part of an autoimmune illness in an adult woman with hypochromic anaemia. Autoantibodies directed against the transferrin receptor were identified in the serum of the patient, but the anaemia with its attendant sideropenia ultimately responded to a combination of steroids and azathioprine therapy; the titre of transferrin receptor autoantibodies of peripheral blood cells diminished. The extent to which this phenomenon occurs generally during the course of autoimmune disorders associated with anaemia is unknown.

Secondary iron storage disease (secondary haemochromatosis)

This is a worldwide problem. It occurs when excess iron is absorbed from the intestine or obtained by the breakdown of transfused red cells in the mononuclear phagocyte system. Each transfused unit of blood contains 200 to 225 mg of iron as haemoglobin. There are instances of iron storage disease occurring in patients who have received oral iron therapy over many years as medicinal tonics or as treatment for refractory anaemia. However, it is unknown if this would occur in the absence of another disorder, such as homozygosity for mutant alleles of the *HFE* gene that predisposes to iron storage disease or underlying bone marrow disease. Conversely, iron excess may develop spontaneously in patients with haemolytic (and especially dyserythropoietic) anaemias alone, although it most commonly results from transfusion with or without underlying bone marrow disease (Table 1).

Table 1 Anaemias associated with iron storage disease

Congenital dyserythropoietic anaemia types I and II
β-Thalassaemia including the intermediate phenotype (non-transfusion dependent)
Sideroblastic anaemia (congenital or acquired)
Hereditary spherocytosis (in association with one or more mutant alleles of the *HFE* gene)
Megaloblastic anaemia (especially pernicious anaemia)
α-Thalassaemia (haemoglobin H disease)

Each millilitre of human blood contains the equivalent of 0.5 mg of elemental iron complexed with protoporphyrin. Iron present in transfused red cells is eventually retrieved after their breakdown in the macrophage system as a result of the actions of haem oxygenase, which releases bilirubin, carbon monoxide, and one atom of iron per haem molecule; thus each molecule of haemoglobin A yields four iron atoms. Although it is the mononuclear phagocyte system in which significant iron storage is first detected in transfused individuals, continued delivery of iron by its route leads to the excess of iron-loaded ferritin and its breakdown product, haemosiderin, in parenchymal cells throughout the body, with ensuing tissue injury and functional impairment. After the transfusion of 15 to 20 units of blood (representing around 5 g of elemental iron), iron toxicity occurs.

In dyserythropoietic anaemias such as thalassaemia and sideroblastic anaemia, symptoms and signs of iron storage disease may develop early in life and are related to increased dietary iron absorption by the intestine. Although some patients with β-thalassaemia intermedia are treated by occasional transfusion, much of the excess iron stored in the body originates from ingested rather than transfused iron. Iron absorption in healthy adults amounts to 1 to 2 mg/day, but in β-thalassaemia intermedia this may be increased more than fivefold. In regularly transfused patients with β-thalassaemia major, the massive expansion of the erythropoietic marrow may be suppressed to render absorption of iron normal or near normal. However, in patients with thalassaemia who are transfused only intermittently, erythroid hyperplasia persists and excessive absorption of iron from the diet contributes significantly to the iron storage derived from transfused cells; several grams of additional iron may thus be acquired each year.

Patients with hypochromic anaemias due to sideroblastic change in the marrow are particularly at risk because they may be misdiagnosed as suffering from chronic or recurrent iron-deficiency anaemia; they thus receive long-term supplementation with oral iron that serves merely to exacerbate the iron-loading state. It is noteworthy, however, that patients with haemolytic anaemia due to sickle-cell haemoglobin C disease do not commonly develop iron overload as a result of enhanced iron absorption: iron storage disease is thus generally restricted to transfused patients with chronic anaemias. Particular difficulties arise in refractory anaemias in which there is a hyperplastic bone marrow with ineffective erythropoiesis which appears to drive the inappropriate absorption of iron by the intestine.

In the South African Bantu people, the excess iron is ingested in an unusually bioavailable form in beers and other alcoholic drinks prepared by fermentation in iron pots (kaffir beers). Soluble complexes of readily bioavailable iron in these drinks contribute to secondary haemochromatosis, which is common in men in this population and other related sub-Saharan African populations. Although much of the iron is at first detected in the mononuclear phagocyte system (and is seen particularly in Kupffer cells on liver biopsy), associated hypogonadism and vitamin C deficiency later induce scurvy and osteoporosis. Dietary adjustment and iron chelation therapy may relieve the disorder, which is becoming less common after its recognition in the early 1950s. It is of interest that family studies point to a genetic component which predisposes individuals to this secondary iron storage disease within given pedigrees.

The nature of the stimulus leading from the excess iron turnover that accompanies hyperplastic bone marrow to the intestinal disturbance is unknown. The degree of excess iron absorption is however related to the extent of expansion of the red-cell precursor population: blood transfusions, which suppress the marrow, decrease the absorption of food iron. The toxic properties of iron appear to be related to its capacity to participate in free radical-generating reactions that form reactive oxygen and nitrogen intermediates implicated in tissue injury.

Clinical features

The clinical features of secondary iron storage disease in children with chronic anaemias closely resemble hereditary forms of juvenile haemochromatosis (see Chapter 11.7.1). Iron accumulates rapidly in the liver and in the endocrine glands. The several hundred gonadotrophs present within the anterior pituitary gland appear to be particularly susceptible to iron toxicity and hypogonadotrophic hypogonadism results. Iron also accumulates in the β-cells of pancreatic islets, leading to diabetes; in the zona glomerulosa of the adrenal glands, leading to early-onset adrenocortical failure; and in the parathyroid glands, ultimately causing hypoparathyroidism. Secondary iron storage disease also has a predilection for the myocardium. This causes sudden death as a result of tachyarrythmias and injury to cardiac conducting tissue or cardiomyopathy which causes intractable cardiac failure. Secondary iron storage disease in β-thalassaemia and congenital dyserythropoietic anaemias is thus characterized by progressive myocardial disease, endocrine failure, and infantilism.

Untreated iron storage disease is the most common cause of death in these disorders. Similar manifestations of iron toxicity are observed in other patients with secondary iron storage in which the accumulation of iron is less rapid. A picture resembling full-blown adult haemochromatosis ultimately supervenes with complications of diabetes and cirrhosis (sometimes complicated by transfusion-related viral hepatitis and the formation of hepatocellular carcinomas) in the presence of deep skin pigmentation. Secondary iron storage disease represents a significant threat to well-being and prognosis in the chronic anaemias. Once cardiac arrythmias have developed, the outlook is usually bleak and urgent chelation therapy with parenteral desferrioxamine is indicated.

Diagnosis

Secondary iron storage disease should be suspected when the saturation of serum transferrin is greater than 60 per cent. In established secondary iron storage disease, there is a raised non-transferrin iron-binding fraction which may contribute to the tissue injury, since the amount of circulating iron may exceed the binding capacity of circulating transferrin. Under these circumstances, transferrin saturation is usually measured at greater than 90 to 95 per cent and is accompanied by an elevation of serum ferritin which, in the absence of active liver disease, faithfully reflects the extent of iron storage disease and the risks of iron-mediated damage.

Iron chelation therapy should probably be introduced at serum ferritin concentrations greater than 1000 μg/l or if there is biopsy evidence of excess iron storage or a transfusion load of more than 15 units of exogenous red blood cells. Diagnostic evidence of iron storage may be obtained from biopsies of the liver or myocardium; skin biopsy shows excess iron in the sweat gland acini and perifollicular apocrine glands together with increased melanin deposition. In biopsy samples of the liver and heart, histochemical iron storage can be quantified by chemical iron estimations: often the liver iron content exceeds 2 per cent of tissue dry weight (normally less than 0.14 per cent or 7 mg of iron per gram dry weight). Iron concentrations may exceed 5 per cent in affected tissues such as endocrine glands and the pancreas. Liver biopsy may facilitate staging of the disease, particularly in relation to coincidental viral hepatitis where the presence of fibrosis and cirrhosis combined with iron deposits in the parenchymal cell may contribute useful prognostic information. In patients in whom tissue biopsy determinations are not possible, an estimate of body iron overload may be gained by injection of a single dose of 500 mg of desferrioxamine intramuscularly and collection of urine for 24 h in an iron-free plastic container; the daily excretion of more than 2 mg of the coloured ferrioxamine–iron complex indicates iron excess.

Although serum ferritin concentrations generally reflect the amount of iron stored in the tissues, there is a poor correlation between the levels of ferritin in iron-overloaded subjects and clinical outcome. Ferritin concentrations in serum are subject to wide variations; as a result of infection or inflammation (when as an acute reaction it is spuriously elevated), and ferritin concentrations may be reduced when vitamin C is deficient. In contrast, since the liver is the principal site of the iron storage, hepatic iron concentrations provide useful guidance as to prognosis overall, including outcomes from iron-induced cardiac injury, fatal complications of which are usually observed in patients when tissue iron exceeeds 1.5 per cent of dry liver weight. In specialized centres, non-invasive methods have been developed to measure liver iron concentrations, including whole-body magnetic susceptibility techniques but neither this nor sophisticated T_2-weighted magnetic resonance imaging of the heart or liver has been generally accepted in practice. Conventional T_2-weighted imaging may provide a crude assurance that iron storage is either present or under control but is too insensitive to contribute to serial monitoring of secondary iron storage disease—except for the investigation of potential complications such as hepatocellular carcinoma.

Treatment

Patients with homozygous β-thalassaemia and related conditions who are transfusion dependent require adequate blood transfusion to maintain a normal or near normal haemoglobin concentration combined with desferrioxamine as an iron-chelating agent. Long-term studies provide compelling evidence that survival in iron-loaded β-thalassaemic subjects is greatly enhanced by treatment with subcutaneous desferrioxamine, which prevents and reverses the cardiac manifestations of iron storage disease. It must be noted, however, that full compliance with this demanding treatment is required for benefit to accrue, which requires equal commitment from the patient and attending medical and nursing personnel alike. Splenectomy or bone marrow transplantation may be considered in certain cases but is beyond the scope of this article (see Chapter 22.5.7). The overall outcome and prognosis for β-thalassaemia has also been improved by screening donor blood for HIV and hepatitis B and C viruses, as well as other pathogens. These factors are ancillary but may potentiate the development of secondary iron storage disease.

The preferred route for desferrioxamine administration is by slow subcutaneous infusion over 12 to 16 h for up to 7 days per week; this is usually done on an ambulatory basis in adults but nocturnal administration is used particularly in children. Nocturnal administration relies on the use of slow clockwork or battery-operated infusion devices. Although electrical syringe pumps are in common use (such as the Graseby driver device), smaller quieter infusion devices (such as the Cronoject) are now available. Light precharged balloon pumps manufactured by Baxter, though expensive, are also in use. The total daily dose of desferrioxamine is usually set at 20 to 30 mg/kg of body weight with the maximum usually determined by the extent to which near-saturated solutions of the drug can be tolerated by the patient. In patients without cardiac disease it has been shown that the daily oral administration of ascorbic acid at 2 to 3 mg/kg increases the amount of iron that can be chelated by desferrioxamine. Serial determinations of serum ferritin concentrations, combined with regular clinical monitoring and assessment of cardiac, hepatic, and endocrine function assist in the assessment of iron storage disease and the efficacy of iron chelation therapy. Periodic echocardiograms and electrocardiography, with 24-h ECG monitoring, are desirable aspects of management. Urinary excretion of the coloured ferrioxamine complex can be easily measured by light spectroscopy. Desferrioxamine promotes not only urinary excretion of iron but also chelates iron from the body stores, which is excreted into the faeces via the biliary system.

Several studies show that patients with β-thalassaemia maintained on adequate transfusion regimes who are able to tolerate their infusions of subcutaneous desferrioxamine, grow and develop normally and have a better prognosis than those who either default from or do not comply fully with the chelation regimen. When treatment is initiated, careful monitoring is needed using 24-h urine collections for iron measurements to judge the excretion of iron as the dose of desferrioxamine is escalated. Daily doses of desferrioxamine may be increased to about 50 mg/kg of body weight; this usually represents the maximum that can be tolerated. In infants and growing children, unless severe cardiac disease or iron overload is present, the dose should not exceed 35 mg/kg per day over 5 nights each week. Thereafter, most well-transfused patients with β-thalassaemia can be maintained in negative iron balance by the use of not more than 40 mg/kg. For patients who receive blood transfusions, a single intravenous infusion of desferrioxamine given separately from but at the same time as each blood transfusion, at a dose of approximately 150 mg/kg of body weight, also contributes to the control of iron storage disease. In patients who develop endocrine failure, prompt replacement of deficient hormones should be introduced. Sex-steroid hormone replacement may relieve infantilism and improve self-esteem in developmentally arrested adolescents and children.

Desferrioxamine is usually well tolerated and, apart from minor skin reactions, is remarkably non-toxic. These reactions can usually be controlled by lowering the concentration of the drug in the infusion and by alternating sites of infusion; hydrocortisone in doses of up to 10 mg has been reported to reduce severe cutaneous reactions. Very high doses of desferrioxamine, particularly those used for treatment of life-threatening cardiac iron overload and given by intravenous rather than subcutaneous infusion (see below), have been associated with retinal injury and lens opacities as well as hearing loss. Since high-tone hearing loss may occur also, it may be prudent to monitor visual acuity and auditory function at intervals during treatment over the years for which desferrioxamine is required. Minor gastroenterological disturbances, myalgia, and very rarely anaphylaxis may occur; rapid administration of desferrioxamine may be associated with hypotension, especially when given intravenously. Desferrioxamine interacts unfavourably with phenothiazines and coma may result from its use in patients receiving these agents. Some patients receiving desferrioxamine develop infections with micro-organisms such as *Yersinia* and fungi such as *Mucor* that have fastidious requirements for iron. Iron-overloaded patients may also develop other systemic microbial infections and are particularly susceptible to infections with the marine vibrio, *V. vulnificus*. It seems likely that under these circumstances the desferrioxamine may serve, as nature intended, as a source of iron for uptake by microbial siderophore systems.

In patients with acute or subacute cardiac manifestations of iron overload, there are encouraging reports of the effects of high-dose intravenous desferrioxamine: desferrioxamine may reverse cardiac failure and life-threatening tachyarrythmias. An oral iron chelator of a different chemical class from the naturally occurring bacterial agent desferrioxamine has recently been licensed for treatment of iron overload in patients unable to tolerate desferrioxamine or in whom it is contraindicated. This drug, of the hydroxpyridone class, Deferiprone, is used at a dose of 25 to 100 mg/kg of body weight daily in three divided doses; the agent is not recommended for children under the age of 6 years.

Deferiprone appears to induce overall negative body iron balance in patients with severe homozygous β-thalassaemia with attendant reductions in serum ferritin concentrations and clearly represents the first newly licensed oral drug with this important indication. In a proportion of patients, however, negative iron balance does not appear to be maintained and the drug may cause serious toxicity including neutropenia and the occasional incidence of agranulocytosis which appears to be mediated by an immune mechanism. The use of Deferiprone appears to be somewhat controversial following a recent report that its continued administration may be associated with progressive hepatic fibrosis. Conversely, despite the inconvenience of its use, long-term studies of patients receiving desferrioxamine for iron storage disease in homozygous β-thalassaemia show that it is largely safe; moreover desferrioxamine improves cardiac function and life expectancy and arrests hepatic fibrosis in secondary haemochromatosis. Safety information and a side-effect profile on the use of Deferiprone at a daily dose of 75 mg/kg is available.

Other aspects of care

The single most important aspect of care is compliance with iron chelation therapy and monitoring—especially for infants and other young patients with iron-loading anaemias such as thalassaemia. Regular attendance of special clinics is advisable so that wide-ranging professional support from familiar personnel can be given to reinforce medical care delivered with attention to continuity and the nurturing of independence.

Patients with secondary iron overload should be monitored not only for the progression of their iron storage as determined by parameters of iron metabolism but also clinically for the presence of iron-mediated tissue injury. Regular echocardiography, electrocardiography, hormone measurements, and physical examinations are required to search for the presence of endocrine failure, including hypoparathyroidism and adrenocortical failure, both of which may be very difficult to detect. Patients with evidence of hypogonadism should be treated with hormone supplementation to ensure normal sexual characteristics and vigilance should be maintained for the development of diabetes mellitus. Psychological difficulties are prevalent in children and adolescents receiving iron-chelation therapy and transfusion for chronic anaemias and appropriate counselling is often needed over long periods to build up trust with them and their families and to maintain compliance with treatment. Patients with established infantilism and stunted growth frequently develop skeletal disease in addition to that related to their marrow disorder and investigations should be carried out to search for osteopenia and osteoporosis for which additional therapy will be needed. Bone disease and growth arrest may be caused by the overenthusiastic use of desferrioxamine in young infants, and in these patients the daily dose of desferrioxamine should be reduced to below 40 mg/kg, which usually restores growth velocity to normal.

Finally, patients with secondary iron storage disease should be advised to moderate their dietary intake of iron-rich foods such as meat: some investigators advocate the drinking of strong tea at meal times, especially in patients with thalassaemia intermedia. This tannin-rich drink has been shown to decrease bioavailability of dietary iron and should improve overall iron balance in this at-risk group. As far as possible, the blood haemoglobin concentration should be maintained in the normal range to ensure growth and responsiveness to hormone supplements; patients with significant transfusion requirements should be considered for splenectomy when they reach an age of over 5 years. As with patients who are not iron overloaded, splenectomized individuals should be treated appropriately by immunization and antimicrobial prophylactic therapy as far as possible to reduce the risk of intercurrent bacterial infection. This risk is potentiated by systemic iron storage.

Treatment of severe cardiac manifestations of iron storage disease

Continuous intravenous infusions of desferrioxamine not exceeding 50 to 60 mg/kg daily are now recommended for life-threatening heart disease. High-dose intravenous infusions may cause unacceptable toxic injury, especially in the retina and inner ear. Desferrioxamine given continuously through a permanent indwelling portable catheter within the superior vena cava, with careful attention to sepsis, is a satisfactory method for securing reversal of cardiac disease in high-risk patients with serum ferritin concentrations that persist at greater than 2500 μg/l or who have hepatic iron concentrations that exceed 1.5 per cent of dry liver weight. Improved outcomes have been reported with the use of anticoagulation induced by warfarin, and scrupulous attention to cutaneous needle re-siting and skin care to reduce the risk of thrombosis and complicating infections.

Pregnancy

Desferrioxamine therapy is not recommended by the manufacturer during pregnancy but despite this, many successful pregnancies have been reported without fetal injury. The drug should probably be avoided during the middle trimester and should almost certainly be avoided, because of unknown teratogenicity, in early pregnancy or at the time of any planned conception. None the less, it may be reasonable to restart desferrioxamine therapy in the final trimester of pregnancy if the risks to the mother from iron storage disease are high. No information is available on Deferiprone in pregnancy and it should probably not be used until more experience with the drug is forthcoming.

Prognosis and outcome

The principal causes of death in secondary iron storage disease include cardiac failure and arrythmias, endocrine failure and the consequences of diabetes mellitus, infection, and hepatocellular carcinoma. Unless treated, secondary haemochromatosis is a rapidly fatal disease when associated with transfusion therapy and intestinal hyperabsorption of iron in the chronic anaemias. Less than one-third of those unable to comply with iron chelation therapy survive with β-thalassaemia major to the age of 25 years. However, the outcome of iron storage disease in patients with chronic anaemia is now greatly improving, with enhanced life quality and duration. One study has indicated that 95 per cent of patients with β-thalassaemia who administer desferrioxamine subcutaneously more than 250 times each year will survive to 30 years; whereas only 12 per cent of those who do not will survive to this age. In the United Kingdom the overall survival is 50 per cent at 35 years, but at one specialist centre the actuarial survival in more than 100 patients was 80 per cent at 40 years. This again emphasizes the benefits of care administered at a dedicated treatment centre. Several reports also show that the frequency of hypogonadism, diabetes, and growth retardation is significantly reduced by effective iron chelation. Continuous intravenous desferrioxamine can be claimed to reverse life-threatening arrythmias in cardiac iron overload and also improve or reverse left ventricular or biventrical heart failure in a majority of cases. One report describes the actuarial survival of more than 60 per cent at 13 years of patients with life-threatening disease and β-thalassaemia so treated; this outcome appears to be accompanied by improved cardiac tissue iron signals on magnetic resonance imaging.

Further reading

Adamkiewicz TV *et al.* (1998). Infection due to *Yersinia enterocolitica* in a series of patients with β-thalassaemia: incidence and predisposing factors. *Clinical Infectious Disease* **27**, 1362–6.

Andrews NC (1999). Disorders of iron metabolism. *New England Journal of Medicine* **341**, 1986–95.

Bothwell T *et al.* (1989). Nutritional iron requirements and good iron absorption. *Journal of Internal Medicine* **226**, 357–65.

Chen FE *et al.* (2000). Genetic and clinical features of haemoglobin H disease in Chinese patients. *New England Journal of Medicine* **343**, 544–50.

Cohen AR *et al.* (2000). Safety profile of the oral iron chelator Deferiprone: a multi-centre study. *British Journal of Haematology* **108**, 305–12.

Cox TM (1998). Iron salts, iron–dextran complex and iron–sorbitol citrate. In: Dollery CT, ed. *Therapeutic drugs: a clinical pharmacopoeia*, 2nd edn, Vol 2, pp 178–83. Baillière Tindall, Edinburgh.

Dallman PR (1989). Iron deficiency: does it matter? *Journal of Internal Medicine* **226**, 367–72.

De Maeyer EM (1989). *Preventing and controlling iron deficiency anaemia through primary health care.* World Health Organization, Geneva.

De Maeyer EM, Adiels-Tegman M (1985). The prevalence of anaemia in the world. *World Health Statistics Quarterly* **38**, 302–16.

Finch C (1994). Regulations of iron balance in humans. *Blood* **84**, 1697–702.

Gordeuk VR, Boyd D, Brittenham G (1986). Dietary iron overload persists in rural sub-Saharan Africa. *Lancet* **i**, 1310–13.

Kent S (2000). Iron deficiency and anaemia of chronic disease. In: Kiple KF, Ornelas KC, eds. *The Cambridge world history of food*, pp 919–39. Cambridge University Press, Cambridge.

McCance RA, Widdowson EM (1937). Absorption and excretion of iron. *Lancet* **223**, 680–4.

Modell B *et al.* (1982). Survival and desferrioxamine in thalassaemia major. *British Medical Journal* **284**, 1081–4.

Moore DF, Sears DA (1994). Pica, iron deficiency and the medical history. *American Journal of Medicine* **97**, 390–3.

Olivieri NF *et al.* (1994). Survival in medically treated patients with homozygous β-thalassaemia. *New England Journal of Medicine* **331**, 574–8.

Olivieri NF *et al.* (1998). Long-term safety and effectiveness of iron-chelation therapy with Deferiprone for thalassemia major. *New England Journal of Medicine* **339**, 417–23.

Pippard MJ (1989). Desferrioxamine-induced iron excretion in humans. *Baillière's Clinical Haematology* **2**, 323–43.

Pippard MJ, Weatherall DJ (1984). Iron absorption in iron-loading anaemias. *Haematologia* **17**, 407–14.

Pippard MJ, Weatherall DJ (2000). Oral iron chelation therapy for thalassaemia: an uncertain scene. *British Journal of Haematology* **111**, 2–5. [A useful review of iron chelation and a dispassionate evaluation of the emerging role of deferriprone.]

Porter JB (2001). Practical management of iron overload. *British Journal of Haematology* **115**, 239–52. [An excellent contemporary review with abundant practical as well as theoretical and scientific information.]

Roche M, Layrisse M (1966). The nature and cause of hookworm anaemia. *American Journal of Tropical Medicine* **15**, 1029–102.

22.5.5 Normochromic, normocytic anaemia

D. J. Weatherall

A mild normochromic anaemia is one of the commonest findings in every branch of clinical practice. It is important to decide whether the anaemia is of significance and how far it should be investigated.

The first decision to be made is whether the blood findings represent 'anaemia' for the particular patient. The haemoglobin level varies considerably at different ages and there is a wide range of 'normal' values for any particular age. Knowledge of any previous blood count is particularly useful since a haemoglobin value in the lower range of normal may represent anaemia in a patient previously known to have a higher haemoglobin when in good health.

Most of the normochromic, normocytic anaemias are secondary to other diseases; a minority reflect a primary disorder of the blood. The most common causes are summarized in Table 1.

Anaemia of chronic disorders (ACD)

This is the rather unsatisfactory phrase used to cover the most common of the normochromic, normocytic anaemias, namely, those found in association with chronic infection, all forms of inflammatory diseases, and in malignant disease. It is very important for clinicians to be able to identify the main features of this type of anaemia. Although it may be extremely mild and asymptomatic, the presence of this blood picture should always alert the clinician to the possibility of there being a serious underlying disease.

Pathogenesis

The precise mechanism of the anaemia of chronic disorders is still not understood. Several different pathological processes that occur in response to inflammation conspire to cause a defective proliferation of red cell progenitors. In addition, at least in some cases, there may be a mild haemolytic component.

The most constant feature of ACD is a low serum iron level despite adequate iron stores in the reticuloendothelial elements of the bone marrow. This abnormal accumulation of iron in the storage cells, together with a low serum iron level in the blood, suggests that there is a block in the release of iron to the developing red cell precursors. This phenomenon may be observed within 24 h after major surgery, for example. There is also a reduced concentration of transferrin, and turnover studies suggest that this reflects a decreased rate of production.

Several studies have found a mild shortening of the red cell life span in ACD, which appears to be due to an extra corpuscular factor and not to an intrinsic abnormality of the red cells. The red cell survival is not grossly shortened; if marrow function were normal it should be able to compensate for the reduced red cell survival. However, there is a defect in the proliferation of red cell progenitors in ACD. This may reflect inadequate iron delivery or the effect of cytokines produced as a response to infection, or both. There also seems to be a subnormal erythropoietin response for the degree of anaemia, possibly arising from the action of various cytokines.

Recent studies have identified a number of cytokines that inhibit haemopoiesis in bone marrow culture and reduce the output of erythropoietin in hepatoma cell lines. The relevance of these *in vitro* studies to the generation of ACD in patients with such a diversity of associated disorders is uncertain. It is very unlikely that one mechanism will be found to account for such diverse abnormalities. Rather, it appears that ACD is a by-product of the acute phase reaction, probably augmented by a variety of different cytokine responses.

Clinical and laboratory findings

The anaemia of chronic disorders is usually mild. In patients with severe inflammation the haematocrit may fall to levels at which symptoms are experienced. Although the anaemia is usually normocytic and normochromic there may be mild hypochromia with a slight reduction in the MCH and MCV, particularly in children. Occasionally there may be marked microcytosis. Microcytosis should prompt consideration of concomitant iron deficiency, especially in patients who might have gastrointestinal bleeding, for example individuals with inflammatory bowel disease or rheumatoid arthritis on aspirin. The reticulocyte count is in the normal range.

The most important finding is a reduction in the serum iron concentration. Because there is a concurrent reduction in the level of transferrin, the per cent saturation of the iron binding capacity is usually normal or only slightly reduced. This observation clearly distinguishes ACD from true iron deficiency anaemia (Table 2). This distinction can also be confirmed by measuring the serum ferritin level, which is usually in the normal range or slightly elevated in patients with ACD while it is low in those who are iron deficient.

The bone marrow appearance is unremarkable. There may be a slight deficiency of red cell progenitors. Iron staining shows a paucity of iron in the red cell precursors and an accumulation of iron in the storage elements of the marrow. Again, this distinguishes ACD from true iron deficiency in which there is an absence of both sideroblasts and storage iron. The abnormal distribution of iron in an adequately stained sample, together with the low serum iron level, is the true hallmark of ACD and a finding that should always be followed up by a search for an underlying inflammatory or neoplastic condition.

Table 1 Some normochromic, normocytic anaemias

Anaemia of chronic disorders
inflammation
neoplasia
Renal failure
Endocrine failure
hypothyroidism
hypopuitarism
Marrow failure
pure red-cell aplasia
aplastic anaemia
infiltration
Acute blood loss
Polymyalgia rheumatica

Table 2 Distinction between iron-deficiency anaemia and anaemia of chronic disorders

	Iron deficiency	Anaemia of chronic disorders
Red cells	Hypochromic microcytic	Normochromic or slightly microcytic
Bone marrow		
Sideroblasts	Absent	Absent
Storage iron	Absent	Present or increased
Serum iron	Low	Low
Total iron-binding capacity	Normal or high	Low or normal
Percentage saturation	Low	Normal
Serum ferritin	Low	Normal

Other forms of normochromic, normocytic anaemia

Other causes of this type of blood picture are summarized in Table 1.

Renal failure

Normochromic, normocytic anaemia is a common presenting feature of renal disease. The features of the anaemia of renal failure are discussed in more detail in the section on blood changes in systemic disease.

Endocrine disease

The hypometabolism observed in hypopituitary and hypothyroid states reduces demand for oxygen in the tissues and, therefore, output of erythropoietin. This is probably the major factor in the development of the mild normochromic, normocytic anaemia which is observed in some patients with these conditions.

Bone marrow failure

Non-specific anaemia is a common feature of bone marrow failure. It may occur in the pure red cell aplasias or as part of aplastic anaemia.

Acute blood loss and early iron deficiency

Blood loss from the gastrointestinal or genitourinary tract may be sufficient to cause anaemia but as long as the iron stores are sufficient to maintain an output of normal red cells the anaemia is normochromic and normocytic. This picture is seen in early cases of bleeding or intermittent bleeding. There is usually a slight increase in the reticulocyte count, reflecting an increased rate of proliferation of red cell progenitors.

Polymyalgia rheumatica and giant cell arteritis

Polymyalgia rheumatica (see Chapter 18.10.4) is nearly always associated with a moderate normochromic, normocytic anaemia together with a marked increase in the erythrocyte sedimentation rate. However, particularly in elderly patients, anaemia may be the presenting feature. The symptoms of polymyalgia or cranial arteritis may be minimal or even absent. This common variant of the polymyalgia syndrome should always be considered in old people with anaemia and a very high sedimentation rate who do not have paraprotein in the blood. The anaemia responds quite dramatically to corticosteroids.

Management

Mild, non-specific anaemias should always be investigated because they may be the first indication of a serious underlying disease. It is important to try to distinguish ACD from iron deficiency or other non-specific normochromic, normocytic anaemias. In ACD, the serum iron level is low and there is a normal saturation of the iron binding capacity. It is worth carrying out a bone marrow examination to study the distribution of iron between the red cell precursors and the storage cells. If the pattern of ACD is observed, it is important to carry out a careful search for chronic inflammation or neoplastic disease. The commonest causes of ACD which give rise to diagnostic problems are low-grade urinary infections, chronic sinus infection, and occult malignancy.

The treatment of anaemias of this type is essentially that of the underlying disease. In the subgroup of elderly patients presenting with this type of anaemia in association with a very high sedimentation rate, in whom underlying blood dyscrasias and paraproteinaemias have been ruled out, it is justifiable to give a therapeutic trial of corticosteroids; and to proceed to further investigations only if there is no immediate and dramatic response characteristic of the polymyalgia syndromes. Early recognition of the true diagnosis may save weeks of fruitless investigation for a non-existent neoplasm.

The major problem for the management of this condition is encountered in those case in which it is impossible to correct the underlying disorder, patients with advanced malignant disease or intractable rheumatoid arthritis, for example. It has been found that the quality of life is undoubtedly improved for many patients of this type if the haemoglobin level is raised. This may be achieved by instituting a regular blood transfusion regimen. As an alternative approach, a number of disorders of this type have been treated with erythropoietin at varying doses. A limited number of trials, some of which were placebo-controlled, have suggested that at least some patients with malignant disease, rheumatoid arthritis, or AIDS experience a useful rise in the haemoglobin level using this approach. In view of the cost of this treatment, further studies of its efficacy are required.

Further reading

Gardner LB, Benz EJ (2000). Anemia of chronic diseases. In: Hoffman R, Benz EJ, Shattil SJ, Furie B, Cohen HJ, Silberstein LE, McGlave P, eds. *Hematology, basic principles and practice*, 3rd edn, pp. 383–8. Churchill Livingstone, New York and London.

22.5.6 Megaloblastic anaemia and miscellaneous deficiency anaemias

A. V. Hoffbrand

Introduction

The megaloblastic anaemias are a group of disorders characterized by a macrocytic anaemia and distinctive morphological abnormalities of the developing haemopoietic cells in the bone marrow. In severe cases, the anaemia may be associated with leucopenia and thrombocytopenia. Megaloblastic anaemia arises because of inhibition of DNA synthesis in the bone marrow, usually due to deficiency of one or other of two water-soluble B vitamins, vitamin B_{12} (B_{12}, cobalamin) or folate. B_{12} deficiency may also cause a severe neuropathy but whether this occurs with folate deficiency is controversial. In a minority of cases, megaloblastic anaemia arises because of a disturbance of DNA synthesis due to a drug or a congenital or acquired biochemical defect that causes a disturbance of B_{12} or folate metabolism or affects DNA synthesis independent of B_{12} or folate. B_{12} and folate are discussed first and the other rare megaloblastic anaemias are mentioned at the end of this chapter.

Biochemical and nutritional aspects of vitamin B_{12} and folate

Vitamin B_{12}

Biochemistry

Four major forms of the vitamin exist in man, all with the same cobalamin nucleus, which consists of a planar corrin ring (hence the term 'corrinoids' for B_{12} compounds) attached at right-angles to a nucleotide portion, 5,6-dimethylbenzimidazole joined to ribose-phosphate (Fig. 1; Table 1).

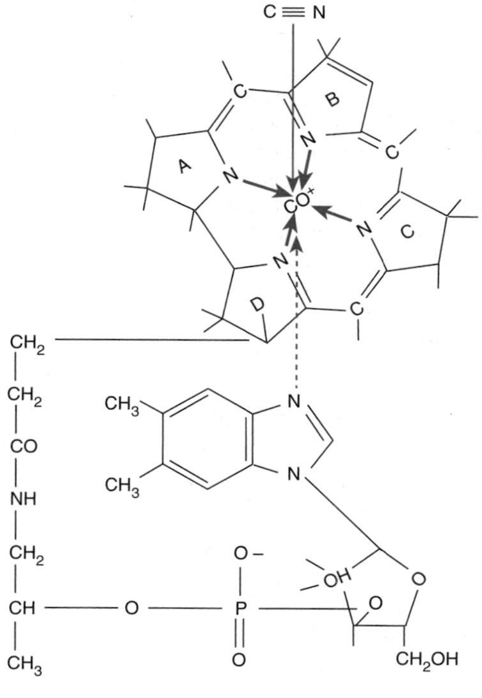

Fig. 1 The structure of cyanocobalamin.

Table 1 Vitamin B_{12} and folate

	Vitamin B_{12}	Folate
Parent form	Cyanocobalamin (cyano-B_{12}), mol. wt. 1355	Folic acid (pteroyglutamic acid), mol. wt. 441.4
Crystals	Dark-red needles	Yellow, spear-shaped
Natural forms	Deoxyadenosylcobalamin Methylcobalamin Hydroxocobalamin	Reduced (di- or tetrahydro-), methylated, formylated, other single carbon additions; mono- and polyglutamates
Foods	Animal produce (especially liver) only	All, especially liver, kidney, yeast, greens, nuts
Adult daily requirements	2 μg	100 μg
Adult body stores	2–5 mg	6–20 mg
Length of time to deficiency	2–4 years	4 months
Daily diet content	5–30 μg	About 200–250 μg
Cooking	Little effect	Easily destroyed
Absorption	Intrinsic factor (+ neutral pH + Ca^{2+}) via ileum	Deconjugated, reduction, and methylation via duodenum and jejunum
Plasma transport	Tightly and specifically bound to transcobalamins	One-third loosely bound albumin, other proteins; ?specific protein
Enterohepatic circulation	3–9 μg/day	60–90 μg/day

5′-deoxyadenosyclobalamin (ado-B_{12}) accounts for about 80 per cent of B_{12} inside human and other mammalian cells and is mainly in mitochondria; methyl-cobalamin (methyl-B_{12}) is a minor component in cells but the main form in plasma. Both are extremely light-sensitive and are photolysed to hydroxocobalamin (hydroxo-B_{12}) within 10 s of exposure to daylight; hydroxo-B_{12} is present in small amounts in tissues and plasma and is available commercially for therapeutic use. The fourth form, cyanocobalamin (cyano-B_{12}), is present only in traces in nature, but is stable and is used radioactively labelled with cobalt-57 or cobalt-58 for *in vitro* and *in vivo* studies of B_{12} metabolism. Hydroxo- and cyano-B_{12} are converted, after two reduction steps in cells of the body, to the two biochemically active forms. The fully reduced compounds are termed Cob(I)alamins, and the oxidized compounds Cob(III)alamins. Analogues of B_{12} (pseudo-B_{12}s) exist in nature and have a different sugar (cobamides) or no nucleotide portion (cobinamides), or alterations in the corrin ring. The source and identity of analogues in human serum is unclear. Endogenous production is suggested by their presence in all sera (including fetal serum) and their fall in parallel with physiologically active B_{12} in B_{12} deficiency.

B_{12} is known to be involved in only three reactions in human tissues: as ado-B_{12} in the isomerization of methylmalonyl CoA to succinyl CoA and of α-leucine to β-leucine, and as methyl-B_{12} in the methylation of homocysteine to methionine, a reaction that also requires methyltetrahydrofolate (Fig. 2). In some bacteria, but not in man, B_{12} has a direct role in DNA synthesis by virtue of its involvement in ribonucleotide reductase.

Nutrition

Vitamin B_{12} is synthesized by micro-organisms; animals obtain it by eating parts of other animals or animal produce (milk, cheese, eggs, etc.), or vegetable foods contaminated by bacteria. Clean vegetables, fruit, nuts, and cereals do not contain B_{12}; cooking has little effect on it. A normal mixed diet contains between 5 and 30 μg daily, the amount increasing with the quality. In some species, but not in man, B_{12} is absorbed after synthesis by bacteria in the large intestine. Total B_{12} in man is about 3 to 5 mg, which is mainly stored in the liver (about 0.7–1.1 μg/g). Adult daily losses are related to body stores; to maintain normal body stores, daily requirements are of the order of 2 μg. It takes 3 to 4 years, on average, for deficiency to develop if supplies are totally cut off by malabsorption. There is an enterohepatic circulation for B_{12}, variously estimated at 3 to 9 μg daily, that is intact in vegans, which may partly account for their tendency to maintain low body stores without progressing to severe deficiency. The body is unable to degrade B_{12} and deficiency has not been shown to be due to excess utilization or loss.

Absorption

About 15 per cent of food B_{12} is available for absorption. It is released from protein binding in food by proteolytic enzymes, heat, and acid, and combines one molecule to one molecule with a glycoprotein 'R' B_{12}-binding protein (also called 'haptocorrin') in gastric juice. This protein is related to plasma transcobalamin I. It binds food B_{12} but does not facilitate its absorption. Pancreatic trypsin is needed to degrade this protein and so release B_{12} for attachment to intrinsic factor (IF) and subsequent absorption. The 'R' binder, unlike IF, also binds B_{12} analogues in food. IF is a glycoprotein produced by the parietal, and possibly other, cells of the stomach (Table 2). The IF gene has been localized to chromosome II. Glycosylation of IF is not required for its B_{12} or ileal receptor binding but may play a part in protecting it from digestion by pancreatic proteases in the intestinal lumen. The normal stomach produces a vast excess of IF, measured in units (1 unit binds 1 ng B_{12}). B_{12} in bile is also attached to IF and reabsorbed

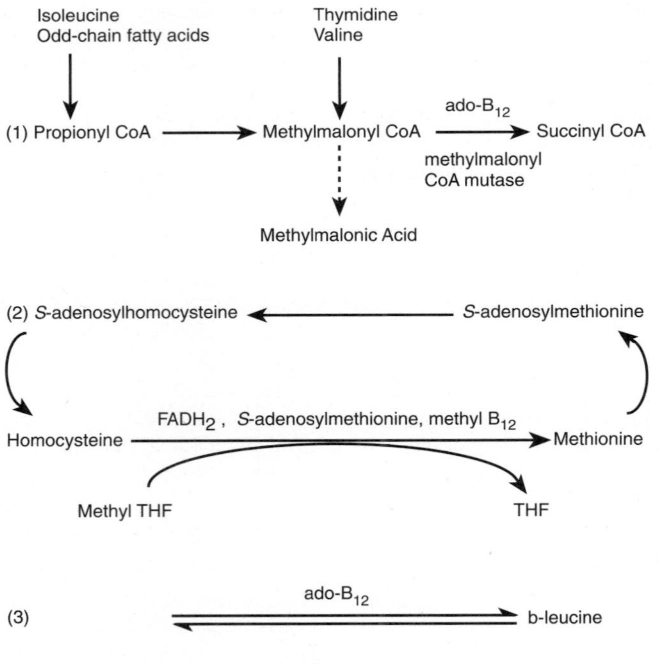

Fig. 2 Biochemical reactions of vitamin B_{12} in human tissues.

Table 2 Vitamin B_{12}-binding proteins

	Intrinsic factor	Transcobalamin I and III[1]	Transcobalamin II
Present in	Gastric juice	Plasma	Plasma, cerebrospinal fluid
Source	Gastric parietal cell	Granulocytes ? other organs	Macrophages, liver parenchyma, ileum
Molecular weight	45 000	60 000	45 500
Structure	Glycoprotein (15% sugar)	Glycoprotein	Polypeptide
Normal total binding capacity	30–110 μg/l	700–800 ng/l	900–1000 ng/l
B_{12} content	No B_{12}	300–400 ng/l B_{12}	30–60 ng/l B_{12}
Function	B_{12} absorption (not itself absorbed)	? storage of B_{12} ? protection of B_{12} Binding of B_{12} analogues	B_{12} delivery to marrow, placenta, brain, and other tissues, B_{12} absorption

[1] Related 'R' binders (haptocorrins) occur in other tissues and secretions, e.g. milk, gastric juice, saliva, and tears.

through the ileum. At neutral pH, in the presence of calcium ions, the B_{12}–IF complex attaches passively to a specific IF receptor, cubulin, on the brush border of the mucosal cells of the terminal ileum. Cubulin is a 460-kDa, 3597 amino acid, peripheral membrane protein present in the epithelium of intestine and kidney. It shows high-affinity, calcium- and cobalamin-dependent binding of IF–cobalamin. The cDNA encodes a precursor protein that undergoes proteolytic processing due to cleavage at a recognition site (Arg^7-Gen^8-Lys^9-Arg^{10}) for the trans-Golgi proteinase furin. The gene is on the short arm of chromosome 10.

After cubilin-mediated endocytosis, IF undergoes lysosomal degradation. After a delay of 3 to 5 h, B_{12} appears in portal blood, with a peak level 8 h after ingestion, complexed with transcobalamin (TC)II secreted into the circulation from the basolateral side of the intestinal cells. IF itself is digested by the cell and is not absorbed. Ileal absorption of B_{12} is limited, by the number of ileal receptors, to a few micrograms daily and although 80 per cent of a single dose of 1 to 2 μg may be absorbed, the proportion diminishes steeply at higher doses. A small (less than 1 per cent) trace of a large (1 mg or more) dose of B_{12} can be absorbed passively and rapidly through the buccal, gastric, and duodenal mucosae without IF participating.

Transport

Vitamin B_{12} in plasma is 70 to 90 per cent attached to a glycoprotein, TC I, which does not enhance cell uptake of B_{12} (see Table 2). It is one of a group of glycoproteins, the 'R' binders or haptocorrins (see above), that are present in many tissues and fluids (e.g. gastric juice, saliva, tears, milk, and colostrum) and have the same amino acid composition but differ in the composition of the carbohydrate moiety. The haptocorrins may have the role of binding analogues of B_{12} derived from food or intestinal organisms and transporting them to the liver for excretion in the bile. A closely related haptocorrin, TC III, also occurs in human plasma and is probably derived from specific granules of neutrophils. It normally carries only 0 to 10 per cent of plasma B_{12}.

The most important plasma B_{12}-binding protein, TC II, is synthesized in macrophages, liver, the ileum and possibly endothelium. TC II gains B_{12} from the ileum and by release of free B_{12} from the liver and other organs. It is normally almost completely unsaturated; however, it actively enhances uptake of B_{12} by bone marrow, placenta, and other tissues of the body that contain receptors for it. The receptor is a dimer of molecular weight 124 000. TC II–B_{12} is internalized by endocytotosis; B_{12} is split off in lysosomes but TC II is not reutilized (Table 1). TC II accounts for most of cell B_{12} uptake; it has 20 per cent amino acid homology and greater than 50 per cent nucleotide homology with human TC I and with rat IF. The regions of homology common to all three proteins are located in seven domains and it is likely that one or more of these are involved in cobalamin binding. Presumably three-dimensional differences at the ligand-binding site of the proteins exist to explain the different affinities of these proteins (TC I < TC II < IF) for cobalamin analogues. At least five genetic variants of TC II exist, distinguished by their electrophoretic mobility, probably reflecting autosomal polymorphism with many codominant alleles at one locus. Serum TC II is normally higher in women than men and in blacks than whites. The concentration of B_{12} in cerebrospinal fluid is low, with a mean of 10 ng/l in normal subjects. Most of this is attached to TC II. There is virtually no B_{12} in normal urine.

Folate

Biochemistry

This vitamin exists in nature in over 100 forms, all of which are derivatives of folic acid (pteroylglutamic acid), which consists of a pteridine, a *para*-aminobenzoic acid moiety and L-glutamic acid (Fig. 3). Natural folates may differ from folic acid by:

(1) being reduced in the pteridine ring to di- or tetrahydo- forms;

(2) having a single carbon moiety attached at positions N_5 or N_{10} (e.g. methyl, formyl, etc.); and

(3) having a chain of glutamate moieties attached by γ-peptide bonds to the L-glutamate moiety.

In human and other mammalian cells, the number of glutamates is mainly four, five, or six. Metabolism of pteroylmonoglutamates to polyglutamates by the enzyme folylpoly-γ-glutamate synthetase allows tissues to concentrate folates. In addition, folypolyglutamates are the active coenzyme forms with increased affinity or lowered K_m values for most of the enzymes of one-carbon metabolism. In body fluids (plasma, cerebrospinal fluid, bile, milk, etc.), however, folates are invariably monoglutamate derivatives. In plasma, 5-methyltetrahydrofolate (methyl-THF) predominates.

The biochemical reactions of folates are shown in Table 3. In each there is transfer of a single carbon group, methyl ($-CH_3$), formyl (–CHOH), methenyl (≡CH), methylene ($=CH_2$), or formimino (=CHNH), from one compound to another. Three of the reactions are concerned with synthesis of DNA precursors (two in purine and one in pyrimidine synthesis). During thymidylate synthesis, oxidation of folate to the dihydro state occurs; the enzyme dihydrofolate reductase, the major target for the antifolates methotrexate and pyrimethamine, returns folate to the active tetrahydro state (Fig. 4). During its reactions, folate is not completely reutilized, some degradation at the C_9–N_{10} bond occurs to non-folate compounds. Thus, folate ultilization is increased and folate deficiency likely when cell turnover and DNA synthesis are increased.

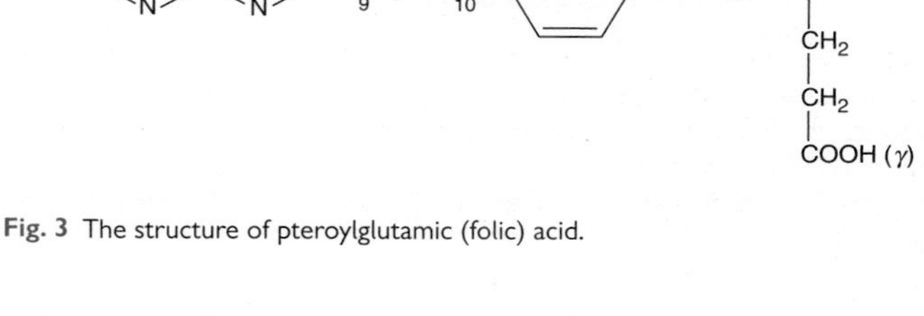

Fig. 3 The structure of pteroylglutamic (folic) acid.

Nutrition

Folate occurs in most foods, the highest concentrations (more than 30 μg/100 g wet weight) being found in liver (where, like B_{12}, its is easily destroyed by cooking, particularly if large volumes of water and high temperatures are used); vitamin C protects it from oxidative destruction so reheating of food is particularly likely to reduce the folate content. Recent studies of a Western diet suggest an average normal daily intake of 250 μg, with 50 per cent or more in the polyglutamate form. Body stores are about 10 to 12 mg, with a mean liver concentration of about 7 μg/g. Primitive or rapidly growing tissues have higher folate concentrations than corresponding mature tissues. Normal adult requirements are about 100 μg daily, although estimates as low as 50 μg and as high as 200 μg have been made.

Absorption

Folates are absorbed rapidly, mainly through the duodenum and jejunum. Polyglutamates are deconjugated to the monoglutamate in the intestinal lumen, at the brush border, and possibly in lysosomes of intestinal cells by the enzyme, 'folate conjugase' (γ-glutamylcarboxypeptidase, pteroylpolyglutamate hydrolase). They are then completely reduced to the tetrahydro state and methylated at the N_5 position so that methyl-THF enters portal plasma whatever food folate is ingested (Table 1). Folic acid itself, which is not present in food, but is used therapeutically, enters the portal blood largely unchanged at doses of more than 100 to 200 μg, as it is a poor substrate for reduction by dihydrofolate reductase. It does, however, share a specific folate uptake process through the intestine, as in the rare disorder, specific malabsorption of folate, there is failure of absorption of all folates including folic acid. The small intestine has a large capacity to absorb folate; on average 50 per cent of natural folate is absorbed whatever the dose. If excessive amounts are fed, the excess is largely excreted in urine as folates or their breakdown products after cleavage of the C_9–N_{10} bond. There is a substantial enterohepatic circulation for folate, estimated to contain up to 90 μg folate daily. If this is broken, plasma folate falls to about a third within 24 h.

Transport

Folate is transported in plasma, two-thirds unbound and about one-third loosely bound to albumin and possible other proteins. An active transport mechanism exists, however, for getting folates into cells. This is closely linked to the rate of folate polyglutamate synthesis and occurs by a carrier-mediated process, that is saturable, pH and energy dependent, with a greater preference for reduced than oxidized folates. In most cells, the folates then remain until the cells die but the liver can release folate from intact cells. Folate-binding proteins are present in human placenta, brush-border membranes of kidney tubular cells, and other cells. They are linked to membranes by a glycosyl-phosphatidyl anchor and play a part in cell uptake of folates and antifolates. Their level is regulated by extracellular and intracellular folate concentration. Milk protein, however, may enhance intestinal folate uptake. In plasma, the binding protein may take oxidized

Table 3 Biochemical reactions of folates

Reaction	Enzyme
1. **Conjugation or deconjugation**	
Hydrolysis of poly- to monoglutamates	Folate 'conjugase' (α-glutamylcarboxypeptidase; pteroylpolyglutamate hydrolase)
Conjugation of monoglutamates to polyglutamates	Folate-polyglutamate synthetase
2. **Oxidation–reduction**	
Oxidized or dihydrofolates, converted to tetrahydrofolates	Dihydrofolate reductase
3. **Amino acid interconversions**	
(*a*) homocysteine → methionine[1]	++
+ +	5-Methyl THF methyltransferase
methyl THF → THF	
(*b*)5-formiminoglutamic acid → glutamic acid	Figlu transferase
(Figlu)	
+ +	
THF → formimino THF	
(c)serine → glycine	Serine–hydroxymethyltransferase
++	
THF → 5,10-methylene THF	
4. **DNA synthesis**	
Purine synthesis:	
(a) GAR → formyl GAR	GAR transformylase
+ +	
5,10 methenyl THF → THF	
(b) AICAR → inosinic acid	AICAR transformylase
+ +	
10-formyl THF → THF	
Pyrimidine synthesis:	
Deoxyuridine monophosphate (dUMP) → thymidine monophosphate (TMP)	Thymidylate synthetase
5,10-methylene THF → THF	
5. **Formate fixation**	
Formic acid + ATP + THF → 10-formyl-THF + ADP	THF formylase
6. ? **Methylation of biogenic amines**	
e.g. dopamine → epinine	? dopamine methyltransferase
++	
methyl THF → THF	

[1] See Figs 2 and 4.

THF, tetrahydrofolate; DHF, dihydrofolate; GAR, glycinamide ribotide; AICAR, 5-amino-4-imidazolecarboxamide ribotide.

Reaction (6) has been demonstrated only *in vitro* and may not take place *in vivo*.

folates and breakdown products of folates to the liver for excretion or reconversion back to functional folates. Plasma folate is filtered by the glomerulus and mostly reabsorbed unless the renal tubular maximum is exceeded. Normal urine folate is 0 to 13 μg in 24 h. Folate is secreted into cerebrospinal fluid (which has a mean concentration of 24 μg/l) and is present in bile. Human milk has a concentration of 50 μg/l. Prostate-specific membrane antigen is a folate hydrolase carboxypeptidase which can release glutamates in either α or γ linkages. The physiological significance of this is unknown.

Biochemical basis of megaloblastic anaemia

All known causes of megaloblastic anaemia, whether drugs, deficiencies, or inborn errors of metabolism, inhibit DNA synthesis by reducing the activity of one of the many enzymes concerned in purine or pyrimidine synthesis or by inhibiting DNA poymerization from its precursors. Folate deficiency, by reducing supply of the coenzyme 5,10-methylene-THF inhibits thymidylate synthesis, a rate-limiting reaction in DNA synthesis. B_{12} does not have a direct role in this or any other reaction in mammalian DNA synthesis. B_{12} deficiency inhibits DNA synthesis indirectly by its effect on folate metabolism.

Clinical, laboratory, and biochemical observations have all shown that B_{12} deficiency disturbs folate metabolism. Patients with severe B_{12} deficiency may show a haemaotological response to folic acid in large doses. Cell folate tends to be low, formiminoglutamic acid (FIGLU) and 5-amino-4-imidazole carboxamide excretion raised, and serine–glycine interconversion reduced in B_{12} deficiency, as in folate deficiency. The deoxyuridine blocking test suggests a defect in thymidylate synthesis in B_{12} deficiency

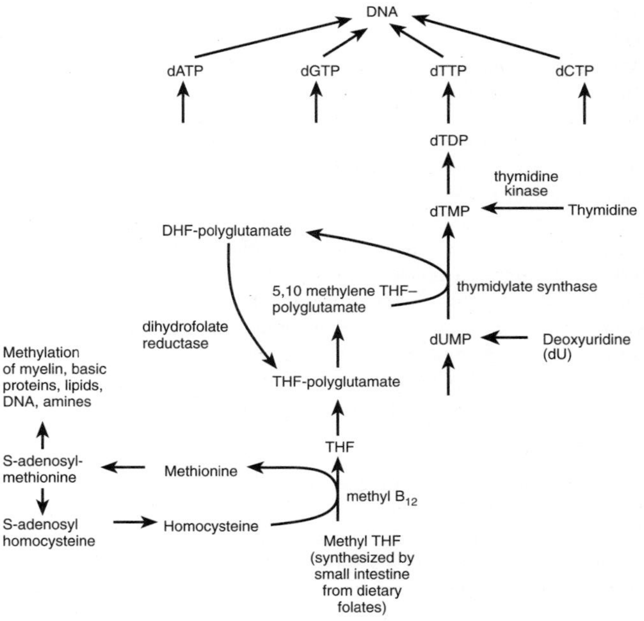

Fig. 4 Suggested mechanisms by which B_{12} deficiency affects folate metabolism and interferes with DNA synthesis. Indirect involvement of B_{12}, as methyl-B_{12}, in DNA synthesis is suggested by the 'methylfolate' trap ('tetrahydrofolate starvation') hypothesis. Methyl-B_{12} is involved in formation of intracellular THF from plasma methyl-THF. THF and/or its formyl derivative, but not methyl-THF, are the 'ground substances' from which all folate coenzymes are made by glutamate addition and single carbon unit transfer (see text). 5,10-Methylene-THF polyglutamate is involved in thymidylate synthesis. D, deoxyribose; A, adenine; G, guanine; T, thymine; C, cytosine; TP, triphosphate; DP, diphosphate; U, uridine; THF = tetrahydrofolate.

that can be corrected *in vitro* by THF as well as by B_{12}. On the other hand, cell uptake of methyl-THF is reduced and serum folate raised in B_{12} deficiency. The most anaemic patients with B_{12} deficiency, as in folate deficiency, show the lowest levels of serum and red-cell folate, and the greatest disturbance of folate biochemical reactions.

An explanation for these effects of B_{12} deficiency on folate metabolism is provided by the 'methylfolate trap' or tetrahydrofolate starvation hypothesis. This suggests that in B_{12} deficiency, folate is 'trapped' as methyl-THF, the form circulating in plasma, because of the need for methyl-B_{12} in the conversion of methyl-THF to THF. The 'trap' is supposed to lower the intracellular supply of THF, the most active of the folate compounds from which the other folate coenzymes are made. The natural folate coenzymes are the reduced derivatives of the folate polyglutamates rather than monoglutamates. Methyl-THF cannot act as a substrate for synthesis of these folate polyglutamates in human cells whereas THF (and formyl-THF) can.

The result is that B_{12} deficiency or inactivation puts a block between methyl-THF entering cells from plasma and the formation of intracellular folate polyglutamate coenzymes (Fig. 4). This causes the rise in plasma folate, a low level of intracellular folates, and reduced activity of all reactions requiring folate coenzymes, including those involved in DNA synthesis. The DNA defect has been ascribed to thymidine starvation. Thymidine corrects *in vitro* apoptosis of folate-deficient cells. Misincorporation of uracil, because of the pile up of deoxyuridine monophosphate and hence of deoxyuridine triphosphate, has been proposed to contribute to the cell abnormality.

Clinical features and causes of megaloblastic anaemia

Although pernicious anaemia is only one of the many causes of megaloblastic anaemia (Tables 4, 5, and 6), it is convenient to describe the general clinical features of the anaemia under this heading because it is the most

Table 4 Causes of B_{12} deficiency and malabsorption of B_{12}

1. **Causes of severe B_{12} deficiency**
   - (a) Nutritional:
     - vegans
     - long-continued extremely poor diet (rarely)
   - (b) Malabsorption:
     - gastric causes
       - acquired (addisonian) pernicious anaemia
       - congenital intrinsic-factor deficiency or abnormality
       - total and partial gastrectomy
       - destructive lesions of stomach
     - intestinal causes
       - gut flora associated with (jejunal diverticulosis, ileocolic, fistula, anatomical blind loop, stricture, Whipple's disease, scleroderma, HIV disease)
       - ileal resection and Crohn's disease
       - chronic tropical sprue
       - selective malabsorption with proteinuria
       - irradiation to cervix
       - HIV disease
       - fish tapeworm
       - transcobalamin II deficiency
2. **Causes of malabsorption of B_{12} usually without severe B_{12} deficiency**

Simple atrophic gastritis, gastric bypass, severe chronic pancreatitis

Zollinger–Ellison syndrome, adult gluten-induced enteropathy, giardiasis

Drugs:

- PAS, colchicine, neomycin, slow K, ethanol, metformin, phenformin, anticonvulsants

Deficiencies of folate, B_{12}, protein

frequent cause of megaloblastic anaemia in Western countries. The laboratory findings and treatment of pernicious anaemia and other megaloblastic anaemias are discussed later.

Table 5 Causes of folate deficiency

1. **Poor diet**
Especially poverty, psychiatric disturbance, alcoholism, dietary fads, scurvy, kwashiorkor, goat's milk anaemia, partial gastrectomy, other gastrointestinal disease
2. **Malabsorption**
Gluten-induced enteropathy (child or adult or associated with dermatitis herpetiformis)
Tropical sprue
Congenital specific malabsorption
Minor factor: partial gastrectomy, jejunal resection, inflammatory bowel disease, lymphoma, systemic infections
Drugs: cholestyramine, sulphasalazine, methotrexate, ? others (see (5) below).
3. **Excessive requirements**
Physiological
Pregnancy
Prematurity and infancy
Pathological:
(a) Malignancies—leukaemia, carcinoma, lymphoma, myeloma, sarcoma, etc.
(b) Blood disorders—haemolytic anaemia (especially sickle-cell anaemia, thalassaemia major), chronic myelosclerosis
(c) Inflammatory—tuberculosis, malaria, Crohn's diseases, psoriasis, exfoliative dermatitis, rheumatoid arthritis, etc.
(d) Metabolic—homocystinuria (some cases)
4. **Excess urinary excretion**
Congestive heart failure, acute liver damage, chronic dialysis
5. **Drugs**
Mechanism uncertain
Anticonvulsants (diphenylhydantoin, primidone, barbiturates)
? nitrofurantoin
? alcohol
Also drugs causing malabsorption of folate (see (2) above)
6. **Liver disease**
Mixed causes above, and poor storage

Table 6 Megaloblastic anaemia not due to vitamin B_{12} or folate deficiency

1. **Abnormalities of B_{12} or folate metabolism**
Congenital
Transcobalamin II deficiency or functional abnormality
Inborn errors of folate metabolism e.g. methylfolate transferase deficiency
Homocystinuria and methylmalonic aciduria (some cases)
Acquired
Nitrous oxide
Dihydrofolate reductase inhibitors: methotrexate, pyrimethamine, trimethoprim, ?pentamidine, triamterene
2. **Independent of B_{12} or folate**
Congenital
Orotic aciduria, (responds to uridine)
Lesch–Nyhan syndrome, ? responds to adenine
Thiamine-responsive
Some cases of congenital dyserythropoietic anaemia
Acquired
AML FAB M_6, other myeloid leukaemias (some cases)
Myelodysplasia
Drugs
Antimetabolites: 6-mercaptopurine, cytosine arabinoside, hydroxyurea, 5-fluorouracil, azathioprine, etc.

Acquired pernicious anaemia (addisonian pernicious anaemia, Biermer's anaemia)

Definition

A disease of unknown origin in which there is atrophy of the stomach leading to severely reduced or absent IF secretion with consequent severe malabsorption of B_{12} and B_{12} deficiency.

Aetiology and associated diseases

Although a disease of the stomach, pernicious anaemia is considered with blood diseases because it usually presents with anaemia; it is indeed the most common cause of megaloblastic anaemia in many countries. It is a disease of older persons, less than 10 per cent of patients are under 40 years, with an incidence of 127/100 000 in Caucasians. There is a female:male ratio in most (but not all) series of about 1.6:1. There is a higher incidence (about 44 per cent compared to 40 per cent) of blood group A compared with controls in Britain. No overall association between pernicious anaemia and HLA type has been found, but those with an endocrine disease also have a greater incidence of HLA-B8, -B12, and -BW15. There are regional differences in incidence in the United Kingdom, with over 200 cases per 100 000 in Scotland but less than 60 per 100 000 in south-east England. It occurs in all races including African, Indian, Native American, and Chinese, as well as Caucasians. There is an association with early greying and blue eyes and a higher incidence in close relatives, of either sex, of an affected person. Family history is positive in about 30 per cent of cases. Those with a positive family history exhibit a younger mean age at presentation (55 years) than those without (66 years), but the type of inheritance is not clear.

Carcinoma of the stomach occurs in about 4 per cent of patients with pernicious anaemia, about three times the control rate. Pernicious anaemia may also be associated with other 'autoimmune' diseases, particularly primary myxoedema, thyrotoxicosis, Hashimoto's disease, Addison's disease, and vitiligo. About 55 per cent of patients show thyroid antibodies and 33 per cent with primary myxoedema have parietal-cell antibody. Close relatives also may show these diseases or their associated antibodies. There is probably no significant association with diabetes mellitus. Other evidence for an immune aetiology of the gastritis of pernicious anaemia is the improvement in mucosal appearance and function with corticosteroid therapy, the presence of antibodies in serum and gastric juice directed against parietal cells and IF, and of cell-mediated immunity to IF (see Chapter 5.2). Parietal-cell antibody is present in the serum of 85 to 90 per cent of patients. The autoantigens are the α- and β-subunit of the gastrin proton pump (H^+, K^+ATPase). Two antibodies to IF exist in serum. Type I ('blocking') occurs in about 50 per cent and is directed against the B_{12}-binding site. Type II (to the ileal binding site) occurs in 30 to 35 per cent but only if type I antibody is also present. Antibodies to IF exist in gastric juice and here they may neutralize the action of remaining IF. The incidence of parietal-cell and IF antibodies in serum in pernicious anaemia may be different in different groups of patients, younger patients having a lower incidence of parietal-cell antibody while Blacks and Hispanics may have a higher incidence of IF antibodies.

The antibodies to IF are virtually specific for pernicious anaemia but parietal-cell antibody occurs in many subjects with atrophic gastritis without pernicious anaemia. Cell-mediated immunity to IF can be demonstrated in all cases of pernicious anaemia. Lymphocyte populations in IF antibody-positive patients show a CD4 to CD8 ratio higher than in controls of those negative for IF antibody. Antibody to IF may cross the placenta and cause temporary deficiency of the factor in the newborn infant. An autoantibody to the gastrin receptor may also occur in serum in pernicious anaemia.

The anaemia may also be associated with hypgogammaglobulinaemia or with selective IgA deficiency when it tends to present at an early age, and antibodies to parietal cell and IF may then be absent. The gastric lesion then includes atrophy of the antrum in contrast to classical pernicious anaemia without hypogammaglobulinaemia. Serum gastrin concentrations are normal whereas these are raised above 200 μg/l in 90 per cent of patients with pernicious anaemia and serum pepsinogen (PG) concentrations are below 30 μg/l in 92 per cent of such patients with a low PGI/PGII ratio.

The relationship of pernicious anaemia to simple gastric atrophy, which occurs in about 15 per cent of people between 40 and 60 years and in 20 to 30 per cent of the older population, is not clear. In many cases, simple gastric atrophy does not progress to the anaemia after 10 or more years of follow-up. In a minority, however, deficiency of IF severe enough to cause malabsorption of B_{12} and megaloblastic anaemia, glossitis, or B_{12} neuropathy occurs. In these people, the development of antibody to IF in the gastric juice may be important.

Pathology

There is a gastritis in which all layers of the body and fundus of the stomach are atrophied with loss of normal gastric glands, mucosal architecture, and absence of parietal and chief cells, but mucous cells lining the gastric pits are well preserved. An infiltrate of plasma cells and lymphocytes with an excess of CD8 cells occurs and intestinal metaplasia may be present. The antral mucosa is remarkably well preserved except in hypogammaglobulinaemia, and, like the fundus, shows an increased number of gastrin-secreting cells.

Clinical features

The general features of megaloblastic anaemia are similar, whatever the underlying cause. Particular clinical features may point to the underlying disease, whether pernicious anaemia or some other cause. In pernicious anaemia, the anaemia usually develops gradually, perhaps over several years, and symptoms may not occur until it is severe. The most common complaints are due to the anaemia, while loss of mental and physical drive, numbness, or difficulty in walking suggest neuropathy. Psychiatric disturbances are common and range from mild neurosis to severe organic dementia. They may occur in the absence of anaemia or macrocytosis. Mild jaundice is frequent. Loss of appetite and weight, indigestion, and episodic diarrhoea are frequent. An intercurrent infection may precipitate severe anaemia and thus symptoms. Older patients may present with congestive heart failure. In a few patients, bruising due to thrombocytopenia is marked. On the other hand, many patients are diagnosed because a routine blood test is made.

The typical patient with pernicious anaemia has fair hair (prematurely grey), with blue eyes, and wide cheekbones. Physical signs, if present, are those of anaemia, perhaps with mild jaundice, giving the patient a so-called lemon-yellow tint. A few patients with either B_{12} or folate deficiency develop a widespread brown pigmentation, affecting nail beds and skin creases particularly, but not mucous membranes, which is reversible with the appropriate therapy. The biochemical basis for this is not clear, nor for the depigmentation that also occurs rarely. The tongue may be red, smooth, and shiny, occasionally with ulcers. A mild pyrexia up to 38°C is common in patients with moderate to severe anaemia. The liver may be enlarged while the cardiovascular system shows changes due to anaemia. Patients with pernicious anaemia may also have features of an associated disorder on presentation, most commonly myxoedema. Other thyroid disorders, vitiligo, carcinoma of the stomach, Addison's disease, and hypoparathyroidism, may precede, occur simultaneously with, or follow the onset of the anaemia.

Vitamin B_{12} neuropathy

B_{12} deficiency may cause a symmetrical neuropathy affecting the lower limbs more than the upper (Section 24), which usually presents with paraesthesiae or with ataxia, particularly in the dark. In some cases, loss of cutaneous sensation, muscle weakness, urinary or faecal incontinence, an optic neuropathy, or psychiatric disturbance dominates. The neuropathy is due to severe B_{12} deficiency judged by serum B_{12} levels or methylmalonic acid excretion, but may occur with mild or no anaemia. It may be due to any cause of severe B_{12} deficiency, most commonly pernicious anaemia. A similar neuropathy has been described in dentists and others repeatedly exposed to nitrous oxide (N_2O) which inactivates methionine synthase. The biochemical explanation for the neuropathy is not clear. A defect in fatty acid metabolism in myelin tissue has been suggested. Studies in N_2O-treated monkeys have also suggested that the neuropathy results from accumulation of *S*-adenosyl homocysteine (caused by the block in conversion of homocysteine to methionine) with inhibition of transmethylation reactions in the brain. Methionine has been shown to prevent the neuropathy caused by N_2O in experimental animals. Defective methylation has yet to be shown in B_{12} neuropathy occurring clinically in man, however, or induced experimentally by dietary deficiency in fruit bats or by N_2O exposure of monkeys or rats. The role of B_{12} and folate in brain metabolism has been extensively reviewed (see Further reading list).

General tissue effects of B_{12} and folate deficiencies

Both deficiencies cause macrocytosis and other abnormal features of proliferating epithelial cells throughout the body (e.g. bronchial, bladder, buccal, and uterine cervix), with glossitis and angular cheilosis, a mild malabsorption syndrome, and reduced regeneration of damaged liver cells. In both sexes, sterility (reversible with B_{12} or folate therapy) may result from effects on the gonads. It is possible that the deficiencies in children affect overall body growth. Nutritional B_{12} deficiency in infants long term causes failure to thrive and poor brain growth with poor intellectual outcome. There does seem to be a real association of maternal folate deficiency with prematurity.

Generalized, reversible melanin pigmentation occurs in a few patients with B_{12} or folate deficiency, the cause of which is uncertain. Defective bactericidal activity of phagocytes due to impaired intracellular killing has been described in B_{12} deficiency but not in folate deficiency. B_{12} deficiency reduces serum levels of the osteoblast-related proteins alkaline phosphatase and osteocalcin but whether clinically important bone disease occurs is unknown.

Neural tube defects (NTD)

Studies by Hibbard and Smithells and coworkers in the 1960s suggested that NTD was associated with reduced maternal folate status and their early studies showed an apparent prevention of NTD by periconceptional vitamin supplementation. It is now established that folic acid supplements at the time of conception and in the early (first weeks) stage of pregnancy reduce the incidence of NTDs (anencephaly, encephalocele and spina bifida) in the first pregnancy and in subsequent pregnancies where such a malformation has occurred previously. The prophylactic daily dose used in a Medical Research Council (MRC) study was 4 mg and this reduced recurrence from 21 to six among 1195 randomized women studied; in a Hungarian first-pregnancy study, 0.8 mg daily preconception reduced the incidence from six to zero among 5000 women.

The explanation for the effect of folic acid on NTD is not certain. Women carrying NTD fetuses have lower serum folate and B_{12} levels and higher serum homocysteine levels than matched controls. There is a linear relationship when plotted on logarithmic scales between prevalence of NTD births and maternal red-cell folate, indicating that an increase in red-cell folate of a given amount is associated with a constant, proportional decrease in the birth prevalence of NTD from any given point on the red-cell folate distribution even within the accepted normal range. Folic acid prevention of NTD despite normal serum and red cell folate levels suggests that folic acid is overcoming a metabolic abnormality in folate metabolism. Only one such defect, a mutated tetrahydofolate reductase, has been identified so far.

Mutated 5,10 methylene tetrahydrofolate reductase (MHTFR) A common thermolabile variant (677C → T) (Ala 225 Val) of the enzyme

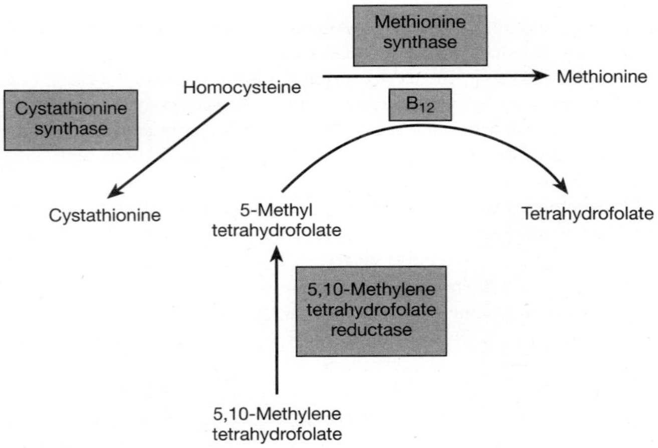

Fig. 5 The role of three enzymes (cysathione synthase, methionine synthase, and MHTFR) and three vitamins (B_{12}, B_6, and folate) in homocysteine metabolism.

MHTFR is associated with lower serum and red-cell folate levels and with higher plasma homocysteine levels than in controls in the general population. The incidence of the homozygous state in the population is approximately 5 per cent; the incidence in the parents and fetuses with NTD is approximately 13 per cent. The presence of this mutation can therefore account for only a small proportion of NTDs.

Cardiovascular disease

McCully (1969) first implicated homocysteine as a cause of atherosclerosis. This was based on pathological studies of children or young adults with congenital homocystinuria, whether due to a defect of cystathionine synthase, methionine synthase, or MHTFR (Fig. 5). In these children, plasma homocysteine levels are raised to 10 to 100 times normal. It is now apparent that even mild rises in plasma homocysteine are associated with coronary or peripheral arterial disease, with stroke and deep vein thrombosis. Determinants of plasma homocysteine include age, sex, renal function, protein intake, vitamin B_6, folate, and vitamin B_{12} status, the presence of the thermolabile variant MHTFR, smoking, and alcohol consumption, as well as intake of various drugs. Folate deficiency assessed by serum or red cell folate or by dietary folate intake is also associated with coronary vascular disease, myocardial infarct, or peripheral vascular disease. Meta-analysis, however, does not confirm an association of the presence of the thermolabile variant of MHTFR with coronary artery disease.

It seems likely that homocysteine is a cause of vascular disease rather than an associated abnormality. Folic acid fortification of the diet reduces plasma homocysteine levels. It has been estimated that fortification of the British diet with folic acid will result in 10 000 fewer annual deaths from myocardial infarct. Trials of folic acid therapy aimed at reducing the incidence of myocardial infarct are now in progress. Preliminary results of electrocardiographic studies and of coronary restenosis after coronary angioplasty in patients with coronary arterial disease receiving folic acid are encouraging.

Other causes of vitamin B_{12} deficiency

Juvenile pernicious anaemia

A few cases of pernicious anaemia with gastric atrophy, achlorhydria, and IF antibodies have occurred in children. They may show associated ('autoimmune') conditions, for example myxoedema, hypoparathyroidism, Addison's disease, or chronic mucocutaneous candidiasis.

Congenital deficiency or structural abnormality of intrinsic factor

About 40 cases have been reported of a child being born with absent or non-functioning IF but an otherwise normal stomach on biopsy and normal secretion studies (e.g. of acid). Inheritance is autosomal recessive. In some cases, IF is present in the gastric juice that is susceptible to acid degradation, cannot bind B_{12}, or that binds B_{12} but cannot attach it to ileal receptors. These children tend to present with irritability, vomiting, diarrhoea, and loss of weight, and are found to have megaloblastic anaemia. The usual age of diagnosis is about 2 years, although a few have been diagnosed as early as 4 months and others only in their teens.

Total gastrectomy

All patients who have this operation will develop B_{12} deficiency, which usually presents between 2 and 6 years postoperatively. They should be treated with prophylactic B_{12} injections from the time of the operation.

Partial gastrectomy

Iron deficiency usually accounts for the anaemia that occurs in up to half of subjects after this operation. Subnormal serum B_{12} levels develop in about 18 per cent of patients from about 2 years postoperatively. About 6 per cent develop megaloblastic anaemia due to the deficiency. In most of these patients, malabsorption of B_{12} is due to an abnormal jejunal flora. The exact incidence of B_{12} deficiency depends mainly on the size of the remnant, which tends to be smaller if the operation is subtotal and the peptic ulcer gastric rather than duodenal. Vagotomy and pyloroplasty is not a cause of B_{12} deficiency.

Small-intestinal lesions

Colonization of the upper small intestine with colonic bacteria, if sufficiently heavy as in the stagnant-loop syndrome, leads to malabsorption of B_{12}. The most common causes are listed in Table 4. It appears that the bacteria destroy IF. Infestation with the fish tapeworm (*Diphyllobothrium latum*) has a similar effect but is now almost completely eradicated; infestation is only sufficiently marked in Finland and around the lakes of Russia to frequently cause megaloblastic anaemia.

Human immunodeficiency virus (HIV) infection

Serum B_{12} levels fall progressively in HIV-infected patients and subnormal serum levels occur in 10 to 35 per cent of patients with the acquired immune deficiency syndrome. Increased levels of TC II are usual and malabsorption of B_{12}, normally not corrected by IF, has been found in some of these patients. An abnormal small-intestinal flora is the most likely cause of B_{12} malabsorption. Megaloblastic anaemia due to B_{12} deficiency is, however, rare.

Resection of a metre or more of terminal ileum

This causes severe malabsorption of B_{12}. Other diseases that may affect ileal structure and function include: tropical sprue, in which severe B_{12} deficiency with anaemia or, rarely, neuropathy is a manifestation only in the chronic phase; gluten-induced enteropathy in which megaloblastic anaemia, if it occurs, is always due to folate deficiency (and B_{12} deficiency, if it occurs, is mild); in Crohn's disease malabsorption of B_{12} is frequent but severe B_{12} deficiency is unusual unless an ileal resection, fistula, or stagnant loop occurs.

Selective malabsorption of vitamin B_{12} with proteinuria (Imerslund's disease, Imerslund–Gräsbeck syndrome, recessive megaloblastic anaemia, MGA1)

This congenital disorder with autosomal recessive inheritance is the most common cause of megaloblastic anaemia due to B_{12} deficiency in non-vegan children. The child secretes IF normally but is unable to transport B_{12} across the ileum to portal blood. Most Finnish patients with MGA1 carry the disease specific mutation P1297L (FM1) in cublin. This mutation increases the K_d for IF–B_{12} binding several fold, so that is there is substantial loss of affinity of the FM1 mutant for B_{12}. A second less frequent mutation (FM2) activates a cryptic splice site with insertion of multiple stop codons in the CUB6 domain. The proteinuria, present in over 90 per cent of cases, is benign, non-specific, and persists after B_{12} therapy. The clinical presentation of the disease is identical to that of congenital IF deficiency. The disease may be heterogeneous, encompassing defects of the ileal IF receptor or subsequent steps in transfer of B_{12} to TC II.

Other causes of malabsorption of vitamin B_{12}

A number of other conditions and drugs may cause malabsorption of B_{12} but rarely cause B_{12} deficiency of clinical severity. *p*-Aminosalicylate, colchicine, neomycin, 'slow' potassium tablets, metformin, and phenformin have all been reported to cause malabsorption of B_{12}. In chronic pancreatitis and the Zollinger–Ellison syndrome, there is failure to release B_{12} from R protein due to absence of or inactivation of pancreatic trypsin. Malabsorption of B_{12} also occurs in inherited TC II deficiency.

Malabsorption of B_{12} occurs temporarily after total-body irradiation before bone marrow transplantation. If chronic graft-versus-host disease affecting the gut develops, malabsorption of B_{12} is usual, due to the abnormal gut flora as well as any ileal defect. Irradiation to the ileum during radiotherapy treatment for carcinoma of the cervix has also been reported to cause B_{12} malabsorption.

Dietary vitamin B_{12} deficiency

This occurs most commonly in Hindus who omit all animal produce from their diet. The incidence of overt megaloblastic anaemia is much lower than the incidence of subclinical deficiency assessed by the serum B_{12} assay. These individuals have low B_{12} stores. In India, babies have been born B_{12} deficient with megaloblastic anaemia caused by severe B_{12} deficiency (due to poor diet or sprue) in the mother. Dietary deficiency of B_{12} also occurs in non-Hindu vegans, and rarely in non-vegetarian people living on inadequate diets because of poverty.

Folate deficiency

Clinical features

The main clinical features of megaloblastic anaemia due to folate deficiency are similar to those when the anaemia is due to B_{12} deficiency, except that a severe neuropathy does not occur and the underlying aetiology tends to be different. Folate deficiency may develop rapidly, and although many mildly deficient patients do not progress for months or years, in some patients the deficiency may lead to a severe pancytopenia ('arrest of haemopoiesis') over a short period, particularly if an infection supervenes.

Folate deficiency is less well established as a cause of an organic neuropathy than B_{12} deficiency but in some studies a mild peripheral neuropathy has been found in as many as 20 per cent of patients, with spinal cord dysfunction less frequently. Neurological abnormalities do occur with inborn errors of folate metabolism and may be precipitated by antifolate drugs. The suggestion that folate therapy may precipitate fits in epileptics has not been confirmed by double-blind trials. Methyl-THF donates a methyl group to homocysteine to form methionine, which passes it on to *S*-adenosyl-methionine involved in methylation of biogenic amines (e.g. dopamine), proteins, phospholipids, and neurotransmitters in the brain. This may explain some of the psychiatric disturbances, such as depression, that seem to be equally common in folate as B_{12} deficiency.

Nutritional folate deficiency

Minor degrees of nutritional folate deficiency are frequent in most countries, but severe folate deficiency may account for about 17 per cent of all cases of megaloblastic anaemia in Britain. It occurs mainly in the old and poor and psychiatrically disturbed living alone on an inadequate diet from which liver, fruit, and fresh vegetables are omitted; in many, barbiturate or alcohol consumption or a physical abnormality—partial gastrectomy, rheumatoid arthritis, or tuberculosis for example—may aggravate the effect of a poor diet. A few cases have developed because a special diet is taken, such as for pheonylkentonuria or for slimming. Scurvy is usually accompanied by severe folate deficiency while goat's milk anaemia is a nutritional folate deficiency due to the low (6 μg/l) folate content of goat's milk. In some countries, nutritional folate deficiency may be the main cause of megaloblastic anaemia, often presenting in pregnancy (e.g. in Burma, Malaysia, Africa, or India). Among Hindus, nutritional B_{12} deficiency is also common, however, and in many countries—Caribbean islands, Sri Lanka, and South-East Asia for example—tropical sprue (see Section 14.9) is an important cause of both deficiencies and is difficult to distinguish from 'pure' nutritional deficiency.

Malabsorption (see Section 14.9)

Gluten-induced enteropathy

Folate deficiency occurs in virtually all untreated patients, the serum folate being subnormal whether or not megaloblastic anaemia is present; red-cell folate is subnormal in 80 per cent or more. Anaemia occurs in about 90 per cent of adult cases, due to folate deficiency alone in 30 to 50 per cent and to mixed iron and folate deficiency in the remainder. Mild B_{12} deficiency may also occur but it is not a cause of anaemia in uncomplicated cases. Spontaneous atrophy of the spleen occurs in most of the patients; in about 10 to 15 per cent of cases, the blood film shows the presence of Howell–Jolly bodies, siderotic granules, and target and crenated cells that do not disappear with either folic acid or a gluten-free diet. Malabsorption of folic acid and of folate polyglutamates has been demonstrated in almost all untreated patients. A gluten-free diet produces a spontaneous rise in serum and red-cell folate and improved folate absorption in those patients who respond.

Malabsorption of folate also occurs in children with gluten-induced enteropathy and virtually all show subnormal serum and red-cell folate levels; anaemia is most often due to combined iron and folate deficiency but 'pure' megaloblastic anaemia also occurs.

Patients with dermatitis herpetiformis almost all show some degree of gluten-induced duodenal and jejunal abnormality; the severity of folate malabsorption and deficiency correlates with the severity of the intestinal lesion.

Tropical sprue (see Section 14.9)

Malabsorption of folate occurs in all severe, untreated patients in the acute phase and megaloblastic anaemia due to folate deficiency may develop within a few months. Not only does the anaemia respond to folate therapy but in many patients all the clinical features, and malabsorption of xylose, fat, B_{12}, and other substances, improve on folate therapy alone. Favourable responses to folic acid are most frequent in the first year of the disease, when about 60 per cent of patients appear to be cured by folic acid alone. Long-standing cases are more likely to be B_{12} deficient and thus to require B_{12} as well as folate and antibiotic therapy.

Congenital specific malabsorption of folate

This is a rare, autosomal recessive abnormality. Affected children all showed features of damage to the central nervous system (mental retardation, fits, athetotic movements) and present with megaloblastic anaemia responding to physiological doses of folic acid given parenterally but not orally. All forms of folate are poorly absorbed. Low levels of folate in cerebrospinal fluid also suggest a defect of folate transport through the choroid plexus.

Other causes

Absorption of folate is impaired by systemic infections. Mild degrees of folate malabsorption have also been reported after jejunal resection or partial gastrectomy, with Crohn's disease, and with lymphoma. In the intestinal stagnant-loop syndrome, folate levels tend to be high due to absorption of bacterially produced folate. Alcohol, anticonvulsants, oral contraceptives, antituberculous drugs, nitrofurantoin, sulphasalazine, bile-salt metabolites, and sodium bromosulphapthalein have been suggested, on variable evidence, to cause malabsorption of folate in some subjects but none is definitely established except sulphasalazine.

Increased folate utilization

A general mechanism of increased folate utilization in conditions of increased cell turnover has emerged. This consists of partial degradation of folate at the C_9–N_{10} band rather than complete recycling of the folate coenzymes required in DNA synthesis.

Pregnancy (see also Section 13)

This, associated with poor nutrition, is probably the most common cause of megaloblastic anaemia world-wide, unless folic acid supplements are taken. The frequency of the anaemia was about 0.5 per cent in most Western cities and up to 50 per cent in some areas of Asia and Africa until the introduction of prophylactic folic acid. The incidence increases with parity, is higher in twin pregnancies, and in some but not all series has been highest at the end of the winter. Folate requirements in a normal pregnancy are thought to be increased to about 300 to 400 μg daily, some 200 to 300 μg above normal. Serum and red-cell folate tend to fall as pregnancy progresses, and to rise spontaneously about 6 weeks after delivery. Lactation may prove an additional cause of folate deficiency, however, which may precipitate megaloblastic anaemia post partum.

The cause of the deficiency in pregnancy is increased degradation of folate due to hydrolysis at the C_9–N_{10} bond. Folate transfer to the fetus may play a minor part. Malabsorption of folate and increased urine folate excretion may be minor factors in some patients; in a few, megaloblastic anaemia of pregnancy is the first sign of adult coeliac disease. The statistical association of iron and folate deficiencies in pregnancy is probably due to a poor quality of the diet in certain women.

Prophylactic folic acid should now be given routinely in pregnancy; 400 μg daily is recommended (see earlier) and intake in women who may become pregnant should be at least this amount daily from food or supplements. Larger doses (4–5 mg daily) should be used if there has been a previous infant with a neural-tube defect. Conventional doses of 5 mg daily are satisfactory generally but have the theoretical drawback of being more likely to mask anaemia in the rare pregnant subject with untreated pernicious anaemia and thus might allow B_{12} neuropathy to develop.

Prematurity

Newborn infants have higher serum and red-cell folate concentrations than adults. These fall to a lowest value at about 6 weeks of age because utilization (and possibly excessive urinary loss) exceed intake. In premature infants, the fall in folate levels after birth is particularly steep and a number of such infants have developed megaloblastic anaemia, particularly if infections, feeding difficulties, or haemolytic disease with exchange transfusion have occurred. Prophylactic folic acid (e.g. 1 mg weekly for the first 3–4 weeks of life) may be given, particularly to those babies weighing less than 1.5 to 1.8 kg at birth.

Malignant diseases

Mild folate deficiency is frequent in patients with cancer (Table 5). In general, the severity correlates with the extent and degree of dissemination of the underlying disease. Patients with megaloblastic anaemia due to folate deficiency are unusual and folic acid might 'feed the tumour'; it should be withheld unless there is a real indication for its use, for example gross megaloblastosis causing severe anaemia, leucopenia, or thrombocytopenia.

Blood disorders

Chronic haemolytic anaemia Requirements for folate are increased in patients with increased erythropoiesis, particularly when there is ineffective erythropoiesis with a high turnover of primitive cells. Occasional patients, presumably those with a poor folate intake, develop megaloblastic anaemia, particularly in sickle-cell anaemia, thalassaemia major, hereditary spherocytosis, and warm-type autoimmune haemolytic anaemia, Prophylactic folic acid is usually given in these disorders.

Chronic myelofibrosis Megaloblastic haemopoiesis was reported in as many as one-third of patients in a series in London (England) with this disease but a lower incidence occurred in a large series in the United States. Circulating megaloblasts, increased transfusion requirements, severe thrombocytopenia, or pancytopenia may be the first indication that folate deficiency has developed. Polycythaemia vera is not a cause of folate deficiency.

Sideroblastic anaemia Folate deficiency, usually mild, may occur in about half of acquired cases. Megaloblastosis, refractory to folate or B_{12}, also occurs in the acquired form as in other myelodysplastic diseases.

Inflammatory diseases

Folate deficiency has been described in patients with tuberculosis, malaria, Crohn's disease, psoriasis, widespread eczema, and rheumatoid arthritis. The degree of deficiency is related to the extent and severity of the underlying disorder. Increased demand for folate probably is a factor but reduced appetite is also important in those who develop megaloblastic anaemia.

Metabolic

Homocystinuria (see Section 11) Patients with the most common form of this disorder, due to cystathionase deficiency, may show folate deficiency, possibly due to excess conversion of homocysteine to methionine and thus excess utilization of the folate coenzyme concerned.

Excess urinary loss of folate

Urine folate excretion of 100 μg a day or more occurs in some patients with congestive cardiac failure or active liver disease causing necrosis of liver cells. It is presumed that losses are due to release of folate from damaged liver cells. Haemodialysis and peritoneal dialysis remove folate from plasma. Folic acid (e.g. 5 mg weekly) is now usually given prophylactically to patients with renal failure who require long-term dialysis.

Drugs

Dihydrofolate reductase (DHFR) inhibitors

Methotrexate, aminopterin, pyrimethamine, and trimethoprim all inhibit DHFR but have different relative activities against the human, malarial, and bacterial enzymes. Methotrexate is converted to polyglutamate forms, which increases its activity against DHFR and also increases its retention in cells. They cause varying degrees of impairment of folate metabolism in man. Trimethoprim, used as an antibacterial agent, may aggravate pre-existing folate or B_{12} deficiency but does not of itself cause megaloblastic anaemia.

Alcohol

Folate deficiency may occur in spirit-drinking alcoholics. The main factor is poor nutrition and it is likely that alcohol interrupts the enterohepatic circulation for folate. It also has a direct effect on haemopoiesis, causing vacuolation of normoblasts, impaired iron utilization, sideroblastic changes, macrocytosis, megaloblastosis, and thrombocytopenia, even in the absence of folate deficiency. Beer drinkers seem relatively immune to folate deficiency because of the high folate content of beer. The usual macrocytosis in less severe, non-anaemic alcoholics is not related to folate deficiency.

Anticonvulsants, barbiturates

Diphenylhydantoin, primidone, and barbiturate therapy may be associated with some degree of folate deficiency. The more severe deficiency is associated with poor dietary intake of folate and usually prolonged drug therapy at high doses. The mechanism for the deficiency is undetermined. Malabsorption of folate, excess utilization due to induction of folate-requiring enzymes, displacement of folate from its binding protein, or competition for folate-requiring enzymes have all been suggested but not proven.

Other drugs

Nitrofurantoin, triamterene, proguanil, and pentamidine have been suggested to cause folate deficiency. Homofolates and carboxypeptidase G are two folate antagonists that have not been used in man.

Liver disease

Folate deficiency occurs most commonly in alcoholic cirrhosis where alcohol, poor nutrition, poor storage, and excess urine losses may all be important. The deficiency is less frequent in other types of liver disease.

Table 7 Laboratory diagnosis of megaloblastic anaemia

1. **General tests**
Peripheral blood film and count
Bone marrow
Serum bilirubin, iron, LDH
2. **Tests for B_{12} or folate deficiency**
Serum B_{12} and folate; red-cell folate
Serum homocysteine and methylmalonic acid levels
Deoxyuridine suppression test
3. **Tests for cause of B_{12} or folate deficiency**
B_{12} deficiency:
Serum antibodies to parietal cell, intrinsic factor
Serum immunoglobulins
Gastric secretion; intrinsic factor, acid,
Endoscopy, gastric biopsy
Barium meal + follow-through
Radioactive B_{12} absorption tests (alone, with intrinsic factor, after antibiotics, with food)
Proteinuria, fish tapeworm ova, intestinal flora, etc.
Folate deficiency:
Small-intestinal function
Xylose, glucose, vitamin A, fat, B_{12} absorption
Duodenal or jejunal biopsy
Barium follow-through
Tests for many underlying conditions

Laboratory investigation of megaloblastic anaemia

This consists of three stages: (i) recognition that megaloblastic anaemia is present; (ii) distinction between B_{12} or folate deficiency (or rarely some other factor) as the cause of the anaemia; (iii) diagnosis of the underlying disease causing the deficiency (Table 7).

Recognition of megaloblastic anaemia

The peripheral blood

There is a raised mean corpuscle volume (MCV) to between 100 fl and 140 fl. Oval macrocytes are seen in the blood film. In mild cases, macrocytosis is present before anaemia has developed. Poikilocytosis and anisocytosis are marked in severe cases. Cabot rings (composed of arginine-rich histone and non-haemoglobin iron) and occasional Howell–Jolly bodies (DNA fragments) may occur due to extramedullary haemopoiesis in the liver and spleen. The MCV may be normal if there is associated iron deficiency, when the blood film appears dimorphic, or if the anaemia (usually due to folate deficiency or antimetabolite drug therapy) develops acutely over the course of a few weeks. The MCV is also normal in some severely anaemic cases involving excess red-cell fragmentation. The reticulocyte count is low for the degree of anaemia, usually of the order of 1 to 3 per cent.

The peripheral blood also shows hypersegmented neutrophils (which have nuclei with more than five lobes) (Plate 1) and the leucocyte count is often moderately reduced in both neutrophils and lymphocytes, although the total leucocyte count rarely falls to less than 1.5×10^9/l. The lymphocyte CD4/CD8 ratio is reduced. The platelet count may be moderately reduced but rarely falls below 40×10^9/l.

Biochemical changes

These are confined to the anaemic patient and include a slight rise in serum bilirubin (up to 50 μmol/l), mainly unconjugated, a rise in serum lactic dehydrogenase of up to 10 000 IU/l, with less marked rises in serum lysosyme and serum transaminases. The serum iron is also raised and falls within 12 to 24 h of effective treatment; the serum ferritin is mildly raised and falls over the first few days of therapy. The serum cholesterol is low and alkaline phosphatase mildly reduced. Absence of haptoglobins is usual. In severe cases, free haemoglobin may be present in plasma, Schumm's test for methaemalbumin in serum is positive, and haemosiderin and fibrin degradation products are present in urine. The direct Coombs' test is weakly positive in some patients, due to complement.

Bone marrow

The bone marrow is hypercellular in moderate or severely anaemic cases and expanded along the lengths of the long bones. The myeloid–erythroid ratio is often reduced or reversed. The erythroblasts are larger than normal and show a number of morphological abnormalities; there is asynchronous maturation of nucleus and cytoplasm, nuclear chromatin remaining primitive with an open, lacy, fine granular pattern despite normal maturation and haemoglobinization of the cytoplasm. Fully haemoglobinized cells with incompletely condensed nuclei may be seen. Excessive numbers of dying cells, and nuclear remnants including Howell–Jolly bodies, mitoses, and multinucleate cells may be present. Because of death (by apoptosis) of later cells, there is a disproportionate accumulation of early cells. Giant and abnormally shaped metamyelocytes and megakaryocytes with hypersegmented nuclear lobes are also usually present (Plate 2). Studies with labelled thymidine have shown an increase of cells in G_2 and mitosis, and of cells with intermediate amounts of DNA between 2C and 4C but not synthesizing DNA, and presumably destined to die.

The severity of these changes tend to parallel the degree of anaemia. In milder cases, changes, described as 'intermediate', 'transitional', or 'moderate', are principally in the size and nuclear chromatin pattern of the individual developing erythroid cells, with giant metamyelocytes present; hypercellularity and gross dyserythropoiesis may be absent. In very mild cases, megaloblastic changes are difficult to recognize. In patients with severe anaemia but only mild megaloblastic changes, some additional cause for the anaemia should be sought.

Deoxyuridine suppression test

This is an *in vitro* biochemical test for B_{12} or folate deficiency based on the presence of a block in thymidylate synthesis (see Fig. 2). Deoxyuridine added to normoblastic cells reduces the incorporation of radioactive thymidine into DNA. The deoxyuridine is converted into deoxyuridine monophosphate (dUMP) and hence to mono-, di-, and tri-thymidine phosphates, which inhibit thymidine kinase and so reduce uptake of the labelled thymidine. Uptake of labelled thymidine into DNA is not blocked as much by deoxyuridine in cells from patients with B_{12} or folate deficiency as in normoblastic cells because of the block in conversion of dUMP to dTMP (thymidine monophosphate) in megaloblasts. Correction of the test *in vitro* with B_{12} or methyl-THF can be used to differentiate the two deficiencies as B_{12} will correct in B_{12} deficiency whereas methyl-THF does not; the reverse occurs in folate deficiency. The test is normal in cells from patients with megaloblastosis due to a block in DNA synthesis other than at thymidylate synthetase.

Chromosomes

Changes found in marrow and other proliferating cells include: (a) random chromatin breaks; (b) exaggeration of centromere constriction; and (c) thin, elongated, uncoiled chromosomes.

Ineffective haemopoiesis

The increased cellularity of the marrow with degenerate forms, and the low reticulocyte count, account for the degree of anaemia and suggest that many developing cells are dying in the marrow. This occurs by apoptosis, especially of late erythroblasts. Red-cell survival is moderately shortened, and radio-iron studies show rapid clearance, with increased plasma iron turnover but poor red-cell iron utilization. The raised uncongugated serum bilirubin, lactic dehydrogenase, and lysosyme are all due to ineffective haemopoiesis.

Differential diagnosis

Other causes of macrocytosis include a high reticulocytosis (e.g. haemolytic anaemia or regeneration of blood after haemorrhage), aplastic anaemia, red-cell aplasia, liver disease, alcoholism and myxoedema, the myelodysplastic syndromes, myeloid leukaemias, cytotoxic drug therapy, chronic respiratory failure, myelomatosis, and other causes of a leucoerythroblastic anaemia. Once a bone marrow biopsy has been done, the principal differentiation is from other causes of megaloblastosis, particularly myelodysplasia. Other causes of megaloblastic anaemia not due to B_{12} or folate deficiency are listed in Table 6.

Some patients with rapidly developing megaloblastic anaemia, particularly due to folate deficiency, may develop almost complete aplasia of the red-cell series, and the peripheral blood and bone marrow may resemble that of acute myeloid leukaemia.

Diagnosis of vitamin B_{12} or folate deficiency

The peripheral blood and bone marrow appearances are identical in folate or B_{12} deficiency. Special tests are, therefore, needed to distinguish between the two deficiencies. The deoxyuridine suppression test has been described already (see above), and is used for reliable and rapid diagnosis in some laboratories but it is not widely available.

Vitamin B_{12} deficiency

The assay of the B_{12} content of serum is now usually done by immunoassay. The normal ranges have been reported to be higher with the immunoassays (e.g. 200–1200 ng/l) than the previously used microbiological assays (e.g. 160–900 ng/l). Subnormal levels are found in cases of megaloblastic anaemia due to B_{12} deficiency, being extremely low in B_{12} neuropathy. Subnormal serum B_{12} concentrations in the absence of tissue B_{12} deficiency have been reported in pregnancy, in severe nutritional folate deficiency, in subjects taking large doses of vitamin C, and occasionally in iron deficiency.

Raised serum B_{12} levels, if not due to therapy or a contaminated serum, are most commonly caused by a raised B_{12}-binding capacity due to a rise in TC I as in a leucocytosis due to a myeloproliferative disease—chronic myeloid leukaemia, polycythaemia rubra vera, or in eosinophilic leukaemia for example. Raised levels of 'R' binder also occur in association with some tumours, especially hepatoma and fibrolamellar tumour of the liver. In benign leucocytosis, the rise is mainly of TC III and this is often not accompanied by a high serum B_{12}. Raised levels of TC II occur in conditions where macrophages are stimulated; for example autoimmune diseases such as systemic lupus erythematosus, rheumatoid arthritis, in Gaucher's disease and in some monocytic or monoblastic leukaemias, in histiocytic lymphomas, and inflammatory bowel disease. In active liver diseases, serum B_{12} leaks from the liver with saturation of the serum B_{12} binders.

A third and less widely used test for B_{12} deficiency is the measurement of the serum concentration of methylmalonic acid (MMA) or 24-h urine excretion of MMA. Serum MMA levels and excretion of MMA are raised in B_{12} deficiency but not in folate deficiency but raised levels may occur in renal failure. Rare cases of congenital methylmalonic aciduria have been described, owing to a variety of enzyme defects.

A sensitive method of measuring MMA in serum has been introduced and combined with serum homocysteine assay for the diagnosis of B_{12} or folate deficiency. Savage, Lindenbaum, Stabler, Allen, and others have used the serum MMA concentration to diagnose B_{12} deficiency in the absence of macrocytes or anaemia in patients with neuropathy and serum B_{12} concentration of more than 200 ng/l. Most find that patients with B_{12} neuropathy show haematological changes of B_{12} deficiency and there are not substantial numbers of patients with undiagnosed pernicious anaemia with normal haematological findings and borderline or even normal serum B_{12} levels.

Folate deficiency

Direct tests include the serum and red-cell folate assay. In most laboratories immunoassays are now used. The serum folate is always low in folate deficiency (and is normal or raised in B_{12} deficiency unless folate deficiency is also present). The serum folate does not accurately measure the severity of folate deficiency. Raised levels occur after folate therapy and also in B_{12} deficiency and in the stagnant-loop syndrome. Red-cell folate is a better guide than the serum folate to tissue folate stores but is also low in a proportion of patients with megaloblastic anaemia solely due to B_{12} deficiency. Serum homocysteine levels are usually raised in folate deficiency, but also in B_{12} deficiency and many other situations.

Diagnosis of the cause of vitamin B_{12} deficiency

Although the clinical and family history and the clinical findings may point to pernicious anaemia or some other cause of B_{12} deficiency, it is important to establish this for certain. A brief dietary history will rapidly establish whether or not the patient is a vegan or takes a very inadequate diet. Radioactive B_{12} absorption tests are valuable to demonstrate malabsorption of B_{12} and to differentiate gastric from small-intestinal lesions as the cause. The patient, after an overnight fast, is fed an oral radioactively labelled dose of cyanocobalamin, usually 1 μg cobalt-57 B_{12}. Absorption can be measured by whole-body counting or by 24-h urinary excretion after a non-radioactive, parenteral flushing dose of 1 mg B_{12} (Schilling test). Hydroxocobalamin, instead of cyanocobalamin as originally described, can be used to flush absorbed, labelled B_{12} into urine.

Normal subjects absorb more than 30 per cent of the 1-μg dose. In patients with a gastric cause, malabsorption is corrected when the labelled B_{12} is given with IF, whereas if the lesion is small intestinal, the absorption does not improve with IF. Treatment with broad-spectrum antibiotics may improve the absorption in the stagnant-loop syndrome. In some patients with pernicious anaemia, the absorption with IF only improves substantially after weeks of B_{12} therapy, possibly due to slow recovery of ileal function from the effects of B_{12} deficiency. A combined test 'Dicopac' was available in which B_{12} labelled with cobalt-57 is given simultaneously with cobalt-58 B_{12} attached to IF. This has been withdrawn because human IF cannot be guaranteed to be virus or prion free. A double isotope test has also been developed in which cobalt-58 B_{12} is incorporated *in vitro* in egg yolk; cobalt-58 B_{12} is given in crystalline form. It is aimed to give a more accurate guide to food B_{12} absorption. Some patients with atrophic gastritis, or after partial gastrectomy and low serum B_{12} levels, may show normal absorption of crystalline B_{12} but reduced absorption of food B_{12}. Patients with pernicious anaemia show malabsorption of both forms.

Gastric secretion studies after pentagastrin stimulation in pernicious anaemia reveal achlorhydria (resting pH 7.0 and not falling by more than 1.0 unit on stimulation) and grossly reduced or absent IF in gastric juice.

Endoscopy and gastric biopsy will show features of gastric atrophy and help to exclude gastric carcinoma. Follow-through radiographic examination of the small intestine will help to exclude a small-intestinal lesion, duodenal or jejunal diverticulosis for example.

The serum gastrin level is raised in most patients with gastric atrophy and the serum is tested for antibodies to IF, parietal cells, and thyroid; serum immunoglobulins are measured in view of the association with hypogammaglobulinaemia.

Diagnosis of the cause of folate deficiency

An inadequate diet is usually at least partly implicated, but an exact estimate of dietary intake from the clinical history is impossible because of variation in folate content of foods, losses in cooking, and size of portions. Often it is the general social circumstances that suggest a poor intake. Drug intake, particularly of barbiturates, is important. Many underlying inflammatory or malignant diseases may exaggerate the tendency to folate deficiency in patients with inadequate diets. The main cause of malabsorption of folate is gluten-induced enteropathy; in patients with severe folate deficiency, tests for antiendomysial and antigliadin antibodies and a duodenal biopsy are usually necessary. In certain tropical countries, sprue may cause a generalized malabsorption syndrome in which folate deficiency commonly occurs. Tests of folate absorption have been devised, either by measuring the rise in serum folate after an oral dose of folic acid or of more natural folate derivatives (e.g. folate polyglutamates), or by measuring urinary or faecal excretion of radioactivity after feeding one or other labelled folate compound. None of these tests has achieved routine use.

Treatment of megaloblastic anaemia

Therapy is aimed at correcting the anaemia, completely replenishing the body of whichever vitamin is deficient, treatment of the underlying disorder, and prevention of relapse. In most cases, it is possible to diagnose which deficiency is present before starting therapy.

Vitamin B_{12} deficiency

Hydroxocobalamin 1000 μg intramuscularly given six times at several days' interval over the first few weeks will restore normal B_{12} stores. There is no evidence that patients with B_{12} neuropathy derive greater benefit from more frequent doses, although many physicians use these for 6 months or so.

Response to therapy

The patient feels better within 24 to 48 h, and the mild fever, if not due to infection, falls to normal. A painful tongue and unco-operative, disorientated state may also be improved in 48 h. The reticulocyte count begins to rise on the second day with a peak after 5 to 7 days. The white-cell count becomes normal by the third to seventh day and the platelet count rises and may reach levels of 500 to 1000 × 10^9/l before falling to normal at about 10 to 14 days. The bone marrow reverts to normoblastic by 36 to 48 h, although giant metamyelocytes persist for 10 to 12 days. The serum iron falls within 24 h, usually to subnormal levels, while the serum lactic dehydrogenase falls more slowly during the first 14 days of therapy.

The neuropathy always improves with therapy but residual deficits remain in some patients, particularly those with the longest histories and the most severe manifestations.

Maintenance

Hydroxocobalamin, 1000 μg intramuscularly, is given once every 3 months for life in pernicious anaemia and most other causes of B_{12} deficiency to prevent relapse. The life expectancy in pernicious anaemia once treated, is as good as that in the general population in women, and slightly lower in men, probably due to the increased incidence of carcinoma of the stomach. In a few patients with B_{12} deficiency, the underlying cause can be reversed; for example expulsion of the fish tapeworm, improvement of vegan diet, surgical correction of an intestinal stagnant loop. A few micrograms of B_{12} can be absorbed each day in pernicious anaemia from oral doses of 1000 μg or more by passive diffusion, but this maintenance therapy is usually reserved for those who cannot have injections—for example those with a bleeding disorder, or who refuse them—and for the extremely rare individual who is allergic to all injectable forms of B_{12}. Vegans may be maintained on much smaller oral doses of B_{12} each day, such as 50 μg as a tablet or syrup.

Prophylactic maintenance

B_{12} therapy should be given from the time of operation after total gastrectomy or after ileal resection if a B_{12} absorption test postoperatively reveals malabsorption of the vitamin. Patients with pernicious anaemia tend to develop iron-deficiency anaemia and they may also develop thyroid disorders or carcinoma of the stomach. It is advisable that a regular blood count be made once a year. Routine, regular endoscopy is not warranted but these diseases must be particularly borne in mind if relevant symptoms or signs develop.

Folate deficiency

This is corrected by giving 5 mg folic acid by mouth daily. It is essential to exclude B_{12} deficiency so that precipitation of a neuropathy is avoided. It is usual to continue for at least 4 months until there is a completely new set of red cells, although body stores will theoretically be normal within a few days of therapy. In patients with severe malabsorption of folate, larger oral doses of folic acid (e.g. 5 mg three times daily) may be used but it is not necessary to give parenteral folate except for those unable to swallow tablets. The response to therapy is as described for B_{12}. The decision whether or not to continue folic acid beyond 4 months depends on whether or not the cause can be corrected. In practice, long-term folic acid is usually needed only in patients with severe haemolytic anaemias (e.g. sickle-cell anaemia and thalassaemia major), myelofibrosis, and in gluten-induced enteropathy when a gluten-free diet is either unsuccessful or not feasible. In patients on a gluten-free diet, assessment of folate status is one simple way of following the improvement in absorption.

Prophylactic folic acid

This should be given to all pregnant women (doses of 300 to 400 μg daily are used, often combined with an iron preparation) and, if the diet is poor, to all women likely to become pregnant. Larger doses are given if there has been a previous neural tube-deficit infant. Folic acid is given to patients undergoing regular haemodialysis or peritoneal dialysis, to premature infants weighing less than 1.5 kg at birth, and to selected patients in intensive care units or receiving parenteral nutrition.

Folate therapy has been shown to improve chromosomal stability in the fragile X syndrome, even though these patients do not have folate deficiency or a demonstrable defect of folate metabolism.

Food fortification

Fortification of cereals and grains with folic acid (140 μg/100 g cereal grain) began in the United States in 1996. Median serum folate in clinical specimens in United States rose from 12.6 to 18.7 μg/l between 1997 and 1998. There was also a reduction of plasma homocysteine in patients with coronary heart disease by consumption of a breakfast cereal fortified with folic acid. These results are consistent with those of the Framingham study which found a rise in serum folate and fall in serum homocysteine in the subjects taking a fortified diet from 1997 to 1998. In one study, addition of 400 μg folic acid daily over a 6-month period resulted in a rise in mean red-cell folate in young adult females from 295 to 571 μg/l, sufficient to reduce the incidence of NTD by 58 per cent. It is also hoped that there will be a significant reduction of deaths from cardiovascular disease by food fortification with folic acid. The theoretical side-effects of fortification are largely in patients with unsuspected B_{12} deficiency who theoretically might present with neuropathy if the extra folate consumed prevents the development of anaemia due to B_{12} deficiency. There is, however, no definite evidence for this at the supplemental doses given in the United States and proposed in Britain. In Britain fortification of flour with folic acid 240 μg per 100 g flour has been recommended but not yet implemented.

Folinic acid (5-formyl-THF)

This reduced folate is used to prevent or treat toxicity due to methotrexate or other dihydrofolate reductase inhibitors.

Severely ill patients

Some patients, usually elderly, are admitted to hospital severely ill with megaloblastic anaemia, perhaps in congestive heart failure or with pneumonia. In this case, it is necessary to commence therapy immediately after obtaining blood for B_{12} and folate assay and aspirating bone marrow, before it is known which deficiency is present. Both vitamins should be given simultaneously in large doses. Heart failure and infection should be treated in conventional fashion but blood transfusion should be avoided, except in cases of extreme anaemia, when 1 to 2 units of packed cells may be given slowly, accompanied by removal of a similar volume of blood from the other arm, and diuretic therapy.

Other therapy

Hypokalaemia may occur during the response to therapy and oral potassium supplements should be given to those with initial heart failure or if severe hypokalaemia is demonstrated, but are not needed routinely. An attack of gout has been reported on the sixth to seventh day of therapy. Most patients develop hyperuricaemia at this stage but the clinical disease probably only occurs in those with a strong gouty tendency. Iron deficiency commonly develops in the first few weeks of therapy and this should be treated initially with oral ferrous sulphate in the usual way.

Megaloblastic anaemia due to inborn errors of folate or vitamin B_{12} metabolism

Folate

A number of babies have been described with congenital deficiency of one or other enzyme concerned in folate metabolism: 5-methyltetrahydrofolate, methylene THF-reductase, FIGLU-transferase, methenyl-THF cyclohydrolase. Some of the babies had multiple congenital defects including the heart and cerebral ventricles and nearly all showed impaired mental development. In the methylfolate transferase deficiency, megaloblastic anaemia was present.

Vitamin B_{12}

Congenital deficiency of TC II was first reported in 1971 in two siblings who developed megaloblastic anaemia requiring therapy with large daily doses of B_{12} at 3 and 5 weeks of age. Similarly affected families have been described in which neuropathy developed in the absence of adequate therapy. A spectrum of loss of TC II occurs and functionally inactive TC II has been detected in some cases, often presenting later in life. The serum B_{12} level is usually normal, B_{12} being bound to TC I. Absorption of B_{12} is impaired. Treatment is with massive doses of B_{12} (e.g. 1000 μg intramuscularly three times each week). In contrast, in subjects with rare, inherited, low levels of TC I, low serum B_{12} levels occur, but haemopoiesis is normal.

Children with one form of congenital methylmalonic aciduria, which responds to B_{12} therapy in large doses, have been shown to have a defect in conversion of hydroxocobalamin to ado-B_{12}. They do not show megaloblastic anaemia. In a few, this defect has been associated with a defect of formation of methyl-B_{12} and with homocystinuria, but some of the children have also surprisingly not shown megaloblastic anaemia. Neurological abnormalities are usual. Homocystinuria and megaloblastic anaemia without methymalonic aciduria have also been reported. In some cases, the defect appears to be in maintaining B_{12} bound to methionine synthase in the reduced state.

Megaloblastic anaemia due to acquired disturbances of folate or vitamin B_{12} metabolism

Folate

Therapy with dihydrofolate reductase inhibitors may cause megaloblastic anaemia. This is usual with methotrexate and less likely with pyrimethamine unless high doses are used or the patient is already folate deficient. Trimethoprim and triamterene are very weak folate antagonists in man, but may precipitate megaloblastic anaemia in patients already B_{12} or folate deficient (see earlier).

Vitamin B_{12}

Nitrous oxide (N_2O)

This anaesthetic gas oxidizes B_{12} from the active fully reduce cob(I)alamin form to the inactive cob(II)alamin and cob(III)alamin forms, inactivating methyl-B_{12} and hence methionine synthase. Megaloblastosis develops within several hours in man and a fault in thymidylate synthase can be demonstrated by the deoxyuridine suppression test in human marrow exposed to N_2O. This recovers over several days when exposure to N_2O is discontinued. After many weeks exposure to N_2O, monkeys develop a neuropathy resembling B_{12} neuropathy in man; peripheral neuropathies have also been described in humans (e.g. dentists and anaesthetists) repeatedly exposed to the gas. When N_2O is used as anaesthetic for patients with low B_{12} stores, megaloblastic anaemia or neuropathy may be precipitated months later, due to failure to replenish B_{12} stores by absorption. Recovery from N_2O exposure needs new cobalamin and also synthesis of new apoenzyme (methionine synthase) because this protein is also damaged by active oxygen derived from the N_2O–cobalamin reaction. Methylmalonic aciduria has not been found in animals or humans exposed for short periods to N_2O, as methylmalonic CoA mutase does not need reduced B_{12}.

Megaloblastic anaemia not due to folate or vitamin B_{12} deficiency or metabolic defect

Congenital

Orotic aciduria

This is a rare, recessive disorder involving two consecutive enzymes (orotidylic pyrophosphatase and orotidylic decarboxylase) in pyrimidine synthesis and presents with megaloblastic anaemia in the first few months of life. The diagnosis is made if needle-shaped, colourless crystals of orotic acid are found in the urine, daily excretion ranging from 0.5 to 1.5 g. Heterozygotes excrete slightly raised amounts of orotic acid but show no haematological disorder. Treatment with uridine (1–1.5 g daily) leads to a haematological response, restoration of normal haemopoiesis and growth, and reduction in orotic acid excretion.

Lesch–Nyhan syndrome

A few patients with this rare disorder of purine synthesis have shown megaloblastic change but whether this was due to associated folate deficiency or a direct result of reduced purine synthesis is not certain (see Section 11).

Vitamin E deficiency

This has been reported to cause megaloblastosis in a group of children with kwashiorkor. However, many were also folate deficient.

Vitamin C deficiency

Megaloblastic appears to be due to associated folate deficiency.

Thiamine responsive

About 12 cases have been well documented. They have also shown sideroblastic change and a defect in phosphorylation of thiamines has been implicated. Diabetes mellitus and semineural deafness are additional features.

Responding to large doses of vitamin B_{12} and folate

A single patient has been reported who needed both vitamins in large doses but the site of the defect was not elucidated.

Congenital dyserythropoietic anaemia

Some cases of congenital dyserythropoietic anaemia show megaloblastic changes not due to B_{12} or folate deficiency.

Acquired

Megaloblastic changes are often marked in acute myeloid leukaemia/M6 and less commonly in other forms of acute myeloid leukaemia. They also occur in about 50 per cent of patients with primary acquired sideroblastic anaemia and in other myelodysplastic syndromes. The exact site of block in DNA synthesis in these syndromes is unknown.

Drugs that directly inhibit purine or pyrimidine synthesis (e.g. cytosine arabinoside, 5-fluorouracil, hydroxyurea, 6-mercaptopurine, or azathioprine) may cause megaloblastic anaemia. Alcohol has also been found to have a direct effect on the bone marrow, causing megaloblastosis in some cases even in the absence of B_{12} or folate deficiency. On the other hand, drugs that inhibit mitosis (e.g. colchicine or daunorubicin) or alkylate preformed DNA (e.g. cyclophosphamide, chlorambucil, or busulfan) do not cause megaloblastosis.

Other deficiency anaemias

Vitamin C

Anaemia is usual in scurvy but the pathogenesis is complicated. It is likely that vitamin C has a direct effect on erythropoiesis but folate and iron deficiencies, haemorrhage, or haemolysis often complicate the picture.

Biochemical and nutritional aspects

Vitamin C is needed for collagen synthesis by its involvement in the hydroxylation of protein and for maintenance of intercellular substance of skin, cartilage, periosteum, and bone. It may also have a general role in oxidative–reduction systems, for example glutathione, cytochromes, pyridine, and flavin nucleotides. Although vitamin C is also thought to be needed for maintaining body folates in the reduced active state, the exact reactions involved are unclear. Vitamin C has a particular role in iron metabolism, iron excess causing increased utilization of vitamin C and in extreme cases clinical scurvy, whereas iron deficiency is associated with a raised leucocyte ascorbate concentration. Vitamin C is needed for incorporation of iron from transferrin into ferritin and for iron mobilization from ferritin. Vitamin C therapy increases iron excretion in patients receiving subcutaneous desferrioxamine infusions and also, at least in experimental animals, affects iron distribution by increasing parenchymal relative to reticuloendothelial iron. Minimum adult daily requirements for vitamin C are about 10 mg but 30 to 70 mg is recommended; utilization, and therefore requirement, are relatively higher in infants, children, and pregnant and lactating women. Vitamin C may be excreted as such but is also broken down to oxalate.

Vitamin C is present in food as its reduced (ascorbic acid) and oxidized (dehydroascorbic acid) forms, the highest concentrations occurring in greens, fruits, tomatoes, liver, and kidney. Potatoes are not a rich source but provide a substantial proportion of normal dietary intake. Cooking, particularly in alkaline conditions with large volumes of water, destroys the vitamin, which is also lost on storage with exposure to the air. Absorption occurs through the length of the small intestine and deficiency is never solely due to malabsorption.

The anaemia of scurvy is typically normochromic, normocytic with a slightly raised reticulocyte count to 5 to 10 per cent and a normoblastic marrow with erythroid hyperplasia. This suggests a direct role for vitamin C in erythropoiesis but not all patients with clinical scurvy are anaemic. Extravascular haemolysis with mild jaundice and increased urobilinogen excretion occurs in many of the patients. Moreover, in many the anaemia is complicated by folate deficiency (due to inadequate folate intake) with a megaloblastic marrow, or in a few by iron deficiency due to external haemorrhage, reduced diet intake, and possibly reduced iron absorption. In a few patients placed on a low folate diet, response of megaloblastic haemopoiesis to vitamin C alone has been described. In others, response of the megaloblastic anaemia to folic acid alone on a low vitamin C diet has occurred but in most such cases, both vitamin C and folic acid have been found necessary.

Vitamin B_6

This, as its coenzyme form pyridoxal-5-phosphate, is involved in many reactions of the body, especially transaminases and decarboxylases. It is also a cofactor in the important rate-limiting reaction in haem synthesis, δ-aminolaevulinic acid (ALA)-synthetase (see Section 11). It occurs in natural tissues in three major forms: pyridoxine, pyridoxamine, and pyridoxal phosphate. Red cells are capable of interconverting them. Anaemia due purely to vitamin B_6 deficiency has been produced in animals. It is hypochromic and microcytic with a raised serum iron and increased iron in erythroblasts, with some partial or complete ring sideroblasts. A similar anaemia has occurred in humans with malabsorption, pregnancy, or haemolysis but has not been fully documented to respond to physiological doses of vitamin B_6 alone. Vitamin B_6-responsive anaemia is, however, well documented among patients with sideroblastic anaemia of all types. Pyridoxine responses occur particularly in the inherited form (when it is assumed that a fault in one or other enzyme of haem synthesis, for example ALA-synthetase, increases the need for pyridoxal phosphate as cofactor) and when sideroblastic anaemia occurs in patients receiving pyridoxine antagonists, such as antituberculous drugs. The value of pyridoxine dietary supplements in lowering serum homocysteine and reducing the incidence of cardiovascular disease has yet to be explored.

Riboflavin

On the basis of studies in experimental animals and humans fed a deficient diet together with a riboflavin antagonist, deficiency of this vitamin is known to cause a normochromic, normocytic anaemia associated with a low reticulocyte count and red-cell aplasia in the marrow, sometimes with vacuolated normoblasts. The exact biochemical basis is undecided. Clinically, a similar anaemia may occur in pure form but is usually associated with the anaemia due to protein deficiency, as in kwashiorkor or marasmus. Other clinical features of riboflavin deficiency—dermatitis, angular cheilosis, and glossitis for example—may be present.

Thiamine

For discussion, see under megaloblastic anaemia not due to folate or B_{12} deficiency or metabolic defect.

Nicotinic acid, pantothenic acid, and niacin

Deficiencies of these vitamins cause anaemia in experimental animals but anaemia purely due to one or other of these deficiencies has not been established to occur in man.

Vitamin E

This vitamin is needed for preventing peroxidation of cell membranes. A haemolytic anaemia responding to vitamin E has been reported in premature infants. Less well documented is a macrocytic anaemia due to vitamin E deficiency in protein-calorie-deficient infants and aggravation of anaemia in patients with thalassaemia major because of vitamin E deficiency.

Protein deficiency (see Section 10)

Anaemia is usual in both 'pure' protein deficiency, kwashiorkor, and in protein-calorie malnutrition (marasmus). It has been reported in many parts of the world where malnutrition, especially in children and pregnant women, is common. The anaemia also occurs in patients with gastrointestinal disease and severe malabsorption. The anaemia is typically normochromic, normocytic, and of the order of 8.0 to 9.0 g/dl. The reticulocyte count is usually reduced and the marrow may show a selective reduction in erythropoiesis. Experimental studies in animals suggest that the anaemia is largely due to reduced serum erythropoietin levels consequent on a lack of stimulus for erythropoietin secretion. Lack of amino acids for synthesis of erythropoietin or globin is not the cause. In many patients, the anaemia is complicated by infection, folate or iron deficiency, and possibly other vitamin deficiencies (e.g. riboflavin, vitamin E) and then it may be more severe and show additional morphological abnormalities in the blood and marrow.

Further reading

General

Chanarin I (1989). *The megaloblastic anaemias*, 3rd edn. Blackwell Science, Oxford. [The major textbook dealing with all aspects.]

Green R (1995). Metabolite assays in cobalamin and folate deficiency. *Clinical Haematology* **8**, 533–66. [Measurements of MMA and homocysteine in plasma are discussed as diagnostic tests for cobalamin and folate deficiencies.]

Green R, Miller JW (1999). Folate deficiency beyond megaloblastic anemia: hyperhomocysteimia and other manifestations of dysfunctional folate status. *Seminars in Hematology* **36**, 477–64. [An excellent review of the non-haematological aspects of folate deficiency.]

Hoffbrand AV, ed. (1976). Megaloblastic anaemia. *Clinical Haematology* **5**, 471–69. [A collection of 12 major reviews dealing with vitamin B_{12} and folate.]

Rosenblatt DS, Hoffbrand AV (1999). Megaloblastic anaemia and disorders of cobalamin and folate metabolism. In: Lilleyman J, Hann I, Blanchette V, eds. *Pediatric hematology*, pp.167–84. Churchill Livingstone, London. [A recent review of inborn errors of B_{12} and folate.]

Savage DG, Lindenbaum J, Stabler SP, Allen RH (1994). Similarities of serum methylmalonic acid and total homocysteine determinations for diagnosing cobalamin and folate deficiencies. *American Journal of Medicine* **96**, 239–46. [Reviews the value of these assays for diagnosing the deficiencies even in patients with normal serum levels of B_{12} and folate.]

Wickramasinghe SN, ed. (1995). Megaloblastic anaemia. Baillieres *Clinical Haematology* **8**, 441–703. A volume containing 12 major articles reviewing different aspects of vitamin B_{12} and folate. [This volume also contains reviews of different aspects of vitamin B_{12} and folate.]

Wickramasinghe SN (1999). The wide spectrum and unresolved issues of megaloblastic anemia. *Seminars in Hematology* **36**, 3–18. [An excellent general update on megaloblastic anaemia.]

Vitamin B_{12}

Carmel R (1995). Malabsorption of food cobalamin. *Clinical Haematology* **8**, 639–56. [This review brings together a large literature.]

Chanarin I, Metz J (1997). Diagnosis of cobalamin deficiency: the old and the new. *British Journal of Haematology* **97**, 695–700. [Discusses whether vitamin assays or measurement of serum methylmalonic acid or homocysteine should be used to diagnose the deficiencies.]

Fish DT, Dawson DW (1983). Comparison of methods used in commercial kits for the assay of serum vitamin B_{12}. *Clinical and Laboratory Haematology* **5**, 272–7. [A useful review of the different methods of assaying serum B_{12}.]

Gleeson PA, Toh BH (1991). Molecular targets in pernicious anaemia. *Immunology Today* **12**, 233–8. [Details the gastric antigens as targets for parietal cell antibody.]

Hewitt JE, Gordon MM, Taggart RT, *et al.* (1991). Human gastric intrinsic factor: characterization of cDNA and genomic changes and localization to human chromosome II. *Genomics* **10**, 432–40. [A major study of genetic aspects of intrinsic factor.]

Kondo H, Kolhouse JF, Allen RH (1980). Presence of cobalamin analogues in animal tissues. *Proceedings of the National Academy of Sciences, USA* **77**, 817–21. [Describes the nature and origin of cobalamin analogues.]

Kozyraki R, Kristiansen M, Silahtaroglu A, *et al.* (1998). The human intrinsic factor—vitamin B_{12} receptor, cubilin: molecular characterization and chromosomal mapping of the gene to 10p within the autosomal recessive megaloblastic anemia (MGA1) region. *Blood* **91**, 3593–600. [The identification of cubilin as the IF.B12 receptor.]

Kristiansen M, Aminoff M, Jacobsen C, *et al.* (2000). Cubulin P1297L mutation associated with hereditary megaloblastic anemia 1 causes improved recognition of intrinsic factor—vitamin B12 by cubilin. *Blood* **96**, 405–9. [Identification of the most frequent mutation underlying MGA1.]

Regec A, Quadros EV, Plalica O, *et al.* (1995). The cloning and characterization of the human transcobalamin II gene. *Blood* **85**, 2711–19. [Important report of genetic aspects of TCII.]

Remacha AF, Riera A, Cadafalch J, Grimferrer E (1991). Vitamin B_{12} abnormalities in HIV-infected patients. *European Journal of Haematology* **47**, 60–4. [Describes the incidence of malabsorption of B_{12} and of B_{12} deficiency in HIV-infected patients.]

Rothenberg SP, Quadros EV (1995). Transcobalamin II and the membrane receptor for the transcobalamin II-cobalamin complex. *Clinical Haematology* **8**, 499–514. [A major review of the structure of TCII, the other transcobalamins, and intrinsic factor.]

Savage DG, Lindenbaum J (1995). Neurological complications of acquired cobalamin deficiency: clincal aspects. *Clinical Haematology* **8**, 657–78. [This review deals with the effects of folic acid at different doses on haematological and neurological aspects of cobalamin deficiency.]

Weir DG, Scott JM (1997). Brain function in the elderly: role of vitamin B_{12} and folate. *British Medical Bulletin* **55**, 669–82. [A large review of this important topic.]

Folate

Antony AC (1992). The biological chemistry of folate receptors. *Blood* **79**, 2807–20. [All aspects of folate receptors are discussed.]

Bailey L, ed. (1994). *Folate in health and disease.* Marcel Decker, New York. A collection of articles about all aspects of the vitamin.

Clarke R, Smith AD, Jobst KA, *et al.* (1998). Folate, vitamin B_{12} and serum total homocysteine levels in confirmed Alzheimer's disease. *Archives of Neurology* **55**, 1449–55. [An important study suggesting folate deficiency may predispose to Alzheimer's disease.][

Giovannucci E, Stampfer MJ, Colditz GA, *et al.* (1998). Multivitamin use, folate and colon cancer in women in the nurses' health study. *Annals of Internal Medicine* **129**, 517–24. [A large study implying but not proving that folate deficiency predisposes to colon cancer.]

Heston WD (1997). Characterization and glutamyl carboxypeptidase functions of prostate-specific membrane antigen: a novel folate hydolase. *Urology* **49** (Suppl. 3A), 104–12. [Demonstration that prostate-specific antigen is a folate hydrolase.]

Hoffbrand AV, Weir DG (2001). The history of folic acid. *British Journal of Haematology* **113**, 579–89. [A comprehensive review of all aspects of folate since the original discovery of the vitamin by Lucy Wills.]

Selhub J, Jacques PF, Wilson PWF, *et al.* (1993). Vitamin status and intake as primary determinants of homocysteinaemia in an elderly population. *Journal of the American Medical Association* **270**, 2693–8.[A study showing the importance of folate status in determining plasma homocysteine levels.]

Shane B (1989). Folylpolyglutamate synthesis and role in regulation of one-carbon metabolism. *Vitamins and Hormones* **45**, 263–335. [An important review of folate metabolism with emphasis on folate polyglutamates.]

Neural tube defect

Botto L, Moore CA, Khoury MJ, *et al.* (1999). Neural-tube defects. *New England Journal of Medicine* **341**, 1509–18. [A major review of all aspects of neural tube defects.]

Czeizel AE, Dundas I (1992). Prevention of the first occurrence of neural tube defects by periconceptional vitamin supplementation. *New England Journal of Medicine* **327**, 1832–5. [The first demonstration of prevention of first occurrence of NTD by folic acid.]

Daley LE, Kirke PN, Molloy A, *et al.* (1995). Folate levels and neural tube defects: implications for prevention. *Journal of the American Medical*

Association **274**, 1698–702. [Demonstration of close relation between incidence of NTD and red cell folate levels in the Irish population.]

Daley S, Mills JL, Molloy AM, *et al.* (1997). Minimum effective dose of folic acid for food fortification to prevent neural tube defects. *Lancet* **350**, 1666–9. [Study of the effects of different supplemental doses of folic acid daily over a 6-month period on red cell folate levels.]

Hibbard EM, Smithells RS (1965). Folic acid and human embryopathy. *Lancet* **i**, 1254. [The first suggestion that folate deficiency may predispose NTD.]

Lawrence JM, Petitti DB, Watkins M, *et al.* (1999). Trends in serum folate after food fortification. *Lancet* **354**, 915–16. [Analysis of folate levels in the United States population after food fortification with folic acid.]

Molloy A, Sean D, Mills JL, *et al.* (1997). Thermolabile variant of 5,10-methylene tetrahydrofolate reductase associated with low red cell folates: implications for folate intake recommendations. *Lancet* **349**, 1591–3. [Identification of low red cell folate in normal subjects with mutated MHTFR.]

MRC Vitamin Study Group (1991). Prevention of neural tube defects: results of Medical Research Council Vitamin Study. *Lancet* **238**, 131–7. [The first study to establish that folic acid therapy periconception substantially reduces the incidence of recurrence of NTD births.]

Smithells RW, Shephard S, Schorah CJ, *et al.* (1980). Possible prevention of neural-tube defects by periconceptional vitamin supplementation. *Lancet* **i**, 339–40. [The first data to suggest that folic acid supplements may prevent NTD.]

Cardiovascular system

Boushey CJ, Beresford SAA, Omenn GS, *et al.* (1995). A quantitative assessment of plasma homocysteine as a risk factor for vascular disease: probable benefits of increasing folic acid intakes. *Journal of the American Medical Association* **274**, 1049–57. [An important study predicting the benefits on incidence of cardiovascular disease of food fortification with folic acid.]

Brattsom L, Wilcken DE, Ohrvik J, *et al.* (1998). Common methylenetetrahydrofolate reductase gene mutation leads to hyperhomocysteinaemia but not to vascular disease: the result of a meta-analysis. *Circulation* **98**, 2520–6. [Meta-analysis showing mutated MHTFR is not a risk factor for vascular disease.]

Christen WG, Ajoni UA, Glynn RJ, Hennekens CH (2000). Blood levels of homocysteine and increased risks of cardiovascular disease. Causal or casual? *Archives of Internal Medicine* **160**, 422–34. [A discussion of whether or not raised homocysteine levels cause vascular disease.]

Den Heijer M, Koster T, Blom HJ, *et al.* (1996). Hyperhomocysteinemia as a risk factor for deep vein thrombosis. *New England Journal of Medicine* **334**, 759–62. [The only published study showing a raised plasma homocysteine is associated with venous thrombosis.]

Frosst P, Blom HJ, Milos R, *et al.* (1995). A candidate genetic risk factor for vascular disease: a common mutation in methylenetetrahydrofolate reductase. *Nature Genetics* **10**, 111–13. [The demonstration of the gene defect underlying thermolabile MHTFR.]

Graham IM, Daly LE, Refsum HNM, *et al.* (1997). Plasma homocysteine as a risk factor for vascular disease: the European Concerted Action Project. *Journal of the American Medical Association* **277**, 1775–81. [A meta-analysis of the association of homocysteine and vascular disease.]

Haynes WG (2000). Homocysteine and artherosclerosis: potential mechanisms and clinical implications. *Proceedings of Royal College of Physicians of Edinburgh* **30**, 114–22. [A useful large review of this topic.]

Homocysteine Lowering Trialists Collaboration (1998). Lowering blood homocysteine with folic acid based supplements: meta-analysis of randomised trials. *British Medical Journal* **316**, 894–8. [An important meta-analysis of trials aimed at lowering plasma homocysteine with folic acid supplements.]

Jacques PF, Selhub J, Borton AG, *et al.* (1999). The effect of folic acid fortification on plasma folate and total homocysteine concentrations. *New England Journal of Medicine* **340**, 1449–53. [The Framlingham study of the effect of adding folic acid to the diet on plasma homocysteine and folate levels.]

McCully KS (1969). Vascular pathology of homocysteinemia. *American Journal of Pathology* **56**, 111–28. [The first suggestion that homocysteine leads to vascular disease.]

Malinow MR, Duall PB, Hess DL, *et al.* (1998). Reduction of plasma homocyst(e)ine levels by breakfast cereal fortified with folic acid in patients with coronary heart disease. *New England Journal of Medicine* **338**, 1009–15. [Study showing that food fortification with folic acid reduces plasma homocysteine levels.]

Morrison HI, Schaubel D, Desmeules M, *et al.* (1996). Serum folate and risk of fatal coronary heart disease. *Journal of American Medical Association* **275**, 1893–6. [A large Canadian study relating folate status to incidence of myocardial infarct.]

Perry DJ (1999). Hyperhomocysteinaemia. *Clinical Haematology* **12**, 451–78. [A major, authorative review of the causes and associations of a raised plasma homocysteine level.]

Rimm EB, Willett WC, Hu FB, *et al.* (1998). Folate and vitamin B_6 from diet and supplements in relation to risk of coronary heart disease among women. *Journal of the American Medical Association* **279**, 359–64. [A retrospective study of the effects of folic acid supplements on the risk of coronary artery disease.]

Robinson K, Arheart K, Refsum H, *et al.* (1998). Low circulating folate and vitamin B_6 concentrations: risk factors for stroke, peripheral vascular disease and coronary artery disease. *Circulation* **97**, 437–43.[A major study relating folate levels to stroke and peripheral vascular disease as well as to coronary artery disease.]

Schnyder MD, Roffi M, Pin R, *et al.* (2001). Decreased rate of coronary restenosis after lowering of plasma homocysteine levels. *New England Journal of Medicine* **345**, 1593–1600. [Demonstrated that a combination of folic acid, vitamin B_{12}, and pyridoxine significantly decrease the rate of restenosis and need for revascularization after coronary angioplasty. There was also a reduction of major cardiac events.]

Verhoef P, Stampfer MJ, Bursing E, *et al.* (1996). Homocysteine metabolism and risk of myocardial infarction: relation with vitamin B_6, B_{12} and folate. *American Journal of Epidemiology* **143**, 845–59. [A major study relating plasma homocysteine to vitamin status and myocardial infarct.]

Vermeulen EGJ, Stenhauwer CDA, Twisk JWR, *et al.* (2000). Effect of homocysteine-lowering treatment with folic acid plus vitamin B_6 on progress of subclinical atherosclerosis: a randomised, placebo controlled trial. *Lancet* **355**, 517–22. [The first study to show a benefit, albeit on electrocardiographic abnormalities, of dietary supplementation with folic acid and vitamin B_6, in patients with atherosclerosis.]

Wald NJ, Watt HC, Law MR, *et al.* (1998). Homocysteine and ischemic heart disease: results of a prospective study with implications regarding prevention. *Archives of Internal Medicine* **158**, 862–7. [A valuable, prospective study quantifying the increased risk of ischaemic heart disease with incremental rises in plasma homocysteine.]

Welch GN, Loscalzo J (1998). Homocysteine and artherothrombosis. *New England Journal of Medicine* **338**, 1042–50. [A useful review of the association of homocysteine and atherosclerosis.]

Miscellaneous

Adams EB (1970). Anemia associated with protein deficiency. *Seminars in Hematology* **7**, 55–66. An excellent review of the role of protein deficiency in causing anaemia.

Cox EV (1968). The anaemia of scurvy. *Vitamins and Hormones* **26**, 635–52. An excellent review of the role of vitamin C in haemopoiesis.

Rindi G, *et al.* (1994). Further studies of erythrocyte thiamin transport and phosphorylation in seven patients with thiamin-responsive megaloblastic anaemia. *Journal of Inherited Metabolic Diseases* **17**, 667–77. This study shows the mechanism of thiamine responsive anaemia.

22.5.7 Disorders of the synthesis or function of haemoglobin

D. J. Weatherall

Disorders of the synthesis or structure of haemoglobin may be either inherited or acquired. The inherited disorders of haemoglobin are the commonest single gene disorders in the world population. Figures compiled by the World Health Organization suggest that there are hundreds of millions of carriers. Each year 200 000 to 300 000 severely affected homozygotes or compound heterozygotes are born. In many of the developing countries, the very high mortality from infection and malnutrition in the first year of life causes these conditions to be under-appreciated as an important public health problem. However, once economic conditions improve and infant and childhood death rates fall, the genetic disorders of haemoglobin start to place a major burden on the health services. This phenomenon has already been observed in parts of the Mediterranean region and Southeast Asia.

As a result of mass migrations of populations from high incidence areas for the haemoglobin disorders these conditions are being seen with increasing frequency in parts of the world where they have not been recognized previously. Some of them, particularly sickle cell anaemia and the more severe forms of thalassaemia, can produce life-threatening medical emergencies. It is thus important for clinicians to have a working knowledge of their clinical features, management, and prevention.

Haemoglobin disorders have also become of particular interest in recent years because they were the first group of diseases to be analysed by the methods of recombinant DNA technology. More is known about their molecular pathology than any other genetic disorders. Their study has given us a good idea of the repertoire of mutations that underlie inherited diseases in man.

Before describing the haemoglobin disorders it is necessary to discuss briefly the structure, function, and synthesis of haemoglobin and the way that it is genetically determined.

The structure, function, genetic control, and synthesis of haemoglobin

Structure

Human haemoglobin is heterogeneous at all stages of development; different haemoglobins are synthesized in the embryo, fetus, and adult, each adapted to the particular oxygen requirements.

Each human haemoglobin has a tetrameric structure made up of two different pairs of globin chains, each attached to one haem molecule (Fig. 1). Adult and fetal haemoglobins have α chains combined with β chains (Hb A, $\alpha_2\beta_2$), δ chains (Hb A_2, $\alpha_2\delta_2$), or γ chains (Hb F, $\alpha_2\gamma_2$). In embryos, α-like chains, called ζ chains, combine with γ chains to produce Hb Portland ($\zeta_2\gamma_2$), or with ε chains to make Hb Gower 1 ($\zeta_2\varepsilon_2$), and α and ε chains combine to form Hb Gower 2 ($\alpha_2\varepsilon_2$). Fetal haemoglobin is itself heterogeneous; there are two kinds of γ chains which differ in their amino acid composition at position 136, where they have either glycine ($^G\gamma$) or alanine ($^A\gamma$). The $^G\gamma$ and $^A\gamma$ chains are the products of separate ($^G\gamma$ and $^A\gamma$) loci.

Function

The well-known sigmoid shape of the oxygen dissociation curve, which reflects the allosteric properties of haemoglobin, ensures that oxygen is rapidly taken up at high oxygen tensions in the lungs, and that it is released readily at the lower tensions encountered in the tissues. The shape of the curve is due to co-operativity between the four haem molecules. When one takes on oxygen, the affinity for oxygen of the remaining haems of the tetramer increased dramatically. This is because haemoglobin can exist in two configurations, deoxy (T) and oxy (R) (T and R stand for tight and relaxed states, respectively). The T form has a lower affinity than the R form for ligands such as oxygen. During the sequential addition of oxygen to the four haems, transition from the T to R configuration occurs and the oxygen affinity of the partially liganded molecule increases rapidly.

The position of the oxygen dissociation curve can be modified in many ways. First, oxygen affinity is decreased with increasing CO_2 tensions, the Bohr effect. This facilitates oxygen delivery to the tissues, where a drop in pH due to CO_2 influx lowers oxygen affinity. The opposite effect occurs in the lungs. Oxygen affinity is also modified by the level of 2,3-diphosphoglycerate (2,3-DPG) in the red cell. Increasing concentrations move the curve to the right, reducing oxygen affinity. Diminishing concentrations have the opposite effect. The 2,3-DPG mechanism plays an important role in response to hypoxia. Increased levels of DPG, with an associated decrease in P_{50} (partial pressure at which haemoglobin is 50 per cent saturated), occur in anaemia, alkalosis, hyperphosphataemia, hypoxic states, and in association with a number of red cell enzyme deficiencies.

Genetic control

The arrangement of the two main families of globin genes is illustrated in Fig. 2. The β-like globin genes form a linked cluster on chromosome 11, that spans about 60 kb (kb = kilobase or 1000 nucleotide bases); they are arranged in the order 5′-ε-$^G\gamma$-$^A\gamma$-$\psi\beta$-δ-β-3′. The α-like globin genes form a linked cluster on chromosome 16, in the order 5′-ζ-$\psi\zeta$-$\psi\alpha$-α2-α1–3′. The $\psi\beta$, $\psi\zeta$, and $\psi\alpha$ genes are pseudogenes; their sequences resemble the β, ζ,

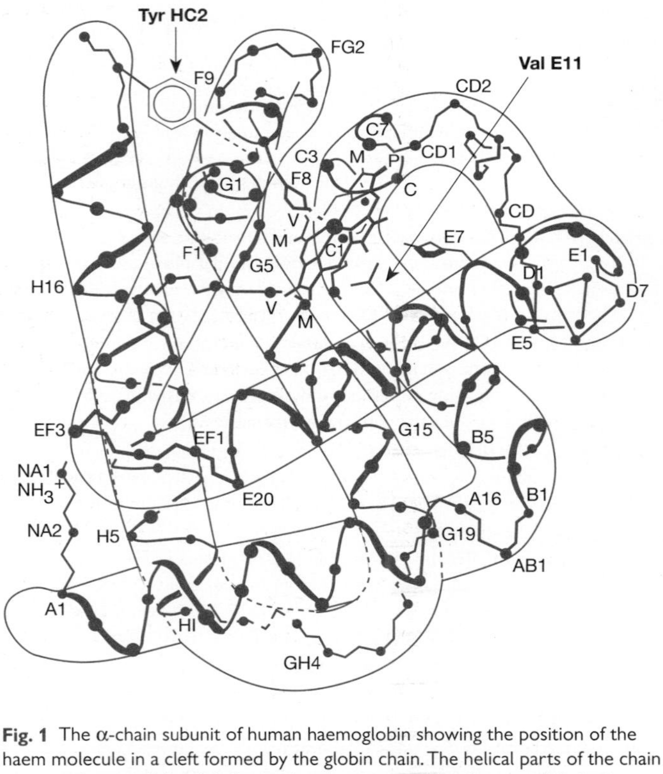

Fig. 1 The α-chain subunit of human haemoglobin showing the position of the haem molecule in a cleft formed by the globin chain. The helical parts of the chain are given letters of the alphabet and each amino acid residue in each helical region has a specific number, for example val E11 is the eleventh amino acid in the E helical region. The non-helical regions of the amino- and carboxyl-terminal ends of the chains are labelled NA and HC respectively. (Reproduced by permission of Dr MF Perutz and the editors of the Cold Spring Harbor Symposia for Quantitative Biology.)

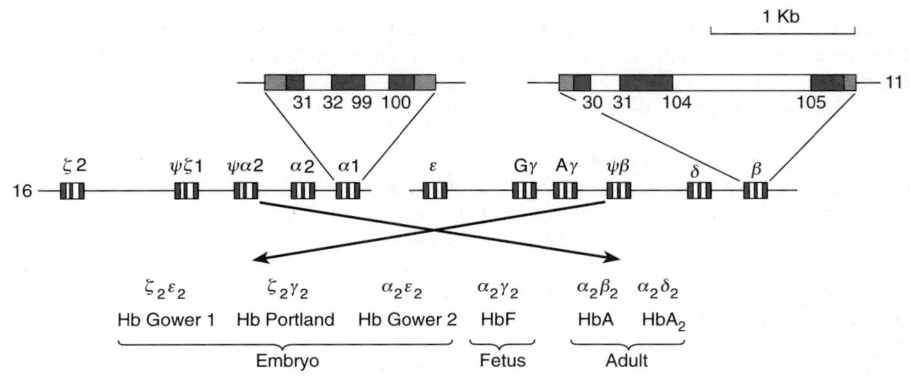

Fig. 2 The genetic control of human haemoglobin. Two of the genes are enlarged to show the introns (unshaded) and exons (dark staining). 1 kb = 1000 nucleotide bases.

or α genes but contain mutations which prevent them from functioning as structural genes. They may be 'burnt out' remnants of genes which were functional at an earlier stage of evolution.

Some of the important structural aspects of the globin genes and their flanking sequences are illustrated in Figs 2 and 3. Like most mammalian genes, the globin genes are interrupted by one or more non-coding regions called intervening sequences (IVS) or introns. The non-α globin genes contain two introns of 122 to 130 and 850 to 900 base pairs between codons 30 and 31 and 104 and 105, respectively. Similar though smaller introns are found in the α and ζ globin genes. In the 5′ flanking regions of the globin genes there are blocks of nucleotide homology which are found in analagous positions in many species. The first, the ATA box, is about 30 bases upstream (to the left) of the initiation codon. The second, called the CCAAT box, is found about 70 base pairs upstream from the 5′ end of the genes. There is a third region of this kind, about 100 base pairs upstream. These regions, called promoters, are involved in the initiation of transcription and hence play an important role in the regulation of the structural genes. As we shall see later, mutations which involve them can reduce the output of the related genes. In the 3′ non-coding regions of all the globin genes there is a sequence AATAAA (Fig. 3) which is the signal for polyA addition to RNA transcripts; we shall discuss the significance of this when we consider the disorders of globin chain synthesis.

The globin gene clusters also contain other types of regulatory elements that interact to promote erythroid-specific gene expression and to co-ordinate changes in globin gene activity during development. They include enhancers, regulatory elements that increase gene expression despite being located at a variable distance from the genes, and master sequences upstream from the clusters which render them transcriptionally active. All these regulatory regions contain sequences to which an array of regulatory molecules called transcription factors are able to bind, some of which are specific for erythropoiesis, while others are ubiquitous in their tissue distribution.

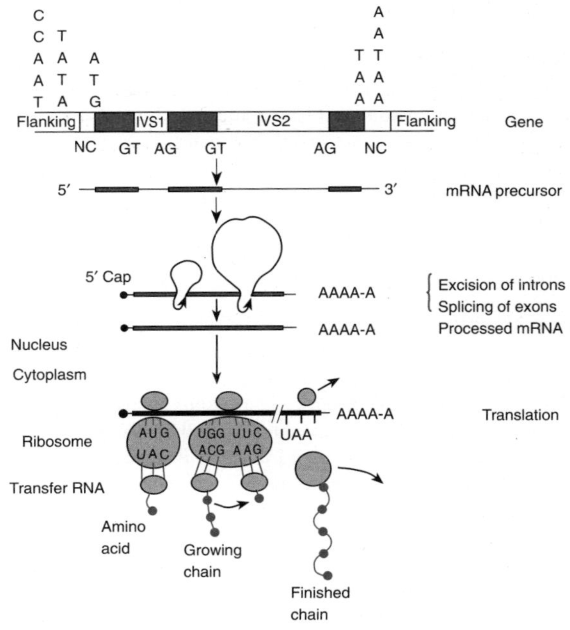

Fig. 3 Globin gene structure, mRNA processing, and globin synthesis. Each of the structures and steps illustrated is described in the text and in Section 5.

Synthesis

When a globin gene is transcribed a messenger RNA molecule is synthesized from one of its strands by the action of an enzyme called RNA polymerase. The primary transcript of the globin genes is the large messenger RNA precursor molecule which contains both introns and the coding regions or exons. While in the nucleus, this molecule undergoes a number of modifications (Fig. 3). First, the introns are removed and the exons are joined together, a process called splicing. The exon/intron junctions always have the sequence GT at their 5′ end, and AG at their 3′ end. This appears to be essential for accurate splicing and if there is a mutation in these sites normal splicing cannot occur. The messenger RNAs are chemically modified (capped) at their 5′ end, and at their 3′ end a string of adenylic acid residues (polyA) is added. The processed messenger RNA now moves into the cytoplasm to act as a template for globin chain production.

Globin mRNA is transported from the nucleus to the cytoplasm where it associates with ribosomes, tRNA, and proteinaceous translation factors. These complexes, called polyribosomes, translate the information encoded in the globin mRNA into the primary amino acid sequence of each globin chain. Individual globin chains combine with haem, which is synthesized through a separate pathway, and with themselves, to form definitive haemoglobin molecules.

Classification of the disorders of haemoglobin

The main groups of disorders of haemoglobin are shown in Table 1. The genetic disorders are divided into those in which there is a reduced rate of production of one or more of the globin chains, the thalassaemias, and those in which a structural change in a globin chain leads to instability or to abnormal oxygen transport. In addition, there is a harmless group of mutations, known collectively as hereditary persistence of fetal haemoglobin, that interfere with the normal switching of fetal to adult haemoglobin production. The acquired disorders of haemoglobin can also be subdivided into those characterized by defective synthesis of the globin chains and those in which the structure of the haem molecules is altered, leading to inefficient oxygen transport.

Like all biological classifications, this way of splitting up the haemoglobin disorders is not entirely satisfactory. For example some structural variants are synthesized in reduced amounts and hence produce the clinical picture of thalassaemia.

The thalassaemias

Historical introduction

The thalassaemias are the commonest of the inherited haematological disorders and, indeed, are the commonest single gene disorders in the world population. The condition was first recognized in 1925 by a Detroit physician called Thomas B. Cooley who described a series of infants who became profoundly anaemic and developed splenomegaly over the first year of life. A milder form was described independently in the same year by an Italian physician, Fernando Rietti. Subsequently, further cases were identified and the disorder was variously called von Jaksch's anaemia, splenic anaemia, erythroblastosis, Mediterranean anaemia, or Cooley's anaemia. In 1936, George Whipple and Lesley Bradford recognized that many of their patients came from the Mediterranean region and hence they invented the word 'thalassaemia' from the Greek θαλασσα, meaning 'the sea'. Although it was realized later that the disorder occurs throughout the world and is not localized to the Mediterranean region, the name has stuck.

Thalassaemia is extremely heterogeneous. Its clinical picture can result from the interaction of many different genetic defects. This chapter concentrates mainly on the clinical and haematological aspects; readers who wish to learn more about the molecular pathology and population genetics of thalassaemia are referred to several reviews and monographs which are cited at the end of this chapter.

Definition and classification

The thalassaemias are a heterogeneous group of genetic disorders of haemoglobin synthesis, all of which result from a reduced rate of production of one or more of the globin chains of haemoglobin. They are divided into the α, β, δβ, or εγδβ thalassaemias, according to which globin chain is produced in reduced amounts (Table 2). In some thalassaemias, no globin chain is synthesized at all, they are called α° or β° thalassaemias. In others, the α^{+} or β^{+} thalassaemias, globin chain is produced but at a reduced rate. Thalassaemia occurs in populations in which structural haemoglobin variants are common. It is not at all unusual for an individual to inherit a thalassaemia gene from one parent and a gene for a structural haemoglobin variant from the other. Both α and β thalassaemia occur commonly in some countries and hence individuals may receive genes for both types. These different interactions produce an extremely complex and clinically diverse series of genetic disorders which range in severity from death *in utero* to extremely mild, symptomless hypochromic anaemias.

Table 1 Disorders of haemoglobin

Genetic
Thalassaemia
Structural variants
Hereditary persistence of fetal haemoglobin
Acquired
Methaemoglobin
Carbonmonoxyhaemoglobin
Sulphaemoglobin
Defective synthesis
haemoglobin H/leukaemia
other neoplastic disorders

Table 2 The thalassaemias

α Thalassaemia
α°
α^{+}
β Thalassaemia
β°
β^{+}
δβ Thalassaemia
$(\delta\beta)^{\circ}$
Haemoglobin Lepore $(\delta\beta)^{+}$
$(\varepsilon\gamma\delta\beta)^{\circ}$ Thalassaemia
δ Thalassaemia

The thalassaemias are inherited in a simple mendelian fashion. Heterozygotes are usually symptomless, although they can be easily recognized by simple haematological analysis. More severely affected patients are either homozygotes for α or β thalassaemia, compound heterozygotes for different molecular forms of α or β thalassaemia, or compound heterozygotes for thalassaemia and a structural haemoglobin variant. Clinically, the thalassaemias are classified according to their severity in major, intermediate and minor forms. Thalassaemia major is a severe transfusion-dependent disorder. Thalassaemia intermedia is characterized by anaemia and splenomegaly though not of such severity as to require regular transfusion. Thalassaemia minor is the symptomless carrier state. While these descriptive terms do not have a precise genetic meaning, they remain useful in clinical practice.

The β thalassaemias

The β thalassaemias are the most important types of thalassaemia because they are very common and produce severe anaemia in their homozygous and compound heterozygous states (Table 3).

Distribution

The β thalassaemias occur widely in a broad belt ranging from the Mediterranean and parts of north and west Africa through the Middle East and Indian subcontinent to Southeast Asia (Fig. 4). The high incidence zone stretches north through Yugoslavia and Romania and the southern parts of the former USSR and includes the southern regions of the People's Republic of China. The disease is particularly common in Southeast Asia where it occurs in a line starting in southern China and stretching down through Thailand and the Malay peninsula through Indonesia to some of the Pacific islands. In these populations, and in some of the Mediterranean island and mainland countries, gene frequencies for the various forms of β thalassaemia range between two and 20 per cent. It should be remembered that β thalassaemia is not entirely confined to these high incidence regions; it occurs sporadically in every racial group.

Molecular pathology

The precise molecular lesions responsible for the defective synthesis of the β globin chains have been determined for many patients with β thalassaemia. The disease is extremely heterogeneous. About 200 different mutations can produce the clinical phenotype of β thalassaemia. Some completely inactivate the β globin genes leading to β° thalassaemia; others cause a reduced output from the genes and hence the picture of β^{+} thalassaemia.

The main classes of mutations that cause β thalassaemia are summarized in Fig. 5. With the exception of a deletion of about 600 bases at the 3' end of the β globin gene, which is only found in certain populations of northern India, deletions are an uncommon cause of β thalassaemia. Most of the mutations are single base changes or small deletions and insertions of one or two bases. As shown in Fig. 5, they occur in both introns and exons, and also outside the coding regions.

Table 3 The β, δβ, and γδβ thalassaemias

Type of thalassaemia	Findings in homozygote	Findings in heterozygote
β°	Thalassaemia major[1,2] Hbs F and A_2	Thalassaemia minor Raised Hb A_2
$β^+$	Thalassaemia major[1,2] Hbs F, A, and A_2	Thalassaemia minor Raised Hb A_2
δβ	Thalassaemia intermedia Hb F only	Thalassaemia minor Hb F 5–15%; Hb A_2 normal
$(δβ)^+$ (Lepore)	Thalassaemia major or intermedia Hbs F and Lepore	Thalassaemia minor Hb Lepore 5–15 per cent; Hb A_2 normal
εγδβ	Not viable	Neonatal haemolysis Thalassaemia minor in adults, with normal Hbs F and A_2

[1] Occasionally have thalassaemia intermedia phenotype.

[2] Many patients with thalassaemia are compound heterozygotes for different molecular forms of β° or $β^+$ thalassaemia.

Many of the exon mutations are nonsense mutations, that is the substitution of a single base in a codon produces a stop codon in the middle of the coding part of the messenger RNA (Fig. 6). Some mutations result in frame shifts; because the information carried by messenger RNA is in the form of a triplet code, the loss of one, two, or four bases throws the reading frame out of phase (Fig. 6). Another important class interfere with splicing. They may alter the invariate GC/AG dinucleotides at the intron/exon junctions, in which case they usually cause β° thalassaemia. Alternatively, they may activate so-called cryptic splice sites, providing an alternate splice site so that both normal and abnormal messenger RNA species are produced (Fig. 7). These lesions cause a $β^+$ thalassaemia, the severity of which depends on the relative usage of the normal and abnormal splice site and hence the quantity of normal and abnormal β globin messenger RNA that is produced.

Many single base substitutions have also been found in the flanking regions of the β globin genes. They alter either the proximal promoter regions or adjacent sequences, causing down regulation of β globin gene transcription to a varying degree. They are usually associated with milder forms of $β^+$ thalassaemia.

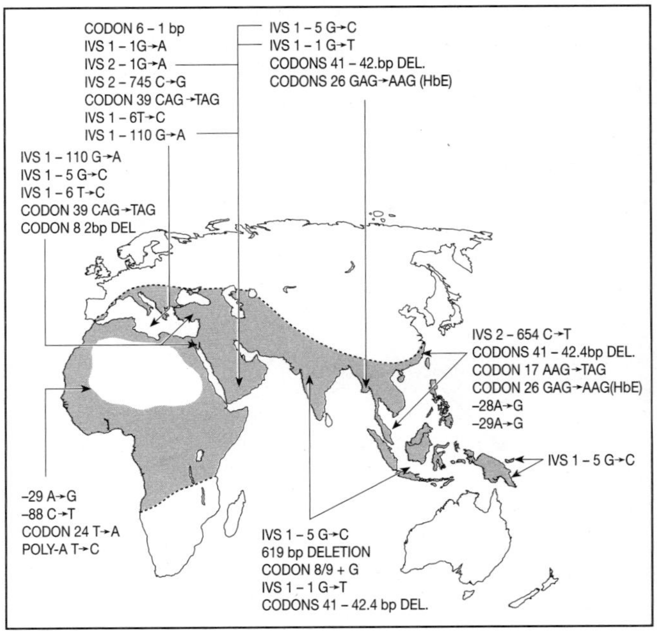

Fig. 4 World map showing the distribution of the different β thalassaemia mutations.

Because there are so many different β thalassaemia mutations it follows that many patients who are apparently homozygous for β thalassaemia are, in fact, compound heterozygotes for two different molecular lesions.

Pathophysiology

The mutations that cause β thalasaemia result in absent or reduced β chain production. Alpha chain synthesis proceeds at a normal rate and hence there is imbalanced globin chain synthesis (Fig. 8). In the absence of their partner chains the excess α chains are unstable and precipitate in the red cell precursors, forming large intracellular inclusions. These interfere with red cell maturation, and hence there is a variable degree of intramedullary destruction of red cell precursors, that is ineffective erythropoiesis. Those red cells which mature and enter the circulation contain α chain inclusions which interfere with their passage through the microcirculation, particularly in the spleen. These cells are prematurely destroyed. Thus the anaemia of β thalassaemia results from both ineffective erythropoiesis and a shortened red cell survival. The mechanisms of the destruction of red cell precursors and their progeny are extremely complex and are not simply a reflection of mechanical damage to the red cells. Free α chains and their degradation products, particularly haem and iron, cause severe oxidative damage to the red cell membrane proteins. The end result is a dehydrated, rigid erythrocyte with a markedly shortened survival.

The anaemia acts as a stimulus to increased erythropoietin production, causing massive expansion of the bone marrow which may lead to serious

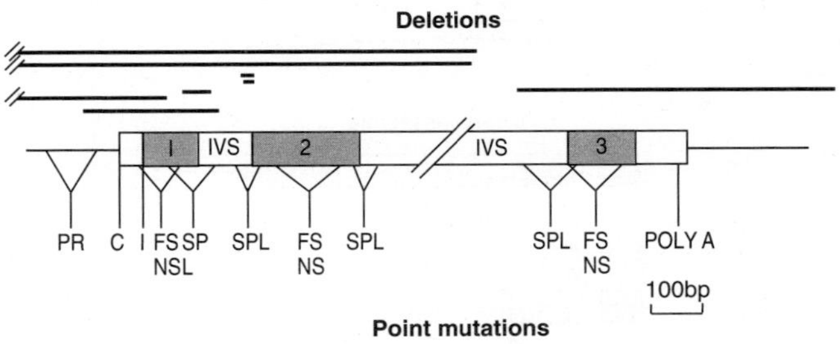

Fig. 5 Some of the mutations that produce β thalassaemia. The β globin gene is divided into three exons (hatched) and two introns (IVS; unshaded). The different deletions are shown at the top of the figure while below the general position of the different point mutations is represented. PR, promoter; C, CAP site; I, initiation site; FS, frameshift; NS, nonsense; SPL, splice-site mutation; polyA, RNA cleavage and polyA addition site.

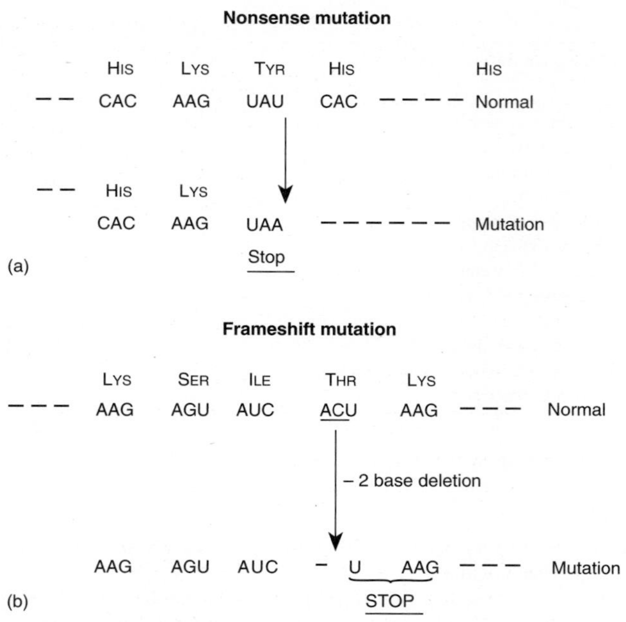

Fig. 6 Point mutations that cause β° thalassaemia: (a) premature stop codon (nonsense mutation); (b) frameshift mutation. See text for further details.

deformities of the skull and long bones. Because the spleen is being constantly bombarded with abnormal red cells, it hypertrophies. The resulting splenomegaly and bone marrow expansion gives rise to an increase in the plasma volume which, together with pooling of the red cells in the enlarged spleen, causes an exacerbation of an already severe degree of anaemia.

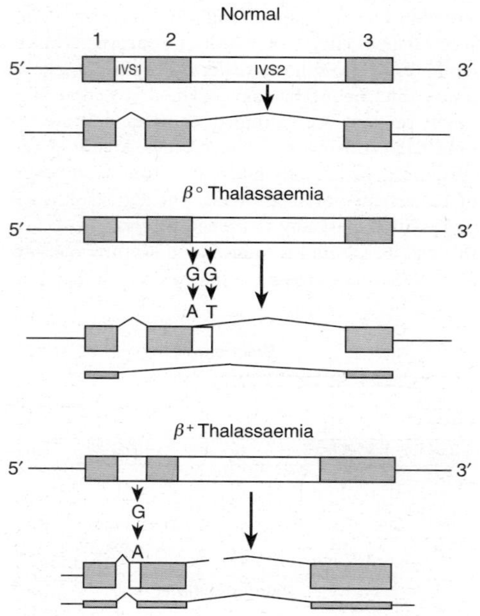

Fig. 7 A representation of the consequences of different splice-site mutations. In β° thalassaemia two different mutations are shown, one that inactivates the normal splice site, and another that produces a new splice site. Two abnormal mRNA molecules are produced. In the β⁺ thalassaemia case a new splice site is produced in the first intron. Both normal and abnormal mRNAs are produced, the latter in greater amounts.

As mentioned previously, fetal haemoglobin production largely ceases after birth. However, some adult red cell precursors (F cells) retain the ability to produce a small number of γ chains. Because the latter can combine with excess α chains to form haemoglobin F, cells which make relatively more γ chains in the bone marrow of β thalassaemics are partly protected against the deleterious effect of α chain precipitation. Red cell precursors which produce haemoglobin F are selected in the marrow and peripheral blood of these patients. Thus, they have relatively large amounts of haemoglobin F in their red cells. Furthermore, because δ chain synthesis is unaffected, the disorder is characterized by a relative or absolute increase in haemoglobin A_2 ($\alpha_2\delta_2$) production. These interactions are summarized in Fig. 7.

If the anaemia is corrected with blood transfusion the erythropoietic drive is reduced, growth and development are improved, and bone deformities do not occur. On the other hand, each unit of blood contains 200 mg of iron; with regular transfusion there is steady accumulation of iron in the liver, endocrine glands, and myocardium. Even though well-transfused thalassaemic children grow and develop normally, they die of iron overload unless steps are taken to remove iron.

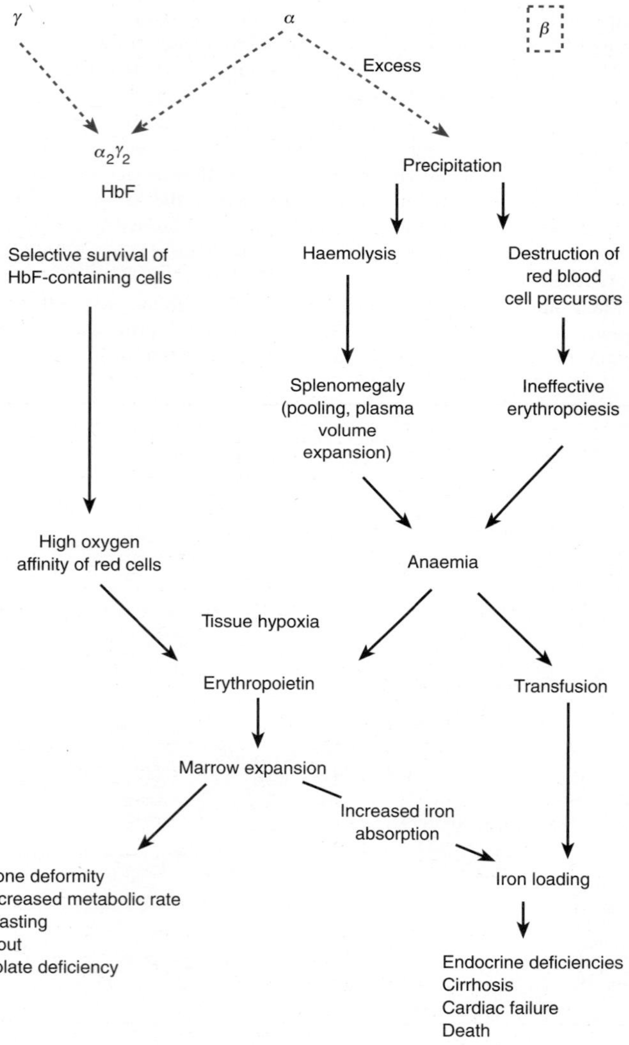

Fig. 8 The pathophysiology of β thalassaemia.

The severe homozygous or compound heterozygous forms of β thalassaemia

These are the commonest and most important forms of thalassaemia and give rise to a major public health problem in many parts of the world.

Clinical features

Most severe forms of β thalassaemia present within the first year of life, as fetal haemoglobin declines, with failure to thrive, poor feeding, intermittent bouts of fever, or failure to improve after an intercurrent infection. At this stage the affected infant looks pale. In many cases splenomegaly is already present. There are no other specific clinical signs. Diagnosis depends on the haematological changes outlined below. If the infant is established on a regular transfusion regimen at this stage, early development is normal. Further symptoms do not occur until puberty, when the effects of iron loading start to appear. If, on the other hand, the infant is not adequately transfused, the typical clinical picture of homozygous β thalassaemia develops. Thus the clinical manifestations of the severe forms of β thalassaemia have to be described in two contexts, that is the well-transfused child and the child with chronic anaemia throughout early life.

In the well-transfused thalassaemic child, early growth and development is normal. Splenomegaly is minimal. However, there is a gradual accumulation of iron. The effects of tissue siderosis start to appear by the end of the first decade. The normal adolescent growth spurt fails to occur. Hepatic, endocrine, and cardiac complications of iron overloading produce a variety of problems including diabetes, hyopoparathyroidism, adrenal insufficiency, and progressive liver failure. Secondary sexual development is delayed or does not occur at all. Short stature and lack of sexual development may lead to serious psychological problems. By far the commonest cause of death, which usually occurs toward the end of the second or early in the third decade, is progressive cardiac damage. Ultimately these patients die due to either protracted cardiac failure or suddenly due to an acute arrhythmia.

There is now good evidence that children who have been both adequately transfused and chelated may grow and develop normally, pass through a normal puberty, and survive to adult life in excellent condition. However, it is becoming apparent that even children who have been well managed in this way still tend to suffer from complications as they get older, particularly delayed sexual maturation, growth disturbances, and osteoporosis. It seems likely that many of these problems are due to subtle damage to the hypothalamic/pituitary axis with secondary hypogonadism. In addition, some of the growth disturbances may reflect toxicity of the chelating agents used to remove iron (see below).

The clinical picture in children who are inadequately transfused is quite different. Early childhood is interspersed with a series of distressing complications. The overall rates of growth and development are markedly retarded. There is progressive splenomegaly; hypersplenism may cause a worsening of the anaemia, sometimes associated with thrombocytopenia and a bleeding tendency. Because of the bone marrow expansion there may be deformities of the skull with marked bossing and overgrowth of the zygomata giving rise to the classical mongoloid facial appearance of β thalassaemia (Fig. 9(a) and (b)). These findings are reflected by radiological changes which include a lacy, trabecular pattern of the long bones and phalanges and a typical 'hair on end' appearance of the skull (Fig. 10). These bone changes may be associated with recurrent fractures. There is increased susceptibility to infection which may cause a catastrophic drop in the haemoglobin level. Because of the massive marrow expansion, these children are hypermetabolic, run intermittent fevers, lose weight (Fig. 8(b)), have increased requirements for folic acid, and may become acutely folate depleted with worsening of their anaemia. Increased turnover of red cell precursors occasionally gives rise to hyperuricaemia and secondary gout. There is a bleeding tendency which, partly due to thrombocytopenia secondary to hypersplenism, may be exacerbated by liver damage associated with iron loading and extramedullary haemopoiesis. There is also an increased risk of thrombotic complications, possibly reflecting procoagulant properties of the abnormal red cell membranes. The bone deformities of the skull can cause distressing dental complications with poorly formed teeth and malocclusion, and inadequate drainage of the sinuses and middle ear which may lead to chronic sinus infection and deafness. If these unfortunate children survive to puberty, they develop the same complications of iron loading as the well-transfused patients. In this case, some of the iron accumulation results from an increased rate of gastrointestinal absorption as well as that derived from the inadequate transfusion regimen.

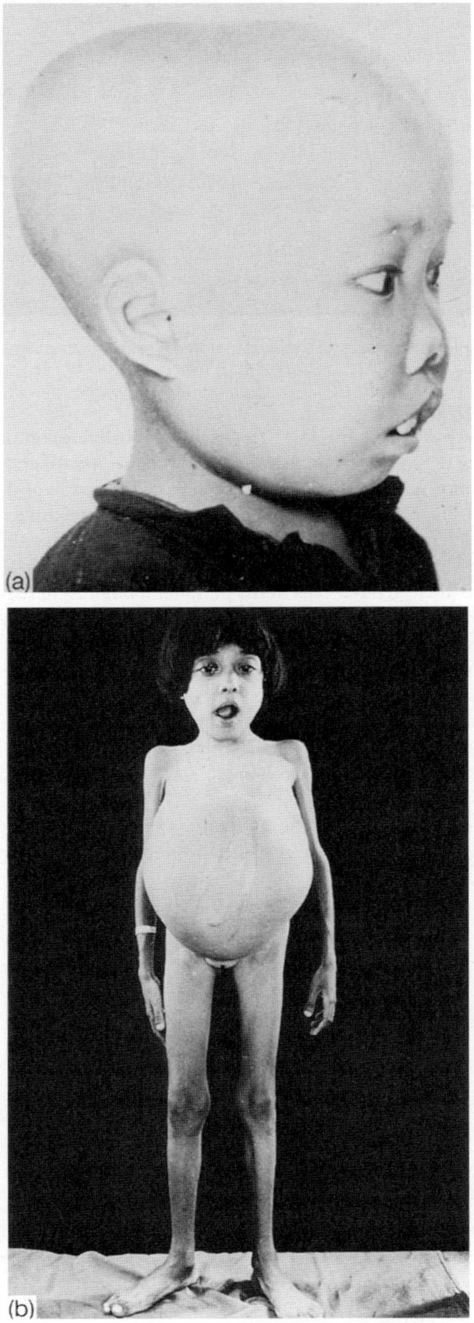

Fig. 9 Homozygous β thalassaemia: (a) skull and facial deformity due to bone marrow expansion; (b) gross wasting of the limbs and hepatomegaly in an undertransfused child.

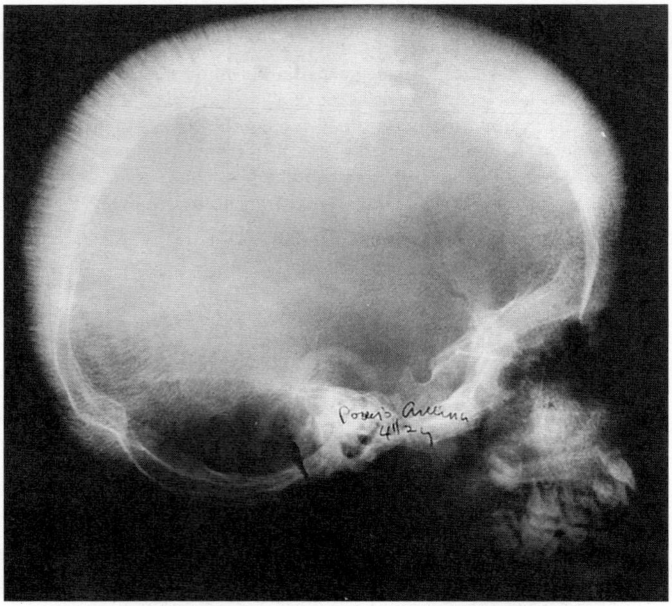

Fig. 10 Radiological changes of the skull in homozygous β thalassaemia.

Haematological changes

There is always a severe anaemia. The haemoglobin values on presentation range from 2 to 8 g/dl. The appearance of the stained peripheral blood film is grossly abnormal (Fig. 11). The red cells show marked hypochromia and variation in shape and size. There are many hypochromic macrocytes and misshapen microcytes, some of which are mere fragments of cells. There is a moderate degree of anisochromia and basophilic stippling. There are always some nucleated red cells in the peripheral blood. After splenectomy, these are found in large numbers. In the postsplenectomy film, many of the nucleated cells and mature erythrocytes show ragged inclusions after incubation of the blood with methyl violet. There is usually a slight elevation in the reticulocyte count. The white cell and platelet counts are normal unless there is hypersplenism in which case they are reduced. The bone marrow shows marked erythroid hyperplasia, with a myeloid/erythroid (M/E) ratio of unity or less. Many of the red cell precursors show ragged inclusions after incubation with methyl violet.

There are biochemical changes of increased haemolysis and progressive iron loading. The bilirubin level is usually elevated and haptoglobins are absent. The ^{51}Cr red cell survival is shortened. The serum iron rises progressively. Most transfusion-dependent children have a totally saturated iron binding capacity. This change is mirrored by a high plasma ferritin level. Liver biopsies show a marked increase in hepatic iron, which may be distributed both in the reticuloendothelial and parenchymal cells (Fig. 12).

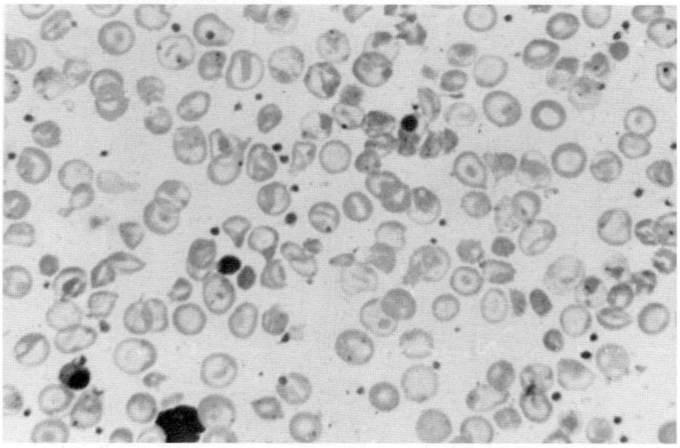

Fig. 11 Peripheral blood film in homozygous β thalassaemia (×630, Leishman stain).

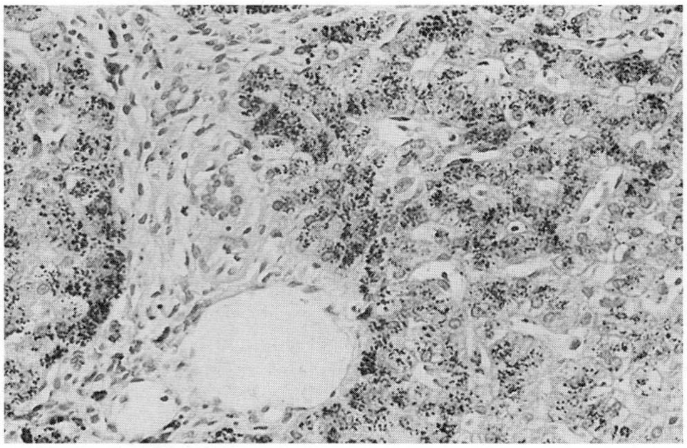

Fig. 12 Histological appearances of the liver in homozygous β thalassaemia showing gross iron deposition (×270, iron stain).

Other biochemical changes

Many thalassaemic children are vitamin E and ascorbate depleted. Folic acid deficiency has already been mentioned. Frank diabetes may develop and endocrine function tests may reveal parathyroid or adrenal insufficiency, or inappropriate response by the pituitary to various release hormones; growth hormone levels are usually normal.

Haemoglobin changes (Table 3)

The haemoglobin F level is always elevated. In β° thalassaemia there is no haemoglobin A and the haemoglobin consists of F and A_2 only. In $β^+$ thalassaemia the level of haemoglobin F ranges from 30 to 90 per cent of the total haemoglobin. The haemoglobin A_2 level is usually normal and is of no diagnostic value.

Heterozygous β thalassaemia

Carriers for β thalassaemia are usually symptom free except in periods of stress such as pregnancy, when they may become more anaemic than normal women. Splenomegaly is rarely present.

Haematological changes

There is a mild degree of anaemia with haemoglobin values in the 9 to 11 g/dl range. The red cells show hypochromia and microcytosis with characteristically low MCH and MCV values. The reticulocyte count is usually normal. The bone marrow shows moderate erythroid hyperplasia.

Haemoglobin changes

The characteristic finding is an elevated haemoglobin A_2 level in the 4 to 6 per cent range. There is a slight elevation of haemoglobin F in the 1 to 3 per cent range in about 50 per cent of cases. A less common form occurs in which the haemoglobin A_2 is not elevated.

β thalassaemia in association with haemoglobin variants

In many populations where there is a high incidence of both β thalassaemia and various haemoglobin variants it is common for an individual to inherit a β thalassaemia gene from one parent and a gene for a structural haemoglobin variant from the other. Although numerous interactions of this type have been described, in clinical practice only three are of importance, that is sickle cell β thalassaemia, haemoglobin C β thalassaemia, and haemoglobin E β thalassaemia.

Sickle cell β thalassaemia

The clinical manifestations which result from the interaction of the β thalassaemia and sickle cell genes vary considerably from race to race. In African populations, there are mild forms of $β^+$ thalassaemia which, when they interact with the sickle cell gene, produce a condition characterized by mild anaemia and few sickling crises. This condition is compatible with normal survival and is often ascertained by chance haematological examination. On the other hand, in Mediterranean populations it is quite common for an individual to inherit a β° or severe $β^+$ thalassaemia determinant from one parent and a sickle cell gene from the other. These interactions are often associated with a clinical picture which is indistinguishable from sickle cell anaemia.

The diagnosis of sickle cell thalassaemia rests on the clinical features of a sickling disorder found in association with a peripheral blood picture with typical thalassaemic red cell changes, that is a low MCH and MCV. In the more severe forms of sickle cell β° thalassaemia, there may be an elevated reticulocyte count and sickled red cells are found on the peripheral blood film. The diagnosis can be confirmed by haemoglobin electrophoresis, which in sickle cell $β^+$ thalassaemia shows haemoglobin S together with 10 to 30 per cent haemoglobin A and an elevated haemoglobin A_2 value. In sickle cell β° thalassaemia, the haemoglobin consists mainly of haemoglobin S with an elevated level of haemoglobins F and A_2. To confirm the diagnosis it is necessary to examine the parents; one should have the sickle cell trait and the other the β thalassaemia trait.

Haemoglobin C thalassaemia

This disorder is restricted to West Africans and some North African and southern Mediterranean populations. It is characterized by a mild haemolytic anaemia associated with splenomegaly. The peripheral blood film shows numerous target cells and thalassaemic red cell changes with a moderately elevated reticulocyte count. Haemoglobin electrophoresis shows a preponderance of haemoglobin C. The diagnosis is confirmed by finding the haemoglobin C trait in one parent and the β thalassaemia trait in the other.

Haemoglobin E β thalassaemia

This is a very common form of thalassaemia in Southeast Asia and throughout the Indian subcontinent. Haemoglobin E is inefficiently synthesized. Thus, when a haemoglobin E gene is inherited together with a β° or severe $β^+$ thalassaemia determinant, that are the commonest types of β thalassaemia in Southeast Asia, there is a marked deficiency of β chain production. The resulting clinical picture can closely resemble thalassaemia major.

The clinical and haematological changes in haemoglobin E thalassaemia are variable. There is usually a marked degree of anaemia and splenomegaly with typical thalassaemic bone changes (Fig. 13). Although not always transfusion dependent, patients with this disorder usually have low haemoglobin values in the 4 to 9 g/dl range with an average of 5 to 7 g/dl. The blood film shows typical thalassaemic red cell changes and the bone marrow shows marked erythroid hyperplasia with α chain inclusions in many of the red cell precursors. Although very little is known about the natural history of this disorder, it seems likely that in many parts of Southeast Asia and India it causes a very high mortality in the early years of life. Complications include a marked susceptibility to infection, secondary hypersplenism, progressive iron loading, a variety of neurological lesions (due to tumours caused by extramedullary erythropoiesis extending in from the inner tables of the skull or vertebrae), folate deficiency, and recurrent pathological fractures. On the other hand, some patients with haemoglobin E thalassaemia grow and develop normally with few complications and there are many recorded cases of pregnancy in women with this disorder.

The diagnosis of haemoglobin E thalassaemia is confirmed by finding haemoglobins E and F and little or no haemoglobin A on haemoglobin electrophoresis and by demonstrating the haemoglobin E trait in one parent and the β thalassaemia trait in the other.

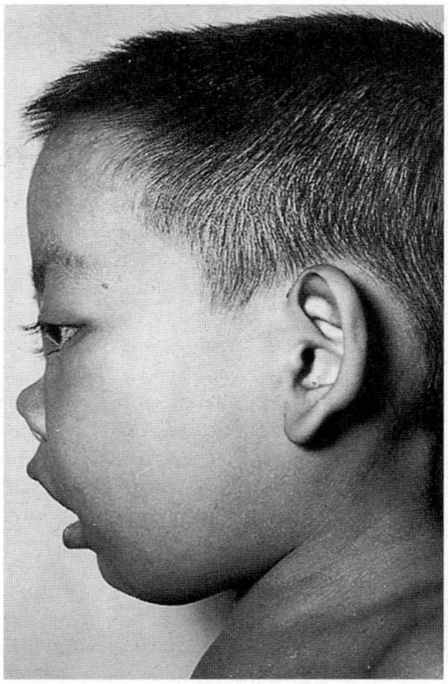

Fig. 13 Bossing of the skull in haemoglobin E thalassaemia.

Other β thalassaemia variants

It is not uncommon to encounter patients with the clinical and haematological features of heterozygous β thalassaemia who do not have an elevated haemoglobin A_2 level. Many of these individuals are heterozygotes for both β and δ thalassaemia. It is important to recognize this interaction because, if it is inherited together with a typical β thalassaemia gene, it can produce a severe transfusion-dependent disorder. Hence this variant is important in antenatal screening programmes. It can only be identified for certain by globin chain synthesis or gene analysis in a specialized laboratory. Families are encountered occasionally in which there is a more severe form of heterozygous β thalassaemia associated with anaemia, jaundice, and splenomegaly. In some of these families it is apparent that the affected individuals are in fact compound heterozygotes for β thalassaemia and the so-called 'silent' β thalassaemia gene, that is a determinant which cannot be identified haematologically in heterozygotes. In other families, a severe form of β thalassaemia behaves as a single gene disorder with full expression in heterozygotes, that is it follows a dominant form of inheritance. In most of these families, the disorder results from the synthesis of a highly unstable β globin chain.

The δβ thalassaemias (Table 3)

Molecular genetics and classification

Disorders due to reduced β and δ chain synthesis are much less common than those due to defective β chain production. They are remarkably heterogeneous at the molecular level. In some cases they result from deletions of the β and δ globin genes, while in others there appears to have been mispaired synapsis and unequal crossing over between the δ and β globin gene loci with the production of δβ fusion genes. The latter produce δβ fusion chains which combine with α chains to form haemoglobin variants called the Lepore haemoglobins (Lepore was the family name of the first patient to be recognized with this disorder). Hence it is usual to classify this group of conditions into the $(\delta\beta)^{\circ}$ thalassaemias and the haemoglobin Lepore or $(\delta\beta)^{+}$ thalassaemias.

Clinical and haematological changes

The $(\delta\beta)^{\circ}$ thalassaemias have been reported in many populations although there are no high frequency areas. In the homozygous state there is a mild degree of anaemia with haemoglobin values of 8 to 10 g/dl. There is often a moderate degree of splenomegaly but these patients are usually symptomless except during periods of stress such as infection or pregnancy. Haemoglobin analysis shows 100 per cent haemoglobin F. Heterozygous carriers have thalassaemic blood pictures, elevated levels of haemoglobin F of 5 to 20 per cent, and normal levels of haemoglobin A_2.The homozygous state for haemoglobin Lepore is characterized by a clinical picture which is usually similar to that of homozygous β thalassaemia although in some cases it may be milder and non-transfusion dependent. The haematological findings are similar to those of β thalassaemia. The haemoglobin consists of F and Lepore only. Heterozygous carriers have thalassaemic blood pictures associated with about 5 to 15 per cent haemoglobin Lepore.

The $(\varepsilon\gamma\delta\beta)^{\circ}$ thalassaemias

There are several rare forms of thalassaemia which result from long deletions of the β globin gene cluster which, as well as removing or inactivating the β genes, involve the δ, γ, and embryonic ε genes. They also involve the main regulatory sequence upstream of the β globin gene cluster, the locus control region. This means that there is no output of globin chains from this gene cluster at all. Clearly, the homozygous state for these disorders would not be compatible with survival. Heterozygotes often have severe haemolytic disease of the newborn with anaemia and hyperbilirubinaemia. If they survive the neonatal period they grow and develop normally; in adult life they have the haematological picture of heterozygous β thalassaemia with mild anaemia, hypochromic microcytic red cells, and a haemoglobin pattern consisting of haemoglobin A, no elevation of haemoglobin F, and a normal level of haemoglobin A_2.

Hereditary persistence of fetal haemoglobin

There is a complex family of conditions characterized by persistent fetal haemoglobin synthesis into adult life associated with no major haematological abnormalities. In some cases they result from long deletions of the β globin gene cluster, similar to those which cause δβ thalassaemia. Indeed, they form a continuum with this condition; homozygotes have 100 per cent fetal haemoglobin, elevated haemoglobin levels and no clinical findings. Other forms result from point mutations in the promoter regions of the γ globin genes. In this case there is increased γ chain production together with reduced β chain production on the affected chromosome. Hence, homozygotes have markedly elevated levels of haemoglobin F but also produce some haemoglobin A. Finally, there is a group in which persistent low levels of haemoglobin F, in the 3 to 10 per cent range, are observed. There is increasing evidence that they may result from mutations either within the β globin gene cluster or on other chromosomes.

The only clinical importance of this complex group of conditions is that they may interact with the thalassaemias or structural haemoglobin variants and reduce the severity of different phenotypes by increasing the amount of haemoglobin F that is produced.

The α thalassaemias

Although the α thalassaemias are commoner on a global basis than the β thalassaemias they pose less of a public health problem. This is because the severe, homozygous forms cause death *in utero* or in the neonatal period and the milder forms do not produce major clinical problems.

Distribution

The α thalassaemias occur widely through the Mediterranean region, parts of West Africa, the Middle East, parts of the Indian subcontinent, and throughout Southeast Asia in a line stretching from southern China through Thailand, the Malay peninsula, and Indonesia to the Pacific island populations (Fig. 14). For reasons which will become apparent when we consider the molecular pathology of these disorders, the serious forms of α thalassaemia are restricted to some of the Mediterranean island populations and Southeast Asia.

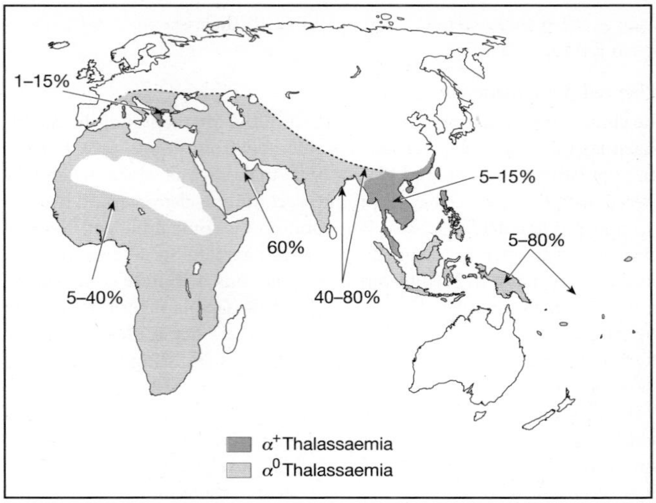

Fig. 14 World map showing the distribution of the α thalassaemias.

Inheritance and molecular pathology

The genetics of α thalassaemia is complicated, and has generated a confusing nomenclature over the years.

Because both haemoglobins A and F have α chains, genetic disorders of α chain synthesis result in defective fetal and adult haemoglobin production. In the fetus, deficiency of α chains leads to the production of excess γ chains which form γ_4 tetramers, or haemoglobin Bart's (Fig. 15). In adults, a deficiency of α chains leads to an excess of β chains which form β_4 tetramers, or haemoglobin H, the adult counterpart of haemoglobin Bart's. Thus, the presence of haemoglobins Bart's or H in red cells is the hallmark of α thalassaemia. For reasons which are not yet clear, a critical level of globin chain imbalance is required before detectable amounts of haemoglobins Bart's or H appear in the red cells. Unfortunately for clinicians, in persons with mild forms of α thalassaemia this level is not reached; significant amounts of these variants only occur in the red cells of patients who

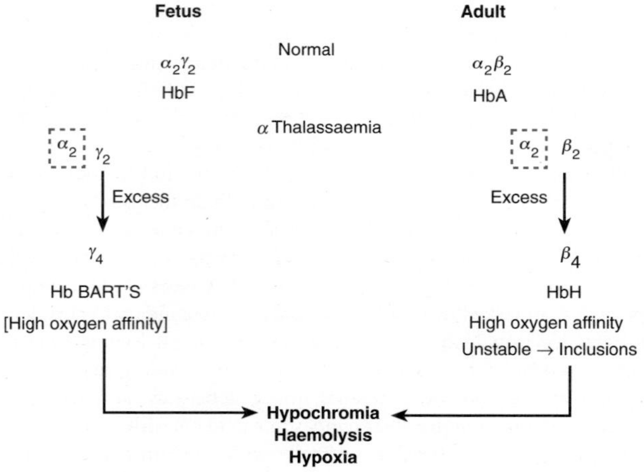

Fig. 15 The pathophysiology of α thalassaemia.

Table 4 The α thalassaemias

Type	Homozygotes	Heterozygotes
α^0	Hb Bart's hydrops	Thalassaemia minor
α^+(deletion)	Thalassaemia minor	Normal blood picture[2]
α^+(non-deletion)	Hb H disease[1]	Normal blood picture[2]

[1] Haemoglobin H disease more commonly results from the compound heterozygous inheritance of α^0 and either variety of α^+ thalassaemia.

[2] There may be very mild red-cell hypochromia.

have a severe degree of α chain deficiency. This means that the carrier states for different forms of α thalassaemia are difficult to diagnose.

Because normal individuals receive two α globin genes from each of their parents, αα/αα, the genetics of the α thalassaemias is more complicated than that of the β thalassaemia. It is useful to define these conditions in heterozygotes. First, there is a more severe form which is called α^0 thalassaemia, which results from loss of both of the linked α globin genes, – –/αα. The second type is almost completely silent in carriers; their red cells are normal or are only slightly hypochromic. This condition is due to the deletion, –α/αα, or reduced activity due to a mutation, $\alpha^T\alpha/\alpha\alpha$, of one of the linked α globin genes. Because there is still some output of α globin from the affected chromosome this is called α^+ thalassaemia. To put it in another way, the terms α^0 and α^+ thalassaemia describe haplotypes, that is the products of two linked α globin genes on one of a pair of homologous chromosomes 16.

In clinical practice we encounter two symptomatic types of α thalassaemia, the haemoglobin Bart's hydrops syndrome and haemoglobin H disease (Table 4). The former results from the homozygous inheritance of α^0 thalassaemia. On the other hand, haemoglobin H disease usually results from the coinheritance of both α^0 and α^+ thalassaemia. We now know that there are many different molecular types of both α^0 and α^+ thalassaemia. These genetic interactions are summarized in Fig. 16.

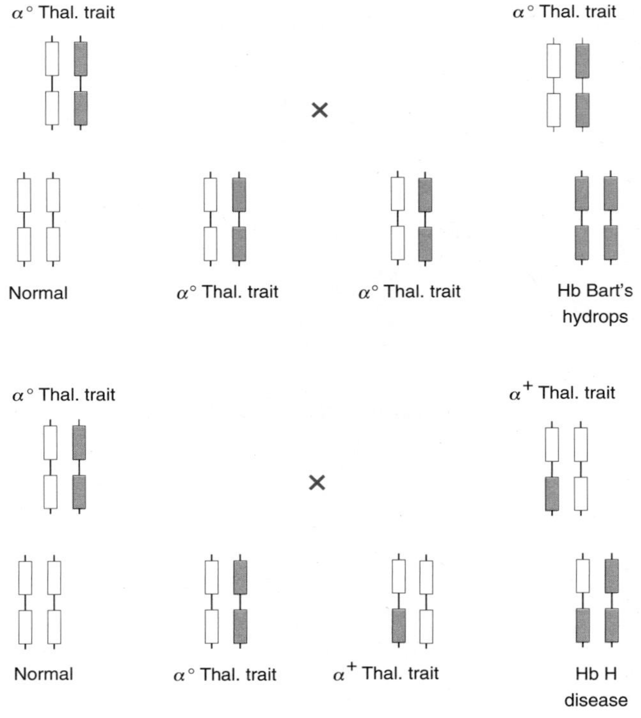

Fig. 16 The genetics of α thalassaemia. The black α genes represent gene deletions or otherwise inactivated genes. The open α genes represent normal genes. α^0 Thalassaemia and α^+ thalassaemia are defined in the text.

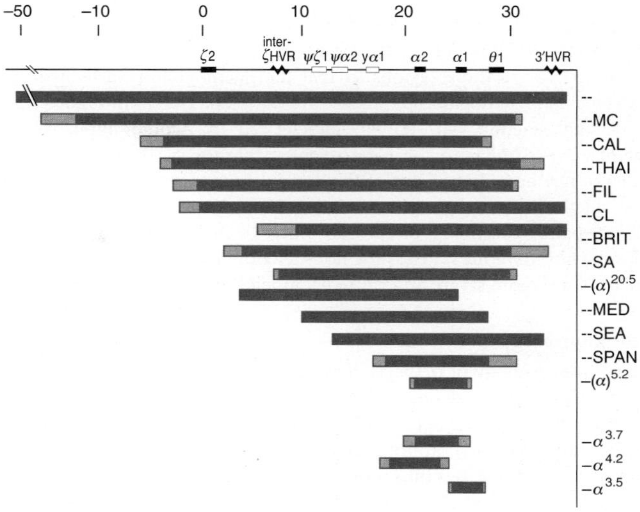

Fig. 17 The different-sized deletions responsible for some forms of α^0 or α^+ thalassaemia. The α globin gene cluster is shown at the top of the figure. Two highly variable regions (HVR) are shown. The abbreviations on the right-hand side indicate the source of origin of patients with the deletions: MED, Mediterranean; SEA, Southeast Asia. The three smaller deletions at the bottom of the figure show some of the main classes of α^+ thalassaemia. The superscripts 3.7, 4.2, and 3.5 indicate the size of the deletions.

Like the β thalassaemias, the α thalassaemias are extremely heterogeneous at the molecular level. Many different sized deletions can remove either both the α globin genes or the main regulatory regions of the α globin gene cluster and cause α^0 thalassaemia, but there are only two which are common. One is found in Southeast Asia. The other occurs mainly in Mediterranean populations (Fig. 17). Similarly, there are several different sized deletions that remove a single α globin gene to produce the deletion forms of α^+ thalassaemia; the commonest are those that remove either 3.7 kb or 4.2 kb of the α gene cluster. There are also many different mutations that can produce the non-deletion forms of α^+ thalassaemia. Many of them are similar to those which produce β thalassaemia. A particularly common form of non-deletion α^+ thalassaemia, found in up to 5 per cent or more of some Southeast Asian populations, results from a single base change in the α globin chain termination codon UAA, which changes to CAA. The latter is the code word for the amino acid glutamine. When the ribosomes reach this point, instead of the chain terminating, they read through messenger RNA that is not normally translated until another stop codon is reached. An elongated α chain variant is synthesized, but the messenger RNA is destabilized by read through of sequences which are not normally translated and so the variant is also produced at a reduced rate. It is called haemoglobin Constant Spring after the name of the town in Jamaica in which it was first discovered. Several other chain termination mutations of this type occur, with different base changes in the terminating codon and hence different amino acids at the beginning of the extension of the α globin chain.

Genotype/phenotype relationships

Molecular studies explain much of the clinical variability of α thalassaemia in different populations. Since the haemoglobin Bart's hydrops syndrome requires the homozygous inheritance of α^0 thalassaemia (– –/– –), this condition only occurs in populations in which α^0 thalassaemia is common. It is mainly confined to Southeast Asia and the Mediterranean islands, populations in which the haemoglobin Bart's hydrops syndrome causes a public health problem. Most forms of haemoglobin H disease are due to the inheritance of α^0 thalassaemia from one parent and α^+ thalassaemia from the other (–α/– – or $-\alpha^T$/– –). Thus, haemoglobin H disease is also restricted mainly to Mediterranean and Oriental populations. On the other hand, α^+

thalassaemia occurs very commonly throughout parts of West Africa, the Indian subcontinent, and the Pacific island populations. α° Thalassaemia does not occur in these regions so that the haemoglobin Bart's hydrops syndrome and haemoglobin H disease are not seen. The homozygous state for α^{+} thalassaemia ($-\alpha/-\alpha$) is characterized by a mild hypochromic anaemia, very similar to the heterozygous state for α° thalassaemia; the results of having only two out of the normal four α genes seem to be the same whether the two genes are missing from the same chromosome or opposite pairs of homologous chromosomes. To complicate matters, sometimes the homozygous state for the non-deletion forms of α^{+} thalassaemia, $\alpha^{T}\alpha/\alpha^{T}\alpha$, are more severe and cause haemoglobin H disease.

Pathophysiology

The pathophysiology of α thalassaemia is different to that of β thalassaemia. A deficiency of α chains leads to the production of excess γ chains or β chains which form haemoglobins Bart's and H respectively (Fig. 15). These more soluble tetramers do not precipitate to any great extent in the bone marrow. Erythropoiesis is thus more effective than in β thalassaemia, that is there is less intramedullary destruction of red cell precursors. However, haemoglobin H is unstable and precipitates in red cells as they age. The large inclusion bodies produced in this way are trapped in the spleen and other parts of the microcirculation leading to a shortened red cell survival. Furthermore, both haemoglobins Bart's and H have a very high oxygen affinity; because they have no α chains there is no haem/haem interaction and their oxygen dissociation curves resemble myoglobin. Thus the pathophysiology of severe forms of α thalassaemia is based on defective haemoglobin production, the synthesis of homotetramers which are physiologically useless, and a haemolytic component due to their precipitation in older red cells. Furthermore, excess β chains cause a different pattern of damage to red cell membrane proteins than free α chains; the red cells tend to be overhydrated in α thalassaemia.

The haemoglobin Bart's hydrops syndrome

This condition is a common cause of fetal loss throughout Southeast Asia and in Greece and Cyprus. Affected infants produce no α chains and hence can make neither fetal nor adult haemoglobin.

The clinical picture is very characteristic (Fig. 18). Infants are usually stillborn between 28 and 40 weeks. Liveborn infants take a few gasping respirations and then expire within the first hour after birth. They show the typical picture of hydrops fetalis with gross pallor, generalized oedema, and massive hepatosplenomegaly. There is a high frequency of other congenital abnormalities, and a very large, friable placenta, all due to severe intrauterine anaemia. The haemoglobin values are in the 6 to 8 g/dl range and there are gross thalassaemic changes of the peripheral blood film with many nucleated red cells. The haemoglobin consists of approximately 80 per cent haemoglobin Bart's and 20 per cent of the embryonic haemoglobin, Portland ($\zeta_2\gamma_2$). It is believed that these infants survive to term because they continue to produce embryonic haemoglobin at this level; haemoglobin Bart's is, as mentioned above, useless as an oxygen carrier.

This syndrome is also characterized by a high incidence of maternal toxaemia of pregnancy and considerable obstetric difficulties due to the presence of the large, friable placenta. Both parents have thalassaemic red cell changes with normal haemoglobin A_2 values, that is the characteristic finding of the heterozygous state for α° thalassaemia.

Haemoglobin H disease

As mentioned earlier, haemoglobin H is a tetramer of normal β chains with the formula β_4. It is produced when there is a marked reduction of α chain synthesis. Haemoglobin H disease usually results from the inheritance of α° thalassaemia from one parent and α^{+} from the other. It may also result from the inheritance of α° thalassaemia and haemoglobin Constant Spring or from the homozygous state for a severe, non-deletion form of α thalassaemia. The latter form of inheritance is particularly common in Saudi Arabia.

There is a variable degree of anaemia and splenomegaly but it is most unusual to see severe thalassaemic bone changes or the growth retardation characteristic of homozygous β thalassaemia. Patients usually survive into adult life although the course may be interspersed with severe episodes of haemolysis associated with infection, or worsening of the anaemia due to progressive hypersplenism. Oxidant drugs such as sulphonamides may increase the rate of precipitation of haemoglobin H and therefore exacerbate the anaemia.

Haemoglobin values range from 7 to 10 g/dl. The blood film shows typical thalassaemic changes. There is a moderate reticulocytosis. Incubation of the red cells with brilliant cresyl blue generates numerous inclusion bodies by precipitation of the haemoglobin H under the redox action of the

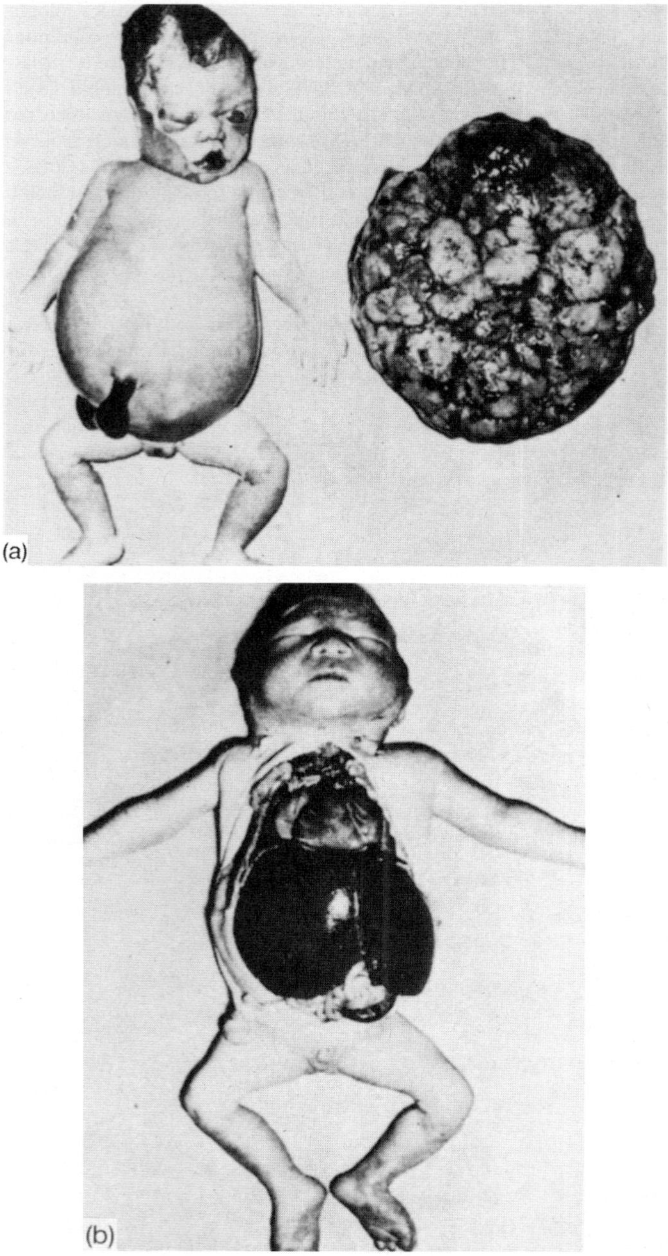

Fig. 18 The haemoglobin Bart's hydrops syndrome: (a) a hydropic infant with massively enlarged placenta; (b) autopsy findings with an enlarged liver. (Reproduced by permission of Professor P. Wasi.)

dye. After splenectomy large, preformed inclusions can be demonstrated on incubation of blood with methyl violet. The haemoglobin consists of from 5 to 40 per cent haemoglobin H together with haemoglobin A and a normal or reduced level of haemoglobin A_2.

Usually one parent is heterozygous for α° thalassaemia and the other for α^{+} thalassaemia, the deletion or non-deletion varieties. Less commonly, both parents are heterozygous for a non-deletion form of α^{+} thalassaemia.

The haematological findings in the α° and α^{+} thalassaemia traits are summarized in Table 4. They can only be identified with certainty by analysis of the α globin genes.

α Thalassaemia and mental retardation

There is an increasingly important group of α thalassaemias which are not restricted to individuals from tropical backgrounds. They are observed in all racial groups and have been best characterized in those of north European origin. These conditions are characterized by variable degrees of mental retardation, dysmorphic features, and α thalassaemic blood pictures. They follow a completely different form of inheritance to the commoner genetic forms of α thalassaemia and constitute a increasingly heterogeneous group of disorders. There are two major varieties of this condition. The first is due to lesions that involve the α globin gene cluster on chromosome 16, ATR-16. There is another group that result from mutations on the X chromosome, ATR-X.

The ATR-16 disorders are characterized by a very variable degree of mental retardation and equally variable dysmorphic features. The blood film shows mild α thalassaemic changes and some cells which contain typical haemoglobin H inclusion bodies. It is now clear that they have a heterogeneous molecular pathology. In some cases the condition results from long deletions which remove the end of the short arm of chromosome 16 and extend for one to two megabases. Occasionally they also include the genes that are involved in tuberous sclerosis and adult polycystic disease of the kidney. In other cases, the loss of the end of the short arm of chromosome 16 is the result of an inherited cytogenetic abnormality, including translocations and other rearrangements.

The ATR-X syndrome is characterized by a much more consistent series of dysmorphic features and more severe mental retardation. These infants often suffer from convulsions after birth. They develop typical facial features, genital abnormalities, and a very mild form of haemoglobin H disease. This condition is inherited as a typical sex-linked disorder which affects males. It results from mutations of a gene on the X chromosome called *ATR-X* which is now known to act as a regulator of transcription via an effect on the structure of chromatin. Female carriers may show a very small proportion of red cells containing haemoglobin H bodies. This condition should be thought of in any child with severe mental retardation and dysmorphic features whose blood film shows evidence of a very mild form of α thalassaemia.

Thalassaemia intermedia

Definition and pathogenesis

The term thalassaemia intermedia is used to describe patients with the clinical picture of thalassaemia which, although not transfusion dependent, is associated with a much more severe degree of anaemia than that found in carriers for α or β thalassaemia. Many of the conditions which have been described previously in this section follow this clinical course, for example haemoglobin C or E thalassaemia, the various δβ thalassaemias and haemoglobin Lepore disorders, and the wide variety of conditions which can result from the interactions of the different β and δβ thalassaemia determinants. However, some children with this condition have parents with typical heterozygous β thalassaemia blood pictures and elevated haemoglobin A_2 levels. These patients appear to be homozygous for β thalassaemia, yet they run a much milder course than is usually the case with this condition. Some of them have inherited an α thalassaemia determinant as well as being homozygous for β thalassaemia. This reduces the overall degree of globin chain imbalance and consequently the severity of the dyserythropoiesis which usually accompanies homozygous β thalassaemia; hence these children run a milder clinical course. In other cases, particularly in African races, relatively mild forms of homozygous β thalassaemia seem to reflect the action of less severe β thalassaemia mutations. Finally, some intermediate forms of β thalassaemia seem to result from the coinheritance of a gene for unusually effective haemoglobin F production.

Clinical and haematological changes

The clinical features of the intermediate forms of thalassaemia are extremely variable. At one end of the spectrum are patients who are virtually symptom free except for moderate anaemia. At the other end there are patients who have haemoglobin values in the 5 to 7 g/dl range and who develop marked splenomegaly, severe skeletal deformities due to expansion of bone marrow, and, as they get older, become heavily iron loaded because of increased intestinal absorption of iron. Recurrent leg ulceration, folate deficiency, symptoms due to extramedullary haemopoietic tumour masses in the chest and skull (Fig. 19), gallstones, and a marked proneness to infection are particularly characteristic of this group of thalassaemias.

Because of the heterogeneity of these disorders, it is only possible to determine the course that is likely to evolve in any individual patient by following the disorder very carefully from early childhood.

Differential diagnosis of the thalassaemias

There are few conditions which are likely to be confused with the more severe forms of homozygous β thalassaemia or haemoglobin H disease. The racial background of the patient, the presence of anaemia from early life, and the characteristic haematological changes make the diagnosis relatively easy. Once thalassaemia is suspected, the parents and near relatives should be examined for the carrier states for α or β thalassaemia. Both disorders can be distinguished from simple iron deficiency by the finding of a normal

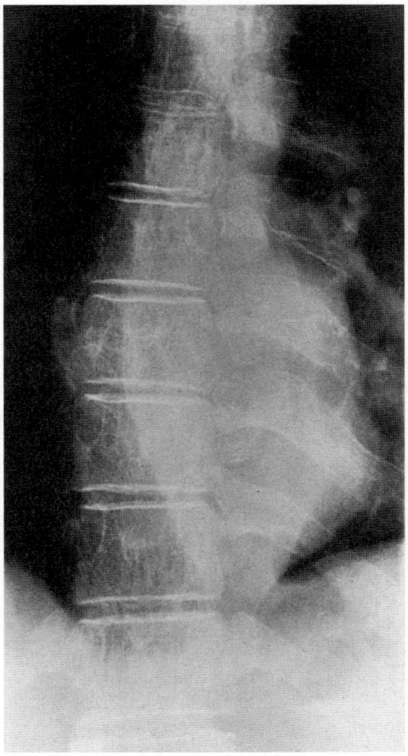

Fig. 19 An extramedullary haemopoietic mass in a patient with β thalassaemia intermedia.

serum iron or ferritin level and by the associated changes in the haemoglobin pattern. It should be remembered, however, that in some groups iron deficiency and heterozygous thalassaemia frequently occur together in the same person, particularly during pregnancy. The sideroblastic anaemias can be easily distinguished from thalassaemia by the morphological appearances of the red cells and the presence of ring sideroblasts in the bone marrow. It should be remembered that there are some rare forms of acquired haemoglobin H disease in elderly patients with leukaemia.

The laboratory diagnosis of thalassaemia

The thalassaemias should be suspected when a typical thalassaemic blood picture is found in an individual of an appropriate racial group. The homozygous states for the severe forms of β thalassaemia are easily recognized by the haematological changes associated with very high levels of haemoglobin F; haemoglobin A_2 values vary so much that they are of no diagnostic help. The heterozygous states are recognized by microcytic hypochromic red cells and an elevated level of haemoglobin A_2. The δβ thalassaemias are characterized by the finding of 100 per cent haemoglobin F in homozygotes and 5 to 15 per cent haemoglobin F together with a normal level of haemoglobin A_2 in heterozygotes (see Table 3).

When β thalassaemia is diagnosed, a quantitative haemoglobin electrophoresis should be carried out to exclude the presence of an abnormal haemoglobin variant such as haemoglobin E or Lepore.

The haemoglobin Bart's hydrops syndrome is recognized by the finding of a hydropic infant with a severe anaemia, a thalassaemic blood picture, and 80 per cent or more haemoglobin Bart's on haemoglobin electrophoresis. Haemoglobin H disease is identified by the finding of a typical thalassaemic blood picture with an elevated reticulocyte count, generation of multiple inclusion bodies in the red cells after incubation with brilliant cresyl blue, and the finding of variable amounts of haemoglobin H on haemoglobin electrophoresis. There are no really useful, simple diagnostic tests for the different α thalassaemic carrier states although α° thalassaemia heterozygotes usually have typical thalassaemic red cell changes with a normal haemoglobin A_2 value. It is essential for counselling purposes to diagnose the different carrier states for α thalassaemia, blood samples should be referred to a laboratory that can carry out DNA analysis of the globin genes.

Prevention and treatment

Thalassaemia produces a severe public health problem and a serious drain on medical resources in many populations. Since there is no definitive treatment, most countries in which the disease is common are putting a major effort into programmes for its prevention.

Prevention

There are two major approaches to the prevention of the thalassaemias. Since the carrier states for the β thalassaemias can be easily recognized, it is at least theoretically possible to screen populations and provide genetic counselling about the choice of marriage partners. If β thalassaemia heterozygotes marry other carriers, one in four of their children will have the severe, transfusion-dependent homozygous disorder. While large-scale programmes of this type have been set up in Italy, the results are not yet available, and in smaller pilot studies in Greece the outcome has not been encouraging. Until more is known about the usefulness of this form of prospective genetic counselling, most countries are developing screening programmes at antenatal clinics. When heterozygous carrier mothers are found, the husbands are tested and if they are also carriers the couple are offered the possibility of prenatal diagnosis and termination of pregnancies carrying fetuses with severe forms of thalassaemia.

Prenatal diagnosis

Prenatal diagnosis can be offered to couples at risk for having children with severe forms of β thalassaemia. Because of the serious obstetric complications and the trauma of carrying a hydropic fetus to term there is also a good case for prenatal diagnosis for the haemoglobin Bart's hydrops syndrome. Termination of pregnancies at risk for milder forms of thalassaemia is also undertaken, but should only be considered after very careful counselling of the parents. Some children with intermediate forms of thalassaemia are symptom free and develop normally; others have more severe anaemia and bone deformity. There has been some success in determining which particular molecular defects and interactions are associated with these different clinical courses. When in doubt, parents should be referred for expert analysis of their variety of thalassaemia and appropriate counselling.

Prenatal diagnosis of thalassaemia can be carried out in several ways. The diagnosis can be made by globin-chain-synthesis studies of fetal blood samples obtained by fetoscopy at 18 to 20 weeks gestation. The diagnosis can also be made by fetal DNA analysis on amniotic fluid cells obtained by amniocentesis earlier in the second trimester. More recently, it has been possible to carry out prenatal diagnosis of thalassaemia and sickle cell anaemia by direct analysis of fetal DNA obtained by chorion biopsy at about the 12th week of gestation. This approach has largely replaced fetal blood sampling or amniocentesis for the prenatal diagnosis of the thalassaemias. First trimester diagnosis is much more acceptable to many women. This reduces the long period of uncertainty, during which the fetus is growing and the mother and her relatives and friends are coming to accept that she is to have a child, and because late second trimester terminations are often difficult. Prenatal diagnosis of thalassaemia is now carried out in many countries, and in Sardinia, Greece, and Cyprus has significantly reduced the number of new cases of thalassaemia in the community.

Because prenatal diagnosis of thalassaemia is now well established it is very important to discuss the genetic implications of the condition when carriers are detected by chance, regardless of the individuals's racial background. They should also be given a letter explaining, in simple terms, the pattern of inheritance and the dangers for their children. This approach should always be followed, even for sporadic cases in low incidence regions, such as northern Europe. Because of the increasing movements of populations they might still marry another carrier and have severely affected children.

Symptomatic treatment

The symptomatic management of severe β thalassaemia requires regular blood transfusion, the judicious use of splenectomy if hypersplenism develops, and the administration of chelating agents to reduce iron overload. When the diagnosis of severe β thalassaemia is suspected during the first year of life, the infant should be followed for several weeks to make sure that the haemoglobin level is fallen to a level at which regular transfusion will be necessary. It is difficult to be dogmatic about exactly when transfusions should be started. A severely anaemic infant who is feeding poorly, inactive, or otherwise failing to thrive, will almost certainly need to be transfused. The object is to maintain the pretransfusion haemoglobin level at about 9.5 g/dl. This usually requires transfusion of 10 to 15 mg/kilo red cells every 4 weeks. Washed red cells should be used. Whole blood should be avoided because of the danger of sensitization to serum or white cell components. The rate of transfusion should not exceed 4 to 5 ml/kg per h. In patients who are profoundly anaemic or show evidence of cardiac insufficiency, the rate should be no more than 2 ml/kg per h. It is important to calculate the annual blood consumption by dividing the total volume of blood transfused over 12 months by the patients weight in the middle of the year. If it is higher than 200 ml/kg body weight, splenectomy should be considered. All blood should be screened for hepatitis B and C, and for HIV.

Hypersplenism is becoming much less common if children are maintained on an adequate transfusion regimen. Increasingly blood requirements, or evidence of hypersplenism, pancytopenia for example, should prompt one to consider splenectomy. It should be avoided before the age of 6 years because of the particularly high incidence of infection in asplenic children. Two to three weeks before splenectomy the child should be given:

(1) pneumococcal vaccine; (2) *Haemophilus influenzae* type B vaccine; (3) meningococcal A and C vaccine. After the operation the children should be maintained on oral penicillin V, 125 mg twice daily, increasing to 250 mg twice daily for older children. For those who are allergic to penicillin, erythromycin should be given.

The only effective chelating agent for the prevention or treatment of iron overload in thalassaemia is desferrioxamine (Desferal). It is now clear that this drug should not be given too soon because toxic effects are observed at low body iron loads. Ideally, the hepatic iron concentration should be measured at about 1 year after regular transfusion has started. Chelation should be initiated in patients with hepatic iron concentrations of above 7 mg/g liver dry weight. Where this is not possible, the drug should be given when the serum ferritin value has reached or exceeded 1000 μg/l although it is becoming increasingly clear that the serum ferritin level is a very imprecise estimate of body iron load. The initial dose should not exceed 25 to 35 mg/kg body weight per 24 h. Iron excretion is potentiated if children receive 100 mg vitamin C by mouth on the days of the infusion. Ideally, progress should be monitored by regular estimates of the hepatic iron concentration but if this is not possible the serum ferritin level should be maintained below 2000 μg/l. In patients who become iron loaded, it is possible to increase the rate of iron excretion considerably but the daily dose of desferrioxamine should not exceed 15 mg/kg body weight. Patients should be monitored continuously for side effects of desferrioxamine; these include retinal damage, ototoxicity, and interference with growth.

There are no entirely satisfactory alternatives to desferrioxamine as a chelating agent. The most widely studied, the oral chelator deferiprone (L1), does not appear to control iron accumulation in a proportion of patients, and causes neutropenia in about 5 per cent of cases. Its long-term toxicity and true place in the management of thalassaemia remains to be determined.

It is very important to monitor transfusion-dependent patients for hepatitis B and C and HIV infection. The management of these conditions is considered elsewhere in this book. Other complications relating to iron load, including hypoparathyroidism, diabetes, and delayed puberty and hypogonadism, require expert endocrinological assessment with appropriate replacement therapy.

Increasing experience with bone marrow transplantation has suggested that, if done early with adequate HLA matching, the results are extremely good. Patients who have become iron loaded and who have liver damage have a less good prognosis but, as more experience has been gained, there appears to be a place for transplantation in older patients.

The intermediate forms of thalassaemia should be treated by careful observation, folic acid supplementation, and, in the face of a falling haemoglobin and increasing spleen size, the judicious use of splenectomy. It is important to monitor the iron status regularly because some of these patients become iron loaded due to increased intestinal absorption later in life and chelation therapy may be necessary.

Currently, a number of experimental approaches to the treatment of the thalassaemias are being pursued, including the use of intrauterine or later stem cell therapy, the stimulation of fetal haemoglobin production, and, in the longer term, the possibility of somatic gene therapy.

Structural haemoglobin variants

Over 400 structural haemoglobin variants have been described, most of which result from single amino acid substitutions. Many of them are harmless and have been discovered during surveys of the electrophoretic patterns of human haemoglobin. Of course, this approach underestimates the number of variants because it only identifies those in which the amino acid substitution alters the charge of the haemoglobin molecule.

Single amino acid substitutions cause clinical disorders only if they alter the stability or functional properties of the haemoglobin molecule. A classification of these diseases is shown in Table 5. They include the sickling disorders, chronic or drug-induced haemolytic anaemia associated with unstable haemoglobins, and polycythaemia or congenital cyanosis, associated with high and low oxygen affinity haemoglobin variants, respectively. There is a rare group of haemoglobin variants that produce methaemoglobinaemia. We shall consider the different varieties of genetic methaemoglobinaemias at the end of this chapter.

Table 5 Clinical disorders due to structural haemoglobin variants

Disorder	Variants
Haemolysis and tissue damage	Haemoglobin S
Drug-induced haemolysis	Haemoglobin Zürich and other unstable haemoglobins
Chronic haemolysis	Unstable haemoglobin variants
	Haemoglobin C
Congenital polycythaemia	High-affinity variants
Congenital cyanosis	Haemoglobin(s) M
	Low-affinity variants
Hypochromia: thalassaemic phenotype	Haemoglobin E
	Haemoglobin Constant Spring

Nomenclature

Originally, the structural haemoglobin variants were named by letters of the alphabet. By the late 1950s there were none left; it was decided to designate new haemoglobin variants by the place of origin of the first patient in whom they were characterized. It is customary to call the heterozygous carrier state the 'trait' and the homozygous condition the 'disease'. For example, haemoglobin S heterozygotes (genotype AS) are said to have the sickle cell trait, while those homozygous for the sickle cell mutation (genotype SS) are said to have sickle cell disease. In practice it is very important to distinguish between the carrier state and the homozygous or compound heterozygous state for a haemoglobin variant; carriers are usually asymptomatic.

The sickling disorders

Sickling disorders (Table 6) consist of the heterozygous state for haemoglobin S, sickle cell trait (AS), the homozygous state or sickle cell disease (SS), and the compound heterozygous state for haemoglobin S together with haemoglobins C, D, E, or other structural variants. Several disorders result from the inheritance of the sickle cell gene together with different forms of thalassaemia.

Pathogenesis

Haemoglobin S differs from haemoglobin A by the substitution of valine for glutamic acid at position 6 in the β chain. Although this has been known for nearly half a century, it is still not absolutely clear how it gives rise to the sickling phenomenon. The latter appears to be due to the unusual solubility characteristics of haemoglobin S which undergoes liquid crystal (tactoid) formation as it becomes deoxygenated. In this state, aggregates of sickled haemoglobin molecules arrange themselves in parallel, rod-like fibres, made up of a complex solid core about 21 nm in diameter, composed of 14 filaments arranged as seven pairs of double filaments. Much is now known about the complex interactions whereby the β6 valine

Table 6 The major sickling disorders

Disorder	Genotype (normal = αα/αα.β/β)	
SS disease (sickle-cell anaemia)	αα/αα	β^S/β^S
SC disease	αα/αα	β^S/β^C
SD disease	αα/αα	β^S/β^D
S-β thalassaemia	αα/αα	$\beta^S\beta^\circ$ or β^S/β^+
S-hereditary persistence of fetal Hb	αα/αα	$\beta^S/-$[1]
S-α thalassaemia	α–/αα or α–/α–	β^S/β^S

[1] Indicates β gene deletion.

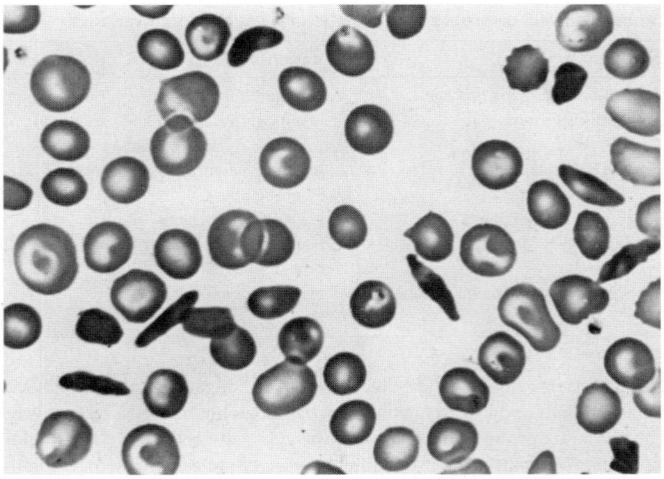

Fig. 20 Irreversibly sickled cells in the peripheral blood (×1000, Leishman stain).

substitution stabilizes the molecular stacks in the deoxy configuration of haemoglobin. There is considerable variation in the extent to which different haemoglobins are able to participate with haemoglobin S in the sickling process. This accounts for some of the clinical variability of the different sickling conditions. For example haemoglobin F is almost completely excluded from the sickling process; increasing concentrations in the red cell reduce the rate of sickling.

The pathophysiology of sickling is an extremely dynamic process. Red cells containing sickle haemoglobin at a high concentration endure a series of cycles of sickling and desickling with progressive membrane damage and loss of plasticity. Finally these dry, rigid cells become irreversibly sickled (Fig. 20). Sickling of this type has two main effects. First, sickled erythrocytes have a shortened survival leading to a chronic haemolytic anaemia. Second, and more importantly, these abnormal red cells tend to adhere to the various receptors on the walls of small blood vessels with the production of aggregates, blockage of the vessels, vascular stasis, and, ultimately, tissue damage.

Distribution

The sickling disorders occur very frequently in African populations and, sporadically, throughout the Mediterranean region and the Middle East. There are extensive pockets in India but the disease has not been seen in Southeast Asia. The high frequency of the sickle cell gene occurs because carriers are more resistant than normal individuals to *P. falciparum* malaria.

Clinical features

Except in conditions of extreme hypoxia, such as flying in an unpressurized aircraft the sickle cell trait causes no clinical disability. However, it is possible for individuals to suffer vaso-occlusive episodes if they become oxygen deprived under anaesthesia. Therefore all individuals of the appropriate racial background should have a sickling test (see below) before receiving an anaesthetic. If the test is positive, the anaesthetic should be given with adequate oxygenation and special care should be taken to avoid post-operative dehydration.

Sickle cell anaemia runs an extremely variable clinical course. At one end of the spectrum it is characterized by a crippling haemolytic anaemia interspersed with severe exacerbations, or crises. On the other hand, it may be extremely mild and only found by chance on routine haematological examination. The reason for these remarkable differences in phenotypic expression, which are only partly understood, include the level of haemoglobin F, coinheritance of α thalassaemia, climate, and, probably most important, socioeconomic factors such as availability of early treatment of infection.

Typically, sickle cell anaemia presents in infancy with symptoms related to anaemia or infection. A common presenting symptom is the hand and foot syndrome. It occurs early in infancy and is characterized by a painful dactylitis with swelling of the fingers or feet. Epiphyseal damage during one of these episodes may lead to chronic shortening of a digit. Infants are anaemic from about the third month of life. During early development they often have significant splenomegaly that gradually resolves due to repeated infarction. Indeed, it is most unusual to feel the spleen after the end of the first decade. Typically, the haemoglobin levels are in the 6 to 8 g/dl range with a reticulocyte count of 10 to 20 percent. There is chronic, mild icterus with an elevated bilirubin level. Examination of the peripheral blood film shows anisochromia and poikilocytosis with a variable number of sickled erythrocytes (Fig. 20). As the children grow older the haematological changes of hyposplenism develop with the appearance of pits on the surface of the red cells, Howell–Jolly bodies, and distorted red cells. The white cell and platelet counts are usually normal or slightly elevated.

Growth and development are usually otherwise normal although there may be some skeletal deformities, including frontal bossing of the skull due to expansion of the bone marrow. In some series, children have tended to be short for their age, while postadolescents were usually tall. Inequalities between upper and lower segments, stressed in the early literature, are unusual. The only other physical finding is chronic leg ulceration; this is discussed below.

Complications

The chronic haemolysis of sickle cell disease is interspersed with acute exacerbations of the illness called sickling crises. Furthermore, there are a series of serious and life-threatening, long-term complications which develop in many patients with sickle cell anaemia.

The different forms of sickle cell crises are summarized in Table 7. The commonest is the painful crisis. This is sometimes precipitated by infection, dehydration, or exposure to cold, although quite often no underlying cause can be found. The episode starts with vague pain, often in the back or bones of the limbs. The pain gradually worsens and its bizarre distribution may cause a major diagnostic puzzle. The pain is almost certainly due to blockage of small vessels with sickled erythrocytes; aspiration over areas of bone tenderness has shown infarction of marrow tissue. Occasionally, abdominal pain is the major symptom and this may be associated with distension and rigidity, a picture very similar to an acute abdominal emergency. The diagnostic difficulties in distinguishing between an abdominal crisis and a surgical abdomen are compounded by the fact that the bowel sounds are often diminished during abdominal crises. Two other serious forms of thrombotic crisis are known as the 'chest' and 'brain' syndromes. The 'chest' syndrome, characterized by acute dyspnoea and pleuritic pain together with infiltrates on the chest radiograph, is due to sequestration of sickle cells in the pulmonary circulation. It is sometimes accompanied by a fall in the PCV and platelet count which also may reflect sequestration of sickled cells in the pulmonary vessels. Neurological involvement may present in a variety of ways including fits with or without focal neurological

Table 7 Acute exacerbations ('crises') in sickle-cell (SS) disease

1. Thrombotic
Generalized or localized bone pain
Abdominal
Pulmonary
Neurological
2. Aplastic
3. Haemolytic
4. Sequestration
Spleen
Liver
?Lung
5. Various combinations of above

signs. Cerebral infarction is commoner in children, while haemorrhage, due to microaneurysms which develop round infarctions ('moya moya') is commoner in adults.

During painful crises there may be a marked increase in the rate of haemolysis with a fall in the haemoglobin level. Such haemolytic episodes are uncommon. Much more serious are periods of transient bone marrow aplasia called aplastic crises. These seem to result from intercurrent infection, particularly due to parvovirus, and frequently affect more than one sibling in the same family.

Finally, and most serious, are the sequestration crises. Occurring mainly in babies and young children, they are characterized by a rapid enlargement of the spleen or liver, which become engorged with sickled erythrocytes. As the crisis progresses a large proportion of the total red cell mass may be trapped in the spleen or liver. Death may occur due to profound anaemia. These episodes show a tendency to recur in the same individual. Hepatic sequestration, which may occur in adults, is easily overlooked if the liver size is not monitored carefully.

The commonest cause of death in sickle cell anaemia appears to be a sequestration crisis or acute infection, or both. It is not absolutely clear why patients with this disorder are so prone to infection although reduced splenic function may play a role. Abnormalities of the alternate pathway of complement activation have also been described. A variety of organisms are involved, particularly the pneumococcus, and, mainly in tropical countries, typhoid infection of bone infarcts leads to typhoid osteomyelitis. Despite the relative resistance of heterozygotes to *P. falciparum* malaria, deaths due to malaria are extremely common in Africa.

Pregnancy may be uneventful, or associated with an increased incidence of painful crises. There is slightly increased incidence of maternal mortality and a definite increase in the rate of fetal loss.

Chronic complications

The chronic complications of sickle cell anaemia result largely from infarcts following repeated episodes of vascular occlusion. Almost any organ can be involved. Those at particular risk are areas which rely largely on small vessels for their blood supply. The bones are particularly prone to infarction. Aseptic necrosis of the humeral or femoral heads may lead to gross deformity of the shoulder and hip joints (Fig. 21). Bone infarcts may result in chronic sequestra formation which may become secondarily infected with the production of osteomyelitis. Infarction of the bone marrow does not seem to have any long-term sequelae, although occasionally pieces may break off and embolize to the lungs. Chronic leg ulceration is a common problem.

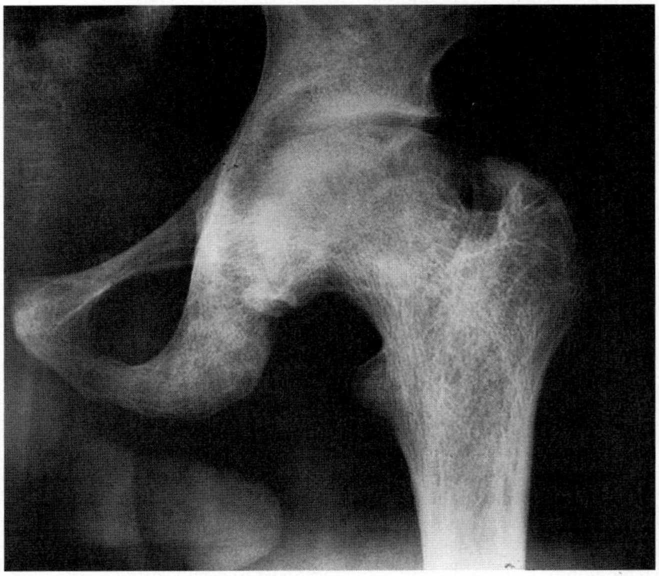

Fig. 21 Aseptic necrosis of the left femoral head in sickle-cell thalassaemia. (Reproduced by courtesy of Dr Graham Serjeant.)

Another organ at particular risk is the kidney. During early childhood renal function may be impaired but this can be corrected by blood transfusion, suggesting that it is due to reversible changes in the renal vasculature. These alterations in renal function are not reversible in later life. Chronic renal failure due to damage of the renal vessels is one of the commonest causes of death in adults with sickle cell anaemia. A typical nephrotic syndrome may develop at some stage during the illness. Pulmonary infarction occurs quite frequently, but repeated episodes leading to severe pulmonary hypertension and right heart failure are unusual, although this complication has been well documented.

There is usually some degree of cardiomegaly. A variety of flow murmurs may be heard but most of these signs seem to be the result of chronic anaemia. Myocardial infarction or fibrosis is not a feature of the disease. Recurrent attacks of painful priapism may lead to permanent deformity of the penis. Occular manifestations are also relatively common in sickle cell anaemia although they tend to be more serious in haemoglobin SC disease; they will be considered with the later disorder in a later section. Finally, there is increased evidence that, unless the neurological crises are treated energetically, permanent brain damage may result.

Course and prognosis

There are still large gaps in our knowledge about the natural history of sickle cell anaemia. Prognosis seems to depend on the racial background of the patient, socioeconomic and ill-defined genetic factors, and, especially the availability of good paediatric care in the early years.

In rural East Africa, the disease still has a high mortality in the first year or two of life. In Jamaica there appears to be a 10 per cent mortality in the early years although survival into adult life and old age is common. This is also the case in some urban parts of Africa and in the United States and Europe. Data from the United States Cooperative Study of Sickle Cell Disease suggest that the median age at death for males is 42 years and for females 48 years. In Saudi Arabia and India, a particularly mild form of the condition occurs. Mortality is extremely low in childhood and a normal survival seems to be common. It is becoming increasingly apparent that the commonest cause of death in the first year or two of life is infection, often associated with splenic sequestration. Later in life infection is still a frequent cause of death, although studies in Jamaica indicate that chronic, progressive renal failure may be responsible for a significant number of deaths. The introduction of prophylactic penicillin has made a major inroad into early deaths from infection (see below).

Laboratory diagnosis

Sickle cell trait causes no haematological changes and is diagnosed by the finding of a positive sickling test together with haemoglobins A and S on electrophoresis (Fig. 22). Sickle cell anaemia is diagnosed by the finding of a variable degree of anaemia, an elevated reticulocyte count, sickled erythrocytes on the peripheral blood film, a positive sickling test, and a haemoglobin electrophoresis pattern characterized by the absence of haemoglobin A and a preponderance of haemoglobin S with a variable amount of haemoglobin F (Fig. 22). The diagnosis is confirmed by finding sickle cell trait in both parents.

There is a variety of simple sickling tests available. For ward laboratories the simplest it to take a drop of blood, mix it with two volumes of freshly prepared 2 per cent sodium metabisulphite, place a coverslip over the mixture, seal the edges with vaseline, and examine the slide for sickling after 1 h.

Control and management

There is very little experience of prospective genetic counselling and education of communities as an approach to reducing the number of carriers of sickle cell disease. Although prenatal diagnosis of sickle cell disease can be carried out by DNA analysis following chorion villus sampling, it has not been taken up as extensively as is the case for the thalassaemias. We

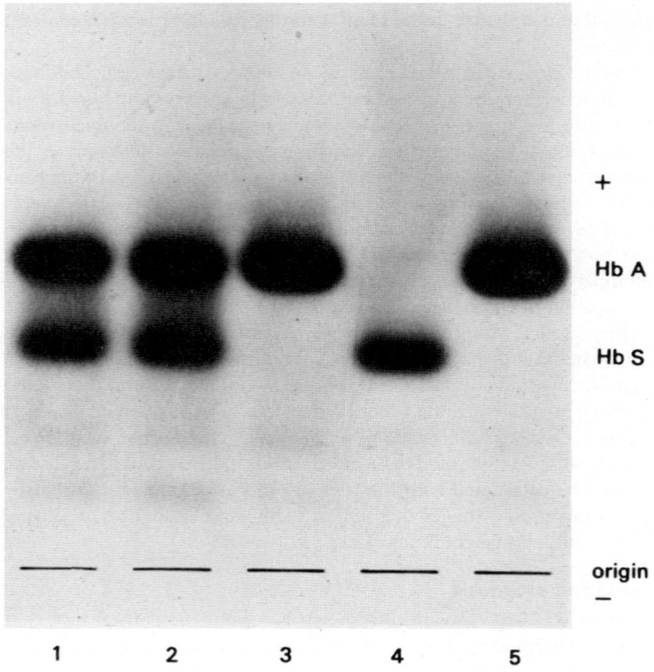

Fig. 22 The haemoglobin pattern in the sickling disorders (starch gel electrophoresis, protein stain, pH 8.5). The following are shown (left to right): (1 and 2) the sickle-cell trait; (3) normal; (4) sickle-cell anaemia; (5) normal.

need to know a great deal more about the factors which modify the clinical prognosis before the place of prenatal diagnosis is clarified.

It is very important that the babies of 'at risk' pregnancies are screened at birth and that the diagnosis is made as early as possible. This is because early deaths due to infection and the frequency of crises may be reduced by the administration of oral penicillin. This should be given to all affected babies at a dosage of 62.5 mg three times a day, up to 1 year of age, 125 mg twice a day from the age of 1 to 3 years, and 250 mg twice a day thereafter. It is also now standard practice for these babies to receive pneumococcal vaccine; in many centres they also receive vaccines against meningococcus and *Haemophilus influenzae*.

Patients with sickle cell anaemia adapt well to their low haemoglobin levels and regular blood transfusion is not required. Particularly in populations in which the diet is low in folate, regular folate supplements should be given. Patients should be given access to a centre that has expertise in the management of this disorder and advised to present at the first sign of a painful crisis. They should also be given a card to carry which states their haemoglobin genotype.

All but the mildest painful crisis should be managed in hospital. Patients should be examined in detail at regular intervals for evidence of underlying infection and given adequate rehydration, oxygen, antibiotics where appropriate, and, in particular, analgesia. The haemoglobin level and reticulocyte count should be estimated at frequent intervals to anticipate an aplastic crisis or pulmonary sequestration episode. While a mild crisis may be managed with first-line analgesics, stronger pain relief is often necessary. There has been concern about the possible dangers of the use of pethedine; it has become fashionable to administer diamorphine by slow, titratrated intravenous infusion. This has to be done under constant surveillance with regular monitoring of respiration and blood gases. It is very unusual for a painful crisis to last more than a few days.

Pulmonary sequestration requires urgent treatment in an intensive care unit. Oxygen should be administered and the blood gases monitored. An exchange transfusion should be initiated unless the haemoglobin level is lower than 4 to 5 g/dl, when the same result can be achieved by rapid transfusion up to 10 to 12 g/dl. Similarly, cerebral complications should be treated by exchange or top-up transfusion. There is evidence that this complication may be prevented by regular Doppler analysis of cerebral blood flow followed, where appropriate, by regular transfusion. Transfusion therapy also prevents recurrence of the cerebral episodes. Hypertransfusion or exchange transfusion should also be used to cover major surgical emergencies or for patients who are having recurrent crises. Occasionally, and most often in young children, the spleen may enlarge to such a degree that secondary hypersplenism develops and splenectomy is required. Splenic sequestration crises require urgent transfusion. Because they tend to recur, they may require splenectomy.

There is no special management required during pregnancy. Occasionally, if the haemoglobin level falls to a value at which symptoms of anaemia occur, or if there are recurrent crises, a regular transfusion regimen should be started to cover pregnancy and delivery.

Ocular manifestations, particularly proliferative retinopathy, require expert ophthalmological treatment. The current place for prophylactic zenon arc or argon laser therapy remains uncertain. Chronic disability due to aseptic necrosis of the femoral head may require hip replacement, although results are often disappointing and this complication requires a great deal more study. Surgical procedures should be undertaken with great caution. It is vital to maintain adequate oxygenation and hydration; limb torniquets should be avoided. Major procedures are best carried out after exchange transfusion. Haeamaturia usually resolves without treatment. Terminal renal failure should be managed as for any other form of renal insufficiency; renal transplantation has been shown to be successful in several studies.

Recurrent priapism is a major problem. Nearly two-thirds of major episodes are preceded by stuttering attacks and therefore it has been suggested that effective therapy at this stage may reduce the risk of sustaining a major attack, with danger of permanent deformity of the penis. Several approaches to management have been suggested although none have been studied in sufficient detail. One approach has been to commence stilboestrol, 5 mg daily, during the stuttering phase. Other forms of treatment at this stage that have been reported to give benefit are the use of opioid analgesics with benzodiazepine or pseudoephedrine hydrochloride. As well as these approaches, the patient should be hydrated, given analgesia, and, possibly, exchange transfusion. Centres with experience of this complication suggest that conservative treatment should be restricted to 24 h at the most. If there is no improvement, surgical correction is recommended, with a cavernosus–spongiosum shunt, a relatively minor procedure that may produce a good cosmetic result.

The management of leg ulcers is unsatisfactory. They may heal with bed rest and debridement but often relapse. Skin grafting does not always give good results and controlled trials have shown that transfusion does not appear to increase the rate of healing.

Experimental forms of treatment have shown some promise. Bone marrow transplantation has been carried out with reasonably good results. However, because of the inherent risks, and the uncertainty of the prognosis, the precise indications are not yet clear. Other studies have been directed at trying to elevate fetal haemoglobin. In a placebo-controlled trial involving adult patients it was found that the administration of hydroxyurea caused a significant reduction in the number of painful crises. This may have resulted from the modest elevation in fetal haemoglobin in response to the drug but other factors such as the reduced white count and increased red cell volume may have played a role. Currently, this drug has been licensed for treatment by the Federal Drug Administration in the United States for adult patients. It has also been used effectively in children but because of its possible leukaemogenic effects its use earlier in life is still restricted to clinical trials.

Other sickling disorders

The other sickling disorders include the interaction of haemoglobin S with haemoglobins C, D, and some of the rarer haemoglobin variants. The interactions with the different forms of β thalassaemia were described above. In many of these conditions, the clinical manifestations are little different from the sickle cell trait, but haemoglobin SC disease and SD disease more closely resemble sickle cell anaemia.

Haemoglobin SC disease

This disease is found in West Africa and less frequently in North Africa. Characterized by a milder anaemia than sickle cell disease, it often goes unrecognized until adult life. It may present with a complication resulting from damage to the microvasculature, probably because of the relatively high haemoglobin level and the combined effects of sickling and red cell rigidity caused by haemoglobin C (see below). Aseptic necrosis of the femoral or humeral heads and unexplained haematuria are the most common complications. Widespread thrombotic episodes, particularly involving the lungs, may occur during intercurrent infection or in pregnancy or the puerperium. Repeated blockage of the retinal vessels may lead to retinitis proliferans, retinal detachment, and permanent blindness.

Haemoglobin SC disease is diagnosed by finding a mild anaemia with splenomegaly and characteristic morphological changes of the red cells, including many target forms, intracellular crystals, and sickle cells. The sickling test is positive and haemoglobin electrophoresis shows haemoglobins S and C in about equal proportions. One parent shows the sickle cell trait and the other the haemoglobin C trait.

Severe thrombotic episodes, particularly in pregnancy, should be treated by exchange transfusion. The role of anticoagulants has never been established. Retinal disease is treated by laser.

Haemolysis due to other common haemoglobin variants

After haemoglobin S the second commonest variant in West Africa is haemoglobin C. Haemoglobin C, because of its relatively low solubility, appears to exist in a precrystalline state in red cells causing their rigidity and premature destruction in the microcirculation. The homozygous state, haemoglobin C disease, is characterized by a mild haemolytic anaemia with splenomegaly, and 100 per cent target cells on the blood film. Haemoglobin analysis shows haemoglobin C with small amounts of haemoglobin F. This is a mild disorder and no specific treatment is required.

The commonest haemoglobin variant throughout Southeast Asia and the Indian subcontinent is haemoglobin E. The homozygous state for this variant, haemoglobin E disease, is characterized by a very mild degree of anaemia with a slight reticulocytosis. The blood film shows mild morphological changes of the red cells which are hypochromic and microcytic, resembling the changes seen in β thalassaemia. No treatment is required.

Haemoglobin variants which migrate in the position of haemoglobin S but which do not sickle have been given the general title of haemoglobin D. There are several different molecular varieties of this variant; the commonest is haemoglobin D Los Angeles. The homozygous state is associated with moderate anaemia, splenomegaly, and a mild degree of haemolysis. The compound heterozygous state with haemoglobin S produces a disorder very similar to sickle cell anaemia. It is diagnosed by finding one parent with the haemoglobin D trait and the other with the sickle cell trait.

The unstable haemoglobin disorders

The unstable haemoglobin disorders are a rare group of inherited haemolytic anaemias which result from structural changes in the haemoglobin molecule that cause intracellular precipitation with the formation of Heinz bodies. Their true incidence is not known. There have been several well-documented families in which patients with one of these haemoglobin variants have had no affected relatives, suggesting that the condition has arisen by a new mutation.

Aetiology and pathogenesis

Most of the unstable haemoglobin variants result from single amino acid substitutions at critical areas of the molecule. For example substitutions in or around the haem pocket can disrupt the normal anatomy and allow in water with subsequent oxidative damage to haem which leads to precipitation of the haemoglobin. Some substitutions, such as those involving proline residues, cause a marked disruption of the secondary structure of a globin chain. A few of these variants result from deletions of either single or several amino acid residues. For example in haemoglobin Gun Hill, five amino acids are missing including the haem binding site. As the unstable haemoglobins precipitate in the red cells or their precursors, they produce intracellular inclusions, or Heinz bodies, which make the cells more rigid causing their premature destruction in the microcirculation (Fig. 23). The degradation products of the precipitated haemoglobin, notably haem and iron, cause oxidative damage to the red cell membrane proteins in much the same way as the excess α and β chains produced in the thalassaemias.

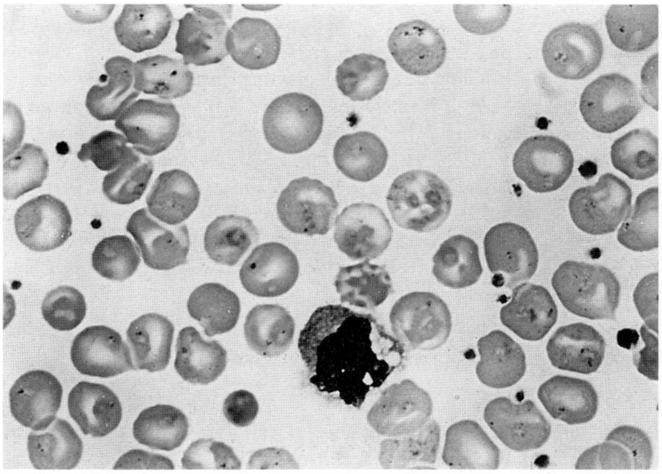

Fig. 23 The peripheral blood film of a patient with an unstable haemoglobin disorder, haemoglobin Hammersmith. This is a postsplenectomy film, which shows small inclusions in many of the red cells (×1000, Leishman stain).

Clinical features

All these conditions are characterized by a haemolytic anaemia of varying severity and splenomegaly. There may be a history of the passage of dark urine, particularly during episodes of infection. Like all chronic haemolytic anaemias, there is an increased incidence of pigment gallstones. The condition may become worse during periods of intercurrent infection. In the more severe forms, such episodes are associated with life-threatening anaemia. Patients with unstable haemoglobins are at particular risk of haemolytic episodes following the administration of oxidant drugs. Apart from intermittent icterus and splenomegaly there are no characteristic physical findings.

Laboratory diagnosis

This condition should be thought of in any familial haemolytic anaemia, particularly if a red cell enzyme deficiency cannot be demonstrated. The peripheral blood film shows the features of haemolysis but the red cell morphology may be relatively normal. Occasionally there is a mild degree of hypochromia and microcytosis. Unless splenectomy has been carried out, Heinz bodies are not seen in the peripheral blood (Fig. 23).

The most characteristic feature of the unstable haemoglobins is their heat instability. If a dilute haemoglobin solution is heated at 50°C for 15 min, most of the unstable haemoglobins precipitate as a dense cloud. A similar phenomenon can be induced by isopropanalol. Some variants can be identified by haemoglobin electrophoresis but others, because they result from the substitution of a neutral amino acid, produce no electrophoretic changes and can only be demonstrated by the heat precipitation test.

Treatment

Because these conditions are so rare there has been very little experience of the effects of splenectomy. From the information that is available, and from the author's personal experience, it appears that if a child has had several life-threatening episodes of anaemia or is running a steady-state haemoglobin level which is impairing development or well-being, splenectomy should be undertaken. It is interesting to note that some of these haemoglobin variants produce a 'right shift' in the oxygen dissociation curve, and a measurement of the P_{50} as part of the presplenectomy assessment may help to decide whether to proceed to surgery; a marked right shift, that is an increased P_{50}, indicates that the anaemia should be more easily tolerated than if the oxygen dissociation curve is moved in the opposite direction with a low P_{50}. An accurate history from the child or its parents is probably more helpful, however.

Haemoglobin variants which cause abnormal oxygen binding

In 1966, an 81-year-old man presented at Johns Hopkins Hospital, Baltimore with mild angina and a haemoglobin value of 19.9 g/dl. No cause could be found for his polycythaemia but it was noted that he had an abnormal haemoglobin. The oxygen dissociation curve of his blood was found to be displaced to the left. This suggested that the abnormal haemoglobin might have a high oxygen affinity and that the patient's increased red cell count might be compensating for a primary defect in oxygen unloading. Further studies showed that this was the case, documenting a new cause for secondary polycythaemia. Since then over 40 haemoglobin variants of this type have been defined, all associated with familial polycythaemia.

Aetiology

The high-oxygen-affinity haemoglobin variants result from single amino acid substitutions at critical parts of the haemoglobin molecule which are involved in the configuration changes that underlie haem/haem interaction and the production of a sigmoid oxygen dissociation curve. Many occur at the junctions between the α and β subunits. Others involve the amino acids which are involved with the binding of 2,3-diphosphoglycerate (2,3-DPG) to haemoglobin. As mentioned earlier, increasing concentrations of 2,3-DPG tend to push the oxygen dissociation curve to the right; fetal haemoglobin has a high oxygen affinity (left-shifted curve) because it cannot interact with 2,3-DPG; mutations of the DPG binding sites have a similar effect.

Pathophysiology

The high-oxygen-affinity variants have a left-shifted oxygen dissociation curve with a reduced P_{50}. Thus the variant haemoglobin holds on to oxygen more avidly than normal haemoglobin. This leads to tissue hypoxia. This in turn causes an increased output of erythropoietin and an elevated red cell mass.

Clinical features

Many patients with high-oxygen-affinity variants are completely healthy and are only found to carry the variant when a routine haematological examination shows an unusually high haemoglobin level or packed cell volume. There have been one or two reports of arterial or venous occlusive disease in these patients. However, this is uncommon. Most patients are asymptomatic. There is no splenomegaly and no other associated haematological findings. Although it might be expected that a high-oxygen-affinity haemoglobin would cause defective oxygenation of the fetus none of the reported families has had a history of frequent stillbirths.

Diagnosis

The condition should be suspected in any patient with a pure red cell polycythaemia associated with a left-shifted oxygen dissociation curve. The diagnosis can be confirmed by haemoglobin analysis.

Treatment

In asymptomatic patients with high-oxygen-affinity haemoglobin variants no treatment is necessary. The difficulty arises if the patient has associated vascular disease with symptoms of coronary or cerebral artery insufficiency. There is insufficient published information to make any dogmatic statements about how this complication should be managed. The author has seen several patients of this type who seem to have responded to venesection; more experience is required before this form of treatment can be recommended however. These patients require a high haemoglobin level for oxygen transport; half their haemoglobin is physiologically useless.

Low-oxygen-affinity variants

At least six haemoglobin variants with reduced oxygen affinity have been reported. The first to be described, haemoglobin Kansas, was found in a mother and son with unexplained cyanosis. The subjects were asymptomatic and had normal haemoglobin levels without any evidence of haemolysis. Like many of the high affinity variants, the amino acid substitution in this variant was at the interface between the α and β globin chains. For reasons which are not clear, some substitutions in this region give rise to variants with a relatively low oxygen affinity. This condition should be thought of in any patient with an unexplained congenital cyanosis; the differential diagnosis is considered below.

Methaemoglobinaemia, carboxyhaemoglobinaemia, and sulphaemoglobinaemia

Methaemoglobinaemia is a condition characterized by increased quantities of haemoglobin in which the iron of haem is oxidized to the ferric (Fe^{3+}) form. Carboxyhaemoglobinaemia (carbonmonoxyhaemoglobinaemia) results from the binding of carbon monoxide to the haem molecules. Sulphaemoglobinaemia is a rare condition in which there is a mixture of haemoglobin derivatives whose structure is poorly characterized but which can be defined by their specific spectral characteristics.

Pathogenesis

As mentioned earlier, each haemoglobin molecule has four haem moieties. At first sight it is not clear why the oxidation of a proportion of the iron atoms, or the fact that they are liganded to carbon monoxide, should cause such profound changes in oxygen transport. However, oxidation of 30 per cent of the haem molecules has a much more serious effect on tissue oxygenation than a reduction of the haemoglobin level by the same amount. This is because, if a single haem is oxidized, it so alters the conformation of the haemoglobin molecule that the oxygen affinity of the other three haems is increased. Thus methaemoglobin, carboxyhaemoglobin, and cyanmethaemoglobin all have very high oxygen affinities with 'left shifted' oxygen dissociation curves, and hence are associated with impaired unloading of oxygen to the tissues.

Methaemoglobinaemia

Methaemoglobin causes a variable degree of cyanosis. It should be suspected in any patient with significant central cyanosis in whom there is no evidence of cardiorespiratory disease. The degree of cyanosis produced by 5 g/dl of deoxygenated haemoglobin can be produced by 1.5 g/dl methaemoglobin and 0.5 g/dl of sulphaemoglobin. Methaemoglobin concentrations of 10 to 20 per cent are tolerated quite well. It is useless as an oxygen carrier; levels above this are thus often associated with dyspnoea and headache. Much depends on the rapidity at which it is formed; many patients with life-long methaemoglobinaemia are asymptomatic while individuals who have accumulated a similar level of methaemoglobin acutely may be acutely dyspnoeic. For reasons which are not clear, it is unusual for patients with chronic methaemoglobinaemia to have an increased haemoglobin level or red cell count.

Methaemoglobinaemia may arise as a result of a genetic defect in red cell metabolism or haemoglobin structure, or may be acquired following the ingestion of various oxidant drugs and toxic agents.

Genetic methaemoglobinaemia

There are two forms of inherited methaemoglobinaemia. The first results from a deficiency of red cell NADH-diaphorase, the second from a structural alteration in either the α or β globin chains of haemoglobin.

NADH-diaphorase catalyses a step in the major pathway for methaemoglobin reduction. The enzyme reduces cytochrome b_5 using NADH as a hydrogen donor. The reduced cytochrome b_5 reduces, in turn, methaemoglobin to haemoglobin. There are several different molecular forms of NADH-diaphorase deficiency which have been identified by electrophoretic analysis of NADH-diaphorase in the red cells of affected patients. The condition is inherited as an autosomal recessive. Homozygotes have elevated levels of methaemoglobin and are cyanotic from birth. Heterozygotes do not have elevated levels of methaemoglobin but seem to be unusually susceptible to the oxidant action of drugs. For example severe cyanosis has been precipitated by the use of antimalarial drugs.

There are several abnormal haemoglobin variants which are associated with genetic methaemoglobinaemia, all of which are designated haemoglobin M, and further identified by their place of discovery, for example haemoglobin M Boston, M Milwaukee. These variants usually result from amino acid substitutions near the haem pocket. Normally, haem lies between two histidine residues, one called the proximal histidine to which it is attached, and the other called the distal histidine. Oxygen is bound to haem at a site opposite to the distal histidine. If the latter is substituted by tyrosine, as occurs in the α chain variant haemoglobin M Boston and in the β chain variant M Saskatoon, a stable bond is formed between the haem iron and the phenolic ring of the tyrosine. The iron atom is 'fixed' in the Fe^{3+} state. These variants are associated with cyanosis which is present from early life. In the case of the α chain variants it is present from birth, while the β chain haemoglobin variants only produce cyanosis after the first few months of life as adult haemoglobin synthesis becomes established. Unlike NADH diaphorase deficiency, which is inherited as a recessive trait, the haemoglobin Ms have a dominant form of inheritance. Thus it is very simple to make the diagnosis of genetic methaemoglobinaemia and to determine the likely molecular basis by taking a good history; even the affected globin chain can be ascertained!

The diagnosis is confirmed by spectroscopic examination of the blood and by determination of methaemoglobin levels. The precise cause can be established by an assay of NADH-diaphorase or by haemoglobin analysis under appropriate conditions.

Genetic methaemoglobinaemia due to NADH-diaphorase deficiency is readily treated by the administration of ascorbic acid, 300 to 600 mg daily by mouth in divided doses, or by the administration of methylene blue, either intravenously (1 mg/kg body weight) or by mouth 60 mg three to four times daily. On the other hand, the genetic methaemoglobinaemias due to structural haemoglobin variants do not respond to ascorbic acid, methylene blue, or any other treatment. Most affected individuals go through life asymptomatic and require no treatment.

Acquired methaemoglobinaemia

Acquired methaemoglobinaemia usually results from the administration of drugs or exposure to chemicals which cause oxidation of haemoglobin. There are many agents which are capable of exceeding the red cells' ability to reduce methaemoglobin. They include ferricyanide, bivalent copper, chromate, chlorate, quinones, and certain dyes with a high oxidation–reduction potential. Nitrite, often used as a preservative, is one of the most common methaemoglobin-forming agents. Nitrates, after conversion to nitrites in the gut, may cause serious methaemoglobinaemia in infants. Other agents which commonly cause methaemoglobinaemia include phenacatin, primaquine, sulfonamides, and various analine dye derivatives.

If any of the agents listed above is given in low dose over a long period of time it may lead to chronic methaemoglobinaemia with or without a haemolytic anaemia. However, after exposure to a large amount of these agents, and the development of in excess of 50 to 60 per cent methaemoglobin, the symptoms of acute anaemia develop because methaemoglobin lacks the capacity to transport oxygen. Thus the clinical picture may be characterized by vascular collapse, coma, and death.

Methaemoglobinaemia with haemolytic anaemia

The haemolytic action of oxidant drugs is described elsewhere. Chronic methaemoglobinaemia with haemolytic anaemia, characterized by Heinz body formation and fragmented red cells, occurs commonly in patients receiving dapsone, salazopyrine, or phenacatin. This condition is usually innocuous and can be modified by adjusting the dose of the drug.

Occasionally, acute intravascular haemolysis associated with methaemoglobinaemia and intravascular coagulation occurs. It usually follows the ingestion or infusion of a strong oxidizing agent such as chlorate or arsine. There is gross intravascular haemolysis and methaemoglobinaemia together with evidence of disseminated intravascular coagulation. The haemoglobin level may fall very rapidly and may be complicated by renal failure.

Treatment

In cases of chronic acquired methaemoglobinaemia, the drug or chemical agent should be removed where possible. If continued therapy is required, it should be administered at a lower dose.

Acute toxic methaemoglobinaemia presents a serious medical emergency. Methylene blue should be administered in a dose of 1 to 2 mg/kg intravenously over a 5-min period. Repeated doses may be needed. Toxicity is uncommon although doses of over 15 mg/kg may cause haemolysis in young infants. The drug should not be used if the methaemoglobinaemia is due to chlorate poisoning as it may convert the chlorate to hypochlorite which is an even more toxic compound. In cases of acute methaemoglobinaemia with intravascular haemolysis, haemodialysis with exchange transfusion is the treatment of choice.

Carboxyhaemoglobinaemia

Carbon monoxide (CO) has an affinity for haemoglobin approximately 210 times that of oxygen. Following acute exposure it is so tightly bound that it takes about 4 h for an individual with normal ventilation to expel half of it. At levels of 5 to 10 per cent there may be no symptoms, but above 20 per cent there is usually headache and weakness. Levels of 40 to 60 per cent or more lead to unconsciousness and death.

Carbon monoxide poisoning is discussed in Chapter 8.1 and secondary polycythaemia due to chronic exposure is considered elsewhere in this chapter.

Sulphaemoglobinaemia

This poorly-defined condition derives its name from the fact that it can be produced *in vitro* by the action of hydrogen sulphide on haemoglobin. It has not been reported as a genetic disorder. It is usually associated with the administration of drugs, particularly sulfonamides or phenacetin. It has also been reported in patients with chronic constipation or malabsorption syndromes (enterogenous cyanosis) although its relationship to these disorders is far from clear.

Other acquired abnormalities of the structure or synthesis of haemoglobin

Glycosylated haemoglobin, haemoglobin AIc

Haemoglobin may undergo post-translational modification in patients with diabetes. The abnormal haemoglobin, haemoglobin AIc, is formed by the non-enzymic combination of glucose with the N-terminus of the β chain, forming first a Schiff base which then undergoes a rearrangement to form a stable ketoamine. The level of haemoglobin AIc is raised in diabetics and is related to the blood sugar level over the previous weeks. The value of the estimation of haemoglobin AIc as an index of the control of diabetes is considered elsewhere.

Haemoglobin Pb

Some children with lead poisoning develop a modified haemoglobin which migrates rapidly on alkaline electrophoresis. The precise structural alteration is not known but, if present, this variant is a useful indicator of severe lead poisoning.

Fetal haemoglobin production in adult life

A number of haematological disorders are associated with a reversion to fetal haemoglobin production after the neonatal period. These include juvenile myeloid leukaemia, other forms of leukaemia, and congenital hypoplastic anaemias. Haemoglobin F may also appear transitorily during rapid regeneration of the bone marrow after drug induced hypoplasia, virus infection, or bone marrow transplantation.

Further reading

Ballas SK (1998). Sickle cell disease: clinical management. *Clinical Haematology* **11**, 185–214.

Bunn HF (1997). Pathogenesis and treatment of sickle cell disease. *New England Journal of Medicine* **337**, 762–9.

Cao A, Galanello R, Rosatelli MC (1998). Prenatal diagnosis and screening of the haemoglobinopathies. *Clinical Haematology* **11**, 215–38.

Dover GJ, Platt OS (1998). Sickle cell disease. In: Nathan DG, Orkin SH, eds. *Hematology in infancy and childhood*, pp. 762–801. WB Saunders, Philadelphia.

Forget BG, Higgs DR, Nagel RL, Steinberg MH, eds (2001). *Disorders of hemoglobin.* Cambridge University Press, New York.

Higgs DR (1993). α-thalassaemia. In: Higgs DR, Weatherall DJ, eds. *Baillière's clinical haematology. International practice and research: the haemoglobinopathies*, pp. 117–50. Baillière Tindall, London.

Higgs DR, Sharpe JA, Wood WG (1998). Understanding α globin gene expression: a step towards effective gene therapy. *Seminars in Hematology* **35**, 93–104.

Olivieri N (1998). Thalassaemia: clinical management. *Clinical Haematology* **11**, 147–62.

Weatherall DJ, Clegg JB (2001). *The thalassaemia syndromes*, 4th edn. Blackwell Science, Oxford.

Weatherall DJ, Clegg JB, Higgs DR, Wood WG (2001). The haemoglobinopathies. In: Scriver CR, Beaudet AL, Sly WS, Valle D, eds. *The metabolic basis of inherited disease*, 8th edn, pp. 3417–84. McGraw-Hill, New York.

22.5.8 Anaemias resulting from defective red cell maturation

James S. Wiley

Erythroid cell maturation is specialized towards the co-ordinated synthesis of large amounts of haem and globin necessary to attain the high concentration of haemoglobin found in the mature red cell. Hereditary or acquired defects in the production of either of these cause a maturation block, which leads to ineffective erythropoiesis in which many of the developing nucleated erythroblasts are destroyed in the marrow before they can reach the circulation. Thus in thalassaemia, defective synthesis of either α or β globin leads to unbalanced production of the other chain which precipitates and leads to destruction of the precursor erythroblast. Defective haem synthesis in the sideroblastic anaemias also leads to an anaemia which is characterized by ineffective erythropoiesis (Table 1). Abnormalities of DNA synthesis in the developing erythroid cells, such as produced by vitamin B_{12} or folic acid deficiency, blocks cell division required for erythroid maturation and produces morphological and biochemical evidence of ineffective erythropoiesis.

Table 1 Anaemias with defective red cell maturation and ineffective erythropoiesis as a major cause

Inhibition of erythroid DNA synthesis
megaloblastic anaemias (vitamin B_{12} or folate deficiency)
drugs blocking DNA synthesis (e.g. hydroxyurea, 6-mercaptopurine)
Clonal disorders of erythropoiesis
refractory anaemia
acquired idiopathic sideroblastic anaemia (refractory anaemia with ring sideroblasts)
acute erythroleukaemia (acute myeloid leukaemia: FAB-M6)
Genetic disorders of erythropoiesis
thalassaemia syndromes
hereditary sideroblastic anaemias
congenital dyserythropoietic anaemias
Miscellaneous
alcohol
drugs
heavy metal poisoning
falciparum malaria

Ineffective erythropoiesis may be recognized by the characteristic erythroid hyperplasia of the bone marrow with normal or only slight increase in reticulocyte numbers. Some other features of ineffective erythropoiesis may be variably present: a mild increase in bilirubin, decrease in haptoglobin, and increased serum lactic dehydrogenase activity. As a result, iron absorption is increased, serum iron and ferritin become elevated, and, after many years, iron overload develops which is indistinguishable from idiopathic haemochromatosis. However, the degree of iron overload does not depend on either the severity of the anaemia or the presence of the characteristic mutation (Cys282Tyr) of the *HFE* gene associated with genetic haemochromatosis.

The sideroblastic anaemias

Sideroblastic anaemias are a group of hereditary or acquired anaemias of varying severity diagnosed by the finding of ring sideroblasts in the bone marrow aspirate. The peripheral blood film shows hypochromic red cells which are microcytic in the hereditary form (Fig. 1), but are often macrocytic in the acquired forms of the disease. Normochromic and normocytic red cells are also present which gives the film a dimorphic distribution of red cell sizes. The diagnostic procedure is bone marrow aspirate followed by staining of the smear with Prussian Blue iron reagent. Ring sideroblasts are diagnostic (Fig. 2) and are defined as erythroblasts containing iron-positive granules arranged in a perinuclear location around one-third or more of the nucleus. Electron microscopy reveals that the iron-containing granules are mitochondria containing precipitated ferric phosphate and ferric hydroxide. The sideroblastic anaemias have diverse aetiologies (Table 2) but have in common an impaired biosynthesis of haem in the erythroid cells of the marrow. Most sideroblastic anaemias are acquired as a clonal disorder of erythropoiesis, with varying degrees of myelodysplasia. The hereditary forms are uncommon. Most are found in males with an X-linked pattern of inheritance. A number of drugs have been associated

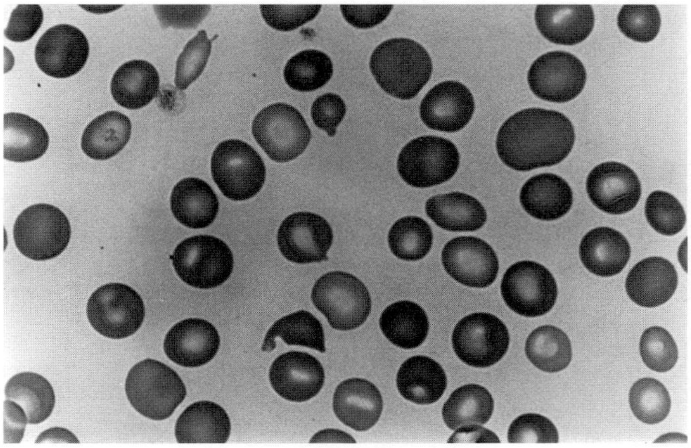

Fig. 1 Peripheral blood smear in hereditary sideroblastic anaemia showing a population of hypochromic and microcytic erythrocytes. (By courtesy of Gillian Rozenberg.)

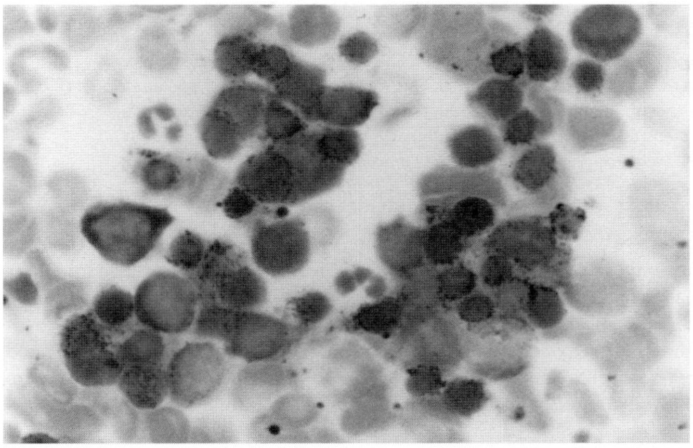

Fig. 2 Bone marrow smear stained with Prussian blue, showing the ring sideroblasts (arrow). (By courtesy of Gillian Rozenberg.)

Table 2 Classification of sideroblastic anaemias

Hereditary	
	X-linked[a]
	autosomal dominant or recessive[a]
Acquired	
	refractory anaemia with ring sideroblasts[a] (acquired idiopathic sideroblastic anaemia)
	associated with previous chemotherapy, irradiation
	'transitional' myelodysplasia/ myeloproliferative diseases
Drugs	
	alcohol
	isoniazid, cycloserine, pyrazinamide
	chloramphenicol
Rare causes	
	erythropoietic protoporphyria
	Pearson's syndrome
	copper deficiency or zinc overload
	hypothermia

[a] Trial of pyridoxine indicated.

with reversible sideroblastic anaemia, chiefly in patients with alcohol abuse (Table 2).

Hereditary sideroblastic anaemias

Aetiology and pathogenesis

Haem biosynthesis occurs by a cascade of eight enzymes (Fig. 3). In man, mutations affecting the first enzyme of this pathway produce hereditary sideroblastic anaemia. Inborn errors that occur in later enzymes in this pathway result in metabolic disorders known as the porphyrias (Fig. 3). The pathway begins with the condensation of glycine with succinyl CoA to form 5-aminolaevulinic acid (ALA), a step which is under the control of the mitochondrial enzyme ALA synthase. This enzyme requires pyridoxal phosphate as a cofactor. Two isoenzymes of ALA synthase have been identified. One is found in liver and other tissues (ALAS 1). The second is confined to erythroid cells of the bone marrow (ALAS 2). The gene for the erythroid-specific ALAS 2 isoenzyme resides on the X chromosome and is now known to be the site of most mutations giving rise to X-linked hereditary sideroblastic anaemia. Several dozen different mutations have been described in different families. All result from a single amino acid alteration arising from a point mutation in the ALAS 2 coding region of DNA. In nearly half the families with hereditary sideroblastic anaemia, the structure of the ALAS 2 gene is normal, suggesting that other defects may be involved, such as the import of ALAS 2 from the cytosol or its anchoring within the mitochondrial matrix. In most families, males are affected with an X-linked pattern of inheritance consistent with a mutation on the X chromosome (Fig. 4). However, occasionally the disease is transmitted as an autosomal dominant; there are even well-documented families in which only females are affected.

Clinical and laboratory features

Typically the anaemia presents in infancy or childhood but when the anaemia is mild, the diagnosis may not be made until adult life. Occasionally, such patients may present with features of iron overload such as diabetes or cardiac failure. Others may be found in family surveys, which should be undertaken when this anaemia is diagnosed. Slight enlargement of the liver or spleen may occur. The degree of anaemia is variable, ranging from severe (less than 80 g/l haemoglobin) to mild (more than 100 g/l haemoglobin) but even with mild or no anaemia the mean corpuscular volume (MCV) is below the normal range. Blood film shows a population of cells with hypochromic, microcytic morphology. Female carriers may show the characteristic red cell dimorphism. White cell counts are normal while platelet counts are normal or slightly elevated. Serum iron and ferritin concentrations are invariably increased and transferrin shows an increased percentage saturation with iron. The differential diagnosis includes idiopathic haemochromatosis, since both diseases have evidence of iron overload. Examination of the blood film, the MCV, and the bone marrow should establish the diagnosis.

Treatment and prognosis

A trial of pyridoxine, 100 to 200 mg/day taken orally, is indicated for 3 months in all patients with proven or suspected hereditary sideroblastic anaemia. About 25 per cent of patients experience a full or partial correction. This vitamin should be continued lifelong in responders but at a lower maintenance dosage. Regular transfusions of packed red cells are the mainstay of treatment of severe anaemia. These should be given to relieve symptoms and allow normal childhood development. Splenectomy is contraindicated in this condition. Iron overload progresses rapidly once transfusions begin. Chelation therapy with desferrioxamine should thus be commenced after the first 10 to 20 transfusions. Iron removal may greatly benefit patients with mild or moderate anaemia and evidence of iron overload. Intermittent phlebotomy of 100 to 200 ml blood should be attempted as this is more effective than chelation therapy in removing iron and should be continued if symptoms allow until the serum ferritin becomes normal.

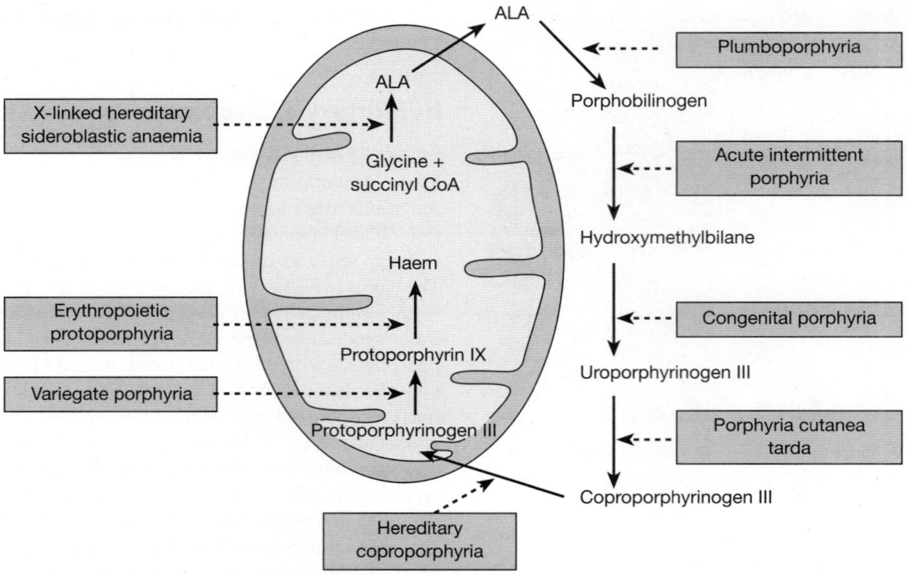

Fig. 3 Pathway of haem biosynthesis in mammalian cells. The first step in the pathway is catalysed by ALAS and occurs within the mitochondrion using pyridoxal 5'-phosphate as a cofactor. ALA then leaves the mitochondrion and is converted by ALA dehydratase to give a monopyrrole, porphobilinogen. Four molecules of this are converted by porphobilinogen deaminase to a linear tetrapyrrole, hydroxymethylbilane. This molecule is then cyclized by uroporphyrinogen III synthase to uroporphyrinogen III, which is then decarboxylated to coproporphyrinogen III. This molecule enters the mitochondrion and is oxidized in succession by coproporphyrinogen III oxidase and protoporphyrinogen III oxidase. The product is protoporphyrin IX, a substrate for ferrochelatase, which catalyses the insertion of Fe^{2+} to form haem. The defective steps associated with specific porphyrias and X-linked hereditary sideroblastic anaemias are shown. (Reproduced from Hoffman R *et al.*, eds. (1999). *Hematology: basic principles and practice*, 3rd edn. WB Saunders Co., Philadelphia, with permission.)

Finally, patients should avoid alcohol and ascorbic acid supplements, both of which enhance iron absorption.

Acquired idiopathic sideroblastic anaemia (refractory anaemia with ring sideroblasts)

Acquired idiopathic sideroblastic anaemia is a refractory anaemia with a hypercellular marrow containing ring sideroblasts which may either be idiopathic or develop following chemotherapy or irradiation (Table 2). Since nearly all cases also show evidence of dyserythropoiesis, this anaemia is now classified as one of the myelodysplastic syndromes and termed refractory anaemia with ring sideroblasts by the French–American–British Group. This classification is supported by the demonstration that the defective haematopoiesis is clonal, both in acquired idiopathic sideroblastic anaemia and the other myelodysplastic syndromes. Clonal haematopoiesis has also been shown in acute erythroleukaemia, in which bizarre dysplastic changes and ineffective erythropoiesis are seen in the developing erythroblasts. These comprise a majority (more than 50 per cent) of all nucleated marrow cells. The fact that more than 20 per cent of the myeloid cells are blasts distinguishes acute erythroleukaemia from one of the myelodysplastic syndromes.

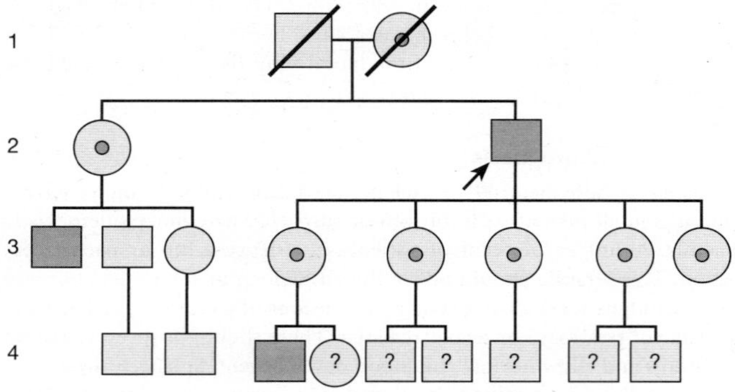

Fig. 4 Pedigree of a family with pyridoxine-responsive sideroblastic anaemia showing X-linked recessive inheritance. ■ affected; ○carrier; ? unknown status. Diagonal lines indicate deceased members. The pedigree has been abbreviated to show only the affected branches of the family. The arrow indicates the proband. (Copyright 1994 Massachusetts Medical Society. All rights reserved. Reproduced with permission.)

Aetiology and pathogenesis

The cause of the defective haem synthesis in acquired sideroblastic anaemia is unclear. Recent reports indicate that levels of ALAS in bone marrow are normal. Indirect evidence points to an acquired defect in the mitochondrial respiratory chain that impairs the reduction of Fe^{3+} to Fe^{2+} since ferrous iron is essential for the terminal ferrochelatase reaction (Fig. 3). Clonal haematopoiesis has been demonstrated in this anaemia by both molecular and karyotypic analysis. Thus a single glucose-6-phosphate dehydrogenase (G6PD) isoenzyme was found in erythrocytes of a woman heterozygous for G6PD who expressed two isoenzymes in her somatic tissues. Clonal chromosome changes are also found in bone marrow cells in many patients with acquired sideroblastic anaemia. Characteristic changes include monosomy 7, trisomy 8, deletions involving chromosomes 5, 7, 11, 13, or 20, and a number of translocations. When sideroblastic anaemia is acquired secondary to chemotherapy or irradiation, chromosomal changes are nearly always found and tend to be multiple. However, they are probably a late event in the course of this anaemia and may be preceded by the expansion of a clone of genetically unstable stem cells.

Clinical and laboratory features

Acquired sideroblastic anaemia typically has an insidious onset. Most patients are middle aged or elderly, but young adults can be affected. Mild splenomegaly may be present. White cell and platelet counts are usually normal; some patients may have thrombocytosis. The bone marrow shows erythroid hyperplasia with varying degrees of dyserythropoiesis, including irregular nuclear contour, nuclear fragmentation (karyorrhexis), bi- or trilobed nuclei, and internuclear bridges. Iron stain of the aspirate shows ring sideroblasts which should total more than 15 per cent of the nucleated erythroid cells to make the diagnosis. Dysplasia of myeloid precursors or megakaryocytes may be present. When associated with leucopenia and/or thrombocytopenia the more descriptive term 'refractory cytopenia' is sometimes used. If the overall blast count exceeds 5 per cent or the peripheral blood monocyte count exceeds 1.0×10^9/l, the condition falls within a different category of the myelodysplastic syndrome. Thus, ring sideroblasts may be seen in other myelodysplastic conditions such as refractory anaemia with excess blasts. Distinguishing acquired idiopathic sideroblastic anaemia from a mild hereditary sideroblastic anaemia presenting in adult life can be difficult. However, careful examination of the marrow for dysplastic changes, the MCV, possible response to pyridoxine, and a family survey all help to distinguish these two entities.

Treatment and prognosis

Transfusions of packed red cells should be given for relief of symptomatic anaemia. A trial of pyridoxine, 100 to 200 mg/day for 3 months, is worthwhile but few patients respond to this vitamin. Acquired idiopathic sideroblastic anaemia and the closely related refractory anaemia have the most favourable outlook among the myelodysplastic syndromes, with a median survival of 42 to 76 months and a 3 to 12 per cent incidence of progression to acute leukaemia. A simple prognostic scoring system has been developed in which two or more of the following place the patient in a poor prognostic category:

(1) haemoglobin less than 100 g/l;

(2) neutrophils less than 1.5×10^9/l;

(3) platelets less than 100×10^9/l; and

(4) blasts more than 5 per cent.

Karyotypic analysis of marrow aspirates is valuable since a normal karyotype confers a favourable prognosis. The karyotype is now included in an international prognostic scoring system.

Defective red cell maturation secondary to alcohol and drugs

Alcohol has a direct toxic effect on erythropoiesis, manifested by the macrocytosis which characterizes red cells of subjects chronically ingesting alcohol in excess. Malnourished and anaemic alcoholics may exhibit ring sideroblasts in the bone marrow as well as vacuolation of erythroblasts. These manifestations gradually disappear over 4 to 12 days when alcohol is withdrawn, although the macrocytosis may take several months to normalize. The antibiotic chloramphenicol when given in dosages greater than 2 g/day produces a reversible inhibition of erythropoiesis associated with ring sideroblasts and vacuolation of erythroblasts. This effect, due to inhibition of mitochondrial protein synthesis, is quite separate from the rare idiosyncratic side-effect of aplastic anaemia. Protracted exposure to the antituberculous drug isoniazid has been occasionally associated with development of a sideroblastic anaemia.

Defective red cell maturation secondary to lead, arsenic, or zinc ingestion or copper deficiency

Patients suffering lead poisoning show clinical and laboratory evidence of reduced haem biosynthesis. Basophilic stippling of red cells is prominent. Mild hypochromic, microcytic anaemia may develop. Red cell protoporphyrin, increased due to inhibition of the terminal step in the haem pathway, provides a sensitive measure of lead exposure. The peripheral neuropathy of lead poisoning may be a result of reduced haem biosynthesis, as in the porphyrias. Acute or chronic arsenic ingestion can cause anaemia with marked dyserythropoiesis. Basophilic stippling of red cells is characteristic while neutropenia and thrombocytopenia may be present. Copper deficiency has been described only in malnourished premature infants or in patients receiving long-term, parenteral hyperalimentation. This syndrome consists of anaemia and neutropenia associated with marrow findings of ring sideroblasts and vacuolated erythroid and myeloid precursors. Large quantities of ingested zinc interfere with copper absorption and reproduce the sideroblastic anaemia and neutropenia characteristic of copper deficiency.

Congenital dyserythropoietic anaemias (CDA)

This rare group of inherited refractory anaemias are characterized by gross multinuclearity of erythroid precursors in the marrow, ineffective erythropoiesis, and associated iron overload. Three types have been described based on morphology of the bone marrow and serological features. The most common, Type II, is also known as HEMPAS (hereditary erythroblast multinuclearity with positive acidified serum test) since red cells are lysed by acidified (pH 6.8) serum from about 30 per cent of normal subjects. In CDA Type II, a defect in glycosylation of erythroblast membrane proteins has been identified. Most patients are diagnosed in late childhood or adolescence with mild to moderate anaemia, with intermittent jaundice or in older patients with manifestations of iron overload. Splenomegaly or hepatomegaly may be variably present. CDA carries a good prognosis with few patients requiring transfusions. The degree of iron overload should be monitored and treated when appropriate.

Further reading

Bennett JM *et al.* (1982). Proposals for the classification of the myelodysplastic syndromes. *British Journal of Haematology* **51**, 189–99.

Bottomley SS *et al.* (1999). Sideroblastic anaemia. In: Lee GR *et al.*, eds. *Wintrobes clinical haematology*, pp. 832–71. Williams and Wilkins, Baltimore.

Cazzola M *et al.* (1988). Natural history of idiopathic refractory sideroblastic anemia. *Blood* **71**, 305–12.

Cotter PD *et al.* (1995). Late-onset X-linked sideroblastic anemia. Missense mutations in the erythroid δ-aminolevulinate synthase (ALAS2) gene in two pyridoxine-responsive patients initially diagnosed with acquired refractory anemia and ringed sideroblasts. *Journal of Clinical Investigation* **96**, 2090–6.

Cox TC *et al.* (1994). X-linked pyridoxine-responsive sideroblastic anemia due to a THR^{388}- to –SER substitution in erythroid 5-aminolevulinate synthase. *New England Journal of Medicine* **330**, 675–9. Shows a typical response of hereditary sideroblastic anaemia to pyridoxine.

Gattermann N *et al.* (1997). Heteroplasmic point mutations of mitochondrial DNA affecting subunit 1 of cytochrome c oxidase in two patients with acquired idiopathic sideroblastic anemia. *Blood* **90**, 4961–72.

Greenberg P *et al.* (1997). International scoring system for evaluating prognosis in myelodysplastic syndromes. *Blood* **89**, 2079–88.

Juneja SK *et al.* (1983). Prevalence and distribution of ringed sideroblasts in primary myelodysplastic syndromes. *Journal Clinical Pathology* **36**, 566–9.

Kibbelaar RE *et al.* (1992). Combined immunophenotyping and DNA *in situ* hybidization to study lineage involvement in patients with myelodysplastic syndromes. *Blood* **79**, 1823–8.

Marks PW, Mitus AJ (1996). Congenital dyserythropoietic anaemias. *American Journal of Hematology* **51**, 55–63. Recent review.

Mufti GJ *et al.* (1985). Myelodysplastic syndromes: a scoring system with prognostic significance. *British Journal of Haematology* **59**, 425–33.

Nusbaum NJ (1991). Concise review: genetic basis for sideroblastic anemia. *American Journal of Hematology* **37**, 41–4.

Raskin WH *et al.* (1984). Evidence for a multistep pathogenesis of a myelodysplastic syndrome. *Blood* **63**, 1318–23.

Roberts PD, Hoffbrand AV, Mollin DL (1966). Iron and folate metabolism in tuberculosis. *British Medical Journal* **2**, 198–202.

Savage D, Lindenbaum J (1986). Anemia in alcoholics. *Medicine* **65**, 322–38.

Weatherall DJ, Abdalla S (1982). The anaemia of *P. falciparum* malaria. *British Medical Bulletin* **38**, 147–51.

Wiley JS, Moore MR (2000). Heme biosynthesis and it disorders: porphyrias and sideroblastic anemias. In: Hoffman R, *et al.*, eds. *Hematology: basic principles and practice*, pp. 428–45. Churchill Livingstone, New York,

22.5.9 Haemolytic anaemia—congenital and acquired

Frank J. Strobl and Leslie Silberstein

Introduction

The mechanisms of haemolysis

Following release into the circulation, normal red cells survive for approximately 120 days. As the circulating red-cell mass decreases (anaemia), less oxygen is transported from the lungs to other tissues of the body. In response, the kidneys increase their synthesis and secretion of erythropoietin, which stimulates erythropoiesis, in order to restore normal red-cell mass and oxygen delivery. A deficient red-cell mass results from inadequate production (hypoplasia), loss (haemorrhage), or premature destruction (haemolysis) of the red cells. In cases where red-cell survival is reduced to such an extent that normal bone marrow cannot compensate, a haemolytic anaemia results. The haemolytic anaemias are either genetically determined or acquired. As will be described in this chapter, premature destruction of red cells occurs through two primary mechanisms. First, decreased erythrocyte deformability secondary to membrane defects, metabolic abnormalities, exogenous oxidizing agents, or pathological antibodies provokes red-cell sequestration and extravascular haemolysis in the spleen and other components of the reticuloendothelial system. Second, exposure to pathological antibodies, activated complement, mechanical forces, chemicals, and infectious agents may lead to red-cell membrane damage and intravascular haemolysis.

The consequences of haemolysis

The clinical and laboratory changes associated with haemolysis reflect the physiological mechanisms responsible for restoring red-cell mass and removing free haemoglobin from the plasma. These changes are outlined in Table 1. Within several days of the onset of haemolysis and the development of anaemia, increased erythropoiesis results in erythroid hyperplasia (decreased myeloid/erythroid ratio) in the bone marrow and reticulocytosis (polychromasia and macrocytosis) in the peripheral blood. The peripheral blood film will also often exhibit microspherocytes, fragmented red blood cells, and nucleated red blood cells. If the haemolysis and anaemia begin early in life and persist, extramedullary erythropoiesis can develop in the spleen, liver, and lymph nodes. Chronic anaemia and the resulting marrow hyperplasia can also result in long-bone deformities. Free haemoglobin in the circulation binds to the serum protein haptoglobin. Haptoglobin–haemoglobin complexes are removed from the intravascular space by the reticuloendothelial system. If the rate of haemolysis is greater than the liver's ability to synthesize haptoglobin, serum haptoglobin levels fall. In patients with severe haemolysis, haemoglobinaemia and haemoglobinuria may develop. At low plasma haemoglobin levels, much of the free haemoglobin is reabsorbed in the proximal renal tubules. The renal tubular cells catabolize the haemoglobin converting iron into haemosiderin, which is eventually shed along with renal tubular cells into the urine resulting in haemosiderinuria. Haemosiderinuria is a reliable indicator of chronic intravascular haemolysis. At higher levels, free haemoglobin is found in the urine. Within the reticuloendothelial system, haemoglobin is metabolized and released into the serum as unconjugated bilirubin. The bilirubin is conjugated in the liver, excreted in the gut, converted to faecal urobilinogen, partially reabsorbed, and excreted by the kidneys as urinary urobilinogen. The intracellular enzyme lactate dehydrogenase is released from lysed red cells into the plasma.

Table 1 The main features of haemolytic anaemia

Increased red cell production	
	Reticulocytosis
	Polychromasia
	Macrocytosis
	Erythroid hyperplasia
	Bone changes
Increased red cell destruction	
	Decreased haemoglobin levels
	Increased unconjugated bilirubin levels
	Decreased haptoglobin levels
	Increased faecal and urinary urobilinogen
	Haemoglobinaemia
	Haemoglobinuria
	Haemosiderinuria
	Splenomegaly
	Increased plasma LDH levels
	Microspherocytes
	Fragmented red blood cells
	Nucleated red blood cells

Congenital anaemias

Congenital anaemias result from inherited defects in the red-cell membrane, red-cell enzymes, or haemoglobin. The haemoglobinopathies and thalassaemias are discussed in Chapter 22.5.7.

Disorders of the red-cell membrane

Introduction

The strength and flexibility required of the red-cell membrane is provided by the lipid bilayer and a proteinaceous, membrane-bound cytoskeleton. The membrane skeleton forms an underlying lattice which both supports and stabilizes the plasma membrane. Figure 1 provides a schematic model of the erythrocyte membrane and membrane-skeleton. The major, integral membrane proteins are band 3 and the glycophorins. Band 3 functions as a transmembrane channel for the diffusion of anions and glucose. The

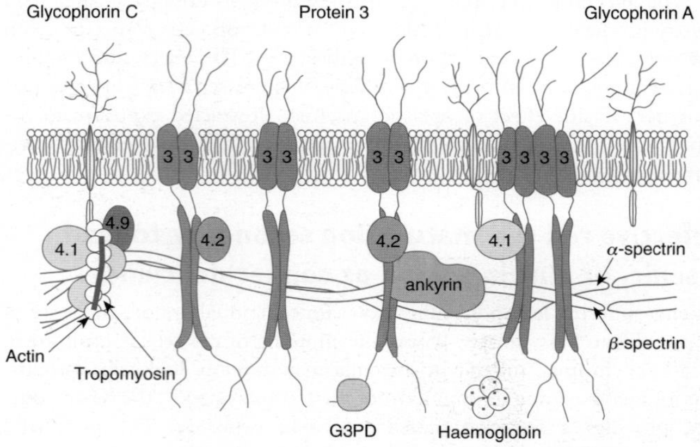

Fig. 1 Schematic illustration of the major components of the red-cell membrane and membrane skeleton. (Reproduced from Lux SE (1989). Hereditary disorders of the red-cell membrane skeleton. *Trends in Genetics* **5**, 222–7, with permission.)

physiological role of the glycophorins is unknown. Cytoplasmic proteins located adjacent to the plasma membrane include spectrin, actin, band 4.1, ankyrin, and band 4.2. Spectrin, a heterodimeric protein composed of α and β subunits, is the principal component of the membrane-skeleton. The heterodimers of spectrin are bound to each other, head-to-head, to form heterotetramers and larger oligomers. The spectrin tetramers are cross-linked at their ends by actin. This interaction is strengthened by band 4.1. Band 4.1 also binds the cytoplasmic domain of glycophorin to spectrin. Ankyrin binds band 3 to the β chain of spectrin. Band 4.2 probably strengthens this interaction. A deficiency in any of these cytoskeletal proteins would be expected to result in defects in erythrocyte shape and deformability.

Hereditary spherocytosis

Aetiology

Hereditary spherocytosis is inherited primarily in an autosomal dominant manner. Up to a quarter of cases, however, exhibit a non-dominant or recessive pattern of inheritance. The disorder is characterized by small spherocytic red cells with reduced deformability. The increased rigidity results in entrapment of the spherocytes, primarily in the microcirculation of the spleen. The aetiology of hereditary spherocytosis appears to be heterogeneous. In most cases, the abnormal deformability is associated with defects in α- and β-spectrin or the proteins that bind spectrin to the plasma membrane: ankyrin, band 3, band 4.1, and band 4.2.

Clinical features

Hereditary spherocytosis occurs in all races but is most common in individuals of northern European descent. The prevalence of hereditary spherocytosis is estimated at 1:5000. Patients usually present in childhood with mild to moderate haemolysis. The main clinical features are anaemia, jaundice, and splenomegaly. The peripheral smear shows reticulocytosis and a variable degree of spherocytosis (Fig. 2). The red cells demonstrate increased osmotic fragility. The persistently elevated serum bilirubin levels often lead to the formation of bilary calculi and recurrent cholecystitis. Infrequent complications include ulcers, dermatitis, extramedullary haematopoietic tumours, cardiomyopathy, mental retardation, renal tubular acidosis, and neurological/muscular abnormalities. Less than 5 per cent of patients have severe disease. Severe haemolytic episodes are associated with infection. Rare aplastic crises are associated with parvovirus infection. Rare megaloblastic crises are associated with folate deficiency, especially during pregnancy.

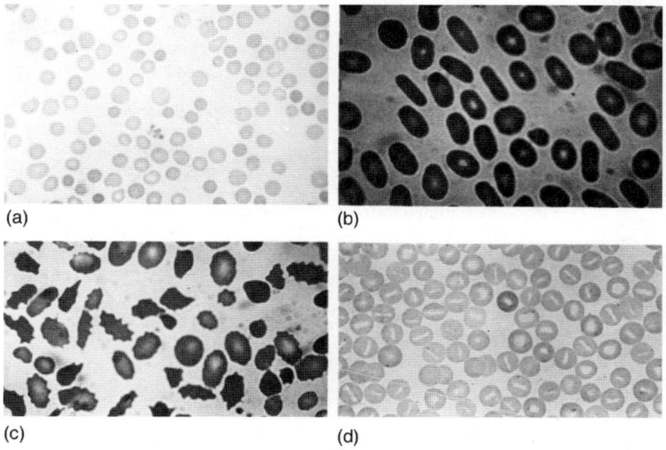

Fig. 2 Altered red-cell morphology: (a) spherocytes; (b) elliptocytes; (c) poikilorytes; (d) stomatocytes.

Treatment

The shortened red-cell survival and resulting anaemia of hereditary spherocytosis can be corrected in almost all cases by splenectomy. In patients with severe hereditary spherocytosis, the haemolysis may only be partially corrected following splenectomy. Except for asymptomatic patients, splenectomy should be performed as early as possible after the age of 3 years. Although erythrocyte survival returns to normal, red-cell morphology and deformability remain abnormal following splenectomy. All patients undergoing splenectomy should receive pneumococcal, meningococcal, and *Haemophilus influenzae* vaccinations several weeks preoperatively. Postsplenectomy, antibiotic therapy to protect against pneumococcal sepsis is also recommended. All patients with haemolytic anaemia should take 1 mg of folic acid each day to prevent folate deficiency. Typically, regular red-cell transfusions are only required for patients with severe disease. Phototherapy and/or exchange transfusions can be used to treat hyperbilirubinaemia in the neonatal period.

Hereditary elliptocytosis

Aetiology

Hereditary elliptocytosis is a genetically heterogeneous disorder characterized by elliptical red cells and haemolysis. Autosomal dominant and rare autosomal recessive forms of the disease have been identified. The clinical severity ranges from an asymptomatic condition to a severe haemolytic anaemia (see hereditary pryopoikilocytosis below). In most cases, defects in both α-spectrin and β-spectrin have been implicated. These point mutations or deletions, which occur at the N-terminus of α-spectrin and the C-terminus of β-spectrin, interfere with spectrin self-association. Partial and complete deficiencies of membrane protein 4.1 are also associated, respectively, with mild and severe forms of hereditary elliptocytosis.

Clinical features

Hereditary elliptocytosis is most common in individuals of African and Mediterranean ancestry with a prevalence of approximately 1:2500. Less than 10 per cent of cases exhibit significant haemolysis. Symptomatic individuals with hereditary elliptocytosis exhibit moderate to severe anaemia, splenomegaly, and reticulocytosis. The peripheral blood smear contains elliptocytes, 'pencil cells', and other abnormally shaped red cells (Fig. 2). The osmotic fragility is normal in mild hereditary elliptocytosis but increased in more severe forms of hereditary elliptocytosis with significant poikilocytosis. Rarely, neonates with hereditary elliptocytosis experience severe haemolysis, which gradually improves during the first year of life. This improvement shadows the normal loss of fetal red cells during infancy. Increased concentrations of 2,3 diphosphoglycerate in fetal red cells probably interfere with spectrin-protein 4.1 interactions, thereby further destabilizing the red-cell membrane.

Treatment

Asymptomatic individuals with hereditary elliptocytosis require no treatment. Symptomatic individuals often obtain some degree of benefit from splenectomy. Recommendations for folate administration, presurgical immunizations, and antibiotic prophylaxis noted earlier for hereditary spherocytosis are similar for patients with hereditary elliptocytosis.

Hereditary pyropoikilocytosis

Hereditary pyropoikilocytosis is inherited in an autosomal recessive fashion. Individuals with hereditary pyropoikilocytosis demonstrate severe haemolytic anaemia characterized by marked red-cell fragmentation, microcytosis, poikilocytosis, and spherocytosis (Fig. 2). The osmotic fragility of red cells is increased. These heat-sensitive cells undergo fragmentation and haemolysis when warmed to greater than 41°C. Red cells from normal individuals do not undergo haemolysis or fragmentation until the temperature nears 50°C. Hereditary pyropoikilocytosis results from homozygosity or compound heterozygosity for the α-spectrin defects involved in hereditary elliptocytosis.

Hereditary spherocytic elliptocytosis

This form of hereditary elliptocytosis is characterized by mild to moderate haemolytic anaemia with both elliptocytes and spherocytes. The molecular basis of this disorder has yet to be identified. The osmotic fragility is increased. Splenectomy may be useful in symptomatic individuals.

Hereditary stomatocytosis

Several families have been identified with members exhibiting moderate to severe anaemia and circulating stomatocytes (Fig. 2). This rare, autosomal dominant disorder results from a defect in membrane permeability that allows increased Na^+ and H_2O influx and results in cellular swelling and increased osmotic fragility. An integral membrane protein, stomatin (band 7.2b), has been reported to be decreased or absent in affected individuals. Symptomatic individuals may obtain some benefit from splenectomy. A number of patients with hereditary stomatocytosis, however, have developed hypercoagulability and thrombosis following splenectomy. Stomatocytosis and mild to moderate haemolytic anaemia are also seen in rare individuals who have either absent (Rh_{null}) or markedly reduced Rh antigen expression.

Hereditary xerocytosis

Hereditary xerocytosis is a rare, autosomal dominant disorder characterized by red-cell dehydration and decreased osmotic fragility. The cellular dehydration appears to be caused by a defect in membrane K+ permeability that leads to intracellular K^+ and H_2O loss. The crenated cells are cleared by the reticuloendothelial system resulting in moderate to severe haemolysis. Splenectomy may provide therapeutic benefit. As with hereditary stomatocytosis, the risk of hypercoagulability and thrombosis are increased following splenectomy in patients with xerocytosis.

Acanthocytosis

Acanthocytes or spur cells are red cells with many thorn-like projections of the membrane surface. Changes in the composition of membrane lipids within the membrane lipid bilayer appear to be responsible for the development of acanthocytosis. Acanthocytosis and haemolytic anaemia are seen in severe liver disease, abetalipoproteinaemia, and the McLoed syndrome. Infrequently, patients with severe liver disease accumulate free cholesterol in the outer leaflet of the red-cell membrane resulting in spur cell shape, trapping of the acanthocytes in the spleen, and rapidly progressive anaemia. Abetalipoproteinaemia is an autosomal recessive disorder characterized by acanthocytosis (>50 per cent on peripheral blood film), fat malabsorption, mild anaemia, retinitis pigmentosa, and progressive ataxia. The McLoed syndrome is characterized by variable acanthocytosis and mild anaemia. The disorder is X-linked and affected individuals appear to lack a membrane precursor of the Kell red-cell antigen that also acts as an integral membrane transporter.

Disorders of red-cell enzymes

Introduction

Erythrocytes circulate throughout the body for approximately 4 months lacking a nucleus, mitochondria, and ribosomes. As a result, red cells cannot synthesize protein nor take advantage of oxidative metabolism. Glucose metabolism is necessary to maintain the integrity of both the erythrocyte membrane and haemoglobin. In red cells, glucose is metabolized to lactate primarily through the anaerobic, Embden–Meyerhof pathway (Fig. 3). Eleven enzymes are required to break glucose down to lactate generating 2 moles of ATP and reducing 2 moles of NAD^+ to NADH. ATP is used primarily by membrane-associated ATPases which pump Na^+ and K^+ against their concentration gradients. NADH prevents the oxidation of iron in haemoglobin. 2,3-diphosphoglycerate (2,3-DPG) which binds to the β-subunits of haemoglobin and facilitates the release of oxygen is also a product of the Embden–Meyerhof pathway. In red cells, the production of 2,3-DPG is exaggerated in order to maintain intracellular concentrations equimolar with the concentration of haemoglobin. The production of 2,3-DPG occurs in a side pathway referred to as the Rapaport–Luebering shunt that branches from the main glycolytic pathway after the formation of 1,3-DPG. The other major red-cell energy pathway is the hexose–monophosphate shunt, which results in the reduction of $NADP^+$ to NADPH (Fig. 4). NADPH maintains adequate levels of reduced glutathione, which protects the red cells against oxidative damage.

Many enzyme deficiencies are associated with haemolytic anaemia. Most of these enzyme deficiencies are not limited to the erythrocyte and, thus, are associated with multisystem disease (Table 2). The remaining enzyme deficiencies associated with haemolytic anaemia are clinically specific to the red cell. The majority of these enzyme deficiencies are rare, having been found in only a few families (Table 3). The two most common red-cell enzyme deficiencies—glucose-6-phosphate dehydrogenase deficiency and pyruvate kinase deficiency—are described below.

Glucose-6-phosphate dehydrogenase (G6PD) deficiency

Aetiology

G6PD catalyses the first step in the hexose–monophosphate shunt, which is responsible for reducing $NADP^+$ to NADPH. NADPH along with glutathione reductase maintains adequate supplies of reduced glutathione.

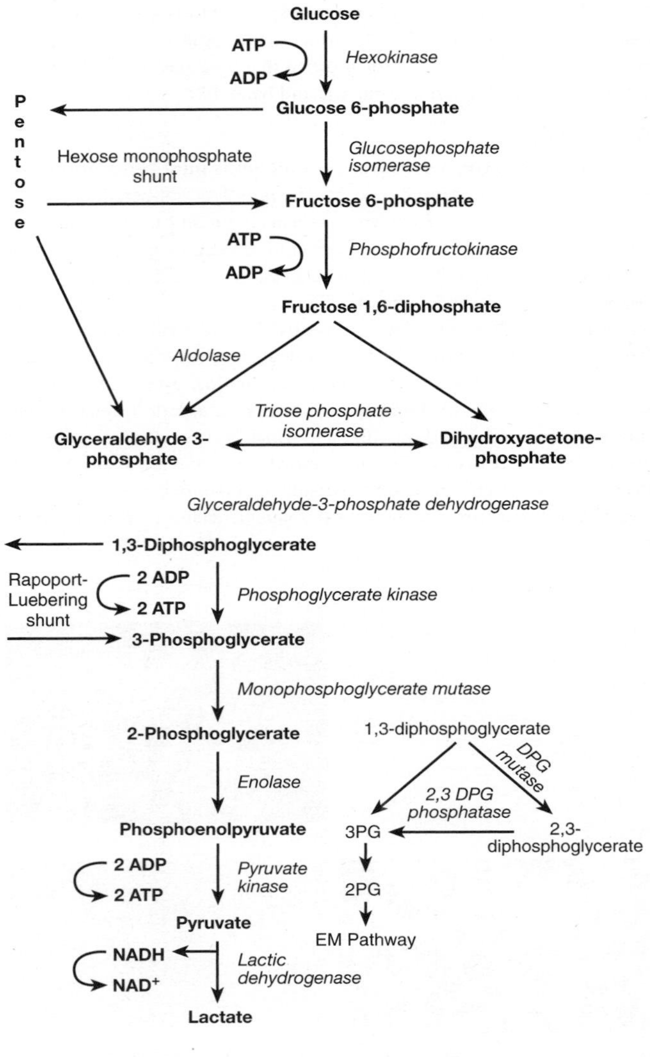

Fig. 3 The relationship between the main red-cell glycolytic pathway (Embden–Meyerhof) and the other metabolic pathways. The insert shows the production of 2,3-DPG in the Rapoport–Luebering shunt.

Reduced glutathione is used by catalase and glutathione peroxidase to convert hydrogen peroxide to water. Oxygen radicals generated either through normal metabolism or by external oxidizing agents are converted to hydrogen peroxide, a highly oxidative agent. Therefore, through this series of enzyme reactions (Fig. 5) haemoglobin and other red-cell proteins are protected from oxidative damage. On the other hand, red cells deficient in G6PD are extremely sensitive to the oxidative actions of chemicals, drugs, infectious agents, and the bean *Vicia faba* (favism). G6PD deficiency is the most common hereditary enzyme deficiency of man affecting hundreds of millions of people world-wide. The disorder results from the X-linked, recessive inheritance of any one of a number of G6PD variants. The gene encoding G6PD is located on the long arm of the X chromosome (Xq28) and consists of 13 exons and greater than 18 kilobases. The G6PD protein is 514 amino acids long. The wild-type G6PD enzyme has been designated G6PD B. Nearly all G6PD mutations are the result of single point mutations that result in single amino acid substitutions. The rare exception consists of multiple point mutations or larger deletions. The altered protein structure most commonly results in decreased enzyme stability or, less commonly, decreased enzyme function. Males inheriting a mutant G6PD gene are affected. In female carriers, the levels of G6PD vary considerably as a result of random inactivation (lyonization) of the X chromosome. Female heterozygotes have two populations of red cells, those deficient in G6PD and those with normal levels of G6PD.

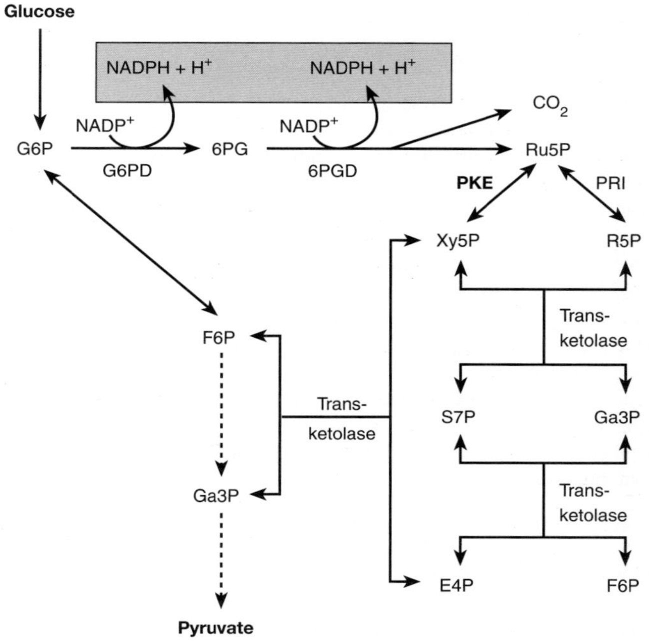

Fig. 4 The hexose monophosphate pathway. Intermediates: G6P, glucose 6-phosphate, F6P, fructose 6-phosphate; Ga3P, glyceraldehyde 3-phosphate; 6PG, 6-phosphogluconate; Ru5P, ribulose 5-phosphate; R5P, ribose 5-phosphate; Xy5P, xylulose 5-phosphate; S7P, sedoheptulose 7-phosphate; E4P, erythrose 4-phosphate. Enzymes: G6PD, glucose 6-phosphate deyhdrogenease; 6PGD 6-phosphogluconate dehydrogenase; PKE, epimerase; PRI, phosphoribose isomerase. Cosubstrates: $NADP^+$ and $NADPH + H^+$, oxidized and reduced forms of nicotinamide-adenine dinucleotide phosphate.

Table 2 Red-cell enzyme deficiencies associated with multisystem disease

Pathway	Enzyme	Clinical features
Embden–Meyerhof	Phospho-fructokinase	Mild HA; myopathy; gout
	Triosephosphate isomerase	Moderate HA; neurological abnormalities
	Phospho-glycerokinase	Severe HA; mental retardation
	Aldolase	Mild HA; mental retardation
Hexose monophosphate shunt	Glutathione synthetase	HA; +/– metabolic acidosis; +/– neutropenia
	Glutamyl cysteine synthetase	HA; +/– neurological abnormalities

HA = haemolytic anaemia.

Table 3 Other rare, red-cell enzyme deficiencies

Pathway	Enzyme	Type of haemolytic anaemia
Embden–Meyerhof	Hexokinase	Mild to severe
	Glucose phosphate isomerase	Mild to severe
Hexose monophosphate shunt	Glutathione peroxidase	Oxidant-sensitive
	Glutathione reductase	Oxidant-sensitive
Nucleotide metabolism	Pyrimidine-5′-nucleotidase	Mild to moderate (basophilic stippling)
	Adenylate kinase	Mild

Clinical features

Since carriers of G6PD deficiency are more resistant to *Plasmodium falciparum* infection, the disorder has a geographical distribution similar to the haemoglobinopathies. G6PD deficiency is widespread in Africa, the Mediterranean, the Middle East, and Southeast Asia. More than 300 G6PD variants have been identified. Although most are clinically insignificant, a number of G6PD variants are associated with chronic anaemia or acute intermittent haemolysis. The two most common clinical forms of G6PD deficiency are an African variant (G6PD A-) and a family of Mediterranean variants. The African variant is synthesized in normal quantities, but is unstable and its levels decline slowly as the red cells age. Only the most senescent red cells are substantially lacking in enzyme activity. The Mediterranean variant has reduced enzyme activity, which also decreases with age. Newly released reticulocytes have significantly reduced G6PD activity, while mature erythrocytes lack any measurable enzyme activity. Both the African and the Mediterranean type are associated with little to no haematological abnormality under normal circumstances, but severe haemolysis and anaemia occur during periods of oxidant stress. Since only a small fraction of the circulating red cells are G6PD deficient in individuals with the African variant, the disorder is usually self-limited. In contrast, since all of the circulating red cells in the Mediterranean variant are G6PD deficient, these individuals may experience acute, life-threatening haemolysis. The onset of intravascular haemolysis often occurs within 24 h of exposure to

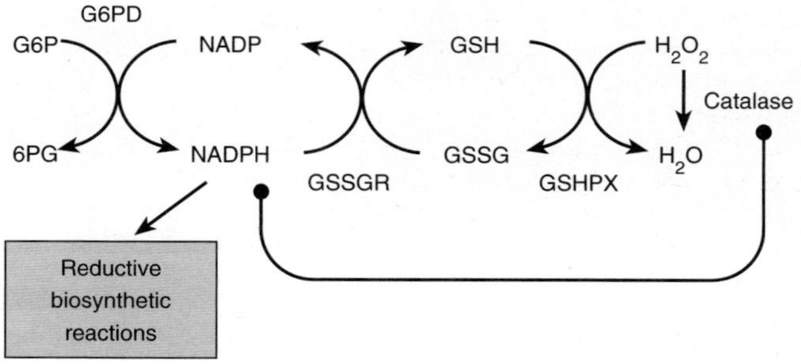

Fig. 5 The role of G6PD in red-cell metabolism: NADPH plays a dual role in (i) regeneration of glutathione (GSH) and (ii) stabilization of catalase (see also Chapter 22.5.12).

the oxidizing agent and is accompanied by malaise, weakness, and abdominal/back pain. Within 2 to 3 days the patient develops anaemia, jaundice, haemoglobinuria, and, on rare occasions, acute renal failure. The peripheral smear often exhibits both anisocytosis and poikilocytosis, including spherocytes and blister cells (Fig. 6). Oxidant damage induces the formation of disulphide bridges within haemoglobin and leads to decreased solubility. Supravital staining with methylviolet demonstrates the presence of Heinz bodies. These intraerythrocytic inclusions consist primarily of denatured and precipitated haemoglobin. Favism is most common in areas where the *Vicia faba* bean grows, such as the Mediterranean and the Middle East. Two fava bean metabolites, divicine and isouramil, are believed to be oxidants. Favism occurs at any age, but is more common in children. Not all G6PD variants are susceptible to favism. Furthermore, every case of fava bean ingestion does not result in haemolysis. Mild haemolysis may also occur during the first weeks of life in G6PD-deficient infants. Occasionally, the jaundice is severe enough to cause kernicterus. Marked haemolysis can also occur in G6PD-deficient individuals during periods of illness, particularly during bacterial and viral infections. Rarely, G6PD deficiency is associated with chronic extravascular haemolysis and anaemia. These individuals retain both their sensitivity to oxidizing agents and, therefore, their risk of acute intravascular haemolysis.

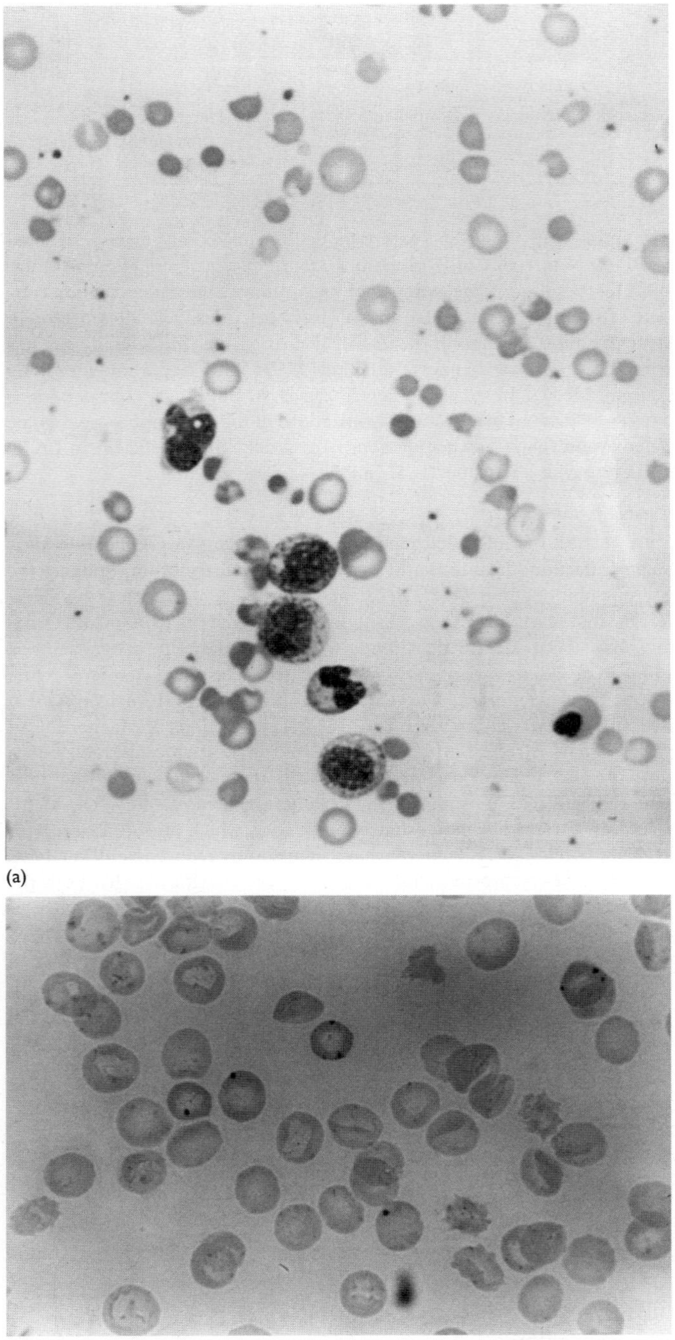

(a)

(b)

Fig. 6 Blood film in a case of acute haemolytic anaemia in a G6PD-deficient patient (favism). (a) Romanovsky stain, showing marked poikilocytosis, polychromatic macrocytes, bite cells, nucleated red cells, and a shift to the left in the granulocytic series. (b) Supravital stain with methyl violet, showing characteristic Heinz bodies.

Treatment

The diagnosis of G6PD deficiency depends on the demonstration of decreased red-cell G6PD activity. A rapid fluorescent screening assay is available to test at risk or suspected individuals during non-haemolytic periods. False-negative results can occur, especially following the resolution of an acute haemolytic episode when reticulocytes with increased enzyme activity predominate. All positive screening results should be confirmed by a quantitative spectrophotometric test based on the generation of NADPH from NADP. Molecular methods can be used accurately to diagnose female carriers heterozygous for G6PD deficiency. G6PD-deficient individuals should avoid substances known to induce haemolysis (Table 4). In newborns, severe jaundice should be treated with phototherapy and/or exchange transfusion. In all patients, blood transfusion should be considered during severe haemolytic episodes. Splenectomy may provide benefit in rare individuals with chronic haemolysis. Transfusion-dependent

Table 4 Some drugs which may induce haemolysis in G6PD-deficient individuals

Antimalarials	**Sulfones**
Primaquine	Thiazolesulfone
Pamaquine	Dapsone
Pentaquine	
Chloroquine	**Nitrofurans**
Quinidine	Nitrofurantoin
Quinine	Nitrofurazone
Quinacrine	Furazolidone
Sulfonamides	**Antipyretics/analgesics**
Sulfanilamide	Acetanilide
Sulfacetamide	Aspirin
Sulfapyridine	Acetominophen
Sulfamethoxazole	Phenacetin
Sulfafurazole	Aminopyrine
Sulfamethoxypyridazine	
Sulfoxone	**Other drugs**
Sulfadiazine	Methylene blue
Sulfamerizine	Nalidixic acid
Sulfisoxazole	Chloramphenicol
Sulfadimidine	Doxorubicin
	Dimercaprol
Other chemicals	Probenecid
Napthalene	Vitamin K analogues
Trinitrotoluene	Phenazopyridine
Toluidine blue	P-aminosalicylic acid
	Ciprofloxacin
	Norfloxacin

individuals should be carefully monitored for haemosiderosis and iron chelation should be initiated early.

Pyruvate kinase deficiency

Aetiology

Pyruvate kinase converts phosphoenol pyruvate to lactate and in the process generates ATP (Fig. 3). Therefore a deficiency in pyruvate kinase impairs the glycolytic pathway resulting in decreased production of ATP. An inadequate energy supply presumably leads to premature destruction of the red cells, particularly in the spleen and liver. There are four pyruvate kinase isoenzymes: M_1, M_2, L, and R. The R isoenzyme is unique to erythrocytes and is a product of the pk gene located on chromosome 1q21. Pyruvate kinase deficiency is inherited in an autosomal recessive fashion. The molecular basis of pyruvate kinase deficiency is quite heterogeneous, including single nucleotide substitutions, deletions, and insertions. Heterozygotes are unaffected, with variable but adequate levels of pyruvate kinase activity in their red cells. Homozygotes have little to no pyruvate kinase activity and exhibit haemolytic anaemia and splenomegaly. Many clinical homozygotes are actually compound heterozygotes with two different genetic lesions.

Clinical features

Pyruvate kinase deficiency occurs most commonly in individuals of northern European descent. The degree of haemolysis varies considerably with individuals and is often exacerbated by physiological stress such as pregnancy or infection. Severe pyruvate kinase deficiency usually presents at birth with haemolysis and jaundice. The haemolysis, anaemia, and jaundice continue throughout life, eventually resulting in splenomegaly, gallstones, and aplastic anaemia. Pyruvate kinase-deficient individuals appear to tolerate their anaemia better than individuals with comparable levels of anaemia due to other aetiologies. It is postulated that since the block in glycolysis occurs after the Rappaport–Leubering shunt, there is increased synthesis of 2,3-DPG in pyruvate kinase-deficient red cells. Increased synthesis of 2,3-DPG encourages the release of oxygen and thus more efficient oxygenation of tissues. The diagnosis of pyruvate kinase-deficiency is best confirmed by the detection of specific mutations at the genomic level.

Treatment

There is no specific therapy for pyruvate kinase deficiency. Periods of active haemolysis are treated with red-cell transfusions. Splenectomy often lessens the degree of haemolysis and anaemia. Splenectomy should be delayed until after the age of 3 years to reduce the risk of pneumococcal and meningococcal infections.

Acquired haemolytic anaemias

Immune haemolytic anaemias

Immune haemolysis may occur when IgG, IgM, or IgA antibodies and/or complement bind to the erythrocyte surface. The red-cell-bound antibodies may induce extravascular haemolysis, intravascular haemolysis, or both. Red cells coated with IgG typically undergo extravascular haemolysis during their transport through the reticuloendothelial system. Interactions between the Fc portion of IgG and surface Fc receptors allow the macrophages to phagocytose the coated erythrocytes. IgM, IgA, and, occasionally, IgG activate and fix complement to the erythrocyte surface. Macrophages also have receptors for the activated complement component C3b and, probably, phagocytose red cells through this pathway. The fixed complement can also induce intravascular haemolysis through activated membrane complex-mediated lysis.

The direct antiglobulin test or direct Coombs' test detects the presence of IgG antibody or complement on the red-cell surface. IgM and IgA antibodies are not directly detectable with standard testing methods. Rather, their presence is indirectly demonstrated by the detection of complement on the erythrocyte. In rare cases, the haemolytic anaemia is due to non-complement-fixing IgM or IgA antibodies. In this situation the direct antiglobulin test will be falsely negative. Eluates can be obtained from the antibody-coated red cells to determine the specificity of the antibody. Alternatively, the antibody may be free in the serum and its specificity determined by the indirect antiglobulin test or indirect Coombs' test. The presence of antibody or complement on the red cell, however, need not reflect ongoing haemolysis. Rather, the diagnosis of haemolytic anaemia rests on clinical findings and other laboratory data, such as red-cell morphology, haemoglobin, bilirubin, haptoglobin, LDH levels, reticulocyte count, and the presence or absence of haemoglobinaemia, haemoglobinuria, or haemosiderinuria. The serological findings provide information as to whether an immune basis exists and what type of immune haemolytic anaemia may be present. Autoantibodies, alloantibodies, and drugs may induce immune haemolytic anaemias.

Autoimmune haemolytic anaemia

Haemolytic antibodies directed against the individual's own red cells may arise as a primary/idiopathic event or may be secondary to lymphoid malignancies, connective tissue disorders, and infection. Autoimmune haemolytic anaemia is best classified according to the temperature at which the antibody optimally binds to the erythrocyte. The four major types of autoimmune haemolytic anaemia are warm autoimmune haemolytic anaemia, cold agglutinin syndrome, paroxysmal cold haemoglobinuria, and mixed-type autoimmune haemolytic anaemia

Warm autoimmune haemolytic anaemia

Aetiology The offending antibody in warm autoimmune haemolytic anaemia is typically IgG and can be found on the red cell, in the serum, or both. The exact specificity of the antibody is often difficult to determine. With very rare exception, warm-reactive autoantibodies bind to all red cells tested, while others appear to have broad specificity within the Rh system. Occasionally, warm reactive autoantibodies will have relative specificity against an individual antigen such as Rh(D), Rh(C), or Kell.

Clinical features Warm autoimmune haemolytic anaemia can arise at any age but is more common in older individuals, probably because of its association with lymphoid malignancies. Females are affected slightly more often than males. The direct antiglobulin test is positive for IgG and/or complement. In its mildest form the direct antiglobulin test is positive but red-cell survival is not significantly affected. Symptomatic patients present with anaemia, jaundice, and splenomegaly. Most patients with warm autoimmune haemolytic anaemia have a chronic, stable anaemia (haemoglobin < 8 g/dl). In its severest form, patients present with fulminant intravascular haemolysis, progressive anaemia, congestive heart failure, respiratory distress, and neurological abnormalities. As with other haemolytic anaemias, the peripheral smear often demonstrates anisocytosis and reticulocytosis with spherocytes and macrocytes (Fig. 7). The platelet count is usually normal except in patients with Evan's syndrome where the autoantibody destroys both red cells and platelets.

Treatment Corticosteroids, which presumably block macrophage Fc receptor activity and inhibit antibody production, are the primary therapy for autoimmune haemolytic anaemia. Prednisone at a dose of approximately 1 to 2 mg/kg body weight in divided doses is effective in most patients. Higher doses rarely provide additional benefit, but do increase the number and severity of side-effects. Treatment continues until the haemoglobin levels stabilize. The initial dose of prednisone can then be tapered at a rate of 5 to 10 mg per week. Once a dose of 10 mg/day is reached, the steroid taper should progress more slowly in order to determine the minimum controlling dose. Side-effects may be reduced by using an alternate-day schedule. Splenectomy should be performed only in steroid-refractory patients or patients requiring unacceptably high doses of prednisone to maintain remission. Alternative therapies including azathioprine, cyclophosphamide, intravenous immunoglobulin (IVIG), danazol, and plasma exchange should be reserved for patients unfit for splenectomy or who have failed to respond to steroids and surgery.

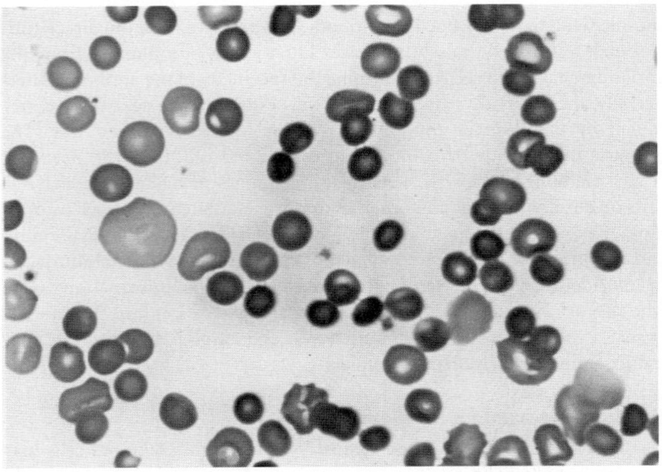

Fig. 7 The peripheral blood changes in autoimmune haemolytic anaemia. There is marked anisocytosis and anisochromia with many macrocytes and microspherocytes. The macrocytes reflect the reticulocytosis (×1000, Leishman stain).

Transfusion with ABO and Rh compatible cross-match least incompatible red cells should be performed in patients with symptomatic anaemia. Transfusion should not be withheld because of serological incompatibility. Active serum autoantibodies, however, can mask the presence of clinically significant alloantibodies. Therefore, the most important consideration prior to transfusion is to confirm the presence or absence of alloantibodies in the patient's serum. Various autologous and allogeneic red-cell absorption techniques exist to remove the autoantibody from a sample of the patient's serum and allow identification of any existing alloantibodies. If clinically significant alloantibodies are present, red cells lacking the corresponding antigen(s) should be selected for transfusion. If the autoantibody has a definite specificity, red cells lacking that antigen may be selected. Transfusions in life-threatening situations should not be delayed if the above tests are not readily available or completed.

Cold agglutinin syndrome

Aetiology Cold agglutinin syndrome accounts for approximately a quarter of all cases of autoimmune haemolytic anaemia. The disorder occurs as an acute or chronic condition. In cold autoimmune disorders the signs and symptoms of disease result from either the agglutination of red cells or from haemolysis. The autoantibodies are typically IgM and are most active at low temperatures. Rare examples of IgG and IgA cold-reactive autoantibodies have been reported. In the lower temperatures of the peripheral circulation, the IgM autoantibodies bind to red cells and activate complement. In warmer areas of the circulation, the IgM dissociates from the erythrocyte leaving activated complement fixed to the red-cell surface. The severity of the disorder depends on both the titre of the antibody and the thermal range at which it is most active. The autoantibody specificity in cold agglutinin syndrome is usually anti-I. Anti –i specificity is associated with infectious mononucleosis.

Clinical features Acute cold autoimmune haemolytic anaemia is commonly seen in adolescents and young adults following infection with *Mycoplasma pneumoniae* or infectious mononucleosis. Haemolysis occurs approximately 1 to 2 weeks following infection and is most commonly associated with a rise in polyclonal anti-I IgM antibody with *Mycoplasma pneumonia* or polyclonal anti-i IgM antibody with infectious mononucleosis. Chronic cold autoimmune haemolytic anaemia occurs most commonly in the elderly, either idiopathically or associated with lymphoma, chronic lymphocytic leukaemia, or Waldenstrom's macroglobulinaemia. Patients may experience chronic intravascular haemolysis and anaemia that are exacerbated by cold temperature. Patients are often also plagued by episodes of Raynaud's phenomenon. Monoclonal IgM antibodies with kappa light chains and anti-I specificity usually cause the red-cell agglutination and haemolysis in this condition. Examination of the peripheral smear shows red-cell agglutination. The direct antiglobulin test is positive for complement.

Treatment Treatment involves keeping the patient in a warm environment (>37°C). Steroids and splenectomy are of little benefit. Severe cold autoimmune haemolytic anaemia secondary to a B-cell neoplasm can be treated with chlorambucil, cyclophosphamide, or α-interferon. Blood transfusion should be avoided. In situations of life-threatening anaemia, the blood should be given slowly through a blood warmer. Plasma exchange is often helpful, but its effects should be expected to be temporary. Hypothermia must be avoided during surgery (especially surgical procedures involving extracorporeal circuits) in patients with cold autoimmune haemolytic anaemia.

Paroxysmal cold haemoglobinuria

Aetiology Paroxysmal cold haemoglobinuria is the rarest form of autoimmune haemolytic anaemia. The disorder is caused by the complement-fixing Donath–Landsteiner IgG antibody. In the cold, this antibody binds to, and irreversibly fixes, complement to the red-cell membrane. Upon return to warmer temperatures, the antibody dissociates from the red cell leaving activated complement to lyse the cell. The Donath–Landsteiner antibody appears to have an anti-P specificity allowing it to bind to practically all red cells.

Clinical features Patients present with acute intravascular haemolysis, abdominal pain, peripheral cyanosis, Raynaud's phenomenon, haemoglobinaemia, and haemoglobinuria after exposure to cold. In the past, paroxysmal cold haemoglobinuria was commonly associated with congenital syphilis but most cases are now associated with viral infections in children or are idiopathic in adults. During or shortly after a haemolytic episode, the direct antiglobulin test is positive for complement but negative for IgG.

Treatment No specific therapy for paroxysmal cold haemoglobinuria exists; steroids are not useful. Most postinfectious cases of paroxysmal cold haemoglobinuria are self-limited and require only supportive care. Avoidance of cold ambient temperatures can help prevent recurrent attacks in patients with chronic paroxysmal cold haemoglobinuria. Transfusion is indicated only for severe haemolysis and life-threatening anaemia. Since the Donath–Landsteiner antibody rarely causes agglutination, most random donor blood units will be compatible with patient sera. Transfusions with extremely rare P-antigen-negative blood should be reserved only for those patients who do not respond to random donor blood. The use of a blood warmer should be considered.

Mixed-type autoimmune haemolytic anaemia

Aetiology Approximately 8 per cent of all autoimmune haemolytic anaemias are of the mixed type. Both IgG and complement are present on the red cells. Both warm-reactive IgG autoantibodies and cold-reactive agglutinating IgM autoantibodies are present in the serum. The warm-reactive IgG autoantibodies are indistinguishable from antibodies encountered in warm autoimmune haemolytic anaemia. The IgM autoantibodies are unlike those in cold-agglutinin syndrome in that they generally have low titres at 4°C and have high thermal amplitudes, reacting at 30°C or above. These IgM autoantibodies usually have no distinguishable specificity, but on occasion have I or i specificities.

Clinical features Mixed-type autoimmune haemolytic anaemia may be idiopathic or secondary, most commonly associated with systemic lupus erythematosus. The haemolytic anaemia is often severe and chronic with intermittent exacerbations. Exposure to cold does not increase the haemolysis.

Treatment Steroids, splenectomy, or cytotoxic agents often provide therapeutic benefit in mixed-type autoimmune haemolytic anaemia. If blood transfusions are necessary, selection of blood should adhere to transfusion guidelines outlined earlier for warm autoimmune haemolytic anaemia. Administration of blood through a warmer should be considered.

Drug-induced haemolytic anaemia

Drugs may induce antibodies to bind to the erythrocyte surface resulting in a positive direct antiglobulin test or haemolysis. There are four mechanisms by which drugs can cause a positive direct antiglobulin test: (1) drug hapten, (2) immune complex formation, (3) autoantibody production, and (4) non-specific adsorption. Only the first three mechanisms are associated with haemolysis. Treatment and prevention are as straightforward as drug avoidance.

Drug hapten Certain drugs bind to the red-cell membrane with a high affinity. Association of the drug with the membrane constituents allows the drug to act as a hapten. The antibodies produced are commonly IgG and are directed predominantly against the drug. Extravascular haemolysis develops gradually, but may be life-threatening if left untreated. After the offending drug is identified and withdrawn, the positive direct antiglobulin test and the haemolysis may persist for several weeks. Serum from these patients will not react with other red cells unless the drug is also present. Penicillin and the cephalosporins are the most notorious examples of this phenomenon. Approximately 3 per cent of patients receiving large doses of penicillin (millions of unit per day) intravenously will develop a positive direct antiglobulin test. Only the rare patient develops haemolytic anaemia.

Immune complex Other drugs induce the binding of IgM or IgG antibodies that activate complement and cause intravascular haemolysis. The antibodies appear to recognize both the drug and a component of the red-cell membrane. The direct antiglobulin test is often positive for complement but not antibody. Haemoglobinaemia and haemoglobinuria are common. Renal failure occurs in about half of the cases. Once the offending drug is withdrawn, the haemolysis stops. Serum from these patients will lyse normal red cells only in the presence of the drug. Quinine, quinidine, phenacetin, chlorpropamide, and sulfonylureas are examples.

Autoantibodies Some drugs stimulate the synthesis of red-cell autoantibodies. Patient serum and red-cell eluates react with normal red cells in the absence of the drug. The autoantibodies are indistinguishable from those found in warm autoimmune haemolytic anaemia. The direct antiglobulin test usually becomes positive after 3 to 6 months of drug administration. The haemolysis typically ceases within 2 weeks after the withdrawal of the drug, but the direct antiglobulin test can remain positive for up to 2 years. α-methyldopa, L-dopa, procainamide, mefenamic acid, and sulindac are examples of drugs that can stimulate the production of red cell autoantibodies.

Non-specific protein adsorption Often a drug-induced positive direct antiglobulin test reflects non-immunological adsorption of protein, including immunoglobulins. First-generation cephalosporins were originally associated with this phenomenon. More recently, other drugs, including suramin, cisplatin, and sulbactam, have also been implicated. This mechanism is not associated with reduced red-cell survival.

Alloimmune haemolytic anaemias

Acute haemolytic transfusion reactions

Aetiology The most catastrophic cases of alloimmune haemolysis occur following the transfusion of ABO-incompatible red cells. Naturally occurring IgM anti-A and anti-B antibodies bind to the incompatible red cells and activate complement resulting in intravascular haemolysis. Human error leading to the misidentification of patients, their blood samples, or the units of red cells to be transfused is responsible for virtually all cases of ABO incompatibility. Only rarely, do other non-ABO IgG alloantibodies cause acute, severe haemolysis.

Clinical features Symptoms of an acute haemolytic transfusion reaction may begin after the infusion of as little as 10 ml of incompatible blood. The signs and symptoms include fever, chills, nausea, vomiting, hypotension, respiratory distress, haemoglobinuria, and chest or flank pain. Despite treatment, acute haemolytic transfusions reactions can result in renal failure, disseminated intravascular coagulation, and even death.

Treatment Once an acute haemolytic transfusion reaction is suspected, the blood transfusion should be stopped immediately. Aggressive treatment of the hypotension with intravenous fluids and pressor agents (that is low-dose dopamine) is crucial. Other critical measures include monitoring the urine output and promoting renal blood flow with diuretics (furosemide or mannitol). Either heparin or the administration of platelets, plasma, and cryoprecipitate can be used to treat organ or life-threatening bleeding secondary to disseminated intravascular coagulation.

Delayed haemolytic transfusion reactions

Aetiology Approximately 2 to 3 per cent of transfusion recipients become alloimmunized to non-ABO red-cell antigens. Haemolysis is not generally seen during the primary immune response since the transfused red cells often disappear from the circulation before antibody titres reach clinically significant levels. In the absence of further antigenic stimuli antibody titres may diminish to undetectable levels. Subsequent transfusion of red cells possessing the offending antigen, however, will induce an anamnestic response with reappearance of the IgG antibodies within hours to days. Binding of the IgG antibody to the transfused antigen-positive red cells results in a positive direct antiglobulin test and possibly mild to moderate extravascular haemolysis.

Clinical features Most patients experiencing a delayed haemolytic transfusion reaction present with fever, jaundice, and decreasing haemoglobin levels 1 to 2 weeks following the transfusion of incompatible red cells. Delayed haemolytic transfusion reactions are often discovered during evaluation for fever of unknown origin or when the haemoglobin level fails to increase following transfusion.

Treatment Treatment is rarely necessary; acute renal failure or disseminated intravascular coagulation are uncommon. If a delayed haemolytic transfusion reaction is suspected, both the patient's serum and an eluate from the circulating red cells should be tested for alloantibodies. If alloantibodies are present, their specificities should be determined. Donor red-cell units lacking the offending antigen should be selected for subsequent transfusions.

Passenger lymphocyte haemolysis

Aetiology Recipients of a haematopoietic or a solid-organ transplant may experience delayed extravascular haemolysis. In this circumstance, lymphocytes of donor origin produce haemolytic antibodies against ABO or other red-cell antigens possessed by the recipient.

Clinical features Haemolysis due to passenger lymphocytes is most commonly seen in out-of-group yet ABO-compatible liver and bone marrow transplants (group A or group B recipients of group O tissue) but can also occur in recipients of lung, heart, and kidney transplants. This haemolysis can begin within several days after the transplant and continue for several months.

Treatment If significant ABO haemolysis occurs, patients should be transfused with group O red cells. If non-ABO haemolysis is present, elution of the patient's red cells may help to identify the antibody specificity and allow transfusion of antigen-negative red cells.

Haemolytic disease of the newborn (HDN)

Haemolytic disease of the newborn occurs when maternal IgG antibodies cross the placenta and bind to fetal red cells resulting in extravascular haemolysis. Usually these antibodies possess specificities within the Rhesus or ABO blood group systems. Occasionally the antibodies are directed against other red-cell antigens such as the Kell, Kidd, and Duffy. In the mildest cases, anaemia develops several weeks after birth and is of little clinical consequence. In more severe cases the neonate develops progressive anaemia and jaundice within the first week of life. If left untreated, bilirubin levels may reach levels associated with kernicterus causing brain damage and death. In the most severe cases, the fetus develops profound anaemia as early as the fifth month of gestation and may be stillborn or delivered grossly oedematous (hydrops fetalis). An infant with hydrops fetalis also has ascites, hepatosplenomegaly, and erythroblastosis and usually dies shortly after birth.

Rhesus D incompatibility

Haemolytic disease of the newborn is most common and severe in rhesus-D-negative women carrying a rhesus-D-positive fetus. The mother develops anti-D IgG antibodies following exposure to the D antigen during a previous pregnancy, or as a result of the transfusion of D-antigen-positive red cells. One half of all cases of rhesus D alloimmunization are due to transplacental haemorrhage from the fetus at the time of delivery. Spontaneous transplacental haemorrhage can also occur during gestation, particularly during the third trimester. The risk of transplacental haemorrhage increases with ectopic pregnancy, spontaneous or therapeutic abortion, chorionic villus sampling, caesarean section, and trauma. Approximately 8 per cent of untreated D-negative women who deliver a D-positive child will become alloimmunized to the D antigen.

It is essential to identify pregnant women at risk for rhesus D haemolytic disease of the newborn and to prevent sensitization. All pregnant women should have their ABO and rhesus types identified as early as possible. Their serum should be screened for alloantibodies against the D antigen and other red-cell antigens. Pregnant women who are D-antigen-negative and have an initial negative antibody screen should have their serum retested for alloantibodies at 28 weeks gestation. If the initial antibody screen is found positive, antibody titres should be followed at 2 to 4-week intervals to determine whether further sensitization is occurring. The presence of an antibody, however, does not indicate on going haemolysis in all cases.

Naturally occurring IgM antibodies are common during pregnancy but do not cross the placenta. Furthermore, fetal red cells may lack the antigen corresponding to the mother's antibody. Molecular typing of the father's DNA or even fetal DNA is available for several red-cell antigens including D, E/e, C/c, Jk^a/Jk^b, and K1/K2. A rising titre of anti-D antibody or other clinically significant red-cell alloantibodies indicates ongoing sensitization and possible haemolytic disease of the newborn.

From 18 weeks of gestation and onward, ultrasonography and fetal blood sampling can be used to assess the severity of haemolysis. After 28 weeks of gestation amniocentesis can be performed. If the fetus is experiencing significant haemolysis and anaemia, clinical intervention must be prompt. Prior to 34 weeks of gestation intrauterine transfusion with blood lacking the offending antigen should be performed. After 36 weeks gestation induced labour should be considered. Upon birth of a 'at risk' fetus a sample of cord blood should undergo a direct antiglobulin test and have measurements of haemoglobin and bilirubin performed. If the direct antiglobulin test on the cord blood sample is positive and the mother's antibody screen remains negative, haemolytic disease secondary to ABO incompatibility or antibodies against low-incidence red-cell antigens should be considered.

Infants with severe anaemia (haemoglobin <12 g/dl) or severe jaundice (bilirubin >14 mg/dl) should undergo exchange transfusion. Phototherapy can also be used to decrease bilirubin levels. A non-sensitized D-antigen-negative mother's blood should also be tested to determine the amount of fetomaternal haemorrhage at delivery. Administration of 300 μg of IgG anti-D (RhIg) within 72 h of delivery will protect 99 per cent of D-antigen-negative mothers from developing anti-D antibodies. Prophylactic administration of RhIg at 28 weeks gestation and following invasive procedures or traumatic events will virtually eliminate the chance of alloimmunization. Patients with large transplacental haemorrhages quantitated by the Kleihauer–Betke acid-elution technique should receive additional RhIg at a dose equivalent to 300 μg for every 15 cc of fetal red blood cells.

ABO incompatibility

Although 15 per cent of pregnancies are ABO incompatible, haemolytic disease of the newborn due to ABO incompatibility is rare. Mild to moderate haemolysis and hyperbilirubinaemia due to ABO incompatibility occurs in about 1.5 per 1000 pregnancies. Group A and group B infants of group O mothers are at greatest risk. Unlike with rhesus D antigen, ABO-haemolytic disease of the newborn occurs during the first pregnancy as often as subsequent pregnancies. Exchange transfusion with group O red cells is rarely required. Hydrops fetalis never occurs.

Non-immune acquired haemolytic anaemias

Red-cell survival may also be reduced by a number of non-inherited, non-immune mechanisms. As red cells circulate they are vulnerable to a variety of insults that may cause structural or metabolic alterations. These changes generally result in reduced red-cell deformability leading ultimately to extravascular haemolysis. These insults include infection, mechanical trauma, and exposure to chemicals, heat, or venom. They often also cause intravascular haemolysis by directly lysing the red-cell membrane. Other less understood causes of acquired non-immune haemolytic anaemias are listed in Table 5.

Infection

Infectious causes of haemolysis are primarily parasites and bacteria. Direct parasitization of red cells by *Plasmodium falciparum*, *Plasmodium vivax*, and *Plasmodium malariae* causes both intravascular haemolysis due to direct membrane destruction and extravascular haemolysis due to membrane alteration and activation of the reticuloendothelial system. Infrequently, *in utero* infection of the fetus with *Toxoplasma gondii* resembles severe haemolytic disease of the newborn. Infants are born hydropic and severely anaemic. Premature delivery and stillbirth are common. *Babesia microti*, endemic in areas of the Northeast and Midwest in North America, is transmitted by ticks and causes severe haemolysis during the erythrocytic phase of its life cycle. Bacterial infections, particularly Gram-negative organisms which produce endotoxin or proteolytic enzymes, may produce mechanical haemolysis by inducing disseminated intravascular haemolysis or red-cell membrane damage via degradation of membrane phospholipids and proteins. *Bartonella bacilliformis* endemic to western South America causes Oroya fever characterized by fever, chills, musculoskeletal pain, and acute intravascular haemolysis.

Chemical

Drugs and chemicals known to cause haemolysis through direct oxidative damage are summarized in Table 6. In most cases the strong oxidant activity of these chemicals overwhelm normally functioning reduction mechanisms responsible for protecting haemoglobin and the red-cell membrane. Variability in the absorption of the chemical or its metabolism determine whether a particular individual will develop chemical-induced haemolytic anaemia. Often it is the chemical's metabolite that is responsible for inducing haemolysis. The red cells of newborns do not have functional reduction mechanisms and thus are more sensitive to oxidant activity.

Table 5 Other causes of acquired haemolytic anaemia

Paroxysmal nocturnal haemoglobinuria
Lipid disorders
Liver disease
Hepatitis
Cirrhosis
Gilbert's disease
Chronic alcoholism (Zieve's syndrome)
Wilson's disease
Vitamin E deficiency
Hypersplenism
Hyperbaric oxygen therapy
Total body irradiation
Chronic large granular lymphocytic leukaemia
Renal disease
Cardiopulmonary bypass
Freshwater/saltwater drowning

Table 6 Chemicals that cause haemolysis

Oxidative haemolysis	
Nitrofurantoin	Arsine gas
Sulfonamides	Chlorate
Sulfones (dapsone)	*p*-Aminosalicylic acid
Phenazopyridine	*p*-Nitroaniline
Phenacetin	Nitrobenzene derivatives
Phenylhydrazine	Vitamin K analogues
Phenothiazine	Paraquat
Isobutyl nitrate	Naphthalene (mothballs)
Amyl nitrite	Hydrogen peroxide
Non-oxidative haemolysis	
Copper	Lead

Mechanical

Mechanical fragmentation of erythrocytes can occur when foreign material is placed within the vasculature, when fibrin strands or platelet thrombi obstruct small blood vessels, or when direct physical forces compress superficial blood vessels.

Foreign material

Mechanical haemolysis occurs most commonly with artificial valvular prostheses, particularly when accompanied by turbulent blood flow. Bacterial endocarditis and associated valvular vegetations can also cause fragmentation of red cells. Haemolysis also occurs in up to 10 per cent of patients with transjugular intrahepatic portosystemic shunts (TIPS). Increased cardiac output as a result of anaemia, exercise, or medications can increase the rate of red-cell fragmentation. The peripheral smear usually demonstrates schistocytes and microspherocytes. Severe haemolysis usually requires surgical repair.

Microangiopathic haemolytic anaemia (MAHA)

MAHA describes a spectrum of disorders characterized by mechanical destruction of red cells resulting from thrombi that occlude the microvasculature. The red cells are probably fragmented during their forced passage through the meshwork of fibrin strands that make up the microthrombi. The degree of anaemia is variable. The peripheral smear reveals findings typical of mechanical haemolysis including schistocytes, microspherocytes, and a reticulocytosis (Fig. 8). The absence of a positive direct antiglobulin test along with significant thrombocytopenia helps to confirm the diagnosis. Two other major forms of MAHA are haemolytic uraemic syndrome and thrombotic thrombocytopenic purpura (TTP).

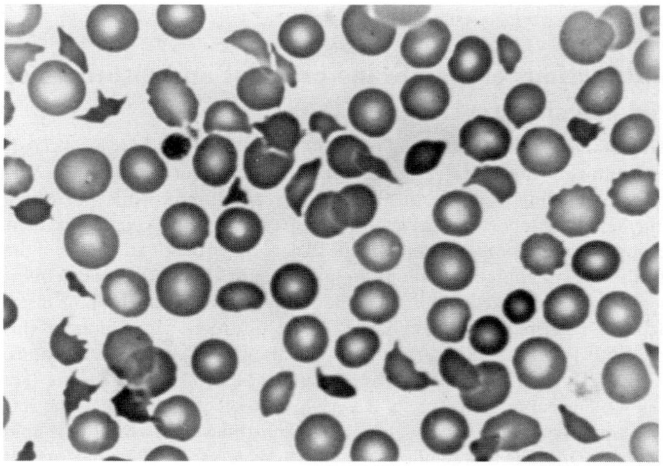

Fig. 8 The peripheral blood changes in microangiopathic haemolytic anaemia. This patient had recurrent thrombocytopenic purpura and the marked fragmentation of the red cells together with microspherocytosis is evident on the blood film (× 1000, Leishman stain).

Haemolytic uraemic syndrome Haemolytic uraemic syndrome is primarily, but not exclusively, a disease of childhood. The disorder consists of widespread damage to the vascular endothelium and fibrin deposition. These pathological changes are frequently most severe in the renal arterioles and glomerular capillaries. The disorder usually develops following a febrile illness. Numerous reports have documented the development of haemolytic uraemic syndrome following infections with toxin-secreting strains of *Escherichia coli* (strain O157:H7) or shigella. Initial nausea, vomiting, and diarrhoea can develop into severe abdominal pain and bloody diarrhoea. Acutely, the child may develop hypertension, oliguria, purpura, bleeding, and anaemia. If left untreated, convulsions, coma, and death may occur. Mortality rates as high as 10 per cent have been associated with haemolytic uraemic syndrome. The peripheral smear exhibits schistocytosis and thrombocytopenia. Therapy consists mainly of supportive care, transfusion, control of blood pressure, and dialysis.

Thrombotic thrombocytopenic purpura (TTP) TTP is caused by either a congenital deficiency of, or an acquired inhibitor to, a serum metalloprotease which is responsible for cleaving unusually large multimers of von Willibrand's factor. Left uncleaved, the large von Willibrand's factor multimers induce TTP by causing the agglutination of circulating platelets. Most episodes of TTP occur without an obvious inciting event. However, TTP has been associated with infection, pregnancy, transplantation, AIDS, and drugs such as mitomycin C, ticlopidine, cyclosporine, and tacrolimus (FK506). TTP occurs mainly in adults and more commonly involves the central nervous system. The onset is often sudden with fever, purpura, petechiae, anaemia, thrombocytopenia, and neurological abnormalities. The neurological sequelae include convulsions, coma, paralysis, delirium, and stroke. The peripheral smear demonstrates schistocytes, thrombocytopenia, and a reticulocytosis. During acute episodes front-line therapy includes steroids and daily plasma exchange with fresh frozen plasma or virally-inactivated solvent-detergent plasma (SD plasma). Plasma exchange probably accomplishes one or more of the following:

(1) removes the antibody to the protease;

(2) removes large multimers of von Willibrand's factor; or

(3) replenishes normal protease.

In patients who do not initially respond to plasma exchange with fresh frozen plasma, cryopoor-supernatant is often used as the replacement fluid. Cryopoor-supernatant contains markedly reduced levels of normal von Willibrand's factor which is believed to enhance the formation of microthrombi in some patients. Individuals with drug-induced TTP appear to be less responsive to therapy. Additional therapies in refractory or relapsing patients include vincristine, cytoxan, cyclosporine, and splenectomy. Anecdotal evidence suggests that platelet transfusion can exacerbate the disorder. Therefore, platelet transfusions should be avoided unless absolutely necessary to treat haemorrhage.

March haemoglobinuria

Haemoglobinuria can occur in soldiers or joggers following extended periods of marching or running on a hard surface or in karate or conga drummer enthusiasts following practice. This mechanical haemolysis appears to be the result of red-cell compression in superficial blood vessels during the period of contact between the extremity and the hard surface. The peripheral smear is normal. Treatment is unnecessary as the syndrome is otherwise symptomless and lacks significant clinical sequelae.

Thermal haemolysis

Normal red cells undergo fragmentation and lysis when heated to temperatures of 49°C or higher. The two most common clinical situations associated with heat-induced red-cell lysis are the use of faulty blood warmers during transfusion or patients who have sustained extensive burns.

Venom

Haemolysis has been observed following bee and wasp stings, spider bites, and snake bites. The haemolysis occurs secondary to disseminated intravascular coagulation or as a result of proteolytic enzymes contained within the venom.

Further reading

Agre P *et al.* (1985). Partial deficiency of erythrocyte spectrin in hereditary spherocytosis. *Nature* **314**, 380–3.

Bowman JM (1986). Fetomaternal ABO incompatibility and erythroblastosis fetalis. *Vox Sanguinus* **50**, 104–6.

Brecher ME (1996). Hemolytic transfusion reactions. In: Rossi EC *et al.*, eds. *Principles of transfusion medicine*, pp. 747–63. Williams and Wilkins, Baltimore.

Conboy JG *et al.* (1993). An isoform specific mutation in the protein 4.1 gene results in hereditary elliptocytosis and complete deficiency of protein 4.1 in erythrocytes but not in nonerythroid cells. *Journal of Clinical Investigation* **91**, 77–82.

Davidson RJL (1969). March or exertional hemoglobinuria. *Seminars in Hematology* **6**, 150.

Freedman J (1987). The significance of complement on the red cell suface. *Transfusion Medicine Reviews* **1**, 58–70.

Furlan M *et al.* (1998). Von Willebrand factor-cleaving protease in thrombotic thrombocytopenic purpura and the hemolytic-uremic syndrome. *New England Journal of Medicine* **399**, 1578–84.

Garratty G (1987). The significance of IgG on the red cell surface. *Transfusion Medicine Reviews* **1**, 47–57.

Hows J (1986). Donor-derived red blood cell antibodies and immune hemolysis after allogeneic bone marrow transplantation. *Blood* **67**, 177–81.

Judd WJ *et al.* (1990). Prenatal and perinatal immunohematology: recommendations for serologic management of the fetus, newborn infant and obstetric patient. *Transfusion* **30**, 175–83.

Leger RM, Garraty G (1999). Evaluation of methods for detecting alloantibodies underlying warm autoantibodies. *Transfusion* **39**, 11–16.

Liu SC, Palek J, Prchal J (1982). Defective spectrin dimer-dimer association in hereditary elliptocytosis. *Proceedings of the National Academy of Science* **79**, 2072–6.

Marsh GW, Lewis SM (1969). Cardiac hemolytic anemia. *Seminars in Hematology* **6**, 133–45.

Prchal JT, Gregg XT (2000). Red cell enzymopathies. In: Hoffman R *et al.*, eds. *Hematology: basic principles and practice*, pp. 561–76. Churchill Livingstone, Philadelphia.

Ramsey G (1991). Red cell antibodies arising from solid organ transplants. *Transfusion* **31**, 76–86.

Savvides P *et al.* (1993). Combined spectrin and ankyrin deficiency is common in autosomal dominant hereditary spherocytosis. *Blood* **82**, 2953–60.

Schrier SL (2000). Extrinsic nonimmune haemolytic anemias. In: Hoffman R *et al.*, eds. *Hematology: basic principles and practice*, pp. 630–8. Churchill Livingstone, Philadelphia.

Shepard KV, Bukowski RM (1987). The treatment of thrombotic thrombocytopenic purpura with exchange transfusions, plasma infusions, and plasma exchange. *Seminars in Hematology* **24**, 178–93.

Shulman NR, Reid DM (1993). Mechanisms of drug-induced immunologically mediated cytopenias. *Transfusion Medicine Reviews* **7**, 215–29.

Tsai H-M, Lian EC-Y (1998). Antibodies to von Willebrand factor-cleaving protease in acute thrombotic thrombocytopenic purpura. *New England Journal of Medicine* **399**, 1585–94.

Vengelen-Tyler V *et al.*, eds (1999). *Technical manual*, 13th edn. American Association of Blood Banks, Bethesda.

Vulliamy TJ, Beutler E, Luzzatto L (1993). Variants of glucose 6-phosphate dehydrogenase are due to missense mutations spread throughout the coding region of the gene. *Human Mutation* **2**, 159–67.

22.5.10 Disorders of the red cell membrane

Patrick G. Gallagher, Sara S. T. O. Saad, and Fernando F. Costa

The red cell membrane

Composition and function

Although the primary structure and a number of the important functions of the red cell membrane have been known for several years, its study continues to yield important insights into our understanding of membrane structure and function. The red cell membrane is composed of three major structural elements: a lipid bilayer primarily composed of phospholipids and cholesterol; integral proteins embedded in the lipid bilayer that span the membrane; and a membrane skeleton on the internal side of the red cell membrane.

The membrane and its skeleton provide the erythrocyte with the ability to undergo significant deformation without fragmentation or loss of integrity during its travel through the microcirculation. The membrane also assembles and organizes the proteins of the lipid bilayer and the membrane skeleton, allowing the red cell to participate in a wide range of functions. These include influencing cellular metabolism by selectively and reversibly binding and inactivating glycolytic enzymes, retaining organic phosphates and other vital compounds, removing metabolic waste, and sequestering the reductants required to prevent corrosion by oxygen. During erythropoiesis, the membrane responds to erythropoietin and imports the iron required for the synthesis of haemoglobin. The lipid bilayer provides an impermeable barrier between the cytoplasm and the external environment and helps maintain a slippery exterior so that erythrocytes do not adhere to endothelial cells or aggregate in the microcirculation. The membrane also participates in erythrocyte biogenesis and ageing. Finally, the membrane participates in the maintenance of pH homeostasis by participating in chloride–bicarbonate exchange.

Interactions of membrane proteins and disorders of red cell shape

Membrane protein–protein and protein–lipid interactions have been classified into two categories, vertical and horizontal interactions (Fig. 1). Vertical interactions stabilize the lipid bilayer membrane while horizontal interactions support the structural integrity of erythrocytes after their exposure to shear stress. The interactions between proteins and lipids of the erythrocyte membrane are more complex than this simplistic model, but it serves as a useful starting point for understanding red cell membrane interactions, particularly in membrane-related disorders. According to this model, hereditary spherocytosis (HS) is a disorder of vertical interactions. Although the primary molecular defects in HS are heterogeneous (see below), one common feature of HS erythrocytes is a weakening of the vertical contacts between the skeleton and the lipid bilayer. As a result, the lipid bilayer membrane is destabilized, leading to release of lipids in the form of skeleton-free lipid vesicles, which in turn results in membrane surface area deficiency and spherocytosis. In this model, hereditary elliptocytosis is a defect of horizontal interactions, primarily those involving spectrin dimer self-association. Defects of horizontal interactions disrupt the membrane

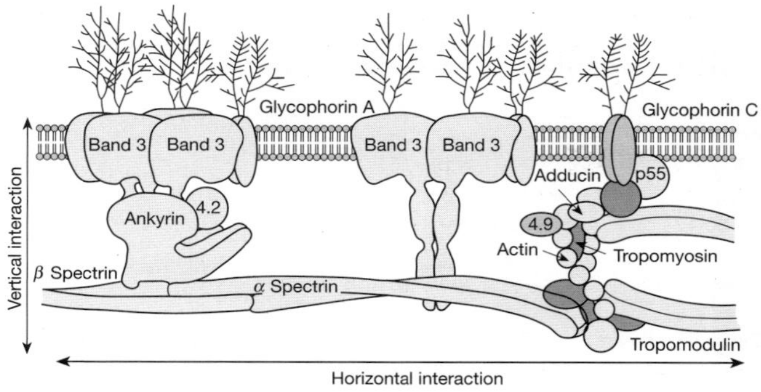

Fig. 1 Schematic diagram of the red cell membrane (not to scale). Membrane–protein and membrane–lipid interactions can be divided into two categories: (1) vertical interactions, which are perpendicular to the plane of the membrane and involve spectrin–ankyrin–band 3 interactions, spectrin–protein 4.1–glycophorin C interactions, and weak interactions between spectrin and the lipid bilayer, and (2) horizontal interactions, which are parallel to the plane of the membrane. (Reprinted from Tse and Lux, 1999, with permission.)

skeletal lattice leading to elliptocytic shape in mild cases and skeletal instability and cell fragmentation in severe cases.

Table 1 Characteristics of hereditary spherocytosis

Clinical manifestations
Anaemia
Splenomegaly
Intermittent jaundice
from haemolysis
from biliary obstruction
Haemolytic, aplastic, and megaloblastic crises
Inheritance
dominant ~75%
non-dominant ~25% *de novo* or recessive
Rare manifestations
leg ulcers, gout, chronic dermatitis
extramedullary haematopoietic tumours
thrombosis
neuromuscular disorders
cardiomyopathy
spinocerebellar abnormalities
Excellent response to splenectomy
Laboratory characteristics
Reticulocytosis
Spherocytosis
Elevated mean corpuscular haemoglobin concentration
Increased osmotic fragility
Normal direct antiglobulin test

Hereditary spherocytosis

Introduction

Hereditary spherocytosis (HS) refers to a group of inherited disorders characterized by the presence of spherical-shaped erythrocytes on peripheral blood smear. HS occurs in all racial and ethnic groups. It is the most common inherited anaemia in individuals of northern European descent, affecting approximately 1 in 2500 individuals in the United States and England. It is much more common in Caucasians than in individuals of African descent. Clinical, laboratory, biochemical, and genetic heterogeneity characterize the spherocytosis syndromes.

Aetiology and pathogenesis

The primary defect in HS is loss of membrane surface area relative to intracellular volume, accounting for the spheroidal shape and decreased deformability of the red cell. This loss of surface area results from increased membrane fragility due to defects in erythrocyte membrane proteins. Increased fragility leads to membrane vesiculation and membrane loss. Splenic destruction of these non-deformable erythrocytes is the primary cause of haemolysis experienced by HS patients. Physical entrapment of erythrocytes in the splenic microcirculation and ingestion by phagocytes have been proposed as mechanisms of destruction. Furthermore, the splenic environment is hostile to erythrocytes. Low pH, glucose, and ATP concentrations, and high local concentrations of toxic free radicals produced by adjacent phagocytes, all contribute to membrane damage.

Membrane loss is due to defects in several membrane proteins, including ankyrin, band 3, α-spectrin, β-spectrin, and protein 4.2. Combined spectrin and ankyrin deficiency is the most common defect observed, followed by band 3 deficiency, isolated spectrin deficiency, and protein 4.2 deficiency. The genetic defects underlying HS are heterogeneous. Multiple genetic loci are implicated and various abnormalities, including point mutations, defects in mRNA processing, and gene deletions, have been described. Except for a few rare exceptions, HS mutations are private, that is each individual kindred has a unique mutation.

Clinical features

The clinical manifestations of the spherocytosis syndromes vary widely. The typical picture of HS combines evidence of haemolysis (anaemia, jaundice, reticulocytosis, gallstones, and splenomegaly) with spherocytosis (spherocytes on peripheral blood smear, positive osmotic fragility) and a positive family history (Table 1). Mild, moderate, and severe forms of HS have been defined according to differences in haemoglobin, bilirubin, and reticulocyte counts correlated with the degree of compensation for the haemolysis (Table 2). Initial assessment of a patient with suspected HS should include a family history and questions about history of anaemia, jaundice, gallstones, and splenectomy. Physical examination should seek signs such as scleral icterus, jaundice, and splenomegaly. After diagnosing a patient with HS, family members should be examined for the presence of HS.

HS typically presents in childhood, but may present at any age. In children, anaemia is the most frequent presenting complaint (50 per cent), followed by splenomegaly, jaundice, or a positive family history. Two-thirds to three-quarters of HS patients have incompletely compensated haemolysis and mild to moderate anaemia. The anaemia is often asymptomatic except for fatigue and mild pallor. Jaundice is seen at some time in about half of patients, usually in association with viral infections. When present, it is acholuric, that is there is unconjugated hyperbilirubinaemia without detectable bilirubinuria. Palpable splenomegaly is detectable in most (75–95 per cent) older children and adults. Typically, the spleen is modestly enlarged but it may be massive.

About 20 to 30 per cent of HS patients have 'compensated haemolysis,' that is erythrocyte production and destruction are balanced. Although the erythrocyte life span may only be about 20 to 30 days, these patients adequately compensate for their haemolysis with increased marrow erythropoiesis. They are not anaemic and are usually asymptomatic. Many of these individuals escape detection until adulthood, when they are being evaluated for unrelated disorders or when complications related to anaemia or chronic haemolysis occur. Haemolysis may become severe with illnesses that cause splenomegaly, such as infectious mononucleosis, or may be exacerbated by other factors such as pregnancy. Because of the asymptomatic course of HS in these patients, diagnosis of HS should be considered during evaluation of splenomegaly, gallstones at a young age, or anaemia from viral infection.

Approximately 5 to 10 per cent of HS patients have moderate to severe anaemia. Patients with 'moderately severe' disease typically have a haemoglobin of 6 to 8 g/dl, reticulocytes about 10 per cent, bilirubin 2 to 3 mg/dl, and 40 to 80 per cent of the normal red cell spectrin content. This category

Table 2 Clinical classification of hereditary spherocytosis

	Trait	Mild spherocytosis	Moderate spherocytosis[1]	Severe spherocytosis
Haemoglobin (g/dl)	Normal	11–15	8–12	≤ 8
Reticulocytes (%)	1–3	3–8	≥ 8	≥ 10
Bilirubin (mg/dl)	0–1	1–2	> 2	> 3
Spectrin content[2] (% of normal)	100	80–100	50–80	20–80
Peripheral smear	Normal	Mild spherocytosis	Spherocytosis	Spherocytosis and poikilocytosis
Osmotic fragility				
fresh	Normal	Slightly increased	Distinctly increased	Distinctly increased
incubated	Slightly increased	Distinctly increased	Distinctly increased	Markedly increased

[1] Values in untransfused patients.

[2] In most patients ankyrin content is decreased to a comparable degree. A minority of hereditary spherocytosis patients lack band 3 or protein 4.2 and may have mild to moderate spherocytosis with normal amounts of spectrin and ankyrin.

includes patients with both dominant and recessive HS and a variety of molecular defects. Patients with 'severe' disease, by definition, have life-threatening anaemia and are transfusion-dependent. They almost always have recessive HS. Most have isolated, severe spectrin deficiency. In addition to the risks of recurrent transfusions, these patients often suffer from haemolytic and aplastic crises and may develop complications of severe uncompensated anaemia including growth retardation, delayed sexual maturation, or aspects of thalassaemic faces.

The parents of patients with recessive HS are clinically asymptomatic and do not have anaemia, splenomegaly, hyperbilirubinaemia, or spherocytosis on peripheral blood smears ('Trait', Table 2). Most have subtle laboratory signs of HS including: slight reticulocytosis and slightly elevated osmotic fragility. The incubated osmotic fragility test is probably the most sensitive measure of this condition, particularly the 100 per cent lysis point (0.43 ± 0.05 g NaCl/dl compared to control 0.23 ± 0.07). It has been estimated that at least 1.4 per cent of the population are silent carriers.

Inheritance

The genes responsible for HS include ankyrin, β spectrin, band 3 protein, α spectrin, and protein 4.2. In approximately two-thirds to three-quarter of HS patients, inheritance is autosomal dominant. In the remaining patients, inheritance is non-dominant due to autosomal recessive inheritance or a *de novo* mutation. Cases with autosomal recessive inheritance are due to defects in either α spectrin or protein 4.2. A surprising number of *de novo* mutations have been reported in the HS genes. A few cases of 'double dominant' HS due to defects in band 3 or spectrin that result in fetal death or severe haemolytic anaemia presenting in the neonatal period have been reported. In general, affected individuals of the same kindred experience similar degrees of haemolysis.

Complications

Gallbladder disease

Chronic haemolysis leads to the formation of bilirubinate gallstones, the most frequently reported complication in HS patients. Although gallstones have been detected in infancy, most occur between 10 and 30 years of age. Management should include interval ultrasonography to detect gallstones, as many patients with cholelithiasis and HS are asymptomatic. Timely diagnosis and treatment will help prevent complications of symptomatic biliary tract disease including biliary obstruction, cholecystitis, and cholangitis.

Haemolytic, aplastic, and megaloblastic crises

Haemolytic crises are usually associated with viral illnesses and typically occur in childhood. They are generally mild and are characterized by jaundice, increased splenomegaly, decreased haematocrit, and reticulocytosis. Intervention is rarely necessary. When severe haemolytic crises occur, there is marked jaundice, anaemia, lethargy, abdominal pain, and tender splenomegaly. Hospitalization and erythrocyte transfusion may be required.

Aplastic crises following virally-induced bone marrow suppression are uncommon, but may result in severe anaemia with serious complications including congestive heart failure or even death. The most common aetiological agent in these cases is parvovirus B19. Parvovirus selectively infects erythropoietic progenitor cells and inhibits their growth. Parvovirus infections are frequently associated with mild neutropenia, thrombocytopenia, or even pancytopenia. During the aplastic phase, the haemoglobin and the production of new red cells fall, the cells that remain age, and microspherocytosis and osmotic fragility increase. Aplastic crises usually last 10 to 14 days (about half the life span of HS red cells), the haemoglobin typically falls to half its usual level before recovery occurs. In patients with severe HS, the anaemia may be profound, requiring hospitalization and transfusion. As the marrow recovers, granulocytes, platelets, and, finally, reticulocytes return to the peripheral blood. Aplastic crisis brings many patients to medical attention, particularly asymptomatic HS patients with normally compensated haemolysis. Because parvovirus may infect several members of a family simultaneously, leading to aplastic crises, there have been reports of 'outbreaks' of HS.

Megaloblastic crisis occurs in HS patients with increased folate demands, for example the pregnant patient, growing children, or patients recovering from an aplastic crisis. With appropriate folate supplementation, this complication is preventable.

Diagnosis

The laboratory findings in HS are heterogeneous. Initial laboratory investigation should include a complete blood count with peripheral smear, reticulocyte count, Coombs' test, and serum bilirubin. When the peripheral smear or family history is suggestive of HS, an incubated osmotic fragility should be obtained. Rarely, additional, specialized testing is required to confirm the diagnosis.

Peripheral blood smear

Erythrocyte morphology is quite variable. Typical HS patients have blood smears with obvious spherocytes lacking central pallor (Fig. 2(a)). Less commonly, patients present with only a few spherocytes on peripheral smear or, at the other end of the spectrum, with numerous small, dense spherocytes and bizarre erythrocyte morphology with anisocytosis and poikilocytosis (Fig. 2(b)). Specific morphological findings have been identified in patients with certain membrane protein defects such as pincered erythrocytes (band 3) or spherocytic acanthocytes (β spectrin).

Erythrocyte indices

Most patients have mild to moderate anaemia. The mean corpuscular haemoglobin concentration is increased (between 35 and 38 per cent) due to relative cellular dehydration in approximately 50 per cent of patients, but all HS patients have some dehydrated cells. The Technicon H1 blood counter and its successors (Technicon, Tarrytown, NY) provide a histogram of mean corpuscular haemoglobin concentration that has been claimed to be accurate enough to identify nearly all HS patients. Finally, the mean corpuscular volume (MCV) is usually normal except in cases of severe HS, when it is slightly decreased.

Osmotic fragility

In the normal erythrocyte, membrane redundancy gives the cell its characteristic discoid shape and provides it with abundant surface area. In spherocytes, there is a decrease in surface area relative to cell volume, resulting in their abnormal shape. This change is reflected in the increased osmotic fragility found in these cells (Fig. 3). Osmotic fragility is tested by adding increasingly hypotonic concentrations of saline to red cells. The normal erythrocyte is able to increase its volume by swelling, but spherocytes, which are already at maximum volume for surface area, burst at higher saline concentrations than normal. Approximately 25 per cent of HS individuals will have a normal osmotic fragility on freshly drawn red cells, with the osmotic fragility curve approximating the number of spherocytes seen on peripheral smear. However, after incubation at 37°C for 24 h, HS red cells lose membrane surface area more readily than normal because their membranes are leaky and unstable. Thus incubation accentuates the defect in HS erythrocytes and brings out the defect in osmotic fragility, making incubated osmotic fragility the standard test for diagnosing HS. When the spleen is present, a subpopulation of very fragile erythrocytes, which have been conditioned by the spleen, form the 'tail' of the osmotic fragility curve; this disappears after splenectomy (Fig. 3). Osmotic fragility testing suffers from poor sensitivity as about 20 per cent of mild cases of HS are missed after incubation. It is unreliable in patients with small numbers of spherocytes, including those who have been recently transfused. It is abnormal in other conditions where spherocytes are present.

Additional testing

Other investigations, such as the autohaemolysis test, the hypertonic cryohaemolysis test, and the acidified glycerol test, suffer from lack of specificity and are not widely used. Specialized testing, such as membrane protein quantitation, ektacytometry, and genetic analyses, are available for studying difficult cases or cases where additional information is desired.

Other laboratory manifestations in HS are markers of ongoing haemolysis. Reticulocytosis, increased bilirubin, increased lactate dehydrogenase, increased urinary and faecal urobilinogen, and decreased haptoglobin reflect increased erythrocyte production or destruction.

Differential diagnosis

HS should be able to be distinguished from other haemolytic anaemias by additional diagnostic testing, such as autoimmune haemolytic anaemia via a Coombs' test. Other causes of haemolytic anaemia (Table 3) should be viewed in the appropriate clinical context. Occasional spherocytes are also seen in patients with a large spleen (such as in cirrhosis, myelofibrosis) or in patients with microangiopathic anaemias, but the differentiation of these conditions from HS is not usually difficult.

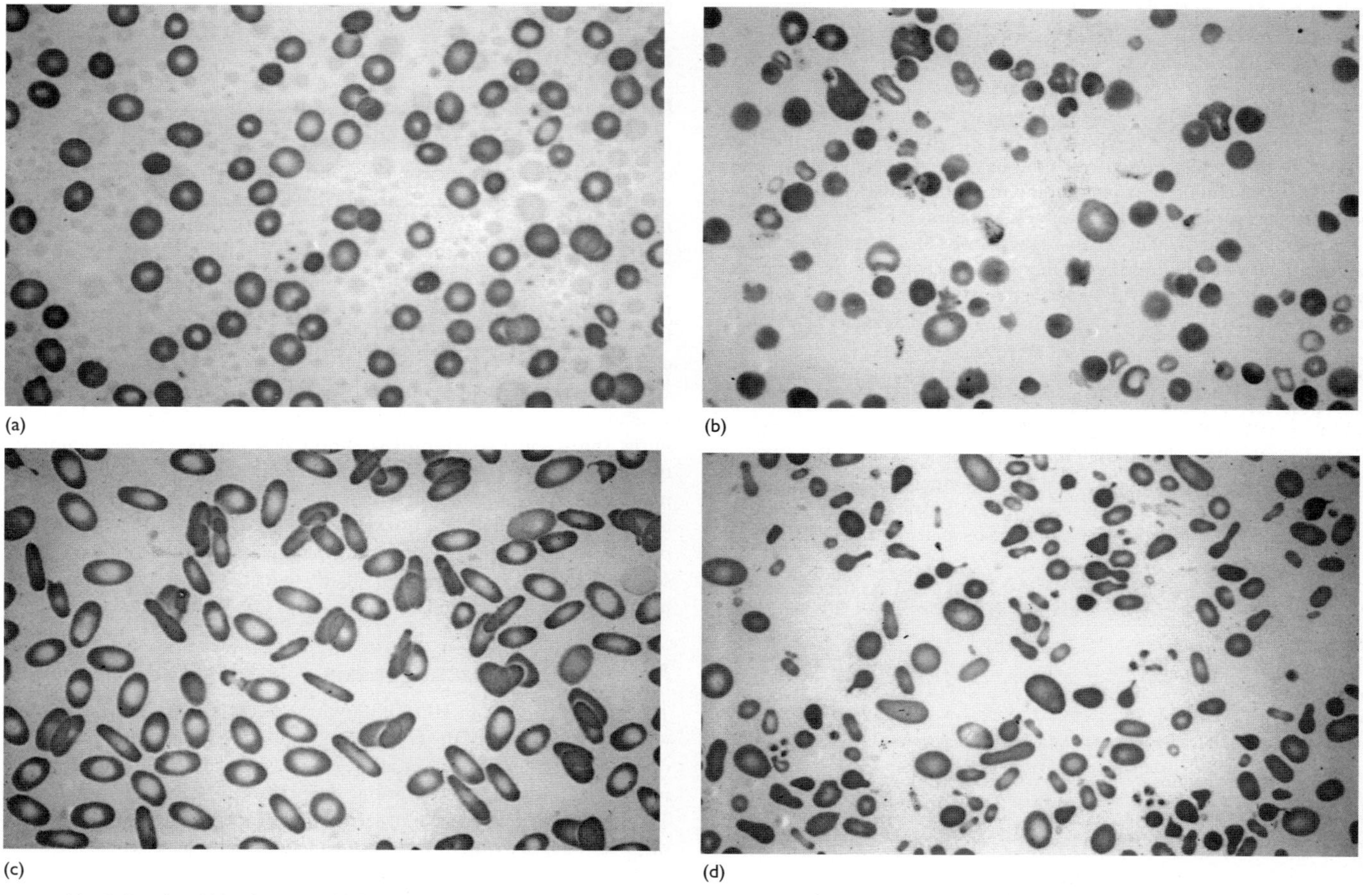

Fig. 2 Peripheral blood smears. (a) Typical hereditary spherocytosis. (b) Severe, recessively-inherited spherocytosis. (c) Hereditary elliptocytosis. (d) Hereditary pyropoikilocytosis.

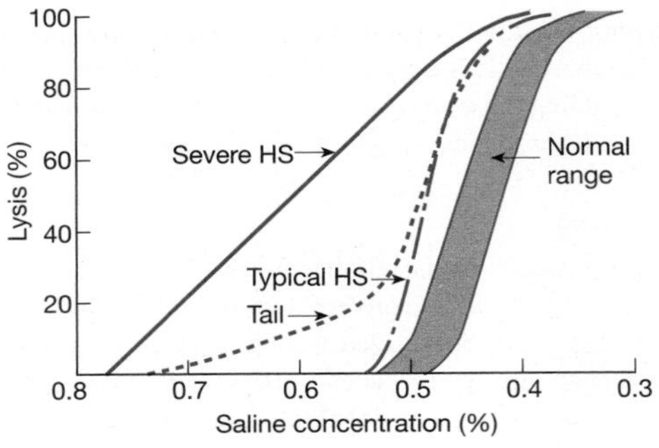

Fig. 3 Osmotic fragility curves in hereditary spherocytosis. The shaded region is the normal range. Results representative of both typical and severe spherocytosis are shown. A tail, representing very fragile erythrocytes that have been conditioned by the spleen, is common in many spherocytosis patients prior to splenectomy.

Treatment

Splenectomy

Splenic sequestration is the primary determinant of erythrocyte survival in HS patients. Thus splenectomy cures or alleviates the anaemia in the overwhelming majority of patients, reducing or eliminating the need for transfusions and decreasing the incidence of cholelithiasis. Postsplenectomy, spherocytosis and altered osmotic fragility persist, erythrocyte lifespan nearly normalizes, and reticulocyte counts fall to normal or near normal levels. Typical postsplenectomy changes, including Howell–Jolly bodies, target cells, and acanthocytes, become evident on peripheral smear. Postsplenectomy, patients with the most severe forms of HS still suffer from shortened erythrocyte survival and haemolysis, but their clinical improvement is striking.

Early complications of splenectomy include local infection, bleeding, and pancreatitis due to injury to the tail of the pancreas incurred during surgery. Overwhelming postsplenectomy infection (OPSI), typically from encapsulated organisms, is an uncommon but significant late complication of splenectomy, especially in the first few years of life. The introduction of pneumococcal vaccines and the promotion of early antibiotic therapy for febrile children who have had a splenectomy have led to decreases in the incidence of OPSI.

Indications for splenectomy

In the past, splenectomy was considered routine in HS patients. However, the risk of OPSI and the recent emergence of penicillin-resistant pneumococci have led to a re-evaluation of the role of splenectomy in the treatment of HS. Considering the risks and benefits, a reasonable approach would be to splenectomize all patients with severe spherocytosis and all patients who suffer from significant signs or symptoms of anaemia including growth failure, skeletal changes, leg ulcers, and extramedullary haematopoietic tumours. Other candidates for splenectomy are older HS patients who suffer vascular compromise of vital organs.

Whether patients with moderate HS and compensated, asymptomatic anaemia should have a splenectomy remains controversial. Patients with mild HS and compensated haemolysis can be followed and referred for splenectomy if clinically indicated. The treatment of patients with mild to moderate HS and gallstones is also debatable, particularly since new treatments for cholelithiasis, including laparoscopic cholecystectomy, endoscopic sphincterotomy, and extracorporal choletripsy, lower the risk of this complication.

When splenectomy is warranted, laparoscopic splenectomy is the method of choice as it results in less postoperative discomfort, shorter hospitalization, and decreased costs. Partial splenectomy via laparotomy has been advocated for infants and young children with significant anaemia associated with HS. The goals of this procedure are to allow for the palliation of haemolysis and anaemia while maintaining some residual splenic immune function. Long-term follow-up data for this procedure are lacking.

Prior to splenectomy, patients should be immunized with vaccines against pneumococcus, *Haemophilus influenzae* type b, and meningococcus, preferably several weeks preoperatively. The use and duration of prophylactic antibiotics postsplenectomy is controversial. Presplenectomy, and in severe cases, postsplenectomy, HS patients should take folic acid to prevent folate deficiency.

Table 3 Conditions with spherocytes on peripheral blood smear

Hereditary spherocytosis
Autoimmune haemolytic anaemia
Liver disease
Thermal injury
Microangiopathic and macroangiopathic haemolytic anaemias
Transfusion reaction with haemolysis
Clostridial sepsis
Severe hypophosphataemia
Poisoning from certain snake, spider, bee, and wasp venoms
Heinz body anaemias
Hypersplenism
ABO incompatibility (neonates)

Elliptocytosis, pyropoikilocytosis, and related disorders

Introduction

Hereditary elliptocytosis (HE) is characterized by the presence of elliptical or cigar-shaped erythrocytes on peripheral blood smears of affected individuals. The world-wide incidence of HE has been estimated to be 1 in 2000 to 4000 individuals. The true incidence of HE is unknown because most patients are asymptomatic. It is common in individuals of African and Mediterranean ancestry, presumably because elliptocytes confer some resistance to malaria. In parts of Africa, the incidence of HE approaches 1 in 100. HE is typically inherited in an autosomal dominant pattern. Rare cases of *de novo* mutations have been described.

Hereditary pyropoikilocytosis (HPP) is a rare cause of severe haemolytic anaemia with erythrocyte morphology reminiscent of that seen in severe burns. Initial studies of erythrocytes from these patients revealed abnormal thermal sensitivity compared to normal erythrocytes. HPP occurs predominantly in patients of African descent. There is a strong relationship between HPP and HE. Approximately one-third of parents or siblings of patients with HPP have typical HE. Many patients with HPP experience severe haemolysis and anaemia in infancy that gradually improves, evolving toward typical HE later in life.

Aetiology and pathogenesis

The principle defect in HE/HPP erythrocytes is an intrinsic mechanical weakness or fragility of the erythrocyte membrane skeleton due to a defect of horizontal interactions (see above). This is due to defects in the red cell membrane proteins α spectrin, β spectrin, protein 4.1, or glycophorin C. The majority of defects occur in spectrin, the principal structural protein of the membrane skeleton. A variety of mutations in the genes encoding these proteins have been described, with several mutations identified in a number of individuals on the same genetic background, suggesting a 'founder effect' for these mutations.

Clinical features

The clinical presentation of HE is heterogeneous, ranging from asymptomatic carriers to patients with severe, transfusion-dependent anaemia. Most patients with HE are asymptomatic and are typically diagnosed incidentally during testing for unrelated conditions. The erythrocyte life span is normal in most patients. The 10 per cent of patients with decreased red-cell lifespan are the ones who experience haemolysis, anaemia, splenomegaly, and intermittent jaundice. Many of these symptomatic patients have parents with typical HE and thus are homozygotes or compound heterozygotes for defects inherited from each of the parents. Symptomatology may vary between members of the same family, indeed, it may vary in the same individual at different times. To explain these observations, modifier alleles have been hypothesized to influence spectrin expression and clinical severity. One such allele, α^{LELY} (low expression Lyon), has been identified and characterized.

Diagnosis

The hallmark of HE is the presence of elliptocytes on peripheral blood smear (Fig. 2(c)). These normochromic, normocytic elliptocytes number from a few to 100 per cent. The degree of haemolysis and anaemia do not correlate with the number of elliptocytes present. A few ovalocytes, spherocytes, stomatocytes, and fragmented cells may also be seen. Elliptocytes may be seen in association with several disorders including megaloblastic anaemias, hypochromic microcytic anaemias (iron deficiency anaemia and thalassaemia), myleodysplasic syndromes, and myelofibrosis; however, elliptocytes are generally less than one-third of red cells in these conditions. History and additional laboratory testing usually clarify the diagnosis of these disorders. In addition to the peripheral blood smear findings found in HE, HPP erythrocytes are bizarre-shaped with fragmentation and budding (Fig. 2(d)). Microspherocytosis is common and the MCV is frequently decreased (50–65 mm^3).

The osmotic fragility is abnormal in severe HE and HPP. Other laboratory findings in HE are similar to those found in other haemolytic anaemias and are non-specific markers of increased erythrocyte production and destruction. When indicated, specialized testing, such as membrane protein quantitation, ektacytometry, spectrin analyses, and genetic studies can be performed.

Treatment

Therapy is rarely necessary. In rare cases, occasional red blood cell transfusions may be required. In cases of severe HE and HPP, splenectomy has been palliative. The same indications for splenectomy in HS can be applied to patients with symptomatic HE or HPP. Postsplenectomy, patients with HE or HPP experience increased haemoglobin, decreased haemolysis, and improvement in clinical symptoms.

During acute illnesses, patients should be followed for signs of haematological decompensation. Ultrasonography at regular intervals to detect gallstones should be performed. In patients with significant haemolysis, folate should be administered daily.

South-east Asian ovalocytosis (SAO)

SAO is characterized by the presence of oval erythrocytes with a central longitudinal slit or transverse bar on peripheral blood smears of affected individuals. It is common in parts of the Philippines, Indonesia, Malaysia, and New Guinea and is inherited in an autosomal dominant fashion. Incredibly rigid, SAO erythrocytes are resistant to invasion by malaria parasites. The underlying defect is a mutation in a critical region of band 3. Haematologically, patients with SAO are asymptomatic, with little or no evidence of haemolysis or anaemia. Osmotic fragility is normal. The finding of characteristic ovalocytes in the peripheral blood of an asymptomatic individual from one of the above mentioned ethnic backgrounds is highly suggestive of the diagnosis. Biochemical and DNA diagnostic techniques are available to detect this condition.

Stomatocytosis

The hereditary stomatocytosis syndromes are a heterogeneous group of disorders characterized by mouth-shaped (stomatocytic) erythrocyte morphology on peripheral blood smear (Fig. 4). The clinical severity of stomatocytosis patients is variable; some patients experience haemolysis and anaemia, while others are asymptomatic. The red blood cell membranes of stomatocytosis patients usually exhibit abnormal permeability to the cations sodium and potassium, with consequent modification of intracellular water content, ranging from dehydrated to overhydrated erythrocytes. The underlying defect(s) leading to abnormal cation permeability and red cell dehydration in these patients is unknown.

Other conditions

Other conditions associated with hereditary stomatocytosis include the Rh deficiency syndromes and familial deficiency of high-density lipoproteins. Acquired stomatocytosis has been observed in a large number of conditions, particularly hepatobiliary disease and acute alcoholism. Acquired stomatocytosis has also been seen in patients with various malignant neoplasms, cardiovascular disease, and after the administration of vinca alkaloids.

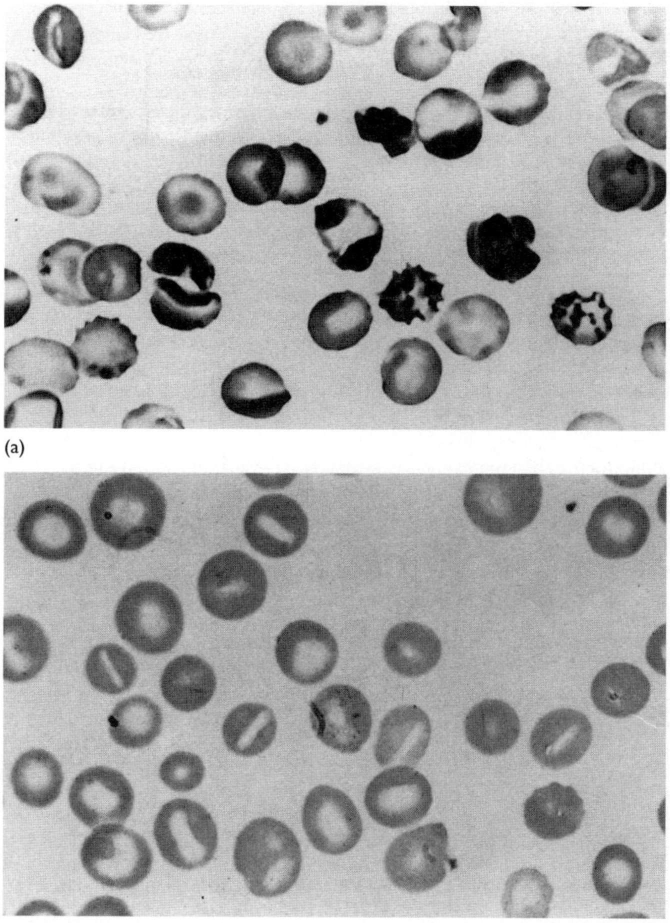

(a)

(b)

Fig. 4 Peripheral blood smears. (a) Dehydrated stomatocytosis. (b) Overhydrated stomatocytosis. (Reprinted from Lande and Mentzer, 1985, with permission.)

Further reading

Conboy J (1999). The role of alternative pre-mRNA splicing in regulating the structure and function of skeletal protein 4.1. *Proceedings of the Society for Experimental Biology and Medicine* **220**, 73–8.

Delaunay J, Dhermy D (1993). Mutations involving the spectrin heterodimer contact site: clinical expression and alterations in specific function. *Seminars in Hematology* **30**, 21–33.

Delaunay, J, Stewart G, Iolascon A (1999). Hereditary dehydrated and overhydrated stomatocytosis: recent advances. *Current Opinion in Hematology* **6**, 110–4.

Eber SW, Armbrust R, Schroter W (1990). Variable clinical severity of hereditary spherocytosis: relation to erythrocytic spectrin concentration, osmotic fragility, and autohemolysis. *Journal of Pediatrics* **117**, 409–16.

Eber SW, *et al.* (1996). Ankyrin-1 mutations are a major cause of dominant and recessive hereditary spherocytosis. *Nature Genetics* **13**, 214–8.

Gallagher PG, Forget BG, Lux SE (1998). Disorders of the erythrocyte membrane. In: Nathan D, Orkin S, eds. *Hematology of infancy and childhood*, pp. 544–664. WB Saunders, Philadelphia.

Hassoun H, *et al.* (1997). Characterization of the underlying molecular defect in hereditary spherocytosis associated with spectrin deficiency. *Blood* **90**, 398–406.

Jarolim P, *et al.* (1995). Mutations of conserved arginines in the membrane domain of erythroid band 3 lead to a decrease in membrane-associated band 3 and to the phenotype of hereditary spherocytosis. *Blood* **85**, 634–40.

Lande WM, Mentzer WC (1985). Haemolytic anaemia associated with increased cation permeability. *Clinical Haematology* **14**, 89–103.

Lux SE, Palek J (1995). Disorders of the red cell membrane. In: Handin RI, Lux SE, Stossel TP, eds. *Blood: principles and practice of hematology*, pp. 1701–816. JB Lippincott, Philadelphia.

Miraglia del Giudice E, *et al.* (1998). High frequency of de novo mutations in ankyrin gene (ANK1) in children with hereditary spherocytosis. *Journal of Pediatrics* **132**, 117–20.

Morrow JS, *et al.* (1997). Of membrane stability and mosaics: The spectrin cytoskeleton. In: Hoffman J, Jamieson J, eds. *Handbook of physiology*, pp. 485–540. Oxford University Press, London.

Tse WT, Lux SE (1999). Red blood cell membrane disorders. *British Journal of Haematology* **104**, 2–13.

Tse WT, *et al.* (1997). Amino-acid substitution in alpha-spectrin commonly coinherited with nondominant hereditary spherocytosis. *American Journal of Hematology* **54**, 233–41.

Wichterle H, *et al.* (1996). Combination of two mutant alpha spectrin alleles underlies a severe spherocytic hemolytic anemia. *Journal of Clinical Investigation* **98**, 2300–7.

Wilmotte R, *et al.* (1993). Low expression allele alpha LELY of red cell spectrin is associated with mutations in exon 40 (aV/41 polymorphism) and intron 45 and with partial skipping of exon 46. *Journal of Clinical of Investigation* **91**, 2091–6.

Yawata Y (1994). Red cell membrane protein band 4.2: phenotypic, genetic and electron microscopic aspects. *Biochimica et Biophysica Acta* **16**, 131–48.

22.5.11 Erythrocyte enzymopathies

Ernest Beutler

Erythrocytes are living cells that contain a large number of enzymes required to carry out a variety of metabolic processes. Some inherited deficiencies of these enzymes are called red-cell enzymopathies. They may cause haematological disorders, including haemolytic anaemias, polycythaemia, and methaemoglobinaemia. Other deficiencies do not produce haematological disorders, but instead mirror important metabolic disorders such as galactosaemia and are therefore of diagnostic value. Some deficiencies, for example those of lactate dehydrogenase or inosine triphosphatase (ITPase) are, as far as has been determined, 'non-diseases'.

This section deals with those red-cell enzyme defects that cause haemolytic anaemia. Many have been described; most are rare but some are sufficiently common that several hundred cases have been documented. Although the enzymatic bases of these defects are very different, the clinical presentation is similar and relatively nondescript. It is impossible to differentiate the enzymatic defects from one another by clinical or routine laboratory methods.

Red-cell metabolism

The two major pathways of red-cell glucose metabolism are illustrated in (Fig. 1).

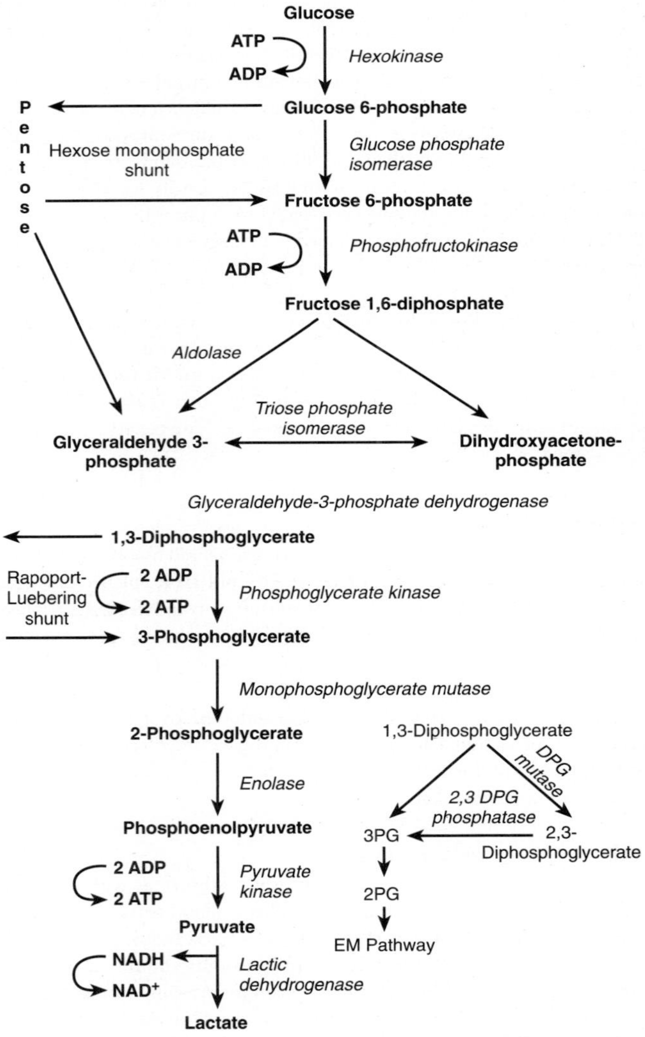

Fig. 1 The relationship between the main red-cell glycolytic pathway (Embden–Meyerhof) and the other metabolic pathways. The insert shows the production of 2,3-DPG in the Rapoport–Luebering shunt.

Glucose is phosphorylated to glucose-6-phosphate in the hexokinase reaction. It is then either metabolized in the anaerobic Embden–Myerhoff pathway or is oxidized in the glucose-6-phosphate dehydrogenase (G6PD) reaction, entering the hexose monophosphate pathway.

Anaerobic metabolism of glucose reduces NAD and, by phosphorylating ADP to ATP, provides energy to maintain erythrocyte shape and to transport molecules into and out of erythrocyte . The hexose monophosphate pathway serves to maintain glutathione and protein sulphydryl groups in the reduced state. These pathways are similar in red cells, as in other tissues and in lower organisms. However, the 2,3-diphosphoglycerate (2,3 DPG) shunt is a unique feature of the Embden–Myerhoff pathway in erythrocytes. This 'energy clutch' of erythrocyte metabolism not only allows flexibility in the amount of ATP that is generated in glycolysis, but also provides a source of 2,3-DPG, the key modulator of haemoglobin oxygen affinity. The pathway also reduces NAD to NADH, which serves to reduce methaemoglobin to haemoglobin. The hexose monophosphate pathway, on the other hand, reduces NADP to the NADPH needed to maintain sulphydryl compounds in the reduced state. There are, in addition, many other metabolic functions that the erythrocyte must carry out. Among these are the synthesis of glutathione, the synthesis and degradation of nucleotides and nucleosides, the detoxification of active oxygen radicals, and the transport of small molecules into and out of the cell.

Genetics

Half of the normal activity of red-cell enzymes is generally sufficient for normal function. Thus, haemolytic anaemias due to red-cell enzyme deficiencies occur as autosomal recessive or sex-linked disorders. Only two of the deficiencies, those of G6PD and phosphoglycerate kinase are encoded by genes on the X chromosome; all of the others are autosomal. Extensive mutation analysis at the DNA level has been performed on patients with some of the enzyme defects; notably, deficiencies of G6PD, pyruvate kinase, glucosephosphate isomerase, and triosephosphate isomerase. The vast majority of mutations of the genes encoding these enzymes are missense mutations or nonsense mutations, but a few deletions, insertions, and splicing mutations have been described. So far, with the possible exception of one mutation of triosephosphate isomerase, no regulatory mutations have been documented. DNA-based diagnosis has assumed an increasingly valuable role in the diagnosis of these disorders.

Specific red-cell abnormalities that may cause haemolytic anaemia

Table 1 summarizes a some of the clinical and genetic characteristics of red-cell enzyme deficiencies.

The more common red-cell enzyme abnormalities

G6PD deficiency

This enzymopathy is described in Chapter 22.5.12.

Pyruvate kinase deficiency

Pyruvate kinase deficiency can be considered the clinical prototype of the non-spherocytic haemolytic anaemias caused by red-cell enzymopathies. The severity of the anaemia varies greatly from patient-to-patient. At one extreme, the anaemia can be quite mild; at the other, the patient may be entirely transfusion-dependent. Indeed, the circulating red cells in such patients may have normal pyruvate kinase activity because there are scarcely any of the patient's own cells present; it appears that most of the patient's cells are destroyed before they leave the marrow and it may be only the transfused cells that are sampled and sent to the laboratory for diagnosis. Pyruvate-kinase-deficient patients have the usual stigmata of haemolytic anaemia; that is, pallor, lack of energy, jaundice, and sometimes gallstones. In those patients who are transfusion-dependent, haemochromatosis occurs with some frequency, probably more so than in patients with many other types of haemolytic anaemia. Patients with pyruvate kinase deficiency usually enjoy a fairly good response to splenectomy. This response is less complete than is observed in hereditary spherocytosis, but may be clinically quite helpful, particularly in reducing the requirement for transfusions.

Pyruvate kinase deficiency is probably the most difficult of all of the red-cell enzymopathies to diagnose, because the enzyme is a complex one with allosteric properties. The residual enzyme activity is not always greatly reduced. Cases have been described in which the residual pyruvate kinase activity is actually higher than is found in normal individuals. In such cases, establishing the diagnosis may depend upon showing that the level of 2,3 DPG or of 3-phosphoglyceric acid in the erythrocytes is greatly elevated, a finding that is characteristic of pyruvate kinase deficiency. It is also useful to measure the thermal stability of the residual enzyme; mutant enzymes are very often unstable on heating. Many different mutations have been documented in patients with pyruvate kinase deficiency. In European populations, the most common of these is a G→ A mutation at nucleotide 1529 coding for a Arg→Gly substitution at amino acid 510. This mutation has not been detected among Asians with pyruvate kinase deficiency; among Gypsies the characteristic mutation is a deletion of exon 11.

The less common red-cell enzyme abnormalities

Glucosephosphate isomerase deficiency

Patients with glucosephosphate isomerase deficiency generally have a milder haemolytic disorder than patients with pyruvate kinase deficiency. The response to splenectomy is usually satisfactory. Although milder in general, this enzymopathy seems to be associated with hydrops fetalis more frequently than the other red-cell enzyme defects. Diagnosis is generally straightforward. A fluorescent screening test can be used to detect the deficiency. Several different mutations have been documented. With few exceptions, they are different in each family.

Pyrimidine 5′-nucleotidase deficiency

Basophilic stippling is the hallmark of pyrimidine 5′-nucleotidase deficiency. Interestingly, this enzyme is very sensitive to inhibition by lead. The stippling that is so characteristic of lead poisoning may be the consequences of inhibition of this enzyme. Pyrimidine 5′-nucleotidase is the most age-sensitive all of the red-cell enzymes; this one alone is decreased in activity in aplastic anaemia or other disorders, such as transient erythroblastopenia of childhood, in which the mean red cell age is greatly increased. This can lead to misdiagnosis; while it is not uncommon to encounter enzyme activities of one-half normal in patients with decreased erythropoiesis, these patients do not suffer from clinically significant pyrimidine 5′-nucleotidase deficiency. Accumulation of pyrimidine nucleotides, which can be documented by measuring the ultraviolet absorption spectrum, does not occur in such patients.

Triosephosphate isomerase deficiency

Triosephosphate isomerase deficiency is the most devastating all of the red-cell enzymopathies. With few exceptions, patients with this abnormality die by the time they are 4 years of age. All tissues are affected, and death is usually due to cardiopulmonary complications. It is been suggested, on the basis of enzyme activities and genetic studies, that the heterozygous state for this deficiency is very common among African-Americans. This has not been confirmed. Many different mutations have been detected in patients with triosephosphate isomerase deficiency; one, at genomic nucleotide

1591, accounts for approximately 50 per cent of the patients with this disorder. Polymorphic changes occur in the promoter region of the triosephosphate isomerase gene, but the significance of these mutations is not yet clear. No treatment has been effective.

The rare red-cell enzyme deficiencies

Hexokinase deficiency

Hexokinase deficiency is one of the more difficult red-cell enzymopathies to diagnose, because the activity of this enzyme is much higher in young red cells than in older erythrocytes. As a result, red-cell hexokinase activity is usually increased in patients with haemolytic anaemia of any type. In patients with hexokinase deficiency, this often gives rise to the anomalous finding that the red-cell hexokinase activity in the affected patient is normal, usually higher than that found in the heterozygous parents. The diagnostic hallmark is normal, rather than elevated, hexokinase activity in the face of a high reticulocyte count and high levels of other red-cell enzymes.

Enzymes of glutathione synthesis

Erythrocytes synthesize glutathione from the amino acids glutamate, cysteine, and glycine in two consecutive enzymatic reactions, each of which utilizes ATP. In the first step, catalysed by γ-glutamylcysteine synthetase, a peptide bond is formed between the γ-carboxyl group of glutamic acid and cysteine. Several patients deficient in this enzyme have been found. In addition to haemolytic anaemia, spinocerebellar degeneration was documented in the initial patient described, but neurological symptoms have not been present in subsequent patients. Defects of the second step of glutathione synthesis, the formation of a peptide link between γ-glutamylcysteine and glycine, catalysed by the enzyme glutathione synthetase, appear in two clinical forms. In some patients, the deficiency is limited to

Table 1 Red-cell enzyme abnormalities leading to haematological disease

Enzyme	Clinical features	Inheritance[a]	Red cell morphology	Response to splenectomy[b]	Prevalence[c]
Hexokinase	HNSHA[d]	AR	Unremarkable	++	Rare
Glucose phosphate isomerase	HNSHA Neurological abnormalities (?)	AR	Unremarkable	+++	Unusual
Phosphofructokinase	HNSHA and/or muscle glycogen storage disease	AR	Unremarkable	0	Rare
Aldolase	HNSHA and mild liver glycogen storage; ? mental retardation	AR	Unremarkable	?	Very rare
Triosephosphate isomerase	HNSHA and severe neuromuscular disease	AR	Unremarkable		Rare
Phosphoglycerate kinase	HNSHA; myoglobinuria; behavioural disturbances	SL	Unremarkable	++	Rare
Bisphosphoglycerate mutase	HNSHA; polycythaemia	AR	Unremarkable		Rare
Pyruvate kinase	HNSHA	AR	Usually unremarkable; occasional contracted echinocytes	++	Unusual
Glucose-6-phosphate dehydrogenase	HNSHA; drug or infection-induced haemolysis; favism	SL	Usually unremarkable; rarely 'bite cells'	±	Very common
Glutathione reductase (complete)	Drug sensitive haemolytic anaemia and favism	AR	Unremarkable	?	Very rare
γ-Glutamyl cysteine synthetase	HNSHA; drug- or infection-induced haemolysis; spinocerebellar degeneration (?)	AR	Unremarkable	?	Very rare
Glutathione synthetase	HNSHA; drug- or infection-induced haemolysis; neurological defect and 5-oxoprolinuria in some cases	AR	Usually unremarkable	0	Rare
Pyrimidine-5′-nucleotidase	HNSHA; ? mental retardation in some cases	AR	Prominent stippling	0	Rare
Adenosine deaminase (increased activity)	HNSHA	AD	Unremarkable		Rare
Adenosine deaminase (decreased activity)	Immunodeficiency	AR	Unremarkable		Rare
NADH-diaphorase (cytochrome b_5 reductase)	Methaemoglobinaemia; sometimes with mental retardation	AR	Unremarkable		Unusual

[a] AR = autosomal recessive; AD = autosomal dominant; SL = sex linked.

[b] On a scale of 0 to 4+ where 4+ is a complete response. In many cases data are meagre.

[c] Very common if incidence is greater than 5 per cent. Unusual if more than 100 cases reported. Rare if 10 to 100 cases reported. Very rare if less than 10 cases reported.

[d] Hereditary non-spherocytic haemolytic anaemia.

the erythrocytes. Haemolytic anaemia appears to be the sole clinical manifestation. In other patients, the deficiency is generalized. These patients excrete large amounts of pyroglutamic acid (5-oxyproline); this product of γ-glutamylcysteine degradation is overproduced in the absence of the feedback inhibition of γ-glutamylcysteine synthetase by glutathione. Patients with the generalized defect have severe neuromuscular manifestations in addition to haemolytic anaemia.

Glutathione reductase deficiency

Only a single family with a severe, hereditary deficiency of glutathione reductase has been described. No haemolysis was present except after the ingestion of fava beans. Low activity of red-cell glutathione reductase, a flavin enzyme, are found when the intake of riboflavine is suboptimal, but this mild or moderate enzyme deficiency has no clinical consequences.

Phosphofructokinase kinase deficiency

Erythrocytes contain two types of genetically distinct phosphofructokinase subunits, L (liver) and M (muscle). Deficiency of the M subunit causes haemolysis, but the haemoglobin level in the blood is often normal or even higher than normal because of the diminished 2,3 DPG levels that are characteristic of this disorder. Muscle enzyme activity is also compromised and a myopathy results. This disorder is sometimes designated Tarui disease or type VII glycogenosis. Deficiency of the L subunit of phosphofructokinase has also been reported, but did not have any clinical consequences.

Aldolase deficiency

A few cases of aldolase deficiency been reported. An association with mental retardation was noted in one case, but it is not clear whether a cause-and-effect relationship exists.

Phosphoglycerate kinase deficiency

Phosphoglycerate kinase shares with G6PD deficiency the distinction of being an X-linked enzymopathy. In addition to haemolytic anaemia, behavioural disturbances have been noted.

Diphosphoglycerate mutase deficiency

The result of diphosphoglycerate mutase deficiency is more frequently erythrocytosis than haemolytic anaemia, because a lack of this enzyme prevents the formation of 2,3 DPG. Consequently, the oxygen affinity of the red cells is increased, stimulating erythropoiesis.

High adenosine deaminase activity

Haemolytic anaemia, inherited as an autosomal dominant disorder, has rarely been found to be associated with greatly elevated red-cell adenosine deaminase levels. The adenosine deaminase that is formed appears to be normal. The abnormality that causes this tissue-specific increase in enzyme activity has not yet been discovered.

Adenylate kinase deficiency

A number of patients with familial haemolytic anaemia have been documented to have markedly decreased levels of red-cell adenylate kinase. However, one very well-studied patient with virtually absent enzyme activity had no clinical disorder. The relationship between this enzyme deficiency and haemolytic anaemia remains unclear.

Specific red-cell abnormalities that do not cause haemolytic anaemia

Severe deficiencies of many red-cell enzymes do not produce haematological abnormality or, indeed, in many cases, no clinical abnormality of all. Included are deficiencies of 6-phosphogluconate dehydrogenase, δ-aminolevulinic acid dehydrase, acetylcholinesterase, AMP deaminase, carbonic anhydrase, catalase, galactokinase, galactose-1-phosphate uridyltransferase, glutathione peroxidase, hypoxanthine-guanine phosphoribosyltransferase, ITPase, and phosphoglucomutase. Discussion of these enzyme deficiencies is beyond the scope of this chapter.

Diagnosis

The diagnosis of red-cell enzymopathies has been carried out at four levels: morphological observations, study of autohaemolysis, quantification of red-cell enzyme activity, and DNA analysis.

Morphological observations

The appearance of erythrocytes on a stained blood film may be useful in determining whether haemolytic anaemia is present and in ruling out some causes of haemolysis, such as hereditary spherocytosis, ovalocytosis, or microangiopathic haemolytic anaemia. The presence of prominent red-cell stippling suggests a diagnosis of pyrimidine 5′ nucleotidase deficiency.

The autohaemolysis test

The autohaemolysis test is performed by incubating sterile, whole blood with and without glucose for 24 h and observing the degree to which the red cells are lysed. This test outlived its usefulness as a tool for differentiating enzymatic cause of haemolytic anaemia many years ago. Although it is true that the haemolysis of pyruvate-kinase-deficient red cells occurring *in vitro* after incubation for 24 h is not usually corrected by glucose, this is by no means always the case, nor is this pattern specific for pyruvate kinase deficiency.

Qualitative and quantitative estimations of red-cell enzyme activity

The most generally useful means for differentiating red-cell enzyme defects from one another and from defects other than known enzyme deficiencies is to semiquantitate or quantitate the red-cell enzyme activities. Fluorescent screening tests have been developed that allow the non-specialized laboratory to detect decreases in the activity of enzymes such as G6PD, pyruvate kinase, glucosephosphate isomerase, or triosephosphate isomerase with a high degree of reliability. The accumulation of pyrimidine nucleotides can be detected by measuring the ultraviolet spectrum of a perchloric acid extract of red cells. This can be used by non-specialized laboratories to detect this abnormality.

Quantification of red-cell enzyme activities is a more specialized task that can be accomplished by the use of standardized techniques in an experienced laboratory. There are a number of caveats that must be taken into account, both with respect to the performance of red-cell enzyme assays and the interpretation of the results. Leucocyte pyruvate kinase and red-cell pyruvate kinase are encoded by different genes. Moreover, the activity of the white cell enzyme is very high. Thus, contamination of a red-cell suspension with a relatively small number of white cells may obscure the diagnosis of red-cell pyruvate kinase deficiency. The interpretation of the results of red-cell enzyme assays may also be confounded by the fact that the blood of patients with haemolytic anaemia is enriched with reticulocytes and young erythrocytes. Since many of the mutations that cause red-cell enzymopathies result in the production of unstable enzymes, the young erythrocytes that circulate may actually contain normal or near-normal levels of enzyme. It is therefore essential to take into account the age of the circulating cells. It may be helpful to obtain blood samples from parents or children of the patient to determine whether half normal activities can be documented.

Problems in interpretation may also arise when the activity of an enzyme as measured *in vitro* does not accurately reflect its intracellular *in vivo* activity. This comes about because of the necessity of using unphysiologically high substrate concentrations for *in vitro* assays. This difficulty is particularly prone to arise in the case of pyruvate kinase deficiency, because this is a complex allosteric enzyme that not only has binding sites for two substrates, ADP and phosphoenolpyruvate, but also for fructose diphosphate, an allosteric effector.

Finally, there is the confounding effect of red-cell transfusions. It is clearly best to wait until just before a transfusion to draw blood for testing.

DNA-based diagnosis

With the development of PCR-based technologies for the detection of mutations, and for the sequencing of DNA, mutation analysis at the DNA level has played an increasing role in the diagnosis of red-cell enzyme defects. DNA is extracted from peripheral blood leucocytes and the exons of the gene of interest are amplified. Alternatively, RNA may be reverse transcribed and the cDNA amplified. Because the stability of DNA is greater than that of RNA, and samples may need to be transported to distant, specialized laboratories, direct DNA amplification of genomic DNA rather than of cDNA is generally the preferred technology. DNA-based diagnosis is not particularly difficult to perform in laboratories experienced with the techniques involved. It has some advantages over enzyme assay-based diagnosis. First of all, DNA is very stable, even before it is purified. Therefore, shipping of blood is less of a logistical problem. Transfused red cells do not pose a problem in performing DNA-based diagnosis, since transfused leucocytes do not persist in the circulation. Once the mutation has been established, family studies are more readily performed; heterozygote detection using quantitative enzyme levels is often of a dubious reliability. Prenatal diagnosis, too, is more readily accomplished utilizing DNA-based diagnosis.

There are some major disadvantages in DNA-based diagnosis of red-cell enzymopathies. While it is quite straightforward to identify a known mutation in the coding region of one of the red-cell enzymes, doing so by examining the genes that encode all of the enzymes that may be involved as a cause of haemolytic anaemia would be a daunting task. Even if the entire coding region of the enzyme is sequenced, one cannot be certain that the mutation was not be in a promoter, an enhancer, or in a splice site.

A general approach to diagnosis of red-cell enzymopathies

The first step is to make certain that the patient has a haemolytic anaemia. The reticulocyte count should be elevated, unless it has been temporarily suppressed by infection. If the patient's history suggests that the anaemia is chronic in nature, a positive family history can be very helpful. Dominant inheritance suggests that an enzymopathy is not the cause; only the very rare anaemia caused by elevated adenosine deaminase levels falls into this category. Instead, dominant inheritance suggests that the patient either has an unstable haemoglobin or hereditary spherocytosis. Sex-linked inheritance may also appear as though it is dominant, but is excluded if there is father-to-son transmission. G6PD deficiency and phosphoglycerate kinase deficiency are the only red-cell enzymopathies that are sex-linked. Often there is no clear-cut family history. Before trying to establishing whether or not a red-cell enzymopathy is present, hereditary spherocytosis, haemoglobinopathies, and other disorders, such as a paroxysmal nocturnal haemoglobinuria, should be excluded.

Fluorescent screening tests are appropriate starting points for the diagnosis of the red-cell enzymopathies. Screening tests for G6PD deficiency, pyruvate kinase deficiency, glucosephosphate isomerase deficiency should be carried out. If the patient is a child with neuromuscular disease, a fluorescent test for triosephosphate isomerase deficiency is also indicated. Stippling of the red cells suggests that the patient may have pyrimidine 5′ nucleotidase deficiency. In this instance the ultraviolet spectrum of a perchloric acid of extract of the red cells should be examined. A clear-cut positive screening test for one of the red-cell enzymopathies, carried out with appropriate controls, is adequate for diagnosis. Quantitative assays for red-cell enzymes can be performed by specialized laboratories and the may include those enzymes for which no screening tests have been developed.

When a diagnosis has been established, either by performing a screening test or by quantitative assay, it is sometimes useful to identify the mutation at the DNA level. This need not be done in every case, but is particularly useful in the case of young couples who hope to have more children and desire genetic counselling and prenatal diagnosis.

Further reading

Baronciani L, Bianchi P, Zanella A (1998). Hematologically important mutations: Red cell pyruvate kinase (2nd update). *Blood Cells, Molecules, and Diseases* **24**, 271–7. [Compilation of the PK mutations.]

Baronciani L, Zanella A, Bianchi P, *et al.* (1996). Study of the molecular defects in glucose phosphate isomerase-deficient patients affected by chronic hemolytic anemia. *Blood* **88**, 2306–10. [The GPI gene and mutations that affect it.]

Beutler E, Blume KG, Kaplan JC, *et al.* (1977). International committee for standardization in haematology: Recommended methods for red-cell enzyme analysis. *British Journal of Haematology* **35**, 331–40. [Standardized methods for the enzymatic diagnosis of red cell enzymopathies.]

Bianchi M, Magnani M (1995). Hexokinase mutations that produce nonspherocytic hemolytic anemia. *Blood Cells, Molecules, and Diseases* **21**, 2–8. [Description of the first hexokinase mutation at the DNA level.]

Fujii H, Miwa S (1999). Red blood cell enzymes and their clinical application. *Advances in Clinical Chemistry* **33**, 1–54. [A good review.]

Jacobasch G, Rapoport SM (1996). Hemolytic anemias due to erythrocyte enzyme deficiencies. *Molecular Aspects Medicine* **17**, 143–70. [A good review.]

Lenzner C, Nürnberg P, Jacobasch G, *et al.* (1997). Molecular analysis of 29 pyruvate kinase-deficient patients from Central Europe with hereditary hemolytic anemia. *Blood* **89**, 1793–9. [Clinical and molecular analysis of PK mutations.]

Lestas AN, Kay LA, Bellingham AJ (1987). Red cell 3-phosphoglycerate level as a diagnostic aid in pyruvate kinase deficiency. *British Journal of Haematology* **67**, 485–8. [The value of intermediate levels in the diagnosis of pyruvate kinase deficiency.]

Schneider A, Cohen-Solal M (1996). Hematologically important mutations: Triosephosphate isomerase. *Blood Cells, Molecules, and Diseases* **22**, 82–4. [Compilation of the TPI mutations]

Schneider A, Forman L, Westwood B, *et al.* (1998). The relationship of the -5, -8, and -24 mutations in African-Americans to triosephosphate isomerase (TPI) enzyme activity and to TPI deficiency. *Blood* **92**, 2959–62. [The TPI promoter mutations and their effect on enzyme activity.]

Tarui S, Okuno G, Ikura Y, *et al.* (1965). Phosphofructokinase deficiency in skeletal muscle. A new type of glycogenosis. *Biochemical and Biophysical Research Communications* **19**, 517–23. [Original description of phosphofructokinase deficiency as a glycogen storage disease.]

Valentine WN, Paglia DE (1990). Erythroenzymopathies and hemolytic anemia: The many faces of inherited variant enzymes. *Journal of Laboratory and Clinical Medicine* **115**, 12–20. [A good review.]

22.5.12 Glucose-6-phosphate dehydrogenase (G6PD) deficiency

Lucio Luzzatto

Definition

Glucose-6-phosphate dehydrogenase (**G6PD**) is a key enzyme in redox metabolism. G6PD deficiency is an inherited condition in which red cells have a markedly decreased activity of G6PD, which predisposes to haemolytic anaemia.

Epidemiology

G6PD deficiency is distributed worldwide. Areas of high prevalence are found in Africa, Southern Europe, the Middle East, South-East Asia, and Oceania. In the Americas and in parts of Northern Europe, G6PD deficiency is also quite prevalent as a result of migrations that have taken place in relatively recent historical times.

Genetics

The inheritance of G6PD deficiency has long been known to have a mendelian X-linked pattern, and the gene encoding G6PD has been mapped to the telomeric region of the long arm of the X chromosome (band Xq28), physically very close to the genes for haemophilia A, dyskeratosis congenita, and colour blindness. At the genomic level, the G6PD gene consists of 13 exons and spans some 18.5 kb (kilobases). Structural and functional studies have revealed features of a 'housekeeping gene'; this is in accord with the fact that G6PD is found in all cells.

X linkage of the G6PD gene has important implications. First, as males have only one G6PD gene (being hemizygous for this gene), they must be either normal or G6PD deficient. By contrast, females, having two G6PD genes, can be either normal or deficient (homozygous), or intermediate (heterozygous). Moreover, as a result of the phenomenon of X-chromosome inactivation, heterozygous females are genetic mosaics, and this in turn has clinical implications. Indeed, in most other (autosomal) enzyme deficiencies, heterozygotes are asymptomatic because cells with an enzyme level close to 50 per cent of normal are biochemically normal. But in the case of G6PD, as a result of X inactivation, the abnormal cells of a woman heterozygous for G6PD deficiency are just as deficient as those of a hemizygous deficient man, and therefore just as susceptible to pathology. Thus, although G6PD deficiency is still often referred to as an X-linked recessive trait, this is a mismomer because a recessive trait is, by definition, not expressed in a heterozygote; instead, G6PD deficiency is expressed in heterozygotes both biochemically and clinically—although it is true that heterozygotes are generally less severely affected.

Clinical manifestations

Acute haemolytic anaemia

In view of the large number of people who carry a G6PD deficiency gene, it is fortunate that the vast majority remain clinically asymptomatic throughout their lifetime. However, they are all at risk of developing acute haemolytic anaemia in response to three types of triggers: (i) drugs (Table 1), (ii) infections, and (iii) broad (fava) beans. Typically, a haemolytic attack starts with malaise, sometimes associated with more or less profound weakness, and abdominal or lumbar pain. After an interval of several hours to 2 or 3 days (usually the onset is more abrupt in children) the patient develops jaundice and dark urine, due to haemoglobinuria. In the majority of cases the haemolytic attack, even if severe, is self-limiting and tends to resolve spontaneously. In the absence of additional or pre-existing pathology the bone marrow response is prompt and effective. Depending on the proportion of red cells that have been destroyed (reflected in the severity of the anaemia), the haemoglobin level may be back to normal in 3 to 6 weeks. The most serious threat in adults is the development of acute renal failure (this is exceedingly rare in children). The anaemia is usually normocytic and normochromic, and it varies from moderate to extremely severe (haemoglobin levels of 4 g/dl or less have been recorded); it is due largely to intravascular haemolysis, and hence it is associated with haemoglobinaemia, haemoglobinuria, and low or absent plasma haptoglobin. The blood film shows anisocytosis, polychromasia, and other features associated with acute haemolysis, including spherocytes (Fig. 1); in severe cases the poikilocytosis is very marked, with bizarre forms, numerous red cells that appear to have unevenly distributed haemoglobin ('hemighosts'), and red cells that appear to have had parts of them bitten away ('bite cells' or 'blister cells'). Supravital staining with methyl violet, if done promptly, reveals the presence of 'Heinz bodies', consisting of precipitates of denatured haemoglobin (Fig. 1; apart from the rare cases when they are formed because of a genetic haemoglobin abnormality, Heinz bodies can be regarded as a signature of oxidative damage to red cells). The white blood cell count may be elevated, with predominance of granulocytes. The platelet count may be normal, increased, or moderately decreased. The unconjugated bilirubin is elevated but the 'liver enzymes' are usually normal.

Favism

This is perhaps the most spectacular form of acute haemolytic anaemia associated with G6PD deficiency; it can occur at any age, but more commonly in children. The child initially becomes very fractious; then he may develop fever, abdominal pain, diarrhoea, and sometimes vomiting; then he may become lethargic. Haemoglobinuria develops within 6 to 24 h from the onset of symptoms. Physical examination reveals pallor, tachycardia, jaundice, and an enlarged spleen; in severe cases there may be evidence of hypovolaemic shock or, more rarely, of high-output heart failure. The cause of favism is the presence in broad beans (or fava beans: *Vicia faba*) of vicine and convicine, two β-glycosides having as aglycones the substituted pyrimidines divicine and isouramil, which produce free radicals in the course of their auto-oxidation. Thus, haemolysis is highly specific for broad beans; other beans are safe. G6PD-deficient subjects (especially when they are adults) do not develop an acute attack of favism every time they eat broad beans; the reasons for this are not yet clear, but important factors are the

Table 1 Drugs and other agents that can cause haemolysis in people with G6PD deficiency

Drugs	Definite association	Possible or doubtful association[1]
Anti-malarials	Primaquine Pamaquine Pentaquine	Chloroquine Quinacrine Quinine
Sulphon-amides	Sulphanilamide Sulphacetamide Sulphapyridine	Sulphamethoxypyridazine Sulphoxone Sulphadiazine Sulphamerizine Sulphisoxazole
Sulphones	Thiazolesulphone Dapsone	
Nitrofurans	Nitrofurantoin	
Antipyretic/ analgesic	Acetanilide	Aspirin Aminopyrine Paracetamol Phenacetin
Other drugs	Nalidixic acid Niridazole Methylene blue Phenazopyridine	Ciprofloxacin Para-aminosalicylic acid Norfloxacin L-Dopa Chloramphenicol Doxorubicin Vitamin K analogues Probenecid Ascorbic acid Dimercaprol
Other chemicals	Naphthalene Trinitrotoluene Toluidine blue	

[1] These drugs can probably cause haemolysis only when given at high doses.

quantity and quality of broad beans consumed. On the other hands, the widespread notion that favism occurs only with some G6PD-deficient variants and not with others is incorrect. For instance, favism has now been well documented with the 'African' variant A–, and even with G6PD Seattle, a variant associated with milder enzyme deficiency.

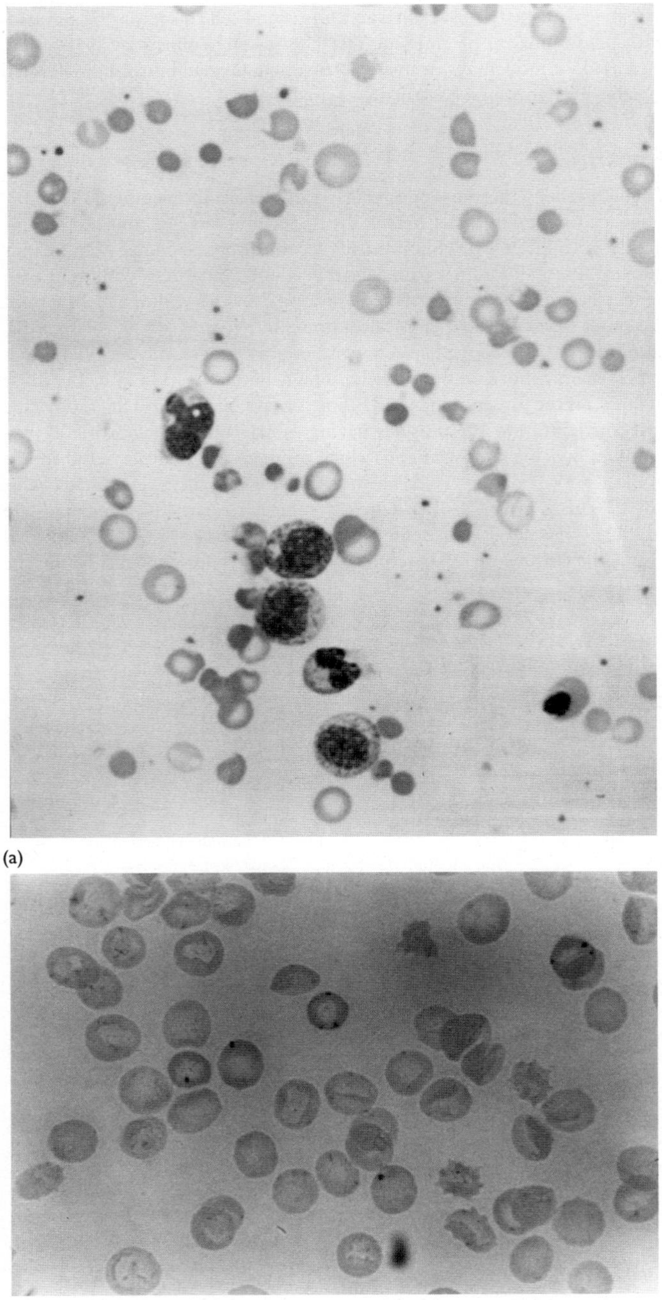

(a)

(b)

Fig. 1 Blood film in a case of acute haemolytic anaemia in a G6PD-deficient patient (favism). (a) Romanovsky stain, showing marked poikilocytosis, polychromatic macrocytes, bite cells, nucleated red cells, and a shift to the left in the granulocytic series. (b) Supravital stain with methyl violet, showing the characteristic Heinz bodies.

Neonatal jaundice

Not every G6PD-deficient baby becomes jaundiced after birth; however, the risk of developing neonatal jaundice is much greater in G6PD-deficient than in G6PD-normal neonates. The extent of the association between G6PD deficiency and neonatal jaundice appears to vary greatly in different populations. The clinical picture of neonatal jaundice related to G6PD deficiency differs from the 'classic' Rhesus-related neonatal jaundice in two main respects: (i) it is very rarely present at birth, and the peak incidence of clinical onset is between day 2 and 3; and (ii) jaundice is more prominent than anaemia, and the anaemia is very rarely severe. The severity of G6PD-related neonatal jaundice varies enormously, from subclinical to overlapping with 'physiological jaundice' to imposing the threat of kernicterus if not treated. The reasons for this are not clear, but prematurity, infection, and environmental factors (for instance, naphthalene–camphor balls used in babies' bedding and clothing) certainly play a part in making neonatal jaundice more severe and more dangerous. From the point of view of public health, it is important to realize that in some parts of the world G6PD deficiency is the commonest cause of severe neonatal jaundice; in addition, if not correctly managed, severe neonatal jaundice can produce permanent neurological damage.

Chronic non-spherocytic haemolytic anaemia

In contrast to the large majority of G6PD-deficient subjects who have minimal and subclinical haemolysis in the steady state, a small minority have chronic anaemia of very variable severity. The patient is always male, and in general he presents because of unexplained jaundice. Frequently the onset is at birth, and a diagnosis is made of neonatal jaundice (Fig. 2), which may be severe enough to require exchange transfusion. Subsequently the anaemia recurs and the jaundice fails to clear completely; or the patients is only reinvestigated much later in life, perhaps because of gallstones in a child or in a young adult. Usually the spleen is moderately enlarged in small children, and subsequently it may increase in size sufficiently to cause mechanical discomfort, or hypersplenism, or both. The severity of anaemia ranges in different patients from borderline to transfusion dependent. The anaemia is usually normochromic but somewhat macrocytic; because a large proportion of reticulocytes (up to 20 per cent or more) will cause an increased mean corpuscle volume and a shifted, wider than normal, size-distribution curve. The red cell morphology is not characteristic, and for this reason it is referred to in the negative as being 'non-spherocytic'. The bone marrow is normoblastic, unless the increased requirement of folic acid associated with the high red cell turnover has caused it to become

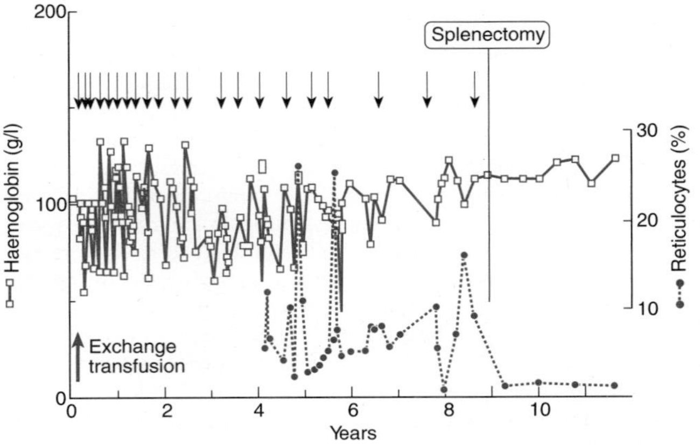

Fig. 2 Clinical course of a patient with chronic non-spherocytic haemolytic anaemia caused by severe G6PD deficiency, illustrating the high transfusion requirement, which was alleviated after splenectomy.

megaloblastic. There is chronic hyperbilirubinaemia, decreased haptoglobin, and increased lactate dehydrogenase. In this condition, unlike in the acute haemolytic anaemia described above, haemolysis is mainly extravascular. However, the red cells of these patients are naturally also vulnerable to acute oxidative damage, and therefore the same agents that can cause acute haemolytic anaemia in people with the ordinary type of G6PD deficiency will cause severe exacerbations with (sometimes massive) haemoglobinuria in people with the severe form of G6PD deficiency.

Laboratory diagnosis

Although the clinical picture of favism and of other forms of acute haemolytic anaemia associated with G6PD deficiency is quite characteristic, the final diagnosis must rely on the direct demonstration of decreased activity of this enzyme in red cells. With neonatal jaundice and chronic non-spherocytic haemolytic anaemia the differential diagnosis is much wider, and therefore this test is even more important. The most popular screening tests are the dye decolorization test, the methaemoglobin reduction test, and the fluorescence spot test. Any of these, provided it is properly standardized and subjected to quality control, is perfectly adequate for diagnostic purposes in patients who are in the steady state; but these semiquantitative tests are not adequate for patients in the acute haemolytic or in the post-haematolytic period, or with other complications; nor can they be expected to identify all heterozygotes. Ideally, every patient found to be G6PD deficient by screening should then be retested for confirmation by a quantitative assay. In normal red cells the range of G6PD activity, measured at 30°C, is 7 to 10 iu/g of haemoglobin. In G6PD-deficient males (or homozygous females) the level of G6PD in the steady state is, by definition, less than 50 per cent of normal; but with most variants it is less than 20 per cent and with some it is practically undetectable. In heterozygous females the level is intermediate and extremely variable; therefore, in some cases the diagnosis may be difficult without family studies or DNA analysis. However, for practical purposes it is most unlikely that a woman will have clinical manifestations if her G6PD level is more than 70 per cent of normal.

Biochemistry and pathophysiology

Red cells are very vulnerable to oxidative damage for two reasons. First, oxygen radicals are generated continuously from within the red cells as haemoglobin cycles from its deoxygenated to its oxygenated form. Second, red cells are directly exposed to a variety of exogenous oxidizing agents. Oxygen radicals produced by such compounds are converted by superoxide dismutase to hydrogen peroxide, which is itself highly toxic. G6PD, the first enzyme of the pentose phosphate pathway (Fig. 3), catalyses the conversion of glucose-6-phosphate (G6P) and NADP to 6-phosphogluconolactone and NADPH. The most important product of the G6PD reaction, certainly in red cells, is NADPH because, by producing glutathione via glutathione reductase, it is crucial for the operation of glutathione peroxidase; in addition, it stabilizes catalase: these are the two enzymes able to detoxify hydrogen peroxide (by converting it to water). Normally, G6PD activity in red cells is such that NADPH is maintained at a high level and there is practically no NADP: the NADPH/NADP ratio plays a large part in the intracellular regulation of G6PD activity.

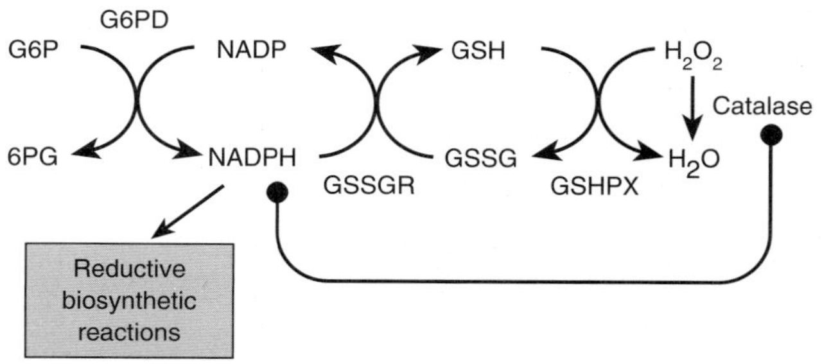

Fig. 3 The role of G6PD in red cell metabolism: NADPH plays a dual role in (i) regeneration of glutathione (GSH) and (ii) stabilization of catalase.

The enzymatically active form of G6PD is either a dimer or a tetramer of a single protein subunit of 514 amino acids with a molecular mass of 59 096 Da. Some regions of the molecule critical for its functions have been identified because they are highly conserved in evolution. The G6P-binding site and the active centre of the enzyme are located near lysine 205. Recently the three-dimensional structure of G6PD has been solved. In the dimer structure the two subunits are symmetrically located across a complex interface of β-sheets. The NADP binding site is near the N-terminus, and bound NADP is important for the stability of G6PD.

Acute haemolytic anaemia associated with G6PD deficiency clearly results from the action of an exogenous factor on intrinsically abnormal red cells. Although the sequence of events ending in haemolysis is not completely understood, we know that oxidative agents cause glutathione depletion in G6PD-deficient red cells. This is followed by oxidation of sulphydryl groups and consequent denaturation of haemoglobin (hence the Heinz bodies) and probably of other proteins, which eventually causes irreversible damage to the membrane of red cells and hence their destruction, partly in the bloodstream and partly through phagocytosis by macrophages. An important feature of haemolysis in G6PD-deficient patients depends on the fact that G6PD decays gradually during red cell ageing (for instance, in normal blood, reticulocytes have about five times more activity than the 10 per cent oldest red cells), and this process is accelerated with many G6PD variants. Thus, a haemolytic attack selectively destroys older red cells because they have a more severe shortage of G6PD. This phenomenon can be so marked with certain G6PD variants that patients in the posthaemolytic state are found to have a significant increase in G6PD activity (hence the risk of misclassification), sufficient to make them relatively resistant to further challenge. By contrast, with some other variants the steady-state level of G6PD is so low that, even in the absence of any oxidant challenge, it becomes limiting for red cell survival: this is the case in patients with chronic non-spherocytic haemolytic anaemia, who may have a red cell lifespan of between 10 and 50 days.

Molecular basis of G6PD deficiency

Since the discovery of G6PD deficiency, one might have expected that some mutations would be located in regulatory regions of the gene, producing a reduction in the amount G6PD produced, without changes in its structure (analogous to thalassaemias); whereas others would be located in the coding region of the gene, thus producing qualitative (or structural) as well as quantitative changes in G6PD (analogous to structural haemoglobinopathies). In fact, whenever G6PD from G6PD-deficient individuals has been subjected to careful biochemical characterization (for example by analysing electrophoretic mobility, substrate affinity constants, or thermostability), qualitative differences have invariably been detected, predicting structural mutations.

By sequencing the G6PD gene from G6PD-deficient subjects it has been verified that all mutations are structural (Fig. 4). The current database of some 130 mutants consists, with few exceptions, of single point mutations in the coding region of the gene, entailing single amino acid replacements in the G6PD protein. The exceptions have been small deletions of one to eight amino acids, and a few instances in which two point mutations rather than one are present (for instance, in G6PD A-, the variant most commonly encountered in Africa). Regulatory mutations have not yet been discovered. Amino acid replacements can cause G6PD deficiency either by affecting its catalytic function or by decreasing the *in vivo* stability of the protein, or by both of these mechanisms. Enzyme instability is the most common mechanism (Table 2). The molecular basis of chronic non-spherocytic haemolytic anaemia associated with G6PD deficiency is highly specific, in the sense that the underlying mutations, while still within the coding region of the G6PD gene, are not the same as those underlying asymptomatic G6PD deficiency. The more severe clinical phenotype can be ascribed in some cases to adverse qualitative changes (for instance, a decreased affinity for the substrate, glucose-6-phosphate); or simply to the fact that the enzyme deficit is more extreme, because of severe instability of the enzyme. For instance, a cluster of mutations map to the dimer interface, and it is clear that they severely compromise the formation of the dimer.

Because the G6PD gene is X linked, frequencies of G6PD deficiency in males are identical to gene frequencies, and they are as high as 20 per cent or more in some of the areas just mentioned. The frequency of homozygous females is of course lower, but the frequency of heterozygous females is higher (according to the Hardy–Weinberg rule) than that of G6PD-deficient males. Different G6PD variants underlie G6PD deficiency in different parts of the world: for instance, G6PD Mediterranean on the shores of this sea, in the Middle East, and in India; G6PD A- in Africa and in Southern Europe; G6PD Mahidol in South-East Asia; G6PD Canton in China; and G6PD Union worldwide. It is also important to realize that in some populations several different polymorphic variants coexist. The overall geographical distribution of G6PD deficiency and its heterogeneity, together with findings from clinical field studies and *in vitro* experiments, strongly support the view that this common genetic trait has been selected by *Plasmodium falciparum* malaria, by virtue of the fact that it confers a relative resistance to heterozygotes against this highly lethal infection.

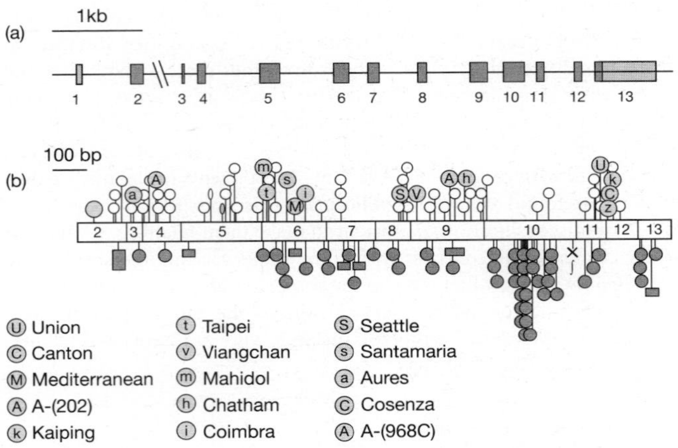

Fig. 4 Hetereogeneity of G6PD deficiency. The 13 exons of the *G6PD* gene are drawn approximately to scale; the introns (not drawn to scale) are shown by thin lines connecting the exons. The location of the mutations for the variants listed in Table 2 are shown; plus that of G6PD Sunderland, as example of an English sporadic variant associated with chronic non-spherocytic haemolytic anaemia and due to a deletion of a triplet of bases, corresponding to codon 35.

Management

Prevention

The acute haemolytic anaemia of G6PD deficiency is largely preventable by avoiding exposure to triggering factors of previously screened subjects. Of course, the practicability and cost-effectiveness of screening depends on the prevalence of G6PD deficiency in each individual community. Favism is entirely preventable by not eating broad beans. Prevention of drug-induced haemolysis is possible in most cases by choosing alternative drugs. A common practical problem is the need to give primaquine for eradication of malaria due to *Plasmodium vivax* or *P. malariae*; in these cases the administration of a lower dose of the drug for a longer time is the recommended approach: this will still cause haemolysis, but of an acceptably mild degree.

Treatment of acute haemolytic anaemia and favism

A patient with acute haemolytic anaemia may present a diagnostic problem, that once solved, does not require any specific treatment at all; or he or she may be present as a medical emergency requiring immediate action. With severe anaemia, immediate blood transfusion is definitely indicated. If there is acute renal failure, haemodialysis may be necessary. Recovery is the rule.

Management of neonatal jaundice

This does not differ from that of neonatal jaundice due to other causes than G6PD deficiency. In most cases, prompt phototherapy is highly effective and sufficient; but with bilirubin levels above 300 μmol/l (or even less in babies who are premature, or who have acidosis or infection), exchange blood transfusion is imperative to prevent neurological damage.

Management of chronic non-spherocytic haemolytic anaemia

In general terms, this does not differ from that of chronic non-spherocytic haemolytic anaemia due to other causes, for example pyruvate kinase deficiency. If the anaemia is not severe, regular folic acid supplements and regular haematological surveillance will suffice. It will be important to

Table 2 Genetic heterogeneity of G6PD deficiency

Variant class	Clinical expression	Degree of enzyme deficiency	Examples	Amino acid replacements	Populations where prevalent	Mechanism of enzyme deficiency
I	Chronic non-spherocytic haemolytic anaemia	Usually less than 10% of normal	Harilaou	216 Phe→Leu	All class I variants are sporadic	Unstable
			Barcelona	Not yet known		Abnormal kinetics
II	Acute haemolytic anaemia triggered by broad beans or infection	Less than 10% of normal	Mediterranean	188 Ser→Phe	Mediterranean, Middle East, India	Unstable
			Mahidol	163 Gly→Ser	South-East Asia	Unstable
			Canton	459 Arg→Leu	China	Unstable
			Union	454 Arg→Cys	Worldwide	?
III	As for class II	10 to 50% of normal	A–	68 Val→Met 126 Asn→ASP	Africa, Southern Europe	Unstable
			Seattle	282 Asp→His	Europe	?
IV	None	More than 60% of normal	A	126 Asn→Asp	Africa	None

avoid exposure to potentially haemolytic drugs, and blood transfusion may be indicated when exacerbations occur, mostly in conjunction with intercurrent infection. In rare patients the anaemia is so severe that regular blood transfusion is necessary, probably at approximately 2-month intervals, in order to keep the haemoglobin in the 8 to 10 g/dl range. A hypertransfusion regimen aiming to maintain a normal haemoglobin level is not indicated (as there is no ineffective erythropoiesis in the bone marrow). However, in patients requiring regular transfusions, appropriate iron chelation should be instituted by the age of 2 years, and must be continued as long as transfusion treatment is necessary; sometimes the transfusion requirement may decrease after puberty. Although, unlike in hereditary spherocytosis, there is no evidence of selective red cell destruction in the spleen, splenectomy has proved beneficial in severe cases. When a diagnosis of chronic non-spherocytic haemolytic anaemia is made, the family must be given genetic counselling, and an effort should be made to establish whether the mother is a heterozygote; if she is, the chance of recurrence is 1:2 for every subsequent male pregnancy. Prenatal diagnosis can be made by DNA analysis if the mutation is first identified in an affected relative.

Further reading

Beutler E (1978). Glucose-6-phosphate dehydrogenase deficiency. In: Beutler E ed. *Hemolytic anemia in disorders of red cell metabolism*, p 23. Plenum Medical, New York.

Beutler E (1991). Glucose-6-phosphate dehydrogenase deficiency. *New England Journal of Medicine* **324**, 169–74.

Dacie JV (1985). Hereditary enzyme deficiency haemolytic anaemias. Deficiency of glucose-6-phosphate dehydrogenase. In: Dacie JV, ed. *Haemolytic anaemias*, III: *The hereditary haemolytic anaemias*, p 364. Churchill Livingstone, London.

Luzzatto L (1993). Glucose-6-phosphate dehydrogenase deficiency and hemolytic anemia. In: Nathan DG, Oski FA, eds. *Hematology of infancy and childhood*, p 674. Daunders, Philadelphia.

Vulliamy T, Mason P, Luzzatto L (1992). The molecular basis of glucose-6-phosphate dehydrogenase deficiency. *Trends in Genetics* **8**, 138–43.

Vulliamy TJ, Beutler E, Luzzatto L (1993). Variants of glucose-6-phosphate dehydrogenase are due to missense mutations spread throughout the coding region of the gene. *Human Mutation* **2**, 159–67.

22.6 Haemostasis and thrombosis

22.6.1 The biology of haemostasis and thrombosis

Harold R. Roberts and Gilbert C. White

Introduction

Fluid blood is contained within the vascular tree, but as a result of minor trauma that occurs during the wear and tear of everyday living, leaks occur in the vessel wall that must be sealed by a solid, impermeable fibrin clot in order to prevent significant blood loss. The clot is formed from factors in flowing blood and is located and restricted to the site of the leak without dissemination throughout the vascular tree. This is the process of haemostasis, an exquisitely controlled mechanism that requires components of the vessel wall, blood platelets, and soluble procoagulant and anticoagulant proteins. The haemostatic plug consists of a mass of platelets, red blood cells, and leucocytes enmeshed in interlocking strands of fibrin fibres that plug the leak.

Once formed, the haemostatic plug is gradually replaced by new tissue that results in wound healing. This process requires lysis of the blood clot by the fibrinolytic system and subsequent ingrowth of new cells. Thus, haemostasis is not an isolated phenomenon, but is one component of the defence mechanisms that include inflammation and eventual wound healing.

Thrombosis, as opposed to haemostasis, is a pathological state in which the normal clotting system is disturbed to the extent that a clot is formed that partially or completely obstructs the flow of blood within the blood vessel and sometimes dislodges to become an embolus.

To understand the biology of haemostasis and thrombosis, it is necessary to know the roles of the vessel wall, the platelets, the coagulation and fibrinolytic systems, and their respective inhibitors.

Blood vessel wall

The anatomy of the wall of both an artery and a vein is shown schematically in Fig. 1. All blood vessels are lined by an intima consisting of a monolayer of endothelial cells that rest upon a loose network of tissue called the extracellular matrix. In addition to the intima, larger and intermediate arteries contain two other layers: the media, composed mostly of smooth muscle cells, and the adventitia, consisting largely of connective tissue, nerves, and nutrient vessels. While these three layers also exist in veins, the media and adventitia are much less distinct and are not visible in the smaller arterioles and capillaries.

Endothelial cells

Endothelial cells form the basis of vascular development and are derived from embryonic mesoderm. Embryonic endothelial cells (angioblasts) develop under the influence of growth hormones including basic fibroblast growth factor and vascular endothelial growth factor, both of which interact with receptors on the cell membrane termed receptor tyrosine kinases. These early blood vessels expand into a vascular tree under the influence of two major hormones, angiopoietin 1 and 2, that bind to a family of tyrosine kinase receptors called tie-1 and tie-2 (tyrosine kinase plus Ig and epidermal growth factor-like domains) on endothelial cells. To fully develop into an intact vascular tree, endothelial cells must interact with the extracellular matrix and other cells, a process that requires cell–cell adhesion that is dependent upon cell surface cytoadhesive molecules such as platelet–endothelial cytoadhesive molecule-1, and vascular endothelial cell cadherin. Endothelial cell structure is also dependent upon the integrin family of molecules and interactions with the extracellular matrix.

Endothelial cells are heterogeneous in appearance, function, and genetic regulation. In the brain, endothelial cells form very tight junctions with one another to preserve the blood–brain barrier; in the spleen and liver, the interendothelial gaps are wide, permitting soluble and cellular trafficking between blood and the extravascular space. Not all endothelial cells synthesize the same proteins. Tissue plasminogen activator is synthesized by

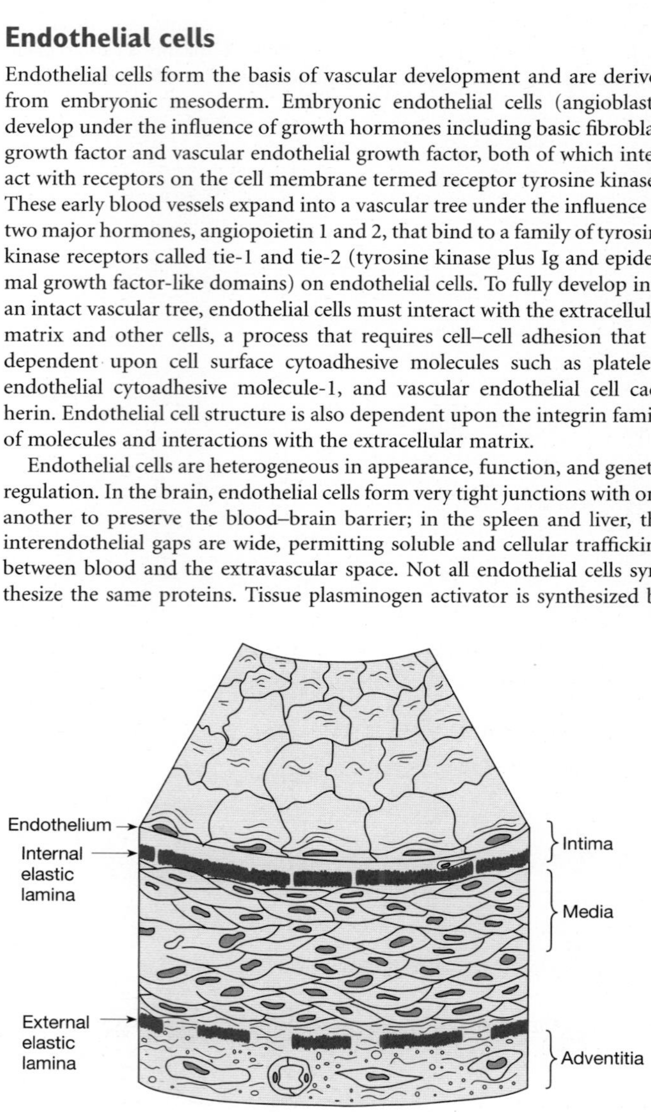

Fig. 1 A schematic diagram of a vessel wall consisting of the intima, the media (smooth muscle cells), and the adventitia. The intima consists of a layer of endothelium that is exposed to the circulating blood. The subendothelial matrix lies below the endothelium and is separated from the media by the internal elastic membrane. See text for detailed description of each layer. (Reprinted by permission, *Robbins pathological basis of disease*, 4th edn, (1989), p.554, WB Saunders Co.)

Table 1 Vasoregulatory substances produced by endothelial cells

Vasoregulatory substance	Action
Vasodilators	
Nitric oxide (NO)	↑cGMP in SMC
Prostacyclin (PGI_2)	↑cyclic AMP in platelets
Monoamine oxidase (MAO)	↓catecholamines
Vasoconstrictors	
Endothelin	activates Ca^{++} channels in SMC
Angiotensin 2	converts angiotensin 1 to 2 by ACE
Prostaglandin G_2,H_2 (PGG_2, PGH_2)	acts on SMC

SMC = smooth muscle cells; AMP = adenosine-monophosphate (converted to adenosine); ACE = angiotensin-converting enzyme on endothelial cells.

only about 3 per cent of cells. Von Willebrand factor, often regarded as a specific marker for endothelial cells, is not expressed in all cells. The microenvironment also plays an important role in regulating endothelial cell function. Haemodynamic forces, including hydrostatic pressure, and shear stresses and strains can influence endothelial cell structure and function. Haemodynamic forces can even regulate endothelial cell gene expression. For example there is a shear stress response element in the gene governing the synthesis of the β chain of the platelet-derived growth factor. Other endothelial cell genes responsive to shear forces include those for: tissue plasminogen activator, intercellular adhesion molecule, and vascular cell adhesion molecule-1.

Endothelial cells contribute to haemostasis by their contributions to vascular tone, procoagulant, anticoagulant, fibrinolytic, and antifibrinolytic activities.

Vascular tone

Vasoregulatory substances produced by endothelial cells are shown in Table 1. The most important vasoregulators are nitric oxide, previously known as endothelial cell-derived relaxation factor and prostacyclin. Nitric oxide and prostacyclin are also important antiplatelet agents. On the other hand, the most important vasoconstrictors are endothelin and angiotensin 2. Endothelin is also a mitogen for smooth muscle cells.

Procoagulant properties

Procoagulant properties of the endothelial cell are depicted in Table 2. von Willebrand factor is synthesized constitutively by endothelial cells and is essential for platelet adhesion to the vessel wall and as a carrier for blood clotting factor VIII. von Willebrand factor is stored in Weibel–Palade bodies, as depicted in Fig. 2. It is released into the circulation in multimers of heterogeneous molecular weight ranging from one to about 20 million. Endothelial cells also secrete very large von Willebrand factor multimers abluminally into the extracellular matrix.

Table 2 Procoagulant and anticoagulant properties of endothelial cells

Procoagulant and anticoagulant	Synthesis	Action
Procoagulants		
von Willebrand Factor (vWF)	Constitutive	Carrier of Factor VIII; platelet adhesion to vessel wall
Tissue Factor (TF)	Inducible	Receptor for Factor VII
Anticoagulants		
Prostacyclin (PGI_2)	Constitutive	Inhibits platelet aggregation
Nitric oxide (NO)	Constitutive	Vasodilation
Thrombomodulin (TM)	Constitutive	TM/thrombin complex, activates protein C
Tissue factor pathway inhibitor (TFPI)	Constitutive	Inhibits TF–VIIa–Xa complex
Glycosoaminoglycans (GAG)	Constitutive	Antithrombins
CD 39	Constitutive	Inhibits platelet aggregation
Tissue plasminogen activator (t-PA)	Constitutive	Converts plasminogen to plasmin

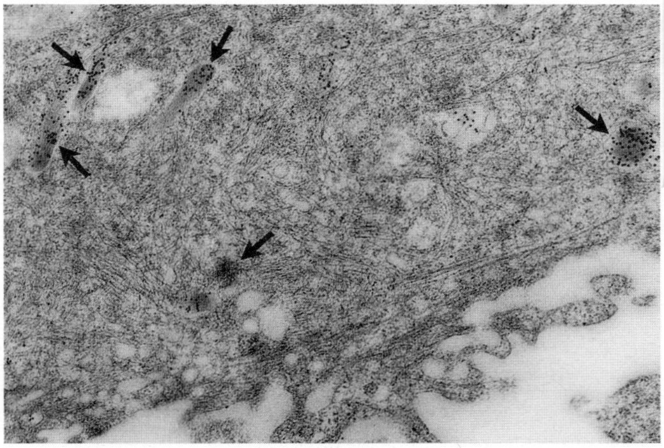

Fig. 2 Electron micrograph of an endothelial cell. Weibel–Palade bodies containing multimers of von Willebrand factor are depicted by the arrows.

Tissue factor acts as a binding protein for factor VII and is essential for the initiation of coagulation. It is not constitutively produced by endothelial cells, but it can be induced by tissue necrosis factor, endotoxin, and other inflammatory substances.

Anticoagulant properties

Anticoagulant properties of the endothelial cells are also shown in Table 2. Prostacyclin not only causes vasodilation, but it is a potent inhibitor of platelet aggregation. Nitric oxide has a similar effect. An important anticoagulant function of endothelial cells is due to the expression of thrombomodulin, a transmembrane-bound protein that acts as a receptor for thrombin. The thrombomodulin/thrombin complex is the physiological activator of protein C, which inactivates clotting factors Va and VIIIa to turn off coagulation. Tumour plasminogen activator (t-PA) is also synthesized by endothelial cells and serves to convert plasminogen to plasmin, the active fibrinolytic enzyme.

Endothelial cells contribute to the control of coagulation by synthesizing tissue factor pathway inhibitor (TFPI), which inhibits the tissue factor-mediated initiation of the clotting reactions. They also secrete glycosaminoglycans, such as heparan sulphate and other proteoglycans that inhibit thrombin. In addition, they express vascular adenosine triphosphate diphosphohydrolase, otherwise known as CD39, on their surface. CD39 acts in concert with 5‘ectonucleotidase to convert ATP/ADP to AMP and then to adenosine, which inhibits platelet aggregation.

Receptor function

The receptor function of endothelial cells plays an important role in haemostasis and thrombosis (Table 3). They express a thrombin receptor termed protease-activated receptor 1 (PAR-1). Thrombin cleaves the carboxyterminal end of the receptor, which then binds to the remaining cell-associated protein (a so-called tethered ligand) and triggers intracellular signalling through G proteins, resulting in activation of endothelial cells. The thrombin–thrombomodulin complex not only activates protein C, but also activates a protein known as the thrombin-activatable fibrinolytic inhibitor (TAFI), a procarboxypeptidase that functions to inhibit fibrinolysis. Endothelial cells also express a protein C receptor different from thrombomodulin that acts to modulate the activity of activated protein C. Urokinase plasminogen activator receptors are not found on resting endothelial cells, but are found on those involved in angiogenesis. There are a

Table 3 Receptor function of endothelial cells

Receptor	Ligand
Protease activated receptor 1 (PAR-1)	Thrombin
Thrombomodulin	Thrombin
Protein C receptor	Protein C
Urokinase plasminogen activator receptor (u-PAR)	Urokinase
Adhesive receptors	
Intercellular cytoadhesive molecule (ICAM) 1, 2	Integrins $\alpha_1\beta_2$; $\alpha_m\beta_2$
Vascular cytoadhesive molecule (VCAM)	$\alpha_1\beta_2$; $\alpha_4\beta_1$
P-selectin	Sialyl–Lewis antigen
E-selectin	

number of adhesive receptors on the surface of endothelial cells as shown in Table 3. The adhesion of neutrophils is dependent upon the expression of P-selectin. P-selectin is rapidly internalized by the endothelial cell, but this is followed by expression of another cytoadhesive molecule, E-selectin, which is necessary for continued adherence and rolling of neutrophils along the endothelial cell surface. Intercellular adhesion molecule and vascular cell adhesion molecule are receptors for leucocytes and are important for the interaction of leucocytes and the vessel wall.

Extracellular matrix

The extracellular matrix is a complex, heterogeneous structure beneath the endothelium with many interactions related to haemostasis and thrombosis. The matrix consists of a network of collagens, elastins, proteoglycans, and glycoproteins, including fibronectin, vitronectin, laminin, tenascin, thrombospondin, von Willebrand factor, and osteopontin, among others, as shown in Table 4. The matrix proteins promote platelet adhesion, cellular migration, cell proliferation, and endothelial and smooth muscle cell interactions.

Collagens are the most abundant proteins in subendothelial connective tissue. Collagen types I, II, III, IV, V, VI, and VII have been identified in various matrix tissues. The collagens are synthesized by endothelial cells, smooth muscle cells, and by adventitial fibroblasts. The various collagens contribute to the integrity of the vessel wall, but they also play a role in platelet activation and, in some instances, coagulation. For example collagen IV has been shown to be a specific high-affinity binding protein for

Table 4 The extracellular matrix

Structural proteins
collagens
I, III, IV, V, VI, VII
elastin
Adhesive proteins
fibronectin
vitronectin
laminin
Von Willebrand factor
Antiadhesive
tenascin
thrombospondin
Ground substance
hyaluronic acid
proteoglycans
chondroitin sulphate
dermatan sulphate
heparan sulphate
others
Degradation and repair
matrix metalloproteinases

Table 5 Matrix metalloproteinases (MMP)

MMP number	Activity	Substrate
MMP-1	collagenase	collagen I, II, III, VII, VIII, X
MMP-2	gelatinase	collagen IV, V, VII, X
MMP-3	stromelysin	microglycans
MMP-8	collagenase	–
MMP-7	matrilysin	fibronectin, laminin, collagen IV
MMP-9	gelatinase	elastin, fibronectin
MMP-10	stromelysin	fibronectin, laminin, elastin, various collagens
MMP-11	stromelysin	fibrinogen, fibrin
MMP-12	elastase	elastin
MMP-14	–	collagen IV, progelatinase A
MMP-15	–	gelatin

Modified from Plow EF, Ugarova T, Miles LA (1998). In: Localzo J, Shafer AI, eds. *Thrombosis and hemorrhage*, 2nd edn, ch. 18, p. 381. Williams and Wilkins, Baltimore.

blood coagulation factor IX, although the function of this complex is not known.

The proteoglycans constitute a heterogeneous group of molecules composed of a core protein attached to a glycosoaminoglycan. These include decorin, biglycan, heparan sulphate, dermatan sulphate, and others. Heparan sulphate, for example, can combine with antithrombin III and inhibit thrombin. The precise role of all of the protoglycans is not known, but some attach to collagen and are necessary for maintaining the structure of the vessel wall.

The matrix also contains elastin, which is secreted by endothelial and smooth muscle cells as tropoelastin that is converted to mature elastin in the matrix where it is assembled into fibres. One function of elastin is simply to maintain the elastic structure of the vessel wall. This substance is found interspersed between smooth muscle cells as well as the matrix. It may also function in cell migration from the vessel wall to the extravascular space.

Fibronectin, vitronectin, and laminins are also components of the extracellular matrix which function in fibrinolysis and platelet adhesion.

Within the extracellular matrix there are a number of matrix metalloproteinases (MMP), which are a group of enzymes useful in matrix degradation and repair. They are secreted as proenzymes and converted to active enzymes that are zinc- or calcium-dependent. They have several functions, as listed in Table 5. Their activities in matrix degradation and repair are controlled by tissue inhibitors of metalloproteinases.

Smooth muscle cells

The smooth muscle cell layer, found in medium and larger sized vessels and more prominently in arteries, has several functions related to the biology of haemostasis and thrombosis. Smooth muscle cells possess contractile, biosynthetic, and proliferative functions. Contractile properties, governed by such substances as nitric oxide, prostacyclin, and endothelin, play important roles in vasodilation and vasoconstriction, respectively. Smooth muscle cells, like endothelial cells, synthesize growth factors such as vascular endothelial growth factor, insulin-like growth factors, epidermal growth factors, activins, and others that are important in smooth muscle cell generation. Smooth muscle cell proliferation is a hallmark of the atherosclerotic lesion. Biosynthetic products of the smooth muscle cells include various types of collagens, elastin, glycoproteins, and proteoglycans. When exposed to injury, smooth muscle cells can also produce tissue factor.

The adventitia

The adventitia is composed of a loose network of cells consisting of fibroblasts, adipocytes, and mast cells. Collagens I and III, glycoproteins, and elastin are synthesized by fibroblasts. Fibroblasts also contain tissue factor. Adipocytes secrete collagen I and III and synthesize lipids.

Platelets

Platelets are the smallest of the circulating blood cells, about 0.5 μ in diameter. They are derived from the cytoplasm of megakaryocytes and are an essential component of the haemostatic plug. Although they are anucleate and appear to be single cells composed of cytoplasm, a surface canalicular system, and storage granules (δ or dense granules and α granules); they are, nevertheless, complicated cells with a variety of very important functions essential for normal haemostasis. These can be broadly divided into the following:

(1) platelet adhesion, defined as platelets adhering to the damaged area of the vessel wall where subendothelial matrix tissue is exposed;

(2) platelet activation, both by agents within the matrix as well as by soluble agonists;

(3) platelet aggregation, defined as platelets sticking to one another in an aggregated mass, forming a platelet plug.

The following sections describe each of these broad areas of platelet function in more detail.

Platelet adhesion

The initial platelet response to vascular injury is adhesion to the vessel wall. Resting, non-activated platelets are not attracted to the vessel wall. However, following vascular damage, platelets rolling along the endothelium rapidly adhere to the subendothelial interstitial matrix. A number of matrix proteins, such as von Willebrand factor, fibronectin, fibrinogen, and thrombospondin, are also present in platelet granules and circulate in plasma.

Platelets possess numerous mechanisms for adhering to the subendothelial matrix (Fig. 3). Adhesion is accomplished by a number of protein receptors on the surface of platelets as described below.

Glycoprotein Ib–IX–V (CD42a–d)

The main function of the platelet membrane glycoprotein Ib–IX–V complex is to act as a receptor that mediates von Willebrand-dependent binding of platelets to collagen, resulting in adhesion of platelets to the vessel wall. Glycoproteins Ibα, Ibβ, IX, and V are members of the leucine-rich glycoprotein family and are characterized by the presence of a common structural motif in the extracellular domain composed of a leucine-rich sequence, PXXLLXXXXXLXXLXLSXNXLXXL*. GPIbα contains seven leucine-rich repeats, GPV contains 15 leucine-rich repeats in the extracellular domain, while GPIbβ and GPIX each contain a single leucine-rich repeat, all in the extracellular domains. GPIbα, GPIbβ, GPIX, and GPV are synthesized as separate gene products which coassociate in a ratio of 2:2:2:1 during transit through the endoplasmic reticulum. Coassociation of GPIbα, GPIbβ, and GPIX, but not GPV, is required for the complex to be expressed on the surface of cells. The role of GPV, a substrate for thrombin, in the function of the complex is uncertain, and mice deficient in GPV bind von Willebrand factor normally and have normal platelet adhesion.

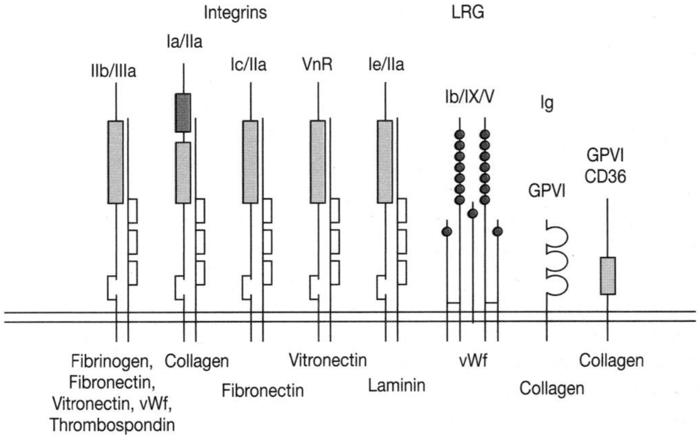

Fig. 3 Receptors mediating the interaction of platelets with subendothelial matrix proteins. Adhesion receptors on platelets include members of the integrin family, leucine-rich glycoproteins (LRG), members of the immunoglobulin (Ig) family, and others. Integrins on the surface of platelets are glycoproteins (GP) IIb/IIIa, which binds multiple ligands; GPIa/IIa, a collagen receptor, GPIc/IIa, which binds fibronectin; VnR, which is a receptor for vitronectin; and GPIc'/IIa, a laminin binding site. Glycoproteins Ib/IX/V are leucine-rich glycoproteins. Glycoprotein VI (GPVI) is a member of the immunoglobulin family and a collagen receptor. Glycoprotein IV (GPIV, CD36) is also a collagen receptor.

Adhesion to von Willebrand factor-coated surfaces through GPIb–IX–V is increased by shear, which is thought to induce a structural change in the receptor that enhances the interaction with von Willebrand factor. The A1 domain of von Willebrand factor forms the principal site that interacts with GPIb. The site in GPIb that binds von Willebrand factor is less well defined. Binding occurs in the amino-terminal, 45-kDa, tryptic fragment from GPIbα. Within this region of GPIbα, an anionic site, YDYYPEE[282], containing two sulphated tyrosine residues at tyrosines 278 and 279, has been further implicated in von Willebrand factor binding. The A3 domain of von Willebrand factor mediates the interaction with collagens type I and III. A model derived from the crystal structure of the von Willebrand factor A3 domain suggests that the von Willebrand factor–collagen interaction is primarily between negatively-charged residues in the A3 domain and positively-charged residues in collagen. Plasma von Willebrand factor does not interact with unstimulated circulating platelets. For binding to occur, platelets have to be activated and plasma von Willebrand factor must undergo a conformational change. After secretion by endothelial cells, von Willebrand factor binds to underlying connective tissue matrix, providing an active surface for platelet attachment after the vessel wall is damaged.

Glycoprotein IIb–IIIa (αIIb/β3)

Under conditions of low shear, platelets can adhere to matrix-bound von Willebrand factor through a mechanism that involves platelet GPIIb–IIIa. GPIIb and IIIa are members of the integrin superfamily, a conserved family of heterodimeric surface receptors, each composed of a larger two-chain α subunit and a smaller β subunit, bound non-covalently. Integrins were initially identified by an ability to bind adhesive glycoproteins containing a tripeptide sequence, arginine–glycine–aspartic acid (RGD), although subsequent work has identified other ligand sequences recognized by integrins. The interaction of von Willebrand factor with GPIIb–IIIa is mediated by an RGD sequence in the C1 domain of von Willebrand factor. GPIIb–IIIa is also able to bind fibronectin, thrombospondin, and vitronectin and may therefore represent an adhesion receptor with broad specificity.

Glycoprotein Ia–IIa (α2β1)

GPIa–IIa is a receptor for types I and IV collagen and mediates platelet adhesion to the vessel wall independent of von Willebrand factor. The integrin sequences that mediate the interaction with collagen reside in a broad sequence called the I domain in the extracellular portion of the molecule. GPIa–IIa is constitutively active and does not require activation to interact with collagen.

Glycoprotein VI–Fc receptor γ-chain complex

GPVI–FcRγ is the major platelet receptor mediating collagen-induced activation of platelets. GPVI is a member of the immunoglobulin superfamily

*A – Alanine, C – Cysteine, D – Aspartic acid, E—Glutamic acid, F—Phenylalanine, G – Glycine, H – Histidine, I – Isoleucine, K – Lysine, L – Leucine, M – Methionine, N – Asparagine, P – Proline, Q – Glutamine, R – Arginine, S – Serine, T – Threonine, V – Valine, W – Tryptophan, Y – Tyrosine, X – any Amino acid

and is characterized by immunoglobulin domains, a transmembrane domain, and a short cytoplasmic tail that lacks known signalling components. GPVI is associated on the platelet surface with FcRγ, apparently in a 1:1 stoichiometry. The complex binds collagen and mediates collagen-generated signals, presumably through the ITAM (or immunoglobulin receptor tyrosine-based activation motif) of FcRγ. Crosslinking of GPVI–FcRγ leads to tyrosine phosphorylation of the ITAM sequence by Src kinase. Syk, another tyrosine kinase, binds to the phosphorylated ITAM sequence through Syk sulphydryl domains, initiating a signal that leads to tyrosine phosphorylation of phospholipase Cγ2 and the generation of inositol phospholipids.

Glycoprotein IV (CD36)

CD 36 is a highly glycosylated transmembrane protein present on platelets, monocytes, endothelial cells, and nucleated erythrocytes, which binds thrombospondin and collagen. The thrombospondin-binding site has been mapped to a single disulphide loop in the extracellular domain of GPIV, but the collagen-binding site is unknown. Although GPIV is a receptor for collagen *in vitro*, individuals with a deficiency of GPIV have no apparent defect in platelet function.

Other adhesion receptors

Platelets can also adhere to subendothelial matrix through glycoprotein Ic–IIa (VLA-5, α5β1), glycoprotein Ic'–IIa (VLA-6, α6β1), or the vitronectin receptor (αvβ3, VnR). GPIc–IIa is a constitutively active receptor for fibronectin that does not require cell activation. There are two sequences in fibronectin which interact with GPIc–IIa: an RGD sequence in the tenth type III repeat which interacts primarily with the GPIIa (β1) subunit and a synergy sequence in the adjacent ninth type III repeat which interacts primarily with the GPIc (α5) subunit. GPIc'–IIa is a laminin receptor which is expressed on platelets. Immunoprecipitation studies suggest that GPIc'–IIa may exist on the cell surface in a complex with proteins with four transmembrane domains, so-called TM4 proteins, such as CD9, CD81, and NAG-2. The nature of these interactions is presently unclear. GPIc'–IIa recognizes a sequence in the long arm E8 fragment of laminin obtained after elastin digestion. The binding requires the presence of divalent cations which bind to specific sites on the integrin α subunit. Small numbers of the vitronectin receptor are expressed on platelets.

Current evidence indicates that all of these adhesion mechanisms may be important. The redundancy in adhesion receptors may:

(1) provide backup mechanisms to protect against blood loss;

(2) generate different signals in response to interaction with different matrix proteins; or

(3) represent different systems at work in different parts of the vascular tree.

An example of the latter might be the relative roles of GPIb–IX–V and GPIIb–IIIa in the von Willebrand factor-mediated adhesion of platelets to collagen. Under high shear conditions, as found in capillaries and small arterioles, GPIb–IX–V may be the predominant mechanism mediating platelet adhesion to collagen and von Willebrand factor-dependent adherence whereas, under low shear conditions, like those found in large veins and in arteries, GPIb–IX–V may be less effective and other mechanisms that require a shorter residence time of platelets on the subendothelial matrix, including GPIc–IIa interaction with fibronectin and GPIa–IIa interaction with collagen, may be important. The presence of multiple receptors for collagen on the platelet surface, including GPIb–IX–V, GPIIb–IIIa, GPIa–IIa, GPIV, and GPVI, is interesting and raises the possibility of different collagen responses. Vitronectin also appears to be important for adhesion at high shear, and can bind to both GPIIb–IIIa and specific vitronectin receptors. Recent evidence suggests that platelet adhesion to collagen types I and III in flowing blood is dependent on both von Willebrand factor and fibronectin. Collagen types I, II, and III have been shown to bind von Willebrand factor.

Platelet activation

Following adhesion and in response to soluble agonists such as thrombin, platelets undergo a series of complex biochemical reactions leading to cell activation. As a result, platelets undergo changes in shape, alterations in surface lipid composition leading to the generation of platelet coagulant activity and thrombin generation, and secretion of the contents of intracellular granules leading to the release of ADP. The thrombin generated at the platelet surface and ADP secreted from platelet granules lead to activation of additional platelets. These reactions involve the metabolism of membrane inositol phospholipids, changes in cellular levels of calcium, activation of contractile proteins, stimulation of heterotrimeric and low molecular weight GTP-binding proteins, and tyrosine and serine–threonine phosphorylation of proteins, among other events. These biochemical reactions initiate second messenger signals that drive the functional changes that occur in platelets which transform them from the resting state to an activated one, and which play a crucial role in haemostasis. Some of these signalling pathways are described in the following sections (see Fig. 4).

Phospholipid metabolism

Metabolism of membrane phospholipids is one of the first signalling pathways identified in platelets and remains one of the most important. Platelet stimulation by a variety of agonists results in activation of membrane-associated phospholipases, including phospholipases C, A2, and D, which cleave fatty acids from the phospholipid. The lipid products generated by these pathways are signalling compounds which are important for changes in cytoplasmic calcium and activation of kinases and phosphatases.

The most intensively studied of these pathways is the metabolism of inositol phospholipids through phospholipase C. Membrane phosphatidylinositol (PI) exists in multiple phosphorylation states: PI, PI-P, PI-P2 which is phosphorylated in the 3,4 or 4,5 positions, and PI-P3 which is phosphorylated in the 3,4,5 positions. Phosphatidylinositol-specific kinases and phosphatases maintain pools of phosphorylated phosphoinositides in a proper concentration range. Platelets contain several isoforms of phospholipase C which are activated by different mechanisms. All cleave phosphatidylinositol 4,5-bisphosphate (PI 4,5-P2) and, later, phosphatidylinositol, as well as phosphatidylinositol 4-phosphate (PI 4-P), to yield diglyceride and inositol trisphosphate (IP3). Phospholipase Cα and Cβ are coupled to heterotrimeric G proteins where phospholipase Cγ is coupled to growth factor receptors. Inositol trisphosphate (IP_3) generated by phospholipase C cleavage of inositol phospholipids has been implicated in the release of calcium from intracellular storage sites in the platelet-dense tubular system. The other product of phospholipase C cleavage, diacylglycerol, activates protein kinase C, which phosphorylates pleckstrin, a 47 000-dalton protein, and other proteins.

Phospholipase A2 is linked to G-protein coupled receptors and cleaves fatty acids in the *sn*-2 position in membrane phospholipids, primarily phosphatidylcholine. In most individuals in western society, the fatty acid in this position is arachidonic acid. Arachidonic acid, liberated by the action of phospholipase A2, is converted to a variety of possible products by the microsomal enzymes, cyclo-oxygenase and lipoxygenase. Cyclo-oxygenase converts arachidonic acid to prostaglandin endoperoxides, prostaglandins F_2, E_2, and D_2, whose main fate in platelets is rapid conversion to thromboxane A_2 by thromboxane synthase. Thromboxane A_2 is believed to play an important role in the release of intracellular granules by acting as a membrane fusogen, fusing granule membranes with the membrane of the surface connected canalicular system and permitting secretion of the granule contents to the outside of the cell. Thromboxane A_2 is also an exceptionally potent constrictor of vascular smooth muscle and a strong platelet-aggregating agent.

Inhibition of the arachidonate pathway has been a primary target for platelet inhibition. Cyclo-oxygenase is irreversibly inhibited by aspirin, which acetylates serine 340, and reversibly inhibited by non-steroidal anti-inflammatory agents. Inhibition of cyclo-oxygenase inhibits thromboxane formation and results in inhibition of the release of intracellular granules. The mechanism by which aspirin is thought to act as an anti-atherosclerosis agent is by inhibition of the release of platelet-derived growth factor.

Phospholipase D acts primarily on phosphatidylcholine to produce choline and phosphatic acid. Protein kinase C and PI-P2 play an important role in activation of phospholipase D. Phosphatidic acid is an intracellular messenger which is proposed to play a role in platelet activation. In addition, phosphatidic acid can be converted to lysophosphatidic acid through the action of phospholipase A2. Like phosphatidic acid, lysophosphatidic acid is an intracellular messenger which is involved in phospholipase activation, ras signalling, and cytoskeleton reorganization.

Calcium metabolism

In resting platelets, the cytoplasmic concentration of calcium is maintained at a low level by active transport of calcium both outside the cell and into the dense tubular system, a sarcoplasmic reticulum-like fraction in platelets. This transport is accomplished by a plasma membrane sarcoplasmic-

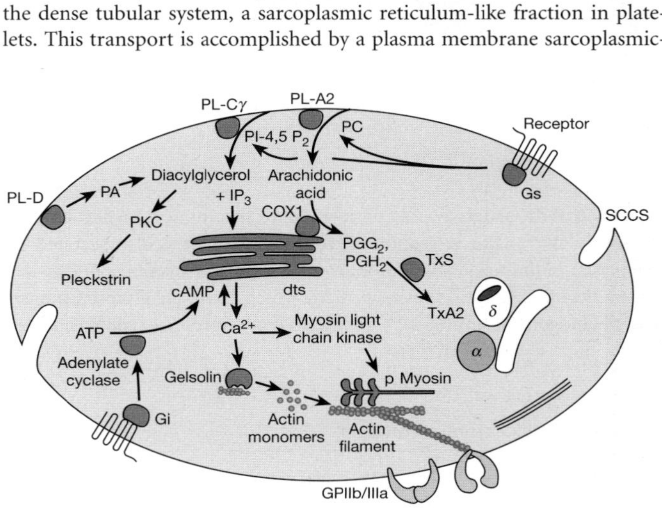

Fig. 4 Signalling pathways involved in platelet activation. Following the interaction of agonist with receptor, there is G protein (Gs)-coupled activation of phospholipid metabolic pathways through phospholipase A_2 (PL-A2), phospholipase Cγ (PL-Cγ), and phospholipase D (PL-D) leading to generation of thromboxane A_2 (TXA2), inositol trisphosphate (IP_3), diacylglycerol, and phosphatidic acid (PA). Arachidonic acid generated by the action of phospholipase A_2 is converted by cyclo-oxygenase-1 (COX-1) to prostaglandin endoperoxides G_2 (PGG_2) and H_2 (PGH_2) which are, in turn, converted to thromboxane A_2 through the action of thromboxane synthase (TXS). Thromboxane generated through arachidonate metabolism is thought to play a role in secretion, through the fusion of α-granule (α) and dense granule (δ) membranes with the membrane of the surface-connected canalicular system (SCCS). Granule contents, including adenosine diphosphate, are emptied into the SCCS and make their way to the outside of the cell. Diacylglyerol stimulates activation of protein kinase C (PKC), resulting in serine–threonine phosphorylation of proteins such as pleckstrin. Inositol trisphosphate stimulates calcium release from storage sites in the dense tubular system (dts). The release of calcium from the dense tubular system is antagonized by cyclic AMP, generated through G protein (Gi)-coupled inhibitory receptor activation of adenylate cyclase. Calcium, released in response to IP_3, activates gelsolin, an actin-capping and -severing protein, which generates actin monomers that then serve as nucleation sites for formation of actin filaments and assembly of the activation-dependent cytoskeleton. Assembly of the cytoskeleton and interaction of the cytoskeleton with surface integrins such as glycoproteins IIb and IIIa (GPIIb/IIIa) may be involved in integrin activation. Calcium also activates myosin light chain kinase which phosphorylates myosin light chain-generating actinomyosin contraction, important for changes in platelet shape and the secretion process.

endoplasmic-reticulum-like calcium ATPase (SERCA2-b), a dense tubular system SERCA3, a sodium-calcium exchange pump in the plasma membrane, and passive calcium fluxes. During platelet activation, inositol trisphosphate (IP_3), generated by metabolism of membrane inositol phospholipids, induces the rapid release of calcium stored in the dense tubular system. This increase in cytoplasmic calcium is essential for platelet activation, and agents that inhibit increases in cytoplasmic calcium inhibit platelet activation while agents that increase cytoplasmic calcium stimulate platelet activation.

Calcium functions as a major intracellular messenger in platelets, mediating calcium-dependent reactions important in almost all phases of platelet activation. An increase in the concentration of cytoplasmic free calcium activates gelsolin, the calcium-dependent actin capping and severing protein, which plays an important role in reorganization of the cytoskeleton. Calcium also activates the calcium and calmodulin-dependent myosin light chain kinase, leading to phosphorylation of myosin light chains, activation of actin-stimulated myosin ATPase activity, and the development of contractile forces. The contraction generated by actin and myosin mediates changes in platelet shape and is important for events leading to platelet secretion. In the absence of calcium ions, tropomyosin inhibits the interaction of myosin with actin, and this may be an additional regulatory role of calcium in platelets. Calpain, a calcium-dependent thiol protease, hydrolyzes numerous proteins involved in platelet signalling. Activation of calpain is believed to be important both for regulation of cytoskeletal events and integrin-mediated signalling.

Cytoskeletal reorganization

Resting platelets are discoid in shape and feature a cellular cytoskeleton that consists of a network of actin filaments that fill and shape the cytoplasm of the cell and a single microtubule coil at the margin of the disc. Upon activation, platelets undergo remarkable morphological changes (Fig. 5). There is an initial change from the normal discoid shape of the resting platelet to a sphere as calcium levels in the cell increase. Filamentous actin appears in the form of stress fibres, and the cellular content of filamentous actin increases. Membrane ruffles form as well as long cellular projections called pseudopodia. Actin cables are present in these pseudopodia, extending to the end of the projections. Also during activation, microtubules contract and 'squeeze' granules toward the centre of the cell.

The energy for contraction is provided by a magnesium ion-dependent ATPase present in myosin and stimulated by actin. Contraction occurs by actin filaments and myosin rods sliding over one another. Myosin light-chain phosphatase may switch off myosin. Membrane glycoproteins GPIIb–IIIa, GPIb–IX–V, and other membrane proteins are associated with the cytoskeleton and provide direction for the contractile process. This activation-dependent cytoskeleton is more than just a structural scaffold for platelet shape changes. Numerous signalling proteins are incorporated into the cytoskeleton and may function in specialized compartments by virtue of their association with the cytoskeleton.

Platelet coagulant activity (platelet factor 3)

Platelet membranes have an asymmetrical distribution of phospholipids, with almost all of the acidic (negatively charged) phospholipids, such as phosphatidyl serine and phosphatidyl inositol, located in the inner leaflet of the plasma membrane. After platelet activation, the acidic phospholipids are translocated to the outer half of the membrane, while phosphatidylcholine moves to the inner half, in a phenomenon known as a 'flip-flop' reaction. This transbilayer movement of phospholipids in the platelet membrane is not well understood, but evidence for a 'flipase' which enzymatically contributes to it has been presented. There is also a translocase enzyme that works in the opposite way and is capable of restoring the acidic phospholipids to the inner leaflet of the membrane bilayer.

The exposed phosphatidyl serine and other negatively-charged phospholipids account for some of the activity traditionally known as platelet factor 3 by contributing to surface properties for binding of factor X and

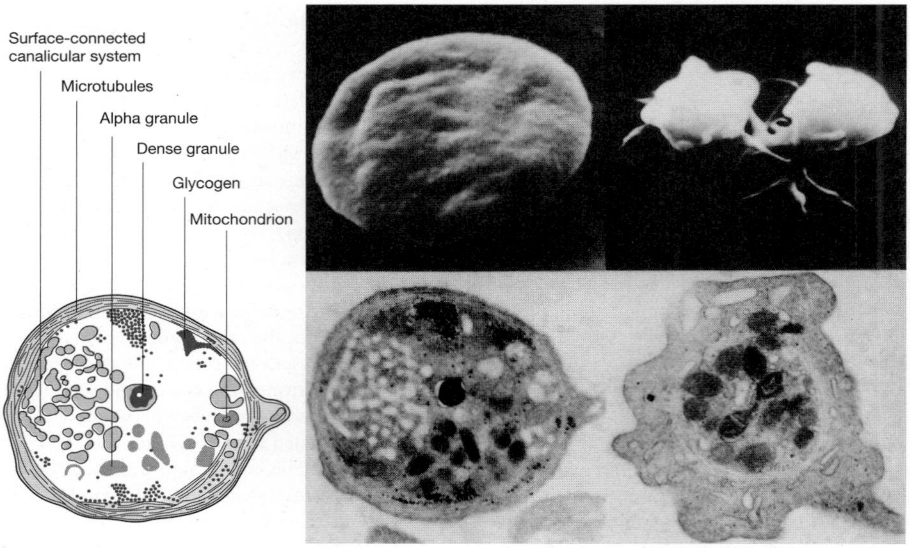

Fig. 5 Platelet morphology. Platelets are small, anucleate cells. In the resting state (a), platelets are ducoid shaped and contain a marginal rim of microtubreles. After activation (b), platelets undergo changes in shape, becoming more rounded and extending cytoplasmic projections, called pseudopods, outward.

prothombin activation complexes. This interaction with platelet phospholipids increases the rate of factor X activation and prothrombin activation nearly a thousand fold. In addition to phospholipids on the platelet membrane, there appear to be other specific binding proteins for blood clotting factors.

Secretion

A primary endpoint of platelet activation is the secretion of platelet granule contents to the outside of the cell. During platelet activation, the granules are 'squeezed' to the centre of the cell where the granules fuse with the surface-connected canalicular system, a series of intracellular canals that are connected to the cell surface. The contents of the granules make their way to the outside of the cell. Secretion requires prostaglandin metabolism and is dependent on contractile events. Products of prostaglandin metabolism, primarily thromboxane A2, may act in the fusion of the granule membrane with that of the surface-connected canalicular system.

Platelets possess two types of storage granules (Table 6), both of which are involved in secretion of active ingredients that modulate platelet function. One type is the dense granule, so called because it is dense by electron microscopy. The other type is the α-granule.

Dense granules contain adenine nucleotides, calcium, and serotonin. Adenine nucleotides are sequestered in the dense granules mainly as adenosine diphosphate (ADP) and adenosine triphosphate (ATP) in a complex with calcium ions and pyrophosphate, and are not interchangeable with the nucleotides involved in general cell metabolism. ADP released from platelet-dense granules activates additional platelets and recruits them to the growing platelet thrombus. Serotonin, a potent modulator of vascular tone and integrity, is also a constituent of dense granules.

α-Granules contain platelet-derived growth factor, β-thromboglobulin, platelet factor 4, fibrinogen, factor V, von Willebrand factor, and thrombospondin. Platelet-derived growth factor is mitogenic for smooth-muscle cells and when released from platelets at a site where the vessel wall is damaged, it stimulates proliferation and migration of smooth-muscle cells in the intima, contributing to the atherosclerotic process. β-Thromboglobulin and platelet factor 4 are basic, lysine-rich proteins which interact with glycosaminoglycans such as heparan sulphate, dermatan sulphate, and chondroitin sulphate, which are components of the endothelial cell surface. Platelet factor 4 has a strong heparin-neutralizing activity and has been implicated in the aetiology of heparin-induced thrombocytopenia. Thrombospondin is a major α-granule glycoprotein, but it is also secreted by fibroblasts, endothelial, and smooth-muscle cells. Thrombospondin is a high-molecular-weight adhesive protein which binds to glycosaminoglycans, fibrinogen, plasminogen, histidine-rich glycoprotein, type V collagen,

Table 6 Platelet granule contents

α Granules	
α_2-Antiplasmin	Immunoglobulin
Albumin	Multimerin
β-Amyloid precursor	Plasminogen activator
β-Thromboglobulin (β-TG)	Platelet-derived growth factor (PDGF)
Clusterin	Platelet factor 4 (PF4)
Endothelial cell growth factor (ECGF)	P-selectin (GMP-140)
Factor V	Transforming growth factor (TGF)-α
Fibrinogen	Transforming growth factor (TGF)-β1
Fibronectin	Vitronectin
Granule membrane protein (GMP) 33	von Willebrand factor
Dense (δ) granules	
Adenosine diphosphate (ADP)	Granulophysin
Adenosine triphosphate (ATP)	Pyrophosphate (PPi)
Calcium	Magnesium
Guanosine diphosphate (GDP)	Serotonin (5-hydroxytryptamine)
Guanosine triphosphate (GTP)	
Lysosomal (γ) granules	
β-Galactosidase	Elastase
β-Glucuronidase	Endoglucosidase
β-Glycerophosphatase	LAMP-1
β-Hexosaminidase	LAMP-2
Cathepsins	LIMP-CD63
Collagenase	*N*-acetylglucosaminidase

and calcium ions. It associates with cell surfaces and extracellular matrices and facilitates cell–cell and cell–matrix interactions.

cAMP pathway

The major mechanism for down-regulation of platelet function is the stimulation of adenylate cyclase, which increases cAMP concentrations. Adenylate cyclase is mainly localized in microsomal fractions and is stimulated by adenosine, prostacyclin, and prostaglandin E_1. cAMP inhibits platelet aggregation, platelet secretion, and platelet adhesion to the vessel wall. These effects are probably exerted by inhibiting calcium flux and/or promoting calcium reuptake.

Activation by soluble agonists

In addition to activation through interaction with subendothelial connective tissues, platelets may also be activated by soluble agonists. These include adenosine diphosphate (ADP), epinephrine, and thrombin. In general, this activation occurs through the interaction between soluble agonist and specific receptors on the platelet surface.

Thrombin is one of the most powerful of platelet agonists. Generated during blood coagulation, thrombin activation of platelets occurs through a novel family of receptors called protease-activated receptors (PARs). These are G protein-coupled, seven-membrane-spanning molecules which are activated by proteolysis. Thrombin cleaves the amino terminal exodomain, unmasking a new amino terminal, which functions as a tethered peptide agonist. The tethered peptide binds intramolecularly to the remainder of the receptor to trigger activation. Four members of the PAR family of receptors have been identified. PAR 1 and PAR 4 mediate activation of human platelets by thrombin.

Thrombin interacts with other proteins on the surface of platelets, but the nature of these interactions is uncertain. Glycoprotein V, part of the GPIb–IX–V complex is a substrate for thrombin although the absence of GPV does not appear to inhibit thrombin activation of platelets. GPIb is an equilibrium binding site for thrombin. Patients with a deficiency of GPIb have been reported to have changes in the rate of activation of platelets by thrombin which is overcome at higher concentrations of agonist.

There are at least three receptors for ADP on platelets, all members of the seven membrane-spanning purinergic (P2) receptor family, either P2Y (G-protein-coupled purinergic receptors) or P2X (ligand-gated channel receptors). One receptor, designated P2Y1, is coupled to phospholipase C, probably through Gq. A second receptor, $P2T_{AC}$, is coupled to adenylate cyclase, probably through Gi. The third receptor, P2X1, is coupled to rapid calcium influx and is a member of the intrinsic ion channel family. Full platelet activation by ADP probably involves an interaction of ADP with all three receptors. ADP-induced activation of the GPIIb-IIIa on platelets requires both P2Y1 and $P2T_{AC}$ and concomitant signalling through GTP-binding proteins, Gq and Gi.

Platelet aggregation

Platelet aggregation, the interaction of one platelet with another, is a major function of platelets and is very important in the haemostatic process. The formation of an aggregated platelet-mass at the site of injury provides a physical plug that occludes the defect in the vessel wall and prevents blood loss.

Aggregation is mediated by two glycoproteins on the platelet surface, GPIIb–IIIa, which constitute a receptor for fibrinogen–fibrin. Thus, GPIIb–IIIa on one platelet binds fibrinogen or fibrin which, by virtue of its dimeric structure, interacts with GPIIb–IIIa on another platelet. On resting platelets, GPIIb–IIIa is in an inactive state and is unable to bind fibrinogen. Following platelet activation, GPIIb–IIIa becomes activated through a process that involves calcium, protein kinase C, and heterotrimetric G proteins. Activation of GPIIb–IIIa requires energy and is a multistep process. Fibrinogen binding to GPIIb–IIIa occurs through a carboxy-terminal dodecapeptide sequence, HHLGGAKQAGDV, in the γ chain of fibrinogen where the AGDV sequence has been suggested to have structural similarity to the RGD sequence.

Blood coagulation

The blood coagulation system consists of a number of zymogens (proenzymes) that are proteolytically converted to active enzymes in a series of steps involving activators and cofactors. The coagulation reactions are initiated by tissue factor in complex with activated factor VII (VIIa). The tissue factor /VIIa complex then activates both factor IX and factor X, which, in the presence of their respective cofactors (factors VIII and V), lead to the rapid conversion of prothrombin to thrombin. The latter converts fibrinogen into a solid fibrin clot that finally undergoes cross-linking by activated factor XIII to become a stable haemostatic plug. Platelets are essential in several steps of the clotting mechanism and form the surface for activated clotting factors, which lead to the explosive generation of thrombin.

Understanding the modern concept of the clotting reactions requires a detailed knowledge of each factor. Table 7 depicts the clotting factors and their inhibitors, including the vitamin K-dependent clotting proenzymes, the non-vitamin K-dependent zymogens, the cofactors, the inhibitors of the clotting factors, and the structural proteins.

The vitamin K-dependent zymogens

The vitamin K-dependent blood clotting zymogens include: prothrombin, factor VII, factor IX, factor X, and protein C; their characteristics are listed in Table 7 and their schematic structures in Fig. 6. A common feature of all these clotting factors is the presence of gamma carboxyglutamic acid (Gla) domains in the amino terminal region of the molecules. Glutamic acid residues in these proteins undergo carboxylation, a post-translational event that is effected by hepatic carboxylase that requires reduced vitamin K as a cofactor. The vitamin K-dependent factors are highly homologous in terms of amino acid sequence. Factors VII, IX, X, and protein C have a similar domain structure with a Gla domain, two epidermal growth factor-like (EGF) domains, and a catalytic domain (Fig. 6). Prothrombin differs from other vitamin K-dependent factors in that it has two kringle domains (Fig. 6). Both factor X and protein C are secreted as two-chain zymogens while the others are single-chain proteins.

The Gla domains of these factors are necessary for binding to phospholipid membranes. Calcium ions occupy the Gla domain to result in a conformational change in the protein that favours binding to platelet membrane surfaces. Phosphatidylserine is the major phospholipid in these reactions.

The vitamin K zymogens are all serine proteases with the typical active site: a serine/histidine/aspartic acid triad. Exposure of the active site requires that the zymogen be activated by cleavage of specific arginyl residues. As a result, all the activated vitamin K-dependent zymogens become two-chain enzymes linked by disulphide bonds, as depicted in Fig. 6. Despite the high degree of sequence homology of these proteins, they are highly specific in their interaction with their cofactors and substrates.

Prothrombin

Prothrombin is synthesized in the liver and has a molecular weight of about 72 000 daltons. The molecule has 10 Gla residues that play a role in the binding of the prothrombin to the surface of activated platelets where it is converted to the active enzyme, thrombin, by the so-called 'prothrombinase complex' consisting of factors $Xa/Va/Ca^{++}$ on the platelet surface. Thrombin is a potent enzyme with a molecular weight of about 38 000 that rapidly converts fibrinogen to a fibrin clot. Thrombin also has many other actions including its role as: a potent activator of platelets; an activator of factor V, VIII, and XIII; an activator of protein C in the presence of its cofactor, thrombomodulin; an activator of procarboxypeptidase to form a thrombin-activatable fibrinolytic inhibitor (TAFI); and as a growth factor. The primary inhibitor of thrombin is antithrombin III.

Factor VII

Factor VII is synthesized in the liver and has a molecular weight of about 50 000 daltons. It has a very short half-life of about 3.5 h. The specific receptor for factor VII is tissue factor found on the surface of many cells such as fibroblasts, activated monocytes, and many other cell types. The physiological activator of factor VII is unknown, although it has been suggested that it might be activated by factor Xa. The factor VII/tissue factor complex activates both factors IX and X. The factor VII–tissue factor –Xa complex is inhibited by tissue factor pathway inhibitor (TFPI). Factor VIIa is not appreciably inhibited by antithrombin III except in the presence of heparin.

Table 7 Characteristics of coagulation proteins

Protein	Plasma concentration (μg/ml)	Biological half-life (hours)	Chromosome
Vitamin K- dependent zymogens			
Prothrombin	100–150	60–70	11p11–q12
Factor VII	0.5	3–6	13q34
Factor IX	4–5	18–24	Xq27.1–q27.2
Factor X	8–10	30–40	13q34
Protein C	4–5	6	2q13–q14
Non-vitamin K dependent zymogens			
Factor XI	5	72	4q32–q35
Factor XII	30	60	5q33
Prekallikrein	50	35	4q35
Factor XIII-A chain[1,2]	10	240	6p24–p25
Soluble cofactors			
Factor V[2]	5–10	12	1q21–q25
Factor VIII	0.1–0.2	8–12	Xq28
von Willebrand factor	10	12	12p13.2
Protein S[3]	25	42	3p11.1–q11.2
Protein Z	2.9	?	13q34
High molecular weight kininogen	70	150	3q26
Factor XIII-B chain[1]			1q31–q32.1
Cellular cofactors			
Tissue factor	–	–	1p21–p22
Thrombomodulin	–	–	20p12–cen
Structural protein			
Fibrinogen	2000–4000	72–120	
Aα chain			4q23–32
Bβ chain			4q23–q32
γ chain			4q23–q32
Inhibitors			
Antithrombin III	150–400	72	1q23–q25
Tissue factor pathway inhibitor	0.1		2q31–q32.1
Protein Z-dependent protease inhibitor (ZPI)			

[1]All of the plasma factor XIII-A chain is in complex with factor XIII-B chain; only half of factor XIII-B chain is in complex with factor XIII-A chain, the rest is free in plasma.

[2]Platelets carry significant amounts of factor XIIIA (roughly half of the total factor XIII activity) and factor V (20 per cent of circulating factor V). The B chain of factor XIII is not in platelets.

[3]Some protein S is in complex with C4b binding protein.

(Reprinted by permission of McGraw-Hill Companies from Roberts HR *et al.* (2001). Molecular biology and biochemistry of the coagulation factors. *Williams Hematology*, 6th edn, p.1460.)

Factor IX

Factor IX is synthesized by hepatocytes and has a molecular weight of about 57 000 daltons. Its plasma half-life is 18 to 24 h. The molecule has 12 Gla residues. About 40 per cent of the factor IX molecules carry a β-hydroxyaspartic acid at position 64 of the molecule. It is activated by VIIa–tissue factor and by activated factor XI, both of which cleave an arginyl bond at position 145 and 180 of the molecule to release an activation peptide of about 10 000 daltons. Factor IXa in complex with its cofactor, activated factor VIII, cleaves factor X to Xa. Antithrombin III will inhibit factor IXa, but the inhibition is not as rapid as the antithrombin III inhibition of thrombin or factor Xa.

Factor X

Factor X is also synthesized by hepatocytes and has a molecular weight of 59 000. It is secreted as a two-chain molecule linked by disulphide bonds. It has 11 Gla residues. When activated by factor IXa or VIIa–tissue factor, an activation peptide is cleaved from the heavy chain to expose the serine-active site on the heavy chain. Factor Xa, in the presence of its cofactor (factor Va), rapidly converts prothrombin to thrombin. The primary inhibitor of factor Xa is AT III.

Protein C

Protein C, unlike the other vitamin K-dependent zymogens, is not a procoagulant, but, when activated by the thrombin–thrombomodulin complex on the surface of endothelial cells, it becomes an anticoagulant by proteolytically cleaving factors Va and VIIIa, thus inhibiting coagulation. To function in this way as an anticoagulant, activated protein C (APC) requires a cofactor, protein S. Protein C is synthesized in the liver and has a very short half-life of about 6 h. It contains nine Gla residues and has a molecular weight of 59 000 daltons. The primary inhibitor of APC is the protein C inhibitor (PCI), also known as plasminogen activator inhibitor-3 (PAI-3).

The non-vitamin K-dependent zymogens

Factor XI

Factor XI is synthesized in the liver as a dimeric protein composed of identical subunits. It has a molecular weight of 160 000 daltons and a plasma half-life of about 72 h (Table 7). In plasma, factor XI circulates in complex with high molecular weight kininogen (HK), a non-enzymatic cofactor. The physiological activator of factor XI is thought to be thrombin, although *in vitro*, this factor can be activated by factor XIIa. The main function of factor XIa is to boost thrombin generation by activating factor IX on the surface of platelets, over and above the factor IX activated by the VIIa–tissue factor complex. Some patients with factor XI deficiency have no bleeding tendency, and those who do usually exhibit mild bleeding when compared to severely affected haemophilic patients.

Factor XII and prekallikrein (PK)

These factors have been collectively referred to as contact factors since it appears that activation of factor XII is enhanced by contact with a surface. Factor XII and PK are zymogens, which, when activated, expose a serine-active site (Table 7). HK is a non-enzymatic protein cofactor that circulates in complex with factor XI and PK. All of these factors are synthesized in the liver. Unlike the vitamin K-dependent proteins, factors XI, XII, and prekallikrein all possess so-called 'apple domains' that have specific functional characteristics. Deficiencies of factor XII and PK are not associated with bleeding tendencies in patients with complete deficiency of these factors. However, deficiency of each factor is associated with a marked prolongation of the partial thromboplastin time (PTT). In this test and in the presence of glass, ellagic acid, or some inert earth material, factor XII can activate factor XI. These factors may not play a major physiologic role in haemostasis, but there is evidence that they do participate in inflammatory responses that involve blood coagulation, fibrinolysis, and kinin generation.

The cofactors

Some of the cofactors are soluble and exist in circulation, namely protein S, protein Z, factors V and VIII, high molecular weight kiningen (HK), and von Willebrand factor (Table 7). Others are cell-bound, such as tissue factor and thrombomodulin.

Protein S

Protein S is synthesized in the liver and endothelial cells. It circulates in plasma and is also found in platelets. It has a molecular weight of 75 000 daltons and a plasma half-life of about 42 h. It contains 11 Gla residues in the amino terminal region. In structure, protein S differs dramatically from the other vitamin K clotting factors in that the carboxy terminal end is homologous to growth hormone. Protein S acts as a cofactor for activated protein C. Protein S exists in two forms: one form is bound to C4b-binding protein and the other exists as a free form in the circulation. Free protein S is a cofactor for protein C and is in equilibrium with the bound form.

Protein Z

Protein Z is synthesized in the liver and has a molecular weight of 62 000 daltons. There is now convincing evidence that when protein Z is incubated with factor Xa, the activity of the latter is reduced. The inhibition of factor Xa activity is due to the presence of a protease inhibitor that requires protein Z as a cofactor. Whether protein Z has other functions is unknown.

Factor V

Factor V is synthesized in the liver and has a biological half-life reported to be between 12 and 36 h. It is a large glycoprotein with a molecular weight of 330 000 daltons. Factor V is highly homologous to factor VIII. A schematic diagram of the structure is shown in Fig. 7. As can be seen, it is composed of A, B, and C domains. The A domains are homologous to the copper-binding protein, ceruloplasmin, so it is not surprising that this domain of factor V is involved in binding to calcium and copper. The C domains are homologous to fat globule proteins and are involved in the binding of factor V to phospholipid-rich platelet membranes. The A and C domains are homologous to similar domains in factor VIII, but the B domain is completely different from that of factor VIII. For factor V to act as a cofactor for factor Xa, it must be activated by thrombin with cleavage of arginyl bonds at positions 708, 1018, and 1545 as shown in Fig. 7. It is inactivated by activated protein C that cleaves bonds at 306 (slow) and 506 (fast).

Factor VIII

Like factor V, factor VIII is synthesized in the liver. It is a large glycoprotein with a molecular weight similar to that of factor V. Again, like factor V, factor VIII has A, B, and C domains with the A domain homologous to caruloplasmin and the C domain homologous to fat globule proteins (Fig. 8). The A domain of factor VIII is essential for binding to phospholipid membranes. The B domain of factor VIII is cleaved during activation

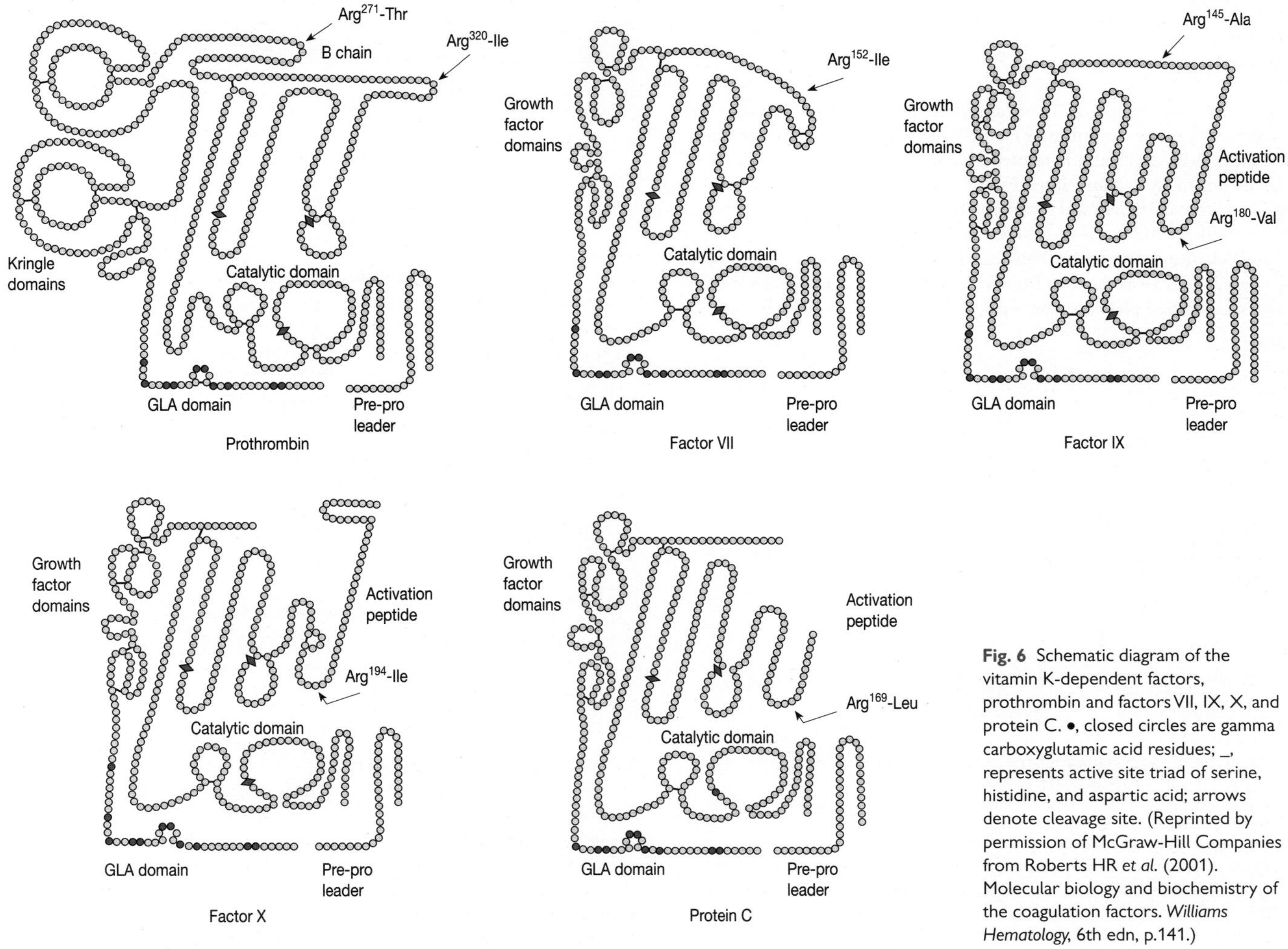

Fig. 6 Schematic diagram of the vitamin K-dependent factors, prothrombin and factors VII, IX, X, and protein C. •, closed circles are gamma carboxyglutamic acid residues; _, represents active site triad of serine, histidine, and aspartic acid; arrows denote cleavage site. (Reprinted by permission of McGraw-Hill Companies from Roberts HR *et al.* (2001). Molecular biology and biochemistry of the coagulation factors. *Williams Hematology*, 6th edn, p.141.)

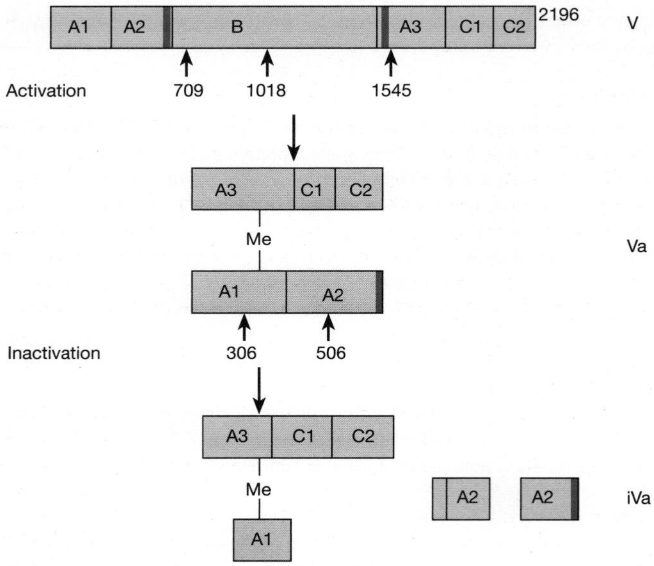

Fig. 7 Schematic diagram of factor V. Factor V is activated by thrombin to factor Va. Factor Va is inactivated by activated protein C (i Va). Activation of factor V by thrombin results in loss of the B chain and formation of a heterodimeric molecule covalently linked by metal ions (Me). Inactivation is by activated protein C that cleaves arginyl bonds at positions 306 and 506. (Reprinted by permission of McGraw-Hill Companies from Roberts HR *et al.* (2001). Molecular biology and biochemistry of the coagulation factors. *Williams Hematology*, 6th edn, p.1419.)

and has no known function. To act as a cofactor for factor IXa, factor VIII must be activated by thrombin or factor Xa. Unlike activated factor V, activated factor VIII exists as a heterotrimer composed of A1, A2, and C1-C2 domains linked by calcium ions. Factor VIII circulates in a non-covalent complex with von Willebrand factor and has a biologic half-life of 8 to 12 h. In the complete absence of von Willebrand factor, such as occurs with type III von Willebrand disease, the half-life of factor VIII is less than 1 h. When activated factor VIII is released from von Willebrand factor, it binds to the surface of activated platelets where it interacts with factor IXa.

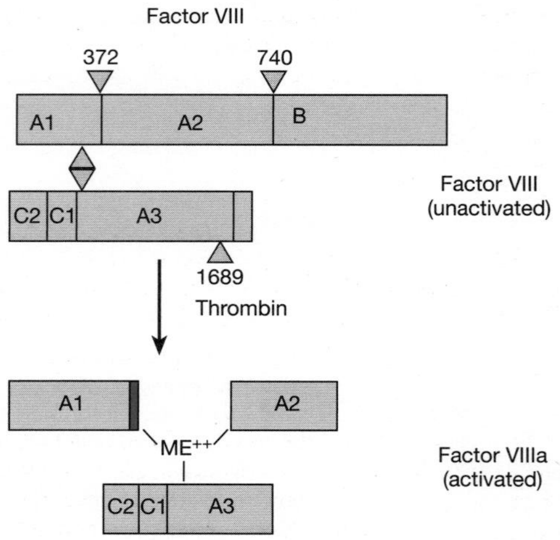

Fig. 8 Schematic representation of factor VIII. Activation by thrombin (or factor Xa) results in a heterotrimer non-covalently linked by metal ions (Me). Like factor Va, factor VIIIa is inactivated by activated protein C. (Reprinted by permission of McGraw-Hill Companies from Roberts HR *et al.* (2001). Molecular biology and biochemistry of the coagulation factors. *Williams Hematology*, 6th edn, p.1420.)

von Willebrand factor

von Willebrand factor is synthesized by endothelial cells and stored in Weibel–Palade bodies. It binds to glycoprotein Ib on platelets and is required for normal platelet adhesion to components of the vessel wall such as collagen. A schematic diagram of von Willebrand factor is shown in Fig. 9. Although synthesized as a prepolypeptide with A, B, C, and D domains, it is secreted into the plasma in multimeric form with molecular weights ranging from 1 million to 15 to 20 million. Higher molecular weight forms of von Willebrand factor are secreted to the abluminal surface of the endothelial cell as one component of the extracellular matrix. The higher molecular weight multimers are very effective in promoting platelet adhesion. von Willebrand factor is also important in platelet aggregation. A major function of von Willebrand factor is to act as a carrier protein for factor VIII. Factor VIII is associated with von Willebrand factor multimers of all sizes.

High molecular weight kininogen (HK)

High molecular weight kininogen circulates in plasma, and part is bound to factor XI and prekallikrein. HK is a cofactor for both of these zymogens. Deficiency of HK is not associated with a bleeding tendency, although the partial thromboplastin times of affected subjects are prolonged.

Tissue factor

Tissue factor, unlike other cofactors, is associated with cell surfaces. It is composed of 263 amino acids and with a 219-amino acid extracellular

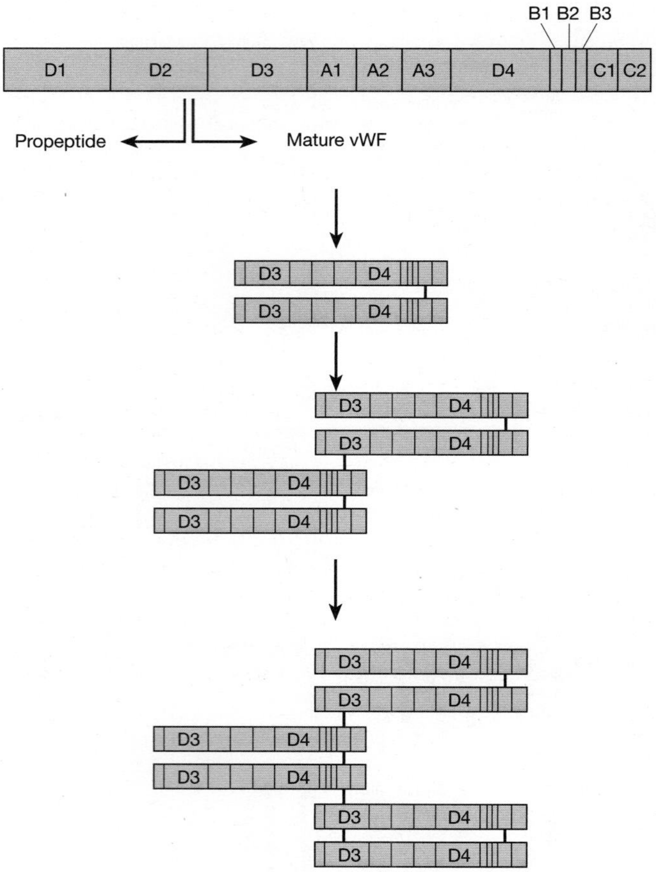

Fig. 9 Schematic diagram of von Willebrand factor. The formation of multimeric forms of von Willebrand factor occurs through links of dimers via D_3 domains. (Reprinted by permission of McGraw-Hill Companies from Roberts HR *et al.* (2001). Molecular biology and biochemistry of the coagulation factors. *Williams Hematology*, 6th edn.)

domain, a 23-amino acid transmembrane domain, and a 21-amino acid intracytoplasmic domain. The characteristics of tissue factor are shown in Table 7. It has a molecular weight of about 46 000 and is constituitively expressed on several extravascular tissues such as fibroblasts and smooth muscle cells. It is not constitutively expressed on cells exposed to the circulating blood, but can be induced in endothelial cells by certain inflammatory cytokines and certain bacterial products such as endotoxin. It can also be induced in blood leucocytes. Tissue factor functions as a receptor for factor VII. When factor VII binds to tissue factor, it is rapidly converted to factor VIIa, although the precise mechanism for its activation is not clear. The VIIa–tissue factor complex is now thought to be the main physiological initiator of blood coagulation by activating both factor IX and factor X, each of which plays a distinct role in subsequent coagulation reactions as described below. On some cells, tissue factor exists in a 'latent' form sometimes referred to as 'encrypted tissue factor' as suggested by the fact that tissue factor antigen levels on cells may be higher than tissue factor functional activity. 'De-encryption' can be accomplished by exposure of cells to agents such as calcium ionophores and various cytokines, but the physiological mechanism by which this process takes place is not known.

Thrombomodulin

Thrombomodulin is a transmembrane protein synthesized by and localized to endothelial cells although it has also been found on mesothelial cells, monocytes, and squamous epithelial cells. It has a molecular weight of about 78 000 daltons. A chondroitin sulphate moiety is attached to thrombomodulin via a serine residue. The major characteristics of thrombomodulin are depicted in Table 7. It serves as a receptor on endothelial cells for thrombin. Thrombin bound to thrombomodulin undergoes a structural transformation such that it no longer activates platelets or clots fibrinogen, but rather activates protein C. The principle function of the thrombomodulin /thrombin complex is to prevent the extension of the haemostatic clot past the site of a break or leak in the vessel wall and as such represents an important control mechanism to restrict the haemostatic plug precisely to the point of injury. Thus, under normal conditions, clot formation does not occur on the endothelial cell surfaces.

Fibrinogen

Fibrinogen is synthesized in the liver and has a molecular weight of 340 000 daltons. It is a dimeric glycoprotein consisting of two sets of identical chains, the α, β, and γ chains. The synthesis of each fibrinogen chain is governed by a separate gene as depicted in Table 7. The normal plasma half-life of fibrinogen is about 3 to 5 days. It is also found in the α granules of platelets as a result of endocytosis. Fibrinogen is the soluble plasma precursor of the solid fibrin clot that is so necessary for haemostasis and normal wound healing. The dimeric structure of fibrinogen is composed of two monomers, each containing disulphide-linked α, β, and γ chains. A schematic diagram of fibrinogen is shown in Fig. 10. It is a triodular structure with a central E domain that includes the disulphide-linked amino termini of all six polypeptide chains. The E domain is linked to the carboxyterminal domains referred to as the D domains.

Fibrinogen conversion to fibrin is accomplished by thrombin cleavage of two fibrinopeptides (fibrinopeptide A and fibrinopeptide B) from each of the two α and β chains, respectively, leading to the formation of the fibrin monomer. The molecular weight of each fibrinopeptide A and B is about 2500 daltons. The soluble fibrin monomer then undergoes spontaneous polymerization by forming side-to-side and end-to-end anastomoses, resulting in protofibrils that aggregate into a visible fibrin clot composed of thicker, branched fibres. During fibrin clot formation, other proteins are occluded in the clot, including plasminogen, fibronectin, thrombospondin, and von Willebrand factor. The fibrin polymerization is enhanced by calcium ions, but the polymerization process alone does not lead to a stable and impermeable fibrin clot since the fibres are held together weakly by hydrogen bonds and electrostatic forces. A stable fibrin clot requires cross-linking of the α and γ chains of fibrin by the action of activated factor XIII.

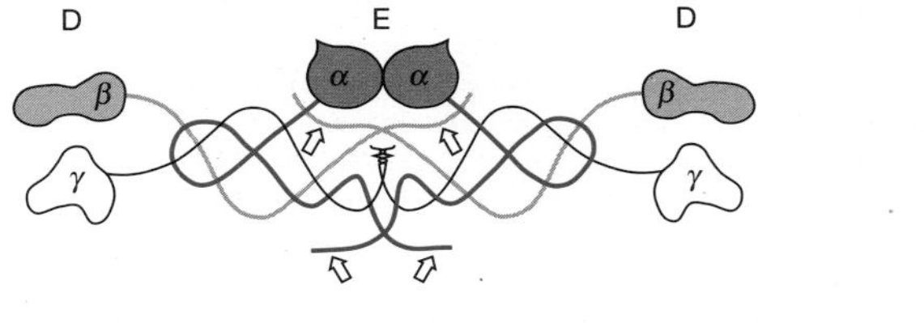

Fig. 10 A diagram of the structure of fibrinogen. The three chains, α, β, γ, are shown. The E domain occurs at the amino termini while the D domains are found at the carboxytermini. Arrows represent cleavage sites for fibrinopeptide A from the α chain and fibrinopeptide B from the β chain.

Factor XIII

Factor XIII is a proenzyme which circulates in the plasma as a heterotetramer composed of two A chains and two B chains (Table 7). Factor XIII has a molecular weight of 320 000 daltons and has a half-life of about 10 days. It circulates in plasma in association with fibrinogen. The A chain contains the active site cysteine, while the B chain is enzymatically inactive and serves as a carrier for the A chain. The A chain is found in platelets where it is not associated with the B chain. Upon activation by thrombin, the A and B chains are separated. In addition, thrombin cleaves the A chain so as to expose the active site cysteine. The active component then cross-links the α and γ chains of fibrin to form a stable, impermeable fibrin clot resistant to lysis by plasmin.

Inhibitors of the coagulation reactions

Tissue factor pathway inhibitor (TFPI)

TFPI is synthesized by endothelial cells. It has a molecular weight of about 34 000 to 40 000 daltons and serves to inhibit the initiation of coagulation (Table 7). TFPI can inhibit factor Xa in a slow reaction and also inhibits the VIIa–tissue factor–Xa complex. It exists in the circulation in at least three pools. One is bound to plasma lipoproteins; one pool is bound to proteoglycans on the vessel wall; and one exists in platelets. The TFPI bound to proteoglycans can be released by heparin. TFPI is a Kunitz-type inhibitor that is essential for control of coagulation.

Antithrombin III

The characteristics of antithrombin are also depicted in Table 7. Antithrombin belongs to a family of protease inhibitors known as 'serpins' that inhibit many proteases with a serine-active site. It is synthesized in the liver and has a plasma half-life of approximately 65 h. Its major function is to inhibit thrombin and factor Xa, although it will also inhibit the other coagulation serine proteases less well. The inhibitory action of antithrombin III is greatly enhanced by heparin, which accelerates the rate of inhibition of the serine proteases.

Protein Z-dependent protease inhibitor

This inhibitor inhibits factor Xa in the presence of calcium, phospholipids, and protein Z. It has a molecular weight of about 72 000 daltons. It, like antithrombin III, is also a member of the serpin family of serine protease inhibitors.

Other inhibitors of clotting factors

The major inhibitor of factor XIa is thought to be α-1-antitrypsin since it has the highest affinity for the enzyme. However, other inhibitors, namely C-1 esterase inhibitor, will also inhibit factor XIa. The other inhibitors that are of some importance in coagulation are also listed in Table 7.

The coagulation pathways

The coagulation reactions have been viewed as a sequential series of steps in which a enzymatic precursor (zymogen) clotting factor is converted to an

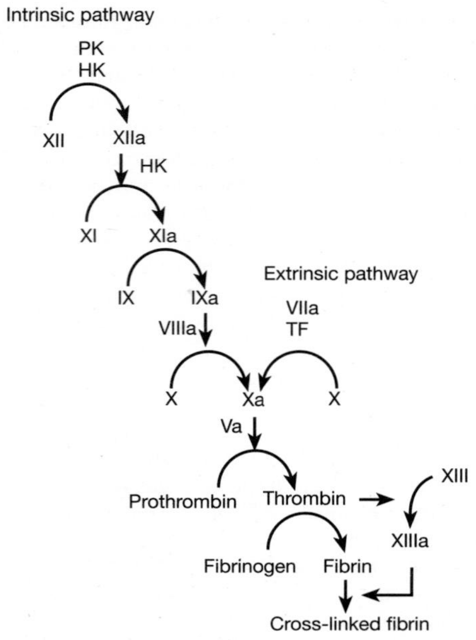

Fig. 11 An earlier model of blood coagulation reactions. The cascade or waterfall hypothesis of coagulation. (Reprinted by permission of McGraw-Hill Companies from Roberts HR *et al.* (2001). Molecular biology and biochemistry of the coagulation factors. *Williams Hematology*, 6th edn.)

active enzyme which, in turn activates another precursor, finally ending in the rapid conversion of prothrombin to thrombin. Early models of the coagulation reactions are shown in Fig. 11. As can be seen, when viewed in this manner, the clotting reactions appear as a waterfall or cascade, hence the terms waterfall or cascade hypotheses. Since tissue factor was extrinsic to the blood stream, the activation of factor X by the VIIa–tissue factor complex was termed the extrinsic system. The intrinsic system consisted entirely of clotting factors within the circulation and, upon conversion of factor IX to IXa by factor XIa, the factor IXa–VIIIa complex could also convert factor X to Xa in the presence of phospholipids. While this concept of coagulation was essentially correct, it did not explain why patients with factor XII deficiency had no bleeding tendency nor why factor XI-deficient patients had only a mild bleeding tendency. It was also pointed out that defects in the intrinsic system could lead to haemorrhage in affected patients even though the extrinsic system was intact and vice versa. The demonstration that the VIIa–tissue factor complex could activate both factor IX and factor X led several groups to conclude that the clotting reactions were, in fact, initiated by VIIa–tissue factor and that the intrinsic and extrinsic systems did not exist *in vivo*. Further work demonstrated that the clotting reactions leading to a haemostatic plug were controlled, in large part, by cell surfaces which modulated the reactions.

The role of the tissue factor cell

When a blood vessel is injured or ruptured, flowing blood is exposed to tissue factor, which is bound through a transmembrane and cytoplasmic tail to cells exposed as the result of injury, for example fibroblasts and other connective tissue cells. Factor VII binds to the tissue factor-bearing cell and is activated. As a result, the VIIa–tissue factor complex on the tissue factor cell activates both factor IX and factor X as shown in Fig. 12(a). The factor Xa and IXa formed in the milieu of the tissue factor cell play very different and distinct roles in subsequent reactions.

The role of factor Xa on the tissue factor cell

Factor Xa, in concert with its cofactor Va (which is found in the vicinity of tissue factor cells) then converts prothrombin to very small amounts of thrombin as shown in Fig. 12(b). This amount of thrombin, though insufficient to clot fibrinogen, can, however, act as a 'primer' of subsequent coagulation reactions to accomplish the following: activate platelets; activate more factor V; dissociate factor VIII from von Willebrand factor and activate factor VIII; and activate factor XI as shown in Fig. 12(b). Factor Xa alone and in complex with VIIa–tissue factor is then inhibited by TFPI. The activated cofactors resulting from the priming amount of thrombin in the milieu of the tissue factor cell then occupy binding sites on the activated platelet as shown in Fig. 12(b). Thus the main function of factor Xa formed

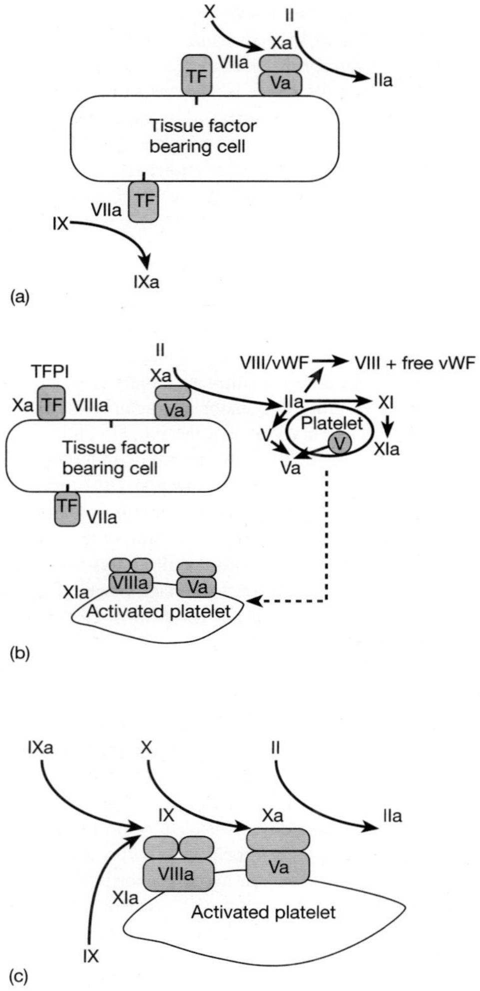

Fig. 12 (a) Tissue factor, a transmembrane protein expressed on tissue factor-bearing cells, acts as a receptor for factor VII, which is rapidly converted to factor VIIa. The tissue factor–VIIa complex then accomplishes two major functions: (1) activation of factor X to Xa and (2) activation of factor IX to IXa. Factor Xa activates factor V on the tissue factor-bearing cell and the resulting Xa–Va complex converts small amounts of prothrombin to thrombin. (b) This small amount of thrombin formed in the vicinity of the tissue factor cell acts as a 'primer' for coagulation by: (1) activating platelets; (2) dissociating factor VIII from von Willebrand factor and activating factor VIII; (3) activating factor V; and (4) activating factor XI. The activated platelets then adhere to the site of vascular injury and bind the cofactors, factors VIIIa and Va. Factor XIa also binds to platelets. The tissue factor–VIIa–Xa complex is then inhibited by TFPI (tissue factor pathway inhibitor). (c) Factor IXa formed by the tissue factor–VIIa complex associates with VIIIa on the platelet surface and recruits additional factor X from plasma to form factor Xa. The factor Xa then associates with its cofactor, factor Va, on the platelet surface to rapidly convert prothrombin to large amounts of thrombin sufficient to clot fibrinogen.

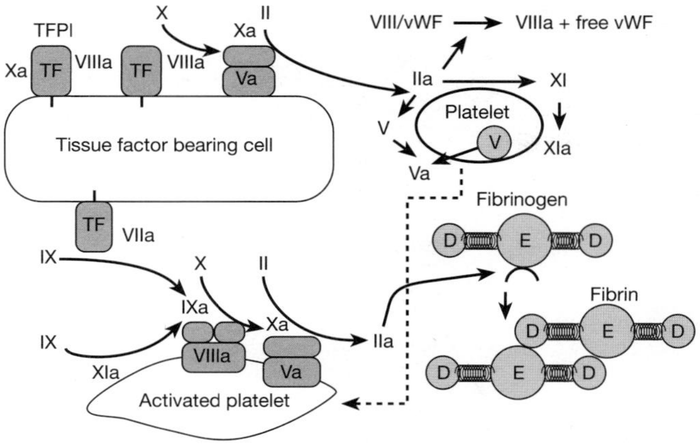

Fig. 13 The clotting reactions summarized. After thrombin formation, fibrinogen is converted to fibrin.

as the result of the VIIa–tissue factor complex is to furnish a priming amount of thrombin sufficient to initiate further subsequent reactions which take place on the activated platelet surface.

The role of factor IXa on the tissue factor cell

Factor IXa formed by the VIIa–tissue factor on the tissue factor-bearing cell diffuses away from the tissue factor cell and occupies a site on the activated platelet adjacent to its cofactor VIIIa (Fig. 12(c)). This factor IXa then plays a primary role in the subsequent burst of thrombin generation on platelet surfaces as noted below.

The role of the activated platelet

The activated platelet mass is the primary site of thrombin generation, which is highly dependent upon the amount of factor IXa formed both by the VIIa–tissue factor cell and factor XIa, which also occupies sites on the platelet. Factor IXa in the presence of its cofactor VIIIa then recruits more factor X from solution and activates it on the activated platelet surface. This factor Xa in the presence of its cofactor Va then converts large amounts of prothrombin to thrombin sufficient to clot fibrinogen. All of these reactions are summarized in Fig. 13. The mass of aggregated platelets upon which these reactions take place is localized to the damaged area of the vessel wall.

The role of the endothelial cells, vessel wall, and inhibitors

The mass of platelets interspersed with fibrin forms a plug at the site of a leak in the vessel wall where the endothelial cell monolayer is disrupted. The question arises as how the haemostatic plug is confined to the damaged area of the vessel wall. A schematic diagram of these events is shown in Fig. 14. The endothelial cells express thrombomodulin, which traps thrombin

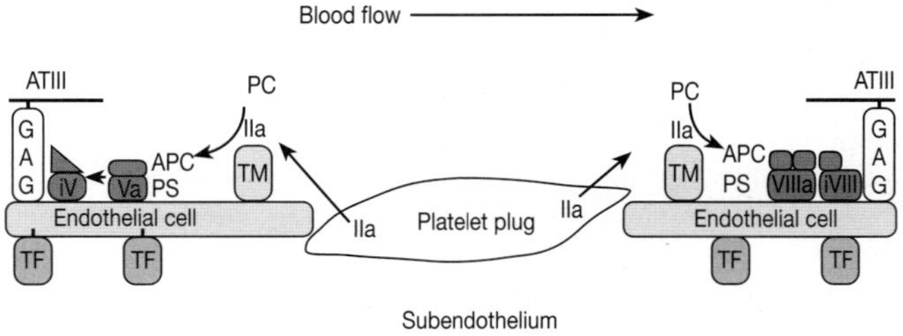

Fig. 14 A diagram of the haemostatic plug and the control mechanisms that restrict this plug to the site of injury and prevent extension of the clot to normal endothelium. TM, thrombomodulin; IIa, thrombin; GAG, glycosoaminoglycans; PC, protein C; APC, activated protein C; PS, protein S; TF, tissue factor; Platelet plug = haemostatic plug. iVa and iVIIIa refer to inactivated Va and VIIIa by APC.

to form thrombomodulin–thrombin complex that controls the procoagulant stimulus by activating the protein C system, resulting in inactivation of both factors Va and VIIIa on the endothelial cell surface. In addition, endothelial cells contain glycosoaminoglycans, some of which inhibit thrombin. Antithrombin III also circulates in solution to inhibit any thrombin that escapes from the haemostatic plug. In this way the fibrin clot sealing a leak in a blood vessel wall is confined precisely to that site such that extension of the clot does not occur under normal circumstances.

On-going coagulation *in vivo*

It is well known that products of the coagulation reactions are found in the circulation under normal (basal) conditions. Small, but definite levels of fibrinopeptides A and B can be measured. Fragment 1+2 derived from the amino terminal portion of prothrombin after thrombin is formed can also be detected. Activation peptides from several of the coagulation factors as well as complexes of activated factors with their inhibitors can also be found in the circulation. These observations strongly suggest that small leaks in blood vessels that occur during the stress and strain of everyday living are repaired by the on-going formation of haemostatic fibrin clots. This has been termed 'basal' coagulation, a process that allows the blood to remain fluid within the vascular tree and at the same time permitting small, exquisitely controlled and confined fibrin clots to plug small leaks in the vasculature without dissemination. The fibrin plug is then removed by the fibrinolytic system following the formation of new tissue.

The fibrinolytic system

The fibrinolytic system is shown schematically in Fig. 15. The components of the system and their characteristics are depicted in Table 8. The active enzyme in the fibrinolytic system is plasmin, which is derived from its precursor, plasminogen. Plasminogen is activated to plasmin by activators. The physiological activator is single-chain tissue plasminogen activator (t-PA), which cleaves plasminogen into two-chain plasmin. Another activator of plasminogen *in vivo* is single-chain urokinase, but this appears to be more important for degradation of matrix proteins. The physiological inhibitor of plasmin is α_2-antiplasmin.

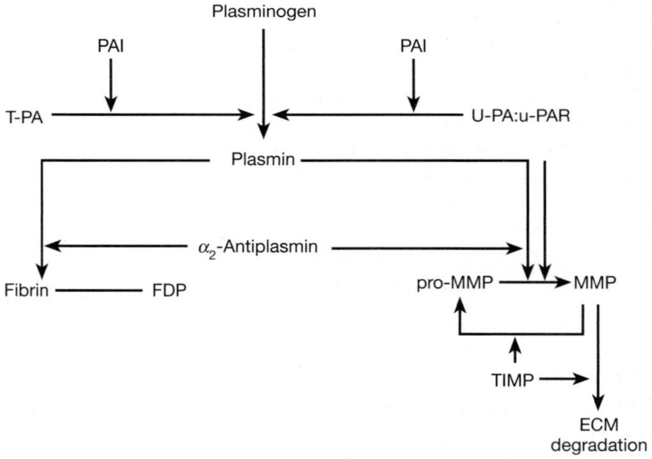

Fig. 15 The fibrinolytic system. Plasminogen is converted to plasmin by activators, including plasminogen activators (t-PA) and urokinase (u-PA). The activators are inhibited mainly by plasminogen activator inhibitor-1 (PAI-1). Plasmin degrades fibrin and activates matrix metalloproteinases (MMP), which degrades extracellular matrix (ECM). Plasmin is inhibited by α_2-antiplasmin. FDP, fibrin degradation product; TIMP, tissue inhibitors of metalloproteinases; U-PAR urokinase protease-activated receptor. (Reprinted by permission of FK Schatter from Collen D. (1999). The plasminogen (fibrinolytic) system. *Thrombosis and Hemostasis* **82**, 261.)

Plasminogen and t-PA associate in the circulation with fibrinogen. Thus when fibrinogen is converted to fibrin, the clot is rich in both of these proteins, which are protected from the inhibitory action of α_2-antiplasmin. Thus, clots can be lysed without interference from inhibitors, yet free plasmin in the circulation will be rapidly inhibited by its inhibitor.

Plasminogen

Plasminogen is synthesized in the liver and has a molecular weight of about 92 000 daltons. It is composed of a single chain and exists in two forms in the circulation: glu-plasminogen and lys-plasminogen. Glu-plasminogen has an amino-terminal glutamic acid and is a larger molecular weight than lys-plasminogen, which is formed in the circulation by plasmin cleavage of an arginyl bond at position 78 of the Glu form, leaving lysine as the amino-terminal residue. Lys-plasminogen rapidly binds to fibrin via lysine binding sites. Thus, lys-plasminogen is in close proximity to fibrin and protected from the action of antiplasmin. When activated, plasminogen is converted to active two-chain plasmin with a serine-active site on the heavy chain that is connected to the light chain by disulphide bonds.

The proteolytic action of plasmin is usually characterized by the proteolysis of fibrinogen and fibrin, but it can also degrade several other proteins including factor VIII, factor V, von Willebrand factor, and others. The cleavage of fibrinogen and fibrin leads to the formation of fibrin(ogen) degradation products. Fibrin(ogen) fragments resulting from plasmin cleavage are shown in Fig. 16. Fragment X is the first and largest fragment of plasmin digestion of fibrinogen. It is still clottable by thrombin, although much slower than native fibrinogen. Fragment X gives rise to fragment Y and D, and fragment Y is further proteolyzed to give rise to a second fragment D plus fragment E. These fragments can be detected in a simple laboratory test using antifibrinogen antibodies coated on latex particles. However, the test is non-specific and does not distinguish between the fibrinogen or fibrin degradation products which are quite similar, since the only difference between fibrin and fibrinogen is the absence of the small fibrinopeptides A and B in fibrin. A better test for detection of fibrin fragments is the so-called D-dimer test, which detects D-dimers resulting from the cross-linking of fibrin by factor XIIIa.

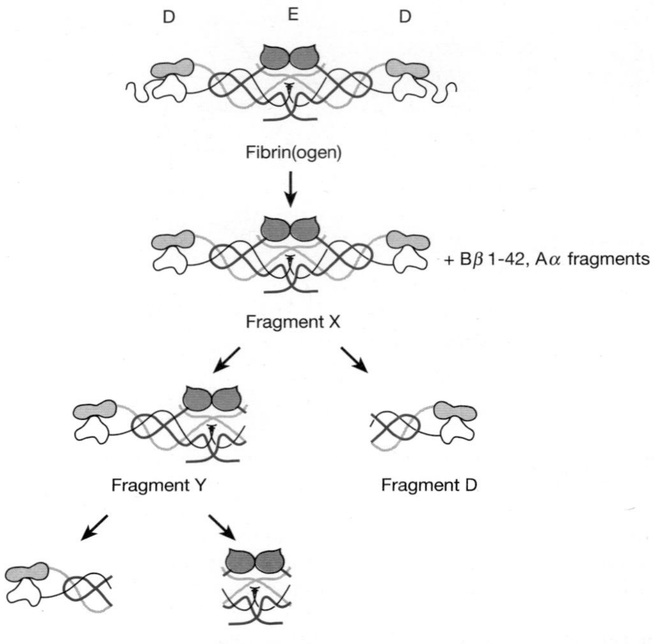

Fig. 16 Plasmin digestion of fibrin(ogen) results in fibrin degradation products: X, Y, D, and E. The final protolytic fragments resulting from plasmin degradation of fibrin are two molecules of fragment D and one of E. (Reprinted by permission from Francis CW, Marder VJ. In: Colman RW *et al.*, eds. *Hemostasis and thrombosis: basic principles and clinical practice*, 3rd edn. JP Lippincott and Co.)

Tissue plasminogen activator (t-PA)

Tissue-type plasminogen activator is considered to be the physiological activator of plasminogen. It is synthesized in endothelial cells and has a molecular weight of about 68 000 daltons. It has high affinity for plasminogen. T-PA circulates for the most part in complex with its inhibitor, plasminogen activator inhibitor-1 (PAI-1). The t-PA–PAI-1 complex can be dissociated during the process of coagulation, and free t-PA associates with fibrin, which enhances t-PA activity. Single-chain t-PA has catalytic activity, but when activated to the two-chain form by plasmin, the activity is increased by three-fold.

Urokinase plasminogen activator

Urokinase plasminogen activator exists as a single-chain zymogen and is found in the kidney, the urine, and fibroblast-like cells. It activates plasminogen by proteolysis of an arginyl residue at position 561. Its main function is in wound healing and vasculogenesis, and it is active in proteolysis of the extracellular matrix. Urokinase plasminogen activator associates with the urokinase plasminogen-activator receptor.

Table 8 Characteristics of the fibrinolytic system

	Plasma Mr (kDa)	Concentration (mg/l)	Chromosomal location
Plasminogen	92	20	6
Plasmin	85	–	
t-PA	68	0.005	8
u-PA	54	0.008	10
α_2-antiplasmin	70	200	18
PAI-1	52	70	7
PAI-2	47, 60	0.0518	18
u-PAR	50, 60		

Plasminogen activator inhibitor-1 (PAI-1)

PAI-1 is the physiological inhibitor of t-PA. It belongs to the serpin family of inhibitors. It is synthesized in endothelial cells and has a molecular weight of 52 000 daltons. Elevated levels of this inhibitor have been associated with arterial and venous thromboses. PAI-2, found in the placenta, also inhibits t-PA, but not as efficiently as PAI-1. PAI-3 is also known as the protein C inhibitor and inhibits plasminogen activators less efficiently than PAI-1.

α_2-Antiplasmin

α_2-Antiplasmin is the physiological inhibitor of plasmin. It has a molecular weight of about 58 000 daltons and is synthesized in the liver. As an inhibitor, it has three major functions: to inhibit plasminogen binding to fibrin; to inhibit the proteolytic activity of plasmin; and to bind to fibrin in a covalent manner by the action of factor XIIIa. By binding to fibrin, α_2-antiplasmin competitively inhibits the binding of plasminogen to fibrin. However, when plasminogen within the fibrin clot is converted to plasmin, the latter is protected from inhibition by antiplasmin. On the other hand, free plasmin formed in the circulation is rapidly inhibited.

Thrombin-activatable fibrinolytic inhibitor (TAFI)

TAFI is also known as plasma procarboxypeptidase B, and it is activated to carboxypeptidase B by large amounts of thrombin in a reaction dependent upon thrombomodulin. TAFI down-regulates fibrinolysis after clot formation and serves as an important regulatory mechanism for the fibrinolytic system. TAFI acts primarily by reducing the number of high-affinity plasminogen binding sites on fibrin, the end result of which is decreased fibrinolysis.

The fibrinolytic and coagulation systems are closely interrelated. Under normal conditions, fibrin clot formation is always accompanied by fibrinolysis. The formation of the fibrin clot leads to localization of t-PA and plasminogen leading to activation of the fibrinolytic system. It also appears that activated factor XI and factor XII enhance fibrinolytic activity. The action of the protein C system to decrease thrombin formation down-regulates the thrombin activatable fibrinolytic inhibitor which would favour increased fibrinolysis. Although much is still unknown, it is generally accepted that both the coagulation and fibrinolytic systems are related to the general process of inflammation involving several other host defence mechanisms.

Further reading

Andrews RK *et al.* (1999). The glycoprotein Ib-IX-V complex in platelet adhesion and signaling. *Thrombosis and Haemostasis* **82**, 357–64.

Brass LF *et al.* (1997). Signaling through G proteins in platelets: to the integrins and beyond. *Thrombosis and Haemostasis* **78**, 581–9.

Cines DB *et al.* (1998). Endothelial cells in physiology and in the pathophysiology of vascular diseases. *Blood* **91**, 3527–61.

Collen D (1999). The plasminogen (fibrolytic) system. *Thrombosis and Haemostasis* **82**, 259–70.

Coughlin SR (1999). Protease-activated receptors and platelet function. *Thrombosis and Haemostasis* **82**, 353–6.

Fay PJ (1999). Regulation of factor VIIIa in the instrinsic factor Xase. *Thrombosis and Haemostasis* **82**, 193–200.

Fox JEB (1999). On the role of calpain and rho proteins in regulating integrin-induced signaling. *Thrombosis and Haemostasis* **82**, 385–91.

Gimbrone MA (1999). Endothelial dysfunction, hemodynamic forces, and artherosclerosis. *Thrombosis and Haemostasis* **82**, 722–26.

Hartwig JH (1999). The elegant platelet: signals controlling actin assembly. *Thrombosis and Haemostasis* **82**, 392–8.

Kroll MH, Schafer AI (1989). Biochemical mechanisms of platelet activation. *Blood* **74**, 1181–95.

Loftus JC and Liddington RC (1997). New insights into integrin-ligand interaction. *Journal of Clinical Investigation* **99**, S77–81.

Majerus PW (1983). Arachidonate metabolism in vascular disorders. *Journal of Clinical Investigation* **72**, 1521–5.

Mann KG (1999). Biochemistry and physiology of blood coagulation. *Thrombosis and Haemostasis* **82**, 165–74.

Roberts HR *et al.* (1998). Newer concepts of blood coagulation. *Haemophilia* **79**, 306–9.

Roberts HR, Monroe DM, Hoffman M (1999). Molecular biology and biochemistry of the coagulation factors and pathways of hemostasis. In: Beutler E *et al.*, eds. *Williams' hematology*, 6th edn. McGraw-Hill, New York.

Roth GJ (1991). Developing relationships: arterial platelet adhesion, glycoprotein Ib, and leucine rich glycoproteins. *Blood* **77**, 5–19.

Ruggeri ZM (1999). Structure and function of von Willebrand factor. *Thrombosis and Haemostasis* **82**, 576–84.

Schmaier AH, Rojkjaer R, Shariat-Madar Z (1999). Activation of plasma kallikrein/kinin system on cells: a revised hypothesis. *Thrombosis and Haemostasis* **82**, 226–33.

Shattil SJ, Kashiwagi H, Pampori N (1998). Integrin signaling: the platelet paradigm. *Blood* **91**, 2645–57.

Smyth SS, Joneckis C, Parise LV (1994). Regulation of vascular integrins. *Blood* **81**, 2827–43.

Solum NO (1999). Procoagulant expression in platelets and defects leading to clinical disorders. *Arteriosclerosis, Thrombosis and Vascular Biology* **19**, 2841–6.

Ware J (1998). Molecular analyses of the platelet glycoprotein Ib-IX-V receptor. *Thrombosis and Haemostasis* **79**, 466–78.

Ware JA, Heistad DD (1995). Platelet-endothelium interactions. *New England Journal of Medicine* **328**, 628–35.

Watson SP (1999). Collagen receptor signaling in platelets and megakaryocytes. *Thrombosis and Haemostasis* **82**, 365–76.

22.6.2 Evaluation of the patient with a bleeding diathesis

Gilbert C. White, II, Harold R. Roberts, and Victor J. Marder

Introduction

The approach to the bleeding patient should be designed to determine if the bleeding tendency is inherited or acquired, systemic or local, and due to coagulation, platelet, or vessel wall defects (see Box 1). One should use the history, physical examination, and laboratory tests to derive answers to these questions.

The history

A history of both recent and remote bleeding should be sought. The nature of the bleeding, including the site or sites, severity, duration, association with trauma including surgical or dental procedures, and necessity for treatment of the bleeding, should be determined. Cutaneous, soft tissue, nasal, oropharyngeal, bronchial, genitourinary, gynaecological, joint, and intestinal bleeding should all be included in the history, as well as other more unusual sites. How much blood was lost? Were transfusions required? Was supplemental iron needed? If the bleeding followed surgery, what type of surgery? Excessive bleeding following tonsillectomy is common even in normal individuals and is harder to interpret than excessive bleeding following an appendicectomy. Spontaneous bleeding is more indicative of a

Box 1 Questions to answer in the evaluation of a bleeding diathesis

Is the bleeding acquired or congenital? Patients with congenital bleeding will often give a history of lifelong bleeding. This may be spontaneous or may be in the setting of previous surgical procedures or trauma. With acquired bleeding disorders, the onset of bleeding is usually recent and the patient often remarks that remote surgical procedures and trauma were not associated with bleeding. The family history is also important in determining if the bleeding is acquired or congenital. It is important to determine if unusual bleeding occurs in parents, grandparents, siblings, aunts, uncles, and children. A positive family history for bleeding favours a congenital disorder.

Is the defect systemic or local? Bleeding from multiple sites suggests a systemic defect, whereas bleeding from a single site may result from local abnormalities.

Is there a coagulation, platelet, or vessel wall defect? Bleeding due to coagulation defects tends to be in joints, soft tissues, or internal organs. Poor wound healing may suggest a disorder of fibrinogen or factor XIII. Platelet disorders are characterized by the presence of purpura and petechias.

bleeding diathesis than bleeding following a surgical or dental procedure, although persistent bleeding following trauma or surgery is often a sign of a coagulation abnormality.

The site of bleeding may provide clues to the cause. Joint bleeding is typical of haemophilia A and B and is much less common in other congenital and acquired bleeding disorders. Umbilical vein bleeding at birth is characteristic of factor XIII and fibrinogen deficiencies. Recurrent intestinal bleeding may be seen in hereditary haemorrhagic telangiectasia (Rendu–Osler–Weber disease) and is also seen in von Willebrand's disease and with certain platelet defects, but intestinal bleeding in general is most commonly due to a structural lesion. Recurrent bleeding from the same site is more consistent with a structural defect, whereas bleeding from multiple sites suggests a systemic haemostatic disorder.

The pattern of bleeding is also important. Delayed bleeding is typically seen with factor XIII deficiency and with α_2-antiplasmin deficiency. The initial clot forms normally, but is unstable and breaks down with normal fibrinolysis, causing bleeding after several days. With mild and moderate forms of haemophilia A and B, there is delayed bleeding and wound healing may be impaired, causing wound breakdown 5 to 7 days after surgery or injury.

The whole picture is more informative than a single event. An individual who has a lifelong history of easy bruising, bleeding following extraction of several teeth, recurrent epistaxis, and a long-standing history of menorrhagia is more likely to have a bleeding disorder than an individual that bled excessively following tonsillectomy but has no history of bruising and no bleeding with other dental or surgical procedures.

A family history is very important. It is not enough to ask if individuals in the family bleed. One should ascertain the number of brothers, sisters, aunts, uncles, parents, and grandparents who are known and determine bleeding histories for each person. In the evaluation of a male with possible haemophilia, a single brother who does not have a bleeding history is not very informative; if there are 10 brothers who have no bleeding history, the diagnosis is questionable. It is also important to determine haemostatic stresses in family members. A brother who has undergone an appendicectomy and suffered internal injuries from a motor vehicle accident without bleeding is more informative than a brother who has had no haemostatic stresses. The pattern of inheritance is also important. A sex-linked pattern of inheritance suggests haemophilia A or B. An autosomal pattern suggests other forms of inherited bleeding.

While the bleeding history is important and may provide clues to the nature of the disorder, it can also be misleading. Normal individuals will often report easy bruising that can be indistinguishable from that reported by individuals with congenital disorders. Epistaxis is frequent in children with nasal allergies whether or not there is an underlying bleeding defect and may suggest a congenital defect when there is none. Even bleeding following surgical and dental procedures can be misleading. For example, blood loss during and after tonsillectomy can be especially prominent, even in normal individuals. Blood loss after dental procedures can also be prominent, especially in individuals with poor dental hygiene.

The physical examination

The skin is a window to the blood coagulation system and careful examination of the skin is important in the evaluation of a bleeding diathesis. Ecchymosis, purpura, petechias, telangiectasia, the appearance of scars, and other cutaneous changes may provide an indication of the presence and type of bleeding disorder. The bleeding manifestations of patients with vascular disorders, thrombocytopenia, or functional platelet disorders mainly occur as spontaneous subcutaneous and mucous membrane haemorrhage and petechiae. In contrast, patients with clotting factor defects such as haemophilia develop deep, spreading haematomas, joint bleeding, and retroperitoneal bleeding.

The term 'purpura' is is a general term used to describe cutaneous extravasations of blood (Plate 1). The smallest of these are petechiase, pinpoint extravasations of blood that are round and do not blanch with pressure. They are most commonly found on the lower extremities where hydrostatic pressure is the greatest. Petechias in which there is a characteristic perifollicular distribution are typical of severe scurvy, or vitamin C deficiency. Patients with scurvy may also have excessive bleeding from multiple sites including the gums, alimentary tract, joints, and brain. More extensive cutaneous bleeding is called 'ecchymosis', or bruising, and may be seen with clotting factor abnormalities as well as platelet and vascular abnormalities.

Telangiectases are dilated small blood vessels that may be found in the skin and in the mucous membranes of the nose, lips, mouth, the whole of the gastrointestinal tract, urinary tract, and vagina in various forms of chronic liver disease, hereditary haemorrhagic telangiectasia (Rendu–Osler–Weber disease), and with hyperoestrogen syndromes. Bleeding from telangiectasia may cause recurrent epistaxis or prolonged and progressive gastrointestinal bleeding from multiple sites, which leads to refractory chronic iron-deficiency anaemia. Other cutaneous abnormalities with which bleeding may be associated are cavernous haemangiomas—large thin-walled venous abnormalities. These may precipitate chronic activation of the coagulation mechanism, causing chronic diffuse intravascular coagulation.

Cutaneous changes also characterize connective tissue disorders, including the Ehlers–Danlos syndrome, pseudoxanthoma elasticum, osteogenesis imperfecta, and Marfan's syndrome, that can all present or be associated with defects of primary haemostasis because of abnormal interactions of platelets with vessel wall connective tissue elements. The characteristics of cutanous scars may provide a clue to an underlying bleeding disorder. Congenital dysfibrinogenaemia and factor XIII deficiency may be associated with proliferative scars or keloids. Characteristic 'cigarette paper'-like scars are seen in the Ehlers–Danlos syndrome. Characteristic thickened skin papules and plaques are also seen with pseudoxanthoma elasticum, along with angioid streaks in the ocular retina.

Primary and secondary amyloid can both cause skin purpura, called 'pinch-purpura' because of the characteristic appearance on the cheeks. Amyloid may be found infiltrating the small blood vessels and has also been shown to cause platelet functional abnormalities due to membrane coating by the amyloid fibrils. The lesions often show a propensity for the periorbital tissues and on the skin may be distributed in linear streaks. Splenomegaly may also cause a mild thrombocytopenia. Occasionally there is evidence of factor X deficiency, secondary to binding to the abnormal amyloid fibrils.

Long-term administration of corticosteroids causes atrophy of the collagen fibres that support the blood vessels in the skin. This causes widespread purpura and bruises, usually on the extensor surfaces on the hands, arms, and thighs. The purpura is similar in aetiology to the senile type. A similar distribution may also be seen in Cushing's syndrome.

Certain acute infections may be associated with a purpuric eruption. The bacterial infections include meningococcal septicaemia, streptococcal septicaemia, and diphtheria. In meningococcal infection, the haemorrhage may extend to the adrenal cortex causing the Waterhouse–Friderichsen syndrome associated with acute adrenal insufficiency. If the purpuric lesions are extensive, purpura fulminans may develop with the skin lesions becoming necrotic and the patient entering an acute, shock-like state. An acute diffuse intravascular coagulation may occur, as bacterial products such as endotoxin or immune complexes will directly activate the clotting system. Immune complexes may also coat the platelet membrane causing an immune-mediated platelet destruction and interfering with platelet function. Several acute viral infections, including smallpox, chickenpox, and measles, as well as more recently described haemorrhagic fevers caused by Ebola virus, Rift valley virus, and Lassa virus may also cause similar purpuric lesions. These patients have a grossly prolonged bleeding time, thrombocytopenia, and abnormalities of platelet function.

Various allergic vasculitic purpuras are caused by inflammation and infiltration of the blood vessel wall as an anaphylactic reaction to a variety of agents including chemicals, toxins, infections, and physical stimuli.

Henoch–Schönlein purpura is probably the most common and involves skin, joints, alimentary tract, kidneys, heart, and central nervous system. There is often a preceding upper respiratory tract infection caused by a β-haemolytic streptococcus producing a rising antistreptolysin-O titre. Epidemics may occur in young children, with a fever followed by a purpuric rash that is often raised to the touch and classically affects the fronts of the legs, thighs, and buttocks. In addition, the patient may develop acute arthritis, gastrointestinal pain, and nephritis associated with proteinuria. The skin lesions may continue to form over several weeks. The most serious acute complications are central nervous bleeding, acute intussusception, or renal failure. The disease is usually self-limiting but the symptoms and purpura may respond to steroid therapy. Tests of haemostasis including studies of platelet function are usually within normal limits.

Bizarre bleeding and purpuric problems are reportedly associated with several psychological factors, so-called 'psychogenic purpura'. These include self-induced bleeding, hysterical bleeding, religious stigmas, and autoerythrocyte sensitization. Most of these patients have a disturbed or overanxious personality and very often the diagnosis is only suspected after numerous investigations have been made with all the results within the normal range. Autoerythryocyte sensitization is frequently associated with severe pain preceding the onset locally of skin bleeding and bruising. The lesion may be produced by the injection of a weak solution of the patient's own washed red cells or free haemoglobin solution subcutaneously into an area of the body, such as the back, with which the patient cannot directly interfere. To distinguish this condition from self-induced injury, it is important to include a negative saline control injection.

Purpuric lesions frequently occur in normal people, usually women. Single or multiple bruises appear spontaneously, mainly on the arms or legs, which rapidly resolve without any specific treatment. Senile purpura is frequent in older people, usually on areas exposed to mild but recurrent trauma such as the backs of the hands, the forearms, and the face. The purpura is caused by atrophy of the subcutaneous tissue with progressive loss of collagen and elastin fibres in the skin leading to inadequate support of the subcutaneous blood vessels. The lesions retain their dark colour, often for several weeks. There are no abnormalities in the haemostatic screening tests.

Laboratory tests

Laboratory investigations are required to identify the precise nature of an underlying bleeding disorder after a patient with a suspected haemorrhagic state has been clinically evaluated. Laboratory tests can be conveniently divided into screening tests and special tests, with the latter applied to the study of any individual patient according to the nature and clinical circumstances of the bleeding, and following the results of prior screening assays.

Screening tests

The most common screening tests performed in the initial assessment of a bleeding tendency are the activated partial thromboplastin time (**aPTT**), prothrombin time (**PT**), thrombin clotting time (**TCT**), platelet count, and bleeding time. Tables 1 and 2 show the results of screening tests in inherited and acquired clotting factor abnormalities.

The aPTT measures the intrinsic clotting system and the 'common pathway', the latter being the confluence of intrinsic and extrinsic systems at the point of prothrombin (factor II) conversion to thrombin (IIa). The aPTT is prolonged by deficiencies or abnormalities of high-molecular-weight kininogen, prekallikrein, factors XII, XI, IX, VIII, X, V, and II (prothrombin), fibrinogen, and by inhibitors of blood coagulation, such as the 'lupus inhibitor', heparin, and fibrin/fibrinogen degradation products. The aPTT is sensitive to activities of about 20 per cent or less of the factors listed above.

The prothrombin time measures the extrinsic clotting system. The prothrombin time is normally about 12 ± 2 s. The prothrombin time is prolonged with deficiencies of plasma factors VII, X, V, and II (prothrombin) and fibrinogen, and by inhibitors of these factors, whether iatrogenic (such as with heparin administration—acting through antithrombin III) or pathological (such as with antibodies against factor V). The test is affected by a decrease in factor VII more than by a decrease in prothrombin or fibrinogen in that it is not significantly prolonged with a fibrinogen level of about 100 mg/dl or with a prothrombin concentration above 30 per cent, but is significantly prolonged when factor VII, V, or X is less than 50 per cent of normal.

The thrombin clotting time measures the thrombin-induced conversion of fibrinogen to fibrin. A normal result requires effective release of fibrinopeptides from fibrinogen and unimpeded polymerization of fibrin monomers to form a polymer gel. The TCT is normal even in the presence of severe coagulation abnormalities that involve the coagulation pathway leading to but not including the conversion of fibrinogen to flbrin. Thus, it is normal in haemophilia (factor VIII or IX deficiency) and factor VII deficiency, and even with a decrease in multiple factors associated with vitamin

Table 1 Screening tests in hereditary bleeding disorders

Clotting factor deficiency	Prothrombin time (PT)	Activated partial thromboplastin time (aPTT)	Thrombin clotting time (TCT)	Bleeding time (BT)	Platelet count	Comments
Fibrinogen (I)						
Afibrinogen	∞	∞	∞	↑	N	Rare
Dysfibrinogen	↑	↑	↑	N	N	
Prothrombin (II)	↑	↑	N	N	N	Rare
Factor V	↑	↑	N	↑	N	Mild to severe bleeding
Factor VII	↑	N	N	N	N	Mild to severe bleeding
Factor VIII	N	↑	N	N	N	X-linked inheritance
Factor IX	N	↑	N	N	N	X-linked inheritance
Factor X	↑	↑	N	N	N	Mild to severe bleeding
Factor XI	N	↑	N	N	N	Mild bleeding
Factor XII	N	↑	N	N	N	No bleeding
Prekallikrein	N	↑	N	N	N	No bleeding
HMW kininogen	N	↑	N	N	N	No bleeding
Factor XIII	N	N	N	N	N	Clot dissolves in 5 mol urea
α_2-Antiplasmin	N	N	N	N	N	Short euglobulin lysis time

N, normal.

Table 2 Screening tests in acquired coagulation disorders

Disorder or condition	PT	PT mix	PTT	PTT mix	TCT	TCT mix	BT	Platelet count	Comments
Liver disease	↑	N	↑	N	↑	N	N to ↑	N to ↓	Factor VIII high; liver function tests abnormal
Diffuse intravascular coagulation	↑	N	↑	N	↑	N	↑	↓	Consumable factors ↓
Heparin	↑	↑	↑	↑	↑	↑	N	N	Reptilase time normal
Coumadin	↑	N	↑	N	N	N	N	N	
Thombocytopenia	N	N	N	N	N	N	↑	↓	
Inhibitors									
Factor V	↑	↑	↑	↑	N	N	↑	N	Often associated with use of topical thrombin
Factor VII	↑	↑	N	N	N	N	N	N	Rare
Factor VIII	N	N	↑	↑	N	N	N	N	Time/temperature
Factor IX	N	N	↑	↑	↑	N	N	N	dependent inhibitor
Factor X	↑	↑	↑	↑	N	N	N	N	Immediate-acting inhibitor
Factor XI	N	N	↑	↑	N	N	N	N	Rare
Factor XII	N	N	↑	↑	N	N	N	N	Usually with autoimmune diseases
Factor XIII	N	N	N	N	N	N	N	N	Usually with autoimmune diseases
Lupus inhibitor	↑	↑	↑	↑	N	N	N	N	Clot soluble in 5 mol urea

The PT mix, PTT mix, and TCT mix may be mildly prolonged in liver disease and diffuse intravascular coagulation. This is due in part to the presence of descarboxy γ-carboxyglutamic acid (Gla)-containing vitamin K-dependent clotting factors in liver disease and to the presence of fibrin degradation products in diffuse intravascular coagulation.

K deficiency. However, the TCT is abnormal in patients with hypofibrinogenaemia or afibrinogenaemia, whether acquired or congenital, or dysfibrinogenaemia, and in the presence of inhibitors such as heparin, myeloma proteins, and fibrin/fibrinogen degradation products, which block either thrombin cleavage of fibrinopeptides or fibrin monomer polymerization.

Mixing studies using either the aPTT or the prothrombin time are used to detect the presence of an inhibitor of coagulation. If normal plasma, containing 1 unit/ml of a given clotting factor, is mixed with an equal volume of deficient plasma containing less than 0.01 unit/ml of that factor, the resulting mix will have 0.5 units/ml of the factor, and the aPTT or prothrombin time of the mixed plasmas will be normal since these tests are not sensitive to clotting factor levels of 40 per cent or above. Conversely, if normal plasma is mixed with plasma containing an inhibitor, the inhibitor will neutralize most of the factor in the normal plasma. As a result, the mix will have less than 0.5 units/ml of the factor, and.the aPTT or prothrombin time of the mixed plasmas will be prolonged. Thus, a prolonged mix is characteristic of an inhibitor, whether in the form of a non-specific inhibitor such as heparin or a lupus inhibitor or a specific inhibitor against a specific coagulation factor.

Although a prolonged mixing study is characteristic of an inhibitor, some inhibitors, especially those against factor VIII and V, display aberrant behaviour in that the aPTT mix may not be immediately prolonged. In such cases, demonstration of the inhibitor may require incubation of the mixed plasmas at 37°C for 1 to 2 h. Thus, inhibitors to factor VIII or V are said to be time- and temperature-dependent. This incubated aPTT forms the basis for the Bethesda assay for quantification of factor VIII inhibitors. Occasionally, the lupus inhibitor may display time and temperature dependence.

The platelet count is a simple first step for evaluating the cellular aspects of haemostasis. Although there is no absolute relationship between the platelet count and the frequency and severity of bleeding, spontaneous bleeding without evidence of trauma is not usually manifest unless the platelet count is less than 10 000/μl, and serious bleeding after trauma or from a local lesion is unusual at counts above 50 000/μl. If platelet-type bleeding occurs when the platelet count is above 50 000/μl, a functional platelet defect of a congenital or acquired nature may be present.

The bleeding time evaluates primary haemostatic competency and therefore reflects both platelet number and function. The bleeding time measures the interval required for haemostasis following a standard superficial incision (1 to 2 mm deep and up to 5 mm long) in the skin of the forearm, while venous pressure is maintained at 40 torr. Prolongation of the bleeding time from a normal between 4 and 7 min usually occurs at a platelet count of 35 000 to 50 000/μl, with progressive prolongation noted with greater decreases in number. At counts below 10 000/μl, the bleeding time is often 15 min or longer: The bleeding time is prolonged in thrombocytopenic states of any aetiology. The bleeding time is also prolonged in various congenital and acquired qualitative platelet disorders, such as Glanzmann's thrombasthenia, Bernard–Soulier syndrome, storage-pool disease, and drug-induced thrombocytopathies (for instance, non-steroidal anti-inflammatory agents, most commonly aspirin). In von Willebrand's disease, the bleeding time is usually prolonged, but to a variable degree, as a result of a decrease or abnormality of plasma von Willebrand factor, which is involved in the binding of platelets to matrix proteins or to other cells. The bleeding time is also prolonged in severe hypofibrinogenaemia, as fibrinogen is the principal ligand for binding platelets to each other.

Although the bleeding time is a useful test of platelet function, it is difficult to standardize. The platelet function analyser (**PFA**)-100 has recently been proposed as a sensitive and reproducible test of platelet function, which may be used as an *in vitro* bleeding time. Citrated whole blood is passed through a standardized hole in a disc made of collagen–epinephrine or collagen–ADP. The time to platelet closure of the hole is measured. The PFA-100 has been reported to be useful in the diagnosis of von Willebrand's disease and qualitative platelet defects.

Some bleeding disorders are not associated with any abnormality of the screening tests. Patients with deficiencies of factor XIII and α_2-antiplasmin have normal prothrombin time, aPTT, and TCT values, but specific assays for these respective proteins are available for definitive diagnosis. Since deficient factor levels of 20 to 25 per cent or less may be needed to prolong a screening test, patients with mild deficiencies may also have normal screening tests, and diagnosis is possible only by direct assay of the factor. The screening tests are also normal in disorders of the vessel wall, such as hereditary haemorrhagic telangiectasia.

Specific tests

Depending on the assessment of both the clinical facts and the screening laboratory assays, individual factor assays and other special tests may be chosen to isolate the cause of the haemostatic disorder. Specific assays for all of the clotting and fibrinolytic factors are usually available in standard coagulation laboratories. In general, functional clotting factor assays are based on the one-stage aPTT using deficient plasmas or a two-stage assay using chromogenic substrates. Immunological assays are also used to measure total levels of fibrinogen, von Willebrand factor, and proteins C and S. Interesting differences have been found between the one-stage and chromogenic assays in the measurement of levels of recombinant factor VIII that may be important in the treatment of haemophilia. The fibrinolysis system includes the inactive precursor protein, plasminogen, promoters of fibrinolysis such as tissue plasminogen activator, the serine protease plasmin, and inhibitors of both activator (plasminogen activator inhibitor) and of plasmin (α_2-antiplasmin). The total concentration of each protein can be measured immunologically or by functional assay, usually by fibrinolytic or chromogenic assay. Clot lysis times measure the action of plasminogen activators and plasmin in the blood and are usually performed on clots formed from the euglobulin fraction of plasma or whole blood. Abnormally short lysis times (less than 2 h for plasma euglobulin) reflect acute episodes of excessive fibrinolysis that accompany a variety of acquired disorders or that result from the administration of plasminogen activators such as streptokinase, urokinase, or tissue plasminogen activator. The degree of fibrinolysis can be assessed indirectly by the measurement of fibrin degradation products.

Aggregation of platelets is measured photometrically by changes in light transmission of a suspension of platelets in plasma following the addition of selected agonists, usually adenosine diphosphate (ADP), thrombin, adrenaline, collagen, arachidonic acid, and ristocetin. Specific patterns of response to these agonists are observed in patients with storage-pool disease, Glanzmann's thrombasthenia, and Bernard–Soulier syndrome. The evaluation of platelet granule contents and secretion relies on specialized assays for quantifying adenosine nucleotides, serotonin (both dense-body constituents), and trace quantities of platelet factor 4, β-thromboglobulin, or adhesive proteins that have counterparts in plasma such as fibrinogen, fibronectin, thrombospondin, and von Willebrand factor (α-granule components). Tests of a specific platelet enzyme system involved in the arachidonic acid pathway (such as prostaglandin synthesis) and calcium transport are usually not available outside research laboratories.

The assessment of von Willebrand's disease bridges the gap between plasma coagulation factor analysis and platelet function tests, since such patients often present with a long bleeding time and a low plasma factor VIII activity. Most such patients have an abnormal and/or decreased plasma von Willebrand factor. Since the latter serves as a carrier protein for factor VIII, the concentration of factor VIII usually parallels the decrease in plasma von Willebrand factor. The protein concentration and type of von Willebrand factor multimer may be measured immunologically by Laurell rocket electrophoresis and by a combined electrophoresis/radioautograph or immunoblot procedure, respectively. Functional assessment of von Willebrand factor activity is performed by the ristocetin cofactor assay, in which ristocetin is added to a standard source of preserved (formalinized) platelets in the presence of the test plasma, and the degree and rate of platelet aggregation are compared with those of normal plasma. Collagen binding assays are also used to measure the function of von Willebrand factor. Usually a defective von Willebrand factor is associated with a deficiency in 'ristocetin cofactor activity', although some patients have von Willebrand factor with high activity, and rare patients (those with 'pseudo-von Willebrand's disease') have von Willebrand factor-hyperactive platelets. Inhibitors to von Willebrand factor may also account for acquired von Willebrand's disease, and von Willebrand factor may also be depleted by virtue of adsorption on to cells, as in some patients with lymphoid tumours.

Special problems

Sometimes, in patients with central venous catheters or arterial lines that are flushed with small amounts of heparin, blood drawn through the catheter may become contaminated with heparin. It thus becomes necessary to distinguish a systemic coagulopathy from heparin contamination. The first clue that the abnormal clotting screens might be due to heparin contamination is the finding of a prolonged TCT and aPTT with a normal or nearly normal prothrombin time. Mixing studies will be prolonged. The easiest way to demonstrate heparin contamination is to redraw the sample, either through a peripheral vein or through the catheter, discarding the initial 5 to 10 ml. If tests on the repeat sample are normal, it can be assumed that the initial sample was contaminated with heparin. The presence of heparin in the sample can be confirmed by a reptilase time. Reptilase is a snake venom that clots fibrinogen; unlike thrombin, reptilase is not inhibited by heparin. Thus, with the effect of heparin, the TCT is prolonged, but the reptilase time is normal.

The diagnosis of diffuse intravascular coagulation also requires a special set of tests ('DIC screen'). Screening tests in diffuse intravascular coagulation will show prolonged clotting times (prothrombin time, aPTT, TCT), a decreased platelet count, and usually a low fibrinogen. Ancillary tests include fibrin degradation products, fibrinopeptide A, and fibrin D-dimer, all of which will be increased in diffuse intravascular coagulation. Fibrin degradation products are also elevated in many other disorders and are not specific for the diagnosis of diffuse intravascular coagulation. In liver disease, which may be complicated by and confused with diffuse intravascular coagulation, factor VII is decreased while factors V and VIII and fibrinogen are less affected and may even be normal.

Application of clinical observations and laboratory studies to diagnosis: illustrative cases

Case 1

A middle-aged man is admitted for surgery. A careful history reveals that on three previous occasions, dental extraction was associated with rebleeding that required repacking on several occasions. He has had no other operative procedures and no trauma of significance. The family history is negative. Because of the history of mild bleeding, coagulation screens are performed and reveal: aPTT 120 s (control 38 s), prothrombin time 12 s (control 12 s), TCT 12 s (control 12 s), platelet count 200 000/μl, and bleeding time 9 min (normal 4 to 7 min). An incubated aPTT mix reveals patient aPTT 112 s, control 36 s, mix 38 s; specific factor assays reveal: factor XII 105 per cent, factor XI 86 per cent, factor IX 94 per cent, factor VIII 5 per cent, von Willebrand factor antigen 40 per cent, and von Willebrand factor activity 25 per cent. Tests of prekallikrein and high-molecular-weight kininogen are normal.

One of the most common laboratory abnormalities is an isolated increase in aPTT. Initially, the test should be repeated, and it should be determined whether the patient is receiving small doses of heparin (minidose or heparin flushes), which can produce an aPTT prolongation. To induce the marked prolongation of aPTT in this case (120 s), relatively large amounts of heparin would be required, and other screening coagulation tests (prothrombin time and TCT) should also be prolonged. If the prolongation of the aPTT is reproducible, further laboratory studies should focus on components of the intrinsic pathway, including prekallikrein, kininogen, factors XII, XI, IX, and VIII, and inhibitors of these factors. If the patient is asymptomatic, four major possibilities should be considered: the patient may have a 'lupus' inhibitor or be deficient in high-molecular-weight kininogen, prekallikrein, or factor XII. These familial syndromes, especially high-molecular-weight kininogen and factor XII deficiency, can give a remarkably prolonged PTT in patients who have no clinical bleeding. Such an occurrence may unnecessarily deter a surgeon from operating.

If the patient has a bleeding diathesis, one should consider factor VIII, IX, or XI deficiency, or von Willebrand's disease. In this case, an incubated aPTT mix ruled out an inhibitor, and specific factor assays showed diminished levels of factor VIII and von Willebrand factor antigen and activity, data consistent with a diagnosis of von Willebrand's disease. An isolated prolongation of the aPTT is relatively common. In contrast, an abnormal prothrombin time as an isolated finding is unusual and, if the disorder is congenital, signifies factor VII deficiency. In contrast, an abnormal prothrombin time and aPTT is a common combination that may be due to isolated deficiencies of factors II, V, and X or fibrinogen and more complex conditions, such as vitamin K deficiency, warfarin therapy, diffuse intravascular coagulation, therapeutic fibrinolysis, and liver disease. Specific assays for factors II, V, and X and measurement of the thrombin time and fibrinogen degradation products may be used to define these problems. The combination of an abnormal aPTT and a long bleeding time suggests von Willebrand's disease, with the long aPTT caused by a low factor VIII level and the decrease in von Willebrand factor activity accounting for the long bleeding time, while other patients with von Willebrand's disease may have normal factor VIII activity and a normal aPTT but a long bleeding time. Variations in the same patient may even occur, which make this diagnosis more difficult in certain instances. In patients with no abnormalities of the screening tests but clinical evidence of a systemic bleeding state, one must consider factor XIII deficiency, α_2-antiplasmin deficiency, and other mild disorders.

This case raises several other important issues. First, should preoperative coagulation screening tests be performed routinely? The argument has been advanced that if a properly taken history is negative, coagulation screens should not be performed in all preoperative patients. This is a cost–benefit argument that presumes an adequate history is obtained, but too frequently this is not done. Therefore the question of routine screening tests is something that must be worked out individually at each institution. In this hypothetical case, the history was suggestive of a mild bleeding disorder, and this necessitated screening tests. Although all three components of the factor VIII complex were abnormal in this patient, the laboratory expression in von Willebrand's disease is highly variable; had the factor VIII antigen and von Willebrand factor activity been normal, von Willebrand's disease would still have been a possibility. Exclusion of von Willebrand's disease with certainty may require determinations on multiple occasions, as well as analysis of multimeric patterns and testing of family members. As for therapy, newer therapeutic modalities such as desmopressin make it possible to avoid transfusion of plasma products in some patients and thus reduce the risk of transfusion-mediated disorders such as hepatitis and AIDS.

Case 2

A 75-year-old man with severe coronary artery disease is admitted for bypass surgery. He has no history of a bleeding tendency and underwent gallbladder surgery 3 years previously without complication. Preoperative evaluation reveals a normal platelet count and normal coagulation screening tests. Surgery is without complication until the fourth hour, about 30 min after coming off the bypass pump, when increased oozing from the surgical site is noted. The activated whole-blood clotting time, which has been maintained at around 300 s during the course of surgery, is found to be greatly prolonged. Studies indicate a platelet count of 22 000/μl, aPTT more than 150 s, and TCT more than 60 s. A reptilase time is markedly prolonged, indicating that heparin alone does not account for the prolonged clotting tests. The blood smear shows about 20 schistocytes per high-power field. The presumptive diagnosis of diffuse intravascular coagulation is confirmed by factor assay, which revealed fibrinogen 75 mg/dl, factor VIII 15 per cent, and factor V 12 per cent, but factor VII 95 per cent.

The initial step in the evaluation of severe intraoperative or postoperative bleeding is to determine whether a systemic haemostatic disorder is present. The screening tests are very important in this determination because the history is often limited to immediate observations of the site, amount, and time of bleeding. If the screening tests are normal and the patient is bleeding briskly, it is unlikely that the bleeding is due to a haemostatic defect, and attention should then be turned to bleeding due to local causes. On the other hand, if the screening tests are abnormal but the patient appears to have highly localized bleeding, a structural defect may still be the cause, aggravated by the haemostatic defect. If the patient is bleeding from numerous sites, including non-operative sites, it is likely that a haemostatic defect exists.

Cardiac surgery in particular can have several effects on the haemostatic system. Coagulation defects may result from haemodilution, especially in cases in which blood loss is massive and replacement with plasma is inadequate relative to other fluids, from heparin administration during cardiac bypass, from diffuse intravascular coagulation and acute fibrinolysis, and from platelet defects or destruction as a result of interaction with the bypass circuit. In the present case, the screening tests showed marked abnormalities. Although heparin can cause similar abnormalities, the prothrombin time was greatly prolonged, and this occurs only with large heparin doses. The reptilase time, which is not sensitive to heparin, was prolonged. The normal factor VII level provided evidence against haemodilution. Although thrombocytopenia could result from consumption after cardiac bypass, it is more likely to be part of a general consumptive coagulopathy. Treatment for diffuse intravascular coagulation was initiated.

Case 3

A 25-year-old woman is referred for evaluation of lifelong easy bruising. While many of these episodes are associated with mild trauma, bruises develop without known trauma as well. There is a predilection for the extremities, but she also has noticed bruises on the trunk. Menses are heavy, and she has been given supplemental iron. Her only surgical procedure was extractions for orthodontic work at the age of 12. Six teeth were extracted over a 2-month period, and two required repacking because of bleeding. The patient's mother and a sister also bruise easily, although the mother underwent uncomplicated gallbladder surgery at the age of 50. Physical examination reveals several small bruises in various stages of healing on the arms and legs, scattered petechias, and scars on the knees from childhood trauma, which are normal in appearance. Coagulation screens reveal: aPTT 36 s, prothrombin time 12 s, TCT 13 s, platelet count 179 000/μl, and bleeding time 36 min. The blood smear shows adequate numbers of platelets that are normal in size and staining characteristics. Additional studies are obtained as follows: factor VIII 75 per cent, von Willebrand factor antigen 110 per cent with multimeric pattern normal, von Willebrand factor activity 86 per cent, and salicylate level 0. Platelet aggregation studies show a normal response to ristocetin, but adrenaline and low concentrations of ADP produce only a single wave of aggregation, and collagen and arachidonic acid produce shape change but no aggregation response. The patient is referred to a platelet research laboratory. The ADP and ATP content of platelets is normal, electron microscopy reveals normal numbers of dense granules and α-granules, and the production of prostaglandin endoperoxides and thromboxane from radiolabelled arachidonate is greatly diminished.

Easy bruising is a common symptom that is seen in patients with coagulation defects, platelet disorders, and vascular and endocrine disorders, but it is also seen in people with no underlying haemostatic defect. In the present case the initial screening tests revealed a prolonged bleeding time with a normal platelet count, indicating a qualitative platelet defect, von Willebrand's disease, or a vessel wall disorder. Some patients with von Willebrand's disease present with an isolated prolongation of the bleeding time, but this is uncommon. Defects of the vessel wall are rare but possible in patients with a prolonged bleeding time, normal platelet count, persistently normal von Willebrand factor studies (including those of family members), and normal *in vitro* platelet function. The most common cause of a long bleeding time with normal von Willebrand factor evaluation is a platelet disorder.

One can approach the diagnosis of a patient with a normal platelet count and a prolonged bleeding time in two ways. One approach studies platelet aggregation and secretion for a primary platelet abnormality, and the other measures factor VIII activity, von Willebrand factor, and ristocetin cofactor activity to diagnose von Willebrand's disease. A diverse array of normal and abnormal findings in factor VIII activity, von Willebrand factor content and multimer distribution, and ristocetin cofactor activity can exist in patients with von Willebrand's disease, but the key observation is the documentation of a plasma protein abnormality that mitigates against a primary platelet disorder of aggregation and/or release. The finding of a total absence of aggregation response to agonists such as ADP, adrenaline, and collagen is consistent with the diagnosis of Glanzmann's thrombasthenia, which can be confirmed by studies that document a defect or deficiency of the glycoprotein IIb–IIIa complex. An isolated absent response of platelet-rich plasma to ristocetin suggests von Willebrand's disease or the Bernard–Soulier syndrome, while an enhanced response occurs in the type 2B variant of von Willebrand's disease. Simple microscopic examination of the platelets may show the large size that is characteristic of the former. Impairment or lack of a second wave of aggregation and decreased dense-granule secretion (ATP or serotonin) may be due to a deficiency in dense-granule contents that may additionally be accompanied by α-granule disorders or by an abnormality in the mechanism of secretion, such as occurs with defects in thromboxane synthesis. The contents of α-granules and dense granules can be measured directly, as can the pathway of thromboxane synthesis, to identify more precisely the specific nature of the defect.

In this case, platelet aggregation studies suggested a release defect with typical inhibition of collagen and arachidonate responses. Further studies indicated that the granule compartment of the platelets was normal, as evidenced by the normal nucleotide levels and the normal electron-microscopic appearance of the platelets. Studies with labelled membrane lipids indicated that there was a defect in lipid metabolism with failure to generate prostaglandin endoperoxides or thromboxane A_2 in response to appropriate agonists. This suggests a defect in arachidonate metabolism as the cause of the release defect. Since radiolabelled arachidonate was not metabolized normally to prostaglandin endoperoxides, the most likely cause is a cyclo-oxygenase deficiency.

Case 4

A young rubber-company worker presents to the emergency department with a 2-week history of spontaneous bruising, intermittent epistaxis, and gum bleeding after tooth brushing. Four hours before admission he developed haematuria. His only medication is frusemide for hypertension. Coagulation screening tests reveal a prothrombin time of more than 60 s, aPPT more than 90.1 s, and TCT 12.8 s. The platelet count is 302 000/μl and the bleeding time is 3 min. Mixing studies reveal a prothrombin time of more than 60 s, mix 12 s. Liver function tests are normal. Specific factor assays are performed and are normal except for factor II 7 per cent, factor VII less than 1 per cent, factor IX 4 per cent, and factor X 2 per cent. A plasma coumadin level is 0. On further questioning, the patient denies the use of anticoagulants and does not have rat poison at home. Despite administration of vitamin K_1 in a dose of 15 mg subcutaneously and 2 mg intravenously twice daily, the prothrombin time and aPTT remain prolonged. The dose of vitamin K is increased to 5 mg intravenously every 4 h. Further history reveals that a new rodenticide containing a long-lasting coumarin, brodifacoum, has recently been used at the rubber-tyre company. Plasma is obtained that reveals the presence of brodifacoum at a level of 162 μg/ml. Although a supervised search of the patient and his room failed to reveal any suspicious material, his clotting times improved and eventually returned to normal after 25 days of isolation.

This case of surreptitious coumarin abuse illustrates some of the difficulties in establishing the diagnosis. Typically seen in health-care workers, the markedly prolonged prothrombin time and aPTT with a normal TCT are characteristic. The diagnosis is further suggested by the finding of reduced plasma levels of the vitamin K-dependent clotting factors in the absence of liver disease. Confirmation of the diagnosis, although strongly suggested by the previous constellation of findings, may require chemical demonstration of the drug in plasma. It is not unusual in such patients for self-administration of the drug to continue in the hospital. Once the question of surreptitious coumarin abuse is raised, one must be suspicious of the patient and family members, as well as friends and individuals at work. Psychiatric evaluation may be essential and, in cases where it is suspected that someone is trying to poison the patient, police involvement may be advised.

Brodifacoum is a member of a family of coumarin compounds termed 'super-warfarins'. They are used in rodenticides and are so termed because of their potency and very long biological half-life. For example, brodifacoum is about 100 times as potent as warfarin and has a half-life of about 22 days in humans, compared with warfarin's half-life of 1 day. As a result, a single dose of 1 to 2 mg of brodifacoum can produce a prothrombin time prolongation for up to 70 to 80 days.

In this case, plasma levels of brodifacoum were markedly increased, but a warfarin level was undetectable. The chemical structure of the coumarin compounds is such that many assays in commercial use are specific for a single compound and will not detect other coumarins. One must therefore have some clue to the agent in use and request a specific assay.

Case 5

A 60-year-old man with coronary artery disease presents with a 1-week history of easy bruising. He was initially seen 4 months earlier with new onset of atrial fibrillation. Following cardioversion, he was started on quinidine with maintenance of a stable cardiac rhythm. He denied other medications and had no history of viral or other illnesses. Laboratory evaluation reveals normal coagulation screens and a bleeding time of 14 min. The platelet count is 12 000/μl with a haematocrit of 42 and a white count of 6700/μl. A bone marrow examination is performed and is normocellular with adequate numbers of megakaryocytes. A test for antinuclear antibodies is negative. Platelet antibody testing is as follows: direct antiplatelet antibodies, 7450 molecules IgG/platelet (normal 0 to 2500); indirect antiplatelet antibodies, 1130 molecules IgG/platelet (normal 0 to 2500); and indirect antiplatelet antibodies in the presence of quinidine, 7140 molecules IgG/platelet.

Thrombocytopenia is a common cause of bleeding and easy bruising. The first step in the evaluation of a patient with thrombocytopenia is to determine if the defect is a failure of platelet production, increased platelet destruction, or splenetic sequestration. Liver disease and other potential causes of splenic enlargement should be considered and a careful examination should be made for splenomegaly. While a normal haematocrit and white count militate against global bone marrow failure, this condition can be excluded only by a bone marrow aspirate and biopsy. The biopsy in particular may be required to rule out aplastic anaemia and infiltrative processes. Other causes of thrombocytopenia, such as leukaemia, myeloma, and megaloblastic anaemias, can be diagnosed by an aspirate. If the marrow contains a normal number and distribution of cells and a reasonable quantity of morphologically normal megakaryocytes, the cause of the thrombocytopenia is unlikely to be reduced production, and one should look for causes of increased peripheral destruction.

Immune thrombocytopenia is diagnosed by the demonstration of a normal bone marrow, the absence of an enlarged spleen, and the absence of non-immune causes of thrombocytopenia. The presence of elevated levels of antiplatelet antibodies confirms the diagnosis, but elevated platelet antibodies may be seen in other causes of thrombocytopenia, and some cases of immune thrombocytopenia may not have elevated platelet antibodies. Immune thrombocytopenia may be seen in lupus erythematosus, chronic lymphocytic leukaemia, with certain drugs, especially quinidine, and by exclusion in idiopathic thrombocytopenic purpura (ITP).

Quinidine is one of the most common causes of drug-induced ITP. Patients may develop thrombocytopenia months or years after starting the drug, but re-exposure to quinidine may produce explosive thrombocytopenia. Although the diagnosis of quinidine purpura should be considered in any patient with thrombocytopenia and a history of exposure to the drug, the diagnosis can be established by either the demonstration of quinidine-dependent antiplatelet antibodies, as in this case, or by improvement in the platelet count on discontinuation of the drug. Typically, the platelet count improves within 4 to 5 days, but it may take up to 6 weeks.

Case 6

A 38-year-old woman is admitted for gallbladder surgery. Preoperative coagulation screens and platelet count are normal. Surgery is performed without complication. On the seventh postoperative day, she develops pain and swelling in the right leg, and a contrast venogram confirms the diagnosis of deep vein thrombosis. A bolus of 5000 units of heparin is given followed by infusion of 1000 units/h to maintain the aPTT in the range of 45 to 60 s. On the thirteenth postoperative day, 6 days after starting heparin, she experiences the sudden onset of increasing pain in the right arm. The arm is cool and dusky distally and the radial and ulnar pulses are markedly diminished. A platelet count is 40 000/μl. A transoesophageal echocardiogram demonstrates no evidence for a mural thrombus or for akinesis. The patient's plasma, but not normal plasma, induces aggregation of normal platelet-rich plasma in the presence of heparin, but not in the absence of heparin and contains heparin-dependent antibodies to platelet factor 4. Based on these findings, a diagnosis of heparin-induced thrombosis with thrombocytopenia is made and heparin is discontinued. The patient is started on argatroban and on warfarin. A white thrombus is successfully removed from the right brachial artery by Fogarty catheter. The platelet count improves steadily over the next 10 days. Following achievement of a therapeutic prothrombin time on warfarin, the argatroban is discontinued and the patient is discharged on warfarin for 3 months with the admonition that she should never again receive heparin.

Among the various complications of heparin, heparin-induced thrombosis with thrombocytopenia is one of the most catastrophic and dramatic. This uncommon complication of heparin therapy typically occurs 5 to 14 days after starting heparin, occurs more frequently with beef lung heparin than with porcine intestine heparin, and resolves when the heparin is discontinued. The usual presentation is isolated thrombocytopenia, but occasionally (as in this case) there is a complicating (arterial) thrombotic event, either arterial or venous. This thrombosis is unique in that it is typically a white thrombus composed predominantly of platelets and little fibrin.

While thrombosis and thrombocytopenia are dramatic complications of heparin, they are rare. The most common complication of heparin therapy is haemorrhage, which may occur in any tissue. In general, the longer the aPTT, the greater the likelihood of haemorrhage. Heparin may also aggravate haemorrhage from structural lesions, such as colonic carcinoma or gastric ulcer. For this reason, bleeding from the gastrointestinal, respiratory, or urinary tract in patients on heparin should prompt a search for a potential source of the bleeding.

The question of how to maintain adequate anticoagulation in an individual with thrombosis who cannot take heparin is an important one. Alternatives to heparin include warfarin, other antithrombotic agents such as dextran, ancrod, novel antithrombin inhibitors such as hirudin or its synthetic analogues, prepared by recombinant technology or peptide synthesis, low-molecular-weight heparinoids, and the peptide inhibitor of thrombin, argatroban. Argatroban is easiest to use since therapy is monitored using the aPTT, in a manner analogous to heparin. Hirudin and its analogues are effective, but monitoring is with a special assay using the snake venom, ecarin, because of the very high affinity of hirudin for thrombin. Low-molecular-weight heparinoids have a risk of cross-reaction with the heparin-dependent antibody. The clinical situation largely determines which agent is used. For example, if gastrointestinal bleeding from an ulcer or polyp occurs on preventative doses of heparin (so-called 'mini-dose' heparin), the easiest course may be simply to discontinue the heparin. In the case presented, the presence of a recent deep vein thrombosis and the complicating arterial occlusion are indications to continue antithrombotic treatment.

Further reading

Collen D (1999). The plasminogen (fibrinolytic) system. *Thrombosis and Haemostasis* **82**, 259–70.

Garvey B (1998). Management of chronic autoimmune thrombocytopenic purpura (ITP) in adults. *Transfusion Science* **19**, 269–77.

George JN, *et al.* (1998). Drug-induced thrombocytopenia: a systematic review of published cases. *Annals of Internal Medicine* **129**, 886–90.

Kingston ME, Mackey D (1986). Skin clues in the diagnosis of life threatening infections. *Review of Infectious Diseases* **8**, 1–11.

Kyle RA, Bayrd ED (1975). Amyloidosis: review of 236 cases. *Medicine* **54**, 271–99.

Lak M *et al.* (1999). Bleeding and thrombosis in 55 patients with inherited afibrinogenemia. *British Journal of Haematology* **107**, 204–6.

Levi M *et al.* (1999). Disseminated intravascular coagulation. *Thrombosis and Haemostasis* **82**, 695–705.

Lundblad RL *et al.* (2000). Issues with the assay of factor VIII in plasma and factor VIII concentrates: A brief review and comments. *Thrombosis and Haemostasis* **84**, 942–8.

Mann KG (1999). Biochemistry and physiology of blood coagulation. *Thrombosis and Haemostasis* **82**, 165–74.

McMillan R (2000). The pathogenesis of chronic immune (idiopathic) thrombocytopenic purpura. *Seminars in Hematology* **37** (Suppl. 1), 5–9.

22.6.3 Disorders of platelet number and function

Kathryn E. Webert and John G. Kelton

Introduction

Platelets are the smallest of the circulating blood cells and their numbers in healthy individuals range from 150×10^9/litre to 450×10^9/litre. Platelets are released from the megakaryocytes in the bone marrow and circulate for 5 to 10 days before being cleared by the cells of the reticuloendothelial system. Disorders of platelet number and function are frequently encountered in medical patients.

Platelets are discoid cells that average 4 μm in diameter. The external membrane is a glycocalyx surface covering a phospholipid bilayer. Penetrating the membrane and traversing the platelet is a tubular system termed the open canalicular system. This system is continuous with the surface membrane and acts as a conduit for the release and uptake of substances. The platelet cytoskeleton is composed of three filamentous systems consisting of microtubules, microfilaments, and intermediate filaments. These tubules maintain the platelet's shape and participate in shape change, a complex process that occurs following platelet activation.

Platelets contain a number of organelles including alpha-granules, dense granules, lysozymes, peroxisomes, and mitochondria. The alpha-granules are the most numerous platelet granules (approximately 50 granules per platelet) and contain proteins synthesized by megakaryocytes, including β-thromboglobulin, platelet factor 4, thrombospondin, and von Willebrand factor. Alpha-granules also contain plasma-derived proteins such as fibrinogen, albumin, immunoglobulin G (**IgG**), and factor V. On the alpha-granule membrane are a variety of proteins including P-selectin and glycoprotein IIb/IIIa. Dense granules are far fewer in number than alpha-granules (four to eight per platelet) and are smaller. Dense granules are important for platelet activation and contain adenosine triphosphate, serotonin, calcium, magnesium, pyrophosphate, and granulophysin. Their membranes also contain a number of platelet proteins including P-selectin, glycoprotein Ib, and glycoprotein IIb/IIIa. Lysosomal granules contain proteolytic enzymes.

Platelet surface structures

Penetrating the platelet membrane are platelet glycoproteins. Most of these glycoproteins can be classified as one of five supergene families: integrins, leucine-rich glycoproteins, immunoglobulin domain molecules, selectins, and quadraspanins. The integrin family is the most common with glycoprotein IIb/IIIa being the most abundant integrin. Glycoprotein IIb/IIIa, also known as $\alpha_{IIb}\beta_3$, is present in high numbers (40 000 to 50 000 surface copies per platelet) and is the key binding site for platelet aggregation. Glycoprotein Ib/IX complex is the second most abundant platelet glycoprotein with an average of 20 000 surface copies per platelet. Glycoprotein Ib is a binding site for von Willebrand factor. A variety of other platelet glycoproteins are present in lower numbers such as glycoprotein Ia/IIa, the receptor for collagen. Finally, platelets carry 400 to 4000 copies of an IgG crystallizable fragment receptor, which is important in heparin-induced thrombocytopenia.

Thrombopoiesis

Pluripotent stem cells produce precursors of the red and white cells and the platelets. The platelet precursor is the megakaryocyte. Megakaryocytes undergo repeated nuclear replication without cytoplasmic division. This produces very large cells with four to 12 times the nuclear material of other cells of the body. Platelets bud off the cytoplasm of the megakaryocytes and are released into the circulation. The mean platelet volume can be measured on a cell counter and is approximately correlated with the number of nuclei in the megakaryocyte. Thrombocytopenia leads to increased proliferation of megakaryocytes and large platelets.

The primary regulator of megakaryopoiesis and platelet production is thrombopoietin. Thrombopoietin, an erythropoietin-like hormone, is primarily produced in the liver, with secondary sites including the kidney, bone marrow, brain, smooth muscle cells, and testes. The receptor for thrombopoietin, c-Mpl, is present on stem cells, megakaryocytes, and platelets. Binding of thrombopoietin to c-Mpl activates a variety of pathways resulting in the proliferation of megakaryocyte progenitors, an increased rate of megakaryocyte maturation, an increase in megakaryocyte nuclear mass and ploidy, and increased platelet release. The circulating level of thrombopoietin is primarily determined by the platelet mass. Platelets bind the thrombopoietin, internalize it, and degrade it. Consequently, less is available to stimulate platelet production. When the platelet count falls, less thrombopoietin is bound to platelets resulting in increased circulating levels of thrombopoietin and increased platelet production. Platelet production is also regulated by a number of other cytokines including interleukins 6 and 11.

The role of platelets in haemostasis

Platelets play a critical role in haemostasis. When the wall of the blood vessel is damaged, platelets adhere to exposed collagen and other components of the subendothelium. The key receptor is glycoprotein Ib linked to the vessel wall through von Willebrand factor. Other adhesive receptors include glycoprotein Ia/IIa, which binds collagen. The adhesion of the platelets to the vessel wall results in platelet activation. Agonists such as thrombin or adenosine diphosphate are released from their granules. The prostaglandin pathway is also activated during platelet activation; arachidonic acid is released from the platelet membrane where it is converted by a number of enzymes into platelet activating agents including thromboxane A_2. A key, rate-limiting step in this pathway is catalysed by the cyclo-oxygenase enzyme. Aspirin, an antiplatelet agent, irreversibly inactivates this enzyme. Following platelet activation, glycoprotein IIb/IIIa undergoes conformational changes making it able to bind fibrinogen. This process is termed platelet aggregation and results in the formation of the haemostatic plug. Activated platelets also contribute to the clotting cascade by serving as the phospholipid membrane surface needed for many reactions leading to thrombin generation, especially the activation of factor X by a complex of factors IXa and VIIIa and the activation of prothrombin by a complex of factors Xa and Va.

Disorders of platelet number

Thrombocytopenia

Thrombocytopenia is defined as a reduction in the number of circulating platelets to less than the laboratory's normal count (typically $< 150 \times 10^9$/litre). Bleeding is uncommon unless the platelet count falls below 10–20×10^9/litre or unless there is an abnormality in platelet function.

Classification of thrombocytopenia

It is convenient to classify disorders of thrombocytopenia into problems of underproduction, increased destruction, and sequestration (Table 1). Since megakaryocytes originate from stem cells it is rare to see a deficit in platelet production without abnormalities also occurring in other cell lines. Although isolated underproduction of platelets can occur, isolated thrombocytopenia usually suggests increased platelet destruction. Platelet sequestration is usually due to splenomegaly and can cause isolated thrombocytopenia, but also causes mild leukopenia or anaemia.

History and physical examination of the thrombocytopenic patient

The physician must investigate the risk of the thrombocytopenia as well as determine the underlying cause. It is important to elicit the duration of the haemostatic impairment to determine if the patient has recently ingested an antiplatelet agent such as aspirin or alcohol, which interferes with platelet function and can trigger bleeding.

The history should be guided by the potential mechanism of thrombocytopenia. For example, if increased destruction is considered, then the patient should be questioned about drugs including prescription drugs, over-the-counter medications, herbal remedies, and illicit drugs. Secondary associations of thrombocytopenia, which include systemic lupus erythematosus, human immunodeficiency virus (**HIV**) infection, and lymphoproliferative disorders (Table 2), will lead to other questions. Finally, one should obtain information about any family members with a history of thrombocytopenia or bleeding disorders.

Physical evaluation focuses on evidence of haemostatic impairment and signs of an underlying cause of the thrombocytopenia. Many patients with thrombocytopenia are asymptomatic. Only at low platelet counts will one see petechiae, which are tiny, red collections of red cells found on dependent parts of the body and sites of trauma. Petechiae are specific for thrombocytopenia. Large bruises or purpura can be observed on the limbs and trunk and have a lower specificity. The risk of bleeding increases progressively from asymptomatic patients, to patients with petechiae and purpura, to patients who have mucous membrane bleeding, which is typically manifest by blood blisters in the mouth. Blood blisters usually occur on the bite margins of the oral mucosa and on the tongue. They indicate that the patient is at significant risk for bleeding and treatment is urgently required. The physical examination should focus on the examination of the joints, lymph nodes, spleen, and liver since abnormalities indicate a secondary cause of the thrombocytopenia.

Laboratory evaluation of the thrombocytopenic patient

One of the most important first steps is to review the peripheral blood film looking for pseudothrombocytopenia. Pseudothrombocytopenia is a laboratory artifact that causes spontaneous platelet agglutination and results in platelet clumps in the peripheral smear. Automated determination of the platelet count will be inaccurate, as the machine will not recognize the larger platelet aggregates as platelets. Pseudothrombocytopenia commonly occurs because of agglutination of the patient's platelets in ethylenediaminetetra-acetic acid. This disorder occurs in 0.1 per cent of blood samples and is caused by a clinically insignificant autoantibody that agglutinates platelets at low calcium concentrations. This can be avoided by using an anticoagulant other than ethylenediaminetetra-acetic acid to collect the blood sample.

Table 1 Classification of thrombocytopenia by aetiology

Aetiology of thrombocytopenia	Relative frequency
Decreased platelet production	
Acquired	
Marrow infiltration: metastatic cancer, haematological malignancies (leukaemia, lymphoma, myeloma), myelofibrosis, storage disorders (Gaucher's disease etc.), granulomatous disorders (sarcoidosis)	+++
Marrow aplasia: aplastic anaemia, postchemotherapy or radiation	+++
Amegakaryocytic thrombocytopenia	++
Ineffective thrombopoiesis: myelodysplasia, secondary to toxins (alcohol), folate and vitamin B_{12} deficiency, paroxysmal nocturnal haemoglobinuria	+
Congenital	+
Wiskott–Aldrich syndrome and variants	
Bernard–Soulier syndrome	R
May–Hegglin anomaly	R
Alport syndrome and variants	R
Other	R
Increased platelet destruction	
Immune mechanisms	
• Autoimmune	
Idiopathic thrombocytopenic purpura	+++++
Evan's syndrome	++
Secondary to other disorders	
Lymphoproliferative disorders, systemic lupus erythematous, HIV infection, thyroid dysfunction, hypogammaglobulinemia, antiphospholipid antibody syndrome	+++
• Alloimmune	
Neonatal alloimmune thrombocytopenia	++
Post-transfusion purpura	+
Refractoriness to platelet transfusions	+++
Immune complex mediated	
Drug-induced	++
Non-immune mechanisms	
Disseminated intravascular coagulation	++
Thrombotic thrombocytopenic purpura	++
Haemolytic uraemic syndrome	++
Sepsis	++++
Malignant hypertension	++
Hypertensive disorders of pregnancy	+++
Hypersplenism	+++
Abnormal vascular surfaces	++
Decreased numbers of circulating platelets (sequestration)	
Splenomegaly	++++
Extracorporeal circulation	++++
Dilutional disorders	++
Hypothermia	++

+ to +++++ indicates the relative frequency. R indicates it is rare.

Table 2 Secondary associations of immune thrombocytopenia

Infections	
Human immunodeficiency virus	
Varicella	
Epstein–Barr virus	
Collagen vascular disease	
Systemic lupus erythematosus	
Rheumatoid arthritis	
Lymphoproliferative disorders	
Chronic lymphocytic leukaemia	
Hodgkin's disease	
Non-Hodgkin's lymphoma	
Other	
Antiphospholipid antibody syndrome	
Autoimmune thyroid dysfunction	
Sarcoidosis	
Post bone marrow transplantation	

The patient's haemoglobin and white blood cell count should be evaluated. Cytopenias involving other cell lines are suggestive of disorders involving the bone marrow such as myeloproliferative or myelodysplastic diseases. The platelet count helps to determine the patient's risk of bleeding. Patients with mild thrombocytopenia (platelet count $> 50 \times 10^9$/litre) have a low risk of bleeding. Patients with severe thrombocytopenia (platelet count $< 20 \times 10^9$/litre) have a higher risk of bleeding and can experience spontaneous bleeding. The peripheral smear may lead to the diagnosis of the condition causing the thrombocytopenia. Fragmented red cells or schistocytes may be seen in thrombotic thrombocytopenic purpura, haemolytic uraemic syndrome, disseminated intravascular coagulation, and renal graft rejection. Leukoerythroblastic changes in the peripheral smear, such as teardrop-shaped red blood cells, nucleated red blood cells, and immature white cells suggest infiltration of the bone marrow. The presence of abnormal circulating cells such as lymphoblasts or myeloblasts suggests a malignant process. Typical changes on the peripheral smear such as megaloblastic red blood cells and hypersegmented neutrophils suggest vitamin B_{12} or folate deficiency. The finding of atypical lymphocytes should cause one to consider the diagnosis of a viral infection. Finally, the finding of giant platelets on the peripheral smear suggests the diagnosis of certain congenital thrombocytopenias. Examination of the bone marrow should be considered if the aetiology of the thrombocytopenia is uncertain after the initial evaluation. Additionally, one should perform a bone marrow examination when abnormalities are seen on the peripheral blood smear or when multiple blood cell lineages are affected. The finding of normal or increased numbers of megakaryocytes in the marrow is supportive of a diagnosis of peripheral destruction or sequestration of the platelets. Other laboratory investigations that may be indicated include antinuclear antibody, rheumatoid factor, thyroid stimulating hormone, and testing for HIV infection.

Disorders of increased platelet destruction

Disorders of increased platelet destruction can be subdivided into two major categories: immune and non-immune. Non-immune causes include disseminated intravascular coagulation, and a variety of schistocytic or haemolytic anaemias such as thrombotic thrombocytopenic purpura. For the majority of thrombocytopenic disorders caused by non-immune mechanisms, the underlying cause is apparent and the patient's clinical presentation indicates the correct diagnosis (i.e. fever and clinical septicaemia suggest infectious causes of thrombocytopenia, fragmentation haemolysis suggests thrombotic thrombocytopenic purpura or haemolytic uraemic syndrome).

Immune mediated platelet disorders

Immune mediated disorders can be caused by autoantibodies, for example idiopathic thrombocytopenic purpura; alloantibodies, exemplified by post-transfusion purpura; and immune complexes, as demonstrated in heparin-induced thrombocytopenia. The majority of immune mediated platelet disorders are caused by IgG antibodies that bind to the platelet membrane.

Autoimmune thrombocytopenia

Autoimmune thrombocytopenia is mediated by antibodies that bind to individual platelet glycoproteins, most frequently glycoprotein IIb/IIIa. The autoimmune thrombocytopenia is classified as primary if there are no underlying conditions and secondary if it is associated with a systemic disease.

Primary autoimmune thrombocytopenia (idiopathic thrombocytopenic purpura) Idiopathic thrombocytopenic purpura (ITP) is one of the most common autoimmune disorders that physicians manage. iIdiopathic thrombocytopenic purpura is a disorder of both children and adults. In young children, frequently under the age of 5, the disease presents abruptly with dramatic evidence of haemostatic impairment. At least 80 per cent of children will have a spontaneous remission of their disease. Girls and boys are affected equally. In contrast, 80 per cent of adults who present with idiopathic thrombocytopenic purpura will have chronic disease. The disorder is typically seen in young and middle-aged adult women.

Adults with idiopathic thrombocytopenic purpura can present in one of three ways. Many patients will be asymptomatic and will have thrombocytopenia discovered incidentally. Other patients will give a history of easy bruising that may have occurred for many years and, frequently, worsened with ingestion of a substance which interferes with platelet function, such as aspirin or alcohol. Finally, patients may have an acute onset of petechiae, purpura, and mucous membrane bleeding.

Treatment of idiopathic thrombocytopenic purpura The most important decision is whether the patient requires any treatment. If the patient has mild or moderate thrombocytopenia (platelet count > 50 × 10^9/litre) and no history of haemostatic impairment, we would monitor this patient with periodic platelet counts every few weeks. These patients usually maintain a consistent platelet count that tends to drop only if the patient has an immune stimulus such as an infection. The decision is more difficult in patients with more severe thrombocytopenia (platelet count (20–50) × 10^9/litre) and who have modest signs of haemostatic impairment such as occasional bruising. We often do not treat these patients, but would alert the patient that the platelets should be raised before a haemostatic challenge such as a tooth extraction or surgery. Patients with severe thrombocytopenia (platelets < 10 × 10^9/litre) usually require treatment, especially if they have clinical signs of haemostatic impairment. The first line of treatment is corticosteroids, typically prednisone (1 mg/kg). Corticosteroids are effective in two-thirds of patients, but have predictable side-effects (Cushing's syndrome, hypertension, diabetes mellitus, osteoporosis). Corticosteroids should be given for as short an interval as possible, tapering the dose once the platelet count has reached haemostatically safe levels (> 100 × 10^9/litre). Patients who have a relapse of their thrombocytopenia may require more definitive treatment such as splenectomy.

Reticuloendothelial blockade through high-dose intravenous immunoglobulins (1 g/kg delivered over 6 h on two consecutive days) or anti-D in a rhesus positive individual (75 μg/kg) will result in a more rapid rise in the platelet count than corticosteroids and are indicated when platelets must be urgently raised. The major disadvantage of these treatments is that they are significantly more expensive than corticosteroids; however, they have fewer side-effects. There is a strong correlation between the response of a patient to high-dose intravenous immunoglobulins and response to a subsequent splenectomy. At least 80 per cent of patients will respond to reticuloendothelial blockade with the peak platelet count occurring in about a week and lasting for 4 to 8 weeks.

Splenectomy Splenectomy should be considered for patients who require ongoing medical management. Patients needing splenectomy should be vaccinated 2 weeks prior to the procedure with pneumococcal, meningococcal, and probably *Hemophilus influenzae* vaccines. The platelet count should be raised to safe levels prior to the procedure. Because of its reduced morbidity and significantly shortened hospital stay, laparoscopic splenectomy is the preferred approach. Splenectomy will result in a long-term remission or cure in about two-thirds of patients.

Second-line therapies As many as one-third of patients will not respond to splenectomy and will require an alternative therapy. Danazol, an attenuated anabolic steroid, will induce a dose-dependent rise in platelet count in some refractory patients. The typical dose ranges from 200 to 1200 mg/day. Unfortunately, it has adverse effects including liver enzyme abnormalities and virilization. Vincristine or vinblastine have been used in refractory patients. However, if a rise in platelet count does occur, it is generally transient. Hence, the drug needs to be given repeatedly, which invariably causes dose-dependent neurotoxicity. Patients with refractory idiopathic thrombocytopenic purpura who require ongoing therapy may need aggressive immunosuppression that includes oral chemotherapy such as cyclophosphamide or azathioprine, intermittent high-dose intravenous immunoglobulins, or intermittent corticosteroids.

Emergency treatment of idiopathic thrombocytopenic purpura Patients with idiopathic thrombocytopenic purpura who have severe bleeding require aggressive therapy including platelet transfusions, high-dose intravenous immunoglobulins, and high-dose corticosteroids, in addition to standard resuscitation including blood replacement if required.

Idiopathic thrombocytopenic purpura during pregnancy Idiopathic thrombocytopenic purpura occurs in young women and frequently these young women will become pregnant. The majority of these patients can successfully carry a child without excessive morbidity or mortality. Typically, the platelet count falls across the pregnancy and the mother may require treatment. We use high-dose intravenous immunoglobulins since corticosteroids may be associated with an increased risk of hypertensive disorders in pregnancy. About 10 per cent of the infants born to these mothers will be thrombocytopenic with the platelet nadir occurring several days after delivery. Very severe thrombocytopenia is uncommon (< 1 per cent) and should suggest an alternative diagnosis such as alloimmune neonatal thrombocytopenia. Infant thrombocytopenia cannot be predicted by any maternal factor or serological test with the possible exception of a history of a previously affected infant. We manage these mothers with routine vaginal delivery unless there is an obstetrical indication for caesarean section.

Secondary immune thrombocytopenias A variety of medical disorders cause secondary immune thrombocytopenia (Table 2). The treatment for secondary immune thrombocytopenia is similar to that of idiopathic thrombocytopenic purpura.

Thrombocytopenia complicating systemic lupus erythematosus Thrombocytopenia can occur in up to 25 per cent of patients with systemic lupus erythematosus. The thrombocytopenia is usually caused by autoantibodies. Some patients will have concomitant platelet dysfunction characterized by increased bleeding and bruising. The treatment is similar to that for idiopathic thrombocytopenic purpura.

A subset of patients with systemic lupus erythematosus or lupus-like disorders have antibodies which interfere with phospholipid-dependent coagulation reactions, commonly detected by an unexplained prolongation of the patient's partial thromboplastin time. These antibodies are immunoglobulins with specificity for negatively charged phospholipids and are also called lupus anticoagulant antibodies. They tend to be heterogenous in their epitope specificity with most binding protein complexes including β_2-glycoprotein I. Another class of antibodies, the anticardiolipin antibodies, is detected by an enzyme-linked immunosorbent assay using cardiolipin as the antigen. Cardiolipin is the same antigen that is detected in the venereal disease research laboratory (VDRL) test for syphilis, which explains the false positive VDRL test in these patients. The two classes of antibodies are distinct, but have overlapping specificities. Most anticardiolipin antibodies recognize an epitope on β_2-glycoprotein I. The term 'antiphospholipid antibodies' applies to both sets of antibodies.

Antiphospholipid antibodies are associated with venous and arterial thrombosis. The antiphospholipid antibody syndrome includes any combination of arterial and venous thrombosis, recurrent fetal losses and thrombocytopenia. Many of these patients will also have a vascular rash termed livedo reticularis. Patients can have haematological abnormalities including mild thrombocytopenia, platelet dysfunction, autoimmune haemolytic anaemia and leucopenia. As the thrombocytopenia is usually mild, treatment is rarely necessary. Many patients require long-term anticoagulation therapy to prevent recurrent thrombotic events.

Thrombocytopenia secondary to lymphoproliferative disorders Immune thrombocytopenia commonly complicates chronic lymphocytic leukaemia. This should be differentiated from thrombocytopenia of underproduction, which is seen in the spent stage of chronic lymphocytic leukaemia. Immune thrombocytopenia is often seen in patients with Hodgkin's disease and can predate or postdate the illness and is not a marker of disease activity.

Alloimmune thrombocytopenia

Alloimmune thrombocytopenia is caused by alloantibodies against platelet glycoproteins. There are two typical alloimmune thrombocytopenic disorders, alloimmune neonatal thrombocytopenia and post-transfusional purpura.

Alloimmune neonatal thrombocytopenia Alloimmune neonatal thrombocytopenia is mediated by alloantibodies in maternal plasma directed against fetal platelet glycoproteins inherited from the father. This disorder causes severe and often life-threatening fetal thrombocytopenia that can occur *in utero*. The most common alloantibody to cause this disorder is targeted against a platelet glycoprotein called PL^{A1} (HPA-1a) located on platelet glycoprotein IIIa.

Post-transfusion purpura In cases of post-transfusion purpura the patient, usually a woman, develops severe thrombocytopenia 5 to 12 days after receiving a transfusion of a blood product containing platelets. The thrombocytopenia is often very severe (platelet count $< 10 \times 10^9$/litre). Post-transfusion purpura occurs when a patient produces an alloantibody to a specific platelet antigen that she lacks, usually PL^{A1}. The syndrome most commonly occurs in multiparous women because previous pregnancies lead to their sensitization. Patients, including men, who have previously been transfused are also at risk.

The diagnosis of post-transfusion purpura is made by the identification of a platelet-specific antibody in a patient with acute onset of thrombocytopenia 5 to 12 days after receiving a transfusion of a blood product. Although post-transfusion purpura is most commonly seen after transfusion of packed red blood cells, all blood products, including plasma, can cause the reaction. Post-transfusion purpura is self-limited with recovery occurring within 1 to 3 weeks. However, because the condition can be lethal, treatment with plasmapheresis or intravenous immunoglobulins should be considered. Platelet transfusions should be avoided except in cases of life-threatening haemorrhage.

Drug-induced thrombocytopenia

Many drugs can cause thrombocytopenia. These medications most commonly implicated include heparin, quinidine, sulfonamides, and gold. However, virtually every medication has been associated with thrombocytopenia.

Patients with drug-induced thrombocytopenia typically have moderate to severe thrombocytopenia. Thrombocytopenia is usually seen 1 to 2 weeks after beginning a medication, but it may occur in patients who have been taking the medication for several years. The platelet destruction is usually IgG-mediated. The thrombocytopenia usually resolves within days of stopping the causative drug. In cases of severe thrombocytopenia, the drug should be discontinued and the patient treated with reticuloendothelial blockade using either intravenous immunoglobulins or intravenous anti-D immune globulin. Treatment with corticosteroids is less effective. In cases of life-threatening haemorrhage, platelet transfusions may be required. Patients should not take the drug causing the thrombocytopenia again as it will cause thrombocytopenia with subsequent exposure.

Heparin-induced thrombocytopenia Heparin-induced thrombocytopenia develops between 5 and 8 days after the initiation of heparin therapy but if the patient has been exposed to heparin within the last 3 months, it can occur earlier. Patients develop moderate thrombocytopenia (platelet counts $(40–80) \times 10^9$/litre). Patients with heparin-induced thrombocytopenia frequently develop thrombotic complications, especially deep venous thrombosis and pulmonary embolism. Other clinical associations include arterial thrombosis, skin lesions, and uncommon thrombotic events such as adrenal gland thrombosis and haemorrhage.

Heparin-induced thrombocytopenia is caused by an IgG antibody, which recognizes a complex of heparin and platelet factor 4. The platelet factor 4/heparin/IgG immune complexes bind to platelet crystallizable fragment receptors causing platelet activation and microparticle formation resulting in activation of coagulation.

The frequency of heparin-induced thrombocytopenia varies among clinical settings. The risk of thrombocytopenia appears to be related to the type, dose, and duration of heparin administration. For example, unfractionated heparin is more immunogenic than low-molecular-weight heparin. Also, different patient populations have different risks of forming heparin-induced thrombocytopenia IgG. For example, the risk of heparin-induced thrombocytopenia IgG is higher in orthopaedic patients than in medical patients.

The diagnosis of heparin-induced thrombocytopenia should be considered in all patients receiving heparin therapy who develop thrombocytopenia or thrombotic complications. Serological tests can be used to confirm the diagnosis of heparin-induced thrombocytopenia. Enzyme assays measure the binding of platelet antibodies to a complex of heparin and platelet factor 4. The gold standard tests are biological assays, such as the serotonin release assay.

Treatment of heparin-induced thrombocytopenia involves discontinuation of heparin. The patient should be treated with an agent that inhibits thrombin generation, such as hirudin or argatroban. Warfarin should not be used to treat acute heparin-induced thrombocytopenia because it can trigger warfarin-induced limb gangrene.

Gold-induced thrombocytopenia Gold-induced thrombocytopenia occurs in as many as 3 per cent of patients treated. There appears to be a genetic predisposition to the syndrome with HLA DR3 occurring in up to 80 per cent of affected patients. The thrombocytopenia usually occurs within the first several months of therapy and can range from mild to severe. Treatment involves stopping the drug and providing supportive treatment. The thrombocytopenia can persist for many months after the discontinuation of gold. This is probably due to persistence of an autoantibody, but may be due to the prolonged release of gold from tissue stores. Rapid correction of the thrombocytopenia may be achieved with intravenous immunoglobulins; however, a relapse of the thrombocytopenia may occur in 2 to 4 weeks. Patients also respond to corticosteroids. Some patients with persistent thrombocytopenia may respond to splenectomy. There is less experience using gold-chelating agents such as deferoxamine or dimercaprol.

Non-immune platelet disorders

Destructive thrombocytopenia and schistocytic haemolysis

Certain disorders are associated with both thrombocytopenia and schistocytic or fragmentation haemolysis. These disorders include thrombotic thrombocytopenic purpura, haemolytic uraemic syndrome, and disseminated intravascular coagulation.

Thrombotic thrombocytopenic purpura Thrombotic thrombocytopenic purpura is a syndrome consisting of thrombocytopenia, microangiopathic haemolytic anaemia, renal impairment, fever, and neurological findings secondary to ischaemia. Thrombotic thrombocytopenic purpura is an uncommon disorder, but its recognition is important because it is usually fatal if not treated.

Most patients who develop thrombotic thrombocytopenic purpura are young to middle-aged with slightly more females affected than males. The presentation of illness may be insidious or acute. Typically, the patient has a several day history of generalized malaise, fatigue, or focal ischaemic problems. The focal ischaemic events usually involve the central nervous system and can include sudden weakness, paraesthesiae, and confusion. Approximately 50 per cent of patients will have a neurological event.

Most adult patients with thrombotic thrombocytopenic purpura do not have an associated underlying condition. Nonetheless, the initial evaluation of a patient with thrombotic thrombocytopenic purpura should exclude diseases associated with thrombotic thrombocytopenic purpura (Table 3). Thrombotic thrombocytopenic purpura can develop spontaneously, but is often triggered by an infection, pregnancy, or vaccination.

All patients with thrombotic thrombocytopenic purpura have destructive thrombocytopenia. The thrombocytopenia is the best indicator of disease activity. Additional laboratory investigations demonstrate abnormalities of microangiopathic haemolytic anaemia, such as anaemia, fragmented red blood cells, and increased reticulocyte count. Serum lactate dehydrogenase and bilirubin levels are elevated. Other abnormalities include elevated serum creatinine, proteinuria, and abnormal liver function tests. Investigators have identified the presence of abnormal von Willebrand factor multimers in patients with thrombotic thrombocytopenic purpura.

Thrombotic thrombocytopenic purpura is treated with plasmapheresis. This treatment has reduced the mortality from 80 per cent to 20 per cent. Plasma exchange of at least one to two volumes of plasma should be performed daily. Plasma should be replaced with cryosupernatant plasma or fresh frozen plasma. Cryosupernatant plasma may be more beneficial because it is depleted of von Willebrand factor. Plasmapheresis should be continued until the platelet count and serum lactate dehydrogenase have normalized. This generally occurs after three to ten exchanges. Plasma exchange is better than plasma infusion alone. However, when plasmapheresis is not immediately available, patients should be treated initially with plasma infusion. If the initial response to plasma exchange is poor, other therapies such as glucocorticoids may be added. Additionally, the volume of plasma exchange may be increased. Other treatments, such as antiplatelet agents, are of uncertain benefit. With discontinuation of plasma exchange, exacerbation of disease occurs in about a third of patients. This risk of relapse can be reduced by splenectomy.

Table 3 Classification of thrombotic thrombocytopenic purpura

Primary (no associated disease)
Primary but triggered by a disorder or condition
Vaccination
Viral infection
Secondary
Pregnancy
Idiopathic thrombocytopenic purpura
Human immunodeficiency virus infection
Collagen vascular disease
Carcinoma (typically adenocarcinoma)
Drug associated:
Allergic: quinidine, ticlopidine
Dose-related toxicity: mitomycin C, cyclosporin, pentostatin, gemcitabine
Bone marrow transplantation (allogeneic)

Haemolytic uraemic syndrome Haemolytic uraemic syndrome includes renal failure, microangiopathic haemolytic anaemia, and thrombocytopenia. Different types of haemolytic uraemic syndrome have been identified including classic epidemic, sporadic, hereditary and sporadic in association with non-infectious conditions. Epidemic haemolytic uraemic syndrome is seen primarily in children and occurs after a diarrhoeal illness caused by enterohaemorrhagic or verotoxigenic *Escherichia coli* serotype O157:H7 or *Shigella dysenteriae* serotype I. Haemolytic uraemic syndrome may be also associated with other bacterial, viral, and rickettsial infections. Patients have been reported to develop haemolytic uraemic syndrome after receiving immunizations.

Laboratory investigations demonstrate severe anaemia and thrombocytopenia. Examination of the peripheral smear shows fragmented red blood cells, burr cells, and spherocytes. Haemoglobinaemia and haemoglobinuria may be severe. Serum lactate dehydrogenase levels and other markers of red blood cell destruction are elevated. The serum creatinine is usually increased.

In children, the treatment of haemolytic uraemic syndrome focuses on providing supportive care with careful attention paid to fluid status and electrolyte levels. Plasma exchange should be considered in children with severe haemolytic uraemic syndrome. In adults, treatment of haemolytic uraemic syndrome generally includes plasmapheresis. Other therapies including antiplatelet agents, fibrinolytic therapy, and heparin therapy have not been shown to be beneficial, and are not recommended.

Disseminated intravascular coagulation Disseminated intravascular coagulation is a disorder in which clotting occurs within the circulation. Disseminated intravascular coagulation is characterized by large amounts of thrombin that overwhelm the physiological inhibitors of coagulation. The thrombin causes platelet aggregation resulting in thrombocytopenia and fibrinogen cleavage into fibrin, which forms the microthrombi. The most common cause of disseminated intravascular coagulation is sepsis, but disseminated intravascular coagulation is associated with a large number of disorders including trauma and obstetric conditions (Table 4). The clinical presentation is variable, but patients with disseminated intravascular coagulation are usually very unwell presenting with fulminant bleeding and organ dysfunction. Some patients have thrombotic events. Occasionally, disseminated intravascular coagulation can be subclinical and

Table 4 Causes of disseminated intravascular coagulation

Infections
Bacterial (Gram-negative bacilli, staphylococci, streptococci, pneumococci, meningococci, others)
Viral (herpes, rubella, varicella, hepatitis, variola, arboviruses, others)
Parasitic (malaria, kala-azar, others)
Rickettsial (Rocky Mountain spotted fever, others)
Fungal (histoplasmosis, aspergillosis, others)
Neoplasms
Adenocarcinomas (prostate, breast, pancreas, lung, ovary, others)
Metastatic carcinoid, rhabdomyosarcoma, neuroblastoma, others
Obstetric complications
Abruptio placenta, retained dead fetus, second trimester abortion, amniotic fluid embolism, others
Haematological disorders
Acute promyelocytic leukaemia, intravascular haemolysis, histiocytic medullary reticulosis
Vascular disorders
Kasabach–Merritt syndrome (giant haemangioma), aortic aneurysm
Tissue injury
Crush injuries, burns, hypothermia, head injury
Miscellaneous
Fat embolism, acute glomerulonephritis, snake bite, extracorporeal circulation, allograft rejection, anaphylaxis, graft versus host disease, many others

detected only with laboratory tests. The diagnosis of disseminated intravascular coagulation is supported by the laboratory finding of thrombocytopenia in association with fragmented red blood cells, decreased fibrinogen level, and elevated fibrinogen and fibrin degradation products such as D-dimers. Coagulation studies often show a prolonged international normalized ratio, partial thromboplastin time, and thrombin time. Disseminated intravascular coagulation is best managed by identifying and treating its cause. If the patient is bleeding, replacement therapy with fresh frozen plasma, cryoprecipitate, and platelets is indicated. Heparin therapy may be of benefit in patients with clinical evidence of ongoing microvascular thrombosis.

Sepsis and infection

Transient thrombocytopenia occurs with systemic infections. Thrombocytopenia occurs in 50 to 75 per cent of patients with bacteraemia or fungal infections. It also occurs in association with viral infections, including HIV. The thrombocytopenia is generally mild to moderate and is not usually associated with symptoms of bleeding. The mechanism leading to the lowered platelet count is multifactorial including activation of platelets by bacterial products or mediators of inflammation; destruction due to immune mechanisms; or destruction due to chemokine-induced macrophage ingestion of platelets. Additionally, severe viral infections may lead to suppression of platelet production. Resolution of the platelet count occurs with eradication of the infection.

Thrombocytopenia associated with HIV is common, occurring in at least 20 per cent of patients with symptomatic disease. Various mechanisms contribute to the thrombocytopenia. Some patients have immune mediated destruction of platelets. Patients also have a defect in platelet production due to direct infection of megakaryocytes and the suppressive effects of medications. The platelet count can improve with antiretroviral therapy. Patients with severe thrombocytopenia should be treated similarly to patients with idiopathic thrombocytopenic purpura including the performance of a splenectomy.

Haemophagocytic syndrome

This rare syndrome is caused by phagocytosis of haematological cells by macrophages. Adult patients can present with an acute illness consisting of fever, weight loss, hepatosplenomegaly, pancytopenia, and increased liver enzymes. Bone marrow aspiration is diagnostic and shows morphological evidence of phagocytosis of platelets, red blood cells, and granulocytes by macrophages. The haemophagocytic syndrome may be associated with infections, particularly with the Epstein–Barr virus, T-cell lymphoma, histiocytosis, or immune disorders such as systemic lupus erythematosus and Still's disease. Treatment is directed at the underlying disorder.

Decreased platelet production

Platelet production is impaired by conditions affecting megakaryocyte progenitor cells, megakaryocytes, or the bone marrow stroma. It is rare to see a deficit in platelet production without abnormalities in the production of other cell lines as well. Decreased platelet production can occur when the bone marrow is aplastic, dysplastic, or infiltrated with other cells. Diagnosis of a defect in platelet production is usually made by evaluation of the bone marrow. Disorders causing decreased platelet production may be classified as congenital or acquired.

Congenital disorders causing decreased platelet production

Thrombocytopenia in infancy is usually due to increased platelet destruction and is only rarely due to decreased production. However, various congenital disorders may result in decreased platelet production. These disorders include congenital amegakaryocytic thrombocytopenia, thrombocytopenia with absent radii syndrome, Wiskott–Aldrich syndrome, May–Hegglin anomaly, Epstein's syndrome, Fechtner's syndrome, and Sebastian platelet syndrome. Bernard–Soulier syndrome is also associated with moderate thrombocytopenia.

Acquired disorders causing decreased platelet production

Toxins A variety of drugs and toxins may cause bone marrow suppression and subsequent thrombocytopenia. Chemotherapy and irradiation cause direct destruction of megakaryocytes and other cells of the marrow. Other medications causing marrow aplasia are numerous and include chloramphenicol, non-steroidal anti-inflammatory drugs, antiepileptic medications, and gold.

Alcohol Thrombocytopenia is the most common haematological abnormality associated with alcohol abuse. The thrombocytopenia can be due to hypersplenism (described subsequently) or alcohol suppression of the marrow. Alcohol induced marrow suppression can cause very severe thrombocytopenia requiring treatment by platelet transfusions. Elimination of alcohol intake will result in an increase of the platelet count within days to weeks. Associated haematological abnormalities include megaloblastic anaemia and ringed sideroblasts.

Nutritional deficiencies Thrombocytopenia may occur with folate or vitamin B_{12} deficiency. The degree of thrombocytopenia is variable and may be severe. Associated haematological abnormalities include megaloblastic anaemia and hypersegmented neutrophils. Replacement of the deficient vitamin will result in recovery of the platelet count. Iron deficiency has also been associated with thrombocytopenia, although more frequently with thrombocytosis. Replacement of iron generally corrects the platelet count.

Infiltration of the bone marrow The bone marrow may become infiltrated with non-haematopoietic or non-stromal cells. Conditions that may lead to marrow infiltration include metastatic cancer, haematological malignancies (leukaemia, lymphoma, myeloma), myelofibrosis, storage disorders, and granulomatous disorders (sarcoidosis, tuberculosis).

Acquired amegakaryocytic thrombocytopenic purpura Bone marrow aplasia is characterized by hypocellularity of the marrow. Aplasia involving more than one lineage of haematopoietic cells is called aplastic anaemia. When isolated decreased platelet production occurs, it is called amegakaryocytic thrombocytopenic purpura. This rare condition frequently progresses to aplastic anaemia. Bone marrow examination reveals absent or severely decreased numbers of megakaryocytes. The disorder may be secondary to various aetiologies including drugs, toxins, and infections, but most frequently it is idiopathic. Treatment varies with the suspected aetiology and typically is supportive, but can include intravenous IgG, corticosteroids, and immunosuppressive therapies.

Myelodysplastic syndromes Myelodysplastic syndrome can present with isolated thrombocytopenia. Examination of the bone marrow usually demonstrates abnormal megakaryocyte morphology and cytogenetic analysis reveals chromosomal abnormalities.

Disorders of platelet distribution and platelet sequestration

Splenomegaly and hypersplenism

Decreased numbers of circulating platelets may be seen in patients with splenomegaly. Normally, one-third of the circulating platelets are pooled in the spleen. With splenomegaly the size of the pool of platelets sequestered in the spleen increases, decreasing the number of circulating platelets. Increased destruction of the platelets may also occur. The thrombocytopenia is usually moderate (platelets $> 40 \times 10^9$/litre). Bone marrow examination reveals normal numbers of megakaryocytes. Other laboratory abnormalities include leucocytosis with a normal differential and mild anaemia. Splenomegaly may be demonstrated by ultrasound or a liver–spleen scan. The diagnosis of hypersplenism can be confirmed by performing an autologous platelet survival test. This test will show a reduced recovery of transfused platelets (usually < 30 per cent) with a normal platelet survival. The thrombocytopenia is rarely severe enough to require treatment; however, splenectomy is curative.

Haemodilutional disorders

A low number of circulating platelets may also be seen in patients who have received large volumes of crystalloid solutions or blood products. This type of thrombocytopenia is commonly seen immediately after surgery and is transient. If treatment is required, the patient should receive platelet transfusions.

Extracorporeal circulation

Patients undergoing cardiopulmonary bypass commonly develop mild thrombocytopenia. The cause of the decreased platelet count is multifactorial; adherence of platelets to synthetic surfaces causes activation and damage to the platelets, haemodilution, and blood loss. The thrombocytopenia is usually mild. Generally, the platelet count recovers within 3 to 4 days to levels greater than the count preoperatively.

Hypothermia

Hypothermia is associated with transient thrombocytopenia. Decreased body temperature results in pooling of platelets in the peripheral circulation. Hypothermia may be seen in cases of environmental exposure, after prolonged surgery, and after transfusions of massive amounts of inadequately warmed blood products.

Thrombocytosis

Thrombocytosis is defined as a platelet count greater than 600×10^9/litre. An elevated platelet count may be primary (essential) or secondary to other disorders.

Thrombocythaemia

Primary thrombocytosis also known as thrombocythaemia is a chronic myeloproliferative disorder. Other chronic myeloproliferative disorders such as polycythaemia vera, myeloid metaplasia, and chronic myelogenous leukaemia can also cause an increase in platelet count.

Incidence and epidemiology

The true incidence of thrombocythaemia has been estimated as approximately two patients per 100 000 population per year. The average age at diagnosis is 60 to 80 years with males and females equally affected. Young women in their thirties may present with thrombocythaemia.

Aetiology and pathogenesis

Thrombocythaemia is probably a clonal process originating at the stem cell level leading to sustained proliferation of megakaryocytes with increased numbers of circulating platelets. Thrombopoietin may also play a role in the pathogenesis of the disorder. Studies have shown reduction of c-Mpl protein and messenger RNA expression. This may reflect an intrinsic defect of c-Mpl transcription or decreased receptor expression that results in ineffective clearance of thrombopoietin.

Clinical findings

Two-thirds of patients have symptoms at the time of diagnosis, typically thrombotic or bleeding. Thrombotic events are common, occurring in 20 to 30 per cent of patients. The thrombosis involves the microvasculature and patients present with headache, transient ischaemic attacks or strokes, paraesthesiae of extremities, distal extremity gangrene, and erythromelagia (burning pain and redness of the toes or fingertips). Patients with essential thrombocythaemia have an increased risk of angina pectoris and myocardial infarction. Patients at greatest risk for thrombotic events are older and have a history of thrombosis. Major bleeding complications are rare, but bruising is common.

Laboratory findings

Patients have an unexplained elevation of their platelet count, typically above 800×10^9/litre. Examination of the peripheral smear can reveal megathrombocytes and leucocytosis with immature myeloid precursor cells. Mild eosinophilia and basophilia can occur. Bone marrow evaluation shows increased cellularity, marked megakaryocytic hyperplasia, and clustering of megakaryocytes. In addition the megakaryocytes often are morphologically bizarre with nuclear pleomorphism. Bone marrow karyotypes are usually normal. The Polycythaemia Vera Study Group has suggested criteria for the diagnosis of essential thrombocythaemia (Table 5).

Table 5 Criteria for diagnosis of essential thrombocytosis

All of the following:
Platelet count > 600×10^9/l on two different occasions, separated by a 1-month interval
Absence of identifiable cause of thrombocytosis, such as infections, inflammatory disorders, or non-haematological malignant disorders
Normal red cell mass (males < 36 ml/kg; females < 32 ml/kg)
Absence of significant fibrosis of the marrow
Absence of the Philadelphia chromosome and the fusion *BCR/ABL* gene
Plus three of the following:
Splenomegaly
Bone marrow hypercellularity seen on biopsy (megakaryocytic hyperplasia present with aggregates of megakaryocytes)
Absence of iron deficiency, as documented by the presence of stainable marrow iron and/or normal serum ferritin
Females: demonstration of clonal haematopoiesis using restriction fragment length polymorphism analysis of genes present on the X chromosome
Presence of abnormal bone marrow haematopoietic progenitor cells, as determined by the formation of endogenous erythroid and/or megakaryocytic colonies
Abnormal platelet aggregation studies in response to epinephrine and adenosine diphosphate when the patient is not taking any drug that might impair platelet function

From: Murphys S *et al.* (1997). *Seminars in Hematology* **34**, 29–39.

Management

Untreated, asymptomatic patients with thrombocythaemia can have a near normal life expectancy. Furthermore, the thrombotic risk in asymptomatic patients younger than 60 years of age with no history of thrombosis is not increased. Therefore, young, asymptomatic patients do not require treatment. Possible indications for treatment to lower platelet count include patients with a history of thrombotic events, patients with cardiovascular risk factors, elderly patients, and patients in whom platelet counts remain very high (> 1000×10^9/litre).

Low-dose aspirin can be used to prevent thrombosis and it may relieve symptoms such as headache and erythromelagia. However, aspirin may unmask bleeding tendencies so it should be avoided in patients with a history of bleeding. Hydroxyurea will lower the platelet count and usually reduces thrombohaemorrhagic complications. Adverse affects include myelosuppression and possibly an increased risk of leukaemic transformation. Anagrelide can effectively lower the platelet count, but its efficacy at reducing complications has not been definitively established. Interferon-α may also be used to lower platelet counts. Unfortunately, side-effects including flu-like symptoms, anorexia, and neuropsychiatric symptoms are severe enough to cause discontinuation of therapy in up to 25 per cent of patients.

Prognosis

The life expectancy of patients with thrombocythaemia is near normal. However, patients do have a high rate of morbidity secondary to thrombotic events. Three to four per cent of patients develop leukaemia. This occurs predominantly in patients who have been treated with alkylating agents.

Secondary thrombocytosis

Essential thrombocythaemia must be differentiated from reactive or secondary thrombocytosis. Causes of secondary thrombocytosis include infections, malignancy, chronic inflammatory bowel disease, rheumatoid arthritis, iron deficiency, and hyposplenism. Reactive thrombocytosis is not associated with symptoms related to the elevated platelet count. Reactive thrombocytosis is not harmful and does not require treatment, although the underlying cause should be determined.

Disorders of platelet function

Congenital disorders of platelet function

Patients with congenital disorders of platelet function often present with a history of easy bruising, epistaxis, menorrhagia, and prolonged bleeding after surgery or dental procedures. Some of these patients may have family members with similar problems. The various platelet abnormalities may be classified functionally into disorders of platelet adhesion, aggregation, secretion, and procoagulant activity.

Disorders of platelet adhesion and aggregation

Platelet function disorders include Bernard–Soulier syndrome which is caused by a deficiency or abnormality of platelet glycoprotein Ib/IX and Glanzmann's thrombasthenia, caused by a deficiency of glycoprotein IIb/IIIa. Both are inherited in an autosomal recessive fashion and are very rare.

Disorders of platelet secretion

Disorders of platelet secretion occur when there are abnormalities of the platelet secretory pathways or if there is a deficiency of platelet granules. Grey platelet syndrome occurs when the alpha granules are decreased or absent. Dense granule deficiency or platelet storage pool deficiency is due to a deficiency of dense granules. In alpha delta storage pool deficiency, both the alpha and dense granules are deficient.

Disorders of platelet procoagulant activity

Platelets play an important role in haemostasis by providing a phospholipid membrane on which various coagulation reactions occur. In disorders such as Scott syndrome, abnormalities of the platelet membrane impair its procoagulant activity.

Treatment

There are no definitive therapies for any of the congenital disorders of platelet function. Administration of 1-desamino-8-D-arginine vasopressin induces the release of von Willebrand factor from endothelial cells and will improve bleeding time and haemostasis. An effect is seen within 1 to 2 h and lasts for up to 12 h. Antifibrinolytic agents, such as aminocaproic acid, may improve haemostasis. Menorrhagia may be controlled by oral contraceptive medications and perhaps by antifibrinolytic medications. In cases of life-threatening bleeding, platelet transfusions may be necessary. However, platelet transfusions can cause immunization against the platelet receptors and should be avoided.

Acquired disorders of platelet function

The most common acquired causes of platelet dysfunction are medications and toxins, systemic disorders, and haematological diseases.

Drugs

There are numerous drugs that have been shown to affect platelet function (Table 6). Aspirin has been demonstrated to cause a significant increase in bleeding. Aspirin acts by irreversibly inhibiting platelet cyclo-oxygenase resulting in decreased formation of thromboxane A_2, an agonist for platelet aggregation. Non-steroidal anti-inflammatory agents affect platelet function by inhibiting cyclo-oxygenase. Ticlopidine and clopidrogel inhibit platelet function by inhibiting the action of platelet adenosine diphosphate. Glycoprotein IIb/IIIa inhibitors block platelet aggregation by directly inhibiting the platelet receptor for fibrinogen, glycoprotein IIb/IIIa. β-lactam antibiotics may bind to and modify the platelet membrane resulting in abnormal platelet aggregation with adenosine diphosphate, epinephrine, and collagen. Nitrates inhibit platelet aggregation. Calcium channel blockers and β-blockers affect platelet aggregation by unknown mechanisms. Other drugs that may adversely affect platelet function include antiepileptic medications, tricyclic antidepressants, and phenothiazines.

Table 6 Medications affecting platelet function

Aspirin
Non-steroidal anti-inflammatory medications
Glycoprotein IIb/IIIa inhibitors
Ticlopidine and clopidrogel
Dipyridamole
Antibiotics
β-lactam antibiotics (penicillins, cephalosporins)
Nitrofurantoin
Cardiovascular medications
Nitrates
β-blockers
Calcium channel blockers
Antiepileptic medications
Psychotropic drugs
Phenthiazines
Tricyclic antidepressants
Anaesthetics
Local anaesthetics
Halothane
Plasma expanders
Dextrans, pentastarch
Antihistamines
Clofibrate
Chemotherapeutic drugs
Mithramycin
Daunorubicin
BCNU (carmustine)

Chronic renal failure

Patients with chronic renal failure or uraemia have platelet dysfunction including defects in adhesion, aggregation, secretion, and procoagulant activity. The bleeding time may be prolonged. The pathogenesis of the platelet dysfunction is unknown, but is probably secondary to toxins present in the uraemic plasma. Treatment of a bleeding uraemic patient includes prompt dialysis. 1-desamino-8-D-arginine vasopressin will improve haemostasis. Maintenance of a normal haematocrit may decrease the bleeding tendency.

Cardiopulmonary bypass surgery

Excessive bleeding occurs in approximately 5 to 20 per cent of patients undergoing cardiopulmonary bypass surgery. Studies have demonstrated decreased platelet aggregation, altered platelet surface membrane proteins, selective depletion of platelet alpha granules, and evidence of *in vivo* platelet activation. An extrinsic platelet defect may occur resulting from thrombin inhibition by high doses of heparin. The aetiology of these abnormalities could be related to the hypothermia of the procedure and damage to the platelets as they pass through the pump system. The haemostatic abnormalities improve within hours after surgery.

Chronic myeloproliferative disorders and myelodysplastic syndromes

Disorders such as chronic myelogenous leukaemia, essential thrombocythaemia, polycythaemia vera, and myeloid metaplasia may be associated with abnormalities of platelet number and function. Abnormalities of platelet function include impaired aggregation with epinephrine, abnormal arachidonic acid metabolism, and storage pool defects. The bleeding tendency responds to treatment of the underlying disorder and correction of the associated thrombocytosis.

Dysproteinaemias

Patients with a paraproteinaemia, such as multiple myeloma or Waldenström's macroglobulinaemia, can have abnormalities in both platelet number and function. Non-specific binding of the paraproteins to the platelet membrane may interfere with membrane surface receptors. Treatment of the disorder causing the paraproteinaemia will usually correct the bleeding problem. Acutely, measures such as plasma exchange may be necessary.

Further reading

George JN (2000). How I treat patients with thrombotic thrombocytopenic purpura-hemolytic uremic syndrome. *Blood* **96**, 1223–9.

George JN *et al.* (1997). Diagnosis and treatment of idiopathic thrombocytopenic purpura: recommendations of the American Society of Hematology. *Annals of Internal of Medicine* **126**, 319–26.

George JN *et al.* (1998). Drug-induced thrombocytopenia: a systematic review of published case reports. *Annals of Internal Medicine* **129**, 886–90.

Gill KK, Kelton JG (2000). Management of idiopathic thrombocytopenic purpura in pregnancy. *Seminars in Hematology* **37**, 275–89.

Lankford KV, Hillyer CD (2000). Thrombotic thrombocytopenic purpura: new insights in disease pathogenesis and therapy. *Transfusion Medicine Reviews* **14**, 244–57.

McMillan R (1997). Therapy for adults with refractory chronic immune thrombocytopenic purpura. *Annals of Internal Medicine* **126**, 307–14.

Nurden AT (1999). Inherited abnormalities of platelets. *Thrombosis and Haemostasis* **82**, 468–80.

22.6.4 Genetic disorders of coagulation

Eleanor S. Pollak and Katherine A. High

Haemostasis, the physiological process of blood clot formation, involves a co-ordinated interaction between the wall of the blood vessel, platelets, and blood coagulation proteins. The haemostatic mechanism maintains a state of readiness to respond to a multitude of haemostatic stressors to prevent haemorrhage while also preventing inappropriate clot formation. Although acquired diseases of the coagulation system frequently occur with liver disease and other pathological disease states, this chapter will specifically focus on genetic disorders resulting from abnormalities and/or deficiencies of the blood coagulation proteins. More specifically, this chapter will cover haemophilia, von Willebrand disease, and deficiencies/abnormalities of fibrinogen and factors II, V, VII, X, XI, XII, and XIII. The role of an inherited increased risk for excess clotting will also be addressed. These conditions may result from either the loss of function of anticoagulant proteins (antithrombin III, protein C, and protein S) or a gain of function of procoagulant proteins (factor V Leiden and prothrombin 20210 G to A).

The coagulation cascade as a haemostatic mechanism

The human blood coagulation system involves a co-ordinated array of reactions which generate a stable fibrin clot when needed and prevent unnecessary clot formation. The system involves numerous proteins which interact, principally on phospholipid surfaces, to create a meshwork of fibrin fragments entrapping haematopoietic cells (Fig. 1). The majority of coagulation enzymatic complexes involve protease enzymes. Many of these enzymes are serine proteases, and a subset of these have the distinguishing feature that their functional synthesis requires vitamin K to enable post-translational modification of glutamic acid residues in the NH_2 terminal region; this property provides the basis of the therapeutic mechanism by which the drug warfarin prevents proper synthesis of functional factors. The principal enzyme balancing the pro- and anticoagulant forces is prothrombin, thought to be the evolutionary forerunner of the mammalian coagulation proteins. In addition to its procoagulant functions, prothrombin, once activated, provides anticoagulant and cellular mobility functions as well.

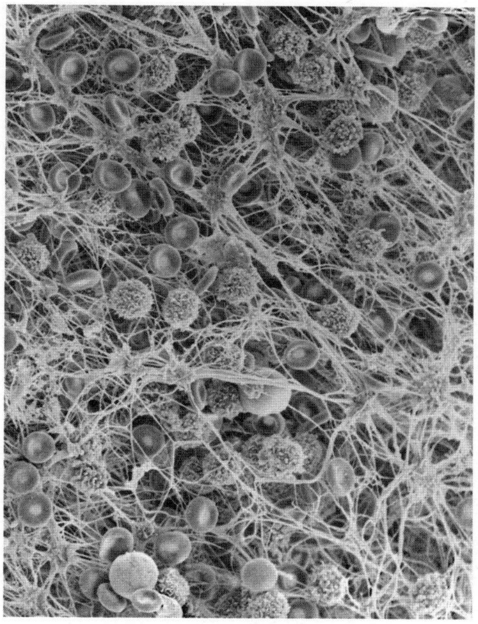

Fig. 1 Scanning electron micrograph of a whole blood clot. There is a meshwork of fibrin fibres emanating from platelet aggregates in which erythrocytes, lymphocytes, and other cells are trapped. (By courtesy of John W. Weisel and Chandrasekaran Nagaswami, Department of Cell and Developmental Biology, University of Pennsylvania School of Medicine, Philadelphia, PA, United States.)

In 1905, Morawitz first described the importance of thrombin, thromboplastin, and calcium in cleaving fibrinogen to create a fibrin clot. In the early 1930s and 1940s laboratory tests were developed that relied on *in vitro* fibrin clot formation to analyse the adequacy of a patient's clotting system. The waterfall cascade of sequential activation steps resulting in a fibrin clot was elegantly described in the early 1960s delineating separate pathways to account for the prothrombin time and the partial thromboplastin time which the earlier laboratory tests measure. However, the set of activation steps is now better described as an interwoven, reinforcing set of reactions (Fig. 2). The unique specificities of the coagulation enzymes summarized in the classical coagulation cascade have been found to be more versatile in activating diverse proteins under varied conditions. However, the separate pathways, now termed the tissue factor (extrinsic) and the intrinsic pathways, help define the steps involved in the principal tests used in clinical medicine for evaluation of haemostatic proteins. For the series of reactions and specific factors involved, the time to clot formation defines the principal parameter used in clinical evaluation of the health of a patient's coagulation system. The assays (the prothrombin time, the activated partial thromboplastin time, and activity levels of specific individual clotting factors) compare the time needed for clot formation in a patient's plasma with that in a control pool of plasma from normal donors.

Endothelial injury and tissue damage first trigger clot formation. The response of the platelets forms the primary phase of healing by temporarily patching the site of vascular injury. Subsequent to this initial platelet phospholipid patch, a fibrin clot provides a more solid framework for the necessary but slower cellular repair. Secondary haemostasis begins with injury-induced exposure of the integral membrane protein tissue factor to plasma proteins enabling formation of the active enzymatic complex tissue factor–factor VIIa. The generation of tissue factor–factor VIIa then catalyses clotting by activating both factor X to factor Xa and factor IX to factor IXa. This activation primarily involves the cleavage of an arginine–

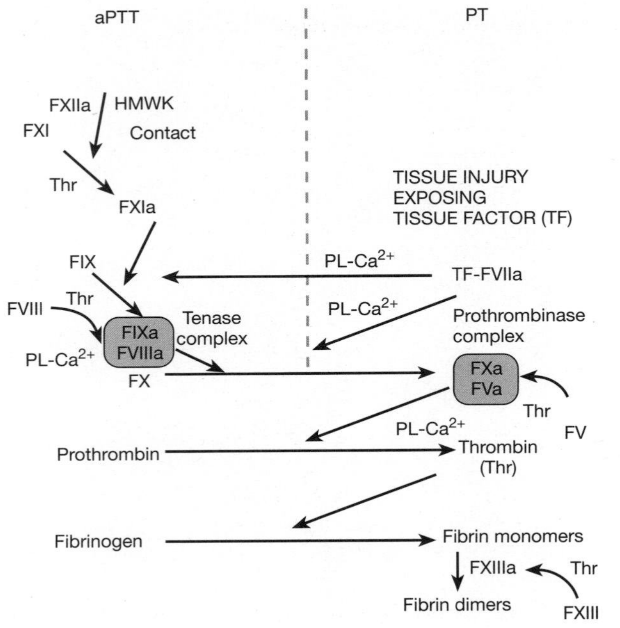

Fig. 2 Schematic representation of the enzymatic reactions involved in blood clot formation. Thr, thrombin; PL-Ca^{2+}, phospholipids/calcium; PT, prothrombin time; aPTT, activated partial thromboplastin time.

isoleucine bond in a secreted plasma protein zymogen to form a two-chain active protein. Thus, once tissue injury has signalled the need for fibrin clot formation and tissue factor–factor VIIa has initiated coagulation, the haemostatic process amplifies through the generation of factor IXa, which is ten times more abundant than factor VII and consequently leads precipitously to thrombin generation. Among thrombin's numerous roles is the activation of the essential procoagulant cofactors factors V and VIII. This process then further amplifies clotting by generating more thrombin through the active cofactors Va and VIIIa which then form the tenase (factor IXa/factor VIIIa) and prothrombinase (factor Xa/factor Va) complexes (see Fig. 1). Thrombin also activates the crosslinking enzyme, factor XIII, the fibrinolytic inhibitor, TAFI, and triggers platelet recruitment. Importantly, thrombin generation simultaneously counterbalances its procoagulation activities by inciting lysis of the clot via the release by endothelial cells of tissue plasminogen activator converting plasminogen to plasmin, the enzyme responsible for lysis of fibrin clots. Thrombin also dampens the clotting process by activating protein C that actively breaks down the critical procoagulant cofactors factors Va and VIIIa.

The basis for initiating clot formation in the prothrombin time and activated partial thromboplastin time test is titration of calcium into an anticoagulated plasma specimen along with a source of phospholipid. In addition, in the prothrombin time test, the source of phospholipid is a thromboplastin reagent which provides tissue factor to enable the tissue factor–factorVIIa complex to catalyse clot formation. In the activated partial thromboplastin time test the phospholipid reagent lacks tissue factor and thus prevents formation of the tissue factor–factor VIIa complex. An activator, such as silica particles, also greatly decreases the time required for clot formation through activation of factor XII via the contact activation system.

Deficiencies of specific clotting proteins

Haemophilia

Deficiency of either factor VIII (haemophilia A) or factor IX (haemophilia B), which together make up the factor VIIIa/factor IXa intrinsic tenase enzymatic complex, results in the clinical phenotype commonly known as haemophilia. A sex-linked bleeding diathesis, now thought to be haemophilia, was described in Talmudic writings as a cause of fatal haemorrhage at circumcision. In the modern era, the disease may cause bleeding at circumcision, but haemophilia principally presents with haematoma formation, easy bruising, and bleeding at the site of venepuncture during the toddler period. The disease exists in severe, moderate, and mild forms classified as such on the basis of a clinical laboratory blood coagulation test performed to assess the level of functional coagulant protein (per cent activity of factor VIII or factor IX). The pathological problem in both haemophilia A, factor VIII deficiency, and haemophilia B, factor IX deficiency (also called Christmas disease), is the inability to form a functional tenase complex to activate factor X to factor Xa. Although factor X can still be activated to factor Xa by tissue factor–factor VIIa, the available quantities of factor VII (400 ng/ml) do not allow sufficient activation of factor X to enable clotting to occur in a physiologically timely fashion. Although patients with haemophilia may have some difficulties with immediate haemorrhage subsequent to a cutaneous or superficial injury, they characteristically have joint and deep tissue bleeding problems as discussed below. The severity of disease is very well predicted by an *in vitro* assay for evaluation of the deficient protein level such that patients with severe disease have levels of factor activity of less than 1 per cent, patients with moderate disease have activity levels of 1 to 5 per cent, and patients with mild disease have activity levels of 6 to 30 per cent. Normal factor VIII and IX levels are 50 to 200 per cent and 75 to 125 per cent respectively.

Numerous genetic mutations have been described accounting for the factor deficiencies causing haemophilia. In part because of the considerable difference in size between the factor VIII gene (186 kbp), and the factor IX gene (34 kbp), the ratio of the frequency of factor VIII to factor IX deficiency is between four and five to one (approximately 186/34 kbp). Thus, the frequency of haemophilia A is approximately one in 5000 to 6000 and that of haemophilia B is approximately one-fifth of that. Among affected cases, approximately one in three to one in four patients presents spontaneously without a familial inheritance pattern. One of the only differences between factor VIII and IX deficiencies is the frequency of severe disease, which occurs more commonly in factor VIII deficiency (60 per cent of cases as compared with 45 per cent in haemophilia B). This difference is largely attributed to the frequency of mutation due to a factor VIII gene inversion in intron 22 of the 26 exon long factor VIII gene. At this locus of the factor VIII gene, a region of homology to sequences telomeric to the factor VIII gene, a recombination event results in the inability to synthesize any functional factor VIII, thus leading to severe disease (less than 1 per cent functional protein activity). In both factor VIII and factor IX deficiency, milder disease is commonly due to missense mutations.

The clinical features of haemophilia predominantly include bleeding into joints and soft tissues. The incidence of central nervous system bleeding has dramatically decreased with concentrate therapy. The life expectancy of people with severe haemophilia had increased from 11 years at the beginning of the twentieth century to approximately 60 years in the early 1980s, before the devastating effects of bloodborne viral disease again shortened average life expectancy.

In the untreated patient with severe disease, haemophilic arthropathy and joint deformity are inevitable complications. In decreasing order of involvement, the most commonly affected joints include the knee, elbow, ankle, shoulder, wrist, and hip. Recurrent bleeding episodes create a hypertrophic synovial lining with chronic inflammation; however, the pathophysiology responsible for recurrent joint bleeding remains unknown. Arthropathies commonly necessitate replacement of affected joints for pain control and improvement of mobility. Soft tissue haemorrhages frequently complicate haemophilia; further complications due to these haemorrhages include compartment syndrome, neurological damage, and extensive blood loss from retroperitoneal bleeds. Haematoma formation, a frequent complication of haemophilia, may arise spontaneously or with trauma and require extensive factor replacement and fasciotomy, the necessity for

Table 1 Coagulation laboratory testing, plasma concentrations, and chromosomal location of coagulation proteins

Clotting factor	PT	aPTT	Half-life of protein	Plasma concentration	Inheritance (chromosome)
Fibrinogen	Increased	Increased	2–4 days	200–400 mg/dl	Autosomal (1)
Prothrombin (factor II)	Increased	Increased	3 days	100 μg/ml	Autosomal (11)
Factor V	Increased	Increased	36 h	10 μg/ml	Autosomal (1)
Factor VII	Increased	Normal	2–6 h	0.5 μg/ml	Autosomal (13)
Factor VIII	Normal	Increased	8–12 h	0.1 μg/ml	X-linked (X)
von Willebrand factor	Normal	Mildly increased in approximately 50% of cases	Several hours	10 μg/ml	Autosomal (12)
Factor IX	Normal	Increased	24 h	5 μg/ml	X-linked (X)
Factor X	Increased	Increased	40 h	10 μg/ml	Autosomal (13)
Factor XI	Normal	Increased	60–80 h	5 μg/ml	Autosomal (4)
Factor XII	Normal	Increased	50 h	30 μg/ml	Autosomal (5)
Factor XIII	Normal	Normal	9–19 days	10 μg/ml	Autosomal (6, α chain, and 1, β chain)
Protein C	Normal	Normal	6 h	5 μg/ml	Autosomal (2)
Protein S	Normal	Normal	30 h	25 μg/ml	Autosomal (3)
Antithrombin III	Normal	Normal	48 h	150 μg/ml	Autosomal (1)

Abbreviations: PT, prothrombin time; aPTT, activated partial thromboplastin time.

which can be assessed by mean arterial pressure in a compartment. Intracranial haemorrhage, occurring in approximately 5 per cent of patients, warrants immediate evaluation and treatment within the first 6 to 8 h of presentation; however, the majority of children presenting to an emergency room with central nervous system symptoms have not suffered from intracranial haemorrhage.

A pseudotumour, an encapsulated collection of blood most commonly originating in bone or soft tissues, is a very rare but extremely serious consequence of haemophilia occurring in approximately 2 per cent of patients. This complication is difficult to manage but may sometimes be treated with surgery at specialized haemophilia centres.

Frequently, patients with haemophilia have haematuria, the severity of which may range from self-limited episodes to gross haematuria with significant blood loss. Protease inhibitors for HIV therapy may lead to haematuria with flank pain or renal stones. Physicians should be aware of the possibility of nephrotic syndrome in patients placed on immune tolerance regimens.

Dental procedures warrant involvement of a haemophilia specialist. Factor replacement levels of 25 to 100 per cent are suggested depending on the complexity of the dental procedure. Antifibrinolytics such as ε-aminocaproic acid or tranexemic acid and fibrin sealants may be a helpful adjuvant to replacement therapy.

Due to the sex-linked inheritance pattern, haemophilia is rarely found in women unless extensive lyonization takes place in the normal gene. Normal vaginal delivery is considered to be relatively safe in the case of a haemophilic infant; however, vacuum extraction and midcavity forceps deliveries and invasive fetal monitoring should be avoided due to the increased risk of formation of subgaleal and cephalic haematomas.

The laboratory diagnosis of haemophilia is based on a modification of the classic activated partial thromboplastin time assay used as a standard test for the haemostatic system. Normally patients are evaluated due to bleeding symptomatology or because of a prolonged activated partial thromboplastin time result. The activated partial thromboplastin time is a very sensitive but poorly specific screening test for haemophilia. All patients, even those with mild disease, will normally have a prolonged activated partial thromboplastin time unless there is a problem with specimen acquisition or the insensitivity of the activated partial thromboplastin time reagent. Once suspected, haemophilia can be evaluated by an inhibitor screen which involves performing a 50:50 mix of patient and normal plasma to evaluate whether the prolongation is due to a deficiency of a clotting protein or alternatively to the presence of an inhibitor. There are many causes of a prolonged activated partial thromboplastin time other than haemophilia (see Table 1). Classically, a phospholipid inhibitory antibody, called a lupus anticoagulant, will cause a prolongation of the activated partial thromboplastin time of the 50:50 mix due to the effect of the phospholipid inhibitory antibody on the normal pooled plasma. A lupus anticoagulant which causes a prolonged activated partial thromboplastin time may also result in a low factor VIII or factor IX level. In such cases, further testing for a lupus anticoagulant is necessary to rule out a low factor VIII due to a lupus anticoagulant as opposed to a deficiency.

Management of haemophilia predominantly involves administering the missing protein (factor VIII or factor IX) to a patient. Factor replacement therapy is most commonly administered in a so-called 'on-demand' regimen, when a patient's symptomatology necessitates treatment. However, prophylaxis is indicated during surgery or at times of expected injury. Prophylactic therapies during early childhood are now recommended when feasible after the first major bleeding episode as a means of preventing arthropathies in patients with severe disease. Prophylactic administration during the first few years of life requires special consideration due to the need for repeated intravenous access generally requiring an indwelling line. These have been associated with high rates of sepsis, particularly in children under the age of 3. Before the development of stringent purification and virucidal procedures, the transmission of viral disease was almost inevitable as each vial of plasma-derived concentrate was pooled from approximately 60 000 to as many as 400 000 donors, although the number has recently been reduced to 15 000. Tragically, the majority of patients with severe disease treated before 1985 developed HIV. Rates of development of hepatitis B and C are also extremely high. Although drastically reduced; the potential for transmission of infectious disease has not been totally eliminated. Many recombinant preparations are prepared with human serum albumin thus leaving a possible source of transfusion of a bloodborne disease.

Treatment

Acute bleeding episodes

Safe and effective treatment options continue to improve for the management of acute bleeding episodes for patients with haemophilia A and B. Blood products available include fresh frozen plasma which contains both factors VIII and IX, prothrombin complex concentrates containing factors II, VII, IX, and X, activated prothrombin complex concentrates (factors IIa, VIIa, IXa, Xa), monoclonal-antibody purified factor VIII and factor IX, and recombinant factor VIII and factor IX. Recombinant factor VIIa is now approved for use in patients with inhibitors during acute bleeds. Currently trials using gene therapy approaches are under way and may provide a method for continuous prophylaxis against bleeding. Recombinant or highly purified products are the optimal therapy because of the great benefit to risk ratio. Availability, ease of administration, cost, viral safety, and thrombotic risk, particularly in patients undergoing high-dose therapy or procedures with a high risk of thrombotic complications, dictate the choice of product. Cryoprecipitate, made from the precipitate of thawed frozen plasma, contains factor VIII but does not contain factor IX. Cryoprecipitate and fresh frozen plasma should only be used in the haemophilia patient in an emergency setting where concentrates are not available. Inhibitor formation, the development of antibodies to the deficient protein, arises subsequent to transfusion of a blood product or factor replacement and is the major complication of treatment. An inhibitor presents an extremely difficult situation for patient management (see Complications of therapy below).

Several immunoaffinity purified plasma-derived factor VIII and factor IX products are available in the United States and Europe and currently have excellent records of viral safety, efficacy, and lack of thrombogenicity. When concentrate is unavailable, fresh frozen plasma is readily available in most emergency settings. Virucidal methods using solvent detergent treatment may now be applied in production of fresh frozen plasma; furthermore, each unit is from a single screened donor, thus the risk of transfusion-transmitted disease is low.

Recombinant factor VIII and factor IX have been licensed for nearly a decade. These proteins are produced in cultured mammalian cells and purified from conditioned medium. Recombinant factor IX is devoid of human plasma whereas the recombinant factor VIII concentrates utilize human plasma-derived albumin for stabilization. Because *in vivo* coagulant activity of recombinant factor IX is only 80 per cent of *in vitro* estimates used for labelling of product in IU/mg, it is recommended that the calculated factor IX dosage be multiplied by a factor of 1.2 for dose calculation when using recombinant factor IX. A plausible explanation for this discrepancy is a difference in post-translational modifications compared with plasma-derived factor IX.

During severe and critical bleeds it is optimal to achieve 50 to 100 per cent factor activity levels for 7 to 10 days (for example for pharyngeal, retropharyngeal, retroperitoneal, and central nervous system bleeds). More modest levels of 20 to 50 per cent for 2 to 7 days are generally adequate for dental extractions, haematuria, intramuscular or soft tissue bleeds with dissection, or bleeds of the mucous membranes. Levels of 20 to 30 per cent for 1 to 2 days are recommended for uncomplicated haemarthroses, superficial muscle, or soft tissue bleeds. The frequency of dosing is every 12 to 24 h for factor IX concentrates and every 8 to 12 h for factor VIII concentrates. At 24 h for factor IX and 12 h for factor VIII, the calculated amount to infuse would be one-half the initial amount of factor IX, as the half-life of factor IX is approximately 18 to 24 h.

The timing of factor level determination should be 15 to 30 min after the loading dose and immediately prior to subsequent doses for appropriate dose adjustments. When factor concentrates are used for patients with inhibitors, higher doses will most likely be required. Additionally, some authors have also reported good success and reduced cost with constant infusion regimens.

Calculation of the optimal factor concentration for administration

The number of IU (International Units) of factor required is equal to:

body weight (kg) × desired % increase in factor VIII or IX level × C.

C is a constant depending on the product and the source of the product: C is equal to 0.5 for administration of plasma-purified and recombinant factor VIII, C is equal to 1 for administration of plasma-purified factor IX,* and C is equal to 1.2 for administration of recombinant factor IX.†

Surgery in patients with haemophilia

When possible, treatment should be instituted by caregivers aware of major and minor adverse reactions and complications occurring in the haemophiliac population. Care should also be given in association with an experienced reference laboratory able to provide timely evaluation of a patient's response to treatment. Therapeutic factor levels should be obtained prior to surgery. Depending on the type of surgery, the factor level should reach levels of 50 to 100 per cent of normal and should be maintained 2 to 7 days postprocedure. In addition to factor concentrates, fibrin glue has been recommended with circumcision, antifibrinolytics with dental procedures, aprotinin with cardiac procedures, and recombinant factor VIIa and/or apheresis in patients with high-titre inhibitors. The use of aprotinin, however, has been proposed to increase the risk of thrombogenicity. A factor level approaching 100 per cent is recommended for brain or prostate surgery, because of a higher risk of bleeding. In patients with milder haemophilia A administration of the synthetic octapeptide desmopressin (**DDAVP**) may be helpful in increasing factor levels. However, this is not the case for haemophilia B.

Complications of therapy

The main adverse outcomes related to treatment with concentrates include transmission of viruses when using plasma-derived products and development of inhibitory antibodies seen with both recombinant and plasma-derived products. Thrombosis has also been a complication of early complex concentrates used for patients with inhibitors.

The development of purification schemes which inactivate viruses, and the development of recombinant products, has dramatically decreased the incidence of transmission of viral disease. Early preparations of prothrombin complex concentrates presented a significant risk of thrombotic complications, but this risk has now been markedly reduced.

Inhibitor formation—the development of antibodies that inhibit clotting activity—occurs subsequent to transfusion of a blood product or factor replacement. An inhibitor presents a difficult situation for patient management. Therapeutic strategies largely rely on the ability to bypass the factor VIIIa–factor IXa tenase complex. Inhibitor formation almost exclusively arises in severely affected patients and occurs in approximately 7 to 52 per cent of patients with haemophilia A but in only about 1 to 3 per cent of patients with haemophilia B. This difference in inhibitor formation is not completely understood, but possible explanations include the higher incidence of severe disease in haemophilia A, prenatal exposure to maternal factor IX but not factor VIII antigens due to the former's ability to pass the placenta, the structural similarity between factor IX and other vitamin K-dependent proteins, the higher plasma levels of factor IX, and the greater inherent immunogenicity of factor VIII due to its larger size. One very rare but severe complication that may occur with the development of a factor IX inhibitor is the development of a potentially life-threatening anaphylactic complication following first treatment.

Therapeutic strategies for treatment of an inhibitor include acute management of the bleeding episode as well as a longer-term treatment directed toward suppression of antibody production. Quantification of the titre of factor inhibitor involves mixing the patient's plasma with test plasma containing a known amount of factor, normally from a pool of healthy donors. After incubation, factor activity levels present in the patient's incubation mixture are compared with that in a control mixture so that the amount of inhibitory antibody can be calculated. The Bethesda unit (**BU**), the standard unit used to report a titre of factor inhibitor, represents the amount of inhibitor that inactivates 50 per cent of factor activity. Acute management of bleeding in a patient with an inhibitor relies first on quantifying the BU of the inhibitor. With low-titre inhibitors (less than 5 BU), it may be possible to overwhelm the inhibitor with aggressive concentrate therapy. With high-titre inhibitors, it is usually necessary to bypass the inhibitor using either prothrombin complex concentrates, activated prothrombin complex concentrates, porcine factor VIII, or, more recently, recombinant factor VIIa. These bypassing agents, with the exception of porcine factor VIII, largely work by directly activating factor X to factor Xa, thus bypassing the need for the intrinsic tenase complex. With porcine factor VIII, it is wise to first perform testing to ensure that the patient's inhibitor does not cross-react with the porcine factor VIII. Because of the life-threatening bleeding complications in patients with inhibitor, immune tolerance regimens have been designed with the aim of eradicating the inhibitor in the long term.

Therapeutic regimens such as the Malmö protocol involve infusion of high-dose factor concentrates along with immunosuppressive agents enabling a tolerance to the deficient factor. This protocol is highly effective in approximately 80 per cent of patients.

Viral diseases

Severely affected patients treated with plasma-derived concentrates before 1985 had an extremely high rate of viral disease. Over the course of a 70-year lifespan, a patient with severe haemophilia may be exposed to donations from 70 million individuals due to the pooling of thousands of donor units for concentrate production. Specific laboratory tests to screen for HIV, hepatitis C, and hepatitis B, in addition to much improved donor screening procedures, have dramatically limited the number of contaminations from individuals carrying viral diseases. Solvent detergent treatment procedures, which inactivate enveloped viruses (HIV and hepatitis viruses B, C, D, and G), and heat treatment procedures used to eliminate non-enveloped viruses (hepatitis A and E viruses and parvovirus B19) have radically decreased the risk of viral infection from plasma-derived products. The viral inactivation procedures in current use include pasteurization, vapour heating, high-dry heating, and nanofiltration. Recently, β-propiolactone ultraviolet inactivation has been discontinued due to ineffective virucidal technique.

HIV In the late 1970s and early 1980s, HIV, the human immunodeficiency virus, appeared in the blood supply before routine laboratory testing was developed to detect its presence. The leading cause of death in American haemophilia patients in 1982 was haemorrhage; however, contaminated blood products during the period between 1979 to 1983 led to a sharp rise in viral disease shortly thereafter. A large proportion of patients with haemophilia became infected with HIV and have subsequently died from AIDS. Risk factors for infection included the severity of the disease (severely affected patients were much more commonly affected than those with moderate or mild disease), the type of concentrate used (factor VIII versus factor IX concentrate), the viral inactivation procedures used in product preparation, and the geographical location of the patient with regard to percentage of blood products contaminated.

The incidence of HIV infection in American patients who received plasma-derived concentrates between 1979 and 1984 was lower in patients receiving factor IX complex concentrates (55 per cent) than in those receiving factor VIII concentrates (approximately 90 per cent). Despite the devastating consequences of HIV for affected individuals and families, the projected impact on births of patients with haemophilia over the next two centuries is small (1.79 per cent reduction).

Hepatitides Contaminated plasma-derived products also led to significant morbidity and mortality due to hepatitis viruses. Effective virucidal techniques have greatly reduced the incidence of hepatitic viral disease in this population. In the United States in the late 1980s 87 per cent of the 345 HIV negative, and more than 99 per cent of the HIV-positive patients showed evidence of prior infection with hepatitis B, hepatitis C, or hepatitis D viruses. Infection due to hepatitis A virus has rarely been reported in patients with haemophilia in the United States. Solvent/detergent inactivation of concentrates has been associated with a high prevalence of antibodies to hepatitis A virus.

Hepatitis B was commonly seen in patients with haemophilia until routine screening of liver enzymes and the subsequent availability of hepatitis-specific antibody and antigen tests in the 1980s. Most patients are now vaccinated against hepatitis B so that it is difficult to estimate hepatitis B infection from concentrate administration. The hepatitis delta virus, dependent on coinfection with hepatitis B virus, has also been a significant cause of morbidity in patients with haemophilia; its prevalence is largely attributed to the administration of prothrombin complex concentrates.

Routine testing for hepatitis C, instituted in the early 1990s, has reduced but not eliminated hepatitis C contamination in the donor pool. A variable susceptibility and morbidity is seen in response to hepatitis infection; cirrhosis was estimated at approximately 20 per cent and liver failure at 10 to 20 per cent 20 years after infection. Concurrent infection with HIV can accelerate complications of hepatitis C virus. There is also an increased likelihood of hepatocellular carcinoma with long-term infection with viral hepatitis.

Other infectious agents The vast majority of patients with haemophilia have antibodies to parvovirus B19. Parvovirus B19 is a small, non-lipid enveloped, highly heat-resistant virus found to contaminate plasma-derived products. Methods that inactivate other non-lipid enveloped viruses in products have not proven to be routinely effective against this virus. Although parvovirus B19 infection is often mild and self-limited, infection with parvovirus B19 has the potential to severely compromise the health of an infected immunodeficient patient.

There is experimental evidence in animal models that cellular blood components, plasma, and plasma components have a potential, though minimal, risk of transmitting the prion disease Creutzfeldt–Jacob disease. To date, no definitive direct infection of a recipient of a blood product or blood product concentrate has been documented, although transmission has been reported from corneal and dura mater grafts and cadaveric pituitary hormones. The American Red Cross currently administers a questionnaire to screen donors for risk of prion disease. There is now concern that transmission of new variant Creutzfeldt–Jacob disease may differ from classical CJD and could potentially be transmitted through plasma-derived concentrates. This new variant has been associated with outbreaks of bovine spongiform encephalopathy, potentially from dietary exposure. Experimental evidence shows that bovine spongiform encephalopathy and new variant Creutzfeldt–Jacob disease are caused by the same infectious agent, and prion-related protein has been found in lymphoid tissue of patients with new variant Creutzfeldt–Jacob disease. In Europe, particular lots of concentrate have been removed from the market due to the development of new variant Creutzfeldt–Jacob disease in product donors.

Treatment of patients infected with hepatitis virus and/or HIV

Vaccination against hepatitis A and B is highly recommended for patients who receive concentrates and lack viral antibodies indicative of past infection. Treatment of hepatitis C with interferon-γ is associated with significant improvement in approximately half of patients in many but not all studies. Liver transplantation has been successful in many cases for patients with liver failure who are unresponsive to treatment. The liver transplant fortuitously corrects the deficiency of clotting protein due to synthesis of clotting factors by the orthotopic liver. However, the possibility of reinfection with viral disease is significant and must be included in management decisions.

Drug-related hepatitis in haemophilia patients has been reported subsequent to treatment of HIV, particularly in response to indinavir. Additionally, complications in HIV-positive haemophilia patients taking protease inhibitors include haematuria, intracranial bleeds, and excessive bleeding often requiring hospitalization and administration of higher than expected doses of factor concentrate to correct the bleeding. Protease inhibitor therapy should not be withheld from HIV-positive individuals with haemophilia. A 6-month, prospective study of 20 haemophilia patients receiving protease inhibitors revealed only one unusual bleed which was corrected by factor infusion.

Gene transfer as a method of treating haemophilia

The development of clotting factor concentrates resulted in a dramatic improvement in life expectancy for individuals with haemophilia. None the less this treatment strategy has a number of disadvantages. The protein must be infused intravenously, and has a relatively short half-life in the circulation. This makes chronic prophylaxis difficult, especially in small children where venous access may present a problem. In addition, the product is expensive so that only about one-third to one-half of the world's haemophiliacs (those in the developed world) have access to the product. Although current viral inactivation techniques have largely eliminated the risk of HIV and hepatitis, there are ongoing concerns about the risk of other bloodborne diseases (Creutzfeld–Jacob disease, transfusion-transmitted viruses) that are not easily eradicated using current techniques. These factors have fuelled interest in the development of a gene transfer approach to the treatment of haemophilia. Such an approach, if successful, would result in continuous production of a level of clotting factor adequate to prevent bleeds rather than treating bleeds after they have occurred. The level of clotting factor required for this goal can be predicted based on a generation of experience with clotting factor concentrates. Thus in Swedish prophylaxis studies, it has been shown that maintenance of trough factor levels in the range of 1 to 3 per cent are adequate to prevent all the life-threatening bleeds and most of the joint bleeds in boys with severe haemophilia. The validity of a target of 1 to 3 per cent is further confirmed by the natural history of the disease; individuals with factor levels of less than 1 per cent are severely affected, whereas those with levels of 1 to 5 per cent have a moderately severe phenotype with a considerably lower incidence of spontaneous bleeding episodes.

Successful gene transfer approaches require three elements: a therapeutic transgene, a means of delivering it, i.e. a vector, and an appropriate target cell type in which gene transfer and expression will exert a therapeutic effect. Of the inherited diseases for which gene transfer approaches have been attempted, haemophilia has a number of advantages. First, tissue-specific expression is not required. Although clotting factors are normally synthesized in hepatocytes, biologically active material can be synthesized in a variety of tissues, including fibroblasts, muscle cells, and endothelial cells. This allows latitude in the choice of target cell. Second, the therapeutic window is wide, since even small increases in circulating levels of factor are likely to result in some improvement in symptoms, and increases to 100 per cent would still leave the patient within normal limits. Excellent small and large animal models of the diseases exist (murine and canine), and determination of therapeutic efficacy is in the case of haemophilia relatively straightforward, since levels of circulating factor correlate well with symptoms of the disease.

A number of different strategies for gene therapy for haemophilia are under active investigation in preclinical studies, and three clinical trials are currently under way, with two more in late planning stages. The plethora of approaches suggests that there will be more than one successful combination of vector and target tissue that is safe and effective for haemophilia. The ongoing trials include an *ex vivo* approach in which fibroblasts from a patient are isolated from a skin biopsy, cells are expanded in culture, transduced with a retroviral vector expressing factor VIII, and then reimplanted onto the patient's omentum. Early data from this trial show safety in the first six patients treated, with evidence of gene transfer and expression in three out of six. In a second trial, a retroviral vector expressing B-domain deleted factor VIII is infused intravenously. This trial has enrolled 13 subjects with severe haemophilia A. There has been no evidence of safety concerns to date. Finally a third trial involves intramuscular injection of an adenoassociated viral vector expressing factor IX. This approach has been demonstrated to be safe and effective in animal models of haemophilia and is currently being tested in patients with severe haemophilia B. Two other planned trials both use liver as the target cell; one uses a gutted adenoviral vector to express factor VIII, and the other uses an adenoassociated viral vector to express factor IX in liver. The trials will determine whether any of these approaches will be safe and effective in patients with haemophilia.

Von Willebrand disease

In 1926 Erik von Willebrand first described what we now know as von Willebrand disease upon finding an autosomally inherited bleeding diathesis in a large kindred on the Aland Islands in the Gulf of Bothnia between Sweden and Finland. Although the bleeding disorder in this family resulted in haemorrhagic death in multiple family members, the bleeding diathesis in patients with von Willebrand disease is usually much milder. Most commonly, patients with von Willebrand disease manifest mucosal platelet-type bleeding tendencies of varying severity. Nose bleeds, menorrhagia, and easy bruising are the most common manifestations.

The pathophysiology of von Willebrand disease involves a functional deficiency of von Willebrand factor, a 270 kDa monomer that forms a large multimeric plasma glycoprotein of several subunits up to 100 subunits. von Willebrand factor, synthesized in the megakaryocyte and endothelial cell and stored in subcellular granules, enables proper two-chain factor VIII formation and serves as a carrier, thus preventing degradation of factor VIII and lengthening the half-life of the labile factor VIII protein to around 8 h. von Willebrand factor secreted by endothelial cells also binds to heparin glycosaminoglycan and to the platelet glycoprotein complex Ib–IX enhancing platelet activation and further platelet recruitment at sites of tissue damage. The interaction between platelets and von Willebrand factor is thought to provide the explanation for the mucosal bleeding phenotype occurring in patients with von Willebrand disease. Patients with von Willebrand disease frequently have reduced levels of factor VIII. However, the remaining factor VIII is normally sufficient to prevent the haemophilia-type symptomatology of arthropathy and deep tissue bleeding.

The gene for von Willebrand factor is located on chromosome 12, is 180 kbp in length, and consists of 52 exons. There are three types of von Willebrand disease: types 1, 2, and 3. Types 1 and 3 are quantitative deficiencies of the von Willebrand factor while type 2 is a qualitative deficiency due to binding defects of the von Willebrand factor. The inheritance of types 1 and 3 are autosomal dominant and autosomal recessive, respectively. However, rare reports of an autosomal dominant inheritance pattern for type 3 have been published. There are four principal subtypes of type 2 classified as follows: 2A, absence of high molecular weight von Willebrand factor species causing decreased platelet-dependent function; 2B, increased affinity of von Willebrand factor for platelet glycoprotein Ib–IX; 2M, platelet functional defect not caused by the absence of high molecular weight multimers; and 2N, a factor VIII binding abnormality.

Laboratory diagnosis of von Willebrand disease involves assaying the plasma for von Willebrand factor. The two principal tests are an antigenic test (von Willebrand factor anitigen) and an activity test (von Willebrand factor RCo) in which formalin-fixed platelet aggregation is induced due to the ristocetin-enhanced von Willebrand factor binding to glycoprotein complex Ib–IX. Comparison of the tests helps identify the enhanced ristocetin-induced aggregation seen in type 2B von Willebrand disease where von Willebrand factor ristocetin cofactor is typically much lower than von Willebrand factor antigen. Other tests performed in the evaluation of von Willebrand disease include the level of factor VIII, which is often decreased, and the activated partial thromboplastin time, which is elevated in approximately half of cases of von Willebrand disease due to the low activity of factor VIII. Non-reducing gel immunoelectrophoresis is employed to assay the distribution of multimeric subunits of von Willebrand factor with a gel containing antibody to von Willebrand factor antigen. This assay is particularly relevant for visualization of the presence of low, intermediate, and high molecular weight von Willebrand factor subunits. The intermediate and high molecular weight species are markedly decreased in subtypes of type 2 disease. A decreased normal pattern is seen in type 1 disease, although the decreased visual intensity may be difficult to quantitate. Type 3 disease shows near absence of all subunit molecular weights. The lower limit of the normal range of von Willebrand factor varies with blood type (A, B, O, AB). Thus, symptomatology must be evaluated based on normal ranges for each blood type. The bleeding time in a patient with von Willebrand disease is most often prolonged; however, the test is no longer routinely necessary because of the non-specific nature of a positive result and the higher specificity of other testing.

The specific treatment for von Willebrand disease varies with a patient's symptomatology, the circumstances of the need for treatment, the subtype of von Willebrand disease, laboratory results indicating the potential success of increased von Willebrand factor with non-protein based treatment, and the clinical experience with a particular patient and his or her biological family members. When possible, treatment based on non-blood products is preferred The mainstay of treatment for mild disease is treatment with the synthetic octapeptide DDAVP, desmopressin. DDAVP causes release of factor VIII and von Willebrand factor from endothelial cells raising the plasma von Willebrand factor by approximately two- to tenfold. Thus treatment with DDAVP relies on a partial quantitative deficiency of von Willebrand factor. Intravenous and nasal preparations are available. The nasal preparation allows a patient to self-administer medication at either regular intervals or on an as-needed basis. The phenomenon of tachyphylaxis, the decreased effectiveness of repeated doses of the compound, does occur, and there is usually little response after three consecutive doses. In the past, DDAVP was considered contraindicated in type 2B von Willebrand disease because of the thrombocytopenia sometimes observed with DDAVP infusion. However, this recommendation is controversial and should be assessed on a case-by-case basis. Patients with type 3 von Willebrand disease may lack sufficient intracellular reserves for effective therapy; thus alternative measures for such patients are usually necessary.

A trial of effectiveness of DDAVP is often indicated, particularly prior to prophylactic surgical use of the compound. The trial is normally performed after subtyping the von Willebrand factor disease to ensure that DDAVP is not contraindicated, as in type 2B. Optimally, the test should not be given within 24 h of the last DDAVP infusion nor at a time of environmental stress in order to minimize problems associated with tachyphylaxis or depletion of intracellular reserves. A therapeutic trial entails measurement of von Willebrand factor antigen before and 1 h after DDAVP infusion of 0.3 μg/kg. The patient should be watched carefully during this period because of possible flushing, mild anaphylactoid reactions, and possible hyponatraemia.

ε-aminocaproic acid is frequently administered in the setting of dental surgery to inhibit fibrinolysis. However, care must be taken in administration to patients with a predisposition to thrombosis because of the potential deleterious effects of ε-aminocaproic acid in this setting. Other compounds which may be administered include oestrogens in women because of the natural positive regulation of synthesis of von Willebrand factor with oestrogen compounds. This may ameliorate menorrhagia in such patients. Components in cryoprecipitate include factor VIII, fibrinogen, and factor XIII, in addition to von Willebrand factor. Cryoprecipitate had been the mainstay of plasma-based therapy until the recent availability of factor VIII concentrates with preserved von Willebrand factor protein such as Alphanate and Humate P. The use of cryoprecipitate, which does not undergo viral inactivation, has thus fallen out of favour.

Treatment of von Willebrand disease with DDAVP is the method of choice in patients who respond to this therapy. DDAVP for intravenous or subcutaneous use is supplied as either a 4 μg/ml 10 ml vial or a 15 μg/ml 1 or 2 ml vial preparation. The recommended dose is 0.3 μg/kg, mixed in 30 ml normal saline, infused slowly over 30 min or 0.4 μg/kg subcutaneously. This dose may be repeated after 12 to 24 h. A DDAVP nasal spray is available in a metered dose pump which delivers 0.1 ml (150 μg) per actuation. The bottle is at a concentration of 1.5 mg/ml and contains 2.5 ml with a nasal spray pump which can deliver 25 150 μg or 12 300 μg doses. For administration, patients who weigh less than 50 kg should deliver one 150 μg spray in one nostril. For those weighing over 50 kg, one spray should be delivered in each nostril for a total dose of 300 μg. Administration may be repeated after 24 h. Precautions to take with the medication include administration no more than every 24 h or for three consecutive days unless under the supervision of personnel from a haemophilia treatment centre. The medication should not be used in pregnant women or in children under 2 years of age. The medication should be used with caution in the elderly and in individuals with a history of cardiovascular disease.

Factor XI deficiency

Factor XI deficiency is an autosomal recessive bleeding diathesis of variable severity. It was first described in 1953 as a third type of haemophilia and is thus sometimes referred to as haemophilia C or alternatively Rosenthal syndrome. The deficiency predominantly occurs in Eastern European Ashkenazi Jews, accounting for more than 50 per cent the cases. In Ashkenazi Jews the disorder is reported to occur in 5 to 11 per cent of individuals in the heterozygous state and 0.1 to 0.3 per cent in the homozygous state. Genetically, the mutations are grouped into three types: type I, abnormalities in the intron–exon splice boundaries; type II, mutations that result in a premature stop in translation; and type III, mutations resulting from a missense mutation.

The protein itself is an 80 000 kDa protein that circulates in the plasma as a zymogen in a non-covalent association with high molecular weight kininogen. It contains four apple domains in its protein structure, and although factor XIa is a cleaving protease, its structure differs from the serine protease coagulation proteins. Factor XI is principally activated by factor XIIa in the presence of a negatively charged surface (contact activation). The lack of any bleeding diathesis related to a severe deficiency of factor XII suggests the importance of thrombin as an alternative mechanism of *in vivo* factor XI activation.

The *in vitro* factor XI activity level does not correlate well with clinical phenotype. Family history of the bleeding complications and the specific mutated sites are more predictive. Bleeding manifestations are rare in heterozygotes and occur in approximately 50 per cent of homozygous patients.

Factor XI activity levels are assayed in an activated partial thromboplastin time based test. Bleeding problems include easy bruising, epistaxis, haematuria, postpartum haemorrhage, haematomas, and menorrhagia. Haemophilia symptoms, including haemarthroses and intramuscular bleeding, are rare. Bleeding most frequently occurs after trauma or surgery. Damage to tissues rich in fibrinolytic activity, such as oral mucosa and the prostate, are more commonly associated with bleeding problems.

Therapy for patients with factor XI deficiency is indicated for symptomatic bleeding and prophylactically for surgery in patients with markedly reduced levels (i.e. below 20 per cent), unless there is no personal or family history of any bleeding complication. Fresh frozen plasma should be readily available at surgery for infusion in case of a bleeding emergency. Factor XI has a half-life of 60 to 80 h; 10 ml plasma/kg/day is usually adequate for maintaining haemostasis. Prophylactic therapy for most surgery includes replacement of factor XI with plasma at a loading dose of 15 ml/kg followed by 3 to 6 ml/kg every 24 h. The protective level for surgical prophylaxis is suggested as 45 per cent for major surgery and 30 per cent for minor surgery.

Antifibrinolytic therapy with ε-aminocaproic may be a helpful adjunct to plasma therapy; however, antifibrinolytics should be avoided in patients with haematuria or bleeding in the bladder because of possible obstruction by clots.

Deficiencies of proteins in the tissue factor and common pathways

The autosomally inherited deficiencies of factors II, V, VII, and X result in bleeding diatheses of varying severity. Such deficiencies of coagulation factor correlate poorly with tests of *in vitro* factor activity; these are thus quite different disorders from haemophilia, in which *in vitro* assessment predicts the clinical phenotype very well. These factor deficiencies can best be assessed by an initial screen using the prothrombin time as a measurement of the tissue factor pathway. Although the activated partial thromboplastin time may be prolonged with deficiencies of factors II, V, and X, but not VII, the prothrombin time is most often much more sensitive.

Factors II, VII, and X, are structurally homologous containing a signal peptide, a propeptide region necessary for recognition by the post-translationally modifying enzyme γ-glutamyl carboxylase, an intermolecular binding region (two epidermal growth factor (EGF) domains in factors VII, IX, and X and two kringle domains in the prothrombin molecule), and a catalytic domain in the carboxy terminal of the molecule.

Deficiency of prothrombin (factor II) results from a lack of prothrombin or a malfunctional prothrombin protein. Deficiencies result in haemorrhagic manifestations. All reported patients with a prothrombin deficiency retain some prothrombin, thus suggesting that complete prothrombin deficiency is incompatible with life. This is consistent with the knockout mouse model which results in embryonic lethality at 9.5 to 11.5 days postcoitum in over 50 per cent of fetuses; however, for some unknown reason, some murine fetuses are able to survive to birth but promptly die within 2 days due to haemorrhage. Patients with heterozygous prothrombin deficiency most commonly are either asymptomatic or have minimal bleeding. Bleeding symptomatology includes easy bruising, soft tissue haemorrhage, excessive postoperative bleeding, epistaxis, and menorrhagia in women. Haemarthroses are uncommon.

Congenital disease is characterized by a lifelong and a family bleeding history. Levels of 20 to 30 per cent prothrombin normally prevent bleeding symptomatology. When necessary, administration of plasma is recommended at doses of 15 to 20 ml/kg followed by 3 ml/kg every 12 to 24 h. Prothrombin complex concentrates can be administered for serious bleeds and as a prophylactic before surgery. Transmission of viral disease and thromboembolic phenomena are risks of the administration of prothrombin complex concentrates.

Factor V deficiency occurs in fewer than one in a million individuals. Approximately 20 per cent of the body's factor V reserve resides in the platelets. Thus, it is not surprising that patients with factor V deficiency tend to have mucosal bleeding manifestations including epistaxis, gastrointestinal bleeds, and menorrhagia in women. Haemarthroses, although a possible complaint, are much less common than in haemophilia. Mild to moderate bleeding may be treated by raising the factor V activity to about 20 per cent of normal with a plasma dose of approximately 15 to 20 ml/kg followed by 3 to 6 ml/kg every 24 h. Because of the large amount of factor V stored in platelet alpha granules, platelet transfusions may be an appropriate therapy. However, patients should be monitored for the possibility of generation of antiplatelet antibodies.

Factor VII deficiency presents as a variable bleeding disorder ranging from mild to severe, with a possibility of fatal intracranial haemorrhage. Patients with homozygous or compound heterozygous mutations manifest symptoms similar to those of a patient with haemophilia. However, unlike the correlation between activity levels and severity of disease in haemophilia, the *in vitro* factor VII activity clotting test provides only a relative indication of possible disease manifestations. Manifestations include haemarthrosis, arthropathies, haematoma formation, and retroperitoneal bleeding. Fatal intracranial haemorrhage is estimated to occur in approximately 16 per cent of patients with severe disease. Levels below 10 per cent activity most often result in bleeding manifestations. Therapy includes replacement of factor VII levels to 10 to 25 per cent for patients undergoing most types of surgery. Therapy includes plasma at 5 to 10 ml/kg for 6 to 12 h for 1 to 2 days for minor episodes. For surgery, the recommended dose is administration of 15 to 20 ml/kg followed by maintenance doses of 3 to 6 ml/kg every 12 h.

Prothrombin complex concentrates may frequently be used to supply the factor VII along with the other vitamin K-dependent proteins. Although thrombogenicity has not been a recent problem, this does remain a potential complication. Recombinant factor VIIa has been used in Europe for several years and was approved for use in the United States in 1999 for treatment of haemophilia with inhibitors. Although the product has not yet been officially approved for use in factor VII-deficient patients in the United States, recombinant factor VIIa is therapeutically effective in this setting at a dose of 25 μg/kg for acute bleeds, a significantly lower dose than that used for treatment of haemophiliac patients with inhibitors. However, the possible development of a factor VII inhibitor must be considered, as this has been reported. The product is administered every 2 h for prophylaxis during surgery for the first 24 h, then reduced to every 3 h 24 to 48 h postoperatively, and then further reduced according to patient symptomatology and necessity, depending on the risk of bleeding into the surgical site.

Factor X deficiency may present with symptomatology similar to that of a patient with severe haemophilia. Haemarthroses, soft tissue haemorrhages, retroperitoneal bleed, central nervous system haemorrhages, pseudotumours, and menorrhagia may occur. Therapy with fresh frozen plasma includes a loading dose of 10 to 15 ml/kg followed by approximately 50 per cent of that at 24 h.

Deficiency of the contact activating factors, factor XIII, and fibrinogen

Although the activated partial thromboplastin time is grossly prolonged (often more than150 s) with deficiencies of the contact activating factors—factor XII, high molecular weight kininogen, and prekallikrein—these deficiencies are not associated with bleeding manifestations and will not be covered further here.

Factor XIII deficiency often presents shortly after birth with bleeding of the umbilical cord. Patients with clinical manifestations typically have factor levels of less than 1 per cent. Factor XIII is a transglutaminase that crosslinks fibrin monomers, thus stabilizing a forming fibrin clot. Patients with deficiency of factor XIII therefore have delayed wound healing and often suffer from soft tissue haemorrhages, haemarthroses, haematomas, and excessive bleeding from poorly healed wounds. Up to 25 per cent of individuals deficient in factor XIII may experience intracranial bleeding. For unknown reasons, affected males may have oligospermia and affected women may suffer from repeated spontaneous abortions. Since routine clotting tests are normal in factor XIII deficiency, a physician must specifically request a test for factor XIII deficiency which entails a clot solubility test using 2 per cent chloroacetic acid on a formed clot. Treatment of factor XIII deficiency involves administration of small amounts of factor XIII required to minimize bleeding complications. Prophylaxis includes using 2 to 3 ml/kg of fresh frozen plasma every 4 to 6 weeks or one bag of cryoprecipitate per 10 to 20 kg every 3 to 4 weeks. To prevent spontaneous abortions, products containing factor XIII can be administered every 14 to 21 days.

Afibrinogenaemia may cause dangerous haemorrhagic episodes. However, it is somewhat surprising that the mutation does not lead to embryonic death in light of the fact that the blood is incoagulable *in vitro*. The lack of necessity for fibrinogen during fetal development is supported by the viable fibrinogen knockout mouse model. Prolonged bleeding from the umbilical cord often permits early recognition of an affected child. The leading cause of death in afbrinogaemia is intracranial haemorrhage. Haemorrhages from mucous membranes occur frequently, and haemarthroses occur in approximately 20 per cent of patients. Pregnancy related problems include first trimester abortion, placental abruption, and postpartum bleeding complications and may be markedly reduced by administration of fibrinogen. However, fibrinogen replacement may cause thromboembolic phenomena. The target fibrinogen level for replacement therapy is approximately 50 to 100 mg/dl. One bag of cryoprecipitate contains approximately 250 mg of fibrinogen; thus dosing of cryoprecipitate usually necessitates 5 to 10 bags per 70 kg person. Therapeutic complications include allergic reactions and the development of antifibrinogen antibodies. Thromboembolic phenomena may occur in conjunction with fibrinolytic inhibitors or oral contraceptives.

Dysfibrinogaemia results from a functional deficiency of fibrinogen associated with a malfunctional molecule, although some degree of antigen remains present. Approximately 55 per cent of patients with dysfibrinogaemia remain asymptomatic, 25 per cent have a bleeding tendency, and 20 per cent may experience thrombotic episodes ranging from mild to fatal events.

Numerous combined deficiencies have been described; the underlying mutation for several of these combined deficiencies has been determined. Combined deficiency of the two structurally similar proteins factor V and factor VIII is an autosomal recessively inherited disorder of variable bleeding severity. The mechanism responsible for the disorder results from a mutation in ERGIC-53, a 53 kDa transmembrane component of the endoplasmic reticulum–Golgi intermediate compartment. Mutations at this site are associated with factor levels of 4 to 30 per cent of normal factor V and factor VIII activity and generally show mucocutaneous and postsurgical bleeding of a severity similar to that seen in individuals with a single protein deficiency at the same level. Other combined deficiencies for which a genetic mechanism has been described include deficiency of factors II, VII, IX, and X caused by a mutation in the γ-glutamyl carboxylase gene, required for a critical post-translational modification in vitamin K-dependent factors.

Hypercoagulable disease due to deficiencies of anticoagulant

Pathological diseases resulting from inappropriate clot formation in either the arterial or venous circulation are a major cause of morbidity in the Western world. The genetic contribution to this pathophysiology, particularly to thrombosis in the arterial circulation, is not well understood. Clearly cardiovascular disease represents a complex multifactorial process. The contribution of genetic causes to venous thrombotic disease is better understood; it may be associated with either an isolated deficiency of an anticoagulant protein, a malfunctional procoagulant protein, or a combination of these processes. The functional deficiencies become particularly relevant during times of increased environmental stress such as in the puerperium or in postsurgical, traumatic, or immobilized states. In addition to deficiency states, several common mutations involving a gain of function have also been described which can disrupt the delicate balance of coagulation by shifting the balance toward greater procoagulant function.

Procoagulant and anticoagulant plasma proteins interact with platelets and cellular phospholipids to promote physiological coagulation. Regulation of the formation of thrombin is the key step in the proper balance between pro- and anticoagulant functions. Anticoagulant proteins are particularly important in areas where there may be prolonged exposure of procoagulant factors and platelet phospholipids to the vessel wall, predisposing an individual to thrombotic disease. Deficiencies of anticoagulant proteins thus place a patient at an increased risk for thrombosis in the slowly flowing venous circulation. In the rapidly flowing arterial circulation, laminar flow largely prevents prolonged interaction between platelets and vessel walls.

The principal anticoagulant proteins that keep the procoagulant proteins in check include thrombomodulin, tissue factor pathway inhibitor, antithrombin III, protein C, and protein S. Thrombomodulin, an integral membrane protein expressed by endothelial cells, plays a key role in tempering the action of thrombin. Despite attempts to discover mutations in the thrombomodulin gene, only rare reports have implicated thrombomodulin in the pathophysiology of disease, although some recent studies suggest the existence of polymorphic regulation variants in the promoter region. Recently, a mutation in the small but critical protein known as tissue factor pathway inhibitor, which inhibits procoagulant function by binding to factor Xa either alone or in association with tissue factor–factor VIIa, has been suggested to be associated with a ninefold increased risk of venous thrombosis.

Deficiencies leading to a hypercoagulable state are most frequently caused by deficiencies of antithrombin III, protein C, and protein S. These anticoagulant deficiencies result from either a quantitative deficiency (type I) or a qualitative deficiency (type II). Deficiencies of any of these factors may cause life-threatening deep venous thromboses and pulmonary emboli, or may be asymptomatic. Clinical presentation relates to physical sequelae in the affected organ. In addition to deep venous thromboses and pulmonary emboli, symptomatology may include superficial thrombophlebitis, mesenteric vein thrombosis, and cerebral vein thrombosis.

Antithrombin III deficiency

A deficiency of antithrombin III was the first anticoagulant protein deficiency described which was associated with an increased risk of thrombosis. Antithrombin III is a 60 kDa glycoprotein found at high concentrations in the plasma—150 μg/ml: approximately 15- to 30-fold higher than that of many other pro- and anticoagulant proteins. Antithrombin III primarily inhibits thrombin but also inhibits factors IXa, Xa, XIa, XIIa, kallikrein, and plasmin. The ability to inhibit thrombin requires interaction with heparin, which increases the inhibitory activity several thousandfold. Historically, the risk of thrombosis in individuals deficient in antithrombin III has been thought to be higher than that seen with deficiencies of protein S or protein C, or than that seen with increased functionality of the procoagulant proteins factor V and prothrombin. Clearly the influences of gene–gene and gene–environment interactions contribute to this risk. A normal activity range for most procoagulant/anticoagulant proteins may be as low as 50 per cent. However, the critical requirement for antithrombin III can be surmised from the 80 per cent lower limit of a normal antithrombin III level, significantly higher than that for other coagulation proteins. This makes the diagnosis of antithrombin III deficiency particularly difficult in the post-thrombotic period when patients frequently have lower levels of antithrombin III due either to consumption of antithrombin III during clot formation or to the decreased function seen with heparin administration. Additionally, the presence of homozygous disease of antithrombin III deficiency has only been reported with rare type II deficiencies resulting from impaired heparin binding mutations. No homozygous type I deficiencies have been reported, probably due to their incompatibility with life.

The frequency of antithrombin III deficiency in patients with thrombophilia varies widely between studies. The cause of these widely differing frequencies has recently been carefully addressed by van Boven and colleagues. Their study clearly shows the strong influence of acquired and genetic factors which modulate the baseline risk due to one specific genetic mutation, highlighting the role of additional factors when combined with genetics. In thrombophilic family studies, the risk of thrombosis is 20 times greater than in control populations. The most frequent presentation is deep venous thrombosis with a pulmonary embolism, particularly after an inciting environmental influence such as surgery or immobilization in men or the start of oral contraceptives or pregnancy/postpartum in women. The average age of first onset is 33 years. In patients deficient in antithrombin III without a known acquired risk, the rate of incidence of thrombosis was less than 1 per cent per year.

Therapy for antithrombin III deficiency includes prophylactic treatment with warfarin, low molecular weight heparin, and treatment of an acute event with heparin or another anticoagulant therapy, for example administration of a fibrinolytic agent in the patient presenting early enough during an acute episode. Antithrombin III concentrate may be administered for therapy of deficiency during an acute event or as a prophylactic treatment to prevent further disease.

Deficiencies of proteins C and S

Deficiencies of proteins C and S present with thrombotic manifestations similar to those seen with antithrombin III deficiency. However, in protein C deficiency an additional condition includes warfarin-induced skin necrosis and dangerously life-threatening purpura fulminans in the homozygous or compound heterozygous protein C deficient neonate. A diagnosis of protein C deficiency is found in approximately 33 per cent of individuals with warfarin-induced skin necrosis, a condition which leads to skin necrosis several days after initiation of warfarin therapy. The proposed mechanism for this condition is due to the earlier decrease in protein C compared with decreases in procoagulant proteins following initiation of warfarin therapy (due to the short half-life of protein C, approximately 6 h). It is thus 'normal' clinical practice to begin warfarin only after a patient has first been anticoagulated with heparin or another immediately acting anticoagulant therapy.

Protein C acts in concert with its cofactor protein S to inactivate the active forms of the procoagulant cofactors, factors Va and VIIIa. Protein C is a vitamin K-dependent serine protease structurally similar to factors VII, IX, and X. Protein S is also vitamin K-dependent because of conserved NH2 terminus but lacks enzymatic function because of the existence of a sex-hormone binding globulin domain instead of a catalytic domain at the COOH terminus. Thrombin activates protein C to activated protein C when bound to thrombomodulin, a protein which acts like an endothelial cell receptor for thrombin. Symptomatic manifestations of protein C or protein S deficiencies are similar to that of antithrombin III deficiency. Deep venous thombosis with or without pulmonary embolism occurs in 50 per cent of patients by the age of 30 to 45, depending on the study population. Environmental and gene–gene interactions are particularly important. As with antithrombin III deficiency, superficial thrombophlebitis, cerebral vein thrombosis, and mesenteric vein thrombosis are all possible complications. Postphlebitic syndrome presents as a complication after deep venous thombosis in up to 50 per cent of patients.

Factor V Leiden and the prothromibn 20210 mutation

Since 1994, two additional common mutations have been described leading to an increased risk of thrombosis. These mutations, unlike the anticoagulant protein deficiencies, are due to gain of function mutations causing either an increased resistance to inactivation in factor V (factor V Leiden) or increased levels of a procoagulant protein (prothrombin) which results in higher levels of thrombin formation.

Activated protein C (APC) resistance was first described by Dahlback in a 42-year-old man with a history of recurrent thromboses. Dahlback noted an absence of prolongation of the activated partial thromboplastin time, found after addition of APC, which is normally prolonged due to inactivation of factors Va and VIIIa. Soon thereafter, Poort and colleagues identified a single mutation as the principal cause of APC resistance in the vast majority (over 90 per cent) of patients. The mutation leads to a decreased ability of APC to inactivate the cofactor Va due to an amino acid substitution (arginine for glutamine) at a critical hydrolysis point in the factor Va protein normally enabling inactivation. Other non-factor V Leiden causes of APC resistance include a haplotype in the factor V molecule, the H2 haplotype.

Factor V Leiden leads to thrombotic disease as described for hypercoagulable states due to deficiencies of anticoagulant protein. Because of the extremely high incidence of factor V Leiden in the Caucasian population (approximately 5 per cent), gene–gene interactions play a particularly important role in manifestation of disease. It should be noted that the frequency of factor V Leiden in most non-Caucasian populations is low.

The prothrombin 20210 mutation reported in 1996 results in an increased concentration of prothrombin, also tipping the balance towards excess thrombin formation. The cause of this increase is associated with a guanine to adenine mutation at the last base of the 3‘ untranslated region in the factor V gene. The mechanism by which this influences prothrombin levels is not understood.

Further reading

General articles about coagulation

Colman RW *et al.* (1994). Overview of hemostasis. In: Colman RW *et al.*, eds. *Thrombosis and hemorrhage*, pp 3–18. JB Lippincott, Philadelphia.

Davie EW and Ratnoff OD (1964). Waterfall sequence for intrinsic blood clotting. *Science* **145**, 1310–12.

Furie B, Furie BC (1992). Molecular and cellular biology of blood coagulation. *New England Journal of Medicine* **26**, 800–6.

MacFarlane RG (1964). An enzyme cascade in the blood clotting mechanism and its function as a biochemical amplifier. *Nature* **202**, 498–9.

Roberts HR, Lozier JN (1992). New perspectives on the coagulation cascade. *Hospital Practice* **27**, 97–105, 109–12.

Haemophilia and von Willebrand disease

Djulbegovic B, Goldsmith GH Jr (1995). Guidelines for management of hemophilia A and B. *Blood* **85**, 598–9.

Furie B, Furie BC (1990). Molecular basis of hemophilia. *Seminars in Hematology* **27**, 270–85.

Furie B, Limentani SA, Rosenfield CG (1994). A practical guide to the evaluation and treatment of hemophilia. *Blood* **84**, 3–9.

Ginsburg D, Bowie EJ (1992). Molecular genetics of von Willebrand disease. *Blood* **79**, 2507–19.

Gitscher J *et al.* (1991). Genetic basis of hemophilia A. *Thrombosis and Haemostasis* **66**, 37–9.

Larson PJ, High K (1992). Biology of inherited coagulopathies: factor IX. *Hematology—Oncology Clinics of North America* **6**, 999.

Ljung R *et al.* (1992). Factor VIII and factor IX inhibitors in haemophiliacs. *The Lancet* **339**, 1550.

Management Association of Hemophilia Clinic Directors of Canada (1995). Hemophilia and von Willebrand's disease. *Canadian Medical Association Journal* **153**,147.

Roberts HR (1993). Molecular biology of hemophilia B. *Thrombosis and Haemostasis* **70**, 1.

Sadler JE (1994). A revised classification of von Willebrand disease. For the Subcommittee on von Willebrand Factor of the Scientific and Standardizaion Committee of the International Society of Thrombosis and Haemostasis. *Thrombosis and Haemostasis* **71**, 520–5.

Triemstra M *et al.* (1995). Mortality in patients with hemophilia. Changes in a Dutch population from 1986 to 1992 and 1973 to 1986. *Annals of Internal Medicine* **123**, 823.

Administration of factor concentrates

Aronson DL (1987). Thrombogenicity of factor IX complex: *in vivo* investigation. *Developments in Biological Standardization* **67**, 149.

Blanchette VS *et al.* (1997). Central venous access devices in children with hemophilia: an update. *Blood Coagulation and Fibrinolysis* **8** (suppl. 1), S11.

Ewenstein BM (1997). Nephrotic syndrome as a complication of immune tolerance in hemophilia B. *Blood* **89**, 1115–16.

Federici AB (1998). Optimizing therapy with factor VIII/von Willebrand factor concentrates in von Willebrand disease. *Haemophilia* **4**, 7.

Goudemand JNC, Ounnoughene N, Sultan Y (1998). Clinical management of patients with von Willebrand's disease with a VHP vWF concentrate: the French experience. *Haemophilia* **4**, 48.

Mannucci PM (1993). Clinical evaluation of viral safety of coagulation factor VIII and IX concentrates. *Vox Sanguinis* **64**, 197.

Warrier I *et al.* (1997). Factor IX inhibitors and anaphylaxis in hemophilia B. *Journal of Pediatric Hematology/Oncology* **19**, 23.

White GC 2nd and Nielsen B (1997). Recombinant factor IX. *Thrombosis and Haemostasis* **78**, 261–5.

Infectious diseases associated with haemophilia therapy

Bruce ME *et al.* (1997). Transmissions to mice indicate that 'new variant' CJD is caused by the BSE agent. *Nature* **389**, 498.

Baxter T, Black D, Birks D (1998). New-variant Creutzfeldt–Jakob disease and treatment of haemophilia. *The Lancet* **351**, 600.

Centers for Disease Control and Prevention (1996). Hepatitis A among persons with hemophilia who received clotting factor concentrate–United States, September–December 1995. *Journal of the American Medical Association* **275**, 427.

Craven BM, Stewart GT, Khan M (1997). AIDS: safety, regulation and the law in procedures using blood and blood products. *Medicine, Science and the Law* **37**, 215.

Eyster ME *et al.* (1993). Natural history of hepatitis C virus infection in multitransfused hemophiliacs: effect of coinfection with human immunodeficiency virus. The Multicenter Hemophilia Cohort Study. *Journal of Acquired Immune Deficiency Syndromes* **6**, 602–10.

Kupfer B *et al.* (1995). Beta-propiolactone UV inactivated clotting factor concentrate is the source of HIV-infection of 8 hemophilia B patients: confirmed. *Thrombosis and Haemostasis* **74**, 1386.

Lee CA, Sabin CA (1997). The natural history of chronic hepatitis C in haemophiliacs. *British Journal of Haematology* **96**, 875.

Makris M *et al.* (1996). The natural history of chronic hepatitis C in haemophiliacs. *British Journal of Haematology* **94**, 746.

Gene therapy in haemophilia

Herzog RW *et al.* (1999) Long-term correction of canine hemophilia B by gene transfer of blood coagulation factor IX mediated by adeno-associated viral vector *Nature Medicine* **5**, 56–63.

Herzog RW, High KA (1999). Adeno-associated virus-mediated gene transfer of factor IX for treatment of hemophilia B by gene therapy. *Thrombosis and Haemostasis* **82**, 540–6.

Mannucci PM, Tuddenbam EG (1999). The hemophilias: progress and problems. *Seminars in Hematology* **36** (suppl. 7), 104–17.

Park F, Ohashi K, Kay MA (2000). Therapeutic levels of human factor VIII and IX using HIV-1-based lentiviral vectors in mouse liver. *Blood* **96**, 1173–6.

Thompson AR (2000). Gene therapies for the hemophilias. *Molecular Therapy: the Journal of the American Society of Gene Therapy* **2**, 5–8.

White GC 2nd, Roberts HR (2000). Gene therapy for hemophilia: a step closer to reality. *Molecular Therapy: the Journal of the American Society of Gene Therapy* **1**, 207–8.

Thrombotic disease

Bates SM, Hirsch J (1999). Thrombotic disorders and their treatment: treatment of venous thromboembolism. *Thrombosis and Haemostasis: State of the Art* **82**, 870–931.

Bucciarelli P, Rosendaal FR, Tripodi A (1999). Risk of venous thromboembolism and clinical manifestations in carriers of antithrombin, protein C, protein S deficiency, or activated protein C resistance: a multicenter collaborative family study. *Arteriosclerosis, Thrombosis, and Vascular Biology* **19**, 1026–33.

Koster T, Rosendaal FR, Briet E (1995). Protein C deficiency in a controlled series of unselected outpatients: an infrequent but clear risk factor for venous thrombosis (Leiden thromobophilia study). *Blood* **10**, 2756–61.

Lane DA, Mannucci PM, Bauer KA (1996). Inherited thrombophilia: part 1. *Thrombosis and Haemostasis* **76**, 651–62.

Lane DA, Manucci PM, Bauer KA (1996). Inherited thrombophilia: part 2. *Thrombosis and Haemostasis* **76**, 824–34.

Rivard GE, David M, Farrell C (1995). Treatment of purpura fulminans in meningococcemia with protein C concentrate. *Journal of Pediatrics* **126**, 646–52.

Rohrer MJ, Andrew M, Michelson AD (1998). Hemorrhage, thrombosis, and antithrombotic therapy in children. In: Loscalzo J, Shafer A, eds. *Thrombosis and Hemorrhage*, pp. 1027–63. Williams and Wilkins, Baltimore.

Sanz-Rodriguez C, Gil-Fernandez JJ, Zapater P (1999). Long-term management of homozygous protein C deficiency: replacement therapy with subcutaneous purified protein C concentrate. *Thrombosis and Haemostasis* **81**, 887–90.

van Boven HH *et al.* (1999). Gene–gene and gene–environment interactions determine risk of thrombosis in families with inherited antithrombin deficiency. *Blood* **94**, 2590–4.

22.6.5 Acquired coagulation disorders

T. E. Warkentin

A 'coagulopathy' is a disorder associated with an abnormal coagulation assay result, such as a prolonged prothrombin time (**PT**) (often expressed as the international normalized ratio, or **INR**), activated partial thromboplastin time (**aPTT**), or thrombin clotting time (**TCT**). Coagulopathies can be associated with either bleeding or thrombosis, and have many causes (Table 1). The importance of the clinical context is illustrated by two patient scenarios that have in common a prolonged INR (6.0; usual therapeutic range, 2.0–3.0) during oral anticoagulant therapy: patient A has a life-threatening intracranial haemorrhage complicating warfarin therapy given for a prosthetic heart valve; in contrast, patient B, who was treated for deep-vein thrombosis (**DVT**) complicating heparin-induced thrombocytopenia (**HIT**), has the limb-threatening complication of warfarin-induced venous limb gangrene, caused by microvascular thrombosis.

Table 1 Coagulopathies that cause bleeding or thrombosis

Associated with bleeding	Associated with thrombosis
Vitamin K deficiency	Heparin-induced thrombocytopenia[a,d]
Coumarin-induced supratherapeutic INR	Chronic DIC secondary to adenocarcinoma[a]
Liver disease	
Severe haemodilution/massive transfusion	Antiphospholipid antibody syndrome ('lupus anticoagulant')[a]
Acute DIC (e.g. pregnancy-associated)	Thrombotic microangiopathic haemolysis[c]
Acquired coagulation factor inhibitor	Coumarin-induced skin necrosis[b]
Heparin or heparin-like anticoagulants	Coumarin-induced venous limb gangrene[b]
Paraprotein-induced coagulopathies	Purpura fulminans (neonatal, idiopathic, post-varicella, or associated with septicaemia/DIC)[b]
Hyperfibrinolysis	
Snake envenomation	

[a]Usually causes thrombosis of large veins and arteries.
[b]Usually causes thrombosis of the microcirculation, including postcapillary venules.
[c]Usually causes arteriolar thrombosis.
[d]Significant prolongation of INR and/or hypofibrogenaemia occurs in <10 per cent of patients.

Table 2 lists common screening tests for coagulopathy. Only a few bleeding disorders give normal results in all these tests (for example, α_2-antiplasmin deficiency, factor XIII deficiency, type 2a von Willebrand syndrome associated with aortic stenosis). A drawback of these assays is that only procoagulant *haemo*static pathways are assessed. Thus, deficiency of a natural anticoagulant such as antithrombin or protein C must be determined by specific testing.

Treatment approaches

Blood products are usually indicated for the treatment of patients with coagulopathies who are bleeding or who require a major invasive procedure. *Fresh-frozen plasma* (**FFP**), which contains all the *haemo*static factors at concentrations between 0.7 and 1.0 U/ml, is appropriate for liver disease, *haemo*dilution from massive transfusion, disseminated intravascular coagulation (**DIC**), reversal of coumarin anticoagulation, and replacement of isolated factor deficiency when specific-factor replacement is unavailable. For a 70-kg adult with a 3-litre plasma volume, 1 litre of FFP will increase the coagulation factors by about 0.25 U/ml. In most patients, this should lead to levels greater than the minimum required for adequate *haemo*stasis (>0.30 U/ml for most factors). Repeat FFP transfusion (for example, 500 ml every 6 h) is necessary if the *haemo*stasis defect is ongoing. FFP is being supplanted by cryosupernatant as a replacement fluid for thrombotic thrombocytopenic purpura (**TTP**). Solvent-detergent-treated plasma (**SD**-plasma), in which most blood-borne pathogens are inactivated (but not hepatitis A, parvovirus B19, or the agent that causes Creutzfeldt–Jakob disease, a theoretical bloodborne pathogen), has become available recently, but is limited by its high cost.

Cryoprecipitate contains fibrinogen (0.10–0.25 g per unit), factors VIII and XIII, von Willebrand factor (**vWF**), and fibronectin. Its major indication is the treatment of hypofibrinogenaemia, where it increases fibrinogen levels using just one-quarter of the volume of blood product compared with FFP. Cryoprecipitate is appropriate for patients with significant hypofibrinogenaemia, for example DIC, primary fibrinolysis, congenital hypofibrinogenaemia. For a bleeding patient whose fibrinogen level is about 0.5 g/l, 10 to 20 U of cryoprecipitate would probably increase the fibrinogen to above 1.0 g/l, although a lower than expected increment could occur if the patient had a higher volume of distribution (for example, a cirrhotic patient with ascites).

Specific-factor concentrates are available for use in patients with an isolated deficiency in certain factors, such as VIII or IX. Additionally, some factor IX concentrates, known as prothrombin complex concentrates (**PCC**), contain all four vitamin K-dependent procoagulant factors, and are appropriate for the rapid reversal of severe coagulopathy related to coumarin use. Activated PCC (for example, **FEIBA** (factor VIII inhibitor bypassing activity)) and factor VIIa are other specialized blood products with specific uses, for instance to manage a bleeding patient with an acquired factor VIII inhibitor.

Pharmacological therapies include the antifibrinolytic agents ε-aminocaproic acid (**EACA**), tranexamic acid (**TA**), and aprotinin. EACA and TA bind to the lysine-binding sites of plasminogen; paradoxically, although increasing the susceptibility of plasminogen to proteolysis by plasminogen activator, these lysine analogues also prevent plasminogen from binding to fibrin, thus impeding fibrinolysis. Oral dosing for EACA is about 7 g (100 mg/kg) initially, followed by 3.5 g (50 mg/kg) every 4 h; similar doses are used for intravenous administration. For tranexamic acid, 1.0 to 1.5 g is given every 8 h by mouth; the dose is reduced to between 0.5 and 1.0 g every 8 h if given intravenously. Both drugs are available in 500-mg capsules. These drugs are appropriate for the treatment of hyperfibrinolysis, for instance bleeding following thrombolytic therapy or cardiac surgery. These drugs are generally contraindicated in patients with DIC, however, as blocking secondary fibrinolysis could lead to microvascular thrombosis. Aprotinin is discussed below in the section on cardiopulmonary bypass surgery.

Desmopressin, or 1-desamino-8-D-arginine vasopressin (**DDAVP**), a synthetic vasopressin analogue, leads to an increase in factor VIII and vWf levels that peak between 45 and 90 min after intravenous infusion (0.3 μg/kg in 50 ml normal saline over 20–30 min; maximum dose, 20 μg). Although repeat DDAVP can be given at 12- to 24-h intervals, the drug becomes less effective over time (tachyphylaxis) as endothelial stores of vWf are depleted. Blood pressure elevation, free-water retention leading to hyponatraemia, flushing, and angina are occasional side-effects.

Table 2 Screening haemostasis tests

Assay	Comment
Prothrombin time (PT), often expressed as international normalized ratio (INR)	Screen for deficiency of factors VII, X, V, II, and/or fibrinogen (e.g. vitamin K deficiency/coumarin therapy, liver disease)
Activated partial thromboplastin time (aPTT)	Screen for deficiency of factors VIII, IX, X, V, II, contact factors, and/or fibrinogen; detect antithrombins, e.g. heparin
Thrombin clotting time (TT or TCT)	Screen for hypofibrinogenaemia and/or presence of heparin; some TCT assays are also sensitive to FDPs
Serum fibrin(ogen) degradation products (FDPs)	Requirement to clot blood sample can lead to false- positive results due to incomplete blood clotting (e.g. residual heparin)
Crosslinked fibrin assay (d-dimer)	Detects fibrin degradation products generated after thrombin, factor XIII, and plasmin have acted upon fibrinogen (marker for DIC)
Paracoagulation assay (e.g. protamine sulphate test)	Positive paracoagulation assay often means DIC is clinically significant and may require blood products or anticoagulant therapy
Bleeding time	Assesses primary haemostasis, i.e. vWF-mediated platelet adhesion to endothelium with secondary aggregation of platelets within haemostatic plug
Complete blood count; blood film examination	Platelet enumeration, and assessment of causes for thrombocytopenia, e.g. red cell fragments indicating microangiopathy

Prohaemorrhagic acquired coagulation disorders

Vitamin K deficiency disorders

Vitamin K-dependent coagulation factors

Vitamin K is required for the post-translational modification of six *haemostatic* factors, four with procoagulant activity (factors II, VII, IX, and X), and two with anticoagulant activity (protein C, protein S). The physiological relevance of a seventh factor, Factor Z, remains unclear. The enzyme, vitamin K-dependent γ-glutamylcarboxylase, adds a carboxyl group to each member of a cluster of glutamyl residues, thereby forming the γ-carboxyglutamyl residues crucial for enabling these six haemostatic factors to interact with phospholipid membranes in a calcium-dependent fashion. During this γ-carboxylation reaction, the reduced form of vitamin K (vitamin KH_2) is oxidized to vitamin K epoxide; oral anticoagulants inhibit the two enzymes (vitamin K epoxide reductase and vitamin K reductase, respectively) that act in sequence to regenerate the reduced form of vitamin K.

Diet and absorption of vitamin K

Vitamin K_1 (phylloquinone) is exclusively derived from plants; vitamin K_2 (menaquinone) is synthesized by bacteria. Green, leafy vegetables, such as broccoli, lettuce, cabbage, and spinach, are very good dietary sources of vitamin K (100–500 μg/100 mg). Vitamin K is fat-soluble, and absorption occurs primarily in the small bowel. Serum vitamin K levels are only between 150 and 800 pg/ml and, as hepatic storage is limited ($t\frac{1}{2}$, just a few days), a regular daily intake of about 0.1 to 0.5 μg/kg is required. Although bacterial synthesis is not a major source of vitamin K to humans, antibiotic treatment nevertheless predisposes to vitamin K deficiency.

Vitamin K deficiency

Malabsorption of fat-soluble vitamins caused by biliary tract disease, or primary bowel disorders such as coeliac or inflammatory bowel disease, can cause vitamin K deficiency. An inadequate diet, particularly when combined with antibiotic therapy, is another cause. Indeed, coagulopathy can arise during a brief period of decreased intake, for example 1-week postoperatively.

A disproportionately prolonged PT/INR in the appropriate clinical setting suggests vitamin K deficiency (Table 3). The diagnosis is usually confirmed by assessing the response to vitamin K administration. Compared with the treatment of a coumarin overdose, small amounts of vitamin K are effective: for example, 1 mg vitamin K_1 given subcutaneously or by slow

Table 3 Results of screening haemostasis assays in various clinical settings

	PT/INR	aPTT	Fibrinogen	TCT	FDPs	Platelets
Vitamin K deficiency or antagonism (coumarin)	↑↑	↑	N	N	N	N
Liver disease	↑, ↑↑	N, ↑	↓, N, ↑	N, ↑	N, ↑, ↑↑	N, ↓, ↓↓
Heparin	N, sl ↑	↑↑	N	↑↑	N	N, ↓
LMWH, danaparoid	N	N, sl ↑	N	N, sl ↑	N	N
Thrombin inhibitors	↑	↑	N	↑↑	N	N
Thrombolytic	sl ↑	N	↓	↑↑	↑	N, ↓
Renal disease	N	N	N	N	N	N, sl ↓
Acute DIC	↑, ↑↑	↑, ↑↑	N, ↓, ↓↓	N, ↑, ↑↑	↑, ↑↑*	↓, ↓↓
Chronic DIC	N, ↑	N, sl↑	N, ↓	N, ↑	↑, ↑↑*	N, ↓, ↓
Primary fibrinolysis	N, sl↑	N, sl↑	↓, ↓↓	↑, ↑↑*	↑, ↑↑*	↓, N
Lupus anticoagulant	N, sl ↑	N, ↑, ↑↑	N	N	N	N, ↓
Factor VIII inhibitor	N	↑, ↑↑	N	N	N	N
Haemodilution	↑	↑, ↑↑	↓, ↓↓	↑, ↑↑	N	↓
Ancrod (snake venom)	sl ↑	sl ↑	↓↓	↑, ↑↑	N	N

*Crosslinked fibrin degradation products (D-dimer) are greater in patients with DIC, compared with primary fibrinolysis.

intravenous infusion (over at least 30 min to minimize risk of an anaphylactoid reaction). For serious bleeding, FFP or especially PCC provides a more rapid correction of the coagulopathy.

Coumarin overanticoagulation

Oral anticoagulants (for example, coumarins such as warfarin and phenprocoumon) are widely used to prevent and treat thrombosis via their vitamin K antagonism. An INR target range between 2.0 and 3.0 is appropriate for most clinical indications, although a higher therapeutic range (INR, 2.5–3.5) is appropriate for patients at very high risk for thrombosis (for instance, mechanical prosthetic heart valves; thrombosis complicating the antiphospholipid antibody syndrome).

Bleeding is the major complication of coumarin, with minor and major bleeding episodes occurring in about 6 to 10 per cent and 1 to 3 per cent of patients/year respectively; the intracranial haemorrhage rate is between 0.25 and 1 per cent/year. Changes in diet or alcohol consumption, poor patient compliance, and the introduction of new drugs (Table 4) can cause bleeding by producing coumarin overanticoagulation. In contrast, recurrent gastrointestinal or urinary tract bleeding at therapeutic levels of anticoagulation often indicates an occult gastrointestinal or renal lesion, respectively.

The treatment of non-therapeutic (elevated) INRs depends on the clinical situation (Table 5). Oral vitamin K_1 use is appropriate in many non-urgent situations as it avoids the risk of anaphylactoid reactions to intravenous use, and has more predictable effects than subcutaneous injection. Much larger and prolonged vitamin K dosing (100–150 mg/day) is required to treat accidental or deliberate overdoses of long-acting, second-generation rodenticides ('superwarfarins'), such as brodifacoum.

Liver disease

Most haemostatic factors are produced exclusively by the liver. Exceptions include factor VIII (hepatic and extrahepatic synthesis), vWf (endothelium, megakaryocytes), and several factors produced by endothelium (for example, plasminogen activator, plasminogen activator inhibitor type I (**PAI-1**)). Table 6 lists the multiple effects on haemostasis caused by liver disease. Often, bleeding is primarily related to anatomical factors, such as oesophageal varices or gastric/duodenal ulcers, though reduced hepatic coagulation-*factor* synthesis can be a contributing factor. Increased susceptibility to DIC via superadded illness (for example, bacterial peritonitis), impaired clearance of activated coagulation factors, and hyperfibrinolysis are other factors.

A prolonged PT/INR is the most frequent laboratory abnormality (Table 3). The fibrinogen level is usually normal or increased; when hypofibrinogenaemia occurs, it generally indicates severe liver disease or hyperfibrinolysis. Fibrin(ogen)-degradation product (**FDP**) and D-dimer levels are often increased; thus, the laboratory picture can resemble that of disseminated intravascular coagulation even in a patient who is otherwise clinically stable.

Management of hepatic coagulopathy should include a trial of vitamin K_1 (for instance, 10 mg subcutaneously for 3 days), although this will not benefit most patients. Fresh-frozen plasma should be given to bleeding patients with a prolonged INR, or who require major invasive procedures. Retrospective studies suggest that minor invasive procedures (for example,

Table 4 Drugs and foods for which there is highest (level I) evidence for interaction with warfarin (taken with permission from Hirsh *et al.* 1998)

Potentiation of warfarin's anticoagulant effect	Inhibition of warfarin's anticoagulant effect
Antibiotics: co-trimoxazole, erythromycin, fluconazole, isoniazid, metronidazole, and miconazole	*Antibiotics*: griseofulvin, rifampin, and nafcillin
Cardiac drugs: amiodarone, clofibrate, propafenone, propranolol, and sulfinpyrazone (biphasic with later inhibition)	*CNS active drugs*: barbiturates, carbamazepine, and chlordiazepoxide
Miscellaneous drugs: anabolic steroids; phenylbutazone; piroxicam; alcohol (if concomitant liver disease); cimetidine; and omeprazole	*Miscellaneous drugs*: cholestyramine; sucralfate
	Foods or enteral feeds that are high in vitamin K; large amounts of avocado

paracentesis, pleurocentesis) can usually be performed safely with an INR as high as 1.8. For patients suspected to have significant fibrinolysis, antifibrinolytic therapy can be tried. PCCs should only be used in emergency situations, given their prothrombotic potential in this patient population. Platelet transfusions usually provide minimal increase in the platelet count in patients with platelet sequestration caused by hypersplenism. DDAVP improves haemostasis in patients with prolonged bleeding time secondary to hepatic platelet dysfunction.

Table 5 Management of non-therapeutic INRs

Clinical situation	Guidelines[a]
INR above the therapeutic range but<5.0, no significant bleeding	Lower the dose; or omit the next dose, and resume therapy at a lower dose when the INR is within the therapeutic range; if the INR is only slightly above the therapeutic range, dose reduction may be unnecessary
INR >5.0 but <9.0, no significant bleeding	Omit the next dose or two, monitor INR more frequently, and resume therapy at a lower dose when the INR is within the therapeutic range
	Alternatively, omit a dose and give vitamin K_1 (1 to 2.5 mg orally especially if the patient is at an increased risk of bleeding),
	Patients requiring more rapid reversal before urgent surgery: vitamin K_1 (2–4 mg orally); if INR remains high at 24 h give an additional dose of vitamin K_1 (1–2 mg orally)
INR >9.0, no clinically significant bleeding	Omit warfarin; give vitamin K_1 (3–5 mg orally); closely monitor the INR; if the INR is not substantially reduced in 24 to 48 h, monitor the INR more often, giving additional vitamin K_1, if necessary Resume therapy at a lower dose when the INR is within the therapeutic range
INR >20; serious bleeding	Omit warfarin; give vitamin K_1 (10 mg, slow IV infusion), supplemented with fresh-frozen plasma or prothrombin-complex concentrate, depending on urgency; vitamin K_1 injections can be repeated every 12 h
Life-threatening bleeding	Omit warfarin; give prothrombin-complex concentrates with vitamin K_1 (10 mg by slow IV infusion); repeat if necessary, depending on the INR
Continuing warfarin therapy indicated after high doses of vitamin K_1	Give heparin until the effects of vitamin K_1 have been reversed, and until the patient is responsive to warfarin
	If continuing warfarin therapy is indicated after high doses of vitamin K_1, heparin can be given until the effects of vitamin K1 have been reversed and the patient becomes responsive to warfarin therapy

[a]Guidelines as given by the Sixth American College of Physicians Conference on Antithrombotic Therapy (2001).
IV, intravenous.

Table 6 Causes of bleeding and thrombosis in liver disease

Predispose to bleeding
Effects of portal hypertension:
- oesophageal varices (bleeding site)
- splenomegaly (thrombocytopenia)

Decreased procoagulant factor synthesis
Abnormal coagulation factor synthesis:
- dysfibrinogenaemia (increased sialic acid content)
- descarboxylated vitamin K-dependent factors

Decreased clearance of plasmin, plasminogen activators, and fibrin(ogen) degradation products
Vitamin K malabsorption
Platelet dysfunction
Increased susceptibility to adverse hepatic effects of alcohol or other drugs
Decreased α_2-antiplasmin synthesis (predisposes to hyperfibrinolysis)

Predispose to thrombosis
Decreased natural anticoagulant synthesis
Decreased clearance of activated coagulation factors
Physician reluctance to prescribe antithrombotic therapy

Haemodilution and massive transfusion

Coagulopathies occur in most patients who receive crystalloids, colloids, or red cell concentrates (**RCCs**) following trauma, surgery, or fluid resuscitation for other major illnesses. In many patients, no bleeding results despite moderate abnormalities in the INR, aPTT, TCT, and platelet count. The reason is that all the individual coagulation factors remain at haemostatically effective levels, even though the laboratory assays are abnormal when all the factor levels are uniformly reduced.

Massive transfusion is defined as the transfusion of blood products equivalent to the patient's total blood volume within 24 h. RCCs do not provide significant amounts of platelets or coagulation factors. Thus, platelet, FFP, and, sometimes, cryoprecipitate infusions are often needed as well. Although 'formulas' to guide transfusion therapy have been devised, individualized assessment that takes into account clinically evident bleeding, risk factors for haemorrhage, supervening DIC or fibrinolysis, acute liver insult, and laboratory test results, is preferable.

Disseminated intravascular coagulation

Disseminated intravascular coagulation, or DIC, is a group of clinicopathological syndromes characterized by widespread activation of coagulation; there results intravascular generation of thrombin, formation of fibrin, and reactive fibrinolysis. Clinical consequences range from coagulation factor and platelet depletion, resulting in generalized haemorrhage, to widespread microvascular thrombosis, predisposing to multisystem organ dysfunction or limb necrosis. 'Acute' DIC, caused by septicaemia, trauma, and obstetrical complications, is most frequent; 'chronic' DIC, typically caused by malignancy, is often associated with a dramatic hypercoagulable state (Table 7). Although DIC is usually a systemic process, sometimes a localized abnormality (such as a vascular malformation or aortic aneurysm) leads to the regional activation of coagulation and resulting in the depletion of haemostatic factors.

DIC is usually triggered by the extrinsic coagulation pathway: tissue factor and factor VIIa (Fig. 1). The proinflammatory cytokine, interleukin-6 (**IL-6**), is a principal mediator of DIC in septicaemia and other systemic inflammatory responses, and impairs natural anticoagulant and fibrinolytic pathways. For example, a sustained increase in PAI-1 impairs plasmin formation despite intravascular fibrin generation.

Diagnostic and treatment approach to DIC

One or more prolonged clotting times and thrombocytopenia in a patient with one of the disorders listed in Table 7 suggests DIC. However, similar test results are seen in patients following major surgery, emphasizing the need to interpret the laboratory data in the appropriate clinical context.

Table 7 Main causes of DIC

Acute DIC
Trauma, burns, shock
Infection
Obstetrical complications:
placental abruption
amniotic fluid embolism
pre-eclampsia/eclampsia
puerperal sepsis
saline-induced abortion
Malignancy, promyeloctic anaemia
Allergic reactions
Severe haemolysis
Chronic DIC
Malignancy
Obstetrical complications:
dead fetus syndrome
Chronic liver disease
Vascular anomalies:
giant haemangioma (Kasabach–Merritt syndrome)
aortic aneurysm

Typically, crosslinked fibrin-degradation products (D-dimers) are significantly increased in DIC. The protamine sulphate 'paracoagulation' test, based on visual detection of gelling of patient plasma after the addition of protamine sulphate, is a rapid test for fibrin monomers; the lower sensitivity of the test is helpful, as a positive result usually indicates clinically significant DIC associated with bleeding or thrombosis. Sometimes, specialized haemostasis assays are useful, for example protein C activity levels in purpura fulminans.

The cornerstone of DIC management is treating its underlying cause and providing supportive measures. For bleeding patients, replacement of depleted haemostatic factors with FFP, cryoprecipitate, and platelet transfusions may be needed. Recently, drotrecogin alfa (recombinant activated protein C) became available in some jurisdictions to treat severe septicaemia. Heparin can benefit patients with large-vessel thrombosis or acral ischaemia. The routine use of vitamin K and folate will avoid coagulation and platelet count disturbances in some patients.

Trauma and shock

Tissue injury due to trauma, burns, or hypoperfusion can cause DIC, especially when organs rich in tissue thromboplastin (for example, the brain) are injured.

Infection

Gram-negative and Gram-positive bacteria can cause DIC, either from procoagulant bacterial components (for instance, endotoxin, *Staphylococcus aureus*-toxin) or via the host response to infection (for example, IL-6). The clinical spectrum ranges from prominent thrombocytopenia with minimal activation of coagulation, to marked coagulation factor and natural anticoagulant depletion. Certain infections, such as meningococcaemia, *Capnocytophaga canimorsus* (from dog bites), sometimes produce severe acquired consumptive protein C deficiency, which leads to widespread ischaemic necrosis of the extremities (purpura fulminans). However, postvaricella purpura fulminans can be caused by acquired antiphospholipid antibodies that interfere with protein S.

Obstetrical complications

Acute DIC can be caused by thromboplastin-like materials released during placental abruption or amniotic fluid embolism. Pre-eclampsia too can be accompanied by DIC, although there can be clinical and laboratory overlap with other life-threatening complications of pregnancy (for example, fatty liver of pregnancy; HELLP syndrome (haemolysis, elevated liver enzymes, low platelets). Bleeding due to hypofibrinogenaemia is often prominent in pregnancy-associated DIC. Chronic DIC can be caused by fetal death.

Acute haemolysis

Haemolysis caused by incompatible blood transfusions, certain infections (for example, *Clostridium perfringens* septicaemia), or microangiopathic disorders such as TTP and HELLP, can sometimes be associated with DIC.

Immunological disorders

Severe allergic reactions (such as anaphylaxis), transplant rejection, glomerulonephritis, and other vasculitic disorders are sometimes associated with DIC.

Vascular anomalies

Giant haemangiomas cause overt DIC in about 25 per cent of affected patients (Kasabach–Merritt syndrome). Although activation of coagulation and fibrinolysis is localized to the vascular anomaly, depletion of haemostatic factors produces a clinical and laboratory profile indistinguishable from DIC. Eradication of haemangioma by radiation, embolization, or surgery is curative. Medical therapies have included heparin, antifibrinolytic

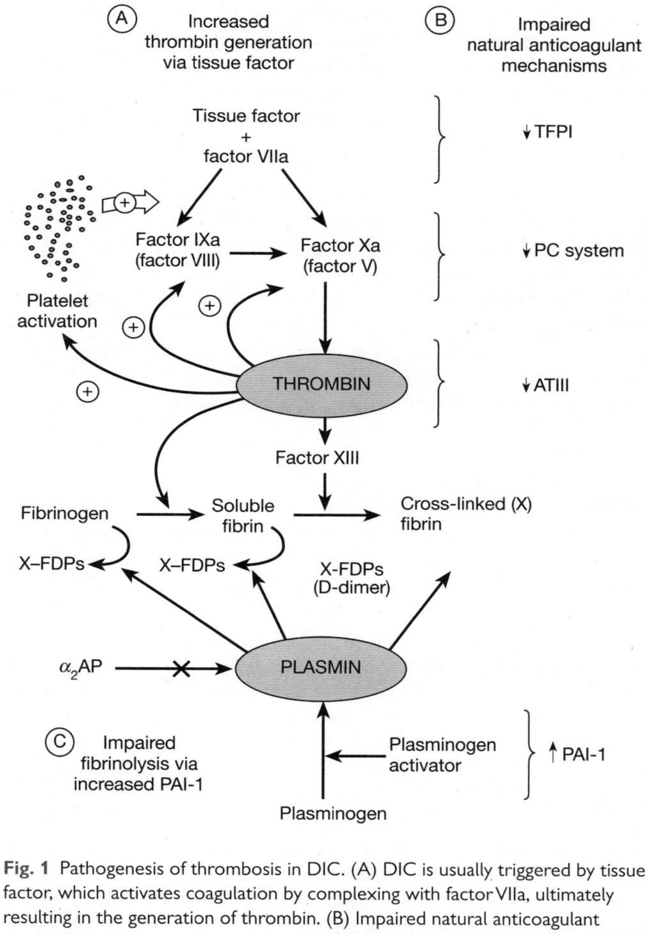

Fig. 1 Pathogenesis of thrombosis in DIC. (A) DIC is usually triggered by tissue factor, which activates coagulation by complexing with factor VIIa, ultimately resulting in the generation of thrombin. (B) Impaired natural anticoagulant mechanisms (e.g. excessive consumption of natural anticoagulants, or cytokine-mediated downregulation of natural anticoagulant pathways) predispose to microvascular thrombosis. (C) Impaired fibrinolysis via increased PAI-1 leads to greater microvascular thrombosis. Sometimes, hyperfibrinolysis is caused by increased plasminogen activator release, or low levels of β_2-antiplasmin. Abbreviations: α_2AP, α_2-antiplasmin; ATIII, antithrombin III; fDPs, fibrinogen degradation products; FDPs, fibrin degradation products; PAI-1, plasminogen activator inhibitor type 1; PC, protein C; TFPI, tissue-*factor* pathway inhibitor.

drugs (combined with cryoprecipitate to thrombose the vascular tumour), glucocorticoids, and interferon.

DIC also occurs in about 0.5 to 1 per cent of patients with abdominal aortic aneurysms, which usually contain adherent thrombi.

Immunoglobulin-mediated factor deficiency

Coagulation-*factor* inhibitors are usually IgG antibodies that bind to specific coagulation factors, and either neutralize their activity (most coagulation-factor inhibitors) or result in accelerated clearance (for example, antiprothrombin antibodies associated with the antiphospholipid antibody syndrome). Acquired inhibitors against coagulation factors are rare in otherwise normal (non-haemophilic) individuals. Even the most common autoimmune coagulation-factor deficiency (factor VIII) has an estimated incidence of only 1 per 1 000 000 per year.

Acquired factor VIII inhibitor

Acquired factor VIII deficiency should be suspected in a patient with spontaneous bleeding, or bleeding following minor trauma, that occurs in association with a prolonged aPTT and a normal PT/INR (Table 3). Most commonly, muscle or cutaneous haematomas occur, but life-threatening retroperitoneal or intracranial haemorrhages are described; haemarthrosis is uncommon (cf. congenital haemophilia). The disorder occurs most commonly in the elderly (median age, 60 years), affects men and women equally, and is idiopathic in 50 per cent of cases. Other autoimmune disorders (for instance, systemic lupus erythematosus, **SLE**), lymphoid and other malignancies, penicillin treatment, or the postpartum state, have been observed in some patients. About 20 per cent of patients die of bleeding, often from their initial bleeding episode.

A rapid screening test for a coagulation-factor inhibitor is performed by repeating the aPTT after mixing patient plasma 50:50 with normal pooled plasma. An inhibitor is suggested by more than a 4-s prolongation time over the control, although some inhibitors require a 2-h incubation at 37 °C to show inhibition. Confirmation is obtained by a specific-factor assay showing reduced levels of factor VIII; inhibitor quantitation is most often performed by Bethesda assay, in which various dilutions of patient plasma are mixed with normal plasma and incubated for 2 h at 37 °C: a Bethesda unit (**BU**) is defined as the reciprocal of the plasma dilution that yields a 50 per cent reduction in residual factor VIII activity in the test system. Unfortunately, the Bethesda assay tends to underestimate the amount of inhibitor in non-haemophilic patients with acquired factor VIII inhibitors.

Therapy of bleeding depends upon its severity and the amount of inhibitor present, if known. For patients with minor bleeding, and low inhibitor levels (<5 BU), desmopressin (DDAVP) can be tried. Peak factor VIII levels occur between 45 and 90 min post-DDAVP, and repeat levels should be measured to assess efficacy. In other patients with low inhibitor levels but with more severe bleeding, purified human factor VIII concentrates are usually effective. One approach is to give an initial intravenous bolus of 100 U/kg, followed by a continuous infusion of factor VIII at 10 U/kg per h, with factor VIII levels measured again 4 to 6 h later. Careful clinical and laboratory assessment for response is needed, since inhibitor levels may have been underestimated, or higher inhibitor levels stimulated by factor VIII use.

Porcine factor VIII should be considered for bleeding patients in whom the inhibitor titres are not yet known, or to those with high inhibitor levels. This is because crossreactivity of the autoantibodies against porcine VIII is usually substantially less than with human factor VIII. After a loading dose of between 50 and 100 U/kg, repeat doses are given every 8 to 12 h, or further porcine VIII is given by constant intravenous infusion (4 U/kg per h).

Either PCCs or recombinant factor VIIa can be given for patients refractory to human or porcine factor VIII. Activated PCCs (for example, FEIBA or Autoplex) may be somewhat more effective than non-activated PCCs, but their risk for causing thrombosis is greater. Factor VIIa is preferable for perioperative management, given its low risk for inducing thrombosis. In desperate situations, extracorporeal immunoadsorption using Staphylococcal protein A may be helpful in removing the antibodies.

Spontaneous disappearance of the inhibitor occurs in about 10 to 30 per cent of patients. Nevertheless, the unpredictable clinical course, and the potential for life-threatening bleeding, means that immunosuppressive therapy should be given to most patients, either with high-dose intravenous IgG (1 g/kg for 2 days, or 0.4 g/kg for 5 days) or corticosteroids (for instance, 1 mg/kg per day). For refractory patients, the substitution or addition of cyclophosphamide can be effective. Other options include combination chemotherapy (prednisone, cyclophosphamide, vincristine) or ciclosporin. Even partial remission can help reduce bleeding. Women with postpartum factor VIII inhibitors usually develop remission within 30 months, and usually do not develop recurrent factor VIII inhibitors with later pregnancies. They also may be less likely to respond to corticosteroids or other immunosuppressive therapy.

Other acquired coagulation-factor deficiencies

Hypoprothrombinaemia should be suspected in patients with the antiphospholipid antibody syndrome, particularly if bleeding occurs or the PT/INR is prolonged. Typically, these pathogenic anti-factor II antibodies are non-neutralizing, and therefore mixing patient plasma 50:50 with normal pooled plasma can produce correction of the aPTT, in contrast to other coagulation-factor inhibitors.

Thrombin inhibitors are rare, but may cause severe bleeding. More often, patients have antibodies that react preferentially against bovine thrombin: these are formed following the use of 'fibrin glue', which contains various bovine clotting factors. Patients have prolonged PT/INR, aPTT, and TCT (especially using bovine thrombin). However, it is more likely that any bleeding is the result of clinically significant anti-bovine factor V antibodies.

Factor V inhibitors

Rarely, IgG antibodies against factor V arise spontaneously or following treatment with topical bovine thrombin used at surgery. FFP usually does not provide enough factor V to treat bleeding; however, platelet transfusions are usually effective, as platelet activation causes factor V to be released into haemostatic plugs.

Factor XIII inhibitors

These inhibitors, which sometimes occur in association with isoniazid therapy, cause bleeding via impaired factor XIII-mediated crosslinking of fibrin. Factor XIII should be measured in a patient with unexplained bleeding and normal results of screening coagulation assays.

Factor X inhibitors

Factor X inhibitors are a rare cause of bleeding in patients with prolonged PT/INR and aPTT. The differential diagnosis also includes amyloidosis of the **AL** (amyloid light chain) variety, caused by adsorption of factor X to amyloid fibrils.

Factor IX inhibitors

In non-haemophilic patients, factor IX inhibitors are rare and usually associated with autoimmune disease. Treatment includes PCCs or purified factor IX, and immunosuppression. The differential diagnosis of acquired, isolated, factor IX deficiency includes the nephrotic syndrome (urinary loss of factor IX).

Factor XI inhibitors

These rare inhibitors are most often observed in association with systemic lupus erythematosus, and usually do not cause bleeding or require specific treatment.

Factor VII inhibitors

Factor VII inhibitors are extremely rare, and usually do not cause bleeding or require treatment. The diagnosis is suggested by an isolated prolonged PT/INR in the absence of coumarin or vitamin K deficiency.

Plates for Section 18

Chapter 18.3 Clinical investigation (rheumatological disorders)

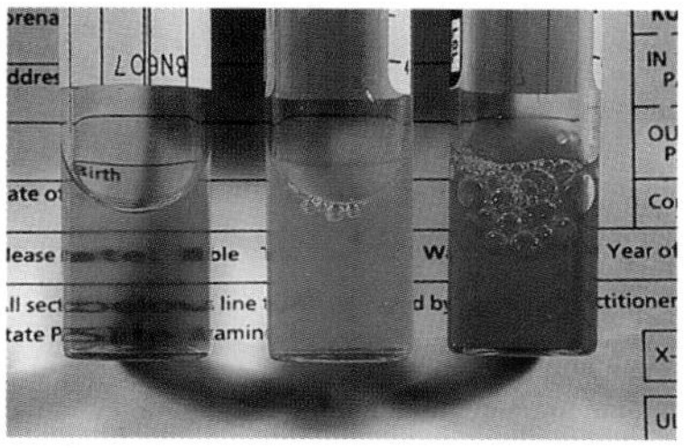

Plate 1 Different macroscopic appearances of synovial fluids: (a) on the left, clear straw-coloured fluid from an osteoarthritic knee (easy to read writing behind it); (b) less viscous, turbid (high cell count) 'inflammatory' fluid from a rheumatoid knee; and (c) uniform bloodstaining (haemarthrosis) due to acute pseudogout.

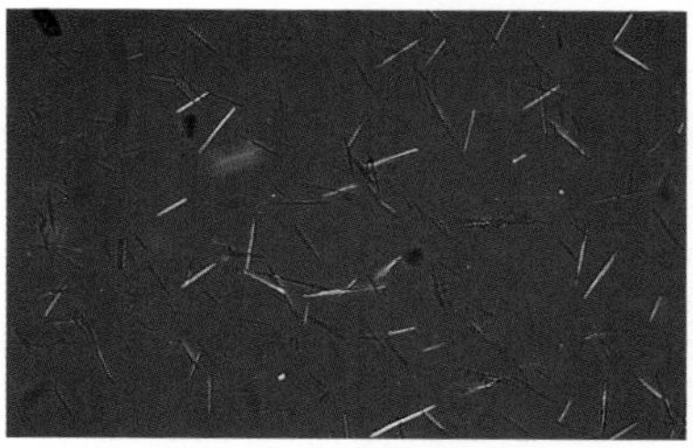

Plate 2 Monosodium urate crystals viewed by compensated polarized light microscopy (×400) showing bright birefringence (negative sign) and needle-shaped morphology.

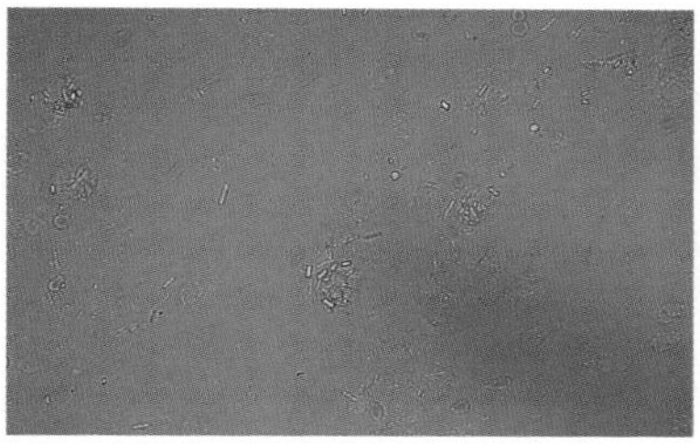

Plate 3 Calcium pyrophosphate crystals viewed by polarized light microscopy (×400) showing weak birefringence (positive sign), scant numbers, and a predominantly rhomboid morphology. These are clearly more difficult to detect than urate crystals.

Chapter 18.5 Rheumatoid arthritis

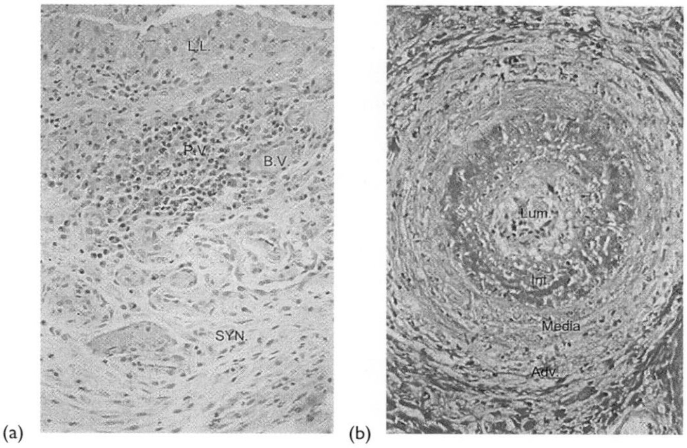

Plate 1 Histology of rheumatoid arthritis. (a) Rheumatoid arthritis synovitis. L.L., lining layer; P.V., perivascular aggregate of lymphocytes and macrophages; B.V., blood vessel; SYN, synoviocytes; (haematoxylin and eosin staining). (b) Small vessel arteritis. Lum., lumen; Int., Intima; P.V., perivascular inflammation; Adv., adventitial tissue. Arterial wall shows a thrombosed vessel with intimal hyperplasia, destruction of internal elastic lamina, and mononuclear cell infiltration of media and perivascular tissue (methylene blue and safranine staining).

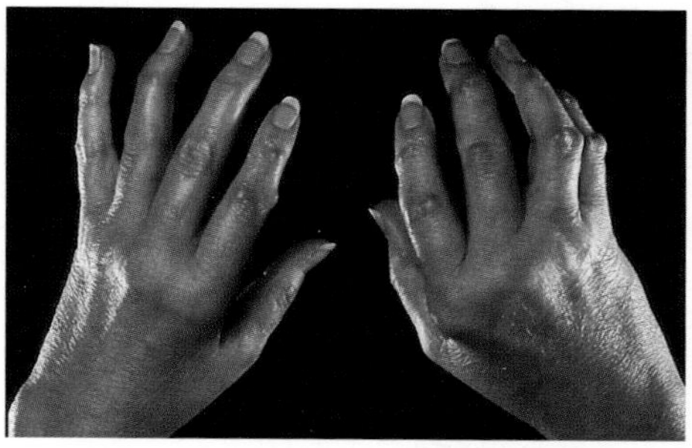

Plate 2 The hands of a person suffering from rheumatoid arthritis. Features to note include symmetrical soft tissue swelling of the second and third metacarpophalageal joints, early swan-neck deformity of the left ring finger, ulnar deviation at the metacarpophalageal joints, and wasting of the small muscles of the hand. In addition, several small rheumatoid nodules are present.

Chapter 18.6 Spondyloarthritides and related arthritides

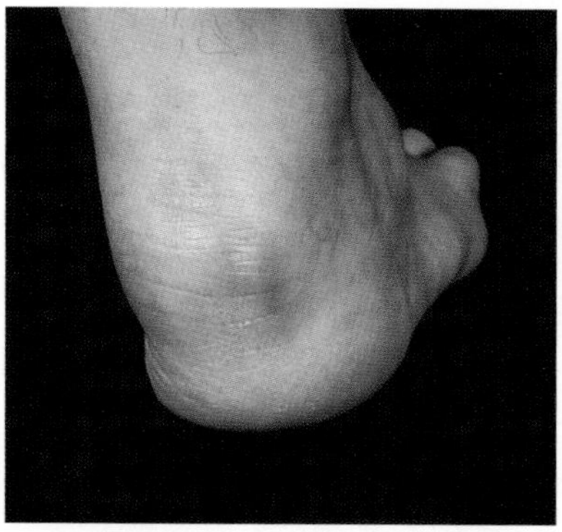

Plate 1 Enthesitis at the insertion of the Achilles tendon in a patient with reactive arthritis.

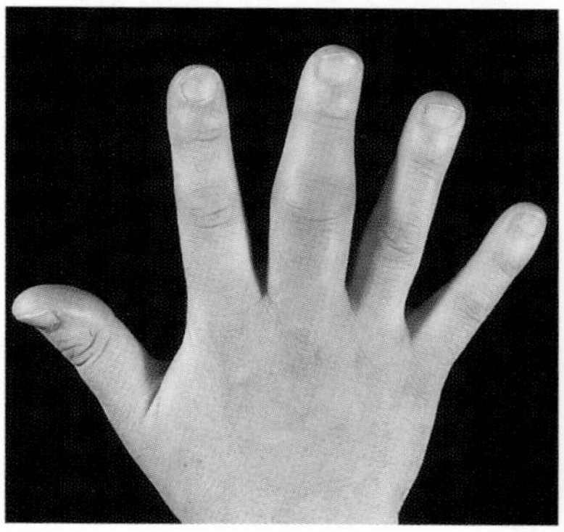

Plate 2 Dactylitis of the third finger of the right hand in a patient with undifferentiated spondyloarthropathy.

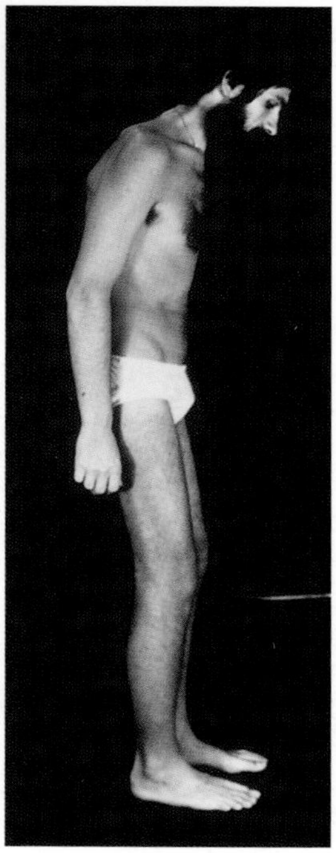

Plate 3 30-year-old man with rapidly progressive ankylosing spondylitis (disease of 5 years duration).

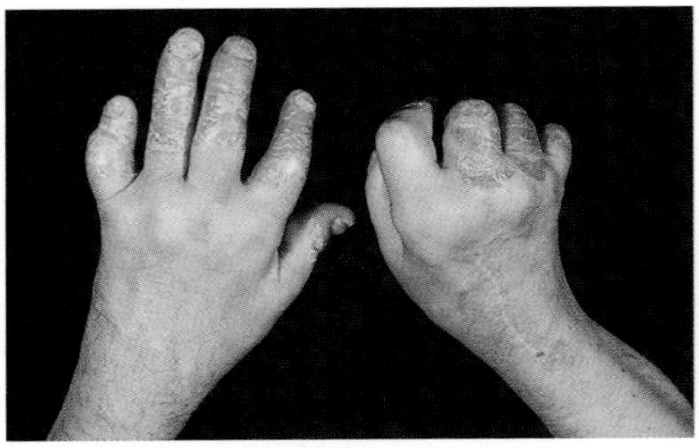

Plate 4 Severe psoriatic arthritis (arthritis mutilans).

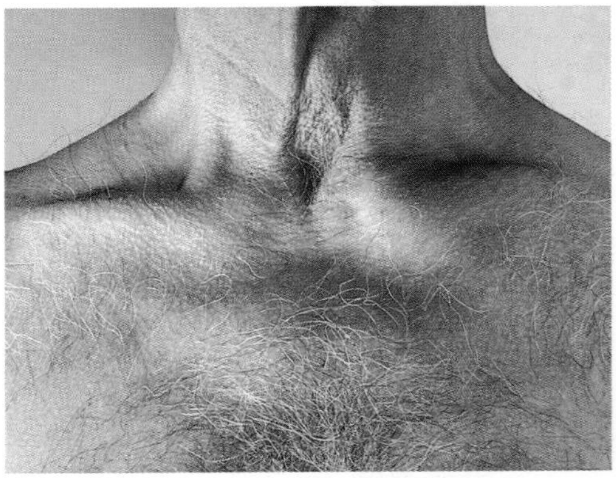

Plate 5 Arthritis/hyperostosis of the left sternoclavicular joint in a 52-year-old man with SAPHO syndrome.

Chapter 18.10.2 Systemic lupus erythematosus and related disorders

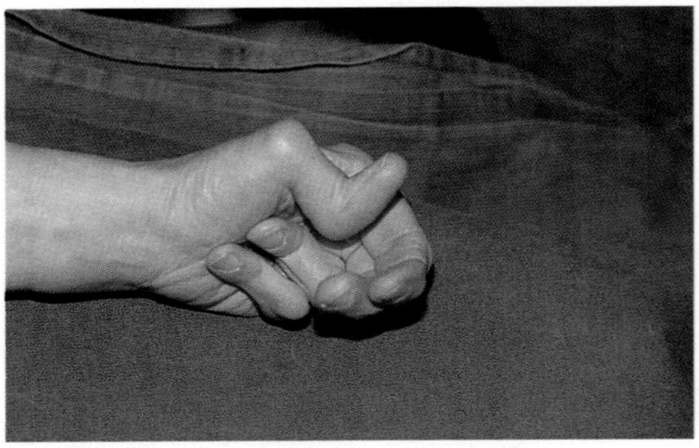

Plate 1 Deforming Jaccoud's arthropathy.

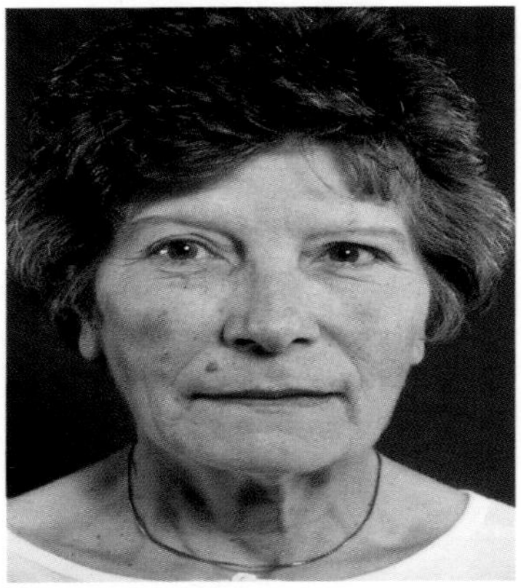

Plate 2 Malar "butterfly" rash.

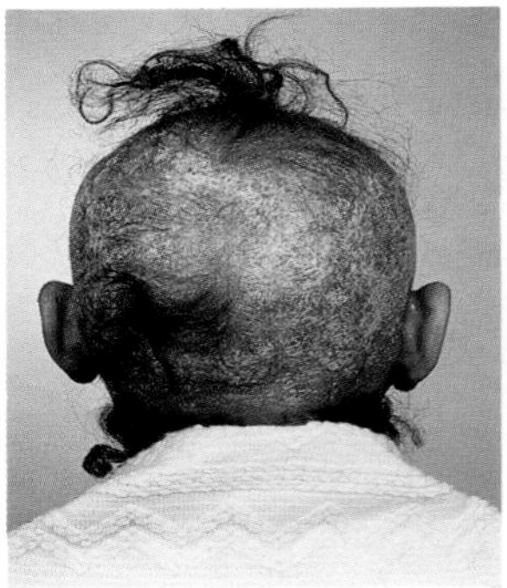

Plate 3 Severe scarring alopecia.

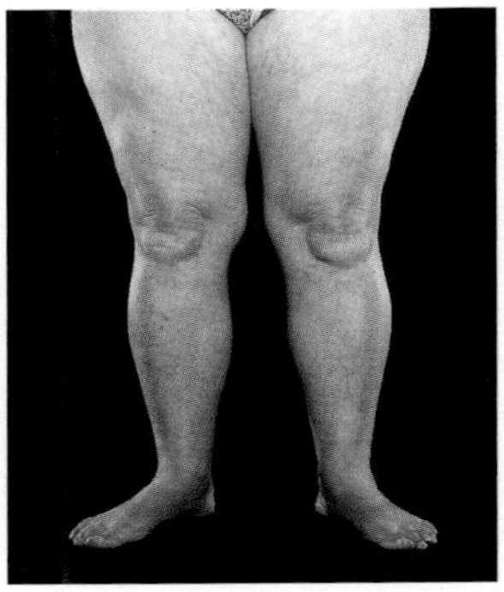

Plate 4 Livedo reticularis.

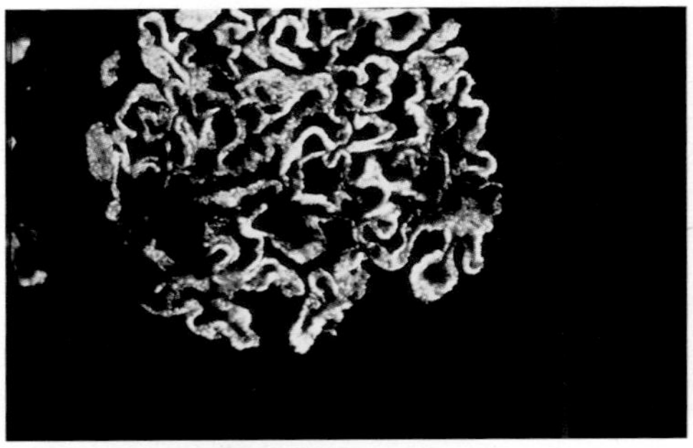

Plate 5 Immunofluorescence microscopy showing deposition of IgG in the glomerulus of a patient with lupus nephritis.

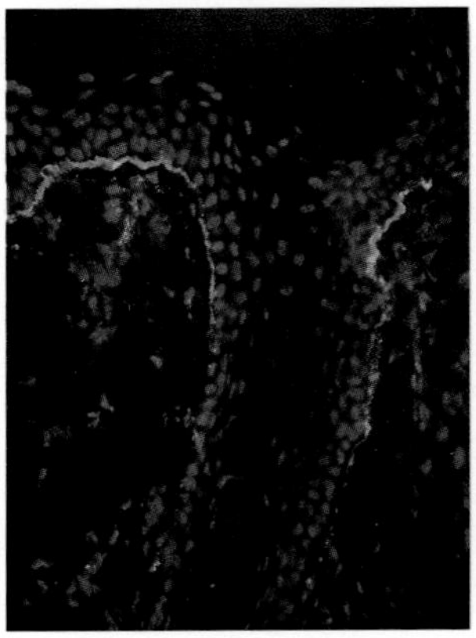

Plate 6 Immunofluorescence microscopy showing deposition of IgG at the dermo-epidermal junction in the skin of a patient with systemic lupus erythematosus (sometimes called the lupus band test).

Chapter 18.10.4 Polymyalgia rheumatica and giant cell arteritis

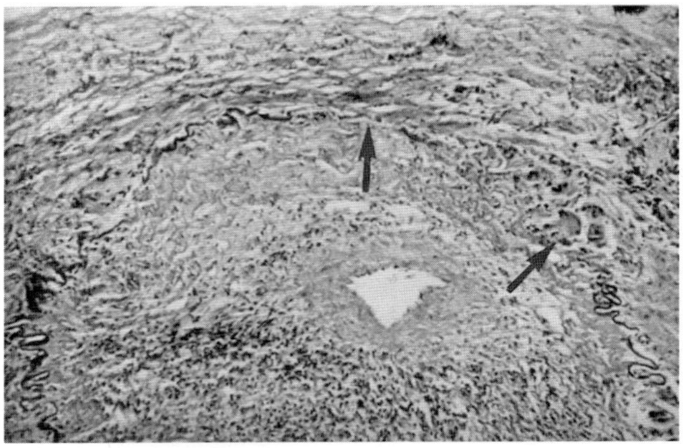

Plate 1 Photomicrograph of a temporal artery biopsy showing giant cells, mononuclear infiltrate, and disruption of the internal elastic lamina.

Chapter 18.10.7 Polymyositis and dermatomyositis

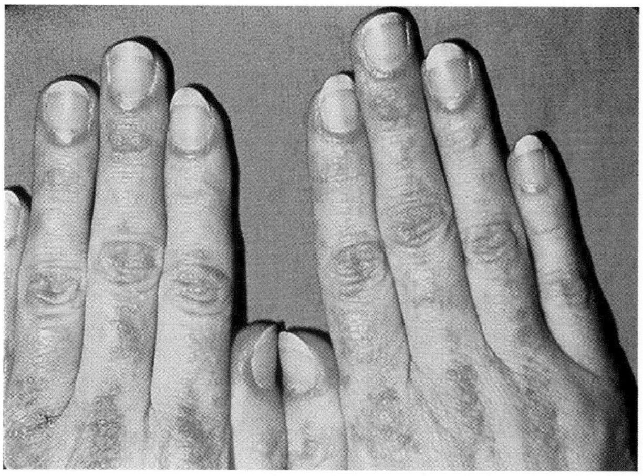

Plate 1 Gottron's sign. Roughened, violaceous papules over the dorsal surfaces of several metacarpophalangeal and proximal interphalangeal joints. Note also the erythema at the bases of the fingernail, caused by capillary loop dilatation.

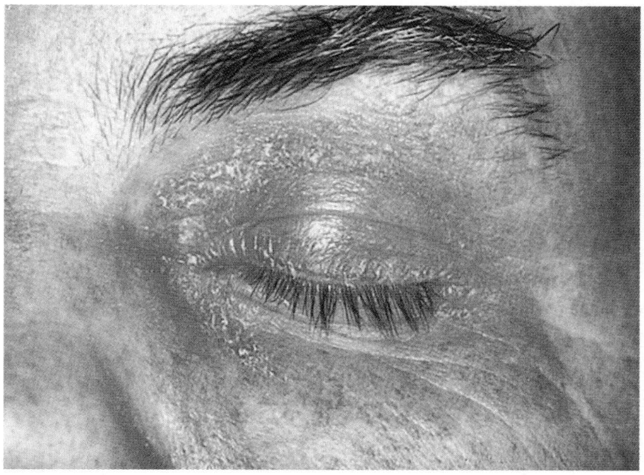

Plate 2 Heliotrope rash. An erythematous (often lilac-coloured) rash over the eyelids in a patient with dermatomyositis (reproduced from Mousari HC, Wigley FM (2000). *Journal of Rheumatology* **27**, 1542-5 with permission).

Chapter 18.10.8 Kawasaki syndrome

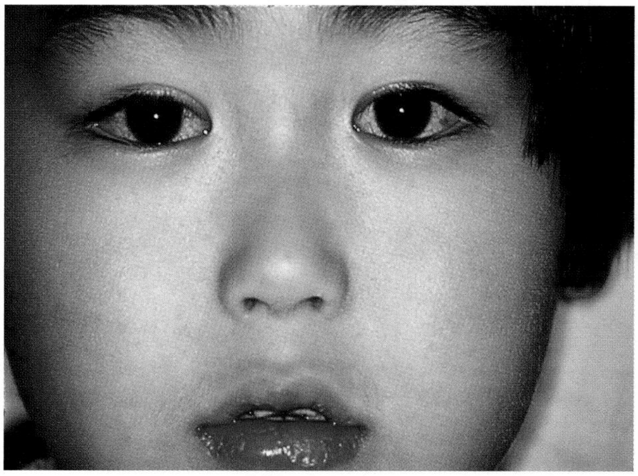

Plate 1 Typical appearance of a patient with Kawasaki disease; note the red eyes and red lips (picture of a 5-year-old boy, taken on the fourth day of illness).

Chapter 18.11 Miscellaneous conditions presenting to the rheumatologist

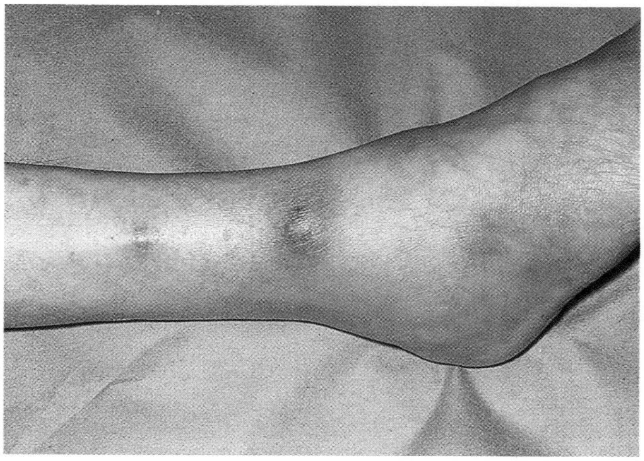

Plate 1 Pyoderma gangrenosum.

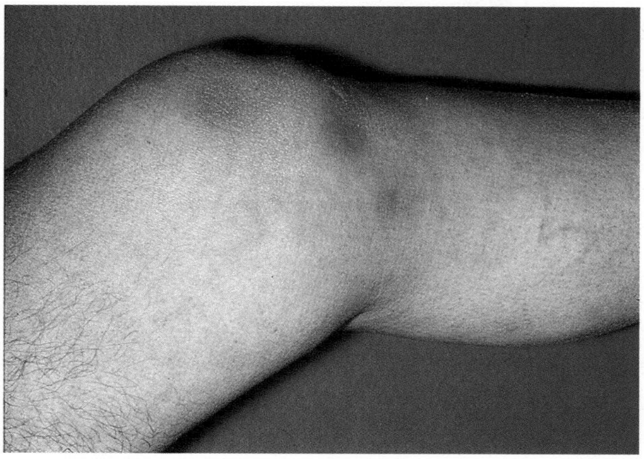

Plate 2 Erythema nodosum.

Plates for Section 19

Chapter 19.2 Inherited defects of connective tissue: Ehlers Danlos syndrome, pseudoxanthoma elasticum, and Marfan syndrome

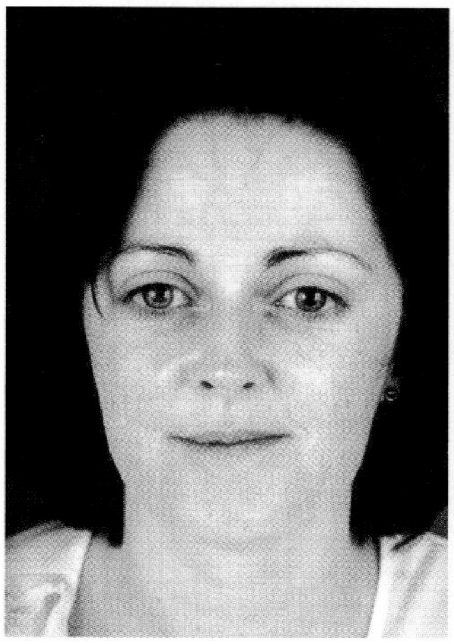

(a)–(b)

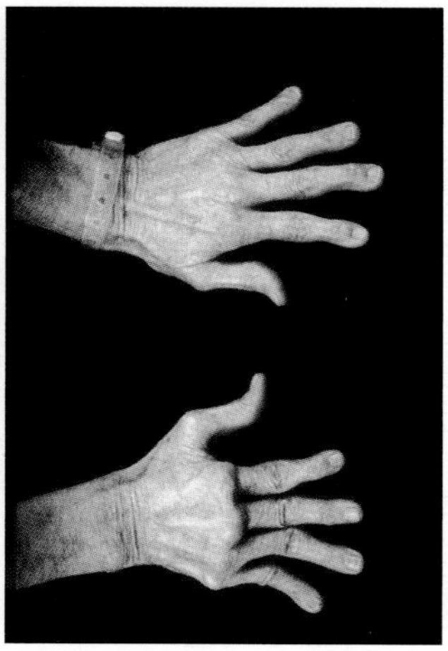

(c)–(d)

Plate 1 *See caption overleaf.*

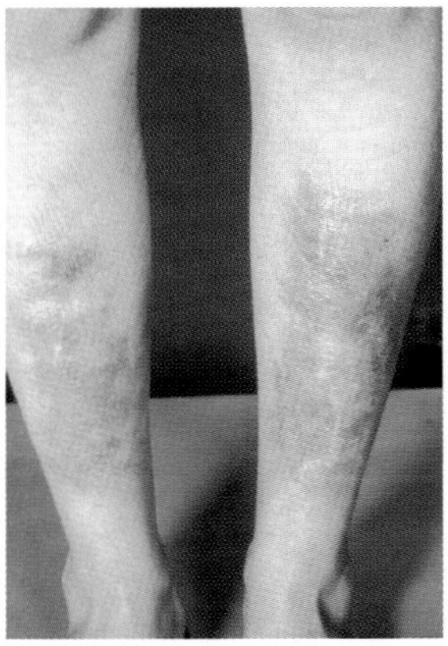

(e)

Plate 1 EDS type IV (vascular type). (a) Acrogeria–a specific clinical feature of EDS IV. Note the large eyes and thin (b) nose (Madonna facies) with periorial wrinkling. (c) Premature wrinkling of the skin on the dorsum of the hands; note also the joint contractures (d) superficially resembling rheumatoid arthritis. (e) Pretibial bruising and haemosiderosis.

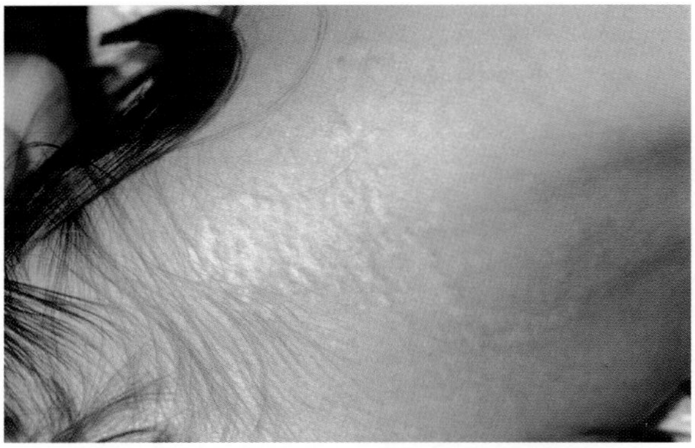

(a)

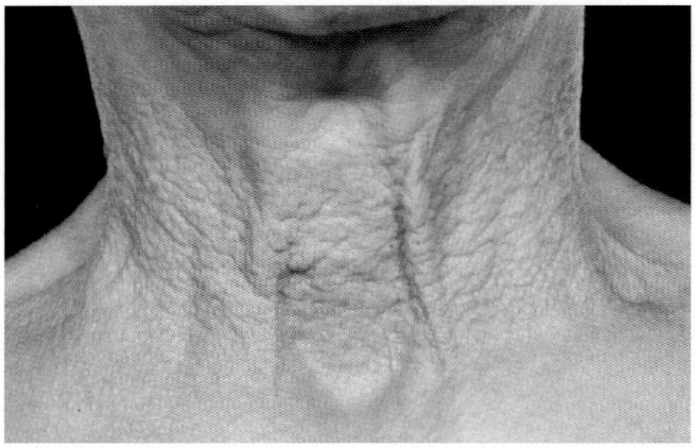

(b)

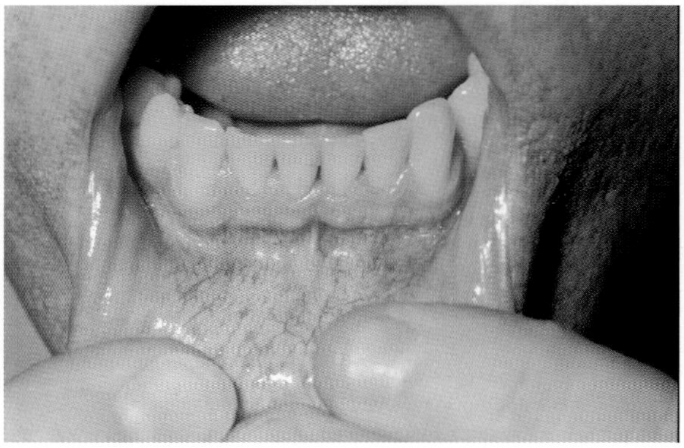

(c)

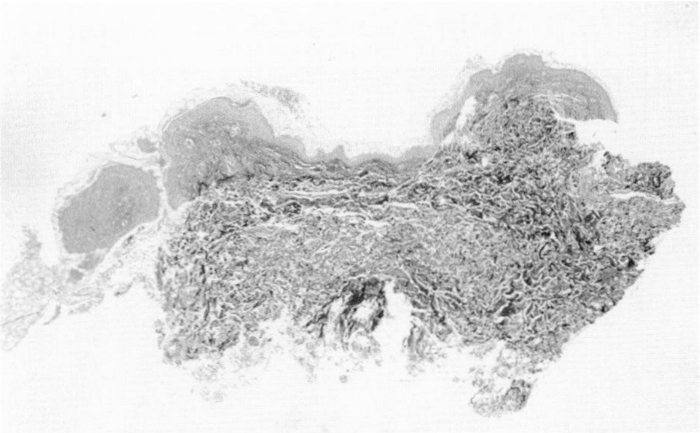

(d)

Plate 2 Skin lesions in pseudoxanthoma elasticum (PXE). (a) Typical flexural skin lesions of PXE of the lateral neck. (b) Widespread cutis laxa in PXE. (c) Mucosal infiltration of the lower lip in PXE. (d) Elastic van Giessen stain of skin section showing mid-dermal elastic fragmentation and degeneration.

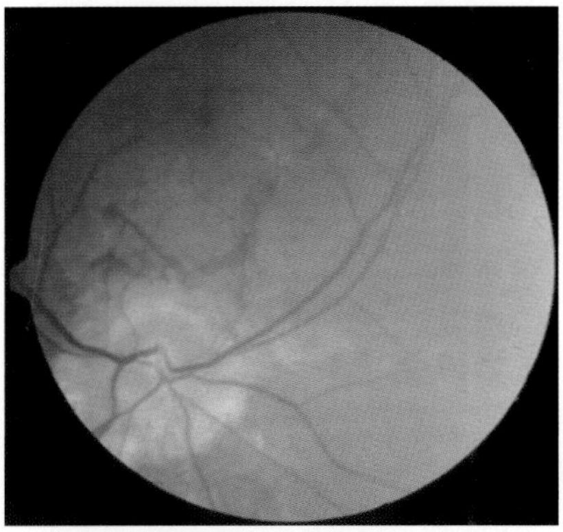

(a)

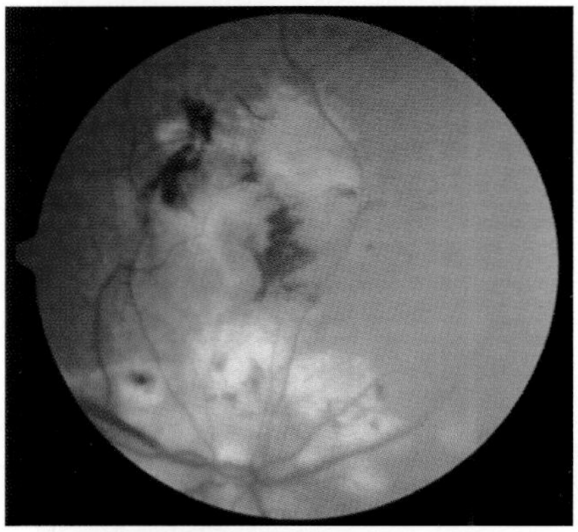

(b)

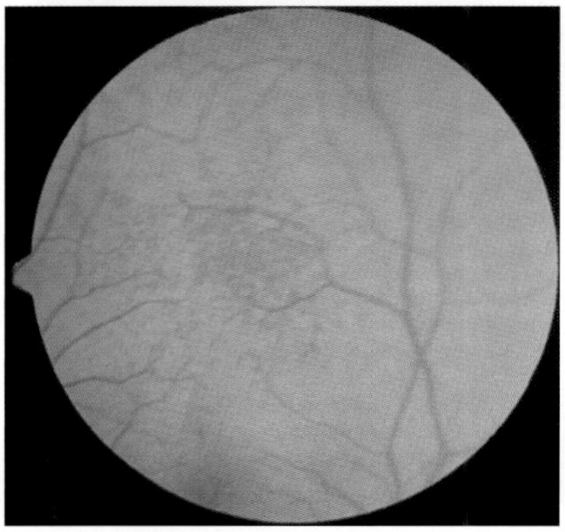

(c)

Plate 3 *See caption overleaf.*

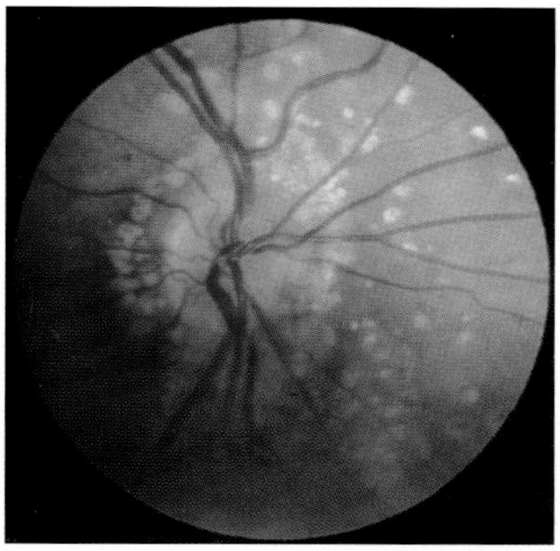

(d)

Plate 3 Retinal changes in PXE. (a) Angioid streaks caused by fracture of the retroretinal Bruch's membrane—an early feature. (b) Macular haemorrhage with consequential choroideretinitis. (c) Specked *peau d'orange* mottling. (d) Salmon spotting and drusen.

Plates for Section 20

Chapter 20.3.2 Clinical investigation of renal disease

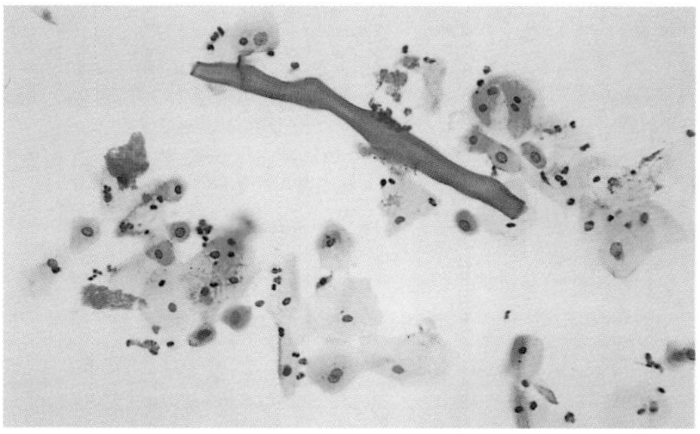

Plate 1 Papanicolaou-stained urine showing a hyaline cast with both normal transitional and squamous cells (blue) and renal tubular cells (pink). (By courtesy of Dr Deery.)

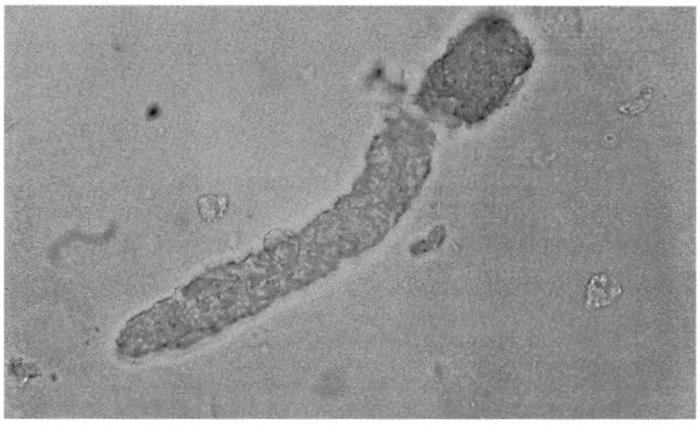

Plate 2 Unstained urine specimen showing a granular cast.

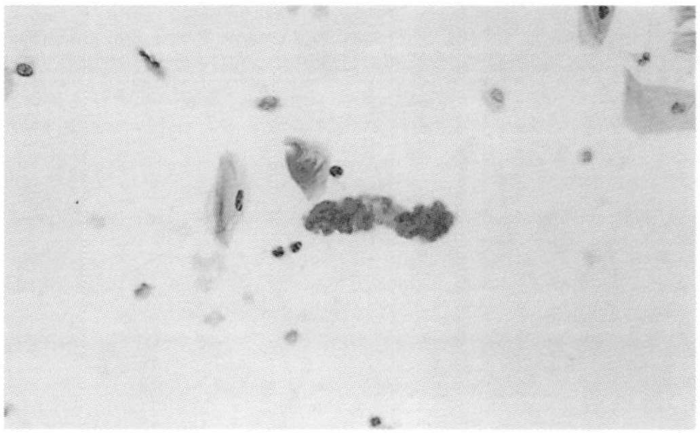

Plate 3 Papanicolaou-stained urine deposit showing a red cell cast.

Chapter 20.7.2 IgA nephropathy and Henoch-Schönlein purpura

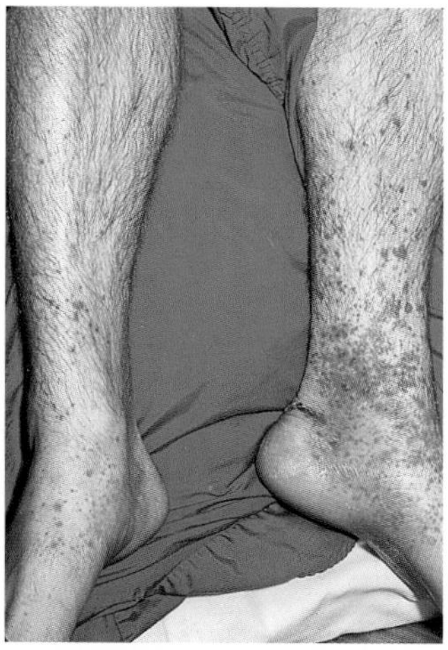

Plate 1 Characteristic purpuric rash affecting the lower limbs in Henoch-Schönlein purpura.

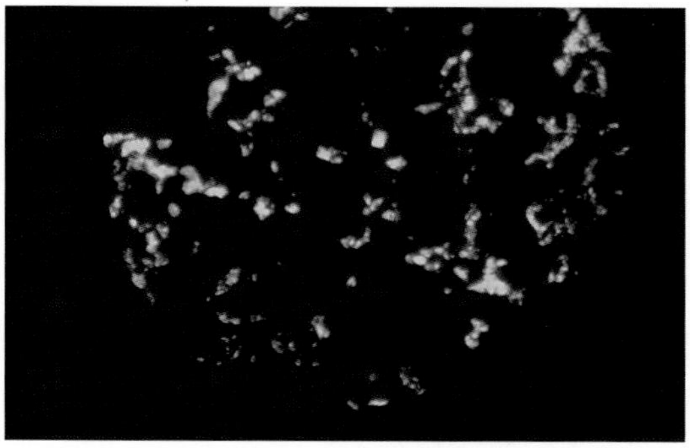

Plate 2 Immunofluorescence of a glomerulus in IgA nephropathy. Bright fluorescent staining is seen within the mesangium with labelled antibodies to IgA. In some cases similar staining is also seen on along capillary walls. A similar distribution of staining for C3 is commonly present (anti-human IgA, × 375).

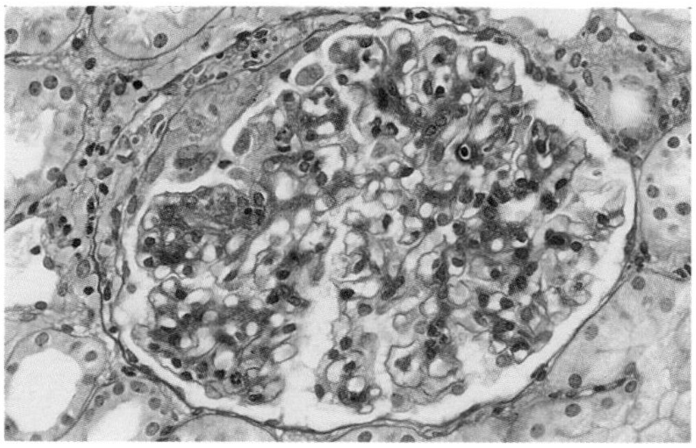

(a)

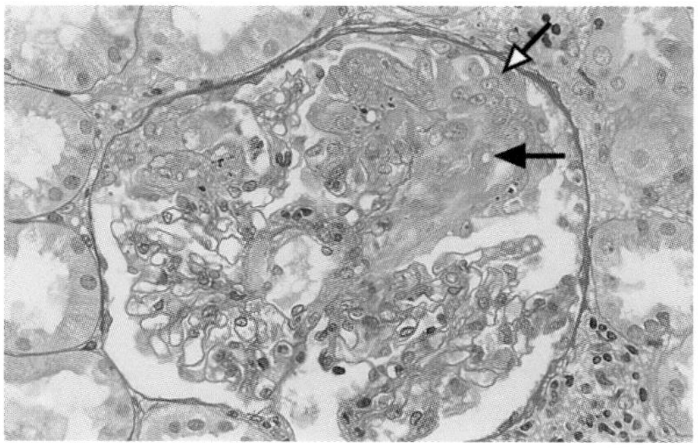

(b)

Plate 3 *See caption overleaf.*

(c)

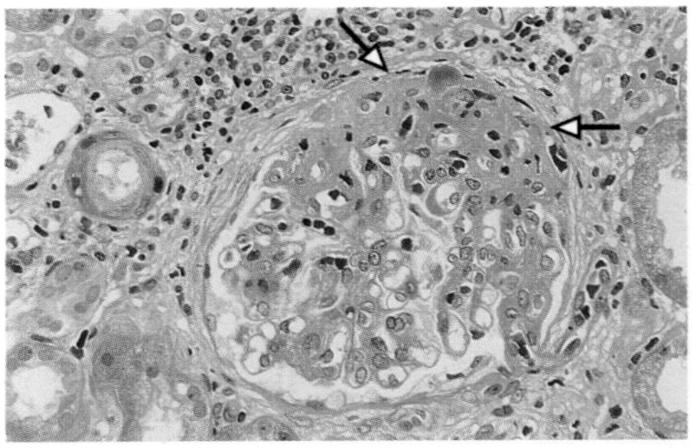

Plate 3 Light microscopic appearances of IgA nephropathy. (a) Glomerulus showing global increase in mesangial matrix and cellularity. (Alcian Blue/PAS stain × 375). (b) Glomerulus showing segmental increase in mesangial matrix and hypercellularity with fibrinoid necrosis (solid arrow) and synechia formation (open arrow) between the segmental lesion and parietal epithelium of Bowman's capsule (Alcian Blue/PAS stain, × 375). (c) Glomerulus showing segmental increase in mesangial matrix, segmental sclerosis with synechia formation (open arrows) to overlying Bowman's capsule (Masson Trichrome stain, × 375).

Chapter 20.7.4 Minimal change nephropathy, focal segmental glomerulosclerosis, and membranous nephropathy

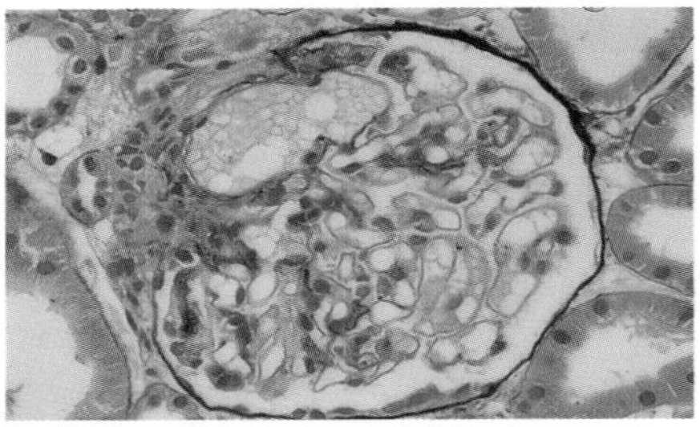

Plate 1 Minimal-change nephropathy. The glomerulus looks normal on light microscopy. Periodic acid-methenamine silver staining (64 ×). (By courtesy of Dr A.J. Howie.)

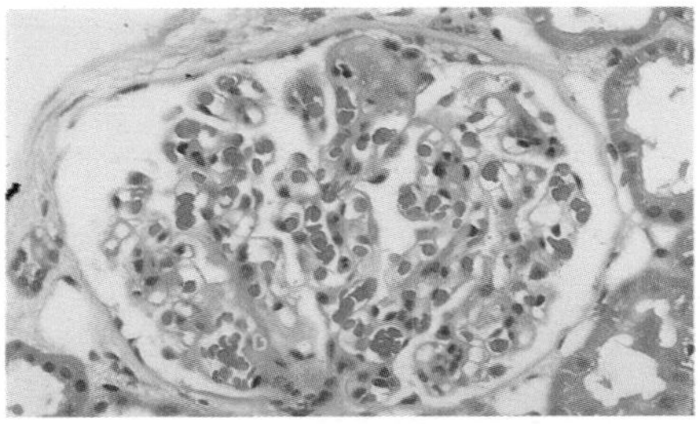

Plate 2 Classical segmental sclerosing glomerulonephritis at an early stage. The glomerulus shows an erratic increase in mesangium with a segmental area of foamy cells and sclerosis opposite the vascular pole, next to the tubular origin. Haematoxylin and eosin staining (50 ×). (By courtesy of Dr A.J. Howie.)

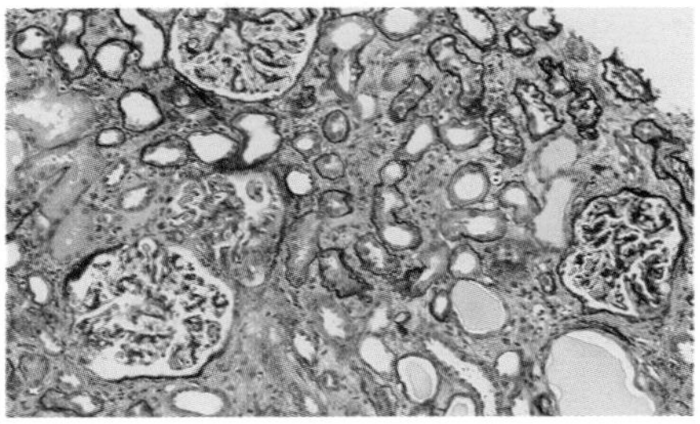

Plate 3 Classical segmental sclerosing glomerulonephritis at a late stage. Four glomeruli show an erratic increase in mesangium and segmental lesions at various sites. Periodic acid-methenamine silver staining (× 64). (By courtesy of Dr A.J. Howie.)

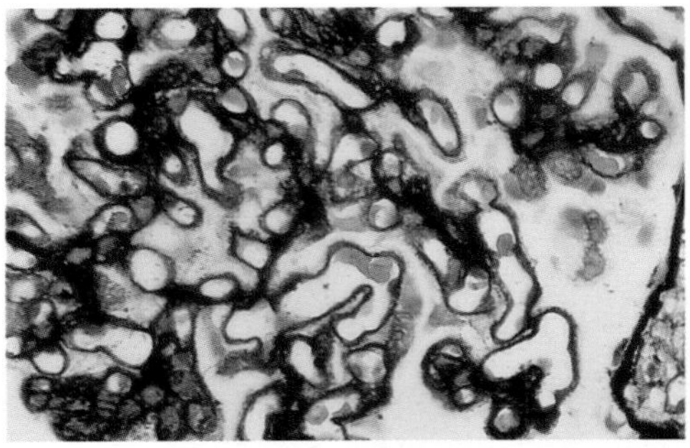

Plate 4 Membranous nephropathy. There are regular short spikes on the outside of glomerular capillary loops. Periodic acid-methenamine silver staining (80 ×).

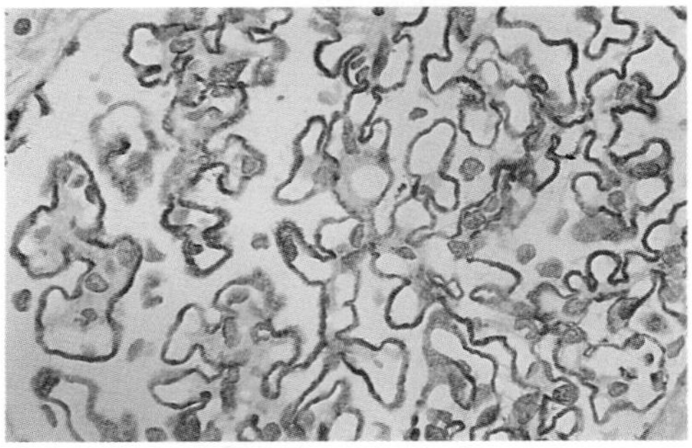

Plate 5 Membranous nephropathy. Immunoperoxidase staining shows uniform granular deposits of IgG on the epithelial side of glomerular basement membranes (80 ×). (By courtesy of Dr A.J. Howie.)

Chapter 20.7.5 Proliferative glomerulonephritis

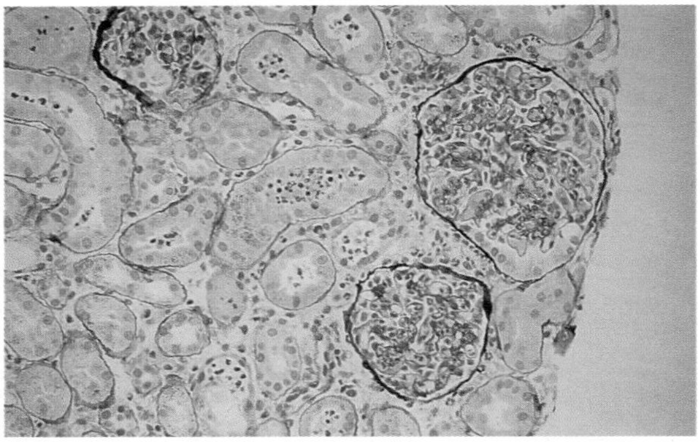

Plate 1 Poststreptococcal glomerulonephritis.

Chapter 20.7.6 Mesangiocapillary glomerulonephritis

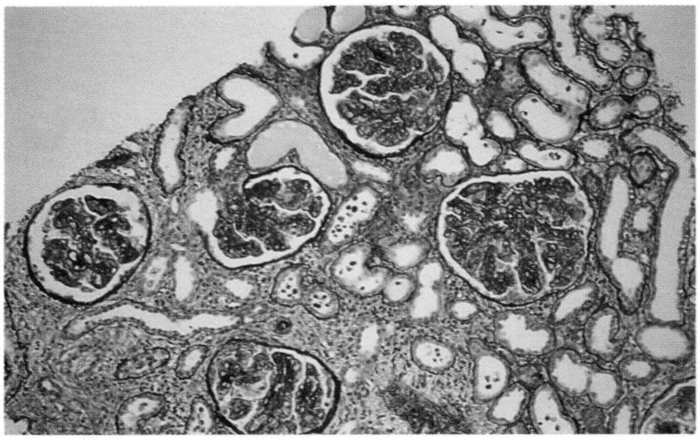

Plate 1 Mesangiocapillary glomerulonephritis. Note characteristic appearance of expanded glomerulus.

Chapter 20.7.7 Antiglomerular basement membrane disease

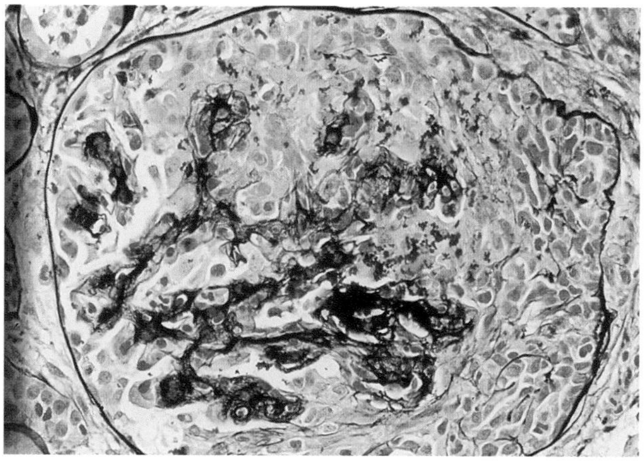

(a)

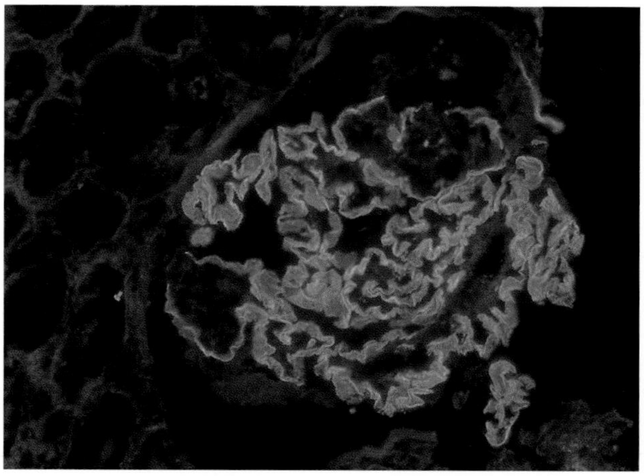

(b)

Plate 1 Renal biopsy from a patient with Goodpasture's disease. (a) Light microscopy showing a single glomerulus with cellular crescent and focal necrosis (silver stain). (b) Immunoflourescence of a single glomerulus with linear deposition of IgG along the GBM. (Figure by courtesy of Dr H.T. Cook.)

Chapter 20.7.8 Infection-associated nephropathies

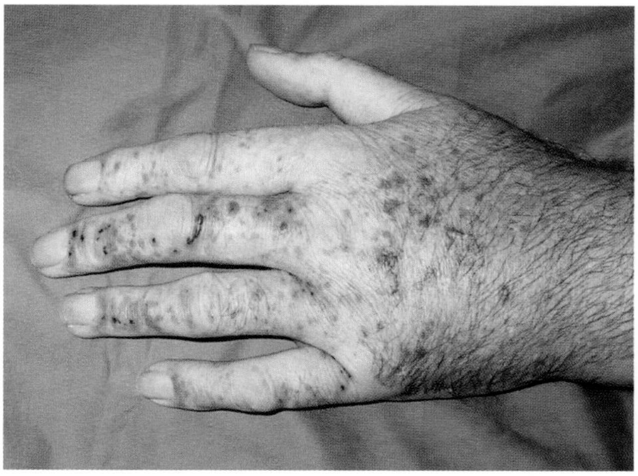

Plate 1 Cutaneous vasculitis in a patient with *Staphylococcus aureus* endocarditis.

Chapter 20.9.1 Acute interstitial nephritis

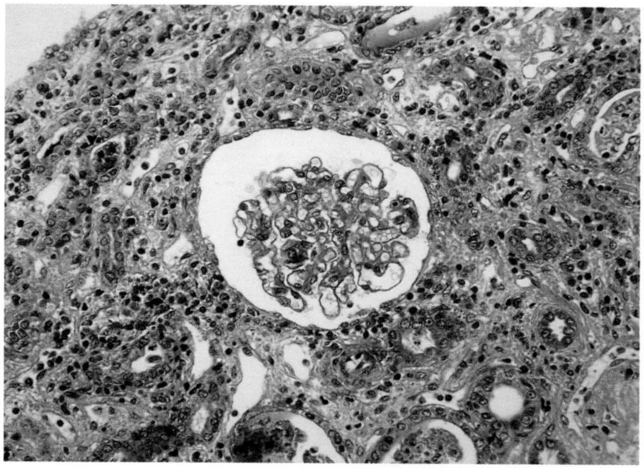

Plate 1 Acute interstitial nephritis. The renal interstitium is invaded by numerous mononuclear cells. The glomerulus is normal. Mason's trichrome 250×.

Chapter 20.10.3 Vasculitis and the kidney

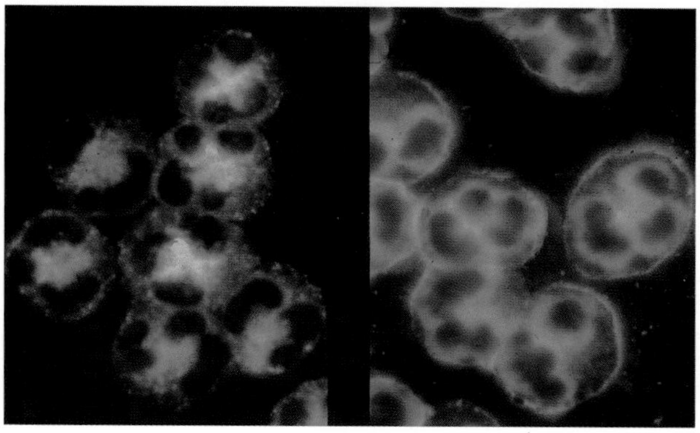

(a) (b)

Plate 1 Indirect immunofluorescence assay for ANCA. (a) Typical staining of cytoplasmic ANCA that is usually due to antibodies to proteinase 3. (b) Typical staining pattern of perinuclear ANCA most often due to antimyeloperoxidase antibodies.

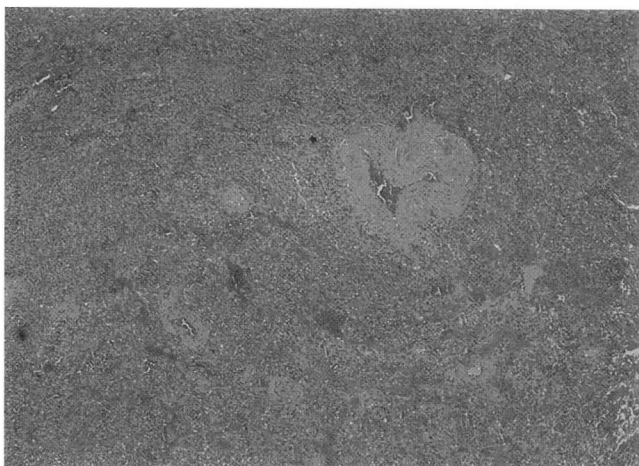

Plate 2 Morphological appearances of pulmonary granulomas in a specimen obtained by video-endoscopic lung biopsy from a patient with Wegener's granulomatosis.

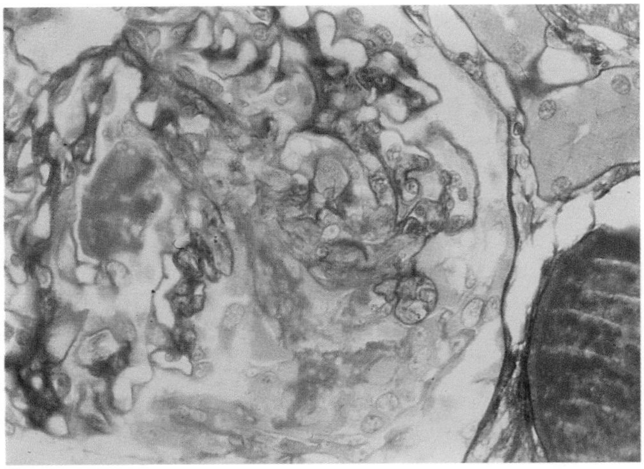

(a)

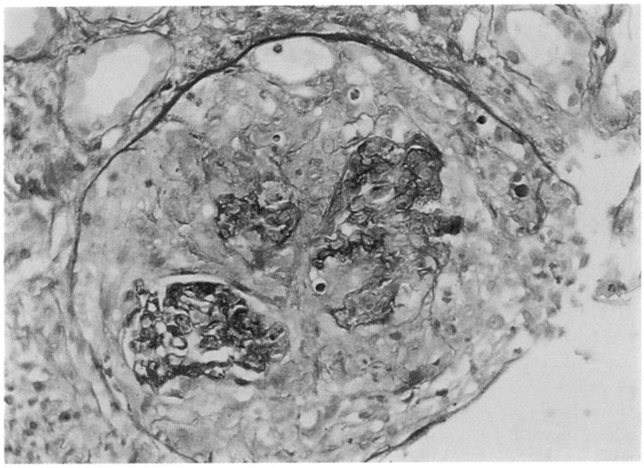

(b)

Plate 3 Morphological appearances on a renal biopsy from a patient with pauci-immune focal necrotizing glomerulonephritis. (a) An early lesion with necrosis of one glomerular segment. (b) A much more florid lesion with the whole glomerular tuft surrounded by a crescent.

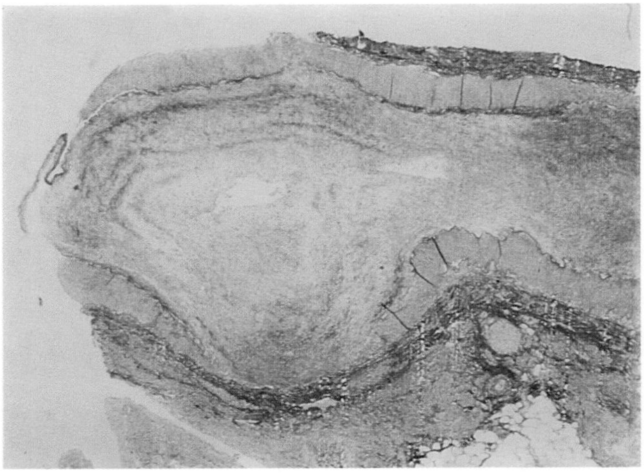

Plate 4 Morphological appearances of a renal artery from a patient with polyarteritis nodosa. The elastic lamina has been destroyed and the artery has become aneurysmal.

Chapter 20.10.4 The kidney in rheumatological disorders

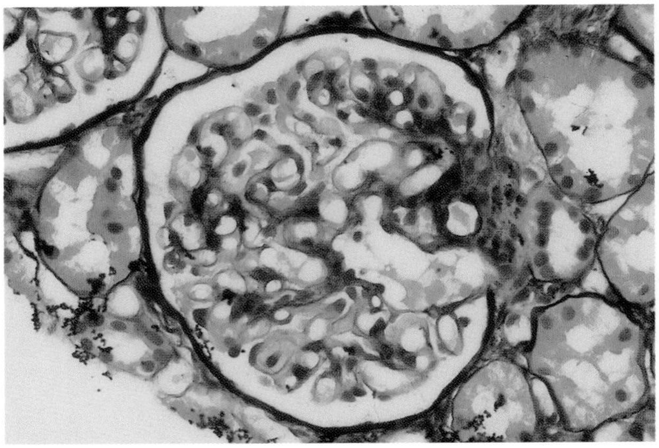

Plate 1 Lupus nephritis. The glomerulus has mild mesangial increase (WHO class II). Periodic acid-methenamine silver staining (×50). (By courtesy of Dr A.J. Howie.)

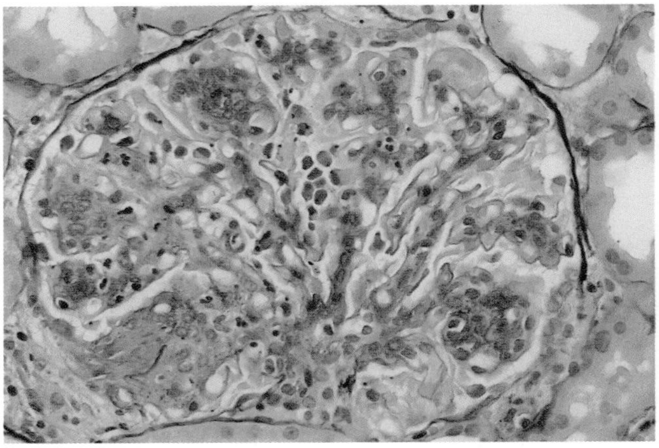

Plate 2 Lupus nephritis. The glomerulus has marked mesangial increase with wire loops, a few doubled basement membranes and segmental lesions (WHO class IV). Periodic acid-methenamine silver staining (×40). (By courtesy of Dr A.J. Howie.)

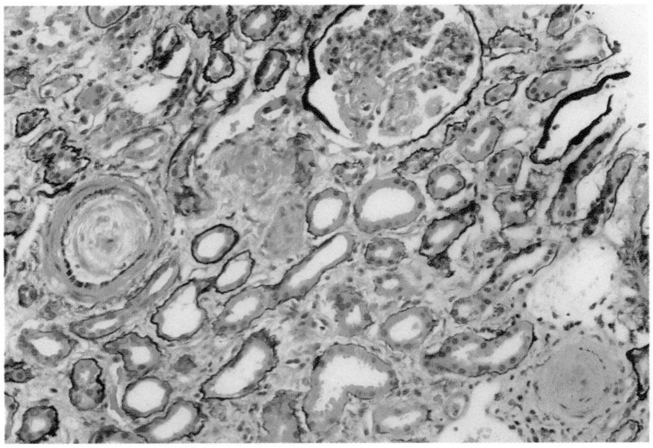

Plate 3 Scleroderma kidney. A small artery has concentric mucoid intimal thickening, an arteriole has thrombosis and fibrinoid necrosis, and tubules and a glomerulus have ischaemic damage. Periodic acid-methenamine silver staining (×25). (By courtesy of Dr A.J. Howie.)

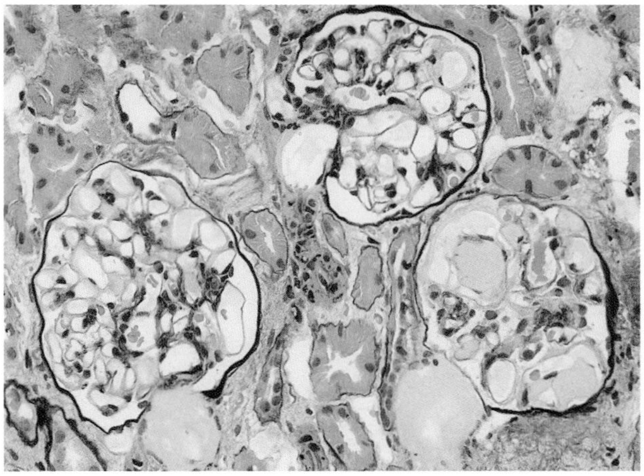

Plate 4 Amyloidosis in rheumatoid arthritis. Arterioles and glomeruli contain acellular masses of amyloid. Periodic acid-methenamine silver staining (×40). (By courtesy of Dr A.J. Howie.)

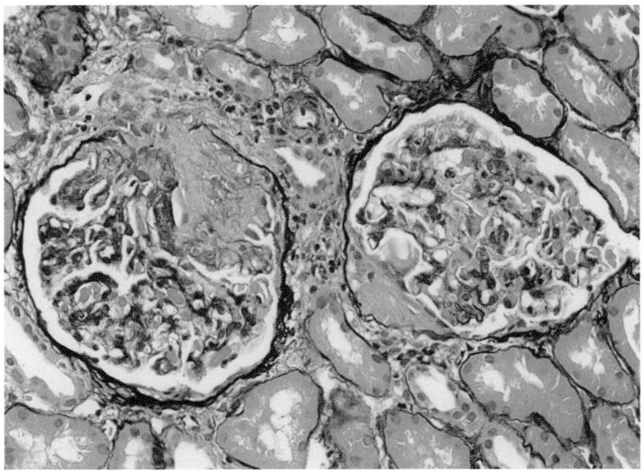

Plate 5 Vasculitic glomerulonephritis in rheumatoid arthritis. Two glomeruli have sharply defined segmental lesions where there has been disruption of the tuft and partial obliteration of Bowman's space. Periodic acid-methenamine silver staining (×32). (By courtesy of Dr A.J. Howie.)

Chapter 20.10.5 Renal involvement in plasma cell dyscrasias, amyloid and fibrillary glomerulopathies, lymphomas, and leukaemias

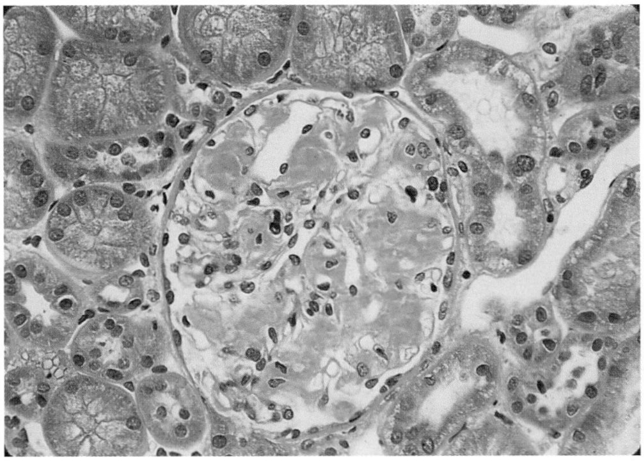

(a)

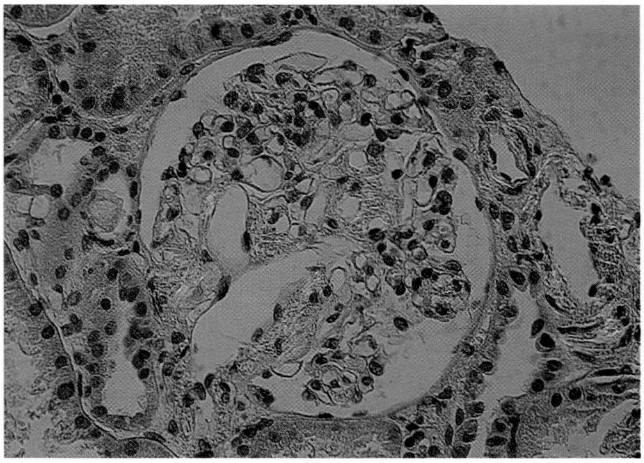

(b)

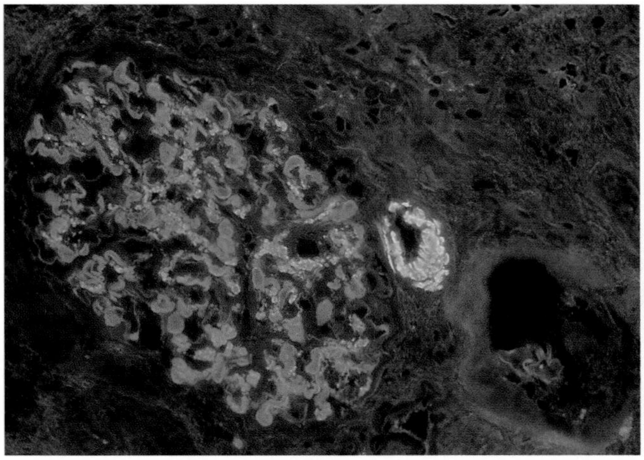

(c)

Plate 1 Light-chain amyloidosis. (a) Amyloid deposits in a renal glomerulus (Masson's trichrome stain, ×312). (b) Congo red stain. Apple-green/yellow dichroism under polarized light (×312). (c) Immunofluorescence with anti-λ antibody. Note glomerular and arteriolar deposits (×312). (From Béatrice Mougenot's personal collection.)

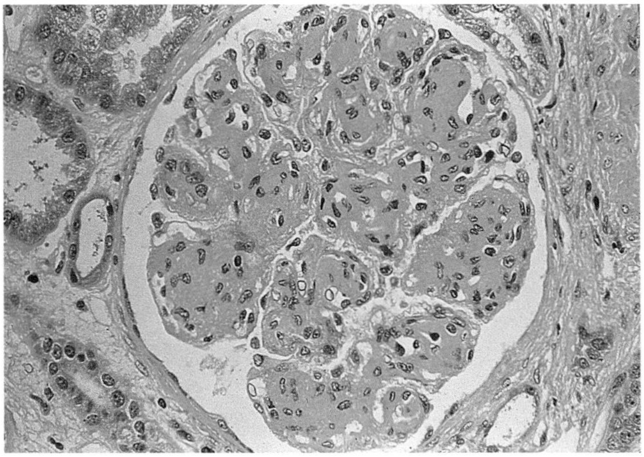

(a)

Plate 2 *See caption overleaf*

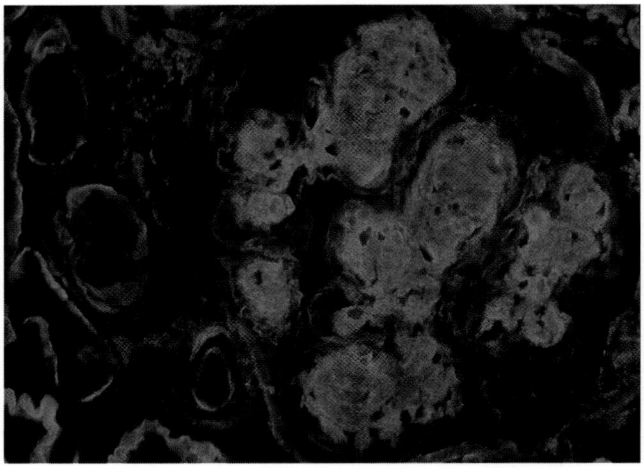

(b)

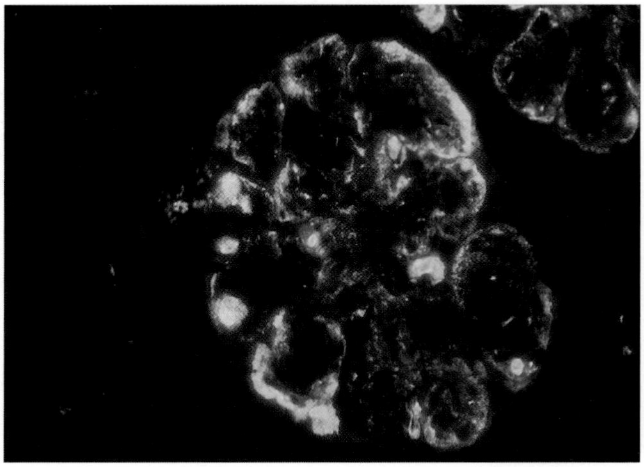

(c)

Plate 2 Cryoglobulinaemic glomerulonephritis. (a) The glomerulus shows a marked endocapillary hypercellularity with massive infiltration of mononuclear leucocytes (Masson's trichrome stain, ×500). (b) Frequent double-contour aspect, and intraluminal thrombi (periodic acid-Schiff stain, ×312). (c) Thrombi and segments of glomerular basement membrane are brightly stained with anti-IgM antibody (immunofluorescence, ×312). (From Béatrice Mougenot's personal collection.)

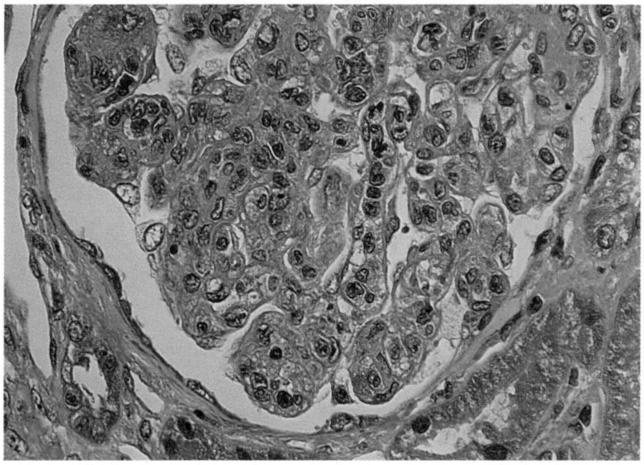

(a)

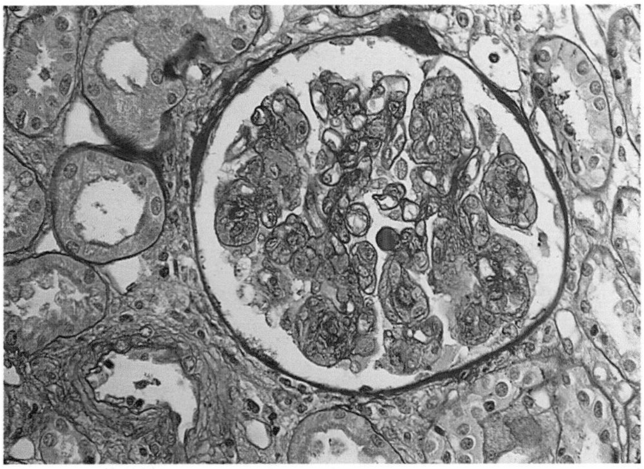

(b)

Plate 3 Monoclonal immunoglobulin deposition disease. (a) Typical nodular glomerulosclerosis. Note the membrane-like material in the centre of the nodules and nuclei at the periphery. Some glomerular capillaries show double contours. Note also thickening of the basement membrane of atrophic tubules (Masson's trichrome stain, ×312). (b) Bright staining of tubular basement membranes and mesangial nodules and, to a lesser extent, of glomerular basement membrane with anti-κ antibody in a case of κ light-chain deposition disease (immunofluorescence, ×312).

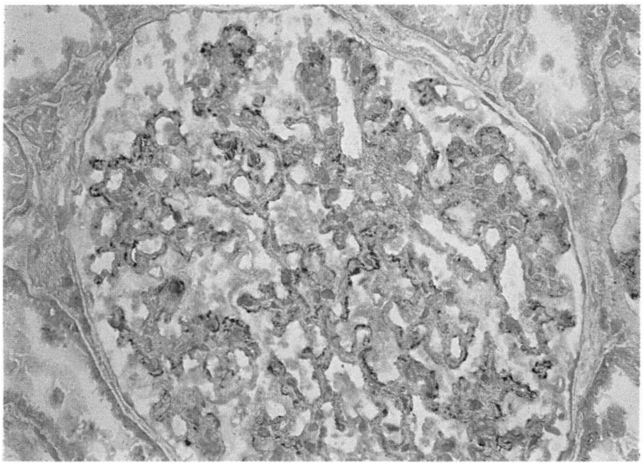

(a)

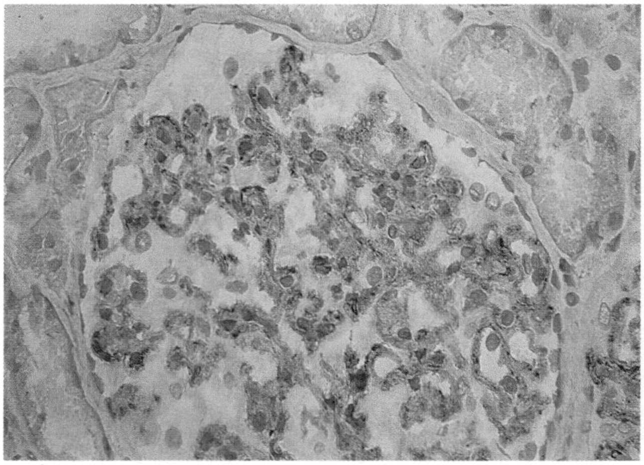

(b)

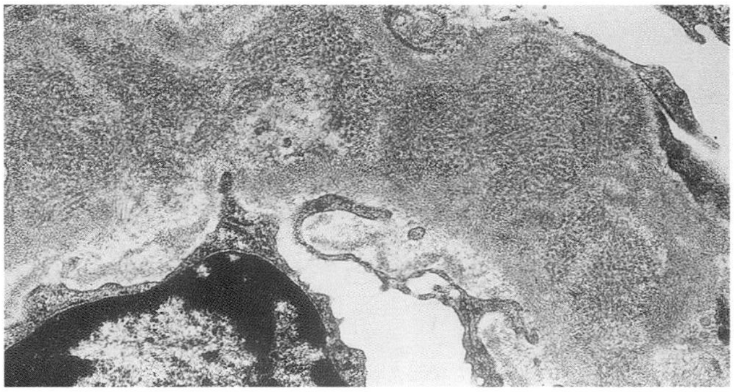

(c)

Plate 4 Immunotactoid glomerulopathy in a patient with chronic lymphocytic leukaemia. A typical membranous glomerulonephritis showing exclusive staining of the deposits with anti-γ (a) and anti-κ (b) antibodies (immunohistochemistry, alkaline phosphatase, $\times$ 312). (c) Electron micrograph of glomerular basement membrane, showing the microtubular structure of the subepithelial deposits (uranyl acetate and lead citrate, $\times$12 000). (From Béatrice Mougenot's personal collection.)

Chapter 20.10.6 Haemolytic uraemic syndrome

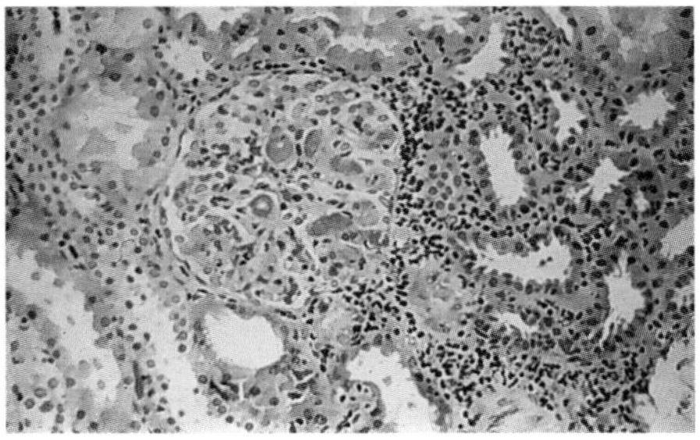

Plate 1 Typical changes of glomerular thrombotic microangiopathy in a patient with HUS (figure kindly provided by Dr Marie O'Donnell).

Plates for Section 21

Chapter 21.5 Infections and other medical problems in homosexual men

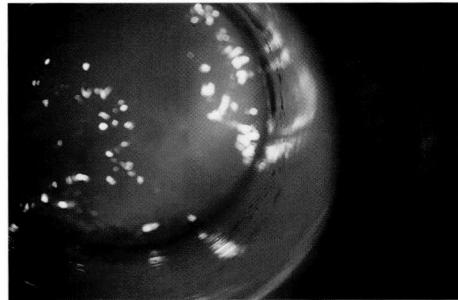

Plate 1 Gonococcal proctitis.

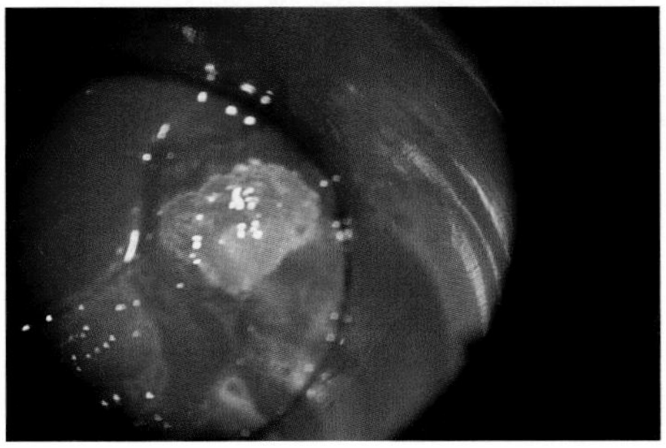

Plate 2 Condylomata acuminata of anal canal.

Chapter 22.3.4 Acute myeloblastic leukaemia

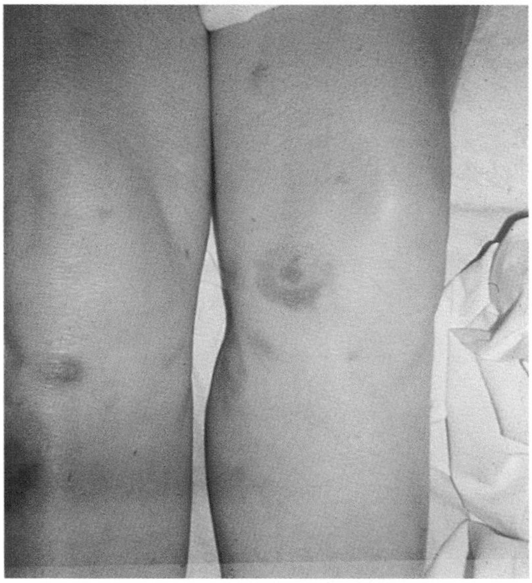

Plate 1 Target purpura. Classic target appearance of purpura formed by infarction of an arteriole by a dividing cluster of leukaemic myeloblasts. Typically, a deep, firm nodule can be felt in the pale centre of the lesion.

Chapter 22.3.5 Chronic lymphocytic leukaemia and other leukaemias of mature B and T cells

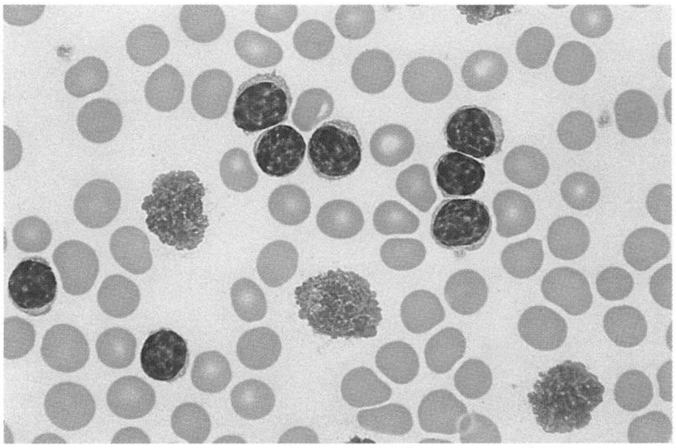

(a)

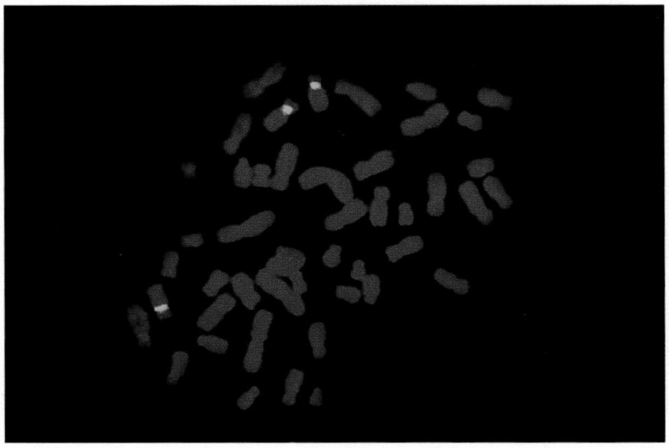

(b)

Plate 1 (a) Peripheral blood film from a case of chronic lymphocytic leukaemia showing small lymphocytes and smear cells. (b) Lymphocyte metaphase demonstrating trisomy 12 by *in situ* hybridization with a centromeric probe shown as single fluorescent dots in three chromosomes no. 12.

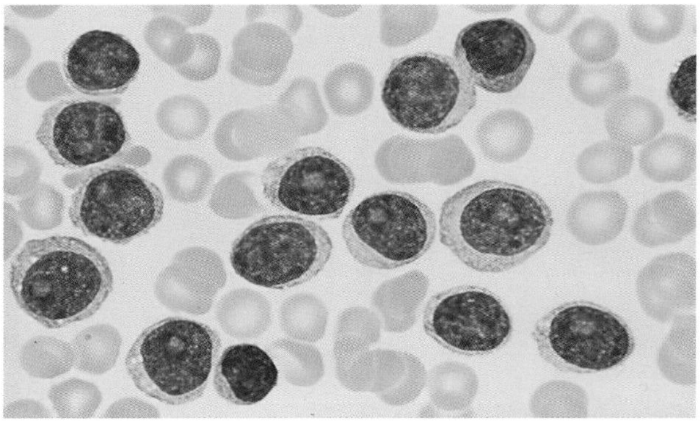

Plate 2 Peripheral blood film from a case of B-prolymphocytic leukaemia with characteristic nucleolated prolymphocytes.

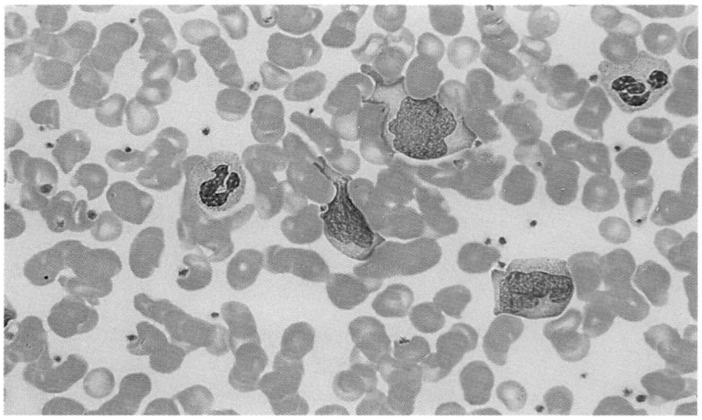

Plate 3 Circulating lymphocytes from a case of mantle-cell lymphoma.

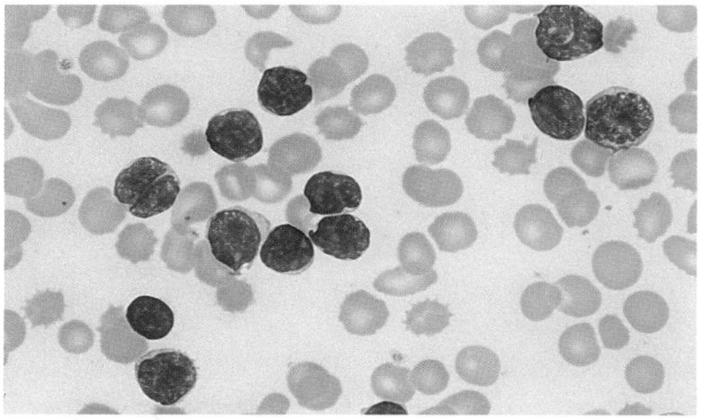

Plate 4 Peripheral blood cells from a case of folicular lymphoma presenting with leukaemia and a high leucocyte count.

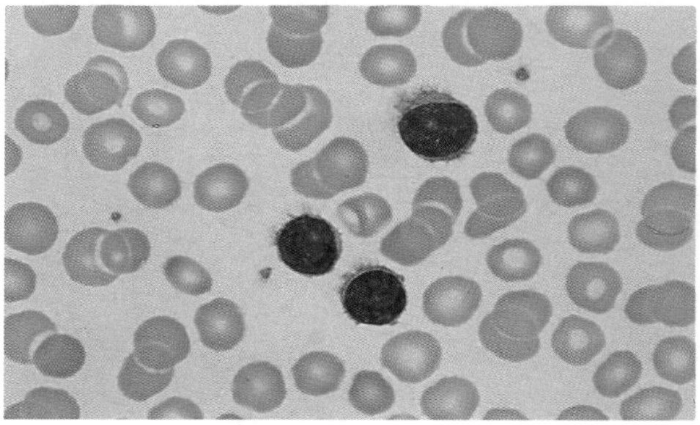

Plate 5 Peripheral blood lymphocytes with short villous projections from a case of splenic lymphoma with villous lymphocytes.

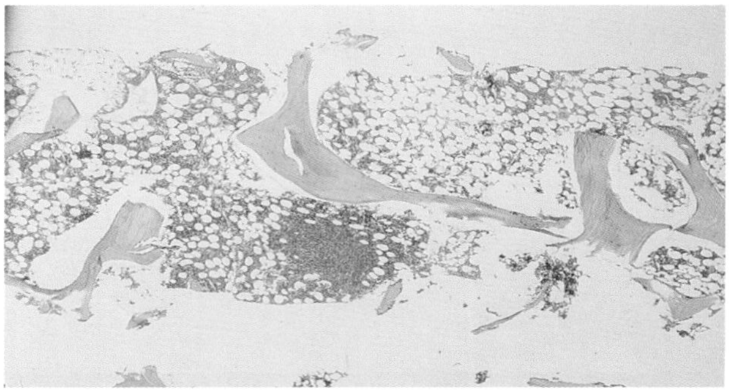

Plate 6 Nodular lymphocytic infiltration pattern in a bone marrow section from a case of mantle-cell lymphoma.

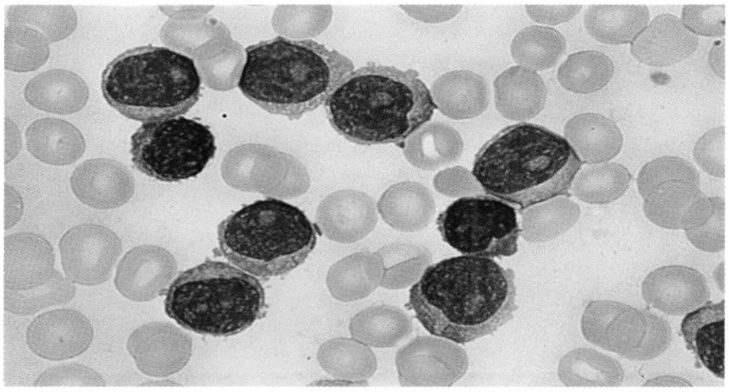

Plate 7 Peripheral blood from a case of T-cell prolymphocytic leukaemia.

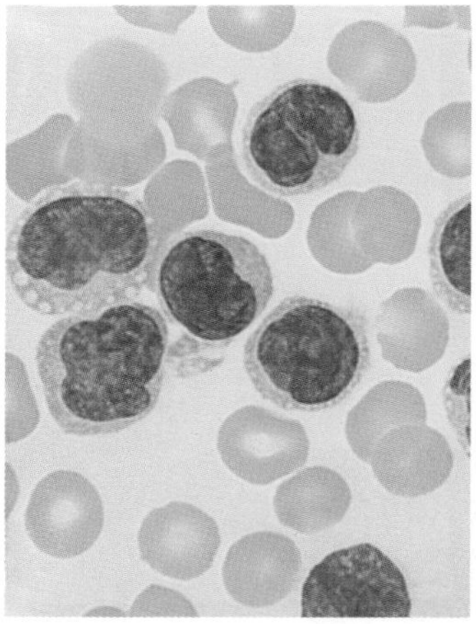

Plate 8 Circulating convoluted T cells from a Caribbean-born patient with adult T-cell leukaemia/lymphoma.

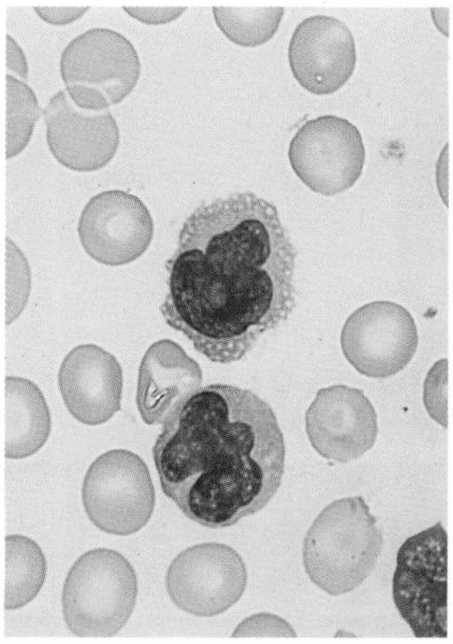

Plate 9 Cerebriform cells from a case of Sezary syndrome evolving with erythroderma and a high lymphocyte count.

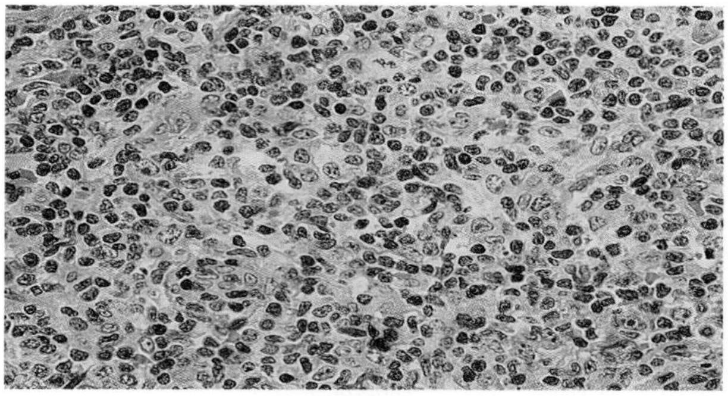

Plate 10 Lymph node section from a case of adult T-cell leukaemia/lymphoma showing diffuse infiltration with pleomorphic small, medium, and large cells.

Chapter 22.3.6 Chronic myeloid leukaemia

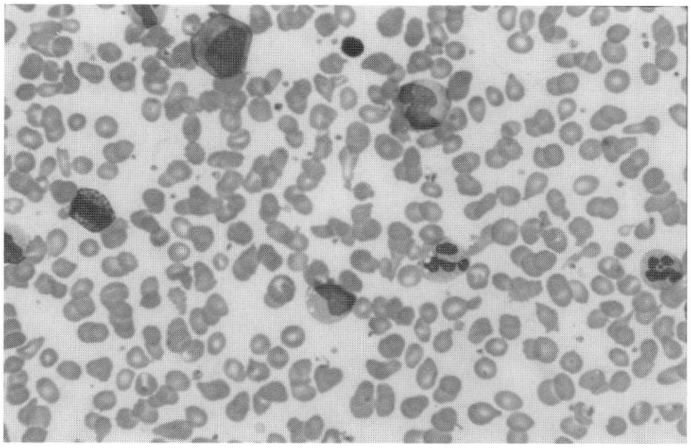

Plate 1 Peripheral blood film from a patient with CML in chronic phase. (Photograph kindly provided by Professor Barbara Bain, Imperial College London.)

Chapter 22.4.1 Leucocytes in health and disease

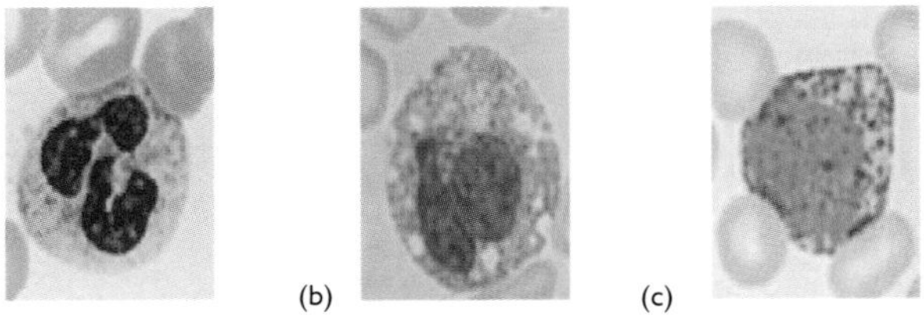

(a) (b) (c)

Plate 1 Peripheral blood granulocytes. (a) Polymorphonuclear leucocyte (neutrophil). (b) Eosinophil. (c) Basophil.

Chapter 22.4.7 Histiocytoses

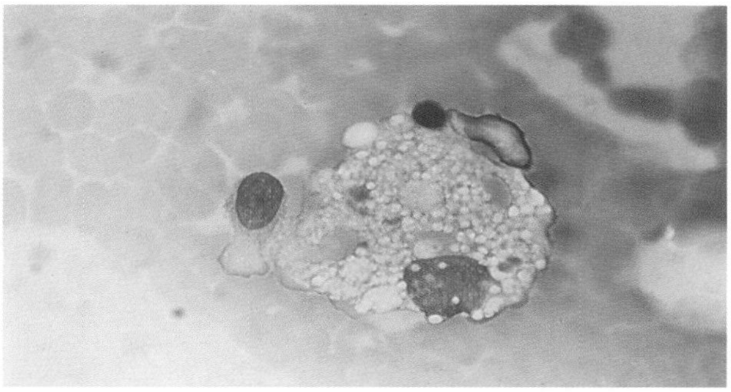

Plate 1 Macrophage exhibiting haemophagocytosis in the bone marrow of a child with haemophagocytic lumphohistiocytosis.

Chapter 22.5.6 Megaloblastic anaemia and miscellaneous deficiency anaemias

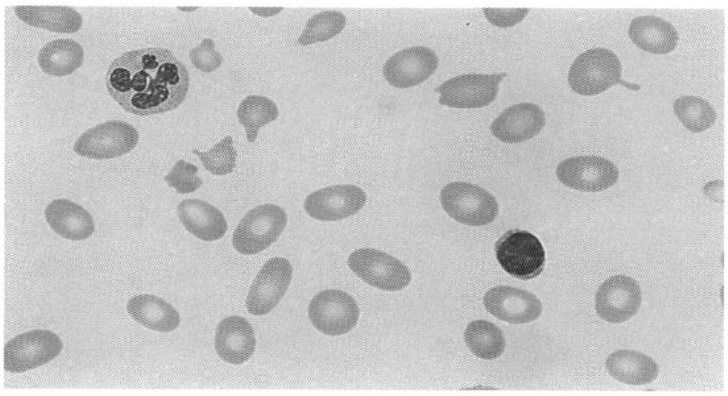

Plate 1 Megaloblastic anaemia. Hb 4.0 g/dl, MCV 120 fl. Hypersegmented neutrophil, oval macrocytes, and a small lymphocyte to show size of macrocytes. The fragmentation of advanced megaloblastosis is present. Thrombocytopenia is marked.

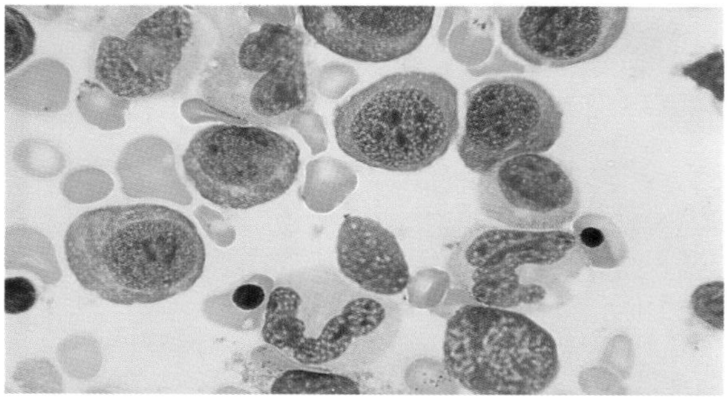

Plate 2 Megaloblastic anaemia. Bone marrow aspirate showing mainly intermediate megaloblasts and four giant metamyelocytes.

Chapter 22.6.2 Evaluation of the patient with a bleeding diathesis

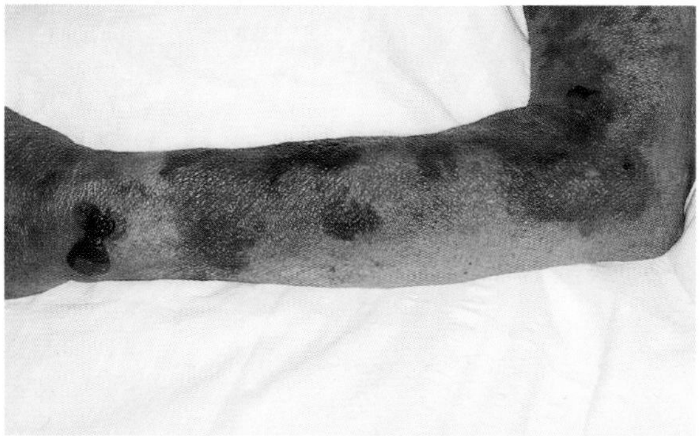

(a)

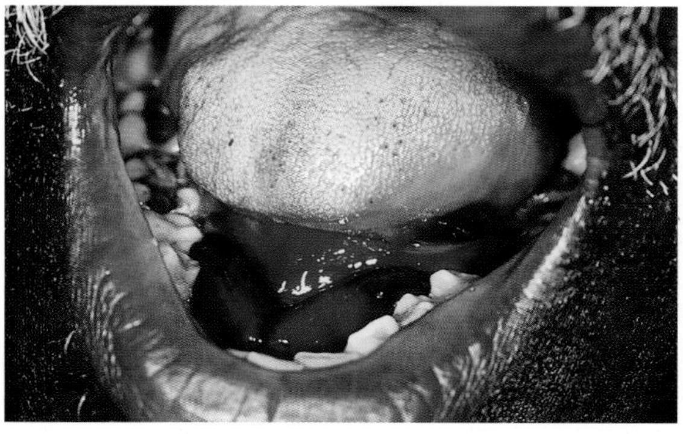

(b)

Plate 1 *See caption overleaf.*

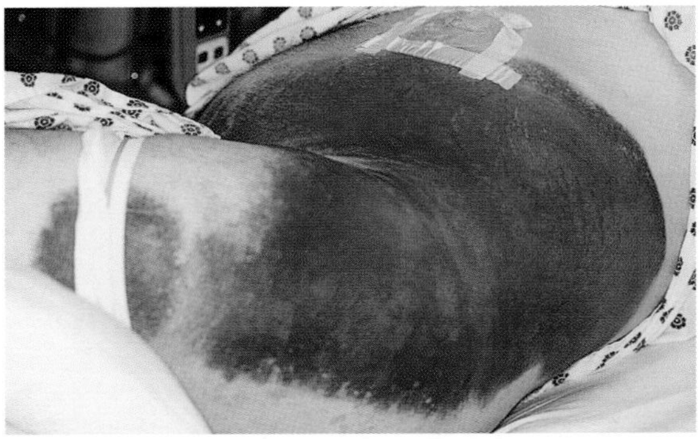

(c)

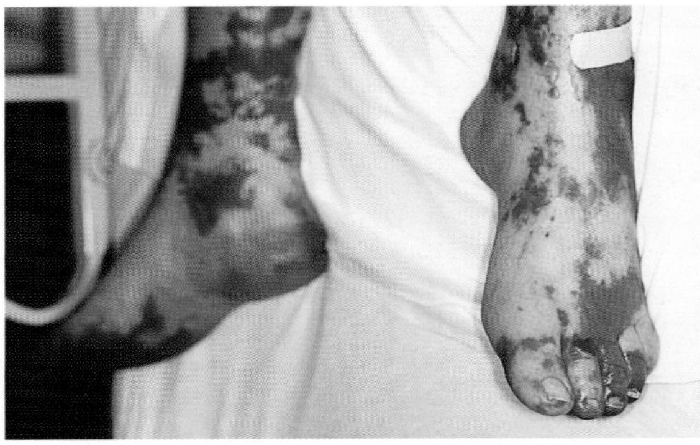

(d)

Plate 1 Purpura. (a) Confluent ecchymoses of varying size and age on the upper arm in an individual with an acquired factor VIII inhibitor. (b) Spontaneous sublingual haematoma in an individual with severe haemophilia A. (c) Blunt trauma-induced left flank and hip ecchymosis and haemotoma in an individual with severe haemophilia A. (d) Gangrenous ecchymoses in an individual with diffuse intravascular coagulation.

Chapter 22.7 The blood in systemic disease

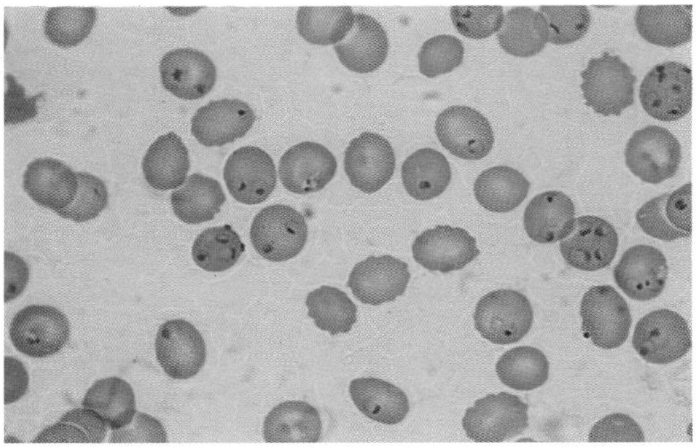

Plate 1 Malaria. Blood film showing fatal *Plasmodium falciparum* infection in a Gambian child.

Plates for Section 23

Chapter 23.1 Diseases of the skin

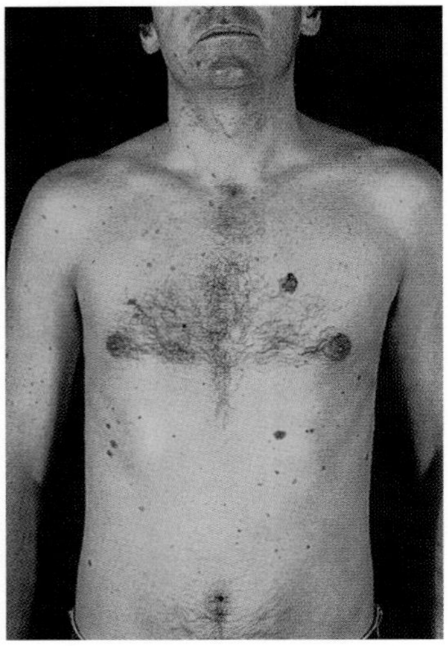

(a)

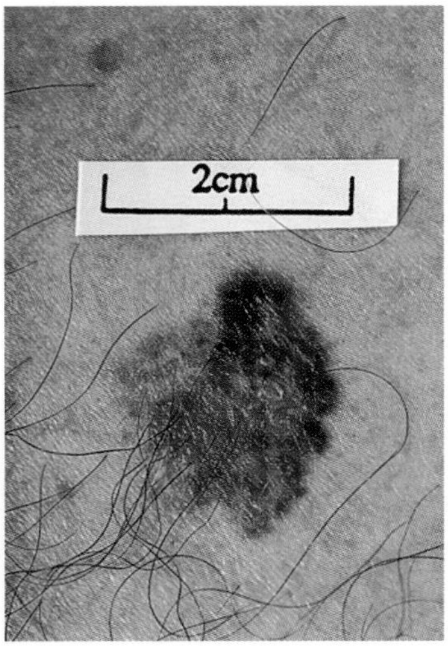

(b)

Plate 1 (a) In a patient with multiple atypical naevi one may stand out as different from the others and can be seen to be a melanoma. (b) It has an irregular outline and contains numerous different shades of brown pigmentation.

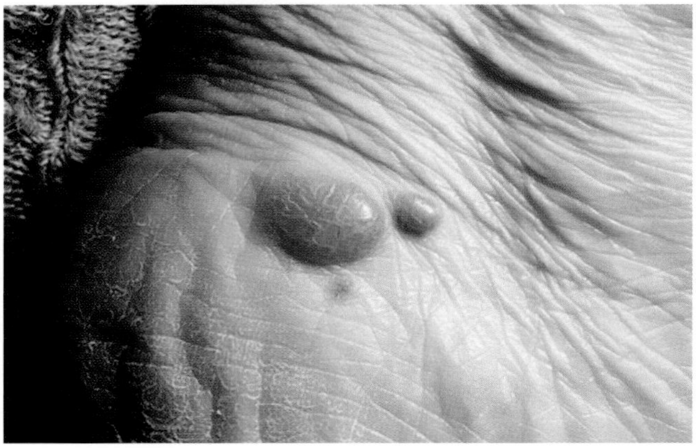

(a)

Plate 2 *See caption next page.*

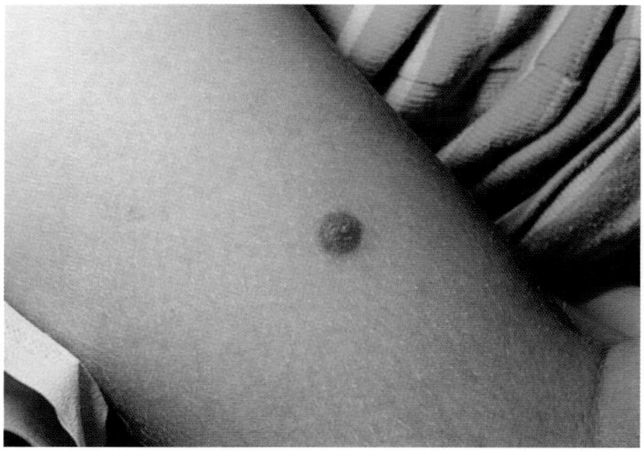

(b)

Plate 2 (a) Most primary melanomas will have some pigmentation, even so-called amelanotic melanoma. (b) Spitz naevi were formerly called juvenile melanoma because of their histological resemblance to melanoma, but their biological behaviour is benign.

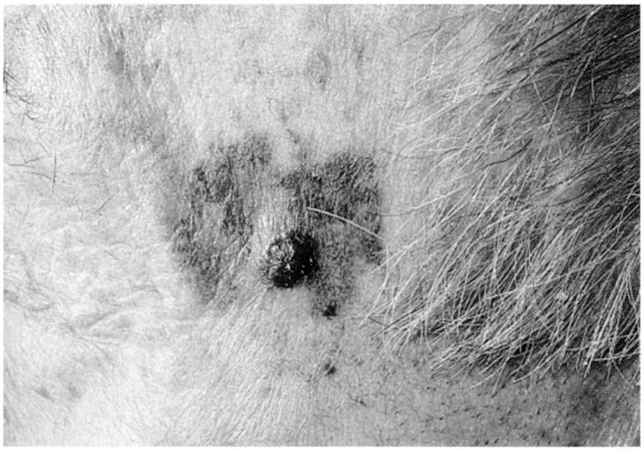

Plate 3 Nodular melanoma arising in a macular lentigo maligna (lentigo maligna melanoma).

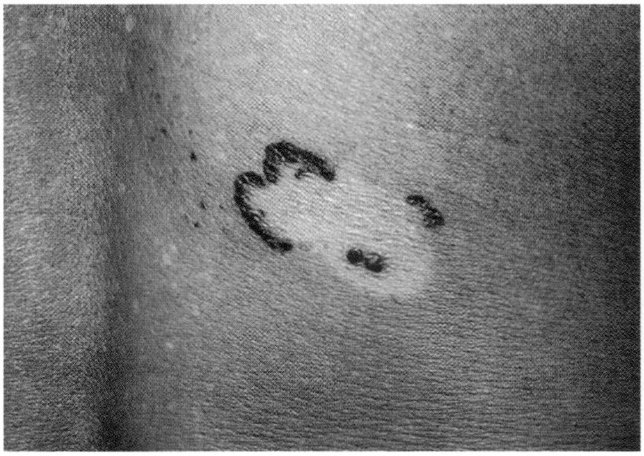

Plate 4 Regression in a melanoma making histological assessment of prognosis impossible.

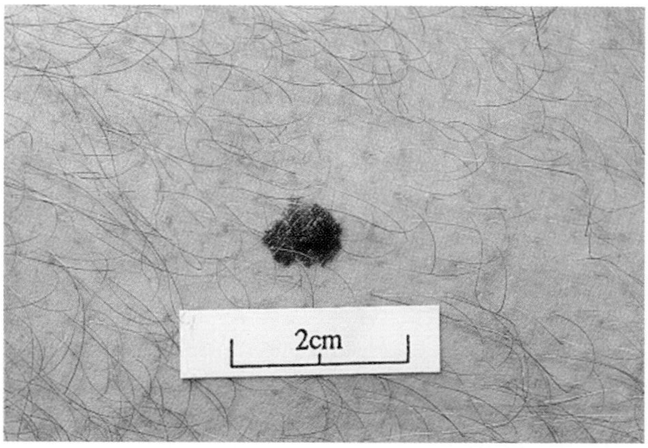

Plate 5 Melanoma most often arises *de novo* on normal skin and grows radially as well as vertically. Early detection requires identification of atypical morphology of smaller lesions.

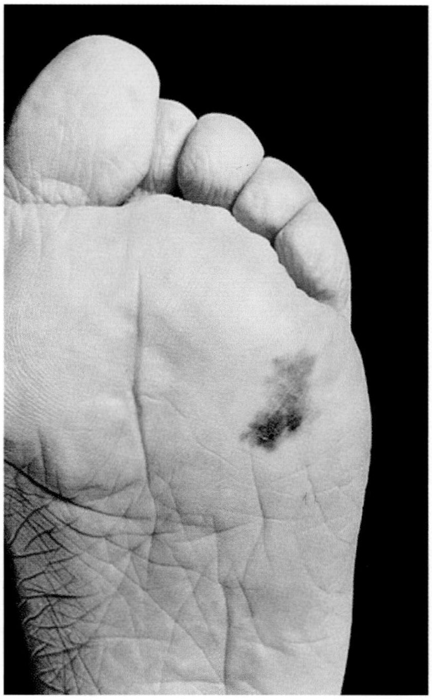

Plate 6 Acral lentigenous melanoma can be difficult to distinguish from benign junctional naevi on the palms and soles.

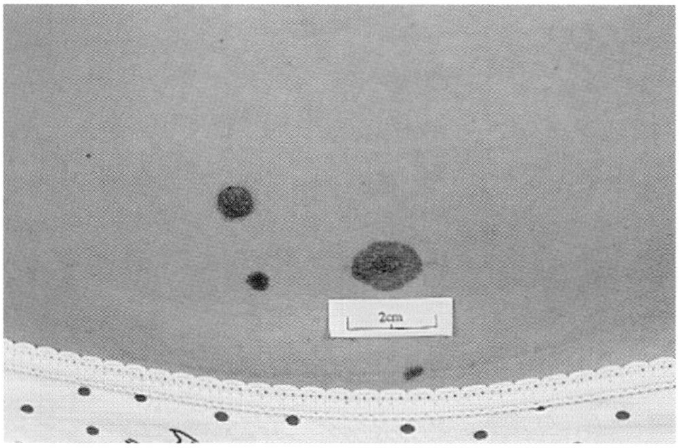

(a)

Plate 7 *See caption overleaf.*

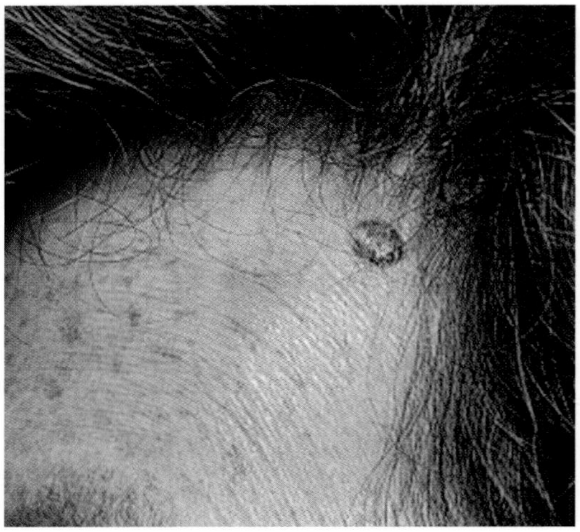

(b)

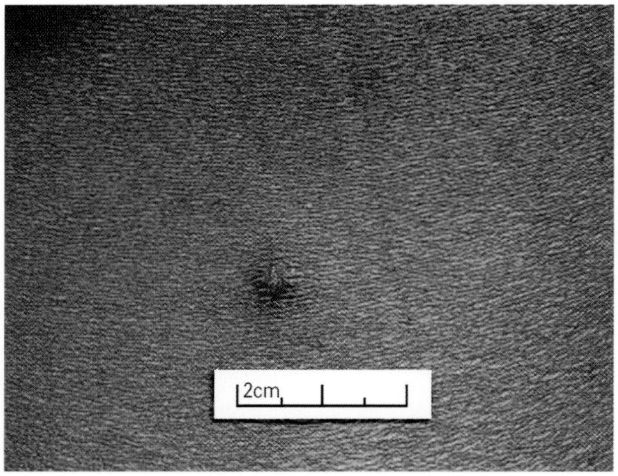

(c)

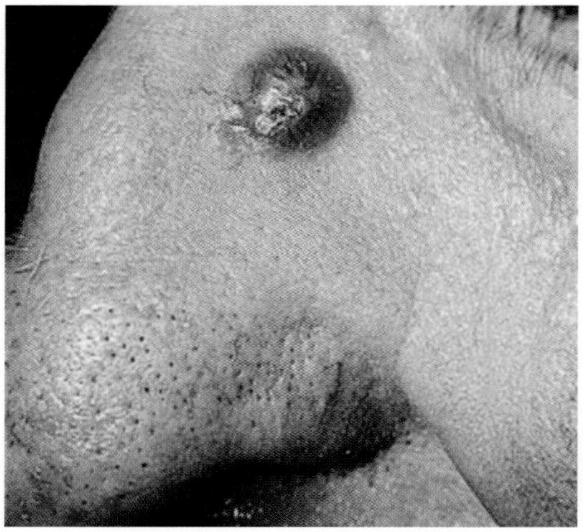

(d)

Plate 7 Lesions commonly confused with melanoma include (a) naevus *en cocarde*, which are central compound naevi with a surrounding macular junctional component, giving the appearance of a fried egg. Blue naevi (b) are often deeply pigmented, but the pigmentation is uniform and a blue tinge is discernible. Dermatofibromas (c) are sometimes easier to diagnose on palpation as they are hard and tethered to the skin. They may feel like a split pea. Pigmented basal cell epitheliomas (d) often have a rolled edge; however, sometimes biopsy provides this unexpected diagnosis.

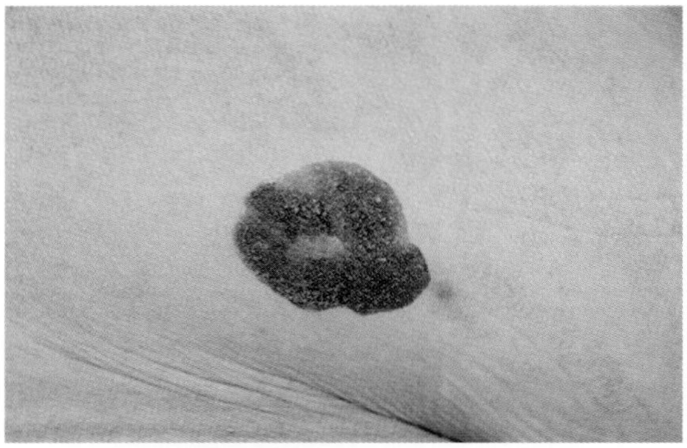

(a)

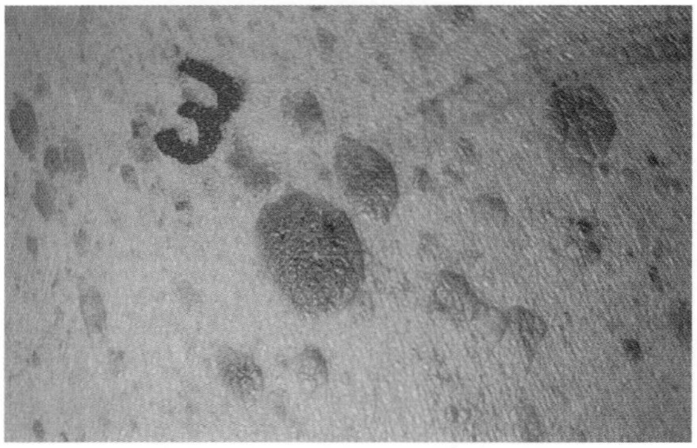

(b)

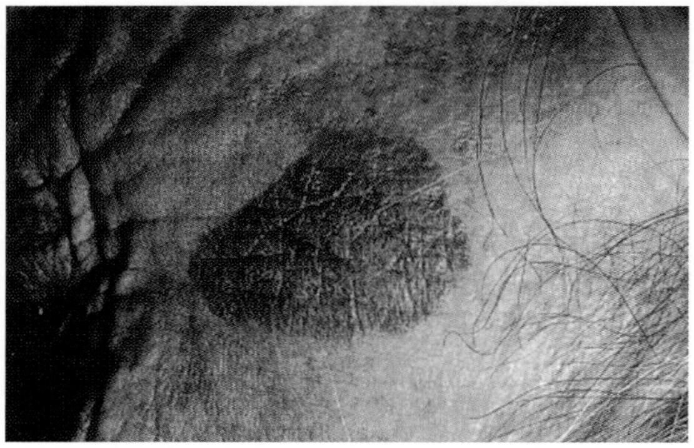

(c)

Plate 8 Seborrhoeic warts are often numerous and come in a variety of shapes and sizes. They may be deeply pigmented and elevated (a) or pale (b). They may also be macular (c). Characteristically they have a waxy surface and a 'stuck on' appearance.

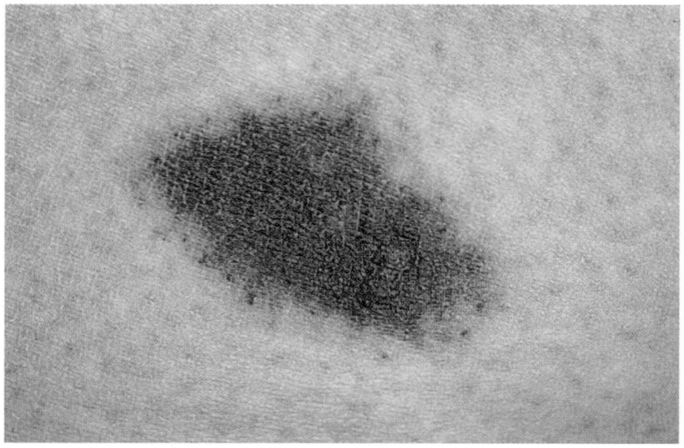

Plate 9 Congenital naevi are often larger than acquired naevi, but are usually evenly pigmented. They have a greater risk of malignant change.

Chapter 23.2 Molecular basis of inherited skin disease

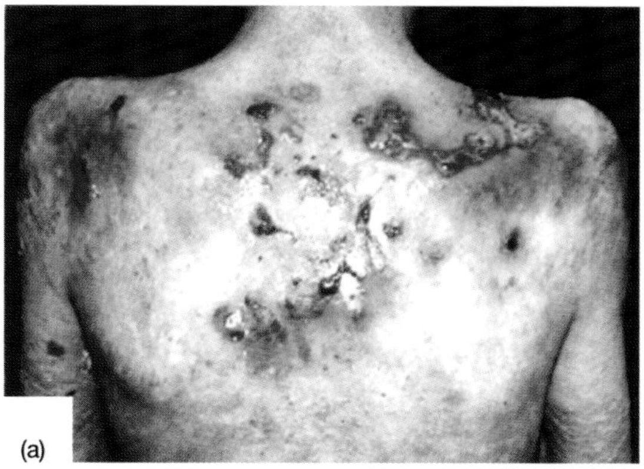
(a)

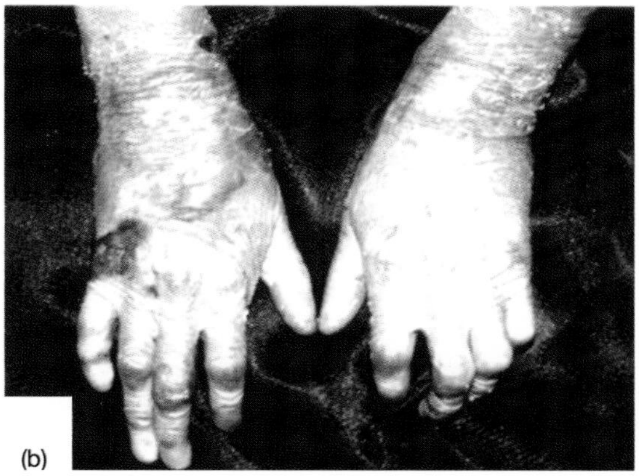
(b)

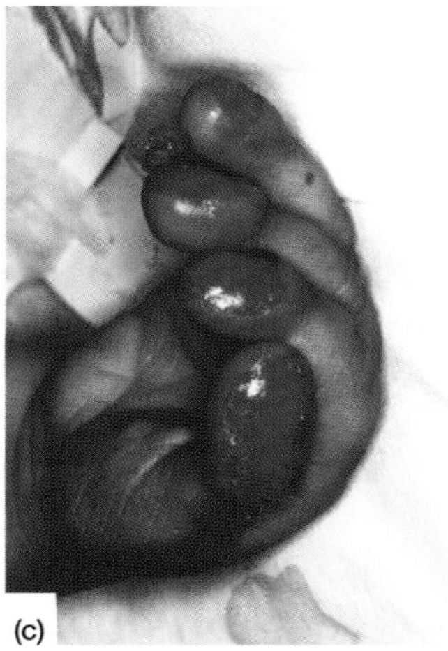
(c)

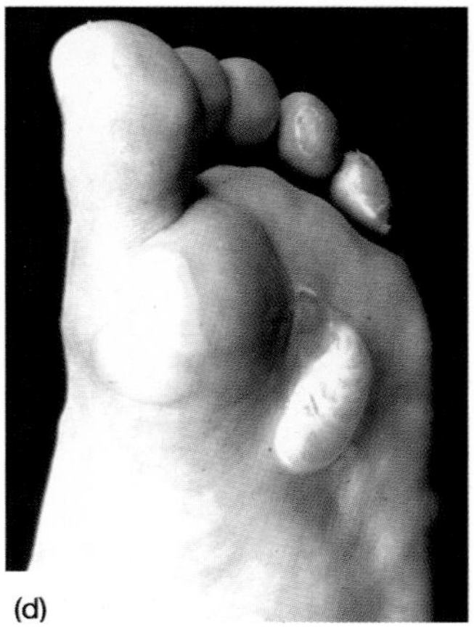
(d)

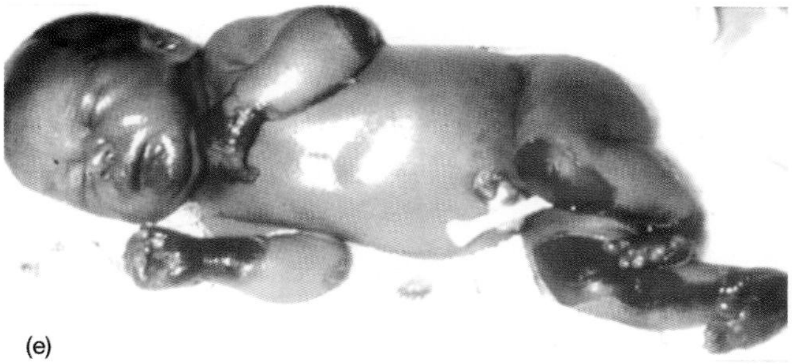
(e)

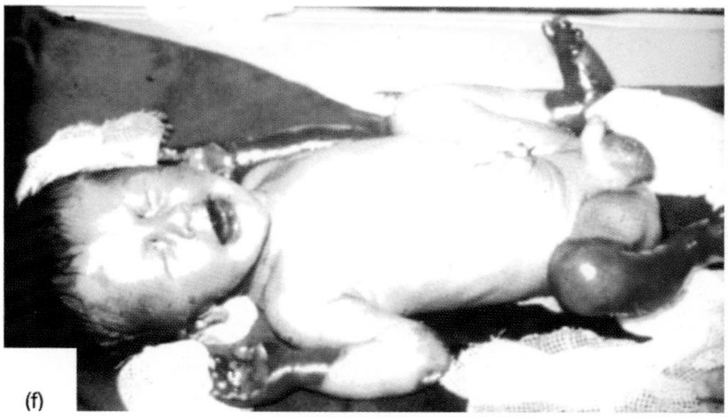
(f)

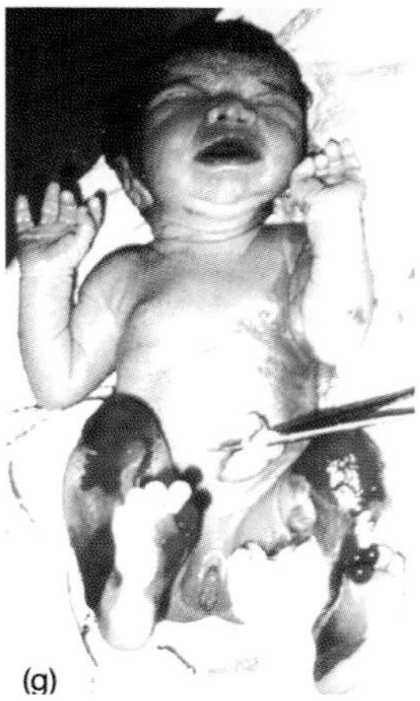
(g)

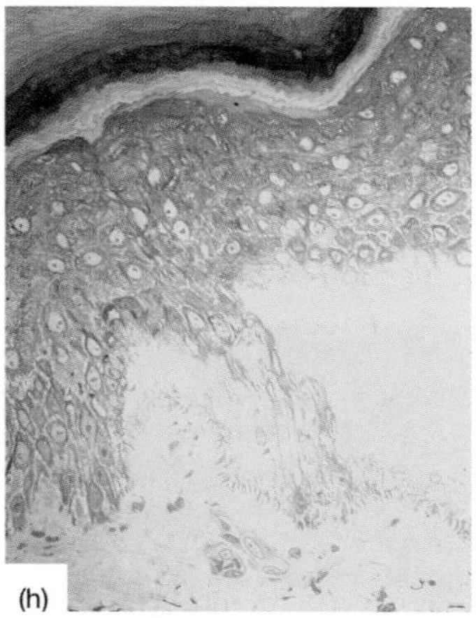
(h)

Plate 1 Clinical photographs of the different forms of epidermolysis bullosa. (a) and (b) a patient with Hallopean–Siemans dystrophic epidermolysis bullosa; (c) the hand of an infant with Herlitz junctional epidermolysis bullosa; (d) blister on the foot of a patient with epidermolysis bullosa simplex; (e) baby with epidermolysis bullosa simplex Dowling–Meara; (f) baby with Herlitz junctional epidermolysis bullosa; (g) baby with Hallopean–Siemans dystrophic epidermolysis bullosa; (h) intraepidermal blister from a Weber Cockayne epidermolysis bullosa simplex patient. Skin section stained with Richardson's stain.

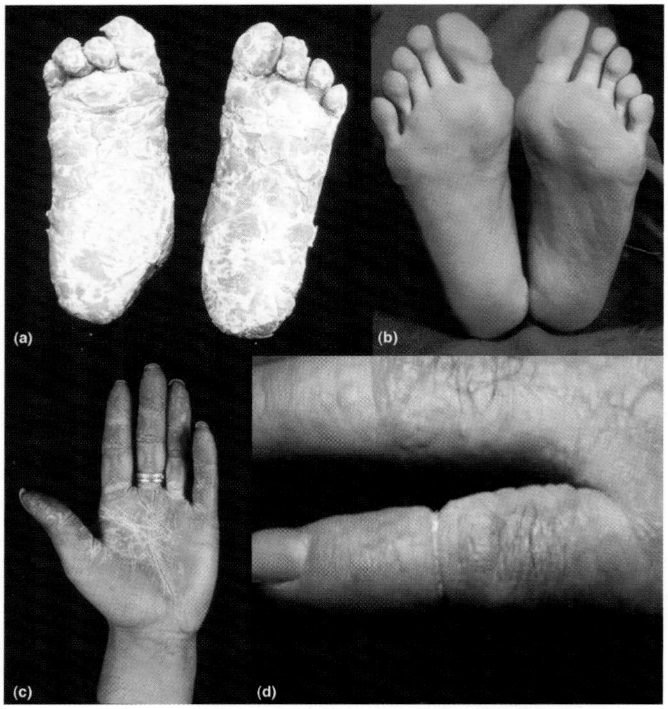

Plate 2 Clinical photographs of: (a) bullous ichthyosiform erythroderma (BIE) and three types of keratoderma; (b) focal palmoplantar keratoderma (PPK) associated with a keratin 16 mutation; (c) striate palmoplantar keratoderma associated with a desmoglein 1 mutation; and (d) constriction around the digit from an individual with Vohwinkel's syndrome associated with a C×26 mutation.

Plates for Section 24

Chapter 23.13.3 Epilepsy in later childhood and adults

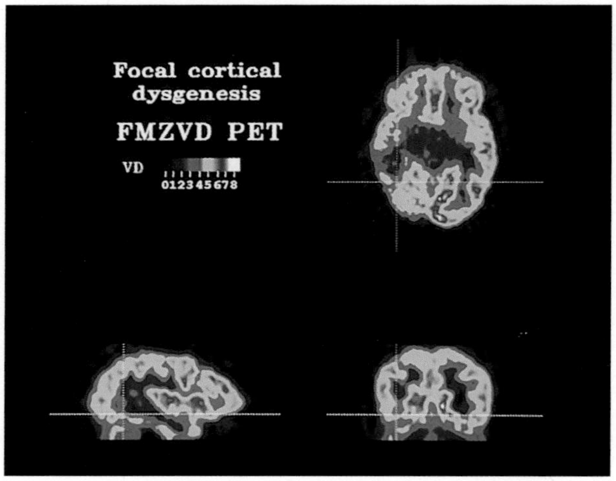

Plate 1 FMZVD PET scan showing a region of probable cortical dysplasia in the right temporal lobe. The 11C-fluamzenil volume of distribution (FMZVD) is an index of $GABA_A$ receptor density.

Chapter 24.13.9 Human prion disease

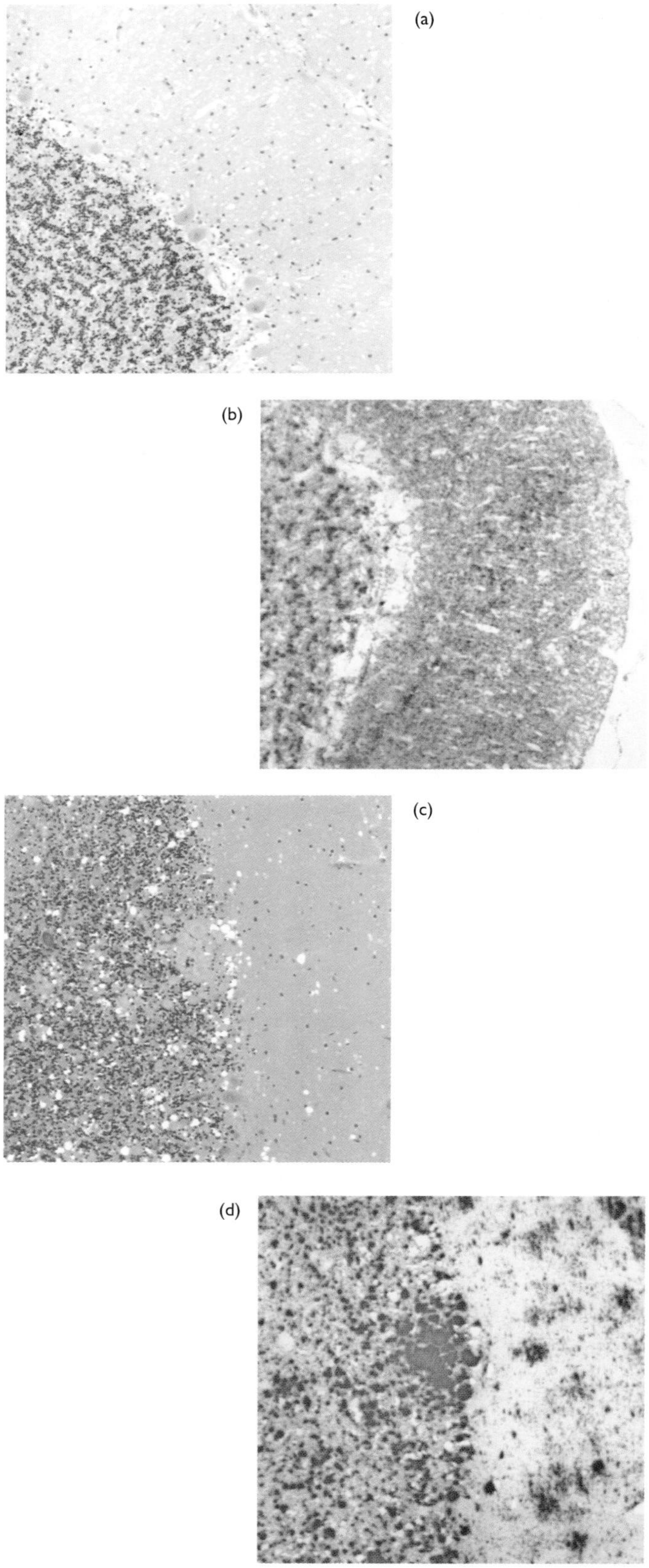

Plate 1 *See caption next page.*

Plate 1 (a) The cerebellum in sporadic CJD shows widespread spongiform change in the molecular layer, with no plaques visible. Haematoxylin and eosin × 250. (b) PrP immunocytochemistry in the cerebellum in sporadic CJD shows a fine granular (synaptic) pattern of deposition in the molecular layer (right) with coarser deposits visible in the granular layer (left). No plaques are visible and the Purkinje cells are unstained. Kg9 monoclonal antibody × 250. (c) The cerebellum in variant CJD shows a group of florid plaques (centre) comprising rounded amyloid deposits surrounded by spongiform change. Spongiform change is also present in the molecular layer (right). Haematoxylin and eosin × 250. (d) Immunocytochemistry for PrP in the cerebellum in variant CJD shows strong staining of the large amyloid plaques (centre) but there is widespread positivity in the form of multiple smaller plaques, with amorphous 'feathery' deposits in the molecular layer (right). Kg9 monoclonal antibody × 250.

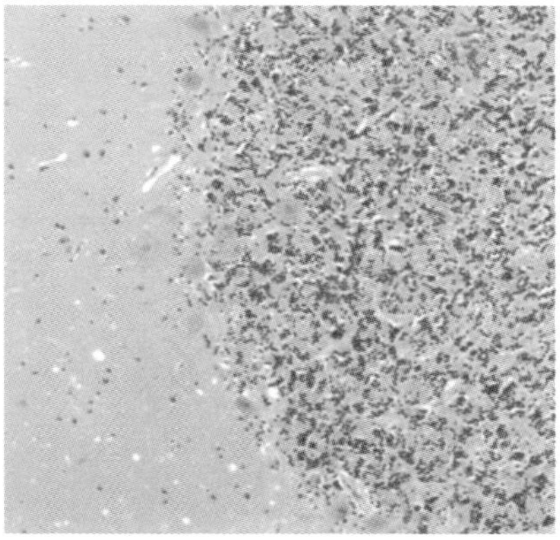

(a)

(b)

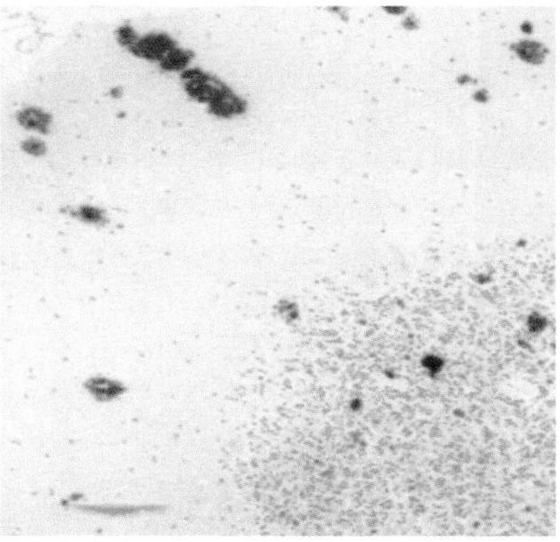

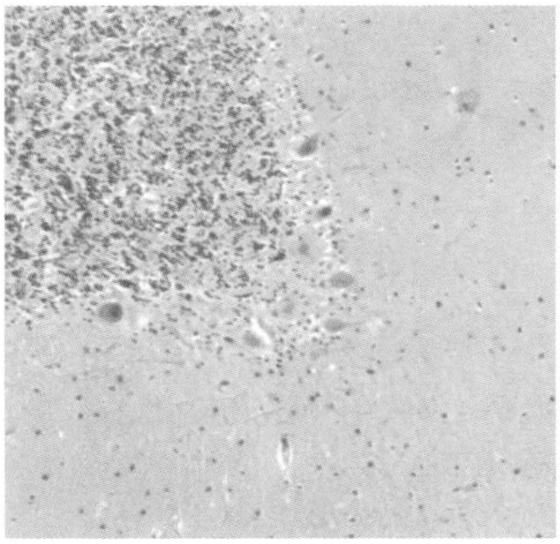

(c)

(d)

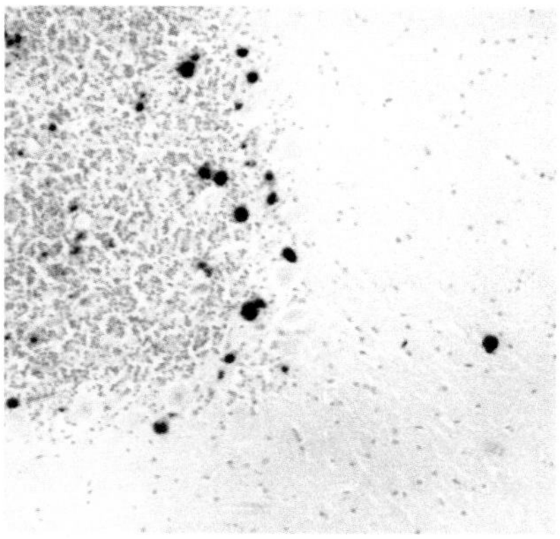

Plate 2 (a) The cerebellum in GSS contains multiple multicentric plaques (centre) which are present both in the molecular layer and in the granular layer. Spongiform change is also present focally in the molecular layer (left). Haematoxylin and eosin × 250. (b) Multicentric plaques in GSS are more easily visualized in the cerebellum using immunocytochemistry for PrP, which shows large deposits of varying size in both the molecular and granular layers. Kg9 monoclonal antibody × 250. (c) The cerebellum in kuru contains typical plaques (the so-called kuru plaques) which are comprised of a rounded structure with a dense centre and a loose fibrillary periphery (centre). Spongiform change is only present to a minimal degree in the molecular layer. Haematoxylin and eosin × 250. (d) Immunocytochemistry for PrP in the cerebellum in kuru shows strong staining of the larger plaques and in addition demonstrates multiple smaller plaques which are not evident on routinely stained preparations. Kg9 monoclonal antibody × 250.

Chapter 24.14.1 Bacterial meningitis

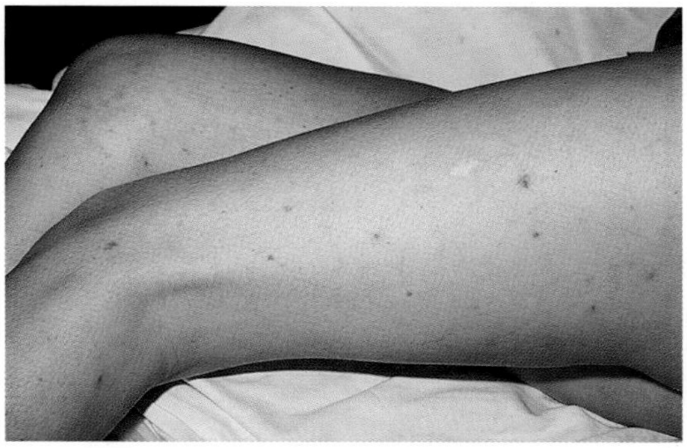

Plate 1 Cutaneous petechiae in a patient with acute meningococcal meningitis. (Copyright D.A. Warrell.)

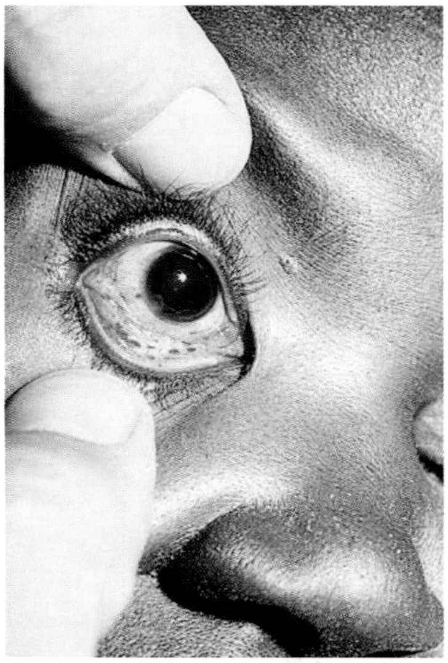

Plate 2 Conjunctival petechiae in a Nigerian boy with meningococcal meningitis. (Copyright D.A. Warrell.)

(a)

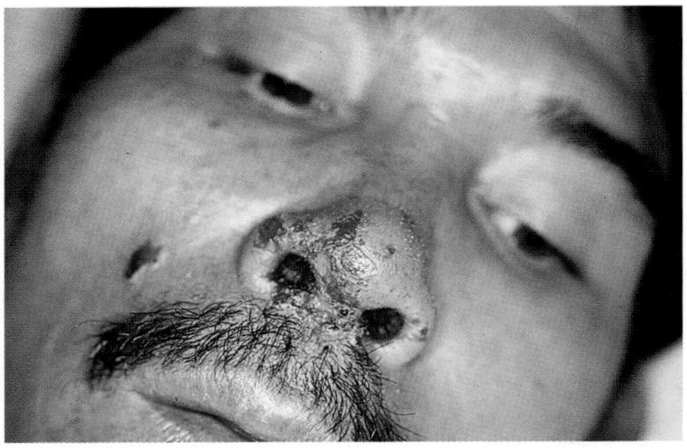

(b)

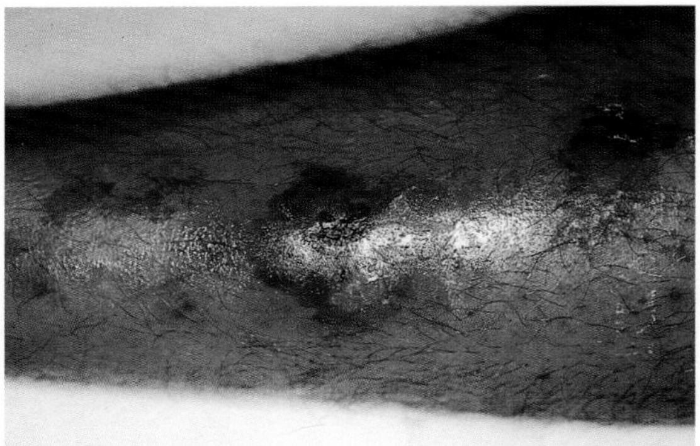

Plate 3 Haemorrhagic lesions on the face (a) and shin (b) of a 63-year-old Thai man with *Streptococcus suis* meningitis. (Copyright the late Prida Phuapradit.)

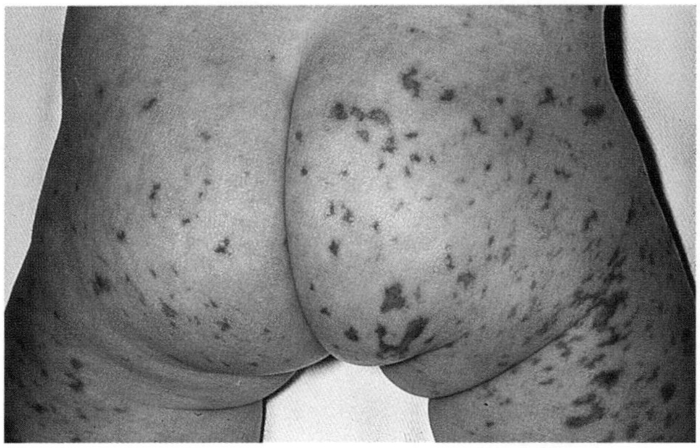

Plate 4 The rash of meningococcal septicaemia in an English child.

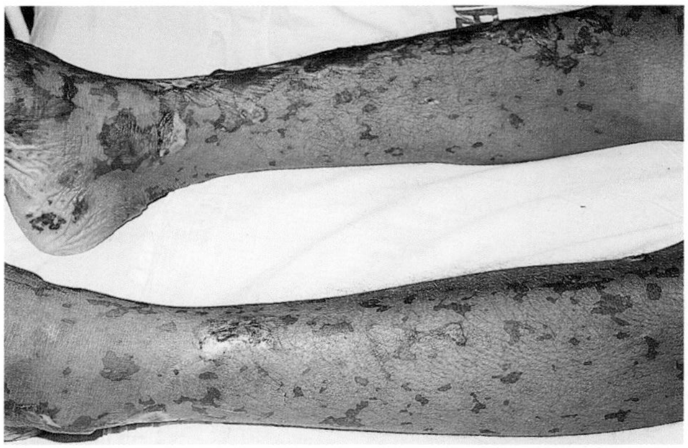

Plate 5 Healing vasculitic rash in a Brazilian boy with meningococcal meningitis and meningococcaemia. (Copyright D.A. Warrell.)

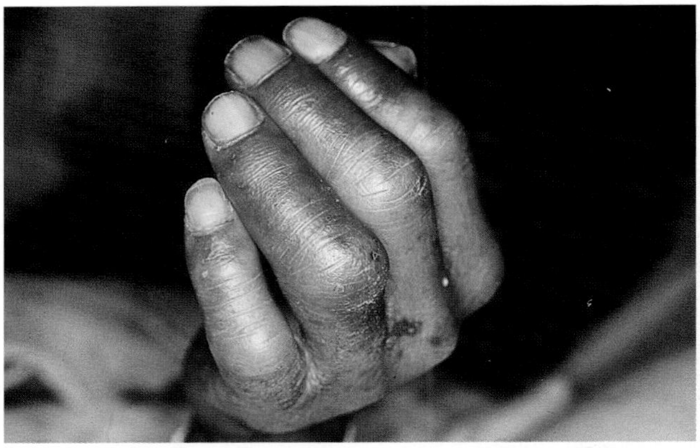

Plate 6 Septic arthritis of the interphalangeal joints in a 73-year-old Thai man with *Streptococcal suis* meningitis. (Copyright the late Prida Phuapradit.)

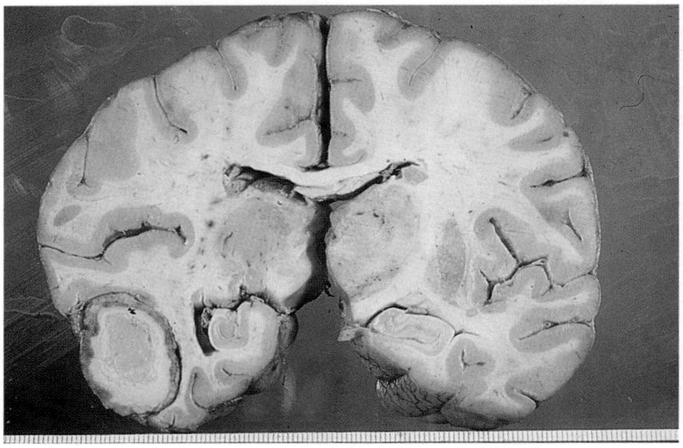

Plate 7 Tuberculoma in the brain. (Copyright Gareth Turner.)

(a)

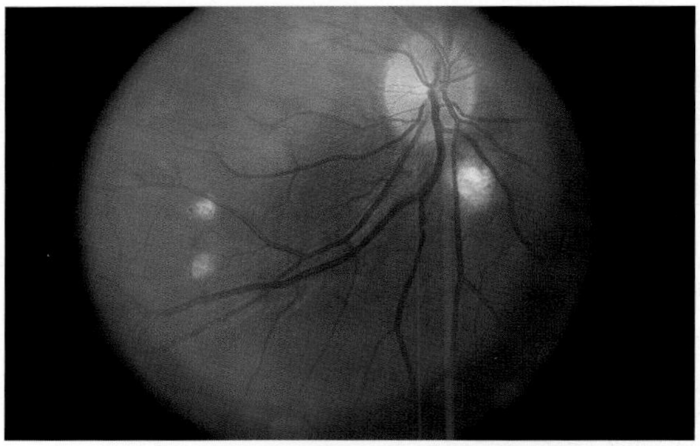

(b)

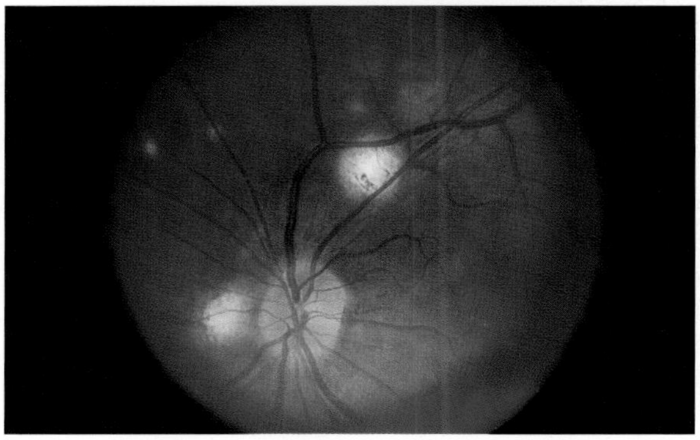

Plate 8 (a and b) Tuberculous choroiditis in a 23-year-old Thai woman. (Copyright the late Prida Phuapradit.)

Plates for Section 25

Chapter 25 The eye in general medicine

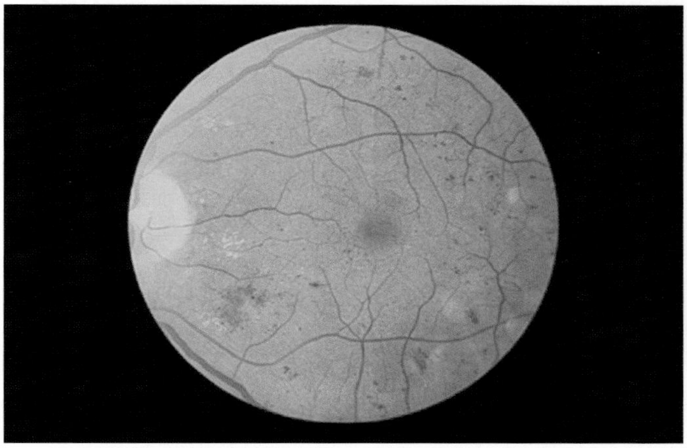

Plate 1 Diabetic, background retinopathy. The hallmarks of background retinal changes are red dots (either microaneurysms or small haemorrhages) and blots (larger haemorrhages) together with glinting hard exudates and. These are no closer than one disc diameter from the central fovea and vision is normal.

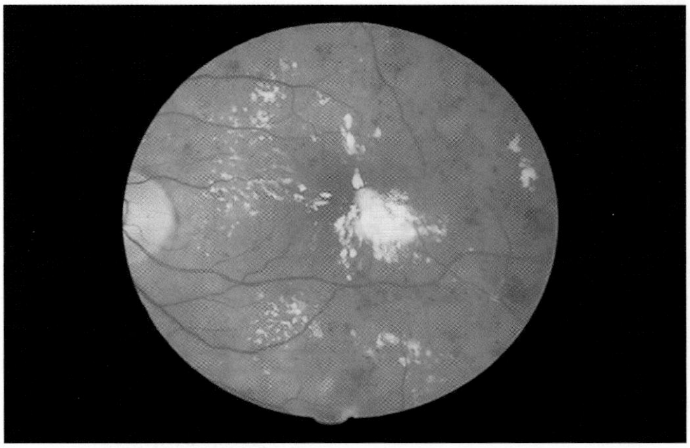

Plate 2 Diabetic, maculopathy. Hard exudate, containing lipid and protein which has leaked from damaged retinal capillaries, has congregated at the fovea. Central vision is irretrievably impaired. Diabetes may present in this way, especially in the elderly.

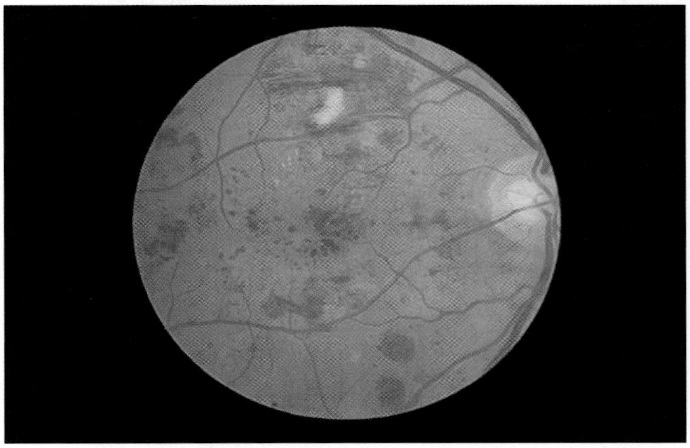

Plate 3 Diabetic, ischaemic retinopathy. Capillary ischaemia creates multiple cotton wool spots—microinfarcts within the nerve fibre layer. Other features are dilatation of retinal veins and multiple blot haemorrhages. Frank proliferation of new vessels is almost inevitable and the retinal changes must be carefully observed.

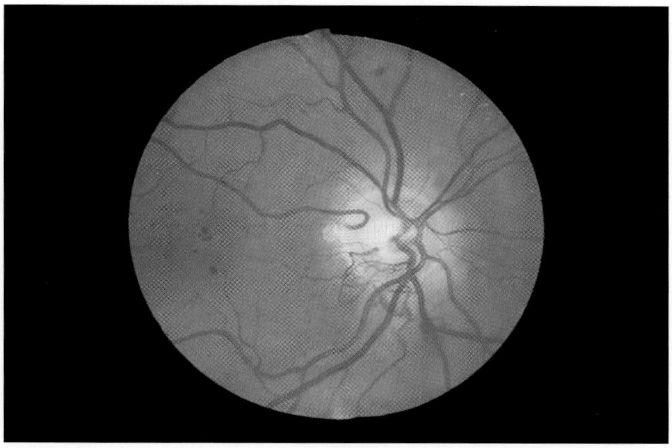

Plate 4 Diabetic, proliferative retinopathy. New vessels have formed on the inferior part of the optic disc. They are fine, looping, and aimless. There may be others in the peripheral retina. If the vessels bleed, vision will become acutely obscured by 'floaters'.

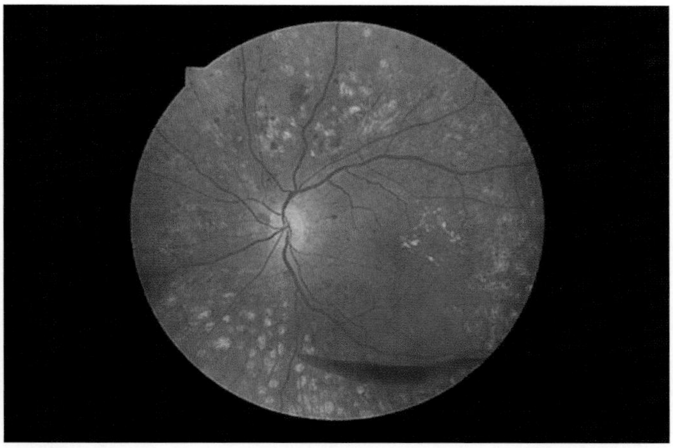

Plate 5 Diabetic, preretinal haemorrhage and laser scars. Neovascular fronds may bleed in front of the retina or into the vitreous, obscuring vision acutely. Here blood has sedimented into a characteristic 'boat' shape and multiple laser scars have been placed outside the major vascular arcades. There are haemorrhages and hard exudate temporal to the fovea.

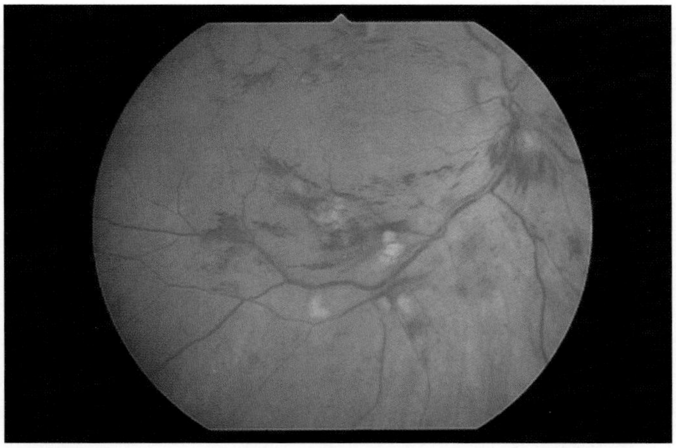

Plate 6 Hypertension, accelerated. Multiple flame shaped haemorrhages, microinfarcts, and swelling of the optic disc margin are characteristic features of accelerated hypertension. Vision may be normal, yet the changes dictate immediate treatment to reduce blood pressure. The diastolic level is usually greater than 110 mmHg and proteinuria is to be expected.

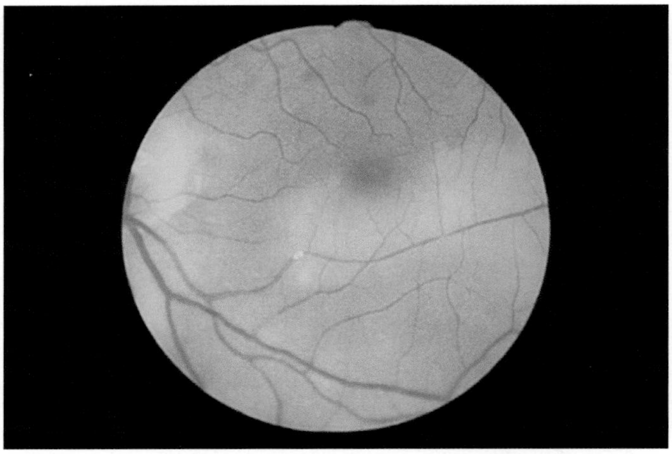

Plate 7 Branch retinal artery occlusion. A small white embolus is lodged at the third bifurcation of the superotemporal branch retinal artery, occluding it. The local retina is oedematous and non-functioning, producing an acute superior scotoma in the left eye. The likely origin is from the ipsilateral carotid or the heart.

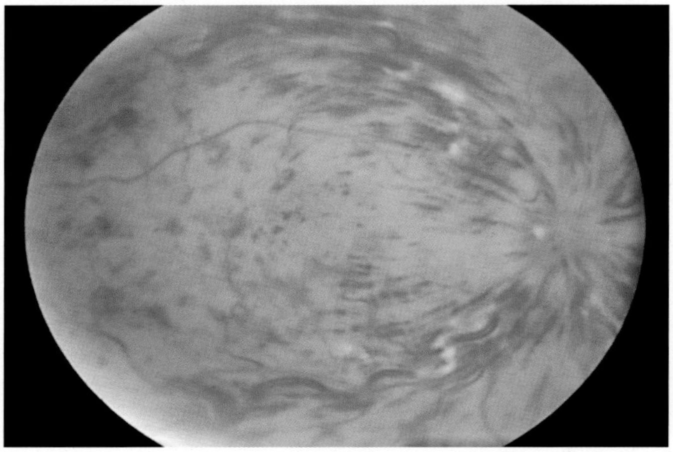

Plate 8 Central retinal vein occlusion. Blockage of the draining central retinal vein results in a 'bloodstorm' appearance with profuse flame haemorrhages forming between the nerve fibres in all quadrants. Cotton wool spots representing micro-infarcts are often also present. Vision is acutely blurred as the fovea becomes oedematous.

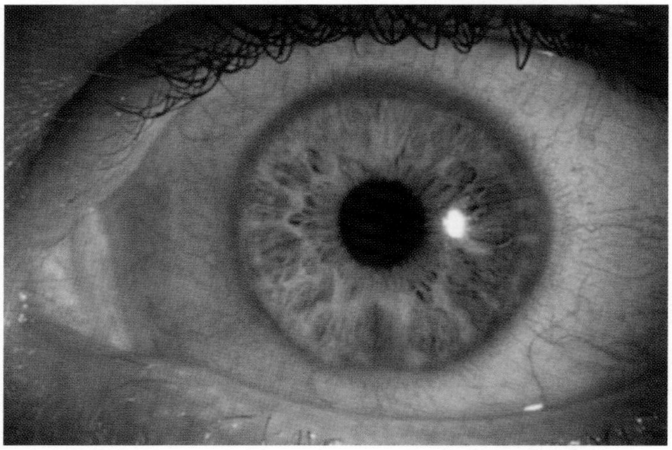

Plate 9 Behçet's hypopyon iritis. The eye is red, painful and photophobic. White cells within the anterior chamber have sedimented into a characteristic hypopyon at the base. If bacterial endophthalmitis is excluded, Behçet's syndrome is a likely cause of this acute, intense, sterile iritis.

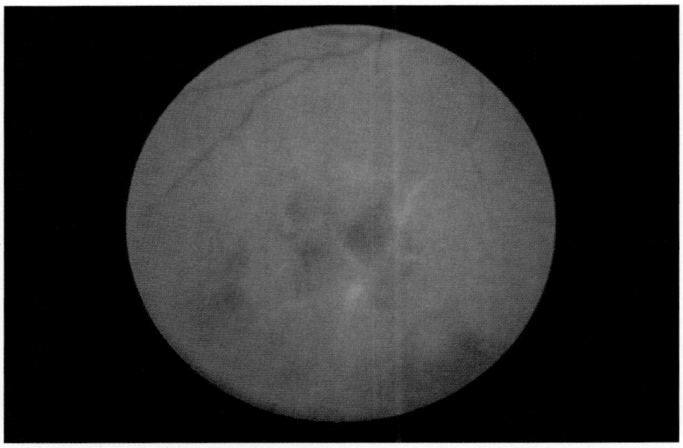

Plate 10 Behçet's retinitis. Occlusion of blood vessels, usually venous, in the peripheral retina produces a wedge of haemorrhage with whitening of the vascular wall. The view is hazy due to inflammatory cells within the vitreous. The retina is ischaemic, function is lost, and neovascularization may occur. Repeated episodes may damage vision irretrievably.

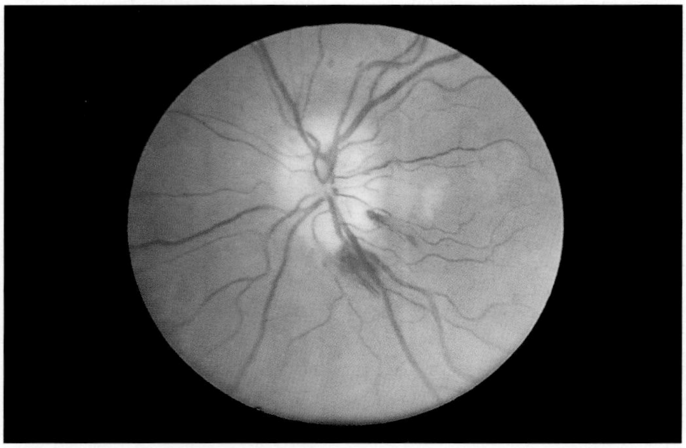

Plate 11 Giant cell arteritis, optic disc infarction. The optic nerve head is infarcted, due to occlusion of multiple ciliary branch arterioles which supply it. The disc is pale and swollen, and juctapapillary haemorrhage has formed. Vision is poor and will not recover. The other eye is at immediate risk unless the systemic inflammatory process is controlled.

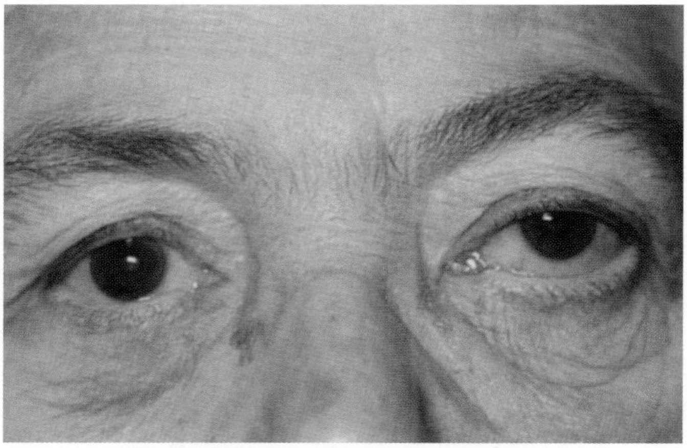

Plate 12 Wegener's granulomatosis of the orbit. An inflammatory mass behind the left eye has displaced it forwards and upwards and the eye moves poorly due to involvement of motor nerves within the orbit. The optic nerve may also be involved. Biopsy confirmed granulomatous vasculitis and ANCA was positive. The adjacent sinuses were involved, with bone loss demonstrated on CT scan.

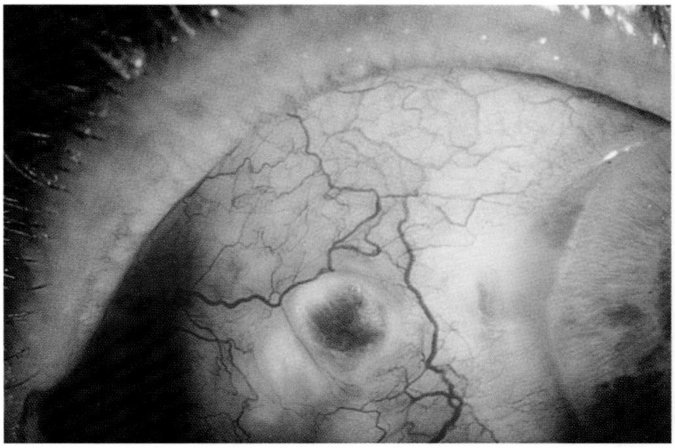

Plate 13 Scleromalacia in rheumatoid arthritis. Vasculitis results in focal ischaemia, with translucency and thinning of the sclera: the coat of the eye may perforate. The most common associated systemic disorder is rheumatoid arthritis. The eye is usually red, and pain may be intense.

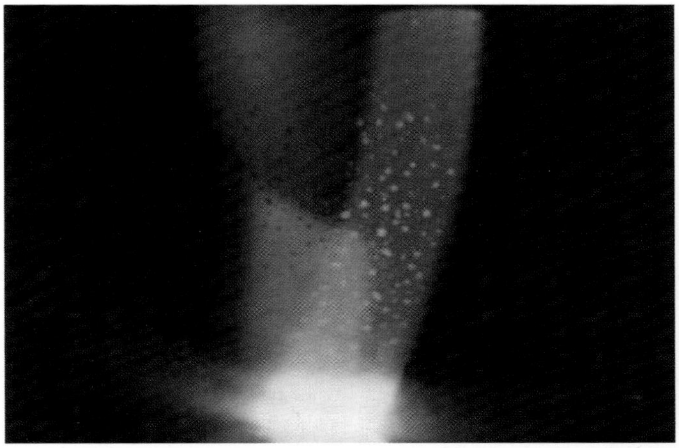

Plate 14 Iritis in ankylosing spondylitis. The slit lamp displays cells within the anterior chamber which have sedimented on to the interior surface of the cornea as white keratic precipitates. These are the hallmarks of iritis (anterior uveitis). The eye is usually red and painful. A frequent association is with ankylosing spondylitis and HLA B27 haplotype.

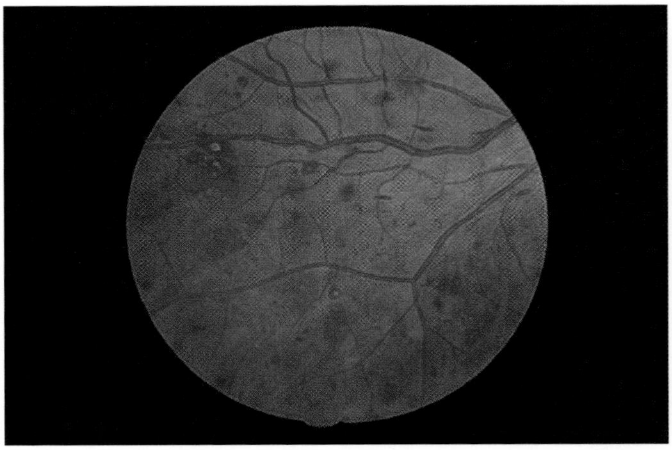

Plate 15 Retinal haemorrhages in leukaemia. Multiple and bilateral retinal haemorrhages suggest a blood dyscrasia, if underlying diabetes and hypertension are excluded. In this case, the peripheral lymphocyte count was considerably raised, consistent with chronic lymphocytic leukaemia. Some haemorrhages have a white centre (Roth spot).

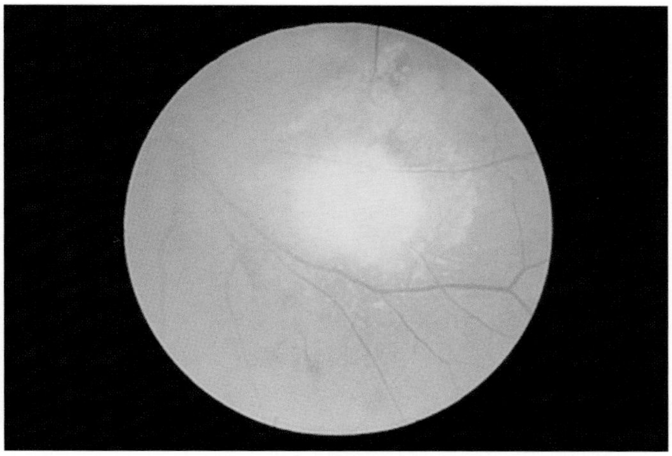

Plate 16 Metastatic staphylococcal endophthalmitis. Blood borne organisms may settle in the eye, forming a focal abscess in the choroid, breaking through the adjacent retina into the vitreous which becomes hazy with inflammatory cells. This patient had poorly-controlled diabetes and a staphylococcal skin infection.

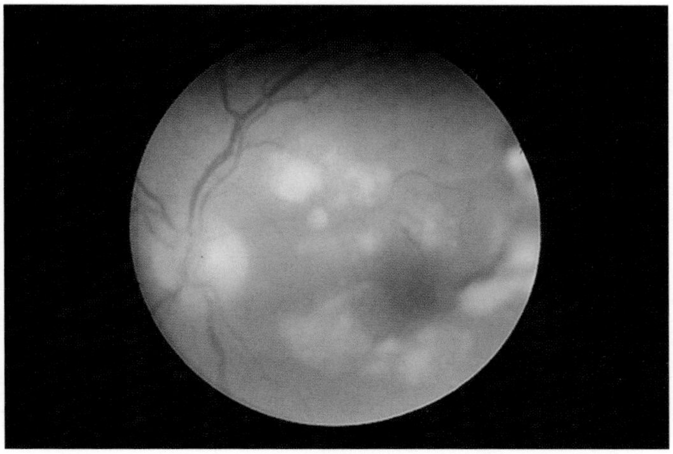

Plate 17 Candida endophthalmitis. Fungal infection of the eye interior forms white 'snowballs' within the vitreous and retina. The organism is usually blood borne and may enter the circulation with intravenously injected agents, including heroin. Infection is indolent, with a relatively white eye and little pain. Vitrectomy and intravitreal antimicrobial treatment may be necessary.

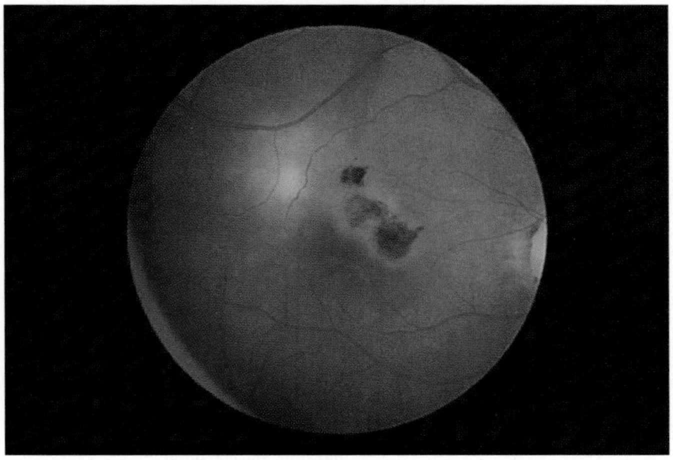

Plate 18 Toxoplasmosis. A fluffy fresh focus of infection within the choroid and retina is found adjacent to an old pigmented scar, typical of toxoplasmosis. The organism encysts within the retina and may reactivate sporadically in this way.

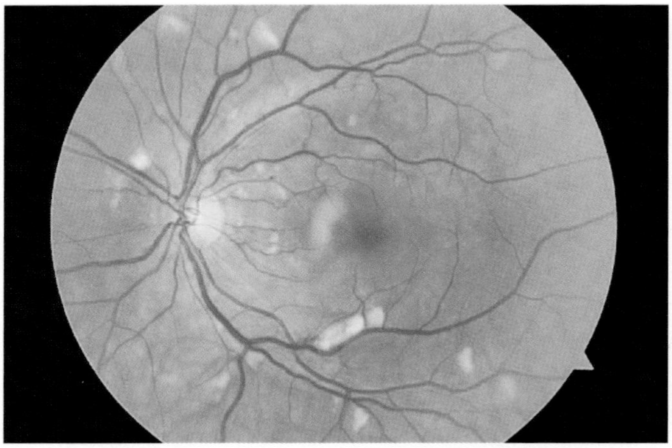

Plate 19 Cotton wool spots. Retinal microinfarcts are due to occlusion of capillaries which supply the nerve fibre layer. These multiple 'cotton wool spots' are found associated with microemboli, as after cardiac surgery employing bypass. In patients with AIDS they may form especially at the time of pulmonary infection, for instance with *Pneumocystis carinii*.

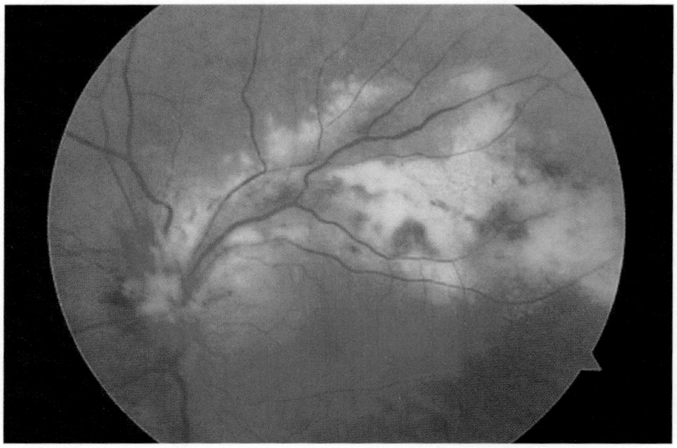

Plate 20 CMV retinitis. The appearance of focal, fluffy, pale retinal necrosis with haemorrhages is characteristic of infection with cytomegalovirus. The area expands relentlessly, spreading along the branch vessels, unless treatment with virustatic agent is instituted or the CD4 lymphocyte count can be improved. The usual underlying disorder is AIDS.

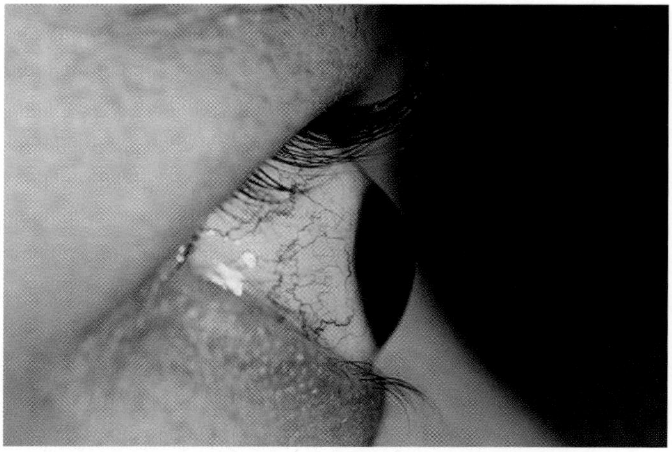

Plate 21 Thyroid eye disease with exophthalmos. Inflammation of orbital tissues—fat and muscles—causes protrustion of the eye—exophthalmos or proptosis. The eyelids also become swollen and the conjunctiva congested. Autoimmune thyroid disease (Graves' disease) is the most common underlying disorder.

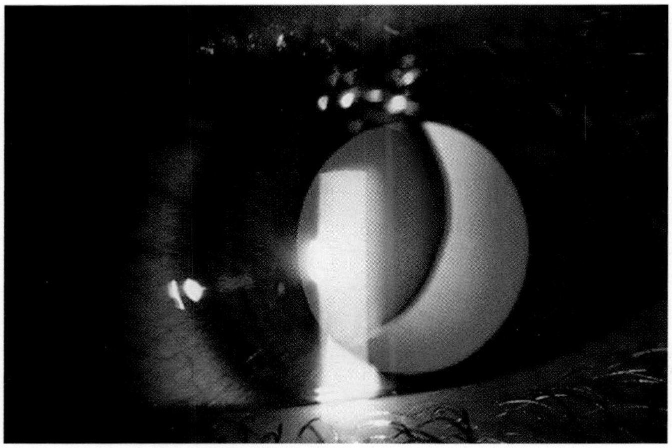

Plate 22 Marfan's syndrome. Dislocation of the lens is sometimes easily visible, though lesser degrees may need careful examination using the slit lamp after dilatation of the pupil. The lens may also be unstable, trembling on eye movement. The most common underlying cause is Marfan's syndrome, with deficiency of fibrillin in the suspensory fibres and upward displacement.

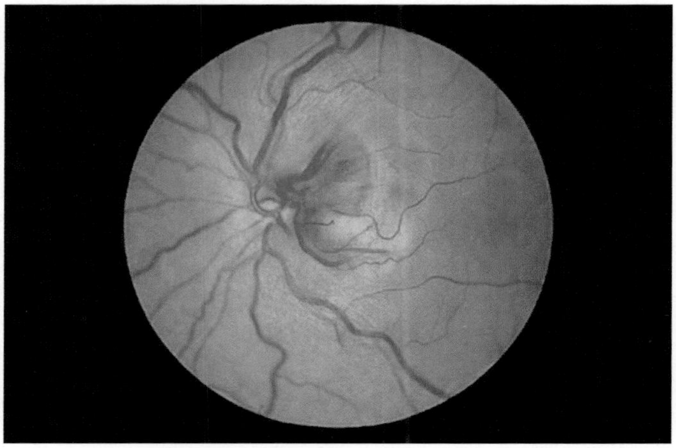

Plate 23 Von Hippel Lindau. Angiomas of the retina are an important early feature of this dominantly inherited condition. They begin as small red lesions which expand. Here the angioma is next to the optic disc, a characteristic position which makes management difficult and visual prognosis poor.

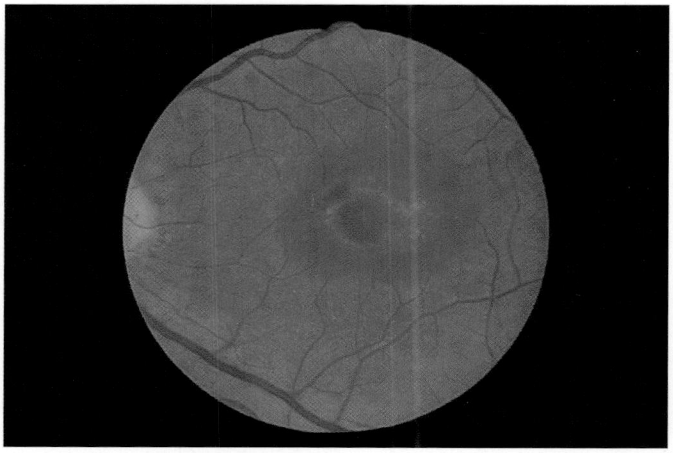

Plate 24 Bull's eye maculopathy. Toxicity at the macula caused by chloroquine results in a concentric target-like pigmentary appearance. The features are reversible in the early, asymptomatic, stages, but once loss of central visual acuity occurs, this may progress despite stopping the drug. Hydroxychloroquine appears to carry a lesser risk.

Acquired von Willebrand syndrome

Rarely, bleeding is caused by a severe acquired deficiency of vWF, most often in the setting of a monoclonal gammopathy, benign or malignant. Typically, there is disproportional deficiency of the largest vWF multimers due to antibody-mediated clearance (acquired type 2a von Willebrand syndrome (vWD)). Aortic stenosis and obstructive cardiomyopathies are other causes of type 2a von Willebrand syndrome: this probably explains why aortic valve replacement has been reported to cure recurrent gastrointestinal haemorrhage in patients with colonic angiodysplasia.

Heparin and acquired heparin-like anticoagulants

Bleeding is a complication of heparin treatment, particularly when the aPTT is above the therapeutic range. In patients with massive accidental or deliberate heparin overdose, intravenous protamine should be given to treat bleeding complications.

Rarely, patients with spontaneous bleeding and prolonged aPTT and TCT measurements have circulating heparin-like anticoagulants. Usually associated with multiple myeloma and other plasma-cell dyscrasias, the coagulopathy does not necessarily respond even to large-dose protamine infusion, and fatal haemorrhage can ensue. Circulating dermatan sulphate glycosaminoglycan appeared to explain the bleeding in a patient with renal failure.

Coagulopathies secondary to plasma-cell dyscrasias

Multiple myeloma, macroglobulin*aemi*a, and other plasma-cell dyscrasias such as primary amyloidosis can cause various coagulopathies (Table 8). Usually, the TCT is prolonged, most often because of paraprotein-induced interference with fibrin polymerization. A long bleeding time suggests inhibition of platelet function by paraprotein; rarely, acquired von Willebrand syndrome is the cause. Apheresis can improve haemostasis by quickly reducing paraprotein levels, as antineoplastic chemotherapy is initiated.

Hyperfibrinolysis

Activation of fibrinolysis occurs normally when fibrin clots are formed during physiological or pathological haemostasis. However, primary fibrinolysis (Table 3) is sometimes the major cause for bleeding, and requires specific treatment.

Thrombolytic therapy

About 0.5 to 0.7 per cent of patients with myocardial infarction who receive thrombolysis with either streptokinase or tissue plasminogen activator (**t-PA**) develop an intracranial haemorrhage. The thrombolytic agent should be stopped immediately in any such patient, and they should receive cryoprecipitate and an antifibrinolytic drug (for instance, EACA); platelets and FFP can help to increase factor V and VIII levels that may have been reduced by plasmin generated by thrombolysis. It can take between 24 and 36 h for fibrinogen levels to recover after stopping thrombolytic therapy.

Table 8 Haemostatic abnormalities associated with dysproteinaemias

Interference with fibrinogen polymerization
Isolated factor deficiency:
factor X, fibrinogen, or α_2-antiplasmin deficiency (amyloidosis)
acquired von Willebrand's disease (benign monoclonal gammopathy)
Hyperviscosity (comprising vascular integrity)
Circulating glycosaminoglycans (heparin-like inhibitor)
Thrombocytopenia secondary to marrow:
marrow failure (disease- or treatment-related)
autoimmune thrombocytopenia
Platelet dysfunction

Malignancy

Cancer-associated DIC usually causes a hypercoagulable state. However, promyelocytic leuk*aemi*a (**PML**) and prostatic adenocarcinoma are two malignancies commonly associated with prominent hyperfibrinolysis. Laboratory abnormalities include prolonged PT/INR, aPTT, and TCT, and a hypofibrinogen*aemi*a. The use of all-*trans*- retinoic acid (**ATRA**) during induction chemotherapy of PML has reduced the frequency of life-threatening bleeding. Antifibrinolytic therapy can control bleeding in cancer-associated fibrinolysis, but there is a risk of thrombosis if tissue factor-induced DIC, rather than the release of plasminogen activator by the tumour, is primarily responsible for the coagulopathy.

Cardiopulmonary bypass surgery

Excess bleeding, defined as more than 1 litre per procedure, is a common problem following heart surgery utilizing cardiopulmonary bypass (extracorporeal circulation). About 20 per cent of all red cell concentrates in the United States are given for cardiac surgical bleeding. About 5 per cent of patients require urgent resternotomy for critical rates of blood loss (defined as: >500 ml in the first h; >400 ml/h in the first 2 h; >300 ml/h in the first 3 h; or >1 litre in 4 h). Re-exploration reveals bleeding vessels in two-thirds of patients; the remainder have diffuse oozing.

Thrombocytopenia, transient platelet dysfunction, and hyperfibrinolysis are the major haemostatic defects. Typically, the platelet count falls by between 30 and 60 per cent mainly from haemodilution, although platelet losses from bleeding and within the extracorporeal perfusion device also occur. The thrombocytopenia persists for 3 to 4 days, followed by recovery of the platelet count to values exceeding the preoperative baseline. Marked prolongation of the bleeding time (>30 min) quickly improves to under 15 min shortly after surgery, and to normal several hours later. Some platelet function defects are 'extrinsic' and reversible (for example, hypothermia, heparin), whereas others indicate longer-lasting 'intrinsic' changes (surface glycoprotein deficiency, acquired-granule depletion). Preoperative treatment with aspirin or abciximab also increases bleeding.

The importance of hyperfibrinolysis in postcardiac surgical bleeding is suggested by meta-analysis of studies of high-dose aprotinin, a plasmin inhibitor derived from bovine lung: a two-thirds reduction in blood transfusion, and 50 per cent reduction in resternotomy. Other antifibrinolytic drugs that reduce bleeding include the lysine analogues, tranexamic acid (for example, 10 mg/kg bolus pre-cardiopulmonary bypass (**CPB**); then 1 mg/kg per h, although dosing regimens vary widely) and EACA (total dose, up to 20 g). Although these therapies are usually given before CPB, they may also provide benefit when used postoperatively for bleeding patients.

Management of postcardiac surgical bleeding also includes blood transfusions, especially platelets and fresh-frozen plasma, although their benefit is unproven. Residual heparin, including heparin 'rebound', can respond to additional protamine. Desmopressin probably is ineffective. No universally accepted algorithm for management exists.

Liver disease

Hyperfibrinolysis complicating liver disease is discussed elsewhere.

Venom-induced coagulopathies (snake bites) (see also Chapter 8.2)

Envenomations can harm or kill humans generally through systemic effects, for instance profound hypotension. Sometimes, however, life-threatening coagulopathies result.

Snake bites

In the United States, about 8000 bites from venomous snakes occur each year, resulting in 10 to 20 deaths. This relatively low mortality reflects the less lethal character of New World snakes, as well as the victim's usual close proximity to medical facilities and antivenin therapy. Pit vipers (rattlesnakes, copperheads, cottonmouths, massasaugas) account for 99 per cent of snakebite poisonings in the United States. Worldwide, about 30 000 to 40 000 people die from snakebite, about half in India. Although death usually results from multiple mechanisms (such as circulatory shock, rhabdomyolysis, renal failure, pulmonary failure, neurotoxicity), bleeding is sometimes the major factor.

Venoms contain multiple digestive enzymes with a broad spectrum of activity that can include effects on human haemostasis (Table 9). Within a species, haemostatic effects of envenomation vary with snake age, diet, and other factors. North American rattlesnakes typically cause the 'defibrination syndrome'; despite even profound hypofibrinogen*aemia*, bleeding is uncommon. In contrast, venom from Old World vipers frequently cause generalized activation of the coagulation system (DIC), with a greater chance for bleeding or microvascular thrombosis. Bleeding can also result from platelet inhibitors present within venom; for example, the platelet fibrinogen receptor antagonist, echistatin (*Echis carinatus*), or 'haemorrhagins' such as jararhagin (*Bothrops jararacussu*) that damage endothelium.

Immediate treatment of a snake bite includes efforts to limit the venom spread (immobilizing and placing a constriction band proximal to the bite site). Rapid transport to medical facilities is crucial since antivenin therapy is the mainstay of treatment. Antivenin treatment is indicated for patients with significant pain or swelling, as well as suspected or proven haemostasis abnormalities, as these indicate envenomation rather than a 'dry bite'. Hypersensitivity testing to the antivenin should be performed to rule out pre-existing hypersensitivity to horse serum. The treatment of snake bite is discussed in Chapter 8.2.

Coagulation studies should include: complete blood count (including platelets), PT/INR, aPTT, TCT, fibrinogen, and FDPs. Abnormal results indicate envenomation, and are an indication for antivenin therapy. The bedside assessment of defibrination involves placing a few millilitres of blood in a clean, dry test tube at room temperature for 20 min; incoagulable blood indicates defibrination. Usually, blood products should only be given to patients with bleeding. A small clinical trial found that heparin was ineffective in patients with DIC caused by a Russell's viper bite.

Laboratory and therapeutic uses of snake venoms

Snake-venom fractions are useful for certain laboratory assays. For example, the thrombin-like enzyme, batroxobin (Reptilase®, *Bothrops atrox moojeni*), cleaves fibrinopeptide A from fibrinogen even in the presence of heparin. Thus, a prolonged Reptilase time indicates hypofibrinogen*aemia* even in heparin-containing plasma.

Ecarin activates prothrombin irrespective of its γ-carboxylation status; thus, it can be used to detect **PIVKA** (proteins induced by vitamin K antagonists) to document vitamin K deficiency or dysprothrombin*aemia*. An ecarin clotting time (**ECT**) is superior to the aPTT for monitoring therapy with hirudin, particularly the high doses used for heart surgery. Differences in phospholipid dependency of venom prothrombin activators has led to the use of a Textarin®/ecarin ratio to detect lupus anticoagulants; a ratio over 1.3 is a sensitive and relatively specific test for lupus anticoagulants.

Russell's viper venom contains a potent activator of factor X (**RVV-X**); the dilute Russell's viper venom time (**dRVVT**), performed by adding RVV-X and diluted rabbit brain phospholipid to test plasma prior to recalcification, measures the rate of formation and activity of the phospholipid-dependent prothrombinase complex in producing thrombin. The dRVVT is thereby prolonged in the presence of a lupus anticoagulant.

A commercially available protein C activator (Protac®) from *Agkistrodon contortrix contortrix* (the southern copperhead) has greatly simplified assays for protein C activity, as well as in screening for defects in the protein C anticoagulant pathway.

The defibrinogenating snake venom, ancrod (Arvin®, derived from the Malayan pit viper, *Calloselasma [Agkistrodon] rhodostoma*), which proteolyses fibrinopeptide A, has been used for antithrombotic therapy, including the management of heparin-induced thrombocytopenia (**HIT**), acute stroke, thrombotic nephropathy, and priapism. The inability to control thrombin generation is a potential drawback of this therapy. Batroxobin (Defibrase®) is another defibrinogenating venom that has seen limited clinical applications.

Prothrombotic acquired coagulation disorders

Some acquired coagulation disorders are characterized by an increased risk for thrombosis, rather than bleeding. Accordingly, the appropriate treatment usually involves anticoagulant therapy, even if there are abnormal coagulation or platelet count values.

Macrovascular thrombosis

Some acquired coagulation disorders typically cause thrombosis in large veins and arteries, although small-vessel thrombi can also result.

Heparin-induced thrombocytopenia

Heparin-induced thrombocytopenia (**HIT**) is caused by IgG antibodies that recognize multimolecular complexes of platelet factor 4 (**PF4**) and heparin. Thrombosis results from IgG-induced platelet activation (via platelet Fc receptors), resulting in the generation of procoagulant, platelet-derived microparticles, tissue-factor expression by endothelium, and inactivation of heparin by PF4 released from platelets. Increased thrombin–antithrombin complex levels indicate DIC in almost all patients with HIT, although a prolonged INR or low fibrinogen level occur in less than 10 per cent of cases.

Typically, the fall in platelet count begins 5 to 10 days after starting heparin; however, in patients who received heparin within the past 100 days, the platelet count can fall abruptly upon resuming heparin therapy, probably because of residual circulating HIT antibodies. HIT occurs in as many as 5 per cent of certain high-risk populations: for example, postoperative orthopaedic patients receiving unfractionated heparin. HIT is less frequent in patients initially treated with low-molecular-weight heparin (**LMWH**).

Most patients with HIT develop venous or arterial thrombosis (Fig. 2), most commonly a deep-vein thrombosis (**DVT**), pulmonary embolism, major limb artery thrombosis, stroke, or myocardial infarction. Acute or chronic adrenal failure from bilateral adrenal haemorrhagic necrosis has been described. The thrombocytopenia is typically moderate in severity (median platelet count nadir, 60×10^9/l), but in only 10 per cent of patients does the platelet count fall to less than 20×10^9/l. In at least 10 per cent of patients, the platelet count never drops below 150×10^9/l (Fig. 2).

Laboratory testing for HIT antibodies includes activation and antigen assays. The former assays detect antibodies via their heparin-dependent, platelet-activating properties. Commercially available antigen assays detect antibodies that bind to surface-immobilized PF4 complexed to heparin or polyvinylsulphonate.

Treatment includes stopping heparin and instituting alternative anticoagulation. Coumarin alone should not be given to patients with acute HIT, particularly to those with associated DVT, as there is a risk for inducing progression to venous limb gangrene. The dramatic natural history of HIT, with a risk for subsequent thrombosis of about 50 per cent even after stopping heparin, means that an alternative anticoagulant, together with DVT surveillance, should be considered for all patients with suspected HIT. Suitable anticoagulants with a rapid-onset of action include danaparoid (a low-molecular-weight heparinoid with predominant anti-factor Xa activity), lepirudin (a recombinant hirudin with potent antithrombin activity derived from leech salivary glands), and argatroban (a synthetic, small-molecule, direct thrombin inhibitor). Among patients with HIT, LMWH treatment has a high risk for clinical crossreactivity, and should be considered a contraindicated treatment for acute HIT. Many patients will

Table 9 Venom-induced coagulopathies (selected examples)

Animal source of venom	Main biological effects (trivial name of venom component in bold)	Comments	Main distribution
Venomous snakes			
Family Viperidae			
SUBFAMILY CROTALINAE (PIT VIPERS*)			
Crotalus adamanteus (Eastern diamondback rattlesnake)	**Crotalase**: cleaves FPA, but not FPB, from fibrinogen (decreased fibrinogen, plasminogen; increased FDPs)	'Thrombin-like' based upon fibrinopeptide A cleavage, but does not activate platelets or factor XIII; despite 'defibrination syndrome', bleeding is uncommon	USA (coastal plain from Florida to Mississippi)
Crotalus atrox (Western diamondback rattlesnake)	**Catroxobin**: cleaves FPA from fibrinogen; other fibrinogenase activities	Also causes defibrination syndrome, usually without bleeding; venom also contains catrocollastatin-C (platelet inhibitor)	USA (California to Arkansas); Mexico
Calloselasma [Agkistrodon] rhodostoma (Malayan pit viper)	**Ancrod**: cleaves FPA from fibrinogen	Purified ancrod used as an antithrombotic agent	Southeast Asia
SUBFAMILY VIPERINAE (TRUE VIPERS)			
Echis carinatus (saw-scaled viper)	**Ecarin**: activates prothrombin and platelets	Causes DIC, often with bleeding; most common cause of snake-bite mortality in the African savannah	India, Africa, Asia
Daboia russelli (Russell's viper, formerly, *Vipera russelli*)	**Russell's viper venom**: activates factor X	Causes DIC, often with bleeding; venom also causes direct nephrotoxicity	Far East
Bothrops jararacussu (jararacucu, lance-headed pit viper)	**Botrocetin**: platelet agglutination via vWF; **Jararhagin**: haemorrhagin	Venom also contains thrombin-like and factor Xa-activating enzymes, and can cause severe bleeding	Brazil
Family Elapidae**			
Notechis scutatus (tiger snake)	**Notecarin**: activates prothrombin	Fatal haemorrhage has been reported	Australia
Family Colubridae***			
Non-snake envenomations that cause coagulopathy			
Lonomia achelous (caterpillar)	Proteolysis of factor XIII; reduced fibrinogen, factor V, plasminogen, and increased FDPs also observed	Severe bleeding in humans (wound site, mucous membranes, and internal haemorrhage)	Venezuela, Brazil
Loxosceles reclusa (brown recluse spider)	Activation of endothelium, with resulting dysfunction of interactions with PMNs	Potential for severe skin lesions; systemic effects (DIC,haemolytic anaemia) occur in small minority of patients	Midwest USA

Two other families of venomous snakes (Hydrophiidae and Atractaspididae) do not cause coagulopathies.

*Pit vipers are New World snakes named for the heat-sensitive pit located between the eye and the nostril that enables the snake to detect warm-blooded prey even in darkness: the three genera of the Crotalidae family that inhabit the US are *Crotalus* (rattlesnakes), *Agkistrodon* (moccasins, including the copperheads and cottonmouths), and *Sistrurus* (massasaugas and pigmy rattlesnakes).

**With the exception of several Australian species, such as taipan, tiger snakes, brown snakes, and black snakes, elapid snake bites usually cause neurotoxicity, and only occasionally result in haemostatic abnormalities.

***The colubrid family includes: boomslang, vine snake, keel backs, and the South American 'green snake,' which can also cause bleeding.

Abbreviations: DIC, disseminated intravascular coagulation; FPD(s), fibrin(ogen) degradation product(s); FPA, fibrinopeptide A; PMNs, polymorphonuclear leucocytes; vWF, von Willebrand factor.

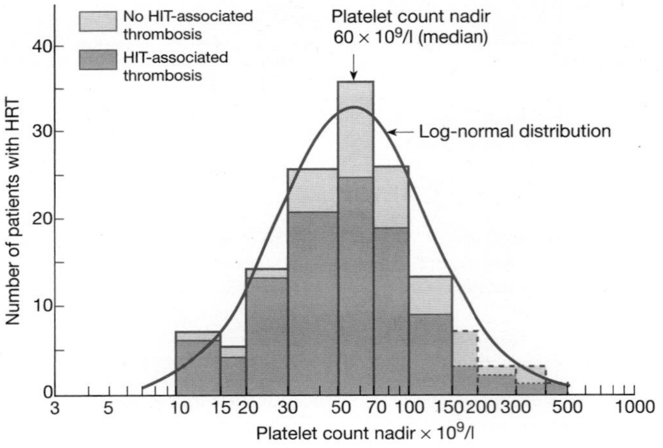

Fig. 2 Thrombosis in relation to the severity of thrombocytopenia in patients with HIT. The magnitude of thrombocytopenia in HIT shows a log-normal distribution. Thrombocytopenia is typically mild-to-moderate (between 20 and 150 × 10^9/l in about 80 per cent of patients; median platelet count nadir, about 60 × 10^9/l). Thrombosis occurs in 50 per cent or more of patients with HIT, irrespective of the platelet count nadir, including patients whose platelet count never falls below 150 × 10^9/l. (Reprinted with permission from Warkentin, 1998.)

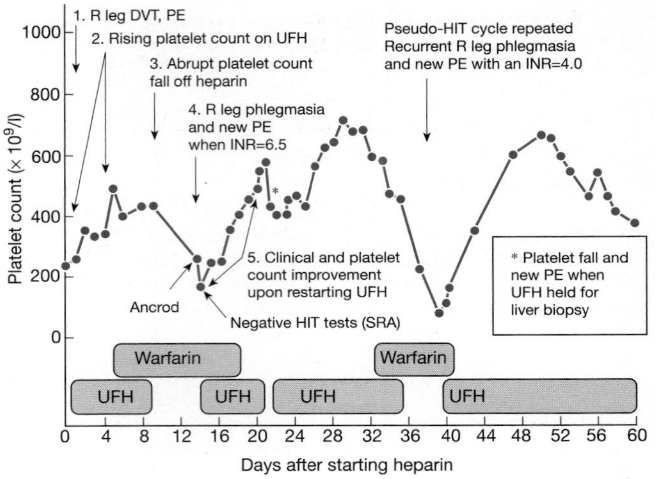

Fig. 3 Pseudo-HIT. Adenocarcinoma with thrombocytopenia and phlegmasia cerulea dolens after stopping unfractionated heparin (UFH). The timing of thrombocytopenia onset suggested HIT, prompting the use of an alternative anticoagulant (ancrod). Heparin was restarted when HIT antibodies were not detected by activation assay (serotonin-release assay, SRA). Subsequently, heparin discontinuation led to the recurrence of thrombocytopenia and warfarin-associated phlegmasia cerulea dolens (repeat of pseudo-HIT cycle). Abbreviations: DVT, deep venous thrombosis; INR, international normalized ratio; PE, pulmonary embolism.

benefit from selected adjunctive treatments, for instance surgical thromboembolectomy for acute arterial thrombosis of a limb.

Adenocarcinoma-associated chronic DIC

Metastatic adenocarcinoma sometimes presents as venous or arterial thrombosis accompanied by DIC. The diagnosis is suggested by an unexpected rise in the platelet count during heparin treatment, followed by an abrupt platelet count fall, together with new or progressive thrombosis, when heparin is stopped, despite therapeutic anticoagulation with warfarin. The clinical situation can mimic HIT ('pseudo-HIT'), but HIT antibodies are absent, and the platelet count recovers during resumption of heparin (Fig. 3). Oral anticoagulants are ineffective, and may even cause venous limb gangrene (discussed subsequently). Heparin, especially LMWH, is the preferred treatment. Tissue factor-containing tumour vesicles, and factor Xa-activating enzymes found in tumour extracts, are two possible explanations for these procoagulant effects of adenocarcinoma.

Antiphospholipid antibody syndrome ('lupus anticoagulant')

This clinicopathological syndrome is characterized by large-vessel venous and/or arterial thrombosis, recurrent miscarriages, and thrombocytopenia. An associated 'lupus anticoagulant' (or 'non-specific inhibitor') is a prolonged aPTT that results from the interference by antibodies against phospholipid-dependent coagulation reactions; these antiphospholipid antibodies are usually directed against protein cofactors such as β_2-glycoprotein I (**β2GPI**) and prothrombin. Sometimes, a prolonged PT/INR is caused by non-neutralizing antiprothrombin antibodies that cause hypoprothrombinaemia by increased prothrombin clearance.

Despite these laboratory abnormalities, bleeding is unusual, since severe thrombocytopenia or hypoprothrombinaemia is uncommon. More often, antiphospholipid antibodies are associated with intermittent thrombosis; rarely, the abrupt onset of life-threatening multiple vascular occlusions occurs ('catastrophic antiphospholipid antibody syndrome'). The explanation for the paradoxical association with thrombosis remains elusive, but it could be caused by antibody interactions with other protein cofactors described (for example, activated protein C, protein S, thrombomodulin). Many patients have a thrombocytopenia that is typically mild and intermittent. Other less common complications include cardiac valvulitis and microvascular thrombosis, which can manifest as acrocyanosis, digital ulceration/gangrene, and livedo reticularis.

Antiphospholipid antibodies are detected by enzyme-linked immunosorbent assays (**ELISA**) using purified phospholipids as the target antigen, for example the anticardiolipin antibody assay. Lupus anticoagulant activity is shown by demonstrating inhibition of phospholipid-dependent coagulation assays. Several assays should be performed, as anti-β_2GPI antibodies especially interfere with the conversion of prothrombin to thrombin (that is, best detectable by dRVVT), whereas antiprothrombin antibodies interfere most with global coagulation assays (for instance, kaolin clotting time). The coagulation times remain prolonged following mixing with normal plasma; confirmation involves adding excess phospholipid to neutralize the effects of the antiphospholipid antibodies. Not all aPTT reagents are sensitive to antiphospholipid antibodies, and so these phospholipid-dependent coagulation assays should be performed in the appropriate clinical situation, even if the aPTT is normal.

The term 'lupus anticoagulant' refers to the frequent occurrence of these antibodies in patients with systemic lupus erythematosus; nevertheless, most patients with the antiphospholipid antibody syndrome do not have SLE. Some patients have other autoimmune disorders, malignancy, infections, or procainamide treatment, but usually no associated condition is identified (primary antiphospholipid antibody syndrome). Many patients require long-term anticoagulation, although the optimal agents and therapeutic level of anticoagulation remain to be defined. Corticosteroids can benefit patients with bleeding caused by hypoprothrombinaemia.

Microvascular thrombosis

Some disorders of haemostasis are characterized by small-vessel thrombi, affecting either arterioles (for example, TTP) or small venules (for example, coumarin-induced necrosis).

Thrombotic microangiopathy

Thrombotic microangiopathy is a clinicopathological syndrome of microangiopathic haemolysis and thrombocytopenia carrying a risk for arteriolar occlusion by microaggregates of platelets and vWF, particularly affecting the kidneys and central nervous system. Microangiopathic red cell changes are characteristic, for example 'helmet cells' (schistocytes) and small, triangle-shaped, red cell fragments. The prototypic illness is thrombotic thrombocytopenic purpura (**TTP**), which typically affects adults and is idiopathic. However, familial and secondary forms of TTP also exist. The haemolytic-uraemic syndrome is a nephrotropic variant of TTP with a distinct pathogenesis, including its association with verocytotoxin-producing *Escherichia coli* acquired from eating undercooked meat (hamburger disease).

The pathogenesis of TTP involves the formation of platelet–vWF microaggregates in high shear situations (arterioles). Platelet-bound vWF levels are increased during TTP. Patients with familial TTP have ultra-large multimers of vWF during remission; these very large multimers disappear during active disease. Recently, a constitutional deficiency of a vWF-cleaving metalloproteinase has been identified in patients with familial TTP. In patients with non-familial TTP, an IgG autoantibody, which inhibits the vWF-cleaving metalloproteinase, has been identified that disappears in remission.

The mainstays of treatment for acute TTP are corticosteroids and fresh-frozen plasma given by infusion or apheresis. Corticosteroids, often given as prednisone 200 mg/day, may treat the autoimmune component of TTP. Provision of either fresh-frozen plasma, or the cryoprecipitate-depleted fraction of plasma (cryosupernatant), has greatly reduced mortality in TTP, possibly by providing limited disulphide-bond reductase activity that facilitates vWF cleavage. Furthermore, apheresis may help cleave the pathogenic autoantibody and large vWF multimers.

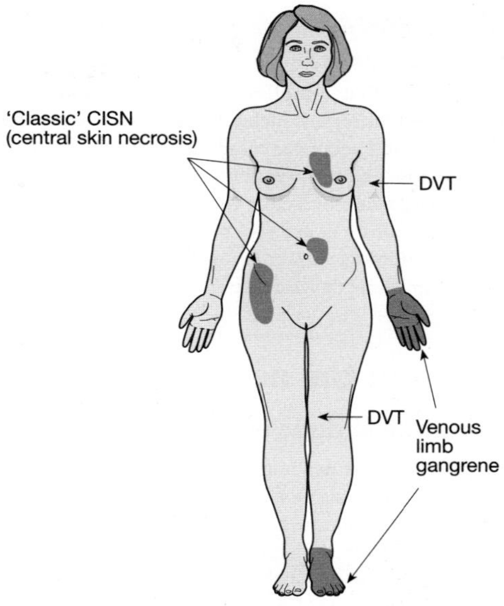

Fig. 4 Coumarin-induced skin necrosis: 'classic' syndrome (usually affecting central tissue sites) and coumarin-induced venous limb gangrene. Typically, an active deep-vein thrombosis (DVT) subtends the distal extremity affected by venous limb gangrene. (Reprinted with permission from Warkentin, 1996.)

Coumarin-induced skin necrosis

Coumarin-induced skin necrosis (**CISN**) is characterized by necrosis of the skin and underlying subcutaneous tissues that typically begins 3 to 6 days after commencing warfarin or coumarin anticoagulants. CISN results from failure of the protein C natural anticoagulant system to downregulate thrombin generation in the microvasculature. The relatively short half-life of protein C, compared with prothrombin, explains the temporal profile of CISN—that is to say, a transient period of disproportionately reduced protein C activity soon after starting coumarin (Table 10). Furthermore, a relatively high proportion of affected patients have a hereditary abnormality of the protein C anticoagulant pathway, especially protein C deficiency. Other disorders associated with CISN include congenital deficiency in protein S or antithrombin, factor V Leiden, and HIT. The pathology is a predominantly non-inflammatory, small-vessel thrombosis affecting the subcutaneous postcapillary venules and small veins.

CISN characteristically affects central (non-acral) sites with substantial underlying fatty tissues, such as the breast, buttocks, hips, and thighs (Fig. 4). Less common areas include the anterior abdomen, flank, back, penis, legs, arms, and face. About 75 per cent of patients are women; one-third have multiple lesions that can be symmetrical. The earliest features are localized pain, induration, and erythema; over the next few hours, the skin lesions progress to central purplish or black discoloration, with blistering, subsequently demarcating to full-thickness skin necrosis. CISN is rare (1/10 000 patients treated with warfarin).

Prompt reversal of anticoagulation with vitamin K may prevent incipient CISN if recognized early. However, the diagnosis is usually not made until necrosis is established; at this point, it is unknown whether vitamin K, fresh-frozen plasma, or protein C concentrates alter its natural history. In patients without HIT, warfarin is usually replaced by heparin. Many patients require surgical treatment, such as skin grafting or tissue amputation. Following recovery, it is usually safe to reintroduce warfarin provided certain precautions are taken, for example the gradual initiation of oral anticoagulation.

Table 10 Half-lives of vitamin K-dependent procoagulant and anticoagulant factors

Procoagulant factors	Half-life (h)	Anticoagulant factors	Half-life (h)
Factor II, or prothrombin	60	Protein C	9
Factor X	40	Protein S	40–60
Factor IX	24		
Factor VII	4–6		

The longer half-life of the major procoagulant vitamin K-dependent zymogen (factor II, or prothrombin), compared with the major natural anticoagulant factor (protein C), is relevant to the pathogenesis of CISN (see text).

Coumarin-induced venous limb gangrene

Venous limb gangrene involves the acral (peripheral) regions of the body—most often the toes, feet, and legs, but sometimes also the fingers, hands, and arms—usually in association with DVT. The severity ranges from an initial stage of phlegmasia caerulea dolens ('swollen, blue, painful' limb) to extensive venous limb gangrene requiring limb amputation. Two disorders predispose to coumarin-induced venous limb gangrene: HIT and cancer-associated DIC. Recent data suggest that the supratherapeutic INR (typically, >3.5) that characterizes venous limb gangrene is caused by a severe reduction in factor VII, which parallels a severe reduction in protein C activity that explains the microvascular thrombosis underlying this syndrome. Essentially, coumarin interferes with the protein C anticoagulant pathway, while at the same time it is unable to control the increased thrombin generation characteristic of HIT or cancer-associated DIC.

Purpura fulminans

Purpura fulminans is a rare syndrome of DIC and microvascular thrombosis that results in multicentric ischaemic necrosis of the skin and subcutaneous tissues, predominantly affecting the extremities. The most common cause is overwhelming septicaemia, especially with meningococcus. A severe, acquired reduction in protein C activity complicating DIC is the most likely cause for the microvascular thrombosis, and some experts recommend treatment with protein C concentrates, if available. Autoantibodies against protein S have been implicated in patients with postvaricella purpura fulminans. In other patients with apparent 'idiopathic' purpura fulminans, autoantibodies that interfere with the protein C anticoagulant system have been described.

Septicaemia and other systemic inflammatory response syndromes

Multiple organ failure often complicates septicaemia and other systemic inflammatory disease syndromes, including adult respiratory distress syndrome, fat embolism, and acute pancreatitis. Thrombocytopenia and coagulopathy are common, and some patients have DIC that could contribute to organ dysfunction via microvascular thrombosis. However, a prothrombotic basis for organ failure is usually speculative, as microthrombosis is rarely documented pathologically, and non-thrombotic microvascular disturbances that impair tissue oxygen delivery also occur.

Haemostasis in the newborn

Neonatal vitamin K deficiency

Haemorrhagic disease of the newborn caused by vitamin K deficiency was once a relatively common cause of bleeding during the first week of life, particularly in breast-fed infants. Low vitamin K levels in mother's milk, and insufficient colonization of the newborn bowel by vitamin K-producing bacteria, predispose to the inability to meet the infant's vitamin K requirements (1 μg/kg per day). The routine administration of vitamin K, either 1 mg given intramuscularly immediately after birth, or three oral doses of vitamin K, has led to the near-disappearance of this problem. Bleeding within 24 h of birth can occur in certain high-risk settings, for example mothers receiving anticonvulsants or warfarin; in these cases, the mother should receive vitamin K, 10 mg by mouth, each day for 2 weeks prior to delivery. Vitamin K deficiency occurring later in infancy despite appropriate neonatal vitamin K prophylaxis can indicate hepatobiliary or bowel disease.

Neonatal disseminated intravascular coagulation

DIC commonly complicates neonatal infection, asphyxia, respiratory distress syndrome, aspiration of meconium or amniotic fluid, maternal hypertensive syndrome, hypothermia, and brain injury. This condition poses a significant risk of bleeding or thrombosis, as the immature liver has an impaired capacity to synthesize coagulation factors, and the reticuloendothelial system has a limited ability to clear activated coagulation factors. Treatment is aimed at the underlying cause of the DIC, with blood product given for the bleeding.

Neonatal purpura fulminans

Purpura fulminans can begin within hours or days following birth, often first affecting the heels or venepuncture sites. The underlying cause is usually a congenital abnormality affecting the protein C anticoagulant system (homozygous deficiency of protein C or protein S; homozygous factor V Leiden), although infection with group B β-haemolytic streptococcus is described. Fresh-frozen plasma given every few days prevents a recurrence in some patients.

Further reading

Ansell J, *et al.* (2001). Managing oral anticoagulant therapy. *Chest* **119**, 22S–38S. [Discusses the management of non-therapeutic (elevated) INRs in patients receiving oral anticoagulants (Recommendations of the Sixth American College of Chest Physicians Consensus Conference on Antithrombotic Therapy).]

Asherson RA, *et al.* (1998). Catastrophic antiphospholipid syndrome. Clinical and laboratory features of 50 patients. *Medicine* (Baltimore) **77**, 195–207. [Describes clinical presentations of multiorgan failure in patients with antiphospholipid antibodies.]

Bevan DH (1999). Cardiac bypass haemostasis: putting blood through the mill. *British Journal of Haematology* **104**, 208–19. [Excellent review of cardiopulmonary bypass surgery and approaches to bleeding.]

Bossi P, *et al.* (1998). Acquired hemophilia due to factor VIII inhibitors in 34 patients. *American Journal of Medicine* **105**, 400–8. [Summarizes the presentation and clinical course of this disorder.]

Cole MS, Minifee PK, Wolma FJ (1988). Coumarin necrosis—a review of the literature. *Surgery* **103**, 271–7. [Comprehensive review of coumarin-induced skin necrosis.]

Hirsh J, *et al.* (1998). Oral anticoagulants. Mechanism of action, clinical effectiveness, and optimal therapeutic range. *Chest* **114**, 445S–469S. [Lists drugs and foods that interact with warfarin.]

Hutton RA, Warrell DA (1993). Action of snake venom components on the haemostatic system. *Blood Reviews* **7**, 176–89. [Good synthesis of clinical and laboratory aspects of snake envenomation.]

Kitchens CS (1992). Hemostatic aspects of envenomation by North American snakes. *Hematology/Oncology Clinics of North America* **6**, 1189–95. [The focus is on envenomation by North American snakes, resulting in defibrination rather than true DIC syndromes.]

Levi M, Ten Cate H (1999). Disseminated intravascular coagulation. *New England Journal of Medicine* **341**, 586–92. [Recent review.]

Levine JS, Branch DW, Rauch J (2002). The antiphospholipid syndrome. *New England Journal of Medicine* **346**, 752–63. [Recent review.]

Manco-Johnson MJ, *et al.* (1996). Lupus anticoagulant and protein S deficiency in children with postvaricella purpura fulminans or thrombosis. *Journal of Pediatrics* **128**, 319–23. [Provides evidence that purpura fulminans following varicella infection is usually caused by autoantibodies to protein S.]

Marsh NA (1998). Use of snake venom fractions in the coagulation laboratory. *Blood Coagulation and Fibrinolysis* **9**, 395–404. [Discusses many laboratory uses of snake venom fractions.]

Meier J, Stocker K (1991). Effects of snake venoms on hemostasis. *Critical Reviews in Toxicology* **21**, 171–82. [Reviews multiplicity of effects of snake venoms on hemostasis.]

Moake JL, Chow TW (1998). Thrombotic thrombocytopenic purpura: understanding a disease no longer rare. *American Journal of Medical Sciences* **316**, 105–19. [Excellent summary of new concepts of TTP, including role for abnormalities in vWF-cleaving metalloproteinase and the autoimmune pathogenesis of TTP.]

Ortel TL, *et al.* (1994). Topical thrombin and acquired coagulation factor inhibitors: clinical spectrum and laboratory diagnosis. *American Journal of Hematology* **45**, 128–35. [Summarizes acquired coagulation inhibitors that occur following treatment with topical bovine thrombin preparations ('fibrin glue').]

Sane DC, *et al.* (1989). Bleeding during thrombolytic therapy for acute myocardial infarction: mechanisms and management. *Annals of Internal Medicine* **111**, 1010–22. [Describes the management of post-thrombolytic hemorrhage.]

Warkentin TE, *et al.* (1997). The pathogenesis of venous limb gangrene associated with heparin-induced thrombocytopenia. *Annals of Internal Medicine* **127**, 804–12. [Indicates that an oral anticoagulant (warfarin) can cause deep-vein thrombosis to progress to venous limb gangrene in patients with heparin-induced thrombocytopenia.]

Warkentin TE, *et al.* (1995). Heparin-induced thrombocytopenia in patients treated with low-molecular-weight heparin or unfractionated heparin. *New England Journal of Medicine* **332**, 1330–5. [Provides evidence that HIT is a prothrombotic state associated with venous and arterial thrombosis that occurs less frequently with low-molecular-weight heparin.]

Warkentin TE (1996). Heparin-induced thrombocytopenia IgG-mediated platelet activation, platelet microparticle generation, and altered procoagulant/anticoagulant balance in the pathogenesis of thrombosis and venous limb gangrene complicating heparin-induced thrombocytopenia. *Transfusion Medicine Reviews* **10**, 249–58. [Compares and contrasts the pathogenesis and clinical profile of coumarin-induced skin necrosis and coumarin-induced venous limb gangrene.]

Warkentin TE (1998). Clinical presentation of heparin-induced thrombocytopenia. *Seminars in Hematology* **35**(Suppl. 5), 9–16. [Summarizes the clinical features of HIT.]

Warkentin TE (2001). Venous limb gangrene during warfarin treatment of cancer-associated deep venous thrombosis. *Annals of Internal Medicine* **135**, 589–93. [Implicates warfarin in the pathogenesis of venous limb gangrene complicating cancer-associated DIC.]

Warkentin TE (2001). Pseudo-heparin-induced thrombocytopenia. In Warkentin TE, Greinacher A, eds. *Heparin-induced thrombocytopenia*, 2nd edn, pp. 271–89. Marcel Dekker, New York. [Describes disorders that clinically mimic heparin-induced thrombocytopenia.]

Wells PS, *et al.* (1994). Interactions of warfarin with drugs and food. *Annals of Internal Medicine* **121**, 676–83. [Identifies drugs and foods that interact with warfarin.]

22.7 The blood in systemic disease

D. J. Weatherall

There are few diseases that do not produce some alteration in the blood. Here, some of the haematological changes associated with general systemic diseases will be summarized. Many of these topics are discussed elsewhere in this book but they are brought together in order to emphasize how blood changes may give the first indication of the presence of non-haematological disorders. It should be remembered that the haematological consequences of systemic disease vary considerably depending on the age of the patient. Recent reviews which deal specifically with this topic in children and the elderly are cited at the end of this chapter.

Malignant disease

The most common haematological finding in malignant disease (Table 1) is the anaemia of chronic disorders, which was described in Chapter 22.5.3. It may occur together with localized or widespread malignancy and is sometimes associated with an elevated erythrocyte sedimentation rate (ESR). It is found in patients with practically every type of carcinoma or reticulosis, is refractory to haematinics, but may respond to successful removal of a primary tumour.

The anaemia of patients with carcinoma, particularly of the gastrointestinal tract, may be complicated by chronic blood loss and superimposed iron deficiency. Chronic bleeding of this type is often associated with a mild thrombocytosis.

Disseminated malignancy

The most common haematological change with disseminated malignancy is a leucoerythroblastic picture characterized by the presence in the blood of immature myeloid cells together with some nucleated red cells, and, sometimes, a mild reticulocytosis. The red cells often show a moderate degree of anisocytosis and poikilocytosis. This finding is very commonly accompanied by the presence of tumour cells in the bone marrow. Clinically, it can cause confusion with the diagnosis of primary myelosclerosis; but splenomegaly is unusual in patients with disseminated carcinoma.

Occasionally, widespread carcinoma leads to a leukaemoid reaction with white-cell counts in the range seen in chronic myeloid leukaemia. The differentiation between these two conditions was described earlier.

The microangiopathic haemolytic anaemia of disseminated malignancy is most frequently found in association with a mucin-secreting adenocarcinoma, particularly of the stomach, breast, and lung.

Less common forms of anaemia associated with cancer

Autoimmune haemolytic anaemia is sometimes found in patients with an underlying lymphoma. It is much less common in other forms of malignancy except for the association with tumours of the ovary. However, there have been reports of autoimmune haemolysis occurring with a wide variety of tumours, including lung, stomach, breast, kidney, colon, and testis.

Pure red-cell aplasia may occasionally be the presenting feature in a patient with a tumour of the thymus. There have been occasional reports of

Table 1 Principal haematological changes in malignant disorders

Haematological change	Malignancy
Erythrocytes	
Anaemia of chronic disorders	All forms
Iron-deficiency anaemia	Gastrointestinal; cervix, uterus
Leucoerythroblastic anaemia	Stomach, breast, thyroid, prostate, bronchus, kidney
Microangiopathic haemolytic anaemia	Mucin-secreting tumours; stomach, bronchus, breast
Secondary myelosclerosis	As for leucoerythroblastic; also reticuloses
Selective red-cell aplasia	Thymus, lymphoma, bronchus
Immune haemolytic anaemia	Ovary; lymphoma; other carcinomas
Megaloblastic anaemia	Stomach; rarely others
Sideroblastic anaemia	Myelodysplastic syndrome
Polycythaemia	Kidney, liver, posterior fossa, uterus
Leucocytes	
Leucocytosis	All forms
Leukaemoid reactions	As for leucoerythroblastic anaemia
Eosinophilia	Miscellaneous carcinomas and reticuloses
Monocytosis	All forms
Basophilia	Myeloproliferative disease; mastocytosis
Lymphopenia	Carcinoma, reticuloses
Platelets	
Thrombocytosis	Gastrointestinal with bleeding; bronchus and others without bleeding
Thrombocytopenia	As for the microangiopathies
Acquired thrombocytopathy	Macroglobulinaemia; other paraproteinaemias
Coagulation	
Disseminated intravascular coagulation	Prostate, many others
Primary activation of fibrinolysis	Prostate
Selective impairment of coagulation (see Table 2)	
Thrombophlebitis	All forms
Miscellaneous	
Abnormal proteins—cryofibrinogens	Prostate, others
Fetal proteins	α-fetoprotein—liver and others Carcinoembryonic antigen (CEA)—gastrointestinal neoplasms Fetal haemoglobin—leukaemia, other tumours
Circulating tumour cells	All forms
Effects of cytotoxic drugs	All forms

this type of anaemia occurring in patients with carcinoma of the bronchus or lymphomas.

Finally, it should be remembered that there is an association between pernicious anaemia and carcinoma of the stomach. A patient may present with a megaloblastic anaemia associated with a malignancy of this type. In the early literature on sideroblastic anaemia, an association with carcinoma was well documented. Since acquired sideroblastic anaemia has been classified as part of the myelodysplastic syndrome there seem to have been no further reports of this association and its significance remains uncertain.

Polycythaemia

The relation between secondary polycythaemia and an underlying neoplasm is discussed in Chapter 22.4.14. It has been found in patients with renal tumours, hepatomas, hamartomas of the liver, uterine fibroids, vascular tumours and cystic adenomas of the cerebellum, and carcinoma of the lung.

Changes in the platelets and blood coagulation

An otherwise unexplained thrombocytosis may be the first indication of an underlying malignancy. It is important to remember that this is not always associated with chronic blood loss; bronchial carcinoma may present in this way. Thrombocytopenia may sometimes occur with bone marrow infiltration by tumour cells, but is seen most frequently as a side-effect of chemotherapy. Autoimmune thrombocytopenia has been observed most commonly in association with lymphoid malignancies, but it can also occur in association with tumours of the lung, breast, and testes.

Generalized haemostatic failure associated with disseminated carcinoma is considered in detail elsewhere (Figs 1 and 2).

Some bleeding disorders associated with cancer seem to be due to selective impairment of coagulation. This may result from pathological inhibitors of different parts of the coagulation system or from isolated factor deficiencies. The mechanism is unknown. If the bleeding disorder is not characterized by consumption of clotting factors or fibrinolysis, a detailed analysis of the activities of the intrinsic and extrinsic pathways must be made in case a correctable lesion is present (Table 2).

Patients with cancer have an increased tendency to thrombosis. Apart from debilitation and periods of prolonged bed rest there is undoubtedly a hypercoaculable state associated with many tumours. This seems to involve a variety of procoagulants including fibrinogen and factors V, VII, VIII, IX, and XI. Low-grade, disseminated, intravascular coagulation can consume anticogulants such as anti-thombin III, protein C, and protein S. Cancer cells can initiate clotting by releasing a tissue factor, a phenomenon which is described in patients with lung, kidney, colon, and breast cancers. The

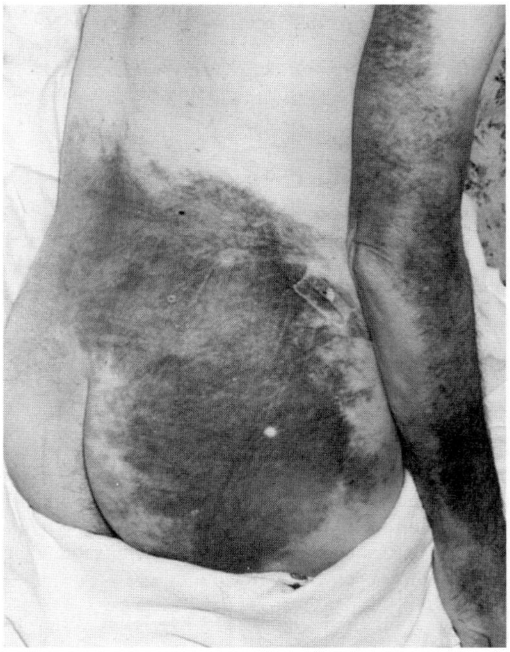

Fig. 1 Disseminated intravascular coagulation in association with carcinoma of the prostate. The patient started to bleed extensively from the iliac-crest marrow biopsy site and from venesection sites. Marrow biopsy showed widespread tumour metastases. (Reproduced from Hardisty RM, Weatherall DJ (ed.) (1982). *Blood and its disorders*, 2nd edn. Blackwell Scientific, Oxford, with permission.)

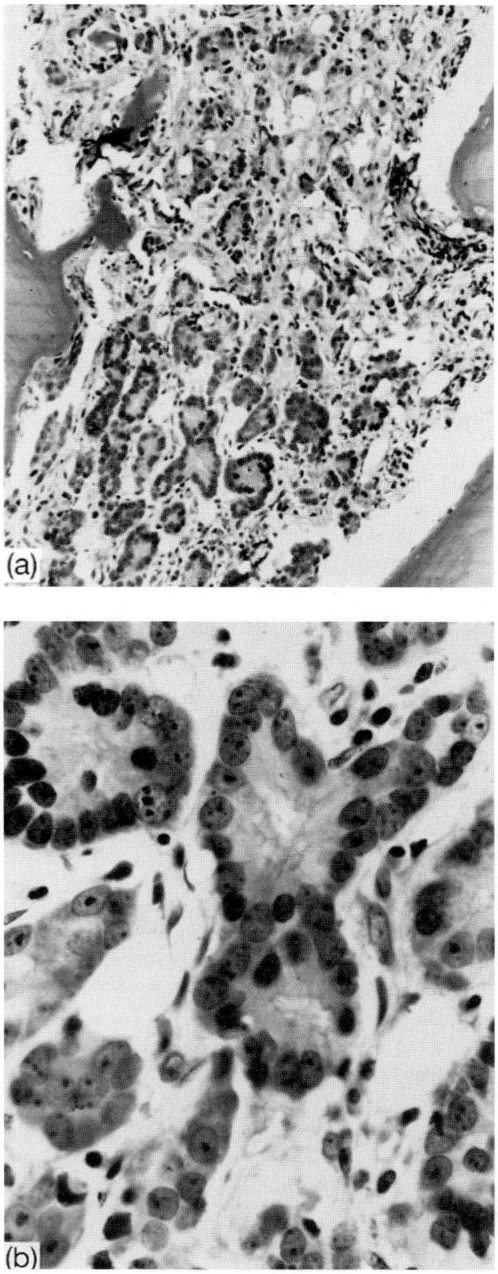

Fig. 2 Section prepared from Gardner-needle biopsies from bone marrow infiltrated with neoplastic cells; the primary tumour was in the prostate. (Reproduced from Hardisty RM, Weatherall DJ (ed.) (1982). *Blood and its disorders*, 2nd edn. Blackwell Scientific, Oxford, with permission.) (a) H and E stain ×230; (b) H and E stain ×920.

Table 2 Selective impairment of coagulation in cancer

Coagulation impairment	Disorder
Inhibitors	
Paraproteins	Plasma-cell disorders
Lupus-like	Hodgkin's disease, lymphoma, myelofibrosis, carcinoma
Factor IX inhibitor	Cancer of colon or prostate
Factor VII inhibitor	Bronchogenic carcinoma
Heparin-like	Bronchogenic carcinoma, myeloma
Isolated factor deficiencies	
Factor XIII	Acute leukaemia, chronic myeloid leukaemia
Factor XII	Chronic myeloid leukaemia
Factor XI	Melanoma
Factor X	Myeloma with amyloid
Factor VIII	Macroglobulinaemia, chronic lymphatic leukaemia, Wilms' tumour
Factor V	Chronic myeloid leukaemia, polycythaemia vera

Modified from Goldsmith (1984).

syndrome of non-bacterial thrombotic endocarditis, characterized by cerebral embolic strokes and extensive fibrin/platelet vegetations on the mitral and aortic valves, is most commonly associated with cancers of the lung, prostate, and pancreas.

White-cell abnormalities

In addition to the leukaemoid reaction, there are several white-cell changes that should make the clinician think about an underlying malignancy. For example a persistent monocytosis or eosinophilia may be associated with Hodgkin's disease or with bronchial carcinoma. Persistent lymphopenia may occur in patients with Hodgkin's disease.

Haematological changes due to cancer chemotherapy

Many agents used in cancer chemotherapy depress the bone marrow causing varying periods of neutropenia and thrombocytopenia associated with a variable anaemia. The bone marrow may also show marked myelodysplastic features. Haemolytic reactions have been associated with a number of drugs, including mitomycin C, and bleomycin–cisplatin. In some cases these drugs are associated with a syndrome of microangiopathic haemolytic anaemia resembling the haemolytic uraemic syndrome. Circulating immune complexes have been observed in some cases and there have been reports of response to plasma exchange and immunosuppression. Some chemotherapeutic agents appear to cause a warm antibody type of haemolytic anaemia. In patients who are glucose-6-phosphate dehydrogenase deficient, the administration of doxorubicin can produce a haemolytic reaction.

Haemophagocytic syndrome

This disorder, which is described in a later section in its association with viral illness, has now been reported in patients with cancer, lymphoma, and acute leukaemia. It is characterized by pancytopenia, fever, and splenomegaly; the bone marrow resembles histiocytosis with intense haemophagocytosis by macrophages.

Infection

Most of the important haematological changes in association with infection are considered in Section 7. Just a few points of particular haematological relevance are summarized below.

Acute bacterial infection

Most acute bacterial infections are associated with a neutrophil leucocytosis. This may be so marked, and associated with a 'shift to the left' with production of myelocytes in the blood, that the condition may present a leukaemoid type of reaction. Occasionally, in patients who are severely ill with acute bacterial infection, the neutrophil response seems inadequate. Some may be frankly neutropenic. A number of these individuals will prove to have an underlying haematological disorder or a debilitating condition such as alcoholism, but many who recover from their infection show no such underlying abnormality. A marrow examination usually reveals a paucity of mature granulocytes. This clinical picture is particularly common in newborn infants, especially those born prematurely. Some infections seem to be particularly prone to association with a reduced white-cell count. They include salmonellosis, brucellosis, pertussis, rickettsial infections, disseminated tuberculosis (in some cases), and disseminated histoplasmosis.

Other leucocyte changes are less common in acute infection. Monocytosis has been reported in patients with typhoid fever and sometimes in brucellosis or subacute bacterial endocarditis. In endocarditis a monocytosis may be associated with the presence of undifferentiated reticuloendothelial cells in the blood that show erythrophagocytosis.

Some degree of anaemia is found almost invariably in patients with bacterial infection. It usually presents a picture of the anaemia of chronic disorders. Haemolytic anaemia may occur in severe septicaemias and is usually associated with disseminated intravascular coagulation. Some organisms, *Clostridium welchii* for example, produce an α-toxin that acts as a lecithinase and causes fulminating intravascular haemolysis.

Disseminated intravascular coagulation is a common accompaniment of severe bacterial infection. Many mechanisms have been suggested, including vascular injury with activation of factor XII or the generation of procoagulants from white cells by the action of endotoxin. Thrombocytopenia is also common in patients with septicaemia. Although this may sometimes reflect disseminated intravascular coagulation, the mechanism is probably more complicated. There may be quite dramatic thrombocytopenia without any other evidence of a consumption coagulopathy. Several mechanisms are involved, including suppression of platelet production by the bone marrow, damage to circulating platelets by immune complexes, endothelial damage, and direct interaction of the platelets with bacteria; phagocytosis of bacteria by platelets may provoke the rapid disappearance of platelets from the circulation.

Chronic bacterial infection

Chronic bacterial infection is usually associated with the anaemia of chronic disorders. Some particularly interesting haematological changes are sometimes ascribed to tuberculosis (Table 3). While the most common change is a mild, normochromic, normocytic anaemia with a raised ESR; more spectacular blood changes have been reported, particularly in association with disseminated tuberculosis. These clinical pictures include leukaemoid reactions, pancytopenia, myelofibrosis, and even polycythaemia. The main problem in assessing these associations is whether the reported patients had infections due to atypical mycobacteria superimposed on an underlying blood disease, or whether disseminated tuberculosis can occasionally produce a clinical picture similar to leukaemia or a myeloproliferative disease. In practice, any patient who presents with an atypical myeloproliferative disorder, and who is going downhill for no apparent cause, should be investigated for tuberculosis. Attempts should be made to grow the organism from bone marrow cultures.

Virus infections

Haematological changes occur quite commonly in association with many virus illnesses. Changes associated with specific viral infections such as infectious mononucleosis are considered in Section 7.

Many virus infections are associated with a modest neutropenia and often with a relative or absolute lymphocytosis. Atypical lymphocytes are

Table 3 Haematological changes in tuberculosis

Type of tuberculosis or therapy	Haematological changes
Type of tuberculosis	
Pulmonary	Anaemia of chronic disorders; iron-deficiency anaemia; anaemia due to therapy; high ESR
Ileocaecal	Anaemia of chronic disorders; megaloblastic anaemia due to vitamin B_{12} or folate deficiency; high ESR
Cryptic miliary (aregenerative)	Leukaemoid reaction; myelosclerosis;[1] pancytopenia; polycythaemia,[1] anaemia of chronic disorders
Antituberculous drugs	
PAS or streptomycin allergy	Fever, lymphadenopathy, eosinophilia
INAH, cycloserine	Sideroblastic anaemia
Rifampicin	Thrombocytopenic purpura

[1]These reports may well represent cases of disseminated tuberculosis in patients with underlying haematological disorders (see text).

characteristic of patients with infectious mononucleosis but they may also be found in association with many other virus infections.

Rubella, acquired in childhood or adult life, is often associated with a leucocytosis and an atypical lymphocytosis. A small proportion of patients develop an acute fulminating thrombocytopenic purpura approximately 4 days after the appearance of the rash. It is usually self-limiting but fatalities have been reported. Thrombocytopenia is also common in infants with congenital rubella. This condition is also characterized by a non-immune haemolytic episode shortly after birth. Thrombocytopenia has also been reported in association with measles. In particularly severe forms of rubella and morbilli, severe haemorrhagic states due to disseminated intravascular coagulation have been seen. Similar changes occur occasionally in patients with varicella infections.

Haematological changes very similar to those seen in infectious mononucleosis can occur in patients with cytomegalovirus (CMV) infection. Infants may exhibit hepatosplenomegaly with purpura and anaemia. The anaemia is characterized by a haemolytic picture with many normoblasts in the peripheral blood. This form of anaemia may last for several weeks and may be associated with severe thrombocytopenia. There are well-documented cases of an infectious mononucleosis-like disorder occurring after transfusion with fresh blood or after perfusion for open heart surgery. This self-limiting syndrome usually occurs 1 to 3 months after blood transfusion and resolves within a few weeks. It is characterized by a moderate rise in temperature, with hepatosplenomegaly, lymphadenopathy, and transient maculopapular rashes, and a lymphocytosis indistinguishable from that of infectious mononucleosis.

Haematological problems are common in patients with AIDS. Lymphopenia is particularly common; neutropenia occurs in 0 to 30 per cent of HIV antibody-positive asymptomatic individuals, and in 20 to 65 per cent of patients with AIDS. Thrombocytopenia occurs in 5 to 20 per cent of asymptomatic HIV-1 infected persons and rises to 25 to 50 per cent in patients with AIDS. There is also a strong association of thrombotic thrombocytopenic purpura with HIV infection. Anaemia is also common. Bone marrow examination often reveals dyserythropoiesis with a variable degree of erythrophagocytosis. There have been a number of reports of the presence of lupus anticoagulant in the blood of patients with AIDS. In addition to these haematological complications, there is the added risk of drug-induced marrow hypoplasia, associated particularly with treatment with zidovudine (AZT).

Haematological complications of infectious hepatitis are rare but can be extremely severe. Coombs' positive haemolytic anaemia has been reported. There is also considerable literature on the occurrence of aplastic anaemia. This disorder seems predominantly to affect young males; the onset of aplasia is usually about 9 weeks after the onset of hepatitis. The condition is associated with a mortality in excess of 90 per cent. In those patients who recover, the period to complete haematological normality ranges between 3 and 20 months.

Many viruses are capable of provoking severe bleeding due to intravascular coagulation. Why viruses can fire off the coagulation cascade is far from clear. Activation of factor XII due to vascular injury or damage to platelets with the release of coagulants have been suggested as possible mechanisms.

The human parvovirus has a particular affinity for red-cell progenitors. It probably causes transient red-cell aplasia quite commonly but this only gives rise to a symptomatic anaemia in patients who have a markedly shortened red-cell survival. Thus parvovirus infection appears to be responsible for the aplastic crises in patients with sickle-cell anaemia, pyruvate kinase deficiency, or other congenital haemolytic anaemias. Viruses can cause acute damage to the bone marrow in immunesuppressed patients as part of the virus haemophagocytic syndrome.

The haematological changes associated with the virus haemorrhagic fevers are described in detail in Section 7.

Parasitic disease

The major haematological accompaniments of the parasitic diseases are described in Section 7. Those which produce important haematological changes will be briefly summarized here.

Toxoplasmosis

Congenital toxoplasmosis can produce a condition identical to erythroblastosis fetalis. The clinical picture is of a pale, hydropic infant with a large spleen and liver associated with severe anaemia, thrombocytopenia, and a leucocytosis, often with a marked eosinophilia. In adult life the acquired forms of toxoplasmosis produce a clinical disorder resembling infectious mononucleosis.

Malaria (Plate 1)

Malarial infection produces a variety of haematological abnormalities. The most severe changes occur during *Plasmodium falciparum* infection. In acute infections in non-immune individuals, there is usually minimal anaemia at the onset of the illness. During the 2 to 3 weeks after treatment there may be a steady decline in haemoglobin level. On the other hand, individuals with chronic malaria, some degree of immunity, and low-level parasitaemias, may be severely anaemic at presentation with an inappropriately low reticulocyte count. The bone marrow is often hyperplastic and shows a marked degree of dyshaemopoiesis (Fig. 3).

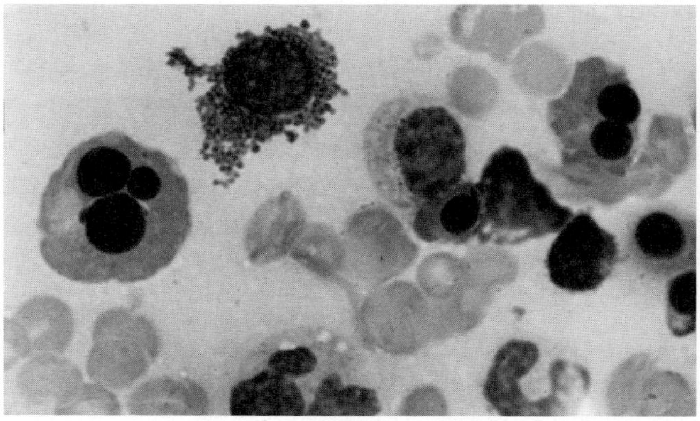

Fig. 3 Bone marrow appearances in *P. falciparum* malaria. There is marked dyserythropoiesis with several multinucleate red-cell precursors (Giemsa stain ×800).

The precise details of the pathophysiology of the anaemia of malaria are still unclear. There is no doubt that in acute attacks there may be massive destruction of parasitized red cells but, curiously, there is strong evidence that the survival of non-parasitized cells is also shortened. Although there is some indirect evidence for an immune basis for red cell destruction, particularly in children, little solid evidence exists for immune destruction in non-immune adults. There is growing evidence that the lack of marrow response may be, at least in part, due to the high levels of tumour necrosis factor (TNF) that are produced during malarial infection. TNF suppresses proliferation of erythroid progenitor cells *in vitro*. Chronic malaria has several features that augment this effect. Large numbers of pigment particles are ingested by the resident macrophages of the spleen and marrow, providing the possibility of a sustained stimulus for TNF production at the site of erythropoiesis.

In some patients with severe *P. falciparum* infections, there may be marked intravascular haemolysis and haemoglobinuria. The mechanism is not certain. Some of these patients may be glucose 6-phosphate dehydrogenase deficient but this is by no means the whole story. It has been suggested that some patients with fulminating malaria have disseminated intravascular coagulation. This is probably uncommon and plays very little part in the pathophysiology of either the anaemia or haemorrhagic phenomena that occur. Thrombocytopenia is extremely common but is only rarely associated with evidence of consumption of blood-clotting factors. In most forms of malarial infection there is a neutropenia. Monocytosis has also been described.

Several interesting haematological manifestations are associated with unusual forms of malaria. In the tropical splenomegaly syndrome, there may be anaemia, thrombocytopenia, and neutropenia, all secondary to hypersplenism. Congenital malaria infection is contracted in intrauterine life from the mother; newborn babies have a febrile illness associated with profound anaemia that appears to result from the combination of haemolysis and bone marrow suppression.

Leishmaniasis

Visceral leishmaniasis, or kala azar, is associated with hepatosplenomegaly, lymphadenopathy, and a pancytopenia, particularly in young children. Early in the course of the disease there is often marked neutropenia. The marrow may be grossly infiltrated with parasitized macrophages. The anaemia is due mainly to a short red-cell survival; there is also an inappropriate marrow response and a variable degree of hypersplenism.

Hookworm

The haematological changes of hookworm infestation are described in Chapter 22.5.3. It is one of the most common causes of iron-deficiency anaemia in the world population. During the systemic phase of the illness, when the larvae invade the lungs, there may be a marked eosinophilia. During this phase the bone marrow shows a remarkable increase in the percentage of eosinophilic myelocytes, which may be out of proportion to the eosinophilia observed in the peripheral blood.

Visceral larva migrans

This condition is characterized by striking haematological changes including anaemia, a marked leucocytosis with eosinophilia, and changes in the titre of anti-A and anti-B blood-group antibodies.

Schistosomiasis

In the chronic phase of *S. mansoni* and *S. japonicum* infections there may be severe portal hypertension, splenomegaly, and the typical picture of hypersplenism.

Other trematode infestations, including clonorchiasis and paragonamiasis, are associated with eosinophilia and anaemia. Antibodies to the P_1 blood-group antigen may be found in grossly elevated titres in the blood of many patients with acute fascioliasis.

Rheumatoid arthritis and related disorders

In patients with rheumatoid arthritis, anaemia is extremely common. It usually follows the general pattern of anaemia of chronic disorders. It is occasionally complicated by genuine iron deficiency, which may result from a variety of causes including poor diet and chronic blood loss due to the effects of treatment, particularly ingestion of salicylates and non-steroidal anti-inflammatory agents or corticosteroids. Furthermore, significant bleeding into actively inflamed joints can occur. It has been estimated that if only two knee joints were affected, the annual blood loss through this mechanism could amount to as much as 2500 ml. It is not certain how much of the iron derived from this blood is available for reutilization for haemoglobin synthesis. The diagnosis of iron deficiency complicating rheumatoid arthritis may not be straightforward; levels of serum iron and iron-binding capacity may be difficult to interpret because of coexisting inflammation. Determination of marrow stores and estimation of serum ferritin may be more helpful. Although the last two are elevated in inflammatory conditions, a low level suggests genuine iron deficiency.

There are no particular changes in the neutrophil response in uncomplicated rheumatoid arthritis; a marked leucocytosis may reflect a response to corticosteroid therapy or a superadded infection such as a septic arthritis. The platelet count is elevated in between 20 and 50 per cent of patients with rheumatoid arthritis. The degree of thrombocytosis parallels the degree of activity of the illness and cannot be accounted for on the grounds of associated intestinal blood loss due to drug therapy.

The haematological changes of Felty's syndrome are summarized in Section 18. There is anaemia, thrombocytopenia, and marked neutropenia. Although many of these changes are features of hypersplenism, recent studies on the neutropenia in this disorder indicate that it has a complex basis. Immune destruction of neutrophils may play a major part.

A variety of haematological changes are due to drug therapy for rheumatoid arthritis and related disorders. Salicylates may produce chronic blood loss, while drugs containing phenacetin produce methaemoglobinaemia and Heinz-body haemolytic anaemia that may sometimes be preceded by a marked eosinophilia. Phenylbutazone produces pancytopenia, which may be severe and irreversible; this drug has now been discontinued in the United Kingdom. Oxyphenylbutazone and penicillamine may also cause severe marrow depression. The administration of gold occasionally causes marked thrombocytopenia or pancytopenia.

The management of the haematological manifestations of rheumatoid arthritis and Felty's syndrome is unsatisfactory. The anaemia generally reflects the activity of the disease. If there is genuine iron deficiency, iron replacement therapy is indicated. The vexed question of whether intramuscular iron administration has some non-specific effect on the anaemia of rheumatoid arthritis, even in the absence of reduced body iron stores, remains unresolved. Similarly, there is controversy about the best way to manage Felty's syndrome. After splenectomy there is sometimes a dramatic rise in the neutrophil and total leucocyte counts, but this is not always associated with a decreased incidence of infection. Some patients show no change in the white-cell count after surgery. It is difficult to advise about the best approach to the management of this condition; only if there are recurrent, life-threatening infections should splenectomy be done. Patients require extremely careful surveillance after the operation. There may be some place for the use of prophylactic antibiotics in those whose neutrophil counts do not respond.

Recent studies have suggested that the anaemia of rheumatoid arthritis, and related inflammatory states, may respond to erythropoietin given in the higher therapeutic dose range. This treatment is extremely expensive and has only been evaluated in a few clinical trials. Its use should be reserved for those patients who have severe anaemia which is refractory to treatment of the underlying inflammatory disorder by any other means.

Systemic lupus erythematosus and other collagen disorders

It is quite common for systemic lupus erythematosus (SLE) to present with a haematological disorder. This is not the case in the other collagen–vascular disorders.

The most common blood change in SLE is anaemia, which occurs in nearly all patients at some stage of the illness. It is usually a mild anaemia of chronic disorders, which may be complicated by blood loss from analgesics or anti-inflammatory medication, renal impairment, or haemolysis. Acquired autoimmune haemolytic anaemia may be the sole presenting feature in SLE and may antedate the appearance of other typical features by many years. The incidence of this complication varies in reported series but occurs overall in approximately 5 per cent of cases. The Coombs' test is invariably positive with anticomplementary reagents and is positive with anti-IgG during episodes of acute haemolysis. Other forms of anaemia in SLE include those associated with hypersplenism due to splenomegaly, and the occasional occurrence of a hypocellular bone marrow, probably due to involvement of small vessels by the disease process.

The most consistent finding in the white-cell count in SLE is leukopenia, which occurs in up to half the patients at some time during the illness. This is often a combined neutropenia and lymphopenia. Mild eosinophilia occurs occasionally, particularly in association with skin involvement.

A mild thrombocytopenia occurs in 10 to 25 per cent of all cases of SLE. More severe thrombocytopenia, producing a picture almost indistinguishable from idiopathic thrombocytopenic purpura, occurs in a small proportion of patients and may be the sole presenting feature in some. Although early reports indicated that splenectomy might be associated with a flare-up of the systemic symptoms of SLE in patients with thrombocytopenia, this has now been shown to be incorrect.

Lupus anticoagulant

This is an antibody that prolongs phospholipid-dependent coagulation tests *in vitro*. Although it received its name because it was found in patients with SLE, it occurs more frequently in patients without this disease and is associated with thrombosis rather than with bleeding. It is particularly common in patients with lupus-like autoimmune disorders without the associated criteria for the diagnosis of SLE. Originally it was thought to occur in approximately 10 per cent of patients but using more sensitive assays it is now clear that it occurs in about 50 per cent.

Both lupus anticoagulants and associated anticardiolipin antibodies are immunoglobulins which react with phospholipid and other molecules (platelet factor IV). They may be associated with venous thromboembolism, arterial thromboembolism, an increased fate of fetal loss, or thrombocytopenia. They are discussed in detail in Section 18.11.

Other collagen disorders

The haematological changes in the other collagen–vascular diseases are much less impressive. They are all associated with the anaemia of chronic disorders. Polyarteritis nodosa may be characterized by an eosinophilia.

The interesting syndrome of polymyalgia rheumatica and temporal arteritis may present to the haematologist (Section 18.11). Haematological changes are characterized by a severe anaemia of chronic disorders with a marked elevation of the ESR. The leucocyte count is usually normal, although there may occasionally be a mild eosinophilia. There is a marked increase in the α_2- and γ-globulins, although this is polyclonal in type. This blood picture can very closely resemble that of multiple myeloma or disseminated malignancy.

Renal disease

Almost all forms of renal disease are associated with haematological changes. However, by far the most important is the severe refractory anaemia that accompanies chronic renal failure.

Anaemia

Anaemia is an important and intractable complication of chronic renal failure. The correlation between the blood urea nitrogen and the haemoglobin level is inconsistent. Although erythropoietin deficiency is an important component, the anaemia has an extremely complex aetiology, which is only partly understood. The red cells of patients with chronic renal disease have a shortened survival, although they survive normally when injected into healthy recipients. Similarly, normal red cells have a shortened survival in uraemic recipients. The nature of the intracorpuscular defect has not been determined. Most red-cell enzymes are present at normal levels and the intracellular level of ATP is elevated. However, changes in membrane function have been demonstrated, in particular decreased activity of the Na^+–K^+ pumps; the toxic substances that cause these changes have not been identified.

There is also impaired red-cell production in the anaemia of chronic renal failure. The fact that the anaemia of chronic renal failure can be corrected by the administration of recombinant erythropoietin suggests that the ineffective production of this hormone due to renal damage is the major aetiological factor in the anaemia of renal failure. However, it has been found that the serum from patients on haemodialysis also inhibits the proliferation of erythroid progenitors. The suppressive activity is found in serum fractions containing material of molecular weights ranging from 47 000 to above 150 000. Interestingly, patients on continuous ambulatory peritoneal dialysis (CAPD) have higher haemoglobin levels than those on haemodialysis. It is possible this reflects the more effective removal of middle molecular-weight molecules of this type by CAPD. Patients on haemodialysis with low haemoglobin concentrations are more likely to have fibrous replacement of their bone marrow. This has been correlated with secondary hyperparathyroidism, suggesting a role for parathyroid hormone in the bone marrow unresponsiveness and fibrosis (see Section 20).

The anaemia of chronic renal failure may be exacerbated by deficiency of iron resulting from blood loss due to excessive blood sampling, incorrect haemodialysis procedures, or bleeding due to defective platelet function (see below). A small proportion of patients with chronic renal failure develop splenomegaly and hypersplenism. Folate deficiency is found occasionally in patients on haemodialysis. There have been a few reports of nephrosis leading to severe urinary loss of transferrin and hence to a low plasma iron-binding capacity. Some patients with renal disease have chronic inflammatory lesions, which may lead to a superadded anaemia of chronic disorders.

The type of renal lesion is also an important factor in determining the severity of anaemia. For example the renal failure of polycystic disease of the kidneys is associated with a relatively higher haemoglobin level than other forms of renal failure. Interestingly, the shrunken kidneys of some patients on long-term dialysis programmes develop cysts and this phenomenon is also associated with a rise in haemoglobin level. It seems likely that both these conditions are associated with a relative increase in the output of erythropoietin.

The anaemia of chronic renal failure is normochromic and normocytic unless there is associated iron deficiency. The red cells show characteristic deformities with multiple tiny spicules and contracted poikilocytes. The capacity of the red cells for oxygen transport does not seem to be impaired. There is often an increased intracellular concentration of 2,3-diphosphoglycerate (2,3-DPG) in response to anaemia and hyperphosphataemia, and the oxygen affinity of haemoglobin is decreased. This right shift in the oxygen dissociation curve may be augmented by uraemic acidosis. However, part of the advantage of the acidosis is cancelled out by the direct effect of low pH on glycolysis and 2,3-DPG production. Intensive dialysis may cause a reduction in the concentration of intracellular phosphate, which has the effect of increasing the oxygen affinity of haemoglobin. This effect may play a part in the so-called dialysis disequilibrium syndrome.

In patients with chronic renal failure who have associated iron deficiency, the red-cell indices are typical of this condition; the reduced mean corpuscle haemoglobin and volume are corrected by iron therapy.

The bone marrow in chronic renal failure shows normoblastic erythropoiesis but the degree of erythroid hyperplasia is not compatible with the degree of anaemia, indicating suppression of erythropoiesis.

White cells

The total and differential white-cell count is usually normal in patients with chronic renal failure. However, the phagocytic activity of granulocytes may be reduced and complement activation by haemodialysis membranes may cause stasis of white cells in the pulmonary circulation with temporary granulocytopenia. Cell-mediated immunity is also depressed.

Platelets and coagulation

There is a variety of haemostatic defects in different forms of renal disease. Most forms are associated with a bleeding tendency, which is seen in its most florid form in acute renal failure. The main features are purpura, and mucosal and gastrointestinal bleeding associated with abnormal platelet function and a prolonged bleeding time; these changes are reversible by dialysis. Various mechanisms have been proposed. These include a direct action of metabolites on platelet function and a disturbance of prostaglandin balance because of a deficiency of a renal factor that modifies vascular production of prostacyclin and/or platelet endoperoxide and thromboxane synthesis. These changes result in an abnormality of the control of platelet cAMP causing the platelets to become refractory to aggregation agents. Many conditions that lead to renal failure are also associated with thrombocytopenia. For example the circulating immune complexes found in patients with acute glomerulonephritis, polyarteritis nodosa, or lupus nephritis may be responsible for platelet activation and the release of aggregating agents. Thrombocytopenia may also be aggravated by heparin therapy or the use of immunosuppressant drugs in patients who have received kidney grafts. Mild thrombocytopenia is well recognized in patients with functioning renal allografts. This has also been found to be associated with an inability to clear the immune complexes. Graft rejection is associated with enhanced platelet aggregation and thrombocytopenia.

The nephrotic syndrome is characterized by a marked tendency to thrombosis. This also has a complex pathogenesis. Both platelet aggregation and release reactions have been shown to be enhanced in this condition. Protein loss in the urine may also play a part. It has been found that an increased loss of antithrombin III is related to thrombotic episodes. Conversely, coagulation factors IX and XIII are also lost in the urine of patients with a nephrotic syndrome; the deficiency of factor IX may be sufficient to induce bleeding.

The haematological changes associated with the haemolytic uraemic syndrome and thrombotic thrombocytopenic purpura were considered earlier in this section.

Polycythaemia

The polycythaemias associated with renal lesions and following renal transplantation are discussed elsewhere.

Treatment of the haematological complications of renal disease

The management of the anaemia of chronic renal failure, which has been revolutionized by the availability of recombinant erythropoietin, is considered in Section 20. The management of bleeding in patients with acute renal failure is based on correction of uraemia by dialysis and appropriate replacement therapy. Peritoneal dialysis is probably more effective in reversing abnormalities of platelet function, although there is no definite evidence that one form of dialysis is superior to another. If there is severe thrombocytopenia, platelet transfusions should be given.

Gastrointestinal and liver disease

Many of the haematological changes that occur in gastrointestinal and liver disease are described in Section 14. Here we will simply summarize the haematological manifestations of those disorders that present frequently with anaemia or defective haemostasis.

Gastrointestinal blood loss

Blood loss in excess of 20 ml/day will always result in a negative iron balance and ultimately in iron-deficiency anaemia, the time taken depending on the body stores of iron when the bleeding started.

The haematological picture shows the typical changes of iron-deficiency anaemia, with hypochromic, microcytic red-cell morphology. Occasionally, there are some clues that this blood picture is associated with chronic blood loss. Quite frequently there is a mild to moderate thrombocytosis, and if iron is being taken there may be a dimorphic blood picture (Fig. 4), red-cell polychromasia, and a low-grade reticulocytosis. It is always worth examining the peripheral blood film very carefully as it may give some clue as to the site of the blood loss. For example the presence of target cells may indicate liver disease, whereas the presence of distorted cells and Howell–Jolly bodies suggests malabsorption due to adult coeliac disease complicated by hyposplenism.

The diagnosis of the site of acute upper intestinal bleeding is considered in Section 14. The investigation of chronic gastrointestinal blood loss may be difficult. First, it is essential to determine whether iron deficiency anaemia is due to a defective intake or due to excessive loss of iron. If gastrointestinal blood loss is suspected the first step is to confirm that this is occurring, by examination of several stool specimens for occult blood. Currently, the most commonly used method is the Haemoccult card which contains a filter paper impregnated with guaiac, or a similar commercial kit. The peroxidase activity of red blood cells releases a free oxygen radical from hydrogen peroxide (the developer) which then reacts with the guaiac to produce a blue colour. This test is simple, easy to perform following a rectal examination, and is quick. Nevertheless, it is relatively insensitive, since blood loss must exceed 20 ml daily for 80 to 90 per cent of tests to be

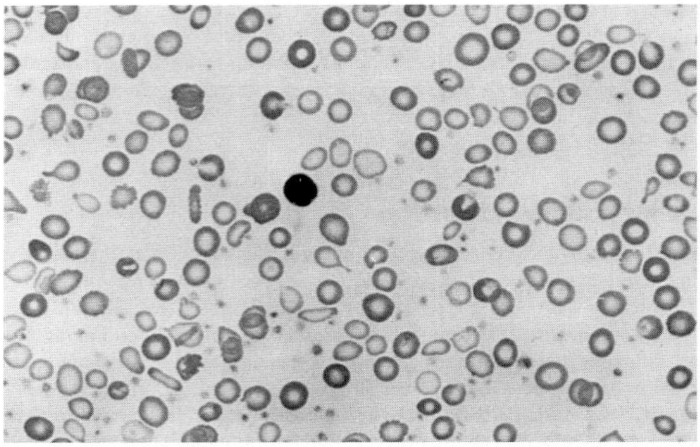

Fig. 4 Peripheral blood picture associated with gastrointestinal bleeding. The red cells show a dimorphic picture with hypochromic and normochromic forms. The platelet count is elevated, a typical finding in bleeding (Giemsa stain × 600).

positive (the normal loss in a healthy individual is 0.5–1.2 ml daily as measured by ^{51}Cr-labelled red cells). False positive results may result from peroxidase or non-specific oxidants in the diet. Thus in many screening programmes, subjects are requested to omit red meat, fresh fruit, cauliflower, swede, turnip, tomatoes, horseradish, and vitamin C supplements from their diet during the 3 days prior to testing. Non-steroidal anti-inflammatory drugs and aspirin may also give positive results but, since the increased blood loss is in the upper gastrointestinal tract, the haemoglobin is metabolized in the small intestine and is therefore not detected in stools by Haemoccult unless blood loss is considerable. Iron therapy does not affect guaiac-based tests. Many newer tests, which are said to be even more sensitive, are being developed but their role in clinical practice is not yet established.

Once having established that there is gastrointestinal blood loss the next step is to determine the site. This requires a detailed history and clinical examination as outlined in the introduction to this section. The next step is a careful endoscopy, followed by sigmoidoscopy and colonoscopy. If these investigations do not provide a diagnosis, and there is persistent bleeding, the duodenum and small bowel should be studied radiologically. Occasionally it is necessary to resort to coeliac or superior mesenteric angiography, which may be useful for showing duodenal or ileal varices, bleeding from Meckel's diverticulum or non-specific ulcers of the ileum, small bowel tumours, and vascular lesions. However, small lesions can only be visualized if there is active bleeding at the time of the examination, probably at a rate of at least 0.5 ml/min.

Inflammatory diseases of the bowel

A mild anaemia of chronic disorders is a common accompaniment of inflammatory disease of the ileum, caecum, and colon. It is observed frequently in patients with Crohn's disease, ileocaecal tuberculosis, ulcerative colitis, and other forms of proctocolitis. In many of these conditions the anaemia of chronic disorders is complicated by intermittent blood loss or dietetic iron deficiency. In some cases of extensive Crohn's disease there may be an added factor of malabsorption. Anaemia occurs in about one-third of these patients and it may be complicated by reduced vitamin B_{12} or folic acid absorption. In one large survey of patients with Crohn's disease, anaemia was present in 79 per cent of the males and 54 per cent of females. Forty-six out of a total of 63 patients had bone marrow biopsies, and of these 39 per cent were megaloblastic. Of this group, 11 were folate deficient, six vitamin B_{12} deficient, and one had both deficiencies. On the other hand, macrocytic anaemia is unusual in patients with ulcerative colitis and the anaemia is usually hypochromic due to blood loss. Interestingly, there have been occasional reports of autoimmune haemolytic anaemia occurring in association with ulcerative colitis; in several cases the autoantibodies showed rhesus specificity.

The anaemia of intestinal inflammatory disease may be made worse by drugs used in its management. Patients who receive salazopyrine for colitis occasionally develop an acute haemolytic anaemia associated with Heinz-body formation. Bone marrow depression may occur in patients receiving immunosuppressive treatment for colitis or Crohn's disease. Ileocaecal tuberculosis may be associated with any of the bizarre haematological manifestations of tuberculosis described above, and it may be complicated by the side-effects of antituberculous drug therapy.

Whipple's disease may produce a clinical picture and blood changes that can mimic several primary haematological disorders. The typical clinical triad of diarrhoea, arthropathy, and enlarged lymph nodes is usually associated with a mild normochromic, normocytic anaemia, a raised ESR, and a polymorphonuclear leucocytosis. Quite often there is associated lymphopenia or eosinophilia. Some cases present less typically. When the spleen is enlarged the condition may closely mimic a primary reticulosis. Malabsorption of vitamin B_{12} or folic acid may occasionally be encountered in this disorder (see Chapter 14.9.6).

Structural disease of the stomach, and small and large bowel

The structural changes and resulting abnormalities of absorption associated with gastritis are described in detail in Section 14. Similarly, the various anatomical abnormalities of the small-gut and malabsorption syndromes that lead to vitamin B_{12} and folate deficiency are reviewed earlier in this section. The relation between gastric surgery and iron and vitamin B_{12} metabolism is discussed in Section 14.

Most anatomical lesions of the small bowel present to the haematologist as a macrocytic anaemia with a megaloblastic bone marrow due to vitamin B_{12} or folate deficiency or as a refractory iron-deficiency anaemia. Several abnormalities of the small gut are associated with the production of a relatively profuse bacterial flora that utilize vitamin B_{12}. These conditions include surgically produced blind loops, strictures, anastomoses between loops of small bowel, fistulae between various sections of the bowel, diverticula of the small bowel, malfunctioning gastroenterostomies, interference of gut motility in conditions such as scleroderma, Whipple's disease, post-vagotomy, and after extensive gut resection, where the disorder may also produce malabsorption. All these conditions are associated with defective vitamin B_{12} absorption, which can be partly corrected by the administration of broad-spectrum antibiotics but not by intrinsic factor.

Megaloblastic anaemia due to intestinal malabsorption is fully reviewed in Section 14.9. It should be remembered, however, that the malabsorption syndromes may present to the haematologist in other ways. For example there is a very high incidence of iron-deficiency anaemia in this group and, particularly in childhood, this is the much the more common form of presentation than a megaloblastic anaemia. The peripheral blood changes of hyposplenism are quite frequently associated with an underlying malabsorption syndrome, which itself may also present with a bleeding disorder due to defective absorption of vitamin K. Patients with malabsorption syndrome frequently have biochemical evidence of vitamin E deficiency; although this may produce a slightly shortened red-cell survival, there is no evidence that vitamin E deficiency alone produces a significant degree of anaemia.

Liver disease

There is usually a moderate degree of anaemia in patients with chronic liver failure (Table 4). The red cells are normochromic or slightly macrocytic with mean corpuscle volume values ranging from 100 to 115 fl. Target cells and a variable degree of polychromasia with a slightly elevated reticulocyte count are often found. The degree of macrocytosis and target-cell formation corresponds reasonably well with the degree of liver failure. The bone marrow tends to be hypercellular with erythroid hyperplasia and macronormoblastic changes.

The actual mechanism of the anaemia of liver failure is uncertain. However, there may be many complicating factors that cause a worsening of the anaemia in this condition. Nutritional folate deficiency is very common in patients with liver disease, particularly the alcoholic form. Secondary iron deficiency is also common and usually results from chronic intestinal blood loss associated with a poor dietetic intake. Interestingly, in patients with severe portal hypertension and cirrhosis, or in those who have undergone portacaval shunt surgery, there may be some increase in iron absorption with marked haemosiderosis of the liver.

A variety of different forms of haemolytic anaemia occur in patients with liver disease. In Zieve's syndrome there is jaundice, hyperlipidaemia, and haemolytic anaemia that follows an excessive alcohol intake. Other forms of haemolytic anaemia may occur. Acute haemolysis has been well documented in patients with viral hepatitis, particularly those who are glucose 6-phosphate dehydrogenase deficient. An acquired haemolytic anaemia with a positive Coombs' test may occur occasionally in patients with chronic active hepatitis. Another form of haemolytic anaemia in liver disease, usually alcoholic cirrhosis, has been observed in which there are

Table 4 Haematological changes in liver disease

Virus hepatitis
Haemolytic anaemia, hypoplastic anaemia
Chronic active hepatitis
Immune haemolytic anaemia, hyperglobulinaemia
Chronic liver failure
Chronic anaemia is often complicated by:
- (a) blood loss and iron deficiency
- (b) alcohol, direct effect on marrow
- (c) folate deficiency
- (d) portal hypertension and hypersplenism
- (e) acute haemolytic episodes (e.g. Zieve's syndrome, spur-cell syndrome)

Thrombocytopenia, leucopenia, haemorrhagic diathesis due to:
- (a) deficiency of vitamin K-dependent factors
- (b) portal hypertension and hypersplenism
- (c) increased fibrinolysis
- (d) thrombocytopenia

Portal hypertension
Anaemia, leucopenia, thrombocytopenia, bleeding from varices
Obstructive jaundice
Mild anaemia, target-cell formation, masking of hereditary spherocytosis
Tumours
Polycythaemia, leukaemoid reactions, α-fetoprotein production
Liver transplantation
Haemorrhagic and hypercoagulable states

marked red-cell abnormalities with burr and spur-shaped forms predominating.

Bleeding and haemostatic failure are extremely common accompaniments of liver failure. They have a complex aetiology including diminished hepatic synthesis of coagulation factors V, VII, IX, X, and XI, prothrombin and fibrinogen. In some forms of liver disease there may be malabsorption of vitamin K with reduction in the K-deficient clotting factors, and reproduction of a dysfunctional form of fibrinogen has been reported in some patients with cirrhosis and hepatocellular carcinoma. In some forms of liver failure there is enhanced fibrinolysis, due to decrease synthesis of α_2-plasmin inhibitor. In severe liver failure disseminated intravascular configuration may occur. Thrombocytopenia is extremely common in liver disease, sometimes due to hypersplenism but in other cases its pathogenesis is not clear.

The management of bleeding in liver diseases is considered in Section 14.21.

The haematological effects of alcohol

Because excessive consumption of alcohol is so common, it is important for clinicians to appreciate the remarkably diverse haematological manifestations that it causes.

Anaemia is particularly common in chronic alcoholics. It has an extremely complex aetiology including a deficient diet, chronic blood loss, hepatic dysfunction, and the direct toxic effects of alcohol on the bone marrow.

Macrocytosis is particularly common in chronic alcoholics. An unexplained macrocytic blood picture should always raise the possibility of alcoholism, although its absence does not rule out the diagnosis. It may be associated with normoblastic or megaloblastic erythropoiesis. In moderately severe alcoholics who are maintaining a reasonable diet, it probably reflects the direct toxic action of alcohol on the bone marrow. The normoblasts may show vacuolation or there may be no specific changes on light microscopy. Megaloblastic anaemia is usually seen in severe alcoholics who are poorly nourished, and is due to folate deficiency. While a folate-poor diet is the major factor, there is some evidence that alcohol plays a more direct part in interfering with folate metabolism by an unknown mechanism. It should be remembered that macrocytosis can also occur in alcoholics during a reticulocytosis in response to bleeding or alcohol withdrawal. It may also reflect coexistent liver disease. The occurrence of sideroblastic anaemia in severe alcoholics was mentioned in an earlier chapter. It is often associated with a macrocytosis or a dimorphic blood picture and occurs in severe alcoholics. The sideroblastic changes revert to normal after stopping alcohol.

Simple iron deficiency is also found commonly in alcoholics and probably reflects both a poor diet and chronic blood loss due to gastritis or bleeding varices. It may be associated with folate deficiency; the blood film is then dimorphic with macrocytes, microcytes, and hypersegmented neutrophils. Alcoholics with chronic pancreatitis may develop iron loading due to increased absorption. These changes, which are specific for alcohol, may be accompanied by any of the haematological manifestations of liver disease.

Alcohol has deleterious effects on the white cells. Severe alcoholics are prone to infection. The neutropenia of alcoholism may reflect both the toxic effect of alcohol on the marrow and folate deficiency. There is also some evidence that alcohol can interfere with neutrophil locomotion and with their ability to ingest foreign material including micro-organisms.

Thrombocytopenia is commonly seen in chronic alcoholics and may occur without accompanying folate deficiency or splenomegaly. Megakaryocytes may be normal or diminished in number. Following withdrawal of alcohol the platelet count usually returns to normal, although it may become markedly elevated for a few days.

Chest disease

(See also carcinoma and tuberculosis, above, and secondary polycythaemia, Chapter 22.3.8).

Pneumonia

Most bacterial pneumonias are associated with a neutrophil leucocytosis. Two relatively common forms of pneumonia are associated with more specific haematological changes. In mycoplasma pneumonia, cold agglutinins can usually be detected in increased amounts towards the end of the first week in up to 80 per cent of cases. The cold antibodies are polyclonal IgM to the red-cell I antigen. Although a positive Coombs' test and an increased reticulocyte count have been described in these cases, serious haemolysis is rare. Occasionally, the condition is complicated by disseminated intravascular coagulation.

There is increasing evidence that in patients with pneumonia caused by *Legionella pneumophila* (Legionnaires' disease) there may be severe thrombocytopenia and, sometimes, lymphopenia. Several cases have been reported to be complicated by disseminated intravascular coagulation.

Pulmonary eosinophilia (see also Section 17.11)

This term refers to a group of disorders that have in common a raised eosinophil count in the peripheral blood in association with pulmonary infiltrates on the chest radiograph. The exact nature of many of the disorders that constitute this syndrome is uncertain. In its simplest form there may be a brief period of respiratory distress in association with eosinophilia. This condition is sometimes called Löffler's syndrome. At the other end of the spectrum there is a severe illness associated with widespread pulmonary infiltrates and eosinophilia, which may culminate with the features of polyarteritis nodosa.

The transient disorder described by Löffler probably represents a heterogeneous group of conditions, which in many cases are associated with parasitic infection. Many parasitic disorders can cause this type of illness, including ascariasis, ankylostomiasis, trichiuriasis, taeniasis, and fascioliasis. A similar condition has been well documented as part of a hypersensitivity reaction to drugs. The most common is *p*-aminosalicylic acid but similar reactions have been observed in patients receiving penicillin, sulphonamides, and nitrofurantoin. A similar clinical picture is associated with the syndrome of allergic alveolitis, including farmer's lung, bird fancier's lung, and a variety of other occupational disorders. Another condition characterized by a marked eosinophilia with pulmonary infiltrates goes under the general term tropical eosinophilia. There is considerable evidence that this disorder is due to occult filarial infection. Pulmonary eosinophilia may also be due to hypersensitivity to fungi, particularly *Aspergillus fumigatus*.

Idiopathic pulmonary haemosiderosis and Goodpasture's syndrome

These disorders occasionally present as a refractory anaemia that has the characteristics of the anaemia of chronic disorders, although it may become markedly hypochromic and microcytic due to chronic blood loss.

Skin diseases

Megaloblastic anaemia and the skin

The whole relation between skin disease and megaloblastic anaemia is extremely complex and much of the work in this field is still controversial. The subject is discussed elsewhere (see Section 23).

A proportion of patients with various dermatoses show evidence of folate depletion, at least biochemically, and in some cases, haematologically. This has been reported in patients with erythroderma, psoriasis, or extensive eczema. There is a well-documented association between malabsorption and dermatitis herpetiformis. Although megaloblastic anaemia is not found frequently in association with disorders of the skin, some patients with these conditions do have mild megaloblastic changes. Earlier reports suggested that a significant proportion of them had abnormalities of small-intestinal function and structure, leading to the descriptive term 'dermatogenic enteropathy'. This concept has been questioned and it is now agreed that a completely flat small-bowel mucosa is rarely seen in these conditions. The relation between dermatitis herpetiformis and malabsorption of the coeliac type seems to be a special case. Several series have shown a high incidence of small-bowel changes of coeliac disease in patients with this condition. Furthermore, there appears to be a high incidence of splenic hypoplasia with typical haematological changes of defective function of the spleen (see Chapter 22.4.4).

Other dermatological disorders

Several dermatological diseases have a major haematological component. Of particular importance are the systemic mast-cell syndromes, Sezary syndrome and cutaneous T-cell lymphomas, hereditary telangiectasia, and some of the inherited disorders of collagen.

Endocrine disease

Pituitary deficiency

A mild, normochromic, normocytic anaemia is very common in patients with anterior pituitary deficiency. The mechanism is not absolutely clear, although the anaemia has many features in common with that of hypothyroidism and is fully responsive to appropriate replacement therapy.

Thyroid disease

Hypothyroidism is associated with a variety of haematological changes. Anaemia is common and may be normocytic, microcytic, or macrocytic.

Severe microcytic anaemia in hypothyroidism is most commonly seen in women who have menorrhagia, which is a frequent complication of this condition. Severe macrocytosis in hypothyroidism usually indicates an associated vitamin B_{12} deficiency; there seems to be a genuine association between pernicious anaemia and myxoedema. It has been suggested that mild macrocytosis may occur in hypothyroidism in the absence of vitamin B_{12} or folate deficiency, although published series of studies have shown a remarkable variability in the incidence of this phenomenon. Some patients with severe hypothyroidism have a small proportion of misshapen red cells on their peripheral blood films.

The anaemia of uncomplicated myxoedema is normochromic and normocytic. The mechanism is still uncertain. Recent studies have shown that T_3, T_4, and reverse T_3 can all potentiate the effect of erythropoietin on the formation of erythroid colonies *in vitro*. This effect appears to be mediated by receptors with β_2-adrenergic properties. It appears that the thyroid hormones have a direct effect in altering the erythropoietin responsiveness of erythroid progenitors. It has also been suggested that part of the normochromic anaemia of hypothyroidism may be a physiological adaptation to reduced oxygen requirements by the tissues.

Curiously, patients with hyperthyroidism do not have elevated haemoglobin levels. There is some recent evidence that there may be a mild increase in the red-cell mass in hyperthyroidism, but that this is compensated for by an increase in plasma volume. In some patients with severe hyperthyroidism, there is a mild anaemia associated with abnormal iron utilization.

Adrenal disease

A mild, normochromic, normocytic anaemia together with neutropenia, eosinophilia, and lymphocytosis is observed in some patients with Addison's disease. There is a variety of haematological changes following the administration of corticosteroids or endogenous overproduction of these agents. These include granulocytosis, reduced lymphocyte count, involution of lymphatic tissues, and a decrease in the eosinophil and monocyte count.

Parathyroid disease

Primary hyperparathyroidism is occasionally associated with anaemia, which responds to removal of the parathyroid glands. The relation between parathyroid disease and marrow fibrosis is discussed in Section 12.

Diabetes mellitus

The structural changes that occur in the haemoglobin of diabetic patients are discussed in Chapter 12.11.1. There have been recent reports that there may be an increase in the red-cell volume of patients with severe diabetes. The mechanism and significance of this observation remains to be clarified. Severe diabetic acidosis is associated with a marked leucocytosis, even when there is no underlying infection. Hyperosmolarity impairs neutrophil function; reduced neutrophil migration has been observed in patients with diabetic ketoacidosis or poorly controlled hyperglycaemia. Because of the high incidence of atheroma in patients with diabetes, both platelet function and vessel-wall metabolism have been studied in considerable detail in this condition. Synthesis of prostaglandin I_2 in biopsy specimens of forearm veins is reduced. A variety of changes in platelet reactivity and survival have been observed. The relation of these changes to the vascular disease of diabetes requires further clarification.

Neuropsychiatric disease

Anorexia nervosa

About a third of patients with severe anorexia nervosa have a mild, normochromic, normocytic anaemia. In patients who are severely malnourished there may be mild neutropenia. There have been reports of the finding of irregularly shaped red blood cells in this condition. The platelet count is usually normal but there may be mild thrombocytopenia and in one study there was a marked increase in the rate of platelet aggregation.

Trauma

The brain is rich in thromboplastin activity. Acute disseminated intravascular coagulation occurs quite commonly after severe head or brain injury.

Myasthenia gravis

The association between myasthenia gravis and pure red-cell aplasia is described in Section 24.22. An immune neutropenia has also been described as part of the myasthenia–thymoma syndrome.

Lesch–Nyhan syndrome

This X-linked recessive disorder is described in detail in Chapter 11.4. There have been occasional reports of the development of severe megaloblastic anaemia, presumably resulting from defective nucleic acid synthesis; the condition has been reversed by the administration of large doses of adenine.

Abetalipoproteinaemia

This condition is characterized by an ataxic neurological disease, retinitis pigmentosa, fat malabsorption, and the absence of chylomicrons and low-density lipoproteins. It is caused by the failure to synthesize or secrete lipoprotein-containing products of the apolipoprotein B gene. It is characterized by the presence of from 50 to 90 per cent of acanthocytes in the peripheral blood. These are abnormal, spiky red cells, which have a moderately shortened survival. Despite these changes there is only a mild haemolytic anaemia.

Acanthocytosis with neurological disease and normal lipoproteins (amyotrophic chorea-acanthocytosis)

This syndrome is characterized by marked acanthocytosis associated with a progressive neurological disease, beginning in adolescence or adult life, which includes orofacial dyskinesia, lip and tongue biting, choreaiform movements, sensorimotor polyneuropathy, distal muscle wasting, and hypotonia. Because it has been found to follow both dominant and recessive forms of inheritance it is likely that this is a heterogeneous disorder. The cause is unknown.

Cardiac disease

There are several important haematological manifestations of cardiac disease, all of which are dealt with in more detail in Section 15. The severe haemolytic anaemia that occasionally follows the insertion of prosthetic valves, particularly the aorta, is described in Chapter 15.7.

A variety of abnormalities of coagulation are found in patients with cyanotic congenital heart disease. These include thrombocytopenia, low plasma fibrinogen levels, defective clot retraction, a deficiency of factors V and VII, and increased levels of fibrin degradation products. Overall, the severity of these abnormalities correlates with the degree of secondary polycythaemia. The exact mechanism is not known. In addition to the quantitative changes in blood platelets, there may also be qualitative abnormalities of platelet function. These include defects in both aggregation and release. They may be associated with a prolonged bleeding time. Again, the mechanism is not understood.

The striking haematological changes that may accompany bacterial endicarditis were mentioned earlier in this chapter. Dressler's syndrome may be associated with the anaemia of chronic disorders, atypical lymphocytes in the peripheral blood, and, certainly in the earlier descriptions of the disease, an eosinophilia of varying degree. Similar changes have been observed in the postpericardiotomy syndrome.

Further reading

Boxer H, Ellman L, Geller R, Wang C-A (1977). Anemia in primary hyperparathyroidism. *Archives of Internal Medicine* **137,** 588–90.

Castaldi PA (1984). Hemostasis and kidney disease. In: Ratnoff OD, Forbes CD, eds. *Disorders of hemostasis*, pp. 473–84. Grune and Stratton, Orlando, FA.

Colman N, Herbert V (1980). Hematologic complications of alcohol. *Seminars in Hematology* **17**, 164–72.

Dainiak N (2000). Hematologic complications of renal disease. In: Hoffman R *et al.*, eds. *Hematology. Basic principles and practice*, 3rd edn, pp. 2357–73. Churchill Livingstone, New York.

Erslev AJ (1995). Traumatic cardiac hemolytic anemia. In: Beutler E, Lichtman MA, Coller BS, Kipps TJ, eds. *Williams hematology*, 5th edn, pp. 663–5. McGraw-Hill, New York.

Goldsmith GH, Jr (1984). Hemostatic disorders associated with neoplasia. In: Ratnoff OD, Forbes CD, eds. *Disorders of hemostasis*, pp. 351–66. Grune and Stratton, Orlando, FA.

Hamblin TJ, ed. (1987). Haematological problems in the elderly. *Bailliere's Clinical Haematology* **1,** 271–596.

Hardcastle JD, Thomas WM (1989). Screening an asymptomatic population for colorectal cancer. In: Mortensen N, ed. *Ballière's clinical gastroenterology*, Vol. 3, pp. 543–66. Ballière Tindall, London.

Herbert V, ed. (1980). Hematologic complications of anemia in alcoholic patients. *Seminars in Hematology* **17**, vols 1 and 2.

Hoxie JA (2000). Hematologic manifestations of HIV infection. In: Hoffman R *et al.*, eds. *Hematology. Basic principles and practice*, 3rd edn, pp. 2430–57. Churchill Livingstone, New York.

Hughes GRV (1983). The lupus anticoagulant. *British Medical Journal* **287,** 1088–9.

Parker RI, Metcalf DD (2000). Basophils, mast cells and systemic mastocytosis. In: Hoffman R *et al.*, eds. *Hematology. Basic principles and practice*, 3rd edn, pp. 830–46. Churchill Livingstone, New York.

Ratnoff OD (1984). Hemostatic defects in liver and biliary tract diseases. In: Ratnoff OD, Forbes CD, eds. *Disorders of hemostasis*, pp. 451–72. Grune and Stratton, Orlando, FL.

Rosenthal DS (2000). Hematologic manifestations of infectious disease. In: Hoffman R *et al.*, eds. *Hematology. Basic principles and practice*, 3rd edn, pp. 2420–30. Churchill Livingstone, New York.

St John DJB, Young GP, *et al.* (1993). Evaluation of new occult blood tests for detection of colorectal neoplasia. *Gastroenterology* **104,** 1661–8.

Stockman JAI, Ezekowitz RA (1998). Hematologic manifestations of systemic diseases. In: Nathan DG, Oski FA, eds. *Hematology of infancy and childhood*, 5th edn, pp. 1841–91. Saunders, Philadelphia.

Weatherall DJ, Kwiatkowski D (1998). Hematologic manifestations of systemic diseases in children of the developing world. In: Nathan DG, Oski FA, eds. *Hematology of infancy and childhood*, 5th edn, pp. 1893–914. Saunders, Philadelphia.

Weinstein IM, Rosenbloom DE (2000). Hematologic problems in patients with cancer and chronic inflammatory disorders. In: Hoffman R *et al.*, eds. *Hematology. Basic principles and practice*, 3rd edn, pp. 2410–20. Churchill Livingstone, New York.

Zaroulis CG, Kourides JA, Valeri CR (1978). Red cell 2, 3-diphosphoglycerate and oxygen affinity of hemoglobin in patients with thyroid disorders. *Blood* **52,** 181–5.

22.8 Blood replacement

22.8.1 Blood transfusion

P. L. Perrotta and E. L. Snyder

Blood transfusion is important for the care of patients with severe anaemia, haemorrhage, thrombocytopenia, and coagulation disorders. Advances in the understanding of red cell, platelet, and leucocyte antigen structure, as well as the immune responses to these antigens, have vastly improved transfusion therapy. Routine blood bank procedures, including ABO typing, antibody screening, and compatibility testing, identify most patients at risk for serious immune-mediated red cell transfusion reactions. One of the most important technological improvements in transfusion therapy was the development of sterile, disposable, and flexible plastic containers that allow separation of whole blood into cellular and non-cellular components, including red blood cells, platelets, and plasma. Anticoagulants and additives currently used in blood collection containers allow storage of liquid red cells for up to 42 days. These advances have essentially eliminated the use of whole blood.

Individual components are stored under optimal conditions. Only that portion of blood required by the patient is transfused. Plasma separated from whole blood can be further fractionated into coagulation factor concentrates, albumin, or gamma globulin. Cell separators capable of collecting platelets, plasma, granulocytes, peripheral blood stem cells, and, more recently, red blood cells, are also in widespread use across the United States and Europe. Changes in recruiting and screening blood donors, as well as advances in the testing of donor blood have reduced the risk of viral transmission in Europe and the United States. All units of blood collected in the United States and Britain are tested for hepatitis B, hepatitis C, HIV-1, HIV-2, HTLV-1, and syphilis. Nucleotide testing for HIV and hepatitis C is now performed in most European countries and in the United States. Other risks of transfusion therapy include acute and delayed haemolytic, febrile non-haemolytic, allergic, and septic reactions. Premedication before transfusions, and leucoreduction of blood components have reduced these risks.

Although the hazards of blood transfusion are relatively small, the expected benefit of a transfusion must outweigh any risk to the patient. Therefore, a thorough understanding of the indications and complications of blood transfusion are required to minimize exposure to unnecessary allogeneic blood products and to prevent wastage of limited blood resources.

Blood group systems

ABO system

Over 250 distinct antigens have been identified on the surface of red blood cells. The most clinically important belong to the ABO system. The codominantly expressed A and B genes, located on chromosome 9, code for glycosyl transferases that add either *N*-acetyl-D-galactosamine (A gene) or D-galactose (B gene) to the common precursor H antigen (Table 1). The O gene is structurally similar to the A gene except for a single base deletion that eliminates production of a functional enzyme. The AB antigens are of critical importance because individuals who lack the A and/or B antigens form IgM and IgG antibodies directed against the missing antigen(s). Circulating A and B antibodies can fix complement and cause intravascular haemolysis. Anti-A and Anti-B antibodies are 'naturally occurring', that is, they are formed without prior clinical antigenic stimulation. Presumably, individuals become immunized following exposure to carbohydrate ABO antigenic determinants commonly found in the bacterial environment. Accordingly, group A persons produce anti-B, group B produce anti-A, and group O produce both anti-A and anti-B. Circulating A and B antibodies are of critical importance in blood therapy because they are of high titre, can fix complement to C9, and are responsible for the vast majority of major haemolytic transfusion reactions.

Table 1 ABO blood group system

ABO type	Gene(s)	Enzyme coded by gene	Resulting antigen	Antibody present in plasma	Frequency (white population)
O	*H*	L-fucosyl transferase	H	Anti-A and Anti-B	0.43
A	*A*	*N*-acetyl-D-galactosamine transferase	A	Anti-B	0.45
B	*B*	D-galactosyl transferase	B	Anti-A	0.09
AB	*A* and *B*	*N*-acetyl-D-galactosamine and D-galactosyl transferase	AB	None	0.04

Table 2 Wiener and Fisher–Race Rh system nomenclature

Serological reactivity					Most likely genotype	Most likely genotype
C	c	D	E	e	(Wiener)	(Fisher–Race)
+	+	+	0	+	*R1r*	*CDe/ce*
+	0	+	0	+	*R1r1*	*CDe/Ce*
0	+	+	+	+	*R2r*	*cDE/ce*
0	+	+	+	0	*R2R2*	*cDE/cDE*
+	+	+	+	+	*R1R2*	*CDe/cDE*
0	+	+	0	+	*R0r*	*cDe/ce*
0	+	0	0	+	*rr*	*ce/ce*
+	+	0	0	+	*r1r*	*Ce/ce*
0	+	0	+	+	*r11r*	*cE/ce*
+	+	0	+	+	*r1r11*	*Ce/cE*

Rh system

The Rh blood group system is composed of at least 44 distinct antigens. The five major antigens in the Rh system (D, C, c, E, and e) are responsible for the vast majority of Rh-related transfusion problems. It is now known that the D polypeptide is encoded at the *RHD* locus, whereas the CcEe polypeptide is coded by alleles at the *RHCE* locus. Based on the D gene frequency in North America and Europe, approximately 15 per cent of individuals will not produce D antigen and are 'Rh negative'. The most common nomenclatures used to classify the Rh antigens include those developed by Weiner and Fisher–Race (Tables 2 and 3). Each of these systems has its advantages and limitations. Very rare individuals who lack all Rh antigens are termed 'Rh-null'. Rh-null red cells are morphologically abnormal and typically have shortened survival, resulting in a mild haemolytic anaemia. The successful cloning of the RhD gene potentially allows application of molecular techniques to determine fetal RhD status.

The most clinically important Rh antigen is D because it is highly immunogenic—the likelihood of a D-negative person developing anti-D following exposure to as little as 0.1 ml of D-positive red cells is extremely high. Approximately 80 per cent of Rh-negative individuals transfused with a single unit of Rh positive red cells will develop anti-D. Anti-D is responsible for immune reactions including haemolytic disease of the newborn (HDN) and immune-mediated transfusion reactions. Despite widespread use of Rh immune globulin, anti-D remains the most common cause of serious HDN. Rh-negative women most commonly produce anti-D following exposure to D-positive red cells during pregnancy, a miscarriage, or abortion. The anti-D formed is of the IgG class and therefore can cross the placenta where it may cause a potentially fatal intrauterine HDN in an Rh-positive fetus.

Other blood groups

There are a large number of other well-characterized red cell blood group systems. Antibodies directed against some of these antigens may be naturally occurring and of little clinical significance (e.g. Lewis, Ii). Other antibodies may form following exposure to the corresponding antigen (e.g. Kell, Duffy, Kidd). Some of these antibodies are clinically significant in that they are associated with immune-mediated red cell destruction of transfused cells and HDN (Table 4). In most cases, compatible blood can be found for patients with significant red cell alloantibodies. Based on the high incidence of some red cell antigens on the cells of specific donor populations, some patients may be difficult to transfuse if they have developed multiple antibodies. This is particularly true in patients with sickle cell disease and other red cell disorders who require frequent transfusions. There have been recent advances in the understanding of the molecular genetics of many blood group antigens. These advances will eventually be used to resolve blood group discrepancies, screen for red cells of specific antigen makeup, and to identify fetuses who are at risk for HDN.

Table 3 Rh blood groups antigens

Fisher–Race (CDE) antigen	Wiener (Rh–Hr) antigen	Antigen frequency (white population)
D	Rh_0	0.85
C	rh'	0.70
E	rh"	0.30
c	hr'	0.80
e	hr"	0.98
C^w	rh^{w1}	0.01
V	hr^v	<0.01

The Kell (K) blood group system is clinically important because antibodies to Kell system antigens can cause haemolytic transfusion reactions and HDN. Only the D antigen is more immunogenic than the K antigen, the major antigen of the system. Kell is present in about 10 per cent of white individuals. Therefore, a K-negative blood recipient is unlikely to receive K-positive red cells during transfusion. The Kell blood group is linked to chronic granulomatous disease, a congenital disease resulting in decreased oxidative capacity of neutrophils, which leads to recurrent, severe bacterial infections. The genetic defect seen in chronic granulomatous disease is located on the X chromosome near the Kx Kell locus. The red cells of patients with chronic granulomatous disease are acanthocytic and are prone to mild haemolytic destruction. Systemic abnormalities described in chronic granulomatous disease include cardiomyopathy, areflexia, skeletal myopathies, and muscle wasting.

The Duffy (Fy) blood group is composed of six antigens, of which Fy^a and Fy^b are most important to transfusion practice. Fy^a antibodies have caused severe haemolytic transfusion reactions and severe HDN. Fy^b antibodies have more rarely been associated with these complications, and antibodies against the remaining Duffy antigens are rarely clinically important. Antibodies against Fy^a and Fy^b are reasonably common in diverse populations because the antigen frequency varies dramatically across racial groups. Fy^a and Fy^b antigens are present in 66 per cent and 83 per cent of white blood donors, respectively. These antigens have a much lower incidence in African populations. The Duffy system has an interesting association with malaria. Specifically, $Fy^{(a-b-)}$ negative red cells are resistant to *Plasmodium vivax* and *Plasmodium knowlesi* infection. Red cells from most West African blacks are $Fy^{(a-b-)}$ and therefore, resistant to these forms of malaria.

The Kidd (Jk) system is composed of three antigens (Jk^a, Jk^b, Jk^3). Jk^a and Jk^b antigens are found on approximately 75 per cent of white donor red cells. Anti-Kidd antibodies have caused severe haemolytic reactions and milder forms of HDN. Kidd antibodies are formed following exposure to Jk antigens during transfusion or pregnancy. They are unusual in that once formed, these antibodies often fall to non-detectable levels, and may not be detected in an already immunized patient. In this situation, transfusion of additional Kidd-positive red cells may cause a rapid immunological response, leading to formation of high-titre anti-Kidd, and subsequent haemolysis.

Detection of blood group antibodies

Antibody screening and antibody identification

Prior to receiving a blood transfusion, patients' red cells are typed for ABO and Rh status using commercially available reagents. During 'front typing', the donor's red cells are reacted with antibodies directed against the A, B, and D antigens. Blood grouping is confirmed during 'back typing' in which donor serum is tested for the presence of anti-A and anti-B antibodies. Following blood grouping, recipient serum or plasma is screened for red cell antibodies. Antibody screening is typically performed by incubating a patient's serum with two to four group O red cells sources that, in sum, contain all the common and clinically significant red cell antigens. If an antibody is present in the serum, it will react with the screening cell and cause red cell agglutination. Naturally occurring ABO antibodies do not

Table 4 Clinically significant blood groups

Red cell antigen	Antigen frequency1	Risk of haemolysis (immediate or delayed)	Risk of HDN
A, B	Variable	High (immediate)	Moderate (anti-A) Low (anti-B)
Rh	Variable	High (immediate and delayed)	Variable High to low
K	0.09	High (immediate and delayed)	High
Fy^a	White 0.66 Black 0.90	High (delayed)	Low
Fy^b	White 0.83 Black 0.73	Low (delayed)	None
Jka	0.77	Moderate (immediate and delayed)	Rare
Jkb	0.73	Moderate (immediate and delayed)	None
M	0.78	Low	Rare
N	0.72	None	None
S	0.55	Moderate (immediate and delayed)	Rare
s	0.89	Low (delayed)	Rare

[1]Antigen frequency in white population unless otherwise specified.

interfere with antibody identification because screening cells are type O. Antibody screening is commonly performed at room temperature (immediate phase), after incubating patient serum and test red cells at 37°C, and after incubation with antihuman globulin serum (Coombs phase). Some blood banks screen samples after adding various antigen–antibody enhancing substances including polyethylene glycol, low-ionic strength saline, and albumin. Each has certain advantages and disadvantages in terms of sensitivity and specificity in detecting clinically significant antibodies. Most blood banks still perform 'tube testing' in which red cell agglutinates are identified in standard test tubes. There are a number of newer systems that are being used to detect antigen–antibody reactions. These include gel systems based on the differential mobility of red cell agglutinates through gel columns, and capture systems in which test red cells are immobilized on microtitre plates. Newer automated and semiautomated systems will probably replace tube testing for the majority of ABO grouping, Rh typing, antibody screening, and crossmatching.

If a patient's serum reacts with one or more screening cells, additional tests are performed to identify the antibody(ies). In most cases, the serum is tested against a larger commercial 'panel' of group O red cells of known antigen profile. Based on the reactivity pattern, the antibody can usually be identified. There are a large number of techniques used to identify red cell antibodies. Many are based on using materials that either enhance or suppress the reactivity of a specific antibody. In some cases, a patient's serum may react with all panel cells. These 'panagglutinins' can be caused by: (1) a single antibody directed against a high incidence antigen present on all panel test red cells; (2) multiple antibodies that in total react with all test cells; or (3) an autoantibody. Autoantibodies are often found in autoimmune haemolytic anaemias, in which case the patient's serum will also react with his or her own red cells (see section on autoantibodies, below).

Compatibility testing

Routine compatibility testing is typically performed on red cell units before being transfused to a patient. Specifically, donor red cells are reacted with patient serum and if no reaction is observed, the unit is considered 'compatible'. In emergency situations, there may be insufficient time to perform compatibility testing. Many hospitals will supply group O Rh-negative red cells until a patient sample is obtained and tested. If a patient's ABO Rh status is known with certainty, then type-specific non-crossmatched blood can be provided. In either case, compatibility testing is performed on these transfused units as soon as possible. It is important to realize that supplies of O negative blood are often limited. A 'computer crossmatch' has been instituted at hospitals in North America. Patients with known ABO and Rh typing, and who have a negative antibody screen are provided ABO compatible blood while omitting the crossmatch step described above. Although a true serological crossmatch is not performed, the computer crossmatch is safe in the vast majority of transfusions.

Autoantibodies

Autoantibodies consist of immunoglobulins that react with a wide range of self-antigens including membrane and intracellular components, adsorbed plasma proteins, and nuclear antigens. Patients with warm autoimmune haemolytic anaemia often require transfusion. In this case, the blood bank may have difficulty finding a 'compatible' unit of red cells because the patient's serum not only reacts with his or her own red cells, but also those of all donor red cells. Additional time may be required by the blood bank to exclude the presence of a significant underlying alloantibody that is obscured by the autoantibody. Upwards of 25 per cent of previously transfused autoimmune haemolytic anaemia patients may have an underlying alloantibody. An underlying alloantibody may result in accelerated red cell destruction. Therefore, transfusion therapy must be carefully planned in these patients. Autoimmune antibodies often appear to have specificity for Rh antigens (e.g. anti-e), but the transfusion of antigen negative red cells (e.g. e-negative) is not indicated as *in vivo* red cell survival of antigen negative cells is usually no better than antigen positive cells.

Clinical use of blood components

Red blood cells

Red blood cells account for approximately 75 per cent of the annual cost of transfusion therapy in the United Kingdom. Red blood cells, prepared from whole blood by removing most of the plasma, are indicated for patients with both acute haemorrhage and chronic anaemias (Table 5). Earlier solutions, composed of citrate, dextrose, and phosphate buffers allowed storage of red cells from 21 to 35 days. It was later observed that the addition of adenine to the preservative solution improved cell viability by increasing intracellular ATP levels. The haematocrit of red cell units varies from 70 per cent (citrate, phosphate, dextrose, adenine (CPDA-1)) to 55 to 60 per cent (additive solution, AS). Citrate contained in blood preservatives binds calcium to inhibit clotting and may cause hypocalcaemia and alkalosis in neonates and massively transfused patients. Red blood cells or AS units refrigerated at 1 to 6°C have a shelf-life of 35 (red blood cells) to 42 (AS units) days depending on the ingredients of the preservative. During storage, the following changes are observed in red cell units: (1) a fall in pH; (2) decreases in red cell ATP and 2,3-diphosphoglycerate; (3) increased supernatant potassium; and (4) decreased supernatant glucose. Leucocytes can be removed from the product at the blood centre collection site (prestorage

Table 5 Use of common blood transfusion components

Component	Indication for use
Red blood cells	Symptomatic acute and chronic anaemias
Red blood cells frozen and deglycerolized	Symptomatic anaemia, storage of red cells of rare antigen composition for up to 10 years
Leucocyte-reduced components (red blood cells and platelets)	Symptomatic anaemia, reduce febrile reactions from leucocyte antibodies, alternative to CMV seronegative components, prevent HLA alloimmunization
Washed components (red blood cells and platelets)	Remove harmful plasma antibodies
Platelet components (pooled platelets and pheresis platelets)	Thrombocytopenia with bleeding, prophylactic transfusion, platelet function abnormalities
HLA matched/selected platelets and crossmatch compatible platelets	HLA-alloimmunized thrombocytopenic patients with decreased platelet survival
Fresh frozen plasma	Replacement of labile and stable plasma coagulation factors for which specific factor concentrates are not available, liver disease, DIC, hypofibrinogenaemia, TTP
Cryoprecipitate	Fibrinogen and factor XIII replacement, factor VIII and vWF replacement when recombinant and virus-inactivated concentrates are not available
Granulocytes by pheresis	Neutropenic patient with infection unresponsive to antibiotics

leucodepletion), in the hospital blood bank prior to release, or at the patient's bedside using leucoreduction filters. Red blood cells with uncommon antigen profiles can be frozen within 6 days of collection and stored for up to 10 years. They are frozen with approximately 40 per cent glycerol to avoid cell dehydration and damage during the freezing process. Frozen red cells are no longer used as a leucoreduced product.

The patient's overall clinical status and laboratory parameters should both be considered when deciding to transfuse a patient. A decision should not be based on the haematocrit alone. Younger patients will usually tolerate a given degree of hypoxaemia and hypotension better than older patients who may have underlying coronary or myocardial disease. Evidence of symptomatic anaemia include excessive fatigue, malaise, headache, tachycardia, hypotension, and end-organ damage. Hypovolaemic shock typically ensues with acute loss (<24 h) of over 30 per cent of total blood volume. Initially, the haematocrit will be falsely elevated in acute haemorrhage, but will then fall with fluid resuscitation. Slowly developing, chronic anaemias are usually better tolerated then rapid onset anaemias due to the ability of the body's fluid compensatory mechanisms. Transfusion is rarely indicated when the haemoglobin (Hb) is greater than 10 g/dl, and is often not considered until the Hb is less than 7 g/dl. A patient's cardiac and pulmonary status must be considered when determining transfusion thresholds. Patients with unstable angina or acute myocardial infarction may require transfusion when the Hb is less than 10 g/dl. In the absence of active red cell destruction, transfusing a single unit will typically increase the Hb by 1 g/dl (haematocrit by 3 per cent).

Platelets

The availability of plastic primary collection bags with attached satellite containers allows the harvesting of platelets as a by-product of red cell separation. In the United States, platelets are prepared by the platelet-rich plasma method, whereas the buffy coat method is used in Europe. Each unit of 'random donor' platelets prepared by differential centrifugation of a single whole blood collection typically contains at least 5.5×10^{10} platelets suspended in 50 ml of plasma. Platelets stored under agitation at 20 to 24°C in plastic containers that allow oxygen diffusion have a shelf-life of 5 days. The risk of bacterial growth and development of platelet function abnormalities (platelet storage defect) preclude storage longer than 5 days. 'Random donor' platelets are usually administered in pools of 4 to 6 units. In the absence of conditions associated with decreased platelet survival, each unit can be expected to raise the recipient's platelet count by 5000 to 10 000/μl. Single donor platelets prepared by apheresis contain more than 3×10^{11} platelets suspended in about 200 ml plasma, equivalent to 6 average random donor platelet units. Platelets are not normally crossmatched with the recipient's serum. ABO type-specific platelets should be provided whenever possible because transfusion of out-of-type platelets may result in a postplatelet increment 10 to 20 per cent less than that expected for ABO type-specific platelets. Rh antigens present on the small number of contaminating red cells found in platelet concentrates are capable of immunizing a Rh negative recipient. If Rh negative platelet concentrates are not available for an Rh negative patient, Rh positive platelets can be transfused followed by administration of Rh immune globulin within 72 h of transfusion.

Platelets are provided to thrombocytopenic patients who are bleeding or to severely thrombocytopenic patients as a prophylactic precautionary measure. Spontaneous bleeding is rare when a patient's platelet count is over 20 000/μl, and studies suggest that patients who receive chemotherapy can tolerate platelet counts as low as 5 to 10 000/μl. Postsurgical patients may require platelet transfusions to control or prevent postoperative bleeding when the platelet count is over 50 000/μl. Overall coagulation status should also be considered because patients with plasma coagulation factor disorders are more likely to bleed at marginal platelet counts. Actively bleeding patients on aspirin, an irreversible inhibitor of platelet function, may require transfusions at higher platelet counts, although transfused platelets will also be affected if the patient remains on aspirin.

Platelet refractoriness is a major problem for patients who are dependent on platelet transfusions. The corrected count increment (CCI) is used to identify patients who are refractory to platelet transfusions through either HLA or platelet (HPA) alloimmunization. The CCI is calculated as follows:

$$\text{CCI} = \frac{\text{Post (/ml)} - \text{Pre (/ml)} \times \text{BSA (m}^2\text{)}}{\text{plts} \times 10^{-11}}$$

where Pre = pretransfusion platelet count, Post = post-transfusion platelet count drawn 1 to 4 h after completion of the transfusion, plts = number of platelets transfused (1 U 'random donor' platelets ~ 0.7×10^{11} plt; 1 U single donor platelets ~ 3 to 4×10^{11} plt), and BSA = body surface area in m^2.

Causes of a platelet refractory state include disseminated intravascular coagulation (DIC), sepsis, and circulating immune complexes. After documenting a low CCI (<5000), crossmatch-compatible platelets or HLA-matched single donor platelets should be considered. These products are not readily available in most blood banks. Increasing the dose of standard platelet concentrates can be considered until compatible platelets are identified. Leucocyte reduction filters, as well as UV-B irradiation, decrease the rate of HLA alloimmunization to platelets. Leucocyte reduction filtered blood products should be provided to patients who will require many platelet transfusions.

Granulocytes

There is renewed interest in granulocyte transfusion kindled by improvements in apheresis collection techniques and the use of steroids and/or growth factors to improve granulocyte yields. Granulocytes are primarily transfused to neutropenic oncology patients who develop Gram positive or Gram negative bacterial sepsis unresponsive to antibiotic therapy for a minimum of 24 to 48 h. Granulocytes collected from non-stimulated healthy donors by apheresis contain at least 1×10^{10} neutrophils/unit and can be stored for only 24 h at 20 to 24°C. Higher numbers of granulocytes can be collected when donors are stimulated by steroids and/or growth factors. They contain large numbers of red cells (20–50 ml) and must be crossmatched with the recipient's serum. Granulocytes should be irradiated (2500 cGy) because of the large number of lymphocytes present in the product. They are considered for the above patients provided they also have an absolute neutrophil count less than 500/μl and a reasonable chance of marrow recovery. Because of their short half-life, granulocytes are usually provided daily until the patient can maintain an absolute neutrophil count greater than 500/μl without transfusion or until the infection resolves. Infusion of larger numbers of granulocytes does allow measurable increases in recipient neutrophil counts, but the optimal dose and frequency remain undefined. Febrile reactions to granulocytes are common, the reactions being more severe when amphotericin is infused near the time of granulocyte transfusions. Overall, the additional benefit of granulocyte transfusions for these neutropenic patients as compared to antibiotic treatment alone is unclear. The collection of granulocytes, or any blood component, by apheresis is not an entirely innocuous process. The donor is at risk for uncommon, but potentially serious, adverse reactions including hydroxyethyl starch-related hypertension and anaphylaxis, and citrate-induced hypocalcaemia. Minor, but typically tolerable, side-effects of pretreating granulocyte donors with dexamethasone (insomnia, flushing) and/or G-CSF (bone pain, headaches, insomnia) occur in a substantial number of donors.

Plasma, cryoprecipitate, and plasma derivatives

Plasma therapy began in the late 1940s with the development of fractionation techniques in which large pools of human plasma collected from many donors could be separated into specific plasma proteins. Plasma is separated from whole blood by centrifugation and frozen within 8 h of collection in order to maintain the activity of labile coagulation factors, factors V and VII. Fresh frozen plasma (FFP) contains all coagulation factors, plasma proteins, and complement. FFP should not be transfused for volume expansion because of the risk of transfusion-transmitted disease and the availability of other, safer non-plasma substitutes. The primary indications for FFP transfusion include deficiency of multiple coagulation factors as seen in liver disease and DIC. It is often used to reverse warfarin anticoagulation urgently. One unit of clotting factor activity is defined as the amount of activity in 1 ml of normal plasma. FFP is not particularly effective in replacing individual clotting factors because of the large volumes that would be required to obtain adequate factor levels. The patient's fluid and cardiovascular status may preclude the use of large amounts of plasma.

FFP is no longer the treatment of choice for coagulopathies where virally inactivated or recombinant products exist, such as for deficiencies of factor VIII (haemophilia A) or factor IX (haemophilia B). Fears of transmitting infectious disease with plasma transfusion remain of concern, particularly for pooled products. In addition to donor screening and testing, other strategies to decrease infectious risk include photoinactivation and solvent/detergent treatment technologies. Solvent and detergent treated plasma prepared from 500 l plasma pools (2500 donors) is available in the United States. This treatment effectively removes lipid enveloped viruses including HIV and HCV, but does not eliminate non-enveloped viruses such as parvovirus B-19 and, possibly, other unrecognized non-lipid-enveloped pathogens.

Cryoprecipitate is prepared by thawing FFP between 1 and 6°C. Each 10 to 20 ml unit contains 100 to 350 mg fibrinogen/unit, at least 80 IU/unit factor VIII, and some von Willebrand factor. Use of cryoprecipitate is generally reserved for patients with von Willebrand's disease or those with severe hypofibrinogenaemia (<100 mg/dl). Cryoprecipitate and thrombin are combined to make 'fibrin glue.' This biological sealant works well but exposes the recipient to the risks of transfusion-transmitted disease due to the use of cryoprecipitate.

Albumin is available as a 5 or 25 per cent solution and is used to treat hypovolaemia and hypoalbuminaemia, primarily in surgical settings. Albumin is virally inactivated by heat treatment plus other viral inactivation steps, and is tested for HCV RNA. Properly processed albumin is not considered to transmit viral disease. Readily available non-plasma colloidal solutions have replaced albumin in many situations requiring volume expansion. Intravenous immunoglobulin (IVIg) is used to treat patients with immune thrombocytopenia, Guillain–Barre syndrome, and autoimmune haemolytic anaemias. Prompt and adequate doses of Rho (D) immunoglobulin (RhIG) available in intramuscular and IV preparations are used to prevent alloimmunization in D-negative patients who are exposed to D-positive red cells through transfusion or pregnancy. Rapid advances in molecular techniques led to the cloning and purification of recombinant clotting factors. Recombinant factor VIII, IX, and factor VIIa are available.

Complications and management of transfusion therapy (Table 6)

Acute intravascular haemolytic reactions

Acute intravascular haemolytic transfusion reactions (AIHTR) are one of the most serious transfusion complications. These reactions occur in blood recipients who have developed antibodies directed against antigens present on the transfused red blood cells. ABO incompatibility remains the most common cause of immediate intravascular haemolytic reactions. Donor erythrocytes carrying either A and/or B red cell antigens bind to the recipient's naturally occurring anti-A and/or anti-B antibodies, resulting in complement fixation, formation of the C5b-9 membrane attack complex, and subsequent haemolysis. Biological response modifiers, such as proinflammatory cytokines (IL-1, TNF-α), chemokines (IL-8), and complement fragments (C3a, C5a), also play a role in the pathophysiology of AIHTRs. AIHTRs are typified by the sudden onset of back pain, hypotension, tachycardia, fever, chills, diaphoresis, and dyspnoea. The symptoms usually begin soon after the transfusion is started in immunocompetent recipients. Laboratory studies reveal an increase in unconjugated bilirubin (typically to 2–3 mg/dl) and marked elevation of lactate dehydrogenase. Other evidence of intravascular haemolysis include haemoglobinuria and haemoglobinaemia. The direct antiglobulin test (direct Coombs) becomes reactive due to the coating of donor red cells with the recipient's antibodies.

AIHTRs are usually caused by transfusions of ABO incompatible blood resulting from patient identification or clerical errors, but they can also be caused by incompatibility within other blood group systems (Duffy, Kidd). Proper labelling of clots used by the blood bank for compatibility testing and careful identification of patients are the best ways to prevent potentially fatal reactions. AIHTRs are medical emergencies and treatment consists of

Table 6 Major risks of blood transfusion therapy

Immune complications	Non-immune complications
Acute haemolytic transfusion reactions	Transfusion-associated bacterial sepsis
Delayed extravascular haemolytic reaction	Circulatory overload, cardiac failure
Febrile transfusion reaction	Viral transmission (Hepatitis A, B, C, cytomegalovirus, parvovirus)
Allergic transfusion reaction (urticaria and anaphylaxis)	Iron overload
Transfusion associated sepsis	Hypocalcaemia
Alloimmunization	Hypothermia
Transfusion-associated graft-versus-host disease	Dilutional coagulopathy due to factor depletion, thrombocytopenia
Transfusion-associated acute lung injury	

Table 7 Symptoms, signs, and management of transfusion reactions

Reaction	Symptoms and signs	Management/treatment
Acute intravascular haemolytic reaction	Back pain, fever, hypotension, shock, dyspnoea, haemoglobinuria, haemoglobinaemia, positive direct Coombs	Stop transfusion, IV fluids, vasopressor support, maintain dirurесis, corticosteroids, dialysis if indicated
Delayed extravascular haemolytic reaction	Anaemia, jaundice, fever, positive direct Coombs	Stop transfusion, fluid support, follow lab results (Hct, LDH, bilirubin)
Febrile reaction	Fever, chills, rigors, mild dyspnoea	Stop transfusion, antipyretics, consider leucoreduced product for subsequent transfusions
Allergic (mild)	Pruritis, urticaria	Antihistamines, may continue transfusion if symptoms improve in <30 min, otherwise stop transfusion
Allergic (anaphylactic)	Urticaria, bronchospasm, dyspnoea, nausea, hypotension	Stop transfusion, antihistamines, vasopressor support, corticosteroids, consider premedication or washed RBCs for subsequent transfusions
Septic reaction	Rapid onset of chills, fever, hypotension	Stop transfusion, culture sample from product and patient, vasopressor support, IV fluids, broad spectrum antibiotics

immediately stopping the transfusion, close monitoring of vital signs, cardiac and airway support, and maintenance of urine output with saline diuresis with or without a loop diuretic (Table 7). Dialysis must be considered in patients with renal failure.

Delayed extravascular haemolytic reactions

Delayed haemolytic transfusion reactions (DHTRs) generally occur in patients who have a negative antibody screen on pretransfusion testing, but who then experience accelerated destruction of transfused red cells 7 to 14 days post-transfusion. In most cases, red cell destruction is caused by an antibody that is initially of a titre below the limits of detection on routine screening. The antibody then rapidly forms on secondary exposure to the offending antigen. Only rare DHTRs are caused by primary allosensitization in which a patient synthesized a new antibody. The antibodies typically fix complement to C3 and stop, thus, resulting in extravascular as opposed to intravascular haemolysis. Antibodies most commonly implicated in DHTRs include those directed against Rh (E, c), Kell, Duffy, and Kidd blood group antigens. DHTRs can be diagnosed by an unexpected post-transfusional fall in haematocrit, development of unconjugated hyperbilirubinaemia, and appearance of a positive direct antiglobulin test. There is usually a delay of 3 days to 2 weeks between transfusion and onset of extravascular haemolysis. Only rarely do delayed reactions cause intravascular haemolysis with associated haemoglobinaemia and haemoglobinuria.

Febrile non-haemolytic reactions

Febrile non-haemolytic transfusion reactions (FNTRs) to red blood cell and platelet transfusion are very common. They are caused by the development of antibodies in the recipient directed against HLA and/or leucocyte-specific antigens on donor white blood cells and platelets. Reactions between leucoagglutinins present in the transfused product and recipient leucocyte antigens can also occur. Subsequent formation of leucocyte antigen–antibody complexes results in complement binding and release of endogenous pyrogens such as IL-1, IL-6, and TNF-α. Cytokines generated by leucocytes during platelet and red cell storage may also contribute to FNTRs. Symptoms occur during or several hours after the transfusion, and typically include low-grade (> 1°C rise) and high grade fevers, accompanied by shaking chills. Rarely, vomiting, dyspnoea, hypotension, and decreased oxygen saturation may develop. The severity of symptoms is often directly related to the number of leucocytes in the product or the rate or volume of transfusion. Leucoreduction of blood components decrease the frequency of febrile transfusion reactions. Premedication with an antipyretic such as acetaminophen can ameliorate mild febrile transfusion reactions. Antihistamines are not helpful in preventing or treating febrile transfusion reactions. Corticosteroids can also minimize febrile transfusion reactions if they are administered several hours before the transfusion. Intramuscular or subcutaneous meperidine will usually resolve severe rigors in a matter of minutes. If symptoms do not resolve in less than 4 h or are especially severe, other complications such as sepsis due to contaminated blood products or a haemolytic reaction should be considered.

Allergic reactions

Allergic reactions to plasma, platelets, and red blood cells are relatively common. They present as pruritis and/or urticaria in the absence of fever. Allergic reactions are usually IgE mediated and most symptoms are attributed to histamine release. It may be difficult to distinguish allergic and febrile transfusion reactions when urticarial symptoms are accompanied by low-grade fever. Common symptoms and signs include erythema, papular rashes, wheals, and pruritis. Severe anaphylaxis resulting in bronchospasm and hypotension are possible. As in other allergic responses, symptoms are not dose-related and severe manifestations can occur following small exposures. Treatment of mild allergic reactions consists of stopping the transfusion and administering diphenhydramine or other antihistamines. In a mild allergic reaction with only pruritis and hives, it is acceptable to continue transfusing the same unit providing the symptoms promptly resolve and there is no fever or vasomotor instability. If symptoms recur after the transfusion is restarted, a new unit should be obtained. Severe anaphylactic reactions with bronchospasm and cardiovascular collapse are rare and should be treated like any other anaphylactic reaction with steroids, vasopressors, and airway support. Washed red blood cells in which the residual donor plasma has been removed and replaced by saline may benefit patients with repeated or severe allergic reactions. Leucocyte reduction filters are not helpful because they do not remove the implicated soluble mediators.

Septic reactions

Blood products can become contaminated by bacteria if a donor is bacteraemic at the time of collection or if improper arm preparation occurs during venipuncture. Transfusion of blood products contaminated by bacteria is particularly dangerous and can result in profound hypotension and shock. There are no laboratory screening tests commonly used to detect bacterial contamination and contaminated units cannot be easily identified by inspection. The risk of septic transfusion reactions is higher for platelet transfusions than other blood components because platelets are stored at room temperature. Common organisms implicated in septic transfusion reactions include Gram-positive (*Staphylococcus* sp.) and Gram-negative (*Enterobacter, Yersinia, Pseudomonas* sp.) bacteria. Blood cultures should be obtained from patients who develop high fevers following or during transfusion, especially if they become hypotensive. A Gram stain of the suspected contaminated product may be helpful but is often negative, and the product should be cultured if possible. Other symptoms attributed to preformed endotoxin and cytokines include skin flushing, severe rigors, and rapid-onset cardiovascular collapse. The symptoms may occur during, or minutes to hours after the transfusion is completed. Treatment includes fluids, cardiorespiratory support, and broad-spectrum antibiotics. Febrile transfusion reactions can usually be distinguished from septic transfusion reactions by the former's self-limited nature and lack of profound hypotension.

Transfusion-related acute lung injury

Transfusion-related acute lung injury (TRALI) is a serious complication of blood transfusion therapy that presents as non-cardiogenic pulmonary oedema. It typically occurs within 6 h of transfusion. It is clinically identical to the adult respiratory distress syndrome (ARDS). The most common clinical findings are rapid-onset symptoms including dyspnoea, tachypnoea, cyanosis, fever, and hypotension. Lung auscultation reveals diffuse, crackly, and decreased breath sounds. Invasive cardiac monitoring demonstrates normal cardiac pressures and function with hypoxaemia and decreased pulmonary compliance. Radiographic findings include diffuse, fluffy infiltrates typical of pulmonary oedema. The aetiology is believed to involve immune-mediated reaction of HLA antibodies or other leucoagglutins with white cells resulting in leucocyte activation. Granulocytes are first activated by HLA or other Ag–Ab complexes and then migrate to the lungs. The activated leucocytes bind to the pulmonary capillary bed via integrins and other cell adhesion molecules where they release proteolytic enzymes that destroy tissue, resulting in a capillary leak syndrome and pulmonary oedema. More recently, reactive lipid products released from donor cell membranes have been associated with the development of TRALI. TRALI should be suspected in patients with severe and rapid-onset respiratory distress following transfusion therapy, or, more specifically, pulmonary oedema without hypervolaemia. Definitive diagnosis requires identification of HLA and/or granulocyte antibodies in either the donor's or recipient's serum, as well as the corresponding antigens on the recipient's or donor's leucocytes. This testing is performed in a few specialized laboratories. Approximately 80 to 90 per cent of patients with TRALI will survive with supportive care including aggressive respiratory support, supplemental oxygen, and mechanical ventilation. Based on the presumed pathogenesis of TRALI, leucoreduced blood products could theoretically decrease the incidence of TRALI. Drugs used to treat TRALI have included corticosteroids and diuretics.

Transfusion-associated graft-versus-host disease

Acute graft-versus-host disease (GVHD) is a rare complication of blood transfusion, but is fatal in approximately 90 per cent of patients. TA-GVHD occurs when donor immunocompetent T and NK cells attack immunoincompetent recipient cells because these recipient cells appear foreign due to differences in major or minor histocompatibility antigens. GVHD is commonly seen following allogeneic bone marrow transplant but may also rarely occur in immunodeficient or immunosuppressed patients following blood transfusion. Removal of T cells from a donor graft can prevent acute GVHD in oncology patients, but is associated with increased graft failure and a decrease in a 'graft-versus-leukaemia' effect. The risk of TA-GVHD is related to the number of viable T lymphocytes transfused, the recipient's immune status, and the HLA disparity between donor and host. Therefore, multiply transfused patients who receive cells from donors who share HLA haplotypes with the recipient are at greatest risk. Clinically, TA-GVHD is characterized by the acute onset of rash, abdominal pain, diarrhoea, liver abnormalities (elevated liver enzymes, hyperbilirubinaemia), and bone marrow suppression 2 to 30 days following transfusion. The maculopapular rash seen is similar to that observed in acute GVHD following bone marrow transplant, and biopsy of the skin may help to confirm the diagnosis. Pancytopenia may be severe and is attributed to destruction of recipient marrow stem cells by donor lymphocytes. Immunosuppressive therapy with prednisone and cyclosporine has had little effect in TA-GVHD. Fortunately, TA-GVHD can be prevented by irradiating products prior to transfusion. Specifically, irradiation of cellular blood products with 2500 cGy inactivates donor lymphocytes and is the most effective method for preventing TA-GVHD.

Transfusion-transmitted disease

Despite major improvements in blood safety during the past 20 years, there remains a relatively small risk of transfusion-transmitted disease. The use of volunteer donors and predonation screening questionnaires were the first steps taken to reduce the risk of transfusion-related hepatitis and HIV. These risks continue to drive mandated pretransfusion testing requirements in developed countries. The advent of enzyme immunoassays in the 1970s, and more recent nucleotide testing, have further decreased the risk of transfusion-transmitted disease (Table 8). Transfusion-transmitted disease is a persistent problem in parts of the world that do not have access to screening tests.

Pretransfusion testing typically includes screening for syphilis, hepatitis B (HBsAg, anti-HBc), hepatitis C (anti-HCV), human immunodeficiency virus (anti-HIV-1/2, HIV-1 p24 antigen), human T cell lymphotropic virus (anti-HTLV-1/2), and syphilis. Serum alanine aminotransferase is measured in most European countries as a non-specific surrogate marker of hepatitis. When positive, these tests are typically confirmed by supplemental or confirmatory testing. Current estimates of the risk of transfusion-related HIV range from 1:500 000 to 1:750 000 units transfused. Despite improvements in tests used to detect HIV antibodies in donors, the 'window period' in which HIV could be transmitted by an infected, but HIV seronegative, donor remained in 1996 at about 25 days. The introduction of screening for HIV-1 p24 antigen in 1997 decreased the window period to approximately 15 days.

Genomic testing for hepatitis C virus (HCV) RNA was implemented in the United States and Europe to detect seronegative, yet infectious units.

Table 8 Organisms potentially transmitted by blood transfusion

Agent/organism	Estimated risk per unit transfused (United States)	Pretransfusion testing
Hepatitis B virus	1:65 000	HBsAg, anti-HBc, ALT
Hepatitis C virus	1:100 000 (pre-nucleotide testing) 1:500 000 (post-nucleotide testing)	anti-HCV, nucleotide testing
HIV-1/2	1:500 000–1:750 000	anti-HIV-1/2, p24 antigen
HTLV-1/2 virus	1:650 000	anti-HTLV-1/2
CMV	1:10–1:20 (see text)	Some units tested for anti-CMV antibodies
Parvovirus B19	Unknown	None
Bacterial contamination	1:1500	None
Treponema pallidum	Rare	RPR
Parasites (*Plasmodium* sp., *Ehrlichia* sp., *Babesia microti*)	Rare	None
New-variant Creutzfeld–Jacob disease	Theoretically possible	Deferral based on history

Nucleotide testing (NAT) for hepatitis C and HIV is typically performed on small pools of samples. The importance of hepatitis C transmission in blood therapy has been confirmed in many countries by retrospective review. During these 'look backs', recipients of blood components from donors later found to be positive (since anti-HCV screening was only instituted in 1991) are examined. A large percentage of these recipients, up to 75 per cent, are found to be anti-HCV positive. The majority of those who seroconvert will develop chronic liver disease. NAT testing will decrease the transfusion-related hepatitis C by decreasing the window period, from approximately 60 to 80, to 10 to 20 days. Hepatitis G virus has been transferred by blood transfusion, but its significance is unclear in that transfusion-acquired HGB infection has not been associated with acute or chronic hepatitis.

Several techniques have been developed to inactivate viruses in plasma including solvent and detergent treatment, and photochemical inactivation using psoralens and long wavelength UV light. Methods to inactivate infectious pathogens in cellular blood components, including platelets and red cells, are not currently available but are under development. Due to the low risk of viral infection by transfusion and the fact that most patients who receive plasma also receive cellular blood components, the cost-effectiveness of virally-inactivated plasma is very low. Albumin, immune globulin, factor concentrates, and other plasma derivatives are also virally attenuated, following standard treatment protocols.

Other pathogens, such as CMV and parvovirus B19, are common in the general donor population, and may pose a serious threat in immunocompromised patients. Approximately 40 to 60 per cent of blood donors have been exposed to CMV during their lifetime and subsequently are CMV seropositive. Only about 2 per cent of CMV seropositive donors, however, are actively infected and transfusion of their blood to an immunocompromised recipient could cause potentially serious disease. The actual risk of post-transfusion seroconversion to a CMV negative recipient who receives CMV-untested blood depends on the prevalence of CMV seropositivity in the donor population.

A number of parasitic diseases are known, or are suspected to be transmitted by blood transfusion. These include malaria, Chagas' disease, babesiosis, leishmaniasis, and toxoplasmosis. Transmission of Lyme disease (*Borrelia borgdorferi*) by transfusion has not been documented. The risk of new-variant Creutzfeldt–Jakob disease (nvCJD), first described in the UK in 1996, is unknown. It is unclear whether nvCJD is transmissible by blood transfusion and this form of transmission has not been reported. Fears of transmitting nvCJD, however, have resulted in implementation of a universal white blood cell reduction policy in the United Kingdom. There is a risk of acquiring babesiosis by blood transfusion, and infections with this organism can be dangerous in at risk populations (e.g. splenectomized patients) if untreated.

Use of special blood products

Leucoreduction

Leucocytes contained in blood components can provoke febrile non-haemolytic reactions, induce HLA alloimmunization, and transmit cytomegalovirus (CMV) to at-risk recipients. Leucocytes are most effectively removed from red cell and platelet concentrates by leucocyte reduction filters. Third-generation leucocyte reduction filters remove 3 to 4 $\log_{10}$ of the total intact leucocytes found in red cell and platelet concentrates. American Association of Blood Bank standards require that units labelled leucoreduced in the United States contain less than 5×10^6 white blood cells. Red cells are either leucoreduced shortly after blood collection (prestorage leucodepletion), following refrigerated storage (poststorage leucodepletion), or at the bedside during transfusion. Filters are similarly used to leucoreduce platelet concentrates—apheresis devices have been designed to collect leucoreduced platelets directly (process leucoreduction). Quality control measures must be in place in order to verify adequate leucoreduction of transfused products.

Leucoreduction has been shown to reduce the prevalence and severity of febrile transfusion reactions and to decrease the risk of HLA alloimmunization. Leucoreduced products are less likely to stimulate the HLA alloantibodies implicated in both febrile transfusion reactions and antibody-induced platelet refractoriness. Other generally accepted benefits of white blood cell reduction include reducing platelet refractoriness, and decreasing the risk of transmitting white blood cell-related infectious agents including CMV and HTLV-I/II. Prestorage leucoreduced products are preferable because they are also devoid of cytokines and other biological response modifiers which play a role in transfusion complications. Many of these proteins are not efficiently removed by leucocyte reduction filters. With the dramatic decrease in the risk of viral transmission, investigators are focusing on the immunomodulatory effects of blood transfusion. These effects specifically deal with associations between allogeneic transfusion and bacterial infection, tumour progression, and tumour recurrence. Universal white blood cell reduction of both red blood cells and platelets has been required and/or is being implemented in a number of countries including the United Kingdom, Canada, France, Ireland, Portugal, and the United States.

Irradiation

Blood components are irradiated to prevent potentially lethal transfusion-associated graft-versus-host disease by interfering with the ability of lymphocytes to proliferate. Irradiation of supportive blood components is indicated in bone marrow or peripheral blood stem cell transplant recipeints, patients with congenital immunodeficiency states, neonates, premature infants, and during intrauterine exchange transfusion. Patients with AIDS commonly receive irradiated components, although there is no clear increased risk of transfusion-associated graft-versus-host disease in this population. Standard guidelines recommend irradiating red blood cells, platelets, and granulocytes with a minimum dose of 2500 cGy. Platelets and red cells are not adversely affected by this exposure. It is not necessary to irradiate FFP or cryoprecipitate because they do not contain viable leucocytes. Bone marrow or peripheral blood stem cells must never be irradiated prior to transplant.

Cytomegalovirus-safe

Cytomegalovirus (CMV) infection is a leading cause of morbidity and mortality in marrow and solid organ transplant patients. Most serious CMV infections that develop in these populations are a result of latent reactivation of recipient CMV, but CMV can also be transmitted by blood transfusion. Therefore, blood banks supply products that have a low potential of transmitting CMV. The available products include CMV seronegative units prepared from donors who are CMV antibody negative, and leucodepleted components. The latter refers to blood components leucoreduced in a blood centre or laboratory using cGMP techniques. Depending on the donor population, however, as many as 80 to 90 per cent of blood donors may be CMV seropositive. Thus, the demand for CMV seronegative products may exceed supply. In addition, CMV seronegative products can transmit CMV disease. Studies suggest that CMV seronegative and leucodepleted filtered products are equivalent in preventing CMV transmission. Many transfusion specialists consider cGMP leucodepleted units as CMV 'safe' in that they are unlikely to transmit CMV disease. In addition to CMV seronegative marrow and solid organ transplant recipients, CMV seronegative or safe components are generally indicated for premature infants, during intrauterine transfusions, for patients with congenital immunodeficiencies, CMV seronegative pregnant females, and seronegative patients with HIV. The British Committee for Standards in Haematology has concluded that leucoreduced components are an 'effective alternative' to seronegative products for preventing CMV transmission by transfusion.

Alternatives to blood component therapy

Autologous transfusion

Commonly used forms of autologous transfusion include preoperative blood donation, acute normovolaemic haemodilution, and autologous blood salvage. Many blood centres provide autologous preoperative blood donation services in which a patient's blood is drawn and stored for later use, usually during a surgical procedure. The criteria for autologous donations are less stringent than those for allogeneic donors. Preoperative blood donation can be utilized in elderly patients, although there is a higher risk of anaemia and more serious cardiovascular complications associated with the donation. Although the use of autologous blood decreases the risk of viral infection, the risk of bacterial contamination remains. Acute normovolaemic haemodilution is performed by removing blood from a patient immediately before surgery and replacing the blood volume with crystalloid or colloid solutions to maintain haemodynamic stability. The withdrawn blood is then later reinfused. Autologous blood salvage is performed by collecting and then returning blood lost during or shortly following operative procedures using intraoperative salvage devices. This technique is primarily employed in cardiac and orthopaedic surgery.

Growth factors

Haematopoietic growth factors used in transfusion therapy are designed to limit the exposure of patients to allogeneic blood. The isolation, characterization, and subsequent synthesis of erythropoietin by recombinant technology (rHuEPO) was one of the most important advances in decreasing red cell transfusions. Use of rHuEPO has dramatically reduced the transfusion needs of patients with renal failure and various anaemias. rHuEPO has also been employed to increase the yield of autologous donations and to stimulate erythropoiesis following surgery. Granulocyte colony stimulating factor (G-CSF) has been shown to decrease infection rates in neutropenic patients undergoing chemotherapy, replacing marginally effective granulocyte transfusions. There is rapid growth in the use of other growth factors including FLT-3 ligand, c-MPL ligand (thrombopoietin, TPO) and various combinations of growth factors. These growth factors have been shown to reduce thrombocytopenia following non-myeloablative chemotherapy. Thrombopoietic growth factors also have the potential to stimulate platelet apheresis donors, increase stem cell harvest yields, and to expand progenitor cells *ex vivo*. Development of neutralizing antibodies against endogenous thrombopoietin has plagued clinical testing of thrombopoietic growth factors.

Blood substitutes

Red cell substitutes currently in development include haemoglobin-based oxygen carriers (HBOCs), perfluorocarbon emulsions (PFCs), and liposome-encapsulated haemoglobin. The two major types of blood substitutes, HBOCs and PFCs, are in phase II and III clinical trials. HBOCs are artificially derived products with oxygen carrying properties. They are structurally similar to haemoglobin but do not contain red cell stroma which is toxic and leads to renal damage. Development of HBOCs has been hampered by the relatively short half-life of these oxygen carriers in the circulation. PFCs are synthetic hydrocarbons that have the ability to carry dissolved oxygen. The particles circulate for only a few hours until they are removed by the reticuloendothelial system. Research efforts to modify or remove red blood cell antigens from donor units is proceeding slowly, but a truly universal compatible red cell unit may one day be within reach.

Further reading

BCSH Blood Transfusion Task Force (1996). Guidelines on gamma irradiation of blood components for the prevention of transfusion-associated graft-versus-host disease. *Transfusion Medicine* **6**, 261–71.

Bowden RA, *et al.* (1995). A comparison of filtered leukocyte-reduced and cytomegalovirus (CMV) seronegative blood products for the prevention of transfusion-associated CMV infection after marrow transplant. *Blood* **86**, 3598–603.

Chapman J, *et al.* (1998). Guidelines on the clinical use of leucocyte-depleted blood components. *Transfusion Medicine* **8**, 59.

Cohn E, *et al.* (1950). A system for separation of components of human blood. *Journal of the American Chemical Society* **72**, 465–74.

Contreras M (1998). The appropriate use of platelets: an update from the Edinburgh Consensus Conference. *British Journal of Haematology* **101** (Suppl 1), 10–12.

Corash L (1999). Inactivation of viruses, bacteria, protozoa, and leukocytes in platelet concentrates: current research perspectives. *Transfusion Medicine Review* **13**, 18–30.

Daniels G, *et al.* (1996). Blood group terminology: from the ISBT Working Party. *Vox Sanguinis* **71**, 246.

Dike AE, *et al.* (1998). Hepatitis C in blood transfusion recipients identified at the Oxford Blood Centre in the national HCV look-back programme. *Transfusion Medicine* **8**, 87–95.

Dobroszycki J, *et al.* (1999). A cluster of transfusion-associated babesiosis cases traced to a single asymptomatic donor. *Journal of the American Medical Association* **281**, 927–30.

Dodd RY (1998). Transmission of parasites by blood transfusion. *Vox Sanguinis* **74**, 161–3.

Ereth MH, Oliver WC, Jr, Santrach PJ (1994). Perioperative interventions to decrease transfusion of allogeneic blood products. *Mayo Clinic Procedings* **69**, 575–86.

Friedberg RC, Donnelly SF, Mintz PD (1994). Independent roles for platelet crossmatching and HLA in the selection of platelets for alloimmunized patients. *Transfusion* **34**, 215–20.

Goldberg MA (1995). Erythropoiesis, erythropoietin, and iron metabolism in elective surgery: preoperative strategies for avoiding allogeneic blood exposure. *American Journal of Surgery* **170**, 37S–43S.

Goodnough LT, *et al.* (1999). Transfusion medicine. Second of two parts–blood conservation. *New England Journal of Medicine* **340**, 525–33.

Hasley PB, Lave JR, Kapoor WN (1994). The necessary and the unnecessary transfusion: a critical review of reported appropriateness rates and criteria for red cell transfusions. *Transfusion* **34**, 110–5.

Hebert PC, *et al.* (1999). A multicenter, randomized, controlled clinical trial of transfusion requirements in critical care. Transfusion Requirements in Critical Care Investigators, Canadian Critical Care Trials Group. *New England Journal of Medicine* **340**, 409–17.

Heuft HG, *et al.* (1998). Epidemiological and clinical aspects of hepatitis G virus infection in blood donors and immunocompromised recipients of HGV-contaminated blood. *Vox Sanguinis* **74**, 161–7.

Issitt PD, Anstee DJ, eds (1998). *Applied blood group serology*, 4th edn. Montgomery Scientific, Durham.

Jackson MR, *et al.* (1996). Fibrin sealant: current and potential clinical applications. *Blood Coagulation and Fibrinolysis* **7**, 737–46.

Klein HG, Strauss RG, Schiffer CA (1996). Granulocyte transfusion therapy. *Seminars in Hematology* **33**, 359–68.

Krishnan LA, Brecher ME (1995). Transfusion-transmitted bacterial infection. *Hematology and Oncology Clinics of North America* **9**, 167–85.

Kuter DJ (1998). Thrombopoietins and thrombopoiesis: a clinical perspective. *Vox Sanguinis* **74**, 75–85.

Lackritz EM, *et al.* (1995). Estimated risk of transmission of the human immunodeficiency virus by screened blood in the United States. *New England Journal of Medicine* **333**, 1721–5.

Liles WC, *et al.* (1997). A comparative trial of granulocyte-colony-stimulating factor and dexamethasone, separately and in combination, for the mobilization of neutrophils in the peripheral blood of normal volunteers. *Transfusion* **37**, 182–7.

Lo YM, *et al.* (1998). Prenatal diagnosis of fetal RhD status by molecular analysis of maternal plasma. *New England Journal of Medicine* **339**, 1734–8.

Lundberg G (1994). Practice parameter for the use of fresh-frozen plasma, cryoprecipitate, and platelets. Fresh-Frozen Plasma, Cryoprecipitate, and Platelets Administration Practice Guidelines Development Task Force of the College of American Pathologists. *Journal of the American Medical Association* **271**, 777–81.

Marcus DM (1969). The ABO and Lewis blood-group system. Immunochemistry, genetics and relation to human disease. *New England Journal of Medicine* **280**, 994–1006.

Murphy MF (1999). New variant Creutzfeldt-Jakob disease (nvCJD): the risk of transmission by blood transfusion and the potential benefit of leukocyte-reduction of blood components. *Transfusion Medicine Review* **13**, 75–83.

Murphy S, Heaton WA, Rebulla P (1996). Platelet production in the Old World and the New. *Transfusion* **36**, 751–4.

Novotny VM (1999). Prevention and management of platelet transfusion refractoriness. *Vox Sanguinis* **76**, 1–13.

Pehta JC (1996). Clinical studies with solvent detergent-treated products. *Transfusion Medicine Review* **10**, 303–11.

Popovsky MA, Moore SB (1985). Diagnostic and pathogenetic considerations in transfusion-related acute lung injury. *Transfusion* **25**, 573–7.

Przepiorka D, *et al.* (1996). Use of irradiated blood components: practice parameter. *American Journal of Clinical Pathology* **106**, 6–11.

Race R (1944). An 'incomplete' antibody in human serum. *Nature* **153**, 771.

Reid ME, Yazdanbakhsh K (1998). Molecular insights into blood groups and implications for blood transfusion. *Current Opinions in Hematology* **5**, 93–102.

Schreiber GB, *et al.* (1996). The risk of transfusion-transmitted viral infections. The Retrovirus Epidemiology Donor Study. *New England Journal of Medicine* **334**, 1685–90.

Silliman C (1999). Transfusion-related acute lung injury. *Transfusion Medicine Review* **13**, 177–86.

Snyder EL (1995). The role of cytokines and adhesive molecules in febrile non-hemolytic transfusion reactions. *Immunological Investigations* **24**, 333–9.

Turner ML, Ironside JW (1998). New-variant Creutzfeldt-Jakob disease: the risk of transmission by blood transfusion. *Blood Review* **12**, 255–68.

Vengelen-Tyler V, ed (1996). *Technical manual,* 12th edn. American Association of Blood Banks, Bethesda.

Vogelsang GB, Hess AD (1994). Graft-versus-host disease: new directions for a persistent problem. *Blood* **84**, 2061–7.

Wandt H, *et al.* (1998). Safety and cost effectiveness of a 10×10(9)/L trigger for prophylactic platelet transfusions compared with the traditional 20×10(9)/L trigger: a prospective comparative trial in 105 patients with acute myeloid leukemia. *Blood* **91**, 3601–6.

Wiener A (1943). Genetic theory of the Rh blood types. *Procedings of the Society for Experimental Biology Medicine* **54**, 316.

Williamson LM, Warwick RM (1995). Transfusion-associated graft-versus-host disease and its prevention. *Blood Review* **9**, 251–61.

Winslow RM (1999). New transfusion strategies: red cell substitutes. *Annual Review of Medicine* **50**, 337–53.

Yamamoto F, *et al.* (1990). Molecular genetic basis of the histo-blood group ABO system. *Nature* **345**, 229.

22.8.2 Haemopoietic stem cell transplantation

E. C. Gordon-Smith

Introduction

The idea that haemopoietic stem cells from the bone marrow could be transferred from a normal individual to a patient to replace defective bone marrow has a long history. With the exception of rare instances where marrow was obtained from an identical twin, such attempts in humans universally failed until a clear understanding of the immune processes involved in tolerance and rejection became available. Much of the pioneering work in making possible human bone marrow transplantation was carried out by E. Donald Thomas and colleagues in the United States, work for which Thomas received the Nobel Prize jointly in 1990. In the post-Second World War era, experiments on inbred mice showed that lethally irradiated animals could be rescued by transfusion of bone marrow from unirradiated mice and that this protection was the result of engraftment of the normal marrow in the recipient. Successful engraftment depended upon the donor marrow being genetically acceptable by the recipient mouse or the recipient mouse being sufficiently immunosuppressed. Successful engraftment when there was immunological disparity between the donor and recipient was followed after a period of 2 weeks or so by a 'secondary' disease in which the recipient failed to thrive and developed gastrointestinal disorders and skin abnormalities manifest by poor further development and eventual death from infection. This so-called 'runt disease' is the murine equivalent of graft-versus-host disease (**GVHD**) in humans in which immunocompetent cells from the immunologically disparate donor mount an attack against recipient tissues. From these and other experiments in outbred animals it was recognized that transplantation of bone marrow would carry the special risk of GVHD and that histocompatibility would be a critical requirement for successful transplantation.

Further work in animals demonstrated that certain treatments, in particular total body irradiation and cyclophosphamide, were sufficiently immunosuppressive to permit engraftment, and that GVHD could be controlled to some extent, where there was not great disparity between the histocompatibility antigens of donor and recipient, with methotrexate. The elucidation of the major histocompatibility locus on chromosome 6 in humans, with the identification of the histocompatibility antigens at the A, B, or C (class I) and DR (class II) loci of the HLA system, finally allowed the identification of appropriate donors for human transplantation. The paramount importance of histocompatibility in haemopoietic stem cell transplantation has been confirmed subsequently by extensive clinical practice. The first successful transplant from a non-identical, but HLA compatible, sibling was carried out in 1968 for a patient with severe combined immune deficiency where the underlying disease prevented rejection. Successful allogeneic transplantation from sibling donors in patients who required conditioning with total body irradiation and cyclophosphamide to permit engraftment was carried out in 1969 in Seattle by the group led by Thomas. Many thousands of such transplants have been carried out subsequently, though it would be fair to say that the indications for transplantation, particularly in malignant disease, are not always as clear as they might be and the problems of GVHD, graft failure, and infection remain hazards which contribute to transplant-related mortality. On the other hand, better support with blood products and antibiotics, improved tissue typing techniques, and the introduction of less toxic ways of controlling rejection and GVHD, as well as better selection of recipients, have improved outcomes steadily over the last 30 years.

Histocompatibility complex and haemopoietic stem cell transplantation

The organization of the major histocompatibility complex (**MHC**) on chromosome 6, and its importance in transplantation, is described in detail in Chapter 5.7. The closeness of the relevant genes in the complex means that within families there is little crossing-over in germ line cells and inheritance more or less follows the autosomal pattern, so that the chances of a sibling having the same HLA type as a patient is about 1:4. This is genotypic identity, in which many unidentified sequences are identical by descent between siblings. At each HLA locus there are large numbers of possible alleles in humans leading to a potential of many millions of different histocompatibility profiles. However, within populations, certain HLA alleles tend to be associated and segregate together, 'genetic disequilibrium', so that it is theoretically and practically possible to find phenotypically identical pairs within an unrelated population.

The identification of phenotypes was originally based upon serological testing for A, B, and DR antigens. The introduction of molecular techniques for identifying DNA sequences directly has shown that there may be a large number of HLA gene products whose cognate protein molecules are assigned to the same phenotype by serological methods. Some of these differences are moreover of considerable importance in terms of immunological incompatibility. These observations on the MHC within the population have made possible the establishment of large volunteer donor pools of individuals prepared to supply haemopoietic stem cells, but also highlight the difficulties of unrelated transplants from an immunological point of view. Indeed, even where there appears to be close identity in an unrelated pool, there are likely to be many fine genetic variations. Selection of donors by improved typing techniques has reduced the risks associated with unrelated transplants, but selection has also restricted the range of appropriate donors. It has also become clear that there are very wide variations in the linkage disequilibria at MHC loci between different populations of the world so that a donor pool of one ethnic type may have a much reduced chance of providing donors for another.

Where there is a histocompatibility disparity between donor and recipient, haemopoietic stem cell transplants may be possible, but the incidence of complications rises steadily as the degree of disparity increases. It is also apparent that the antigens of the MHC are not the only antigens which are important in determining the presence or absence of GVHD. GVHD is mediated by CD4+ and CD8+ cytotoxic T lymphocytes, but the role of specific HLA antigens and minor antigens in determining the attack, and the part played by recipient antigens in susceptibility to the disease, have not been worked out in detail. As discussed later, the immunological attack on normal tissues which produces GVHD seems to be linked to an ability to attack abnormal tissues, particularly malignant, producing a graft-versus-leukaemia (**GVL**) effect. Much effort has gone into trying to identify the cells which mediate GVL and to see if they can be separated from those that produce GVHD. So far the results are inconclusive. The problems and benefits of immunological disparity obviously only apply in the allogeneic transplantation procedures and are absent when autologous stem cells are used to restore haemopoiesis after intensive chemotherapy.

Haemopoietic stem cells

The idea that there was a cell in the haemopoietic system which was capable of giving rise to all lineages of the haemopoietic system for life through a process of self-renewal, proliferation, and differentiation of progeny became current in the early part of the twentieth century. Experiments by Till and McCulloch in mice demonstrated that there were individual cells which could give rise to colonies of different haemopoietic lineages in the spleen of irradiated and transplanted mice. Subsequently it was shown that the passage of small numbers of early precursor cells could repopulate the haemopoietic system serially in lethally irradiated mice. It seems probable that a single stem cell can repopulate an entire animal in terms of haemopoiesis and the immune system. In animals, stem cells can be identified by immunophenotyping, purifying this population of cells, and showing that they are capable of haemopoietic reconstitution in a series of lethally irradiated animals. Such experiments in humans are impossible, but the best *in vitro* techniques have suggested that the human haemopoietic stem cell is closely related to precursors that carry an antigen designated CD34, lack other haemopoietic markers including CD33, and have no lineage-specific markers. Whether such cells are truly the most primitive cells that are capable of giving rise to both haemopoetic and immunological precursors is not of practical importance since successful haemopoietic reconstitution, both in allogeneic and autologous transplants, is closely related to the number of such cells present in the donation. The CD34+, CD33- cells represent some 1×10^{-3} to 10^{-4} of the cells of normal human haemopoietic marrow.

Sources of haemopoietic stem cells

In the first 20 years or so of haemopoietic stem cell transplantation virtually all donations were collected from the bone marrow. Animal experiments had demonstrated that marrow infused intravenously into a recipient was capable of repopulating the marrow and this method of delivery was practised from the beginning in human transplantation. Within normal marrow, haemopoietic stem cells are located in specific areas, usually close to the bony trabeculas in the haemopoietic spaces. The observation that marrow infused into the circulation could find its way to the marrow cavity indicated that haemopoietic stem cells were capable of trafficking through the circulation and homing to the appropriate part of the marrow microenvironment. It was also recognized that there were small numbers of stem cells in normal circulating blood, and that this number was increased during the marrow recovery following cytotoxic chemotherapy. The discovery of haemopoietic growth factors and their subsequent production by recombinant technology led to their use in clinical practice. Administration of many of these cytokines, particularly granulocyte colony-stimulating factor (**G-CSF**), granulocyte–macrophage colony-stimulating factor (**GM-CSF**), and stem cell factor increases the number of circulating colony-forming cells and CD34+ cells enormously, such that for a period of a few days following treatment there would be more than adequate numbers in the circulation to use as a source of transplant cells. Homing and mobilization of haemopoietic stem cells seems to be a continuous, dynamic process—even under normal conditions.

In the early development of the fetus, haemopoiesis takes place in the liver, and fetal liver cells have been used as a source of haemopoietic stem cells, mainly for the treatment of inherited disorders characterized by severe combined immune deficiency. The logistics of such transplants, which require 11-week-old fetal livers, make this an impractical approach. However, research on embryonic stem cells suggests that there may be other important sources of stem cells, not only for haemopoiesis but for other types of tissue replacement. Of more immediate practical importance was the finding that cord blood contained large numbers of haemopoietic cells with high proliferative potential and characteristics of stem cells. Cord blood has become a third practical source of donor cells. Each of these sources—bone marrow, peripheral blood, and cord blood—have advantages and disadvantages that impinge on clinical management. A critical requirement for successful transplantation is that there should be a sufficient number of stem cells—the ability to expand stem cells *ex vivo* would solve this and other requirements, but so far this has not proved to be practical for clinical use.

Haemopoietic stem cells from bone marrow

Until about 1993 most transplants were conducted using bone marrow stem cells. Much of the data concerning the success and problems of stem cell transplantation are derived from the use of bone marrow and this remains the principal source of stem cells in allogeneic transplants. Bone marrow is harvested with the patient under general anaesthetic by aspiration from the posterior, superior iliac crests, and if necessary the sternum. Experience showed that some 3×10^8 nucleated cells/kg from the bone marrow were required for successful engraftment and this usually involved collecting 1 to 1.5 litres of bone marrow mixed, of course, with blood. Donors usually have a unit of blood collected before harvesting, which is returned at the end of the procedure to ameliorate the anaemia. The procedure takes 1 to 2 h and the donor usually requires brief admission to hospital to recover. Serious complications are very rare and are those associated with the general anaesthetic or local complications such as osteomyelitis or abscess formation. The advantage of this source of stem cells from the donor's viewpoint is that collection is rapid with a maximum of

48 h involvement. The disadvantage is the need to have an anaesthetic and the pain or discomfort that follows the procedure.

Haemopoietic stem cells from peripheral blood

Haemopoietic stem cells may be mobilized into the peripheral blood following exposure to granulocyte colony-stimulating factor. For allogeneic transplantation, donors receive G-CSF (filgrastim or lenograstim) at a dose of 10 μg/kg subcutaneously daily for 5 days. The peripheral granulocyte count rises to 30×10^9/l or higher and CD34+ cells appear in the peripheral blood reaching a maximum 5 to 6 days after the start of treatment. Leucocytes are collected by cytopheresis with the objective of reaching more than 2×10^6 CD34+ cells/kg body weight of the recipient. Sufficient cells can usually be collected in one procedure. Attempts to increase the circulating stem cell concentration still further using additional cytokines, such as stem cell factor, have not proved to be sufficiently safe for general use. The main disadvantages for donors of this type of stem cell collection is that of bone pain or ache following the injections of G-CSF and the procedure of cytopheresis. The advantage is the avoidance of admission to hospital and an anaesthetic. When autologous collection of stem cells is required, the concentration of CD34+ cells may be increased further by giving cyclophosphamide (or some other chemotherapeutic agents, such as etoposide) before starting the G-CSF. The recovery from the marrow suppression so produced leads to mobilization of stem cells even without G-CSF. This procedure is used mainly for patients with malignant disease for whom the stem cells can be used to rescue them from the effects of further chemotherapy.

The use of peripheral blood for harvesting stem cells for allogeneic transplants provides high numbers of CD34+ cells and more rapid engraftment than that seen with bone marrow-derived stem cells. On the other hand, peripheral blood contains more T cells than bone marrow and, whilst original concerns that acute GVHD would be unacceptably severe unless T cells were removed has not proved to be the case, chronic GVHD does seem to be more prevalent. Nevertheless, the ease of collection and advantages of rapid engraftment have meant that most autologous transplants, and an increasing proportion of allogeneic, are sourced from the peripheral blood.

Haemopoietic cells from umbilical cord blood

Sourcing haemopoietic stem cells from umbilical cord blood has several theoretical and practical advantages.

Umbilical cord blood is widely available with no risk to mother or infant, there is low viral contamination, the immaturity of the immune cells reduces the risk of GVHD, and the cells may readily be stored frozen. Furthermore, a balance of umbilical cord blood stem cells from different ethnic groups to take advantage of genetic disequilibrium can be achieved and specific HLA types can be targeted. A disadvantage is the relatively small numbers of haemopoietic stem cells that are present, so that cells derived from umbilical cord blood are mainly suitable for child recipients rather than adults; a further difficulty is the lack of any back-up source of cells should the transplant fail or relapse occur. There is also the theoretical risk that the umbilical cord blood stem cells carry some latent genetic defect which might appear years after the transplant.

Plasticity of stem cells

It has become apparent that there are present in the bone marrow, and in other tissues, cells which are totipotent in their capacity to develop into differentiated cells depending upon the molecular and cellular microenvironment to which they are exposed. Thus bone marrow-derived cells may differentiate to cardiac muscle cells, nerve cells, striated muscle fibres, and many other tissues, whether they be ectodermal, mesodermal, or endodermal in origin. This potential is also present in embryonic stem cells. The reconstitution of a whole animal from a single somatic nucleus reinserted into an enucleated oocyte (cloning) is the ultimate indication of plasticity. In the future, haemopoietic stem cells may be used to repair neurological or muscle defects and other sources of stem cells used to prepare haemopoietic deficiencies.

Donors for allogeneic stem cell transplantation

Problems of transplant-related morbidity and mortality, graft rejection, GVDH, and infection increase with increasing donor disparity. HLA-matched sibling donors are not only phenotypically matched for the MHC, but have genotypic identity throughout most of the MHC. This does not eliminate transplant-related morbidity and mortality, but reduces the incidence and severity of the problems compared with unrelated volunteer donors matched phenotypically for the MHC. Sibling donors are therefore preferred. Same sex donors are more successful than mismatched, and transplantation from male donors is more successful than female. HLA-matched sibling donors are only available for about 1 in 3 recipients in populations with an average of two or three children per family. To overcome this shortfall, volunteer donor banks have been established, now including some 3 million typed donors worldwide. This pool can provide HLA-suitable matches for about 80 per cent of recipients with the same genetic disequilibrium as the donor pool, though finding the right match may take several weeks. Even with fully matched donors, either sibling or volunteer, extensive immunosuppression of the recipient is required pre-transplant to prevent graft rejection and post-transplant to control GVHD. New methods of immunosuppression which allow the stepwise development of donor marrow may produce a greater degree of tolerance and permit successful engraftment of haemopoietic stem cells with some degree of HLA disparity. Volunteer donor stem cells were the source of about a quarter of all allogeneic transplants in 1999 and this proportion is increasing.

Stem cells from umbilical cord blood banks have been used successfully in transplants for genetic abnormalities, particularly Fanconi anaemia, and also for children with malignant disease. However, this source has proved difficult for adults mainly because of the low numbers of stem cells in the cord blood.

Management of recipients for haemopoietic stem cell transplantation

The treatment of recipients pretransplant includes measures to induce immunosuppression and irradication of diseased bone marrow. This was the theory behind the so-called conditioning regimens used during the first 30 years of stem cell transplantation. For haemopoietic stem cell transplantation for malignant disease, most protocols contained cyclophosphamide combined either with total body irradiation (single dose or fractionated) or with busulphan. For non-malignant conditions, particularly acquired aplastic anaemia, cyclophosphamide in higher dosage, either alone or combined with antilymphocyte globulin (ALG), was the major immunosuppressive agent. Some of the more widely used regimens are indicated in Table 1. The incidence and severity of GVHD was reduced by giving methotrexate intermittently post-transplant. The introduction of cyclosporin to reduce graft failure and ameliorate GVHD greatly improved the results of transplantation. Such conditioning regimens, particularly for malignant and genetic disorders, carry considerable delayed as well as acute toxicity, particularly for children. Where radiation is used and to a lesser extent busulphan, infertility is usual, growth is retarded, and other endocrine functions may be impaired. Late onset of solid tumours also occurs.

Table 1 Outline of examples of conditioning regimens for allogeneic haematopoietic stem cell transplantation

	Indications
Myeloablative	
Cyclophosphamide at 120 mg/kg + TBI of 750 to 1400 cGy	Acute leukaemia Chronic myeloid leukaemia Relapsed lymphoma
Cyclophosphamide at 120 mg/kg + busulphan at 16 mg/kg	As above Thalassaemia major Other congenital bone marrow disorders
Cyclophosphamide at 200 mg/kg ± antilymphocyte globulin (ALG)	Acquired aplastic anaemia
Cyclophosphamide at 25 to 100 mg/kg + TBI of 200 cGY	Fanconi anaemia
Non-myeloablative	
Fludarabine at 30 mg/m^2 + ALG or Campath 1H + low-dose cyclophosphamide or melphalan	Fanconi anaemia Congenital disorders of haemopoiesis or immune system Acquired aplastic anaemia
With DLI	Malignant disorders

TBI, total body irradiation. Lower doses given in single fraction, higher doses fractionated.
DLI, donor lymphocyte infusions. Given 6 weeks or longer postinfusion to provide GVL or graft-versus-tumour effect.

Where transplantation was used for patients who had already received irradiation or chemotherapy to the central nervous system, for example patients with a relapsed acute lymphoblastic leukaemia, intellectual impairment as well as the above problems are common.

Subsequently it has been recognized that much of the success of stem cell transplantation in certain malignant conditions, most notably chronic myeloid leukaemia but also acute myeloid leukaemia, is related to the immunosuppressive attack (GVL), provided by donor lymphocytes. Likewise the repopulation of marrow by donor haemopoietic stem cells does not require the immediate abolition of recipient marrow. Conditioning regimens have been introduced which do not rely on cytotoxic measures to obliterate recipient marrow and immune system, but which have increasing immunosuppressive effects to allow the gradual reintroduction of donor marrow. Such regimens include fludarabine, a highly immunosuppressive drug that is not very cytotoxic, together with antilymphocyte globulin or monoclonal antibodies that have a specific immunosuppressive effect. Depletion of T cells in the donor preparation, with subsequent later add-back of donor lymphocytes, is also employed. Some examples of these so-called non-myeloablative regimens are included in Table 1. Results using this approach have been encouraging, but long-term follow-up will be necessary to confirm these advantages.

Removal of T cells from donor preparations has long been used as a way of preventing GVHD. Unfortunately, survival rates are not generally improved by T-cell depletion. The benefit of reducing GVHD is balanced by an increasing graft failure and, in malignant disease, by an increase in cancer relapse.

Graft-versus-host disease (GVHD)

Acute GVHD may develop at any time within the first 6 weeks post-transplant. The typical features and classification of severity are shown in Table 2. Grades III and IV of GVHD are an important cause of transplant-related morbidity and mortality. The immunosuppressive effect of GVHD may lead to reactivation of latent viruses, particularly cytomegalovirus, as well as death from fungal or bacterial infections. Liver failure, catastrophic diarrhoea, and gastrointestinal haemorrhage are other direct causes of death from GVHD. Chronic GVHD mainly affects the skin. It may follow acute GVHD or arise *de novo* 6 weeks or so post-transplant. The rash may vary from a mild dryness of the skin in localized areas to a major extensive scleroderma-like illness with progressive ulceration and scarring. Extensive and chronic GVHD is associated with a poor outcome. Examples of acute and chronic GVHD are shown in Fig. 1.

Table 2 Clinical analysis of acute graft-versus-host disease

Clinical staging: Stage	Organ involvement*		
	Skin	Liver	Gut
+	Maculopapular rash < 25 per cent of body surface	Bilirubin 30 to 50 μmol/l (2 to 3 mg/dl)	Diarrhoea 0.5 to 1 litre/day and/or persistent nausea
++	Maculopapular rash 25 to 50 per cent of body surface	Bilirubin 50 to 100 μmol/l (3 to 6 mg/dl)	Diarrhoea 1 to 1.5 litre/day
+++	Generalized erythroderma	Bilirubin 100 to 250 μmol/l (6 to 15 mg/dl)	Diarrhoea > 1.5 litre/day
++++	Desquamation and bullae	Bilirubin > 250 μmol/l (> 15 mg/dl)	Pain +/– ileus

Clinical grade: Grade	Stage			
	Skin	Liver	Gut	Functional impairment
0 (none)	0	0	0	0
I (mild)	+ to 2+	0	0	0
II (moderate)	+ to 3+	+	+	+
III (severe)	2+ to 3+	2+ to 3+	2+ to 3+	2+
IV (life threatening)	2+ to 4+	2+ to 4+	2+ to 4+	3+

*Confirmation may require biopsy.

Amelioration of GVHD with cyclosporin plus or minus methotrexate has already been discussed and the role of T-cell depletion mentioned. The optimal regime for prevention has yet to be elucidated. Treatment depends on the use of corticosteroids together with specific anti-T-cell monoclonal

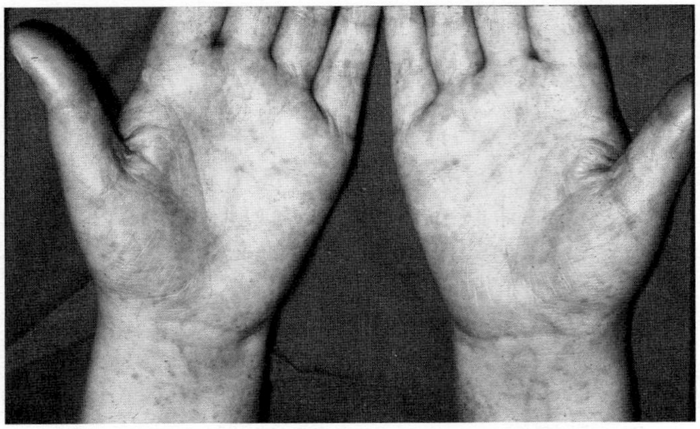

(a) Acute

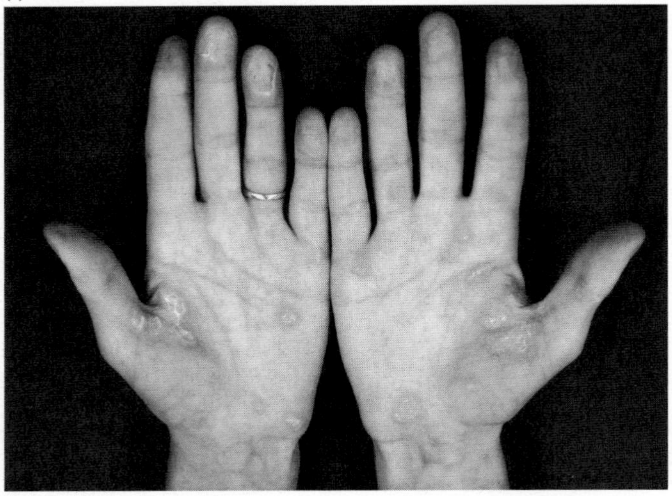

(a) Chronic

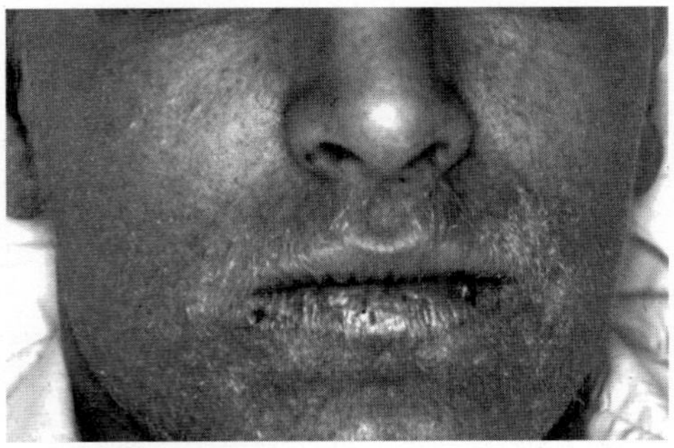

(b) Acute

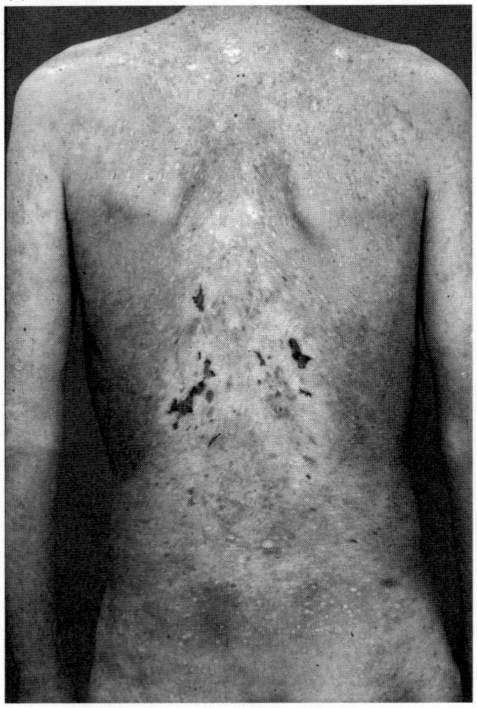

(b) Chronic

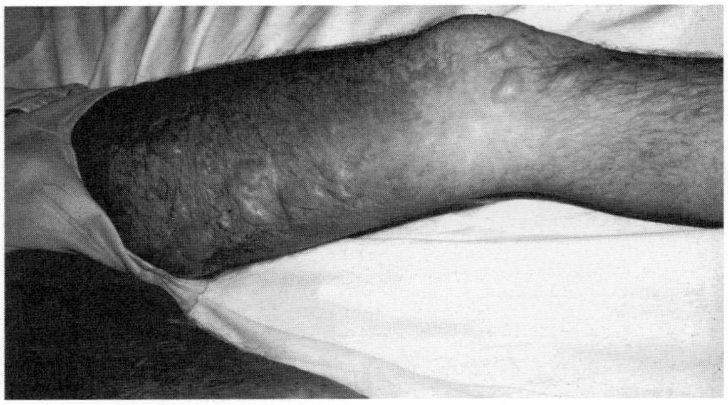

(c) Acute

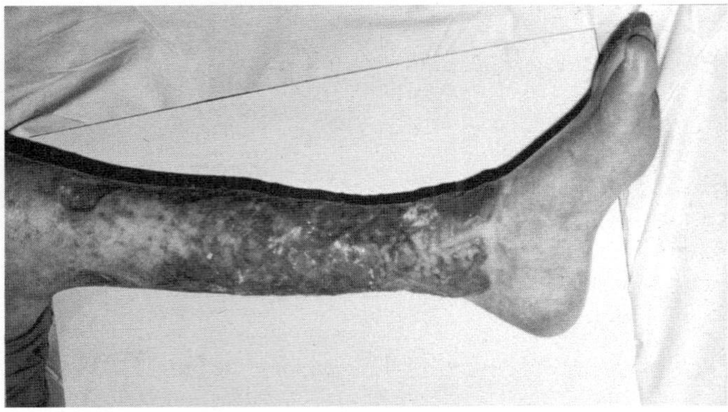

(c) Chronic

Fig. 1 Skin manifestations of acute and chronic graft-versus-host disease. Acute GVHD: (a) Grade I, skin +, showing typical palmer maculopapular rash (recovered); (b) Grade IV, skin 4+, generalized erythroderma with early exfoliation; liver 3+, bilirubin > 250 μmol/l (fatal); (c) Grade III, skin 4+, bullous desquamation (recovered). Chronic GVHD: (a) Scleroderma-like plaques on hands; (b) Sclerotic scarring on back; (c) Severe ulceration and contracting scleroderma-like skin involvement.

antibodies. Management of chronic GVHD with thalidomide has also been tried.

Graft versus leukaemia (GVL)

The observation that patients with leukaemia, particularly chronic myeloid leukaemia, who had allogeneic transplants and developed acute and/or chronic GVHD had considerably less relapse, though not better survival, than patients without GVHD led to the idea that there was a specific GVL effect (Fig. 2). This was confirmed when it was found that patients with chronic myeloid leukaemia who relapsed post-transplant could be put back into cytogenetic and molecular remission by giving them donor lymphocytes in increasing dosage. Sometimes this was associated with an increase of GVHD, but by no means in every case. There seems to be a hierarchy of susceptibility to GVL effect: chronic myeloid leukaemia being the most clear-cut, some effect in acute myeloid leukaemia, less in acute lymphoblastic leukaemia, and uncertain in lymphoma and myeloma. It is not yet clear whether the cells responsible for GVL are identical to those which produce GVHD or whether it is a separate population. Donor lymphocyte infusions now form part of the management plan post-transplant both for the management of relapse and for some of the non-myeloablative regimes.

Table 3 Main disorders for which haematopoietic stem cell transplantation may be appropriate*

Malignant disorders:		
	Haematological malignancies	Acute leukaemias
		Chronic myeloid leukaemia
		Non-Hodgkin's lymphoma
		Hodgkin's lymphoma
		Myeloma and other plasma cell dyscrasias
		Chronic lymphocytic leukaemia
	Solid tumours	Malignant teratoma
		Ewing's sarcoma
		Renal cell carcinoma
Bone marrow failure syndromes		Myelodysplasias
		Myeloproliferative disease
		Aplastic anaemia
		Paroxysmal nocturnal haemoglobinaemia
Congenital disorders:		
	Haematological	Fanconi anaemia
		Diamond Blackfan anaemia
		Kostmann's syndrome
	Immunological	Severe combined immune deficiency
	Metabolic	Malignant osteopetrosis
		Lysosomal diseases

*Stem cell transplantation may be considered an option according to availability of a suitable donor, the stage or severity of the disease, and the availability and effectiveness of other forms of management.

Indications for haemopoietic stem cell transplantation

The indications for haemopoietic stem cell transplantation fall broadly into two groups. In the first, donor stem cells are used for replacement therapy—a rather crude form of gene therapy for inherited disorders and the re-establishment of marrow function in non-malignant bone marrow failure syndromes. The main indications in this group are shown in Table 3. In the second group, donor stem cells are used as an adjunct to chemotherapy, both through additional cytotoxicity and biological modification through the GVL effect, in malignant disease. It is in this group that uncertainties remain as to the most appropriate timing as well as effectiveness of allogeneic transplantation. Randomized controlled trials have proved difficult to mount and much of the evidence is placed upon registry data or historical controls. At the same time that the results of haemopoietic stem cell transplantations have improved, the results of chemotherapy have also become better. Nevertheless, particularly in children and younger adults, allogeneic transplantation is widely used with some success, particularly for relapsed conditions. There is a very marked inverse relationship between success of transplantation and age, children having much less transplant-related morbidity and mortality due to reduction in infection and GVHD. Children also tolerate a higher degree of HLA mismatching than adults. The upper age limit for allogeneic transplant has continued to rise as results improve and in some conditions where transplantation is the only hope of cure, for example chronic myeloid leukaemia, patients aged more than 60 years have been successfully transplanted. However, the transplant-related morbidity and mortality at this age is very marked. As would be expected, results of allogeneic transplantation are best in low-risk groups, in first complete remission or with chemosensitive disease, and are worst in relapsed and resistant disease. However, it was in this last group that the potential benefits of allogeneic transplantation were first clearly demonstrated by Thomas and his group in Seattle. In most protocols for the management of leukaemias the inclusion of allogeneic transplantation, where a suitable sibling donor is available, is considered either up-front or as a form of rescue in younger patients. The results of unrelated donor transplants consistently lag behind those of matched sibling donors and whilst HLA antigen-mismatched stem cells are used in desperate situations, success rates decline as transplant-related morbidity and mortality increases.

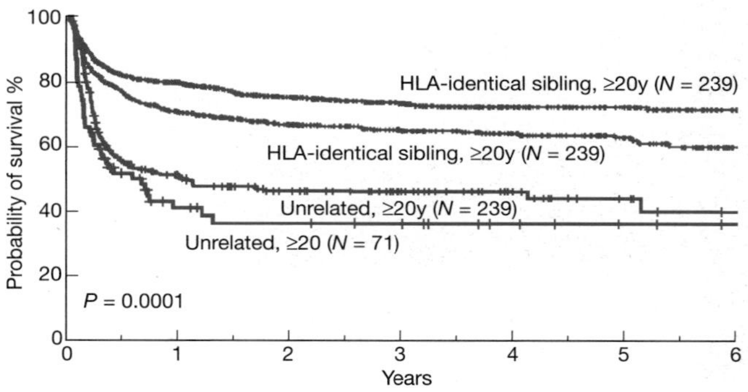

Fig. 2 Probability of survival after allogeneic bone marrow transplantation for severe aplastic anaemia by donor type and recipient age (1991 to 1997). Data from 2064 transplants from the International Bone Marrow Transplant Registry, reproduced with permission.

Indications for autologous transplantation

The use of autologous haemopoietic stem cells for treatment of malignant disease can only be considered a form of rescue from increased chemotherapy since the allogeneic effects which produce GVL do not exist. Where there may be tumour antigens that are amenable to immune suppression, attempts have been made to induce specific immunotoxicity, so far without clear-cut benefit. On the other hand, autologous stem cell rescue does allow greatly increased chemotherapy regimens for lymphoma, myeloma, and a variety of solid tumours with shortening of hospital stay—indeed in some cases treatment can be managed in an outpatient setting—and a prolonged course of therapy with repeated rescue from stored cells. Autologous stem cells will also provide the vehicle for gene therapy once techniques for gene insertion and long-term expression become practical.

Future directions for haemopoietic stem cell transplantation

Transplant-related morbidity and mortality should continue to decline as management of infections, particularly viral and fungal infections, improve. Undoubtedly the plasticity of totipotent stem cells will be explored to treat non-haemological or oncological conditions and both autologous and allogeneic stem cells will be used for specific gene therapy for both acquired and inherited disorders.

Further reading

Laughlin MJ (2001). Mini-Review. Umbilical cord blood for allogeneic transplantation in children and adults. *Bone Marrow Transplantation* **27**, 1–6.

Przepiorka D *et al.* (1995). 1994 consensus conference on acute GVHD grading. *Bone Marrow Transplantation* **15**, 825–8.

Rubinstein P *et al.* (1998). Outcomes among 562 recipients of placental blood transplants from unrelated donors. *New England Journal of Medicine* **339**, 1565–77.

Thomas ED, Blume KG, Forman SJ, eds. (1999). *Haematopoietic cell transplantation*, 2nd edn. Blackwell Scientific Inc., Malden MA.

23

Diseases of the skin

23.1 Diseases of the skin

T. J. Ryan and R. Sinclair

Introduction

Dermatology is concerned not only with skin diseases but with the Greek ideal of beauty, being confident of 'looking good'. Dermatologists observe the attitudes of parents, schoolteachers, spouses, employers, beauticians, nurses, and others to stigma. Whether it be incipient baldness, the wrinkles of ageing, or tattoos, there are cultural factors to be understood, and a cost of not treating. When is ugliness illness; how much is disfigurement worth in a court of law, and on what does wellbeing depend?

Throughout this section, the impairment, disability, and handicap of skin failure will be emphasized. . Dermatology is made difficult by its great variety of physical signs. It is an encyclopaedic subject with more than 3000 named entities. Fortunately, fewer than 10 diseases represent 70 per cent of dermatological practice—acne; bacteriological, viral, and fungal infections; tumours; dermatitis; psoriasis; leg ulcers; and warts.

Good physicians look at the skin while listening to the patient or eliciting physical signs. Recognizing minor details depends not merely on seeing but of knowing their significance. Unfortunately, so much of recognition is the naming of physical signs, and dermatologists have accumulated an enormous amount of jargon. Physicians should know enough to recognize a life-threatening physical sign, such as a melanoma, the malignant pustule of anthrax, or the eroded blisters in the mouth in pemphigus vulgaris. Furthermore, they should recognize signs that are significant indications of systemic disease, such as erythema nodosum, splinter haemorrhages, arsenical keratoses, and the white macules of tuberous sclerosis.

There is no branch of medicine more dependent on observation and less dependent on the laboratory than that of dermatology. However, in few other branches of medicine is there a requirement for the specialist to be so experienced in histopathology. One advantage is that a biopsy can be sent away to experts together with a photograph of the clinical lesion. It is also ideal for telemedicine, easily transmissible to specialist opinion.

In spite of the advances in antimicrobial and corticosteroid therapy, which have completely altered the nature of skin clinics in technically advanced countries, there is no diminution in the number of patients attending for help with skin problems. There is an increase in skin cancer, in the demand for cosmetic treatment, and in the number of environmental agents that damage the skin and cause dermatitis. In developing countries the overwhelming demand is for better management of bacterial and parasitic skin infections, but this is complicated by poverty, malnutrition, poor housing, and water shortage..

The structure of the skin

The skin consists of the epidermis and its supporting dermis lying on a layer of fat (Fig. 1). It is similar to mucosal surfaces where the surface epithelium is separated from its underlying lamina propria by a basement membrane zone which, in turn, is separated from the submucosal fat by the muscularis mucosa.

Unlike in the mucosa or skin of most animals, a subdermal muscle layer only exists in human skin in the areola and scrotum. The epithelium gives rise to all the cutaneous appendages, including: the eccrine sweat glands found over the entire cutaneous surface, but which are more numerous in the palms and soles; the apocrine sweat glands found in the axilla, groin, and beneath the breasts; the hair; and oil-producing sebaceous glands on the upper chest and back.

The epidermis is a stratified squamous epithelium (Fig. 2) comprising a germinative basal layer that is adherent to the basement membrane zone. Through cell division, the basal layer gives rise to successive layers of differentiating cells whose principal function is to synthesize the insoluble protein, keratin. In the process, these cells ultimately die and are shed from the skin surface. Keratins are the intermediate filaments of the epithelial-cell cytoskeleton, which serve as a scaffold in these cells and contribute to cell integrity.

The epidermis is infiltrated by a number of dendritic cells, including melanocytes, Langerhans, and indeterminate cells. The function of the indeterminate cells is unknown. Skin pigmentation is due to melanin fed into the basal keratinocyte rather than to that stored within the melanocyte. Skin colour is partly due to melanocyte numbers and activity, and partly a reflection of how melanin is stored and processed in the keratinocyte. Melanin is produced from tyrosine and dopamine and acts as a free-radical scavenger.

The rich vasculature has a generous reserve to meet the requirements of wounding and repair, so common at the skin surface. Vasodilatation can increase blood flow by a factor of 200, essential for thermoregulation. Macromolecules and cells leave the dermis through the lymphatic system,

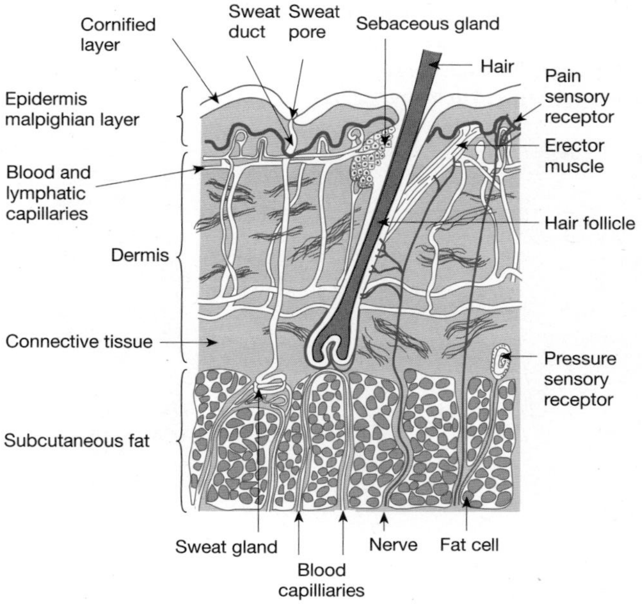

Fig. 1 The structure of human skin.

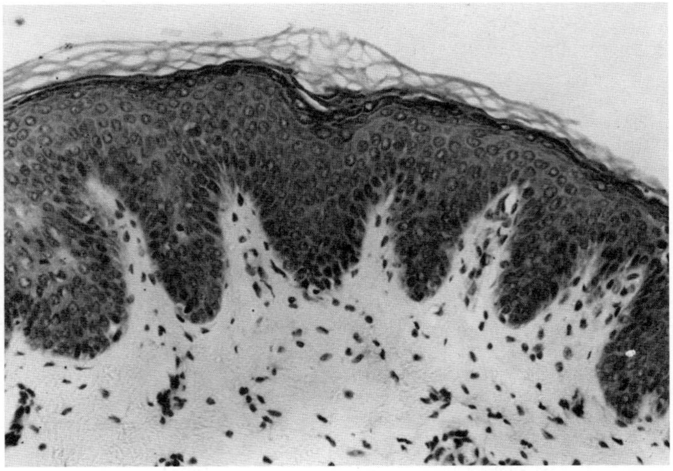

Fig. 2 A section of skin showing the epidermis and upper dermis. Note that the epidermis and the dermal projections interdigitate. The epidermal cells lose their nuclei as they approach the surface.

which is initiated in an elastic network at the junction of the upper and middle dermis (Fig. 3). The lymphatic system is responsive to hydrostatic forces and to movement of the solid elements of the dermis by massage or compression. The dermis also supports the extremely complex neural network necessary for touch and for sensing danger. All the main constituents of the dermis, collagen, and elastic fibrous proteins embedded in the mucopolysaccharide ground substance, are secreted by fibroblasts.

The two functions of basal cells, repair or reduplication and the production of keratin, require that the epidermis should turn over in a controlled way and die in an orderly fashion. Turnover takes about 30 days from the time of reduplication at the basal layer to its loss from the surface. Whereas the lower layers of the epidermis depend on oxygen for mitosis and migration, cells in the upper differentiating layers are anaerobic with no mitochondria. The optimal temperature for epidermal metabolism is probably lower than that for most body cells. Both lipids and carbohydrates provide the energy for epidermal cell metabolism.

Functions of the skin and 'skin failure'

Like the heart, lungs, and liver, the skin can also fail with disastrous consequences. It is the largest organ of the body and, being on the surface, is continuously exposed to injury.

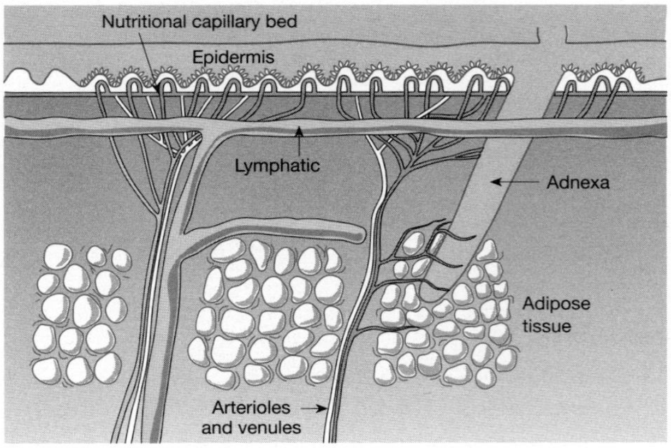

Fig. 3 The lymphatics are the exits from the skin for cells and macromolecules. They control hydrostatic and oncotic pressure and they are one pathway for antigen presentation.

Skin has to be both supple and strong because it is fondled, bent, stretched, trodden upon, and compressed, as well as scratched and prodded. Not only must skin have the capacity to rapidly repair itself to form a physical barrier impervious to excess water loss and to the absorption of damaging environmental agents, it must resist wear and tear. These functions are impaired in people with skin diseases, making them more vulnerable and less able to repair damage, and causing them social embarrassment.

Langerhans cells take up antigens and load protein-derived peptides on the major histocompatibility complex (**MHC**), travel to the lymph nodes, and present the antigens to lymphocytes that are preprogrammed to return to the skin. Depletion of these cells, by ultraviolet radiation, prevents contact dermatitis mediated by delayed cellular immunity. This network of cells is the primary immunological defence system of the skin and is termed the 'skin-associated lymphoid tissue' (**SALT**), analogous to the **MALT** (mucosa-associated lymphoid tissue) found in the bowel. The sensation of pain, so finely mediated by the precise innervation of the epidermis, has a similar warning function, helping us to recognize the environment and to itch in the presence of smaller invaders and to follow this with an accurate scratch response. The skin is capable of the presystemic metabolism of drugs and other substances applied topically. It is also capable of forming toxic metabolites. Skin can synthesize vitamin D from calciferol in the presence of sunlight, and contains the enzyme to metabolize it to 1,25-dihydroxycholecalciferol. There is an interaction between the cells in the dermis and those in the overlying epidermis. This interaction is mediated by cytokines, those important in the skin include: interleukins 1, 2, 3, 6, 8, and 10; interferons α, β, and γ; and multiple growth factors including epidermal growth factor (**EGF**), fibroblast growth factors (**FGF**) 1 and 2, insulin growth factors (**IGF**) 1 and 2, vascular endothelial growth factors (**VEGF**) 1 to 5, transforming growth factors (**TGF**) α and β, and neurotrophins. Furthermore, a range of peptides, complement factors, eicosanoids, and platelet-activating factors in the epidermis are involved in intracellular communication.

The epidermis contains very high levels of interleukin-1 (**IL-1**), 100 000 times greater than the content of most other tissues. Most IL-1 is produced by keratinocytes and, although this is a continuous process, levels are increased in the presence of ultraviolet light and endotoxins. There is a large intrakeratinocyte preformed pool of IL-1 and a predominantly intracellular inhibitor as a controlling factor by competing for receptors, which are normally scarce in the epidermis but can be induced by ultraviolet rays, trauma, or γ-interferon.

The dermis supports the epidermis and its adnexa. Like bone, the skin resists distortion. It is subjected to compression and shearing strains and many mechanical stresses are transduced into biochemical signals. Skin is more supple than bone, and hydrostatic forces or swelling pressure are more finely sensed and distributed.

The dermis, in addition to being a supporting structure, determines many of the characteristics of the epidermis. It is an essential inducer and controller of hair, sweat, and sebum, and provides a selective environment whereby hormones such as oestrogen and testosterone can influence some, but not all epithelial functions; for example, in the pathogenesis of acne hirsutism and androgenic alopecia.

Sexual attraction, being subject to whim and advertising, is an important function on which the fortunes of the cosmetic industry are founded. The social anthropologist has done much to draw attention to what denotes sex appeal; for instance, colouring or decolouring, tattooing, distorting, stretching, and, of course, adorning with jewellery and clothing are all involved. Sex appeal depends on the skin not being too greasy, too matt, or too wrinkled. The White adolescent wants a preparation to reduce a greasy forehead; the Black person wants grease to rid him of any degree of powdery exfoliation. One person must have a beauty spot, and another must not. Some scents attract, while the stink of sweaty feet and rotting shoes repels.

The influence of the psyche

Blushing, cold sweats, and pallor are skin reflections of the mind. Any group of students shown a mite under the microscope will laugh at the sudden awareness of itching it induces in one of their number. The acute inflammatory process mediating a weal or any exudation can be enhanced by anxiety or diminished by relaxation. While a 'neurotic' basis for urticaria, prurigo nodularis, or lichen simplex is no longer overemphasized by terms such as 'angioneurotic oedema' or 'neurodermatitis', modern Western scientific medicine has made such terms unpopular. This is because the influence of the psyche cannot be measured, is mainly subjective, and therefore, by some, is not to be believed. Practitioners of alternative medicine, as well as almost every lay person, recognize a link between anxiety and skin disease.

The principal anxieties resulting from skin disease are the fear of being infectious, unclean, and, ultimately, unwelcome. As with sexually transmitted diseases, a person's upbringing and religious and social mores will often determine their reaction to skin disease.

Few patients will accept that our largest organ can simply wear out or be worn down like the heels of a leather shoe, which after all is only skin. They will, however, believe that their skin disease is due to a malfunction of the liver, an impurity in the blood, to worry, or to a dietary indiscretion. Such beliefs must be countered with tactful explanation.

Occasionally, problems with the psyche will manifest on the skin; for example, Picker's nodules, neurotic excoriations, acne excorieé, trichotillomania, and even onychomania. The relationship of the problem to the psyche is usually acknowledged by the patient; however, patients who refuse to admit to their artefactual dermatitis can be challenging both diagnostically and therapeutically.

A common frustration of patients seeking advice or help is being told their skin problem is trivial. However, when the effect of all chronic or trivial diseases on well being is measured, it is found that the degree of handicap has been belittled. Not all skin disease is psychosomatic.

The handicap of skin disease

Common skin diseases, such as dermatitis and psoriasis, affect the following 'functional specificities' on which personal autonomy depends:

- to move around in and manipulate the environment (Figs 4 and 5);
- to service oneself;
- to resist normal stresses and traumas;
- to groom oneself;
- to be intimate; and
- to organize oneself emotionally.

Some diseases, for instance leprosy, affect other faculties such as sight. To have personal and economic independence it is necessary to perform effectively in any situation. Skin diseases affecting the hands and feet prevent the patient from getting out and about or from moving around the home (Figs 4 and 5). Skin disease, for a variety of reasons, may prevent or threaten the expected care of the home, self, or family, and it often interferes with education and employment.

The threat to life

Absence of skin, as in burns and ulcers, is a common cause of disability and death. Isolation due to rejection by a community is associated not only with poverty, but with infanticide, suicide, and a greater loss of life especially during childbirth. Skin disease does sometimes constitute an emergency and may cause death. Fatal melanoma is not rare, and only human immunodeficiency virus (**HIV**) infection and accidents worldwide are more common causes of death in males aged between 20 and 30 years. There is a 10 per cent incidence of metastasis from squamous epithelioma of the lip, a problem which may increase as actinic damage supersedes pipe-smoking as the major aetiological factor.

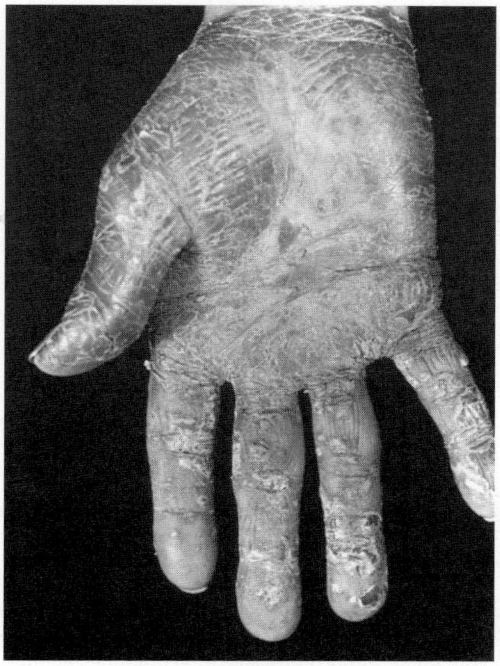

Fig. 4 Psoriasis of the hands interferes with dexterity and makes patients unwelcome in many occupations, such as food handling or public relations.

Angio-oedema of the upper respiratory tract is the most frightening of dermatological emergencies, accounting for the deaths of most cases of the very rare hereditary angio-oedema due to C1-esterase inhibitor deficiency and other much more common causes of urticaria.

Respiratory obstruction is recorded in other diseases such as epidermolysis bullosa (due to inhalation of 'casts') and Behçet's disease (due to ulceration of the larynx).

Many chronic skin diseases cause death by impairing the skin's ability to protect against adverse climatic conditions, environmental irritants, and infective agents, which all result in fluid loss or increased demands being placed on internal organs such as the heart. Blistering disorders, such as toxic epidermal necrolysis (**TEN**), pemphigus vulgaris, widespread impetigo, or epidermolysis bullosa, are especially threatening.

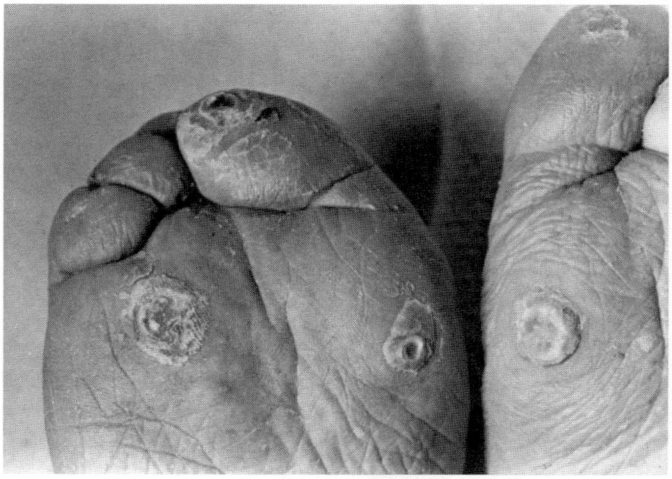

Fig. 5 A callus or corn is common in ageing skin and pain can make walking very difficult. The patient can be more handicapped than an amputee with a comfortable prosthesis.

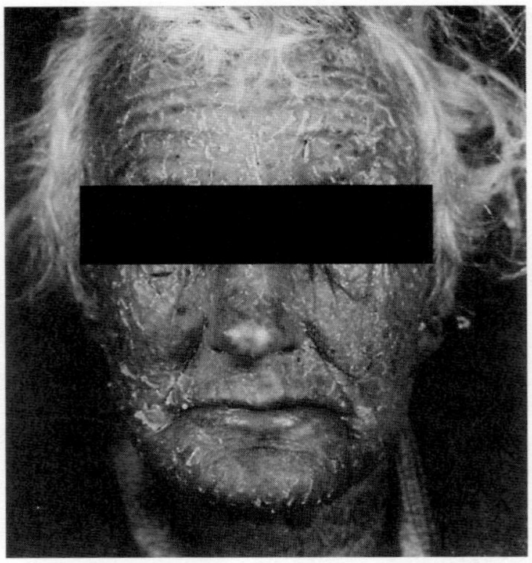

Fig. 6 Some diseases are a threat to life. Exfoliative dermatitis is life-threatening because of fluid loss, heart failure, and loss of temperature control. This patient died following perforation of the small intestine while being treated with steroids.

Erythroderma due to eczema (Fig. 6), psoriasis, or lymphoma commonly results in failure of body temperature control, in a high cardiac output, and, more rarely, in uncontrollable protein-losing enteropathy. Fluid loss and prerenal failure are important and particularly relevant factors in hot countries. In the tropics many die from uncontrolled dermatitis and commonly associated superinfections.

Restricting employment

Not to be able to resist normal stresses and traumas is a common inconvenience. It accounts for the need for sufferers from atopic eczema, even when in remission, to avoid occupations such as hairdressing, nursing, food handling, and mechanical engineering. Unemployment may be the consequence. Wear and tear of the skin is the most common consequence of work and those who have lowered resistance are unable to work. Some skin diseases present as blisters or as psoriasis in response to even minimal trauma—known as the Koebner phenomenon.

To communicate and to be welcome

The skin is involved in display. Through it we make contact with others. It is observed and touched. If there are defects in a person's skin, observers may not like what they see and will not touch it. Many children with such defects experience insults from other children who refuse to hold hands or play with them. Adults experience more subtle signals, which may prevent a normal sex life and interfere with employment (Fig. 7). Isolation causes premature death.

The greatest handicap of all is to be unwelcome. Whether real or merely perceived, it is the commonest social effect of skin disease. The whiteness of the skin of vitiligo, the blood on the sheets, and scale on clothing and furniture left by the person with psoriasis are huge disadvantages. Albinos are outcasts in Africa, while those with severe psoriasis are rejected in the United Kingdom.

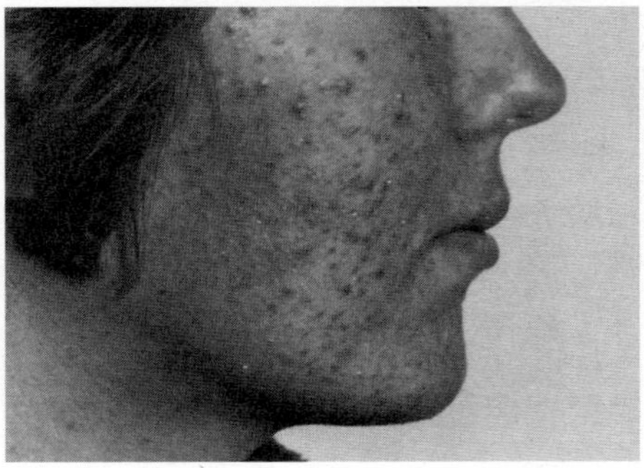

Fig. 7 Acne vulgaris is a cosmetic disability that makes a teenager feel very self-conscious and unwelcome.

Prevalence

An examination of more than 20 000 Americans aged between 1 and 74 years revealed that 60 per cent had significant skin disease (least frequent among children and most common in the old), which often persisted for more than 5 years. In about 10 per cent of cases the condition was a physical handicap: diseases of the hand being the greatest and most frequent handicap. It has been estimated that 6.8 million Americans are handicapped in their social relationships because of a skin condition. Diseases of the skin account for almost half of all reported cases of industrial illness in the United States.

The interview, examination, and investigations

The interview

The following questions form a suitable basis for conducting a dermatological interview:

1. How long have you had it; exactly when did it start; have you had it before?
2. Which part of your skin was first affected; where were you when it started; what were you doing?
3. How did it progress, to what sites, and what was there before?
4. Does it come and go; how long does each individual lesion last?
5. Does it itch; is it painful, tender, numb?
6. Does it develop blisters or clear fluid?
7. Does anything make it better?
8. Does anything make it worse?
9. Have you consulted any one about this? What was their diagnosis?
10. What ointments, creams, lotions, or bath oils have you used? Have you had any medicine or injections?
11. Has anyone else you know got it; does it run in your family; do any other diseases like asthma, eczema, or hay fever run in your family?
12. Have you had any previous illnesses?

The examination

Clinical examination

Undressing, removal of bandages, and, in some countries, even the removal of a hat may be difficult to achieve. In such cases more will be learnt by generally looking at the patient than trying to force compliance. However, the patient must undress when the diagnosis is in doubt.

One should keep looking until something is recognized. Often much of a rash is atypical, but somewhere there should be a classical physical sign. Good lighting is essential; sunlight is best. A magnifying glass is essential for detecting nail-fold telangiectasia, scabies, or crab lice.

Touch assures the patient there is no abhorrence and that contagiousness and uncleanliness are insignificant. Papules are palpable, macules are not. Compression distinguishes purpura from telangiectasia and reveals much about the depth of the lesion and its hardness.

Skin scrapings for fungal mycelia

Skin scrapings are best taken from moist areas since mycelia in dried scales or in the nails may be too desiccated. Scrapings should be placed on a slide and covered with 10 per cent potassium hydroxide, this helps to clear the keratin of extraneous material which obscures the fungus. Gentle heating is helpful, but not essential. In hot climates the rate of evaporation from potassium hydroxide is such that crystals form and it is best to renew the solution regularly.

Finding parasites

A microscope is essential for the diagnosis of mycelia, lice, and other parasites. Vaseline placed over the aperture of a 'boil' raised by bot or tumbu fly larvae may force their emergence since they cannot survive without oxygen. If onchocerciasis is suspected, a new itchy papule can be picked up on the end of a needle, quickly snipped, placed in saline, and examined under the microscope to see whether microfilariae swim out. Scabies mites can be picked out of the end of the burrow on the fronts of the wrists and between the fingers.

Wood's light

Ultraviolet-A rays (UVA, 360 nm) (Wood's lamp) highlight white areas in white skin, as in tuberous sclerosis, and are helpful for identifying *Microsporum audouini* and *M. canis*, which fluoresce green. Erythrasma due to *Corynebacterium minutissimum* fluoresces coral red. Porphyrins in teeth or urine fluoresce pink, and anaerobes such as *Bacteroides melanogenicus* in wounds and ulcers fluoresce red.

Biopsy investigations

The lesion chosen for biopsy should not be modified by excoriation, therapy, or secondary infection. For interpretation, the histopathologist will need some history, such as the site, duration, and appearance of the rash (macular, papular, vasculitic, vesicular), whether it is itchy, and whether the lesion is recent, established, or resolving. A drug history is of particular importance. If possible, a provisional diagnosis and one or two differential diagnoses should be provided. Multiple biopsies from different sites taken from lesions in different stages of development are helpful.

Collection and transport of biopsy samples

Samples for direct immunofluorescence

Direct immunofluorescence is useful for the diagnosis of cutaneous lupus erythematosus (biopsy preferably taken from the centre of the lesion) and vesiculobullous disorders (preferably perilesional skin for suspected bullous pemphigoid, or non-lesional skin for pemphigus or dermatitis herpetiformis).

It is best to provide the biopsy material as a separate specimen rather than dividing it for use in other investigations, this prevents the histological appearance of a crush artefact. The specimen must be received fresh (not in formalin), either in saline-soaked gauze or in an empty container placed inside a larger container containing ice. Ideally, the specimen should be received by the laboratory within 4 h of its removal. A biopsy can remain preserved in saline-soaked gauze for up to 24 h; however, the longer the time, the greater is the risk of a false-negative result. As a last resort, honey is a good preservative.

Samples for microbiology

If infection is suspected, a separate biopsy from the lesion should be submitted fresh in a sterile container. Ideally, it should be placed in sterile, saline-soaked gauze and received by the laboratory within 4 h.

Histological terminology and definitions

The histological report may include the following terms:

- *Hyperkeratosis*: thickening of the horny layer usually resulting from the retention and increased adhesion of epidermal cells.
- *Parakeratosis*: cell nuclei in the horny layer usually resulting from a high rate of cell turnover as in psoriasis.
- *Spongiosis*: separation of cells within the spinous layer by oedema fluid, i.e. the epidermis looks like a sponge—a feature of eczema. Severe spongiosis produces vesicles that may coalesce into blisters.
- *Acantholysis*: loss of cohesion between prickle cells and isolation, and balloon-like appearance of individual epidermal cells, a feature of the blistering disorder pemphigus.
- *Liquefaction*: degeneration and rupture of basal cells—characteristic of lupus erythematosus, lichen planus, and erythema multiforme.
- *Pigmentary incontinence*: the shedding of melanin from the epidermis into the dermis following injury to the basal layer.
- *Elastotic degeneration*: changes in dermal collagen that occur in light-exposed and ageing skin; whorled masses of disorganized elastin-staining fibres replace normal collagen.
- *Fibrinoid degeneration*: deposition of eosinophilic material resembling fibrin.
- *Necrobiosis*: a type of focal necrosis of collagen that leads to the formation of a palisading granuloma, i.e. macrophages lining up like a fence around the necrotic material.
- *Lichenoid*: a heavy infiltrate of white cells hugs the epidermal interface with the dermis and fills the upper dermis.

The basis of rashes

The skin is not homogeneous. It varies in its thickness, rate of epidermal turnover, amount and quality of hair, sebaceous glands, sweat, etc. Some rashes follow the distribution of a particular skin component; for example, of hair follicles in folliculitis (Fig. 8), sweat glands in prickly heat, sebaceous glands in acne vulgaris, dermatomes in herpes zoster, or annular and reticulate patterns as in some rashes determined by the vascular anatomy.

Inflammation near the surface of the skin usually damages the epidermis so that vesiculation scaling or erosion become a feature of the response. In contrast, deep dermal or subcutaneous inflammation merely produces 'lumps' known as nodules, and swelling or redness with intact skin markings and no distortion of the epidermis may be the only feature. Rashes may be fundamentally classified into epidermal conditions and dermal conditions: those causing epidermal rashes are included in Table 1, and conditions causing deep dermal rashes are shown in Table 2.

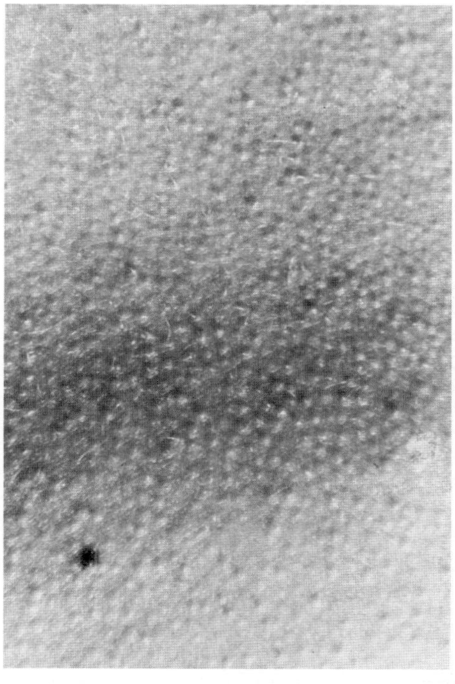

Fig. 8 Perifollicular hyperkeratosis having the distribution of the hair follicle.

Pityriasis lichenoides, pityriasis rubra pilaris, mycosis fungoides, lichen planus, discoid lupus erythematosus, and Darier's disease are examples of epidermal rashes with specific histology. A biopsy to confirm the diagnosis is recommended if these disorders are suspected. The management of some of these disorders is complex, and a pretreatment biopsy is helpful to document the diagnosis histologically before the morphology of the rash is altered by treatment.

Almost all dermal rashes will require a biopsy to confirm the diagnosis. Occasionally, rashes will be polymorphous with various sites showing epidermal and others dermal change. This is common in epidermal rashes, particularly when they are partly treated. By definition, dermal rashes show no epidermal change whatsoever, even if only 5 per cent of the rash shows epidermal involvement it is still considered an epidermal rash.

The rate of development of the rash is often determined by the type of inflammatory response—oedematous weals or blisters are more acute than white-cell infiltration, purpura, or pustules, and ischaemic necrosis and exfoliation are late responses.

The clinician is a detective and in assessing physical signs must know the sequence of events leading up to what can be seen. The distribution of the rash and its minutest morphology are important. Some classical distributions are shown in Figs 9 and 10, while Table 3 illustrates some well-known morphological terms and Figs 11 and 12 show some other shapes.

The management of skin disease requires the elimination of possible agents causing injury and the recognition and treatment of altered host responses. Endogenous rashes tend to be symmetrical, whereas biting insects and fleas, for example, will produce groups of bites quite indiscriminately. Unlike the rashes of secondary syphilis, the site of the primary chancre is not influenced by host symmetry (Fig. 12). Fungus infections such as cattle ringworm or even *Trichophyton rubrum* in humans are frequently more obvious on one side of the body than another, whereas psoriasis is usually exactly symmetrical.

Injury to the skin from contact dermatitis usually has the distribution of contact; in cases due, for example, to mascara, gloves, or shoes, there will be symmetry (Fig. 13), but casually brushing against a noxious plant will produce bizarre asymmetrical patterns. Scratching spares the centre of the back, and a completely clear area between the shoulder blades when the rest of the body is covered with scratch marks (Fig. 14(a)) suggests that the cause of the rash is the injury done by such scratching. Scabies mites do not seem to like climbing about in hairy areas, so usually spare the head but favour between the fingers, the front of the wrists, or the glans penis.

External irradiation from the sun spares skin beneath the lobes of the ear and under the chin (Fig. 14(b)), whereas an airborne pollen dermatitis will not spare such areas but may have a similar cut-off point below the collar. Small islands of normal skin in a generalized erythroderma are characteristic of pityriasis rubra pilaris (Fig. 14(c)).

Recognizing the signs of exogenous injury make it easier to eliminate the cause. Unfortunately, much skin disease is due to altered host responses, known as 'vulnerability'.

Table 1 Red scaly rashes

Fungus
Tinea
Candidiasis
Pityriasis versicolor
Dermatitis
Atopic
Discoid
Hand and foot (pompholyx)
Asteatotic (dry)
Stasis
Contact
Erythrodermic
Pityriasis
Pityriasis rosea
Pityriasis versicolor
Seborrhoeic dermatitis
Pityriasis rubra pilaris
Mycosis fungoides
Pityriasis lichenoides
Psoriasis
Plaque psoriasis
Guttate psoriasis
Flexural psoriasis
Palmoplantar psoriasis
Erythrodermic psoriasis
Pustular psoriasis
Lichen planus
Discoid lupus erythematosus
Darier's (and other acantholytic) disorders
Drug eruptions
Scabies
Neoplasia
Acrodermatitis enteropathica
Acrokeratosis verruciformis
Warts

Table 2 Dermal rashes

Granulomas		
Infectious	Tuberculosis, syphilis, deep fungal infection, bacterial botryomycosis	
Non-infectious	Sarcoid, granuloma annulare, necrobiosis lipoidica, rosacea	
Infiltrates		
Non-cellular	Solar elastosis, porphyria, colloid milium, amyloid, mucin, xanthoma	
Cellular	Polymorphs:	Sweet's syndrome
	Mast cells:	mastocytosis
	Plasma cells:	plasmacytoma
	Eosinophils:	insect bites, Well's syndrome
	Lymphocytes:	T-cell and B-cell lymphomas, leukaemia, lymphocytoma cutis, Jessner's, lupus erythematosus
	Histiocytes:	Histiocytosis X and non-X
Vascular	Vasculitis	
	Panniculitis	
	Kaposi's sarcoma	
Erythema	Annular erythema	
	Toxic erythema	
	Urticaria	
	Livedo reticularis	
	Erythema nodosum	
	Cellulitis	
Neoplasia	Primary	
	Secondary	

Vulnerability

This is a common characteristic in skin disease, and is seen in dermatitis due to the irritants affecting vulnerable atopic skin. It is seen in the haematogenous localization of immune complexes or other agents at sites altered by previous injury. It is also seen in the Koebner phenomenon, a term used to describe the development of psoriasis, warts, or lichen planus when the skin is injured to a degree that, in most people, would produce no more than a temporary wound but in predisposed individuals results in a recognizable skin disease.

Vulnerability is well worth recognizing because it may be possible to treat the predisposition when it may not be possible to eliminate the trigger. Thus, those whose skin breaks down too easily from unavoidable exposure

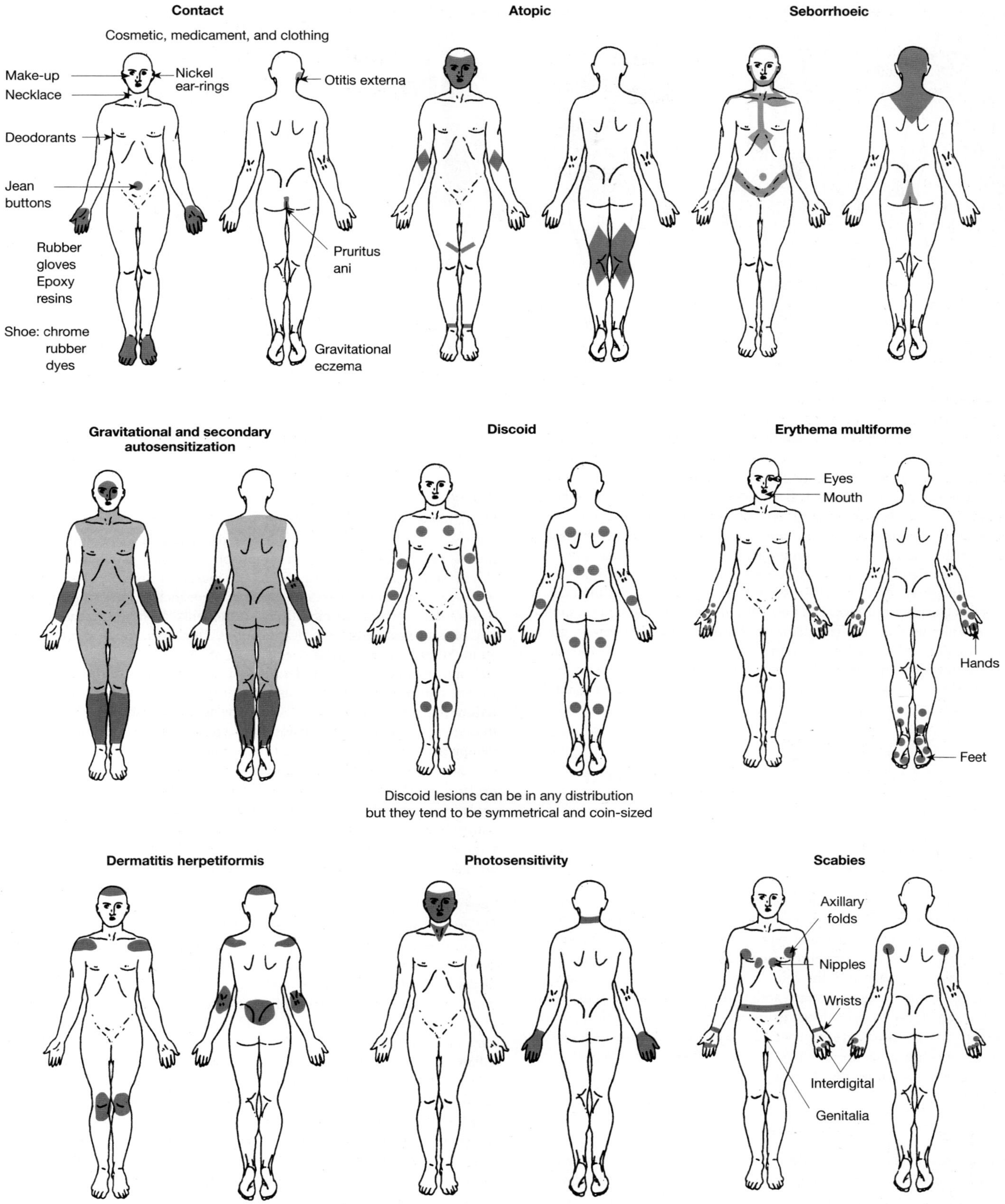

Fig. 9 Distribution of rashes.

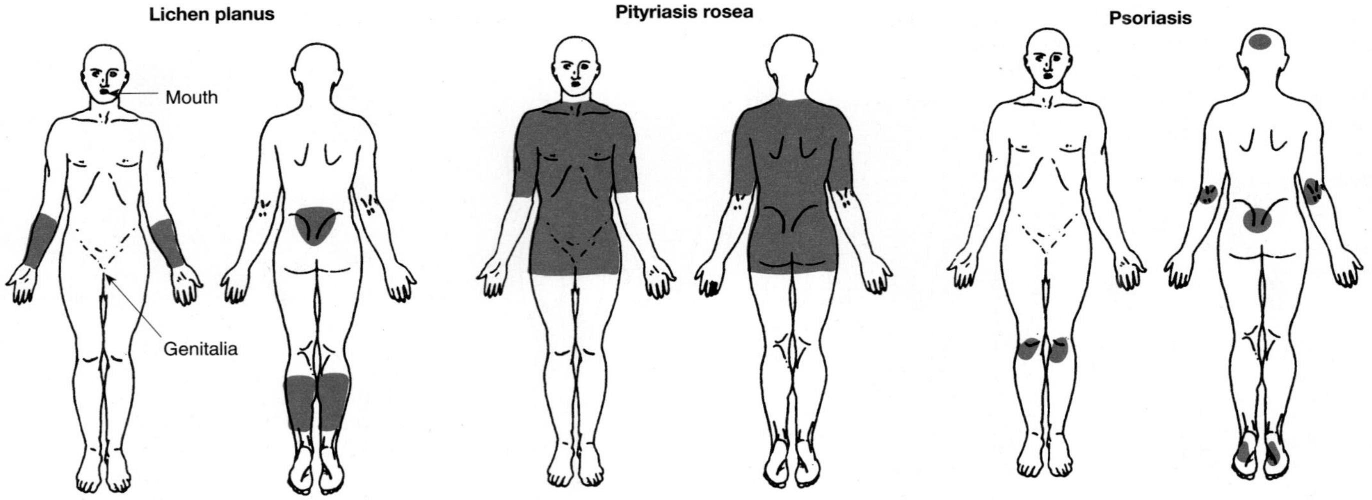

Fig. 9 Distribution of rashes.

to solvents may be helped to retain their job by liberally applying emollients.

Recurrent episodes of vasculitis in the legs due to immune complexes may be reduced by more frequent elevation of the legs, the use of supportive bandages, and the avoidance of cold environments. Vulnerability in the legs is due to the chronic stress of blood stasis and venous hypertension, which can be shown to cause inhomogeneity of capillary vessel patterns, adhesiveness of endothelium to leucocytes, and reduced fibrinolysis.

The ecology of the skin, with its integrated, well-balanced interaction between bacteria and surface secretions, also determines the skin's response at its interface with the environment. Erythrasma, pitted keratolysis, pityriasis versicolor, and seborrhoeic eczema are partly constitutional and partly due to exogenous organisms. The seborrhoeic diathesis is poorly understood but such persons seem especially vulnerable to colonization by immunogenic organisms.

Factors determining or modifying skin disease

Changes of skin with age, gender, and race

Newborn–childhood

Birthmarks are usually first noticed in the newborn but some, like cavernous haemangiomas, may not be present on the first day of life. Certain epidermal or so-called 'congenital-type' pigmented naevi do not appear until puberty. In type 1 neurofibromatosis, café-au-lait macules and Lisch nodules may not appear until the child is 5 years of age, axillary freckling is uncommon before the age of 3 years, and neurofibromas tend not to appear until puberty. Only the plexiform neurofibromas present at birth. Some birthmarks have important diagnostic significance indicating serious systemic disease. Examples are the hypopigmented lesions of tuberous sclerosis (see Fig. 65) and the telangiectatic lesion of the Sturge–Weber syndrome.

Puberty

Secondary sexual characteristics develop at puberty, and at the same time an increase in susceptibility to apocrine diseases, sweating, and blushing is characteristic. Acne vulgaris is mainly a problem for the teenager. Certain diseases such as ichthyosis and eczema tend to improve, while others such as herpes simplex infection and psoriasis are more common. Naevi, particularly pigmented ones, tend to become more prominent.

Pregnancy

See Chapter 13.13.

Old age

Skin diseases in old age are common and reduce the quality of life. Most elderly people have multiple skin problems, including seborrhoeic eczema, intertrigo, and dermatophytosis. Probably the principal characteristic of elderly skin is its inhomogeneity or the increased diversity that develops with age. Some changes are endocrine-related, such as hirsutism and baldness. Others are more specifically age-related, like dryness, decreased sweating, or poor healing of superficial wounds. Dry, scaly, rough skin occurs in about 80 per cent of people over the age of 75, as well as disparities in the size and thickness of the epidermis and in its pigmentation. Seborrhoeic warts are universal and actinic injury, Campbell di Morgan spots, and dilatation and derangement of superficial venules are common. For reasons that are still obscure, some diseases are age-related: for example, pruritus, pemphigoid, and lichen sclerosus et atrophicus.

Degenerative disease and the cumulative exposure to solar radiation explains neoplasia of the skin. Degenerative disease of the vascular system explains venous ulcers and arterial ischaemic diseases. In one study, after controlling for age, sex, and sun exposure, premature wrinkling increased with years of smoking. Heavy smokers were 4.7 times more likely to be wrinkled than non-smokers.

Race

Differences in populations are partly explained by genetic factors, but so much adaptation to the environment occurs that customs and diet may determine some attributes. Although it is frequently reported that certain diseases are absent in tropical climates, this is probably because they have never been looked for or recognized. Erythema is violaceous so that purpura may be difficult to detect in people with dark skins; minor skin problems may not be complained of in the tropics, where many neoplastic and inflammatory diseases are so florid and attendance for advice is so often delayed. A move to a more temperate climate is often associated with urbanization, which can equally influence the skin. The most easily recognized difference between one person and another is their skin colour, and the consequences of sun exposure are much reduced in those with dark skins. Vitiligo is probably more common in the Caucasian races of the Middle East, North Africa, and India. The Japanese rather readily seem to develop a slate-blue or ashy discoloration of the trunk following inflammatory disease. On the other hand, acne vulgaris is uncommon in Japanese people, while both acne and rosacea seem to be uncommon in those with black skins. However, comedone formation due to cosmetics without full-blown acne is common in black skin. Blackness is due to more evenly dispersed, larger and less degradable pigment granules. The stratum corneum of black skin is more compact with a higher lipid content and is subject to less penetration by irritants. Another easily recognized factor is hair size and shape. Facial hirsutism is rare in Japanese women and relative sparseness of hair is a feature of mongoloid races. On the other hand, Mediterranean and some Indian races seem to be particularly hirsute (Fig. 15). The shininess of black skin is partly due to sebum and partly to thermal stress which encourages increased eccrine sweating. Such skins tend to become rather dry in a temperate climate. Scales show up on dark skins. Keloids are a considerable problem for Afro-Caribbeans and can sometimes be massive. Susceptibility to infection depends on immunological factors and on previous exposure. As with malaria or syphilis, some populations seem to acquire a genetic resistance to tuberculosis and leprosy.

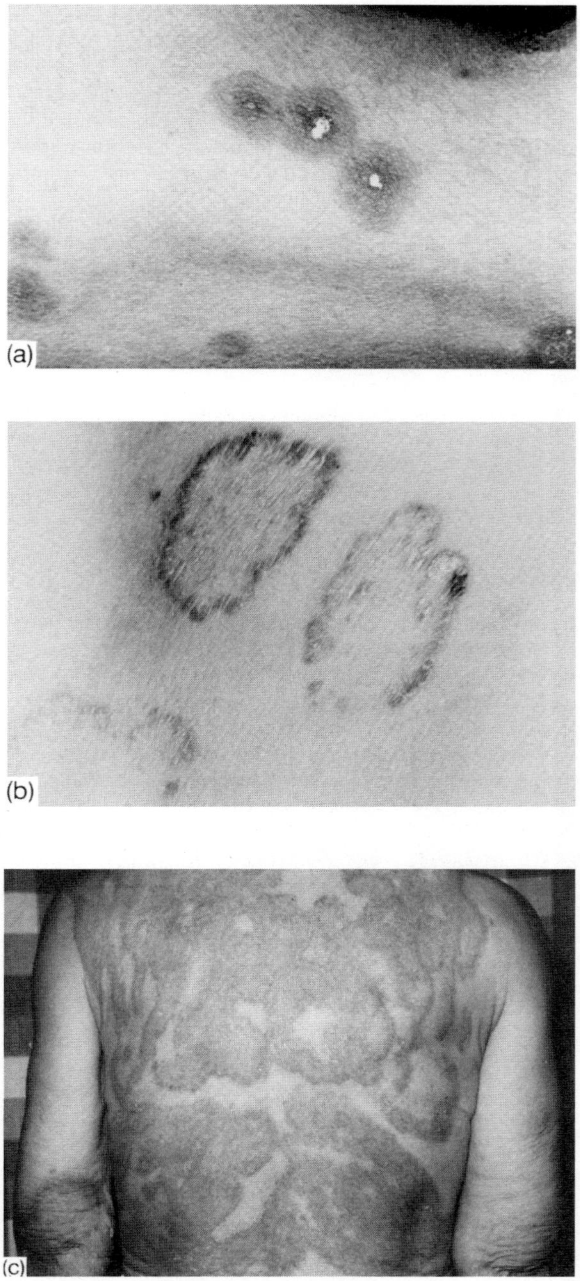

Fig. 10 (a) An example of the 'target' lesion of erythema multiforme. (b) Healing of the centre of the lesion is a feature of many skin diseases, including fungus infections and, in this case, psoriasis. (c) Annular erythema in lupus erythematosus with Ro antibody. This pattern of widespread erythema is also observed in association with underlying malignancy.

Table 3 Some morphological terms

Macules	are flat with no changes in surface marking or texture—they may be merely areas of redness, purpura, or melanin
Papules	are circumscribed, palpable elevations or thickenings of the epidermis or of the upper dermis by infiltration or oedema
Plaques	are disc-shaped lesions, often resulting from the coalescence of papules
Nodules	are circumscribed palpable masses larger than 1 cm in diameter, usually consisting of oedema or malignant or inflammatory cells filling the dermis or subcutaneous tissue. Some are small and painful (Table 4) others are juxta-articular (Table 5)
Vesicles and bullae	are visible accumulations of fluid (often the lay person uses the term 'blister' to include wealing, in which there are no visible accumulations other than swelling). Vesicles are small, while bullae are larger than 1 cm
Annular lesions	result from spreading infiltrations or a healing centre, often with refractoriness due to such factors as raised tissue pressure or scarring preventing vasodilatation or leakiness in the centre of the lesions. Vascular patterns in the skin have a reticular or annular anatomical distribution (Table 6)
Linear lesions	are due to external scratches, or to a developmental or anatomical distribution of lymphatics, blood vessels, or nerves (Table 7)

Is it contagious (Tables 1–7)?

Physicians are often asked whether a skin disease is 'infectious'. The questioner really means, 'Did I catch it?' 'Can I give it to someone else?' 'Is the treatment of choice a simple antiseptic or antibiotic regimen?' The physician may ask, 'Am I missing something which is a danger to other patients in the the ward or to my nursing staff?' Infections are often present in several members of the family at the same time (Fig. 16).

There are many infections, dealt with elsewhere in this textbook, in which a highly virulent organism has broken the defences of a normally resistant host, but there are also organisms that are usually harmless but occasionally, because of immunosuppression or other changes in the host, produce a rash. Pityriasis versicolor, candidiasis, erythrasma, and trichomycosis axillaris, all discussed in Section 7, are examples. More difficult is the relationship with staphylococcal or streptococcal bacteria—although these generally sit in silence on the skin, they are unwelcome in a ward full of more susceptible and vulnerable patients. Psoriasis is not infectious, but the massive exfoliation from such a patient is a great source of cross-infection. Bacterial spread by skin scales is generally considerable and the basis of surgical gowning. Few would feel bound to treat every patient with psoriasis for bacterial infection, but the same degree of infection in atopic eczema is thought to be contributory to the disease, perhaps through a bacterial superantigen effect.

Pathology from skin infection is more common in hot humid climates, and erosions from scratching, prickly heat, and other infections (such as lice or scabies) predispose to boils and other patterns of pyoderma, especially in the groins and axillas.

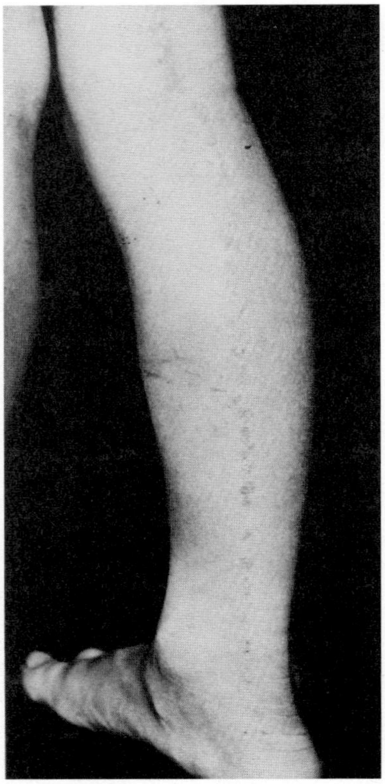

Fig. 11 Example of a linear distribution, in this case lichen planus. The distribution does not conform to a dermatome and the exact cause of the linear lesions remains largely unexplained.

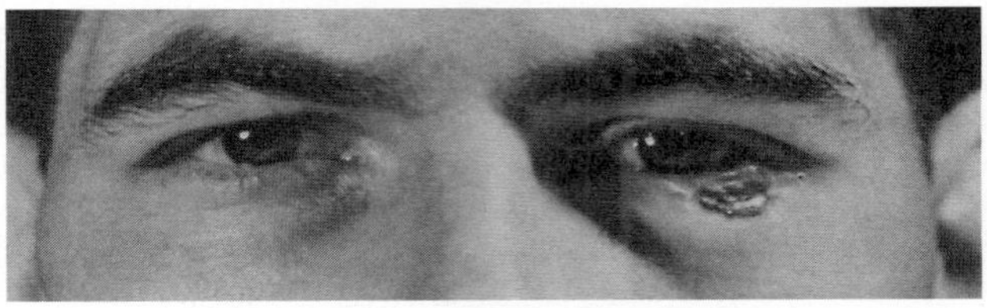

Fig. 12 A primary chancre of the lower left eyelid illustrating how skin diseases due to exogenous causes are often asymmetrical.

The primary pathology of infection is often asymmetrical, but an immune response attempting to get rid of it is usually exactly symmetrical and takes 5 to 10 days to develop.

The most difficult diagnostic problem is that of viral disease. The hospital doctor is not well placed to recognize its variety. Rather, it is the general practitioner called to the patient's home who sees virus disease in its early stages or in its transient phase. It is essential to know what rashes are currently endemic.

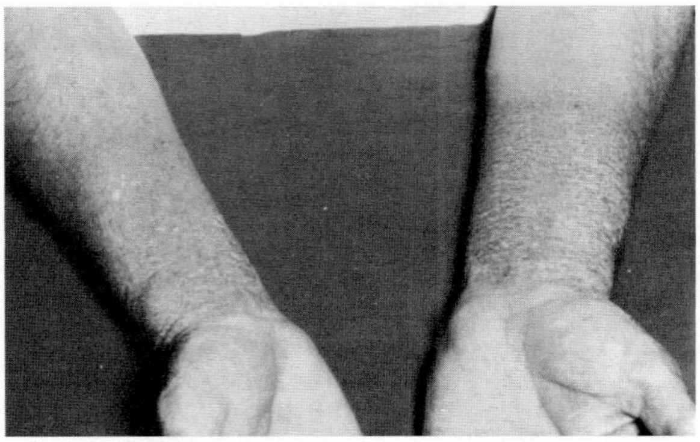

Fig. 13 Occasionally, symmetry in the distribution of contact may be due to a symmetrical application as in the case of this glove dermatitis.

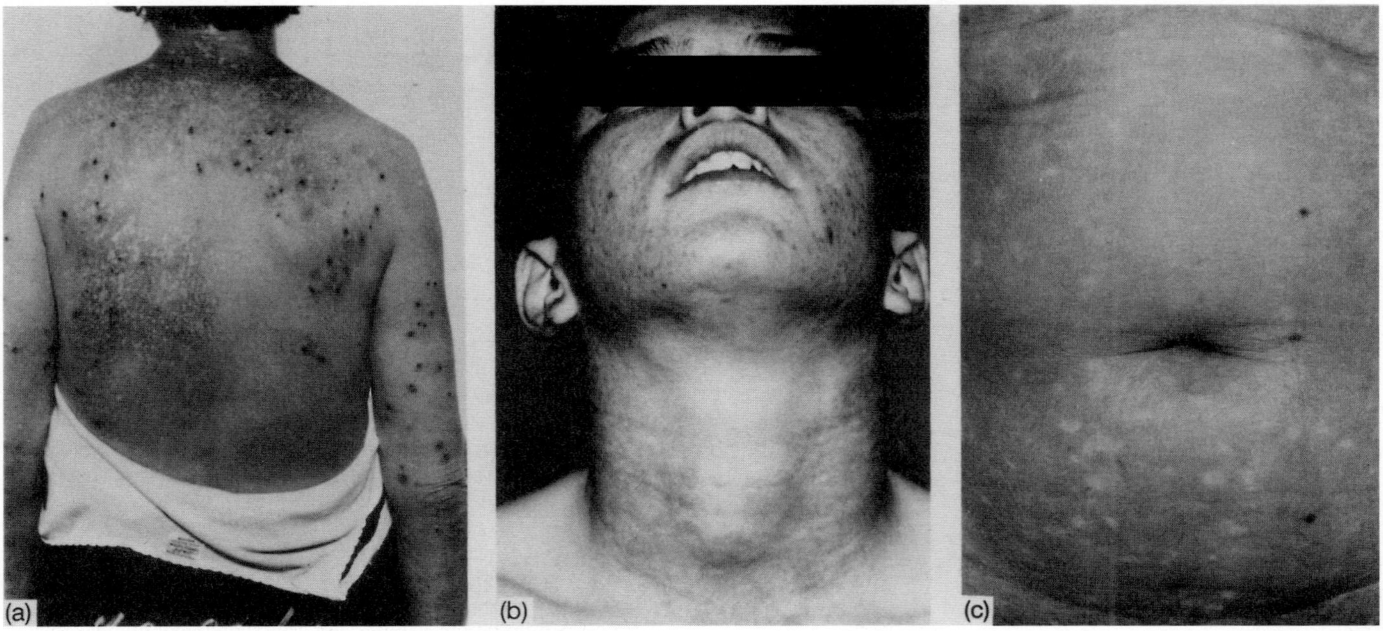

Fig. 14 (a) The central area of the back is spared from this dermatosis induced by scratching, simple because the patient is unable to reach the site. (b) External irradiation from the sun spares the area beneath the lobes of the ear and under the chin in this case of solar dermatitis. (c) Small islands of unaffected skin scattered throughout a generalized redness and keratoderma are characteristic of pityriasis rubra pilaris.

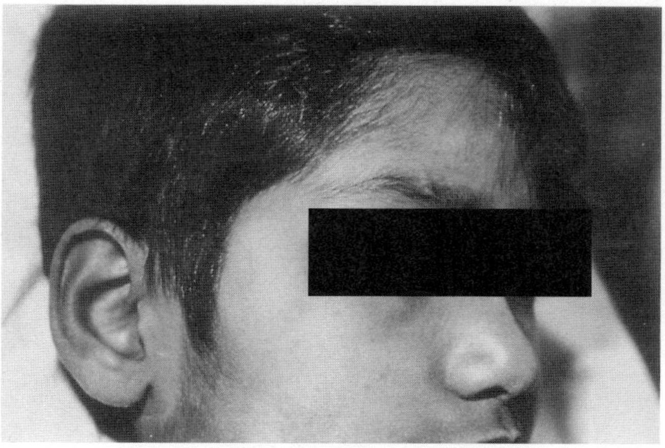

Fig. 15 Hair growth on the forehead of an Indian child. This is entirely within normal limits and is of racial origin.

People with rashes due to infection commonly have an associated fever, lymphadenopathy, coryza, diarrhoea, vomiting, hepatomegaly, or headache. However, the abrupt sterile pustulation of generalized pustular psoriasis (Fig. 17) or the painful deep swelling of delayed-pressure urticaria or vasculitis will also be accompanied by high fever and a neutrophil leucocytosis, but usually there is no lymphadenopathy in these non-infectious processes. Erythema multiforme, Sweet's disease, and toxic epidermal necrolysis similarly show great systemic effects. Since people with widespread skin disease may be unable to control their body temperature, high fever in such persons is not necessarily a sign of infection.

When the diagnosis is in doubt, good practice is to take adequate swabs and specimens for culture and histological examination, and to treat and touch the patient as his or her comfort requires. Washing the hands suffices to avoid the transmission of scabies, fungus, and most bacterial diseases as

Table 4 Severe pain on compression of a small dermal papule or nodule is a well-recognized symptom of the following lesions. If there is doubt, excision is the treatment of choice, so that a definitive histological examination can be made

Glomus	Eccrine spiradenoma
Leiomyoma	Angiolipoma
Neuroma	Chondrodermatitis (of the outer helix)

Table 5 Juxta-articular nodules

Rheumatoid nodules	Granuloma annulare
Gouty tophi	Multicentric reticulohistiocytosis
Xanthomas	Synovial cysts, ganglia, or Heberden's nodes

Table 6 Some annular lesions

Impetigo	Urticaria
Dermatophytosis	Lichen planus (Fig. 49)
Syphilis	Lupus erythematosus (Ro antibody) (Fig. 10(c))
Leprosy	Purpura
Lupus vulgaris	Seborrhoeic eczema
Pityriasis rosea	Sarcoidosis
Erythemas:	Mycosis fungoides
toxic, urticarial, and multiforme (Fig. 10(a))	Granuloma annulare/multiforme
Psoriasis (Fig. 10(b))	Glucagonoma

Table 7 Linear lesions with dermatomal distributions include the well-recognized herpes zoster. Many linear lesions follow a pattern that does not exactly conform to innervation or blood supply, especially when it extends the whole way up the leg or arm

Lichen striatus	Artefacta scratching
Lichen planus[a] (Fig. 11)	Focal dermal hypoplasia
Psoriasis[a]	Incontinentia pigmenti
Epidermal naevi	Papular mucinosis
Darier's disease[a]	Sarcoid[a]
Morphea	Warts[a]
Porokeratosis of Mibelli	Molluscum contagiosum
Contact dermatitis[a]	Syringoma
Phytophotodermatitis	

[a] May be a reaction to a scratch (Koebner phenomenon).

Note: some linear nodules are determined by lymphatic drainage: mycobacteria, sporotrichosis, neoplasm, coccidioidomycosis.

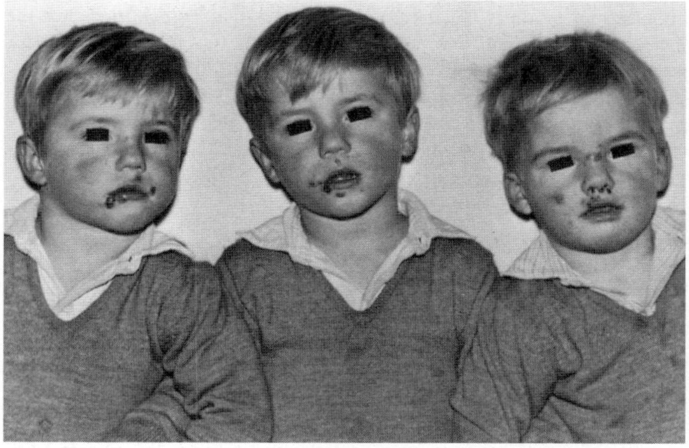

Fig. 16 Infections such as impetigo are highly contagious and tend to be found in more than one member of the family, as in these triplets.

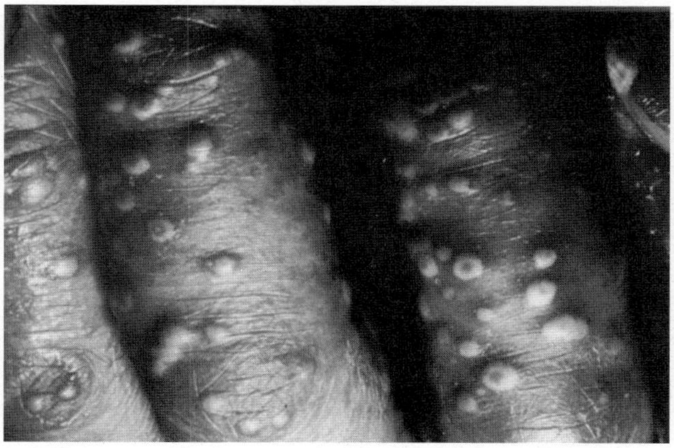

Fig. 17 Pustules are not necessarily due to infection. These pustules are from pustular psoriasis and are sterile.

well as warts and syphilis. However, practitioners should take the utmost care to avoid inoculating their skin when taking scrapings or biopsies. Patients with much exfoliation should not be nursed on a general ward, but in a single cubicle.

Pustules need not be caused by infection; for instance, the primary lesions are always sterile in psoriasis or an irritant folliculitis from oils. Vesicles need not be due to viruses since they are a feature of papular urticaria, dermatitis hepetiformis, and vasculitis (see Fig. 83). Dark skins exposed to much oil and cosmetics often have a chronic pustular dermatosis of the lower legs that may be sterile.

Humidity is a principal cause of profuse skin infection, and treatment by cooling and drying has always been a standard therapy for infected eczema. The fact is that drying is promoted by the use of wet dressings and the consequent evaporation. Wet dressings that are occlusive and changed infrequently encourage infection: ideally, they should be changed every 2 to 4 h. Occlusive surfaces, for instance between the toes, the groins, and the breasts, need to be treated with drying agents (such as those commonly present in deodorants (aluminium chloride)) or with powders. Dry mopping of the ear in otitis externa is similarly helpful.

In some parts of the world, skin clinics are overwhelmed by massive numbers of patients suffering from scabies (Fig. 18), staphylococcal and streptococcal infection, and dermatophytosis. Control is impossible because reinfection is inevitable. Soap and water do much to reduce the incidence of common dermatoses, but water is too valuable to use for washing when there is a drought.

In Mediterranean countries, ringworm of the scalp would be easy to manage (Fig. 19) were it not that the population explosion provides more children for infection than it is possible to treat, and that subclinical infections are difficult to recognize.

Is it hereditary?

See Chapter 23.2 for a complete discussion.

Is it due to malnutrition?

Skin diseases resulting from malnutrition have been termed the 'dermatoses of the poor'. Although they are common in starving communities, they are also seen in those living only on drugs or alcohol, those suffering from malabsorption syndromes, and those debilitated by neoplasia or severe chronic infections. Increasingly, elderly patients suffering from dementia are responsible for more cases in Western urban communities. Poor personal hygiene and lack of, or failure to use, water supplies contribute to some aspects of skin diseases in malnutrition, as well as to the infections of both skin and mouth which often accompany them.

The skin makes up 8 per cent of body weight and uses up about one-eighth of the body's protein; hence it is affected early in malnutrition.

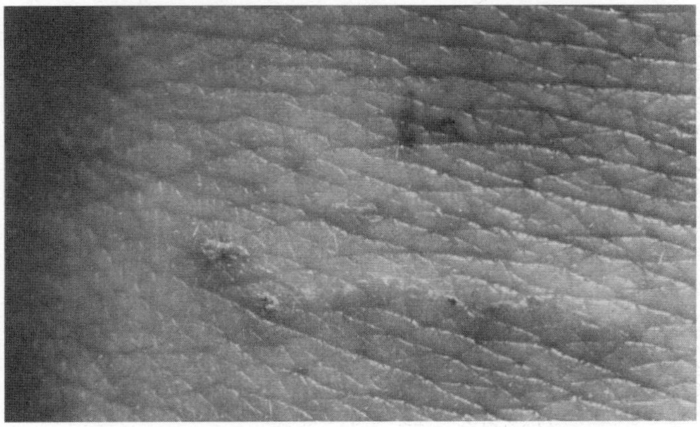

Fig. 18 The diagnostic feature of scabies. The burrow of the mite in the horny layer of the epidermis. The dark spots are haemoglobin in the belly of the mite.

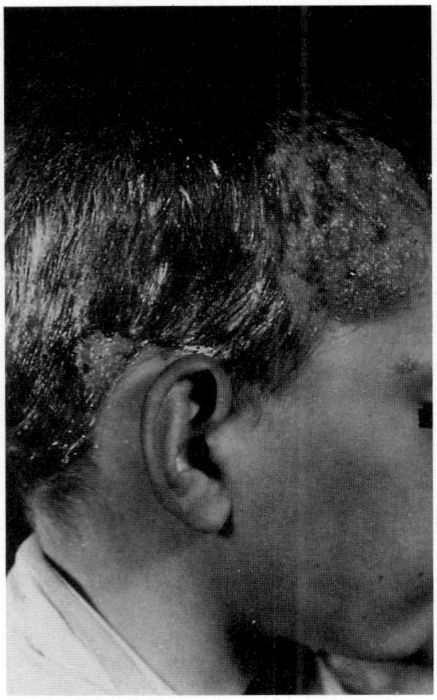

Fig. 19 Multiple exudative lesions due to tinea capitis.

In experimental malnutrition and in studies of people during the Second World War, early signs were dryness of the skin and hyperpigmentation. At birth, malnutrition is seen as loss of vernix and maceration. At all ages the skin is wrinkled and peeling with deficient subcutaneous fat. Older persons proceed to a mild ichthyosis and the associated hyperkeratosis is often a sign of slow turnover. The dry scale is well knit and retains pigment, and histologically may be dense and homogenized. The stratum corneum is unsupple and cracks appear in the horny surface, particularly on the front of the legs (Fig. 20). It is known as eczema craquelée and such eczema that

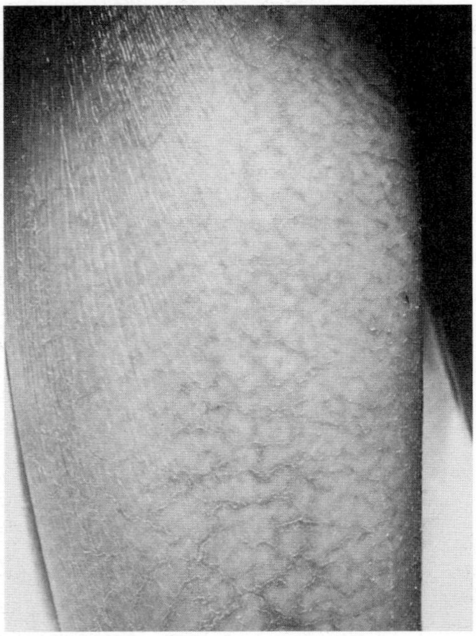

Fig. 20 An early and common sign of malnutrition of the skin, especially in the elderly, is cracking of a well-made stratum corneum giving a pattern of eczema craquelée.

develops is often well marginated, unlike other forms of endogenous eczema.

Most malnutrition is a consequence of mixed deficiencies including protein loss. There is weight loss, weakness, and emaciation. Anaemia, oedema, sore tongue, and dry, thin hair are often features.

Vitamin A deficiency should be thought of when there is significant dryness of the eyes and perifollicular hyperkeratosis. It is the commonest preventable cause of blindness.

Vitamin B deficiency causes a dermatitis that has a seborrhoeic distribution, particularly of the nasolabial folds, scrotum, and vulva. The lips are dry, cracked, crusted, or ulcerated; the tongue is sore and smooth.

Nicotinic acid deficiency or pellagra causes the well-known triad of dementia, diarrhoea, and dermatitis. Early signs are prominent sebaceous follicles of the nose. The light-sensitivity dermatosis is also exacerbated by heat, friction, and pressure. The erythema is a characteristic dusky brown and the dermatitis is well marginated. In dark skins the lesions are relatively depigmented but equally well marginated.

Vitamin C deficiency causes perifollicular haemorrhages, painful bruising, or woody oedema of the legs. This means that they look oedematous but are hard to the touch. In a dark skin it may appear that the skin is stretched and shiny. Although coiled hairs are an early sign, they are common in the normal population, especially in the elderly. Swollen and bleeding gums are an important sign but occur only in those with teeth. Vitamin C deficiency should be considered in any non-healing wound.

Protein deficiency is common in all forms of malnutrition. However, a characteristic disease is recognizable when the protein deficiency is supplemented by carbohydrate and there is no active starvation. In children this is typified by kwashiorkor. Features of protein deficiency include:

(1) erythema as in a second-degree burn;
(2) dry hyperkeratotic hyperpigmented scales;
(3) peeling like enamel paint, cracking like crazy paving;
(4) skin signs are maximal over pressure areas; and
(5) there is straightening and reddening of the hair.

In some dark skins, raised annular patches of pigmented scales on the trunk are an early sign of malnutrition. This is known as pityriasis rotunda.

Management includes avoiding secondary deficiencies, since the sudden provision of some but not all the necessary foods may precipitate conditions like blindness from vitamin A deficiency. In malnutrition, zinc may be lacking or poorly absorbed, leading to alopecia, diarrhoea, glossitis, and an eroded perioroficial rash called acrodermatitis enteropathica. Some improvement in the rash of kwashiorkor has been described using local zinc ointments, and with the prescription of other trace elements such as selenium.

Is there an association with a systemic disease?

There is a number of associations of skin disease with diseases of the gastrointestinal tract and haematological, cardiovascular, respiratory, renal, and central nervous systems. However, no completely satisfactory system for listing these has been devised. Many of the skin diseases are discussed more fully in other sections.

Gastrointestinal system

Oral mucosa

Leucoplakia may be associated with Darier's disease, pachyonychia congenita, or simple white sponge naevus. It is premalignant in dyskeratosis congenita. In mucocutaneous candidiasis oral candida is associated with nail dystrophy, alopecia areata, and endocrinopathy. Oral hairy leucoplakia is a sign of the acquired immunodeficiency syndrome (**AIDS**). Major aphthous ulcers are a feature of Beçhet's syndrome, while minor aphthae are found in systemic lupus erythematosus, Crohn's disease, as well as iron and folate deficiency states.

Oesophagus

Bullae are common in epidermolysis bullosa, and occasionally the entire epithelial lining of the oesophagus may be coughed up as a cast. Bullae also occur in pemphigus and mucocutaneous pemphigoid. The superficial erosions that follow rupture of the bullae in pemphigus heal without scarring, while scarring and stricture formation complicate healing in mucocutaneous pemphigoid and epidermolysis bullosa. Stiffness and loss of peristalsis frequently occur as an early sign in scleroderma, best demonstrated by a prone barium swallow. Carcinoma of the oesophagus has been associated with plantopalmar hyperkeratosis (tylosis). Webbing of the postcricoid region with anaemia is associated with dyskeratosis congenita—an atrophy of the skin and nails.

Stomach

Pernicious anaemia is an organ-specific autoimmune disease leading to atrophy of parietal cells that clusters with vitiligo and alopecia areata. Carcinoma may present with acanthosis nigricans (Fig. 105) and tripe palms. Gastric polyposis is associated with perioral and finger lentiginoses in the Peutz–Jeghers syndrome, as well as with nail dystrophy and alopecia in the Canada–Cronkite syndrome.

Gastrointestinal bleeding is a consequence of telangiectasia in hereditary haemorrhagic telangiectasia as well as in acrosclerosis with telangiectasia. It may also occur in disorders of elastic tissues such as Ehlers–Danlos syndrome or pseudoxanthoma elasticum. Henoch–Schönlein purpura usually causes lower gastrointestinal bleeding.

Malignant atrophic papulosis (Degos' disease) is a rare vasculitis of the skin, gastrointestinal tract, and brain. The skin lesion is a porcelain-white punctate scar and the viscera suffer from infarction.

Small bowel

Regional ileitis may present with granulomatous swelling of the buccal mucosa or lips as well as with perianal granulomas and fistulas (Fig. 21). Erythema nodosum, oral aphthous ulcers, and pyoderma gangrenosum are also associated with Crohn's disease, along with any secondary skin changes due to malabsorption.

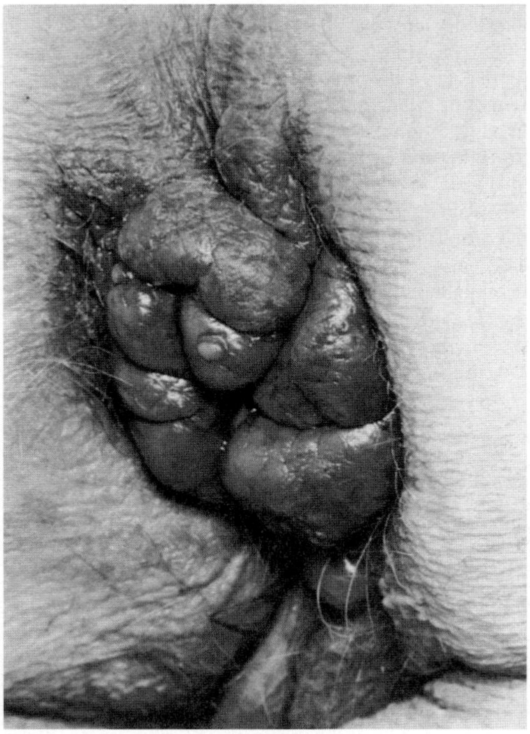

Fig. 21 Perianal granuloma in Crohn's disease.

Dermatitis herpetiformis is associated with subclinical coeliac disease and may be complicated by small bowel lymphoma. Pigmentation and malnutrition of the skin is particularly recorded in Whipple's disease. Bowel bypass syndrome due to anatomical blind loops may present with widespread pustules and vasculitis ulcers. Metastatic carcinoid syndrome produces characteristic flushing.

Colon

Ulcerative colitis is responsible for many disorders of the skin and mouth, but aphthous ulcers are more common here. Rashes include erythema multiforme, erythema nodosum, and pyoderma gangrenosum. Perianal abscesses and fistulas are also common associations.

Dermatomyositis is most commonly associated with carcinoma of the large bowel.

Pancreas

Paraneoplastic migratory thrombophlebitis (Trousseau's sign) is most likely to be associated with carcinoma of the pancreas. Acute fat necrosis of the trunk or limbs is a consequence of acute pancreatitis. There is an increased electrolyte concentration in the sweat of patients with cystic fibrosis.

Glucagonoma produces the characteristic eruption of necrolytic migratory erythema. The skin lesions are dusky red, annular, and scaly with a vesicopustular element due to epidermal-cell necrosis in the most superficial layers of the epidermis. In addition to the skin changes seen as a complication of diabetes, diabetes mellitis is directly associated with a number of skin disorders. Diabetic dermopathy produces hyperpigmented dull-red papules with superficial scale on the shins of 30 to 60 per cent of patients with diabetes. It heals with atrophic brown scars. Diabetic thick skin is also common, and may manifest as a generalized process in 20 per cent of cases or be localized to the neck and upper back (scleroedema of Bushcke), the fingers (Huntley's papules), or the back of the hands (cheirarthropathy). Acanthosis nigricans and anogenital pruritis are common in obese insulin-resistant diabetic patients, while generalized granuloma annulare, diabetic bullae, lipoatrophy, diabetic yellow skin, and perforating disorders are all uncommon.

Necrobiosis lipoidica diabeticorum (**NLD**) (see Fig. 114) is a characteristic eruption consisting of yellowish to red-brown plaques on the shin, which eventually become atrophic in the centre and may ulcerate. Potent topical steroids or intralesional injection of triamcinolone may be required to control NLD, but care is required as they have a tendency to aggravate the atrophy. NLD occurs in 0.3 per cent of diabetic patients and pre-dates diabetes in 30 per cent.

Although diabetes may be complicated by skin infections such candida or bacterial furuncles, a dermatophytic infection is no more common than in non-diabetic patients. Hyperlipidaemia may be associated with xanthoma, neuropathy with foot deformity and ulceration, and angiopathy with cold, pale hairless legs. NLD, diabetic dermopathy, the erysipelas-like erythema seen on the legs and feet of elderly people with diabetes, and the diabetic rubeosis of the face are all thought to be due to microangiopathy.

Liver

The skin consequences of liver disease include spider naevi, palmar erythema, purpura and bruising, white nails, and clubbing of the fingers. There is loss of hair in the beard, axillas, and pubic region. Gynaecomastia, acne, Dupuytren's contracture, xanthoma, jaundice, pruritus, and pigmentation are other features.

A number of patients presenting with porphyria cutanea tarda or lichen planus will be found to be infected with the hepatitis C virus. Hepatitis B infection is associated with polyarteritis nodosa and the childhood exanthem of pink palpable lesions named the Giannoti Crosti syndrome. A proportion of patients with non-infectious or autoimmune hepatitis will have cutaneous features of lupus or sarcoidosis. Haemochromatosis produces diffuse skin pigmentation and patients may develop hepatocellular carcinoma.

Other systemic manifestations in the skin

These include renal disease in cutaneous vasculitis and lupus erythematosus. Cardiovascular disease and skin disease occur with carcinoid, or secondary to amyloid, scleroderma, as well as subacute bacterial endocarditis, which may produce nodules in the skin—Osler's nodes. Myxoma is recorded with pigment anomalies of the skin in the **LAMB** (lentigenes, atrial myxoma, mucocutaneous myxomas, blue naevi) and **NAME** (naevi, atrial myxoma, myxoid neurofibroma, ephelides) syndromes. Disease occurring in the CNS is observed in Beçhet's syndrome, sarcoid, lupus erythematosus, and with vascular stenosis and livedo reticularis (Sneddon's syndrome). There is also respiratory failure in sarcoid, Churg–Strauss vasculitis, and asthma is common in atopy. Haematological associations include Sweet's acute febrile neutrophilic dermatoses, pyoderma gangrenosum, leukaemia-associated genodermatoses, leukaemia cutis, B-cell lymphoma, and Hodgkin's disease.

Is climate responsible?

Heat, cold, food, and water are all dependent on the climate. The management of skin disease requires washing, soaking, and adequate nutrition as well as control of body temperature. Children and the newborn are particularly susceptible.

Humidity explained why, 70 per cent of lost combat man-days in Vietnam during the rainy season were through skin disease. The distribution of water determines the ecology of many human parasites, such as biting insects that thrive in the rainy season. Wet clothing can cause severe discomfort (particularly inside a boot, around the waist, or between the legs) while marching. Even in the Arctic, occlusive clothing can accumulate much sweat and make walking impossible. 'Immersion foot' and 'paddy foot' can bring a military campaign to an end. In Kuwait, outbreaks of industrial dermatitis were blamed on the absorption of allergens by the skin that become moisturized in certain seasons, while in Scandinavia a low humidity in some factories accounted for drying of the epidermis and consequent irritant dermatitis.

Seasonal variations not only account for increased bacterial injury and epidemics of viral exanthems, but also for eczema; for example, in the atopic patient sensitive to sunlight, or the allergic contact dermatitis due to handling plants seen so often in market gardeners and florists. Sweaty feet in hot weather increase the dermatitis from footwear, and sweat-pore occlusion encourages widespread bacterial infections in extreme heat. The incidence of some disease is influenced by height above sea-level and by the thickness of the atmosphere. People are less likely to be sun-burned at the low level of the Dead Sea where UVA greatly predominates over UVB, but actinic dermatitis is common in Mexico and in the Andes. Many infections are most exuberant at sea-level. At the slightly higher level of 600 to 1500 m, transmission of leishmaniasis and onchocerciasis by flies is more common. Many of the skin diseases caused by infections with a unique geographical distribution are discussed in Section 7, including pinta, buruli ulcer, or deep mycoses. In this chapter they are only mentioned if they are important in the differential diagnosis of some physical sign, such as depigmentation, wartiness, and blisters.

Both cold weather and low humidity predispose to irritant dermatitis; for instance, the high incidence of dry skin in hospital is explained by the central heating and the very light clothing worn. Pediculosis is encouraged when people huddle together to keep warm.

While much is said about changes in the world's climate, less is said about changes in the skin's microclimate. These are brought about by changes in home heating and bed linen, as well as by clothing, including footwear. Duvets encourage perspiration and can exacerbate nocturnal itch and scratch. Plastic-soled shoes also increase foot temperature and perspiration and lead to tinea, pitted keratolysis, or juvenile plantar dermatosis. The skin, like antique wooden furniture, suffers from contemporary Western overheating and the resultant drying out. Dermatitis is one consequence. The second commonest environmental cause of neonatal mortality is hypo- or hyperthermia.

Cold

Every polar explorer who is inadequately protected will suffer frostbite, snow blindness, and even death. Although the majority of people in more temperate climates do not die of cold, individual susceptibility to its effects varies. A high incidence of skin disease can be attributed to inadequate protection against minor degrees of cold injury. Vasoconstriction and increased blood viscosity mediate internal disease.

It is often noted that residents of the United Kingdom have pink cheeks and blue hands to a degree not seen in, for instance, Australia or the United States. This is because of chronic exposure to cooling. In Canada or Scandinavia where the winters are a danger to the unprotected, there would be no such exposure of the schoolchild or teenager as seen during the winter in the United Kingdom, where 10 per cent of the population are affected by chilblains, acrocyanosis, Raynaud's phenomenon, and the various manifestations of perniosis, an incidence never approached in most other parts of the world.

Chronic cold causes thickening of the subcutaneous and dermal tissues, as in pigs. During the miniskirt era, girls' thighs regularly became fatter in temperate climates. Fat insulates the surface of the skin from the inside, so cooling of the surface is obvious. Chronic cooling causes telangiectasia, which is often perifollicular, and sometimes even angiokeratoma. Pink cheeks are one consequence, but similar changes may be seen over the fat of the calf or upper arm. Cooling causes stasis in the venules so that circulating noxious agents, such as immune complexes and bacteria, usually localize and deposit at such sites.

The anatomy of the skin vasculature is such that cooled skin often shows a pink and blue mottling known as cutis marmorata. If the changes are fixed and do not reverse with warmth, for example in a hot bath, it is then known as livedo reticularis (Fig. 22(a)). This is commonly seen in collagen vascular diseases such as lupus erythematosus. Much disease is localized in the venules of such damaged vasculature. Chilblains or perniosis is essentially a cold-induced ischaemia. Pressure from tight clothing often encourages the damage done by cooling (Fig. 22(b)).

Ultraviolet radiation and the sun

The sun emits electromagnetic rays comprising a continuous spectrum of short to long waves. Only a narrow range of wavelengths between 400 nm and 770 nm react with photocells in the retina and observed as the various colours of the rainbow. Beyond red (770 nm) is infrared. Heat is due to infrared radiation, which can be felt. Below violet (400 nm) are the ultraviolet (200–400 nm) and X-rays. Most short wavelengths, that can neither be seen nor felt, are filtered out by the Earth's thick atmosphere which includes ozone and water vapour. Therefore, as there is less atmosphere above mountain tops, the danger of radiation exposure is greater. The content of water vapour in the atmosphere varies, which accounts for protection from sunburn in winter, cloudy days, the early morning, or late evening sun. The thick atmosphere of the low-lying Dead Sea in Israel and Jordan is also protective against UVB radiation. Glass filters out wavelengths below 320 nm, so that the closed windows of a car will protect even in a tropical desert unless one is sensitive to the longer wavelengths of ultraviolet radiation. Porphyria is, for example, a disease triggered by UVA radiation and is thus difficult to protect against by shade, cloud, or glass.

Ultraviolet radiation (**UVR**) is arbitrarily divided into UVC (200–280 nm), UVB (280–320), and UVA (320–400 nm). The principal effects of ultraviolet light on the skin are elastic fibre damage and cutaneous ageing, apoptosis, immunosuppression, suntan, sunburn, and carcinogenesis. While each subclass of UVR can produce all of these effects, UVC is relatively more likely to cause cancer, UVB relatively more likely to produce burning, and UVA relatively more likely to produce ageing. UVA is estimated to be 10 times less effective than UVB at producing a suntan and 100 times less effective than UVB at producing non-melanoma skin cancer. This is the basis of so-called 'safe tanning' using UVA light in solariums. However, high-dose UVA does cause non-melanoma skin cancer. In addition, the spectrum responsible for producing melanoma has not been established and may include UVA.

UVR immunosuppression may lead to the reactivation of herpes simplex. It may also suppress tumour surveillance and thereby enhance carcinogenesis. The immunosuppressive, and hence anti-inflammatory, action spectrum has been defined for psoriasis at 312 nm. UVA is only effective for the treatment of psoriasis when the phototoxicity is augmented by a photosensitizer such as psoralen. The action spectrum for the suppression of atopic dermatitis has not been defined, but the skin of patients may improve when exposed to both UVA and UVB. However, a number of related factors influence the response of atopic dermatitis to sunlight and artificial UVR, including ambient humidity (which tends to moisten skin) and heat (which lowers the threshold to itch and scratch).

The diagnosis of UVR damage is determined by recognizing the distribution of the rash as being typical of exposure. Thus the head, nose, and

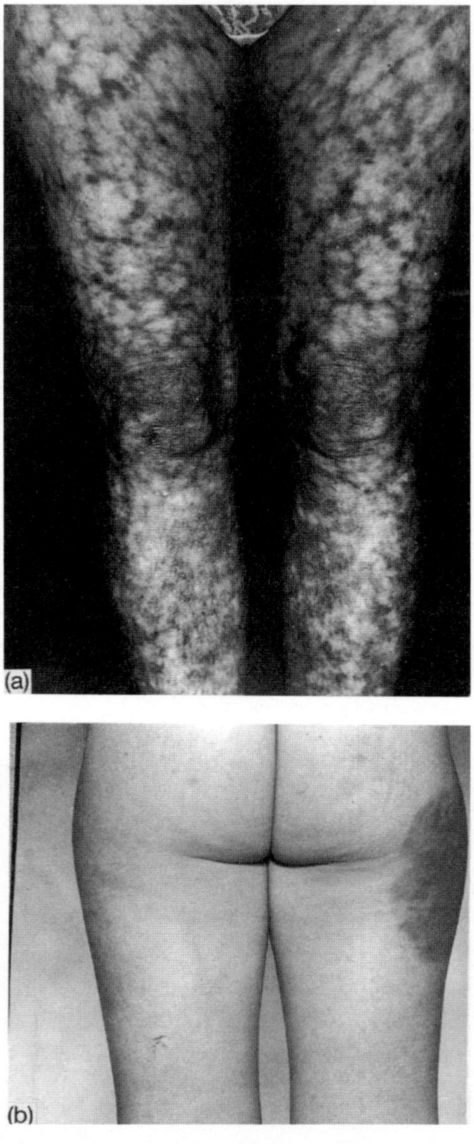

Fig. 22 (a) Chronic vascular disease, especially if inflammatory, summates with the physical effects of cooling to produce livedo reticularis. A non-inflammatory variety associated with cerebrovascular disease is known as Sneddon's syndrome. (b) An equestrian chilblain is due to the combination of the insulating effect of fat and pressure from tight jeans in a young girl riding on a damp and frosty morning.

cheeks are principally affected, but there is often sparing below the eyebrows, under a forelock, beneath and behind the ears, and below the chin (see Fig. 14(b)). The sides and back of the neck are picked out, but there is a sharp border to the sun damage where the collar shields the skin from sunlight. Much, of course, depends on the style of clothing as well as on the direction of irradiation. The backs of the hands and dorsum of the feet are often caught by the sun; however, there may be some tolerance of such skin previously exposed and tanned so that skin not so tolerant is clearly more prone to burning. Mediation of sunburn erythema is partly due to the generation of prostaglandins. Plant dermatitis often produces a rash having the distribution of sun exposure. Phytophotodermatitis is a rash in the distribution of actual contact with plant juices on which the sun then acts and produces a burn. The pattern of such casual contact is often streaky and bizarre. Some perfumes containing berloque or musk ambrette are also responsible (see Fig. 53).

White skin and the sun

Over the past 50 years, hats, parasols, long skirts, and shawls as well as shady verandas have been replaced by bikinis, solariums, and reckless sun-worshipping. Even redheads and blondes attempt to get a suntan. Only recently through public education has this trend been slowed.

Exposure to sunlight is a major cause of skin ageing and of the epidermal and dermal degenerative diseases that accompany ageing (Fig. 23). In Australia, South Africa, and the south-western United States solar keratosis, basal-cell carcinoma (**BCC**), chronic solar cheilitis, and squamous-cell carcinoma (**SCC**) (Fig. 24) are the commonest reasons for referral to a dermatologist (Table 8). Some two out of every three Australians will develop one or more non-melanoma skin cancers during their lifetime; in Queensland, the lifetime risk of developing a melanoma is 10 per cent. Even children are not completely immune, and persons who burn easily and still persist in exposing themselves regularly to the sun will inevitably suffer gross skin changes, even at an early age. Fortunately, the most common skin cancers have a low potential for metastases.

Disorders

Solar keratosis Solar keratoses are erythematous scaling lesions between 2 and 10 mm in diameter, seen on areas of maximal sun exposure such as the face, dorsum of the hands, forearms, and lower legs. Histologically, these precancerous lesions show dysplasia of the basal keratinocytes. The estimated risk of transformation into either SCC or BCC is very low—1 per cent per annum. Many small lesions resolve spontaneously, particularly with photoprotection. Larger lesions respond to cryosurgery, while patients with multiple lesions may require treatment with topical fluorouracil cream.

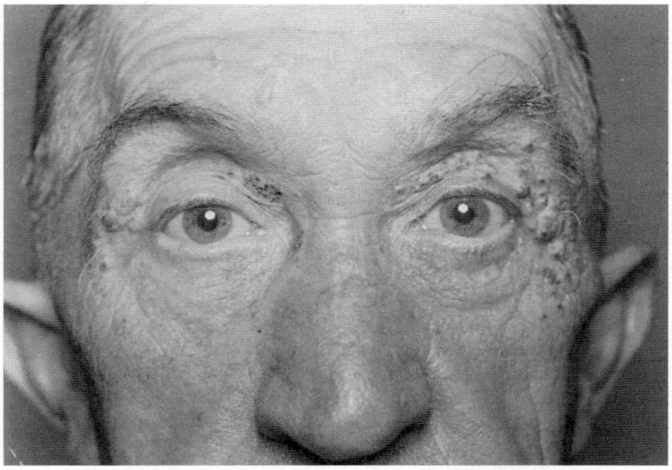

Fig. 23 Prominent sebaceous glands and comedo formation in solar elastosis.

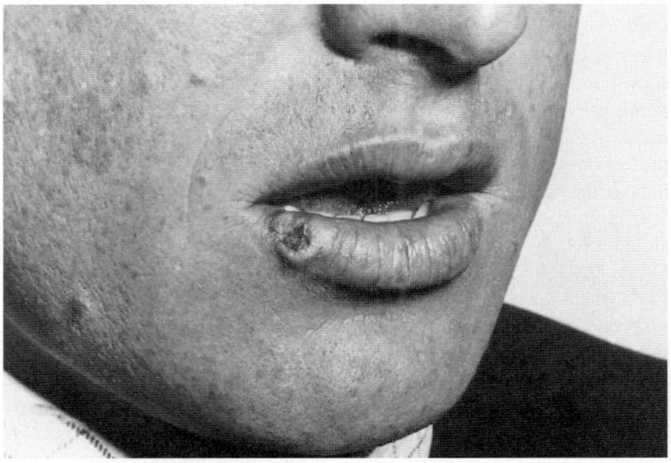

Fig. 24 Squamous epithelioma of the lower lip as a consequence of sun exposure.

Basal-cell carcinoma Basal-cell carcinoma is a slow-growing invasive neoplasm arising from the basal cells of the epidermis or outer root sheath of hair follicles. Some 50 per cent occur on the head and neck, 30 per cent on the upper trunk, and the remainder elsewhere. BCC can be subdivided into nodular, ulcerated (rodent ulcer), morphoeic, pigmented, and superficial forms. They have a tendency to local invasion, but metastasis rarely, if ever, occurs. Local recurrence is most common with morphoeic BCC. Treatments are influenced both by tumour factors (for example, the size, site, margin definition, and subtype of the BCC) and host factors (for example, general infirmity, coexisting illnesses (such as a bleeding diathesis or susceptibility to bacterial endocarditis), access to local facilities, and patient preference). Options include surgical excision, curettage and electrocautery, radiotherapy, cryosurgery, and injection of interferon-α. Topical immunomodulatory creams, such as imiquimod, are also effective in selected cases.

A number of genetic syndromes of increased susceptibility to BCC have been described. These include the Gorlin syndrome, Bazex syndrome, and Rombo syndrome. Exposure to arsenic also increases BCC susceptibility.

Squamous-cell carcinoma Squamous-cell carcinomas are faster growing areas of ulceration or tender nodules that occur on areas of maximal sun exposure, such as the dorsum of the hands, balding scalp, face and neck, upper trunk, and lower legs. While UVR is the principal aetiological factor, other predisposing factors include exposure to radiotherapy, chronic leg ulcers, burn scars or sinuses from osteomyelitis, erythema ab igne, and the porokeratosis of Mibelli. Systemic immunosuppression, as used to prevent organ transplant rejection, increases the susceptibility to SCC by 100-fold. In addition, people with xeroderma pigmentosa, dystrophic epidermolysis bullosa, Rothmund Thomson syndrome, and arsenic exposure have a greater susceptibility to developing SCC. Up to 1 per cent of SCCs will metastasize, most commonly to regional lymph nodes; however, 20 per cent of any metastasis is bloodborne to the liver, lungs, brain, and bone. Survival rates following metastatic SCC are poor, with less than 30 per cent responding to current therapies. High-risk SCCs include rapidly growing tumours, large lesions (>2 cm in size), deeply invading tumours (>4 mm), poorly differentiated tumours or tumours with perineural invasion, recurrent tumours, tumours of the lips or ears or arising within scars, and tumours occurring in immunosuppressed patients.

Following surgery, 75 per cent of local recurrences occur within 2 years, and 95 per cent within 5 years. In addition, patients are at risk of developing a second primary skin cancer. Within 5 years, 12 per cent of patients will have developed a new SCC, 43 per cent a new BCC, and 2 per cent a melanoma.

Melanocytic naevi (moles) Melanocytic naevi are benign neoplasms of melanocytes. Junctional naevi are localized collections of naeval melanocytes found in the epidermis and superficial dermis, they are flat and pigmented. Compound naevi are localized collections in the epidermis and superficial and deep dermis, these naevi are pigmented and raised. Intradermal naevi are localized collections in the deep dermis with no involvement of the epidermis or junctional dermis, such naevi are flat and flesh-coloured. Most naevi are absent at birth. They tend to first appear and increase in number during childhood, reaching their maximum in early adulthood. Naevi counts have been shown to increase at an earlier age in Caucasians who live closer to the equator, where sun exposure and intensity is greatest.

Large numbers of naevi, both common acquired naevi and atypical naevi, are markers of individuals who are susceptible to developing melanoma. Atypical naevi are large (>6 mm) compound naevi often with a surrounding macular erythematous component, irregular in colour or shape, but nevertheless benign. These lesions may or may not show histological evidence of dysplasia, therefore the old term 'dysplastic naevi', which leads to much confusion, is not recommended. Although the clinical differentiation of atypical naevi from melanoma is difficult, it may be facilitated by regular surveillance and clinical photography. The presence of more than five atypical moles on a person has been shown to be a powerful and independent marker of melanoma susceptibility.

'Congenital naevi' is a term applied both to compound naevi present at birth and to acquired naevi that are clinically and histologically similar to moles present at birth. One child in 100 is born with a congenital pigmented naevus, while 6 to 12 per cent of children and adults have a 'congenital type naevus'. The risk of evolution of a small congenital naevus (<2 cm) into invasive melanoma is unknown, but is thought to be much less than 1 per cent. Prophylactic excision is not universally advocated, but rather considered on a case-by-case basis. Large congenital naevi (20 cm) occur in 1 in 500 000 births and probably carry a 4 to 6 per cent risk of progression to melanoma over a lifetime. The melanoma usually develops after puberty and does not always occur in the naevus itself. Unfortunately, removal of large lesions is rarely easy and may involve numerous surgical procedures.

There may be a natural evolution of acquired naevi from junctional to compound to intradermal naevi. The malignant potential of individual lesions is low, therefore prophylactic excision of acquired melanocytic naevi to prevent transformation into melanoma is not advised. Most melanomas arise *de novo* in the absence of any clinical or histological evidence of a pre-existing naevus. Excision of naevi is advocated where it is not possible to clinically exclude a diagnosis of melanoma. The lesion should be totally excised and submitted for histological assessment. Destructive therapy of melanocytic naevi without histological assessment is a recipe for disaster, for clinical diagnosis is not completely accurate and an opportunity to re-excise an incompletely or inadequately removed tumour may be missed. Patients who subsequently present with metastatic melanoma without an identified primary will rightly or wrongly point the finger at the physician who removed the 'naevus', and claim compensation. Therefore, complete removal and histological examination is advocated even when moles are removed for purely cosmetic reasons.

Melanoma Melanoma is a malignant neoplasm of melanocytes, which, although initially confined to the epidermis, later invades deeper layers of

Table 8 Clinical features of chronic sun exposure

Clinical diagnosis	Principal characteristics			Additional features	
Elastosis	Less elastic, more fragile, yellowish, furrowed	Telangiectasia, venous lakes, spider angiomas	Prominent sebaceous glands (Fig. 24)	Linear and stellate scars	Idiopathic guttate melanosis
Keratosis	10% precancerous	Yellow-brown hyperkeratosis on a red telangiectatic background—the scale is not laminated as in psoriasis but firmly psoriasis but firmly painful; unlike lupus erythematosus, it bleeds when the scale is removed	Cutaneous horn common	Annular lesions frequent	Bleed easily when scratched
Solar cheilitis	Lower lip	Yellow-white thickenings	Scaling and crusting	Fissuring	
Basal-cell epithelioma	Central erosion	Telangiectasia runs over the edge	Pearl-like border	Cystic, pigmented, or sclerotic forms	
Squamous-cell vepithelioma	Indurated beyond the visible margin (Plates 1–9)	Ulcerated, hyperkeratotic, or granulomatous	Crusted and horny	Hard, elevated, or undermined edge	
Keratoacanthoma	Rapid growth: 4–6 weeks	Sharply defined, hemispherical	Central horny core which may leave a crater	2–12 months, disappears spontaneously	Scarring may be considerable
Bowen's disease	Often single with a well-defined edge	Usually red scaly or crusted plaques	Often slightly pigmented		
Malignant melanoma	Change in the depth of pigmentation (either darkening or loss), irregular notched border	Growth changes, satellites	Bleeding, itching, or ulceration	Family history of atypical multiple pigmented naevi	

the skin. Melanoma is one of the most common cancers and cause of cancer-related deaths among adult Caucasians. It is caused by childhood exposure (in particular intermittent exposure) to sunlight resulting in sunburn. The incidence of melanoma increases with age, the lifetime risk for people in the United Kingdom being around 1 to 2 per cent. The greater exposure to sunlight experienced by Australians has increased their lifetime risk to between 3 and 10 per cent, depending on their proximity to the equator. Melanoma is rare during childhood and in Blacks and Asians.

Hutchinson's melanotic freckle occurs on the head and neck of older people who have been heavily exposed to sunlight. These are slow-growing *in situ* melanomas with the potential to progress to invasive melanoma and metastasize. Acral lentiginous melanoma, including subungual melanoma, is equally common in all races and therefore does not appear to be caused by exposure to the sun. A tendency to delayed diagnosis gives this variant a generally poor prognosis.

Superficial spreading and nodular melanomas predominately occur on the trunk in men and on the limbs in women, not necessarily at sites heavily exposed to sunlight. The clinical features of a superficial spreading melanoma include a history of a new mole or a change in the size, shape, or colour of an existing mole. Itching and bleeding are late signs. On examination, melanomas are asymmetrical, irregular in outline and colour, and often stand out as different from other moles on the patient's skin. They are frequently over 6 mm in diameter at the time of diagnosis; however, this feature is now less common than in the past due to improved awareness of the early warning signs by at-risk populations. These signs are illustrated in Plates 1 to 7.

The risk of metastasis, and hence the 5-year survival rate, is related to the depth of invasion of the melanoma measured in millimetres from the granular layer of the epidermis, known as the Breslow thickness. Patients with lesions confined to the epidermis (melanoma *in situ*) have a 5-year survival rate of 100 per cent; those less than 0.76 mm, 98 per cent; between 0.76 and 1.5 mm, 95 per cent; between 1.5 and 3 mm, 80 per cent; and lesions of more than 3 mm in depth, 60 per cent.

At presentation, 10 per cent of cutaneous melanomas will have metastasized. In order to identify the primary lesion it is important to look at the entire cutaneous surface—in the eyes, inside the mouth, and the vulva, etc.—and to examine the skin with a Wood's light (see above), for the primary melanoma may have undergone spontaneous regression after giving rise to metastases and only be identified as a hypopigmented patch under such light.

Metastasis is usually to the regional lymph node basin. If a single lymph node is involved the 5-year survival is 45 per cent, if two lymph nodes are involved the survival rate is 28 per cent, but this rate drops to 9 per cent if more than four lymph nodes are involved. The median survival time following metastasis is between 5 and 16 months. Although systemic metastasis is predominately to the lung, liver, brain, and bone, lesions can arise anywhere including bowel, kidney, and muscle. Localized skin metastasis is also common.

In general, there is a low yield from routine investigations for melanoma; moreover, chest radiographs and CT and/or MRI scans are not routinely ordered in asymptomatic patients. However, the investigation of new symptoms results in a high percentage of positive findings, and this policy is the preferred approach. When metastasis does occur, 50 per cent will be within 1 year, 85 per cent within 2 years, and 95 per cent will be within 5 years. The survival rate of such patients increases with disease-free time following removal of a melanoma; the only caveat is that metastasis following thin lesions, albeit rare, may be delayed.

There is no adjuvant therapy that improves survival, and chemotherapy and radiotherapy are only used for palliation. Surgery, when possible, remains the treatment of choice for metastatic melanoma. Initial optimism regarding the use of adjuvant interferon or elective lymph node dissection has now waned. However, the use of lymphoscintography and sentinel-node biopsy to identify high-risk patients for such therapy now seems helpful in finding lymph node metastases, but its use as a tool to improve long-term survival is still uncertain. The only intervention that improves survival is early diagnosis and complete removal of the primary melanoma. Even re-excision of the scar does not improve survival; but it is still recommended with ever-decreasing margins with the sole intention of reducing the incidence of local recurrence/metastasis. Currently, the margins recommended are 0.5 cm for *in situ* melanoma and 1 cm for invasive melanomas with a Breslow thickness of less than 1.5 mm. A minimum margin of 1 cm and a maximum margin of 2 cm of normal skin is recommended for lesions between 1.5 mm and 4 mm deep. Although re-excision of the scar for lesions greater than 4 mm is unlikely to be worthwhile, a minimum margin of 2 cm is recommended.

Rashes due to sun or artificial light and associated ultraviolet rays

Sunburn Initially this is an erythema occurring about 6 to 8 h after exposure, which may progress to blistering and later to skin-peeling. However, redness may begin as early as 2 h if the exposure is excessive. Sunburn tends to resolve, often with peeling, after 24 to 72 h, depending on its severity. Topical corticosteroids and oral non-steroidal anti-inflammatory agents may provide partial relief.

Solar urticaria Here, erythema and wealing occur immediately on exposure to sun, often of sites not habitually exposed to the sun. It is a rare but very disabling condition due to a broad spectrum of wavelengths that rarely responds to sunscreens, although it often does well with plasmapheresis or, paradoxically, phototherapy.

Polymorphic light eruption Polymorphic light eruption is an altered quality of sunburn. Thus instead of erythema there is an itchy papular or eczematous response about 6 to 8 h after exposure, which may persist for several days (Fig. 25). There are several variants including a lymphoma-like pattern with heavy lymphocytic infiltrates.

Actinic prurigo Sun-induced prurigo shares features with atopic eczema, polymorphic light eruption, and persistent light eruption due to photosensitivity agents in the environment. It is uncommon except in genetically susceptible individuals with HLA-A24 and CW4 and the rare subtype DR4 DRB1*0407, which is particularly common among some native Americans. It has a chronic course that is only initially seasonal. Urticarial plaques

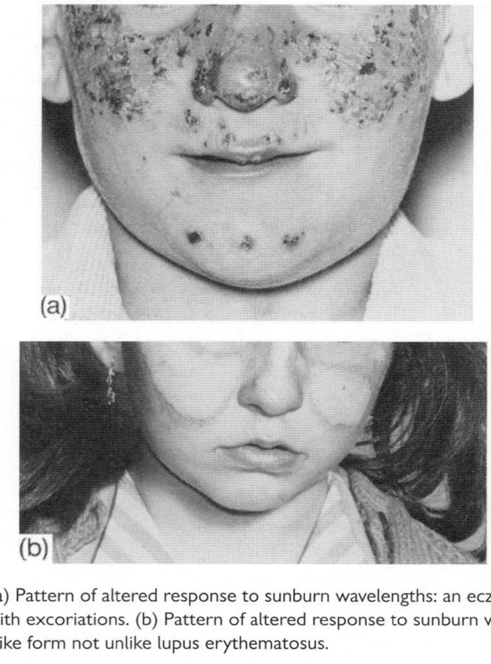

Fig. 25 (a) Pattern of altered response to sunburn wavelengths: an eczematous prurigo with excoriations. (b) Pattern of altered response to sunburn wavelengths: a plaque-like form not unlike lupus erythematosus.

develop a few hours after ultraviolet exposure and are followed by a persistent eczematous rash, which is not always confined to exposed skin.

Exacerbation or localization of other dermatoses in sun-exposed sites This is characteristic of pellagra, Hartnup's disease, lupus erythematosus, dermatomyositis, pemphigus erythematosus/foliaceous, Darier's disease, herpes simplex, rosacea, scleroderma, erythema multiforme, actinic lichen planus, and lymphocytoma. It sometimes occurs in psoriasis, seborrhoeic dermatitis, atopic eczema, acne, and bullous pemphigoid.

Ultraviolet rays may diminish antigen surveillance by reducing the population of Langerhans cells.

Porphyrias See Chapter 11.5 for further discussion.

Drug eruptions and photosensitivity Various drugs can cause acute eruptions of erythema that swell or blister like severe sunburn, which, since UVA is often responsible, are independent of bright sun. The reactions are often dose-dependent, as with psoralens in PUVA therapy. Ingestion of a spinach (Atriplex) also causes photosensitivity (see Table 9). Some eruptions present only as deep pigmentation.

Xeroderma pigmentosum See Chapter 25.2 for further discussion.

Persistent light eruption 'Persistent light eruption' is the term given to a sensitivity to light induced by agents previously applied to the skin, often years before. Drugs eliciting light sensitivity are listed in Table 9.

Investigations

Patients should be asked about their family history, their occupation, drug or food ingestion, and exposure to perfumes, as well as how and when any exposure occurred. It is important to know whether glass is protective. Many patients confuse the effects of heat and sunlight, making it important to clarify whether exposure to an open fire, for example, also exacerbates their condition.

Light-testing has become a useful dermatological tool, with a number of centres having access to a monochromator that specifically evaluates each band of light.

Table 9 Photosensitivity due to drugs

Sulphonamides and related chemicals:	
Antibacterials:	sulfathiazole, long-acting sulphonamides
Diuretics:	chlorothiazide, hydrochlorothiazide, quinethazone
Antidiabetic:	sulphonylureas, carbamides
Rarely:	paraphenylenediamine, procaine group of anaesthetics
Antibiotics	
Tetracyclines:	tetracycline, dimethylchlortetracycline (demeclocycline hydrochloride, Ledermycin®)
Chlortetracycline hydrochloride (Aureomycin®)	
Griseofulvin	
Antiarrhythmic	
Amiodarone	
Phenothiazines	
Chlorpromazine, promazine, trimeprazine, meprazine, promethazine hydrochloride	
Other psychotrophic drugs	
Chlordiazepoxide	
Antihistamines not of phenothiazine structure	
Diphenhydramine	
Antimalarials	
Chloroquine	
Occasional, rare, or of historical interest	
Isoniazid, psoralens, stilbamidine 9-aminoacridine, eosin, trypaflavine, methylene blue, Rose bengal, furosemide, nalidixic acid (Negram®)	

Prophylaxis

Health education in schools should emphasize that burning in the sun is not related to heat or wind, rather it is maximal when the sun is directly overhead. Therefore protection is essential between the hours of 10 am and 2 pm, mainly achieved by covering the head and body and keeping in the shade. Sunscreens are effective only if they are properly used; that is to say, they must be applied evenly and thoroughly and well before exposure, and reapplied at appropriate intervals, but they are no substitute for avoidance. Frequent, uninhibited exposure leads to the accumulation of almost inevitable and irreversible injury, which may only become apparent some 20 years later.

Management

The ill-effects of a cool, sunny, and windy noon must be explained, as well as the relative safety of a hot sunny evening. Ensuring protection for those who are sensitive to UVB includes giving advice on the time of day and season likely to be harmful. Most patients can safely take a swim in the early morning or late afternoon. Those with severe sensitivities, such as xeroderma pigmentosum, can be saved from all ill-effects by diligent protection, including clothing. Indeed, clothing and shade are the best protections for children sensitive to the sun, but a wet T-shirt can transmit ultraviolet rays; tightly woven silks, Lycra, and cottons are more effective than loosely woven yarns or wool. Fluorescent lighting emits small amounts of UVR and is safe for all but the most sensitive. Glass windows are protective against UVB and shorter wavelengths, while Perspex and certain plastics also protect against UVA. Natural pigment and thickening of the epidermis accounts for normal tolerance.

Sunscreens are rated, according to UVB protection, by a solar protection factor (SPF). There is an inverse relationship between SPF and sun protection, such that there is only a minimal difference between SPF 8 and SPF 16 and probably no real difference between SPF 16 and SPF 50. The limiting factor of any sunscreen is correct application and reapplication.

Sun-screening agents include thick reflective pastes or creams such as zinc oxide or titanium dioxide; these filter out both UVA and UVB and also prevent tanning. Sun-screening agents may absorb light, with invisible lotions or creams containing *p*-aminobenzoic acid in 70 per cent alcohol mainly filtering UVB. This allows some tanning due to the effects of UVA.

Is it what I have eaten? Food and drug eruptions

It is generally accepted that much of what we eat is antigenic and that absorption does occur. Usually allergens are complexed with antibodies in the gut wall and tolerance occurs. It is easy to demonstrate that antibodies are made to counteract food allergens and that complexes circulate in the blood as a result of eating. This is not necessarily allergy because resulting inflammation is rare.

Infrequent ingestion is more likely to cause an allergy than tolerance.

Both erythema and acute urticaria can be caused by food, but chronic urticaria is rarely so. In the atopic person, IgE-mediated food allergy is well recognized. Contact urticaria occurs when eggs or milk touch the lips and cause immediate swelling, whereas generalized urticaria and bowel upset result when agents such as fish, nuts, or strawberries are eaten. However, in many patients such eruptions are examples of non-allergic intolerance.

Anaphylactoid reactions are either idiosyncrasies, whereby an individual reacts abnormally to a substance tolerated by most of the population due to some defect in their physiology, or they result from a direct effect or action of a drug on a mast cell, or other cell, often on first exposure to the eliciting substance. Examples of non-allergic responses include C_1-esterase deficiency and angio-oedema, or lactose intolerance and lactase deficiency, causing diarrhoea.

A high iodine level in a diet induces blistering in dermatitis herpetiformis and exacerbates erythema nodosum leprosum. Sources include iodophors used in dairy cleansing, iodine-containing food supplements, and dough improvers in bread, as well as in cough mixtures.

Following the development of toxic erythema and purpura in an extensive epidemic amongst eaters of margarine in The Netherlands and Germany, the possibility that food additives could cause rashes is now well recognized. Urticaria, asthma, and migraine have also been studied in this respect. The total number of food additives exceeds 20 000 and an average person eats about 1.5 kg every year. Salicylates and benzoates as well as many colouring agents present in more than 1000 drugs marketed in the United States partly act through the control of prostaglandin metabolism. Some 10 per cent of people sensitive to aspirin are also sensitive to the colouring agent tartrazine. The mechanism, though suspected to be related to prostaglandin metabolism, has yet to be clarified. It is confusing that some other types of food allergy, perhaps less dependent on IgE and on the release of histamine from mast cells, are prevented by prostaglandin inhibitors: 'If one takes indometacin, one can eat anything'!

Careful studies of food additives have led the authors to the conclusion that food containing additives is very rarely a danger, but food without additives is commonly so. So far as intolerance is concerned, the potentiating effect of psychological tension and unaccustomed or overindulgent eating habits is a probable explanation.

Shellfish and strawberries are well known for not only releasing histamine from mast cells but for causing thrombocytopenic purpura. Usually such agents cause urticaria within hours of ingestion. However, the response is inconsistent, since there may be times or forms of presentation of the same food that avoid this effect. Eggs, nuts, chocolate, fish, shellfish, tomatoes, pork, strawberries, milk, cheese, and yeast are common causes of a sudden transient thrombocytopenia, and sensitivity to food in this way is the basis of the 'thrombo' test. A 20 per cent fall in the platelet count 1 h after ingestion occurs in 70 per cent of persons showing allergy to aspirin, barbiturates, and penicillin. In one series, 203 out of 215 patients with urticaria showed a prolonged bleeding time from the ear lobe 2 h after challenge with a drug, chemical, or food. Bitter lemon or tonic water containing quinine is especially well documented.

In patients with atopic eczema and asthma the problem of food allergy is more complex. These patients seem to be more susceptible to histamine release even from non-allergic sources.

The gut of the newborn with atopy is said to be more immature in its handling of foreign protein; or it may be that the complexing of IgA is less effective so that IgG is brought into play in the immature gut in a manner not usual for the mature immunological system of the adult gastrointestinal system. This is the basis for advocating breast feeding without cows' milk substitution for all babies of atopic parents. Hypoallergic foods are marketed which contain 'predigested' casein, and this is an industry with a strong following. However, minute amounts of antigens from the maternal diet are found in breast milk, so it cannot be assumed that the first experience of a dietary antigen occurs at the time of weaning. Even the fetus is normally supplied by minute samples of the mother's diet. What matters is how much and when.

Another form of food sensitivity is that occurring in nickel-sensitive subjects. Nickel sensitivity is one of the commonest aggravating factors of hand dermatitis, and there seems little doubt that contamination from metal pots and from some green vegetables can contribute to the contact allergic dermatitis in sensitive individuals.

Drug eruptions

The 1975 Boston Collaborative Program of Drug Surveillance observed that adverse reactions accounted for 3 per cent of hospital admissions and 14 per cent of medical resources, and that 30 per cent of hospital patients developed adverse reactions.

It is wise to assume that any drug can cause any rash, but until there are simple, reliable, and specific *in vitro* tests for testing human tissue for hypersensitivity, the diagnosis of drug eruptions will depend entirely on clinical judgement. The physician has to decide whether the rash has some other cause by recognizing certain physical signs, ranging from the mite burrows in scabies to the herald patch of pityriasis rosea. Then if a drug seems a likely cause, there must be an attempt to decide which of the medications currently prescribed, or taken secretly, may be responsible.

Drug rashes are essentially blood borne and therefore often have a symmetrical urticarial, erythematous, or purpuric and ischaemic pattern determined by the vascular anatomy. Less likely is a 'primary epithelial' reaction in the initial stages, and so scaling or even the vesiculation of eczema as a first manifestation of a generalized drug rash would be unusual. The exceptions are well known and include the intraepidermal immunologically induced 'pemphigus' rash of penicillamine, rifampicin, and captopril, especially when the first of these is used to treat rheumatoid arthritis; another is when cell-mediated hypersensitivity to epidermal protein and the drug occurs in a person previously having a contact dermatitis to a local antihistamine or sulphonamide. The psoriasis-like rash of practolol and various other β-blockers as well as the scaly eruption (particularly of the scalp) from methyldopa, are exceptions.

Nevertheless, if a rash looks like eczema, it is probably not caused by a drug. If it is an erythema and urticaria, it may well be. As later stages of the rash are frequently complicated by secondary desquamation and peeling, the diagnosis should be made on the initial manifestation.

Unlikely or likely drugs

It may be helpful to rule out unlikely offenders such as digoxin, paracetamol, steroids, other hormones, and vitamin and electrolyte supplements. In any drug group there are likely and less likely offenders. Thus of the antibiotics, oxytetracycline, nystatin, and erythromycin are not under suspicion, but dichlortetracycline is a common cause of a photosensitivity rash. Moreover, ampicillin is almost invariably responsible for a characteristic bright-pink maculopapular rash in patients with infectious mononucleosis

Sulpha-containing medications such as sulphonamides, thiazide diuretics, oral hypoglycaemic agents, dapsone, and even captopril are capable of causing most rashes. Non-steroidal anti-inflammatory drugs (**NSAIDs**), antibiotics, antiepileptics, gold, penicillamine, allopurinol, halides, and other antihypertensives are all possible candidates worthy of consideration.

Timing

While drug rashes usually relate to newly started medications, this is not always the case. For example, a person may have tolerated multiple courses of a particular antibiotic prior to becoming allergic to it. Maculopapular drug exanthems most commonly begin 7 to 10 days after the drug is commenced, by which time many antibiotic courses will have been completed. The rash often increases in severity with time until the patient stops taking the drug. Once the drug is stopped, the rash may last a further 7 to 14 days and often evolves from a typical maculopapular exanthem to a scaly rash that may resemble the peeling that follows sunburn or even be slightly eczematous. Repeat exposure to that drug, even years later, will usually lead to recurrence of the exanthem within hours to days. Interestingly, some patients do not react on re-exposure, suggesting a toxic rather than an allergic mechanism. This is particularly common in people who react to amoxicillin in the context of infectious mononucleosis.

Other exanthems frequently show a different time course. Anaphylaxis often begins within minutes, while fixed drug eruptions usually begin 30 min to 8 h after rechallenge. Lichenoid drug eruptions often do not begin for many months and sometimes even years. Urticarial reactions are variable: they may start within a few hours with an antibiotic allergy, but may take a week or two to develop following treatment with NSAIDs or angiotensin-converting enzyme inhibitors.

Erythema multiforme, or Stevens–Johnson syndrome, occasionally occurs surprisingly early after a drug's administration, leading to the suspicion that the disease for which the drug was given may have prepared the host in some way.

Many patients do not admit to taking a drug, perhaps because it was never prescribed but borrowed from a family member or neighbour or bought over the counter and therefore considered to be harmless. In general, drug rashes do not persist after withdrawal of the drug—exceptions include pemphigus from penicillamine.

Transient susceptibility

The best example of a susceptibility reaction is urticaria. Many people with chronic urticaria are susceptible to it for a period of many months, during which time the rash may be triggered by prostaglandin synthetase inhibitors, such as aspirin or indometacin. It is possible that certain drug exanthems require both a drug and an infection to provoke the rash, so the underlying disease of the patient should always be taken into account. Patients with infectious mononucleosis or chronic lymphocytic leukaemia are prone to toxic erythema with ampicillin, while people with AIDS are 1000 times more susceptible to developing the Stevens–Johnson syndrome following treatment with sulphonamides. Sometimes immune-complex diseases, such as cutaneous vasculitis from infective organisms, are provoked by interference with immunological mechanisms by certain drugs. The particular set of circumstances, which may not recur, would depend on the formation of antibodies, the nature of the infectious organism, and the taking of the drug at that time. Diseases such as psoriasis or dermatitis herpetiformis may go into spontaneous remission, during which time they are less likely to be provoked by drugs. Dermatitis herpetiformis is provoked by iodine so readily that it should be avoided if possible.

Drug allergy is rarely proven, but overdosage is a frequent well-established fact due to faulty prescribing, attempted suicide, or altered metabolism as in renal or hepatic failure. Interethnic differences in drug metabolism are due to human gene polymorphisms. Drugs may interfere with metabolism, with hormones, they may be deposited, they may react with sunlight, they may modify the ecology of the skin in respect to infective organisms; they may cause reactivity of certain cells such as the mast cell; they may be cytotoxic; and they can act as allergens in the formation of immune complexes, hapten–protein complexes, delayed cellular immunity, and a variety of other mechanisms. Some are not understood, such as the effect of halogens on the formation of granulomas (Fig. 26(a)) and in the causation of an acneiform eruption (Fig. 26(b)). This includes the use of fluoride gel preparations applied to the teeth to prevent dental caries.

Specific drug eruptions

The most common diagnostic problem is a toxic urticated erythema. It begins like measles without the upper respiratory and conjunctival prodromal signs. It usually develops, over a number of hours, as a bright pink indurated papular eruption (Fig. 27) and, unlike urticaria, persists for days, ultimately involving the epidermis and producing scales (Fig. 28). After the first 2 to 3 days the rash tends to be fixed, with the principal changes due to mild bleeding of the skin with overlying slight peeling. Fever and arthropathy may be associated. Common causes are ampicillin, phenylbutazone, phenothiazine, co-trimoxazole, diazides, and sulphonylureas. Exfoliative dermatitis is the end result of this type of reaction (Fig. 29). Gold, phenylbutazone, indometacin, allopurinol, hydantoins, sulphonylureas, ampicillin and amoxicillin, co-trimoxazole, carbamazepine, phenytoin, cefaclor, gentamicin, and *p*-aminosalicylic acid are causative drugs.

Psoriasis β-Blockers can cause a psoriaform scaly eruption that may be modified by basal-cell necrosis. The high turnover as in psoriasis, with the slowing down that results from such necrosis, gives rise to a hyperkeratotic scale that is more adherent than in psoriasis and often slightly yellowish. The palms and soles, elbows, and knees are particularly favoured (Fig. 30).

Labetalol, propranolol, and oxprenolol cause a partly psoriaform and partly lichenoid rash, which is most marked over bony prominences. There is an itchy hyperkeratosis of the palms and soles. Most β-blockers merely exacerbate ordinary psoriasis. Other drugs capable of this include lithium, antimalarials, non-steroidal anti-inflammatories, potassium iodide, amiodarone, and calcitriol, it also occurs on the withdrawal of oral steroids.

Lupus erythematosus Lupus erythematosus, like erythemas or necrotizing vasculitis, is most commonly caused by hydralazine, phenytoin, practolol, penicillamine, and isoniazid. Many other drugs have been incriminated. The drug-induced lupus erythematosus is reversed by withdrawal of the drug, but it recurs when it is readministered. The disease is characterized by antinuclear antibody in high titre with normal DNA binding. Inhibition of C4 underlies the immunological disease induced by hydralazine.

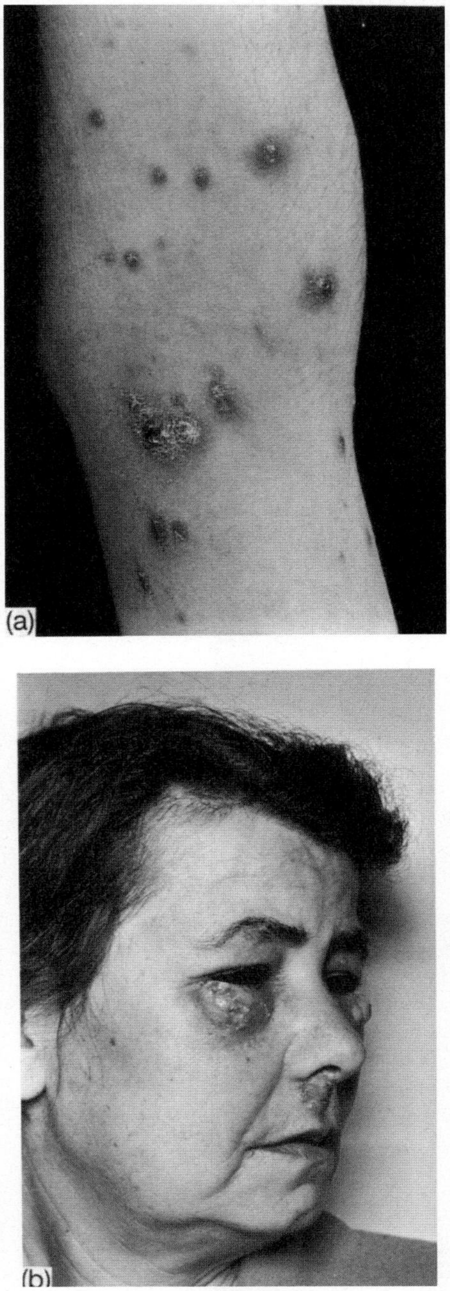

Fig. 26 (a) Iodides and bromides are occasionally responsible for a granulomatous eruption with pseudoepitheliomatous hypertrophy. Potassium iodide in a cough mixture was responsible for the eruption in this patient. (b) Prolonged administration of iodides or bromides causes a particularly inflammatory form of acne which, although commonly in the distribution of acne vulgaris, may be more widespread. This eruption was due to an iodide-containing 'tonic' for the blood.

Scleroderma An epidemic originating from denatured rape-seed oil in Spain caused facial oedema, exanthems, and ultimately a scleroderma-like syndrome.

Fixed drug eruption Although the mechanism is unexplained, the eruption is easy to recognize as it is usually circular and erythematous (Fig. 31), and it frequently blisters. Postinflammatory hyperpigmentation due to pigment incontinence in the dermis is characteristic. It is fixed in site, and whenever the subject takes the causative drug the eruption begins within a few hours in exactly the same site. The tongue and the glans penis are common sites. The affected area can be transplanted without loss of responsiveness in some cases. In pigmented races, very dark pigmentation remains between attacks. In addition to the drugs listed in Table 10, purgatives, blood cleansers and tonics, and many other home remedies containing phenolphthalein, are common causes. Continued ingestion leads to the development of multiple new spots. Skin biopsy is diagnostic in the early stages, and it is safe to rechallenge patients in order to determine the causative agent.

Anticonvulsant hypersensitivity syndrome This severe reaction is characterized by an extensive morbilliform skin rash that often evolves into an exfoliative erythroderma or toxic epidermal necrolysis (TEN), accompanied by fever, lymphadenopathy, hepatitis, nephritis, and leucocytosis with atypical lymphocytes on the blood film. There is a significant mortality and intensive nursing care is required. Other drugs such as allopurinol can produce a similar syndrome.

Management of drug eruptions

The best way is to stop the use of all drugs likely to cause the eruptions. Readministration of the drug is possible for most drug eruptions other than those that cause anaphylactic shock, but it is usually at a risk of considerable morbidity and therefore should be considered only if essential to the patient. Skin tests are unhelpful, as a risk of dangerous anaphylaxis, false-negatives, and lack of knowledge of the antigen, makes skin testing useless.

Blood tests are of no help in trying to find which drug is causing the problem. Various tests, such as the reaction of basophil cells or the release of lymphokines from lymphocytes, have not proved of routine value. Eosinophils may suggest that an eruption is due to a drug, and, as mentioned above, a fall in the platelet level within 1 h or a prolongation of bleeding time 2 h after injection is helpful for some urticarial rashes.

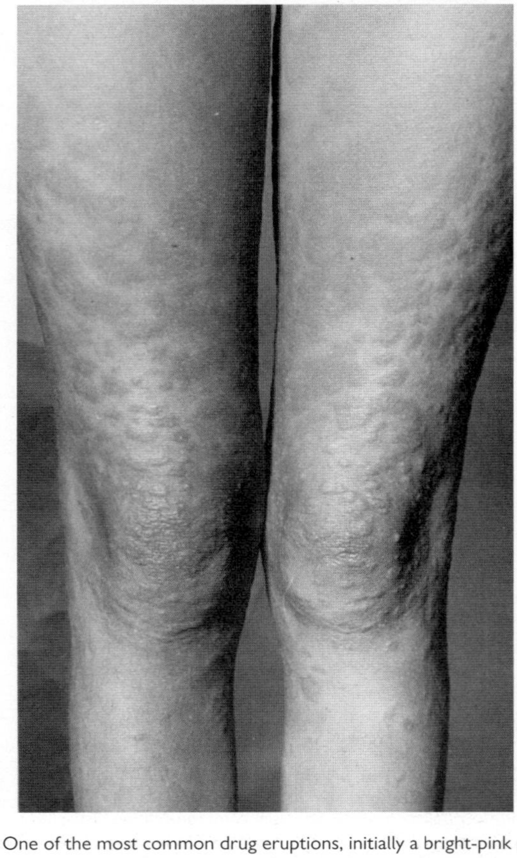

Fig. 27 One of the most common drug eruptions, initially a bright-pink papular eruption, symmetrical, and becoming confluent. This case is due to ampicillin.

Dermatitis

Definition

Dermatitis is a non-specific inflammatory response of the skin to a combination of exogenous and endogenous factors. There is no clear distinction between dermatitis and eczema, and the two terms are interchangeable. Endogenous dermatitis comprises discoid, asteatotic, varicose (or stasis or gravitational), vesicular, hand/foot (pompholyx), atopic, and seborrhoeic dermatitis. Exogenous dermatitis includes irritant contact, allergic contact, phototoxic, and photoallergic dermatitis. However, sometimes there is no clear distinction between these two types.

Clinical features

Dermatitis has both dermal and epidermal components. Some signs are confined to the dermis such as swelling, heat, itchiness, tenderness, and redness, but at the same time the epidermis proliferates and therefore thickens and produces scale. The oedema in the dermis extends to the epidermis, swells the cells, and separates them to give the histological appearance of a sponge, known as spongiosis, and frequently this results in vesicles, which distinguish dermatitis from other proliferative states of the

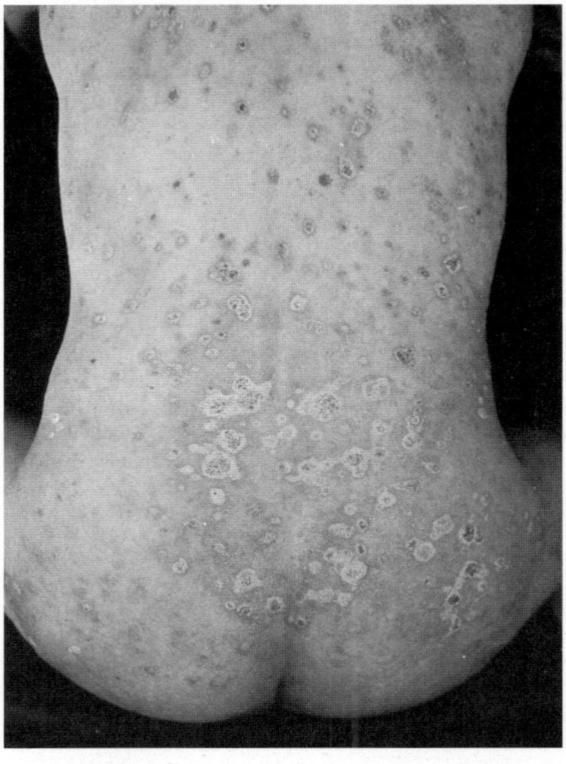

Fig. 28 A later stage of acute drug eruption, in this case due to Myocrisin®. The epidermis is reacting to the dermal inflammation by hyperplasia spreading centrifugally to produce an annular scaly lesion, with the scale exfoliating in the centre of the lesion and attached to the spreading margin.

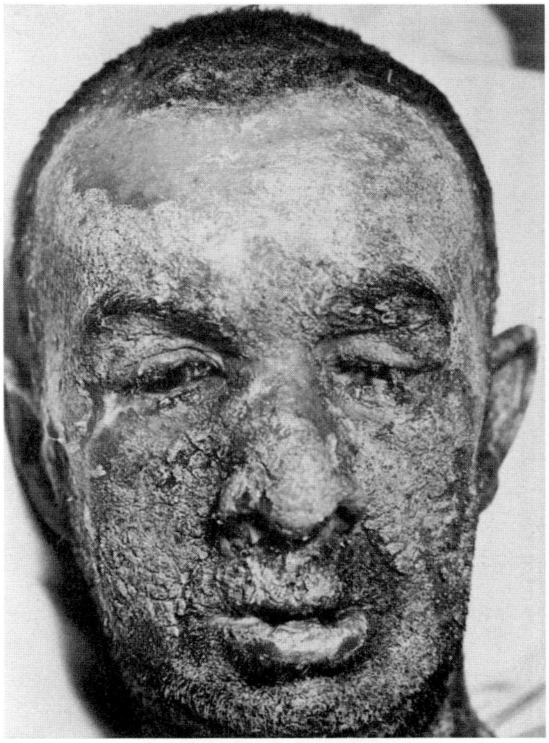

Fig. 29 Severe oedema, crusting, and exfoliation due to dermatitis from arsenicals.

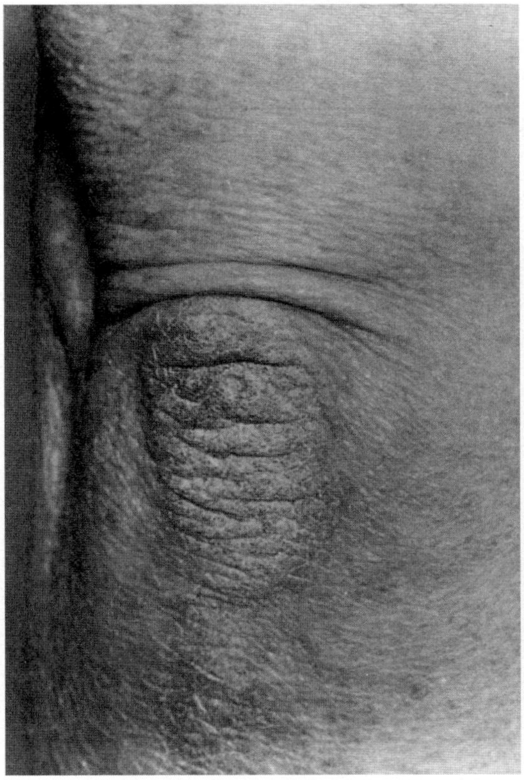

Fig. 30 Hyperkeratosis and slight scaling is a feature of the psoriasiform eruption caused by β-blockers.

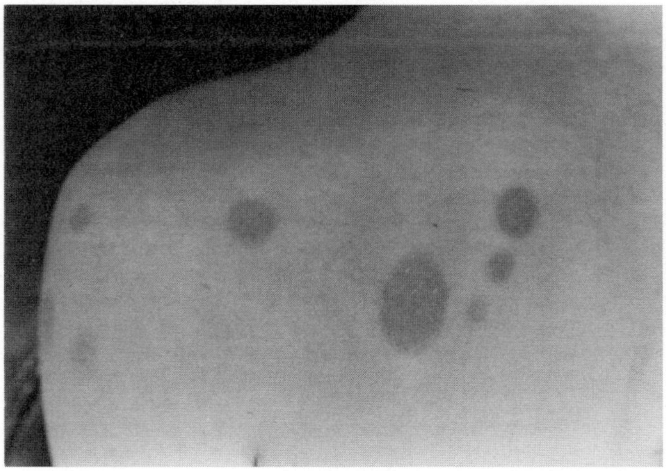

Fig. 31 Fixed drug eruption due to phenolphthalein present in a laxative. Such an eruption characteristically appears within half a day of taking the causative drug and the site affected is the same on every occasion. Violaceous annular lesions are common and may persist for several weeks.

epidermis such as psoriasis. Acute weeping exudation occurs when the vesicles burst (Fig. 32). Itching is usually severe in dermatitis.

The reaction pattern of dermatitis is not homogeneous. It is made up of papular elements of different ages and size, sometimes confluent in the centre (Fig. 33), with widely scattered satellite papules or vesicles. The

Table 10 Drugs causing fixed drug eruptions

Phenazone (synonym: antipyrine), dipyrine
Phenolphthalein
Barbiturates: phenytoin
Sulphonamides
Dapsone, iodides
Quinine and derivatives
Tetracyclines
Oxyphenbutazone, pyrazolones
Chlordiazepoxide

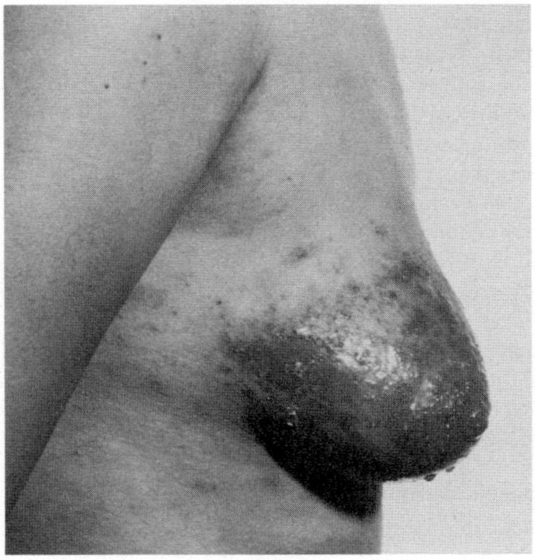

Fig. 32 Acute dermatitis is characterized by an oedematous epidermis in which vesiculation, oozing, and crusting are the principal features. The borders are often ill-defined, while the centre of the lesion is confluent.

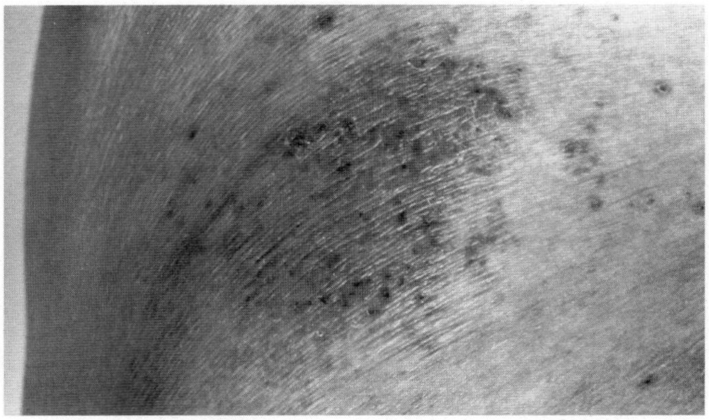

Fig. 33 Dermatitis comprises papules that are confluent in the centre and become vesicular or evidently excoriated. Oedema makes the line markings in the skin more prominent. There are satellite lesions beyond an ill-defined border.

scales are of varied size and broken by excoriation, exudate, and even pinpoint haemorrhages.

A secondary factor prominent in pigmented skin is a loss of melanin, or at least a failure to retain it, in the acute lesion so that the skin is depigmented. In later or more chronic stages the dermis is darkened by pigment 'incontinence', so that thickened chronic epidermal plaques may contain increased pigment in the underlying dermis. Chronically scratched skin has a brownish violaceous colour due to the combination of pigment, vasodilatation, and epidermal thickening.

For unknown reasons, dermatitis of the foot frequently provokes an autosensitization or 'id' response in the hand. Thus, vesicular eczema of the hands often follows a fungus infection of the feet, varicose eczema of the lower legs often spreads to the forearms and face, and a severe allergic contact dermatitis may generalize to the trunk and limbs.

Contact dermatitis

Primary irritant contact dermatitis

An irritant can be defined as a chemical that in most people is capable of producing cell damage if applied for a sufficient time and in a sufficient concentration. Fibreglass spicules rubbed into the skin are a typical example (Fig. 34). Irritant contact dermatitis is caused by exposure to a single or a few contacts with a highly irritating substance such as a concentrated acid, or by chronic low-grade cumulative exposure to substances that are mildly irritating, such as a very dilute acid. A low-grade, cumulative, irritant contact dermatitis can occur after a few months or even several years, depending on the nature of the irritant and the sensitivity of the skin. This is exemplified by housewives' hand dermatitis, which usually recovers slowly or incompletely because of the inability to fully protect the hands against all irritants (Fig. 35). Many people at home or in industry are in daily contact with various chemicals over long periods. They work in wet or extremely dry conditions with skin cleansers, alkalis, acids, cutting fluids, solvents and oxidants, reducing agents, enzymes, and medicaments. The skin is also worn and irritated by cold and heat, sun, pressure, scratching, or friction of various kinds from tools or clothing. Many variables influence the skin's toughness or vulnerability. It can be immature in the newborn or worn out in the aged. The most important cause of lowered resistance is a constitutional disease, such as the ichthyotic skin of old age (Fig. 36), atopic eczema, or psoriasis.

Contact allergic dermatitis

Allergic contact dermatitis is caused by a type IV delayed hypersensitivity reaction to a chemical in contact with the skin. Initial sensitization can occur 7 to 10 days after the first contact with a potent allergen. However, it is more usually a consequence of many months or years of exposure to small amounts of the allergen. Once sensitized, contact with the allergen

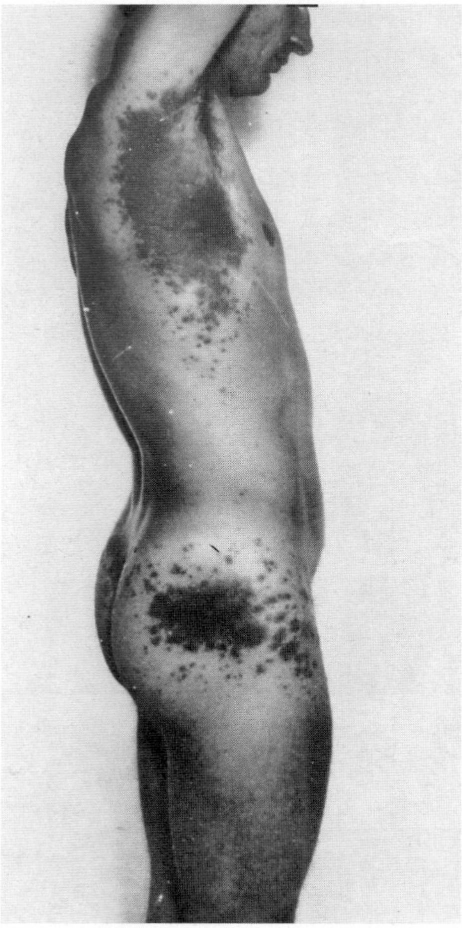

Fig. 34 Primary irritant dermatitis due to small spicules of fibreglass at sites of friction after this patient had insulated a roof.

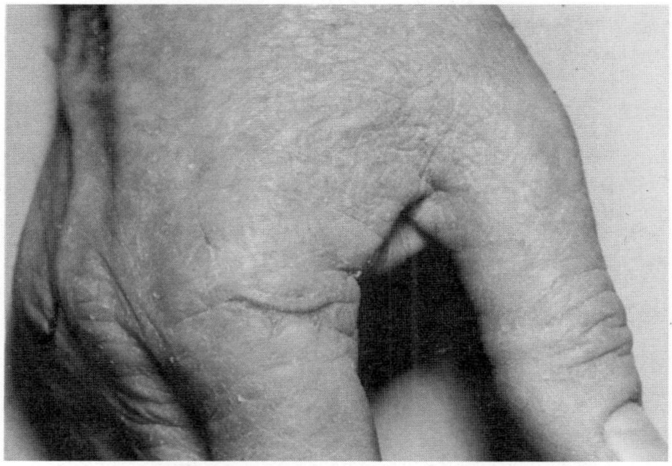

Fig. 35 Chronic dermatitis causes irregular thickening of an inhomogeneous epidermis. The texture of the stratum corneum varies so that it is firmly attached at some points but exfoliates with small scales at others. Loss of moisture causes decreased suppleness, cracking over joints, and exposure of deeper epidermal cells. This causes irritation of the dermis at the bottom of the deep crevasses.

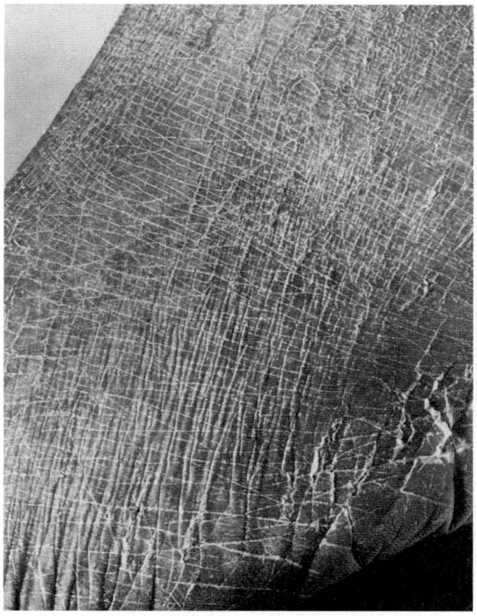

Fig. 36 Chronically thin and slowly turning-over epidermis results in a closely knit stratum corneum which is firmly adherent but cracks excessively. It is characteristic of elderly, malnourished, or ichthyotic skin. Such skin is less resistant to primary irritants.

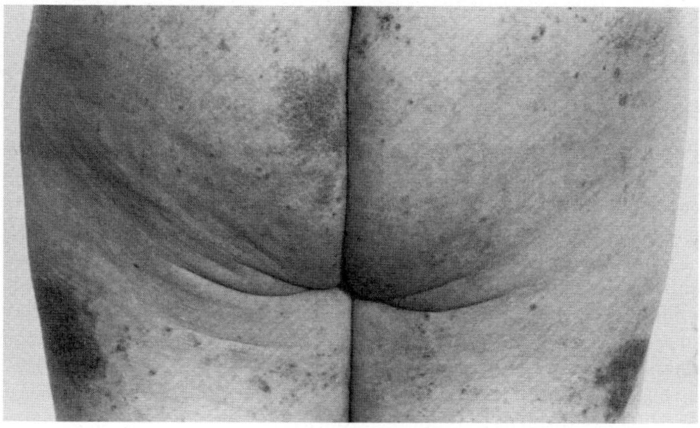

Fig. 37 Contact dermatitis due to garments containing nickel. The diagnosis is made by observing how the distribution of the rash corresponds to the distribution of the contact with the causative agent.

can produce dermatitis within 24 to 48 h and all areas of the body are equally susceptible. Sensitivity can vary due to the amount of exposure, the degree of penetration of the skin, and the tolerance of the immune system.

It is believed that certain allergens, such as nickel and chrome, have a greater affinity for the skin than others. This is partly due to the easier recognition and assimilation by the epidermal antigen-presenting cells known as Langerhans cells. The allergen binds to epidermal microsomal protein, or to some cell-surface marker, or to serum proteins that are plentiful in the epidermis. It is a complex of the allergen with such protein that is recognized as foreign. Although the T lymphocyte ultimately recognizes the complex, the macrophage is a necessary intermediary. Suppression of Langerhans cells by ultraviolet rays diminishes cell-mediated immunity. Genetic factors play a part in the recognition process. Once recognized, T-cell proliferation occurs in the paracortical area of the lymph node, and on re-exposure sensitized lymphocytes release lymphokines. The mechanisms of lymphocyte stimulation include some role for suppressor and effector cells. The role of antibodies, some of which are clearly specific for the same antigen, is also unknown. The inflammatory reaction resulting from recognition is variable and dependent on other pharmacological agents, including secretions from the mast cell, and on prostaglandins. Some of the variation in response, such that persons are consequently labelled as more or less allergic, depends on these secondary factors, and these can be modified by various conditional factors, including anxiety and the hormonal status of the monthly menstrual cycle.

Contact dermatitis sensitizers

In the following, we will concentrate on some specific groups of sensitizers and irritants.

Cosmetics Cosmetics applied to the skin, although more rarely a cause of dermatitis in technically advanced countries where the industry has worked hard to eliminate allergens, are still a source of much disease in developing countries. Perfumes and preparations containing tars, formaldehyde, and Dowicil are increasingly incriminated, and are as commonly irritant as they are allergic.

Vaseline dermatitis in the Bantu is an example. In technically advanced countries, deodorants are a common cause of dermatitis, while in the hair industry, glyceryl monothioglycollate (acid perms) is the most common allergen. Hair bleaches, such as ammonia persulphate, commonly cause immediate, non-immune wealing. When in doubt, because the constituents are so complex, cosmetics should be tested by direct application to the skin, but this can give rise to false-negative results. Hair dyes are now so common that their relative safety can be expected. However, again in developing countries, the dye paraphenylenediamine may produce an acute dermatitis, often first affecting the eyelids and other aspects of the face before showing much evidence of dermatitis on the scalp.

Clothing and textile dermatitis On the whole this is rare, but clips containing metal are quite a common cause of dermatitis (Fig. 37); for example, jeans' buttons can cause dermatitis of the skin below the umbilicus. There is also evidence that the rubber in the elastic of many garments is sometimes the cause of dermatitis. Dyes are usually a problem at sites of friction where there is also moisturization by sweat: the majority of which are azodyes or paraphenylenediamine. In the textile industry, chrome and formaldehyde are important agents causing dermatitis.

Shoe dermatitis is commonly due to chrome or to rubber additives such as mercaptobenzothiazole or butyl phenol formaldehyde. Adhesives and dyes may also be responsible. This form of dermatitis should be considered in every person with eczema of the feet. It often spares the area between the toes as this is the point where the shoe is not in contact with the skin. Much modern footwear has plasticized toecaps and fails to absorb sweat. Increased sweating encourages a shearing strain on the skin, particularly in the athletic child. Frictional dermatitis of the foot is common in such children and is known as juvenile plantar dermatosis.

Foods In technically advanced countries, handling animal feeds containing antibiotics gives more trouble than handling food for human consumption. Elsewhere, plants and fruits such as garlic, cinnamon, onions, and lemons and oranges cause much trouble, as do shellfish and various species of fish that are sometimes contaminated by algae. This is an important hazard for fisherman, which, in the United Kingdom, is known as the 'Dogger Bank' itch.

Plastics An increasingly frequent cause of dermatitis arises from the use of acrylic and epoxy polymers or resins. Acrylics account for dermatitis from adhesive tape, spectacle frames, bonding agents, dentures, hearing aids, bone cement, artificial fingernails, sealants, printing plates, and inks.

Epoxy resins are used as surface coatings for steel pipes and ships, powder paints, electrical insulation adhesives, construction of concrete and steel buildings, and for the surface of roads and bridges. Although they are amongst the most potent sensitizers, they are only active during their initial handling since complete polymerization makes the sensitizing monomer non-available. About 90 per cent of contact dermatitis from epoxy resins is from bisphenol A. Protection in industry depends on common-sense avoidance of handling them and general cleanliness in the workshop, but volatile epoxy resins affecting the face are difficult to avoid.

Rubber Natural as well as synthetic rubbers require the addition of several agents that are strong sensitizers. They make the rubber more malleable and supple, prevent perishing by oxidization, and some speed up the manufacturing processes.

Accelerators include thiuram, mercaptobenzothiazole, and guanides; antioxidants include the monobenzyl ether of hydroquinone. Most cases of rubber sensitivity are due to clothing such as rubber gloves, or to tyres or rubber linings used in the transport industry. Others include the contraceptive sheath, shoes, fingerstalls, masks (particularly motorbike or scuba-diving masks), elastic bands, bicycle or golf-club handles, and rubber sheets or cushions. Anaphylaxis is not rare from a type I sensitivity to rubber latex surgical gloves.

Colophony Rosin is made from pine trees and is used worldwide for paper size adhesives, inks, undersea cables, Elastoplast, violin rosin, and cosmetics. Some medicaments like Zam-Buk®, Secaderm® salve, and ilonium also contain colophony, therefore explaining the contact dermatitis arising from the use of these agents. It is responsible for about 3.5 per cent of positive patch tests in the London contact dermatitis clinics.

Plants and wood Sensitivity to plants and woods accounts for enormous worldwide morbidity and occasional mortality. Some plants release their allergen only when bruised, others when lightly touched, and others by airborne pollen. Some produce a contact non-allergic urticaria (that is, immediate stinging) as with the nettle or cowage (*Mucuna pruritum*); others cause an allergic dermatitis, or even photosensitivity. Many are highly irritant.

In North America the commonest cause is poison ivy, in Europe it is *Primula obconica*. Both produce a severe, streaky blistering eruption from contact allergy mediated by cellular immunity.

Chrysanthemum or ragweed plants, members of the Compositae or daisy family, cause a more diffuse redness and oedema of the face from sesquiterpene lactones. This may look like a photosensitivity and be enhanced by sunlight (see above). Avoidance of the plant may be impossible for someone whose job depends on contact with it, and is a special problem where it is a common environmental weed. In the Poona region of India the weed *Partheneum hysterophorus* can lead to death. Dermatitis resulting from contact with this plant builds up into a severe erythroderma with secondary infection and even pseudolymphoma. In those who are suffering from other diseases it may summate and lead to a very severe illness.

Potentially allergenic plants are most numerous in the cashew family, such as poison ivy, poison oak, poison dogweed, elder or sumac, mango, wax, or lacquer trees, and hence in one form or another they are present worldwide. Attacks can be aborted by washing within an hour of contact. Severe oral dermatitis and acute gastrointestinal systems can be troublesome when sensitivity is due to the mango or cashew nut.

Contamination of other handled agents can also cause outbreaks of dermatitis, as has been recorded with articles of clothing, mail, and even from voodoo dolls.

Wood dermatitis is often due to its resins or its attendant lichens, liverworts, and mosses, and even its insect parasites are occasionally responsible. It is a severe cause of industrial dermatitis in workers in the furniture industry. Furthermore, it can even cause mouth dermatitis in children handling wooden toys, and, in music classrooms, has also been noticed in those playing recorders made of certain woods.

Medicaments

An enormous number of medicaments are now used, often containing unknown constituents. The problem particularly arises where these have been repeatedly applied to the skin over a number of years, and therefore a contact dermatitis is found in patients with leg ulcers, pruritus ani or vulvae, and in those suffering from otitis externa. Local anaesthetics, lanolin and cetylstearyl alcohols, antibiotics and antiseptics, antifungal compounds, and antihistamines are the most significant groups of causative agents. Topical corticosteroids are increasingly recognized as relatively common contact sensitizers (hydrocortisone, hydrocortisone-17-butyrate, budesonide).

An example of the importance of recognizing such sensitivity is illustrated by ethylene diamine; this is a common cause of dermatitis and is present in certain neomycin–nystatin ointment mixtures (for example, Tri-Adcortyl®) and in aminophylline suppositories. It is used as a solvent in many industries and is one cause of coolant-oil dermatitis. This combination of an industrial use and a medicament may mean that a person loses his employment as a result of the previous use of a medicament. Sensitivity to ethylene diamine has serious implications, since it is also sometimes used as a preservative of intravenous aminophylline, and deaths have been recorded.

Metal Beryllium, used in the manufacture of fluorescent lights, causes skin ulcers, dermatitis, and granulomas. Chrome confers hardness to metals, and dermatitis from it is also common in the leather tanning industry. It is a contaminator of cement. In industrial countries it is one of the most common sensitizers in men; most obtain their sensitivity from cement, but their greatest disability is due to the later inconvenience of being unable to wear leather footwear containing chrome. Ferrous sulphate can be used as an additive in cement to convert hexavalent chromium to the less sensitizing trivalent form.

Cobalt sensitivity is commonly found in association with nickel or chrome sensitivity. Jewellery, and possibly metal prostheses for hip replacements, may be responsible.

Nickel is used in various metal alloys, electroplating, enamels, and glass. It is easily absorbed through the skin and its presence in body-piercing rings or studs and in buttons and clips probably accounts for the high incidence of metal dermatitis. Sensitization is particularly common with jewellery made of nickel-containing alloys; gold of 14 carats and above is considered safer. There is a general worldwide trend towards increased nickel sensitivity, which contributes substantially to hand dermatitis. Simply handling nickel-containing money or pots and pans does not seem to be responsible. However, the abrasive cleaning of such in washing-up water releases nickel, and is a reason for blaming this occupation or for recommending the use of running water.

Employment and contact dermatitis It will be seen from the above that many people working in industry are liable to contract specific types of 'contact dermatitis'. Some industries are particularly susceptible.

Hairdressers During their apprenticeship, the hands of hairdressers suffer from the very abnormal wear and tear of frequent shampooing. The skin of atopic subjects almost always break down. Nickel dermatitis is particularly common. When the rash only affects the palmar surfaces, contact dermatitis is more likely than irritant dermatitis. The latter commonly affects the more tender dorsa of the hands and between the fingers.

Bakers Dough, sugars, and fruit and vegetable peels are irritants often causing considerable skin damage in atopic subjects. Many of the flour additives can cause contact urticaria.

Builders Cement is highly irritant but skin quickly hardens. Severe alkaline burns of the lower legs from calcium hydroxide in wet cement is now well recognized, especially in the amateur using ready-mixed cement.

Chrome dermatitis may be very similar to constitutional patterns, including seborrhoeic and stasis eczema, and for this reason anyone in the building industry who has any pattern of eczema should be patch-tested.

Agricultural and horticultural workers Carelessly used fungicides and pesticides are frequent causes of dermatitis. This particularly occurs on isolated farms in developing countries.

Patch-testing

The principle of patch testing is to apply the suspect agent to the patient's skin, but avoiding irritants, and observe its effect on cell-mediated immunity. It involves:

(1) applying the agent on a carrier material such as aluminium foil on filter paper, and covering with adhesive tape;

(2) using a non-irritant concentration of the agent in white soft paraffin in water or ethyl alcohol; for most chemicals this is 0.1 to 1 per cent (in the case of cosmetics or medicaments the concentration used in the whole product is suitable);

(3) applying (1) to the patient's back, which gives a more consistent response than the arms or legs; and

(4) removing the covering adhesive tape and filter paper with aluminium foil 2 h before reading at 2 and 4 days.

Most practitioners obtain reagents from Trolab, Karen Trolle-Lassen, Land, Pharm 6B AN, Hansens Alle, 2900 Hellerup, Denmark, and replace them about every 6 months.

False-positives result from sweat gland occlusion, sensitivity to adhesive tape, irritants, and generally increased irritability of the skin, usually due to active eczema but exposure to ultraviolet irradiation can also be causative.

A positive patch test is a papular and a palpable erythema, which may be vesicular (Fig. 38).

Treatment of contact dermatitis

The level of complaint is often lessened by good industrial relations or a happy home. Those who are well satisfied with life may call their problem merely roughness of the skin; those who are unhappy or dissatisfied may well call their problem dermatitis. Especially in those who have atopic eczema or psoriasis, emotional stress is considered to be a factor worth controlling if possible. Such stresses are often no more than the anxieties and irritations of daily living and employment in a complex society.

Elimination of known irritants or allergens must be attempted but, as in the case of poison ivy in the United States or some of the Compositae in Asia, complete avoidance may be impossible. For less severe allergens, such as chrome or nickel, the skin can settle to a tolerable degree merely by removing obvious sources in clothing or jewellery. Dermatologists can encourage cleanliness and ventilation in working environments and the substitution of less allergenic materials in industrial processes. It is not always advisable to make workers change their jobs; this particularly applies to chrome sensitivity in building industry workers, since once they are sensitized, most other jobs are equally difficult. However, most sufferers can manage by taking a little more care at work and with the help of emollients. Anti-inflammatory agents, such as steroid creams, are always of help and can help the affected person stay at work, particularly where exposure is just short-term (for example, during the training of hairdressers or nurses).

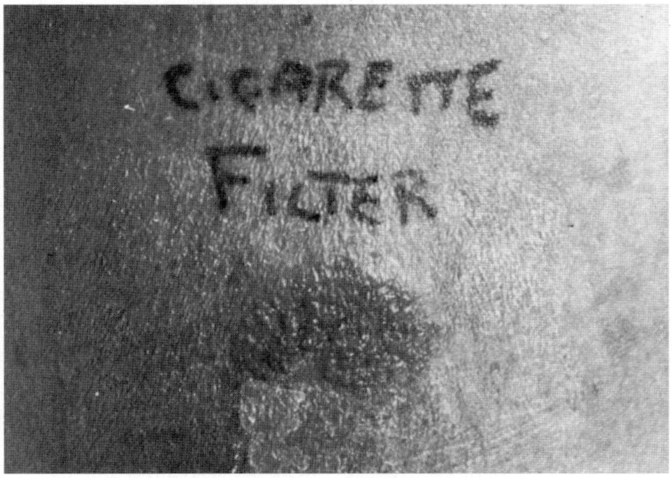

Fig. 38 Contact for about 48 h with the allergen to which the patient is sensitive can be used as a test at any site on the skin. This is the basis of the patch-test reaction. In this case a finger dermatitis due to an allergen in cigarette smoke could be proved by applying a smoked filter paper to the patient's back.

Severe chronic allergy can be relieved by immunosuppressive drugs such as azathioprine. Chelating agents, such as Antabuse®, have been used in cases of severe nickel dermatitis.. Nickel-free diets are complicated but much less unpleasant than drug therapy.

The prognosis for contact dermatitis is often good. Thus 30 per cent of nickel dermatitis of the hands is healed in 6 years. Only 25 per cent of apprentice hairdressers with hand dermatitis have to change their job. Only rarely, as with certain plant allergies, is the problem a persistent and intolerable problem affecting many persons in the community.

Contact urticaria—latex gloves

This is an acute swelling developing within a few minutes to half an hour of contact with certain agents. In atopic eczema there is an particular susceptibility to this phenomenon, but it is also well recognized in non-atopic subjects and is particularly common as a result of the application of cosmetics. Many agents commonly applied to the skin will produce irritation in certain sites, such as the eyelids or scrotum, and this is not always an immunological phenomenon. Urticaria from latex occurs within 15 to 30 min of wearing the glove. It is IgE-mediated. The rash may extend beyond the area of exposure. Doctors and dentists are at particular risk, as are patients frequently exposed to latex gloves such as spina bifida patients who self-catheterize. Patients may crossreact to condoms or medical instruments such as intubation tubes, as well as some fruits and vegetables such as bananas and avocados. Severe sensitivity may induce anaphylaxis and such patients should always carry adrenaline (epinephrine). In extreme cases anaphylaxis can occur to airborne contact with latex particles in procedure rooms, and affected doctors may need to seek an alternative vocation. Diagnosis is by radioallergosorbent testing (**RAST**); prick-testing should only be done where resuscitation equipment is available. Prevention by the use of non-powdered, high-quality rubber gloves or vinyl gloves is prudent, especially when the hands are already damaged.

Atopic eczema

This is a constitutional disorder of the skin affecting about 10 per cent of the population. It is one of the most common diseases of childhood and one of the main reasons for loss of work in industry. It accounts for about 50 per cent of cases of hand eczema. Its inheritance is discussed in Chapter 23.2.

Atopic dermatitis is a multifaceted disease, the cause of which is still unknown. Patients with atopic dermatitis frequently have an elevated IgE level. Allergic respiratory disease affects about 50 per cent of eczema sufferers, and 70 per cent of patients are aware of other family members with the disease. Other associations include dry skin, facial pallor, low finger temperature, pronounced vasoconstriction on exposure to cold, white dermographism, and a susceptibility to cutaneous viral and bacterial infections. Ophthalmological manifestations of atopy include infraorbital folds, infraorbital darkening of the skin, conjunctivitis, keratoconus, and cataract formation. Hyperpigmentation of the lateral neck is known as atopic 'dirty' neck. Drug reactions of the anaphylactic type are more common and abdominal symptoms due to food allergy are frequently described. Contact urticaria is common. Alopecia areata may be more severe and less likely to respond to treatment. Around 60 per cent of patients present within the first year of life, and for 90 per cent the disorder starts within the first 5 years of life. In the majority, the eczema gradually improves but the skin remains vulnerable to physical and chemical irritants throughout life.

Data from the International Study of Asthma in Childhood have shown a global prevalence of 2 to 16 per cent of children aged between 6 and 7 years over a 1-year period.

Pathogenesis

Atopic dermatitis is essentially an exaggerated response to environmental irritants and allergens. The basis of this exaggerated response is immunological, with an altered T-cell response and consequent production of proinflammatory cytokines. In atopic patients, CD4-positive T-helper cells, and in particular class 2 helper cells (T_H2), recognize antigens and secrete IL-4, IL-10, and IL-13, which stimulate B-cell growth and IgE and mast-cell production. In addition, T_H2 cells produce IL-5 which leads to eosinophilia. This may provide atopic patients living in tropical areas with relative protection from parasitic infections. T_H2-derived IL-10 inhibits T_H1 cytokine production, while IL-4 promotes T_H2 differentiation. T_H1 cells produce interferon-gamma (IFN-γ), IL-2, and IL-3. IFN-γ produced by T_H1 cells enhances the development of T_H1 cells and inhibits T_H2 cells. Reduced childhood exposure to infections and intestinal bacteria or parasites, as well as increasing vaccination and immunization, are proposed as causes of T_H1 and T_H2 imbalances favouring atopy.

Epidemiological studies have incriminated a number of allergens that may trigger this immunological response, including pollution, central heating, and house dust mites. Unfortunately, the identification and avoidance of allergens in atopic dermatitis has proven to be more complex than in asthma and hayfever. Skin tests by pricking various antigens into the skin result in weal-and-flare responses that are often multiple and strongly positive. However, there is a poor correlation between the skin-test response and the activity of the eczema, which may even be in remission during, for example, the hayfever season in spite of strong reactivity to skin testing with grasses.

The role of food allergy is difficult to test accurately in such a fluctuating and multifactorial disease. Neither prick tests nor allergen-specific IgE tests can be used to predict those most likely to benefit from dietary elimination. Exclusion diets and food challenges rarely detect meaningful dietary allergens and are therefore reserved for the most severely affected patients. Exclusive breast feeding is of benefit, but is not necessarily due to the avoidance of dietary factors. Breast milk contains much IgA. Complete avoidance of cows' milk during the first 6 months of life in a child born of atopic parents is believed to be beneficial, but nevertheless there are many who fail to benefit.

Humoral immunity

T cells infiltrating the skin in atopic eczema are predominantly IL-4/IL-10/IL-13-producing Thy-2 responses that encourage B cells to produce excessive IgE. IgE reagenic antibody is elevated in over 80 per cent of patients with atopic dermatitis, often to over 2000 units/ml. However, the significance of this finding remains uncertain, since atopic eczema can occur in agammaglobulinaemia and normal levels are found in many actively eczematous patients. Of course, serum levels need not reflect the level of activity of the IgE surrounding the mast cell in the skin itself. Complexes with antigen and the mast cell are often, after all, the basis of the IgE-mediated weal-and-flare response. There is an increased frequency of the presence of specific reaginic IgE antibody also known as the test reagent radioallergoabsorbent test (RAST) to numerous allergens in the sera of atopic people.

Reactivity of the immune system

About 80 per cent of atopic patients demonstrate an excessive reactivity of their immune system, reacting to certain foods and to house dust with immediate itching and swelling of the tissues. The agents to which 90 per cent of atopic patients react differ from those usually encountered in allergic disease—these include a number of animal and vegetable proteins from milk, meat, and corn. Eczema itself is most typically a consequence of delayed or cell-mediated immunity; however, T-cell function seems to be depressed in atopic skin, leading to a greater susceptibility to viral, bacterial, and fungal infections. Herpes simplex, vaccinia, warts, *Staphylococcus aureus*, and *Trichophyton rubrum* infections are most favoured; 90 per cent of atopic subjects carry *Staphylococcus aureus* in their skin, compared to 10 per cent of normal subjects. Fortunately, the atopic subject is not as susceptible to strains responsible for impetigo, toxic epidermal necrolysis, or furunculosis. There is also decreased reactivity to other common allergens such as poison ivy, *Candida* spp., or dinitrochlorbenzene (**DNCB**).

An atopic eczema-like syndrome is also a feature of immune deficiency diseases; for example, the Wiskott–Aldrich syndrome, the hyper-IgE syndrome of Buckley, Jobs, and Jung, and thymic aplasia, as well as the DiGeorge and Nesselof syndromes which also demonstrate high levels of IgE and decreased cell-mediated immunity. It is possible that immaturity of the humoral antibody system results in defective T-lymphocyte regulation, and that IgE production is increased as one consequence.

Characteristics

Atopic patients have an inherently dry and irritable skin. Itch and scratching are responsible for most of the skin changes seen clinically and histologically.

A low itch threshold

A diagnosis should not be made if there is no history of itching. Besides the usual causes of itching, many minor irritants, such as woollen clothing or a change in climate, cause scratching. Scratching causes excoriations and ulceration, as well as thickening of the epidermis and swelling and redness of the underlying dermis. The broken surface is sore and further irritated by soaps, some ointment bases such as sorbic acid, sea-water, or citric fruit juices. It has been found, using intradermal trypsin as a test of itch, that atopic patients have a prolonged itch reaction, although it may be that other patients with other forms of eczema are similarly affected.

Dry and lined skin

In non-excoriated areas the skin is often dry and lined. This is more obvious in hard-water areas in temperate climates. The palms are particularly heavily lined and cause embarrassment even to the fortune teller! About 70 per cent of adult patients have a hand dermatitis that usually spares the palms. In nursing mothers, nipple eczema may be a problem during breast feeding. It seems there is a deficiency in sweating and sebum excretion leading to chapping, wear, and tear, particularly from solvents or water. In industry, people with atopic dermatitis are less tolerant of contact with primary skin irritants and therefore more likely to develop occupational dermatitis. Another feature of atopic dryness is keratosis pilaris, which is a perifollicular hyperkeratosis.

Vasodilatation

The vasculature too readily vasodilates in the popliteal and cubital fossas, thereby heating the skin and hence inappropriately lowering the itch threshold. When scratched, rubbed, or stretched, the skin blanches for a few minutes, beginning 12 to 15 s after injury. This is partly due to upper dermal precapillary shutdown and also to persistent inflammatory oedema. Deeper vessels often dilate so that the skin is warm. This combination of hot but pale skin accounts for the itching as well as the atopic pallor.

Clinical features

Itching is the chief feature and becomes apparent during the first 2 to 6 months of life. The face is usually first affected and scratching begins between the second and third month. Sore lips from licking and chapping as well as conjunctivitis with ectropion are common; 70 per cent of patients have a skin fold or wrinkle just beneath the margin of the lower lid of both eyes (Fig. 39). When the child begins to crawl, exposed surfaces such as the knees and hands become the most involved. The papules are scratched and become exudative and so secondary infection associated with lymphadenopathy is a common finding. Lymphadenopathy can sometimes be so gross as to lead to the suspicion of some dire malignant disease. From 18 months onwards the sites most characteristically involved are the flexures of the elbows, knees, sides of neck, wrists, and ankles (Fig. 40). Local areas of lichenified skin may persist at such sites, and the face, too, may be heavily lichenified. Rubbing the eyes does not fully explain why keratoconus and anterior subcapsular cataracts are featured in severe cases. Seasonal influences on the disease are mainly climatic, due to sunlight and humidity and

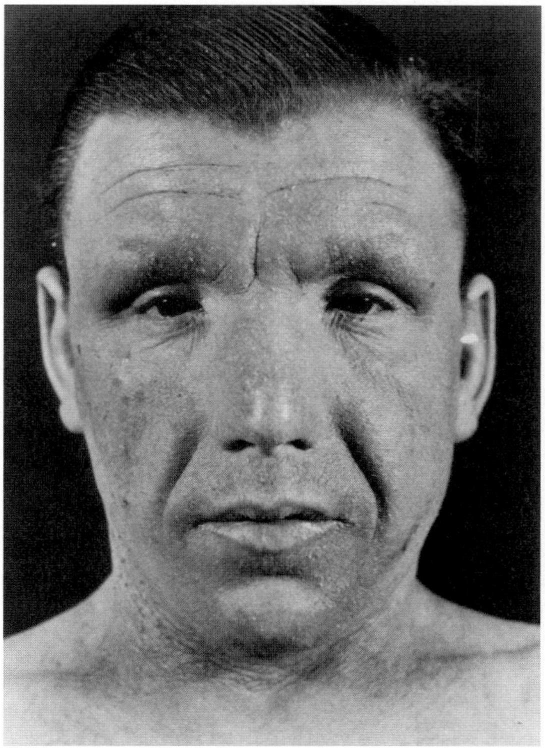

Fig. 39 Atopic eczema in an adult, showing the characteristic skin fold just beneath the lower eyelid and the loss of eyebrow hair, as well as thickening of the skin due to rubbing.

the use of central heating, but are probably also related to seasonal allergies. Pollen is a feature of spring and early summer, while house dust seems to be a feature of late summer allergies.

Prognosis

Most children develop their eczema within the first 6 months of life, but about one-fifth of patients may have a delayed onset, even into adult life. Generally, there is a tendency for gradual improvement, with many children 'growing out' of their atopic dermatitis around the age of 3 to 4 years. Complete clearance without breakdown when in contact with skin irritants is unusual, but most people, in the absence of major irritants, are clear by the time they are teenagers.

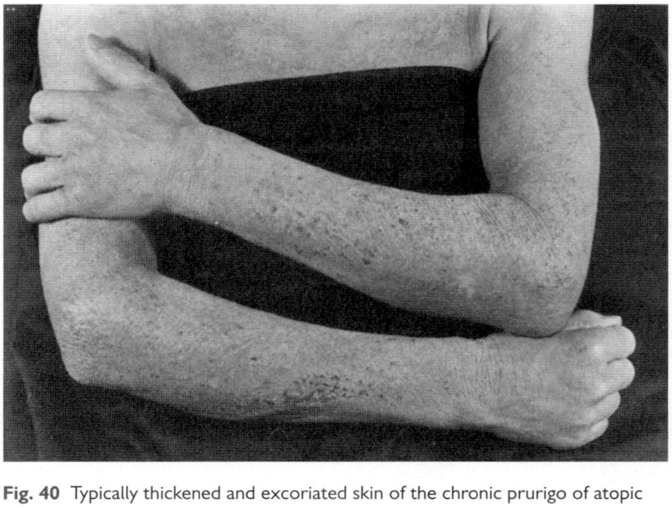

Fig. 40 Typically thickened and excoriated skin of the chronic prurigo of atopic eczema.

Management

In the absence of any treatment that permanently modulates the immune response, the main focus of treatment is to reduce exposure to environmental irritants and to prevent overheating. It is useful for parents to have access both to the doctor and nurse as well as to the literature provided by patient groups. All factors that irritate the skin should be even more avoided by atopic patients, and these include various primary irritants such as soap, wool, and extremes of climate. Moisturization of the skin is good, but evaporation is bad. Wet wrapping is the application of wet dressings over moisturizing creams, which are then covered by dry dressings. Liberal washing with soap substitutes based on emulsifying ointments is mostly helpful, and these are most effective if applied at least four times a day. The common-sense avoidance of jobs involving large amounts of primary irritants should be advised. Attempts should be made to avoid contact with herpes simplex, molluscum contagiosum, and other viruses affecting the skin; however, vaccination poses no particular problems for children with atopic dermatitis and should not be withheld, unless the child is being treated with systemic immunosuppressants. It is still difficult to know how to remedy an immunological defect. While breast feeding is to be recommended for all infants, it may be particularly important for babies with a strong family history of eczema. There is evidence that breast feeding may reduce the incidence of atopic eczema by up to two-thirds, though not all authors agree. It is postulated that a period of transient immune vulnerability exists during early life, during which exposure to food antigens, perhaps by complexing with IgG, IgM, and IgE instead of IgA, results in allergic sensitization and the subsequent development of atopic eczema. The effect of breast feeding may be due to its low antigen load compared to cows' milk. Breast milk is also rich in IgA, which may modify the absorption of food antigens. Breast feeding should continue for an extra 3 to 4 months, since any supplement exposes the immature gut to foreign protein. Especially to be avoided is any supplement given in hospital during the first week of life. Further benefit might be gained by avoiding eggs and cows' milk in the mother's diet, since foreign protein can be transmitted through the mother's milk. When breast feeding is impossible, milk substitutes are second-best since they are expensive and require care to prevent bacterial contamination. Some paediatricians believe cows' milk should be avoided for 1 year and eggs for 18 months.

Some patients appear to benefit from a regime of antigen avoidance, although this is not always the case. Neither RAST tests nor skin-patch tests are reliable in selecting patients who are helped by dietary modification, since even those known to benefit from antigen avoidance may not show specifically raised IgE levels nor positive skin tests.

Elimination diets must be carefully assessed to obtain complete avoidance with, at the same time, adequate nutrition, and since they are not without risk in this respect they should be reserved for the most severely affected children. Some authors recommend the avoidance of eggs, chicken, milk, and artificial colouring agents or preservatives. Goat's milk has lost favour on nutritional grounds. Careful studies of the use of Chinese herbal teas have shown an improvement in generalized dry eczema in children, but users should be aware of the potential hepatotoxicity of these drinks.

Other environmental allergens shown to be important for some children include the house-dust mite. Avoidance includes removing dust-collecting fabrics such as carpets, curtains, bedclothing, and soft-furnishings, and using high-powered vacuum cleaning rather than brushing. A cold and dry environment discourages the mite. Polished floorboards, hydronic rather than ducted heating, blinds rather than curtains, plastic mattress and pillow covers, washable cotton blankets rather than duvets are all appropriate (albeit often expensive) measures in severe cases regardless of whether a house-dust mite allergy is established. Cats and dogs should always be kept off the bed, and avoided all together if contact with them worsens the dermatitis.

Topical therapy

Apart from the liberal use of emollients, steroid creams are effective antipruritic agents. Ointment bases are preferred for dry dermatitis, while creams are used in flexures and for weeping infected or acute dermatitis. Prescribing habits have changed over the past few years. Certainly there was a period when overprescription resulted in systemic side-effects as well as local atrophy of the skin; however, underusage, often encouraged by the dispensing pharmacist, is now far more prevalent. Withholding of steroids deprives the child of the one effective therapy. Short, sharp bursts of effective therapy with strong steroids may be entirely justified, but prolonged daily usage of weaker, partially effective steroids is bound to lead to complications. However, special care is required on the face and flexures. Topical steroids are stored in the skin, and for this reason once-daily application may be sufficient. It seems an inexplicable fact of life that ringing the changes with ointments is of benefit, and a skilled practitioner will always have an alternative preparation on which the worried parents can pin their faith. Secondary infection is so common and bacterial allergy so important that vigorous treatment of infection is justified, and topical antiseptics and systemic antibiotics should be given according to the sensitivities of the bacteria. Erythromycin is particularly valuable; mupirocin, topically, is as effective. The matter of climatic therapy remains unpredictable; undoubtedly a change of climate does effect great improvements in some children, whether it be exposure to sunlight or to the sea or to a mountain top.

Ascomycin macrolactam derivatives formulated as a topical cream inhibit the release of inflammatory cytokines from T cells and show great promise as a topical therapy.

Severe cases of eczema, as with asthma, may have to be controlled by systemic steroids, either in the form of prednisolone or corticosteroid injections. This may be simply to help the patient over an acute period, although a small minority of patients may require long-term therapy for several years. Azathioprine is an effective steroid-sparing agent. Ciclosporin controls severe eczema but provides little long-term benefit. Periodic hospital admission with intensive topical therapy can provide months of respite. Ultraviolet light in air-conditioned cabinets is helpful for many people. An initial worsening often requires cover with prednisolone. Traditional herbal remedies are popular and controlled studies have shown some benefits from Chinese medicinal plants, but it should not be assumed that because they are 'natural' they are safe. Significant hepatic toxicity has been documented and a carcinogenic potential of some of these agents is suspected.

Other patterns of dermatitis

Infected dermatitis

Increasing evidence suggests that bacterial allergy plays a part in the development of an eczematous response in the skin, *Staphylococcus* spp. being particularly implicated. Bacterial allergy may play a part in all types of eczema, but occasionally it is the single cause. This is most frequently seen as a rather well-demarcated patch of eczema with crusting and scaling on an exposed area. There may be small pustules on an advancing edge. It is seen around discharging wounds, around ulcers, and occasionally around a paronychia or in a flexure, subject to sweating and maceration; it is particularly common around the ear or at sites of occlusion such as under a hatband or between the toes. An underlying pediculosis may be one trigger. Black skin commonly seems to develop a similar condition that principally affects the shins. Management includes the use of local antiseptics and wet soaks, or dyes, such as gentian violet, combined with an appropriate systemic antibiotic.

Herpes simplex infection often presents with a sudden inexplicable flare of atopic dermatitis, often monthly, but this may be difficult to prove as vesicles are rapidly excoriated. Swabs for immunoperoxidase staining or viral culture may need to be frequently repeated. A trial of prophylactic oral antiviral therapy can be considered in cases with a suggestive history.

Seborrhoeic dermatitis

Adult seborrhoeic dermatitis is different to the infantile disorder bearing the same name. It mainly affects the scalp and face, but can also involve the upper trunk and flexures including the axillas, groins, scrotum, and anus. The aetiology is unknown but the distribution does appear to be in the areas of sebaceous activity. There is a strong association with neuroleptic-induced parkinsonism, idiopathic parkinsonism, spinal injury, as well as with AIDS. *Pityrosporum orbicularis* may be the responsible pathogen. The oval blastosphere is predominant in AIDS, whereas the hyphal form is increased in pityriasis versicolor. The most characteristic lesion is a dull or yellowish-red and greasy plaque with a marginated scale. On the scalp it produces dandruff. On the face it tends to involve the medial cheeks, nose, nasolabial folds, and eyebrows. It is the most common cause of a 'butterfly rash'. Seborrhoeic dermatitis affects the axillas and groins with well-defined brownish-red scaly areas deep into the folds, on the front of the chest and in the middle of the back there may be small brown follicular papules covered by greasy scales or multiple discrete patches. Rarely, a widespread eruption resembles pityriasis rosea with oval lesions with peripheral scale. Severe cases of seborrhoeic dermatitis develop marked crusting and scaling, particularly of hair-bearing areas and the genitalia. Otitis externa is one manifestation. The disorder tends to recur and may be chronic.

Management includes an attack on local infection and the removal of crusts with wet soaks. Preparations, such as vioform hydrocortisone, sulphur, and ichthammol in a variety of water-miscible bases, usually in 1 to 2 per cent concentrations, have traditionally been prescribed. Lithium succinate ointment is recently favoured. Imidazoles control pityrosporum overproduction, which is thought to play some part in the diathesis. Anti-yeast shampoos with zinc pyrithione or ketaconazole are effective, as are tar shampoos.

Nummular (discoid) eczema

The main feature of this eczema is that it is discoid or composed of rounded lesions scattered, often symmetrically, over the body. They are intensely vesicular and intensely itchy. Undoubtedly endogenous, external influences play little part in their development, although occasionally sensitivity to metals, such as nickel or chrome, may produce a similar picture. Onset is usually in adult life, although Asian children seem prone to this form of dermatitis. Patients are no more likely to be atopic, but dry skin and overheating are important aggravating factors. Secondary infection is common; sometimes nummular eczema is as a reaction pattern to a localized primary irritant such as an insect bite.

Pityriasis alba

This is a pattern of eczema quite common in children, often in those with darker skins, in which a very low-grade dry eczema with shedding of pigment transiently gives rise to a white patch of skin (see Fig. 64). It may be associated with drying out—reduced sebum—around the hair follicles, known as keratosis pilaris.

Itch without rash (pruritus)—mechanisms and causation

'Pruritus' is the term used when itching (the most prominent symptom in skin disease) is the primary complaint, which leads to scratching in the absence of visible evidence of lesions predisposing to itch. Itch is a sensation largely dependent on superficial nerve endings—unmyelinated C fibres—in an intact upper dermis and epidermis. These are very thin fibres, but rich in terminal branching. Thinly myelinated nerves in lateral spinothalamic tracts and secondary neurones to the thalamus relay both pain and itch, and the cerebral cortex can modify these responses. Itch is induced by a number of agents including histamine and histamine releasers such as substance P, opioid peptides, cytokines, bradykinin, bile salts, and proteases, and is potentiated by prostaglandin E. It can be disassociated from pain in hypoalgesia. Central neurological and emotional psychiatric factors control the threshold to itch and pain. Awareness is a complex attribute modifying or intensifying the response to the itch. The itch itself may cause irritability, depression, or invoke the attitude of the masochist who wears a 'hair shirt'.

Itching is usually worse when the skin is heated to normal body temperature and when there is little else to distract the sufferer—a combination common at night. Vasodilatation in the cubital or popliteal fossas partially accounts for the lower itch threshold at such sites in people with atopic dermatitis.

The itching threshold is lowered by isolation, including the common accompaniments of ageing such as blindness, deafness, and loneliness. Endogenous depression is often missed in the elderly and should be treated. Paroxysmal itching may originate in the central nervous system and provoke deep scratching, which is pleasurable but injurious. It is a feature of cocaine addiction.

The itch of different dermatoses evokes different types of scratching. Urticaria is almost never scratched but usually rubbed or pinched, perhaps because the exact site of the itch is difficult to pinpoint. Similarly, excoriations are rare in lichen planus (see 'Localized pruritis', below). Where intense itching is exactly located it is often persistent and deeply excoriated.

A common factor is dryness and desiccation of the stratum corneum, common in the elderly and worse in winter. Sweat retention also causes intense pruritus such as prickly heat. People recently engaged in insulating their roof with fibreglass suffer from pruritus caused by the almost invisible spicules of fibreglass (see above and Fig. 34).

Pruritic conditions

Parasitic causes of itching (scabies) (see Chapter 8.2)

Parasites are an important cause of pruritus, but those experienced at examining the skin will usually observe primary urticarial or papular lesions in amongst the scratches. Onchocerciasis, trichinellosis, and schistosomiasis cause severe pruritus, usually with marked eosinophilia as well as urticaria, prurigo, and depigmentation. In onchocerciasis, loss of elasticity and the development of a leather-like skin hanging in folds is one consequence.

Delusions of parasitosis are common, affected people usually present to pest exterminators and museum entomologists rather than to doctors. This condition is a monosymptomatic delusional disorder, and patients often function well in other aspects of their life. Follie aux deux is common, and the entire family may be drawn into the delusional framework. Referral to a psychiatrist is often resisted. It is best treated with antipsychotic drugs such as pimozide.

Aquagenic pruritus

This occurs after contact with water—fresh, salt, or sweat. In some people it starts from the moment of contact and lasts 15 min. In others, it is less immediate and longer lasting. Treatment with acetylcholine or histamine antagonists or ultraviolet rays sometimes help. A common similar reaction in the elderly, due to rapid drying out after prolonged hydration, is helped by shortening the period of hydration. It is a premonitory sign of myeloproliferative disease.

Generalized pruritus and systemic disease

Hepatic disease

Obstructive jaundice causes severe pruritus. It is particularly an early feature of biliary cirrhosis, and bile salts rather than bilirubin have been held responsible for the itch. The degree of jaundice need not be great. Bile salts in the skin can achieve a relatively higher concentration than may be indicated by serum levels. A bile-salt concentration of 1 mmol/l causes itching when applied to a blister base; dihydroxy salts, especially chenodeoxycholate, are responsible.

Contemporary studies look to opioid metabolism as a cause of the pruritus, and these early studies on bile salts are only part of the story. Oestrogen-induced pruritus of pregnancy or from the contraceptive pill often shows little or no jaundice in spite of intrahepatic biliary obstruction, severe pruritus, and a much increased alkaline phosphatase level. Chlorpromazine and testosterone can have the same effect.

Blood disease

Iron deficiency has also been blamed for itching even when the patient is not anaemic—though in iron deficiency, which is common, itch is rarely found to be so associated. Some thinning of hair is a frequent complaint. Polycythaemia is frequently associated with itching, particularly after a hot bath. It is believed to be related to blood histamine levels and occasionally to iron deficiency, and hence the reported positive response to iron therapy within 2 to 10 days. Lymphatic leukaemia is another cause of pruritus often long-lasting before it becomes clinically overt.

Carcinoma of the internal organs and lymphoma

Carcinoma of the bronchus in particular may very rarely present with generalized pruritus. Pruritus occurs in 25 per cent of patients with Hodgkin's disease, often burning in quality and associated with icthyosis.

Chronic renal failure

No matter how uraemic is the patient, itching is not a feature of acute renal failure or even of malignant hypertension. Patients with chronic pyelonephritis or chronic glomerulonephritis usually suffer greatly from pruritus, which is not necessarily relieved by haemodialysis. Parathyroidectomy, for reasons that remain obscure, may relieve itching in those in whom removal of the gland is necessitated by secondary hyperparathyroidism. The cause of pruritus in renal failure is unknown, but raised histamine levels, endogenous opioids, and dryness of the skin are factors. Mast cell numbers are also increased in patients with chronic renal failure.

Endocrine disease

Pruritus is sometimes a presenting symptom of diabetes mellitus but generally this is principally localized to the vulva. About 1 in 10 patients with hyperthyroidism complain of itching. Dry skin in hypothyroidism often itches.

Drugs

Morphine, allopurinol, or those causing cholestasis should be enquired about.

Management of pruritus

Overheating should be avoided as should vasodilators such as alcohol and hot drinks. Calamine lotion is used as a cooling agent: all topical therapy is more cooling if kept in a refrigerator. Evaporation is increased by the enhanced surface area provided by the powder. Dryness of the skin should be discouraged by the use of emollients. Oily calamine or 0.5 per cent menthol in aqueous cream are preferred when xerosis coexists with itch. In dry conditions, such as the hospital ward, a moist microenvironment can be enhanced by appropriate clothing. A sensation of cooling can be achieved with 1 per cent menthol or camphor and 1 per cent phenol, both of which have a mild anaesthetic effect. Menthol is also an antihistamine. Nails should be kept short and together with occlusive bandaging may reduce the vicious circle of itch and skin damage. In general, woollen clothing is itchy, cotton clothing is not. Too frequent bathing or showering should be discouraged unless emulsifying ointments are added to the bath as soap substitutes. Bath salts should be avoided. Proprietary bath oils are more cosmetically acceptable but tend to be expensive for regular daily use.

Obviously, any known cause of the pruritis should be treated accordingly. Class I antihistamines, which pass the blood–brain barrier, may principally act through their sedative and anticholinergic effects, and they also reduce awareness. Class II antihistamines, which do not pass the blood–brain barrier, cause no sedation; but as histamine is one of the most prominent mediators of itch, they should always be tried and are often most effective in higher dose than indicated in the National Formulary. The role of increased histamine release and its mediation of itch in senile pruritus justifies the prescription of a class II antihistamine. Chlorpromazine may reduce the reactivity to the itch. Plasma exchange has been used to control sweats and pruritus. The anion-exchange resin cholestyramine, 6 to 8 g daily, or oral activated charcoal helps to relieve the pruritus of liver disease and sometimes its use in patients with chronic renal disease or polycythaemia has been helpful. Suberythema doses of UVB irradiation twice weekly, and even natural sunlight, often ameliorate pruritus, reducing mast cells and some of the cytokine activity inducing inflammation; they have also been used to treat the itching associated with uraemia and with certain acute exanthems such as pityriasis rosea. Use of hydroxyethyl rutosides (Paroven®) and thalidomide have been advocated in the treatment of patients in renal failure. Pentoxifylline (oxpentifylline) is reported to relieve the pain and itch of keloids. Opioid activity can be blocked by opioid antagonists or competitors such as codeine; these have been advocated for the treatment of pruritus of liver disease. The H_2-receptor antagonist cimetidine is sometimes helpful in Hodgkin's disease.

Localized pruritus

Localized intensely itchy areas of skin having no obvious causation are a common problem in the dermatology clinic. The nape of the neck, upper back (Fig. 41), genitalia, lower leg, elbow, and outer thigh are easily accessible sites liable to persistent rubbing and scratching. Such injury to the skin results in thickening, purple-brown violaceous coloration due to dilated vessels and postinflammatory pigmentation. The normal line marks of the skin are exaggerated and excoriations are usually numerous. This is termed 'lichen simplex' or 'neurodermatitis', and the fairly well-defined patches cause paroxysms of itching and emotional upsets with anxiety or irritability, which, in themselves, are also promoting factors. Capsaicin ointment, which reduces substance P in the skin, may relieve localized pruritus after several applications. The burning initially induced by this therapy can be reduced by the prior application of local anaesthetic creams (for example, Emla (lidocaine (lignocaine) and prilocaine cream)).

Nodular prurigo is an unexplained reaction to scratching, evoking severe, very localized pruritus. The nodules are 1 to 2 cm in diameter and scattered over accessible areas. It is sometimes a consequence of a partially resolved, more generalized pruritus arising from atopic eczema or parasitic infestation. Freezing with liquid nitrogen is helpful, but this may lead to depigmentation in pigmented races.

Local steroids are helpful and anything that protects the skin from scratching may eventually allow healing. Occlusive tape or bandaging is occasionally helpful but secondary infection is a problem, especially in hot countries.

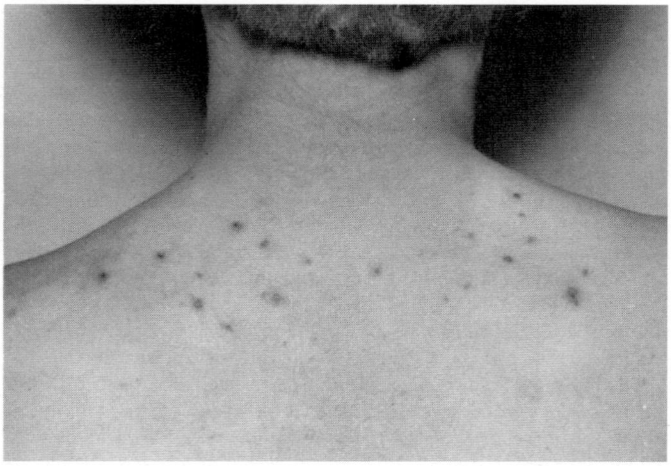

Fig. 41 Prurigo nodularis is a form of scratched lesion which is very exactly localized. The upper back is a common site for such persistent excoriation.

Intralesional injection with triamcinolone causes rapid resolution in some cases but this may be only a temporary response, and where the lesions are large or multiple such inoculation is not without the side-effects of steroid therapy. It is always worth admitting such patients to hospital and treating them with traditional dermatological therapies such as tar bandages. A more recent suggestion is that some of these lesions are an immunological response and this has led to therapies as far ranging as azathioprine and thalidomide.

Pruritus ani

Pruritus ani is common in White adult males. It is rare in Blacks except as a manifestation of infestations such as oxyuris, lice, and scabies. Psoriasis, atopic dermatitis, seborrhoeic dermatitis, tinea cruris, candidiasis, and streptococcal infection can all be found in the anal region, albeit rarely, and should be excluded. Extramammary Paget's disease is a rare cause of itch. People with diabetes are prone to pruritis ani for reasons not entirely clear. An important cause is soiling of the perianal skin. Haemorrhoids, fissures, and fistulas contribute to this problem, as can rectal carcinoma. The anal sphincter relaxes in response to anal distension too readily in some sufferers; in others, incomplete bowel evacuation leaves some residual faeces in the folds of the anus. Because soft stools are more likely to cause irritation, fibre intake needs to be carefully balanced to keep the stool firm while at the same time preventing constipation. Pruritis ani is commonly exacerbated by hot, spicy foods: curry and coffee should be limited. Bacterial and fungal contamination is common, and anxiety may lead to excessive hygiene measures that irritate the skin or result in supervening lichen simplex. Both allergic and irritant contact dermatitis may result from the common use of multiple medication.

Often, the perianal skin needs to be cleaned immediately and an hour or two after the bowels have been opened. Weak- or medium-strength local steroids are the mainstay of treatment, and can be mixed with anticandida or antiseptic agents to deal with or prevent secondary contamination and infection.

Pruritus vulvae and vulvodynia

The vulva has a generous innervation and is highly sensitive. Itch or pain or both are common when the skin is irritated or inflamed. It is socially unacceptable to scratch one's vulva in public and these symptoms are often associated with guilt, a sense of being unclean, dyspareunia, and marital disharmony. Furthermore, sexuality is central to a woman's psyche and primary psychological problems or guilt over an extramarital affair may somatize with a vulval or vaginal complaint. When marital problems exist, a vulval problem may be the justification to reject sexual advances, and sympathy from the doctor rather than a cure may occasionally be sought.

The vulva is a favoured site for candidiasis, tinea cruris, atopic dermatitis, psoriasis, seborrhoeic dermatitis, lichen sclerosis, and lichen planus. In addition, physiological vaginal discharge or semen may irritate inflamed skin. This is much more common when the discharge is altered in nature or amount by an infection such as candidiasis, trichomoniasis, or another sexually transmitted disease. Pruritus ani and vulvae are rare in regions where malnutrition is common, except as a manifestation of an orogenital syndrome due to vitamin B deficiency: the pruritus is then associated with dermatitis and angular cheilitis. Threadworm infection is common in children, while urinary tract infections are common in adults and children and are associated with urethral stinging and burning and will also aggravate a pre-existing complaint of vulval itch or pain. Sexual intercourse, in particular unaroused sexual intercourse, produces local mechanical trauma that rarely initiates dermatitis but invariably aggravates it. Anticipation that vaginal intercourse will be painful leads to further complications such as vaginismus that may continue for many years after the precipitating event has resolved.

Sufferers use a large number of agents to relieve their pruritus, some of which cause contact dermatitis. Pruritus vulvae may also be caused by sensitivity to the rubber of condoms or spermicidal jelly, or even to deodorants. Local anaesthetics and local steroids are much used; however, the latter encourage secondary infections, with fungus usually spreading on to the buttocks and down the thighs. Potent fluorinated steroids may lead to a rosacea-like pustular perioral facial dermatitis.

Management includes a thorough examination to exclude the above and to recognize skin diseases such as psoriasis, seborrhoeic dermatitis, lichen sclerosis, atopic dermatitis, and lichen planus. Vaginal swabs should routinely be taken to look for candidiasis and trichomonas infection, and other sexually transmitted diseases when indicated. Skin swabs and scrapings for the detection of secondary fungal, bacterial, and viral (herpes simplex) infection are useful. A full history of topical medicaments and other preparations should be elicited, and patch-testing performed if required. Detailed instructions regarding local hygiene should be given to patients, including advice on the need to avoid excessive ritual washing, particularly with soap. Counselling regarding sexual intercourse may be needed.

Pruritis vulvae usually responds well to potent topical steroids. The risk of atrophy is small if the itch is confined to the vulva. Secondary infection may be prevented by the concomitant use of a topical antiyeast preparation such as nystatin or antiseptic such as Vioform (clioquinol), which tend to be non-irritating. Maintenance treatment with a weak topical steroid may be required.

Recurrent vaginal candidiasis may be recalcitrant to therapy. It relates to oestrogen levels and is not seen before the menarche or after the menopause, except in women receiving hormone replacement therapy. Long-term oral antifungal agents may be required, particularly when topical preparations irritate the skin. Occasionally, menstruation and endogenous oestrogen production may need to be interrupted by depot medroxyprogesterone acetate (Provera).

Atrophic vaginitis should be sought and treated in postmenopausal women presenting with dyspareunia. Primary vulvodynia has been described with vulval vestibulitis, vulval pain syndrome, and pudenal neuralgia. These are complex and controversial entities for which there is no satisfactory treatment. Tricyclic or one of the newer antidepressants in full dosage may help either in altering sensory perceptions or treating an underlying depression. Compliance is often difficult.

Psoriasis

In temperate zones, psoriasis affects between 1.5 and 3 per cent of the Caucasian population. It is less common in sunny climates and among certain ethnic groups, such as Asians, native Americans, and Samoans. Around 30 per cent of patients have a positive family history and there is 75 per cent concordance among monozygotic twins, compared with 20 per cent concordance with dizygotic twins. It is a polygenic trait with two patterns of inheritance. Type 1, with a strong family history and early onset, shows linkage disequilibrium for human leucocyte antigens CW_6, B_{13}, and BW_{57}. It affects 30 per cent of patients and is possibly an IL-Ira gene defect. Type 2 occurs as a late-onset disorder and is linked with CW_2, B_{27}, and CW_6.

Known triggers for expression in genetically susceptible people include trauma, stress, infection, pregnancy, hypocalcaemia and dialysis, HIV infection, alcohol, and certain drugs such as lithium, β-blockers, antimalarials, NSAIDs, and steroid withdrawal. Paradoxically, sunlight may worsen psoriasis in some individuals.

Pathogenesis

The pathogenesis of psoriasis includes a tenfold increase in the speed of epidermal-cell proliferation. Since the cells pass upwards through the epidermis at a faster rate and do not seem to have time to produce a horny layer, they remain nucleated even when exfoliated. Numerous problems beset the measurement of the cell-cycle time in human epidermis. For example, there are the technical difficulties of counting and the exact recognition of different stages of the cell cycle and differentiation. Do all cells in the germinal layer have the potential to divide or is the potential greater in psoriasis? Is the actual cell cycle faster in psoriasis? The answer is probably that it is and that more cells enter the cycle per unit time in psoriasis. Moreover, cell-cycle inhibitory factors may be reduced and stimulatory factors increased. The kinetics of keratinocyte turnover are clearly essential to our understanding of psoriasis. Probably there is no single cause, but neutrophils, which are attracted in large numbers into the epidermis, may play a part. Streptococcal antigens crossreact with skin antigens, thereby stimulating an autoimmune response. The role of the lymphocyte has long received consideration and has been encouraged by the observations of exacerbations of psoriasis in patients with AIDS, its control by ciclosporin, and the possible immunosuppressive effects of other effective therapies, such as corticosteroids or PUVA. Psoriasis in those with AIDS is most pronounced at intermediate levels of immunodeficiency, and is diminished or lost in terminal profound immunodeficiency states. At the biochemical level, almost every aspect of cell kinetics is a candidate, including the availability of cyclic AMP, increased cyclic GMP, fatty acid deficiency, eicosanoids, phosphorylating mechanisms, polyamines, putrescine, spermidine, and calcium-modulating enzymes such as calmodulin and vitamin D analogues. How cells stick together and how adhesion is modulated during migration and mitosis introduces many other concepts, ranging through the role of interleukins (IL-1, -2, -6, -8), interferons (IFN-γ), transforming growth factors-α and -β, to the interaction with proteases, since in psoriasis the proteinase–antiproteinase balance seems to be disturbed. Psoriasis is not merely a disorder of the keratinocyte. Thus arthritis cannot be explained on such a basis. Within the dermis, some hypothesize that the fibroblast, the mast cell, or even the endothelial cell are prime targets for whatever it is that fires the psoriatic process. Recent greater understanding has added neuropeptides to the list of potential triggers, since they induce mast-cell degranulation and fire the interaction between the fibroblast and keratinocyte.

The lesion-free skin in people with psoriasis is not normal. Psoriasis is readily induced and various medications, such as chloroquine, practolol, and lithium, can produce a flare-up. Oddly, glycogen levels, so high in the psoriatic lesions, may be lower than in the normal surrounding skin. The dermis is not normal, and the earliest signs of any abnormality following injury are infiltration by mast cells and macrophages.

The microvasculature in psoriasis is characterized by tortuous and leaky capillaries, generous protein exudation, and poor clearance through immature lymphatics.

Koebner phenomenon

The 'Koebner phenomenon' is a term given to psoriasis developing in traumatized skin; this occurs at some stage in about half of all the patients with psoriasis, and is most common when the psoriasis is active. It is an all-or-nothing phenomenon on the skin surface. After the initial repair stimulus, the epidermis gradually thickens and there is accentuation of the papillary interdigitations and the rete ridges. An early heavy infiltrate by neutrophils forming microabscesses within the epidermis is preceded by increased numbers of mast cells and macrophages in the dermis. High turnover of the epidermal cells results in a less-compact and still partially nucleated scale known as parakeratosis. The reverse Koebner phenomenon, where trauma initiates clearing of psoriasis can also occur, and is probably more common than the true Koebner phenomenon.

Clinical appearance

Psoriasis can affect all age groups, but has a peak age of onset between the ages of 5 and 9 years in girls and 15 and 19 in boys. The commonest lesion is a sharply marginated plaque with silvery scales (Fig. 42). These mask the underlying redness from the tortuous convoluted capillaries that lie close to the surface of the skin. The edges of the lesion are usually the most active and there is commonly clearing in the centre (Fig. 43). Since itching is

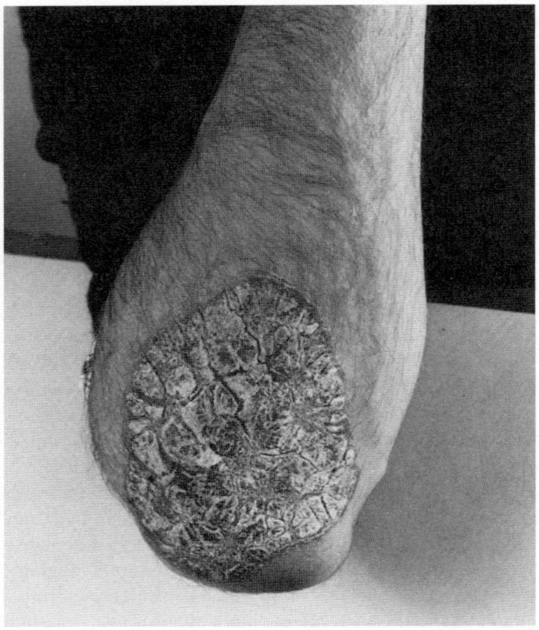

Fig. 42 A psoriasis plaque showing the silvery scales, well-defined border, and predilection for the elbow.

common, scratching may modify the appearance, increasing shedding of scale and causing bleeding.

Sites most commonly affected are the elbows, knees, and scalp, areas that normally have a higher rate of epidermal turnover. The face is less often affected. Spontaneous fluctuations are common and remissions occur in about one-third of cases per annum. As there are several well-recognized patterns, it is important to examine the patient thoroughly until a completely recognizable lesion of psoriasis can be detected. Many lesions and some patterns may be quite atypical, especially during the development of psoriasis (Fig. 44) or during its resolution.

Guttate psoriasis

This term is derived from the Latin *gutta*, meaning a drop. The skin looks as though it has been splashed by the psoriasis. It often follows a streptococcal sore throat or vaccination and is especially common in children. The lesions are scattered over the entire body and tend to be no more than a few millimetres in diameter. They may include the face and are often red slightly scaly spots. Guttate psoriatic lesions appear less well defined and less obviously covered by silvery scales than in classic types of psoriasis. In the absence of a family history the prognosis tends to be good.

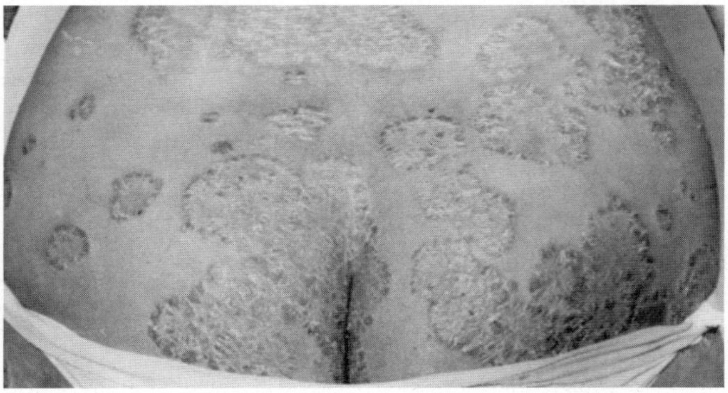

Fig. 43 Psoriasis that is less stable than in Fig. 42. The lesions are erupting and more active at the periphery while healing in the centre.

Nummular discoid

This is probably the commonest form of psoriasis, in which coin-shaped lesions of various sizes (Fig. 45) are scattered over the body in a completely symmetrical distribution. Such lesions are usually well defined and chronic.

Palmar and plantar psoriasis

This may be typical of lesions elsewhere (see Fig. 4), but the psoriasis is often modified due to the nature of the palmar and plantar skin. The scales tend to be more adherent and less silvery and are more likely to develop deep cracks because of the thickness of the epidermis at these sites (Fig. 46). Neutrophils tend to collect into larger abscesses trapped by the thicker surface layers of the stratum corneum, the sterile pustules so formed are often the most obvious feature. Although this pattern may be seen as part of a more generalized disease, in many cases it only affects the hands and feet. There is some evidence that it is a different disease, since the above-mentioned HLA associations are absent and there is no obvious increase in the rate of epidermal turnover. Where the psoriasis is an occasional and acute response to infection, it is known as pustular bacterid.

Psoriasis of the nails

Some 25 per cent of patients with psoriasis have nail disease. Among those with psoriatic arthritis this figure is in excess of 75 per cent. Pin-point pitting is usual but can be seen in other disorders affecting nail growth (see Fig. 66). Onycholysis with brown discoloration of the base of the uplift of the nail, known as brown onychodermal band, is probably even more characteristic. Salmon-pink circular discoloration in the nail-plate, likened to oil drops, are only seen in psoriasis. Sometimes the nail growth is distorted, thickened, and friable and difficult to distinguish from a fungus disorder affecting the nail (see Fig. 69).

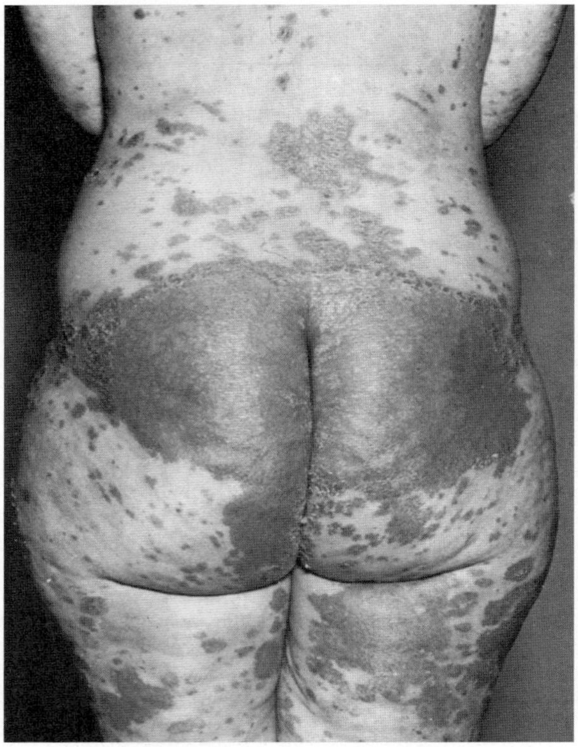

Fig. 44 A still more unstable form of psoriasis, tending to be more exudative and exfoliative and not retaining its rapidly produced scale. While tending to be symmetrical, new ill-defined lesions are erupting. There are some linear lesions on the trunk suggestive of the Koebner phenomenon or a reaction to a skin injury, in this case probably from scratching.

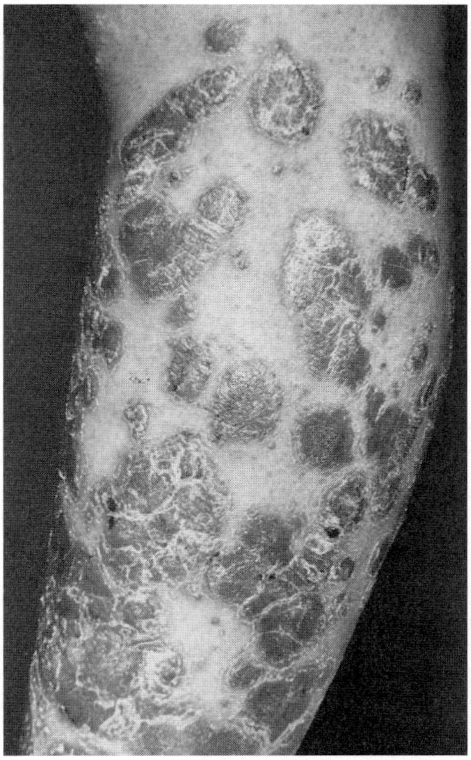

Fig. 45 Discoid lesions still well defined but becoming almost confluent.

Flexural psoriasis

When psoriasis affects the groins, natal cleft, or axillas, it is usually less scaly. The bright-red plaques are shiny and liable to cracking and maceration. They may be very well defined.

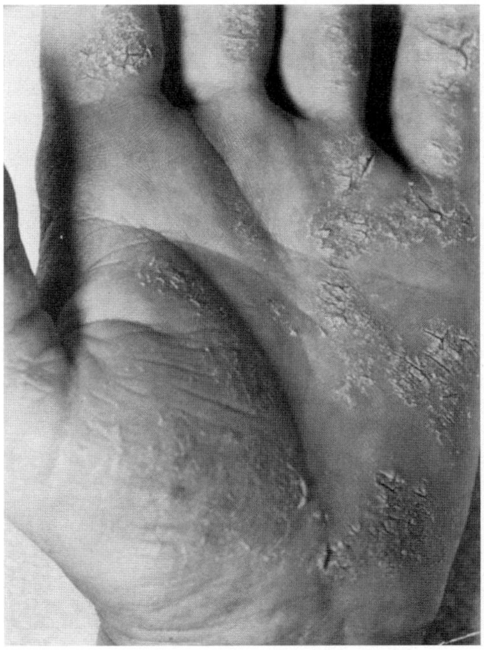

Fig. 46 Psoriasis of the palms may not have the typical scale. It is sometimes pustular or, as in this case, hyperkeratotic with a tendency to form deep cracks (see Fig. 4).

Erythroderma

This may present as a medical emergency due to fluid loss, septicaemia, or lowering of body temperature. The elderly may develop high-output cardiac failure. Oedema is a consequence of capillary leak, low albumin, and heart failure. When psoriasis affects the entire skin there is generalized redness, the well-defined margins are lost, and the scales are profusely exfoliated. The erythroderma may be indistinguishable from that found in eczema or lymphoma. Bacteraemia commonly ensues when the normal protective function of the skin is lost. The loss of water is difficult to estimate and prerenal failure can develop very rapidly. The vasodilatation and the obstruction to the sweat ducts by the proliferating epidermis results in impaired thermoregulation. Hyperthermia is very common in hot climates, while hypothermia can occur in cold climates. Internal organs such as the gut and liver may be impaired and loss of protein both from the skin and the gut is an important complication.

Generalized pustular psoriasis

In this condition, which is relatively rare, waves of bright erythema develop within a few hours together with a fever, arthropathy, and leucocytosis. Myriads of pustules (see Fig. 17) quickly develop and equally quickly disappear. This disorder may occur in the absence of a previous history of psoriasis and even occasionally as a viral exanthem. However, most commonly it is only a complication of psoriasis that has been treated by systemic or local steroids. It is an acute rebound phenomenon of steroid withdrawal.

Acute generalized exanthematous pustulosis occurs in patients with no previous or family history of psoriasis and has been blamed on mercurial drugs and antibiotics. Another rare cause of pustular psoriasis is hypoparathyroidism. Cutaneous drug eruptions may mimic this condition, and any suspected drug should be stopped. Generalized pustular psoriasis is potentially life threatening and therefore admission to hospital is required. Oral retinoids are helpful, as is methotrexate. Oral steroids are best avoided due to the potential for rebound flare when they are stopped.

Arthropathic psoriasis (see Section 18)

The incidence of polyarthritis in those with psoriasis is about 7 per cent in hospital series; 4 per cent of all patients with inflammatory polyarthritis have psoriasis. Up to one-third of patients with pustular psoriasis develop a polyarthritis. There is a long-standing debate concerning the association of psoriasis with inflammatory polyarthritis; it is still uncertain whether it is a chance association, possibly related to a genetic linkage disequilibrium. Since psoriasis is a common disorder, patients with a positive Rose–Waaler test can have coincidental rheumatoid arthritis.

Management

By far the most disabling aspect of psoriasis is its appearance, and patients' lives can be completely taken over by manoeuvres designed to avoid exposing the affected skin to the public eye. Management includes a sympathetic hearing and, when necessary, admission to an outpatient or inpatient unit where others with psoriasis are being treated.

Psoriasis can usually be controlled with therapy. While the skin can be made to return to normal, the inherited susceptibility is fixed, and so patients remain vulnerable to relapse. Some environmental triggers have been identified and should be avoided. These include infection (streptococcal, HIV), trauma to the skin (Koebner phenomenon), psychological stress, and drugs such as lithium, chloroquine, and β-blockers; however, many triggers are unknown and therefore unavoidable.

It is common to combine treatments, either different topicals together, or topical agents with oral preparations or ultraviolet therapy. The response to treatment is variable, and those that were previously effective may no longer be so, and vice versa.

The aims are to depress epidermal cell turnover, suppress skin inflammation, reverse angiogenesis, and remove hyperkeratosis without irreversibly damaging the skin or other organs. It is important that the treatment chosen is appropriate for the type and site of the psoriasis. In mild cases, emollients (for example, 10 per cent glycerine in sorbolene cream) or keratolytics (for example, salicylic acid 3–10 per cent in aqueous cream) may suffice, but disabling or disfiguring psoriasis may warrant the use of systemic antimetabolite or immunosuppressive drugs.

Local steroids

Topical corticosteroids are anti-inflammatory, immunosuppressive, and antiproliferative. Steroid creams and ointments are often used as the first-line treatment for all types of psoriasis because of their ease of use. The stronger halogenated steroids are the most effective. A response may be seen as early as 1 to 2 weeks. Complete resolution generally takes 4 to 6 weeks and occurs in around two-thirds of those who use it. Relapse on cessation of therapy is common and one-third of patients need to continue once- or twice-weekly application. Care is required on the face and flexures to prevent the formation of stria and telangiectasia. Other side-effects associated with continued use are skin atrophy, gradual extension of the psoriasis, and greater instability of the skin so that psoriasis erupts whenever the therapy is partially or completely withdrawn. Eventual widespread usage and systemic absorption complicates the increasing addiction of the skin for the stronger steroids. Some patients so treated show no remission until all such therapy is withdrawn; although in a few this can be done with no immediate worsening of the psoriasis, in most patients withdrawal leads to a rapid worsening of their skin condition.

Tar

Tar is antiproliferative, antipruritic, and anti-inflammatory. Tar has been known to be effective and safe for more than 50 years. Follow-up of patients treated with tar between 1917 and 1937, using the Danish Cancer Registry of all cell cancers from 1943 to 1990, found no overall risk of skin cancer; however, recent rulings by the European Commission have limited its availability in some countries. The smell, colour, and stain of crude coal tar (**CCT**) make it cosmetically unsatisfactory and it may be irritant on more vulnerable skin such as the face and flexures. Less irritating and more cosmetically acceptable varieties of tar include liquor picis carbonis (**LPC**), ichthammol, and oil of Cade; however, these are comparatively less effective than crude coal tar. CCT (2.5–6 per cent) or LPC (2–10 per cent) may be prescribed in a base of aqueous cream, sorbolene cream, or liquid paraffin. A keratolytic such as salicylic acid can be added to augment its efficacy. Many proprietary formulations are available in most countries.

The preparations are applied once or twice daily; but diluted by 50 per cent if they are irritant. Generally little response is seen for 1 to 2 weeks. Complete resolution takes between 6 and 8 weeks; however, subsequent remissions may be prolonged. Occasional patients are allergic to one or more of the constituents. The general principles of when to use a lotion, ointment, or paste are discussed below. Acute or inflamed psoriasis responds to ichthammol, which has a milder action than coal tar.

Dithranol

Dithranol is antiproliferative and mildly anti-inflammatory. It is more effective than coal tar in the treatment of psoriasis, especially if the plaques are large, well-defined, and few in number, but is more irritant, especially to the eyes and genitalia. However, an acceptable diluted concentration can generally be found, and the concentration can then usually be gradually increased. The dithranol is mixed in zinc oxide and salicylic acid paste (Lassar's paste) in a concentration of 0.1, 0.25, 0.5, 1, or 2 per cent. Weaker preparations are used in the more sensitive occlusive flexures. It is safe in pregnancy.

Non-lesional skin may be protected by Vaseline, and it is usual to apply dithranol paste accurately to the active parts of the skin lesion. Powdering fixes the paste and a gauze or nylon dressing protects the overlying clothing from dithranol's staining property. Patients tolerating this regimen are cleared in about 3.5 weeks on average. Staining is inevitable and short lived and is a sign of effectiveness. Irritation, feeling like a mild burn, is treated by stopping treatment for 1 or 2 days. Various proprietary brands are slightly easier to manage and include Vaseline-based preparations and creams or sticks. The 'minute regimen' is a system using 1 to 5 per cent dithranol in Vaseline and 2 per cent salicylic acid. It is only applied for about 80 min, then removed with an oil. Dithranol is suitable for those whose employment requires their skin to be free of ointments for most of the day.

Calcipotriol

Calcipotriol, a vitamin D analogue, is a safe and cosmetically acceptable, effective topical treatment, which inhibits proliferation and enhances epidermal differentiation. It is applied twice daily at a rate of no more than 100 g/week. However, calcipotriol is irritant for about 10 per cent of users, particularly when used on the face. Its combination with betamethasone valerate in popular.

Tazarotene

Tazarotene is a topical synthetic retinoid that also has some efficacy in the treatment of psoriasis. In general, it works best in combination with other topical agents, but is commonly irritating on the skin.

Phototherapy

Natural sunlight is helpful in about 75 per cent of patients and probably accounts for a decreased incidence of psoriasis in sunny climates. Suberythema doses of UVB are a useful substitute, and its effectiveness can be increased by prior bathing or an application of tar which sensitizes the skin to the UVB.

PUVA therapy, which is a combination of long-wave ultraviolet rays (UVA or black light) and 8-methoxypsoralen tablets (0.5 mg/kg) taken 2 h before exposure, produces effective clearance and a bronze skin in most patients. A 15- to 30-min exposure two or three times per week succeeds in clearing the psoriasis in 6 to 10 weeks. The treatment is stopped on clearance of the psoriasis. Patients who relapse quickly may be considered for maintenance therapy either once a week or once every 2 weeks. Recurrences are no less frequent than with other forms of therapy. Dryness, atrophy, and other expected changes of irradiation are a consequence. The risk of skin cancer is as yet difficult to estimate, but it is not insignificant. In male patients receiving more than 200 treatments, the incidence of squamous-cell carcinoma was 30 times greater than that found in the general population in Sweden. As the risk of melanoma in these patients may also be increased, further long-term studies are required. The risk is especially great in those who have arsenical keratoses or other evidence of a previous intake of arsenic. Concurrent treatment with methotrexate is also considered a risk factor.

Broad-band UVB therapy has been used for much longer and is similarly effective as PUVA. Increased carcinogenicity, although not proven, is suspected. Narrow-band UVB (311 mm) is thought to be less irritant and highly specific for psoriasis. By screening out the shorter wavelengths within the UVB spectrum it is assumed to be safer than broad-band treatment.

Climatotherapy is the combination of natural sunlight (or a filtered form of sunlight in the case of the Dead Sea area) with sea salts and/or other constituents—sulphur, black mud, and bromides—present in different geographical regions. It is effective, but no more so than other regimens that provide topical medicaments and mental relaxation. The Dead Sea may be exceptional in the number of its peculiar features, such as low humidity, increased atmospheric pressure, UVB filtration, and minerals in high concentration.

Systemic therapy

When psoriasis is widespread, severe, or causing disfigurement or disability, systemic therapy is indicated. This may take the form of drugs that have antiproliferative or anti-inflammatory, or immunomodulatory effects. The main agents used are acitretin, methotrexate, and ciclosporin. A host of other agents such as hydroxyurea, sulfasalazine, tioguanine, mycophenolate mofeate, tacrolimus, and azathioprine have some efficacy in psoriasis. Human anti-IL-8 antibody may prove to be a new approach to the management of psoriasis.

Acitretin affects cell proliferation and differentiation mechanisms and is also an anti-inflammatory agent. It may be used in psoriasis as monotherapy in the control of palmoplantar and other hyperkeratotic forms of the disease, as well as pustular erythrodermic and atypical presentations of psoriasis, or in combination with phototherapy to augment its efficacy. The usual dose is 0.5 to 1 mg/kg daily; however, many patients cannot tolerate this dose but lower doses may be similarly effective. The major adverse effect of acitretin is teratogenicity, hence contraception is mandatory for women of childbearing age for the duration of therapy and for at least 2 years after the completion of a course of treatment. This makes acitretin undesirable for use among premenopausal women. Other adverse effects of acitretin include all those of hypervitaminosis A; cheilitis, hair fall, photosensitivity, elevation of liver enzymes, and increase of serum lipids.

Methotrexate slows epidermal-cell proliferation and is an immunomodulator. It is the most commonly prescribed antipsoriasis drug. The usual dose is 0.2 to 0.4 mg/kg orally once weekly. Toxicity is more common in the elderly and in patients with reduced renal clearance, therefore lower doses may be required. Patients should abstain from alcohol while being treated with methotrexate. Adverse effects include nausea, pancytopenia, and elevation of liver enzymes. Nausea may be controlled by the concomitant administration of folic acid. Long-term use of low-dose methotrexate may induce liver fibrosis, which seems to be more common in patients treated for psoriasis with methotrexate than in those being so treated for rheumatoid arthritis. Monitoring of patients includes regular full blood and liver function tests. Liver biopsy may be considered in patients with abnormal liver function tests after a cumulative dose of methotrexate between 2 and 4 g to exclude the liver cirrhosis that occasionally complicates the fibrosis.

Ciclosporin A inhibits selectively activated T-helper cells and reduces the production of cytokines. It is very effective in controlling psoriasis at doses between 2 and 5 mg/kg per day. However, ciclosporin A does not produce long remissions and recurrence follows discontinuation. It is not recommended for continuous use beyond 12 weeks, twice per year, because of long-term adverse effects such as hypertension, deterioration of renal function, hypertrichosis, gingival hyperplasia, and the development of neoplasia (specifically, skin squamous-cell carcinoma and lymphoma). It is reserved for the most difficult cases when other treatments have failed or been deemed unsuitable.

On the basis of preliminary reports, one can predict that monoclonal antibody therapy against adhesion molecules and against interleukin-2 receptors will have increasing advocates.

Pityriasis rosea

Pityriasis rosea is a relatively common, self-limiting, inflammatory skin condition that characteristically affects young adults. The cause is thought to be a virus (possibly human herpesvirus-7). The eruption begins with a herald patch that may be mistaken for ringworm. This is followed about 2 weeks later by the development of multiple, scaly, salmon-coloured macules, each about 1 to 2 cm in size and oval in shape. The macules are confined to the trunk and upper limbs and are arranged along the skin creases to create an appearance reminiscent of a Christmas tree. Itch is variable. The rash disappears spontaneously, usually within 6 to 8 weeks.

The aim of treatment is the palliation of any associated itch while awaiting spontaneous resolution. In the absence of itch, reassurance may suffice. First-line therapy to relieve itch consists of topical antipruritic agents such as calamine lotion, 1 per cent menthol in aqueous cream, or a moderately potent topical corticosteroid cream. UVB phototherapy can be used to relieve itch and may hasten resolution of the rash.

Lichen planus and lichenoid eruptions

Lichen planus is an idiopathic inflammatory condition. It may affect the skin, hair, nails, and oral and genital mucosa. Alopecia occurs if the scalp is involved, and nail damage and destruction are seen when the nail matrix is affected. Occasionally lichen planus can be triggered by drug ingestion or hepatitis C infection.

Lichen planus and lichenoid eruptions are characterized by violaceous papules that are usually flat-topped and shiny and heal leaving pigmentation. Histology shows damage to the basal layer of the epidermis and an intense infiltration of lymphocytes and a few histiocytes situated immediately below the epidermis (Fig. 47). A T-cell-mediated CD4+ attack on the epidermis may be triggered by viral, drug, or neoplastic processes. Lichen planus thus presents a model for the elimination of damaged and normal keratinocytes. Cytokines, interferon-γ, and tumour necrosis factor-β play a critical role. Lymphocyte and keratinocyte molecules subserving adhesion are activated and, in the mouse, lichen planus can be blocked by monoclonal antibodies. The disturbances in epidermal growth that result from this damage range from extreme atrophy with ulceration and almost no epidermal-cell turnover to considerable hypertrophy and hyperkeratinization, giving rise to thick nodules meriting the name 'hypertrophic lichen planus'. Most patients are between the ages of 30 and 60 years and it is extremely rare in children. More-erosive forms are seen in the elderly, and pigmented skin tends to develop more hypertrophic varieties.

HLA-A3 and -A5 occur more often in patients with lichen planus than in controls. The graft-versus-host skin reactions following bone marrow transplantation often present with an identical pattern of pathology to that of lichen planus. There is some clinical pathological overlap with the appearance seen in lupus erythematosus. Although immunofluorescence studies show heavy deposits of fibrin and immunoglobulin, these could be entirely non-specific. There is some evidence of defective carbohydrate metabolism and abnormal glucose tolerance, but the basis of this association still has to be explained. A lichen planus-like drug eruption may also be produced by a variety of medications, particularly antihypertensive and antimalarial agents, gold and organic arsenicals, antituberculous therapy, chlorpromazine, as well as from contact with colour developers.

Clinical features

The classical lesion is a shiny, flat-topped papule (Fig. 48) described as polygonal and violaceous. Small white dots or lines in such papules (termed 'Wickham striae') are due to a mixture of oedema, white-cell infiltrate, and

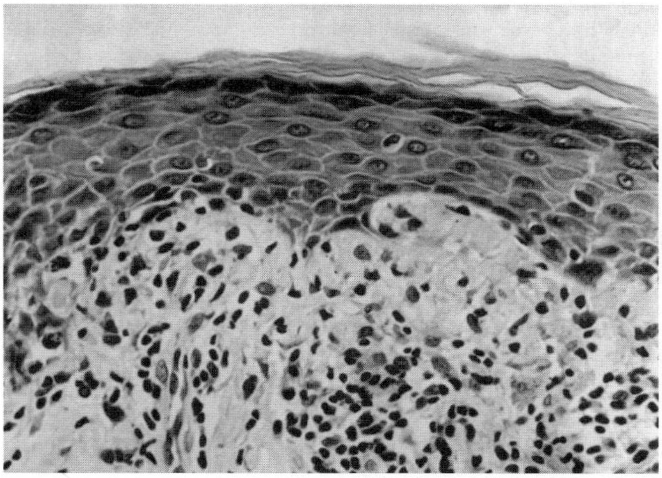

Fig. 47 Lichen planus. There is thickening of the granular layer and necrosis of the basal-cell layer. Pale cells at the lower edge of the epidermis are destroyed epidermal cells. The predominant white cell is a lymphocyte. The infiltrate is often confined to the upper dermis.

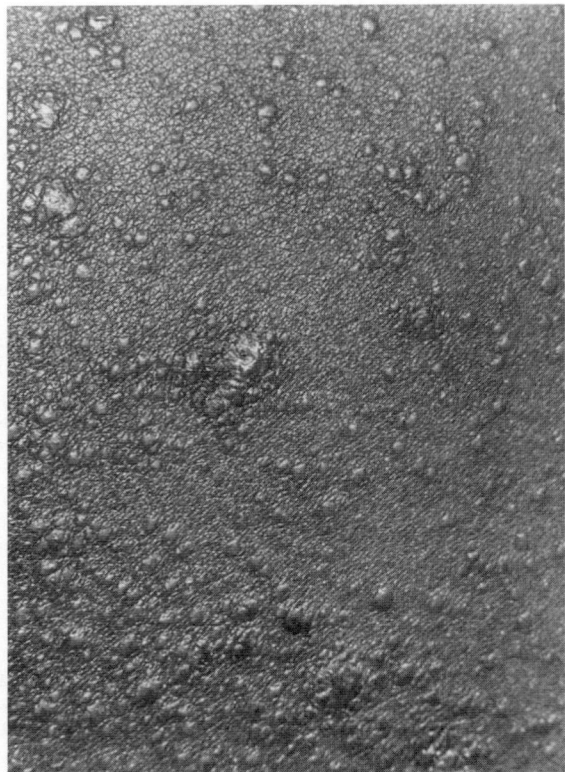

Fig. 48 A black skin affected by the shiny, flat-topped, often polygonal, papules of lichen planus.

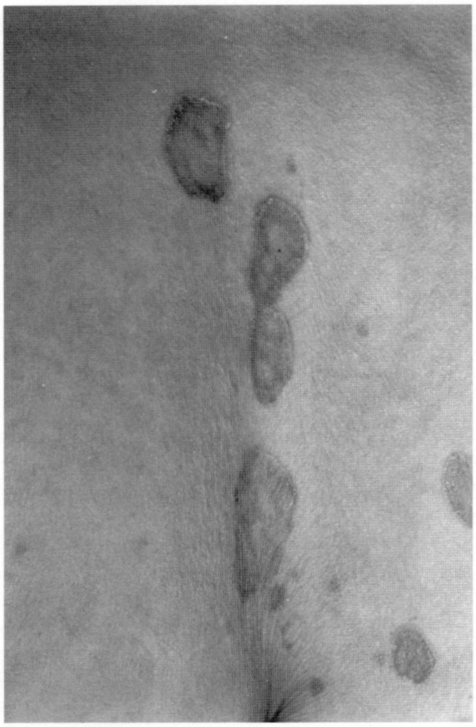

Fig. 49 Lichen planus may heal in the centre, leaving atrophy and pigmentation. The edge is slightly raised; which gives rise to the annular form of the condition.

vasculature disturbances. The papules may become confluent and heal in the centre, giving rise to annular (Fig. 49) lesions or plaques with varying degrees of epidermal response. This may result in either atrophic skin or extreme hypertrophy. A lacy-white appearance (Fig. 50) is common in lesions of the mouth or the glans penis. Hair-follicle involvement may give rise to keratosis pilaris and actual destruction of the hair follicle. Thus, lichen planus is one cause of scarring alopecia. Healing of the lesion is often followed by pigmentation due to melanin in the dermis. Warty hyperkeratotic lesions may be very persistent, as may ulceration, particularly of the peripheries or of the oral mucosa. The initial lesions are commonly found on the front of the wrists, in the lumbar region, or around the ankles. The palms and soles may be involved, in which case the appearance may even suggest a vesicular eruption. Involvement of the mucosa and tongue, which occurs in between 30 and 70 per cent of cases, may extend to the genitalia and perianal area, and has even been described in the rectum, stomach, and larynx. Severe itching is common. Ridging of the nails is essentially due to cessation of nail growth, producing longitudinal linear depressions.

Prognosis

The mean age of onset is during the fifth decade. It may be very explosive or insidious in onset. Most cases clear slowly: 66 per cent of cases take up to a year to clear; 85 per cent clear in 18 months. Mucous membrane lesions or extremely hypertrophic lesions on the legs often persist for years, and there is a risk of squamous epitheliomatous changes, particularly in ulcerated mucosal lesions.

Treatment

Treatment is mainly aimed at relieving the itching, and local steroid creams are perhaps the most effective. Occasionally, a course of prednisolone or ACTH is justified for the treatment of a very severe widespread lichen planus. Probably it does not influence the course of the disease but merely its intensity. As with all itching conditions of the skin, cooling evaporating lotions such as calamine lotion may be helpful. Persistent ulcerated lesions can be excised or grafted. Lesions in the mouth can be treated with local steroid creams, those containing Orabase (a carmellose and gelatin paste) being particularly effective. An asthma-type spray may be a more effective way of administering steroids to the oral mucosa, but must be used without inhalation.

Acne vulgaris

Acne is a common, chronic inflammatory disease of pilosebaceous ducts, that affects a high proportion of the population. An onset around puberty

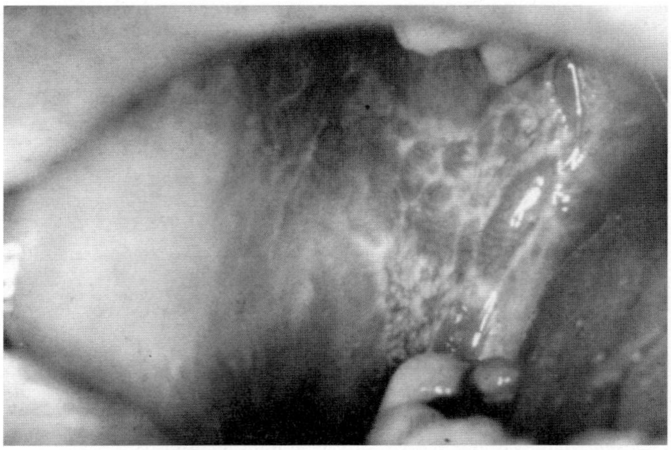

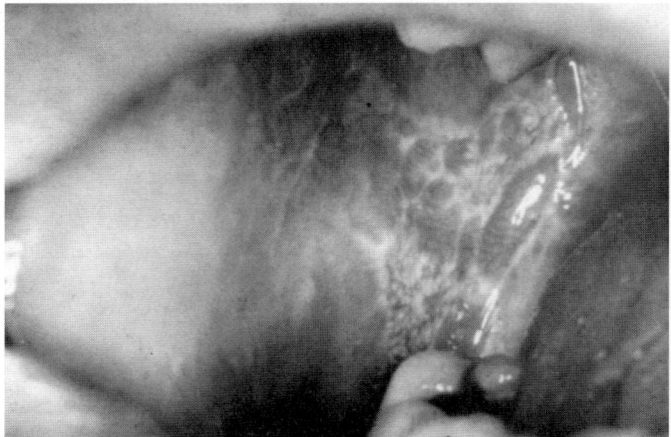

Fig. 50 Lichen planus of the mouth is one cause of mucosal whiteness. Unlike candidiasis the lesions cannot be removed by scraping. They are characteristically 'lacy' in appearance.

is usual and it tends to resolve within 10 years if untreated. Its onset coincides with major changes in the life of an adolescent and may have a negative impact on the psyche of the sufferer and cause profound psychological effects. Physicians should not underestimate the effects acne may have on an individual's body image. Even minor acne may cause depression and negative feelings in particular individuals. It is strongly familial and monozygotic twins show high concordance. It is seen less in some races (Blacks, Japanese, Inuits). The disease may vary at presentation from one to two evanescent lesions occurring at a time, to a severe inflammatory disorder that can result in disfiguring scarring.

Commonly involved areas are those with the highest concentration of sebaceous glands, that is the face, neck, chest, shoulders, and upper back. The primary lesion of acne is the comedo. This non-inflamed lesion may be open (blackhead) or closed (whitehead), and may be accompanied by inflammatory lesions (papules, pustules, and cysts).

Aetiology

The three main processes contributing to acne are: increased sebum secretion; pilosebaceous duct obstruction; and inflammation.

Under the influence of local sex-hormone metabolism, androgens stimulate an increase in the size of the sebaceous glands and, hence, more sebum is produced (see below). These large glands themselves produce more active androgen metabolites through the activity of type 1, 5α-reductase; one effect of these metabolites is to further enlarge the sebaceous glands. Sebum acts in partnership with bacteria to produce keratinization and hence blockage of the pilosebaceous duct and comedo formation.

The principal organism responsible is *Propionibacterium acnes*, which increases in number during flare-ups and is important in the change from non-inflammatory to inflammatory acne. This bacterium produces many inflammatory substances, such as lipases, proteases, hyaluronidases, and chemotactic factors that play a role in producing lesions. Therapy that lowers the *Propionibacterium acnes* count plays a pivotal role in management, but resistance of the bacterium to some antibiotics, especially erythromycin, is an emerging problem in acne therapy.

Acne may also be drug-induced, particularly secondary to anabolic and corticosteroids, iodides, lithium, phenytoin, streptomycin, and isoniazid. Sebum consists of triglycerides, wax esters, squalene, and sterol esters. The fatty acids in sebum are inflammatory and are formed by the lysolytic enzymes of bacteria, even in healthy skin, from unsaturated 14- to 16- or 18-carbon components of the triglycerides. It is possible that acne in people living in the tropics is due to a secondary response in the rate of turnover of the follicular lining, perhaps induced by occlusion under a belt or braces in such hot environments. The acne of Cushing's disease may also be due to an increased rate of such turnover. Chlorinated hydrocarbons also cause acne. Chloracne is an important symptom of poisoning and was present in 168 cases of poisoning in the Seveso industrial accident. The exact way in which the inflammation is produced is uncertain; as the follicle contains fatty acids and bacterial proteases which activate the classical alternative pathway of complement and attract neutrophils, this may be one mechanism.

Sebaceous gland activity is regulated by hormones and, in particular, by androgens from the testes and adrenals, which stimulate, and oestrogens, which seem to suppress activity. In the adult male the glands are normally maximally stimulated, leading to more severe in boys than in girls. The skin itself is a major site for androgenic conversion similar to that observed in the prostate gland and in the male genitalia. Dihydrotestosterone, rather than testosterone, may be the end-organ effector and is formed within the target cells where it stimulates lipogenesis as well as mitosis. Eunuchs do not develop acne. Oestrogens reduce the size of sebaceous glands and sebum production is diminished.

Clinical features

Closed comedones (whiteheads) are the first stage of acne, seen as tiny white nodules below the surface especially when the skin is stretched (see Fig. 7). These may rupture giving rise to irritation of the dermis (that is, inflamed papules) or form the open comedo (blackhead) by pushing open the mouth of the follicle (Fig. 51). Because the black material is melanin, blackheads are blacker in dark skins and white in the albino; melanin is transferred to the keratinocytes before these cells are shed into the sebaceous follicle. Acne cysts (Fig. 52) occur as the result of ballooning of the distended follicle, often leading to destruction of the walls of the cyst and hair and sebaceous apparatus. Adjacent cysts often form fistulas and

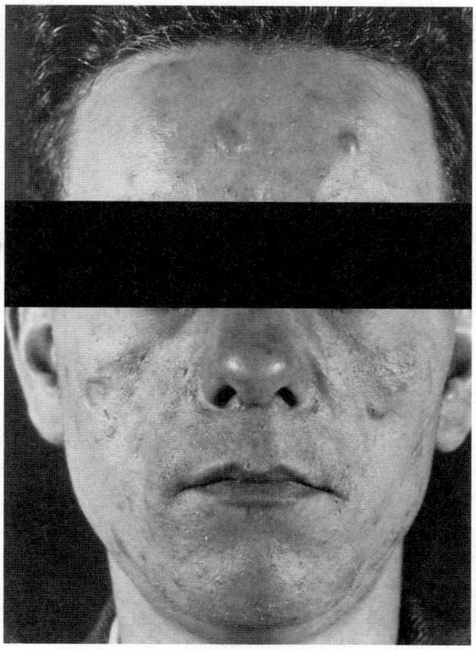

Fig. 51 greasy skin is a common accompaniment of acne, as is comedo formation, or 'blackheads', as seen on the forehead of this young man. Whether either are wholly responsible for the consequent inflammation and scarring also seen in this photograph is debatable.

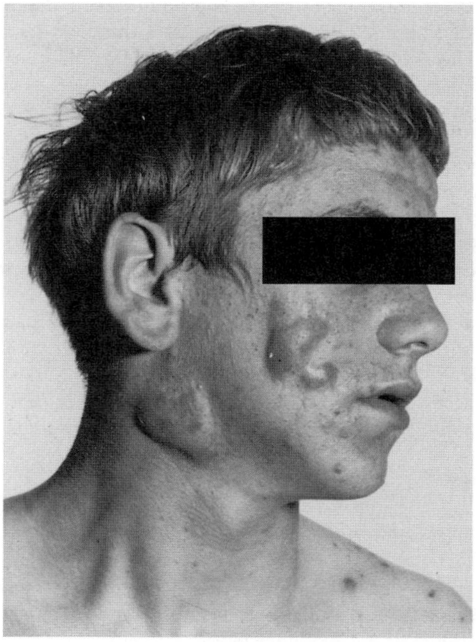

Fig. 52 Large cystic lesions are the most disfiguring aspect of acne vulgaris.

sinuses, which rupture, displacing epithelium in the dermis, and forming irregular channels or foreign-body reactions.

Atrophic or hypertrophic scars of all types may be seen; frequently, excoriations, picking, and squeezing contribute to the irregularities of pigment and to the epidermal or dermal thickening. Rarely, young males develop suppurative and highly inflamed lesions in the skin over the chest with pain, fever, and accompanying polyarthralgia, probably mediated by immune mechanisms and the activation of complement.

Acne usually presents before the menarche and without treatment usually resolves within 8 to 10 years. A more persistent form—particularly affecting the chin—may last until middle age, especially in women who have premenstrual exacerbations. Some women with adult acne also have the polycystic ovary syndrome.

Cosmetics

In many parts of the world cosmetics contribute to acne, the lesions of which may be confined to the site of application. Vaseline-type preparations or medicated oily shampoos used by young men and women with long hair, are a well-known cause.

Management

The withdrawal of aggravating factors such as cosmetics and drugs is paramount where they appear to be involved in the aetiology of acne. Most patients with acne, however, have no such triggers. Trauma, such as picking and vigorously squeezing acne lesions, can aggravate the condition; in some cases of acne excoriée the effect of trauma dominates the clinical picture. Large superficial pustules can be evacuated by gentle pressure without deleterious effect, and the removal of loose comedones with a comedo extractor is commonplace in the practice of dermatology.

Local preparations

All local preparations produce some erythema and occasional pustulation before the acne comes under control. Sulphur is a time-honoured agent, producing local irritation and causing peeling. It is helpful for the treatment of pustules, but may not be so good for comedones which precede pustulation, often by several months. Comedones are reduced by topical retinoids, azelaic acid (20 per cent cream), and by 10 per cent salicylic acid in ethanol. Topical retinoids help the follicle-lining cells to slough off without plugging the follicle. They can be applied in cream, lotion, or gel formulations, and are indicated for comedones rather than for pustules or cysts. Side-effects of the topical retinoids include irritation, redness, and peeling.

Long-acting oxidizing antiseptics such as benzoyl peroxide reduce sebum excretion, reduce comedo production, and inhibit *P. acnes in vitro*. They are the topical treatment of choice, are a mild irritant, and may produce mild peeling after several days' application. It is best to start sparingly with 2.5 per cent preparation, and later to increase the amount applied or the concentration to 5 or even 10 per cent.

Topical antibiotics such as clindomycin (1 per cent), erythromycin (2 per cent), and tetracycline can be used to reduce the population of *P. acnes* in the pilosebaceous duct. In view of emerging bacterial resistance and the possibility of transfer of resistant genes between bacteria via plasmids or transposons, prolonged therapy, and in particular prolonged monotherapy, with these agents is not recommended. When used, they should be combined with topical benzoyl peroxide to inhibit bacterial resistance.

Oral therapy

Antibiotics used include tetracycline, minocycline, doxycycline, erythromycin, and trimethoprim (either trimethoprim alone or as co-trimoxazole). The treatment is prophylactic and the onset of action is delayed for 6 to 8 weeks. Patients can expect a 60 per cent improvement after 3 months and an 80 per cent improvement after 6 months. Relapse is common on cessation of the treatment, however maintenance topical therapy may suffice.

Gastric upset, diarrhoea, and vulvovaginal candidiasis are the most common problems encountered with antibiotics. Photosensitivity to doxycycline and drug-induced hepatitis from minocycline are both uncommon side-effects. Morbilliform drug eruptions due to co-trimoxazole are relatively frequent. Tetracycline may produce discoloration of the teeth in the fetus and in children, hence oral erythromycin is the treatment of choice during pregnancy. Rarely, Gram-negative folliculitis occurs, particularly around the nose or in persistent cysts. This results in sudden worsening with considerable inflammation and may warrant a course of ampicillin.

The oral contraceptive pill is frequently prescribed for women with acne, as the oestrogen component suppresses sebaceous gland activity and decreases the formation of ovarian and adrenal androgens. However, the progestogen component can aggravate acne and therefore contraceptive agents with a low-progestogen dose are preferable. The newer progestogens, such as norgestimate, gestodene, and desogestrel, have less androgenic effects and are therefore the agents sought in a contraceptive pill where an anti-acne effect is desired. Oral contraceptives containing a combination of cyproterone acetate (see below) and an oestrogen (for example, 2 mg cyproterone acetate and 35 μg ethinyl oestradiol), are also an effective treatment of acne in women. While they are more effective than the low-progestogen oral contraceptives, they also have more adverse effects. The onset of action is slow, however they may be suitable for long-term therapy. They are usually more effective when used in combination with other therapies rather than as an isolated treatment. Cyproterone acetate and spironolactone can be used for their antiandrogenic properties in the control of severe acne in women not planning to become pregnant. They are most commonly used when there are associated symptoms of virilization, for example in the polycystic ovarian syndrome.

Where the acne is resistant to treatment or persistently relapses, and in cases of severe cystic acne and acne where scarring is likely, oral isotretinoin (0.5–1 mg/kg) is the treatment of choice. This vitamin-A derivative acts by correcting the keratinization defect in acne, decreasing sebaceous gland activity, and reducing the population of *P. acnes*. It is also anti-inflammatory. A cumulative dose of 120 to 150 mg/kg over a period of 4 to 6 months is usually required and one course is usually sufficient for most patients, although approximately 10 per cent of cases need a further course. Isotretinoin is teratogenic, so strict avoidance of pregnancy is of paramount importance whilst taking the drug and for one full reproductive cycle after discontinuation. Prescription is usually limited to dermatologists. Adverse effects of some degree are universal, including dry skin, eyes, and lips, as well as epistaxis, facial erythema, joint stiffness, myalgia, headaches, in addition to an initial flare of the acne on commencement of the treatment. Prednisolone can be used to ameliorate this initial flare. Other side-effects such as depression and paronychia are rare. The severity of the side-effects are dose-dependent and are generally ameliorated by a reduction in dose. Most adverse effects settle within 2 weeks of discontinuing the drug, and many patients cope better with the annoying adverse effects of cheilitis, xeroderma, and photosensitivity as their course progresses.

Diet

Studies of the effects of starvation in the obese or the malnourished show little evidence of the effect of diet on acne vulgaris, even in pellagra where some plugging of the follicles around the nose is an early sign. Chocolate worsens acne in some individuals, but this has not been shown in trials of larger populations. Nutrition may influence the age of onset of puberty and hence overeating may result in earlier acne.

Acne surgery

Comedo extraction is the expression of a follicle's contents by the application of pressure on the surface, often with a special device called a comedo extractor. The benefits of active attack on the lesions, thereby counteracting stasis and build-up of the contents, has to be weighed against the fact that suppression is always incomplete and a tendency to rupture into the dermis may promote inflammation. Cryotherapy destroys the lining of large cysts. Deep sinuses may require externalization. Solitary inflamed lesions benefit from intralesional inoculation of steroids. Persistent acne cysts sometimes resolve with the injection of small amounts of intralesional triamcinolone.

Pigmentation

The principal pigments in the skin include melanin (black), phaeomelanin (reddish-yellow), haemoglobin (red) and its by-products bilirubin (red) and biliverdin (green), as well as haemosiderin which produce colours of yellow, green, red, and brown. Longer wavelengths such as red penetrate deeper and are absorbed by melanin. Since blue does not penetrate so deeply it is not absorbed and is reflected back, which is why dermal pigment appears blue—hence blue naevus. Although racial causes of pigmentation are common, physical causes are also important since white skin may visibly tan in the sun. Tanning and burning are independent events, with different time courses (albeit overlapping), due to the interaction of ultraviolet radiation with distinct chromophores in the skin. Tanning consists of two phases: (1) immediate pigmentary darkening and (2) delayed pigmentation. Immediate darkening occurs within seconds to minutes of exposure, and is due to oxidation of melanin granules stored within keratinocytes in the skin. Delayed darkening is due to the increased melanin production within melanosomes, increased transfer of melanosomes from melanocytes to keratinocytes, and acanthosis of the epidermis. It begins 8 h after exposure, reaches a maximum at 24 h, and in the absence of re-exposure resolves over days to weeks.

Some pigmented lesions are naevi (Tables 11, 12, and 13, Plates 1–7, Figs 53–58, and see Fig. 106), others result from pigment 'incontinence' which increases the amount of pigment in the dermal macrophages and is commonly postinflammatory.

Pigmentation as a feature of systemic illness is most significantly due to endocrine dysfunction affecting the melanocyte-stimulating hormone. In countries where malnutrition and infections are common, protein and vitamin deficiency, as well as cachexia from a variety of causes, account for disturbances in skin colour.

'Tinea' or pityriasis versicolor is due to a superficial fungus known as *Malassezia furfur*. It usually affects the upper trunk and may spread on to the neck or arms. The lesions are slightly scaly, off-white, pink, and brown. 'Pityriasis' is the term for a bran-like powdery scale and 'versicolor' implies the variation in the colouring (Fig. 58).

In leprosy, hypomelanosis is a feature of tuberculoid and borderline tuberculoid types (See Fig. 59 and Chapter 7.11.24). Light touch and later pinprick sensation are impaired. There is often a lack of sweating and there may be loss of hair. An adjacent enlarged peripheral nerve may be palpable, which may be mistaken for an enlarged lymph node.

Pigmentation of the buccal mucosa, tongue, or fingernails is significant only in white skin since it is a normal finding in dark races.

Depigmentation

'Leucoderma' is a term used for any whiteness of skin, and ranges from a partial hypopigmentation to the complete depigmentation characteristic of vitiligo. Microbial diseases such as pityriasis versicolor (Fig. 58), leprosy (Chapter 7.11.24) (Fig. 59), and syphilis are important infectious causes of hypopigmentation. Pinta should be suspected in people from central or southern America showing a succession of erythematous hyperpigmented lesions progressing to warty or atrophic plaques of depigmented skin. The late stage resembles vitiligo. Naevus anaemicus is a hypovascularity of the skin observed in white skins (Fig. 60); it is not a disorder of melaninization.

Vitiligo

This common, autoimmune skin disease results in the destruction of melanocytes and the total depigmentation of affected skin. However, an association with other autoimmune diseases and a family history of such is found in one-third of cases. The cause is unknown, but the melanocyte seems to be damaged by some, as yet, unidentified antibody or toxin. Although vitiligo is most likely due to an immunological attack on the melanocyte, there are theories based on oxygen free-radical metabolism. In many parts of the world where skins are deeply pigmented, vitiligo is a principal cause of attendances at a dermatology department. Vitiligo affects up to 1 per cent of the United Kingdom population but 8.8 per cent in India. It presents during the first decade of life in 25 per cent of those affected. Except in those people unable to protect themselves from bright sunlight the disability is purely cosmetic, but it causes more concern and social handicap than almost any other common disease.

Occupational vitiligo is a well-recognized effect of exposure to certain chemicals used in the rubber industry—monobenzyl ether of hydroquinone, *p*-tertiary butylcatechol, and *p*-tertiary butylphenol. The hands are usually the first part of the body to be involved along with the genitalia, presumably through contact with the chemical excreted in the urine.

Clinical features

The initial depigmentation often occurs at sites of trauma, particularly the knuckles of the hands, and sometimes forms a white halo around a naevus (Figs 61 and 62). The face and neck are usually affected early. In white-skinned people the first complaint often occurs during the summer when the unaffected skin is at its darkest from sun exposure. There is usually marked symmetry; the axillary folds and genitalia are commonly affected;

Table 11 Localized causes of pigmentation. Light-exposed—especially on the face, and usually due to increased numbers of normal melanocytes in the epidermis

Actinic or senile lentigo	A common grey/brown macule especially of the face and limbs in middle-aged or older persons, usually due to sun exposure in youth. It is without epidermal changes. Spreading pigmented actinic keratoses show slight verrucous changes and can merge into a squamous-cell carcinoma or into a lentigo maligna.
Berloque dermatitis	Brown, often streaky, macules often initially inflammatory with redness, blistering, or scaling at sites exposed to perfumes and sunlight. Several plants may be responsible. The streaky pigmentation may persist for years (Fig. 53).
Freckle-ephelis	Small, brown macules usually numerous in light-exposed skin of genetically fair, blonde, or red-haired and blue-eyed people.
Lentigo maligna	Usually a well-defined, irregular, brown to black mottled macular lesion especially on the face of old people. The melanocytes are dysplastic, vacuolated in the epidermis, and malignant change is common (see Fig. 25).
Melasma or chloasma	Usually brown symmetrical macules of the butterfly area of the face, or crossbow pattern on the forehead. It is common in pregnancy or in those taking oral contraceptives containing oestrogen (see Fig. 55).
Xeroderma pigmentosum	The patchy macular pigmentation is associated with keratoses, telangiectasia, and malignancies. Basal-cell and squamous-cell carcinomas and even melanoma are common. Intolerance to the sun results in excessive sunburn often 72 h after exposure. The disorder begins in early childhood, often as a bright erythema and swelling following exposure to the sun. The aetiology is genetic and concerns a defect in DNA repair, following injury by light (see Chapter 25.2).
De Sanctis–Cacchioni syndrome	Xeroderma pigmentosum, mental deficiency, dwarfism, and neurological disorders.

the eye is not involved. Transient hypopigmentation is sometimes observed in evolving lesions; however, depigmentation of the lesion is ultimately total (Fig. 63) and should cause no confusion with the hypopigmentation of diseases such as leprosy. Such areas are never anaesthetic as in leprosy. Pigment may accumulate and be well defined at the borders of the lesion, giving a hyperpigmented edge. Melanocytes of hair follicles are usually unaffected and repigmentation, when it occurs, is often from such sites (Fig. 63(b)).

The clinician should be aware of associations with diabetes mellitus, pernicious anaemia, Addison's disease, myxoedema, and thyrotoxicosis. Less than one-third of patients show spontaneous repigmentation. In most cases the loss of pigment gradually extends. Depigmentation of the vulva, penis, and neck is sometimes persistent and of a localized variety, but need not necessarily progress to generalized vitiligo. It should be distinguished from the more atrophic lichen sclerosis which may also cause whitening of the skin at those sites.

Management

Patients are usually much distressed by the cosmetic disability. It is helpful to explain that there is a 30 per cent chance of spontaneous cure. Offering advice on camouflage make-up (many dermatology units have advisors specially skilled in this art) gives the patients an opportunity to help themselves, especially for important social occasions. But such camouflage is tedious and difficult to apply effectively for everyday use. There is no special advantage in the purchase of more expensive cosmetics since the basic constituents are cheap. The best effect is achieved from powder and grease mixtures with a powder finish patted gently into the skin after application. Dihydroxyacetone is the basis of many artificial (fake) suntan lotions, but again these are difficult to apply satisfactorily without overpigmenting the adjacent unaffected skin.

Patients should be told to avoid occupations which injure the skin (such as playing with animals that scratch) to prevent vitiligo from the Koebner phenomenon. The cosmetic effect of removing the remaining pigment is

Table 12 Pigmentation more commonly on the trunk

Acanthosis nigricans
Pigmentation affects the axillas and groins. There is a velvety thickening of the skin with skin tags. The condition may be benign when associated with obesity and in the young, but in older persons with oral, facial, or hand pigmentation and thickening, it is more often due to an underlying adenocarcinoma. Pruritus may be associated and indicates underlying carcinoma (see Fig. 105).

Becker's naevus
Large, lightly pigmented, and often hairy macular pigmentation affecting a segment of the trunk, such as the shoulder or one flank. It is often first noticed after puberty. It is entirely benign (Fig. 54).

Dermatosis papulosa nigra
This is a papular variety of seborrhoeic warts, producing discrete but multiple dark lesions of the face and neck. It is the commonest dark lesion in Blacks.

Tinea nigra
A localized, asymptomatic fungus infection causing a brown or black macular lesion on the palm; sometimes when there is no scaling it may be taken for a lentigo.

Erythrasma
This is due to a corynebacterial infection of the groins, axillas, and between the toes. On white skin it is light brown, but in dark skin it may produce a lighter or darker hue. Wood's light shows the coral-red fluorescence.

Tinea versicolor
This is a flat to slightly elevated scaly papule or reticulate plaque producing either a brownish coloration or depigmentation. It affects the upper trunk, upper limbs and neck (Fig. 58).

Urticaria pigmentosum
These are pigmented lesions due to nests of mast cells in the skin. In children they may be quite large, palpable lesions about the size of a thumb, or they may be lentil-sized and numerous. Occasionally, though, there is a diffuse and velvety texture to the skin. The diagnostic feature of the lesion is the wealing that results from scratching.

Café au lait
These lesions resemble large freckles. They are often as large as a thumb or palm, and tend to be oval in shape. There is a variant known as naevus spilus which is speckled with much darker spots. In neurofibromatosis there are usually at least five café au lait spots and generalized freckling extending into the axillas (Fig. 56). Very large, pigmented, unilateral macules with serrated edges are characteristic of Albright's syndrome.

Leopard syndrome
Very numerous and progressive darkening lentigos of the trunk and limbs(Fig. 51) are associated with the following, denoted by the acronym'Leopard': lentigenoses, ECG abnormalities, ocular defects, pulmonary stenosis, abnormalities of genitalia, retardation of growth, deafness

Peutz–Jeghers syndrome
This consists of polyposis of the small intestine. It is associated with numerous small pigmented macules affecting the perioral buccal areas extending quite far beyond the margins of the lips, it also affects the dorsum of the fingers. Note: lentigos of the lips and postinflammatory pigmentation are in themselves quite common and need not be associated with any internal disorder.

Laugier–Hunziker syndrome
An acquired hyperpigmentation of the lips, oral mucosa, nail-bed, fingertips, and genital mucosa, usually sporadic, can be familial.

sometimes preferred by those whose skin is almost completely depigmented. The formulation used by the Sheffield Royal Infirmary is prepared as follows: hydroquinone 30 g; hydrocortisone BP 6 g; retinoic acid 600 mg; butylated hydroxytoluene 300 mg; and methylated spirit and polyethylene glycol in equal parts to 600 ml. Monobenzyl ether of hydroquinone may also be used to induce permanent hypopigmentation.

Psoralens and sunlight are one of the most ancient remedies used in medicine, UVA (black light) and selective UVB are recently developed extensions of the older remedy. Psoralens, methoxy- or tri-psoralen, are taken by mouth 2 h before exposure to light, or they may be applied topically 30 min before exposure. The simplest regimen is a combination of meladinin paint and sunlight. It is necessary to test reactivity with short-time exposure and always to expose the skin at the same time of the day to avoid burning the skin by an unexpectedly high intensity of UVA. The chances of remission are in the order of 50 to 60 per cent, but success may take 2 to 3 years to accomplish. As might be expected from an autoimmune disorder, local steroid preparations are sometimes helpful, particularly in early or evolving disease. Although they have been advocated in combination with psoralens, therapeutic triumphs are difficult to assess, and the requirement to use these agents for years rather than days makes side-effects very likely. Local steroids are sometimes used to stabilize a rapidly progressive early stage of the disease. Cosmetically disabling local patches can be treated with light dermabrasion and the application of autologous split-skin grafts from pigmented skin. In Asia many clinics have treated thousands of patients in this way and there are several traditional herbal remedies prescribed for widespread lesions.

Other forms of pigment loss

Albinism

This is a group of at least 15 genetically distinct syndromes, determined not by absence of melanocytes but by their inability to synthesize melanin (see

Table 13 Disorders of increased pigmentation

Circumscribed brown[a] hyperpigmentation	
Infection:	tinea versicolor; erythrasma
Café-au-lait type:	Albright's syndrome; neurofibromatosis
Lentigo type:	Leopard syndrome; Peutz–Jeghers syndrome
Melasma type (chloasma):	pregnancy; drugs; idiopathic
Miscellaneous:	acanthosis nigricans; postinflammatory; stasis; Becker's naevus; fixed drug eruption; urticaria pigmentosa; Minocin-induced (often black)
Generalized brown[a] hyperpigmentation	
Reticulate:	naevoid; poikiloderma; dyskeratosis congenita
Metabolic:	haemochromatosis; porphyria; chronic liver disease
Endocrine and/or autoimmune:	Addison's disease; pregnancy; pernicious anaemia; myxoedema; thyrotoxicosis; Felty's syndrome; ACTH- and MSH-secreting tumours; scleroderma
Nutritional:	malnutrition; malabsorption
Drugs:	antimalarials; tetracyclines; heavy metals; cancer therapeutic agents; phenothiazines; clofazimine (usually reddish-brown); amiodarone; tricyclic antidepressants
Other types:	postinflammatory; Whipple's disease; catatonic schizophrenia; Schilder's disease
Generalized slate-grey[b] hyperpigmentation	
Haemochromatosis	
Nutritional deficiency	
Drugs:	chlorpromazine; Minocin®; gold; silver

[a] Brown: increased melanin in epidermal cells.

[b] Grey, slate, or blue: increased melanin in dermis.

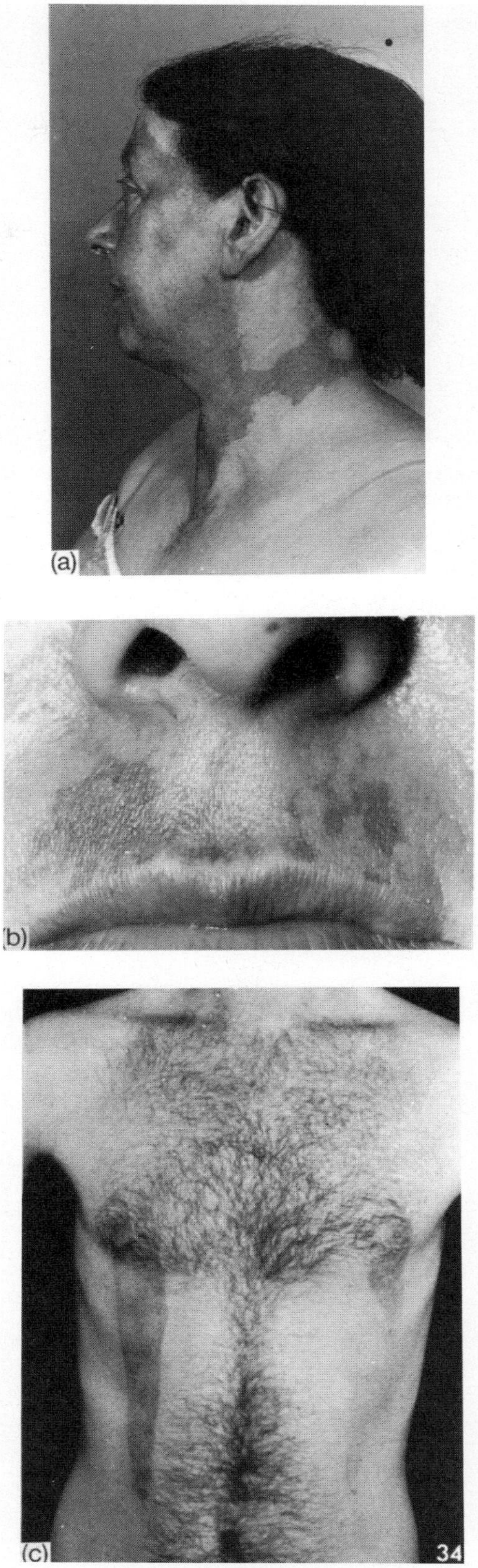

Fig. 53 Pigmentation due to cosmetic agents. Often initially a dermatitis, it is especially induced by exposure to ultraviolet rays. It tends to have the streaky distribution of application. (a) Neck pigmentation from eau de cologne. (b) Lip pigmentation from lanolin. (c) From eau de cologne and sunbathing, the bizarre pattern is characteristic of an exogenous cause.

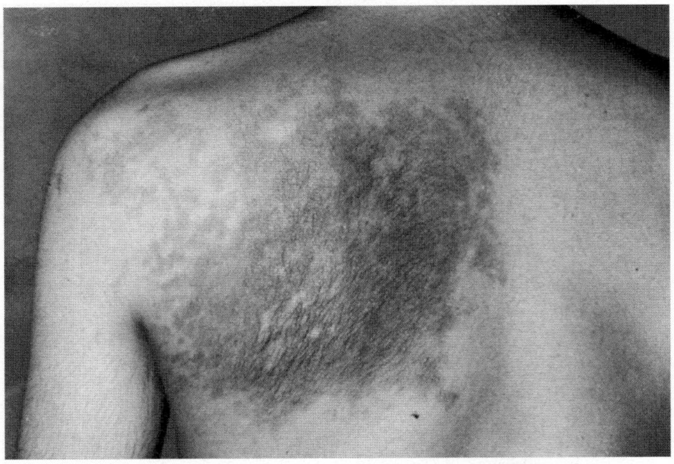

Fig. 54 Becker's naevus is due to melanin in the dermis and is often segmental and usually hairy. It may only become overt after childhood.

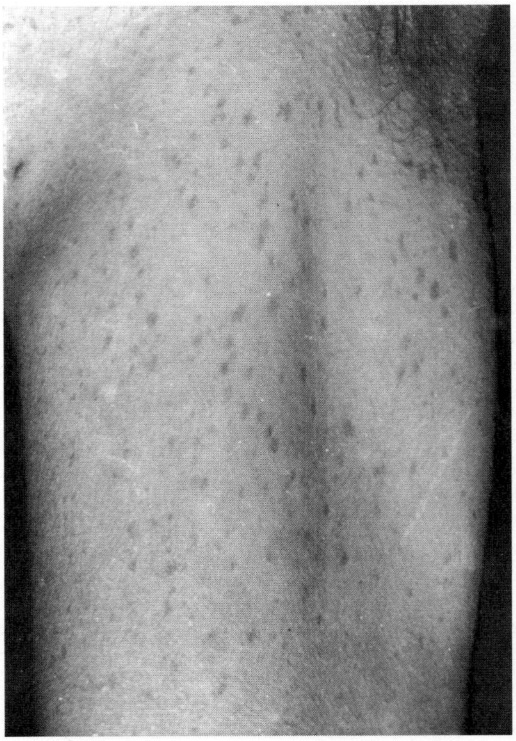

Fig. 56 In neurofibromatosis freckles extend into the axilla. This is a diagnostic feature in incomplete penetrance, important in the genetic counselling of white-skinned, but less reliable in black-skinned, patients.

Chapter 23.2). Since melanin is important not only in the skin but also at such sites as the cochlea and retina, and also because the body's capacity to transfer organelles other than melanin is sometimes impaired, there are a number of associated defects affecting vision, hearing, and the delivery of lysosomes. In some societies where inbreeding is usual, albinism is common (San Blas Islands, Tanzania, southern Nigeria). Albinos in many countries are outcast, poor, underfed, and often die from skin cancer.

Albinism can occur in two forms: partial and complete albinism. Partial albinism occurs in piebaldism and albinoidism, a group of conditions where pale skin is seen without associated eye changes. Complete albinism is subdivided into ocular and oculocutaneous albinism. Skin changes are not seen in ocular albinism, but deafness is common in the autosomal dominant and autosomal recessive forms as well as one of the X-linked recessive forms. Oculocutaneous albinism (pale skin together with eye changes) is subdivided into tyrosinase-positive and tyrosinase-negative forms, according to whether incubation of hair bulbs with tyrosine induces pigmentation. In practice, this test is rarely performed. The tyrosinase-negative forms of albinism are all inherited as an autosomal recessive trait, while the tyrosinase-positive forms may be dominant or recessive.

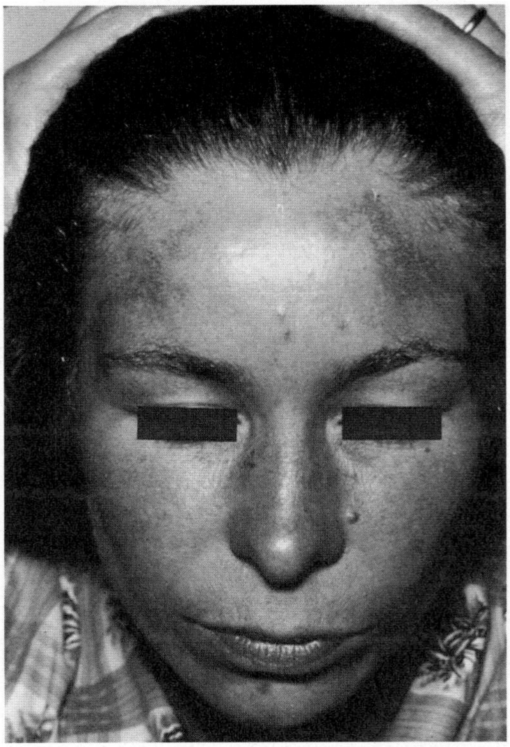

Fig. 55 Crossbow pattern of chloasma in encephalitis, an association that has been described but may be incidental.

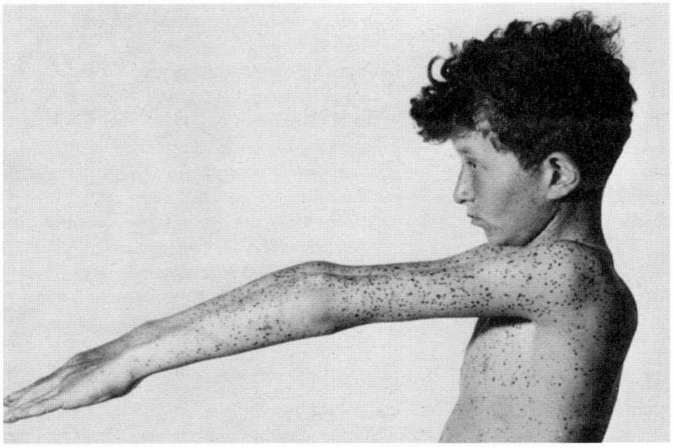

Fig. 57 Syndrome of progressive darkening of numerous lentigos associated with cardiovascular and neurological abnormalities.

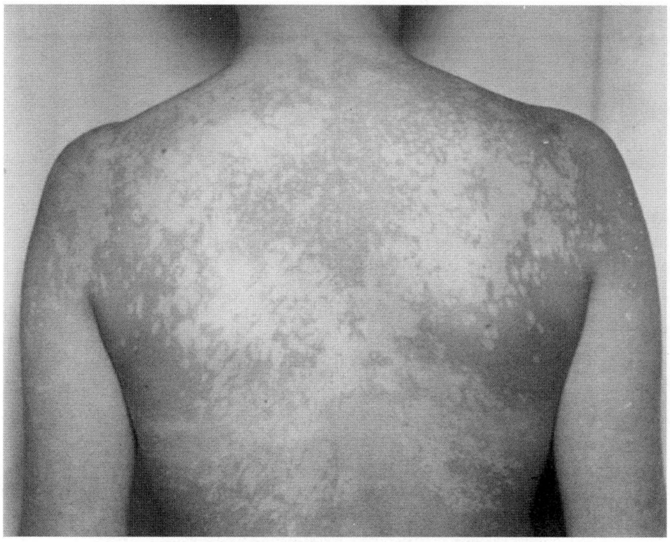

Fig. 58 Pityriasis versicolor due to the organism *Malassezia furfur* causes redness and slight brownish coloration of very pale, white skin, and depigmentation in dark or sallow skin. It favours the upper trunk.

Phenylketonuria

This cause of whiteness should not be forgotten. It results in elevated levels of phenylalanine which compete for tyrosinase.

Halo naevi

These are characterized by a loss of pigment around benign (see Fig. 62), or very rarely, malignant melanocytic naevi. It is a common first sign of vitiligo (see above). The central naevus should be assessed on its merits and need only be removed if there is a progressive enlargement, bleeding, and irregularities in the pigment, shape, or size of the naevus.

Tuberous sclerosis

The oval macules, which look like a thumbprint and are tapered at one end, sometimes known as leaf-like (Fig. 65), are present in about 90 per cent of

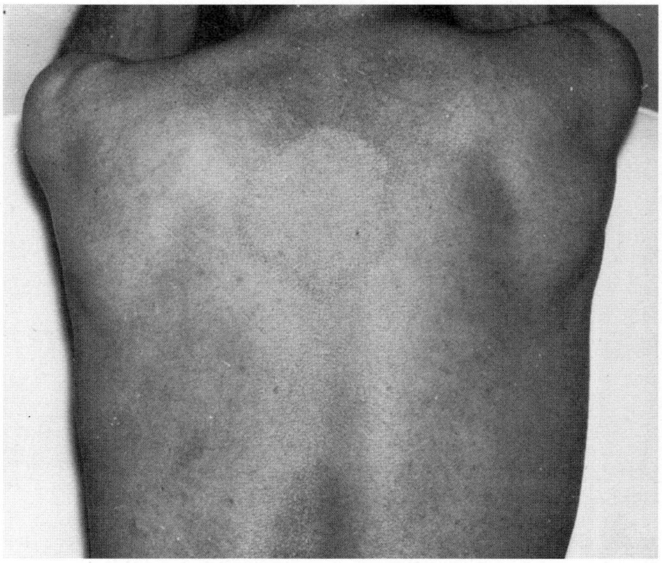

Fig. 59 Hypopigmentation, especially with a hyperpigmented border, should always be tested for loss of sensation. This lesion is typical of tuberculoid leprosy.

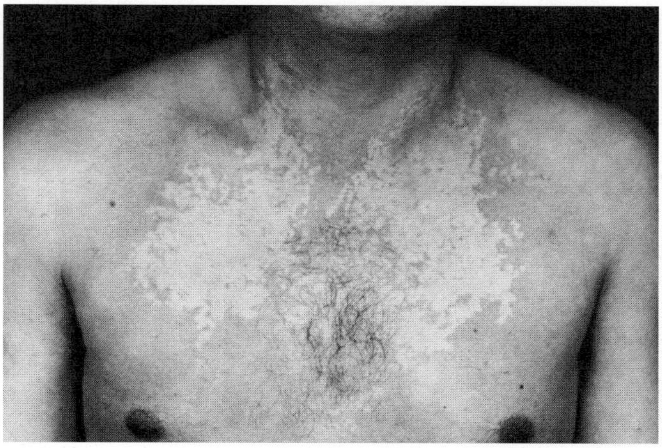

Fig. 60 Not all whiteness is due to loss of pigment. Decreased vasculature has been present since birth in this case of naevus anaemicus.

affected babies. They are easier to see using Wood's light (UVA; see above).

Idiopathic guttate hypomelanosis

This is characterized by small, depigmented, sharply defined, often polygonal macules in light-exposed areas. It is probably caused by sun damage, and is almost universal amongst ageing Whites living in sunny climates.

Postinflammatory depigmentation

This is probably the commonest cause of leucoderma. Pigmented skin retains less pigment when there is accelerated epidermal turnover as in wound repair, eczema, or psoriasis, but the lesions are not as white as in vitiligo. One particular form commonly seen on the face but here illustrated in the cubital fossae is known as 'pityriasis alba' (Fig. 64), which is, in fact, a variant of a dry eczema causing mild hypopigmentation. It may be sharply circumscribed and have a halo of surrounding inflammation. Pityriasis alba is usually slightly scaly and there is follicular prominence due to hyperkeratosis. The cheeks and upper arms are most commonly affected and atopic children are the most frequent sufferers.

Discoid lupus erythematosus (**DLE**) is a common cause of depigmentation in some parts of the world. It is preceded by the itching, deep-violet

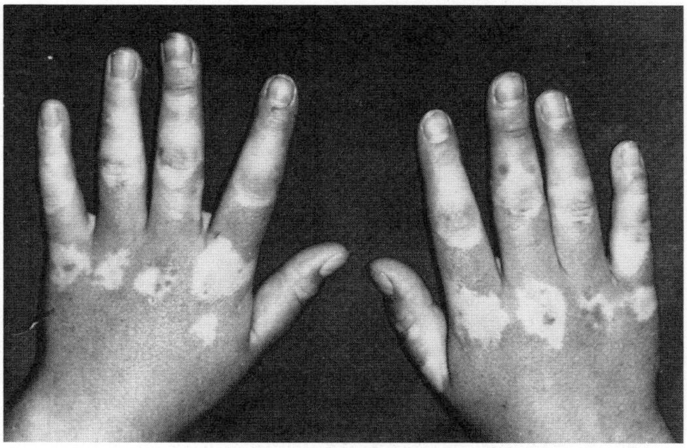

Fig. 61 Vitiligo is complete depigmentation and not merely hypopigmentation; it often begins at sites of minor trauma such as the knuckles. As with all essentially endogenous disorders it is symmetrical.

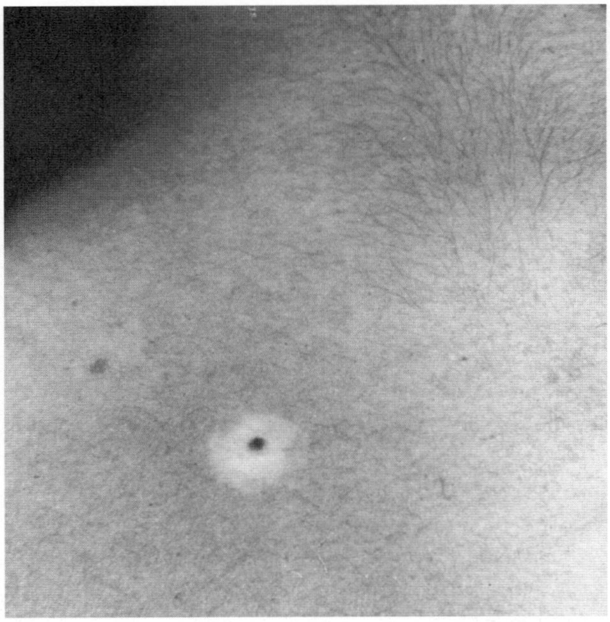

Fig. 62 Vitiligo often begins around a pigmented naevus—a halo naevus.

erythema of light-exposed skin. Hair loss from the scalp is common, usually of the scarring type.

Diseases of nails, hair, and sweat glands

Nails and hair adorn our bodies. In addition, nails aid in picking up small objects. The handicap of disease of hair or nails is greatest in those who are most conscious of their 'looking good'. Beauty is not only in the eyes of the beholder but it is also an image in the mind. Hence, most consultations concerning hair are about too much or too little in comparison to the norm for a particular population. Excessive sweating and body odour is also a cause of great distress.

Nails

Nails grow continuously throughout life. The germinative epithelium is in the nail matrix, which is protected from the environment by a waterproof seal created by the cuticle. The structural integrity of the nail unit requires an intact cuticle and solid adhesion between the nail-plate and the nail-bed. Normal fingernails grow at the rate of approximately 1 cm in 3 months, with toenails taking anything from 9 to 24 months to grow as much. The nails grow more rapidly in psoriasis and more slowly in cold, ischaemia, or severe systemic illness.

There are only a limited number of ways in which injury, infection, inflammation, metabolic disease, and neoplasia may present in a nail. The important physical signs are alterations of the nail-plate, such as thickening, thinning, abnormal curvature, onycholysis (lifting of the nail-plate), pitting (Fig. 66), ridging (Fig 67), discoloration (Fig. 68), and growth changes (Fig. 69). Other possible presentations include paronychia (or inflammation of the skin of the nail-folds) and destruction of the nail unit (Table 14).

Paronychia

Paronychia may be acute or chronic. Acute paronychia is painful and is due to bacterial (usually staphylococcal) or viral (herpes simplex) infection. Chronic paronychia is painless and is a traumatic nail dystrophy. Pushing back the cuticles, or removing the cuticles using keratolytics (as used by manicurists), damages the waterproof seal between the proximal nail-fold and the nail-plate that protects the nail matrix. Once damaged, water and debris can enter the nail matrix and produce inflammation of the undersurface of the proximal nail-fold. Cuticle loss is an essential feature of the diagnosis; if the cuticle is intact, consideration should be given to other causes of swelling of the proximal nail-fold. Habit tic deformity is commonly associated.

Secondary infection with *Candida* spp. is common and for a long time was thought to be important in the initiation of paronychia. Whilst it may aggravate the problem, it does not cause it, and paronychia should be thought of as essentially a problem caused by nail manicure. Chronic paronychia may be aggravated by episodes of acute paronychia caused by secondary infection with staphylococci. The proximal nail-fold becomes painful and pus may be expressed.

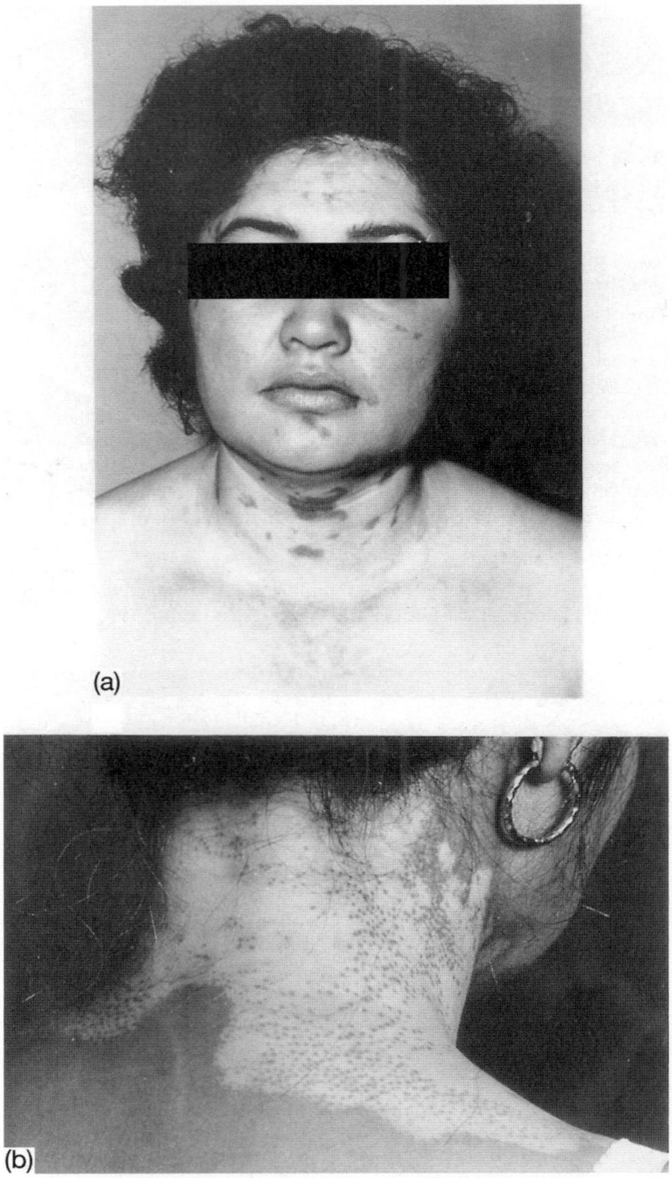

Fig. 63 (a) The pigment loss in this once dark-skinned woman is almost complete. Satisfactory cosmetic management would be depigmentation of the few residual areas of normal skin. (b) Although repigmentation of the skin in vitiligo is usually from the follicles, it is slow, unpredictable, and incomplete.

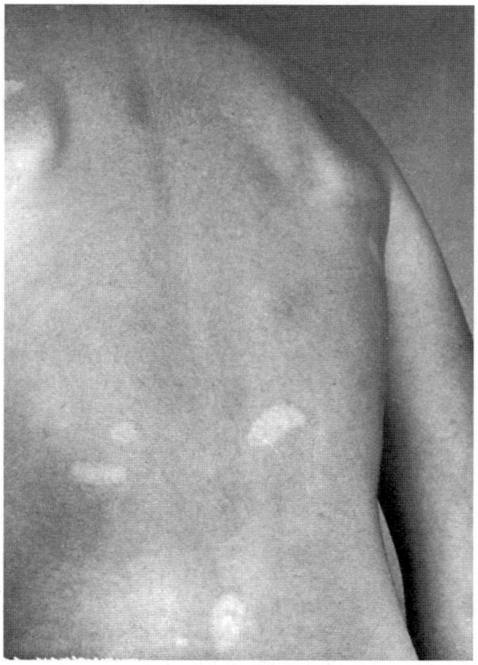

Fig. 65 Typical oval or 'leaf-like' hypopigmented lesions of tuberous sclerosis. They are present at birth.

Treatment involves addressing any associated infection with either topical antifungal preparations or oral antibiotics and antiviral agents.

Tinea unguium (onychomycosis)

See Chapter 7.12.1 for further discussion.

Nail psoriasis

See above 'Psoriasis'

Lichen planus of the nail

See above 'Lichen planus'.

Hair

The hair cycle

Knowledge of the normal hair cycle is fundamental to understanding hair disorders. Hair growth on the scalp is cyclical, with each follicle producing a number of different hairs during a person's lifetime. The anagen growth

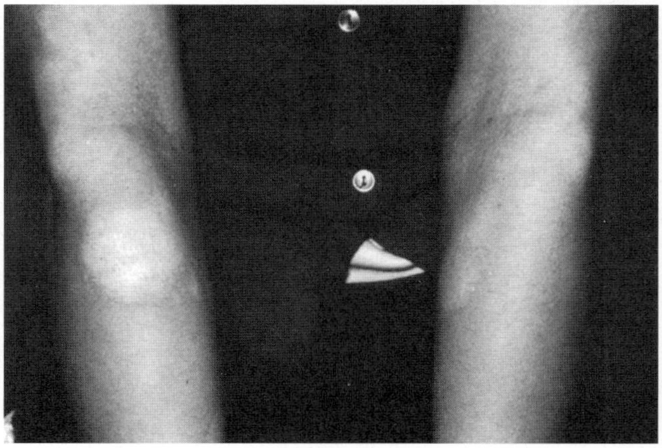

Fig. 64 Pityriasis alba caused by a mild dry eczema. Slightly scaly areas of depigmentation are a common cause of discoloration.

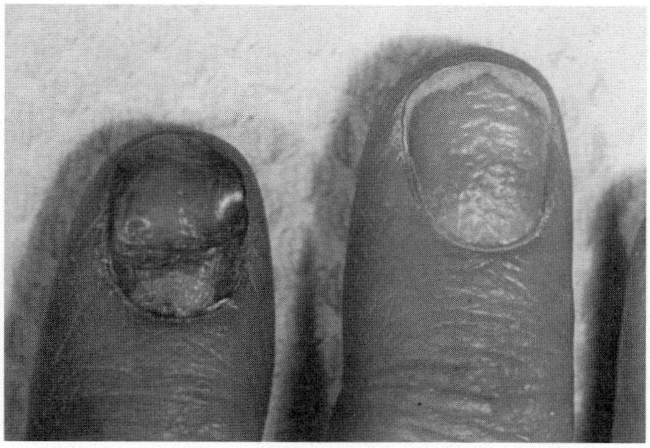

Fig. 66 Pits of the nails are due to very localized accelerations in growth such that the nail keratin is less well knit. Such pits are very common in psoriasis.

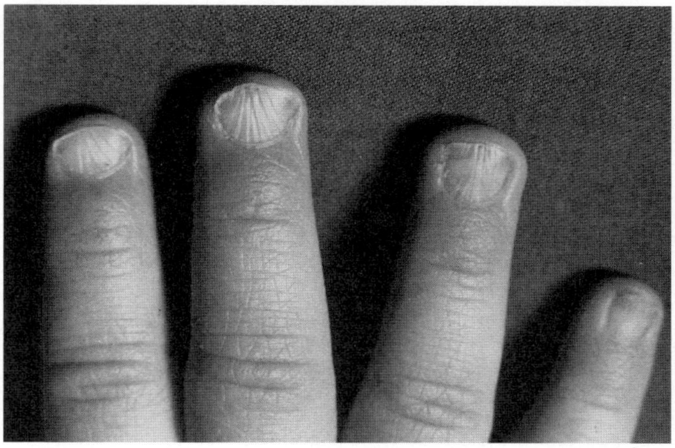

Fig. 67 Longitudinal ridging is usually due to decreased growth, and the nails are often thin and poorly made (idiopathic dystrophy).

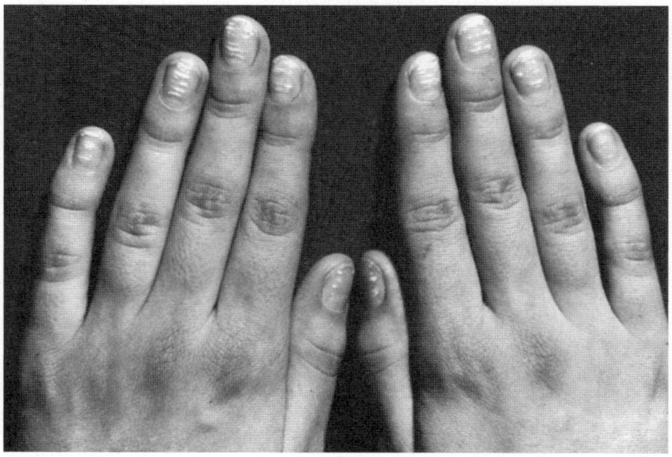

Fig. 68 Transverse white nails, in this case idiopathic, may also indicate arsenical poisoning.

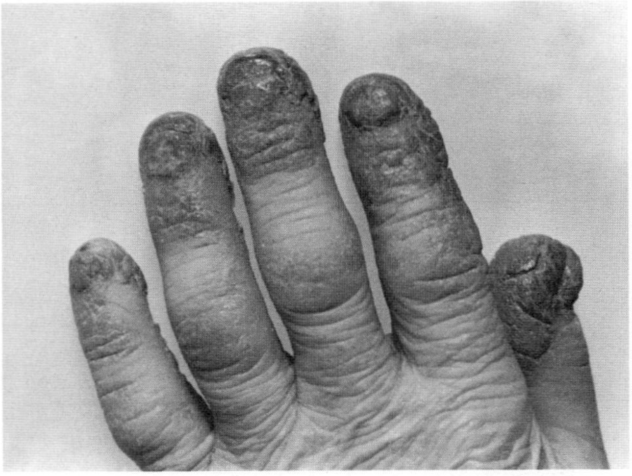

Fig. 69 Severe growth changes of the nail are often a consequence of psoriasis or eczema of the fingertips. The latter may resolve while nail growth disturbance may persist for many months.

phase lasts about 3 to 5 years on the scalp, during this phase hair grows at a rate of approximately 1 cm per month. The duration of anagen varies from person to person and is the prime determinant of how long one's hair will grow if not cut. The length of anagen decreases in androgenetic alopecia on the scalp and increases with hirsutes on the face and body. Lengthening of the eyelashes and eyebrows is seen in AIDS, malnutrition, and in chronic liver disease.

The anagen phase is followed by an involutional stage known as 'catagen', which lasts 2 weeks and leads into a 3-month long dormant phase known as 'telogen'. During telogen the hair remains anchored into the follicle but no longer grows. At the end of telogen the follicle awakens and commences production of the next anagen hair. As the new hair grows it displaces the old telogen hair from the follicle. Thus every 3 to 5 years each of the 100 000 hairs on the scalp is shed and replaced. In animals the growth cycle is synchronized leading to a scheduled moult. In contrast, human hair growth is unsynchronized and so, rather than replacing all scalp hair at the end of the growth cycle, between 50 and 100 hairs are lost every day, most of which go unnoticed.

Examination for other causes of hair loss

The scalp should be examined for evidence of disease such as scaliness, redness, injury, or scarring with its associated loss of follicles (Fig. 70). Severe seborrhoeic eczema, which produces diffuse and excessive dandruff, is often associated with hair thinning. Psoriasis, on the other hand, tends to leave some scalp unaffected and mostly the hair grows well. In very thick plaques, hair may get broken off or its growth is occasionally inhibited. Lichen planus and discoid lupus erythematosus both destroy the hair follicles and, respectively, produce a violaceous or red colour as well as scarring. Tinea capitis (see Fig. 19) is a common cause of hair loss in many parts of the world. The acute, painful, boggy, inflammatory swelling of cattle ringworm, known as kerion, is sometimes mistaken for a bacterial abscess and is inappropriately incised—closer examination would show satellite lesions which are clearly not abscesses. Kerions of the head often heal with scarring and some permanent loss of hair. Equally classic in presentation are groups of children with discoid patches of slightly scaly red areas of broken hairs due to other forms of animal ringworm. Fortunately, most adult scalps are resistant to these fungi, though *Trichophyton tonsurans* infection is on the increase—as are all types of infections—in HIV-positive patients. Tinea capitis is, however, particularly a problem for children. In many parts of the world *T. violaceum* is responsible in black-skinned children, and *M. canis* in white. White scales and scarring in dark heads is often due to favus (a type of tinea capitis). In Africa and the Middle East, favus is due to *T. schoenleinii*. Infection of the scalp with *Streptococcus* spp. or *Staphylococcus* spp. is common in parts of the world where generalized impetigo is common. The scalp may carry a persistent staphylococcus in persons who scratch or pick at their scalp, sometimes known as 'tycoon scalp'. The rash of secondary syphilis often causes a patchy pattern of hair loss scattered over the scalp like numerous 'glades in a wood'. Loss of eyebrows is a feature of lepromatous leprosy (Fig. 71).

Hair pulling (trichotillomania) or twisting with subsequent breaking is a common habit in infants and in people with learning difficulties, or occasionally in those who are psychotic (Fig. 72). It is not always consciously done, and if the hair is then eaten there may be little evidence of where the hairs have disappeared to!

Alopecia areata, alopecia totalis, and alopecia universalis

'Alopecia' is a generic term for hair loss; areata is the plural of area. 'Alopecia areata' is a descriptive term for a disorder characterized by one or more discrete circular areas of hair loss (Fig. 73(a) and (b)) which can

Table 14 Common nail disorders and growth changes (see Fig. 69)

Disorder	Cause
Thickening of the nail plate	tinea, psoriasis, trauma, onychogryphosis, pachyonychia congenita
Thinning of the nail plate (atrophy)	lichen planus, impaired peripheral circulation, twenty-nail dystrophy, wear and tear (repeated immersion in water), artificial fingernails
Abnormal curvature	
koilonychia	juvenile, hereditary, iron deficiency anaemia, haemochromatosis, excessive exposure to solvents, repetitive trauma
clubbing	hereditary, chronic liver disease, chronic suppurative lung disease, congenital hypoxic heart disease, lung cancer and mesothelioma
over curvature	hereditary pincer nail
Lifting of the nail plate (onycholysis)	psoriasis, tinea, trauma, photo-onycholysis
Pitting in the nail plate	psoriasis (Fig. 66), alopecia areata, dermatitis
Grooves in the nail plate	
longitudinal	Heller's median nail dystrophy (Fig. 67), myxoid cyst, angiofibroma, Darier's disease
horizontal	Beau's lines, habit tic, dermatitis (Fig. 68)
Discoloration of the nail plate	
white-striate leuconychia	liver cirrhosis, hypoalbuminaemia
white-longitudinal lines	Darier's disease (Fig. 21) and Hailey Hailey disease
red	splinter haemorrhages, renal failure, congestive cardiac failure
black	haematoma, melanoma, racial pigmentation, naevus, minocycline, cytotoxic drugs
green	pseudomonas infection, aspergillus infection
blue	antimalarial agents, argyria, Wilson's disease
yellow	cigarette smoking, tetracyclines, yellow-nail dystrophy
Swelling of the proximal nail folds(paronychia)	trauma (biting, splits, splinters), manicure (retracting the cuticles), candida infection, staphylococcal infection, herpetic whitlow
Swelling of the lateral nail folds	ingrowing toenails, retinoids, over curvature of the nail plate
Destruction of the nail apparatus	lichen planus, melanoma, Bowen's disease, squamous cell carcinoma, trauma

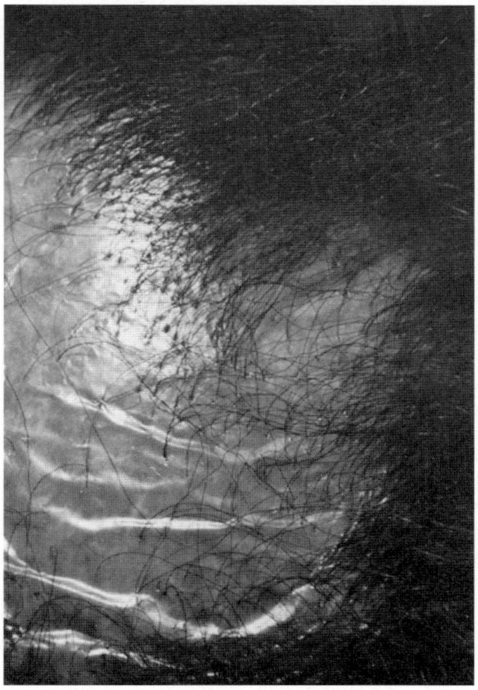

Fig. 70 Scarring is an important prognostic feature because hair loss is irreversible. This pattern of hair loss may be due to a number of chronic inflammatory processes, including lichen planus.

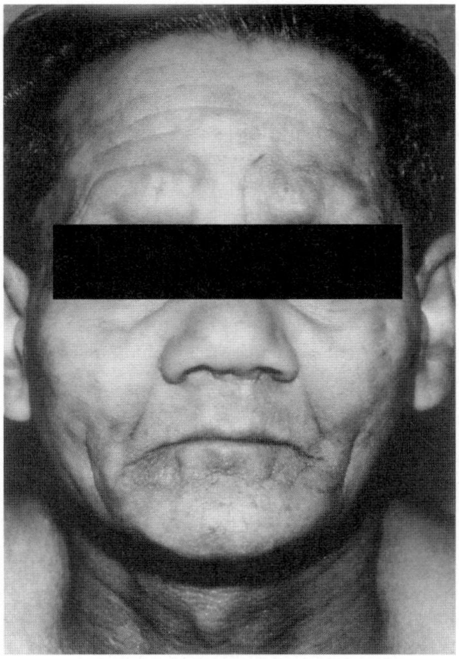

Fig. 71 Loss of eyebrows is a feature of lepromatous leprosy. The skin of the face is thickened but the patient may be unaware of the disease, and for this reason the loss of eyebrows could be the first reason for complaint. Nasal mucosal swelling and erosion is usually obvious.

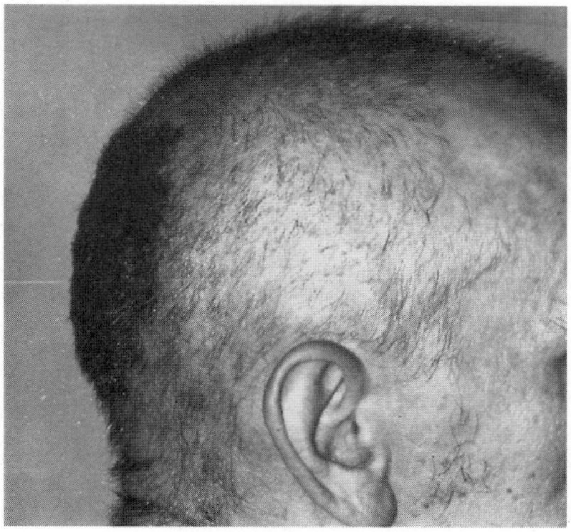

Fig. 72 Trichotillomania, or hair pulling, gives rise to hair loss and the hair length varies because it is broken irregularly. It is a common habit of children, but in the adult it is usually an indication of a personality disorder.

occur anywhere on the body. Alopecia totalis and universalis are variants of alopecia areata, differentiated only by the extent of the hair loss.

Telogen effluvium

Diffuse shedding of telogen hairs from the scalp is common. It occurs when anagen hair growth is interrupted, causing follicular hair production to cease and hairs to enter the telogen rest phase of the hair cycle. The telogen phase lasts 3 months before anagen hair growth is resumed. The new anagen hairs push out the old telogen hairs which are shed *en masse*. An acute telogen effluvium almost invariably occurs after pregnancy and may also follow acute illness, major surgical procedure, a crash diet, or on discontinuing or changing the type of oral contraceptive pill. The shedding occurs 3 months after the trigger and may persist for up to 6 months.

Anagen effluvium

Anagen effluvium is the dramatic and rapid hair loss most commonly seen in association with cancer chemotherapy and radiotherapy to the scalp. Other causes are: high-dose colchicine; thallium, mercury, and arsenic poisoning; and cantharadin. The insult to the hair follicle is sufficiently severe to cause an immediate metabolic arrest with complete cessation of hair production. The hair may come out by the root or, if the insult is brief, the hair shaft will narrow, providing a point of weakness that subsequently snaps off. The follicle may remain in anagen, in which case recovery is quick, or move into telogen, in which case regrowth will be delayed by about 3 months.

Androgenetic alopecia

Androgenetic alopecia is a progressive patterned baldness, which is sufficiently common among both men and women to be considered a secondary sexual phenomenon. It is also called common baldness, male-patterned baldness, and female-patterned alopecia. When it occurs prematurely in a man, it can be an unwanted and distressing event and patients may present for treatment. Among women it is usually both unwanted and unexpected at any age and women commonly present for both diagnosis and treatment.

Hirsutes

While unwanted hair occurs in both men and women, men rarely complain of this to doctors. Unwanted hair in a female or hirsutes is difficult to define objectively due to racial, cultural, and fashion norms. Superfluous hair on a woman in a distribution that mirrors the development of secondary sexual hair in a male is common. Most cases are due to hair-follicle hypersensitivity to normal levels of circulating androgens, while a proportion will be due to elevated levels of circulating androgens. Such patients will usually have other features of systemic androgen excess, such as menstrual irregularity, severe acne, and premature androgenetic alopecia.

Hirsuitism should be distinguished from hypertrichosis (Table 15), which is the widespread overgrowth of non-androgen-dependent hair and that does not respond to antiandrogen therapy. Hypertrichosis may be primary (in which case it is usually apparent prior to puberty) with the hair evenly distributed over the back and limbs. Although prepubertal hypertrichosis is commonly familial, a positive family history is not always found. Secondary causes of hypertrichosis include drugs such as minoxidil, diazoxide, ciclosporin, and phenytoin.

Sweat glands

Apocrine

Apocrine glands occur throughout the skin surface in the embryo, but subsequently disappear to leave just those in the axillas, areolas, and anogenital region in adults. The secretions are formed by the dissolution of apocrine gland cells which are discharged in the hair follicles close to the surface of the skin. They are not active until puberty. Bacterial decomposition accounts for body odour, while the secretions are important in animals for identity and marking out territorial areas. They are also important sexual organs. All such functions are vestigial in man. People sometimes present complaining of body odour. Washing with soap and water is the first phase of management. Deodorants reduce the bacterial flora. Eating garlic and betel nuts should be discouraged since these 'perfumes' are excreted in apocrine sweat. Apocrine sweat is sometimes coloured. If staining is severe and uncontrolled by deodorants, it may be necessary to excise the glands. Retention of apocrine sweat and extreme irritation, known as Fox–Fordyce disease, is similar to prickly heat. Treatment may include the use of topical steroids, destruction with cryotherapy, or excision.

Table 15 Hypertrichosis

Malnutrition	
Anorexia nervosa	
Early	
	Dermatomyositis and scleroderma
	Cutaneous porphyria
	Drugs: diazoxide, minoxidil, phenytoin corticosteroids, ciclosporin
	Various congenital diseases
	Hypertrichosis lanuginosa, either congenital or malignant
Local	
	Congenital pigmented naevi
	Spina bifida: faun tail
	Lichen simplex
	Localized chronic inflammation
	The eye lashes in AIDS
Endocrine causes of generalized hirsutism	
	Polycystic ovary syndrome
	Idiopathic
	Cushing's syndrome
	Congenital adrenal hyperplasia
	Androgen-secreting tumours
	Hypothyroidism
	Acromegaly

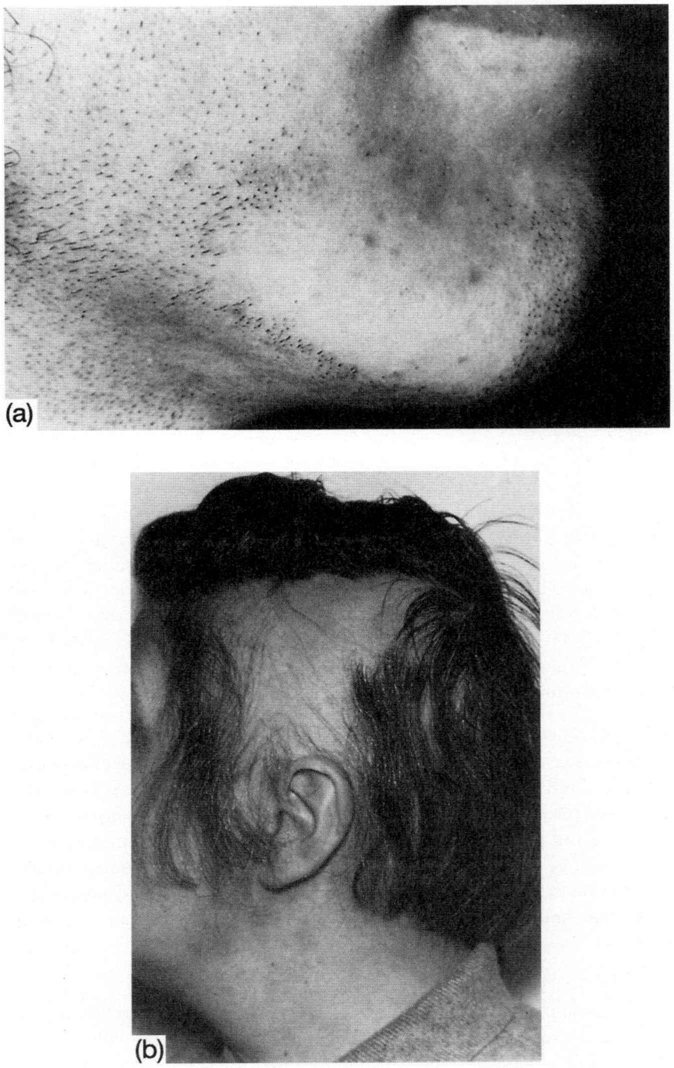

Fig. 73 (a) Alopecia areata is characterized by abortive hair growth and the formation of a short, stubby, 'exclamation mark' hair at the edge of the area of hair loss. (b) Alopecia of the temple or occiput has a poorer prognosis for regrowth.

Hydradenitis suppurativa

This is a relatively common and often misdiagnosed condition of the skin characterized by boils, pimples, sinus formation, and comedones (Fig. 74) in the axilla, groin, and submammary areas. It is also known as apocrine acne, as these are the sites of apocrine glands. The lesions often heal with scarring, which may be pitted and cribriform. It may occur alone or in association with severe cystic acne of the trunk, pilonidal sinus, and dissecting cellulitis of the scalp, which are all part of the follicular occlusion tetrad. Dissecting cellulitis of the scalp is a severe folliculitis rather than a true bacterial cellulitis. Hydradenitis suppurativa is very commonly associated with obesity, and may be seen in women along with other features of androgen excess.

Boils should be treated as they develop and prophylaxis given to guard against the development of new lesions. However, there is considerable person-to-person variation in the severity and frequency of the development of the boils, which will determine the need for prophylaxis. Boils may be incised and drained or injected with steroid as they tend to be inflammatory rather than infective, although a short course of oral antibiotics may be indicated based on the results of culture and sensitivity testing. Antibiotic prophylaxis is modelled on the principles of acne therapy. However, because antibiotic resistance does seem to be a problem, they are generally rotated every 4 to 6 months to prevent the emergence of resistance. Those antibiotics shown to be effective include minocycline, co-trimoxazole, metronidazole, erythromycin, tetracycline, cefalexin, and clindamycin. Other therapies that can be used for resistant cases include cyproterone acetate, spironolactone, and isotretinoin. If these treatments are unsuccessful, wide

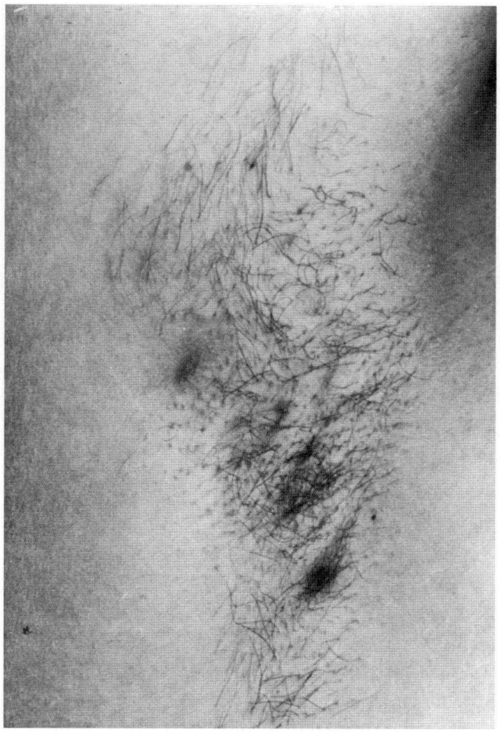

Fig. 74 Axilla showing dusky or violaceous erythema overlying cystic 'blind' boils. The follicular prominence and comedone formation is characteristic of early hydradenitis.

surgical excision or liposuction (which disrupts the glands) may be considered.

Eccrine

Humans possess about 3 to 4 million sweat glands, equivalent in weight to one kidney. The secretory coil produces a plasma-like fluid, which can be secreted at a maximum rate of 2 to 3 l/h. Sodium is reabsorbed in the sweat duct.

While eccrine sweat glands occur in all areas, those in the hands, feet, axillas, and face frequently sweat profusely in the absence of general sweating. Humans rely on evaporation rather than insulation or panting for protection against a hot environment. Generalized sweating occurs when the body temperature rises and is a feature of fever as well as thermoregulation in a warm climate, and when the metabolic rate is increased, as in exercise or thyrotoxicosis.

Eccrine sweat glands are largely innervated by unique postganglionic sympathetic fibres that release acetylcholine at the neuroglandular junction. The control centre is located in the hypothalamus. It is important to consider whether the sweating is appropriate for the degree of stimulus (Table 16).

Emotional- or anxiety-induced sweating is commonly inappropriate for the degree of anxiety. Many teenagers complain of sweaty hands and feet as well as the smell resulting from the bacterial breakdown of skin and clothing. The fear of being unwelcome increases their anxiety and subsequent sweating. It may summate with thermoregulatory sweating and therefore be worse in hot weather or at a dance. Winter clothing is often more troublesome than the loose garments of summer. Sweating of the hands and feet occurs with acrocyanosis and with some forms of keratoderma.

Segmental, unilateral sweating is often due to irritating lesions of the spine and requires a neurological opinion.

Excessive sweating (hyperhidrosis) contributes to tinea pedis and to eczema from footwear.

Table 16 Causes of hyperhidrosis

Hot weather or room
Exercise
Fever: infection or pyrogen
Fear, anxiety, lie detectors
Thyrotoxicosis, acromegaly, diabetes mellitus
Lymphoma
Cancer
Hypoglycaemia; alcohol intoxication
Nausea
Gustatory
Neurological lesions of the sympathetic nervous system, cortex, basal ganglia, or spinal cord

Treatment of hyperhidrosis

A sympathetic listener is helpful, as is simple advice on hygiene, washing, keeping cool, and appropriate clothing. Basic points of management include the avoidance of obesity, relaxation exercises are helpful if the patient is unduly self-conscious. Cotton-fibre clothing, for example, is more appropriate than non-absorbent fibres. Many shoes, including their linings, are now made from materials that prevent the absorption of sweat and keep the foot and sock wet. Frequent changes of socks prevents bacterial overgrowth, and wearing leather shoes or sandals reduces discomfort. Tranquillizers are sometimes helpful and propantheline, 15 mg every few hours, may be of benefit or can be reserved for a social occasion. The abolition of sweating carries a risk of hyperthermia.

Hypohidrosis

This occurs in the newborn and in premature children during the first month of life, and is also seen in infants as a result of sweat-duct occlusion, especially in the flexures of skin folds on the neck. It may also result from exfoliative dermatitis or erythroderma and is a feature of hypohidrotic ectodermal dysplasia (see Chapter 23.2). Such patients are usually male and are susceptible to heat stroke, and therefore early diagnosis of the affected baby in a hot climate is important. Absence of sweating causes loss of skin moisturization and impaired grip. Examination of the palmar surface of the fingers with a magnifying lens will show the absence of duct orifices.

Miliaria, prickly heat

Miliaria crystallina is a superficial obstruction of sweat glands, producing clear vesicles. This may occur when more sweat is produced by the glands than the ducts can absorb. Miliaria is commonly seen in patients with high fever. Deeper obstruction gives rise to red, itchy papules known as prickly heat. Around one in three people exposed to hot climates are affected; while prickly heat sometimes begins within a few days of arrival in hot climes, it is commonly a problem 2 to 6 months later. Occlusion of the skin by impermeable clothing aggravates the condition. Bacteria may play some part in its generation and in the complication of staphylococcal abscesses. It is a contributory factor to extreme thermal stress in unacclimatized people. This is also a feature in people working in hot industries around furnaces or in underground mines. Relief from sweating even for a few hours is essential. Loose, non-occlusive clothing and exposure of the skin folds as much as possible is beneficial. Vitamin C (1 g daily) was advocated by dermatologists in the British Army in Malaysia. It is important to realize that severe hypohidrosis of the trunk and limbs may be missed as a cause of asthenia if the face is sweating. The small particles of powder in calamine shake lotions promote cooling by increasing the surface area. A localized loss of sweating ability may be due to tuberculoid leprosy, syringomyelia, and diabetes mellitus.

Skin disorders affecting the genitalia

A diagnosis of disorders affecting the genitalia cannot be made without looking. Natural shyness on the part of the patient or lack of zeal on the part of the doctor are common. Racial and religious grounds for incomplete examination must be overcome by appropriate selection of the examiner and chaperone, as well as an interpreter.

It may be inappropriate to delve into the sexual, gynaecological, or medical history of the patient, and so initial questioning may be limited until an examination has indicated the nature of the disease. A contact dermatitis may require the most detailed and searching questioning.

Many skin conditions of the vulva or penis can be best diagnosed by examining the rest of the skin. For example the knees, scalp, and elbows in psoriasis, the front of the wrists and shins in lichen planus, the mouth in pemphigus, or the neck, breasts, and wrists in lichen sclerosis et atrophicus.

Infections

Infections are commonly transmitted by sexual intercourse and tend to be associated with vaginal or urinary meatal symptoms (see Chapter 21.7).

The pubic region is commonly affected by nits and crab lice, and viral molluscum contagiosum causes smooth, pearly, umbilicated papules (see Fig. 111).

Genital warts

See Chapter 7.10.18 for further discussion.

Candidiasis

See Chapters 7.11.1 and 21.4 for further discussion.

Herpes simplex

See Chapter 7.10.2 for further discussion.

Adult intertrigo

Obesity and sweating predispose to mixed irritation and infection in the occluded skin under the breasts and in the axillas and groins. The affected area is moist, red, fissured, and malodorous. Attempts at keeping the site dry and free of excessive infection have been improved by preparations such as miconazole and hydrocortisone, and ZeaSORB® powder which acts as a drying agent without too much caking. Washing and gentle drying is the most important therapy. Blind boils and comedones are likely to be due to hidradenitis suppuritiva.

Psoriasis in the flexures is usually well defined, bright red, and, unlike at other sites, is non-scaly. It is worth treating initially for 3 days with a strong steroid because this sometimes clears the psoriasis. More often the lesions persist, in which case strong steroids are then harmful since they cause so much atrophy. Hydrocortisone can be used but is only mildly effective. It is important to protect the skin from excessive infection by regular washing.

Dermatitis of the genitalia is commonly due to contact with the agents listed in Table 17, some of which are added to the bath and inadequately mixed with the water. Certain deodorant sprays may cause a considerable immediate contact swelling. Mixed-type infections may contribute to the problem. Persistent pruritus and scratching is a very common disorder, producing thickening of the skin and a range of colours from white-fissured areas to pigmented and violaceous plaques.

Table 17 Causes of contact dermatitis affecting the genitalia

Antiseptics
Fungicides
Ethylene diamine (usually in Tri-Adcortyl®)
Neomycin
Rubber dermatitis (condoms)
Hexachlorophane
Allergens carried on hands (usually also affect eyelids)
Perfumes, antiseptics in soaps and sprays
Wood dusts, oils, fibreglass; irritants according to occupation

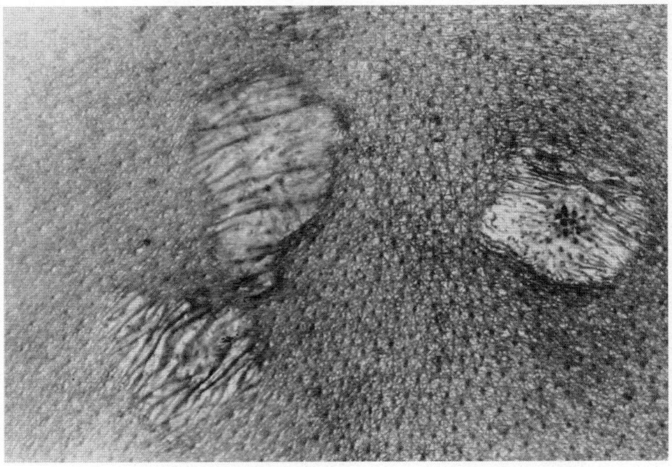

Fig. 75 Lichen sclerosis causes tissue-paper-like crinkling or atrophy of the skin. The border is often violaceous but the centre of the lesion is white.

In uncircumcised adult males a persistent reddish brown, somewhat fixed balanitis, is heavily infiltrated with plasma cells. This benign condition, known as Zoon's balanitis, is cured by circumcision.

Leucoplakia versus the atrophy of lichen sclerosus et atrophicus

This is often confusing, since it is possible for the skin of the genitalia to be thinned but nevertheless to be covered by a thickened scale. The lesion of lichen sclerosus is well defined (Fig. 75), white, and may have a violaceous border. Small haemorrhagic blisters are common, especially in children, and should not be mistaken for sexual abuse. The perianal areas are always involved, especially in children (Fig. 76). Intractable itching, burning, or soreness of the perineum or genitalia is unfortunately common. In young women it usually slowly improves; in older persons it persists. Lichen sclerosus et atrophicus responds well to high-potency local steroids.

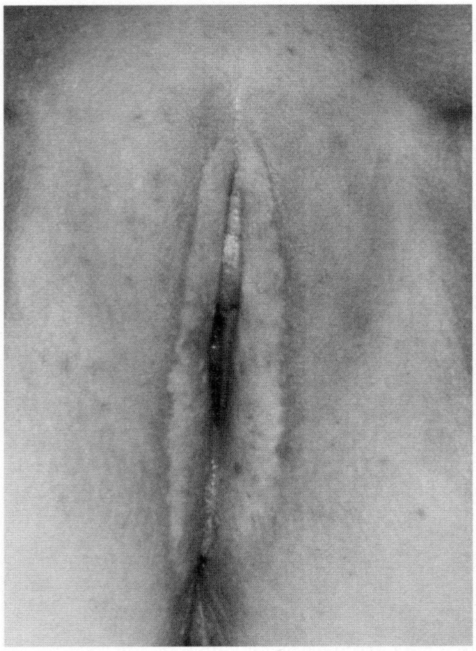

Fig. 76 Lichen sclerosis of the vulva in a child tends to clear at puberty. In the elderly it is a persistent cause of irritation.

Histologically, lichen sclerosus et atrophicus is characterized by an extremely thin epidermis with a thickened scale and an acellular homogenized upper dermis. By contrast, leucoplakia and lichen simplex are composed of a greatly hypertrophied epidermis and usually thickening of the underlying dermis as well. A biopsy should be performed where there is diagnostic doubt, but leucoplakia and lichen sclerosus may coexist in as many as 24 per cent of patients. Although lichen sclerosus et atrophicus, especially when damaged by scratching, may develop a squamous-cell epithelioma, there is no advantage nor relief of discomfort by prospective vulvectomy.

In the case of leucoplakia, vulvectomy is usually advocated as there is much greater chance of the development of a squamous epithelioma. However, since the skin is predisposed to lichen sclerosus in areas well beyond the genitocrural folds, simple vulvectomy is not a satisfactory treatment for lichen sclerosus itself. Attention to hygiene is important, as is exclusion of mixed infections or contact dermatitis. Rarely, perineal discomfort and eczema may be due to vitamin B_2 deficiency. The main treatment of lichen sclerosus is with strong topical steroids.

Well-defined asymmetrical plaques of red pigmented skin should be biopsied to exclude intraepidermal carcinoma to which this site is predisposed.

The term 'kraurosis vulvae' is now obsolete since it does not differentiate senile atrophy from the now well-recognized lichen sclerosus.

Urticaria

Urticaria is a transient swelling and/or flushing of the skin. The underlying vasodilatation and accumulation of tissue fluid in the dermis is due to a succession of inflammatory mediators acting mainly on the small blood vessels. The time taken to bring their effects under control varies, and thus the inflammatory response varies from the very transient to a more persistent inflammation overlapping with vasculitis.

The knowledge that histamine plays a part in immediate-type (anaphylactic) hypersensitivity has led to the widespread misconception that all urticaria must be allergic. A non-immunological pharmacological explanation is more likely in most cases.

Immunology

Allergens of the type commonly incriminated in sufferers from atopic disease bind to IgE antibodies attached to the surface of mast cells or basophils, these cells then release various mediators including histamine, serotonin (5-hydroxytryptamine), and the slow-reacting substance (leucotriene) of anaphylaxis. Such allergens include egg white, cows' milk, house dust, dandruff, feathers, and tomatoes. It is commonly a contact-type reaction, affecting the lips during eating or some other parts of the skin when in contact with animals or house dust. Transfusion reactions and some drug rashes are due to complement-fixing antibodies attached to blood cells.

The urticaria of serum sickness, penicillin reactions, the acute illness of systemic lupus erythematosus, and many infectious diseases are partly due to immune complexes of immunoglobulins and allergen with subsequent complement activation.

Complement activation

Although complement is activated by immunological reactions, it is also activated enzymatically by proteases (such as plasmin) when there are insufficient natural inhibitors of this mediator in the serum and tissues. Congenital or acquired deficiencies in inhibitor levels account for some forms of angioedema, and for hereditary angioedema in particular. The activation of complement by the alternative pathway may explain the aetiology of some non-familial cases.

Histamine liberators

Some drugs and foods release histamine from mast cells, or at least make such release more likely by inhibiting controlling factors: inhibition of prostaglandin activity may be one such mechanism. Examples of mast-cell stimulators include morphine, codeine, thiamine, polymyxin, and D-tubocurarine. Bee venom, strawberries, and shellfish as well as aspirin, salicylates, benzoates, and tartrazine are enhancers of an urticarial tendency, bringing it to the fore in susceptible subjects as well as occasionally initiating the eruption.

Genetic factors

Familial urticaria is a well-recognized phenomenon. There are reports of hereditary angioedema affecting many members of large families. In this condition the angioedema occurs without associated urticaria. The autosomal dominant pattern of inheritance is mediated through an absence of the C_1-esterase inhibitor. Familial cold urticaria is another autosomal dominant disease, and has been described in several families in the United States, France, and The Netherlands. A low level of chymotrypsin inhibitors was detected in one family. Studies of HLA antigens have been rewarding. BW35 has been associated with acute ordinary urticaria, while HLA-B1*04 (DR4) and its associated allele, DQB1*0302 (DQ8), are raised in patients with chronic idiopathic urticaria compared with a control population.

Careful studies have incriminated candidiasis, though it is not so important a factor in the experience of the majority of practitioners.

Types of urticaria

Variations are observed in the number, size, and depth of weals, as well as in the sensation experienced by the patient. Moreover, the lesions vary in their degree of persistence. Such features allow the classification of different types of urticaria, but there is considerable overlap in their aetiology and pathogenesis.

Only a minority of cases are due to an early, avoidable, and identifiable cause. Although some are due to autoantibodies, non-immunological pharmacological causation is not rare. The majority remain of unknown aetiology.

Contact urticaria

This is a weal-and-flare reaction lasting for 20 to 40 min after the application of certain agents to the skin. Some reactions may be IgE-mediated, such as those produced by animal dander, saliva, or seminal fluid, but most are probably non-immunological, as with the nettle or jellyfish sting, or the solar or aquagenic varieties of urticaria. Often there is a consequent or associated dermatitis, as in atopic eczema. Many of the ointments used to treat dermatitis contain bases such as sorbic acid or polyethylene glycol which cause immediate stinging and a slight swelling.

Cholinergic urticaria

Cholinergic urticaria is characterized by numerous, superficial, small swellings that sting, smart, or itch and are surrounded by a blush lasting for only a few minutes (Fig. 77). The cause is unknown. The commonest pattern is found in adolescents and young adults and, like blushing, is brought on by emotion, exercise, and hot baths.

Heat urticaria

This is a rare local response to heat in which histamine is released or complement activated.

Angio-oedema

A few, deep, large swellings, which may be tender and often itchy, sometimes preceded by redness, lasting several hours or even days are characteristic. Proteases such as complement, plasmin, and kinins are incriminated.

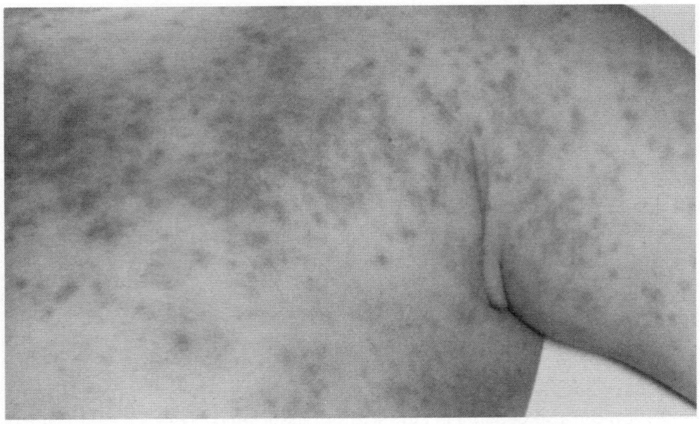

Fig. 77 Cholinergic urticaria is like blushing brought on by emotion, exercise, and heat. It is transient, lasting no more than about 15 min, and may be associated with small, superficial weals with a prominent flush. These tend to sting rather than itch.

Ordinary urticaria or hives

This is characterized by numerous weals of all sizes, and varying degrees of pallor or redness, which itch and last for one or more hours, but not usually for more than a day. Successive lesions may account for long illness: chronic urticaria is arbitrarily defined as continuous or recurrent lesions of more than 3 months' duration. Histamine is the principal mediator. Current evidence supports the view that skin blood vessels have both H_1 and H_2 receptors.

Time of onset

Cholinergic urticaria (see above) develops abruptly and instantaneously within minutes of the triggering event. Ordinary urticaria also develops within minutes of the release of the mediator. However, foodstuffs and certain allergens, or drugs such as aspirin, have to be digested and absorbed before the mediators are released. Ordinary urticaria is often difficult to relate to events in the patient's life for this reason. Delayed onset is a well-recognized phenomenon of some of the physical urticarias (see below). Thus delayed dermographism is the development of redness and slight wealing occurring several hours after scratching the skin. Delayed-pressure urticaria is a tender swelling appearing 2 to 12 h after localized pressure injury to the skin. It is possible that the insult localizes noxious agents such as soluble immune complexes, or that mechanisms such as transient ischaemia and the release of proteases bring to light homeostatic defects (for instance, a deficiency of inhibitors of complement or other proteases).

Physical urticaria

Several types of urticarial eruptions are only caused by specific physical insults: for example, from sunlight, cold, heat, pressure, scratch, or stretch.

Solar urticaria is uncommon. A weal develops within 30 s to 3 min of exposure to the sun; however, tolerance may develop in such habitually exposed sites as the hands and feet. The differential diagnosis of porphyria, lupus erythematosus, or photosensitivity following drug ingestion has to be considered, in which case the urticaria is more persistent, and because the longer, more penetrating ultraviolet rays are responsible, it can occur even on a cloudy day or when the skin is protected by glass, clothing, or sunscreens.

Familial cold urticaria is an autosomal dominant disease, usually presenting in infancy, in which the rash develops up to several hours after exposure to, for example, cold winds. Fever and joint pains accompany the rash and there is a leucocytosis. Low levels of a chymotrypsin inhibitor have been demonstrated. It may not be induced by the application of ice to the skin.

Acquired cold urticaria is the most common form of cold urticaria and occurs within a few minutes of plunging into cold water or after applying ice to the skin; this is one cause of sudden death in young people plunging into ice-cold water. Mast-cell degranulatation is a feature.

Papular urticaria

This is the only form of urticaria to have a persistent epidermal component. Most often papular urticaria is caused by insect bites. The epidermis is either damaged directly or by mediators in the upper dermis which evoke an eczematous response, so that oedema of the epidermis and a proliferative repair effect results in a typical itchy and persistent papule. Such lesions are usually excoriated, whereas most urticarias are not deeply scratched but merely rubbed. They often blister (see Fig. 90).

Scaling is not a feature of urticaria. While acute dermatitis and some erythema initially appear to be urticarial in nature, the development of scaling immediately excludes such diagnoses.

Distribution of the rash

Cholinergic urticaria favours the head and upper trunk. Angio-oedema most commonly involves mucocutaneous junctions such as the lips, eyes, and penis. The physical urticarias clearly relate to sites of exposure; solar urticaria affects the face and the dorsum of the hands, or, if tolerance has developed, at sites exposed for the first time during the summer. Pressure urticaria favours the soles of the feet when walking or digging, or the backs of the thighs or lumbar region when sitting.

Bizarre patterns

Evolving and resolving urticaria inevitably exhibits a changing morphology. The redness of the vasodilatation merges with the veiling pallor of the oedema. Healing in the centre and peripheral spread often produces bizarre gyrate or circinate and serpiginous patterns, but they are transient and never scaly, unlike similar patterns in the erythemas or epidermal diseases such as psoriasis.

Investigations

History-taking is the most effective investigation of urticaria. It is important to establish whether there is urticaria and angioedema, or angioedema alone. In simple cases, the individual weals last for less than 24 h. Persistence beyond 24 h, and in particular resolution with bruising, is highly suggestive of urticarial vasculitis and justifies a biopsy. The chronicity of the urticaria is also important. Acute urticaria lasts less than 6 weeks and investigations are not required, a drug and dietary history generally suffice. If the lesions have been appearing for more than 6 weeks, further questioning is important, and some investigations may be considered. Trigger factors should be specifically asked for to detect the physical urticarias.

Exercise or a hot bath reproduces the lesions of cholinergic urticaria. Intradermal histamine, 1 μg in 0.1 ml saline, produces a weal that should disappear within 1 h. This disappearance is delayed in pressure urticaria and in immune-complex disease. Localization of a noxious agent results in a persistent lesion. In practice, avoidance of cause can be advised only if this is recognized after taking a history and examining the patient. The two most helpful investigations are a full blood count and the erythrocyte sedimentation rate (ESR). An eosinophilia should alert one to parasites such as microfilaria or trichiniasis, while a raised ESR is due to a systemic illness such as sepsis, malignancy, or 'collagen' disease.

Rubbing or scratching the skin with a fingernail produces a weal and flare in the dermographic subject within 5 min. A 4- to 6-kg weight hung for 10 min over the shoulder on a bandage or belt causing a tender swelling 2 to 8 h later, reveals delayed-pressure urticaria. A biopsy at this stage for immunofluorescence studies may confirm the localization of immune complexes. The white cell count at the time of the biopsy may show neutrophilia, especially if there is accompanying fever. A reduction of serum C_1-esterase inhibitor should be looked for in patients with angio-oedema, especially if initiated by minor surgery, associated with abdominal pains, and if other members of the family affected. Complement levels are not a reliable guide to the participation of proteases and hardly influence the management of urticaria.

Chronic urticaria is a known symptom of filariasis and strongyloidosis, but in ascariasis and enterobiasis it occurs, if anything, more often in controls. Urticaria is such a difficult disease to assess that possible aetiological factors, such as parasitic disease, are worth treating in their own right rather than in the expectation of resolution of the eruption.

About 25 per cent of cases of acute hepatitis B present with urticaria.

Foci of infection as a cause of urticaria are statistically difficult to support, but dental and sinus infections continue to be described as aetiological factors based on impressive case histories.

Bee stings

See Chapter 8.2 for further discussion.

When should urticaria be taken more seriously?

Urticaria is life-threatening when it is part of anaphylaxis, when angio-oedema involves the upper respiratory tract, or when it is part of a systemic immune-complex disease and is associated with more dire pathology such as meningococcal septicaemia or lupus erythematosus. The latter type of urticaria is recognized by its more persistent lesion, lasting at least 1 to 2 days, and often tender and ultimately purpuric. It should be remembered that all acute urticaria may be very widespread and be accompanied by joint pains, stomach aches, and fever. However, if the individual lesion lasts for only a few hours it is less likely to be due to a noxious circulating trigger such as an immune complex or infective organisms.

Management

Removal of the known physical factor and the known trigger is helpful, but no cause is found in the majority of adult cases of chronic urticaria. Insect repellents and topical steroids play some part in the management of papular urticaria. Elimination diets require the exclusion of suspected foods for at least a week, followed by their reintroduction for a week; this cycle should be repeated at least three times to be confident of a real effect, which, however, is convincing in only about 5 per cent of patients with urticaria. Functional autoantibodies against the high-affinity IgE receptor (FcεRI), or less commonly IgE, have been demonstrated by autologous-serum skin testing and *in vitro* histamine release from basophils, and Western blotting and an enzyme-linked immunosorbent assay (**ELISA**), in over 30 per cent of patients with chronic 'idiopathic' urticaria. It may respond to immunotherapy. Some European centres rely on studies of the gastrointestinal tract to reveal the presence of *Candida albicans*, *Campylobacter* spp., and other infections as possible causes of urticaria. Food, medicines, and infectious or parasitic diseases are the commonest suspected factors. However, in Europe and the United States physical urticaria accounts for more than half of the patients in some series. Cold, heat, and solar urticaria often respond to the induction of tolerance by subthreshold desensitization. It is useful to try different antihistamines because of much individual variation response and in their side-effects. Antihistamines are often prescribed in too low a dosage to be effective, and patients should be encouraged to rest at home taking a rather higher dosage. The evidence that skin blood vessels possess both H_1- and H_2-receptors has encouraged trials with a combination of their antagonists. At present, the financial cost and large number of pills that have to be taken every day is a disadvantage. Most H_1-antihistamines are cheap and free of serious side-effects. Drowsiness is often troublesome, but the variations in response are considerable. Otherwise, they are effective in the majority of patients, providing they are taken regularly to prevent the urticaria rather than to treat the existing weals. Long-acting antihistamines are worth trying when short-acting ones fail. Although the value of combined H_1- and H_2-blockers (4 mg cyproheptadine and 300 mg cimetidine, four times daily) remains unproven, like all regimens it has resulted in some individual successes. Hydroxyzine (10–25 mg, three times a day) or cetirizine 10 mg, once or twice a day, is often effective in treating dermographism or cholinergic urticaria. Nifedipine in conjunction with antihistamines has its advocates. Avoidance of known urticaria triggers, such as aspirin, tartrazine, benzoate, and other salicylates, often requires a rather complex diet. Prednisolone should be reserved for a few days' treatment for severe acute urticaria or exacerbation of chronic urticaria.

For impending upper respiratory obstruction, adrenaline (epinephrine) 1/1000, 0.5 ml (adult dose), is first given intramuscularly and hydrocortisone 100 mg intravenously. Such an acute emergency requires maintenance of the airway, if necessary by intubation or tracheotomy, and the administration of oxygen.

Management of autosomal dominant hereditary angio-oedema

This should be suspected if there is a family history of angio-oedema or a few long-lasting swellings precipitated by trauma. Signs include a transient erythema followed by the oedema, and a recurring colicky abdominal pain is often a feature. The diagnosis should be confirmed by looking for low serum levels of functional α-neuroaminoglycoprotein, C_1-esterase inhibitor (normal 18 ± 5 mg/100 ml, although levels vary).

Prophylaxis includes care to protect against trauma, especially in the region of the mouth and neck after dental manoeuvres. Danazol or stanazolol prophylaxis may be appropriate if episodes are frequent. Methyltestosterone, 10 mg as linguets after breakfast and another when there is a suspicion of developing oedema, often aborts attacks. Fresh plasma, containing C_1-esterase, may be given before surgery or at the initiation of an attack. Unlike other forms of chronic urticaria, adrenaline (epinephrine), antihistamines, and corticosteroids are of only little benefit. Intravenous Trasylol is an inhibitor of proteases and is sometimes helpful, as is epsilon-aminocaproic acid (**EACA**) 12 to 18 g daily in divided dosage. The most effective treatment is danazol, which may be supplemented by fresh plasma during an attack or, if available, a C_1-esterase inhibitor concentrate.

Cutaneous vasculitis

The broadest definition of vasculitis is 'the response of small blood vessels to injury'. No other definition encompasses its great variety, which ranges from a transient increase in permeability or wealing, to coagulation and necrosis of the vessel wall. It is caused by agents such as immune complexes, toxins, or by physical stimuli such as cold and heat, as well as impaired perfusion.

The term 'vasculitis' includes many diseases described elsewhere in this book, such as Henoch–Schönlein purpura, polyarteritis nodosa, nodular vasculitis, Wegener's granulomatosis, hypersensitivity angiitis, and allergic granulomatosis. Examples of diseases sometimes included within this term are Behçet's syndrome, pyoderma gangrenosum, purpura fulminans, thromboangiitis obliterans, erythema nodosum, chilblains, atrophie blanche, and livedo reticularis.

Vasculitis overlaps with urticaria and with infarction or gangrene. To use some of the older terminology, some authors have described urticaria as the predominant feature of Henoch–Schönlein purpura in children, and a number of vasculitic syndromes have more recently been described in which urticaria is the only skin manifestation. At the other end of the spectrum, 'necrotizing angiitis' and 'polyarteritis nodosa' are labels often given to infarctive or more destructive patterns of vasculitis.

The physical signs of the skin disease are more or less recognizable as distinct patterns. The names they have been given are of dubious value when it comes to managing the disease. It is possible to explain these patterns and to decide what aspects of the physical signs are the most useful clues to pathogenesis.

Pathology and nomenclature

When a vessel is injured a response ensues which removes or neutralizes the cause of the injury, followed by repair. The response depends on the intensity of the injury, on the efficiency of the inflammation, and on the rate and

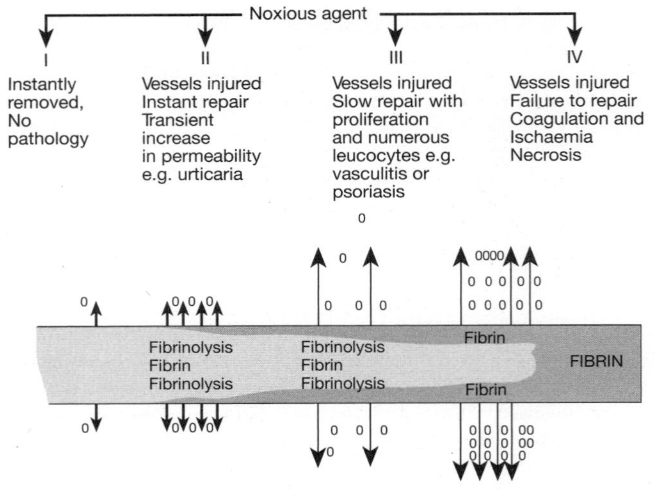

Fig. 78 A spectrum of inflammatory events ranging from a transient wealing, or almost physiological permeability through inflammatory neutrophilic infiltration and oedema, to complete necrosis of the vessel, due to thrombosis, and coagulation or destruction of its wall.

effectiveness of the repair. Herein lies one of the main reasons why a particular injury does not always produce the same rash. The inflammatory response is a very complex sequence of events (Fig. 78), subject to considerable modification by each individual's particular range of mediators. Important factors explaining variability are local-tissue architecture and previous disease experience, such as scarring or even temporary exhaustion of mediators by prior injury. Formerly, authors used to describe sites of lowered resistance. We now know that such sites comprise areas of non-homogeneous blood supply with hypoxia, leakiness, and blood stasis, as well as exhausted mast cells and endothelial cells undergoing various stages of repair, or upgrading of cell-wall adhesion factors for white cells. Paralysis of the mononuclear phagocytic system is also important.

This variation in the inflammatory response can be superficial or deep, and is modified by the distribution of the injury—gravitational, light-exposed, cold-exposed, or at sites of pressure or abrasion; this is one explanation of the physical signs that make up classifiable rashes. A rash with urticarial, purpuric, nodular, pigmented, and necrotic lesions is better not given an eponymous name to any particular combination of physical signs.

Another reason for the later delineation of different syndromes such as Behçet's triad, cutaneous polyarteritis nodosa, or limited Wegener's granulomatosis was the recognition that vasculitis may be confined to either one or more organs. But this, too, is of dubious value: Behçet described mouth, eye, and genital lesions, but the disease is often more widespread; Wegener's granulomatosis affects the respiratory tract but the skin and kidneys are also frequently affected.

One other point of debate is the value of the term 'arteritis'. Smooth muscle in the arterial wall is damaged by ischaemia, which, in most small vessels, is attributable to vasoconstriction, coagulation, and thrombosis, or to obstructed flow due to a more distal vasculitis. Thus 'malignant hypertension', 'coagulation', 'embolism' (Fig. 79), 'thrombotic thrombocytopenia', or 'vasculitis' are often sufficiently appropriate diagnostic terms and are more helpful when considering prognosis, aetiology, or management. The histological diagnosis of arteritis is similarly unsatisfactory. Damaged venules can themselves look like small arteries; even when an artery is clearly involved, it is rarely possible in the same section to see the more distal vasculitis responsible for the obstruction to blood flow and consequent ischaemia.

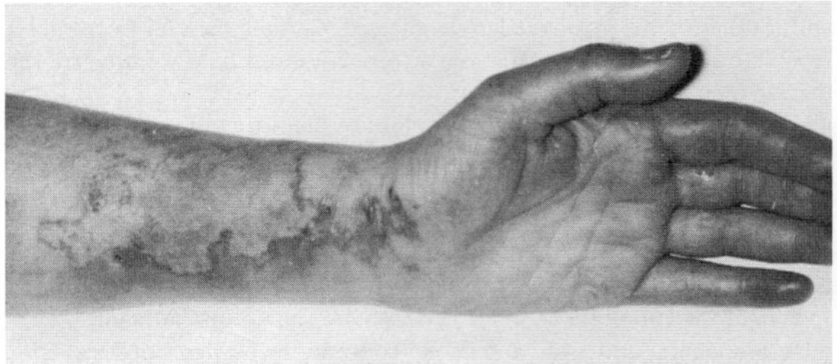

Fig. 79 The white infarct characteristic of embolization or arterial block. Most cutaneous vasculitis labelled as 'arteritis' is, in fact, venular, but the white infarct is characteristic of arterial occlusion.

Harmful agents responsible for vasculitis

Immune complexes, infective agents, drugs, food additives, and circulating particulate matter all injure blood vessels. It is probable that these are present in small amounts in all of us some of the time, but it is likely that the injuries are often so mild as to be imperceptible and quickly repaired.

Immune complexes

The 'defensive' system of antigen-clearing involves complexing the antigen with antibody and complement to make phagocytosis by macrophages more inevitable. As this is a system that is used to remove damaged tissue, it is often difficult to distinguish whether damage preceded or is a consequence of the immune complex. It is the process of complexing that activates complement not the complex itself. Free and poorly complexed antigen may indeed have a greater potential to cause damage than well-complexed material. Trapping antigen in a tissue and its exposure to immunoglobulin and complement is determined by local events having little to do with what circulates in the bloodstream.

Immune complexes follow the ingestion of food, the presence of a fetus in the pregnant, invasion of the body by parasites such as scabies, or a neoplasm such as breast cancer, and can be demonstrated in everyone following the most mild of virus infections. For this reason, the mere demonstration of immune complexes is not enough to blame them for coincidental vasculitis. Excess antigen is released when infections are overwhelming or when tissues are broken down by immune attack or neoplasia, and sometimes as a consequence of food or drugs.

Immune complexes are mostly harmless but become harmful when they are of certain size and shape or composition. Actual harm is observed only when, and as, they are localized at a site ill-equipped to deal with them and slow to repair the damage done by them.

Often an alteration in host response prevents adequate neutralization of even mildly noxious agents. Recent exposure to similar noxious agents, exhaustion, and insufficient time for recovery of fibrinolytic mechanisms or the phagocytic potential, and the secretions of the mononuclear phagocytic system explain why repeated or continuous exposure to harmful agents precipitates vasculitis. Such an explanation most often explains localized recrudescence in the nose, in Wegener's granulomatosis, or in legs affected by gravitational eczema, ulcers, or atrophie blanche. Factors such as severe infection, foods, drugs, diseases promoting coagulation (for example, hepatitis), and malignancy often alter the inflammatory response and need not act as specific triggers. Immune complexes circulating in a patient known to have disseminated lupus erythematosus may suddenly become damaging when any of these other factors affect the patient. Localization of the defective inflammatory process is often determined by environmental factors: cold exposure, abrasion, or pressure on the skin causing mild stasis and ischaemia are well-known examples met clinically; these conditions are also used experimentally to demonstrate the localization of harmful agents from the bloodstream.

In recent years the discovery of congenital defects in complement and other protease inhibitors has explained why harmful agents are inadequately neutralized in some people. Hereditary angio-oedema is a good example of such a disease. There is a congenital absence of a complement inhibitor, but only in certain circumstances is this important. Trauma or infection sets off the sequence of events, which in this case includes the activation of complement by plasmin, dependent in its turn upon the secretion of plasminogen activator by damaged endothelium. Normally this is balanced by other inhibitors and by absorption into small amounts of fibrinogen and fibrin.

Local deficiencies in the sequence of events triggered by injury depend upon blood flow and diffusion, not only of activators but also of inhibitors. Injury usually releases fibrinolysis activators from endothelium, and heparin, histamine, and hyaluronidase, etc., from adjacent mast cells. These increase permeability and diffusion but prevent coagulation and complement activation. Repeated inoculation of histamine can itself cause vasculitis. It is not always necessary to invoke an immunological mechanism. When the mast cells and endothelium are more or less exhausted, and when activating or inhibiting products are released by adjacent epidermal injury, the proteases, complement, kinins, and materials like fibrin or C-reactive substance occur in sufficient quantities to perpetuate the inflammation and to attract white cells in large numbers.

Diagnosis

Almost essential to the diagnosis is the presence of purpura (Fig. 80), but a tender urticarial lesion that lasts for more than 12 h and leaves a slight bruise on resolution falls within the term 'vasculitis' (Fig. 81). The histology of such a lesion often shows more perivascular neutrophils than the common short-lasting urticarial weal. At the other end of the spectrum is obliterative or sclerosing thromboangiitis in which total occlusion of a small vessel often prevents exudation, and because there is no neutrophilic infiltrate, there may not be such acute destruction of the vessel wall. A similar appearance may be observed in disseminated intravascular coagulation (**DIC**) (Fig. 82) and in platelet embolic diseases.

Vasculitis affecting the deep dermis or fat and subcutaneous tissues most commonly produces a nodule, sometimes overlaid with redness or violaceous skin. Blistering and pustulation, when they occur as manifestations of vasculitis, are usually part of a superficial polymorphic eruption in which at least some of the lesions are palpable purpura, thus distinguishing the eruption from other more monomorphic blistering diseases. These physical signs are illustrated in Fig. 83. Very heavy infiltration with eosinophils is a feature of eosinophilic cellulitis, which is sometimes a reaction to arthropod bites.

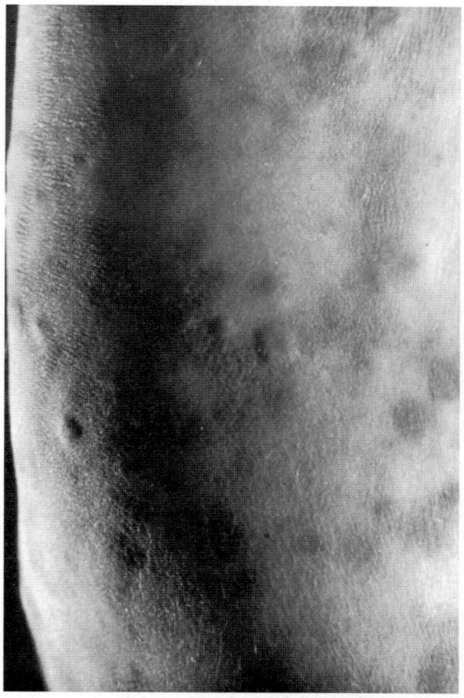

Fig. 81 Typical urticarial initial lesion of vasculitis, often proceeding to purpura and later to necrosis. However, in some types, hypocomplementaemic vasculitis, a persistent urticaria, is the only lesion.

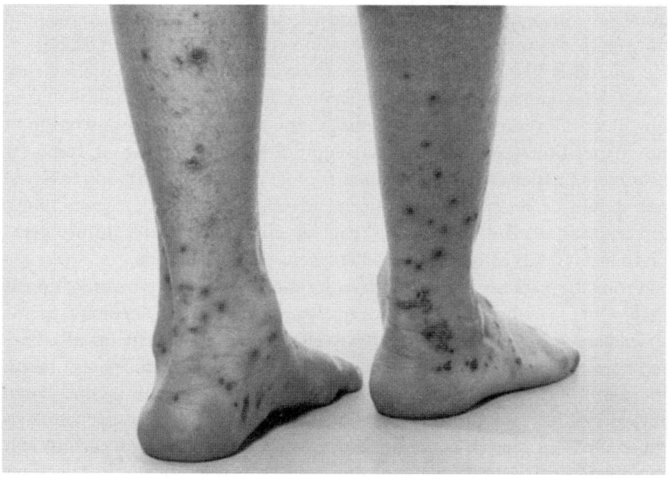

Fig. 80 Typical purpura of the lower leg of adult Henoch–Schönlein purpura. The lesions are palpable and inflammatory.

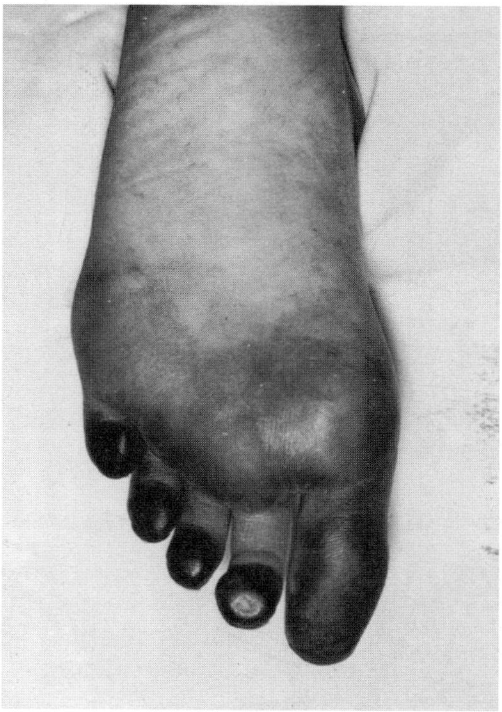

Fig. 82 The blue-to-black discoloration of the extremities in disseminated intravascular coagulation meningococcaemia.

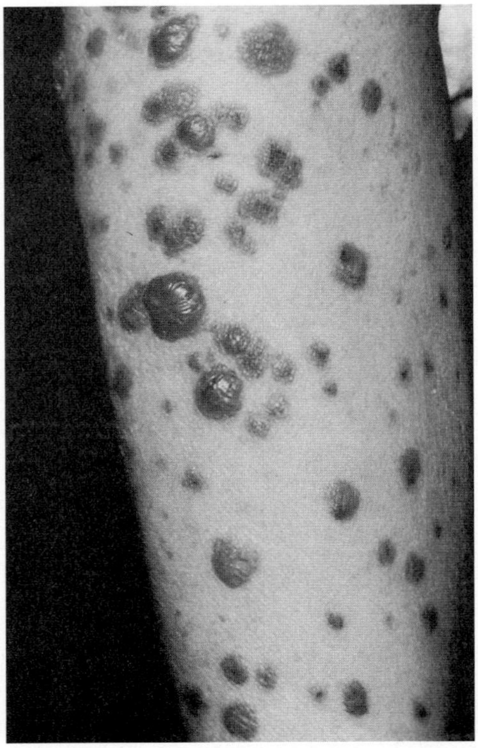

Fig. 83 The presence of blisters in vasculitis is due to the intensity of the oedema in the upper dermis; sometimes it is due to necrosis.

So far as the diagnosis of purpura is concerned, the traditional classification of thrombocytopenia (Fig. 84) versus non-thrombocytopenia is useful. Vasculitis is included within the latter term, and the purpura is more often palpable.

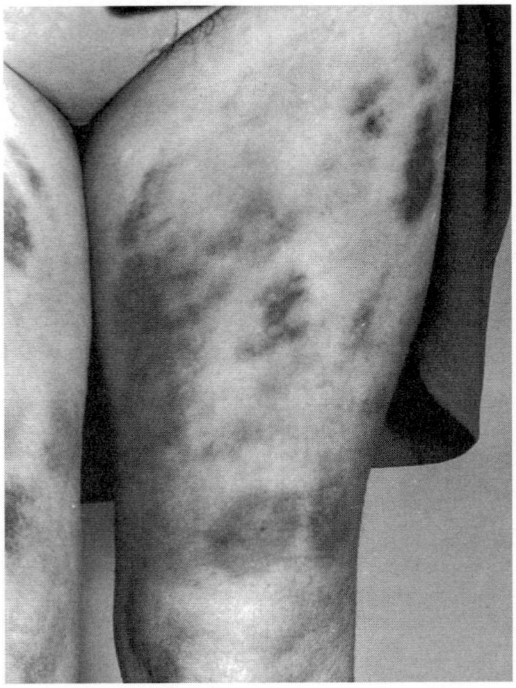

Fig. 84 Bruising or ecchymosis is most commonly due to thrombocytopenic purpura, but it is also a feature of the painful bruising syndrome.

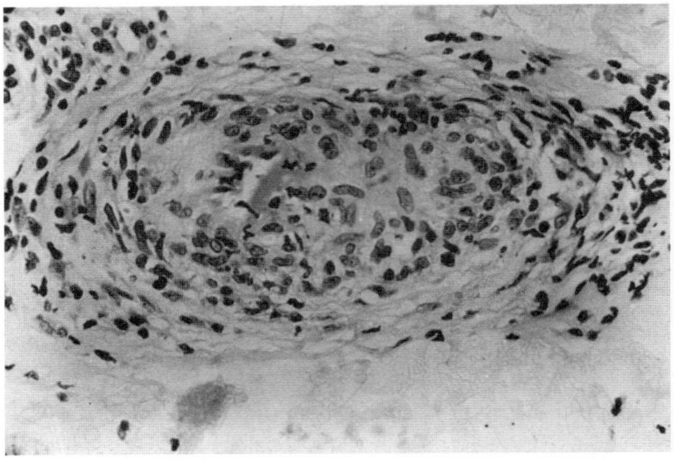

Fig. 85 A damaged vessel surrounded by broken-up neutrophils is typical of the hypocomplementaemic pattern of vasculitis.

Vasculitis in which immune complexes have played a causative role is more likely to be 'leucocytoclastic'—a term used to describe numerous disrupted neutrophils at the site of the damaged vessel (Fig. 85). It is now well recognized that a mononuclear variety of vasculitis also occurs, sometimes termed 'lymphocytic vasculitis', in which complement activation seems less significant but where upgrading of cell-wall adhesion factors is a response to cytokines and other pharmacological agents, such as histamine. It is a feature of drug eruptions and also of damage to vessels sometimes prior to the deposition of immune complexes, that is within 2 h of a cutaneous capillary fragility test. In fact macrophages rather than lymphocytes could be the more injurious infiltrate, depending on the stage of maturation and their secretion. Much of the pathology of vasculitis is that of ischaemia. Whatever the cause of the vessel damage, there is usually some impairment of blood flow. Hypoxia and infarction are quite capable of causing equally extensive pathology.

The significance of eosinophils in some forms of vasculitis is not known and they are no guide to prognosis or therapy.

Detection of cause

The first investigation required is a full blood count to exclude thrombocytopenic purpura. Efforts should also be made to exclude septic vasculitis due to meningococcaemia and gonococcaemia. Other viral, bacterial, and fungal diseases will also need to be considered in the context of AIDS. Allergic vasculitis has a characteristic histology, showing leucocytoclasis and endothelial damage with fibrin deposition. A skin biopsy should be taken for direct immunofluoresence studies at the same time. Demonstration of IgA deposition (usually IgA1) is required for a diagnosis of Henoch–Schönlein purpura. A serum antineutrophil cytoplasmic antibody (**ANCA**) test should be ordered. A perinuclear ANCA indicates microscopic polyarteritis and a need to monitor renal function carefully. A diffuse cytoplasmic ANCA is associated with Wegener's granulomatosis.

From the patients' point of view the most worthwhile investigation is that which results in improved management. Certain noxious agents should always be looked for in order to eliminate them therapeutically. Bacteria are the most important of these: the streptococcal sore throat is still the commonest precursor of vasculitis in children, and otitis media, dental caries, cystitis, and sinusitis occasionally play a role; in many countries tuberculosis or leprosy is the commonest cause; bacterial endocarditis and meningococcal septicaemia are often missed. Other treatable infections occasionally causing vasculitis are syphilis, neisseria, rickettsiae, and mycoplasma. Although viruses cannot usually be eliminated, any history of a recent 'flu-like illness or vaccination may be relevant. Hepatitis B virus is a well-recognized cause.

Screening for connective tissue disease with an ANA and rheumatoid factor is useful. Lupus erythematosus and rheumatoid arthritis are common causes of immune-complex vasculitis. But, as mentioned above, it is the exposure of antigen so that its complexing can activate complement that is important, not the complex itself.

Drugs such as penicillin and sulphonamides, allopurinol, amiodarone, streptokinase, thiazides, and warfarin have often been incriminated, but many other drugs appear less likely to be allergens than modifiers of the host response. Similarly, some foods may act as allergens, while others have a more obscure enhancing action. Enquiries should be directed towards headache pills, throat lozenges, purgatives, health foods, any medicine given for a specific illness, and any recent intake of food or drugs to which the patient is known to be sensitive. Questions should also be asked about recent vaccination, radiological investigation with contrast medium, or radiotherapy.

Cold agglutinins, cold fibrinogens, and cryoglobulins should also be looked for. It is now clear that many patients have cold-precipitated immune complexes. Perhaps even more have soluble immune complexes that are localized by blood stasis due to cold, pressure, vasoconstriction, or prior inflammation. The number of patients in whom an antigen has been isolated is small, and in still fewer has it been possible to eliminate the antigen, except in the case of bacteria sensitive to antibiotics. It is not particularly helpful to find a cryoglobulin; it does not alter management since, in any case, every patient should be kept warm. One of the difficulties is that it is often the antibody to the infective agent that in its turn becomes recognized as foreign. Infection may initiate this problem but after elimination of the organism the antibody persists as an autoantigen.

Even after extensive investigations there will remain a proportion of patients in whom everything appears to be normal and no cause for the vasculitis is found. Most often this is seen in women with cold, fat legs, and some degree of venous insufficiency. In these women there is decreased resistance to the deposition of antigen–antibody complexes and decreased clearance. Sometimes even the normal load of complexes generated by a meal or a trivial viral infection overwhelm the cutaneous defences. In such patients rest and compression stockings are particularly valuable.

Factors that modify the inflammatory response

These are very numerous and include any known chronic illness, such as malnutrition, diabetes mellitus, blood disorders, rheumatoid arthritis or other forms of collagen disease, chronic respiratory disease, disorders of the bowels or liver, and hypertension. Malignancy, whether carcinoma or lymphoma, is not an unusual factor and recent surgery, pregnancy, and unusual anxiety are also included in this list.

The mechanisms involved include coagulation and thrombosis, and, since these are treatable, a full blood count should always include a platelet count and other simple relevant tests, especially estimation of prothrombin time, fibrinogen titre, and fibrin degradation products.

Prognosis

The difficulty of naming a constellation of physical signs may force the physician to produce labels traditionally linked to a poor prognosis. One example is the term 'polyarteritis nodosa', another 'Wegener's granulomatosis'.

For all patterns it is useful to use the term 'vasculitis' supplemented by the terms 'limited' or 'local', implying a mild process affecting one locale or organ, and 'complicated' meaning severe and affecting many organs. Such adjectives, by describing the severity of the disease, give a lead to its management.

Management

Avoid all further injury

This allows healing to take place so preventing further damage to already inflamed tissue. Rest is essential for all cases of acute inflammation, but blood stasis should be counteracted by adequate elevation and movement of the limbs. Cold and direct sunlight should also be avoided since both injure the skin and affect blood flow. Women's legs are particularly at risk, depending on the fashion for long or short skirts or trousers.

Scratching, pinching, pressure, and constriction of the skin by ill-fitting clothing or bandages should be discouraged. Patients lying in bed will develop vasculitis on the buttocks, elbows, and over the greater trochanter unless they shift their position every few minutes. Venepuncture sites become inflamed in some forms of vasculitis, particularly in Behçet's disease and pyoderma gangrenosum, and also in severe generalized leucocytoclastic angiitis.

Eliminate circulating noxious agents, especially if they are antigens

Vasculitis following a severe streptococcal sore throat, meningococcal or gonococcal septicaemia, or tuberculosis should be treated with the appropriate antibiotics. Foci of infection, once so popular, are now too rarely thought of; when found they need to be eliminated, sometimes even by surgery. Certain bacterial diseases, such as bacterial endocarditis or leprosy, are not easily eliminated and require prolonged supervision. Although viral diseases are increasingly incriminated, there is no satisfactory way of dealing with them as yet. Immune-complex disease, sometimes as a manifestation of rheumatoid arthritis or lupus erythematosus but more often having no particular association, is now the most often suspected cause of vasculitis. Usually there are no specific measures for dealing with the problem, but immune complexes become less damaging if the factors localizing them are eliminated. Plasmapheresis is practised by a few specialized units. Drugs and food thought to be responsible can be omitted.

Provide specific treatment

Acute short-lasting itchy weals often respond to antihistamines. Acute tender swelling due to progressive tissue oedema may need to be treated with steroids. Painful swollen joints, acute optic neuritis, temporal (giant cell) arteritis, erythema nodosum, tender persistent weals, and tense painful swellings at the edge of pyoderma gangrenosum all usually respond to corticosteroids.

Fulminant vasculitis affecting more than one organ and brought about by a known trigger (allergens, drugs), should be covered by steroids once the cause has been eliminated. Immunosuppressive drugs such as azathioprine, cyclophosphamide, and methotrexate are used as a last resort in persistent chronic vasculitis, but they are of doubtful value except in granulomatous forms affecting the lung where they are the treatment of choice. Necrosis and gangrene are usually due to ischaemia. While inflammation alone may account for this in small vessels supplying superficial lesions, hypertension, coagulation, and thrombosis, as well as the cause of cardiac or peripheral vascular disease in general, sometimes underlie large areas of necrosis. The causes of vasculitis are also, for the most part, the causes of local or disseminated intravascular coagulation. Heparin is probably the drug of choice when fibrinogen, platelets, and prothrombin have been consumed and the levels of fibrin degradation products are raised. It is probably the most useful anticoagulant in malignant disease. Aspirin's anti-inflammatory effect is well known and is particularly effective when platelet aggregation is suspected. Dapsone, enhancers of fibrinolysis, and potassium iodide have had their successes and failures in recurrent nodular forms of vasculitis. Good management includes giving advice on smoking cessation, oral contraception, high blood pressure, and hyperlipidaemia. The prognosis depends on the presence of complications: particularly important are those affecting the eyes, central nervous system, and kidneys. Examination of the eyes for papilloedema and of the urine for red cells, protein, and casts is imperative.

Other vasculitides

Erythema nodosum

It is convenient to include erythema nodosum under the heading 'Vasculitis', though some still prefer to call it panniculitis. There is injury to small blood vessels in the deep dermis and subcutaneous tissue. However, primary injury to the blood vessels from a noxious agent, such as soluble immune complexes, is difficult to prove. Erythema nodosum is characterized by tender red swellings on the front of the shins (Fig. 86) and often also on the thighs and forearms. Bruising is common, but necrosis, scarring, and atrophy of the tissues are not features.

Erythema nodosum is a reaction pattern to infection (viral, bacterial, and mycotic) and sometimes to drugs. Neoplasia, pregnancy, and sarcoidosis are other causes. The causes are listed in Table 18. By far the commonest is a streptococcal sore throat. Sarcoidosis and tuberculosis are common causes where the incidence of these diseases is high. Ulcerative colitis and Crohn's disease are common associations seen in teaching hospital practice. Worldwide, erythema nodosum is commonly due to lepromatous leprosy. This is a widespread and often very persistent reaction to local antigen and is not typical of erythema nodosum in general. It may become pustular and necrotic. Erythema nodosum is often preceded by or accompanied by fever, malaise, fatigue, loss of weight, and arthralgia. Although it sometimes resolves in 2 to 3 weeks, the presence of persistent and recurrent forms over several months may suggest an alternative diagnosis. It is important not to label the disease as polyarteritis nodosa or rheumatic fever, for instance, merely because it is persistent and the patient is ill for several months, or the ESR is unusually high. The number, size, and chronicity of the lesions is variable. They can be few and as large as a hand, or multiple and the size of a thumbnail. They can be acute, tender, and last only a few days; or they can be chronic, less tender, and migratory, tending to heal in the centre and spread peripherally as a swollen ring. The more chronic lesions are less red and may be violaceous, or any of the colours of a resolving bruise. The front of the leg is a site of poor lymphatic drainage where foreign protein and bacteria are only slowly removed, especially in the deep dermis and adipose tissue. The underlying tibia splints the overlying tissue so that massage of the lymphatics is reduced. Pretibial cellulitis, pretibial myxoedema, and erythema nodosum have similar localizing factors explaining their pathogenesis.

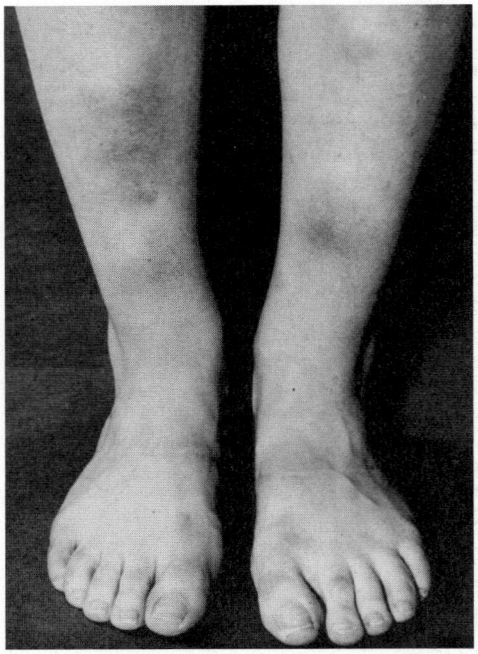

Fig. 86 Tender erythematous swelling on the front of the legs with ill-defined borders is characteristic of erythema nodosum.

Table 18 Some causes of erythema nodosum

Streptococcus spp.	Blastomycosis
Tuberculosis	Coccidioidomycosis
Sarcoidosis	Trichophyton verrucosum
Lymphogranuloma venereum	Ulcerative colitis
Cat-scratch disease	Crohn's disease
Ornithosis	Leukaemia
Epstein–Barr virus	Hodgkin's disease
Tularaemia	Sulphonamides
Histoplasmosis	Bromides
Yersinia spp.	Pregnancy and contraceptive pill
Leprosy	

Investigations

Investigations are required to confirm the diagnosis and extent of disease, to look for a cause, and to ensure the safety of treatment. A skin biopsy will show a lobular panniculitis. Occasionally, granulomas may be seen in patients with sarcoidosis, thus enabling a specific diagnosis to be made. A chase for the source of infection should include a history of possible contacts at home and abroad, human or animal. An anti-DNAase B will demonstrate a recent streptococcal infection. A Mantoux test may have a place, but intradermal testing for sarcoidosis is no longer available. Chest radiography is essential and the most useful for a diagnosis of sarcoid, tuberculosis, or mycoplasma pneumonia. Exclusion of tuberculosis by chest radiography is also useful prior to corticosteroid treatment. A fall in the ESR, which is often initially above 100 mm/h, is a useful guide to complete recovery.

Treatment

This is one of the diseases in which ultimate recovery is to be expected. While for the first 2 to 3 weeks it is possible to keep the patient at rest and to prescribe acetylsalicylic acid, the difficult period is often several weeks after the initial illness when the patient has to be mobilized. Firm support bandages or stockings give some relief for persistent aching and swelling legs. Steroids reduce swelling and fever but do not affect the length of the illness.

Pyoderma gangrenosum

As the name implies this is a necrosis of the tissues, often with a heavy neutrophilic infiltrate; but it is not primarily an infection, rather it is a reaction pattern in which venous and capillary engorgement, haemorrhage, and coagulation feature prominently. The exact pathogenesis is uncertain. In many cases there is an associated depression of the immune system demonstrable by *in vitro* and clinical tests. Failure of macrophages to respond to tissue injury or to clear noxious agents is another feature. Its associations are an important guide to its possible causation, these include ulcerative colitis, Crohn's disease (particularly of the colon), rheumatoid arthritis, seronegative arthritis with paraproteinaemia, Wegener's granulomatosis, and plasma-cell dyscrasias including myeloma. A bullous variety is associated with leukaemia, primary thrombocythaemia, and with myelofibrosis. Nevertheless, up to half of the cases seen in dermatology clinics have no significant association. The clinical features are initially varied, but all ultimately become turgid and ulcerate. These features include a tender red or blue nodule suggestive of erythema nodosum, vesico pustules, or an acneiform folliculitis. The swollen red or blue edge is often acutely tender; blistering may be considerable, especially in the leukaemic variety. The necrosis follows no particular pattern and, like a carbuncle, may have multiple centres. It is usually undermined, and exuberant granulation tissue sprouts from the base of the ulcer. Although the calves, thighs, buttocks, abdomen, and face are favoured, no site is immune.

There is considerable toxicity associated with the acute varieties. Dermatologists see the chronic variety, which is not obviously associated with underlying disease and in which the general health of the patient is not impaired. The ulcerated lesions are not necessarily tender but they are irregular and persistent, often for years. Dermatitis artefacta is often suspected, and the personality of the patient disabled for many months may be consequently affected and encourage the suspicion. Synergistic gangrene is one cause of very similar acute pathology. Unlike pyoderma gangrenosum, which is often multiple, synergistic gangrene is more clearly associated with a recent wound (for example, an operation on the gastrointestinal tract), and the area of gangrene is acute, solitary, and an extension of the wound. Aerobic and anaerobic culture should be performed in any form of pyoderma gangrenosum for amoebiasis, tuberculosis, buruli ulcer, and deep fungus infections such as nocardiosis or blastomycosis. ,

The treatment of choice is oral high-dose corticosteroids. The management of underlying diseases, such as ulcerative colitis or leukaemia, is essential. Any suspicion of an infective causation such as amoebiasis requires the appropriate investigations and treatment. For cases responding poorly to steroids, dapsone 100 mg daily or clofazimine is worth a try. Colchicine, cyclophosphamide, and ciclosporin also have their advocates. Various subacute presentations respond to locally applied steroids by inoculation or under an occlusive dressing.

Behçet's disease

See Chapter 18.10.5 for further discussion.

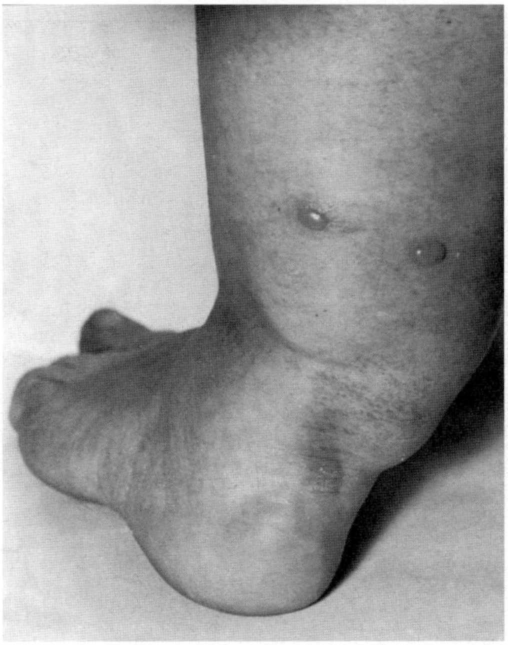

Fig. 87 Urticarial lesions, in this case due to cold; they often blister, especially on the lower legs.

Vesicoblistering diseases

A vesicle is an elevated circumscribed lesion, usually no larger than 0.5 cm in diameter, filled with serum and sometimes blood and pus. Above this size a vesicle is called a bulla or blister.

Predisposing factors

These include congenital diseases such as epidermolysis bullosa and metabolic disorders such as porphyria.

Causes

Friction and minor knocks can produce blisters in the predisposed person or at sites unaccustomed to wear and tear. The hands and feet are most often affected. Friction is increased by damp, sweating skin.

Ischaemia

Prolonged pressure obliterating the blood supply for more than 2 h causes damage to the smooth muscle of small arterioles and to underlying fat. The epidermis can survive more than 6 h of ischaemia, and much longer periods may be survived in cool skin with a decreased metabolism. Unconscious patients or those with sensory loss, especially from barbiturate poisoning, are particularly vulnerable, but most cases occur from peripheral vascular disease with acute interference of blood supply.

Acute sweat-pore occlusion

This occurs especially with fever or in hot climates. Numerous small transparent vesicles are seen, especially in the flexures or in parts of the body in which the stratum corneum is unduly thick. In the fingers or feet this is called pompholyx.

Burns

Burns can occur from cold (Fig. 87), as in frostbite, and by cryotherapy, heat, or ultraviolet irradiation (photosensitivity from plants, porphyria, or pellagra) (Fig. 88). Dermatitis artefacta is often induced by burning the skin; it is clearly self-induced but usually denied, and is often of a bizarre pattern. Cigarette burns are amongst the commonest induced lesions.

Chemicals

These may be toxic, for example mustard gas and cantharidin. Sometimes an allergic dermatitis from contact with chemicals also produces vesicles due to separation of the epidermal cells by inflammatory oedema. Plant dermatitis is amongst the most common of causes; for example, from the primula in Europe and poison ivy in the United States.

Fixed drug eruptions

These can cause erythema and blistering and appear and reappear at the same site whenever the causative drug is ingested; usually itching occurs within 6 h of ingestion.

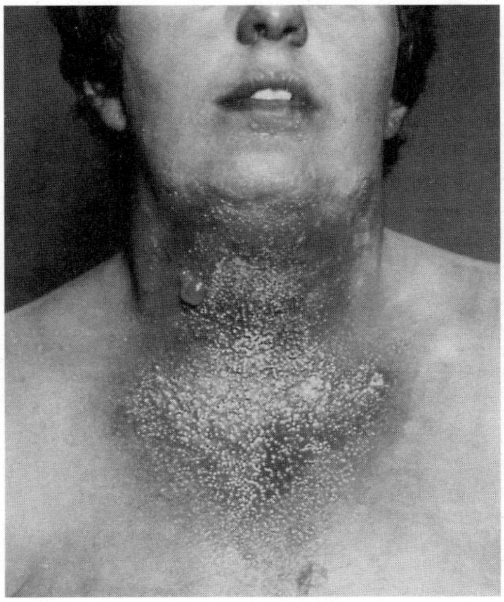

Fig. 88 Blistering on the front of the neck due to an ultraviolet light burn. Self-induced by a home lamp.

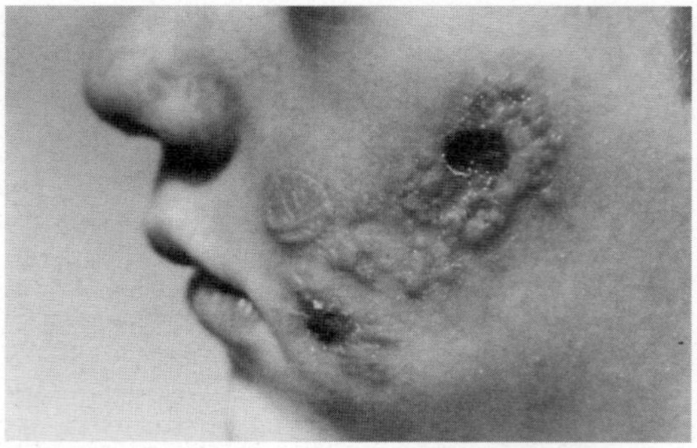

Fig. 89 Blisters on the cheek due to herpes simplex virus infection.

Infections

(See also under the appropriate chapters in Section 7.)
Viral disorders including herpes simplex (Fig. 89), herpes zoster, chickenpox, and smallpox, or bacterial diseases most commonly cause blisters, particularly *Staphylococcus* and *Streptococcus* spp.

Fungus infections commonly present as blistering on the soles of the feet, and insect bites give rise to papular urticaria that often blisters on the lower legs (Fig. 90). Blisters, pruritus, and fever have been described in ornithologists bitten by ticks carried by marine birds on the Middle East coastline. Arthropods, like the brown recluse spider, give rise to necrotic blisters, while the hairy caterpillar, for example, secretes a toxin in its hairs that can produce blistering. Some infarctions can produce a vasculitis or disseminated intravascular coagulation, which may also present as vesicular or haemorrhagic blisters. Where the Cantharidine beetle is common, avoid injury to it when alighting on the skin and let it fly away.

Specific skin disorders

Erythema multiforme

This, as the name implies, can present with a variety of patterns. The classic pattern affects the hands and feet more than the trunk. Such lesions have an erythematous and coin-shaped presentation which is more intense and blistering in the centre—a target-shaped lesion (see Fig. 10(b)). Several toxic erythematous eruptions overlap with the classic pattern and sometimes the classic distribution and even the target lesions are missing. Involvement of the mucosa is common so that the mouth, eyes, and genitalia may be affected in varying degrees. Where the blistering and mucosal lesions are severe, the disease is termed the 'Stevens–Johnson syndrome'

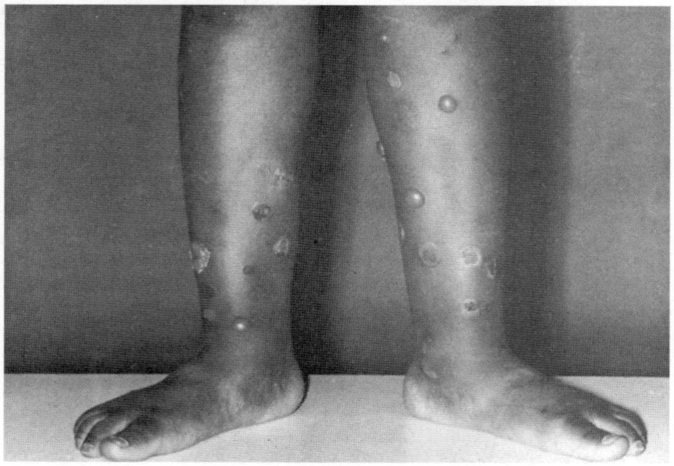

Fig. 90 Typical multiple blisters due to insect bites during the rainy season in India.

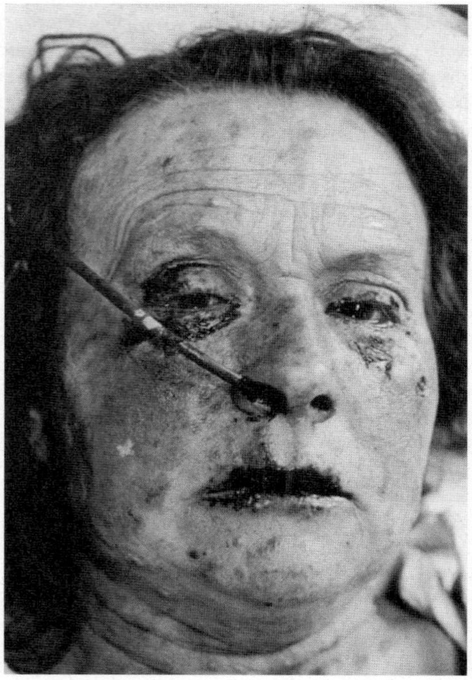

Fig. 91 Stevens–Johnson syndrome, or severe erythema multiforme, resulting in severe erosions of the mouth and conjunctivitis.

(Fig. 91). This is usually associated with high fever and sometimes also with anterior uveitis, pneumonia, renal failure, polyarthritis, or diarrhoea.

Aetiology

The commonest cause is herpes simplex virus infection. Herpes simplex DNA has been demonstrated by polymerase chain reaction (**PCR**) in around 75 per cent of cases. Other infections such as mycoplasma, orf, streptococcus, typhoid, and diphtheria may be incriminated. Drugs also cause this disorder and sulphonamides are amongst the most common. In fact, any infection and any drug can probably give rise to erythema multiforme, usually after a latent period of 1 to 3 weeks. Other causes include neoplasm and its treatment with drugs or radiotherapy, as well as certain other systemic diseases such as AIDS, rheumatoid arthritis, lupus erythematosus, and ulcerative colitis. One of the difficulties is the overlap with the other patterns of toxic erythema and their causation. The erythema of pregnancy may sometimes be called erythema multiforme.

Pathology

There is vacuolar degeneration and apoptosis of the basal cells of the epidermis; vesicles develop between the cells and the underlying basement membrane. Vasodilatation and a lymphocytic infiltrate around the upper dermal vessels are observed.

Treatment

Any known cause should be removed, and systemic steroids prescribed if the patient is very uncomfortable and toxic. Recurrent attacks should also be treated by eliminating the cause if known: for instance, treating the earliest stage of herpes simplex with aciclovir, famciclovir, or valaciclovir and avoiding triggers like bright sunlight. Viral resistance and long-term side-effects of frequent or long-term usage have not, so far, been demonstrated. In the absence of randomized clinical trials, strong debate continues as to whether steroids, plasmapheresis, ciclosporin, and intravenous immunoglobulins are helpful or harmful. Indeed, a combination of high-dose prednisolone with cyclophosphamide given for 3 days each month seems to be effective and almost without side-effects. It is certain that fluid replacement, antimicrobial management, nutritional support, local comfort, and keeping the patient warm are essential life-saving manoeuvres.

Toxic epidermal necrolysis (TEN)

This is a rare variety of erythema with acute epithelial necrosis apoptosis affecting all areas of the skin. This is sometimes called 'scalded skin syndrome' because of its clinical appearance. It is usually acute in onset and may be preceded by various patterns of toxic erythema or blistering. Pressure and shearing stresses on the skin tend to encourage the extension of the blisters. There are two varieties of the disease: the first, originally described by Ritter, is due to a staphylococcus, often phage type 71, and particularly affects children—the blistering and resulting erosions are very superficial and they are due to a split at the level of the stratum granulosum; the second is a drug reaction or a toxic consequence of malignant disease or its therapy. The entire epidermis is necrotic. European physicians have found it of epidemiological value to define TEN as more than 30 per cent of skin detachment and the Stevens–Johnson syndrome as less than 10 per cent, with an overlap syndrome of between 10 and 30 per cent.

Sometimes sulphonamides, barbiturates, phenytoin, pyrazolone derivatives, and phenolphthalein are responsible, while a number of other drugs are also blamed, albeit more rarely.

The use of human intravenous immunoglobulin containing anti-Fas antibodies, and therefore protective against apoptosis, shows promise. Pulse therapy with intravenous gammaglobulin is also under investigation, using 0.4 g/kg for 5 days.

Rarer blistering disorders

These include diseases like pemphigus, pemphigoid, and dermatitis herpetiformis. At one time these were all grouped together, for their pathogenesis has only recently become clearer. The main distinction is in the level of the blister, which determines both clinical and histological features—pemphigus is an intraepidermal blister, whereas the other disorders tend to be subepidermal. Resulting cleavage within the dermis produces dermal inflammation, oedematous papules, infiltration with white cells, as well as bleeding into this blister. The more superficial the blister, the more erosive the appearance: the skin lesions may be red and glistening, whereas deeper dermal blisters tend to be tense and less easily broken. The type and site of immunoglobulin deposition is a further diagnostic feature.

Pemphigus

Pemphigus vulgaris

This is a blistering condition favouring the mucosa as much as the skin. Separation of epidermal cells above the basal layers of the epidermis always occurs in association with an antibody having an affinity with intercellular material in the epidermis. The separated epidermal cell is large, basophilic, and rounded and is termed an 'acantholytic cell'.

Aetiology The pemphigus antibody will cross the placental barrier and promote neonatal blistering. It is also pathogenic *in vitro*. This antibody reacts with a specific 85-kDa protein, plakoglobin, and a 130-kDa protein in pemphigus vulgaris, but in pemphigus foliaceous (see below) it reacts with a 160-kDa protein, an extracellular epitope of desmoglein. The 130-kDa polypeptide is an epidermal cadherin. The loss of adhesion occurs because of the important adhesive role of these components in the desmosome. (See Chapter 23.2, Fig. 1.)

It is assumed to be an autoimmune disease, possibly associated with HLA-A10 and DR4, and is found more commonly in the Jewish race. Moreover, in Asia, it is one of the commonest causes of admission to a skin hospital. The more superficial variety that affects Brazilians may or may not be a separate, genetically determined reaction pattern. The antibody that binds with complement both *in vivo* and *in vitro* is specific for an, as yet unidentified, intercellular material which activates proteases that lyse intercellular adhesive materials. Several investigators have found that the antibody can frequently cause intraepithelial clefting *in vitro* in human, rabbit, and monkey epithelium. There is an association with thymoma as well as with lymphoma and carcinoma. Not surprisingly, therefore, it occurs with lupus erythematosus and myasthenia gravis.

Penicillamine has been responsible for the development of pemphigus in about 9 per cent of patients treated for rheumatoid arthritis. Captopril and rifampicin as well as meprobamate have also been incriminated.

Clinical features Erosions of the mucosa of the mouth are the initial problem in more than half the cases. The erosions are often misdiagnosed as mouth ulcers, but close examination reveals a friable mucosa with no well-defined aphthous ulcers. Actual blisters may be missed because they are so quickly eroded. On the skin, the superficial nature of the blisters also determines that the principal lesion is a more painful erosion and the flaccid blisters quickly burst. The base is red and bleeds easily. The epidermis at the edge of the blister is easily dislodged by sliding pressure (Nikolsky sign). There are many reports of clinical and histological overlap with pemphigus foliaceous or pemphigoid. In all such cases pemphigus vulgaris proves to be the final diagnosis.

Treatment Corticosteroids are lifesaving; without them the disease is one of the most dangerous in dermatology. Very high dosage is required; prednisolone 120 mg daily is a common starting dose and failure to control the eruption within a week merits doubling of even this high dose. As soon as there are no new blisters the steroids are reduced by large increments about every 3 days. Withdrawal is more gradual below 30 mg daily. Most practitioners now add azathioprine, methotrexate, or cyclophosphamide as a steroid-sparing immunosuppressant.

In contrast to the presteroid era, cure now seems possible and many patients are off all treatment after 2 years. However, the side-effects of the therapy are considerable. Death from gastrointestinal haemorrhage is not infrequent. Thromboembolic disease is probably a consequence of the disease as much as the therapy. Steroid-induced osteoporosis with consequent vertebral collapse is a frequent and irreversible side-effect. Bacterial infection of the eroded skin is inevitable and septicaemia is common. The sore mouth and eroded skin require expert nursing—dressings tend to stick to the skin and their removal causes further skin damage. Oral fluids should not be strongly osmotic and soft diets should not include particles that lodge under blister roofs or in crevices.

Pemphigus vegetans

Pemphigus vegetans is a reaction to the erosions in which the repairing epidermis becomes hypertrophic and the dermis is granulomatous; small pustules surround the vegetations. This disease is common in the axillae and groin and the angles of the mouth and nose (Fig. 92). It may be encouraged by steroid dependency.

Pemphigus foliaceous

This is a more benign variant of pemphigus in which the blisters are more superficial. The bullae are subcorneal and scaling and crusting may be a principal feature (Fig. 93). The face and upper trunk are most often

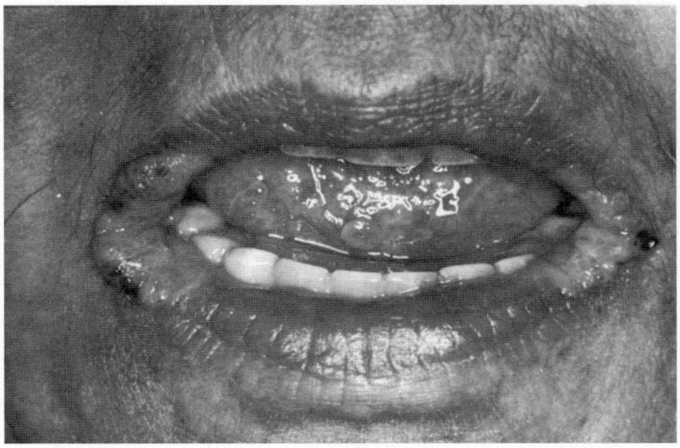

Fig. 92 Pemphigus vegetans showing the typical granulomatous hypertrophy underlying erosions at the angles of the mouth.

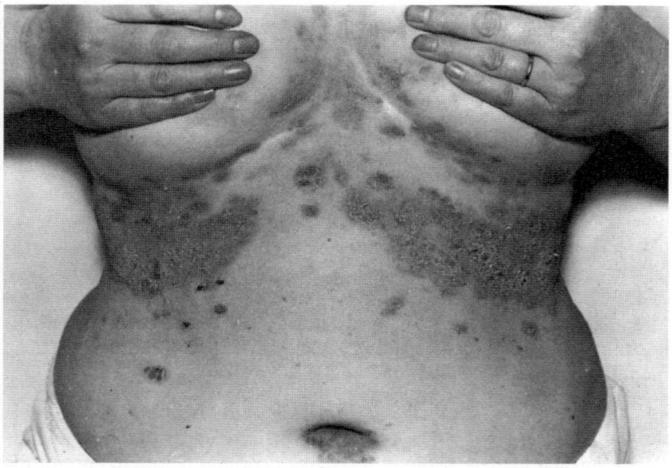

Fig. 93 Pemphigus foliaceous blisters, so superficial that they merely look like crusting of the erosions. In this case it would have to be distinguished from an intertrigo and secondary monilial infection.

affected. Localized forms may look more like seborrhoeic warts because of their chronicity and definition. Oral lesions are unusual. Antibodies against intercellular epithelial material are present as in pemphigus vulgaris, but basement membrane antibody and antinuclear antibody are also frequently observed. An association exists with lupus erythematosus and with thymoma and myasthenia gravis.

Fogo selvagem

This is a form of pemphigus foliaceous is commonly seen in people working in the rural peanut farms of Brazil. Many members of one family may be affected. Progression to a generalized erythroderma is usual and the mortality is almost 50 per cent, due as much to treatment as from the disease. An immunological reaction to an insect vector has been proposed, based on the study of the black-fly bites and the hypothesis of crossreactivity between the epidermal antigens and the antigen of the fly. Topical steroids may be preferable to high-dose systemic therapy in those who cannot be closely supervised.

Pemphigoid

The bullae in pemphigoid are subepidermal and acantholysis is not a feature. About 80 per cent of patients are over 60 years of age. Pemphigoid is about twice as common as pemphigus. There is a specific antibody (usually IgG) for the basement membrane zone of the epidermis and this is present in about 70 per cent of patients. Complement is bound *in vivo*. The basement membrane remains in the floor of the bullae in most cases. Two large epidermal polypeptides are the major antigenic target of bullous pemphigoid (**BP**) antibodies. The *BP230* gene is localized to the short arm of chromosome 6 and the *BP180* gene to the long arm of chromosome 10. Both protein products of these genes are components of the hemidesmosome. BP180 is a transmembrane glycoprotein with an external terminal ectodomain consisting of collagen triple-helical domains, which bind keratin to the hemidesmosome. (See Chapter 23.2, Fig. 1.)

Clinical features

Initial features of pemphigoid are often non-specific and confusing. It can be eczematous or urticarial. The lesions often begin around a site of damage such as a leg ulcer or burn. After 2 or 3 weeks blisters may erupt abruptly. They favour the flexures and are tense and dome-shaped, often containing blood. Small blisters in the mouth are rare and tend not to erode as in pemphigus. Patients with pemphigoid are distressed by itching, and oedema of the skin may be troublesome, but their general health is usually unaffected.

Treatment

The treatment of choice is prednisolone, 60 to 80 mg daily, until there are no new blisters. Since morbidity in the elderly is great, azathioprine, methotrexate, dapsone, minocycline, or cyclophosphamide may be used to allow a lower maintenance dose of the steroid. Osteoporosis, gastric ulceration, and diabetes mellitus are particularly common complications of steroid therapy. However, complete remission after 1 year is common.

Specific disorders

Cicatricial pemphigoid Also called 'benign mucosal pemphigoid', the cause of this disorder is unknown, but its immunology includes autoantibodies to an 180-kDa protein. Although mortality is low, cicatricial pemphigoid is responsible for great discomfort. It affects older adults, and the subepidermal bullae favour the mucosa of the mouth, conjunctiva, and the perineal orifices. The base of the lesions are heavily infiltrated with lymphocytes and plasma cells and there is eventual fibrosis. Those adhesions occurring between the bulbar and palpebral conjunctiva result in eventual shrinkage, and entropion is followed by blindness. The skin is less often involved and the sparse lesions often heal by scarring. The scalp is more often affected than other sites.

Treatment No treatment is very effective, but steroids and azathioprine are usually prescribed.

Dermatitis herpetiformis

This is a vesicobullous disorder associated with the granular deposition of IgA in the dermis and a usually symptomless subtotal villous atrophy of the small intestine. The IgA is believed to be derived from plasma cells in the intestine. As in coeliac disease, HLA-A8/DRW 3 is associated and may be responsible for a defective Fc receptor status. It is probable that gluten hypersensitivity results in circulating immune complexes with an affinity for material in the upper dermis (this is possibly reticulin or transaminases related to gliadin), and that the Fc-receptor dysfunction impairs the removal of the immune material by macrophages. Histology of the skin shows fibrin, neutrophils, and eosinophils in the dermal papillae.

Clinical features

The eruption is characterized by intensely itchy, grouped papular or vesicular lesions that lie on an urticarial or erythematous base. The elbows, knees, sacrum, and shoulders are favoured (see Fig. 9), with the face and scalp more commonly affected than in the case of pemphigus or pemphigoid. The itchy vesicles are quickly excoriated since this relieves the pruritus. The eruption waxes and wanes, sometimes being in remission for many months. However, for most people it remains a lifelong disorder. An increased incidence of lymphoma is well documented.

Treatment

Dapsone (100–200 mg daily) or sulphapyridine (0.5 g, three times daily) are remarkably effective and can be used as a diagnostic test since itchiness is relieved within 48 h. The maintenance dose should be titrated to suit each patient: it may be as low as 50 mg of dapsone per week. Haemolytic anaemia is common on higher dosage and especially when, in some cases, 400 mg of dapsone per day is needed to control the eruption. A gluten-free diet strictly adhered to controls some but not all disease; 70 per cent pf patients can stop taking dapsone after 2 years of such dieting.

Steroid therapy is strangely ineffective and heparin oddly effective. Inorganic arsenicals (Fowler's solution) are effective and were once very popular, and are probably justified in elderly patients much troubled by the disease and unable to tolerate dapsone or sulphapyridine.

Specific disorders

Juvenile bullous pemphigoid This is a bullous disorder characterized by a predilection for the face and perineum. Linear IgA is deposited on the basement membrane of the epidermis. It is neither associated with enteropathy nor with HLA-A8. The response to dapsone, sulphapyridine, or steroids is unpredictable.

Pemphigoid gestationis This differs from the common toxic erythema of pregnancy in having large blisters, often periumbilical, beginning as a degeneration of the epidermal cells. Pemphigoid gestationis is associated with HLA-B8/DR3 and an IgG1 autoantibody that avidly binds C3. Thus, it is a blister above the basement membrane, believed to be due to a specific antibody to the basal cell; the antibody is present in umbilical cord blood and binds with a 180-kDa glycoprotein in the basement membrane of the amnion. This disorder occurs during or immediately after pregnancy and usually ceases fairly abruptly within weeks of parturition. It recurs in subsequent pregnancies and as an effect of oral contraceptives.

Other causes of blistering

Lichen planus and lichen sclerosis et atrophicus both rarely blister. Bullous disease and malignancy are a debated association, since so much bullous disease occurs in an age group in which malignancy is common. However, individual case histories of uncontrollable bullous disease with atypical immunofluorescence are impressive.

Trophoneurotic blisters are another debated association. Unconscious patients seem predisposed to produce these subepidermal blisters even at sites not affected by pressure or shearing forces. This is an important hazard often causing unjustified accusation of mismanagement in the nursing care of such patients.

Diabetes mellitus is a cause of intraepidermal blisters without immunofluorescent material and showing no acantholysis (Fig. 94).

Abnormal vascularity of the skin: angioma and telangiectasia

Patterns of blood vessel development that are inappropriate for the needs of the skin or for thermoregulation include both overgrowth and atrophy. An excess of capillary and venular vessels is a characteristic of wound healing and of many hyperproliferative conditions of the skin (for example, psoriasis). These usually present as redness and individual vessels cannot be seen by the naked eye. Proliferation is still more extreme in strawberry haemangioma, granuloma telangiectaticum, also known as pyogenic granuloma, and in certain malignancies such as Kaposi's sarcoma and angioendothelioma.

On the other hand, telangiectasia is characterized by the dilatation of individual capillaries or venules so that they are visible to the naked eye. There is little evidence that the endothelial cell is at fault and it is more likely that the basic defect is an atrophy or loss of supporting tissue.

Proliferative vasculature is more unstable than that observed in telangiectasia and the natural history is for it to resolve, often completely. Vessels and wounds or angiomas are vulnerable, and the growing phase may be associated with necrosis as a result of thrombosis secondary to a surface injury of the skin. On the other hand, telangiectasia has no tendency to thrombose and the overlying skin rarely ulcerates. The natural history of such dilated vessels is to persist until extreme old age when they may be partially absorbed.

The pulsed dye laser has revolutionized the management of vascular lesions of the skin, but it has also shown the need for a multidisciplinary approach to the diagnosis of cellularity, depth of lesion, haemodynamic changes, and involvement of organs other than the skin. The perfect result is elusive.

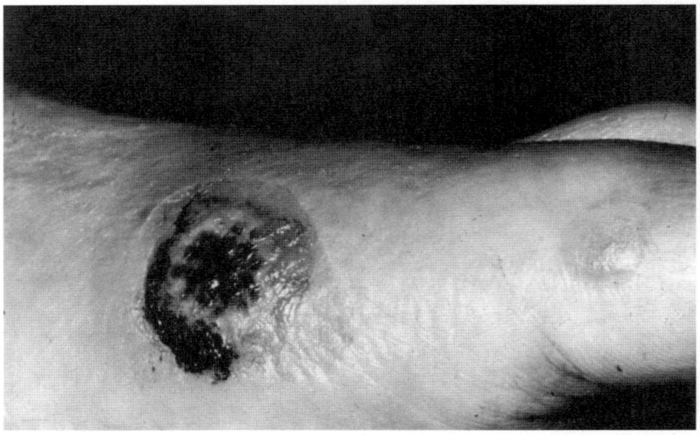

Fig. 94 A haemorrhagic blister on the foot in a patient with diabetes mellitus.

Naevi

Strawberry naevi

Although these are almost never present at birth, they may be preceded by a small area of blanching observed at birth. From a few days after birth the lesion consists of rapidly proliferating nests of granulation tissue. After a few weeks the rate of growth becomes less rapid and some vessels become dilated and cavernous. A stable period of no growth often occurs between about 9 months and about 1 year, after which gradual absorption by fibrosis is to be expected. Management consists of reassuring the parents and emphasizing its satisfactory natural resolution (Fig. 95).

However, there are exceptions to this policy of non-intervention. For example, plastic surgery may be advised where involvement of the eyelid interferes with sight. Some large haemangiomas sequester platelets, thus

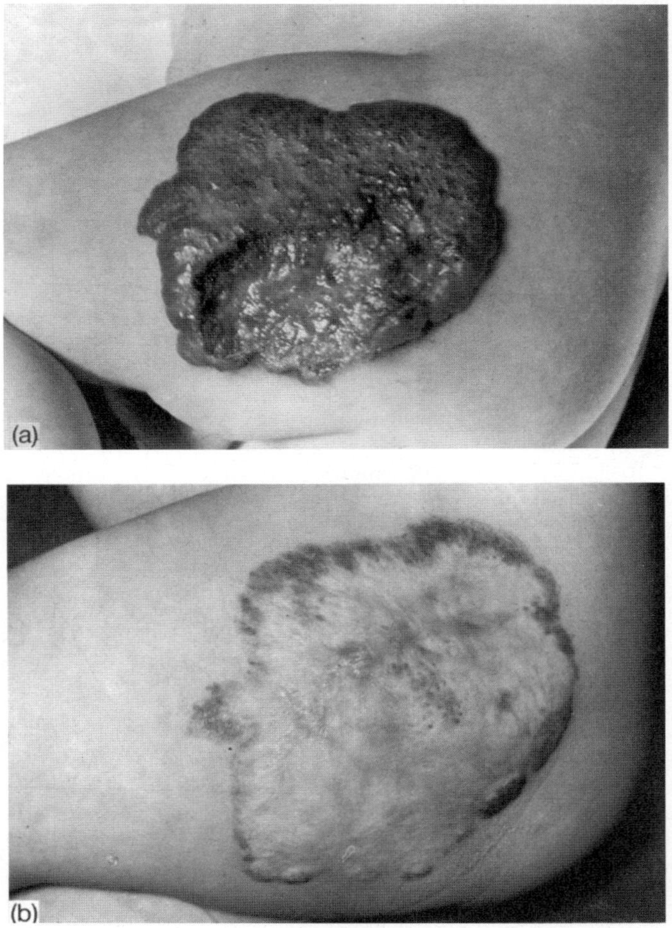

Fig. 95 Strawberry' naevus. (a) A proliferative but benign neoplasia which, after a rapid phase of new growth, stabilizes and eventually regresses. The lesions often ulcerate if traumatized. In this case, ulceration has hastened resolution but there is more residual scarring (b) than usual.

giving rise to a bleeding tendency (the Kassabach–Merrick syndrome). High-dose steroids (3 mg/kg) are lifesaving. On withdrawal, rebound overgrowth may be observed, justifying a second or third course of treatment. Ulceration of the haemangioma is common, especially in the nappy area and when there is a primary irritant rash. Bleeding is easily controlled by light pressure. The ulceration often accelerates resolution.

Sometimes haemangiomas have a deep element in which arteriovenous shunts are a complication. Interference with underlying structures is not common, but joint involvement warrants surgical advice and management.

The treatment of haemangiomas has included radiotherapy; more recently, systemic steroids, interferon-α, pressure pads, excision, and, currently, embolization. The latter requires angiographic control and siting of sclerosing adhesives at the appropriate site. The delineation of vascular endothelial growth factors and their receptors is opening up new approaches to therapy.

Port wine naevi

This is a pattern of vascular birthmark present at birth and is usually segmental. It is unwise to make a prognosis at birth because pale naevi and segmental patterns of erythema may look similar and often fade. The majority of port wine naevi persist for life. Arteriovenous shunts and gravitational stasis often cause some increase in the vasculature during adult life. A pale plaque of macular telangiectasia in the nape of the neck is present in the majority of normal babies, and persists in more than half of those affected.

Variants of port wine naevi affecting deeper vasculature range from the Klippel–Trenaunay disorder causing enlargement of the limb, to a reticulate and more atrophic pattern sometimes associated with shortening of the limb. Asymmetrical gigantisms and disturbances of pigment are associated with some developmental patterns of widespread segmental telangiectasia. Telangiectatic vessels on the upper face and nose may be associated with eye or brain defects, presenting as glaucoma or epilepsy.

Telangiectasia

Telangiectases are enduring dilatations of blood vessels. They are usually less than 1 mm in length and may be point-like or punctate, linear, spider, or stellate, forming flat, square, oblong, or oval plaques, or mat-like with an eccentric punctum. They blanch completely when compressed. Telangiectasia is not new-vessel formation—indeed, new vessels in wounds are not unduly dilated.

Telangiectases are probably always secondary to mesenchymal connective tissue dysplasias. However, they can be congenital and naevoid, acquired and genetic (in other words, familial or inherited), as well as being secondary to 'collagen' diseases such as lupus erythematosus, scleroderma, or dermatomyositis, or the result of radiation damage.

All dilatations of small vessels are made worse by blushing, as is seen in rosacea, carcinoid diseases, and oestrogen and related hormonal imbalances (for example, in pregnancy or liver disease). They are also made worse by a loss of supporting tissue, as in steroid atrophy, solar elastosis, ageing (Fig. 96), and Cushing's syndrome.

Telangiectasia is often associated with increased melanin pigmentation and brown spots may be predominant, even in hereditary haemorrhagic telangiectasia; but poikiloderma is a typical example of atrophy, telangiectasia, and pigmentation. Some telangiectasias may be insufficiently dilated to be recognized by the naked eye. However, if they involve most of the vessels in an affected area they may appear as a persistent erythema (for instance, the red cheeks of young children), or as capillary naevi affecting the eyelids, nape of the neck, or forehead, known as salmon patches or stork bites. The erythema may be pale pink or deep purple in colour. The darker the lesion, the more likely the dilated vessels will be inhomogeneous, making some visible to the naked eye. Naevoid lesions usually affect well-defined segments of the skin, though not necessarily dermatomal or unilateral in pattern (Fig. 97). The best known are naevi affecting the trigeminal nerve (Sturge–Weber syndrome) or sometimes an entire limb.

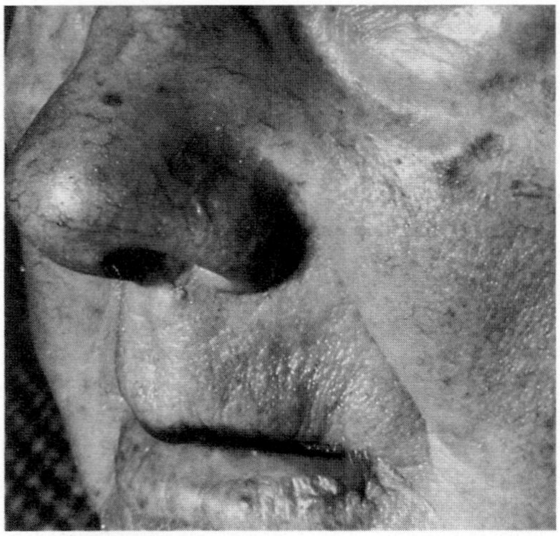

Fig. 96 Ageing is accentuated in light-exposed skins. One feature of ageing is the poor collagen support of skin vasculature. Telangiectasia is a common consequence.

Diffuse polymorphic patterns that develop in childhood or in young adults favour exposed areas such as the face and forearms, probably because sunlight exaggerates connective tissue dysplasia. However, haemodynamic factors such as gravitational stasis of the venous system also play a part, and the distribution of spider naevi may depend on drainage into the superior vena cava. Gravitational stasis particularly determines the patterns of stellate and arborizing telangiectasia on the legs. While 5 per cent of the population has between two and ten telangiectases on the lips, fingers, palms, and soles, grosser patterns of telangiectasia in disease may involve these sites. Dermatomal or unilateral patterns are rare. A high incidence, up to 40 per cent, of telangiectasia affecting the trunk is described in aluminium workers, apparently associated with the electrolytic processes used in the industry.

Although diffuse and acquired patterns of telangiectasia are commonly familial, sporadic cases account for about 20 per cent, even in the well-known hereditary haemorrhagic telangiectasia. A benign variety of this disease is not associated with severe bleeding and is also probably dominantly inherited. Telangiectasia confined to the lips may also present a dominant pattern of inheritance. However, no large-scale study has been undertaken to rule out polygenic inheritance in any of these disorders. The haemorrhagic diathesis has been recorded as a dominant gene, with many large pedigrees described; but even so, 10 per cent of probands with telangiectasia do not bleed. Severe epistaxis and severe bleeding after tooth extraction or cuts and even heavy menstrual bleeding are characteristic of hereditary haemorrhagic telangiectasia. Minor but frequent nose bleeds are common with even the benign forms. Arteriovenous shunts are described commonly in association with hereditary haemorrhagic telangiectasia. These result in

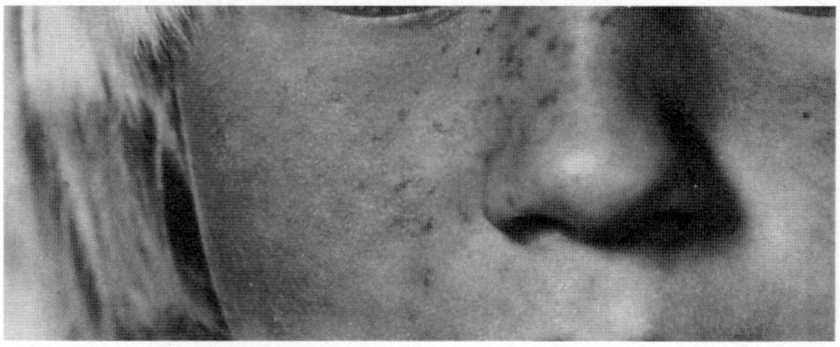

Fig. 97 Segmental telangiectasia of punctate-spider naevoid type.

pulsating nodules of the skin, which may have severe consequences in the lung or brain. Arteriovenous shunts are occasionally seen in the non-haemorrhagic telangiectatic forms of the disease.

Histology

The dilated vessels are unremarkable. However, special studies have helped to show that the vessels are venules (that is, alkaline phosphatase-negative) and that they secrete generous amounts of plasminogen activator. The supporting tissue and overlying epidermis is usually atrophic.

Treatment

Although telangiectases are easy to camouflage with 'covermark' types of preparations, advice may need to be given on its application with respect to the use of cream and powder, blends, and matching of skin colour.

Telangiectases when small and localized can be destroyed by cryotherapy, cautery, electrolysis, or laser therapy; the latter can be endoscopic. Since the laser specifically burns haemoglobin, it is therefore more successful in the treatment of the larger blood-containing dilatations. Sclerotherapy is also possible.

Bleeding should first be treated by the simple first-aid measure of elevation and local pressure. Cautery is most effective only on a dry blanched area controlled by compression. Patients can be taught to inflate a lubricated finger cot tied over the end of a small catheter to immediately control severe epistaxis.

Oestrogen therapy

Oestrogen therapy is sometimes advocated: for instance, ethinyloestradiol 0.25 mg daily, increased to 0.5 mg per day at the end of 4 weeks if epistaxis continues. However, its effectiveness has not been proved in controlled trials.

Percutaneous embolization

This is increasingly used to close unwanted vasculature. However, it requires careful angiographic control and skilled surgeons, and has not overcome the problem of rapid recanalization and opening up of collaterals. Nevertheless, percutaneous embolization is the treatment of choice for severe uncontrolled bleeding from arteriovenous shunts.

Facial erythema (flushing)

In temperate climates the weather-beaten face of the farmer or fisherman is largely a reflection of exposure to cold, as are the rosy cheeks and 'shiny morning face' of the schoolchild. The 'butterfly' area of the cheeks and bridge of the nose pick up hot and cold thermal irradiation. Marked telangiectasia of the cheeks in adults is a common consequence of rosy cheeks in childhood. It may be associated with thickening of the subcutaneous tissues.

Rosacea is usually associated with acneiform pustulation and lymphoedema. For unknown reasons, a keratitis is sometimes associated. Some physicians advocate the elimination of *Helicobacter pylori* with a 1-week course of 20 mg omeprazole twice daily, 400 mg metronidazole twice daily, and 250 mg clarithromycin twice daily. Tetracycline, 250 mg twice daily, or metronidazole gel and lotion are effective therapies for rosacea. A somewhat similar appearance may be seen in sarcoid, especially the lupus pernio variety in which a diffuse granuloma underlies dilated blood vessels filled with slow-flowing blue blood. Mitral or pulmonary stenosis also causes a persistent malar flush. In discoid lupus erythematosus, telangiectasia (Fig. 98(a)) is accompanied by atrophy (Fig. 98(b)), often with well-defined margins and follicular plugging. The borders of rosacea and sarcoid lesions tend to be more diffuse. Asymmetry can be a feature of all disorders.

Telangiectasia due to other collagen diseases varies from the redness and oedema of the orbit, characteristic of dermatomyositis (Fig. 99), to erythema of the backs of the hands and nail-folds, with persistent erythema such that vessels become increasingly inhomogeneous, and quite large dilated forms may be observed.

In scleroderma, especially of the adult acrosclerotic variety, telangiectasia in the form of flat macules, often with square or oblong shapes and fairly well-defined margins, are characteristic. Systemic sclerosis of the face usually causes stiffness and tethering of the skin to deeper structures over the nose and loss of suppleness in the perioral skin. There is, of course, the associated Raynaud's phenomenon and digital ischaemia.

A plethoric complexion is a feature of superior vena cava obstruction, and also of polycythaemia rubra vera and Cushing's syndrome.

Flushing of the face is a common complaint, particularly in the young who may suffer from transient blushing; in older age groups it is characterized by persistent rosacea. Carcinoid should be thought of when there is a prolonged blush associated with a bounding pulse, asthma, abdominal

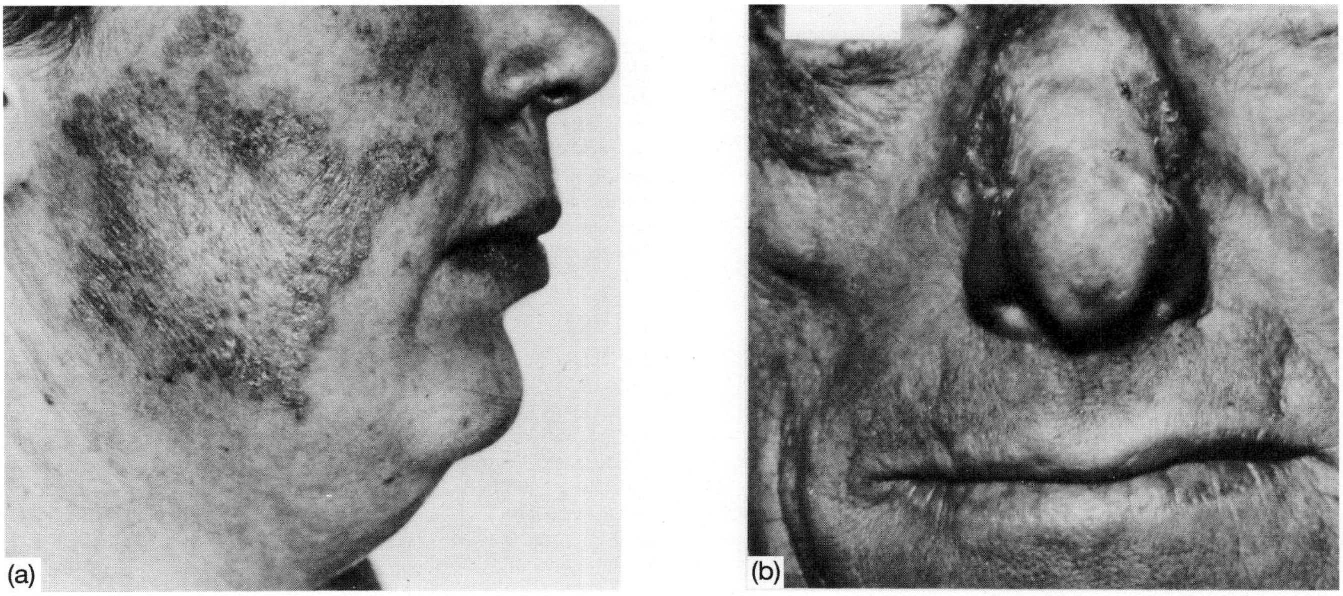

Fig. 98 In lupus erythematosus—chronic discoid type—(a) telangiectasia and (b) erythema is common. There is follicular plugging and destruction of the skin, resulting in pigment loss and scarring.

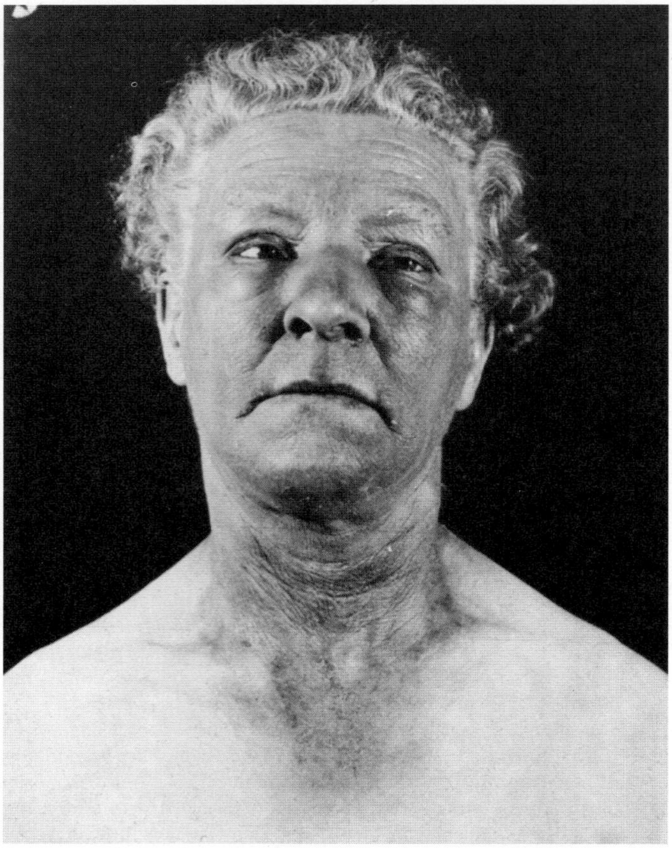

Fig. 99 Bright erythema and oedema of the face, especially periorbitally, is characteristic of dermatomyositis.

pain, and diarrhoea. Frequent applications of steroids to the face for atopic or seborrhoeic eczema produces gross diffuse telangiectasia; rebound eczematous changes often occur on withdrawal (Fig. 100) when the irritation may be severe. Treatment of this condition is the complete withdrawal of all steroids for 3 to 4 weeks, after which the condition tends to settle.

Neurogenic flushing is accompanied by sweating, but this can be dampened with β-blockers. Local heating of the oropharynx is one physiological cause, for which sipping iced water gives relief. Nocturnal overheating causing restlessness and facial flushing; rubbing is another contributory factor.

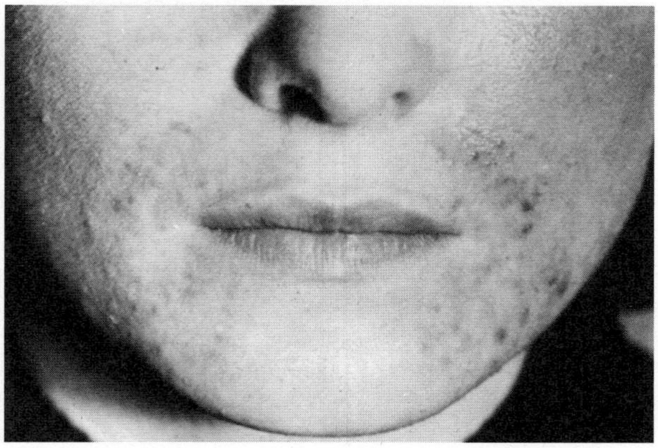

Fig. 100 Perioral dermatitis is a common consequence of the application of fluorinated steroids to the face.

Disorders of collagen and elastic tissue

The metabolism and diseases of collagen are described in Section 19. The fundamental defects are in its chemical structure, its crosslinkage between fibres, and its distribution and quantity.

There are at least 18 collagen types, hence there are many genetic diseases.

Signs of collagen defects

These include:

- Diminished skin thickness and increased transparency mean that deeper structures such as veins and nerves are visible and the sclerae are blue.
- Diminished resistance to shear allows the skin to split and tear, sometimes even without surface breaks. Purpura is usually associated and healing results in white stellate scars. Cutaneous striae are another pattern of skin stretching, with separation in this case. Diminished resistance of the skin is a feature of age; osteoporosis and rheumatoid arthritis are other recognized associations. Steroids are responsible for both stellate scars and cutaneous striae, which is the case whether they are endogenously produced, as in Cushing's disease, or prescribed for other diseases. Local application of steroid cream is probably now the commonest cause of these changes.
- Laxity is the failure of the skin to return rapidly to its former state after distortion by stretch. In some way it is caused by degeneration of elastic tissue but changes in water content and cellularity, as well as increased crosslinkage of collagen, play some part even when the total collagen is reduced.

Diseases due to defective collagen

Solar and senile elastosis

This affects white-skinned races, especially those employed in agricultural or marine work. Chronic exposure to ultraviolet radiation causes abnormal collagen having the histological staining characteristics of elastic tissue but not its properties. It is broken and aggregated and contributes to a thickened, yellow and wrinkled skin, especially on exposed areas during old age. The yellow plaques may be sharply marginated on the face. In the neck deep furrows form a rhomboidal network. The sebaceous glands and ducts are poorly supported, dilated, and patulous, forming giant comedones. On the neck the goose pimple, or plucked-bird, appearance is due to the protection provided by hair follicles shading the dermis against ultraviolet rays. Colloid milium is the abnormal production of a scleroprotein by fibroblasts giving rise to yellowish translucent papules or plaques in light-exposed skin. It may begin in childhood.

Striae

These are common but imperfectly understood; stretch is always a factor. The epidermis is thin and elastic fibres are scanty. Striae are seen on the back and thighs of adolescents during growth, especially when there has been a spurt and the child is athletic. It occurs more in girls than in boys. Striae are a feature of pregnancy and especially affect the abdomen and breasts, usually caused by excessive adrenocortical activity. Incomplete fibroblasts inhibition causes atrophy of collagen in response to glucocorticoids. When the collagen is ageing or degenerate, as follows irradiation or in diseases such as cutis laxa or the Ehlers–Danlos syndrome, striae are uncommon and may not appear even in the pregnant or those with Cushing's syndrome. Striae have also been described in those with chronic infections such as tuberculosis. They are only a diagnostic problem when they are newly formed, in which case they may appear to be weal-like and raised.

Later they flatten and become bluish-red and still later, white and depressed.

Localized fibrosis, keloids, and hypertrophic scars

The connective tissue response to cutaneous injury exceeds the need for appropriate repair at that site, commonly giving rise, a few weeks later, to hypertrophic scars. If the scar continues to hypertrophy and extends beyond the limits of the injured skin site, especially after a period of 3 months after the injury, it is often then termed a keloid. Such scars tend to be more tender than hypertrophic scars. Keloids tend to be familial and are commoner in Blacks. They are rare in infancy and old age and tend to be less severe after the age of 30. Significant factors are the presence of foreign material in the wound and tension. Preferred areas are the ear lobes, chin, neck, shoulders, upper trunk, and lower legs. Keloids in their early stages may respond to strong local steroids applied locally or intralesionally. Compression therapy is sometimes helpful, as is cryotherapy in the early stages. Re-excision and radiotherapy to the edges of the wounds is now the treatment most preferred.

Pseudoxanthoma elasticum

This is a hereditary disorder of elastic tissue; of which there are four distinct types:

Dominant type I

Here, small, yellowish papules form linear or reticulate plaques, which in older persons are soft, lax, and hang in folds, they are flexually distributed, especially in the groins, axillas, and neck (Fig. 101). There is a severe degeneration of Bruch's membrane giving rise to the slate-grey, poorly defined 'angioid' streaks that form an incomplete ring or radiating lesions around the optic disc of the retina. There is early blindness. Vascular complications include intermittent claudication and coronary artery disease.

Dominant type II

The small, yellowish papules are fewer and flatter than in dominant type I disease. There is increased extensibility of the skin. Vascular and retinal changes are mild. The sclerae are blue and there may be a high arched palate and myopia.

Recessive type I

This resembles dominant type I pseudoxanthoma elasticum, but the vascular and retinal degeneration is mild. Haematemesis is especially common, and women are more often affected than men.

Recessive type II

This is a very rare form, but the skin changes are extensive and generalized. There tends to be no systemic complications. The pathology of pseudoxanthoma elasticum includes a deposition of calcium on the elastic fibres. The mid-dermal elastic tissue is fragmented and swollen.

Perforating elastoma

This is a condition of elastic fibre degeneration in the upper dermis, with a resulting foreign body reaction and extrusion through the overlying epidermis. This reaction gives rise to papules that develop a central plaque of extruded material. There is a tendency for the formation of annular and serpiginous patterns, particularly over the back and neck region. The disorder is associated with mongolism, Marfan syndrome, Ehlers–Danlos syndrome, pseudoxanthoma elasticum, and osteogenesis imperfecta.

Ehlers–Danlos syndrome: cutis hyperelastica

Ehlers–Danlos syndrome is a rare inherited disorder of connective tissue (see Chapter 19.2). The condition is usually recognized when the child begins to walk since there is hyperextensibility of the joints. Trivial cuts form gaping wounds and heal poorly. The skin feels soft and can be

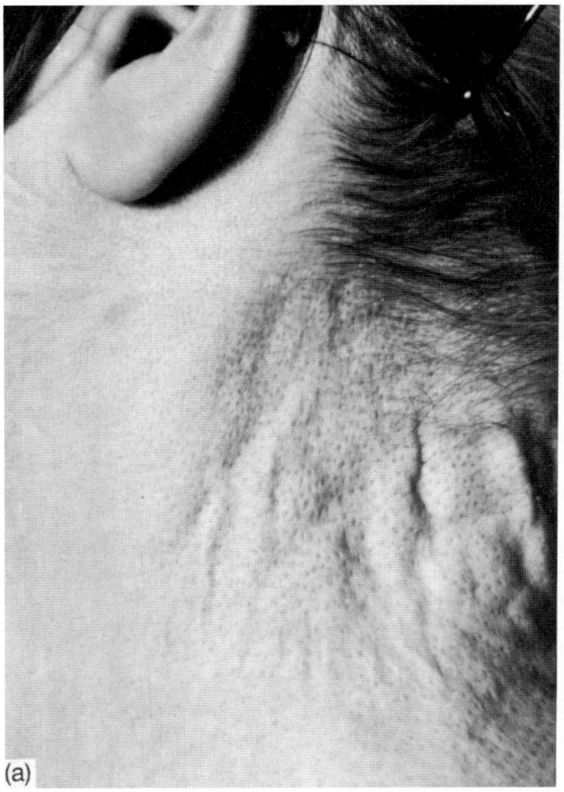
(a)

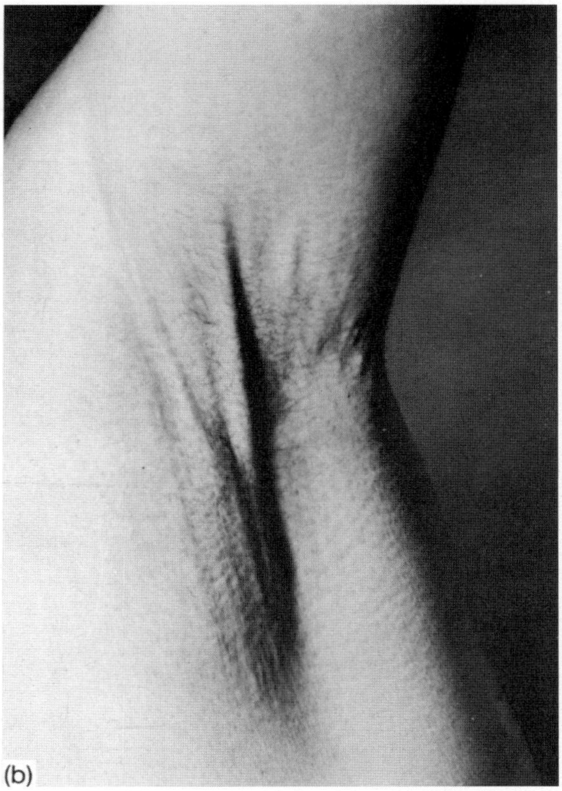
(b)

Fig. 101 (a) Yellowish papules and loss of elasticity of the skin of the neck in pseudoxanthoma elasticum. This may be a clue to gastrointestinal bleeding or even blindness. (b) Yellowish papules and loss of elasticity of the skin of the axillas in pseudoxanthoma elasticum. This may be a clue to gastrointestinal bleeding or even blindness.

stretched, particularly over the knees and elbows. Arterial rupture, aortic dissection, and intestinal perforation have been described in severely affected individuals with deletions in the *COL3A1* gene on chromosome 3 affecting the length of collagen type 3.

Cutis laxa

This is a rare disease in which the skin hangs in loose folds due to the loss of elastic tissue. Severely affected individuals have associated pulmonary emphysema. Both dominant and recessive patterns of inheritance are seen (Fig. 102).

Atrophy

Atrophy is characterized by thinning, loss of elasticity, loss of hair follicles, and a smooth surface to the skin. When pinched gently the skin produces fine wrinkles and may be compared to tissue paper. The upper dermal atrophy causes poor support to an atrophic vasculature and telangiectasia is often observed. At the same time there tends to be increased pigmentation within the dermis. Atrophy may be a consequence of inflammation following acute bacterial (particularly elastase-producing organisms) infection vasculitis or pancreatitis. It may be widespread, as in the chronic scarring of leprosy or onchocerciasis. Some circumscribed atrophies follow an urticarial vasculitic process, probably caused by an infection that destroys elastic tissue. Perifollicular atrophy or postacne atrophy is similarly due to elastase-producing strains of staphylococci. Syphilis is another cause of destruction of elastic tissue. Non-infectious causes include lupus erythematosus and localized scleroderma with its variants.

Poikiloderma

The combination of pigmentation, telangiectasia, and atrophy is known as poikiloderma (see Fig. 108), causes of which include irradiation, lymphoma, and collagen diseases such as lupus erythematosus and dermatomyositis. A congenital form is associated with light sensitivity, skin cancers, and dwarfism. It may follow lichen planus or stasis eczema. Poikiloderma is common on light-exposed areas of the neck and may be aggravated by cosmetics. It is also described in graft-versus-host diseases.

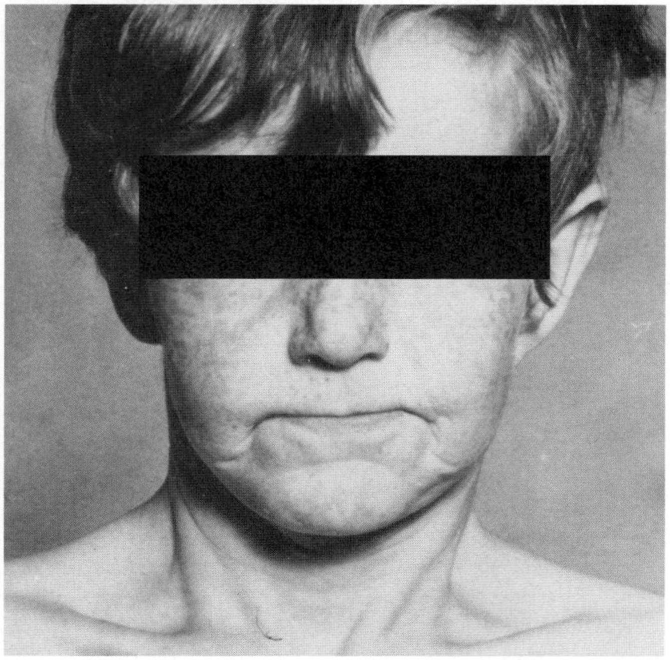

Fig. 102 Drooping of the facial skin of a 9-year-old boy is due to premature loss of elasticity. The diagnosis is cutis laxa.

Morphea

Morphea is a localized form of scleroderma with a good prognosis for complete recovery (Fig. 103). It is not associated with any systemic disease, though subsets in Europe due to *Borrelia burgdorferi* cannot be ruled out. Occasionally a generalized form produces such tightness of the chest wall that breathing may be impaired. The generalized form of morphea also greatly restricts the limbs, and a combination of ischaemia and lymphoedema may result in ulceration of the peripheries.

Deep dermal and subcutaneous atrophy

The skin loses its subcutaneous or deep dermal tissue in a number of conditions. Such skin is waxy in colour and may be yellow, pigmented, or bluish with a loss of connective tissue. Deeper vessels may become more obvious, resulting in either telangiectasia or obvious cutaneous atrophy and linear stretch marks that are initially red and which sometimes protrude above the surface of the skin, but later there is always marked atrophy.

The atrophic skin may be tethered to underlying tissue or more obviously scarred. Such skin may feel hard or sclerosed (Table 19).

Other causes of deep dermal atrophy include the injection of insulin—this is commonly seen on the thighs or arms of diabetics. 'Anetoderma' is a term used for very discrete, round idiopathic losses of dermis.

Hemi- or generalized atrophy of a non-inflammatory origin is mainly of unknown aetiology. Partial lipodystrophy is associated with glomerulonephritis, hypocomplementaemia, and protease inhibitors. The Lawrence–Seip syndrome, or total lipoatrophy (with acanthosis nigricans, genital hypertrophy, resistant diabetes, and hepatomegaly), is a condition affecting infants. Atrophie blanche (Fig. 104) is an obliteration of single capillaries in the upper dermis, leading to very localized scarring, the causes of which are listed in Table 20.

Malignant disease

Infiltrations of the skin presenting as papules, *peau d'orange*, nodules, plaques, or ulcerating tumours of the dermis with destruction of overlying epidermis are a common terminal event of malignancy. Such lesions may arise from localized spread, as from a carcinoma of the breast, when they tend to be single or grouped and asymmetrical. More widespread haematogenous spread but with multiple lesions are a still more common terminal event. Certain metastases have diagnostic features, such as the scarring alopecia of breast carcinoma affecting the scalp or the pedunculated tumour of hypernephroma.

Signs of underlying malignancy

The three 'P's of pallor, pigmentation, and pruritus are common terminal events in malignant disease, any of which can also be a presenting sign, albeit rarely in the case of pruritis. Defective immunosurveillance predisposes to infections such as candidiasis or herpes simplex and herpes zoster. Although disseminated intravascular coagulation is a common terminal event of malignancy, it may be a presenting sign of lymphoma, leukaemia, or carcinoma of the pancreas. Rarer diseases associated with malignancy are given in Table 21, and include:

- Acquired ichthyosis, in which the skin becomes progressively drier and more scaly. The surface stratum corneum may crack, giving rise to reactive patterns of eczema craquelée (Fig. 20). Increasing scale eventually overlaps with exfoliative dermatitis but, unlike the exfoliative dermatitis due to drugs or psoriasis, the scale is more adherent, in other words it is less exfoliative. There is usually accompanying atrophy of the skin.

- Dermatomyositis is commonly caused by malignancy in white-skinned adults. In children or in Blacks it is more often a manifestation of autoimmune (collagen) disease. The muscle weakness is proximal. The skin signs include erythema (see Fig. 99), lichenoid, or psoriaform eruptions, and itching or tenderness may be considerable. Periorbital swelling and redness, as well as a streaky erythema on the backs of the fingers and ragged telangiectatic nail-folds, are other features.
- Acanthosis nigricans is the pigmentation and wartiness of the axillas and groins. There is a velvety brown thickness of the skin of the hands and at mucocutaneous junctions such as the lips (Fig. 105).
- Acquired hypertrichosis lanuginosa is a generalized increase in terminal hair. It should be distinguished from hirsutes, which is an increase in hair in sites normally associated with hair growth, such as the chin.
- Acute onset of multiple irritable seborrhoeic warts is known as the sign of Leser–Trélat.
- Superficial thrombophlebitis or migrating thrombophlebitis is particularly associated with carcinoma of the pancreas.
- Bullous pyoderma gangrenosum is a feature of leukaemia and myeloma.
- Bullous disease of erythema multiforme type, or occasionally more suggestive of pemphigoid, is more likely to be associated with malignancy if the oral mucosa is involved or if immunofluorescence studies are negative.
- Erythema gyratum repens (Fig. 106) is one of many patterns of erythema forming repeated concentric rings. The more bizarre and rapidly evolving the process, the more likely it is to be associated with malignancy. This is particularly so when it is generalized, oedematous, or scaling (see also Fig. 10(c)).
- Palmar keratoses are found in association with cancer of the bladder or lung.

Cutaneous lymphoma

Few aspects of dermatology have been more confusing than those concerning lymphoma. In some respects it has been simplified by the recognition and identification of B and T lymphocytes and the realization that terms such as 'reticulosis', 'prereticulosis', and 'reticulum cell' were misapplied. T cells normally traverse through the epidermis and upper dermis, producing a horizontal infiltrate and flat patches. B cells prefer the mid and deep dermis, and produce nodules. Expression on the keratinocyte of $\alpha3\beta1$ integrin chains possibly explains epidermotropism. The Hassall's corpuscle in the thymus may have features in common with the cells of the epidermis, which explain helper T-cell, Langerhans-cell, and epidermal interaction. The epidermis also produces cytokines, which may account for lymphocyte behaviour—attraction, differentiation, and proliferation. Classification

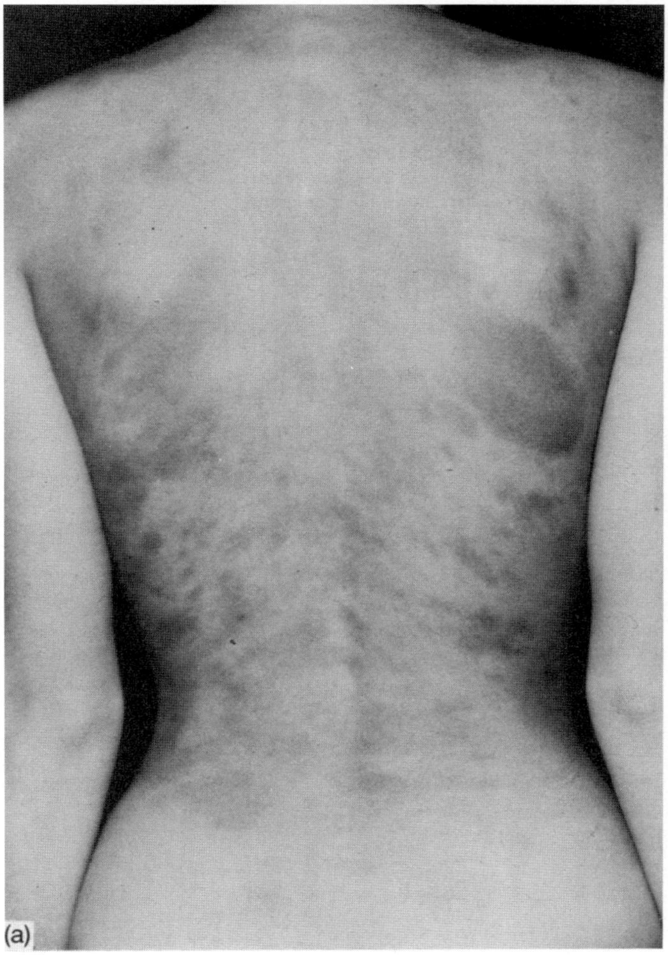
(a)

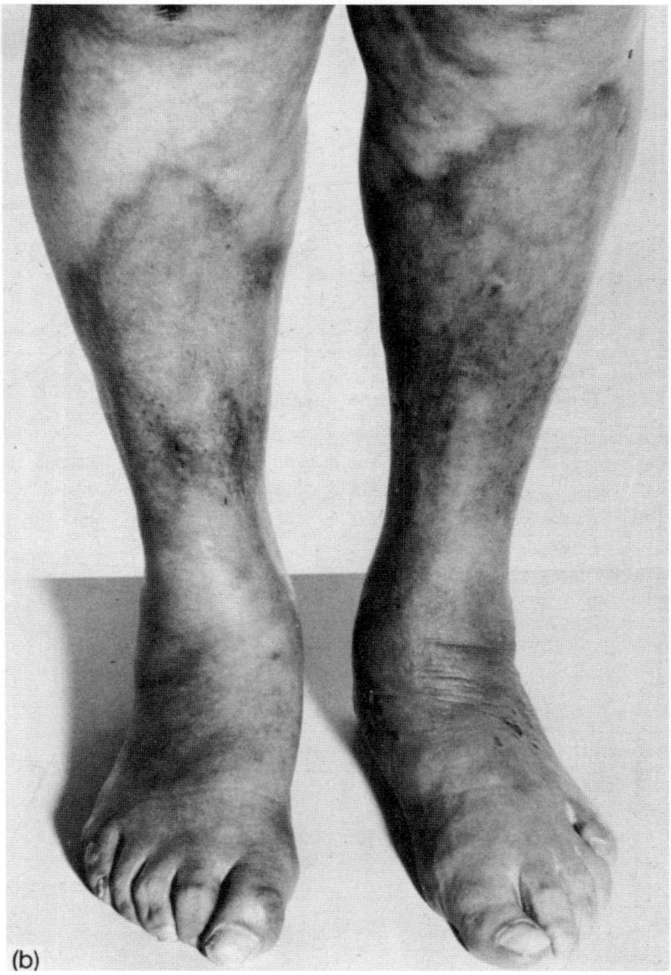
(b)

Fig. 103 (a) Widespread hardness of the skin and brownish or violaceous plaques that are often atrophic are features of morphea—a localized form of scleroderma. (b) Pseudoscleroderma, identical to morphea, is also a consequence of post-thrombophlebitic fibrosis of the lower limbs.

and staging procedures are complex, and evolving with improved technology. The simplest classification into B-cell, T-cell, and non-B and non-T-cell lymphoma, with a single subgrouping into small cells indicating low-grade malignancy, and large cells indicating high-grade malignancy, is now largely accepted. However, neither morphology nor a panel of monoclonal antibodies have provided a system of identification by which treatment can be planned with absolute certainty and prognosis reliably determined.

Enzymatic, cytochemical, immunological, monoclonal antibody, gene rearrangement analysis, functional, and ultrastructural methods used in research are not routinely available for aiding clinical diagnosis, but they indicate that conditions in which the epidermis is eczematous, scaly, or crusting are usually infiltrated with T cells, especially of Thy-2 lineage and with reduced IFN-γ signalling, as in mycosis fungoides, Sézary syndrome, and pagetoid reticulosis. This may explain the reduced capacity to control

Table 19 Conditions causing sclerosis

Scleroderma

Dermatomyositis

Eosinophilic fasciitis (Schulman's syndrome)
This resembles scleroderma but the onset of oedema and induration of the extremities is accompanied by eosinophilia. A variant known as the eosinophil-myalgic syndrome follows the ingestion of L-tryptophan

Scleromyxoedema (lichen myxoedematosus)
A deposition of mucin associated with a paraprotein, an abnormal lambda light chain affecting face, limbs with thickened skin and exaggeration of natural contours or ridges, and flexion of the fingers. The deposition is papular and often linear

Progeria
Associated with alopecia and bird-like facies as well as arteriosclerosis

Porphyria cutanea tarda
The scleroderma is associated with hypertrichosis, skin fragility, blistering and scarring in light-exposed areas

Graft-versus-host reactions
A history of bone marrow or thymus transplant precedes the lichenoid rash and scleroderma

Carcinoid disease and mast-cell disorders
The release of serotonin and histamine over a prolonged period is sometimes associated with fibroblast proliferation and sclerosis

Pseudoscleroderma
This is due to infiltration occurring in amyloid, breast carcinoma, leprosy, lipoid proteinosis, mucopolysaccharide storage disorders, myxoedema. Thickening of the tissues is a feature of acromegaly

Scorbutic pseudoscleroderma
In the Bantu this is described as smooth, very dark skin, tightly stretched and hard on the lower aspects of the legs. It has abnormal iron pigment in histological material

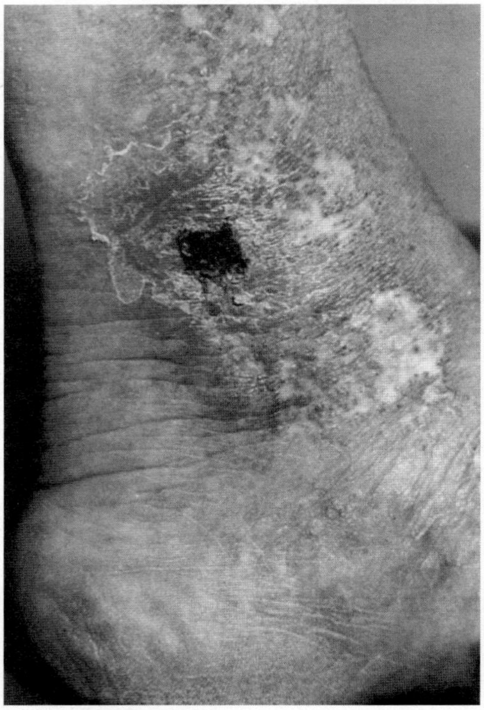

Fig. 104 Atrophie blanche is an obliteration of the capillaries in the upper dermis, causing sclerosis. Residual vessels are elongated and coiled. They are liable to thrombosis and overlying ulceration is a consequence.

Table 20 Atrophie blanche: list of associated diseases

Pigmented purpuric eruptions	Rheumatoid arthritis
Gravitational stasis	Hashimoto's disease
Thrombophlebitis	Sickle-cell anaemia
Thromboangiitis obliterans	Anterior poliomyelitis
Polyarteritis nodosa	Sjögren's syndrome
Diabetes mellitus	Capillary naevi
Scleroderma	Drug eruptions
Lupus erythematosus	Trauma, cuts
Dermatomyositis	Carcinoma

Table 21 Classification of cutaneous paraneoplastic syndrome

Autosomal dominant paraneoplasias	Skin markers	Internal malignancies	Coincidence (%)
Basal-cell naevus syndrome (Gorlin)	Multiple basal-cell carcinomas	Brain medulloblastoma	–20
Birt–Hogg syndrome	Trichodiscoma	Gastrointestinal tract	?
Carney syndrome	Lentigines, blue naevi	Heart myxoma, testes	>75
Cowden syndrome	Trichilemmoma, fibroma	Breasts, thyroid	70
Gardner's syndrome	Cysts, osteoma, pigmented ocular fundus	Colon	100
Howel–Evans syndrome (tylosis)	Palmoplantar keratomas	Oesophagus	100
Multiple endocrine neoplasia syndrome (MEN 2b)	Neuroma (lips and tongue)	Thyroid, phaeochromocytoma	>85
Dysplastic naevus syndrome	Multiple dysplastic naevi	Melanoma, testes, eyes	?
Peutz–Jeghers syndrome	Lentigines on lips	Ovaries, testes	rare
Torre–Muir syndrome	Sebaceous tumours	Gastrointestinal tract, lung, urinary	–100%

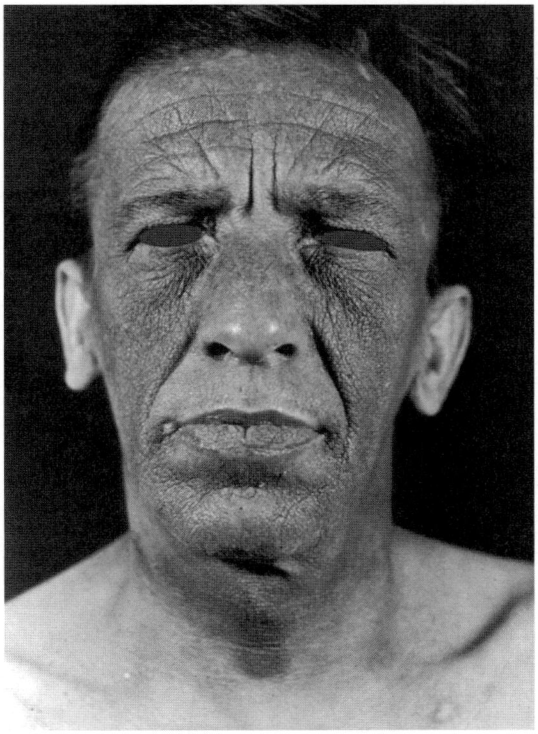

Fig. 105 Acanthosis nigricans: a darkening and thickening of the skin with a tendency to papilloma formation. The angles of the mouth are often involved, as in this patient with carcinoma of the lung.

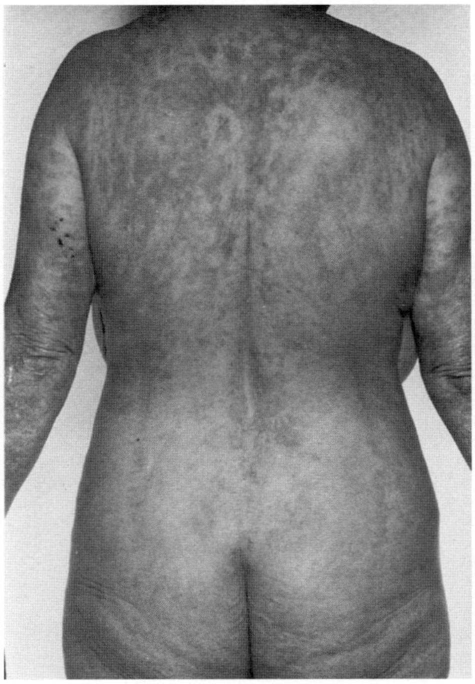

Fig. 106 Erythema gyratum repens in a patient with adenocarcinoma of the colon.

infection and secondary malignancies. Mononuclear phagocytes, including the Langerhans cells and eosinophils, often infiltrate the upper dermis. Most of the purple-red tumours that show no involvement of the epidermis and produce sharply demarcated infiltrates in the middle or deep dermis are due to B-cell proliferation. The late tumour stage is reflected in the progression to large, anaplastic, lymphoblastic cells.

The previously labelled reticulosarcomas starting as dome-shaped, deep-red solitary tumours are now thought to be lymphoblastic, more often B cell than T cell. Such less differentiated blast cells also give rise to heavy infiltrates in the whole dermis, and are less inclined to produce the nests of cells within the epidermis that are a feature of mycosis fungoides. There is destruction of blood vessels and fibrous tissue, whereas blood vessels are well preserved in mycosis fungoides and often characterized by prominent epithelioid endothelial cells as in postcapillary venules of lymph nodes. Benign lesions show a well-defined germinal centre.

All types of lymphoma may affect any organ, including lymph nodes and the blood, but mycosis fungoides, Sézary's syndrome, and pagetoid reticulosis favour the skin and often seem confined to it. The leonine facies is a peculiar, diffuse, deep nodular feature more often seen in B-cell lymphoma, as in chronic lymphatic leukaemia.

During the early stage of mycosis fungoides, the behaviour of the T cell cannot be proven to be malignant, and some suggest that it is merely hyperreactive or overstimulated. The source of this stimulus could even be the skin macrophage known as the Langerhans cell, which increase in number in mycosis fungoides. Exactly when 'overstimulus' becomes 'lymphoma' has been debated, but no conclusions can be reached. Environmental infections such as retroviruses and *B. burgdorferi* as well as genetic susceptibility are possible incriminating factors.

The distinctive cell found in the tissues and blood of patients with the Sézary syndrome and in the epidermis of those with mycosis fungoides is a T cell with an usually, but not invariably, hyperconvoluted cerebri-form nucleus. This cell is also observed in a variety of non-lymphomatous dermatoses and should be equated more with the 'overstimulus' concept rather than with malignancy.

Clinical features of lymphoma

Dermatologists have long grappled with the problem of skin diseases suspected of culminating, often years later, in a malignancy of the lymphoid tissue. These diseases have features of chronic dermatitis and psoriasis (parapsoriasis) because there is a chronic reaction in the dermis and epidermis that is often indistinguishable from other causes of such a reaction. One feature that causes anxiety is a lack of symmetry in an atypical distribution; there is also inhomogeneity within the lesion. Infiltration with white cells suggesting tumour formation is another feature. Yet another, is the combination of atrophy or thinning of the dermis, telangiectasia, and pigmentation known as poikiloderma. Persistent superficial dermatitis, previously known as parapsoriasis in plaque (benign type), consists of flat, symmetrical, slightly scaly, red patches on the trunk or limbs that persist for years. They are round, oval, or finger-like and sometimes yellowish (Fig. 107). This is now thought to be a benign condition.

Poikiloderma atrophicans vasculare, previously known as parapsoriasis (large plaque or lichenoides), resembles radiodermatitis in that there is atrophy, telangiectasis, and reticulate pigmentation (Fig. 108). It favours areas not exposed to natural sunlight such as the breasts or buttocks. Poikilodermal lesions may be composed of small papules or large plaques of any shape. Although the expected outcome, often many years later, is the cutaneous T-cell lymphoma known as mycosis fungoides, Hodgkin's disease is also a possibility.

B-cell lymphomas, when present in the skin, form firm pink-red or skin-coloured tumours, often in groups coalescing to produce annular or other patterns (Fig. 109).

Lipomelanic reticulosis is a non-specific enlargement of lymph nodes associated with widespread dermatitis or erythroderma.

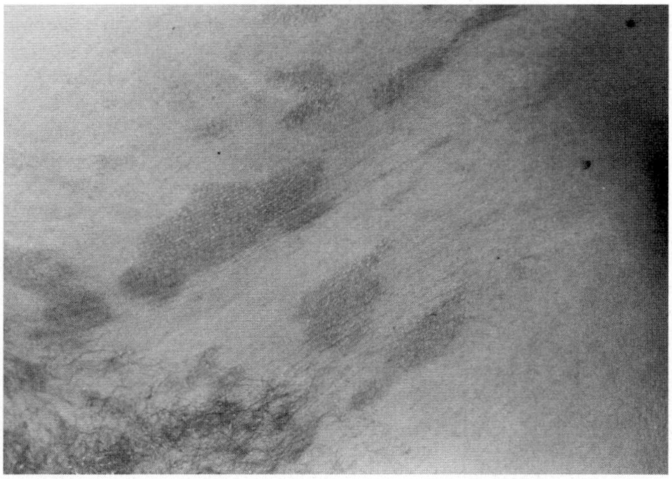

Fig. 107 Lower abdominal, persistent superficial dermatitis (parapsoriasis). These are fixed and persistent digitate (finger-like) patterns, erythematous, and slightly scaly.

Although mycosis fungoides is often initially no more than a non-specific dermatitis or, more commonly, poikiloderma atrophicans vasculare, occasionally it is a tumour from the start. The lesions may be symptomless, but severe pruritus is common. Affected areas become more infiltrated, scaly, and reddened (Fig. 110), and often they are annular, serpiginous, or have other bizarre shapes. Erythroderma and widespread ulceration is the final stage of the disease. The diagnostic histological feature is invasion of the epidermis by atypical lymphocytes, often in clusters—Pautrier abscesses—and a heavy pleomorphic infiltration of the upper dermis hugging the epidermis but causing less necrosis of individual epidermal cells than in lichen planus.

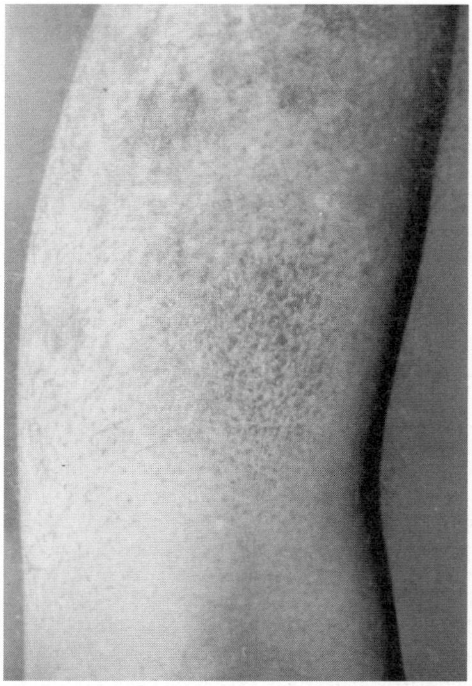

Fig. 108 Poikiloderma; atrophy, pigmentation, and telangiectasia, commonly preceding the development of lymphoma in the skin. The clinical appearance resembles radiodermatitis.

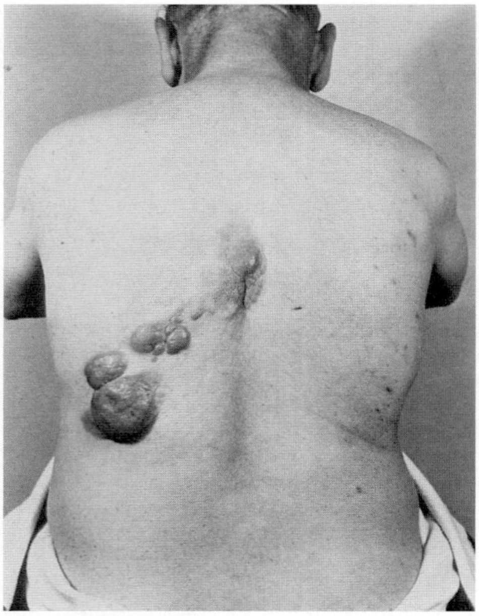

Fig. 109 Fleshy tumours grouped and arising in the dermis without epidermal hyperplasia. This is characteristic of B-cell lymphomas.

Skin manifestations of Hodgkin's disease include infiltration of the skin with nodules of the disease. Pigmentation and pruritus are common. Prurigo with deep excoriations and secondary infection is one of its most distressing manifestations. Ichthyosiform atrophy as part of the terminal wasting disease is common. The scaling is often as severe as an exfoliative dermatitis, but shedding of the scale is less than that of psoriasis. Hair loss, herpes zoster, and, rarely, erythema nodosum are other complications.

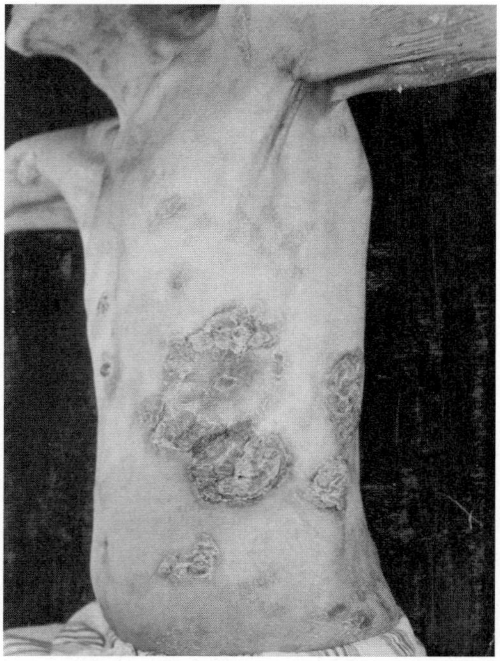

Fig. 110 Marked irregular epidermal reactivity is a characteristic response to T-cell lymphoma of the mycosis fungoides type.

Management of cutaneous lymphoma

The rate of progression is highly variable but usually slow. There is still no clear picture of the natural history of mycosis fungoides. With so many new therapeutic possibilities it should not be forgotten that Samman treated a series of patients conservatively and that only 45 out of 212 patients died of mycosis fungoides. Most of those who died had tumours, skin ulcers, or palpable lymph nodes at the time of presentation, and in the absence of these the prognosis tends to be very good. In patients with benign patterns of the disease it is important not to overtreat. 'Staging' is an attempt to record the extent and progression of the disease in the skin and lymph nodes using multiple biopsies and scanning of internal organs. Some localized forms of lymphoma, even when anaplastic, can be cured by excision. Extensive disease, when confined to the skin, responds well to radiotherapy and topical medication.

Radiotherapy

Small-field orthovoltage radiation has been standard therapy for many years and is very useful for controlling plaques and tumours resistant to other modalities. It is not unusual for patients to require a small dose of radiation to only one area at as little as yearly intervals. Electron-beam therapy is recommended for most patients with extensive infiltrated plaques or tumours. Although a high initial response rate can be expected in the majority of patients, they only remain free of disease for about 3 years.

Topical nitrogen mustard (mechlorethamine, HN_2)

This is a useful treatment for patients who have less-infiltrated skin lesions. Clinical response may be slow and maintenance therapy may be required for at least 2 years. The chief side-effect is allergic contact dermatitis, occurring in about 30 to 60 per cent of patients. Desensitization can be attempted but is difficult to effect. Although there is some debate as to whether an aqueous or ointment-based preparation is best, the latter probably produces fewer hypersensitivity reactions.

PUVA

Several reported series of the good effects of PUVA have resulted in most academic departments using this as a first-line therapy for widespread superficial lesions. However, PUVA penetrance is limited so that deep tumours are unlikely to be cleared. Erythrodermic (Sezary) patients do well with extracorporeal photochemotherapy.

Systemic chemotherapy

On the whole this is reserved for palliation in patients with systemic disease and deep tumours. There is usually some initial response, but clearance for more than 1 year is unusual. Cutaneous lymphoma is susceptible to immunosuppression and this is a rich field of investigation at the present time.

Viral warts

Warts are caused by the papovavirus (see Chapter 7.10.17), which enters the skin through small abrasions, particularly if the skin is moist and warm. Virus is found by electron microscopy in the differentiating cells of the upper epidermis rather than in the proliferating basal-cell layer. The incubation period is probably several months. A number of strains of wart virus give rise to different types of warts—common, plantar, mosaic, plane, and anogenital. Molluscum contagiosum is caused by a pox virus (Fig. 111).

The incidence of warts is increased in immunosuppressed patients, either from drugs or associated with lymphoma. However, cell-mediated immunity is more certainly a factor than humoral immunity. The peak incidence is in children between 12 and 16 years of age, and in recent years there seems to be an increase in infection rate in people living in Europe and the United States compared to Asia, Australia, and Africa.

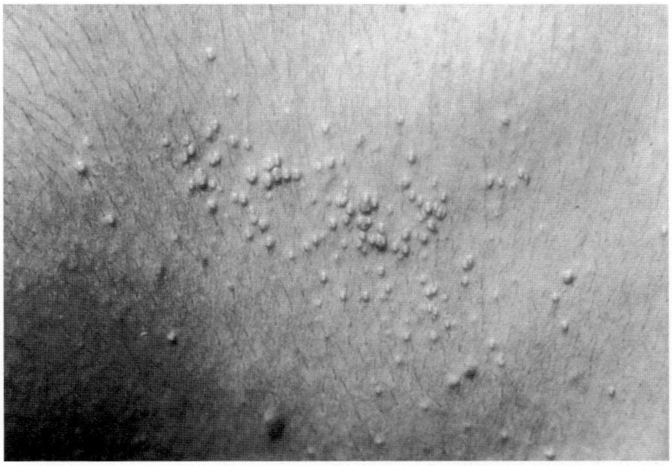

Fig. 111 Molluscum contagiosum: groups of virus-induced papules characterized by a central punctum.

Trauma may account for the distribution of warts on the hands and feet. Nail-biting in children and shaving in men, as well as ill-fitting shoes in adults, are all relevant factors. Some 20 per cent of warts disappear within 6 months and 65 per cent in 2 years, although plane warts and mosaic warts are slow to clear.

Common warts are firm papules with a rough horny surface. They occur singly or coalesce into large masses. The knuckles and nail-folds are particularly favoured, as are the knees and, more rarely, the penile shaft. They should be differentiated from warty tuberculosis, which is usually a solitary plaque with an erythematous border. Granuloma annulare of the knuckles does not have a horny surface. A persistent wart on the toes or fingers may be a reaction to a subungual exostosis. Squamous epitheliomas or keratoacanthomas are usually solitary and found in an older population.

Plane warts are smooth, flat, or slightly elevated and affect the face or back of hands. They may coalesce or form linear lesions in scratch marks. Lichen planus may be difficult to distinguish from plane warts but is unusual on the face and prefers the flexor surface of the wrists as well as the oral mucosa. The histology of plane warts is unexciting, whereas lichen planus shows destruction of the basal-cell layer of the epidermis and a heavy infiltrate of mononuclear cells.

Filiform and digitate warts are common in the beard area, on the lips, and in the nasal vestibule.

A plantar wart begins as a small 'sago-grain' papule. As it enlarges, paring the surface with a scalpel distinguishes the wart from the surrounding horny ring of normal epidermis and reveals the small capillaries in the tips of the elongated papillae. Most warts occur over pressure points. Clusters of small warts make up a mosaic. A wart which shows numerous thrombosed capillaries and is darker than usual is probably regressing. The fourth interdigital space is a common site for soft corns due to pressure of the little toe on the head of the metatarsal caused by a tightly fitting shoe, these are often seen in ballet dancers. Soft warts or even condylomata lata have been described at such sites.

Treatment

Most human papillomavirus (**HPV**) infections in the vagina and cervix are invisible to the naked eye but can be identified by painting the area with acetic acid (3–5 per cent); however, the demonstration of latent virus is of uncertain biological significance. Although infection with HPV is not sufficient to cause cancer, it may act as a promoter. There is no successful means of eliminating HPV. Warts should be treated on the basis that they are unaesthetic and uncomfortable.

Spontaneous resolution is to be expected. Overall, 12 weeks is the usual time required to cure warts irrespective of the treatment used, and most standard treatments do no better or worse than this. Podophyllin and formalin or salicylic acid are standard therapies.

Podophyllin, 10 to 20 per cent in liquid paraffin or in tincture benzoic compound, is painted on to anogenital warts and the area then powdered. The podophyllin is irritant and some patients need to wash it off in 2 h, others feel no such discomfort. However, podophyllin should not be used during pregnancy since absorption sufficient to damage the fetus is a possibility. The treatment is repeated at intervals of 1 to 3 weeks.

Formalin (as a 10 per cent solution) can be applied as a soak to multiple warts on the soles of the feet, but dryness and fissuring may be troublesome.

Salicylic acid is the most reliable chemical for treating warts. Paints or plasters containing 20 to 40 per cent salicylic acid are best applied after a 5-min soak with warm soapy water and preferably after excess surface keratin has been removed.

Imiquimod, which induces interferon-α and other cytokines, is now available as a topical agent and is effective against anogenital warts and molluscum contagiosum.

Freezing is with liquid nitrogen, either in a special spray or by application from a cotton-wool bud on the end of an orange stick. The wart should be whitened for at least 20 to 30 s and blistering is a common consequence.

Local anaesthetic injected into the base of a wart to lift it up from the dermis can be followed by curettage. Compression with the thumb on immediate adjacent tissue prevents bleeding while silver nitrate is applied. The rim of horny tissues around the wart side should be cut away using scissors.

Curettage of molluscum contagiosum may be made painless in the majority of children, except at mucocutaneous junctions, by the use of a eutetic mixture of local anaesthetics (**EMLA**) applied under occlusion for 60 min.

Granulomas and other infiltrations of the skin

A granuloma is a compact accumulation of cells, comprising mainly monocytes or their variants, macrophages, epithelioid cells, and giant cells. Often there is subsequent fibrosis. Lymphocytes are more numerous in granulomas due to allergens to which the host is sensitive. Degeneration or the presence of foreign bodies encourage neutrophil and eosinophil participation.

Granulomas are classified as high or low turnover:

- *high turnover:* tissue-destructive, induced by toxic irritants or delayed hypersensitivity, continuous recruitment of macrophages and many mitoses, and frequent epithelioid and giant cells;
- *low turnover:* space-occupying but not destructive, induced by inert (bacterial) and non-degradable irritants, no continued recruitment but long survival of macrophages and few mitoses, and few epithelioid and giant cells.

The clinical features of granulomas are either space-occupying nodules lying in the dermis or, if close to the skin surface, they may be seen as yellow or brownish-red and sometimes translucent areas. The chronic changes in blood supply associated with the lesion cause a bluish colour and sometimes telangiectasia. If they are located in the upper dermis, there may be overlying epithelial hyperplasia or ulceration with extrusion of some of the granulomatous material. On the other hand, thinning of the epidermis may be considerable. In dark skins, pigmentary changes may include hypo- or hyperpigmentation.

A common cause of granulomas is persistent irritation of the skin by external trauma causing ulceration and pseudoepitheliomatous hyperplasia. Examples include granuloma fissuratum of the ear or nose due to ill-fitting spectacles. The ingrowing toenail, the pilonidal sinus, or the presence of extrafollicular but intradermal hair (as is seen in the interdigital clefts of barbers, and cattle or horse dealers) are other examples.

Granuloma gluteal infantum is seen in the nappy area due to incomplete resolution of an irritant rash to which steroid creams have been too extravagantly applied. Numerous agents acting as foreign bodies are causes of chronic granulomas in the skin. They include sea-urchin spines, silicates, cactus allergen, grit, and various chronic infections such as *Candida albicans*, *Trichophyton verrucosum* (Fig. 112(a)), coccidioidomycosis, atypical mycobacteria from fish tanks or swimming pools, tuberculosis (Fig. 112(b)), leprosy (Fig. 112(c)), leishmaniasis (Fig. 112(d)), and halogen granulomas (see Fig. 26).

Sarcoidosis

See Chapter 17.11.6 for further discussion.

Urticaria pigmentosa or mastocytosis

Mast cells are normally present in the skin but the numbers vary greatly, with up to 80 per mm^3 found in the upper dermis. In mastocytosis they are greatly increased in number, and may be found as a single isolated mastocytoma, or as numerous nests scattered over the entire body (that is, the classic urticaria pigmentosa) or diffusely throughout the entire skin. Occasionally there is systemic infiltration of all tissues including the liver, spleen, and bone marrow. A very rare leukaemic variety is also recognized.

The mast cell releases histamine, leucotrienes, and heparin, all of which may have systemic effects. However, it is increasingly realized that the local contribution to mastocytosis is through the secretion of proteases from these cells.

In the infant, mastocytosis may present as blisters; more commonly, the lightly pigmented swellings in the skin are noted and observed to swell when scratched or following a hot bath or exercise. Rarely, there is generalized flushing and itching. The condition is most common during the first year of life or at birth, and an onset at this age is a good prognosis for eventual complete resolution by adolescence.

In adults, a late onset is associated with diffuse plaques and telangiectasia.

The systemic variety presents in 10 per cent of adult cases, causing osteoporosis or osteosclerosis. The spleen may be enlarged, and bleeding disorders are the consequence of either thrombocytopenia or from the effects of heparin. Involvement of the gut causes a variety of symptoms including colic and diarrhoea. Right-sided heart failure due to pulmonary hypertension is recorded. Urinalysis for histamine or prostaglandin D_2 may help to confirm the diagnosis when the skin lesions are absent.

Treatment

Treatment is unsatisfactory, but the increasing use of various combinations of H_1- and H_2-antagonists is proving beneficial in some cases. The prognosis for eventual resolution is good in children. A solitary or troublesome single lesion in an adult can be excised. The cosmetic appearance of pigmented lesions is helped by sun exposure or by the use of UVA and psoralens, but the number of mast cells is not reduced. Disodium cromoglycate helps some patients with systemic mastocytosis. The number of mast cells can be suppressed by high-potency steroids applied under occlusive dressings.

Cutaneous manifestations of histiocytosis X

The cutaneous lesions of histiocytosis X are small yellow-brown keratotic scaling papules. These coalesce to form a diffuse seborrhoeic dermatitis that is ulcerative, crusting, and purpuric. Granulomatous eroded plaques that are particularly found in the flexures and in the external auditory meatus cause great discomfort. The hair margins are commonly involved. The common association of diabetes insipidus and hepatosplenomegaly is described elsewhere. The diagnosis is confirmed by demonstrating pale-

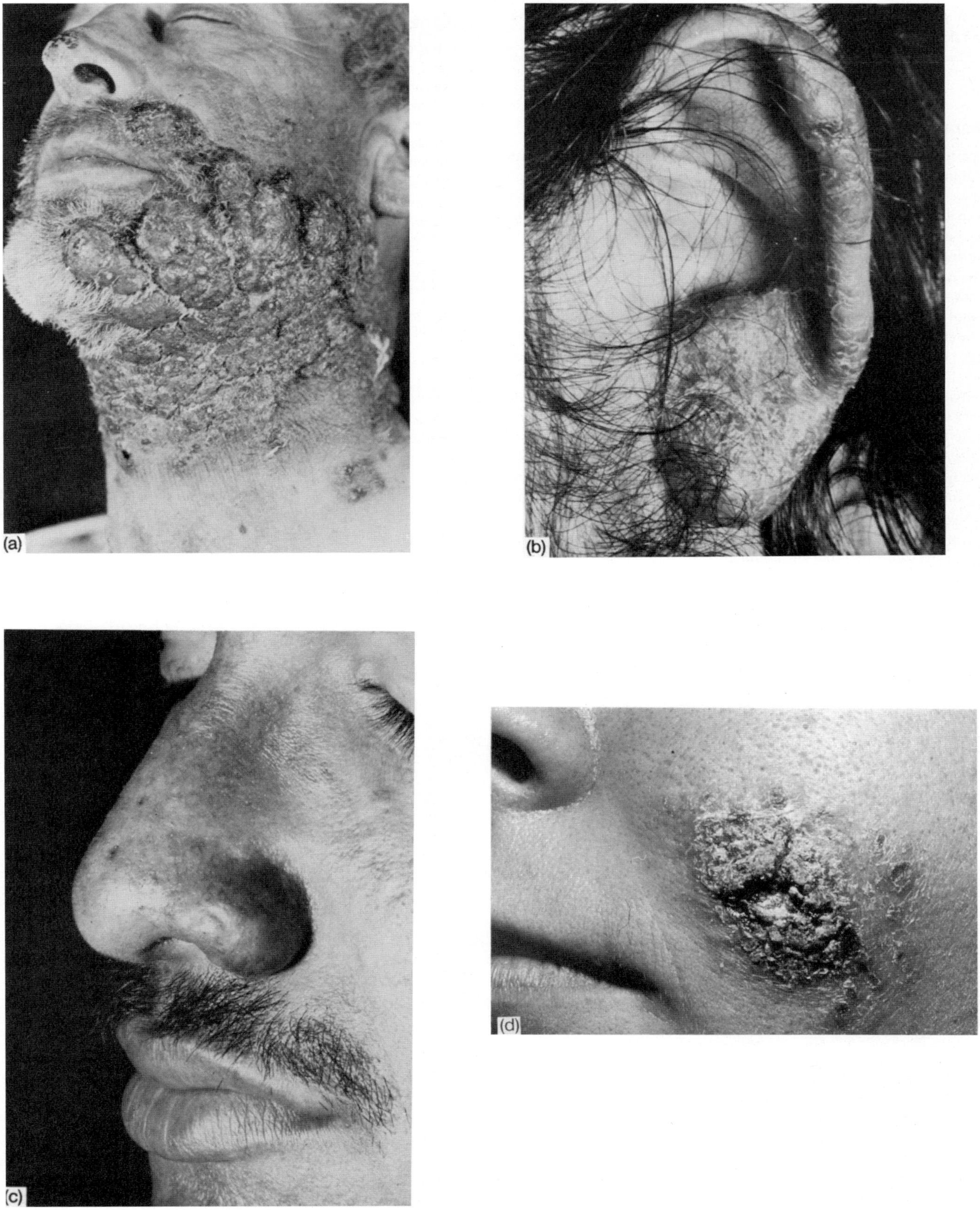

Fig. 112 (a) Chronic granulomas due to cattle ringworm: *Trichophyton verrucosum.* (b) The ear involved by lupus vulgaris (tuberculosis); a brownish-red granuloma inducing irritation in the overlying epidermis. (c) The nose is a common site for the granuloma of lepromatous leprosy. (d) Chronic granuloma due to leishmaniasis following a sandfly bite presenting as an ill-defined cresting and wartiness.

staining histiocytes devoid of lipid, which contain the Langerhans-cell granules.

Fibrosis, eosinophils, and giant cells are features of a more benign process.

Granuloma annulare and necrobiosis lipoidica

A partial necrosis of collagen- and connective-tissue cells associated with immunoglobulin and complement deposition results in a lymphocytic and histiocytic response known as a 'palisading granuloma'. This is entirely reversible over many months and years in patients with granuloma annulare, but in those with necrobiosis lipoidica it tends to result in fibrosis and scarring. The association with insulin-dependent diabetes mellitus and with AIDS is unpredictable, but is to be expected in more widespread forms, in older age groups with granuloma annulare, and in about 75 per cent of cases of necrobiosis lipoidica.

In children, granuloma annulare commonly appears on the knuckles (Fig. 113), fingers, and dorsum of the feet. Ears and elbows are quite frequently affected. Granuloma annulare may be mistaken for warts but the overlying epidermis, if closely inspected, is rarely papilliferous. The tendency to heal in the centre and spread centrifugally over many weeks gives rise to the annular appearance.

Necrobiosis lipoidica is commonly found on both shins (Fig. 114). Widespread forms of granuloma annulare may often be of the giant type, forming large violaceous plaques or rings. No treatment is necessary since eventual resolution of granuloma annulare is expected in 75 per cent of cases within 2 years, but intralesional steroids probably speed resolution, particularly sometimes aborting necrobiosis lipoidica. These disorders may respond to PUVA therapy.

Cutaneous amyloidosis

Systemic amyloidosis is described elsewhere. A waxy appearance of the skin and the ease with which purpura develops within the lesions on slight trauma are suggestive of the diagnosis.

Lichen amyloidosis consists of discrete, firm, hemispheroidal papules. Hyperkeratosis and pigmentation is common, suggesting a waxy infiltrated lichen simplex. The lower legs and outer thighs are involved (Fig. 115(a)). There is no systemic implication.

Macular amyloid is a common pigmented variant, often in a rippled pattern (Fig. 115(b)), affecting the shoulders and backs of Asian peoples. Local high-potency steroids under occlusive dressings have a temporary good effect.

Crohn's disease

This is a well-recognized cause of chronic granulomatous infiltration occurring perianally (see Fig. 21) or in the buccal mucosa.

Management of skin disease

Recent advances in treatment have been many. The understanding of cell recognition, adhesion, and the role of interleukins, tumour-necrosis factor, and interferons have led to the development of significantly successful antagonists, though they are not without side-effects. The skills of the dermatological surgeon have been refined, and laser therapy has provided a tool that can be both well and badly used. There will be gene guns in the future. The long reign of steroids may be coming to an end as more specific anti-inflammatory agents with less side-effects are trialled. It has to be said, however, that the basis of dermatological therapy is still empirical and randomized controlled trials rare. The principal symptom of itch remains

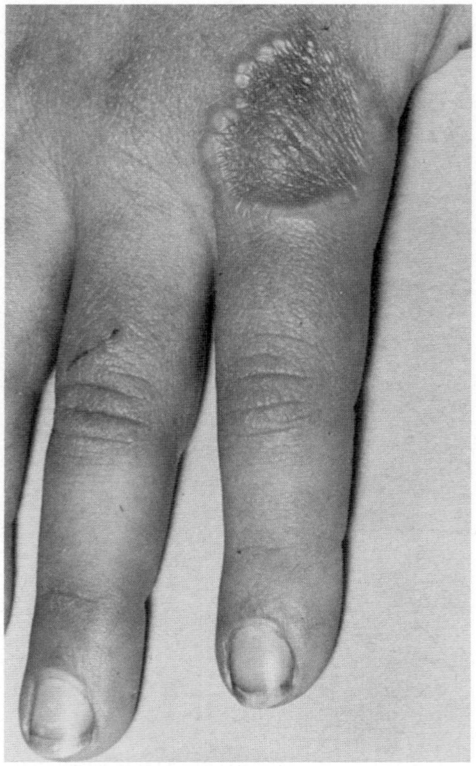

Fig. 113 Papules of granuloma annulare forming a ring around a now healed, but previously affected, area on the knuckle.

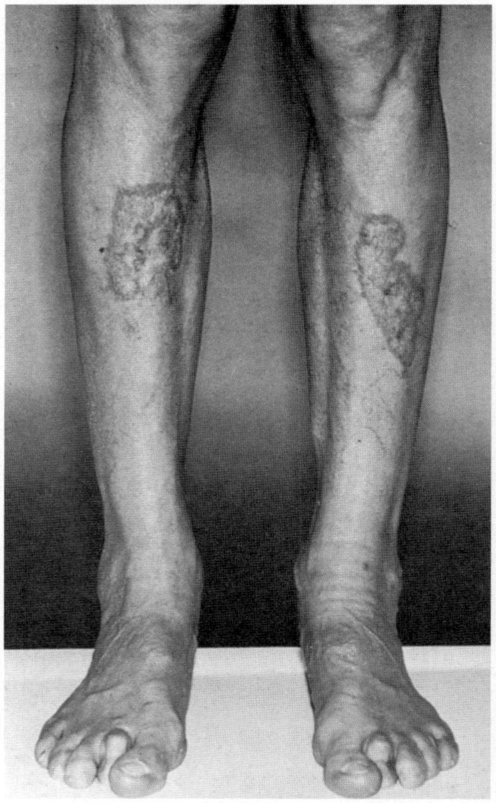

Fig. 114 Necrobiosis lipoidica usually affects the skin of the shins. The yellowish atrophic plaques are associated with diabetes mellitus.

poorly understood, and the 'look good, feel good' factor that contributes to well being is elusive.

Conventional dermatology is not the only resource for patients with skin problems: alternative and complementary medicine, some of it based on long tradition, has become increasingly popular.

General principles

Acute lesions require rest and elevation because this reduces swelling. Dressings should be applied lightly and evenly to the surface, and should support the inflamed area without drag or compression. All agents applied to the skin should be no stronger than necessary. It is very easy for instance, to make a potassium permanganate solution too strong or to use poorly mixed and inhomogeneous medicaments. Preferably, only substances whose components are known and prescribed by experts should be applied to the skin. This is particularly relevant to indigenous medicine. A simple agent used well and which is familiar to the prescriber is always safer than the haphazard prescription of a range of new and poorly tested agents.

Some of the oldest remedies, such as calamine lotion and tar preparations appearing in the *British national formulary* or *The WHO essential drugs list*, do least harm, but patients with chronic skin disease are unlikely to persevere with these unless they are educated and encouraged. This takes time. Remember, patients spend more time listening to other patients in the waiting room than they do to the doctor—and are often in a more receptive frame of mind then. Make sure that the advice given in the waiting room is correct by handing out leaflets and teaching groups of patients, for example with audiovisual aids. Many patients do best with printed sheets of instructions so that they can read at their own pace quietly, and away from the physician. When appropriate, they should be told that their disease is neither contagious nor cancer, nor passed on to their offspring by their genes.

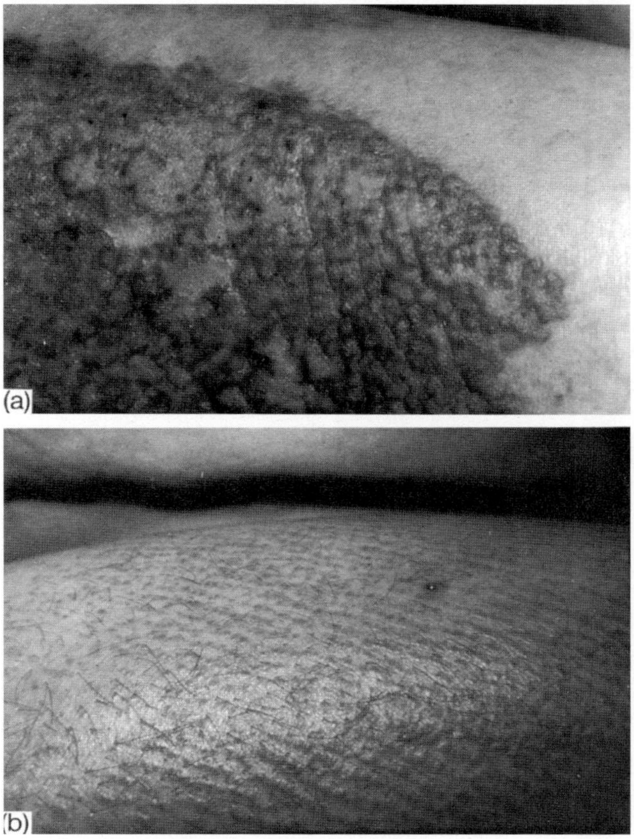

Fig. 115 (a) Lichen amyloidosis commonly affects the shins or outer aspects of the thighs. The brownish, waxy, lichenified skin is pruritic. (b) Rippled pigmentation of macular amyloid.

There are a number of supporting organizations of value in the management of skin disease. A high proportion of patients with skin problems are found to be suffering from the stresses of their domestic environment (confused elderly relatives or delinquent teenage children, for example). For these patients the help of a medical social worker is often very successful. The British Red Cross Society in the United Kingdom now provides a 'beauty care' service that has been extended to the provision of camouflage make-up. Patients' associations often provide a great deal of education and support.

In hospital practice, inpatient treatment is only occasionally necessary and can be greatly reduced by adequate provision of a good outpatient service. Some units link this to their inpatient department in order to provide a service outside the unit's normal working hours—it is clearly more convenient for a working person to attend a department that is open in the evening.

Elimination of primary irritants or known allergens, or of infection, should be the aim of treatment. However, it is fruitless to attempt to make the skin and its diseases sterile at all times. Restoration of the skin barrier and the prevention of cracks and heaping up of scales and exudate reduces bacterial penetration. Scratching, rubbing, wrongly applied dressings, and unsuitable local medications are reasons for worsening of the skin condition and for the impairment of natural defences and repair mechanisms.

Chronic skin conditions are more difficult to cure, and a correct diagnosis is even more important. Spontaneous healing may not occur without the cause being eliminated, and therefore the chronic inflammation may be self-perpetuating. A biopsy for histological analysis is often helpful and bacterial or mycological analysis is clearly indicated where chronic infection is a possibility.

The handicap of the chronic lesion includes a feeling of being unwelcome, often leading to the accusation of being 'unclean' and to being 'outcast'. The physician and nurse can sometimes do more to alleviate the skin condition by paying attention to this aspect of the handicap, rather than using more specific measures. Sympathetic questioning along the lines indicated earlier will help to relieve the patient's suspicion that the dermatology team is not interested in the problem. Touching the skin during examination often does more to make the patient feel that the physician cares than any other manoeuvre.

When treating any skin disease, the overall objective is to create the body image that the patients hope for—not that which is perceived as ideal by the attendant—and when this fails, to help them to live with their problem and expect less. Every effort should be made to ensure that children remain willing to go to school, adults stay at work, and the old are kept comfortable. Remedies should be convenient and cosmetically acceptable, and if this is not possible, the social support should be that much more intensive. Attention to diet, camouflage measures, and regular careful attention to the skin can be very irksome for the patient, but can be made less so through cooperation with the doctor, nurse, or patient association, for example the obesity clinic supported by a weightwatchers' group.

It is essential that the skin be protected from further injury. Homely advice such as 'keep warm and out of the sun' and 'rest as much as possible with your feet up' is appropriate for much acute or severe skin disease, but the skin does not normally experience sustained rest. It is best to encourage movement such as intermittent stretching or compression. For a normal and healthy skin, movement promotes blood supply, lymphatic drainage, and a well-balanced structure that is water-containing and to which a well-attached epidermis is attached and supported by appropriately distributed fibres as skeletal support. The best movements are natural and not too vigorous, but they should provide a full range of flexion and extension over the joints.

Some chronic and incurable skin diseases become easier to tolerate when time is given to the education of the patient, thereby increasing patient understanding, satisfaction, and self-help.

The priorities of the patient with skin disease differ from those of the therapist. Thus the patient equates severity with social ostracism or the subjective itch, rather than with the percentages of body involved or systemic complications. Other people who should be drawn into the management of the patient with skin disease include parents, school teachers, employers, hairdressers, and the sporting fraternity—for example, swimming-pool attendants. A school report that, without these discussions, refers to weeping sores and scratching which interfere with the work of other children, should be a thing of the past.

Many chronic skin conditions are either hypertrophic or atrophic. Hypertrophic conditions require suppressive therapy, as described above in the section on psoriasis. Common suppressants are corticosteroids or radiotherapy. However, these are less suitable for treating atrophy. Another adage worth paying attention to is: 'If it is wet, dry it, and if it is dry, wet it!'

The management of skin disease in technically developed countries usually assumes regular follow-up. In developing countries in Africa or India, or with the nomads of the Middle East, there is almost no possibility of follow-up. Treatments with a high risk of side-effects or exacerbations on withdrawal are therefore not ideal. Because malnutrition and infection are so common, dietary supplements and antibiotics are of value in almost any disease in which host or constitutional vulnerability is a factor. Health education is always difficult, but the mother with children is usually the most receptive pupil.

New technologies—lasers and narrow-band UVB

The management of skin diseases is usually low-technology and low-cost. Economic forces have encouraged dermatologists to purchase high-technology equipment, some of which provides an advance in management for those who can afford it: laser therapy has proved excellent for vascular and pigmented lesions, and for the removal of hair. The technology requires a wavelength that is selective for a specific subcellular target, delivered in pulses with sufficient energy to be destructive for that target without at the same time damaging surrounding tissues. As the pulse is so short, there is no time for surrounding tissues to be heated. Many treatments are needed for some of the more troublesome conditions (for example, pigmentation), while some therapies (such as hair removal) are not permanent but partial. The technology has been improved by photodynamic therapy, whereby an agent such as protoporphyrin is added to the subcellular structure, which is then irradiated. Several tumours have been treated in this way. Dermatologists have always used ultraviolet light, either from sunlight or from ultraviolet lamps. The most recent innovation is the use of narrow-band UVB, which is as effective as UVA in the prophylactic management of polymorphic light eruption and is used in a number of other sun-induced dermatoses. While narrow-band ultraviolet light has been found to induce malignancy in animals, the lower dose required in humans compared to other forms of light seems to induce remissions without significant tumour risk. It has been given to children and patients who are pregnant, but it is probably too early to say that it is entirely safe.

Local topical treatment

The fingertip unit

The 'fingertip unit' is the amount of ointment expressed from a tube with a 5-mm diameter nozzle, applied from the distal crease to the tip of the index finger—1 unit weighs 0.49 g and covers 286 cm^2 in men, and 0.43 g which covers 257 cm^2 in women. One unit will cover an area equivalent to twice the area of the hand, thus four hands is equivalent to two finger units, which is equivalent to about 1 g.

Drugs are dissolved or suspended in bases, which have properties of their own quite independent of the active ingredient. As shown in Table 22, bases were originally either powder, water, or grease. However, modern processes have prepared bases that are essentially much more complex than this, although they still retain the objectives of the primary agents. Powder may repel water or absorb it and allow further evaporation. Modern powders tend not to cake and abrade the skin as much as the original talc or starch. Watery lotions evaporate and cool, as well as wet and dissolve. Various agents, such as alcohol or glycerine, may be added to increase any one of these properties. Creams and emulsions of oil and water (aqueous or milky) or water in oil (butter or oily) are cooling, moisturizing, and emollient. The penetration of active agents through the skin is aided by the aqueous (vanishing) oil and water creams. Ointments based on Vaseline or paraffin are more occlusive and less quickly absorbed. They are better at softening dry surface scales.

There are various other water-soluble preparations, such as macrogels or emulsifying ointment in which a wax or animal fat is mixed with mineral oil. Pastes are powder and oil mixtures, such as talc and Vaseline, which are more occlusive and protective. They are useful for allowing the slow release of agents (such as dithranol) at the skin surface. As the addition of an active

Table 22 Bases and their properties

Base	Application site	Effect	Disadvantage	Examples
Watery and shake lotions (powder in water)	Acutely inflamed, wet and oozing	Drying, soothing, and cooling	Tedious to apply; frequent changes(lessened by polyethylene occlusion); powder in shake lotions may clump	Fuller's earth solution; Lotio Terra silica; saline solution BPC; potassium permanganate(1/8000–1/18 000); 0.5% acetic acid in water; Eusol in chlorinated lime; boric acid solution; calamine lotion
Creams	Both moist and dry	Cooling, emollient, and moisturizing	Short shelf- life; fungal and bacterial growth in base; sensitivities to preservatives and emulsifying agents	Oily cream BP. Aqueous cream BP, i.e. variants on water, oil, and water mixes
Fatty acid, propylene, glycol	Both moist and dry	Emollient and moisturizing	May sting when applied; occasional sensitivity to propylene glycol	FAPG base
Ointments	Dry and scaly	Occlusive and emollient	Messy to apply and soils clothing; removed with an oil	Soft white paraffin; Vaseline; hydrous wool fat (lanolin); emulsifying ointment BP
Pastes; powder/ ointment mixture	Dry, lichenified, and scaly	Protective and emollient; delays absorption of grease	Messy and tedious to apply (linen or calico needed)	Zinc compound paste BP, Lassar's paste BP
Dusting powders	Flexures; may be slightly moist	Lessens friction	If too wet, clumps and irritates	Talcum dusting powder BPC; zinc, starch, and talc dusting powder BPC

ingredient to a base often makes it unstable, various other agents are added as a preservative or to control pH. Further dilution usually makes the preparation still more unstable (that is, shortens its shelf-life). Much of the skill in preparing an ointment, cream, or paste lies in the use of the homogenizer by the pharmacist.

The actions and side-effects of topical steroids are listed in Table 23. Tar and dithranol preparations were discussed above in the section on psoriasis. Tacrolimus is a new topical immunomodulating agent related to ciclosporin. However, unlike ciclosporin, it can be used topically to treat conditions such as pyoderma gangrenosum or the more common psoriasis and atopic eczema. A new oral agent, mycophenolate mofetil—another immunomodulatory agent (1 g orally, twice daily) for psoriasis, pyoderma gangrenosum, bullous pemphigoid, pemphigus vulgaris, and systemic vasculitis—also shows some promise as a topical agent.

Table 23 Topical steroids

Active constituents	Include hydrocortisone and synthetic halogenated derivatives of prednisolone such as betamethasone 17-valerate, triamcinolone acetonide, and fluocinolone acetonide. Halogenation increases topical activity
Bases	Available in lotions, creams, fatty acid propylene glycol base, and ointments. Over 100 preparations listed in MIMS
Penetration	Readily penetrate skin via the horny layer and appendages. Form a reservoir in the horny layer. Polyethylene occlusion and the use of higher concentrations increase penetration
Metabolism	Some, though probably minor, metabolism in epidermis and dermis (for example, hydrocortisone conversion and other metabolites). Leave skin via dermal vascular plexus and enter general metabolic pool of steroids. Further metabolism in liver
Excretion	As sulphate esters and glucuronides
Action	Anti-inflammatory Vasoconstrictors Decrease permeability of dermal vessels Decrease fibrin deposition Decrease kinin formation Decrease prostaglandin synthesis Depress fibroblastic activity Stabilize lysosomal membranes Reduce cytokine activity Immunosuppressive: antigen–antibody interaction unaffected but inflammatory consequences lessened (above mechanisms) Decrease rate of epidermal turnover
Side-effects	Thinning of epidermis Thinning of dermis Telangiectasia and striae (due to thinning of epidermis and dermis) Bruising (due to thinning of dermis and vascular wall fragility) Hirsutism Folliculitis and acneiform eruptions May worsen or disguise infection (bacterial, viral, and fungal) Systemic absorption (rare but, for example, occurs in infants, when applied in large quantities under polyethylene pants) Allergy to hydrocortisone is well documented
Uses	Eczema. Psoriasis in a few instances (facial, flexural, and palms/soles). Many non-infective pruritic dermatoses

Currently there are at least 60 different topical corticosteroids available in the United Kingdom which can be classified into four groups: mild, moderate, potent, and very potent. When treating skin disease, the doctor should select one from each group and test its efficacy and limitations; this should cover all contingencies. The least potent corticosteroids that gives good control should be used, starting with a mild preparation and increasing potency as required. With experience more potent corticosteroids can be used appropriately from the outset. If a very potent agent is required, it should be remembered that more than 50 g/week leads to measurable adrenal suppression. Because of the reservoir, once daily application is recommended, supplemented by frequent emollients.

Skin cleaning

It is naïve to attempt to sterilize the skin, and the long-term consequences of obsessive washing or the use of local antibiotics are always worse than the original state of the skin. Antibiotic regimens are essential for acute complications such as cellulitis, or for specific infections such as erysipelas. Washing is important for reducing smell and for removing debris, but this is best done by soaking rather than scrubbing. Soaking is, in fact, one of the most effective of skin treatments for oozing exudative conditions. Management of skin conditions requires clean water fit for drinking; this can be obtained by a variety of sterilizing procedures, including boiling, pasteurizing for prolonged periods in the sun, adding antiseptics, charcoal, and other forms of filtering. Soaps irritate because they are alkaline and degreasing agents, and some patients are sensitive to perfumes and other additives in the soaps. Most skin will tolerate some soaping, but the amounts needed to degrease in hard-water areas can cause considerable dryness and cracking of the skin. Soft rainwater or boiled milk should not be despised. Bran is an ancient and harmless water softener: about a pound of bran or oatmeal tied into a muslin bag and soaked in boiling water produces a very thin, starchy emulsion. Because cold causes the stratum corneum to dry, shrink, and crack, cold water is not therapeutic for the skin. Dry skin is best treated at body temperature.

Emulsifying ointment is a useful soap substitute; it can be made into 'cakes of soap' or spooned out of a pot and mixed with hot water to soften it. Liberally applied it is a useful softener of crusts.

Bathing in water, often for prolonged periods several times a day, is an effective remedy for a generalized sore skin. However, the skin tends to dry excessively when all grease is removed and this can enhance pruritus. For this reason, emulsifying ointments and proprietary (oilatum) oils are usually added to the bath.

Although the use of antiseptics in the bath is of dubious value, weak solutions of potassium permanganate 1/8000 to 1/16000 are often used. Patients often use these agents too extravagantly. High concentrations of antiseptics poured into a bath may lie on the bottom of the bath and burn the skin, especially in sensitive areas such as the scrotum.

Bacteria are best dealt with by removing crusts and other debris, soaking does this even without the addition of antiseptics. In intertriginous areas soaking should be followed by drying. Organisms thrive in moist crevasses, for instance under the breasts, in the groins, and between the toes. Non-caking powders are helpful in drying such areas, and many proprietary brands of powders such as ZeaSORB® can be recommended. Like leather, treatment with grease prevents cracking and penetration by undesirable agents.

Softening crusts and exudates

Crusts and exudates (for example, as observed in impetigo, fungus infections, acute dermatitis, and psoriasis) require softening by prolonged contact with a wetting or greasing agent. The problem with wetness is that it quickly evaporates and dries. Wet soaks require absorbent dressings, but modern hospitals often supply only gauze, which is not particularly wettable. Old-fashioned linen or cotton sheets are ideal for wet dressings; usually these are applied in several layers and covered with a light ventilated dressing such as a hand towel or tubular gauze. Occlusive dressings are too heating. Polythene occlusion should not be used. Less rapidly drying agents include the ancient boric and starch poultice—30 g of starch and 4 g of boric acid mixed in 568 ml (1 UK pint) of water, cooled, and smeared on to linen strips to thickly impregnate them. This wet dressing is applied to the crusted area and changed every 4 hours. Vaseline ointments are also suitable for softening scales, as in psoriasis. Where the skin is dry and non-exudative, scaling is best softened with a paste made of 50 per cent Vaseline and 50 per cent talc (talc slowly releases the Vaseline over a number of hours).

Other treatment

Smell

Malodorous necrotic skin is always very difficult to deal with, but the removal of debris and dead tissues is essential. Antibiotics and local antiseptics cut down bacterial degradation, which is a cause of smell. Metronidazole 400 mg three times daily is sometimes used to reduce the smell of tumours as it is effective against various anaerobic bacteria. Charcoal dressings are also helpful. Social intercourse out of doors can be encouraged, while perfumes may be helpful indoors. Washing removes dirt debris and excess bacteria, making the skin less attractive to biting insects.

Diet

Widespread skin disease is a cause of water and protein loss. The tongue and degree of thirst are a good guide to water loss, as is the specific gravity of urine. High-protein diets are necessary, especially when there is great exfoliation.

Retinoids

The greatest advance in dermatological therapeutics of the last decade has been the introduction of systemic retinoids. The main retinoids available are *cis*-retinoic acid and acitretin. These modulate cell differentiation and growth, inhibit polymorphonuclear-cell chemotaxis, inhibit polyamine formation, and inhibit eicosanoid formation. They are effective in the treatment of acne, psoriasis, and genetic dyskeratoses. Their side-effects include teratogenesis, hyperostosis, lipidaemia, hepatitis, and the various minor skin, bowel, and neurological problems previously recorded with vitamin A prescribing. Retinoids are prescribed in combination with other topical therapies or PUVA therapy in an attempt to reduce their dosage and consequent side-effects.

Mood-controlling drugs

Apart from the value of psychotherapeutic drugs to control the secondary emotional reactions to skin disease (many such drugs are used to control skin symptoms), antipruritics are often sedative, but hydroxyzine and alimemazine (trimeprazine) are favoured. Delusions of parasitosis and obsessive concern with pruritus is relieved by pimozide.

The placebo

For many skin conditions, such as alopecia areata, there is no specific treatment, and for some patients the available effective remedies are inappropriate, such as the painful treatments for warts in very young children. Nevertheless, to do nothing at all is to encourage despair. Placebos such as mild lotions for alopecia areata or warts should be harmless, cheap, and given knowingly without self-deception.

Subjective symptoms such as itchiness are intolerable for some patients, but can sometimes be relieved by inert agents such as calcium lactate or vitamin B pills given with assurance and confidence.

Bed rest

It is hard for patients with skin disease to play the sick role, especially when they are otherwise well. When told to rest at home, sitting on a couch and pottering about are often only a partial acceptance of the sick role. Admission to hospital and complete bed rest often switches off skin disease such as atopic eczema within 2 or 3 days; for psoriasis, 2 or 3 weeks is often required.

Irritable and distraught, the patient and his family may need rest from each other as well as the knowledge that the illness is genuine and severe enough to take to bed. The patient's bed should be placed where there is no danger to other patients from cross-infection (exfoliative skin disease is a rich source of staphylococcal infection), which means that neighbouring patients should be selected both for their likely resistance to infection and for their likely good companionship. Modern hospitals include a high proportion of single cubicles for patients with skin disease, together with a day room for social mixing once the skin dressings have been completed.

Intertrigo

The treatment of intertrigo is essentially undertaken to protect the area from chafing and secondary infection, and to encourage dryness. Underlying disorders such as diabetes mellitus or obesity must be managed along traditional lines. Infection from bacteria, *Candida* spp., or fungi requires monitoring by appropriate swabs and scrapings. Bed rest and nudity are helpful. In hot climates a fan encourages evaporation and drying. Skin folds should be kept apart by ventilated loose-weave dressings. Acute eczema requires bland wet lotions, steroid creams, and simple antibacterial agents such as gentian violet or vioform cream. When dry, powdering is to be encouraged. Frequent bathing is always helpful.

Hand dermatitis

To provide healing and to prevent relapse of dermatitis of the hands, patients should use lukewarm water and emulsifying ointments when washing. If possible, running water is better than a prolonged soak in a bowl of detergent soap. Soap should be used sparingly and the hands thoroughly rinsed and dried carefully with a clean towel. As far as possible there should be no direct contact with detergents and other strong cleansing agents, shampoos, polishes, and stain removers. Oranges, lemons, grapefruit juices, and various other irritant vegetables should be avoided. Rings should not be worn during housework or other work even when the dermatitis has healed, because irritants often collect under them. Rings should be frequently cleaned on the inside with a brush and left in ammonia (one tablespoon (20 ml) to 500 ml of water) overnight, then rinsed thoroughly. If gloves are used for washing dishes and clothes, they should be made of plastic and not rubber since the latter often causes dermatitis. They should not be worn for more than 15 to 20 min at a time. If water happens to enter a glove, it must be taken off immediately. The gloves should be turned inside out and rinsed several times a week. Sprinkling with talc before they are used helps to dry them. Cotton gloves can be used under the plastic ones. They should only be worn a few times before they are washed.

Vulnerability

The skin in many diseases is vulnerable. This is manifested as the tendency to produce disease even from minor trauma. It is seen in the primary irritant dermatitis of the atopic eczema sufferer, the Koebner phenomenon of psoriasis, lichen planus, the hyperreactivity of the skin to needle puncture or pressure localization in vasculitis, and in the skin ulceration that results from minor knocks to the legs in gravitational stasis. The skin's vulnerability is severe in epidermolysis bullosa.

In all these diseases advice has to be given about protection of the skin. It can be given in the form of information sheets detailing the care of the hands or legs, or in booklet form for mothers of children with epidermolysis bullosa. The various patient associations produce excellent literature in this respect.

Management of leg ulceration

The cause of ulceration should be identified and, if possible, eliminated. However, the aetiology of an ulcer in an elderly woman living in a city is likely to be different to that of a young man in a rural area in Central Africa. The causes of ulceration are listed in Table 24.

Elevation

The leg being below the level of the heart, there is always a tendency to develop venous hypertension and stasis. Deep vein thrombosis, absence of valves in the deep veins, and shunting of blood from the deep veins to the superficial veins via perforators are a significant cause of congestive changes in the microcirculation supplying the epidermis.

Healing of leg ulceration is always helped by elevation. If there is a major degree of arterial disease, so that there are absent peripheral pulses, then the leg should not be raised more than about 23 cm above the level of the heart. In every other case, emptying of the distended veins and superficial venules is helped by lying the patient in a prone position and elevating the legs to an angle of at least 45°. This is best done by placing an object such as a chair under the mattress (Fig. 116). It is also best to elevate the leg during the day, because the patient cannot sustain such a position when asleep and will curl up into a bundle at the top of the bed.

When stiff hips, heart failure, and obesity are factors preventing elevation of the legs, a compromise includes the use of compression bandages and attempts to make the most of any muscle pump in the lower leg. Intermittent positive pressure inflatable bags are commercially available. These are leggings that blow up and squeeze the legs at a pressure and rate that can be regulated.

Elevation is also a requirement for the treatment of lymphoedema, but the protein collecting in the tissues of a swollen leg usually fails to clear satisfactorily via the lymphatics. Movement such as massage, vibration, or ankle exercise is necessary to hasten the passage of protein out of the tissues into the lymphatics. Provided the solid elements of the skin (that is, collagen fibres) are moved, the massage or vibration need not be very sophisticated. In the absence of lymphatics the only other way protein can be removed from the tissues is by proteolysis and macrophages. To control venous hypertension, the pressure at the ankle should be 40 mmHg and there should be a gradient of decreasing pressure as one moves proximally. This gradient is aided by the increasing circumference of the calf. Each layer of bandage doubles the compression.

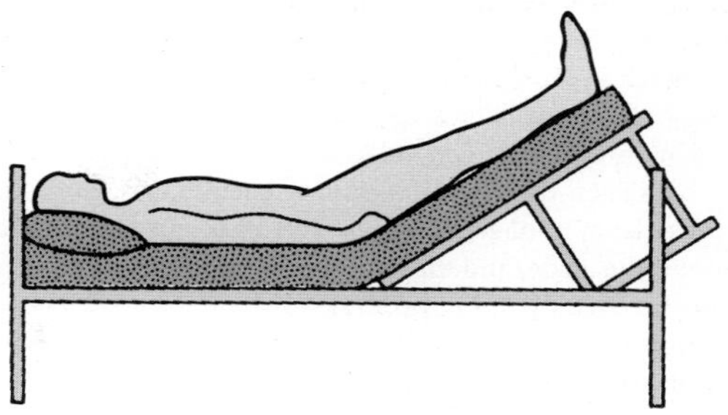

Fig. 116 Elevation of legs above the heart, necessary in the treatment of leg ulcers. A chair can be used to prop up the end of the mattress.

Table 24 Causes of leg ulceration

Trauma	External injuries, burns, scalds, chemical, self-inflicted, artefacts, contact dermatitis
Infections	
Viral	
Bacterial	Acute: 'desert sore', gas gangrene Chronic: buruli ulcer, tuberculosis, leprosy, swimming pool granuloma
Anaerobic	Meleney's ulcer, synergistic gangrene
Streptococcal	
Mycotic	Superficial or deep fungus
Spirochaetal	Syphilis, yaws
Leishmaniasis	
Infestations, bites	Spiders, scorpions, snakes
Metabolic	Diabetes
Vasculitis	Collagen disease, immune complex disease
Pyoderma gangrenosum	
Perniosis erythrocyanosis	
Venous	Stasis, congenital absence of veins, post-thrombotic
Atrophie blanche	
Necrobiosis lipoidica	
Neoplastic	Epithelioma, Kaposi's sarcoma, leukaemia, reticulosis, melanoma
Arteriovenous anastomoses	
Ischaemic	Scars, fibrosis, radiodermatitis
Arterial	Hypertension, temporal arteritis, atherosclerosis
Thrombosis, embolism, platelet agglutination	
Blood diseases	Coagulation, platelet disorders; impaired fibrinolysis Thrombocythaemia, polycythaemia Dysglobulinaemia, spherocytosis, sickle-cell anaemia
Neuropathic	Diabetes mellitus, leprosy
('trophic')	Tabes dorsalis, syringomyelia, alcoholic neuropathy

Arterial disease should always be excluded by examining the arterial system, especially by taking the blood pressure in the legs and arms or by an arteriogram. Stopping smoking and keeping walking is essential therapy.

Wound dressings should encourage moist wound healing, which favours epithelial migration and the development of granulation tissue.

Movement

Inflammation is aimed at removing injurious agents and promoting healing. In acute infection or injury there is often a need for immobilization. However, such immobilization should be localized to the site of injury. Gentle passive movement of the joints and active movement of the main muscles of the leg are encouraged by wriggling the toes or ankles, or by quadriceps exercises.

Unfortunately, many patients with leg ulceration continue to be immobile and to dread any movement that causes pain, long after any need for immobilization to contain the inflammation. Stiffness of the ankle and contractures at the joints are common and delay healing as well as considerably add to crippling.

Deep vein thrombosis is a consequence of immobilization, and this too contributes to morbidity as well as mortality. Thus, in general terms, the maintenance of mobility is essential in the management of leg ulcers.

Exercises in bed can be followed by exercises in the standing position aimed at maintaining an upright posture and ankle mobility, as well as strengthening the muscles of the calves which are so important in pumping blood through and away from the deep veins. For those who are able, walking should be encouraged. Special instruction should be given concerning the harm done by sitting with the legs dependent or crossed, or standing without movement at the ankle. Even a soldier standing to attention needs to maintain venous return by imperceptible, but nevertheless effective, wriggling of the toes. 'March at the sink' is a suitable war cry in the home.

Dressings and bandages

The objective of bandaging is to hold the dressing in position, to protect the leg from further injury, and to provide a sleeve against which movement of the underlying muscles can compress and empty the superficial veins.

The superficial vessels of the skin of the leg are often distorted and congested from chronic inflammation and gravitational stasis. Such vessels are often damaged and cause ischaemic ulceration as a result of external injury, arising from the kinks, wrinkles, and inequalities of an ill-fitting bandage, etc. It should be remembered that a leg that swells can develop severe ischaemia beneath a constricting bandage, even when it was quite loose before the leg became swollen. Large, swollen legs, as in lymphoedema or after deep vein thrombosis, can tolerate unskilled bandaging and tight compressive bandages. By contrast a thin, ischaemic or ageing skin suffers greatly from carelessly applied bandages. The leg is an awkward shape, particularly around the ankle, and many of the twists and the bulk of the bandage tends to be over the bony prominences where the skin is thin and ulcers are common. One system of bandaging is to use two layers—one as a dressing and the other as a cover. The bandage used as a dressing is made from strips of material, no longer than 1.5 times the leg circumference, that are impregnated with a paste. These strips may be applied from a bandage that is cut whenever the direction of the bandaging requires a change. Above the ankle, the bandage is folded at the side of the leg and reversed so as not to completely encircle the leg. Any strips of materials such as calico or linen similarly impregnated will do as well. The overlying covering bandage should be more stretchable than cotton—plasticity rather than elasticity is necessary for a thin leg. Large lymphoedematous legs may be covered by a stronger inelastic material (short stretch). This provides a low resting pressure that increases on desirable activity. Immobile patients may do better with a frequently reapplied, long-stretch elastic bandage, such bandages should be reapplied over orthopaedic padding.

The control of infection—what should be put on the ulcer?

If the cause of ulceration is eliminated, then healing should take place. However, healing depends on healthy epidermis at the edge of the ulcer. Often this is damaged by proteolytic enzymes from slough and infection. Unhappily common is the damage resulting from irritation or sensitivity to medicaments. For this reason, simple bland therapy aimed at reducing debris should be used. Debris will float off if softened. Hard adherent crusts are usually dry. The most effective remedy is wetness: saline is perfectly adequate, provided it is applied very frequently as a wet dressing. Surgical debridement should be performed with a scalpel or scissors if there is any non-viable tissue. This is not difficult as long as it is remembered that dead tissue has no sensation. In other words, trim away anything the patient is unaware of, provided the diseases causing neuropathy (for example, leprosy and diabetes mellitus) have been excluded, in which case only necrotic and non-adherent tissue should be removed. Antiseptics such as eusol, 0.5 per cent acetic acid (a 5-ml teaspoon of vinegar in 500 ml (about a UK pint of water)), or 0.5 per cent silver nitrate in aqueous solution are other wetting agents; however, while helpful for removing slough, they inhibit granulation tissue and are less often recommended.

Many antibiotics are applied to ulcers and they rarely control infection. It is naïve to believe that an ulcer can be made sterile. Antibiotics are commonly and rapidly inhibited by serum and debris under a bandage. It is also common for such agents to do damage to the epidermis. In this respect, it is sometimes forgotten that the health of the surrounding epidermis is more important for healing than the state of the ulcer bed. Tropical phagedenic ulcers often follow trauma, and relative avascularity encourages invasion by fusospirochaetal organisms.

Contact dermatitis

Healing is often delayed and ulcers may be enlarged by damage to the surrounding epidermis. Such dermatitis, so often evident around the ulcer, occurs either because of medicaments, bacterial toxins, or allergy. Table 25 is a list of common causes of contact dermatitis.

Toenails

Poor sight, apathy, stiff hips, and obesity are all reasons why toenails are uncut. It is surprising how the Western world has come to expect 'professionals' to deal with this problem when, in fact, toenail cutting is something any good neighbour can do. Clippers rather than scissors are to be recommended because they cut or fracture hard, thickened nail more effectively. The nails should be softened by soaking them in warm water for 10 min. Only the distal part of the nail protruding beyond the toe needs be cut. Good positioning of the cutter and patient and adequate light are essential. Only very distorted nails or the foot with arteriosclerosis and the consequences of diabetes mellitus need the attention of a chiropodist, where such is available.

Table 25 Common causes of contact dermatitis in leg ulcers

Ointment bases and preservatives	*Additives in bandages*
Wool alcohols (lanolin)	Ester gum resin
Parabens	Azo disperse yellow No. 3
Propylene glycol	Colophony
Chlorocresol	Mercaptobenzothiazole thiuram
Ethylene diamine	(rubber)
Antibacterial agents	*Self-medication*
Sodium fusidate	Caine mix (local anaesthetics)
Gentamicin sulphate	Antihistamine creams
Neomycin	Dettol®
Soframycin®	Germolene®
Quinoline mix (Vioform®)	

Corns

These are due to thickening of the epidermis due to external pressure, or from pressure from underlying bony prominences. It should be possible to avoid external pressure by making adjustments to footwear and skilful padding, so that the weight is taken on less bony areas of the foot. Surgery is sometimes necessary to remove bony prominences. Skin thickening is self-perpetuated, but is greatly helped by careful paring away of excess keratin, avoiding damage to underlying blood capillaries which often project upwards to near the surface.

Carcinoma

Carcinoma develops in the hypopigmented margin of ulcers that have persisted for many years. Such ulcers often invade bone but rarely metastasize. Local excision and grafting is often preferable to amputation.

Surgery

Whereas in technically developed countries, amputation and a good prosthesis may help a disabled person regain their mobility, amputation is objected to by certain races (for example, the Bantu) and religions (such as the Hindu). It inevitably causes them to be rejected so that they are unemployable and outcast. Consideration of amputation must take into account social circumstances and the degree of subsequent aftercare, both available and needed for successful rehabilitation.

Injection of superficial veins with sclerosants (or their removal) is indicated only when the deep veins are patent. If the deep veins are blocked, then the superficial veins are the only venous drainage of the legs and should be preserved. Assessment of the proportion of flow returned through the superficial veins is greatly facilitated by the Doppler flowmeter. Surgical debridement and skin grafting is often a means of quickly healing ulceration but is outside the scope of this textbook.

The decubitus ulcer

The decubitus ulcer is a consequence of tissue distortion, often due to pressure obstructing blood flow. It occurs especially in patients with neurological disease, where painful stimuli from tissue distortion or ischaemia is not recognized. Because the pathogenesis of decubitus ulcers includes impaired blood perfusion, anything that affects the blood supply can contribute to the problem. Thus, in general, old patients who are ill or dying, and especially if they have vascular disease, are most likely to develop sores. Such sores are unusual in those with a purely motor neurological disease and no sensory loss, or in the very old who have a healthy vascular system.

Because it is distortion of the tissues rather than simply pressure that induces sores, shearing forces on the sacral area and heels also need to be taken into account. Such forces are increased by moisture from sweating or incontinence. Distortion of the tissues is enhanced by deformities such as kyphoscoliosis or contractures.

While the basis of management is the relief of tissue distortion by the frequent relaxation of stresses and strains on the tissues, best brought about by movement, attention must also be paid to factors contributing to poor perfusion. These include intercurrent illness causing hypoxia, hypotension, immobility, dehydration, and impairment of consciousness or peripheral sensation. Most acute illnesses requiring admission to hospital provide the necessary criteria for the development of a decubitus ulcer within the first hours or days. The chronic sickness that determines prolonged bed rest at home rarely produces this degree of tissue ischaemia, and thus the hospital nurse gets blamed for what has never occurred at home. The blame is partly misdirected because, for example, an old woman with a fractured hip may develop decubitus ulcers while immobile in the ambulance, on a hard trolley waiting for a bed, or on the operating table. All attendants should be taught the causes of decubitus ulcer.

All ill patients are best nursed in bed. Some of the worst pressure sores can occur while sitting in a collapsed state in a day room or during the postoperative phase of 'mobilization'. The basis of management is regular shifting of position, which has arbitrarily become the practice of turning the patient every 2 hours or intermittent shifts in the surface on which the patient is lying. The combination of heavy and uncooperative patients, together with inadequate staffing levels, especially at night, often result in a failure to prevent bed sores. Good equipment to modify pressure on the mattress is important, and may include a fleece under the patient's heels and buttocks, a bed cradle to take the weight of the bedclothes, a variety of soft surfaces, and a ripple bed to provide alternating pressure, preferably one with large ripples.

In countries where such equipment is unavailable, there is often a large contingent of relatives at the bedside whose attentiveness can be mobilized to assist in frequently turning and massaging the patient.

A long, severe illness is difficult to manage outside an intensive care unit because, as implied by the word 'intensive', there is a requirement for vigilance of all aspects of the patient's physical, conscious, and activity level. It is for this reason that some nursing schools demand that a checklist, known as the Norton pressure sore score, is regularly completed. But even this becomes less accurate each day as a long illness drags on. Once an ulcer has developed it becomes a problem of wound healing. Removal of dead tissue is essential, often by surgical debridement. The development of granulation tissue and re-epithelialization will follow only if the patient's general health improves and their blood supply is adequate. There are so many agents advocated for the healing of wounds that it is important to realize that none are essential and many are harmful to healthy tissue. Those that will remove slough may inhibit living cells. Granulation tissue is the best protection against infection but is discouraged by many of the strongest antiseptics. All wound dressings should aim to reduce debris, to keep the wound moist, and to promote granulation tissue perfused by an adequate supply of normal blood.

Further reading

General

Champion RH, *et al*, eds (1999). *Rook, Wilkinson and Ebling textbook of dermatology*, 6th edn. Blackwell Scientific, Oxford.

Cotterill JA, Millard (1999). Psychocutaneous disorders. In: Champion RH, *et al.*, eds. *Rook, Wilkinson and Ebling textbook of dermatology*, 6th edn, pp 2715–814. Blackwell Scientific, Oxford.

Demis JD (1999). *Clinical dermatology*, 26th revision. Lippincott, Williams and Wilkins, Baltimore.

Fitzpatrick TB, *et al.* (1999). *Dermatology in general medicine*, 6th edn. McGraw-Hill, New York.

Goldsmith LA (1991). *Physiology and biochemistry of the skin*, 2nd edn. Oxford University Press.

Graham-Brown R, Bourke JF (1998). *Mosby's color atlas and text of dermatology.* Mosby London.

McKee PH (1999). *Pathology of the skin with clinical correlations*, 2nd edn. Mosby Wolfe, London.

Oumeish YO (1998). Environmental dermatology. *Clinics in Dermatology* 16, 1–184.

Panconesi E (1985). Stress and skin diseases. Psychosomatic dermatology. *Clinics in Dermatology* **2**, 1–282.

Parrish LC, Millikan LC (1994). Contemporary tropical dermatology. *Dermatology Clinics* **12**, 1–840.

Schaefer H, Redelmaier TE (1996). *Skin barrier, principles of percutaneous absorption.* Karger, Basel.

Weinstock MA (1995). Dermatoepidemiology. *Dermatology Clinics* **13**, 1–716.

The interview, examination, and investigations

Ackerman AB (1978). *Histologic diagnosis of inflammatory skin diseases*, p 863. Lea and Febiger, Philadelphia.

Ackerman AB (1995). *Resolving quandaries in dermatology, pathology and dermatopathology*, pp 1–327. William and Wilkins, Baltimore.

Ashton RE (1995). Teaching non-dermatologists to examine the skin: a review of the literature and some recommendations. *British Journal of Dermatology* **132**, 221–5.

Elder D, Jaworsky C, Johnson B, eds. (1997). *Lever's histopathology of the skin*, 8th edn, pp. 1–1073. Lippincott, Philadelphia.

McKee PH (1999). *Pathology of the skin with clinical correlations*, 2nd edn. Mosby Wolfe.

Weedon D (1992). *The skin: systemic pathology*, 3rd edn, Vol. 9, pp. 1–1095. Churchill Livingstone, New York.

Factors determining or modifying skin disease

Breathnach SM (1999). Drug reactions. In: Champion RH, *et al.*, eds. *Rook, Wilkinson and Ebling textbook of dermatology*, 6th edn, pp 3349–518. Blackwell Scientific, Oxford.

La Ruche G, Cesarini JP (1992). Histologie et physiologie de la peau noire. *Annales de Dermatologie et de Venerologie* **119**, 567–74.

Parish LC, Millikan LE (1994). *Global dermatology.* Springer-Verlag, New York.

Dermatitis

Burton JL, Holden CA (1999). Eczema, lichenification and prurigo. In: Champion RH, *et al.*, eds. *Rook, Wilkinson and Ebling textbook of dermatology*, 6th edn, pp 629–80. Blackwell Scientific, Oxford.

Holden CA, Parish WE (1999). Atopic dermatitis. In: Champion RH, *et al.*, eds. *Rook, Wilkinson and Ebling textbook of dermatology*, 6th edn, pp 681–708. Blackwell Scientific, Oxford.

Rietschel RL, Fowler JF (2001). *Fischer's Contact dermatitis*, 5th edn., pp. 1–862. Lippincott Williams and Wilkins, Philadelphia.

Rycroft RJG (1999). Occupational dermatoses. In: Champion RH, *et al.*, eds. *Rook, Wilkinson and Ebling textbook of dermatology*, 6th edn, pp 861–82. Blackwell Scientific, Oxford.

Wilkinson JD, Shaw S (1999). Contact dermatitis, allergic. In: Champion RH, *et al.*, eds. *Rook, Wilkinson and Ebling textbook of dermatology*, 6th edn, pp 733–820. Blackwell Scientific, Oxford.

Williams HC (2000). *Atopic eczema. The epidemiology, causes and prevention of atopic eczema.* Cambridge University Press, Cambridge.

Pruritus

Fleischer AB (2000). *The clinical management of itching.* The Parthenon Publishing Group.

Psoriasis

Camp RDR (1999). Psoriasis. In: Champion RH, *et al.*, eds. *Rook, Wilkinson and Ebling textbook of dermatology*, 6th edn, pp 1589–650. Blackwell Scientific, Oxford.

Acne

Cunliffe WJ, Simpson NB (1999). Disorders of the sebaceous glands. In: Champion RH, *et al.*, eds. *Rook, Wilkinson and Ebling textbook of dermatology*, 6th edn, pp 1927–84. Blackwell Scientific, Oxford.

Pigmentation

Behl PN (1994). *Asian clinics in dermatology*, Vol. 1, No. 1. Vitiligo Update. The Skin Institute, Greater Kailash, New Delhi.

Bleehan SS (1999). Disorders of skin colour. In: Champion RH, *et al.*, eds. *Rook, Wilkinson and Ebling textbook of dermatology*, 6th edn, pp 1753–816. Blackwell Scientific, Oxford.

Njoo MD (2000). Treatment of vitiligo. Thela thesis. University of Amsterdam.

Wasserman HP (1974). *Ethnic pigmentation*. Excerpta Medica, Amsterdam.

Nails

Baran R, Dawber RPR, eds. (1994). *Diseases of the nails and their management*, 2nd edn. Blackwell Scientific, Oxford.

Samman PD (1986). *The nails in disease*, 4th edn. Heinemann, London.

Hair

Rook A, Dawber RPR (1991). *Diseases of hair and scalp*, 2nd edn. Blackwell Scientific, Oxford.

Sinclair R, Banfield C, Dawber R (1999). *Handbook of diseases of the hair and scalp*. Blackwell Scientific, Oxford.

Skin disorders affecting the genitalia

Ridley, M. and Neill, S. (1998) *The vulva*. Blackwell Scientific, Oxford.

Vesicoblistering diseases

Wojnarowska F, Eady RAJ, Burge SM (1999). Bullous eruptions. In: Champion RH, *et al.*, eds. *Rook, Wilkinson and Ebling textbook of dermatology*, 6th edn, pp 1817–99. Blackwell Science, Oxford.

Angioma and telangiectasia

Colver GB, Ryan TJ (1996). Vascular disorders. In: Harper J, ed. *Inherited skin disorders*, pp 182–200. Butterworth and Heinemann, Oxford.

Mulliken JF, Young AE (1988). *Vascular birthmarks*. WB Saunders, Philadelphia.

Connective tissue

Burton JL, Lovell CR. (1999). Disorders of connective tissue. In: Champion RH, *et al.*, eds. *Rook, Wilkinson and Ebling textbook of dermatology*, 6th edn, pp 2003–171. Blackwell Science, Oxford.

Lymphoma

MacKie RM (1999). Cutaneous lymphomas and lymphocytoma. In: Champion RH, *et al.*, eds. *Rook, Wilkinson and Ebling textbook of dermatology*, 6th edn, pp 2373–402. Blackwell Scientific, Oxford.

Worret IF (1993). Skin signs and internal malignancies. *International Journal of Dematology* **32**, 1–5.

Warts

Storling JC, Kurt JB (1999). Human papilloma virus. In: Champion RH, *et al.*, eds. *Rook, Wilkinson and Ebling textbook of dermatology*, 6th edn, pp 1029–50. Blackwell Scientific, Oxford.

Granulomatous disease

Chu AC (1999). Histocytoses. In: Champion RH, *et al.*, eds. *Rook, Wilkinson and Ebling textbook of dermatology*, 6th edn, pp 2311–36. Blackwell Scientific, Oxford.

Cunliffe WJ (1999). Necrobiotic disorders. In: Champion RH, *et al.*, eds. *Rook, Wilkinson and Ebling textbook of dermatology*, 6th edn, pp 2297–310. Blackwell Scientific, Oxford.

Ryan TJ (1978). Lymphatics of the skin. In: Jarrett A, ed. *Physiology and pathophysiology of the skin* Vol 5, pp 1755–808. Academic Press, New York.

Management of skin diseases

Arndt KA (1995). *Manual of dermatologic therapeutics*, 5th edition. Little Brown, Boston.

Lebwohl MG, Heymann WR, Berth-Jones J, Coulson I (2000). *Treatment of skin diseases*, pp. 1–693. Mosby, London.

Maddin S, McClean D (1993). Dermatologic therapies. *Dermatology Clinics* **11**, 1–224.

Management of leg ulcers

Westerhof W (1993). *Leg ulcers. Diagnosis and treatment.* Elsevier, Amsterdam.

Decubitus ulcers

Parish LC, Witkowski JA, Crissey JT (1997). *The decubitus ulcer in clinical practice*, pp 1–241. Springer, Berlin.

US Department of Health and Human Services (1994). *Treatment of pressure ulcers*. Clinical practice guideline number 15. AHEPR Publication No 96 – 0652.

23.2 Molecular basis of inherited skin disease

Irene M. Leigh and David P. Kelsell

Introduction

Most patients referred by the general practitioner to the dermatology clinic will be seeking advice and treatment for a few common skin disorders including psoriasis, eczema, and acne. Although the genetic basis of these disorders is complex, putative susceptibility gene variants for some of these diseases have been identified, including the mast cell chymase gene in atopic eczema and the corneodesmin gene in the HLA-linked component of psoriasis vulgaris. In addition, several genes have been identified which predispose to malignancies of the skin including p16 and CDK4 in melanoma and the Patched gene involved in Gorlin's syndrome, in which mutation carriers have an elevated risk of basal cell carcinomas. There are a myriad of rarer epidermal disorders and syndromes for which the genetic basis has been elucidated. Here, we describe the current molecular understanding of these rarer traits which include blistering disease, ichthyosis, palmoplantar keratodermas, and the ectodermal dysplasias.

Structure of the epidermis

To understand the diseases it is first necessary to understand the basic biology of the epidermis and associated basement membrane zone. The basic structure of the epidermis is illustrated in Fig. 1. The epidermis is a stratified squamous epithelium comprised predominantly of keratinocytes. The remaining small percentage of intraepidermal cells are resident melanocytes, Langerhans cells, and migratory leucocytes. The keratinocyte undergoes a process of terminal differentiation which results in a stratum corneum, the critical component for the function of the epidermis as a barrier. It is a highly insoluble, non-viable cell made up of a cornified envelope enclosing keratin macrofibres separated by a highly lipid-rich, intercellular layer. This lamellated lipid is the predominant component of the barrier and is secreted into the extracellular space from membrane-coating granules synthesized in the stratum granulosum. The epidermis is separated from the underlying dermis by a complex basement membrane zone.

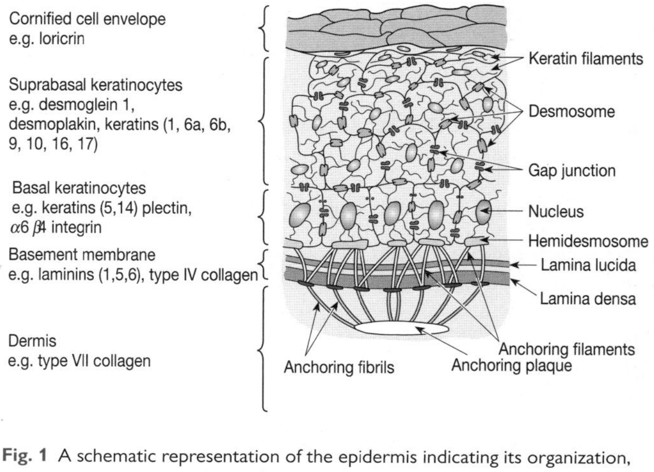

Fig. 1 A schematic representation of the epidermis indicating its organization, important structures, and site of expression of a number of skin-disease-associated proteins.

The basement membrane zone

When studied ultrastructurally, the basement membrane zone of the epidermis contains four distinct layers:

(1) the basal cell membrane of the basal keratinocyte which contains electron-dense adhesion plaques called hemidesmosomes;

(2) the electronlucent lamina lucida which is traversed by anchoring fibrils;

(3) the electron dense lamina densa;

(4) within the sublamina densa region the lamina fibroreticularis contains distinct anchoring structures called anchoring fibrils which insert into the lamina densa and loop around bundles of connective tissue collagens.

The hemidesmosome

Although ultrastructurally this organ appears to resemble desmosome morphology (see below), there are clearly differences in biochemical composition. Two major hemidesmosomal-associated proteins were identified initially by the characterization of autoantibodies arising in bullous pemphigoid, an autoimmune mechanobullous disease of late adult life. These proteins are known as bullous pemphigoid antigen 1 (230 kDa) and bullous pemphigoid antigen 2 (180 kDa). Bullous pemphigoid antigen 2 has been identified as a unique transmembrane collagen, type XVII collagen, which has an extracellular domain containing the immunodominant epitope of bullous pemphigoid. Bullous pemphigoid antigen 1, like plectin, a further component of hemidesmosomes, is a member of the plakin family of proteins. These proteins have been thought to contribute to plaque structures within hemidesmosome. Other members of the plakin family, including desmoplakin, envoplakin, and periplakin, are found associated with the desmosome. Plectin and bullous pemphigoid antigen appear to interact with keratin intermediate filaments as they course towards the hemidesmosome and bind them into the hemidesmosome structure, acting as a protein clamp. This appears to provide a stable link between the intermediate filament cytoskeleton and the basement membrane zone. Basal keratinocytes also express a number of integrins which are a super family of receptors for extracellular matrix proteins. The major hemidesmosomal integrin is $\alpha6\beta4$ integrin, although other areas of the basal cell membrane express $\alpha6\beta1$, $\alpha5\beta1$, $\alpha3\beta1$, and $\alpha2\beta1$ integrins.

The lamina lucida appears to contain a complex of laminin molecules, particularly laminins 5 and 6. It is thought that laminin 5 is the major component of the anchoring filament. The lamina densa is constructed of a meshwork of interacting type IV collagen. From this arise the anchoring fibrils of the basement membrane complex which are made of aggregates of antiparallel dimers of type VII collagen.

Keratins

The cytoskeleton of all epithelial cells contains a number of filamentous systems including actin, microfilaments, microtubules, and intermediate filaments. The protein characteristic of intermediate filaments of all epithelial cells is the keratin family of proteins. Keratin polypeptides segregate in two dimensional gel electrophoresis into acidic and basic polypeptides. Nineteen keratins can be identified by this procedure, with each protein being the product of an independent gene. The type II keratin gene family encodes the basic keratin polypeptides and the type I family the acidic keratin polypeptides. Each keratin is expressed in a body-site and cell-type-specific manner, for example K9 is only expressed in the suprabasal layer of the palmoplantar epidermis. The keratin genes are clustered in two chromosomal regions in the human genome: the type I keratins mapping to 17q12–q21 and the type II keratins to 12q11–q13.

A keratin filament comprises both type I and type II keratins. The fundamental building block of a keratin filament is a heterodimer, aligned along the length of its helical backbone, comprising four helical regions separated by non-helical linker regions with a non-helical head and tail domain. These heterodimers aggregate in a complex, antiparallel fashion to form the intact intermediate filament which associates with both hemidesmosomes and desmosomes to provide stability and integrity of the cell. In addition to keratin mutations associated with human disease, *in vitro* and transgenic models of keratin genes harbouring mutations have shown that there are critical regions for filament assembly; these are located particularly at the helix initiation and termination motifs. The function of the head and tail domains is not entirely clear.

Desmosomes

Desmosomal proteins form a complex structure which interfaces between adjacent epithelial cells. The desmosomal plaques of electron dense material run along the cytoplasm parallel to a junctional region in which three ultrastructural bands can be seen. The plaques contain plakoglobin (which is also found in adherens junctions and also thought to be important in cell signalling), desmoplakin, and plakophilin 1. In addition, the desmosomal cores are enriched in calcium binding glycoproteins, called desmogleins and desmocollins. The desmogleins and desmocollins are the adhesive proteins of the desmosome and are similar to the classical cadherins in their general structure, with five extracellular repeats that contain Ca^{2+}-binding sites, a single transmembrane region, and a cytoplasmic domain. To date, six human desmosomal cadherins have been identified and these are clustered in the chromosomal region 18q11–q12. The cytoplasmic domain has binding sites for plakoglobin, plakophilin 1, and desmoplakin, linking them to the intermediate filaments. Desmoglein 1 has been identified as the target antigen for the autoimmune bullous disease pemphigus variatious, and desmoglein 3 for pemphigus vulgaris.

Gap junctions

Gap junctions provide a mechanism of synchronized cellular response to a variety of intercellular signals by regulating the diffusion of small molecules (< 1 kDa), such as metabolites and ions, directly between the cytoplasm of adjacent cells. Connexins are the major proteins of gap junctions and these are encoded by a large gene family. All connexins have four transmembrane domains and two extracellular loops with the amino- and carboxy-terminus located in the cytoplasm. Each connexin assembles into hexameric hemichannels (termed connexons) in the endoplasmic reticulum and these are then transported into the lipid bilayer of the plasma membrane. A connexon then docks with a connexon of an adjacent cell to form a dodecameric, aqueous channel. These intercellular channels cluster in the cell to form the gap junctions. Connexons can form either homotypic or heterotypic channels, with various channel types having distinct molecular permeabilities. The majority of connexins have a wide tissue distribution. Those expressed in the skin include connexin 26, 31, and 43.

Diseases associations with the above structural proteins have provided a molecular classification of disease to complement the classical, morphological description of hereditary blistering diseases and disorders of keratinization, some of which are described below.

Table 1 Genetics of epidermolysis bullosa

Type of epidermolysis bullosa: site of blistering	Genetic defect (chromosome)	Associated disorder
Simplex:	Keratin 5 (12q11–q13)	
basal cells	Keratin 14 (17q12–q21)	
Hemidesmo-somal:	Plectin (8q24)	Muscular
basal cells/ lamina lucida	Integrin α6 (2q24–q31)	dystrophy
	Integrin β4 (17q24)	Pyloric atresia
	Type XVII collagen (10q24)	
Junctional:	Laminin α3 (18q11)	
lamina lucida	Laminin β3 (1q32)	
	Laminin γ2 (1q25–q31)	
Dystrophic:	Type VII collagen (3p21)	
sublamina densa		

Epidermolysis bullosa

The genetic analysis of the heterogeneous group of mechanobullous disorders has given rise to enormous progress in understanding the function of proteins in the basement membrane at the dermo–epidermal junction and the role of keratins in the cytoskeleton (Table 1). The clinical phenotypes of epidermolysis bullosa correspond to different levels of separation within the basement membrane zone or basal keratinocyte, identified via electron microscopic examination. All cases of epidermolysis bullosa are skin disorders characterized by blistering of mucocutaneous sites following minor trauma, which are classified by a combination of laboratory and clinical criteria.

Epidermolysis bullosa simplex

In epidermolysis bullosa simplex, tissue separates within the basal keratinocyte, with or without aggregation of keratin intermediate filaments. This is the most common form of epidermolysis bullosa and is usually autosomal dominantly inherited. Mutations in the genes encoding the basal-cell-specific keratins K5 and K14 have been found to underlie epidermolysis bullosa simplex described, and these probably lead to cytoskeletal weakness and a tendency of cells to rupture on pressure. Three types of epidermolysis bullosa simplex are described below and clinical pictures are shown in Fig. 2 and Plate 1.

Epidermolysis bullosa simplex Weber Cockayne

The soles and palms are mainly affected, rarely in other sites. The blistering occurs from infancy (with walking) and is exacerbated by heat and ameliorated by cold. The blister heals without scarring.

Epidermolysis bullosa simplex Koebner

The blisters are widespread on scalp, trunk, arms, and legs in addition to the palmoplantar. These cases may represent autosomal recessive inheritance. Nail dystrophy, oral blisters, and dental caries are common.

Epidermolysis bullosa simplex Dowling–Meara (herpetiform epidermolysis bullosa simplex)

The blistering may be very severe and is potentially fatal in infancy. The blisters occur in groups on an erythematous bed, which heals without scarring but hyperpigmentation and milia formation may occur. Patchy keratoderma develops in later life.

Junctional epidermolysis bullosa

In junctional epidermolysis bullosa, the epidermis separates from the dermis through the lucida of the basement membrane zone. Most mutations

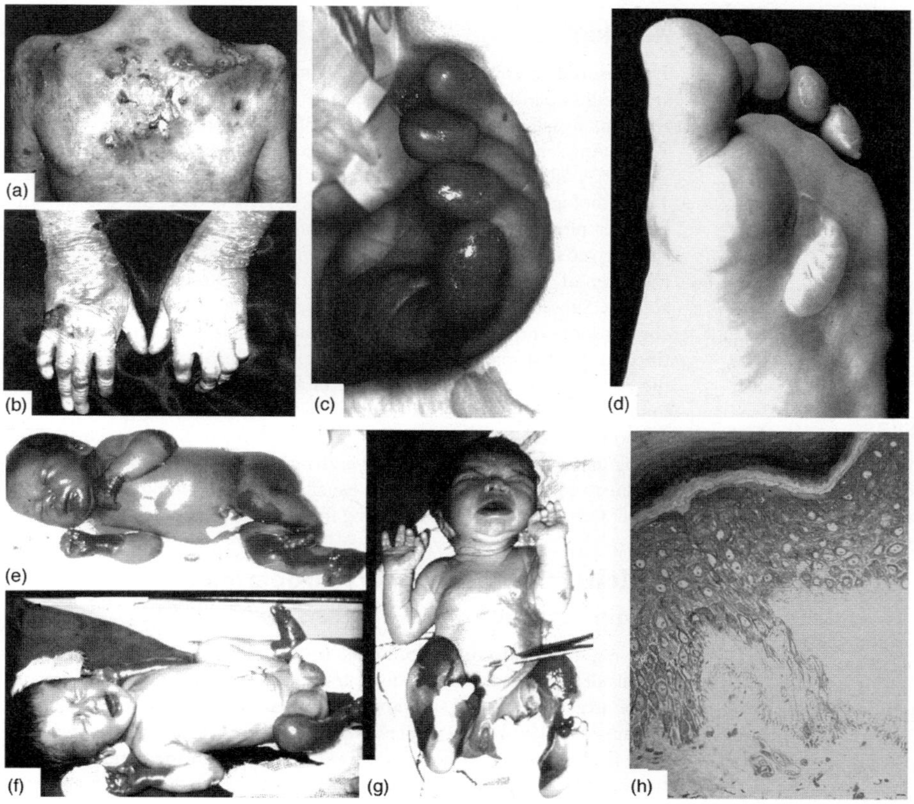

Fig. 2 Clinical photographs of the different forms of epidermolysis bullosa. (a) and (b) a patient with Hallopean–Siemans dystrophic epidermolysis bullosa; (c) the hand of an infant with Herlitz junctional epidermolysis bullosa; (d) blister on the foot of a patient with epidermolysis bullosa simplex?; (e) baby with epidermolysis bullosa simplex Dowling–Meara; (f) baby with Herlitz junctional epidermolysis bullosa; (g) baby with Hallopean–Siemans dystrophic epidermolysis bullosa; (h) intraepidermal blister from a Weber Cockayne epidermolysis bullosa simplex patient. Skin section stained with Richardson's stain. (See also Plate 1.)

lie within genes encoding the three subunit polypeptides of laminin 5 (*LAMA3*, *LAMB3*, *LAMC2*). Clinically this disease has been subdivided into two main categories—Herlitz (lethal) and non-Herlitz (non-lethal) forms.

Herlitz junctional epidermolysis bullosa

Blistering and erosions are present at birth and become widespread as the skin is so fragile that it peels away on contact. The resulting lesions are slow healing and tend to persist, becoming infected. The oropharyngeal mucosa is involved, often making feeding difficult. If the infant survives for a few months typical, crusted lesions will be seen on the nose, mouth, and jaw and across the rest of the skin in patches. The teeth have abnormal enamel and are lost easily, as are the nails. Infants usually die from overwhelming infection.

Non-lethal junctional epidermolysis bullosa

The patients show generalized skin fragility and blistering but mucosae are less severely affected. The lesions do heal leaving atrophic scars (generalized atrophic benign epidermolysis bullosa (GABEB)). Poor hair and tooth development occur and nails are dystrophic. Large hyperpigmented patches are seen.

Dystrophic epidermolysis bullosa

In recessive and dominant forms of dystrophic epidermolysis bullosa, separation occurs below the dermoepidermal region at the level of the anchoring fibrils and a large number of mutations have been discovered in the type VII collagen gene (*COL7A1*), which encodes the constituent protein of anchoring fibrils. In dystrophic epidermolysis bullosa, scarring and dystrophy are prominent features in addition to skin fragility and blistering.

Severe generalized recessive dystrophic epidermolysis bullosa

This is the most severe form of dystrophic epidermolysis bullosa and is very disabling in view of the deformities produced by scarring. Blisters are present at birth and recur readily at sites of trauma especially the hands, feet, neck, shoulders, and sacrum. They heal slowly with scarring and milia formation producing a 'mitten-like deformity' and clubbed feet. The severe oral lesions lead to microstoma and inability to protrude the tongue or open the mouth. Poor dentition leads to feeding problems. Scalp blistering and scarring gives permanent hair loss; eye involvement gives corneal erosions and opacities and general physical development is retarded. Oesophageal and perianal strictures lead to difficulty in swallowing and constipation. Although children often survive into adult life, multiple squamous cell carcinomas may develop in the chronically scarred skin and progress rapidly.

Dominant dystrophic epidermolysis bullosa

The skin is less fragile than recessive dystrophic epidermolysis bullosa and blistering much more difficult to provoke and so tends to be localized to bony prominences—knees, elbows, hands, and feet. Localized scarring with milia may replace the nails. Other areas (oral and anal) are much less affected.

Hemidesmosomal epidermolysis bullosa

Rarer forms of epidermolysis bullosa result from inherited defects in three hemidesmosonal components: plectin mutations in epidermolysis bullosa simplex with muscular dystrophy (epidermolysis bullosa simplex muscular dystrophy); type XVII collagen mutations in generalized atrophic benign epidermolysis bullosa; and $\alpha 6\beta 4$ integrin mutations in epidermolysis bullosa with pyloric atresia.

Diagnosis and management of blistering in childhood

Early diagnosis is the key to management and prediction of prognosis. Diagnosis of a baby born with blisters is often difficult on clinical grounds, so diagnosis will rest on electron microscopy of a shave skin biopsy. Immunohistochemistry is likely to be indicative in recessive cases of gene knockout—LH7.2 antibody to type VII collagen and GB3 to laminin 5 being diagnostic reagents. There is no specific treatment for any form of epidermolysis bullosa so the management centres on wound care, avoidance of physical trauma, and general physical and psychological support. Specialist nurses can advise on nursing babies with silk-covered dressing pads and vaseline gauze dressings. Oral hygiene and dental care needs to be life long. High calorie and fibre diet is essential to improve growth. Gastrostomy feeding can also help maintain body weight in children unable to eat. Finger and hand contractures require splinting at night and regular surgical release by an expert surgeon. Now that the genetic basis of epidermolysis bullosa has been identified, prenatal diagnosis by DNA-based techniques and gene therapy by *ex vivo* techniques are being actively explored.

Hailey–Hailey disease and Darier's disease

The genetic basis if these two rare, autosomal dominant, intraepidermal blistering diseases have recently been elucidated and shown to be due to mutations in calcium pumps, *ATP2C1* in Hailey–Hailey disease and *ATP-2A2* in Darier's disease.

Ichthyoses

Ichthyoses manifest as dry, rough skin with persistent scaling over most of the body which may resemble fish scales (ichthys, Greek fish). Congenital ichthyosis may be bullous or associated with other abnormalities (ichthyosiform syndromes). Ichthyosis can be acquired in later life, due to drugs such as hypercholesterolemic agents, chronic hepatic disease, lymphoma and other malignancies, thyroid disease, chronic renal hepatic failure, and malabsorption. It is sometimes difficult when a patient's ichthyosis has improved in adult life and then worsened again in late adult life to be absolutely sure whether they have a congenital or acquired ichthyosis. The progressive understanding of the molecular and cellular biology of the ichthyoses will aid in establishing their classification and potential treatment.

Autosomal dominant ichthyosis vulgaris

This commonest ichthyosis is associated with atopic eczema in up to 50 per cent of individuals. The condition improves in teenagers and young adult life and often worsens again with age. The clinical features present with dryness and scaling in the neonatal period but becoming progressively more obvious in childhood. Scaliness is small, flaky or brawny, and is most pronounced on the extensor arms and lower legs. Facial involvement is often minimal, although patients may have dandruff and they have increased markings on the palms and soles. Hyperlinearity of palm creases may be seen. It is usually very well tolerated symptomatically, with the dryness and roughness only being a problem. Treatments have therefore been aimed at removing the keratotic, retained stratum corneum with keratolytic agents such as salicylic acid (1–5 per cent lactic acid) and other hydroxy acids or buffered urea creams.

Histopathology shows hyperkeratosis with a diminished or absent granular cell layer but otherwise very little abnormality at both light and ultrastructural level. This disease is inherited as an autosomal dominant. However, genetic analysis has been hampered by variable penetrance and difficulties in ascertainment. The molecular basis of autosomal dominant ichthyosis vulgaris has centred on studies of filaggrin, the filament aggregating protein expressed in the keratohyalin granules in the stratum granulosum as a precursor protein, profilaggrin. Studies have shown alterations in the expression of profilaggrin although no disease-associated mutations have been identified in the gene encoding this protein. Therefore the genetic defect(s) underlying ichthyosis vulgaris may be in proteins involved in the synthesis or the degradation of profilaggrin rather than in the profilaggrin gene itself. Further studies are awaited.

X-linked recessive ichthyosis

This disorder is much less common than the autosomal dominant form and predominantly affects the male children of female carriers. The scaling is absent usually within the first week of life and progressively increases. The scaling tends to be prominent on the arms, thighs, and lower leg and very large, adherent, brown scaling may involve the flexures and the face. The pathology shows a normal granular cell layer and normal keratohyalin granules ultrastructurally. The molecular basis of this form of ichthyosis was derived from observations of low urinary oestriol secretion in the third trimester of pregnancy and the presence of reduced steroid sulphatase activity. Subsequently, the steroid sulphatase gene was mapped to the X chromosome and disease-associated mutations in this gene have been identified in the vast majority of patients. Steroid sulphatase mutations lead to the abnormal breakdown of cholesterol sulphate in the stratum corneum lipids, resulting in an increase in stratum corneum thickening. A small proportion of patients will have other manifestations of Kallman's syndrome, hypogonatrophic, hypogonadism, and neurological abnormalities. These are due to contiguous gene defects, usually a large deletion on the short arm of the X chromosome encompassing the steroid sulphatase locus.

Bullous ichthyosiform erythroderma or epidermolytic hyperkeratosis

This is a rare, autosomal dominant ichthyosis. At birth, there is a mild erythroderma and, at sites of minor trauma, blisters and peeling may occur. Large areas of denuded skin are often apparent after a difficult birth. In infancy, a yellow-brown hyperkeratosis develops, particularly at sites of joint flexures with cobble-stone keratoses present on the hands, feet, and trunk. Ridged scale may accumulate in skin creases, which are highly susceptible to bacterial and/or fungal infections leading to a pungent body odour. Histologically, there is lysis and clumping of the keratin filaments in the granular layer of the epidermis. Intercellular spaces are often apparent due to the rupture of suprabasal keratinocytes. Immunohistochemical studies revealed the specific aggregation of the suprabasal keratins of the epidermis, Keratin 1 and 10. Subsequently, mutations in either K1 or K10 have been shown to underlie the disease in many bullous ichthyosiform erythroderma patients. A clinical photograph of the feet of a bullous ichthyosiform erythroderma patient is shown in Fig. 3(a), and Plate 2.

Ichthyosis bullosa of Siemans

This is a rarer form of bullous ichthyosis. Neonatal disease is much milder with episodic, superficial blistering occurring throughout childhood, sometimes into adulthood. This blisters occur mainly on the flexures, lower limbs, and abdomen. At these sites, a rippled, grey hyperkeratosis may occur. Plate-like scaling and a focal peeling (Mauserung) are usually found. There is an absence of palmoplantar keratoderma and erythroderma. Mutations in another suprabasal keratin, K2e, have been identified as the genetic basis of this condition. This type II keratin is expressed in many of the higher suprabasal keratinocytes.

Netherton's syndrome

Netherton's syndrome is a severe, autosomal recessive disorder, often resulting in infant mortality, which is characterized by ichthyosis with erythroderma and trichorrhexis invaginata (hair shaft abnormalities often termed 'bamboo' hair). Hair anomalies are a characteristic feature seen in patients with Netherton's syndrome. From scanning electron microscopy, plucked hairs from patients often display trichorrhexis invaginata, tortion nodule, pili torti, and trichorrhexis nodosa. Also, light microscopy reveals invaginated hair cuticle into the cortex. Recently, a genome scan of families with Netherton's syndrome mapped the disease to a locus on chromosome 5q32. Mutations in the gene encoding SPINK5, a serine protease inhibitor, have recently been identified.

Sjörgen–Larsson syndrome

Sjörgen–Larsson syndrome is inherited as an autosomal recessive trait and is particularly prevalent in north-western Sweden (1 in 10 000), occurring less frequently elsewhere. The syndrome characteristics include ichthyosis, spastic diplegia, and mild to moderate mental retardation. The skin disease presents as mildly erythrodermic at birth with scaling developing in the first few months. These persist with scaling particularly of the face and limbs. In the flexures, neck, and periumbilical folds, an orange/brown lichenification overlaid with hyperkeratosis is a characteristic of Sjörgen–Larsson syndrome. In early life, neurological defects, including upper motor neurone defects of the limbs, mental disability, and often ocular abnormalities (spots on the retina), are observed. Histologically, the affected skin displays orthohyperkeratosis, acanthosis, and papillomatosis. The genetic defect has been shown to be in the fatty aldehyde dehydrogenase (*FALDH*) gene which affects essential fatty acid metabolism.

Keratodermas

The inherited keratodermas are characterized by thickened skin on the palms and soles. Palmoplantar skin is specialized for high levels of weight bearing and friction, so the stratum corneum is much thicker (hyperkeratotic) than the rest of the epidermis. Keratodermas can be classified clinically according to the pattern of thickening on the palm and sole skin. Three distinct clinical patterns have been observed:

- diffuse—the hyperkeratotic thickening is evenly and symmetrically distributed over the palm and sole; it is usually manifest at birth;
- focal—hyperkeratotic plaques develop particularly at sites of weight bearing and friction; these are usually plaque-like callosites or linear thickening (striate keratoderma);
- punctate—multiple, bead-like keratoses which pepper the palmoplantar skin.

They can have autosomal recessive or dominant inheritance and may occur in syndromes. Keratodermas can be further subgrouped into:

- simple—palmoplantar involvement only;
- complex—associated with lesions of non-volar skin, hair teeth, nails, and sweat glands (including ectodermal dysplasias);
- syndromic—with associated abnormalities of other organs including deafness, cancer, cardiomyopathy, and adrenal insufficiency.

They can also be classified biologically by their recently-discovered genetic defects, for example see Fig. 3 and Tables 2 and 3. This branch of the genodermatoses is genetically heterogeneous with mutations in genes encoding keratins, desmosomal proteins, connexins, and a protease.

Diffuse palmoplantar keratodermas

Simple: diffuse epidermolytic palmoplantar keratoderma (EPPK)

EPPK is characterized by epidemolytic hyperkeratosis with keratin filament clumping in suprabasal keratins. This autosomal dominant disease presents

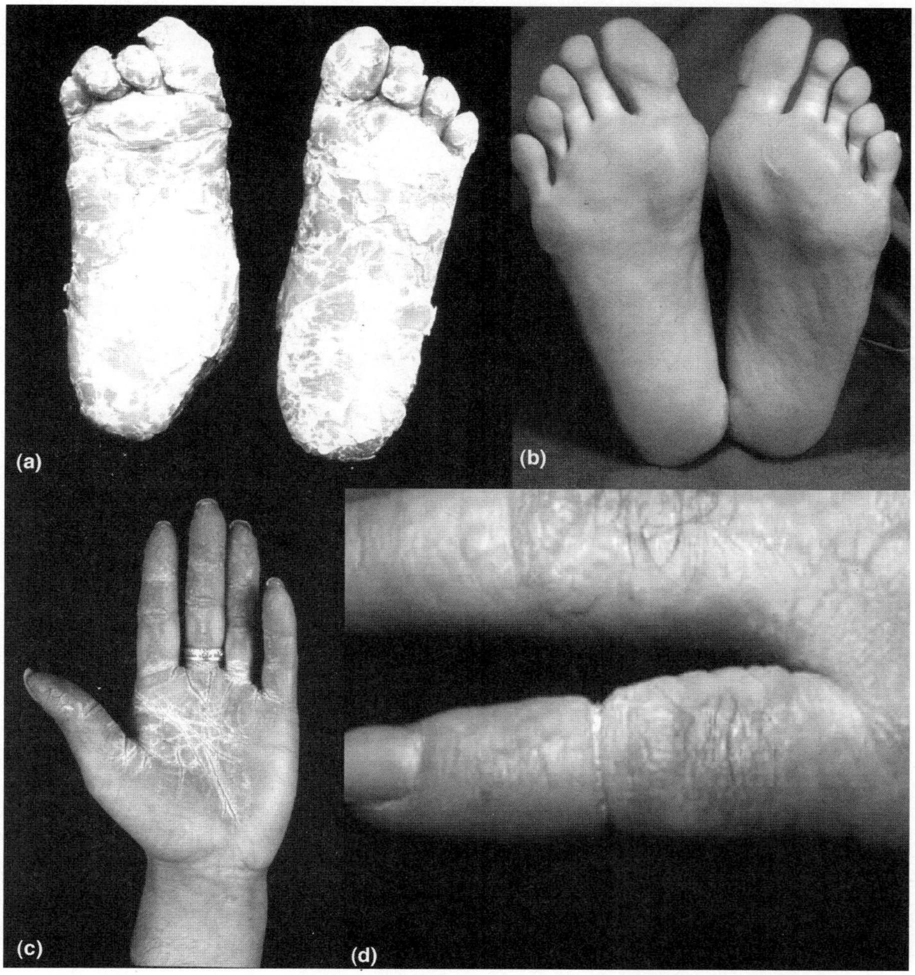

Fig. 3 Clinical photographs of: (a) bullous ichthyosiform erythroderma (BIE) and three types of keratoderma: (b) focal palmoplantar keratoderma (PPK) associated with a keratin 16 mutation; (c) striate palmoplantar keratoderma associated with a desmoglein 1 mutation; and (d) constriction around the digit from an individual with Vohwinkel's syndrome associated with a Cx26 mutation. (See also Plate 2.)

Table 2 Genetics of diffuse palmoplantar keratoderma (PPK)

Type of diffuse PPK	Associated disorder	Genetic defect (map location)
EPPK (epider-molytic PPK)		Keratin 9 (17q12–q21)
NEPPK (non-epidermolytic PPK)	Umbilical hyperkeratosis	Keratin 1 (12q11–q13)
NEPPK		Not known (12q11–q13)
Syndromic NEPPK (Naxos disease)	Woolly hair and cardiomyopathy	Plakoglobin (17q12–q13) Desmoplakin (6p23–p24)
Vohwinkel's syndrome	Sensorineural deafness Ichthyosis	Connexin 26 (13q12) Loricrin (1q21)
Erythrokerato-derma variablis	Generalized erythroderma	Connexin 31 (1p34–p36)
Clouston's syndrome	Alopecia, nail dystrophy, sensorineural deafness	Connexin 30 and connexin 30.3 (13q11–q12)
Hypohidrotic ectodermal dysplasia	Erythroderma, impaired sweating, hair and nail abnormalities	Plakophilin (1q32–q34)
Mal de Meleda	Hyperhidrosis and perioral erythema	SLURP-1 (8q24)

with symmetrical thickening, giving a cracked, crocodile-skin-like surface due to the underlying epidermolysis, which starts in early infancy. The majority of EPPK pedigrees are linked to the type I keratin cluster on chromosome 17q12–q21 and disease is due to mutations in the palmoplantar-specific keratin, K9, the majority clustering in the helix initiation domain of the protein.

Simple: diffuse non-epidermolytic palmoplantar keratoderma (NEPPK)

NEPPK is also inherited as an autosomal dominant trait and is often difficult to distinguish clinically from EPPK, due to the variability of finding epidermolysis by electronmicroscopy in EPPK. There is a waxy, uniform, yellow thickening over the palms and soles which may spread onto the dorsum of hands and wrists with a sharp cut-off. It is commonly aggravated by secondary fungal infection, which may require intermittent, oral antifungal agents. These often improve the keratoderma. In a number of families the defect has been linked to 12q11–q13. A single family has a mutation in the variable head domain of KRT1. However in the majority of NEPPK families, fine mapping of the 12q11–q13 locus has excluded the type II keratin genes, and a number of candidate genes in the area including a keratinocyte-expressed elastase have been excluded by sequencing.

Complex: erythrokeratoderma variabilis

Erythrokeratoderma variabilis is a rare, autosomal dominantly inherited skin disease characterized by diffuse palmoplantar keratoderma and transient, figurate, red patches at various sites and severity. Germline mutations in connexin 31 (*GJB3*) and connexin 30.3 (GJB4) have been identified in the affected members of some erythrokeratoderma variabilis families.

Focal keratoderma

Most focal palmoplantar keratodermas are characterized by discoid lesions and the majority can be regarded as complex palmoplantar keratodermas as they are often associated with abnormalities of hair, nails, teeth, and glands.

Simple: striate palmoplantar keratoderma

This focal palmoplantar keratoderma is characterized by distinctive linear streaks on palms and soles, over the ventral aspects of fingers and extending onto palms; it is often more extreme on the feet. Variable nail and hair involvement, with fragility or splitting, are seen. Recently, mutations in two desmosomal proteins, desmoglein 1 (18q11–12) and desmoplakin 1(6p21), have been described which result in a hemizygous gene knockout, resulting in haploinsufficiency of the gene product.

Complex: pachyonychia congenita type 1/ focal palmoplantar keratoderma with oral mucosal hyperkeratosis

This clinical overlap syndrome presents in childhood with nail changes (pachyonychia), typically a subungual hyperkeratosis trumpet-shaped nail, especially on the thumb and first finger and toe nails. The sole lesions are painful callosites over weight-bearing areas on the feet, with less prominent callosities on the palms. The mucosa shows milky hyperkeratosis over gingiva. Nutmeg-grater-like follicular keratoses also occur. Variable fragility and blistering can be associated with severe pain on walking. Milder nail involvement shows splinter haemorrhages at the onychocorneal bind. The pathological findings of epidermolytic hyperkeratosis with keratin filament clumping suggested that keratin gene mutations underlie this disorder,

Table 3 Genetics of focal palmoplantar keratoderma (PPK)

Type of focal PPK	Associated disorder	Genetic defect (map location)
Focal NEPPK	Follicular and orogenital hyperkeratosis	Keratin 16 (17q12–q21)
Focal NEPPK (tylosis)	Oesophageal cancer, oral and follicular hyperkeratosis	Not known (17q24q25)
Pachyonychia congenita type 1	Nail dystrophy and oral lesions	Keratin 6a (12q11–q13) Keratin 16 (17q12–q21)
Pachyonychia congenita type 2	Epidermal cysts, nail dystrophy, and oral lesions	Keratin 6b (12q11–q13) Keratin 17 (17q12–q21)
Striate PPK		Desmoglein 1 (18q12) Desmoplakin (6p21)
Papillon–Lefevre		Cathepsin C (11q14)
Oculocutaneous tyrosinaemia	Photophobia, corneal ulceration, and mental retardation	Tyrosine aminotransferase (16q22)

confirmed by the identification of mutations in *KRT6a* and *KRT16* in affected individuals from multiple families.

Complex: pachyonychia congenita type 2/ steatocystoma multiplex

The steatocysis palmoplantar keratoderma may be very limited although pachyonychia nail changes present early. Multiple epidermal cysts and steatocysis are seen. Woolly scalp hair and fuzzy eyebrows are seen and natal teeth can occur. The finding of keratin clumps in skin bearing keratin K17, particularly deep outer root sheath, suggested *KRT17* as the candidate gene and autosomal dominant mutations in hot spots have now been described. Mutations in *KRT6b* have also been described. The resulting pathology varies from keratin cysts, vellous hair cysts, to oil filled cysts.

Complex: Papillon–Lefevre syndrome

This focal palmoplantar keratoderma is inherited as an autosomal recessive and is marked by associated severe periodontitis and loss of primary and secondary dentition with opalescent oral mucosa. The inflammatory lesions often result in pocket formation seen pathologically. Linkage to 11q14 was demonstrated in a number of families. Recently, mutations in cathepsin C, a lysosomal protease, have been shown to underlie this disorder. It is postulated that cathepsin C may be important in the processing of key structural proteins, such as keratins, in the epidermis.

Syndromic keratodermas (multiple phenotypic)

Palmoplantar keratoderma and deafness

A number of families with palmoplantar keratoderma and sensorineural deafness have been described, which could have been due to a mutation of a single gene expressed in all affected tissues or cosegregation of two distinct gene mutations. One such disorder is Vohwinkel's syndrome; a mutating palmoplantar keratoderma with constrictions developing around and autoamputating fingers. In a small family with a Vohwinkel's pattern of keratoderma and profound sensorineural deafness, two distinct mutations in the gene encoding the gap junction protein connexin 26 (*GJB2*) were identified. One of the mutations was associated with the profound deafness, the other (*D66H*) segregated with the skin disease. This led to the important discovery that mutations in *GJB2* were causative in both autosomal dominant (DFNA3) and recessive (DFNB1) deafness, accounting for 40 to 60 per cent of hereditary sensorineural deafness world-wide. In other families with Vohwinkel's syndrome, the same palmoplantar keratoderma-associated mutation D66H in *GJB2* has been identified. Mutations in loricrin, a cornified cell envelope component of the stratum corneum, have also been identified in individuals affected with a variant form of Vohwinkel's syndrome, which is associated with ichthyosis and normal hearing. In addition, palmoplantar keratoderma and deafness has also been associated with mitochondrial mutations.

Palmoplantar keratodermas and cancer

Focal NEPPK and oesophageal cancer

Three pedigrees from United Kingdom, United States, and Germany have been studied in which a focal NEPPK with oral hyperkeratosis segregates with a high lifetime risk of squamous cell carcinoma of the oesophagus (40–91 per cent by age 70). In all three families, linkage to DNA markers mapping to 17q24–q25 has localized the disease gene to a region of less than 1 cM. The cornified envelope protein, envoplakin, lies in this region but has been genetically excluded as the candidate gene.

Huriez disease (sclerotylosis)

This is an autosomal dominant disease characterized by palmoplantar keratoderma, nail changes, and scleroatrophy of the distal extremities. Around 15 per cent of individuals develop aggressive squamous cell carcinomas, occurring in their thirties and forties. It is proposed that the scarring resulting from skin fragility predisposes to the squamous cell carcinomas. Recently, the Huriez disease gene has been mapped to chromosome 4q23.

Punctate palmoplantar keratoderma

A weak association between punctate palmoplantar keratoderma and cancer has been observed in a family with a number of epithelial-derived tumours developing in members under the age of 50. As yet, the punctate palmoplantar keratoderma locus has not been genetically mapped though a number of candidate regions, such as the keratins, have been excluded by linkage.

Other palmoplantar keratoderma syndromes

Diffuse NEPPK, woolly hair, and arrhythmogenic venticular cardiomyopathy (which leads to heart failure and arrhythmias) is due to recessive mutations in plakoglobin. Recessive mutations in another desmosomal protein, desmoplakin, underlie a similar syndrome consisting of a striate PPK, woolly hair, and dilated left ventricular cardiomyopathy. In triple A or Allgroves syndrome, individuals have adrencorticotrophic-hormone-resistant adrenal insufficiency, achalasia, and alacrimia with a PPK due to mutations in aladin, a member of the WD-repeat family of regulatory proteins.

Ectodermal dysplasias

There are a very large number of ectodermal dysplasias which display abnormalities of the skin, hair, teeth, nails, and/or sweating. The clinical classification is unsatisfactory but may become more transparent when the genetic basis of a significant number of these complexes have been classified. At present, there is limited genetic understanding. Two major subgroups are hidrotic and non-hidrotic ectodermal dysplasia. The concept of dysplasia in these diseases is developmental rather than premalignant.

Hidrotic ectodermal dysplasia (Clouston's syndrome)

Hidrotic ectodermal dysplasia is characterized by nail dystrophy with thick, slow growing, and discoloured, short nails. Diffuse palmoplantar keratoderma is variable but may be severe and spread to knuckles and finger joints. Scalp hair is sparse, fine, pale, and brittle with thin eyebrows and sparse body hair. The disease is inherited as an autosomal dominant. Disease in a large kindred from Canada was mapped to 13q11–12 which harbours a connexin gene cluster. Mutations in the gene encoding connexin 30 underlie this disorder.

Hypohidrotic ectodermal dysplasia

This X-linked, recessively inherited disease is characterized by a loss of sweat glands causing absent or reduced sweating (hypohidrosis) and total or partial loss of teeth. Patients may be very uncomfortable on exertion and are heat intolerant. The teeth are characteristically conical and the mouth dry. In severe forms, the facial appearance is altered with saddle nose, sunken cheeks, and sparse, dry, fine, short hair with absent eyebrows. The disease maps to Xq12–13.1 and is caused by mutations in the ectodysplasin anhidrotic protein. An autosomal recessive form is due to mutations in the ectodysplasin receptor.

Concluding comments

This chapter has focused on the rarer types of genetic skin diseases rather than the more common, genetically complex disorders such as eczema, psoriasis, and acne. This is largely because only a few potential disease-associated genetic variants have been identified with the more common epidermal disorders. In contrast, great advances have been made in understanding the molecular basis of the rarer blistering diseases, ichthyoses, and the keratodermas, with the identification of a number of important proteins involved in epidermal and also non-epidermal biology. In addition, these studies have revealed genetic heterogeneity with mutations in different proteins causing similar clinical manifestations, for example Vohwinkel's syndrome can be due to mutations in either connexin 26 or loricrin. With the imminent completion of the sequencing of the entire human genome, the capability for high throughput genotyping using to high density single nucleotide polymorphism (SNP) maps and new technology development, it is likely that the genetic basis of the more common epidermal disorders will be elucidated in the near future.

Further reading

Review papers

Aumailley M, Rousselle P (1999). Laminins of the dermo-epidermal junction. *Matrix Biology* **18**, 19–28.

Corden LD, McLean WHI (1996). Human keratin diseases: hereditary fragility of specific epithelial tissues. *Experimental Dermatology* **5**, 297–307.

Kelsell DP, Stevens HP (1999). The palmoplantar keratodermas: much more than palms and soles. *Molecular Medicine Today* **5**, 107–13.

Ruhrberg C, Watt FM (1997). The plakin family: versatile organizers of cytoskeletal architecture. *Current Opinions in Genetics and Development* **7**, 392–7.

Uitto J, Pulkkinen L, McLean WH (1997). Epidermolysis bullosa: a spectrum of clinical phenotypes explained by molecular heterogeneity. *Molecular Medicine Today* **3**, 457–65.

White TW, Paul DL (1999). Genetic diseases and gene knockouts reveal diverse connexin functions. *Annual Review Physiology* **61**, 283–310.

Significant research papers

Armstrong D *et al* (1999). Haploinsufficiency of desmoplakin causes a striate subtype of palmoplantar keratoderma. *Human Molecular Genetics* **8**, 143–8.

Chipev CC *et al* (1992). A leucine-proline mutation in the H1 subdomain of keratin 1 causes epidermolytic hyperkeratosis. *Cell* **70**, 821–8.

De Laurenzi V *et al* (1996). Sjogren-Larsson syndrome is caused by mutations in the fatty aldehyde dehydrogenase gene. *Nature Genetics* **12**, 52–7.

Hilal L *et al* (1993). A homozygous insertion-deletion in the type VII collagen gene (COL7A1) in Hallopeau-Siemens dystrophic epidermolysis bullosa. *Nature Genetics* **5**, 287–93.

Hu Z *et al* (2000). Mutations in ATP2C1, encoding a calcium pump, cause hailey-hailey disease. *Nature Genetics* **24**, 61–5.

Kelsell DP *et al* (1997). Connexin 26 mutations in hereditary non-syndromic sensorineural deafness. *Nature* **387**, 80–3.

Kere J *et al* (1996). X-linked anhidrotic (hypohidrotic) ectodermal dysplasia is caused by mutation in a novel transmembrane protein. *Nature Genetics* **13**, 409–16.

Lamartine J, *et al.* (2000). Mutations in GJB6 cause hidrotic ectodermal dysplasia. *Nature Genetics* **26**, 142–4.

Lane EB *et al* (1992). A mutation in the conserved helix termination peptide of keratin 5 in hereditary skin blistering. *Nature* **356**, 244–6.

Maestrini E *et al* (1996). A molecular defect in loricrin, the major component of the cornified cell envelope, underlies Vohwinkel's syndrome. *Nature Genetics* **13**, 70–7.

McKoy G, *et al.* (2000). Identification of a deletion in plakoglobin in arrhythmogenic right ventricular cardiomayopathy with palmoplantar deratoderma and woolly hair (Naxos disease). *Lancet* **355**, 2119–24.

McLean WHI *et al* (1995). Keratin 16 and keratin 17 mutations cause pachyonychia congenita. *Nature Genetics* **9**, 273–8.

Norgett EE, *et al.* (2000). Recessive mutation in desmoplakin disrupts desmoplakin-intermediate filament interactions and causes dilated cardiomyopathy, woolly hair and keratoderma. *Human Molecular Genetics* **9**, 2761–6.

Reis A *et al* (1994). Keratin 9 gene mutations in epidermolytic palmoplantar keratoderma (EPPK). *Nature Genetics* **6**, 174–9.

Richard G *et al* (1998). Mutations in the human connexin gene GJB3 cause erythrokeratodermia variabilis. *Nature Genetics* **20**, 366–9.

Rickman L *et al* (1999). N-terminal deletion in a desmosomal cadherin causes the autosomal dominant skin disease striate palmoplantar keratoderma. *Human Molecular Genetics* **8**, 971–6.

Rothnagel JA *et al* (1994). Mutations in the rod domain of keratin 2e in patients with ichthyosis bullosa of Siemens. *Nature Genetics* **7**, 485–90.

Sakuntabhai A *et al* (1999). Mutations in ATP2A2, encoding a Ca2+ pump, cause Darier disease. *Nature Genetics* **21**, 271–7.

Smith FJD *et al* (1996). Plectin deficiency results in muscular dystrophy with epidermolysis bullosa. *Nature Genetics* **13**, 450–6.

Toomes C *et al* (1999). Loss-of-function mutations in the cathepsin C gene result in periodontal disease and palmoplantar keratosis. *Nature Genetics* **23**, 421–4.

Vidal F *et al* (1995). Integrin beta 4 mutations associated with junctional epidermolysis bullosa with pyloric atresia. *Nature Genetics* **10**, 229–34.

Yen PH *et al* (1987). Cloning and expression of steroid sulfatase cDNA and the frequent occurrence of deletions in STS deficiency: implications for X-Y interchange. *Cell* **49**, 443–54.

24

Neurology

24.1 Introduction and approach to the patient with neurological disease

Alastair Compston

Clinical neurology uses intuitive conversation, structured examination, and selective investigation to formulate problems into an anatomical and pathological framework. The competent neurologist instinctively senses relevant components of the history, appreciates the most likely underlying mechanism, reliably elicits the physical signs, knows which investigations are necessary and relevant, and communicates the situation accurately and sensitively. This system has evolved over several centuries during which knowledge has accumulated on structure and function, localization in health and disease, the reliability of physical signs and laboratory investigations, and the nosology of disease.

The neurological history

Although patients usually start with an account of that which troubles them most, the neurologist prefers a history of the components in the order in which they occurred. It may take some time to establish this chronology. The first task is to assess the core symptoms and how they cluster. The neurologist asks enough questions to settle whether, for example, a reported episode of difficulty with speech refers to a disturbance of language (aphasia) or articulation (dysarthria); whether there are motor or sensory deficits in a 'heavy' limb; whether alterations of sensation are positive (tingling and paraesthesiae) or negative (numbness) symptoms; whether a disturbance of bladder function suggests neurological or urological disease; and whether double vision actually refers to diplopia or altered acuity. Some questions reflect the peculiarities of neurological anatomy; it may surprise the patient complaining of impaired vision on the right that the symptom is in fact unaltered by sequential closure of either eye—because it is hemianopic; or that awareness of temperature and the appreciation of pain may be disturbed in the 'good' leg in some forms of spinal cord disease (the Brown–Sequard syndrome).

Once the individual symptoms are accurately defined, they can be grouped and from this follows an interpretation of their anatomical basis suggesting the involvement of one or more sites. Recognizing these patterns is fundamental to interpretation of the neurological history and this synthesis directs attention to specific components of the subsequent examination. It is easy to conclude that the patient with cognitive impairment has disease of the cerebral cortex but a more detailed history will additionally indicate whether this is diffuse or focal and reflects involvement of the dominant or non-dominant hemispheres and the frontal, temporal, or parietal cortices. Inco-ordination of more than one motor skill (eye movement, speech, the limbs, and balance) necessarily indicates involvement of brainstem–cerebellar connections. The process causing a hemianopic field defect lies above and that resulting in lower cranial nerve palsies below the tentorium. The combination of motor and sensory symptoms in the limbs with altered sphincter function indicates spinal cord disease; for the male patient with an unreliable bladder, the significance of linking urgency and frequency to impotence and constipation may seem strange. In turn, the coexistence of diffuse distal symmetric motor and sensory symptoms, shoulder and pelvic girdle weakness, or ocular, bulbar, respiratory, and upper limb weakness steers the thinking towards peripheral nerve, primary muscle, and neuromuscular junction disease respectively.

As a generalization, abrupt events are vascular or electrical in origin; subacute symptoms are demyelinating or inflammatory; and symptoms which develop slowly suggest structural deficits or degeneration. The subsequent course also reveals the underlying process; self-limiting events are often vascular; paroxysmal symptoms tend to be electrical or demyelinating, depending on their duration; and progressive syndromes are compressive or degenerative. The circumstances may be suggestive of a particular pathophysiology: trauma, preceding infection, drug exposure, or pregnancy alert the observer to structural, demyelinating, toxic, and venous thrombotic mechanisms respectively. Dangerous for the beginner but nevertheless important to recognize are the inconsistencies of exaggeration, mismatch between the severity of symptoms and altered function, and anatomical impossibilities which usually feature in non-organic neurological disease. Together, these pattern recognitions are the stuff of neurological diagnosis.

The neurological examination

Examination of the patient with neurological disease needs to be structured and organized without exhausting the patient and examiner through obsessive attention to irrelevant detail. Much can be learned by astute observation without formal assessment. Gross defects of cognition do not need to be confirmed by reciting telephone numbers in reverse or assembling lists of former prime ministers; defects of speech will usually be evident in conversation; many neurological diagnoses are immediately apparent from the patient's gait; movement disorders can be observed whilst taking the history. That said, it is best routinely to adopt a basic core examination and do things in order since the detection of one abnormality will determine the interpretation of another. It takes only a few minutes for the experienced and adequately equipped examiner to confirm that corrected visual acuity is normal in each eye, that there is no gross field defect, and that the optic fundi are normal. Although more detailed assessment will sometimes be necessary, a full range of smooth following (pursuit) eye movements in the horizontal and vertical planes can rapidly be established: this will detect obvious ophthalmoplegia and can be supplemented by cover testing of each eye during fixation on the examiner's nose, and rapid gaze from right to left—very few significant defects of eye movement will escape this rapid screen. Movement of the lower face during forced eye closure, voluntary elevation of the palate, and rapid protrusion or side-to-side movement of the tongue take a few seconds to observe and effectively cover all the lower cranial nerves. It is rarely necessary to test the sense of smell or hearing and a tuning fork is most useful for establishing that deafness is conductive and therefore probably not relevant. Before moving to the limbs, it is worth testing neck flexion in patients where the history suggests muscular or neuromuscular disease.

A sufficient routine examination of the arms would start with posture (outstretched with the eyes open and then closed); a quick look for selective muscle wasting; tone in flexion–extension and supination–pronation at the elbow and wrist respectively; strength in flexion and extension at the elbow and wrist, spreading the fingers and abduction of the thumb; co-ordination during movement between the patient's nose and examiner's finger (or both hands if there is gross inco-ordination so as to avoid accidental ocular injury); and the tendon reflexes. This will take the experienced examiner less than a minute. It may be necessary to establish specific patterns of muscle weakness: global loss affecting the hand in cortical disease; selective involvement of extensor groups in upper motor neurone disease; the patterns of C5–T1 nerve root lesions; diffuse distal weakness of both extremities in peripheral neuropathy; and the subtle distinctions between radial, median, and ulnar neuropathies and C7, C8, and T1 root lesions respectively. Detailed sensory examination of the arms rarely achieves more than can be learned from establishing that crude protective sense (recognition of a sharp pin) or discrimination (position sense and the ability to distinguish two points or perform a simple task such as manipulating a button) are intact.

Although this may involve some rearrangement of clothing, it otherwise takes almost no time to swipe the abdominal reflexes in passing, before examining the legs. Here, the structured motor examination is as for the arms although increased tone is more easily detected by lifting the relaxed leg from the couch at the thigh, and testing internal and external rotation at the hip. Characteristic patterns of weakness are the involvement of flexors at all joints and eversion at the ankle in upper motor neurone lesions; the usual diffuse symmetrical distal involvement in peripheral neuropathy at a time when the hands may be normal; and difficulty in distinguishing injury of the lateral popliteal nerve from an L5/S1 root lesion (in which the ankle jerk is lost) in the context of unilateral foot drop. Proximal weakness is best detected by watching the patient walk, and the calf muscles are normally so strong as to be untestable except with the patient standing. As in the arm, co-ordination can only be assessed once the degree of weakness is established. Tendon reflexes in the legs may be brisk in isolation and often spread, so that in an upper motor neurone lesion when one is tapped several may respond—and in either leg. Even non-neurologists rarely forget to elicit the plantar responses.

Sensory examination of the legs tends to be more reliable for protective than discriminative sensation. In mapping a sensory level it is best to move from the relatively anaesthetic to the normal zone noting the band of hypersensitivity which usually exists at the boundary. It is a matter of fact that many patients confuse the examination by exaggeration or elaboration of physical signs; this most usually affects power and the usual clues are a mismatch between the ability to walk and findings on formal assessment of muscle strength (or vice versa) and simultaneous contraction of agonist and antagonist muscles. Sensory testing is subjective and so necessarily vulnerable to inaccurate reporting, but confirming that a sensory level is present both on the abdomen and back, and on the same side on each with a slightly higher level on the trunk, is a simple manoeuvre which may yield surprising discrepancies in the patient with non-organic deficits.

The overall purpose of the history and examination is to assess where and through what mechanism structure and function have been affected. Detecting these patterns becomes routine for the experienced neurologist but the process represents more than just a ritual of clinical neurology. From anatomical localization follows a formulation of likely mechanisms and pathological conditions underlying the patient's symptoms and signs.

Investigation of neurological disease

The investigation of patients with neurological disease was revolutionized in the early 1970s with the introduction of computed axial tomography. Before then, only the most primitive structural details of the central nervous system could be detected by demonstrating indirectly the shape and placement of the ventricles and blood vessels, and usually at some discomfort to the patient. Function in the central and peripheral nervous systems was measured using neurophysiological techniques. Disruption of the blood–brain barrier and immunological activity in the central nervous system were assessed through analysis of the cerebrospinal fluid.

Investigation still does not replace clinical assessment but, as the sections which follow make clear, it is now possible to detect structural changes in most parts of the brain and spinal cord at high resolution; to distinguish many pathological appearances at these sites on the basis of differences in the magnetic resonance signals; to map function within regions of interest using changes in blood flow and the use of metabolic substrates; to show variations in efferent and afferent electrical activity in the central and peripheral nervous systems; and to detect an increasing range of soluble mediators of normal and pathological function in the cerebrospinal fluid. Taken together, these laboratory investigations still do no more than supplement clinical assessments and, in one sense, the high expectations of diagnosis make for additional difficulties in interpreting neurological illness when the images are normal compared with the era when authoritative statements from neurologists could never be validated and necessarily went unchallenged.

The value of many routine investigations lies in confirming normality and endorsing abnormalities already strongly suspected on clinical grounds. Given the increasing sensitivity of techniques for brain imaging, altered appearances which are not necessarily of pathological significance and genuine lesions which are not relevant in the particular clinical context need to be interpreted with common sense. Overall, the trend has been for the pendulum to swing from diagnosis without adequate laboratory evidence to diagnosis made in defiance of clinical intuition. Even when an imaging abnormality has been identified, its nature may require clinical discussion in order to resolve the most likely pathological substrate—the distinction between ischaemic and inflammatory tissue often proving difficult and not all neoplastic tissue being easily identified as such.

The management of neurological disease

The first issue that confronts the doctor looking after a person with neurological disease is when to discuss and name the diagnosis. Most wait until there is sufficient clinical or laboratory evidence to rule out misdiagnosis; telling people that they have a condition when they do not is bound to cause distress and has landed some specialists in the law courts. However, overcaution and avoidance of discussion can be equally damaging and there are many more patients who harbour bitterness over delay in learning the true nature of their illness than those who wish they had not been told so soon, or at all. The majority of individuals cope extremely well even with the prospect of conditions which are known to be life threatening or have a poor prognosis for disability. Advice may be needed on alterations in lifestyle resulting from neurological disease—for example driving in epilepsy, and the use of drugs in pregnancy. There is a basic human need to know why a thing has happened and most patients enquire about causation but, naturally, the uppermost question is whether symptoms can be treated or the natural history of disease usefully modified.

The chapters which follow document specific treatments for particular conditions but judgement is often required in deciding whether to deploy these remedies depending on age, significance of the symptoms for the individual, level of disability, security of the diagnosis, adverse effects, and the patient's own views. Drug treatment may be used, on an intermittent or regular basis, to suppress symptoms—for example, intravenous methyl prednisolone to reduce inflammation, anticonvulsants to suppress epilepsy, γ-aminobutyric acid agonists to deal with spasticity, or anticholinesterases to enhance transmission at the neuromuscular junction. Pharmacological options also exist for interfering with the mechanism of disease, again on an intermittent or routine basis—such as the use of triptans to relieve migraine, or the replacement of dopamine in Parkinson's disease. In other situations, the rationale of treatment is to modify the underlying disease process, for example by suppressing inflammatory processes in acute post-infectious polyneuritis using intravenous gammaglobulin, treating patients with multiple sclerosis using β-interferon, and using immunosuppressants such as methotrexate and cycophosphamide in polymyositis and vasculitis respectively. Many other illustrations could be given confirming that the age-old witticism concerning the therapeutic nihilism of clinical neurology is at best now only of historical interest and was always generally rather ill-informed. Beyond the present pharmacological achievements in drug treatment lie many opportunities for improving handicap and disability through the use of rehabilitation which increasingly assumes centre stage in the management of neurological disease through attention to the person with impairments in a particular social and cultural setting rather than focusing on the pathophysiology of disease in an individual void. For the future, there is the prospect of enhanced regeneration in the context of diseases affecting the central and peripheral nervous systems, restoring structure and function and thereby both limiting and repairing the damage.

24.2 Electrophysiology of the central and peripheral nervous systems

Christian Krarup

Introduction

In clinical neurophysiology, the core investigations in electrophysiological studies of the central nervous system (**CNS**) and peripheral nervous system (**PNS**), comprise electroencephalography (**EEG**), evoked potentials, electromyography (**EMG**), and nerve conduction studies. However, since these provide no direct information about pathological changes, it is often necessary to supplement findings by imaging or other laboratory studies, and it is mandatory to view the results in a clinical context. Furthermore, electrophysiological parameters provide information about changes over time obtained from various anatomical regions that may not be accessible to direct pathological examination.

Additional methods (including cardiovascular reflexes in the study of the autonomic nervous system, respiratory movements and oxygen saturation in polysomnographic studies of sleep disturbances, and recording of force in the study of voluntary muscle) are becoming increasingly important in clinical neurophysiology, recognizing that electrophysiological methods must often be supplemented by other investigations.

Electroencephalography (EEG)

At EEG the spontaneous ongoing activity from the cerebral cortex is recorded through electrodes placed over the scalp. In most routine studies, recordings are carried out over 30 to 60 min. In addition, specialized studies may be performed to diagnose patients with particular types of epilepsy, during carotid artery endarterectomy, or brain death. In patients with poorly described epileptic fits, the clinical features may require that both visual information and EEG evidence are obtained simultaneously (video-EEG). This may, in patients who are candidates for surgical treatment of medically intractable epilepsy, be carried out over many days. In some patients, additional information may be obtained with intracranial subdural or intracerebral depth electrodes. During epilepsy surgery, an electroencephalogram is recorded directly from the cortex, so-called electrocorticography.

Indications

The main indications for obtaining an EEG include paroxysmal events, convulsions, disturbed levels of consciousness, and neuroinfections. EEG is not well suited as a screening procedure in patients with suspected focal cerebral lesions, since deep-seated lesions show no abnormalities at EEG if the cortex itself or its afferent projections are unaffected. However, when the clinical picture in patients with focal brain lesions is complicated by periodic changes in consciousness, convulsions, or unexplained changes in focal weakness, EEG is necessary to establish the presence of secondary paroxysmal events. Furthermore, EEG is often indicated in patients with encephalopathy to ascertain whether the clinical features are complicated by additional ictal discharges.

I am indebted to Dr H. Høgenhaven MD for comments on the manuscript.

Serial EEGs are often necessary to assess the prognosis in patients with diffuse brain lesions. When abnormalities obtained early during a cerebral disorder (for example, cardiac arrest associated with cerebral ischaemia) are followed by further deterioration of the EEG pattern, a poor prognosis is indicated.

Method

The recording takes place with the patient in a comfortable position in a quiet room. After placing surface or needle electrodes over the scalp according to an international, standardized system (the 10–20 system Fig. 1), the technician ensures that the impedance of the electrodes is less than 5 kΩ. The patient's age, clinical state, and medication is indicated on the record, in particular whether the level of consciousness is normal. The session includes recordings while the patient is awake, during activation procedures, and, if possible, during drowsiness and sleep. During the recording the technician makes notes about the patient's awareness and state of consciousness, but fully describes any events that occur during the recording.. Activity is evaluated at different electrode montages, including both bipolar and unipolar recordings. Bipolar recordings are of value for localizing abnormalities in focal brain areas, whereas unipolar recordings are necessary for examining more widespread and generalized disturbances.

During recording the awake patient is asked to relax with closed eyes to assess the background activity. The EEG waveforms are characterized by summated continuous postsynaptic de- and hyperpolarizations of large numbers of cortical cells by input from other brain areas and are, on an empirical basis, described in terms of their frequencies. The frequency contents of the EEG are classified into activity with frequencies of 8 to 13 Hz (α-activity), 3.5 to 7.5 Hz (θ-activity), 3 Hz or less (δ-activity), and activity above 13 Hz (β-activity). Interpretation of the EEG should include a description of the background activity, the presence of abnormal wave forms ('transients') during rest and activation procedures, and whether any changes in the background or the occurrence of abnormal waveforms occur diffusely, synchronously, or in a focal pattern (Figs 1(b), (c), and 2). Advanced algorithms to localize the distribution of waveforms (brain mapping) are now used for both diagnostic purposes and research on epileptic and non-epileptic syndromes, and they are of particular relevance in the temporal and spatial development of transient abnormalities.

Activation procedures include hyperventilation: here the patient breathes deeply at a rate of 20/min for 2 to 4 min and changes are followed up to 2 min after hyperventilation. In children and young adults, this may elicit θ- and δ-activity (activities considered to be abnormal in individuals over 30 years of age), while patients with absences may develop spike-and-(sharp)-wave patterns during hyperventilation (see Fig. 1(c)). The possible epileptogenic effect of photic stimulation is evaluated by stimulating with variable frequencies when the eyes are opened and closed. In susceptible individuals, spike activity limited to the occipital regions is not associated with epilepsy, but spikes or sharp waves in a more widespread distribution are indicators of a lowered epileptogenic threshold.

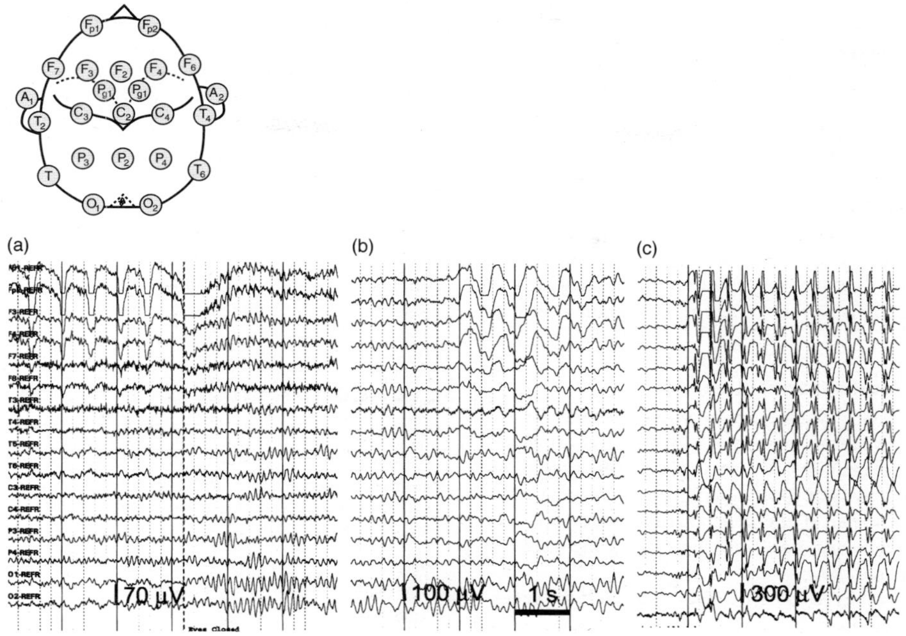

Fig. 1 Examples of EEG curves recorded using a common reference recording montage. The top panel shows the electrode placement using the 10–20 international system (with permission from Niedermeyer and Lopes da Silva). (a) EEG from a 20-year-old normal man (aviation candidate). Eye blinking was carried out to the left of the stippled line. At the stippled line he closed his eyes and the 10-Hz background activity became prominent, mainly over the posterior regions. (b) A 72-year-old female with progressive gait abnormalities, dementia, and urine incontinence. The CT scan showed cerebral atrophy and hydrocephalus. The EEG showed high-amplitude delta waves over the frontal regions. The background activity was slowed to 7 Hz. (c) An 8-year-old boy with absences. The EEG showed generalized 3-Hz spike–wave paroxysms.

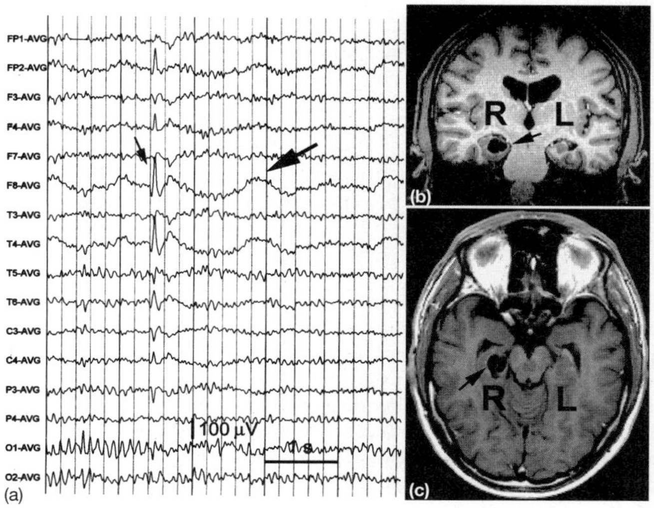

Fig. 2 A 31-year-old man with a history of complex partial seizures. (a) The EEG showed a spike focus over the right pre- and midtemporal regions (small arrow). In addition, there was a slow wave (1–2 Hz) focus over the same regions (large arrow), highly suspicious of a focal brain lesion. An average reference electrode montage was used. (b) Coronal *T*1-weighted MRI after contrast injection. (c) Transverse reconstructed section. Arrows indicate the site of a cystic-ring enhancing lesion in the right hippocampal region. (MRI by courtesy of the Danish Research Centre for Magnetic Resonance, Hvidovre Hospital, Copenhagen University Hospital.)

The normal EEG

The frequency content in the normal subject is highly dependent on age, the level of awareness, and medication. In the normal awake adult with closed eyes, the EEG is dominated by α-activity. The α-activity is most pronounced over posterior parts of the head (Fig. 1(a)), and is subject to modulations by changes in vigilance; for example, it disappears when the subject opens the eyes.

In the newborn, the EEG is characterized by low-frequency activity and variable amplitudes. In premature children, the EEG may be dominated by burst-suppression activity which does not occur in the normal, full-term baby. During maturation, the background frequencies move into the α-range by the early teens. Even in normal young adults, intermittent posterior slowing may be seen over the occipital regions, which becomes enhanced and spreads to other regions during hyperventilation. This slow activity during hyperventilation is augmented by low glucose levels in the blood, so that glucose should be given by mouth to subjects with excessive amounts of slow activity during hyperventilation.

During drowsiness the α-activity is diminished and disappears, first intermittently and subsequently completely, to be replaced by θ-activity (stage-1 sleep). During stage-2 sleep (light sleep), sleep spindles (bursts of 12–14 Hz activity), sharp waves over the vertex, and K-complexes (high-amplitude, slow-wave activity) are recorded in addition to θ-activity. At deeper levels of sleep (stages 3 and 4), increasing amounts of high-amplitude δ-activity are recorded (often designated 'delta sleep'). The EEG may be badly misinterpreted if drowsiness is not recognized during the recording session, therefore the technician must monitor the level of awareness at all times.

The abnormal EEG

The abnormal EEG may be characterized by changes in the background activity, the presence of low-frequency waveforms, epileptiform activity, or by periodic phenomena. The EEG is evaluated for the presence of abnormal frequencies or wave forms, either intermittently or constantly, whether these are localized diffusely or focally, and whether they occur in a synchronous or an asynchronous distribution. Preservation, distortion, or loss of normal background patterns are evaluated.

Abnormal frequencies

Slowing of the normal background activity occurs diffusely in patients with encephalopathy (for example, ischaemic or metabolic brain disease) or degenerative brain disease (for instance, Alzheimer's disease). Focal slowing (see Fig. 2) and attenuation of background activity is highly suggestive of focal brain disease (for example, stroke, tumour, or subdural haematoma).

Generalized, diffuse, and focal abnormalities

Generalized abnormalities occur synchronously throughout the brain, though the amplitudes and wave forms may vary at different recording sites (see Fig. 1(c)). Diffuse abnormalities are also present over large brain areas, but the low-frequency activity or spikes/sharp waves may occur independently. It should be considered if the generalized changes occur in recordings with a single reference electrode, since this may erroneously give rise to the impression of generalization.

These abnormalities are considered to have a central origin if the generalization occurs from the onset, but they may also be due to a focal cortical lesion if generalization occurs as a secondary phenomenon. So-called intermittent rhythmic δ-activity (Fig. 1(b)) may occur over widespread areas of the brain due to raised intracranial pressure and have little localizing value. Diffuse low-frequency abnormalities, often associated with triphasic waves, indicate widespread cortical abnormalities in metabolic encephalopathies.

Spikes, sharp waves, and periodic complexes

The central role of EEG in the diagnosis and follow-up of patients with epilepsy justifies the attention paid to the identification and localization of epileptic discharges. The features characteristic of epileptiform events consist of waves of various forms, usually spikes (potential duration, 70 ms or less) or sharp waves (potential duration, 70 to 200 ms) in a rhythmic pattern, that are of high voltage compared to the background activity and reflect hypersynchronization of neuronal discharges (Fig. 1(c)). Spikes may be followed by a negative wave, the so-called 'spike–wave complex'. Since it is unusual for an epileptic seizure to coincide with the EEG, the diagnosis therefore relies on the presence of epileptiform discharges during interictal recordings: the examination at the first EEG may be negative in up to 50 per cent of patients. Repeat studies or prolonged recordings (possibly under video control) are frequently indicated, and proper activation procedures, such as hyperventilation, photic stimulation, and possibly sleep deprivation or the use of sedatives to ensure sleep during the study, may be needed. The diagnostic yield of repeated EEG studies has accordingly been found to show abnormalities in more than 90 per cent of patients with a clinically established diagnosis of epilepsy.

Paroxysmal discharges may be focal or generalized in distribution according to the underlying aetiology. Recently developed focal epileptic symptoms (Fig. 2) may be evidence of a brain tumour and should be thoroughly investigated with appropriate imaging studies. Epileptic activity may develop abruptly in patients with primary generalized seizures (Fig. 1(c)). It is, however, important to evaluate this development closely to distinguish primary from secondary seizures that develop focally and then spread to adjacent cerebral regions, and possibly with generalization to the whole brain. Detection of focal epileptic activity may require specialized electrode montages. For example, an epileptic focus in the temporal lobe may require recording through electrodes placed over the zygomatic arch or through a needle sphenoidal electrode placed at the foramen ovale. Such focal epileptic activity may, moreover, not become apparent until the patient becomes drowsy or goes to sleep.

The electrophysiological activity is usually not unambiguous for subgroups of epileptic seizures, though the particular combination of clinical characteristics, the EEG changes during seizures, and the interictal activity may be distinctive for epileptic syndromes, hence the term 'electroclinical diagnosis' has been coined. Generalized 3-s spike–wave complexes are considered pathognomonic for generalized absence seizures (petit mal, Fig. 1(c)), and hypsarrhythymia (high-voltage, irregular slow waves interspersed with spikes) occurs almost exclusively in infantile spasms. Periodic, lateralized epileptiform discharges (**PLED**) give a trace of continuous focal spike activity with a frequency of 0.5 to 3 s, seen in connection with acute severe brain disease. Periodic generalized complexes of sharp waves are characteristically seen in patients with Creutzfeldt–Jakob disease, herpes simplex encephalitis, and subacute sclerosing panencephalitis, and may be present in patients with severe brain anoxia.

Evoked potentials

Evoked potentials are specific CNS potentials obtained by stimulation of particular sensory receptors or fibre tracts and are carried out to examine the integrity of afferent and efferent pathways. The sensory pathways routinely examined include the visual system (visual-evoked potentials, **VEPs**), fibre tracts in the brainstem (brainstem auditory-evoked potentials, **BAEPs**), and somatosensory pathways in the dorsal columns (somatosensory-evoked potentials, **SSEPs**). Motor-evoked potentials (**MEPs**) are elicited by magnetic stimulation of the motor cortex and used to study the corticospinal tracts. Methodological questions and pathophysiological findings are discussed below; however, a detailed description of the methods used are considered beyond the scope of this chapter and the reader is referred to the Further reading list.

Near-field and far-field responses

The responses discussed in this chapter are the modality-specific components of the evoked potentials (**EPs**) that reflect the propagation of action potentials in fibre tracts and cortical areas. The so-called 'event-related' potentials, although time-locked to a stimulus, are not modality specific but reflect the activity in neuronal networks involved in cognitive processing (for example, P300), they will not be described further.

The electrical responses recorded close to the source are the so-called 'near-field potentials', which may arise from axons or be of postsynaptic origin. These include action potentials recorded from peripheral nerves, the spinal cord, or cortical areas. However, the activity recorded from scalp electrodes with a non-cephalic reference also reflect activity in deeply located structures, known as 'far-field potentials'. The origin of a number of these EP components is incompletely known, and the latencies and amplitudes of only some of these are of clinical relevance in routine practice.

Indications

The main purpose of evoked-potential studies is to ascertain the presence of pathological processes localized to myelinated fibre tracts or to the synaptic connections through which messages are relayed. The conduction velocity of the fibres is gauged by the latencies of the responses, and these are particularly susceptible to abnormalities in the myelin sheath. Hence, evoked potentials are of particular use in demyelinating disorders, for example multiple sclerosis. However, conduction abnormalities are not specific for a particular disease, and delayed conduction may be seen in a variety of disorders including hereditary diseases, compression of nervous tissue (such as spondylotic myelopathy), and infectious diseases (such as in patients with the acquired immunodeficiency syndrome, **AIDS**). Thus, the constellation of EP abnormalities, the clinical setting, and other paraclinical or laboratory findings are all important factors in a diagnosis.

The amplitudes of responses are influenced by the number of conducting fibres; in disorders characterized by fibre loss without involvement of the myelin sheath, abnormalities may be confined to a reduction in amplitude. However, because of the amplification that occurs at synaptic relays, the amplitude of the evoked potential is a poor indicator of the degree of fibre loss. Thus, a cortical response may still be recordable at SSEP testing in patients with a severe neuropathy and an absent peripheral nerve response. Finally, conduction may be delayed in disorders characterized by axonal loss, possibly related to delays at synaptic transmission. Thus, in patients with amyotrophic lateral sclerosis (**ALS**), the MEP recording often shows a delayed central conduction time even though the disorder is characterized by fibre loss rather than demyelination.

SSEP and MEP investigations have proved to be valuable intraoperative monitoring tools during surgery on the vertebral column for scoliosis and on the spinal cord for tumours or vascular malformations. Both a reduction in amplitudes and a prolongation of latencies have proved reliable indicators of impending damage to the spinal cord, and hence the need to take measures to avoid permanent damage. Additionally, the use of electromyographic recordings from relevant muscles is helpful during scoliosis operations in warning the surgeon that a root may be in danger of damage from screws or other hardware.

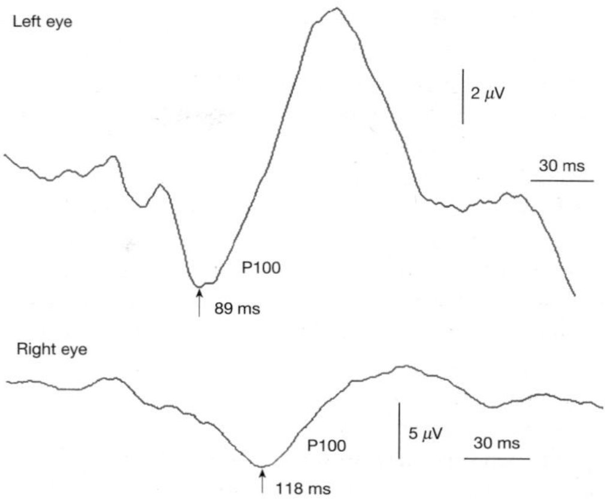

Fig. 3 Pattern-reversal, visual-evoked potentials (checkerboard stimulation) from a 64-year-old man showed a normal pattern-VEP with a P100 latency of 89 ms from the left eye and an abnormal pattern-VEP from the right eye with a latency of 118 ms (27 per cent prolonged, upper normal limit 103 ms). The findings indicated the presence of a right-sided optic nerve lesion.

Visual-evoked potentials

Method

Visual-evoked potentials (VEPs) are evoked by either a diffuse stroboscopic flash (flash-VEP) that stimulates the whole retina or by pattern-reversal stimulation (pattern-VEP), where a black-and-white checkerboard reverses position at a frequency of 2/s. The patient is seated at a distance of 1 m and gazes at the centre of the checkerboard projected either on a screen or a TV monitor. The pattern-VEP is sensitive to the co-operation of the patient, whereas the flash-VEP can be used to ascertain whether functional connections exist between the retina and the occipital lobes. The size of each square is either 9 mm or 18 mm, depending on the visual acuity. The pattern-VEP is generated mainly by the central 10° of vision. The responses are recorded over the occipital lobes. At least 100, and preferably 200, sweeps are averaged to yield responses of adequate resolution.

Each eye is stimulated in turn, and in routine studies the whole visual field is stimulated. In some conditions, however, it is more revealing to stimulate part of the visual field: in which case, the half-field is usually stimulated. Half-field stimulation is particularly useful in conditions where lesions are localized in the visual projections behind the chiasm, but its interpretation requires considerable expertise.

Measurements

The pattern-VEP comprises three main components, of which the positive phase at a latency of about 100 m is the most constant (Fig. 3). In clinical practice, the latency of this phase and the amplitude of the response are measured. In flash-VEP, the latencies of the N70, P90, and N120 phases are measured.

Clinical correlations

Flash-VEP is reduced in patients with retinal disease. It is a useful test in patients with retinosa pigmentosa, and in those who cannot co-operate, in particular in children.

Monocular, full-field, pattern-VEP with prolonged latency to the P100 component in one eye indicates that the lesion is localized anterior to the optic chiasm (Fig. 3). Although this is most frequently due to demyelination of the optic nerve, it may be due to retinal degeneration, optic nerve compression, or glaucoma. In some patients with mild optic neuritis, the latencies only show an abnormal interocular difference. The interpretation is more uncertain if bilateral prolonged latencies are found, since this may be due to lesions anywhere along the visual pathways. Interocular differences in patients with bilateral retrochiasmal lesions (for example, spinocerebellar syndromes) are within the normal range. Marked latency differences in patients with bilateral abnormalities suggest bilateral optic nerve lesions. Retrochiasmal lesions may be further examined by partial-field (half-field) studies of the individual eye.

Electroretinography

The electroretinogram (**ERG**) is the electrical response evoked in the retina by a flash and is due to depolarization of the interstitial Müller cells and pigmented epithelium. The ERG is recorded by a contact-lens electrode or with an infraorbital surface electrode. The state of light and dark adaptation can be used to separate the function of the rods and cones. The ERG is usually carried out when the VEP pattern is missing and it is uncertain whether this may be due to a retinal problem. In such cases, the ERG may be evoked by a routine flash. Dark-adapted ERG is carried out in the differential diagnosis of retinal degenerations and is a specialist task usually carried out in collaboration with a neuro-ophthalmologist.

Brainstem auditory-evoked potentials (BAEPs)

Method

The auditory brainstem response is elicited by passing short-lasting clicks, at an intensity of 75 to 100 dB, through earphones to each ear separately. The responses of interest include the time-locked far-field responses with latencies of less than 10 ms. The brainstem-derived response consists of several phases (usually numbered as positive waves PI–VI), which indicate conduction along peripheral pathways in the cochlear nerve and different relay stations of the lateral lemniscus pathway within the brainstem.

Measurements

The waves of interest are the positive peaks PI to PVI; PI, PIII, and PV are usually recorded, whereas the remaining waves may be missing even in normal subjects. PI is generated in the cochlear nerve, PII in the cochlear nucleus, PIII in the pons, and PV at the midbrain level. For clinical purposes, the latency of PI is measured to ascertain peripheral conduction and that of PI to PIII, PI to PV, and PIII to PV to ascertain the central conduction time within the brainstem.

Clinical correlations

BAEP recording is helpful in investigating the integrity of the brainstem; it is used to confirm brain-death in some laboratories. Its main usefulness lies in the localization of lesions at the cochlear nerve, at the entry into the brainstem (cochlear nucleus), and at different sites within the brainstem. Central abnormalities are found in 50 per cent of patients with multiple sclerosis.

Somatosensory-evoked potentials (SSEPs)

Method

These responses are evoked by repetitive stimulation (2–5/s) of the median nerves at the wrists and the tibial nerves behind the medial malleolus (Fig. 4), using a stimulus duration of 0.2 ms at a strength just sufficient to elicit a slight motor response. Differentiation between peripheral and central disease is obtained after stimulation of the median nerve by recording peripheral nerve responses through surface or subcutaneous needle electrodes at the supraclavicular fossa (Erb's point, designated the N9 response), from the spinal cord at C6 (designated the N13), and over the contralateral hemisphere (the potential is designated N20). On stimulation of the tibial nerves, recordings are carried out from the peripheral nerve at the popliteal fossa (or at the gluteal fold), at Th12 (designated the N23), and over the brain (onset response and P40 response). Up to 1000 responses are averaged depending on the level of noise and the size of the response. The average is carried out in two bins to ensure reproducibility.

Measurements

The latencies to the onsets of the peripheral nerve responses are measured to calculate the peripheral conduction velocities (Fig. 4), to the negative peak of the spinal response, and to the first negative response at the cortex after the median nerve and to the onset and the P40 responses after tibial nerve stimulation.

The central conduction time is calculated as the differences in latencies between the spinal responses at C6 and the peak of the N20 response after median nerve stimulation, and between the spinal responses at Th12 and the onset latency (or the P40 latency) after tibial nerve stimulation. The values are compared to height-matched controls.

Clinical correlations

SSEPs from median and tibial nerves are helpful when very proximal nerve disorders or central nervous system disorders are suspected. A prolonged latency of the spinal responses evoked from the tibial nerves indicates the presence of proximal lumbosacral plexus or root lesions, and may be differentiated from a peripheral neuropathy by a normal peripheral nerve response at the popliteal fossa or the gluteal fold. Similar information is obtained regarding the brachial plexus and cervical roots at C6 from median nerve stimulation. SSEP studies may be extended by dermatomal stimulation in the legs and the arms to diagnose monoradicular lesions. SSEPs are, however, particularly useful for identifying spinal cord disease; the central conduction time obtained separately from the upper and lower limbs may be used to determine the probable localization of myelopathic lesions (Fig. 4(b)). The central conduction time often shows marked prolongation in patients with multiple sclerosis.

Motor-evoked potentials (MEPs)

Motor-evoked potentials are obtained by activating focal motor cortical areas by a short-lasting, strong magnetic pulse of up to 2 tesla, which induces a current within the excitable tissue of the cortex. In some laboratories, electrical stimulation rather than magnetic stimulation is employed. However, electrical stimulation is painful; moreover, the electrical stimulus activates fibres deeper within the cerebrum than does the magnetic stimulus. The two methods therefore yield results that cannot be directly compared. The descending waves from the cortex consist of D-waves from cortical neurones followed by I-waves that arise transynaptically. In addition, stimulation is performed at cervical and lumbar spinal levels. At magnetic stimulation, excitation occurs at the proximal spinal nerves rather than at the spinal cord.

The motor responses are recorded from muscles of the upper and lower limbs (including proximal and distal muscles) using surface electrodes to evaluate the compound muscle action potential (**CMAP**). Facilitation of cortical neurones by slight voluntary contraction is necessary for obtaining 'maximal' motor responses.

Measurements

The amplitudes and latencies of the CMAPs are measured at both cortical and spinal stimulation (Fig. 5). The central conduction time is obtained by calculating the differences of these latencies; however, since excitation at spinal stimulation occurs at the proximal peripheral nerve, the central conduction time includes conduction along the roots. The central conduction time has therefore also been calculated using the F-wave latency to obtain a measure of the peripheral conduction time. In central lesions, the central conduction time is prolonged compared to height- and age-matched controls (Fig. 5(b)). In addition, the CMAP amplitudes of the cortical response may be reduced, indicating central axonal loss, conduction failure, or increased temporal dispersion along corticospinal fibres. The shape of the CMAP recording in patients with multiple sclerosis is often polyphasic, indicating dispersion along demyelinated central pathways.

Clinical correlations

The central motor conduction time is prolonged in demyelinating disorders and the investigation is of particular value in patients suspected of having multiple sclerosis (Figs 5(a) and (b)). However, slowing of central conduction is a non-specific abnormality that may also be seen in patients with other causes of CNS motor disorders. In amyotrophic lateral sclerosis

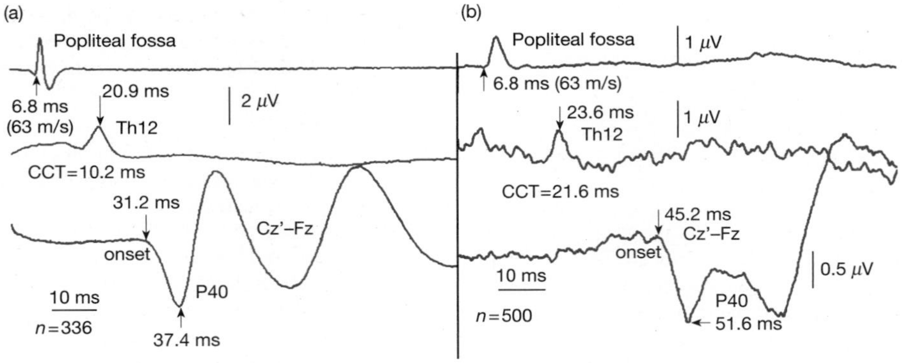

Fig. 4 Somatosensory-evoked potentials from (a) the right leg of a 25-year-old normal woman (a) and (b) the left leg of a 55-year-old man with signs of myelopathy. The tibial nerve was stimulated at the medial malleolus and responses recorded from the peripheral nerve at the popliteal fossa, from the spine (Th12), and the scalp. In both subjects, the peripheral conduction velocities and spinal latencies were normal. The latencies of the cortical responses to both the 'onset' and the P40 were normal in (a) and 31 per cent and 25 per cent prolonged, respectively, in (b). The central conduction time (CCT) was calculated as the difference between the spinal latency and the onset latency. The central conduction time was normal in (a), whereas it was 98 per cent prolonged in (b), consistent with myelopathy.

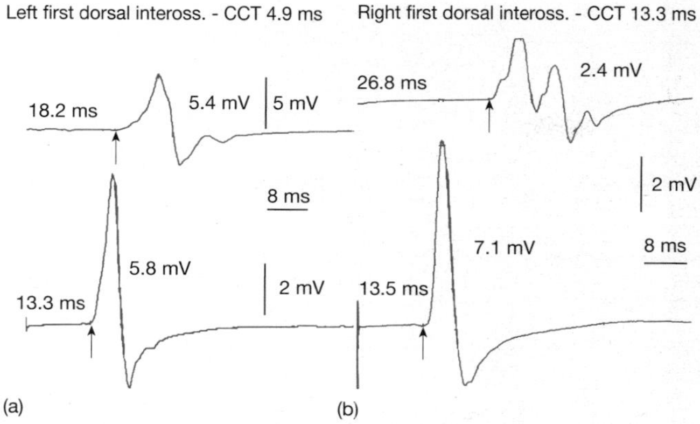

Fig. 5 Motor-evoked potentials obtained by magnetic stimulation from (a) the left and (b) the right first dorsal interosseous muscles in a 60-year-old woman suspected of having multiple sclerosis (the pattern-VEP and the SSEP were also abnormal). Lower traces: compound muscle action potentials (CMAPs) evoked by stimulation of the cervical spine. Upper traces: CMAPs evoked by cortical stimulation. The latencies of the responses (shown above the traces) at spinal stimulation were normal on both sides, whereas cortical latency was normal in (a) and 36 per cent prolonged in (b). The central motor conduction time (CCT, indicated above traces) was calculated as the difference between the cortical and peripheral latencies. The central conduction time in the left arm was normal in (a), whereas it was 86 per cent prolonged in (b), consistent with a central lesion.

for example, the central conduction time is often abnormal in an irregular pattern, though the prolongation is usually only slight. The MEP should therefore be supplemented with other evoked potentials (pattern-VEP and SSEP), MRI, and spinal fluid examinations.

In some patients with peripheral nerve disorders, in particular acute or chronic inflammatory demyelinating neuropathy, the MEP examination may show abnormalities indicating central as well as peripheral nervous system involvement. This may be an erroneous finding due to slowed conduction along spinal roots. Due to the stimulation of peripheral nerves distal to the intervertebral foramen, the conduction along the spinal roots is included in the central conduction time, and slowing at this segment may therefore erroneously be localized to the CNS.

Studies of the peripheral neuromuscular system

Indications

Electromyography (**EMG**) is used to establish whether weakness is due to a primary disease of muscle fibres (myopathy) or to a loss of α-motor fibres (neurogenic disorders). Nerve conduction studies are carried out to ascertain the loss of motor or sensory axons or the disturbed function of myelinated fibres. Both types of studies are usually needed for a differential diagnosis, and since the findings are rarely specific for particular disorders, the interpretation relies on inferences from several criteria of abnormality. The degree to which the findings should be supplemented and confirmed by light or electron microscopy of nerve- or muscle-biopsy specimens and other laboratory studies depends on the clinical setting. EMG and nerve conduction studies should be viewed as an extension of the clinical examination and form part of a neuromuscular consultation. EMG and nerve conduction studies assist in answering specific differential diagnostic questions relating to focal or generalized disorders of the peripheral neuromuscular system. Even though subclinical involvement has important implications in the diagnostic interpretation in several conditions (for example, neurogenic changes in non-weak muscles where amyotrophic lateral sclerosis is a possibility), the use of these studies to 'rule out' neuromuscular involvement in diffuse or focal pain problems should be discouraged.

Disturbances of neuromuscular transmission require specialized studies, including the recording of compound muscle responses evoked by repetitive stimulation of motor nerve fibres. In single-fibre EMG, the action potentials from individual muscle fibres are recorded during voluntary activity or during repetitive stimulation to measure the stability of neuromuscular transmission.

Electromyography

Method

EMG is carried out using needle electrodes. In routine studies, most laboratories either use concentric needle electrodes and a core recording lead with a surface area of 0.07 mm^2 referenced to the cannula, or insulated monopolar needles with a surface recording area of 0.17 mm^2 referenced to a surface electrode. The results obtained with these electrodes differ in regard to the amplitude of the motor-unit potential (**MUP**), whereas its duration only differs slightly. The baseline is somewhat more unstable when recorded with a monopolar electrode than a concentric needle. The signals should be recorded via a high-impedance amplifier with a frequency range of between 2 and 10 kHz.

Measurements

Recordings are carried out at rest, during weak voluntary activity, and during maximal voluntary activity (Table 1).

During rest, both the presence and type of spontaneous activity are characterized. During weak voluntary effort, individual MUPs are recorded without disturbance by other MUPs. The duration and amplitude of the MUP are also measured. The duration of the MUP reflects the activity of muscle fibres of the motor unit at a distance from the recording electrode. In contrast, the very few muscle fibres placed at the tip of the concentric electrode determines the amplitude of the MUP. The mean amplitudes and durations of at least 20 different MUPs recorded from 10 different sites at three different insertions are obtained. The shapes of individual MUPs are evaluated and designated as simple (less than five phases) or polyphasic (five or more phases). The findings are compared to age-matched control values from the investigated muscle, and the percentage deviation is calculated to ascertain whether the findings are normal or consistent with myopathy of chronic partial denervation (Tables 1 and 2).

During a maximal voluntary contraction, all motor units in the muscle are activated. The MUPs from individual motor units cannot therefore be distinguished, but they form an interference pattern which, according to the degree of overlap, is measured semiquantitatively as a 'full', 'reduced', or 'discrete' recruitment pattern. Although a full recruitment pattern occurs in normal muscle, it requires the patient's full co-operation. It should therefore be noted whether the activity is recorded during maximal or submaximal effort. In addition to the degree of overlap, the envelope amplitude of the main activity is measured to distinguish myopathy and neurogenic involvement.

Table 1 EMG limits in normal muscle

	Normal limit
Spontaneous activity recorded at rest	
Number of sites outside endplate region with fibrillation potentials or positive sharp waves	2 sites
Voluntary activity	
1. Weak effort	
Duration of the motor-unit potential (%)	± 20[a]
Amplitude of motor-unit potential (%)	< −50, > +100[a]
Incidence of polyphasic potentials (%)	12[b]
2. Full effort	
Pattern	Full recruitment
Amplitude of envelope curves (mV)	>2 mV, <4 mV

[a]Mean of 20–25 or more MUPs compared to age-matched controls.

[b]In the deltoid and facial muscles, 25%; in the anterior tibial and lateral vastus muscles, 20%.

Table 2 EMG criteria of neuromuscular disease

	Specific criteria	Non-specific criteria
Myopathy		
MUP during weak effort	Reduction in duration (>20% shortened)	Increased incidence of polyphasic potentials (>12%). Reduced amplitude
Recruitment pattern	Full recruitment in a weak and wasted muscle. Reduced amplitude of full recruitment pattern	Reduced recruitment pattern
Activity at rest		Fibrillation activity and positive sharp waves
Peripheral nerve and root disease		
MUP during weak effort	Increase in duration (>20% prolonged). Increase in amplitude	Increased incidence of polyphasic potentials (>12%)
Recruitment pattern	Discrete activity. Increased amplitude	Reduced recruitment pattern
Activity at rest		Fibrillation activity and positive sharp waves (4–10 sites)
Anterior horn cell disease		
MUP during weak effort	Increase in amplitude (>500% increased)	Increase in amplitude of individual MUPs (200%)
Recruitment pattern	Increased amplitude (>8 mV)	
Activity at rest	Fasciculations (malignant, intervals of >3 s)	Fasciculations (benign, intervals <1 s)

(With permission from *Journal of Neurology*.)

Clinical correlations

Recordings at rest

The sarcolemma of the denervated muscle fibre undergoes changes, including a gradual spread of acetylcholine receptors, and the resting membrane potential is reduced. Spontaneous discharges of denervated fibres occur in a cyclical pattern, and they appear as fibrillation potentials or positive sharp waves (Fig. 6). Fibrillation potentials have a triphasic shape and a duration of 5 ms at most, and the discharge pattern may be regular or irregular (Figs 6(a) and (b)). Positive sharp waves are considered as arising from damage to the cell membrane and indicate a propagation block at the needle recording electrode (Fig. 6(b)). No particular pathological significance is assigned to whether the denervation activity consists of fibrillation potentials or positive sharp waves.

Continuous, non-propagated, miniature endplate potentials (**m.e.p.p.**)—and, in addition, irregular, spontaneous, endplate potentials (**e.p.p.**) with negative onset—are recorded from the resting normal muscle within the endplate region. Such single-fibre potentials cannot be distinguished from fibrillation potentials when recorded outside the endplate region. Therefore, spontaneous single fibre activity in normal muscle may be recorded at up to two out of ten recording sites (Table 1).

Denervation activity arises with a delay after the nerve lesion, and the lag is dependent on the length of the distal nerve stump: that is, it occurs within 5 to 10 days at very distal lesions. Similarly, after a nerve root lesion, denervation arises after few days in paraspinal muscles and after 2 to 3 weeks in distal extremity muscles. The presence of denervation activity indicates that the denervation is ongoing, but it may continue for years after occurrence of the lesion if reinnervation does not take place. However, denervation activity also occurs in muscular dystrophy, inflammatory myopathy (polymyositis, dermatomyositis, inclusion body myositis), and some metabolic myopathies (for example, acid maltase deficiency), whereas it is rare or absent in mitochondrial myopathy. In myopathy, denervation is due to segmental muscle-fibre necrosis, thus leaving a segment of the muscle fibre denervated. Denervation activity is a non-specific sign of neuromuscular disease (Table 1).

Whereas denervation activity arises from single muscle fibres, other types of spontaneous activity are due to discharges in groups of muscle fibres, possibly the whole motor unit. These include fasciculations (defined as irregular discharges with short or long intervals of less or more than 3 s (Fig. 7), myotonic discharges (defined as burst of activity with gradually waxing and waning frequencies, often elicited by percussion, needle movement or voluntary activity, and with a decreasing incidence after repeated contractions), complex repetitive discharges (defined as bursts of activity of variable duration with sudden occurrence and drop-out of discharge components that may arise from single fibres), and myokymia (defined as fasciculations, doublets, or triplets occurring with variable and sometimes high frequencies; neuromyotonia belongs in this category of activity).

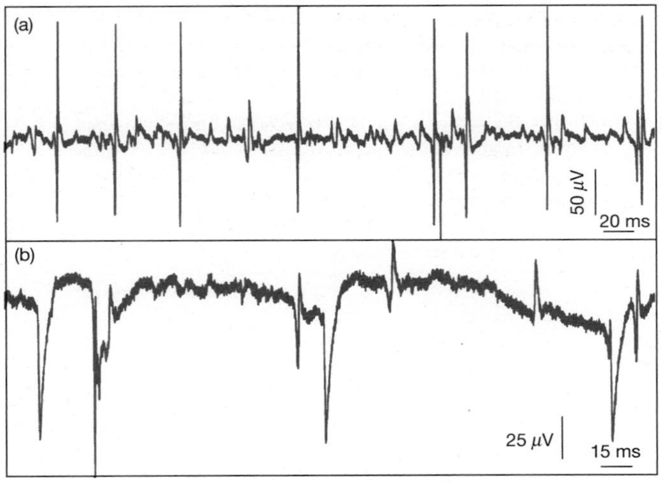

Fig. 6 Fibrillation potentials (a) and (b) and positive sharp waves (b) recorded from a muscle with profuse denervation activity. Fibrillation potentials arise from single muscle fibres and have a triphasic shape, duration of ≤ 5 ms, and variable amplitudes depending on the distance to the recording electrode. Positive sharp waves are thought to arise from damaged muscle fibres with conduction block at the recording electrode.

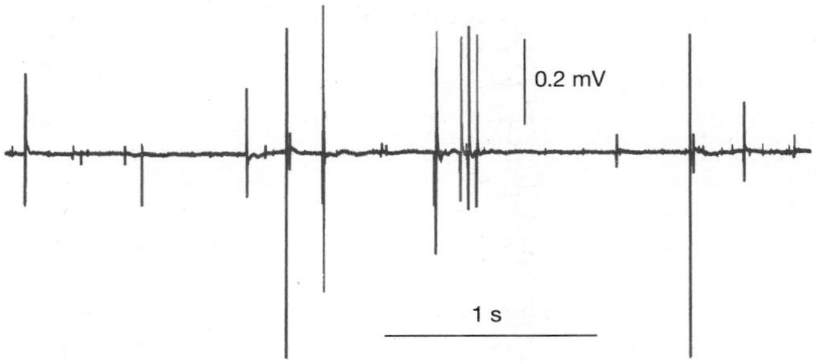

Fig. 7 Fasciculations recorded from the extensor digitorum communis muscle of a patient with multifocal motor neuropathy. The discharges arise from groups of muscle fibres or whole motor units and occur with irregular intervals.

Recording at weak effort

The smallest functional unit in the muscle is the motor unit, which differs quantitatively by several orders of magnitude in different muscles; in lower extremity muscles the motor units have 1000 to 2000 muscle fibres, whereas they have between 5 and 10 in extraocular muscles. The motor units also differ according to the biochemical characteristics of the muscle fibres in fast-contracting motor units (type II fibres) and in slowly contracting motor units (type I fibres). The diagnostic power of EMG mainly depends on the assessment of the structural changes of the motor units as evidenced by evaluation of the MUP. Reliance on the EMG has varied considerably over the years: quantitative measurements of MUPs may be used to gauge the overall size of the motor units and therefore as a diagnostic indicator of whether weakness is due to neurogenic abnormalities or to myopathy; as opposed to qualitative evaluation, which can only give an impression of the MUP changes. The use of quantitative measurements is now more widely used and accepted as the introduction of computerized measurement devices has enabled adequate numbers of MUPs to be sampled. This may increase the use of the MUP to differentiate between neurogenic and myogenic abnormalities.

MUP parameters measured include the duration, amplitude, and shape of the MUPs (Fig. 8). The motor units in myopathic muscle are reduced in size due to the functional loss or degeneration of individual muscle fibres, and this is reflected in reduced durations and amplitudes of the MUPs (Figs 9 and 10). In contrast, the motor units in neurogenic lesions are enlarged due to collateral reinnervation of muscle fibres, and the mean duration of the MUPs is prolonged and the amplitude is increased (Figs 9 and 10). These changes, which indicate the presence of chronic partial denervation, tend to be more pronounced in very chronic conditions. However, in motor neurone disease, MUPs may be gigantic even in muscles without clinical weakness. In specialized multielectrode studies, the motor-unit territory in myopathy is reduced, whereas the territory in neuropathy and amyotrophic lateral sclerosis is increased.

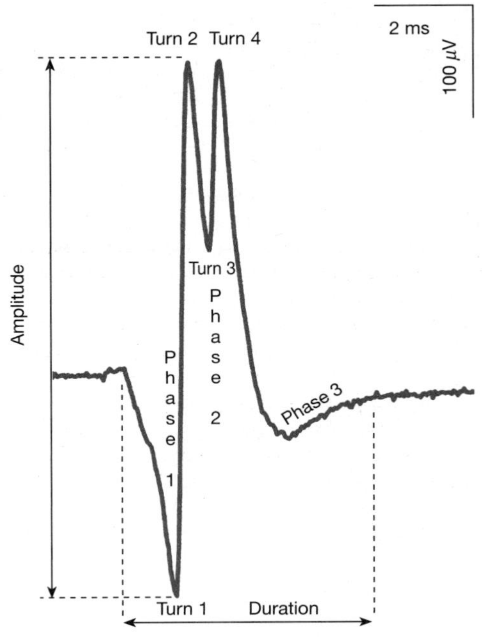

Fig. 8 Motor-unit potential (MUP) to illustrate measurements. The duration is measured from the first deflection from the baseline to the return to baseline. The amplitude (negative sign upwards) is measured peak-to-peak. The MUP has three phases and four turns (potential reversals of >100 µV). This potential is simple in shape (less than five phases). (From Simonetti *et al.*, with permission by Lippincott, Williams & Wilkins.)

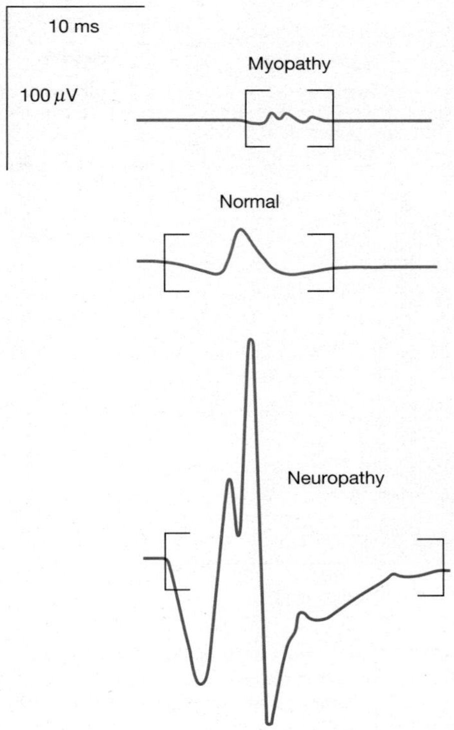

Fig. 9 Examples of MUPs from patient with myopathy (top), normal subject (middle), and neuropathy (bottom).

Whereas the changes in duration and amplitude are specific for either a myopathy or a neurogenic lesion, an increased incidence of polyphasic MUPs occurs both in myopathy and in neurogenic lesions, and is therefore a non-specific sign of neuromuscular involvement (Table 2). It is claimed that long-duration polyphasic MUPs are characteristic of neurogenic lesions, whereas short polyphasic MUPs are seen in myopathy. However, polyphasic MUPs in myopathy have two mechanisms: loss of muscle fibres in the motor unit, which results in short-duration MUPs; and degeneration of muscle fibres followed by regeneration and subsequent reinnervation, resulting in long-duration MUPs. With disease progression, muscle fibre regeneration cannot keep pace with degeneration, and long-duration MUPs become less frequent with advanced disease. The long-duration MUPs in myopathy may obscure the interpretation of the EMG, and it is therefore necessary to calculate the mean duration of simple MUPs (less than five phases) to avoid error.

The EMG examination should include a number of muscles according to the likely clinical diagnosis, since involvement of different muscles may vary in different disorders. In myopathy, proximal muscles in the upper and lower extremities should be examined. Some muscles show clear abnormalities characteristic of the disorder, whereas others show only non-specific changes (for example, fibrillation potentials and increased incidence of polyphasic potentials), and several criteria should therefore be collected. In neurogenic lesions on the other hand, distal muscles are most severely affected and may show abnormalities at an earlier stage than proximal muscles. In this connection it should be considered that some distal muscles may be affected due to focal non-related causes. The extensor digitorum brevis muscle, for example, should be avoided in elderly people due to frequent neurogenic changes caused by compression of the deep peroneal nerve by footwear. In patients suspected of having amyotrophic lateral sclerosis, both clinically weak and non-affected muscles should be studied; as a rule, both show signs of chronic partial denervation often with such pronounced changes that this supports the diagnosis (Table 2). Since amyotrophic lateral sclerosis often has a focal distribution at presentation, it is

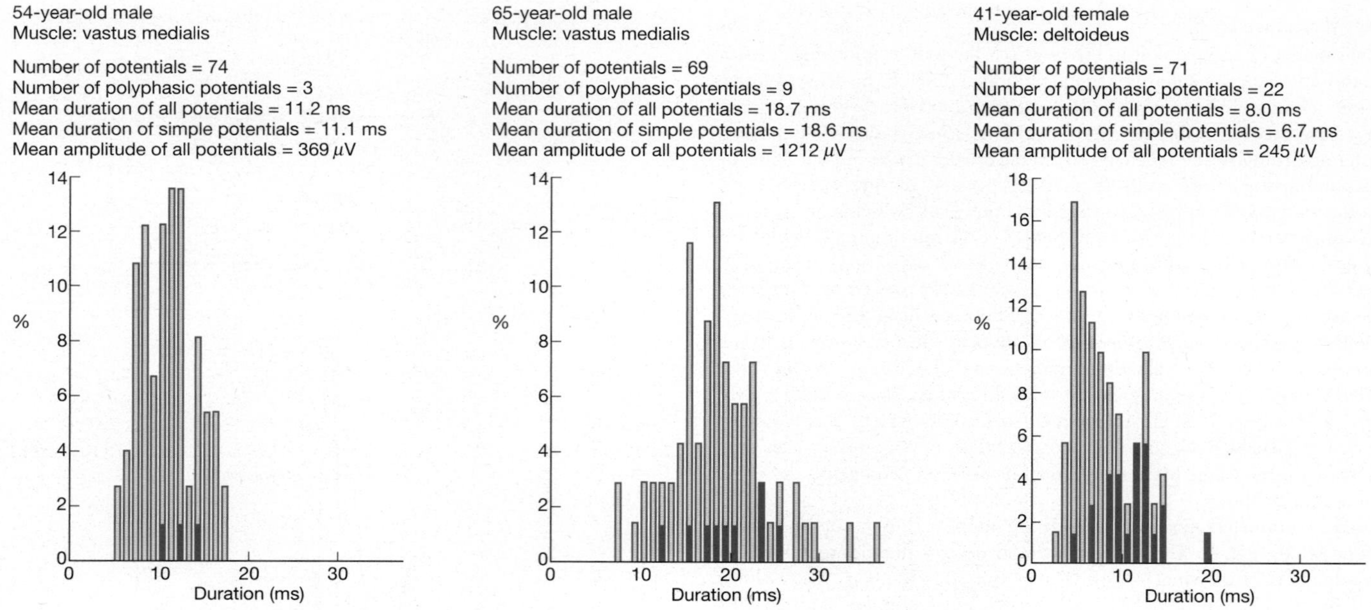

Fig. 10 Quantitative measurements of MUPs from a normal subject (left), a patient with neuropathy (middle), and one with myopathy (right). The total number of MUPs analysed, the number of polyphasic MUPs, the mean duration of all MUPs, the mean duration of simple MUPs, and the mean amplitude of all MUPs are indicated above the histograms. The histograms show the distribution of the durations of simple MUPs (open bars) and of polyphasic MUPs (filled bars). The amplitude and duration were markedly increased (duration, +51 per cent; amplitude, +427 per cent) in the patient with neuropathy. The duration was 29 per cent diminished and the amplitude was normal in the patient with myopathy. The incidence of polyphasic MUPs was slightly (13 per cent and 25 per cent) increased in the patients with neuropathy and myopathy, respectively. (Modified from Simonetti *et al.*, with permission by Lippincott, Williams & Wilkins.)

important to exclude spinal root compression and peripheral nerve lesions as causes of the neurogenic involvement; therefore, it is customary to study several muscles in different extremities to ensure that any changes are widespread.

Maximal voluntary contraction

The number of motor units is normal in myopathy, and therefore the loss of muscle fibres is associated with a full recruitment pattern with reduced amplitude (Table 2). In severely weak myopathic muscle, the loss of muscle fibres may eventually result in a reduced recruitment pattern (see above). Where there is neurogenic involvement, the loss of motor units results in a reduced recruitment pattern, often with increased amplitude due to collateral reinnervation. In advanced denervation, the number of motor units is so depleted that the recruitment pattern becomes discrete (Fig. 11(c)). This is considered a specific sign of neurogenic involvement, whereas a reduced pattern may occur in either myopathy or neurogenic disease. With motor neurone involvement, the reduced or discrete pattern has a markedly increased amplitude, often of more than 8 mV, which is considered typical of motor neurone disease (Table 2; Fig. 11(c)).

Specialized recordings

As indicated in Method section, the amplitudes of the MUPs, in particular when recorded with a concentric needle, are markedly variable and dependent on the distance between the recording area and the closest two or three muscle fibres of the motor unit. An increased or decreased amplitude is therefore a relatively insensitive indicator of motor-unit abnormalities. To record more evenly from the whole motor unit and hence obtain a more reliable measure of the MUP amplitude, the macroelectrode (which consists of 15 mm of the non-insulated cannula of the needle electrode to increase the recording surface area), has been introduced. This has been useful in serial studies designed to follow the disintegration of the motor unit in patients with postpolio syndrome.

In contrast to the macroelectrode, the single-fibre electrode has a small recording area of 25 μm, which allows recording of the action potential from individual muscle fibres in the motor unit. The main use of the single-fibre electrode has been in the recognition of disorders of neuromuscular transmission. The timing of the discharges of two (or more) muscle fibres in the motor unit is followed during repetitive activity. Whereas the discharges are quite stable in normal muscle, they become unstable in myasthenia gravis or the Lambert–Eaton syndrome. The larger variance of the discharges is termed 'increased jitter'; in more severely affected neuromuscular transmission disturbances, some of the discharges may fall out altogether, so-called 'blocking'. Increased jitter is also encountered in myopathy. In neurogenic lesions, where the activity of several muscle fibres may be recorded simultaneously, groups of discharges may become unstable, indicating that conduction along immature terminal sprouts may have a diminished safety factor.

Quantitation of the MUP relies on the ability to distinguish the individual MUP from the activity in other motor units. This may introduce a bias regarding the type of motor unit that a diagnosis is based on. Thus small, fatigue-resistant motor units are recruited during weak effort, whereas large motor units are activated at higher levels of activity. Methods have therefore been developed that quantitate the electrical activity during higher levels of activity. These methods have been used to investigate patients with myopathy and neurogenic involvement, and have been found to supplement the findings obtained using quantitative evaluation of MUPs.

Nerve conduction studies

Motor and sensory nerve conduction studies of peripheral nerves are performed by recording the propagated responses evoked by supramaximal electrical nerve stimulation. The responses reflect the summation of action potentials from individual sensory nerve fibres (the compound sensory action potential, **CSAP**) or motor units (the compound motor action potential, **CMAP**), and their amplitudes represent a semiquantitative measure of the number of activated myelinated fibres. The CSAP amplitude is an

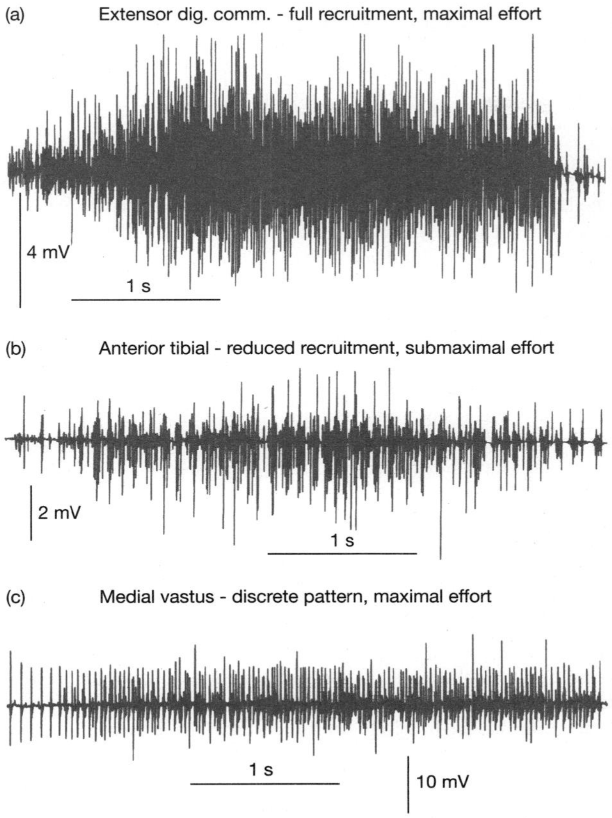

Fig. 11 Electrical activity recorded during voluntary effort. The recruitment pattern in (a) was full and had a normal amplitude of 3.5 to 4 mV, whereas it was reduced in (b) due to incomplete co-operation by the patient (submaximal effort) as shown by the uneven discharges that occurred in bursts. In (c) the recruitment pattern was discrete due to the loss of motor units, and the amplitude was markedly increased to between 8 and 10 mV due to collateral reinnervation (46-year-old man with motor neurone disease).

expression of activity in large fibres with diameters greater than 7 μm, whereas small fibres in the nerve contribute only slightly to the response. The CMAP amplitude is a reflection of the number of α-motor neurones. A reduction of the CSAP or the CMAP amplitudes is an indicator of fibre loss. However, the CMAP amplitude is also influenced by the size of the motor-unit response. During chronic axonal loss, collateral spouting causes an increase of the MUP, which partially or completely may compensate for the fibre loss. Since reinnervation does not have the same effect on sensory nerves, the CMAP is a less sensitive measure for determining the degree of fibre loss in chronic axonal lesions than the amplitude of the CSAP. Conduction studies are supplemented with EMG to ascertain whether motor fibres are affected by the pathological process.

Method

Investigations of motor and sensory fibres are carried out separately.

Motor conduction studies

The nerve is stimulated by an electrical pulse of 0.1- to 0.2-ms duration applied to the nerve at well-defined sites, with the cathode (depolarizing electrode) being placed over the nerve distal to the anode if a longitudinal electrode placement is used. It is essential that the stimulation pulse is supramaximal, defined as being 10 to 20 per cent above the stimulus strength that elicits a maximal CMAP. This stimulation strength requires that the output of the stimulator provides a stimulus at least four times higher than threshold when surface electrodes are used, and ensures that all fibres in the nerve remain activated even though the stimulation electrode may move slightly. The CMAP is recorded from the muscle, preferably using surface electrodes or a subcutaneous needle electrode to ensure that activity from all the muscle fibres in the muscle can be 'seen' by the recording electrode. Usually a belly-tendon montage is used, with the reference electrode being placed over a remote site. Recording of the CMAP with a concentric electrode is usually discouraged since the amplitude is highly dependent on how close the electrode is in relation to the active muscle fibres. However, a concentric needle electrode is useful in very atrophic muscles, as it allows a sharp deflection from the baseline to be measured. The response is amplified at a frequency band between 10 (or 20) Hz and 10 kHz.

Measurements The parameters include latencies, conduction velocities, amplitudes, areas, durations, and shapes of the CMAPs (Fig. 12). The latency is measured to the first deflection from the baseline, which is negative when the CMAP is recorded from the endplate zone. Motor nerve conduction velocities (**MNCV**) between two sites of stimulation are calculated by dividing the distance between stimulation sites by the difference in latencies (Fig. 12).

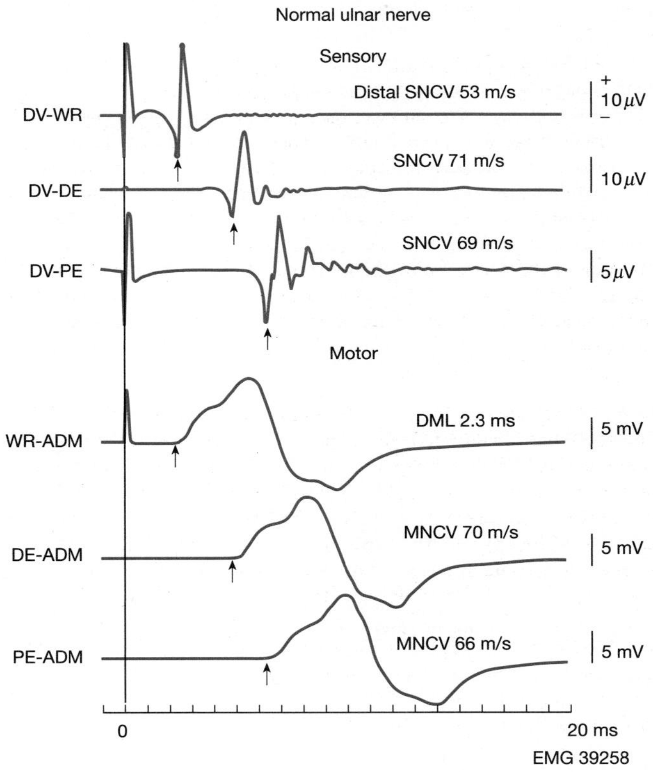

Fig. 12 Motor and sensory conduction studies of a normal ulnar nerve from a patient with diffuse complaints from the arm. Above: compound sensory action potentials, evoked by electrical stimulation at digit V (DV), were recorded via needle electrodes at the wrist (WR), below the elbow (DE), and above the elbow (PE). The latencies were measured to the first positive peak (arrows) and the sensory nerve conduction velocities (SNCV), indicated above the traces, were calculated as indicated in the Method section. Below: compound muscle action potentials, evoked by stimulation at the wrist (WR), below the elbow (DE), and above the elbow (PE) were recorded via a surface electrode over the abductor digiti minimi muscle (ADM). The latencies were measured to the first deflection from the baseline (arrows). DML (distal motor latency) and MNCV (motor nerve conduction velocities), indicated above the traces were obtained as described in the Method section.

$$\frac{\text{Distance between stimulation sites (mm)}}{\text{Difference between distal and proximal latencies (ms)}} = \text{MNCV (m/s)}$$

An MNCV is not calculated for the most distal site of stimulation since the latency includes conduction along terminal motor-axon branches and the neuromuscular transmission delay. In this instance, the delay is designated the distal motor latency (**DML**) (Fig. 12).

The CMAP amplitude (in mV) is measured either at the negative phase or peak-to-peak. The negative phase is usually preferred since it is less subject to influence by the positioning of the reference electrode. The area and duration of the negative phase are useful in evaluating temporal dispersion or conduction block.

Sensory conduction studies

In contrast to the CMAP, the compound sensory action potential (in μV) is recorded directly from active nerve fibres, and it is therefore only about 1/500th to 1/1000th of the CMAP amplitude. The response may be recorded through surface electrodes placed on the skin above the nerve or through needle electrodes placed close to the nerve. Surface electrodes are easy to apply but have a lower sensitivity than needle electrodes. In some normal, elderly people a CSAP from the lower limbs may, therefore, not be recorded through surface electrodes that have a resolution of about 1 μV, whereas near-nerve needle electrodes allow the recording of responses with an amplitude as low as 0.1 μV. In addition, the use of needle electrodes allow simultaneous recording from several sites along the nerve, which are usually not possible using surface electrodes (Fig. 12).

Sensory responses may be recorded antidromically (proximal stimulation, distal recording) or orthodromically (distal stimulation, proximal recording). The recording and reference electrodes may be placed longitudinally in relation to the nerve (bipolar recording), or the reference electrode may be placed transversely at a remote site (unipolar recording). The recording arrangements have advantages and disadvantages: the main advantage of bipolar recording being a smaller stimulus artefact; and the main disadvantage that the potential recorded by the reference electrode influences the CSAP shape and amplitude. Due to the low amplitude of the CSAP, electronic averaging is usually required to obtain a clear response that is suitably free of noise.

Measurements The parameters include latencies, conduction velocities, amplitudes, and shapes of the CSAPs. The latency is measured to the first positive phase of the CSAP. This indicates conduction along the largest fibres in the nerve. Since the conduction path between the sites of stimulation and recording does not include synaptic transmission, a distal sensory nerve conduction velocity (SNCV) may be calculated (Fig. 12):

$$\frac{\text{Distance between stimulation and recording sites (mm)}}{\text{Latency (ms)}} = \text{Distal SNCV (m/s)}$$

When the orthodromically conducted CSAPs are recorded at several sites along the nerve, the SNCV is calculated using a similar procedure as that used to calculate the MNCV:

$$\frac{\text{Distance between proximal and distal recording sites (mm)}}{\text{Differernce between proximal and distal latencies (ms)}} = \text{SNCV (m/s)}$$

In some laboratories, the latency of the CSAP is measured to the first negative phase. This is to be discouraged, since this part of the response is a summation of both large and small fibres. A change in summation due to temporal dispersion therefore precludes measurements to the same group of fibres.

The amplitude of the CSAP (in μV) is measured peak-to-peak. The shape is usually bi- or triphasic. In both axonal and demyelinating neuropathies the shape may become dispersed, and when recorded with a needle electrode, the shape may become polyphasic. Due to temporal dispersion, the conduction distance has a marked influence on the shape of the CSAP. At long conduction distances a polyphasic shape may be normal.

Clinical correlations

The motor and sensory nerve conduction velocities (MNCV, SNCV) are measures of conduction of the largest motor and sensory fibres in the nerve. These limitations should be considered when the results of the studies are interpreted as, for example, a small-fibre neuropathy may escape detection. Similarly, if just a single large motor fibre is preserved, the motor conduction velocity may remain normal, indicating that the conduction velocity cannot be used in isolation to establish the presence of a neuropathy.

Focal nerve lesions

The number of patients referred to the clinical neurophysiology laboratory with possible focal nerve lesions due to compression or entrapment at root level, or along the course of the nerve, far outweighs that for other neuromuscular disorders. In entrapment and focal compression neuropathy, the main pathological abnormalities comprise demyelination at the site of the lesion, which is complicated by axonal loss in advanced lesions. Accordingly, the electrophysiological findings display a disproportionate slowing of conduction at the site of the compression, and also, in some cases, a loss of fibres as demonstrated by reduced amplitudes of the CMAP and the CSAP. This is illustrated in Fig. 13 from a patient with ulnar nerve entrapment at the elbow; the MNCV and SNCV across the elbow were markedly reduced compared to the conduction velocities distal to the elbow, consistent with a focal demyelinating lesion. The CSAP amplitudes were, in addition, markedly diminished, thus indicating axonal loss (Fig. 13(b)), and the slight reduction in SNCV distal to the elbow is commensurate with a loss of large fast-conducting fibres. The apparent sparing of the CMAP

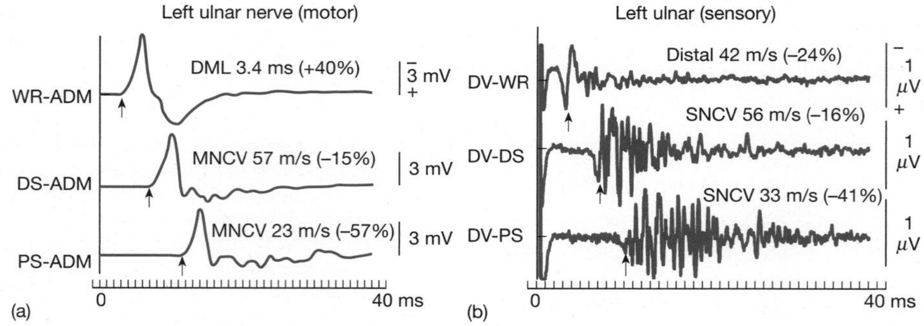

Fig. 13 Conduction studies in a patient with clinical signs of an ulnar nerve lesion. Both (a) motor and (b) sensory conduction showed a marked reduction of conduction velocities across the elbow (57 per cent and 41 per cent reduced between distal to the ulnar sulcus (DS) and proximal to the sulcus (PS), respectively). In addition, there was motor and sensory axonal loss, as indicated by the reduction in amplitudes of the CMAP and the CSAPs. The mild–moderate slowing of conduction distal to the elbow was probably due to a loss of large fibres.

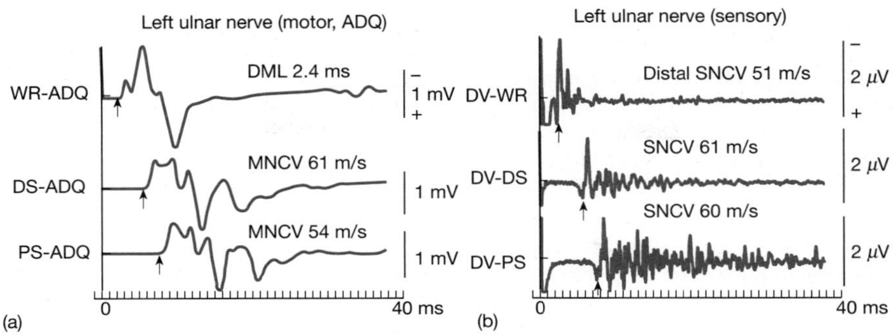

Fig. 14 Conduction studies in a patient with clinical signs of an ulnar nerve lesion that was clinically localized at the brachial plexus or the spinal roots, as indicated by the extent of sensory complaints along the medial forearm and upper arm. Both (a) motor and (b) sensory conduction showed normal conduction velocities distal to and across the elbow. However, the amplitudes of the CMAPs and the CSAPs were markedly decreased, indicating diffuse axonal loss. The loss of sensory fibres is inconsistent with a root lesion and indicates entrapment at the brachial plexus.

amplitude is due to collateral reinnervation masking the motor fibre loss revealed by EMG examination (see above). The slight MNCV reduction distal to the elbow is due to the fibre loss (Fig. 13(a)). Similar methods are used to study focal nerve lesions in patients with compression of the peroneal nerve at the fibular head and in patients with Saturday night palsy (compression of the radial nerve in the spiral groove).

In patients with carpal tunnel syndrome, the distal motor latency of the CMAP to the abductor pollicis brevis muscle, evoked by stimulation at the wrist, is prolonged, indicating a slowing of conduction beneath the flexor retinaculum. However, because it is difficult to stimulate motor fibres distal to the entrapment, differential attenuation of the MNCV is therefore not assessed. To ensure that the median nerve is selectively affected, the latency to the non-affected ulnar nerve should be normal. The SNCV, by contrast, may be tested both distal to and across the carpal tunnel, and is disproportionately reduced along this segment of the nerve compared with that distal to it. Variations on the study paradigm have been devised to increase the sensitivity of the electrophysiological studies.

On the other hand, it is usually not possible to directly study conduction across the compressed nerve segment in patients with very proximal lesions located at spinal roots or the brachial plexus across a cervical rib or band. In these situations, the anatomical distribution of EMG signs of chronic partial denervation is important in the differential diagnosis. For example, EMG findings in patients with apparent involvement of the ulnar nerve due to a C8 lesion or a thoracic outlet syndrome include abnormalities in non-ulnar nerve innervated muscles (for instance, the abductor pollicis brevis and the extensor digitorum communis muscles). This distribution of motor axon loss, and the absence of focal MNCV changes at the elbow (Fig. 14(a)), show that a single nerve lesion is not the cause of the clinical deficit, but it does not distinguish between a radicular and a brachial plexus lesion. By contrast, sensory conduction studies in root lesions usually remain normal, provided that the lesion is located proximal to the dorsal root ganglion, whereas the CSAP from digit V in the thoracic outlet syndrome is diminished due to sensory fibre loss at the level of the brachial plexus (Fig. 14(b)).

Generalized nerve lesions (peripheral neuropathy)

The electrophysiological study in patients with suspected polyneuropathy should document that pathological abnormalities are widely distributed. It is therefore a prerequisite that several motor and sensory nerves in the upper and lower limbs are investigated. However, the study should be individually tailored to delineate the distribution of changes, and the strategy should reflect the symptoms and clinical findings and hence address the question of the differential diagnosis. For example, it may be necessary to investigate certain nerves bilaterally if the symptoms are asymmetrical. This would allow the investigation to show whether the patient may have a mononeuropathy, a multiple mononeuropathy, or a polyneuropathy with asymmetrical features.

Axonal polyneuropathy

The underlying pathology in most patients with peripheral neuropathy is axonal loss in a symmetrical distribution, primarily located at distal nerve segments and more pronounced in the legs than in the arms. The electrophysiological characteristics in these patients are due to a loss of nerve fibres, that is associated with EMG signs of chronic partial denervation and conduction studies that show diminished amplitudes of evoked CMAPs and CSAPs. The remaining fibres in the nerve may conduct normally, and the MNCV and the SNCV in these patients may therefore be normal or show a reduction consistent with a large-fibre loss (Fig. 15). In some patients, the pathological changes may primarily be present at the distal nerve segments, thus studies of these segments will also be required (Fig. 15).

Only motor or sensory fibres are involved in the rarer types of neuropathy, and demonstration of such a distribution may have important implications in the differential diagnosis. A sensory neuronopathy in a 47-year-old woman with profound sensory ataxia is illustrated in Fig. 16. The motor nerve conduction studies and the EMG were normal, but the sensory conduction studies were profoundly abnormal, and the sural nerve biopsy showed a 95 per cent loss of myelinated fibres (Figs 16(a) and (b)). The SNCV was at the lower normal range, consistent with the slightly diminished diameter of the largest remaining fibres being around 10 μm (Figs 16(b) and (c)). These findings were consistent with an autoimmune sensory neuronopathy.

Demyelinating neuropathy

Primary demyelination usually has a hereditary, inflammatory, or autoimmune basis. Although demyelinating neuropathy is rare compared to axonal neuropathy, it has become increasingly important to be able to diagnose acquired demyelinating neuropathy with a high degree of certainty since acute or chronic inflammatory demyelinating neuropathy may respond to immunomodulatory therapy. The primary electrophysiological sign of demyelination is a markedly reduced conduction velocity that is beyond the diminution caused by large-fibre loss. In hereditary motor and sensory neuropathy, type I and III, the MNCV and the SNCV are markedly diminished to less than 50 per cent of the lower limit of normal throughout the nerves, consistent with primary demyelination. In these conditions the amplitudes of the CMAPs and the CSAPs are, however, also markedly reduced and nerve biopsy confirms a marked loss of myelinated nerve fibres. Pure demyelination without axonal loss does not occur in these hereditary conditions and is extremely rare in acquired demyelinating neuropathy. The distinguishing features in acquired demyelinating neuropathy include widespread demyelination, often in a multifocal pattern, as indicated by focal temporal dispersion or conduction block or both of CMAPs and CSAPs. Criteria have been established to assist in the diagnosis of these demyelinating neuropathies (Table 3).

A weakness or sensory loss does not result solely from a diminished conduction velocity, but also as a consequence of nerve fibre loss or a block of conduction between the CNS and the target muscle. Conduction block is a partial or complete inability of fibres to propagate action potentials along a segment of the nerve, and is demonstrated by recording a larger motor or sensory response more distal to than proximal to the site of the block (Fig. 17(a)). This reduction in amplitude should be greater than that associated with a temporal dispersion of the conducting fibres. Therefore to demonstrate a block of motor fibres, the CMAP should show a reduction of at least 50 per cent (Fig. 17(a)). Conduction block may occur in acquired acute or chronic inflammatory demyelinating neuropathy and in some cases of monoclonal gammopathy. It does not occur in hereditary demyelinating neuropathy and probably not in gammopathy with IgM anti-MAG antibodies. However, demyelination due to compression may also cause a conduction block, and in demyelinating neuropathy a conduction block must therefore be demonstrated outside the usual sites of entrapment or compression. The pathophysiological changes in inflammatory demyelinating diseases usually show a multifocal pattern, with some nerves showing pronounced changes while other nerves or nerve segments have normal conduction.

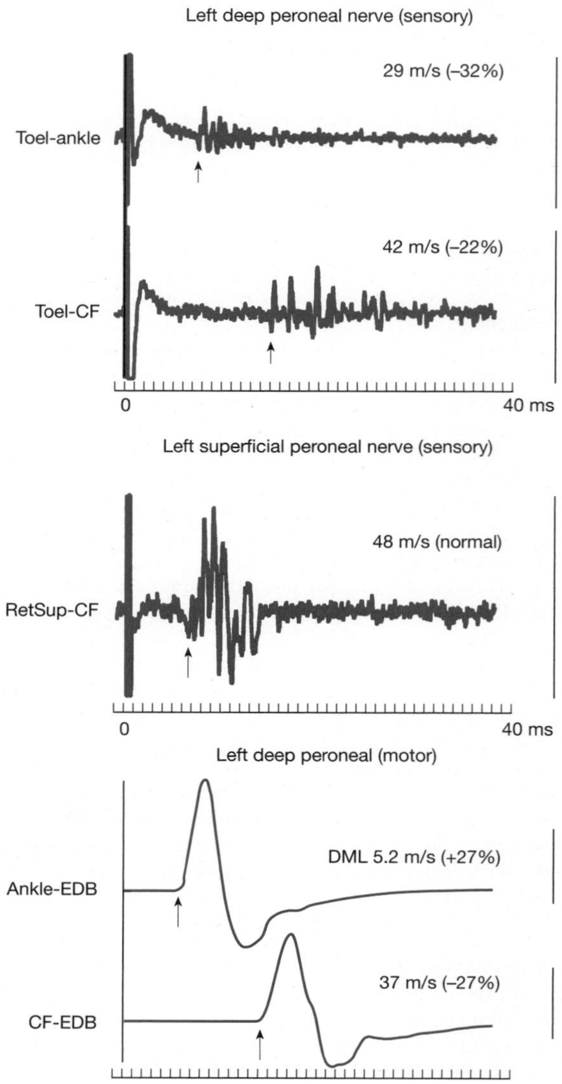

Fig. 15 Motor and sensory conduction studies of the peroneal nerve in a patient with diabetic neuropathy. The findings in this patient were consistent with axonal loss, primarily present in the very distal segment of the nerve. Top panel: orthodromic compound sensory action potentials (CSAPs), evoked at the deep peroneal nerve in the first dorsal interstice (Toel), were recorded at the ankle (ankle) and the fibular head (CF). The amplitudes were more than 95 per cent diminished. The SNCVs were moderately diminished due to large-fibre loss. Middle panel: CSAP of the superficial peroneal nerve evoked at the superior retinaculum (RetSup) at the ankle and recorded at the CF. The amplitude was slightly diminished, and the SNCV was normal. Lower panel: compound muscle action potentials (CMAPs) of the deep peroneal nerve, evoked at the ankle and the fibular head, were recorded at the extensor digitorum brevis muscle (EDB). The distal motor latency (DML) was prolonged and the MNCV was reduced due to fibre loss.

Apparent conduction block may be found in acute neuropathies due to vasculitis. However, conduction along the nerve segment distal to a focal lesion may continue for several days before Wallerian degeneration takes place, and repeated studies should therefore be carried out to exclude this possibility.

Motor disorders (motor neurone disease and motor neuropathy)

Conduction studies in motor neurone disease are normal at early stages of the disease, but at late stages the CMAP amplitudes are reduced. The distal motor latencies of weak and wasted muscles are often prolonged, and the MNCV slightly to moderately reduced due to a loss of large α-motor axons. In ALS, sensory conduction studies are usually normal, though the CSAP amplitudes may be slightly diminished. Therefore, conduction studies are mainly of use in the diagnosis of ALS in that they are normal in the face of widespread neurogenic changes at EMG. However, patients with X-linked bulbospinal muscular atrophy (Kennedy's syndrome) are characterized by a marked reduction of CSAP amplitudes, while the EMG examination shows abnormalities characteristic of motor neurone disease (fasciculations, widespread denervation, markedly enlarged and prolonged MUPs, and discrete high-amplitude recruitment at maximal effort).

Asymmetrical or focal weakness, atrophy, fasciculations (see Fig. 7), without or with only slight sensory symptoms, due to multifocal motor neuropathy may be mistaken for the early stages of spinal forms of motor neurone disease. The course is, however, prolonged over several years, and there is no involvement of bulbar muscles and no signs of corticospinal involvement. The electrophysiological features in these patients are distinct, with conduction block of motor fibres indicating focal demyelination. Usually there is also EMG evidence of chronic partial denervation, indicating fibre loss. The sensory conduction studies through affected nerve segments are normal. These patients frequently have high titres of anti-GM1 antibodies, and often respond clinically and electrophysiologically to intravenous infusions of immunoglobulin. Patients with chronic inflammatory demyelinating neuropathy may have mainly motor symptoms, with only minimal sensory deficits. Motor conduction studies in chronic inflammatory demyelinating neuropathy show signs of mixed demyelination, including conduction block, and fibre loss; sensory conduction studies are abnormal, with small CSAP amplitudes and often reduced SNCV. This is an important distinction, since patients with chronic inflammatory demyelinating neuropathy may respond to treatment with corticosteroids and other immune-modulating strategies that have no effect on multifocal motor neuropathy.

Further reading

Albers JW, Kelly JJ (1989). Acquired inflammatory demyelinating polyneuropathies: clinical and electrodiagnostic features. *Muscle and Nerve* **12**, 435–51.

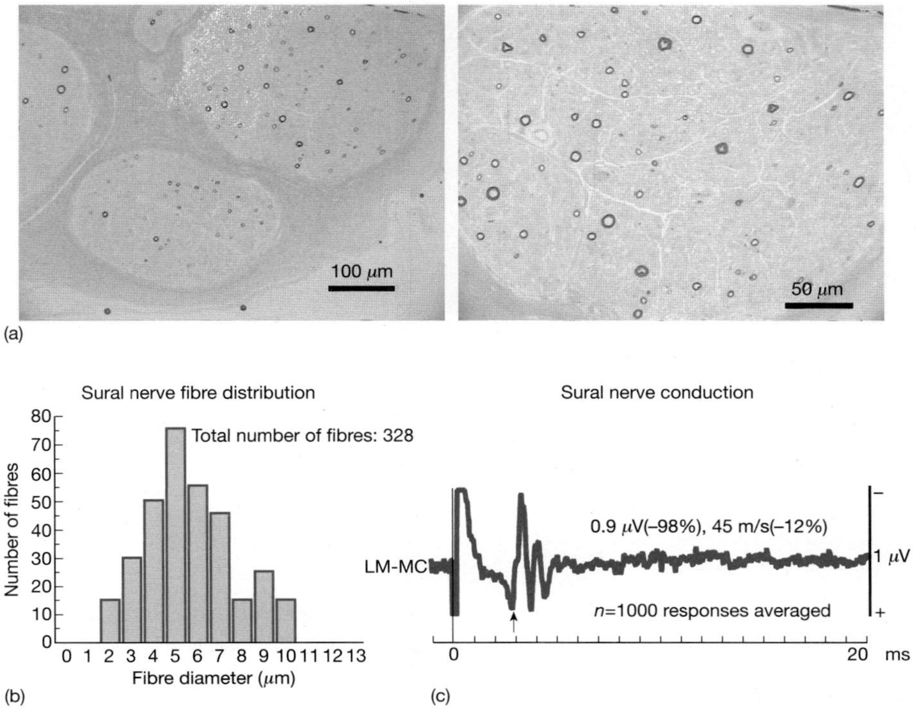

Fig. 16 Morphometric and electrophysiological studies of the sural nerve in a 47-year-old woman with sensory neuronopathy. (a) Transverse semithin sections of the sural nerve showed a generalized severe fibre loss without evidence of degeneration or regeneration. (b) A total of 328 myelinated fibres were counted in the whole nerve. The fibre-diameter distribution showed a loss of both small and large fibres with a maximal diameter of 10 to 11 μm. (c) Conduction studies in the sural nerve showed a pronounced reduction of the CSAP amplitude and a dispersed shape. The SNCV was at the lower normal limit, consistent with the diameters of the largest fibres at morphometry. (Histological studies by courtesy of H. Schmalbruch, University of Copenhagen.)

Table 3 Criteria for the classification of acquired demyelinating polyneuropathies

Nerve conduction parameter	Albers and Kelly, 1989	Ho *et al.*, 1997	Copenhagen values	
			Upper limbs	Lower limbs
Distal motor latency	>115% of UNL (amp. nl.) >125% of UNL (amp. <nl.)	>110% of UNL (amp. nl.) >120% of UNL (amp. <nl.)	4.5 ms 5.4 ms	6.4 ms 7.7 ms
Motor conduction velocity	<90% of LNL (amp. nl.) <80% of LNL (amp. <nl.)	<95% of LNL (amp. >50% of LNL) <85% of LNL (amp. <50% of LNL)	45 m/s 38 m/s	35 m/s 30 m/s
Focal conduction changes	Temporal dispersion (>10–15% increased duration). Proximal/distal amplitude ratio, <0.7	Temporal dispersion		
F-wave latency	>125% of UNL	>120% of UNL		

LNL, lower normal 95 per cent confidence limit; UNL, upper normal 96 per cent confidence limit; amp., amplitude of CMAP; nl., normal.

Binnie CD, *et al.* (1995). EMG, nerve conduction and evoked potentials. In: Osselton JW, ed. *Clinical neurophysiology*, pp. 43–321. Butterworth–Heinemann, Oxford.

Bouche P, *et al.* (1999). Electrophysiological diagnosis of motor neuron disease and pure motor neuropathy. *Journal of Neurology* **246**, 520–5.

Brown WF, Bolton CF, eds. (1993). *Clinical electromyography*, 2nd edn. Butterworth–Heinemann, Boston.

Buchthal F (1957). *An introduction to electromyography*. Scandinavian University Books, København, Stockholm.

Buchthal F (1985). Electromyography in the evaluation of muscle disease. Symposium in Electrodiagnosis. *Neurologic Clinics* **3**, 573–98.

Buchthal F, Kamieniecka Z (1982). The diagnostic yield of quantified electromyography and quantified muscle biopsy in neuromuscular disorders. *Muscle and Nerve* **5**, 265–80.

Chiappa KH, ed. (1997). *Evoked potentials in clinical medicine*, 2nd edn. Lippincott–Raven, Philadelphia.

Fuglsang-Frederiksen A (1981). *Electrical activity and force during voluntary contraction of normal and diseased muscle*. Munksgaard.

Fuglsang-Frederiksen A (2000). The utility of interference pattern analysis. *Muscle and Nerve* **23**, 18–36.

Ho TW, *et al.* (1997). Patterns of recovery in the Guillain-Barre syndromes. *Neurology* **48**, 695–700.

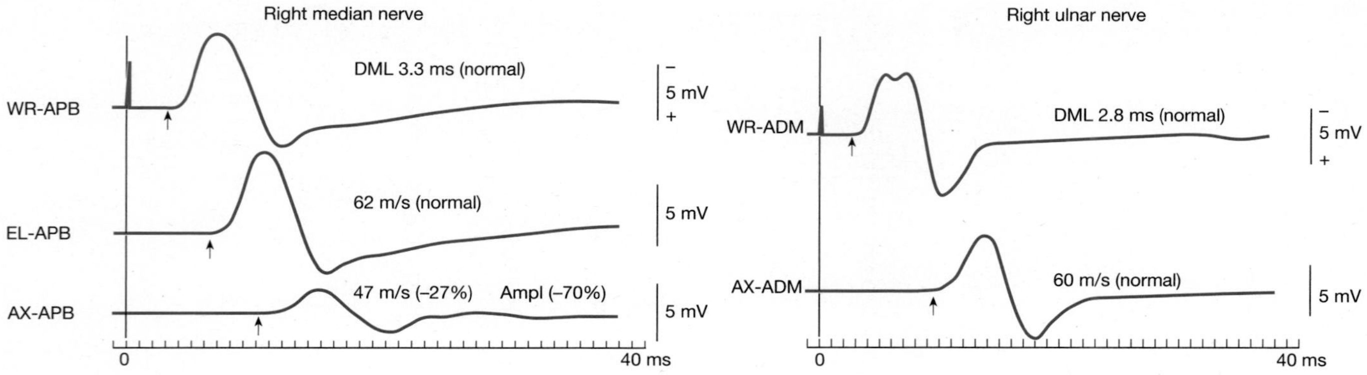

Fig. 17 Motor conduction studies of the median and ulnar nerves of a 29-year-old woman with electrophysiological signs of demyelinating neuropathy and clinical signs of relapsing chronic inflammatory demyelinating neuropathy. Clinical examination showed marked weakness of the thenar and forearm median innervated muscles. The force in ulnar innervated muscles was normal. Left panel: CMAP recorded from the abductor pollicis brevis muscle (APB). Stimulation at the wrist (WR) and elbow (EL) elicited normal CMAPs and the DML and MNCV along the forearm were normal. Stimulation at the axilla (AX) resulted in a markedly reduced CMAP amplitude and a reduced MNCV between the elbow and axilla, consistent with a partial conduction block. Right panel: stimulation of the ulnar nerve at the wrist and axilla evoked CMAPs at the abductor digiti minimi (ADM) of normal amplitudes, DML and MNCV, indicating that motor fibres were not affected.

Kimura J (1989). *Electrodiagnosis in diseases of nerve and muscle. Principles and practice*, 2nd edn. FA Davis, Philadelphia.

Krarup C (1999). Pitfalls in electrodiagnosis. *Journal of Neurology* **246**, 1115–26.

Mauguière F (1995). Evoked potentials. In: Osselton JW, ed. *Clinical neurophysiology*, pp 325–572. Butterworth–Heinemann, Oxford.

Niedermeyer E, Lopes da Silva F, eds (1993). *Electroencephalography. Basic principles, clinical applications, and related fields*, 3rd edn. Williams & Wilkins, Baltimore.

Nuwer MR (1999). Spinal cord monitoring. *Muscle and Nerve* **22**, 1620–30.

Sandberg A, Hansson B, Stålberg E (1999). Comparison between concentric needle EMG and macro EMG in patients with a history of polio. *Clinical Neurophysiology* **110**, 1900–8.

Simonetti S, Nikolic M, Krarup C (1999). Electrophysiology of the motor unit. In: Younger DS, ed. *Textbook of motor disorders*, pp 45–60. Lippincott Williams & Wilkins, Philadelphia.

Stålberg E, Trontelj JV (1979). *Single fibre electromyography.* Mirvalle Press, Old Woking, Surrey.

24.3 Brain and mind: functional neuroimaging

Richard Frackowiak

Introduction

The sensory input to the brain is generally organized into sets of separate, functionally distinct, maps in the cerebral cortex. That much has been known for many years from neurology and animal studies. Can deductions based on non-human primate experiments be assumed to hold true for the brains of humans? For one thing there are obvious differences in the size of the brain between species, and certain areas such as the frontal lobes seem greatly developed in humans. Certain functions, for example spoken language and silent speech, are apparently unique attributes of the human brain. There may be a species-specific organization of specialized cortical areas to account for such human cognitive attributes.

The aim of functional neuroimaging is to describe the activity of neuronal populations and how they are organized into brain networks and systems. This systems-level approach seeks a biological understanding of how integrated brain functions are embodied in the physical structure of the brain. Important areas of enquiry include an understanding of how sensory inputs map onto the brain, and where subsequent signal processing occurs when complex percepts are experienced. Other examples include how sensory and motor systems interact during sense-guided movement, such as reaching under visual control, or how cognitive functions, such as memory and language, are organized and what is the basis for their modification by emotional state.

Functional neuroimaging methods fall broadly into two classes—those that provide information about synaptic activity and those that provide information about neurochemistry or neurotransmission. The former methods usually depend on measurements of the distribution of local cerebral blood flow (often known as perfusion maps) or, when comparisons between successively recorded distributions in different brain states are made, as activation studies. Local perfusion is a surrogate marker for local synaptic activity because of a tight coupling between it and local cerebral glucose metabolism both at rest and with activation. Such measurements can be accomplished with positron emission tomography and with functional magnetic resonance imaging, although in this method the images depend less clearly on perfusion alone as the signal is dependent on blood oxygen level. Radioactivity is not used in functional magnetic resonance imaging, which can therefore be safely repeated an unlimited number of times in any individual. Both positron emission tomography and functional magnetic resonance imaging localize changes in local brain activity to a millimetre or so. The second class of functional neuroimaging methods relies on mapping the distribution of chemical species of interest with positron emission tomography after injection of appropriately specific radiotracers, or by identification of unique magnetic signatures of compounds of interest with magnetic resonance spectroscopy. It is also possible to map non-invasively the distribution of electrical or magnetic signals coming from the brain. The anatomical precision with which this can be done is markedly worse than with positron emission tomography and functional magnetic resonance imaging, but brain activity can be followed millisecond by millisecond, a temporal resolution that is not possible with the other two methods.

There are clinical uses for functional neuroimaging, such as preoperative assessment of the functional integrity of peritumoural tissue and non-invasive assessment of language and memory dominance in patients undergoing temporal lobe surgery for epilepsy. Positron emission tomography and functional magnetic resonance imaging have had an apparently less spectacular impact on clinical practice than have anatomical imaging methods such as computed tomography and conventional magnetic resonance imaging. This is because functional neuroimaging is used to discover disease mechanisms of general significance, relevant to groups of patients, while computed tomography and magnetic resonance imaging provide information of direct relevance to the diagnosis, prognosis, and management of individual patients. Nevertheless, there are some striking examples of the impact of functional neuroimaging on clinical practice. For example, the definition of the haemodynamic and energetic consequences of preclinical and clinical carotid artery disease and the description of the time course of the natural transition from ischaemia to infarction have modified views about surgical treatment and about pharmaceutical approaches to stroke therapy, and have also affected the design of clinical trial protocols. Functional neuroimaging is able to detect preclinical degenerative brain disease and to distinguish between different clinical disorders. Positron emission tomography has also been invaluable in assessing the therapy of Parkinson's disease by monitoring fetal mesencephalic graft survival and the effects of subthalamic and pallidal lesions and chronic subthalamic nucleus stimulation.

From sensation to cognition

The visual system has been relatively well studied by some of the modern neuroimaging methods described above and will be used to illustrate some general principles. A simple imaging experiment to imagine is measurement of the distribution of brain activity during an eyes-open and an eyes-closed state. A comparison of brain activities recorded in each of the two states identifies areas of the brain in which activity is specifically associated with vision. When early sensory processing is the object of study this comparative approach is relatively free of assumptions. When more complex cognitive functions are studied more sophisticated experiments and analyses must be used.

The visual world is mapped from retina to cortex

The visual world depends on patterns of light hitting the retina. The evoked retinal signals are transmitted to the visual cortex in a point to point manner. Signals coming from adjacent patches of retina and hence adjacent parts of the visual field are mapped onto adjacent patches of cortex, a fact that is also deduced from studies of patients with focal lesions of the visual cortex. This retinotopic organization of primary visual cortex (V1) has been clearly confirmed with functional scanning in normal humans. Activity recorded in the brain with peripheral visual targets can be compared with that recorded with central presentation. Each quadrant of the visual field is located in the opposite cerebral hemisphere and quadrant of the visual cortex. The fovea is represented at the pole of the occipital cortex and peripheral vision activates more anterior parts of the calcarine cortex. One can calculate from such data the magnification factor, i.e. the length of cortex that maps a given 'length' of the visual field, and also the borders between specialized extrastriate visual regions.

The extrastriate occipital cortex receives multiple parallel outputs from area V1. This cortex is functionally heterogeneous, different parts activate in association with different aspects of visual perception (for example form, colour, movement, and face recognition). Area V5 is an extrastriate area in which activity is associated with visually perceived motion. The brains of individuals vary one from another quite markedly, not only in shape but also in the disposition of the gyri and sulci of parts of the cortex. However, accurate alignment of functional and anatomical images is a trivial issue with the use of modern computers. It is possible to show precise relationships between structure and function despite considerable individual variability of the normal anatomy of the occipital cortex. V5 is always found in a circumscribed part of the occipital lobe at the junction with the temporal lobe in the angle formed by two occipital gyri—the inferior occipital and the ascending limb of the inferior temporal. This anatomical site is relatively developed in infants with heavy myelination of the associated white matter fibres. In summary, there is a remarkable correlation between developmental factors, functional specialization, and anatomical location, despite considerable variability in the absolute spatial location of the anatomical structure between different individuals. The heavy myelination that is characteristic of area V5 can be demonstrated by high-resolution anatomical magnetic resonance imaging, as can the stria of Gennari, a unique structural characteristic of primary visual cortex (V1).

Activity in V5 occurs with perceived visual motion, whether that motion is real or illusory. One area of extrastriate cortex (V3) shows equivalent activity when real or illusory objects are perceived. Schizophrenic patients with visual delusions show activation of extrastriate areas that determine the content of their delusions. This evidence suggests that the visual brain is constructing an intrerpretation of the visual scene from the information provided. Sometimes that information is appropriate to reality, at other times it has a configuration that, for unknown reasons, elicits activity in an unexpected specialized visual area. The consequent illusory perception is congruent with that experienced when the area is activated by real stimuli. The Kanizsa triangle is an example of a normal visual illusion of this type for which a partial explanation can be proposed. The perception of an apparent triangle in front of a solid body can be ascribed to the fact that in normal visual life we expect to see objects hidden by others that lie in front of them. The triangle illusion is a reflection of this phenomenon. Similarly, activation of the visual motion area (V5) is seen during the waterfall illusion in which looking at a waterfall and looking away results in a temporary illusion of continuing motion. The stimulus–response characteristic of the visual processing machinery is determined in part by genes and in part by experience. At times the experiential component results in a conflict with reality and hence an illusion.

Sometimes two perceptual solutions seem equally likely to the brain, as in the case of ambiguous or bistable figures. These figures can be interpreted in one of two ways. The alternatives flip in a deterministic fashion described by a gamma function so that as long as fixation is maintained conscious control over flip frequency is minimal. Studies with event-related functional magnetic resonance imaging, a new technical development that permits examination of changes in the blood oxygen level-dependent signal due to transient neural or perceptual events, has led to investigation of the mechanisms underlying this phenomenon. A perceptual 'flip' results in a transient activation of extrastriate visual areas (amongst other neocortical sites). At the same time there is a transient deactivation of the pulvinar of the thalamus and V1. This result suggests a subcortical–cortical perceptual system in which the thalamus maintains perceptual stability and the cortex effects a reinterpretation of the perceptual content when the stabilizing influence of the thalamus wanes. The importance of the functionally specialized modules to perceptual content can also be demonstrated non-invasively by temporary, localized, functional lesions using transcranial magnetic stimulation. Thus the perception of visual motion can be temporarily disturbed by a shock at an appropriate time after a moving stimulus excites the retina.

Patients with lesions at functionally specialized sites have syndromes of loss of function and provide additional information about the organization of the visual system.. Thus lesions in the lingual gyrus at the site of V4 lead to the syndrome of achromatopsia (cortical colour blindness). Lesions in the V1 cortex provide a substrate for examining the function of retinocortical pathways that access extrastriate cortex without passage through and processing in V1. Up to 10 per cent of retinofugal fibres are of this type. A patient with a V1 lesion has been described who shows residual perception of high contrast, rapidly moving stimuli in his blind hemifield. This is associated with activation of V5, but not V1, which is destroyed. This finding raises issues about just how much cortex is required to produce a conscious experience and whether consciousness is itself organized in a modular fashion. The importance of such 'minor' pathways has not been well understood. In normal subjects, event-related electrical potential mapping in response to a perceptible moving visual stimulus shows a response in area V5 that preceeds the response in V1 by up to 40 ms. As all specialized areas that send projections to another area receive them from it in return, the conditions are established by which preprocessing of a salient visual motion stimulus in V5 might prime V1 to receive the main neural volley from the same stimulus—a potential feedforward regulatory system.

Beyond the extrastriate cortex

The awareness of the position of an object and knowledge of its physical qualities, leading to recognition, are two visual cognitive functions that depend, at least in part, on a recognition of the object's shape, colour, and direction of motion. Imaging studies suggest that the pathways activated in association with these two attributes of objects overlap substantially, but there is also some segregation relevant to each attribute in brain areas in front of the occipital cortex. Activation of posterior parts of the inferior temporal lobes occurs when objects are recognized, for example to be named. Identification of an object's position in space preferentially activates posterior parts of the parietal lobe. A third pathway, in which activity is associated with visually guided reaching for objects, has been demonstrated in the parietal lobes between those areas activated by recognition and those by awareness of position. The recognition of further pathways is to be expected because, in general, integration of visual signals with behaviour occurs at multiple anatomical levels in the human brain. Each specialized brain area that has connections to another specialized area receives signals back. Each area sends and receives signals to and from multiple other dispersed areas and draws on signals from these areas as the behavioural context demands. Yet signal traffic is not chaotic, a remarkable and often ignored result provided by functional neuroimaging.

Synaesthesia are curious experiential phenomena in which signals of one sensory modality elicit experiences in another. The condition is probably developmental and not uncommon early in life. The most frequent manifestation is the visualization of colours whilst reading or speaking. Certain colours are associated with certain stimuli, for example the first letter of a word. The experiences are not unpleasant but bizarre and are therefore frequently unacknowledged or even denied. Such phenomena provide a paradigm for examination of the interactions between sensory modalities. In aural–colour vision synaesthetes, there is abnormal activation of cortical areas beyond V4 and other early extrastriate visual areas. In fact, activity in V4 may be diminished in association with synaesthesia. Another situation in which crossmodality interactions occur is in blind Braille readers. If blindness is congenital, Braille reading is always more proficient than if it is learned after acquired blindness. Touch stimulation in Braille readers elicits visual cortex activation. However, this phenomenon involves V1 only in people with acquired blindness. It is therefore equally plausible that V1 is recruited for touch processing or that in a primed, previously 'seeing', V1 activity may be due to imagery of letters read through the touch sense. Such people can also provide important information about postperceptual processing. For example, sighted people reading visually, blind people reading with Braille, and blind people hearing spoken words all activate a posterior inferior temporal region implicating it in a supramodal function that involves word processing irrespective of input modality.

Conclusion

The brain is organized according to relatively well-ordered principles. Responses are reproducible and common to most humans. The correlation of behaviour, anatomy, and physiology promises much for an understanding of normal brain function and also for understanding better the symptoms of cerebral disease. Functional neuroimaging and advances in computerized analysis of structural images are breakthroughs for the cognitive neurosciences. It is now possible to analyse thoughts, percepts, actions, and emotions at the level of neuronal populations. Brain activity can be followed over time and in different contexts permitting the study of recovery, attention, and pharmacological modulation of brain function. New methods for measuring connection strengths between brain areas and their modification under different conditions add further opportunities for expanding knowledge as to how the human brain works in health and disease.

Further reading

Frackowiak RSJ *et al.*, eds (1997). *Human brain function.* Academic Press, San Diego.

Zeki S (1993). *A vision of the brain.* Blackwell, Oxford.

Frackowiak RSJ, Gadian DG, Mazziotta JC (2000). Functional neuroimaging. In: Bradley WG *et al.*, eds. *Neurology in clinical practice,* pp 665–75. Butterworth-Heinemann, Boston.

24.4 Investigation of central motor pathways: magnetic brain stimulation

K. R. Mills

The ability to stimulate percutaneously and without pain the central nervous system of awake humans has opened up new areas for neurophysiological investigation both in terms of the early diagnosis of neurological disease and the further understanding of normal and abnormal motor control. Magnetic stimulators are now available that are capable of exciting both upper and lower limb areas of the motor cortex, as well as cranial nerves, motor roots, and deeply sited peripheral nerves.

Magnetic stimulators

The magnetic stimulator is an essentially simple device; a brief pulse of electric current is passed through a coil which then generates an intense magnetic field permeating unattenuated into the surrounding media. Any electrical conductor, such as the brain, in the vicinity of the coil will have currents induced within it; these induced currents are capable of exciting cerebral neurones. Coils are placed on the scalp and may be plane circular, figure of eight, or double cone in geometry, the last being especially effective in exciting leg areas of the motor cortex. Some magnetic stimulators produce a predominantly monophasic field pulse, others produce multiphasic pulses; with the former, the side of the coil next to the scalp determines which hemisphere is predominantly excited, whereas with the latter both hemispheres are about equally excited.

Physiology

If a single anodal shock is applied to the exposed cortex of a monkey and recordings are made from the pyramidal tract, it is seen that, if stimulus intensity is sufficient, an initial wave produced by direct activation of pyramidal tract neurones (the D wave) is followed by a variable number of other waves produced by indirect trans-synaptic activation (I waves) of the same pyramidal neurones. In humans a single weak stimulus to the scalp probably excites pyramidal tract cells trans-synaptically; stronger stimuli may excite the cells directly. The effect of a single stimulus is to cause a high frequency (500 to 1000 Hz) burst of impulses to descend in the fastest fibres of the pyramidal tract; the spinal motoneurones are engaged by these impulses and if their excitability is high enough and there is sufficient temporal and spatial summation, then the motoneurones fire, causing a muscle contraction. There is considerable convergence and divergence of pyramidal tract fibres within motoneurone pools; single spinal motoneurones receive many corticospinal inputs and, conversely, single pyramidal tract fibres branch to supply many spinal motoneurones. Intrinsic hand muscles are the most easily excited from brain stimulation but all voluntary muscles appear to be accessible from cortical stimulation. The amplitude of response of a muscle depends on the intensity of the stimulus, to a lesser extent on coil placement on the scalp, but most potently on the degree of voluntary preactivation of the muscle. Thus the amplitude of response of an intrinsic hand muscle may be 20 to 30 times greater if the subject performs a gentle (5 to 10 per cent maximum) voluntary contraction of the muscle. This facilitation is probably due to both cortical and spinal cord mechanisms, voluntary action increasing the effectiveness of the stimulus at the cortex at the same time as the excitability of spinal motoneurones is increased by other pathways. The latter mechanism predominates in intrinsic hand muscles. Clearly, many factors, including mental set, affect the size of muscle response to the stimulus and it should be emphasized that this phenomenon of response variability contrasts with the identical and reproducible responses obtained from maximal electrical peripheral nerve shocks; central motor conduction studies should not be regarded simply as an extension of nerve conduction measurements.

Single scalp shocks also bring into play inhibitory mechanisms: if a subject maintains a steady voluntary muscle contraction, the initial excitation caused by the stimulus is followed by a silent period. The mechanisms underlying this are still unclear but probably involve inhibition at both cortical and spinal levels.

Safety of magnetic stimulation

A number of studies have looked at the acute effects of magnetic stimuli on animals. It has been shown that magnetic stimuli have little detectable effect on the heart rate, arterial blood pressure, or cerebral blood flow in cats. Magnetic brain stimulation has no acute effects on the human electroencephalogram or on the performance of simple cognitive tests. There have currently been no reports of adverse effects in healthy human subjects, but clearly, workers in the field should remain vigilant, especially for long-term effects.

It has been calculated that the total amount of power dissipated in the brain during magnetic stimulation is 1.8 $\mu J/cm^3$ per stimulus and at the maximal rate of stimulation of 0.3 Hz, the average power dissipation is 53 μW, some five orders of magnitude below the basal metabolic rate of the brain.

It was considered prudent for early users of magnetic stimulation to exclude patients who had a history of epilepsy from their studies. Since then, magnetic stimulation has actually been used to attempt to localize epileptic foci in patients with intractable seizures. However, the risks of provoking a fit are considered small since it had been shown in cats that repetitive stimuli direct to the cortex in animals that had lesions induced by penicillin were only effective at rates above 5 Hz. Despite magnetic stimulation devices being used on many thousands of patients, many of whom must have had a predilection for epilepsy, there have been only a few reports of a fit being related to single-pulse brain stimulation.

Measurement of central motor conduction time

The latency of muscle response has a central and peripheral component and a delay due to synaptic transmission in the spinal cord. There is good evidence that, at least with limb muscle, the connection from the pyramidal tract to spinal motoneurone is monosynaptic. The central component of conduction—central motor conduction time (**CMCT**)—can be estimated by subtracting from the cortex to muscle latency an estimate of the peripheral conduction time obtained either from F wave measurement (see Chapter 24.2) or from responses evoked by root stimulation. In healthy subjects, the mean latency (± standard deviation) of responses in intrinsic hand muscle is 19.7 ± 1.2 ms and the CMCT is 6.1 ± 0.9 ms. The amplitude of responses from brain stimulation is usually compared with that obtained from maximal peripheral nerve stimulation; again there is great variability, but in healthy subjects the response from cortical stimuli is usually at least 15 per cent of that from nerve stimulation. Since many factors can influence these values, each laboratory should develop its own normative database.

Motor roots may be excited by both electrical and magnetic stimulators. The former method is preferable since it is not possible to obtain maximal responses in all healthy subjects with magnetic coils, even with optimal coil geometry, coil orientation, and coil position. Both devices activate motor roots at or just outside the intervertebral foramina and so peripheral conduction time estimated by this method omits conduction in the small segment of motor root within the spinal canal and CMCT is slightly overestimated. The method must be used, however, if F waves are unobtainable.

Compound responses from muscle may be recorded with surface electrodes, or single motor unit responses may be recorded with needle electrodes; the former method is used clinically, the latter is useful in research. A number of parameters of the surface-recorded response are useful: the maximum amplitude, the onset latency with the muscle relaxed or contracted, the threshold for evoking a response, and the variability in latency or amplitude in a series of responses.

Prolongation of CMCT has been reported in many conditions and is not specific. Delay can be produced by a variety of pathological processes: demyelination of central fibres can lead to slowing of impulse propagation in the central motor pathway; desynchronization of descending impulses can lead to loss of temporal summation at the motoneurone and delay in its firing; and loss of corticospinal axons can lead to impairment of spatial summation at motoneurones and can again delay firing.

Multiple sclerosis

In multiple sclerosis, CMCT is prolonged in about 70 per cent of cases when there are clear clinical signs of a pyramidal lesion in the particular limb (Fig. 1). The delay in some cases is very considerable, CMCT may be up to five times longer than in controls. It is likely that, in these cases, demyelination of central fibres is the mechanism leading to delay. In other cases, delay is more modest, only a few milliseconds, and the mechanism is less certain. Abnormal central motor conduction appears to correlate most closely with exaggerated reflexes and spasticity rather than with weakness or cerebellar signs in the limb. Abnormal CMCT from leg areas of motor cortex also correlates with the finding of extensor plantar responses.

Central motor conduction can be abnormal, however, even in the absence of clinical signs. In a large series, it was found that central conduction was abnormal in 20 per cent of cases of multiple sclerosis with no motor signs in the particular limb. The technique can thus be used as a screening test for multiple sclerosis, although it compares unfavourably with visual evoked potentials, which have a higher rate of abnormality in the absence of clinical signs. This may merely reflect the greater accuracy with which the motor system can be examined clinically. Central motor studies may also be helpful in deciding on the importance of equivocal motor signs, such as mild impairment of fine finger movements.

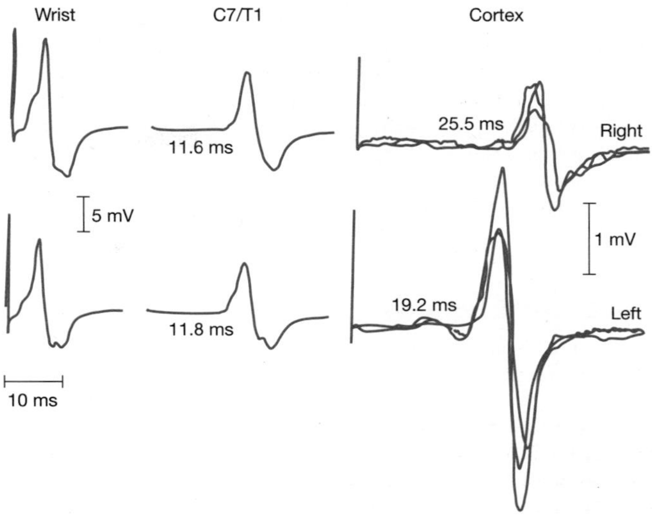

Fig. 1 Slowing of central motor conduction in multiple sclerosis. Compound muscle action potentials are recorded with surface electrodes over the left and right abductor digiti minimi muscles. Stimuli are given to the ulnar nerve at the wrist (left), the C7/T1 motor roots (middle), and the motor cortex (right). Onset latencies are shown and the variability of responses from cortical stimulation can be seen. On the left CMCT is 7.4 ms, but on the right is prolonged at 13.9 ms.

Motor neurone disease

In motor neurone disease, the most common abnormality is a raised threshold for excitation of the motor cortex, although in early cases the threshold may be reduced. In many cases responses cannot be obtained even with the strongest stimuli applied in optimal conditions. CMCT may be prolonged, but usually only modestly, and responses are often reduced in amplitude in comparison with responses evoked by maximal nerve stimulation. The test can be used to confirm an upper motor neurone component to weakness when lower motor neurone signs predominate or for detecting an upper motor neurone lesion in a limb without clinical signs.

Cerebrovascular disease

In stroke, responses in an affected limb may be normal, delayed, or absent, with abnormality grossly paralleling the clinical abnormality. Central motor conduction studies have been used to predict outcome of stroke; if performed within the first 48 h after the ictus, a poor outcome at 6 months is predicted by absent responses and a favourable outcome by normal responses. Whether the prediction is superior to that made purely on clinical grounds is uncertain, but at least the method is quantitative and can be used serially to follow recovery.

Movement disorders

Most studies have shown central motor conduction to be normal in Parkinson's disease, multiple system atrophy, Wilson's disease, Huntington's disease (including at-risk relatives), dystonia, and progressive supranuclear palsy. In some cases of Wilson's disease, central conduction delays have been found. In all these conditions, however, there may be subtle changes in motor cortex excitability detectable as a change in threshold or an abnormal inhibitory response to appropriately timed pairs of cortical stimuli.

Degenerative neurological diseases

A number of rarer degenerative diseases have been investigated with the technique: Friedreich's ataxia often shows delayed and dispersed responses, as does early-onset cerebellar ataxia with retained reflexes, the severity of the abnormalities reflecting disease duration. In late-onset cerebellar degeneration on the other hand, the responses are normal in 62 per cent of cases. In hereditary spastic paraparesis and tropical spastic paraparesis, responses from upper limb muscles are usually normal, whereas those from the lower limbs are delayed or absent. Abnormalities of central motor conduction have also been described in some cases of hereditary motor and sensory neuropathy types I and II, the abnormalities being found especially in those patients with additional upper motor neurone signs. Central motor conduction abnormalities have also been described in a family with hereditary motor and sensory neuropathy with pyramidal signs (HMSN type V).

Spinal cord lesions

Magnetic brain stimulation has been used to assess the completeness of spinal cord injury. A variety of facilitating techniques must be used; the modulation of flexion reflexes by brain stimuli has been shown to be useful in establishing whether injury is complete; in 4 of 26 patients evidence of incomplete lesions was found in patients with clinically complete spinal cord injuries. In compressive myelopathy, by recording from a variety of upper limb muscles, CMCT can be used to localize more accurately the compressed cord segment.

Paediatric applications

The central conduction time in a group of 457 normal subjects between the ages of 32 weeks and 55 years has been determined. It was found that central conduction time decreases rapidly over the first 2 years of life and then remains constant at the adult value. In contrast, peripheral conduction increases in proportion to arm length after the age of 5 years. It is suggested that this constant central delay could be useful during the acquisition of motor skills. Central motor conduction has been studied in a range of neurological diseases in children. For example, in 13 of 20 children with an upper motor neurone syndrome of varied aetiology, the central conduction time was abnormal, but magnetic resonance imaging and/or computed tomography scans showed focal abnormalities in only seven. In 15 children with extrapyramidal syndromes, the central conduction time was normal.

Use of brain stimulation for neurosurgical monitoring

Although somatosensory motoring has been shown to be of use during neurosurgical procedures to alert the surgeon of the possibility of cord damage, the use of motor monitoring is far more relevant since paraplegia is one of the most feared, although rare, outcomes of surgery near the cord. Electrical brain stimulation and recording from the cord by epidural electrodes has been achieved; responses consist of a series of waves analogous to the D and I waves recordable in primates. Magnetic stimulation appears to produce I waves but the responses are very sensitive to the depth of anaesthetic agents, especially nitrous oxide. If the aim of monitoring is merely to stimulate the motor cortex, there seems little to be gained by using magnetic stimuli in favour of the electrical method since the pain of the procedure is not a factor.

Conclusion

Non-invasive magnetic brain stimulation has shown itself to be a powerful technique in the diagnosis and prognosis of disorders of the central motor system, as well as providing new insights into the normal control of human voluntary movement. It can be used serially to monitor progress or the effects of drugs, can be used safely in neonates and children, and can be used to demonstrate short- or long-term plasticity in the human nervous system after injury.

Further reading

Levy WJ *et al.*, eds (1991). Magnetic motor stimulation: basic principles and clinical experience. *Electroencephalography and Clinical Neurophysiology*, Suppl 43.

Mills KR (1999). *Magnetic stimulation of the human nervous system.* Oxford University Press.

Rothwell JC *et al.* (1991). Stimulation of the human motor cortex through the scalp. *Experimental Physiology* **76**, 159–200.

24.5 Imaging in neurological diseases

Andrew J. Molyneux and Philip Anslow

Introduction

The modern imaging techniques of X-ray computed tomography (**CT**) and magnetic resonance imaging (**MRI**) for the demonstration of structural neurological disease have developed rapidly over the last 20 years. They have done more than any other single development to revolutionize the diagnosis and treatment of structural neurological disease. More recently, a variety of functional imaging techniques have been developed that enable functional and biochemical information to be obtained from the living brain.

Current techniques for neuroimaging

Computed tomography (CT)

X-ray computed tomography was developed by the British scientist and engineer Godfrey Hounsfield during the early 1970s. CT was the first technique to provide non-invasive and cross-sectional images of the brain. It was introduced into clinical usage at the Atkinson Morley Hospital in Wimbledon, London, in 1972 and results were published in 1973. This was the start of a complete revolution in radiological imaging, for which Hounsfield received the Nobel prize for medicine in 1979.

CT rapidly became the mainstay of the diagnosis of structural brain disease until the advent of magnetic resonance imaging (MRI) into widespread clinical use during the late 1980s and early 1990s. However, CT remains an extremely valuable and essential tool, particularly in the acute situation and in countries and regions where the cost of MRI systems is prohibitively expensive.

CT produces a series of cross-sectional images, usually in the axial plane (hence the acronym CAT scan, standing for computed axial tomography). During exposure to an X-ray beam, a detector array spins around the patient and measures the absorption coefficients of tissues within the beam. It is the different coefficients that provide contrast.

Magnetic resonance imaging (MRI)

Magnetic resonance imaging is a fundamentally different method of obtaining images. It relies on a powerful static magnetic field and the various properties of the protons (hydrogen ions) in the different tissues. When a strong magnetic field is subjected to certain radio waves of a specific frequency (radiofrequency) the protons will resonate at an exact frequency that depends on the field strength of the magnet. The radio signal emitted back by the protons when the radiofrequency is switched off can be detected in a receiver coil and a detailed image built up. The resolution of modern MRI scanners is extremely high, as is the sensitivity of the images obtained for the detection of intracranial anatomy and pathology.

Many different radio-pulse sequences are of use in MRI, which are determined by the way the radio signals are timed. They detect different aspects of tissue properties by what is called 'the relaxation times of the protons'; times that will vary according to the proton-containing tissue and the relative mobility of the water molecules. The most commonly used sequences are what are termed '*T*1-weighted and *T*2-weighted sequences'. The appearances of these scans are quite different: for example, cerebrospinal fluid (**CSF**) is white on *T*2 and dark on *T*1 images (Figs 1 and 2). Some tissues such as fat and some blood breakdown products (for instance, methaemoglobin) will appear bright on *T*1- and *T*2-weighted images.

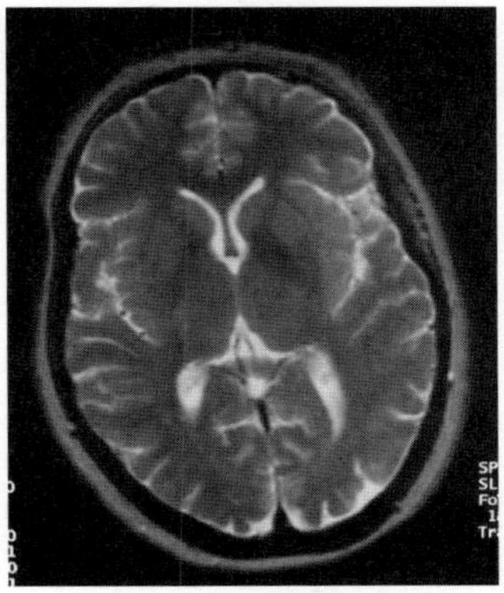

Fig. 1 Normal axial *T*2-weighted image of a brain at the level of the ventricular system. Note that the cerebrospinal fluid is white, the white matter is dark, and the grey matter is lighter than the white matter. This is the most commonly used MRI sequence and it is usually the most sensitive in the detection of pathological processes.

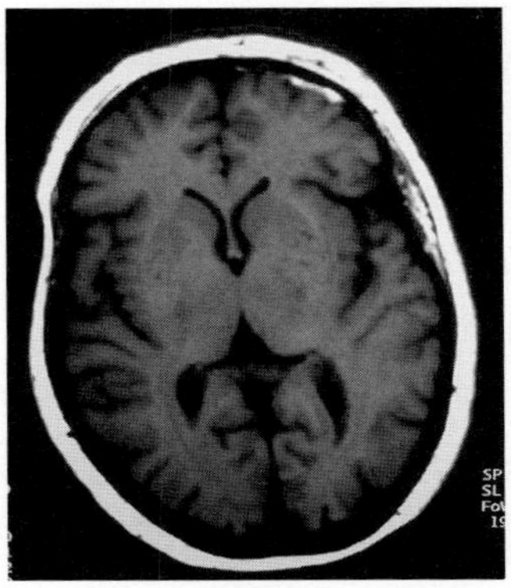

Fig. 1 Axial *T*1-weighted unenhanced MRI image at the similar level of the ventricles as in Fig. 1, showing the CSF dark and the white matter lighter than the grey matter.

Contrast enhancement in brain imaging

Intravenous contrast in brain imaging is frequently used to determine the vascularity of structures and whether the blood–brain barrier is intact. It will show the extent and patterns of enhancement in tumours, infarcts, and inflammatory lesions. For CT scanning, the same iodinated contrast agents that are used in general vascular imaging are used. In MRI, gadolinium-labelled compounds, which shorten the *T1* relaxation time, are used. These provide extremely useful information and show the same patterns of enhancement as the iodinated contrast media used for CT scanning, although the sensitivity of MRI contrast agents are significantly greater.

Cerebral angiography

This is used to demonstrate the intra- and extracerebral vessels. The procedure is nearly always performed by transfemoral catheterization of the neck vessels. Before the introduction of CT it was the main means of diagnosing intracranial pathology, particularly of masses and stroke-causing lesions such as vessel occlusions or haemorrhages. The main indication now for angiography is intracranial haemorrhage or suspected extracranial carotid or vertebral stenosis. Non-invasive methods, such as Doppler ultrasound of the neck vessels and magnetic resonance angiographic imaging (which does not require contrast media), has reduced the number of patients requiring invasive intra-arterial angiography, particularly for suspected ischaemic cerebrovascular disease.

Other imaging techniques including functional imaging

Although these are used less frequently, nuclear medicine studies using radioactive labelled isotopes—generally with technetium-99m and **HMPAO** (hexamethylpropylene amine oxide) as the ligand—and a gamma camera can be used to produce perfusion imaging scans of the brain. This technique is known as single-photon computed tomography (**SPECT**). Positron emission tomography (**PET**) scanning requires a cyclotron to produce the very short-lived isotopes of carbon and oxygen, and is primarily used as a research tool for investigation of the functional imaging of the brain.

Functional MRI and spectroscopy

High-field MRI 1.5 tesla or greater, up to 4 tesla, magnetic fields can also be used to provide functional information on brain function and biochemistry (spectroscopy from either hydrogen or phosphorous nuclei). These techniques are not yet in routine clinical use.

Imaging of common neurological diseases

Cerebrovascular disease and stroke

The most frequent neurological presentation is that of acute stroke. Patients presenting with a sudden onset of neurological deficit should be deemed to have suffered a vascular event until proved otherwise. In practice the clinical diagnosis of stroke is very accurate, provided an adequate history is available. The primary role of imaging in patients with acute stroke is to identify whether it is ischaemic or haemorrhagic in origin, or where there is doubt about the underlying pathology based on the clinical history. CT scanning provides a completely reliable way of excluding primary intracerebral haemorrhage as a cause of acute stroke, provided it is performed within about a week of onset. In ischaemic stroke, depending on the timing of the examination relative to the onset of neurological deficit, it will variably detect acute infarction.

Cerebral infarction

Early appearances

Within hours of a stroke, the CT scan may show a vague low attenuation or slight swelling and effacement of the sulci in the area of damage, or it may be normal. Standard MRI imaging may also be normal at this stage. However, certain more recently introduced MRI techniques, known as 'diffusion-weighted imaging', can show abnormalities even within less than an hour of onset that reflect alterations in the state and mobility of the protons in tissue water.

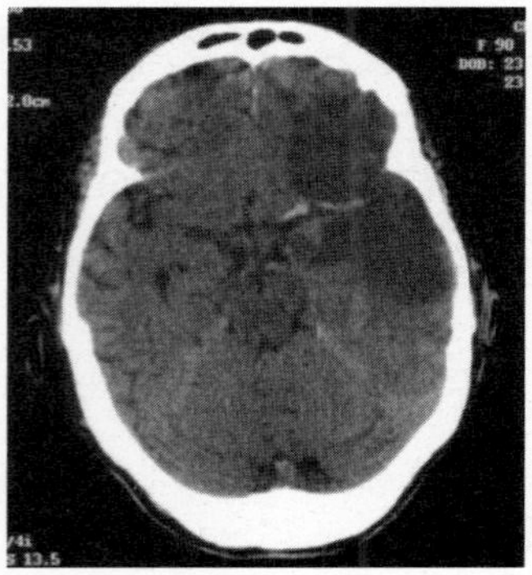

Fig. 3 CT scan showing an acute middle cerebral territory infarction within a few hours of onset of the neurological deficit. (Note the increased density in the left middle cerebral artery representing a thrombus.)

It should be emphasized that a negative CT or MRI scan in a patient with a clinical acute stroke does not mean that the patient has not had a stroke. It just means that imaging has not detected an area of infarction (Figs 3 and 4).

Later imaging findings

There is progressive development of a low-attenuation area on CT scanning, or a high *T2* signal area on MRI scanning, in the area of damage. There may also be some swelling around the area, representing oedema with effacement of sulci and ventricles. It may be impossible to identify those areas that are truly infarcted and the area, which is ischaemic and may recover, called the 'ischaemic penumbra'. Over a period of a week or more the area of infarction matures with the development of a progressively better defined area of low attenuation, and loss of volume in the damaged area over time.

Intravenous contrast is frequently used when the nature of pathology in patients with cerebral infarction and its differential diagnosis from a mass lesion is in doubt. This will demonstrate increased vascularity of tissues and areas where the normal blood–brain barrier is disrupted; normal cerebral tissue will not enhance and the tight junctions of the normal blood–brain barrier will not allow contrast into the cerebral tissues. In areas of ischaemia or infarction there is diffuse cortical enhancement in ischaemic/infarcted areas. It is possible to confuse these appearances with tumours.

Intracranial haemorrhage

Primary intracranial bleeding (**PICH**) into the brain parenchyma is easily detected on CT scanning. Blood appears as an area of high attenuation on CT imaging (Fig. 5).

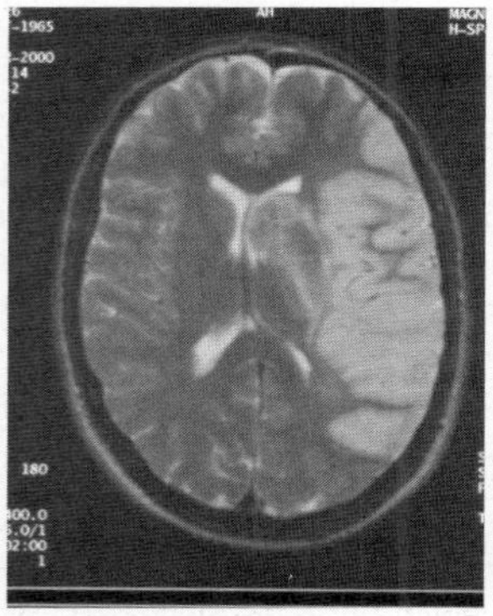

Fig. 4 *T2*-weighted MRI scan of the same patient as in Fig. 3 showing the extensive high *T2* signal affecting grey and white matter in the left middle cerebral artery territory.

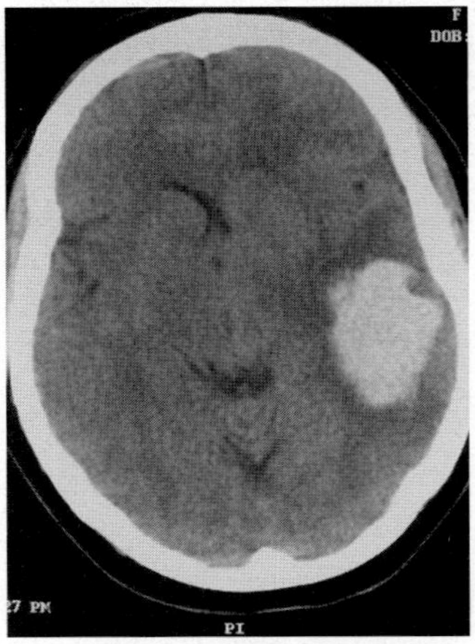

Fig. 5 CT scan of a patient with an acute stroke due to a large intracerebral haemorrhage in the left temporal lobe.

Blood in the subarachnoid space may be visible around the base of the brain as a white layer, in contrast to the normal dark outline of CSF in the basal cisterns. If a scan is carried out within 24 h of a subarachnoid haemorrhage (**SAH**) it will usually be positive for the presence of blood (about 90 per cent of the time); with a large SAH, the scan will remain positive for 3 to 4 days (Fig. 6).

However, the lack of visible blood on CT scanning does not exclude the diagnosis of a subarachnoid haemorrhage. Lumbar puncture is essential if this diagnosis is suspected and if CT is negative or equivocal. The key clinical differential diagnosis is of acute meningitis or a very small subarachnoid haemorrhage undetectable on CT, which may result from rupture of an intracranial aneurysm.

After an intracranial haemorrhage, a decision must be made whether to investigate patients in more detail for the presence of an underlying lesion responsible for the haemorrhage, such as an intracranial aneurysm or vascular malformation. Selection of which patients should undergo cerebral angiography is sometimes difficult. However, all patients under about 50 years of age with primary intracranial bleeding but without a typical hypertensive bleed should probably undergo cerebral angiography to search for an underlying vascular malformation. All patients who survive a primary subarachnoid haemorrhage and who are in good condition should undergo cerebral angiography to detect the presence of an berry aneurysm that may be responsible for the haemorrhage. Recently ruptured aneurysms have a high likelihood of re-bleeding, as much as 30 per cent in the first 4 weeks after the haemorrhage. Without treatment there is a 50 per cent mortality by 6 months. These lesions should be detected and treated if possible,

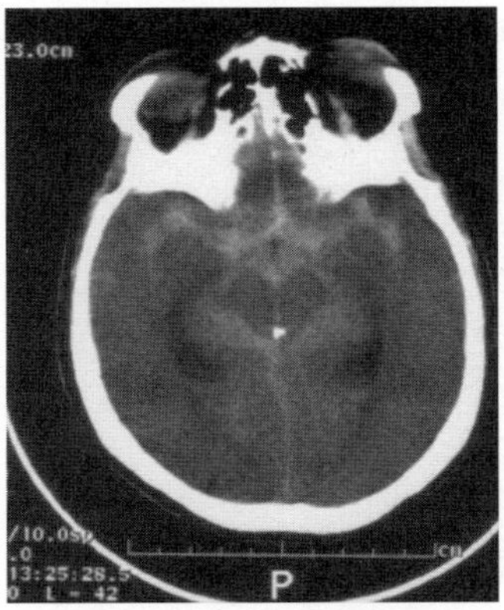

Fig. 6 CT scan of a patient with a subarachnoid haemorrhage. Note that the CSF surrounding the brainstem and in the basal cisterns is high attenuation (bright) compared with normal CSF, which on CT would be dark.

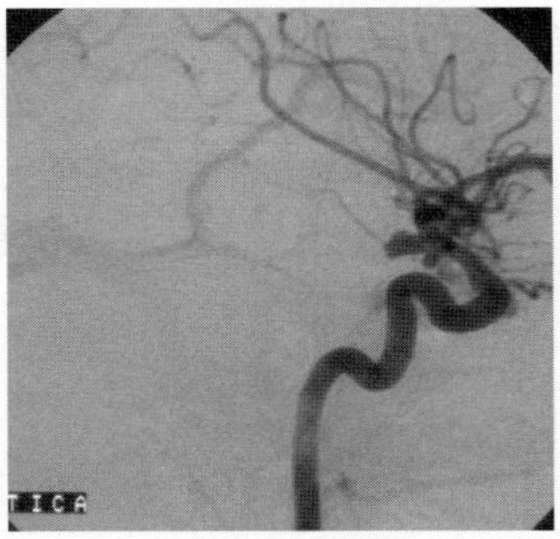

Fig. 7 Digital subtraction cerebral angiogram showing two aneurysms arising from the internal carotid artery that had recently ruptured.

either by surgical clipping or the newer endovascular techniques using detachable platinum coils (Figs 7 and 8). A recent large multicentre randomized trial has reported improved 1 year outcomes following coil treatment compared with surgical clipping.

Other vascular diseases

Cerebral venous sinus thrombosis

This uncommon, potentially fatal, condition presents with severe headache, confusion, variable neurological deficits, and sometimes seizures. Since it can be difficult to detect on CT scanning, the diagnosis is best made on MRI scanning, where a lack of flow void is seen on some sequences (*T*2-weighted) and a high signal on *T*1-weighted sequences is seen in affected dural sinuses. Flow-sensitive MRI sequences demonstrate the obstructed sinus well. Anticoagulation treatment is urgently required since progression of the thrombosis can lead to intracerebral haemorrhage and fatal venous infarction (Figs 9 and 10).

Inflammatory diseases of the nervous system

Multiple sclerosis

The most common neurological disease after stroke is multiple sclerosis. Imaging plays a crucial role in the diagnosis of this condition. However, it is important to understand that MRI alone cannot provide the diagnosis. The investigation must be placed in the context of the clinical presentation and the history and findings on neurological examination.

When patients present with symptoms of spinal cord disease, MRI of the brain and spine is indicated. The whole spinal cord is imaged to ensure that no spinal cord compressive lesion is responsible for the neurological condition. An inflammatory plaque will be seen in the spinal cord, particularly in the cervical cord, in a number of cases (Fig. 11); although failure to identify such a lesion does not mean that one is not present. Current imaging will not detect all spinal or indeed all brain lesions. However, imaging of the brain in patients with a spinal cord lesion is helpful in determining the presence of further lesions in the brain, thereby indicating a multifocal pathology. The difficulty comes in older patients over 45 years of

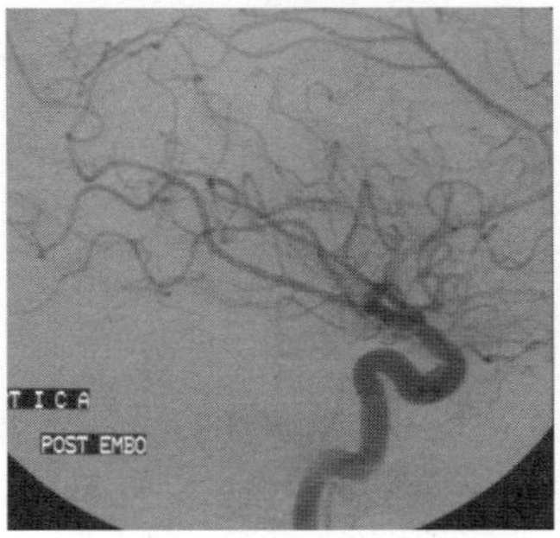

Fig. 8 Digital subtraction cerebral angiogram following placement of detachable platinum coils in the aneurysm to occlude the flow and prevent re-bleeding.

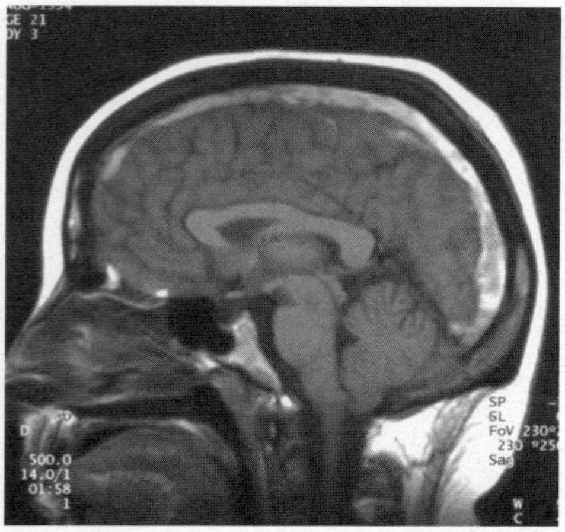

Fig. 9 Sagittal *T*1-weighted MRI scan showing a high signal in the superior sagittal sinus representing an extensive clot throughout the sinus. This 30-year-old woman presented with severe headaches, a depressed level of consciousness, and papilloedema.

age, where the frequency of incidental lesions in the brain presumed to be due to age-related vascular pathology becomes much more common. The pattern and extent of the white-matter lesions in patients with multiple sclerosis often characteristically affect the corpus callosum and deep white matter. However, it has again to be emphasized that the diagnosis of multiple sclerosis must not be based purely on imaging findings, attacks must be disseminated in time as well as location in the nervous system. An incorrect diagnostic label has profound consequences for the patient (Figs 12 and 13).

Neoplasms

Primary intracranial tumours

Primary intracranial tumours can be divided into those arising outside the brain and those arising in the cerebral substance (intra-axial or extra-axial). The range of pathology of the two locations is fundamentally different, as is often the prognosis. The primary objective of neuroimaging is to establish whether a mass lesion is present and to determine whether the lesion is intra- or extra-axial.

Extrinsic brain tumours

The most common tumours arising from structures outside the brain are meningiomas and acoustic schwannomas arising from the VIIIth nerve (frequently called 'acoustic neuroma'). Both these tumours are usually benign and present with symptoms of local pressure: VIIIth cranial nerve tumours can produce sensorineural deafness and/or sometimes dizziness, while meningiomas over the cerebral convexity may cause seizures.

The imaging characteristics of meningiomas and acoustic neuromas are similar. CT scans usually show a slight hyperdense mass causing local displacement of cerebral tissue. Masses generally enhance uniformly following the administration of intravenous contrast, although they may occasionally contain areas of low attenuation that may represent necrosis or occasionally cyst formation within the tumour (Figs 14 and 15).

Although MRI shows lesions that give a uniform intermediate signal on *T*1 and *T*2-weighted sequences, gadolinium administration yields uniform similar but intensely enhanced images (Fig. 16). Differentiation between

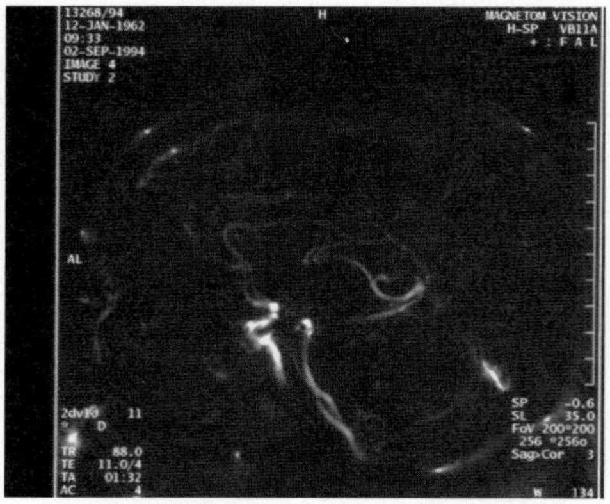

Fig. 10 Sagittal magnetic resonance venogram image showing the lack of flow in the superior sagittal sinus. This sequence is sensitive to flow and is useful in demonstrating whether a venous sinus or artery is blocked, if it is unclear from the normal sequences.

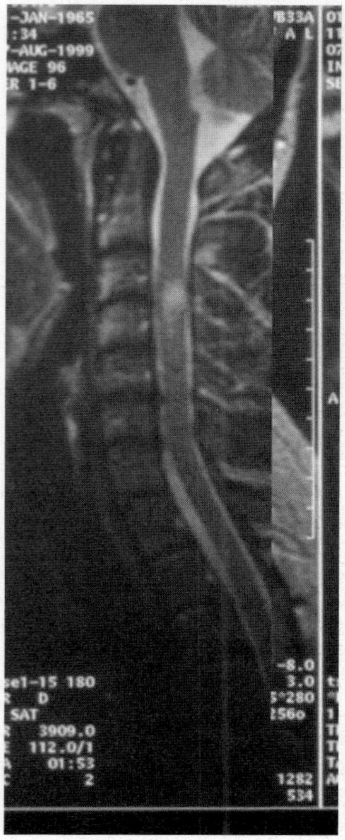

Fig. 11 Sagittal *T*2-weighted image of the cervical cord showing a high-signal lesion lying at the C3 level with some associated swelling of the cord. This is typical for acute demyelination.

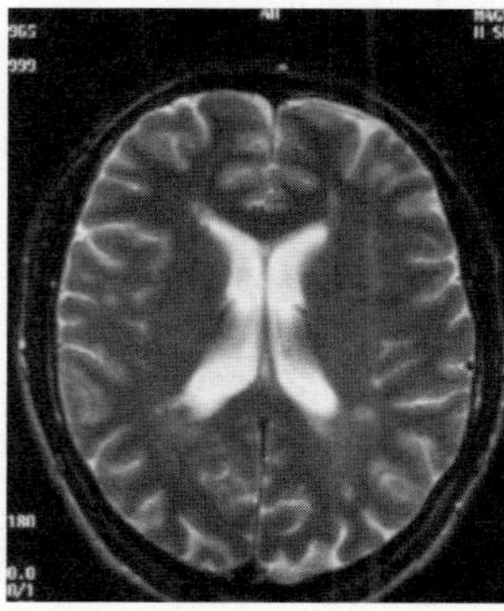

Fig. 12 Axial *T*2-weighted MRI showing high-signal lesions in the white matter around the ventricles and in both hemispheres.

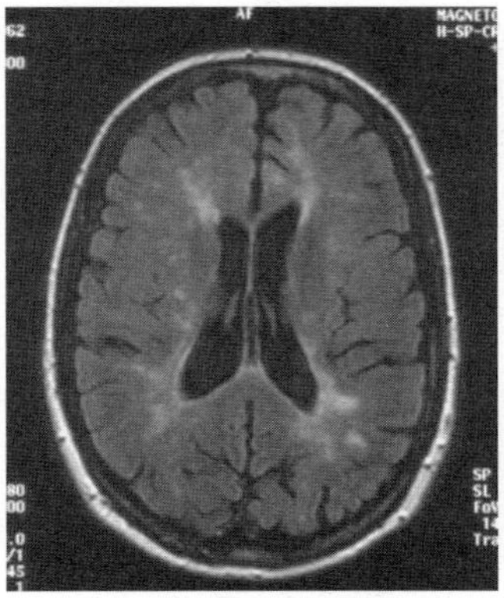

Fig. 13 This is known as a 'Flair sequence'. It detects lesions that give a high *T2* signal but suppresses the signal from the CSF in the ventricles, so that lesions adjacent to the ventricles are more evident.

intrinsic and extrinsic lesions is usually easier on MRI than on CT scanning because of the multiplanar capability of MRI compared with CT. MRI is also superior for surgical planning purposes, to establish the relationship of the tumour to adjacent structures such as the venous sinuses or the skull base.

Screening for acoustic schwannomas The most frequent presentation of an acoustic schwannoma is sensorineural hearing loss, but only a small percentage of patients with these symptoms will have an acoustic neuroma. Nevertheless, such patients should be screened to exclude the presence of a tumour. This is best achieved by a limited MRI scan, either a high-resolution *T2*-weighted or a 3D sequence. A modern MRI scanner can perform such a scan in less than 15 min.

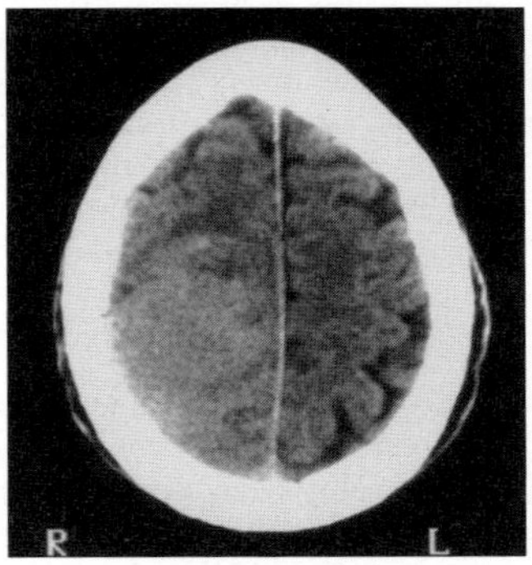

Fig. 14 Typical appearance of a meningioma. CT scan without contrast showing a high-attenuation mass lying over the surface of the brain.

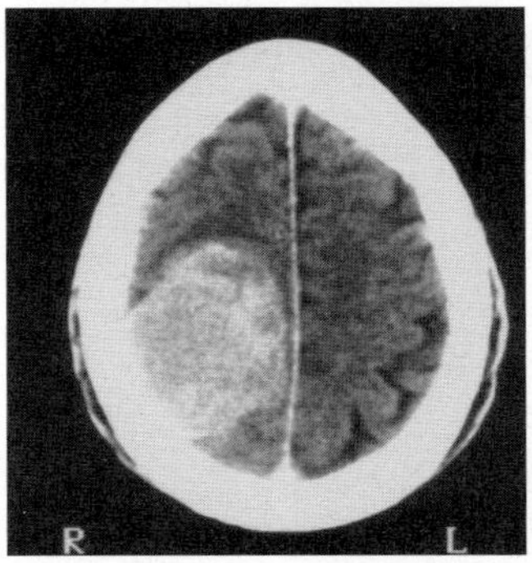

Fig. 15 CT scan after intravenous contrast showing the uniform enhancement of the mass lying over the surface of the brain.

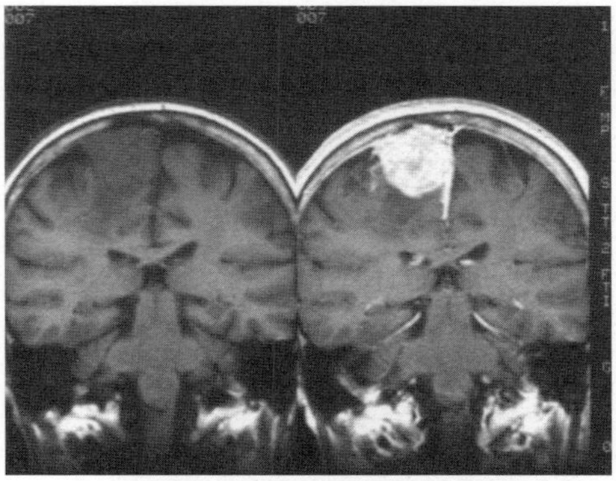

Fig. 16 Coronal *T1*-weighted MRI scan showing the typical appearances of a meningioma before and after intravenous gadolinium.

Intrinsic cerebral tumours

When a mass lesion arises from the brain substance, the range of tissues of origin is completely different. Most tumours arise from glial cells and are therefore classified as gliomas in broad terms. However, the range of biological behaviour of these tumours is very wide. Similarly, the imaging findings can vary greatly, reflecting this biological behaviour. The most common single brain tumour is the malignant glioma or glioblastoma multiforme. These tumours are also referred to as high-grade gliomas.

Glioblastoma multiforme These tumours show widespread infiltration and a mass effect on CT and MRI, with a high *T2* signal on MRI and a low attenuation on CT. The distinction between oedema and tumour infiltration may be difficult on imaging grounds.

However, the pattern of glioblastoma multiforme is usually very characteristic on imaging, with extensive enhancement following contrast on both CT and MRI scanning. Irregular margins of low-signal areas due to tumour necrosis are common. It is also common for cysts to form in association with both glioblastoma multiforme and lower grade gliomas (Fig. 17). Figures 18, 19, and 20 show the MRI appearances of a glioblastoma.

Astrocytoma These tumours are less aggressive than glioblastoma multiforme and range from benign lesions, which may remain stable for many years, to aggressive malignant lesions. Astrocytomas often form cysts and are seen in children as what are termed 'pilocytic astrocytomas'. These are often benign. The imaging findings show a diffuse mass effect on CT and

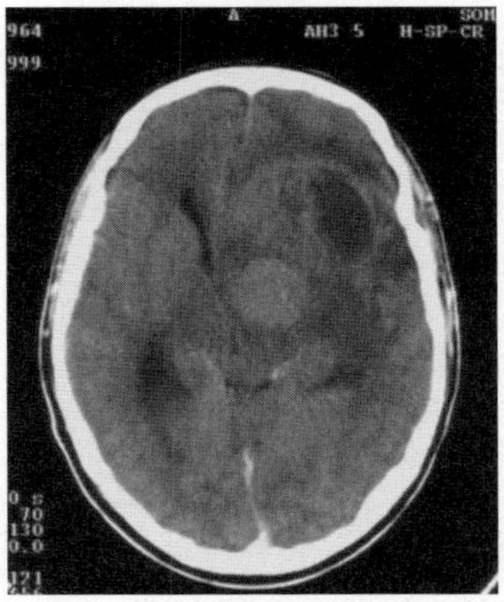

Fig. 17 Contrast-enhanced CT scan showing a large, deeply situated mass in the left hemisphere, with considerable enhancement postcontrast and a cystic or necrotic component with a low-attenuation area. This lesion was confirmed as a glioblastoma multiforme.

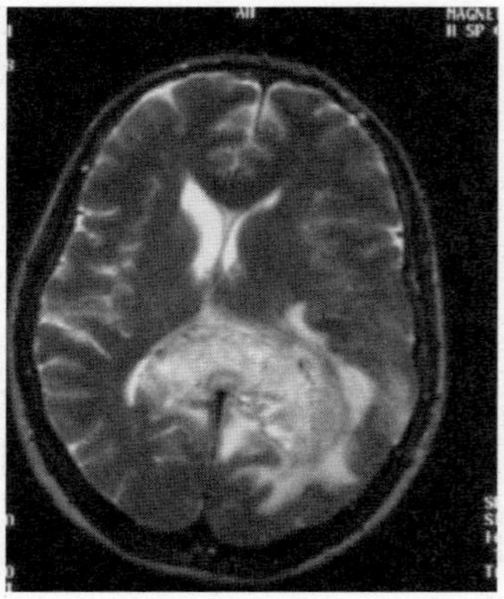

Fig. 18 Axial *T*2-weighted image of a large glioblastoma involving the corpus callosum.

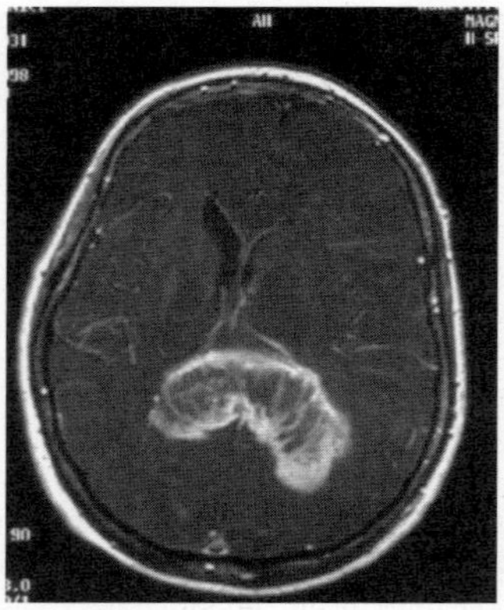

Fig. 19 Contrast-enhanced axial *T*1-weighted MRI image of glioblastoma showing marked irregular contrast enhancement of the margins of the tumour, with lack of central enhancement reflecting the extensive necrosis that is often a feature of these tumours.

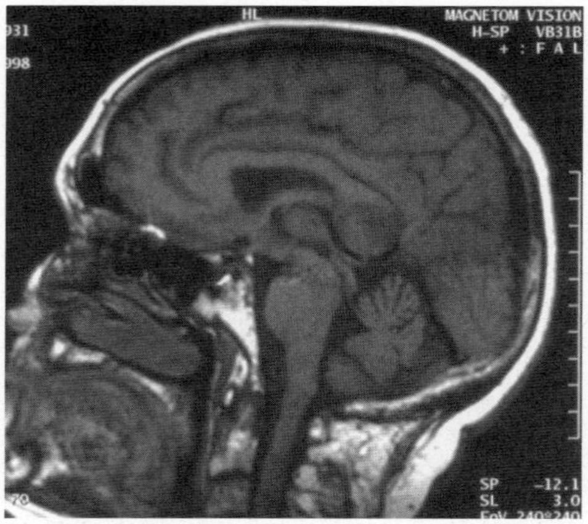

Fig. 20 Sagittal *T*1-weighted image without contrast showing the marked enlargement of the splenium of the corpus callosum depicted in the same patient as Figs 18–19.

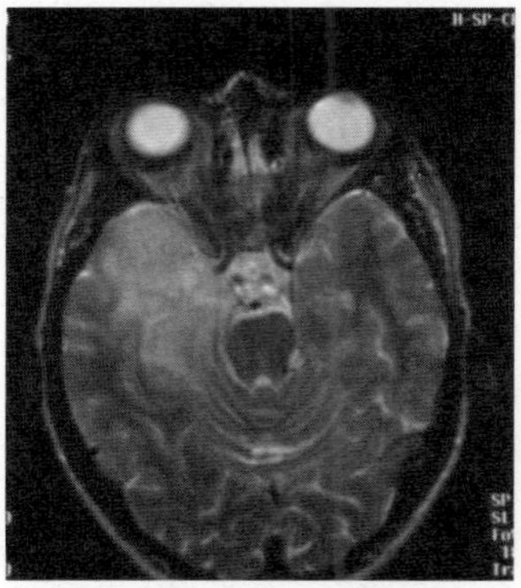

Fig. 21 Axial *T*2-weighted MRI showing a diffuse high-signal lesion in the right temporal lobe with a diffuse mass effect and sulcal effacement. These are typical appearances for a low-grade glioma. Although the differential diagnosis includes herpes encephalitis, the clinical presentation is completely different.

MRI, with low attenuation on CT and on *T*1-weighted MRI sequences but a high signal on *T*2-weighted MRI. Enhancement is very variable; sometimes there is considerable enhancement in pilocytic astrocytoma in children but often little in the way of enhancement in many low-grade astrocytomas in adults (Fig. 21).

Oligodendroglioma These tumours are the most benign of the intrinsic cerebral tumours. They often present with seizures rather than neurological deficit. Their radiological hallmark is calcification, best detected on CT scanning. Calcification may be invisible on MRI. The time course of these tumours may be very long, often evolving over 10 to 20 years. Oligodendrogliomas may remain static for long periods (Figs 22 and 23).

Posterior fossa tumours Intrinsic posterior fossa tumours are the most common intracranial tumours in children. The most common lesion is a medulloblastoma (Fig. 24). These usually arise in or near the midline posterior fossa in relation to the cerebellar vermis, they account for about 75 per cent of posterior fossa tumours in children. Other tumours commonly encountered are ependymomas and pilocytic astrocytomas, both of which have a better prognosis than medulloblastomas. Medulloblastomas and ependymomas commonly metastasize down the spinal canal, producing what are known as 'drop metastases' to the lumbar or sacral region.

Other intracranial tumours *Colloid cyst* This is a very characteristic benign lesion that arises at the foramen of Munro and causes obstructive hydrocephalus. Colloid cysts are usually readily detectable on CT and MRI and absolutely characteristic in their position, though the attenuation and signal characteristics can vary quite widely (Fig. 25).

Pituitary region tumours MRI is the investigation of choice for suspected pituitary lesions. CT is a second best imaging modality.

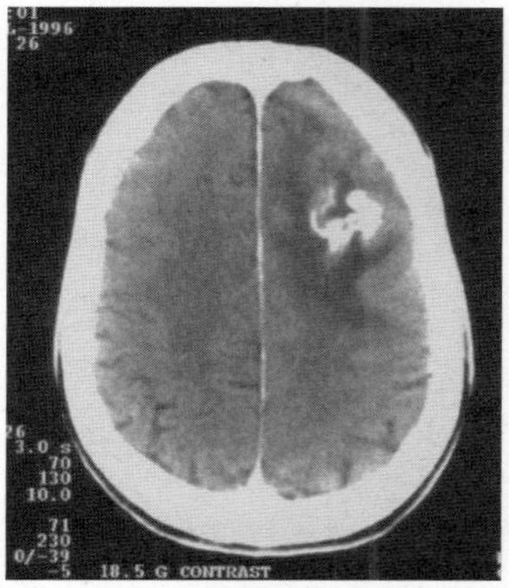

Fig. 22 CT scan of a partially calcified oligodendroglioma in the left frontal lobe.

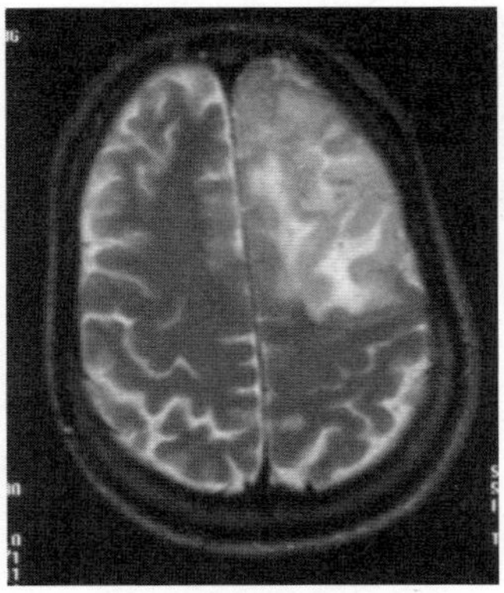

Fig. 23 MRI scan of the same pathology as in Fig. 22 with a diffuse high signal throughout the left frontal lobe.

These tumours, which arise outside the brain itself, are associated with a characteristic range of pathology. The most common lesion is a non-functioning pituitary adenoma, followed by hormonally active tumours, namely Cushing's disease (producing ACTH), prolactinomas, growth-hormone-secreting tumours (acromegaly). All these have similar characteristics, but their size varies widely: ACTH-secreting adenoma are usually very small and may not be detectable even on high-quality MRI imaging. Non-functioning adenomas tend to present late, often with visual loss and/or pituitary failure due to the large size and optic chiasmal compression (Figs 26 and 27).

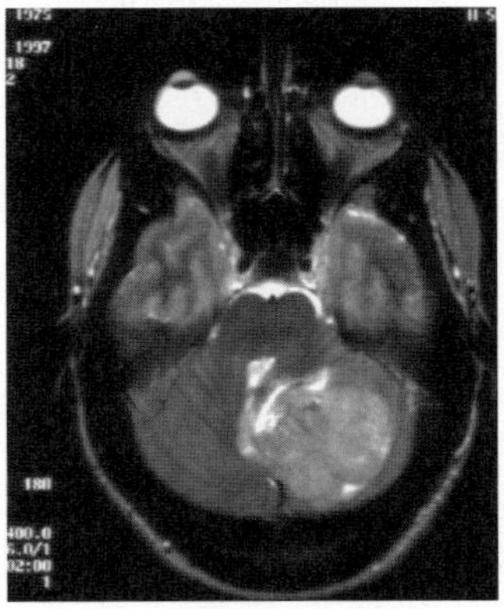

Fig. 24 Large medulloblastoma in the left cerebellar hemisphere demonstrated on *T*2-weighted MRI causing severe compression of the fourth ventricle.

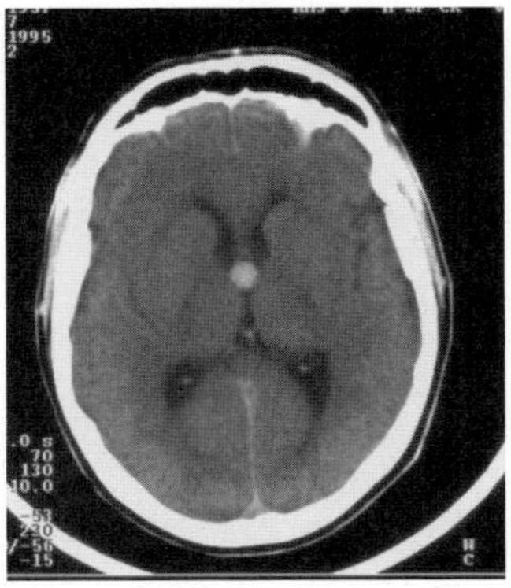

Fig. 25 CT scan showing the typical appearance of a colloid cyst arising at the foramen of Munro.

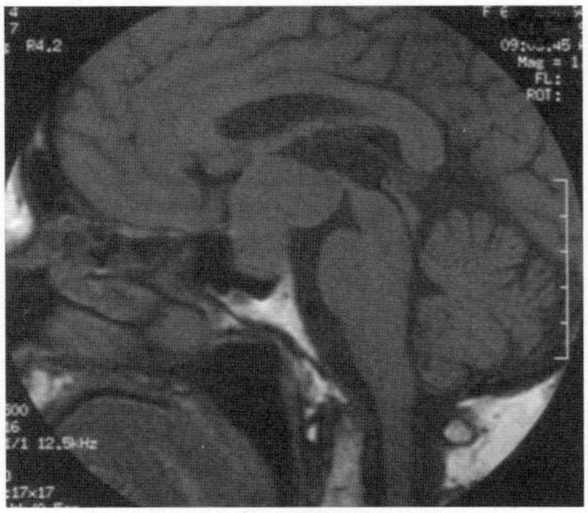

Fig. 26 Sagittal *T*1-weighted MRI showing a large pituitary adenoma extending into the suprasellar cistern.

Craniopharyngioma This specific benign tumour arises in the hypothalamic region usually in young patients, and presents with either visual loss and/or pituitary failure. The characteristic findings on CT are calcification, which may also be seen on plain skull films. There is often a cystic as well as a solid component to the lesion.

Brainstem gliomas These relatively uncommon tumours occur at a relatively young age. However, because of their location there is no prospect of any surgical approach and if any treatment is appropriate, it is usually radiotherapy. Brainstem gliomas may vary widely in their aggressiveness, from rapidly progressive lesions behaving like glioblastomas to indolent lesions that may remain static for many years (Fig. 28).

Secondary cerebral tumours

These are amongst the most common intracranial tumours and may be the presenting feature in some patients. Lung, breast, and gastrointestinal tumours as well as melanomas especially metastasize to the brain.

Secondary tumours may be solitary or multiple and are fairly characteristic on the imaging, with intracranial masses surrounded by oedema and frequently with enhancement after intravenous contrast (Fig. 29). The differential diagnosis of multiple ring-enhancing lesions in the brain is between cerebral metastases and abscesses. Sometimes this distinction cannot be made on imaging grounds and other evidence of the underlying cause must be sought; if necessary, biopsy or aspiration may be required.

Meningeal deposits of primary or secondary tumours are relatively uncommon, but they do occur and may be difficult to detect. MRI with gadolinium enhancement is the most sensitive detection method if the cerebrospinal fluid examination is negative for abnormal cells.

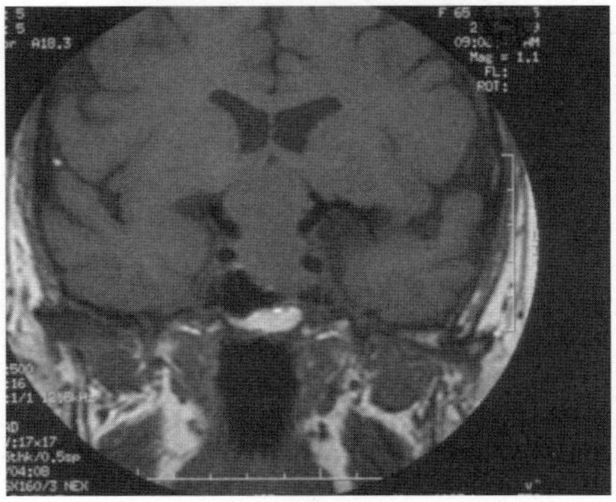

Fig. 27 Coronal *T*1-weighted MRI showing a large pituitary adenoma extending into the suprasellar cistern.

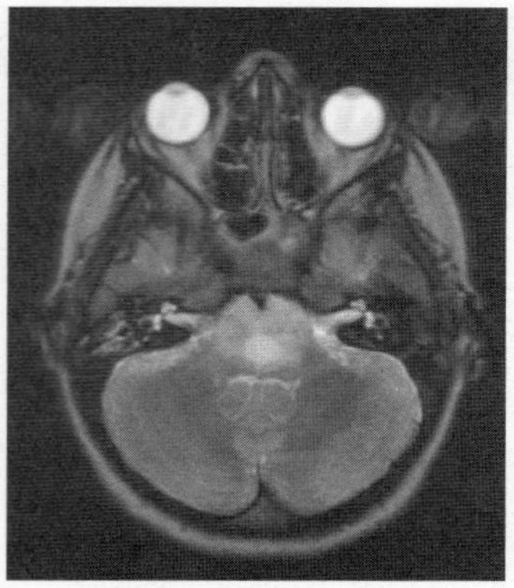

Fig. 28 Brainstem glioma shown on axial *T2*-weighted MRI with a diffuse high signal within the pons causing a local mass effect.

Intracranial infections

Although intracranial infections are less common than tumours, it is vitally important that they be detected as urgent and definitive diagnosis and treatment is essential to their effective management.

Bacterial infections

Pyogenic brain abscesses may be single or multiple. In the early stage they may not be particularly well defined, but by the time they present for scanning they often show a characteristic ring-enhancing mass surrounded by oedema (Fig. 30). If a pyogenic abscess is suspected then burr-hole aspiration is mandatory to establish the diagnosis and to drain the abscess. Abscesses may be seen at various stages of evolution if associated with a septicaemic illness. The source is either due to blood spread, or direct spread from the infection in the paranasal sinuses or the mastoid.

Meningitis is not usually diagnosed by CT or MRI and lumbar puncture remains the method of choice. If imaging is performed, however, it may show a mild communicating hydrocephalus and enhancement of the meninges following intravenous contrast. Note that mild communicating hydrocephalus is not a contraindication to lumbar puncture (see below).

Subdural empyema

This is rare, but important, intracranial infection due to spread from a paranasal sinus infection. Pus accumulates in the subdural space causing a spreading cortical thrombophlebitis. Empyema is usually due to the anaerobic bacterium, *Streptococcus milleri.* Such abscesses are rapidly fatal if they are not treated aggressively with antibiotics and neurosurgical drainage. CT findings are those of a thin subdural collection of fluid, which spreads over

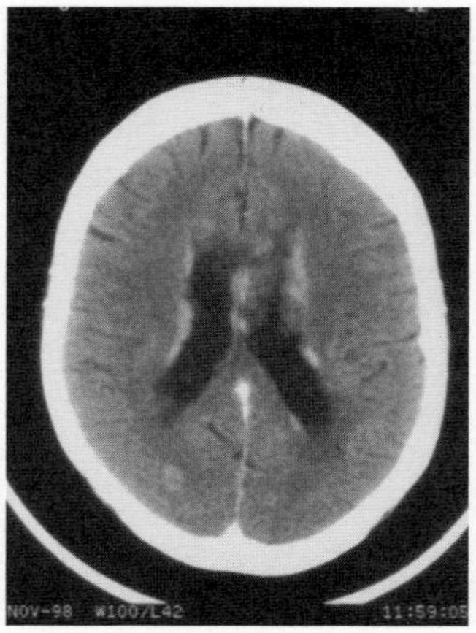

Fig. 29 Enhanced CT of a brain showing extensive secondary deposits around the cerebral ventricles from an oat-cell carcinoma of the bronchus.

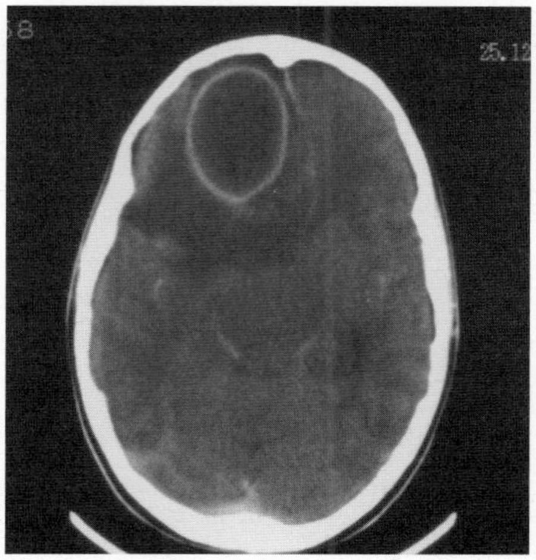

Fig. 30 Enhanced CT scan showing a large ring-enhancing frontal mass due to a pyogenic abscess. The differential diagnosis for these appearances is from a metastasis, or a glioma can occasionally appear similar.

the surface, and often alongside the falx. MRI is more sensitive in the detection of the small subdural collections, but it is unnecessary if the diagnosis is clear on CT scans (Fig. 31).

The underlying brain appears swollen and tight with the sulci obliterated, it will show moderate meningeal enhancement following intravenous contrast.

Tuberculosis

This may manifest itself as either abscesses or granulomas in the brain or a basal meningitis. If the meninges are involved there is almost invariably a degree of hydrocephalus.

Viral encephalitis

The most common cerebral viral infection is herpes simplex encephalitis (**HSE**). The imaging findings are often fairly typical, though CT scan changes may be very subtle during the early phase. CT scans show a mild swelling in the temporal region and diffuse low attenuation, as the focus of the pathology in HSE lies in the hippocampal region and medial temporal structures. MRI detects the disease more accurately and earlier and is the investigation of choice. When the disease is advanced or only partially treated it can present with a quite marked mass effect and irregular enhancement simulating an aggressive tumour.

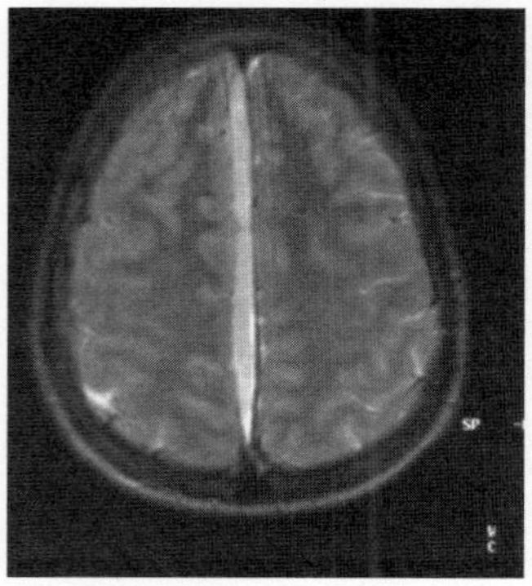

Fig. 31 Axial *T2*-weighted MRI showing a collection of fluid alongside the falx in a patient with a large subdural empyema.

Hydrocephalus

An understanding of hydrocephalus and its two main types is important to knowing whether it is 'safe to carry out a lumbar puncture' in a patient or not.

Obstructive or non-communicating hydrocephalus

This is the term given to enlargement of the ventricles caused by an obstruction, usually a mass lesion in the cerebrospinal fluid pathways within the brain (that is, between where the CSF is produced from the choroid plexus in the lateral ventricles and the outflow from the fourth ventricle). It is usually caused by a tumour pressing on the CSF pathways.

Communicating hydrocephalus

If cerebrospinal fluid escapes from the fourth ventricle but there is disturbance of flow around the basal cisterns over the cortex, or there is a failure of absorption of CSF, this is termed 'communicating hydrocephalus'. Communicating hydrocephalus occurs most commonly with a subarachnoid haemorrhage or meningitis and usually does not require treatment. However, because cerebrospinal fluid escapes from the fourth ventricle and circulates round the spinal CSF spaces, it means that it is safe to perform a lumbar puncture to measure and, if appropriate, lower CSF pressure. Lumbar puncture or drainage may also relieve intracranial pressure after a subarachnoid haemorrhage.

Congenital anomalies and paediatric imaging

Any detailed discussion of this subject is beyond the scope of this chapter, and the reader is directed to a specialist text such as Scott, Atlas.

Where available, MRI is the investigation of choice in infants and children presenting with suspected congenital anomalies of the brain. It provides the most information and avoids exposure of young patients to ionizing radiation. The main drawback in this age group is the need for sedation or anaesthesia. The most common indication for imaging in such patients is developmental delay or seizure disorders. It also plays a vital role in the imaging of a suspected, neonatal, hypoxic ischaemic insult and in elucidating the cause of cerebral palsy. CT is a reasonable alternative, but cannot be relied to detect all relevant pathology, particularly in hypoxic ischaemic injury.

A wide variety of congenital anomalies are possible. These range from minor abnormalities of neuronal migration, or localized areas of dysplastic cortex, to major anomalies of the whole brain and encephaloceles where there is an associated defect of the skull or spine such as a spina bifida. The most frequent is the Chiari malformation of the posterior fossa associated with cerebellar ectopia, the cerebellar tonsils lie below the foramen magnum.

Summary

Modern imaging techniques have revolutionized the diagnosis of neurological disease in the last 20 years. The techniques are likely to become more sophisticated and accurate with further extension into functional imaging techniques, both with magnetic resonance and nuclear medicine single-photon emission tomography (SPECT) and positron emission tomography (PET).

The contribution of these techniques to the efficient and effective diagnosis of intracranial and spinal pathology, together with the ability to effectively exclude structural disease, has had a huge impact on clinical practice. The development of interventional neuroradiological techniques for the treatment of vascular disease in the brain, particularly the endovascular coil treatment for intracranial aneurysms, may soon represent a further revolution in the management of patients with subarachnoid haemorrhages and intracranial aneurysms.

Further reading

Scott, Atlas (1996). *Magnetic resonance imaging of the brain and spine.* Lippincott-Williams and Wilkins, Philadelphia.

24.6 Inherited disorders

24.6.1 Inherited disorders

P. K. Thomas

There are many genetically determined neurological disorders, and other multifactorial disorders in which a genetic component can be detected. Inherited movement disorders, disorders of the peripheral nerves and muscles, and those aminoacidurias that are associated with neurological involvement are considered elsewhere, as is the question of genetic factors in the aetiology of conditions such as developmental abnormalities of the nervous system, epilepsy, migraine, Alzheimer's disease, and multiple sclerosis.

Hereditary ataxias

The classification of the hereditary ataxias remains a matter of controversy. A spinocerebellar degeneration may develop in disorders with a known metabolic basis. This category includes abetalipoproteinaemia (see Section 11), ataxia telangiectasia, and xeroderma pigmentosum (see Section 23). In general, the inherited cerebellar and spinocerebellar degenerations can be divided into examples having an early onset (under the age of 25 years), which are usually of autosomal recessive inheritance and of which Friedreich's ataxia is the commonest example, and the later onset cases of cerebellar degeneration that are most often dominantly inherited.

Early onset hereditary ataxias

Friedreich's ataxia

This disorder is an example of a spinocerebellar degeneration and is dominated by progressive ataxia with an onset in childhood or adolescence. The condition is inherited as an autosomal recessive trait and affects males and females approximately equally. The gene responsible has been localized to chromosome 9q13–q21 and is due to a trinucleotide repeat in a non-coding region of the gene for frataxin, a mitochondrial protein. Degeneration of the larger dorsal root ganglion cells occurs with consequent loss of the larger myelinated fibres in the peripheral nerves and degeneration in the dorsal columns. Degeneration is also evident in Clarke's column, in the spinocerebellar tracts, and in the corticospinal pathways. There is variable loss of Purkinje cells in the cerebellum.

The average age of onset is 11 to 12 years, but cases of later onset may occur. The initial symptom is almost invariably ataxia of gait, although foot or spinal deformity may antedate this. At first it is noted that the child walks awkwardly with a tendency to stumble and fall readily; in cases of early onset, walking may never have been normal. As the disease progresses, the gait slowly becomes more irregular and clumsy. The patient walks on a broad base and tends to lurch from side to side. Involvement of the upper limbs develops later, at first giving rise to clumsiness of fine movements, subsequently for all movements. A coarse intention tremor becomes obvious. The trunk is also affected, leading to oscillation of the body when standing or sitting unsupported. A regular tremor of the head (titubation) occasionally appears. Nystagmus is present in about one-quarter of the cases. Dysarthria of cerebellar type develops and may become severe enough to make speech almost unintelligible.

Initially weakness is not obtrusive, but this develops as the disease advances, beginning in the legs and later involving the upper limbs. It results from degeneration in the corticospinal pathways and tends to vary in severity between cases. The plantar responses become extensor, but tone is not usually increased because of the accompanying disturbance of the afferent fibres from muscle spindles. There may be mild wasting of the anterior tibial and small hand muscles related to loss of anterior horn cells. Bladder and bowel function is usually unaffected.

Loss of the larger dorsal root ganglion cells leads to impairment of the sense of joint position, vibration, and to some extent of touch–pressure sensibility, initially distally in the limbs. The impairment of proprioception superimposes a sensory element on the cerebellar ataxia. The tendon reflexes are depressed or absent.

Apart from occasional nystagmus, the ocular movements are usually intact. The pupils are unaffected. Optic atrophy is present in about one-third of cases and 10 per cent of cases develop sensorineural deafness with particular difficulty in speech discrimination.

Associated skeletal deformities are common, in particular foot deformities (pes cavus and pes equinovarus) and kyphoscoliosis. Contractures of the knees may develop in the later stages. Electrocardiography demonstrates widespread T-wave inversion and ventricular hypertrophy in nearly 70 per cent of patients. Echocardiography may suggest the presence of hypertrophic obstructive cardiomyopathy, but these findings are not specific and the ECG is a more sensitive investigation for the detection of cardiomyopathy. The ECG changes are present early in the disease and tend not to be associated with symptoms. Cardiac failure occurs late and is usually precipitated by supraventricular arrhythmias.

Although progressive dementia is not a feature of the disease, reduced intelligence is present in some cases. There is an increased incidence of diabetes mellitus in Friedreich's ataxia (10 per cent).

The disease is slowly progressive, the average age of death being in the latter part of the fourth decade. The foot and spinal deformities may require orthopaedic correction. Ultimately patients become bedridden. Death is usually from an intercurrent infection or cardiac failure.

Later onset hereditary ataxias (ADCA)

Autosomal dominant cerebellar ataxia

This comprises the main group of disorders within the adult onset hereditary ataxias. The age of onset usually ranges from the third to the fifth decades. Clinically, these disorders can be divided into three categories. Autosomal dominant cerebellar ataxia (ADCA) type I consists of a multisystem disorder with varying combinations of cerebellar ataxia, dementia, optic atrophy, disturbances of eye movement, pyramidal and extrapyramidal features, and peripheral neuropathy. Autosomal dominant cerebellar ataxia type II consists of these features plus pigmentary macular degeneration. Autosomal dominant cerebellar ataxia type III is a relatively pure cerebellar degeneration. Molecular genetic studies have identified a number of different mutations underlying autosomal dominant cerebellar ataxia, designated spinocerebellar ataxia, at present running from spinocerebellar ataxia 1 to spinocerebellar ataxia 7. Amongst these, spinocerebellar ataxia 1 to 4 and spinocerebellar ataxia 6 correspond to autosomal dominant cerebellar ataxia type I, spinocerebellar ataxia 5 (Lincoln ataxia) to autosomal dominant cerebellar ataxia type III, and spinocerebellar ataxia 7 to autosomal dominant cerebellar ataxia type II. Spinocerebellar ataxia 3 is Machado–Joseph disease. A number of these disorders (spinocerebellar ataxias (SCA) 1, 2, 3, 6, and 7) have been shown to be the result of unstable CAG (cytosine–adenine–guanine) trinucleotide repeats.

The category of Marie's delayed cerebellar atrophy was introduced to describe cases of hereditary ataxia with a later onset than Friedreich's ataxia in which the symptoms develop during the third or fourth decades of life or later. It is clear that Marie collected together a heterogeneous group of disorders, but his description served to emphasize the broad subdivision of the hereditary ataxias into the early and later onset groups. Cerebellar degeneration may be a feature in mitochondrial encephalomyopathies. Many instances of late onset cerebellar ataxia, particularly those without ophthalmoplegia or optic atrophy, are probably non-genetic.

Familial episodic ataxia

This comprises two disorders—episodic ataxia 1 mapping to chromosome 12p13 and episodic ataxia 2 mapping to chromosome 19p13. Both involve transient attacks of ataxia together in some cases with paroxysmal kinesogenic choreoathetosis which lasts for seconds to minutes in episodic ataxia 1 and minutes to hours in episodic ataxia 2. Chronic ataxia may develop in episodic ataxia 2. Episodic ataxia 1 has been shown to be due to mutations in K^+ channel genes. In both forms the attacks respond to acetazolamide.

Hereditary spastic paraplegia

Hereditary spastic paraplegia can be subdivided into a 'pure' form (Strümpell's disease) and others in which a variety of other features coexist, some of which are due to mitochondrial dysfunction. Strümpell's disease is genetically heterogeneous. It may display either autosomal dominant inheritance with mutations on chromosomes 14q and 15q or autosomal recessive inheritance. It may present during childhood or even with delayed motor development in infancy; in other cases the onset does not occur until adult life. It gives rise to difficulty in walking because of weakness and spasticity in the legs. The tendon reflexes are exaggerated and the plantar responses are extensor. Foot deformity may be present in cases of early onset. Some patients show a mild degree of cerebellar ataxia and sensory impairment in the legs of posterior column type. The disease progresses slowly and may later affect the upper limbs. Precipitancy of micturition or urinary incontinence may occur. Pathologically there is degeneration of the corticospinal pathways in the lateral columns of the spinal cord and some fibre loss in the gracile fasciculi. An X-linked form of hereditary spastic paraplegia also exists, related to mutations in the gene for proteolipid protein. It is allelic with Pelizaeus–Merzbacher disease.

Severe spasticity, if present, may be alleviated to some extent by oral baclofen or dantrolene. Continuous intrathecal administration of baclofen by an infusion pump is helpful in selected cases. The precipitancy of micturition may be improved by oxybutynin. Surgical correction of foot deformities is sometimes required.

Genetically distinct disorders in which a spastic paraplegia is associated with other clinical features include the Sjögren–Larsson syndrome, a recessively inherited condition which combines congenital ichthyosis and oligophrenia with a childhood onset spastic paraplegia, and the dominantly inherited disorder in which the paraplegia is associated with distal amyotrophy in the limbs resembling peroneal muscular atrophy. Hereditary spastic paraplegia can represent a mitochondrial disorder affecting the gene for paraplegin.

Disorders of lipid metabolism (see also Section 11)

Neurolipidoses

The lipidoses constitute a group of disorders characterized by the intracellular accumulation of a variety of different lipids. Some predominantly involve the nervous system; others primarily affect the reticuloendothelial system, but may also involve nervous tissue. They may be classified in terms of the particular lipid that is stored.

Niemann–Pick disease

This consists of a group of recessively inherited disorders in which there is an accumulation of lipid in 'foam cells' in the reticuloendothelial system. Types A and B, due to mutations on chromosomes p15.1–15.4, are the result of acid sphingomyelinase deficiency resulting in accumulation of sphingomyelin. Types C and D are related to a defect in the intracellular homeostasis of unesterified cholesterol. In type A, progressive mental deterioration and spastic paralysis in association with hepatosplenomegaly appear in the first 6 months of life, leading to death before the age of 3 years. Cherry-red spots are present at the maculae in 50 per cent of cases. Type B does not affect the nervous system. Types C and D resemble type A but the storage material consists of cholesterol and neutral lipids. Sphingomyelinase activity is normal.

Glucosyl ceramide lipidosis (Gaucher's disease)

Three variants exist, all recessively inherited, characterized by hepatosplenomegaly related to the accumulation of glucosyl ceramide in histiocytes as a consequence of a deficiency of the enzyme glucocerebrosidase. The type I adult onset form does not usually affect the nervous system but types II and III, with an infantile and juvenile onset respectively, and a more rapid progression, display widespread cerebral involvement.

Gangliosidoses

These comprise a group of recessively inherited disorders in which there is a combination of progressive dementia, epilepsy, and visual failure. They are related to defective ganglioside degradation. Several GM_1 gangliosidoses exist and are the result of an inherited deficiency of acid β-galactosidase. In the infantile form, which maps to chromosome 3p14.3, there is a generalized storage of GM_1 ganglioside affecting the brain, the viscera, and the skeleton. The onset is at birth or in early infancy, and initially is manifested by a failure to thrive and by hepatosplenomegaly. Later, mental and motor deterioration become evident, and a cherry-red spot may be present at the macula, related to retinal degeneration. Skeletal abnormalities, including abnormal facial features, have led to the condition being referred to as the 'pseudo Hurler syndrome'. Death takes place before the age of 3 years. A juvenile onset variant also exists.

The GM_2 gangliosidoses involve the storage of GM_2 gangliosides, which are largely confined to the nervous system. In the type 1 variety (Tay–Sachs disease), the disorder usually begins within the first 6 months of life. It is encountered most frequently in Ashkenazi Jews. Initially there is retardation of development which is followed by progressive dementia, hypotonic weakness, and blindness. There is a cherry-red spot at the macula. Later, seizures occur and terminally generalized spasticity develops. Death generally takes place in the fourth year of life. The disorder is related to an inherited deficiency of hexosaminidase A and the gene has been localized to chromosome 15q23–q24. Carrier detection is possible by a serum assay, and mass screening programmes have been undertaken in some countries. Antenatal diagnosis by amniocentesis is also possible. There is no specific therapy. The type 2 form (Sandhoff's disease) is similar clinically but involves a combined deficiency of hexosaminidase A and B. A form with juvenile onset also exists, as do phenotypes presenting as spinal muscular atrophy, spinocerebellar degeneration, or as a dystonic syndrome. The gene is localized on chromosome 5q13.

Neuronal ceroid lipofuscinosis

Under this heading are grouped a number of rare disorders in which retinal degeneration, progressive dementia, epilepsy, spasticity, and ataxia occur in various combinations. The age of onset may be infantile (Santavuori), late infantile (Jansky–Bielschowsky), juvenile (Spielmeyer–Vogt or Batten), or adult (Kufs). There is neuronal storage of lipopigment, but the molecular basis for these disorders has not been established. The infantile, late infantile, and juvenile forms are all of autosomal recessive inheritance. The infantile, late infantile, and juvenile forms map to chromosome 1p, 11p, and 16p respectively.

Leucodystrophies

These disorders are characterized by a diffuse disintegration of white matter in the central nervous system and sometimes also by segmental demyelination in the peripheral nerves. The cell bodies of the neurones are generally spared, although both myelin sheaths and axons show destruction in the white matter lesions.

Metachromatic leucodystrophy (sulphatide lipidosis)

The most common variant is the late infantile type which usually begins in the third year of life with weakness and ataxia in the limbs. Subsequently a progressive dementia supervenes, seizures may occur, and in some instances optic atrophy develops. The tendon reflexes may be depressed or absent in those patients in whom peripheral nerve involvement is prominent. Nerve conduction velocity is reduced. Death sometimes occurs after a course of a few months, but occasionally after as long as 5 or 6 years. Terminally the affected children are demented, with a spastic tetraplegia, and are often blind.

The term metachromatic leucodystrophy is derived from the presence of galactosyl sulphatide in the affected tissues. This stains metachromatically with dyes such as cresyl violet and toluidine blue. It may be demonstrated within cells in fresh specimens of urine and also within Schwann cells and macrophages in biopsies of the peripheral nerves or rectal wall. The disorder, which maps to chromosome 22q13–13qter, is inherited in an autosomal recessive manner, and is due to a deficiency of aryl sulphatase A. This can be demonstrated by assay on leucocytes.

Juvenile and adult onset forms of metachromatic leucodystrophy are also encountered, but are rare. Prenatal diagnosis by amniocentesis and assay of aryl sulphatase activity on cultured amniotic fibroblasts is possible in both the late infantile and juvenile forms. Variants related to multiple sulphatase deficiency and to deficiency of activator protein also occur.

Globoid cell leucodystrophy (Krabbe's disease)

This derives its title from the presence of large multinucleate cells containing galactosylceramide in areas of white matter damage. The condition begins at the age of 3 or 4 months as a failure to thrive. Developmental regression then becomes evident and the tendon reflexes are lost. As the disease advances, generalized hypertonus appears, together with various types of seizure, and optic atrophy. Death often occurs in the first year of life or it may be delayed into the second year. There are also rare late onset cases.

The peripheral nerves are affected, biopsies showing segmental demyelination and inclusions within Schwann cells. Nerve conduction velocity is reduced. This can be helpful diagnostically in suspected cases

The disorder is inherited in an autosomal recessive manner and is due to a deficiency of galactosylceramide β-galactosidase. It maps to chromosome 14q21–q31. This may be demonstrated by assays on leucocytes or serum.

Adrenoleucodystrophy and adrenomyeloneuropathy (see Chapter 24.10)

These are a group of conditions that give rise to widespread demyelination in the brain with an onset during childhood, and cases of adrenoleucodystrophy can be separated by virtue of X-linked inheritance and associated adrenal insufficiency with features resembling those of Addison's disease. The disorder maps to chromosome Xq28. The affected boys exhibit a progressive illness characterized by the development of dementia, cortical blindness, ataxia, and spastic weakness in the limbs. A myeloneuropathy is sometimes the presenting deficit, or other phenotypes. Manifesting female carriers may show a mild spastic paraparesis or adrenal insufficiency.

Other rare demyelinating conditions

Pelizaeus–Merzbacher disease is an X-linked recessive disease that appears in early infancy. It maps to chromosome Xq22. Affected males develop ataxia and spasticity. It is due to the defective production of proteolipid protein in central myelin. Canavan's disease also develops in early infancy, is of autosomal recessive inheritance, and gives rise to progressive mental deterioration and megalencephaly associated with spongy degeneration of the white matter. It is related to a deficiency of aspartoacylase. Affected children show excessive urinary excretion of *N*-acetylaspartic acid. Prenatal diagnosis is possible.

Fabry's disease (α-galactosidase A deficiency) (see also Section 11)

This condition, otherwise known as angiokeratoma corporis diffusum, is an inborn error of glycosphingolipid metabolism. Neutral glycosphingolipids are deposited in various tissues as a consequence of a deficiency of the enzyme α-galactosidase A. The disorder is inherited in an X-linked recessive manner and maps to chromosome Xq21.33–q22. Affected hemizygous males develop a mild peripheral neuropathy which is manifested by the occurrence of severe pains in the extremities, often beginning in childhood. Cerebrovascular lesions also occur, either cerebral infarction or haemorrhage. Non-neurological features include corneal opacification, punctate angiectatic lesions over the lower trunk, buttocks, and upper legs, and cardiac and renal lesions. Heterozygous females may display mild manifestations, most usually corneal opacification.

Hereditary lipoprotein deficiency (see also Section 11)

The occurrence of peripheral neuropathy in hereditary high-density lipoprotein deficiency (Tangier disease) is discussed in Section 11. Hereditary abetalipoproteinaemia (Bassen–Kornzweig disease) is a recessively inherited disorder mapping to chromosome 2p24, in which a spinocerebellar degeneration may develop with features that bear some resemblance to Friedreich's ataxia. Other manifestations of this uncommon disorder include intestinal malabsorption, pigmentary retinopathy, and the presence of acanthocytes in the peripheral blood (see Section 22). In addition to the absence of serum low-density lipoproteins, the serum cholesterol level is substantially reduced. There is evidence that the development of the neurological lesions may be prevented by the administration of vitamin E orally, the absorption of which from the gut is impaired. A spinocerebellar degeneration has also been described in individuals homozygous for hereditary hypobetalipoproteinaemia, a genetically separate condition.

Isolated vitamin E deficiency

A spinocerebellar syndrome resembling Friedreich's ataxia has been described in recent years due to vitamin E deficiency in the absence of generalized fat malabsorption. Titubatory head tremor is a particular feature. The disorder is of autosomal recessive inheritance, maps to chromosome

8q13.1–13.3, and is due to a deficiency of an α-tocopherol carrier protein. Treatment is by vitamin E replacement.

Neurocutaneous syndromes

This category encompasses a number of disorders in which a variety of neurological disturbances are associated with cutaneous abnormalities.

Neurofibromatosis

Two major forms of this disorder exist. Both are of autosomal dominant inheritance. The gene for neurofibromatosis type 1 (von Recklinghausen's disease) is on the proximal long arm of chromosome 17 at q11.2. The gene product neurofibromin is a member of the GTPase activating family of proteins. The disorder has a wide range of manifestations, the most constant of which are focal areas of hyperpigmentation (*café au lait* spots), multiple neurofibromas, and Lisch nodules on the iris. Six or more *café au lait* spots are necessary for them to be considered abnormal. Axillary and inguinal freckling is frequent. The cutaneous fibromas are of varying dimensions and can be extremely numerous. At times, giant plexiform neuromas develop in which there is extensive subcutaneous overgrowth of neurofibromatous tissue. Massive mediastinal, pelvic, or retroabdominal plexiform neurofibromas can occur, as well as cervical paraspinal tumours and astrocytomas of the optic nerve, cerebellum, or brainstem. Malignant change occurs in a small proportion of peripheral neurofibromas. Mental retardation due to diffuse cortical dysgenesis is encountered in at least 10 per cent of patients. Other manifestations include congenital glaucoma, phaeochromocytoma, spinal deformity, pathological fractures of limb bones with malunion and pseudoarthrosis, and local gigantism of a limb. The neurofibromas are composed of proliferated Schwann cells and fibroblasts in a collagenous matrix through which course nerve fibres in an irregular manner.

Most cases of neurofibromatosis type 1 require no treatment. Neurofibromas causing pressure symptoms may necessitate excision and others may merit removal for cosmetic reasons. Rapid expansion of a tumour, the development of pain, and loss of neural function, will suggest malignant change. This most often occurs during adolescence or in young adults. The development of hypertension will require investigation for phaeochromocytoma, and spinal deformity may need orthopaedic attention.

The gene for neurofibromatosis type 2 (central neurofibromatosis) has been mapped to chromosome 22q12.2. The gene product merlin has homology with proteins at the plasma membrane/cytoskeleton interface. This disorder is characterized in particular by bilateral acoustic neurinomas (Fig. 1) but tumours may occur on other cranial nerves or spinal roots and also paraspinally. Meningiomas and gliomas may develop. A further feature is the occurrence of juvenile posterior subcapsular lenticular opacities.

Segmental neurofibromatosis affecting a restricted area of the body may be due to somatic mutation.

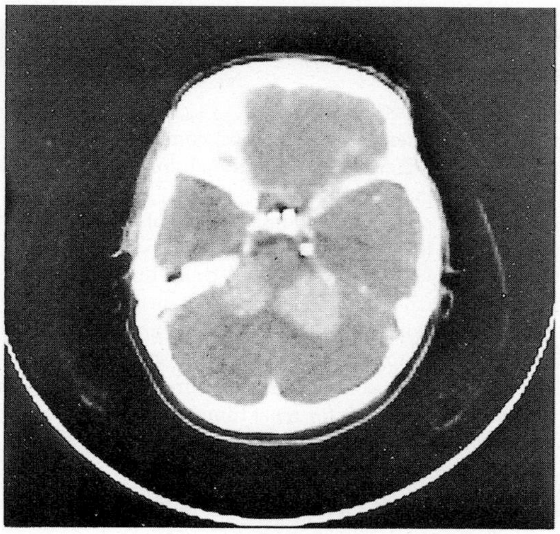

Fig. 1 Computed tomography scan showing bilateral acoustic neurinomas in a patient with neurofibromatosis type 2. She also had an astrocytoma of the thoracic spinal cord.

Tuberous sclerosis (Bourneville's disease, epiloia)

The features of this condition are mental retardation, infantile spasms, epilepsy, and the occurrence of retinal hamartomata and characteristic skin lesions. The disorder is dominantly inherited, but may be transmitted by individuals who are asymptomatic and who show only minimal clinical evidence of the disease. Isolated cases are frequent, comprising as many as 80 or 90 per cent of index cases. Many of them probably represent new mutations: others are transmitted by gene carriers with trivial manifestations. Genetic heterogeneity has now been established, with separate loci on chromosomes 9q34 (*TSC1*) and 16p13.3 (*TSC2*). The gene *TSC2*, which has a more severe phenotype, has been identified and its product, called tuberin, has the structure of a GTPase activating protein.

The earliest cutaneous lesions are irregular foliate areas of depigmentation over the trunk. These patches are readily identified when viewed under ultraviolet illumination using a Woods lamp. Facial angiofibromas ('adenoma sebaceum') are a second type of skin lesion which develop over the cheeks in a 'butterfly' distribution and on the forehead (Fig. 2) with multiple small warty elevations. Finally, a 'shagreen patch' may be present over the lower back. This consists of an area of elevated roughened skin with a yellowish tinge which has been likened to shark skin.

The cerebral changes give rise to mental retardation which is evident in early life and which may be static or involve a slowly progressive cognitive decline, often complicated by behavioural disorder. Infantile spasms or epilepsy with recurrent generalized or focal seizures may occur in association with mental retardation or in individuals of normal intelligence. The cerebral lesions, which are demonstrable by computed tomography or magnetic resonance imaging, are typified by nodular or tuberous masses composed of proliferated glial cells and enlarged distorted neurones. They may become calcified. They are found scattered throughout the cerebral cortex and also extend into the ventricles to produce an appearance that was considered to resemble 'candle guttering' when seen in pneumoencephalograms. Gliomas sometimes arise in these lesions.

Retinal tumours, termed phakomas, may be present, and cardiac rhabdomyomas occasionally arise as well as hamartomas of the lungs and kidneys. Polycystic disease of the kidneys may also be associated.

Treatment consists of control of the epilepsy and the management of the mental retardation and behavioural disorder. Many of the more severe cases require institutionalization.

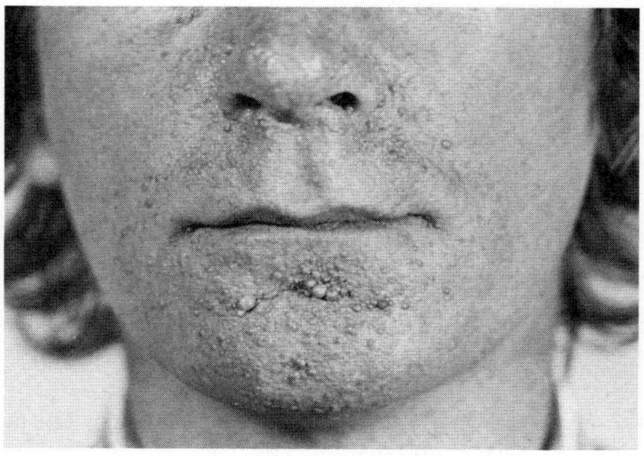

Fig. 2 Adenoma sebaceum in a patient with tuberous sclerosis.

Cerebelloretinal haemangioblastosis (von Hippel–Lindau disease)

This condition comprises the occurrence of vascular tumours in the retina and within the central nervous system, most commonly in the cerebellum and spinal cord. The inheritance is autosomal dominant in pattern. The disorder maps to chromosome 3p25–26.

The retinal lesions consist of angiomatous vascular malformations. The cerebellar lesion is a haemangioblastoma, often cystic, which may slowly expand and present with features of a cerebellar tumour. It may require surgical treatment. Such tumours may be associated with polycythaemia, related to the production of erythropoietin or a similar substance by the tumour. Haemangioblastomas may occur in the spinal cord and rarely in the cerebral hemispheres, as may renal cell tumours and renal and pancreatic cysts. Regular screening for renal tumours in patients and relatives at risk is an important aspect of management.

Ataxia telangiectasia (Louis–Bar syndrome)

The inclusion of this disorder with the neurocutaneous syndromes depends upon the coincidence of a progressive cerebellar degeneration with cutaneous vascular lesions. The inheritance is of autosomal recessive type and the gene is localized on chromosome 11q22.3–q23.1. Ataxia begins in early childhood and choreoathetosis and oculomotor apraxia appear later. Telangiectasia of the conjunctivae is present as a relatively early feature and later becomes evident in the pinnae, over the face, and in the limb flexures. Some patients show an immunoglobulin deficiency and recurrent infections, or the development of malignancies may complicate the clinical picture. Defective DNA repair after irradiation with X-rays is demonstrable in cultured skin fibroblasts. Affected children usually become unable to walk by the age of 12 years and death occurs during the second or sometimes the third decade of life.

Hereditary myoclonic epilepsies (see also Chapter 24.10)

A number of conditions exist in which generalized epileptic seizures and myoclonus are associated with a progressive degenerative neurological disorder occurring on a genetic basis.

Lafora body disease

This is the most clearly defined form of progressive myoclonic epilepsy. It consists of a combination of major seizures, myoclonus, and progressive dementia with an onset in late childhood or early adolescence, with death usually occurring before adult life is reached. Cerebellar signs may appear later in the illness. The condition is characterized by the presence of intracellular inclusion bodies found most consistently in neurones of the cerebral cortex and in the cerebellar dentate nuclei. They are also detectable in the liver, axillary sweat gland, and in skeletal muscles, all of which are convenient sites for biopsy in order to establish the diagnosis. These Lafora bodies are composed of a polyglucosan. The disorder is caused by an autosomal recessive gene, mapping to 6q23–25. Treatment is directed towards control of the epilepsy.

Progressive myoclonic ataxia (Ramsay Hunt syndrome)

This is a heterogeneous group, the best characterized form being Unverricht–Lundborg disease or 'Baltic myoclonus'. Stimulus-sensitive myoclonus develops from the age of 6 to 15 years, associated with mild mental retardation, followed later by dysarthria and ataxia. The disorder is of autosomal dominant inheritance. The gene maps to chromosome 21q22.3 and encodes for cystatin B, a cysteine protease inhibitor.

Mitochondrial encephalomyopathy

Myoclonus and ataxia, along with other features, may occur in mitochondrial disorders.

Sialidosis

The cherry-red spot–myoclonus syndrome consists of two autosomal recessive disorders (types I and II) with an onset in late childhood, adolescence, or early adult life that combine action myoclonus with mental retardation, ataxia, cherry-red spots at the maculae, and cataracts. Both types I and II are related to a deficiency of sialidase. Type II is associated with dysmorphic features.

The myoclonus in these inherited disorders may respond to combination treatment with clonazepam and piracetam.

Hereditary spinal muscular atrophies

The hereditary spinal muscular atrophies constitute a group of disorders that involve a selective degeneration of anterior horn cells and sometimes also of the motor nuclei of the lower cranial nerves. They can be classified in terms of the pattern of involvement and the age of onset. Only the more common varieties will be described.

Hereditary proximal spinal muscular atrophy

Acute infantile spinal muscular atrophy (Werdnig–Hoffmann disease) almost always begins within the first year of life. It may have a prenatal onset and is one cause of the 'rag doll' child syndrome of hypotonic muscle weakness in infancy. Progressive proximal muscular weakness and wasting, later becoming generalized and involving the bulbar musculature, usually leads to death before the age of 4 years. Cases with prolonged survival also occur (chronic childhood form). In hereditary juvenile proximal spinal muscular atrophy (Kugelberg–Welander disease) the onset is during childhood after the age of 2 years or as late as adolescence. The involvement of the proximal limb and trunk musculature mimics limb girdle muscular dystrophy, but fasciculation may be observed. The course is relatively benign, but progressive disability in adult life occurs in some cases; others remain relatively mildly affected. All three forms are of autosomal recessive inheritance and have been mapped to chromosome 5q12.2–q13.3. They appear to be due to allelic genes.

X-linked bulbospinal neuronopathy

This disorder, otherwise known as Kennedy's syndrome, consists of the development, commonly in the third or fourth decades, of progressive limb weakness and, later, a bulbar palsy. Contraction fasciculation of the facial muscles is usually present. Muscle cramps and upper limb postural tremor are often evident from early adult life. About 50 per cent of cases show gynaecomastia and some have diabetes mellitus. The disorder is due to a trinucleotide repeat expansion within the androgen receptor gene on the proximal long arm of the X chromosome at Xq21.3–q22.

Other miscellaneous disorders

A wide variety of other rare inherited conditions exist, of which the following deserve brief mention.

Hereditary optic neuropathy

Dominantly inherited juvenile optic neuropathy

This disorder gives rise to the insidious bilateral onset of optic atrophy during childhood with either mild or severe loss of vision. A central or centrocaecal scotoma may be detected. Electroretinography and visual evoked potentials demonstrate no loss of retinal receptors and suggest that the lesion affects retinal neuronal elements. There are no associated neurological abnormalities.

Leber's hereditary optic neuropathy

This disorder typically gives rise to acute or subacute bilateral visual loss in males between the ages of 18 and 30 years, although earlier and later ages of onset may be encountered. It may remain monocular for months or years. Initially there is enlargement of the blind spot and later this increases to involve central vision, producing a large centrocaecal scotoma. In the acute phase there is swelling in the nerve fibre layer around the optic disc with tortuous retinal arterioles and peripapillary telangiectasias. Later the disc becomes atrophic. In affected females the age of onset tends to be later and a multiple sclerosis-like syndrome may develop (Harding's syndrome). The disease is only transmitted by females and has recently been shown to be due to mutations of mitochondrial DNA.

Mucopolysaccharidoses (see also Section 11)

The mucopolysaccharidoses constitute a group of disorders related to deficiencies of specific lysosomal enzymes, involving an accumulation in various tissues of acid mucopolysaccharides and gangliosides, and the presence of mucopolysaccharides in the urine. In both the recessively inherited Hurler's syndrome and the X-linked recessive Hunter's syndrome, the skeletal and other manifestations may be accompanied by mental retardation and pigmentary retinal degeneration. Spastic weakness in the limbs may develop in Hurler's syndrome. Mental retardation is also seen in the recessively inherited Sanfilippo's syndrome. Entrapment neuropathies are a feature in some forms, related to the skeletal changes.

Subacute necrotizing encephalopathy (Leigh's syndrome)

Typically this label is applicable to a fatal encephalopathy that develops during the first 2 years of life with variable combinations of mental retardation, seizures, optic atrophy, cerebellar ataxia, and central respiratory failure associated with lactic acidosis. Pathologically there are necrotic lesions in the brainstem and a prominence of small blood vessels. Haemorrhage does not occur. The distribution of the lesions bears some resemblance to Wernicke's encephalopathy. Later onset cases with similar pathological changes occur. The disorder is genetically heterogeneous, but may be related to mutations in mitochondrial DNA leading to a deficiency of cytochrome oxidase. Pyruvate dehydrogenase and pyruvate decarboxylase deficiency may also be responsible.

Progressive neuronal degeneration of childhood with liver disease (Alpers–Huttenlocher syndrome)

This disorder, which is probably of autosomal recessive inheritance, begins at 3 to 15 months of age with developmental delay and failure to thrive. Recurrent vomiting and hypotonia are common, followed by intractable seizures. Death occurs at 10 to 90 months. Pathologically there is extensive neuronal loss and astrocytosis, particularly in the cerebral cortex, and fatty degeneration, cell loss, and fibrosis in the liver. An unidentified biochemical defect is assumed.

Infantile neuroaxonal dystrophy (Seitelberger's disease)

This is a rare, probably recessive condition that develops between the ages of 1 and 3 years and gives rise to progressive motor weakness from both upper and lower motor neurone deficits. It maps to chromosome 22q13–qter. Optic atrophy also occurs and death usually ensues before the end of the first decade. Degenerative changes are present in the brain and the spinal cord, the most striking feature of which is the occurrence of large axonal swellings in the grey matter of the brain and spinal cord.

Menkes' syndrome ('kinky' or 'steely' hair)

Menkes' syndrome is an X-linked recessive disorder in which developmental regression begins within a few months of birth. The gene locus is at Xq12–q13. Muscle hypotonus or hypertonus and seizures appear and are associated with abnormal hair. The scalp hair is sparse, stubbly, and greyish in colour. When examined under magnification, the hairs are seen to be twisted and display partial breaks. The serum copper and caeruloplasmin levels are low and the condition probably results from defective absorption of copper from the gut. Prenatal diagnosis is possible.

Lesch–Nyhan syndrome

This is an X-linked recessive disorder (see also Chapter 24.10 and Section 11) related to the absence of an enzyme of purine metabolism, hypoxanthine–guanine phosphoribosyl transferase. It maps to chromosome Xq25–q27.2. The salient features are overproduction of uric acid and consequent hyperuricaemia which are associated with various behavioural and neurological manifestations, including mental retardation, self-mutilation, choreoathetosis, pyramidal signs, and spasticity in the limbs. The neurological abnormalities develop in childhood and death usually occurs in the second or third decade from renal failure. Allopurinol may reduce some of the non-neurological consequences of the hyperuricaemia, but no treatment influences the neurological abnormalities, the mechanism of which is not understood. Prenatal diagnosis and carrier detection are available.

Cockayne's syndrome

This is of autosomal recessive inheritance and consists of the development in childhood of dwarfism, microcephaly, progeria, mental retardation, cataract, pigmentary retinopathy, and ataxia. There is cutaneous sensitivity to ultraviolet light. The cerebral changes are those of a leucodystrophy. A demyelinating neuropathy coexists.

Further reading

Baraitser M (1997). *The genetics of neurological disorders*, 3rd edn. Oxford University Press, Oxford.

Emery AEH and Rimoin DL (1997). *Principles and practice of medical genetics*, 3rd edn. Churchill Livingstone, Edinburgh.

Harding AE (1984). *The hereditary ataxias and related disorders*. Churchill Livingstone, Edinburgh.

Rosenberg RN *et al.*, eds (1997). *The molecular and genetic basis of neurological disease*. Butterworth-Heinemann, Oxford.

24.6.2 Neurogenetics

Nicholas Wood

Introduction

There has been dramatic improvement in our understanding of inherited neurological disease. It is clearly impossible to be comprehensive here, and a few examples have been chosen to illustrate some of these major developments. The genetics of movement disorders, especially Huntington's disease, are discussed in the context of identified genes causing neurological disease. However, the greatest challenge of the next few years will be to identify the genetic factors and environmental interactions involved in complex disorders such as Parkinson's disease.

Table 1 shows a much wider range of disorders. The rapid progress in this area, however, means that it cannot be comprehensive or up to date

Table 1 Inherited neurological disorders

	Gene nomenclature	Mode of inheritance	Locus	Gene	Mutation	Comments
Movement disorders						
Huntington's chorea	HD	AD	4p16.3	Huntingtin	Trinuc	
Wilson's disease	WND	AR	13q14.1	Copper transport-protein	Pm/Del	
Primary torsion dystonia	DYT1	AD	9q34	Torsin A	GAG-Deletion	Early onset, generalized, rarely isolated writer's cramp
X-chromosomal dystonia–Parkinson's syndrome	DYT3	XL	Xq11.2	Unknown	Unknown	Only found on the Philippines
Primary dystonia, mixed type	DYT6	AD	8cen	Unknown	Unknown	At present only described in two families
Primary dystonia, focal type	DYT7	AD	18p13.1	Unknown	Unknown	Founder effect in European populations
Dopa-responsive dystonia	DRD	AD	14q22	GTP-cyclohydrolase I	Pm	No mutations found in some cases
Dopa-responsive dystonia	DRD	AR	11p15.5	Tyrosine hydroxylase	Pm	Individual case reports
Paroxysmal dystonia	FPD1	AD	2q33–35	Unknown	Unknown	
Dentatorubropallidoluysian atrophy	DRPLA	AD	12p13.31	DRPLA protein	Pm	Rare in Europe
Familial Parkinson's disease	PARK1	AD	4q21	α-Synuclein	Pm	Very rare
Autosomal recessive juvenile parkinsonism	PARK2, AR-JP	AR	6q25–27	Parkin	Del, pm, rearrangements	Pathology—no Lewy bodies
Familial Parkinson's disease	PARK3	AD	2p13	Unknown	Unknown	North German founder effect
Familial hyperekplexia	STHE	AD	5q32	Glycine receptor	Pm	
Essential tremor	ETM1	AD	3q13	Unknown	Unknown	
Ataxias						
Friedreich's ataxia	FRDA	AR	9q13–21.1	Frataxin	Trinuc/Pm	
Ataxia with vitamin deficiency	AVED	AR	8q13.1–13.3	α-Tocopherol transfer protein	Pm	
Spinocerebellar ataxia	SCA1	AD	6p21.3	Ataxin 1	Trinuc	SCA1,2, and 3 comprise around 60 per cent of the dominant hereditary
	SCA2	AD	12q23–24.1	Ataxin 2	Trinuc	spinocerebellar
	SCA3/MJD	AD	14q24	Ataxin 3	Trinuc	atrophies
	SCA4	AD	16q22.1	Unknown	Unknown	Individual families
	SCA5	AD	11cen	Unknown	Unknown	Individual families
	SCA6	AD	19p13	Calcium channel	Trinuc	Allelic to FHM and EA2
	SCA7	AD	3p12–21.1	Ataxin 7	Trinuc	
	SCA8	AD	13q21		Trinuc	
	SCA10	AD	22q13	Unknown	Unknown	Pure cerebellar ataxia
	SCA 11	AD	15q	Unknown	Unknown	Pure cerebellar ataxia
Episodic ataxia with myokymia	EA1	AD	12p13	Potassium channel	Pm	
Episodic ataxia without myokomia	EA2	AD	19p13	Calcium channel	Pm	Allelic to FHM and SCA6
Neuromuscular disorders						
Spinal muscular atrophy:	SMA I	AR	5q11.2–13	Survival motor l'enfant (SMN)		
Infantile (Werdnig–Hoffmann)	SMA II	AR	5q11.2–13	SMN	Exon deletion	
Juvenile (Kugelberg–Welander)	SMA III	AR	5q11.2–13	SMN		
Adult	SMA IV	(?)	?			
Duchenne muscular dystrophy	DMD	XL	Xp21.2	Dystrophin	Pm and rearrangements	
Becker muscular dystrophy	BMD	XL	Xp21.2	Dystrophin		
Emery–Dreyfuss myopathy	EDMD	XL	Xq28	Emerin	Pm	
	EDMD-AD	AD	1q11-q23	Lamin A/C	Pm	
Myotonic dystrophy (Curschmann's disease)	DM	AD	19q13.3	Myotonin	Pm	
Fazioscapulohumeral dystrophy	FSHD	AD	4qter	Unknown		

Table 1 ***Continued***

Limb girdle myopathy	LGMD1A	AD	5q22-q31	Unknown		
	LGMD1B	AD	1q11–21	Unknown		
	LGMD2A	AR	15q15-q21	Calpain 3	Pm	
	LGMD2B	AR	2p16-p13	Unknown		
	LGMD2C	AR	13q12	Sarcoglycan	Pm	
	LGMD2D	AR	17q12-q21	Adhalin	Pm	
	LGDM2E	AR	4q12	β-Sarcoglycan	Pm	
	LGMD2F	AR	5q33-q34	Unknown		
	LGMD2G		17q11-q12	Unknown		
Myotubular myopathy	MTM1	Xl	Xq28	Myotubularin	Pm	
Central core diseases	CCO	AD	19q12-q13	Ryanodin receptor	Pm	
Malignant hyperthermia	MH	AD	19q12-q13	Ryanodin receptor	Pm	
Hyperkalaemic periodic paralysis	SCN4A	AD	17q23	Sodium channel	Pm	
Paramyotonia congenita	SCN4A	AD	17q23	Sodium channel	Pm	
Hypokalemic periodic paralysis	HypoPP	AD	1q31–32	Calcium channel	Pm	
Myotonia congenita	CLCN1	AD	7q35	Chloride channel	Pm	
Myotonia congenita (Becker)	CLCN1	AR	7q35	Chloride channel	Pm	
Neuropathies						
Charcot–Marie–Tooth:						
Type Ia	CMT1a	AD	17p11.2	PMP-22	1.5 MB duplication of 17p11.2	
Type Ib	CMT1b	AD	1q22–23	Po	Pm	
Type II (neuronal)	CMT 2a	AD	1p36	Unknown		
	CMT2b	AD	3q13-q22	Unknown		
	CMT2d	AD	7p14	Unknown		
Type IVa	CMT4a	AR	8q	Unknown		
	CMT4b	AR	8q	Unknown		
X-chromosomal	CMTX	XL	Xq13.1	Connexin-32	Pm	
Hereditary sensory neuropathy	HSN I	AD	9q22.1–22.3	Unknown		
Hereditary motor neuropathy	HMN II	AD	12q24	Unknown		
	HMNV	AD	7p	Unknown		
Hereditary neuralgic amyotrophy	HNA	AD	17q24–25	Unknown		
Tomaculous neuropathy (liability to pressure palsies)	HNPP	AD	17p11.2	PMP-22	1.5 MB deletion of 17p11.2	
Bulbospinal neuropathy	XBSN	X	Xq13–22	Androgen receptor	Trinuc	
Inherited tumour syndromes						
Neurofibromatosis 1 (von Recklinghausen's)	NF1	AD	17q11.2	Neurofibromin	Pm/Del	
Neurofibromatosis 2	NF2	AD	22q12.2	Merlin	Pm/Del	
von Hippel–Lindau disease	VHL	AD	3p25		Pm/Del	
Tuberous sclerosis	TSC1	AD	9q34	Hamartin		
	TSC2	AD	16p13	Tuberin	Pm	
Familial Alzheimer's disease	AD1	AD	21q21	Amyloid precursor protein	Pm	
	AD2	AD	19q13.2	ApoE and		
	AD3	AD	14q24.3	Presenilin 1	Pm	
	AD4	AD	1q31-q42	Presenilin 2	Pm	
Frontotemporal dementia with parkinsonism	FTPD-17	AD	17q21	Tau	Pm	
Familial Creutzfeld–Jakob disease	PRNP	AD	20pter-p12	Prion protein	Pm and rearrangements	5 to 10 per cent of CJD cases
Gerstmann-Sträussler syndrome	PRNP	AD	20pter-p12	Prion protein		Part of the CJD spectrum
Fatal familial insomnia	PRNP	AD	20pter-p12	Prion protein		Part of the CJD spectrum
Familial amyotrophic lateral sclerosis	SOD1	AD	21q22	Superoxide dismutase 1	Pm	20 per cent of hereditary ALS

Table 1 *Continued*

Familial spastic paraplegia	SPG1	X	Xq28	L1CAM		Complicated form
	SPG2	X	Xq21	Proteolipid protein	Pm and rearrangements	Allelic to Pelizeus–Merzbacher disease
	SPG3	AD	14q11.2–24.3	Unknown		
	SPG4	AD	2p24-p21	Unknown		
	SPG5	AR	8p12-q13	Unknown		
	SPG6	AD	15q11.1	Unknown		
	SPG7	AR	16q24.3	Paraplegin	Pm	
	SPG8	AD	8q23–24	Unknown		One family
Benign familial neonatal convulsions	EBN1	AD	20q13.3	KCNQ2	Pm	
	EBN2	AD	8q24	KCNQ3	Pm	
Familial nocturnal frontal lobe epilepsy	ADNFLE	AD	20q13	CHRNA4	Pm	
Febrile seizures	FEB1	AD	8q13	Unknown		
Febrile seizures	FEB2	AD	19p13.3	Unknown		
Febrile seizures	GEFS+	AD?	19q13.1	SCN1B		
Juvenile myoclonic epilepsy	EJM1	AD	6p21.3	Unknown		
	EJM2	AD	6p11	Unknown		
	EJM3	AR	15q14	Unknown		
Progressive myoclonic epilepsy of Unverricht–Lundborg type	EPM1	AR	21q22.3	Cystatin B, CSTB	A dodecamer repeat expansion accounts for around 90 per cent of disease alleles worldwide	
Lafora's disease	MELF	AR	6q23-q25	Laforin	Not all families link to 6q	
Neuronal ceroid lipofuscinosis—infantile, variant late infantile, variant juvenile	CLN1	AR	1p32	Palmitoyl protein thioesterase (PPT)		
Neuronal ceroid lipofuscinosis—classic late infantile	CLN2	AR	11p13	Pepstatin-insensitive protease		
Neuronal ceroid lipofuscinosis—juvenile	CLN3	AR	16p12	Novel membrane protein		
Neuronal ceroid lipofuscinosis—Finnish late infantile	CLN5	AR	13q22	Novel membrane protein		
Neuronal ceroid lipofuscinosis—variant late infantile	CLN6	AR	15q21	Unknown		
Neuronal ceroid lipofuscinosis—infantile, variant late infantile, variant juvenile	CLN8	AR	8p23	Novel membrane protein		Finnish disease
CADASIL	CADASIL	AD	19p13.1	Notch3	Pm	
Familial hemiplegic migraine	FHM	AD	19p13	Calcium channel	Pm	Allelic to SCA6 and EA2
Myoclonic epilepsy with ragged red fibres	MERRF	Mat	nt 8344	tRNALys		
Mitochondrial encephalomyo-pathy with lactatacidosis and 'stroke-like episodes'	MELAS	Mat	nt 3243 (nt 3271)	tRNALeu		
Leber's optic neuropathy	LHON	Mat	nt 11778 nt 14484 nt 3460	complex I subunit ND4		

This compilation of inherited neurological disorders is not complete. However, the speed at which progress is made in molecular genetic research causes such tables to become outdated very quickly. In case of doubt it is recommended that current publications, websites, or special centres be consulted.

For many if not for most of the diseases listed here, mutations in other currently unknown genes may also be responsible.

AD, autosomal dominant; AR, autosomal recessive; Del, deletion; Ins, insertion; Mat, maternal (mitochondrial) transmission; Pm, point mutation; Trinuc, trinucleotide-repeat expansion; X, X-chromosomal. CADASIL, cerebral autosomal dominant arteriopathy with subcortical infarcts and leucoencephalopathy.

Table 2 CAG repeat disorders

Disease	Chromosome	Protein
SCA1	6	Ataxin 1
SCA2	12	Ataxin 2
SCA3	14	Ataxin 3
SCA6	19	Calcium channel
SCA7	3	Ataxin 7
Huntington's disease	4	Huntingtin
DRPLA	14	Atrophin
XLBSN (Kennedy's)	X-linked	Androgen receptor

DRPLA, dentatorubropallidoluysian atrophy; XLBSN, X-linked bulbospinal neuropathy.

and current research publications should be consulted for the latest information.

Huntington's disease

This is one of the most common hereditary movement disorders with a prevalence of approximately 1 in 20 000. Onset is usually between the fourth and sixth decades, but onset in childhood and old age can also be seen. The initial mental and cognitive signs may be very subtle and progress insidiously. Family members often report a change in personality, a coarsening of sensitivities, and the expression of new, often antisocial, behaviours. Usually in parallel, but often not even noticed by the relatives, is the onset of choreic movements. These may start as a slight fidgetiness before semi-purposeful jerky movements develop.

As the disease progresses, dementia becomes more pronounced and the chorea more extreme; this may eventually upset balance and resemble an ataxic disorder. Finally, immobility occurs. The mean time from onset to death is approximately 15 years.

Huntington's disease may present with a parkinsonian syndrome and occasionally epilepsy, especially if the onset is early (under 20 years). Later onset may produce a predominant choreic illness with little cognitive disturbance. Before the identification of the gene it had been noted that age of onset and decreased severity increased in successive generations. This 'anticipation' was initially ascribed to bias but there is now a molecular explanation, which is discussed below.

There is no disease-modifying treatment currently available, but controlled trials are now being undertaken. These are largely based on findings from transgenic animals. Choreic movements may be controlled by sulpiride or tetrabenazine, but often patients prefer chorea to the parkinsonism that can result from this medication. Psychiatric disturbances should be treated as appropriate.

Genetics

The disease is autosomal dominant and therefore offspring are at a 50 per cent risk of inheriting the mutant allele. It is highly penetrant and very seldom are gene carriers ultimately unaffected. The gene was cloned in 1993 and was shown to be due to an expanded CAG repeat in exon 1 of a novel gene, subsequently called Huntingtin. The role of the protein is still unknown but progress has been made in evaluating the role of this abnormal CAG triplet repeat. This is in part because the same mutation is found in a group of neurodegenerative diseases (see Table 2). These diseases not only differ in their clinical features but the genes and proteins have very little in common other than this abnormal repeat. The codon CAG encodes glutamine and the term polyglutamine disorders has been coined. All the CAG repeat disorders so far described are the result of a relatively modest expansion within the coding region of the affected gene. Although the exact number of repeats on both the normal and the abnormal allele varies between the different diseases, the normal range of repeats is in the 20s, whereas for the disease-carrying allele, it tends to be over 40. All of these diseases are predominantly adult-onset neurodegenerative disorders, and most show evidence of anticipation. This is particularly seen with paternal transmission. The exact function of the polyglutamine tract remains unknown, but the repeat length is a major determinant of age of onset and probably also partly determines severity. Recent transgenic animal and cell culture studies strongly support the hypothesis of a gain of function for the allele harbouring the CAG expansion. It is unknown how the neuronal specificity of this disorder is brought about as both wild-type and mutant proteins are widely expressed. Moreover, the common link between an expanded polyglutamine tract and toxicity is unknown. There are at least 14 other proteins that interact with Huntingtin. An insight into the toxic pathway has emerged recently since mice transgenic for exon 1 of the human Huntingtin gene carrying over 100 CAG repeats developed abundant intranuclear inclusions. These pathological changes predated the neurological phenotype. Similar findings are reported in several of the other CAG repeat disorders. Identification of a common downstream pathway which could be manipulated by inhibitory drugs might offer the hope of improving the outcome from these disorders.

Dentatorubropallidoluysian atrophy

This is a dominant disorder reported mainly in Japanese families but is found worldwide. It has a variable phenotype including various combinations of ataxia, dystonia, myoclonus, other types of seizure, dementia, and parkinsonism. It may also closely resemble Huntington's disease. Onset ranges from late childhood to late adult life. The pathological features are incorporated in the name of the disease. This disorder was mapped to chromosome 12p in Japan, and the disease mutation is another expanded CAG repeat. The same mutation has now been described in other populations, but the disease is much less frequent than Huntington's disease outside Japan.

Parkinson's disease

There are several akinetic rigid syndromes with a clearly defined genetic basis (see Table 3). Many are of childhood onset and have additional neurological features. Nevertheless, as the table illustrates, there is a growing list

Table 3 Genetically determined akinetic rigid syndromes

Disease	Locus	Protein
Wilson's disease	13q14.3	Cu-binding ATPase
Dopa-responsive dystonia	14q	GTP cyclohydrolase*
Juvenile Huntington's disease	4p	Huntingtin
SCA3/MJD	14q32.1	Ataxin 3
DRPLA	12q23–24.1	Atrophin
Pelizaeus–Merzbacher	X-linked	Proteolipid protein
Ataxia telangectasia	11q	ATM
Lesch–Nyhan syndrome	Xq26	Hgpt deficiency
Hallervorden–Spatz	20p12.3–13	Unknown
Familial prion diseases	20pter-12	PRP
Juvenile parkinsonism (park 2)	6q25.2–27	Parkin
AR Juvenile parkinsonism	11p	Linked to TH
AD parkinsonism (park 1)	4q21–23	α-Synuclein
AD parkinsonism (park 3)	2p.13	Unknown
AR younger-onset parkinsonism	1p	Unknown
AR younger-onset parkinsonism	1p	Unknown
AD parkinsonism	4p.15	Unknown
FTDP/DDPAC/PPND	17q	Tau

* Most cases are autosomal dominant (with reduced penetrance), however autosomal recessive inheritance has been shown to be due to mutations in the tyrosine hydroxylase (TH) gene (chromosome 11p).

AD, autosomal dominant; AR, autosomal recessive; DDPAC, disinhibition–dementia–parkinsonism–amyotrophy–complex; DRPLA, dentatorubropallidoluysian atrophy; FTDP, frontotemporal dementia parkinsonism; Hgpt, hypoxanthine guanine phosphoribosyltransferase; PPND, pallidopontonigral degeneration; SCA 3/MJD, spinocerebellar ataxia type 3/Machado–Joseph disease.

of adult-onset disorders in which parkinsonism may be the presenting feature, in many cases the diagnosis can be confirmed by DNA testing techniques. However, these disorders account for only a small minority of cases of adult-onset parkinsonism, and in the remainder the role of genetic factors is less clear-cut.

Parkinson's disease is a common neurodegenerative disorder among the elderly. In Europe the overall age-standardized prevalence for Parkinson's disease in subjects of 55 years or older is 1.6 per 100, with an increasing frequency up to 4.3 per cent in those aged 85 years and over. Despite intensive efforts, the cause of Parkinson's disease remains largely unknown and treatment is symptomatic with only temporary results. However, there is increasing evidence that genetic factors play an important role in the aetiology of Parkinson's disease. Familial clustering of Parkinson's disease has been reported in many studies. Classic linkage and positional cloning strategies have identified a number of genes and loci responsible for mendelian Parkinson's disease (see Table 3). The α-synuclein gene was the first identified gene in autosomal dominant Parkinson's disease. Since then, a mutation in UCH-L1 and two loci 2p13 and 4p14–16.3 have been implicated in autosomal dominantly inherited Parkinson's disease.

Juvenile Parkinson's disease

This condition differs from Parkinson's disease not only in the age of onset, but also the classic triad of signs (bradykinesia, rigidity, and tremor) is relatively mild, whereas there is more prominent dystonia, postural instability, and hyperreflexia. Additional features include: (i) early onset, typically before the age of 40; (ii) dystonia at onset; (iii) diurnal fluctuations; (iv) slow disease progression; and (v) early and severe levodopa-induced dyskinesias. A gene for autosomal recessive juvenile Parkinson's disease has recently been linked to chromosome 6q25.2–27 and designated *PARK2*. Pathological examination has shown a massive loss of dopaminergic neurones in the pars compacta of the substantia nigra, in the absence of Lewy bodies, the histopathological hallmark of classic Parkinson's disease. A novel gene designated parkin, in which homozygous exon deletions were detected in four Japanese families with autosomal recessive juvenile Parkinson's disease, has been described. The parkin protein is composed of 465 amino acids, shows moderate homology to ubiquitin at the amino terminus, and contains a RING-finger motif at the carboxy terminus, and it has been shown that it has ubiquitin ligase activity. Subsequently, it has been shown that among the patients with isolated Parkinson's disease, mutations were detected in 77 per cent with onset at 20 years or earlier, but they were much more rare in later onset disease accounting for 3 per cent with onset at over 30 years. Multiple mutations have now been described in this gene and it is numerically the most important locus hitherto described for Parkinson's disease.

Very recently two other autosomal recessive loci have been identified (PARK6 and 7).

Other parkinsonian syndromes

There are a number of syndromes incorporating both parkinsonism and additional features. These are summarized in Table 3. Some of the more recent developments are discussed in more detail here.

Chromosome 17-linked tauopathies

There are a number of diseases consisting of parkinsonism complicated by a variety of features, especially cognitive impairment, see Table 3. Recently the genetic mechanisms underlying chromosome 17-linked parkinsonism dementia have been defined. Mutations of the *tau* exon 10 splice site and coding mutations in *tau* have been described which are predicted to lead to an increase in the transcription of four repeat tau isoforms or a disruption of microtubule binding, respectively. This is consistent with the predominant deposition of four repeat tau isoforms in these types of neurodegeneration.

Other tauopathies

Progressive supranuclear palsy and corticobasal degeneration

Progressive supranuclear palsy is a neurodegenerative condition which affects the brainstem and basal ganglia. It is frequently misdiagnosed, most commonly as Parkinson's disease. Patients present with disturbance of balance, a disorder of vertical gaze, and parkinsonism not resposive to levodopa. They usually develop progressive dysphagia and dysarthria leading to death from the complications of immobility and aspiration. Its prevalence is estimated at 1.4 per 100 000 with a median survival of 9 years, but a pathological study showed that 20 per cent of clinically diagnosed cases of Parkinson's disease had alternative pathological diagnoses and progressive supranuclear palsy accounted for about 6 per cent. Treatment for progressive supranuclear palsy remains largely supportive.

Progressive supranuclear palsy is also a tauopathy characterized by deposition of the four-repeat isoform of tau. Analysis of sporadic cases of progressive supranuclear palsy has demonstrated that one allele (A0) of an intronic polymorphism within the *tau* gene occurs more frequently in patients with progressive supranuclear palsy than controls. It appears that this allele increases the risk of developing progressive supranuclear palsy, but is in itself neither necessary nor sufficient to cause the disease. Interestingly this allele (Ao) and its associate haplotype (H1) is also known to be associated with increased risk of developing corticobasal degeneration, another tauopathy. The link between a genetic predisposition to progressive supranuclear palsy and the differential isoform expression of the *tau* gene may be the key to explaining the pathogenesis of these conditions.

Dystonias

Primary torsion dystonia is a clinically and genetically heterogeneous movement disorder. It is characterized by involuntary muscle spasms causing twisting and repetitive movements and postures, and is distinguished from secondary dystonia by the absence of causative exogenous factors (such as drugs, trauma) or other neurological disorders.

Early-onset dystonia (before 28 years) is the most severe and common form of hereditary primary torsion dystonia. It usually begins in a limb and spreads to other limbs within a few years, usually sparing craniocervical muscles. Most cases of early-onset dystonia are caused by an autosomal dominant gene with reduced penetrance (*DYT1*), on human chromosome 9q34. The *DYT1*-associated phenotype is similar in all ethnic communities, with highest prevalence in the Ashkenazi Jewish population. Recently, a 3-base pair (GAG) deletion in the coding sequence of the *DYT1* gene was found in all affected individuals and obligate gene carriers with 9q34-linked primary torsion dystonia, both in the Jewish and non-Jewish populations. About two-thirds of patients with early-onset dystonia carry the *DYT1* 3-base pair deletion. *De novo* GAG deletions in the *DYT1* gene can also occur rarely.

Dopa-responsive dystonia

In classic cases, the disease manifests in early childhood with walking difficulties due to dystonia of the lower limbs. Some 'parkinsonian' features such as reduced facial expression or slowing of fine finger movements frequently accompany the dystonia. Although rare, patients respond very well to small doses of levodopa without the later motor fluctuations seen in Parkinson's disease, suggesting that dopamine biosynthesis may be disturbed. This has implicated the biochemical pathway producing dopamine. Two different genes have been implicated in this disorder, both of which disrupt dopamine production. Most commonly, heterozygote mutations of the GTP cyclohydrolase I gene are found. This is the rate-limiting enzyme in the synthesis of tetrahydrobiopterin. Tetrahydrobiopterin is an essential cofactor for tyrosine hydroxylase, the rate-limiting enzyme in the synthesis of dopamine. Reduced levels of tetrahydrobiopterin lead to the dopamine-deficit syndrome, dopa-responsive dystonia, because of reduced tyrosine hydroxylase activity. The second, much less common, genetic abnormality is due to recessive mutations in tyrosine hydroxylase itself.

Other genes associated with dystonic syndromes are summarized in Table 1.

Paroxysmal movement disorders

Paroxysmal dyskinesias are rare movement disorders that are currently classified into three groups: paroxysmal non-kinesigenic dyskinesia, paroxysmal kinesigenic dyskinesia, and paroxysmal exercise-induced dyskinesia.

Paroxysmal non-kinesigenic dyskinesia (formerly termed paroxysmal dystonic choreoathetosis) is distinguished by attacks, mainly choreoathetotic, lasting from 5 min to 4 h, which are usually precipitated by alcohol, fatigue, coffee, tea, or excitement, but not by sudden movement. Between attacks, neurological examination is usually normal. This disorder is usually inherited in an autosomal dominant fashion, and sporadic cases are rare. It has been linked to a 4 cM area on chromosome 2q33–35, but the responsible gene has not yet been identified.

In paroxysmal kinesigenic dyskinesia, typically the paroxysms consist of dystonic posturing and choreoathetotic or ballistic movements. All attacks are brief (usually less than 2 min) and are precipitated by sudden movements. Frequency may be as high as 100 attacks each day. Patients with this disorder usually respond to anticonvulsants. Linkage of this disorder to chromosome 16 has recently been described, but no genes have yet been cloned.

In paroxysmal exercise-induced dyskinesia, attacks are mainly dystonic and in most cases predominantly involve the legs. They are precipitated by exercise and are not brought on by sudden movements. Response to medication is generally poor. Recently, a novel autosomal recessive syndrome characterized by rolandic epilepsy, paroxysmal exercise-induced dyskinesia, and writer's cramp has been linked to a region on chromosome 16. There appears to be at least two genes causing paroxysmal movement disorders on chromosome 16.

These disorders with their overlap with other paroxysmal movement disorders, epilepsy, and some response to anticonvulsant medication implicate an ion channel disorder.

The ataxias

The clinical features of the inherited ataxias are described in Chapter 24.6.1. Inherited ataxic disorders can be divided according to their mode of inheritance. Most autosomal recessive disorders are of early onset (less than 20 years), and autosomal dominant disorders are usually of later onset (over 20 years). X-linked inheritance of ataxia is exceedingly rare.

Autosomal recessive ataxias

Friedreich's ataxia

Friedreich's ataxia is the most common of the autosomal recessive ataxias and accounts for at least 50 per cent of cases of hereditary ataxia in most large series reported from Europe and the United States. The prevalence of the disease in these regions is similar, between 1 and 2 per 100 000.

Cloning of the gene showed that the predominant mutation was a trinucleotide repeat (GAA) in intron 1. Expansion of both alleles was found in over 96 per cent of patients and the remaining alleles carry point mutations. To date no cases have been reported of two point mutations in a singe case, therefore the absence of a least one expansion is very strong evidence against the diagnosis of Friedreich's ataxia. This has permitted the introduction of a specific and sensitive diagnostic test, as it is a relatively simple matter to measure the repeat size. On normal chromosomes the number of GAA repeats varies from 7 to 22 units, whereas on disease chromosomes, the range is anything from around 100 to 2000 repeats. The number of repeats is a determinant of age of onset and therefore to some degree influences the severity.

The exact mechanism of action of this repeat in intron 1 is not known, but it is possible that this huge expansion disrupts normal splicesome binding and therefore exon 1 is not spliced correctly to exon 2. This results in a reduction in mRNA and protein levels accordingly.

Other autosomal recessive ataxias

The other early-onset ataxias listed in Table 4 are rare.

Autosomal dominant cerebellar ataxias

The autosomal dominant cerebellar ataxias are a clinically and genetically complex group of neurodegenerative disorders divided into three types (see Chapter 24.6.1). Type I is characterized by a progressive cerebellar ataxia and is variably associated with other extracerebellar neurological features such as ophthalmoplegia, optic atrophy, peripheral neuropathy, and pyramidal and extrapyramidal signs. The presence and severity of these signs is, in part, dependent on the duration of the disease. Mild or moderate dementia may occur, but it is usually not a prominent early feature. Type II is clinically distinguished from type I by the presence of pigmentary macular dystrophy, whereas type III is a relatively 'pure' cerebellar syndrome and generally starts at a later age. This clinical classification is still useful, despite the tremendous improvements in our understanding of the genetic basis, because it provides a framework which can be used in the clinic and helps direct the genetic evaluation.

Molecular genetics of the autosomal dominant cerebellar ataxias

The classification of the autosomal dominant cerebellar ataxias is potentially confusing. The progress in our understanding of the genes and mutations has led to an additional classification system, but luckily there are many common features between these disorders. The first autosomal dominant cerebellar ataxia to be linked (to chromosome 6p) was labelled spinocerebellar ataxia type 1 (**SCA1**). Thereafter, each new locus was given a subsequent SCA number; SCA2 to chromosome 12q, and so on. At the time of writing there are currently 13 SCA loci. Of these, mutations have been identified definitively for SCA 1, 2, 3, 6, 7, and 12. SCA 12 has only been described in two families to date. The others have all been described in many different populations. They are all caused by an expansion of an exonic CAG repeat. The resultant proteins all possess an expanded polyglutamine tract and there are now at least eight conditions caused by these expansions. This common mutational scheme is discussed above with reference to Huntington's disease.

Autosomal dominant periodic ataxia

Autosomal dominant periodic ataxia is characterized by the childhood or adolescent onset of attacks of ataxia, dysarthria, vertigo, and nystagmus. Not all patients have affected relatives. There are at least two forms of this disorder.

Episodic ataxia type 1

The attacks tend to be relatively brief (minutes and occasionally hours) and clinically and electrophysiologically myokymia may be seen. Mutations in a potassium channel have been found. These patients may benefit from acetazolamide, and phenytoin has also been reported to be useful. Patients tend to be neurologically normal between the attacks.

Episodic ataxia type 2

The attacks tend to be longer, lasting hours or even days. They are usually associated with vertigo and consequent nausea and vomiting. They tend to be more severe in childhood with associated drowsiness, headache, and fever. Although when the disease first begins the patients are well between attacks, an interictal nystagmus can be seen. As the years pass, a slowly progressive ataxia is seen. MRI may reveal cerebellar atrophy. These patients tend to respond better to acetazolamide therapy than patients with episodic ataxia type 1. Mutations in a calcium channel gene on chromosome 19q have been demonstrated. Other mutations in this gene have been

Table 4 Rare autosomal recessive ataxias

Syndrome	Core features	Additional features	Comments
Early-onset cerebellar ataxia with retained reflexes	The prognosis is better than in classic Friedreich's ataxia. Age of onset between 2 and 20 years. The upper limb and knee reflexes are normal or increased, but the ankle jerks may be absent	Cerebellar atrophy is more frequently found on CT or MRI than in Friedreich's ataxia	Genetically heterogeneous; inheritance is probably autosomal recessive in most cases
Cerebellar ataxia with hypogonadotrophic hypogonadism	Abnormal sexual development is obvious from the time of expected puberty. Onset in the third decade, although the age range is from 1 to 30 years. The disorder comprises dysarthria, nystagmus, and progressive limb and gait ataxia	Less frequent clinical features include mental retardation, dementia, deafness, distal weakness and wasting, choreoathetosis, retinopathy, and loss of vibration and joint position sense	Autosomal recessive
Cerebellar ataxia with myoclonus (Ramsay–Hunt syndrome)	This is a heterogenous syndrome with multiple causes. Overlaps with that of progressive myoclonic epilepsy	Unverricht–Lundborg disease MERRF Sialidosis	Autosomal recessive— gene test available mtDNA point mutation Autosomal recessive
Behr's syndrome	Optic atrophy, spasticity, ataxia, and mental retardation. Optic atrophy and ataxia, with or without mental retardation and deafness, have been described as an autosomal recessive trait	Occasional associated peripheral neuropathy	Autosomal recessive
Marinesco–Sjögren	Ataxia	Cataracts, mental retardation, short stature, delayed sexual development	Autosomal recessive
Vitamin E deficiency	Progressive gait and limb ataxia, areflexia, and large-fibre sensory loss. Onset of symptoms at 3 to 13 years	Isolated vitamin E deficiency Abetalipoproteinaemia	Mutations in a gene encoding α-tocopherol transfer protein (α-TTP) Lipoprotein electrophoresis

described in families with familial hemiplegic migraine and a form of dominant ataxia (SCA6), that is, they are allelic.

Further reading

Bandmann O, Marsden CD, Wood NW (1998). Atypical presentations of DRD mutations. *Advances in Neurology* **78**, 283–90.

Bhatia KP (1999). The paroxysmal dyskinesias. *Journal of Neurology* **246**, 149–55.

Brice A (1998). Unstable mutations and neurodegenerative disorders. *Journal of Neurology* **245**, 505–10.

Conrad C *et al.* (1997). Genetic evidence for the involvement of tau in progressive supranuclear palsy. *Annals of Neurology* **41**, 277–81.

Davies SW *et al.* (1997). Formation of neuronal intranuclear inclusions underlies the neurological dysfunction in mice transgenic for the HD mutation. *Cell* **90**, 537–48.

De Silva R, Khan NL, Wood NW (2000). New developments in the genetics of Parkinson's disease. *Current Opinion in Genetics and Development* **10**, 292–8.

Enevoldson PG, Sanders MD, Harding AE (1994). Autosomal dominant cerebellar ataxia with pigmentary macular dystrophy: a clinical and genetic study of eight families. *Brain* **117**, 445–60.

Harding AE (1984). *The hereditary ataxias and related disorders.* Churchill Livingstone, Edinburgh.

Hutton M *et al.* (1998). Association of missense and 5'-splice-site mutations in tau with the inherited dementia FTDP-17. *Nature* **393**, 702–5.

Kitada T *et al.* (1998). Mutations in the parkin gene cause autosomal recessive juvenile parkinsonism. *Nature* **392**, 605–8.

Ozelius LJ *et al.* (1989). Human gene for torsion dystonia located on chromosome 9q32–34. *Neuron* **2**, 1427–34.

Ozelius LJ *et al.* (1997). The early-onset torsion dystonia gene (DYT1) encodes an ATP-binding protein. *Nature Genetics* **17**, 40–8.

Reddy PH, Williams M, Tagle DA (1999). Recent advances in understanding the pathogenesis of Huntington's disease. *Trends in Neurosciences* **22**, 248–55.

Valente EM *et al.* (1998). The role of DYT 1 in primary torsion dystonia in Europe. *Brain* **121**, 2335–9.

24.7 Lumbar puncture

Robert A. Fishman

Indications

Lumbar puncture should be performed only after clinical evaluation of the patient and consideration of the potential value and hazards of the procedure. The cerebrospinal fluid findings are important in the differential diagnosis of the gamut of central nervous system infections, meningitis, and encephalitis, as well as subarachnoid haemorrhage, confusional states, acute stroke, status epilepticus, meningeal malignancies, demyelinating diseases, and central nervous system vasculitis. Examination of the cerebrospinal fluid is usually necessary in patients with suspected intracranial bleeding to establish the diagnosis, although computed tomography (**CT**), when available, may be more valuable. For example, primary intracerebral haemorrhage or post-traumatic haemorrhage is often readily observed with CT making lumbar puncture an unnecessary hazard. However, in primary subarachnoid haemorrhage lumbar puncture may establish the diagnosis when CT is falsely negative. Lumbar puncture is useful to ascertain that the cerebrospinal fluid is free of blood before anticoagulant therapy for stroke is begun. (However, extensive subarachnoid bleeding is a rare complication of heparin anticoagulation, begun several hours after a traumatic bloody tap. Therefore heparin therapy should not begin for at least an hour after a bloody tap.) Lumbar puncture has limited therapeutic usefulness, for example in intrathecal therapy in meningeal malignancies and fungal meningitis.

Contraindications

Lumbar puncture is contraindicated in the presence of infection in the skin overlying the spine. A serious complication of lumbar puncture is the possibility of aggravating a pre-existing, often unrecognized, brain herniation syndrome (for example uncal, cerebellar, or cingulate herniation) associated with intracranial hypertension. This hazard is the basis for considering papilloedema to be a relative contraindication to lumbar puncture. The availability of CT has simplified the management of patients with papilloedema. If CT reveals no evidence of a mass lesion , then lumbar puncture is usually needed in the presence of papilloedema to establish the diagnosis of pseudotumour cerebri and to exclude meningeal inflammation or malignancy.

Thrombocytopenia and other bleeding diatheses predispose patients to needle induced subarachnoid, subdural, and epidural haemorrhage. Lumbar puncture should be undertaken only if urgently needed when the platelet count is depressed to about 50 000/μl or below. Platelet transfusion just before the puncture is recommended if the count is below 20 000/μl or dropping rapidly. The administration of protamine to patients on heparin and vitamin K or fresh frozen plasma to those receiving warfarin is recommended before lumbar puncture to minimize the hazard of the procedure.

Complications

Complications of lumbar puncture include worsening of brain herniation and spinal cord compression, headache, subarachnoid bleeding, diplopia, backache, and radicular symptoms. Post-lumbar puncture headache is the most common complication, occurring in about 25 per cent of patients and usually lasting 2 to 8 days. It results from low cerebrospinal fluid pressures due to persistent fluid leakage through the dural hole. Characteristically, pain is present in the upright position and is promptly relieved with a supine position. Aching of the neck and low back is common. The headaches are aggravated by cough or strain and may be associated with nausea, vomiting, or tinnitus. They are less likely if a small syletted needle is used and if multiple puncture holes are not made. The management of post-spinal headache depends upon strict bedrest in the horizontal position, adequate hydration, and simple analgesics. If conservative measure fail, the use of a 'blood patch' is indicated. The technique utilizes the epidural injection of autologous blood close to site of the dural puncture to form a thrombotic tamponade which seals the dural hole.

Cerebrospinal fluid

The cerebrospinal fluid pressure should be measured routinely. The pressure level within the right atrium is the reference level with the patient horizontal in the lateral decubitus position. The normal lumbar cerebrospinal fluid pressure ranges between 50 and 200 mmH_2O (and as high as 250 mmH_2O in very obese subjects). With the use of the clinical manometer the arterially derived pulsatile pressures are obscured but respiratory pressure waves reflecting changes in central venous pressures are visible. Low pressures are seen in dehydration, spinal subarachnoid block, following previous lumbar puncture or other cerebrospinal fluid leaks, or may be technical in origin because of faulty needle placement. Increased pressures occur with brain oedema, intracranial mass lesions, infections, acute stroke, cerebral venous occlusions, congestive heart failure, pulmonary insufficiency, and benign intracranial hypertension (pseudotumour cerebri) of diverse aetiology.

Normal cerebrospinal fluid contains no more than five lymphocytes or mononuclear cells per microlitre. A higher white cell count is pathognomonic of disease in the central nervous system or meninges. A stained smear of the sediment is needed for an accurate differential cell count. A variety of centrifugal and sedimentation techniques have been used. A pleocytosis occurs with the gamut of inflammatory disorders. The changes characteristic of the various meningitides are listed in Table 1. The heterogeneous forms of neuro-AIDS also are associated with a wide range of cellular responses. Other disorders associated with a pleocytosis include brain infarction, subarachnoid bleeding, cerebral vasculitis, acute demyelination, and brain tumours. Eosinophilia most often accompanies parasitic infections, for example cysticercosis. Cytological studies for malignant cells are rewarding with some central nervous system neoplasms.

Bloody cerebrospinal fluid due to needle trauma contains increased numbers of white cells contributed by the blood. A useful approximation to a true white cell count can be obtained by the following correction for the presence of the added blood: if the patient has a normal haemogram, subtract from the total white cell count (WBC; per μl) one white cell for each 1000 red blood cells (RBC) present. Thus, if bloody fluid contains 10 000 red cells and 100 white cell/μl, ten white cells would be accounted for by the added blood and the corrected leucocyte count would be 90/μl. If the patient's haemogram reveals significant anaemia or leucocytosis, the following formula may be used to determine more accurately the number of white cells (W) in the spinal fluid before the blood was added:

$$W = \frac{\text{blood WBC} \times \text{cerebrospinal fluid RBC}}{\text{blood RBC}} \times 100.$$

The presence of blood in the subarachnoid space produces a secondary inflammatory response which leads to a disproportionate increase in the number of white cells. Following an acute subarachnoid haemorrhage, this elevation in the white cell count is most marked about 48 h after onset, when meningeal signs are most striking.

To correct cerebrospinal fluid protein values for the presence of added blood due to needle trauma, subtract 0.001 g for every 1000 red blood cells. Thus, if the red cell count is 10 000/μl and the total protein is 1.1 g/l the corrected protein level would be about 1 g/l. The corrections are reliable only if the cell count and total protein are both made on the same tube of fluid.

Blood in the cerebrospinal fluid: differential diagnosis and the three-tube test

To differentiate between a traumatic spinal puncture and pre-existing subarachnoid haemorrhage, the fluid should be collected in at least three separate tubes (the 'three-tube test'). In traumatic punctures, the fluid generally clears between the first and the third collections. This is detectable with the naked eye and should be confirmed by cell count. In subarachnoid bleeding, the blood is generally evenly admixed in the three tubes. A sample of the bloody fluid should be centrifuged and the supernatant fluid compared with tap water to exclude the presence of pigment. The supernatant fluid is crystal clear if the red cell count is less than about 100 000 cells/μl. With bloody contamination of greater magnitude, plasma proteins may be sufficient to cause minimal xanthochromia; this requires enough serum to raise the cerebrospinal fluid protein concentration to about 1.5 g/l.

Following subarachnoid haemorrhage, the supernatant fluid usually remains clear for 2 to 4 h and even longer after the onset of subarachnoid bleeding. The clear supernatant fluid may mislead the physician to conclude erroneously that the observed blood is due to needle trauma in patients who have had a lumbar puncture within 4 h of aneurysmal rupture. After an especially traumatic puncture, some blood and xanthochromia may be present for as long as 2 to 5 days following the initial puncture. In pathological states associated with a cerebrospinal fluid protein greater than 1.5 g/l, and in the absence of bleeding, very faint xanthochromia may be detected. When the protein is elevated to much higher levels, as in spinal block, polyneuritis, and meningitis, the xanthochromia may be considerable. A xanthochromic fluid with a normal protein level or a minor elevation to less than 1.5 g/l usually indicates a previous subarachnoid or intracerebral haemorrhage (rarely the xanthochromia is due to severe jaundice, carotenaemia, or rifampin).

Pigments

Two major pigments derived from red cells may be observed in cerebrospinal fluid—oxyhaemoglobin and bilirubin. Methaemoglobin is only seen spectrophotometrically. Oxyhaemoglobin, released with lysis of red cells, may be detected in the supernatant fluid within 2 h of a subarachnoid haemorrhage. It reaches a maximum in about the first 36 h and gradually disappears over the next 7 to 10 days. Bilirubin, is produced *in vivo* by leptomeningeal cells following red cell haemolysis. Bilirubin is first detected

Table 1 Cerebrospinal fluid findings in meningitis

Meningitis	Pressure (mmH_2O)	Leucocytes/μl	Protein (g/l)	Glucose (mmol/l)
Acute bacterial	Usually elevated	Several hundred to more than 60 000; usually a few thousand but occasionally less than 100 (especially meningococcal or early in disease). Polymorphonuclears predominate	Usually 1 to 5, occasionally more than 10	0.2 to 2.2 in most cases (in the absence of hyperglycaemia)
Tuberculous	Usually elevated; may be low with dynamic block in advanced stages	Usually 25 to 100; rarely more than 500. Lymphocytes predominate except in early stages when polymorphonuclears may account for 80 per cent of cells	Nearly always elevated, usually 1 to 2; may be much higher if dynamic block	Usually reduced; less than 2.5 in three-quarters of cases
Cryptococcal	Usually elevated	0 to 800; average 50. Lymphocytes predominate	Usually 0.2 to 5; average 1	Reduced in most cases; average 1.7 (in absence of hyperglycaemia)
Viral	Normal to moderately elevated	5 to a few hundred; but may be more than 1000, particularly with lymphocytic choriomeningitis. Lymphocytes predominate but there may be more than 80 per cent polymorphonuclears in the first few days	Frequently normal or slightly elevated; less than 1; may show greater elevation in severe cases	Normal (reduced in one-quarter of cases of mumps and herpes simplex)
Syphilitic (acute)	Usually elevated	Average 500. Usually lymphocytes; rarely polymorphonuclear	Average 1	Normal (rarely reduced)
Cysticercosis	Often increased; low with dynamic block	Increased mononuclears and polymorphonuclears with 2 to 7 per cent eosinophilia in about half of cases	Usually 0.5 to 2	Reduced in a fifth of cases
Sarcoid	Normal to considerably elevated	0 to fewer than 100 mononuclear cells	Slight to moderate elevation	Reduced in half of cases
Tumour	Normal or elevated	0 to several hundred mononuclears plus malignant cells	Elevated often to high levels	Normal or greatly reduced (low in three-quarters of carcinomatous meningitis cases)

Cerebrospinal fluid immunoglobulins are commonly increased in all of the above (including carcinomatous meningitis) as well as in multiple sclerosis and central nervous system vasculitis. Cerebrospinal fluid immunoglobulins are assessed by the IgG index: (IgG (cerebrospinal fluid) × albumin (serum))/ (IgG serum × albumin(cerebrospinal fluid)). The normal index is less than 0.65. Oligoclonal bands (with gel electrophoresis) present in cerebrospinal fluid but absent in serum are also a measure of abnormally increased cerebrospinal fluid immunoglobulins synthesized within the CNS).

about 10 h after the onset of subarachnoid bleeding. It reaches a maximum at 48 h and may persist for 2 to 4 weeks after extensive bleeding. The severity of the meningeal signs associated with subarachnoid bleeding correlates with the inflammatory response, i.e. the leucocytic pleocytosis.

Total protein

The total protein level of cerebrospinal fluid ranges between 1.5 and 5 g/l. While an elevated protein level lacks specificity, it is an index of neurological disease reflecting a pathological increase in the permeability of endothelial cells. Greatly increased protein levels, 5 g/l and above, are seen in meningitis, bloody fluids, or cord tumour with spinal block. Polyneuritis (Guillain Barre syndrome), diabetic radiculoneuropathy, and myxoedema may also increase the level to 1 to 3 g/l. Low protein levels, below 0.15 g/l, occur most often with cerebrospinal fluid leaks due to a previous lumbar puncture or traumatic dural fistula.

Immunoglobulins

Although a vast number of proteins may be measured in cerebrospinal fluid only an increase in immunoglobulins is of diagnostic importance. Such increases are indicative of an inflammatory response in the central nervous system and occur with immunological disorders, and bacterial, viral, spirochaetal, and fungal diseases. Immunoglobulin assays are most useful in the diagnosis of multiple sclerosis, other demyelinating diseases, and central nervous system vasculitis. The cerebrospinal fluid level is corrected for the entry of immunoglobulins from the serum by calculating the IgG index (see Table 1). More than one oligoclonal band in cerebrospinal fluid with gel electrophoresis (and absent in serum) is also abnormal, occurring in 90 per cent of multiple sclerosis cases and variably in the gamut of inflammatory diseases including central nervous system vasculitis.

Glucose

The concentration of glucose in cerebrospinal fluid is dependent upon the concentration in the blood. The normal range of glucose concentration in cerebrospinal fluid is between 2.5 and 4.5 mmol/l in patients with a blood glucose between 4 and 7 mmol/l, i.e. 60 to 80 per cent of the normal blood level. Cerebrospinal fluid glucose values between 2.2 and 2.5 mmol/l are usually abnormal, and values below 2.2 mmol/l invariably so. Hyperglycaemia during the 4 h prior to lumbar puncture results in a parallel increase in cerebrospinal fluid glucose. The latter approaches a maximum and the cerebrospinal fluid/blood ratio may be as low as 0.35 in the presence of a greatly elevated blood glucose level and in the absence of any neurological disease. An increase in cerebrospinal fluid glucose is of no diagnostic significance apart from reflecting hyperglycaemia within the 4 h prior to lumbar puncture. The cerebrospinal fluid glucose level is abnormally low (hypoglycorrhachia) in several diseases of the nervous system apart from hypoglycaemia. It is characteristic of acute purulent meningitis, and is a usual finding in tuberculous and fungal meningitis. It is usually normal in viral meningitis, although reduced in about 25 per cent of mumps cases, and in some cases of herpes simplex and zoster meningoencephalitis. The cerebrospinal fluid glucose is also reduced in other inflammatory meningitides including cysticercosis, amoebic meningitis (*Nagleria*), acute syphilitic meningitis, sarcoidosis, granulomatous arteritis, and other vasculitides. The glucose level is also reduced in the chemical meningitis that follows intrathecal injections, and in subarachnoid haemorrhage, usually 4 to 8 days after the bleed. The major factor responsible for the depressed glucose levels is increased anaerobic glycolysis in adjacent neural tissues and to a lesser degree by polymorphonuclear leucocytes. Thus, the decrease in the cerebrospinal fluid glucose level is accompanied by an inverse increase in the cerebrospinal fluid lactate level.

Microbiological and serological reactions

The use of appropriate stains and cultures is essential in cases of suspected infection. Tests for specific bacterial and fungal antigens (countercurrent immunoelectrophoresis) are useful in establishing a specific aetiology. DNA amplification techniques using the polymerase chain reaction have improved diagnostic sensitivity. Serological tests on cerebrospinal fluid for syphilis include the reagin antibody tests and specific treponemal antibody tests. The former are particularly useful in evaluating cerebrospinal fluid because positive results may occur even in the presence of a negative blood serology. There is no basis for applying the specific treponemal antibody tests to cerebrospinal fluid because these antibodies are derived from the plasma where they are present in greater concentration. The search continues for specific diagnostic markers in cerebrospinal fluid in the heterogeneous degenerative diseases of the central nervous system.

Further reading

Fishman RA (1992). *Cerebrospinal fluid in diseases of the nervous system*,2nd edn. WB Saunders, Philadelphia.

24.8 Disturbances of higher cerebral function

Peter Nestor and John R. Hodges

Introduction

Modern scientific study of higher cerebral function began in the late nineteenth century with the case studies of Broca and Wernicke. Their observations of language disorders associated with damage to the left hemisphere gave rise to the notion that specific mental faculties could be dissociated from each other and localized to specific regions within the cerebral hemisphere. Since that time clinicopathological and, more recently, imaging studies have established associations between specific cognitive disorders and focal brain lesions; these studies also show that some lesions do not give rise to highly specific deficits. The field of neuropsychology has offered complementary insights into this area by providing concepts of how cognitive faculties are organized.

The border between psychiatry and neurology has become less distinct; many patients with brain diseases have psychiatric symptoms, cognitive complaints are prominent in depression and schizophrenia, and a biological basis for many 'functional' psychiatric disorders is now well accepted.

Another critical area has been the study of anatomy: the finding that neocortical histology varies by region led to the development of cytoarchitectonic maps such as that of Brodmann. Brodmann's map has become a shorthand way of discussing regional specialization across the cortex. Meanwhile, anatomical studies of neural tracts have provided insights into how topographically distinct regions may interact.

Handedness and hemispheric dominance

The finding of asymmetric functions in the human cerebral cortex led to the introduction of the term hemispheric dominance. Neuroscientists often refer to cognitive processes being a function of the 'dominant' or 'non-dominant' hemisphere; when such terminology is used, the 'dominant' hemisphere is synonymous with that which underpins language function. In right handers, over 95 per cent have left hemisphere dominance: only rarely does aphasia arise from right hemisphere damage in which circumstance it is referred to as 'crossed aphasia'. In left handers, dominance is more complex and language skills are more often shared between the hemispheres although the left hemisphere is relatively dominant in about 70 per cent of individuals. While the left hemisphere usually specializes in language, the non-dominant hemisphere plays an important role in spatial cognition (with damage to the frontoparietal regions resulting in spatial neglect) and particularly in face processing (with damage to the right occipitotemporal junction producing prosopagnosia).

Primary sensory input and motor output

Motor

The primary motor area lies in the precentral gyrus, immediately rostral to the central sulcus. The body is represented 'somatotopically' along the precentral gyrus; the lower limb at the superomedial, and the face at the inferolateral extremity with the upper limb in between. This is of clinical importance as the vascular supply of the superomedial region is from the anterior cerebral artery whilst the rest of the motor cortex is from the middle cerebral artery. Thus middle cerebral artery territory infarction will affect face and upper limb with relative sparing of the lower limb, and the converse will be the case with anterior cerebral territory occlusions.

Vision

After passing from the retina, via optic nerves and tracts to the lateral geniculate body of the thalamus, visual information passes to the striate cortex of the occipital lobes (primary visual cortex) through the optic radiations (see Chapter 24.11). As images presented to the right visual field are represented on the left retina and conveyed to the left occipital lobe, a lesion of the latter will cause a right homonymous hemianopia (and vice versa for right occipital lesions). Fibres in each optic radiation separate such that input from the superior half of the retina (inferior visual field) runs from lateral geniculate to the striate cortex via parietal white matter whilst that from the inferior retina (superior visual field) loops down into the temporal lobe. Consequently, a lesion of the parietal lobe can cause a contralesional inferior quadrantanopic field defect whilst a temporal lobe lesion can cause a contralesional superior quadrantanopia. Large temporoparietal lesions (for example due to middle cerebral artery occlusion) may also cause homonymous hemianopia which may be distinguished from that due to an occipital lesion by preservation of opticokinetic nystagmus in the latter but not the former.

Bilateral lesions to the primary visual cortex lead to 'cortical blindness' in which vision is lost, but unlike blindness secondary to retinal or optic nerve diseases, pupillary reflexes are preserved. Some cortically blind individuals deny they have any visual disorder at all (namely visual anosagnosia)—a condition known as Anton's syndrome. These cases tend to have more extensive lesions involving both striate and adjacent visual association cortices.

Somatosensory

The primary somatosensory cortex occupies the post-central gyrus of the parietal lobe with a somatotopic representation of the body analogous to that of the primary motor area. Sensory deficits due to lesions of the thalamus, or lower components of the sensory system, cause gross abnormalities in the appreciation of touch, pinprick, temperature, and other sensations, and must be excluded before comment can be made on higher sensory function. Parietal lesions cause specific impairment of 'discriminative' sensation, including joint position sense and two-point discrimination. Parietal drift (the patient is asked, with eyes closed, to maintain the upper limbs outstretched in front of the trunk at 90°) is a sign of impairment of the former ability. It is considered specific for a contralateral parietal lesion when the drift is upward, as a downwards drift may also be a consequence of subtle motor weakness. The normal separation distance at which one can discriminate one point from two varies according to body region: fingertips 3 mm, palm 1 cm, and body surface 4 to 7 cm.

Other signs of parietal sensory impairment are an inability to name numbers traced on the palm of the hand (agraphaesthesia), and an inability to name small objects (such as keys and coins) placed in the patient's hand (astereognosis). Obviously there is potential to confuse true astereognosis with a more general deficit of object naming such as due to loss of semantic knowledge or aphasia (see below). However, ambiguous results on parietal sensory testing can largely be avoided if the examiner adopts a methodical approach of: (i) excluding a lesion below the parietal lobe by establishing that the patient can appreciate, for instance, a pinprick or light touch; and (ii) examining from the suspected normal to abnormal side to exclude a more general impairment of cognitive faculties.

Auditory

Auditory information coming from the cochlear nuclei via the inferior colliculus and the medial geniculate nucleus of the thalamus travels to the primary auditory cortex (Heschl's gyrus) in the posterosuperior temporal lobe. Clinically apparent cortical hearing impairment is uncommon due to the bilateral representation of auditory material from each ear by the cerebral cortex. Bilateral lesions of this area (as a result of strokes, prolonged hypotension, or carbon monoxide poisoning) will cause 'cortical deafness', a rare disorder manifest by inability to understand spoken language or recognize sounds although presence or absence of noise can be determined. Unlike Wernicke's aphasia (see below), subjects can understand written text and their language output is normal.

Cognitive domains

Beyond the primary sensory and motor cortices, the neocortex is made up of unimodal and heteromodal association areas. Unimodal association cortices lie adjacent to their respective primary modality while heteromodal association cortex is found in the prefrontal and temporoparietal regions. Moving from primary through unimodal to heteromodal association cortex, the linkage of topographical region to specific functional attribute becomes progressively less tightly defined. Heteromodal association cortices, as the name implies, receive inputs from multiple unimodal areas but also from non-neocortical areas. Anatomically, as the neocortex approaches the diencephalon, upon which the cerebral hemispheres sit, it transforms into a histologically distinct area: the limbic system. These areas also have critical roles in cognition, particularly in the domains of memory and emotion and have reciprocal projections with heteromodal association cortices.

Other brain regions which have important modulatory roles on cognition include: (i) the basal forebrain nuclei, which contain cholinergic neurones that project extensively to limbic and neocortical regions and are known to be important to the successful encoding of memory; (ii) the basal ganglia, which have reciprocal links to frontal association cortices and have important modulatory roles relating particularly to attention and speed of cognitive processing; and (iii) brainstem reticular formation nuclei which project into the hemispheres via the thalami: the most clearly defined role for these projections being at the level of arousal.

Although the remainder of this section discusses various disorders of higher mental function individually, one should not view these specific deficits as a random and independent collection of phenomena. It cannot be overemphasized that one should always follow a logical sequence in assessing cognitive function so as to avoid false-positive diagnoses due to sequential effects. For example, tests of executive function that utilize analysis of complex verbal material would be beyond the grasp of a patient with Wernicke's aphasia due to the fundamental disorder of language comprehension without needing to implicate frontal lobe damage. Likewise, a patient with an acute delirium may be unable to perform even the most basic memory tasks as a consequence of their attention deficit and therefore ought not to be labelled amnesic. Therefore, regardless of the suspected disorder, one should always bear the following sequence in mind: (i) ensure adequate attention to undergo further testing; (ii) as almost all tests are going to be presented with verbal instruction, assess language comprehension; and (iii) as tests of executive function and praxis often require adequate levels of function in all other cognitive domains, these should be left to last. In summary, always ask 'can this apparent disorder be explained in terms of a more elemental deficit?'

Attention

The ability to attend to a specific sensory stimulus, such as a human voice or passage of text, and to maintain attention is an obligatory first step to any further cognitive processing. Humans are continuously bombarded with sensory stimuli from both within and between individual sensory input modalities; loss of ability to focus and sustain attention (or alternatively, block out irrelevant 'noise') renders the individual incapable of following a specific sensory stimulus (such as a conversation) and at the same time vulnerable to random irrelevant environmental stimuli. Although disorders of the frontal lobes, basal ganglia, and ascending reticular formation are associated with poor attention, it is overly simplistic to consider attention as a localizable brain function. The commonest causes of acute attention failure are diffuse brain insults such as a metabolic encephalopathy or closed head injury; breakdown in attentional processing is the central deficit in delirium or acute confusional states, the main features of which are summarized in Table 1.

Digit span is one of the most simple methods of assessing attention, especially in the backwards condition; normal subjects have a forward span of at least six digits and a reverse span one or two digits less. The digits must be presented as individual items (read the string to be repeated at a rate of one digit per second). A common pitfall is to cluster digits as one does when reciting telephone numbers. This inflates span as each cluster becomes an individual item: compare repeating 6953–8127 with 6 ... 9 ... 5 ... 3 ... 8 ... 1 ... 2 ... 7. Ability to persevere at a given task is another way of considering attention; this can be tested by asking the patient to recite the months of the year in reverse order.

Orientation is heavily dependent upon attention and is assessed by questions of time and place. Testing personal orientation adds little, as only profoundly aphasic or hysterical patients are unable to relate their own name. A recent onset of profound disorientation and attention deficit is typical of a delirium. It should be noted that many patients with episodic memory problems (such as early Alzheimer's disease) remain well orientated.

Language and related disorders

Numerous terms are in use to describe aphasic syndromes, although some serve more to confuse than enlighten. The terms 'expressive' and 'receptive'

Table 1 The features of delirium

Onset	Usually acute/subacute
Course	Fluctuating, nocturnal exacerbations
Conscious state	May be impaired, derangement of normal sleep/wake cycle
Cognitive profile	Disorientated in time and place
	Severe impairment of attention (with knock-on effects to other cognitive domains, i.e. due to poor registration etc.)
Psychiatric features	Incoherent and perseverative
	Mood disorders: agitation, apathy
	Visual illusions and hallucinations
	Paranoid ideas common
Physical signs	Asterixis
	May be evidence of general medical illness (pyrexia, signs of hepatic failure etc.)

From Hodges JR, ed. (2001). *Early onset dementia: a multidisciplinary approach*. Oxford University Press, Oxford.

particularly seem to mislead: on the one hand all patients with aphasia have some form of difficulty 'expressing' themselves, and on the other hand 'receptive' aphasia is often, erroneously, taken to mean that patients have difficulty only with incoming language, but can produce their own language perfectly well. Less ambiguous terms for the two principal divisions of aphasia are 'non-fluent' and 'fluent', which correspond in classic aphasia nomenclature to Broca's and Wernicke's aphasia. The classic aphasia syndromes are, however, rarely seen in the acute stages after stroke and do not characterize the language deficits found in the dementias. A better approach is therefore to consider language fluency and paraphasias in spontaneous conversation, comprehension, naming, and repetition.

Examining patients with aphasia

Fluency and paraphasic errors

Speech can be described as fluent if the patient is able to produce some well-formed sentences or phrases even if empty or anomic (such as 'Oh you know, the thing you put the stuff in when you're going somewhere and ...'). Non-fluent language, in contrast, is a consequence of breakdown of the language production and syntactic (grammatical) aspects of language and is the hallmark of damage to Broca's area and the insula. Output is laboured or 'telegraphic', with often as few as two or three words per minute; in spite of which they can convey meaning fairly successfully, for example 'I ... go ... hospital'.

Paraphasic errors are substitutions of a correct word for one related in sound or meaning. The former, known as phonological or phonemic paraphasias, involve the substitution of related sound fragments ('phonemes') such as 'dobble' for 'bottle'. Semantic paraphasic errors involve substitution of words of related meaning; the substituted word is typically a higher frequency example of the same semantic category (such as 'dog' for 'fox') or else of a superordinate category (such as 'animal' for 'fox'). In more extreme circumstances, paraphasic substitutions may not be words at all ('neologisms'); fluent output with virtually continuous neologisms is an utterly incomprehensible state sometimes referred to as jargon aphasia. Patients with lesions to Wernicke's area invariably make a mixture of phonemic and semantic errors. Semantic errors are also very common in Alzheimer's disease and semantic dementia. In Broca's aphasia, phonological errors predominate.

Comprehension

Some degree of impairment of language comprehension can be detected in both fluent and non-fluent aphasia. Patients with fluent aphasia have more overtly impaired comprehension of word meaning (for example ordinary nouns). In mild cases this can be demonstrated with semantically complex language tasks (such as 'Can you point to a source of artificial illumination?') or by defining uncommon words (such as 'What is an aubergine, accordion etc.'). Comprehension of single nouns is preserved in patients with non-fluent aphasia, but comprehension—in addition to production—of complex grammar is impaired. This can be tested with reversible passive sentences (such as 'The lion was eaten by the tiger, who survived?') or by asking the patient to obey syntactically complex commands (such as 'Touch the keys after touching the book').

Anomia

Naming is a complex task that requires the integrity of three basic processes: visual analysis, semantic knowledge (see Memory, below), and word production (phonology). Virtually all patients with aphasia are anomic when tested using items of low familiarity and late age of acquisition. The type of naming error and the ability to circumvent the deficit varies, however, according to the locus of damage. Patients with visuoperceptive deficits that produce visual errors (a 'head' for a 'mushroom' etc.) have retained tactile naming and can give correct responses when asked to put a name to a description ('What do we call the large grey African animal with a trunk?').

A breakdown in the central semantic process causes impairment in naming from all modalities, while phonological deficits produce phonological errors regardless of the mode of input.

Repetition

Lesions involving any of the peri-Sylvian language structures are almost always associated with impaired repetition, although this may not be apparent unless multisyllabic words ('caterpillar', 'fundamental' etc.) and phrases ('no ifs, ands, or buts') are tested. Certain aphasic syndromes (see below) show either disproportionate impairment or preservation of repetition.

Aphasic syndromes

Broca's aphasia

This classic form of non-fluent aphasia is characterized by grossly distorted speech output with impaired production and comprehension of syntax. Phonological paraphasias are common and there is impaired repetition of phrases. It is associated with lesions to the left ventrolateral frontal lobe (Broca's area); owing to its close proximity to the motor cortex, when focal lesions (such as stroke or tumour) cause a Broca's aphasia it is typically associated with a right hemiparesis. The distortion of language output, often described as speech apraxia, is thought to relate to concurrent damage to structures within the insula, which is almost always affected.

Wernicke's aphasia

In Wernicke's aphasia there is fluent although vacuous output with a mixture of semantic and phonological paraphasic errors and often neologisms. There is also impaired comprehension of word meanings and impaired repetition. In contrast to the fundamental loss of word meaning seen in patients with semantic dementia and destruction of the left inferior temporal lobe after herpes simplex encephalitis, patients with Wernicke's aphasia have breakdown in the mapping between speech and meaning systems. Lesions localize to the posterior portion of the left superior temporal gyrus—known as Wernicke's area. As this area overlies the optic radiation, the commonest neighbourhood sign is a right homonymous hemianopia.

Conduction aphasia

This form of aphasia, as the name implies, is due to a disconnection of the two principle language areas. Comprehension is relatively preserved and output is fluent although phonemic paraphasias occur. The striking abnormality is an impairment of repetition even for single syllable words such that attempts at repeating are laboured and contain phonemic errors. Likewise, naming produces phonemic errors even for high frequency items (such as for 'cup': 'cah ... cahb ... cub' etc.). Lesions producing conduction aphasia occur in the region of the supramarginal gyrus, and particularly, the underlying arcuate fasciculus, the tract linking the anterior and posterior language areas.

Global aphasia

In this devastating form of aphasia there is derangement of all aspects of language; patients with global aphasia are non-fluent and have impaired word comprehension, repetition, and naming. Language output is restricted to infrequent unintelligible noises or, at best, a single word or clichéd phrase. As the blood supply to both language areas is from the middle cerebral artery, global aphasia is not uncommon secondary to proximal occlusion of this vessel. Consequently these patients are usually also hemiplegic and hemianopic.

Atypical aphasias and the dementias

The term 'transcortical aphasia' is a legacy of an abandoned neural explanation for a distinct category of aphasia. Although the term is meaningless in its originally coined anatomical sense, it is still sometimes used to describe a distinct syndrome in which a patient with aphasia shows preservation of repetition. Patients with so-called transcortical sensory aphasia are fluent and show profound impairment in word comprehension with preserved repetition; this syndrome is also referred to as amnesic aphasia reflecting the loss of word meaning. It is seen in semantic dementia (the temporal lobe variant of frontotemporal dementia or Pick's disease) and advanced Alzheimer's disease. Earlier in Alzheimer's disease impaired naming with intact fluency and word comprehension (sometimes called anomic aphasia) is commonly seen. Impairment in language output with preserved repetition, transcortical motor aphasia, is most often associated with dorsomedial frontal lesions that involve the supplementary motor area.

Dyslexia

Patients with aphasia show dyslexic difficulties in keeping with their type of aphasia, thus those with fluent aphasia will struggle to understand the meaning of words in printed form, while those with non-fluent aphasia have trouble with grammatical aspects or reading (particularly word endings: -ed, -ing etc.). Within acquired dyslexia, however, dissociations have been defined for reading single words, these syndromes are known as deep and surface dyslexia.

Deep dyslexia and surface dyslexia

There may be a dissociation between ability to read orthographically regular (pronounced as they are spelt) words such as mint, flint, and hat, and irregular words such as pint, cellist, and island. Difficulty reading the latter type is known as surface dyslexia and is one of the hallmarks of semantic dementia; for an irregular word such as 'pint' or 'yacht' to be read correctly, the reader must access knowledge of the word meaning as the graphical representation of the word alone (that is, its 'surface' structure) will not lead to correct pronunciation. If the semantic knowledge base (located in the dominant temporal lobe) breaks down, then the word can only be pronounced according to the rules of graphical to phonological translation and thus 'pint' will be pronounced like 'mint' (known as a 'regularization' error); in other words, analogous to how a normal person would pronounce a non-word, such as 'rint'.

A complimentary syndrome is that of deep dyslexia in which patients produce semantic paralexias when reading (reading 'prison' for 'gaol' or 'beer' for 'pint'), are unable to read non-words, and have greater difficulty with abstract than concrete words. This, simplistically, is thought to represent a loss of the grapheme to phoneme route with intact semantic knowledge (that is,. its 'deep' meaning). Deep dyslexia is typically seen in patients with extensive left hemisphere lesions and global aphasia.

Alexia without agraphia

This syndrome represents a classic disconnection syndrome of visual input from language areas due to a lesion in the left occipital lobe and adjacent splenium (disrupting input form the right occipital lobe); as such, although the right occipital cortex is capable of registering text, the information cannot be decoded by the language hemisphere. Patients are not aphasic and can write normally, they cannot read but can say words spelt out loud to them. Visual field testing shows a right homonymous hemianopia. Patients rapidly relearn how to read by identifying individual letters and reconstructing words by a laborious and slow letter-by-letter reading strategy.

Agraphia

Various acquired disorders of writing occur as homologues of other cognitive deficits. For instance, patients with aphasia make writing errors consistent with their aphasic syndrome (for example patients with a Broca's aphasia will make errors in writing syntax), deep and surface dysgraphia give rise to similar errors as deep and surface dyslexia, and ideomotor apraxia (see below) will cause a disorder in motor execution such that writing will be of poor quality.

Visuospatial and perceptual disorders

The regions of the brain concerned with the higher order analysis of visual information can be divided into a dorsal (occipitoparietal) pathway concerned with spatial information and preparation for reaching, and a ventral (occipitotemporal) pathway concerned with identifying visual stimuli. In other words, the dorsal stream is involved in 'where?' and 'how?' and the ventral with 'what?' information for a given visual stimulus. Some of the most striking neuropsychological syndromes are seen following selective damage to one stream.

The dorsal stream and Balint's syndrome

Constructional apraxia, an inability to draw or copy line drawings such as wire cubes and clock faces, is a common finding in parietal pathology, particularly with right-sided lesions. More severe breakdown in spatial cognition causing individuals to misreach for visually guided targets, to trip on steps, or collide with furniture when walking is seen with bilateral parietal diseases (such as watershed infarction, the biparietal variant of Alzheimer's disease, and venous sinus thrombosis) and results clinically in Balint's syndrome; the features of which are simultanagnosia, optic ataxia, and ocular apraxia. Simultanagnosia is the inability to integrate and make sense of an overall visual scene in spite of preservation in the ability to identify individual elements. Such patients are relatively better at identifying small objects; this can also be demonstrated by an inability to read vertically printed words although they can be read when printed normally. Ocular apraxia describes the inability to direct gaze to a novel visual stimulus, while optic ataxia is the inability to reach accurately for a visually guided target.

Spatial neglect

Although considered under the visuospatial heading, spatial neglect is really a cross-modality disorder that typically involves the neglect of all sensory information (visual, tactile, auditory) from the side contralateral to the lesion. Chronic neglect virtually only occurs in the context of right parietal lobe damage. Right hemispatial neglect following an acute left parietal lesion can occur, but is usually less severe and tends to resolve within days. In addition to being a cross-modality disorder it is not correct to define a 'hemispatial field' in purely retinotopic terms. For instance, if a patient who exhibits neglect on visual field testing has the body turned to face the neglected extrapersonal hemispace (with head and eyes fixed in the original position), then the neglected space is reduced.

Visual neglect is best tested by cancellation (crossing off 'A's on a sheet of paper containing randomly arranged letters), drawing (clock, house, flower), or line bisection tasks. Patients with severe visual neglect may even appear to be hemianopic. A milder form of neglect can be elicited by 'sensory extinction' of the neglected side during bilateral sensory (visual and somatosensory at the bedside, although auditory neglect can be demonstrated experimentally) stimulation. Patients often have associated hemiparesis, although as part of their neglect syndrome they may deny this impairment—a phenomenon known as anosagnosia. When presented with the hemiparetic limb they may even deny that it is their own.

The ventral stream

Lesions to the occipitotemporal pathway give rise to difficulty recognizing visual stimuli that is not a consequence of being unable to appreciate where an object is in space as is the case in simultanagnosia. This deficit is known as visual object agnosia and has been divided further into aperceptual and associative varieties. In aperceptual agnosia, basic aspects of vision (acuity, fields, and contrast sensitivity) are intact, but patients cannot identify, or match identical, objects and have grave difficulty copying line drawings, although knowledge of these objects is intact if tested using other inputs such as describing from name. In contrast, associative agnosia describes a state where loss of object knowledge occurs such that although patients can copy line drawings well and match perceptually identical pictures, they cannot match non-perceptually identical images such as different angles of the same face or, for instance, tell that two different types of clock are both clocks. Associative agnosia is a cross-modality disorder such that knowledge of objects is impaired in non-visual modalities—in other words one component of generalized failure of semantic knowledge (see below). Differentiating these agnosias requires the use of test material only found in neuropsychology laboratories. One component of object knowledge is colour, loss of which (achromatopsia) usually accompanies occipitotemporal lesions and is more accessible to bedside evaluation.

A restricted form of impaired object recognition relates to faces. Known as prosopagnosia, the subject can no longer recognize previously familiar faces but can recognize their voices and have access to knowledge from their names. Usually bilateral lesions of the inferior occipitotemporal junction are responsible, although cases with lesions restricted to just the right side have been described.

Memory

Memory is divided by researchers into implicit and explicit subtypes (also known as non-declarative and declarative, respectively). Implicit memory refers to unconscious memory systems such as that responsible for conditioning as well as memory for motor tasks such hitting a golf ball or playing a piece of music 'by heart'. Explicit memory, in contrast, refers to consciously apprehended memory and is further divided into episodic and semantic memory. In clinical terms, when one refers to memory, it is only the explicit type of memory which is considered. When assessing memory complaints it is useful to apply a theoretically motivated approach to analysing symptoms according to the subcomponent of memory involved. In broad terms, memory subtypes can be considered under the following headings.

Working memory

Working memory refers to the amount of information that can be held by the brain 'on-line' (such as reading a phone number then holding it as the object of one's attention until the number can be dialled, or solving mathematical problems in the head); in the absence of rehearsal, when the focus of one's attention has moved to a novel topic for more than a few seconds, such items are lost. Working memory is also referred to as 'short-term' memory by psychologists, although this latter term is often used by patients and their doctors to describe recently acquired episodic memory (see below); it also involves aspects of attention (see above) so, to avoid confusion, the term 'working memory' is preferable. Slips of working memory are often erroneously seen by patients as the harbinger of dementia and thus these individuals are commonly referred to memory clinics: these lapses of attention (such as forgetting why you opened the refrigerator door or went into the study, or immediately forgetting a new telephone number) are common everyday symptoms which are increased with anxiety, depression, and also occur more commonly with advancing age. Complaints of this type are also common after head injury and in basal ganglia disorders.

Semantic memory

Semantic memory refers to the brain's knowledge store of, for example, objects and word meanings; it is also the term applied to knowledge of facts, such as that Paris is the capital of France, canaries are small yellow birds kept as pets, or that Ronald Reagan was a president of the United States. The inferolateral and polar regions of the temporal lobes (left for word and object meanings, right for face knowledge) are particularly critical to supporting semantic knowledge. Loss of memory for words is the usual complaint in patients with a primary disorder of semantic memory such as semantic dementia (also known as progressive fluent aphasia) and after herpes simplex virus encephalitis. However, it is important to distinguish between the occasional word finding lapse, usually for proper nouns, which occurs normally (especially in later life), and the relentlessly progressive loss of vocabulary, which occurs in association with left temporal lobe pathology. Low frequency words are the most vulnerable and patients with semantic dementia often have some insight into this problem in the early stages. For instance, a carpenter may complain that he can no longer remember the names of tools. Alzheimer's sufferers show a similar phenomenon, although it is usually overshadowed by their profound episodic memory deficit.

Table 2 Causes of the amnesic syndrome

Type	Common aetiologies
Transient	• Transient global amnesia • Transient epileptic amnesia • Closed head injury (may be permament) • After electroconvulsive therapy • Drugs (especially ethanol)
Anatomically defined	
Hippocampus (and adjacent mesial temporal structures)	• • Alzheimer' s disease • Herpes simplex encephalitis • Limbic encephalitis (paraneoplastic) • Watershed infarction: (cardiac arrest, CO poisoning, etc) • Complicating epilepsy surgery
Diencephalon (dorsomedial thalamus, mamillary bodies)	• Korsakoff's psychosis
Basal forebrain	• Infarction (watershed, deep perforator occlusion, 'top of the basilar' syndrome)
Fornix	• Ruptured anterior communicating artery aneurysm
Retrosplenial/posterior cingulate	• Complicating colloid cyst removal from third ventricle
Psychogenic (non-organic)	• Various: tumour, haemorrhage etc.

From: Hodges JR, ed. (2001). *Early onset dementia: a multidisciplinary approach.* Oxford University Press, Oxford.

Breakdown in semantic memory manifests as inability to name objects or drawings with the production of broad superordinate responses (such as 'animal' for 'elephant') and the inability to define the meaning of words. Category fluency (the ability to generate exemplars from a given semantic category such as types of animals or kitchen utensils or birds) is another sensitive measure of semantic memory. Knowledge of famous people can be tested by identifying photographs and names or asking the patient to list prime ministers in chronological order.

Episodic memory

Episodic memory refers to the event-based memories unique to each individual, in other words our recollection of personally experienced episodes (indeed, it is sometimes termed 'autobiographical' memory). Difficulty with the acquisition of new event-based memories (such as inability to recall details of a television programme or conversation with a friend despite good attention at the time) is the hallmark of early Alzheimer's disease and other causes of the amnesic syndrome (Table 2). Lesions that give rise to amnesia involve the limbic system of the brain (especially the hippocampi and their connections; Fig. 1). Although bilateral involvement is

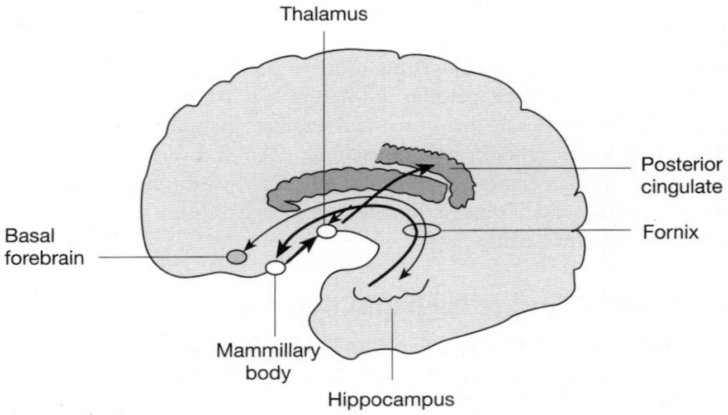

Fig. 1 Principal connections of structures critical to sustaining human memory.

usually required to cause a full-blown amnesic syndrome, neuropsychological testing can often reveal a selective deficit in verbal or non-verbal memory in cases of left- or right-sided damage, respectively. Retrograde memory (established prior to the amnesic insult) is typically better than anterograde (established any time after) in amnesic syndromes and within retrograde memory, very remote memory is classically (although not universally) better preserved than recent memory.

On examination, patients with amnesia have a striking inability to relate anecdotes from their recent life, although in cases of basal forebrain amnesia they may offer confabulations. Amnesia can be assessed in the clinic by asking the patient to learn some information such as a new name and address; patients with amnesic syndromes (including early Alzheimer's disease) typically repeat a name and address perfectly after two to three trials, but show very rapid forgetting and recall little or nothing after a delay of a few minutes of a distracting task.

Amnesia may occur as a temporary state as is seen with transient global amnesia, in which there is a sudden onset of severe amnesia that lasts several hours before resolution; afterwards the patient, characteristically elderly, is left with an islet of amnesia for the hours of the episode. Transient global amnesia typically occurs as a solitary episode; recurrent attacks of self-limiting amnesia occasionally occur as a consequence of epileptic activity, hence the term transient epileptic amnesia.

Apraxia

Apraxia is defined as a loss of ability to carry out skilled motor tasks that cannot be explained in terms of an elementary disorder of motor control (weakness or ataxia), primary sensory disturbance, or a global impairment of cognition. In the early twentieth century Leipmann distinguished three types of apraxia—limb-kinetic, ideomotor, and ideational—and although these terms have suffered from a lack of universally accepted definition they are still widely used today. In an attempt to clear up ambiguity, the terms 'production' and 'conceptual' apraxia are also now used to indicate ideomotor and ideational apraxia according to the definitions below.

Limb-kinetic apraxia refers to the loss of fine motor dexterity that can be seen, for instance, with mild pyramidal lesions (such as after recovery from stroke). In spite of apparently good strength and co-ordination, the subject cannot manage tasks requiring fine motor control such as tying a shoelace or buttoning a shirt. As such, according to the above definition, this is not a 'true' apraxia but rather an artefact of the insensitivity of bedside tests of the motor system: in other words a primary motor deficit is only unmasked by tasks more demanding than routine tests of power and co-ordination.

Ideomotor (production) apraxia refers to the inability to execute the motor programme for a given task (the temporal and spatial organization of movement) in spite of adequate comprehension, as demonstrated, for instance, by the ability to describe the correct execution of the task (such as sharpening a pencil: 'you put the pointed end of the pencil into the hole then turn it') or to identify correctly a task when done by someone else. Patients with ideomotor apraxia also have problems performing meaningless (non-symbolic) gestures.

Ideational (conceptual) apraxia, in contrast, is a loss of knowledge of actions: there is an inability to either perform or recognize a given motor task. There is also an inability to match tools correctly to their actions, thus a subject may select a screwdriver to hammer a nail. Unlike patients with ideomotor apraxia, they do not show disorders of the spatial and temporal aspects of action and thus their tool use, although incorrect, is fluent.

To screen for apraxia, patients should be asked to perform skilled motor tasks to verbal instruction or to imitation including both meaningful and meaningless gestures. If deficits are uncovered, tests such as correctly identifying mimes performed by the examiner and matching tools to functions should be given. Subtle disorders of praxis may be evident only with low frequency tasks (such as using a vegetable peeler or a pencil sharpener as opposed to a knife or a hairbrush). When asked to pantomime an action (such as hair combing or brushing teeth), 'body part as tool' errors are often cited as evidence for apraxia: the patient uses his or her hand as the tool (for example rubbing an extended index finger over the teeth as a toothbrush). It is, however, not uncommon for normal subjects to make these 'body part as tool' errors when asked to perform such tasks, hence it is essential when this type of error is committed to draw it to the subject's attention and reinstruct them accordingly. Normal subjects are able to correct these errors, whilst those with apraxia cannot.

In terms of the neural substrate for production (ideomotor) apraxia, the overwhelming majority of cases follow damage to the left (dominant) hemisphere. More specifically, there is evidence that a motor system incorporating the superior parietal lobule (Brodmann areas 5 and 7) and the premotor area of the left frontal lobe is particularly critical to the temporal and spatial organization of motor programmes. Conceptual apraxia is also indicative of left hemisphere dysfunction in most cases, although whether a more specific site can be identified is contentious. It is also important where a conceptual apraxia is suspected to ensure it is not just one manifestation of a more generalized breakdown of semantic knowledge (see Memory, above)

Buccofacial apraxia represents a specific form of apraxia in which patients are unable to perform tasks such as licking lips or blowing out matches to command. It is particularly associated with non-fluent aphasia, presumably as the motor programming of articulation and non-linguistic buccofacial movements share a common pathway.

Personality and behavioural change

So far, disorders of higher mental function have been considered in quite discrete terms, both in the sense of the cognitive deficit and the cerebral location. Alterations in complex behaviour, personality, and social comportment, however, cannot be so simply defined, but are broadly associated with frontal or anterior temporal lobe pathology. The key to identifying such disorders is the presence of a sustained change from a previous state (thus differing from a lifelong eccentric personality) which cannot be explained by a primary psychiatric diagnosis. The only reliable way to confirm such changes is by taking a separate history from a spouse or other close personal acquaintance with knowledge of the patient's premorbid personality.

Prefrontal syndromes

The prefrontal cortex comprises that part of the frontal lobe rostral to the premotor area; it is classified as heteromodal association cortex and receives extensive inputs from unimodal association areas posterior to the central sulcus. The frontal lobes also have loop projections running to the basal ganglia, then the thalamus, and back to the frontal lobes. Thus lesions along this loop (as seen in conditions such as Huntington's disease or progressive supranuclear palsy) may also share deficits in common with primary frontal lobe disorders. Anatomically, the prefrontal cortex can be divided into dorsolateral, orbital, and medial surfaces; although in many cases damage will not be restricted to just one of these regions, they provide a useful framework for considering prefrontal functions. Broadly, lesions to the dorsolateral surface are responsible for the frontal 'dysexecutive' syndrome, to the orbital surface for the classic frontal behavioural syndrome, and to the medial surface (anterior cingulate) for a profound amotivational state.

The dysexecutive syndrome

The term 'executive' refers to aspects of higher-order brain function, such as problem solving, reasoning, and mental abstraction, which rely upon the dorsolateral prefrontal lobes. It is also associated with impulsivity, susceptibility to distraction, and failure to persevere with the task at hand. Various methods are available to measure these phenomena although no single test offers foolproof sensitivity in this domain, so one should apply as many as possible if the index of suspicion is high.

The combination of letter- and category-based verbal fluency provides much useful information. In letter fluency, the patient is asked to generate as many words as they can think of beginning with a given letter in 1 min. They are instructed not to use proper nouns and not to just change the endings to create new exemplars ('go, goes, going' etc.). Neuropsychologists typically use the letters F, A, and S for this test, so it is best to choose another letter if it is likely that patients are also going to have a formal neuropsychological assessment. In category fluency, patients are asked to produce as many exemplars as possible from a given category in 1 min. Normal subjects usually generate 15 or more words on letter fluency and do slightly better on the 'animal' category. Patients with executive deficits secondary to frontal (or the subcortical loop) pathology show an exaggeration of this relationship, doing poorly on category fluency but even worse on letter fluency (patients with semantic impairments related to temporal lobe diseases such as semantic dementia and Alzheimer's disease typically show the reverse pattern of relatively worse performance on category fluency).

The 'go–no go' test offers a way of assessing impulsivity: the patient is asked to tap the desk once if the examiner does so, but if the examiner taps twice, he should not tap at all. Patients with frontal pathology are often unable to stop themselves from tapping in both conditions. Failure to abstract meaning from proverbs ('What does "too many cooks spoil the broth" mean') is a common test but is influenced by background intellectual ability and is culture bound. The so-called 'cognitive estimates' test is also useful ('What is the height of the post-office tower in London?' or 'How fast does a racehorse gallop?'), as are 'differences and similarities' ('What's the difference between a child and a dwarf?' or 'In what way are a sculpture and a piece of music similar?'). Finally, the susceptibility to irrelevant stimuli mean that the tests of attention discussed above may also be impaired.

Orbitofrontal syndrome

The striking changes in behaviour seen in patients with prefrontal lesions relate particularly to orbital (or ventral) surface damage. Although devastating in their effects on social function, such lesions are notoriously difficult to detect using standard psychometric tests. Patients lack empathy and emotional warmth: for instance, if confronted with something as serious as the admission to hospital of their spouse, their primary concern may be that their mealtime routine will be disturbed. They are disinhibited and oblivious to social mores such that they may be overly familiar with strangers, disregard personal space, and make inappropriate (often of a sexual nature) comments or gestures. They often make rash and irresponsible decisions such as spending money above their means. They may develop stereotyped and ritualistic behaviours such as insisting on always taking a particular route when shopping or repetitively closing doors in the home: these behaviours can be so severe as to constitute a secondary obsessive–compulsive disorder syndrome.

A useful clue is often the presence of a change in eating behaviour. Patients may become fixated on one dish; often they develop a preference for sweet foods. A lack of normal satiety means that they may overeat, often with secondary weight gain.

Imitation and utilization behaviour are dramatic phenomena related to orbital frontal lobe damage. The patient with imitation behaviour unconsciously mimics the examiner's posture and mannerisms regardless of how absurd they are: raising an arm in the air, placing a leg on the desk, or sitting on the floor. Utilization behaviour is even more striking: patients will use any object placed in their grasp. The classic example is the patient offered multiple pairs of spectacles who attempts to wear them all, one on top of another.

Amotivational states

Medial frontal lesions are particularly associated with apathy. Patients lack spontaneity, they will not initiate conversation although can reply to specific questions. Likewise, if left to their own devices, they may not spontaneously move, preferring to sit in a chair staring blankly into space. This apathy has also been termed abulia in the past, in its most extreme form where the individual lies motionless with no speech the term akinetic-mutism has also been applied. The catatonic phenomenon of maintaining postures when the limbs are moved by the examiner may also be seen. Patients with depression also show marked apathy, although it is accompanied by both the biological features of depression (anorexia, diurnal variation etc.) and internal symptoms of mood disturbance (pessimism, suicidal thoughts, anhedonia etc.).

Temporal lobe syndromes

In addition to the cognitive deficits that can occur with temporal lobe lesions such as amnesia and loss of semantic knowledge, behavioural distrubances can also occur. The most severe, secondary to bilateral anterior temporal damage (including the amygdala), is the Klüver–Bucy syndrome, which comprises three characteristic features: placidity, even in threatening situations, indiscriminant hypersexuality, and oral exploration of objects. Other behaviours have been described in temporal lobe dysfunction, particularly, although not exclusively, in association with interictal temporal lobe epilepsy. These include preoccupation with religious or philosophical issues and a tendency to excessive writing.

Further reading

Baddeley AD (1999). *Essentials of human memory.* Psychology press, Hove.

Berrios GE, Hodges JR (2000). *Memory disorders in psychiatric practice.* Cambridge University Press, Cambridge.

Cummings JL (1995). Anatomic and behavioral aspects of frontal-subcortical circuits. *Annals of the New York Academy of Sciences* **769**, 1–13.

Driver J, Mattingley JB (1998). Parietal neglect and visual awareness. *Nature Neuroscience* **1**, 17–22.

Garrard P, Perry R, Hodges JR (1997). Disorders of semantic memory. [Editorial.] *Journal of Neurology, Neurosurgery and Psychiatry* **62**, 431–5.

Graham KS, Patterson K, Hodges JR (1999). Episodic memory: new insights from the study of semantic dementia. *Current Opinion in Neurobiology* **9**, 245–50.

Hodges JR (1994). *Cognitive assessment for clinicians.* Oxford University Press, Oxford.

Hodges JR, Spatt J, Patterson K (1999). 'What' and 'how': evidence for the dissociation of object knowledge and mechanical problem-solving skills in the human brain. *Proceedings of the National Academy of Sciences USA* **96**, 9444–8.

McCarthy RA, Warrington EK (1990). *Cognitive neuropsychology: a clinical introduction.* Academic Press, San Diego.

Mesulam MM (1998). From sensation to cognition. *Brain* **121**, 1013–52.

Patterson K, Lambon-Ralph MA (1999). Selective disorders of reading? *Current Opinion in Neurobiology* **9**, 235–9.

Rothi LJG, Heilman KM, eds (1997). *Apraxia: the neuropsychology of action.* Psychology Press, Hove.

Tulving E, Craik FM, eds (2000). *The Oxford handbook of memory.* Oxford University Press, New York.

Ungerleider LG, Haxby JV (1994). 'What' and 'where' in the human brain. *Current Opinion in Neurobiology* **4**, 157–65.

Walsh K, Darby D (1999). *Neuropsychology: a clinical approach.* Churchill Livingstone, Edinburgh.

24.9 Brainstem syndromes

David Bates

Most of the brainstem syndromes involving both the long tracts of the brainstem and the cranial nerve nuclei occur due to vertebrobasilar ischaemia but were originally described in relation to tumours and other non-vascular disorders. Vascular disorders by their very character often have a rostrocaudal and patchy localization rather than the simplified transverse localization that is usually demonstrated in diagrams. It may not always be possible to identify the cause of specific symptoms and signs in an individual patient and therefore the diagnosis of vascular disorders in the brainstem is more profitably identified by knowledge of brainstem anatomy.

The classic presentation of brainstem syndromes, including the long tracts and deficits of cranial nerve nuclei, commonly causes crossed cranial nerve and motor or sensory long tract deficits; the cranial nerve palsy is ipsilateral to the lesion and the long tract signs contralateral. It is important to assess the.extracranial vascular supply to the posterior circulation, especially to listen for bruits over the subclavian vessels and to record the pulse and blood pressure in both upper limbs, remembering that the vertebral arteries arise from the subclavian vessels. Apart from the crossed cranial nerve and long tract deficits, there may be ataxia, vertigo, the presence of an internuclear ophthalmoplegia and unreactive pupils, the symptoms of diplopia and oscillopsia, and the finding of nystagmus or ocular paresis.

The circulation to the brainstem is supplied by the vertebral arteries, which are the main arteries to the medulla, then the basilar artery, which supplies the pons and midbrain. The vertebral arteries are frequently asymmetrical and commonly give rise to the large posterior inferior cerebellar arteries shortly before they join to form the basilar. The vertebral arteries are susceptible to trauma within the cervical spine, but the most common lesions affecting the vertebral arteries are dissection, which is probably under-recognized, or thrombosis.

The basilar artery supplies branches which may be described as paramedian, supplying the area of the pons close to the mid-line, the short circumferential which supply the lateral two-thirds of the pons, the long circumferential which are the superior and anterior inferior cerebellar arteries, and several interpeduncular branches which arise at the bifurcation of the basilar artery and supply the sub-thalamic and high midbrain regions.

The brainstem syndromes

Thalamic syndrome

Sometimes spontaneously but commonly following a recognized hemiplegic and hemianaesthetic stroke, the patient develops altered sensation in a hemisensory distribution together with unpleasant dysaesthetic burning pain (thalamic pain). The pain may be worsened by stimulation and is associated with hemianaesthesia, sometimes proprioceptive loss, and some evidence of hemiparesis. Anatomically the lesion is usually in the ventroposteriolateral nucleus of the thalamus and is commonly caused either by a vascular event or by a tumour. The investigations required are imaging and therapy is with centrally acting analgesic agents.

Tectal deafness

There is a rare syndrome associated with damage at the level of the inferior colliculi, either due to neoplasia or vascular lesions resulting in bilateral deafness and sometimes associated difficulty in co-ordination, weakness, and vertigo. The condition must be differentiated from conductive bilateral hearing loss, cochlear disorders, bilateral eighth nerve lesions, and pure word deafness. The lesion can be identified by brain imaging.

Thalamic stroke syndrome

Lesions affecting the thalamus are commonly vascular and arise from infarction within the distribution of the posterior communicating artery, the basilar and the anterior and posterior choroidal arteries. There is usually hemiparesis with hemianopia, hemianaesthesia, and sometimes hemiataxia. There is often confusion, disorientation, and there may be language disturbance. On occasion there may be vertical-gaze ophthalmoplegia, loss of pupillary reflexes, and an inability to converge the eyes. There may also be memory impairment and on occasions visual perceptual disturbances are recorded.

Midbrain syndromes

Damage to areas of the midbrain is characterized by long tract signs contralateral to the lesion with defects of the third and fourth cranial nerves ipsilaterally. They can been seen with lesions in the brainstem or as the evolution of symptoms of rostrocaudal deterioration associated with supratentorial brain swelling (Figs 1 and 2). They are characterized by ipsilateral third and fourth cranial nerve palsies together with contralateral hemiparesis, loss of vibration, propriception, and stereognosis, contralateral loss of pain and temperature, and an ipsilateral Horner's syndrome. Ataxia may occur and there can be eyelid ptosis, diplopia, supranuclear

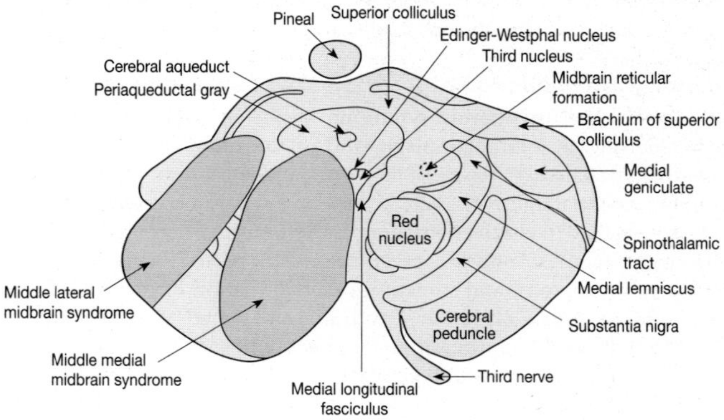

Fig. 1 Midbrain at the superior colliculus level, showing the medial and lateral territories involved with occlusive stroke in this region. (Reprinted with permission from DeArmond SI, Fusco MM, Dewey MM, 1976, *Structure of the human brain*, 2nd edn. Oxford University Press, New York.)

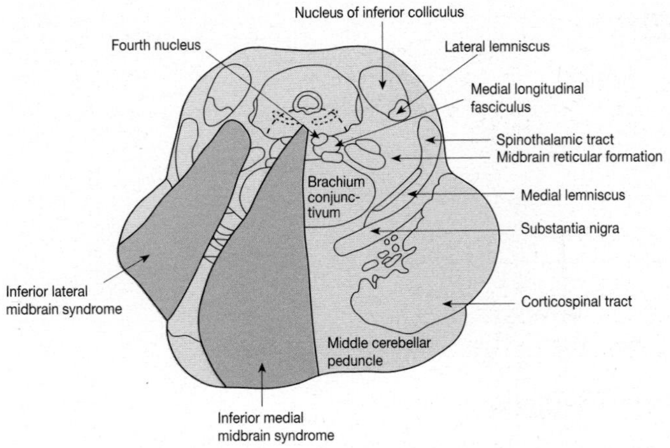

Fig. 2 Midbrain at the inferior colliculus level showing the medial and lateral territories involved with ischaemic stroke syndromes in this area. (Reprinted with permission from DeArmond SI, Fusco MM, Dewey MM, 1976, *Structure of the human brain*, 2nd edn. Oxford University Press, New York.)

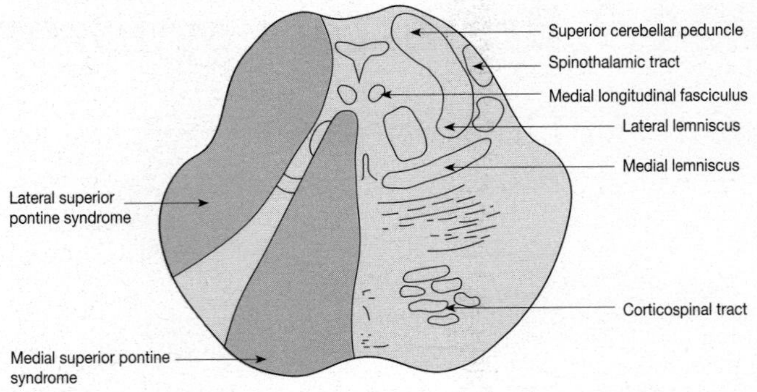

Fig. 3 Superior pontine level, showing the medial and lateral territories involved with occlusive stroke in this region. (Reprinted with permission from Adams RD, Victor M, 1993, *Principles of neurology*, 5th edn. McGraw-Hill, New York.)

horizontal-gaze paresis, and an internuclear ophthalmoplegia. The association of an ipsilateral oculomotor palsy with a crossed hemiplegia due to a lesion at the base of the midbrain is called a Weber syndrome. Claude syndrome causes an ipsilateral oculomotor palsy with contralateral cerebellar ataxia and tremor and is due to a lesion in the tegmentum of the midbrain involving the red nucleus and the third nerve nucleus. Benedikt's syndrome also involves the tegmentum of the midbrain resulting in an oculomotor palsy with contralateral cerebellar ataxia, tremor, and corticospinal signs and can be regarded as a combination of Claude and Weber's syndrome. Nothnagel syndrome occurs with unilateral or bilateral involvement of the third nerve nucleus together with the superior cerebellar peduncles and causes bilateral ptosis, paralysis of gaze, and cerebellar ataxia.

Damage in the region of the dorsal midbrain results in the Parinaud syndrome in which there is paralysis of upward gaze due to damage to the supranuclear mechanisms for upward gaze, loss of accommodation, and fixed pupils. Although this may be seen with ischaemic lesions, it is more commonly seen with pineal tumours.

Pontine syndromes

Lesions in the pons and medulla are commonly identified as involving either the medial or the lateral aspect of the brainstem, depending upon whether the paramedian or short circumferential vessels from the basilar have been involved. In the pons the following three levels of damage can be detected and the basal syndrome can occur at any level.

Superior pontine syndrome

The medial superior pontine syndrome results in ipsilateral cerebellar ataxia, internuclear ophthalmoplegia, and palatal and pharyngeal myoclonus with contralateral paralysis of face, arm, and leg and sometimes loss of sensation contralaterally. The lateral superior syndrome causes ataxia of limbs and gait with dizziness, nausea, and vomiting; there is horizontal nystagmus, paresis of conjugate gaze towards the side of the lesion, loss of optokinetic nystagmus, and sometimes skew deviation of the eyes. There may also be an ipsilateral Horner's syndrome and there is contralateral loss of pain and thermal sensation on the face and limbs with impaired touch, vibration, and position sense (Fig. 3).

The mid-pontine syndrome

The medial, mid-pontine syndrome causes ipsilateral ataxia of the limbs and gait with contralateral paralysis of the face, arm, and leg, deviation of the eyes away from the lesion, and variably impaired sensation contralaterally. The lateral syndrome at this level causes ataxia of the limbs on the side of the lesion together with paralysis of the muscles of mastication and impaired sensation over the face on the same side due to damage to the fifth nerve (Figs 4 and 5).

The inferior pontine syndrome

The medial syndrome causes paralysis of conjugate gaze to the side of the lesion, nystagmus, ataxia of limbs on the same side, and double vision on gaze to that side. Contralaterally there is paralysis of the face, arm, and leg with impaired touch and proprioception over the opposite side of the body. The lateral syndrome involves ipsilateral, horizontal, and vertical nystagmus with vertigo and nausea, ipsilateral facial paralysis, paralysis of conjugate gaze to the side of the lesion, deafness, tinnitus, and ataxia on the side of the lesion with impaired sensation of the face on that side. On the opposite side there is impaired sensation over half of the body (Fig. 6).

Basal pontine syndrome (locked in syndrome)

Bilateral lesions of the paramedian vessels from the basilar, commonly seen in patients with hypertension, result in infarction of the basis pontis causing quadriplegia with loss of the ability to speak. The ascending reticular activating system is intact and consciousness is therefore preserved. Vertical eye movements and eye closure are all that are possible and under voluntary control in the 'locked-in syndrome'.

Pseudobulbar palsy

Bilateral lesions of the long descending tracts in the brainstem can result in pseudobulbar palsy, although this condition is more commonly seen with

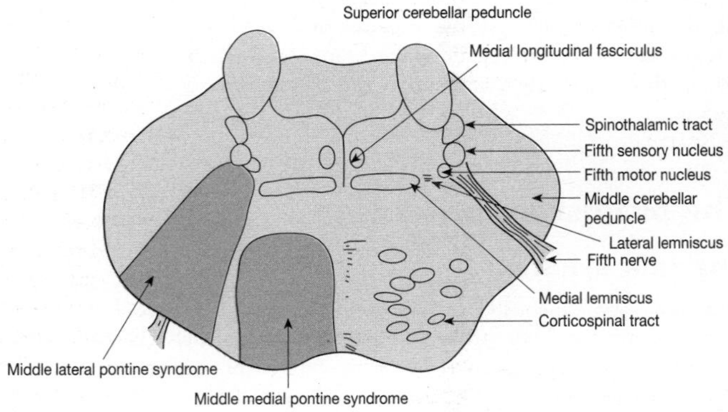

Fig. 4 Mid-pontine level, showing the medial and lateral territories involved with ischaemic stroke syndromes in this locality. (Reprinted with permission from Adams RD, Victor M, 1993, *Principles of neurology*, 5th edn. McGraw-Hill, New York.)

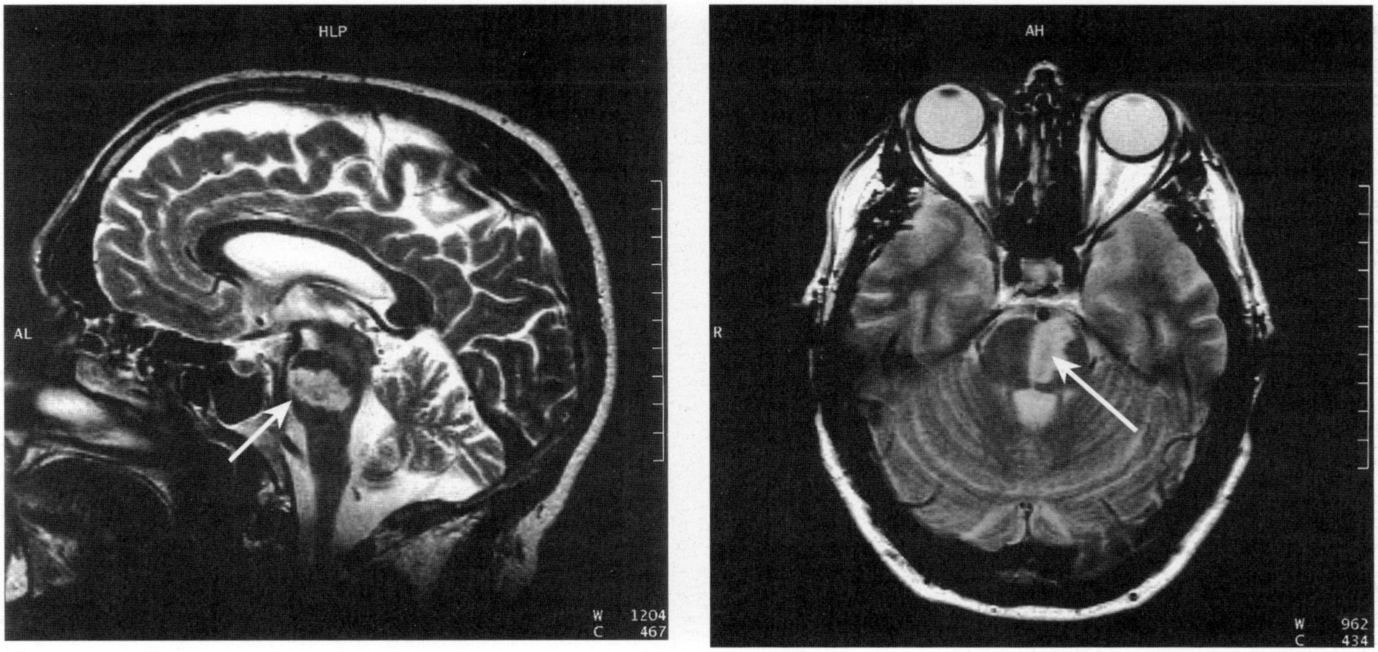

(a) (b)

Fig. 5 MRI scan of a mid-pontine infarction.

lesions higher in the cerebrum. The symptoms are those of spastic dysarthria, dysphagia, bilateral facial weakness with quadriparesis, and emotional lability.

Medullary syndromes

The medial medullary syndrome may occur with occlusion of the vertebral artery or a branch of the lower basilar artery; it causes paralysis and atrophy of the tongue on the side of the lesion with contralateral paralysis of the arm and leg but sparing the face and impaired tactile proprioceptive sensation over the contralateral half of the body. The lateral medullary syndrome occurs most commonly with dissection or occlusion of the vertebral artery, resulting in ischaemia into the posterior, inferior cerebellar artery; this causes pain, numbness, impaired sensation of the ipsilateral half of the face with ataxia of limbs on that side, the symptoms of vertigo and nausea, double vision, and oscillopsia, and the signs of nystagmus. There is an ipsilateral Horner's syndrome, often dysphagia with paralysis of the vocal cord ipsilaterally, and loss of sensation on the arm, trunk, and leg. There is contralateral impaired pain and thermal sensation over half the body and possibly the face (Fig. 7).

A syndrome involving ipsilateral seventh and sixth nerve palsies with a contralateral hemiplegia is called the Millard–Gubler syndrome; the involvement of the tenth cranial nerve causing paralysis of the soft palate and vocal cord with contralateral hemianaesthesia is termed the Avellis syndrome and is due to a lesion in the tegmentum of the medulla. The lateral medullary syndrome is eponymously called the Wallenberg syndrome.

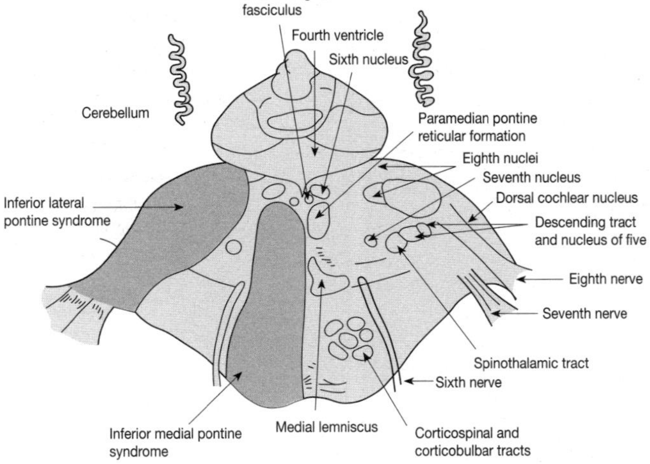

Fig. 6 Inferior pons at the level of the sixth nerve nucleus, showing the medial and lateral territories involved with occlusive stroke in this area. (Reprinted with permission from Adams RD, Victor M, 1993, *Principles of neurology*, 5th edn. McGraw-Hill, New York.)

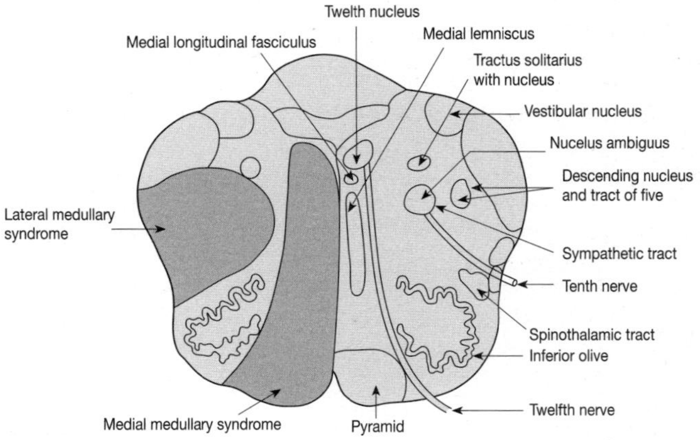

Fig. 7 Cross-section of medulla at the level of the inferior olivary complex, showing the medial and the more common lateral territory involved with ischaemic stroke in this brainstem site. (Reprinted with permission from Adams RD, Victor M, 1993, *Principles of neurology*, 5th edn. McGraw-Hill, New York.)

Investigations and treatment

The clinical identification of lesions lying within the brainstem by a combination of cranial nerve and long tract signs, though important is only the beginning of diagnosis. Such syndromes commonly occur with ischaemic lesions within the brainstem but can also be seen with neoplasia, demyelination, and infective and hamartomatous lesions. The identification of a brainstem syndrome makes imaging, ideally with MRI rather than CT, obligatory and only then, and possibly following other investigations to identify systemic abnormality or cerebrospinal fluid changes, can appropriate therapy be introduced. Vascular lesions within the brainstem often carry a remarkably good prognosis, but if the syndrome appears to be evolving, the possibility of anticoagulation must be considered. In those lesions in which damage affects the medulla it may be important to protect the airway and avoid aspiration during the early phases of the illness.

Further reading

Adams RD, Victor M (1989). *Principles of neurology*, 4th edn. McGraw-Hill, New York.

Caplan LR (1988). Vertebrobasilar system syndromes. In: Vinken PJ, Bruyn GW, Klawans HL, eds. *Handbook of clinical neurology*. Elsevier, Amsterdam.

24.10 Subcortical structures—the cerebellum, thalamus, and basal ganglia

N. P. Quinn

The cerebellum

Structure and function

The cerebellum occupies the greater part of the posterior fossa, reaching from the tentorium rostrally to the foramen magnum caudally, and lying dorsal to the lower pons and medulla, from which it is separated by the fourth ventricle. Its blood supply is derived from posterior circulation via the superior, anterior inferior, and posterior inferior cerebellar arteries. The cerebellum can be divided into cortex, intrinsic nuclei, and interposed white matter (medullary substance). The cortex comprises three cell layers—from the surface inwards these are the molecular layer (3), the Purkinje cell layer (2), and the granular cell layer (1). The only output cells of the cortex are the Purkinje cells. Inputs to the cerebellar cortex comprise either climbing or mossy fibres. The former synapse directly with Purkinje cells. The latter synapse with granule cells in layer 3, whose axons ascend to layer 1 where they form parallel fibres which synapse with Purkinje cell dendrites ascending from layer 2.

The cerebellum can also be divided into: archicerebellum (flocculonodular lobe), with largely vestibular inputs; palaeocerebellum (anterior lobe), with largely spinal cord inputs; and neocerebellum (posterior, largest lobe), with largely pontine inputs from cerebral cortex. Yet another way of dividing the cerebellum is into functional 'units' as follows: the vermal zone, comprising the fastigial nuclei and the midline unpaired portion of cerebellum, projects to vestibular nuclei and controls mainly axial posture, tone and balance, and locomotion; the paravermal zones, comprising the globose and emboliform nuclei and corresponding cerebellar cortex, project via the contralateral red nucleus and other nuclei of the reticular formation to influence ipsilateral limb tone; and the lateral zones, comprising the dentate nuclei and lateral cerebellar cortex, project via contralateral thalamus on to motor cortex to effect ipsilateral motor co-ordination.

The integrating function of cerebellum is evident from the fact that afferent fibres (Fig. 1) heavily outnumber efferent ones by about 40 to 1. Connections travel in three cerebellar peduncles, the lower two mainly afferent and the upper one efferent: the inferior cerebellar peduncle (restiform body) carries spino-, vestibulo-, and olivocerebellar fibres and input from other medullary ('precerebellar') nuclei; the middle cerebellar peduncle (brachium pontis) carries major afferent fibres from the pontine nuclei responsible for relaying and integrating a large input from all areas of the cerebral cortex; the superior cerebellar peduncle (brachium conjunctivum) contains a few afferent spinocerebellar fibres, but most of its bulk comprises cerebellar efferent fibres which originate in the intrinsic cerebellar nuclei and stream up to the contralateral red nucleus, or through it to the thalamus, to influence heavily thalamocortical, and then corticospinal, input. Other cerebellar efferents go to vestibular nuclei and to nuclei in the pontine and medullary reticular formation. These brainstem efferents provide access to the rubrospinal, vestibulospinal, and reticulospinal tracts.

Clinical aspects

There are several theories on the main functions of the cerebellum. Thus it may work as a timing device to control the duration and latency of muscle activities, it may act as a learning device to lay down circuitry for repeating previously performed movements, and it may act as a co-ordinator to harmonize and correctly scale the contribution of several brain areas to an intended movement.

The symptoms and signs resulting from lesions of the cerebellum or its pathways in humans have been based on observations in trauma (particularly gunshot wounds), tumour, stroke, and degenerative and demyelinating diseases.

Midline vermal lesions cause truncal ataxia, often in the absence of limb ataxia. The gait is wide based and particularly precarious on turning or on heel–toe walking. Patients may be unsteady for many reasons, only one of which is ataxia, so the former term is preferable where any doubt exists. Unilateral cerebellar hemispheric lesions cause deviation or falling to the ipsilateral side. Unlike a sensory ataxia, cerebellar ataxia is not made worse by shutting the eyes. Generally, ataxic patients have more problem going down, and those with weakness going up, stairs.

Disease of cerebellar hemispheres or outflow tracts often causes limb ataxia, which is in fact an amalgam of several components. First, there may be dysmetria (misreaching, or past-pointing) evident in the arms on the finger–nose test or in the legs when the heel is first brought to the opposite kneecap. Second, there is the breakdown in force, rate, and rhythm known as dysdiadochokinesia. This can best be sought by asking patients to tap gently, regularly, and rapidly on your hand or a table with their fingers. This breakdown of smooth repetitive movements can even be detected by feel or by sound ('listening to the cerebellum'). The third element is intention tremor. Many individuals claimed to have intention tremor do not actually

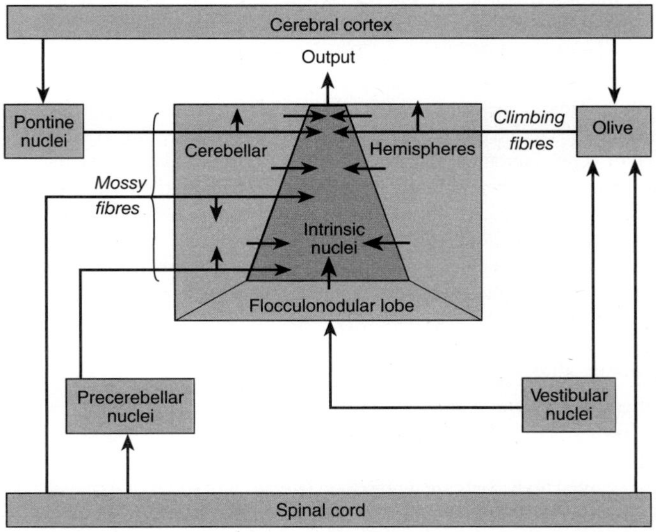

Fig. 1 A simplified diagram showing the principal afferents to cerebellar cortex and to intrinsic cerebellar nuclei. Both mossy (left) and climbing (right) fibre inputs project to both cortex and intrinsic nuclei.

have it, the principal error being to use this term to describe a tremor that simply appears or worsens terminally. Thus, many postural tremors are positionally dependent, and some are only seen when the hands are in a given posture, particularly either outstretched or held in front of the nose. Other non-cerebellar tremors may be present, or appear only during action (action or kinetic tremor). Only if additional signs of cerebellar dysfunction considered above are also present, is it reasonable to use the term intention tremor. Such tremor should augment throughout a movement from inception to completion. A particular form of tremor may be produced by lesions strategically placed in a small area between cerebellum, midbrain, and subthalamus. This tremor has been variously called Holmes', rubral, midbrain, or peduncular tremor, and combines a tremor at rest with a tremor on posture and an intention tremor on movement. Cerebellar lesions may also cause the 'rebound phenomenon' resulting from impaired damping of limbs when suddenly a load is removed or a displacement applied. Finally, any judgement concerning possible limb ataxia can only be made after taking into account any weakness, sensory loss, akinesia, or apraxia that may also be present.

Cerebellar dysarthria may often simply manifest as slurred speech, as if intoxicated. However, in addition some patients may have either scanning or explosive speech, due to an inability to modulate its rate, rhythm, and force appropriately. Dysarthria is usually present with lesions of the vermis, whole cerebellum, or its connections, but may be absent if one lateral hemisphere alone is involved.

Eye movements are frequently abnormal in disease of the cerebellum or its connections. The following may be seen: gaze-evoked, rebound, downbeat, or positional nystagmus, dysmetric voluntary saccades and jerky pursuit, square-wave jerks (macrosaccadic oscillations), impaired vestibulo-ocular reflex suppression, and skew deviation. The presence of diplopia usually implies additional pathology outside the cerebellum proper.

The thalamus

Structure and function

The two thalami sit at the head of the brainstem, their medial borders largely separated by the third ventricle, but often partially fused as the massa intermedia. Their blood supply derives from the posterior circulation via the posterior cerebral arteries and perforators from the terminal part of the basilar artery. They constitute the largest nuclear mass in the diencephalon (the others being the hypothalamus and subthalamus), and occupy a strategic position both anatomically and functionally.

The structure of the thalamus, already complex, is further confused by the existence of different nomenclatures (the one used here is that of Walker). Broadly speaking, there are three nuclear groups (anterior, medial, and lateral). The lateral group is divided into the lateral and ventral masses, each of which contain a number of nuclei. The ventral lateral cell mass is the main region where somatosensory afferents terminate.

The thalamus receives inputs from cerebral cortex, sensory tracts, basal ganglia, and cerebellum. Almost all of its output is to the cerebral cortex, either in the form of reciprocal circuits or of more complex loops (see later) from cortex through other subcortical structures to thalamus and back to cortex again, but there is a small output to striatum.

Thalamic afferents

Somatic and visceral afferents

Somatic and visceral afferents from the body pass via the medial lemniscus and spinothalamic tract into the ventral posterolateral nucleus caudalis, where caudal body parts are represented laterally and rostral parts medially. Inputs from the face (via trigeminothalamic tracts) pass even more medially into the ventral posteromedial nucleus. Somatotopic representation is maintained through the connections to the parietal lobe in the form of the sensory homunculus with legs medially, arms high, and face low over the convexity. Taste afferents feed into ventral posteromedial nucleus parvocellularis, and hearing and vision into the medial and lateral geniculate bodies, respectively.

Basal ganglia input

The medial globus pallidus projects to the centromedian nucleus, to ventral anterior nucleus parvocellularis, and to ventral lateral nucleus oralis and medialis, and its homologue the substantia nigra pars reticulata to the mediodorsal nucleus and ventral anterior nucleus magnocellularis.

Cerebellar input

Afferents from intrinsic cerebellar nuclei ascend to the ventral lateral nucleus caudalis, to the ventral posterolateral nucleus oralis, and to the adjacent zone x.

Thalamic efferents

All the thalamic nuclei project to the cerebral cortex with the exception of important outputs from the intralaminar centromedian-parafascicular nuclear complex to striatum.

Clinical aspects

From the above it is clear that, depending on the nuclei involved, thalamic lesions might influence either sensation or motor function or sometimes both. Most commonly an infarct or haemorrhage (10 to 15 per cent of all intracerebral haemorrhages) causes contralateral sensory loss or impairment. A small lacunar infarct in the ventral posterolateral nucleus may give rise to a pure sensory stroke, sometimes sparing the face. A larger lesion may cause the thalamic syndrome of Dejerine and Roussy, in which an initial mild and transient hemiplegia is accompanied by persisting superficial and deep sensory impairment, mild hemiataxia, and astereognosis. These are commonly accompanied by choreoathetoid movements and severe, persistent, paroxysmal, often intolerable pains on the affected side. When mild, the movements may be pseudoathetotic due to deafferentation; when severe, they suggest that the lesion may extend beyond the thalamus to involve basal ganglia connections. Other movement disorders described after thalamic strokes are myoclonus, asterixis, tremor, dystonia, and a delayed-onset syndrome of choreiform and dystonic movements associated with slow rhythmic jerks at 2 to 3 Hz involving the contralateral arm. A significant, persisting hemiplegia implies either a large thalamic lesion also involving internal capsule or the possibility that the stroke is primarily capsular and not thalamic. A particular form of subcortical aphasia has been described in thalamic lesions.

Finally, surgical lesions have been stereotactically placed in the ventral lateral nucleus caudalis (also known as the ventral intermediate nucleus—Vim in Hassler's nomenclature) to relieve tremor in Parkinson's disease and benign essential tremor, and also rigidity (but not akinesia) in the former. Chronic electrical stimulation of the same area is also effective. However, the thalamus as a target for surgery in Parkinson's disease has now largely been superseded by the subthalamic nucleus (see later) because inactivation of the latter target also improves the other features of parkinsonism.

The basal ganglia

Structure and function

There is no uniform agreement on how many of the subcortical nuclei one should include under the terms basal ganglia and extrapyramidal motor system, but all definitions at least include the neostriatum (caudate nucleus and putamen, often together called simply the striatum) and the palaeostriatum (the lateral and medial globus pallidus with the latter's homologue, the substantia nigra pars reticulata). The term corpus striatum refers to neostriatum plus palaeostriatum, and lentiform nucleus to putamen plus globus pallidus. The substantia nigra pars compacta and the subthalamic nucleus and the limbic amygdaloid complex of archistriatum should also be considered part of the basal ganglia. The claustrum, substantia innominata, red nucleus, pedunculopontine nucleus, and even the thalamus are considered in some classifications to be part of the basal ganglia, but will not be dealt with here under that heading.

The putamen lies lateral to the thalamus, separated from it (and from most of the caudate nucleus, except anteriorally) by the internal capsule. The caudate nucleus, whose head lies anterodorsomedial to the putamen, describes most of a circle as it follows, and progressively tapers with, the lateral ventricles through its body posteriorally, its tail swinging forward until its anteriorly pointing tip terminates in the amygdaloid nucleus. The pallidum lies medial to the putamen but still lateral to the internal capsule, and is divided into lateral and medial pallidal segments. The substantia nigra lies in the midbrain, transversely above the cerebral peduncles. Its pars reticulata, the termination of the striatonigral pathway, is homologous with medial globus pallidus, and its pars compacta contains the dopaminergic neurones which form the nigrostriatal pathway. Below the thalamus, medial to the internal capsule and rostral to the midbrain, is the subthalamic nucleus.

Most of the caudate, putamen, and globus pallidus derive their arterial supply from anterior circulation via the lateral lenticulostriate arteries and branches of the anterior choroidal and anterior cerebral arteries. Like the thalamus, the subthalamic region, and also the substantia nigra, are supplied by posterior circulation.

The basal ganglia and their (inter-) connections, rich in neurotransmitters, have been extensively studied. The 'striopallidal complex' receives a wide variety of inputs from cerebral cortex. Its principal output is to the thalamus, which in turn projects back to the cortex to complete a basal ganglia–thalamocortical circuit. However, it is important to note the existence of additional output to the brainstem in the pallidotegmental tract which terminates in the pedunculopontine nucleus. This structure is believed to play an important role in the control of balance and locomotion, and in the maintenance of rigidity. The caudate and putamen are the afferent, and the globus pallidus and substantia nigra pars reticulata the efferent, parts of the striopallidal complex. There is additional dopaminergic input from substantia nigra pars compacta and the adjacent ventral tegmental area in the midbrain which modulates striatal activity. A highly simplified schema concentrating on the motor circuit is presented in Fig. 2.

The massive cortical inputs into the striatum are largely excitatory, using glutamate as a neurotransmitter. Other inputs come from the intralaminar thalamic nuclei, amygdala, and dorsal nucleus of the raphe. In the nigrostriatal pathway from the substantia nigra pars compacta, dopamine preferentially stimulates dopamine D_1 receptors to activate neurones of the direct pathway to the medial globus pallidus which contain dynorphin, substance P, and GABA, and are therefore inhibitory. Dopamine D_2 receptor stimulation preferentially inhibits the first neurones of the indirect pathway to the lateral globus pallidus which contain enkephalin and GABA. These neurones inhibit subthalamic neurones which in turn, using glutamate, excite cells in the medial globus pallidus and substantia nigra pars reticulata. These in their turn use GABA to inhibit thalamic neurones, which finally complete the loop with an excitatory pathway back to the cortex.

This model can be used to predict the functional consequences of over- or underactivity of individual parts, either in human disease states or in experimental animals. In the latter, 2-deoxyglucose autoradiographic studies can be used to confirm such predictions elegantly and validate the model. Thus, the consequences of cell loss in the substantia nigra pars compacta that occur in Parkinson's disease would be as follows: along the direct pathway there is impaired stimulation of the striatal cells that normally inhibit the neurones of the medial globus pallidus/substantia nigra pars reticulata, so the latter are overactive. Along the indirect pathway, there is impaired inhibition (hence overactivity) of the neurones that inhibit the lateral globus pallidus, which is therefore underactive. However, this leads to less inhibition (hence overactivity) of the subthalamic nucleus, which increases excitatory input to the medial globus pallidus/substantia nigra pars reticulata (already overactive via the direct pathway). This overactivity in turn inhibits thalamic, and then cortical, activity. The model would predict that making a lesion in the overactive subthalamic nucleus or medial globus pallidus might relieve parkinsonism, and indeed this has been demonstrated in MPTP-treated primates and patients with Parkinson's disease, respectively.

The model can also be used to understand hyperkinetic movement disorders. Hemiballism (severe unilateral proximal chorea) is classically caused by a destructive lesion in, or close to, the subthalamic nucleus. In this instance an underactive subthalamic nucleus would release the thalamus and hence the cortex from inhibition by the medial globus pallidus/substantia nigra pars reticulata, and again this sequence has been confirmed by 2-deoxyglucose experiments in animals.

All that has been mentioned so far concerns motor function, traditionally equated with the function of the basal ganglia. However, as the complexity and diversity of basal ganglia anatomy, circuitry, and function has become apparent, the concept of multiple basal ganglia–thalamocortical circuits has developed. Although some overlapping of cortical input to the striatum does indeed occur, rather than cortical inputs being simply funnelled through the circuits, thereafter the loops are increasingly non-overlapping, allowing more separate and independent processing throughout

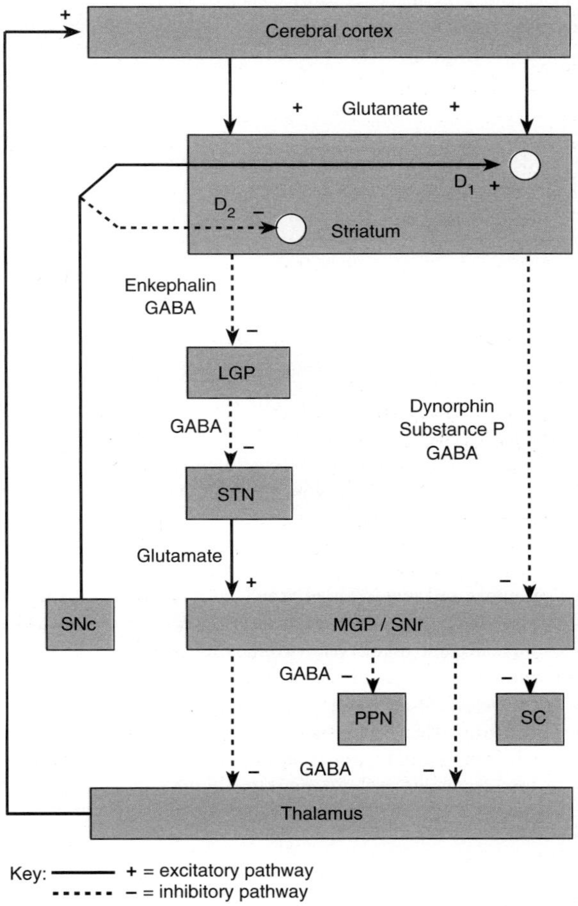

Fig. 2 A simplified schematic diagram showing the principal connections of the basal ganglia. Excitatory synapses are indicated by +, inhibitory ones by –. D^1 signifies dopamine D^1, and D^2 dopamine D^2, receptors. LGP and MGP, lateral and medial globus pallidus; STN, subthalamic nucleus; SNr and SNc, substantia nigra pars reticulata and pars compacta; PPN, pedunculopontine nucleus; SC, superior colliculus.

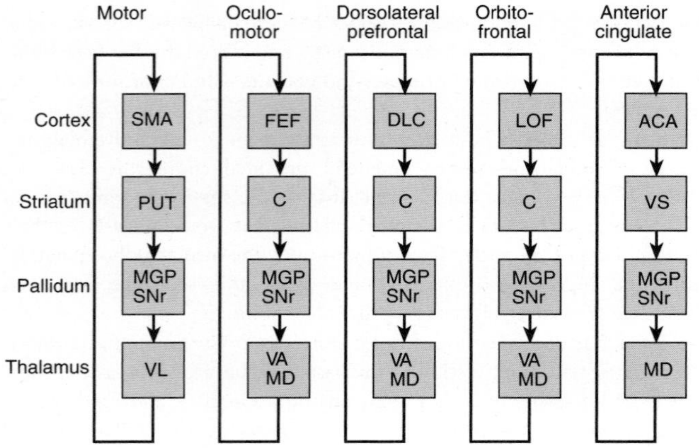

Fig. 3 A highly simplified diagram of proposed basal ganglia–thalamocortical loops (after Alexander *et al.*, 1986, with permission). Same abbreviations as for Fig. 2

the basal ganglia. Five such circuits have been proposed: (i) the motor and (ii) the oculomotor, involved in sensorimotor functions of the body and eyes; (iii) the dorsolateral prefrontal and (iv) orbitofrontal, involved in cognitive aspects of behaviour; and (v) the anterior cingulate circuit, related to limbic functions. A simplified representation of these loops is given in Fig. 3.

The last decade has also seen considerable advances in our knowledge of striatal anatomy and neurochemistry. Morphological techniques have long demonstrated a variety of striatal neuronal types. These are either projection neurones (spiny medium type I, the vast majority, and large type II), or intrinsic neurones (aspiny types I to III). However, the striatum as a whole seemed rather amorphous until neurochemical markers gave a new perspective. Thus, the medium type I spiny projection neurones are the major targets of nigral dopaminergic transmission, and make synaptic contact with large aspiny cholinergic interneurones. The former cells are selectively lost in Huntington's disease, resulting in a loss of their inhibitory transmitter GABA, together with colocalized metenkephalin or substance P. In contrast, type I aspiny interneurones containing neuropeptide Y and somatostatin, and type II aspiny interneurones containing acetylcholine, are largely spared in Huntington's disease.

It is now recognized that striatal neurones are also organized into a mosaic pattern comprising patches or striosomes with high levels of μ-opiate receptors and low levels of acetylcholinesterase, suspended in a matrix of cells containing high levels of aceytlcholinesterase, somatostatin, and calbindin. Patch and matrix receive different inputs from the midbrain, thalamus, and cortex. In particular, deeper levels of prefrontal or limbic cortex tend to project to striosomes and more superficial layers of sensorimotor cortex to matrix. Patches mainly project to substantia nigra pars compacta, whereas matrix neurones may take either the direct or indirect route to the medial globus pallidus/substantia nigra pars reticulata.

Clinical aspects

On the basis of the above evidence, we can no longer assume that basal ganglia pathology produces only motor symptoms and signs. Thus, in patients with Parkinson's disease, Huntington's disease, and progressive supranuclear palsy—all of which principally (but not exclusively) involve basal ganglia— affective disorder, 'subcortical dementia', or 'frontal lobe deficits' may be seen.

Nevertheless, the most striking clinical features of basal ganglia disease remain those in the motor sphere, comprising tremor, rigidity, akinesia, and postural abnormality as evidenced by Parkinson's disease, and hyperkinetic movement disorders such as chorea and dystonia seen, for example, in Huntington's disease and in subjects with Parkinson's disease chronically treated with levodopa preparations.

The classic tremor of Parkinson's disease is slow (4 to 6 Hz), pill-rolling, and disappears and diminishes on movement, to reappear once a new posture has been adopted. In animal studies a nigral lesion seems necessary, but not sufficient, to cause this tremor.

Akinesia is a symptom complex comprising slowness of movement (bradykinesia), poverty of movement, progressive diminution and fatigue of rapid alternating movements, and difficulty in initiating and sequencing movements and in accomplishing simultaneous motor acts. Since changes in neuronal discharge relating to movement seem to occur later in the basal ganglia than in the motor cortex, it has been proposed that the basal ganglia are more concerned with using information from a previous movement to set up the premotor areas to select the correct parameters for running subsequent motor programmes. In Parkinson's disease levodopa strikingly improves akinesia. Lesions or high-frequency deep brain stimulation (which functionally causes inhibition) in the thalamus does not relieve akinesia in humans, but lesions or deep brain stimulation in the internal pallidum or subthalamic nucleus do so.

Rigidity almost always accompanies akinesia. Resistance to passive movement is broadly similar in flexion and extension. It is described as lead-pipe or, if there is superimposed tremor (visible or invisible), as cogwheeling. Abnormalities of the tonic stretch reflex are felt to contribute to its pathophysiology.

As well as akinesia, both tremor and rigidity respond to levodopa. Unlike akinesia, both also respond to thalamotomy, but the lesion needs to be larger for rigidity than for tremor.

Postural instability is another feature of parkinsonism. This is in part due to impairment of anticipatory responses and postural adjustments associated with movement, and problems in controlling body sway. Unlike the above features, this may often be levodopa resistant.

Of the hyperkinetic movement disorders, chorea (in the case of Huntington's disease) and dystonia (when secondary to discernible brain pathology) can be related to basal ganglia disease. Although chorea can be produced by making lesions in the subthalamic nucleus in intact monkeys, or by chronic dopaminergic treatment of primates with a lesioned nigrostriatal tract, it is not usually possible to produce spontaneous chorea in animals solely by making a caudate lesion analogous to that in Huntington's disease. Similarly, although dystonia may be seen in humans after lesions of the putamen (principally), caudate, or thalamus, there is again no good animal model, although it can be induced by dopaminergic drugs in MPTP-treated primates.

Further reading

Albin RL, Young AB, Penney JB (1989). The functional anatomy of basal ganglia disorders. *Trends in Neurosciences* **12**, 366–75. [An excellent synthesis of anatomical and functional aspects of the basal ganglia.]

Alexander GE, DeLong MR, Strick PL (1986). Parallel organization of functionally segregated circuits linking basal ganglia and cortex. *Annual Review of Neuroscience* **9**, 357–81.

Carpenter MB (1991). *Core text of neuroanatomy*, 4th edn. Williams & Wilkins, Baltimore. [The best medium-sized all-round textbook of neuroanatomy.]

Crossman AR (1990). A hypothesis on pathophysiological mechanisms that underlie levodopa - or dopamine agonist-induced dyskinesia in Parkinson's disease: Implications for future strategies in treatment. *Movement Disorders* **5**, 100–8.

Gerfen CR (1992). The neostriatal mosaic: multiple levels of compartmental organisation. *Trends in Neurosciences* **15**, 33–9.

Graybiel AM (1989). Dopaminergic and cholinergic systems in the striatum. In: Crossman A, Sambrook MA, eds. *Neural mechanisms in disorders of movement*, pp 3–15. Libbey, London.

Hassler R (1959). Anatomy of the thalamus. In: Schaltenbrand G, Bailey P, eds. *Introduction to stereotaxis with an atlas of the human brain*, pp. 230–90. G. Thieme, Stuttgart.

Krack P *et al.* (2000). Thalamic, pallidal, or subthalamic surgery for Parkinson's disease? *Journal of Neurology* **247** (suppl. 2:II), 122–34.

Lehericy S, *et al.* (2001). Clinical characteristics and topography of lesions in movement disorders due to thalamic lesions. *Neurology* **57**, 1055–66.

Lera G *et al.* (2000). A combined pattern of movement disorders resulting from posterolateral thalamic lesions of a vascular nature: a syndrome with clinico-radiologic correlation. *Movement Disorders* **15**, 120–6.

Limousin P *et al.* (1998). Electrical stimulation of the subthalamic nucleus in advanced Parkinson's disease. *New England Journal of Medicine* **339**, 1105–11.

Marsden CD (1990). Neurophysiology. In: Stern GM, ed. *Parkinson's disease*, pp 57–98. Chapman & Hall, London. [A clear overview of the physiological mechanisms underlying the clinical features of parkinsonism.]

Marsden CD, Obeso JA (1994). The functions of the basal ganglia and the paradox of stereotaxic surgery in Parkinson's disease. *Brain* **117**, 877–97.

Rothwell JC (1994). *Control of human voluntary movement*, 2nd edn. Croom Helm, London. [A short textbook on the physiology of human motor disorders.]

Walker AE (1938). *The primate thalamus.* University of Chicago Press.

24.11 Visual pathways

Christopher Kennard

Introduction

Diagnosis of disturbances of the visual pathways requires both a thorough knowledge of their anatomy and physiology, as well as the ability to carry out a thorough neuro-ophthalmological examination. It is the examination which should enable the character and extent of the visual disturbance to be documented as well as the topographic localization of the lesion, so that the relevant investigative techniques, such as imaging, can be appropriately requested.

Clinical evaluation of visual function

Examination of visual function initially requires an accurate assessment of the visual acuity. Acuity should be tested separately in each eye using the Snellen or some other optotype chart, which contains rows of letters of diminishing size. If an impairment (> 6/6) is noted, the patient should be allowed to wear glasses or alternatively to view the chart through a pinhole which eliminates any significant refractive error or optic media distortion. If the acuity does not improve, it is necessary to try and distinguish media opacities and retinal abnormalities from optic nerve dysfunction using the swinging flashlight test. In a darkened room each eye is alternatively stimulated with a bright light, which is moved rhythmically from one eye to the other. A dilatation of the pupil of the defective eye when the light is swung from the good eye on to it is termed a 'relative afferent pupillary defect', and signifies optic nerve dysfunction. Another good indicator of an optic nerve disturbance is a defect of colour vision, which may be tested using one of several available booklets of colour plates such as the Ishihara pseudo-isochromatic plates.

The photostress test is a useful test to distinguish a maculopathy from optic nerve dysfunction. The retina of the 'normal' eye is bleached by shining a bright light at the pupil for 10 s, and measuring the time for normal acuity to be re-established. The test is repeated in the 'abnormal' eye and if the difference in recovery time between the two eyes is greater than 60 s, the test is considered abnormal, indicating that the impairment is retinal and not due to an optic nerve disturbance.

Careful fundoscopic examination of the eye is essential to identify abnormalities of the optic media, retina, and optic nerve head.

Finally, examination of the visual fields is essential for topographic localization, since due to the invariate ordering of nerve fibres along the visual pathway, lesions at specific sites produce field defects of specific shapes (Fig. 1). Simple confrontation tests provide a qualitative method of investigating the visual fields. The examiner sits opposite the patient, maintaining a constant distance, and each eye is tested separately. With the patient fixating the examiner's nose, he/she is asked to count stationary fingers presented on either side of the vertical meridian in each quadrant in turn. If the patient cannot identify the fingers in a particular area, the fingers are gently wiggled, and the hand moved towards fixation until they are visible to the patient so mapping out the field defect. To examine the central field a red, 5 to 10 mm hatpin is moved away from or towards the central point of fixation. The patient is asked to describe any changes in the perception of colour or brightness, and whether or not the object disappears at any point. Perimetry provides a quantitative technique for measuring the fields, but a full description is beyond the scope of this chapter.

Abnormalities of the optic disc

Optic disc anomalies

Optic nerve hypoplasia

Hypoplasia of the optic nerve may be mild or severe, unilateral or bilateral, and may be associated with normal or impaired visual function. It may occur in isolation, or be associated with central nervous system anomalies,

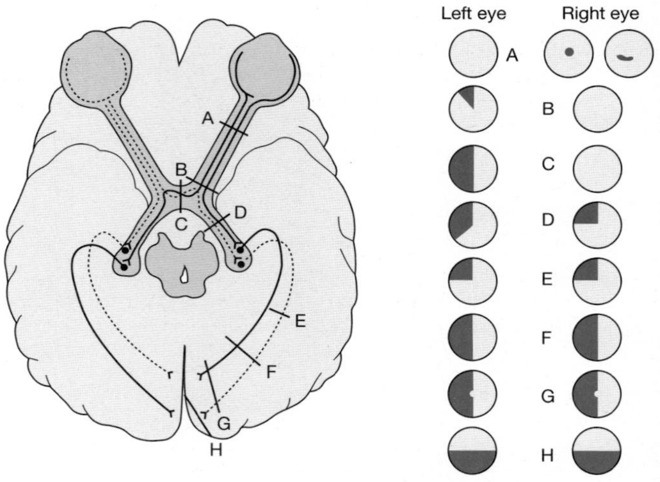

Fig. 1 Patterns of visual field loss due to lesions at different locations along the visual pathway. (a) Optic nerve lesions result in a central scotoma or arcuate defect. (b) Optic nerve lesions just prior to the chiasma produce junctional scotoma due to ipsilateral optic nerve involvement with the inferior contralateral crossing fibres (dashed lines). (c) Chiasma lesions produce bitemporal hemianopia. (d) Optic tract lesions result in incongruous hemianopic defects. (e) and (f) Lesions of the optic radiation result in either homonymous quadrantinopia or hemianopia depending on the extent and location of the lesion (upper quadrant, temporal lobe; lower quadrant, parietal lobe). (g) Lesions of the striate cortex produce a homonymous hemianopia, sometimes with macular sparing, particularly with vascular disturbances. (h) Lesions of the superior or inferior bank of the striate cortex result in inferior or superior altitudinal defects, respectively.

such as the absence of the septum pellucidum in the De Morsier's syndrome (septo-optic dysplasia).

Optic nerve dysplasia

Optic nerve dysplasia presents with a spectrum of abnormalities, including optic nerve colobomas, optic pits, and the morning glory syndrome, all considered to be associated with abnormal closure of the embryonic optic stalk and cup fissure. They are sometimes associated with basal encephaloceles and other forebrain anomalies.

Optic disc colobomas

These are deeply evacuated nerve head anomalies with blood vessels exiting from the margins which are associated with defects in the retinal nerve fibre layer, leading to an appropriate visual field loss.

Optic pits

Optic pits are crater-like depressions in the optic disc with a dark grey hue, usually situated in the temporal disc margin with an accompanying nerve fibre layer defect.

The morning glory syndrome

In this condition, an enlarged dysplastic disc is associated with an elevated centrally retained mass of glial and embryonic glial and vascular material, which radiates outwards in a sunburst pattern.

Tilted discs

An asymmetrically shaped, tilted disc is produced when the optic nerve leaves the globe at an extremely oblique angle. It is often associated with a crescentric zone of exposed sclera along one edge that results in elevation of the superior disc. The disc may appear hypoplastic and patients with this condition often have moderately high myopia and oblique astigmatism.

Optic nerve drusen

Drusen of the optic disc can give rise to an elevation of the optic nerve head. Drusen are intrapapillary, prelaminar refractile concretions that arise from degenerating nerve fibres. Anomalous discs due to drusen are usually smaller than normal, have an absent central optic disc cup, and exhibit an aberrant branching pattern of the central retinal vessels. Initially the drusen are buried with simple elevation of the disc, but become more apparent in later years when they appear to give rise to a typical lumpy disc, with a scalloped margin.

Myelinated nerve fibres

In slightly less than 1 per cent of the population some portions of retinal nerve fibres are myelinated, although normally optic nerve myelination stops at the lamina cribrosa. It appears on fundoscopy as a white area, usually adjacent to the disc, which has a centrifugal feathered edge.

Optic disc swelling

Although optic disc swelling and papilloedema have in the past been used synonymously, it is now usual only to refer to papilloedema as optic disc swelling when it is associated with raised intracranial pressure. Other cases of optic disc swelling are either due to local abnormalities in the optic nerve or orbit, or due to congenital anomalies as described above.

Local causes of optic disc swelling are usually associated with impaired visual acuity and colour vision, central arcuate or altitudinal field defects, and often an afferent pupillary defect. This contrasts with papilloedema when the acuity remains normal, except in the final stages, and is usually bilateral.

Papilloedema

The evolution of the disc changes in papilloedema due to raised intracranial pressure are usually classified into four stages: early, fully developed, chronic, and atrophic.

In early papilloedema there is disc hyperaemia, mild disc swelling with blurring of the fine peripapillary nerve fibre layer striations, dilatation of retinal veins with loss of spontaneous venous pulsations, and occasionally fine splinter haemorrhages at the disc margin.

In fully developed papilloedema, disc elevation is moderate to marked, and there is increased venous distension and tortuosity, an increasing number of peripapillary haemorrhages, cotton wool spots, and dilated capillaries on the disc surface. The retinal blood vessels and disc margin become increasingly indistinct.

In chronic papilloedema, there is resolution of the haemorrhages and exudates leaving a dome-shaped ('champagne cork') disc swelling, which often contains hard exudates. White refractile bodies may appear on the disc surface, known as corpora amylacea. As time goes on there is increasing nerve fibre attrition, leading to progressive visual field loss.

Finally, there is post-papilloedema (consecutive) atrophy, in which the disc acquires a milky opalescence and the retinal vessels are sheathed.

Clinical features

Usually papilloedema is bilateral and there is an absence of visual symptoms. However, unilateral or bilateral transient visual obscurations may occur, which last a few seconds and are often associated with postural changes. Although it has been suggested that such obscurations herald permanent visual loss, there is no evidence to support this view. The longer the papilloedema persists, the more likely there is to be progressive visual field loss, which usually starts as a peripheral field constriction. Occasionally, sudden visual loss occurs in a patient with papilloedema due to ischaemic optic neuropathy.

Pathogenesis

Papilloedema is due to impairment of axonal transport in the retinal nerve fibres, leading to axonal distension which is seen as disc swelling at the level of the prelaminar optic nerve.

Aetiology

There is a vast array of different causes leading to increased intracranial pressure, in particular space-occupying lesions such as tumours (Table 1).

Management

Treatment primarily depends on the underlying cause of the raised intracranial pressure. If due to a mass lesion which cannot be completely

Table 1 Causes of papilloedema

Mass lesions: tumours, aneurysms, granulomas, parasitic cysts
Intracranial haemorrhage: subdural haematoma, epidural haematoma, subarachnoid haemorrhage
Arteriovenous malformations
Intracranial infections: brain abscess, meningitis, encephalitis
Obstructed cranial venous outflow: dural venous sinus thrombosis, dural venous sinus infiltration, jugular vein compression, dural venous sinus arteriovenous malformation
Obstructive hydrocephalus
Brain oedema following trauma
Spinal cord tumours
Benign intracranial hypertension
(i) idiopathic
(ii) secondary to metabolic and endocrine disorders: Addison's disease, diabetic ketoacidosis, thyrotoxicosis, hypoparathyroidism, chronic uraemia
(iii) secondary to toxic causes: tetracycline, nalidixic acid, steroid therapy, lithium, hypervitaminosis A
Guillain–Barré syndrome
Craniostenoses
Mucopolysaccharoidoses
Systemic illness: Behçet's syndrome, status epilepticus, Reye's syndrome, Whipple's disease, systemic lupus erythematosis, systemic hypertension, chronic respiratory insufficiency

removed, or due to a non-surgically remediable cause, then a shunting procedure or medical measures, for example osmotic agents or diuretics such as acetazolamide, may be used. Increasingly, optic nerve sheath fenestration is being used for patients with intractable papilloedema who are developing early visual loss.

Ischaemic optic neuropathy

Ischaemic optic neuropathy is due to infarction of the optic nerve head, and can either be arteritic, as part of giant cell arteritis, or non-arteritic (idiopathic ischaemic neuropathy, anterior ischaemic optic neuropathy), which is the commoner form of the condition.

Non-arteritic ischaemic optic neuropathy

This tends to occur in patients aged between 45 and 80 years, and is characterized by abrupt, painless, and generally non-progressive visual loss, associated with an arcuate or altitudinal visual field loss. In nearly all cases, there is optic disc oedema, often associated with one or more splinter haemorrhages at the disc margin. Although previously considered irreversible, as many as 40 per cent of patients may show some improvement.

There is a 40 per cent chance of involvement of the fellow eye within five years. Optic atrophy rapidly ensues after the ischaemic event. The cause of non-arteritic ischaemic optic neuropathy remains obscure, and there is no treatment of proven benefit. The most important aspect of management is to exclude the possibility of the arteritic form, since in such cases the fellow eye is particularly vulnerable to similar involvement.

Arteritic ischaemic optic neuropathy

The arteritic form of ischaemic optic neuropathy usually occurs in giant cell (cranial, temporal) arteritis, but also rarely occurs in lupus and polyarteritis nodosa. Anyone with non-arteritic ischaemic optic neuropathy over the age of 50 should be suspected of having giant cell arteritis. This often occurs in the context of headache, malaise, weight loss, anorexia, anaemia, proximal muscle ache or stiffness, temporal artery tenderness, jaw claudication, and fever. These symptoms and signs usually precede the visual loss. The disc infarction is similar to that seen in non-arteritic ischaemic optic neuropathy.

A high index of suspicion is required for giant cell arteritis, and if suspected, an urgent erythrocyte sedimentation rate and temporal artery biopsy should be arranged. At the same time as the blood for the erythrocyte sedimentation rate is taken, the patient should be started immediately on systemic steroids (prednisolone at 80 mg daily, plus 200 mg of intravenous hydrocortisone immediately). In most patients the erythrocyte sedimentation rate is markedly elevated, as is the C-reactive protein. Occasionally the erythrocyte sedimentation rate may be normal. A biopsy of the superficial temporal artery should be obtained as soon as possible after the diagnosis has been considered. The biopsy will not be affected by the use of corticosteroids for at least 48 h. A positive temporal artery biopsy confirms the diagnosis of giant cell arteritis, but in 25 per cent of patients skip areas are found in biopsy specimens, and therefore a negative biopsy may sometimes be obtained.

Steroid treatment should not be tapered or withdrawn too early, since a relapse of symptoms is common. The dose of prednisolone can be gradually tapered after 2 to 3 weeks to maintain a normal erythrocyte sedimentation rate and the patient asymptomatic. Treatment should be continued for at least 6 to 12 months.

Optic atrophy

Optic atrophy is the final result of a variety of disturbances to the optic nerve or retina. The disc appears pale, and there is an absence of disc vasculature and retinal nerve fibres (Fig. 1).

Table 2 Causes of optic disc atrophy

Deficiency states
Thiamine ('tobacco–alcohol amblyopia')
B_{12} (pernicious anaemia, 'tobacco amblyopia'?)
Drugs/toxins
Ethambutol
Chloromycetin
Streptomycin
Isoniazid
Chlorpropamide
Digitalis
Chloroquine
Placidyl
Antabuse
Heavy metals
Hereditary optic atrophies
Dominant (juvenile)
Leber's
Associated heredodegenerative neurological syndromes
Recessive, associated with juvenile diabetes
Demyelination
Graves' disease
Atypical glaucoma
Macular dystrophies

Optic atrophy occurs after any disease process that results in death of the retinal ganglion cells with a dying back of their nerve fibres. This can, therefore, be due to diseases that directly involve the ganglion cells themselves or from damage to the axons in the pregeniculate visual pathway, resulting in retrograde atrophy. The development of optic atrophy is usually slow, dependent on its cause. In most instances the optic atrophy is bilateral, the disc appearing chalky-white in colour with clearly defined margins. The differential diagnosis of optic atrophy is considered in Table 2.

Optic neuritis

Optic neuritis is a term used to describe an idiopathic optic neuropathy or one resulting from inflammatory, infectious, or a demyelinating aetiology. In most cases the optic disc is normal on ophthalmoscopy and the term retrobulbar neuritis is used. In those cases in which the optic disc is swollen, the terms papillitis or anterior optic neuritis are used.

Clinical features

It is important to distinguish between those features of typical optic neuritis of idiopathic or demyelinating causation from atypical optic neuritis. In typical optic neuritis there is usually acute unilateral loss of visual acuity and of visual field, which may progress over hours or a few days, reaching its maximal effect within one week. Ninety per cent of patients complain of ocular pain which is noted especially with eye movement, and which may precede the visual impairment by a few days. The visual loss may range from contrast defects with maintained acuity, to no light perception. The patient is usually aged under 40 years, although optic neuritis may occur at any age, and improvement takes place in most patients (90 per cent) to normal or near normal visual acuity over several weeks. There may be persistent subtle residual defects of colour vision, depth perception, and contrast sensitivity, which may continue for several months. Subsequent disc pallor may occur but does not correlate closely with the level of visual recovery. An afferent pupillary defect is present in over 90 per cent of patients with acute optic neuritis. Although optic neuritis is generally associated with a central scotoma, a wide variety of field defects may be found ranging from a central scotoma, to altitudinal and nerve fibre layer defects.

Atypical optic neuritis may involve bilateral simultaneous onset of optic neuritis in an adult patient. There is often lack of pain and there may be

Table 3 Causes of optic neuritis

Unknown aetiology
Multiple sclerosis
Viral infections of childhood (measles, mumps, chicken pox) with or without encephalitis
Viral encephalitides
Postviral, paraviral infections
Infectious mononucleosis
Herpes zoster
Contiguous inflammation of meninges, orbit, sinuses
Granulomatous inflammations (syphilis, tuberculosis, cryptococcosis, sarcoidosis)
Intraocular inflammations

other ocular findings suggestive of an inflammatory process, such as an anterior uveitis. Other features include a worsening of visual function beyond 14 days of onset, in a patient outside the 20- to 50- year age span. They may also have evidence of other systemic conditions, particularly inflammatory or infectious diseases (Table 3).

The evaluation of patients with optic neuritis rather depends on whether or not it is a typical or atypical case. Typical optic neuritis probably does not necessitate any additional laboratory investigations, although an abnormal MRI of the brain significantly increases the likelihood of developing multiple sclerosis.

Those patients with atypical optic neuritis should have a chest radiograph, laboratory tests including a blood count, biochemistry, and tests for collagen and vascular disease and syphilis serology. Examination of the cerebrospinal fluid is probably justified in this group of patients.

Management

Although intravenous methylprednisolone leads to a more rapid visual recovery, at the end of 6 months the visual acuity is no better than without the treatment. Therefore, steroid treatment of patients with typical optic neuritis is unnecessary, unless there is severe ocular pain that cannot be managed with analgesics, or if there is already poor vision in the fellow eye due to some other disease process.

Heredofamilial optic neuropathies

The hereditary optic neuropathies can either be those which are autosomal dominant or recessive, or those which are due to point mutations in mitochondrial DNA. The autosomal conditions usually present in childhood with impaired vision and pale optic discs.

Leber's hereditary optic neuropathy

This mitochondrial disorder develops primarily in males (approximately 14 per cent in women) in the second to third decade of life. It is characterized by an abrupt loss of central vision in one eye, usually followed by a loss of vision in the remaining eye which may occur weeks, months, or sometimes years later. Occasionally visual loss may occur simultaneously in the two eyes. There is no associated pain on eye movement in contrast to acute optic neuritis, and the visual loss is usually permanent with optic atrophy and large absolute central scotomas. However, the fundoscopic picture in the acute phase often shows swelling of the papillary nerve fibre layer, circumpapillary telangiectatic microangiopathy, and tortuosity of the retinal vessels.

There is a maternal pattern of inheritance and point mutations in mitochondrial DNA, particularly at the 11778 nucleotide and less frequently at 3460 and 14484, have been identified. The significance of the point mutation at 14484 is that a much higher percentage (37 per cent as opposed to 4 per cent) of patients show some visual recovery when compared with patients who have a defect at 11778. It is, therefore, appropriate to carry out genetic testing in those individuals presenting with atypical optic neuritis of the appropriate sex and age, even if a positive family history is not available. There is no effective treatment for this condition.

Nutritional and toxic optic neuropathies

Bilateral, slowly progressive central visual loss with centro-caecal scotomas, and usually normal or mild temporal atrophic optic discs characterizes optic nerve failure due to either nutritional deficiency or a toxic cause. Once a family history of one of the hereditary familial diseases has been excluded, this condition should be considered, and is usually due to a combination of alcohol abuse, deficiencies within the B vitamin complex, and frequently a high tobacco consumption. With treatment by abstinence of the likely toxic agents and vitamin supplementation, recovery of vision usually occurs, unless the condition is so long standing that optic atrophy has intervened. Recent epidemics of optic neuropathy in Cuba and in West Africa have probably been related to multiple dietary deficiencies.

Toxic optic neuropathy has been associated with ethambutol, chloramphenicol, halogenated hydroxyquinolones, lead, isoniazid, and vincristine.

Tumours of the optic nerve

Optic nerve sheath meningiomas

Although optic nerve sheath meningiomas may arise directly from the optic nerve sheath, usually in the orbital regions of the nerve, they frequently arise from the tuberculum sellae, sphenoid wing, and olfactory groove, leading to secondary invasion or compression of the nerve. Primary optic nerve sheath meningiomas, most frequently found in middle-aged women, are usually unilateral, but if bilateral raise the possibility of central neurofibromatosis (NF-2). Although most patients will have mild (2 to 4 mm) proptosis at the time of their initial consultation, they complain of dimming of vision and decreased colour vision. Visual loss progresses over years with optic disc swelling gradually being supplanted by optic atrophy, with or without the evolution of optociliary venous (retinochoroidal anastamoses) shunt vessels.

The CT picture in patients with these tumours is most often one of diffuse narrow enlargement of the optic nerve, with bulbous swellings of the nerve in the region of the globe and orbital apex. 'Railroad-track' calcification of the optic nerve sheath in the orbit is a characteristic feature. Use of MRI has enabled optic nerve sheath meningiomas to be distinguished from optic nerve gliomas, where the former but not latter shows that the nerve is readily distinguished from the optic nerve sheath.

Management of patients with optic nerve sheath meningiomas is controversial. While there is general agreement that nerve sheath tumours are most aggressive in children and become progressively more indolent with advancing age, there is no consensus as to the best way to treat these lesions. Clinical resection, particularly when there is intracranial spread, is usually incomplete. These patients rarely die from the meningioma and it is probably best to observe. In some instances radiotherapy has shown to result in some visual improvement.

Optic nerve gliomas

Optic nerve gliomas, which may also involve the chiasma, are of two distinct types. By far the commoner is the benign glioma of childhood, and the other the malignant glioblastoma in adults. Approximately a quarter of cases occur in the setting of NF-1.

Benign optic nerve gliomas usually present within the first two decades of life, with a peak incidence from 1 to 6 years of age. The usual presenting manifestations are proptosis and visual loss, which may be so mild as to be undetectable, although a profound reduction in acuity is more common. The fundus may show either papilloedema or optic atrophy.

The clinical course of childhood optic nerve gliomas is highly variable. In some, tumour enlargement proceeds slowly for a time but then reaches a plateau, while in others the enlargement proceeds unabated. Necropsy has suggested that they are in fact hamartomas rather than true neoplasms. Optic nerve gliomas are generally managed conservatively, although some practitioners favour radiation therapy for lesions with chiasmal involvement and surgery for at least those tumours restricted to the orbit.

Optic nerve gliomas of adulthood are malignant gliomas which usually arise in males aged 40 to 60 years. These patients often present with a rapid onset of visual failure, which on some occasions may mimic acute optic neuritis. The tumour rapidly progresses and the patient usually dies within a short period.

Other optic nerve tumours

Metastatic cancer may lead to optic nerve involvement, either as a result of infiltration of the meninges as occurs with cancer of the breast and lung, or by direct tumour infiltration as with lymphoproliferative disorders and certain types of leukaemia and non-Hodgkin's lymphoma. Paraneoplastic optic neuropathy has also been described in patients with small cell carcinoma of the lung.

Disorders of the optic chiasm

Approximately 25 per cent of all brain tumours occur in the chiasmal region and since half of these cases initially present with visual loss, an appreciation of the various field abnormalities is important. Although there are a number of other causes for the chiasmal syndrome, such as trauma and demyelination, these are rare. The neuro-ophthalmological signs of a compressive optic chiasm lesion are primarily a field defect and deterioration of visual acuity, which depend on the relationship of the chiasm to the pituitary. The classic field defect of a chiasmal lesion is a bitemporal hemianopia. This may be complete or incomplete and may or may not be symmetrical. It is unusual to have a bitemporal hemianopia without some reduction in central visual acuity in at least one eye, due to the optic nerve being compromised in addition to the chiasm.

In large series of patients with pituitary tumours the most common field defect is a bitemporal hemianopia (67 per cent); less common are junctional scotoma (29 per cent), homonymous hemianopia (7 per cent), and prechiasmal field loss (2 per cent). Other signs include optic disc pallor, but its absence usually denotes a virtual complete return of visual function with successful decompression.

Other causes of chiasmal compression in addition to pituitary adenomas (50 to 55 per cent) include craniopharyngiomas (20 to 25 per cent), meningiomas (10 per cent), and gliomas (7 per cent).

Optic tract lesions

The optic tract is the first point in the visual pathways where the ipsilateral temporal and contralateral nasal retinal nerve fibres come together, and so the field defect is usually a partial or complete homonymous hemianopia. When partial, there is often gross incongruity between the visual field defects found in each eye, which may also be found with lesions of the lateral geniculate nucleus and more rarely the optic radiations.

The most frequently encountered lesions causing the optic tract syndrome are aneurysms, craniopharyngiomas, and pituitary tumours.

The optic radiations

As the geniculostriate fibres leave the lateral geniculate nucleus, the ventral fibres (subserving the superior visual field) pass anteriorly around the temporal horn of the lateral ventricle to form Meyer's loop. Lesions in this region usually result in a wedge-shaped congruous homonymous field defect, mainly affecting the superior quadrant. The visual acuity and pupillary responses are both normal. Lesions involving the optic radiation are due to vascular occlusion, tumours (intrinsic or metastatic), or abscesses.

Although lesions of the dorsal optic radiation in the parietal lobe may result in a homonymous hemianopia primarily affecting the lower fields, large lesions usually result in a complete homonymous hemianopia with macular splitting. Damage to the parietal or occipitoparietal cortex may result in the phenomenon in the contralateral visual field called unilateral visual inattention or visual extinction. A test object presented in this field is perceived normally, but when an identical object is similarly presented equidistant from the fixation point in the ipsilateral visual field, the stimulus in the field contralateral to the parietal lobe lesion disappears.

Occipital lobe

On reaching the occipital lobe there is a high degree of order in the fibres of the optic radiation and lesions, which are usually due to infarction, trauma, or tumour, produce homonymous congruent field defects. The only features of the field defect which help localize the lesion to the occipital lobe, rather than the anterior optic radiation, are the presence of sparing of the macula or temporal crescent areas in a homonymous hemianopia.

In macula sparing there is preservation of the visual field within a region of 1 to 2° up to 10° around the fixation point in the hemianopic field. In the more usual situation the hemianopic field is split along the vertical meridian through the fixation point (macula splitting).

Altitudinal (dorsal/ventral) field defects involving either the upper or lower occipital poles may occur as a result of trauma or vascular lesions.

Cortical blindness

Cortical blindness usually indicates selective involvement of the occipital visual cortex. The essential features are: (i) complete loss of all visual sensation, (ii) loss of reflex lid closure to threat, (iii) normal pupillary light reactions, and (iv) normal retina and full extraocular eye movements. The commonest aetiology is hypoxia of the striate cortex.

Disorders of higher visual processing

In the extrastriate cortex there is parallel processing of different aspects of visual information before an organized synthesis of the visual scene can be generated. Specific lesions in one or other of these areas might be expected to give rise to an appropriate specific loss of a visual modality such a colour (achromatopsia), movement (akinetopsia), or faces (prosopagnosia).

Acquired disorders of colour vision due to lesions of the central nervous system are of two types. In one type there is an inability to see colours (dyschromatopsia or achromatopsia). These patients have lesions in the region of the lingual and fusiform gyri, which lies in the anterior inferior region of the occipital lobe. They complain that they cannot see colours and that everything looks grey or in varying shades of black and white. They are unable to identify the figures on pseudo-isochromatic test plates although they are able to name the colours of brightly coloured objects correctly. Other functions such as visual acuity, object recognition, and depth perception are all normal, but there is often an associated visual field defect, usually a bilateral superior homonymous quadrantanopia. In the other type of disorder the colour sense is normal but the naming and recognition of colour is impaired. This can occur as part of an aphasia, such as Wernicke's or anomic, in the syndrome of alexia without agraphia, or as one feature of visual agnosia (see below).

Rare cases of patients who exhibit a selective deficit of movement perception (akinetopsia) have been reported. The patients have bilateral lesions involving the lateral occipito-parieto-temporal junction.

Visual agnosia

The term visual agnosia refers to a rare condition in which there is an inability to recognize, name, or demonstrate the use of an object presented visually, in the absence of a language deficit, general intellectual dysfunction, or attentional disturbances. The patient is, however, able to name the object when using other sensory modalities such as touch or sound.

One classification depends on the specific category of visual material that cannot be recognized. A disturbance of recognition of objects (object agnosia), faces (prosopagnosia), or colour (colour agnosia) may occur in isolation or in various combinations. When patients are able to copy and match-to-sample objects that they fail to name or recognize visually, the agnosia is termed associative; but if there is an inability to perform all these tasks, the agnosia is termed apperceptive.

Prosopagnosia is a specific inability to recognize familiar faces despite a normal ability to recognize everyday objects, and is, therefore, different from visual agnosia. Most cases of prosopagnosia are due to infarction, head injury, or hypoxia resulting in bilateral lesions in the ventromedial aspects of the occipitotemporal region.

Visual illusions

Visual illusions occur when the visually perceived target appears altered in size, shape, colour, position in space, and in number of images. The illusory type of defects may occur in the entire field of vision, or may affect only the object or the background. The term 'dysmetropsia' indicates the apparent smallness (micropsia), largeness (macropsia), or irregularity of shape (metamorphopsia) of objects. Dysmetropsia usually occurs as a result of retinal disease due to distortion of the relative distance between rods and cones.

Visual hallucinations

Visual hallucinations occur under many circumstances, such as drug withdrawal, anoxia, migraine, infection, and schizophrenia, in addition to those related to focal neurological disease in the occipital or temporal lobes. Those in the latter category may be unformed, consisting of flashes of light (coloured or white), lines, or simple shapes, or they may be complex highly organized hallucinations of people or objects.

Palinopsia

Palinopsia is a rare disorder in which there is persistence (perseveration) or recurrence of visual images after the exciting stimulus has been removed.

Further reading

Apple DJ, Rabb MF, Walsh PM (1982). Congenital anomalies of the optic disc. *Survey in Ophthalmology* **27**, 3–41.

Beck RW, ONTT Study Group (1992). A randomised, controlled trial of corticosteroids in the treatment of acute optic neuritis. *New England Journal of Medicine* **326**, 581–8.

Boghen DR, Glaser JS (1975). Ischaemic optic neuropathy: the clinical profile and natural history. *Brain* **98**, 689–708.

Chung SM, Selhorst JB (1992). Cancer associated retinopathy. In: Katz B, ed. *Neuro-ophthalmology in systemic disease. Ophthalmology Clinics of North America* **5**(3), 587–96.

De Renzi E (1997). Prosopagnosia. In: Finberg TE, Farah MJ, eds. *Behavioural neurology and neuropsychology*, pp 245–55. McGraw-Hill, New York.

Dutton JJ (1992). Optic nerve sheath meningiomas. *Survey in Ophthalmology* **37**, 167–83.

Dutton JJ (1994). Gliomas of the anterior visual pathway. *Survey in Ophthalmology* **38**, 427–52.

Horton JC, Hoyt WF (1991). The representation of the visual field in human striate cortex: a revision of the classic Holme's map. *Archives of Ophthalmology* **109**, 816–24.

Humphreys GW, Riddoch MJ (1993). Object agnosias. In: Kennard C, ed. *Visual perceptual defects*, pp 339–59. Baillière Tindell, London.

Kölmel HW (1993). Visual illusions and hallucinations. In: Kennard C, ed. *Visual perceptual defects*, pp 243–64. Baillière Tindell, London.

Liu GT *et al.* (1994). Visual morbidity in giant cell arteritis: clinical characteristics and prognosis for vision. *Ophthalmology* **101**, 1779–85.

Manford M, Anderman F (1998). Complex visual hallucinations: clinical and neurobiological insights. *Brain* **121**, 1819–40.

McDonald WI, Barnes D (1992). The ocular manifestations of multiple sclerosis. I. Abnormalities of the afferent visual system. *Journal of Neurology, Neurosurgery and Psychiatry* **55**, 747–52.

Neetens A, Smets RM (1989). Papilloedema. *Neuro-Ophthalmology* **9**, 81–101.

Riddoch G (1917). Dissociation in visual perceptions due to occipital injuries, with special reference to appreciation of movement. *Brain* **40**, 15–57.

Riordan-Eva P *et al.* (1995). The clinical features of Leber's hereditary optic neuropathy defined by the presence of a pathogenic mitochondrial DNA mutation. *Brain* **118**, 319–37.

Rosenberg MA, Savino PJ, Glaser JS (1979). A clinical analysis of pseudo-papilloedema: I. population, laterality, acuity, refractive error, ophthalmoscopic characteristics, and coincident disease. *Archives of Ophthalmology* **97**, 65–70.

Sadun AA *et al.* (1994). Epidemic optic neuropathy in Cuba: eye findings. *Archives of Ophthalmology* **112**, 691–9.

Sugishita M *et al.* (1993). The problem of macular sparing after unilateral occipital lesions. *Journal of Neurology* **241**, 1–9.

Thompson HS (1966). Afferent pupillary defects. *American Journal of Ophthalmology* **62**, 860–73.

Zeki S (1993). *A vision of the brain.* Blackwell, London.

24.12 Disorders of eye and ear

24.12.1 Eye movements and balance

Thomas Brandt and Michael Strupp

Introduction

The main objective of this chapter is to describe the clinically relevant principles of ocular motor and vestibular disorders. The anatomical and functional overlap of the vestibular and ocular motor systems warrants a joint discussion.

Eye movements

Different types of eye movement can be distinguished, each with particular functions, physiological properties, and specific anatomical substrates. Many abnormalities of eye movement are thus distinctive and often indicate the site and the side of a lesion. This is useful for topographic diagnosis, a method that still frequently proves superior to imaging techniques. It is therefore important that the physician examines in detail the eye movements of a patient suffering from, for example, double vision, oscillopsia, or vertigo, for he can by this means often differentiate between 'peripheral' and 'central' ocular motor or vestibular disorders. In their excellent book *Neurology of eye movements*, Leigh and Zee (1999) correctly state that 'an understanding of the properties of each functional class of eye movements will guide the physical examination; a knowledge of the neural substrate will aid topological diagnosis'.

Normal vision relies on eye movements in two essential ways. On the one hand, eye movements make it possible to shift the gaze and to view objects of interest. On the other, when the head moves during locomotion, the eyes move in a direction opposite to that of the head and compensate for these head movements, thereby preventing involuntary shifts of the visual images projected on the retina. The retinal images are kept steady. Optimal functioning of the eye movements is ensured by the co-operation between the optokinetic reflex and the vestibulo-ocular reflex.

In essence, there are three types of conjugate eye movements: smooth pursuit, saccades, and the vestibulo-ocular reflex. In the following paragraphs we summarize their properties, main function, clinical examination, and pathological findings as well as the typical features of vestibular nystagmus and gaze-evoked nystagmus.

Smooth pursuit keeps the image of a moving object on the fovea. The pursuit system generates smooth tracking eye movements that closely match the pace of a target; its examination is illustrated in Fig. 1. Various anatomical structures (motion-sensitive visual cortex, frontal eye fields, pontine nuclei, cerebellum, vestibular and ocular motor nuclei) are involved in smooth pursuit eye movements. Therefore, topographically impaired smooth pursuit (reduced gain) is an unspecific finding, which may be further influenced by alertness, a variety of drugs, and age. Moreover, vertical smooth pursuit is worse than horizontal, and downward tracking worse than upward. Marked asymmetries of smooth pursuit, however, indicate a central lesion; strongly impaired smooth pursuit is observed in intoxications and degenerative disorders involving the cerebellum or extrapyramidal system.

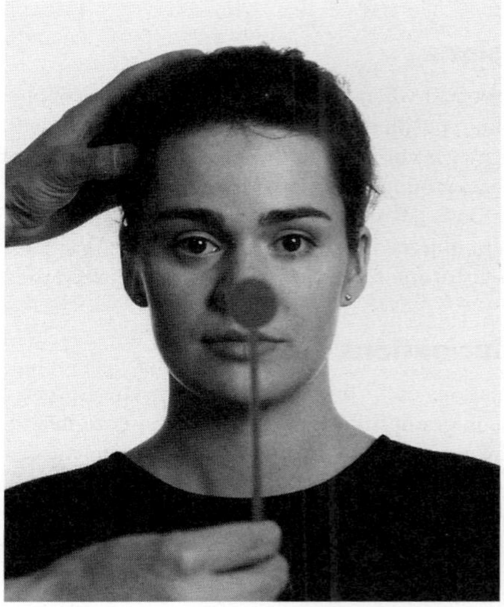

Fig. 1 Clinical examination of smooth pursuit. The patient is asked to track visually an object moving slowly in horizontal and vertical directions (10 to 20°/s) with the head stationary. Look for corrective (catch-up or back-up) saccades; they indicate an inappropriate smooth pursuit gain.

Saccades bring images of objects of interest on the fovea; their clinical examination is illustrated in Fig. 2. Slowing of saccades—often accompanied by hypometric saccades—is also often a side-effect of many types of medications/toxins and is found in neurodegenerative disorders. Slowing of horizontal saccades is observed in brainstem lesions, for example of the ipsilateral paramedian pontine reticular formation; slowing of vertical saccades may be due to a midbrain lesion and is observed in progressive supranuclear palsy. Lesions of the cerebellum or cerebellar pathways may cause hypermetric saccades, followed by corrective saccades that can be easily observed. For example, in Wallenberg's syndrome, a saccadic overshoot toward the side of the lesion is due to an interruption of the inferior cerebellar peduncle; interruption of the superior cerebellar peduncle leads to contralateral hypermetric saccades. In internuclear ophthalmoplegia the adducting saccade is slower than the abducting saccade. Delayed-onset saccades are most often caused by cerebral cortical lesions.

The vestibulo-ocular reflex holds images of the seen world steady on the retina during brief head rotations and locomotion. Halmagyi and Curthoys

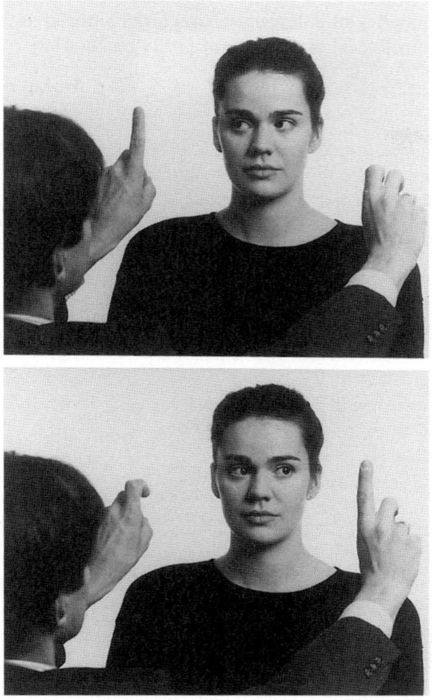

Fig. 2 Clinical examination of saccades. First observe spontaneous saccades to visual or auditory targets. Then ask the patient to glance back and forth between two horizontal and two vertical targets, keeping the head stationary. The velocity, accuracy, conjugacy, and the initiation time of the saccade should be observed. Normal individuals can immediately reach the target with a fast single movement or one small corrective saccade.

(1988) described an important clinical bedside test of the horizontal vestibulo-ocular reflex, which is illustrated in Fig. 3. This simple test allows the physician to find out whether there is a unilateral or a bilateral peripheral vestibular deficit.

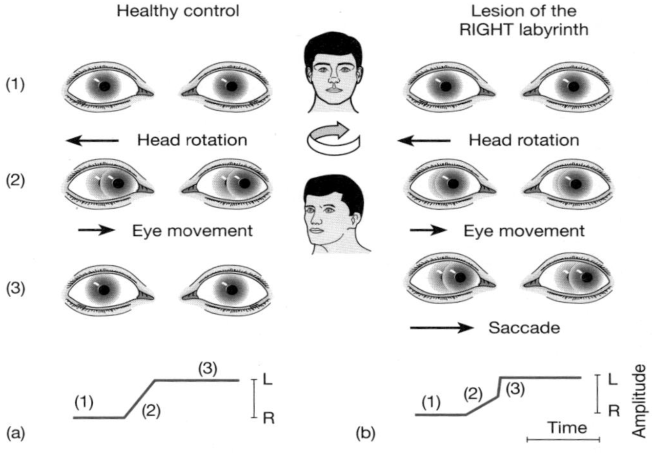

Fig. 3 Clinical bedside testing of the horizontal vestibulo-ocular reflex by the Halmagyi–Curthoys test. Fast 20 to 30° rotations of the head toward the side of the lesion show the dynamic deficit of the horizontal vestibulo-ocular reflex. In contrast to the healthy control (a), the patient is not able to generate a fast contraversive eye movement and has to perform a corrective (catch-up) saccade to fixate the target (b). It is important to instruct the patient to look carefully at the examiner's nose and to apply brief, high acceleration head thrusts to detect a unilateral peripheral vestibular deficit, for example due to vestibular neuritis or acoustic neuroma.

Finally, two clinically important pathological eye movements should be mentioned: gaze-evoked nystagmus and spontaneous nystagmus. As illustrated in Figs 4 and 5, gaze-evoked nystagmus should be observed when the patient is fixating with both eyes. It is most often a side-effect of medication/toxins such as anticonvulsants, hypnotics, or alcohol. Horizontal gaze-evoked nystagmus may be due to structural lesions of the brainstem (medial vestibular nucleus and nucleus prepositus hypoglossi, that is, the neural integrator to maintain gaze position after execution of a gaze shift), or the flocculus. Vertical gaze-evoked nystagmus is observed in midbrain lesions involving the interstitial nucleus of Cajal. A dissociated horizontal gaze-evoked nystagmus (greater in the abducting than the adducting eye) and an adduction deficit are the signs of internuclear ophthalmoplegia due to a lesion of the medial longitudinal fasciculus.

Spontaneous nystagmus indicates a tone imbalance of the vestibulo-ocular reflex which may be central or peripheral; when peripheral—as in

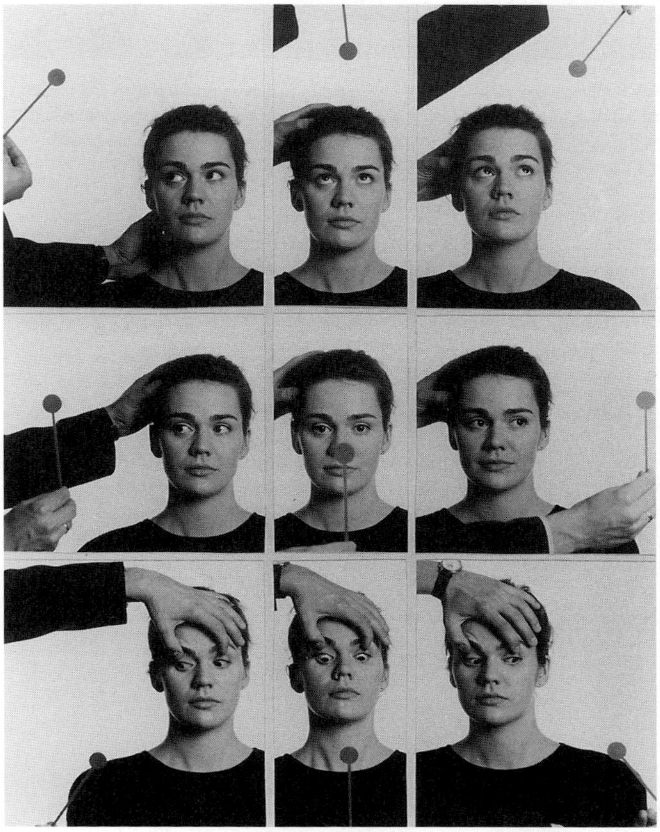

Fig. 4 Clinical examination of the eyes in nine different positions to evaluate ocular alignment, fixation deficits, nystagmus, range of movement, and gaze-holding abilities. The examination can be performed using an object (left) or an examination lamp. In primary position look for (a) abnormal eye movements such as nystagmus (for example, peripheral vestibular: horizontal-rotatory, suppressed by fixation; central vestibular: vertical (upbeat, downbeat), horizontal or torsional, poorly suppressed or even increasing with fixation; congenital: usually horizontal, variable in frequency and amplitude, increasing with fixation); square-wave jerks (small saccades of 0.5 to 5° that cause the eyes to move from the primary position, for example in progressive supranuclear palsy or certain cerebellar syndromes); ocular flutter (intermittent bursts of horizontal oscillations); or opsoclonus (combined horizontal, vertical, and rotatory oscillations); the latter two may have different aetiologies, for example encephalitis, tumours, or drugs/toxins and (b) misalignment of the visual axes. Then establish the range of motion with ductions (one eye viewing) and versions (with both eyes viewing) in the eight end-positions; this can indicate, for example, ocular muscle or nerve palsy. Gaze-holding deficits can be evaluated in eccentric gaze position (Fig. 5).

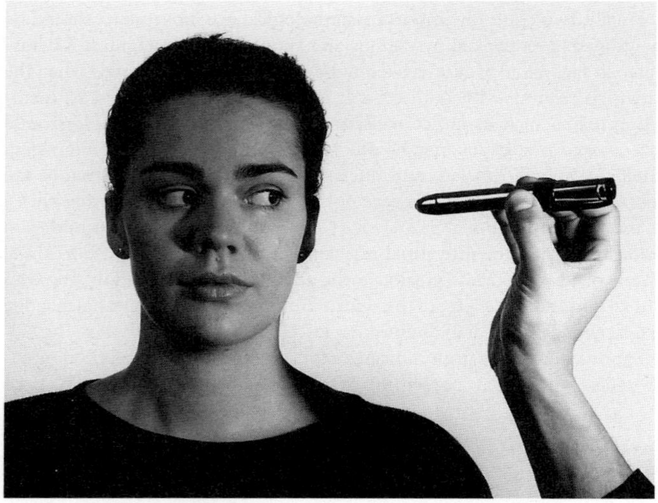

Fig. 5 Clinical examination of the eye positions/movements using an examination lamp. The advantage of the lamp as opposed to an object is that the reflected light on the eye can be observed and thus ocular misalignments can be easily detected. In addition, the patient can fixate with one or both eyes in the end-positions.

vestibular neuritis—it is typically damped by visual fixation. Therefore, spontaneous nystagmus should be examined by Frenzel's glasses (Fig. 6).

As a general rule, it is often necessary to combine the pathological clinical findings of the different eye movement systems to differentiate between a central and peripheral vestibular disorder and to make an exact topographical diagnosis.

Dizziness and vertigo

Vertigo, dizziness, and disequilibrium are common complaints of patients of all ages, particularly the elderly. As presenting symptoms, they occur in 5 to 10 per cent of all patients seen by general practitioners and 10 to 20 per cent of all patients seen by neurologists and otolaryngologists. The clinical spectrum of vertigo is broad, extending from vestibular rotatory vertigo with nausea and vomiting to presyncope light-headedness, from drug intoxication to hypoglycaemic dizziness, from visual vertigo to phobias and panic attacks, and from motion sickness to height vertigo. Appropriate preventions and treatments differ for the various types of dizziness and vertigo; they include drug therapy, physical therapy, psychotherapy, and surgery.

Vertigo usually implies a mismatch between the vestibular, visual, and somatosensory systems. These three sensory systems subserve both static and dynamic spatial orientation, locomotion, and control of posture by constantly providing reafferent cues. The sensory information is partially redundant in that two or three senses may simultaneously provide similar information about the same action. Thanks to this overlapping of their functional ranges, it is possible for one sense to substitute, at least in part,

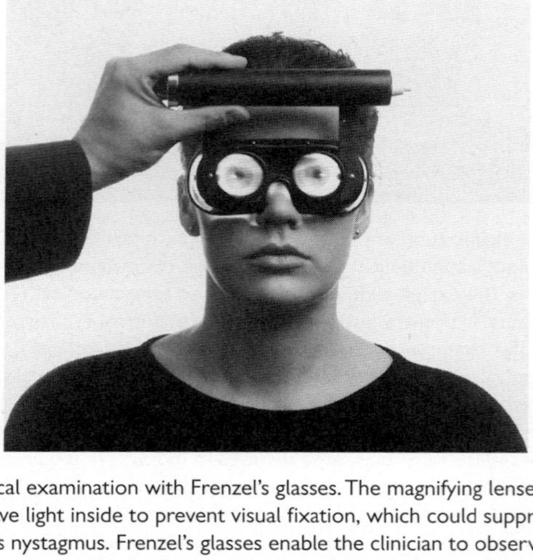

Fig. 6 Clinical examination with Frenzel's glasses. The magnifying lenses (+16 dioptres) have light inside to prevent visual fixation, which could suppress spontaneous nystagmus. Frenzel's glasses enable the clinician to observe spontaneous eye movements better. Examination should include spontaneous and gaze-evoked nystagmus, head-shaking nystagmus (instruct the patient to rotate his head about 20 times and observe eye movements following head shaking), positioning and positional nystagmus, as well as hyperventilation-induced nystagmus.

Table 1 Frequency of different vertigo syndromes in 3695 patients seen in a neurological dizziness unit (1989 to 2001)

Diagnosis	Frequency *n*	%
Benign paroxysmal positioning vertigo	695	18.8
Phobic postural vertigo	556	15.0
Central-vestibular vertigo	497	13.5
Basilar migraine (vestibular migraine)	348	9.4
Menière's disease	261	7.1
Peripheral vestibulopathy (vestibular neuritis)	295	8.0
Bilateral vestibulopathy	127	3.4
Psychogenic vertigo (without phobic postural vertigo)	123	3.3
Vestibular paroxysmia (disabling positional vertigo)	90	2.4
Perilymph fistula	10	0.3
Unknown aetiology	145	4.2
Other (central vestibular syndromes without vertigo)	539	14.2

Table 2 Pharmacological therapies for vertigo

Therapy	Vertigo
Vestibular suppressants	Symptomatic relief of nausea (in acute peripheral and vestibular nuclei lesions), prevention of motion sickness
Antiepileptic drugs	Vestibular epilepsy, vestibular paroxysmia (disabling positional vertigo), paroxysmal dysarthria and ataxia in multiple sclerosis, other central vestibular paroxysms, superior oblique myokymia
β-Receptor blockers	Basilar (vestibular) migraine (benign recurrent vertigo)
Betahistine	Menière's disease
Antibiotics	Infections of the ear and temporal bone
Ototoxic antibiotics	Menière's disease (Menière's drop attacks)
Corticosteroids	Vestibular neuritis, autoimmune inner ear disease
Baclofen	Downbeat or upbeat nystagmus or vertigo
Acetazolamide	Familial periodic ataxia or vertigo

Table 3 Physical therapies for vertigo

Therapy	Vertigo
Deliberate manoeuvres	Benign paroxysmal positioning vertigo
Vestibular exercises	Vestibular rehabilitation, central compensation of acute vestibular loss, habituation for prevention of motion sickness, improvement of balance skills (for example in the elderly)
Physical therapy (neck collar)	Cervical vertigo (?)

Table 4 Surgical interventions for vertigo

Surgery	Vertigo
Surgical decompression of eighth nerve	Tumour (acoustic neuroma) or cyst
Surgical decompression of vertebral artery	Rotational vertebral artery occlusion
Ampullary nerve section or canal plugging	Benign paroxysmal positioning vertigo
Endolymphatic shunt	Menière's disease
Vestibular nerve section or labyrinthectomy	Intractable Menière's disease
Neurovascular decompression?	Vestibular paroxysmia (disabling positional vertigo)
Surgical patching	Perilymph fistula

Table 5 Benign paroxysmal positioning vertigo (typical posterior semicircular canal type, p-BPPV)

Clinical syndrome

Brief attacks of rotational vertigo and concomitant rotatory-linear nystagmus precipitated by rapid head-trunk tilt toward the affected ear or by neck extension (when first lying down in bed, sitting up from a supine position, turning over in bed from one side to the other, extending the neck to look up)

- Latency: vertigo and nystagmus begin 1 s or more after head tilt
- Duration: attacks last less than 40 s
- Nystagmus: linear-rotatory, with the fast phase beating toward the undermost ear or upward
- Reversal: when the patient returns to the seated position, vertigo and nystagmus reoccur in the opposite direction
- Fatigability: repetition of the manoeuvre results in ever-lessening symptoms

Incidence/age/sex

Most common cause of vestibular vertigo that manifests throughout life, particularly in the elderly. Incidence 11 to 64 per 100 000 population per year with incidence peaking in the sixth and seventh decades; females exceed males by 2 to 1

Pathomechanism

'Canalolithiasis' of the posterior semicircular canal; dislodged otoconia (degeneration, trauma) congeal to form a free-floating 'heavy' clot which always gravitates to the most dependent part of the canal during changes in head position, thereby causing push or pull forces on the cupula

Aetiology

- 'Idiopathic' forms (ageing) ~ 50 per cent
- Symptomatic forms ~ 50 per cent (due to head trauma, vestibular neuritis, or prolonged bed rest)

Course/prognosis

- Natural history is considered benign because it resolves spontaneously within days to months in most patients, persists in about 20 to 30 per cent when untreated, and recurs in 30 to 50 per cent after variable periods for years

Management

- Physical liberatory manoeuvres to free the canal of the 'heavy' clot (see Fig. 7)
  - (i) Brandt and Daroff manoeuvres
  - (ii) Semont manoeuvre
  - (iii) Epley manoeuvre

These are successful in almost 100 per cent of the patients within days or weeks

- Surgical procedures (plugging of the posterior canal or posterior ampullary nerve section) are effective but unnecessary in all but a few exceptional cases

Differential diagnosis

Central positional vertigo/nystagmus, vestibular paroxysmia, perilymph fistula, drug or alcohol intoxication, Menière's disease, psychogenic vertigo

From Brandt (1999).

for deficiencies in the others. When information from two sensory sources conflicts, the intensity of the vertigo is a function of the degree of mismatch; it is increased if information from an intact sensory system is lost, as for example in a patient with pathological vestibular vertigo who closes his eyes. The distressing sensorimotor consequences of the mismatch are frequently based on our earlier experiences with orientation, balance, and locomotion, that is, there is a mismatch between the expected and the actually perceived pattern of multisensory input.

Vertigo may thus be induced by physiological stimulation of the intact sensorimotor systems (height vertigo; motion sickness) or by pathological dysfunction of any of the stabilizing sensory systems, especially the vestibular system. The symptoms of vertigo include sensory qualities identified as arising from vestibular, visual, and somatosensory sources. As distinct from one's perception of self-motion during natural locomotion, the experience of vertigo is linked to impaired perception of a stationary environment; this perception is mediated by central nervous system processes known as 'space constancy mechanisms'. Loss of the external stationary reference system required for orientation and postural regulation contributes to the distressing mixture of self-motion and surround motion.

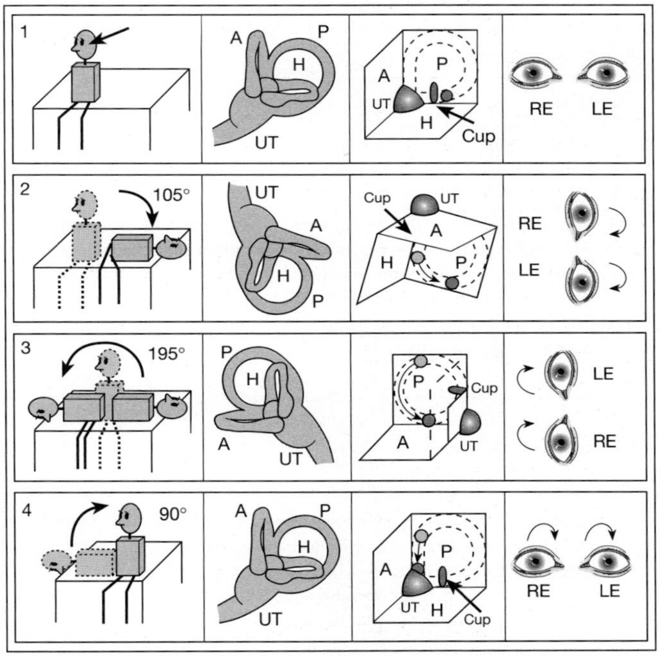

Fig. 7 Schematic drawing of the Semont liberatory manoeuvre in a patient with typical benign paroxysmal positioning vertigo (BPPV) of the left ear. Boxes from left to right: position of body and head, position of labyrinth in space, position and movement of the clot in the posterior canal and resulting cupula deflection, and direction of the rotatory nystagmus. The clot is depicted as an open circle within the canal; a black circle represents the final resting position of the clot. (1) In the sitting position, the head is turned horizontally 45° to the unaffected ear. The clot, which is heavier than endolymph, settles at the base of the left posterior semicircular canal. (2) The patient is tilted approximately 105° toward the left (affected) ear. The change in head position, relative to gravity, causes the clot to gravitate to the lowermost part of the canal and the cupula to deflect downward, inducing BPPV with rotatory nystagmus beating toward the undermost ear. The patient maintains this position for 2 min. (3) The patient is turned approximately 195° with the nose down, causing the clot to move toward the exit of the canal. The endolymphatic flow again deflects the cupula such that the nystagmus beats toward the left ear, now uppermost. The patient remains in this position for 2 min. (4) The patient is slowly moved to the sitting position; this causes the clot to enter the utricular cavity. Abbreviations: A, P, and H: anterior, posterior, and horizontal semicircular canals; Cup, cupula; UT, utricular cavity; RE, right eye; LE, left eye. (From Brandt *et al.* 1994.)

Physiological and clinical vertigo syndromes are commonly characterized by a combination of phenomena involving perceptual, ocular motor, postural, and autonomic manifestations: vertigo, nystagmus, ataxia, and nausea. These four manifestations correlate with different aspects of vestibular function and emanate from different sites within the central nervous system.

1. The vertigo itself results from a disturbance of cortical spatial orientation.
2. Nystagmus is caused by a direction-specific imbalance in the vestibulo-ocular reflex, which activates brainstem neuronal circuitry.
3. Vestibular ataxia and postural imbalance are caused by inappropriate or abnormal activation of monosynaptic and polysynaptic vestibulo-spinal pathways.
4. The unpleasant autonomic responses with nausea, vomiting, and anxiety travel along ascending and descending vestibulo-autonomic pathways to activate the medullary vomiting centre.

About 50 per cent of all patients presenting with dizziness, vertigo, or disequilibrium in a neurological dizziness unit will be suffering from one of the five following common syndromes (Table 1):

(1) benign paroxysmal positioning vertigo;

(2) somatoform vertigo (phobic postural vertigo);

(3) basilar migraine (vestibular migraine);

(4) Menière's disease; or

(5) vestibular neuritis.

A clinician unfamiliar with dizzy patients can most effectively deepen his knowledge by acquainting himself with these five most frequently met and challenging conditions of vertigo. Diagnosis and management of vertigo syndromes always require interdisciplinary thinking, and history taking is still much more important than recordings of eye movements or brain imaging techniques. Although most clinicians welcome the attempts to develop computer interview systems for use with neuro-otological

Table 6 Menière's disease

Clinical syndrome
- Fluctuating hearing loss
- Tinnitus
- Subjective fullness of the ear
- Prolonged vertigo/nystagmus attacks with nausea
- Rare vestibular drop attacks

Monosymptomatic forms possible, variable auditory and vestibular deficits in the intervals between attacks. There is no pathognomonic test to establish the diagnosis unequivocally

Incidence/age/sex
- 50/100 000
- Affects mainly age group from 30 to 50 years
- Incidence in males and females roughly equal
- Rare in children

Pathomechanism
- Endolymphatic hydrops of the labyrinth due to insufficient fluid resorption in the endolymphatic sac or blockage of longitudinal endolymph flow
- Attacks: periodic ruptures of the endolymph membrane with potassium palsy of ampullary nerves and mechanical hearing disturbance
- Intervals: pressure-dependent loss of cochlear and vestibular neurones, distortion of labyrinth structures

Aetiology
- Acquired, 'delayed endolymphatic hydrops'(i.e. labyrinthitis, viral or bacterial; traumatic, temporal bone fracture)
- Embryopathic (e.g. Mondini dysplasia)
- Idiopathic (aetiology not known)

Course/prognosis
- Usually begins in one ear with increasing frequency of attacks and major auditory/vestibular deficit occurring during the first years
- Thereafter spontaneous reduction in vertigo attacks (permanent fistulization?), no further progression of deficit but increasing involvement of the opposite ear (30 to 60 per cent)

Management
- Medical
  - (i) betahistine
  - (ii) diuretics
- Destructive (in rare cases)
  - (i) ototoxic antibiotics (gentamicin)
  - (ii) vestibular nerve section

Differential diagnosis
- Vertigo in migraine (benign paroxysmal vertigo of childhood, basilar (vestibular) migraine, benign recurrent vertigo)
- Perilymph fistula
- Neurovascular compression ('vestibular paroxysmia')
- Vestibular neuritis
- Benign paroxysmal positioning vertigo
- Transient ischaemic attacks
- Familial episodic ataxia
- Cogan's syndrome,
- Syphilitic labyrinthitis
- Vestibular atelectasis
- Hyperviscosity syndrome

From Brandt (1999).

Table 7 Vestibular neuritis

Clinical syndrome

Acute onset of sustained:
- rotatory vertigo
- postural imbalance with falls toward the affected ear
- horizontal-rotatory spontaneous nystagmus (toward the unaffected ear)
- nausea and vomiting
- unilateral hypo- or unresponsiveness in caloric testing

Incidence/age/sex

Third most common cause of peripheral vestibular vertigo that manifests throughout life (affects mainly ages 30 to 60 years; rare in children) without preference of sex

Pathomechanism

Acute partial unilateral loss of labyrinthine function (horizontal and anterior semicircular canal paresis) with a vestibular tone imbalance in yaw and roll planes

Aetiology

Most probably viral infection of the superior division of the vestibular nerve trunk

Course/prognosis

Spontaneous recovery within 1 to 6 weeks due to:
- (contralateral) vestibular, somatosensory, and visual substitution of the vestibular deficit
- central compensation of vestibular tone imbalance
- peripheral restoration of labyrinthine function (incomplete in about 50 per cent)

Better prognosis and higher recovery rate in children

Management

Medical treatment:
- (i) antivertiginous drugs (dimenhydrinate, scopolamine)
- (ii) corticosteroids

Physical therapy (vestibular exercises)

Differential diagnosis
- Acute central brainstem lesions at the root entry zone of the eighth nerve and the vestibular nucleus (multiple sclerosis plaques, small pontomedullary infarcts)
- Peripheral labyrinthine and vestibular nerve disorders, such as vascular (AICA infarcts), inflammatory (Lyme borreliosis), or immunological (Cogan's syndrome) disorders

From Brandt (1999).

patients and expert systems as diagnostic aids in otoneurology, their application in a clinical setting is still quite limited.

Dizziness is a vexing symptom, difficult to assess because of its purely subjective character and its variety of sensations. The sensation of spinning or rotatory vertigo is much more specific; if it persists, it undoubtedly indicates acute pathology of the labyrinth, the vestibular nerve, or the caudal brainstem, which contains the vestibular nuclei.

History taking allows the early differentiation of vertigo and disequilibrium disorders into seven categories that serve as a practical guide for differential diagnosis:

(1) dizziness and light-headedness (such as presyncopal dizziness or drug intoxication);

(2) single or recurrent attacks of (rotatory) vertigo (such as Menière's disease, vestibular migraine);

(3) sustained (rotatory) vertigo (such as vestibular neuritis, Wallenberg's syndrome);

(4) positional/positioning vertigo (such as in benign paroxysmal positioning vertigo, central positional vertigo);

(5) oscillopsia (apparent motion of the visual scene, such as in bilateral vestibulopathy, downbeat nystagmus);

(6) vertigo associated with auditory dysfunction (such as Menière's disease, Cogan's syndrome); and

(7) dizziness or to-and-fro vertigo with postural imbalance (such as phobic postural vertigo, episodic ataxia).

Table 8 Bilateral vestibular failure

Clinical syndrome

Symptoms:

- Unsteadiness of gait (particularly in the dark or on unlevel ground)
- Oscillopsia associated with head movements or when walking
- Episodes of vertigo early in the development of bilateral vestibular failure but not in chronic state

Signs:

- Pathological vestibulo-ocular reflex-bedside test
- Absent vestibulo-ocular reflex with bithermal caloric testing and pendular body rotation in the dark
- Increased postural sway with eyes closed and/or standing on foam rubber

Incidence/age/sex

- Rare condition that manifests throughout life (mean age 52 years)
- Without preference of sex

Pathomechanism

Progressive loss of bilateral labyrinthine and/or vestibular nerve function due to various aetiologies with concurrent somatosensory and visual 'compensation' (substitution) of vestibular function for spatial orientation, ocular stabilization, and postural control

Aetiologies

- Ototoxicity, cerebellar degeneration, meningitis, tumours, immune-mediated inner ear disease, neuropathies, bilateral sequential vestibular neuritis, bilateral Menière's disease, congenital malformation, familial vestibulopathy, vascular disorders, and others
- Idiopathic (> 20%)

Course/prognosis

Bilateral vestibular failure may develop simultaneously or sequentially, take an abrupt or slowly progressive course, be complete or incomplete. Permanent loss of vestibular function is most frequent, but partial recovery is possible, particularly in the idiopathic, post-meningitic, and ototoxic groups

Management

- Prevention of bilateral vestibular failure (ototoxic drugs)
- Recovery from bilateral vestibular failure (immune-mediated inner ear disease)
- Vestibular rehabilitation

Differential diagnosis

- Of the various disorders causing bilateral vestibular failure
- Of disorders similar in symptomatology (unsteadiness and oscillopsia):
  - (i) cerebellar or ocular motor disorders without bilateral vestibular failure
  - (ii) phobic postural vertigo
  - (iii) intoxication
  - (iv) vestibular paroxysmia
  - (v) perilymph fistula
  - (vi) 'cervical vertigo'
  - (vii) orthostatic hypotension
  - (viii) hyperventilation syndrome
  - (ix) visual disorders
  - (x) unilateral vestibular loss

From Brandt (1999).

Management of the dizzy patient

The prevailing good prognosis of vertigo should be emphasized because of the following.

1. Many forms of vertigo have a benign cause and are characterized by spontaneous recovery of vestibular function or central compensation of a peripheral vestibular tone imbalance.

Table 9 Basilar migraine with episodic vertigo as the key symptom ('vestibular migraine')

Clinical syndrome

- Episodes of rotational or (less frequent) to-and-fro vertigo lasting from seconds to days with a duration of a few minutes or several hours most frequently
- Increased sensitivity to motion during the attack ('motion sickness') and increased susceptibility to motion sickness in between the attacks
- In 33 per cent of patients episodic vertigo is not associated with headache
- In 66 per cent of patients episodic vertigo and ocular motor deficits occur without associated (vertebrobasilar) neurological deficits
- In 33 per cent vertigo is associated with visual symptoms, dysarthria, tinnitus, decreased hearing, diplopia, ataxia, bilateral paraesthesia, bilateral paresis, or decreased level of consicousness

Incidence/age/sex

- 5 to 8 per cent of migrainous population, female:male ratio in adults = 1.5:1, first manifestation throughout life with a mean age of about 40 years

Aetiology/pathomechanism

- Genetic transmission, either through recessive gene with high penetrance or autosomal dominant gene with reduced penetrance
- The pathomechanism involves migrainous spreading depression or hypoperfusion

Cause/prognosis

- As in other forms of migraine
- Different forms of migraine attacks occur in alternation or sequentially in the same individual

Management

- Acute migraine attack:
  - (i) analgesics (acetylsalicylic acid, paracetamol, ergotamine, sumatriptan)
  - (ii) antiemetics (metoclopramide, domperadone)
- Prophylaxis for migraine attacks:
  - (i) β-receptor blockers (metoprolol, propranolol)
  - (ii) calcium antagonists (flunarizine)
  - (iii) serotonin antagonists (pizotifen)

Differential diagnosis

- Vestibular paroxysmia (disabling positional vertigo), Menière's disease, transient ischaemic vertebrobasilar attacks, central vestibular ataxia, familial periodic vertigo, vestibular epilepsy

Benign paroxysmal vertigo in childhood and recurrent vertigo in adults are subtypes of basilar migraine

From Brandt (1999).

2. Most forms of vertigo can be effectively relieved by pharmacological treatment (Table 2), physical therapy (Table 3), surgery (Table 4), or psychotherapy.

There is, however, no common treatment, and vestibular suppressants provide only symptomatic relief of vertigo and nausea. A specific therapeutic approach thus requires recognition of the numerous particular pathomechanisms involved. Such therapy can include causative, symptomatic, or preventive approaches.

The essential characteristics are given for benign paroxysmal positioning vertigo (Table 5; see Fig. 7), Menière's disease (Table 6), vestibular neuritis (Table 7), bilateral vestibular failure (Table 8), and vestibular migraine (Table 9).

Further reading

Baloh RW, Halmagyi GM (1996). *Disorders of the vestibular system.* Oxford University Press, Oxford.

Brandt T (1999). *Vertigo—its multisensory syndromes,* 2nd edn. Springer, London.

Brandt T, Steddin S, Daroff RB (1994). Therapy for benign paroxysmal positioning vertigo, revisited. *Neurology* **44**, 796–800.

Bronstein A, Brandt Th, Woollacott M (1996). *Clinical disorders of balance, posture and gait.* Arnold, London.

Halmagyi GM, Curthoys IS (1988). A clinical sign of canal paresis. *Archives of Neurology* **45**, 737–9.

Herdman, SJ (2000). *Vestibular rehabilitation,* 2nd edn. F.A. Davies, Philadelphia.

Leigh RJ, Zee DS (1999). *Neurology of eye movements,* 3rd edn. F.A. Davies, Philadelphia.

24.12.2 Disorders of hearing

Linda M. Luxon

> Our hearing is a choice and dainty sense, and hard to mend, yet soon it may be marred. Blows, falls and noise...all these...breed tingling in the ears and hurt our hearing.
>
> (Physicians of the Medical School of Salerno)

Hearing loss is the most common sensory impairment and the World Health Organization has estimated that at least 120 million people are affected worldwide. In the United Kingdom, about 20 per cent of the adult population are affected and, of these, three-quarters are over the age of 60 years. Age, gender, occupational group, and occupational noise exposure are factors affecting the prevalence of hearing impairment in adults, while a neonatal intensive-care unit history, a family history of childhood hearing loss, and craniofacial abnormalities explain over half of the population of congenitally hearing-impaired children. The most frequent form of acquired hearing impairment in children is a conductive hearing loss due to chronic secretory otitis media, while meningitis, in particular meningococcal meningitis, is the commonest cause of acquired sensorineural hearing loss. In the developing world, many of the preventable causes of hearing impairment remain common: consanguineous marriages, birth trauma, childhood infections, noise exposure, and the unlicensed sale of ototoxic drugs.

Tinnitus, defined as a noise in the head or ears lasting for more than 5 min, increases with age and affects approximately 20 per cent of the population over the age of 60 years, but only 4 per cent of the population complain of this symptom.

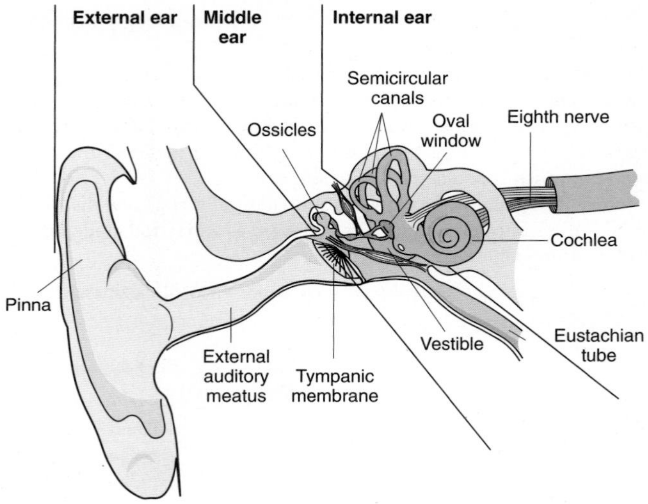

Fig. 1 Diagram to illustrate the anatomy of the peripheral auditory system.

Hearing impairments

Pathophysiology

For clinical purposes the ear is separated into three parts: the external, middle, and internal ear (Fig. 1). The external ear is important in funnelling sound to the tympanic membrane and in the localization of sound. The middle ear ossicles connect the tympanic membrane to the oval window of the cochlea, such that sound waves cause displacement within the fluid-filled compartment of the membranous labyrinth. Within the internal ear, the mechanical activity at the oval window is transduced into neural responses by the hair cells of the Organ of Corti (Fig. 2).

Disorders of the external and middle ear result in abnormalities of the mechanical transmission of sound from the environment to the internal ear, and give rise to a conductive hearing loss. Common examples include impacted wax, serous otitis media (glue ear), chronic otitis media, and disorders of the ossicular chain, for example otosclerosis, and traumatic discontinuity.

Disorders of the internal ear and the VIIIth cranial nerve characteristically give rise to a sensorineural hearing loss, in which the perception of both bone- and air-conducted sounds is reduced and the appreciation of the intensity of sound and the frequency resolution of complex sounds are impaired. Many conditions may affect the cochlea, ranging from inherited, congenital or iatrogenic non-syndromal or syndromal malformations to ototoxic damage (aminoglycoside, antimalarial, loop diuretics), ischaemia including vertebrobasilar ischaemia, diabetic vasculitis, infections (mumps,

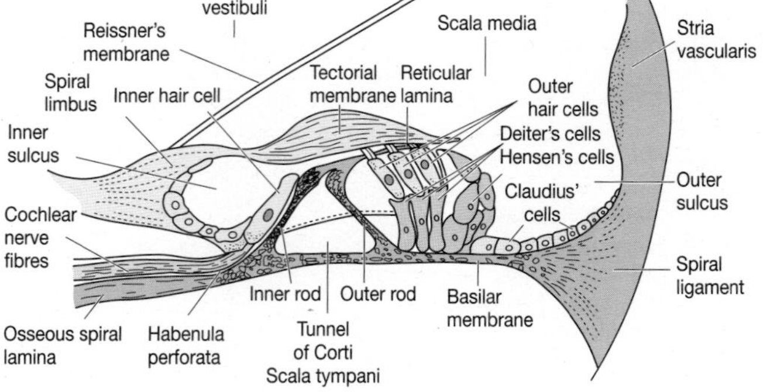

Fig. 2 Diagram of the Organ of Corti.

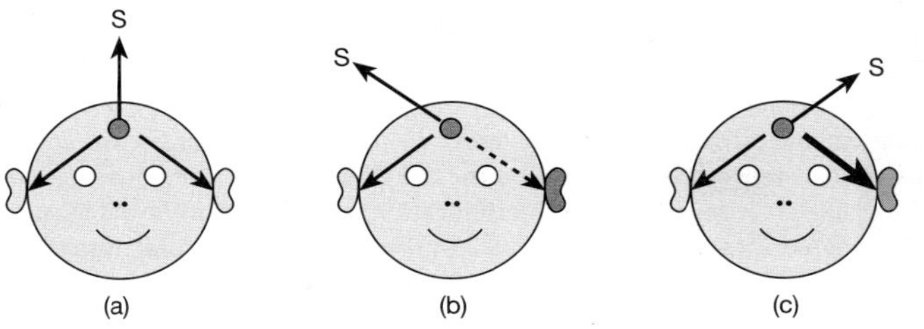

Fig. 3 Diagram to illustrate the Weber tuning fork test in (a) a normal subject, (b) a case of unilateral sensorineural hearing loss, and (c) a unilateral conductive hearing loss, in which the sound is heard more effectively in the affected ear because of the lack of masking by environmental sounds. (s, sound heard; •, tuning fork)

rubella, syphilis, cytomegalovirus), autoimmune disorders, degenerative disorders, trauma, and idiopathic conditions such as Menière's disease. Pathology of the VIIIth nerve leading to hearing impairment has been defined in spinocerebellar degenerations, trauma, cerebellopontine angle tumours, bony disorders such as Paget's disease, infective disorders (meningitis), and inflammatory conditions (sarcoidosis). Much doubt has been cast on so-called 'presbyacusis', which may merely reflect an accumulation of toxic/traumatic insults to the ear over many years, and recent advances in molecular biology and genetics have shown the role of genetic mutations/deletions in late-onset/progressive hearing impairments.

Clinical examination

Clinical examination requires examination of the anatomy of the external ear to define visible signs of congenital ear disease (pits, tags, nodules, or malformations) and evidence of other craniofacial features suggestive of syndromal hearing impairment. In addition, a detailed examination of the tympanic membrane is required to define the presence of pathology within the middle ear. Wax or debris obstructing the external auditory meatus should be removed by or under the supervision of a clinician with experience in this field. Syringing should never be undertaken in the presence of an infection or if it is unknown whether the tympanic membrane may be perforated. Tuning-fork tests remain the most valuable clinical test of auditory function and frequently enable a clinician to distinguish a conductive from a sensorineural hearing loss (Fig. 3). The tests are based on two physiological facts: first, the inner ear is normally more sensitive to sound conducted by air than to that conducted by bone; and second, in the presence of a purely conductive hearing loss the affected ear is subject to less environmental noise, making it more sensitive to bone-conducted sound. A general medical and neurological examination is mandatory to define syndromes and the plethora of general medical conditions associated with hearing impairment.

Investigations

A battery of audiological tests is required to:

- quantify audiometric thresholds at each frequency;
- differentiate a conductive from a sensorineural hearing loss;
- differentiate a cochlear from a retrocochlear abnormality;
- identify central auditory dysfunction in the brainstem, midbrain, or auditory cortex; and
- identify a non-organic component.

Each test can be defined as being subjective (dependent upon patient co-operation) or objective (independent of patient co-operation) in terms of providing auditory data. To differentiate a sensorineural hearing loss of cochlear origin from that of an VIIIth nerve dysfunction or neurological disorder, two pathophysiological phenomena are of importance:

1. *Loudness recruitment* is defined as an abnormally rapid increase in loudness, with an increase in intensity of the stimulus, and is characteristic of disorders affecting the hair cells of the Organ of Corti, but is absent in pathology of the VIIIth nerve.
2. *Abnormal auditory adaptation* is a decline in discharge frequency with time, observed following an initial burst of neural activity in response to an adequate continuing stimulus applied to the Organ of Corti. This phenomenon is characteristic of VIIIth nerve and brainstem auditory dysfunction.

Puretone audiometry is the most widely available, subjective, quantitative test of auditory thresholds. Electronically generated pure tones are delivered by earphones and the subject is required to respond to the quietest tone, at given frequencies between 125 and 8000 Hz in each ear. The sound may be delivered by air conduction (**AC**) or, if the tones are delivered by a bone vibrator on the mastoid process, by bone conduction (**BC**). In the latter test condition, because the intra-aural attenuation for a bone-conducted sound is negligible, masking of the ear not under test with narrow-band noise is mandatory. Bone-conduction thresholds significantly better than air-conduction thresholds indicate a conductive hearing loss, whereas similar bone-conduction and air-conduction thresholds are characteristic of sensorineural hearing loss (Fig. 4).

The stapedius muscle in the middle ear contracts bilaterally in response to loud sound directed into either ear. Using an impedance bridge, the minimum intensity of sound at a given frequency required to produce contraction of the stapedius muscle and thus a movement of the tympanic membrane can be measured (the acoustic reflex threshold). This objective measure enables recruitment and abnormal auditory adaptation to be measured, and allows assessment of middle ear, cochlear, VIIIth nerve, and brainstem auditory function.

Otoacoustic emissions are weak signals that can be recorded in the ear canal and are the result of contractile properties of the outer hair cells of the cochlea. Measurement of otoacoustic emissions thus provides objective information about cochlear function.

Speech audiometry is a subjective test requiring the subject to repeat standard lists of words delivered at varying intensities through headphones. The responses are scored and provide an assessment of auditory discrimination. They are of particular value in assessing the efficacy of hearing-aid provision.

Electrophysiological tests provide the major objective means of assessing auditory function and siting pathology in the auditory system. Electrocochleography enables the measurement of the electrical output of the cochlea and VIIIth cranial nerve in response to an auditory stimulus, while brainstem auditory evoked responses are of particular value in discriminating between cochlear and VIIIth nerve dysfunction. Recordings are obtained by averaging a series of time-locked responses generated by the

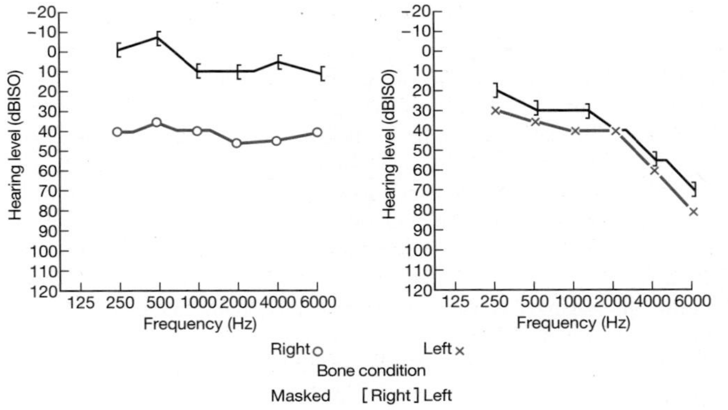

Fig. 4 Pure tone audiograms showing both air- and bone-conduction thresholds and illustrating a right conductive hearing loss (A) and a left sensorineural hearing loss (B).

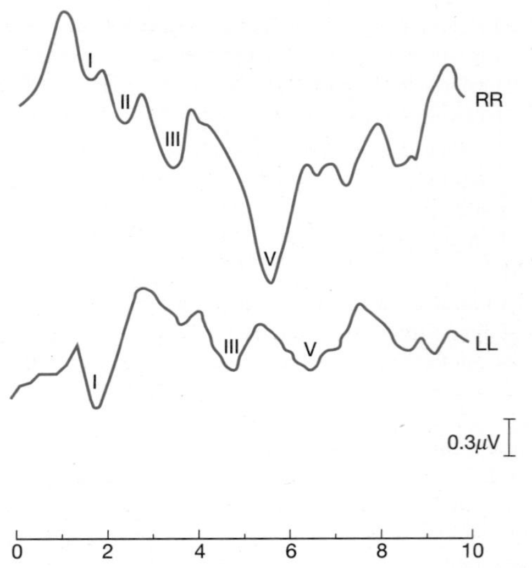

Fig. 5 Illustration of auditory evoked brainstem responses showing normal waves I, II, III, and V from the right ear (RR) and delayed waves III and V from the left ear (LL) in a case of a left acoustic neurinoma.

major processing centres of the auditory system in response to a repetitive sound stimulus (Fig. 5). Analysis of the waveform must be undertaken in conjunction with knowledge of the puretone thresholds if appropriate and valid conclusions about auditory function are to be obtained. Cortical or late-evoked auditory responses are the most effective method of defining auditory threshold at each frequency in an uncooperative patient, and are essential in legal cases in which a non-organic loss should always be excluded.

Management

Appropriate management requires a detailed history and examination to ensure both appropriate management of related general medical conditions and protection from leisure (discotheques) and occupational noise hazards and ototoxic drugs. Auditory rehabilitation is a problem-solving exercise centred on each individual patient, and depends on assessing both the auditory disability of the individual and the relevance of this to other important people in the patient's life. Not only auditory impairment, but also communication skills, including lip-reading ability, the use of visual cues, and the level of speech and language, together with psychological and sociological factors must be considered.

The remedial process may be straightforward in a highly motivated patient in whom there is an uncomplicated hearing loss. However, in the presence of a complicating factor, such as a hearing loss that is difficult to aid or arthritis making hearing aid manipulation difficult, the particular problem must be addressed to ensure optimal use of subsequent hearing-aid provision. In patients who have a negative view of hearing aids, environmental aids and instruction in communication skills prior to the introduction of a hearing aid may facilitate long-term rehabilitation. In general, the provision of a hearing aid is only effective when the patient himself, rather than well-meaning family members, wishes to pursue matters.

Although hearing aids play a pivotal role in audiological rehabilitation, a detailed description of their provision and selection is outside the scope of this short review. For many patients, wearable hearing aids, which bring sound more effectively to the ear, are invaluable, but environmental aids (assisted-listening devices such as amplification systems, alerting warning devices—for example, flashing lights connected to a doorbell or an alarm clock), may be adequate. In addition, sensory substitution systems, for example where visual signals are generated in response to auditory cues such as a telephone or doorbell ringing, or a baby crying, may be helpful to a hearing impaired person.

The general principles of hearing-aid provision include the fitting of a comfortable earmould which provides a secure mounting for the aid and a good acoustic connection between the aid and the ear canal. Hearing-aid selection involves matching the amplification required from the aid at specific frequencies with that required by the user. A particular disability experienced in most hearing-impaired subjects is that of hearing speech in a noisy environment and, although programmable digital processing hearing aids are of some help in this situation, conventional aids provide selective amplification of the frequencies relevant to speech, with minimal amplification at the peak frequency of background noise. Conventional aids may be divided into body-worn and head-worn aids, which can be in spectacles, behind the ear, in the ear, or in the canal in design. The major advantage of body-worn aids is the very high gain and maximum output that can be achieved, whereas the disadvantage is the unsightly nature of the device and the poor microphone placement.

Cochlear implants are electronic devices that convert sound into electrical current for the purpose of directly stimulating residual auditory nerve fibres to produce hearing sensations. The devices are implanted in the cochlea, usually with an electrode array, with an externally worn microphone and processor. Cochlear implants have been used in totally deafened adults and children with good results, and should be considered in all cases of profound acquired hearing loss and in children in whom there is good evidence of auditory nerve preservation in both congenital and acquired hearing impairment.

The value of counselling for the hearing-impaired person by a skilled hearing therapist must be emphasized. Such simple hearing tactics as encouraging the individual to ensure that the light is always on the speaker's face, that he or she places himself so that the better ear is towards the speaker, and sitting close to the sound source thereby minimizing background noise, can greatly improve communication ability. For the profoundly hearing-impaired, psychological problems associated with isolation are significant and it is therefore essential that psychological, medical, and social support are readily available.

Tinnitus

Tinnitus may be defined as a perception of sound, which originates from within the head rather than from within the external world. Rarely, the sound may have an externally detectable component and is then termed 'objective tinnitus' as opposed to the more common 'subjective tinnitus.' The experience of tinnitus is universal, but the complaint of tinnitus is rare.

Many conditions are associated with tinnitus, but it is frequently, although not always, associated with hearing impairment. The proposed pathophysiological mechanisms include:

- decoupling of the stereocilia of the hair cells;
- misinterpretation of auditory neural activity by higher auditory centres;
- self-sustaining oscillation of the basilar membrane;
- spontaneous otoacoustic emissions;
- an abnormality of the spontaneous resting activity of primary auditory nerve fibres, either secondary to the hypo- or hyperexcitability of damaged hair cells or as a direct consequence of the derangement of primary neurones themselves;
- damage to the myelin sheath between auditory nerve fibres allowing ephaptic transmission (cross-talk) between adjacent nerve fibres; and
- derangement of efferent fibres of the vestibulocochlear nerve, producing aberrant auditory behaviour.

A number of studies have demonstrated that tinnitus complaint does not correlate with psychoacoustic features of the tinnitus, but there is a significant correlation between tinnitus complaint and psychological symptoms. Importantly, the onset of tinnitus complaint may be associated with negative life events such as retirement, redundancy, bereavement, and divorce.

The assessment of tinnitus includes a detailed history, clinical examination, and audiometric investigation as outlined for hearing impairment. The commonest causes of objective tinnitus include palatal myoclonus, temporomandibular joint abnormalities, vascular abnormalities such as and arteriovenous fistula, and vascular bruits. Rarely, a patulous auditory tube may give rise to tinnitus in which the patient complains of a blowing sound associated with respiration.

Bilateral subjective tinnitus with evidence of a cochlear hearing loss is associated most commonly with presbyacusis, endolymphatic hydrops, vascular labyrinthine lesions, and noise-induced hearing loss. However, it is also common with head injury, whiplash injury, ototoxicity, barotrauma, surgical intervention, and after such simple clinical practices as syringing. Unilateral subjective tinnitus, with or without an associated sensorineural hearing loss. must be fully investigated to exclude an underlying cerebellopontine angle lesion, in particular an acoustic neurinoma.

Management

The primary management of tinnitus is medical, although surgical intervention is required for the correction of arterial stenoses giving rise to bruits and for glomus jugulari tumours and arteriovenous malformations. Destructive surgery, for example labyrinthectomy or auditory nerve section, has no place in the management of tinnitus as there is no evidence that destruction of the peripheral cochlear elements brings about improvements in tinnitus complaint.

The medical management of tinnitus can be divided into psychological, pharmacological, and prosthetic intervention.

The psychological aspects of tinnitus management include an explanation of tinnitus, reassurance that the symptom will not progressively deteriorate or indeed remain unchanged, the exclusion of sinister pathology to allay fear, and, if necessary, the appropriate formal psychiatric management of depression/anxiety.

In the presence of a hearing impairment, the provision of hearing aids to 'mask' tinnitus with desirable environmental noise may be of value. In the absence of such a loss, tinnitus maskers and noise generators have been advocated to promote 'adaptation', but it must be emphasized that there is no hard evidence that tinnitus maskers are superior to placebo devices.

Pharmacologically, intravenous lidocaine (lignocaine) has been shown to result in the disappearance or amelioration of tinnitus, but no oral preparation has been found to be equally effective. Psychiatric drugs may be required for psychological management, although no single drug has been shown to be uniformly effective.

Tinnitus retraining therapy is a management strategy based on a neurophysiological model of tinnitus. The retraining is a combination of prosthetic and psychological intervention, which in essence provides a structured framework for the various well-established mechanisms of tinnitus management outlined above.

In conclusion, positive reassurance, appropriate psychiatric management, and prosthetic support remain the mainstays of the medical management of tinnitus.

Further reading

Ludman H, Wright T, eds (1998). *Diseases of the ear*, 6th edn. Arnold, London.

Martini A, Prosser S (2002). Disorders of the inner ear in adults. In: Luxon LM, *et al.*, eds. *A textbook of audiological medicine.* Taylor and Francis, London.

24.13 Diseases of the nervous system

24.13.1 The unconscious patient

David Bates

It is important to distinguish transient unconsciousness occurring with syncope, seizures, cardiac arrhythmias, or metabolic abnormalities from unconsciousness that persists and is coma. Prolonged loss of consciousness is seen commonly in three clinical situations: following head injury, after an overdose of sedating drugs, or in the situation of 'non-traumatic coma' where there are many possible diagnoses but the most common are anoxia, ischaemia, systemic infection, and metabolic derangement. It is important that the physician asked to see a patient in 'non-traumatic coma' should remember that the patient may be harbouring delayed effects of trauma such as subdural haematoma or meningitis arising from a basal skull fracture. The possibility of raised intracranial pressure following a parenchymal haematoma in a patient with hypertension, the decompensation of a cerebral tumour, or the collection of pus means that all causes of loss of consciousness must be considered; in the diagnosis of medical coma it is not easy to exclude the possibility of head injury.

Urgent assessment of the patient in coma is required to identify and, where possible, correct the pathological cause, protect the brain from the development of irreversible damage, and identify those patients in whom the prognosis is hopeless. In this last group the institution and continuation of resuscitative measures is inappropriate and will serve only to prolong the anguish of relatives and carers.

Definition

Normal consciousness

Consciousness is the state of awareness of the self and the environment when provided with adequate stimuli; normal consciousness is exhibited by those patients who are fully responsive to stimuli and show appropriate behaviour and speech. Patients who are asleep can be roused and are then able to perform normally. Normal consciousness depends upon the integration of activity in the ascending reticular activating substance of the brainstem and the neuronal connections between areas of the cerebral cortex. The ascending reticular activating substance determines arousal, which is shown by awakening with eye opening, motor responses, and verbal communication. The content of consciousness, which is the combination of psychological responses to feeling, emotions, and mental activity, is mediated by the cerebral cortex. (Fig. 1)

Coma

Coma is a state of unrousable unconsciousness without any psychologically understandable response to external stimuli or inner need. The patient may appear to be asleep but is incapable of responding normally to external stimuli other than by showing eye opening to pain, flexion or extension of the muscles in the limbs to pain, and occasionally grunting or groaning in response to painful stimuli. It occurs when there is damage to the ascending reticular activating substance or bilateral damage to areas of the cerebral hemispheres, or both (Figs 2, 3, 4, and 5).

Confusion

Patients are usually disorientated with lowered attention, an inability to express thoughts, drowsiness, and defects in memory. There is a clouding of consciousness characterized by an impaired capacity to think, understand,

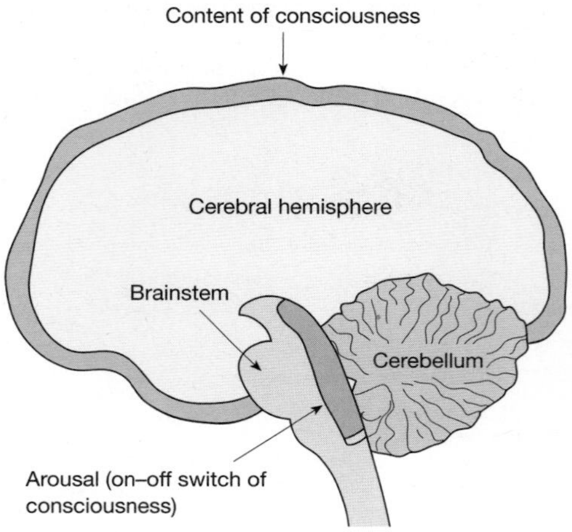

Fig. 1 Normal consciousness.

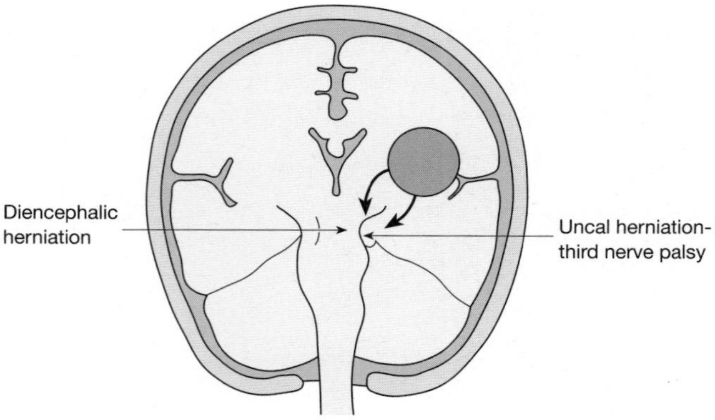

Fig. 2 Supratentorial mass.

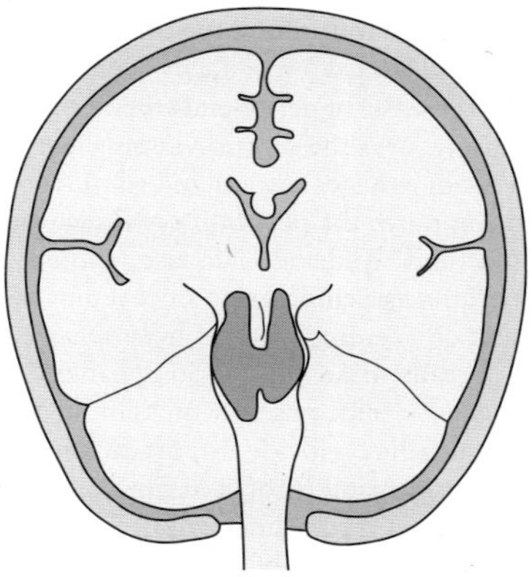

Fig. 3 Brainstem lesion—intrinsic.

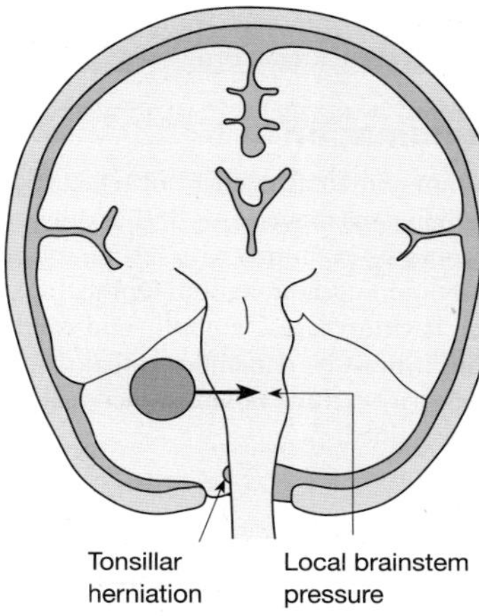

Fig. 4 Brainstem lesion—local pressure.

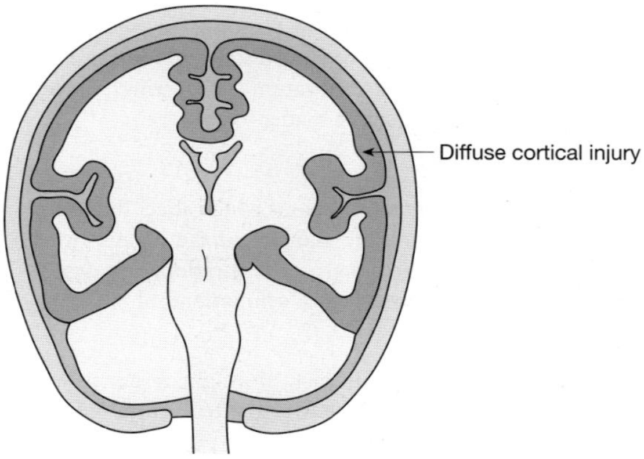

Fig. 5 Bihemispheric damage.

respond to, and remember stimuli. It is important to differentiate acute confusion from dysphasia, amnesia, acute psychosis, severe depression, or dementia. Confusion is most commonly seen as the result of toxic or metabolic disturbances, particularly in the elderly.

Delirium

There is motor restlessness, hallucination, disorientation, and delusion. The patient is often frightened and irritable and the state can be regarded as a more profound example of confusion; both states should alert the doctor to impending coma. Delerium is most commonly seen in patients with toxic or metabolic disorders but can be mimicked by degenerative brain disease, acute psychosis, and hypomania.

Stupor

The patient appears to be asleep and will show little or no spontaneous activity, respond only to vigorous stimulation, then lapse back into somnolence. It may be difficult to differentiate stupor from catatonic schizophrenia or severe retarded depression, but in stupor due to organic disease the electroencephalogram will always be abnormal.

The vegetative state

The patient breathes spontaneously, has a stable circulation, and shows cycles of eye opening and eye closure which may simulate sleep and waking, but they are unaware of self and environment. It can be seen transiently in the recovery from coma or it may persist to death. This state is usually seen in patients with diffuse bilateral cerebral hemisphere disturbance with an intact brainstem, although it can occur with bilateral damage to the most rostral part of the brainstem. It is most commonly seen following head injury or as the result of hypoxic-ischaemic damage following cardiac arrest. The patient appears to be awake but is unaware, a condition that frequently causes distress to carers and relatives (Fig. 6).

The locked-in syndrome

Damage to the ventral portion of the pons below the level of the third nerve nuclei results in the rare condition of total paralysis of the limbs and lower cranial nerves but intact consciousness (Fig. 7). The patient can open, elevate, and depress the eyes but cannot move the eyes horizontally and there is no voluntary movement or speech. The diagnosis is made when the doctor recognizes that the patient is able to open the eyes voluntarily and allow them to close in response to command and can therefore respond to verbal and sensory stimuli by blinking. The commonest cause is infarction of the ventral pons, usually in a patient with hypertension, although it can also be seen with pontine tumours, multiple sclerosis, in central pontine myelin-

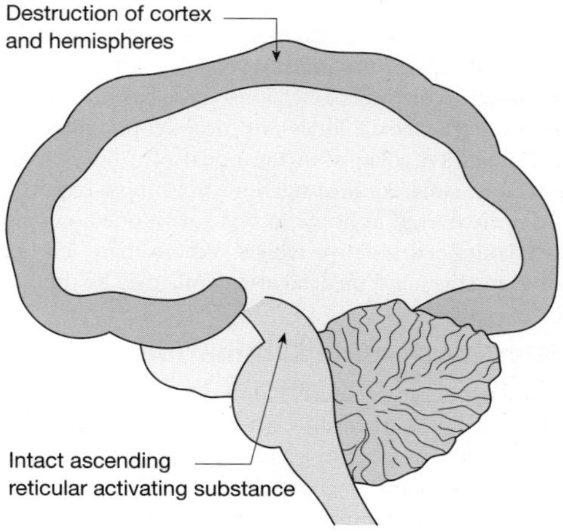

Fig. 6 Vegetative state.

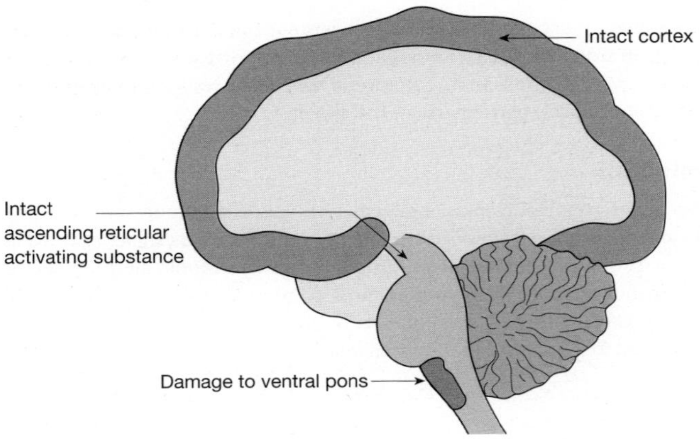

Fig. 7 Locked-in syndrome.

olysis following profound hyponatraemia, and after head injury. The prognosis is poor although some patients recover, usually with residual spasticity. An electroencephalogram may help by showing an alert state, reactive to external stimuli and neurophysiology can be used to exclude similar incapacities occurring in myasthenia gravis or the Guillain–Barré syndrome.

Psychogenic unresponsiveness

The term 'pseudocoma' or psychogenic unresponsiveness is used for patients who appear to be unconscious and in coma but who are not. The simplest way to identify this condition is to undertake oculovestibular testing (see below), which will reveal the presence of nystagmus and indicate that the patient has an intact brainstem and cortex.

The management of patients in coma

History

Once the patient is stable it is important to obtain as much information as possible from those who accompanied the patient to hospital or who observed the onset of coma. The circumstances in which consciousness is lost are of vital importance in helping to identify the diagnosis. Generally, coma is likely to present in one of three ways: as the predictable progression of an underlying illness; as an unpredictable event in a patient with a previously known disease; or as a totally unexpected event. In the first category are patients following focal brainstem infarction who deteriorate or those with known intracranial mass lesions who show similar deterioration. In the second category are patients with recognized cardiac arrhythmia or the known risk factor of sepsis from an intravenous cannula. In the final category it is important to distinguish whether there has been a previous history of seizures, trauma, febrile illness, or focal neurological disturbances. The history of a sudden collapse in the midst of a busy street or office indicates the need for different investigations from those required when the patient has been discovered at home in bed surrounded by empty bottles that previously contained sedative tablets. Where there is uncertainty, a telephone call to relatives and medical attendants may be useful.

Clinical assessment and examination

Estimation of the temperature, pulse, blood pressure, and respiratory rate, and examination of the skin, cardiovascular system, chest, and abdomen may often yield important clues in establishing the cause of a loss of consciousness. Fever, though not diagnostic, will usually indicate the presence of a systemic infection, meningitis, encephalitis, or abscess; seizures increases the likelihood of the latter two diagnoses. Hypothermia is most commonly seen following exposure to low environmental temperatures, intoxication with alcohol or barbiturates, the presence of peripheral circulatory failure, or profound myxoedema. Tachy- or bradyarrhythmias, evidence for valvular heart disease, or peripheral emboli raise the possibility of a cardiogenic cause; bruits over the carotid vessels suggest cerebrovascular disease; and splinter haemorrhages suggest endocarditis or collagen vascular disease. Hypotension raises the possibility of shock, myocardial infarction, or septicaemia and Addison's disease should be considered. Hypertension is less helpful as a clinical sign since it may be seen both as the result of cerebral insult or as an indicator of hypertensive encephalopathy.

The odour of the breath of an unconscious patient may indicate the presence of alcohol, a ketotic fetor raises the possibility of diabetes, and the fetor of hepatic or renal failure provide important clues. Clubbing of the finger nails suggests the possibility of a respiratory or gastrointestinal abnormality, and evidence of tracheal deviation, fluid in the chest, or collapse of the lung suggests the possibility of a respiratory cause. In the abdomen the finding of enlargement of an organ might indicate portal hypertension, polycystic kidneys, and an associated subarachnoid haemorrhage, or abnormality in the blood-forming organs. The general colour of the skin and mucous membranes might reveal anaemia, jaundice, cyanosis, or the pink discoloration of carbon monoxide poisoning. Purpura suggests a bleeding diathesis and bruising around the head indicates the possibility of trauma or a base of skull fracture. A rash may indicate an infective or inflammatory disease and hyperpigmentation raises the possibility of Addison's disease. The evidence of puncture wounds might identify an individual who is diabetic or a recreational drug user.

Neurological examination

This requires observation and an assessment of reflex responses. The position, posture, and spontaneous movements of the patient should be noted; the skull and spine should be examined with testing for neck stiffness and Kernig's sign to identify meningeal irritation. Ophthalmoscopy to identify papilloedema, fundal haemorrhages, emboli, and subhyaloid haemorrhages is important but it must be remembered that the absence of papilloedema does not necessarily exclude raised intracranial pressure. The ears and fauces should be examined.

Level of consciousness

The level of consciousness must be documented by the initial observer and can then be monitored by medical and nursing staff to determine the progress of the patient and identify the need for further investigation, therapy, and decision. The most useful hierarchical grading scale to assess the level of consciousness is the Glasgow coma scale in which the patient's response to graded stimuli of eye opening, motor response, and verbal response are recorded (Table 1); all four limbs are observed for responses to pain and the best response is recorded, although asymmetry should be noted and may be important in identifying lateralization. The scale measures consciousness and it is possible to score gradations from the fully conscious patient (eye opening—4, motor response—6, verbal response—5) to the totally unresponsive patient (eye opening—1, motor response—1, verbal response—1). If the level of consciousness can be shown to be improving, then urgent decisions may be delayed, but if deterioration is occurring, it is imperative that a decision about management be made.

Brainstem function

The brainstem reflexes identify those lesions which affect the reticular activating substance and determine the viability of the patient. Most of the reflexes involve the eyes and the pattern of respiration, although the latter may be compromised by requirements of ventilation.

Pupillary reactions

Unilateral dilatation of a pupil with lack of a light response suggests an uncal herniation of the temporal lobe over the tentorium entrapping the third nerve, although it may also be seen with a posterior communicating artery aneurysm or other third nerve damage. Midbrain lesions typically cause loss of the light reflex with pupils in the mid-position, lesions in the

Table 1 Neurological observation and assessment

Glasgow coma scale	Score
Eye opening	
Spontaneous	4
To speech	3
To pain	2
Nil	1
Verbal response	
Orientated	5
Confused conversation	4
Inappropriate words	3
Incomprehensible sounds	2
Nil	1
Best motor response	
Obeys	6
Localizes	5
Withdraws	4
Abnormal flexion	3
Extension response	2
Nil	1
Brainstem function	
Pupillary reactions	
Corneal responses	
Spontaneous eye movements	
Oculocephalic responses	
Oculovestribular responses	
Respiratory pattern	
Motor function	
Motor response	
Muscle tone	
Tendon reflexes	
Seizures	

pons cause small pupils with retained light responses, and fixed dilatation of the pupils suggests significant brainstem damage but must be differentiated from the fixed dilatation caused by atropine-like agents instilled by earlier observers. A Horner's syndrome may be seen with lesions in the hypothalamus or brainstem but can also be seen when diseases affect the wall of the carotid artery. Small pupils that react briskly to light raise the possibility of metabolic causes of coma such as hepatic or renal failure; drug intoxications tend not to affect the pupillary light responses.

Corneal responses

The corneal reflex is usually retained until very deep coma; if absent in a patient who appears to be otherwise in light coma, there is a distinct possibility that the cause may be drug intoxication. The loss of the corneal reflex in the absence of drug overdose is a poor prognostic indicator.

Spontaneous eye movements

Conjugate deviation of the eyes suggests a focal hemispheric or brainstem lesion, depression of the eyes is seen with damage to the midbrain at the level of the tectum, and skew deviation of the eyes suggests a lesion at the pontomedullary junction. Incoordinate eyes suggests damage to the ocular motor or abducent nerve in the brainstem or pathways, but a minor degree of divergence of the eyes is normal in the unconscious patient. Patients in light coma will often have normal roving eye movements, similar to those of sleep, which may be conjugate or dysconjugate. They cannot be mimicked and, when present, exclude the possibility of psychogenic unresponsiveness, when eye movements are likely to be more jerky.

Reflex eye movements are important in assessing brainstem activity. The oculocephalic response obtained by rotating the patient's head from side to side and observing the position of the eyes is likely to show Doll's eye movements when the brainstem is intact but the eyes will remain in the midposition of the head when the brainstem is depressed. Oculovestibular testing is undertaken by the installation of 50 to 200 ml of ice-cold water into an external auditory meatus. The conscious patient, and those in psychogenic coma, will develop nystagmus with the quick phase away from the side of the stimulation indicating an active pons and intact corticopontine connections. A tonic response with conjugate movement of the eyes towards the stimulated side indicates an intact pons and suggests a supratentorial cause for the coma, whereas a dysconjugate response or no response at all implies a lesion within the brainstem.

Respiration

The techniques of ventilation limit the value of observation of respiration in patients with coma, but if testing is possible before respiration is controlled, then deep breathing suggests acidosis, regular shallow breathing is consistent with drug overdose, long-cycle Cheyne–Stokes respiration suggests damage at the level of the diencephalon, and short-cycle Cheyne–Stokes respiration damage at the level of the medulla. Central neurogenic hyperventilation occurs with lesions in the low midbrain and upper pons, and reflex responses such as yawning, vomiting, and hiccoughing may occur with brainstem disturbances.

Motor function

Motor function is assessed as part of the level of consciousness in the Glasgow coma scale, but lateralizing abnormalities are important and indicate the likelihood of a focal cause, although they may occasionally be seen in the context of hepatic encephalopathy or hypoglycaemia. The presence of generalized or focal seizures implies hemispheric damage and may help in lateralization; multifocal myoclonus suggests a metabolic or anoxic cause with diffuse cortical irritation.

Investigation

After performing the resuscitation, history, examination, and assessment the physician should identify one of the three following states (Table 2).

Coma with focal signs or evidence of head injury

In such patients, whether the focal signs indicate a brainstem or supratentorial problem, a CT scan or MRI should be undertaken. A normal scan may be seen in patients with hypoglycaemia or hepatic coma and the presence of structural pathology will be identified allowing a decision to be made about the indications for surgery or other therapy.

Coma with meningeal irritation but without focal signs

Such patients will most commonly have subarachnoid haemorrhage, acute meningitis, or meningoencephalitis as the cause of their coma. Brain imaging is the ideal investigation to identify the presence of subarachnoid blood and to exclude the possibility of focal collections. Depending upon the results of the scan a lumbar puncture can then be undertaken and may give diagnostic information. If the index of suspicion of meningitis is high then treatment should be commenced and, in the absence of focal signs or pupilloedema, lumbar puncture may precede imaging.

Coma without focal lateralizing neurological signs and without meningismus

Most patients will have suffered diffuse anoxic-ischaemic disease, metabolic derangement, or drug insult. It may be necessary to undertake imaging techniques but the probability of finding a focal abnormality is low and it is more likely that haematological or biochemical tests or a search for toxins in the blood will provide the diagnosis, or help identify an episode of ischaemia or hypoxia in the past. There may occasionally be an indication to undertake a lumbar puncture in such patients to exclude an inflammatory or infective cause. Patients who are in coma as the result of drug overdose will usually be identified from the history and the circumstances of discovery, but the possibility of drug-induced coma should always be considered in patients without focal signs and without meningism. A discrepancy between marked depression of brainstem responses in a patient who appears to be in relatively light coma suggests the diagnosis, the importance

Table 2 Investigations to identify the coma state

Diagnostic category	Investigations	Causes
Coma with focal signs		
± Papilloedema	CT scan or MRI	Haematoma (extradural, subdural, parenchymal)
Hemiparesis	Chest radiograph	Infarction
Brainstem signs		Tumour
Focal seizures		Abscess
		Rarely metabolic
Coma with meningismus		
± Fever	± Imaging	Meningitis
± Fundal changes	Lumbar puncture	Encephalitis
	Blood tests	Subarachnoid haemorrhage
		Diffuse head injury
		Cerebral malaria
		Hypertensive encephalopathy
Coma alone		
History	Blood tests	Drug overdose
Systemic signs	± Lumbar puncture	Hypoxic ischaemia
	Electroencephalogram	Metabolic (diabetes, hepatatic, renal, etc.)
		Toxic (alcohol, carbon monoxide)
		Epilepsy

of which is that such patients have a good prognosis provided that they are given adequate respiratory and circulatory support during the coma.

Prognosis

The prognosis of individual patients depends upon the aetiology, the depth of the coma, the duration of the coma, and certain clinical signs.

Aetiology

Following head injury, prognosis is dependent upon the presence of intracranial haematoma, the age of the patient, and the severity of systemic injury and its effects. Patients in coma following drug overdose have, in general, a good prognosis provided that they are adequately resuscitated and protected. Patients who are in coma as a result of causes other than head injury or drug overdose for a period of more than 6 h have only a 10 per cent chance of making a good recovery. Those who have suffered subarachnoid haemorrhage or stroke have a less than 5 per cent chance of making such a recovery and those with hypoxic or ischaemic injury, typically following cardiac arrest, about 10 per cent. Those with metabolic or infective causes have almost a 30 per cent change of making a good recovery. A vegetative state is most likely to occur after head injury or hypoxic-ischaemic damage.

Depth of coma

Patients with no response to eye opening, no focal response to pain, and a poor response to pain have a poorer outcome than those who respond with eye opening, grunting, and flexion of the limbs.

Duration of the coma

When patients have been in coma for 6 h about 12 per cent may make a good recovery, those who remain in coma for 24 h have only a 10 per cent chance of recovery, and at the end of a week only 3 per cent of patients can be expected to make a good recovery. In general, patients who remain in coma for more than 7 to 14 days either die or enter a continuing vegetative state.

Clinical signs

Brainstem reflexes are the most important clinical signs in defining prognosis; the absence of corneal or pupillary reflexes or of oculovestibular responses for 24 h, in the absence of sedative drugs, is almost incompatible with recovery to independence whatever the cause of coma. Most brainstem reflexes are useful indicators of a poor prognosis but some, such as the development of nystagmus and oculovestibular testing or vocalization of any recognizable word within 48 h, identify patients with a good chance of recovery.

Continuation of care

The long-term care of patients in coma may be undertaken in an intensive care unit, on a specialist ward, in a rehabilitation unit, or long-stay hospital. It is important that those in whom prognosis is hopeless should not be permanently exposed to the rigors of intensive care medicine but should continue to receive basic care within routine hospital wards or a more long-stay environment. So long as patients are considered to have a potential for recovery they should be looked after in an intensive care unit or in a specialist ward. Their respiration, skin, circulation, and bladder and bowel function need attention, seizures must be controlled, and the level of consciousness should be regularly assessed and monitored. It is important that the mobility of joints and circulation to pressure areas are maintained during the long-term care of the patient and the possibility of aspiration pneumonia, peptic ulceration, and other complications of long-term intensive care need to be avoided. Techniques such as mechanical ventilation and steroid therapy should not be used routinely in the management of comatose patients; they do not improve prognosis and may compromise recovery. Investigations are of little help in identifying long-term prognosis because various types of electroencephalogram pattern have been recorded from patients in prolonged coma and CT scans simply show cortical atrophy with ventricular dilatation. Some somatosensory-evoked responses have been reported to show loss of the cortical component in long-term unconsciousness and positron emission tomography (PET) is reported to show metabolic underactivity, but at present, neither test can provide decisive information as to prognosis.

Further reading

Bates D (1991). Defining prognosis in medical coma. *Journal of Neurology, Neurosurgery and Psychiatry* **54**, 569–71.

Bates D (1993). The management of medical coma. *Journal of Neurology, Neurosurgery and Psychiatry* **56**, 589–98.

Fisher CM (1969). The neurological examination of the comatose patient. *Acta Neurologica Scandinavica* **45**(Suppl 46), 1–56.

Plum F, Posner JB (1980). *The diagnosis of stupor and coma*, 3rd edn. Davis, Philadelphia.

Teasdale G, Jennett WB (1974). Assessment of coma and impaired consciousness: a practical scale. *Lancet* **ii**, 81–4.

24.13.2 Headache

Peter J. Goadsby

Headache is perhaps the commonest of human maladies, and while no less interesting, varied, or biologically based than some of its neurological cousins it has been the subject of less attention than its clinical load demands. If only for cynical reasons of practicality, the general reader will need some basis with which to approach the patient with headache. Diagnosis and management of headache is clinically based, offering the doctor the opportunity to be a physician not a filter for test results, with the chance to treat and improve symptoms. Moreover, there is a sufficient biological basis now for headache to satisfy even the most scientific of inquisitors. Here the principles will be set out: the secrets and enjoyment remain, as with anything truly medical, in the clinic.

General principles

A formal classification system exists for headache, and it might surprise the casual observer that this runs to nearly 100 pages. The International Headache Society system is explicit in the sense that it uses features of the headache to make the diagnosis, summing features to make the diagnosis more certain. In clinical practice a broad categorization that serves well, and is consistent with the International Headache Society system, is the concept that there are primary and secondary forms of headache. Such a system is outlined in Table 1. Primary headaches are those in which headache and its associated features are the disease in themselves, and secondary headaches are those caused exogenously, such as headache associated with fever. Mild secondary headache, such as that seen in association with upper respiratory tract infections, is common but only rarely worrisome. The clinical dilemma remains that while life-threatening headache is relatively uncommon in Western society, it is present and requires suitable vigilance by doctors. Primary headache, in contrast, while not life-threatening is often disabling over time.

Secondary headache

Key clinical features of secondary headache

There are certain issues which are vital to establish in the patient presenting with any form of head pain so that important secondary headaches will not be missed. Perhaps the most crucial is the length of the history. Patients with a short history require prompt attention and may require quick investigation and management, whereas patients with a longer history generally require time and patience rather than speedy consultation. There are some important general features, including associated fever or sudden onset of pain (Table 2), and these demand attention. Unless a benign diagnosis can be positively established, patients with a history of headache of recent onset or neurological signs need referral for specialist neurological assessment. A similar rule can be applied to computed tomography (**CT**) or magnetic resonance imaging (**MRI**). Patients with a history of recurrent headache over a period of a year or more, fulfilling International Headache Society criteria for migraine (Table 3) and with a normal physical examination, have positive brain imaging in only about one in a 1000 images. It should be noted that brain tumour is a relatively rare cause of headache, and rarely a cause of isolated long-term histories of headache. The management of secondary headache is generally self-evident—treatment of the underlying condition such as an infection or mass lesion. An exception is the condition of chronic post-traumatic headache in which pain persists for long periods after head injury. This is an interesting generic problem which may be seen after central nervous system infection, trauma, both blunt and surgical, intracranial bleeds, and other precipitants. While the syndrome is generally self-limiting up to 3 to 5 years after the event, it may require treatment of the headache (see Chronic Daily Headache below).

Table 1 Common causes of headache (after data from Rassmussen BK (1995). *Cephalalgia* **15**, 45–68)

Type	Prevalence (%)
Primary headache	
Migraine	16
Tension-type	69
Cluster headache	0.1
Idiopathic stabbing	2
Exertional	1
Secondary headache	
Systemic infection	63
Head injury	4
Subarachnoid haemorrhage	< 1
Vascular disorders	1
Brain tumour	0.1

Table 2 Warning signs in head pain

Sudden onset of pain
Fever
Marked change in the character or timing of pain
Neck stiffness
Pain associated with higher centre complaints
Pain associated with neurological disturbance, such as clumsiness or weakness
Pain associated with local tenderness, such as of the temporal artery

Primary headache syndromes

The primary headaches are a group of fascinating syndromes in which headache and associated features are seen in the absence of any exogenous cause. The common syndromes (Table 1) are tension-type headache, migraine, and cluster headache and the collection of headaches known as primary chronic daily, or frequent, headache. Some other less well known syndromes will be mentioned because they are easily treated when diagnosed.

Pathophysiology of headache

Understanding of headache has advanced considerably over the last decade. The severe primary headaches—migraine and cluster headache—have been studied extensively. In experimental animals the detailed anatomy of the connections of the pain-producing intracranial extracerebral vessels and the dura mater has built on the classical human observations that it is these structures, and not the brain, that are responsible for generating pain

Table 3 Simplified diagnostic criteria for migraine (after Goadsby and Olesen (1996) and adapted from the International Headache Society)

Repeated attacks of headache lasting 4 to 72 h which have the following features, normal physical examination, and no other reasonable cause for the headache

At least two of:
- Unilateral pain
- Throbbing pain
- Aggravation by movement
- Moderate or severe intensity

At least one of:
- Nausea/vomiting
- Photophobia and phonophobia

from within the head. The key structures involved in the nociceptive process are:

- the large intracranial vessels and dura mater;
- the peripheral terminals of the trigeminal nerve that innervate these structures;
- the central terminals and second-order neurones of the trigeminal nucleus.

Together these structures are known as the trigeminovascular system. The cranial parasympathetic autonomic innervation provides the basis for symptoms such as lacrimation and nasal stuffiness that are prominent in cluster headache and paroxysmal hemicrania, and which may also be seen in migraine. It is clear from human functional imaging studies that vascular changes in migraine and cluster headache are driven by these neural vasodilator systems so that these headaches should be regarded as neurovascular. The concept of a primary vascular headache should be abandoned since it neither explains the pathogenesis of what are complex central nervous system disorders nor necessarily predicts treatment outcomes.

Migraine is an episodic syndrome of headache with sensory sensitivity, such as to light, sound, and head movement, probably due to malfunction of aminergic brainstem/diencephalic sensory control systems (Fig. 1). The first of the migraine genes has been identified for familial hemiplegic migraine, in which about 50 per cent of families have mutations in the gene for the α_1 subunit of the neuronal P/Q voltage-gated calcium channel. This finding, together with the clinical features of migraine, suggests that it might be part of the spectrum of diseases known as channelopathies—disorders involving malfunction of voltage-gated channels. Functional neuroimaging has suggested that brainstem regions in migraine, and the posterior hypothalamic grey matter, site of the human circadian pacemaker cells of the suprachiasmatic nucleus in cluster headache, are good candidates for specific involvement in primary headache.

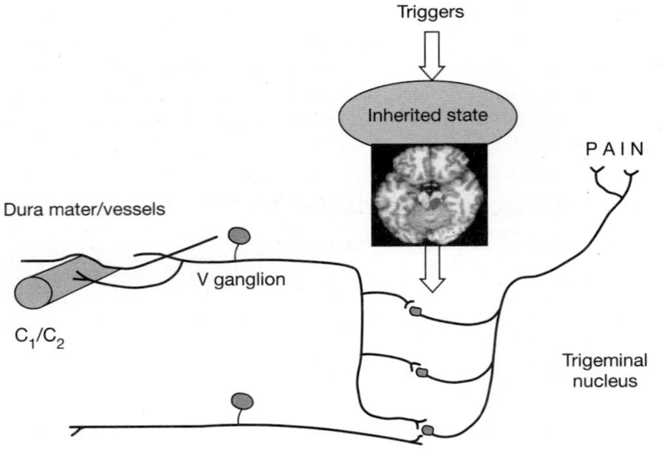

Fig. 1 Illustration of the some elements of migraine biology. Patients inherit a malfunction in brain control systems for pain and other afferent stimuli which can be triggered and are in turn capable of activating the trigeminovascular system as the initiating event in a positive feedback of neurally driven vasodilatation. The trigeminal innervation of pain-producing intracranial structures—dura mater and blood vessels—passes through the trigeminal ganglion (V ganglion) to terminate in the most caudal part of the trigeminal nucleus. Cervical inputs which terminate in the trigeminocervical complex accounts for the non-trigeminal distribution of pain in many patients. Migraine thus has a pain system for its expression and brain centres—modulatory systems—which define the associated symptoms and periodicity of the clinical syndrome. (Brainstem changes after Weiller and colleagues.)

Migraine

Migraine is generally an episodic headache with certain associated features, such as sensitivity to light, sound, or movement, and often with nausea or vomiting accompanying the headache (Table 3). None of the features is obligatory, and indeed given that the migraine aura, visual disturbances with flashing lights or zig-zag lines moving across the visual field or other neurological symptoms, is reported regularly in only about 15 per cent of patients, a high index of suspicion is required to diagnose migraine. A headache diary can often be helpful in making the diagnosis but perhaps more so in measuring the burden of the disease to the individual and then observing the effects of treatment. At a minimum the diary would mark on a calendar each day with headache, the length of the attack, what medication was taken and the doses, and what life events may have been taking place, such as a menstrual period. In differentiating the two main primary headache syndromes seen in clinical practice, migraine at its simplest level is headache with associated features, and tension-type headache is headache that is featureless (see below). Useful rule in practice is that most disabling headache is probably migrainous in biology. As for management, it is preferable to misdiagnose tension-type headache as migraine as opposed to the reverse, since there is so much good that can be done for migraine sufferers and so little for tension-type headache that patients may gain by such a diagnostic bias.

If headache with associated features describes migraine attacks, then 'headachy' describes the migraine sufferer over their lifetime. The migraine sufferer inherits a tendency to have headache that is amplified at various times by their interaction with their environment, the much discussed triggers. The brain of the 'migraineur' seems more sensitive to sensory stimuli and to change; and this tendency is even more notably amplified in females over the course of their menstrual cycle. The migraine sufferer does not habituate to sensory stimuli easily and so is often and adversely stimulated in the world in which they live and work. Migraine sufferers may have headache when they sleep in, when they are tired, when they skip meals, when they are stressed, or when they relax. They are less tolerant to change and part of successful management is to advise them to maintain regularity in their lives in the knowledge of this fluctuating brain sensitivity.

It has been said that migraine can never occur daily, but few biological phenomena respect absolute rules. This author takes the view that there is a very distinct syndrome of Chronic Migraine that is simply the most severe end of a complex phenomenon and often requires referral for specialist advice. Chronic Migraine is part of the group of headaches known as Chronic Daily Headache (see below) whose final nosology will only be settled when there are clearer biologically based development of disease markers. After making a diagnosis the next step in the clinical process is to be sure that the burden of the condition has been understood: how much headache does the patient have and, more important, what can't the patient do; what is their degree of disability? One can ask the patient directly to get a flavour, obtain a diary, or get a quick but accurate estimate using the Migraine Disability Assessment Scale (MIDAS), which is well validated and very easy to use.

Management of migraine

After diagnosis, the management of migraine begins by an explanation of certain things to the patient, notably:

- Migraine is an inherited tendency to headache, and cannot be cured.
- Migraine can be modified and controlled by the adjustment of lifestyle factors and the use of medicines.
- Migraine is not life-threatening nor associated with serious illness, the exception being in females who smoke and receive oestrogenic oral contraceptives, but migraine can make life a misery.
- Migraine management takes time and co-operation when information, such as that from a headache diary, has to be collected or inquiry made concerning the effect of the disease on the patient's life: the disability accrued to the disease.

Non-pharmacological management

Non-pharmacological management of migraine involves helping the patient identify things that aggravate the problem and encouraging them to modify these. Many patients will not find any joy in this approach; they should not be disparaged for this, but for those who do identify such factors, it will be a rewarding strategy. The crucial lifestyle advice is to explain to the patient that migraine is a state of sensitivity of the brain to change. This implies that the migraine sufferer needs to regulate their life with a healthy diet, regular exercise, regular sleep patterns, avoiding excess caffeine and alcohol and, as far as practical, modifying or minimizing changes in stress. A balanced life with fewer extremes will benefit most migraine sufferers. Patients also need to know that the brain sensitivity that is migraine varies, so that triggers will vary in their likelihood of resulting in headache.

Preventative treatments for migraine

The decision to start prophylactic treatment requires consideration from both doctor and patient. The basis for considering preventative treatment from a medical viewpoint is a combination of frequency of acute attacks and the tractability of these attacks. Attacks that are unresponsive to medications for acute management are targets for prevention, while attacks which are simply treated may be less obvious candidates for prevention. The other part of the equation relates to what is happening with time. If a patient diary shows a clear trend to increased frequency it is better to get in early with prevention than wait for the problem to become chronic. A simple rule for frequency might be that for one to two headaches a month there is usually no need to start preventative treatment; for three to four discussion may be needed; and for five or more a month prevention should be considered. Options available for treatment are covered in detail in Table 4 and vary somewhat by country. The problem with preventative treatments is not that there are none, but that they were all developed for other conditions. Often the doses required to reduce headache frequency produce marked and intolerable side-effects. It is not clear how preventatives work, although it seems likely that they modify the brain sensitivity that underlies migraine. Generally each drug should be started at a low dose and gradually increased to a reasonable maximum to determine if there is going to be a useful clinical effect.

Treatments for acute attacks of migraine

Treatments for acute attacks of migraine can be usefully divided into disease non-specific treatments—analgesics and non-steroidal anti-inflammatory drugs—and disease specific treatments—ergot-related compounds and triptans (Table 5). It must be said at the outset that most medications for acute attacks seem to have a propensity to aggravate headache frequency and induce a state of refractory daily or near-daily headache—analgesic-associated Chronic Daily Headache (see below). Codeine-containing compound analgesics are a particularly pernicious problem when available in over-the-counter preparations; the author recommends avoiding their frequent (more than twice a week) use. Many patients who stop taking regular analgesics will have no change to their headache, although some will have a distinct reduction in their headache frequency. Almost all who reduce acute attack medication overuse feel in some way better and will be easier to treat with standard preventatives.

Treatment strategies

Given the array of options for controlling an acute attack of migraine, how does one start? The simplest approach to treatment has been described as 'stepped care'. In this model all patients are treated, assuming no contraindications, with the simplest treatment, such as aspirin 900 mg with an antiemetic. Aspirin is an effective strategy (as proven by double-blind controlled clinical trials) and is best used in its most soluble formulation. The alternative would be a strategy known as 'stratified care', by which the physician determines, or stratifies, treatment at the start based on the likelihood of response to levels of care. An intermediate option may be described as stratified care by attack. The latter is what many headache authorities suggest and what patients often do when they have the options. Patients use simpler options for their less severe attacks relying on more potent options when their attacks or circumstances demand them (Table 6).

Non-specific treatments for acute attacks

Since simple analgesics such as aspirin and paracetamol (acetaminophen) are cheap and can be very effective, they can be employed in many patients. Dosages should be adequate, and the addition of domperidone (10 mg orally) or metoclopramide (10 mg orally) can be very helpful. Non-steroidal anti-inflammatory drugs can very useful when tolerated. Their success is often limited by inappropriate dosing, and adequate doses of naproxen (500 to 1000 mg orally or *per rectum*, with an antiemetic), ibuprofen (400 to 800 mg orally), or tolfenamic acid (200 mg orally) can be extremely effective. Tolfenamic acid has been shown in a double-blind placebo-controlled study to have comparable efficacy to sumatriptan 100 mg, a result that reinforces the general clinical view that non-steroidal anti-inflammatory drugs can be very useful compounds in treating migraine.

Specific treatments for acute attacks

When simple measures fail, or more aggressive treatment is required, the specific treatments are required. While ergotamine remains a useful anti-migraine compound, its place as the treatment of choice has slipped in recent years. There are particular situations in which ergotamine is very useful, but its use must be strictly controlled as ergotamine overuse itself produces severe headache and a host of vascular problems. The triptans have revolutionized the life of many patients with migraine and are clearly the most powerful option available to stop a migraine attack. They can be rationally applied by considering their pharmacological, physicochemical, and pharmacokinetic features, as well as the formulations that are available.

Table 4 Preventative treatments in migraine

Drug	Dose	Selected side-effects
Pizotifen	0.5 to 2 mg daily	Weight gain, drowsiness
Propranolol	40 to 120 mg twice daily	Reduced energy, tiredness, postural symptoms. Contraindicated in asthma
Tricyclics: amitriptyline, dothiepin, imipramine	25 to 75 mg at bedtime*	Drowsiness
Valproate	400 to 500 mg twice daily	Drowsiness, weight gain, tremor, hair loss, fetal abnormalities, haematological and liver abnormalities
Gabapentin	900 to 3600 mg daily	Dizziness, sedation
Methysergide	1 to 4 mg daily	Drowsiness, leg cramps, hair loss, retroperitoneal fibrosis (a 1 month drug holiday is required every 6 months)

Commonly used preventatives are listed with reasonable doses and common side-effects. The local national formulary should be consulted for detailed information.

* Some patients are very sensitive and may only need a total dose of 10 mg, although generally 1 to 1.5 mg/kg body weight is required for a response.

Table 5 Oral treatments for acute migraine

Non-specific treatments (often used with antiemetic/prokinetics, such as domperidone (10 mg) or metoclopramide (10 mg))	Aspirin (900 mg)	
	Paracetamol (1000 mg)	
	NSAIDS:	
		Naproxen (500 to 1000 mg)
		Ibuprofen (400 to 800 mg)
		Tolfenamic acid (200 mg)
Specific treatments	Ergot derivatives:	
		Ergotamine (1 to 2 mg)
	Triptans:	
		Sumatriptan (50 or 100 mg)
		Naratriptan (2.5 mg)
		Rizatriptan (10 mg)
		Zolmitriptan (2.5 mg)
		Eletriptan (40 or 80 mg)

NSAIDS = non-steroidal anti-inflammatory drugs.

Tension-Type Headache

As its name suggests Tension-Type Headache (TTH) is a term that describes the headache form most seeking understanding. One might challenge the reader to define the essence of TTH, which eludes this author, or consider for a moment how hard it is to study something that is commonly considered to be well understood. TTH has two forms, episodic TTH, where attacks occur on less than 15 days a month and chronic TTH where attacks, on average over time, are seen on 15 days or more a month. The latter is part of the broader clinical syndrome of Chronic Daily Headache (see below), but the terms are not equal.

Table 6 Clinical stratification of specific treatments for acute migraine

Clinical situation	Treatment options	
Failed analgesics/NSAIDS	First tier:	
		Sumatriptan 50 or 100 mg orally
		Rizatriptan 10 mg orally
		Eletriptan 40 mg orally
		Zolmitriptan 2.5 mg orally
		Almotriptan 12.5 mg
	Slower effect/better tolerability:	
		Naratriptan 2.5 mg
	Infrequent headache:	
		Ergotamine 1 to 2 mg orally
		Dihydroergotamine nasal spray 2 mg
Early nausea or difficulties taking tablets	Sumatriptan 20 mg nasal spray	
	Rizatriptan 10 mg MLT wafer	
Headache recurrence	Ergotamine 2 mg (perhaps most effective pr/usually with caffeine)	
	Naratriptan 2.5 mg orally	
Tolerating acute treatments poorly	Naratriptan 2.5 mg	
Early vomiting	Sumatriptan 25 mg per rectum	
	Sumatriptan 6 mg subcutaneously	
Menstrually related headache	Prevention:	
		Ergotamine orally at bedtime
		Oestrogen patches
	Treatment:	
		Triptans
		Dihydroergotamine nasal spray
Very rapidly developing symptoms	Sumatriptan 6 mg subcutaneously	
	Dihydroergotamine 1 mg intramuscularly	

Abbreviations: NSAIDS, non-steroidal anti-inflammatory drugs.

Clinical features

TTH has been defined by the International Headache Society both for its episodic and chronic forms, but by the time this chapter is read that definition will have changed. In the initial classification admixtures of nausea, photophobia, or phonophobia in various limited combinations, without clear biological rationale, were permitted in either the episodic or chronic form of TTH. These are being removed as the classification is being revised. A useful clinical approach is to diagnose TTH when the headache is completely featureless: no nausea, no vomiting, no photophobia, no phonophobia, no osmophobia, no throbbing, and no aggravation with movement. Such an approach neatly divides migraine, which has one or more of these features and is the main differential diagnosis, from TTH. For research I would further divide up the patients with attacks of a TTH phenotype who have migraine at other times, a family history of migraine, migrainous illnesses of childhood, or typical migraine triggers to their attacks, to try and understand what the TTH biology alone imparts to the sufferer.

Pathophysiology

The pathophysiology of TTH is incompletely understood. This results from the fact that the name implies to most that it is a product of nervous tension, for which there is no clear evidence, and the definitions employed have undoubtedly admitted patients with migraine to the studies. It seems likely that TTH will be due to a primary disorder of central nervous system pain modulation, to contrast with migraine which is a much more generalized disturbance of sensory modulation. There are data suggesting a genetic contribution to TTH but one must question these since they applied the current, faulty, diagnostic criteria.

Management

Adopting the clinical approach to TTH outlined above results in diagnosing a headache form that is usually less disabling, and more in the category of irritating. Its episodic form is generally amenable to simple analgesics, paracetamol (acetaminophen), aspirin, or NSAIDs, which can be purchased over the counter. There are clear clinical studies to demonstrate that triptans in TTH alone are not helpful, although germane to the above discussion, triptans are effective in TTH where the patient also has migraine. For chronic TTH amitriptyline is the only treatment with a clear evidence base; the other tricylics, selective serotonin reuptake inhibitors, or the benzodiazepines have not been shown in controlled trials to be effective. Similarly, there is no controlled evidence for the use of EMG biofeedback, relaxation therapy, or acupuncture, and both positive and negative studies using botulinum toxin. At the time of writing botulinum toxin is regarded as experimental. Stress management has been shown to be an effective approach in a controlled trial.

Cluster headache

Cluster headache is a rare form of primary headache with a population frequency of 0.1 per cent. Most standard textbooks cover the topic and the reading list contains specialized books on cluster headache. Cluster headache is part of a spectrum of primary headaches with prominent cranial autonomic activation, lacrimation, conjunctival injection or rhinorrhoea, collectively known as the Trigeminal-Autonomic Cephalgias (TACs). Cluster headache is probably the most painful condition known to humans; of more than 500 patients on our data base we are yet to talk with one who has had a more painful experience, including childbirth, severe burns and multiple limb fracture. A neurologist should manage cluster headache, if possible. Its core feature is periodicity, be it circadian or in terms of active and inactive bouts over weeks and months (Table 7). The typical cluster headache patient is male (male:female ratio 3:1) who has one to two attacks of unilateral pain of relatively short duration (30 to 180 minutes) every day

Table 7 Simplified diagnostic criteria for cluster headache (after the International Headache Society)

Episodic attacks of pain lasting 15 to 180 min coming in daily bouts for weeks with the following features
Unilateral often orbital or supraorbital
Attack frequency of one to eight per day
Associated with one or more of:
- Conjunctival injection
- Lacrimation
- Nasal congestion
- Rhinorrhoea
- Ptosis
- Miosis
- Eyelid oedema

for bouts of 8 to 10 weeks a year. Sufferers are generally perfectly well between times. Patients with cluster headache tend to move about during attacks, pacing, rocking, or even rubbing their head for relief. The pain is usually retro-orbital, boring, and very severe. It is associated with a red or watering eye, the nose running or blocking, and eyelid droop, the cranial autonomic symptoms, on the same side as the pain. Cluster headache is likely to be a disorder involving central pacemaker regions of the posterior hypothalamus, which is likely to share much with the other TACs but may be usually differentiated on clinical grounds from them (Table 8).

Management of cluster headache

Cluster headache is managed using treatments for acute attack and preventative agents. Treatments for acute attacks are usually required by all cluster headache patients at some time, while preventatives can almost be life-saving for those patients with chronic cluster headache and are often needed to shorten the active periods.

Preventative treatments

The options for preventative treatment in cluster headache are a little different depending on whether the patient has the episodic or chronic variety of the condition (Table 9). Most experts would now favour verapamil as the first-line preventative treatment, although for some patients with the episodic variety and short bouts limited courses of oral corticosteroids or methysergide can be very useful.

Verapamil has been suggested as a useful option for the last decade and compares favourably with lithium. What has clearly emerged from clinical practice is the need to use higher doses than had initially been considered and certainly higher than those used in cardiological indications. Although most patients will start on doses as low as 40 mg twice daily, doses of up to 960 mg daily and beyond are now employed. Side-effects, such as constipation and swelling of the legs, can be a problem, but the issue of cardiovascular safety is more difficult. Verapamil can cause heart block by slowing conduction in the atrioventricular node, as demonstrated by prolongation of the A–H interval. Given that the PR interval on the ECG is made up of atrial conduction, A–H, and His bundle conduction, it may be difficult to monitor subtle early effects as verapamil dose is increased. This question needs study in this group of patients but at present it seems appropriate to do a baseline ECG and then repeat the ECG 10 days after a dose change, usually 80 mg increments, when doses exceed 240 mg daily.

Treatment of acute attacks

Attacks of cluster headache often peak rapidly and thus require a treatment with a quick onset. Many patients with acute cluster headache respond very well to treatment with oxygen inhalation. This should be given as 100 per cent oxygen at 8 to 12 litre/min for 15 to 20 min. It is important to have a high flow and a high oxygen content. Injectable sumatriptan has been a boon for many patients with cluster headache. It is effective, rapid in onset, and with no evidence of tachyphylaxis. Sumatriptan is not effective when given pre-emptively as 100 mg orally three times daily, although the nasal spray has now been shown to be effective in a placebo-controlled study.

Chronic Daily Headache

Daily headache gives the subspecialty a bad name but can be very rewarding when tackled clinically in a methodical manner. Chronic Daily Headache is not one entity but a collection of very different problems requiring different approaches to their management. Certainly not all daily headache is simply Tension-Type Headache (Table 10), and this is the commonest clinical mistake in headache diagnosis confusing the clinical phenotype with the headache biotype. The current definition for 'Daily Headache' requires pain on 15 or more days a month. Both terms are used here because the subject is under intense discussion. Population based estimates of Daily Headache are remarkable, demonstrating that 4.5 to 4.8 per cent of Western populations, notably in Spain and the United States, have daily or near daily headache. Daily Headache may again be primary or secondary, and it seems useful to consider the possibilities in this way when making decisions about clinical management (Table 10). It should be said that population based studies bear out the impression that many patients with refractory daily headache overuse various over-the-counter analgesic preparations.

Chronic daily headache and migraine

While it is widely accepted that chronic variants exist in some of the primary headaches— notably tension-type headache, cluster headache, and paroxysmal hemicrania—chronic migraine is a somewhat controversial entity in some quarters. Most authorities would agree that migraine may sometimes be chronic in terms of frequency but whether this occurs often or not is frequently argued. The issue of whether patients with frequent

Table 8 Differential diagnosis of cluster headache and related syndromes

Feature	Cluster headache	CPH	SUNCT	ISH	Trigeminal neuralgia	Hemicrania continua	Hypnic headache
Gender	M > F by 3:1	F > M by 3:1	M > F	F > M	F > M	F > M	M = F
Pain:							
Type	Boring	Boring	Stabbing	Stabbing	Stabbing	Steady	Throbbing
Severity	Very severe	Very severe	Moderate/severe	Severe	Very severe	Moderate	Moderate
Location	Orbital	Orbital	Orbital	Any	V2/V3 > V1	Unilateral	Generalized
Duration	15 to 180 min	1 to 45 min	15 to 120 s	Seconds to 3 min	< 5 s	Continyous	15 to 30 min
Frequency	1 to 8 per day	1 to 40 per day	1 per day to 30 per hour	Any	Any	Variable	1 to 3 per night
Autonomic	+	+	+	–	–	+	–
Alcohol	+	–	–	–	–	–	–
Indomethacin	±	+	–	+	–	+	–

Abbreviations: CPH, chronic paroxsymal hemicrania; SUNCT, short-lasting neuralgiform pain with conjunctival injection and tearing; ISH, idiopathic stabbing headache.

Table 9 Preventative management of cluster headache

Episodic cluster headache	Prednisolone Verapamil Methysergide Daily (nocturnal) ergotamine Valproate
Chronic cluster headache	Verapamil Lithium Methysergide Valproate

headache, some of which fulfils standard criteria for migraine and some for tension-type headache, have a single migrainous problem with two phenotypic manifestations is a very vexed one. Given that tension-type headache describes a phenomenon that is indistinct at best it seems unlikely that all such headaches will have a single underlying mechanism.

Considering the population based surveys quoted above, about two-thirds of daily headache patients have chronic tension-type headache and about one-third satisfy the Silberstein–Lipton criteria for 'transformed migraine' (now called Chronic Migraine). The philosophy behind Chronic Migraine is that some patients who inherit a migrainous predisposition end up with Chronic Daily Headache on a migrainous basis. The typical patient will have a dull daily often-featureless pain, punctuated by more severe attacks which would often, in isolation, fulfil standard criteria for migraine. This group is dominant in headache specialty clinics, with about 90 per cent of patients referred to headache clinics having transformed migraine, usually accompanied by overuse of analgesics. It might be that these patients have a more intractable organic problem which explains their over-representation in referral centres. If it is accepted that all other forms of primary headache have chronic counterparts, particularly the typically episodic primary headache, cluster headache, then having frequent migraine is not such a fanciful concept— it can then be called Chronic Migraine, by analogy with the other primary headaches.

Treatment of frequent primary headache with or without migrainous features, whatever view of the biology or nomenclature one takes, requires control of analgesic, ergotamine, or triptan overuse when present and instigation of preventative medicines. It is exceptional for a patient misusing medication to be successfully treated with preventatives unless these other excessive medications are stopped. Preventatives used in episodic migraine are all employed, including tricylics, Valproate (divalproex), Gabapentin, Flunarizine, Methysergide and monoamine oxidase inhibitors. Comorbidity with depression is common in migraine, so that appropriate management of accompanying depression is important. Admission to hospital and treatment with a carefully monitored course of intravenous dihydroergotamine can be a very effective way to break the cycle of persistent headache.

Table 10 Daily* (frequent) headache (after Silberstein SD, Lipton RB, Sliwinski M (1996). *Neurology* **47**, 871–5)

Primary daily headache
Chronic tension-type headache
Transformed or chronic frequent migraine
Chronic cluster headache
Chronic paroxysmal hemicrania
New daily persistent headache
Secondary daily headache
Chronic headache with intracranial pathology, e.g. subdural, brain tumour
Inflammatory disease, such as giant cell arteritis
Chronic headache after dural irritation, such as postinfection or postbleed
Chronic headache after trauma, such as blunt head trauma or neurosurgical procedures
Chronic headache with cerebrospinal fluid pressure abnormalities, e.g. low or raised pressure

* Where headache should be on 15 days per month or more.

Syndromes responsive to indomethacin

There are number of primary headache syndromes with distinct characteristics that respond to treatment with indomethacin. Many share features with cluster headache, and are collectively known as the trigeminal autonomic cephalgias (TACs) (Table 8), while others do not. They deserve some attention because they can often be very easily treated.

Paroxysmal hemicrania

Sjaastad and colleagues first reported eight cases of a frequent unilateral severe but short-lasting headache without remission, coining the term 'chronic paroxysmal hemicrania'. The mean daily frequency of attacks varied from seven to 22 with the pain persisting from 5 to 45 min on each occasion. The site and associated autonomic phenomena were similar to those of cluster headache, but the attacks of chronic paroxysmal hemicrania were suppressed completely by indomethacin. A subsequent review of 84 cases showed a history of remission in 35 cases whereas 49 were chronic. By analogy with cluster headache the patients with remission have been referred to as having episodic paroxysmal hemicrania, and those without can be labelled with chronic paroxysmal hemcrania. Pareja has recorded attacks which swap sides, just as is known for cluster headache, and attacks with autonomic features without pain. This has been observed in cluster headache after trigeminal nerve section, by this author and others, and is excellent evidence for a disorder which is primarily of the central nervous system.

The essential features of paroxysmal hemicrania are:

- Female preponderance.
- Unilateral, usually frontotemporal, with very severe pain.
- Short-lasting attacks (2 to 45 min).
- Very frequent attacks (usually more than five a day).
- Marked autonomic features ipsilateral to the pain.
- Robust, quick (less than 72 h), and complete response to indomethacin.

Other issues

The treatment of paroxysmal hemicrania is complicated by the gastrointestinal side-effects seen with indomethacin, but thus far there is no convincing replacement. The issue of triptan response is not clearly settled and may be both variable and dependent on the length of the attacks. Injection of the greater occipital nerve is not useful in paroxysmal hemicrania. Piroxicam has been suggested to be helpful, although again it is not as effective as indomethacin. By analogy with cluster headache, verapamil has been used in paroxysmal hemicrania, although the response is not spectacular and higher doses require exploration. Paroxysmal hemicrania can coexist with trigeminal neuralgia—paroxysmal hemicrania-tic syndome—just as in cluster-tic syndrome. Similarly, secondary chronic paroxysmal hemicrania has also been reported with a syndrome like Tolosa–Hunt and in patients with a pituitary microadenoma and a maxillary cyst. If there is any doubt regarding the differential diagnosis between paroxysmal hemicrania and cluster headache then either an oral indomethacin challenge, or a formal placebo-controlled indomethacin test by injection, should be completed.

Hemicrania continua

Sjaastad and Spierings reported two patients, a woman aged 63 and a man of 53, who developed unilateral headache without obvious cause. One of these patients noticed redness, lacrimation, and sensitivity to light in the eye on the affected side. Both patients were relieved completely by indomethacin while other non-steroidal anti-inflammatory drugs were of little or no benefit. Newman and colleagues reviewed the 24 previously reported cases and added 10 of their own, including some with pronounced autonomic features resembling cluster headache. They divided their case histories into remitting and unremitting forms. Of the 34 patients reviewed, 22 were women and 12 men with the age of onset ranging from 11 to

58 years. The symptoms were controlled by indomethacin 75 to 150 mg daily. The essential features of hemicrania continua are:

- Unilateral pain.
- Pain is moderate and continuous but with fluctuations.
- Complete resolution of pain with indomethacin.
- Exacerbations may be associated with autonomic features.
- Migrainous features, such as nausea, photophobia or phonophobia, are frequently reported.

Apart from overuse of analgesics as a secondary aggravation, and a report in an HIV-infected patient, the status of secondary hemicrania continua is unclear. Injection of the greater occipital nerve is not useful in hemicrania continua.

Time to treatment response

Antonaci and colleagues proposed the 'indotest' by which the intramuscular injection of 50 mg of indomethacin could be used as a diagnostic tool. In hemicrania continua, pain was relieved in 73 ± 66 min and the pain-free period was 13 ± 8 h. The time elapsing between the thrice daily oral administration of 25 to 50 mg indomethacin and relief varied from 30 min to 48 h and thus a response to treatment can be rapidly assessed in the outpatient setting. Acute treatment with sumatriptan has been employed and reported to be of no benefit.

Idiopathic (Primary) Stabbing Headache

Short-lived jabs of pain, defined by the International Headache Society as Idiopathic (Primary) Jabbing Headache, are well documented in association with most types of primary headache. The essential clinical features are:

- Pain confined to the head, although rarely is it facial.
- Stabbing pain lasting from one to many seconds and occurring as a single stab or a series of stabs.
- Recurring at irregular intervals (hours to days).
- Cranial autonomic symptoms, such as lacrimation, conjunctival injection and rhinorrhoea, are not reported.

Raskin and Schwartz first described these sharp, jabbing pains about the head resembling a stab from an ice-pick, nail, or needle. They compared the prevalence of such pains in 100 migrainous patients and 100 headache-free controls and only three of the control subjects had experienced ice-pick pains compared with 42 of the migraine patients, of whom 60 per cent had more than one attack per month. The pains affected the temple or orbit more often than the parietal and occipital areas and often occurred before or during migraine headaches. The sites of the ice-pick pains generally coincide with the site of the patient's habitual headache.

Pains in the retroauricular and occipital region are also well described and these respond promptly to indomethacin. Ice-pick pains have been described in conjunction with cluster headaches, and are generally experienced in the same area as the cluster pain. Sjaastad described what he called 'jabs and jolts' lasting less than a minute in patients with chronic paroxysmal hemicrania. These longer attacks are almost certainly part of the spectrum of jabbing headache. It is of interest that jabbing pains generally are not accompanied by cranial autonomic symptoms. The response of idiopathic jabbing headache to indomethacin (25 to 50 mg twice to three times daily) is generally excellent. As a general rule the symptoms wax and wane, and after a period of control on indomethacin it is appropriate to withdraw treatment and observe the outcome.

Benign cough headache

Sharp pain in the head on coughing, sneezing, straining, laughing, or stooping has long been regarded as a symptom of organic intracranial disease, commonly associated with obstruction of the cerebrospinal fluid pathways. The presence of an Arnold–Chiari malformation or any lesion causing obstruction of cerebrospinal fluid pathways or displacing cerebral structures must be excluded before cough headache is assumed to be benign. Cerebral aneurysm, carotid stenosis, and vertebrobasilar disease may also present with cough or exertional headache as the initial symptom. The term 'benign Valsalva's manoeuvre-related headache' covers the headaches provoked by coughing, straining, or stooping but 'cough headache' is more succinct and so widely used it is unlikely to be displaced. The essential clinical features of benign cough headache are:

- Bilateral headache of sudden onset, lasting less than a minute, precipitated by coughing.
- May be prevented by avoiding coughing.
- Diagnosed only after structural lesions, such as a posterior fossa tumour, have been excluded by neuroimaging.

Comparing benign cough with benign exertional headache Pascual and colleagues reported that the average age of their patients with benign cough headache was 43 years more than their patients with exertional headache.

Management

Indomethacin is the medical treatment of choice in cough headache. Raskin has reported that some patients with cough headache are relieved by lumbar puncture which is a simple option when compared with prolonged use of indomethacin. The mechanism of this response remains unclear.

Benign exertional headache

The relationship of this form of headache to cough headache is unclear and certainly much is shared. Indeed the relationship to migraine also requires delineation. Credit must be given to Hippocrates for first recognizing this syndrome when he wrote 'one should be able to recognize those who have headache from gymnastic exercises, or walking, or running, or any other unseasonable labour, or from immoderate venery'.

The clinical features are:

- Pain specifically brought on by physical exercise.
- Bilateral and throbbing in nature at onset and may develop migrainous features in those patients susceptible to migraine.
- Lasts from 5 min to 24 h.
- Prevented by avoiding excessive exertion, particularly in hot weather or at high altitude.

The acute onset of headache with straining and breath holding as in weightlifter's headache may be explained by acute venous distension. The development of headache after sustained exertion, particularly on a hot day, is more difficult to understand. Anginal pain may be referred to the head, probably by central connections of vagal afferents, and may present as exertional headache, so-called cardiac cephalalgia. The link to exercise is the main clinical clue. Phaeochromocytoma may occasionally be responsible for exertional headache. Intracranial lesions or stenosis of the carotid arteries may have to be excluded as discussed for benign cough headache. Headache may be precipitated by any form of exercise and often has the pulsatile quality of migraine.

Management

The most obvious form of treatment is to take exercise gradually and progressively whenever possible. Indomethacin at daily doses varying from 25 to 150 mg is generally very effective in benign exertional headache. Indomethacin 50 mg, ergotamine tartrate 1 to 2 mg orally, ergotamine by inhalation, or methysergide 1 to 2 mg orally given 30 to 45 min before exercise are useful prophylactic measures.

Other interesting primary headaches

Hypnic headache

This syndrome was first described by Raskin in patients aged between 67 and 84 who had headache of a moderately severe nature that typically came on a few hours after going to sleep. These headaches last from 15 to 30 min, are typically generalized, although they may be unilateral, and can be throbbing. Patients may report falling back to sleep only to be awoken by a further attack a few hours later with up to three repetitions of this pattern over the night. In the largest series (Dodick's) of 19 patients, 16 (84 per cent) were female and the mean age at onset was 61 ± 9 years. Headaches were bilateral in two-thirds of cases and unilateral in one-third, and in 80 per cent of cases pain was mild or moderate. Three patients reported similar headaches when falling asleep during the day. None of these patients had photophobia or phonophobia and nausea was unusual.

Management

Patients with this form of headache generally respond to a bedtime dose of lithium carbonate (200 to 600 mg) and in those that do not tolerate this verapamil or methysergide at bedtime may be alternative strategies. Two patients who responded to flunarizine 5 mg at night have now been reported. Dodick and colleagues reported that one to two cups of coffee or caffeine 60 mg orally at bedtime were helpful, and this is well worth trying as the first step in Hypnic Headache. This author has controlled a patient poorly tolerant of lithium by using verapamil at night (160 mg).

Short-lasting unilateral neuralgiform headache attacks with conjunctival injection and tearing (the SUNCT syndrome)

It has been remarked (Lance) that as the duration of the pain in the cluster headache-like syndromes becomes shorter, their names become longer! Sjaastad and colleagues reported three male patients whose brief attacks of pain in and around one eye were associated with sudden conjunctival injection and other autonomic features of cluster headache. Attacks lasted only 15 to 60 s and recurred five to 30 times an hour. Attacks could be precipitated by chewing or eating certain foods, such as citrus fruits, and were not abolished by indomethacin. Most cases have some associated precipitating factors, particularly movements of the neck. Of the patients recognized with this problem males predominate and the paroxysms of pain usually last between 5 and 250 s, although longer duller interictal pains are recognized as well as attacks of up to 2 h in two patients. The conjunctival injection seen with SUNCT is often the most prominent autonomic feature and production of tears may be very obvious. SUNCT is more or less intractable to medical management although there is a modest benefit with carbamazepine that is nothing like its effect in trigeminal neuralgia. Recently, we have found that topiramate and lamotrigine are useful in SUNCT syndrome.

Secondary SUNCT and associations

There have been three reported patients with secondary SUNCT syndromes. The first two patients had homolateral cerebellopontine angle arteriovenous malformations diagnosed on MRI. The third patient had a cavernous haemangioma of the brainstem seen only on MRI. These cases highlight the need for cranial MRI in investigating for secondary SUNCT. Just as there is a reported case of chronic paroxysmal hemicrania associated with trigeminal neuralgia there is a single report of a patient with trigeminal neuralgia who developed a SUNCT syndrome.

Benign sex headache

Sex headache may be precipitated by masturbation or coitus and usually starts as a dull bilateral ache while sexual excitement increases, suddenly becoming intense at orgasm. The term orgasmic cephalalgia is not useful since not all sex headache requires orgasm. Three types of sex headache are discussed: a dull ache in the head and neck that intensifies as sexual excitement increases, a sudden severe ('explosive') headache occurring at orgasm, and a postural headache resembling that due to low cerebrospinal fluid pressure developing after coitus. The latter in the author's clinical experience is simply another form of headache due to low cerebrospinal fluid pressure arising from vigorous sexual activity usually with multiple orgasm and might be usefully considered with the secondary chronic daily headaches (Table 10). The essential clinical features of sex headache are:

- Precipitation by sexual excitement.
- Bilateral at onset.
- Prevented or eased by ceasing sexual activity before orgasm.

Headaches developing at the time of orgasm are not always benign. Subarachnoid haemorrhage was precipitated by sexual intercourse in 4.5 per cent of 66 cases reported by Fisher and 12 per cent of 50 cases studied by Lundberg and Osterman. One young man was reported to have developed a brainstem thrombosis and another a left hemisphere infarction.

Sex headache affects men more often than women and may occur at any time during the years of sexual activity. It may develop on several occasions in succession and then not trouble the patient again, although there is no obvious change in sexual technique. In patients who stop sexual activity when headache is first noticed it may subside within a period of 5 min to 2 h, and it is recognized that more frequent orgasm can aggravate established sex headache. About half of patients with sex headache have a history of exertional headaches but there is no excess of cough headache in patients with sex headache. In about 50 per cent of patients sex headache will settle in 6 months. Migraine is probably more common in patients with sex headache.

Management

Benign sex headaches are usually irregular and infrequent in recurrence, so management can often be limited to reassurance and advice about ceasing sexual activity if a milder, warning headache develops. When the condition recurs regularly or frequently, it can be prevented by the administration of propranolol, but the dosage required varies from 40 to 200 mg daily. An alternative is the calcium channel blocking agent diltiazem 60 mg three times daily. Ergotamine (1 to 2 mg) or indomethacin (25 to 50 mg) taken about 30 to 45 min prior to sexual activity can also be helpful.

Thunderclap headache

Severe headache of sudden onset may occur in the absence of sexual activity and it is appropriate to consider the issue here as it may be the sentinel bleed of an intracranial aneurysm and there are some issues that overlap clinically. Day and Raskin reported a woman with three episodes of very severe headache of sudden onset who was found to have an unruptured aneurysm of the internal carotid artery, with adjacent areas of segmental vasospasm. While headaches of explosive onset may certainly be caused by the ingestion of sympathomimetic drugs or tyramine-containing foods in a patient who is taking monoamine oxidase inhibitors, and can also be a symptom of phaeochromocytoma, the relationship between thunderclap headache and aneurysm in the absence of CT scan or cerebrospinal fluid evidence of subarachnoid haemorrhage is difficult. Wijdicks and colleagues followed up 71 patients whose CT scans and cerebrospinal fluid findings were negative for an average of 3.3 years. Twelve patients had further such headache, and 31 (44 per cent) later had regular episodes of migraine or tension-type headache. Factors identified as precipitating the headache were sexual intercourse in three cases, coughing in four, and exertion in 12, while the remainder had no obvious cause. A history of hypertension was found in 11 and of previous headache in 22. Markus compared the presentation of 37 patients with subarachnoid haemorrhage and 189 with a similar thunderclap headache but normal cerebrospinal fluid examination and could not discern any characteristic which distinguished the two conditions on clinical grounds.

Investigation of any severe headache of sudden onset, be it in the context of sexual excitement or isolated thunderclap headache, should be driven by the clinical context. The first presentation should be vigorously investigated with CT and cerebrospinal fluid examination and where possible MRI angiography. Formal cerebral angiography should be reserved to situations of high clinical suspicion. It is worth noting that of diffuse multifocal reversible spasm may be seen in thunderclap headache without there being an intracranial aneurysm.

Further reading

Antonaci F *et al.* (1998). Chronic paroxysmal hemicrania and hemicrania continua. Parenteral indomethacin: the 'Indotest'. *Headache* **38**, 122–8.

Day JW, Raskin NH (1986). Thunderclap headache: symptom of unruptured cerebral aneurysm. *Lancet* **2**, 1247–8.

Dodick DW, Mosek AC, Campbell JK (1998). The hypnic ('alarm clock') headache syndrome. *Cephalalgia* **18**, 152–6.

Ferrari MD *et al.* (2001). Triptans (serotonin, 5-HT1B/1D agonists) in acute migraine treatment – a meta-analysis of 53 trials. *Lancet* **358**, 1668–75.

Fisher CM (1968). Headache in cerebrovascular disease. In: Vinken PJ, Bruyn GW, eds. *Handbook of clinical neurology,* Vol 5, pp 124–6. Elsevier, Amsterdam.

Goadsby PJ, Olesen J (1998). Diagnosis and management of migraine. *British Medical Journal* **312**, 1279–82.

Goadsby PJ, Silberstein SD (1997). Headache. In: Asbury A, Marsden CD, eds. *Blue books in practical neurology,* Vol 17. Butterworth-Heinemann, New York.

Goadsby PJ (2000). The pharmacology of headache. *Progress in Neurobiology* 62, 509–25.

Goadsby PJ (2002). Chronic tension-type headache. In: Barton S, ed. *Clinical evidence,* Vol. 6. BMJ Publishing Group, London, in press.

Goadsby PJ, Lipton RB, Ferrari MD (2002). Migraine: current understanding and management. *New England Journal of Medicine* **346**, in press.

Griggs RC, Nutt JG (1995). Episodic ataxias as channelopathies. *Annals of Neurology* **37**, 285–7.

Kudrow L (1987). Cluster headache. In: Blau JN, ed. *Headache: clinical, therapeutic,conceptual and research aspects.* Chapman and Hall, London.

Kudrow L, Esperanca P, Vijayan N (1987). Episodic paroxysmal hemicrania? *Cephalalgia* **7**, 197–201.

Lance JW (1976). Headaches related to sexual activity. *Journal of Neurology, Neurosurgery and Psychiatry* **39**, 1226–30.

Lance JW, Hinterberger H (1976). Symptoms of pheochromocytoma, with particular reference to headache, correlated with catecholamine production. *Archives of Neurology* **33**, 281–8.

Lundberg PO, Osterman PO (1974). The benign and malignant forms of orgasmic cephalgia. *Headache* **14**, 164–5.

Markus HS (1991). A prospective follow-up of thunderclap headache mimicking subarachnoid haemorrhage. *Journal of Neurology, Neurosurgery and Psychiatry* **54**, 1117–25.

May A *et al.* (1998). Hypothalamic activation in cluster headache attacks. *The Lancet* **351**, 275–8.

May A *et al.* (1999). Correlation between structural and functional changes in brain in an idiopathic headache syndrome. *Nature Medicine* **5**, 836–8.

Newman LC, Lipton RB, Solomon S (1994). Hemicrania continua: ten new cases and a review of the literature. *Neurology* **44**, 2111–14.

Olesen J, Goadsby PJ (1999). In: Olesen J, ed. *Cluster headache and related conditions,* Vol 9. Oxford University Press, Oxford.

Pareja JA (1995). Chronic paroxysmal hemicrania: dissociation of the pain and autonomic features. *Headache* **35**, 111–13.

Pascual P *et al.* (1996). Cough, exertional, and sexual headache. *Neurology* **46**, 1520–4.

Quality Standards Subcommittee of the American Academy of Neurology (1994). The utility of neuroimaging in the evaluation of headache patients with normal neurologic examinations. *Neurology* **44**, 1353–4.

Raskin NH (1988). The hypnic headache syndrome. *Headache* **28**, 534–6.

Raskin NH (1995). The cough headache syndrome: treatment. *Neurology* **45**, 1784.

Raskin NH, Schwartz RK (1980). Icepick-like pain. *Neurology* **30**, 203–5.

Rassmussen BK (1995). Epidemology of headache. *Cephalalgia* **15**, 45–68.

Silberstein SD, Lipton RB, Sliwinski M (1996). Classification of daily and near-daily headaches: a field study of revised IHS criteria. *Neurology* **47**, 871–5.

Sjaastad O *et al.* (1980). Chronic paroxysmal hemicrania (CPH). The clinical manifestations. a review. *Uppsala Journal of Medical Science* **31**, 27–33.

Sjaastad O *et al.* (1989). Shortlasting unilateral neuralgiform headache attacks with conjunctival injection, tearing, sweating, and rhinorrhea. *Cephalalgia* **9**, 147–56.

Sjaastad O, Spierings EL (1984). Hemicrania continua: another headache absolutely responsive to indmethacin. *Cephalalgia* **4**, 65–70.

Stewart WF *et al.* (1999). Reliability of the migraine disability assessment score in a population-based sample of headache sufferers. *Cephalalgia* **19**, 107–14.

Tfelt-Hansen P *et al.* (2000). Ergotamine in the acute treatment of migraine—a review and European consensus. *Brain* **123**, 9–18.

Tzourio C *et al.* (1995). Case-control study of migraine and risk of ischaemic stroke in young women. *British Medical Journal* **310**, 830–3.

Weiller C *et al.*(1995). Brain stem activation in spontaneous human migraine attacks. *Nature Medicine* **1**, 658–60.

Wijdicks EFM, Kerkhoff H, van Gijn J (1988). Long-term follow up of 71 patients with thunderclap headache mimicking subarachnoid haemorrhage. *Lancet* **2**, 68–70.

24.13.3 Epilepsy in later childhood and adults

G. D. Perkin

Definitions

Using guidelines developed by the International League Against Epilepsy (**ILEA**), epilepsy is defined as recurrent (two or more) epileptic seizures, unprovoked by any immediate identifiable cause. Excluded are febrile seizures and neonatal seizures (the latter defined as those occurring in the first 4 weeks of life). Multiple seizures occurring within a 24-h period are considered to represent a single event. The epileptic seizure itself is defined as the clinical manifestation of an abnormal and excessive discharge of a set of brain neurones. The manifestation is a sudden transient phenomenon that may include alteration of consciousness, motor, sensory, autonomic, or psychic events which are perceived either by the individual or by an observer. Problems arise, when using the term epilepsy, with those individuals who may have had only two or three attacks in a lifetime. To take account of this, the terms active and inactive epilepsy are used, the former referring to patients with at least one seizure in the previous 5 years, the latter to patients who have been seizure free over the same period. The definitions are further qualified, for inactive cases, according to whether the individual is on drug therapy.

The idiopathic epilepsies are defined as those epileptic disorders (partial or generalized) which have characteristic clinical and electroencephalographic features coupled with a genetic predisposition. Cryptogenic epilepsy defines cases of partial or generalized epilepsy in which no aetiological factor has been identified. Symptomatic seizures are those occurring in association with a known risk factor. Epileptic syndromes have been defined by the ILEA on the basis of clinical characteristics, age of onset, and electroencephalographic findings.

Epidemiology

Incidence

Most reported incidence rates lie between 40 and 70 per 100 000. Figures for developing countries usually exceed 100 per 100 000. Age-specific rates show a bimodal distribution, with the highest peak in the first decade, falling thereafter until a second peak in later life.

Prevalence

Prevalence figures are more widely available. For adults, rates lie between 1.5 and 57 per 1000, with an average of 10.3 per 1000. Cumulative incidence (or lifetime prevalence) rates, excluding febrile seizures, are higher, producing a figure between 1.5 and 5 per cent (Fig. 1).

Sex

Males have slightly higher prevalence rates than females.

Socio-economic status

Higher prevalence rates have been reported in the lower socio-economic groups, both in developed and developing countries.

Pathophysiology

Inherent in any discussion of epilepsy mechanisms is the need to define a homogeneous population. Generalized tonic–clonic seizures, for example, can occur with many different epileptic syndromes. Epileptic seizures are thought to arise at cortical sites. Partial seizures begin focally in the cortex, generalized seizures infer widespread, bilateral cortical involvement from the beginning. An interictal discharge occurs when a group of pyramidal neurones is synchronously activated. During the discharge, the cells develop a large and prolonged depolarization which is terminated by a hyperpolarizing potential. Seizures develop when any of the inhibitory processes suppressing interictal discharges fail.

The underlying mechanisms behind epileptic discharges have been best defined for absence seizures where a thalamocortical circuit is responsible for generating synchronous burst-firing of neurones. The circuit involves neocortical pyramidal neurones, thalamic relay neurones, and neurones of the nucleus reticularis thalami. The last are exclusively γ-aminobutyric acid (**GABA**) in type. A voltage-dependent calcium channel (T-channel) appears critical in allowing burst-firing of neurones to appear. Following activation, the T-channels acquire repolarization via $GABA_B$ receptors present on thalamic relay neurones. $GABA_A$ receptors also play an important regulatory role in synchronized thalamocortical burst-firing.

Less information is available on the pathophysiological mechanisms of generalized convulsive seizures. Roles for $GABA_A$ receptors and for altered serotonergic neurotransmission have been suggested.

Classification

The ILEA classification scheme, as revised in 1989, is now widely used for epidemiological, management, and research purposes. The scheme divides seizures into focal, generalized, and unclassifiable forms (Table 1).

Though it is widely used, the classification has disadvantages. The ability to determine whether consciousness is preserved, in order to make the distinction between simple and complex partial seizures, is often limited.

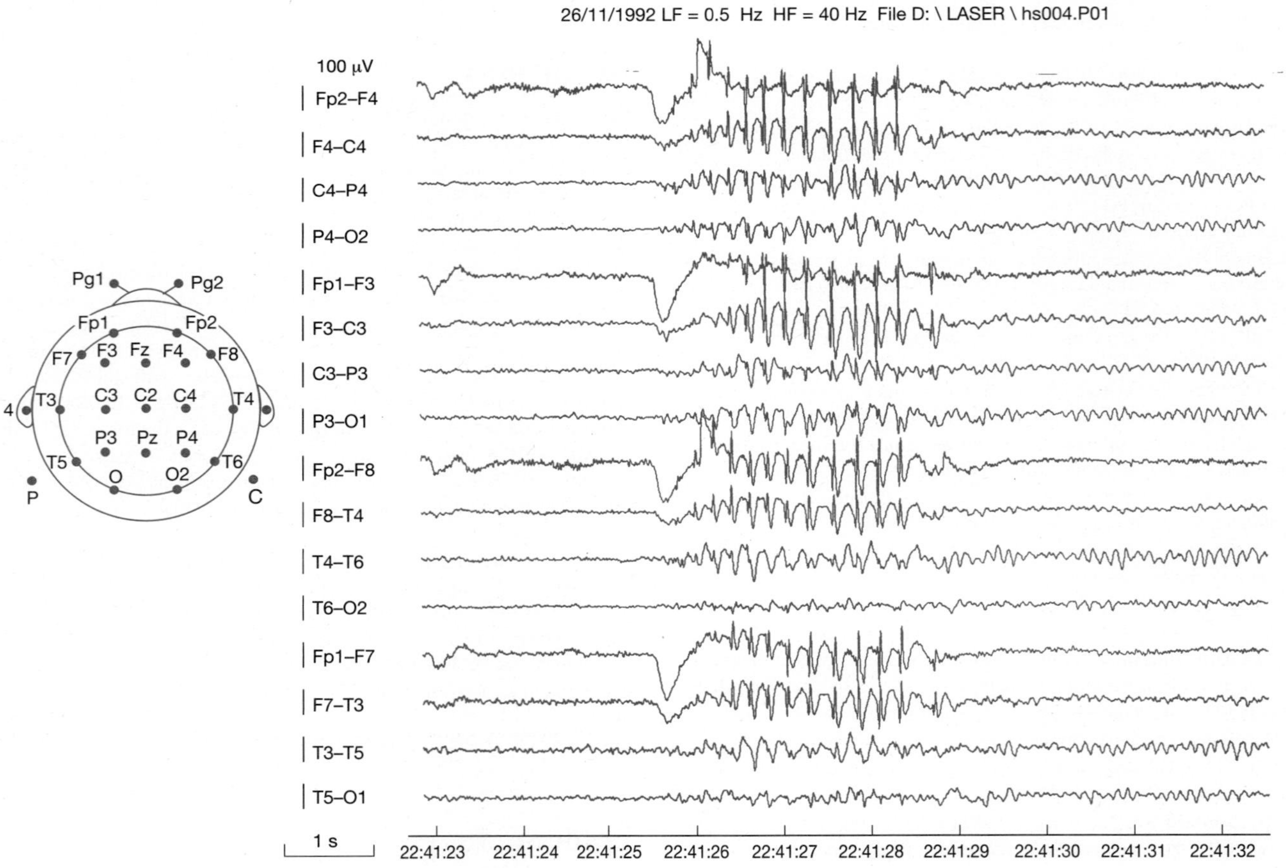

Fig. 1 Electroencephalogram of a typical absence seizure. The first 2.5 s of the record are entirely normal. The event begins with a large downward deflection which records eye closure, immediately followed in all channels by a spike-and-wave discharge at a frequency of 3 cycles/s. The seizure terminates as abruptly as it began. (Record kindly provided by Dr David Fish.)

Table 1 Classification of epilepsy

I. *Partial (focal, local) seizures*
A. Simple partial seizures (consciousness not impaired)
1. With motor symptoms
2. With somatosensory or special sensory symptoms
3. With autonomic symptoms
4. With psychic symptoms
B. Complex partial seizures (with impairment of consciousness)
1. Beginning as simple partial seizures and progressing to impairment of consciousness
(a) With no other features
(b) With features as in simple partial seizures
(c) with automatisms
2. With impairment of consciousness at onset
(a) With no other features
(b) With features as in simple partial seizures
(c) With automatisms
C. Partial seizures evolving to secondarily generalized seizures
1. Simple partial seizures evolving to generalized seizures
2. Complex partial seizures evolving to generalized seizures
3. Simple partial seizures evolving to complex partial seizures to generalized seizures
II. *Generalized seizures (convulsive or non-convulsive)*
A. 1. Absence seizures
2. Atypical absence seizures
B. Myoclonic seizures
C. Clonic seizures
D. Tonic seizures
E. Tonic–clonic seizures
F. Atonic seizures (astatic seizures)
III. *Unclassified epileptic seizures*

Some individuals, though appearing alert, can be shown to have impaired awareness when carefully tested.

An elaboration of the classification consists of a list of epileptic syndromes into which, theoretically, all generalized and partial epileptic seizures can be fitted. The idiopathic generalized seizures are classified according to age of onset and seizure type. The partial seizures, attributed to dysfunction of restricted cortical areas, are predominantly classified according to their clinical features, supplemented by electroencephalographic findings. Much criticism has been made of this syndromic classification. In routine clinical practice many cases (probably the majority) are left in non-specific categories. Moreover, the classification fails to incorporate data derived from CT or MRI.

Partial seizures

Simple partial motor seizures

Any part of the body can be affected by a focal motor seizure, according to the site of origin of the discharge. Sometimes the seizure remains localized to the same area (for example the hand), sometimes it 'marches' along the motor cortex, producing successional jerking of contiguous body parts (jacksonian seizures). During the focal stage, consciousness is preserved. With secondary generalization (that is, diffuse bilateral spread) consciousness is lost. The parts of the body most commonly affected by this type of seizure correlate with their area of representation in the motor cortex. Other focal motor disturbances reflecting epileptic discharges include rotation of head and eyes contralaterally (from the dorsolateral prefrontal cortex), tonic foot movements ipsilaterally (the paracentral lobule), and head turning with arm extension on the same side (supplementary motor cortex). Following such seizures there may be paralysis of the affected part lasting for minutes or hours (Todd's paresis).

Simple partial sensory seizures

Seizures emanating from the sensory cortex produce paraesthesias or numbness. The seizure can march in an analogous fashion to a motor seizure, and similarly, can then become generalized. Where the tongue or face are involved, the symptoms are sometimes felt bilaterally. More complex sensory phenomena may be experienced and with discharges in the second sensory area, the limb sensations can be ipsilateral, contralateral, or bilateral.

Occipital lobe seizures

Visual symptoms predominate, usually as simple rather than complex phenomena. The latter, producing alteration of size, shape, or depth of objects are associated with seizures arising at the occipito-parieto-temporal interface. In addition there may be ocular deviation, jerking, or forced closure of the eyelids. Visual hallucinations may occur.

Frontal lobe seizures

Frontal lobe seizures are commonly nocturnal and frequently associated with turning to a prone position. Vocalization is common and tends to consist of a continuous monotone with moaning or grunting. An aura before the attack is unusual. Other recognized features include pelvic thrusting, rocking of the body, and head movements. Rapid postictal recovery is common.

Simple partial (temporal lobe) seizures

The distinction between simple and complex partial seizures is difficult, based as it is on evidence of altered consciousness with the latter. Olfactory, gustatory, and vertiginous sensations occur. The taste and smell sensations are sometimes pleasurable but often disagreeable. A metallic taste is common. Abdominal sensations also occur, which are typically ill-defined and may ascend to the chest and throat. Psychic symptoms are more often associated with complex partial seizures. There may be intense pleasure or fear ushering in the attack. The patient can experience a sense of loss of personal or environmental reality (depersonalization and derealization, respectively). There may be a sense of intense familiarity (*déjà vu*) or unfamiliarity (*jamais vu*). Epileptic anger is unprovoked and rapidly subsides. Illusions are encountered, in the form of disordered visual perceptions, and visual or auditory hallucinations, sometimes of considerable complexity (Fig. 2).

Where consciousness is disturbed, various automatic activity or movement may occur of which the patient is unaware (automatisms). These may take the form of eating (chewing or swallowing), speaking, gesture, or more elaborate skilled activities. Some of these automatic movements are also seen with absence seizures. When elaborate, the patient may partly undress, or move about from one room to another. The symptomatology of mesial and lateral temporal lobe discharges has been distinguished, the latter having additional somatosensory, visual, or auditory manifestations to the other features mentioned above.

Other, rarer, focal seizure types are confined to childhood. In benign childhood epilepsy with centrotemporal spikes, consciousness is preserved. The sensory phenomena are usually confined to the mouth where motor activity may also occur. Speech arrest occurs if the dominant hemisphere is affected.

Any of the focal epilepsies can lead to secondary generalization. Consciousness is lost, and a tonic–clonic seizure is the usual outcome. Prolonged focal seizures (epilepsia partialis continua) lead to a repetitive or continuous focal motor activity which may last for weeks or months and is most often the consequence of a focal cortical insult.

Generalized seizures

Tonic–clonic seizures (grand mal epilepsy)

Some patients report a premonition for hours or even days before the attack. The symptoms are usually a vague sense of loss of well being and do not imply a focal origin for the attack. An aura, on the other hand, lasting a few seconds before the onset implies a focal origin for the attack, demanding classification as a focal seizure with secondary generalization. The tonic phase is associated with contraction of axial then limb muscles. If upright, the patient falls heavily. Injury is common. Contraction of the jaw can lead to tongue injury. Forcible contraction of the diaphragm results in a sudden gasp or epileptic cry. Cyanosis results from a loss of respiratory activity. Subsequently clonic movements appear and slowly increase in amplitude. Gradually, periods of relaxation intervene between the clonic contractions until finally all movements cease. The patient is then flaccid. Urinary or faecal incontinence or both may occur at this stage. Subsequently the patient is liable to sleep, often heavily. If the patient wakes, initial confusion and disorientation is the norm. Headache and muscle pains are common. Incomplete forms occur in which the clonic or tonic phase predominates.

In addition to injuries incurred in falling, and those resulting from biting of the cheeks or tongue (typically the lateral margin is affected), the seizures may be of such violence that vertebral compression fractures occur. Sudden death occurring soon after a tonic–clonic seizure is a recognized, though rare, complication. Its incidence lies between 1:500 and 1:1000 deaths per person-year.

Absence seizures (petit mal)

Patients are totally unaware of their absence seizures. Activity suddenly ceases but without loss of posture. Adventitious movements occur, for example slight contractions of the eyes or some lip movement. The head may drop slightly. More typically, the patient simply stares blankly and is unresponsive. Attacks last around 10 to 20 s. In some cases more overt limb movement occurs.

Atypical absences are defined as attacks which begin less abruptly, last longer, and frequently lead to loss of postural tone. They usually coincide with other seizure types. Absence seizures begin in childhood and usually cease in adult life, though some 50 per cent of patients will later develop tonic–clonic seizures.

Myoclonic seizures

Myoclonus consists of brief, shock-like contractions of muscle, occurring either in a generalized or focal distribution. Many forms of myoclonus are non-epileptic. Those associated with epilepsy are accompanied by an ictal electroencephalographic discharge. In primary generalized epileptic myoclonus, the myoclonus is accompanied by diffuse cortical epileptic discharges.

Atonic seizures

Atonic seizures result in sudden loss of muscle tone. If the hypotonus is generalized, falls occur, often with substantial injury. The attacks begin in infancy or childhood. The episodes are brief and recovery rapid unless injury has occurred.

Status epilepticus

Status epilepticus is defined as a single seizure lasting more than 30 min or successional seizures without recovery of consciousness between. The seizures are usually tonic–clonic. Both complex partial seizures and absence seizures can occur in the form of status epilepticus. In such cases, alteration of the conscious level is likely to be the major clinical feature with little motor activity, particularly with the latter.

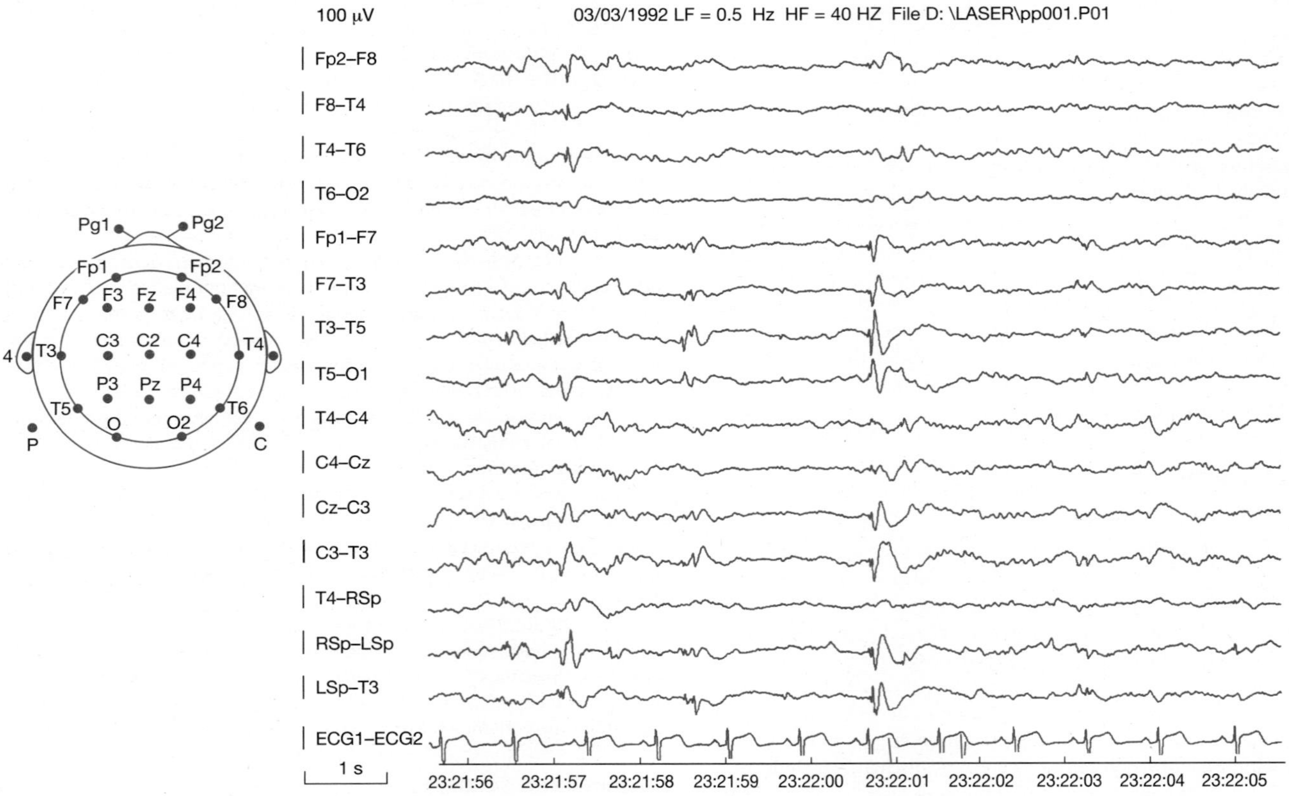

Fig. 2 Interictal spike and slow-wave complex in a patient with complex partial seizures. The discharges are particularly apparent over the left temporal lobe (T3 to T5), but there are some independent discharges over the right temporal lobe (T4 to T6). (Record kindly provided by Dr David Fish.)

Epilepsy syndromes

The need to define epileptic syndromes arises from the fact that individual seizure types may be a manifestation of a number of differing conditions, all with individual characteristics and prognosis. The epileptic syndrome is based on a combination of seizure type, presumed localization (according to clinical features and electroencephalographic characteristics) in the case of the partial seizures, and age of onset. In routine, as opposed to heavily specialized, practice only a third of newly diagnosed epilepsy can be fitted into such a classification system.

Causes of epilepsy

In most surveys, only about a quarter to a third of epilepsy cases have been attributable to a specific cause. With modern imaging methods, this proportion is likely to rise significantly.

Genetically determined

In some genetically determined disorders, epilepsy is only one feature of the condition. Many such disorders have features other than epilepsy and typically produce significant neurological disability. Examples include the forms of progressive myoclonic epilepsy associated with Lafora body disease and Unverricht–Lundborg disease. More relevant, in clinical terms, are those genetically determined conditions in which epilepsy is the sole or major manifestation. Among these are some with simple forms of inheritance, and some with complex forms. The epilepsies occurring with such syndromes may be generalized or partial in nature.

Epilepsy syndromes with simple inheritance

Examples in this category include benign familial neonatal convulsions and benign familial infantile convulsions. Linkage to chromosome 20q has been described for the former, coding for potassium channel proteins.

Epilepsy syndromes with complex inheritance

Examples include juvenile myoclonic epilepsy and benign rolandic epilepsy.

Juvenile myoclonic epilepsy

This epilepsy type usually begins between the ages of 12 and 18. Early morning, sudden myoclonic jerks of the arms and shoulders are characteristic. Subsequently, generalized tonic–clonic seizures occur in the majority of patients. Genes for this disorder, inherited in a dominant manner, have been localized to both chromosome 6 and 15.

Benign rolandic epilepsy

This condition presents between the ages of 5 and 10 years. Unilateral motor or sensory seizures occur in sleep. The condition is associated with centrotemporal spikes on electroencephalography. The epileptiform abnormality may be linked to chromosome 15.

Included within the umbrella of the genetically determined epilepsy syndromes (though often classified separately from the epilepsies) are febrile seizures. These occur in between 2 and 5 per cent of children, typically between the ages of 6 months and 3 years. Simple febrile seizures are generalized and last less than 15 min. Complex febrile seizures either have focal features, are longer lasting, or recur within a 24-h period. About two-thirds of children with a febrile seizure do not have a recurrence. Febrile seizures do not have an adverse effect on development but a proportion of children develop epilepsy at a later age. Inheritance of febrile seizures is considered to be as an autosomal dominant trait.

Migration disorders

Alterations of the migration processes that establish the cellular and laminar organization of the neocortex are now considered to underlie a number of cases of epilepsy, particularly those arising in childhood. The migration disorders may be generalized (such as agyria), hemispheric (hemimegalencephaly), or focal (such as cortical dysplasia). Several forms of the migration disorders are genetically determined, and linked to mutations on the X chromosome. Some of these migration disorders are detectable by high-resolution MRI. The epilepsies produced can be either focal or generalized, and typically are difficult to control.

Trauma

Approximately 70 per cent of those individuals who eventually develop post-traumatic epilepsy will have their first seizure within 2 years of the original injury. Risk factors that predict post-traumatic epilepsy include early seizures (those occurring in the first week), a depressed skull fracture, or evidence of intracranial haemorrhage. There is no justification for the use of prophylactic anticonvulsants in the hope of preventing the development of post-traumatic seizures.

Tumour

Though adult-onset epilepsy is often equated with the presence of tumour, the cause in later life of symptomatic epilepsy is more likely to be cerebrovascular or Alzheimer's disease. The likelihood of a tumour producing seizures increases as the tumour is sited more anteriorly in the hemisphere, so that over 50 per cent of patients with frontal lobe tumours have epilepsy. Adult-onset status, in someone without a history of epilepsy, is particularly suggestive of frontal lobe tumour. Epilepsy is more common with slow-growing tumours and may be generalized or focal in nature.

Cerebrovascular disease

The prevalence of epilepsy after stroke has been reported to lie between 6 and 15 per cent, and appears as likely with cerebral infarction as with cerebral haemorrhage.

Infection

In large-scale surveys, infection has been considered the cause of epilepsy in 3 to 5 per cent of cases. Differences in rate between countries are often attributed to the variable prevalence of certain agents, for example cysticercosis. Other tropical infections which have been considered potential contributors to epilepsy prevalence include malaria, schistosomiasis, and trypanosomiasis. Epilepsy is a recognized feature of bacterial, tuberculous, and fungal meningitis, and of viral encephalitis. Epilepsy is often the first symptom of a tuberculoma.

Cerebral degeneration

Epilepsy is more common in patients with Alzheimer's disease or multi-infarct dementia compared with age-matched controls.

Multiple sclerosis

The prevalence of epilepsy in multiple sclerosis is probably of the order of 2 per cent. Both generalized and focal seizures have been attributed to multiple sclerosis. Rarely, status epilepticus and epilepsia partialis continua have been recorded.

Alcohol

Alcohol lowers seizure threshold. Seizures may occur during binge drinking, or during a period of withdrawal after alcohol excess.

Metabolic disorders

Seizures may occur in association with hypocalcaemia, hypercalcaemia, hypomagnesaemia, hypoglycaemia, hyponatraemia, and hypernatraemia. Severe renal and hepatic failure can both precipitate seizures.

Certain drugs are considered to lower the seizure threshold and are relatively contraindicated in patients with epilepsy. The drugs in question include the tricyclic antidepressants, the phenothiazines, and isoniazid. Rapid withdrawal of barbiturates or benzodiazepines can trigger seizures in those without a history of epilepsy.

Precipitants of epilepsy

Recognized precipitants of epilepsy include inadequate sleep, alcohol abuse, and ingestion of certain drugs. In catamenial epilepsy the attacks are confined to the menstrual period. Seizures confined to sleep are well recognized and indeed sleep electroencephalography recordings are characteristically more likely to register abnormal discharges than recordings made in the alert individual. In reflex epilepsy attacks are virtually inevitably triggered by a particular stimulus. Precipitants include photic stimulation, startle, noise, and movement. Rarer forms of reflex epilepsy have been linked to musical passages, eating, and performance of certain mental tasks.

Differential diagnosis

Syncope

Most individuals who faint experience a characteristic set of symptoms prior to loss of consciousness. These include mental slowing, fading of vision, altered hearing, malaise, and sweating. The process is the result, in varying combination, of bradycardia and profound arterial vasodilatation in skeletal muscle. Unless the individual lies down, loss of consciousness occurs and the patient falls to the ground. Characteristically the fall is gentle, and self-injury relatively uncommon. In falls associated with tonic–clonic or atonic seizures, the fall is precipitate and injury much more likely. Rarely, in complicated faints, there may be brief clonic jerks of the limbs. More commonly, multifocal myoclonus is observed, lasting a few seconds and following the loss of posture. The eyes tend to remain open. Lateral head turns, repetitive movements (such as lip licking), and hallucinations are all recognized features. After the episode there may be brief confusion and feelings of weakness, but these rapidly resolve. If, on the other hand, the upright posture is maintained (typically the individual is a soldier on parade) then stiffness of the limbs or repetitive generalized shaking occurs which is virtually indistinguishable from the movements occurring with epilepsy. Usually, however, a true tonic–clonic sequence does not occur in these circumstances.

Micturition syncope

Micturition syncope occurs predominantly in males, but of any age group. The attacks are almost always nocturnal, typically after an evening of alcohol consumption. Onset is usually during or shortly after micturition. The warning symptoms are often brief. The attacks seldom occur frequently; if they do, then the individual, if male, is advised to micturate in the sitting position.

Cough syncope

Patients with cough syncope effectively perform a Valsalva manoeuvre during a bout of prolonged coughing. Treatment is directed at the underlying chest condition.

Cardiac syncope

A variety of cardiac abnormalities, all having in common the end result of failing output and reduced cerebral perfusion, are associated with syncopal attacks. Mechanisms include complete heart block, paroxysmal ventricular tachycardia or fibrillation, and supraventricular tachycardia or bradyarrhythmia. In addition to disorders of rhythm, abnormalities of ventricular contractility or obstruction of outflow can have a similar outcome, usually when increased output is required during a period of exertion. Rarely, pedunculated masses within the heart, for example an atrial myxoma, cause outflow obstruction when the patient assumes certain postures. Features suggesting that a cardiac lesion may be responsible for a syncopal attack include a history of cardiac disease, palpitations or chest pain in association with the attack, and the finding of cardiac abnormalities on clinical examination.

Separate from these mechanisms are cases of syncope associated with postural hypotension. Autonomic failure resulting in postural hypotension is a feature of: multisystem atrophy; certain neuropathies with autonomic fibre involvement, such as diabetes; and drug therapy, for example with phenothiazines and tricyclic antidepressants. The correct diagnosis is usually readily established from the history.

Carotid sinus syncope

Patients with this condition usually present either with vertigo or with syncopal attacks. The syncopal attacks are sometimes followed by flushing and may be triggered by pressure over the neck, for example during neck rotation. In most patients, the syncope is related to atrioventricular block or asystole. Occasionally, a pure vasodilator reaction occurs, with peripheral pooling of blood.

Transient ischaemic attacks

These attacks should seldom be confused with epilepsy. In some patients with carotid occlusion (or severe stenosis), attacks of limb shaking occur in which involuntary limb movements described as shaking, trembling, or twitching occur, usually for seconds. The movements, which are coarse and irregular, predominate distally. Sometimes the attacks coincide with limb weakness or speech difficulty. The attacks are not influenced by anticonvulsants but can be relieved by endarterectomy where there is an underlying carotid stenosis.

Migraine

Loss of consciousness is a recognized feature of basilar migraine. The condition presents in children or adolescents. The headache is occipital. Visual disturbances are common, along with altered sensations (typically bilateral), ataxia, and dysarthria. Typically the patient, if unconscious, can be roused. Rarely, tonic–clonic seizures are seen with the attacks.

Hyperventilation

Most patients with the hyperventilation syndrome do not develop carpopedal spasm or tetany. Rather, they have a constellation of symptoms which are liable to be confused with other conditions such as epilepsy. Those symptoms include dizziness or vertigo, weakness, paraesthesiase, chest pain, and altered consciousness. Probably some 5 to 15 per cent of patients lose consciousness during hyperventilation, but never with a tonic–clonic progression that would cause real diagnostic difficulty.

Narcolepsy and cataplexy

Narcolepsy is defined as excessive daytime sleepiness, often occurring under unusual circumstances. The onset of sleep is usually preceded by a feeling of tension, tiredness, or a noise in the head. In some patients, onset occurs without warning. At times, patients have periods of semi-automatic behaviour for which they may subsequently be amnesic.

Cataplexy is typically triggered by sudden arousal. Attacks are brief, and may lead to such loss of muscle control that the patient falls. During the attack, the patient is flaccid, the eyes may roll or diverge, and the facial muscles flicker. Despite this, the patient usually remains fully alert.

Drop attacks

Drop attacks are almost confined to women in the last third of life. Typically, while walking, the patient drops to their knees without warning. The patient is aware of the fall, and is usually able to get up quickly, providing there is no injury. The attacks occur in otherwise fit individuals, are not due to vertebrobasilar ischaemia, and eventually remit completely. They are untreatable.

The parasomnias

Parasomnias are largley confined to children. They consist either of abnormal motor activity or excessive autonomic activity. Motor activity includes sleep starts, sleep myoclonus, bruxism, and head banging. Sleep myoclonus produces repetitive leg contraction, typically dorsiflexion of the feet. It increases with age and is usually idiopathic. Head banging, which may coincide with body rocking, is usually only seen in children or infants. The movements, typically occurring in clusters, are often accompanied by various forms of vocalization. In most cases, the child is normal. Sleep terrors usually happen within the first hour or two of sleep, occur in children, and result in a sudden cry followed by anxiety, tachycardia, sweating, and hyperkinesis. The child is not completely aware of the episodes, which sometimes necessitate short-term treatment with benzodiazepines.

Non-epileptic seizures

Non-epileptic seizures sometimes occur in isolation, but sometimes in those with true epilepsy. They account for 20 per cent of the patients referred to specialist epilepsy units, usually with a diagnosis of intractable epilepsy. The vast majority of sufferers are women. They are more likely to have a family history of psychiatric disorders, a past personal history of psychiatric disorder, a history of suicide attempt(s), evidence of sexual maladjustment, and current depressive symptoms. Indeed there is a substantial overlap, in terms of clinical characteristics, between non-epileptic seizures and multiple personality disorder. In addition to the features noted above, up to 90 per cent of patients give a history of sustained trauma, including childhood abuse, which may have been physical or sexual.

Certain features from the history should alert the physician. The attacks usually take place with witnesses present. They develop gradually rather than suddenly and the movements displayed are often unpredictable and bizarre. Attempt to constrain the patient are resisted. Vocalization is common. Incontinence is uncommon and tongue biting particularly so, but self-injury is a recognized feature. Typically the seizures are difficult to control. Serum prolactin levels taken 20 min after the event are normal, in contrast to tonic–clonic seizures where they are commonly, though not inevitably, elevated. Videotelemetry has proved of considerable value in differentiating epileptic from non-epileptic seizures. Management is extremely difficult. Drug withdrawal is resisted by the patient, who often resents suggestions of psychiatric referral and exploration of psychological morbidity.

Investigation

Investigation of a patient with suspected epilepsy (or a single seizure) is performed for three main reasons. The investigation may provide valuable support for the diagnosis, may give an indication as to which part of the brain has initiated the seizure, and finally, imaging may allow a statement as to the underlying structural process, where such exists.

Routine haematological and biochemical tests should be undertaken in all patients with suspected epilepsy although they seldom point to a metabolic disturbance that has not already been recognized.

Electroencephalography

Certain facts about the electroencephalogram must be understood before interpretation is attempted. Epileptiform discharges are encountered in between 0.5 and 4 per cent of individuals who have never had a seizure and who do not do so during a period of follow-up. Furthermore, a routine electroencephalogram in adults with established epilepsy shows epileptiform abnormalities in only some 40 to 50 per cent of cases. With repeat recording, with or without sleep records, the figure rises to 70 or 80 per cent. In other words, some patients with unequivocal epilepsy will have persistently normal or, at least, non-epileptic electroencephalograms. Serial electroencephalographic recording is sometimes helpful in an attempt to define the origin of the seizure and to delineate the seizure type better. If photosensitivity is suspected (10 per cent of individuals with seizures occurring between 1 and 7 years are photosensitive), serial recordings are appropriate, as they are in any individual with atypical status, or in whom cognitive impairment might be due to subclinical epileptic activity. Where surgical intervention is being planned for the epilepsy, routine and sleep recordings are followed by videotelemetry in order to record individual attacks. For some patients, depth electrodes will be needed to establish the seizure source. Magnetoencephalography localizes focal epileptic discharges by measuring the changes in extracranial magnetic fields which these discharges generate. The system costs some 25 times as much as a conventional electroencephalographic system. Depth electrodes are positioned stereotactically at sites determined by clinical and surface electroencephalographic criteria. Depth recordings are more accurate and sensitive in detecting focal discharges than either nasopharyngeal or sphenoidal electrodes.

The electroencephalogram has also been used to attempt prediction of seizure recurrence in individuals after a single seizure of unknown cause. Epileptic discharges, in one series, predicted a seizure recurrence over 2 years of 83 per cent, compared with a 12 per cent rate in individuals with a normal recording. The electroencephalogram has also been used to predict seizure recurrence during or after drug withdrawal in someone whose epilepsy has gone into remission on medication. The predictive value of electroencephalographic abnormalities in such cases has varied widely from series to series.

CT scanning

Neuroimaging is carried out in order to define whether a structural abnormality underlies the patient's epilepsy and, if so, whether some additional treatment, other than anticonvulsants, might be required. CT scanning was originally the most often used imaging process, prior to the more widespread availability of MRI. Some authors advocate MRI in all patients with epilepsy, other than for those epilepsies which are clearly idiopathic (such as absence seizures, juvenile myoclonic epilepsy, and benign rolandic epilepsy). In practice, this is probably unreasonable. For example, a patient with the onset of epilepsy in their 70s or 80s, who has a normal CT (at least, with no evidence of focal pathology) hardly merits MRI if the epilepsy is well controlled.

MRI

MRI is undoubtedly both more sensitive and more specific than CT in detecting small brain lesions and abnormalities of the cerebral cortex thought to be relevant in the genesis of epilepsy (Fig. 3). The most common abnormalities detected are hippocampal sclerosis, malformations of cortical development, vascular malformations, tumours, and acquired cortical damage. MRI is particularly indicated for partial seizures, onset of generalized or unclassified seizures in adult life, patients with fixed focal clinical or neuropsychological deficit, and for those patients with poor seizure control. Quantitative measures of the hippocampi improve the diagnostic sensitivity of MRI for hippocampal sclerosis. MRI is much more sensitive than CT for detecting malformations of cortical development. Magnetic resonance spectroscopy, examining nuclei ^{31}P and ^{1}H, has been used for assessment of patients with complex partial seizures for possible surgery.

Single photon emission computed tomography (SPECT)

This technique allows measurement of cerebral blood flow and of specific brain receptors. Both ictal and interictal studies have been performed. Ictal SPECT can achieve a correct localization of over 90 per cent in unilateral temporal lobe epilepsy.

Positron emission tomography (PET)

PET scanning is used to measure cerebral blood flow, regional cerebral glucose metabolism, and the distribution of specific receptors, such as the benzodiazepine–$GABA_A$ receptor complex (Fig. 4 and Plate 1). The spatial resolution achieved is superior to SPECT. Epileptic foci, studied interictally, display reduced blood flow and reduced glucose metabolism. Typically, the abnormalities found are more extensive than the corresponding pathological lesion. Increasingly it appears likely that MRI and functional MRI will largely replace this technique in patient evaluation.

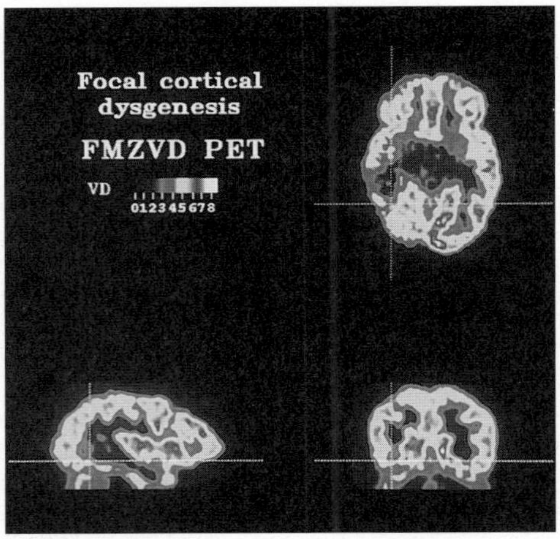

Fig. 4 FMZVD PET scan showing a region of probable cortical dysplasia in the right temporal lobe. The 11C-fluamzenil volume of distribution (FMZVD) is an index of $GABA_A$ receptor density. (See also Plate 1.)

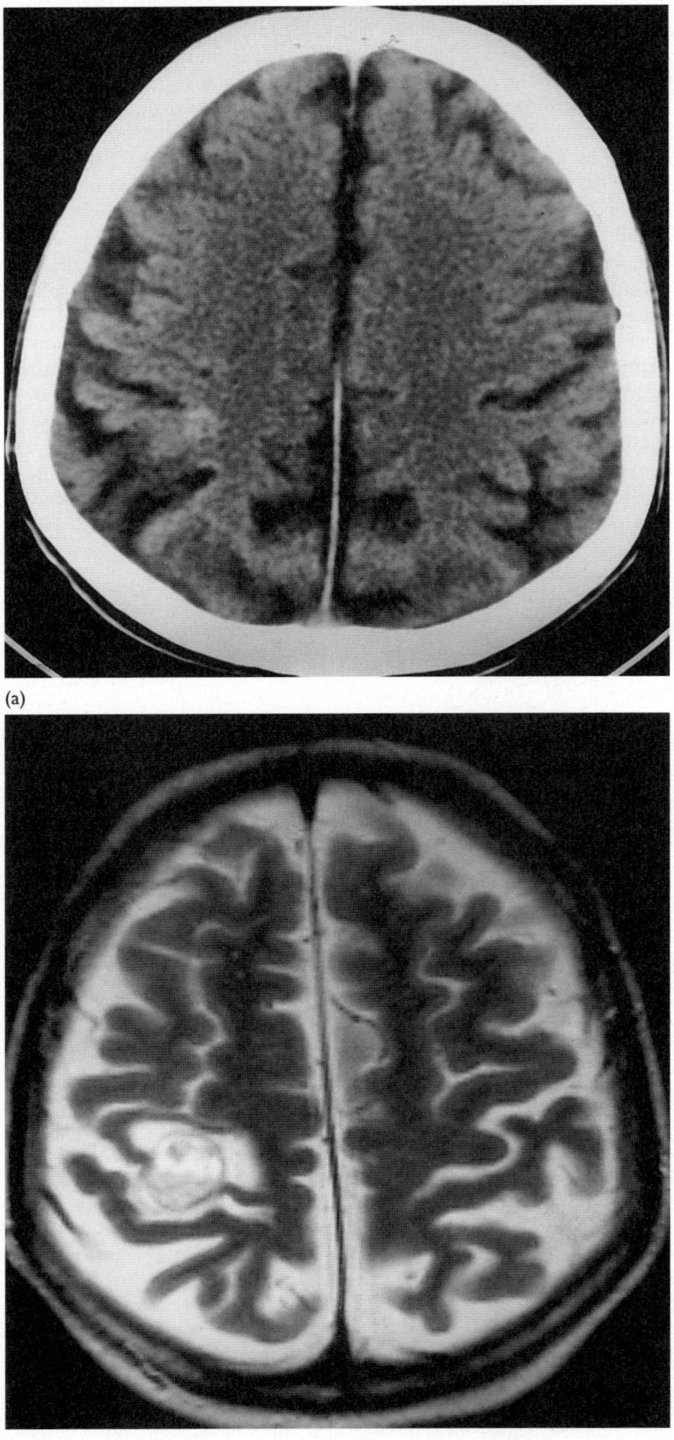

(a)

(b)

Fig. 3 CT scan (a) and MRI scan (b). The readily visible cavernome on MRI is only just visible on CT.

Treatment—drug therapy

Choice of drug therapy

A number of principles can be stated in relation to drug therapy.

Does the patient require anticonvulsants?

The issue of whether isolated seizures should be treated remains unresolved. Seizure recurrence rate after a single seizure reaches 80 per cent in untreated individuals, the vast majority recurring within 2 years of onset. Many patients prefer to defer treatment after a single seizure, a decision substantially influenced by how soon they wish to start driving. For a patient who has very infrequent seizures, say 5 or more years apart, it may seem logical to withhold medication.

Choice of anticonvulsant

An algorithm can provide some guidelines regarding drug treatment (Fig. 5). For generalized seizures (tonic–clonic, absence, or myoclonic) sodium valproate is the drug of choice. Further choices are determined by seizure type. There is no controlled trial data indicating the most appropriate add-on drug or combination of drugs. Myoclonus can be exacerbated by carbamazepine, gabapentin, and lamotrigine and absences by carbamazepine and gabapentin. For partial seizures, with or without generalization, carbamazepine and valproate are probably the drugs of choice, though controlled studies have indicated that phenobarbitone and phenytoin are of comparable value.

In addition, choice of drug will be influenced by the patient's age, sex (regarding the use of oral contraceptives and likelihood of pregnancy), and reliability of adherence to a particular drug regime. The patient should always be started on a single drug.

Dosage

Although standard dose regimes tend to be quoted, many anticonvulsants are sometimes effective in relatively low doses. Accordingly the drug is introduced in low dosage and is then gradually increased according to need and tolerance. Sometimes only dosages that lead to toxic serum levels appear effective. Some patients tolerate such toxic levels without difficulty.

Failure of first drug

When this occurs, a second drug should be gradually introduced without withdrawing the first. If the patient responds, the drug used originally can be slowly withdrawn.

Drug combinations

If drugs given individually have failed then drug combinations should be considered, remembering that they may interact with each other.

Generic prescribing

The bioavailability of the anticonvulsant drugs should be unaffected by whether they are prescribed generically, or as a specific branded product. Patients sometimes disbelieve this assumption and prefer branded products. If they are given generic prescriptions, they should be warned that the appearance of their medication may change from prescription to prescription.

The problem of non-compliance

Non-compliance is a significant problem with the anticonvulsants and is a potent cause of poor control. A full explanation of each drug's side-effect profile and its potential interactions is essential and appears conducive to improved compliance. Drugs that are given once or twice a day are preferred to ones needing more frequent prescriptions. Slow-release preparations allow drug regimes to be simplified.

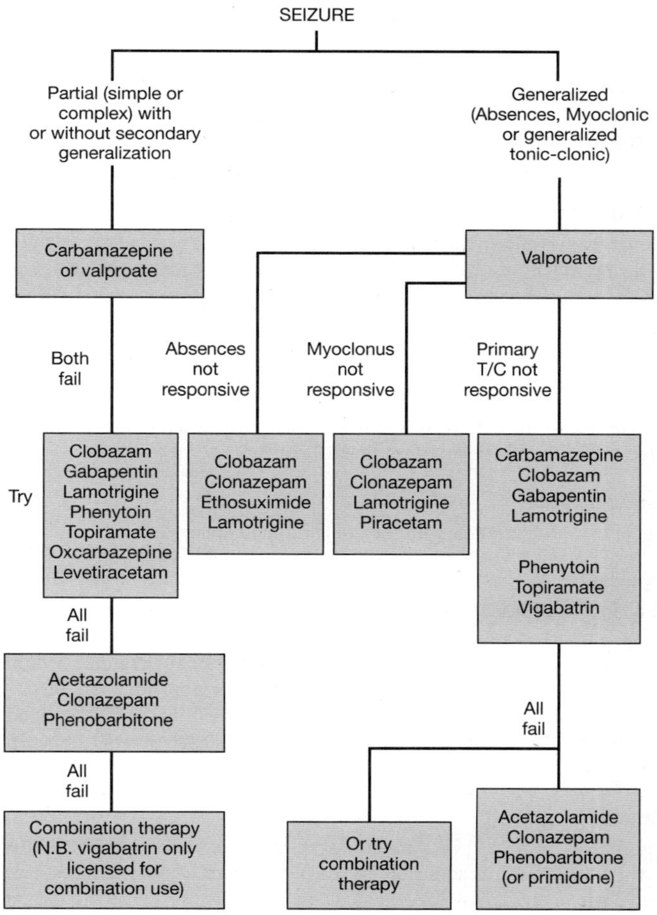

Fig. 5 Choice of anticonvulsant.

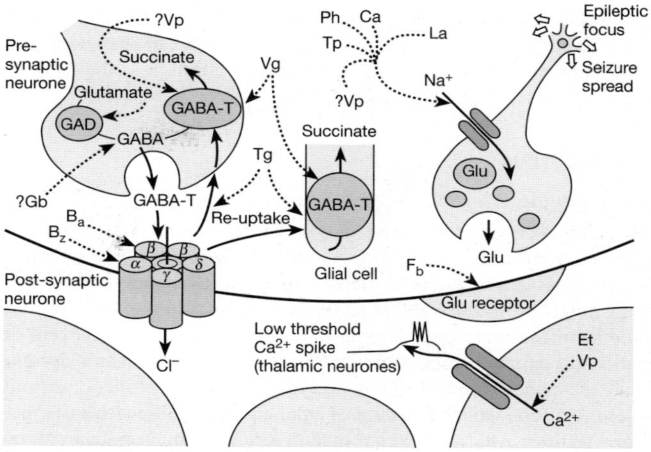

Fig. 6 Mechanism of action of some of the anticonvulsants. Ba, barbiturate; Bz, benzodiazepine; Ca, carbamazepine; Et, ethosuximide; Fb, felbamate; Gb, gabapentin; La, lamotrigine; Ph, phenytoin; Tg, tiagabine; Tp, topiramate; Vp, valproate; Vg, vigabatrin.

Mechanisms of action (Fig. 6)

The prime role of GABA-mediated inhibition in the epileptic process implies that drugs which enhance $GABA_A$-receptor-mediated inhibition will have anticonvulsant activity. The $GABA_A$-receptor complex comprises at least three subunits, α, β, and δ, which appear to combine as a five-membered structure forming an anion-permeable channel. Both barbiturates and benzodiazepines act by potentiating $GABA_A$-mediated inhibition. The barbiturates bind to the β-subunit to potentiate action of endogenous agonist GABA and prolong the opening time of the chloride ion channel. Benzodiazepines bind to the α-subunit to potentiate the action of GABA and increase the frequency of opening of the chloride ion channel. GABA is metabolized by GABA transaminase. Vigabatrin irreversibly binds to GABA transaminase to inhibit degradation of GABA and thereby elevate brain GABA levels. GABA-mediated inhibition can also be enhanced by blocking GABA uptake into glia and neurones after its release into the synaptic cleft during synaptic transmission.

Tiagabine blocks uptake of synaptically released GABA into both presynaptic neurones and glial cells, allowing GABA to remain at its site of action for longer periods. Gabapentin acts presynaptically to promote GABA synthesis or release.

The second major neurotransmitter system involved in the genesis of epileptic activity is excitatory utilizing glutamate and, perhaps, aspartate as neurotransmitters. They act on several different receptors including α-amino-3-hydroxy-5-methylisoxazole-proprionic acid (AMPA) and N-methyl-D-aspartate (**NMDA**). The NMDA receptor is activated by glutamate or aspartate in conjunction with glycine. Blockade of the NMDA receptor results in antiepileptic effects.

Voltage-dependent calcium ion currents are thought to be of importance in the genesis of epileptic events. Ethosuximide acts by inhibition of one class of voltage-dependent calcium ion currents (T currents). Valproate may have a similar role.

Regulation of sodium channels also appears of relevance in the modification of the epileptic process. Phenytoin, carbamazepine, and possibly valproate reduce the rate of recovery from inactivation of depolarized voltage-dependent sodium channels, thereby blocking sustained repetitive firing of action potentials in depolarized neurones. Lamotrigine inhibits glutamate and aspartate release, suggesting it may act at voltage-dependent sodium channels to decrease the presynaptic release of glutamate. Lamotrigine may have additional effects on calcium channels. Oxcarbazepine may act by reducing glutamate release via a blocking action on presynaptic calcium channels. Topiramate influences sodium channel activity, suggesting that its anticonvulsant properties are similar to those of phenytoin. Felbamate probably acts primarily through its effects on the NMDA receptor.

Selected drugs

Carbamazepine

Carbamazepine is a first-line drug for both partial seizures and for generalized tonic–clonic seizures. In its standard form, it needs to be given three times per day, but a slow-release preparation allows twice daily prescribing. Dosage ranges from 300 to 1600 mg/day. Sedation is common and the drug should be introduced slowly. A drug rash occurs in perhaps 3 per cent of patients and demands immediate drug withdrawal. Signs of intoxication include drowsiness, blurred vision, and dizziness. Leucopenia occurs and can lead to a frank aplastic anaemia. Hyponatraemia and oedema are recognized features, associated with a mild degree of inappropriate antidiuretic hormone production. The drug influences atrioventricular conduction and should not be given to patients with atrioventricular conduction abnormalities unless they are already paced. The relationship between dosage and plasma concentrations is linear. Carbamazepine is a liver-enzyme inducer and is teratogenic (see below).

Sodium valproate

Sodium valproate is considered, at least by some physicians, to be the drug of choice for all epilepsy types. It is not enzyme-inducing, and therefore does not influence the metabolism of the oral contraceptive. Liver toxicity is a recognized, though rare, hazard. Elevated liver enzyme levels are more common, but usually return to normal without need for drug withdrawal. Thrombocytopenia occurs rarely. Gastrointestinal effects are fairly common. Nausea and weight loss are seen, but appetite stimulation with weight gain is more common. Tremor occurs, as a dose-related effect. Hair loss, of a mild degree, is not uncommon. After a few months, hair regrowth occurs, often more curly than before. Sedation is less troublesome than with other anticonvulsants. Disturbances of menstruation are recognized. It has been suggested that the drug can trigger polycystic ovarian disease. The dose ranges from 600 to 2500 mg/day and it is given twice or three times per day. A slow-release preparation can be given once daily. Plasma levels are not a useful guide to efficacy.

Other drugs

Phenytoin

Experience with phenytoin is vast and despite its side-effect profile and complex pharmacokinetics, large quantities of the drug continue to be prescribed. A 100 mg tablet, in the United Kingdom, costs approximately one-thirtieth of the price of a comparable dose of lamotrigine. The drug is effective in both generalized tonic–clonic seizures and in the partial seizures. It has a long half-life, and can be given once daily, conveniently at bed time. Sedation is common. Toxic effects, generally dose related, include drowsiness, ataxia, confusion, blurred vision, and dizziness. Most patients who are intoxicated with the drug have nystagmus. Permanent cerebellar ataxia and peripheral neuropathy are recorded. Other side-effects or toxic effects include rashes, gum hypertrophy, thickening of the facial features, chorea, and sleep disturbance. The drug is a potent enzyme-inducer and is teratogenic. The relationship between dosage and plasma concentrations is non-linear. Once the dose exceeds 300 mg/day, increments should be pegged to 50 mg or even 25 mg at a time.

Lamotrigine

Lamotrigine is licensed for both generalized and partial seizures. Occasionally it exacerbates myoclonus. Doses seldom exceed 400 mg/day. A drug rash occurs in about 3 per cent of patients. It interacts with enzyme-inducing anticonvulsants, which lower its plasma level. Valproate enhances lamotrigine levels. The drug can be given once daily. It is said not to be teratogenic.

Phenobarbitone

Phenobarbitone is a very effective anticonvulsant but often badly tolerated. Children may become hyperactive on the drug, adults (and particularly the elderly) heavily sedated. Doses of up to 180 mg/day are used. It has a long half-life and can be given once daily. Rapid withdrawal of phenobarbitone in non-epileptic patients can trigger seizures. Over-rapid withdrawal in someone with epilepsy can trigger status epilepticus. Methyl phenobarbitone is largely converted to phenobarbitone by the liver and phenobarbitone is the main metabolite of primidone, although primidone's other metabolite phenylethylmalonamide probably possesses anticonvulsant activity.

Vigabatrin

Vigabatrin is probably a more potent anticonvulsant than many of the other recently introduced drugs. Increasingly, it has been recognized to cause retinal damage. Up to a third of patients develop concentric constriction of the visual fields, more marked nasally than temporally. The defect is often asymptomatic and probably irreversible. It is now recommended that vigabatrin should only be used as add-on therapy where other combinations have been unsuccessful. Dosage should not exceed 3 g/day. Regular visual field analysis is mandatory.

Gabapentin

Gabapentin is used as add-on therapy for partial seizures with or without secondary generalization. Up to 4.8 g is given in three divided doses. The drug is generally well-tolerated and does not interact with other anticonvulsants. Its anticonvulsant effect appears to be relatively weak.

Ethosuximide

Ethosuximide is seldom used in adults as its role is confined to the treatment of absence seizures. Gastrointestinal disturbances are common along with drowsiness, dizziness, and ataxia. Agranulocytosis or aplastic anaemia have been encountered rarely. The dose range is usually 1 to 1.5 g daily.

Clonazepam

Clonazepam is effective for tonic–clonic seizures but is particularly valuable in the treatment of myoclonic epilepsy. Sedation is a major problem, and the drug must be introduced cautiously. The maximum tolerated dose is about 8 mg/day.

Clobazam

Tolerance to clobazam tends to develop fairly readily. It is sedative. Adult dosage ranges from 30 to 60 mg daily. Used intermittently it can be very effective for the treatment of catamenial epilepsy.

Acetazolamide

Use of this drug is largely confined to childhood epilepsies.

Topiramate

This drug is licensed both for primary generalized tonic–clonic seizures, and as adjunct therapy for partial seizures. It is sedative and must be introduced slowly. The total daily dose (given as a twice daily regime) seldom exceeds 400 mg. Nausea, anorexia, and weight loss are encountered. Behavioural disturbances are reported, including emotional lability, mood change, and aggression. There is an increased incidence of renal stones in those taking the drug.

Tiagabine

Tiagabine is a GABA uptake inhibitor resulting in increased synaptic GABA levels. Initial doses in adults are 4 to 5 mg twice daily. Most studies have used 32 to 56 mg/day, in three divided doses. The drug is licensed as add-on therapy in refractory epilepsy. Side-effects include dizziness, tiredness, tremor, and altered mood.

Oxcarbazepine

This drug is closely related to carbamazepine. It is a less potent hepatic enzyme inducer however. It is licensed as monotherapy or adjunctive therapy, in partial seizures with or without secondary generalization. Its side-effect profile is similar to that of carbamazepine. Patients who are hypersensitive to carbamazepine should not receive oxcarbazepine. The dosage range lies between 600 and 2400 mg daily, in adults.

Levetiracetam

The mode of action of levetiracetam is not understood. It is not metabolized in the liver nor does it inhibit or induce hepatic enzymes. There are no known interactions with the other anticonvulsants. Two-thirds of an oral dose is excreted unchanged in the urine. A quarter is metabolized to an inactive metabolite, also excreted in the urine.

Levetiracetam is licensed as adjunctive therapy in the treatment of partial seizures with or without secondary generalization. The daily dose in adults ranges from 1000 to 3000 mg. The dose needs to be adjusted in the presence of renal impairment. It is not advised for use in pregnancy.

Side-effects include asthenia, somnolence, headache, gastrointestinal disturbances, mood changes, and skin rash.

Other drugs, with very restricted licences, or not yet licensed, include felbamate and zonizimade.

Table 2 Anticonvulsants, dosage range, and serum levels (where appropriate)

Anticonvulsant	Typical adult dose range (mg/24 h)	Therapeutic serum levels (μmol/l)
Sodium valproate	800–2500	
Phenytoin	150–350	40–80
Carbamazepine	600–1600	17–42
Phenobarbitone	60–180	65–170
Lamotrigine	200–400	
Gabapentin	900–3600	
Vigabatrin	1000–3000	
Topiramate	200–400	
Tiagabine	30–45	
Ethosuximide	1000–1500	285–700
Clonazepam	2–8	
Clobazam	30–60	
Oxcarbazepine	600–2400	
Levetiracetam	1000–3000	

Particular issues

Enzyme-induction

Drugs that induce liver enzymes (phenytoin, phenobarbitone, carbamazepine, topiramate, and possibly lamotrigine) will alter the pharmacokinetics of other agents or drugs which undergo hepatic metabolism. Women on an oral contraceptive pill need to take a preparation containing at least 50 μg of ethinyloestradiol. If breakthrough bleeding still occurs, the dose of oestrogen can be increased to a maximum of 100 μg daily. Alternatively, an injectable long-term contraceptive can be used. The interactions between anticonvulsants are complex, another reason for avoiding drug combinations where possible.

All the enzyme-inducing anticonvulsants have the potential for accelerating vitamin D metabolism. Those individuals at risk for developing vitamin D deficiency (for example due to poor nutrition) are at risk of developing osteomalacia or rickets when taking certain anticonvulsants.

Drug monitoring

Anticonvulsant levels are measured far too frequently. There are specific circumstances where their measurement is of value:

(1) to ascertain compliance;

(2) to monitor dosage adjustment with phenytoin; and

(3) to ascertain the unpredictable effect of combining anticonvulsant preparations.

Phenytoin undergoes saturable hepatic metabolism. Regular monitoring of the serum level is advisable, particularly after dose adjustment. Occasionally, measurement of the levels of carbamazepine, phenobarbitone, and ethosuximide aids management, particularly where epilepsy control has been poor. Carbamazepine epoxide, a metabolite of carbamazepine, can sometimes be the cause of carbamazepine toxicity even when carbamazepine levels are in the therapeutic range. There is no value in the routine monitoring of levels of valproate, vigabatrin, lamotrigine, gabapentin, topiramate, clonazepam, or clobazam.

When measuring levels, the same time after the last dose should be used, wherever possible. Examples of therapeutic serum levels are given in Table 2. The therapeutic ranges of the anticonvulsants should be interpreted with caution. Some patients respond to a drug with subtherapeutic levels. Others need toxic levels to achieve seizure control and can often tolerate such levels without overt difficulty.

Pregnancy

There is an increased risk of congenital malformations in women who have taken anticonvulsants during pregnancy (approximately 4 to 8 per cent overall risk). Most evidence has accumulated for phenytoin, phenobarbitone, valproate, and carbamazepine. There are very few data on the newer anticonvulsants, though lamotrigine is said not to be teratogenic. The critical period for development of the major malformations is from 3 to 8 weeks' gestation.

Phenytoin and phenobarbitone

Both these drugs are associated with cardiovascular malformations (2 per cent risk) and cleft lip/palate syndromes (1.8 per cent risk).

Valproate

Valproate leads to a 2 per cent risk of spina bifida compared with a 0.01 to 0.02 per cent risk for all births. Cardiovascular and urogenital malformations are also recognized to occur.

Carbamazepine

Carbamazepine is associated with spina bifida (1 per cent risk) and hypospadias.

A folic acid supplement of 5 mg daily should be given to women with epilepsy who are taking valproate or carbamazepine and who are contemplating pregnancy. Doses of valproate should be less than 1000 mg/day if possible and slow-release forms of the drug prescribed. For women on other anticonvulsants, a dose of 0.4 mg/day of folic acid suffices.

Seizure frequency increases in pregnancy in about a third of patients with epilepsy. Tonic–clonic seizures are associated with an increased risk of miscarriage. Vitamin K at 20 mg/day should be given in the last month of pregnancy in women on enzyme-inducing drugs to reduce the risk of haemorrhagic disease of the newborn baby.

The epilepsy risk in the offspring of an affected patient is around 2 to 4 per cent but higher where the epilepsy of the parent has a strong genetic basis.

Breast feeding

All the commonly used anticonvulsants are present in low concentrations in breast milk. If the mother is on a barbiturate or a benzodiazepine, significant sedation of the baby is possible. If breast feeding then ceases abruptly, a withdrawal reaction can occur in the infant with tremor and agitation.

Drug withdrawal

Generally medication is continued until at least a 2- to 3-year period free of seizures has been established. Approximately two-thirds of patients remain fit free after drug withdrawal. Factors known to predispose towards recurrence include neurological abnormalities on examination, an underlying structural basis for the epilepsy, the need for multiple drug therapy, and a history of difficulty in establishing initial control. The electroencephalogram is of limited value in predicting outcome although rather better in children than adults. Any drug withdrawal should be gradual, say over 3 to 6 months. Absence seizures usually remit spontaneously in late adolescence, but juvenile myoclonic epilepsy tends to recur after drug withdrawal.

Driving

In the United Kingdom, driving must cease for 1 year after any type of seizure. If a nocturnal pattern of seizures has been established for 3 years, driving can then continue even if nocturnal seizures are still occurring. The Driver and Vehicle Licensing Agency prefers patients not to drive during a period of drug withdrawal, and for 6 months after the withdrawal has been completed. For drivers of heavy goods vehicles a 10-year period of freedom must be established, during which there has been no anticonvulsant use. Furthermore, a continuing liability to epilepsy has to be excluded.

Status epilepticus

Status epilepticus has already been defined. The commonest type is tonic–clonic status. The commonest precipitants are sudden anticonvulsant withdrawal, poor compliance in a patient with known epilepsy, and alcohol abuse. The mortality figures for status epilepticus have varied substantially from series to series. In one recently published, prospective, population-based study, the overall incidence was estimated at 41 to 61 per 100 000 person-years with a mortality of 22 per cent. Incidence rises in the elderly, as does mortality. From other series, overall mortality figures lie between 8 and 37 per cent. At least half the cases occur in the absence of previous epilepsy. Although non-compliance and subtherapeutic drug levels are often quoted as causes of status, several studies have established that the majority of individuals with epilepsy who present in status have therapeutic drug levels at or around the time of presentation. Status in the absence of previous epilepsy is followed by unprovoked seizures in about half the cases.

The diagnosis is by no means straightforward. In one study, half the patients transferred to a specialist centre for management of their status were either in pseudostatus or in drug-induced coma. The diagnosis of pseudostatus should be considered if the attacks are atypical or if the status does not respond to initial therapy.

Analysis of immediate management of patients in status suggests that many are given inadequate loading and maintenance doses of anticonvulsants. The patient should be moved away from possible hazard, such as broken glass, an airway established, and oxygen administered. Lorazepam is probably the drug of choice. It is given in a dose of 0.1 mg/kg intravenously at the rate of 2 mg/min. Alternatives included diazepam (Diazemuls) given intravenously in a dose of 10 to 20 mg at a rate of 5 mg/min or clonazepam given in a dose of 1 mg by slow intravenous injection.

Using the intravenous route, 50 per cent glucose should be administered to a total volume of 50 ml after blood has been taken to establish the glucose concentration. Thiamine in a dose of 250 mg (Pabrinex I/V High Potency) should be given by slow intravenous injection over 10 min if there is suspicion of alcohol withdrawal, but remembering that the infusion can produce an anaphylactic response. In addition to plasma glucose measurement, blood should be taken for urea, electrolytes (including calcium and magnesium), acid-base balance, liver function tests, and full blood count. A serum sample should be stored in case anticonvulsant or alcohol levels are required subsequently. Blood cultures should be performed if the patient is febrile.

If immediate therapy is successful and the patient is receiving phenytoin or valproate, those drugs can be given intravenously before reverting to oral therapy. If the patient is not on anticonvulsants, a phenytoin infusion at 20 mg/kg in 0.9 per cent sodium chloride should be given at a maximum rate of 50 mg/min. An alternative is Fos-Phenytoin, a water-soluble drug, which is metabolized to phenytoin with a half-life of 8 to 15 min. It is given intravenously in the same dose at 150 mg/min in order to achieve a comparable effect. The drug is more expensive than phenytoin but causes less phlebitis, less hypotension, and is better tolerated.

Midazolam has been developed for intranasal use and may prove of value where immediate intravenous access is difficult, for example in young children.

If phenytoin infusion is unsuccessful, valproate infusions can be used, with 25 mg/kg as a loading dose delivered at 3 to 6 mg/kg/min. If seizures continue phenobarbital can be considered, given at 20 mg/kg intravenously at 50 to 75 mg/min. Intramuscular or rectal paraldehyde is now seldom used, most experts suggesting a move instead to thiopentone, propofol, or midazolam.

Propofol or midazolam are rapidly metabolized and have less hypotensive effects than the barbiturates. The suggested dose of propofol is 1 to 2 mg/kg followed by a continuous infusion of 2 to 10 mg/kg/h.

For all the therapies used in patients with refractory status, intensive care placement is essential with the patient intubated and haemodynamic monitoring in place.

Sudden death

Patients with epilepsy have an increased risk of death compared with age- and sex-matched controls. Sudden unexpected death in epilepsy predominates in younger age groups and in those with more severe epilepsy. It is likely that most of the deaths are the result of unwitnessed seizures producing either respiratory complications, cardiac arrhythmias, or both.

Surgery

Despite optimal treatment, some 30 per cent of patients with new-onset seizures continue to have attacks. Prerequisite in patient selection for surgery is accurate localization of the epileptic discharge and understanding of circumstances where a resection might prove detrimental in terms of functional deficit.

Assessment for epilepsy surgery demands localization techniques incorporating seizure characteristics, electrophysiological recording, and imaging. Equally important is the recognition by the physician that certain epilepsy syndromes are likely to be resistant to medical therapy and that early rather than delayed referral for surgical opinion is beneficial. Mesial temporal lobe epilepsy, secondary to hippocampal sclerosis, is the commonest cause of medically refractory partial seizures. In most such patients, a unilateral structural abnormality can be confidently established, resection of which leads to a 70 per cent chance of remission. Disabling neurological complications after surgery, such as hemianopia, hemiparesis, or dysphasia, occur in about 2 per cent of patients. Depression and psychosis are recognized complications of temporal lobectomy.

MRI characteristics of mesial temporal sclerosis include atrophy or increased signal on T_2-weighted images. The presence of atrophy is the best predictor for a good surgical outcome. Besides visual inspection, measurement of hippocampal volume and techniques for measuring the T_2 signal change are used to improve sensitivity.

SPECT and PET measure the changes in cerebral blood flow and cerebral glucose metabolism, respectively, which accompany the epileptic process. Both have relatively high sensitivity and moderate specificity for the diagnosis of temporal lobe seizures, but lower sensitivity for epilepsy arising at other sites. Interictal PET and ictal SPECT produce very similar results in predicting outcome after temporal lobectomy.

Proton magnetic resonance spectroscopy can contribute to recognition of the lateralization of the epileptic focus and to the identification of those patients with bilateral changes who are less likely to respond to surgery.

Continuous surface electroencephalographic monitoring is usually undertaken as part of the work-up for patients being considered for surgical intervention. The technique, however, has limitations. It often fails to detect seizure activity arising in areas distant from surface electrodes, such as the orbitofrontal cortex, and may falsely lateralize foci, particularly in the presence of large lesions. For improving electroencephalographic localization, some form of intracranial recording is necessary. Depth electrodes are used to sample deeper structures such as the hippocampus. Electrocorticography is performed at the time of surgery. Subdural electrodes, sometimes with depth electrodes, measure directly from the surface of the exposed brain.

Other less commonly performed surgical procedures include neocortical resections, lesionectomies, hemispherectomies, multilobar resections, and corpus callosotomy. Hemispherectomy is performed when a diffuse epileptogenic region has been localized within one hemisphere, the other hemisphere being normal. Division of the corpus callosum is performed in patients with severe secondary generalized epilepsy who have disabling drop attacks. Cortical dysplasia is increasingly recognized as a cause of intractable epilepsy. MRI criteria have been developed to allow recognition of areas of focal cortical dysplasia and assist in planning the extent of cortical resection.

Vagal nerve stimulation

Vagal nerve stimulation is achieved through the implantation of a small stimulator on the left vagus. The exact mechanism of action remains uncertain. The nucleus of the tractus solitarius, the main terminus for vagal afferents, has projections to the locus caeruleus, raphe nuclei, reticular formation, and other brainstem nuclei. These nuclei have been shown to influence cerebral seizure susceptibility. In patients with chronic partial seizures, there is reduction in the number of seizures, rather than their elimination. The long-term role of this procedure is not yet determined.

Psychiatric aspects of epilepsy

A substantial proportion of patients with poorly controlled epilepsy are likely to have psychiatric symptoms. Those symptoms may partly reflect the underlying structural process in the brain, the effects of repeated seizures, the effects of any social stigma attached to the diagnosis, and as a reaction to the patient's anticonvulsants. Psychiatric symptoms occurring around the time of the seizures tend to be affective or cognitive if before or with the seizure, but psychotic afterwards. Additional psychiatric morbidity is encountered as an interictal phenomenon. It correlates with multiple drug use, the serum concentrations of those drugs, and certain of the anticonvulsants including the newer agents, such as lamotrigine, vigabatrin, and topiramate.

Patients with poorly controlled epilepsy may require referral to a clinical psychologist, partly with a view to helping in the psychological adjustment to the condition, and partly to identify specific areas of cognitive impairment which might require attention.

The role of specialist nurses and the general practitioner

Patients almost inevitably indicate some dissatisfaction with the level of information and support that they receive for their epilepsy. Studies suggest that improvement in these areas can occur using a specialist nurse, working either in general practice or in association with a hospital clinic. Where joint care is to be achieved between general practice and hospital, it is vital that good quality communication and record keeping are achieved. Giving the patient files which document vital information, including their drug regime, is valuable. Patients prefer the continuity of care achievable through seeing the same doctor at each consultation and are more likely to adhere to medical advice under those circumstances.

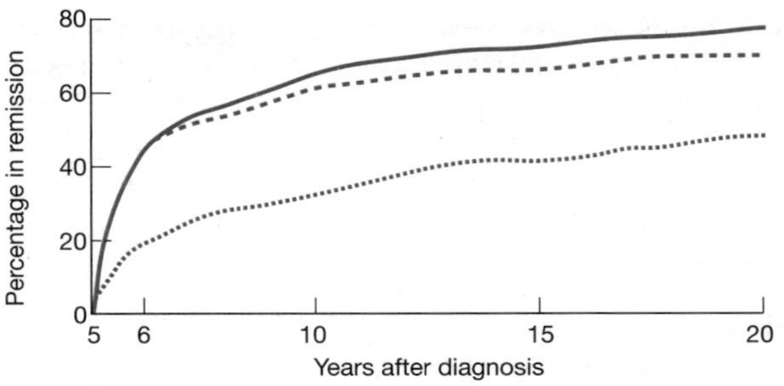

Fig. 7 Probability of seizure recurrence after a first epileptic seizure. (Data from the National General Practice Study of Epilepsy, reproduced by kind permission.)

Prognosis

Prognosis for patients with epilepsy followed in the community is considerably better than for a hospital-based population. Figure 7 records the percentage of patients in remission (defined as being seizure free for 5 years). The top curve indicates the percentage of patients achieving a 5-year period of remission at any time during the 20-year period of follow-up. The middle curve refers to those patients in remission for at least the last 5 years at the time of sampling. The difference between the top and middle curves represents those patients who have relapsed after achieving a 5-year remission. The bottom curve indicates the probability of being in remission whilst not taking anticonvulsants. The curves in Fig. 7 flatten off, indicating that remission becomes less likely the longer the seizures persist. Factors that influence outcome adversely include a combination of complex partial and tonic–clonic seizures, clustering of seizures, abnormal physical signs, and the presence of learning difficulties.

Overall care

For many patients, shared care between hospital, a specialist nurse, and general practice is ideal. Such an arrangement necessitates a reasonable level of epilepsy experience from the general practitioner, allowing many issues to be resolved without recourse to hospital consultation. The complexities of epilepsy care in terms of new drug developments, issues relating to pregnancy, the question of non-epileptic seizures, and the potential for surgery for many patients with poorly controlled epilepsy makes the case for epilepsy clinics manned by physicians with a particular interest in epilepsy.

Further reading

Arruda F *et al.* (1996). Mesial atrophy and outcome after amygdalohippocampectomy or temporal lobe removal. *Annals of Neurology* **40**, 446–50.

Berg AT, Shinnar S (1994). Relapse following discontinuation of anti-epileptic drugs: a meta-analysis. *Neurology* **44**, 601–8.

Berkovic SF, Scheffer IE (1997). Epilepsies with single gene inheritance. *Brain Development* **19**, 13–18.

Bowman ES (1993). Etiology and clinical course of pseudoseizures. Relationship to trauma, depression and dissociation. *Psychosomatics* **34**, 333–42.

Crawford P *et al.* (1999). Best practice guidelines for the management of women with epilepsy. *Seizure* **8**, 201–17.

Dichter MA (1994). Emerging insights into mechanisms of epilepsy: implications for new antiepileptic drug development. *Epilepsia* **35**(Suppl 4), S51–S57.

Duncan JS (1997). Imaging and epilepsy. *Brain* **120**, 339–77. [An excellent review article, covering all aspects of imaging, including MRI, magnetic resonance spectroscopy, single photon emission computed tomography, and positron emission tomography.]

Goldstein LH (1990). Behavioural and cognitive-behavioural treatment for epilepsy: a progress review. *British Journal of Clinical Psychology* **29**, 257–69.

Handforth A *et al.* (1998). Vagus nerve stimulation therapy for partial-onset seizures. A randomised active-control trial. *Neurology* **51**, 48–55.

Lempert T, Bauer M, Schmidt D (1994). Syncope: a videometric analysis of 56 episodes of transient cerebral hypoxia. *Annals of Neurology* **36**, 233–7.

Manford M *et al.* (1992). The national general practice study of epilepsy applied to epilepsy in a general population. *Archives of Neurology* **49**, 801–8.

Mattson RH *et al.* (1985). Comparison of carbamazepine, phenobarbital, phenytoin, and primidone in partial and secondarily generalized tonic–clonic seizures. *New England Journal of Medicine* **313**, 145–51.

Nashef L, Brown SW, eds (1997). Epilepsy and sudden death. Proceedings of an international workshop. *Epilepsia* **38**(Suppl 11), S1–S76.

Raymond AA *et al.* (1995). Abnormalities of gyration, heterotopias, tuberous sclerosis, focal cortical dysplasia, microdysgenesis, dysembryoplastic neuroepithelial tumour and dysgenesis of the archicortex in epilepsy. Clinical, EEG and neuro-imaging features in 100 adults patients. *Brain* **118**, 629–60.

Ridsdale L *et al.* (1997). The effects of nurse-run clinics for patients with epilepsy in general practice. *British Medical Journal* **314**, 120–2.

Sander JWAS, Shorvon SD (1996). Epidemiology of the epilepsies. *Journal of Neurology, Neurosurgery and Psychiatry* **61**, 433–43.

Saygi S *et al.* (1992). Frontal lobe partial seizures and psychogenic seizures: comparison of clinical and ictal characteristics. *Neurology* **42,** 1274–7.

Shorvon S (1994). *Status epilepticus: its clinical features and treatment in children and adults.* Cambridge University Press.

Sperling MR *et al.* (1996). Temporal lobectomy for refractory epilepsy. *Journal of the American Medical Association* **276**, 470–5.

Van Donselaar CA *et al.* (1992). Value of the electroencephalogram in adult patients with untreated idiopathic first seizures. *Archives of Neurology* **49**, 231–7.

Wallace H *et al.* (1997). *Adults with poorly controlled epilepsy.* Royal College of Physicians of London. [An excellent, short, monograph whose title is deceptive. Many issues are covered, including the role of electroencephalography, neuroimaging, and the issues relating to contraception and pregnancy.]

24.13.4 Narcolepsy

David Parkes

The narcoleptic syndrome

The prevalence of narcolepsy in Western Europe is about four per 10 000. Reported rates worldwide vary 100-fold. This variation may result in part from differences in true case ascertainment and broad definitions of 'narcolepsy'. Narcolepsy is as common in men as women. It usually starts in childhood or adolescence, with a second peak at 30 to 40 years. However, the age at presentation extends from under 1 to over 70 years. Narcolepsy is lifelong and spontaneous recovery does not occur.

Narcolepsy has two key features, cataplexy and daytime sleepiness. Cataplexy is unique to the syndrome but daytime sleepiness has many different causes. The presence of both symptoms is essential for a definite diagnosis. The initial symptom is usually sleepiness, followed by cataplexy within 2 years. Very occasionally this order is reversed and the gap may be prolonged to several decades. Cataplexy is provoked by emotional stimuli such as laughter, startle, excitement, or anger. There is a sudden loss of tone in antigravity muscles with a tendency to fall as well as mouth opening, dysarthria, mutism, and phasic muscle jerking around the mouth. Most attacks are mild and last a few seconds but self-injury can occur in more severe episodes. Several attacks may occur each day. Cataplexy is comparable to the atonia of rapid eye movement sleep but without loss of awareness. As cataplexy is seldom witnessed by the physician, an unequivocal history using clear language is essential to establish its presence.

Sleep, automatic behaviour, and failure of self-monitoring all reduce wakefulness. Sleep pressure increases with monotony and sleep attacks have a 3- to 4-h cyclicity throughout the day. Sleepiness is usually more disabling than cataplexy and causes chronic school and work failure, broken relationships, frustration, embarrassment, poor self-image, and depression. Despite daytime sleepiness, the total sleep period over 24 h is normal as multiple nocturnal arousals shorten night sleep. Insomnia, motor disorders bordering sleep, and vivid dream intrusion at the wake–sleep boundary are common. The old concept of four symptoms—sleepiness, cataplexy, sleep paralysis, and hypnagogic hallucinations—needs revision.

The diagnosis of narcolepsy is totally dependent on a clear sleep–wake history, supported by a sleep–wake diary and a disability rating scale such as the Epworth or Ullanlinna. Study in a sleep laboratory is never a substitute (Table 1).

Aetiology

Narcolepsy has a genetic not a psychological basis. Ninety five per cent of Caucasian subjects with narcolepsy have the HLA D-related (DR) serotype DR2 and oligotype DQ B1*0602. The DR association is slightly different in other ethnic groups. The HLA type is not specific to narcolepsy, being present in 25 to 30 per cent of white subjects, only 1 in 500 of whom have narcolepsy. Despite the HLA association there is no present evidence of an immune defect in narcolepsy, or of definite involvement of HLA systems in normal sleep mechanisms. Attempts to identify additional non-HLA genes in humans, with the possible exception of linkage to γ-aminobutyric acid genetic systems on chromosome 4 and the monoamine oxidase X-linked locus, are unconvincing.

An unexpected pathway for sleep has been identified involving hypocretin. The hypocretins are neuropeptides made in the dorsal and lateral hypothalamic areas of the brain, and are implicated in the regulation of feeding and energy (Table 2). A mutation in a hypocretin receptor has been shown in dogs with narcolepsy, but not in DR2 positive humans with the disease. However, in most narcoleptics studied there is a near total absence of

Table 1 Clinical features of narcolepsy

Cataplexy*	Laughter-provoked sudden antigravity muscle atonia
Daytime sleepiness*	Subalertness, automatic behaviour and sleep at 3- to 4-h intervals, most marked in the absence of environmental stimuli
Short night sleep latency†	Sleep within seconds of going to bed
Interrupted night sleep†	Frequent brief nocturnal arousals with complaint of insomnia
Frequent parasomnias†	Sleep paralysis, night terrors, motor restlessness, and other parasomnias are all more common from childhood in narcoleptic than normal subjects
Abnormal time of dream recall†	Dream recall when awake, or at wake–sleep as well as sleep–wake boundary; frequent and vivid dream mentation

* Essential for a definite diagnosis.
† Present in 50 to 95 per cent of all subjects.

Table 2 Properties of hypocretin

- Properties: Hcrt1 and Hcrt2
- Hcrt1 crosses blood–brain barrier and has an affinity for Hcrt1 and Hcrt2 receptors
- Involved in sleep state regulation
- Hcrt neurones control the ascending cortical activating system
- Hcrt neurones project to:

tuberomammillary areas (histamine)
locus caeruleus (noradrenaline)
raphe (5-hydroxytryptamine (serotonin))
penduncle pons (acetylcholine)

Hcrt = hypocretin.

hypocretin in the cerebrospinal fluid and brain tissue. Further understanding here, and of the relationship between HLA and hypocretin systems, will be essential in the development of new treatments for narcolepsy.

Familial narcolepsy does occur but accounts for only 5 to 10 per cent of all cases, some of whom show dominant inheritance.

In the few reported studies of monozygotic twins, disease discordance has been found in up to 70 per cent of pairs. Narcolepsy thus appears to be caused by an environmental agent in a genetically susceptible subject. The nature of this external factor is not known.

Pathophysiology of narcolepsy and sleep laboratory investigation

The normal non-rapid eye movement–rapid eye movement sleep cycle of adults is reversed in narcolepsy, where periods of rapid eye movement occur at the onset of sleep. In addition two characteristics of rapid eye movement sleep, atonia and dreaming, are fragmented and intrude into wakefulness, resulting in cataplexy and vivid recall of dreams. Rapid eye movement sleep is generated in ventral pontine areas contiguous with neurones controlling voluntary eye movements. However, no anatomical defect in this area of the brain has been found in narcolepsy, and pursuit and saccadic eye movements are normal.

The mean sleep latency test measures the pressure for sleep using electroencephalographic parameters at 2-h intervals from 10.00 to 16.00 or 18.00 under standard conditions. A mean latency of under 5 min is usually considered abnormal and of over 10 min normal. Results between 5 and 10 min are in a grey area. Results of the mean sleep latency test do not always mirror behavioural tests of alertness. In addition to sleep latency, a mean sleep latency test will show rapid eye movement activity at sleep onset. However, this activity is not diagnostic of narcolepsy. Timing of rapid eye movement sleep varies with recording position, age, previous sleep deprivation, and drug treatment. Overall, polysomnogram findings are less specific and sensitive in the diagnosis of narcolepsy than a definite history of cataplexy. Diagnosis and treatment should therefore depend on the clinical picture rather than on sleep laboratory findings. In cases with an indefinite history, laboratory findings may add confusion rather than clarity and should never be used alone to establish diagnosis. Likewise, HLA tests will not confirm narcolepsy, although the diagnosis is unlikely if the DR2 antigen is absent.

Symptomatic narcolepsy

Narcolepsy has been associated with a wide range of other disorders. These are mostly uncommon and rarely if ever cause problems in differential diagnosis. In many cases there is obvious brainstem pathology and poor resemblance of symptoms with those of true narcolepsy. The occasional association of narcolepsy with multiple sclerosis may result not from a brainstem lesion but from a common genetic predisposition. There is an over-representation of the same HLA D-related antigen in both conditions.

Differential diagnosis

There are a number of narcoleptic syndrome variants with overlapping clinical features (Table 3).

In narcolepsy the commonest mistake is failure to diagnose, rather than incorrect diagnosis. Daytime sleepiness is never normal and is rarely psychological in origin. It is sometimes wrongly attributed to insomnia and most insomniacs have a low, not high, daytime sleep tendency. The symptom is serious and requires investigation rather than a pseudodiagnosis of laziness.

The second most common mistake is to label all forms of sleepiness as due to narcolepsy or sleep apnoea. Real difficulty lies in cases of apparent narcolepsy presenting before cataplexy and where at best the diagnosis can only be possible or probable, not definite narcolepsy. Follow-up is essential here whatever the sleep laboratory findings. Narcolepsy and sleep apnoea sometimes coexist, particularly in overweight males. Cataplexy is sometimes confused with epilepsy or drop attack, but a careful history will usually separate these.

Hypersomnia without cataplexy or any feature of psychological or physical illness is common. Here exact diagnosis of the cause is often impossible. The idea of idiopathic hypersomnia is based on the concept of abnormal pressure for non-rapid eye movement sleep, with prolonged dream-free deep sleep by night and day, sometimes with a familial or genetic basis. In reality there is little or no distinction in sleep–wake behaviour in different forms of hypersomnia and prolonged follow-up sleep and laboratory studies are needed.

Other causes of sleepiness with medical or psychological illness are unlikely to be confused with narcolepsy. In addition to head injury, hypnotic drug and alcohol abuse, and sleep-related respiratory illness they include:

- depression (insomnia is more common than hypersomnia)
- postviral illness (often Epstein–Barr virus)
- cerebrovascular disease (sometimes with bilateral thalamic infarcts)
- multisystem atrophy
- shift work and circadian delay syndromes
- sleep apnoea treated with continuous positive airway pressure (this rarely completely reverses sleepiness).

Treatment

Treatment of narcolepsy is a problem for both physician and patient. The prescriber may refuse stimulant drugs owing to fear of abuse, or restrict dosage to prevent tolerance. Patients may demand large doses and complete freedom to overdose, not recognizing their own irritability and euphoria.

Most subjects with narcolepsy need a central stimulant drug to improve alertness, and two-thirds need an additional anticataplectic drug to prevent atonia. One drug from each group in Table 4 should be chosen. Dexamphetamine and methylphenidate but not modafinil have a partial anticataplectic as well as an alerting effect. Stimulant drug treatment should be supported by a 15 min nap once or twice a day. Adequate treatment is essential to restore school performance, work, driving ability, and quality of life. This is best achieved with an as-needed, variable dose rather than a fixed dose regime, dependent on factors such as day of the week, activity, and response level. A sleep–wake diary is an important aid to starting and monitoring treatment. Drug response is immediate, while sudden withdrawal may be followed by a severe rebound of sleepiness, cataplexy, or both lasting several days. Stimulant response is the same in hypersomnia as in narcolepsy.

Metabolic tolerance with the need for an increase in dose develops in one-tenth to one-third of subjects. Dose revision, changing to an alternative drug, or a 2-week drug holiday may be necessary. Psychological addiction does not occur and there is no evidence of stimulant abuse in narcoleptics of normal personality. Very occasionally a recreational drug

Table 3 The narcolepsies

	Clinical features	Notes
Idiopathic narcoleptic syndrome DQ B1*0602 positive	Cataplexy and daytime sleepiness	90 per cent of all cases, 5–10 per cent familial Hypocretin deficiency
Idiopathic narcoleptic syndrome DQ B1*0602 negative variant	Identical clinical symptoms to positive cases	Familial cases more common than in positive subjects
'Incomplete' narcolepsy	Cataplexy without daytime sleepiness or vice versa	HLA DR2 positive. Follow-up required to detect development of additional symptoms
Excess daytime sleepiness with sleep paralysis	Mild rather than severe sleepiness; no cataplexy	No HLA association. Sometimes familial, common in black and oriental subjects
'Symptomatic' narcolepsy	Structural brainstem lesion	Glioma, angioma, lymphoma, encephalitis
'Syndromic' narcolepsy	Narcolepsy-like symptoms in gene-determined central nervous system disorders	Moebius, Prader–Willi and Niemann Pick syndromes, Norrie disease
Multiple sclerosis with the narcoleptic syndrome	Sleep and cataplexy with established multiple sclerosis	Possible common genetic HLA-determined susceptibility
Idiopathic hypersomnia	Sleepiness alone	Diagnostic ragbag, unrelated to narcolepsy

user will feign a history of narcolepsy to obtain stimulants and a urinary drug screen may be appropriate.

Serious dose-related or idiosyncratic side-effects are uncommon. However, sweating and irritability with the stronger stimulants, mild headache with modafinil, and sexual side-effects, increased appetite, and weight gain with clomipramine sometimes limit treatment. Acute amphetamine psychosis is not a problem in narcoleptics and a lifetime of treatment does not cause vascular toxicity or hypertension. A poor drug response should lead to re-evaluation of diagnosis and treatment compliance. Management problems include pregnancy, with the need for the safety of mother and baby to be balanced against potential drug teratogenicity and secretion in breast milk, and cardiovascular disease where low- rather than high-dose treatment is indicated. Conventional treatment is unsatisfactory in about one-fifth of narcoleptics. If disability is severe, a therapeutic trial of morning venlafaxine, 37.5 mg with slow increase to 275 mg per 24 h should be considered but this regime must be carefully monitored.

Table 4 Treatment of narcolepsy

	Total 24-h dose range	Notes
Excess daytime sleepiness		
Dexamphetamine	5–60 mg	Tolerance an occasional problem but no evidence of addiction, dependence, or abuse
Methylphenidate	10–80 mg	As dexamphetamine, possibly a smoother response
Mazindol	2–8 mg	Non-amphetamine compound, less potent than above but preferred by some patients
Modafinil	200–400 mg	Different behavioural effect from dexamphetamine
Cataplexy		
Clomipramine	10–150 mg	Most potent anticataplectic drug known but long-term weight gain is a major problem in treatment
Fluoxetine	20 mg	Less potent alternative to clomipramine but limited side-effects

Notes:

Give stimulant drugs at 4- to 8-h intervals on a variable-dose, as-needed basis.

For a sedative anticataplectic, for example clomipramine, give a single evening dose. Stimulant compounds, for example fluoxetine, should be given as a single morning dose. Most 5-hydroxytryptamine (serotonin) reuptake inhibitors and selective serotonin reuptake inhibitors abolish cataplexy and possibly sleep paralysis.

Insomnia if severe may require hypnotic treatment, for example twice weekly zopiclone 7.5 mg. Avoid nightly dosage, review at 3-month intervals.

Further reading

Diagnostic Classification Steering Committee (Thorpy MJ, chairman) (1990). *International classification of sleep disorders: diagnostic and coding manual.* American Sleep Disorders Association, Rochester, MN.

Hublin C *et al.* (1994) The Ullanlinna narcolepsy scale: validation of a measure of symptoms in the narcoleptic syndrome. *Journal of Sleep Research* **3** 52–9.

Johns MW (1991). A new method for measuring daytime sleepiness: the Epworth sleepiness scale. *Sleep* **14**, 540–5.

Ling L *et al.* (1999). The sleep disorder canine narcolepsy is caused by a mutation in the hypocretin (orexin) receptor 2 gene. *Cell* **98**, 365–75.

Nevsimalova *et al.* (2000). Clinical features of hypocretin (orexin) mutation in human narcolepsy. *Neurology* **54**, A30–A31, Suppl. 3.

Parkes JD *et al.* (1998). The clinical diagnosis of the narcoleptic syndrome. *Journal of Sleep Research* **7**, 41–52.

Peyron *et al.* (2000). A mutation in a case of early onset narcolepsy and a generalized absence of hypocretin peptides in human narcoleptic brains. *Nature Medicine* **6**, 991–7.

Thannickal *et al.* (2000). Reduced number of hypocretin neurons in human narcolepsy. *Neuron* **27**, 469–74.

24.13.5 Syncope

L. D. Blumhardt

Definition

Syncope (fainting) is a brief loss of consciousness that results from an acute reduction in cerebral blood flow (from the Greek 'synkoptein' to cut or break). It is the most common cause of recurrent episodes of disturbed consciousness.

Pathophysiology

Although there is a seemingly endless list of causes and predisposing factors (Table 1), the sequence of reflex events, once triggered, is relatively constant. Loss of consciousness (probably ultimately due to hindbrain ischaemia) results from a sudden reduction of cerebral perfusion as compensatory mechanisms fail, due either to a reflex reduction of venous return to the heart, or to an inadequate response of the heart when an increased cardiac output is required.

In the common faint (vasovagal syncope), the reduced venous return is caused mainly by a sudden reflex reduction in the resistance of the peripheral blood vessels with pooling, particularly in the lower limbs and abdomen. There is generally some associated, but less important, slowing of heart rate (hence the term vasovagal, originally coined by Sir Thomas Lewis), but in some individuals, an exaggerated reflex bradycardia or even sinus arrest due to vagal hyperactivity may be the dominant factor in reducing cardiac output (cardio-inhibitory syncope). This is a particular feature of loss of consciousness arising from painful pressure on the eyeball (oculocardiac reflex). In cough syncope, the high intrathoracic pressure generated by violent coughing (which may exceed 250 mmHg), triggers a reflex fall in cardiac output. Similar events underlie syncope associated with the Valsalva manouvre and possibly also contribute to the rare defaecation syncope. The proposed mechanisms responsible for carotid sinus syncope include hypersensitivity of the baroreceptors in a diseased carotid sinus and, possibly, contributions from an exaggerated vagal response or oversensitivity of the sinus node. In syncope associated with eating, a vagally induced bradycardia may be provoked by stretching of the oesophagus (swallow syncope) or by very cold stimuli (ice-cream syncope). In other subjects, critical cardiac slowing can be provoked by rectal stretch (for example during proctoscopy or prostatic massage). In micturition syncope, the mechanism is thought to be a combination of high nocturnal vagal tone, postural hypotension, and the sudden loss of the vasopressor effect of a full bladder.

Table 1 Causes of syncope and predisposing/trigger factors

Type of syncope	Predisposing/trigger factor
Common faints (vasovagal syncope)	Prolonged standing
	Sudden postural change
	Warm environment
	Emotion
	Pain
	Fatigue
	Anaemia
	Hypoglycaemia
Postural hypotension	Elderly
	Convalesence
	Autonomic failure
	Drugs
Valsalva mechanism	Wind instruments
	Defaecation
	Weight-lifting
Micturition syncope	Nocturnal micturition
	Alcohol
Cough syncope	Chronic airways disease
	Smoking
	Defects of atrioventricular conduction
	Arnold–Chiari malformations
Carotid sinus disease	Head posture
	Atherosclerosis
Carotid syncope	
Arrhythmias	Sinus node disease
	Bradyarrhythmias
	Tachyarrhythmias
Structural	Hypertrophic cardiomyopathy
	Valvular stenosis
	Atrial myxoma
	Aortic arch disease
	Pulmonary hypertension
	Constrictive pericarditis
Reflex 'vagal' anoxic seizures (non-epileptic)	Pain
	Minor trauma
	Emotion
Hypovolaemia	Haemorrhage
	Protein loss
	Dehydration
	Addison's disease
Areflexic postural hypotension	Diabetes
	Polyneuropathies
	Tabes dorsalis
	Multisystem atrophy
	High spinal cord disease
Metabolic	Anoxia
	Hypoglycaemia
Hyperventilation	Anxiety
Vertigo	Vestibular disease

Clinical features

In many subjects syncope is preceded by a characteristic sequence of premonitory symptoms (presyncope). A typical history may include lightheadedness, sweating ('clamminess'), sensations of warmth or cold, nausea, and blurring of vision. Subjects may also report tinnitus, receding sounds, 'closing in of peripheral vision', weakness, increased salivation, urgency of micturition, vomiting, diarrhoea, and the need to get fresh air. These symptoms may be proffered in any combination and any, or all, may be missing. It is important to distinguish the usual complaints of dizziness, 'light-headedness', 'muzziness', or giddiness due to hypotension, from vertigo (dizziness with a rotational element) which does not occur in syncope. An eyewitness may report on the sweating, restlessness, excessive yawning, slow sighing respiration, and marked facial pallor. In some individuals the loss of consciousness may be abrupt with little or no warning, whereas in others the symptoms of presyncope may build up slowly. With sufficient warning and insight, some subjects may be able to prevent the syncope by lying down and increasing cardiac return by elevating their legs, but many seem either unaware of this possibility, or are unable to invoke it in time.

If no preventative action is taken, syncope, characterized by a sudden loss of consciousness and collapse with loss of muscular tone, may then follow. The subject is noted to be limp or floppy (no stiffness, rigidity, or tongue biting) and is usually motionless. In some subjects there may be flickering of the eyelids and perhaps an occasional irregular myoclonic twitch or jerk in a limb. Respiration is shallow, the blood pressure low or unrecordable and the pulse thready, rapid, or slow, and often difficult to feel. In uncomplicated syncope, the loss of consciousness usually lasts only seconds and recovery is rapid without confusion. Sweating and profound 'waxy' pallor due to intense vasconstriction of skin vessels may persist well after recovery. If the subject gets up too rapidly, a further episode of syncope may occur.

Most syncope is uncomplicated. Injuries are uncommon, but can occur depending on the circumstances of the faint. If the bladder is full there may be incontinence. If the anoxia is profound, the patient may vomit or be doubly incontinent. If a recumbent posture does not result from the fall, a secondary anoxic seizure may follow (convulsive syncope) in some predisposed individuals. This event is commonly mistaken for epilepsy if the sequence of events is not carefully established from a witness. To complicate matters further, syncope may rarely precipitate a true epileptic seizure.

Main variants of syncope

Vasovagal syncope

The common faint usually occurs for the first time in childhood or adolescence and recurs in well-recognized situations, for example venepuncture, dental procedures, at the sight of blood or injury, sudden emotions, acute pain, postural change, and prolonged standing in stuffy or warm surroundings (school assembly or church). There is almost invariably a postural element—faints occur when standing or sitting and only very rarely when lying (for example in pregnancy). Many secondary factors may increase the risk of faints in the susceptible subject including anaemia, blood loss, convalescence, hypoglycaemia, sleep deprivation, hypotension, cardiac or vascular disease, and drugs. Although there is often a recrudescence of faints later in life, caution should be exercised in diagnosing vasovagal syncope occurring *de novo* in the elderly (check for an earlier history of faints in appropriate circumstances), as the blackouts may be due to cardiac arrhythmias.

Susceptibility to fainting varies widely and some individuals may experience syncope only in association with particular triggers. The diagnosis is usually easy when intense pain such as abdominal colic, glossopharyngeal neuralgia, migraine, or diagnostic manipulation such as venepuncture, oesophagoscopy, or rectal examination provoke attacks. It may be more difficult when syncope complicates a severe vestibular vertigo.

Micturition syncope

The occurrence of loss of consciousness at night during or usually shortly after micturition is highly characteristic of this condition. Contrary to a surprisingly widespread misconception, it is not a complication of prostatism, but occurs almost exclusively in healthy men (some of whom also suffer from vasovagal syncope) with a peak incidence in the third and fourth decades. It does occur in women, but very rarely.

The condition usually responds to advice to mobilize slowly when arising at night and to micturate in the sitting down position.

Cough syncope

This condition is usually associated with chronic obstructive airways disease and smoking. A series of coughs, or sometimes even a single forceful cough, is followed by a collapse with brief loss of consciousness. Afflicted patients often appear unaware of the association between their coughing bouts and the syncope and an account from a witness is required. There may be muscular jerks or twitches during cough syncope and the differentiation from epilepsy is important. Careful clinical assessment is required as cerebellar ectopia with compression of the brainstem and atrioventricular conduction abnormalities may rarely present with similar symptoms. Treatment is usually directed towards the chest condition and education of the patient and relatives into the mechanisms and possible avoidance measures.

Carotid sinus syncope

This is a rare but important cause of syncope as it is potentially treatable. The diagnosis should be considered in elderly patients, usually men with atherosclerotic vascular disease, hypertension, or diabetes when blackouts are associated with a tight collar, head turning, or even the posture or pressure on the neck when shaving. It may also occur with infiltrating cervical tumours or radiation. If suspected, gentle sequential unilateral carotid sinus massage carried out with electrocardiographic control for 6 s per side may result in conduction block or cardiac arrest. Many would accept an asystole of more than 3 s as diagnostic, but the criteria remain controversial. Denervation of the carotid sinus or cardiac pacing is usually effective.

Cardiac syncope

This can be divided into syncope caused by outflow obstruction from the left ventricle and syncope due to disorders of cardiac rhythm. An inability to increase the cardiac output as required, for example during exercise or sexual activity, may cause syncope in hypertrophic cardiomyopathy, aortic stenosis, restrictive pericarditis, left ventricular insufficiency, or atrial myxoma. However, it is more common, even where structural heart disease exists, for loss of consciousness to be caused by an arrhythmia. Syncope may be sudden with no warning (as with with heart block or sinus arrest for example) or there may be dizziness, palpitations, dyspnoea, or chest pain (for example with tachyarrhythmias). The symptoms may closely mimic those of complex partial seizures (temporal lobe epilepsy) which can themselves generate cardiac arrhythmias. After transient cardiac arrest there may be facial flushing as the cardiac output is restored. The clinical presentation of a patient with a slow pulse and syncopal attacks has long been recognized (Stokes–Adams syndrome) and may be due to atrioventricular block, ventricular tachycardia, fibrillation, or standstill. Similar attacks occur with sinus node disease ('sick sinus' or tachycardia–bradycardia syndrome) and the long QT syndrome (see Section 15).

Syncope associated with exercise may also be associated with aortic arch disease, congenital heart disease, and pulmonary hypertension.

Reflex ('vagal') anoxic seizures

This particular form of reflex cardiac arrhythmia can be regarded as one end of the spectrum of fainting disorders. It is important because it is frequently misdiagnosed as epilepsy. In its most common form, a child (the condition may persist into early adult life) has faints that typically are triggered by minor trauma such as a painful knock in the playground. The brief loss of consciousness may be associated with rigidity, pallor, muscular twitching, and sometimes incontinence. There is usually a rapid recovery with little if any confusion. Simultaneous electrocardiographic and electroencephalographic recordings demonstrate that the primary cardiac asystole is followed by secondary anoxic changes (high-amplitude slow waves) on the electroencephalograph with no evidence of epilepsy. The attacks can be provoked in the laboratory by ocular pressure. Treatment if necessary is with long-acting atropine preparations.

Postural hypotension

Convalescent patients may be subject to large reductions of blood pressure on changing their posture. Many drugs, including diuretics, antihypertensives, levodopa, nitrates, major tranquillizers, antidepressants, alcohol, and calcium antagonists may play an important or primary role. Areflexic or 'paralytic' postural hypotension may complicate or be the presenting symptom of diseases affecting the autonomic nervous system, such as diabetes mellitus, idiopathic orthostatic hypotension, extrapyramidal diseases, tabes dorsalis, peripheral neuropathies, and high spinal cord disease. Some otherwise healthy individuals are peculiarly sensitive to mild postural hypotension. A lordotic posture may contribute to syncope in subjects standing to attention on a parade ground.

Diagnostic approach

The essential clues to the diagnosis of syncope are usually found in the history of the immediate circumstances of the collapse and the events leading up to it. A past or family history of similar events, perhaps in more obvious circumstances, will often provide the diagnosis. Factors favouring syncope may be the recent initiation of drugs or a prolonged period of erect posture or postural change. Was there a Valsalva factor present (for example, straining or lifting, or the forceful playing of a wind instrument) or an emotional or painful experience? Are there background factors favouring syncope, such as anaemia, recent convalescence, fatigue, cardiac disease, or blood loss? The history of the attacks themselves needs to be built up in an as much detail as possible including an eyewitness account of events immediately before, during, and after the attack. Was the subject's muscle tone appropriately limp? There should be no tongue biting, rigidity, or rhythmic tonic–clonic movements suggesting seizure activity. If a seizure appears to have occurred in a situation more appropriate to a syncopal episode, a careful history will often establish that the patient's position after the faint did not allow rapid restoration of cerebral blood flow (for example they were propped against a wall or held upright). A secondary anoxic seizure (convulsive syncope) is then the correct diagnosis, rather than epilepsy. Injuries (apart from a bitten tongue) do not particularly favour epilepsy, but confusion is unlikely after syncope, unless there was a complicating head injury or seizure.

Young men who collapse in the bathroom, or on the way back to bed during the night, are at risk of misdiagnosis, particularly if a secondary convulsive syncope has occurred. These circumstances should alert the clinician to the possibility of micturition syncope. The patient with chest disease and blackouts is often peculiarly 'amnesic' for his attacks which he does not associate with his respiratory condition. As for all forms of syncope the eyewitness account is critical to establish the associations, the correct sequence of events, and the diagnosis. The presence of other medical conditions such as chronic airways disease (cough syncope), cardiac disease (arrhythmias), or atherosclerosis (carotid sinus syncope) may provide the main diagnostic clue.

Management

Simple faints require usually require only reassurance, counselling, and education for patients and relatives. They should be instructed in the mechanisms and the avoidance of predisposing situations and trigger factors as well as measures to be taken during presyncopal episodes. Apart from a blood count if anaemia is suspected, or a blood sugar estimation if hypoglycaemia is a possibility, investigations are seldom indicated unless relevant abnormalities are present on history or examination. Investigating all patients with syncope is expensive and produces a low yield. Syncopal episodes occurring *de novo* in adults without obvious triggering factors, or precipitated by exercise, may require electrocardiography, Holter monitoring, treadmill tests, and perhaps sophisticated intracardiac conduction studies. Structural heart disease or failure should be excluded.

Where the diagnosis remains in doubt, or if epilepsy is a possibility, an electroencephalograph and perhaps simultaneous electrocardiographic/electroencephalographic recordings with video monitoring of attacks in a specialist unit may be indicated.

Further reading

deBono DP, Warlow CP, Hyman NM (1982). Cardiac rhythm abnormalities in patients presenting with transient non-focal neurological syndromes. *British Medical Journal* **284**, 1437–9.

Eberhart C, Morgan JW (1960). Micturition syncope. *Journal of the American Medical Association* **174**, 2076–7.

Jaeger FJ, Maloney JD, Fouard-Tarazi (1990). Newer aspects in the diagnosis and management of syncope. In: Rappaport E, ed. *Cardiology update.* Elsevier, New York.

Kapoor WN *et al.* (1982). Syncope of unknown origin. The need for a more effective approach to its diagnostic evaluation. *Journal of the American Medical Association* **247**, 26 787–91.

Kapoor WN, Peterson J, Karpf M (1986). Defecation syncope. *Archives of Internal Medicine* **146**, 2377–9.

Leatham A (1982). Carotid sinus syncope. *British Heart Journal* **47**, 409–10.

Levin B, Posner JB (1982). Swallow syncope. Report of a case and review of the literature. *Neurology* **22**, 1086–93.

Lewis T (1932). Vaso-vagal syncope and the carotid sinus mechanism. *British Medical Journal* **1**, 873–6.

Lipsitz LA (1983). Syncope in the elderly, *Annals of Internal Medicine* **99**, 92–105.

Proudfit WL, Forteza MS (1959). Micturition syncope. *New England Journal of Medicine* **260**, 228–31.

Sharpey-Schafer EP (1956). The mechanism of syncope after coughing. *British Medical Journal* **ii**, 860–3.

Sharpey-Schafer EP (1956). Syncope. *British Medical Journal* **1**, 506–9.

Stephenson JPB (1978). Reflex anoxic seizures ('white breath holding'): non-epileptic vagal attacks. *Archives of Disease in Childhood* **43**, 193–200.

Sugrue DD, Wood DL, McGoon MD (1984). Carotid sinus hypersensitivity and syncope. *Mayo Clinic Proceedings* **59**, 637–40.

24.13.5.1 Head-up tilt-table testing in the diagnosis of vasovagal syncope and related disorders

Steve W. Parry and Rose Anne Kenny

In many patients, the diagnosis of vasovagal syncope or presyncope is evident from their history and physical examination. Where doubt exists, or a definitive diagnosis is needed to clarify atypical presentations or aid decision-making for driving or occupational purposes, head-up tilt-table testing should be considered.

The head-up tilt-table test employs prolonged, controlled orthostatic stress to provoke vasovagal syncope, with characteristic symptoms and concurrent haemodynamic changes confirming the diagnosis. In susceptible patients, head-up tilt causes relative central hypotension through displacement of venous blood to the lower limbs and capacitance vessels, with consequent vigorous left ventricular contraction and inappropriate cardiac mechanoreceptor activation. The resultant afferent neural traffic traverses unmyelinated C-fibres to the nucleus tractus solitarius, which then orchestrates the vagal activation and vasodilatation characteristic of the vasovagal response. In the absence of a 'gold-standard' diagnostic test, estimates of the sensitivity and specificity of head-up tilt-table testing from comparisons with healthy volunteers vary between 32 to 85 per cent and 60 to 90 per cent, respectively. The reproducibility of positive responses in patients with vasovagal syncope is up to 87 per cent in the short term (30 min) and 85 per cent over several days and months. The test's reliability, non-invasive nature, relative cheapness, and safety record make head-up tilt-table testing the current diagnostic test of choice in the investigation of unexplained syncope.

Haemodynamic responses during a positive test may also guide therapeutic strategies, and are divided into vasodepressor (predominant blood pressure fall in the absence of significant bradycardia/asystole), cardioinhibitory (predominant bradycardia/asystole), or mixed (a combination of the two) subtypes. Cardioinhibitory vasovagal syncope may benefit from permanent pacemaker therapy, whereas the predominant vasodepressor subtypes are unlikely to do so. Heart rate responses during tilt may also assist in the choice of medical therapy; for example beta-blockers are useful if pronounced tachycardia antedates symptomatic hypotension/bradycardia.

Head-up tilt-table testing is a relatively benign investigation, with few reported complications worldwide, most of which have anecdotally been related to inappropriate staff training and lack of resuscitation facilities. Relative contraindications include severe coronary or cerebrovascular arterial stenoses, clinically severe left ventricular outflow obstruction, and critical mitral stenosis.

Methodology

Tilt-table testing should be conducted in a quiet, dimly lit environment at a comfortable temperature to minimize confounding autonomic nervous activation. The table should have a foot-plate support, and be capable of smooth, rapid movement between supine and calibrated upright positions between 60° and 80° (lesser or greater angles increase the number of false-negative and false-positive studies, respectively). Subjects should be fasted for no more than 2 h before testing to avoid potential confounding from postprandial hypotension. Intravascular instrumentation is avoided in all but isoproterenol-provoked tilt testing as this markedly lowers the test's specificity. After 10 min rest in the supine position, subjects are strapped

Table 1 The Newcastle protocols for head-up tilt-table testing

Tilt test description	Method
Passive drug-free tilt	40 min (min) at 70°
Isoproterenol (μg) tilt	5 min tilt, 5 min supine 5 min 1μg/min supine, 5 min 1μg/min at 70° Infusion discontinued, supine 2 min 5 min 3 μg/min supine, 5 min 3 μg/min at 70°
Glyceryl trinitrate (GTN) tilt	2 metered doses (800 μg) sublingual GTN spray supine 5 min supine then 20 min at 70°

Patients should remain supine for 20 min prior to testing. Isoproterenol and GTN tilts should follow non-diagnostic, passive, drug-free tilt where the history is suggestive of vasovagal syncope. Tilt should be terminated if symptom reproduction with concomitant hypotension/bradycardia or adverse events develop. See text for further details.

(Reproduced with permission of BMJ Publishing Group, *Heart* 2000, 83, 564–9.)

securely to the tilt table to prevent injury during syncope and collapse, and then tilted to 70° for 40 min.

A summary of the Newcastle protocols for head-up tilt-table testing is provided in Table 1. Continuous blood pressure monitoring is advised during the test, preferably with non-invasive beat-to-beat digital photoplethysmographic devices such as Finapres (Ohmeda, Wisconsin) or Portapres (TNO-TNM Biomedical, Amsterdam), though sphygmomanometric devices are widely used. Electrocardiography should be undertaken at baseline, continuously during symptoms or haemodynamic changes, and every 5 min otherwise. The test should be supervised by a nurse, physician, or technician trained in the management of the test and its potential complications, with advanced resuscitation equipment and a clinician trained in its use immediately available at all times.

The head-up tilt-table test is deemed diagnostic only if arterial hypotension and/or bradycardia are accompanied by symptoms reproducing the patient's syncopal or presyncopal symptoms. Haemodynamic changes without symptom reproduction should not be construed as vasovagal syncope.

Pharmacological and mechanical provocative agents in head-up tilt-table testing

Where the initial prolonged, passive tilt test is negative, several agents may be used to increase the sensitivity of the test.

Isoproterenol provokes the vasovagal response by simulating the catecholaminergic surge seen prior to syncope in susceptible subjects. Isoproterenol should be used with caution in subjects with known arrhythmias, coronary artery disease, significant aortic stenosis, left ventricular outflow obstruction, and uncontrolled hypertension. Tilt-testing should be terminated if sustained tachycardia (>150 beats/minute), hypertension (>180/100), arrhythmia, or intolerable symptoms supervene.

Nitrates, in particular sublingual glyceryl trinitrate, have more recently been used in this context, with nitrate-induced vasodilatation simulating the venous pooling which provokes spontaneous episodes. Nitrate-provoked tilt testing is as specific and sensitive, and better tolerated than, isoproterenol.

Developments incorporating intravenous adenosine and clomipramine are currently being evaluated, but are not yet in routine use.

Mechanical provocation, using a suction chamber to exert a lower-body negative pressure (again simulating venous pooling), has been successfully used in specialist centres.

Non-vasovagal indications for head-up tilt-table testing

Carotid sinus massage in the head-up tilt position (following an initial supine, bilateral, non-diagnostic massage) may increase the diagnostic rate for carotid sinus hypersensitivity by 30 per cent. Head-up tilt testing is used to diagnose orthostatic hypotension in patients unable to stand unaided for 3 min, while the postural orthostatic tachycardia syndrome may similarly be diagnosed during tilt-testing if the patient's heart rate rises by more than 30 beats/min (or to a maximum of 120 beats/min) during the presence of characteristic symptoms in the absence of hypotension. Tilt-table testing may also be useful in the differential diagnosis of apparently epileptiform events. Prolonged asystole during vasovagal syncope may result in myoclonic jerking, tonic–clonic movements, and (rarely) incontinence (urinary and faecal) which can be mistaken for generalized convulsions. The short duration of the event, rapid recovery, and the absence of postictal confusion and neurological signs should prompt tilt testing as part of the diagnostic work-up. Psychogenic and hyperventilation syncope result in symptom reproduction without haemodynamic changes during tilt, with hypocapnia being demonstrated in the latter. Head-up tilt testing may also be useful in demonstrating neurocardiovascular disorders as attributable causes of unexplained falls in older patients (in whom falls and syncope frequently overlap), with amnesia for loss of consciousness prompting a non-syncopal presentation.

Further reading

Benditt DG, *et al.* (1996). Tilt table testing for assessing syncope. ACC Expert Consensus Document. *Journal of the American College of Cardiology* **28**, 263–75.

Kenny RA, *et al.* (1986). Head-up tilt: a useful test for investigating unexplained syncope. *Lancet* **1**, 1352–4.

Kenny RA, O'Shea D, Parry SW (2000). The Newcastle protocols for head-up tilt table testing in the diagnosis of vasovagal syncope and related disorders. *Heart* 83, 564–9.

24.13.6 Brain death and the vegetative state

B. Jennett

Cardiopulmonary resuscitation and intensive care are now commonplace in the developed world, so that life-threatening brain insults may now be followed by complete recovery. Sometimes, however, these interventions do no more than extend the process of dying for hours or days because the patient is brain dead. In others intervention comes too late after cardiorespiratory arrest to save the cerebral cortex and thalamus which are more vulnerable to hypoxia than is the brainstem. In that case, or when head injury has irretrievably damaged the cortical connections, the patient can survive for a long period in a vegetative state.

Brain death

Much of the controversy about brain death arose because it was not appreciated that death is a process rather than an event, with organs failing in various sequences. Most often the heart stops first, followed within minutes by respiratory arrest due to brainstem hypoxia. After primary respiratory arrest there is rapid hypoxic brain failure but the heart may continue to beat for 15 to 20 min. If the brainstem fails first due to an intracranial catastrophe and a ventilator takes over respiration the heart can beat for days (occasionally weeks)—this is the state of brain death.

The crucial lesion is irreversible loss of brainstem function with subsequent lack of downward drive to maintain respiration and of upward activation of the cerebral cortex by the ascending reticular pathways. When systemic hypoxia has not been the initial insult the cerebral cortex may be structurally intact, and islands of electrical activity may be detected on the electroencephalogram. Early definitions of brain death (for example the Harvard Criteria of 1968) implied that the whole nervous system was dead with a flat electroencephalogram and an absence of all motor activity. But the spinal cord is more resistant to hypoxia even than the brainstem, and is unaffected by intracranial catastrophes—so spinal reflexes often persist after brain death. To resolve this confusion the term brainstem death is now preferred in the United Kingdom. Although in the United States the most commonly used diagnostic criteria are those for brainstem death, most guidelines and statutes still refer to whole brain death. About half the cases of brain death result from head injury, after hours or days of intensive treatment following initial resuscitation. About a third have suffered severe non-traumatic intracranial haemorrhage, and the rest a variety of catastrophic intracranial events, including systemic hypoxia associated with cardiac arrest.

Criteria for diagnosis

Undue emphasis on the final confirmation that no residual brainstem function persists has sometimes distracted attention from the stepwise process of diagnosis, for which these tests are only the last stage. Indeed the most important step is the first one, satisfying the preconditions. These require that the patient be apnoeic and in deep coma due to irreversible structural damage to the brain. This implies that reversible causes of brainstem depression have been adequately excluded. It is usually obvious that structural brain damage has occurred—there has been a recent head injury or a classical history of spontaneous intracranial haemorrhage or of some less acute intracranial condition. Establishing the irreversibility of such brain damage depends on failure to improve after the correction of factors such as systemic hypotension and hypoxia and raised intracranial pressure. Other causes of temporary failure of brainstem function are depressant drugs (including alcohol), neuromuscular relaxant drugs, and physiological factors such as hypothermia and gross metabolic imbalance. The first two of these may complicate cases of structural brain damage but it is only in a minority of cases that serious doubts arise about confusing factors. For example, when a patient is found unconscious and no satisfactory history can be discovered it may be necessary to undertake formal screening for drugs. In all cases the diagnosis of brain death should be delayed until sufficient time has passed for the exclusion of all temporary causes of brainstem depression, usually at least 6 h.

The tests applied to indicate lack of brainstem function are simple to carry out and to interpret. There should be no response of the pupils to light, of the eyelids to corneal touching, of the facial muscles to pain, of the throat muscles to movements of the endoctracheal tube, or of the eyes to syringing each external auditory meatus with ice cold water (the caloric or vestibulo-ocular reflex). Only when there has been a negative response to all of these is the final crucial test applied—to verify that there is still apnoea. There must be no respiratory movement after disconnection from the ventilator for long enough to allow the $P\text{aco}_2$ to rise to 6.65 kPa (6.8 kPa in the United States), oxygenation being maintained by delivering 6 litre/min of oxygen down the endotracheal tube. To exclude any possibility of observer error it is required that all these tests are carried out by two doctors and on two occasions.

Action after diagnosis of brain death

There is now wide acceptance of the concept that when the brain is dead the person is dead. In the United Kingdom the legal time of death is when the first tests confirm brainstem death, and not some later time when the heart stops. Some doctors are still reluctant to make this diagnosis explicitly and then to act logically and legally by disconnecting the ventilator. The useless ventilation of a brain dead patient deprives that patient of death with dignity, needlessly prolongs the distress of relatives, wastes resources for intensive care, and is bad for the morale of nursing staff. Moreover the opportunity to offer organs for transplantation is lost because gradual circulatory failure makes such organs useless for donation.

The persistent vegetative state

This term was introduced in 1972 by Jennett and Plum to describe the clinical condition resulting from loss of function in the cerebral cortex with a functioning brainstem. Because of the latter, vegetative patients breathe spontaneously and are not ventilator-dependent; another difference from brain death is that they can survive for many years if adequately fed and nursed. The commonest cause of vegetative survival after acute brain damage is severe head injury, the mechanism being severe diffuse axonal injury severing the subcortical connections over a wide area. Secondary hypoxic brain damage is a contributing factor in some traumatic cases. Most non-traumatic cases result from severe hypoxia/ischaemia of the brain following cardiac arrest, near drowning, or strangulation, whilst a few result from severe hypoglycaemia in diabetics. Other causes are acute intracranial haemorrhage or infection. In adults the vegetative state can evolve gradually during the late stages of chronic dementing conditions, and in children can result from severe congenital malformations of the brain or from progressive metabolic or chromosomal diseases affecting the brain.

At autopsy after acute hypoxic insults there is commonly a widespread loss of cortical neurones. After acute traumatic and non-traumatic damage leading to vegetative survival there is almost always severe bilateral thalamic damage, whilst the cortex may be relatively spared. There is also progressive degeneration over many months of neurones and nerve fibres and their myelin sheaths remote from the site of initial damage, which is reflected during life in progressive enlargement of the ventricles as visualized by computed tomography or magnetic resonance imaging. Findings on the electroencephalogram are variable, but there is often loss of evoked cortical responses to somatic stimuli. Positron emission tomography shows severe depression of glucose metabolism in cortical grey matter, to levels found only in experimental deep barbiturate narcosis.

Diagnosis

In practice the diagnosis depends on characteristic clinical features recorded by skilled observers over a period of time. The patient has long periods of spontaneous eye opening (hence the inappropriateness of calling this condition irreversible or prolonged coma). The eyes may briefly follow a moving object or the head turn reflexly to a sudden noise that may also produce a startle reaction. All four limbs are paralysed and usually spastic, with only reflex posturing and withdrawal from a painful stimulus, and often there is a grasp reflex. The face may grimace and groans may be heard but never words. There is no psychologically meaningful response to external stimuli or any learned behaviour—no evidence of a working mind. There may be emotional behaviours such as smiling, crying, or laughing but these are not related to appropriate external stimuli. It is concluded that although awake these patients are not aware and do not suffer distress or pain. Misdiagnosis by non-experts is not uncommon, and care is needed to exclude the minimally conscious state in which there are very limited responses indicating some cognitive activity. It must also be ascertained that the patient does not have the locked-in syndrome, due to brainstem damage resulting in full awareness but widespread paralysis, leaving the patient able to communicate only by a yes/no code using the sole remaining motor power, blinking the eyelids or moving the eyes.

Prognosis

Patients in a vegetative state for some time can still make some recovery, and persistent does not mean permanent. Of patients in the vegetative state 1 month after an acute insult, about half of the head injured will regain some consciousness, but only a few of the non-traumatic cases do. Most who recover consciousness remain very severely disabled and dependent, particularly if they have been vegetative for several months. After head injury permanence cannot be declared until 12 months, but after non-traumatic insults after 6 months according to United Kingdom criteria and 3 months in the United States. There is a high mortality in the first year after becoming vegetative but once this period is survived patients can live for many years, if tube feeding and good nursing care is maintained and infective complications actively treated.

Action after permanence declared

There is now a consensus in many countries that survival for years in a permanent vegetative state is of no benefit to the patient, and that it is therefore appropriate to withdraw life-sustaining treatment once permanence is declared. Many courts in the United States and the United Kingdom have agreed that artificial nutrition and hydration is medical treatment that can be withdrawn if judged to be no longer of benefit to the patient. Once this is done a peaceful death occurs in 8 to 12 days, and the cause of death is regarded as the original brain damage. Only in the United Kingdom is it a legal requirement to seek court approval before withdrawing such treatment, although this situation is under review.

Further reading

Brain death

Conference of the Medical Royal Colleges and their Faculties in the United Kingdom (1976). Diagnosis of brain death. *British Medical Journal* **2**, 1187–8.

Conference of the Medical Royal Colleges and their Faculties in the United Kingdom (1979). Diagnosis of death. *British Medical Journal* **1**, 322. [Original descriptions of United Kingdom criteria for brainstem death.]

Health Departments of Great Britain and Northern Ireland (1998). *A code of practice for the diagnosis of brain stem death.* Department of Health, London. [Most recent United Kingdom update.]

Quality Standards Sub-committee of the American Academy of Neurology (1995). Practice parameters for determining brain death in adults. *Neurology* **45**, 1012–14. [Widely accepted United States criteria.]

Youngner SJ, Arnold RM, Shapiro R, eds (1999). *The definition of death.* Johns Hopkins University Press, Baltimore. [Review of controversies, clinical, ethical, legal and social—primarily from an American viewpoint.]

Vegetative state

Adams JH, Graham DI, Jennett B (2000). The neuropathology of the vegetative state after an acute brain insult. *Brain* **123**, 1327–38. [Detailed pathology of 35 traumatic and 14 non-traumatic cases.]

Jennett B (2002). *The vegetative state: medical facts, ethical and legal dilemmas.* Cambridge University Press, Cambridge.[Review of medical facts, ethical issues and details of legal cases in several countries.]

Multi-Society Task Force on PVS (1994). Medical aspects of the persistent vegetative state. *New England Journal of Medicine* **330**, 1499–507, 1572–9. [Review of world literature and prognostic data from an American perspective.]

Quality Standard Sub-Committee of the American Academy of Neurology (1995). Practice parameters: assessment and management of patients in PVS. *Neurology* **45**, 1015–18. [Most recent American criteria.]

Wade DT and Johnston C (1999). The permanent vegetative state: practical guidance on diagnosis and management. *British Medical Journal* **319**, 841–4 (see also Editorial by B Jennett on pp 796–7). [Recent United Kingdom review.]

24.13.7 Stroke: cerebrovascular disease

J. van Gijn

Introduction

Cerebrovascular diseases include many pathological conditions: two main categories being infarction, (through occlusion of major arteries, small arteries, or venous sinuses) and haemorrhage (through rupture of small arteries, arterial aneurysms, or capillaries). Intracerebral haemorrhage was first recorded by the Swiss physician Wepfer, and in more detail by Morgagni in Padua. Non-haemorrhagic stroke, 'serious apoplexy', puzzled the medical community until cerebral softening ('ramollissement') was recognized as a pathological entity in 1820 by Rostan in Paris. Initially it was regarded as an inflammatory condition. The relationship of brain softening with arterial occlusion and atherosclerosis gradually dawned on pathologists in the nineteenth century when it was firmly established by Rokitansky and Virchow. Subarachnoid haemorrhages and their usual source, intracranial aneurysms, were first recognized at the beginning of the nineteenth century; the diagnosis could (sometimes) be made during life from the beginning of the twentieth century. In 1931 the Edinburgh neurosurgeon Norman Dott carried out the first intracranial operation for a ruptured aneurysm, by wrapping it in muscle.

Knowledge of cerebrovascular disease has received great impetus from the advent of computed tomography (**CT**) scanning. Previously, observations depended on postmortem studies and on indirect neuroradiological studies such as angiography and pneumoencephalography. CT scanning has allowed the rapid and reliable distinction between haemorrhagic and ischaemic stroke during life. Subsequently, CT and the newer technique of magnetic resonance imaging (**MRI**) have identified several subtypes of stroke, each requiring specific therapeutic measures. Examples are lacunar infarction, intracranial venous thrombosis, arterial dissection, and complications after aneurysm rupture (rebleeding, ischaemia, or hydrocephalus). The rapid increase in diagnostic accuracy coincided with dissemination of the randomized clinical trial and other methodological innovations in medicine. As a result, stroke research is no longer a backwater of medicine but a bustling area.

The consequences of stroke are often devastating. A sudden loss of a large amount of brain tissue affects much more than specific, localizable functions such as movement, sensation, vision, and language. The greater part of the brain has no defined task, but serves to connect and integrate the separate 'functions'. Mood, initiative, sense of humour, and speed of thought are examples of essential aspects of human life that can be severely affected by stroke, but which are often sadly ignored. There are no 'silent' areas in the brain that can be damaged with impunity.

Epidemiology of stroke

Worldwide, stroke is the third most common cause of death after coronary heart disease and all cancer deaths, and stroke is the most important single cause of disability in the Western world. Although the incidence of stroke is not technically difficult to measure, it does require the expenditure of much time and resources. The few reliable studies, mostly from developed countries, show that age- and sex-standardized annual incidence rates for subjects aged 45 to 84 years are between 300 and 500 per 100 000. The pathological type varies, even between studies with a high rate of CT scanning, but a general estimate is 82 per cent infarction, 15 per cent primary intracerebral haemorrhage, and 3 per cent subarachnoid haemorrhage. The incidence of transient ischaemic attacks (**TIAs**) has been rather consistently estimated at 35 per 100 000 of the entire population, or about 80 per 100 000 of subjects between 45 and 84 years of age.

In terms of an average general practice of 2400 people (1000 patients between 45 and 84 years of age), four patients will have a stroke per annum, whilst one will have a TIA. Intracerebral haemorrhage will occur about twice every 3 years, and subarachnoid haemorrhage once every 8 years.

Arterial occlusive disease

The cerebral circulation and its disorders

Brain tissue is critically dependent upon a constant supply of oxygen and glucose. The cerebral blood flow (800 ml/min) accounts for 15 to 20 per cent of the entire cardiac output, whereas the brain (1350 g) accounts for only 2 per cent of the adult body weight. Neurones in the brain require a constant supply of ATP to maintain concentration gradients of ions across their membranes, necessary for the generation of action potentials. The resting brain consumes energy at the same rate as a 20-Watt light bulb.

Whether occlusion of an artery in the brain or in the neck actually leads to ischaemia depends on collateral pathways. If an end artery is occluded and there is no collateral circulation at all, ischaemic symptoms will occur within seconds. Neurones will start dying within minutes, and within hours the entire supply area of the artery will be irreversibly damaged. In contrast, permanent occlusion of a major artery, such as the internal carotid artery, may be symptomless in the presence of an adequate collateral circulation. Broadly speaking, three levels of collateral circulation can be distinguished (Fig. 1; these can be thought of as three lines of defence):

1. *The circle of Willis* (Fig. 2). Even if there is no blood whatsoever flowing to the brain from one or even both internal carotid arteries, collateral flow from the other internal carotid artery or from the basilar artery, via an intact circle of Willis, may ensure an adequate blood supply in the territory of the occluded artery.
2. *Connections between extracranial and intracranial vessels.* If the internal carotid artery is occluded at its origin, collateral channels may develop via the external carotid artery. Branches supplying the outer orbit may connect with branches to the retina, resulting in a reversed flow in the ophthalmic artery. From there, blood reaches the distal part of the internal carotid artery. Similarly, branches of occipital arteries (normally supplying the neck muscles) may fill the basilar artery if this is occluded at its origin.
3. *Leptomeningeal anastomoses.* If, for example, the main stem of the middle cerebral artery is occluded, its terminal branches at the surface of the brain may anastomose with similar branches of the anterior and posterior cerebral arteries; in this way the cerebral cortex in the territory of the occluded artery is spared, partly or wholly, although the deep territory will still be ischaemic.

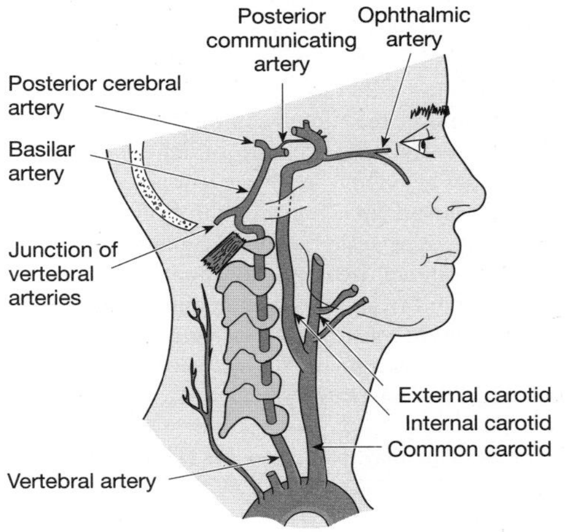

Fig. 1 Arterial supply of the brain. The drawing shows, on the right side, the internal carotid artery, external carotid artery, and vertebral artery. If a main artery is occluded then collateral flow may occur via the circle of Willis (see also Fig. 2

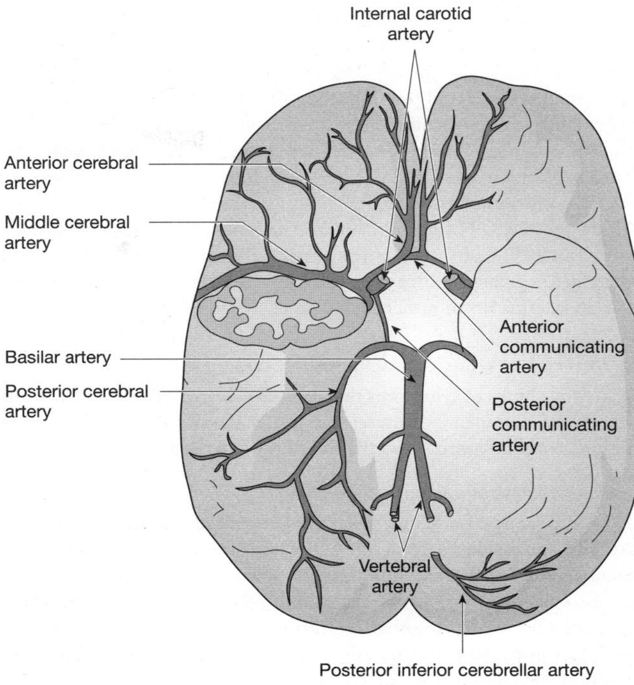

Fig. 2 The arterial circle of Willis, at the base of the brain.

Atherothrombosis is the major cause of occlusion of the major arteries in the brain or in the neck. However, two important qualifications should be made. First, atherosclerosis of the intracranial arteries is relatively uncommon, at least in White people (other than in Black or Oriental people). This means that brain infarction in the West is usually caused by an embolism, in which a thrombus has been dislodged from an upstream lesion. The source can be the internal carotid artery, the aorta, or the heart. Second, atherosclerosis is not a sufficient cause in itself: not everyone with severe atherosclerotic disease suffers an ischaemic stroke. Other factors are irregularity of the plaque, turbulence of blood, platelet aggregation, and the balance of clotting factors.

Diagnosis of transient ischaemic attacks

Transient ischaemic attacks are important to diagnose because they are potential harbingers of stroke. They precede cerebral infarction probably in only 15 to 20 per cent of cases (it is difficult to be certain of the figure because almost all such information has been retrospectively collected in patients once they had suffered a stroke).

Unfortunately the term 'transient ischaemic attack' is rather imprecise, because it tacitly implies three restrictions. To begin with, it refers only to the brain and not to angina pectoris or intermittent claudication. Also excluded is transient ischaemia of the entire brain, for example in syncope or ventricular fibrillation. It is only ischaemia of a part of the brain that is conventionally covered by the term 'TIA'. Finally, how transient is transient? Traditionally the limit has been set at 24 h. Obviously this threshold has more to do with astronomy than with biology or disease. In fact, most TIAs last minutes, not hours. The longer an attack lasts, the greater the chance that CT scanning afterwards will show a relevant ischaemic lesion. In terms of patient management the essential question is not whether the attack has lasted 3 min, 3 days, or 3 weeks, but what its cause is and how recurrences can be prevented.

What actually happens in the brain during a given period of ischaemia can often only be guessed at. The usual assumption is that an embolus, consisting of platelets or loosely organized thrombus, temporarily blocks an intracerebral vessel and then dissolves into smaller fragments. There is scant evidence for this phenomenon, apart from chance observations during fundoscopy, angiography, or operation. Other explanations, applicable only to a minority of cases, include marginal flow, secondary to severe narrowing or occlusion of arteries.

The diagnosis of a TIA is problematic. That one has to rely on the history alone is a first difficulty (it requires time, skill, and patience), but not a unique one. A greater source of interobserver variation is that the term 'TIA' is an interpretation rather than a description.

Main varieties of transient ischaemic attacks

There are four kinds of symptoms that can safely be regarded as TIAs, given that the onset is sudden (within seconds), that all symptoms appear at the same time, without 'march', and that there is no better explanation.

Transient weakness of one half of the body

Apart from weakness there may also have been numbness. Isolated numbness or pins and needles on one side of the body are a rare manifestation of transient cerebral ischaemia; other causes such as overbreathing are more likely. Weakness and numbness are closely related perceptions, and one should not take these or other expressions ('an arm gone dead') for granted. It is important to make sure the problem had to do with moving the limbs or the face on one side (facial weakness on one side often manifests itself through slurred speech or drooling), and not with what it felt like when those body parts were touched or with spontaneous sensations. It is also critical to verify that the problem occurred in at least two of three body areas, and that, in the elderly, it was not just a leg or arm that had 'gone to sleep' after a mid-day nap. All four limbs may be affected at the same time in TIAs of the brainstem.

Transient loss of the ability to find words or to understand them

The medical term for this type of TIA is 'dysphasia' or 'aphasia'; the problem here is not that patients and relatives may not recognize the episode as representing a problem of language, but describe the attack as 'confusion'. It is helpful to ask specific questions about the patient's ability to put thoughts into words (motor dysphasia), and about having been able to understand what was said (sensory dysphasia). If a patient can write sentences but cannot speak, the cause is almost certainly psychological. A frequent problem is the distinction between dysphasia (disorder of language) and dysarthria (disorder of articulation). To ask whether pronunciation was difficult may not be very helpful. After all, in both cases the patient's thoughts are clear and the difference between finding the right words and forming the right sounds is not great. A useful question is whether the words made sense and whether they were in the right order. Dysphasia relates to the left hemisphere in right-handed people, and in 50 per cent of left-handers.

Transient loss of vision in one eye

The difficulty in this case is to distinguish transient monocular blindness from the loss of vision on one side in both eyes (hemianopia). Either type of attack can be experienced as a problem in one eye. The distinction is not academic, as monocular attacks of blindness should lead to investigation of the internal carotid artery in the neck with a view to angiography and operation, whereas hemianopia mostly (in 80 per cent) reflects a disorder in the posterior circulation, in which case treatment will often be medical. The vital question to ask is whether patients have alternately covered each eye during the attack. A surprisingly large proportion of patients have done so, but they will not always offer this information without prompting. On having covered the 'good eye' in case of hemianopia, the patient should still have been able to see with the 'bad eye', though only the nasal half of the visual field. With a monocular disorder the blindness should have been complete.

Table 1 Attacks that should **not** be regarded as TIAs

Any attack with loss of consciousness
Any attack with involuntary jerking
Any attack with positive visual phenomena (bright lights, etc.)
Any attack with *only*:
numbness
dizziness (with or without spinning sensations)
double vision
slurred speech
unsteady walking

Transient loss of vision in one hemifield

Hemianopia reflects dysfunction of the occipital lobe. It is also a common aura in migraine attacks, which may occur without ensuing headache, especially in the elderly. It is therefore important for the physician to enquire about the mode of onset: flashing lights, bright colours, zig-zag lines, and a gradually expanding deficit all argue in favour of a migrainous attack rather than ischaemia in its restricted sense of a stroke warning.

Differential diagnosis of transient ischaemic attacks

Table 1 lists the types of attacks that should not be regarded as TIAs, either because of positive phenomena (such as rhythmic jerking) that are incompatible with the definition of focal ischaemia, or because other causes are much more likely. Especially the tendency to label any episode of 'dizziness' in the elderly as 'vertebrobasilar ischaemia' or, even worse, 'vertebrobasilar insufficiency' should be strongly resisted.

In addition, some specific disorders other than atherosclerosis may cause attacks that are more or less indistinguishable from true TIAs as defined above. They are listed in Table 2. These rare, but important, causes are reason enough for ordering a CT or MRI scan of the brain in patients with cerebral TIAs (not necessarily in those with transient monocular blindness). A chronic subdural haematoma should always be suspected in the elderly, especially if they are taking anticoagulants. Hypoglycaemia should come to mind in diabetic patients. Focal weakness may follow an epileptic seizure (Todd's paralysis) and may be misdiagnosed as TIA if the initial jerking is missed or misinterpreted. Tumours may also cause temporary deficits without focal epilepsy. Transient global amnesia is a disorder of memory probably caused by migrainous vasospasm; although technically ischaemic in nature, it is not associated with an increased risk of stroke or other vascular disease.

Prognostic implications of transient ischaemic attacks

In a population-based study of 184 patients in the United Kingdom after they had one or more TIAs, the actuarial risk of stroke was 12 per cent during the first year after a TIA (13-fold excess risk) and approximately 6 per cent per annum over the subsequent 5 years (sevenfold excess risk). The actuarial risk of death, stroke, or myocardial infarction over the first 5 years after a TIA was between 8 and 9 per cent per annum. Heart disease and stroke each accounted for about one-third of all deaths. Given that most of these patients were treated with aspirin, which reduces the rate of vascular events after cerebral ischaemia by about 15 per cent (see below), the risk of stroke without treatment can be estimated at 14 per cent in the first year and 7 per cent in subsequent years, and the average risk of death, stroke, or myocardial infarction in the first 5 years at 10 per cent per annum. In individual patients, these average risks will be modified by their

Table 2 Disorders that may mimic genuine TIAs

Chronic subdural haematoma
Intracranial tumour (glioma, metastasis, meningioma)
Hypoglycaemia
Focal deficits following a partial epileptic seizure
Transient global amnesia
Myasthenia gravis

age, specific risk factors, coexistent disease, and the interval since their first attack.

Investigations in patients with cerebral ischaemia

There is no great difference between searching for the cause of a TIA and searching for the cause of an ischaemic stroke. Very early CT or MRI scanning is mandatory: mainly to exclude intracerebral haemorrhage and the occasional structural lesion mimicking stroke, not so much to demonstrate infarcts. Table 3 lists the major and contributory causes of TIA and ischaemic stroke, with corresponding investigations. In general, first-line investigations are: a full blood count; erythrocyte sedimentation rate (**ESR**); plasma glucose, creatinine, and electrolytes; plasma lipids; treponemal antibodies; urinalysis; ECG; and unenhanced CT scan of the brain.

Table 3 Major or contributory 'causes' of TIA or ischaemic stroke, with corresponding investigations

Causal factors	Appropriate investigation
Arterial atheroma	
Internal carotid artery in the neck	Duplex ultrasound study[*]
Intracranial arteries	Angiogram (with MR, CT, or catheter)
Small-vessel disease	–
Aorta	Transoesophageal echography
Other arterial disease	
Congenital arterial anomalies	Angiogram (with MR, CT, or catheter)
Moya-moya syndrome	Angiogram (with MR, CT, or catheter)
Arterial dissection	MRI; angiogram (with MR, CT, or catheter)
Giant-cell arteritis[§]	ESR[*], temporal artery biopsy[*]
Systemic vasculitis	Antinuclear antibody[*], tissue biopsy[*]
Embolization from arterial aneurysms	MRI; angiogram (with MR, CT, or catheter)
Cholesterol embolization syndrome	Biopsy of skin, muscle, or kidney
Meningitis, encephalitis	Cerebrospinal fluid[*], brain biopsy[*]
Drugs of abuse	Toxicological screening of urine
Genetic conditions (MELAS, CADASIL, Fabry's disease)	Analysis of mitochondrial or nuclear DNA, alpha-galactosidase A[*]
Irradiation	–
Migraine	–
Embolism from the heart	
Atrial fibrillation	ECG[*]; long-term monitoring of heart rhythm[*]
Recent myocardial infarction	ECG[*]
Rheumatic valvular disease	Echocardiogram[*]
Infective endocarditis	Echocardiogram[*], blood cultures[*]
Open foramen ovale	Venography[*], echocardiogram
Atrial myxoma	Echocardiogram[*]
Haemostatic factors	
Polycythaemia	Haematocrit[*]
Sickle-cell disease	Peripheral blood smear, sickling test
Thrombocytosis	Platelet count[*]
Leukaemia	White cell count[*], morphological analysis[*]
Disseminated intravascular coagulation	Platelet count, prothrombin and activated partial thromboplastin times, fibrinogen, fibrinogen degradation products, D-dimers
Contributing risk factors	
Hypertension	Serial measurement of blood pressure[*]
Diabetes	Fasting glucose[*]
Hypercholesterolaemia	Plasma cholesterol[*]
Hyperhomocystinaemia	Plasma homocysteine level[*]

[*] Investigations with implications for management, either evidence-based or possible.

[§] Only with involvement of the optic nerve or occipital lobe.

CT, computed tomography; ECG, electrocardiogram; ESR, erythrocyte sedimentation rate; MR(I), magnetic resonance (imaging).

Diagnosis of cerebral infarction

Distinction from other types of stroke

From a practical point of view, the first step is to distinguish ischaemic stroke from intracerebral haemorrhage. In the past, when a certain distinction could be made only at operation or autopsy, a decreased level of consciousness and headache were considered typical of intracerebral haemorrhage. After CT scanning became available in the 1970s, it was soon clear that smaller haemorrhages were not associated with headache and drowsiness. Given that 3 out of 20 strokes are haemorrhagic, and on the assumption that two-thirds of all haemorrhages lack distinctive clinical features, a diagnosis of cerebral infarction based on clinical features alone is wrong in every tenth case on average. Even complex clinical scoring methods can hardly improve on this error rate.

CT scanning

Acute parenchymal haemorrhage is of a higher density than normal brain tissue on CT scanning (see Fig. 6). The hyperdensity occurs immediately and is caused by the iron molecules in haemoglobin. Signs of infarction are more difficult to detect at an early stage: in the first decade of CT scanning this was not possible until after 3 days, when frank tissue necrosis caused a hypodense lesion on the scan. With improved CT technology, subtle early signs of cerebral infarction have been recognized, at least with a large area of infarction. These features include loss of outline of the insular ribbon and the lentiform nucleus (Fig. 3), loss of normal differentiation between grey and white matter, and effacement of cortical sulci.

Within the first few days, the area of infarction changes into a slightly hypodense, ill-defined, and somewhat swollen lesion on CT scanning, to become more clearly demarcated and hypodense towards the end of the first week (Fig. 3). Occasionally there may be massive swelling with brain herniation, or haemorrhagic transformation. During the second week the infarct may again gradually increase in density, because the degradation products of necrotic brain tissue more readily absorb X-rays. In the third and fourth week the infarcted area may even become isodense, thereby almost indistinguishable from normal brain, the so-called 'fogging effect'. Eventually a sharply demarcated, atrophic, hypodense (similar to cerebrospinal fluid) defect remains. It is not always possible to tell with certainty how old an infarct is, nor to distinguish it from the scar of a haemorrhage that occurred weeks or years before. Intravenous injection of X-ray contrast will, in the first week, cause some enhancement of gyri (if the lesion involves the cortex).

The proportion of patients in whom CT scanning shows an appropriate infarct depends not only on the time of scanning and the generation of the scanner, but also on the size of the infarct and on its location. With serial CT scanning, eventually more than 90 per cent of infarcts show up.

Magnetic resonance imaging

MRI is especially useful for demonstrating small infarcts and lesions in the posterior fossa; it is also more sensitive than CT scanning in the early phases of brain ischaemia. Signal changes on *T*2-weighted images occur after 6 to 8 h, and on *T*1-weighted images after 16 h. Infarcts of any size are more often and more quickly visible on fluid-attenuated inversion recovery (**FLAIR**) scans and on diffusion-weighted imaging, but these techniques are not widely available. The distinction from intracerebral haemorrhage is less obvious than on CT, but the paramagnetic effects of deoxyhaemoglobin can be identified after a few hours.

Classification of cerebral infarction

Time was often the guiding principle in the classification of stroke in the era before brain imaging and its positive effects on the accuracy of clinical diagnosis. From the point of view of management and prognosis, however, it is rather irrelevant to distinguish 'progressive stroke' from 'completed stroke', or 'permanent stroke' from 'reversible ischaemic neurological deficit' (**RIND**, a kind of 'extended TIA' with complete recovery within 3 or 6 weeks, depending on local convention). What counts is the eventual severity of the functional deficit and, conversely, what remaining function is at stake.

The anatomical classification distinguishes infarcts according to the territory of major cerebral arteries: in the cerebral hemispheres infarcts can be located in the supply areas of the anterior cerebral artery, middle cerebral artery, posterior cerebral artery, or in the border zones between these three main branches; the cerebellum and brainstem are supplied by the vertebral arteries, basilar artery, and their branches. Problems are that there is little if any relationship with function, that there is no distinction between partial and complete infarcts in a given territory, and that the boundaries between different territories vary substantially between individuals.

Classification according to the cause of ischaemic stroke is of interest for studies aiming to describe or influence the pathophysiological background

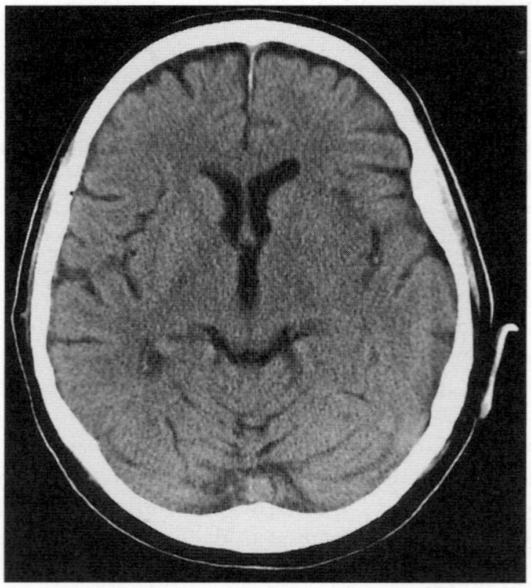

(a)

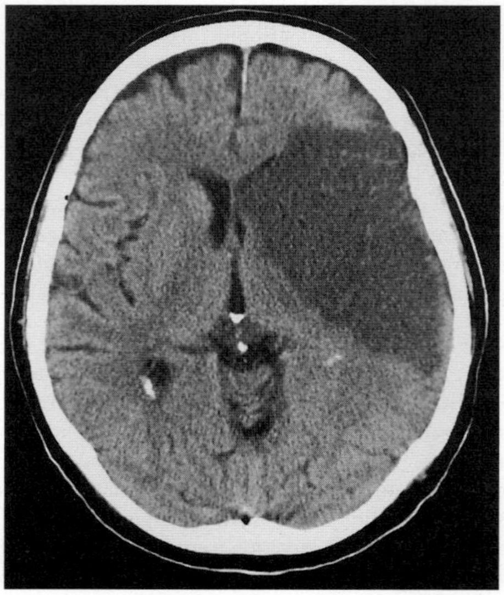

(b)

Fig. 3 Acute cerebral infarction in a 78-year-old man. (a) CT scan about 6 h after symptom onset. In the left brain hemisphere (on the reader's right) there are subtle changes in the region of the basal ganglia: other than on the normal side, it is difficult to distinguish the different brain nuclei and their separation by white matter. (b) CT scan 4 days after symptom onset shows marked hypodensity in the entire territory of the left middle cerebral artery.

of strokes. The so-called 'TOAST (Trial of Org 10172 in Acute Stroke Treatment) classification', for example, distinguishes five subtypes of ischaemic stroke:

(1) large-artery atherosclerosis;

(2) cardioembolism;

(3) small-vessel occlusion;

(4) stroke with other specific cause; and

(5) stroke with undetermined cause.

At present, about 40 per cent of patients would presently end up in the category 'undetermined cause', even in specialized stroke services. Moreover, these distinctions can only be applied after a few days in hospital. Finally, and most important, the system is not suited for assessing the severity of stroke.

Rehabilitation specialists and geriatricians will be more interested in the functional abilities of patients than in the niceties of neurological nosology. They mostly grade patients' disability on a scale for activities of daily life (such as the Barthel scale, which ranks 10 in-house activities in hierarchical order, from bowel continence to taking a bath), or on a scale that includes some elements of social role fulfilment ('handicap'), such as the Rankin scale (Table 4).

A system that strikes a useful compromise between the functional and the anatomical point of view is the classification of the Oxfordshire Community Stroke Project, which distinguishes four categories:

(1) total anterior circulation infarcts (**TACI**), with both cortical and subcortical involvement, representing about one-sixth of all ischaemic strokes in the community;

(2) partial anterior circulation infarcts (**PACI**), with more restricted and predominantly cortical infarcts (one-third of all infarcts);

(3) posterior circulation infarcts (**POCI**), clearly associated with the vertebrobasilar arterial territory (one-quarter); and

(4) lacunar anterior circulation infarcts (**LACI**), confined to the territory of the deep perforating arteries (one-quarter).

Although the classes are anatomically defined, they contain important prognostic information: case fatality is highest by far in the TACI group.

Syndromes of cerebral infarction

Occlusion of the internal carotid artery may cause no symptoms at all or infarction in the entire territory of the ipsilateral anterior and middle cerebral artery (and sometimes of the posterior cerebral artery or contralateral anterior cerebral artery as well), depending on the presence of a complete circle of Willis and other collaterals. If arterial dissection is the cause of carotid occlusion, subadventitial bulging of the artery may cause Horner's syndrome and lower cranial nerve palsies, with or without infarction. Occlusion of the anterior, middle, and posterior cerebral arteries may lead

Table 4 Modified Rankin scale for measuring outcome, for example after stroke (but not exclusively so)

Grade	Description
0	No symptoms
1	Minor symptoms that do not interfere with lifestyle
2	Symptoms that lead to some restriction of lifestyle but do not interfere with the patient's capacity to look after himself
3	Symptoms that restrict lifestyle and prevent totally independent existence
4	Symptoms that clearly prevent independent existence, although no constant attention is required
5	Totally dependent patient requiring constant attention, night and day

to complete or partial infarction in their respective territories, depending on collaterals at the surface of the brain. Obviously, branch occlusions cause smaller infarcts. What follows is a description of syndromes associated with complete infarction in the average territory of the main cerebral arteries.

Infarcts in the area of the anterior cerebral artery

These cause contralateral hemiparesis more marked in the leg than in the arm, with no or only mild sensory deficit. Other frontal lobe features include mutism, incontinence, and apathy or, conversely, disinhibition.

Middle cerebral artery infarcts

If complete, these typically present with contralateral hemiplegia (most marked in the arm), sensory deficit, hemianopia, and cognitive defects such as aphasia (dominant hemisphere) or contralateral neglect (non-dominant hemisphere). Massive infarction of the entire territory of the middle cerebral artery may lead to such a degree of brain swelling that fatal herniation occurs, especially in young patients without cerebral atrophy.

Occlusion of a vertebral artery

Where this involves the origin of the posterior inferior cerebellar artery, such occlusion causes Wallenberg's syndrome, with ipsilateral cerebellar ataxia through infarction of the inferior part of the cerebellum. In addition, it causes a slightly bewildering combination of deficits through infarction of the dorsolateral medulla: decreased skin sensation in the ipsilateral half of the face and the contralateral half of the body, ipsilateral Horner's syndrome, ipsilateral weakness of the soft palate, larynx and pharynx, and rotatory vertigo.

Basilar artery syndrome

The full basilar artery syndrome, with infarction of most of the pons and midbrain, consists of coma, tetraparesis including facial movements, and loss of all eye movements and of pupillary and corneal reflexes. There are two characteristic partial syndromes of the basilar artery. One is the locked-in syndrome (infarction of the base of the pons), with tetraparesis including facial movements and loss of horizontal eye movements. Consciousness is preserved through sparing of the reticular formation, but patients can communicate only through vertical eye movements; these may not always be correctly interpreted or even noticed. The other is the top-of-the-basilar syndrome, with variable combinations of hemianopia or complete cortical blindness (occipital lobes), amnesia (inferior temporal lobes), as well as vertical gaze palsies, pupillary disturbances, and hallucinations (perforating branches to the midbrain).

Posterior cerebral artery syndrome

This may include hemianopia (occipital lobe), amnesia (lower temporal lobe), and oculomotor disorders or disturbances of language or visuospatial function, through the involvement of perforating branches to the thalamus.

Occlusion of a single perforating artery

Such an occlusion, of one of the many arterioles that originate at right angles from a large parent artery to supply a small area in the deep regions of the brain or brainstem (Fig. 4), may be clinically silent, or cause a so-called 'lacunar syndrome'. A necessary condition for the clinical diagnosis of a lacunar syndrome is the absence of 'cortical' deficits, such as aphasia, neglect, hemianopia, and conjugate deviation of the eyes. The most common and archetypal form is pure motor stroke. In these cases the small, deep infarct strategically involves corticospinal fibres (pyramidal tract) to the motor neurones of the limbs, anywhere in its course. Analogous fibres to the facial nucleus in the pons may be affected as well. The infarct can be located in the corona radiata, adjoining the wall of the body of the lateral ventricle, or slightly more caudally, in the posterior limb of the internal capsule, or, less commonly, in the pons or the medulla. Other 'lacunar syndromes' are sensorimotor stroke (corona radiata or internal capsule), pure sensory stroke (thalamus), and ataxic hemiparesis (usually the base of the pons). Lacunar infarcts in the brainstem may lead to an almost infinite range of syndromes, often with the name of a French nineteenth century neurologist attached to it. Often such syndromes consist of an ipsilateral cranial nerve deficit and a contralateral hemiparesis.

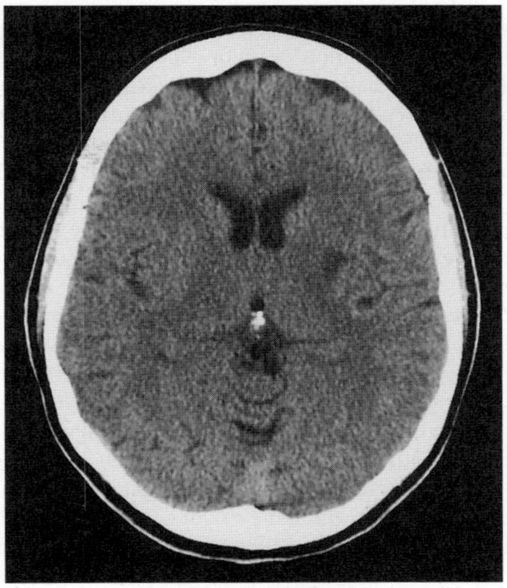

Fig. 4 Small, deep infarct ('lacune') in a 63-year-old woman. CT scanning shows a small area of hypodensity (distinct from sulci) in the left brain hemisphere (on the reader's right), just lateral to the internal capsule.

Treatment of acute cerebral infarction

Several medical interventions aim at dissolving the occluding clot, or at least preventing it from growing: thrombolysis, antiplatelet agents, and anticoagulants. A different strategy, not yet well developed, is to protect ischaemic brain tissue. In addition, some underlying causes of stroke need urgent treatment, such as endocarditis. Before considering these specific measures, it is appropriate to consider the appropriate hospital setting in which stroke patients should be cared for.

Stroke units versus general wards

Specially organized stroke units can be a ward or team that exclusively manages stroke patients (a dedicated stroke unit) or a ward or team that provides a generic disability service (a mixed-assessment or rehabilitation unit). According to a meta-analysis of 20 randomized trials, care in a stroke unit reduces the risk of death or institutionalized care by 13 per cent. The observed benefits are independent of patient age, sex, stroke severity, and types of stroke-unit organization. No single element responsible for the benefits of organized stroke care has so far been identified, and probably there is none. The strength of stroke units lies in the integration of multidisciplinary efforts: stroke physician, nursing staff, physiotherapists, occupational therapists, speech therapists, rehabilitation physicians, and social workers.

Thrombolysis

Restoration of blood flow, to reperfuse the ischaemic brain as soon as possible after the cerebral artery has been occluded, and irrespective of its cause, should theoretically lead to a reduction in the volume of brain damaged by ischaemia and to an improvement in clinical outcome, analogous to myocardial infarction.

The main agents tested so far in the treatment of stroke (17 trials in over 5000 patients) are intravenous recombinant tissue plasminogen activator (**r-tPA**) and intravenous streptokinase, each in about half the patients. Almost all were treated within 6 h of stroke onset. Across all trials there was an excess of symptomatic intracranial haemorrhages (3 per cent in controls versus 10 per cent in treated patients). For every 1000 patients treated this corresponds to 70 extra intracranial haemorrhages, of which 44 are fatal.

However, patients who survived the treatment were, on average, less disabled. For the outcome criterion 'death or dependence at the end of follow up' (3 months for most trials) the proportion was 59 per cent in the control group and 55 per cent among treated patients. This corresponds to a net gain of about 40 patients avoiding death or dependency for every 1000 patients treated with thrombolysis within 6 h, despite the excess haemorrhages.

There are still many unanswered questions about the role of thrombolysis in the treatment of ischaemic stroke. The first of these is the time window. The earlier treatment is given the better, which is confirmed by subgroup analysis of patients treated within 3 h, but inevitably this subgroup is biased towards more severe strokes (these get to hospital quickest). Second, is one agent better than another? For r-tPA alone, the balance of risks and benefits seems more favourable than for all agents together: per 1000 patients treated, an excess of 30 fatal intracranial haemorrhages, and a net result of 60 patients avoiding death or dependence, but the difference with streptokinase treatment is not statistically significant. Third, we can roughly identify patients in whom the risk of haemorrhage in the infarcted tissue is great (those with the most severe deficits and those with early signs of extensive infarction), but the potential benefits are also greatest in this group. More controlled studies are needed. Another question is whether the gains in patients with stroke are not offset by unbalancing the 'worried well' who will be also rushed to hospital, once stroke has been recognized as an emergency. There are many contraindications in view of the risk of cerebral haemorrhage, and only a minority of patients admitted with cerebral infarction can be treated with thrombolysis.

Antiplatelet agents

More than 99 per cent of the evidence from randomized trials in this area relates to the use of aspirin. The pooled results of two trials with aspirin (160–300 mg), started within 48 h of the onset of stroke, concluded that 13 fewer patients die or become dependent for every 1000 patients treated. There was no evidence of a net hazard in some 800 patients who had been inadvertently randomized after a haemorrhagic stroke. Only the combination with thrombolytic treatment should be avoided, because there are indications that aspirin enhances the danger of intracerebral haemorrhage.

Anticoagulants

Anticoagulants tested in clinical trials are standard unfractionated heparin, low molecular weight heparins, heparinoids, oral anticoagulants, and thrombin inhibitors. There is no evidence that anticoagulant therapy reduces the odds of being dead or dependent at the end of follow-up.

Neuroprotective agents

There are many steps in the destructive cascade between vessel occlusion and irreversible cell death where pharmacological intervention might be beneficial, at least theoretically. The pharmaceutical industry has developed several compounds for clinical development and testing. There is no doubt that in animal models many neuroprotective agents, given either before or after the onset of ischaemia, reduce the area of cerebral infarction. So far, none of these agents has been proven to reduce disability in patients, despite dozens of clinical trials. Many other trials are under way, but reduction of disability by neuroprotective drugs is likely to be modest at best.

Surgical decompression of space-occupying infarcts

To prevent brain herniation, some centres in Germany have adopted the procedure of removing large parts of the skull vault in patients with massive supratentorial infarction, but all reports up to now have been uncontrolled. Clearly there is a need for randomized trials, which should take account of the quality of life of both patients and their carers.

With operations for space-occupying infarcts of the cerebellum there is a similar lack of controlled trials, but less controversy. Without operation, swelling of a cerebellar infarct can be fatal, whereas the deficits after surgical evacuation are surprisingly mild. In many patients, however, it is sufficient to relieve obstructive hydrocephalus, by external ventricular drainage.

Secondary prevention of ischaemic stroke

In the management of patients with TIAs or moderately disabling ischaemic strokes, it is often forgotten that the control of primary risk factors is by far the most effective way of diminishing the risk of stroke or other vascular events. First and foremost is blood pressure control, but also important are cessation of smoking, controlling diabetes and hyperlipidaemia, reducing overweight, and daily exercise.

Specific measures to reduce the risk of threatened stroke are discussed below. Drug treatment depends on whether the likely cause is embolism from the heart or arterial disease. With sources in the heart, mostly from atrial fibrillation, anticoagulant therapy (to give an **INR** (international normalized ratio) between 2.5 and 4) is the first choice in the absence of contraindications; no evidence exists for a fixed age limit. In all other patients, aspirin is the mainstay of treatment, but its preventive effect is only modest. Other antiplatelet drugs are only slightly more effective, if at all. Carotid endarterectomy is highly effective in patients with severe, symptomatic carotid stenosis (80–99 per cent reduction of the original lumen diameter), but this is found in less than 10 per cent of all eligible patients with ischaemic events.

Aspirin

The preventive effect of aspirin, in different doses, has been studied in 11 placebo-controlled randomized trials, in over 8000 patients after a TIA or moderately disabling stroke. There is virtually no difference in risk reduction for daily doses between 30 mg and 1300 mg. The overall risk reduction is 13 per cent (95 per cent confidence interval, 6 to 19 per cent). Side-effects, mainly indigestion, nausea, heartburn, or gastrointestinal bleeding are more common as the dose increases, but absolute rates are difficult to compare between studies, owing to differences in criteria.

Thienopyridine derivatives

These antiplatelet agents block the adenosine diphosphate pathway of platelet aggregation. The oldest derivative, ticlopidine, when given in a dose of 250 mg twice daily, is about as effective as aspirin (any dose above 30 mg). The major disadvantages are, however, that it is definitively more toxic (diarrhoea and skin rashes are reported in 15–20 per cent, and neutropenia in about 1 per cent of patients) and that it is much more expensive than aspirin.

Clopidogrel (75 mg daily) was tested in a single trial, which included patients with ischaemic stroke and those who had suffered myocardial infarction or who had peripheral vascular disease. It reduced the risk of the composite outcome event of vascular death, non-fatal stroke, or non-fatal myocardial infarction by 8.7 per cent (95 per cent confidence interval, 0.3 to 16.5). For the stratum of patients with an ischaemic stroke, the advantage was not statistically significant. Again, the cost makes it unattractive as the drug of first choice.

Dipyridamole

The pharmacological actions of this drug on platelets are unclear. Large trials of its efficacy in the secondary prevention of stroke have only tested it together with aspirin. In the analysis of all major vascular events the largest trial showed a benefit for the combination therapy in comparison with aspirin alone, but four earlier, smaller studies did not. The overall analysis shows a marginal difference in favour of the combination therapy, but without further evidence it should not be accepted as standard treatment.

Anticoagulants

So far there is little evidence to support the use of anticoagulants in the secondary prevention of stroke, except in patients with atrial fibrillation. A large trial of patients with cerebral ischaemia who were in sinus rhythm used a target intensity of an INR between 3.0 and 4.5, which is not unusual for preventing arterial thrombosis; patients in the control group were treated with aspirin. The study was prematurely stopped because of a significant excess of bleeding complications, mostly intracerebral. Anticoagulant therapy with an intensity of an INR between 2.0 and 3.0 deserves further study.

Carotid endarterectomy

Although this operation was increasingly performed from the 1960s onwards, it was not until the 1980s that two randomized surgical trials were performed: one in Europe and one in North America. In patients with severe, symptomatic carotid stenosis (80–99 per cent reduction in lumen diameter) the risk of disabling or fatal stroke substantially decreases after surgery. On average, about eight patients need to be operated upon to prevent one ipsilateral ischaemic stroke occurring within 4 years. This basic risk difference varies with age and sex, and it levels off after 3 or more years from randomization (that is, 3½ years after the qualifying event). It should be kept in mind that carotid endarterectomy is indicated in only a minority (less than 10 per cent) of patients with TIAs or moderately disabling ischaemic strokes: the attacks have to be in the carotid territory, the patients should be fit and willing to undergo the operation, and the angiogram should show an accessible stenosis of over 80 per cent at the carotid bifurcation.

Venous occlusive disease

The advent of non-invasive brain imaging methods in the 1970s and 1980s resulted in increased recognition of cerebral venous thrombosis. Before that time, physicians only rarely considered the diagnosis in patients with otherwise unexplained headache, focal deficits, seizures, impaired consciousness, or combinations of these features.

Causal factors

Unlike arterial occlusion, cerebral venous thrombosis is only rarely (some 10 per cent) associated with damage to the vessel wall, by infection, tumour growth, or trauma. Much more frequent causes are inherited disorders of coagulation. The most common form is the factor V Leiden mutation, found in some 20 per cent of patients without other causes. Stagnant flow (completing Virchow's triad of causes of thrombosis), contributes no more than a few per cent. In 20 per cent of patients no causal factors can be identified.

Often there is no single cause but a combination of contributing factors: for example, the postpartum period and protein S deficiency; pregnancy and Behçet's disease; or oral contraceptive drugs and the factor V Leiden mutation. The risk of cerebral venous thrombosis in the postpartum period increases with maternal age and with the performance of a caesarean section.

In neonates, cerebral venous thrombosis is usually associated with acute systemic illness, such as shock or dehydration; in older children, the most frequent underlying conditions are local infection (the leading cause before the antibiotic era), coagulopathy, and, in Mediterranean countries, Behçet's disease.

Diagnosis of cerebral venous thrombosis

The clinical features of cerebral venous thrombosis consist essentially of headache, focal deficits, seizures, and impairment of consciousness, in various combinations and degrees of severity. The symptoms and signs depend on which sinus is affected, and for a large part on whether the thrombotic process is limited to the dural sinus or extends to the cortical veins.

In the case of the superior sagittal sinus, which is affected in 70 to 80 per cent of all cases, cerebral venous thrombosis alone will lead to the syndrome of intracranial hypertension, that is headache and papilloedema. Up to 30 per cent of patients with so-called 'benign intracranial hypertension' may in fact have sinus thrombosis. Papilloedema can cause transient visual obscurations and sometimes irreversible constriction of visual fields, beginning in the inferonasal quadrants. The increased pressure of the cerebrospinal fluid may also give rise to VIth nerve palsies, and sometimes to other cranial nerve deficits. The onset of the headache is usually gradual, but in up to 15 per cent of patients it is sudden and may initially suggest the diagnosis of a ruptured aneurysm.

Involvement of cortical veins causes one or more areas of venous infarction, with or without haemorrhagic transformation. If the affected veins drain into the sagittal sinus the venous infarcts are typically located near the midline in the Rolandic and parieto-occipital regions, often on both sides. In the case of the lateral sinus the venous infarct is usually located in the posterior temporal area.

Clinically, the infarcts manifest themselves through epileptic seizures, or through focal deficits such as hemiparesis or dysphasia. If unilateral weakness develops (with thrombosis originating in the superior sagittal sinus), it tends to predominate in the leg, in keeping with the parasagittal location of most venous infarcts. Obstruction of cortical veins draining into the posterior part of the superior sagittal sinus or into the lateral sinus will commonly lead to hemianopia, dysphasia, or a confusional state. Impairment of consciousness may result from multiple lesions in the cerebral hemispheres, or from transtentorial herniation and compression of the brainstem. Either epilepsy or a focal deficit is a presenting feature in 10 to 15 per cent of patients; in the course of the illness seizures occur in 10 to 60 per cent of reported series, and focal deficits in 30 to 80 per cent.

Involvement of the cortical veins alone, without sinus thrombosis and its associated signs of increased cerebrospinal fluid pressure, is an extremely rare occurrence. Thrombosis of the deep venous system, including the great vein of Galen, may lead to bilateral haemorrhagic infarction of the corpus striatum, thalamus, hypothalamus, the ventral corpus callosum, the medial occipital lobe and the upper part of the cerebellum. In those cases the clinical picture is often dominated by deep coma and disturbance of eye movements and pupillary reflexes.

Investigations

CT

CT scanning will readily show 'venous' infarcts. These do not correspond to a known arterial territory, but often show haemorrhagic transformation (Fig. 5); they are sometimes bilateral, in the parasagittal area, or supra- as well as infratentorial, or they are in the deep regions of the brain. In addition, CT scanning will often provide evidence of the underlying sinus thrombosis: the hyperdense sinus sign or, less reliably, the so-called 'empty delta sign' after injection of intravenous contrast material.

MRI

Magnetic resonance imaging has made catheter angiography redundant in the diagnosis of cerebral venous thrombosis. It is not sufficient to rely on non-visualization of a cerebral sinus on MR venography, since this may represent hypoplasia. Demonstration of the thrombus itself is essential, but this greatly depends on the interval from disease onset. Three stages can be distinguished. In the acute stage (days 1 to 5) the thrombus appears strongly hypointense in *T*2-weighted images and isointense in *T*1-weighted images. In the subacute stage (up to day 15) the thrombus signal is strongly hyperintense, initially on *T*1-weighted images and subsequently also on *T*2-weighted images. The third stage begins 3 or 4 weeks after symptom onset: the thrombus signal becomes isointense on *T*1-weighted images but remains hyperintense on *T*2-weighted images, though often inhomogeneously. Recanalization may occur over months in up to one-third of patients, but persistent abnormalities are common and do not signify recurrent thrombosis.

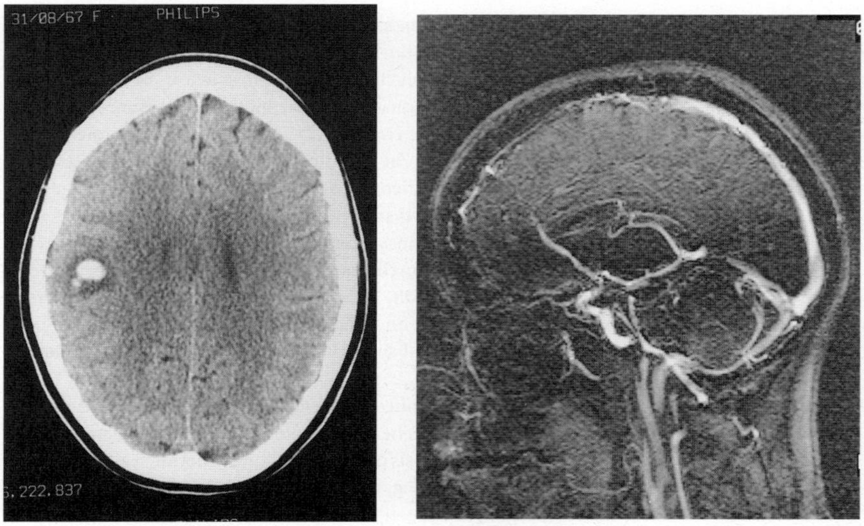

(a) (b)

Fig. 5 Cerebral venous thrombosis in a 27-year-old woman. (a) This CT scan shows a small infarct with haemorrhagic transformation in the right brain hemisphere, adjacent to the top of the lateral ventricle. (b) Magnetic resonance imaging, focused on venous structures, shows non-filling of the frontal part (on the reader's left) of the superior sagittal sinus.

Treatment and prognosis

Anticoagulant treatment is plausible, but the evidence from controlled clinical trials is sparse. In the acute phase, heparin (low molecular weight heparin, either intravenously or subcutaneously) seems preferable to oral anticoagulants, because its intensity can be closely monitored. The totality of the evidence for heparin treatment consists of no more than 80 randomized patients; there is a non-significant trend towards a better outcome in treated patients. At least heparin treatment seems safe, even in patients with haemorrhagic infarcts. Local thrombolysis via endovascular catheters has only been performed in uncontrolled studies.

Death rates in different series range between 5 per cent and 30 per cent, and probably depend more on case mix than on treatment. Residual deficits consist mostly of hemispherical deficits or visual impairment from optic atrophy.

The risk of recurrence has seldom been addressed systematically, but is probably in the order of 10 per cent. It seems wise to advise other means of contraception than 'the pill'. In women with a peripartum episode of cerebral venous thrombosis the available evidence does not warrant the advice to avoid a further pregnancy, although in patients with the factor V Leiden mutation the risk of a recurrent episode is probably higher than average.

Primary intracerebral haemorrhage

Causes of primary intracerebral haemorrhage

In most cases there is no single cause for a primary intracerebral haemorrhage. Even in the classical example of a so-called hypertensive haemorrhage in the region of the basal ganglia, the question is what anatomical or other factors distinguished this patient from others, in whom there were similar degrees and duration of hypertension but no brain haemorrhage. Even a combination of recognized 'causes', such as that of hypertension and anticoagulants, does not invariably lead to intracerebral haemorrhage. In general, therefore, several causal factors combine. These can be broadly distinguished into three categories (Table 5): anatomical factors (lesions or malformations of the brain vasculature), haemodynamic factors (blood pressure), and haemostatic factors (to do with platelet function or with the coagulation system). Abnormalities of the vascular system account for the vast majority of haemorrhages. The type of underlying abnormality varies with age: below the age of 40 years arteriovenous malformations or cavernomas are the most common single causes, whereas between 40 and 70 years the most frequent sources are ruptured perforating arteries (deep haemorrhages); in the elderly one also finds haemorrhages in the white matter ('lobar' haemorrhages), commonly attributed to amyloid angiopathy.

'Hypertensive' intracerebral haemorrhage

'Hypertensive' intracerebral haemorrhage results from degenerative changes in small perforating vessels, in the deep regions of the brain (basal ganglia and thalamus; Fig. 6), or in the cerebellum or brainstem. Microaneurysms occur on these vessels but are not necessarily the site of rupture. It is probable that rupture of a single small artery leads to a cascade of secondary haemorrhages from adjacent arterioles. This might explain the rapid expansion of intracerebral haematomas seen during a single scanning procedure or on serial scanning. A stable phase is usually reached in a matter of hours.

Table 5 Causes of primary intracerebral haemorrhage

Anatomical factors	*Haemodynamic factors*
Lipohyalinosis (complex small-vessel disease) and microaneurysms	Arterial hypertension
Cerebral amyloid angiopathy	Migraine
Saccular aneurysms	Haemostatic factors
Cerebral arteriovenous malformations	Anticoagulants
Cavernous angiomas	Antiplatelet drugs
Venous angiomas	Thrombolytic treatment (for non-neurological indications)
Telangiectasias	Clotting factor deficiency
Dural arteriovenous fistulas	Leukaemia and thrombocytopenia
Haemorrhagic transformation of an arterial infarct	
Intracranial venous thrombosis	*Other factors*
Septic arteritis and mycotic aneurysms	Intracerebral tumours
Moya-moya syndrome	Alcohol
Arterial dissection	Amphetamines
Caroticocavernous fistula	Cocaine and other drugs
	Vasculitis
	Trauma ('Spät- Apoplexie')

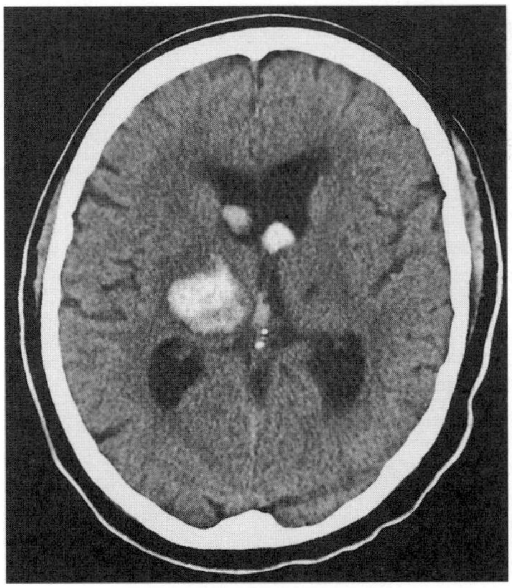

Fig. 6 Primary intracerebral haemorrhage in a 52-year-old man. This CT scan shows a hyperdense lesion in the right thalamus; the haemorrhage has ruptured into the ventricular system.

Deep brain haemorrhages are not always a one-time event. The recurrence rate in the first year is 7 per cent, against 2 per cent per annum over the subsequent 6 years.

Amyloid angiopathy

This condition accounts for about 10 per cent of intracerebral haemorrhages. Its frequency rises with age, but so does that of 'hypertensive' haemorrhage. The underlying abnormality consists of patchy deposits of amyloid in the muscle layer of small- and medium-sized cortical arteries of the occipital, parietal, and frontal lobes. Amyloid can also be found in asymptomatic individuals, the proportion increasing with age. It is not found outside the brain and does not represent generalized amyloidosis. Haemorrhages associated with amyloid angiopathy typically occur at the border of the grey and white matter of the cerebral hemispheres. Recurrent haemorrhage associated with amyloid angiopathy is much more common than with 'hypertensive' small-vessel disease. Autosomal dominant forms of amyloid angiopathy occur in The Netherlands and in Iceland.

Possible manifestations of amyloid angiopathy other than haemorrhage are transient episodes of focal neurological deficits, and also intellectual deterioration, associated with diffuse demyelination of the subcortical white matter (leukoaraiosis).

Cerebral arteriovenous malformations (AVMs)

AVMs are tangles of dilated arteries and veins, without a capillary network between them. On angiography, they are recognizable by large feeding arteries and a rapid shunting of blood to enlarged and tortuous veins via a central nidus of dilated vessels. Haemorrhage is the initial clinical manifestation in 50 to 60 per cent of symptomatic AVMs. Other clinical features include epileptic seizures, headaches, and progressive neurological deficits. Demonstrable AVMs are the most common single cause of intracerebral haemorrhage in patients under 45 years of age (about 30 per cent).

Between 10 and 20 per cent of AVMs are associated with thin-walled saccular aneurysms. These occur on peripheral feeding arteries, not at the classical sites at the circle of Willis, and are likely sources of bleeding. In AVMs in which one or more aneurysms have formed, the annual risk of rebleeding is as high as 7 per cent, against 2 to 3 per cent per annum for other AVMs. If there is no associated aneurysm, the site of rupture is mostly on the venous side of the malformation.

Cavernous angiomas (cavernomas)

Cavernous angiomas consist of sharply demarcated areas with widely dilated and thin-walled vascular channels, without intervening brain tissue. They are often asymptomatic and are encountered in 0.5 per cent of routine postmortems—in the white matter or cortex of a cerebral hemisphere in about one-half of all cases, in the posterior fossa in one-third, and in the basal ganglia or thalamus in one-sixth. If a cavernoma is at all symptomatic, epileptic seizures are at least as common a manifestation as haemorrhage. The annual risk of haemorrhage in patients in whom the lesion presents with seizures or focal deficits is rather low, between 0.25 per cent and 0.6 per cent. After a first rupture, rebleeding is more frequent, around 4.5 per cent per annum. Haemorrhages from a cavernous angioma are rarely fatal.

Familial forms of the disorder occur in several countries around the world, and should be suspected if multiple cavernomas are found.

Diagnosis of primary intracerebral haemorrhage

History

The history sometimes suggests the cause of the haemorrhage. Previous epileptic seizures should raise suspicions about the presence of an arteriovenous malformation, cavernoma, or a tumour. Amyloid angiopathy should come to mind with a history of transient ischaemic attacks, intellectual deterioration, or both. A record of long-standing hypertension indicates small-vessel diseases as the most probable underlying condition in a patient with a haematoma in the basal ganglia or in the posterior fossa; on the other hand, hypertension is so common that it may coexist with other conditions. If the patient is known to have had cancer, haemorrhage into a brain metastasis is a strong possibility. The use of oral anticoagulants is a vital piece of information in patients with intracerebral haemorrhage, because their action should be neutralized as soon as possible. It is equally important to know about the use of recreational drugs, particularly cocaine and amphetamines. Finally, the circumstances preceding an intracerebral haemorrhage may help to identify its cause, such as puerperium (intracranial venous thrombosis, choriocarcinoma), or neck trauma (dissection of the vertebral or carotid artery).

Physical examination

The physical examination will provide rather few clues to the cause of an intracerebral haemorrhage, except for petechiae or bruising, which indicate a generalized haemostatic disorder, signs of malignant disease such as cutaneous melanoma, a collapsed lung or enlargement of the liver or spleen, or telangiectasias in the skin and mucous membranes. Finding a high blood pressure on admission is the rule, but only in about 50 per cent is there is evidence of long-standing hypertension. Retinal haemorrhages indicate intracranial bleeding in general, most often a subarachnoid haemorrhage. Heart murmurs may be coincidental but should at least raise the possibility of infective endocarditis, as should the finding of needle marks in possible drug addicts. The neurological examination will show focal deficits corresponding to the site of the lesion, with or without a decreased level of consciousness.

Investigations

Investigations should start with the usual tests of blood and serum. These will sometimes uncover a cause of intracerebral haemorrhage, such as a low platelet count or massive liver damage. Brain imaging (CT or MRI) is the most important single investigation in patients with suspected intracerebral haematomas. The location of the haematoma may to some extent indicate the underlying cause. Intraventricular extension of the haemorrhage occurs relatively often with deep, 'hypertensive' haemorrhages. The presence of a fluid-blood level within the haematoma strongly suggests an underlying coagulopathy, either iatrogenic or from haematological disease. A grossly irregular margin of a lobar haematoma suggests amyloid angiopathy. Multiple or recurrent haemorrhages in the white matter suggest amyloid angiopathy, at least in the elderly. Intracranial venous thrombosis should be suspected with irregularly shaped haemorrhages in the parasagittal region. Repeat brain CT after injection of contrast may pick up underlying lesions. Sometimes these can only be identified weeks later, when the lesion is no longer obscured by mass effects.

Treatment of primary intracerebral haemorrhage

Factors predicting the prognosis for the survival of patients with primary intracerebral haemorrhage are: level of consciousness (Glasgow Coma Scale); age; volume of haematoma (poor prognosis if supratentorial haematoma >50 ml); and intraventricular extension of haemorrhage (poor prognosis if volume >20 ml). Of course, the possible interventions outlined below apply only to patients who have a chance of survival.

In patients taking oral anticoagulants the first step is the intravenous injection of 10 to 20 mg of vitamin K, at no more than 5 mg/min, followed by infusion of a concentrate of the coagulation factors II, VII, IX, and X, or of fresh-frozen plasma.

Intracranial pressure is often raised. Factors other than the local effects of the haematoma may contribute, such as fever, hypoxia, hypertension, seizures, and elevations of intrathoracic pressure. An unsolved question is the use, in comatose patients, of monitoring and, if judged appropriate, lowering intracranial pressure. There are many believers of this approach but few controlled studies. Insertion of a ventricular catheter may be a definitive measure in patients with cerebellar haemorrhage and no signs of direct compression of the brainstem.

There is insufficient evidence of benefit for the surgical treatment of supratentorial haematoma. Randomized trials have at best been inconclusive, including those employing endoscopic evacuation. In patients with cerebellar haematomas there is no doubt that surgical evacuation can be lifesaving, often with surprisingly few neurological sequelae. Sound indications for evacuation are the combination of a depressed level of consciousness with signs of progressive brainstem compression (unless all brainstem reflexes have been lost for more than a few hours, in which case a fatal outcome is unavoidable), or a haematoma greater than 3 to 4 cm. If the patient has a depressed level of consciousness and hydrocephalus, without signs of brainstem compression and with a haematoma less than 3 cm, ventriculostomy can be carried out as an initial (and sometimes only) procedure.

Subarachnoid haemorrhage

Causes of subarachnoid haemorrhage

Ruptured aneurysms are by far the most common source of non-traumatic subarachnoid haemorrhage (**SAH**), about 85 per cent of cases. Around 10 per cent are non-aneurysmal perimesencephalic haemorrhages, the remaining 5 per cent is made up by rarities (Table 6).

Table 6 Causes of subarachnoid haemorrhage

Cause	Incidence (%)
Ruptured aneurysm	85
Non-aneurysmal perimesencephalic haemorrhage (of venous origin?)	10
Rarities:	5
arterial dissection (transmural)	
cerebral arteriovenous malformation	
dural arteriovenous fistula	
pituitary apoplexy	
mycotic aneurysm	
cardiac myxoma	
sickle-cell disease	
tumours	
spinal arteriovenous malformation or aneurysm	
trauma (without contusion)	
cocaine abuse	

Cerebral aneurysms

Cerebral aneurysms are not congenital, they develop during the course of life. Therefore aneurysmal haemorrhage in a child is extremely rare. The aneurysms are saccular in shape and mostly arise at sites of arterial branching at the base of the brain, at or near the circle of Willis (see Fig. 7). It is largely unknown why some adults develop aneurysms. There are families with two or more affected first-degree relatives, but these account for less than 5 per cent of all SAHs. Many classical risk factors for stroke in general also apply to SAH: smoking, hypertension, heavy drinking, and oral contraceptives. Not all aneurysms rupture. Their prevalence can be estimated from angiographic studies (for other purposes) and autopsy studies at approximately 2 to 3 per cent in middle age, up to 5 per cent at the end of life. On the assumption that this proportion is 1 per cent for a standardized population across all age groups, and given that the incidence of SAH is approximately 6 per 100 000 (of the entire population), the annual risk of rupture of an aneurysm is 0.6 per cent.

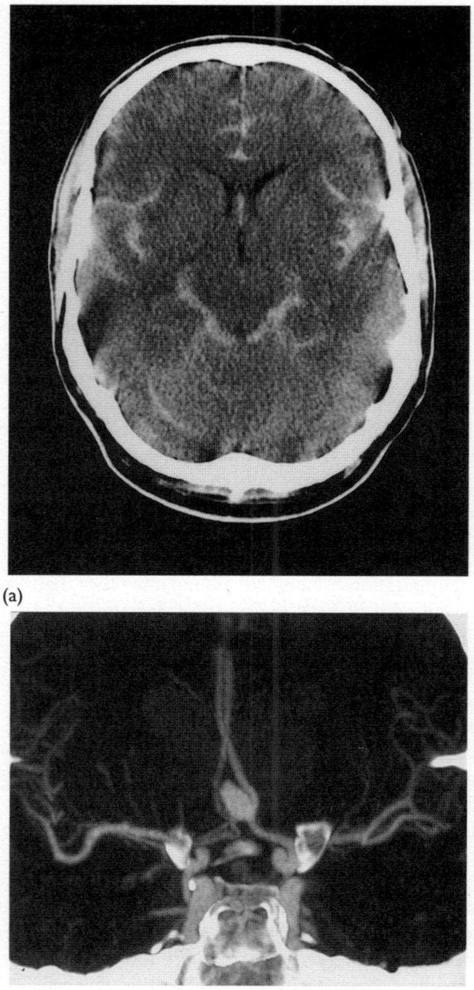

(a) (b)

Fig. 7 Aneurysmal subarachnoid haemorrhage in a 31-year-old woman. (a) CT scanning shows evidence of extravasated blood throughout the basal cisterns. (b) CT angiogram, with intravenous contrast, shows an aneurysm at the anterior communicating artery.

Non-aneurysmal perimesencephalic haemorrhage

This is a distinct and benign variety of subarachnoid haemorrhage, in which the distribution of extravasated blood on the brain CT scan is different from that seen with aneurysms, in the cisterns around the midbrain or ventral to the pons. The angiogram is completely normal, and the long-term outcome is invariably excellent. This subtype constitutes 10 per cent of all subarachnoid haemorrhages and two-thirds of subarachnoid haemorrhages with a normal angiogram.

Diagnosis of subarachnoid haemorrhage

History

The key feature in the history is that of a sudden, severe, and unusual headache. However, 50 per cent of patients lose consciousness at the onset, and the headache may emerge only later. The diagnosis is most difficult in patients with headache as the only feature. In general practice, exceptionally sudden forms of common headaches outnumber ruptured aneurysms. The incidence of aneurysmal haemorrhage being about 6 per 100 000 of the population per year, the average general practitioner will, on average, see one such patient every 8 years. There are no single or combined features of the headache that distinguish reliably, and at an early stage, between SAH and innocuous types of sudden headache. The discomfort and cost of referring the majority of patients for only a brief consultation in hospital is a reasonable price to pay for avoiding misdiagnosis of a ruptured aneurysm.

Physical examination

The physical examination is unhelpful in patients with a headache alone, without loss of consciousness or focal deficits. Neck stiffness takes about 6 h to develop, so its absence soon after the onset does not make the diagnosis of SAH more unlikely.

Investigations

CT scanning is the most important investigation. This will show extravasation of blood in the basal cisterns of the brain in at least 95 per cent of patients with a ruptured aneurysm, if the scan is performed within 3 days (Fig. 7)—after this interval the sensitivity of CT scanning quickly decreases. In patients with a negative CT scan but a convincing history, lumbar puncture is indicated. If the cerebrospinal fluid (**CSF**) is blood-stained, it is essential to distinguish SAH reliably from a traumatic tap. For that purpose at least 6 h, and preferably 12 h, should have elapsed from symptom onset. In cases of SAH, sufficient lysis of red cells will have occurred in the meantime for bilirubin and oxyhaemoglobin to have formed. These pigments give the CSF a yellow tinge after centrifugation (xanthochromia); they are invariably detectable until at least 2 weeks later. The 'three tube test' (a decrease in red cells in consecutive tubes in the case of a traumatic puncture) is notoriously unreliable. If the supernatant seems crystal-clear, the specimen should be stored in darkness until the absence of blood pigments is confirmed by spectrophotometry. Cerebral angiography is necessary for demonstrating or excluding an aneurysm as the source of haemorrhage; catheter methods are rapidly being replaced by CT and MR angiography (Fig. 7).

Treatment of aneurysmal subarachnoid haemorrhage

Several complications may occur after a first episode of an aneurysmal SAH, of which rebleeding and cerebral ischaemia are the most dreaded. Despite advances in surgical and medical management, the population-based case fatality rate is still around 50 per cent, with half of the survivors remaining more or less disabled.

As general nursing measures, continuous observation and an intravenous access are essential. A bladder catheter is necessary for monitoring fluid balance. Headache should be relieved in a step-wise approach, with paracetamol and codeine as first steps. Distressing anxiety can be alleviated with short-acting benzodiazepines. Stools should be kept soft with oral laxatives and also by an adequate intake of fluids.

Prevention of rebleeding is challenging, if only because any effective measure tends to be offset by an increased risk of ischaemia. Moreover, at least 10 per cent of all patients with SAH suffer a further bleed within hours of the initial haemorrhage. Over the next 4 weeks the rate of rebleeding without intervention is at least 30 per cent. The immediate case fatality rate of rebleeding is 50 per cent. Surgical clipping of the aneurysm is the most effective method of treatment, but the earlier the operation is performed, the greater the risk of ischaemic complications. Endovascular treatment ('coiling') is rapidly gaining ground; however, whether the balance between effectiveness and safety is more favourable than with surgery needs to be determined by clinical trials. Antifibrinolytic drugs decrease the rate of rebleeding but do not improve overall outcome.

Delayed cerebral ischaemia occurs in up to 25 per cent of patients with a ruptured aneurysm, mainly between days 5 and 14 after the initial bleed. Understanding its pathogenesis has been impeded by simplistic notions about 'vasospasm' or 'clots around vessels'. Narrowing of the arteries at the base of the brain is a factor, but not a sufficient one. The total amount of subarachnoid blood is a potent risk factor, but only after rupture of an artery, and the distribution of blood in the subarachnoid space does not predict the site of ischaemia. The calcium antagonist nimodipine, in a dose of 60 mg every 4 h by mouth or nasogastric tube, reduces the frequency of cerebral ischaemia and poor outcome by about one-third; its mode of action is incompletely understood. As a rule, hypertension should be left untreated; it is a compensatory reaction to maintain cerebral perfusion. The plasma volume should not be allowed to fall; hyponatraemia is caused by renal sodium depletion, and not, as still often believed, by dilution as a result of inappropriate secretion of antidiuretic hormone. Fluids should therefore be replaced and not restricted. The basic intake should be at least 3 litres per day, with intravenous fluids supplementing oral intake; compensation should be made for fever or a negative fluid balance.

Further reading

Algra A, van Gijn J (1999). Cumulative meta-analysis of aspirin efficacy after cerebral ischaemia of arterial origin. *Journal of Neurology, Neurosurgery and Psychiatry* **66**, 255. [Systematic review of aspirin in the secondary prevention of stroke.]

Antithrombotic Trialists' Collaboration (2002). Collaborative meta-analysis of randomised trials of antiplatelet therapy for prevention of death, myocardial infarction, and stroke in high-risk patients. *British Medical Journal* **324**, 71–86. [Systematic review.]

Bamford J, *et al.* (1991). Classification and natural history of clinically identifiable subtypes of cerebral infarction. *Lancet* **337**, 1521–6. [Proposes a simple classification system for ischaemic stroke that combines anatomical and prognostic information.]

Barnett HJM, *et al.* (1998). Benefit of carotid endarterectomy in patients with symptomatic moderate or severe stenosis. *New England Journal of Medicine* **339**, 1415–25. [One of two trials showing that carotid endarterectomy is indicated for patients with a recent, non-disabling, carotid-territory ischaemic event when the symptomatic stenosis is greater than about 80 per cent.]

Bousser M-G, Ross Russell RW (1997). *Cerebral venous thrombosis.* WB Saunders, London. [Comprehensive monograph.]

Brilstra EH, *et al.* (1999). Treatment of intracranial aneurysms by embolization with coils—a systematic review. *Stroke* **30**, 470–6.

De Bruijn SFTM, Stam J, for the Cerebral Venous Sinus Thrombosis Study Group (1999). Randomized, placebo-controlled trial of anticoagulant treatment with low-molecular-weight heparin for cerebral sinus thrombosis. *Stroke* **30**, 484–8. [Controlled clinical trial in 60 patients, showing that low molecular-weight heparin is safe.]

Dennis M, *et al.* (1990). Prognosis of transient ischemic attacks in the Oxfordshire Community Stroke Project. *Stroke* **21**, 848–53. [Provides a population-based, follow-up study about the outcome after transient ischaemic attacks.]

EAFT (European Atrial Fibrillation Trial) Study Group (1993). Secondary prevention in non-rheumatic atrial fibrillation after transient ischaemic attack or minor stroke. *Lancet* **342**, 1255–62. [Proves the effectiveness of oral anticoagulants.]

European Carotid Surgery Trial Collaborative Group (1998). Randomised trial of endarterectomy for recently symptomatic carotid stenosis: final results of the MRC European carotid surgery trial (ECST). *Lancet* **351**, 1379–87. [One of two trials, see Barnett *et al.* (1998) for comment.]

Gent M, *et al.* (1996). A randomised, blinded, trial of clopidogrel versus aspirin in patients at risk of ischaemic events (CAPRIE). *Lancet* **348**, 1329–39. [Shows a marginal advantage of clopidogrel over aspirin.]

Greenberg SM (1998). Cerebral amyloid angiopathy—prospects for clinical diagnosis and treatment. *Neurology* **51**, 690–4. [Review.]

Gubitz G, Sandercock P, Counsell C (1999). Antiplatelet therapy for acute ischaemic stroke (Cochrane Review). *The Cochrane Library* **Issue 1, 2000**. Update Software, Oxford. [Reviews the evidence from controlled trials (mostly with aspirin).]

Gubitz G, *et al.* (2000). Anticoagulants for acute ischaemic stroke (Cochrane Review). *The Cochrane Library* **Issue 1, 2000**. Update Software, Oxford. [Shows there is no net benefit.]

Hop JW, *et al.* (1997). Case-fatality rates and functional outcome after subarachnoid hemorrhage—a systematic review. *Stroke* **28**, 660–4.

Koudstaal PJ, *et al.* (1992). TIA, RIND, minor stroke: a continuum, or different subgroups? Dutch TIA Study Group. *Journal of Neurology, Neurosurgery and Psychiatry* **55**, 95–7. [Shows how irrelevant it is to strictly distinguish ischaemic episodes of the brain according to their duration.]

Lemesle M, *et al.* (1998). Incidence of transient ischemic attacks in Dijon, France—a 5-year community-based study. *Neuroepidemiology* **17**, 74–9. [A recent study on the incidence of TIAs, summarizing preceding estimates.]

Linn FHH, *et al.* (1996). Incidence of subarachnoid hemorrhage—role of region, year, and rate of computed tomography: a meta-analysis. *Stroke* **27**, 625–9. [Shows the incidence of subarachnoid haemorrhage is lower than was estimated before the introduction of CT scanning.]

Linn FHH, *et al.* (1998). Headache characteristics in subarachnoid haemorrhage and benign thunderclap headache. *Journal of Neurology, Neurosurgery and Psychiatry* **65**, 791–3. [Shows that sudden headaches from a ruptured aneurysm cannot be distinguished from innocuous forms of headache.]

Mathew P, *et al.* (1995). Neurosurgical management of cerebellar haematoma and infarct. *Journal of Neurology, Neurosurgery and Psychiatry* **59**, 287–92. [Narrative review.]

Rinkel GJE, van Gijn J, Wijdicks EFM (1993). Subarachnoid hemorrhage without detectable aneurysm. A review of the causes. *Stroke* **24**, 1403–9. [Lists the causes of subarachnoid haemorrhage other than aneurysms.]

Rinkel GJE, *et al.* (1998). Prevalence and risk of rupture of intracranial aneurysms—a systematic review. *Stroke* **29**, 251–6.

Roos YBWEM, for the STAR Study Group (2000). Antifibrinolytic treatment in subarachnoid hemorrhage—a randomized placebo-controlled trial. *Neurology* **54**, 77–82. [Latest trial of antifibrinolytic drugs after aneurysmal subarachnoid haemorrhage, showing fewer rebleeds but no improvement in outcome.]

Stroke Unit Trialists' Collaboration (1998). Organised inpatient (stroke unit) care for stroke (Cochrane Review). *The Cochrane Library* **Issue 1, 2000**. Update Software, Oxford. [Reviews the evidence from controlled trials.]

Sudlow CLM, Warlow CP (1997). Comparable studies of the incidence of stroke and its pathological types—results from an international collaboration. *Stroke* **28**, 491–9. [Summarizes 11 reliable studies about stroke incidence.]

The Stroke Prevention in Reversible Ischemia Trial (SPIRIT) Study Group (1997). A randomized trial of anticoagulants versus aspirin after cerebral ischemia of presumed arterial origin. *Annals of Neurology* **42**, 857–65. [Shows that high-intensity anticoagulation is not safe for patients with TIA or moderately disabling stroke who are in sinus rhythm.]

Van der Wee N, *et al.* (1995). Detection of subarachnoid haemorrhage on early CT: is lumbar puncture still needed after a negative scan? *Journal of Neurology, Neurosurgery and Psychiatry* **58**, 357–9. [Shows that a few per cent of aneurysmal haemorrhages are missed by CT scanning, even in the first few days after symptom onset.]

van der Zwan A, *et al.* (1992). Variability of the territories of the major cerebral arteries. *Journal of Neurosurgery* **77**, 927–40. [Shows the inter-individual variability of boundaries between the territory of major cerebral arteries.]

Wardlaw JM, del Zoppo G, Yamaguchi T (1999). Thrombolysis for acute ischaemic stroke (Cochrane Review). *The Cochrane Library* **Issue 1, 2000**. Update Software, Oxford. [Reviews the evidence from controlled trials about the balance between risks and benefits.]

Warlow CP, *et al.* (2001). *Stroke—a practical guide to management*, 2nd edn. Blackwell, Oxford. [Comprehensive monograph about cerebrovascular disease, including a chapter about the historical background.]

24.13.8 Alzheimer's disease and other dementias

Clare J. Galton and John R. Hodges

Introduction

The definition of dementia has evolved from one of progressive global intellectual deterioration to a syndrome consisting of progressive impairment in memory and at least one other cognitive deficit (aphasia, apraxia, agnosia, or disturbance in executive function) in the absence of another explanatory central nervous system disorder, depression, or delirium (according to the *Diagnostic and Statistical Manual of Mental Disorders*, 4th edn (**DSM-IV**)). Even this recent syndrome concept is becoming inadequate, as researchers and clinicians become more aware of the specific early cognitive profiles associated with different dementia syndromes. For instance, in early Alzheimer's disease there may be isolated memory impairment many years before more widespread deficits develop.

Since dementia is predominantly a disorder of later life, it represents an increasing problem for individuals and society with the projected increase in the elderly population. It is estimated that the 18 million people with dementia worldwide will increase to 34 million by the year 2025. This increase is most marked in the developing countries, where the 11 million people with dementia in the year 2000 will reach 24 million by 2025. In the developed world, the equivalent figures are 7 million in 2000 and 11 million in 2025. In Europe alone, 4 million people will be affected by the year 2004.

Although the incidence of dementia is difficult to establish, community prevalence studies suggest that about 8 per cent of all people over 65 years of age suffer from dementia, this shows a marked increase with advancing age. The prevalence below 65 years is about 1:1000, this rises to 1:50 to the age of 70 and 1:20 from 70 to 80. Over 80 years of age the prevalence is 1:5.

Dementia has numerous causes that can be classified in many ways (Table 1 shows a classification by aetiology). Although a large number of medical and neurological conditions can occasionally cause a dementia syndrome, most of these are rare and have other neurological features that suggest the diagnosis, for example multiple sclerosis, the acquired immunodeficiency syndrome (**AIDS**) dementia complex, and the vasculitides. Routine investigation (see below) focuses on some of these rarer causes because, although rare, they often result in a reversible dementia. An alternative classification, based on the patterns of cognitive impairment, is that of subcortical and cortical dementias as illustrated in Table 2. This classification shows that disease of diverse cerebral structures can result in dementia but that the resultant patterns of cognitive deficits can be very different. Alzheimer's disease is the prototypical cortical dementia. Subcortical dementias are also discussed further below.

The most common causes of dementia before and after the age of 65 years are shown in Fig. 1. The relative frequencies of causes of dementia differ depending on age, but it is notable that Alzheimer's disease is the most common cause in both groups. The genetic forms of Alzheimer's disease and other rarer causes are more common in the younger age group. Before considering the common and treatable causes of dementia, we discuss the main differential diagnoses to be considered as alternatives to dementia.

Table 1 Causes of dementia

Degenerative disorders
Alzheimer's disease
Frontotemporal dementia
Dementia with Lewy bodies
Parkinson's disease
Huntington's disease
Progressive supranuclear palsy
Corticobasal degeneration
Multisystem atrophy
Progressive myoclonic epilepsy's

Vascular diseases
Multi-infarct disease (large vessel and lacunar infarcts)
Binswanger's disease
Primary cerebral amyloid angiopathy
Hypertensive encephalopathy
Vasculitides:
–systemic lupus erythematosus
–polyarteritis nodosa
–Behçet's disease
–giant-cell arteritis
–primary CNS angitis
CADASIL
Anoxia postcardiac arrest
Sickle-cell disease

Infections
Prion dementias:
–sporadic and familial Creutzfeldt–Jakob disease
–Gerstmann–Straussler–Scheinker syndrome
–familial fatal insomnia
AIDS dementia complex
Progressive multifocal encephalopathy)
Cerebral toxoplasmosis*
Cryptococcal meningitis*
Neurosyphilis
Subacute sclerosing panencephalitis
Progressive rubella encephalitis
Viral encephalitis
Viral, bacterial, and fungal meningitides
Whipple's disease

Neoplastic causes
Primary intracerebral tumours:
–frontal gliomas crossing the corpus callosum (butterfly glioma)
–posterior corpus callosal or midline tumours (thalamic, pineal, third ventricle)
–cerebral lymphoma
Extracerebral tumours:
–frontal meningiomas
–posterior fossa tumours (acoustic neuromas) causing hydrocephalus
Multiple cerebral metastases
Malignant meningitis
Paraneoplastic (limbic) encephalitis

Toxic causes
Alcoholic dementia
Heavy metals:
–lead, mercury, manganese
Carbon monoxide poisoning
Drugs:
–lithium, anticholinergics, barbiturates, digitalis, neuroleptics, cimetidine, propranolol

Acquired metabolic disorders and deficiency states
Chronic renal failure
Dialysis dementia
Portosystemic encephalopathy
Hypothyroidism
Cushing's disease
Addison's disease
Panhypopituitarism
Hypoglycaemia (chronic or recurrent)
Hypoparathyroidism
Vitamin B_{12}, B_1, and folate deficiency
Malabsorption syndromes

Inherited metabolic disorders (that may present in adulthood)
Wilson's disease
Porphyria
Leucodystrophies:
–adrenoleucodystrophy
–metachromatic leucodystrophy
–globoid-cell leucodystrophy
Gangliosidoses
Niemann–Pick disease
Cerebrotendinous xanthomatosis
Adult-onset neuronal ceroid-lipofuscinosis (Kuf's disease)
Mitochondrial cytopathies
Subacute necrotizing encephalopathy (Leigh's disease)

Trauma
Major head injury
Subdural haematoma
Dementia pugilistica

Hydrostatic causes
Hydrocephalus:
–communicating (including normal pressure) and obstructive

Inflammatory
Multiple sclerosis
Sarcoidosis
Acute disseminated encephalomyelitis

* Associated with immunocompromisation.

CADASIL, cerebral autosomal dominant subcortical infarcts and leucoencephalopathy.

Table 2 Cortical and subcortical dementias

Feature Examples	Cortical Alzheimer's disease	Subcortical Parkinson's and Huntington's diseases
Speed of mental processing	Normal	Slowed up
Memory	Severely impaired Recognition and recall affected	Forgetfulness Recognition better
Language	Aphasia common	Normal
Frontal 'executive' abilities	Preserved in early stages	Disproportionately impaired early in disease
Visuospatial and perceptual abilities	Impaired early	Impaired late
Personality	Unconcerned	Apathetic and inert
Mood	Usually normal	Depression common

Differential diagnosis

Pseudodementia

This term has been used to describe two disorders namely: depressive pseudodementia and hysterical pseudodementia. Cognitive symptoms are common in depression, particularly in the elderly population. The main complaints are of poor recent memory and concentration with distractibility. There is often a lack of subjective feelings of depression, thereby making the diagnosis difficult. The telltale signs are the so-called biological features of depression, such as sleep disturbance and a loss of appetite and libido. Other common symptoms are low energy and a lack of interest in hobbies and activities. There may be a past personal or familial history of depression. The cognitive picture is of impaired attention and subsequent patchy performance on memory and frontal tasks. There may be some inconsistency in test performance and patients easily give up on a task. Language output may be sparse but paraphrasic errors are not present. Even after detailed testing it may be difficult to distinguish depression from dementia, indeed there may also be some overlap between the syndromes in the elderly. For this reason, ideal practice would be for all newly presenting patients with dementia to undergo psychiatric assessment, and if any doubt remains a therapeutic trial of antidepressants may be warranted.

Hysterical pseudodementia commonly presents with a rapid onset of memory and/or intellectual impairment. There is loss of personal identity and salient personal and life events, which is unlike organic disorders of memory. There may be an obvious precipitant (such as marital problems, financial problems, or trouble with the law) and a past psychiatric history is common. 'Ganser syndrome' is a name for the condition where the patient gives bizarrely wrong answers to questions. For example, when asked 'How many legs does a horse have', they reply three or five. Even with such functional states, the examiner has to be aware of the potential concomitant organic disorder exaggerating the condition, as in other conversion disorders.

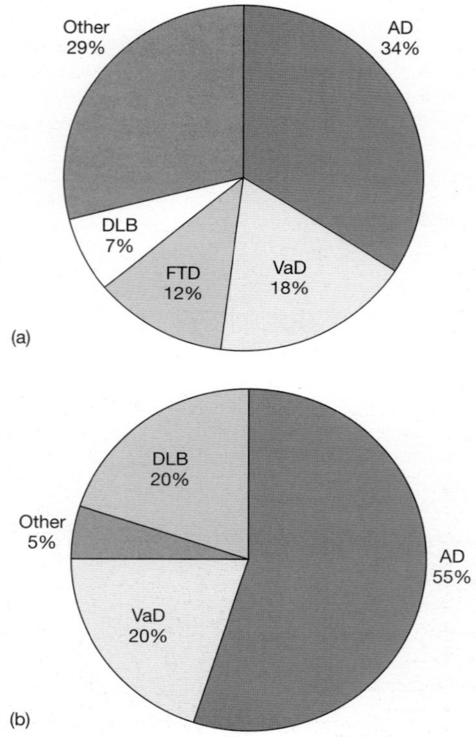

Fig. 1 (a) Relative frequencies of different dementia diagnoses in the under-65-year olds. (b) Relative frequencies of different dementia diagnoses in the over-65-year olds. AD, Alzheimer's disease; VaD, vascular dementia; FTD, frontotemporal dementia; DLB, dementia with Lewy bodies.

Delirium

This clinical syndrome is caused either by a diffuse brain pathology (for example, intracranial infections, head trauma, epilepsy (postictal states and non-convulsive status), raised intracranial pressure, subarachnoid haemorrhage) or is secondary to a large number of systemic illnesses or insults, including infections, metabolic derangements, hypoxia, and drugs.

The clinical features include the acute onset of attentional abnormalities and disturbance of consciousness (from clouding to coma), perceptual distortions, illusions and hallucinations, psychomotor disturbance (hypo- or hyperactivity and rapid shifts between the two), disturbance of the sleep–wake cycle, emotional lability, and marked fluctuations in performance and behaviour. The most consistent abnormality is in attention, with a reduced ability to maintain attention to external stimuli leading to distractibility and difficulty answering questions, and to appropriately shift attention to new stimuli leading to perseverations. The investigation and treatment needs to be focused in each case on the likely precipitants (although in about 5–20 per cent of the elderly no cause is found). Although the course and prognosis depend on the underlying diagnosis, if there is resolution of the precipitant there should be cognitive improvement to the baseline state.

Alzheimer's disease

Definition

Alzheimer's disease (**AD**) is the most common cause of dementia. Of the 5 to 10 per cent of the population aged over 65 years who have some kind of cognitive decline, over 50 per cent of cases will be due to AD and, although accounting for a smaller percentage of presenile cases, AD is still the single largest cause. The initial disease description by Alzheimer in 1907 was of a woman in her fifties with a progressive dementia and behavioural disturbance, who was found to have neurofibrillary tangles and amyloid plaques throughout her cerebral cortex. The term 'Alzheimer's disease' was then applied to similar cases with a presenile dementia, before it was realized that identical pathological changes were seen in the majority of elderly demented patients. Since plaques and tangles are found in a very high proportion of non-demented elderly subjects, debate continues about whether AD represents a continuum or a distinct disease process that increases in

Table 3 The NINCDS-ADRDA criteria for Alzheimer's disease

Probable Alzheimer's disease
Dementia established by clinical examination, documented by the Mini-Mental State Examination (MMSE) or similar and confirmed by neuropyschological tests
Decline in memory and at least one non-memory intellectual function
Decline from previous level and continuing progression
Onset between 40 and 90 years of age
No disturbance in consciousness
Absence of systemic disorders or other brain diseases that in and of themselves could account for the progressive deficits in memory and cognition
Definite Alzheimer's disease
Clinical criteria of probable AD
Histopathological evidence of AD at postmortem or biopsy
Possible Alzheimer's disease
Patient has dementia syndrome with no other cause but clinical variation from typical for AD
Patient has second disorder that is sufficient to produce dementia but not considered the cause of the dementia
Single gradually progressive cognitive deficit in absence of other cause

NINCDS–ADRDA, National Institute of Neurological and Communicative Disorders and Stroke–Alzheimer's Disease and Related Disorders Association.

frequency with age. With recognition of a number of causative gene mutations (see below) AD is now generally believed to be a multifactorial disease with familial and sporadic forms.

Histological diagnosis remains the 'gold standard', but current research criteria, such as the widely used NINCDS-ADRDA (see Table 3), are accurate in up to 90 per cent of cases. Rather than merely being a diagnosis of exclusion, AD is now recognized as a clinicopathological entity amenable to positive diagnosis. Much recent research has focused on methods of early and accurate diagnosis, which is particularly important in view of the advent of potential disease-modifying treatments.

Epidemiology and risk factors

Age is the most important overall risk factor for AD. A positive family history is also a risk factor, although autosomal dominant presentations account for less than 5 per cent of cases. To date, three major causative gene mutations have been established: mutations in the presenilin genes I and II on chromosome 14 and 1, respectively, and involving the amyloid precursor protein (**APP**) gene on chromosome 21. In these families the onset is invariably at an early age (35–55 years), with remarkable consistency within families and, as with Huntington's disease, penetrance is complete. Dementia is rapidly progressive and seizures and myoclonus are common. Individuals with Down's syndrome (trisomy 21) develop Alzheimer's disease during their third and fourth decades. This is thought to be due to the extra copy of the amyloid precursor gene on chromosome 21.

Apolipoprotein E (**ApoE**) is a risk factor rather than a causative gene for AD in both early- and late-onset cases, which at present is thought to be the single most common genetic determinant of a susceptibility to late-onset Alzheimer's disease. ApoE is a component of several classes of plasma and cerebrospinal fluid lipoproteins. The brain is the most important site of ApoE production outside the liver, and ApoE is thought to be important in lipid homeostasis in the brain. There are three common alleles for the *ApoE* gene: $\varepsilon 2$, $\varepsilon 3$, and $\varepsilon 4$. One or two $\varepsilon 4$ alleles confer an increased risk of Alzheimer's disease and lower the age of onset in a 'dose-dependent' fashion.

Many meticulous epidemiological studies have established that women are at an increased risk for AD, even after adjusting for confounding factors such as the increased longevity of women and their over-representation in the elderly population, and the increased vascular disease in men. Possible explanations include hormonal effects and the postmenopausal loss of potential protective effects of oestrogen. Significant head trauma in earlier life is also a risk factor that may summate with ApoE status, and there appears to be a unexplained protective effect of non-steroidal anti-inflammatory drugs.

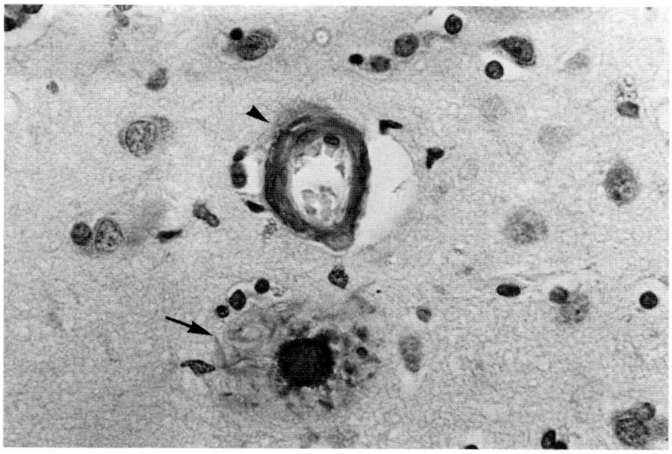

Fig. 2 Amyloid plaque.

Pathology

Pathologically, the macroscopic features of Alzheimer's disease are cortical atrophy, particularly involving the medial temporal lobe and parietotemporal association areas with relative sparing the primary sensory motor and visual cortices. The pathological process is thought to start in the entorhinal cortex, hippocampus, and other medial temporal lobe structures before spreading to the temporoparietal neocortex and basal frontal cortex, and then to the other association areas. The histological hallmarks are the senile plaques and neurofibrillary tangles (see Figs 2 and 3, respectively). Neither lesion is specific for Alzheimer's disease, as both are found to a lesser extent in the ageing brain; neurofibrillary tangles are also seen in a range of diseases, including progressive supranuclear palsy, encephalitis lethargica, postencephalitic parkinsonism, cerebral trauma, and dementia pugilistica.

Neurofibrillary tangles are formed from bundles of paired helical filaments that replace the normal neuronal cytoskeleton. The central core of the paired helical filaments is the microtubule-associated protein tau. The abnormal phosphorylation of the tau protein causes the microtubular abnormalities and the subsequent collapse of the cytoskeleton. The neurofibrillary tangles are seen as intensely staining intraneuronal inclusions with silver stains or specific anti-tau immunochemistry.

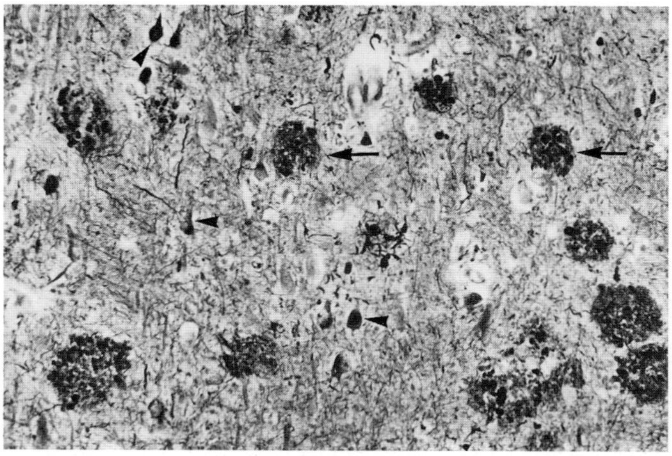

Fig. 3 Neurofibrillary tangle.

A variety of amyloid plaques are observed in Alzheimer's disease. Diffuse amyloid plaques have a loose accumulation of β/A4 amyloid without surrounding abnormal neurites, and are considered to be precursors to neuritic plaques. The mature neuritic plaque consists of a dense core of β/A4 amyloid surrounded by a halo and ring of abnormal neurites, before this stage the plaque is a loose accumulation of β/A4 amyloid surrounded by abnormal neurites. A hypermature plaque has a dense core of β/A4 amyloid surrounded by reactive astrocytes but without abnormal neurones. The role of microvascular pathology in AD remains controversial. Cerebral congophilic angiopathy can be seen in a high proportion of cases and almost certainly contributes to the hyperintense lesions commonly seen on *T*2-weighted magnetic resonance imaging (**MRI**) scans.

Besides a reduction in synaptic loss from neurones, which may explain some cognitive sequelae of the pathology, there is a major loss of neurotransmitters—especially of acetylcholine. The 'cholinergic hypothesis' of neurotransmitter loss causing attentional and mnemonic dysfunction has been much investigated. There is certainly evidence of severe neuronal loss in the nucleus basalis of Meynert in the basal forebrain, the major site of cholinergic neurones, and the current therapies are armed at improving cognitive function through inhibition of anticholinesterases. There is also disruption to other neurotransmitters including the serotonin system.

Pathophysiology

The increased understanding of the genetics of Alzheimer's disease has led to some advances in theories of the molecular basis of this condition. The β/A4 amyloid is formed from the cleavage of a larger molecule, amyloid precursor protein (APP) of approximately 700 amino acids. Mutations in either the presenilin gene (presenilin I and II) or the amyloid precursor protein gene affect APP and its metabolism, supporting the amyloid cascade hypothesis of Alzheimer's disease pathogenesis (see Fig. 4). APP is cleaved by beta- and gamma-secretases to produce β/A4 amyloid at a length of between 39 and 43 amino acids: the shorter fragments remain in solution, while longer peptides, the result of abnormal cleavage sites, are more prone to aggregate and form insoluble amyloid deposits. Besides mutations in the *APP* gene altering the cleavage site, there is evidence that presenilin genes affect the gamma-secretase-mediated cleavage of the transmembrane section of APP. The amyloid hypothesis suggests that accumulation of beta-amyloid, by overproduction or failure to break down, leads to amyloid deposition, thereby causing amyloid plaques, and leading to neurofibrillary tangles and cell death. There is evidence that insoluble β/A4 amyloid is toxic and that this may disrupt calcium homeostasis and enhance the production of glutamate. This hypothesis is still controversial; it explains rare familial cases and the association with trisomy 21, but the role of tau pathology, the formation of neurofibrillary tangles, and ApoE are not yet fully incorporated into a unifying model.

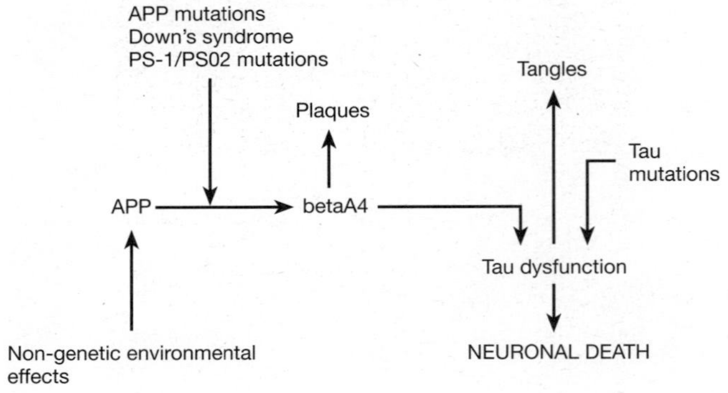

Fig. 4 Proposed pathogenesis of Alzheimer's disease.

Clinical features

The earliest cognitive deficit is impairment of so-called episodic memory (memories for events or episodes, including day-to-day memory and new learning), which is thought to reflect the earliest site of pathology in the medial temporal lobe structures. 'Minimal or mild cognitive impairment' (**MCI**) is a term increasingly used for people who are impaired on episodic memory tasks but who do not otherwise fit the criteria for a diagnosis of dementia. It is becoming clear that many, if not all, such people are in the predementia or early stage of AD, but progression to a full-blown dementia syndrome can take several years. The main clinical features at this stage are severe forgetfulness with often repetitive questioning and impairments in social function or job performance particularly concerning the retention of new information. As the disease progresses to mild Alzheimer's disease, memory function worsens, particularly affecting recall (for example, forgetting recent visits or family events), increasing disability in managing complex day-to-day activities such as finances and shopping, mental inflexibility and poor concentration, which reflects involvement of attentional and executive function. Insight is variably affected, often patients retain a partial awareness into their difficulties but underestimate the extent of the problem. Remote memory is relatively well preserved with a temporally graded pattern (that is, sparing of most distant memories). As the disease continues to progress patients often develop impairments in language, most typically word-finding difficulties, a shrinking vocabulary, and poor understanding of complex words and concepts. Visuospatial impairments and apraxia, which may develop at this stage, are particularly disabling, causing difficulty in dressing, cooking, and performing other daily activities. In a small subgroup of patients, language or visuospatial difficulties can be the first or most prominent presenting feature. As the cognitive deficits progress there is worsening of language function and semantic memory, and behavioural problems can be prominent.

Neuropsychiatric symptoms are also common in the earliest stages of AD, particularly apathy, anxiety, and mood disturbance. Delusions and hallucinations occur in up to 50 and 30 per cent of patients, respectively, in the later stages. Agitation, restlessness, wandering, and disinhibition also cause considerable carer burden. The final stages of the disease are characterized by reduced speech output (or mutism), ambulatory difficulties, dependence, and incontinence. Seizures and myoclonus are common late features. There is considerable variation in the time to this stage, but the average time from diagnosis to death is around 10 years.

Neurological examination is unremarkable in the early stages, although increased tone (often frontal resistant, or gegenhalten, in type) and mild extrapyramidal features can occur as the disease progresses. Reflex changes such as extensor plantar responses (Babinski reflex) and—in contrast to frontotemporal dementia—pout, snout, and grasp reflexes occur late. In the final stages, there can be greatly increased rigidity and joint contractures.

Investigation

The aims of neuropsychological, imaging, and laboratory investigations in Alzheimer's disease are twofold: first to exclude other potentially reversible causes of dementia, and second to confirm the diagnosis of probable Alzheimer's disease. The extent and nature of investigation obviously needs to be tailored to the individual, but all patients should undergo brain imaging and have a neuropsychological assessment to confirm the diagnosis of dementia. The neuropsychological profile can also be informative in the differential diagnosis of dementia (see Table 2). Particularly characteristic is early impairment in delayed verbal recall of new material, followed by reduced category fluency (in which subjects are asked to generate exemplars from a given category, for example 'animals'), impaired naming of low-frequency words, and difficulty with complex visuospatial tasks such as copying complex figures or block design from the revised Wechsler Adult Intelligence Scale (**WAIS-R**).

Table 4 Recommended investigations in dementia

Routine
Full blood count and ESR
Biochemical profile:
–urea or creatinine, electrolytes, calcium, liver function
Serum vitamin B12 and RBC folate levels
Thyroid function
Serological tests for syphilis
Chest radiography
CT scan of brain
Other tests which may be indicated in certain cases
EEG (e.g. Creutzfeldt–Jakob disease and subacute sclerosing panencephalitis)
MRI
SPECT
Neuropsychological examination (confirm dementia and pattern of disease)
CSF examination
Immunological tests for vasculitides
Screening for cardiac sources of emboli
Slit-lamp examination for Kayser–Fleischer rings and caeruloplasmin estimation (Wilson's disease)
Specific blood and/or urine tests for inherited metabolic disorders
Screening for HIV infection
Genetic screening for HD mutation/ specific AD mutations if familial dementia
Cerebral biopsy

ESR, erythrocyte sedimentation rate; RBC, red blood cells; CT, computed tomography; EEG, electroencephalogram; MRI, magnetic resonance imaging; SPECT, single-photon emission computed tomography; CSF, cerebrospinal fluid; HD, Huntington's disease; AD, Alzheimer's disease.

The basic laboratory investigations required in all patients, particularly to exclude treatable causes of dementia, and some of the other investigations that may be indicated in certain cases depending on the patient's age, family history, or specific medical history are shown in Table 4. Research into biological markers of AD is yet to yield a consistent biological or surrogate marker. Screening for specific gene mutations in young-onset familial cases is only available in specialist centres.

Magnetic resonance imaging scans of patients with Alzheimer's disease in the earliest stages (including MCI) show evidence of atrophy of the hippocampus and entorhinal cortex (parahippocampal gyrus) reflecting the pathology (Fig. 5). Unfortunately, the variability in size of these structures in normal elderly subjects means that, at present, these imaging abnormalities are not specific enough to be of predictive value. The co-registration of serial MRIs appears capable of detecting abnormal rates of brain atrophy, even before the onset of clear-cut cognitive symptoms in at-risk familial cases, but it remains a research instrument. *T*2-weighted MRI often reveals periventricular high-signal changes even in 'pure' early-onset cases. Single-photon emission computed tomography (**SPECT**) scans similarly demonstrate typical abnormalities in the parietotemporal regions but the specificity is again low in individual cases. More recent technological developments, such as perfusion MRI, magnetic resonance spectroscopy (**MRS**), and photon emission tomography (**PET**) scans may enhance diagnostic accuracy but are expensive and not yet suitable for routine clinical use.

Management and prognosis

The management of a patient with dementia involves many sensitive issues. It is crucial to provide medical and psychological support to patients as well as to their families and carers. During the progression of the disease there will be different treatment goals at different stages, ranging from aiding failing memory in the setting of independent living to managing behavioural problems and aggression, and eventually full supportive nursing care. There is great variation in the rate of progression, young-onset cases and those with prominent aphasia appear to deteriorate most rapidly. On average, patients spend several years in the mild or minimal stages

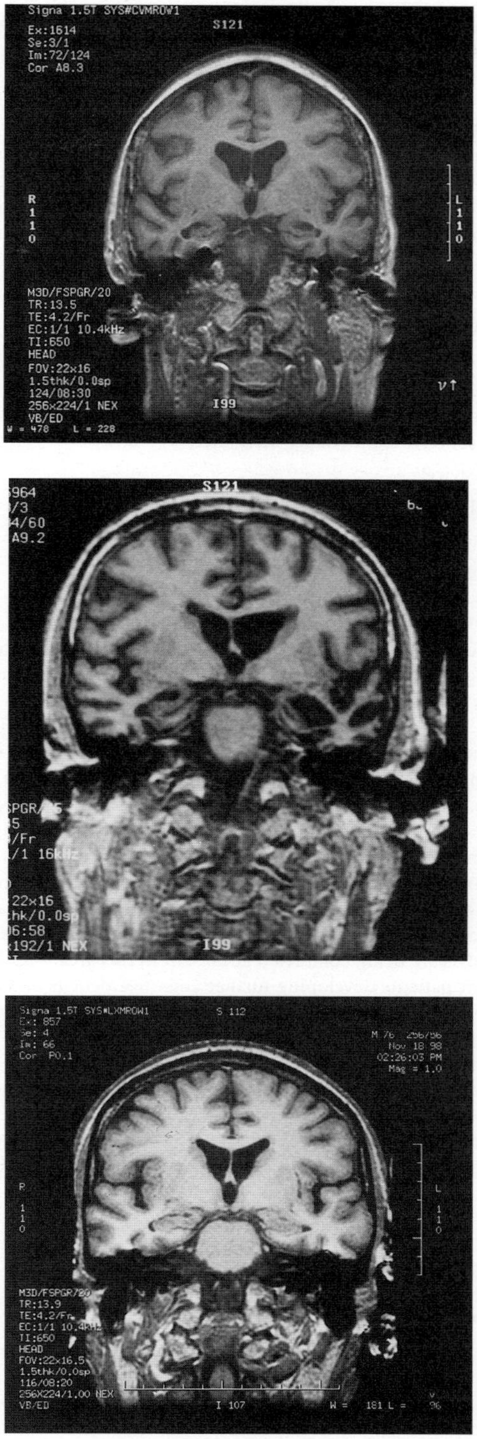

(a) (b) (c)

Fig. 5 (a) Coronal *T*1-weighted MRI scan of a patient with early Alzheimer's disease showing bilateral early hippocampal atrophy. (b) Coronal *T*1-weighted MRI image of a patient with FTD showing left temporal atrophy. (c) Coronal *T*1-weighted MRI scan of a normal subject.

(although it can be as long as 5 to 10 years), between 4 and 5 years in the moderate disease stages, and depending on the quality of care in the dependant stages, a year or more requiring full nursing care.

Non-pharmacological treatment

The mainstay of treatment is social support and increasing assistance with day-to-day activities. Issues such as driving and planning for future financial affairs are important and should be discussed early in the course of the disease. Throughout the course of the illness there will be differing requirements for the support services listed below:

- information and education;
- carer support groups;
- community dementia team, including home nursing and personal care;
- community services such as meals-on-wheels, community transport services, home maintenance assistance;
- sitter service;
- day centre;
- respite care; and
- residential/nursing home.

Pharmacological treatment

Pharmacological treatments can be divided into symptom- and disease-orientated approaches. Symptom modification relates to the treatment of depression, agitation, and psychotic phenomena and requires the input from a specialist psychiatrist. The cholinesterase inhibitors donepezil and rivastigmine are the only disease-specific drugs licensed for use in the United Kingdom. The importance of acetylcholine depletion in AD is established; these cholinesterase inhibitors generally achieve modest improvements in cognition in 25 to 50 per cent of the patients studied. However, the disease-modifying effects of these drugs remain controversial. Antioxidants (such as vitamin E), ginkgo biloba, and monoamine oxidase-B (**MAO-B**) inhibitors have shown benefits in some clinical trials, although again their long-term benefit is yet to be established. Pilot trials and experimental studies are being conducted at present in this area. Ideally, the goal is to prevent patients developing further cognitive deficits and to prevent those with MCI from progressing to dementia. The epidemiological findings of protection from cognitive decline in women using hormone-replacement therapy (**HRT**) is of interest in developing preventive strategies, and a trial is in progress to look at the effect of HRT in preventing or delaying the onset of dementia. Further research on the role of the amyloid and tau proteins in the pathogenesis of Alzheimer's disease will be the spur to both curative and preventive treatment for this common dementia.

Frontotemporal dementia

Definition

Frontotemporal dementia (**FTD**) is now preferred to the older term 'Pick's disease', to describe patients with focal frontal and/or temporal focal atrophy, since the underlying pathology of these syndromes can be variable. Arnold Pick (1851–1924) first described patients with both progressive aphasia, associated severe left temporal cortical atrophy at postmortem, and patients with behavioural disturbances associated with frontal lobe atrophy. In 1910, Alzheimer described the histological changes in patients with focal lobar degeneration as distinct from the syndrome that bears his name. Alzheimer described both argyrophilic intracytoplasmic inclusions (Pick bodies) and diffusely staining ballooned neurones (Pick cells). More recently it has become clear that these pathological changes are not the only features that accompany the clinical syndromes of frontal and temporal dementias; some patients have non-specific changes of neuronal loss, spongiosis, and gliosis only, while others have rather different ubiquitin-positive neuronal inclusions. The concept, therefore, has been broadened to accommodate differing underlying neuropathological features.

Epidemiology

FTD is increasingly recognized as a common cause of dementia, particularly in the younger age groups (see Fig. 1(a))—the peak incidence of onset being 45 to 65 years of age. In hospital series, the ratio of FTD to Alzheimer's disease has been found to vary from 1:5 to 1:20, with men and women being equally affected. Many cases are familial with up to 40 per cent having an affected family member.

Pathology and aetiology

The gross pathological appearance of FTD is that of profoundly atrophied frontotemporal regions that may be so severe as to produced the so-called knife-edged gyri and deep widened sulci. The histopathological hallmarks are widespread cortical and subcortical gliosis and loss of large cortical nerve cells. Severe astrocytosis with swollen neurones (Pick cells) and inclusions (Pick bodies), that are both tau- and ubiquitin-positive, are seen in about 20 per cent of cases. Pick bodies are intracytoplasmic argyrophilic neuronal inclusions composed of straight filaments, microtubules, and occasional paired helical filaments. In other patients there may be spongiform degeneration or microvacuolation of the superficial neuropil (cortical layer II) with no inclusions. Frontotemporal dementia can be seen with motor neurone disease, in which the histological changes above are combined with loss of anterior horn cells and motor neurone cells, particularly of the hypoglossal nuclei.

The aetiological basis of this disease is presently unknown. In some familial cases there is a mutation in the microtubule-associated protein tau gene on chromosome 17.

Clinical features

The presentation of frontotemporal dementia mirrors the neuropathological areas of disease; in the early stages frontal and temporal presentations can be distinguished.

Frontal presentations

Patients present with insidiously progressive changes in personality and behaviour that reflect the early locus of pathology in ventromedial frontal lobes. There is often impaired judgement, an indifference to domestic and professional responsibilities, and a lack of initiation and apathy. Social skills deteriorate and there can be socially inappropriate behaviour, fatuousness, jocularity, abnormal sexual behaviour, or theft. Many patients are restless with an obsessive–compulsive behaviour, such as hoarding food. Emotional lability and mood swings are seen, but other psychiatric phenomena such as delusions and hallucinations are rare. Patients become rigid and stereotyped in their daily routines and food choices. A change in food preference towards sweet foods is very characteristic. Of importance is the fact that simple bedside cognitive screening tests such as the Mini-Mental State Examination (**MMSE**) are insensitive at detecting frontal abnormalities. More detailed neuropsychological tests of frontal function (such as the Wisconsin Card Sorting Test or the Stroop Test) usually show abnormalities. Speech output can be reduced with a tendency to echolalia (repeating the examiner's last phrase). Memory is relatively spared in the early stages, although it does deteriorate as the disease advances. Visuospatial function remains remarkably unaffected. Primary motor and sensory functions remain normal. Primitive reflexes such as snout, pout, and grasp develop during the disease process. Muscle fasciculations, or wasting particularly affecting the bulbar musculature, can develop in the FTD subtype associated with motor neurone disease.

Temporal presentations

Temporal lobe degeneration presents with a form of progressive fluent aphasia, also known as semantic dementia, in which there is a profound loss in conceptual knowledge (or semantic memory) causing anomia and impaired comprehension of words, objects, or faces. The patient typically complains of 'loss of memory for words' and has fluent, empty speech with substitutions such as 'thing' 'one of those' etc., but the grammatical aspects are preserved. Naming is impaired with semantically based errors (such as 'animal' or 'horse' for zebra). Patients are unable to understand less frequent words and fail on a range of semantically based tasks such as matching words to pictures and matching pictures according to their meaning. Repetition of words and phrases is normal even though patients are unaware of their meaning. Unlike patients with Alzheimer's disease, day-to-day memory (episodic memory) with good visuospatial skills and non-verbal problem-solving ability is relatively preserved, at least in the early stages.

Another form of progressive focal atrophy, described by Mesulam, produces progressive non-fluent aphasia. Such patients present with a gradual loss of expressive abilities and gross impairments in the phonological (sound-based) and grammatical aspects of language production. This leads to non-fluent, agrammatical, and poorly articulated speech with multiple phonological errors (for example, sitter for sister or fencil for pencil). Repetition of multisyllabic words and phrases is impaired but, in contrast to semantic dementia, word comprehension and object recognition are well preserved.

Diagnosis

The diagnosis of frontotemporal dementia is based on the clinical, neuropsychological, and imaging assessments. The consensus broad clinical criteria are shown in Table 5. The differences between the various syndromes described above is obvious early in the disease, but there is increasing overlap between the temporal and frontal syndromes as the disease progresses. MRI demonstrates a characteristic pattern of frontal and/or temporal lobe atrophy: in contrast to Alzheimer's disease, the changes involve the polar and lateral temporal structures and are asymmetrical, commonly involving the left side to a greater extent (see Fig. 5). The functional imaging (single-photon emission tomography (**SPECT**) or positron emisson tomography (**PET**)) findings mirror the structural imaging results, with reduced frontotemporal perfusion and hypometabolism.

Management and prognosis

There is no curative treatment at present, thus the general management of the dementia sufferer and their family, as discussed above, is of prime importance. The prognosis can be variable with differing rates of progression between individuals. The disease is progressive and the average duration from diagnosis is around 5 to 10 years.

Dementia with Lewy bodies

Definition

Since the discovery in the 1960s that patients with Lewy bodies (ubiquitin-positive inclusions) in the cortex have a distinctive pattern of dementia with features of both Parkinson's and Alzheimer's disease, it has been increasingly recognized as an important cause of dementia. The terminology has been confusing with multiple designations including: Lewy body dementia, dementia of Lewy body type, diffuse Lewy body disease, and cortical Lewy body disease. The consensus clinical criteria for 'dementia with Lewy bodies' (**DLB**), the term now preferred, are shown in Table 6.

Epidemiology

Dementia with Lewy bodies is a common cause of dementia in the elderly population, although the true prevalence remains unclear. As many as 12 to 36 per cent of patients with a clinical diagnosis of Alzheimer's disease reach the pathological criteria for a diagnosis of dementia with Lewy bodies.

Table 5 The clinical diagnostic features of frontotemporal dementia (FTD)

Frontal syndrome		
I	*Core features*	
A	Insidious onset and gradual progression	
B	Early decline in social contact	
C	Early impairment in personal conduct	
D	Early emotional blunting	
E	Early loss of insight	
II	*Supportive features*	
A	Behavioural	
	i.	Decline in personal hygiene and grooming
	ii.	Mental rigidity and inflexibility
	iii.	Distractibility and impersistence
	iv.	Hyperorality and dietary changes
	v.	Perseverative and stereotyped behaviour
	vi.	Utilization behaviour
B	Speech and language	
	i.	Altered speech output: –aspontaneity and economy of speech –pressure of speech
	ii.	Stereotypic speech
	iii.	Echolalia
	iv.	Perseveration
	v.	Mutism
C	Physical signs	
	i.	Primitive reflexes
	ii.	Incontinence
	iii.	Akinesia, rigidity, and tremor
	iv.	Low and labile blood pressure
D	Investigations	
	i.	Neuropsychology: significant impairment on frontal lobe tests in the absence of severe amnesia, aphasia or perceptuospatial disorder
	ii.	Electroencephalography: normal on conventional EEG despite dementia
	iii.	Brain imaging (structural and or functional): predominant frontal and/or anterior temporal abnormality
Semantic dementia		
I	*Core features*	
A	Insidious onset and gradual progression	
B	Language disorder characterized by:	
	i.	Progressive, fluent, empty spontaneous speech
	ii.	Loss of word meaning, manifest by impaired naming and comprehension
	iii.	Semantic paraphrasias;
	and/or	
C	Perceptual disorder characterized by:	
	i.	Prosopagnosia: impaired recognition of identity of familiar faces; *and/or*
	ii.	Associative agnosia: impaired recognition of object identity
D	Preserved perceptual matching and drawing reproduction	
E	Preserved single word repetition	
F	Preserved ability to read aloud and write to dictation orthographically regular words	
II	*Supportive diagnostic features*	
A	Speech and language	
	i.	Pressure of speech
	ii.	Idiosyncratic word use
	iii.	Absence of phonemic paraphrasias

Table 5 continued

	iv.	Surface dyslexia and dysgraphia
	v.	Preserved calculation
B	Behaviour	
	i.	Loss of sympathy and empathy
	ii.	Narrowed preoccupations
	iii.	Parsimony
C	Physical signs	
	i.	Absent or late primitive reflexes
	ii.	Akinesia, rigidity, and tremor
D	Investigations	
E	Neuropsychology	
	i.	Profound semantic loss, manifest in failure of word comprehension and naming, and/or face and object recognition
	ii.	Preserved phonology and syntax, and elementary perceptual processing, spatial skills, and day-to-day memory
F	Electroencephalography normal	
G	Brain imaging (structural and/or functional): –predominant anterior temporal abnormality (symmetrical or asymmetrical)	
Progressive non-fluent aphasia		
I	*Core diagnostic features*	
A	Insidious onset and gradual progression	
B	Non-fluent spontaneous speech with at least one of the following: –agrammatism, phonemic paraphrasias, anomia	
II	*Supportive diagnostic features*	
A	Speech and language	
	i.	Stuttering or oral apraxia
	ii.	Impaired repetition
	iii.	Alexia, agraphia
	iv.	Early preservation of word meaning
	v.	Late mutism
B	Behaviour	
	i.	Early preservation of social skills
	ii.	Late behavioural changes similar to FTD
C	Physical signs: –late contralateral primitive reflexes, akinesia, rigidity, and tremor	
D	Investigations	
	i.	Neuropsychology: non-fluent aphasia in the absence of severe amnesia or perceptuospatial disorder
	ii.	Electroencephalopathy: normal or minor asymmetrical slowing
	iii.	Brain imaging (structural and/or functional): asymmetrical abnormality predominantly affecting dominant (usually left) hemisphere

(Adapted with permission from Neary *et al.* (1998). Frontotemporal lobar degeneration: a consensus on clinical diagnostic criteria. *Neurology* **51,** 1546–54.)

Pathology

Pathological criteria require the presence of cortical and subcortical Lewy bodies. Confusingly, there is considerable overlap with the histological features of both Parkinson's and Alzheimer's diseases, although the distribution of pathology is the key to distinguishing these conditions. Lewy bodies are intracytoplasmic eosinophilic neural inclusions formed from altered cytoskeleton components that can be seen on haematoxylin and eosin staining, but are more prominently shown using anti-ubiquitin immunohistochemistry. Cortical Lewy bodies are found in the temporal lobe, insular cortex, and cingulate gyrus, and are always accompanied by typical 'core and halo' Lewy bodies in the substantia nigra (the pathological hallmark of Parkinson's disease). Dystrophic ubiquitin-positive neurites are also seen in the hippocampus, amygdala, nucleus basalis of Meynert, and other brainstem nuclei.

Alzheimer changes—neurofibrillary tangles and amyloid plaques—are seen in up to 50 per cent of cases, raising nosological issues with Alzheimer's disease. The distribution of changes is of importance in distinguishing the conditions: for example, neurofibrillary tangles in DLB commonly spare the hippocampus, which is severely affected in Alzheimer's disease.

The neurotransmitter changes in DLB reflect the areas of pathology, with severe dopamine depletion in the basal ganglia and marked reduction in acetylcholine throughout the cortex.

Table 6 Clinical features of dementia with Lewy bodies

Dementia in association with:
Fluctuations in cognition (especially attention and alertness)
Visual hallucinations (typically well formed)
Mild spontaneous parkinsonism
Supportive features:
Repeated or unexplained falls, syncope, or transient loss of consciousness
Neuroleptic sensitivity syndrome
Hallucinations in other modalities
Systematized delusions

(Adapted with permission from McKeith *et al.* (1996). Consensus guidelines for the clinical and pathologic diagnosis of dementia with Lewy bodies (DLB): report of the consortium on DLB International Workshop. *Neurology* **47,** 1113–24.)

Clinical features

Patients typically present with a progressive cognitive decline paralleling that seen in those with Alzheimer's disease. There are, however, a number of characteristic and distinguishing features. First, there is a tendency to marked spontaneous fluctuations in cognitive abilities, particularly alertness and attention, producing a delirious state lasting days or even weeks. Second, visual hallucinations, illusions, and fleeting misidentification phenomena occur in 50 to 80 per cent of sufferers even at an early stage and without drug provocation. The hallucinations are commonly well-formed images of people or animals. The marked cholinergic deficit is postulated to be the cause of their tendency to visual hallucinations. Third, is the occurrence of spontaneous parkinsonism, which is usually mild in the early stages. Rigidity, gait disturbance, and bradykinesia are all common, although in contrast to patients with Parkinson's disease the tremor is usually mild and atypical (with postural and action components) and symmetrical. Repeated falls also occur. In the later stages the akinetic rigid syndrome can cause severe disabilities in mobility and swallowing an increase in the number of falls. Fourth, there is often an exquisite sensitivity to neuroleptic medication, producing the malignant neuroleptic syndrome (delirium, hyperpyrexia, muscle rigidity, massive elevation of creatine phosphokinase, and renal failure).

Diagnosis

Neuropsychologically there is a mixture of subcortical and cortical features, with prominent cognitive slowing plus impairment of executive (planning and organizational abilities) and visuoperceptual abilities. Compared with patients with Alzheimer's disease, those with DLB tend to have greater deficits in attention and visuospatial processing. Memory loss may be less prominent than in Alzheimer's disease. There is no diagnostic test for this condition and the diagnosis *in vivo* relies on the clinical features described above and in Table 6. Brain imaging demonstrates similar changes to Alzheimer's disease, although there is a suggestion that medial temporal lobe atrophy is less pronounced.

Management

The symptomatic management of this disorder is complicated by the presence of both hallucinations and an akinetic rigid syndrome. Patients are notoriously sensitive to the side-effects of dopamine-enhancing medications used for the treatment of the akinetic rigid syndrome. However, although dramatic motor improvements are not to be expected, a cautious medication trial is worth attempting. Even though neuroleptic drugs should be avoided whenever possible, neuropsychiatric features, if severe, can be ameliorated with the newer atypical neuroleptics such as clozapine and olanzapine, without exacerbation of the parkinsonism. Thus the main aim is to maintain a balance between the patient being mobile and lucid.

Of considerable interest is the anecdotal improvement in the marked attentional cognitive deficits to treatment with cholinesterase inhibitors such as donepezil and rivastigmine. Although there have been no controlled trial reports as yet, patients with DLB may respond better than those with Alzheimer's disease to this drug therapy.

Vascular dementia

Definition and epidemiology

Vascular dementia can be defined as a dementia resulting from a cerebrovascular disorder. This is obviously a broad categorization and many different aetiologies may be included in this rubric, for example multiple infarcts from cardiac emboli, vasculitides including systemic lupus erythromatosus, primary cerebral amyloid angiopathy, and cerebral autosomal dominant arteriopathy with subcortical infarcts and leucoencephalopathy (CADASIL). The term 'multi-infarct dementia' was introduced in the 1970s to emphasize the contribution of multiple cerebral infarcts to clinical dementia syndromes and to replace the older label of 'atherosclerotic dementia', although it is now apparent that diffuse small-vessel disease contributes significantly in the absence of clinically overt strokes. Traditionally regarded as the second commonest cause of dementia, it is increasingly difficult to estimate the true contribution of vascular disease. Postmortem studies of patients with multi-infarct dementia show that Alzheimer's changes commonly coexist. Conversely, the advent of sensitive instruments for detecting cerebral vascular lesions *in vivo* (magnetic resonance imaging), has revealed that presumed vascular changes are common in patients with the clinical diagnosis of Alzheimer's disease, even in young patients with known gene mutations, and that the presence of vascular lesions may be contributing to the severity of Alzheimer's disease. Finally, it is increasingly apparent that traditional risk factors for vascular dementia—including hypertension, diabetes, hypercholesterolaemia—are also factors which increase the likelihood of developing Alzheimer's disease.

Clinicopathological vascular syndromes

The variety of vascular diseases that affect the brain are legion, and the resultant clinical features and underlying pathology widely different (see Table 1). The most important vascular syndromes will be considered below.

Large infarcts

Recurrent cerebral infarcts involving multiple main arterial territories (for example, posterior or middle cerebral artery territories), resulting from thrombosis or embolism, can cause dementia with a step-wise cognitive decline. There is commonly a history of atherosclerotic risk factors (for example, hypertension, smoking, and hypercholesterolaemia), other evidence of atherosclerotic cardiac or peripheral vascular disease, and neurological signs on examination (for example, spasticity, hyperreflexia, extensor plantor responses, and a pseudobulbar palsy). There are often asymmetries on the neurological examination, and gait apraxia and/or bladder dysfunction can be early features. The cognitive picture is characterized by cortical features and is dependent on the sites of the lesions. There is often severe language impairment, visuospatial disturbance, amnesia, and dyspraxia, related to lesions in the middle and posterior cerebral artery distributions. Specific syndromes can result from discrete lesions: for example, lesions of the left angular gyrus result in a fluent aphasia, agraphia, acalculia, right–left disorientation, and finger agnosia or Gerstmann's syndrome.

Lacunar infarcts

The small multiple lacunar lesions are caused by occlusion in the deep penetrating arterial branches. The underlying pathogenic mechanism is a distinct small-vessel arteriopathy with replacement of the muscle and elastin in the arterial wall by collagen, leading to tortuous vessel and microaneurysm formation as a result of long-standing hypertension. The basal ganglia, thalamus, and deep white matter are common sites for lesions, due to the nature of the arterial supply. These lacunes may coexist with the larger infarcts (described above) thereby contributing to a mixed picture. However, the typical presentation of the lacunar state is with a more subcortical syndrome causing impaired attention and frontal executive malfunction, forgetfulness, apathy, and emotional lability. Thalamic lacunes can result in a speech disorder and, if bilateral, in amnesia. Examination features are similar to those seen with larger infarcts, with rigidity, gait disturbance, and extrapyramidal and pyramidal signs.

Small-vessel disease (Binswanger's disease)

'Binswanger's disease' (or 'diffuse leucoaryosis') is the term applied to the radiologically defined syndrome of confluent subcortical and corpus callosal demyelination and loss of the cerebral white matter, which again typically complicates severe or accelerated hypertension. The clinical features are similar to those of the lacunar state described above. On CT there is symmetrical diffuse low-density periventricular hypodensity, which can be accompanied by ventricular dilatation. This is visualized with great sensitivity on *T*2-weighted MRI as a diffuse white-matter of high intensity. Pathologically, there is demyelination, axonal loss, and gliosis, thought to be due to diffuse ischaemia in the territory of the long perforating arteries.

Cerebral amyloid angiopathy

Amyloid is deposited in the cerebral vessels both with increasing age and in a proportion of cases with ordinary Alzheimer's disease. However, there is also a rare and sometimes familial form of cerebral amyloidosis that produces recurrent cerebral haemorrhages and an Alzheimer's type dementia. Amyloid deposition in the vessel walls causes structural weakness leading to intracerebral haemorrhages and narrowing of the vessel to produce ischaemia. The haemorrhages tend to be lobar and can be recurrent.

Cerebral autosomal dominant arteriopathy with subcortical infarcts and leucoencephalopathy (CADASIL)

This recently established disorder may be a commoner cause of vascular dementia than previously realized. Patients present in their early twenties with migraine-like headaches and subsequently develop stroke-like episodes, which are sometimes ascribed to migraine or may mimic the attacks of acute demyelination. A subcortical dementia syndrome develops during their fifth and sixth decades. MRI shows multiple subcortical infarcts and diffuse white-matter disease. Other clues to the diagnosis are the absence of risk factors for atherosclerotic disease and the strong family history. Pathologically there is a distinctive non-amyloid, non-atherosclerotic angiopathy of the leptomeningeal and perforating arteries of the brain, with eosinophilic granular substance replacing smooth muscle. The diagnosis can be also confirmed with the finding of the same pathological changes in the cutaneous blood vessels in a skin biopsy. Mutations in the *notch3* gene on chromosome 19 have been reported in patients with CADASIL.

Treatment of vascular dementia

The treatment should be directed to the amelioration of any underlying cause of the vascular disorder, such as reducing cardiac embolism and treating vasculitides and hypertension. The potential for altering the progression of the disease is alluring. Nevertheless, efforts directed at altering atherosclerotic risk factors tend to produce disappointing results. The course of vascular dementia can be as severe as or even more rapid than that of Alzheimer's disease.

Subcortical dementias

Despite shortcomings, the differentiation between cortical and subcortical dementias continues to be useful in clinical practice. This classification highlights the fact that, although disease of diverse cerebral structures can result in dementia, the resultant patterns of cognitive deficits are very different. Alzheimer's disease is the prototypical cortical dementia, vascular syndromes can present with a spectrum of features from cortical to subcortical, as can dementia with Lewy bodies. Purer forms of subcortical dementia result from pathology of the basal ganglia and white matter, the prototypical examples being Huntington's disease and progressive supranuclear palsy (Steele–Richardson–Olszewski syndrome). The typical cognitive pattern is that of attentional and executive dysfunction with marked cognitive slowing (bradyphrenia) causing problems with mentation and information retrieval. Memory is moderately impaired due to reduced attention and poor registration, but is not as severely impaired as in Alzheimer's disease. There is often an associated personality change and mood disturbance with prominent apathy. Spontaneous speech is impoverished and slow.

Huntington's disease

Huntington's disease is an autosomal dominant inherited disorder with an incidence of about 4 per 100 000. The mutation is an expansion of the trinucleotide repeat (CAG) in the IT-15 gene on chromosome 4, which encodes the polyglutamine protein, huntingtin, essential for nervous system development. There is a clear dose-response relationship between the length of the CAG repeat and the age of onset of the disorder. Psychiatric symptoms, such as depression, irritability, and personality changes often precede the motor disorder, which is typically choreiform. The other cognitive changes that develop over the next 10 to 20 years are of a subcortical pattern, with deficits in attention and concentration, executive function, and retrieval from memory.

Progressive supranuclear palsy

Progressive supranuclear palsy (**PSP**) is a rare, but increasingly recognized, disorder with an incidence of 1 to 2 per 100 000. The subcortical dementia is accompanied by an atypical parkinsonian syndrome. The motor deficits are symmetrical in onset, with severe rigidity in the axial muscle groups and bulbar symptoms. A supranuclear gaze palsy invariably develops, but in the early stages the only feature may be slowing of fast downward movement (saccadic slowing). Another early feature is a marked tendency to falls. The pathological features are neurofibrillary tangles, neuropil threads, and neuronal loss and gliosis in the subthalamic nucleus, red nucleus, substantia nigra, and dentate nucleus. The main neurotransmitter deficit is in dopamine. Unlike Parkinson's disease, progressive supranuclear palsy does not respond well to levodopa. The disease progresses rapidly with an average time course of around 5 years.

Parkinson's disease

Subcortical dementia occurs in about one-third to one-half of patients with Parkinson's disease, which develops at a late stage in the motor disorder in contrast to dementia with Lewy bodies.

Corticobasal degeneration

Corticobasal degeneration is a rare cause of a dementia and motor signs. Patients present with an asymmetrical akinetic rigid syndrome together with limb apraxia, and the almost pathognomic feature of alien limb phenomenon in which the hand(s) act as if 'with a will of their own'. Myoclonus and dystonia also occur. Dementia is common in the later stages and there is considerable overlap with frontotemporal dementia. The pathology is focused in the frontal and parietal cortices as well as the substantia nigra, basal ganglia, and thalamus.

Treatable causes of dementia

Normal-pressure hydrocephalus

Normal-pressure hydrocephalus has a classic triad of presenting features: cognitive impairment, gait disturbance, and incontinence. The cognitive features are typically those of a subcortical dementia with frontal features and psychomotor slowing. The gait disorder is a dyspraxia and may show the pathognomonic feature of 'being stuck to the floor', although there is an absence of signs when the patient is examined in the supine position. The condition may be secondary to a prior disturbance of cerebrospinal fluid flow (resulting from, for example, a head injury, meningitis, or a subarachnoid haemorrhage), but often no cause is found in the elderly. Neuroimaging shows ventricular enlargement disproportionate to the degree of cortical atrophy. The presence of periventricular lesions can make the distinction from vascular dementia difficult. The investigation and management of these patients should be undertaken by the neurosurgeons, the definitive treatment being ventricular shunting. If treated early the prognosis is good.

Chronic subdural haematomas

This treatable cause of dementia is caused by head trauma. It is common in individuals at risk of recurrent head injuries, such as the elderly, alcoholics, and people with epilepsy. Risk is also increased by coagulation disorders, either pathological or iatrogenic. The clinical features are of a subacute dementia with symptoms of raised intracranial pressure and fluctuating cognitive performance and focal neurological signs. Diagnosis is confirmed by neuroimaging, the peripheral mass lesions may be of varying signal density on CT, depending on the age of the lesion. If the lesions are isodense with the brain tissue, the diagnosis can be easily overlooked. Treatment is by neurosurgical evacuation, except in clinically insignificant collections. Although the outcome is good, about 10 to 40 per cent of patients have a recurrence that may require a further drainage.

Benign tumours

Subfrontal meningiomas are the classic tumours that present with features of a frontal dementia. The onset is usually insidious with personality changes and other frontal features. Besides the neuropsychological abnormalities there may be anosmia or unilateral visual failure and optic atrophy. Other relatively benign midline tumours occasionally present with hydrocephalus and cognitive impairment secondarily to this (for example, colloid cysts of the third ventricle and non-secretory pituitary tumours).

Metabolic and endocrine disorders

Metabolic derangements can give rise to acute-onset cognitive impairments, but the features are invariably those of a delirium rather than a dementia. Chronic hypocalcaemia and recurrent hypoglycaemia can result in a dementia often accompanied by ataxia and involuntary movements. Endocrine disorders can more frequently present with a dementia syndrome, with or without psychiatric features (for example, hypothyroidism,

Addison's disease, and hypopituitism). The prominent complaints common to most disorders are mental slowing, apathy, and poor memory. Cushing's disease can present with psychiatric features, although a dementia syndrome is rarer. Although not strictly an endocrine disorder, Hashimoto's encephalopathy is a recently recognized cause of chronic delirium or dementia, often accompanied by seizures and fluctuating focal neurological signs. The diagnosis is made by finding extremely high levels of anti-thyroid antibodies despite a euthyroid state. Patients respond well to high-dose steroid therapy.

Deficiency states

Vitamin B12 deficiency can cause the classic picture of subacute combined degeneration of the spinal cord and a dementia. The dementia can be variable in severity and it is unusual to present without some features of peripheral neurological disease, at least, diminished vibration sense in the lower limbs and/or sensory ataxia. Reflexes can be increased, decreased, or mixed. Although most patients have a macrocytic anaemia, neurological manifestations can occasionally occur in the absence of haematological features. Severe thiamin (vitamin B1) deficiency results in the Wernicke–Korsakoff syndrome, with delirium, ataxia, and ophthaloplegia. The commonest causes are alcoholism and recurrent prolonged vomiting, such as hyperemesis gravidarum. If not promptly treated a chronic amnesic syndrome can occur.

Infections

Neurosyphilis, once a common cause of dementia, is now rare. The associated neurological features include pupillary abnormalities, optic atrophy, ataxia, and pyramidal signs. The diagnosis is confirmed with serology and examination of cerebrospinal fluid. Treatment with penicillin can result in some improvement. Those at increased risk are people inadequately treated for syphilis and those infected with the human immunodeficiency virus (**HIV**). HIV infection is an increasingly common cause of dementia in some parts of the world. The encephalopathy (AIDS–dementia complex) is characterized by psychomotor slowing, personality change, and other features of a subcortical dementia. Examination of the cerebrospinal fluid can show a pleocytosis and increased protein and oligoclonal bands. White-matter changes are visible on neuroimaging. Cognitive changes in patients with HIV may also be due to opportunistic infections such as cerebral toxoplasmosis and cryptococcal meningitis and progressive multifocal leucoencephalopathy, which all require specific treatment.

Further reading

American Psychiatric Association (1994). *Diagnostic and statistical manual of mental disorders (DSM-IV).* Washington DC.

Bak TH, Hodges JR (1998). The neuropsychology of progressive supranuclear palsy. *Neurocase* **4**, 89–94.

Berrios GE, Markova IS, Girala N (2000). Functional memory complaints: hypochondria and disorganisation. In: Berrios GE, Hodges JR, eds. *Memory disorders in psychiatric practice*, pp 384–99. Cambridge University Press, Cambridge.

Braak H, Braak E (1991). Neuropathological staging of Alzheimer-related changes. *Acta Neuropathologica (Berlin)* **82,** 239–59.

DeLeon M, *et al.* (1997). Frequency of hippocampal formation atrophy in normal aging and Alzheimer's disease. *Neurobiology of Aging* **18,** 1–11.

Galton CJ, Hodges JR (1999). The spectrum of dementia and its treatment. *Journal of the Royal College of Physicians London* **33,** 234–9.

Gauthier S (1999). *Clinical diagnosis and management of Alzheimer's disease.* Martin Dunitz, London.

Goedert M, Spillantini MG, Davies SW (1998). Filamentous nerve cell inclusions in neurodegenerative diseases. *Current Opinion in Neurobiology* **8,** 619–32.

Greene JDW, Hodges JR (2000). The dementias. In: Berrios GE, Hodges JR, eds. *Memory disorders in psychiatric practice*, pp 122–63. Cambridge University Press, Cambridge.

Gregory CA, Hodges JR (1996). Frontotemporal dementia: use of consensus criteria and prevalence of psychiatric features. *Neuropsychiatry, Neuropsychology, and Behavioural Neurology* **9,** 145–53.

Harvey J, *et al.* (1998). Genetic dissection of Alzheimer's disease and related dementias: amyloid and its relationship to tau. *Nature Neuroscience* **1,** 355–8.

Harvey RJ (2001). Epidemiology of pre-senile dementia. In: Hodges JR, ed. *Early onset dementia*, pp. 1–23. Cambridge University Press, Cambridge.

Hodges JR, Patterson K (1995). Is semantic memory consistently impaired early in the course of Alzheimer's disease? Neuroanatomical and diagnostic implications. *Neuropsychologia* **33,** 441–59.

Hodges JR, *et al.* (1992). Semantic dementia: progressive fluent aphasia with temporal lobe atrophy. *Brain* **115,** 1783–806.

Hodges JR, *et al.* (1999). The differentiation of semantic dementia and frontal lobe dementia (temporal and frontal variants of fronto-temporal dementia) from early Alzheimer's disease: a comparative neuropsychological study. *Neuropsychology* **13,** 31–40.

Jellinger K, *et al.* (1990). Clinicopathological analysis of dementia disorders in the elderly. *Journal of Neurological Sciences* **95,** 239–58.

Kalaria RN, Ballard C (1999). Overlap between pathology of Alzheimer's disease and vascular dementia. *Alzheimer's disease and Associated disorders* **13,** S115–S123.

Linn RT, *et al.* (1995). The 'preclinical phase' of probable Alzheimer's Disease. *Archives of Neurology* **52,** 485–90.

McKeith IG, *et al.* (1996). Consensus guidelines for the clinical and pathologic diagnosis of dementia with Lewy bodies (DLB): report of the consortium on DLB International Workshop. *Neurology* **47,** 1113–24.

McKhann G, *et al.* (1984). Clinical diagnosis of Alzheimer's disease: report of the NINDS-ADRDA Work Group under the auspices of the Department of Health and Human Services Task Force on Alzheimer's disease. *Neurology* **34,** 939–44.

Mesulam MM (1982). Slowly progressive aphasia without generalized dementia. *Annals of Neurology* **24,** 17–22.

Neary D, *et al.* (1998). Frontotemporal lobar degeneration: a consensus on clinical diagnostic criteria. *Neurology* **51,** 1546–54.

Rahman S, *et al.* (1999). Specific cognitive deficits in early frontal variant frontotemporal dementia. *Brain* **122,** 1469–93.

Reisberg B, *et al.* (1997). Diagnosis of Alzheimer's disease. Report of an International Psychogeriatric Association Special Meeting Work Group Under the Cosponsorship of Alzheimer's Disease International, the European Federation of Neurological Societies, the World Health Organisation, and the World Psychiatric Association. *International Psychogeriatrics* **9,** S11–S38.

Rockwood K, *et al.* (1999). Subtypes of vascular dementia. *Alzheimer's disease and Associated disorders* **13,** S59–S65.

Roman GC, *et al.* (1993). Vascular dementia: diagnostic criteria for research studies. Report of the NINDS-AIREN International Workshop. *Neurology* **43,** 250–60.

Sano M, *et al.* (1997). A controlled trial of selegiline, alpha-tocopherol, or both as treatment for Alzheimer's disease. *New England Journal of Medicine* **336,** 1216–22.

Snowden JS, Neary D, Mann DMA (1996). *Fronto-temporal lobar degeneration: fronto-temporal dementia, progressive aphasia, semantic dementia.* Churchill Livingstone, Hong Kong.

Welsh K, *et al.* (1991). Detection of abnormal memory decline in mild cases of Alzheimer's disease using CERAD neuropsychological measures. *Archives of Neurology* **48,** 278–81.

24.13.9 Human prion diseases

R. G. Will

Introduction

Prion diseases, also known as transmissible spongiform encephalopathies, are fatal disorders of the central nervous system affecting both animals and humans (Table 1). The clinical features and patterns of occurrence of these diseases vary, but they are linked by a number of characteristics including experimental and natural transmissibility, shared neuropathological features, prolonged incubation periods measured in years, and the deposition of prion protein, which may be the causal agent, in the brain of the host. Prion diseases have become the subject of intense scientific and public interest because of the likelihood that they are caused by a new disease mechanism and because of the implications for public health following the identification of a new human prion disease, variant Creutzfeldt–Jakob disease, and the accumulating evidence that it is caused by the transmission of the cattle prion disease, bovine spongiform encephalopathy, to humans.

The causal agent

Scrapie was first transmitted experimentally from sheep to sheep in 1936 and to laboratory mice in 1961, but laboratory transmission of human prion diseases was not achieved until 1966 (kuru) and 1968 (Creutzfeldt–Jakob disease). The seminal discovery that apparently neurodegenerative diseases were transmissible stimulated extensive research into the nature of the infectious agent. No bacterium or virus has been isolated in these diseases and there is no immunological response to infection. This is of central importance as there is, as yet, no serological test to identify the presence of infection during the incubation period of any prion disease. The transmissible agent is remarkably resistant to inactivation procedures, including those that disrupt nucleic acids. Prusiner proposed in 1982 that the protein deposited in the central nervous system in these diseases was itself the causal agent. Purified infectious fractions of brain contain prion protein (for proteinacious infectious particle) which is a major, and perhaps the only, component of the infectious agent. This membrane-associated glycoprotein is present in all mammalian species. The normal function of prion protein is unknown. In prion diseases a post-translationally modified form of the protein, partially resistant to protease digestion, is deposited in the brain and is associated with neuronal dysfunction and death.

Table 1 The spongiform encephalopathies

Disorder	Species
Sporadic Creutzfeldt–Jakob disease	Human
Inherited Creutzfeldt–Jakob disease (includes Gerstmann–Straussler–Scheinker and fatal familial insomnia)	Human
Iatrogenic Creutzfeldt–Jakob disease	Human
Kuru	Human
Variant Creutzfeldt–Jakob disease*	Human
Scrapie	Sheep/goat/moufflon
Transmissible mink encephalopathy	Mink
Chronic wasting disease	Deer/elk
Bovine spongiform encephalopathy*	Cattle
Feline spongiform encephalopathy*	Cat/cheetah/puma/ ocelot/tiger
Spongiform encephalopathy of captive exotic ungulates*	Kudu/nyala/oryx/ gemsbok/eland

* These disorders are associated with the same infectious agent (bovine spongiform encephalopathy).

There is a range of experimental evidence supporting the hypothesis that the disease-associated form of prion protein is the causal agent in prion diseases, most notably a series of elegant studies in transgenic rodents. Cellular expression of prion protein is necessary for the development of the neuropathological changes and the disease. Hereditary forms of human prion disease are associated with, and perhaps caused by, mutations of the prion protein gene. However, the occurrence of multiple strains of the infectious agent and the stability of the transmission characteristics of the bovine spongiform encephalopathy agent in the laboratory following cross-species transmission are not readily explained by the prion theory. The importance of prion protein as a determinant of disease expression has become increasingly clear in human prion disease. The phenotype of different clinicopathological subtypes of Creutzfeldt–Jakob disease is related to the deposition in the brain of different molecular isotypes of prion protein, probably reflecting distinct tertiary protein structures, despite the identical amino acid sequences of the normal and disease-associated forms of prion protein.

In experimental transmission of prion diseases there are a number of key determinants of the efficiency of transmission, as judged by the incubation periods in recipient animals and the proportion of these animals that develop disease. The route of inoculation influences these variables. The intracerebral route is the most efficient. Intravenous, intraperitoneal, and oral routes are decreasingly efficient. The incubation period is inversely related to the infective dose, while the strain of the infectious agent influences both the incubation period and whether recipient animals develop disease. In some transmission studies, for example transmission of bovine spongiform encephalopathy to hamsters or transmission of scrapie to chimpanzees, recipient animals do not develop disease even after intracerebral inoculation of high levels of infectivity. Within-species transmission is more efficient than cross-species transmission and this 'species barrier' to transmission is influenced by characterisitics of both the host and the infective agent. The relative homology of amino acid sequences of prion proteins between species is not the only determinant of the species barrier. The relative efficiency of transmission between species cannot be predicted.

After ingestion, the agent replicates in the lymphoreticular system, including the spleen and lymph nodes, before entering the thoracic spinal cord or brainstem, probably via the autonomic nervous system, and then spreading caudally to the brain. Moderate levels of infectivity plateau in the lymphoreticular system and are not associated with organ dysfunction, while in the spinal cord and brain high levels of infectivity develop, for example 10^{12} infectious units per gram of brain in one model of hamster scrapie, leading to neuronal death and clinical disease. In some experimental and natural prion diseases infectivity in the lymphoreticular system can be detected at about one-third of the total incubation period by inoculation of tissues of the lymphoreticular system, such as spleen, into recipient animals. The implication is that, in the absence of an *in vivo* serological test for the presence of infectivity, animals or humans incubating a prion disease may harbour significant infectivity in some organs or tissues but cannot be identified as being infected. This has important implications for the control and public health implications of prion diseases.

Human prion diseases

Human prion diseases may be classified as sporadic, inherited, or acquired (Table 2).

Sporadic Creutzfeldt–Jakob disease

Sporadic Creutzfeldt–Jakob disease is a rare disease, with an annual incidence of about 1 case per million population. The disease occurs worldwide and the cause is unknown, with no convincing evidence of an environmental source of infection and in particular no proven link with the animal prion diseases. The regional clusters of cases identified in some countries are unusual and may reflect the chance aggregation of a rare phenomenon.

Table 2 Human prion diseases

Sporadic	Creutzfeldt–Jakob disease
Inherited	Familial Creutzfeldt–Jakob disease
	Gerstmann–Straussler–Scheinker syndrome
	Fatal familial insomnia
Acquired	Iatrogenic Creutzfeldt–Jakob disease
	Variant Creutzfeldt–Jakob disease
	Kuru

Overall the geographical and temporal distribution of cases of sporadic Creutzfeldt–Jakob disease appear to be random and case control studies have demonstrated no consistent risk factors for the development of disease, with no good evidence of an increased risk through occupation, dietary factors, or animal contact. The current favoured hypothesis is that sporadic Creutzfeldt–Jakob disease is caused by a spontaneous mutation of prion protein to the abnormal form, which acts as a template for protein self-replication and eventual disease.

Clinically sporadic Creutzfeldt–Jakob disease presents with a rapidly progressive dementia associated with a range of neurological signs, most commonly myoclonus of the limbs, cerebellar ataxia, and rigidity. Less common features include dysphasia, pyramidal or extrapyramidal signs, primitive reflexes, cortical blindness, and lower motor neurone signs. Despite the predominantly cortical neuropathology epilepsy is rare. The rapidity of the progression of neurological deficits and cognitive decline is distinct from most other causes of dementia and the mean survival is only about 4 months from clinical onset, although in about 10 per cent of cases the illness is more prolonged and a small minority of patients survive for 2 years or more (Fig. 1). Terminally there is often a state of akinetic mutism.

Although the clinical presentation in sporadic Creutzfeldt–Jakob disease is relatively stereotyped, a minority of cases present atypically, for example acutely mimicking stroke, with cortical blindness, or with an initially pure cerebellar syndrome.

The neuropathological characteristics of sporadic Creutzfeldt–Jakob disease include spongiform change, neuronal loss, and astrocytosis in the cerebral and cerebellar cortex, in accordance with the neurological signs seen in life (Plate 1). Neuropathological changes are widespread and deposition of prion protein can be detected with immunocytochemical techniques. In about 10 per cent of cases there are cortical deposits of prion protein in the form of amyloid plaques. There is heterogeneity in the distribution and morphology of the neuropathological changes, which correlate in part with the clinical phenotype and with two isotypes of prion protein which can be distinguished on Western blot of brain tissue (Fig. 2).

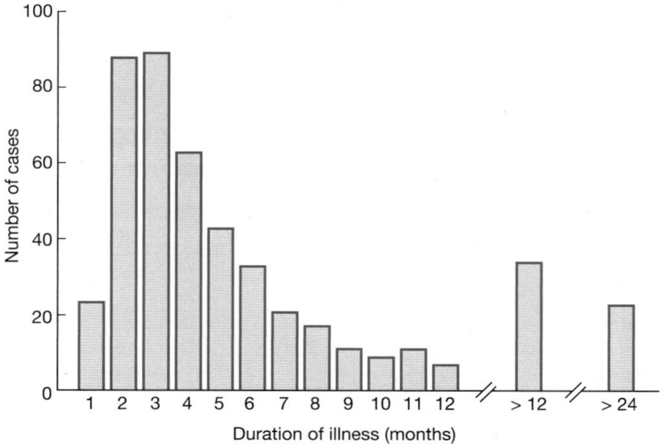

Fig. 1 Sporadic Creutzfeldt–Jakob disease—survival.

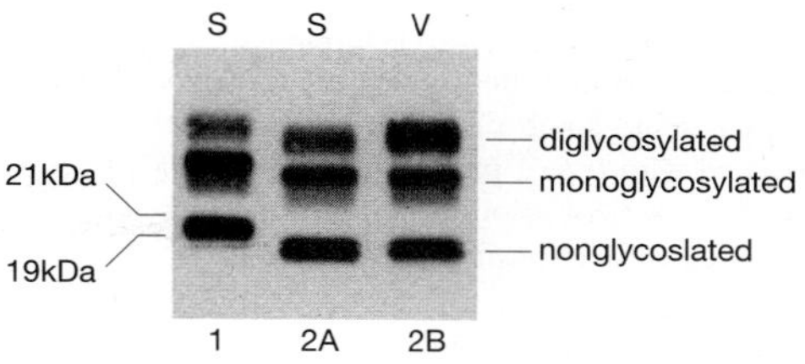

Fig. 2 Western blot of brain tissue showing type 1 and type 2 prion proteins. Lane 1 is sporadic Creutzfeldt–Jakob disease, lane 2A is sporadic Creutzfeldt–Jakob disease and lane 2B is variant Creutzfeldt–Jakob disease. Type 2A and type 2B have the same mobility but are differentiated by the relative proportions of different glycoforms—in variant Creutzfeldt–Jakob disease there is an excess of the diglycosylated form.

Sporadic Creutzfeldt–Jakob disease is mainly a disease of late middle age (Fig. 3) with a mean age at death of 66 years. In most systematic studies males and females are affected with equal frequency.

The human prion protein gene is situated on chromosome 20 and contains a polymorphic region at codon 129, which expresses either methionine or valine. Methionine homozygosity (MM) at codon 129 increases susceptibility to sporadic Creutzfeldt–Jakob disease (Table 3). The genotype distribution in sporadic cases is MM 80 per cent, valine homozygous (VV) 15 per cent, and heterozygous (MV) 5 per cent in contrast to the genotype distribution in the normal Caucasian population. There is accumulating evidence that the disease phenotype in sporadic Creutzfeldt–

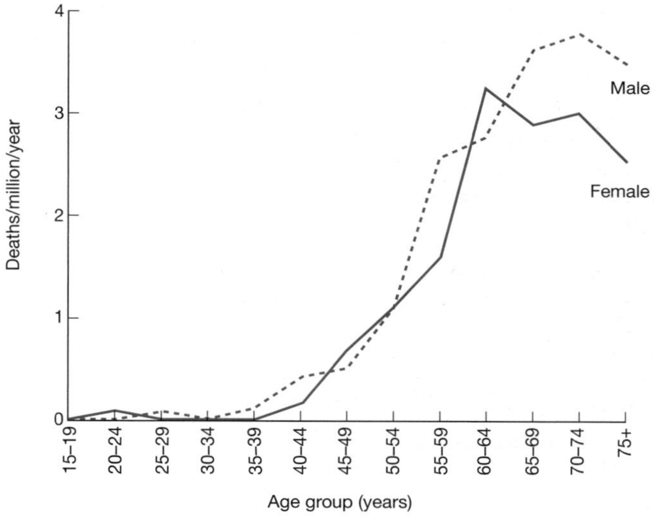

Fig. 3 Age- and sex-specific mortality rates from sporadic Creutzfeldt–Jakob disease in the United Kingdom, 1995 to 2000.

Table 3 Percentage of codon 129 genotypes in the normal population and in different forms of Creutzfeldt–Jakob disease, and in Kuru

	Genotype		
	MM	**MV**	**VV**
Normal population	39	50	11
Sporadic Creutzfeldt–Jakob disease	70	13	17
Iatrogenic Creutzfeldt–Jakob disease			
central	74	20	6
peripheral	48	21	32
Variant Creutzfeldt–Jakob disease	100	0	0
Kuru	30	45	25

Jakob disease, as well as susceptibility, is influenced by an interplay between the codon 129 genotype and the prion protein isotype. The classical form of sporadic Creutzfeldt–Jakob disease, representing the great majority of cases, is associated with type 1 prion protein and an MM genotype, while alternative combinations of prion protein isotype and codon 129 genotype are often associated with atypical phenotypes.

Hereditary prion diseases

Familial clusters of Creutzfeldt–Jakob disease account for about 10 per cent of all cases and within pedigrees there is a dominant pattern of inheritance. The paradox of a transmissible disease that is also inherited was clarified by the identification of a mutation at codon 102 of the prion protein gene in two families affected by Gerstmann–Straussler–Scheinker syndrome (GSS), a condition known to be a human prion disease on the basis of the neuropathology and laboratory transmissibility. More than 20 prion protein gene mutations, including point and insertional mutations, have now been identified in familial Creutzfeldt–Jakob disease or Gerstmann–Straussler–Scheinker syndrome (Table 4), and all cases of hereditary human prion disease to date have been found to have a mutation of the prion protein gene. Fatal familial insomnia was first identified as a prion disease following the identification of a mutation at codon 178 of the prion protein gene in affected family members and it was only later that transmission in the laboratory confirmed the status of fatal familial insomnia as a prion disease. The current hypothesis is that mutations of the prion protein gene lead to an instability in the structure of prion protein and an increased chance of a spontaneous transformation of prion protein to the abnormal self-replicating disease-associated form. With the exception of the prion disease associated with a mutation at codon 200 of the prion protein gene, all hereditary human prion diseases are fully penetrant.

The incidence of Creutzfeldt–Jakob disease in localized areas of Slovakia and in Libyan-born Israelis was discovered many years ago to be 60 to 100 times greater than expected. Possible explanations for these clusters included excessive dietary exposure to sheep scrapie and a high coefficient of inbreeding. Following the identification of the mutations of prion protein in human disease, genetic studies have shown that in both clusters there is a high population frequency of mutations at codon 200 of the prion protein gene and that the excess of cases of Creutzfeldt–Jakob disease is due to an excess of familial cases, with an expected background incidence of sporadic cases.

Table 4 Inherited prion diseases—mutations of the prion protein gene

Creutzfeldt–Jakob disease phenotype
D178N-129V
V180I-129M
T183A-129M
E200K-129M
H208R-129M
V210I-129M
M232R-129M
Fatal familial insomnia phenotype
D178N-129M
Phenotype of GSS syndrome
P102L-129M
P102L-129M-219K
P102L-129V
P105L-129V
A117V-129V
Y145STOP-129M
F198S-129V
Q212P
Q217R-129V
Heterogeneous phenotype: insertional mutations
Ins 24 bp-129M
Ins 48 bp-129M
Ins 96 bp-129M
Ins 96 bp-129V
Ins 120 bp-129M
Ins 144 bp-129M
Ins 168 bp-129M
Ins 192 bp-129V
Ins 216 bp-129M

GSS: Gerstmann–Straussler–Scheinker.

Overall the age at death in hereditary prion diseases is about 5 to 10 years earlier than in sporadic Creutzfeldt–Jakob disease, but the duration of clinical illness is often more prolonged and the clinical features vary with the underlying mutation. With some mutations, notably the codon 200 mutation, the clinical course is similar to sporadic Creutzfeldt–Jakob disease, but cases of hereditary prion disease may present with ataxia, for example Gerstmann–Straussler–Scheinker syndrome, or with a highly atypical phenotype such as fatal familial insomnia in which the early clinical features include dysautonomia and insomnia. There may be variation in the clinical phenotype both within and between families even if these are associated with the same underlying mutation in the prion protein gene.

Neuropathologically there is great heterogeneity in hereditary prion diseases, and as with the clinical phenotype there is an overall relationship between the neuropathological features and the specific prion protein gene mutation, although there can be great variation within and between pedigrees (Plate 2). The neuropathology can be similar to sporadic Creutzfeldt–Jakob disease but in a significant proportion of hereditary prion diseases there is amyloid plaque formation and in fatal familial insomnia gliosis and neuronal loss may be restricted to the thalamus.

In some forms of hereditary prion disease the codon 129 genotype may influence clinical characteristics, including age at death, and the neuropathology. Variation at this locus has a profound effect on the disease phenotype in association with mutations at codon 178 of the prion protein gene. Cases with a codon 178 mutation and a methionine at codon 129 of the prion protein gene develop fatal familial insomnia, whereas with valine at codon 129 the phenotype is similar to sporadic Creutzfeldt–Jakob disease.

Iatrogenic Creutzfeldt–Jakob disease

Creutzfeldt–Jakob disease has been transmitted accidentally in the course of medical treatment by neurosurgical instruments, corneal grafts, cadaveric dura mater grafts, and human pituitary derived hormones (Table 5). The presumption is that infection from individuals with Creutzfeldt–Jakob disease was transmitted to uninfected individuals via these procedures and there is strong circumstantial evidence that this has occurred. In two of the transmissions by corneal grafts the donors died of sporadic Creutzfeldt–Jakob disease and in the neurosurgical transmissions there was a clear temporal link between surgical procedures on Creutzfeldt–Jakob disease cases and patients operated on using the same instruments who subsequently developed Creutzfeldt–Jakob disease. It is presumed that some human dura

Table 5 Iatrogenic Creutzfeldt–Jakob disease worldwide

Mode	No. of cases	Mean incubation period (years)	Clinical
Neurosurgery	5	1.6	Visual/cerebellar/ dementia
Depth electrodes	2	1.5	Dementia
Corneal transplant	2	15.5*	Dementia
Dura mater	114	6	Visual/cerebellar/ dementia
Human growth hormone	139	12	Cerebellar
Human gonadotrophin	4	13	Cerebellar

* Range 1.5 to 26.5 years.

mater grafts and human pituitary hormones came from individuals suffering from Creutzfeldt–Jakob disease and there may have been cross-contamination in the production process leading to dissemination of infection. Infection via human pituitary growth hormone has been demonstrated in laboratory transmission studies. All cases of iatrogenic transmission of Creutzfeldt–Jakob disease have involved surgical instruments, grafts, or hormonal products potentially contaminated by central nervous system tissue and, by implication, high levels of infectivity.

There is a distinction between the clinical features in iatrogenic Creutzfeldt–Jakob disease which depends on the route of inoculation. In exposures in or adjacent to the nervous system (neurosurgical instruments, dura mater grafts, and corneal transplants) the majority of cases present with a progressive dementia similar to sporadic Creutzfeldt–Jakob disease. With a peripheral route of exposure to infection (pituitary hormones) there is a progressive cerebellar ataxia and cognitive impairment develops late in the clinical course, if at all.

The incubation period also varies according to the route of exposure to infection. With central exposure the mean incubation period ranges from about 18 months, similar to the incubation periods in primates after experimental intracerebral inoculation, to 6 years with dura mater grafts. With a peripheral route of exposure the mean incubation period is about 12 years, but may extend to over 30 years, which is similar to the extended incubation periods in kuru, a human prion disease also caused by a peripheral route of exposure to infection.

Homozygosity at codon 129 of the prion protein gene, either MM or VV, increases susceptibility to human growth hormone related Creutzfeldt–Jakob disease and heterozygosity may lead to a more prolonged incubation period. In dura mater related Creutzfeldt–Jakob disease 81 per cent of cases have an MM genotype, similar to the proportion of sporadic cases with this genotype, but the codon 129 genotype does not influence the incubation period.

Reducing the risks of iatrogenic transmission of Creutzfeldt–Jakob disease

Measures to reduce the risk of iatrogenic transmission of Creutzfeldt–Jakob disease have been introduced in many countries. There are strict selection criteria for obtaining corneal grafts, recombinant growth hormone replaced human growth hormone in 1985, and human dura mater grafts have not been licensed in the United Kingdom since the early 1990s. There is no evidence that Creutzfeldt–Jakob disease has been transmitted iatrogenically through non-central nervous system tissues such as blood, blood products, or organ transplantation, but continued vigilance is necessary as many of the mechanisms of iatrogenic transmission of Creutzfeldt–Jakob disease were not predicted. The possibility of secondary transmission of variant Creutzfeldt–Jakob disease through blood transfusion, the use of fractionated blood derivatives, organ transplantation, or contaminated surgical instruments is a matter of continuing concern.

Variant Creutzfeldt–Jakob disease

Bovine spongiform encephalopathy was identified in 1986 as a novel prion disease in cattle in the United Kingdom, and is thought to have been caused by feeding cattle material contaminated with sheep scrapie or, perhaps, to have been a previously unrecognized endemic prion disease of cattle. Bovine to bovine recycling of infection through cattle feed amplified the epidemic and there have now been over 180 000 cases of bovine spongiform encephalopathy in the United Kingdom. Small numbers of cases of bovine spongiform encephalopathy have been identified in other countries, mainly in Europe.

In 1996 ten cases of a novel form of human prion disease, variant Creutzfeldt–Jakob disease, were identified in the United Kingdom and a causal link with bovine spongiform encephalopathy was proposed as this was a new disease occurring only in the United Kingdom, the country with the greatest potential human exposure to bovine spongiform encephalopathy. Up to January 2002 there have been 114 cases of variant Creutzfeldt–Jakob disease in the United Kingdom, five in France, and one in the Republic of Ireland. The mean age at death in variant Creutzfeldt–Jakob disease is 29 years (range 15 to 74 years, Fig. 4) contrasting with a mean age at death in sporadic Creutzfeldt–Jakob disease of 66 years. The hypothesis that variant Creutzfeldt–Jakob disease is caused by the bovine spongiform encephalopathy agent has been supported by the consistent disease phenotype, and in particular the neuropathology which is distinct from other human prion diseases, the failure to identify similar cases in the past either in the United Kingdom or elsewhere, and laboratory transmission studies which have shown a remarkable similarity between the transmission characteristics of bovine spongiform encephalopathy and variant Creutzfeldt–Jakob disease in mice.

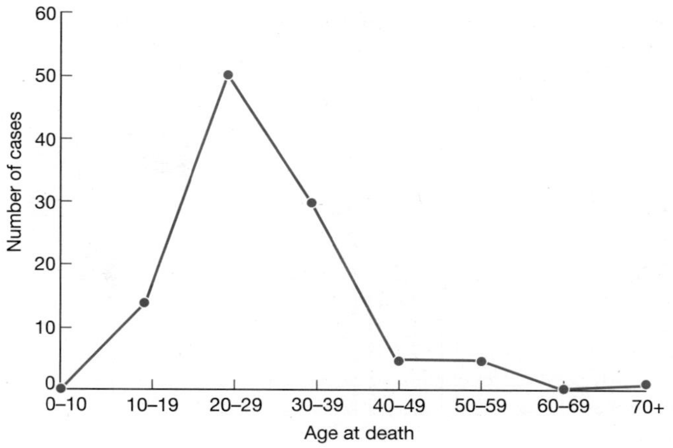

Fig. 4 Age distribution of cases of variant Creutzfeldt–Jakob disease in the United Kingdom (January 2002).

The clinical features of variant Creutzfeldt–Jakob disease are relatively distinct from other forms of human prion disease, including sporadic and iatrogenic Creutzfeldt–Jakob disease. Patients present with psychiatric symptoms, including depression, withdrawal, and anxiety, followed after a period of months by progressive ataxia, dementia, and choreiform or dystonic involuntary movements, which often evolve into myoclonus. The terminal stages are similar to sporadic Creutzfeldt–Jakob disease, but the overall duration of illness, mean 14 months, is significantly more prolonged. The distinctive neuropathological characteristic of variant Creutzfeldt–Jakob disease is the widespread deposition of deposits of prion protein with a halo of spongiform change, so-called florid plaques, throughout the cerebral and cerebellar cortex, in addition to the spongiform change, neuronal loss, and gliosis seen in other human prion diseases.

Cases of variant Creutzfeldt–Jakob disease have been identified from throughout the United Kingdom and risk factors include residence in the United Kingdom and an MM genotype at codon 129 of the prion protein gene. All the United Kingdom cases and the case diagnosed in the Republic of Ireland had been resident in the United Kingdom during the 1980s to early 1990s when human exposure to bovine spongiform encephalopathy was likely to have been maximal. Three of the French cases had never visited the United Kingdom, implying that exposure to bovine spongiform encephalopathy must have occurred in France from indigenous bovine spongiform encephalopathy or export from the United Kingdom of cattle or food products. A case control study has not yet demonstrated any significant dietary risk factor in variant Creutzfeldt–Jakob disease, although the favoured hypothesis is that transmission of bovine spongiform encephalopathy to humans was through contamination of food, probably with tissues from the central nervous system such as brain or spinal cord which are known to contain high levels of infectivity in cattle affected with bovine spongiform encephalopathy. All tested cases of variant Creutzfeldt–Jakob

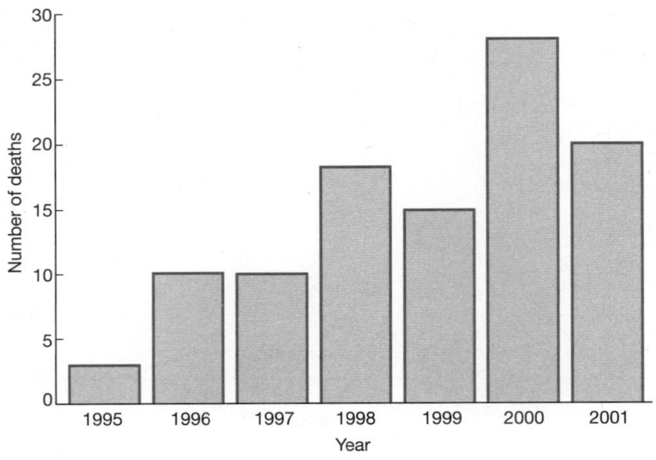

Fig. 5 Variant Creutzfeldt–Jakob disease—number of deaths per annum in the United Kingdom (January 2002).

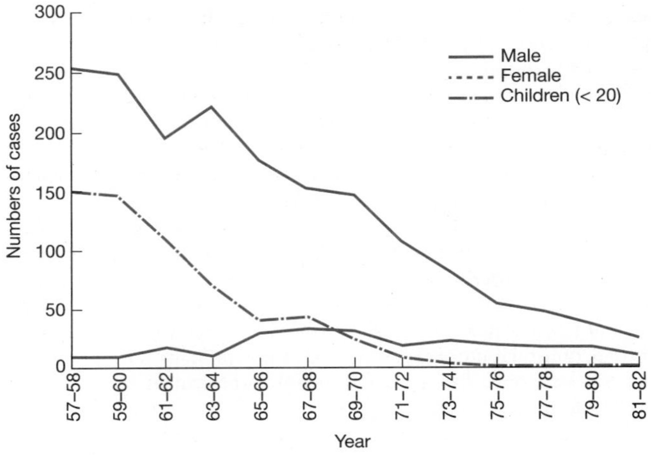

Fig. 6 Kuru—numbers of cases by age, sex, and time.

disease to date have been MM homozygotes at codon 129 of the prion protein gene. This genotype is also present in about 80 per cent of cases of sporadic Creutzfeldt–Jakob disease and may represent a susceptibility factor for the development of variant Creutzfeldt–Jakob disease. Variation at this locus can, however, influence the incubation period and disease phenotype and it is possible that cases of human infection with bovine spongiform encephalopathy may yet be identified in individuals with a VV or MV genetic background.

The possible future number of cases of variant Creutzfeldt–Jakob disease is unknown, but there has been an increase in the annual number of deaths from variant Creutzfeldt–Jakob disease in the United Kingdom (Fig. 5) and statistical analyses, taking into account delays in referral and confirmation, have shown a significant increase in the temporal incidence of cases since 2000. Long-term predictions have estimated a total of 100 to over 136 000 cases of variant Creutzfeldt–Jakob disease in the United Kingdom. This wide range reflects the many uncertainties including the mean incubation period of bovine spongiform encephalopathy in humans, the level of the species barrier between bovines and humans, and the extent of human exposure to the bovine spongiform encephalopathy agent.

Kuru

The transmissibility of human prion diseases was first demonstrated in 1966 with the transmission of a spongiform encephalopathy to chimpanzees 18 to 21 months after intracerebral inoculation of a brain extract from a patient who had died of kuru. This seminal experiment followed years of clinical, epidemiological, and anthropological research in the Fore region of Papua New Guinea where kuru was endemic. In the early 1960s kuru caused over half of all deaths in the affected population and there have been more than 3000 deaths from kuru in the at-risk population of 30 000 people.

The epidemiological characteristics of kuru are unusual with familial aggregation of cases and a high incidence of disease in women and children in the early years of the epidemic. Since 1960 there has been a decline in the incidence, particularly in women and children (Fig. 6), and there have been no cases in children born after 1959. After extensive investigation into a possible genetic or toxic origin, anthropological research established that kuru was transmitted in the course of ritual cannibalism. As a mark of respect, relatives consumed affected individuals and virtually all tissues were consumed, including the brain and viscera. Although men took part in these rituals, women and children are thought to have consumed the internal organs such as the brain which contained the highest levels of infectivity. It is also possible that there was transcutaneous transmission through rubbing of tissue on the skin. Detailed investigation of individual cannibalistic events has shown that a number of members of the same family, including those who came from different areas, developed kuru after attending a single cannibalistic rite. Ritual cannibalism ceased by 1960, explaining the subsequent decline in incidence of kuru, but there are still occasional cases with incubation periods exceeding 40 years. It is of interest that at the height of the epidemic many hundreds of women were affected by kuru during pregnancy and breastfed their children, but none of these children later developed kuru.

Clinically kuru presented with a cerebellar syndrome, initially truncal ataxia and titubation, followed by ataxia of gait and dysarthria. A prodromal phase of headache and limb pain was common and hypotonia was a prominent early feature. Involuntary movements such as myoclonus and rigidity of the limbs did not occur, in contrast to other forms of human prion disease. Terminally patients became immobile and communication was often impossible because of severe dysarthria. Dementia did not occur, and even in the terminal akinetic and mute state patients could obey simple commands. In children the clinical features were similar, but in the early stages there were often brainstem signs such as strabismus, nystagmus, and ptosis. The total duration of illness ranged from 12 to 18 months in adults and 3 to 12 months in children.

In kuru, neuropathological changes were most apparent in the cerebellum, consistent with the clinical features. Neuronal loss and intense cerebellar astrocytosis were uniform findings and about three-quarters of cases had amyloid plaque deposition, particularly in the granule cell layer of the cerebellum. The cerebral cortex showed mild spongiform change. The similarity of the neuropathology of kuru to scrapie was commented on by Hadlow in 1959, prompting the transmission studies which later demonstrated that kuru, like scrapie, was experimentally transmissible.

By using stored samples, analysis of the influence of the codon 129 polymorphism of the prion protein gene on susceptibility to kuru has shown that homozygosity, either MM or VV, increases susceptibility and that heterozygotes may have a more prolonged incubation period. The analysis of codon 129 genotype in kuru is complicated by the limited number of tested cases and the possible effect of the high mortality rate on the codon 129 distribution in a closed population.

The diagnosis of human prion diseases

Human prion diseases are rare, but the high public profile of Creutzfeldt–Jakob disease and variant Creutzfeldt–Jakob disease has resulted in an increase in the number of cases in which the diagnosis of one of these diseases is suspected. Accurate diagnosis of any condition, including patients suffering from a human prion disease, is essential but the exclusion of a

Table 6 Diagnostic criteria for sporadic Creutzfeldt–Jakob disease

I	Rapidly progressive dementia
IIA	Myoclonus
IIB	Visual or cerebellar problems
IIC	Pyramidal or extrapyramidal features
IID	Akinetic mutism
III	Typical electroencephalogram
Definite	Neuropathologically/immunocytochemically confirmed
Probable	I + two of II + III or Possible + positive 14-3-3
Possible	I + two of II + duration less than 2 years

diagnosis is also important, particularly for a fatal and untreatable condition. Although symptomatic treatment, for example for involuntary movements, can be helpful in human prion diseases there is currently no available treatment that influences the clinical course nor any treatment to prevent the development of neurological disease after infection. An important objective is to improve diagnostic accuracy in human prion diseases and in particular to allow early diagnosis. In the absence of a test for the presence of the infectious agent, diagnosis depends on the recognition of the clinical characteristics of human prion diseases supported by a range of investigations, some of which have been developed in recent years. Diagnostic criteria for sporadic, iatrogenic, familial, and variant Creutzfeldt–Jakob disease have been formulated and validated (Tables 6 and 7). In all human prion diseases a definite diagnosis can only be made by the examination of brain tissue, usually at post-mortem.

In the majority of cases of sporadic Creutzfeldt–Jakob disease the diagnosis is made in life because of the multifocal neurological deficits, the development of myoclonus, and in particular the rapidity in the progression of cognitive impairment. The clinical picture is distinct from more common forms of dementia. In forms of sporadic Creutzfeldt–Jakob disease with early focal neurological features such as a cerebellar syndrome the rapid evolution of other neurological deficits and dementia suggests the diagnosis of Creutzfeldt–Jakob disease. Diagnosis can be difficult in cases of sporadic Creutzfeldt–Jakob disease with atypical features such as long duration of illness, and in these cases investigations such as magnetic resonance imaging of the brain can be helpful. There is increasing evidence that cases of sporadic Creutzfeldt–Jakob disease may be atypical if there is an underlying MV or VV codon 129 prion protein genotype.

Table 7 Diagnostic criteria for variant Creutzfeldt–Jakob disease

IA	Progressive neuropsychiatric disorder
IB	Duration of illness more than 6 months
IC	Routine investigations do not suggest an alternative diagnosis
ID	No history of potential iatrogenic exposure
IIA	Early psychiatric symptoms*
IIB	Persistent painful sensory symptoms†
IIC	Ataxia
IID	Myoclonus or chorea or dystonia
IIE	Dementia
IIIA	Electroencephalogram does not show the typical appearance of sporadic Creutzfeldt–Jakob disease (or no electroencephalogram performed)‡
IIIB	Bilateral pulvinar high signal on magnetic resonance scan
IVA	Positive tonsil biopsy
Definite	IA + neuropathological confirmation of variant Creutzfeldt–Jakob disease§
Probable	I + four out of five of II + IIIA + IIIB
Probable	I + IVA
Possible	I + four out of five of II + IIIA

* Depression, anxiety, apathy, withdrawal, delusions.

† This includes both frank pain and/or unpleasant dysaesthesia.

‡ Generalized triphasic periodic complexes at approximately one per second.

§ Spongiform change and extensive deposition of prion protein with florid plaques, throughout the cerebrum and cerebellum.

Hereditary prion diseases are often suspected because of a family history of a similar disorder, but in a significant proportion of cases of Creutzfeldt–Jakob disease associated with a prion protein gene mutation there is a family history of another neurodegenerative disorder or no relevant family history. The gradual clinical progression in many forms of hereditary human prion disease makes accurate diagnosis difficult and the diagnosis may only be recognized in life after prion protein gene analysis. Genetic testing should only be carried out with fully informed consent.

The diagnosis of iatrogenic Creutzfeldt–Jakob disease depends on the identification of a relevant risk factor, for example previous treatment with human growth hormone, and an assessment of the neurological presentation. Most patients with growth hormone related Creutzfeldt–Jakob disease present with a cerebellar syndrome, while after central iatrogenic exposure to infection the clinical picture is usually similar to that of sporadic Creutzfeldt–Jakob disease. The utility of specialist investigation in iatrogenic Creutzfeldt–Jakob disease is uncertain because of the rarity of these forms of Creutzfeldt–Jakob disease and limited information on investigations.

The clinical picture in the later stages of variant Creutzfeldt–Jakob disease is similar to that of sporadic Creutzfeldt–Jakob disease and, although the recognition of the diagnosis in the first cases of this new disease was difficult, the clinical phenotype is now well known and the diagnosis is usually apparent after neurological signs develop, often in young patients in an age group in which dementia is very unusual. Diagnosis in the early stages is, however, difficult as there is a period of many months in which the clinical picture is dominated by psychiatric symptoms, including depression, anxiety, and withdrawal. Clues to the possibility of variant Creutzfeldt–Jakob disease include cognitive impairment, subtle gait ataxia, and persistent painful sensory symptoms in combination with the psychiatric symptoms.

Investigations in human prion disease

Many of the investigations carried out in suspected cases of human prion disease do not show any specific disease related abnormality, but help to exclude other diagnoses, some potentially treatable. The interpretation of the results of investigations depends on the clinical picture because the sensitivity and specificity of surrogate markers for prion disease, such as 14-3-3 cerebrospinal fluid analysis (see below), depend on clearly defining the characteristics of the patients in which the test has been carried out.

Routine haematological and biochemical tests are usually normal. About a third of cases of sporadic or variant Creutzfeldt–Jakob disease may have minor abnormalities in liver function tests.

The electroencephalogram shows periodic triphasic complexes at about 1 per second in 60 to 70 per cent of cases of sporadic Creutzfeldt–Jakob disease (Fig. 7) and in some cases of iatrogenic Creutzfeldt–Jakob disease after central exposure to infection. These electroencephalogram changes are relatively specific, but similar appearances can be seen in hepatic encephalopathy, lithium or metrizamide toxicity, metabolic disturbance, and rarely in other forms of dementia such as Alzheimer's disease.

There is no cerebrospinal fluid pleocytosis in any form of human prion disease, and cerebrospinal fluid protein is elevated in about a third of cases. Elevation of the 14-3-3 cerebrospinal fluid protein, a marker for neuronal damage, has a sensitivity and specificity of about 90 per cent in the diagnosis of sporadic Creutzfeldt–Jakob disease, but is less useful in the diagnosis of variant Creutzfeldt–Jakob disease.

A computed tomography scan of the brain is usually normal, but can show non-specific cerebral atrophy. Magnetic resonance imaging of the brain shows a high signal on T_2-weighted images in the caudate nucleus

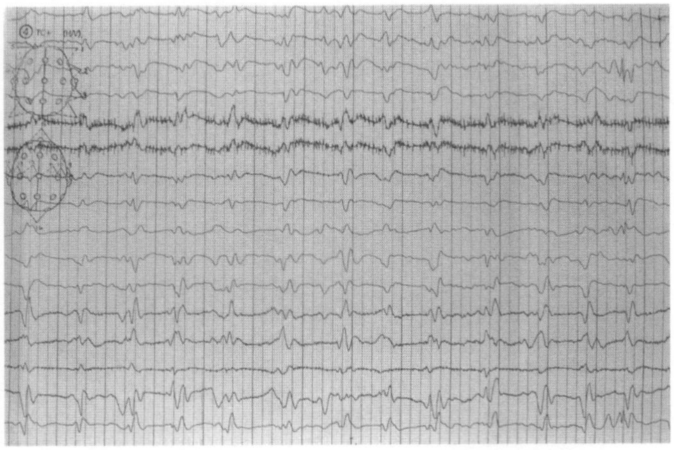

Fig. 7 Typical electroencephalogram in sporadic Creutzfeldt-Jakob disease.

and putamen in about 70 per cent of cases of sporadic Creutzfeldt–Jakob disease (Fig. 8), but the sensitivity and specificity of these abnormalities has not been formally assessed. In variant Creutzfeldt–Jakob disease about 80 per cent of cases show a high signal on T_2-weighted images (and PD and FLAIR sequences) in the pulvinar region of the posterior thalamus (Fig. 9) and in the appropriate clinical context these abnormalities have a high sensitivity and specificity for the diagnosis of variant Creutzfeldt–Jakob disease. To date all cases of variant Creutzfeldt–Jakob disease classified as 'probable', a diagnosis requiring the abnormalities on magnetic resonance imaging, that have come to post-mortem examination have been confirmed as variant Creutzfeldt–Jakob disease.

Brain biopsy can allow the confirmation of the diagnosis of a human prion disease in life, but this investigation has risks and is mainly carried out when there is a realistic possibility of an alternative diagnosis. Tonsil biopsy in variant Creutzfeldt–Jakob disease can also increase the likelihood of the diagnosis in life, but this procedure is also invasive and, although early diagnosis is important for the relatives of the patient and for clinicians, it does not benefit the patient.

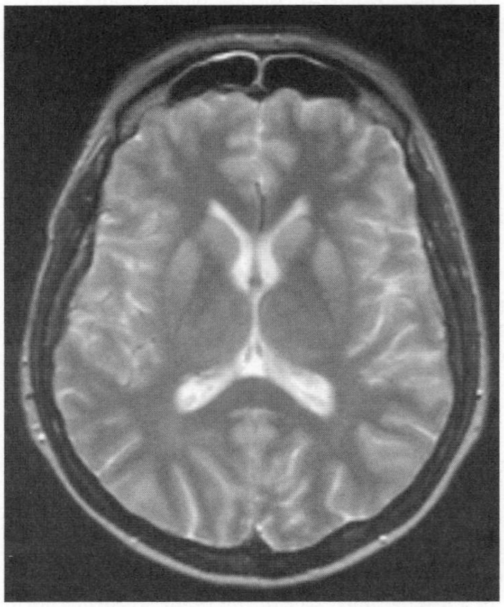

Fig. 8 MRI image of sporadic Creutzfeldt–Jakob disease showing high signal changes symmetrically in the caudate and putamen.

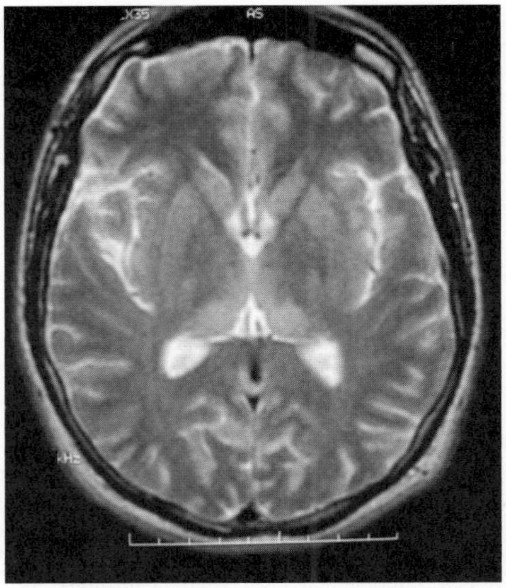

Fig. 9 MRI image of variant Creutzfeldt–Jakob disease showing high signal symmetrically in the posterior thalamus.

Conclusion

There have been remarkable scientific advances in the understanding of prion diseases and it is hoped that this may lead to the identification of a diagnostic test in life for the presence of infection and to therapies to prevent the development of disease. Human prion diseases have attained a public notoriety disproportionate to the overall burden of disease caused by these rare conditions. However, the transmission of an animal prion disease, bovine spongiform encephalopathy, to humans has been a tragedy and the prolonged incubation periods characteristic of this group of diseases indicate that the eventual consequences of bovine spongiform encephalopathy for public health both in the United Kingdom and in other countries are unpredictable.

Further reading

Brown P *et al.* (2000). Iatrogenic Creutzfeldt–Jakob disease at the millennium. *Neurology* **55**, 1075–81.

Collinge J, Palmer MS (1997). Human prion diseases. In: Collinge J, Palmer MS, eds. *Prion diseases*, pp 18–56. Oxford University Press, New York.

DeArmond SJ, Ironside JW (1999). Neuropathology of prion diseases. In: Prusiner SB, ed. *Prion biology and diseases*, pp 585–652. Cold Spring Harbor Laboratory Press, New York.

Donnelly CA, Ferguson NM (1999). Predictions and scenario analysis for vCJD. In: Donnelly CA, Ferguson NM, eds. *Statistical aspects of BSE and vCJD*, pp 163–94. Chapman and Hall, London.

Gajdusek DC (1990). Subacute spongiform encephalopathies: transmissible cerebral amyloidoses caused by unconventional viruses. In: Fields BN, Knipe DM, eds. *Fields virology*, pp 2289–324. Raven Press, New York.

Gambetti P *et al.* (1999). Inherited prion diseases. In: Prusiner SB, ed. *Prion biology and diseases*, pp 509–83. Cold Spring Harbor Laboratory Press, New York.

Parchi P *et al.* (1999). Classification of sporadic Creutzfeldt–Jakob disease based on molecular and phenotypic analysis of 300 subjects. *Annals of Neurology* **46**, 224–33.

Prusiner SB (1994). Prion diseases of humans and animals. *Journal of the Royal College of Physicians of London* **28** (suppl.), 1–30.

Prusiner SB (1999). Development of the prion concept. In: Prusiner SB, ed. *Prion biology and diseases*, pp 67–112. Cold Spring Harbor Laboratory Press, New York.

Will RG *et al.* (1999). Infectious and sporadic prion diseases. In: Prusiner SB, ed. *Prion biology and diseases*, pp 465–507. Cold Spring Harbor Laboratory Press, New York.

24.13.10 Parkinsonism and other extrapyramidal diseases

Donald B. Calne

The concept of extrapyramidal disease

The concept of extrapyramidal disease arose at the start of the twentieth century. Nineteenth-century anatomists, physiologists, and neurologists established the importance of the pyramidal pathway, but they later recognized that pathology outside this system also led to major disturbances of voluntary movement. It was concluded that alternative pathways within the central nervous system contribute to the control of movement and the term 'extrapyramidal system' was coined. Pathology in this extrapyramidal system was associated with involuntary movements, which became the hallmark of what were called 'extrapyramidal diseases'. Over the course of the twentieth century, however, the notion of a pyramidal pathway was criticized. In consequence, the idea of disease involving an extrapyramidal pathway was also discredited, so the term 'movement disorders' became fashionable, and is now widely used.

In spite of these changes in nomenclature, there is general agreement that certain structures, deep in the brain, play an important part in the planning and execution of voluntary movement. In particular, it has been shown through clinicopathological correlation, that the basal ganglia are linked to motor control. The basal ganglia comprise the caudate nucleus, the putamen, and the globus pallidus. In addition, certain nuclei feeding into this system, such as the substantia nigra, are usually included. Myoclonus and ataxia will not be discussed in this review, because their pathology does not involve the basal ganglia.

Parkinson's disease

Definition

The terms 'paralysis agitans', 'the shaking palsy', 'Parkinson's disease', 'idiopathic parkinsonism', and 'idiopathic Parkinson's disease' have all been used, at various times, to describe the same entity. The definition of this entity is, however, fraught with difficulties. Initially, it was thought that the presence of Lewy bodies in the substantia nigra was the pathological *sine qua non* for the distinction of Parkinson's disease from other disorders. However, it has recently been recognized that Lewy bodies are quite non-specific, occurring in such diverse entities as Hallervorden–Spatz disease, certain forms of dementia, and subacute sclerosing panencephalitis. Furthermore, it has also been recognized that some patients who looked in every way as if they had Parkinson's disease during life, proved to have degeneration of cells in the substantia nigra with tangles rather than Lewy bodies.

There have been different approaches to resolving the dilemma created by this difficulty with definition. Perhaps the most satisfactory solution, for the present, is the use of the term 'Parkinson's syndrome' until we understand the aetiology, or, more likely, the many aetiologies of 'Parkinson's disease'. But the old terminology persists in most of the current literature, so the term 'Parkinson's disease' will be used here for the idiopathic syndrome of parkinsonism.

Aetiology

We already know that several distinct aetiologies are responsible for Parkinson's disease. For example, genetic factors have been identified, including mutations of the α-synuclein gene, the parkin gene, and a gene located on chromosome 2. Genetic causes of parkinsonism tend to produce symptoms at a younger age than sporadic Parkinson's disease. Most cases are sporadic, and are likely to have environmental aetiologies.

We are left with the unproven probability that there exist several different causes for Parkinson's disease, just as there exist several different causes for meningitis, or peripheral neuropathy.

Epidemiology

The prevalence of Parkinson's disease is around 200 to 300 per 100 000. The incidence is about 20 per 100 000 per year. These figures apply to the United Kingdom, Canada, and the United States. Studies on the geographical distribution indicate a low rate in Africa, China, and Japan. Prevalence rises with age, and Parkinson's disease is slightly commoner in males. The prevalence also increases with distance from the equator. A recent Canadian study suggests that Parkinson's disease is commoner in healthcare workers, teachers, and those who share cramped living conditions for sleeping (for example, miners and loggers working in camps)—while those who live more secluded lives have a low prevalence. These finding suggest the possibility that a viral infection might contribute to causation in some cases.

Pathology

The classical hallmark of Parkinson's disease is the relatively selective degeneration of the dopaminergic nigrostriatal pathway. In particular, the ventral tier of the zona compacta of the substantia nigra undergoes degeneration, and there is a reduction of dopamine in the striatum with a characteristic spatial distribution. The loss is predominantly posterior in the putamen, extending, to a lesser extent, forward into the anterior putamen and the caudate. In most cases of Parkinson's disease, Lewy bodies can be found in the substantia nigra.

Clinical features

The principal clinical features of Parkinson's disease are resting tremor, rigidity, and bradykinesia. In addition, postural reflexes are impaired, though this is a rather non-specific finding. These clinical features can be regarded as the inclusion criteria for a diagnosis. There are also exclusion criteria, for Parkinson's disease should not be considered if pyramidal signs, cerebellar signs, gaze palsies, or autonomic deficits are prominent. As Parkinson's disease progresses, many patients develop dementia.

It is usual to find asymmetry in the clinical presentation of patients with Parkinson's disease, and they almost always respond to dopaminomimetic treatment if there are no dose-limiting side-effects.

Natural history

Parkinson's disease starts several years before patients first notice symptoms. The full extent of this 'preclinical phase' has not been defined. However, we do know that the loss of dopaminergic nigral cells is slow, and that some 50 per cent of the nigrostriatal pathway is lost when symptoms first become apparent. Pathological observations, positron emission tomography, and clinical examination all indicate that the rate of progression of neuronal loss decreases over the course of Parkinson's disease.

The mean duration of Parkinson's disease depends on the time of onset. In general, progression is slower when Parkinson's disease presents in younger patients; it may run a course of over 35 years in these circumstances. In older patients, although the duration is shorter, life expectation is still only slightly reduced. Primarily, the patient is faced with a reduction in the quality, rather than the quantity, of life. Nevertheless, the late stage of the illness can entail cruelly protracted and profound disability.

Differential diagnosis

The most common disorder that can be confused with Parkinson's disease is essential tremor. While the classical description of a resting tremor has been employed to characterize Parkinson's disease, the early stage of the illness is often accompanied by a rather low-amplitude postural tremor, similar to that seen in essential tremor. This phase in the evolution of Parkinson's disease only lasts for a year or two. In contrast, postural tremor is present for many years in essential tremor, and it is only in advanced stages of essential tremor that a resting tremor appears.

Drug-induced parkinsonism is another important consideration in the differential diagnosis of Parkinson's disease. All drugs that block dopamine receptors or deplete dopamine in the brain are capable of producing a parkinsonian syndrome. While the major tranquillizing drugs used to treat psychosis are most frequently responsible, other drugs such as metoclopramide, used to control nausea and modify gastrointestinal motility, are now an important cause of parkinsonism.

The most common serious neurodegenerative disorder to be confused with Parkinson's disease is progressive supranuclear palsy (Steele–Richardson syndrome). It may take a year or two before the importance of gaze palsies, nuchal rigidity, dementia, and impaired balance all lead to the realization that one is not dealing with classical Parkinson's disease.

Multiple system atrophy is also easily mistaken for Parkinson's disease. Again, the clinician may have to wait until the autonomic deficits or cerebellar features of multiple system atrophy become prominent. Drugs used to treat Parkinson's disease tend to induce orthostatic hypotension, compounding the difficulty in differential diagnosis. The task of determining whether orthostatic hypotension is part of the underlying illness or a consequence of treatment often poses a challenge.

Treatment

Medical treatment

There is no convincing evidence that any current treatment slows down the course of Parkinson's disease, so all treatment is directed at reducing symptoms and improving quality of life. The cornerstone of treatment is dopaminomimetic therapy, to overcome the impact of reduced dopamine in the striatum. The standard therapy for many years has been levodopa, combined with a peripheral decarboxylase inhibitor. Evidence is now accumulating that for initial treatment in the younger parkinsonian patient, the new artificial dopamine agonists give the best initial results. A recent 5-year study has shown advantages with ropinirole—because of a substantially reduced prevalence of dyskinesia. Other artificial dopamine agonists seem have similar benefits.

Drugs that inhibit the enzyme catechol-*O*-methyltransferase (COMT) are also useful in the management of Parkinson's disease because of their ability to extend the duration of action of levodopa.

Most patients develop a fluctuating response to levodopa after 3 to 6 years. This may be a deterioration in symptoms at the end of the interval between doses (wearing-off reactions) or unpredictable loss of mobility (on–off reactions). COMT inhibitors smooth out wearing-off fluctuations. The first COMT inhibitor, tolcapone, helped many patients. Unfortunately, it produced very rare fatal hepatic toxicity, so its use is restricted. Another COMT inhibitor, entacapone, has recently been introduced and this drug does not damage the liver.

Ropinirole

Ropinirole, a non-ergot dopamine agonist, is usually started at a dose of 0.25 mg three times a day, after food. The regimen is then increased to a four-times a day schedule, with individual doses gradually built up 8 mg daily. All dopaminomimetics can cause nausea and hypotension. Taking drugs after meals reduces nausea, which can generally be abolished by the addition of 10 mg domperidone, 30 to 60 min before each dose of dopaminomimetic agent. Increasing the intake of salt and fluids usually alleviates hypotension. The response to ropinirole varies from individual to individual, and sometimes the dose has to be increased further, up to 24 mg daily. All dose adjustments should be undertaken slowly. Psychiatric reactions, in particular visual hallucinations, are commoner than with levodopa. The main advantage of ropinirole is that it produces less dyskinesia than levodopa.

A disadvantage of ropinirole is a propensity to cause somnolence during the day, which may exceed the sleepiness associated with levodopa and the ergot derivatives, bromocriptine and pergolide. This problem of daytime sleepiness is shared with the other new dopamine agonist, pramipexole (see below).

Pramipexole

Pramipexole is another non-ergot dopamine agonist. The usual starting dose is 0.375 daily, but this is slowly increased to a range between 1.5 and 6 mg daily in four divided doses. The benefits and side-effects of pramipexole are similar to those of ropinirole, but there has been no controlled comparison of the two drugs. Just as with ropinirole, daytime sleepiness can be a problem. In some countries, physicians have been instructed by government regulatory agencies to warn patients taking pramipexole of the dangers of driving when receiving the drug—several motor accidents have been reported. In rats, pramipexole can increase sleep, and it has been suggested that this effect is produced by excessive stimulation of dopamine D3 receptors.

Bromocriptine

Bromocriptine was the first artificial dopamine agonist to be used for Parkinson's disease. It is an ergot derivative, and, in common with other ergots, can rarely cause pleural or pulmonary fibrosis, pleural effusion, and erythromelalgia. It is useful to obtain a baseline chest radiograph before starting treatment—for comparison if dyspnoea later develops. The usual starting dose of bromocriptine is 0.25 mg once daily, gradually building up to a dose of 20 to 30 mg daily, distributed in four doses, after food, as for all antiparkinson drugs. Occasionally the dose of bromocriptine may need to be increased further, to 40 or 50 mg daily.

Pergolide

Pergolide, another ergot derivative, was the second artificial dopamine agonist to be introduced for the treatment of Parkinson's disease. The usual starting dose is 0.15 mg daily, which may be increased up to 6 mg daily. The benefits and side-effects of pergolide are similar to those of bromocriptine. Pergolide is an agonist at D1 and D2 dopamine receptors, in contrast to bromocriptine, which is an agonist at D2 receptors and an antagonist at D1 receptors. These differences in pharmacological profile do not seem to be reflected by corresponding differences in therapeutic results, so D1 agonism may not be achieved at the dose levels of pergolide that are employed therapeutically.

Cabergoline

Cabergoline is the newest ergot-derived dopamine agonist. It has the unusual properties of a plasma half-life extending beyond 60 h, so that one dose a day suffices for treatment. The dose range is between 0.25 and 4 mg daily. While it is certainly useful to have a drug with a long duration of action, side-effects will, of course, persist longer than with other dopaminomimetic agents.

Levodopa

Levodopa is prescribed in combination with a decarboxylase inhibitor that does not cross the blood–brain barrier. Sinemet®, a combination of levodopa and carbidopa (co-careldopa), is marketed worldwide. Madopar® (or Prolopa®), a combination of levodopa and benserazide (co-beneldopa), is marketed in many countries. The usual starting regimens for levodopa/carbidopa and levodopa/benserazide is 50 mg of levodopa with 12.5 mg of the decarboxylase inhibitor, administered twice daily, increasing, at 3- to 5-day intervals, to 150 mg of levodopa four times daily. Levodopa, combined with a decarboxylase inhibitor, has the lowest prevalence of early side-effects—but with the artificial dopamine agonists, levodopa can cause nausea and hypotension. Over a longer period, levodopa frequently causes dyskinesia and fluctuations in mobility. While psychiatric side-effects can occur with levodopa, they are less common than with the artificial dopamine agonists.

Preparations of Sinemet and Madopar with prolonged action

Sinemet CR and Madopar HBS have both been marketed as formulations with longer plasma half-lives than standard Sinemet and Madopar. Because these longer acting preparations are often incompletely absorbed, a higher dose has to be given to achieve the same effect as the standard preparations. The increase is about 30 per cent, but there is considerable variation between patients—a usual dose would be 200 mg four times a day The longer acting preparations of Sinemet and Madopar are most useful in patients who have 'wearing-off' reactions.

Entacapone

Entacapone is a new COMT inhibitor given together with levodopa (plus a decarboxylase inhibitor), and the combination extends the plasma half-life of levodopa. Thus patients who have 'wearing-off' reactions get prolongation of the 'on period'. The usual dose is 200 mg with each dose of levodopa. Since entacapone can exacerbate dyskinesia, it is often necessary to reduce the dose of levodopa when introducing entacapone. A reduction of 20 to 30 per cent usually suffices.

Early medical treatment

Most neurologists tend to start elderly patients with Parkinson's disease on a combination of levodopa with a decarboxylase inhibitor, often using the long-acting preparations. This treatment achieves quite a rapid improvement in symptoms with minimal early side-effects. Unfortunately, with prolonged treatment, dyskinesia and fluctuations in mobility may develop and ultimately become significant problems. However, with older and frailer patients, the early period of excellent therapeutic response is given first priority.

With younger patients neurologists tend to place more emphasis on the long-term results. In these circumstances it is usual to start treatment with an artificial dopamine agonist, because of the lower risk for the development of fluctuations in mobility and dyskinesia.

Late medical treatment

After 2 or 3 years, patients who started treatment with an artificial dopamine agonist need the addition of levodopa. For most of the duration of their disease, therefore, parkinsonian patients take a combination of an artificial dopamine agonist and levodopa.

Surgical treatment

Some 30 to 40 years ago, there was widespread interest in achieving suppression of tremor by placing a lesion in the ventrolateral or the ventral intermediate nucleus of the thalamus. With the advent of levodopa this procedure was performed less often, but recently there has been a resurgence of interest in stereotactic surgery. Lesions placed in the globus pallidus consistently alleviate dyskinesia and also help tremor. To a lesser extent, pallidotomy can improve rigidity and bradykinesia.

The trend in surgery is now changing from producing lesions to electrical stimulation. 'Deep brain stimulation' produces good results, with less risk of unwanted consequences. Furthermore, deep brain stimulation of the subthalamic nucleus seems to result in greater benefit than stimulation of the pallidum. At present, the surgical treatment of Parkinson's disease is going through a period of active research extending to the transplantation of cells that produce dopamine or levodopa.

Other parkinsonian syndromes

Progressive supranuclear palsy

The classical diagnostic feature of progressive supranuclear palsy is paresis of conjugate gaze. Initially there is a problem with looking up and down on command, and as the condition advances there is difficulty in following objects up and down. Vertical movement of the eyes can only be achieved by central visual fixation while the neck is flexed and extended. Although the disturbance with gaze is first apparent in the vertical plane, ultimately horizontal gaze also becomes affected. There is over-reaction of the frontalis muscles and extension of the neck to compensate for the weakness of upward conjugate eye movement. Patients with supranuclear palsy usually have an akinetic syndrome involving all limbs, with prominent rigidity of the neck and impairment of righting reflexes. As the condition advances there is intellectual impairment. Progressive supranuclear palsy usually presents in middle or late life, and it advances more rapidly than Parkinson's disease. There is sometimes a family history suggesting autosomal dominant inheritance.

Neuronal loss occurs with neurofibrillary tangles and gliosis. Atrophy of the tectum may be seen on brain imaging. The pathology extends to the substantia nigra, globus pallidus, subthalamus, dentate nucleus, and periaqueductal grey matter.

In the early stages of clinical evolution, there may be some response to dopaminomimetic therapy. Ultimately, however, this is lost. Once it has been appreciated that a patient has an atypical form of parkinsonism with prominent gaze palsies, the differential diagnosis is vascular disease of the brainstem. During life, it is often difficult to distinguish between progressive supranuclear palsy and vascular disease.

Multiple system atrophy

The term 'multiple system atrophy' was coined by Oppenheimer. Included within this entity are three syndromes that usually overlap: (1) strionigral degeneration leading to parkinsonism; (2) autonomic failure; and (3) olivopontocerebellar degeneration.

Multiple system atrophy is a sporadic disorder that generally presents in later life. The pathology may be widespread, involving the basal ganglia, the dorsal nucleus of the vagus, Onuf's nucleus, the cerebellum, and the intermediolateral column of the thoracic spinal cord.

Multiple system atrophy runs a briefer course than Parkinson's disease. While there may be some initial response to dopaminomimetic drugs, these often exacerbate orthostatic hypotension, and hence are seldom useful in advanced illness. It is usually necessary to use agents such as fludrocortisone and midrodrine in an effort to raise the blood pressure, but sometimes the supine blood pressure is so high that treatment becomes extremely difficult.

Stridor, loud snoring, and sleep apnoea are frequently encountered in multiple system atrophy. Sometimes tracheostomy is necessary.

Drug-induced parkinsonism

Drugs that block dopamine receptors, or deplete the storage of dopamine, can produce a syndrome clinically indistinguishable from Parkinson's disease. Almost always, withdrawal of the offending drug leads to a restoration of normal motor function. In patients who are disabled by psychotic symptoms, it may be impossible to stop treatment in order to alleviate the parkinsonian syndrome. In these circumstances, the treatment of choice is clozapine, which has fewer tendencies to produce parkinsonism than any other antipsychotic agent. Clozapine carries a risk of bone marrow depression, so regular blood counts are mandatory when this drug is employed.

Essential tremor

Essential tremor is probably more common than all the other movement disorders put together. Sometimes the adjective 'benign' is attached to the disorder, but this can be quite misleading. Essential tremor may be severe and disabling, though it seldom evolves to produce other neurological deficits—an exception is the quite frequent occurrence of ataxia in long-standing essential tremor among the elderly.

Although essential tremor most often involves the hands, the neck is also vulnerable, so that the head shakes from side to side, or up and down. Sometimes the voice is affected and there may also be a tremor of the chin. Uncommonly, essential tremor can occur in the legs.

The characteristic feature of essential tremor is a postural shake that is sustained during movement. Essential tremor can start at any age, and it may interfere with work, for example in cases where dexterity is important. It is also troublesome when tremor, in front of the public, leads to difficulty in job performance. The impact of essential tremor is amplified through stress, for when a patient particularly wants to control the shaking, circumstantial anxiety leads to exacerbation of the tremor.

Essential tremor can progress to have a serious effect on the quality of life. For example, eating and drinking can become so difficult that patients will no longer eat in the company of others. Essential tremor tends to get worse in the later stages of life, when it can become prominent at rest, mimicking the resting tremor of Parkinson's disease. There may also be some 'cog-wheeling', when testing passive resistance to movement of the wrist. Thus essential tremor can easily be confused with early Parkinson's disease.

In about half the patients with essential tremor it is possible to obtain a family history, indicating autosomal dominant inheritance: genes have been identified on chromosomes 2 and 3. We do not know the site of the pathology of essential tremor, but interest has been focused on the internal olive, the red nucleus, and the dentate nucleus.

The treatment of essential tremor is usually difficult. Some 30 per cent of patients respond to β-blocking drugs, and benzodiazepines such as clonazepam can be helpful. Sometimes primidone is useful. Although essential tremor is characteristically alleviated by alcohol, it is obviously inadvisable for patients to use alcohol on a regular basis to stop the shaking.

When essential tremor is severe, and it is impossible to achieve an adequate response with drugs, improvement can usually be obtained by performing a thalamotomy. Recently, encouraging results have been achieved with deep brain stimulation using an electrode implanted into the ventrolateral nucleus of the thalamus. Deep brain stimulation carries less risk than thalamotomy.

Dystonia

The term 'dystonia' is used to describe a pattern of abnormal movements in which there is sustained contraction of muscles, which may last for several seconds and can induce distorted postures. If a joint can twist, dystonia usually produces torsion—hence the term 'torsion dystonia'. Superimposed on these slow muscle contractions are often quick involuntary movements, which may be regularly repetitive in space and time, or quite irregular.Dystonia is often exacerbated by voluntary movement.

In addition to the term 'dystonia' being applied to these physical signs, it is also used for the 'disease' where no cause can be found. If dystonia is limited to one group of muscles, it is termed 'focal dystonia', and when the entire body is involved it is termed 'generalized dystonia'.

Generalized idiopathic dystonia

This condition usually starts in childhood or early adult life. It is dominantly inherited and the gene responsible, *DYT1*, has been identified on chromosome 9. This form of dystonia is particularly common in Ashkenazim Jews. Dystonia generally progresses over several years and then reaches a plateau. Treatment is difficult; high doses of anticholinergic drugs such as trihexyphenidyl are most effective.

Dopa-responsive dystonia

In any patient with generalized dystonia it is most important to consider the possibility of dopa-responsive dystonia (hereditary progressive dystonia, Segawa's disease), because treatment for this disorder is so effective. Low doses of dopaminomimetic drugs are therapeutic throughout the life of the patient.

The pathogenesis of dopa-responsive dystonia has been worked out with considerable precision. Several mutations—about 60—can be responsible, all on chromosome 14, and all associated with the production of the cofactor for tyrosine hydroxylase, tetrahydrobiopterin. When this cofactor is lacking, tyrosine cannot be converted to dopa, so there is inadequate dopamine available in the striatum. This condition of dopamine depletion leads to dystonia, and in addition these patients usually have some parkinsonian features. Indeed, when dopa-responsive dystonia presents in late life, the parkinsonian features may overshadow the dystonia.

Hemidystonia

Dystonia involving one side of the body is often caused by a structural lesion in the contralateral basal ganglia. Infarcts are most often responsible, but brain imaging should be undertaken to exclude tumours.

Focal dystonia

The commonest form of dystonia is localized to the neck muscles; known as cervical dystonia or spasmodic torticollis. Sometimes there is a genetic basis for this condition, but usually it presents sporadically. Cervical dystonia generally responds to local injections of low concentrations of botulinum toxin. Blepharospasm is another focal dystonia that responds well to botulinum toxin, and dystonia of the vocal cords also responds, in many cases, to small injections of this toxin.

Tardive dyskinesia

Tardive dyskinesia is a syndrome of involuntary movements induced by long-term exposure to dopamine-blocking drugs. Major tranquillizers are usually responsible, but drugs employed to treat nausea, such as metoclopramide, are more recent culprits. While dystonic features usually predominate in tardive dyskinesia, there may also be obvious chorea.

Tardive dyskinesia is a chronic condition, and while it sometimes resolves spontaneously in younger patients, it is generally permanent in the elderly. Paradoxically, there is frequently an exacerbation—or initial appearance—of tardive dyskinesia when the drug responsible is reduced or stopped.

Treatment for tardive dyskinesia is withdrawal of the drug responsible when possible, and the administration of tetrabenazine. Unfortunately, tetrabenazine can cause depression, and is therefore contraindicated when tardive dyskinesia develops in a psychotic patient with depressive features. In this setting, serious psychotic disease with tardive dyskinesia is often managed by increasing the dose of the causal drug.

Chorea

The term 'chorea' derives from the Greek word for dancing. The physical sign of chorea is quick involuntary movement, irregular in space and time, generally most prominent in the extremities. Chorea is closely related to ballism, which is a high-amplitude displacement of the proximal muscles. In patients who develop ballism due to a stroke, the natural history of spontaneous improvement progresses through a phase of chorea, followed by a final resolution of the chorea.

Huntington's chorea

Huntington's chorea is an inexorably progressive disorder featuring a combination of chorea and dementia. The pathology primarily involves the caudate nucleus, but it extends beyond this initial focus.

Huntington's chorea is dominantly inherited; it is caused by a mutation on chromosome 4—the huntingtin gene—characterized by an expansion of CAG repeats.

Huntington's chorea generally starts in mid-adult life, around the age of 35 years. However, it can start in childhood, when it tends to have a more rigid presentation resembling parkinsonism. This is known as the Westphal variant. Sometimes Huntington's chorea can present in late-adult life, over the age of 70.

There is no effective treatment for Huntington's chorea. Tetrabenazine will reduce the involuntary movements, but the progressive dementia is resistant to all therapy.

Other forms of chorea

Neuroacanthocytosis is a rare autosomal recessive disorder associated with hypogammaglobulinaemia. It produces involuntary movements, of which the commonest is chorea—but neuroacanthocytosis can also cause parkinsonism or dystonia.

Sydenham's chorea is associated with rheumatic fever; both are now rare conditions, although they still occasionally occur in children. The chorea runs a benign course, with spontaneous remission usually taking place within 3 to 6 months.

Rarely, chorea can occur during pregnancy, or with exposure to oestrogens. Occasionally other drugs such as phenytoin and digoxin can cause chorea. Severe thyrotoxicosis may produce choreatic movements, as may systemic lupus erythematosus.

Tic

Although tics are usually quick involuntary movements, they may be more prolonged; the term 'dystonic tic' has been coined for the slow variety. Patients feel a compulsion to move, and the characteristic feature of all tics is the patient's ability to suppress them for brief periods of 30 to 60 s.

Tics confined to a single muscle group often persist through life. When tics move around from one part of the body to another, they are termed 'chronic multiple tic', or Gilles de la Tourette disease.

Gilles de la Tourette disease

Gilles de la Tourette disease is dominantly inherited, though the penetrance is variable, so that often a positive family history cannot be obtained. Gilles de la Tourette disease affects boys more often than girls, and it generally starts before the age of 15 years. Tics persist, waxing and waning in severity, over several years, though they often disappear in mid-adult life. In addition to the common movements of the face, shoulders, and hands, there are often truncal movements, and sometimes there are involuntary noises, such as excessive sniffing, throat clearing, or barking. Words may be uttered inappropriately and often these are expletives. Similarly, affected individuals may make obscene gestures.

The pathological basis of tics is not known, but they generally respond to drugs that decrease dopaminergic transmission. In the past, major tranquillizing drugs have been used, but these carry a risk of causing tardive dyskinesia, which, may itself, be expressed as a tic. Tetrabenazine is the most satisfactory treatment for most patients. Unfortunately, sedation can be a troublesome side-effect, particularly for children who are attending school. Depression can also develop and the drug should be withdrawn if this happens. It is therefore best to try to manage patients without using drugs, explaining that educating family, friends, employers, and teachers may help patients to cope. Sometimes, however, Gilles de la Tourette can cause severe tics and noises that are socially disruptive, and in such cases a minimal but therapeutic dose of tetrabenazine must be sought, usually between 12.5 and 100 mg daily.

Gilles de la Tourette disease is often associated with obsessive–compulsive behaviour and attention disorder with hyperactivity; in such cases psychiatric advice is necessary. Clomipramine or fluoxetine may be helpful in these circumstances.

Other conditions

The spectrum of movement disorders is extensive, and space does not permit consideration of all. For a more comprehensive survey, the reader is referred to Jankovic and Tolosa (1998), which provides descriptions of Creutzfeldt–Jakob disease, Hallervorden–Spatz disease, cortical basal ganglionic degeneration, dentatorubropallidoluysian atrophy, olivopontocerebellar atrophy, paroxysmal dystonia, restless leg syndrome, myoclonus, and ataxia. This source also describes the neurology of Wilson's disease, but for a discussion of the metabolic disturbance and treatment of Wilson's disease the reader is referred to Chapter 11.7.2.

Further reading

Calne DB (2000). Parkinson's disease is not one disease. *Parkinsonism and Related Disorders* **7**, 3–7.

Frucht S, *et al.* (1999). Falling asleep at the wheel: motor vehicle mishaps in persons taking pramipexole and ropinirole. *Neurology* **52**, 1908–10.

Gasser T, *et al.* (1998). A susceptibility locus for Parkinson's disease maps to chromosome 2p13. *Nature Genetics* **18**, 262–5.

Higgins JJ, Jankovic J, Patel PI (1998). Evidence that a gene for essential tremor maps to chromosome 2p in four families. *Movement Disorders* **13**, 972–7.

Ichinose H, *et al.* (2001). Dopa-responsive dystonia: from causative gene to molecular mechanism. *Advances in Neurology* **86**, 173–7.

Jankovic J, Tolosa E, eds. (1998). *Parkinson's disease and movement disorders.* Williams and Wilkins, Baltimore.

Johnson RH, *et al.* (1966). Autonomic failure due to intermedio-lateral column degeneration. *Quarterly Journal of Medicine* **35**, 276.

Kitada T, *et al.* (1998). Mutations in the Parkin gene cause autosomal recessive juvenile parkinsonism. *Nature* **392**, 605–8.

Krack P, *et al.* (1998). Treatment of tremor in Parkinson's disease by subthalamic nucleus stimulation. *Movement Disorders* **13**, 907–14.

Kurtzke JF, Goldberg ID (1988). Parkinsonism death rates by race, sex, and geography. *Neurology* **38**, 1558–61.

Largos P, *et al.* (1998). Effects of the D3 preferring dopamine agonist pramipexole on sleep and waking, locomotor activity and striatal dopamine release in rats. *European Neuropsychopharmacology* **8**, 113–20.

Lee CS, *et al.* (1994). Clinical observations on the rate of progression of idiopathic parkinsonism. *Brain* **117**, 501–7.

Marion S (2001). The epidemiology of Parkinson disease. *Advances in Neurology* **87**, 163–73.

Polymeropoulos MH, *et al.* (1997). Mutation in the α-synuclein gene identified in families with Parkinson's disease. *Science* **276**, 2045–7.

Rajput AH, *et al.* (1989). Parkinsonism and neurofibrillary tangle pathology in pigmented nuclei. *Annals of Neurology* **25**, 602–6.

Rascol O, on behalf of the 056 Study Group (1999). Ropinirole reduces risk of dyskinesia when used in early PD. *Parkinsonism and Related Disorders* **5**, S83. [Abstract]

Rinne UK and the PKDS009 Collaborative Study Group (1999). A five year double blind study with cabergoline versus levodopa in the treatment of early Parkinson's disease. *Parkinsonism and Related Disorders* 5, S84. [Abstract]

Rojo A, *et al.* (1999). Clinical genetics of familial progressive supranuclear palsy. *Brain* **122**(Pt 7), 1233–45.

Samii A, *et al.* (1999). Reassessment of unilateral pallidotomy in Parkinson's disease. A 2 year follow up study. *Brain* **122**, 417–25.

Schulzer M, *et al.* (1994). A mathematical model of pathogenesis in idiopathic parkinsonism. *Brain* **117**, 509–16.

Singer C, Sanchez-Ramos J, Weiner WJ (1994). Gait abnormality in essential tremor. *Movement Disorders* **9**(2), 193–6.

Tanner CM, *et al.* (1999). Parkinson's disease in twins: an etiologic study. *Journal of the American Medical Association* **281**, 376–8.

Tasker RR (1998). Deep brain stimulation is preferable to thalamotomy for tremor suppression. *Surgical Neurology* **49**, 145–53.

Tsui JKC, Calne DB, eds. (1995). *Handbook of dystonia*. Marcel Dekker, New York.

Tsui JKC, *et al.* (1999). Occupational risk factors in Parkinson's disease. *Canadian Journal of Public Health* **90**, 334–5.

24.13.11 Disorders of movement (excluding Parkinson's disease)

Roger Barker*

Movement disorders typically result from diseases of the basal ganglia and can be classified into one of five main categories: dystonia, chorea, tremor, tics, and myoclonus (see Table 1 for definitions). Each type of abnormal movement may occur in several diseases and many treatments are empirical. However, the study of molecular genetics and the use of functional imaging has revealed subtle neurochemical abnormalities which should facilitate development of more rational therapies.

In this section, attention is drawn to abnormal movements that are a principal manifestation of the disease. Movement disorders have been divided into hyperkinetic and hypokinetic conditions; however, this classification may be misleading because a given disease often evolves with time. It is probably more useful to classify movement disorders by type.

The dystonias

Definition

Dystonias are characterized by prolonged muscle contractions, causing abnormal movements and postures.

Classification

When no symptomatic cause for dystonia can be discovered, the syndrome is described as idiopathic or primary dystonia, and if generalized then the disorder is synonymous with idiopathic torsion dystonia. Secondary dystonia is due to a defined exogenous, structural, or metabolic disorder. 'Dystonia plus' syndrome constitutes dystonia in combination with other abnormalities (for example myoclonic dystonia) and heredodegenerative dystonia occurs when there is an underlying brain degeneration. Dystonia may affect the whole body (generalized dystonia), adjacent parts such as an arm and neck (segmental dystonia), or may be restricted to one part (focal dystonia) as in spasmodic torticollis, dystonic writer's cramp, blepharospasm, oromandibular dystonia, and laryngeal dystonia.

Idiopathic dystonia is frequently inherited (see below), but the focal dystonias usually occur sporadically in middle life. However, focal dystonias may be isolated fragments of the syndrome of idiopathic torsion dystonia.

Aetiology

The many metabolic and other inherited or sporadic diseases that can cause dystonia (Table 2) usually produce other neurological symptoms and signs. A symptomatic cause for dystonia is found in about 50 per cent of children with the condition, but is rare in those with adult onset. In adults, dystonia is most likely to remain confined to its site of origin as a focal dystonia, and the legs are rarely affected. Children often develop symptoms in the legs and frequently develop segmental or generalized dystonia.

* We acknowledge the contribution of the late Professor C. D. Marsden to this chapter in the third edition of the textbook. Much of his text provides a basis for this chapter.

Table 1 Movement disorders*

Dystonia	Sustained spasms of muscle contraction which distort the limbs and trunk into characteristic postures—the twisted (torticollis), flexed (antecollis) or extended neck (retrocollis), the arched (lordosis) or twisted back (scoliosis), the hyperpronated arm, and plantar-flexed inverted foot. The spasms typically occur on willed action (action dystonia). Dystonic spasms may be intermittent, producing dystonic movements, which may be repetitive to give a rhythmic character, or sustained to hold a fixed dystonic posture
Athetosis	Athetosis was originally used to describe the sinuous, writhing digital movements that may follow a stroke; it later became synonymous with cerebral palsy, resulting from perinatal anoxia or kernicterus. Affected infants are floppy, exhibit delayed motor milestones, and before the age of 5 years develop athetoid movements—athetoid cerebral palsy, or 'athetosis'
Tremor	A rhythmic sinusoidal movement of a body part caused by regular muscle contractions
Chorea	A continuous flow of irregular, jerky, and explosive movements, that flit randomly from one part of the body to another. Each muscle contraction is brief, often appearing as a fragment of what might have been a normal movement, and unpredictable in timing or site (see Fig. 5).
Myoclonus	Rapid shock-like muscle jerks, often repetitive and sometimes rhythmic
Tics	Similar to myoclonic jerks, but are repetitive, stereotyped movements that can be mimicked voluntarily and can be held in check by an effort of will. Simple tics are confined to a few muscles; complex tics may include quasipurposeful movements.

* Nearly all dyskinesias disappear in sleep, are aggravated by anxiety, and improved by relaxation. Many movement disorders merge: for example Huntington's disease may show chorea and dystonia giving the appearance of 'hanging chorea'.

The recent identification of mutations in genes responsible for forms of dystonia gives hope for understanding its basis (see Table 2). Abnormalities within the basal ganglia and associated cortical motor areas have been found in some patients with secondary dystonia.

Idiopathic (torsion) dystonia

Symptoms

Idiopathic (torsion) dystonia may present in childhood, when it is frequently inherited as an autosomal dominant trait, or in adult life, when a family history is unusual. In many families with early onset disease, genetic linkage studies have localized the abnormal gene mutation to the *DYT1* locus on chromosome 9q34 which codes for torsin A, a protein of unknown function expressed in the brain (including the substantia nigra). Ashkenazi Jews are particularly prone to this condition. It usually presents in children with dystonic spasms of the legs on walking, or sometimes of the arms, trunk, or neck. The condition is usually progressive when it commences in childhood; the spasms spread to all body parts, leading to severe disability within about 10 years. The intellect is preserved and there are no signs of pyramidal or sensory deficit. Speech is often spared, permitting the pursuit of intellectual employment despite severe physical disability. A spontaneous remission of symptoms occurs in about 10 to 20 per cent of patients, usually within 5 years of onset. There is no way of predicting who will remit or when such a remission will occur. Most remissions are transitory, lasting a matter of weeks or months, but occasionally they may persist.

In adults, the condition usually presents as a focal dystonia (blepharospasm, oromandibular dystonia, spasmodic dysphonia, torticollis, axial dystonia, or dystonic writer's cramp). The legs tend to be spared, and progression is slow, with the dystonia remaining confined to its site of origin. Segmental dystonia develops in some cases.

Treatment

Dystonia is distressing and difficult to treat. Every child and young adult with dystonia should receive a trial of levodopa (for example, Sinemet-Plus up to two tablets three times a day for 3 months), for they may have the condition of dopa-responsive dystonia-parkinsonism (see below).

The drugs which most patients find helpful, and continue to take to suppress muscle spasm, are benzodiazepines such as diazepam, often in a large dose of 20 to 50 mg daily, and an anticholinergic such as benzhexol, again in large doses (up to as much as 120 mg/day). Fifty per cent of children and 10 per cent of adults will be helped, but adults are more sensitive to anticholinergic side-effects. Phenothiazines and other neuroleptics, such as haloperidol, may also help some patients, as may tetrabenazine, but often at the expense of drug induced parkinsonism. Unfortunately, dystonia is far less responsive to neuroleptics than is chorea. Many other drugs have been tried in dystonia, but none has gained wide acceptance.

The recent interest in neurosurgery for movement disorders has extended to the treatment of dystonia, especially when the disease is advanced and disabling. Originally the thalamus was targeted for surgery but pallidotomy has recently been favoured in the management of patients with generalized dystonia (whereas selective denervation procedures have been used in focal dystonia—see below). In general, patients with generalized torsion dystonia respond erratically to this procedure and at present there is little evidence to support its use.

Dopa-responsive dystonia-parkinsonism (Segawa's syndrome)

This condition is inherited as an autosomal dominant condition with incomplete penetrance and has as its defect mutations in the guanosine triphosphate cyclohydrolase 1 gene. This generates a cofactor for maintaining the normal activity of tyrosine hydroxylase, the rate limiting step in the catecholamine biosynthetic pathway. Homozygous deficiency of this enzyme severely inhibits tyrosine hydroxylase activity and produces mental retardation, seizures, and truncal hypertonia. However, the more common partial deficiency in tyrosine hydroxylase results in dystonia affecting the legs which becomes worse as the day goes on. Rest without sleep does not help, but sleep relieves the dystonia. Many patients also have features of parkinsonism, although focal dystonia may be the presenting feature. The disease can easily be mistaken for cerebral palsy (given its lower limb predominance) or an unexplained 'spastic paraparesis'.

Table 2 Causes and classification of dystonia: (a) Idiopathic primary dystonias: hereditary

Disease	Symbol	Inheritance	Gene	Clinical features
Idiopathic torsion dystonia	*DYT1*	Autosomal dominant	9q34 (torsin A)	Late childhood. Limb then generalized
	DYT6	Autosomal dominant	8q21–22	Early adulthood. Craniocervical dystonia becoming generalized
			18p	Adulthood. Focal cervical dystonia and spasmodic dysphonia
X-linked dystonia-parkinsonian syndrome (Phillipines; lubag disease)	*DYT3*	X linked	Xq12–13.1	
Adult onset focal dystonia	*DYT7*	Autosomal dominant	18p31	Torticollis. Spasmodic dysphonia
Alcohol responsive myoclonic dystonia		Autosomal dominant	?	Myoclonic jerks compounded by dystonia. Young adults. Non-progressive, relieved by alcohol
Dopa responsive dystonia (Segawa's syndrome)		Autosomal dominant	14q22.3 (GTP cyclo-hydrolase 1)	Childhood. Lower limb dystonia with parkinsonism. Worse at end of day
		Autosomal recessive	11p 15.5 (tyrosine hydroxylase)	Very rare
Paroxysmal kinesogenic or non-kinesogenic dystonia		?Autosomal dominant	2q	Episodes of dystonia or chorea that last for seconds with movement or startle (kinesogenic). Non-kinesogenic episodes last for minutes to hours and are provoked by stress and certain agents

(b) Idiopathic primary dystonias: non-hereditary

1. Sporadic generalized dystonia
2. Sporadic paroxysmal choreoathetosis/dystonia
3. Focal dystonia
   - (a) Cranial dystonia
     - Meige's syndrome
     - Blepharospasm ± oromandibular dystonia
   - (b) Spasmodic torticollis—simple and complex
   - (c) Dystonic writer's cramp
   - (d) Other occupational dystonias
   - (e) Spasmodic dysphonia
   - (f) Others

(c) Symptomatic secondary dystonias

1. Inherited metabolic (e.g Wilson's disease)
2. Acquired metabolic (e.g. kernicterus)
3. Inherited possible metabolic (e.g. Hallervorden–Spatz disease)
4. Other inherited causes (e.g. neuroacanthocytosis, Huntington's disease)
5. Miscellaneous causes (e.g. Parkinson's disease and its treatment, progressive supranuclear palsy, trauma including head trauma, cervical cord and peripheral nerve injury, anoxia/ischaemia, tumours of the basal ganglia, toxins, and drug induced)
6. Psychogenic

There is a reduction in turnover of dopamine due to the abnormality in tyrosine hydroxylase activity; patients respond well to low doses of levodopa without showing any of the long-term complications encountered in Parkinson's disease.

Spasmodic torticollis

Symptoms

Spasmodic torticollis may be the presenting feature of dystonia in childhood, but isolated spasmodic torticollis usually occurs in the middle aged or elderly. The onset is usually insidious, often with initial pain, and sometimes appears to be precipitated by trauma. The dystonic spasms affect sternomastoid, splenius, and other neck muscles to cause the head to turn to one side (torticollis) (Fig. 1), or occasionally to extend (retrocollis) or to flex (antecollis) the neck. The spasms may be repetitive to cause tremulous torticollis, or sustained to hold the posture. The trunk commonly shows a compensatory lordosis.

The condition is usually lifelong, but remissions of a year or more occur in about one-fifth of cases. Most patients are otherwise normal apart from their torticollis, although some may exhibit a postural tremor similar to that of benign essential tremor, and a minority may develop dystonia elsewhere. As with all types of dystonia, the frequency and intensity of the muscle spasms vary considerably, being particularly worse in conditions of mental or emotional stress. A feature characteristic of spasmodic torticollis is the 'geste antagonistique', in which the patient discovers some particular manual act which controls the deviation of the head. A touch of the forefinger to the jaw may suffice, but other more complex and bizarre actions are common.

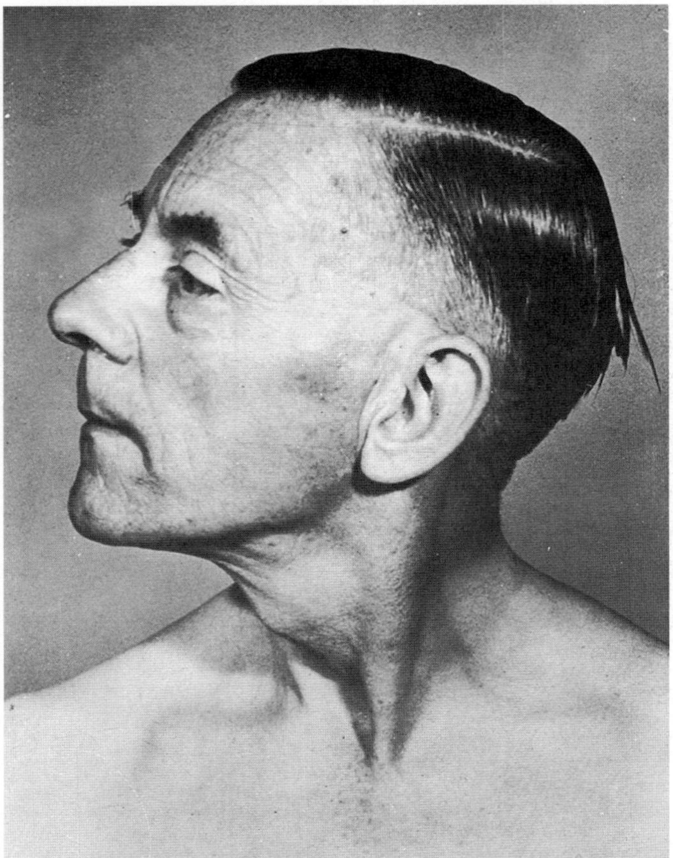

Fig. 1 Spasmodic torticollis in a 57-year-old man. The hypertrophy of the sternomastoid muscle is evident.

Treatment

Spasmodic torticollis, like other types of adult onset focal dystonia, does not usually benefit from conventional drug therapy. The best treatment is injection of botulinum toxin A into the most affected muscles. Botulinum toxin prevents the release of acetylcholine and causes functional denervation with localized muscle weakness. Identification of the overactive muscles is a prerequisite to the administration of localized injections of botulinum toxin which, in the case of torticollis, typically involves injections into the sternomastoid and splenius muscles. These injections usually have an effect within a week although the maximum benefit is not apparent until several weeks later. Repeat injections are required approximately every 3 months as relapse, by terminal sprouting, occurs. In about 10 to 20 per cent of patients, antibodies eventually develop to the botulinum toxin A making it less effective with time. In these cases a switch to a botulinum toxin type F or B may be desirable; the long-term efficacy of this manoeuvre is under investigation.

Surgery is sometimes practised and local denervation procedures are still considered in patients with otherwise intractable cervical dystonias.

Dystonic writer's cramp

Symptoms

Inability to write (or to type, play a musical instrument, or wield any manual instrument) has many causes but in most patients no objective neurological deficit is found other than abnormal posturing of the hand and arm on writing. Typically, the pen is gripped with great force and driven into the paper (Fig. 2). However, in some patients the arm adopts a typical dystonic posture and in such cases of dystonic writer's cramp, other manual acts such as wielding a knife or screwdriver are similarly affected. Such dystonic writer's cramp may be the initial symptom of generalized torsion dystonia, but in adults it often remains as an isolated disability. The same considerations apply to other occupational cramps, such as pianist's cramp.

Treatment

Writer's cramp, and related conditions, are usually permanent disabilities. Advice to write with the opposite hand allows most to cope with everyday events, but approximately 1 patient in 20 then develops the same problem in the non-dominant hand. Drugs (such as bezhexol and diazepam) are rarely of benefit but botulinum toxin injections into the muscles of the affected forearm may help some patients.

Blepharospasm and oromandibular dystonia (cranial dystonia)

Symptoms

Blepharospasm refers to recurrent spasms of eye closure. The orbicularis oculi forcibly contracts for seconds or minutes, often repetitively and sometimes so frequently as to render the patient functionally blind (Fig. 3). Spasms of eye closure commonly occur while reading or watching television, or in bright light; they often decrease or disappear when the subject is alerted or under scrutiny. Oromandibular dystonia refers to recurrent spasms of muscle contraction affecting the mouth, tongue, jaw, larynx, and pharynx, causing spasms of lip protrusion or retraction, jaw closure or opening (Fig. 4), and difficulty in speech and swallowing. Such patients may lacerate their lips and tongue or even dislocate their jaw, and are usually unable to cope with dentures. Speech may take on a characteristic, forced strained quality, and chewing and swallowing may be impaired.

These two conditions are closely related, for the patient with blepharospasm may develop oromandibular dystonia and vice versa. The term Brueghel syndrome is often used when the dominant (or only) feature is a dystonically opened jaw, whilst Meige syndrome has blepharospasm as its central feature. Both conditions may occur in generalized torsion dystonia,

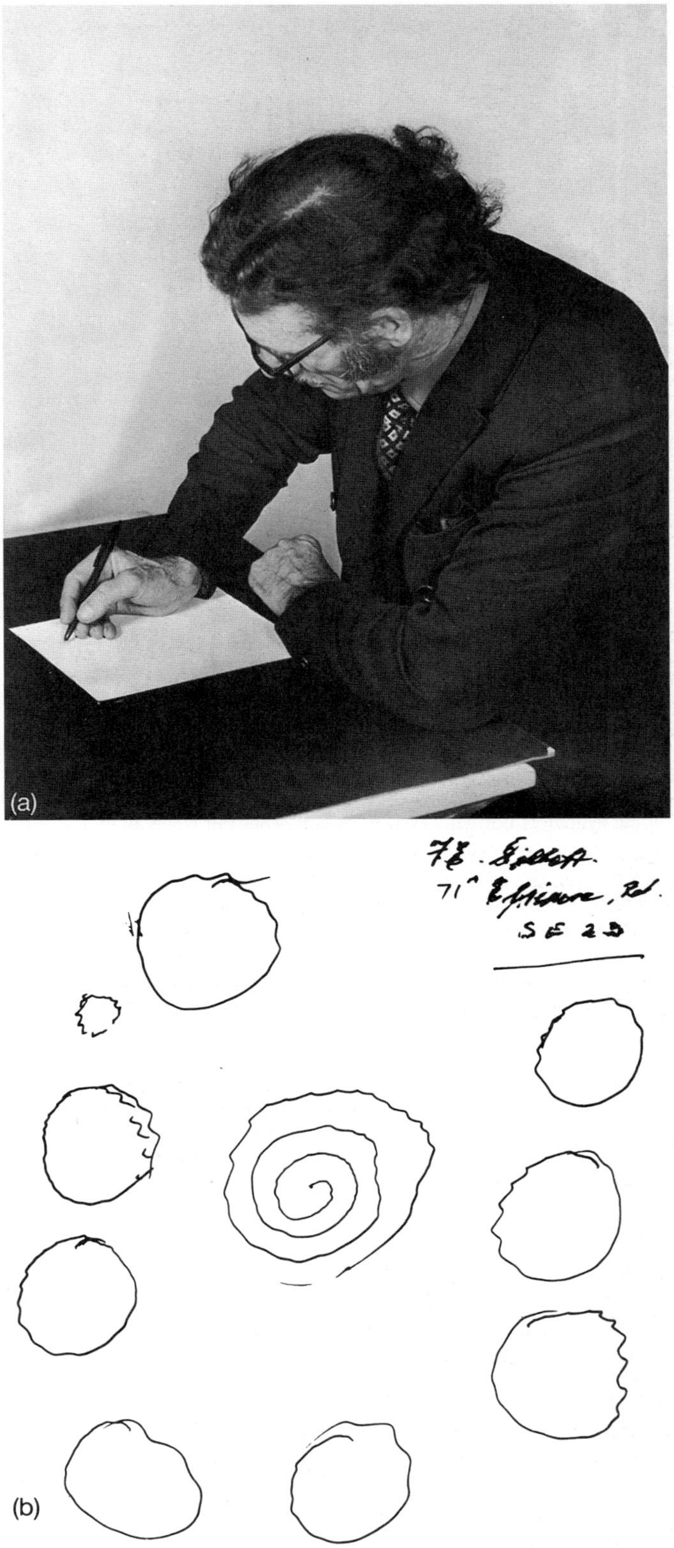

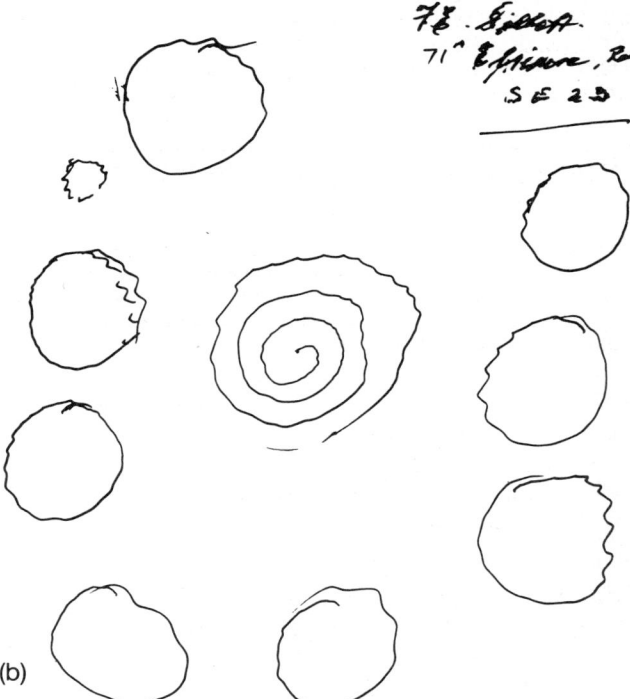

Fig. 2 (a) Dystonic writer's cramp in a 52-year-old man, whose right elbow rises and whose fingers grip the pen so tightly that they slide off. (b) Example of writing and drawing in this patient showing difficulty in executing the task and thus legibility of script and ability to copy simple figures.

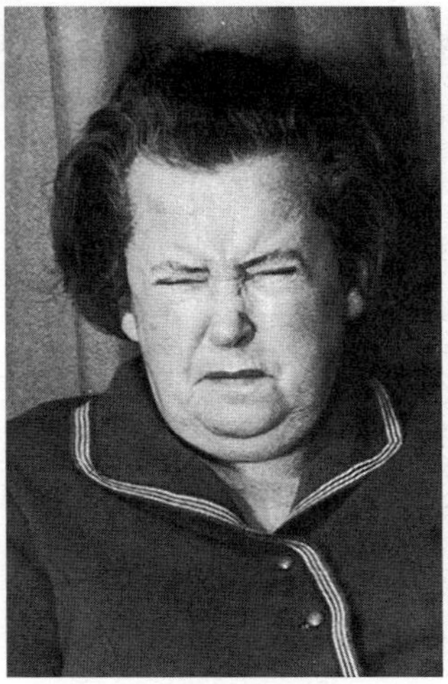

Fig. 3 Blepharospasm in a 57-year-old woman. Her jaw also is forcibly clamped shut, biting her gums, and some spasm of orbicularis oris is evident, in addition to the obvious spasm of orbicularis oculi.

or result from drugs; they also appear in isolation in late life without evident cause.

Treatment

Unfortunately, both blepharospasm and oromandibular dystonia are notoriously difficult to control with drugs (for example benzhexol, diazepam, and/or a neuroleptic). Surgery cannot improve oromandibular dystonia but can relieve blepharospasm. The best treatment for blepharospasm is to inject botulinum toxin into the orbicularis oculi which gives relief in about 70 to 80 per cent of cases, thereby restoring normal vision for about 3 months. The injections can be repeated as necessary. Botulinum toxin injections can be used to control some jaw spasms.

Spasmodic dysphonia

Dystonic spasms of the muscles controlling the vocal cords cause spasmodic dysphonia, which impairs speech and singing, and may be severe enough to prevent communication. The most common type involves the adductor muscles, leading to a strangled speech with pitch breaks and stops. Less common is abductor dysphonia which produces a breathy, low-

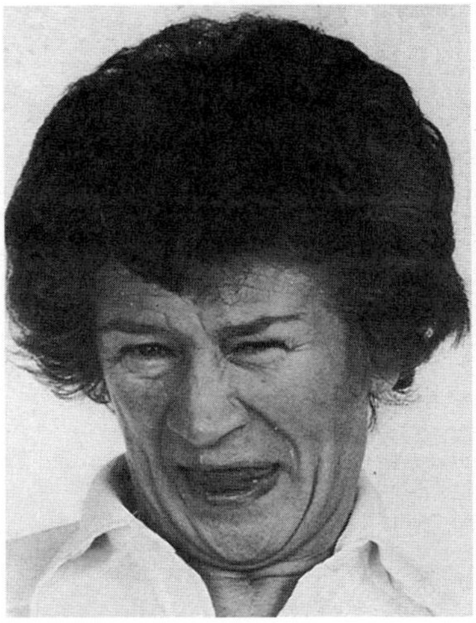

Fig. 4 Oromandibular dystonia in a 42-year-old woman. The spasm of forced jaw opening with tongue protrusion is evident.

volume voice. The diagnosis can be established by direct non-invasive visualization of the vocal cords during talking. Spasmodic dysphonia may occur in association with cranial or generalized dystonia, or may appear as an isolated focal dystonia in adult life. Speech can be restored by injection of botulinum toxin into the overactive vocal muscles, identified by electromyography.

Paroxysmal dystonia

Focal dystonias often commence with the appearance of a dystonic posture or spasm only on one motor act (action dystonia), but there are rare, usually familial, disorders in which dramatic dystonia occurs intermittently in attacks, the patient being normal in between. These conditions are thought to be caused by mutations in genes encoding ion channels. Several families with paroxysmal dystonic choreoathetosis have now shown linkage to chromosome 2q35–37, where a number of candidate genes have been identified for study.

Chorea

Chorea is seen in many disorders (see Table 3, Fig. 5), but the most common cause other than the treatment of Parkinson's disease is Huntington's disease. There are also several non-inherited conditions in which chorea can occur and in which treatment is beneficial.

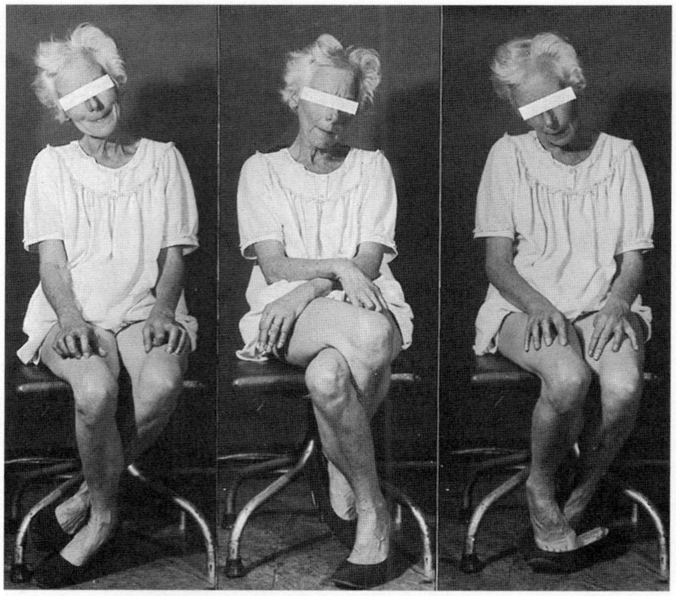

Fig. 5 Chorea due to polycythaemia rubra vera in a 57-year-old woman. The characteristic fleeting choreic movements are captured in these three sequential frames.

Huntington's disease

Definition

A dominantly inherited, relentlessly progressive disease, usually of middle life, characterized by chorea and dementia. It was first described in 1872 by George Huntington, a year after he had qualified in medicine, in a handful of families of English descent in a region of Long Island, New Jersey.

Aetiology

The prevalence of the disease is about 1 in 10 000 and it occurs in all ethnic groups worldwide. The condition is inherited as an autosomal dominant trait with full penetrance. The genetic defect is now known, can be tested for, and consists of an abnormal cytosine–adenine–guanine triplet repeat in the gene encoding huntingtin on chromosome 4 and represents one of a number of triplet repeat disorders causing neurological disease. Triplet repeat sequences normally exist in several genes but when an excess number of repeats occurs a disease state is produced. This pathological triplet (or trinucleotide) repeat occurs in the coding region of the huntingtin gene and the consequence of a large unstable DNA sequence is that the triplets can expand during mitosis and meiosis, resulting in longer triplet repeat sequences (dynamic mutation). The most likely time for triplet expansion is during spermatogenesis and subsequent fertilization/embryogenesis; this has two major implications. First, longer repeats tend to occur in the offspring of affected men, and secondly longer repeats tend to occur in the subsequent generations. This results in an earlier onset and more severe form of the disorder in subsequent generations—a phenomenon known as genetic anticipation; i.e. longer repeat sequences are associated with younger onset, more severe forms of the disease.

Table 3 Chorea

Hereditary	Autosomal dominant
	Huntington's disease
	Spinocerebellar ataxias
	Autosomal recessive
	Neuroacanthocytosis
	Wilson's disease
	Other
	Leigh's syndrome
Drug induced	Neuroleptics
	Anti-convulsants
	Anti-Parkinson's medication
	Oral contraceptive (often with a history of previous Sydenham's chorea
Toxins	Carbon monoxide poisoning
Metabolic	Hyperthyroidism
	Pregnancy
Infection	Sydenham's chorea
Immunological	Systemic lupus erythematosus
Vascular	Infarction
	Polycythaemia
Tumours	
Trauma	Cerebral palsy
	Acquired
Age related	Senile chorea
Paroxysmal	
Psychogenic	

The abnormal expansion of the cytosine–adenine–guanine repeat in Huntington's disease (more than 36 repeats) causes a new gain of function in the mutant huntingtin. This new protein acquires a unique function that is central to the evolution of the neurodegenerative process. Furthermore this protein is known to interact with a number of other proteins (for example huntingtin associated protein 1), which may be critical for the development of selective pathology. Inclusion bodies resulting from the polymerization of polyglutamine sheets in the mutant huntingtin protein develop in neurones but the exact mechanism by which selective neuronal death at specific sites occurs is unknown.

The chorea of Huntington's disease appears to result from relative overactivity of dopamine mechanisms in the brain, perhaps because the intact dopaminergic nigrostriatal pathway is releasing approximately normal quantities of dopamine on to only a few remaining striatal neurones. Positron emission tomographic studies using ^{18}F-labelled deoxyglucose have revealed a profound reduction of glucose metabolism in the striatum, even in patients without discernible cerebral atrophy.

Pathology

The brain is generally atrophic, with conspicuous damage to the cerebral cortex and corpus striatum, where there is loss of nerve cells and reactive gliosis without inflammatory changes associated with extensive neurotransmitter changes.

Coronal section of the brain characteristically shows dilated lateral ventricles, in which the floor becomes concave rather than convex, due to marked caudate atrophy; commonly, cortical atrophy is also evident. The main histological abnormality is found in the caudate and putamen, where there is extensive loss of small neurones, leading to shrinkage, and a false impression of gliosis, although such changes are found elsewhere. More recently attention has focused on the early stages of the condition, as the identification of the genetic defect involved has allowed for the disease to be diagnosed with certainty. In early cases and in mice transgenic for the mutant human huntingtin protein the earliest histological findings are the neuronal inclusions, which precede the cell loss.

Symptoms

The onset is typically insidious, usually between the ages of 30 and 50 years, and can be with motor, cognitive, and/or psychiatric symptoms and signs. The initial symptoms are frequently those of a change in personality and behaviour, but chorea may be the first sign. At this stage the patient often retains distressing insight, fully aware of what is in store. Serious depression is common and suicide is a risk. Erratic behaviour at work or in society may lead to psychiatric referral, or rarely a frank schizophrenic-like psychosis may develop. As the disease progresses, cognitive deficits become more pronounced and chorea more severe with walking, speech, and the use of the hands are impaired. As the disease progresses, many patients develop increasing rigidity and akinesia, with reduction of the chorea. Finally the patient becomes bedridden with marked weight loss; death occurs on average about 14 years from the onset. Huntington's disease does not always present in this fashion, and a number of variants are recognized including an akinetic-rigid parkinsonian syndrome (the Westphal variant), which is most frequent in children.

Diagnosis

Despite the diverse clinical manifestations of Huntington's disease, with genetic testing the diagnosis is now straightforward. However, in some cases the characteristics of the disease are not obvious and a history is not available, which can mean that the diagnosis is overlooked (see Table 3).

Treatment

There is currently no cure for Huntington's disease. Drugs that modify the dopaminergic input to the striatum can be used (for example tetrabenazine and sulpiride) to treat the chorea but rarely provide a sustained benefit—in fact most patients with Huntington's disease rarely complain of their chorea. Other drugs may be required for psychiatric symptoms including selective serotonin reuptake inhibitors for depression, neuroleptics for psychotic symptoms, and carbamazepine and sodium valproate as mood stabilizers.

A further recent intervention in Huntington's disease has involved the use of neurotrophic factors, such as ciliary neurotrophic factor as well as neuroprotective therapies (for example coenzyme Q); the benefits of these measures are uncertain. Surgical treatment for chorea is poorly documented but there has been increasing interest in the possibility of neural transplantation in Huntington's disease.

Sooner or later chronic hospital care is required for patients with Huntington's disease. Increasing nursing problems may require admission to hospital where dietary advice (including gastrostomy for feeding) and physiotherapy may be of benefit. Particular attention should be directed towards supporting the family, for the nature of the disease poses great ethical and emotional problems.

Genetic testing

Predictive testing programmes are now available for individuals at risk, provided by multidisciplinary teams specializing in this condition and often directed by an experienced neurogeneticist.

Sydenham's chorea

Definition

Chorea (St Vitus's dance) associated with psychological disturbance due to rheumatic fever (rheumatic chorea) in childhood and adolescence was first described by Thomas Sydenham in 1686.

Aetiology and pathology

Sydenham's chorea was associated with many streptococcal infections, but it is now most frequently associated with acute rheumatic fever, and as a result is rare in most parts of the world. The mechanism is thought to be antibody mediated, against epitopes within structures of the basal ganglia, which would help explain the characteristic radiological lesions seen within the basal ganglia of affected patients. Antineural antibodies have been isolated in cases of Sydenham's chorea and may result from cross-reactivity with elements of group A streptococcal membranes, although the pathogenic nature of these antibodies has not been demonstrated unequivocally.

Symptoms

About three-quarters of cases occur between the ages of 7 and 12 years. The onset is usually gradual, but may be abrupt. The initial symptoms are often psychological, with irritability, agitation, disobedience, and inattentiveness. A frank organic confusional state occurs in about 10 per cent of patients. Generalized chorea then appears and may worsen for a few weeks; speech is impaired in about a third of patients. The chorea is predominantly unilateral in about 20 per cent of patients, and in severe cases is accompanied by flaccidity and subjective weakness (chorea mollis). Although cardiac disease may be found, the child usually has no fever or other manifestations of rheumatic fever.

The chorea and psychological disturbance recover over 1 to 3 months, rarely up to 6 months, but recurrences occur in about a quarter of patients over the next 2 years. About a third of patients will show evidence of rheumatic cardiac involvement at the time of the illness, and about the same proportion later develop chronic rheumatic heart disease. Those who have suffered one or more attacks of Sydenham's chorea are at particular risk of developing chorea in adult life during pregnancy (chorea gravidarum), or when exposed to drugs including oral contraceptives, digoxin, or phenytoin. Although usually self-limiting, more persistent neurological deficits occasionally occur in Sydenham's chorea.

Treatment

Treatment as for rheumatic fever is necessary. The chorea may be controlled with diazepam, haloperidol, or tetrabenazine. A course of penicillin should be given, and prophylactic oral penicillin should be continued until about the age of 20 years to prevent further streptococcal infection.

Hemiballism (hemichorea)

Hemiballism refers to wild flinging or throwing movements of one arm and leg. These movements, like those of chorea, are irregular in timing and force, but involve the large proximal muscles of the shoulder and pelvic girdle. The occasional child or adolescent with Sydenham's chorea may present with hemiballism, but the syndrome usually occurs in elderly hypertensive and/or diabetic patients as a result of a stroke. The vascular lesion usually affects the subthalamic nucleus, although lesions at other anatomical sites may be responsible. It may appear as the hemiplegic weakness improves, when it is often accompanied by thalamic pain, although in other patients the hemiballism appears abruptly without weakness or sensory deficit. The intensity of the movements varies from mild to a severity that causes injury and requires urgent treatment.

Hemiballism due to stroke usually remits over 3 to 6 months. Treatment with a phenothiazine, haloperidol, or tetrabenazine will often control hemiballism until recovery occurs, but interventional neurosurgery is occasionally required and may be beneficial.

Tremor

Three types are generally recognized—static, postural, and action tremors (Table 4). Static tremor occurs when a relaxed limb is fully supported at rest. Postural tremor appears when a part of the body is maintained in a fixed position and may also persist during movement. Kinetic or action tremor occurs specifically during active voluntary movement of a body part. If the amplitude of such an action tremor increases as goal-directed movement approaches its target, this is an intention tremor. Psychogenic tremors are generally rare. They are often of sudden onset with a variable but rarely remitting clinical course and typically affect the trunk or limb with standing and/or using the limb respectively.

Physiological tremor has a frequency in the 7 to 11 Hz band and is typically symptomatic in states of increased sympathetic nervous activity and is increased by stimulation of peripheral β_2-adrenergic receptors in muscle. The fine postural tremors associated with stress and anxiety states along with thyrotoxicosis fall into this category and usually respond to β-adrenergic blocking drugs. Symptomatic postural tremors occur in association with many neurological disorders and can be shown to differ from physiological tremor by frequency analysis.

Benign essential (familial) tremor

Definition

A condition characterized by postural tremor of the arms and head which can present at any age, although usually in early adult life. It is only slowly progressive, generally causes mild disability, and is not associated with dystonia or parkinsonism.

Aetiology

The cause of benign essential tremor is unknown. A positive family history is obtained in over half of such patients with a pattern of inheritance that indicates an autosomal dominant trait.

Table 4 Classification and types of tremor

Static or rest tremor
Parkinson's disease
Parkinsonism (including drug induced, postencephalitic)
Other extrapyramidal diseases
Multiple sclerosis
Postural tremor
Physiological tremor
Exaggerated physiological tremor, as in:
Thyrotoxicosis
Anxiety states
Alcohol
Drugs (e.g. sympathomimetics, antidepressants, sodium valproate, lithium)
Heavy metal poisoning (i.e. mercury—the 'hatter's shakes')
Structural neurological disease, as in:
Severe cerebellar lesions ('red nucleus tremor')
Wilson's disease
Neurosyphilis
Peripheral neuropathies
Benign essential (familial) tremor
Task-specific tremors (e.g. primary writing tremor)
Kinetic or action (including intention) tremor
Brainstem or cerebellar disease, as in:
Multiple sclerosis
Spinocerebellar degenerations
Vascular disease
Tumours
Psychogenic tremors

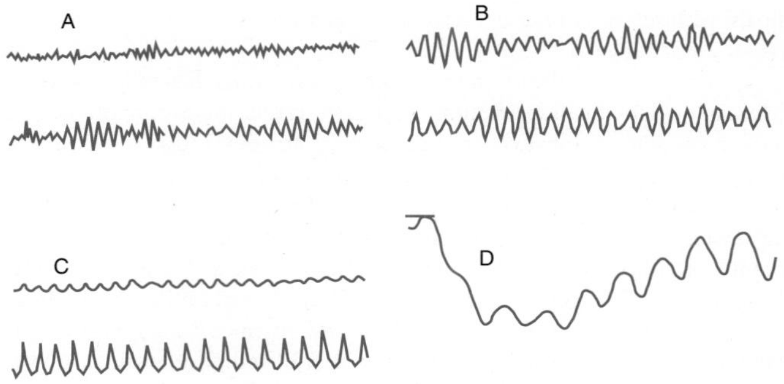

Fig. 6 Recordings of tremor with accelerometers placed on the right arm (above) and the left arm (below) in (a) a patient with enhanced physiological tremor of the outstretched arms (frequency 9 to 10 Hz), (b) a patient with benign essential tremor with the arms outstretched (frequency 7 Hz), (c) a patient with left-sided Parkinson's disease at rest (frequency 5 Hz), and (d) a patient with severe cerebellar disease and marked intention tremor attempting to touch his nose with the right hand (frequency 2 to 3 Hz). All recordings are of 4 s duration. (By courtesy of Dr M. Gresty.)

Pathophysiology

No pathological or biochemical abnormality has been identified in benign essential tremor, but few cases have come to autopsy. Essential tremor is usually of a frequency of 5 to 8 Hz (Fig. 6). Recent functional imaging studies indicate abnormal activation of the cerebellum, red nucleus, and thalamus.

Symptoms

Tremor is present in one or both hands on maintaining a posture, as when holding a cup or glass. Handwriting becomes untidy and tremulous (see Fig. 7). There is no tremor at rest, but a rhythmic oscillation develops when the patient holds the arms outstretched. On movement, as in finger–nose testing, the tremor continues but does not get strikingly worse, as is the case with cerebellar intention tremor. Tremor of the head (titubation) and jaw is present at about 50 per cent of cases, and tremor of the legs occurs in about a third. Despite the tremor, tests of co-ordination are usually normal, walking is unaffected, and there are no other neurological abnormalities.

Two other factors are characteristic of this disorder. First, a family history and, secondly, the observation that small or moderate doses of alcohol may suppress the tremor. The illness is static or only slowly progressive in most patients, causing predominantly a social disability, but individuals dependent upon manual skill may be disabled.

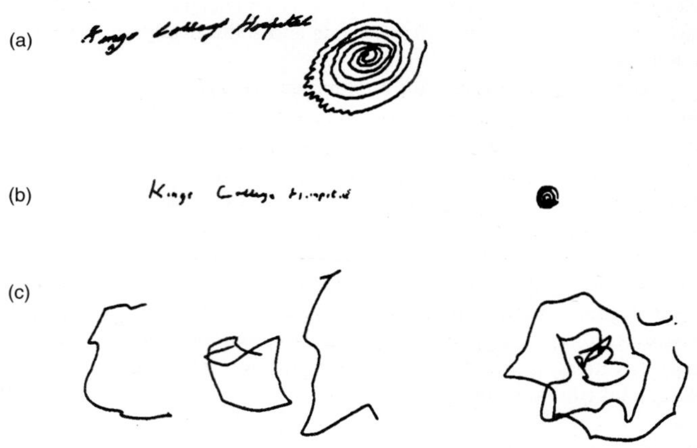

Fig. 7 Samples of handwriting and spiral drawings from (a) a 50-year-old woman with benign essential tremor, (b) a 38-year-old man with Parkinson's disease, and (c) a 20-year-old man with torsion dystonia (who attempts to write COLLEGE).

Table 5 Tics

Simple tics	Transient tic of childhood
	Chronic simple tic
Multiple tics	Chronic multiple tics
	Gilles de la Tourette syndrome
Symptomatic tics	Encephalitis lethargica
	Drug induced tics
	Neuroacanthocytosis

Other variants of the syndrome are occasionally encountered. Thus isolated, inherited head tremor may occur, with either 'yes–yes' or 'no–no' movements, and tremulous 'writer's cramp' (primary writing tremor) is recognized. Tremor of the legs on standing, at around 5 to 8 Hz (orthostatic tremor), may occur as an isolated syndrome or in the context of essential tremor.

Treatment

Although alcohol may suppress the tremor effectively, and can be of value if used wisely, there is a risk of patients becoming alcoholics. Benzodiazepines, such as diazepam, may give some relief at times of stress, but have no major effect on the tremor. Thirty to 40 per cent of patients respond satisfactorily to a β-adrenergic receptor antagonist such as propranolol (up to a dose of 240 mg/day). Primidone, in standard anticonvulsant dosages, also helps some. Stereotaxic thalamotomy or deep brain stimulation of the thalamus may be required in the very small number of patients whose tremor is severe.

Tics

Tics occur in several disorders (see Table 5) and are defined as simple or complex. A simple tic is a sudden, rapid twitch-like movement always of the same nature and at the same site and occurs in about a quarter of all children, disappearing within a year or so (transient tic of childhood). Sometimes these persist into adult life, but are rarely considered as abnormal (chronic simple tic) such that only a minority seek assistance. Tics that are more widespread and severe, and take the form of complicated stereotyped patterns of motor action, are termed complex tics.

Characteristically, complex and simple tics can be suppressed voluntarily although this causes mounting inner tension which can only be relieved by expression of the tics. Complex multiple tics accompanied by vocal utterances, particularly swear words (coprolalia), and compulsive thoughts constitute the Gilles de la Tourette syndrome, which is an organic cerebral disease of unknown aetiology.

Gilles de la Tourette syndrome

Aetiology

George Gilles de la Tourette described the syndrome of chronic multiple tics with vocalizations in 1885, although Itard had described an earlier case. The condition appears to be inherited as an autosomal dominant trait, with variable penetrance. In affected families the genetic abnormality may be expressed as the full syndrome, as chronic multiple tics alone, or as an obsessive–compulsive neurosis (see below). Whilst the cause of this bizarre condition is unknown, the basal ganglia are believed to be involved because abnormalities within the striatum (and paralimbic areas) have been detected using positron emission tomography. Subtle abnormalities within the caudate and pallidum have been reported at post-mortem. Furthermore, drugs acting on the basal ganglia, such as haloperidol, may control the symptoms.

Symptoms

The illness usually begins between the ages of 5 and 15 years, with multiple involuntary repetitive muscular tics which vary in site, number, frequency, and severity with time. These particularly affect the upper part of the body, especially the face, neck, and shoulders, more than the limbs and trunk. Typical initial symptoms are eye blinking, head nodding, sniffing, or stuttering. With time other more complex tics affecting other parts of the body appear. The motor tics are often preceded by a sensory urge (sometimes called a sensory tic), and they can be controlled, albeit temporarily, by an effort of will. Eventually, however, the patient has to 'let the tics go'.

Sooner or later, most patients with multiple tics make involuntary noises, such as grunting, squealing, yelping, sniffing, or barking. Indeed, the coexistence of such noises with multiple tics is an essential feature of Gilles de la Tourette syndrome. In about 60 per cent of cases the noises become transformed into swear words (coprolalia). About a third of patients also exhibit echolalia—an involuntary tendency to repeat words or sentences just spoken to them. A smaller proportion of patients also exhibit copropraxia (involuntary obscene gesturing) and echopraxia (involuntary imitation of the movements of others), as well as palilalia (involuntary repetition of their own words or sounds).

Many patients with Gilles de la Tourette syndrome also exhibit features of an obsessive–compulsive disorder. These psychiatric manifestations of the condition may be even more disabling than the tics. A hyperactive attentional disorder is common in children.

Once established, Gilles de la Tourette syndrome is usually lifelong, although its severity waxes and wanes. A small proportion of cases, probably less than 1 in 20, experience spontaneous remission of symptoms after adolescence, but in most the multiple tics and the vocalizations persist, although they usually become less prominent in adults. No other neurological abnormality develops; intellect and motor co-ordination are retained.

Diagnosis

Patients with tics and vocal utterances, which are essential components of Gilles de la Tourette syndrome, are often initially considered to have a psychiatric disorder or, if organic disease is considered, chorea or dystonia are diagnosed. Once coprolalia is evident there is no difficulty in establishing the correct diagnosis, although other diseases such as Wilson's disease with onset in childhood require consideration.

Treatment

The multiple tics and the vocalizations of coprolalia cause considerable distress, social isolation, and psychological harm. Neuroleptic drugs such as haloperidol or pimozide may satisfactorily control tics, noises, and coprolalia. The effective dose requires careful and gradual titration as there is risk of side-effects, especially the emergence of a tardive dyskinesia after months or years of therapy (see below). Since treatment must usually be for life, the harm must be carefully balanced against the need for any form of therapy. The obsessive-–compulsive symptoms of the illness may improve with drugs such as clomipramine or fluoxetine. In extreme cases psychosurgery has been undertaken with limbic leucotomies.

Myoclonus

Myoclonus is a feature of many neurological diseases and can be classified according to its aetiology (see Table 6).

Generalized or multifocal myoclonus can occur in four clinical settings:

(i) as the solitary feature of the illness (essential myoclonus);

(ii) as a dominant feature of a progressive brain disease (progressive myoclonic encephalopathy);

(iii) as a residual feature of some transient brain insult (static myoclonic encephalopathy); or

(iv) as a feature of obvious epilepsy (myoclonic epilepsy).

Benign essential myoclonus

This condition consists of widespread myoclonus affecting all four limbs, trunk, neck, and face, occurring at about 10 to 50 per minute, enhanced by

Table 6 Myoclonus

Generalized myoclonus
Essential myoclonus
*Progressive myoclonic encephalopathies**
• With demonstrable metabolic cause (e.g. Lafora body disease, mitochondrial encephalomyopathy)
• Hereditary myoclonus with no known metabolic cause (e.g. familial myoclonic epilepsy (Unverricht–Lundborg disease))
• Other sporadic diseases (e.g. subacute sclerosing panencephalitis, Creutzfeldt–Jacob disease, Alzheimer's disease)
• Metabolic myoclonus (e.g. porta-systemic encephalopathy, CO_2 narcosis)
Static myoclonic encephalopathies† (e.g. Postanoxic action myoclonus (Lance–Adams syndrome)
Myoclonic epilepsies‡
Focal myoclonus
Spinal myoclonus (secondary to spinal cord lesion, e.g. demyelination)
Propriospinal myoclonus
Palatal myoclonus (lesions of dentatorubro-olivary tract)
Ocular myoclonus
Hemifacial spasm
Cortical myoclonus
Epilepsia partialis continua

* Obvious myoclonus (with or without seizures) clearly as part of a progressive encephalopathy.

† Obvious myoclonus after some acute and now static cerebral insult.

‡ Obvious epilepsy as the main problem, with myoclonus.

action and sensory stimuli, often in the context of a positive family history. Onset is usually in childhood or adolescence, but disability is strikingly mild, there is no progression, intellect is normal, fits do not occur, and no other deficit appears. Some patients report that alcohol helps their jerks, and many respond to a β-adrenergic antagonist such as propranolol.

Progressive myoclonic encephalopathies

Most of the diseases causing a progressive myoclonic encephalopathy are described in detail elsewhere, particularly the lysosomal storage disorders and other metabolic disorders as well as the spinocerebellar degenerations. A discussion of other associated conditions lies outside the scope of this chapter.

Static myoclonic encephalopathies : postanoxic action myoclonus (Lance–Adams syndrome)

This is a distinct entity that may appear after a period of cerebral anoxia, typically respiratory arrests in the context of an acute asthmatic attack. After recovery of consciousness, such patients exhibit muscle jerks affecting the face, trunk, and limbs, often provoked by sensory stimuli, and strikingly elicited by willed voluntary action. The condition has been associated with abnormalities of brain 5-hydroxytryptamine, as 5-hydroxytryptophan produces a marked improvement in some patients. However, the side-effects of this therapy, in particular the development of the eosinophilia myalgia syndrome, have meant that other treatments such as clonazepam, piracetam, and sodium valproate are more commonly used

Myoclonic epilepsies

In the myoclonic epilepsies, epileptic seizures are the obvious and dominant feature of the condition. There is some confusion in separating the many conditions that may cause this syndrome, which occurs particularly in children. A convenient, if arbitrary, distinction is based on the age of onset and is discussed in more detail in the section on epilepsy.

Focal myoclonus

There are a number of conditions in which myoclonic muscle jerking may be restricted to one part of the body. Some pathological processes may cause focal myoclonus limited to those segments innervated by the part of brainstem or spinal cord affected (segmental myoclonus). Palatal myoclonus, with rhythmic contractions 60 to 180 per minute is an unusual variant. Sometimes this spreads to the pharynx and larynx and speech is disturbed; the ocular muscles maybe involved. Similar pathologies causing cerebral damage, particularly to the cerebral cortex, may cause rhythmic repetitive focal muscle jerking associated with electrical evidence of epileptic cortical discharge in the electroencephalogram (epilepsia partialis continua).

Spinal myoclonus

Repetitive, often rhythmical, myoclonic jerking restricted to a limb, or even to a few muscles of an arm or leg, may occur with myelitis, spinal cord tumour, or angioma, or after spinal cord trauma. The rhythmic muscle jerking occurs spontaneously, at 20 to 180 per minute, is not affected by peripheral stimuli, often persists in sleep, and is not associated with any change in the electroencephalogram. Anticonvulsants may help, but such segmental myoclonus is often very difficult to control.

Epilepsia partialis continua

Encephalitis, tumour, abscess, infarct, haemorrhage, or trauma to the cerebral cortex may rarely cause repetitive, rhythmic muscle jerking once or twice a second, confined to one collection of muscles, persisting even in sleep for days, weeks, or months. Usually the damage involves not only the cerebral cortex, but also deeper structures including the thalamus. Because of its large cortical representations, the most common site of epilepsia partialis continua is the hand. Typical Jacksonian focal motor fits, and grand mal seizures may also occur in such patients. The surface electroencephalogram usually shows a spike discharge over the opposite motor cortex preceding each jerk by a short interval. Treatment is with anticonvulsants, but may be difficult.

Hemifacial spasm

Hemifacial spasm occurs at a frequency of about 1 in 100 000 people and most commonly affects middle-aged or elderly women, and usually appears without obvious cause. Rarely, it may be symptomatic of demonstrable facial nerve compression. The condition consists of irregular, but repetitive clonic twitching of the muscles of one side of the face. Usually those around the eyes are first involved, producing a feeling identical to the benign myokymia of the lower eyelid which occurs in normal people when fatigued. However, the repetitive twitching spreads slowly to involve the whole face, each spasm closing the eye and drawing up the corner of the mouth. At this stage, a mild facial weakness and contraction becomes evident, but a frank facial palsy never develops. Facial sensation is normal and there are no other physical signs in idiopathic hemifacial spasm. The disorder is so distinctive and unilateral that it is rarely confused with other conditions. True facial myokymia, due to brainstem tumour or demyelination, consists of a continuous rippling contraction of the facial muscles, giving the appearance of a 'bag of worms'.

Treatment with drugs is usually unrewarding. Posterior fossa exploration, with separation of blood vessels from the seventh nerve gives long-lasting relief and failure, when it occurs, is normally evident within the first few months after surgery. However, injection of botulinum toxin into the facial muscles, repeated every 3 to 4 months, is a simpler and effective treatment.

Other movement disorders

Restless leg syndrome (Ekböm's syndrome)

This is a common and poorly understood condition in which patients have a desire to move their extremities often in association with paresthesiae and dysaesthesiae. This is made worse by rest and so is often mainly present at the end of the day and at night and is relieved by activity such as walking around. It is commonly associated with periodic limb movements during sleep. The aetiology of the condition is unknown, but may be due to abnormal cerebellar and thalamic activation. It can be seen with peripheral neuropathies, uraemia, pregnancy, iron deficiency, rheumatoid arthritis, and spinal cord lesions. In some cases there is a family history suggestive of an autosomal dominant inheritance. It responds to a number of drugs including L-dopa, dopamine agonists, baclofen, carbamazepine, clonazepam, clonidine, and opioid drugs.

Stiff man syndrome

This term includes a range of rare conditions which are characterized by muscle rigidity with or without spasms. This includes the stiff man syndrome which is characterized by axial rigidity involving the paraspinal muscles which leads to a hyperlordotic posture of the back and an abnormal gait often described as walking through treacle. These patients often have muscle spasms in response to sensory stimuli with an exaggerated startle response. The patients characteristically have antiglutamic acid decarboxylase antibodies which may account for the high incidence of diabetes mellitus and other autoimmune disorders in this condition. Treatment is usually with baclofen and diazepam, although clonazepam, sodium valproate, and vigabatrin have all been used successfully. Immunosuppressive therapy is often disappointing, although it may benefit some patients.

Hyper-rekplexia

Startle is a sterotypic response that involves a complex series of movements including eye closure, facial grimacing, and a typical body posture. In certain conditions it is exaggerated, and termed hyper-rekplexia. It can be seen in a number of conditions and with a range of central nervous system lesions as well as occurring in isolation. In some cases the condition is inherited in an autosomal dominant fashion and in these cases mutations in the glycine receptor are found. In general the condition responds to clonazepam.

Drug induced movement disorders

The extensive use of antipsychotic neuroleptic drugs has led to much iatrogenic extrapyramidal disease. These drugs, all of which block dopamine receptors in the basal ganglia and elsewhere, are used widely to control acute psychotic behaviour, whatever its cause, and to prevent relapse of schizophrenia. They also are employed as antiemetics, as are other similar drugs such as metoclopramide, and to treat vertigo. The major neurological complications of these drug therapies are summarized in Table 7.

Akathisia refers to an irresistible and unpleasant sensation of motor restlessness, and the inability to sit or stand still, all of which may be mistaken for a recurrence of psychotic behaviour. Akathisia remits if the offending neuroleptic is withdrawn, or if the dose can be reduced sufficiently: It does not usually respond to anticholinergic drugs, but may be helped by a benzodiazepine or propranolol.

Anticholinergic drugs may also be used to treat drug induced parkinsonism if the causative neuroleptic has to be continued for psychiatric reasons, although anticholinergics are not routinely administered to those on neuroleptics.

Acute dystonic reactions commonly consist of oculogyric crises, trismus, neck retraction, or torticollis, and may be mistaken for tetanus or meningitis. Although uncommon, acute dystonic reactions pose a repeated diagnostic problem in casualty departments. Such reactions rapidly disappear after intravenous injection of an anticholinergic drug such as Kemadrine or a benzodiazepine.

Chronic tardive dyskinesias are the most serious of the drug induced movement disorders for they usually persist despite drug withdrawal. About 20 per cent of those receiving chronic neuroleptic therapy will exhibit a tardive dyskinesia. The characteristic syndrome is one of orofacial mouthing, with lip smacking and tongue protrusion (orobuccolingual dyskinesia), accompanied by trunk rocking and distal chorea of the hands and feet. In younger patients the picture may be dominated by axial and cranial dystonia (tardive dystonia), a condition which persists and is largely refractory to treatment although is less likely to occur if the offending drug is discontinued within 5 years of being instituted.

Tardive dyskinesias usually appear after at least 6 months' neuroleptic drug therapy, and their incidence increases with exposure to the drugs and also with the age of the patients, although some of the more recent atypical antipsychotic drugs have less of a propensity to cause this condition. Tardive dyskinesias often get worse in the weeks immediately after stopping the offending drug, or may appear then for the first time. After drug withdrawal, tardive dyskinesias disappear in about 60 per cent or more of patients over the next 3 years, but continue unaltered in the remainder. They are difficult to treat and whilst the offending agent ideally should be stopped this is often not possible. Anticholinergic drugs tend to worsen orobuccolingual dyskinesia, but may relieve tardive dystonia. Baclofen may help some patients.

Other drugs that cause dyskinesias include levodopa in patients with Parkinson's disease. It seems likely that most such drug induced dyskinesias are due to pharmacological effects on dopamine mechanisms in the basal ganglia, resulting in dopaminergic overactivity, in contrast to the akinetic-rigid syndrome produced by dopamine depletion or blockade.

Further reading

General

Marsden CD, Fahn S, eds. (1982). *Movement disorders*, vol. I. Butterworth, London.

Table 7 Drug-induced extrapyramidal disease

Disorder	Drugs responsible	Susceptible age group	Incidence	Onset after initiation of therapy	Effect of withdrawal of drug	Treatment
Tremor	Bronchodilators, tricyclics, lithium carbonate, caffeine	Any	Dose-dependent, about 35%	Rapid	Disappears	Withdraw drug
Parkinsonism	Reserpine, tetrabenazine, neuroleptics	Any but increases with age	Dose-dependent, about 50%	Gradual, within first months	Disappears slowly, may take a year	Anticholinergics
Acute dystonia	Neuroleptics, diazoxide	Children, young adults	2–5%	Acute, within first few hours or days	Disappears	Anticholinergics, diazepam
Akathisia	Neuroleptics	Any	About 30%	Gradual, within first months	Disappears	Anticholinergics
Tardive dyskinesia	Neuroleptics	Increases with age	20–40%	Delayed, but increases	May get worse; persists in about 40%	Withdraw drug, tetrabenazine

Marsden CD, Fahn S, eds. (1987). *Movement disorders*, vol. II. Butterworth, London.

Marsden CD, Fahn S, eds. (1994). *Movement disorders*, vol. III. Butterworth, London.

Watts RL, Koller WC (1997). *Movement disorders. Neurologic principles and practice.* McGraw-Hill, New York.

Dystonia

Marsden CD, Quinn NP (1990). The dystonias. *British Medical Journal* **300**, 139–44.

Berardelli, A *et al.* (1998). The pathophysiology of primary dystonia. *Brain* **121**, 1195–212.

Dauer WT *et al.* (1998). Current concepts on the clinical features, aetiology and management of idiopathic cervical dystonia. *Brain* **121**, 547–60.

Nygaard TG, Wooten GF (1998). Dopa-responsive dystonia. *Neurology* **50**, 853–5.

Warner TT, Jarman P (1998). The molecular genetics of the dystonia. *Journal of Neurology, Neurosurgery and Psychiatry* **64**, 427–9.

Chorea

Harper PS (1996). *Huntington's disease*, 2nd edn. WB Saunders, Philadelphia.

Nausieda PA *et al.* (1980). Sydenham's chorea: an update. *Neurology* **30**, 331–4.

Reddy PH, Williams M, Tagle DA (1999). Recent advances in understanding the pathogenesis of Huntington's disease. *Trends in Neuroscience* **22**, 248–55.

Vidakovic A, Dragasevic N, Kostic VS (1994). Hemiballism: report of 25 cases. *Journal of Neurology, Neurosurgery and Psychiatry* **57**, 945–9.

Tremor

Bain P (1993). A combined clinical and neurophysiological approach to the study of patients with tremor. *Journal of Neurology, Neurosurgery and Psychiatry* **69**, 839–44.

Elble RJ (1986). Physiological and essential tremor. *Neurology* **36**, 225–31.

Hubble JP, Busenbark KL, Koller WC (1989). Essential tremor. *Clinical Neuropharmacology* **12**, 453–82.

Myoclonus and tics

Brown P *et al.* (1991). The hyperekplexias and their relationship to the normal startle reflex. *Brain* **114**, 1903–28.

Fahn S, Marsden CD, Van Woert M (1986). Myoclonus. *Advances in Neurology* **43**, 1–709.

Lees AJ (1987). *Tics.* Churchill Livingstone, London.

Pranzatelli MR (1994). Serotonin and human myoclonus. Rationale for the use of serotonin receptor agonists and antagonists. *Archives of Neurology* **51**, 605–17.

Robertson MM (1989). The Gilles de la Tourette syndrome: the current status. *British Journal of Psychiatry* **154**, 147–69.

Singer HS, Walkup JT (1991). Tourette syndrome and other tic disorders. Diagnosis, pathophysiology and treatment. *Medicine* **70**, 15–32.

Other movement disorders

Barker RA *et al.* (1998). Review of 23 patients affected by the stiff man syndrome: clinical subdivision into stiff trunk (man) syndrome, stiff limb syndrome and progressive encephalomyelitis with rigidity. *Journal of Neurology, Neurosurgery and Psychiatry* **65**, 633–40.

Gershanik OS (1993). Drug-induced movement disorders. *Current Opinions in Neurology and Neurosurgery* **6**, 369–76.

Rajendra S, Schofield PR (1995). Molecular mechanisms of inherited startle syndromes. *Trends in Neuroscience* **18**, 80–2.

Walters AS, group organizer and correspondent (1995). Toward a better definition of the restless legs syndrome. *Movement Disorders* **10**, 634–42.

24.13.12 Ataxic disorders

Nicholas Wood

Introduction

The term 'ataxia', derived from the Greek, means 'irregularity' or 'disorderliness'. Unsteadiness can result from a number of causes, including poor vision, impaired postural reflexes, or a deficiency of sensory input, that is sensory ataxia. This chapter is devoted to the symptoms, signs, and the pathological and clinical features of the disorders of the cerebellum (and its connections). There are two basic clinical rules which can be applied: (1) lesions of the vermis generally cause ataxia of midline structure (that is, truncal and gait ataxia); (2) output from the cerebellar hemisphere is to the contralateral cerebral hemisphere, which provides output to the contralateral limbs, therefore cerebellar hemisphere lesions are ipsilateral. It should, however, be noted that clinical assessment is complicated by the fact that few patients with ataxia have pure cerebellar disease as there is often additional pathology in the brainstem, spinal cord, or elsewhere.

Symptoms of ataxic disorders

The history is extremely important. A clarification of what patients mean should also be sought. Many refer to 'giddiness' or 'dizziness' when they really mean unsteadiness of gait without associated vertigo or light-headedness. The age and speed of onset and development of other features provides important aetiological clues. Rate of progress and any precipitating or relieving factors should be noted. There has been a tremendous improvement in our understanding of the genetic basis of many ataxia disorders and a detailed family history is paramount.

Disturbances of gait

This is the most frequent presenting feature in ataxic disorders. Patients may report an inability to walk in a straight line and a tendency to bump into things. This may be significantly worse in the dark, thus indicating a sensory ataxia. Sudden changes of direction are particularly difficult and problems turning may be reported. The duration of the gait disturbance should be established, and it is worth asking about early motor milestones and athletic ability at school that may bring out a much longer history than previously appreciated. Collateral history should be sought especially if an insidious onset is suspected, as this may be difficult for a patient to report. A question as to diurnal variation particularly a history of morning unsteadiness that wears off later in the day, often associated with morning headache, suggests raised intracranial pressure even if examination is normal.

Limb incoordination and tremor

Clumsiness of the arms is often noted later in the course of their illness. Generally a tremor that is worse on action is reported and as this worsens patients notice clumsiness carrying objects and deterioration of their handwriting. This is more common in multiple sclerosis than in degenerative disease. Disturbance to the midline structures may result in titubation, and this, in combination with action tremor in the upper limbs and little in the way of gait disturbance, should raise the suspicion of Wilson's disease.

Dysarthria

This may be noted by friends and relatives before the patient. Classically described as having a staccato quality, it is a useful symptom or sign as it points against a purely sensory ataxia.

Visual and ocular motor symptoms

Visual symptoms are relatively rare in pure cerebellar disease and if present is more often associated with brainstem disturbance, especially episodic or persistent diplopia associated with ataxia. Vertical oscillopsia suggests downbeat nystagmus, and a structural foramen magnum lesion should be suspected. Acute or subacute oscillopsia, with chaotic involuntary eye movements observed by relatives, may be mentioned in the history of patients with viral cerebellitis, paraneoplastic cerebellar degeneration, and the dancing-eyes syndrome (opsoclonus). There are some very rare degenerative ataxias with gradual visual loss, due to either optic neuropathy or retinopathy.

Other symptoms

Details of any headache or vomiting should be sought, the presence of which may suggest a posterior fossa mass lesion. An acute history suggests cerebellar haemorrhage. If longer standing then a tumour becomes more likely. It should also be remembered that infections, especially an abscess, can cause similar symptoms. Intermittent symptoms and perhaps associated fever and malaise raise the possibility of posterior fossa cysticercosis, and a detailed travel history over the last 20 years should be sought.

Vertigo is more suggestive of neoplastic, inflammatory, and vascular disease rather than the more slowly progressive degenerative processes.

Direct questioning should cover the urinary system, skeletal deformities, cardiac disease, and assessment of cognitive abilities since many ataxias can be associated with disease in other systems (see Table 1).

A detailed enquiry of drug ingestion (for both medical and recreational purposes, including alcohol) and occupational exposure is also required.

Signs of cerebellar disease

This section covers the examination in the sequence that it appears to the physician.

Gait and posture

A patient walking into the consulting room may have a broad-based gait with a poor turn, and there is often a lurching quality to the overall sequence. More detailed assessment of mild gait ataxia may be obtained by asking the patient to tandem walk (heel–toe). Asking the patient to stand still may reveal the broad base and unless there is additional proprioceptive loss or vestibular disease, this instability is not aggravated by eye closure.

Speech

It is often stated that cerebellar speech is very distinctive with an explosive quality, so-called scanning dysarthria. Although when this is heard it is characteristic, more often a combination of spastic and cerebellar features can be heard. Additional signs such as a slow moving tongue and brisk jaw jerk support the latter.

Muscle tone

Many textbooks state firmly that cerebellar disease gives rise to hypotonia, and some even include it within the symptoms. Not only do patients never complain of hypotonia but this is rarely detectable clinically in symmetrical slowly progressive or chronic disorders. Pendular knee jerks are also difficult to detect without the eye of faith and many patients with 'cerebellar' ataxic disorders have disease of the spinal cord, peripheral nerves, or both, which complicates the clinical picture.

Limb ataxia

Limb ataxia usually results from a combination of dysmetria and dysdiadochokinesis. Dysmetria refers to errors in the range and force of movement resulting in an erratic, jerky movement which may under- or

Table 1 Differential diagnosis of ataxic disorders: associated general physical signs

Short stature	
Mitochondrial encephalomyopathy, ataxia telangiectasia, Sjögren–Larsson syndrome, Cockayne syndrome	
Hypogonadism	
Recessive ataxia with hypogonadism, ataxia telangiectasia, Sjögren–Larsson syndrome, mitochondrial encephalomyopathy, adrenoleucomyeloneuropathy	
Skeletal deformity	
Friedreich's ataxia, Sjögren–Larsson syndrome, many other early-onset inherited ataxias, hereditary motor and sensory neuropathy	
Immunodeficiency	
Ataxia telangiectasia, multiple carboxylase deficiencies	
Malnutrition	
Vitamin E deficiency, alcoholic cerebellar degeneration	
Hair	
Argininosuccinicaciduria	Brittle hair
Giant axonal neuropathy	Tight curls
Thallium poisoning, hypothyroidism, adrenoleucomyeloneuropathy	Hair loss
Foramen magnum lesions	Low hairline
Skin	
Ataxia telangiectasia	Telangiectases, particularly: conjunctiva, nose, ears, flexures
Xeroderma pigmentosum	Extreme light sensitivity, tumours
Hartnup disease	Pellagra-type rash
Cholestanolosis	Tendinous swellings
Hypothyroidism, Cockayne syndrome, Refsum's disease	Dry skin
Adrenoleucomyeloneuropathy	Pigmentation
Eyes	
Ataxia telangiectasia	(see Skin)
Wilson's disease	Kayser–Fleischer rings
Cerebellar haemangioblastoma	Retinal angiomas in von-Hippel–Lindau disease
Congenital rubella, cholestanolosis, Sjögren–Larsson syndrome	Cataract
Gillespie syndrome	Aniridia
Fever	
Abscess, viral cerebellitis, cysticercosis, dominant periodic ataxia, intermittent metabolic ataxias	Fever may precipitate neurological deterioration in last two
Haemorrhage, infarction, demyelination, posterior fossa mass lesions, intermittent metabolic ataxias	Vomiting
Hepatosplenomegaly	
Niemann-Pick disease type C, some childhood metabolic ataxias, Wilson's disease, alcoholic cerebellar degeneration	
Heart disease	
Mitochondrial encephalomyopathy	Conduction defects
Friedreich's ataxia	Cardiomegaly, murmurs, arrhythmias, late heart failure, abnormal ECG

overshoot the target. Dysdiadochokinesis is demonstrated by asking the patient to tap one hand on the other, alternately pronating and supinating the tapping hand, or rapidly opening and closing the fist. The tapping out of simple rhythms (with the hand or foot) is also useful in assessing both the rhythmicity and force of the tap.

Classically, testing of coordination is undertaken after the motor and sensory tests as the presence of weakness or sensory loss can confuse the picture. There is also a natural asymmetry in cerebellar function, with better performance, particularly for rapid alternating movements, in the dominant limb. About 40 per cent of patients with vermis lesions do not have limb ataxia but have striking gait ataxia.

Tremor

Intention tremor is present if a rhythmical side-to-side oscillation is seen on finger-to-nose testing. A combination of gross intention tremor and a postural component is often called rubral or red nucleus tremor, although peduncular tremor is probably a more accurate label. It is most commonly seen in multiple sclerosis and occasionally in late-onset degenerative ataxias. A nodding head tremor (titubation) with a frequency of 3 to 4 Hz may be seen with midline cerebellar disease.

Eye movements

Square wave jerks may be seen in the primary position; these are inappropriate saccades that disrupt fixation and are followed by a corrective saccade within 200 ms. Assessment of pursuit may see a jerkiness with saccadic intrusions. Additional isolated or multiple lesions of the third, fourth, or sixth cranial nerves suggests brainstem pathology. Examination of the saccadic system can reveal hypo- or hypermetric saccades. An internuclear ophthalmoplegia may be found whilst examining this system, suggesting a diagnosis of multiple sclerosis, but it can rarely be associated with some degenerative ataxias. The vestibulo-ocular reflex (doll's head manoeuvre) should then be examined to look for any supranuclear component. An inability to suppress this reflex is evidence of pathology involving the vestibulocerebellum.

Acute or subacute presentation of almost any of the above eye movements, especially if associated with alcohol abuse or vomiting, raises the possibility of Wernicke's encephalopathy and requires urgent treatment with thiamin.

Gaze-evoked nystagmus is the most common type of nystagmus associated with cerebellar disease; eccentric gaze cannot be maintained, and the slow phase of the nystagmus is toward the primary position, with rapid corrective movements. It does not have much localizing value. Although downbeat nystagmus should raise the suspicion of a foramen magnum lesion, this is also seen in degenerative cerebellar disease.

Positional nystagmus in a patient with vertigo and unsteadiness should be attributed to benign labyrinthine disease only if it is transient, torsional, and fatiguable; if it does not have these features, a posterior fossa lesion should be suspected.

Other neurological signs and general examination

As the causes of ataxia are numerous, a large variety of other neurological and general physical signs may be found on examination. Table 1 lists the various signs and their possible diagnostic significance.

Disorders of the cerebellum

Numerous pathological processes can affect cerebellar function, some of which such as multiple sclerosis and neoplasia are discussed elsewhere. This section will approach the diseases with approximate reference to the time-course (acute, subacute, chronic) and the nature of the course of the disease.

Developmental disorders

The cerebellum has a long developmental period and is not fully mature until about 18 months of age. It is therefore susceptible to a large number of insults, including intrauterine infections, ischaemic damage, toxins, and genetically determined syndromes (see Table 2). Some of these developmental anomalies, such as dysgenesis or agenesis of the vermis, the cerebellar hemispheres, or parts of the brainstem, give rise to congenital ataxia. These are non-progressive disorders, and in most cases coordination improves with age.

Cerebellar dysfunction in an infant or young child may be overlooked, as it often gives rise to a relatively non-specific abnormal motor development. Later there is nystagmus, obvious incoordination on reaching for objects, and truncal ataxia when first attempting to sit. Associated mental retardation is common but unhelpful diagnostically.

Ataxia of acute or subacute onset

Cerebellar ataxia of extremely acute onset has two main causes: cerebellar haemorrhage (usually associated with headache, vertigo, vomiting, altered consciousness, and neck stiffness); and cerebellar infarction (in which cerebellar signs are usually combined with signs of brainstem ischaemia, and the presentation may mimic that of haemorrhage). Diagnosis should be made as a matter of urgency and imaging is required to clarify these two possibilities.

Subacute, reversible ataxia may occur as a result of viral infection in children between 2 and 10 years of age. There is usually pyrexia, limb and gait ataxia, and dysarthria developing over hours or days. Although recovery occurs over a period of weeks and is usually complete, it can take up to 6 months.

In older patients the possibility of a postinfectious encephalomyelitis, particularly that related to varicella infection, should be considered. The postinfectious Miller Fisher variant of the Guillain-Barré syndrome may present with a triad that includes subacute ataxia, areflexia, and ophthalmoplegia. Nerve conduction studies and examination of cerebrospinal fluid (**CSF**) may be helpful, but the former are often normal. Other infective

Table 2 Congenital inherited ataxic disorders

Syndrome	Additional features	Mode of inheritance
Joubert's syndrome	Episodic hyperpnoea, abnormal eye movements, and mental retardation	Autosomal recessive
Gillespie's syndrome	Mental retardation and partial aniridia	Uncertain inheritance
Congenital ataxia with mental retardation and spasticity	Includes pontoneocerebellar and granule-cell hypoplasia	Autosomal recessive, autosomal dominant, and X- linked
Disequilibrium syndrome		Autosomal recessive
Paine's syndrome	Spasticity, mental retardation, and microcephaly	X-linked recessive ataxia

(Adapted with permission from Harding AE, *et al.* (1984). Autosomal recessive late-onset multisystem disorder with cerebellar cortical atrophy at autopsy: report of a family. *Journal of Neurology, Neurosurgery and Psychiatry* **47**, 853–6.)

Table 3 Infections causing cerebellar disease

Viruses	Others
Echo	*Mycoplasma pneumoniae*
Coxsackie groups A and B	Legionella pneumoniae
Herpes simplex	Lyme disease
Polio	*Toxoplasma gondii*
Epstein–Barr	Typhoid fever
Varicella	*Plasmodium falciparum*
Congenital rubella	Tick paralysis
	Prion disease

agents are shown in Table 3. Viral titres and CSF examination may be helpful, although serological evidence of viral infection may be difficult to establish.

Other causes of subacute ataxia include hydrocephalus, foramen magnum compression, posterior fossa tumour (primary or secondary), abscess, or parasitic infection in any age group. A number of important toxins and drugs also need to be considered, including thallium, lead, barbiturates, phenytoin, piperazine, alcohol, solvents, and antineoplastic drugs.

Vascular disorders of the cerebellum

Cerebrovascular disease is dealt with in detail in Chapter 24.13.7. Transient ischaemic attacks involving the vascular supply to the cerebellum rarely produce ataxia and dysarthria alone, usually there are associated symptoms of brainstem dysfunction. Cerebellar infarction (from embolus or, more commonly, vertebrobasilar occlusive disease) and haemorrhage (usually on a background of hypertension or, less commonly, secondary to a vascular malformation or tumour) are relatively rare. Imaging is often necessary for early diagnosis as the later the diagnosis the worse the prognosis. Both infarction and haemorrhage may be amenable to surgical therapy.

Ataxia with an episodic course

These attacks can be considered bizarre and some patients are misdiagnosed as hysterical. However, a good history can usually distinguish between the main causes (listed in order of approximate frequency): drug ingestion, multiple sclerosis, transient vertebrobasilar ischaemic attacks, foramen magnum compression, intermittent obstruction of the ventricular system due to a colloid cyst or cysticercosis, and dominantly inherited periodic ataxia. Autosomal dominant periodic ataxia is characterized by childhood or adolescent onset of attacks of ataxia, dysarthria, vertigo, and nystagmus; not all patients have affected relatives.

There are at least two forms of this disorder: episodic ataxia-1 and -2. Episodic ataxia-1 (**EA1**) is typified by brief attacks (minutes and occasionally hours) and clinically and electrophysiologically myokymia may be seen. Mutations in a potassium-channel gene (*Kv1.1*) have been found. These patients may benefit from treatment with acetazolamide or phenytoin. Patients tend to be neurologically normal between the attacks. In episodic ataxia-2 (EA2) the attacks tend to be longer lasting, hours or even days, usually associated with vertigo and consequent nausea and vomiting. The attacks tend to be more severe in childhood with associated drowsiness, headache, and fever. Although when the disease first begins the patients are well between attacks, an interictal nystagmus can be seen. A slow deterioration in the ataxia is seen as the disease progresses. MRI may reveal cerebellar atrophy. These patients tend to respond better to acetazolamide therapy than patients with EA1. Point mutations in a calcium-channel gene (*CACNA1A*) have been demonstrated in some families with this disorder.

In children and young adults a metabolic disorder should be suspected, particularly defects of the urea cycle, aminoacidurias, Leigh's syndrome, and mitochondrial encephalomyopathies. Screening investigations include blood ammonia, pyruvate, lactate and amino acids, and urinary amino acids.

Ataxia with a chronic progressive course

Chronic alcohol abuse is the commonest causes of progressive cerebellar degeneration in adults. Thiamin deficiency is probably the main (but not sole) explanation for the chronic progressive cerebellar syndrome found in alcoholics. Patients with this syndrome are almost invariably malnourished. Ataxia may develop during periods of abstinence, and identical cerebellar degeneration has been observed in non-alcoholic patients with severe malnutrition. Cerebellar ataxia is common in the Wernicke–Korsakoff syndrome, and the pathological features of both this syndrome and a cerebellar degeneration frequently coexist. With administration of thiamin some improvement may occur in early cases of alcoholic cerebellar degeneration, but if the patient is already chair-bound the response to treatment is limited.

Other deficiency disorders can give rise to a progressive ataxia. There is a rare syndrome associated with zinc deficiency which responds to oral replacement therapy. Deficiency of vitamin E, either genetic (for example, isolated vitamin E deficiency due to mutations in the α-tocopherol transfer protein, or abetalipoproteinaemia) or acquired, due to malabsorption, may also produce a progressive ataxia. Establishing the diagnosis of vitamin E deficiency is important as treatment with vitamin E may prevent progression of the neurological syndrome and can, in rare circumstances, lead to some improvement.

A number of toxic agents can produce progressive cerebellar dysfunction, including pharmaceutical products, solvents, and heavy metals. The most common cause of a cerebellar syndrome due to drug toxicity seen in neurological practice is that associated with anticonvulsant medication, particularly phenytoin. Transient ataxia, dysarthria, and nystagmus usually develop when serum concentrations of phenytoin, carbamazepine, or barbiturates are above the therapeutic range, and remit when they return to within the therapeutic range. Chronic phenytoin toxicity is reported to cause persistent cerebellar dysfunction, and this is associated pathologically with a loss of Purkinje cells. A persistent cerebellar deficit, with dysarthria and limb and gait ataxia and cerebellar atrophy on CT scan, has also been described as a sequel to the acute encephalopathy of lithium toxicity that is usually precipitated by fever or starvation. Serum lithium levels are not always raised in such cases.

Recreational or accidental exposure to a number of solvents, including carbon tetrachloride and toluene, causes cerebellar ataxia along with other neurological problems, including psychosis, cognitive impairment, and pyramidal signs in the case of toluene. The neurological deficit is potentially reversible but may persist after prolonged exposure in solvent abusers. Exposure to heavy metals including inorganic mercury, lead, and thallium can also produce cerebellar damage.

Structural lesions such as posterior fossa tumours, foramen magnum compression, or hydrocephalus must be excluded by imaging studies. Tumours which may involve the posterior fossa include: astrocytoma, ependymoma, haemangioblastoma, and cranial nerve neuromas.

Paraneoplastic cerebellar degeneration related to carcinomas of the lung or ovary or to the reticuloses usually follows a subacute course, with patients losing the ability to walk within months of onset. A variety of antineuronal antibodies may be found in these patients and help to confirm the diagnosis. Approximately half of patients with paraneoplastic cerebellar degeneration (**PCD**) have demonstrable antibodies directed against neurones in their serum and CSF. The most common antibody seen in PCD is called anti-Yo, and it specifically stains Purkinje cell cytoplasm. If antineuronal antibodies are detected then a search for the underlying malignancy should then be undertaken involving imaging and analysis of tumour markers. Presentation with ataxia precedes diagnosis of the malignancy in 70 per cent of cases and is usually subacute, progressing to severe disability over several months or even weeks, and then arresting. Onset may be acute and is sometimes accompanied by vertigo, mimicking a vascular event. There is severe truncal, gait, and limb ataxia and dysarthria. Opsoclonus may be combined with myoclonus, producing a disorder in adults similar to the dancing eyes syndrome of childhood, and which is sometimes associated with neuroblastoma. There is currently no evidence of a useful response either to immunosuppressant therapy or to plasma exchange. However, there are anecdotal reports of some improvement or stabilization following removal of the primary tumour. The best method of screening for the underlying malignancy is debated, but standard magnetic resonance imaging (**MRI**) may be complemented by whole-body positron emission tomography (**PET**) scanning. Searching for primary tumour markers may also be useful.

Rarely, infectious agents can cause slowly progressive ataxia (see Table 3), these include the chronic panencephalitis of congenital rubella infection in children and, in adults, Creutzfeldt–Jakob disease (**CJD**), the iatrogenic form of which should be particularly considered. A specific enquiry regarding potential risk-factor exposure should be sought, especially growth-hormone replacement. It is now known that the so-called variant form of CJD may also cause ataxia, often in association with psychiatric disturbance. Multiple sclerosis only exceptionally presents as an isolated chronic progressive cerebellar syndrome.

Some conditions that are not generally considered primarily as ataxic disorders may present with clumsiness, tremor, or definite cerebellar signs, particularly in childhood or adolescence. These include Wilson's disease and several inherited neuropathies, such as hereditary motor and sensory neuropathy (**HMSN**; Charcot–Marie–Tooth disease, including the so-called Roussy–Levy syndrome). Although intention and postural tremor are quite frequent in the demyelinating type of HMSN (type I), dysarthria and pyramidal signs do not occur. Other chronic demyelinating neuropathies, such as chronic inflammatory and paraproteinaemic neuropathies and Refsum's disease, may give rise to prominent tremor and ataxia; the same applies to giant axonal neuropathy.

Superficial siderosis is a rare disorder that causes slowly progressive cerebellar ataxia, mainly of gait, and sensorineural deafness, often combined with spasticity, brisk reflexes, and extensor plantar responses. The diagnosis may not be suspected clinically, but the neuroradiological abnormalities are striking, MRI showing a black rim of haemosiderin around the posterior fossa structures and spinal cord, and less often the cerebral hemispheres, on *T*2-weighted images. Superficial siderosis is most commonly secondary to chronic leaking of blood into the subarachnoid space. Treatment relies on identifying the source of bleeding; chelation therapy does not appear to be effective.

After excluding acquired causes of ataxic disorders, there remains a considerable number of patients with degenerative ataxias, not all of which are overtly genetically determined. The inherited ataxias can largely be classified according to their clinical and genetic features (see below), and in a small proportion of cases a recognizable metabolic defect can be detected. It is important to make as accurate a diagnosis as possible in these disorders for the purposes of prognosis, genetic counselling, and, occasionally, specific therapy.

Progressive metabolic ataxias

Ataxia may be a minor feature of storage and other metabolic neurodegenerative disorders developing in early childhood. Some enzyme deficiencies that usually give rise to diffuse neurodegenerative disorders in which ataxia is a feature, either developing in infancy or early childhood, include the sphingomyelin lipidoses, metachromatic leucodystrophy, galactosylceramide lipidosis (Krabbe's disease), and the hexosaminidase deficiencies. Also included within this group is adrenoleucomyeloneuropathy, a phenotypic variant of adrenoleucodystrophy. This is diagnosed by estimation of very long-chain fatty acids. Although X-linked, approximately 10 per cent of carrier females may manifest neurological abnormalities. The role of diet and dietary supplements (for example, oleic acid and Lorenzo's oil) remains to be established. Ataxia may be prominent in Niemann–Pick disease type C (juvenile dystonic lipidosis), combined with a supranuclear gaze palsy. Sphingomyelinase activity is normal, but foamy storage cells are found in the bone marrow.

Cholestanolosis (also called cerebrotendinous xanthomatosis, **CTX**) is a rare autosomal recessive disorder caused by defective bile salt metabolism, due to a deficiency of mitochondrial sterol 27-hydroxylase. It gives rise to ataxia, dementia, spasticity, peripheral neuropathy, cataract, and tendon xanthomas in the second decade of life. Treatment with chenodeoxycholic acid appears to improve neurological function.

Various phenotypes classifiable as hereditary ataxias have been described in the mitochondrial encephalomyopathies, many of which are associated with a defect of mitochondrial DNA. These include late-onset ataxic disorders associated (for example, the Kearns–Sayre syndrome) with such features as dementia, deafness, and peripheral neuropathy. These features overlap with the syndrome of progressive myoclonic ataxia, which may also be caused by ceroid lipofuscinosis, sialidosis, and Unverricht–Lundborg's disease or so-called Baltic myoclonus. Most of these disorders can now be distinguished with appropriate gene tests or enzyme estimations.

Acquired metabolic and endocrine disorders causing cerebellar dysfunction

These include hepatic encephalopathy, pontine and extrapontine myelinolysis related to hyponatraemia, and hypothyroidism. The last of these is only very rarely a cause of a cerebellar syndrome in both children and adults.

Ataxic disorders associated with defective DNA repair

There are a number of rare conditions associated with a reduced capacity to perform excision repair of DNA damaged by ultraviolet light and some chemical carcinogens. The commonest is ataxia telangiectasia (**AT**). Clinically related conditions include xeroderma pigmentosum and Cockayne's syndrome. Characteristically, motor development is often delayed and ataxia noted at the time of first walking. Growth retardation and delayed sexual development are frequent, and there is mild mental retardation in some cases. A mixed movement disorder may be seen, often with a combination of ataxia, dystonia, and chorea. The cutaneous telangiectasia of AT tend to develop on the conjunctivas between the ages of 3 and 6 years, but occasionally are inconspicuous or absent in adult life. Ataxia telangiectasia is associated with abnormalities of both humoral and cell-mediated immunity. The gene for AT has now been cloned and is called *ATM*.

Degenerative disorders

The degenerative cerebellar and spinocerebellar disorders are a complex group of diseases, most of which are genetically determined. In some there is an underlying metabolic disorder, and it is important to diagnose these as there may be important implications for treatment and genetic counselling. There has been a rapid growth in our knowledge of the genetic basis of many of the spinocerebellar degenerations. The next phase will be to understand how these genes and the abnormal proteins they produce cause cell-specific neuropathology. Inherited ataxic disorders can be divided according to their mode of inheritance (Tables 4 and 5). Most autosomal recessive disorders are of early onset

Table 4 Ataxic disorders of unknown aetiology: autosomal recessive ataxias (onset usually before 20 years of age)

Friedreich's ataxia
Early-onset cerebellar ataxia with:
- retained tendon reflexes
- hypogonadism
- myoclonus (progressive myoclonic ataxia, Ramsay Hunt syndrome)
- childhood deafness
- congenital deafness
- optic atrophy with or without mental retardation (including Behr's syndrome)
- cataract and mental retardation (Marinesco–Sjögren's syndrome)
- pigmentary retinopathy

Autosomal recessive late-onset ataxia

(before 20 years of age), while autosomal dominant disorders are usually of later onset (over 20 years of age).

Autosomal recessive ataxias

Friedreich's ataxia is the most common of the autosomal recessive ataxias (see Table 4), accounting for at least 50 per cent of cases of hereditary ataxia in most large series reported from Europe and the United States. The prevalence of the disease in these regions is similar, between 1 and 2 per 100 000.

The onset of symptoms, generally with gait ataxia, is usually between the ages of 8 and 15 years. However, an onset between 20 and 30 years of age, but fulfilling all other diagnostic criteria, have been described. In addition to the progressive ataxia, a number of variable features are seen, including dysarthria and pyramidal tract involvement. Initially, this latter feature may be mild, with just extensor plantar responses, but invariably a pyramidal pattern of weakness in the legs is seen after 5 or more years' duration of the disease. Eventually this can lead to paralysis. Distal wasting, particularly in the upper limbs, is seen in about 50 per cent of patients with Friedreich's ataxia. Skeletal abnormalities are also commonly found, including scoliosis (85 per cent) and foot deformities typically pes cavus, in approximately 50 per cent of patients. Additional clinical support for a suspicion of Friedreich's ataxia include optic atrophy, which can be seen in 25 per cent of patients; however, it is rare (<5 per cent) for Friedreich's ataxia to produce major visual impairment. Deafness is found in less than 10 per cent of cases, but rather more have impairment of speech discrimination. Nystagmus is seen in only about 20 per cent, but the extraocular movements are nearly always abnormal, with broken-up pursuit, dysmetric saccades, square-wave jerks, and failure of fixation suppression of the vestibulo-ocular reflex.

Investigation of patients reveals an axonal sensory neuropathy; an abnormal ECG in 65 per cent of patients with widespread T-wave inversion. Diabetes mellitus occurs in 10 per cent of patients with Friedreich's ataxia, and a further 10 to 20 per cent have impaired glucose tolerance.

The gene encoding frataxin (*X25*) was cloned in 1996. The predominant mutation is a trinucleotide repeat (GAA) in intron 1 of this gene. Expansion of both alleles is found in over 96 per cent of patients. The remaining patients have point mutations in the frataxin gene. This was the first autosomal recessive condition found to be due to a dynamic repeat and, as it is a relatively simple matter to measure the repeat size, it has permitted the

Table 5 Autosomal dominant cerebellar ataxia (ADCA): clinicogenetic classification

Clinical features	Genetic loci[a] and	chromosomal location	Normal allele[b]	Pathological allele[b]
ADCAI				
Cerebellar syndrome plus: pyramidal signs	***SCA1***	6p22–23	6–44	39–83
supranuclear ophthalmoplegia	***SCA2***	12q23–24.1	13–33	32–77
extrapyramidal signs	***SCA3***	14q32.1	12–40	54–89
peripheral neuropathy	*SCA4*	16q24-ter	–	–
dementia	*SCA8*[c]	13q21	16–91	110–130
	SCA12[d]	5q31		
	SCA13	19q13.3		
ADCAII				
Cerebellar syndrome plus: pigmentary maculopathy	***SCA7***	3p12–21.1	4–35	36–306
Other signs as **ADCAI**				
ADCAIII				
'Pure' cerebellar syndrome	*SCA5*	Cent 11	–	
Mild pyramidal signs	***SCA6***[e]	19p13	4–18	20–33
	SCA10	22q	–	–
	SCA11	15q14–21.3	–	–
EA1	K channel *Kv1.1*	12q	Point mutations	
EA2	Ca channel *CACNA1A*[e]	19p13	Point mutations	
Periodic autosomal dominant ataxia				

[a] Cloned *SCA* genes are shown in bold type.
[b] Size ranges are given for normal and pathological alleles observed in the different SCAs.
[c] Note that combined CTG/CTA repeat sizes are given for *SCA8*. The pathogenicity of *SCA8* is still not established.
[d] *SCA12* has only been reported in one family and is due to an expanded CTG repeat.
[e] *SCA6* and *CACNL1A* are allelic variants.
SCA, spinocerebellar ataxia; EA, episodic ataxia.

introduction of a specific and sensitive diagnostic test. On normal chromosomes the number of GAA repeats varies from 7 to 22 units, whereas on disease chromosomes the range is anything from around 100 to 2000 repeats. The length of the repeat is a determinant of the age of onset and therefore to some degree influences the severity, in that early-onset cases tend to progress more rapidly.

There is accumulating evidence that frataxin is mitochondrially located and may be involved in iron transport. Clinically, this fits; a syndrome of ataxia and neuropathy, in association with diabetes, cardiomyopathy, deafness, and optic atrophy, has the hallmarks of a mitochondrial disease.

Other autosomal recessive ataxias are individually rare and are listed in Table 4.

Autosomal dominant ataxias

The autosomal dominant cerebellar ataxias (**ADCAs**) are a clinically and genetically complex group of neurodegenerative disorders (see Table 5). ADCA type I is characterized by a progressive cerebellar ataxia and is variably associated with other extracerebellar neurological features such as ophthalmoplegia, optic atrophy, peripheral neuropathy, and pyramidal and extrapyramidal signs. The presence and severity of these signs is, in part, dependent on the duration of the disease. Although mild or moderate dementia may occur, it is usually not a prominent early feature. ADCA type II is clinically distinguished from the ADCA type I by the presence of pigmentary macular dystrophy, whereas ADCA type III is a relatively 'pure' cerebellar syndrome and generally starts at a later age. This clinical classification is still useful, despite the tremendous improvements in our understanding of the genetic basis (see below), because it provides a framework which can be used in the clinic and helps direct the genetic evaluation.

The genetic loci causing the dominant ataxias are given the acronym *SCA* (spinocerebellar ataxia). At the time of writing 17 *SCA* loci have been identified. Of these, the genes are established for *SCA1*, *-2*, *-3*, *-6*, *-7*, *-10*, *-12*, and *-17*. The last three are all extremely rare. *SCA12*, *-36*, and *-7* are all caused by a similar mutational mechanism, an expansion of an exonic CAG repeat. The resultant proteins all possess an expanded polyglutamine tract, and at least eight conditions caused by these expansions are now known. Other types of ADCA are exceedingly rare.

Idiopathic degenerative late-onset ataxias

About two-thirds of cases of degenerative ataxia developing over the age of 20 years are singleton cases, and they represent a significant clinical problem; it is difficult even to know how to label them. The literature is confusing, mixing pathological terms such as 'olivopontocerebellar atrophy' (**OPCA**) with clinical terms, I prefer to use the term 'idiopathic late-onset cerebellar ataxia' (**ILOCA**). A proportion of patients in this group, progress to develop the features of multiple system atrophy (**MSA**). These patients may have, or develop, facial impassivity and extrapyramidal rigidity, whilst others present with features of autonomic failure such as postural hypotension, impotence, bladder dysfunction, and a fixed cardiac rate. A cerebellar presentation occurs in about 15 per cent of patients with MSA. The distinction of idiopathic late-onset cerebellar ataxia from MSA may therefore be difficult clinically at presentation.

Most patients with idiopathic late-onset cerebellar ataxia lose the ability to walk independently between 5 and 20 years after onset, and their lifespan is slightly shortened by immobility. Those who go on to develop MSA have a particularly poor prognosis. Investigations, apart from those excluding acquired causes of cerebellar degeneration such as malignancy and hypothyroidism, tend to be unhelpful. Electrophysiological evidence of a sensory peripheral neuropathy is found in about 50 per cent of cases, which can be a useful pointer to the presence of a degenerative multisystem disorder. CT or MRI scan may show cerebellar and brainstem atrophy, or pure cerebellar atrophy. The prognosis is worse in patients with clinical and radiological evidence of brainstem involvement, compared to those with a pure cerebellar syndrome and cerebellar atrophy alone on MRI.

Further reading

Anderson NE, Rosenblum MK, Posner JB (1988). Paraneoplastic cerebellar degeneration: clinical-immunological correlations. *Annals of Neurology* **24**, 559–67.

Bootsma D, *et al.* (2001). Nucleotide excision repair syndromes: xeroderma pigmentosum, Cockayne syndrome and trichothiodystrophy. In: Scriver CR, *et al.*, eds. *The metabolic basis of inherited disease*, 8th edn, pp 245–74. McGraw Hill, New York.

Campuzano V, *et al.* (1996). Friedreich's ataxia: autosomal recessive disease caused by an intronic GAA triplet repeat expansion. *Science* **271**, 1423–7.

De Michele G, *et al.* (1989). Late onset recessive ataxia with Friedreich's disease phenotype. *Journal of Neurology, Neurosurgery and Psychiatry* **52**, 1398–403.

Enevoldson PG, Sanders MD, Harding AE (1994). Autosomal dominant cerebellar ataxia with pigmentary macular dystrophy: a clinical and genetic study of eight families. *Brain* **17**, 445–60.

Fearnley JM, Stevens JM, Rudge P (1995). Superficial siderosis of the central nervous system. *Brain* **118**, 1051–66.

Hanna MG, Wood NW, Kullmann D (1998). The neurological channelopathies. *Journal of Neurology, Neurosurgery and Psychiatry* **65**, 427–31.

Harding AE (1981). Friedreich's ataxia: a clinical and genetic study of 90 families with an analysis of early diagnostic criteria and intrafamilial clustering of clinical features. *Brain* **104**, 589–620.

Harding AE (1984). *The hereditary ataxias and related disorders.* Churchill Livingstone, Edinburgh.

Harding AE, Diengdoh JV, Lees AJ (1984). Autosomal recessive late-onset multisystem disorder with cerebellar cortical atrophy at autopsy: report of a family. *Journal of Neurology, Neurosurgery and Psychiatry* **47**, 853–6.

Klockgether J, *et al.* (1990). Idiopathic cerebellar ataxia of late onset: natural history and MRI morphology. *Journal of Neurology, Neurosurgery and Psychiatry* **53**, 297–305.

Klockgether T, *et al.* (1998). The natural history of degenerative ataxia: a retrospective study in 466 patients. *Brain* **121**, 589–600.

Marsden CD, *et al.* (1990). Progressive myoclonic ataxia (the Ramsay Hunt syndrome). *Archives of Neurology* **47**, 1121–5.

Muller DP, Lloyd JK, Wolff OH (1983). Vitamin E and neurological function. *Lancet* **i**, 225–8.

Peterson K, *et al.* (1992). Paraneoplastic cerebellar degeneration. I. A clinical analysis of 55 anti-Yo antibody-positive patients. *Neurology* **42**, 1931–7.

Quinn NP, Marsden CD (1993). The motor disorder of multiple system atrophy. *Journal of Neurology, Neurosurgery and Psychiatry* **56**, 1239–42.

Stewart GE, Ironside JW (1998). New variant Creutzfeldt–Jakob disease. *Current Opinion in Neurology* **11**, 259–62.

Woods CG, Taylor AMR (1992). Ataxia telangiectasia in the British Isles: the clinical and laboratory features of 70 affected individuals. *Quarterly Journal of Medicine* **298**, 169–79.

24.13.13 The motor neurone diseases

Michael Donaghy

Introduction

The motor neurone diseases result from selective loss of function of the lower and/or upper motor neurones controlling the voluntary muscles of the limbs or bulbar region. The term 'motor neurone disease' is best used to describe a family of diseases within which there is extensive differential diagnosis; in the past the term has been used synonymously with amyotrophic lateral sclerosis, one of the most serious of these diseases. Precise diagnosis is essential for advising patients about prognosis, for identifying those diseases with genetic implications, and to offer immunosuppressant therapy to patients with some acquired lower motor neurone syndromes.

In practice, differential diagnosis requires clinical and electrophysiological classification as to whether the disease involves the upper or the lower motor neurones, or both. This anatomical differentiation is augmented by the age of onset, the rate of deterioration, and familial occurrence (Table 1). Sensation and cognition are normal on simple clinical assessment in the motor neurone diseases.

The clinical signs of lower motor neurone involvement consist of muscle wasting, fasciculations, and flaccid weakness. The tendon reflexes are often retained until profound denervation or fibrous replacement have affected the muscle. Fasciculations are visible flickerings within the muscle belly which are insufficient to produce movement around the joint; electromyography shows that they correspond to simultaneous discharge of all the muscle fibres within a diseased motor unit. Nerve conduction studies will exclude peripheral neuropathy. Electromyography helps to distinguish denervation from myopathy. Muscle biopsy is often required to exclude myopathy, particularly in syndromes causing slowly progressive proximal limb weakness, and bulbar weakness, such as inclusion body myositis.

Upper motor neurone involvement produces spasticity, clonus, extensor plantar responses, and weakness. Extensor plantar responses or clonus may be obscured by coexisting leg muscle atrophy. The abdominal reflexes are often preserved in motor neurone diseases involving the upper motor neurones. This contrasts with their loss in spinal cord disease due to tumours, compression, or demyelinating disease. Sphincter control and sexual function are usually preserved in motor neurone disease, although trunk and abdominal wall weakness may make excretion slow and awkward.

Motor neurone diseases are incurable for the most part and therefore treatment must aim to overcome, or minimize, the various sources of disability. Malnutrition due to dysphagia can be circumvented by nasogastric tube feeding or percutaneous endoscopic gastrostomy. Various forms of assisted respiration offset respiratory muscle weakness, including continuous positive airways pressure via a facial mask. Limb spasticity can be reduced by baclofen, dantroline, or diazepam. Wheelchairs and arm appliances may overcome inadequate limb function. Electronic communication devices should be supplied to those whose speech is incomprehensible. Amitriptyline may help contain the embarrassing emotional lability of pseudobulbar palsy. Housing and workplace modifications can allow patients to maintain independence despite their disability.

Table 1 Classification of the motor neurone diseases

	Disease	Inheritance	Age of onset*
Combined upper and lower motor neurone syndromes	Amyotrophic lateral sclerosis:		
	Sporadic	Not inherited	Adult, elderly
	Familial adult onset	Autosomal dominant	
	Familial juvenile onset	Autosomal recessive	Childhood
Lower motor neurone syndromes	Proximal hereditary motor neuronopathy:		
	Acute infantile form (Werdnig–Hoffmann)	Autosomal recessive	Infantile
	Chronic childhood form (Kugelberg–Welander)	Autosomal recessive	Infantile, childhood
	Adult onset	Autosomal recessive	Adult
	Adult onset	Autosomal dominant	Childhood, adult
	Hereditary bulbar palsy:		
	With deafness (Brown–Violetta–Van Laere)	Inherited (?mode)	Childhood, adult
	Without deafness (Fazio–Londe)	Autosomal recessive	Childhood
	X-linked bulbospinal neuronopathy (Kennedy syndrome)	X linked	Adult, elderly
	Hexosaminidase deficiency	Autosomal recessive	Childhood, adult
	Multifocal motor neuropathies	Not inherited	Adult, elderly
	Post-polio syndrome	Not inherited	Elderly
	Post-irradiation syndrome lumbosacral radiculopathy	Not inherited	Adult, elderly
	Monomelic, focal, or segmental spinal muscular atrophy	Not inherited	Adult
Upper motor neurone syndromes	Primary lateral sclerosis	Not inherited	Adult, elderly
	Hereditary spastic paraplegia	Autosomal dominant	Adult, elderly
	Lathyrism	Not inherited	Adult
	Konzo	Not inherited	Adult

* Adult: 15 to 50 years; elderly: more than 50 years.

Combined upper and lower motor neurone syndromes

Amyotrophic lateral sclerosis

Amyotrophic lateral sclerosis occurs worldwide, usually with an incidence of 1 to 1.5 per 100 000 population and a prevalence of 4 to 6 per 100 000. It is commoner in men and the incidence increases with advancing age; it is unusual before the fifth decade of life. The cause of the common sporadic form of amyotrophic lateral sclerosis is quite unknown. Its incidence is particularly high in areas of the Western Pacific, particularly in Guam and the Japanese Kii Peninsula where it tends to occur in younger adults and can be associated with dementia or parkinsonism. Autosomal dominant inheritance is evident in approximately 5 per cent of patients with adult onset amyotrophic lateral sclerosis. Roughly 20 per cent of familial amyotrophic lateral sclerosis is associated with the 40 different missense mutations of the Cu/Zn superoxide dismutase (*SOD1*) gene on chromosome 21 which catalyses conversion of toxic superoxide anion radicals to hydrogen peroxide. The disease associated with various *SOD1* mutations shows varying degrees of penetrance and a variable phenotype. It tends to begin earlier in adulthood and may involve minor sensory symptoms. A rare juvenile onset autosomal recessive form of amyotrophic lateral sclerosis with prominent bulbar involvement has been described from North Africa and a rare juvenile onset autosomal dominant form without bulbar involvement occurs in the United States.

Pathology

Lower motor neurones are lost from clinically affected areas of the spinal cord and brainstem. Surviving neurones may show intracytoplasmic inclusions (Bumina bodies) and proximal axonal accumulations of neurofilaments (spheroids). The motor cortex is depleted of Betz cells and the pyramidal tracts degenerate. It is becoming increasingly recognized that other populations of neurones can also degenerate in motor neurone disease even though this is not usually evident clinically. These include peripheral sensory neurones and Clarke's column neurones. Up to 10 per cent of patients may eventually develop a mild dementia, often of frontal lobe type. These recent findings show that amyotrophic lateral sclerosis is either a generalized neurodegenerative disorder, in which the motor neurones take the vast brunt of the disease, or that it sometimes overlaps with other neurodegenerations. However, for the practical purpose of clinical diagnosis early in the disease, amyotrophic lateral sclerosis should be regarded as having purely motor manifestations.

Clinical features

At presentation, patients either have bulbar or spinal symptoms, although both usually become evident as the disease progresses.

The bulbar form causes dysphagia, dysphonia, and inhalation of foodstuffs due to weakness of the tongue, pharynx, and larynx. The tongue is wasted, weak, and fasciculating, palatal movements are reduced, and the ability to cough explosively is lost due to vocal cord paralysis. This bulbar palsy is usually accompanied by, or even preceded by, varying degrees of pseudobulbar involvement. The tongue is spastic and immobile with 'hot potato' speech and difficulty in inhibiting emotional responses such as laughing or crying. Ventilatory respiratory failure may develop due to weakness of the diaphragm and intercostal muscles. Occasionally, amyotrophic lateral sclerosis can present with dyspnoea. Diaphragm weakness can be detected clinically by noting that the upper abdomen is drawn inwards, rather than outwards, during the second half of inspiration. Furthermore, the forced vital capacity is substantially lower when the patient is lying down compared with standing, because the weight of the liver no longer assists diaphragmatic descent.

The spinal form of amyotrophic lateral sclerosis usually presents with wasting and weakness of one limb, usually as intrinsic hand muscle wasting or foot drop. Occasionally the initial weakness predominantly affects the musculature of the shoulder girdle. Asymptomatic involvement of other limbs is often evident on examination. It is diagnostically important to demonstrate combined upper and lower motor neurone signs in at least two limbs. Wasted fasciculating muscles also exhibiting clonus or hyperreflexia are a helpful finding. With time the limbs become useless due to progressive denervation. Patients become wheelchair- or bedbound, or unable to use their arms for grooming or feeding. Despite enforced recumbency, decubitus ulcers are relatively unusual because autonomic regulation of skin blood flow and secretion is unaffected. Sphincter control is not affected, although practical difficulties in excretion may result from immobility and because abdominal wall weakness prevents the exertion of intra-abdominal pressure.

Prognosis

Amyotrophic lateral sclerosis progresses relentlessly, both in the severity and the extent of muscular involvement. Death commonly results from ventilatory respiratory failure, from choking, or from inhalational pneumonia; malnutrition often contributes. The median survival from first symptoms in those with bulbar onset is approximately 20 months, with only 5 per cent surviving 5 years. The alternative diagnosis of X-linked bulbospinal neuronopathy should be considered in these long survivors. The median survival for those with spinal onset is approximately 29 months with nearly 15 per cent surviving 5 years. Although a subacute and reversible syndrome resembling spinal amyotrophic lateral sclerosis has been described, this is so extraordinarily rare that it should not influence the physician's prognostications.

Differential diagnosis and investigation

A diagnosis of amyotrophic lateral sclerosis is usually depressingly obvious on simple clinical grounds. Often only electrophysiological investigation is necessary to confirm denervation and to exclude a potentially treatable myopathy or demyelinating neuropathy. Sometimes upper motor neurone involvement is not clinically demonstrable, particularly in patients with absent Babinski responses due to severely denervated toe extensor muscles. Unfortunately measurement of central motor conduction following electromagnetic stimulation of the brain is less reliable for revealing upper motor neurone involvement in such cases than had been hoped. If patients present with the combination of arm denervation and upper motor neurone signs in the legs, the cervical spinal canal should be imaged with magnetic resonance scanning to exclude a compressive lesion, most often spondylitic radiculomyelopathy.

The usual diagnostic problem lies in differentiating amyotrophic lateral sclerosis from other motor neurone diseases. A lack of upper motor neurone involvement should raise the possibility of alternative diagnoses. The post-polio syndrome causes slow deterioration in limb or bulbar function some decades after acute poliomyelitis. X-linked bulbospinal neuronopathy is much more slowly progressive than bulbar amyotrophic lateral sclerosis; grimacing usually evokes characteristic lower facial contractions; gynaecomastia, diabetes mellitus, or abnormal sensory nerve conduction are often evident; and other male family members may be affected. Multifocal motor neuropathy or neuronopathy usually develops insidiously, characteristically produces marked weakness with little wasting, predominantly affects the arms, may be associated with paraproteinaemia or antiganglioside antibodies, and may involve motor nerve slowing or conduction block. Adult onset proximal hereditary motor neuronopathy is very slowly progressive, with early and symmetric involvement of proximal muscles, and rarely involves bulbar muscles.

Giving the diagnosis

Doctors or relatives are sometimes tempted on compassionate grounds not to tell patients about their diagnosis of amyotrophic lateral sclerosis. But when patients eventually detect this conspiracy of secrecy it can lead to serious loss of trust at a time when death looms and trustworthy relationships are of inestimable value. When given the opportunity, patients usually indicate that they wish to know the name of the disease and the likely outcome, and they may even wish a detailed discussion of likely modes of death. Of course questions should be answered honestly, although sometimes it may be preferable to discuss them in stages with the spouse present so as to soften the blow early on in the course of the disease. Once a patient has been told the diagnosis, the doctor must address the particular issues presented by that patient's own brand of amyotrophic lateral sclerosis before they become upset by the summary information which they may glean from lay reference books, journalism, or the Internet.

Treatment

No treatment is known to cure amyotrophic lateral sclerosis. Trials of drug therapy have concentrated upon slowing the downhill progression of disability or improving survival. The antiglutamate agent riluzole, administered orally, has been licensed for treatment of amyotrophic lateral sclerosis. The 100 mg dosage improved the chance of tracheostomy-free survival at 18 months by an extra 35 per cent although there was no significant benefit on muscle function. Criticisms of this study have included the nature of the Cox model statistical adjustment, and it should be noted that more of the placebo group had bulbar features at entry to the study. Riluzole is generally well tolerated by patients; nausea, gastrointestinal upset, and raised transaminase enzyme levels may occur and usually resolve with reduction in dose. Ineffective therapeutic trials have included mixtures of branched chain amino acids, dextromorphan, total lymphoid irradiation, and the free radical scavenger acetylcysteine.

Much can be done to overcome disability and alleviate distress by the care team of speech therapist, physiotherapist, occupational therapist, social worker, and physician. The Motor Neurone Disease Association is often able to provide equipment promptly. Severe dysphagia is most effectively bypassed by percutaneous endoscopic gastrostomy. Preferably the patient or their carer should have good hand function and vision so that they can change nutrient bags at home. If video-swallow shows that cricopharyngeal spasm is responsible for dysphagia, cricopharyngeal myotomy may help. Speech failure can be circumvented by computer-assisted communication devices operated through a practical modality, such as pressure, blowing, head nodding, or blinking depending upon which muscles remain strong.

Decisions regarding the advisability of instituting assisted respiration pose complex practical and ethical dilemmas. Patients with diaphragm weakness and nocturnal dyspnoea may be helped by continuous positive airways pressure delivered by a facial mask. Endotracheal intubation and ventilation are rarely recommendable in a disease causing such ubiquitous irreversible weakness.

Lower motor neurone syndromes

These forms of motor neurone disease generally follow a much more benign course than amyotrophic lateral sclerosis. They include syndromes previously described as spinal muscular atrophy and progressive muscular atrophy. Differential diagnosis within the lower motor neurone syndromes depends principally upon attention to the age of onset, the pattern of the weakness, and a possible family history.

Proximal hereditary motor neuronopathy

Acute infantile form (Werdnig–Hoffmann disease)

This is one of the commonest fatal autosomal recessive disorders of children. The disease frequency of approximately 1 in 25 000 in England results from a gene frequency of 1 in 160. Acute infantile spinal muscular atrophy has been linked to chromosome 5q11.2–13.3. Within this region two candidate genes have been isolated, *SMN* (survival motor neurone) and *NAIP* (neuronal apoptosis inhibitory protein). Mutations in these genes occur in up to 98 per cent (*SMN*) and 20 to 50 per cent (*NAIP*) of patients. Although a valuable aid to diagnosis, and potentially for prenatal diagnosis, it should be noted the *SMN* gene mutations occasionally occur in healthy relatives of an affected proband, and that these same mutations, particularly *SMN*, are also found in milder or later onset forms of spinal muscular atrophy including Kugelberg–Welander disease.

Before the age of 6 months, babies become inactive, weak, hypotonic, feed poorly, and are slow to attain motor milestones. They may be born with limb deformities, and in retrospect, fetal movements have been often absent or sparse. The tongue is weak and may fasciculate. Head control is poor and the infant's areflexic and proximally wasted limbs tend to assume a frog-like position. Respiratory movements are decreased with prominent involvement of intercostal muscles. Half the infants die by 6 months, and almost all have succumbed by 18 months, usually to respiratory complications.

Chronic childhood form (Kugelberg–Welander disease)

This form develops at any time from infancy to the early teens. It is also autosomal recessive, may be genetically heterogeneous, and may commence discordantly within families. It may resemble Werdnig–Hoffmann disease if the onset is early, but follows a comparatively benign course. More than 90 per cent of patients are able to walk or to sit unsupported at some time, although these abilities are often lost eventually. Tongue involvement occurs in only half, and significant dysphagia is unusual. Some patients develop respiratory insufficiency as a result of intercostal muscle involvement. The proximal limb weakness and wasting is only slowly progressive and may stabilize spontaneously. Those with severe early weakness often develop secondary spinal and joint deformities. The prognosis varies, although survival into middle age is usual. It is important, although initially difficult, to differentiate those with infantile onset and no family history from Werdnig–Hoffmann disease.

Adult onset forms

The autosomal recessive adult form starts from 15 to 60 years of age, usually in the fourth decade. Slowly progressive proximal limb weakness ensues, but significant disability for walking does not usually occur until the sixth or seventh decade. Life expectancy is only slightly reduced. Distal muscles can be involved too, the tendon reflexes are usually lost, but bulbar involvement is uncommon. The lack of upper motor neurone signs or of bulbar involvement, and the rather indolent progression, distinguish this from amyotrophic lateral sclerosis.

Autosomal dominant forms are rare, and fall into two groups with onset in childhood and in early middle age respectively. The limb weakness is predominantly proximal. Bulbar involvement does occur, although it is unusual. The childhood form may stabilize at adolescence and some patients retain walking ability into middle or old age. The adult onset form causes more severe disability. The lack of upper motor neurone signs distinguishes these conditions from hereditary amyotrophic lateral sclerosis.

X-linked recessive bulbospinal neuronopathy (Kennedy syndrome)

This disorder occurs only in men, with onset in the third to fifth decades of life. It is due to a mutation causing CAG (cytosine–adenine–guanine) repeat sequences of increased length within the androgen receptor gene. Molecular genetic analysis now forms the basis of a diagnostic test. Weakness usually first affects hand or pelvic girdle muscles and the bulbar symptoms may not be evident until 20 years later, if at all. Fasciculations are usually visible in the limb, tongue, and facial muscles. Characteristically, muscle contractions around the chin are induced by pursing the lips or grimacing. The disorder is only slowly progressive. Most patients survive into their seventh or eight decades except when bulbar involvement is unusually severe. The disorder is often misdiagnosed as amyotrophic lateral sclerosis until the unusually slow deterioration is questioned. Unlike amyotrophic lateral sclerosis, there are no upper motor neurone signs and patients commonly show gynaecomastia, diabetes mellitus, and absent sensory nerve action potentials.

Hexosaminidase deficiency

Autosomal recessive GM2 gangliosidosis presents a variable neurological picture, occasionally as a pure motor neurone syndrome due to lower and, rarely, upper motor neurone involvement. More usually there are also other neurological abnormalities such as cerebellar ataxia or dementia. Hexosaminidase assays should be reserved for those patients with early onset of unusual motor neurone disorders, particularly in Ashkenazi Jews.

Hereditary bulbar palsy of infancy and childhood

The Brown–Violetto–van Laere syndrome presents in the teens with bilateral sensorineural deafness, followed some years later by bulbar, facial, limb, and sometimes respiratory muscle weakness. Fazio–Londe disease is an autosomal recessive bulbar palsy of childhood, without deafness, and respiratory muscle involvement may lead to death within a few years.

Monomelic, focal, or segmental motor neuronopathies

This condition is also known as chronic asymmetric or focal spinal muscular atrophy, or monomelic motor neurone disease. Although most commonly described from Asia, especially Japan, it is seen regularly elsewhere in the world. It usually occurs sporadically and most patients are young adult males. It presents with distal wasting and weakness of one hand or forearm. This progresses steadily for the first 2 years before either stabilizing, or settling to a slow rate of subsequent progression. Initially there may be concern that this is the first presentation of amyotrophic lateral sclerosis, but the expected upper motor neurone and bulbar involvement fail to materialize, and spread to other limbs is unusual. Nerve conduction studies are necessary to exclude focal entrapment neuropathies, or multifocal motor neuropathy with conduction block. Magnetic resonance imaging of the cervical spine will detect syringomyelia or other spinal cord disease.

Post-irradiation lumbosacral radiculopathy

This may follow months or years after inclusion of the lower thoracic and upper lumbar spine in irradiation fields treating testicular tumours or lymphoma. It usually affects both legs, or occasionally one, and later causes mild symptoms affecting the sphincters and sensation. It is painless, and electrophysiology does not reveal the myokymic discharges or abnormal sensory nerve action potentials of irradiation plexopathy. The normal imaging of the lumbosacral plexus and cauda equina, and the absence of pain, exclude tumour recurrence.

Post-polio syndrome

After two or more decades, very slowly progressive weakness may affect muscles previously involved by acute paralytic poliomyelitis. Although this predominantly affects the limbs, approximately half of cases also have mild choking or dysphagia and weakness of the respiratory muscles which may lead to hypercapnic respiratory failure. The sluggish deterioration, lack of upper motor neurone involvement, and previous history serve to distinguish post-polio syndrome from amyotrophic lateral sclerosis. Electromyography reveals the giant motor units typical of extensive reinnervation during recovery from previous acute poliomyelitis. At least equally commonly, late deterioration after polio is due to a secondary degenerative arthritis or fibromyalgia.

Multifocal motor neuropathy and neuronopathy

Patients with these conditions may present at any stage of adult life with multifocal and slowly progressive muscle weakness for as long as 20 years. The clinical picture is immensely variable. Distal limb muscles are mainly involved, often notably asymmetrically. The first symptoms and most severe weakness usually affect the arms. Characteristically, severely weakened muscles show little or no wasting. Reflex loss is generally restricted to affected muscles. The condition is neurophysiologically heterogeneous, ranging from muscle denervation to multifocal conduction block in motor nerves, and occasionally a diffusely demyelinating pure motor peripheral neuropathy. Serum antibodies to GM1 gangliosides are detectable in a third of cases, but are of no proven pathogenetic significance. This antibody assay currently lacks specificity since positives are sometimes found in other neurological diseases. Paraproteinaemia is common, particularly immunoglobulin G. These motor neuropathies usually progress insidiously, sometimes in a stepwise manner, and occasionally spontaneous remissions occur. It is important to detect the subgroup of patients with multifocal motor conduction block, or with diffuse demyelinating neuropathy, because improvement may follow immunosuppressant therapy. Although cyclophosamide is reportedly effective, its potential toxicity should limit its use to those patients with severely disabling and progressive weakness. High-dose intravenous human immunoglobulin therapy can produce dramatic improvement lasting 6 to 8 weeks and repeated administration is the mainstay of treatment in severely symptomatic patients. Unfortunately, steroid therapy does not improve multifocal motor neuropathy, and may precipitate further deterioration.

Upper motor neurone syndromes

The pure upper motor neurone syndromes are the rarest forms of motor neurone disease. They should be considered only after magnetic resonance imaging has excluded structural or demyelinating disease of the spinal cord, foramen magnum, or brain. Spasticity is often severe in the purely upper motor neurone diseases, but unfortunately antispasticity medications are often relatively ineffective. Rarely, similar upper motor neurone syndromes may be seen with syphilis, Lyme disease, and HTLV-I infection.

Primary lateral sclerosis

This rare sporadic form of motor neurone disease has an average age of onset of 50 years, and slow progression thereafter for an average of 15 years. The clinical features are all attributable to symmetric degeneration of the upper motor neurones destined for the spinal cord and the bulbar motor neurones. Spasticity and weakness usually commence insidiously in the legs and ascend ultimately to involve the bulbar muscles. Less commonly patients present with an isolated spastic dysarthria, a symptom of pseudobulbar palsy. Pseudobulbar emotional lability may be distressing for these patients, given their normal cognition, and it often responds well to amytriptiline. Bladder function is generally preserved, at least until the later stages. Electromyography does not reveal the muscle denervation to be expected in predominantly upper motor neurone forms of amyotrophic lateral sclerosis. Magnetic resonance imaging may reveal atrophy of the precentral gyrus motor cortex reflecting loss of the Betz cells from which the pyramidal tract originates. Central motor conduction is notably delayed following electromagnetic stimulation of the motor cortex.

Autosomal dominant 'pure' familial spastic paraplegia

Various forms of slowly progressive symmetric spastic paraparesis may be inherited with linkage to chromosomes 2, 14, or 15, most usually on an autosomal dominant basis with onset in the fourth to sixth decades. The degree of leg spasticity often outweighs the severity of the weakness. Bulbar involvement is very rare, and arm function may be well preserved despite severe leg involvement. The condition is slowly progressive. It may remain asymptomatic in some family members, coming to light only when a familial basis for the disease is sought. Sphincter control is not impaired, but sexual impotence can develop. Sometimes varying combinations of other clinical features have been associated with hereditary spastic paraplegia, particularly with recessively inherited forms: distal amyotrophy, mental retardation, dementia, pigmentary retinopathy, optic atrophy, extrapyramidal features, sensory neuropathy, or ataxia.

Lathyrism

Neurolathyrism is a spastic paraparesis caused by regular consumption of the chickling pea (*Lathyrus sativus*) for some months. It is endemic in parts of India and may be epidemic in times of famine. Patients present either subacutely or chronically with a spastic paraparesis and a characteristic scissoring gait in which the balls of the feet take most of the weight. Once it has developed, neurolathyrism is usually not progressive, but little or no recovery occurs even after chickling pea consumption ceases.

Konzo

Konzo is a form of tropical myelopathy which can occur in epidemics at times of famine in several parts of Africa, including Zaire. It seems to be due to dietary cyanide exposure resulting from insufficient soaking of the cassava roots used to produce flour. There is an abrupt onset of symmetric spastic paraparesis which is non-progressive but permanent. Blood cyanide levels are raised at the onset of disease.

Further reading

Bowen J *et al.* (1997). The post-irradiation lower motor neurone syndrome. Neuronopathy or radiculopathy? *Brain* **119**, 1429–39.

Cochrane G, Donaghy M (1993). Motor neuron disease. In: Greenwood RJ *et al.*, eds. *Neurological rehabilitation*, pp 571–85. Churchill Livingstone, Edinburgh.

Donaghy M *et al.* (1994). Pure motor demyelinating neuropathy: deterioration following steroid therapy and improvement with intravenous immunoglobulin. *Journal of Neurology, Neurosurgery and Psychiatry* **57**, 778–83.

Donaghy M (2001). The motor neuron diseases. In: Donaghy M, ed. *Brain's diseases of the nervous system*, 11th edn, pp. 444–60. Oxford University Press, Oxford.

Gregory RP, Mills KR, Donaghy M (1993). Progressive sensory nerve dysfunction in amyotrophic lateral sclerosis: a prospective clinical and neurophysiological study. *Journal of Neurology* 240, 309–14.

Harding AE (1993). Inherited neuronal atrophy and degeneration predominantly of lower motor neurones. In: Dyck PJ *et al.*, eds. *Peripheral neuropathy*, 3rd edn, ch.55. WB Saunders, Philadelphia.

Howard RS, Wiles CM, Loh L (1989). Respiratory complications and their management in motor neuron disease. *Brain* **112**, 1155–70.

Lacomblez L *et al.* (1996). Dose-ranging study of Riluzole in amyotrophic lateral sclerosis. *The Lancet* **347**, 1425–31.

La Spada AR *et al.* (1991). Androgen receptor gene mutations in X-linked spinal and bulbar muscular atrophy. *Nature* **352**, 77–9.

Le Febvre S *et al.* (1998). The role of the SMN gene in proximal spinal muscular atrophy. *Human Molecular Genetics* **7**, 1531–6.

Ludolph AC *et al.* (1987). Studies on the aetiology and pathogenesis of motor neuron diseases. I Lathyrism: clinical findings in established cases. *Brain* **110**, 149–66.

McShane MA *et al.* (1993). Progressive bulbar paralysis of childhood. A reappraisal of Fazio–Londe disease. *Brain* **115**, 1889–900.

Olney RK, Aminoff MJ, So YT (1991). Clinical and electrodiagnostic features of X-linked recessive bulbospinal neuronopathy. *Neurology* **41**, 823–8.

Pestronk A *et al.* (1990). Lower motor neuron syndromes defined by patterns of weakness, nerve conduction abnormalities, and high titres of antiglycolipid antibodies. *Annals of Neurology* **27**, 316–26.

Pringle CE *et al.* (1992). Primary lateral sclerosis. Clinical features, neuropathology and diagnostic criteria. *Brain* **115**, 495–520.

Rabin BA *et al.* (1999). Autosomal dominant juvenile amyotrophic lateral sclerosis. *Brain* **122**, 1539–50.

Riluzole for amyotrophic lateral sclerosis (1997). *Drug and Therapeutics Bulletin* **35**, 11–12.

Rosen DR *et al.* (1993). Mutations in Cu-Zn superoxide dismutase gene are associated with familial amyotrophic lateral sclerosis. *Nature* **362**, 59–62.

Sonies BC, Dalakas MC (1991). Dysphagia in patients with the post-polio syndrome. *New England Journal of Medicine* **324**, 1162–7.

Tandan R, Bradley WG (1985). Amyotrophic lateral sclerosis: Part 1. Clinical features, pathology, and ethical issues in management. *Annals of Neurology* **18**, 271–80.

Tandan R, Bradley WG (1985). Amyotrophic lateral sclerosis: Part 2. Etiopathogenesis. *Annals of Neurology* **18**, 419–31.

Tylleskär T *et al.* (1992). Cassava cyanogens and Konzo, an upper motor neuron disease found in Africa. *The Lancet* **339**, 208–11.

24.13.14 Diseases of the autonomic nervous system

Christopher J. Mathias

Introduction

The autonomic nervous system has two principal efferent pathways, sympathetic and parasympathetic, that innervate and influence every organ in the body (Fig. 1). Autonomic actions are predominantly involuntary and automatic, as indicated by the term 'autonomic' first proposed by Langley in 1898. The structure of the autonomic system, with numerous synapses centrally and peripherally as well as its multiple neurotransmitters, provides flexible control of organ function locally and in an integrated manner—as in the maintenance of systemic blood pressure and body temperature. Disease of the autonomic nervous system may cause local or systemic effects.

Basic principles

The autonomic nervous system is primarily a visceromotor system, in which each efferent pathway is influenced in a variety of ways. Feedback and central integration is important and virtually every sensory pathway can influence its activity. For example, in spinal cord lesions, activation of visceral, skin, and muscle receptors below the level of the lesion influences autonomic activity and blood pressure through spinal pathways while heart rate responses to classic afferent baroreceptor pathways are retained. Key cerebral autonomic centres are in the hypothalamus, midbrain (Edinger–Westphal nucleus and locus ceruleus), and brainstem (nucleus tractus solitarius and vagal nuclei), and through intracerebral connections. Many other areas affect autonomic activity. Examples are the insular cortex, anterior cingulate gyrus, and amygdala, that are important in processing of emotion and autonomic effects. Parasympathetic efferent pathways are craniosacral and sympathetic efferents are thoracolumbar; each has pre- and postganglionic fibres. The sympathetic ganglia are placed further from target organs than are the parasympathetic ganglia.

Autonomic nerve terminals at target organs vary in complexity; they have the capacity to synthesize neurotransmitters and a host of mechanisms affect uptake and interaction with local or bloodborne chemicals (Fig. 2(a and b)). There are differences between organs, especially the gastrointestinal system, in which the enteric nervous system is considered as a third autonomic division. The multiplicity of neural pathways, transmitters, and modulators results in selective control of responses in specific vascular territories and organs, making it a highly complex but precisely regulated and integrated system.

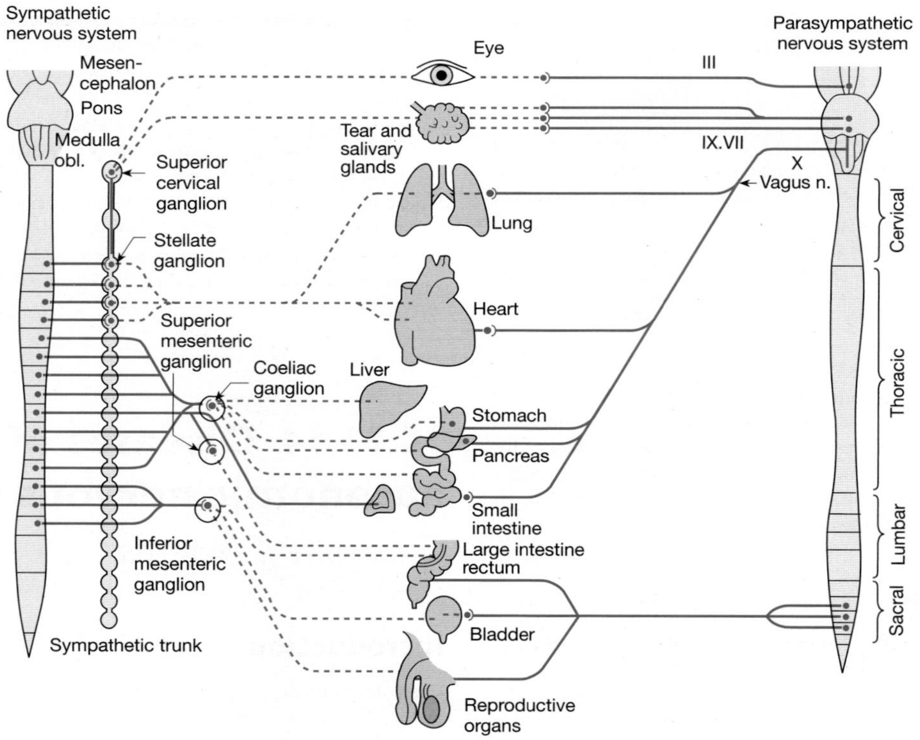

Fig. 1 Sympathetic (thoracolumbar) and parasympathetic (cranial and sacral) pathways that innervate a variety of organs. Janig W (1995). In: Schmidt RF and Thews G, eds. *Physiologie des Menschen*, 25th edn, pp 340–69. Springer Verlag, Heidelberg.

Classification

Diseases of the autonomic nervous system may be primary without a known cause, or secondary with specific abnormalities (dopamine β-hydroxylase deficiency) or strong associations with other diseases (Holmes–Adie syndrome or diabetes mellitus) (Table 1). Drugs are a common cause of autonomic dysfunction (Table 2). Neurally mediated syncope is an intermittent autonomic abnormality. Orthostatic intolerance is listed separately.

Classification may be considered in various ways. Dysfunction may be localized (Table 3) or widespread. Diseases may result from lesions that are central (multiple system atrophy), spinal (spinal cord transection), peripheral (pure autonomic failure), or from a highly specific biochemical deficit (dopamine β-hydroxylase deficiency). Some are age-related, with presentation at birth (Riley–Day syndrome), second decade (vasovagal syncope), or adulthood (familial amyloid polyneuropathy). Autonomic failure commonly causes underactivity, but the reverse, overactivity, causes paroxysmal hypertension during autonomic dysreflexia in high spinal cord injuries. In neurally mediated syncope there is a combination of vagal overactivity and sympathetic withdrawal.

Clinical features

Sympathetic adrenergic failure causes orthostatic hypotension and ejaculatory failure in men, while sympathetic cholinergic failure causes anhidrosis. Parasympathetic failure results in a fixed heart rate, a sluggish urinary bladder and large bowel, and in the male erectile failure. With overactivity there may be hypertension, tachycardia, and hyperhidrosis; while parasympathetic overactivity causes bradycardia. In autonomic disorders there are many clinical manifestations and this may cause diagnostic difficulties, especially when the disorder is generalized.

The presenting complaints often provide clues. Palmar hyperhidrosis or gustatory sweating may indicate a localized disorder, or be a harbinger of widespread autonomic impairment, as the latter may complicate diabetes mellitus. A cardinal feature is orthostatic (postural) hypotension (defined as a decrease in systolic blood pressure of more than 20 mmHg and in diastolic pressure of less than 10 mmHg on standing or head-up tilt, Fig. 3); this impairs perfusion of vital organs, such as the brain. The symptoms vary from fainting (syncope, loss of consciousness) sometimes with ensuing injury, to fatigue and lethargy. Numerous factors in daily life enhance or reduce hypotension (Table 4). Some patients recognize these, with the self-introduction of corrective measures. Large meals, refined carbohydrate, and alcohol, which enhance postprandial hypotension, are avoided. Many sit down, lie flat, or assume curious postures, such as squatting or stooping, that now are recognized to raise blood pressure (Fig. 4). With time, symptoms of orthostatic hypotension wane, for reasons that include improved cerebrovascular autoregulation. In neurally mediated syncope, venepuncture or pain (in vasovagal syncope) or cervical movements and pressure (in carotid sinus hypersensitivity) cause hypotension and bradycardia. A history of impaired sweating and temperature intolerance, urinary disturbances, sexual dysfunction (in men) and gastrointestinal derangement (constipation), especially in combination with orthostatic hypotension, should suggest a generalized autonomic disorder (Table 5).

In the Riley–Day syndrome (familial dysautonomia) there is a history of consanguinity, usually in the Ashkenazi Jewish population. A family history often is elicited in vasovagal syncope, and is expected in familial amyloid polyneuropathy. A drug history including exposure to chemicals, toxins, and poisons is important.

A detailed clinical examination is necessary. Pupillary and associated ocular abnormalites occur in Horner's syndrome. To assess orthostatic hypotension, blood pressure should be measured with the patient lying flat, and after standing (or sitting if not possible). A fall in systolic blood pressure of less than 20 mmHg in the prescence of appropriate symptoms does

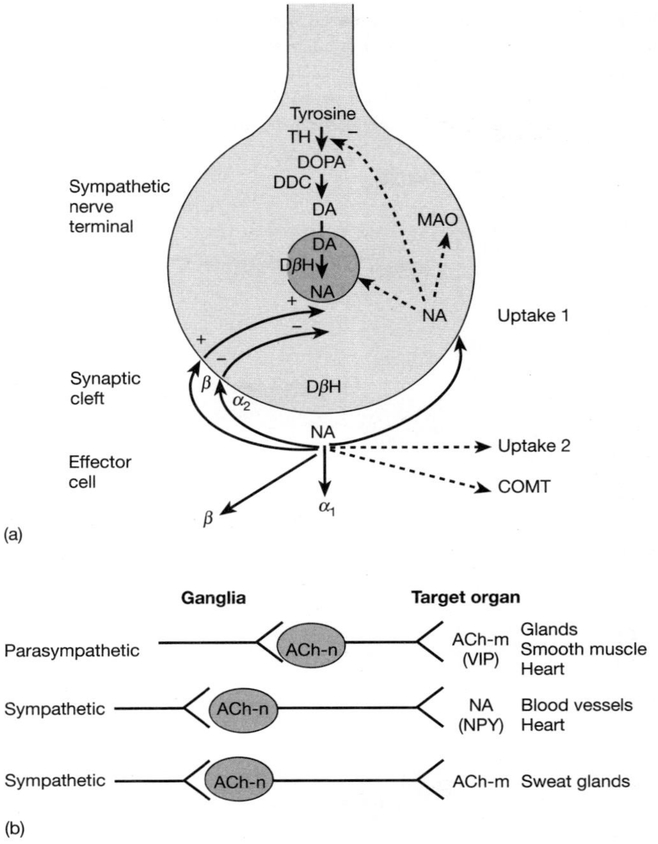

Fig. 2 Schema of some pathways in the formation, release, and metabolism of noradrenaline from sympathetic nerve terminals. Tyrosine is converted into dihydroxyphenylalanine (**DOPA**) by tyrosine hydroxylase (TH). DOPA is converted into dopamine (DA) by dopa decarboxylase (DDC). In the vesicles, dopamine is converted into noradrenaline (NA) by dopamine β-hydroxylase (DβH). Nerve impulses release both dopamine β-hydroxylase and noradrenaline into the synaptic cleft by exocytosis. Noradrenaline acts predominantly on α_1-adrenoceptors but has actions on β-adrenoceptors on the effector cell of target organs. It also has presynaptic adrenoceptor effects. Those acting on α_2-adrenoceptors inhibit noradrenaline release; those on β-adrenoceptors stimulate noradrenaline release. Noradrenaline may be taken up by a neuronal process (uptake 1) into the cytosol, where it may inhibit further formation of DOPA through the rate-limiting enzyme tyrosine hydroxylase. Noradrenaline may be taken into vesicles or metabolized by monoamine oxidase (MAO) in the mitochondria. Noradrenaline may be taken up by a higher-capacity but lower-affinity extraneuronal process (uptake 2) into peripheral tissues, such as vasular and cardiac muscle and certain glands. Noradrenaline is also metabolized by catechol-*O*-methyl transferase (COMT). Thus, noradrenaline measured in plasma is the overspill not affected by these numerous processes. (From: Mathias CJ (2000). Disorders of the autonomic nervous system. In: Bradley WG *et al.*, eds. *Neurology in clinical practice*, 3rd edn, pp 2131–65. Butterworth-Heinemann, Boston.) (b) Outline of the major transmitters at autonomic ganglia and postganglionic sites on target organs supplied by the parasympathetic and sympathetic efferent pathways. The acetylcholine (ACh) receptor at all ganglia is of the nicotinic subtype (ACh-n). Ganglionic blockers such as hexamethonium thus prevent both parasympathetic and sympathetic activation. Atropine, however, acts only on the muscarinic (ACh-m) receptor at postganglionic parasympathetic and sympathetic cholinergic sites. The cotransmitters, along with the primary transmitters, are also indicated—NA, noradrenaline; VIP, vasoactive intestinal peptide; NPY, neuropeptide Y. (From: Mathias CJ (1998). Autonomic disorders. In: Bogousslavsky J, Fisher M, eds. *Textbook of neurology*, pp 519–45. Butterworth-Heinemann, Massachusetts.)

Table 1 Classification of disorders resulting in autonomic dysfunction.

Primary (aetiology unknown)
Acute/subacute dysautonomias:
Pure pandysautonomia
Pandysautonomia with neurological features
Pure cholinergic dysautonomia
Chronic autonomic failure syndromes:
Pure autonomic failure
Multiple system atrophy (Shy–Drager syndrome)
Autonomic failure with Parkinson's disease
Secondary
Congenital:
Nerve growth factor deficiency
Hereditary:
Autosomal dominant trait:
Familial amyloid neuropathy
Porphyria
Autosomal recessive trait:
Familial dysautonomia (Riley–Day syndrome)
Dopamine β-hydroxylase deficiency
Aromatic L-amino acid decarboxylase deficiency
X-linked recessive:
Fabry's disease
Metabolic diseases:
Diabetes mellitus
Chronic renal failure
Chronic liver disease
Vitamin B_{12} deficiency
Alcohol-induced
Inflammatory:
Guillain-Barré syndrome
Transverse myelitis
Infections:
Bacterial—tetanus, leprosy
Viral—human immunodeficiency virus infection
Parasitic—Chagas' disease
Prion—fatal familial insomnia
Neoplasia:
Brain tumours—especially of the third ventricle or posterior fossa
Paraneoplastic, to include adenocarcinomas of lung, pancreas, and Lambert–Eaton syndrome
Connective tissue disorders:
Rheumatoid arthritis
Systemic lupus erythematosus
Mixed connective tissue disease
Surgery:
Regional sympathectomy—upper limbs, splanchnic denervation
Vagotomy and drainage procedures—'dumping syndrome'
Organ transplantation—heart, kidney
Trauma:
Spinal cord transection
Miscellaneous:
Subarachnoid haemorrhage
Syringobulbia and syringomyelia
Neurally mediated syncope
Vasovagal syncope
Carotid sinus hypersensitivity
Micturition syncope
Swallow syncope
Associated with glossopharyngeal neuralgia
Drugs
See Table 2

From Mathias CJ (2000).

Table 2 Drugs, chemicals, poisons, and toxins causing autonomic dysfunction

Decreasing sympathetic activity
Centrally acting:
Clonidine
Methyldopa
Moxonodine
Reserpine
Barbiturates
Anaesthetics
Peripherally acting:
Sympathetic nerve endings (guanethidine, bethanadine)
α-Adrenoceptor blockade (phenoxybenzamine)
β-Adrenoceptor blockade (propranolol)
Increasing sympathetic activity
Amphetamines
Releasing noradrenaline (tyramine)
Uptake blockers (imipramine)
Monoamine oxidase A inhibitors (tranylcypromine)
β-Adrenoceptor stimulants (isoprenaline)
Decreasing parasympathetic activity
Antidepressants (imipramine)
Tranquillizers (phenothiazines)
Antidysrhythmics (disopyramide)
Anticholinergics (atropine, probanthine, benztropine)
Toxins (botulinum)
Increasing parasympathetic activity
Cholinomimetics (carbachol, benthanechol, pilocarpine, mushroom poisoning)
Anticholinesterases
Reversible carbamate inhibitors (pyridostigmine, neostigmine)
Organophosphorus inhibitors (parathion, sarin)
Miscellaneous
Alcohol, thiamine (vitamin B deficiency)
Vincristine, perhexiline maleate
Thallium, arsenic, mercury
Mercury poisoning ('Pink' disease)
Ciguatera toxicity
Jellyfish and marine animal venoms
First dose effects of drugs (prazosin, captopril)
Withdrawal of chronically used drugs (opiates, clonidine, alcohol)

From Mathias CJ (2000).

Table 3 Examples of localized autonomic disorders

Holmes–Adie pupil
Horner's syndrome
Crocodile tears (Bogorad's syndrome)
Gustatory sweating (Frey's syndrome)
Reflex sympathetic dystrophy
Idiopathic palmar/axillary hyperhidrosis
Chagas' disease[a]
Surgical procedures[b]
Sympathectomy—regional
Vagotomy and gastric drainage procedures in 'dumping syndrome'
Organ transplantation—heart, lungs

From Mathias CJ (2000).

[a] Listed here as it targets intrinsic cholinergic plexuses in the heart and gut.

[b] Surgery may cause some of the disorders listed above such as Frey's syndrome following parotid surgery.

not exclude autonomic failure. Indeed, orthostatic hypotension may be unmasked, or enhanced, by factors such as food ingestion and exercise. Furthermore, in the presence of vascular disease (such as carotid artery stenosis) even a small fall in blood pressure results in cerebral ischaemia. Lack of additional neurological features favour pure autonomic failure

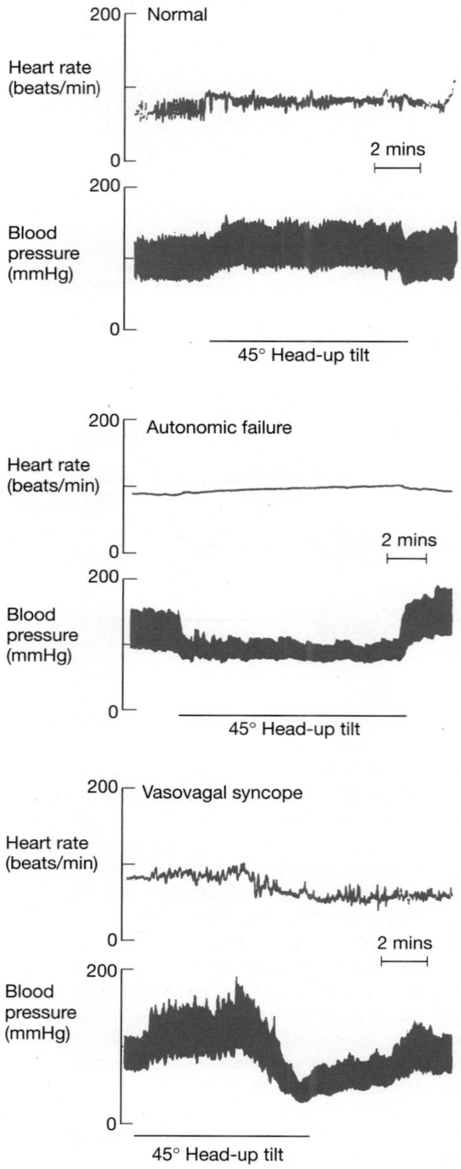

Fig. 3 Blood pressure and heart rate before, during, and after head-up tilt in a normal subject (uppermost panel), a patient with chronic autonomic failure (middle panel), and a patient with vasovagal syncope (lowermost panel). In the normal subject there is no fall in blood pressure during head-up tilt, unlike the patient with autonomic failure in whom blood pressure falls promptly and remains low with a blood pressure overshoot on return to the horizontal. In the patient with autonomic failure there is only a minimal change in heart rate despite the marked blood pressure fall. In the patient with vasovagal syncope there was initially no fall in blood pressure during head-up tilt; in the latter part of tilt, as indicated in the record, blood pressure initially rose and then markedly fell to extremely low levels, necessitating the return of the patient to the horizontal. (From Mathias CJ, Bannister R (1999). Investigation of autonomic disorders. In: Mathias CJ, Bannister R, eds. *Autonomic failure: a textbook of clinical disorders of the autonomic nervous system*, 4th edn, pp 169–95. Oxford University Press, Oxford.)

Table 4 Factors influencing orthostatic hypotension

Speed of positional change
Time of day (worse in the morning)
Prolonged recumbency
Warm environment (hot weather, central heating, hot bath)
Raising intrathoracic pressure—micturition, defaecation, or coughing
Food and alcohol ingestion
Water ingestion[a]
Physical exertion
Manoeuvres and positions (bending forward, abdominal compression, leg crossing, squatting, activating calf muscle pump)[b]
Drugs with vasoactive properties (including dopaminergic agents)

Adapted from Mathias CJ (2000).

[a] Raises supine blood pressure in chronic autonomic failure.

[b] These manoeuvres usually reduce the postural fall in blood pressure, unlike the others.

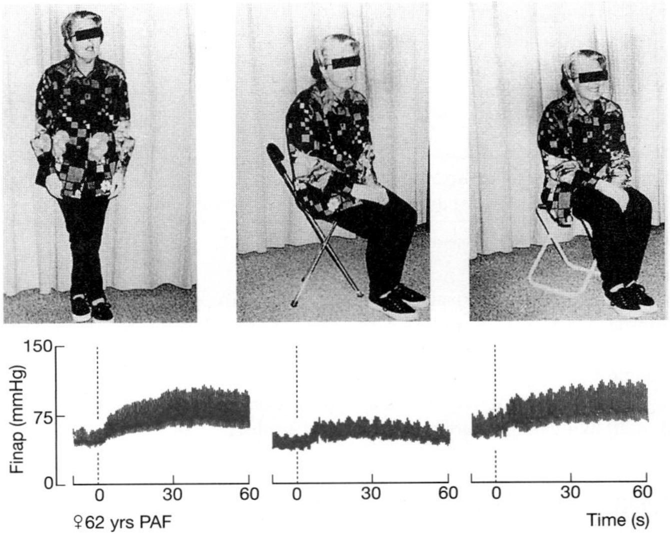

Fig. 4 The effect on finger arterial blood pressure (Finapres) of standing in the crossed-leg position with leg muscle contraction (left), and sitting on a Derby chair (middle), or fishing chair (right) in a patient with orthostatic hypotension. Orthostatic symptoms were present initially when standing and disappeared on crossing legs and sitting on the fishing chair. Sitting on a Derby chair caused the least rise in blood pressure and did not relieve the patient's symptoms completely (From Smith AAJ, Hardjowijono MA, Wieling W (1997). Are portable folding chairs useful to combat orthostatic hypotension? *Annals of Neurology* **42**, 975–8.)

Table 5 Some of the clinical manifestations and possible presentations in primary chronic autonomic failure syndromes[a]

Cardiovascular	Orthostatic hypotension
Sudomotor	Anhidrosis, heat intolerance
Gastrointestinal	Constipation, occasionally diarrhoea, oropharyngeal dysphagia
Renal and urinary bladder	Nocturia, frequency, urgency, incontinence, retention
Sexual	Erectile and ejaculatory failure in the male
Ocular	Aniscoria, Horner's syndrome
Respiratory	Stridor, involuntary inspiratory gasps, apnoeic episodes
Other neurological deficits	Parkinsonian and cerebellar/pyramidal features

[a] Certain features, such as oropharyngeal dysphagia and respiratory abnormalities (including those resulting from laryngeal cord paresis), occur in multiple system atrophy rather than in pure autonomic failure (from Mathias 1997).

(with a good prognosis) while associated parkinsonism or cerebellar dysfunction is suggestive of multiple system atrophy. Several disorders causing a peripheral neuropathy result in autonomic impairment. Basic bedside testing for glycosuria (in diabetes mellitus), or proteinuria (in systemic amyloidosis), provides important information.

Investigation

When an autonomic disorder is suspected, the first step is to determine if autonomic function is normal or abnormal. Autonomic screening tests (Table 6) have their value, but also limitations. The majority are directed towards cardiovascular assessment and to exclude autonomic underactivity. Tests of other systems increasingly are being made available. Normal screening results do not necessarily exclude an autonomic disorder, as on the basis of the history and clinical examination, additional tests such as

Table 6 Investigations in autonomic failure

Cardiovascular

Physiological:
- Head-up tilt, standing; Valsalva manoeuvre
- Pressor stimuli—isometric exercise, cutaneous cold pressor, mental arithmetic
- Heart rate responses—deep breathing, hyperventilation, standing, head-up tilt
- Liquid meal challenge
- Exercise testing
- Carotid sinus massage

Biochemical:
- Basal plasma noradrenaline, adrenaline, and dopamine levels
- Plasma noradrenaline—supine and standing
- Basal urinary catecholamines
- Plasma renin activity
- Plasma aldosterone

Pharmacological:
- Noradrenaline—α-adrenoceptors, vascular
- Isoprenaline—β-adrenoceptors, vascular and cardiac
- Tyramine—pressor and noradrenaline response
- Edrophonium—noradrenaline response
- Clonidine—growth hormone response
- Atropine—heart rate response

Sweating

Thermoregulatory—increase core temperature by 1°C

Sweat gland response to intradermal acetylcholine

Sympathetic skin response

Gastrointestinal

Barium studies, videocinefluoroscopy, endoscopy, gastric-emptying studies, anal sphincter electromyography

Renal function and urinary tract

Day and night urine volumes and sodium/potassium excretion

Urodynamic studies, intravenous urography, ultrasound examination, urethral sphincter electromyography

Sexual function

Penile plethysmography

Intracavernosal papaverine

Respiratory

Laryngoscopy

Sleep studies to assess apnoea/oxygen desaturation

Eye

Lacrimal function—Schirmer's test

Pupillary function—pharmacological and physiological

From Mathias and Bannister 1999.

carotid sinus massage may be needed in patients with syncope. If autonomic tests are abnormal, further evaluation will determine the site and extent of the autonomic lesion, the functional deficit, and whether it results from a primary or secondary disorder, as an accurate diagnosis is essential for prognosis and for appropriate management. Thus, a 24-h ambulatory blood pressure profile and the effects of stimuli in daily life (such as food and exercise) aid management of orthostatic hypotension; while plasma catecholamine measurements (Fig. 5) and the clonidine growth-hormone stimulation test may separate the different primary autonomic failure syndromes. Investigations may be needed to diagnose underlying diseases, and include neuroimaging studies (MRI or CT scanning), sural nerve biopsy (with specific staining with monoclonal antibodies), and genetic testing. These tests should be combined with non-neurological investigations depending on the suspected diagnosis.

Management

This varies depending upon the autonomic disease, the systems affected, the functional autonomic deficit, and whether the disorder is primary or secondary. Treatment should take account of the underlying condition, for example in parkinsonian syndromes, where autonomic features may be worsened by antiparkinsonian therapy. In some diseases simple intervention is effective, such as unblocking a urinary catheter to resolve autonomic dysreflexia in high spinal cord lesions. Complex procedures such as hepatic transplantation are needed to reduce variant transthyretin levels in familial amyloid polyneuropathy. Multidisciplinary expertise may be needed, as in the Riley–Day syndrome and multiple system atrophy, to prevent complications, enhance survival, and improve quality of life. A combined approach is needed to reduce orthostatic hypotension, overcome urinary incontinence, alleviate gastrointestinal disturbances, and treat sexual dysfunction.

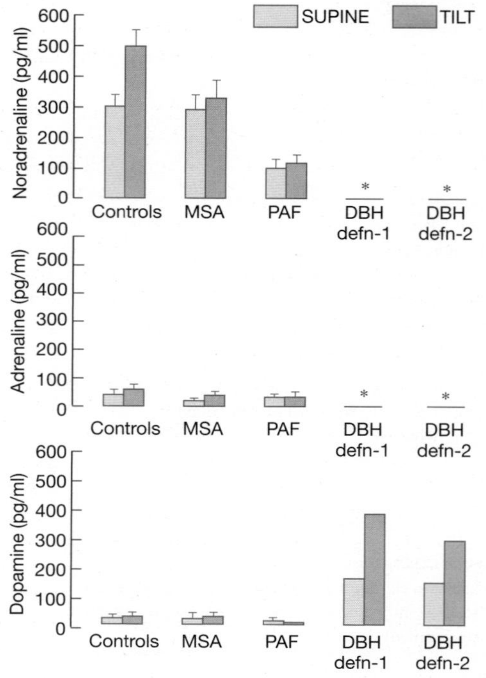

Fig. 5 Plasma noradrenaline, adrenaline, and dopamine concentrations (measured by high-pressure liquid chromatography) in normal subjects (controls), patients with multiple system atrophy (MSA), patients with pure autonomic failure (PAF), and two individual patients with dopamine β-hydroxylase deficiency (DβH defn) while supine and after head-up tilt to 45° for 10 min. The asterisk indicates levels below the detection limits for the assay, which are less than 5 pg/ml for noradrenaline and adrenaline and less than 20 pg/ml for dopamine. Bars indicate ± SEM. (Adapted from Mathias CJ, Bannister R (1999). Investigation of autonomic disorders. In: Mathias CJ, Bannister R, eds. *A textbook of clinical disorders of the autonomic nervous system*, 4th edn, pp. 169–95. Oxford University Press, Oxford.)

Table 7 Outline of non-pharmacological and pharmacological measures in the management of postural hypotension due to neurogenic failure

Non-pharmacological measures
To be avoided:
Sudden head-up postural change (especially on waking)
Prolonged recumbency
Straining during micturition and defaecation
High environmental temperature (including hot baths)
'Severe' exertion
Large meals (especially with refined carbohydrate)
Alcohol
Drugs with vasodepressor properties
To be introduced:
Head-up tilt during sleep
Small, frequent meals
High salt intake
Judicious exercise (including swimming)
Body positions and manoeuvres
To be considered:
Water ingestion
Elastic stockings
Abdominal binders
Pharmacological
Starter drug—fludrocortisone
Sympathomimetics—ephedrine or midodrine
Specific targeting—octreotide, desmopression, or erythropoietin

Adapted from Mathias and Kimber 1998.

The management of orthostatic hypotension is outlined in Tables 7 and 8; in individual disorders modification is needed.

Individual autonomic disorders

Primary autonomic failure

The onset is usually slow and insidious (chronic autonomic failure) unlike the acute–subacute dysautonomias.

Chronic autonomic failure

The most common is multiple system atrophy where there is additional neurological disease, unlike pure autonomic failure. Patients usually are middle aged at presentation although, with increasing awareness, diagnosis is being made in younger patients.

In pure autonomic failure, diagnosis usually is considered because of orthostatic hypotension. Nocturia (rather than incontinence) is frequent, presumably because fluid shifts from the peripheral to the central compartment elevate blood pressure and improve renal perfusion. Constipation often occurs. In temperate climates, hypohidrosis may not be recognized, unlike tropical areas where heat intolerance and collapse may occur. In the male, impotence is common. The clinical and laboratory findings indicate widespread sympathetic failure, usually with parasympathetic deficits. Physiological and biochemical tests, along with limited neuropathological data, indicate a peripheral autonomic lesion. Management is directed predominantly towards reducing orthostatic hypotension. Although recovery does not occur, the overall prognosis in pure autonomic failure is good.

The most common neurodegenerative disease affecting the autonomic nervous system is multiple system atrophy. It is a non-familial and sporadic disorder with autonomic features and additional neurological (parkinsonian, cerebellar, and pyramidal) features (Table 5) that occur at any stage and in any combination, in an unpredictable manner. Thus, patients initially

Table 8 Drugs used in the treatment of orthostatic hypotension

Site of action	Drugs	Predominant action
Plasma volume: expansion	Fludrocortisone	Mineralocorticoid effects—increased plasma volume Sensitization of α-adrenoreceptors
Kidney: reducing diuresis	Desmopressin	Vasopressin$_2$-receptors on renal tubules
Vessels: vasoconstriction (adrenoceptor-mediated)	Ephedrine	Indirectly-acting sympathomimetic
Resistance vessels	Midodrine[a], phenylephrine, methylphenidate	Directly-acting sympathomimetics
	Tyramine	Release of noradrenaline
	Clonidine	Postsynaptic α_2-adrenoceptor agonist
	Yohimibine	Presynaptic α_2-adrenoceptor antagonist
	DL-DOPS and L-DOPS	Prodrug resulting in formation of noradrenaline
Capacitance vessels	Dihydroergotamine	Direct action on α-adrenoceptors
Vessels: vasoconstriction (non-adrenoceptor mediated)	Triglycyl-lysine-vasopressin (glypressin)	Vasopressin$_1$-receptors on blood vessels
Vessels: prevention of vasodilatation	Propranolol	Blockade of β_2-adrenoceptors
	Indomethacin	Prevents prostaglandin synthesis
	Metoclopramide	Blockade of dopamine receptors
Vessels: prevention of post-prandial hypotension	Caffeine	Blockade of adenosine receptors
Heart: stimulation action	Pindolol, xamoterol	Intrinsic sympathomimetic
Red cell mass: increase	Erythropoietin	Stimulates red cell production

From Bannister and Mathias 1999.

[a] Through its active metabolite.

may consult a range of specialists. It is randomly progressive, which adds to the difficulty of diagnosis. It is synonymous with the previously used term, Shy–Drager syndrome.

In multiple system atrophy the additional neurological features are predominantly parkinsonian; in a smaller number they are cerebellar and as the disease advances there is usually a mixture of features (Fig. 6). The neuropathological findings include striatonigral degeneration in multiple system atrophy (parkinsonian) and olivopontocerebellar degeneration in multiple system atrophy (cerebellar), with both changes often seen in either form. There is cell loss in various brainstem nuclei (that include the vagal nuclei), in the intermediolateral cell mass in the thoracic and lumbar spinal cord, and in Onuf's nucleus in the sacral spinal cord that accounts for the various autonomic and allied abnormalities. The paravertebral ganglia and visceral (enteric) plexuses are spared. A specific feature is the presence of intracytoplasmic argyrophyllic oligodendrocyte inclusion bodies, within the brain and spinal cord. Most patients with multiple system atrophy have

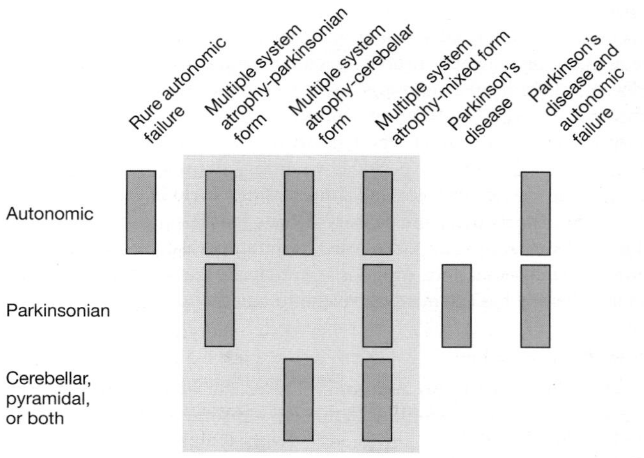

Fig. 6 Schematic representation of the major clinical features of primary chronic autonomic failure syndromes that include the three major neurological forms of multiple system atrophy (adapted from Mathias CJ (1997). Autonomic disorders and their recognition. *New England Journal of Medicine* **310**, 721–4).

parkinsonian features and distinguishing multiple system atrophy from idiopathic Parkinson's disease, especially in the early stages, is difficult. Thus, the true prevalence and incidence of multiple system atrophy is not known. At autopsy up to a quarter of patients previously considered to have Parkinson's disease, have the characteristic neuropathological features of multiple system atrophy.

In multiple system atrophy (parkinsonian), bradykinesia and rigidity is often bilateral, with minimal or no tremor, unlike Parkinson's disease; however, this may not be a useful discriminator in an individual. Lack of a motor response to L-dopa is not indicative of multiple system atrophy, as two-thirds respond initially, although refractoriness and side-effects eventually reduce the benefit. The presence of autonomic failure (especially orthostatic hypotension) and unexplained genitourinary symptoms with sphincter disturbance should alert one to the possibility of multiple system atrophy in patients with parkinsonian or cerebellar signs. Oropharyngeal dysphagia and respiratory abnormalities favour multiple system atrophy, although these often occur later. The combination of cardiovascular autonomic failure and an abnormal urethral/anal sphincter electromyogram, with characteristic clinical features are virtually confirmatory of multiple system atrophy. Additional evaluation includes neuroimaging studies using MRI, positron emission tomography, and proton magnetic resonance spectroscopy of the basal ganglia, which are abnormal, at least in established cases. Clonidine growth-hormone testing, based on α_2-adrenoceptor stimulation of the hypothalamus with release of human growth-hormone releasing factor, distinguishes central from peripheral autonomic failure and separates Parkinson's disease from multiple system atrophy (Fig. 7); whether this is the case in the early stages of parkinsonism and in patients on dopaminergic agents (that are growth hormone secretagogues), remains to be resolved.

The prognosis in multiple system atrophy is poor compared with idiopathic Parkinson's disease and pure autonomic failure. Akinesia and rigidity often worsen, with increasing refractoriness and side-effects (including orthostatic hypotension), to antiparkinsonian therapy. As the disease advances there is often considerable immobility and difficulty in communication. In multiple system atrophy (cerebellar), worsening truncal ataxia causes falls and an inability to stand upright; orthostatic hypotension compounds the disabilities. Incoordination of the upper limbs, speech defects, and nystagmus result in further handicaps.

Respiratory complications include obstructive apnoea (due to laryngeal abductor cord paresis) and central apnoea may necessitate tracheostomy. Oropharyngeal dysphagia enhances the risk of aspiration, especially when vocal cord paresis is present; a percutaneous feeding gastrostomy may be needed. Urinary bladder dysfunction is distressing, and its management, together with that of constipation and, if appropriate, treatment of sexual dysfunction, is important in improving quality of life. There is often a need for specialist therapists, including speech therapists, physiotherapists, dietitians, and occupational therapists. As the neurological decline is inexorable, supportive therapy is crucial in management of multiple system atrophy, and should incorporate the family, carers, and community along with the primary care medical practitioner and therapists.

There is a smaller group of patients with Parkinson's disease, often successfully treated with dopaminergic therapy for many years, who develop severe orthostatic hypotension and other features of autonomic failure. They differ from most patients with Parkinson's disease in whom autonomic dysfunction, if present, is relatively mild and mainly compounded by drug therapy. In Parkinson's disease with autonomic failure, the autonomic lesions appear peripheral (and thus similar to pure autonomic failure)—a conclusion based on low plasma noradrenaline levels and other studies that suggest cardiac sympathetic denervation. Whether in patients with Parkinson's disease complicated by autonomic failure there is a coincidental association of a common condition with an uncommon disease (pure autonomic failure), vulnerability to autonomic degeneration in a subgroup of Parkinson's disease, a link with increasing age, chronic drug therapy, or an inherent metabolic susceptibility—or a combination of these factors—is unknown.

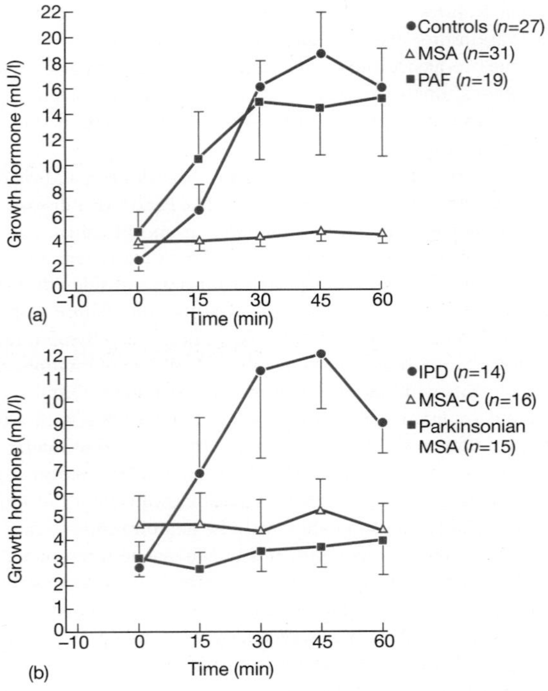

Fig. 7 (a) Serum growth hormone (GH) concentrations before (0) and at 15-min intervals for 60 min after clonidine (2 μg/kg.min) in normal subjects (controls) and in patients with pure autonomic failure (PAF) and multiple system atrophy (MSA). GH concentrations rise in controls and in patients with pure autonomic failure with a peripheral lesion; there is no rise in patients with multiple system atrophy with a central lesion. (From Thomaides T *et al.* (1992). The growth hormone response to clonidine in central and peripheral primary autonomic failure. *Lancet* **340**, 263–6.) (b) Lack of serum GH response to clonidine in multiple system atrophy (the cerebellar form and the parkinsonian form) in contrast to patients with idiopathic Parkinson's disease with no autonomic deficit (IPD), in whom there is a significant rise in GH levels. (From Kimber JR, Watson L, Mathias CJ (1997). Distinction of idiopathic Parkinson's disease from multiple system atrophy by stimulation of growth hormone release with clonidine. *Lancet* **349**, 1877–81.)

Acute/subacute dysautonomias

These disorders are relatively rare and consist of three main varieties: pure pandysautonomia (with features of both sympathetic and parasympathetic failure); pandysautonomia with additional neurological features usually indicative of a peripheral neuropathy; and pure cholinergic dysautonomia. The prognosis in pandysautonomias is variable, with substantial recovery in some. Recovery in two patients following immunoglobulin therapy favours an immunological basis, and the possibility of a Guillain–Barré syndrome variant. In pure cholinergic dysautonomia, described mainly in children and young adults, there is widespread parasympathetic failure with blurred vision, dry eyes, xerostomia, dysphagia with middle and lower oesophagus involvement, severe constipation, and urinary retention. Clinical findings include dilated pupils, an elevated heart rate, dry and warm skin, a distended abdomen, and a palpable urinary bladder. Anhidrosis may result in hyperthermia. The term 'cholinergic' is used because parasympathetic and also cholinergic sympathetic pathways (to sweat glands) are affected. Sympathetic vasoconstrictor function is preserved and orthostatic hypotension does not occur. Recovery is poor, but the prognosis is good if the condition is detected early. Management includes supportive therapy and adequate fluid and nutrient replacement of losses due to gastrointestinal and sudomotor failure. Barium studies should be avoided because contrast medium accumulates in the atonic colon. The differential diagnosis includes exposure to drugs, poisons, and toxins with anticholinergic effects. Similar autonomic features occur in thorn apple (*Datura stramonium*) seed poisoning; the poisoning is associated with hallucinations, hyperreflexia, and clonic jerking movements and recovery occurs in a few days. Botulism B affects cholinergic but spares motor systems and substantial recovery is expected within 3 months of the exposure.

Secondary disorders

Many disorders are associated with autonomic failure; a few are described.

Riley–Day syndrome (familial dysautonomia)

This is a recessive genetic defect characterized by absent lingual fungiform papillae, lack of corneal reflexes, absence of overflow emotional tears, decreased deep tendon reflexes, and a diminished response to pain and temperature; the disease occurs typically in children of Ashkenazi Jewish extraction. An abnormal intradermal histamine skin test (absent axon flare) and pupillary hypersensitivity to cholinomimetics provide diagnostic confirmation. Prenatal diagnosis is possible with the genetic markers linked to chromosome 9 (q31). Autonomic underactivity and overactivity include lability of blood pressure (hypertension and orthostatic hypotension), intermittent hyperhidrosis, periodic vomiting, dysphagia, constipation, and diarrhoea. The neurological abnormalities include emotional and behavioural disturbances, and sensory deficits that result in injury to skin and joints. Skeletal problems (scoliosis), respiratory (aspiration), and renal failure contribute to a poor prognosis. Anticipation of complications and adequate therapy has extended survival into adulthood.

Amyloid neuropathy

Deposition of amyloid into autonomic nerves can occur in reactive systemic amyloidosis (in chronic inflammatory disorders) or in immunoglobulin light chain (AL) amyloidosis (with lymphomas). In familial amyloid polyneuropathy, sensory, motor, and autonomic abnormalities result from deposition in peripheral nerves of mutated variant transthyretin, produced mainly in the liver. Symptoms of a sensory and motor neuropathy often begin in adulthood in the lower limbs in Portuguese, Japanese, and Swedish forms (familial amyloid polyneuropathy I), and in upper limbs in Indian/Swiss and German/Maryland forms (familial amyloid polyneuropathy II). These and other forms are now classified by the chemical and molecular nature of abnormal fibrillary protein, immunologically related to transthyretin. The most common is based on the first point mutations in the transthyretin gene associated with familial amyloid polyneuropathy—methionine 30 is the Portuguese form. The cardiovascular system, gut, and gastrointestinal and urinary systems are affected at variable stages, with the disease progressing relentlessly. Autonomic symptoms and signs may be dissociated, leading to underrecognition of the autonomic deficit. Hepatic transplantation reduces variant transthyretin levels and prevents progression of neuropathy. Its ability to reverse neuropathy is unclear, emphasizing the need for intervention before nerve damage occurs.

Dopamine β-hydroxylase deficiency

This rare disorder (with seven patients reported, two of which are siblings) was recognized in the 1980s. Enzymatic deficiency probably occurs at birth but presentation is often in childhood. Orthostatic hypotension has been the clue to recognition. The clinical features indicate sympathetic adrenergic failure, with sparing of sympathetic cholinergic and parasympathetic function; thus sweating is preserved and urinary bladder and bowel function appear normal. In the male, erection is possible but ejaculation difficult to achieve. Basal levels of plasma noradrenaline and adrenaline are undetectable but dopamine is abnormally elevated. Sympathetic nerve terminals, except for the enzymatic and functional defect, are otherwise intact, as demonstrated by electron microscopy, immunohistochemistry, and sympathetic microneurography. Effective treatment is with the prodrug l-dihydroxyphenylserine, that has a structure similar to noradrenaline and is converted by the enzyme dopa-decarboxylase (abundantly present in extraneuronal tissue such as liver and kidneys) to noradrenaline (Fig. 2(a)).

Diabetes mellitus

In patients with long-standing diabetes, especially those on insulin, there is a high incidence of peripheral and autonomic neuropathy. Vagal denervation occurs earlier, impairing heart rate variability. Reduced sympathetic activity, for example in the feet, may increase blood flow substantially at an early stage before detection of neuropathy. Orthostatic hypotension may be enhanced by insulin. There may be sweating abnormalities (gustatory sweating), delayed stomach emptying (gastroparesis diabeticorum), impaired urinary bladder function (diabetic cystopathy), and impotence. Diarrhoea may be extremely distressing.

Spinal cord injuries

Autonomic dysfunction affecting many systems occurs in spinal injuries, depending upon the lesion level and the degree of completeness. Cardiovascular dysfunction may be life threatening, especially in high lesions, in the acute phase in spinal shock, since lack of sympathetic activity with increased vagal tone may cause bradycardia and cardiac arrest (Fig. 8). After a few weeks, spinal shock passes and isolated spinal reflex activity returns; in cervical and high thoracic lesions, abnormal spinal activation results in the syndrome of autonomic dysreflexia. This is induced by cutaneous, skeletal muscle, or visceral stimuli below the level of the lesion. Thus, severe muscle spasms, an anal fissure, or a blocked urethral catheter can result in paroxysmal hypertension (due to increased spinal sympathetic nerve activity, independent of normal cerebral pathways) with associated bradycardia (because of preserved baroreceptor afferents and vagal efferent pathways (Fig. 9). Patients with lesions below T6 are spared. Patients with high lesions also are prone to orthostatic hypotension which compounds difficulties in management, especially shortly after injury.

Drugs

Dysfunction may result from an autonomic neuropathy (as induced by alcohol, vincristine, and perhexiline maleate) or through pharmacological effects. The latter may be expected with the sympatholytic agents, or may be a minor unexpected effect in susceptible individuals. An example of this is the anticholinergic bladder effects of disopyramide, which may cause urinary retention in patients with prostatic hyperplasia. A variety of toxins and poisons, including mushroom toxicity and botulism, as well as nerve gases such as sarin, affect the autonomic nervous system. The first-dose effect of ACE-inhibitors and prazosin may be mediated by the Jarisch–Bezold reflex. Autonomic overactivity occurs during withdrawal of clonidine, alcohol, and opiates.

Neurally mediated syncope

This is an intermittent abnormality with increased cardiac parasympathetic (causing severe bradycardia, cardio-inhibition) and sympathetic withdrawal (causing hypotension vasodepression) that results in fainting. The episodes may be cardio-inhibitory, vasodepressor, or mixed (Fig. 10(a and

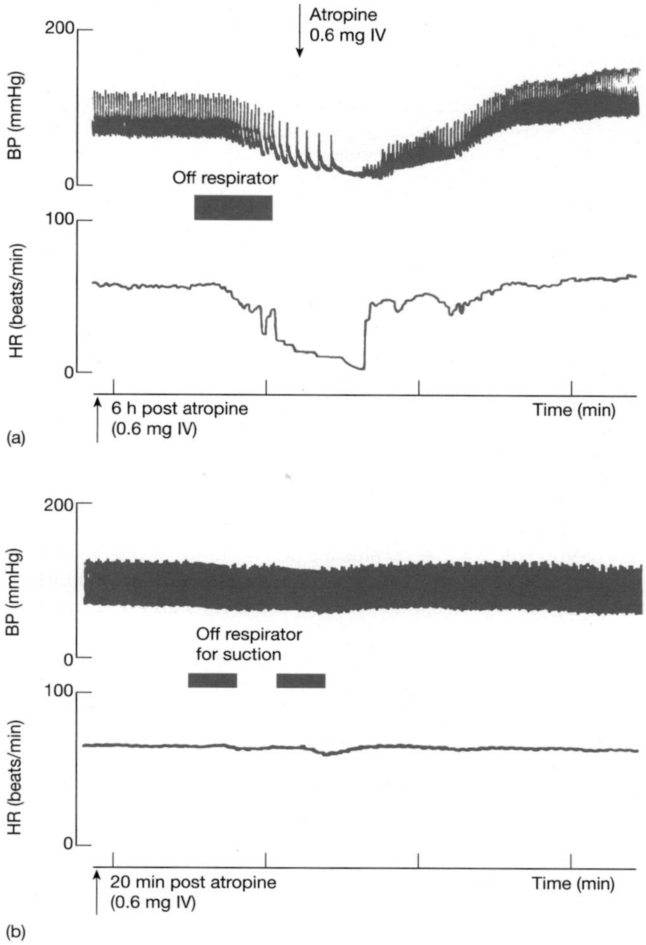

Fig. 8 (a) The effect of disconnecting the respirator (as required for aspirating the airways) on the blood pressure (BP) and heart rate (HR) of a recently injured tetraplegic patient (C4/5 lesion) in spinal shock, 6 h after the last dose of intravenous atropine. Sinus bradycardia and cardiac arrest (also observed on the electrocardiograph) were reversed by reconnection, intravenous atropine, and external cardiac massage. (From Frankel HL, Mathias CJ, Spalding JMK (1975). Mechanisms of reflex cardiac arrest in tetraplegic patients. *Lancet* **ii**, 1183–5.) (b) The effect of tracheal suction 20 min after atropine. Disconnection from the respirator and tracheal suction did not lower either heart rate or blood pressure (From Mathias CJ (1976). Bradycardia and cardiac arrest during tracheal suction—mechanisms in tetraplegic patients. *European Journal of Intensive Care Medicine* **2**, 147–56.)

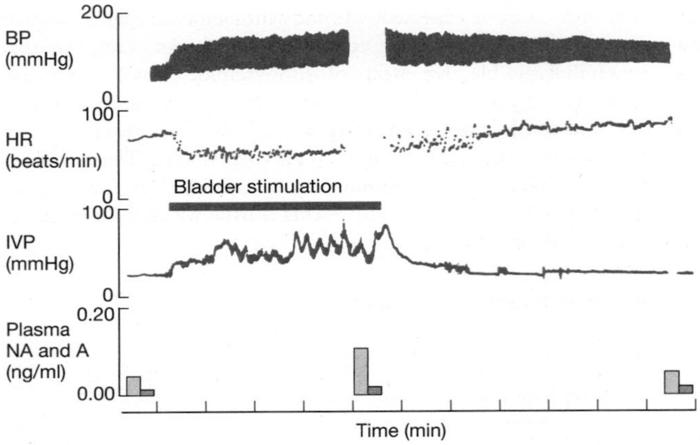

Fig. 9 Blood pressure (BP), heart rate (HR), intravesical pressure (IVP), and plasma noradrenaline (NA) and adrenaline (A) concentrations in a tetraplegic patient before, during, and after bladder stimulation induced by suprapubic percussion of the anterior abdominal wall. The rise in BP is accompanied by a fall in heart rate as a result of increased vagal activity in response to the rise in blood pressure. The level of plasma noradrenaline (open histograms), but not adrenaline (filled histograms), rises suggesting an increase in sympathetic neural activity independently of adrenomedullary activation. (From Mathias CJ, Frankel HL (1986). The neurological and hormonal control of blood vessels and heart in spinal man. *Journal of the Autonomic Nervous System* **Suppl.**, 457–64.)

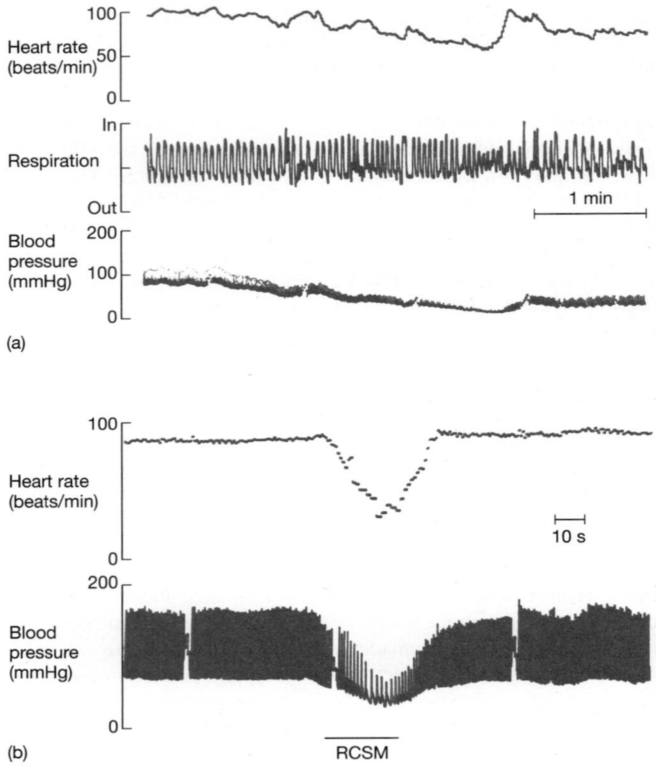

Fig. 10 (a) Blood pressure changes towards the end of a period of head-up tilt in a patient with recurrent episodes of vasovagal syncope. Blood pressure that was previously maintained begins to fall. There is also a reduction in heart rate. Initially there are relatively minor changes in respiratory rate. The patient was about to faint and was replaced to the horizontal (indicated by elevated time signal below) and then to 5° head-down tilt. Blood pressure and heart rate recover but still remain lower than previously. This patient had no other autonomic abnormalities on detailed autonomic testing. Blood pressure was measured non-invasively by the Finapres. (From Mathias CJ, Bannister R (1999). Investigation of autonomic disorders. In: Mathias CJ, Bannister R, eds. *Autonomic failure: a textbook of clinical disorders of the autonomic nervous system*, 4th edn, pp 169–95. Oxford University Press, Oxford.) (b) Heart rate and blood pressure before, during, and after right carotid sinus massage (RCSM) in a patient with syncopal episodes. There is a fall in heart rate and blood pressure during carotid sinus massage, typical of the mixed (cardio-inhibitory and vasodepressor) form of this disorder. The breaks in the record indicate interval calibration by the Finapres machine. (From Mathias CJ (2000). Autonomic dysfunction. In: Grimley-Evans J *et al.*, eds. *Oxford textbook of geriatric medicine*, 2nd edn, pp 833–52. Oxford University Press, Oxford.)

b)). Between episodes, screening autonomic tests usually reveal no abnormalities. In the young, a common cause is vasovagal syncope. This is often familial and more likely in females; it often presents in the early teenage years and is induced by stimuli such as fear, sight of blood, and venepuncture, and at times even discussion of venepuncture. Hypotension is more likely in the upright position and may occur whilst standing still, especially in warm weather when salt and fluid depletion occurs. Testing includes prolonged head-up tilt, or a provocative stimulus such as venepuncture during head-up tilt. A variety of physiological (head-up tilt plus lower body negative pressure) or pharmacological (isoprenaline infusions) stimuli have been used to unmask an episode. Cardiac conduction disorders and other causes of syncope (such as neurological or metabolic) should be excluded. Treatment includes reducing or preventing exposure to precipitating causes and behavioural psychotherapy in patients with phobias. Added salt, fluid repletion, and exercise are often useful. Drugs such as fludrocortisone, vasopressor agents, and antidepressants such as the serotonin-uptake release inhibitors have been used. The long-term prognosis is favourable.

In the elderly, carotid sinus hypersensitivity is increasingly recognized, especially in those with falls of otherwise unknown cause. A classic history of syncope induced by head movements or collar tightening may be provided, although in many the precipitating factors are unclear. Carotid sinus massage should be performed in the laboratory with requisite precautions, ideally using continuous blood pressure and heart rate recordings, with the subject also tilted head-up, because hypotension is more likely to occur when sympathetic activation is needed. Treatment, especially of the cardio-inhibitory forms, includes a cardiac demand pacemaker; vasodepressor forms may require pressor agents. Surgical denervation of the carotid sinus has been used successfully, especially where unilateral hypersensitivity occurs.

A variety of other stimuli, acting through short-lived autonomic mechanisms, also can cause syncope. This may be in conjunction with factors such as heat or drugs that cause vasodilatation or reduce intravascular volume, thus increasing the tendency to hypotension and syncope. Examples include syncope associated with glossopharyngeal neuralgia (caused by swallowing), or induced by micturition, defaecation, coughing, laughing, and playing wind instruments.

Orthostatic intolerance without hypotension

This disorder is increasingly recognized, mainly in women below the age of 50 years. Dizziness on postural change or with modest exertion occurs usually without syncope. The symptoms appear to disrupt their lives, almost disproportionately. There is a substantial rise in heart rate (over 30 beats/min or to 120 beats/min) without orthostatic hypotension, hence the term postural (orthostatic) tachycardia syndrome. Associated features may include those of a partial autonomic neuropathy, chronic fatigue syndrome, mitral valve prolapse, and hyperventilation. It is unclear whether other factors such as vestibular dysfunction contribute. The relationship of this syndrome to previously described psychosomatic disorders such as Soldier's heart (da Costa's syndrome) is not known. Treatment includes salt and fluid repletion, exercise, and β-adrenergic blockers. Many recover within a year.

Further reading

Appenzeller 0, Oribe E (eds) (1997). *The autonomic nervous system*, 5th edn. Elsevier Biomedical, Amsterdam.

Low PA. (ed.) (1997). *Clinical autonomic disorders*, 2nd edn. Little Brown & Company, Boston.

Mathias CJ (2000). Disorders of the autonomic nervous system. In: Bradley WG, Daroff RB, Fenichel GM, Marsden CD, eds. *Neurology in clinical practice*, 3rd edn, pp. 2131–65. Butterworth-Heinemann, Boston.

Mathias CJ, Bannister R (1999). *Autonomic failure: a textbook of clinical disorders of the autonomic nervous system*, 4th edn. Oxford University Press, Oxford.

Mathias CJ, Kimber JR (1999). Postural hypotension —causes, clinical features, investigation and management. *Annual Review of Medicine* **50**, 317–36.

Mathias CJ, Deguchi K, Schatz I (2001). Observations on recurrent syncope and presyncope in 641 patients. *Lancet* **357**, 348–53.

24.13.15 Disorders of cranial nerves

P. K. Thomas

The olfactory nerve

Loss of the sense of smell (anosmia) is most commonly encountered as a sequel to head injury and is probably related to severance of the central processes of the neurones of the olfactory mucosa as they pass through the cribriform plate to the olfactory bulb. It is usually permanent. Distortion of olfaction (parosmia) may occur and may be persistent. The sense of smell is occasionally congenitally absent or may be acutely and permanently lost after a coryzal infection. Bilateral anosmia is frequently accompanied by impairment of taste related to reduced detection of the volatile substances that impart flavours to foods. Unilateral anosmia may occur in olfactory groove meningiomas or other subfrontal tumours. This is usually not detected by the patient.

The central connections of the olfactory pathways are complex and include projections to the temporal lobes, hypothalamus, the septal region, and the amygdaloid nuclei. Olfactory hallucinations are well known to occur as a manifestation of temporal lobe epilepsy. Identification of odours may be impaired after bilateral medial temporal lesions and may be defective in multiple sclerosis, possibly as the result of demyelination in the olfactory tracts. Complaints of hypersensitivity of the sense of smell commonly have a psychoneurotic basis and persistent olfactory hallucinations may be reported by psychotic patients. Persistent parosmia is sometimes produced by lesions of the temporal lobe.

Third, fourth, and sixth cranial nerves

The third, or oculomotor, nerve supplies all the external ocular muscles with the exception of the superior oblique and lateral rectus. It also carries the parasympathetic innervation of the preganglionic pupilloconstrictor fibres of the iris. A complete third nerve lesion produces a dilated and unreactive pupil, complete ptosis, and loss of upward, downward, and medial movement of the eye. The eye becomes deviated downwards and laterally. Diplopia is only experienced when the lid is held up.

The fourth or trochlear nerve supplies the superior oblique muscle. Following a lesion of this nerve, there is extorsion of the eye when the patient looks outwards. When the patient looks downwards and medially, diplopia is experienced. This is particularly disturbing because of its occurrence on looking downwards and produces difficulty in walking and in descending stairs. The patient may compensate for this by tilting the head to the opposite side.

The sixth or abducens nerve supplies the lateral rectus. A lesion of this nerve causes convergent strabismus, inability to abduct the affected eye, and diplopia which is maximal on lateral gaze to the affected side.

The third, fourth, and sixth nerves may be affected singly or in combination, and the paralysis may be complete or partial. In some instances, the lesion is within the brainstem, where it may affect either the nuclei or intramedullary portion of the nerve fibres. In older patients, the commonest causes are vascular disease and neoplasms of the brainstem.

Extramedullary lesions of the third, fourth, and sixth nerves are more frequent and may occur at any point along their course, either intracranially or within the orbit. A third nerve palsy may develop in the region of the tentorial hiatus as a false localizing sign related to displacement of the brainstem produced by supratentorial space-occupying conditions. Unilateral or bilateral sixth nerve palsies may also arise as a consequence of raised intracranial pressure, probably caused by traction, again secondary to brainstem displacement. These nerves can be involved singly or together in conditions such as chronic basal meningitis or carcinomas of the skull base. Gradenigo's syndrome comprises a sixth nerve palsy and pain of trigeminal distribution. It is produced by a lesion at the apex of the petrous temporal bone. As this syndrome was most commonly infective in origin and related to chronic middle ear disease, it is now encountered considerably less frequently.

The third, fourth, and sixth nerves traverse the cavernous sinus, as do the first and second divisions of the trigeminal nerve. In this situation, they are most commonly damaged by an intracavernous aneurysm of the internal carotid artery. The third nerve is affected more often than the fourth and sixth. The consequent internal and external ophthalmoplegia is frequently accompanied by pain, and sometimes sensory loss and paraesthesiae, in the corresponding frontal region related to compression of the first division of the trigeminal nerve, and occasionally in the cheek from damage to the maxillary division. In the superior orbital fissure syndrome, caused for example by a tumour invading the fissure, a total ophthalmoplegia may result, associated with pain and sensory loss in the distribution of the first division of the trigeminal nerve. The eye is often proptosed because of obstruction of the ophthalmic vein. The Tolosa–Hunt syndrome consists of a painful external ophthalmoplegia related to a granulomatous angiitis. Within the orbit, the third, fourth, and sixth nerves may be affected by conditions such as tumours and granulomas. They may be damaged as a result of trauma at any point along their course and may be affected singly or in combination or as part of a cranial neuropathy, of which diabetes, the Miller–Fisher syndrome, Lyme borreliosis, and sarcoidosis are the most important examples. Internal and external ophthalmoplegias are common and this list of causes is by no means exhaustive.

Pupillary abnormalities

Constriction of the pupil (miosis) occurs as a result of paralysis of the sympathetic innervation of the pupillodilator fibres of the iris and may be accompanied by the other features of Horner's syndrome, namely mild ptosis and vasodilatation and anhidrosis of the face on the same side. The ocular manifestations may be encountered alone if the damage is restricted to the intracranial portion of the sympathetic plexus around the carotid artery. Raeder's syndrome consists of these components of Horner's syndrome together with involvement of the first division of the trigeminal nerve. It may be caused by tumours of the skull base. Miosis may also be produced by the local action of cholinergic drugs and by morphine and related compounds.

Pupillary dilatation may be caused by lesions of the third nerve, although it is of interest that the isolated third nerve palsies of presumed vascular origin that may occur in diabetes mellitus, in contradistinction to compressive lesions of the nerve, characteristically spare the pupil. Anticholinergic drugs such as atropine and related substances give rise to pupillary dilatation, as does cocaine.

The Argyll–Robertson pupil is small, fails to react to light, but constricts on ocular convergence, and, if bilateral, the pupils are frequently unequal in size (anisocoria). The pupil may be irregular in outline and it does not dilate fully in response to mydriatics. Argyll–Robertson pupils are almost always related to neurosyphilis but somewhat similar pupils are occasionally encountered in diabetic neuropathy and in some hereditary neuropathies.

The myotonic pupil (Holmes–Adie syndrome) reacts abnormally slowly both to light and on convergence, but particularly so for the response to illumination. A very bright light may be required to demonstrate any pupillary constriction, or if the patient remains in a dark room for some minutes, the pupil slowly dilates. The condition may be unilateral or bilateral and is commoner in women than men. Myotonic pupils may be associated with absence or depression of the tendon reflexes and occasionally with anhidrosis in the limbs.

Trigeminal nerve

The fifth cranial nerve is predominantly sensory in function, but also innervates the muscles of mastication. It emerges from the pons and runs forwards to the Gasserian ganglion which is situated in Meckel's cave near the apex of the petrous temporal bone. The three sensory divisions of the nerve run anteriorly from the ganglion. The first or frontal division passes through the cavernous sinus and the superior orbital fissure. Its branches supply sensation to the anterior part of the scalp, the forehead, and the eye, including the conjunctiva and cornea. The second or maxillary division leaves the skull through the foramen rotundum, traverses the infraorbital canal, and supplies the cheek. The mandibular division emerges from the skull through the foramen ovale to reach the infratemporal fossa with the motor root with which it unites to form a single trunk. It is distributed to the lower lip, chin, and the lower part of the cheek, and its auriculotemporal branch supplies part of the ear and temporal area. It also supplies the inner aspect of the cheek and the anterior two-thirds of the tongue, and its lingual branch carries taste fibres from the anterior two-thirds of the tongue which leave it in the chorda tympani to join the facial nerve. It is important that the skin over the angle of the jaw is supplied from the second cervical nerve root, and the absence of this 'trigeminal notch' may be useful in distinguishing hysterical or feigned loss of sensation on the face which usually follows the angle of the jaw. The motor root innervates temporalis, masseter, pterygoids, mylohyoid, the anterior belly of the digastric, and also tensor tympani and tensor palati muscles. With unilateral paralysis of the masticatory muscles, the jaw deviates towards the affected side on opening because of the action of the unopposed external pterygoid on the unaffected side.

The trigeminal nerve may be affected by intramedullary lesions, it may be damaged during the intracranial part of its course, or its branches may be compromised extracranially. An acoustic neurinoma may compress the nerve in the posterior fossa or the nucleus of the descending root may be affected by direct compression of the brainstem by this tumour. Loss of corneal sensation is usually the earliest feature. Reference has already been made to involvement of the nerve in association with damage to the sixth nerve at the apex of the petrous temporal bone (Gradenigo's syndrome), as has involvement of the first and second divisions in the cavernous sinus, or the first division in the superior orbital fissure.

Trigeminal neuralgia

Symptoms

This condition is characterized by paroxysms of intense pain strictly confined to the distribution of the trigeminal nerve. In most cases the cause is unknown. It is generally encountered in individuals over the age of 50 years. In younger patients it may be due to multiple sclerosis. Rarely, compression of the nerve, for example by tumours in the cerebellopontine angle, is responsible.

The salient feature of the disorder is pain which is usually unilateral and is felt either within the territory of one division of the nerve only, or may involve two adjacent divisions or affect the whole territory of the nerve. Less commonly it is bilateral.

The pain occurs in brief searing paroxysms, each attack lasting only a matter of seconds. The pain is often described as piercing or knife-like. Its intense quality may cause the patient to screw up their face in agony, hence the use of the term 'tic doloureux' to describe the condition. The paroxysms may be spontaneous or provoked by movements of the face and jaw, by touching the skin, or by draughts of cold air on the face. Eating and speaking may become extremely difficult. 'Trigger spots' on the skin of the face may be present, the touching of which provokes the paroxysms. The attacks may be followed by less severe pain of a dull, boring character and by tenderness of the skin in the affected area. Fortunately the attacks usually cease at night.

The quality of the pain is characteristic, and when trigeminal neuralgia is present, the diagnosis is not usually missed, especially if a paroxysm is witnessed. The usual mistake is to regard as trigeminal neuralgia pain that is due to some other cause, and since there are many conditions that give rise to facial pain, the opportunities for error are numerous. Pain that is of a continuous character is not trigeminal neuralgia and some other cause must be sought. Absence of provocation by eating, talking, or the touching of trigger spots also makes the diagnosis unlikely. Once the diagnosis is accepted, it is essential to exclude compressive lesions affecting the nerve.

In the early stages, remissions lasting for months or years are usual, but in older patients remissions, if they occur, are likely to be brief. In all cases the remissions tend to become shorter as time goes on, and without treatment the condition persists for the rest of the patient's life.

The distribution of the pain is usually in one or two divisions of the nerve. The first division is rarely affected primarily, but pain may spread into it from the second division. If the pain begins in the second division it may, after a time, affect the third, and vice versa.

Treatment

The introduction of carbamazepine revolutionized treatment of this distressing condition. In a high proportion of cases, the paroxysms can be abolished or reduced. A dosage of 200 mg three to five times per day is employed. Ataxia and drowsiness may be troublesome side-effects with higher dosages, and aggravation of ataxia even with modest dosages may impede treatment in cases of multiple sclerosis. Hypersensitivity reactions producing skin rashes or, rarely, bone marrow depression may develop but are, fortunately, uncommon.

If carbamazepine is not successful, or if the patients fail to tolerate it, other drugs such as phenytoin or clonazepam can be tried, but they are rarely effective. In this event, thermocoagulation of the ganglion may have to be considered. This should be undertaken only if the disorder is established so that a prolonged natural remission is unlikely to occur. It should also not be undertaken unless the patient is completely unable to tolerate the disorder, despite analgesics and sedation, and if they are fully aware of the consequences. The persistent analgesia and sometimes dysaesthesiae may subsequently be troublesome, and when the first division is made anaesthetic, damage to the conjunctiva leading to corneal scarring has to be avoided. It may be possible to limit the anaesthesia to the affected area, sparing, for instance, the eye if the first division is not involved by the pain. If thermocoagulation fails, section of the sensory root by a posterior fossa approach employing a microsurgical technique is indicated.

Ophthalmic herpes zoster

In elderly individuals, the fifth nerve is prone to involvement in herpes zoster, the first division being most vulnerable, giving rise to the distressing condition of ophthalmic herpes. The clinical features and treatment of herpes zoster are considered elsewhere (see Section 7). An unfortunate sequel may be visual impairment from residual corneal scarring. Particularly in older subjects, post-herpetic neuralgia may also be a sequel. This gives rise to persistent and unremitting spontaneous pain associated with cutaneous hyperaesthesia in the affected area. Treatment is difficult. Analgesics, sedation, and antidepressive preparations to combat the secondary depression that is frequently present may be of some assistance.

Isolated trigeminal neuropathy

Rarely, a chronic isolated unilateral or bilateral affection of the trigeminal nerve may occur as a manifestation of Sjögren's sicca syndrome, or progressive systemic sclerosis or amyloidosis, although most cases are idiopathic. Extensive nasal scarring and tissue loss may occur secondary to repeated injury from picking and scratching.

Facial nerve

The seventh cranial nerve is largely motor. The nerve traverses the facial canal in the petrous temporal bone in close relationship to the middle ear and emerges at the stylomastoid foramen. Its branches pass forward through the parotid gland to be distributed to the muscles of the face, including the platysma. Within the petrous bone, a branch is given to the stapedius muscle. The chorda tympani, carrying the taste fibres from the anterior two-thirds of the tongue, joins the nerve within the facial canal and a small branch supplies cutaneous sensation to the region of the external auditory meatus. The nerve also carries preganglionic parasympathetic fibres destined for the lachrymal gland.

The distinction between upper and lower motor neurone lesions of the facial muscles is usually easy. In general, with upper motor neurone lesions there is a relative preservation of power in the upper facial muscles, because these have a bilateral innervation from the cerebral hemispheres. There is no loss of tone with upper motor neurone lesions, so that the sagging of the face that is an unsightly feature of lower motor neurone palsy does not occur.

In common with the trigeminal nerve, the facial nerve may be affected by tumours in the cerebellopontine angle. In the past, it was often involved in middle ear infections. It may be involved in meningeal carcinomatosis, fractures, and tumours of the skull base, in a variety of cranial neuropathies, and cephalic herpes zoster, but the most common lesion by far is Bell's palsy. More peripherally, the nerve may be implicated in tumours of the parotid gland.

Bell's palsy

This term describes a usually unilateral facial paralysis of relatively rapid onset related to a lesion of the nerve within the facial canal. Taste may also be affected. It may develop at any age, most commonly between 20 and 50 years, and affects both sexes equally. Its causation is unknown. In the acute stage, the nerve is swollen and compression within the facial canal may contribute to the damage to the nerve fibres.

The onset is rapid and is frequently heralded or accompanied by aching pain below the ear or in the mastoid region. This clears within a few days and is not present in every case. The paralysis usually reaches its maximum severity after 1 or 2 days but occasionally progresses over the course of several days. Complete paralysis may occur. In the lower face, this may cause a mild dysarthria and some difficulty in eating because of food collecting between the gums and the inner sides of the cheek and the escape of fluid when drinking. The face sags and on smiling is drawn across to the unaffected side. Paralysis of orbicularis oculi renders voluntary eye closure impossible and, particularly in the older subject, ectropion develops. This can result in conjunctival injury from foreign bodies or conjunctivitis. If the paralysis is partial, the lower face is usually affected to a greater extent than the upper.

In the more severe cases, loss of taste over the anterior two-thirds of the tongue is often present, and paralysis of the stapedius muscle may result in a lack of tolerance for high-pitched or loud sounds.

Bell's palsy has to be distinguished from selective lesions of the facial nerve within the brainstem, in which instance taste will not be affected. A facial paralysis superficially resembling Bell's palsy may occur in multiple sclerosis, in which event evidence of more widespread neurological disease may well be detected on examination, or the history may indicate episodes of neurological disturbance in the past. With respect to peripheral lesions, middle ear disease requires exclusion. Facial paralysis related to cephalic herpes zoster is discussed above. A lesion of the facial nerve may represent a mononeuropathy from some generalized disorder of which diabetes, Lyme borreliosis, and sarcoidosis are the most important. Bell's palsy is rarely bilateral and the occurrence of bilateral facial paralysis would raise the possibility of Guillain–Barré syndrome. This may begin with facial weakness, or the weakness may remain restricted to the facial musculature. The occurrence of bilateral facial weakness would also raise the possibility of sarcoidosis.

In approximately 85 per cent of cases of Bell's palsy, the paralysis is the result of a local conduction block within the facial canal without axonal degeneration and this is effectively the situation in all instances of mild weakness. The conduction block is presumably the consequence of segmental demyelination. Providing that such cases do not progress to more severe weakness, all recover fully within a few weeks. In cases where there is total paralysis, a proportion of these will be the result of a conduction block, but in about 15 per cent axonal degeneration will have occurred. Those with a conduction block will again recover satisfactorily within a few weeks. In patients with a degenerative lesion, recovery has to take place by axonal regeneration. Evidence of reinnervation does not appear in under 3 months and the ultimate recovery is often incomplete or may fail to occur altogether. Synkinesis is frequent after reinnervation so that blinking, for example, results in a simultaneous contraction of the angle of the mouth. Aberrant parasympathetic reinnervation may also occur, leading for instance to gustatory lachrymation ('crocodile tears').

Axons remain excitable distal to the lesion for 3 or 4 days after interruption. It is therefore not possible to be certain from electrodiagnostic tests whether axonal degeneration has taken place until after this time. At that stage, electrical stimulation of the facial nerve at the stylomastoid foramen with brief pulses will still elicit a muscle contraction if the paralysis is due to conduction block, whereas none will be obtained if axonal degeneration has taken place.

In the early stages, the main endeavour of treatment should be to prevent either a partial lesion, or complete paralysis related to a conduction block, progressing to a degenerative lesion. There is some evidence that corticosteroids may be advantageous by reducing oedema in the nerve. Thus it is justifiable to treat all cases with corticosteroids if seen within a few days of onset, providing no contraindication to such treatment exists. A course of a week's duration with an initially high dosage is recommended.

Surgical decompression of the nerve has been advised. To be effective, this would have to be performed at the outset, which is not justifiable as 85 per cent of cases will recover satisfactorily without treatment. So far there are no means of predicting which cases will progress to a degenerative lesion. If this were available, decompression could be undertaken selectively in such cases.

It is helpful to perform electrodiagnostic studies at about 1 week after the onset. If this reveals a degenerative lesion, it is then known that recovery will be delayed. A prosthesis attached to the teeth to elevate the angle of the mouth to reduce facial deformity may be helpful. In patients with severe ectropion, a lateral tarsorrhaphy to protect the eye may be required. Electrical stimulation of the paralysed facial muscles has no effect on the ultimate prognosis.

In those cases in which regeneration fails to occur, operation may be desirable for cosmetic reasons to counteract the facial deformity. The angle of the mouth may be elevated by a fascial sling attached to the temporalis fascia, but the result is never highly satisfactory. Restoration of facial tone may be achieved by anastomosis of the hypoglossal nerve to the facial, but at the expense of denervation of the tongue on that side. Any operation should not be contemplated before an adequate length of time has been allowed for regeneration. This should be of the order of 9 months.

Facial paralysis related to 'geniculate' herpes zoster (Ramsay–Hunt syndrome)

Facial paralysis of rapid onset accompanied by severe pain in and around the external auditory meatus and in the throat may accompany 'cephalic zoster'. Vesicles may be detectable in the ear and ulceration in the fauces, or anywhere on the head. Occasionally there is concomitant vertigo, tinnitus, and some deafness with involvement of the eighth nerve ('otic herpes zoster'). Prognosis for recovery of the facial paralysis is stated to be less good than in Bell's palsy.

Hemifacial spasm

This consists of a unilateral disturbance affecting the facial muscles, producing irregular clonic or twitching movements of the facial muscles, usually of insidious onset. It most commonly occurs in middle-aged women. There may be a mild degree of facial weakness, but severe paralysis does not occur. Usually no underlying cause is demonstrable. The condition selectively affects the facial nerve, within the brainstem or in the posterior fossa.

It begins with intermittent twitching of the facial muscles such as around the eye or at the angle of the mouth. These movements gradually become more frequent and extend to involve the rest of the facial muscles, often gradually advancing over the course of some years. If they become severe, the face is contorted by irregular clonic spasms which may keep the eye closed for prolonged periods. The facial distortion is often a considerable embarrassment to the patient, who finds that the spasms tend to be aggravated by emotional stress.

The condition must be distinguished from benign fasciculation of the face, which usually occurs around the eyes, related to fatigue or emotional tension, and from the myokymic twitching that is occasionally encountered as a manifestation of multiple sclerosis. The latter consists of a persisting irregular rippling movement of the facial muscles that usually subsides after a week or two. These conditions can be distinguished by electromyography (see Chapter 24.2.5).

No satisfactory treatment is available. If exaggeration by emotional factors is evident, the administration of diazepam or a similar preparation may produce a marginal improvement. In severe cases, injections of botulinum toxin may be helpful, although these have to be repeated. Neurosurgical intervention to relieve compression of the nerve by aberrant vessels in its intracranial course has been advocated and may be helpful in selected cases.

Glossopharyngeal nerve

The ninth cranial nerve leaves the skull through the jugular foramen, closely related to the tenth nerve. It supplies the stylopharyngeus muscle and the constrictor muscles of the pharynx. Parasympathetic fibres are supplied to the parotid gland. Sensory fibres are carried from the posterior third of the tongue, the ear, the fauces, and the nasopharynx, and chemoreceptor and baroreceptor afferents from the carotid sinus.

The glossopharyngeal nerve is rarely affected in isolation. Lesions usually occur in conjunction with involvement of the vagus and give rise to some dysphagia, impaired pharyngeal sensation, and loss of taste over the posterior third of the tongue. It may be affected in the jugular foramen syndrome (Vernet's syndrome), along with the tenth and eleventh nerves, of which glomus tumours or metastatic carcinoma are the commonest causes. The nerve may also be involved in diphtheritic neuropathy and in a polyneuritis cranialis.

Glossopharyngeal neuralgia is a rare form of neuralgia within the distribution of the glossopharyngeal nerve. Its features are otherwise strictly comparable with those of trigeminal neuralgia in the quality and severity of the pain, its occurrence in brief paroxysms, its provocation by actions such as speaking or swallowing, and the remissions in its course. As with trigeminal neuralgia, it is most often encountered in elderly subjects, and the pain may initially be confined to individual branches. Thus it may be felt deep in the ear, related to the tympanic branch, or in the throat, related to the pharyngeal branches. It also usually responds to treatment with carbamazepine.

In treatment, carbamazepine may be effective. In instances of severe pain unrelieved by this preparation, surgical treatment, usually avulsion of the nerve, may be required.

Vagus nerve

The tenth cranial nerve is structurally complex. Within the skull it is joined by the cranial division of the eleventh nerve. It leaves the skull through the jugular foramen. Cutaneous sensory fibres are carried from the external ear and visceral afferent fibres are carried from the pharynx, larynx, trachea, oesophagus, and the thoracic and abdominal viscera. Motor fibres are supplied to the striated musculature of the palate and pharynx and through the external and recurrent laryngeal nerves, to the muscles of the larynx. Parasympathetic fibres are provided to innervate the parotid gland (through the glossopharyngeal nerve), the heart, and the abdominal viscera.

The important symptoms of damage to the vagal nerve are those relating to pharyngeal and laryngeal innervation. The cells of origin in the nucleus ambiguus of the medulla may be damaged in the lateral medullary syndrome, in motor neurone disease, and in acute bulbar poliomyelitis, leading to dysphagia and dysphonia. Involvement along with the glossopharyngeal nerve in the jugular foramen syndrome has already been mentioned. The recurrent laryngeal nerve may be damaged during operations on the thyroid gland or by tumours within the neck, or within the thorax, usually by carcinoma of the bronchus. The nerve on the left is vulnerable to damage from aneurysm of the aortic arch. Isolated and unexplained lesions of the recurrent laryngeal nerve are not uncommon.

Nuclear or high vagal lesions, as well as involving the larynx, cause palatal and pharyngeal paralysis. If unilateral, there are no symptoms from palatopharyngeal paralysis. The uvula is pulled up to the opposite side on phonation and pharyngeal sensation is impaired on the affected side. With bilateral paralysis, the palate is paretic leading to nasality of the voice and nasal regurgitation of liquids on attempts at swallowing. Bilateral palatopharyngeal paralysis may be encountered in motor neurone disease, bulbar poliomyelitis, diphtheritic neuropathy, and polyneuritis cranialis.

Unilateral intrinsic laryngeal paralysis from lesions of the recurrent nerve may be asymptomatic or give rise to hoarseness of the voice. If the superior laryngeal nerve is also involved leading to paralysis of the cricothyroid muscle, the affected cord lies in a paramedian or cadaveric position. The effects of bilateral lesions of the recurrent laryngeal nerves depend upon the degree of approximation of the vocal cords. Lesions of insidious onset tend to give rise to dysphonia and also to stridor on exertion. In partial lesions, close approximation of the cords may result from selective paralysis of the abductor muscles, giving rise to limitation of the airway and sometimes necessitating tracheostomy. With bilateral lesions involving both the recurrent and superior laryngeal nerves, both cords are paralysed and in the cadaveric position. Phonation is impossible.

Spinal accessory nerve

The spinal accessory portion of the eleventh cranial nerve arises from the upper cervical cord and the lower medulla. The nerve passes through the foramen magnum and joins the cranial portion of the nerve before emerging from the skull through the jugular foramen. The spinal accessory nerve then separates and supplies the sternomastoid and trapezius muscles, the latter also receiving an innervation from the cervical plexus.

The nerve may be affected by lesions in the region of the jugular foramen, but more commonly it is damaged by injuries to the neck or by operations for the removal of cervical glands, particularly as it crosses the posterior triangle of the neck. Isolated and unexplained lesions of the nerve are occasionally encountered.

Unilateral paralysis of the sternomastoid usually passes unnoticed by the patient. The muscle does not stand out when the head is turned to the opposite side. Paralysis of the trapezius, on the other hand, causes difficulty in lifting the arm above the horizontal, in shrugging the shoulder, and in approximating the scapula to the midline and therefore also in carrying the extended arm backwards. The shoulder droops when the arm is hanging at the side and there is moderate winging of the scapula which is accentuated when the patient attempts to elevate the arm laterally.

The hypoglossal nerve

The twelfth cranial nerve supplies all the muscles of the tongue, both intrinsic and extrinsic. It leaves the skull through the anterior condyloid foramen. A unilateral lesion of the hypoglossal nerve causes weakness and atrophy of the tongue on the affected side. When protruded, the tongue deviates to the affected side. Articulation is unaffected. The nerve may be affected by tumours in the region of the anterior condyloid foramen, or by tumours or penetrating injuries in the neck. If the lesion is the result of a unilateral lower brainstem lesion, it may be combined with a crossed hemiplegia.

Bilateral lesions give rise to generalized atrophy of the tongue. Protrusion becomes impossible and articulation is disturbed. The commonest cause is motor neurone disease (progressive bulbar palsy variant). The wasting of the tongue is usually accompanied by fasciculation.

Further reading

Adour WEK *et al.* (1972). Prednisone treatment for idiopathic facial paralysis (Bell's palsy). *New England Journal of Medicine* **287**, 1268–75.

Asbury AK *et al.* (1970). Oculomotor palsy in diabetic mellitus: a clinicopathological study. *Brain* **93**, 555–66.

Brodal A (1965). *The cranial nerves*, 2nd edn. Blackwell Scientific, Oxford.

Bruyn GW (1983). Glossopharyngeal neuralgia. *Cephalgia* **3**, 143–9.

Cogan DG (1956). *Neurology of the ocular muscles*, 2nd edn. CC Thomas, Springfield, IL.

Cogan DG (1966). *Neurology of the visual system.* CC Thomas, Springfield, IL.

Dyck PJ *et al.*, eds. (1993). *Peripheral neuropathy*, 3rd edn. WB Saunders, Philadelphia.

Esslen E (1977). *The acute facial palsies. Investigations on the localization and pathogenesis of meato-labyrinthine facial palsies.* Springer, New York.

Farrell DA, Medsger A (1982). Trigeminal neuropathy in progressive systemic sclerosis. *American Journal of Medicine* **73**, 57–61.

Katusic S *et al.* (1990). Incidence and clinical features of trigeminal neuralgia. *Annals of Neurology* **27**, 89–95.

Lecky BRF, Hughes RAC, Murray NMF (1987). Trigeminal sensory neuropathy. A study of 22 cases. *Brain* **110**, 1463–86.

Rush JA, Younge BR (1966). Paralysis of cranial nerves III, IV and VI: causes and prognosis of 1000 cases. *Archives of Ophthalmology* **99**, 76–89.

24.13.16 Diseases of the spinal cord

L. D. Blumhardt

Anatomy

The spinal cord extends from its junction with the brainstem (medulla oblongata) at the foramen magnum (opposite the odontoid peg at C1) to the lower border of the first lumbar vertebra. It is enclosed within the arachnoid and dura mater, which extend below the termination of the spinal cord (conus medullaris) into the sacral canal.

The clinically important upper motor neurones run in the corticospinal tract which crosses at the level of the pyramids and then runs caudally in the lateral white matter of the cord. The uncrossed sensory fibres in the posterior columns of the cord convey the sense of joint position and two-point discrimination. Fibres transmitting pain and temperature sensation enter the cord in the posterior spinal roots and ascend three or four segments in the dorsolateral funiculus before decussating through the central grey matter to the contralateral side, where they ascend in the spinothalamic tracts of the anterior and lateral columns. Ascending and descending autonomic fibres involved in sphincter control are in close proximity to the spinothalamic pathways.

The blood supply of the spinal cord is made up of an arterial plexus that is supplied mainly from the anterior spinal artery in the anterior fissure and the two posterior spinal arteries in close proximity to the posterior columns. The anterior plexus is the most extensive and supplies the majority of the cord including the anterior and lateral columns, the corticospinal and spinothalamic tracts, and the anterior grey matter. The posterior system supplies the posterior columns and grey matter. The plexus receives variable supplies from the vertebral arteries, thyrocervical trunk, and multiple spinal medullary arteries arising from the intercostal arteries. The most constant and important contribution to the anterior spinal artery arises from the tenth left intercostal artery ('artery of Adamkiewicz').

Anatomical localization

The sensory and motor pathways of the cord can be damaged by disease anywhere in their long spinal course. Clues to the segmental level of a lesion may be provided by sensory or motor levels, or by involvement of the spinal and superficial cutaneous reflexes. Spastic upper motor neurone weakness in all four limbs arises from involvement of the motor pathways at the cervical level and of the lower limbs at the thoracic level. Loss or reduction of a deep tendon reflex may indicate damage to a particular arc within a segment of the cord, or the appropriate spinal root. By convention, the biceps and supinator jerks are considered C5–C6, the triceps jerk C7, the knee jerk L(3)4, and the ankle jerk S1. Sensory loss, muscle wasting and weakness, or pain within a spinal segment, may also have localizing value. In addition, the loss of superficial reflexes (abdominal D7 to D12, cremasteric L2, plantar S1) has potential localizing value: thus the superficial abdominal reflexes will be abolished by lesions at D6 or above, whereas the upper abdominal reflexes should be retained when the lesion is at D10 or below.

If there is complete transection of the cord, motor power and all sensation is lost below the level of the segment involved. In addition, there will be retention of urine with overflow incontinence. If the condition develops suddenly a state of spinal shock occurs in which there is flaccid paralysis of both skeletal and smooth muscle with loss of sensation and reflex activity below the level of the lesion. Partial lesions result in a variable syndrome of motor and sensory signs. There is often loss of coordination of bladder contraction and sphincter relaxation with consequent urgency and incontinence. If the cord damage is unilateral, the Brown–Séquard syndrome will result in ipsilateral loss of posterior column function combined with contralateral upper motor neurone signs and symptoms and spinothalamic irritation, or impairment. There is a level on the trunk usually several segments below the lesion. Light touch sensation is generally relatively preserved. Superficial abdominal reflexes are generally lost below the level of the lesion. The syndrome is often partial or incomplete.

A spastic paraparesis (upper motor neurone weakness and spasticity in the lower limbs) may be associated with loss of reflexes in the arms, typically asymmetric C5–C6 loss or reduction in cervical spondylotic myelopathy, Damage to the C5–C6 reflex arc may be associated with weakness of shoulder abduction and elbow flexion, reduced biceps and supinator jerks, and enhanced triceps jerks, with spastic weakness below this level. Syringomyelia is usually associated with general upper limb areflexia with a spastic paraparesis and dissociated sensory loss (see below). Lesions at the level of the foramen magnum (meningioma or developmental abnormalities) that involve the cervical enlargement may be confusingly associated with wasting of the small muscles of the hands. Respiratory involvement may complicate high cervical lesions through paralysis of the muscles of the thoracic wall or diaphragm.

Symptoms of spinal cord disease

Lesions of the upper and lower motor neurones cause characteristic patterns of symptoms. Lower motor neurone weakness and wasting often goes unnoticed by patients in the early stages when it will already be obvious to an examiner. By contrast, in the earliest stages of upper motor neurone involvement, symptoms may be present in the absence of signs. Upper motor neurone weakness, which is usually responsible for the first symptoms of a myelopathy, may be described as involving sensations of heaviness, dragging, 'numbness', stiffness, tripping, scuffing, lack of control, clumsiness, or loss of dexterity. Rapid repetitive movements are particularly impaired. Associated spasticity may cause extensor spasms and clonus, which may be described as a vibration of the foot usually noticed when negotiating stairs or kerbs. Lesions of the spinothalamic tracts result in a sensory level on the trunk with loss or reduction of pain and temperature sensation on the opposite side below the lesion (usually two or three segments below, because of the ascending course of the fibres prior to sensory decussation). Partial or irritative spinothalamic lesions cause a variety of unpleasant sensory symptoms, including burning pains, increased sensitivity to touch, feelings of wetness, or the sensation of movements under the skin (formication). Posterior column involvement can lead to tingling paraesthesiae and tight constricting feelings around joints, as well as sensory ataxia. Stretching or movement of the cervical cord on neck flexion may cause shooting paraesthesiae ('electric shocks') down the back into the lower limbs ('Lhermitte's symptom'). This can be associated with any pathology in the cervical canal but is most often seen with multiple sclerosis. Autonomic involvement may cause hesitancy, urgency, and urge incontinence of bladder and bowel.

Acute and subacute myelopathy

Rapidly developing weakness in the lower limbs (over minutes, days, or weeks) requires immediate referral to a neurological unit for diagnosis and management. The urgent problem is to establish the site of the weakness (spinal cord or peripheral nerve) and the cause (intrinsic or extrinsic spinal cord disease or acute polyneuritis). It is essential to exclude a compressive cause requiring emergency decompression. An acute transverse myelopathy, with absent deep tendon reflexes, non-elicitable plantar responses, and paralysed, flaccid limbs (so-called 'spinal shock'), may superficially mimic acute Guillain–Barré syndrome, but retention of urine and a sensory level on the trunk will indicate the correct pathological localization in the spinal cord.

An acute or subacute spinal cord syndrome may be due either to extrinsic cord compression (Table 1) or to intrinsic pathology. If compressive, the prognosis for recovery may depend on how rapidly the spinal cord can be decompressed. There are many intrinsic causes of an acute myelopathy, including multiple sclerosis, acute disseminated encephalomyelitis, viral myelitis, systemic lupus erythematosus, sarcoidosis, Behçet's disease, paraneoplastic syndrome, and spinal cord infarction or haemorrhage. Unless there are other clues from the history, or from general or neurological examination, it is not usually possible to make a reliable distinction between intrinsic and extrinsic causes. It is vitally important to relieve bladder retention and to search for a primary focus of infection or underlying neoplasia that may have led to metastasis. Neuroimaging of the spinal cord (preferably magnetic resonance imaging) must be carried out as an emergency procedure. Lumbar puncture should be avoided until compression has been excluded, as worsening of the myelopathy may be precipitated by reduction of cerebrospinal fluid pressure below an obstruction.

Chronic progressive myelopathy

The first symptoms of a slowly progressing spinal cord lesion, particularly a compressive lesion, are often due to the insidious development of upper motor neurone weakness. There may be a barely noticeable deterioration in ambulation with the onset of subtle difficulties (heavy limbs, dragging foot or leg), at first only apparent when running or during long walks. At first there may be little in the way of objective signs, and symptoms may progress very slowly over months or years A careful history and examination in

Table 1 Main causes of compressive myelopathy

Trauma
Spinal fracture or dislocations
Haematoma
Infection
Epidural abscess
Parasitic disease (e.g. shistosomiasis, cysticercosis, echinococcus)
Inflammation
Arachnoiditis
Sarcoidosis
Ankylosing spondylitis
Rheumatoid subluxation
Vascular
Spinal haemorrhage
Epidural haematoma
Neoplastic-associated ishaemia
Degenerative and skeletal
Cervical spondylotic myelopathy
Spinal stenosis
Prolapsed intervertebral disc
Osteoporosis
Paget's disease of bone
Fluorosis
Kyphoscoliosis
Congenital anomalies
Arnold–Chiari malformation
Spinal dysraphism
Basilar impression
Achondroplasia
Klippel–Feil syndrome
Neoplastic
Benign tumours (meningioma, neurofibroma)
Lymphoma
Metastases
Extramedullary haematopoiesis
Congenital skeletal abnormalities
Arnold–Chiari malformation
Syringomyelia

anyone who complains of walking difficulties is mandatory. Upper motor neurone weakness is frequently missed by incomplete examination as it primarily involves flexor movements in the legs and extensors in the arms. As for acute myelopathy, the cause may be intrinsic or extrinsic, and neuroimaging is indicated without delay. Common compressive causes are cervical spondylotic myelopathy, prolapsed intervertebral dorsal disc, neurofibroma, meningioma, and ependymoma. Multiple sclerosis is the most common intrinsic cause in the United Kingdom, but motor neurone disease, hereditary spastic paraplegia, HTLV-I myelopathy, vitamin B_{12} or folate deficiency, and, rarely, thyroid disease may present in this way and require exclusion.

Cervical spondylotic myelopathy

This is a spinal cord compression syndrome that typically occurs in the sixth decade or later. It usually presents as a chronic progressive spastic paraparesis, but an acute or subacute ascending myelopathy can also occur. Radicular symptoms (pain and sensory impairment or paraesthesiae) may or may not be present, but typically, there is coexisting radiculopathy and the C5–C6 reflexes are found to be depressed or absent and the C7 reflexes brisk ('inverted supinator jerk'). Magnetic resonance imaging of the cervical spine is the investigation of choice. Those affected have constitutionally narrower cervical canals. Coexisting ischaemic demyelination due to compression is often present in the centre of the cord, but a statistical association with multiple sclerosis has also been described.

Spinal epidural abscess

Pain with signs of spinal cord compression may occur acutely with a spinal epidural abscess, and often with little in the way of systemic disturbance. Staphylococcal and streptococcal organisms are frequently responsible and septicaemia may be present. Treatment is with appropriate antibiotics and surgical drainage procedures.

Tuberculosis

Tuberculosis is primarily an infection of the spinal vertebral bodies and intervertebral discs. Compression of the cord often results from vertebral collapse. Infection may spread through the meninges to involve the spinal cord directly, or there may be associated arterial occlusions. Management is by antituberculous drugs and, where appropriate, surgery for decompression or spinal stabilization.

Syringomyelia

A rare condition (prevalence approximately 7 per 100 000) in which an irregular fluid-filled cavity (syrinx) causes a central cord syndrome. The cavity usually begins in the cervical area, initially localized to a segment or two, but may extend the whole length of the cord. Adjacent structures including the decussating fibres destined for the spinothalamic tracts, the anterior horn cells, and the pyramidal tracts may become involved, although the posterior columns are characteristically spared.

Typically in early adult life the patient notices weakness and wasting of an upper limb and/or loss of the sensation of pain. Painless injuries often occur and may lead to dramatic symptoms (one of the author's patients was a butcher who lost the ends of his fingers in a mincer before noticing). There is usually areflexia in the arms, a spastic paraparesis, and a 'dissociated' sensory loss (retention of common touch and proprioception sense with loss of pain and temperature sensation) in the upper limbs with extension on the trunk in the forequarter ('cape') area. Associated features may include Horner's syndrome, upper limb pain, and a mild dorsal scoliosis. The syrinx and the presence of any associated abnormality at the foramen magnum are now easily established by magnetic resonance imaging, sometimes before a typical clinical syndrome develops. Tumours and Tangier's disease can also result in a central cord syndrome. The condition can be static for years, but often progresses irregularly. Rostral extension into the brainstem (syringobulbia) may cause dysarthria, dysphagia, wasting of the tongue, and sensory loss in the face (sparing the central areas such as the mouth and nose until last).

A syrinx is often associated with an Arnold–Chiari malformation, but can be secondary to an intrinsic spinal cord tumour or spinal cord injury. Treatment by surgery is controversial and outcomes are complicated by the variable natural history. If there is an associated cerebellar ectopia and hypodevelopment of the posterior fossa, decompression of the foramen magnum may successfully relieve pain and halt progression. Drainage of the syrinx by various shunt procedures may also be helpful if it is carried out before moderate or severe disability has resulted.

Spinal arachnoiditis

Any inflammatory process can result in a progressive fibrosis of the subarachnoid space. The most common causes include myelographic contrast media, subarachnoid haemorrhage, surgery, trauma, and infection. Complications include cystic compression and ischaemic damage to the spinal cord and/or spinal nerve roots, often with intractable pain and blockage of cerebrospinal fluid pathways. Once initiated, arachnoiditis can be progressive and there is no effective treatment. Attempts at surgical correction may cause further fibrosis and deterioration.

Schistosomiasis (bilharziasis)

A chronic infection with a trematode worm (in South America, Asia, and Africa) occasionally causes spinal cord or root compression or a transverse myelitis due to a granulomatous inflammatory reaction to the parasite's eggs. Granulomas may be intrinsic or extrinsic and there may be associated meningoencephalitis and intracranial granulomas. Treatment is with praziquantel. Other worms including cysticercosis and echinococcus may also (rarely) cause spinal cord compression.

Demyelinating diseases

Involvement of the spinal cord is almost invariable in multiple sclerosis. In the early stages of the disease, acute or subacute episodes of partial myelopathy often occur with partial or complete recovery (relapsing–remitting disease). Lhermitte's symptom is common, but non-specific for demyelination. In the later stages (secondary progressive multiple sclerosis) a chronic progressive myelopathy associated with spasticity, sensory loss, and ataxia is characteristic. Eighty five per cent of patients with primary progressive multiple sclerosis present as an insidious progressive myelopathy, mostly in middle age. Diagnosis is established by clinical history and examination, magnetic resonance imaging of the spinal cord and brain, evoked potentials, examination of the cerebrospinal fluid (intrathecal oligoclonal bands), and blood tests to exclude other causes of myelopathy.

Perivenous inflammation and demyelination also occur in the white matter of the brain and spinal cord following vaccination or an acute childhood viral infection such as measles, mumps, rubella, or chicken pox (acute disseminated encephalomyelitis), but the triggering infection is not always identifiable. The illness is usually monophasic, but recurrent symptoms indicate that the initial bout was the onset of multiple sclerosis.

Acute/subacute transverse myelitis

An acute or subacute spinal cord syndrome may occur as a monophasic, spontaneous illness with no obvious cause, or may follow a viral infection or vaccination. It is characterized by a sensory level on the trunk (usually thoracic) to all modalities with retention of urine and faeces and severe symmetrical paraplegia. The myelogram may be normal or show a swollen cord. The spinal fluid shows an inflammatory reaction with an excess of white cells and raised protein. High-dose intravenous steroids are usually administered. There may be a full or partial recovery, or permanent paraplegia may result.

Many conditions can give rise to a similar clinical picture, including infections (sarcoidosis, syphilis, Lyme disease, spinal tuberculosis, brucellosis), collagen vascular diseases, viruses (Epstein–Barr, herpes zoster, herpes simplex, rubella), and multiple sclerosis. However, unlike the acute or subacute partial spinal cord syndromes, multiple sclerosis develops in only a small proportion and the cause most often remains obscure, even after many years of follow-up.

Paralytic poliomyelitis

After an incubation period of 1 to 2 weeks, a viraemia is associated with fever, vomiting, and headache. Replication of the virus in the anterior horn cells of the spinal cord and the motor nuclei of the brainstem is usually associated with signs of meningitis and pains in the spine and limbs ('preparalytic phase'). Recovery may then occur, but some patients may go on to develop a highly variable, asymmetric, patchy muscle weakness. Reflex loss, fasciculation, and muscle wasting are early features, but sensation remains normal. A minority of patients develop bulbar complications including respiratory failure. A variable degree of recovery may occur. Management is supportive with control of frequently associated infections. Widespread vaccination has virtually eliminated this condition.

Human immunodeficiency syndrome (AIDS) myelopathy

A subacute to chronic progressive myelopathy characterized by vacuolar changes in myelin sheaths with relative axonal preservation and an emphasis on the dorsolateral thoracic spinal cord is the most common form of myelopathy in AIDS. Spasticity, weakness, loss of the sense of joint position, and sphincter dysfunction develop over weeks or months. Magnetic resonance imaging usually shows the spinal cord to be normal or nonspecifically atrophic. There may be coexisting dementia or neuropathy. Treatment is limited to management of symptoms.

Myelitis in AIDS may result from a variety of causes including infection with herpes simplex, cytomegalovirus, varicella zoster, HTLV-I and -II, syphilis, or tuberculosis. Vitamin B_{12} deficiency, lymphoma, and spinal epidural abscess may also cause an acute or subacute myelopathy in this situation.

HTLV-I associated myelopathy ('tropical spastic paraparesis')

Retroviral infection results in a chronic slowly progressive myelopathy characterized by paraesthesiae (often painful) in the lower limbs, sphincter dysfunction, and spastic paraparesis. Some cases may also have cerebellar ataxia, optic neuritis, and signs of a peripheral neuropathy. There is positive HTLV-I serology in the blood and cerebrospinal fluid.

Nutritional deficiencies

Subacute combined degeneration of the spinal cord due to vitamin B_{12} deficiency has become rare with the early diagnosis and treatment of pernicious anaemia. Presenting complaints are persistent paraesthesiae in the feet and later in the hands with unsteadiness of gait. There may be signs of peripheral nerve damage (distal sensory loss and loss of ankle jerks). Unless treatment is initiated early, weakness in the lower limbs becomes more marked with extensor plantar responses and ataxia indicating largely irreversible damage to the pyramidal tracts and posterior columns. There may be additional loss of memory and cognition, reduced vision with central scotomas, and sphincter disturbance. The patients are usually middle aged and there may be no evidence of anaemia or changes in the blood film. The serum level of vitamin B_{12} is almost invariably markedly reduced. Treatment with hydroxycobalamin should be started immediately to prevent irreversible damage. Motor symptoms usually respond better than sensory symptoms, and paraesthesiae may persist indefinitely. Rarely, a similar syndrome may be associated with folate deficiency.

Low levels of vitamin E may cause a spinocerebellar syndrome with pyramidal signs, with or without peripheral nerve involvement and ophthalmoplegia. Patients present with an unsteady gait and weakness with limb ataxia, and loss of reflexes, proprioception, and vibration sense. The cause is often malabsorption due to gastrointestinal disease (see also Section 14).

Vascular disease

Haemorrhage into the parenchyma of the spinal cord is rare and may be spontaneous, or a complication of arteriovenous malformations, trauma, and clotting abnormalities, including anticoagulant therapy. Infarction of the spinal cord may result from aortic disease (atherosclerosis, dissecting aneurysm, surgery), thoracic or cardiac surgery, or cardiac arrest (hypotension). The resulting paraplegia is often ushered in by acute pain at the level of the infarction. As the anterior spinal artery is most often involved, loss of pain and temperature sensation occurs below the level of the infarction with preservation of common sensation and proprioception. Infarction of one-half of the cord results in the Brown–Séquard syndrome. Rarely, the whole cord can be infarcted below the occlusion. Recovery from infarction is variable and unpredictable. Embolism may occur in decompression sickness or bacterial endocarditis and ischaemic damage in the context of autoimmune vasculitic diseases such as systemic lupus erythematosus and Sjögrens disease. Spinal arteries may be secondarily involved during bacterial meningitis or syphilitic leptomeningitis, or by neoplasia.

Drug abuse, particularly of heroin or cocaine, may cause an acute myelopathy. The clinical picture resembles an anterior spinal artery occlusion with paraplegia, sensory level and bladder dysfunction, and sparing of posterior column function. The causes include particulate emboli, vasculitis, and watershed infarction from hypotension.

Decompression sickness arising from bubbles of gas in the bloodstream caused by too rapid decompression following exposure to high atmospheric pressures (usually due to diving) may cause ischaemic damage to the spinal cord. Generally within minutes of a return to normal atmospheric pressure a widely variable syndrome of paraesthesiae, sensory loss, pain, and weakness in the limbs develops, that either recovers on rapid recompression, or progresses to a permanent spastic paraparesis.

Venous thrombophlebitis may cause a patchy, asymmetric, and rapidly ascending subacute necrotic myelitis. This may occur as a result of intra-abdominal or pelvic sepsis, but often no cause can be found. The prognosis is poor.

Spinal arteriovenous malformations are congenital abnormalities of blood vessels supplying the spinal cord and may cause either an acute or chronic progressive spinal cord syndrome. There may be various combinations of spinal cord compression, venous infarction, vascular 'steal' due to shunting, haemorrhage, or progressive fibrosis. Pain may worsen with exercise. Haemorrhage into the cerebrospinal fluid can cause sudden confusion, headaches, and neck stiffness. Cord compression may result from a secondary haematoma. Auscultation over the spine should be performed in all patients with undiagnosed myelopathy, although bruits are only present in a minority. The arteriovenous malformation may be demonstrated by magnetic resonance imaging or myelography and its vascular supply established by spinal angiography, which is not without risk. They may be inoperable, or amenable to embolization or surgical removal in expert hands.

Subacute necrotizing myelitis is a rare condition in which a flaccid paraplegia results from extensive cord involvement below the highest segment. There may be a stepwise development with ascending levels. The lesion can be associated with vascular abnormalities, but no cause can usually be identified, treatment is not effective, and the prognosis is poor.

Spirochaetal infections

Acute vascular cord lesions including an anterior spinal artery occlusion may be the presentation of meningovascular syphilis. Damage to the spinal cord can also arise from chronic inflammatory changes in the cervical meninges (leptomeningitis) involving spinal nerve roots and spinal cord. Symptoms and signs of wasting of the small hand muscles (C8–T1) with and without upper motor neurone signs may be present.

The diagnosis is often suspected when high cell and protein levels are found and confirmed by serology in the blood and cerebrospinal fluid.

The classical chronic progressive neurological disorder tabes dorsalis has become very rare due to improved recognition and early treatment of syphilis. Clinical features may include an ataxic steppage gait, lancinating pains in the legs, skin ulcers, hypotonicity, and painless arthritis. Damage starts in the dorsal root ganglion cells and particularly involves the central processes extending into the posterior columns. Classic 'lightning' pains or electric shock-like sensations in the lower limbs and eventually loss of deep pain sensation usually occur. Further damage to the spinal roots leads to loss of reflexes and hypotonicity of the limbs. Hypermobility of joints with loss of pain sensation may lead to a progressive painless destruction of knee, ankle, or elbow joints ('Charcot's joints'). Damage to the pyramidal tracts eventually results in extensor plantar responses ('taboparesis'). Additional findings may include analgesic patches on the trunk and inner arms, loss of sphincter control with a dilated atonic bladder, optic atrophy, small light near-dissociated pupils (Argyll–Robertson pupils), and ptosis. Painful autonomic attacks ('crises') affecting the bladder, rectum, stomach, or larynx, may also be a feature.

Toxic damage

X-ray therapy to the thorax or neck, particularly directed at the bronchi or oesophagus, may occasionally result in damage to the spinal cord (radiation myelopathy). The risk is dose related. An acute transient form of myelopathy characterized by paraesthesiae and Lhermitte's symptom comes on soon after exposure and usually remits. The mechanism is probably demyelination of the posterior columns. The delayed myelopathy that comes on 6 months to several years after treatment is due to a vasculopathy with cord necrosis and atrophy leading to a progressive spinothalamic sensory loss and disabling paraplegia. Magnetic resonance imaging excludes other possibilities, including compression from metastases and paraneoplastic subacute necrotizing myelitis.

The neurotoxin β-*N*-oxalylamino-L-alanine, a glutamine receptor agonist, contained in the pulse *Lathyrus sativus* (chickling pea) may cause an acute or chronic paraparesis, often with prominent muscle spasms, which usually occurring in outbreaks during periods of famine (lathyrism). Chronic cyanide poisoning from ingesting the roots of the cassava plant may result in pyramidal signs, usually combined with a painful peripheral neuropathy.

Neuronal degenerations

Hereditary spastic paraplegia

This is a relatively rare condition, in which degeneration of the pyramidal tracts and posterior columns causes a slowly progressive spastic paraparesis of varying severity. It is essential to take a family history and examine relatives carefully, as mild cases may be asymptomatic, causing misdiagnoses and an underestimate of the true prevalence. There are dominant (70 to 80 per cent of cases) and recessive forms. Genetic studies of the autosomal dominant variant have identified loci on at least three chromosomes that account for about half the cases. Type I hereditary spastic paraplegia comes on in childhood or adolescence with clumsiness and poor athletic performance caused by spasticity. Weakness is usually slight or absent. Sensory loss tends to be mild and late and usually involves proprioception. Abdominal reflexes are often retained and significant bladder involvement is relatively uncommon until the later stages. Pes cavus is often present. Type II hereditary spastic paraplegia has similar clinical features, but an onset after the age of 35 years. Recessive forms tend to be more rapidly progressive and are often misdiagnosed. Other causes of spastic paraparesis must be excluded.

Motor neurone disease

The full-blown picture of amyotrophic lateral sclerosis with mixed lower and upper motor neurone features is unmistakeable, but individual cases can sometimes resemble other diseases, particularly cervical spondylotic myelopathy and primary progressive multiple sclerosis. A minority of cases present with a pure upper motor neurone spinal cord syndrome with a spastic paraparesis ('primary lateral sclerosis') and no evidence of lower motor neurone wasting or weakness. The clinical picture is of a slowly progressing spastic paraparesis or quadraparesis. The differential diagnosis is extensive and many of the conditions listed in Table 2 need to be considered and excluded. Investigations may include magnetic resonance imaging, electromyography, muscle biochemistry, evoked potentials, and examination of the cerebrospinal fluid. Prolonged clinical follow-up may be required to clarify the diagnosis.

Friedrich's ataxia

This is a rare, progressive, autosomal recessive condition that begins in childhood or adolescence and leads, usually by the third decade, to limited

Table 2 Main causes of non-compressive myelopathy

Demyelinating
Multiple sclerosis
Acute disseminated encephalomyelitis
Devic's disease
Familial and degenerative
Hereditary spastic paraplegia
Friedrich's ataxia
Motor neurone disease
Metabolic
B_{12} deficiency (subacute combined degeneration of the cord)
Folate deficiency
Hyperthyroidism
Vitamin E deficiency
Nicotinic acid deficiency
Adrenoleukodystropy
Infections
Viral
Herpes zoster
AIDS
HTLV-I
Spirochaetal
Syphilis
Lyme disease
Parasitic
Schistosomiasis
Trichinosis
Gnathostomiasis
Vascular and inflammatory
Collagen vascular disease (Sjögrens, systemic lupus erythematosus)
Venous thrombophlebitis
Arteriovenous malformations
Sarcoidosis
Arachnoiditis
Injury
Radiation
Decompression sickness
Iatrogenic (epidural analgesia, sympathetic blocks)
Toxic
Lathyrism
Cyanide poisoning (e.g. cassava)
Nitrous oxide
Clioquinol (SMON)
Intravenous drug abuse
Paraneoplastic
Necrotizing myelopathy
Limbic encephalomyelitis
Syringomyelia

mobility and death a few years later. Presentation is usually with unsteadiness and clumsiness. Features include dysarthria, inco-ordination of the limbs, gait ataxia, impaired proprioception, and areflexia.

Adrenomyeloleucodystrophy

This is an X-linked recessive disorder in which demyelination in the brain and spinal cord occurs as a result of the accumulation of very long chain fatty acids. Adult males develop a spastic paraparesis with or without mild sphincter involvement and sensory loss. A very slowly progressive mild spastic paraparesis with sphincter and sensory loss may also be found in heterozygote females. Associated adrenal insufficiency may be very mild. The condition may be mistaken for multiple sclerosis, although the magnetic resonance abnormality, when present, usually shows widespread symmetrically distributed lesions often in the posterior white matter more appropriate to a leucodystrophy. A locus has been demonstrated at chromosome Xq28. There are increased levels of very long chain fatty acids in the serum.

Further reading

Fink JK, Heineman-Patterson T (1996). Hereditary spastic paraplegia: advances in genetic research. *Neurology* **46**, 1507.

24.13.17 Spinal cord injury and its management

M. P. Barnes

Introduction

Spinal cord injury is a prime example of the improvement in survival and quality of life that can follow from the application of modern rehabilitation techniques. In the early part of the last century around 9 out of 10 people with a spinal cord injury died within 1 year and only 1 per cent survived in the long term. The situation greatly improved with the advent of spinal cord injury centres, particularly pioneered in the United Kingdom by Sir Ludwig Guttmann at Stoke Mandeville. The co-ordinated, multidisciplinary care provided at these centres significantly reduced mortality and improved quality of life. However, even in the 1960s there was still a 35 per cent mortality associated with tetraplegia, and it has only been in the last decade or so that modern rehabilitation techniques have reduced mortality to less than 5 per cent. Life expectancy has improved such that the major causes of late death in spinal injury are now those experienced by the general population, such as cancer and myocardial infarction. However, there is no room for complacency. Deaths from renal failure or respiratory infection in those with tetraplegia are still too common. Although life expectancy in those with paraplegia is only modestly reduced, people with tetraplegia still have a significantly reduced survival rate. A 20-year-old male would normally be expected to have a further 56 years' life expectancy, but this is reduced to about 45 years in those with paraplegia, and those with tetraplegia only have an expected survival of a further 33 years.

Although this chapter will concentrate on the medical management of spinal cord injury and its complications, it would be incomplete without a mention of the acute and emergency management.

Epidemiology

The annual incidence of spinal cord injury, at least in Western Europe, is around 10 to 15 cases per million of the population per annum. The mean age of injury is about 33 years, although the mode is 19 years. Most injuries occur in males (around 82 per cent). The commonest cause is road traffic accidents (about 40 per cent). Regrettably, spinal cord injury from violence (either self-harm or criminal assault) is increasing, particularly in the United States. In the older age group, falls become a more common cause. Table 1 summarizes the leading causes in the United Kingdom and United States.

Table 1 Causes of spinal cord injury—comparison of causes in the United Kingdom and United States

Cause	UK (%)	USA (%)
Road traffic accidents	35	43
Violence	7	19
Sports injuries	21	11
Falls (domestic and industrial)	36	19
Other	1	8

The proportion of injuries from road traffic accidents has seen a modest reduction in recent years, probably due to the introduction of seat-belt legislation and improved safety features on cars. Hopefully, the improved safety of vehicles and improved traffic regulation, particularly speed control in urban areas, will further reduce the incidence in coming years. There is some evidence in the last decade that the incidence of spinal injury has plateaued, having been increasing in previous decades. Regrettably, the commonest result of injury is tetraplegia (around 60 per cent), which, compared to paraplegia, is still increasing.

Early acute management

The appropriate management of the individual at the scene of an accident is vital to avoid unnecessary worsening of a spinal cord injury. If the individual is unconscious then it should be assumed there is an injury to the cervical spine until proven otherwise. Until this diagnosis can be ruled out the head and neck should, as far as possible, be held firmly in a neutral position. This is normally achieved at the scene of an accident by immobilization in a semi-rigid collar, but if this is not available alternative improvised methods of stabilizing the head and neck should be initiated. The individual should not be placed in the coma position as this will rotate the cervical spine, but is best placed, if other injuries allow, in a lateral position with the head kept in line with the spine by the underlying arm. If any movement is necessary the person should be 'log rolled' to ensure their spine is kept in a straight and neutral position at all times. Usually, transportation is on a spinal board with a head immobilizer. Speed of evacuation is important, particularly if there are other life-threatening injuries. Preferably, the individual should be transferred to the Regional Spinal Injuries Unit; but obviously the individual may need to be resuscitated, and other life-threatening injuries may need treatment at the nearest casualty department. It is worth recalling that the diagnosis of intra-abdominal injury can be very difficult in people with spinal cord injuries. The initial phase of spinal shock will tend to give rise to paralytic ileus and abdominal distension, which can further confuse the situation if an abdominal injury is suspected.

Obviously, a general and neurological examination is vital—particularly to determine the neurological level of the lesion. Figure 1 illustrates the myotomes, dermatomes, and reflexes as an *aide mémoire*. Table 2 summarizes the likely functional outcome according to lesion level.

Spinal injury, however, can not be determined solely by examination and often there are very few local signs. There may be some bruising, tenderness, or deformity, but equally there may be no clue on examination as to the actual nature and extent of the underlying bone injury. Thus, although radiological investigation is essential, it should preferably only be undertaken in a unit familiar with the management of those with spinal injury. In a radiology department it is still important to remember that spinal movement must be minimal. Usually, radiography will clearly reveal the fracture or dislocation, although bony abnormalities are occasionally minimal or absent. This is particularly true in older people with underlying cervical spondylosis when tetraplegia can result from a hyperextension injury without fracture or dislocation. Radiological examination can also be normal in children when a spinal traction injury can occur without evidence of bony damage.

Initial management of people with injuries to the cervical spine usually consists of skeletal traction applied through skull callipers. Traction will help to stabilize and splint the spine and can also reduce fractures and dislocations. A number of different callipers are available, of which the Gardner–Wells calliper is but one type (Fig. 2).

The amount of traction applied will vary according to the type and extent of injury, but it will be in the order of 2 kg for upper cervical injuries and somewhat more, around 4 kg, for lower cervical spinal injuries. Sometimes, if the spine is dislocated, reduction is achieved by incrementally increasing the weight of traction every few hours. Once the neck has reduced, a halo brace is a useful alternative to skull traction in many people and will allow early mobilization.

The standard treatment for thoracic and lumbar injuries is simple support of the individual in the correct posture, usually with a pillow under the lumbar spine to maintain the normal lordosis.

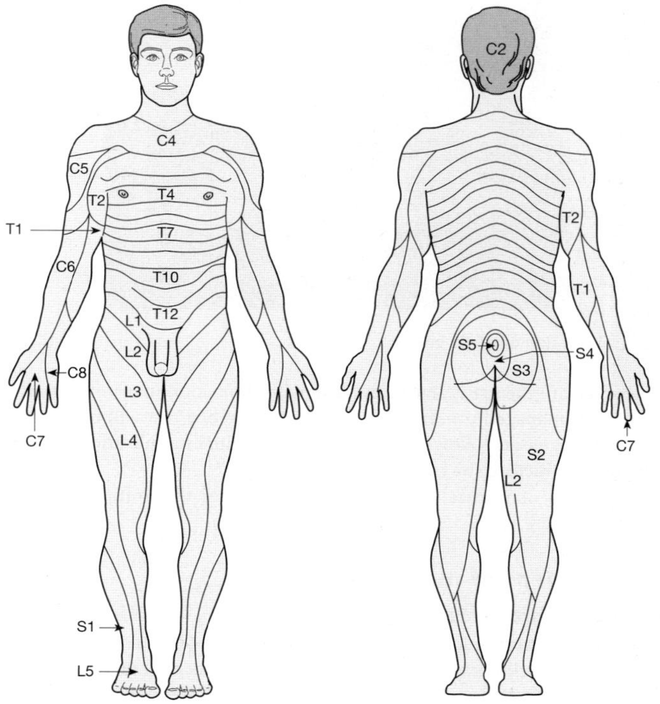

Myotomes	**Reflexes**	
Muscle group	*Nerve supply*	
Diaphragm	C(3), 4 (5)	
Shoulder abductors	C5	
Elbow flexors	C5, 6	Biceps jerk C5, 6
Supinators/pronators	C6	Supinator jerk C6
Wrist extensors	C6	
Wrist flexors	C7	
Elbow extensors	C7	Triceps jerk C7
Finger extensors	C7	
Finger flexors	C8	
Intrinsic hand muscles	T1	Abdominal reflex T8-12
Hip flexors	L1, 2	
Hip adductors	L2, 3	
Knee extensors	L3, 4	Knee jerk L3,4
Ankle dorsiflexors	L4, 5	
Toe extensors	L5	
Knee flexors	L4, 5 S1	
Ankle plantar flexors	S1, 2	Ankle jerk S1, 2
Toe flexors	S1, 2	
Anal sphincter	S2, 3, 4	Bulbocavernosus reflex S3, 4 Anal reflex S5 Plantar reflex

Fig. 1 An *aide mémoire* to examination—summary of the dermatomes, myotomes, and associated reflexes.

Surgical versus conservative treatment

In most cases, skull traction for cervical injuries and conservative postural treatment for thoracolumbar injuries is quite sufficient and operative intervention is unnecessary. It has long been a source of controversy whether

Table 2 Expected residual functional ability according to the level of lesion

Level of injury—complete lesions	
Lesion below C3	Dependent on others for all care Diaphragm paralysed, needs permanent ventilation or diaphragm pacing Chin-, head-, or breath-controlled electric wheelchair
Lesion below C4	Dependent on others for all care Can breathe independently using diaphragm Can shrug shoulders Can use electric wheelchair with chin control Can type/use computer with a mouth stick Environmental control system operated by shoulder shrug or mouthpiece
Lesion below C5	Can move shoulders and flex elbows Can eat with a feeding strap/universal cuff Can wash face, comb hair, clean teeth—using feeding strap/universal cuff Can write using individually designed splint and wrist support Can help in dressing upper half of body Can push manual wheelchair short distances on the flat provided that pushing gloves are used with capstan rims on the wheels May be able to transfer across level surfaces using sliding board and a helper Electric wheelchair needed for functional mobility
Lesion below C6	Can extend wrists Still needs strap to eat and for self-care Can write using individually designed splint but may not need wrist support Can dress upper half of body unaided Can help in dressing lower half of body Can propel wheelchair up gentle slopes Can be independent in bed, car, and toilet transfers Can drive with hand controls
Lesion below C7	Full wrist movement and some hand function, but no finger flexion or fine hand movements Can do all transfers, eat, and dress independently Can drive with hand controls
Lesion below C8	All hand muscles expect intrinsics preserved Wheelchair independent, but difficulty in going up and down kerbs Can drive with hand controls
Lesion below T1	Complete innervation of arms Totally independent wheelchair life Can drive with hand controls

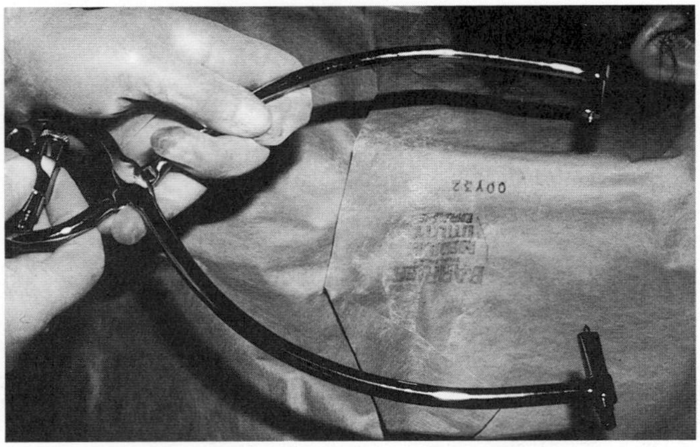

Fig. 2 Skull traction using Gardner–Wells calliper.

operative intervention and fusion aids neurological recovery. Practice varies from country to country and indeed from centre to centre. In a broad-based survey in the United States 60 per cent of people underwent spinal surgery. Most individuals underwent fusion and internal fixation, but increasing numbers also now undergo anterior or posterior decompression of the spinal cord with or without internal fixation and fusion. However, practice in the United States tends to be more oriented towards surgical intervention than in the United Kingdom and other parts of Western Europe. In the United Kingdom, surgical intervention will tend to be reserved for those with unstable displaced fractures, whereas conservative management would be the normal practice for stable and/or undisplaced fractures. However, if the neurological symptoms are deteriorating then many spinal centres would now recommend surgical intervention.

Use of steroids

Another treatment intervention that can be considered in the very early stages after injury is a short course of high-dose methylprednisolone. There is some evidence that such intervention, started within 8 h of injury, improves the neurological outcome. However, this is not totally accepted and such practice not uniform. The results of further trials are awaited.

Management in the spinal cord injury centre

Initial management will consist of resuscitation, treatment of associated injuries, and stabilization of the spine, either conservatively or by surgical intervention. However, the individual should be transferred to a recognized spinal injury centre as soon as possible. There is clear evidence that the outcome is maximized, both physically and psychologically, if individuals are managed in such centres as opposed to a less co-ordinated and less experienced approach in another hospital setting.

Management of the spine

As mentioned above, the injured person will either be managed conservatively or surgically. The advantage of surgery is that the individual can be mobilized more quickly. If a conservative approach is adopted, mobilization and active rehabilitation is obviously difficult in the first few weeks. Cervical spine traction is normally maintained for around 6 weeks and then monitored for signs of bony union and stability. Once the fracture site is stable the individual can be gradually sat up in bed whilst continuing with cervical support. A profiling bed, which enables a more natural seated position to be adopted, is most useful. In the early few weeks a halo brace can be used instead of skull traction. The advantage of this brace (see Fig. 3) is to allow early mobilization. The halo brace is kept on for between 10 and 12 weeks until the site is stable. In those with thoracolumbar injuries, who are usually managed conservatively, the period of bed rest will usually last from 8 to 12 weeks followed by bracing and gradual mobilization, assuming that the fracture site is stable.

A number of medical problems can occur over this initial period of immobilization.

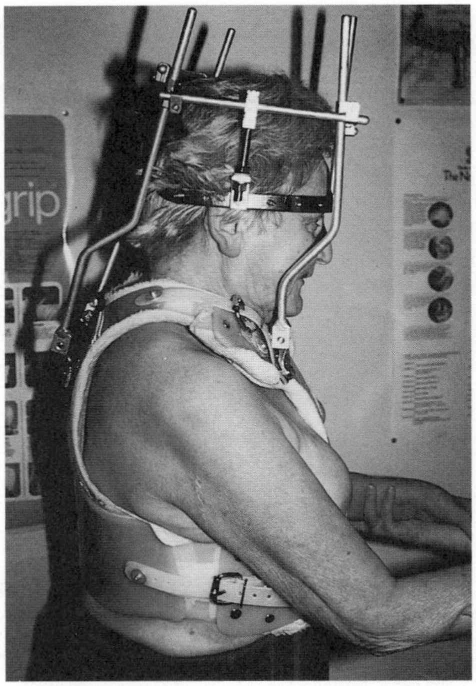

Fig. 3 Illustration of a halo brace.

Management of medical problems

Respiratory problems

Respiratory insufficiency can occur in people with cervical cord injuries. Intercostal muscles may be paralysed, and in high cervical lesions the diaphragm can also be paralysed. However, even in people with lower lesions, respiratory problems can still occur from associated injuries such as rib or sternal fractures. Since respiratory function can decline several hours or even days after injury, probably due to the development of spinal cord oedema, respiratory function should therefore be monitored carefully and ventilation provided if required. Regular chest physiotherapy is vital at this time. Since pulmonary embolism is also a risk, particularly in those immobilized, anticoagulation is advisable prior to mobilization.

Pressure sores

Regrettably, the development of pressure sores still occurs even with high-quality care. Sores are commonest where there are bony prominences near the skin: such as the ischial tuberosity, greater trochanter, sacrum, heel, and sometimes at the back of the head in those with skull traction. A key to prevention is awareness of the potential problem, with vigilance, regular changes of position in bed, and regular lifting in the wheelchair. A large range of commercial mattresses and wheelchair cushions are available that relieve pressure. Shear forces should be avoided as far as possible when lifting or positioning the patient; and obviously the individual should never be dragged over sheets or from the wheelchair. The skin should be kept clean, with particular care taken to avoid any urine or faecal soiling. If a sore does occur then the area must be kept clean, any dead tissue be removed, and there should be complete relief of pressure from that area until it is fully healed. Occasionally, surgery is indicated for larger or deeply infected sores that otherwise would take too long to heal. Education of the injured person and their family is essential. Despite awareness of the problem around 25 per cent of people still develop a pressure sore during the rehabilitation phase. About 15 per cent of people will develop a pressure sore in the first year following discharge—a figure that increases still further with time, such that by year 10 about 15 per cent of those with incomplete lesions and 28 per cent of those with complete lesions will have developed at least one pressure sore. Septicaemia from pressure sores is still responsible for around 10 per cent of deaths in people with spinal injury.

Bladder problems

In the early part of this century, problems, usually infection, of the urinary system were responsible for at least half the deaths of those with spinal injury. Although very significant progress has been made in the management of bladder and kidney problems, nevertheless urinary tract complications are still the leading residual cause of mortality and morbidity.

During the period of spinal shock the bladder is usually non-contractile, so that catheterization may be appropriate at this time. Once spinal shock begins to wear off the commonest problem is of detrusor hyperreflexia, which usually gives rise to the frequent passage of small quantities of urine associated with urgency. However, other possibilities include detrusor sphincter dyssynergia and detrusor hyporeflexia. The latter will tend to occur when there is damage to the S2, 3, and 4 sacral nerves.

The management of urinary problems usually involves obtaining satisfactory answers to three questions:

- Is there impairment of renal function?
- Is there a failure of bladder emptying?
- Is there detrusor hyperreflexia?

Is there impairment of renal function?

Screening of the upper urinary tract is important both in the short and long term. Intravenous urography should be used in the early months after injury, but long-term follow-up can often be carried out by renal ultrasound scanning or plain abdominal radiography. Late complications are possible, such as renal calculi. Cystometrography is also vital for determining the exact nature of the underlying bladder and sphincter problems.

Is there a failure of bladder emptying?

A residual urine volume greater than 100 ml is generally accepted as the level at which intervention is necessary. Residual urine can predispose to infection and stone formation, and contributes to impairment of renal function, particularly if the failure to empty is associated with a high intravesical pressure and back-pressure up to the kidney. Occasionally, failure of emptying can be managed by artificial stimulation such as suprapubic tapping or perineal stimulation. However, in most cases failure of bladder emptying requires mechanical drainage. The most useful method is intermittent, clean self-catheterization. This is carried out by the disabled person, or sometimes by a carer, four or five times every 24 h such that volumes in the bladder are kept to less than 500 ml. Intermittent self-catheterization has revolutionized the management of bladder problems in those with spinal injury. Anticholinergic drugs, such as propantheline, oxybutynin, or imipramine, may sometimes help to reduce detrusor activity. Condom drainage in the male is helpful in preventing leakage between catheterizations. A silastic indwelling catheter might need to be used if intermittent self-catheterization is impossible. However, suprapubic catheterization is far better in the long term and is associated with less problems. Regrettably, there are many problems of catheterization, including leakage, blockage, stone formation, and infection.

Is there detrusor hyperreflexia?

A small number of people can control minor problems with the detrusor hyperreflexia by rigid bladder drill, emptying the bladder at frequent and regular intervals. However, most people need some form of oral medication and, as above, anticholinergics are the most effective, and oxybutynin the most common—propantheline and imipramine are alternatives. Once again, protection against the embarrassment of leakage is often necessary and is more readily achieved in men with the use of condom drainage. A variety of absorbent pads can be worn by women. Advice from a specially trained nurse continence advisor can be invaluable whatever the nature of the problem.

A whole variety of surgical techniques may be applicable in particular circumstances. An endoscopic distal sphincterotomy can be useful for those with reflex bladder emptying. The technique of bladder augmentation with an ileocystoplasty can also be helpful to allow for sufficient capacity for intermittent, clean self-catheterization. Fortunately, urinary diversion techniques are now needed less frequently. Recent advances include artificial urinary sphincters for treating neuropathic incontinence. Some centres also now employ sacral anterior nerve root stimulators that can be used in some people with suprasacral cord lesions. For instance, the bladder can be emptied by activating a radio-linked implant to stimulate the S2, S3, and S4 anterior nerve roots. Occasionally, a similar implant can also be used to assist in defecation and in obtaining a penile erection.

Incontinence can be a major disability and handicap, and, indeed if not treated properly, the complications can be life-threatening. Long-term follow-up is essential, and proper management can make significant reductions in long-term risks and produce major improvements in the quality of life.

Bowel care

During the initial period of spinal shock the bowel remains flaccid and should not be allowed to overdistend, with the attendant risk of constipation and overflow incontinence. Manual evacuation is usually carried out until bowel activity returns. Eventually, reflex emptying can occur in those with predominant upper motor neurone lesions, but the bowel can remain flaccid in those with lower motor neurone involvement. In the former, bowel evacuation can usually be triggered by glycerin suppository or by anal digital stimulation. In those with flaccid bowel there is a continuing need to evacuate manually or by straining using abdominal muscles. Advice on proper diet is also required, with a good-quality, high-fibre diet being the most helpful.

Autonomic dysreflexia

This is a potentially fatal problem most commonly seen in those with cervical cord injuries above the sympathetic outflow, but it can occur in those with high thoracic lesions above T6. Autonomic dysreflexia is characterized by an exaggerated autonomic response to a stimulus below the level of the lesion. Stimuli can include distension of the pelvic organs such as the bladder, colon, and rectum: such distension induces sympathetic activity resulting in vasoconstriction and hypertension. Other stimuli include catheterization, urinary infections, sexual intercourse, pressure sores, and even tight clothing; surgical procedures can also induce the reflex. Symptoms include headaches, sweating, vasodilatation, nasal obstruction, paraesthesia, and anxiety. Significant hypertension also occurs. The problem occurs in around 50 to 80 per cent of those at risk, with most cases occurring between 2 and 12 months' postinjury. Other than awareness of the problem and avoidance of the necessary stimuli, attention is directed to reducing blood pressure. Sublingual nifedipine can be used, or intravenous hydralazine in more severe cases. Chlorpromazine, nitroprusside, and diazoxide are also possibilities. Occasionally, the sympathetic reflex activity may have to be blocked by spinal epidural anaesthetic.

Spasticity and contractures

Spasticity occurs in an upper motor lesion with intact spinal reflex arcs below the level of the lesion. It is usually worse in those with incomplete lesions. Spasticity can be functionally useful and the individual can sometimes use flexor or extension spasms as an aid to dressing. However, spasticity usually produces functional problems as well as causing pain. In the long term there is a significant risk of muscle contractures. Initial management focuses on removing any unnecessary exacerbating factors such as pressure sores, tight catheter leg bags, or even urinary infections and constipation. Treatment should always involve an expert neurological physiotherapist who will advise on appropriate positioning and seating. In the early stages, passive stretching of the spastic muscles and regular standing regimes can be helpful; in the longer term, such regimes can often be taken on by the disabled person and their carers. Although antispastic drugs should always be used with care as they induce significant tiredness and weakness, they can provide some useful background antispastic effect. Baclofen, dantrolene, and tizanidine are the commonest prescribed. The latter is a more recently introduced drug, at least in the United Kingdom, and is an effective antispastic agent that appears to produce less weakness than the other available drugs. However, spasticity is often localized and focal treatment is more appropriate. Nerve blocks with phenol and alcohol can be used, but intramuscular botulinum toxin has recently proved very useful in the management of spasticity. The toxin is injected directly into the muscle and blocks the release of acetylcholine from nerve endings, which, over 2 or 3 days, produces a muscle relaxation that lasts for 2 to 3 months. Occasionally, more severe spasticity will need other treatment measures, such as the use of intrathecal baclofen. If contractures have resulted, surgical correction by tenotomy, tendon lengthening, or muscle division is often the only way to get the limb back into a functionally useful position. Aggressive early management of spasticity is important in order to maximize any neurological recovery and prevent unnecessary complications.

Heterotopic ossification

This term is used when bone develops in an abnormal anatomical position in soft tissues. The prevalence in spinal cord injury is reported to vary between 5 and 50 per cent. Heterotopic ossification commonly occurs around the hips and knees, causing a decrease in the range of movement as well as localized swelling and joint effusion. It normally occurs during the first few months after the injury and will only rarely begin later than 1-year postinjury. Unfortunately treatment is difficult. Etidronate disodium (Didronel) is probably the most useful treatment. Surgical intervention can be required in severe cases, but is usually unsatisfactory. Some centres now use prophylactic etidronate disodium for about a year.

Deep venous thrombosis

Deep venous thrombosis still remains a significant complication after spinal injury, with a small risk of death from pulmonary embolism. Heparin is generally used as a prophylactic but some centres now use external pneumatic calf compression.

Pain and dysaesthesia

Peripheral pain is quite common in the early weeks after injury. Although, burning pain can, unfortunately, also continue for some months, it usually responds reasonably well to the use of carbamazepine, tricyclic antidepressants, or gabapentin. Pain from other sources such as osteoarthritis can also occur. It should be remembered that people with spinal cord injury do not always appreciate pain or that it is manifested in different ways, such as autonomic dysreflexia or worsening of spasticity. Treatment modalities—for example, transcutaneous nerve stimulation, acupuncture, and psychological techniques, such as relaxation and hypnotherapy or alleviation of depressive illness—can all help. Spinal cord stimulation is occasionally used, as are surgical techniques, such as dorsal-root, entry-zone radiofrequency coagulation. Other causes of pain such as nerve root compression should also be borne in mind.

Rehabilitation

There is no evidence that rehabilitation can promote natural recovery, but there is ample evidence that a co-ordinated multidisciplinary team can improve functional outcome for the person with a spinal cord injury. The team can ensure that functional abilities are maximized and that physical and psychological complications are kept to a minimum. The co-ordinated team input is vital during the early weeks and months after injury, but it is equally important that the team maintains contact over the period of discharge and indeed into the longer term.

Principles of rehabilitation

There is no room in this chapter to dwell on the basic principles of rehabilitation. However, it is important to state that modern rehabilitation practice is somewhat different from other medical specialties. It is based on the principles of education and is a process in which the disabled person and the family must be involved for it to have any meaning. Rehabilitation should go beyond the narrower confines of physical disease to also deal with the psychological consequences of physical disability and with the social milieu in which the disabled person has to operate.

Rehabilitation is based around the concepts of impairment, disability, and handicap as outlined by the World Health Organization in 1980. 'Impairment' is simply a term that describes a loss or abnormality of psychological, physiological, or anatomical structure or function. Rehabilitation must go beyond impairment and should place such impairment within a functional context—the 'disability'. 'Handicap' describes the social context of disability. Rehabilitation can be defined as an active and dynamic process by which a disabled person is helped to acquire knowledge and skills in order to maximize physical, psychological, and social function.

The basic nature of rehabilitation is to work with the disabled person and their family in partnership. The professional should impart accurate information and advice, give guidance on prognosis and natural history, and help the individual to establish realistic goals in an appropriate social context.

A key to successful rehabilitation is goal-setting. The first goal should be a long-distance strategic aim. In the context of spinal cord injury this could, for example, include enabling the person to return to their previous home fully competent in wheelchair use. The overall strategic goal can also have a number of long-term subgoals in different spheres of life such as employment, home, and leisure. Once the long-term goal has been determined, steps will need to be defined to achieve that goal, which in turn will involve setting a number of short- and medium-term goals. These shorter term aims should be clearly stated. A useful mnemonic is SMART: that is, the goals should be specific, measurable, achievable, relevant, and time-limited. The implication of goal-setting is that the team, and indeed the disabled person, should know when the goals have been achieved. Thus, valid and reliable outcome measures are important tools; but it is neither possible nor desirable to outline such tools. The outcome measures will depend on the goals set. However, it is often useful to employ a general disability measure such as the Functional Independence Measure or, in the short term, the more physically oriented Barthel Score. Some of the standard scales employed in the field of spinal cord injury are frankly of little value in monitoring progress. First to be developed was the Frankel Score. This has now been largely superseded, at least in the United States, by the 1992 revised American Spinal Injury Association Classification (see Table 3). Although this scale is now widely quoted in the spinal cord literature (mainly in terms for helping to determine natural history and prognosis), it is not a tool for monitoring goal attainment.

Rehabilitation team

Medical input is obviously vital to the team, particularly during the early acute stages of management. Spinal cord injury consultants are now trained rehabilitation specialists who do not necessarily have surgical qualifications. However, spinal cord injury centres will always need input from spinal surgeons, as well as assistance from urologists and a variety of other medical consultants. Because of their 24-h daily contact with the injured person, nursing staff on the ward are clearly vital team members, many of whom possess additional spinal cord injury or other specialist qualifications; for example, in giving continence advice or in the management of sexual problems.

Table 3 American Spinal Injury Association Classification

Grade A	Complete	No sensory or motor function preserved in sacral segments S4/5
Grade B	Incomplete	Sensory, but not motor, function is preserved below the neurological level and extends through the sacral segments S4/5
Grade C	Incomplete	Motor function is preserved below the neurological level, and the majority of key muscles below the neurological level have a muscle grade less than 3
Grade D	Incomplete	Motor function is preserved below the neurological level, and the majority of key muscles below the neurological level have a muscle grade greater than or equal to 3
Grade E	Normal	Sensory and motor function is normal

The key muscles are C5 (elbow flexors), C6 (wrist extensors), C7 (elbow extensors), C8 (finger flexors), T1 (small-finger adductors), L2 (hip flexors), L3 (knee extensors), ankle dorsiflexors, long-toe extensors, and ankle plantar flexes.

The physiotherapist's role during the very early stages of management is to minimize chest complications, particularly in those with high cervical cord lesions. Physiotherapy advice is helpful to ensure the patient is correctly positioned in bed and to prevent the complication of spasticity. Once a patient is beginning to mobilize the physiotherapist is the key person to advise on the choice of wheelchair and for teaching the individual to become familiar with all aspects of its control. A number of advanced wheelchair skills will eventually be learnt, such as back-wheel balancing, to allow manoeuvrability over rough ground and up kerbs, and sideways jumping for manoeuvrability in a limited space. In people with lower cord lesions the physiotherapists can be involved in providing limited gait training using callipers and crutches. Orthotic devices, such as the reciprocating-gait orthosis (**RGO**) and hip-guidance orthosis (**HGO**), may be considered in some cases. The physiotherapist can also help in the context of handicap by encouraging and assisting with the development of sporting activities. However, this assistance clearly overlaps with the role of the occupational therapist.

The occupational therapist is usually concerned with assisting people to reach their highest level of physical and psychological independence, particularly with regard to personal care and appropriate adaptation of the home, work, and leisure environments. For example, the occupational therapist will be involved in the design of appropriate splinting (for example, writing or typing splints and feeding straps) to assist those with high cord lesions. Many increasingly sophisticated assistive technology devices are now available to enable even those with profound disabilities to remain reasonably independent. For instance, environmental control equipment will enable an individual to operate a door intercom, turn lights on and off, turn the pages of a book, control the television, and use a telephone and computer, etc. Even people with high tetraplegia can control these devices using mouth sticks or breath control. The occupational therapist will often be involved in giving such advice, particularly at the time of discharge back into the home environment.

If necessary, a psychologist may be particularly useful in enabling the person to make an emotional adjustment to their new disability.

The social worker is likely to be involved with the family as a whole, and only a small part of the job is to advise on disability benefits. Most of the social worker's task is to ensure that the disabled person and family integrate and adapt to the new disability as smoothly as possible.

At some point, others, such as vocational advisors, specialist nurses, and dieticians, will all need to be part of the comprehensive spinal injury team.

Long-term issues in spinal cord injury

Discharge home

A particularly difficult time for the injured person is discharge home. Often the person will have spent several weeks or months in a spinal cord centre and returning home can be a traumatic process both for the injured person and their family. Brief, trial home visits will almost certainly have been carried out beforehand. These visits are particularly important for ensuring that the house is appropriately adapted. Obviously in some cases a new house or bungalow will need to be purchased. A number of adaptations regarding access, both internal and external, hoisting gear, adaptations to the toilet, bathroom, and kitchen may all be required before the individual can return home. Environmental control equipment may need to be prescribed and installed. Psychological support is also vital over this period not only for the injured person but for their family. Anxiety and depressive illness are both quite common and will need active intervention. The community services and the primary care team will need to be involved. Planned discharges are vital and should involve a case conference between the hospital and community staff to ensure a smooth hand-over. However, at this time many spinal cord injured people will wish to move away from the more paternalistic hospital care that was important during the first few weeks' postinjury. Most will choose to live as independently as possible, albeit with the help of their family or a personal assistant. Advice on the available financial support is important. If financial compensation from a personal injury claim is ongoing then a solicitor can be helpful at this point to arrange interim payments from the Court towards the costs of home adaptations, transport, and personal care.

Emotional problems

Obviously there are profound changes in one's life following spinal cord injury. The refocusing of life ambitions can be a frustrating, anxious, or depressing time. The attitude of family and friends will have a further bearing over the period of adjustment. Regrettably, clinical depression is common and occurs at some point in at least 50 per cent of individuals. Suicide can also occur. Whilst such problems are not always preventable, anxiety, depression, and adjustment problems can be alleviated by appropriate intervention. Although the role of medication, at least in the short term, can be helpful, probably most assistance can be provided by cognitive therapy or other forms of counselling and psychological support. Contact with others in similar circumstances can often be helpful and may be facilitated through the various peer support groups.

Sexual life

Sexual ability depends on the level and completeness of the spinal lesion. Sexual readjustment is an important part of the rehabilitation process both for the injured person and their partner, regardless of gender. Self-image and self-confidence can be severely affected. Individuals should be counselled about the totality of sexuality as there is a tendency for discussions to focus on penetrative sexual intercourse. In both sexes, absence of genital sensation can be compensated for by the use of other erogenous zones such as the breasts, neck, and mouth. Orgasm is sometimes possible even in those with complete spinal cord lesions. In women, problems can result from the lack of vaginal lubrication. In men, various techniques and devices are available to restore erectile capacity. Most people with complete upper motor neurone lesions will have reflex but not psychogenic erections; however, these are often not always sustained or strong enough for intercourse. Reflex erections are usually impossible in those with parasympathetic lesions. A satisfactory erection can often be achieved either by the use of intracavernosal drugs or mechanical means such as vacuum erection aids and compressive retainer rings. However, the recent introduction of sildenafil (Viagra) is beginning to reduce the need for mechanical or injected assistance.

Fertility

Fertility is not usually reduced in women, although some can go through a time of amenorrhoea. However, fertility is generally reduced in men who have low sperm counts with diminished motility. Sometimes if ejaculation is not possible during intercourse it can be induced by direct stimulation or by electroejaculation. Fertility can also be improved by some of the modern assistive conception techniques such as *in vitro* fertilization and intracytoplasmic sperm injection. Women with spinal cord injury who become pregnant may have some problems in labour, particularly if the lesion is complete above T10. Autonomic dysreflexia is also a risk during labour. However, spinal cord injury is not by itself an indication for caesarean section.

Later medical complications

All the complications listed above in the acute phase can, of course, occur later. This is why it is so important for the multidisciplinary team to keep an overview of the individual in the long term. However, a few other problems are more likely to occur in the long term:

- Pathological fractures—there is a higher risk of osteoporosis in paralysed limbs and thus pathological fractures may occur with minimal trauma. For example, a minor fall from a chair or even a flexor spasm secondary to spasticity can result in a fractured leg. Treatment should usually be conservative.
- Post-traumatic syringomyelia—this occurs in about 4 per cent of people and consists of an ascending myelopathy due to secondary cavitation in the central part of the spinal cord. The problem is commonly delayed several years' postinjury. It presents with pain in the arm with a characteristic disassociated sensory loss: reduced pain and temperature sensation but preservation of proprioception. Motor loss of the lower motor neurone type occurs and occasionally sensory loss can spread up to the face (syringobulbia). Surgical treatment including decompression and drainage of the cavity may be necessary.
- Respiratory management—those with high cervical cord lesions with lost diaphragmatic function obviously require long-term ventilatory support. Modern portable ventilators can be readily mounted on a wheelchair. Speech is entirely possible with an uncuffed tracheostomy tube that allows air to escape to the larynx. In some people it is possible to implant a phrenic nerve stimulator to achieve diaphragmatic ventilation. Regrettably, it is still the case that individuals with long-term, ventilator-dependent requirements have significantly more morbidity and mortality than those with lower lesions.

Leisure pursuits

A wide variety of leisure pursuits are now possible for those with spinal cord injury. Although integration to able-bodied clubs and pursuits is obviously to be encouraged, a reasonable range of sports and other clubs exists for those with spinal injuries. Wheelchair skills can be finely tuned to develop expertise in a variety of sports. Physical access to leisure and social outlets is improving, albeit very slowly. Recent legislation, such as the Disability Discrimination Act in the United Kingdom, should further improve the situation.

Driving

Access to a motor vehicle is vital in modern society. Driving should be entirely possible for people with spinal cord injury, with the probable exception of those with very high cervical cord lesions. Automatic transmission is vital and hand controls are usually essential. Hand controls enable the individual to control the accelerator and brake functions from a lever or other device near the steering wheel. A variety of infrared devices to control secondary functions such as windscreen wipers, lights, and horn are now available. Very light-powered steering makes life easier for those with weak grip. Those with higher cord lesions who can still retain some useful shoulder and upper arm function can still drive a car using a variety of commercial devices attached to the steering wheel. A number of techniques can be taught to stow wheelchairs safely for those with paraplegia, and for those with higher lesions there are a number of mechanical wheelchair stowage devices. It is also quite possible to adapt a suitable vehicle to enable people to drive from their wheelchair. Financial advice is often required, combined with advice on the range and type of possible adaptations. The United Kingdom now has a number of driving assessment centres, often attached to rehabilitation centres.

Employment

Between 25 and 35 per cent of people with spinal cord injuries return to work, either in their original occupation or, after a period of retraining, to a new job. The chances of employment are higher in the younger population and in those who already had a job at the time of injury. There is also a positive correlation with the number of years of education. Fortunately, employment should become more prevalent as the ability to work at home becomes more readily acceptable. The individual should be encouraged to contact disablement employment advisors who can provide both advice and financial help for a return to work. In other cases, careers' advice or retraining to obtain new qualifications may be more appropriate.

Information

The key to independence is access to good-quality information. In most countries there are now voluntary organizations that can provide such information and advice. These organizations can also act as pressure groups, many of which have been instrumental in promoting increased awareness and improved legislation for disabled people. The Internet now provides an excellent source of information and advice, and training in computer literacy should certainly be encouraged by the rehabilitation team.

Conclusions

The management of spinal cord injury can pose a range of challenges to the multidisciplinary rehabilitation team. Although we cannot yet promote natural recovery in spinal cord injury, such interventions may be possible in the future. However, our failure to influence the natural history of a spinal cord injury should certainly not inhibit active and dynamic rehabilitation to enable the individual to resume as normal a life as possible. The application of modern rehabilitation practice, together with greater social awareness and understanding, has led to significant improvements in the overall survival and quality of life of people with spinal cord injuries.

Useful addresses

Spinal Injuries Association, 76 St James Lane, London N10 3DF. Tel: +44 (0) 181 444 2121. This association, for spinal cord injured people and all involved in their care, produces an excellent quarterly newsletter.

Further reading

Archives of Physical Medicine and Rehabilitation (1999). Spinal cord injury—current research outcomes from the model spinal cord injury care systems. *Archives of Physical Medicine and Rehabilitation* **80**, Special issue. [An entire edition of the journal devoted to spinal cord injury and current research outcomes from the model spinal cord injury care systems. A comprehensive review of the whole subject.]

Barbeau H, *et al.* (1999). Walking after spinal cord injury: evaluation, treatment and functional recovery. *Archives of Physical Medicine and Rehabilitation* **80**, 225–35. [A useful review article regarding modern developments to promote ambulation after spinal injury.]

Barnes MP, Ward AB (2000). *Textbook of rehabilitation medicine.* Oxford University Medical Publications, Oxford. [General background text in rehabilitation medicine for the undergraduate and junior postgraduate.]

Berkowitz M, *et al.* (1992). *The economic consequences of traumatic spinal cord injury.* Demos, New York.

Ditunno JF (1999). Predicting recovery after spinal cord injury: a rehabilitation imperative. *Archives of Physical Medicine and Rehabilitation* **80**, 361–3. [An up-to-date source of references regarding natural history.]

Giménez y Ribotta M, Privat A (1998). Biological interventions for spinal cord injury. *Current Opinion in Neurology* **11**, 647–54. [A useful and brief review article covering future possible interventions to promote natural recovery following spinal cord injury.]

Grundy D, Swain A (1996). *ABC of spinal cord injury,* 3rd edn. BMJ Publishing Group, London. [A very useful general text.]

Rehabilitation Institute of Chicago Procedure Manual (1994). *Spinal cord injury—medical management and rehabilitation.* Aspen, Maryland.[A thorough text on medical aspects of spinal cord injury.]

Trieschmann RB (1988). *Spinal cord injuries—psychological, social and vocational rehabilitation,* 2nd edn. Demos, New York. [One of the few volumes to thoroughly discuss the psychological, social, and vocational problems after spinal injury.]

Wade DT (1992). *Measurement in neurological rehabilitation.* Oxford University Press, Oxford. [An invaluable textbook outlining a number of important and useful outcome scales.]

World Health Organization (1980). International classification of impairments, disabilities and handicaps. World Health Organization, Albany, NY.

World Health Organization (1998). *The world health report—1998. Life in the 21st century vision overall.* WHO, Geneva. [A useful reference for a number of world health issues and in particular includes a discussion of the new classification of impairments, activities, and participation.]

24.13.18 Traumatic injuries of the head

24.13.18.1 Intracranial tumours

Jeremy Rees

Introduction

Intracranial tumours comprise primary tumours that originate from the brain, cranial nerves, pituitary gland, or meninges and secondary tumours (metastases) that arise from organs outside the nervous system. These tumours present to many different specialists and their management is difficult because of their location and their variable clinical manifestations.

Aetiology

There are no known risk factors apart from prior irradiation to the skull and a few rare neurogenetic syndromes, such as neurofibromatosis (optic nerve glioma, meningioma, vestibular schwannoma) (Fig. 1), von Hippel–Lindau syndrome (haemangioblastoma), and Li–Fraumeni syndrome (glioma).

Epidemiology

Intracranial tumours represent the sixth most common neoplasm in adults (approximately 8 per cent of all primary neoplasms) and the second most common neoplasm in children. After stroke, intracranial tumours are the leading cause of death from neurological disease in the United Kingdom.

Based on a recent Scottish study, the crude annual incidence for primary intracranial tumours is 15.3 per 100 000 and for secondary tumours 14.3 per 100 000 population. There is evidence that the incidence is increasing, particularly in elderly patients. Different tumour types present at different ages. Supratentorial gliomas are uncommon below the age of 30 years but become increasingly prevalent thereafter. The most frequent tumours of middle life (third and fourth decades) are astrocytomas, meningiomas, pituitary adenomas, and vestibular schwannomas, while glioblastoma multiforme and metastases are more frequent in the fifth and six decades of life. In contrast, children tend to have infratentorial tumours: 70 per cent of childhood primary intracranial tumours originate below the tentorium cerebelli, whereas in adults the figure is only 25 per cent. There is a strong female preponderance of meningiomas and schwannomas, whereas slightly more men have astrocytomas.

Pathogenesis

Certain genetic lesions are associated with brain tumours. Chromosomal deletions—particularly chromosome 10, which contains multiple tumour suppressor genes—are found in astrocytic tumours, occurring in up to 70 per cent of glioblastomas. Mutations of a tumour suppressor gene *p53*, located on chromosome 17p, have also been reported in approximately 40 per cent of astrocytic tumours. In general the accumulation of predictable genetic alterations is associated with increasing malignant progression.

Clinical features

With increasing sophistication of neuroimaging, tumours are being detected at an earlier stage than before. Patients typically present with one or more of four clinical syndromes:

- progressive neurological deficit
- seizures
- raised intracranial pressure
- altered mental states.

The particular combination of clinical features varies depending on the location, histology, and rate of growth of the tumour. For instance, patients with low-grade gliomas present typically with a seizure disorder that may remain static for many years, while patients with malignant gliomas typically develop a rapidly progressive neurological deficit and raised intracranial pressure

Progressive neurological deficit

Focal neurological symptoms due to brain tumour are typically subacute and progressive with over 50 per cent of patients having focal signs by the time of diagnosis. Cortical tumours produce contralateral weakness, sensory loss, dysphasia, dyspraxia, and visual field loss depending on their location. Posterior fossa tumours cause ataxia and cranial nerve palsies. Vestibular schwannomas cause progressive unilateral deafness followed by ipsilateral facial sensory loss. Pituitary tumours may cause a bitemporal hemianopia if there is chiasmal compression or endocrine disturbances due to either hypopituitarism or hypersecretion of specific hormones.

Seizure disorder

Brain tumours account for about 5 per cent of epilepsy cases although they are over-represented in cases of intractable epilepsy. Seizures are the presenting symptom in 25 to 30 per cent of patients with gliomas and are present at some stage of the illness in 40 to 60 per cent overall. Approximately half the patients have focal seizures and the other half have secondarily generalized seizures. Low-grade gliomas are associated with seizures in over 90 per cent of cases and these frequently remain the only complaint for many years. Conversely, malignant gliomas have a lower frequency of seizures, presumably because of their more rapid growth and destructive characteristics. In these patients, seizures are associated with a better prognosis. Seizures are also common initial manifestations of meningiomas (40 to 60 per cent) and metastases (15 to 20 per cent). Supratentorial tumours and those superficially located are particularly likely to cause seizures, particularly in the frontal and temporal lobes. A Todd's paresis, which may persist, is an uncommon but characteristic feature of tumour-associated epilepsy. About 10 per cent of patients presenting *de novo* in status epilepticus have an underlying tumour.

Raised intracranial pressure

Intracranial tumours increase intracranial pressure either by a direct mass effect, by provoking cerebral oedema, or by producing obstructive hydrocephalus. The most common symptom of raised intracranial pressure is headache, which is the presenting symptom in 25 to 35 per cent of patients; papilloedema is found in up to 50 per cent of patients with headache due to tumours. The classic picture of headache, vomiting, and visual obscurations (transient fogging of vision usually on rapid changes in posture) due to raised intracranial pressure is well known and easily recognized, but most patients present before this develops. Less than 1 per cent of patients presenting with isolated headache has a brain tumour.

Most brain tumour headaches are intermittent and non-specific and may be indistinguishable from tension headaches. Supratentorial tumours typically produce frontal headaches, while posterior fossa tumours usually result in occipital headache or neck pain. Certain features of a headache are suggestive but not pathognomic of raised intracranial pressure. These include headaches that wake the patient at night or are worse on waking and improve over the course of the day.

Mental state changes

These are an uncommon presentation of brain tumours occurring in about 20 per cent of patients at diagnosis. Personality changes may initially be quite subtle and may show themselves as an inability to cope at work. In

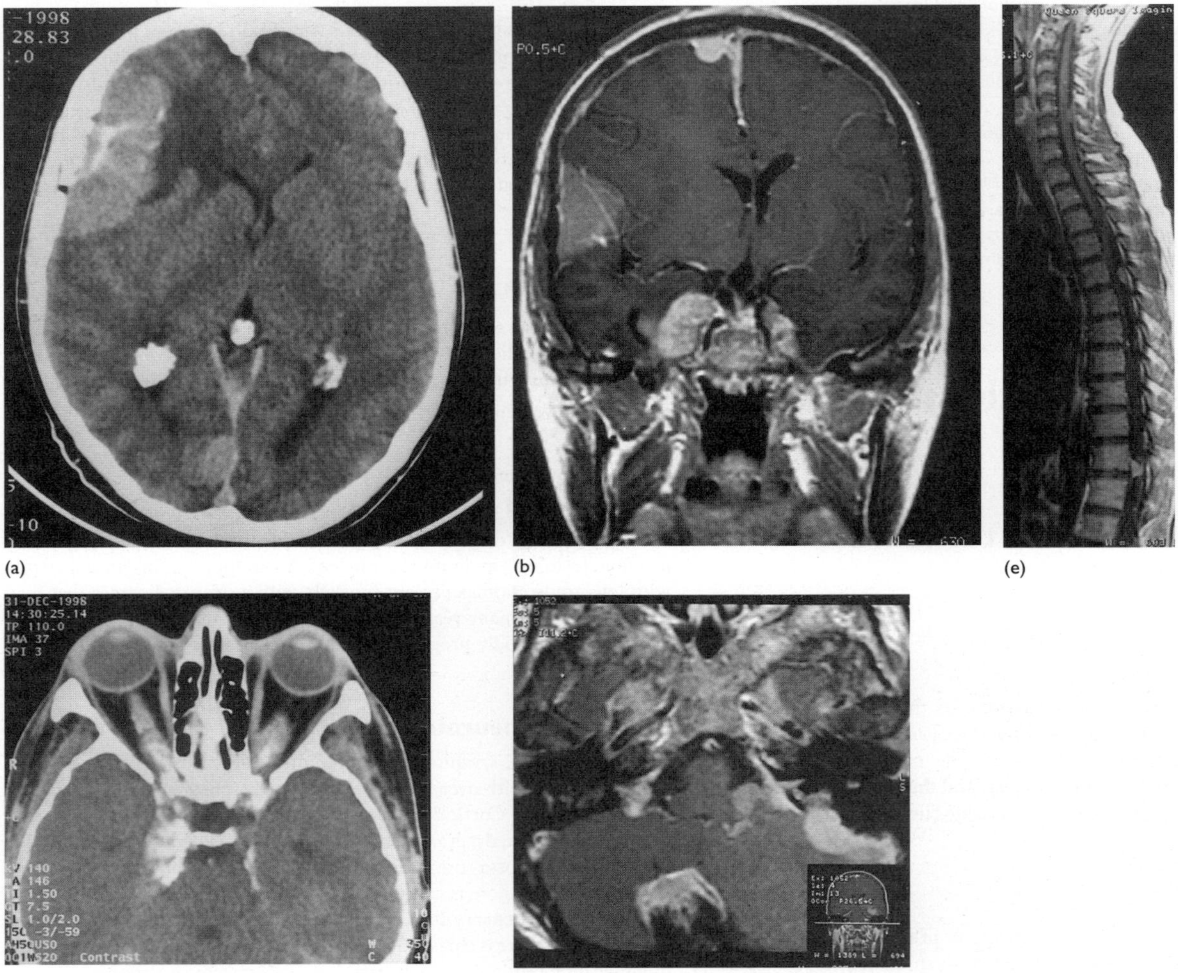

Fig. 1 Contrast-enhanced CT and MR scans of a patient with neurofibromatosis type 2 and multiple intracranial tumours. (a) CT of the brain with gadolinium enhancement showing a large right parietal convexity meningioma surrounded by vasogenic oedema exerting considerable mass effect. There is also a smaller falx meningioma in the right occipital region. (b) Coronal T_1-weighted MRI of the brain with gadolinium enhancement showing multiple meningiomas in the right temporoparietal region, right parafalcine region, and both cavernous sinuses. (c) Contrast-enhanced CT scan of the orbits showing bilateral optic nerve sheath meningiomas with intracranial extension into the right cavernous sinus causing a partial right third nerve and sixth nerve palsies. (d) Axial T_1-weighted MRI of the brain with gadolinium enhancement showing bilateral vestibular nerve schwannomas, and a large fourth ventricle tumour. (e) Sagittal T_1-weighted MRI of the spinal cord with gadolinium enhancement showing three discrete meningiomas encroaching on the spinal column at mid-cervical, mid-thoracic, and upper lumbar levels.

these cases it is essential to obtain a collateral history from relatives or colleagues at work.

Pathology

Neuroepithelial tumours (predominantly gliomas) account for approximately 50 to 60 per cent of all primary brain tumours. The other common types are meningiomas (20 per cent), pituitary adenomas (15 per cent), vestibular schwannomas (5 per cent), and primary central nervous system lymphomas (5 per cent). The most common sites of origin of secondary tumours are lung (50 per cent), breast (15 per cent), melanoma (10 per cent), and unknown (15 per cent).

The gliomas are a family of neoplasms that arise from astrocytes, oligodendrocytes, and ependymal cells. Astrocytomas are the most common type of glioma and are infiltrating neoplasms composed of fibrillary astrocytes. Almost all of these tumours have the propensity to undergo anaplastic change to a more malignant lesion. Thus a fibrillary astrocytoma (Fig. 2) progresses to an anaplastic astrocytoma (Fig. 3) and then to the most malignant form, glioblastoma multiforme. This process occurs more often and more rapidly in older patients. The grading systems that have been used have attempted to describe degrees of anaplastic change and thereby correlate the histological appearances with prognosis. The most widely accepted classifications of gliomas are the World Health Organization three-tiered system and the St Anne–Mayo grading system as shown in Table 1. These systems have been retrospectively applied to large series of patients and have been shown to provide reproducible and prognostically useful information. A rare type of astrocytoma is the oligodendroglioma characterized by the presence of uniform round nuclei with small nucleoli. This also has the propensity to undergo anaplastic change but unlike anaplastic astrocytomas, oligodendrogliomas are frequently chemosensitive (see below).

Diagnosis

The diagnosis of a brain tumour is made by a combination of CT/MR scanning and pathological examination of either a biopsy or resection specimen. Newer techniques include magnetic resonance spectroscopy and metabolic imaging (single photon and positron emission tomography). These may permit a non-invasive method of differentiating between low-grade and high-grade gliomas and between tumour recurrence and radiation damage.

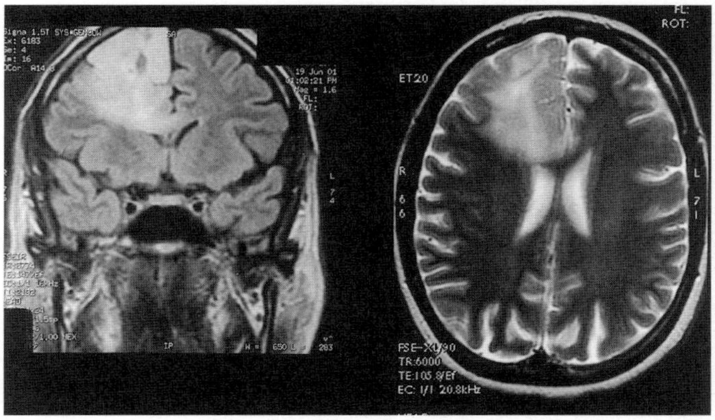

Fig. 2 Coronal and axial T_2-weighted MRI of the brain showing a diffuse lesion in the right frontal lobe which returns high signal. It is seen extending from the cortex into the deep white matter and infiltrating across the corpus callosum. There is mass effect causing compression of the frontal horn of the lateral ventricle. The tumour did not enhance with gadolinium. This patient presented with generalized seizures and has remained well after 3 years of follow-up. Biopsy revealed a fibrillary astrocytoma (WHO Grade II).

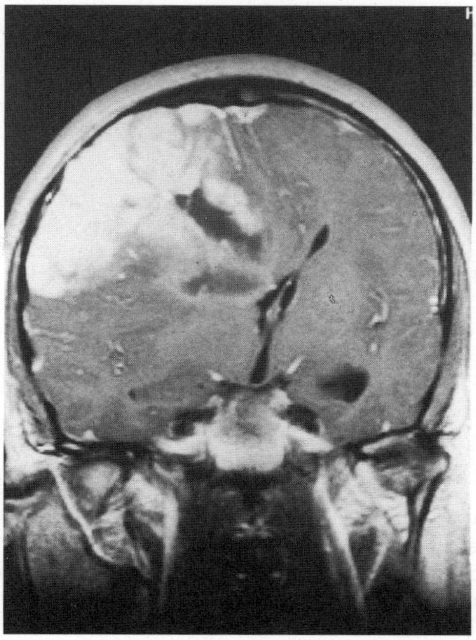

Fig. 3 Coronal T_1-weighted MRI of the brain with gadolinium enhancement showing a large heterogeneous enhancing tumour arising from the right frontal lobe exerting considerable mass effect in a patient presenting with a 2-month history of complex partial seizures, headaches, and papilloedema. The lesion was resected and shown to be an anaplastic astrocytoma.

Treatment

The three methods of treatment for brain tumours are surgery, radiotherapy, and chemotherapy. The use of each is dictated by the location of the tumour, the likely histology, and the patient's age and general condition.

Surgery

Recent advances in tumour neurosugery include the use of computerized neuronavigation techniques, improved pre- and intraoperative mapping of eloquent brain areas using functional magnetic resonance imaging (fMRI), and cortical mapping. These have all contributed to improving the morbidity and mortality of neurosurgery but an effect on overall survival has not been demonstrated.

Surgery is indicated as a first-line treatment for meningiomas, non-secreting pituitary adenomas, and vestibular schwannomas. The role of surgery in the management of primary intracranial tumours, particularly gliomas, is more controversial. Some types of glioma, for example pilocytic astrocytomas, can be cured by surgical resection. For most types, however, removal is not curative. While surgery is of undoubted benefit in relieving the symptoms and signs of raised intracranial pressure or an evolving focal deficit, there are no prospective randomized data to support its use for prognostic purposes alone. However, it may be beneficial in a subgroup of patients who are young, fit, and who have a tumour in a non-eloquent region, such as the non-dominant frontal lobe. Overall, about 50 per cent

Table 1 Pathological classification of astrocytomas

	WHO	St. Anne–Mayo*
Pilocytic astrocytoma	I	1 (0 variables)
Diffuse/fibrillary astrocytoma	II	2 (1 variable*)
Anaplastic astrocytoma	III	3 (2 variables*)
Glioblastoma multiforme	IV	4 (3 or 4 variables*)

* Based on presence or absence of four variables: nuclear atypia, mitoses, vascular proliferation, and necrosis. In practice, grade 2 lesions contain nuclear atypia, grade 3 mitoses, and grade 4 either or both vascular proliferation and necrosis.

of patients with medically refractory seizures derive considerable seizure reduction from surgery.

There is evidence that a combination of surgery and radiotherapy offers a survival advantage over radiotherapy alone for the treatment of solitary metastases in patients whose systemic cancer is well controlled.

Radiotherapy

Radiotherapy is the only treatment which has been proved to extend survival in patients with primary malignant brain tumours. Radiotherapy provides useful palliation in patients with low-grade gliomas, but there is no evidence to suggest that early radiotherapy prolongs overall survival compared with radiotherapy given at the time of tumour progression. Meningiomas are also partially radioresponsive and should be treated with radiotherapy where there is atypical or malignant histology or where there is recurrent tumour which is not surgically accessible.

Advances in technology have allowed greater accuracy of radiotherapy delivery and, in particular, the use of stereotactic frames which permit the focusing of radiation to a small tumour with minimal dosage to the surrounding normal tissue. This can be done either in a single high dose (stereotactic radiosurgery) or in smaller fractions (stereotactic radiotherapy) and is predominantly indicated for lesions less than 3 cm in diameter which are well circumscribed, extra-axial, and more than 5 mm away from vital structures.

Chemotherapy

There has been increased awareness of the chemosensitivity of certain tumours, particularly anaplastic oligodendrogliomas and primary lymphomas of the nervous system in adults and diencephalic gliomas in children. Approximately two-thirds of anaplastic oligodendrogliomas respond dramatically to a combination of treatment with procarbazine, lomustine, and vincristine, and this is now the first-line treatment for these tumours, particularly in the group who have combined deletions of chromosomes 1p and 19q. The addition of methotrexate-based chemotherapy to cranial irradiation markedly improves disease control and survival of patients with primary lymphomas. Adjuvant nitrosurea chemotherapy is used in patients with malignant gliomas although it offers only a marginal survival advantage. Recently, a new oral alkylating agent, Temozolomide, has been approved for use as a second-line treatment for recurrent malignant glioma. There is no chemotherapy that is effective for the treatment of meningiomas.

Prognosis

Neither earlier diagnosis of tumours nor advances in treatment over the last decade have significantly changed the overall prognosis of primary brain tumours. The median survival of glioblastoma multiforme without treatment is 3 months and with radiotherapy about 1 year. Anaplastic astrocytomas are associated with a median survival of 18 months. Young age and good performance status are the most important prognostic factors.

The outlook for patients with low-grade gliomas is considerably better with a median survival of 5 to 10 years depending on age, performance status, and histology. Oligodendrogliomas are more chemosensitive than astrocytomas and have a more indolent course, so their prognosis is correspondingly better with patients surviving 10 to 15 years after diagnosis.

At least 40 per cent of primary intracranial tumours are extra-axial (not arising from within the brain substance itself) and are thus readily treatable, if not curable. Some tumours such as meningiomas and pituitary adenomas are associated with 10-year survival of over 90 per cent if diagnosed before irreversible neurological damage has occurred.

Further reading

Cairncross JG *et al.* (1998). Specific genetic predictors of chemotherapeutic response and survival in patients with anaplastic oligodendrogliomas. *Journal of the National Cancer Institute* **90**, 1473–9. [First study to show definitive correlation between molecular genetic analysis and chemoresponsiveness of brain tumours.]

Counsell CE, Collie DA, Grant R (1996). Incidence of intracranial tumours in the Lothian region of Scotland, 1989–90. *Journal of Neurology, Neurosurgery and Psychiatry* **61**, 143–50. [Epidemiological study in Scotland showing incidence rates more than twice those previously reported in the United Kingdom.]

Daumas-Duport C *et al.* (1988). Grading of astrocytomas, a simple and reproducible method. *Cancer* **62**, 2152–65. [A 15-year follow-up study of a previously used grading system showing very good correlation between histological critieria and survival.]

DeAngelis LM *et al.* (1992). Combined modality therapy for primary CNS lymphoma. *Journal of Clinical Oncology* **10**, 635–43. [Non-randomized study showing significant improvement in disease-free survival in patients treated with chemotherapy in addition to radiotherapy.]

Forsyth P, Posner JB (1993). Headaches in patients with brain tumours, a study of 111 patients. *Neurology* **43**, 678–83. [Descriptive study of 111 patients with brain tumour headaches showing that the 'classic' early morning brain tumour headache is uncommon.]

Greig NH *et al.* (1990). Increasing annual incidence of primary malignant brain tumours in the elderly. *Journal of the National Cancer Institute* **82**, 1621–4. [Study showing up to a 500 per cent increase in incidence rates of malignant brain tumours in the elderly from the early 1970s to the mid-1980s, which may be despite more extensive uptake of imaging.]

Kleihues P, Burger PC, Scheithauer BW (1993). *Histologic typing of tumours of the central nervous system.* Springer-Verlag, New York. [Definitive pathological typing system for brain tumours.]

Patchell RA *et al.* (1990). A randomised trial of surgery in the treatment of single metastases to the brain. *New England Journal of Medicine* **322**, 494–500. [Randomized trial of surgery and radiotherapy against radiotherapy alone showing increased survival in surgical patients (median 40 compared with 15 weeks).]

Quigley MR, Maron JC (1991). The relationship between survival and extent of the resection in patients with supratentorial malignant gliomas. *Neurosurgery* **29**, 385–9. [Meta-analysis of over 5000 patients with malignant gliomas treated surgically showing little correlation between extent of resection and survival.]

Shaw EG, Scheithauer BW, O'Fallon JR (1997). Supratentorial gliomas, a comparative study by grade and histological type. *Journal of Neuroncology* **31**, 273–8. [Detailed analysis of survival and correlation with histology in over 500 patients with gliomas.]

Walker MD *et al.* (1978). Evaluation of BCNU and/or radiotherapy in the treatment of anaplastic gliomas. A cooperative clinical trial. *Journal of Neurosurgery* **49**, 333–43. [First randomized trial confirming survival benefit of patients with malignant gliomas treated with radiotherapy.]

24.13.18.2 Traumatic injuries of the head

Laurence Watkins and David G. T. Thomas

Epidemiology

It is estimated that each year in the United Kingdom approximately 1 million people attend hospital after a head injury. Almost half of these are children under 16 years old. Head injuries cause 9 deaths per 100 000 population per year in the United Kingdom. This represents 1 per cent of all deaths, but 15 to 20 per cent of deaths for those between 5 and 35 years old. Since mainly young people are affected, the prevalence of disability caused is very significant, with an estimated 135 000 people in the United Kingdom dependent on care after brain trauma.

In 1986, the Royal College of Surgeons of England published guidelines on the provision of surgical services for patients with head injuries. More recently, there have been concerns that inappropriate treatment might be leading to unnecessary death and disability. This possibility, together with increasing public expectation, led to a further working party which published updated guidelines in 1999. The availability of CT scanning has also increased, so that now it is considered essential for all hospitals which admit patients with head injuries to have 24-h CT scanning facilities.

Basic concepts

Primary and secondary injury

Primary injury is the damage caused to the brain at the moment of impact. It encompasses diffuse axonal injury and focal contusions. Medicine has little to offer for primary injury; prevention, however, is a major concern for health and safety legislation, town planning, and traffic laws (such as the compulsory wearing of seat belts and crash helmets). The focus of medical intervention is the prevention of secondary damage.

The causes of secondary brain damage can be divided into extracranial (hypoxia and hypotension) and intracranial (haematoma, brain swelling, and infection).

Grading the severity of injury

Only 20 per cent of patients are admitted to hospital and most of these are discharged in less than 48 h. About 1 in 500 of the patients attending hospital will develop intracranial haemorrhage. The doctor's task is to manage patients in such a way that the few with preventable causes of secondary injury are identified and treated effectively.

The British Society of Rehabilitation Medicine defines three broad groups depending on their Glasgow Coma Score (**GCS**) after initial resuscitation:

(1) Mild—GCS 13 to 15;

(2) Moderate—GCS 9 to 12; and

(3) Severe—GCS 3 to 8.

This is a useful categorization for decision-making in head injury management. It should not be confused with other schemes, which are generally retrospective and used for epidemiological and statistical purposes.

The golden hour

Taking into account the practicalities of CT scanning, interhospital transfer, and preparation for theatre, the time available for initial assessment, resuscitation, and treatment of other injuries in the emergency department is less than 1 h. This is sometimes referred to as 'the golden hour' in which rapid action is critical to the patient's outcome.

In a typical series of patients who had surgery for acute subdural haematoma, over 70 per cent had a functional recovery (good recovery or moderate disability) if the delay from injury to operation was less than 2 h. If the delay was between 2 and 4 h, just over 60 per cent made a functional recovery. In contrast, for those whose operation was more than 4 h after the injury, less than 10 per cent made a functional recovery (Fig. 1).

Patients who 'talk and die'—the importance of deteriorating conscious level

A classic paper, by Jennett and his team, coined the phrase 'talk and die' to describe patients whose primary injury was mild, but who succumbed to secondary injury: usually an intracranial haematoma. Deterioration in conscious level is an urgent clinical sign that requires immediate action.

The Glasgow Coma Score (Table 1) is now widely used in the United Kingdom and elsewhere, giving objective recording of conscious level, with a high correlation between different observers. Any deterioration is thus more likely to be noticed. When communicating about a patient with head injury, it is good practice to specify observations of each parameter, rather than to use the corresponding numerical scores, which are open to misinterpretation.

Change in conscious level is the most useful clinical sign in head injury assessment. Generally, a patient with primary brain injury shows a gradually improving conscious level. A patient whose conscious level deteriorates is very likely to be suffering secondary brain injury and therefore requires further investigation and treatment. Conscious level must therefore be assessed at the earliest opportunity, and then reassessed at frequent intervals.

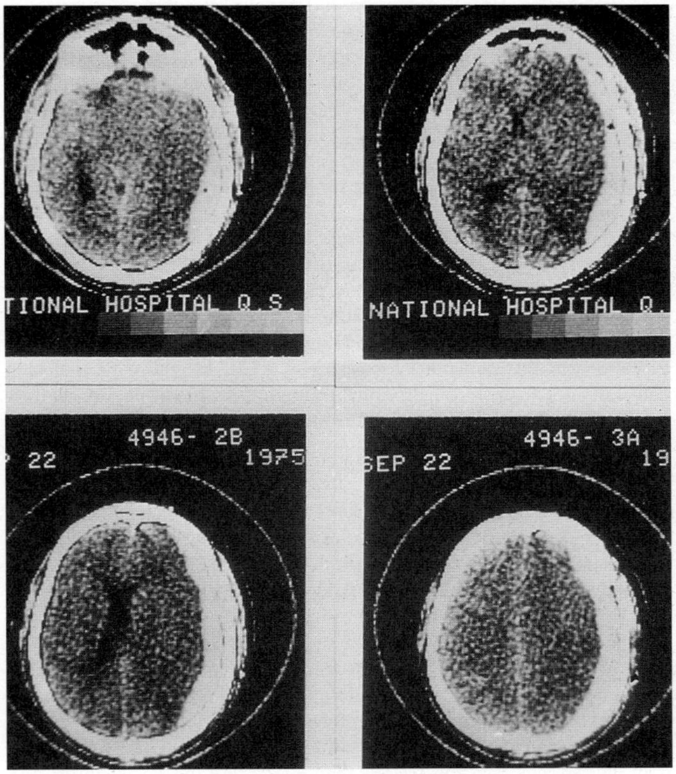

Fig. 1 Typical CT scan appearances of acute subdural haematoma. Fresh haemorrhage appears hyperdense (white). A subdural haemorrhage conforms to the surface of the brain, typically in a thin crescent. There is effacement of the lateral ventricle on the side of haematoma and midline shift away from it. An extradural haematoma, in contrast, usually appears biconvex, with well-defined edges since it is confined between the bone and dura.

Table 1 The Glasgow Coma Score

Motor function:	
Obeying commands	6
Localizing	5
Flexion	4
Abnormal flexion	3
Extension	2
None	1
Verbal response:	
Orientated	5
Confused	4
Inappropriate words	3
Incomprehensible	2
None	1
Eye opening:	
Spontaneous	4
To speech	3
To pain	2
None	1

Early management of the patient with head injuries

Extracranial injuries

Life-threatening extracranial injuries always take priority over the head injury. However severe the head trauma, the patient needs to be stabilized for safe transfer. Also, hypotension and hypoxia are important causes of secondary brain injury. Time-consuming definitive surgery such as the internal fixation of limb fractures should, however, be postponed if possible.

Airway, breathing, and circulation are the first priorities. Management should follow the general recommendations taught in the Advanced Trauma Life-Support (ATLS) courses. In particular, assessment should include consideration of respiratory problems, shock, and possible internal injuries.

All patients with head injury should be assumed also to have a cervical spine injury until proven otherwise. Cervical immobilization should be established, unless the patient is fully conscious, co-operative, and able to convince the examining doctor that he has no neck pain or tenderness, a full range of cervical movement, and no neurological deficit. There are rare exceptions to this guideline: for example, a patient with a fixed flexion deformity due to ankylosing spondylitis might present with a cervical fracture; in that circumstance placing the neck in a 'neutral' position, in a cervical collar, might actually produce neurological injury.

Initial management of head injuries

After initial assessment, resuscitation, and stabilization of extracranial injuries, the patient is graded for the severity of their head injury. These categories then give a useful broad guide to management.

Severe

If the head injury is severe (GCS 3 to 8) then a member of the team should immediately refer to a neurosurgical unit. If the patient's best motor response is localization or obeying, then they may not necessarily require ventilation, provided that oxygen saturation can be maintained at more than 95 per cent, the $P\text{CO}_2$ at less than 6 kPa, and the $P\text{O}_2$ at more than 12 kPa on 40 per cent inspired oxygen. If the patient's best motor response is flexion or worse, or if any of the above criteria are not met, then the patient should be electively intubated and ventilated prior to transfer. Ventilation should be adjusted to maintain the $P\text{CO}_2$ in the range 4.0 to 4.5 kPa. At this stage, the intracranial pressure is unknown, but should be assumed to be high; therefore a mean arterial pressure of at least 90 mmHg should be maintained.

Whether a CT scan is performed at the referring hospital or on arrival at the neurosurgical unit will depend on the local availability of scanning facilities. This decision is based on whichever pathway is likely to produce the fastest response, given local conditions.

If, after discussion with the neurosurgical unit, a patient is accepted for transfer, they should be accompanied by personnel able to insert and manage an endotracheal tube and ventilation.

Moderate

If the head injury is moderate (GCS 9 to 13), then an urgent CT scan would be advisable. If the CT scan detects an intracranial abnormality, then urgent neurosurgical referral is appropriate and the immediate management will be similar to that for severe head injuries given above. If no abnormalities are detected on CT scan, care should be taken to exclude metabolic and other causes of reduced conscious level (such as hypoglycaemia or drug overdose). If it appears that diffuse brain injury is the only cause of depressed conscious level, then the care of the patient is discussed with the neurosurgical unit. In some cases transfer will be advised, while in others observation under the care of the emergency department will be appropriate. This will depend on local resources and practices. In either situation, if conscious level remains depressed at 48 h, the patient should be transferred to a neurosurgical unit for further assessment.

Mild

Most head injuries are mild (GCS 14 to 15). After initial assessment, the next decision is whether further investigation is required and whether this should be a skull radiograph and/or CT scan.

Patients who have a GCS of 15, have no history of loss of consciousness, and have none of the following criteria for investigation may be considered for discharge according to the local head injury protocol. They must be under the supervision of a responsible adult and written information must be provided concerning symptoms and signs which would warrant seeking further urgent medical advice.

In this context, the criteria for skull radiography include:

- GCS 14
- history of loss of consciousness or amnesia
- scalp swelling
- scalp laceration (to bone or more than 5 cm in length)
- high-energy mechanism of injury
- headache and/or vomiting which is not improving with time
- significant maxillofacial injuries.

In children, additional criteria include:

- fall from a height greater than twice the height of the child
- fall on to hard surface
- tense fontanelle
- any suspicion of non-accidental injury.

If no skull fracture is detected, then the patient should be observed until conscious level is normal and associated symptoms have resolved. If a fracture is seen on skull radiography, then the patient will require CT scanning and admission to hospital.

In addition to the presence of a skull fracture on the plain radiograph, the following are indications for CT scanning:

- focal neurological deficit
- Battle sign (bruising over the mastoid)
- periorbital haematoma ('raccoon eye' bruising)
- subconjunctival haemorrhage with no posterior limit
- blood or cerebrospinal fluid in ears or nostrils
- suspicion of penetrating injury
- seizure
- anticoagulation or known coagulopathy
- difficulty in assessment, whether due to extremes of age (very young or very old) or intoxication.

If the CT scan shows no abnormality, the patient should be admitted for observation for at least one night, and longer if symptoms persist. If the CT scan does show an intracranial abnormality, the care of the patient should be discussed with the neurosurgical unit. In most cases, transfer to the neurosurgical unit will be advised.

Management of intracranial complications

Intracranial haematoma

In almost all cases of intracranial haematoma, urgent evacuation is indicated, bearing in mind that the longer the delay, the greater the risk of death or disability. The above guidelines for observation/skull radiograph/CT scan/transfer to neurosurgical unit are all aimed at the earliest diagnosis of the minority of patients with an intracranial haematoma.

The risk of a traumatic intracranial haematoma depends on conscious level and whether a skull fracture is present (Table 2).

Table 2 The risk of intracranial haematoma

Risk factor	Risk of haematoma
No skull fracture:	
Orientated	1:5983
Not orientated	1:121
A skull fracture:	
Orientated	1:32
Not orientated	1:4

Infection

Meningitis and brain abscess can develop following any head injury in which a communication has been made between the environment and the intracranial contents. The most obvious example is a compound depressed fracture, where comminuted bone fragments have been forced inwards, breaching the dura. With some penetrating injuries (such as a fall on to a sharp object or assault with a pointed weapon) the visible wound may be small and appear insignificant. Since the injury may have been low velocity, the patient may have a deceptively normal conscious level. Such patients should always be referred for neurosurgical assessment.

A closed depressed fracture does not require surgery except for cosmetic reasons if it is on a visible part of the skull.

Cerebrospinal fluid rhinorrhoea or otorrhoea indicates that a skull base fracture has breached the dura. This places the patient at risk of meningitis while the cerebrospinal fluid leak continues. Ninety per cent of such cases close spontaneously within 2 weeks, and usually neurosurgical intervention is not considered until this time has elapsed. An exception is a fracture of the posterior wall of the frontal sinus, visualized on CT scan. Such cases should be discussed with the neurosurgeon or the craniofacial team (if one exists locally) with a view to possible early anterior fossa repair.

The use of antibiotics in cerebrospinal fluid leaks is controversial. In practice, most neurosurgical units still prescribe a penicillin or cephalosporin for 1 week or until the cerebrospinal fluid leak stops (which ever is longer). A working party reviewing the literature, however, concluded that the available evidence does not support the use of prophylactic antibiotics in patients with cerebrospinal fluid fistulas.

Follow-up and late complications of head injury

Cognitive symptoms

After head injury there is a variable period before memory function returns and ongoing memories again begin to be stored. This period is referred to as post-traumatic amnesia and is a useful measure of the severity of brain damage. For example, when questioned after recovery, a patient may not remember the accident but clearly recalls being placed on a stretcher and taken into the ambulance: this would suggest a relatively short post-traumatic amnesia of a few minutes. The post-traumatic amnesia is fixed for a given injury and memories of this period do not later 'recover'.

It is also common for a patient to lose memory of events immediately before the injury. This is known as retrograde amnesia. Unlike post-traumatic amnesia, the period of retrograde amnesia often progressively reduces as the patient recovers.

Incomplete recovery following head injury has behavioural, cognitive, emotional, social, and economic effects. For adults with severe head injuries, 85 per cent remained disabled at 1 year following the accident. In the intermediate group, 63 per cent remained disabled at 1 year. Even those with so-called 'minor' injuries can face considerable problems: at 3-month follow-up 79 per cent still have headaches, 59 per cent have symptomatic memory impairment, and 34 per cent have not returned to work.

The most widely used measure of outcome after head injury is the Glasgow Outcome Scale (Table 3). These are broad categories, which miss the subtleties of impairment in many who have had mild injuries, but its wide adoption and recognition make the Glasgow Outcome Scale invaluable for statistical comparisons.

Table 3 The Glasgow Outcome Scale

Good recovery	Able to resume preinjury lifestyle
Moderate disability	Independent, but unable to resume full preinjury activities
Severe disability	Dependent on the care of others for the activities of daily living
Vegetative	No sign of psychologically mediated responses
Dead	

Even 'mild' injuries, with early brief loss of consciousness and an initial GCS of 14 to 15, can lead to significant symptoms that can interfere with return to previous activities. These 'postconcussional symptoms' include headache, dizziness, poor concentration, memory impairment, and personality change. The patient's relatives often report personality changes, such as 'bad temper' and lack of motivation. Such symptoms usually improve over 6 months, especially if the patient and family are warned to expect such problems and reassured that they are eventually likely to resolve.

Rehabilitation after severe head injury requires multidisciplinary input from rehabilitation neurology, physiotherapy, occupational therapy, speech therapy, and neuropsychology. Other specialists and therapy services are accessed as appropriate for each individual patient. At least as far as the Glasgow Outcome Scale is concerned, 60 per cent of patients reach their final outcome category by 3 months after the injury. Ninety per cent reach their final score by the end of 6 months.

Epilepsy

Epilepsy is more common if there has been an intracranial haematoma, a depressed skull fracture, or post-traumatic amnesia of more than 24 h. A single seizure, within 1 week the injury, is of less significance than repeated seizures or those occurring after the first week. Any patient who has had a seizure, a craniotomy, or depressed skull fracture should be advised not to drive or operate dangerous machinery. They should also contact the Driving and Vehicle Licensing Authority.

Chronic subdural haematoma

The initial injury may have seemed very minor and may have occurred many weeks previously. The most common symptom is headache, progressively worsening and eventually accompanied by vomiting. There may also be a focal deficit, which can vary in severity. Increasing intracranial pressure may lead to cognitive impairment and eventually a depressed level of consciousness.

Whatever the pathophysiology, the treatment of choice is evacuation of the subdural collection and irrigation with isotonic saline at body temperature. This is a relatively small operation, which can even be performed under local anaesthetic, so even advanced age and general frailty do not contraindicate its use.

Hydrocephalus

Hydrocephalus occasionally occurs after head injury, particularly if there has been traumatic subarachnoid or intraventricular haemorrhage. It can be distinguished from post-traumatic cerebral atrophy by the CT scan appearances: in hydrocephalus, the sulci will be small or effaced relative to the large ventricles and there may be periventricular lucency due to interstitial oedema.

Further reading

American College of Surgeons Committee on Trauma (1997). *Advanced trauma life-support for doctors. Student course manual*, 6th edn. American College of Surgeons, Chicago.

British Society of Rehabilitation Medicine (1998). *Rehabilitation after traumatic brain injury.* British Society of Rehabilitation Medicine, London.

Commission on the Provision of Surgical Services (1986). *Report of the working party on head injuries.* Royal College of Surgeons, London.

Infection in Neurosurgery Working Party of the British Society for Antimicrobial Chemotherapy (1994). Antimicrobial prophylaxis in neurosurgery and after head injury. *Lancet* **344**, 1547–51.

McMillan T, Greenwood R (1991). *Rehabilitation programmes for the brain injured adult: current practice and future options in the UK.* A Discussion Paper for the Department of Health. Department of Health, London.

Mendelow AD, Teasdale GM, Jennett B (1983). Risks of intracranial haematoma in head injured adults. *British Medical Journal* **287**, 1173–6.

Reilly PL *et al.* (1975). Patients with head injury who talk and die. *Lancet* **ii**, 375–7.

Rimel RW *et al.* (1981). Disability caused by minor injury. *Neurosurgery* **9**, 221–8.

Seelig JM *et al.* (1981). Traumatic acute subdural haematoma. Major mortality reduction in comatose patients treated within 4 h. *New England Journal of Medicine* **304**, 1511–18.

Teasdale GM (1995). Head injury. *Journal of Neurology, Neurosurgery and Psychology* **58**, 526–39.

Working Party on the Management of Patients with Head Injuries (1999). Report of the Working Party on the Management of Patients with Head Injuries. Royal College of Surgeons, London.

24.13.19 Benign intracranial hypertension

N. F. Lawton

Synonyms

Pseudotumour cerebri and idiopathic intracranial hypertension are synonymous with benign intracranial hypertension.

Definition

Benign intracranial hypertension is a syndrome of raised intracranial pressure occurring in the absence of an intracranial mass lesion or enlargement of the cerebral ventricles due to hydrocephalus. The synonyms pseudotumour cerebri and idiopathic intracranial hypertension have both been preferred because the outcome is not invariably benign. Although rarely life-threatening, the rise in intracranial pressure may result in permanent visual loss due to optic nerve damage.

Incidence

Benign intracranial hypertension is a rare disease. The incidence is approximately 1 in 100 000 in the general population but rises to 19 in 100 000 in obese women of childbearing age. The disease is certainly more common in females, the preponderance over males ranging from 3:1 to 8:1. Although benign intracranial hypertension may occur in infants and the elderly, it is primarily a disease of young women between the ages of 17 and 44 years. Very rarely, it is familial and may occur in more than one generation.

Clinical features

It is the hallmark of benign intracranial hypertension that presenting symptoms and signs are those of raised intracranial pressure alone. The diagnosis should not be entertained in the presence of neurological features which suggest a focal lesion. Furthermore, there is a remarkable preservation of consciousness and intellectual function rarely encountered in patients with mass lesions or hydrocephalus. A history of epilepsy, either generalized or focal, virtually excludes the diagnosis of benign intracranial hypertension, although seizures may occur in the small group of patients with venous sinus thrombosis (see below). Preservation of cerebral function also distinguishes benign intracranial hypertension from acute viral or bacterial meningoencephalitis. Patients with benign intracranial hypertension routinely present to outpatient departments and become a medical emergency when papilloedema is seen.

Headache

This is the most common symptom and is present to some degree in virtually every case. Characteristically the headache is typical of raised intracranial pressure. It is then generalized, throbbing, worse on waking, and aggravated by factors which temporarily increase cerebrospinal fluid pressure such as straining, coughing, or changing posture. Not infrequently, however, headache is mild and non-specific so that the distinction from common tension headache may be difficult. At presentation, headache has usually been present for weeks, although sometimes for months. Although up to 50 per cent of patients complain of nausea, typical early morning projectile vomiting is rare.

Obesity

Among the medical conditions associated with benign intracranial hypertension, obesity is sufficiently common to be a characteristic feature. Up to 90 per cent of patients in reported series are overweight, although a history of rapid weight gain immediately prior to the onset is unusual.

Papilloedema

This is a virtually universal finding and the importance of fundus examination in every patient with headache cannot be overemphasized. Papilloedema is usually moderate and may be unilateral. Occasionally the appearance of the optic discs may be equivocal, and fluorescein angiography is indicated to demonstrate the characteristic leakage of dye in true papilloedema.

The classic symptom of papilloedema, which is not specific to benign intracranial hypertension, is a transient obscuration of vision, often described as a fleeting greyness, a halo, or a more vivid episode of 'Catherine wheels' lasting for a few seconds. Obscurations may be provoked by straining or a change in posture, but may also occur spontaneously. Persistent blurring of vision may also occur and patients may describe scotomas in the field of vision associated with optic nerve damage. Occasionally, sudden and permanent loss of vision results from infarction of the optic nerve.

Visual obscurations, persistent blurring, or scotomas are reported by 30 to 70 per cent of patients. A history of obscurations is often only elicited by direct questioning.

Visual field defects

Visual field analysis is the essential investigation in the examination and follow-up of patients with benign intracranial hypertension. The most common defects are enlargement of the blind spots, generalized constriction of the fields, and scotomas caused by optic nerve damage. There may be a predilection for visual field loss in the inferior nasal quadrants.

Diplopia

About 30 per cent of patients complain of horizontal diplopia due to sixth nerve palsy, which may be bilateral. The cause is a false localizing sign of raised intracranial pressure.

Aetiology

In the majority of patients with benign intracranial hypertension no cause can be identified. Many clinical associations have been reported, but these may have occurred by chance. Preceding minor head injury and intercurrent infections come into this category. Furthermore, the known associations are rare with the exceptions of obesity and the predilection for females. A positive family history, vitamin deficiency, and drugs are each a factor in less than 2 per cent of cases.

Dural sinus thrombosis

Before the advent of antibiotics, benign intracranial hypertension was frequently associated with chronic middle-ear disease complicated by dural sinus thrombosis. The term 'otitic hydrocephalus' was coined to describe this syndrome on the erroneous assumption that ventricular enlargement was present.

Although true 'otitic hydrocephalus' is now rare, the syndrome of benign intracranial hypertension may still occur following venous thrombosis in dural sinuses or in the extracranial jugular system. Sinus thrombosis may complicate pregnancy, the use of oral contraceptives, head injury, venous occlusive disease due to hypercoagulability states, dehydration due to any cause, or mediastinal obstruction. Sinus thrombosis should be suspected clinically when the onset of headache is sudden and accompanied by focal signs or impaired consciousness. Occasionally, the syndrome of benign intracranial hypertension is a late presentation of undiagnosed sinus thrombosis. In the majority of patients, however, venous obstruction is not the predisposing cause and the cerebral venous system is normally patent.

Menstrual disorders

Apart from the complication of venous thrombosis, benign intracranial hypertension is associated with pregnancy *per se*. It is not clear whether an association with menstrual irregularity is more than would occur by chance in obese young women. An association with menarche has been reported.

In spite of the clinical associations which suggest an underlying disorder of female endocrinology, hormonal studies have not shown a consistent abnormality. The pituitary–adrenal axis is intact and occasional abnormal responses may be due to obesity rather than benign intracranial hypertension. Thyroid function and prolactin secretion both appear to be normal. Cerebrospinal fluid vasopressin levels are raised, but this is not specific and may occur in a variety of neurological diseases. Reports of a specific increase in cerebrospinal fluid oestrone, which might link benign intracranial hypertension with obesity because adipocytes are the major source of oestrone, have not been confirmed.

Deficiency states

A rare cause of benign intracranial hypertension in children is hypovitaminosis A due to generalized nutritional deficiency or malabsorption. In such cases the condition responds specifically to vitamin A supplements. Poisoning with vitamin A due to excessive consumption of fish or animal liver may also cause benign intracranial hypertension.

Drug-induced benign intracranial hypertension

Both tetracycline and the retinoids isotretinoin and etretinate, which are vitamin A derivatives, may cause benign intracranial hypertension during long-term treatment for acne. These drugs should not be used in combination. All-*trans*-retinoic acid in the treatment of acute promyelocytic leukaemia is also a cause in this category. Other drugs occasionally responsible for the syndrome include nalidixic acid, nitrofurantoin, and lithium. Corticosteroids may lead to benign intracranial hypertension during their withdrawal after chronic treatment and the syndrome may occur in Addison's disease.

Empty sella

It has been suggested that this association in about 4 per cent of cases is caused by raised intracranial pressure in combination with incompetence of the diaphragma sellae. The theory is supported by the finding of raised pressure at lumbar puncture in some patients with empty sella, suggesting chronic benign intracranial hypertension as the underlying cause. Clinical hypopituitarism does not occur, but occasionally the empty sella may harbour a prolactinoma.

Pathogenesis

The mechanism by which intracranial pressure rises is poorly understood and the contribution of various factors controversial. Since the intracranial contents are housed in a rigid container, an increase in cerebrospinal fluid pressure may result from an increase in blood volume, swelling of the brain parenchyma, or an increase in the cerebrospinal fluid volume due to overproduction or malabsorption. There is little evidence to suggest that increased blood volume or cerebrospinal fluid production are important factors.

Swelling of the brain parenchyma

Direct evidence of a swelling due to cerebral oedema is slight and a single report of oedematous changes in brain biopsies has not been confirmed. However, the tendency for the ventricles to be small may indicate an increase in cerebral volume secondary to leakage from the cerebral vascular bed rather than transudation of cerebrospinal fluid from the ventricular system. Brain imaging in benign intracranial hypertension does not show the periventricular leakage of cerebrospinal fluid that occurs in hydrocephalus. Although there is currently no direct evidence for vasogenic cerebral oedema, this factor cannot be ignored, because it is one mechanism for raised pressure which does not anticipate some degree of hydrocephalus.

Decreased absorption of cerebrospinal fluid

A defect of cerebrospinal fluid absorption is widely regarded as the important factor in the pathogenesis of benign intracranial hypertension. Apart from those cases in which there is dural sinus thrombosis, it is assumed that the defect lies in the arachnoid villi of the superior sagittal sinus where the bulk of cerebrospinal fluid absorption takes place. The delayed clearance of radio-iodinated human serum albumin from the ventricular system after injection into the lumbar subarachnoid space is indirect evidence of reduced cerebrospinal fluid absorption. Simultaneous cannulation of the superior sagittal sinus and the subarachnoid space has shown increased resistance to cerebrospinal fluid absorption in the majority of cases. Manometry has shown consistent hypertension in venous sinuses but it is not clear whether this is primary or secondary to raised intracranial pressure. Finally, vitamin A deficiency in rats and cows produces a rise in intracranial pressure associated with diminished absorption of cerebrospinal fluid and histological changes in the arachnoid villi which are reversible with vitamin A supplements.

The absence of hydrocephalus in benign intracranial hypertension has been cited as an objection to the theory of reduced cerebrospinal fluid absorption. It is probably more significant, however, that sinus thrombosis may cause the syndrome of benign intracranial hypertension by preventing cerebrospinal fluid absorption, and is similarly associated with normal or small ventricles.

Investigations

The diagnosis of benign intracranial hypertension can only be confirmed by measurement of cerebrospinal fluid pressure, but in suspected cases it is essential to exclude a mass lesion or hydrocephalus before proceeding to lumbar puncture.

Radiology

Characteristically, CT scanning shows small and slit-like cerebral ventricles which may increase in volume as intracranial hypertension resolves. A similar appearance is seen on magnetic resonance imaging. Sagittal sinus thrombosis may be visualized on CT scanning as the characteristic 'empty delta' sign due to clot within the sinus. MRI is far superior to CT and provides graphic images of sinus thrombosis. Occasionally MR or CT angiography may be needed to exclude sinus thrombosis or conventional venography if thrombolytic therapy is contemplated.

Cerebrospinal fluid pressure

At lumbar puncture the opening pressure is greater than 200 mm cerebrospinal fluid, but it is important to note that in simple obesity the cerebrospinal fluid pressure may be as high as 250 mm. The diagnostic significance of cerebrospinal fluid pressure must therefore be correlated with the clinical picture. In the few patients whose cerebrospinal fluid pressure is equivocal, continuous monitoring may demonstrate intermittent peaks of raised pressure.

Cerebrospinal fluid analysis

The composition of the cerebrospinal fluid in benign intracranial hypertension is entirely normal, and the presence of white cells or a raised protein concentration cast serious doubt on the diagnosis. An exception to this rule is the rare syndrome resembling benign intracranial hypertension which occurs in association with postinfective polyneuropathy and with spinal tumours. Both conditions may lead to raised intracranial pressure with papilloedema and normal-sized ventricles but a marked rise in cerebrospinal fluid protein. The syndrome may also complicate cryptococcal meningitis and meningoradiculopathy in HIV infection.

Management

Patients given a diagnosis of benign intracranial hypertension are usually bewildered and frightened. It is important to provide a simple explanation of the nature of the condition and the rationale for treatment. Anticoagulation with heparin may be effective in the treatment of acute sinus thrombosis, emphasizing the importance of angiographic diagnosis in this small group of patients. With the further exception of rare cases due to drug treatment, the management of benign intracranial hypertension is aimed at the symptomatic reduction of intracranial pressure to protect vision and relieve headache. The methods available are difficult to evaluate because of the high spontaneous remission rate and the lack of controlled trials. Choice of treatment is further complicated by the absence of reliable risk factors for visual loss. In particular, the height of the cerebrospinal fluid pressure at diagnosis is of no prognostic significance.

In the past, repeated therapeutic lumbar puncture every 2 to 5 days has been shown to reduce cerebrospinal fluid pressure temporarily and may occasionally lead to spontaneous remission. When acute medical treatment is indicated, prednisolone (40 to 60 mg daily) is effective in relieving headache and visual obscuration due to papilloedema. However, steroids are unsatisfactory as long-term treatment because of their complications, especially in obese young females. For this reason diuretics are widely used in patients with mild symptoms. Acetazolamide or a thiazide diuretic may relieve headache, but the efficacy of diuretics in preventing slowly progressive visual loss is unproven.

Because of the limitations of medical treatment, an increasing number of patients are treated surgically, progressive visual field loss and unrelieved headache being the indications for operation. Because of the difficulty of tapping small cerebral ventricles, a lumboperitoneal shunt is usually favoured. Unfortunately, the technical failure rate of lumboperitoneal shunts is high and surgical revision may be required in up to 20 per cent of patients. For this reason the alternative operation, in which the optic nerve sheath is decompressed, has recently been revived, particularly in North America. This procedure produces rapid improvement in papilloedema, occasionally in both eyes after unilateral surgery. It is not clear whether long-term improvement is due to the creation of a cerebrospinal fluid fistula into the orbit or fibrosis of the meninges preventing transmission of the high cerebrospinal fluid pressure to the optic nerve head. However, headache is often unrelieved by this procedure, and lumboperitoneal shunting may not be avoided. There is also a risk of further visual loss postoperatively, which is much less common after a shunt procedure.

Currently it would seem reasonable to begin treatment with diuretics, reserving steroids as a temporary medical treatment in patients with severe symptoms. If surgery becomes necessary, lumboperitoneal shunting seems a logical procedure, with resort to optic nerve sheath decompression in the event of repeated shunt failure. Occasionally, subtemporal decompression may be a last therapeutic resort.

Although the efficacy of weight loss *per se* has not yet been established, a weight-reducing diet is recommended in obese patients. In patients with extreme obesity, gastric bypass surgery has reportedly relieved intracranial hypertension.

Pregnancy

The main threat is to the fetus and the rate of spontaneous abortion is increased. Spontaneous remission of benign intracranial hypertension during pregnancy has been the rule, although the number of reported cases is small. It would seem reasonable to begin treatment with diuretics, although steroids and shunt operations may occasionally be required.

Prognosis

Benign intracranial hypertension is a chronic condition in most patients, but spontaneous relapse and remission of symptoms is common. There is evidence that raised intracranial pressure may be found at follow-up lumbar puncture in patients whose symptoms have been in remission for several years. Mortality from benign intracranial hypertension is nil in most series, although an underlying sagittal sinus thrombosis may lead to a fatal outcome. Permanent visual loss occurs in up to 50 per cent of patients and is a significant disability in 10 per cent. Because the choice of treatment is determined primarily by progression of optic nerve damage, serial visual field analysis is the important yardstick of clinical progression.

Further reading

Ahlskog JE (1982). Pseudotumour cerebri. *Annals of Internal Medicine* **97**, 249–56.

Corbett JJ, Thompson HS (1989). The rational management of idiopathic intracranial hypertension. *Archives of Neurology* **46**, 1049–51.

Janny P *et al.* (1981). Benign intracranial hypertension and disorders of CSF absorption. *Surgical Neurology* **15**, 168–74.

McComb JG (1983). Recent research into the nature of cerebrospinal fluid formation and absorption. *Journal of Neurosurgery* **59**, 369–83.

Rush JA (1980). Pseudotumour cerebri: clinical profile and visual outcome in 63 patients. *Mayo Clinic Proceedings* **55**, 541–6.

Sergott RC, Savino PJ, Bosley TM (1988). Modified optic nerve sheath decompression provides long term visual improvement for pseudotumour cerebri. *Archives of Ophthalmology* **106**, 1384–90.

24.14 Infections of the nervous system

24.14.1 Bacterial meningitis

*D. A. Warrell, J. J. Farrar, and D. W. M. Crook**

Bacterial meningitis, also known as pyogenic, purulent, or cerebrospinal meningitis, is an inflammation of the leptomeninges with infection of the cerebrospinal fluid (**CSF**) within the subarachnoid space of the brain and spinal cord, and the ventricular system.

Anatomy of the subarachnoid space

In the absence of pathological blockages, bacteria entering the subarachnoid space at any point can spread over the surface of the brain and into the perivascular spaces of Virchow–Robin. After reaching the basal cisterns they can pass through the foramina of Luschka and Magendie into the fourth ventricle, and thence through the cerebral aqueduct of Sylvius to reach the third ventricle, and through the interventricular foramina of Monro to the lateral ventricles. Subdural empyema (pachymeningitis interna) or effusion complicating leptomeningitis can also spread freely because the arachnoid membrane and dura mater are almost entirely separated. By contrast, because of the tight application of the dura mater to the periosteum of the skull, epidural collections of pus are localized. In the spinal column, however, the epidural space is loose and contains fat, permitting the extension of a posterior spinal epidural abscess over several vertebral segments. Within the subarachnoid space and intraventricular system, infection may produce blockages of CSF circulation, especially at the various foramina or in the aqueduct, causing obstructive hydrocephalus or spinal block. If reabsorption of CSF across the subarachnoid granulations is prevented by a subarachnoid haematoma or empyema or thrombosis of the intracranial veins and venous sinuses, communicating hydrocephalus will result. In patients with meningitis, intracranial hypertension may be the result of cerebral oedema, the ventricular dilatation of hydrocephalus, or subdural or epidural collections of pus. Obstructive hydrocephalus and intracranial collections of pus carry a special risk of producing brain herniation after lumbar puncture.

Because they cross the inflamed basal meninges, the cranial nerves and cerebral blood vessels may be damaged. Cranial nerves may be compressed by intracranial hypertension (VI) or brain herniation (III) or suffer ischaemic damage from vasculitis. Cerebral veins and arteries may thrombose.

Acute bacterial meningitis

Classification

Pyogenic bacterial meningitis occurs in a number of clinical situations, each of which is associated with a particular pattern of infecting organisms, clinical presentation, and outcome. Spontaneous meningitis is the most important category and can be divided into neonatal meningitis or meningitis of childhood and adulthood. Post-traumatic meningitis follows neurosurgery or fractures of the skull. Device-associated meningitis complicates the use of CSF shunts and drains. Infection may also be considered as community acquired or nosocomial (hospital acquired) (Table 1).

Aetiological agents and epidemiology

The bacterial species that cause meningitis vary by geographical region and according to the categories mentioned above. Age and local social conditions influence the attack rate and mortality of spontaneous meningitis.

Neonatal meningitis is usually caused by three species: group B streptococci (*Streptococcus agalactiae*); K1 capsulate *Escherichia coli*; and *Listeria monocytogenes*. A wide range of other organisms has been reported to cause the disease. Infection mostly occurs in the postpartum period, but can occur as late as 6 weeks after birth. Prolonged rupture of membranes and low birth weight are important risk factors.

Spontaneous community-acquired meningitis in children (under 14 years of age) is usually caused by *Neisseria meningitidis*, *Streptococcus pneumoniae*, or *Haemophilus influenzae*. However, national implementation of conjugated *H. influenzae* type b (**Hib**) capsular vaccine immunization programmes by many countries during the 1990s has dramatically reduced, or nearly eliminated, Hib meningitis. The introduction of the conjugate vaccine against *Neisseria meningitidis* Group C in 1998 reduced the incidence of meningococcal meningitis in England and Wales. Similarly, pneumococcal conjugate vaccination in the United States is reducing the incidence of pneumococcal meningitis in this age group. The highest attack rate of all three bacterial species is in children under 1 year of age and falls off rapidly with increasing age. The decrease in susceptibility with increasing age results from the acquisition of protective immunity, mainly as a result of nasopharyngeal carriage.

In most countries, more than 50 per cent of cases of spontaneous community-acquired meningitis in adults are caused by *N. meningitidis* and *S. pneumoniae* (Table 1). *Listeria monocytogenes,* aerobic Gram-negative bacilli (such as *Escherichia coli*), *H. influenzae*, and *Staphylococcus aureus* cause most of the remaining cases. The attack rate of endemic *N. meningitidis* meningitis is usually low (1–5 cases/10^5 persons per year), but occasionally the incidence of the infection may increase and even reach epidemic proportions (for example, >300 cases/10^5 persons per year). Crowding is thought to play a role in the epidemics occurring in military recruits, South African miners, and other groups of people crowded together in closed environments. The attack rate of *N. meningitidis* disease may increase secondarily to epidemics of influenza A. However, the precise origin of the major epidemics affecting countries such as Brazil (in the 1970s) and regions such as sub-Saharan Africa remains unexplained. The bacterial capsule plays a role in determining the pattern of invasive disease caused by *N. meningitidis.* Capsulate serogroups A, B, and C occur sporadically and cause outbreaks of invasive disease, while serogroups Y, W, Z, W-135, and 29-E cause only occasional cases.

* Contains material contributed to OTM3 by the late Prida Phuapradit.

Table 1 Causative organisms in spontaneous community-acquired single episodes of adult meningitis in the United States, Malawi, and Vietnam

Organism	Massachusetts General Hospital Boston, USA 1962–88 *n* = 253		Queen Elizabeth Central Hospital Blantyre, Malawi 1997–1999 *n* = 351		The Centre for Tropical Diseases Ho Chi Minh City, Vietnam 1998–2001 *n* = 500	
Streptococcus pneumoniae	97	38%	88	25%	38	8%
S. suis	0		0		65	13%
Gram-negative bacilli	9	4%	22	6%	11	2%
Neisseria meningitidis	35	14%	64	18%	9	2%
Streptococcal species	17	7%	6	2%	11	2%
Staphylococcus aureus	13	5%	0		3	1%
Listeria monocytogenes	29	11%	0		0	
Haemophilus influenzae	9	4%	0		7	1%
Mixed bacterial species	6	2%	0		5	1%
Mycobacterium tuberculosis culture confirmed					46	9%
Probable tuberculous meningitis			44	13%	210	42%
Other probable bacterial meningitis	4	2%	59	17%	5	1%
No confirmation of bacteria	34	13%	68	19%	90	19%

The attack rate of *S. pneumoniae* meningitis (1–2 cases/10^5 persons per year) is remarkably constant around the world. It increases in patients over 70 years of age. A high proportion of pneumococcal cases exhibit an associated infective focus. Otitis media or sinusitis is found in approximately 30 per cent of cases and pneumonia in up to 25 per cent. Hypogammaglobulinaemia (primary or secondary, for example in nephrotic syndrome and chronic lymphocytic leukaemia), sickle-cell disease, splenic dysfunction, and previous trauma to the skull (see below) are risk factors for developing pneumococcal meningitis.

Streptococcus suis (Group R haemolytic streptococcus) serotype 2 is an important cause of meningitis (and rarely infective endocarditis, and septicaemia) in the Far East (Hong Kong, Thailand, Vietnam) and in other countries. Infection is related to occupational contact with pigs or pork, but the precise epidemiology remains poorly understood. In Holland the incidence of *S. suis* meningitis among abattoir workers and pig breeders was 3.0/100 000 per year. It is now the commonest cause of adult bacterial meningitis in Hong Kong and Vietnam. Possible routes of entry include skin abrasions, found in 40 per cent of patients, and upper respiratory and gastrointestinal tracts. Splenectomized patients are particularly at risk, as with other capsulated Gram-positive organisms.

Worldwide, *Listeria monocytogenes* accounts for few cases of meningitis, with an attack rate of approximately 0.2 to 0.4 cases/10^5 persons per year or 1 to 5 per cent of the cases of meningitis. Increased attack rates have been associated with contaminated foods such as unpasteurized soft cheeses, pâté, and poorly refrigerated precooked chicken. People at the extremes of age, pregnant women, and those with altered host defence mechanisms from prolonged immunosuppression with corticosteroids or alkylating agents such as azathioprine are at increased risk of listeriosis. *Staphylococcus aureus* causes 1 to 5 per cent of the cases with spontaneous meningitis and usually occurs in association with infective endocarditis. Spontaneous cases of *H. influenzae* meningitis, both capsulate type b and non-capsulate strains, account for up to 5 per cent of adult cases of meningitis. Aerobic Gram-negative (for example, *E. coli*) meningitis occurs especially in aged, debilitated, and diabetic people. The source in these infections is usually thought to be the renal tract.

Post-traumatic meningitis occurs in patients with skull or spinal injuries (for example, skull fractures) or in those who have undergone head and neck or spinal surgery. It usually arises in association with a CSF leak and soon after injury, but may occur many years after the trauma. The risk of developing meningitis is as high as 25 per cent with a clinically apparent CSF leak. The aetiology depends on whether the infection is acquired nosocomially or in the community. The majority of hospital-acquired infections are caused by aerobic Gram-negative bacilli, such as *E. coli, Klebsiella pneumoniae,* other Enterobacteriaceae, *Acinetobacter* spp., and *Pseudomonas* spp. Less commonly, *S. pneumoniae, H. influenzae, S. aureus,* and other normal upper respiratory tract flora cause meningitis in patients in hospital. Post-traumatic meningitis acquired in the community is caused mainly by *S. pneumoniae* (>90 per cent) and *H. influenzae.*

Device-associated meningitis is a well-recognized entity occurring in patients with CSF drains and CSF shunts. Most infections are nosocomial and are caused by coagulase-negative staphylococci (50–60 per cent) and *S. aureus* (15–30 per cent). Aerobic Gram-negative bacilli, *Streptococcus* spp., *Corynebacteria* spp., and *Propriobacterium acnes* are encountered. These infections usually present within a few months of inserting the device. Occasionally, *S. pneumoniae, N. meningitidis,* and *H. influenzae* are responsible.

Recurrent meningitis is an unusual (<10 per cent of meningitis) but well-recognized clinical category. Such cases frequently have either an underlying anatomical defect (for example, CSF leak or spina bifida) or an immunological defect. The immune deficiencies that most often predispose to recurrent meningitis are hypogammaglobulinaemia and complement deficiencies. Consideration should be given to vaccinating such patients against the most common pathogens.

The increasing incidence of human immunodeficiency virus (**HIV**) infection has altered the presentation and pattern of aetiological agents causing meningitis. A large series of adult patients with meningitis who presented to the Queen Elizabeth Central Hospital in Blantyre, Malawi, was reported in 1975. At that time, meningitis comprised 2.5 per cent of medical admissions, the most common pathogens being *N. meningitidis* and *S. pneumoniae.* Since then, the population of Malawi has been very severely affected by the **AIDS** (acquired immunodeficiency syndrome) pandemic, and the HIV seroprevalence of antenatal women has climbed steadily through the 1980s to the present level of more than 30 per cent. The changed overall pattern in this series is probably due to the influence of HIV infection; in a survey of 153 patients with invasive pneumococcal disease, HIV seroprevalence was 95 per cent. In South Africa, HIV-infected children have more antibiotic-resistant isolates and a different clinical presentation compared to HIV-uninfected children. In adults, the HIV epidemic was found to be responsible for increasing chronic infections such as tuberculous and cryptococcal meningitides.

Pathogenesis

The acquisition of infection and mode of invasion of the CSF vary with the type of meningitis. However, once infection is established, the inflammatory injury and pathophysiology are remarkably similar in all types of meningitis. Important steps in the pathogenesis of spontaneous meningitis are nasopharyngeal colonization and mucosal adherence and invasion involving receptors, bacterial fimbriae or pili, encapsulation, and other virulence factors that are blocked by secretory IgA and other host defences such as the complement system. Within the subarachnoid space, these defences are inadequate as there is no complement and concentrations of IgG antibodies are low. The cell walls of Gram-positive bacteria and lipopolysaccharides of Gram-negative bacteria cause inflammatory change, thereby increasing vascular permeability and leading to the development of cerebral oedema.

The organisms that cause neonatal meningitis are acquired by the baby from the vagina and perineum during delivery, or from the environment soon after birth. The three main infecting species, *S. agalactiae* (group B streptococci), *E. coli*, and *L. monocytogenes*, invade the host, cause septicaemia, and, as a result, produce meningitis. An unusual feature of *E. coli* and many *S. agalactiae* strains (capsular types K1 and III, respectively) is that their capsules consist of polysialic acid. The association of this unusual type of capsule with two virulent strains suggests a role in the pathogenesis of neonatal meningitis.

Causative organisms of spontaneous meningitis, *S. pneumoniae*, *H. influenzae*, and *N. meningitidis*, are acquired by person-to-person spread. Replication in the nasopharynx is the essential first step before invasion. Asymptomatic carriage implies a stable and well-adapted relationship between microbe and host. Fortunately, this is the usual outcome. Invasion and infection of the host resulting in disease represents a rare and potentially catastrophic breakdown in the relationship between the bacterium and host. Invasion of the host is particularly likely to occur early after acquisition of the organism, before the host has developed protective immunity. Carriage is sufficient to produce immunity and resistance to disease. The greatest risk of disease, therefore, is in the first few years of life, at a time when the non-immune host first encounters these pathogens. The precise anatomical site of invasion is not known for all three pathogens. Animal studies suggest that the nasopharynx is the probable site of systemic invasion for *H. influenzae* meningitis, associated with escape into the bloodstream of a single organism that multiplies and produces septicaemia. In a proportion of these bacteraemic cases, bacteria then gain access to the CSF. Invasion of the CSF is probably dependent on the concentration of organisms in the blood and on the species causing bacteraemia (for example, bacteria such as enterococci can cause high-intensity bacteraemia under some conditions but the organisms seldom enter the CSF, whereas *N. meningitidis*, *H. influenzae*, and *S. pneumoniae* frequently invade the CSF). The choroid plexus, a highly vascular tissue, is probably the site of CSF invasion. Once organisms have entered the CSF and multiplied, purulent meningitis is inevitable.

Organisms causing post-traumatic meningitis invade the CSF directly through an anatomical defect. Bacteraemia, which is common, is secondary to the meningitis. Shunt-associated meningitis is caused mainly by organisms that colonize the skin and contaminate the surgical wound and prosthetic material at the time of surgery. The infected shunt becomes coated with a film of adherent bacteria, commonly referred to as a 'biofilm', which is not susceptible to clinically achievable levels of antibiotic. Such infections are usually incurable unless the foreign material is removed.

Once bacteria have gained access to the subarachnoid space they multiply in the CSF relatively uninhibited by host defences. Neutrophils, which rapidly accumulate in the infected CSF, have little inhibitory effect on the growth of the infecting bacteria in experimental animals. Complement is found in such low concentrations in CSF that it is unlikely to have an antibacterial effect. Investigation of the mediators of this inflammatory response is incomplete, but studies of pneumococcal and *H. influenzae* meningitis have identified important features of this inflammatory reaction. The pneumococcal cell wall has been shown to be a potent inducer of inflammation. Since this reaction can be attenuated by cyclo-oxygenase inhibitors, prostaglandins are believed to be important. The role of cytokines in the CSF has not been fully elucidated in this type of meningitis. However, the pneumococcal cell wall is a potent inducer of systemic interleukin-1 (**IL-1**), but not of tumour necrosis factor (**TNF**). The exact role of these mediators in pneumococcal meningitis remains unresolved. The main bacterial component responsible for inducing inflammation in *H. influenzae* type b is lipopolysaccharide (**LPS** or endotoxin), a potent inducer of cerebrospinal fluid TNF and IL-1 which have been shown to mediate the inflammatory response in the subarachnoid space. There is a suggestion of a dose–response effect between lipopolysaccharide and the inflammatory mediators, and so interventions that release lipopolysaccharide may exacerbate the inflammatory reaction. It has also been suggested that certain antibiotics which produce an enhanced lipopolysaccharide release may temporarily exaggerate the inflammatory reaction in a type of Jarisch–Herxheimer reaction.

The inflammatory reaction in meningitis is associated with a number of severe alterations in the normal physiology of the CNS. First, permeability of the blood–brain barrier increases. This is best measured by the increased penetration of the CSF by albumin. Also, antibiotic penetration of the CSF is greatly enhanced. Second, increased intracranial pressure results from cerebral oedema secondary to an accumulation of interstitial fluid, and communicating hydrocephalus is caused by decreased CSF re-absorption and cellular swelling secondary to cell injury. Third, a vasculitis may affect mainly the large vessels traversing the subarachnoid space. This vascular injury may not only disrupt the normal autoregulation of cerebral blood flow, but, in severe cases, the vessel may become obstructed with thrombus, causing a cerebral infarct. The major impact of increased intracranial pressure and vasculitis is decreased cerebral perfusion, causing general hypoxic brain injury.

Pathology

There is diffuse acute inflammation of the pia-arachnoid, with migration of neutrophil leucocytes and exudation of fibrin into the CSF. Pus accumulates over the surface of the brain, especially around its base and the emerging cranial nerves, and around the spinal cord. The meningeal vessels are dilatated and congested and may be surrounded by pus. Pus and fibrin are found in the ventricles and there is ventriculitis, with loss of ependymal lining and subependymal gliosis. Dilatation of the ventricular system may result from obstructive or communicating hydrocephalus. Other abnormalities include subdural effusion or empyema, septic thrombosis of the cerebral venous sinuses, subarachnoid haematomas, compression of intracranial structures as a result of intracranial hypertension, and herniation of the temporal lobes or cerebellum. Gross changes, such as pressure coning, which would provide an obvious cause of death, are rarely found. In some cases death may be attributable to related septicaemia (Fig. 1), although the familiar finding of bilateral adrenal haemorrhage (Waterhouse–Friederichsen syndrome) may well be a terminal phenomenon rather than a cause of fatal adrenal insufficiency as was once imagined. Patients with meningococcal septicaemia may develop acute pulmonary oedema. Myocarditis was a common finding in some series of patients. Histological appearances were of an acute interstitial myocarditis, occasionally with myocardial necrosis and thrombosis of small arterioles. Pericarditis and pericardial effusion were features, particularly of group C meningococcal infections. Myocarditis and Waterhouse–Friederichsen syndrome also occur, less frequently than in meningococcal septicaemia, in septicaemia caused by *H. influenzae*, pneumococcal, streptococcal, and staphylococcal infections.

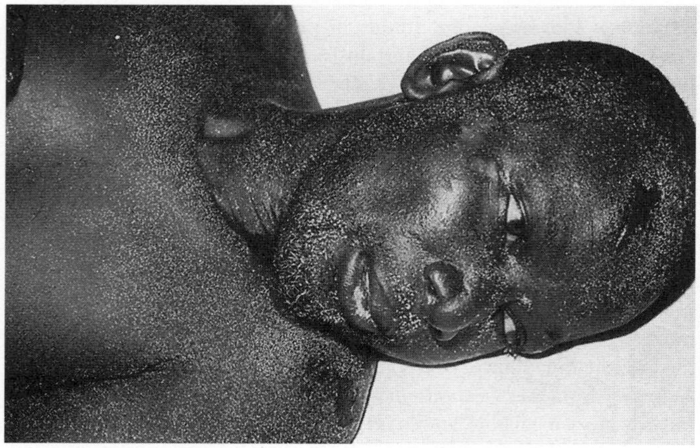

Fig. 1 Nigerian patient with pneumococcal meningitis and septicaemia who developed 'urea frost' and later died of renal failure. This illustrates the importance of septicaemic complications outside the central nervous system in determining mortality. (Copyright D.A. Warrell.)

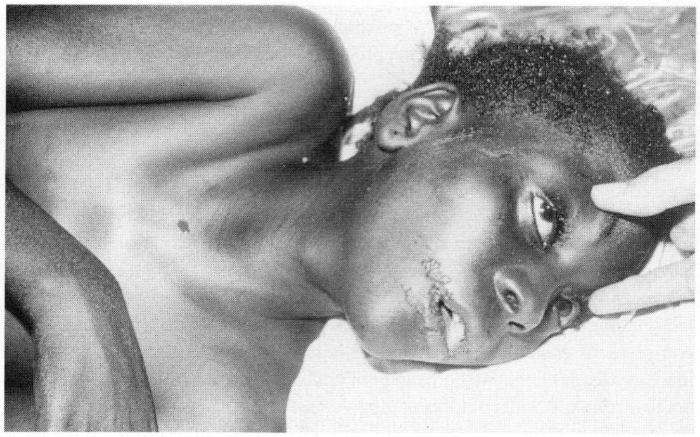

Fig. 2 Nigerian girl in coma with severe meningococcal meningoencephalitis. Note head retraction, dysconjugate gaze, and herpes labialis. (Copyright D.A. Warrell.)

Clinical features

Acute bacterial meningitis carries a mortality in untreated patients of between 70 and 100 per cent. Delay in treatment greatly increases the risk of permanent neurological sequelae. The early diagnosis of this condition is, therefore, a formidable challenge to clinical acumen, but early clinical suspicion of meningitis may be impossible in many cases, especially in neonates and small children. When meningitis is secondary to infection elsewhere, such as pneumococcal pneumonia or *H. influenzae* otitis media, the presenting symptoms may be those of the original infection. The incubation period is only a few days. Progression is occasionally so rapid (*N. meningitidis*) that the patient becomes comatose within a few hours after the first symptoms. Early manifestations include non-specific malaise, apprehension, or irritability, followed by fever, usually without rigors, headache, myalgias, and vomiting. Convulsions occur in infants and children and meningitis must always be included in the differential diagnosis of childhood febrile convulsions. Photophobia, drowsiness, or more severe impairment of consciousness usually develop later. Headache quickly becomes more severe and is the dominant symptom. In older children and adults the symptoms most suggestive of meningitis are irritability, severe headache, and vomiting, but in the case of meningococcal infection, diarrhoea is a common non-specific symptom and the vasculitic rash is a crucial sign. An early symptom of meningococcal septicaemia is pain in the calves.

There is rarely any doubt that the child or adult with meningitis is severely ill and distressed. Meningism is best elicited by gentle passive flexion or rotation of the neck with the patient lying supine. If patients can shake their heads vigorously they are unlikely to have meningitis! To elicit Kernig's sign the lower limb is flexed at the hip. The patient with meningism will resist extension of the knee by contracting the hamstring muscles. Brudzinski's neck sign is best elicited while the patient sits up in bed with the legs stretched out. Gentle flexion of the neck will induce a compensatory flexion of the hips, knees, and sometimes the upper limbs. Later, the patient with marked meningism lies in a characteristic position with the neck and back fully extended (Fig. 2) as in tetanic opisthotonos. Local causes of neck stiffness, such as local sepsis (for example, in the nuchal muscles or cervical lymph nodes), cervical spondylitis (particularly common in the elderly), temporomandibular arthritis, dental problems, and pharyngeal lesions, should be considered. Meningism is not uncommon in patients without meningitis who have other febrile conditions such as pyelonephritis. Meningism may be reduced or absent in patients who are immunosuppressed. The optic fundi should be examined as a prelude to lumbar puncture. Papilloedema is suggestive of cerebral oedema or an intracranial space-occupying lesion, such as a cerebral abscess or a subdural or epidural collection of pus. The absence of papilloedema does not, however, exclude cerebral oedema and, if in doubt, and cerebral imaging is available, that investigation must precede a lumbar puncture. Retinal vein pulsation excludes intracranial hypertension. Hypertensive retinopathy will suggest hypertensive encephalopathy, and subhyaloid haemorrhages a subarachnoid haemorrhage. Patients with meningococcal meningitis associated with meningococcal antigenaemia have a petechial rash (Plate 1) which may appear first on the shins or volar surface of the forearms. Petechiae may be visible on the bulbar and tarsal conjunctivas (Plate 2) and palate. An identical rash is occasionally seen in patients with echovirus type 9, leptospirosis, *S. aureus, S. pneumoniae, S. suis* (Plate 3) *H. influenzae, Salmonella typhi,* and other infections, especially in those associated with infective endocarditis. The brownish or reddish geometrical, vasculitic rash of fulminant meningococcaemia is unmistakable (Plates 4 and 5) and, characteristically, the toes and fingers become necrotic (Fig. 3). There is associated profound hypotension, shock with peripheral cyanosis, and spontaneous systemic bleeding. Herpes labialis is commonly seen in all forms of bacterial meningitis, because a fever is the rule and recurrences are provoked by fever (see Figs 2 and 4). Physical examination must exclude otitis media, sinusitis, mastoiditis, and nasopharyngeal and other possible sites of sepsis. In patients with recurrent bacterial meningitis, a search should be made for a congenital dermal sinus, which is usually in the midline between the head and coccyx and is often marked by a tuft of long hairs. Watery discharge from the nose or ears should be collected and tested

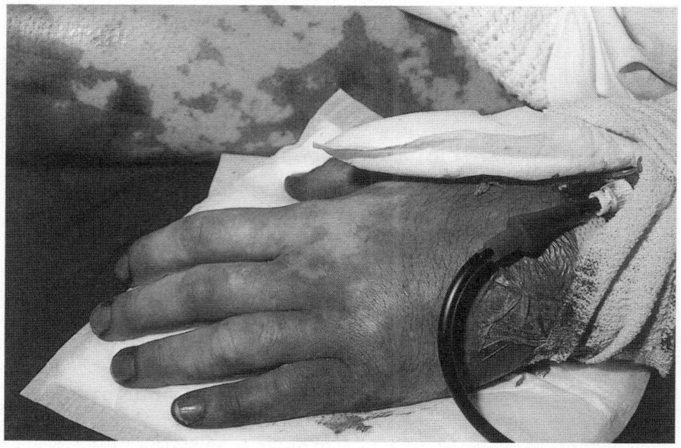

Fig. 3 Gangrene of the fingers in a man with fulminant meningococcaemia. Eventually, three of his limbs had to be amputated. (Copyright D.A. Warrell.)

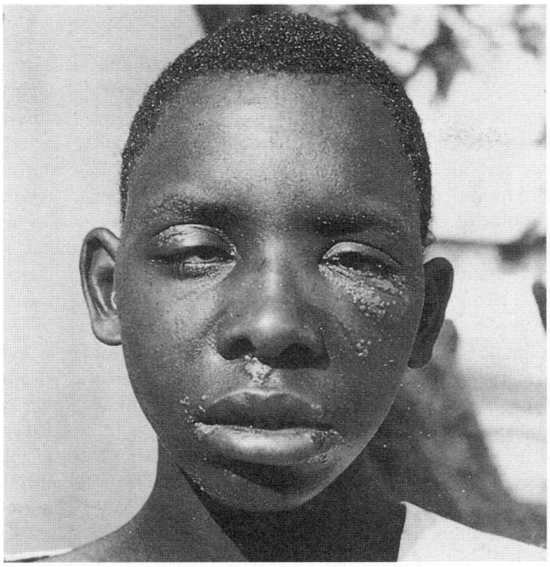

Fig. 4 Nigerian man recovering from meningococcal meningitis. Note right VIth nerve lesion and herpes labialis. (Copyright D.A. Warrell.)

for glucose; the possibility of a basal skull fracture with cerebrospinal fluid leak should be excluded.

Cranial nerve lesions may become evident as the disease progresses. The commonest are VI (Fig. 4), III, VII, VIII, and II. Patients who become deeply comatose (meningoencephalomyelitis) may lose all signs of meningism and develop focal neurological signs, focal epileptiform convulsions, dysconjugate gaze, upper motor neurone signs, and involuntary movements. Vascular lesions may produce hemiparesis or quadriparesis, speech disorders, and visual field defects. Bilateral sensorineural deafness develops early, 2 to 9 days after the start of symptoms, in the majority of patients with *S. suis* type 2 meningitis. Initially associated with tinnitus and vertigo, this may progress to complete deafness within 24 h. Bacteria probably invade the cochlea via the cochlear aqueduct from the subarachnoid space to produce suppurative labyrinthitis and acute deafness. Associated clinical features of *S. suis* meningitis include third nerve palsy, septic arthritis (Plate 6), and purpuric skin lesions (Plate 3).

Papilloedema, with or without other symptoms and signs of intracranial hypertension (vomiting, postural headache, coma, high blood pressure, bradycardia, etc.) and localizing neurological signs, suggests a subdural effusion or empyema. This is particularly common in children under 2 years old with *H. influenzae* meningitis.

Neonates and infants

Meningitis is particularly difficult to diagnose in this age group. Infants may become irritable or lethargic, stop feeding, and are found to have a bulging fontanelle, separation of the cranial sutures, meningism, and opisthotonos, and they may develop convulsions. These findings are uncommon in neonates, who sometimes present with respiratory distress, diarrhoea, or jaundice.

Post-traumatic meningitis

This is often indistinguishable clinically from spontaneous meningitis. However, in obtunded or unconscious patients who have suffered a recent head injury, few clinical signs may be present. A fever and a deterioration in the level of consciousness or loss of vital functions may be the only signs of meningitis. Finding a CSF leak adds support to the possibility of meningitis in such patients, but this is undetectable in many cases.

Infections of CSF shunts

Patients may present with clinical features typical of spontaneous meningitis, especially if virulent organisms are involved. The more usual presentation is insidious, with features of shunt blockage such as headache, vomiting, fever, and a decreasing level of consciousness. Fever is a helpful sign, but is not a constant feature and may be present in as few as 20 per cent of cases. Shunts can be infected without causing meningitis, in which event the features of the infection will be determined by where the shunt drains. Infection of shunts draining into the venous system produces a disease similar to chronic right-sided infective endocarditis together with glomerulonephritis (shunt nephritis), while infection of shunts draining into the peritoneal cavity produces peritonitis.

Diagnosis

Examination of cerebrospinal fluid (see Chapter 24.7)

Examination of CSF is crucial for the diagnosis of meningitis. The main risk of lumbar puncture, fatal pressure coning, is greatest in patients with space-occupying lesions or post-traumatic cerebral oedema. Fortunately, it is a rare complication in cases of spontaneous meningitis, but caution should be exercised when contemplating spinal puncture. Patients with clinical features suggesting raised intracranial pressure (for example, papilloedema, loss of retinal vein pulsation, focal neurology, bradycardia, and coma) should be examined by CT or MRI of the head, if available, to exclude a space-occupying lesion or severe cerebral oedema. In meningitis, the CSF opening pressure is usually raised (>200 mm of CSF), and occasionally it is markedly raised (>500 mm of CSF), suggesting the potential danger of pressure coning. Other contraindications to lumbar puncture include local skin sepsis at the site of puncture and any clinical suspicion of spinal cord compression.

Frank turbidity of the first drop of CSF emerging from the lumbar puncture needle instantly suggests the diagnosis of bacterial (pyogenic) meningitis. Microscopic examination of CSF for white cells, red cells, and organisms; the measurement of glucose and protein; and culture are important investigations in a case of possible meningitis. A raised CSF white blood cell (**WBC**) count is present in the majority of patients with bacterial meningitis but, rarely, the count may be normal (<6 WBC/μl, all lymphocytes) but the CSF may still appear turbid becuase of the vast numbers of bacteria. A majority of cases (>90 per cent) present with a count of more than 100 WBC/μl. The white cell differential count is helpful. Most cases (>80 per cent) have over 80 per cent of neutrophils. A predominance of lymphocytes is occasionally found and is reported especially in early bacterial meningitis, in association with *L. monocytogenes* infection and in partially treated patients. Red blood cells and xanthochromia are sometimes present. A wide range of non-bacterial infections and non-infectious conditions lead to pleocytosis of the CSF. In this respect, early viral meningitis, parameningeal septic foci, meningeal or cerebral tumours, cerebral infarction, chemical meningitis, aseptic meningitis complicating immunoglobulin replacement, cerebral vasculitis, and demyelination may be indistinguishable from bacterial meningitis.

Detection of bacteria in CSF confirms the diagnosis of bacterial meningitis. Gram-staining of the CSF will reveal organisms in 50 to 80 per cent of cases. The Gram-stain appearance of bacteria may be characteristic of a particular species, but caution must be exercised for up to 10 per cent of smears are misinterpreted. It is prudent, therefore, to administer appropriate empirical therapy initially and to change to specific therapy only when the infecting organism has been isolated and identified. Culture of organisms has a sensitivity of approximately 80 per cent in untreated cases, and is aided by the culture of good volumes of CSF and minimizing the delay between the lumbar puncture and setting up of the culture. Organisms are recovered much less often from partially treated cases. Isolation of an organism is not only helpful in establishing the diagnosis, but allows the identification and susceptibility testing of the aetiological agent. The culture result can also be used to decide on the need for antibiotic prophylaxis, contact tracing, and other public health control measures.

Measurement of CSF glucose is helpful in making the diagnosis of bacterial meningitis. A glucose concentration below 40 mg per cent is considered low and is found in 50 to 70 per cent of cases. In many cases, glucose may even be undetectable. As the CSF glucose concentration is a function of the serum glucose, a more reliable measure of hypoglycorrhachia (low CSF glucose) is the ratio of serum to CSF glucose concentration. A ratio below 0.31 for glucose concentrations of simultaneously obtained serum and CSF indicates hypoglycorrhachia. A few other conditions may lead to a reduced CSF glucose level. They are: tuberculous, syphilitic, parasitic, fungal, or mumps meningitis; herpes simplex encephalitis; carcinomatous meningitis; meningeal sarcoidosis; post-subarachnoid haemorrhage; severe systemic hypoglycaemia; and rare forms of central nervous system vasculitis.

An elevated CSF protein concentration is a common, but non-specific, finding. Similarly, measurement of CSF lactate is sensitive, but non-specific for meningitis. A range of rapid bacterial antigen tests may be helpful in detecting the presence of bacterial capsular polysaccharide antigens of pneumococci, meningococci, *H. influenzae*, and group B streptococci. These tests may reach a sensitivity and specificity of 90 per cent or greater for detecting specific causes of bacterial meningitis. However, in our experience these tests seldom add to the diagnostic yield of a good Gram stain performed on an adequate volume of CSF. PCR is also used.

The interpretation of the CSF test results depends on the clinical presentation and course of the disease. Acute viral meningitis is the most common differential diagnosis of bacterial meningitis. The CSF in viral meningitis typically contains a preponderance of lymphocytes, less than 1000 WBC/μl, and a normal glucose level. Fortunately, most patients with acute bacterial meningitis will exhibit a combination of clinical and CSF findings sufficiently characteristic to allow a reliable diagnosis. However, in some cases, it may be impossible to distinguish between aseptic meningitis, chronic meningitis, partially treated bacterial meningitis, and early acute bacterial meningitis. In these circumstances it may be necessary to initiate empirical antibiotic treatment. Depending on the clinical course of the patient, it may also be necessary to repeat the spinal tap and monitor the changes in glucose, lactate, and cell count in the CSF. These dynamic changes are particularly helpful now that antimicrobial resistance is an increasing problem and delayed response to treatment might occur requiring an early change of therapy. It is important to appreciate that CSF abnormalities secondary to bacterial meningitis, such as neutrophil pleocytosis, and raised protein levels, may persist for up to a week or longer, although the glucose and lactate levels should show signs of improvement within 48 to 72 h in patients receiving appropriate antibiotics. Since the pleocytosis and hypoglycorrhachia typical of acute bacterial meningitis may persist for a few days after treatment is started, it can be possible to diagnose partially treated meningitis despite negative Gram stain and culture. The difficulty arises when the neutrophil response switches to a lymphocytic one and the glucose starts to normalize after starting treatment for pyogenic meningitis. At this point it can be extremely difficult to distinguish partially treated bacterial meningitis from early tuberculous meningitis (**TBM**)). In these situations the importance of the clinical history (longer than 7 days—TBM), physical signs (lower cranial nerve signs—TBM), peripheral blood white cell count (elevated—pyogenic meningitis), and meticulous Gram and Ziehl–Neelsen stain of the CSF are crucial.

Other tests

Blood cultures should be obtained for all patients with suspected meningitis, as the aetiological agent may be grown. In patients with associated rash, a Gram stain and culture from fluid aspirated from the skin lesions may secure a microbiological diagnosis. A small amount of sterile saline should be injected under the lesion and immediately aspirated for staining and culturing. Radiological imaging of the central nervous system may be helpful. CT scanning can indicate whether or not a shunt is obstructed. Skull fractures or parameningeal septic foci (for example, sinusitis, spinal epidural abscess, or brain abscess) may also be detected by scanning.

Differential diagnosis

Meningeal irritation is seen in many acute febrile conditions, especially in children. Local infections of the nasopharynx, cervical lymph nodes, muscles, and spine may produce convincing neck stiffness. Tetanus may be easily confused with meningitis if the persisting rigidity and recurrent spasms go unnoticed. In all these conditions the CSF will be normal. Subarachnoid haemorrhage can present with sudden headache, neck stiffness, and deteriorating consciousness, and a less dramatic progression of symptoms is seen in patients with some intracranial tumours. Tuberculous and cryptococcal and other fungal meningitides usually develop more slowly than acute bacterial meningitis. They may be distinguished by examining CSF. Cryptococci and free-living amoebae may be mistaken for lymphocytes in the CSF unless an India-ink preparation is examined to reveal the capsule of cryptococcus and the characteristic movements of amoebae. Aseptic meningitis comprises a large number of conditions, many of them caused by viruses, in which there are clinical signs of meningism and the CSF is found to be abnormal. This group includes partially treated bacterial meningitis and the chemical meningitides, resulting from the introduction of irritants into the subarachnoid space (contrast media, antimicrobial agents, and contaminants of lumbar puncture and spinal anaesthesia). The CSF glucose concentration may be very low. Discharge of a tuberculoma may produce a sterile tuberculin reaction, and the discharge of the contents of a craniopharyngioma or epidermoid cyst into the CSF can also cause chemical meningitis. Lead encephalopathy may present with meningism, lymphocyte pleocytosis, and an increase in CSF protein.

Recurrent purulent meningitis

This usually suggests a congenital or traumatic defect providing access to the subarachnoid space, such as congenital occult spina bifida or fracture of the base of the skull. A CSF leak may be apparent in about 50 per cent of the cases with post-traumatic recurrent meningitis. The head trauma may have occurred many years earlier and a connection with the subarachnoid space may be clinically inapparent. *S. pneumoniae* and *H. influenzae* are the predominant aetiological agents for community-acquired cases. Gram-negative aerobic bacilli or *S. aureus* are the main causes in nosocomial cases.

Rarely, recurrent meningitis may arise from episodes of recurrent sepsis of a parameningeal focus (for example, sinusitis or mastoiditis) or from a complement deficiency. Deficiency in a number of the components of the complement pathway has been detected in patients with recurrent meningitis. *N. meningitidis* meningitis caused consecutively by different serogroups is the usual presentation in these cases.

Mollaret's meningitis (benign recurrent aseptic meningitis or benign recurrent lymphocytic meningitis) is mentioned here because it is an important differential diagnosis of recurrent bacterial meningitis. It is a sporadic condition presenting between the ages of 5 and 60 years. The symptoms are typical of acute meningitis—malaise, fever, vomiting, neck stiffness, convulsions, and coma. There is complete spontaneous recovery, usually within a few days, and symptom-free intervals lasting from a few days to years. About half the patients develop other neurological disturbances including hallucinations, diplopia, cranial nerve lesions, and signs of an upper motor neurone lesion. Pleocytosis is usually less than 3000/μl, with a predominance of lymphocytes, monocytes, and large endothelial ('Mollaret's') cells, but occasionally neutrophils are in the majority. The CSF protein level is mildly increased, with increased gammaglobulin. CSF glucose concentration may be decreased. Recently, evidence of herpes simplex type 1 and 2 has been obtained, using polymerase chain reaction (**PCR**) technology. Other causes of recurrent meningitis include Behçet's syndrome, Vogt–Koyanagi–Harada syndrome, sarcoidosis and systemic lupus erythematosus, and undiagnosed viral meningitis (for example, that due to encephalomyocarditis virus).

Management

Bacterial meningitis progresses rapidly and has a high mortality. Antimicrobial treatment must therefore be started as soon as possible after the diagnosis is suspected clinically. This is vitally important in meningococcal meningitis/septicaemia. If this condition is suspected by the practitioner (and in Britain the first doctor the patient meets is usually the general practitioner), the patient should **without delay** be given benzylpenicillin (intravenous or intramuscular (**IV/IM**)), cefotaxime (IV/IM), or ceftriaxone (IV). Although it is desirable that antibiotics are given following a blood culture their administration must not be delayed while waiting for the culture to be taken (Table 2). These drugs should be carried by general practitioners in their emergency bags. Antigen may still be detectable in the CSF later in hospital. Patients with no papilloedema or lateralizing neurological signs to suggest a space-occupying lesion, and with no other contraindications (see above), should undergo an immediate lumbar puncture. Again antimicrobial treatment should be started as soon as bacterial meningitis is suspected clinically and, if necessary, before the lumbar puncture is performed.

Antimicrobial treatment

Successful antimicrobial treatment of meningitis (Tables 3 and 4) depends on the agents crossing the blood–brain barrier and achieving a concentration of more than tenfold the minimum bactericidal concentration in the CSF (a level which predictably sterilizes the subarachnoid space). Before the aetiological agent has been isolated, empirical treatment that will be effective against the likely bacterial causes should be started immediately the diagnosis is made. Once the pathogen has been isolated, specific treatment based on the susceptibility of the isolate can be substituted for the empirical regimen.

Table 2 Recommended immediate antimicrobial treatment that should be given by general practitioners in cases of suspected meningococcal meningitis/septicaemia

Antibiotic	Route	Adults and children		Infants
Dose/day		>10 years	1–9 years	<12 months
Benzylpenicillin	IV/IM	1.2 g	600 mg	300 mg
Cefotaxime	IV/IM	1.0 g	500 mg	250 mg
Ceftriaxone	IV/IM	2.0 g	100 mg/kg	100 mg/kg
Chloramphenicol	IV	1.0 g	500 mg	250 mg

IV, intravenous; IM, intramuscular.

Table 3 Empirical treatment of meningitis

Type	Drug	Dose	Frequency	Duration
Spontaneous meningitis				
Neonatal	Ampicillin plus aminoglycoside (e.g. gentamicin) or cefotaxime	Dose depends on age		Until organism is isolated or 2 weeks
Child	Cefotaxime	200 mg/kg per day, divided IVI	6 hourly	Until organism is isolated **or** 2 weeks
	Ceftriaxone	100 mg/kg per day, given IVI	1 daily	
Adult	*Prevalence of intermediate penicillin-resistant organisms low and* Staph. aureus *unlikely*			
	Penicillin	2.4 g IVI	4 hourly	
	Prevalence of intermediate penicillin-resistant organisms >5% and Staph. aureus *unlikely*			
	Cefotaxime **or**	2 g IVI	4 hourly	Until organism is isolated **or** 2 weeks
	Ceftriaxone	2 g IVI	12 hourly	
	High prevalence of penicillin-resistant pneumococci (MIC >1 mg/ml)			
	Cefotaxime **or**	1 g IVI	12 hourly	
	Ceftriaxone **plus**		(measure	
	Vancomycin		levels)	
	Underlying immunosuppression, pregnancy, or age >65 years			
	Ampicillin **plus**	2 g IVI	4 hourly	Until organism is isolated **or** 3 weeks
	Cefotaxime	2 g IVI	4 hourly	
	or Ceftriaxone	2 g IVI	12 hourly†	
Post-traumatic meningitis				
Community acquired	Treat as for spontaneous meningitis in adults			Until organism is isolated **or** 2 weeks
Nosocomial	*Probability of* Pseudomonas *spp. high*			
	Ceftazidime	2 g IVI	8 hourly	Until organism is isolated **or** 3 weeks
	Meropenem	2 g IVI	8 hourly	
	Probability of Pseudomonas *spp. low*			
	Cefotaxime	2 g IVI	4 hourly	Until organism is isolated **or** 3 weeks
	or Ceftriaxone	2 g IVI	12 hourly†	
Shunt-associated meningitis				
Insidious onset	Vancomycin	1 g IVI **and** 5–10 g intrathecally	12 hourly 48–72 hourly	Until organism is isolated **or** 2 weeks
Acute onset	Treat as for nosocomial post-traumatic meningitis			

Empirical treatment should be started immediately the diagnosis is made, and in this table does not take into account Gram stain of antigen test results. Cultures of blood can usually be obtained before antibiotics are given. If CSF has not already been sampled, it should be obtained as soon as possible after starting treatment.

IVI, intravenous injection/infusion.

† Once the patient is improving and stable, 2 g IVI may be given once a day.

Table 4 Specific treatment of meningitis

Type	Drug	Dose	Frequency	Duration
Pneumococcal	Penicillin	2.4 g IVI	4 hourly	2 weeks
	or Ceftriaxone	2 g IVI	12 hourly	
	or Cefotaxime	2 g IVI	4 hourly	
	or Vancomycin	1 g IVI	12 hourly	
Meningococcal	Penicillin	1.4 g IVI	4 hourly	7 days
	or Ampicillin	2 g IVI	4 hourly	7 days
	or Ceftriaxone	2 g IVI	12 hourly	7 days
	or Cefotaxime	2 g IVI	4 hourly	7 days
Haemophilus influenzae	Ampicillin	2 g IVI	4 hourly	14 days
	or Ceftriaxone	2 g IVI	12 hourly	14 days
	or Cefotaxime	2 g IVI	4 hourly	14 days
Gram-negative bacillary (e.g. *Escherichia coli*)	Ceftriaxone	2 g IVI	12 hourly	3–4 weeks
	or Cefotaxime	2 g IVI	4 hourly	3–4 weeks
	or Meropenem	2 g IVI	8 hourly	3–4 weeks
Pseudomonas aeruginosa	Ceftazidime	2 g IVI	8 hourly	3–4 weeks
	Meropenem	2 g IVI	8 hourly	3–4 weeks
Listeria monocytogenes	Ampicillin	2 g IVI	4 hourly	3 weeks
	plus Gentamicin	1 mg/kg IVI	3 hourly	2 weeks
	or Trimethoprim/ sulfamethoxazole*	5 mg/kg trimethoprim IVI	12 hourly	3 weeks
Staphylococcus aureus	Flucloxacillin	2 mg IVI	4 hourly	4 weeks
	or Nafcillin	2 mg IVI	4 hourly	4 weeks

Choice of drug depends on susceptibility tests.

* Trimethoprim/sulfamethoxazole is formulated in a fixed ratio of one part trimethoprim and five parts sulfamethoxazole.

IVI, intravenous injection/infusion.

Empirical regimens (Table 3) depend on the clinical circumstances of the case and the local pattern of aetiological agents and their antibiotic susceptibility patterns. Neonatal meningitis is largely caused by group B streptococci, *E. coli*, and *L. monocytogenes*. Initial treatment, therefore, should consist of an aminoglycoside and penicillin or ampicillin; alternatively, a third-generation cephalosporin, preferably cefotaxime or ceftriaxone, **and** penicillin or ampicillin (to cover *L. monocytogenes*) should be used.

In the community, children are at risk of meningitis caused by *N. meningitidis*, *S. pneumoniae*, and, rarely in Hib-vaccinated children, *H. influenzae*. Antimicrobial resistance has emerged among the three major bacterial pathogens causing meningitis. Recently, chloramphenicol resistance in the meningococcus has been described, and although intermediate penicillin resistance is common in some countries, the clinical importance of penicillin resistance in the meningococcus has yet to be established. β-Lactamase-producing *H. influenzae* are relatively common, and chloramphenicol resistance is emerging. Third-generation cephalosporins are required to treat meningitis caused by these resistant strains. Pneumococci resistant to penicillin and to chloramphenicol are widespread, and resistance to third-generation cephalosporins is found in many parts of the world. Correct management of these strains includes the addition of vancomycin or rifampicin to therapy with third-generation cephalosporins. It is crucial to have up-to-date information on the resistance patterns of these common pathogens within communities to guide antibiotic prescribing. Spontaneous meningitis in adults is usually caused by *S. pneumoniae* or *N. meningitidis*; however, in older patients (>50 years of age) and chronically immunosuppressed patients, there is an increased risk of *L. monocytogenes* and infection caused by Enterobacteriaceae (for example, *E. coli*). If infection with *L. monocytogenes* is possible, penicillin or ampicillin should be used. In all age groups, patients presenting with features of meningococcaemia should receive parenteral penicillin (for example, 2.4 g or 4 million units) immediately. *S. suis* remains sensitive to the β-lactams and should be treated with penicillin, cefotaxime, or ceftriaxone.

Community-acquired, post-traumatic meningitis is caused mainly by *S. pneumoniae*, *H. influenzae*, and a wide range of other bacterial species. Cefotaxime (2 g intravenously, every 6 h), ceftriaxone (2 g intravenously, every 12 h), or chloramphenicol (1 g, every 6 h) plus ampicillin (2–3 g intravenously, every 6 h) should be given. Nosocomial post-traumatic meningitis is mainly caused by multiresistant hospital-acquired organisms such as *K pneumoniae*, *E. coli*, *Pseudomonas aeruginosa*, and *S. aureus*. Depending on the pattern of susceptibility in a given hospital unit, ceftazidime (2 g intravenously, every 8 h), cefotaxime, ceftriaxone, or meropenem should be chosen. If *P. aeruginosa* infection seems likely, ceftazidime or meropenem is the preferred antibiotic.

Device- and shunt-associated meningitis is caused by a wide range of organisms, including methicillin-resistant staphylococci (mostly coagulase-negative staphylococci), multiresistant aerobic bacilli, and *Candida* sp. Cases with shunts and an insidious onset are probably caused by organisms of low pathogenicity, and empirical therapy is a less urgent requirement. For postoperative meningitis the first-line empirical therapy should be cefotaxime (3 g intravenously, every 8 h), or ceftriaxone (2 g intravenously, every 12 h), or meropenem (2 g intravenously, every 8 h). If the patient has received broad-spectrum antibiotics recently or if *P. aeruginosa* is suspected, ceftazidime (2 g intravenously every 8 h) or meropenem should be given. Meropenem should be used if an extended-spectrum, β-lactamase organism is suspected, and flucloxacillin or vancomycin if *S. aureus* is likely. The infected shunt or drain will almost certainly have to be removed urgently.

Once the aetiological agent has been isolated and its susceptibilities determined, the empirical treatment should be changed, if necessary, to an agent or agents specific for the isolate (Table 4). The optimal duration of treatment has not been determined by rigorous scientific investigation; however, treatment regimens that are probably substantially in excess of the minimum necessary to achieve cure have been arrived at through wide clinical experience.

Treatment of brain abscess (see Chapter 24.14.3)

Brain abscesses may arise as a result of direct spread from contiguous anatomical structures, following injury or local infection or metastasis from a distant source. Whenever an abscess is suspected a detailed search for the source of the infection is important. The middle ear and mastoid cavity and frontal, paranasal, ethmoidal, and sphenoidal sinuses are common sites for the primary focus. Metastatic abscesses can spread from foci in the heart (endocarditis), the lungs (bronchiectasis), dental abscesses, the pelvis, and gastrointestinal tract. Once diagnosed, surgical drainage remains the treatment of choice for almost all abscesses. Empirical therapy can be guided by consideration of the likely primary focus of the infection, but it should include penicillin or a third-generation cephalosporin (cefotaxime of ceftriaxone), and metronidazole. For abscesses complicating trauma, flucloxacillin or vancomycin should be added. It is unclear if there are any benefits to be gained by instilling antibiotics into the abscess cavity during drainage. Treatment should continue for a minimum of 6 weeks.

General management and treatment of complications

General treatment

In the conscious patient, the severe headache may need treatment with opiates and the associated pyrexia may require treatment with antipyretics or cooling with tepid sponging or fanning. Many patients are unconscious and should be managed accordingly. Their airway should be maintained and they may need intubation to protect the airway and maintain ventilation. A urethral catheter should be inserted.

The associated septicaemia in patients with meningitis may result in septicaemic shock. These patients require careful monitoring and treatment of shock. A combination of fluid administration to expand the intravascular volume, pressors, and inotropic support is needed. Multiple end-organ failure may develop, requiring intensive medical support, including ventilation and renal dialysis.

Treatment of complications

Raised intracranial pressure is a serious complication of meningitis. Clinically, altered consciousness, poorly reactive unequal or dilated pupils, cranial nerve palsies, bradycardia, and hypertension suggest its onset. Various measures can be used to lower a raised intracranial pressure, including elevation of the head of the bed to 30°, administration of mannitol, and endotracheal intubation and mechanical hyperventilation. These measures may be used to maintain an adequate perfusion pressure monitored by continuous intra-arterial and intracranial pressure monitoring. The effect of these measures on the outcome of patients with raised intracranial pressure have not been evaluated systematically. The role of corticosteroids in reducing intracranial pressure remains unresolved and no consistent approach to their use is accepted.

The use of corticosteroids aimed at reducing the sequelae of meningitis has received support from a number of studies. The most pronounced effect has been the reduction of deafness in children infected with *H. influenzae* and treated with cefuroxime (a less effective cephalosporin for meningitis than cefotaxime or ceftriaxone). In three recent studies of bacterial meningitis (mainly *H. influenzae*) in children treated with ceftriaxone, dexamethasone (0.4 mg/kg intravenously, every 12 h for 2 days starting 10 min before the first dose of antibiotic) reduced the incidence of neurological and audiological sequelae. Studies in Cairo suggested that dexamethasone significantly reduced the mortality and incidence of permanent sequelae in adult patients with pneumococcal meningitis but in Malawi, this drug did not prove to be an effective ancillary treatment in children with acute bacterial meningitis.

Seizures occur in as many as 40 per cent of patients with meningitis and subclinical fitting should be considered in patients with persisting coma. A prophylactic anticonvulsant might be justified in pneumococcal meningitis. Rapid control of seizures can be achieved by administering intravenous diazepam or lorazepam, but respiration may be depressed. Phenytoin should be used for the longer term control of seizure activity. Severe cases that fail treatment with these antiepileptic agents should undergo endotracheal intubation and receive high-dose phenobarbital.

Many patients with meningitis develop hyponatraemia as a result of the syndrome of inappropriate antidiuretic hormone secretion (**SIADH**). Such cases may require fluid restriction. Complications such as cerebral venous sinus thrombosis and cavernous sinus thrombosis may occur, but may be difficult to detect. Anticoagulants or fibrinolytics may be used in such patients with the hope of improving the outcome (Chapter 24.13.7).

Prognosis and sequelae

In Europe and North America the overall mortality of patients with meningitis caused by *N. meningitidis* is about 7 to 14 per cent; for *H. influenzae,* 3 to 10 per cent; *Strep. pneumoniae,* 15 to 60 per cent; and for group B streptococci and *L. monocytogenes* meningitis, above 20 per cent. The mortality is much higher in the very young and old, and in patients with debilitating illnesses. A study in Zaria, Nigeria, demonstrated that the mortality of pneumococcal meningitis was 32 per cent in patients who were fully conscious on admission, 40 per cent in those who were confused, 54 per cent in semiconscious patients, and 94 per cent in those who were comatose. In Vietnam, in a prospective study of 250 cases of adult bacterial meningitis, the overall mortality rate was 13 per cent.

Permanent neurological sequelae include mental retardation, deafness and other cranial nerve deficits, and hydrocephalus. The reported incidence of sensorineural deafness after meningitis ranges from 5 to 40 per cent. A large proportion of patients recover within a few months. *N. meningitidis* and *H. influenzae* are the main causes of this complication. Permanent deafness occurs in more than 50 per cent of patients with *S. suis* meningitis. It may be bilateral, complete, and associated with vestibular involvement. *H. influenzae* used to be the major cause of acquired mental retardation in the United States. This complication was found in 30 to 50 per cent of children who had suffered from *H. influenzae* meningitis.

Prevention

Vaccination

Vaccines to the three major pathogens causing community-acquired meningitis are available. *H. influenzae* type b capsular conjugate vaccines are in wide use and are dramatically reducing the incidence of *H. influenzae* type b meningitis. In most countries where the *H. influenzae* type b meningitis vaccine has been introduced, Hib invasive disease has been essentially eliminated. A 7-valent pneumococcal conjugate vaccine is now widely available in the developed world, the efficacy of which is supported by a Californian Kaiser Permenete study in children. Studies in adults are being carried out in the developing world. A conjugate, type C meningococcal vaccine is available and has been used in the United Kingdom immunization schedule, producing a dramatic decline in group C meningococcal invasive disease including meningitis.

The purified capsular polysaccharide vaccines directed at *N. meningitidis* (serogroups A, C, Y, and W135) and *Strep. pneumoniae* (23-valent) are less effective than conjugate vaccines, especially in children under 2 years of age. No effective vaccine exists for *N. meningitidis* serogroup B. Vaccination of groups of adults at high risk, such as close contacts, military recruits, and migrant miners in Africa, has been highly effective in preventing meningococcal meningitis caused by serogroups A and C. The trials designed to assess the efficacy of population-based vaccination against *N. meningitidis* (serogroups A, C, Y, and W135) and *Strep. pneumoniae* are awaited with interest. The annual Muslim pilgrimage to Mecca (The Haj) is frequently associated with meningitis in returning travellers. It is advisable for people travelling to Mecca to be vaccinated with the polyvalent vaccine against *N. meningitidis* groups A, C, W135, and Y.

Since 1905, major epidemics of meningococcal meningitis have occurred in sub-Saharan Africa every few years, culminating in a massive epidemic in

1996 in which nearly 200 000 cases were reported. For epidemic meningitis control in sub-Saharan Africa, the World Health Organization recommends a strategy of emergency vaccination with meningococcal A+C polysaccharide vaccine when epidemic thresholds are exceeded. A recently derived model of how to respond to such epidemics has concluded that, given the relatively poor routine-vaccination coverage in this region, current strategies of vaccination campaigns that achieve higher coverage would generally be more effective and less costly than model routine-scheduled programmes, assuming that campaigns can be rapidly implemented. Until a better vaccine is available, countries in this region should aim to speed up the response times to outbreaks, perhaps through improved surveillance, and to bolster existing vaccination infrastructures.

Vaccination should be considered in all patients with recurrent meningitis, traumatic head injury, and in splenectomized patients.

Chemoprophylaxis

The attack rate of meningitis is higher in the immediate contacts of an index case of meningococcal (up to 1000-fold) or *H. influenzae* type b meningitis (500-fold only in children under 4 years of age) than in the population at large. The administration of rifampicin or ciprofloxacin eliminates the carrier state and is assumed to eliminate the risk of secondary cases of meningitis. A major preventive effect of sulfadiazine chemoprophylaxis has been shown in large outbreaks of meningococcal meningitis among military recruits; however, meningococci are now usually resistant to sulphonamides. Rifampicin and ciprofloxacin are assumed to produce a similar effect. Close adult contacts of meningococcal disease are given either rifampicin (300 mg, every 12 h for 2 days) or a single oral dose of ciprofloxacin (750 mg) (ciprofloxacin is still to be avoided in children, but is now accepted for prophylaxis). Contacts of *H. influenzae* type b disease (including adults) are given rifampicin for 4 days, and Hib vaccine is given to unvaccinated children under 4 years of age. However, in those countries where Hib vaccination has been implemented, the need for chemoprophylaxis is under review. Doctors, nurses, and other healthcare workers need not be given chemoprophylaxis unless they have given mouth-to-mouth resuscitation.

Although antibiotics are administered prophylactically to many cases of skull fracture with CSF leak, there is no evidence of benefit. Surgical closure of the leak is the only effective means of preventing meningitis in such cases. However, since many acute leaks heal spontaneously, this is necessary only in cases with large defects or in those with recurrent meningitis.

The prevention of device-associated meningitis relies on rigorous infection control. Ventricular and lumbar drains should be removed as soon as possible. Shunt insertion should be performed while adhering to a strict aseptic technique, and surgical antibiotic prophylaxis may also help to reduce shunt infection.

Tuberculous meningitis

Epidemiology

Tuberculous meningitis (**TBM**) has been a major problem and cause of death in developing countries. Human *Mycobacterium tuberculosis* is responsible for most cases. In Western countries, its incidence has fallen in parallel with tuberculosis as a whole. For example, in the late 1940s there were 2000 cases/year in England and Wales, accounting for 10 to 20 per cent of cases of bacterial meningitis; but by the early 1970s this had fallen to less than 4 per cent.

Most cases of TBM are in young children, but primary infection can be acquired at a later age and, in recent years, a larger proportion of patients with this condition have been adults. The disease is uncommon, but severe, in pregnant women.

There has been an increase in the incidence of tuberculosis in many parts of the world related to the epidemic of HIV infection. HIV-infected patients with tuberculosis are at increased risk of meningeal involvement. In some areas of endemic tuberculosis, TBM is an important complication in patients with HIV infection.

Pathogenesis

Small caseous microtubercles develop in the brain, meninges, or, less commonly, in the bones of the skull and vertebrae close to the meninges. This infection seeds through the bloodstream from the primary lesion or a site of chronic infection. Many patients develop miliary tuberculosis at the stage of haematogenous spread. Infection of the meninges results from rupture of a microtubercle with discharge of tuberculoprotein and mycobacteria into the subarachnoid space. This event will be marked by an episode of fever and meningeal irritation caused by the intrathecal tuberculin reaction. Subacute inflammation, especially of the basal meninges, then develops, producing cranial nerve lesions, cerebral arteritis causing infarction, impairment of CSF absorption, or obstruction to the CSF circulation causing hydrocephalus, and, in the spinal cord, spinal arachnoiditis, producing multiple radiculopathy or myelopathy.

Pathology

Meningeal miliary tubercles may be found on the brain surfaces of most victims of miliary tuberculosis. They are usually few in number and occur in the region of the sylvian fissure, while there may be larger caseous plaques deeper in the sulci. The brains of patients dying of TBM are usually oedematous. A mass of thick, greyish exudate encases the base of the brain, filling the basal cisterns. Within the ventricular system there is ependymitis with a similar exudate choking the choroid plexus. The exudate consists of lymphocytes, plasma cells, giant cells, and foci of caseation, but mycobacteria are usually scanty. At the base of the brain the cranial nerves and the internal carotid artery and its branches are trapped and damaged by the exudate. Arteries are obliterated by an endarteritis, with resulting ischaemia and infarction of superficial areas of the brain, internal capsule, basal ganglia, and brainstem. There is congestion and phlebitis of the meningeal veins. Both the inflammatory exudate and the arteritis are probably a delayed hypersensitivity reaction to the tuberculoprotein. Some degree of hydrocephalus develops in most cases. Usually the hydrocephalus is communicating in type and is caused by obliteration of the basal cisterns. Less commonly, blockage of the foramina of Luschka and Magendie in the fourth ventricle, or the aqueduct, causes obstructive hydrocephalus. The exudate may extend into the spinal cord, enveloping the nerve roots and spinal cord and producing spinal arachnoiditis and spinal block. Tuberculomas, single or multiple and varying in size, may be found in virtually any part of the brain (Plate 7).

Clinical features

Symptoms of meningitis are preceded by 2 to 8 weeks of non-specific prodromal symptoms which are unlikely to raise the suspicion of TBM. This phase of vague malaise, irritability, insomnia, lethargy, anorexia, headache, abdominal pain, vomiting, and behavioural changes may develop after a head injury, surgical operation, or common childhood infection such as measles, influenza, or otitis media, suggesting that meningeal infection may be precipitated by these conditions. By the time patients have developed obvious symptoms and signs of meningitis, the disease is well advanced. They usually have low-grade fever, but severe pyrexia can occur. Half of the patients will have symptoms and signs of tuberculosis in the lungs or elsewhere. Rarely, TBM presents dramatically as an acute encephalopathy with severe headache, neck stiffness, vomiting, and seizures, mimicking acute bacterial meningitis, viral encephalitis, and subarachnoid haemorrhage.

During the second stage there is evidence of meningeal irritation (headache, vomiting, neck stiffness), cranial nerve damage, evolving hydrocephalus, and cerebral endarteritis. Infants are irritable with opisthotonos and a tense fontanelle. Cranial nerve lesions, seen in 25 per cent of cases, involve one or more of the following: II, III, IV, VI, VII, and VIII. The pupils may be dilated, unequal, and unresponsive, and many patients have a VIth nerve palsy (Fig. 5). Fundal examination reveals papilloedema in 40 per cent of cases and sometimes evidence of optic atrophy. Choroid tubercles are occasionally seen (Plate 8). Bilateral visual failure with optic atrophy is a feature of arachnoiditis in the cistern of the optic chiasm. Raised intracranial pressure, a common and serious complication of TBM, results from obstruction of the CSF circulation in the basal cisterns by the exudates or, less commonly, obstruction of the outlets of the fourth ventricle. Increasing headache, vomiting, and impairment of conscious level are mainly the result of intracranial hypertension rather than the meningeal irritation. Hydrocephalus, which often accompanies the increased intracranial pressure, is common and should be suspected in all patients with TBM. They often have severe headache, ocular palsy, pyramidal signs in the lower limbs, and incontinence of urine. If left untreated, the patients become stuporose or comatose and develop signs of brainstem damage, such as decerebrate rigidity, irregular breathing, and impairment of brainstem reflexes. About 20 per cent of the patients develop focal neurological signs such as hemiparesis, hemianaesthesia, aphasia, and hemianopia. These are the results of cerebral infarct, caused by the arteritis. Convulsive disorders are common in children but rare in adults. About 10 per cent of the patients develop symptoms and signs of spinal arachnoiditis (Fig. 6), which vary from radicular pain, radicular weakness of the lower limbs, and urinary retention, to paraplegia with sensory loss on the trunk. SIADH is common in patients with severe TBM. It produces impairment of consciousness, but decerebrate rigidity or other signs of brainstem damage are not found. Other uncommon neurological abnormalities include internuclear ophthalmoplegia, hemichorea, and hypothalamic disorders leading to loss of control of blood pressure and body temperature and diabetes insipidus.

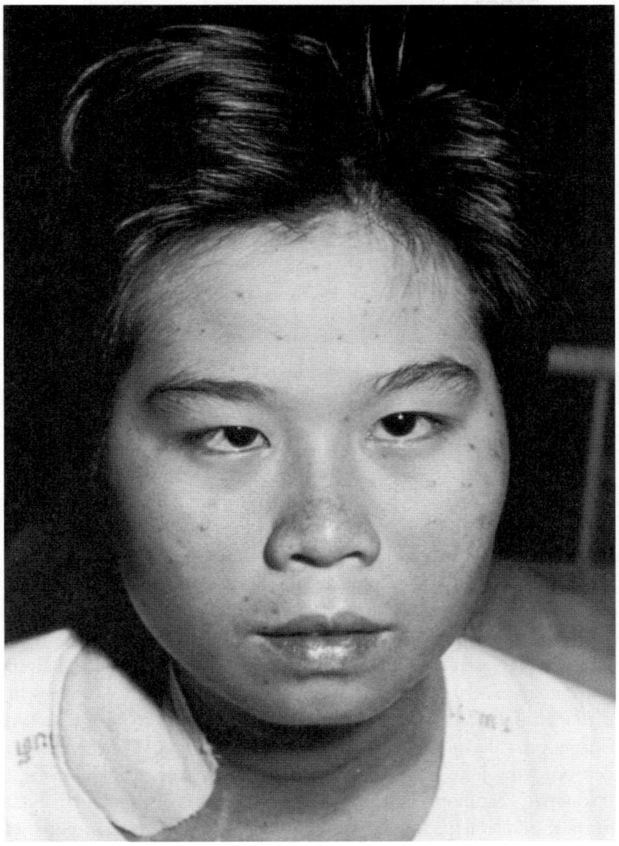

Fig. 5 Bilateral VIth nerve palsies in a Thai girl with TBM. The cervical node biopsy was positive for acid-fast bacilli. (Copyright the late Prida Phuapradit.)

HIV-infected patients with tuberculosis are at a higher risk of developing the meningitis than non-HIV-infected patients. In HIV-infected patients, peripheral, intrathoracic, and intra-abdominal lymphadenopathy is more common, but the clinical manifestations of TBM do not seem to be modified by the HIV infection.

Diagnosis

The blood count is usually normal, but marked leucocytosis of more than 20 000/μl ('leukaemoid picture') may occasionally be found in TBM and miliary tuberculosis. Examination of CSF is crucial. Lumbar puncture does not seem to pose the same dangers as in acute bacterial meningitis and, apparently, lumbar puncture has been repeated safely as a treatment of raised intracranial pressure in patients with TBM even when there is papilloedema. The CSF opening pressure is raised in the majority of patients,

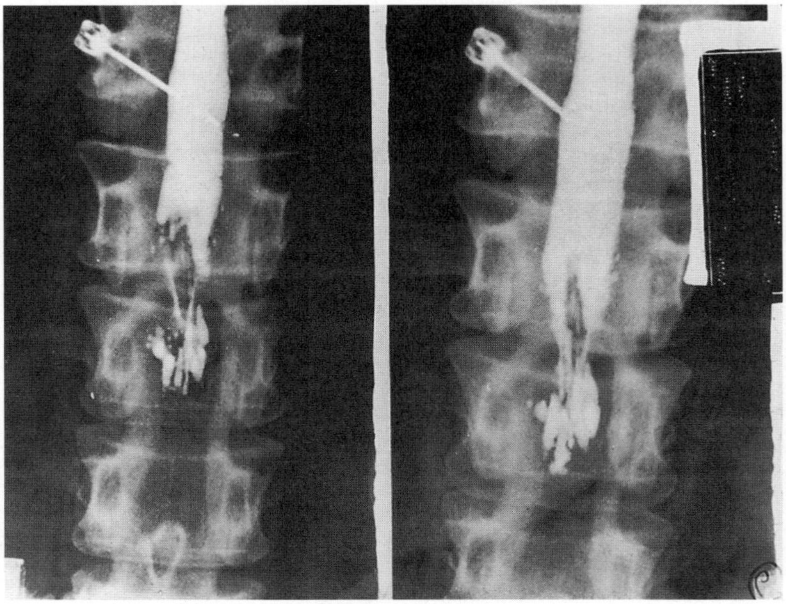

Fig. 6 Spinal arachnoiditis revealed by myelography in a Thai patient with TBM. (Copyright the late Prida Phuapradit.)

but it may be low or fall in those developing block from spinal arachnoiditis. The CSF is clear or slightly turbid, and may form a spider's web clot on standing. The mechanism of the cobweb formation is unclear, but it does not appear to be caused by the high protein concentration *per se.* In patients with spinal block the fluid may be xanthochromic with a very high protein concentration and may quickly form a jelly (Froin's syndrome). Total cell counts range between 10 and 1000/μl. Both lymphocytes and neutrophils are present and the latter can be as high as 70 per cent of the total. In 90 per cent of the patients the white cell count is less than 500/μl. Rarely, the cell count exceeds 1000/μl. The CSF glucose concentration of the initial CSF sample is low in about 90 per cent of the patients. Although non-specific, this finding is of great practical use, because it is a simple test that differentiates TBM presumptively from most cases of viral meningitis. Indeed, TBM must be strongly suspected in any patient who presents with lymphocytic meningitis and a low CSF glucose concentration. The CSF protein concentration is usually raised, and ranges from normal to 5 g/l. Levels of more than 5 g/l suggests a spinal block. Success in detecting tubercle bacilli in CSF by Ziehl–Neelson staining can, in some hands, be increased from the usual average of 10 to 20 per cent by centrifuging a large volume of CSF (10–20 ml) and carefully examining the sediment under a microscope. Repeated lumbar punctures increase the chance of finding tubercle bacilli and of observing the characteristic changes in CSF composition. Marked neutrophil pleocytosis of the CSF may be seen transiently in association with abrupt deterioration of the headache, increased neck stiffness, and fever, suggesting bacterial meningitis. The phenomenon is self-limited, and is thought to be the result of a rupture of a microtubercle into the subarachnoid space. Culture of mycobacteria is successful in 40 to 60 per cent of cases. Specimens other than CSF (for example, sputum, gastric washings in children, urine, etc.) should also be cultured. Since it can take up to 2 months or longer for the mycobacteria to grow in the standard cultures, a number of methods for the rapid diagnosis of TBM have therefore been developed. The bromide partition test is not of practical use, because it lacks specificity and is abnormal in other types of meningitis and even in cerebral malaria. It is no more useful than the CSF glucose concentration. Tests for detecting membrane antigen of tubercle bacilli in CSF by enzyme immunoassay and latex-particle agglutination are disappointing because they are not reproducible and do not have sufficient sensitivity and specificity to be of clinical use. Detection of tuberculostearic acid (a lipid component of the mycobacterial cell wall) in the CSF by gas chromatography and mass spectroscopy is highly specific and sensitive, but the apparatus is very expensive and technically too complicated for clinical use. Detection of the genome of *M. tuberculosis* in the CSF by PCR can be specific and sensitive in the rapid diagnosis of TBM. Recent studies in centres of excellence suggest a sensitivity of 75 per cent and a specificity of 94 per cent; however, further work on larger sample sets are still required to establish the utility, reproducibility, and cost-effectiveness of this approach. Cell-mediated immunity should be assessed. The tuberculin test is positive in 50 to 95 per cent of patients with TBM. Reactivity is suppressed in debilitated or immunosuppressed patients. Serological tests for HIV infection and a CD4 cell count should, if possible, be performed in every case. Immunological assays based on the production of γ-interferon following stimulation with *M. tuberculosis*-specific antigens (ESAT6 and CFP10) (ELI-SPOT TEST) have shown promise as a diagnostic tool among contacts of patients with TB. Their potential role in TB meningitis has not yet been established. A search for evidence of tuberculosis elsewhere in the body is useful. Chest radiographs are normal in about half of the patients, and miliary mottling is seen in only a minority.

The advent of computed tomography (**CT**) scanning and magnetic resonance imaging (**MRI**) has provided insight into disease progression, and gives prognostic and diagnostic information. Both CT and MRI of the brain will reveal hydrocephalus, basilar meningeal thickening, infarcts, oedema, and tuberculomas (Figs 7 and 8).

In a CT study of 60 cases of TBM in adults and children, only three had normal brain scans. Hydrocephalus was reported in 87 per cent of children and 12 per cent of adults. The incidence of hydrocephalus is greater in the young, and increases with duration of the illness. In children, hydrocephalus is invariably present after 6 weeks of illness. Infarcts are seen on CT scanning in 28 per cent, with 83 per cent occurring in the middle cerebral artery territory. The basal ganglia are the most commonly affected region. Poor prognosis has been associated with enhancing basal exudates and periventricular lucency.

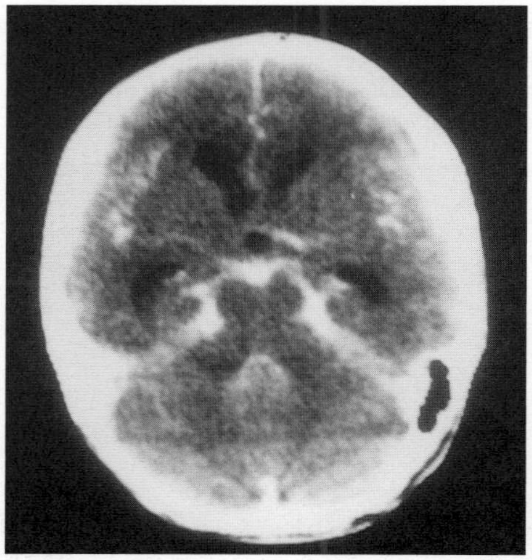

Fig. 7 CT scan with enhancement showing thick basal exudates and hydrocephalus. (Copyright the late Prida Phuapradit.)

MRI has increased sensitivity in detecting the distribution of meningeal inflammatory exudate. Gadolinium-enhanced, *T*1-weighted images highlight the exudate, and reveal parenchymal infarcts as hyperintense areas. MRI may provide more diagnostic information than CT when assessing space-occupying lesions. Cerebral miliary TB, with multiple small intraparenchymal granulomas, produces moderate perilesional oedema and contrast enhancement. Larger tuberculomas are initially non-enhancing, but later demonstrate marked enhancement.

CT and MRI are sensitive for the changes of TBM, particularly hydrocephalus and basal meningeal exudates, but they lack specificity. The radiological differential diagnosis includes cryptococcal meningitis, cytomegalovirus encephalitis, sarcoidosis, meningeal metastases, and lymphoma. The major role of neuroradiology has been in the management and,

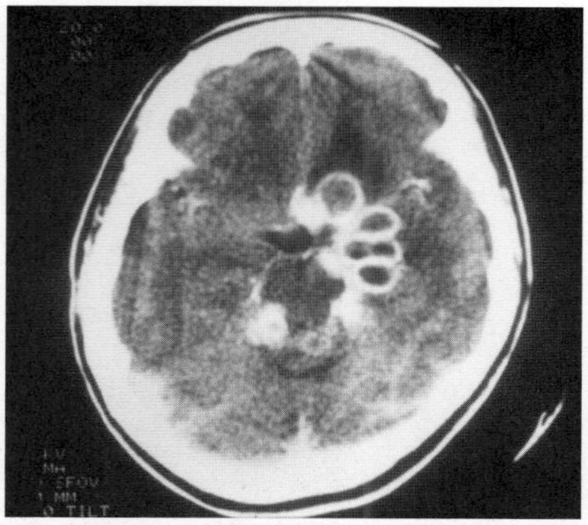

Fig. 8 CT scan with enhancement of a patient with TBM showing multiple tuberculomas developing near the basal cisterns (Copyright the late Prida Phuapradit.)

in particular, in the diagnosis and follow-up of those complications requiring neurosurgery.

Differential diagnosis

Although a few patients with TBM present acutely, the majority show a subacute or chronic progression. Clinically, the differential diagnosis should include cryptococcal meningitis and various subacute or chronic meningitides, including partially treated bacterial meningitis, parameningeal infections, neoplastic and granulomatous infiltrations of the meninges (for example, carcinomas, leukaemias, lymphomas, sarcoidosis), and cerebral tumours. Fungal meningitides (with *Cryptococcus* spp., Coccidioides, *Histoplasma* spp., *Candida* spp.) may present like TBM. Other conditions that have caused confusion in particular clinical or geographical settings are meningovascular syphilis, toxoplasma meningitis in immunosuppressed patients (notably in those with AIDS), cysticercosis, amoebic meningoencephalitis, African trypanosomiasis, and schistosomal myelopathy. In most of these cases, CSF examination, including cytology, an India-ink preparation, immunodiagnostic tests (for example, cryptococcal latex agglutination), serological tests, and microbial cultures will allow differentiation.

Treatment

The untreated mortality of TBM is close to 100 per cent. Full treatment must be started when the diagnosis is suspected on clinical grounds, immediately after adequate samples have been taken for microscopy, culture, and immunodiagnosis. The choice of antituberculosis drugs has been based mainly on their pharmacokinetic and antibacterial properties. Isoniazid, pyrazinamide, ethionamide, and cycloserine freely distribute into the CSF. Penetration is limited, but still adequate during the first few months of the meningitis, in the case of rifampicin, ethambutol, and streptomycin. *p*-Aminosalicylic acid should not be used because it does not enter the CSF. At least two drugs to which the organism is sensitive should be used. During the first 2 months, however, intensive chemotherapy with three or four antituberculosis drugs should be given: the impairment of the blood–brain barrier during the active stage of meningitis allows most antituberculosis drugs to enter the CSF in amounts sufficient to kill the organism, and offers a good chance of eliminating mycobacteria from the CSF after a short period of treatment. The combination of isoniazid and rifampicin for 12 months, with pyrazinamide and streptomycin during the first 2 months, is an effective regimen that has been widely used. In adults, daily single doses of 300 mg of isoniazid, 600 mg of rifampicin, and 1500 mg of pyrazinamide provide adequate levels in the sera and CSF of patients with active TBM. Higher doses of these drugs are unnecessary and may result in a higher incidence of hepatotoxicity. The incidence of adverse reactions of antituberculosis drugs in TBM is acceptable and is similar to that encountered in the treatment of pulmonary tuberculosis.

In countries where rifampicin cannot be afforded, triple therapy with isoniazid, pyrazinamide, and streptomycin should be tried. TBM in HIV-infected patients should be similarly treated as the meningitis in those not infected. Responses to treatment and the outcome of TBM are similar in the two groups. Drug-resistant isolates of *M. tuberculosis*, which have been found increasingly, poses problems in the treatment now and in the future. Ethionamide, kanamycin or amikacin, and cycloserine should be considered in this situation. Development of new effective antituberculosis drugs is urgently needed.

Response to antituberculosis chemotherapy is slow, particularly in patients who are not given corticosteroids. There may be an increase in temperature and CSF protein concentration as well as a transient neutrophil pleocytosis during the first 2 months after starting optimal chemotherapy. However, some signs of clinical improvement are usually seen within the first few weeks. Early clinical evidence of response is an improvement of the headache, sense of general well being, and a decrease in the elevated intracranial pressure. A rapid return to normal in CSF composition within a few days virtually excludes the diagnosis of TBM, in which case antituberculosis treatment should be stopped. Usually it would take at least a few weeks to a few months for the cells, CSF glucose, and protein levels to return to normal. However, the high protein concentration persists in some patients.

'Trial' of chemotherapy is justified when there is clinical suspicion of TBM, particularly when diagnostic facilities are limited. Treatment should be continued for 12 months unless there is rapid improvement in the patient's condition and CSF composition, suggesting another cause for aseptic meningitis. In some severely ill patients who present acutely with features of acute bacterial meningitis (for example, neutrophil pleocytosis) but in whom initial laboratory results are unhelpful, it may be necessary to initiate 'blind' treatment for acute bacterial and TBM simultaneously. In these, fortunately rare cases, isoniazid, rifampicin, and streptomycin or ethambutol, together with penicillin or a third-generation cephalosporin, can be given.

There is conflicting evidence regarding the length of treatment. The current United Kingdom guidelines recommend 12 months in uncomplicated cases of TBM (including cerebral tuberculoma without meningitis), extending to 18 months should pyrazinamide be omitted. No guidelines exist for the components and duration of treatment in the case of multi-drug-resistant TBM. Treatment for 12 months is probably a conservative estimate of the time required for bacterial cure. Different regimes, incomparable patient groups, and the variable use of adjuvant steroid therapy, makes meta-analysis from the trials impossible. Some suggest that TBM should be treated for a minimum of 2 years. Evidence from 781 cases of TBM treated for 2 years revealed that 35 patients had a recrudescence; however, nearly all patients with relapse had received less than 6 months' therapy, indicating that therapy should continue in excess of this period. In South Africa, 95 children were treated for 6 months with a combination of isoniazid 20 mg/kg, rifampicin 20 mg/kg, pyrazinamide 40 mg/kg, and ethionamide 20 mg/kg. Some 96 per cent of these cases presented in either stage II or III TBM. The doses of both isoniazid and rifampicin used were considerably higher than those recommended in the United Kingdom, but no serious adverse reactions were reported. The study provides good evidence for the adequacy of short-course intensive chemotherapy, but the lack of a control group does not allow conclusions to be drawn regarding the optimal dosages. Studies using 9 months' chemotherapy (2 months' isoniazid, rifampicin, pyrazinamide, streptomycin, followed by 7 months' rifampicin and isoniazid) at lower doses produced similar outcomes.

Treatment of complications

The complications of TBM are common, some of which are often serious enough to cause severe morbidity and death in spite of active treatment with antituberculosis drugs. Increased intracranial pressure, found in about 90 per cent of the patients and often associated with communicating hydrocephalus, is usually caused by the basal arachnoiditis. Less commonly, it is caused by diffuse cerebral oedema which compresses the small lateral ventricles. In these patients, conservative treatment by repeated lumbar punctures in combination with acetazolamide, with or without furosemide (frusemide), and corticosteroids should be tried. Within the first 4 to 6 weeks of treatment, the CSF pressures in the majority of the patients return to normal and the transependymal oedema (periventricular lucency on the CT scan) disappears. However, the sizes of the ventricles usually remain unchanged during the first 4 to 6 weeks of treatment. This is a state of arrested hydrocephalus. Usually, it would take up to 6 months for the ventricular size to return to normal. In a few centres, intrathecal hyaluronidase, which might resolve the basal exudates, has been shown to be beneficial in the treatment of communicating hydrocephalus and spinal arachnoiditis. If these conservative measures fail, surgical treatment will be needed for the hydrocephalus. Patients with communicating hydrocephalus who are very ill with impairment of consciousness should receive early temporary external ventricular shunting. Shunt surgery, as a first-line treatment, should be reserved for patients with non-communicating hydrocephalus.

Corticosteroids might be expected to reduce the inflammatory reaction and the fibrotic organization of exudate in the brain and spinal cord. A recent Cochrane review analysed six trials comprising a total of 595 patients. Steroids were associated with fewer deaths (relative risk (**RR**) 0.79; 95 per cent confidence interval (**CI**) 0.65 to 0.97) and a reduced incidence of death and severe residual disability (RR, 0.58; 95 per cent CI, 0.38 to 0.88). Subgroup analysis suggested an effect on mortality in children (RR, 0.77; 95 per cent CI, 0.62 to 0.96), but the results in a smaller number of adults were inconclusive (RR, 0.96; 95 per cent CI, 0.50 to 1.84). There is little evidence that the severity of disease influences the effects of steroids on mortality. The conclusion of the Cochrane reviewers was that adjunctive steroids might be of benefit in patients with TBM. However, existing studies were small, and publication bias may account for the positive results. The data are stronger for the use of steroids in children than in adults. No data are available on the use of steroids in HIV-positive patients. The usual regimen is intramuscular dexamethasone (16 mg/day in adults and 0.5 mg/kg per day in children) in divided doses, or oral prednisolone 60 mg/day for adults, 2 mg/kg per day for children, given in a tapering course over 3 to 6 weeks. There is no evidence that corticosteroids interfere with the penetration of antituberculosis drugs into the CSF. Intrathecal injection of corticosteroids is unnecessary.

Fluid, electrolyte, and acid–base disturbances are common, the result of vomiting, inadequate fluid intake, and SIADH. Progressive loss of vision caused by fibrosing exudate around the optic chiasma may respond to surgical decompression. Cerebral tuberculomas may occasionally develop during the course of the treatment of TBM. Characteristically, the lesions are thick-walled nodules of small or moderate size in clusters, and develop in the surface of the brain near the basal cisterns, such as the interpeduncular cistern and cistern of the optic chiasm (Fig. 8). They should be treated conservatively and the response to antituberculosis treatment assessed by CT scan. Biopsy or surgical intervention is unnecessary and may be harmful. Tuberculomas usually respond very slowly to antituberculosis drugs and it usually takes at least 24 months or longer for the lesions to disappear. Nursing care is very important during the acute illness, when there are the usual problems presented by unconscious patients, and during the prolonged phase of convalescence and rehabilitation. Anticonvulsants are often needed, especially in children.

Prognosis and sequelae

In Western industrialized countries, the mortality from TBM is still high, at about 15 to 30 per cent, and in developing countries it remains between 30 and 50 per cent. The prognosis is worst and the risk of sequelae highest in those admitted in coma with signs of brainstem damage, in the very young and very old, pregnant women, and those with malnutrition or other diseases. The outcome of TBM in HIV-infected patients is similar to that in patients without HIV infection. There are permanent sequelae in 10 to 30 per cent of survivors. Intellectual impairment is especially common in infants and young children. As many as 60 per cent of patients who have seizures during the illness will suffer recurrences. Up to 25 per cent of survivors will have cranial nerve deficits, including blindness, deafness, and squints. Some 10 to 25 per cent of survivors have some residual weakness after hemiparesis or paraparesis. About 10 per cent of patients develop CSF spinal block at some stage of the illness, but this will recover completely in at least half of them. Occasionally neurological deficit may progress or appear months after the illness as the subarachnoid exudate becomes fibrotic and calcified.

Prevention (see also Chapter 7.11.22)

BCG vaccination at birth reduces the risk of infection by at least 80 per cent, but this seems to vary in different countries. It is recommended for all infants born into communities where tuberculosis is prevalent, including Asians living in Britain and expatriates living in tropical countries. To prevent the development of TBM in household contacts of newly diagnosed cases of pulmonary tuberculosis, prophylaxis with isoniazid 10 mg/kg daily for 6 to 12 months is recommended for all Mantoux-positive children under the age of 5 years.

Further reading

Acute bacterial meningitis

Anonymous (2000). The management of neurosurgical patients with postoperative bacterial or aseptic meningitis or external ventricular drain-associated ventriculitis. *British Journal of Neurosurgery* **14**, 7–12.

Bisno AL (1994). Infections associated with indwelling medical devices. In: Bisno AL, Waldvogel FA, eds. *Infections associated with indwelling medical devices*, 2nd edn, pp 93–109. American Society Medical Press, Washington DC.

Christie AB (1980). *Infectious diseases: epidemiology and clinical practice*, 3rd edn, pp 605–46. Churchill Livingstone, Edinburgh.

Durand ML, *et al.* (1993). Acute bacterial meningitis in adults. *New England Journal of Medicine* **328**, 21–8.

Girgis NI, *et al.* (1990). Dexamethasone for the treatment of children and adults with bacterial meningitis. *Reviews of the Infectious Diseases* **12**, 963–4.

Gordon SB, *et al.* (2000). Bacterial meningitis in Malawian adults: pneumococcal disease is common, severe and seasonal. *Clinical Infectious Diseases* **31**, 53–7.

Gray LD, Fedorko DP (1992). Laboratory diagnosis of bacterial meningitis. *Clinical Microbiological Reviews* **5**, 130–45.

Infection in Neurosurgery Working Party of the British Society for Antimicrobial Chemotherapy. (2000). The rationale use of antibiotics in the treatment of brain abscess. *British Journal of Neurosurgery* **14**, 525–30.

Kay R, Cheng AF, Tse CY (1995). *Streptococcus suis* infection in Hong Kong. *Quarterly Journal of Medicine* **88**, 39–47.

Molyneux EM, *et al.* (2002). Dexamethasone treatment in childhood bacterial meningitis in Malawi: a randomised controlled trial. *Lancet* **360**, 211–18.

Rathore MH (1991). Do prophylactic antibiotics prevent meningitis after basilar skull fracture? *Pediatric Infectious Disease Journal* **10**, 87–8.

Schaad UB, *et al.* (1993). Dexamethasone therapy for bacterial meningitis in children. *Lancet* **342**, 457–61.

Scheld WM, Whitley RJ, Durack DT (1997). *Infections of the central nervous system*, 2nd edn. Lippincott-Raven, Philadelphia.

Tedder DG, *et al.* (1994). Herpes simplex virus infection as a cause of benign recurrent lymphocytic meningitis. *Annals of Internal Medicine* **121**, 334–8.

Tugwell P, Greenwood BM, Warrell DA (1976). Pneumococcal meningitis: a clinical and laboratory study. *Quarterly Journal of Medicine* **45**, 583–601.

Tuberculous meningitis

Alarcon F, *et al.* (1990). Tuberculous meningitis: short course chemotherapy. *Archives of Neurology* **47**, 1313–17.

Berenguer J, *et al.* (1992). Tuberculous meningitis in patients infected with the human immunodeficiency virus. *New England Journal of Medicine* **327**, 668–72.

Donald PR, *et al.* (1988). Intensive short course chemotherapy in the management of tuberculous meningitis. *International Journal of Tuberculosis and Lung Disease* **2**, 704–11.

Girgis NI, *et al.* (1991). Dexamethasone adjunctive treatment for tuberculous meningitis. *Pediatric Infectious Disease Journal* **10**, 179–83.

Goel A, Pandya S, Satoskar A (1990). Whither short-course chemotherapy for tuberculous meningitis. *Neurosurgery* **27**, 418–21.

Joint Tuberculosis Committee of the British Thoracic Society (1998). Chemotherapy and management of tuberculosis in the United Kingdom: recommendations 1998. *Thorax* **53**, 536–48.

Kaojarern S, *et al.* (1991). Effect of steroids on cerebrospinal fluid penetration of antituberculosis drugs in tuberculous meningitis. *Clinical Pharmacology and Therapeutics* **49**, 6–12.

Parsons M (1988). *Tuberculous meningitis. A handbook for clinicians*, 2nd edn. Oxford University Press, Oxford.

Phuapradit P, Vejjavjiva A (1987). Treatment of tuberculous meningitis: role of short-course chemotherapy. *Quarterly Journal of Medicine* **62**, 249–58.

Prasad K, Volmink J, Menon GR (2000) Steroids for treating tuberculous meningitis (Cochrane review). *Cochrane Database Systematic Reviews* (3), CD002244.

Schoeman JF, *et al.* (1985). Intracranial pressure monitoring in tuberculous meningitis: clinical and computerized tomographic correlation. *Developmental Medicine and Child Neurology* **27**, 644–54.

Schoeman JF, *et al.* (1991). Tuberculous hydrocephalus: comparison of different treatments with regard to intracranial pressure, ventricular size and clinical outcome. *Developmental Medicine and Child Neurology* **33**, 396–405.

Shankar P, *et al.* (1991). Rapid diagnosis of tuberculous meningitis by polymerase chain reaction. *Lancet* **337**, 5–7.

Tartaglione T, *et al.* (1998). Diagnostic imaging of neurotuberculosis. *Rays* **23**, 164–80.

Thwaites G, *et al.* (2000) Tuberculous meningitis. *Journal of Neurology, Neurosurgery, Psychiatry* **68**, 289–99.

Visudhiphan P, Chiemchanya S (1989). Tuberculous meningitis in children: treatment with isoniazid and rifampicin for twelve months. *Journal of Pediatrics* **114**, 875–9.

24.14.2 Viral infections of the central nervous system

*D. A. Warrell and J. J. Farrar**

Viruses invade and damage the central nervous system in two ways: directly, by infecting the leptomeninges, brain, and spinal cord; and, indirectly, by inducing an immunological reaction resulting in para- and postinfectious diseases. In both cases, the terms 'meningitis', 'encephalitis', and 'myelitis' are used alone or in combination. Meningitis implies inflammation of the meninges without alteration of consciousness, convulsions, or the production of focal neurological abnormalities; in encephalitis there is impairment of cerebral function, usually with an altered state of consciousness and often with convulsions and focal neurological signs; while myelitis indicates involvement of the spinal cord. Retroviral and prion diseases of the central nervous system are dealt with elsewhere (see Chapters 7.10.21–23 and Chapter 24.13.9).

Virology

There is considerable geographical and seasonal variation in the kinds of viruses causing meningitis, myelitis, and encephalitis. However, compared with bacterial infections of the central nervous system, there is less variation with age and immunocompetence.

Enteroviruses are responsible for 80 to 90 per cent of diagnosed cases of viral meningitis. Almost all the serotypes have been implicated in sporadic cases, and outbreaks have been associated with coxsackieviruses A7 and 9, all the coxsackie B types, and many of the echoviruses, especially 4, 6, 9, 11, 14, 16, and 30. Recently, echovirus 13, a rare type, has caused cases in the United States, Australia, and Europe and there has been an increase in echovirus 30 cases. Mumps is responsible for about 10 to 20 per cent of cases of viral meningitis. Other less common causes include herpes zoster, herpes simplex virus (predominantly type 2, HSV-2), measles, adenoviruses, Epstein–Barr virus and, in the United States, togaviruses, such as St Louis, eastern and western equine encephalitis, and West Nile and bunyaviruses, such as California (La Crosse) encephalitis viruses.

* Contains some material contributed by PGE Kennedy to OTM3.

Poliovirus has long been considered the major cause of viral 'paralytic' myelitis throughout the world, but has now been virtually eliminated from the Americas. A confusingly similar syndrome of acute flaccid paralysis caused by Japanese encephalitis (**JE**) has now been reported from Vietnam. Coxsackie A7 (AB IV) has caused occasional small outbreaks, and other coxsackie A and B viruses, echoviruses, enterovirus 70, and flaviruses (tick-borne encephalitis) have all been implicated as causes of flaccid paralysis. Herpes zoster, paralytic rabies, Epstein–Barr, and *Herpes simiae* B viruses can cause myelitis or ascending paralysis, and HSV-2 can cause lumbosacral myeloradiculitis.

Viruses causing encephalitis vary from country to country. JE virus is the most widespread human togavirus infection in the world and is the major cause of encephalitis throughout Asia. There are at least 50 000 cases of JE with 15 000 deaths annually. The virus is transmitted by Culex mosquitoes and is endemic across much of southern Asia and the Indian subcontinent. It is spreading through the Pacific rim to New Guinea, Torres Strait Islands, and Cape York Peninsula, in northern Australia. Dengue viruses have been implicated as a cause of encephalitis in South-East Asia.

In 1999 an outbreak of an encephalitic illness among pig farm and abattoir workers was reported from Singapore and Malaysia. There were 258 cases of encephalitis, with a case fatality rate of almost 40 per cent. The causative agent was a new paramyxovirus, Nipah virus, closely related to the Hendra and Manangle viruses described in Australia. Nipah virus encephalitis is a zoonosis infecting pigs and flying foxes (*Pteropus* spp.). Almost all patients infected in this outbreak had direct contact with pigs. Hendra virus has caused a few cases of equine and human encephalitis (Chapter 7.10.6.1).

In North America, herpes simplex virus is the most common cause of sporadic fatal viral encephalitis, followed by the California encephalitis group, St Louis encephalitis virus, herpes zoster, enteroviruses, mumps, measles, and, most recently, the West Nile virus. In the United States, herpes simplex encephalitis has an estimated incidence of 2.3 per million population each year; HSV-1 accounts for 95 per cent of cases; HSV-2 causes encephalitis mainly in neonates and those who are immunosuppressed, such as transplant patients and those with human immunodeficiency virus (**HIV**) infection. In 1999 there was an outbreak of West Nile infection in the eastern United States with a cluster of cases of encephalitis in New York and, since then, 16 human deaths. West Nile virus is a mosquito-borne flavivirus closely related JE. It has been known to cause encephalitis in Africa, the Middle East, and southern and eastern Europe, but this was the first appearance of this virus in the New World. In endemic areas, infection with West Nile virus is usually asymptomatic or associated with a mild 'flu-like' illness. Only occasionally does it cause encephalitis, with a case fatality rate for patients admitted to hospital in New York of 12 per cent. The virus has now become established in migrant bird populations along the Atlantic coast of the United States and has killed hundreds of thousands of crows.

In the United Kingdom, mumps is the most frequently diagnosed viral encephalitis, followed by echoviruses, coxsackieviruses, measles, herpes simplex virus, herpes zoster virus, Epstein–Barr virus, and adenoviruses (especially adenovirus 7). Louping ill is the only indigenous arthropod (tick)-borne encephalitis in Britain. In Central and Eastern Europe and Scandinavia, tick-borne encephalitis virus and Russian spring–summer encephalitis viruses are endemic. Usutu, a flavivirus, has been isolated in birds in Austria. In many developing countries rabies is an important cause of viral encephalitis. Other regional causes are Rift Valley fever virus in Africa and the Middle East, arenaviruses (Junin, Guanarito, Sabiá, Lassa, and Machupo) in Latin America and Africa, Marburg and Ebola viruses in Africa, Colorado tick fever virus in North America, and Murray Valley encephalitis virus in Australia.

Postinfectious encephalomyelitis most commonly follows measles, vaccinia, varicella, rubella, mumps, and influenza. Guillain-Barré syndrome, a sensorimotor polyneuropathy (see Chapter 24.19), has been associated with infections by Epstein–Barr virus, cytomegalovirus, coxsackie B, and herpes zoster virus. Nervous-tissue vaccine against rabies may give rise to postvaccinal encephalitis (see below), while vaccination against influenza, rabies, hepatitis B, measles, and poliomyelitis has been complicated by Guillain-Barré syndrome.

Immunodeficient patients are particularly vulnerable to some viral infections. Those with depressed cell-mediated immunity (Hodgkin's disease) may develop herpes zoster encephalitis, and cytomegalovirus may cause a subacute encephalitis in patients with acquired immunodeficiency syndrome (**AIDS**). In children or adults with hypogammaglobulinaemia, enteroviruses, including live-attenuated polio vaccine, may produce a progressive and fatal meningoencephalitis. Progressive multifocal leucoencephalopathy, a chronic and fatal papovavirus infection in patients with impaired cell-mediated immunity, is described below. HIV infection of the brain and meninges may be responsible for acute meningoencephalitis at the time of seroconversion and for subacute chronic encephalopathies and dementia in patients with AIDS (see Chapters 7.10.23 and 24.14.4).

Epidemiology

Many viral infections of the central nervous system occur in seasonal peaks or as epidemics, while others, such as herpes simplex encephalitis, are sporadic. Epidemics of Japanese encephalitis occur in the summer or rainy season in northern India, Nepal, northern Thailand, Korea, Taiwan, and China. However, in southern Vietnam, Indonesia, Malaysia, southern India, and the Philippines the disease can occur all the year round, although the peak is at the start of the rainy season. This variation in the incidence of disease is an important consideration when recommending vaccination. In endemic areas it is mostly a disease of children, but as the disease spreads to new regions, or non-immune travellers visit endemic regions, non-immune adults are also affected. The major vector is *Culex tritaeniorhynchus* mosquitoes which have been infected by first feeding on the bird (cattle egrets, herons) or mammal reservoir species. Indigenous children and non-immune (immigrant) adults are most susceptible. Tick-borne encephalitides occur in spring and early summer when the ticks are most active. Mumps encephalitis is commonest in the late winter or early spring, while enterovirus infections occur most often in the summer and early autumn. Rodent-related encephalitides, such as the arenaviruses, are most common when the rodent population is at its peak, either in the fields (Machupo and Junin viruses) or in the home (lymphocytic choriomeningitis virus). Zoonotic viral infections, such as Rift Valley Fever, survive periods of cold weather, during which the invertebrate–vertebrate cycle is suspended by 'overwintering' in their arthropod vectors (for example, in the bottom of dried-up ponds) or hibernating vertebrate reservoirs.

Invasion of the central nervous system seems to be a rare event in most viral infections. In the case of some togavirus infections, such as JE, there may be only one case of encephalitis for every 500 to 1000 asymptomatic infections. Eastern equine encephalitis virus produces a much higher proportion of encephalitic cases than other togaviruses.

Infections by many neurotropic viruses are most frequent and severe in children and the elderly. Herpes simplex encephalitis affects all age groups but shows peaks of incidence in those aged between 5 and 30 years and over 50 years. When HSV-2 invades the central nervous system it is likely to cause a benign lymphocytic meningitis in adults, but in neonates it usually produces a severe encephalitis. Among mosquito-borne epidemic encephalitides, California encephalitis and JE are most common in children, St Louis and West Nile encephalitis in the elderly, while eastern and western equine encephalitis affect both the very young and the elderly. Postinfectious encephalitis is most frequent in children, for it complicates the common childhood exanthematous viral infections. It is the most common demyelinating disease in the world.

Pathogenesis

Most viral infections reach the central nervous system from the primary site of infection and multiplication via the bloodstream, but the rabies virus enters peripheral nerves through acetylcholine and other receptors and travels to the CNS in axoplasm, employing the microtubular dynein motor system. Viruses inoculated through the skin include those transmitted by arthropods, rabies virus, herpes simplex virus, *Herpes simiae* B, and lymphocytic choriomeningitis virus. Arthropod-borne viruses are presumed to replicate in local lymph nodes, vascular endothelium, and circulating fixed macrophages, in order to sustain viraemia. Rabies virus may multiply locally in the cytoplasm of muscle cells before entering peripheral nerves. Viruses that enter through the respiratory tract (for example, measles, mumps, varicella) or gut (enteroviruses) multiply in local lymphoid tissue before entering the bloodstream. Viraemia is a feature of most viral infections, yet invasion of the central nervous system is rare in most cases. The explanation for this is not known, but the CNS contains a number of intrinsic physical barriers to infectious agents such as viruses. These include the blood–brain barrier with its 'tight junctions', virus-resistant cells, and the absence of lymphatic drainage. Non-specific mechanisms at or near the site of virus entry, such as gastric acidity and cilia in the respiratory tract, also play a protective role. In the case of rabies, herpes simplex, and herpes zoster viruses, the virus enters the central nervous system through the peripheral nerves. Although the subarachnoid space surrounding the olfactory nerves projects through the cribriform plate and is directly beneath the nasal mucosa, this route of infection seems to be extremely rare in humans and has been proven only in a few cases of inhaled rabies virus infection and herpes simplex encephalitis. Viruses have been inoculated directly into the central nervous system by infected corneal transplant grafts (rabies) and prions through infected brain-surface electrodes (Creutzfeldt–Jakob disease). Herpes simplex encephalitis may complicate primary herpes simplex virus infection in children and young adults, but in most cases of herpes simplex encephalitis the cause is thought to be reactivation of latent virus (HSV-1) in the trigeminal nerve, autonomic nerve roots, or brain.

Some viruses, such as the enteroviruses and mumps, usually infect the meninges rather than the parenchyma of the central nervous system, whereas others, such as the togaviruses, usually cause encephalitis. Different neural cells are selectively vulnerable to different neurotropic viruses. Examples are the predilection of polioviruses for motor neurones of the anterior horns of the spinal cord, and of rabies for neurones of the limbic system and cerebellar Purkinje cells. The pathological effects of viral infections on the central nervous system include:

(1) the destruction and phagocytosis of neurones (neuronophagia) as a result of either viral invasion *per se* or immune lysis;

(2) demyelination;

(3) inflammatory oedema with the compressive effects of raised intracranial pressure; and, in some cases,

(4) vascular lesions.

In rabies, a universally fatal encephalitis, neuronolysis is relatively mild. However, rabies virus may interfere with neurotransmission at central and peripheral synapses. It also produces severe systemic effects, following its centrifugal spread (for example, myocarditis and cardiac arrhythmias) or its focal effects on vasomotor and respiratory centres in the brainstem and in the temporal (lobes and amygdala (cf. Klüver–Bucy syndrome) (Chapter 7.10.9).

Postinfectious encephalitis and the Guillain-Barré syndrome are thought to result from sensitization to central and peripheral myelin, respectively. The animal model for the former is experimental allergic encephalomyelitis, which can be produced in a variety of animals following immunization with myelin basic protein. A similar animal model for Guillain-Barré syndrome is known as experimental allergic neuritis. It is uncertain how the preceding viral infection induces this autoimmune response. In the case of postvaccinal encephalomyelitis resulting from old-fashioned nervous tissue antirabies vaccines containing homogenized animal brain, the mechanism is still not clear. The anti-myelin basic protein is not always present and is probably not the direct cause of demyelination.

The host's immune responses to viruses play a crucial role in combating infection. They may be directed against either the virus particle or the virus-infected cell, and may be humoral- or cell-mediated. An important local immune response at infected surfaces is provided by IgA antibody, which is present in secretions in the gut, saliva, and respiratory tract. This is important, for example, in the early stages of poliovirus infection where the antibody neutralizes the virus by combining with viral surface proteins. The systemic viral infection may also be limited by means of circulating IgG and IgM antibodies, which can neutralize the virus in a variety of different ways. Immune responses may also occur locally within the CNS, where local synthesis of immunoglobulins in response to virus infection, sometimes in an oligoclonal pattern, may be evident. Such antibody elevations may be of considerable diagnostic value (see below). Under certain conditions immune responses to viruses may themselves set in train immunopathological processes leading to disease. This may occur in a number of different ways, such as through the deposition in blood vessels of immune complexes formed between an antiviral antibody and viral antigen. In other cases, such as lymphocytic choriomeningitis virus infection, the induction of virus-specific cytotoxic T lymphocytes is itself responsible for the production of encephalitis.

Pathology

Meningitis

The basal leptomeninges, ependyma, and choroid plexus are infiltrated with mononuclear cells but the parenchyma is normal. In mumps meningitis there may be exfoliation of ependymal cells.

Poliomyelitis

Virus is distributed widely throughout the brain and spinal cord, possibly even in non-paralytic cases, but usually the only cells to suffer chromatolysis and phagocytosis are motor neurones in the anterior horns of the spinal cord, medulla, and grey matter of the precentral gyrus.

Encephalitis

Most viral encephalitides are characterized by lymphocytic infiltration of the meninges and perivascular cuffing (in Virchow–Robin spaces) in the cortex and underlying white matter, by lymphocytes, plasma cells, histiocytes, and some neutrophils, and proliferation of microglia with the formation of glial nodules. Neuronolysis and demyelination are variable in their degree and location. Infected neurones may show characteristic inclusion bodies in their nuclei (measles, herpes simplex virus, and adenoviruses) or cytoplasm (Negri bodies in rabies). Microhaemorrhages and foci of necrosis may be found.

Herpes simplex encephalitis

Characteristic features of this condition are gross cerebral oedema and severe haemorrhagic and necrotizing encephalitis, which is often asymmetrically localized to the inferior and medial parts of the temporal lobe, the insula, and the orbital part of the frontal lobe. Histological sections show eosinophilic Cowdry type A intranuclear inclusions with margination of chromatin in neurones, oligodendrocytes, and astrocytes, inflammatory and haemorrhagic perivascular reactions, but no demyelination. Cowdry type A inclusions are also found in herpes zoster virus and cytomegalovirus encephalitides. The unique cerebral localization of herpes simplex encephalitis has not been satisfactorily explained, but is probably the result of viral spread along specific neural pathways rather than a differential susceptibility of particular cell populations. A popular idea is that herpes simplex virus spreads along olfactory pathways to the base of the brain and temporal lobes, but it is also possible that virus may spread from the trigeminal ganglia through sensory fibres innervating the dura near these regions. This latter mechanism is consistent with the discovery of latent HSV-1 in the trigeminal, superior cervical, and vagal ganglia in a high proportion of normal individuals, irrespective of whether they have a history of mucocutaneous herpes infections ('cold sores'). Latent HSV-1 might be reactivated by a variety of stimuli, such as sunlight, fever, trauma, and stress; however, the actual mechanisms underlying its latency and reactivation in the nervous system are not yet fully understood. If herpes simplex encephalitis is caused by the reactivation of latent virus, its rarity, despite ubiquitous asymptomatic infection in humans, is hard to explain.

Japanese encephalitis

Microscopical appearances are typical of other viral encephalitides: there is oedema, congestion, and focal haemorrhages of the brain and meninges, and perivascular cuffing, neuronophagia, and glial nodules of the brain parenchyma. Neuronolysis and neuronophagia are unusually widespread in the thalamus, basal ganglia, brainstem, cerebellum (where there is marked destruction of Purkinje cells), and the spinal cord. Viral antigen is localized to neurones, especially in the brainstem and thalamus.

Nipah virus encephalitis

Pathological studies on the brains of fatal cases demonstrated that the endothelium of small blood vessels in the central nervous system was particularly susceptible to infection. This led to disseminated endothelial damage and syncytium formation, vasculitis, thrombosis, ischaemia, and microinfarction. There was also evidence of neuronal infection by the virus that may have contributed to neurological dysfunction.

West Nile virus encephalitis

Pathological studies from the outbreak of this encephalitis in New York showed varying degrees of neuronal necrosis in the grey matter, with infiltrates of microglia and polymorphonuclear leucocytes, perivascular cuffing, neuronal degeneration, and neuronophagia. Viral antigens were demonstrated in neurones and in areas of necrosis. No antigen was detected in other major organs, including lung, liver, spleen, and kidney. The major pathological lesions were seen in the brainstem and spinal cord.

Enterovirus 71

Pathological studies of patients who died of enterovirus 71 infection showed severe perivascular cuffing, parenchymal inflammation, and neuronophagia in the spinal cord, brainstem, and diencephalon, and in focal areas in the cerebellum and cerebrum. Although no viral inclusions were detected, immunohistochemistry showed viral antigen in the neuronal cytoplasm. Inflammation was often more extensive than neuronal infection, suggesting that other indirect factors may be involved in tissue damage in addition to the effects of direct viral invasion.

Postinfectious encephalomyelitis

This is a perivenous microglial encephalitis with demyelination. Fibrinoid necrosis of arterioles is an associated lesion in a more severe form designated 'acute haemorrhagic leucoencephalitis'.

Clinical features

Meningitis

A prodromal influenza-like illness, followed by a brief remission of symptoms, is typical of lymphocytic choriomeningitis viral infection and some outbreaks of enteroviral meningitis (for example, echovirus 9), but in most cases of viral meningitis, symptoms start suddenly. As with bacterial meningitis, there is fever, headache, a stiff neck, and vomiting, especially in children. Compared with bacterial meningitis, headache is less severe and tends to be frontal or retrobulbar (eye movements may be painful) and neck stiffness is less marked. Nausea, anorexia, abdominal pain, myalgias, and sore throat are particularly common in enteroviral meningitis. Myalgia is particularly severe with coxsackie B infections. As in acute bacterial meningitis, infants usually present with vague irritability and a tense fontanelle, and young children with fever and irritability or lethargy. Conjunctival injection, pharyngitis, and cervical lymphadenopathy may be found. Macular or petechial exanthems or enanthems are seen with coxsackie A and B and echovirus infections (especially echovirus 9). Vesicles on the hands, feet, and mouth have been reported with coxsackie A16 and enterovirus 71 infections. By definition, the level of consciousness is normal in simple meningitis. Neurological features include vertigo, nystagmus, cerebellar ataxia, facial spasms, and involuntary movements.

The specific cause of viral meningitis may be suggested by characteristic signs outside the nervous system, such as genital or rectal vesicles in the sexually active age group (HSV-2), herpes zoster skin lesions, swelling in the parotid region (mumps, and occasionally coxsackie, lymphocytic choriomeningitis, and Epstein–Barr viruses), orchitis (mumps and lymphocytic choriomeningitis virus), and arthritis (lymphocytic choriomeningitis virus). However, potentially helpful features, such as gastrointestinal symptoms associated with enteroviral infections and parotitis associated with mumps, may be completely absent in patients with meningitis.

Paralytic poliomyelitis

The infection (see Chapter 7.10.7) is acquired by droplet spread from the respiratory tract or by the faecal–oral route. The 'minor illness', coinciding with viraemia, is a non-specific episode of influenza-like symptoms—fever, headache, sore throat, malaise, and mild gastrointestinal symptoms—which resolves in a few days. Most of those infected have no further symptoms but, in a minority, the 'major illness' follows, sometimes after a few days' remission of symptoms. The features are those of viral meningitis: muscle pain, spasms, and sensory disturbances may precede or accompany the development of lower motor neurone (flaccid) paralysis. Any combination of motor unit deficits may be seen (Fig. 1). It is most unusual for paralysis to extend after the first 3 days or after the temperature has fallen (Fig. 2). Respiratory and bulbar paralysis is life-threatening. Encephalitis is rare. The commonest causes of death are aspiration and airway obstruction, resulting from bulbar paralysis, and paralysis of respiratory muscles.

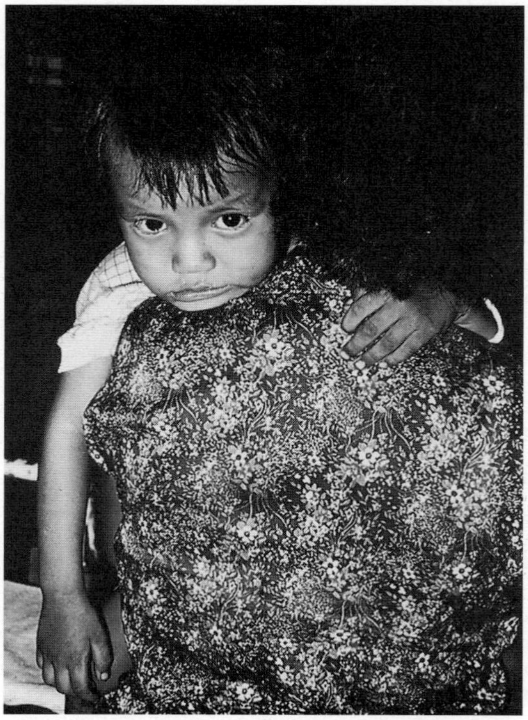

Fig. 1 Paralytic poliomyelitis in a 3-year-old Thai child. Note systemic illness and paralysis of right arm. (Copyright D.A. Warrell.)

Disturbances of respiratory and cardiac rhythm, thought to be the result of damage to medullary vasomotor and respiratory centres, are extremely uncommon. Other complications include impaired control of body temperature and blood pressure, gastrointestinal haemorrhage, aspiration pneumonia, and paralysis of the bladder and bowel.

Encephalitis

Most patients with viral encephalitis present with the symptoms of meningitis (fever, headache, neck stiffness, vomiting) followed by altered consciousness, convulsions, and sometimes focal neurological signs, signs of raised intracranial pressure, or psychiatric symptoms.

Herpes simplex encephalitis

This relatively common sporadic encephalitis may occur in any age group. In neonates, it is caused by HSV-2.

As well as the usual clinical features of a severe viral encephalitis, patients with herpes simplex encephalitis have symptoms related to the focal nature of the encephalitis (frontal and temporal cortex and limbic system). These include behavioural abnormalities, olfactory and gustatory hallucinations, anosmia, amnesia, expressive aphasia, and temporal lobe seizures. Herpetic skin or mucosal lesions are rarely found, except in the case of acute genital HSV-2 infection, or proctitis, and a past history of 'cold sores' does not affect the chances of the infection being due to herpes simplex virus. Effects of cerebral oedema are unusually severe. Patients usually lapse into coma towards the end of the first week and most deaths occur within the first 2 weeks. This condition is also discussed in Chapter 7.10.2.

Japanese encephalitis

After an incubation period of 7 to 14 days, patients develop non-specific prodromal symptoms (fever, headache, malaise, and nausea) lasting 2 to

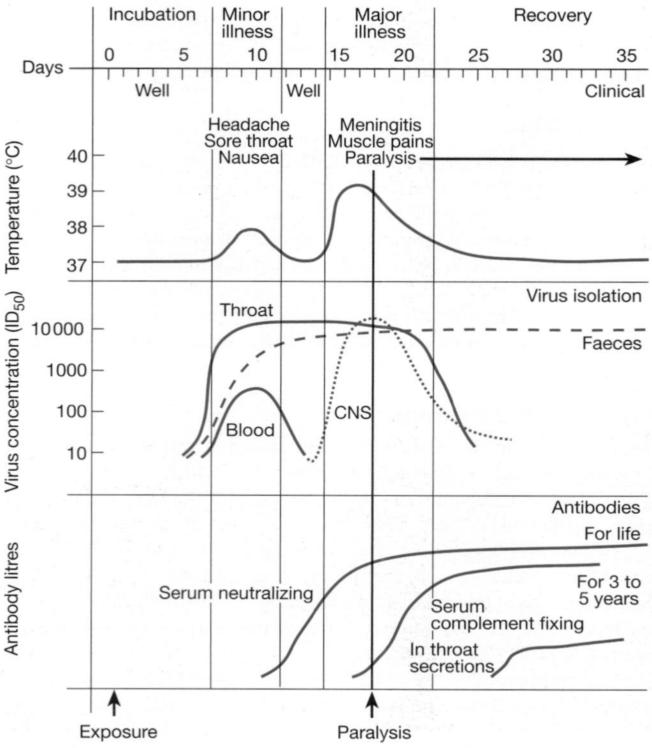

Fig. 2 The course of a paralytic poliomyelitis infection. (Reproduced from Christie (1981). *Medicine International*, **1**, 139. Adapted from Bodian, D. (1957). Mechanisms of infection with polio viruses. In *Cellular biology, nucleic acids, and viruses*. New York Academy of Sciences, by permission.)

3 days. Neurological symptoms begin suddenly, with increasing headache, deteriorating level of consciousness, and generalized convulsions, which may result in status epilepticus. There is meningism and mask-like facies, with upper motor neurone signs or a myelitic pattern, cranial nerve lesions (for example, lower motor neurone VII), flaccid paralysis, ataxia, involuntary movements (Fig. 3), and, in severe cases, prolonged coma, hemi- or quadriparesis, decerebrate rigidity, and respiratory failure. Fever persists for 6 to 7 days and, in survivors, neurological symptoms may persist for several weeks. Parkinsonian and extrapyramidal features occur frequently and choreoathetoid movement disorders or severe dystonias can last for many months. The case fatality rate is 30 per cent in those admitted to hospital. Most deaths occur in the first 7 to 10 days from respiratory failure, aspiration pneumonias, intracranial hypertension, and uncontrolled seizures. Up to 50 per cent of survivors suffer from intellectual impairment, psychiatric problems, persistent epilepsy, or a vegetative state with spastic quadriparesis and evidence of basal ganglia involvement, such as dystonia of the limbs and trunk, rigidity, and tremor (Fig. 3).

Nipah virus encephalitis

The main clinical features of Nipah virus encephalitis are fever, headache, dizziness, reduced consciousness, and prominent brainstem dysfunction. Distinctive signs included myoclonus, areflexia, hypotonia, hypertension, and tachycardia, suggesting extensive brainstem and spinal cord involvement. MRI imaging during the acute illness shows widespread focal lesions in subcortical and deep white matter and, to a lesser extent, in grey matter on T_2-weighted sequences (Fig. 4).

West Nile virus encephalitis

The most common clinical features are encephalitis, meningitis, fever, weakness, and headache following an incubation period of 3 to 15 days. Infection usually results in an acute febrile episode with no CNS involvement. In unusual cases or, as in the United States, when the virus is introduced into a naïve population, the incidence of encephalitis rises particularly in the elderly. An erythematous rash of the neck, trunk, and limbs is present in 20 per cent of cases. Patients over 50 years of age were most at risk of developing encephalitis during the New York outbreak, but all age groups are affected in endemic areas. Muscle weakness, areflexia, and diffuse flaccid paralysis in association with an axonal polyneuropathy was also reported. MRI imaging of the brain demonstrated enhancement of the meninges and periventricular areas. There is no specific treatment.

Enterovirus 71

As the goal of poliomyelitis eradication appears more achievable, another enterovirus is emerging as a significant cause of acute neurological disease in Asia. Enterovirus 71 (**EV71**) was first recognized in 1969 and is responsible for a variety of clinical manifestations, including: hand, foot, and mouth disease; aseptic meningitis; meningoencephalitis; and acute flaccid paralysis. In an outbreak of hand, foot, and mouth disease in Malaysia; a

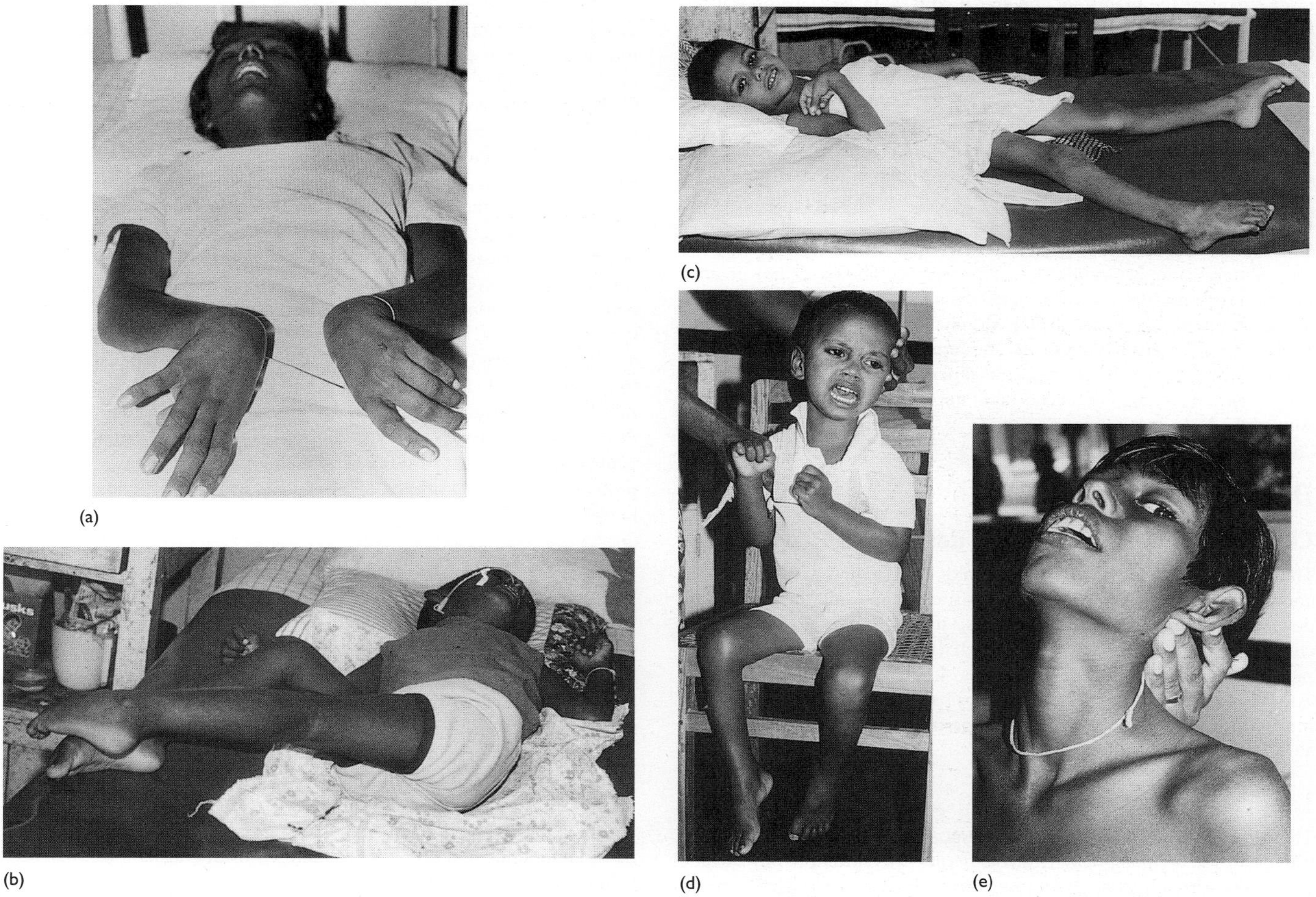

Fig. 3 Japanese encephalitis in Anuradhapura, Sri Lanka. (a) Comatose female patient showing symmetrical chorioathetotic movements of the upper limbs. (b) Comatose child showing dystonic movements of the upper and lower limbs. (c) Convalescent child, conscious but with residual dystonia of all four limbs. (d) Convalescent child with floppy head and involuntary movements of all four limbs. (e) Convalescent boy with residual weakness of the neck flexors. (All figures by courtesy of Dr D.T.D.J. Abeysekera.)

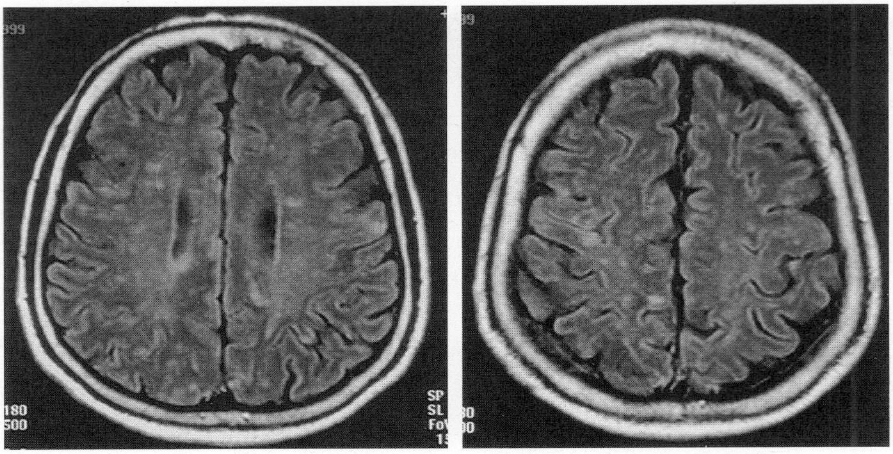

(a) (b)

Fig. 4 (a) and (b) Acute Nipah virus encephalitis. MR brain images in a 57-year-old pig farmer showing multiple focal lesions in the grey–white matter junction. These are areas of infarction secondary to vasculitis. (By courtesy of Drs B.J. Abdullah and Sazilah Sarji, Kuala Lumpur.)

number of young children developed fatal encephalomyelitis, dying within a few hours of presentation with cardiovascular instability and severe pulmonary oedema. Postmortem examination in four cases revealed major involvement of the brainstem and spinal cord, with EV71 being isolated from brain tissue in all cases; there was no apparent cardiac pathology and virus was not isolated from the myocardium. Molecular characterization of these four viruses and others isolated concurrently suggest that at least two potentially virulent EV71 strains were circulating during the outbreak. An adenovirus was also thought to have complicated the infection in 60 per cent of the children dying with a similar clinical picture. It is possible that co-infection with the two viruses may have resulted in severe disease.

Postinfectious encephalomyelitis

Sudden convulsions, coma, fever, or pareses appear 10 to 14 days after the start of vaccination (vaccinia or nervous tissue rabies vaccine) or after infection with measles, varicella, rubella, mumps, or influenza. In the case of measles, varicella, and rubella, encephalitic symptoms develop 2 to 12 days after the rash has appeared, and in mumps before or after parotid swelling. Involuntary movements, cranial nerve lesions (VII, III), pupillary abnormalities, nystagmus, ataxia, and upper motor neurone signs are common

Diagnosis

Clinical and epidemiological details

The time of year, known current epidemics, the patient's age, occupation, animal contacts, and countries or states visited recently may help to narrow down the possibilities. A specific diagnosis may be suggested by distinctive clinical features of the encephalitis itself (for example, hydrophobia in rabies, temporal lobe features in herpes simplex encephalitis) or of the associated infection (for example, mumps parotitis; measles rash; skin and mucosal lesions of herpes viruses; and gastrointestinal symptoms associated with enteroviral infections).

Laboratory investigations

These should aim to demonstrate a specific viral agent (particularly important for the potentially treatable herpesvirus infections) or exclude potentially treatable non-viral causes of meningitis or encephalomyelitis (Table 1). The most important investigation is examination of the cerebrospinal fluid (**CSF**). Contraindications to lumbar puncture are the same as for acute bacterial meningitis (Chapter 24.7 and Chapter 24.14.1). If there are lateralizing neurological signs or evidence of raised intracranial pressure, a computed tomography (**CT**) or magnetic resonance imaging (**MRI**) scan should be performed to exclude an intracranial mass lesion before contemplating a lumbar puncture. CSF pressure is especially increased in herpes simplex encephalitis, where there is intense cerebral oedema. Pleocytosis ranges from tens to thousands of cells/µl. Lymphocytes and other mononuclear cells predominate, except in the early stages of some infections (for example, enteroviruses, herpes simplex encephalitis). The CSF contains erythrocytes or is xanthochromic in haemorrhagic encephalitides such as herpes simplex encephalitis and acute necrotic leucoencephalitis. Protein concentration is usually increased in the range of 50 to 150 mg/dl with an increasing proportion of IgG as the disease progresses. Leakage of serum IgG into the CSF and intrathecal IgG synthesis, indicated by a monoclonal band, are responsible. CSF glucose concentration is usually normal or increased towards the level in a blood sample taken simultaneously, but low levels are occasionally reported, especially in mumps and lymphocytic choriomeningitis virus infections. Measurement of lactate, C-reactive protein, lactic dehydrogenase, creatine kinase (CK-BB), muramidase, and various cytokines in the CSF have not proved helpful in distinguishing viral from other infections. CSF examination may be misleading if it is normal: as it is at the first examination in 10 to 15 per cent of patients with herpes simplex encephalitis; if there is a predominantly neutrophil pleocytosis; or if the glucose concentration is low. Myelin basic protein may be found in the CSF of patients with postinfectious encephalomyelitides.

Virology

Full laboratory resources allow a specific virus to be implicated in 70 to 75 per cent of cases of lymphocytic meningitis and in 30 to 40 per cent of patients with meningoencephalitis (Table 2). At appropriate stages of the illness, a rapid diagnosis by direct immunofluorescence may be made of herpes simplex virus (skin and brain), herpes zoster virus (skin lesion scrapings), rabies (skin sections and brain), measles (nasopharyngeal aspirate), and some non-viral causes such as Rocky Mountain spotted fever (skin). Electron microscopy of skin lesions will identify a herpesvirus. Some viruses can be isolated from the CSF (for example, mumps, enteroviruses, lymphocytic choriomeningitis virus, Central European encephalitides, Louping ill, and HIV). Virus cultured from a distant site may help with the diagnosis (for example, polio and other enteroviruses from stool, or arthropod-borne viruses from blood culture), but they may not be related to the neurological symptoms (for example, cytomegalovirus from the pharynx or urine, herpes simplex virus from skin or mucosa or adenovirus seen in stool by electron microscopy). Specific viral IgM can be

Table 1 Causes of aseptic meningitis[a], with or without encephalitis or myelitis, other than viruses and postinfectious/postvaccinal syndromes

Cause	Diagnostic clinical feature or investigation
Bacteria	
Acute bacterial meningitis (partially treated)	CSF antigen detection (CIE, LA), repeated CSF examination
Intracranial/spinal abscess or empyema (parameningeal infections)	Physical examination (exclude otitis media, trauma, dermoid sinus, etc.), radiographs, CT/MRI scans, myelogram
Brucella	CSF, blood culture, serology
Cat-scratch disease bacillus	Warthin–Starry stain of skin and lymph-node, skin test
Mycobacteria	CSF microscopy, LA, culture; Mantoux test, chest radiograph
Mycoplasma	CSF and serum IgM (IFA)
Spirochaetes	
Leptospira	Serology
Relapsing fevers	Blood smear, mouse inoculation
Lyme disease	Serology (EIA, IFA), culture, skin biopsy, CSF IgG(EIA IFT)
Syphilis	Serology (FTA-ABS) serum and CSF
Spirillum minus	Microscopy of wound or lymph-node aspirates, mouse inoculation
Rickettsiae	
(Rocky Mountain spotted fever, murine, epidemic, scrub typhus)	Serology (Weil–Felix), skin biopsy IFT (RMSF)
Fungi	
Blastomyces	CSF culture, EIA, demonstration at other sites, lung, skin, biopsy
Candida	CSF culture (repeated)
Coccidioides	CSF-CFT, culture, microscopy
Cryptococcus	CSF India ink, LA—beware false-positive with surface condensate on agar
Histoplasma	CSF culture (repeated), demonstration at other sites, blood smear (buffy coat) serum, urine, CSF antigen detection (RIA)
Protozoa	
Amoeba (Acanthamoeba, Naegleria, Balamuthia)	CSF microscopy (fresh wet preparation + India ink), culture
Malaria (cerebral)	Blood smears
Toxoplasma	(Immunocompromised patients—AIDS) CSF animal inoculation, serology, brain biopsy
Trypanosomiasis (African and South American)	Blood smear (buffy coat), lymph node aspirate, CSF microscopy, and IgM, serology, xenodiagnosis
Helminths	
Angiostrongylus cantonensis	CSF larvae, eosinophilia
Cysticercosis	CT/MRI scan, radiographs, examination for subcutaneous cysts, CSF-CFT, histology
Gnathostoma spinigerum	Cutaneous migratory swelling, CSF eosinophilia
Hydatid disease	Casoni test, serology, CT/MRI scan, radiographs
Paragonimus	CSF ova, eosinophils, serology, CT/MRI scan or skull radiograph, histology
Schistosomiasis	Low transverse myelitis, ova in urine or stool, CT/MRI scan, CSF eosinophilia, myelogram, histology
Sparganosis	Histology, CT/MRI scan
Strongyloides stercoralis	(Immunocompromised patients) larvae, ova in stool, duodenal fluid, etc.
Behçet's syndrome	Clinical syndrome
Carcinomas, cysts, leukaemias, lymphomas	CSF cytology, evidence of condition elsewhere
Chemical	Recent lumbar puncture, spinal anaesthesia, myelography, isotope cisternography
Drugs	Non-steroidal anti-inflammatory agents immunomodulators, antimicrobials (e.g., trimethoprim)
Kawasaki's disease	Clinical features, echocardiography, coronary angiography, etc.
Lead encephalopathy	Blood lead, blood smear, urinary coproporphyrins
Mollaret's meningitis	Recurrence, CSF 'Mollaret's' cells (PCR for HSV)
Sarcoidosis	Histology, Kveim test, Mantoux test, serum Ca^{2+}, ACE
Systemic lupus erythematosus and other collagen/vascular diseases	Antinuclear antibodies, DNA antibodies, lupus erythematosus cells
Vogt–Koyanagi–Harada syndrome	Clinical syndrome
Whipple's disease	Clinical features, jejunal histology

[a] Aseptic meningitis: CSF pleocytosis but no bacteria stainable by Gram's method and no growth on standard bacterial culture media.

ACE, angiotensin-converting enzyme; CSF, cerebrospinal fluid; CFT, complement fixation test; CIE, countercurrent immunoelectrophoresis; EIA, enzyme immunoassay; FTA-ABS, fixed Treponema antigen–antibody slide test; IFA, immunofluorescent antibody; LA, latex agglutination; RIA, radioimmunoassay; RMSF, Rocky mountain spotted fever.

detected in serum for mumps, Epstein–Barr virus, cytomegalovirus, or measles, or, using a μ-capture technique, in the CSF for JE virus. This method is being used increasingly to detect IgM to other viruses. The viraemia associated with JE is very brief and isolation from CSF difficult. Virus can occasionally be isolated from postmortem material. A viral diagnosis is often delayed until a rising convalescent antibody titre is found by an appropriate technique. This is usually the case for mumps, coxsackieviruses, and most arthropod-borne viruses.

An important diagnostic advance has been the introduction of polymerase chain reaction (**PCR**) technology for the routine diagnosis of a viral infection of the CNS. PCR greatly amplifies the amount of viral nucleic acid in the test sample, enabling the identification of herpes simplex virus in the CSF of suspected cases of herpes simplex encephalitis within a short time of the onset of symptoms. PCR is now the investigation of choice for the rapid diagnosis of HSV encephalitis, having a sensitivity of 95 per cent and a specificity of 100 per cent. The application of microchip and real-time PCR technology may further aid the rapid diagnosis of encephalitis. It is hoped that molecular techniques may aid the early diagnosis of a greater variety of CNS viral infections in the future (Table 2).

Brain biopsy

For the rapid diagnosis of viral encephalitides such as progressive multifocal leucoencephalopathy there is still no substitute for brain biopsy, but few would regard this inherently risky procedure as being justified. Electroencephalography, CT or MRI scans, angiography, or technetium scans can help to direct the surgeon towards the affected area of brain.

Imaging of the brain and spinal cord

CT and MRI scans of the brain and spinal cord can be extremely useful for the diagnosis of the site, nature, and extent of mass lesions and associated oedema, sub- and epidural empyemas, meningitis, cerebritis, and ventriculitis, the presence of intracranial hypertension, hydrocephalus, cerebral and brainstem herniation, demyelination, and other anatomical abnormalities (see Chapter 24.5).

CT scans are superior for bony details and calcifications, are quicker to perform, and are less dependent on the patient being able to lie motionless for prolonged periods. The resolution of MRI is greater for parenchymal lesions, but MRI cannot be performed in patients with pacemakers and may be dangerous in those with metal clips in cerebral blood vessels. Some viral encephalitides do have characteristic lesions on MRI. Some 94 per cent of patients with HSV have high-signal T_2-hyperintense lesions in the medial and inferior temporal regions, and JE is associated with characteristic lesions in the basal ganglia. More discrete high-signal intensity 2- to 7-mm lesions, particularly in the subcortical and deep white matter of the cerebral hemispheres, have been associated with the recently described Nipah virus infection (Fig. 4). However, these classical descriptions often overlap and the general features of oedema, infarction, and high signal on the T_2-weighted images are commonly seen in a variety of viral infections of the CNS.

Differential diagnosis

Viral infections of the CNS must be distinguished from the many other conditions that produce similar clinical features and CSF abnormalities

Table 2 Specimens for the virological diagnosis of acute meningitis or meningoencephalomyelitis

	Specimens for virus isolation/identification						Serology	
	Throat swab	Stool	CSF	Blood	Other specimens	PCR CSF	Acute	Convalescent
Adenovirus	++[a]	+	–		?[b]	?[b]	+	
Arenavirus								
Lymphocytic choriomeningitis	–	–	+++	+		?[b]	+	+2–3 months
Enteroviruses								
Polioviruses	+	+++	–	–		++[c,d]	+	+
Coxsackie and echoviruses[f]	+	+++	+++	–		+	+	+
Herpesviruses								
Cytomegalovirus	–	–	–	–	Urine[a]	+	+[a]	+
Epstein–Barr	+[a]	–	–	–		+	+[a]	+
Herpes simplex								
type 1	+[a]	–	+	–	Brain	+++	+[a]	
type 2	–	–	+	–	Vesicular fluid	+	+[a]	+
Herpes simiae (B)	–	–	–	–	Vesicular fluid	–	+[a]	+
Herpes varicella/zoster	–	–	+	–	Vesicular fluid	+[b]	+[a]	+
Mumps	+++	–	++	–	Saliva, urine	?[b]	+	+
Rhabdoviruses								
Rabies	–	–	+	–	Skin biopsy, saliva, brain	+	+	+
Retroviruses								
HIV-1	–	–	+	+++		+++[e]	+++	–
HIV-2	–	–	+	+++		?	+++	–
HTLV-1	–	–	+	–		+	+++	–
Togaviruses	–	–	+	++		+[e]	+	+

[a] Isolations or antibody responses may represent non-specific activation.
[b] Too few data to indicate general usefulness in diagnosis.
[c] Also serum/blood.
[d] Also stool.
[e] Also brain tissue.
[f] Some coxsackie A serotypes (especially A1–6) cannot be grown on cells.

(Table 1). The differential diagnosis of viral meningitis includes the other causes of aseptic meningitis, such as partially treated bacterial meningitis, tuberculous meningitis, spirochaetal infections (leptospirosis, borreliosis, Lyme disease, and syphilis), fungal, amoebic, neoplastic, granulomatous, and idiopathic meningitides. Viral myelitides must be distinguished from other causes of transverse myelitis and the Brown–Séquard syndrome. These include spinal compression by tumours, abscesses, helminths or their ova, or vertebral disease.

The differential diagnosis of paralytic poliomyelitis includes: postinfectious and other immunopathic polyneuroradiculopathies, such as Guillain-Barré syndrome and Landry's ascending paralysis; metabolic neuropathies such as acute porphyria; paralytic rabies; neoplastic polyradiculopathies; and rarities, such as tick paralysis and *Herpes simiae* B virus infection. The lack of objective sensory loss in poliomyelitis usually distinguishes it from these other entities.

The differential diagnosis of viral encephalitis includes other infective encephalopathies: bacterial, fungal, protozoal, and parasitic; intracranial abscesses and neoplasms; toxic and metabolic encephalopathies; and heat stroke. The diagnosis of 'viral encephalitis' should not be made too hastily, as it may condemn the patient with concealed cerebral malaria or some other curable encephalopathy to delayed treatment or even death.

Treatment

Antiviral chemotherapy

Aciclovir and, to a lesser extent, vidarabine (cytosine arabinoside) have proved effective in treating herpes simplex encephalitis. This subject is also discussed in Chapter 7.10.2. The nucleoside analogue acycloguanosine (that is, aciclovir) is only taken up by cells infected by herpes simplex virus and is therefore non-toxic to normal, uninfected cells. In view of this remarkable lack of serious toxicity, treatment can be started as soon as herpes simplex encephalitis is suspected clinically. Although there is still some controversy in the United States regarding the role of brain biopsy in herpes simplex encephalitis, virtually all clinicians in the United Kingdom now start therapy with aciclovir immediately on suspicion of encephalitis without attempting to confirm the diagnosis by brain biopsy. Aciclovir has also been used to treat herpes zoster virus encephalitis, but there is no convincing evidence for its efficacy in cytomegalovirus infections of the CNS. The rare, but very dangerous, encephalomyelitis caused by *Herpes simiae* B virus should be treated with aciclovir. Ribavirin is effective against some RNA viruses, such as those causing Lassa fever, haemorrhagic fever with renal syndrome, and possibly Argentine haemorrhagic fever, Rift Valley fever, and Congo Crimean haemorrhagic fever.

Interferons have been used by intravenous, intrathecal, or intraventricular routes in the treatment of rabies, herpes zoster virus, and other herpesvirus encephalitides, but have not proved effective. Although initial pilot studies of the use of interferon in JE were encouraging, the efficacy of this expensive treatment is awaited from randomized controlled trials.

Hyperimmune plasma given within 8 days of the start of symptoms has reduced the mortality of Argentine haemorrhagic fever (Junin virus) from between 20 and 30 to 1 and 3 per cent. Hyperimmune human globulin has also proved effective in the treatment of Congo Crimean haemorrhagic fever.

Supportive treatment

Corticosteroids have been used in the treatment of most of the viral encephalomyelitides, both in an attempt to combat cerebral oedema (especially in herpes simplex encephalitis) and for their other anti-inflammatory effects. Convincing evidence of benefit from controlled trials is lacking, but the immunosuppressive effects of corticosteroids have not led to obvious clinical deterioration, except perhaps in some cases of diffuse myelitis. Corticosteroids or ACTH have also been used for postinfectious and postvaccinal encephalomyelitides, but the evidence for their efficacy is not convincing and, since they may exacerbate latent rabies in experimental animals, should be used only in life-threatening cases of rabies postvaccinal encephalomyelitis. Severe intracranial hypertension should be treated with intravenous mannitol or mechanical hyperventilation. Nursing and general care are the same as for acute bacterial meningitis (Chapter 24.14.1) and tuberculous meningitis. Seizures must be controlled with phenytoin or phenobarbital, fever lowered by cooling, respiratory failure treated by mechanical ventilation, and attention given to fluid, electrolyte, and acid–base balance. Hyponatraemia is attributable to inappropriate secretion of antidiuretic hormone in some cases.

Paralytic poliomyelitis

Most authorities recommend rest and even mild sedation during the preparalytic stage of the 'major illness', because of the suspicion that exercise increases paralysis. The severe muscle pains and spasms reported in patients in some parts of the world are treated with mild analgesics, such as salicylate, and with hot-water bottles. During the phase of developing paralysis, patients must be observed closely and, if possible, assessed objectively for the development of life-threatening bulbar and respiratory paralysis. Those with weakness of swallowing should be nursed on their sides to prevent aspiration. The need for a cuffed tracheostomy tube may be avoided by careful positioning, frequent observations, and suction. Indications for mechanical ventilation are a progressive decline in ventilatory capacity to less than 30 to 50 per cent of normal, hypoxaemia, or gross disturbances of respiratory rhythm (Cheyne–Stokes respiration, long apnoeic intervals, etc.) suggesting damage to the respiratory centres. Respiratory weakness without bulbar paralysis may be treated in a tank respirator or rocking bed, which do not require tracheostomy. However, patients with severe or rapidly progressing respiratory paralysis need urgent tracheostomy and intermittent positive-pressure ventilation. Overventilation must be avoided. Assisted ventilation may be required for long periods. In the Copenhagen epidemic of the 1940s, this was achieved by manual ventilation. Attempts should be made to wean patients off the ventilator as soon as their condition becomes stable. Severe fluctuations in body temperature and blood pressure, reminiscent of those in severe tetanus and rabies, may require intensive care. The paralysed patient may have to lie in bed for many months and will develop complications from this prolonged immobilization. These include bed sores, osteomalacia, hypercalciuria leading to renal calculi, recurrent urinary tract infections resulting from chronic urethral catheterization, respiratory infections, and contractures of muscles and tendons leading to severe musculoskeletal deformities that will require orthopaedic correction. Some of these can be prevented by passive movement of the joints and splinting. Physiotherapy and psychological support are needed during the prolonged phase of rehabilitation.

Prognosis and sequelae

Viral meningitis has an excellent prognosis, but some patients with HSV-2 infection have recurrent attacks with spinal cord or nerve root involvement. Case fatality rates of some viral encephalomyelitides are as follows: rabies, 100 per cent; herpes simplex encephalitis (untreated), 40 to more than 75 per cent (highest in neonates and those over 30 years old); eastern equine encephalitis, 50 per cent; Japanese encephalitis, 10 to 40 per cent; measles, 10 to 20 per cent; varicella, 10 to 30 per cent; western equine encephalitis, 8 per cent; St Louis encephalitis, 3 per cent; California encephalitis, Venezuelan encephalitis, and mumps, less than 1 per cent. The mortality of paralytic poliomyelitis increases from 5 per cent in young children to more than 20 per cent in adults. Postinfectious and postvaccinal encephalomyelitides carry case fatalities of 15 to 40 per cent.

Neurological sequelae are found in 5 to 75 per cent of survivors of Japanese encephalitis and herpes simplex encephalitis, and are especially common in infants. They include mental retardation, loss of memory, speech abnormalities (including subtle expressive aphasias), hemiparesis, ataxia, dystonic brainstem and cranial nerve lesions, recurrent convulsions, and various behavioural and personality disturbances. Sequelae are common with postinfectious encephalomyelitis. An unusual sequel to paralytic poliomyelitis developing after an interval of many years is a condition characterized by progressive muscle weakness and wasting, attributable to depletion of anterior horn cells, which has some similarities to motor neurone disease.

Prevention

Prophylactic vaccination against poliomyelitis and measles has virtually eradicated encephalitides caused by these viruses in many communities. Postexposure rabies vaccination has also proved effective in preventing rabies encephalitis, and tissue-culture rabies vaccines are used increasingly for pre-exposure prophylaxis. A formalin-inactivated, adult mouse-brain vaccine is manufactured in Osaka for JE. It is effective and carries a very low risk of objective neurological complications (one in a million courses). An alternative live-attenuated vaccine has been developed in China, and has been shown to be both safe and effective in over 100 million Chinese children. Promising future vaccine candidates are currently being evaluated in non-human primate models, including a chimeric live-attenuated JEV/yellow fever virus combination and two poxvirus-vectored recombinant JE vaccines. Travellers to endemic regions should be vaccinated.

Since the outbreak of West Nile infection in the United States, several vaccine candidates have already been identified and immune protection against infection demonstrated in several animal models: human trials have been planned. There have been no reports of such success against Nipah virus. Vaccines for use in humans have been prepared against a number of other arthropod-borne viruses (for example, European tick-borne encephalitis).

Hyperimmune immunoglobulin has been used for prophylaxis (and in some cases attempted treatment) of measles, herpes zoster virus, HSV-2, vaccinia, rabies, and some other infections in high-risk groups. Immunocompromised patients, such as those with leukaemia, who are household contacts of a case of herpes zoster virus infection, should be given prophylactic hyperimmune globulin and, if they develop skin lesions, they should be treated with aciclovir to prevent the development of severe disease.

Interferons have been used with some success to prevent herpesvirus infections, for example cytomegalovirus in high-risk groups such as renal transplant recipients. However, the evidence does not yet justify their recommendation.

Caesarean section before rupture of the membranes in a full-term pregnant woman with genital herpes may prevent HSV-2 encephalitis in the neonate. If the herpetic lesions are discovered during or after vaginal delivery, topical aciclovir should be applied to the eyes of the neonate, as they are the most likely portal of entry.

Arthropod-borne viral encephalitides can be prevented by avoiding or controlling the arthropod vectors (for example, by the use of mosquito nets, insect repellents, insecticides, etc.), by attempting to control the numbers of wild vertebrate reservoir species, or by immunizing domestic animals, such as horses (eastern and western equine encephalitides) and pigs (JE). To control rabies, the principal wild mammalian vectors can be immunized (for example, wild foxes, racoons, and black-backed jackals have been immunized by distributing oral vaccine in bait). Domestic dogs and cats should be vaccinated. To prevent the viral encephalitides transmissible from laboratory animals (for example, lymphocytic choriomeningitis from mice and rats, *Herpes simiae* B from monkeys) their screening, quarantine, handling, and housing should be strictly controlled.

Reye's syndrome

Reye's syndrome is an acute encephalopathy affecting children between the ages of 2 and 16 years. It is rapidly fatal in 10 to 40 per cent of cases. The defining characteristics are sudden impairment of consciousness, increase in serum aminotransferase concentrations (or, if a biopsy is done, a fatty liver), and the exclusion of other diseases. Symptoms develop a few days after varicella or an upper respiratory tract or gastrointestinal illness. Clusters of cases (median age 11 years) have been associated with influenza B epidemics, while sporadic cases (median age 6 years) have followed varicella, coxsackie, dengue, and other viral infections. Studies in the United States have demonstrated an association between Reye's syndrome and the use of salicylates, but not of paracetamol, during the preceding viral illness. This has led the United Kingdom Committee on Safety of Medicines to recommend that aspirin should not be given to children under 12 years of age, unless specifically indicated for childhood rheumatic conditions. Aflatoxin has been implicated in Thailand. In the United States, the annual incidence of Reye's syndrome in those under 18 years old is 0.42 per 100 000 urban dwellers and 1.8 per 100 000 rural and suburban dwellers.

The child is nauseated and retches or vomits for 1 or 2 days before becoming confused or comatose and requiring admission to hospital. Most are afebrile and have hepatosplenomegaly but no jaundice at presentation. Fever develops later. The CSF is usually normal or contains a few mononuclear cells. Irritability, extreme agitation, aggression, and delirium are succeeded by coma and death in 2 to 3 days. Decorticate and decerebrate posturing and convulsions may be partly attributable to hypoglycaemia, which occurs in the majority of cases. There is rapid neurological deterioration with loss of pupillary and oculovestibular reflexes, evidence of increased intracranial pressure, deepening coma, and death. Neurological sequelae are common in survivors. Blood ammonia is increased above the normal limit of 48 μg/dl in almost all cases. The characteristic histological abnormality is fatty droplets in the liver cells. Mitochondrial abnormalities, but no inflammatory changes, have also been seen in neurones and hepatocytes.

The differential diagnosis includes acute hepatic encephalopathy, especially associated with poisoning, infective encephalopathies such as cerebral malaria (usually distinguishable by a positive blood smear) or bacterial, viral, and fungal meningoencephalitides (distinguished by characteristic CSF abnormalities).

There is no specific treatment, but mortality can be reduced by treating hypoglycaemia, cerebral oedema, respiratory failure, fluid and electrolyte disturbances, and other complications. These measures are also considered in Chapter 24.14.1.

Other viral infections or disorders in which viruses play a role in the pathogenesis of neurological disease

Subacute sclerosing panencephalitis

This disorder (see also Chapter 7.10.6) is a form of subacute encephalitis affecting children and young adults due to persistent infection with the measles virus. The cumbersome title, usually abbreviated to **SSPE**, is derived from the conditions formerly known as subacute sclerosing leucoencephalitis and inclusion-body encephalitis, now known to be the same disease.

Aetiology

An infective cause was long suspected and there is now conclusive evidence to incriminate the measles virus. Measles virus antibody titres are extremely high in the blood and CSF, measles antigen has been demonstrated in the brain, and the virus has sometimes been isolated, but only with difficulty. Most affected children have had measles at an unusually early age and there is a mean interval of some 6 years between infection and the onset of encephalitis. The disease can occur in children vaccinated with live measles virus, but the risk is much lower than that following the natural disease.

The measles virus in subacute sclerosing panencephalitis appears to be incomplete, as the matrix (**M**) protein required to attach the nucleocapsid to the cytoplasmic membrane prior to budding is deficient or absent. It is not known whether the absence of M protein from the brain is the result of an abnormality of the virus or of the host, and, if the latter, whether inborn or acquired. Current thought is that during the long symptom-free interval between infection and appearance of disease, viral material accumulates, eventually leading to cell damage. The paradox of high antimeasles antibodies, except against M protein, and persistent virus has not been explained. The comparatively early age of clinical measles in affected children, often below the age of 2 years, suggests that the immature immune system permits entry and persistence of the virus in the brain.

Pathology

As its name implies, both grey and white matter show the changes of encephalitis, with perivascular cuffing and more diffuse cellular infiltration, neuronal loss and myelin destruction, with variable glial scarring or sclerosis. Acidophilic nuclear inclusion bodies are never profuse and may not be detected. No visceral lesions are found.

Clinical features

In the great majority, the onset is in the first two decades, but young adults may also be affected. The disease is twice as common in boys as in girls. Incidence has fallen sharply in countries where measles vaccination is at a high level; the annual incidence in England and Wales has fallen from 20 to around 5. Subacute sclerosing panencephalitis remains relatively common in parts of eastern Europe, Egypt, and the Lebanon. No convincing predisposing factors have been identified and, in particular, immunosuppressed children are not at special risk but they may occasionally develop acute measles inclusion-body encephalitis.

The speed of onset is extremely variable, but there is usually a prolonged period of altered behaviour, mild intellectual deterioration, and loss of energy and interest, often misinterpreted as sloth or neurosis. After some weeks or months increasing clumsiness or the appearance of focal neurological symptoms draws attention to the organic nature of the disease. Periodic involuntary movements then appear, the commonest form being myoclonus, consisting of a stereotyped jerk or lapse of posture involving the limbs, often asymmetrically, occurring every 3 to 6 s. The myoclonus may result in sudden falls, which are occasionally the presenting symptom. Visual signs may be prominent, with papilloedema, retinitis, optic atrophy, or cortical blindness. Choroidoretinal scarring is present in 30 per cent of cases. In other cases the onset is relatively abrupt with no recognizable prodromal stage. There is no fever or other evidence of systemic infection.

Further progression is marked by intellectual deterioration, rigidity and spasticity, and increasing helplessness. Some 40 per cent of patients die within a year, but a similar proportion survive for more than 2 years. A period of apparent arrest is common and in some patients, particularly at the upper end of the age range, substantial remission and prolonged survival occur. Even in such cases there may be radiological evidence of continued cerebral damage and it is probable that the disease is always eventually fatal.

Investigation

There is no significant pleocytosis in the cerebrospinal fluid and total protein is not increased, but there is evidence of intrathecal synthesis of immunoglobulin and oligoclonal bands of IgG. Although the measles antibody titres in blood and CSF are usually raised to high levels, occasionally they overlap control values. In established disease, the electroencephalogram (**EEG**) shows highly characteristic periodic discharges, synchronous with the myoclonus, but persisting in the absence of the movements. The CT scan shows low-density, white-matter lesions and cerebral atrophy.

Treatment

There is no effective treatment for subacute sclerosing panencephalitis. Inosiplex, 100 mg/kg daily by mouth in divided doses, possibly prolongs survival, particularly in older patients with disease of slow onset, but adequately controlled trials are naturally difficult to mount. Interferon given by intraventricular catheter has been reported to induce partial remission.

Progressive multifocal leucoencephalopathy (see also Chapter 24.14.4)

This disease is caused by opportunistic infection by papovaviruses, most commonly JC virus and the simian virus SV40. A high proportion of normal adults have antibodies to the former and the agent appears to be ubiquitous. The reservoir of SV40 is in monkeys and the agent was apparently transmitted in early types of poliomyelitis vaccine, without evident ill-effects. These viruses are potentially oncogenic, but are non-pathogenic for humans unless the immune system has been compromised.

Progressive multifocal leucoencephalopathy thus occurs in patients already affected by such conditions as lympho- or myeloproliferative diseases, sarcoidosis, and other chronic granulomatous diseases, or, more recently, AIDS, and also in those therapeutically immunosuppressed. Most patients are over 50 years old but, with the spread of AIDS, younger people are being affected, with a male preponderance, and the disease is no longer rare.

Pathology

The virus particularly invades the nuclei of the oligodendroglia and, as a result, there is demyelination of the white matter of the cerebral hemisphere, spreading from numerous foci. The cerebellum and brainstem are less often involved and the spinal cord is spared. Abnormal giant forms of oligodendrocytes with eosinophilic inclusions are seen microscopically, and arrays of intranuclear virus particles can often be identified by electron microscopy. JC virus antigen can be identified by immunofluorescence or immunohistochemistry. DNA probing has revealed unintegrated virus in oligodendrocytes, astrocytes, endothelial cells, and in extraneural organs such as kidney, liver, lung, spleen, and lymph nodes.

Clinical features

The onset is usually with progressive signs of a focal lesion of one cerebral hemisphere; limb weakness, aphasia, or visual field defect such as homonymous hemianopia. More widespread signs gradually develop, leading to personality changes, intellectual deterioration, dysarthria or fluent aphasia, and bilateral weakness. Fits are rare. There is no systemic evidence of infection. Spontaneous temporary arrest or partial remission are common but eventual progression causes death in 6 to 12 months, although much more chronic cases are on record, with survival, exceptionally, to 5 years.

Investigation

The CSF is normal apart from occasionally a mild elevation of protein and slight pleocytosis, and is not under increased pressure. The EEG shows a bilateral excess of slow activity. The CT scan may at first show little abnormality, but eventually large, non-enhancing, low-density lesions appear in the cerebral white matter. MRI is more sensitive. Serum antibodies are of no diagnostic help but the response in the CSF has not been fully evaluated. The diagnosis can be confirmed only by cerebral biopsy, but it is essential that white matter is included in the specimen. This may be important to distinguish lymphoma and, rarely, herpes simplex encephalitis involving white matter.

Treatment

No treatment is of proven value, but cytosine arabinoside has sometimes appeared to induce partial remission.

Progressive rubella panencephalitis

This extremely rare disorder (see also Chapter 7.10.12) may follow congenital rubella or rubella in early childhood. It evolves insidiously some 10 years after the original illness and is characterized by progressive mental retardation with behaviour changes, fits, ataxia, spasticity, optic atrophy, and macular degeneration. Pathological changes are those of encephalitis with perivascular infiltration. The CSF may show a slight rise in white cell and protein content, elevation of gammaglobulin and of antirubella antibodies to an extent greater than the rise in the serum level, suggesting local production of antibody within the CNS. The EEG may show changes similar to those seen in subacute sclerosing panencephalitis due to measles virus. The mechanism responsible for the appearance of this disorder is unknown and there is no effective treatment.

Vogt–Koyanagi–Harada syndrome

The cause of this rare syndrome is thought to be an inflammatory autoimmune reaction to an unidentified viral infection. The disorder affects tissues having a common embryological origin, the uvea and leptomeninges and the melanoblasts, ocular pigments and auditory labyrinth pigments originating from the neural crest. The dermatological features consist of patchy whitening of eyelashes, eyebrows, and scalp hair, alopecia, and vitiligo. Neurological manifestations include meningoencephalitis, raised intracranial pressure, neurosensory deafness, tinnitus, nystagmus, ataxia, ocular palsies, and focal cerebral deficits. Ocular features are those of uveitis with pain and photophobia, more generalized inflammation of the eye, retinopathy, and impaired visual acuity. The condition tends to be self-limiting but may result in serious permanent ocular and neurological deficits. Steroids and immunosuppressive drugs have been used and are said to arrest the progression of at least some features of the disorder.

Viral causes of psychiatric illness

Mental changes are common in patients with encephalitis. Influenza, infectious mononucleosis, and infectious hepatitis are sometimes followed by psychiatric sequelae, in particular a depressive reaction. Psychosis following encephalitis lethargica has been reported on occasions.

Other possible virus infections in which the nervous system is involved

Acute disseminated encephalomyelitis is considered in Chapter 24.16. Reye's syndrome is discussed above and Behçet's syndrome in Chapter 18.10.5. Mollaret's meningitis is discussed in Chapter 24.14.1.

Further reading

Boos J, Esiri MM (1986). *Viral encephalitis: pathology, diagnosis and management.* Blackwell Scientific, Oxford.

Cardosa MJ, *et al.* (1999). Isolation of subgenus B adenovirus during a fatal outbreak of enterovirus 71-associated hand, foot, and mouth disease in Sibu, Sarawak. *Lancet* **354**, 987–91.

Christie AB (1980). *Infectious diseases: epidemiology and clinical practice,* 3rd edn. Churchill Livingstone, Edinburgh.

Goh KJ, *et al.* (2000). Clinical features of Nipah virus encephalitis among pig farmers in Malaysia. *New England Journal of Medicine* **342**, 1229–35.

Griffiths JF (1985). SSPE and lymphocytes. *New England Journal of Medicine* **313**, 952–3.

Jackson AC, Johnson RT (1989). Aseptic meningitis and acute viral encephalitis. In: Vinken PJ, *et al.*, eds. *Handbook of clinical neurology,* Vol. 12, ch. 56, *Viral diseases,* pp. 125–48. Elsevier, Amsterdam.

Johnson RT, *et al.* (1985). Japanese encephalitis: immunocytochemical studies of viral antigen and inflammatory cells in fatal cases. *Annals of Neurology* **18**, 567–73.

Krupp LB, *et al.* (1985). Progressively multifocal leukoencephalopathy: clinical and radiological features. *Annals of Neurology* **17**, 344–9.

Nash D, *et al.* (2001). The outbreak of West Nile virus infection in the New York City area in 1999. *New England Journal of Medicine* **344**, 1807–14.

Pattison EM (1965). Uveomeningoencephalitic syndrome (Vogt–Koyanagi–Harada). *Archives of Neurology* **12**, 197–205.

Price RW, Plum F (1978). Poliomyelitis. In: Vinken PJ, *et al.*, eds. *Handbook of clinical neurology,* Vol. 34, *Infections of the nervous system,* pp 93–132. North Holland, Amsterdam.

Scheld WM, Whitley RJ, Durack DT, eds. (1997). *Infections of the central nervous system,* 2nd edn. Lippincott-Raven, New York.

Solomon T, *et al.* (1988). Poliomyelitis-like illness due to Japanese encephalitis virus. *Lancet* **351**, 1094–8.

Solomon T, *et al.* (2000). Neurological manifestations of dengue infection. *Lancet* **355**, 1053–9.

Townsend JJ, *et al.* (1975). Progressive rubella panencephalitis—late onset after congenital rubella. *New England Journal of Medicine* **292**, 990–3.

24.14.3 Intracranial abscess

P. J. Teddy

Intracranial abscesses may occur within the extradural or subdural space, or may be intracerebral. Occasionally, abscesses exist in more than one tissue plane. Intracerebral and subdural abscesses may rupture into the subarachnoid space and be accompanied by meningitis; intracerebral pus may rupture into the ventricular system and produce ventriculitis.

Aetiology

Extradural abscesses are usually related to focal osteomyelitis of the skull, mastoiditis and nasal sinusitis, penetrating injuries of the skull, and are a rare complication of craniotomy.

Subdural empyema is related most commonly to infection of the paranasal sinuses and middle ear. Other causes include septicaemia related to cyanotic congenital heart disease, lung abscess, trauma, and intracranial surgery.

The most common intracranial abscess is found within the intracerebral compartment, with about 60 per cent related to middle-ear infection and 20 per cent to frontal sinusitis. Other established causes are septicaemia related to congenital heart disease with a right-to-left shunt, lung abscess, bronchiectasis, penetrating injuries of the head, and bacteraemia following tooth extraction. In about 10 per cent of cases no primary source of infection can be identified. Owing to their strong connection with sinus and middle-ear disease, most intracerebral abscesses are found within the frontal or temporal lobes, or within the cerebellum. Infection disseminated through the bloodstream from more distant sites may result in multiple abscesses in any part of the brain.

Microbiology

The most common organisms associated with subdural empyema are aerobic, anaerobic, and micro-aerophilic streptococci, *Staphylococcus aureus*, and *Bacteroides* spp.

Cerebral abscesses associated with otitis media, mastoiditis, and nasal sinusitis usually show a mixed growth of anaerobes and aerobic organisms including anaerobic and micro-aerophilic streptococci and *Bacteroides. Streptococcus viridans and Staph. aureus* are frequently seen. *Listeria* spp. tend to produce areas of focal cerebritis rather than true abscess.

Pathology

Infection within an accessory air sinus or the petrous bone may cause an area of localized osteitis just above the dura, which can then spread intracranially. Initially it may be entirely confined to the extradural space, but will eventually penetrate the dura and spread subdurally or, if the adjacent arachnoid is stuck to the inflamed patch of dura, then it will spread into the subarachnoid space to give meningitis. If the subarachnoid space has been obliterated, it may penetrate the brain to produce initially a focal cerebritis. Usually after about 10 days the area of cerebritis becomes enclosed within an area of gliotic brain, and after about 3 weeks a firm capsule forms around the pus. Large intracerebral abscesses may rupture into the ventricular system, producing a ventriculitis.

Cerebral abscesses are usually surrounded by areas of oedematous brain, which may exert a considerable mass effect.

Clinical features

These will depend upon the site, size, and number of lesions, and the involvement of neighbouring structures such as the cerebral ventricles and the venous sinuses. The signs are therefore legion, but the diagnosis should be considered in any case where there is an obvious primary source of infection associated with evidence of raised intracranial pressure, focal neurological signs, epileptic seizures or meningeal irritation, or any combination of these.

Extradural abscess may be difficult to detect clinically, but is sometimes manifest by severe, unremitting, localized headache in association with sinusitis or mastoiditis. Patients with subdural empyema frequently appear toxic, with a swinging pyrexia, severe headache, a depressed level of consciousness, contralateral hemiparesis, papilloedema, meningeal irritation, and seizures. There is usually an accompanying frontal sinusitis with tenderness of the forehead and redness and swelling of the eyelids, or mastoiditis or scalp infection.

Diagnosis

If a brain abscess is suspected, predisposing sources of infection, including possible distant sites, should be carefully sought, as intracranial abscesses derived by haematogenous spread are often more fulminating in their course than those associated with local cranial disease. If CT is available, scans of the skull base, including views of the mastoids and other skull sinuses, should be performed. Otherwise, skull radiography with sinus views is necessary. Chest radiographs should be obtained.

The investigations of choice for all forms of suspected intracranial abscess are either CT scanning, with and without contrast, or MRI. CT will normally demonstrate both extradural and subdural empyema, may demonstrate diffuse cerebritis in early cases, and will normally show intracerebral abscesses as ring-enhancing lesions with low-attenuation centres (see Fig. 1). Nevertheless, there are pitfalls, particularly in the early stages both of subdural empyema and of cerebral abscess. Subdural empyema may initially be fairly thinly spread over the cerebral cortex, producing relatively little midline shift, and may be virtually isodense with brain on CT. Under such circumstances, contrast-enhanced MRI (particularly with coronal views) is of great value.

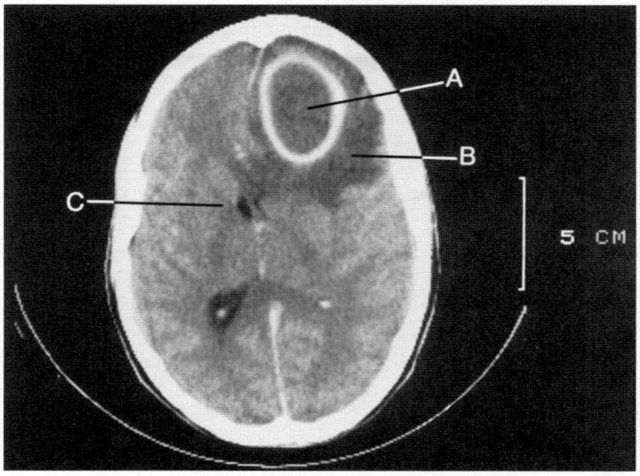

Fig. 1 Contrast CT scan showing large right frontal cerebral abscess (A) with surrounding oedema (B) and ventricular compression (C).

The principal differential diagnoses in an intracranial abscess are meningitis, subdural haematoma, and intracranial tumour. It is not always possible to differentiate between intracerebral abscess and tumour on CT scan, particularly when there is an appearance of ring enhancement, and it is largely for this reason that the biopsy of suspected cerebral tumour is advocated in nearly all such cases. MRI, however, tends to show a low-signal capsule on T_2-weighted images and may be helpful in making this differentiation.

One obvious concern is to differentiate between bacterial meningitis and intracerebral abscess. Both may present with pyrexia, neck stiffness, and with some focal signs, but if there is any evidence whatsoever of raised intracranial pressure, or any other supportive evidence of cerebral abscess, a lumbar puncture should be strictly avoided until a neurosurgical opinion has been sought. Lumbar puncture in the presence of cerebral abscess can lead to tonsillar or tentorial herniation, and in any event, the cerebrospinal fluid can be entirely normal.

Management

Except in a few cases of multiple or inaccessible abscess, and the occasional patient whose general medical condition is such that surgery is precluded, treatment of the intracranial infection requires evacuation of pus and high-dose intravenous antibiotic therapy.

The single, main factor in securing a good outcome is early diagnosis. Early management includes taking specimens for blood culture and culture of any extracranial infective lesion, setting up an intravenous infusion, administration of anticonvulsant agents, and, in cases of grossly depressed level of consciousness and massive cerebral oedema seen on CT scan, giving intravenous dexamethasone.

Pus from the suspected primary site of infection should be collected immediately and both aerobic and anaerobic cultures obtained. The intracranial pus must be similarly cultured. Antimicrobial treatment, using massive intravenous doses, should be commenced immediately without waiting for the culture report, and subsequently changed in the light of the sensitivity findings. The antimicrobial regimen should include penicillin (4 mega units 4-hourly), metronidazole, ampicillin, and either gentamicin or chloramphenicol depending on the likely source of infection and the infective agent. Intravenous antimicrobials should be continued for at least 1 week before reverting to oral medication.

Most supratentorial abscesses can be sterilized by aspiration through a burr hole, and the direct instillation of antibiotics is sometimes employed. Aspiration must usually be repeated several times, but in about 30 per cent of cases a single aspiration will suffice. Once the abscess is sterile, the capsule will shrink and finally form an irregular gliotic scar within the brain. Shrinkage of the abscess must be checked by serial CT scan. Subdural empyema should be evacuated through a craniotomy rather than burr holes, as very often the pus can spread widely, and particularly alongside the falx cerebri. Extradural empyema is evacuated through a burr hole, or through a craniotomy for larger collections.

Cerebellar abscess, when diagnosed early, may be aspirated through a burr hole, but immediate total excision is often recommended because the small volume of the posterior cranial fossa leaves little latitude in terms of tonsillar herniation and death.

Prognosis

The mortality is around 10 per cent, but the main problems remain those of late diagnosis and resistant bacteria. Even with an otherwise good outcome, epilepsy may continue in about 30 per cent of cases, particularly in patients with temporal-lobe abscess and subdural empyema.

Further reading

Lorber B (1997). Listeriosis. *Clinical Infectious Diseases* **24**,1–9.

Mathisen GE, Johnson JP (1997). Brain abscess. *Clinical Infectious Disease*, **25**, 763–79.

Report of the Quality Standards Subcommittee of the American Academy of Neurology.(1998). Evaluation and management of intracranial mass lesions in AIDS. *Neurology*, **50**, 21–6.

24.14.4 Neurosyphilis and neuroAIDS

Hadi Manji

Neurosyphilis

Introduction

Syphilis remains a public health problem in certain areas of the United States, Eastern Europe, and in the developing world. The incidence of primary and secondary syphilis in the United Kingdom (excluding Scotland) increased from 109 cases in 1995 to 259 cases in 2000 – an increase of 138 per cent. Since syphilis, like other ulcerating genital infections such as herpes and chancroid, is an independent risk factor for the acquisition and transmission of infection with the human immunodeficiency virus (**HIV**), the disease has once again come under scrutiny. In addition, there are recent anecdotal reports of *Treponema pallidum* being more neurovirulent and with a greater risk of treatment failure in those dually infected with HIV.

Invasion of the central nervous system occurs early in the course of syphilis infection. *T. pallidum* has been isolated from the cerebrospinal fluid of up to 40 per cent of neurologically asymptomatic patients with untreated primary and secondary syphilis. Despite this, cohort studies of untreated patients suggest that symptomatic late syphilis (neurosyphilis, cardiovascular syphilis, and gummas) occurs in 15 to 40 per cent of such individuals; the Oslo study documented an incidence of clinical neurosyphilis in 9.4 per cent. Thus, it would seem as if, at least in the immunocompetent patient, *T. pallidum* has a low virulence for the central nervous system.

Clinical features (see Table 1)

Acquired syphilis is divided into an early, potentially infectious stage (primary, secondary, and early latent where less than 2 years have lapsed since infection) and a late, non-infectious stage (late latent where more than 2 years have lapsed, gummatous, cardiovascular, and neurosyphilitis). Although there is a rough time course to the development of the various neurological syndromes, there is considerable overlap; these syndromes are, in reality, part of a spectrum of disease.

Neurosyphilis may include meningitis (acute and chronic), a myeloradiculopathy due to a pachymeningitis and granulomatous lesions (gummas) that present as space-occupying lesions within the brain, the spinal cord, or the epidural space causing compression. Meningovascular syphilis involves the small- and medium-sized arteries, typically causing an endarteritis (Heubner's endarteritis obliterans) resulting in infarction. The so-called late manifestations of neurosyphilis result from a low-grade meningoencephalitis. In patients with general paralysis (also called general paralysis of the insane or dementia paralytica) the focus is on the frontotemporal cortex. Therefore, during the early stages, vague symptoms may include personality and mood changes, with impaired faculties of concentration and attention being the presenting features; memory difficulties develop later.

In tabes dorsalis (taboparesis), which may coexist with general paralysis, the clinical presentation results from involvement of the dorsal roots and ganglia as well as the posterior columns within the spinal cord, with the resultant emphasis on a sensory ataxia. Diabetes may produce a similar clinical picture with a neuropathy and pupillary abnormalities (diabetic pseudotabes).

The optic nerve may be involved with or without other evidence of neurosyphilis, but must always be treated as if it were part of a systemic infection. A uveitis, chorioretinitis, optic neuritis, papillitis, and optic atrophy have all been reported at different stages of the disease. Extraocular presentations include nerve palsies involving the eye muscles and a superior orbital fissure syndrome. Although the Argyll Robertson pupil may occur in any form of the disease, it is generally encountered in tabes dorsalis. The pupils are small and irregular, being unreactive to light, but constrict normally to accommodation and convergence. Unilateral involvement is rare. The light/near dissociation is the result of gliosis in the periaqueductal grey midbrain tegmentum, which may also account for the bilateral ptosis seen in some individuals.

Diagnosis

Neurosyphilis has a myriad of neurological manifestations and therefore the diagnosis enters the differential of most neurological conditions (Table 1). Treatment in the early stages of the disease (that is, of the meningitic and meningovascular syndromes) may well result in recovery, whereas the late forms—with general paralysis and tabes dorsalis—may only respond partially, if at all. These common neurological presentations include stroke, especially in younger patients, chorioretinitis, optic neuropathy of unknown cause, and single or multiple cranial neuropathies, particularly those involving the VIIIth nerve with vertigo and sensorineural

Table 1 Clinical features of neurosyphilis

	Syphilitic meningitis		Meningovascular	General paralysis	Tabes dorsalis
Time course	Acute	Within first year; may occur during secondary syphilis	Months to years after infection, average 7 years	15–20 years	20–25 years
	Chronic	20–25 years			
Clinical features	Acute	Cranial nerve palsies (III, VI, VII, VIII), hydrocephalus	Stroke (hemiparesis, dysphasia), seizures, cranial nerve palsies, encephalitic syndrome, anterior spinal artery syndrome	Frontal-temporal dementia, psychiatric symptoms (delusions, apathy), personality change, seizures, dysarthria, tremor (tongue, face, hands), AR pupils, optic atrophy	Lightning pains (limbs, viscera); loss of pain and temperature(Charcot's joints), joint position (sensory ataxia, positive Romberg's sign), areflexia, sluggish pupils(early), autonomic and sphincter dysfunction
	Chronic	Myeloradiculopathy			

deafness. Syphilis serology should be routinely performed in patients with dementia and psychiatric illnesses.

The serum reaginic tests, Venereal Diseases Research Laboratory test (**VDRL**) and rapid plasma reagin test (**RPR**), are usually positive in secondary syphilis when the first neurological complications may be encountered. However, a false-negative result may occur due to the prozone phenomenon if undiluted serum is used. This occurs in 1 to 2 per cent of cases of secondary syphilis and is due to blockage of agglutination caused by the saturation of antigenic sites by excess antibody. The specific serological tests (*Treponema pallidum* haemagglutination test (**TPHA**), *T. pallidum* particle agglutination test (**TPPA**), fluorescent treponemal antibody absorption test (**FTA-abs**), and the treponemal enzyme immunoassay (**EIA**)) are invariably positive.

In late syphilis (meningovascular syphilis, gummatous, general paralysis, and tabes dorsalis), the serum VDRL/RPR tests are negative in 30 per cent of untreated cases. All the specific tests have a sensitivity approaching 100 per cent, so that a negative treponemal antigen test has an extremely high predictive value for excluding neurosyphilis.

It is recommended that all patients with positive syphilis serology who have ocular and or neurological symptoms and signs should undergo cerebrospinal fluid (**CSF**) examination, as should patients with latent infection of unknown duration. In order for these tests to be correctly interpreted it is important that the CSF is not significantly (macroscopically) contaminated with blood.

In patients with neurosyphilis there is usually a lymphocytic pleocytosis (>5 cells/μl), with an elevated protein (>0.4 g/l). In the late stages, particularly in tabes, the CSF may be quiescent. A reactive CSF-VDRL establishes the diagnosis of active neurosyphilis, but a non-reactive test does not exclude it. The sensitivity of the CSF–VDRL is 50 per cent, with a specificity of 100 per cent. A non-reactive CSF-FTA-abs or TPHA excludes the diagnosis. However, a reactive CSF-FTA-abs or TPHA does not establish the diagnosis because the presence of treponemal antibodies in the CSF could result from the passive transfer from the blood, or may result from a previous episode of treated syphilis. The sensitivity for the CSF-FTA-abs is 100 per cent, with a specificity of 30 per cent.

The role of the polymerase chain reaction (**PCR**) in the diagnosis of neurosyphilis is unclear at present, for technique cannot discriminate between viable and non-viable organisms. *T. pallidum* DNA has been detected in CSF up to 3 years after intravenous treatment with penicillin.

Treatment

In patients with symptomatic neurosyphilis or ocular disease, the World Health Organization/United Nations Programme on HIV/AIDS (**WHO/UNAIDS**) as well as the Centers for Disease Control (**CDC**) recommend treatment with penicillin G (2–4 mU intravenously every 4 h for 14 days). In the United Kingdom the preference is for procaine penicillin (1.8–2.4 million IU intramuscularly once daily, plus probenecid 500 mg by mouth four times daily, for 17–21 days). The alternative is intravenous benzyl penicillin (3–4 million units intravenously every 4 h for 17–21 days). In patients with a history of penicillin allergy one option is to perform skin testing to confirm the allergy and to then consider desensitization. The other is to treat with doxycycline 200 mg by mouth four times daily for 28 days.

Following treatment of neurosyphilis, a repeat lumbar puncture should be performed at 6-month intervals until the cell count is normal. This should be decreased by 6 months and be entirely normal by 2 years. The CSF-VDRL may take years to become non-reactive.

Syphilis in the era of HIV

Since the onset of the AIDS epidemic there have been numerous reports of an accelerated course of syphilis and of treatment failures in patients who are dually infected. Compared to non-immunosuppressed individuals there certainly does seem to be a higher than expected rate of cases of syphilitic meningitis and meninogovascular syphilis. To date, however, there are no denominator data. Since cell-mediated immunity, which is necessary to eradicate *T. pallidum*, may be impaired in HIV infection this seems plausible.

As a result of altered B-cell function there has been concern regarding serological tests. However, these are usually positive or may show a delayed response in the occasional case.

There is still debate as to whether or not patients with HIV and early syphilis who are neurologically asymptomatic should have a CSF examination. Any CSF cytochemical abnormalities could be either be due to HIV or syphilis. In view of the treatment failures reported with benzathine penicillin some authorities suggest that all HIV patients with early syphilis should be treated with neurosyphilis treatment regimens.

NeuroAIDS (or neurological complications of HIV infection)

Introduction

Soon after the onset of the AIDS epidemic in 1981, it became clear that the nervous system was frequently involved. However, opportunistic infections such as toxoplasmosis and cryptococcal meningitis as well as neoplasms (such as primary central nervous system lymphoma (**PCNSL**)) accounted for only 30 per cent of the neurological problems encountered. It also became evident that in the later stages of the AIDS illness, patients developed neurological complications due to the human immunodeficiency virus itself. This included a progressive decline in cognitive function in association with motor abnormalities—the HIV–dementia complex.

Neurological disorders are the AIDS-defining illness in up to 20 per cent of cases. Over the course of the illness the prevalence of neurological complications increases up to 70 per cent. These include other opportunistic infections and tumours, as well as the HIV-related problems of dementia, vacuolar myelopathy, and distal sensory peripheral neuropathy.

At postmortem more than 90 per cent of the brains from patients dying of AIDS show evidence of HIV encephalitis and of one of the opportunistic infections such as cytomegalovirus (**CMV**) and tumours.

During the last 5 years, with the introduction of the highly active antiretroviral therapies (**HAART**), there has been a dramatic decline in the incidence of neurological opportunistic infections as well as HIV related disorders such as HIV dementia. However, these are expensive drugs and are out of reach of the majority of HIV-infected individuals worldwide.

Clinical approach

All areas of the neuraxis are vulnerable in individuals infected with HIV. Not infrequently do differing pathological processes occur simultaneously in various parts of the nervous system. Thus, Occam's Razor—the principle of diagnostic parsimony, often used in medicine—does not always apply. Another aspect is the possibility of simultaneous infection with more than one organism: for example, meningitis due to *Mycobacterium tuberculosis* and *Cryptococcus neoformans*. Mass lesions in the brain, with some not responding to antitoxoplasma therapy, could be due to lymphoma or another infective cause such as a tuberculoma.

The nervous system is involved early in the course of infection, as evidenced by neurological seroconversion illnesses such as an aseptic meningitis, encephalitis, and the Guillain–Barré syndrome. Furthermore, during the asymptomatic phase of the illness (that is, when patients are well) the cerebrospinal fluid shows abnormalities in up to 60 per cent of cases. This may be a lymphocytic pleocytosis of up to 50 cells/mm^3, an elevated protein, or the presence of oligoclonal bands. The CSF glucose level is usually normal. Therefore, these cytobiochemical markers are unhelpful in making a diagnosis of a meningitic or an encephalitic illness. Reliance is therefore placed on specific markers such as the cryptococcal antigen or antibody tests like the CSF-VDRL or TPHA.

As a result of the impaired immune response, a rise in antibody titres to specific infections may not occur, especially during the later stages of HIV infection. Furthermore, the typical clinical picture—the presentation of which, at least in some infections like meningitis, are due to a brisk inflammatory response such as fever—may not occur. In cryptococcal meningitis, only one-third of patients exhibit the classical signs of meningism: namely, neck stiffness, photophobia, and a positive Kernig's sign.

The specific type of opportunistic complications encountered is dependent on a number of factors, including the degree of immunosuppression. During the early stages when subjects are relatively immunocompetent, with CD4 counts above 500/μl, autoimmune disorders such as demyelinating neuropathies may occur. Between CD4 counts of 200 and 500/μl multidermatomal herpes zoster infections may present. Once the level declines below 200/μl, patients are vulnerable to all the major opportunistic infections and the complications due to HIV itself. Symptomatic infection with cytomegalovirus tends to occur at very low levels below 50/μl.

In different parts of the world, some infections may be more prevalent than others. The incidence of toxoplasmosis in France is significantly higher than in the United Kingdom because of a higher background seroprevalence, due to differing dietary habits and the greater prevalence of raw meat consumption.

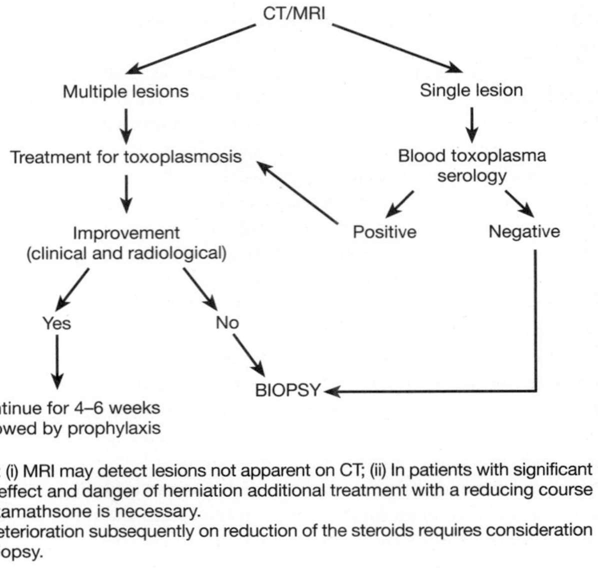

Fig. 1 Management of mass lesions in AIDS

Opportunistic infections

Toxoplasmosis

Toxoplasma gondii, whose definitive host includes members of the cat family with humans the intermediate hosts, is an obligate intracellular protozoan. Human infection occurs through the ingestion of tissue cysts in undercooked meat. Variations in dietary habits therefore explains the differing seroprevalence rates worldwide—90 per cent in French adults compared to 50 per cent of residents in the United Kingdom. Symptomatic toxoplasmosis is usually due to a reactivation of latent infection in individuals with HIV. The risk of an HIV-infected patient who is seropositive for IgG *T. gondii* antibody developing toxoplasmosis is around 25 per cent.

Toxoplasmosis is the most common cause of mass lesions in the brains of patients with HIV infection. The clinical presentation is variable, but headache, confusion, seizures, and focal neurological deficits such as hemiplegia, dysphasia, and visual field defects are the most common. Other presentations described include: a variety of movement disorders (choreoathetosis, dystonia, and hemiparkinsonism); psychiatric illness such as depression; brainstem syndromes; and a rapidly progressive diffuse encephalitis. Rarely, the spinal cord may be involved with a myelitis or a cauda equina syndrome.

A definitive diagnosis of toxoplasma encephalitis can only be made by brain biopsy. With increasing experience and pragmatism, it is now standard practice to treat any HIV-infected individual who has a low CD4 count and multiple lesions on imaging with antitoxoplasma therapy (Fig. 1). A response, clinically and radiologically, confirms the diagnosis. Although a negative blood toxoplasma serology result makes the diagnosis less likely, it may occur in up to 17 per cent of cases. This loss of seropositivity may be the result of impaired antibody synthesis with increasing immunosuppression. It is useful therefore to document an individual's toxoplasma serostatus on first diagnosis of HIV-positivity. For similar reasons, the expected rise in IgM and IgG levels does not occur. A single lesion on magnetic resonance imaging (**MRI**) is most likely to be due to lymphoma. A single lesion on computed tomography (**CT**) scanning should, if possible, be followed by MRI, which is a more sensitive method of detecting lesions particularly in the posterior fossa (Fig. 2).

The main differential diagnosis is that of primary CNS lymphoma, which presents at similar CD4 counts and with a similar presentation both clinically and on imaging studies (Table 2).

A response is seen in 90 per cent of patients by the second week of treatment (Table 3). It is necessary to reimage 2 weeks after treatment even if there is clinical evidence of improvement, since it is not uncommon for some lesions to improve but others due to, for example *Mycobacterium tuberculosis*, to enlarge which then makes it necessary to consider a biopsy. The radiological improvement generally lags behind the clinical improvement.

Patients infected with HIV who are seropositive for IgG against *T. gondii* should be offered primary prophylaxis with 980 mg of co-trimoxazole (trimethoprim and sulfamethoxazole) when their CD4 count falls below $100/mm^3$. This will confer cross-protection against *Pneumocystis carinii* pneumonia.

Cryptococcus neoformans

This encapsulated yeast is a ubiquitous organism in the environment acquired by humans through inhalation. Although disseminated infection can involve the skin, bones, lungs, eyes, and prostate, symptomatic infection with *C. neoformans* most often presents as a meningitis.

Cryptococcal infection is the most common infectious cause of meningitis in patients with AIDS (Table 4). The presentation may be acute, but it is usually subacute with symptoms of malaise, headache, fever, and vomiting. The classical signs of meningism—neck stiffness, photophobia, and

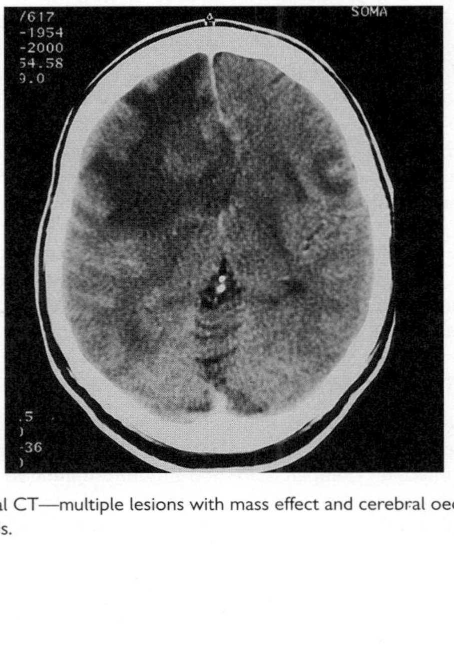

Fig. 2 Cranial CT—multiple lesions with mass effect and cerebral oedema due to toxoplasmosis.

Table 2 Focal neurological syndromes

Infections	
Toxoplasma gondii (abscesses, encephalitis)*	
JC virus (PML)*	
Mycobacterium tuberculosis (tuberculoma)*	
Fungal microabscesses (*Cryptococcus neoformans, Histoplasma capsulatum, Candida albicans, Aspergillus fumigatus*)	
Cytomegalovirus	
Neoplasms	
Primary CNS lymphoma*	
Metastatic tumours (non-Hodgkin's lymphoma, Kaposi's sarcoma)	
Cerebrovascular	
Ischaemic stroke (coagulopathies)	
Embolic stroke (bacterial and non-bacterial endocarditis)	
Vasculitis (meningovascular syphilis, herpes varicella zoster)	

* Most common.

Kernig's sign—are present in only one-third of patients. Other, less common symptoms include altered mental status, seizures, and focal neurological signs. The latter are due to parenchymal cryptococcal abscesses.

Brain imaging is usually normal, although the basal meningitis may result in hydrocephalus or sometimes, particularly on MRI, small abscesses—cryptococcomas—may be visualized.

Cerebrospinal fluid examination is essential for the diagnosis, with culture of the fungus being the 'gold standard'. The cytochemical markers in the CSF may be normal. India-ink staining of the CSF will reveal the fungal hyphae in 70 to 80 per cent of cases and cryptococcal antigen is detected in over 90 per cent. Cryptococcal antigen is also detected in the blood in over 90 per cent of patients, and should be measured in conjunction with the CSF level since in occasionally reported cases of fulminant cryptococcal meningitis the CSF may be negative and the blood positive. The blood antigen measurement may be used as a screening test in patients presenting with symptoms of early infection such as headache. However, it should be appreciated that a negative result does not completely exclude the diagnosis of cryptococcal meningitis.

Treatment with amphotericin B remains the drug of choice for the treatment of severe cases of cryptococcal meningitis. The mortality rate still remains around 10 per cent. Features that have been identified with a poor outcome include a relapse infection, abnormal mental status, CSF cryptoccal antigen titre over 1:1024, CSF white cell count <20 cells/mm^3, positive India-ink staining, hyponatraemia, and positive culture from an extrameningeal site. A CSF opening pressure of greater than 250 mmH_2O is also a marker of poor prognosis. In milder cases, where none of these features are present, oral fluconazole may be used. Although combination with 5-flucytosine has been shown to improve outcome in non-AIDS patients, this has not been confirmed in patients with AIDS. However, the combination should be considered in fulminant cases.

A specific complication that requires close monitoring is the development of raised intracranial pressure due to obstruction of the arachnoid

Table 3 Treatment of neurological opportunistic infections

Infection	Drug	Dose	Duration	Side-effects	Notes
Toxoplasmosis					
Acute	Pyrimethamine	Loading dose of 200 mg, then 75 mg orally	4–6 weeks	Myelosuppression	
	+				
	Sulfadiazine	6–8 g/day orally or intravenously	4–6 weeks	Nephrotoxicity, renal calculi, crystalluria	Clindamycin 2.4 g/day oral or IV is an alternative to sulfadiazine. Side-effect pseudomembranous colitis
	+				
	Folinic acid	15 mg/day orally	4–6 weeks		To counteract the myelosuppressive effects of pyrimethamine
Maintenance	Pyrimethamine	25–50 mg/day orally	Indefinitely		
	+				
	Sulfadiazine	2 g/day orally	Indefinitely		Clindamycin 1.2 g/day
	+				
	Folinic acid	15 mg/day orally	Indefinitely		
Primary prophylaxis	Trimethoprim + Sulfamethoxazole	80 mg/day orally; 400 mg/day orally		Nausea, Stevens–Johnson syndrome, neutropenia, thrombocytopenia	CD4 count <200/μl and toxoplasma serology positive
Cryptococcal meningitis					
Acute	Amphotericin B	0.6–1.0 mg/kg per day intravenously	At least 2–4 weeks until symptoms resolve and CSF culture negative	Hypokalaemia, renal failure, anaemia	Via central line because of thrombophlebitis. In mild cases fluconazole400 mg initially IV then continued orally
	+/–				
	5-Flucytosine	100 mg/kg per day orally	2–4 weeks	Myelosuppression	
Maintenance	Fluconazole	200–400 mg/day orally	Indefinitely	Nausea, vomiting, abnormal liver function tests	Amphotericin 1 mg/kg per week if intolerant or relapse on fluconazole

Table 4 Meningitis in HIV infection

Infections	*Cryptococcus neoformans* *Mycobacterium tuberculosis* *Listeria monocytogenes* *Treponema pallidum*
Neoplasms	Metastatic non-Hodgkin's lymphoma

villi and cerebral oedema. This should be managed with repeated lumbar puncture or, if necessary, by the insertion of a lumbar or ventricular drain.

Maintenance therapy is essential, with relapse rates approaching 100 per cent if secondary prophylaxis with oral fluconazole is not adhered to. The serum cryptococcal antigen titre is not useful in predicting relapse.

JC (Jamestown canyon) virus

Progressive multifocal leucoencephalopathy (**PML**) is caused by the reactivation of latent JC virus, which is acquired by the majority of the population during childhood as a banal upper respiratory infection. Prior to the AIDS epidemic, PML was a rare condition encountered in patients immunosuppressed as a result of haematological malignancies, drugs used in the treatment of post-transplant patients, autoimmune disorders such as systemic lupus erythematosus (**SLE**), and granulomatous disorders such as sarcoidosis. Nowadays, underlying HIV infection accounts for 85 per cent of cases.

Prior to the introduction of HAART, the incidence of PML was 4 per cent. The clinical presentation is subacute, with progressive focal neurological deficits such as a hemiparesis, visual field defects, and a cerebellar syndrome. The disorder is not restricted to the white matter since patients may also develop dysphasia and seizures. Occasional patients may present with a progressive dementia with focal neurological signs.

MRI characteristically shows multiple areas of high signal on T_1-weighted images and a low signal on T_2-weighted ones (Fig. 3). There is little or no enhancement, with no mass effect or oedema around the lesions. Blood serological testing is unhelpful since 80 per cent of the general population is seropositive. Recently it has become possible to confirm the diagnosis of PML by isolating JC-viral DNA in cerebrospinal fluid by PCR techniques. This has a sensitivity of 75 per cent with a specificity of 95 per cent. In PCR-negative cases it may be necessary to either repeat the CSF examination or to perform a brain biopsy. The typical histological features show areas of focal demyelination, bizarre enlarged astrocytes, and abnormal oligodendrocytes with inclusion bodies that stain for JC viral antigens.

There is, to date, no specific treatment. Cytosine arabinoside, both intravenous and intrathecal, has been shown to be ineffective. Trials are underway to examine the efficacy of cidofovir, an anti-CMV drug, and interferon-α. However, improving immune function with HAART has been shown to improve survival times from a median survival of 10 weeks to 40 weeks.

Cytomegalovirus (CMV)

The neurological complications from this herpesvirus results from reactivation in severely immunocompromised patients. Almost all patients infected with HIV are seropositive for cytomegalovirus. Postmortem studies of the brains of patients who died from AIDS show evidence of CMV in 25 per cent of cases. However, clinical CMV disease, apart from CMV retinitis, is rare.

CMV retinitis is the most common manifestation of CMV disease and can affect up to 20 per cent of patients with AIDS. The slowly progressive necrotizing retinitis results in characteristic white irregular lesions with central necrosis and haemorrhages—the cheese and tomato ketchup appearance. Retinal detachment may occur in patients with extensive retinal involvement. The retinitis presents with symptoms of reduced visual acuity, floaters, and loss of peripheral vision. Since the condition may be asymptomatic in the early stages, regular ophthalmological screening is recommended for high-risk patients with CD4 counts below 50 cells/µl.

A necrotizing ventriculoencephalitis has been described, usually in patients with evidence of CMV disease elsewhere (Table 5). The onset is subacute over a period of days or weeks with confusion, seizures, and brainstem signs such as internuclear ophthalmoplegia, ataxia, and cranial nerve palsies. Imaging studies typically show periventricular enhancement.

CMV polyradiculopathy presents over a period of days with back pain, leg weakness, sensory impairment, and sphincter disturbance. The differential diagnosis includes syphilitic polyradiculopathy and infiltration with metastatic lymphoma. The cerebrospinal fluid reveals a polymorphonuclear leucocytosis which is unusual for a viral infection. Early recognition and treatment is necessary to stabilize and, in some cases, improve the neurological impairment.

Drugs licensed for the treatment of CMV disease include ganciclovir, cidofovir, and foscarnet. Oral ganciclovir is prescribed for secondary prophylaxis.

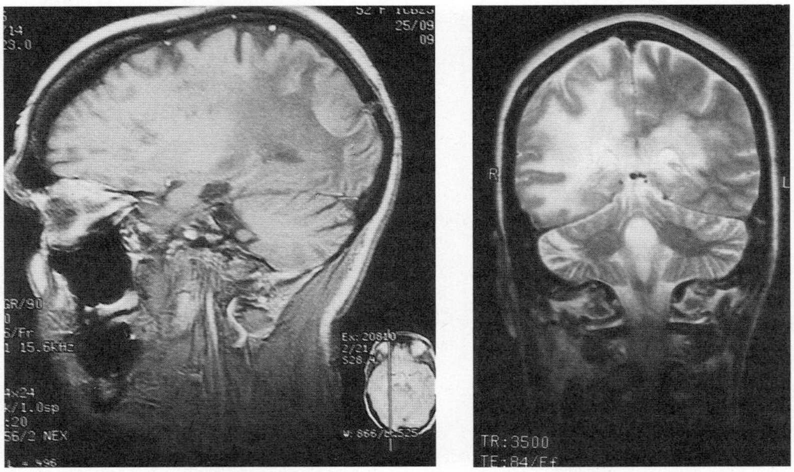

(a) (b)

Fig. 3 (a) T_2 weighted and (b) T_1 weighted MRI in a patient with PML.

Opportunistic tumours

Primary CNS lymphoma (**PCNSL**) is the second most common cause of mass lesions after toxoplasmosis in adults, and the most common in paediatric patients with AIDS. Histologically, this a high-grade, non-Hodgkin's, B-cell lymphoma. Recent evidence suggests that the Epstein–Barr virus is causally linked to PCNSL, with the identification of the viral DNA incorporated into that of the neoplastic cells.

The common presenting symptoms are those of headache with focal neurological deficits, altered level of consciousness, and seizures.

Brain imaging reveals enhancing mass lesions with surrounding oedema and mass effect. These are similar to those found in toxoplasmosis. PCNSL is more likely to present as a single mass lesion than toxoplasmosis and is also more likely to invade the ventricular walls. Recent studies using thallium-201 single-photon emission computed tomography (**SPECT**) suggest that it may be possible to differentiate between an abscess and a tumour, with the former having little uptake compared with the high uptake of the mitotically active lymphoma.

There is no effective treatment for PCNSL. Whole brain radiotherapy provides, at best, only a modest benefit, with most patients succumbing within 2 months.

HIV-associated neurological disorders

HIV–dementia complex

Before the introduction of HAART (and in areas of the world where they are still unavailable) approximately 15 to 20 per cent of individuals infected with HIV developed a variably progressive dementia with associated motor deficits. In children, a similar HIV-1 associated progressive encephalopathy occurs more frequently than with opportunistic infections. This usually occurs within the context of severe immunosuppression in those with a CD4 count of less than 200/mm^3. In around 3 per cent of cases, HIV-dementia is the AIDS-defining illness. Large cohort studies, using clinical, MRI, and neuropsychological methods, have largely discounted the early reports of evidence of cognitive changes in asymptomatic HIV-positive patients.

The clinical presentation in the early stages is with vague symptoms of apathy, mood changes, and difficulty with memory and concentration. These are features of a subcortical dementia with no features of cortical involvement such as language, visuospatial or calculation difficulties. This picture may be mimicked by depression, metabolic encephalopathy, and drugs, both therapeutic and recreational. At this stage, there may be few physical signs apart from brisk reflexes, impaired fine finger movements, and unsteady gait.

Later, the memory impairments are obvious, as is the psychomotor retardation—which may progress to frank mutism and a global dementia. Some patients develop seizures. The motor signs due to the associated vacuolar myelopathy with a spastic paraparesis and sphincter disturbances are also present in a significant number of patients (Table 6). In addition, some patients will have the HIV-related distal sensory peripheral neuropathy. Thus, this group will have absent ankle jerks and extensor plantar responses.

The diagnosis of the HIV–dementia complex is made by clinical assessment—there are usually no focal signs and the tempo of the disorder is an insidious one. Investigations are performed to exclude other infection or neoplastic pathologies, and therefore necessitate imaging, preferably with MRI, and a CSF examination. MRI may show evidence of cerebral atrophy with compensatory ventricular dilatation, a diffuse white-matter high signal on T_2-weighted images with no enhancement. A CSF examination may be non-specifically abnormal with a pleocytosis, elevated protein level, and oligoclonal bands. It important to exclude cryptococcal and tuberculous meningitis as well as neurosyphilis. The HIV RNA-viral load in cerebrospinal fluid correlates with the severity of clinical dementia, but there is too much overlap between non-demented and demented subjects for the measurement to be of use as a diagnostic aid. There is no correlation between the plasma HIV RNA-viral load and dementia. Electroencephalography (**EEG**) may be normal in the early stages, with non-specific diffuse slowing being shown later.

Table 5 Encephalitis in HIV

Virus	Cytomegalovirus Herpes simplex Herpes zoster ?Human herpesvirus 6
Protozoa	Toxoplasmosis

Table 6 Myelopathy in HIV

Infections	HIV-associated vacuolar myelopathy* Herpes zoster* Cytomegalovirus HTLV-1 (co-infection) *Treponema pallidum* Toxoplasmosis Epidural abscess
Neoplasm	Metastatic non-Hodgkin's lymphoma
Other causes	Vitamin B12, vitamin E deficiency

HTLV-1, human T-cell leukaemia/lymphoma virus-1.
* Most common.

The pathology of the HIV–dementia complex is a spectrum ranging from diffuse myelin pallor, microglial nodules—which are non-specific and may be found in CMV encephalitis—to multinucleated giant cells that are indicative of productive brain infection and cortical neuronal loss. There is no clear correlation between the clinical and pathological findings.

The mechanisms of disease in the HIV–dementia complex are still unclear. It is, however, evident that HIV predominantly infects the microglial and astrocytic cells rather than neurones or oligodendrocytes. One hypothesis for the entry of the virus into the CNS is the 'Trojan horse' theory, with invasion occurring by infected peripheral blood monocytes penetrating a blood–brain barrier that has been disrupted by damage to the capillary endothelial cells. Neuronal damage is subsequently caused by virotoxins (for example, Gp120) and cytokines (for example, tumour necrosis factor-α) released from activated macrophages.

After the introduction of zidovudine in 1987, there was a dramatic reduction in the incidence of HIV-associated dementia. One clinical study looking specifically at the effect of zidovudine on cognitive function confirmed its beneficial effect, albeit at dosages much higher than those currently used. With the introduction of the newer antiretroviral drugs—the majority of which have poor penetration into the CSF and presumably the brain—there is concern that, despite the reduction of plasma HIV viral loads, the CNS may develop into a safe sanctuary for the virus from which reinfection could occur. However, recently published studies do suggest that these newer therapies improve cognitive function and it seems prudent, until further data become available, to use drugs that best penetrate the CSF to treat HIV dementia complex.

Since macrophage activation resulting in the release of neurotoxic factors also has a role in the pathophysiological mechanism, trials are underway to assess the therapeutic benefits of drugs such as the **PAF** (platelet-activating factor) antagonist, lexipafant, and the **NMDA** (*N*-methyl-D-aspartate) antagonist, memantine.

HIV-associated neuropathy

The most common neurological complication encountered in patients infected with HIV is distal sensory polyneuropathy (**DSPN**), which may occur in 30 per cent of those with AIDS (Table 7). It is a significant cause of morbidity.

Typically, patients complain of numbness of the soles of the feet together with shooting pains and parasthesias developing over a period of months.

Table 7 Peripheral nerve complications in HIV infection

HIV related	
Axonal neuropathy (distal sensory peripheral neuropathy)*	
Demyelinating neuropathy—acute (Guillain-Barré syndrome), chronic (chronic inflammatory demyelinating neuropathy (CIDP))	
Vasculitic (mononeuritis multiplex)	
Diffuse inflammatory lymphocytic syndrome (DILS)	
Lower motor neurone syndrome (resembling motor neurone disease)	
Drugs	
Antiretrovirals (ddI, ddC, d4T)*	
Isoniazid	
Thalidomide	
Dapsone	
Metronidazole (high dose)	
Vincristine	
CMV related	
Vasculitic (mononeuritis multiplex)	
Lumbosacral polyradiculopathy	
Others	
Syphilis (polyradiculopathy)	
Metastatic non-Hodgkin's lymphoma (polyradiculopathy)	
Ganglioneuritis	
Autonomic neuropathy	

* Most common.

There is little or no weakness. The hands are infrequently involved. The ankle jerks are depressed or absent. Sensory testing reveals impaired pain and temperature perception as well as vibration.

Further investigations are usually unnecessary in a patient with a CD4 count below 200 and showing the typical clinical picture, but it is always worth checking the blood sugar, vitamin B_{12} level, and syphilis serology. It is important to enquire about alcohol intake and the possibility of an excess intake of vitamin B_6.

Neurophysiological and pathological studies suggest this to be a length-dependent axonal neuropathy. Productive HIV infection has not been found in pathological specimens and the underlying mechanisms, like those for HIV dementia, are linked to macrophage activation products.

Since antiretroviral therapy has no benefit, treatment is symptomatic with the use of tricyclic antidepressants and anticonvulsant drugs such as gabapentin.

The nucleoside analogues didanosine (**ddI**), zalcitabine (**ddC**), and stavudine (**d4T**) cause a dose-dependent sensory neuropathy that may be indistinguishable from distal sensory polyneuropathy. Clues to this drug-induced neuropathy include the shorter history of weeks rather than months, and the improvement on stopping the offending drug. However, there may be a continued worsening of symptoms for a period of 4 to 8 weeks after stopping—the phenomenon of 'coasting'. The underlying mechanism appears to be the impairment of mitochondrial protein synthesis.

Further reading

Brew B (2001). *HIV neurology.* Oxford University Press, Oxford.

Clinical Effectiveness Group (1999). National guideline for the management of early syphilis. *Sexually Transmitted Infections* **75**(Suppl 1), S29–S33.

Clinical Effectiveness Group (1999). National guideline for the management of late syphilis. *Sexually Transmitted Infections* **75**(Suppl 1), S34–S37.

Harrison MJ, McArthur JC (1995). *AIDS and neurology.* (*Clinical Neurology and Neurosurgery Monographs*). Churchill Livingstone, Edinburgh.

Seminars in Neurology (1999). **19,** Thieme Medical Publishers. [Whole volume devoted to HIV neurology.]

Swartz MN, Healy BP, Musher DM (1999). Late syphilis. In: Holmes KK, *et al.*, eds. *Sexually transmitted diseases*, pp 487–509. McGraw-Hill, New York.

24.15 Metabolic disorders and the nervous system

Neil Scolding and C. D. Marsden*

In general, the term metabolic diseases of the nervous system covers the neurological consequences of systemic disorders of metabolism. This alone is an enormous field, ranging from common disorders, such as diabetes, chronic and acute alcohol poisoning, and renal disease, to less common but no less important disorders such as pontine myelinolysis and critical illness polyneuropathy.

Metabolic complications of major organ disease

Cardiovascular disease/anoxia

Cerebral anoxia may be due to insufficient cerebral blood flow, reduced oxygen availability, reduced oxygen carriage by the blood, metabolic interference with the utilization of oxygen, or combinations of these events. Thus, acute cardiovascular insufficiency as a consequence of cardiac arrest is a relatively common cause of severe global cerebral anoxia; others as diverse as suffocation, anaesthetic catastrophes, drowning, or acute carbon monoxide poisoning can produce similar results.

A brief period of global ischaemic anoxia causes syncope. If the episode is prolonged, myoclonic jerks or tonic–clonic seizures may occur. Still more protracted insults may precipitate a period of confusion and residual amnesia.

Persisting acute severe anoxia rapidly leads to loss of consciousness, generalized fits, dilated pupils, and bilateral extensor plantar responses. Periods of anoxia up to perhaps 5 min may cause transient coma with recovery of consciousness. A delayed postanoxic encephalopathy, characterized pathologically by demyelination in the hemispheres and in the basal ganglia, may follow within 1 to 2 weeks, often commencing with increasing irritability, apathy, and confusion. Frank dementia may emerge, or an amnesic syndrome in less severe cases, and there may also be pseudobulbar palsy and other pyramidal signs, gait ataxia, and incontinence, and/or an akinetic–rigid syndrome with or without dystonia. Some patients may be severely disabled by action myoclonus—dramatic muscle jerking on attempted movement. The residual deficits following prolonged cerebral anoxia with survival may be permanent; in other patients they gradually recover, often to a very considerable degree, although over months or years. In yet other patients, the condition may progress over a matter of some weeks or months.

If oxygen deprivation lasts longer than a few minutes, permanent or prolonged but reversible brain damage occurs. Irreversible coma is accompanied by flaccidity and loss of all reflex function except heart beat and tendon jerks. The pupils remain fixed and dilated and the electroencephalogram is flat on repeated examination. (Drugs and hypothermia may cause a flat electroencephalogram, but recovery is possible.) Such patients may be said to have suffered irreversible brain death if all signs of brainstem function are absent on repeated examination over 12 to 24 h. Other, less severely affected patients show partial recovery of brainstem reflex function, such as pupillary responses, reflex eye movements, and muscle tone, and may breathe spontaneously. However, no sign of consciousness or intelligent response to the external world occurs, and they may remain in such a 'persistent vegetative state' for months or years.

Subacute or gradual anoxia may occur in severe anaemia, heart failure, pulmonary disease, or exposure to high altitude ('mountain sickness'). It produces inattentiveness, fatigue, headache, and intellectual deterioration, followed by memory difficulties and ataxia.

Cerebral anoxia is also the main cause of neurological symptoms in a number of other systemic conditions. Disseminated intravascular coagulation (see Section 22), resulting from platelet aggregation and fibrin formation, can be produced by a number of illnesses, including sepsis and malignancy. Patients complain of headache and difficulty in concentration, vertigo, blurred vision, and speech difficulties. Such confusion and disorientation may progress to stupor and coma with focal or generalized signs of brain disturbance. Spontaneous bleeding is common, in the form of petechiae in the skin or optic fundus, purpura, and even intracranial haemorrhage. Cerebral malaria (see Chapter 7.13.2) should always be borne in mind as a cause of unexplained coma in patients recently returning from an infective area. Most patients describe chills and fever for a few days prior to the onset of lethargy, stupor, and finally coma. The diagnosis is established by finding the parasite in fixed smears of the blood.

Fat embolism follows severe trauma, particularly to the limbs, but may also be a complication of burns and other severe system disturbance. Multiple pulmonary microemboli of fat may lead to progressive hypoxia and respiratory failure. Multiple cerebral microemboli produce confusion, lethargy, stupor, and finally coma. Symptoms often begin hours to days after the original injury, and are accompanied by fever and hyperventilation. A characteristic petechial rash usually develops over the upper half of the body on the second to third day after injury. There may also be fundal haemorrhages. The respiratory features range from the appearance of linear streaks radiating from the hilar region or patchy opacities on the chest to the fully developed adult distress syndrome (see Section 16). Clotting abnormalities range from mild thrombocytopenia to acute disseminated intravascular coagulation (see Section 22). Management consists of correcting hypoxia, in severe cases with positive end-expiratory pressure (PEEP) ventilation, and correction of the coagulation disorder (see Section 16). Cardiac surgery, at least in the earlier days of bypass pump oxygenation, produced frequent transient neurological damage in many patients. Improvements in technique, such as the introduction of filters in blood perfusion lines to remove debris, have greatly reduced neurological complications of the procedure. However, some patients still emerge from the anaesthetic with signs of diffuse or focal brain damage. If they survive the acute episode, the prognosis usually is good.

* It is with regret that we must report the death of Professor C.D. Marsden since the publication of the third edition of this textbook. Much of his text for that edition has been retained here.

Hepatic failure

Patients with liver disease of whatever cause (see Section 14) may develop acute hepatic coma or a more chronic form of hepatic encephalopathy with behavioural disturbance and other neurological symptoms.

Acute hepatic coma

This occurs with massive liver necrosis due to severe hepatitis or poisons such as paracetamol. In other patients, who may have relatively well-preserved liver function but extensive portosystemic shunts, coma may be precipitated by a sudden intake of nitrogenous substances as occurs with gastrointestinal bleeding, infections, or high-protein diets. Personality and cognitive changes proceed if unchecked to confusion, apathy, and lack of concentration, or occasionally excitement requiring sedation, and are rapidly followed by stupor and coma in a matter of a few hours or days. Characteristic findings are asterixis ('liver flap'), in which the outstretched hands show postural lapses or negative myoclonus, and hepatic fetor. Chorea and pyramidal signs may appear as the patient lapses into coma. Decerebrate posturing is common at this stage, and focal deficits such as hemiplegia may occur. Nystagmus, conjugate deviation of the eyes, skew deviation, and even disconjugate eye movements may be evident, but reflex eye movements and pupillary responses are preserved, until the patient becomes totally unresponsive and dies. Paroxysmal and later persistent high-voltage triphasic slow waves are present in the electroencephalogram until death is imminent.

Many metabolic abnormalities may contribute to the cause of hepatic coma, including hyperammonaemia (more than 145 μmol/l or 200 mg/dl), which results from the products of intestinal digestion bypassing the urea-synthesizing mechanisms of the liver. However, hypoglycaemia and hyperventilation producing a respiratory alkalosis are also nearly always present. Altered amino acids and neurotransmitters (especially α-aminobutyric acid), formation of toxic amines such as octopamine, and short-chain fatty acids have also been incriminated. Intravascular coagulation occurs, as do other coagulation defects, leading to secondary vascular damage to the brain; cerebral oedema can raise intracranial pressure seriously or even fatally.

Hepatic coma carries a high mortality, but if the patient can be kept alive, liver regeneration and recovery may occur. Treatment includes correcting where possible the precipitant, sterilizing the bowel, correction of metabolic and bleeding abnormalities, the administration of lactulose, and haemoperfusion or other techniques to remove toxins (see Chapter 14.21.3). The benzodiazepine antagonist flumazenil may have a useful role. Intracranial pressure monitoring is fraught with hazards, not least the coagulopathy, but mannitol (though not dexamethasone) is of proven benefit in lowering intracranial pressure in this context.

Chronic hepatic encephalopathy

This refers to the development of changes in intellect, cognitive function, and consciousness, often accompanied by other neurological signs (such as tremor or chorea, an akinetic–rigid syndrome, ataxia, or even spastic paraparesis) occurring in those with chronic liver failure, and particularly in those with extensive portosystemic anastomoses. (For Wilson's disease see Chapter 11.7.2.) The exact nature of the substances responsible for chronic hepatic encephalopathy has not been established. Characteristically, the disorder fluctuates, with episodes of marked confusion, excitement, or frank hepatic coma. In addition, intellectual changes, parkinsonism, ataxia, or spasticity may gradually progress. Treatment consists of a low-protein diet and antibiotics to sterilize the gut, and the administration of lactulose.

Respiratory disease

Hyperventilation causes hyocarbia and alkalosis, resulting in parasthesias, especially perioral, light-headedness and unsteadiness, visual disturbances, and occasionally carpopedal spasm; syncope may follow.

More seriously, chronic respiratory failure causes what is essentially a low-grade chronic hypoxia and hypercarbic encephalopathy, with the defining features of confusion and headache accompanied by a myoclonic or asterictic tremor and papilloedema. Mechanical devices for delivering domiciliary oxygen have transformed the management of this disorder, and the quality of life of its sufferers.

Obstructive sleep apnoea is characterized by conspicuous snoring and an often obese habitus. Early morning headache and inattentiveness or irritability with excessive daytime sleepiness should suggest this disorder.

Critical illness polyneuropathy

This disorder develops subacutely but often asymptomatically in (often anaesthetized) patients on intensive care units receiving intensive support for multiorgan failure and/or sepsis, only revealing itself as they otherwise improve. It is axonal in nature, but of still unknown aetiology. The prognosis is variable; it may slowly improve in patients whose underlying disease allows sufficient time for recovery.

Renal failure

Renal failure (see Section 20) is associated with a variety of neurological complications. Uraemic encephalopathy was common before the use of dialysis. Patients become progressively drowsy, stuporose, and finally lapse into coma. Hyperventilation, multifocal myoclonus, tremor, asterixis, tetany, and generalized fits are common. Eye movements and pupillary reactions are not affected. Uraemia, metabolic acidosis, hyperkalaemia, disorders of calcium, sodium, and water balance, and hypertensive encephalopathy all contribute to the clinical picture. Dialysis rapidly reverses the metabolic abnormalities of uraemia, but the encephalopathy may take days to clear. Other complications of chronic renal failure include myopathy due to chronic hypocalcaemia, and a symmetrical sensorimotor polyneuropathy, often subacutely progressive and disabling. It may be resistant to dialysis, but renal transplantation has been associated with a slow and sustained improvement.

Iatrogenic disease in renal failure

Some patients develop the dialysis disequilibrium syndrome during correction of their uraemic abnormalities. Rapid correction of the metabolic changes, possibly through osmotic shifts, leads to the emergence of asterixis, myoclonus, delirium, generalized convulsions, stupor, and even coma. Raised intracranial pressure with papilloedema may occur. Chronic dialysis—perhaps 3 to 7 years—may precipitate dialysis dementia if dialysate with a high aluminium content has been used. Such patients begin to develop speech hesitancy and arrest, then intellectual and cognitive abnormalities, convulsions, myoclonus, and sometimes focal neurological abnormalities. Death follows with a year.

Wernicke's encephalopathy (see below) can occur, due to chronic dialysis without thiamine supplements.

Patients with renal disease are particularly prone to develop toxic complications of drugs normally excreted in the urine—peripheral neuropathy due to nitrofurantoin, labyrinthine damage due to streptomycin, or optic atrophy due to ethambutol.

Metabolic disorders due to endocrine disease (see Section 12)

Adrenal disease

Phaeochromocytoma

Phaeochromocytoma causes paroxysms of anxiety, tremor, headache, and palpitations, together with the consequences of malignant hypertension. Fits may occur. The associations with von Hippel–Lindau disease, multiple endocrine neoplasia syndromes, ataxia telangiectasia, and Sturge–Weber syndrome should not be overlooked.

Cushing's syndrome

Endogenous Cushing's syndrome in two-thirds of cases is due to a pituitary ACTH-secreting adenoma—conventionally termed Cushing's disease. Ectopic ACTH-secreting malignant neoplasms and ACTH-independent adrenal tumours represent the other principal causes of endogenous disease; iatrogenic hyperadrenalism produces similar neurological symptoms. The systemic features are described in Chapter 12.7.1. Neurological complications include: (i) proximal myopathy, which can be severe and painful; (ii) psychiatric disorders, ranging from mild mood disturbance through moderate depression (common) to severe psychosis; (iii) a benign intracranial hypertension-like picture; and (iv) direct consequences of a pituitary tumour, particularly optic chiasmal compression.

Adrenal insufficiency

Hypoadrenalism due to primary adrenal failure (Addison's disease) or ACTH deficiency (from pituitary disease or chronic steroid treatment) causes weakness, lassitude, nausea and diarrhoea, and stupor or coma may be precipitated by surgical procedures or other acute illness. Hypotension (especially postural), hyponatraemia, hyperkalaemia, and often hypoglycaemia (see Chapter 12.11.1) occur: each may be symptomatic—indeed, attacks of hyperkalaemic periodic paralysis may occur. Amnesic deficits, depression, and impaired concentration progressing to confusion are relatively common. Addisonian crises may be accompanied by generalized convulsions, which are attributed to hyponatraemia and water intoxication. Benign intracranial hypertension with papilloedema and a proximal myopathy may also occur.

X-linked adrenoleukodystrophy is discussed in Section 12.7.

Thyroid disease

Thyroid disease carries one set of neurological complications directly related to abnormal thyroxine levels; another sharing the same autoimmune origin (and eponyms)—Hashimoto's encephalopathy and Grave's ophthalmopathy. Here only the former will be considered.

Thyrotoxicosis

The features of hyperthyroidism include anxiety, tremor, tachycardia, and insomnia. Chorea or mania may occur. A severe proximal myopathy is not uncommon, and rarely myasthenia gravis is seen. Thyroxine-responsive hypokalaemic periodic paralysis is well reported.

Myxoedema

Hypothyroidism may present with lethargy, even progressing to a toxic confusional state or a subacute hypothermic, hypotensive coma. The latter (which may be provoked by infection, trauma, exposure to cold, or sedation), together with the occasionally seen psychosis or dementing illness ('myxoedema madness') responds to (judicious) thyroxine hormone replacement. Ataxia occurs in 5 to 10 per cent of patients with hypothyroidism, and improves with thyroxine replacement.

Hypothyroid myopathy is characterized by proximal weakness with stiffness, aching, and cramps, and pseudomyotonic delayed muscle relaxation evident on tapping tendons or muscle bellies (with percussion-induced muscle ridging). Muscle hypertrophy (Hoffmann's syndrome) is rare. The carpal tunnel syndrome may occur due to deposits of myxoedematous tissue around the median nerve of the wrist, and rarely this may cause a diffuse peripheral neuropathy.

Diabetes mellitus

Diabetes mellitus (Chapter 12.11.1) causes a wide variety of neurological disturbances. Centrally, stupor or coma may be produced by hyperosmolality, ketoacidosis, lactic acidosis, spontaneous (prediabetic) or iatrogenic hypoglycaemia, uraemia, or hypertensive encephalopathy. Transient ischaemic attacks and stroke due to cerebral arteriosclerosis and hypertension are common in patients with diabetes.

Peripherally, nerve damage may occur in patients with established diabetes, or may be the presenting feature of the illness; it is described in more detail in Chapter 24.19. The following syndromes are recognized.

1. Single painful nerve lesions (mononeuritis) such as isolated ocular nerve palsies, Bell's palsy, a lateral popliteal nerve palsy, or an intercostal neuropathy are common and may result from haemorrhage or infarction of the nerve.
2. Carpal tunnel syndrome, an ulnar nerve palsy, or other compression neuropathies may result from the undue susceptibility of peripheral nerves in diabetes to pressure.
3. Mononeuritis multiplex may occur, with a microvascular basis.
4. Diabetic amyotrophy refers to a proximal motor neuropathy causing the subacute weakness and wasting, often with pain, affecting quadriceps muscles, usually asymmetrically. It is probably due to ischaemia or haemorrhage in the femoral nerve or lumbosacral plexus.
5. A distal symmetrical peripheral neuropathy in diabetes may take the form of a mild asymptomatic sensory neuropathy with loss of vibration sense in the feet and absent ankle jerks. Less commonly, there is severe and progressive sensorimotor neuropathy affecting the legs before the arms.
6. Autonomic neuropathy is common, producing impotence, diarrhoea, loss of sweating, and abnormal pupils. The last may be irregular, and unreactive to light, mimicking Argyll Robertson pupils. Autonomic neuropathy causes orthostatic hypotension, syncope, and sometimes abrupt cardiac arrest in patients with diabetes.

It should be recalled that diabetes may occur as a feature of a number of genetically determined neurological diseases, including Friedreich's ataxia, X-linked spinomuscular atrophy, mitochondrial cytopathies, myotonic dystrophy, and the Wolfram syndrome; it is also associated with the stiff man syndrome.

Hypoglycaemia

Hypoglycaemic coma can be difficult to diagnose and dangerous. In any case of coma, stupor, or confusion of unknown cause, and often in newly presenting status epilepticus, blood should be drawn for glucose analysis and insulin levels, and then 25 g of glucose (with thiamine) should be administered intravenously. Such an injection can do no harm and may save life.

The commonest cause of hypoglycaemia is insulin overdose, or excessive hypoglycaemic drug intake. Hyperinsulinism due to an adenoma of the islets of Langerhans in the pancreas is uncommon, as is hypoglycaemia due to prediabetes or a retroperitoneal sarcoma. Hypoglycaemia may also occur in alcoholism and liver disease, after gastric surgery, and in a variety of rare metabolic conditions.

Hypoglycaemia presents in four ways: (i) as an organic toxic confusional state, sleepy confusion, bizarre behaviour, or mania; (ii) as unexplained coma with brainstem dysfunction, including decerebrate spasms and neurogenic hyperventilation, but with preserved oculocephalic reflexes and pupillary responses; (iii) as a stroke-like illness with focal deficit; and (iv) as epilepsy. Hyperinsulinism, very rarely, also causes predominantly motor peripheral neuropathy.

Hypoglycaemia is established by measurement of the blood glucose concentration, and by clinical response to intravenous glucose replacement. Hyperinsulinism is difficult to diagnose on occasion, but can be established by satisfying the criteria for Whipple's triad, namely symptoms of hypoglycaemia, associated with a low blood sugar and a disproportionately high serum insulin, and clinical response to glucose replacement. A 72-h fast, measuring morning blood sugar and insulin levels, will detect nearly all pancreatic islet cell adenomas (see Chapter 12.10).

Metabolic disorders due to ionic or acid–base abnormalities

Hyponatraemia or 'water intoxication'

Sodium is the most abundant serum cation, so that hyponatraemia is almost always the cause of hypo-osmolality. Serum osmolality is approximately equal to double the serum sodium concentration plus 10, provided glucose and urea levels are normal. Normal serum osmolality is 290 ± 5 mosmol/kg; serum osmolality below about 260 or above about 330 mosmol/kg is likely to produce cerebral changes. Hyponatraemia means that body water is increased relative to solute, resulting in water excess in the brain. Rapid changes in serum sodium osmolality produce much greater neurological effects than does slowly developing chronic hyponatraemia. Hyponatraemia occurs in renal disease, as a result of excessive intravenous water infusions, due to excessive diarrhoea, vomiting, or sweating, or may result from the inappropriate secretion of antidiuretic hormone that occurs in bronchial carcinoma, focal hypothalamic damage due to neoplasm or infection, or diffuse acute brain disease resulting from head injury, meningitis, or encephalitis, or subarachnoid haemorrhage. (It is, however, noteworthy that in the latter acute situations, salt-wasting may also cause hyponatraemia, in which circumstances fluid restriction exacerbates the problem: hypovolaemia distinguishes salt-wasting from the eu- or hypervolaemia of vasopressin excess.) Patients with hyponatraemia become confused and restless, and develop asterixis, multifocal myoclonus, generalized convulsions, stupor, and coma. Symptoms may appear when the plasma sodium drops below about 120 mmol/l, and fits and coma usually are associated with plasma sodium values below 110 mmol/l. A few patients with chronic hyponatraemia may develop the syndrome of central pontine myelinolysis (see below). Treatment is by water restriction; infusions of hypertonic saline are not advised.

Central pontine myelinolysis

This is a rare disease, often associated with hyponatraemia, and in particular with rapid attempts to correct serum sodium by parenteral hypertonic fluids: elevation by no more than 0.55 mmol/l per hour is allegedly safe. It is also seen in alcoholics, in severe liver and renal disease, and other metabolic disturbances. The disease is characterized by a rapidly progressive flaccid or spastic quadriplegia, with involvement of bulbar muscles producing dysarthria and dysphagia. Consciousness and eye movement may remain intact. At worst the patient may be unable to speak or swallow, or to move any muscle except those of the eyes. Death is common but remarkable recovery may occur.

Hypernatraemia

The common cause of hyperosmolality is diabetes, producing severe hyperglycaemia. Hyperosmolality due to hypernatraemia is rare, except in those who dehydrate in hot climates. Chronic uncompensated water loss in untreated diabetes insipidus may result in mild hypernatraemia, but such patients only develop severe hypernatraemia if they fail to drink. Patients with simple diabetes insipidus usually maintain thirst, but if intercurrent illness leads to excessive water loss and restricted water intake, they may become dehydrated, drowsy, stuporose, and unconscious. Simple diabetes insipidus may be due to pituitary surgery, trauma, or pituitary tumours. If pathology extends into the hypothalamic region, not only may secretion of vasopressin be deficient, but thirst regulation may also be abolished. Hypothalamic damage causing severe hypernatraemia may occur in large pituitary tumours, craniopharyngiomas, hypothalamic tumours, sarcoidosis, or Hand–Schüller–Christian disease. Loss of thirst in such patients often precipitates hypernatraemic coma with serum sodium rising above 160 to 170 mmol/l. Hypernatraemia may also occur as a result of severe water depletion, particularly in children with intense diarrhoea.

Hypercalcaemia (see Chapter 12.6)

A high serum calcium concentration may be due to primary hyperparathyroidism, immobilization, sarcoidosis, vitamin D intoxication, or multiple bony metastases. Symptoms include anorexia, nausea, vomiting, intense thirst, polyuria, and polydipsia. Muscle weakness, lassitude, and a mild encephalopathy are common. The latter may produce delusions and changes in mood so that many such patients are initially treated for a psychiatric condition. A toxic confusional state with lethargy and stupor, sometimes with generalized or focal seizures and papilloedema, also may occur. A more severe syndrome with pyramidal signs, ataxia, and an internuclear ophthalmoplegia is also described.

Hypocalcaemia (see Chapter 12.6)

Reduced serum calcium concentration may be caused by parathyroid or thyroid surgery, chronic renal failure, or chronic anticonvulsant drug treatment. It also occurs in primary idiopathic hypoparathyroidism (when the serum parathormone level is low), and in pseudohypoparathyroidism (in which the serum parathormone level is normal or high, and there is no response to parathyroid hormone; skeletal deformities and dysmorphism also are present). Pseudopseudohypoparathyroidism is a syndrome with similar skeletal and dysmorphic abnormalities but normal serum calcium and parathormone levels. Hypocalcaemia causes neuromuscular irritability, tetany with a positive Chvostek's sign, and a mild encephalopathy. Severe degrees of hypocalcaemia produce generalized convulsions, psychotic behavioural disturbances, stupor, and coma. Raised intracranial pressure with papilloedema may occur in hypoparathyroidism. Hypocalcaemia is commonly misdiagnosed as mental retardation, dementia, or epilepsy. Skin changes and cataracts are characteristic. Calcification in basal ganglia on skull radiograph or CT scan may be evident. Rarely, basal ganglia calcification may be associated with extrapyramidal disorders.

Magnesium

Renal disease may impair the ability to excrete magnesium, which is cardiotoxic. Hypomagnesaemia, due to inadequate intake or excessive renal or gastrointestinal loss, causes secondary hypocalcaemia; the former rarely occurs without the latter, and the neurological complications often attributed to low magnesium are precisely those of hypocalcaemia. Hypermagnesaemia may cause an encephalopathy with decreased or absent tendon jerks; the latter may progress to a flaccid paralysis.

Potassium

Hypokalaemia, not uncommonly caused by diuretics, is associated with myalgia and a proximal myopathy; if severe, rhabdomyolysis can occur. Hyperkalaemia can precipitate an areflexic flaccid paralysis, which may be fully reversible with correction of the serum potassium. The periodic paralyses are discussed in Chapter 24.22.5.

Acid–base disturbances

Systemic acidosis and alkalosis (see Section 11) occur in many diseases causing metabolic coma, but of the four disorders of acid–base balance (respiratory or metabolic acidosis or alkalosis), only respiratory acidosis acts as a direct cause of stupor and coma. Hypoxia associated with respiratory acidosis may be important in producing neurological abnormalities. Metabolic acidosis, by itself, usually only causes delirium or, at most, drowsiness. The reason why even severe disorders of systemic acid–base balance usually do not interfere with the function of the brain is that it possesses powerful mechanisms for protecting its own acid–base balance, including respiratory compensation, changes in cerebral blood flow, and cellular buffering in nervous tissue. Coma in metabolic acidosis due to diabetic ketosis or hyperosmolality, lactic acidosis, uraemia, alcohol poisoning, or intake of ethylene glycol, methyl alcohol, or paraldehyde is usually due to associated metabolic abnormalities or direct effects of other toxins in these conditions. Severe respiratory acidosis produces a reduction in alertness parallel to the degree of acidosis. Respiratory alkalosis, although constricting cerebral arterioles and decreasing cerebral blood flow, rarely interferes with cerebral function. A patient in coma with respiratory alkalosis due to hyperventilation has some other condition such as sepsis, hepatic disease, pulmonary infarction, or salicylate overdose. Even severe metabolic alkalosis only produces a confusional state rather than stupor or coma.

Alcohol and the nervous system

Alcohol damages the nervous system in many ways. Some are the result of acute or chronic poisoning, while others are a consequence of associated vitamin deficiency. This section will mainly address the neurological consequences of chronic, excessive alcohol intake, not the acute transient effects of alcohol.

Delirium tremens

This develops several days after ethanol abstinence in chronic abusers. Usually rapid in onset, there is an agitated confused state, with signs of sympathetic overactivity. Circulatory collapse may contribute to the 5 to 10 per cent mortality. It is generally distinguished from the less severe alcohol withdrawal syndrome, characterized by broadly similar symptoms that occur sooner—within hours of withdrawal—and are usually self-limiting. Ethanol withdrawal seizures represent a not uncommon cause of late-onset fits. Benzodiazepines have transformed the management of delirium tremens and the alcohol withdrawal syndrome, and significantly reduced its mortality.

The Wernicke–Korsakoff syndrome

Aetiology

Inadequate intake of thiamine, of whatever cause, may lead to foci of marked hyperaemia with multiple small haemorrhages affecting particularly the upper brainstem, hypothalamus, and thalamus adjacent to the third ventricle, and the mamillary bodies. Histologically there is a proliferation of dilated capillaries with perivascular haemorrhage in these areas. There may be associated alcohol-induced damage to the cerebral cortex, cerebellum, and peripheral nerves.

Such pathology can be produced in animals by a diet deficient in thiamine. Thiamine deficiency can be demonstrated in patients with the Wernicke–Korsakoff syndrome, and administration of thiamine can reverse many of the symptoms and signs of this syndrome. (Wernicke's and Korsakoff's syndromes probably represent the acute and chronic consequences of the same pathological process.) Thiamine and its pyrophosphate are cofactors to at least four enzymes—pyruvate decarboxylase, α-ketoglutarate dehydrogenase, the branched-chain ketoacid decarboxylase system, and transketolase. Thiamine deficiency results in reduced conversion of pyruvate to acetyl coenzyme A, causing elevated plasma and tissue pyruvate levels, with decreased flux through the Krebs cycle, reducing ATP production, and impairing energy supply. In addition, there is a shortage of one-carbon groups for biosynthetic pathways.

Alcoholism with an inadequate diet is the most frequent cause of the Wernicke–Korsakoff syndrome today. Malnutrition in prisoners of war, or at times of famine, may also be responsible. Chronic vomiting, for example during pregnancy or due to gastrointestinal disease, systemic malignancy, prolonged intravenous feeding, and anorexia nervosa are rarer causes.

Clinical features

The onset may be insidious or subacute with increasing lethargy and inattentiveness, which develops into a typical confusional state with disorientation in time and place, loss of memory, and altered consciousness. Ophthalmoplegia develops with diplopia. The most common eye signs are nystagmus on lateral or vertical gaze, sixth-nerve palsies, or defects of conjugate gaze. Retinal haemorrhages may occur. Most patients who are alcoholics will also have signs of a peripheral neuropathy, and many exhibit ataxia—the third classically described feature. Hypothermia may appear. Wernicke's encephalopathy is a medical emergency: untreated, the patient lapses into stupor and then coma, and dies—the mortality untreated is 20 per cent.

In less acute cases, or in those recovering from the acute confusional phase, the characteristic features of the Korsakoff psychosis or amnesic syndrome will appear. The patient has an often very severe gross defect of memory for recent events, such that new information cannot be retained for more than a matter of minutes or hours. The patient is disorientated in time and place, but alert. Despite the severe defect of recent memory, he or she can recall events in the remote past. Gaps in memory are filled by giving imaginary and often graphic accounts of events (confabulation).

Diagnosis

Diagnosis is essentially clinical. The cerebrospinal fluid is usually normal, although the protein may be slightly raised. Brain scanning can be normal, although patients who are alcoholic (who fall often) may have subdural haematomas. Demonstration of reduced red cell transketolase activity, or of raised plasma pyruvate levels, is often invalidated by intake of food as soon as the patient comes under supervision.

Treatment

The Wernicke–Korsakoff syndrome must be considered in any individual with unexplained confusion, stupor, or coma, particularly in the presence of eye signs, a peripheral neuropathy, or a history of alcoholism or excessive vomiting. Thiamine should be given to all such patients. High-potency vitamin injections should be given daily until oral vitamin B complex preparations can be taken.

A particular problem arises commonly in the emergency department when patients exhibiting stupor or coma of unknown cause are admitted. All such patients should be given high-dose thiamine and glucose parenterally—if glucose is given without thiamine to a patient with Wernicke–Korsakoff syndrome, rapid deterioration and death can follow. Those who are thiamine deficient cannot handle the glucose load.

Effective treatment will restore consciousness and reverse eye signs, the latter usually within hours, but unfortunately the Korsakoff amnesia syndrome frequently does not resolve. The earlier the treatment, the better the chances of recovery, so suspicion or possibility of this diagnosis represents a medical emergency.

Alcoholic peripheral neuropathy (see also Chapter 24.17)

Aetiology

Although thiamine deficiency has long been held responsible for the peripheral neuropathy associated with chronic alcoholism, a direct toxic effect has more recently been proposed. Pathologically the picture of peripheral nerve damage is very similar to that seen in beriberi. There is predominantly axonal neuropathy of the 'dying back' type, affecting the somatic and sometimes the autonomic nerves.

Clinical features

Alcoholic peripheral neuropathy predominantly involves sensory nerves, producing distal parasthesias in the feet, followed by the hands, and characteristic pain. The last may be intense and agonizing. Squeezing the calves or scratching the soles of the feet may cause severe discomfort. At a later stage, weakness and wasting of the distal limb muscles follows. Tendon reflexes are lost. Evidence of autonomic neuropathy may be seen in abnormal pupillary reactions and tachycardia, although postural hypotension is rare and the sphincters are usually spared.

Treatment

Alcohol must be proscribed and high-potency vitamin B given parenterally for some 10 days and then orally. The prognosis depends on how early treatment is initiated. Symptoms may take weeks to subside and in more severe cases recovery may take many months or may be incomplete.

Alcoholic cerebellar degeneration

Some patients who are alcoholic may develop a relatively pure syndrome of midline cerebellar ataxia, with a progressive unsteadiness of gait and of leg movements, and little or no involvement of the arms. Speech is not affected, and nystagmus is not present. Many such patients also have evidence of alcoholic peripheral neuropathy. Pathologically there is degeneration of the cerebellar cortex, particularly of the Purkinje cells, and also of the olivary nuclei. Changes in the cerebellum characteristically affect the anterior and superior parts of the vermis and hemispheres. This complication of alcoholism does not seem to be due to thiamine deficiency. However, withdrawal of alcohol and vitamin replacement can lead to recovery.

Alcoholic dementia (see Section 26)

In the past, there has been much debate over whether alcoholism produces dementia. However, it is now clear that a large proportion of those who habitually take excessive alcohol develop cognitive deficits. These can vary from mild changes to severe diffuse global dementia, and are associated with atrophy of the cerebral cortex and enlargement of the cerebral ventricles.

The dementia has the usual features of personality change, loss of memory, impairment of intellect, and emotional instability. Patients who are alcoholic commonly fail at work or in personal relationships. The gradual drift into destitution is well described in the literature and all too familiar on the streets. Head injuries in alcoholic bouts and epilepsy may occur and contribute to the overall final picture. The fully developed case of the 'down and out' is an antisocial demented individual, with dysarthric speech, tremor, an ataxic gait, and a peripheral neuropathy, who still forlornly or aggressively clutches the bottle and a bag of residual belongings.

The dementia of alcoholism is not directly related to thiamine deficiency alone. Treatment by withdrawal of alcohol, if possible, and vitamin replacement can lead to improvement. Indeed, some degree of reversal of evidence of cerebral atrophy on CT brain scan can be seen after 'drying out'. However, the prognosis is generally poor, not least because of the difficulties of persuading those addicted to alcoholic to stop drinking.

Marchiafava–Bignami disease

This rare disease was first described in Italian drinkers of crude red wine, but occurs in other patients who are alcoholic. It presents as a subacute dementing illness, which progresses rapidly to fits, spasticity or rigidity, and paralysis, culminating in coma and death within a few months. Pathologically there is widespread demyelination and axonal damage in the corpus callosum and the central white matter of the cerebral hemispheres, as well as in the optic chiasma and middle cerebellar peduncles. Abstinence stabilizes but rarely reverses the syndrome.

Alcoholic myopathy

Acute alcohol poisoning can produce a dramatic toxic myopathy. There is severe pain, muscle tenderness, oedema, and weakness, which may be associated with myoglobinuria, renal damage, and hyperkalaemia. Arrhythmias may occur. The syndrome is reversible if the necessary intensive support is available. A subacute painless myopathy resolving after withdrawal of alcohol has also been described. Chronic alcoholism is associated commonly with a painless myopathy, occasionally with coexistent cardiomyopathy; again abstinence can cure the disorder.

Tobacco–alcohol amblyopia

Another uncommon complication of alcohol occurs in combination with strong tobacco. The patient develops sudden or subacute bilateral visual failure, associated with bilateral centrocaecal scotomas. The condition has been attributed to cyanide in tobacco causing a disorder of vitamin B_{12} metabolism. Visual failure and optic atrophy may occur in patients with pernicious anaemia, particularly those who smoke. A related condition is tropical amblyopia, occurring in Africa. This has been related to excessive consumption of cassava root containing cyanide. Treatment of these conditions is with hydroxycobalamine injections.

Superficial siderosis of the central nervous system

Superficial siderosis is an unusual disorder of the nervous system that has been recognized only recently. The four principal clinical manifestations are: progressive ataxia; cranial polyneuropathy, particularly sensorineural deafness; myelopathy causing a spastic tetraparesis; and progressive dementia. Headaches occasionally feature. Cerebrospinal fluid examination reveals xanthochromia which, importantly, persists with repeated examination. MRI is diagnostic, with low signal intensity on T_2-weighted images apparent at the surface of the cerebellum, cranial nerves, brainstem, spinal cord, and more deeply on the borders of the dentate and basal ganglia. Iron deposition can be shown by high-strength MRI, corresponding to pathological descriptions of siderotic deposits in the meninges. Repeated subarachnoid haemorrhage, cerebral tumours, or past surgery are recognized causes of this syndrome, but often none is historically evident; repeated subclinical haemorrhage is postulated but not proven. No treatments are of proven benefit.

Porphyria

Porphyrias affect predominantly the liver (acute intermittent porphyria (AIP), variegate porphyria, hereditary coproporphyria, and porphyria cutanea tarda) or the blood (for example erythropoietic protoporphyria). AIP spares the skin. Certain drugs (sulphonamides, barbiturates, oral contraceptive pill), starvation, alcohol, and other insults can precipitate 'crises' in AIP, hereditary coproporphyria, and variegate porphyria characterized by: (i) a predominantly motor, often proximal areflexic peripheral neuropathy, occasionally mimicking the Guillain–Barré syndrome; (ii) abdominal pain and cardiovascular instability caused by autonomic involvement; and (iii) confusion or psychosis. Fits may occur and acute attacks are commonly accompanied by progressive severe hyponatraemia due to inappropriate secretion of vasopressin. Increased urine and faecal porphyrins lead to the diagnosis. Acute attacks are treated largely symptomatically with benzodiazepines or opiates and major tranquillizers, and cardiorespiratory support. Carbohydrate loading may be beneficial.

Further reading

Metabolic complications of major organ disease

Bolton CF, Young GB (1990). *Neurological complications of renal diseases.* Butterworth Heinemann, Stoneham, Massachusetts.

Jones EA, Weissenborn K (1997). Neurology and the liver. *Journal of Neurology, Neursurgery, and Psychiatry* **63**, 279–303.

Metabolic disorders due to endocrine disease

Shaw P (1998). Neurological complications of thyroid disease. In: Goetz CG, Aminoff MJ, eds. *Handbook of clinical neurology* **26** (70) *Systemic diseases Part II*, pp. 81–110. Elsevier Science BV, Amsterdam.

Watkins PJ, Thomas PK (1997). Diabetes mellitus and the nervous system. *Journal of Neurology, Neursurgery, and Psychiatry* **65**, 620–32.

Metabolic disorders due to ionic or acid–base abnormalities

Abrams GM, Jay C (1998). Neurological complications of mineral metabolism and parathyroid disease. In: Goetz CG, Aminoff MJ, eds. *Handbook of clinical neurology* **26** (70) *Systemic diseases Part II*, pp 111–129.

Gocht A, Colmant HJ (1997). Central pontine and extrapontine myelinolysis: a report of 58 cases. *Clinical Neuropathology* **6**, 262–70.

Alcohol and the nervous system

Harper C (1983). The incidence of Wernicke's encephalopathy in Australia—a neuropathological study of 131 cases. *Journal of Neurology, Neurosurgery, and Psychiatry* **46**, 593–8.

Harper C, Giles M, Finlay-Jones R (1986). Clinical signs in the Wernicke–Korsakoff complex: a retrospective analysis of 131 cases diagnosed at necropsy. *Journal of Neurology, Neurosurgery, and Psychiatry* **49**, 341–5.

Miles MF, Diamond I (1998). Neurological complications of alcoholism and alcohol abuse. In: Goetz CG, Aminoff MJ, eds. *Handbook of clinical neurology* **26** (70) *Systemic diseases Part II*, pp 339–57.

Miscellaneous metabolic and deficiency disorders of the nervous system

Bruyn RPM, Bruyn GW (1998). Superfical siderosis of the central nervous system. In: Goetz CG, Aminoff MJ, eds. *Handbook of clinical neurology* **26** (70) *Systemic diseases Part II*, pp 65–80.

Young GB (1995). Neurologic complications of systemic critical illness. *Neurologic Clinics* **13**, 645–58.

24.16 Demyelinating disorders of the central nervous system

Alastair Compston

Clinicians suspect demyelination when episodes reflecting damage to white matter tracts within the central nervous system occur in young adults. The diagnosis of multiple sclerosis becomes probable when these symptoms and signs recur, affecting different parts of the brain and spinal cord. Demyelination also underlies many postinfectious neurological conditions affecting the central nervous system.

Neurobiology of demyelination

Glial development and myelination

Glial progenitors migrate from germinal zones around the lateral ventricles, the fourth ventricle, and in the ventral spinal cord, and differentiate either into astrocytes or oligodendrocytes. Oligodendrocyte precursors can be recovered from the adult nervous system. These behave as stem cells, dividing asymmetrically (at least *in vitro*) to produce one daughter precursor cell and one oligodendrocyte—providing a potential pool of new oligodendrocytes.

Growth, differentiation, and survival of glial progenitors and their progeny are orchestrated by growth factors. These are produced by neurones, astrocytes, and microglia. Those factors involved in rodent development (where most is currently known: glial-derived nerve growth factor, fibroblast growth factor 2, platelet-derived growth factor, insulin-like growth factors 1 and 2, nerve growth factor, neurotrophin 3, ciliary neurotrophic factor, retinoic acid, glial growth factor, interleukin 6, and leukaemia inhibitory factor) are not yet shown to be relevant in development of the human central nervous system.

Myelination occurs when the membraneous processes of mature oligodendrocytes contact and ensheathe axons and compact to form the myelin lamellae needed for saltatory axonal conduction. The number of surviving oligodendrocytes is matched to local axon density. Compact myelin consists of a condensed membrane, mainly composed of lipid (cholesterol, phospholipid, and galactolipid) with some protein, wrapped spirally many times around axons to form a segmented sheath. The glycoproteins are galactocerebroside, myelin-associated glycoprotein, and myelin oligodendrocyte glycoprotein (**MOG**). The two major proteins are proteolipid protein (**PLP**) and myelin basic protein (**MBP**). A further structural component is the myelin-specific enzyme 2′,3′-cyclic nucleotide 3′-phosphohydrolase (CNP-ase). It is periodically interrupted along the course of the axon at the (unmyelinated) nodes of Ranvier, where electrical resistance is low due to the high concentration of sodium channels, and depolarization thereby facilitated. In myelinated axons, the action potential generates electrical currents which preferentially trigger depolarization at the next node of Ranvier. This saltatory conduction is considerably more rapid than continuous propagation of the nerve impulse.

Pathophysiology of demyelination

Myelin injury blocks saltatory conduction through myelinated pathways in the central nervous system. Although function may be preserved by redundancy in individual systems or tracts, strategically placed pathways lose their safety factor for conduction resulting in neurological symptoms and signs. Most clinical manifestations of demyelination merely reflect abnormalities to be expected from any process that disrupts physiological performance at that site. However, saltatory conduction may be compromised by partial demyelination in ways which account for specific features of multiple sclerosis and related disorders.

Partially demyelinated axons cannot transmit fast trains of impulse. This may explain symptoms that reflect physiological fatigue. Depolarization may traverse the lesion but at reduced velocity. This accounts for the characteristic delay in arrival of potentials evoked by sensory stimuli and recorded over appropriate cortical receptor zones. Partially demyelinated axons may discharge spontaneously. This explains distortions of sensation reported by a high proportion of patients. Increased mechanical sensitivity manifests as movement-induced symptoms including flashes of light on eye movement, and the electric sensation that spreads down the spine, limbs, or anterior chest wall after neck flexion—Lhermitte's symptom and sign. Increased temperature sensitivity, with a reduction in the safety factor for conduction in partially demyelinated axons, explains the temporary increase in severity of pre-existing symptoms experienced by many patients after exercise or immersion in hot water. Cold may improve performance—some patients adopting complicated water-cooled systems and others reporting that, for example, vision improves after eating ice cream. Ephaptic transmission occurs between neighbouring and partially demyelinated axons giving rise to paroxysmal symptoms of demyelination usually manifesting as trigeminal neuralgia, ataxia, and dysarthria, or tonic brainstem seizures. These are often triggered by touch or movement.

There are several mechanisms of symptom recovery early in the course of multiple sclerosis. These include the resolution of conduction block in nerve fibres which were never demyelinated, re-establishment of conduction in persistently demyelinated axons, functional reorganization of surviving pathways, and remyelination. Onset and recovery of conduction block and clinical impairments match the phase of acute inflammation. Transient symptoms depend on reversible conduction block caused by direct action of cytokines and inflammatory mediators (especially nitric oxide) on normal or hypomyelinated axons (Fig. 1). Function may be restored after demyelination by rearrangement of sodium channels providing a variety of alternative patterns of ordered or partially disordered conduction. There is probably also a contribution from the remyelination seen in acute lesions. Experimentally, remyelinated axons restore conduction of the nerve impulse and motor function.

Inflammation and the brain

Demyelinating disease includes conditions in which myelin fails to develop (leucodystrophies) or is lost through inflammatory (multiple sclerosis and related conditions) and metabolic (central pontine myelinolysis) mechanisms. Outstandingly the most common group is inflammatory demyelination. In all but the most severe forms, perivascular inflammation evolves through stages of acute axonal injury, demyelination, oligodendrocyte

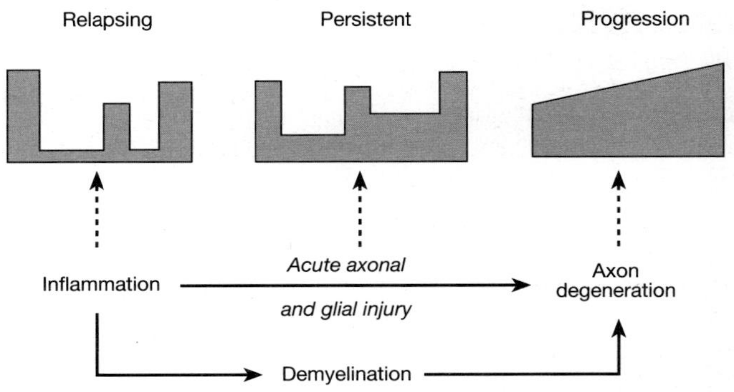

Fig. 1 Inflammatory mediators cause reversible symptoms in multiple sclerosis. Inflammation drives demyelination, which explains persistent symptoms. Progression depends mainly on axon degeneration, which causes acute axonal inury and continues throughout the course, but is conditioned by the amount of early inflammation.

depletion, remyelination, astrocytosis, and axon chronic degeneration. The order and relationship of these separate components is still debated. The resulting plaques are widely distributed but concentrated around venous networks, the ventricles, and in the corpus callosum, the optic nerve, brainstem, and cervical cord.

Conditions required for inflammatory cell penetration of cerebral vessels include slowing of the circulation and the establishment of electrostatic force which allows adhesion between circulating and lining cells. Endothelial cells extend microvillar processes in response to injury and these entangle inflammatory cells as they pass along the vessel wall. Infiltrating lymphocytes which are not activated against brain antigen either return to the circulation or (in common with immune cells that have outlived their purpose elsewhere) die by apoptosis. Activated T cells that encounter antigen persist within the nervous system.

Outward migration of cells from the inflammatory nidus is promoted by local production of chemokines interacting with specific receptors on migrating cells, and by metalloproteases which degrade tissue barriers. Proinflammatory cytokines (especially interferon-γ) amplify the immune response. Microglia are activated, leading to the release of yet more T-cell derived interferon-γ, and the recruitment of additional naive microglia. Contact is established between activated microglia and the oligodendrocyte–myelin unit if the latter is opsonized with ligands for (Fc and complement) receptors activated on the surface of microglia. Demyelinated axons are coated with anti-MOG antibody in the lesions of acute multiple sclerosis. This may be a key antigen in attracting degradation of the oligodendrocyte–myelin unit by activated microglia. Adherent activated microglia deliver their lethal signal to the target oligodendrocyte using tumour necrosis factor-α bound to the cell surface. Together, these inflammatory processes lead to disruption of the myelin membrane with increased spacing, vesicular disruption, splitting, vacuolation, and fragmentation of the lamellae.

Much emphasis has been placed on the role of axon degeneration as a pathological feature. In hyperacute multiple sclerosis, large confluent zones of demyelination are associated with extensive axonal loss and surrounding oedema but little inflammation. In many other lesions, immunohistochemical staining for the amyloid precursor protein shows that axonal injury is initiated as part of the acute demyelinating episode. However, it is not certain when axons actually die. Acute damage to axons with transection appears early and the circumstantial evidence suggests vulnerability of recently demyelinated axons to the inflammatory environment of acute lesions; but there is also a chronic attrition which may be degenerative and secondary to loss of trophic support normally provided by myelin.

Acute lesions sometimes show an increase in the number of oligodendrocytes indicating microglia-associated loss of healthy oligodendrocytes and recruitment of new progenitors which then undergo differentiation. Axons are remyelinated in acute shadow plaques. Remyelination is associated with inflammation and reactive astrocytes which deliver cytokines and growth factors. The morphological criteria for remyelination are inappropriately thin myelin lamellae for the corresponding axon, with a short internode and myelin embedded in a satellite cell. Experimentally, remyelination can restore structure, conduction of the nerve impulse, and function, but—in a clinical context—new myelin may not survive repeated injury. The source of remyelinating cells is presumed to be the oligodendrocyte progenitor which is found in the lesions of multiple sclerosis.

Isolated demyelinating syndromes

The clinical expression of demyelination may be focal and monophasic even when imaging shows multiple lesions. The distinction between multiple sclerosis and isolated demyelinating disorders can therefore reliably only be made when more than one episode has occurred, affecting two or more sites, and not merely on the basis of anatomical dissemination of lesions.

Acute disseminated encephalomyelitis

Typically, acute disseminated encephalomyelitis develops within days or a few weeks after an infectious illness. It is usually but not invariably a disease of children. Formerly, acute disseminated encephalomyelitis affected 1 in 1000 children with exanthematous illnesses, the risk being slightly lower following pertussis and scarlet fever than measles and rubella, but these childhood illnesses, and hence their complications, are now less prevalent. A greater variety of causative organisms has been implicated in adult-onset acute disseminated encephalomyelitis, but in both groups a presumptive diagnosis often has to be made in the absence of an identifiable preceding infection.

The disorder is usually diffuse, and with a cerebral flavour, but the clinical manifestations may be restricted to the brainstem, optic nerves, or spinal cord. About 50 per cent of cases occurring after varicella infection present with a pure cerebellar syndrome. Headache, drowsiness, meningeal irritation, signs of systemic infection, focal or generalized fits, and combinations of lesions indicating damage to the cerebrum, optic nerves, brainstem, or spinal cord evolve over the course of a few days. The cerebrospinal fluid contains a mixture of polymorphonuclear cells and lymphocytes with raised protein and slight reduction in glucose; oligoclonal bands may be present. Whilst there is an appreciable mortality, the majority of patients survive, sometimes with persistent neurological deficits. Magnetic resonance imaging shows changes similar to those occurring in multiple sclerosis but the lesions are more extensive and symmetrical; they persist long after recovery of the clinical illness.

The hyperacute form of acute disseminated encephalomyelitis (Hurst's disease) starts with headache and progresses over hours to disorientation, confusion, drowsiness, and coma; events move quickly and the illness often proves fatal before the diagnosis has been established. The combination of pyrexia and a marked cerebrospinal fluid pleocytosis with a predominantly neutrophil response mimics pyogenic infection of the central nervous system, but the course is not influenced by antimicrobial treatment. Occasionally, the clinical and pathological features of acute haemorrhagic leucoencephalitis are focal and suggest a rapidly expanding tumour or herpes simplex encephalitis.

The outcome in acute disseminated encephalomyelitis is probably influenced by early use of high-dose intravenous steroids, but anecdotally, there may be a more favourable response to intravenous immunoglobulin. A proportion of patients recovering from the initial attack subsequently relapse. In some, although the illness remains monophasic, separate sites are involved sequentially over several weeks but the disorder does not recur. In others, the illness is subsequently shown to be the encephalopathic presentation of multiple sclerosis, which then follows the typical relapsing–remitting course. The nosological status of multiphasic disseminated encephalomyelitis—based on a history of episodes and atypical imaging appearances for multiple sclerosis—has not gained general acceptance.

Postvaccinial encephalomyelitis has become a rare disorder and the definitive series were collected several decades ago when vaccination against smallpox was necessary. The illness develops within 2 to 3 weeks of vaccination with a skin rash and systemic symptoms, followed by cerebral or myelitic signs which usually recover spontaneously, in due course.

Optic neuritis

Optic neuritis presents with pain on eye movement, followed by blurred vision which evolves over hours or days, sometimes to complete blindness; patients may be aware of selective loss of colour vision and flashes of light (phosphenes) on eye movement. The pain disappears within a few days; vision improves in 90 per cent of patients over months, but defects of colour perception frequently persist. Optic neuritis may present with progressive visual failure in one or both eyes, but in these situations care must be taken to exclude compression of the anterior visual pathway. Transient visual loss, mimicking optic neuritis, also occurs in ischaemic optic neuropathy, sarcoidosis, or Eales' disease and a family history should be taken since the presentation of visual failure in Leber's hereditary optic neuropathy is similar to bilateral sequential optic neuritis in men. The lesion responsible for optic neuritis can be imaged *in vivo*; inflammation within the intracanalicular portion of the nerve and long lesions are associated with delayed or incomplete recovery of vision. Correlations between imaging, symptoms, and neurophysiological changes indicate that the visual deficits in optic neuritis arise at the time of altered blood–brain barrier permeability. They are associated with conduction block and precede demyelination or axonal degeneration.

The frequency with which the optic nerve is involved leads to anxiety in the informed patient that an episode of optic neuritis is likely to be the first manifestation of multiple sclerosis. The risk is highest in the first 5 years, but the proportion of cases having recurrent demyelination continues to rise thereafter and life-table analysis suggests that up to 80 per cent eventually convert. In children, optic neuritis is commonly bilateral and recurrent demyelination affecting other parts of the nervous system rarely occurs. Bilateral simultaneous optic neuritis in adults, although less common than in children, also carries a low risk of multiple sclerosis. Recurrent optic neuritis is associated with an increased risk and this is marginally higher in females than males. MRI abnormalities in the periventricular white matter are found in more than 60 per cent of patients with optic neuritis, and the risk of developing multiple sclerosis is substantially increased for those having two or more such lesions at presentation; conversely, the absence of cerebral lesions is a good prognostic sign. The presence of oligoclonal bands on cerebrospinal fluid electrophoresis during the acute phase is also a significant risk factor.

Transverse myelitis

The spinal cord is vulnerable to postinfectious inflammatory damage, but as with acute disseminated encephalomyelitis in adults, the precipitating cause is often not identified. Transverse myelitis presents with pain at the site of the lesion, followed by weakness in the legs, sensory symptoms, and sphincter involvement. The weakness increases and the clinical picture is that of spinal shock—features rarely seen in acute cord lesions due to multiple sclerosis. Sphincter control is lost, but unlike patients with multiple sclerosis, there is usually difficulty in emptying rather than filling the bladder. The need to exclude a structural abnormality in patients with transverse myelitis means that many patients undergo radiological investigation which may demonstrate cord swelling. The spinal fluid shows an increased mononuclear cell count, numerically intermediate between the marked pleocytosis of acute necrotizing myelitis and the marginal abnormalities seen in multiple sclerosis; total protein is raised and oligoclonal bands may be present on electrophoresis, but the glucose is usually normal. Transverse myelitis is more common in adults than children; there is a high frequency of persistent disability, but a much lower conversion to multiple sclerosis than following optic neuritis.

Acute necrotizing myelitis causes rapidly progressive flaccid areflexic paraplegia with anaesthesia and loss of sphincter control. The intensity of inflammation results in severe pain with meningism, pyrexia, and systemic symptoms. The condition mimics cord compression; the cerebrospinal fluid changes resemble pyogenic or tuberculous infection of the central nervous system. For these reasons, treatment with high-dose intravenous steroids, which may usefully influence mortality and limit long-term disability, is often withheld. Acute necrotizing myelitis has been described in association with herpes virus infection, and as a complication of acute lymphocytic leukaemias, lymphoma, carcinoma, and acquired immune deficiency syndrome.

Devic's disease (neuromyelitis optica)

Devic's disease is characterized by massive confluent demyelination in the anterior visual pathway together with equally severe spinal cord damage, occurring simultaneously or sequentially and in either order, the episodes usually separated by weeks or months. Cellular reaction in the cerebrospinal fluid more usually involves polymorphonuclear cells than lymphocytes, but often lacks oligoclonal bands. Cerebral white matter abnormalities tend to be frontotemporal and the spinal lesion is long, extending over several segments, in contrast to the several short lesions which characterize spinal MRI in multiple sclerosis.

The distinction from multiple sclerosis is partly confused by definitions. Demyelinating disease often follows the Devic pattern in Japanese and African patients, where multiple sclerosis is otherwise rare. Cases are described complicating pulmonary tuberculosis, especially in African patients. European patients with bilateral simultaneous optic neuritis and transverse myelitis often show manifestations of widespread demyelination and multiple events occur in due course. There is a better prognosis for recovery when the optic nerves and spinal cord are affected in rapid sequence, but the outcome is generally poor with an appreciable mortality, especially in relapsing patients with more than two episodes.

Isolated brainstem syndromes

The clinical symptoms and signs of isolated brainstem syndromes typically consist of disequilibrium, disturbed eye movements, facial numbness, and dysarthria, but there may be severe headache which rightly leads to early investigation in order to exclude a structural lesion. The majority of patients progress to clinically definite multiple sclerosis; as with other isolated demyelinating syndromes, abnormal MRI outside the affected site at presentation is a poor prognostic sign for clinical conversion.

Multiple sclerosis

Aetiology

The aetiology of multiple sclerosis involves an interplay between genes and the environment. It is a disease of northern European people and occurs less frequently in other racial groups. The familial recurrence rate is approximately 15 per cent. Meta-analysis amongst relatives of probands from three population-based series shows that the age-adjusted risk is highest for siblings (3 per cent), then parents and children (2 per cent), with lower rates in second- and third-degree relatives. Recurrence in monozygotic twins is around 35 per cent. Conversely, the frequency of multiple sclerosis in adoptees is similar to the population risk for Europeans. The age-adjusted risk for half-siblings is intermediate between social and biological relatives. Recurrence is higher in the children of conjugal pairs with multiple sclerosis (age-adjusted 20 per cent) than the offspring of single affecteds (2 per cent) (Fig. 2).

Population studies demonstrate an association between the class II MHC alleles (DR15 and DQ6) and their corresponding genotypes. A specifically

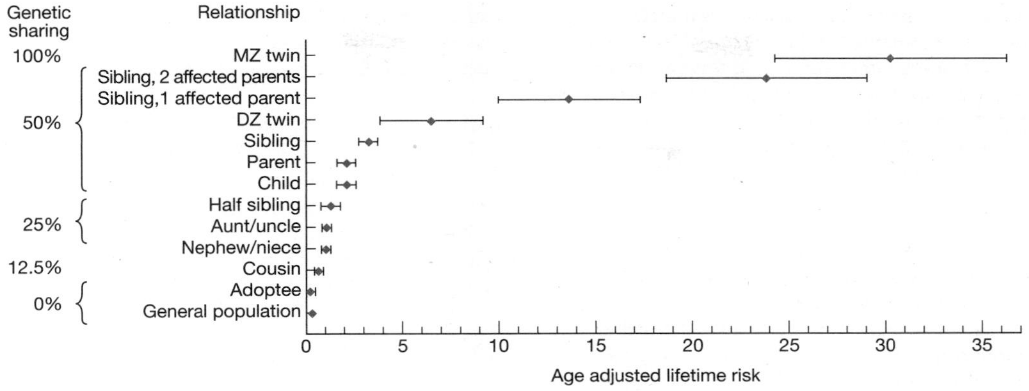

Fig. 2 Lifetime risk for multiple sclerosis amongst European people and in biological and social relatives of affected individuals. The increased risk with relatedness implicates genetic factors whereas the incomplete concordance in identical twins reflects the contribution made by environmental conditions.

different association in seen in Mediterranean populations (DR4). Extensive searches, using association and linkage studies over many years, have yielded very few additional candidates for susceptibility. To date, eight genome screens have failed to identify a major susceptibility locus using identity by descent analysis in sibling pairs and enough markers to provide around a 10 centiMorgan map. The possible reasons are that no such gene exists, it has been missed, or heterogeneity has obscured the picture. Whole genome association screens dependent on linkage disequilibirum are in progress. Genetic analyses assume that multiple sclerosis is one disease, but this may not be true. Mutations of mitochondrial DNA are responsible for a multiple sclerosis-like illness characterized by disproportionate involvement of the anterior visual pathway, although mitochondrial genes do not contribute generally to susceptibility in multiple sclerosis. Conditioning the United Kingdom genome screens for DR15 shows clustering of regions of interest within subsets of families. A major part of future studies in the genetics of multiple sclerosis will be to resolve the question of disease heterogeneity.

The distribution of multiple sclerosis cannot be explained only on the basis of population genetics. In white South African people and in Australia, prevalence rates are half those documented for many parts of northern Europe. There is a gradient in frequency, both in Australia and in New Zealand, which does not follow genetic clines. The risk is higher for English-speaking white people migrating into South Africa as adults than in childhood. Multiple sclerosis occurs at a low frequency in the Caribbean poulation, but the risk increases substantially in their first-generation descendants raised in the United Kingdom. Over and above the effect of racial predisposition, migration influences distribution of the disease. Surveys of multiple sclerosis have prompted speculation on the occurrence of post-Second World War epidemics in Iceland, the Orkney and Shetland Islands, and the Faroes, but others prefer the interpretation that these merely reflect improved case recognition.

The risk of developing multiple sclerosis is increased for individuals exposed to measles, mumps, rubella, and Epstein–Barr virus infection relatively late in childhood or adolescence. These studies suggest that an age-linked period of susceptibility to viral exposure exists in those who are constitutionally at risk of developing the disease. Attempts to implicate specific environmental agents are frustrating. Putative candidates of current interest are human herpes virus 6 and *Chlamydia pneumoniae.*

Clinical symptomatology

Special senses

Visual involvement is almost invariable and most commonly affects the optic nerve (see above). The post-chiasmal visual pathway is occasionally involved resulting in hemianopic field defects. Deafness occurs in multiple sclerosis, sometimes at presentation. Feelings of unsteadiness are common. Acute brainstem demyelination causes severe positional vertigo, vomiting, ataxia, and headache. Taste may be subjectively abnormal but ageusia is rarely described. Anosmia is reported in a high proportion of asymptomatic patients examined with more than usual thoroughness.

Motor symptoms and signs

Impaired mobility affects the majority of patients with multiple sclerosis usually as a result of spinal disease. Movements are slow, weakness differentially affecting extensors in the arms and flexors in the legs, and there are the expected signs of upper motor neurone lesions. Spasticity may be more problematic than weakness and all aspects of immobility are frequently complicated by fatigue. Cerebellar involvement causes incoordination of speech, bulbar control, eye movements, the individual limbs, or balance, usually in combination with corticospinal damage. Damage to the superior cerebellar peduncle or red nucleus produces a disabling proximal wild flinging tremor, and many other movement disorders have been described. Lower motor neurone signs occur when there is extensive demyelination adjacent to the dorsal root entry zone.

Sensory symptoms and signs

Altered sensation occurs at some stage in nearly every patient with multiple sclerosis. Damage to the posterior columns in the cervical cord produces tight, burning, twisting, tearing, or pulling sensations, which are usually unpleasant. Associated loss of proprioception severely compromises function. Spinothalamic tract involvement leads to loss of thermal and pain sensation. Non-specific tingling without accompanying signs is often described and the commonest physical sign found in the absence of symptoms is impaired vibration sense in the legs.

Demyelination of the dorsal or lumbar segments of the spinal cord produces paraesthesias and numbness in the legs, ascending to the trunk, and sometimes associated with sacral sparing, although a characteristic sensory syndrome seen in patients with multiple sclerosis is numbness of the perineum and genitalia with disturbed sphincter function.

Autonomic involvement

Autonomic symptoms occur in most patients with multiple sclerosis. Bladder symptoms are most common in women, whereas impotence occurs frequently in males. Loss of inhibition of reflex bladder emptying, normally mediated by cholinergic neurones that contract the detrusor and relax the internal sphincter, results in urgency and frequency with incontinence when combined with immobility. With conus lesions, the problem is impaired bladder emptying. Failure to fill and empty may coexist, resulting in detrusor contractions against a closed sphincter.

Impaired control of the rectal sphincter is much less of a problem than failure of emptying. Some impotent males with multiple sclerosis retain reflex erections, in which case psychogenic factors are often invoked; others have erectile failure due to spinal cord disease. Mechanical difficulties, spasticity, altered sensation, skin excoriation, and in-dwelling catheters affect sexual performance in both sexes. Other autonomic features in multiple sclerosis include: loss of thermoregulation leading to inappropriate sweating, fever, and hypothermia; Horner's syndrome; abnormalities of cardiac rhythm and vascular responses with acute pulmonary oedema; weight loss; and inappropriate secretion of vasopressin.

Eye movements

Abnormalities of eye movement are routine in multiple sclerosis. They are often asymptomatic but may manifest as double vision and oscillopsia. The commonest sign is first-degree symmetrical horizontal jerking nystagmus. Weakness of the lateral rectus is more common than isolated third and fourth nerve palsy. Internuclear ophthalmoplegia is often bilateral and may coexist with gaze paresis to produce the 'one and one half' syndrome.

Vertical up-beating nystagmus is always associated with bilateral internuclear ophthalmoplegia. Down-beating nystagmus has other important causes which can be confused with multiple sclerosis. Ocular flutter consists of horizontal saccadic oscillations without an intersaccadic interval. Opsoclonus, in which the movements occur in all directions, is equally disabling. Ocular bobbing describes an initial rapid downward eye movement followed by slow return to the neutral position and denotes cerebellar involvement. Abrupt displacement from the primary position during central fixation (square wave jerks) occurs with severe cerebellar deficits.

Other brainstem manifestations

Facial weakness, indistinguishable from Bell's palsy, occurs in patients with multiple sclerosis, alone or in association with other signs of brainstem disease including hemifacial spasm and diffuse rippling of muscle fibres (myokymia). Exceptionally, there may be unilateral involvement of the hypoglossal and recurrent laryngeal nerves. Extensive brainstem demyelination may produce disturbances of consciousness and respiratory failure distinct from the narcolepsy syndrome which is seen more frequently in patients with multiple sclerosis than expected by chance—an observation of immunogenetic interest in view of their shared HLA DR2 association. Occasional manifestations include the locked-in state, persistent hiccup, and the lateral medullary syndrome.

Paroxysmal symptoms are invariably brief but repetitive and last a few months before remitting. Symptomatic trigeminal neuralgia may begin in the first division or bilaterally, at a younger age than the idiopathic condition, and with associated signs of trigeminal involvement including motor weakness and sensory loss. It is usually associated with demyelinating lesions of the dorsal root entry zone, but may coexist with compression of the fifth cranial nerve by ectatic vessels. Other than trigeminal neuralgia, isolated involvement of the fifth nerve is rare. Paroxysmal dysarthria and ataxia with a clumsy arm, complex disturbances of sensation, and painful tetanic posturing of the limbs lasting 1 or 2 min are often triggered by movement and preceded by positive sensory symptoms on the side opposite to the muscular spasm. These are easily recognized and treated. Bursts of pain and paraesthesias, sensory distortion, itching, cough and hiccup, painful extensor spasm, akinesia, kinesogenic choreoathetosis, and complex gaze palsies—any of which may respond to anticonvulsants, especially carbamazepine—also appear to be paroxysmal manifestations of multiple sclerosis.

Cognitive and affective symptoms

Defects of visual and auditory attention occur in multiple sclerosis, sometimes at an early stage, and these are also detectable in patients with isolated demyelinating lesions. An overall impairment in intelligence quotient relates more to duration of disease, and onset of the progressive phase, affecting memory rather than language skills. Specific cognitive deficits due to hypothalamic involvement including the Korsakoff state and the syndrome of bulimia, lack of social restraint, mental interia, and mutism are sometimes seen. Psychotic behaviour is rare, but depression occurs more frequently than in patients with comparable neurological disability; hypomania is occasionally seen but should not be confused with pathological laughter and crying, arising from loss of central inhibition of facial and bulbar reflexes in association with extensive brainstem disease.

Rare manifestations of multiple sclerosis

The list of rare clinical manifestations (some already described) includes massive cerebral lesions, aphasia, headache, fever, movement disorders, epilepsy, hypothalamic and pituitary symptoms, respiratory failure, and peripheral neuropathy. Narcolepsy, Sjögren's syndrome, ankylosing spondylitis, type I neurofibromatosis, and autoimmune thyroid disease have periodically been associated with multiple sclerosis.

Childhood multiple sclerosis

In retrospect, symptoms attributable to recurrent demyelination often affect individuals with multiple sclerosis as teenagers, but onset in the first decade also occurs; 2 per cent of patients with multiple sclerosis present before the age of 10, and 5 per cent before 16 years. Children with multiple sclerosis are usually girls. The individual episodes are often severe but the long-term prognosis surprisingly good. Fever and meningism, impaired conscious level due to cerebral oedema with swollen optic discs, and seizures are regular features and the distinction from acute disseminated encephalomyelitis can often only be made by the later occurrence of remission and relapse.

Clinical course and prognosis

The majority (80 per cent) of patients present with relapsing–remitting disease. Typically, the illness passes through the three phases of relapse with full recovery, relapse with persistent deficits, and secondary progression. One patient may spend several years or even a few decades in each, whereas another moves rapidly to a condition of fixed progressive disability. About 25 per cent of patients have multiple sclerosis in a form which is not disabling. In 5 per cent, relapses occur frequently and do not recover, leading rapidly to disability and early death from respiratory failure when the medulla is affected and from massive cerebral or spinal demyelination. Up to 15 per cent become severely disabled within a short time.

Episodes occur at random frequency but initially average about 1.5 per year and decrease steadily thereafter. Recovery from each attack is invariably slower than onset and may be incomplete. Self-evidently, secondary progressive multiple sclerosis tends to affect whichever system has previously been involved. Progression may follow directly upon a severe relapse and be interrupted by further episodes. In 20 per cent, multiple sclerosis is progressive from onset. The spinal cord bears the brunt of progressive multiple sclerosis, but optic nerve, cerebral, and brainstem disease may also advance slowly. Primary progressive spinal disease is the usual mode of presentation when multiple sclerosis develops beyond the fifth decade. Life expectancy is at least 25 years, and a high proportion of patients die from unrelated causes.

The prognosis is relatively good when sensory or visual symptoms dominate the illness and there is complete recovery from individual episodes; this pattern in most common in young females. Conversely, motor involvement, especially when co-ordination or balance are disturbed, has a less good prognosis. The outlook is also poor in later-onset patients and these are often males. Frequent, prolonged relapses with incomplete recovery and a short interval between the initial episode and first relapse carry a worse prognosis, but the main determinant of disability is onset of the progressive phase.

Prospective studies show that 9 per cent of upper respiratory (adenovirus) and gastrointestinal infections occurring in patients with multiple sclerosis are followed by relapse and 27 per cent of new episodes are related to infection. The emerging evidence suggests that disease activity is not increased by vaccination. Relapse rate is affected by pregnancy. There is a reduction in the prepregnancy relapse rate for each trimester with approximately a threefold higher risk in the puerperium, and the attacks may be more severe. The clinical course is uninfluenced by breast feeding or epidural anaesthesia. There is no evidence that trauma ever triggers the first or recurrent clinical manifestations of multiple sclerosis in someone who has the underlying disease process, or alters the course in individuals who have already experienced symptoms. A study of 170 patients studied prospectively for 8 years showed that (with the possible exception of electric shock) all forms of trauma are negatively correlated both with clinical exacerbations and disease progression.

Laboratory investigations

Investigations are used for four purposes in patients with multiple sclerosis: to demonstrate the anatomical dissemination of lesions; to provide evidence for intrathecal inflammation; to demonstrate that conduction is altered in a form consistent with demyelination; and to exclude conditions that mimic demyelinating disease. That said, the diagnosis can often reliably be made using clinical criteria and without laboratory support.

Electrophysiology

Demyelination can be detected in clinically unaffected pathways using visual, auditory, somatosensory, central motor, and event-related potentials; their latencies are characteristically delayed whereas, except in acute lesions, the amplitude is unaffected. Evoked potentials add little in situations where the pathway under investigation is clinically affected. Since they provide qualitatively different information, evoked potentials remain useful as an adjunct to diagnosis despite the advent of imaging techniques.

Magnetic resonance imaging

Low-density lesions, corresponding to areas of demyelination, may be seen using contrast-enhanced computed tomography and these occasionally have the appearances of cerebral tumour or abscess, but this technique is insensitive compared with MRI. More than 95 per cent of patients with clinically definite multiple sclerosis have periventricular lesions and more than 90 per cent also show discrete white matter abnormalities. Focal demyelination can be imaged in the optic nerve, brainstem, and spinal cord.

Variations in the imaging protocol are beginning to distinguish separate components of the underlying pathological process. Imaging can distinguish inflammation (gadolinium–DTPA enhancement of T_1-weighted lesions, indicating that the lesion is of recent origin), demyelination (magnetization transfer ratio), astrocytosis (T_2-weighted lesions, the signal arising from increased water content), and axonal damage (reduction in diffusion tensor imaging anisotrophy and *N*-acetyl-aspartate spectra with chemical shift imaging, or the presence of focal atrophy and T_1-weighted black holes). The evolving lesion starts with increased blood–brain barrier permeability which lasts for up to 4 weeks and precedes the onset of T_2-weighted magnetic resonance changes. These lesions may disappear but reactivation is sometimes seen, the cycles lasting about 8 weeks. The periventricular lesions, which best characterize multiple sclerosis, correlate with areas of persistent demyelination and astrocytosis. A mixture of new, evolving, and recovering lesions may be seen in an individual patient at any one time. Magnetic resonance lesions occur about 15 times more frequently than new clinical events. Eventually, there is a reduction in the frequency of new lesions as patients switch from the relapsing to progressive phases of the disease and evidence for atrophy is then more apparent. The number or volume of lesions correlates poorly—if at all—with disease severity or course, but there is less cerebral involvement in patients who present with primary progressive disease compared with those having similar disability from secondary progression. The imaging abnormalities of multiple sclerosis are not specific and similar changes occur with inflammatory or vascular lesions and with advancing age (Fig. 3).

Imaging is not always necessary for diagnostic purposes in patients with a history of relapsing disease affecting multiple sites within the central nervous system. The major practical use is in the investigation of individuals with isolated demyelinating lesions, recurrent episodes at a single site, or progressive disease affecting the spinal cord. In all these situations the first requirement is to exclude a structural lesion, especially since these can present with relapsing symptoms. Imaging any region of the nervous system, clinically affected in isolation, will reliably exclude a structural lesion that might mimic multiple sclerosis and may show changes consistent with focal demyelination, but will not distinguish the syndromes of isolated demyelination from multiple sclerosis. Once the clinically affected part has proved negative for a structural lesion, the diagnosis of multiple sclerosis also requires the demonstration of anatomically separate lesions, ideally with enhancement to identify recent lesions, or the accumulation of new imaging abnormalities over time even if these are not expressed clinically.

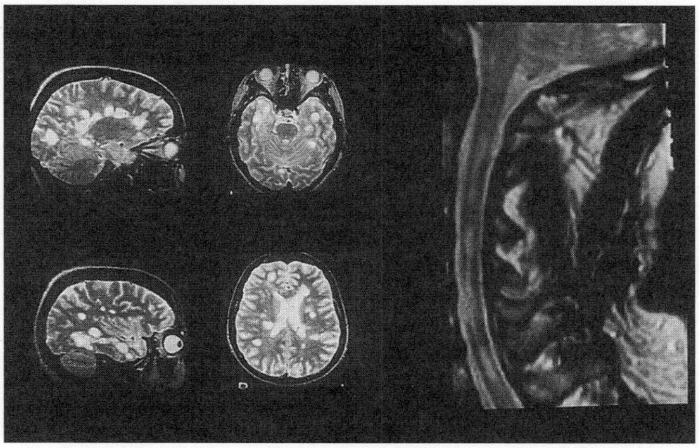

Fig. 3 T_2-weighted MRI abnormalities diffusely affecting the cerebrum and spinal cord in multiple sclerosis.

Cerebrospinal fluid

Cerebrospinal fluid analysis provides information which is complementary to imaging abnormalities and specifically useful in elderly patients suspected of having multiple sclerosis. The cell count rarely exceeds 50 lymphocytes/ml, even during periods of clinical activity, and is normal in more than 50 per cent of patients. There is a rise in total protein with a specific increase in the immunoglobulin concentration and the presence of oligoclonal bands on protein electrophoresis in more than 90 per cent of cases, after correction for leakage of serum proteins through the blood–brain barrier, providing evidence for synthesis of immunoglobulin within the central nervous system. As with the imaging abnormalities, these are sensitive but not specific. Although some antibodies are directed against components of the oligodendrocyte or its myelin membranes, and others recognize extrinsic antigens including viruses, collectively these specificities only account for a minority of the bands. In each clinical situation a number of additional investigations will be required to exclude conditions which mimic multiple sclerosis.

Differential diagnosis

The commonest error in clinical practice is to make the diagnosis of multiple sclerosis in patients with progressive spinal disease in whom a structural lesion has not been adequately excluded. Rarely, spinal tumours present with intermittent symptoms creating difficulties for the unwary; it is just not safe to assume the diagnosis of multiple sclerosis in patients with symptoms and signs restricted to a single site whatever the clinical course. Lesions at the foramen magnum are particularly well placed to cause confusion through appearing to produce evidence for independent spinal and brainstem lesions. Errors also arise with progressive and relapsing manifestations of brainstem or spinal arteriovenous malformations.

Care must be taken in the diagnosis of multiple sclerosis when several members are affected within one family. Hereditary spastic paraplegia mimics familial multiple sclerosis and this should also be considered in isolated cases of progressive spastic paraplegia when pyramidal manifestations occur in isolation and with disproportionate spasticity. Other familial disorders confused with multiple sclerosis include the hereditary ataxias, adult-onset leucodystrophies, and vasculopathies (CADASIL). Pedigrees with affected males and maternal inheritance may be examples of X-linked adrenoleucodystrophy and individuals with the phenotype of multiple sclerosis occur in families with the clinical and genetic features of Leber's hereditary optic atrophy (Harding's disease).

Clinical, immunological, and imaging abnormalities indistinguishable from multiple sclerosis occur with granulomatous and vasculitic diseases of the brain, especially the cerebral variant of systemic lupus erythematosus which often occurs in the absence of systemic manifestations or informative serology. Sarcoidosis may present with clinical involvement of the central nervous system, typical magnetic resonance and cerebrospinal fluid abnormalities, and without pulmonary or cutaneous manifestations; uveitis also occurs in multiple sclerosis and so is not necessarily a useful discriminator. Orogenital ulceration in a patient with the clinical manifestations of multiple sclerosis suggests the diagnosis of Behçet's disease.

Alternative diagnoses need to be considered when multiple sclerosis is diagnosed in African or Asian people in whom progressive spinal disease, sometimes with visual involvement, is more probably due to HTLV1-associated tropical spastic paraplegia or neuromyelitis optica (see above). Infections of the nervous system can mimic the isolated demyelinating syndromes and multiple sclerosis. These include tuberculous and other chronic meningitides, and the neurological manifestations of acquired immunodeficiency syndrome and Lyme disease; borreliosis can also cause a chronic or relapsing disorder of the central nervous system, but this is usually preceded by the characteristic painful polyradiculitis and facial palsy that epitomizes Lyme disease. Similarities between multiple sclerosis and neurosyphilis should not be forgotten in the context of opportunistic infection complicating HIV infection. The age distribution and clinical manifestations usually make it easy to distinguish subacute combined degeneration of the spinal cord from multiple sclerosis, but focal spinal lesions, accompanied by Lhermitte's sign, occur in vitamin B_{12} deficiency.

The high public profile which multiple sclerosis currently enjoys leads many individuals with vague sensory symptoms or dizziness to consider the diagnosis for themselves. Many are easily reassured when these transient symptoms are unaccompanied by physical signs; these understandable anxieties differ from the syndromes fabricated by individuals seeking the dignity of a neurological diagnosis in the setting of psychiatric disease, which are much more difficult to manage.

Treatment of demyelinating disease

Management of the acute episode

Corticosteroids are effective in abbreviating acute episodes in multiple sclerosis. There is no difference in early or eventual response to treatment using high-dose oral or intravenous regimens. Most neurologists prefer the intravenous route despite the practical advantage of oral therapy. There may be a role for intravenous immunoglobulin in patients with severe acute deficits which do not respond to corticosteroids, although this strategy has not been assessed in clinical trials. Plasma exchange given up to 1 month after onset in the context of failed response to intravenous corticosteroids may reduce persistent deficits, although this does not prevent subsequent disease activity.

The treatment of symptoms

Several manifestations of multiple sclerosis can be improved symptomatically. Urgency or frequency of micturition respond to drugs with anticholinergic activity (oxybutinin or propantheline). A simple means for intermittently reducing urine volume, and hence the desire to micturate, is to use intranasal desmopressin spray. When detrusor and sphincter function become uncoupled, causing impaired bladder emptying with failure to fill, the preferred treatment is self-intermittent catheterization, which is easily adopted by motivated patients with adequate vision and arm function and ensures complete bladder emptying often with unimagined advantages to social activities and sleep. Other options include subtrigonal injections to reduce bladder sensation, a suprapubic catheter with closure of the lower urinary tract, urinary diversion through an ileal conduit, insertion of an artificial mechanical sphincter, or electrical stimulation of the spinal nerve roots in an attempt to synchronize sphincter contraction and relaxation. These may be preferable to an indwelling urethral catheter or, worse still, constant dribbling incontinence, which usually leads to skin excoriation.

Constipation in multiple sclerosis is managed by dietary alteration and the use of bulk laxatives, avoiding agents that act directly on the bowel wall. Loperamide may be useful where the predominant complaint is rectal urge incontinence. Psychological factors contribute to impotence in males with multiple sclerosis, but in most cases the complaint is a direct consequence of spinal demyelination. Trends in management have shifted from the use of semirigid prostheses and vacuum pump-induced tumescence, and self-administered cavernous injection of papaverine or prostaglandin E_1 applied through the urethra, to oral treatment with sildenafil (Viagra)—a phosphodiesterase inhibitor which acts by increasing local production of nitric oxide in response to sexual stimulation.

The mainstay of pharmacological treatment for tremor is β-blockers; alternatives include anticonvulsants, isoniazid, ondansetron, and hyoscine. Physical restraint is rarely successful. Stereotactic procedures involving stimulation of the ventrolateral nucleus produce results comparable to destructive procedures, but the dividend is small. Unsteadiness arising from altered vestibular input may improve with the use of a vestibular sedative.

Fatigue may improve with amantadine or modetanil. Use of the aminopyridines in this and other contexts is limited by adverse effects including the risk of convulsions, although they can improve vision and muscle strength. Baclofen is still the most widely used effective antispastic agent. Benzodiazepines also reduce spasticity by increasing presynaptic spinal inhibition. Dantrolene sodium acts by uncoupling excitation–contraction mechanisms in individual muscle fibres. It is claimed that Tizanidine reduces spasticity without increasing weakness. Patients report that spasticity and pain improve with the use of cannabis and this is now formally being evaluated. Intrathecal baclofen carries the potential advantage of selectively reducing muscle tone in affected muscles whilst leaving others intact. It is mainly appropriate for patients with advanced disease and does not seem to have any additional adverse effects compared with systemic administration. Another approach is to use local injection of botulinum toxin. There may be a role for surgical interruption of the reflex pathways or tenotomy and peripheral nerve block with phenol or alcohol.

The paroxysmal manifestations of multiple sclerosis usually stop abruptly with the use of carbamazepine; this and other anticonvulsants, especially gabapentin, may also relieve trigeminal neuralgia or the more refractory forms of pain arising from spinal demyelination. Nerve block and chemical or surgical destruction of nerve fibres are sometimes an acceptable method for reducing pain in multiple sclerosis. All these sensations are coped with less well in the context of impaired mood and can respond usefully to antidepressants.

For those who develop significant disabilities and impairments, comprehensive care includes access to physical and occupational therapists, social workers, and other health-care staff with expertise in the management of chronic neurological illness. Complications are best prevented by awareness and anticipation since they usually develop quickly yet take months to resolve. Minimizing handicap by attention to social, vocational, marital, sexual, and psychological aspects of the illness remains more important to most patients than drug treatment. In situations where the natural history has already led to loss of mobility, the early use of mechanical aids and home adaptations should be encouraged despite the associated stigma.

Immunological treatment in multiple sclerosis

The use of non-specific agents in multiple sclerosis proved the concept that immunosuppression is a valid approach to treatment even if the magnitude of the effect often failed to establish a role for any one drug. The modern era began with meta-analysis of trials evaluating azathioprine showing a reduction in relapse rate but with a more modest effect on disability. The conclusion that the effect was of doubtful value to the individual patient and potentially posed serious long-term risks, meant that azathioprine was never routinely used to treat patients with multiple sclerosis. More recently introduced drugs appear to offer better adverse effects profiles but only achieve comparable efficacy. Some have already disappeared because of a poor showing in initial or confirmatory phase III trials, and due to unexpected toxicity. Casualties include linomide, cladribine, methotrexate, anti-CD4 monoclonal antibody, anti-TNFα antibody, oral myelin, altered myelin basic protein peptide, T cell vaccination, sulfasalazine, and intravenous imunoglobulin. For example, despite the apparent therapeutic rationale, a fusion protein linked to the soluble TNFα receptor produces a dose-dependent increased relapse rate, reduced time to relapse, and longer and more severe episodes—results which presumably have their explanation in the complex interacting networks of pro- and anti-inflammatory cytokines. Only a minority of patients receiving one or more well tolerated courses of a chimeric anti-CD4 antibody, sufficient partially to suppress the CD4 count, demonstrated clinical and imaging effects. Thus, the available anti-CD4 monoclonals used in isolation appear not to have a therapeutic future in multiple sclerosis. The two trials of altered myelin basic protein peptide ligand therapy in multiple sclerosis, designed to tolerize against auto-aggressive myelin basic protein-reactive T cells, either promoted relapses of multiple sclerosis or caused intolerable allergic adverse effects.

Several drugs, however, are now licensed in Europe and the United States for use in defined groups of patients with multiple sclerosis. Mitoxantrone achieves a higher conversion to disease inactivity (clinical and enhanced magnetic resonance imaging) in patients with active disease receiving monthly injections of methyl prednisolone—at least in the short term—but treatment is limited by the cumulative potential for cardiotoxicity. Glatiramer acetate (Copaxone) has been used in multiple sclerosis on the basis that disease activity can be suppressed by mimicking the antigenic challenge initiating brain inflammation. There is a reduction in relapse rate, more relapse free patients, and a delay in time to relapse but a less clear-cut effect on disability. Copaxone is associated with a change in cytokine production from a pro-inflammatory Th-1 to an anti-inflammatory Th-2/3 profile.

The therapeutic rationale for use of the β-interferons rests on the argument that IFN-β may limit inflammation by inhibiting antigen presentation, promoting a Th-2 immune phenotype, restricting migration of cells across the blood-brain barrier, reducing parenchymal cytokine production, and enhancing growth factor protection of axons; but it seems intrinsically unlikely that so many desirable properties, many characterized *in vitro* using experimental systems, are all relevant *in vivo*. BetaferonTM (IFN-β1b) is given by alternate day subcutaneous injection (8 million international units [miu]); AvonexTM (IFN-β1a) by weekly intramuscular injection (30 μg); and RebifTM (IFN-β1a) by alternate day subcutaneous injection (12 or 30 miu). IFN-β1a and IFN-β1b both reduce relapse rate by about one third and significantly reduce the accumulation of lesion load on magnetic resonance imaging in relapsing-remitting multiple sclerosis. The main adverse effects of IFN-β1b and IFN-β1a are local injection site reactions, flu-like symptoms and hyperthermia; contraindications include the use of IFN-β in pregnancy, and in patients with epilepsy or depression. Complications are not necessarily immediate and may occur 2 to 3 years after starting treatment. Between 15 and 40 per cent of patients receiving IFN-β develop neutralizing activity. Antibodies to IFN-β1a and IFN-β1b are immunologically and biologically cross-reactive. Subsequent attention has turned to whether there are dose response effects, a role for patients already in the progressive phase, and clinically useful delays in conversion to multiple sclerosis when IFN-β is given after a first episode of demyelination.

Comparisons of the licensed regimens do not show obvious dose effects or superiorities but some would rank high-dose Rebif above Betaseron and then Avonex for efficacy; whereas Avonex may have the edge over the other products for convenience and adverse effects. Although IFN-β1b was shown to delay progression in patients with secondary progressive multiple sclerosis, it seems likely that this mainly reflects suppression of superimposed new inflammatory lesions rather than an effect on other components of the pathogenesis contributing to secondary progression – and trials of the other products have shown no benefit; at best, IFN-β is only indicated in patients with secondary progressive multiple sclerosis also having frequent and clinically significant relapses. As predicted from the initial demonstrations of reduced relapse rate, IFN-β increases the time to a second and hence defining episode for multiple sclerosis in patients with isolated episodes of demyelination but this does not mean that these drugs have been shown to prevent multiple sclerosis.

Much effort has gone into the design of humanized monoclonal antibody and small molecule treatments for multiple sclerosis which either remove lymphocytes from the systemic circulation or prevent their migration into the central nervous system. Pulsed anti-α4 integrin antibody treatment in relapsing-remitting or progressive disease reduces active magnetic resonance lesions in the short term and is being studied in phase III trials. The humanized anti-CDw52 (CAMPATH-1H) antibody was originally shown to suppress radiological markers of cerebral inflammation by more than 90 per cent after a 1-week course and for at least 18 months during which relapses also stopped. However, 50 per cent of patients became progressively disabled from deficits acquired prior to treatment; these showed brain atrophy with evidence for axon degeneration on magnetic resonance spectroscopy. Clinical progression and atrophy correlated with the amount of brain inflammation in the pretreatment phase but occur in the absence of ongoing disease activity. The reduction in brain inflammation was associated with alteration in the immune response from a Th-1 pattern of cytokine release but, unexpectedly, this exposed autoimmune thyroid disease in one-third of patients. This drug is in phase II trials.

These observations support the hypothesis that inflammation is necessary for new lesion formation and conditions axon degeneration. The implication is that immunological therapies will best prevent progression of disability if given early in the course and before the cascade of events leading to axon degeneration is irretrievably established. This may explain the present limitations of immunotherapy in patients with secondary progressive multiple sclerosis but raises the dilemma of exposing individuals who may never develop disabilities from multiple sclerosis to the unpredictable hazards of prolonged immunosuppression.

Central pontine myelinolysis

Central pontine myelinolysis is associated with metabolic disturbances induced by alcohol with and without Wernicke's encephalopathy, non-alcoholic cirrhosis, Wilson's disease, following hepatic transplantation, as a complication of uraemia and haemodialysis, after prolonged vomiting, and in the context of diuretic therapy. In each of these situations, affected individuals have usually been hyponatraemic before the onset of neurological symptoms. Central pontine myelinolysis seems to result from overzealous correction of a low (and occasionally also a high) serum sodium. Demyelination correlates both with the degree of hyponatraemia and rate at which this is corrected; starting levels of less than 110 mmol/l or rates of correction of more than 2 mmol/l per hour substantially increase the risk of central pontine myelinolysis. Rapid changes in sodium are better tolerated in acute than chronic hyponatraemia.

The illness affects central pontine pathways and spreads centrifugally. The fully evolved clinical picture is of flaccid paralysis with facial and bulbar weakness, disordered eye movements, loss of balance, and altered consciousness. Features of hyponatraemia, such as epilepsy, are not usually present since pontine demyelination follows correction of the serum sodium. The recent literature emphasizes the extrapontine manifestations including movement disorders and other features of extrapyramidal disease. The clinical features are distinctive and present no diagnostic difficulties unless the reduction in serum sodium has been overlooked; the acute changes of central pontine myelinolysis can be imaged and abnormalities persist after clinical recovery. Prognosis depends on the underlying metabolic disorder. With stabilization of the serum sodium and management of bulbar failure, neurological recovery is often complete and the condition does not recur spontaneously.

Childhood and adult-onset leucodystrophies

The leucodystrophies are characterized by non-inflammatory demyelination. They include a heterogeneous group of conditions. Increasingly, these are being shown to result from mutations affecting genes which determine the synthesis, maintenance, and structure of myelin. Although rare even in paediatric practice, these need to be considered in young adults with atypical syndromes combining physical and intellectual deficits, sometimes with peripheral nerve involvement, in whom imaging shows confluent lesions confined to white matter.

Diffuse sclerosis (Schilder's disease)

The term diffuse cerebral sclerosis was originally used to identify a heterogeneous group of diseases affecting cerebral white matter. Of the diseases previously classified under this heading, familial sudanophilic diffuse sclerosis, Pelizaeus–Merzbacher disease, Krabbe's diffuse sclerosis (globoid cell leucodystrophy), Canavan's diffuse sclerosis (spongy degeneration of the white matter), Alexander's disease, and metachromatic leucodystrophy are dysmyelinating leucodystrophies. Conversely, Binswager's subcortical encephalopathy is now considered a consequence of diffuse cerebral arteriosclerosis—although some cases may have been examples of CADASIL; and Balo's concentric sclerosis is now considered within the spectrum of multiple sclerosis. Many male patients previously classified as having diffuse sclerosis were probably suffering from adrenoleucodystrophy. Some of the relapsing disorders were probably Leigh's disease associated with mutations of mitochondrial DNA. But even after separating these newly recognized conditions, the nosological status of diffuse sclerosis remains uncertain and some consider that, between them, acute childhood multiple sclerosis and adrenoleucodystrophy account for all the cases.

Krabbe's disease

Globoid cell leucodystrophy usually presents as an early infantile disorder. Late-onset globoid cell leucodystrophy is uncommon—almost all patients becoming symptomatic before the age of 5 years and so almost never leading to confusion with childhood multiple sclerosis. The clinical picture is dominated by behavioural changes with startle, progressive intellectual and motor deterioration, epilepsy, visual failure, and peripheral neuropathy leading to severe disabilities; pyrexia and other autonomic features usher in the onset of a vegetative state. Visual evoked potentials are delayed and the spinal fluid has a raised protein level but does not contain oligoclonal bands. MRI shows periventricular lesions subsequently extending into extensive white matter changes. The deficiency of α-galactocerebrosidase, best demonstrated in peripheral blood leucocytes or skin fibroblasts, leads to the accumulation of galactocerebroside, the neurotoxic molecule psychosine, and the myelin-laden macrophages or globoid cells.

Adrenoleucodystrophy

An important group of disorders is characterized by deposition of saturated fatty acids in the brain and other lipid-containing tissues as a result of defective very-long-chain fatty acyl-CoA synthetase activity in peroxisomes. The molecular defect may result from failure of the adrenoleucodystrophy gene product to anchor very-long-chain fatty acids into the peroxisomal membrane or translocate these into peroxisomes.

Four related syndromes share this biochemical abnormality: childhood adrenoleucodystrophy and adult-onset adrenomyeloneuropathy are X linked; neonatal adrenoleucodystrophy and Zellweger's syndrome are autosomal recessive disorders.

X-linked childhood adrenoleucodystrophy presents with behavioural disturbance, dementia, and epilepsy followed by involvement of special senses and motor systems. Although a significant proportion of children later develop adrenal insufficiency, Addison's disease may precede the neurological manifestations by several years. Treatment has been proposed with a dietary supplement containing a 4:1 mixture of glyceryl trioleate and trieructate, popularly known as Lorenzo's oil. This lowers the plasma levels of very-long-chain fatty acids, but does not appear to influence the phenotype in individuals with established neurological disease, although there may be a prophylactic role. Bone marrow transplantation is successful in early symptomatic cases and, in view of the inflammatory reaction, trials of immunosuppression are in progress.

Adrenomyeloneuropathy presents in adult men with spastic paraparesis and sensory loss in the legs; attention is drawn to an unusual cause for this otherwise common neurological problem by the associated peripheral neuropathy, but the diagnosis is frequently overlooked if adrenal insufficiency is not obvious at presentation. Identification of the peroxisomal defect in easily sampled body tissues has led to the description of cases with obscure clinical manifestations; these include focal cerebral lesions, Kluver–Bucy syndrome, dementia, and spinocerebellar degeneration. Mild spastic paraparesis with sphincter involvement and peripheral neuropathy may occur in obligate heterozygote female carriers with elevated very-long-chain fatty acids. The gene has been mapped to Xq28, close to that for glucose-6-phosphate dehydrogenase deficiency and colour blindness.

Autosomal recessive adrenoleucodystrophy presents in infancy with seizures, hypotonia, retardation, retinal degeneration, and hepatic involvement; females are more commonly affected than males. Although the clinical manifestations and mode of inheritance are similar in neonatal adrenoleucodystrophy and Zellweger's syndrome, these are thought to be separate disorders.

The sensitivity and specificity of routine assays for very-long-chain fatty acids show that the level of hexasanoic acid and its ratios to tetrasanoic and docosanoic acids are fully discriminating in homozygote males, irrespective of the clinical phenotype, from the day of birth if dietary supplements have not been given, providing an opportunity for mass screening; there is a false-negative rate of 15 per cent for heterozygotes.

Metachromatic leucodystrophy

The separation of metachromatic leucodystrophy from the heterogeneous group of diffuse sclerosis occurred when metachromatic material was first detected in urinary deposits. It subsequently became clear that the diagnosis can be confirmed by demonstrating increased urinary sulphatide excretion with a deficiency of arylsulphatase A in urine, peripheral blood leucocytes, and skin fibroblasts, or showing metachromatic material in peripheral nerve biopsies having segmental demyelination and remyelination. There is diffuse white matter involvement due to non-inflammatory demyelination with loss of oligodendrocytes, axon preservation, and reactive astrocytes which, together with macrophages, contain the metachromatic material, especially in the most extensively demyelinated areas.

The clinical phenotype varies with the amount of surviving arylsulphatase A depending on heterozygosity of the mutant allele; pseudodeficiency refers to those individuals with low levels of arylsulphatase A that are sufficiently high not to display a clinical phenotype. Some affected individuals have a genetic defect of the arylsulphatase A activator and this is associated with a more complex pattern of sphingomyelin storage, biochemically and in terms of the tissue distribution.

The most common form of metachromatic leucodystrophy develops in late infancy with delayed walking due to the neuropathy, which may be painful. There are also features of brainstem involvement and the emergence of diffuse upper motor neurone signs with reduced intellectual development, optic atrophy, and death within about 5 years from presentation. In later-onset childhood cases, after several years normal development, there are behavioural changes with poor school performance, anticipating cerebellar and upper motor neurone disability which then follows much the same course as in younger patients, although with less evidence for neuropathy. The early adult form of metachromatic leucodystrophy is rare, or perhaps seldom diagnosed, and tends to present with intellectual or emotional abnormalities. Onset with dementia and behavioural disorders is usual with ataxia, paralysis, and optic atrophy only developing at late stages; the presentation is occasionally with paraparesis or cerebellar ataxia and the condition can then more easily be mistaken for multiple sclerosis. Clinical evidence for peripheral neuropathy may be revealed by slowed nerve conduction. Treatments have included dietary manipulation with reduced vitamin A and sulphur-containing substances, and bone marrow transplantation, but the successes are limited.

Multiple sulphatase deficiency combines the features of metachromatic leucodystrophy with mucopolysaccharidosis. It also has neonatal, early childhood, and juvenile forms. The pattern of combined motor and mental regression or lack of development reflecting widespread dysmyelination with peripheral neuropathy is associated with dysmorphic features and organomegaly. The more severe phenotype also reflects extensive neuronal loss due to the combination of stored sulphatide, sulphated steroids, and mucopolysaccharides. The enzyme defects are complex involving many sulphatases including arylsulphatase A.

Pelizaeus–Merzbacher disease

The three phenotypes of X-linked Pelizaeus–Merzbacher disease usually present in childhood. The clinical features which may distinguish the otherwise ubiquitous motor and developmental delay with epilepsy are abnormal eye movements, dystonia and choreoathetosis, and laryngeal paralysis. Affected individuals often stabilize with severe disabilities and live into early adult life. Some cases do not manifest until early adult life, but here the blur with specifically different disorders becomes more apparent. MRI either fails to show myelin or depicts myelin which is immature with an atrophic brain.

The molecular defect is a mutation of the gene for proteolipid protein (encoded on X-q21.2). Proteolipid protein is normally involved in stabilizing the lamellar structure of central myelin. Over 30 mutations have been described resulting in expression of truncated forms of proteolipid protein sufficient to cause extensive oligodendrocyte loss and failure of myelination. The pedigree is not always X linked in the early-onset connatal form and, in these situations, a genetic defect other than proteolipid protein mutation is presumably involved.

Adult-onset dominant leucodystrophies

Forms of dominantly inherited leucodystrophy also occur exclusively in adults and may closely resemble chronic progressive multiple sclerosis. MRI shows diffuse, non-discrete, white matter disease and there are no oligoclonal bands in the spinal fluid. It remains uncertain whether all the adult-onset dominant leucodystrophies are one and the same disorder, and many are difficult to distinguish from the heterogeneous group of hereditary spastic paraplegias. The various phenotypes are gradually being classified as their biochemical and genetic defects are characterized. A family with spastic paraparesis, ataxia, and mild dementia presenting in adulthood, but with onset in childhood, has been described; diffuse white matter abnormalities were present on cerebral magnetic resonance, whereas pathognomic features of the other leucodystrophies were absent. The most recent addition to this group involves two siblings with behavioural abnormalities progressing to dementia with extensive white matter abnormalities on MRI in whom brain biopsy showed glycolipid inclusions in macrophages unlike any other lysosomal storage disease.

Further reading

Barnes D *et al.* (1997). Randomised trial of oral and intravenous methylprednisolone in acute relapses of multiple sclerosis. *Lancet* **349**, 902–6. [No difference between these two regimens for management of acute relapse.]

Bauer HJ, Hanefeld FA (1993). *Multiple sclerosis: its impact from childhood to old age.* Saunders, London. [The definitive monograph on childhood multiple sclerosis.]

Brex PA *et al* (2002). A longitudinal study of abnormalities on MRI and disability from multiple sclerosis. *New England Journal of Medicine* **346**, 158–64. [Long term follow-up of patients with isoloated demyelinating lesions.]

Coles AJ *et al.* (1999). Monoclonal antibody treatment exposes three mechanisms underlying the clinical course in multiple sclerosis. *Annals of Neurology* **46**, 296–304. [Clinical evidence for the complex pathogenesis of multiple sclerosis.]

Comi G *et al.* (2001). Effect of early interferon treatment on conversion to definite multiple sclerosis: a randomised study. *Lancet* **357**, 1576–82. [Delay to second episode in patients with isolated demyelination treated with β-interferon.]

Compston DAS *et al.* (1998). *McAlpine's multiple sclerosis.* WB Saunders, London. [The most recent monograph on multiple sclerosis.]

Compston DAS, Coles AJ (2002). Multiple sclerosis (seminar) *Lancet* **359**, 1221–31. [A comprehensive review of the pathogenesis and treatment of multiple sclerosis.]

Confavreux C *et al.* (1998). Rate of pregnancy-related relapse in multiple sclerosis. *New England Journal of Medicine* **339**, 285–91. [A prospective study of disease activity in pregnancy.]

Confavreux C *et al* (2001). Vaccinations and the risk of relapse in multiple sclerosis. Vaccines in Multiple Sclerosis Study Group. *New England Journal of Medicine* **344**, 319–26. [Evidence that vaccinations do not increase activity in multiple sclerosis.]

Ebers GC *et al.* (2000). The natural history of multiple sclerosis: a geographically based study. 8: familial multiple sclerosis. *Brain* **123**, 641–9. [The clinical features and natural history of multiple sclerosis in a population-based cohort described (to date) in a series of eight papers.]

Edan G *et al.* (1997). Therapeutic effect of mitoxantrone combined with methylprednisolone in multiple sclerosis: a randomised multi-center study of active disease using MRI and clinical criteria. *Journal of Neurology, Neurosurgery, and Psychiatry* **62**, 112–18. [Trial defining the role of mitoxantrone in multiple sclerosis.]

European Study Group on Interferon β-1b in Secondary Progressive MS (1998). Placebo-controlled multicentre randomised trial of interferon β-1b in treatment of secondary progressive multiple sclerosis. *Lancet* **352**, 1491–7. [Suggestive evidence for the role of interferon-β in progressive multiple sclerosis.]

Genain CP *et al.* (1999). Identification of autoantibodies associated with myelin damage in multiple sclerosis. *Nature Medicine* **5**, 170–5. [The putative autoantigen in multiple sclerosis.]

Hohlfeld R (1997). Biotechnical agents for the immunotherapy of multiple sclerosis: principles, problems and perspectives (review). *Brain* **120**, 865–916. [The present and future basis for treatment in multiple sclerosis.]

Jacobs LD *et al.* (1996). Intramuscular interferon β-1a for disease progression in relapsing multiple sclerosis. *Annals of Neurology* **39**, 285–94. [The pivotal trial of interferon-β1a in multiple sclerosis.]

Jacobs LD *et al.* (2000). Intramuscular interferon β-1a therapy initiated during a first demyelinating event in multiple sclerosis. *New England Journal of*

Medicine **343**, 898–904. [Delay to second episode in patients with isolated demyelination treated with β-interferon.]

Jeffery ND, Blakemore WF (1997). Locomotor deficits induced by experimental spinal cord demyelination are abolished by spontaneous remyelination. *Brain* **120**, 27–37. [Experimental evidence that remyelination restores function.]

Johnson K *et al.* (1998). Extended use of glatiramer acetate (Copaxone) is well tolerated and maintains its clinical effect on multiple sclerosis relapse rate and degree of disability. *Neurology* **50**, 701–8. [Evidence that copolymer-1 has a clinical effect in multiple sclerosis.]

Luchinetti C *et al.* (1999). A quantitative analysis of oligodendrocytes multiple sclerosis lesions: a study of 117 cases. *Brain* **122**, 2279–95. [New ideas on the cellular pathology of multiple sclerosis.]

McDonald WI *et al* (2001). Recommended diagnostic criteria for multiple sclerosis: guidelines from the International Panel on the diagnosis of multiple sclerosis. *Annals of Neurology* **50**, 121–7. [Revised diagnostic criteria for multiple sclerosis.]

Miller DH *et al.* (1999). Effect of interferon-β1b on magnetic resonance imaging outcomes in secondary progressive multiple sclerosis: results of a European multicenter, randomised, double-blind placebo-controlled trial. *Annals of Neurology* **46**, 850–9. [Interferon-β1b may only suppress residual inflammation in secondary progressive multiple sclerosis.]

Miller HG, Stanton JB, Gibbons JL (1956). Parainfectious encephalomyelitis and related syndromes. *Quarterly Journal of Medicine* **25**, 427–505. [The classic account of acute disseminated encephalomyelitis.]

Moser HW (1997). Adrenoleukodystrophy: phenotype, genetics, pathogenesis and therapy. *Brain* **120**, 1485–508. [Review of adrenoleucodystrophy: the Gordon Holmes lecture.]

Paty DW, Li DKB, The IFNβ Multiple Sclerosis Study Group (1993). Interferon β-1b is effective in relapsing–remitting multiple sclerosis. MRI results of a multicenter, randomized, double-blind, placebo-controlled trial. *Neurology* **43**, 662–7. [The pivotal study of interferon-β1b in multiple sclerosis.]

PRISMS Study Group (1998). Randomised double-blind placebo-controlled study of interferon β-1a in relapsing/remitting multiple sclerosis. *Lancet* **352**, 1498–504. [The second pivotal study of interferon-β1a in multiple sclerosis.]

PRISMS-4 (2001). Long-term efficacy of interferon-β-1a in relapsing MS. *Neurology* **56**, 1628–36. [Late follow-up results for patients in the phase II trial of Rebif.]

Secondary Progressive Efficacy Clinical Trial of Recombinant Interferon-β-1a in MS (SPECTRIMS) Study Group (2001). Randomized controlled trial of interferon-β-1a in secondary progressive MS: MRI results. *Neurology* **56**, 1505–13. [No evidence for efficacy of β-interferon in secondary progressive multiple sclerosis.]

Sibley WA, Bamford CR, Clark K (1985). Clinical viral infections and multiple sclerosis. *Lancet* **i**, 1313–15. [Prospective study of infections and disease activity in multiple sclerosis.]

Sibley WA *et al.* (1991). A prospective study of physical trauma and multiple sclerosis. *Journal of Neurology, Neurosurgery, and Psychiatry* **54**, 584–9. [Prospective study of trauma and disease activity in multiple sclerosis.]

The IFNβ Multiple Sclerosis Study Group, the University of British Columbia MS/MRI Analysis Group (1995). Interferon β-1b in the treatment of multiple sclerosis: final outcome of the randomised controlled trial. *Neurology* **45**, 1277–85. [Final result on the pivotal study of interferon-β1b in multiple sclerosis.]

The Lenercept Multiple Sclerosis Study Group, the University of British Columbia MS/MRI Analysis Group (1999). TNF neutralisation in MS. Results of a randomised, placebo-controlled multicenter study. *Neurology* **53**, 457–65. [Suppressing tumour necrosis factor-α makes multiple sclerosis worse: surprising result.]

Trapp BD *et al.* (1998). Axonal transection in the lesions of multiple sclerosis. *New England Journal of Medicine* **338**, 278–85. [Rediscovery of the axonopathy in multiple sclerosis.]

Turbridy N *et al.* (1999). The effect of anti-α4 integrin antibody on brain lesion activity in MS. *Neurology* **53**, 466–72. [Minimal effect of anti-adhesion monoclonal antibody in active multiple sclerosis.]

van Oosten BW *et al.* (1997). Treatment of multiple sclerosis with the monoclonal anti-CD4 antibody cM-T412; results of a randomised, double-blind, placebo-controlled, MR monitored phase II trial. *Neurology* **49**, 351–7. [Trivial effect of anti-CD4 monoclonal antibody in multiple sclerosis.]

Wingerchuk DM *et al.* (1999). The clinical course of neuromyelitis optica (Devic's syndrome). *Neurology* **53**, 1107–14. [Definitive recent series of Devic's disease.]

Youl BD *et al.* (1991). The pathophysiology of acute optic neuritis: an association of gadolinium leakage with clinical and electrophysiological deficits. *Brain* **114**, 2437–50. [Classic study of the pathophysiology of inflammation in human demyelinating disease.]

24.17 Disorders of the neuromuscular junction

David Hilton-Jones and Jackie Palace

Introduction

Two fundamentally different pathological processes are associated with disease at the neuromuscular junction. First, acquired disorders in which autoantibodies are directed against nerve or muscle ion channels. Second, and much rarer, inherited conditions in which the defect may be pre- or postsynaptic. These acquired and inherited conditions share some symptomatology. The most important are the autoimmune diseases: myasthenia gravis, the Lambert–Eaton myasthenic syndrome, and acquired neuromyotonia—disorders for which therapy is available.

The pharmacological and neurophysiological complexities of the neuromuscular junction can be simplified to a level that permits ready understanding of the pathogenesis and treatment of these various conditions and will reduce the frequency of misdiagnosis and/or mismanagement.

Neuromuscular transmission

Anatomically there are three main components to the neuromuscular junction (Fig. 1). The presynaptic component is the motor nerve terminal, which contains packages (quanta) of acetylcholine, each of which contains several thousand molecules of acetylcholine. This is separated from the postsynaptic acetylcholine receptors, which sit atop the terminal expansions of the junctional folds of the muscle fibre membrane, by the synaptic space. The nerve fibre membrane contains voltage-gated sodium, potassium ,and calcium channels. Voltage-gated sodium channels are also present postsynaptically, at the base of the clefts of the junctional folds.

The nicotinic acetylcholine receptor is a pentameric structure composed of four different subunits—α, β, γ, and δ in fetal muscle, and α, β, ε, and δ in adult muscle. It is configured to produce a central ion channel. Structurally and functionally there are similarities to voltage-gated ion channels, but the acetylcholine receptor is a ligand-gated channel, the ligand being acetylcholine.

Depolarization of the motor nerve terminal is dependent upon voltage-gated sodium channels. Repolarization is the result of inactivation of these sodium channels and opening of voltage-gated potassium channels. During depolarization, voltage-gated calcium channels open—the influx of calcium ions into the nerve terminal triggers release (by exocytosis) of quanta of acetylcholine.

The acetylcholine binds to the α-subunits of the acetylcholine receptors. This alters the conformation of the channel allowing cations (mainly sodium) to enter the muscle fibre. This influx generates the end-plate potential, which in turn activates voltage-gated sodium channels. These trigger the action potential which is propagated through the muscle fibre and initiates contraction. Spontaneous release of individual quanta of acetylcholine, as opposed to mass release triggered by a nerve action potential, gives rise to miniature end-plate potentials, which can be recorded by microelectrode. These are of insufficient amplitude to trigger an action potential in the muscle fibre membrane.

The action of acetylcholine on acetylcholine receptors is terminated by the hydrolysis of acetylcholine by the enzyme acetylcholinesterase, which is anchored to the basal lamina by a collagen-like molecule, ColQ.

The acquired myasthenic disorders are associated with antibodies directed against one of the ion channels (Table 1). That there are three autoimmune disorders known to affect such a small region may be explained by the fact that the neuromuscular junction, unlike the peripheral nerves, is not contained within the blood–nerve barrier, which stops just short of the nerve terminal, and is thus potentially exposed to immune-mediated attack. The inherited disorders may affect presynaptic processes (acetylcholine resynthesis, packaging, or release), acetylcholinesterase binding, or

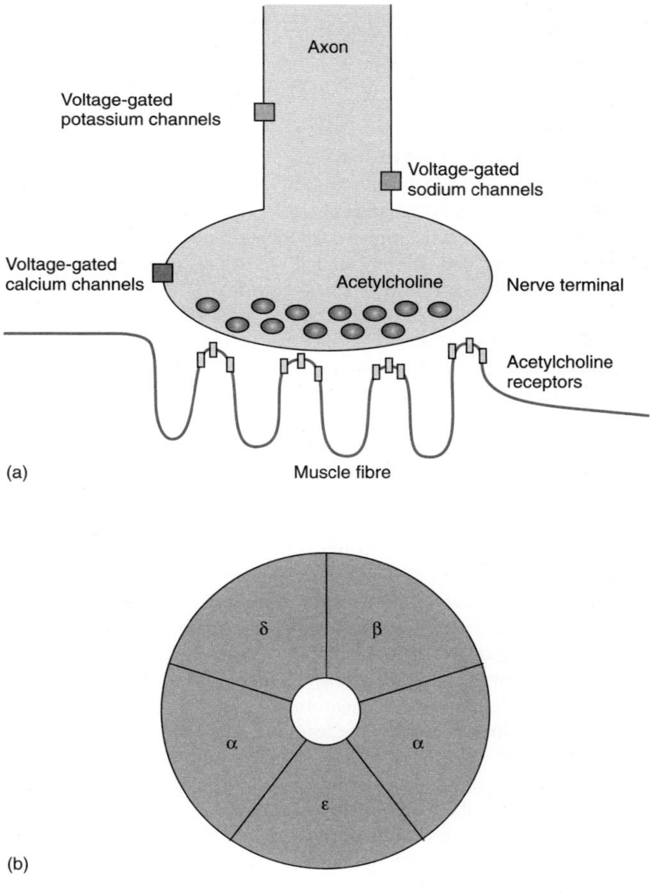

Fig. 1 (a) VGNC, voltage-gated sodium channel; VGCC, voltage-gated calcium channel; VGKC, voltage-gated potassium channel; ACh, acetylcholine. (b) Cartoon of the organization of the subunits of the nicotinic acetylcholine receptor (see text).

Table 1 Ion channels responsible for the different clinical disorders

Ion channel	Clinical disorder
Acetylcholine receptor	Myasthenia gravis
Voltage-gated calcium channel	Lambert–Eaton myasthenic syndrome
Voltage-gated potassium channel	Acquired neuromyotonia

postsynaptic function (point mutations in acetylcholine receptor subunits). Pathogenetic mechanisms are considered in more detail when discussing individual disorders.

Myasthenia gravis

This is by far the most common of the conditions to be discussed in this section and responds favourably to treatment. In general, over 90 per cent of patients can be returned to normal function, although in most this represents a pharmacological remission and the patient remains dependent on treatment.

Epidemiology

All ethnic groups are affected. The annual incidence is about 4 per million population, and the prevalence about 8 per 100 000. All ages may be affected. Overall, women are more frequently affected, in a ratio of about 3:2. The female bias is even more marked in younger-onset cases, whereas over the age of 50 years male cases predominate. A rather different pattern is seen in people of Asian origin; prepubertal onset is very common, the disease is often purely ocular, and there is a strong association with HLA DRw9.

Pathogenesis

The fundamental disorder in myasthenia gravis is loss of functional acetylcholine receptors consequent upon binding of anti-acetylcholine receptor (**anti-AChR**) antibodies. IgG class antibodies can be detected, by the standard assay used for diagnostic purposes, in 85 per cent of patients with generalized myasthenia and about one-half of those with purely ocular myasthenia (so-called seropositive cases). Antibodies mostly bind to the main immunogenic region of the α-subunits of the acetylcholine receptor. Patients who do not have antibodies detected by this assay are called seronegative. However, there is overwhelming evidence even in these patients that their disease is immune mediated, possibly by IgG antibodies that bind to other regions within the end-plate area or to other IgM class antibodies; their clinical characteristics are similar to seropositive patients, they respond to plasma exchange and immunosuppressant therapy, their plasma can induce neuromuscular transmission dysfunction when injected into animals, and the infants of such mothers may be born with neonatal myasthenia (see below) indicating transplacental transfer of a humoral component.

Loss of functional acetylcholine receptors by antibody binding is due to complement-mediated lysis, acceleration of internalization and degradation, and blocking of acetylcholine binding. Morphological consequences include widening of the synaptic cleft and a marked reduction of the postsynaptic folds of the muscle fibre membrane.

Although the efferent limb of the immune response, described above, has been reasonably well characterized, numerous questions remain to be answered about the afferent limb. Susceptibility to myasthenia gravis is associated with particular immune response genes, with correlation to different haplotypes relating to the age of onset of the disease. These observations are not of immediate relevance to routine clinical practice. In contrast, knowledge about involvement of the thymus is relevant to classification and management.

In early-onset, seropositive patients there is hyperplasia of the thymic medulla, with germinal centres surrounded by a T-cell zone. The acetylcholine receptor is expressed on thymic myoid cells and there is enrichment of acetylcholine receptor-specific T cells. In addition, the thymus has a key role in the process of inducing immune tolerance, by removal of self-antigen T-cell clones. On the basis of these observations, and the beneficial response to thymectomy, there seems little doubt that the thymus is involved in the pathogenesis of myasthenia gravis, but exactly how has yet to be elucidated. Identification of the mechanism may well be important in developing immune-specific treatment.

In late-onset cases and seronegative patients, the thymus is typically normal or atrophic, although some pathological changes have been noted.

Thymomas occur in about 10 per cent of cases. They are locally invasive (notably affecting the pleura and pericardium) and may seed within the pleural cavity. These patients are almost invariably seropositive. Surgical excision is required because of local tumour invasiveness, but in contrast to those patients with thymic hyperplasia, this does not usually ameliorate the myasthenic symptoms.

Based on the presence or absence of antibodies detected by the routine clinical assay and the state of the thymus gland, four main subgroups of patients can be identified (Table 2). Penicillamine-induced myasthenia, which generally recovers following drug withdrawal, is clinically similar to the idiopathic disease and the patients are seropositive.

Clinical features

Myasthenia gravis causes skeletal muscle weakness but the most characteristic feature is fatiguability. The term fatigue causes some confusion because it may have different meanings to a clinician, physiologist, and lay person. Thus, the fatigue of chronic fatigue syndrome is quite different from that of myasthenia. Simply, fatigue in myasthenia gravis manifests itself by increasing, demonstrable weakness precipitated by repeated or sustained muscular activity. Symptoms fluctuate from day to day and week to week, which may in part explain the common delay in diagnosis and suspicions as to its genuineness. Other factors which can exacerbate the weakness include heat, emotional factors, menstruation, intercurrent infections, and drugs that interfere with neuromuscular transmission (aminoglycoside antibiotics, quinine, quinidine, β-blockers, procainamide, and neuromuscular-blocking drugs related to anaesthesia).

In over one-half of patients the presenting symptoms relate to extraocular muscle weakness (diplopia and ptosis); these muscles will be involved in over 90 per cent of patients at some stage during the disease. The next most frequent presentation is with limb-girdle weakness. Typically, as the disease worsens, the weakness spreads from the extraocular muscles to the lower facial and bulbar muscles (causing dysarthria and dysphagia), to the neck, and then to the limbs. However, there are many variations on this theme. A relatively common presentation in older patients, typically men, is with selective weakness of neck extension—as they walk their head drops forwards and they arrive in the clinic holding up their head with a hand under the chin. Relatively selective weakness of finger extension and abduction is common.

On examination, weakness may or may not be evident—fatigue can be demonstrated in limb muscles, but is often most striking around the eyes and with respect to bulbar muscles. Fatiguable ptosis is a striking sign (Fig. 2). As the patients give their history, the fatigue of bulbar muscles may be revealed by increasing dysarthria. A potentially misleading sign is 'pseudo-internuclear ophthalmoplegia', which may be bilateral—failure of adduction due to weakness of the medial recti. Eye movements may show

Table 2 The four main subgroups of myasthenia gravis

	Age of onset (years)		Thymoma	Seronegative
	< 40	> 40		
Thymus	Hyperplasia	Atrophy	Thymoma	?Normal/atrophy
Anti-AChR antibody titre	High	Low	Intermediate	Absent

striking fatigue. With increasing severity, the weakness at rest may be so marked that it is difficult to demonstrate fatigue. Respiratory muscle weakness may be out of proportion to limb weakness—it is best assessed by measuring the vital capacity (not peak flow), and the effects of it by monitoring oxygen saturation. Muscle wasting is only seen in undertreated patients with long-established disease. The tendon reflexes are normal, and indeed often rather brisk. There are no abnormal sensory signs.

There is an increased incidence of other autoimmune diseases, particularly thyroid disease (about 3 per cent of patients) and less frequently rheumatoid arthritis, systemic lupus erythematosus, polymyositis, Lambert–Eaton myasthenic syndrome, and acquired neuromyotonia.

Natural course

This is very variable. In some patients the disorder remains confined to the extraocular muscles (ocular myasthenia gravis). If that is the case for more than 2 years, and particularly if the patient is seronegative, the development of generalized disease is unlikely. Older studies, before the introduction of immunosuppressive therapies, suggest that the disease reaches maximum severity within 7 years. In one study, the interval between onset and the first episode of maximal weakness ('myasthenic crisis') was less than 36 months in over 80 per cent of patients. Permanent, spontaneous remission occurs, but is rare—in the order of 1 per cent per annum. On the other hand, particularly early in the course of the disease, there may be protracted periods of spontaneous remission, sometimes lasting several years.

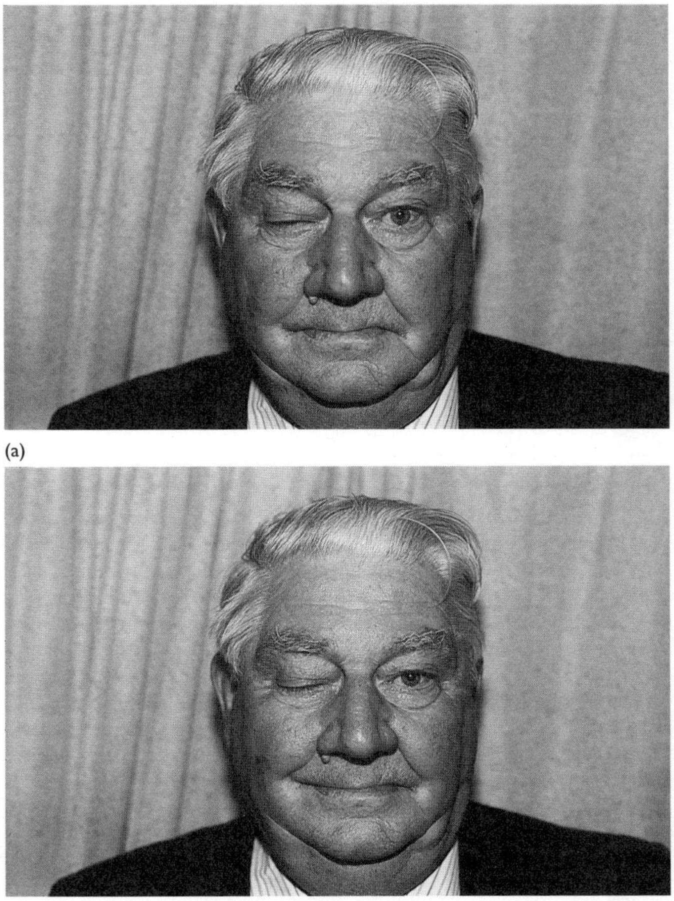

(a)

(b)

Fig. 2 Fatiguable ptosis in myasthenia gravis.

Diagnosis

This is based on the clinical picture, supported by appropriate laboratory results. For practical purposes, the presence of anti-AChR antibodies is confirmatory and no further diagnostic investigations are required. In seronegative patients, electromyography and the intravenous edrophonium (Tensilon®) test are helpful. Although the edrophonium test has a long pedigree and sound pharmacological basis (it is a short-acting cholinesterase inhibitor), there are concerns about its use, particularly by the inexperienced. The patient is given 600 µg of atropine intravenously—this blocks the potentially unpleasant muscarinic effects of the edrophonium and also acts as a single-blind placebo for the patient. The test dose of 2 mg of edrophonium follows, which in some patients is sufficient to give a diagnostic response. If not, a further 8 mg of edrophonium is given. There must be an easily assessable measure of improvement—most commonly degree of ptosis. The test is therefore likely to be of most use in patients with purely ocular symptoms and signs. Rarely, cardiorespiratory collapse may occur. False-negative and false-positive results are not uncommon.

The conventional electromyographic measure for diagnosing myasthenia gravis is the demonstration of a decremental response of the compound muscle action potential in response to repetitive nerve stimulation at 3 Hz. More sensitive, but not specific and only available in specialist centres, is the presence of increased jitter and blocking, as assessed by single-fibre electromyography.

The presence of a thymoma is best assessed by computed tomography or magnetic resonance imaging of the thorax.

Differential diagnosis

There are few difficulties in the presence of extraocular muscle involvement and readily demonstrable fatigue, although there can be confusion with the Lambert–Eaton myasthenic syndrome and the congenital myasthenic syndromes. Diagnostic difficulties can occur when, as occasionally happens, eye signs and fatigue are absent. Amyotrophic lateral sclerosis with little wasting may be suspected. Conversely, in long-established myasthenia, muscle wasting may be misleading. More difficult is seronegative, purely ocular myasthenia—the most important differential diagnosis is mitochondrial cytopathy, in which increased jitter may also occur. Other diagnoses to consider include oculopharyngeal muscular dystrophy and thyroid ophthalmopathy.

Botulism, caused by food poisoning, an infected wound, or clostridial overgrowth in the gastrointestinal tract in infants, may need to be considered. Features of autonomic malfunction are usually present.

Treatment

As noted, thymomas require excision, but this in itself will not improve the myasthenia. Management of patients with thymic tumours follows the same guidelines given below.

Anticholinesterase drugs, by reducing acetylcholine breakdown, give symptomatic improvement in most patients, and may be sufficient in those with very mild disease. Pyridostigmine is the drug of choice, given orally four or five times daily, starting at 30 mg per dose and increasing if required to 60 mg. Abdominal cramping is a common side-effect, relating to muscarinic overstimulation, and responds to propantheline, ideally taken 30 min before each dose of pyridostigmine. If an adequate response is not obtained at this dose, then further increases should not be made and other forms of therapy should be considered. The management of ocular myasthenia differs somewhat from the generalized form of the disease, the latter also depending upon age of onset and antibody status.

Ocular myasthenia

If anticholinesterase drugs have given an inadequate response, alternate-day prednisolone therapy should be introduced. A suitable starting daily dose is 5 mg, increasing by 5 mg every fourth dose (or weekly) until an adequate response has been obtained (often, for an adult, a dose of around

30 mg) or a maximum acceptable dose (around 0.75 mg/kg body weight) has been reached. Once remission has been achieved, the pyridostigmine can be withdrawn, and then the prednisolone reduced slowly— initially by 5 mg per month, but when down to 20 mg by as little as 1 mg, each month). Azathioprine may be added if there is an inadequate response or the minimal effective dose of prednisolone is deemed to be unacceptably high. Ocular muscle surgery can be beneficial if there is a poor or incomplete response to treatment and if the defect appears to be fixed.

Early-onset, seropositive myasthenia

Many, but not all, of these patients benefit from thymectomy. Up to one-third enter remission, and a further one-half improve. These benefits are occasionally rapid, but more typically develop over the following 1 to 2 years, possibly longer. The conventional approach is through a sternal split. There is concern that less invasive surgical procedures risk leaving behind thymic remnants which will negate the benefits of the operation. Thymectomy should be performed in centres experienced in such surgery and with the support of appropriately trained anaesthetists and neurologists.

For those patients who do not respond adequately to anticholinesterase drugs and thymectomy, immunosuppression with prednisolone and azathioprine is indicated. A controlled trial has shown the benefits of the addition of azathioprine (2.5 mg/kg body weight per day)—the starting dose is 25 or 50 mg daily, increased by 25 or 50 mg daily, each week (or more rapidly as an in-patient) until the target dose is reached. During introduction, weekly tests of full blood count and liver function are required. When established, testing can be reduced gradually to 3-monthly. Introduction of prednisolone may exacerbate myasthenic weakness and should generally be done in hospital. The starting dose is 10 mg on alternate days, increasing by 10 mg per dose until the patient reaches the target dose of 1 to 1.5 mg/kg body weight per dose. When remission has been achieved the dose is slowly reduced, as for ocular myasthenia, until the minimal effective dose has been established.

For those who do not respond to, or are intolerant of, prednisolone and/or azathioprine, other immunosuppressant drugs such as cyclosporin, methotrexate, or cyclophosphamide may be used.

Late-onset and seronegative myasthenia

Although not formally assessed, it appears that these patients do not benefit significantly from thymectomy. Most respond to the immunosuppressant regime described above.

Myasthenic crisis

Intubation and assisted ventilation may be required. Plasma exchange and intravenous immunoglobulin may both lead to a rapid improvement (within 1 to 2 weeks) in strength, but the beneficial effects start to wear off within about 8 weeks. However, this gives useful time in which to establish an immunosuppressant regime, as discussed above.

Plasma exchange and intravenous immunoglobulin are also useful in preparing myasthenic patients for thymectomy and may reduce the likelihood of deterioration consequent upon the introduction of prednisolone.

Osteoporosis is an important concern in patients receiving long-term, high-dose prednisolone. A bone density determination should be carried out before starting such therapy, and repeated periodically, as appropriate. Local guidelines should be followed—these will advise on general physical measures, assess dietary calcium intake, and indicate the need to introduce calcium/vitamin D or a bisphosphonate, and the place of hormone replacement therapy for postmenopausal women.

Prognosis

The outlook for most patients with myasthenia is good, with over 90 per cent achieving near-normal functional recovery. Death is most likely to occur during a myasthenic crisis early in the course of the disease. The response to thymectomy has been noted. Unwanted effects relating to the immunosuppressant drugs may have an important influence on the outcome.

Myasthenia in pregnancy

Pregnancy has no significant long-term effect on myasthenia, but relapse may be more common in the puerperium. Some 10 per cent of infants born to myasthenic mothers have transient neonatal myasthenia due to transplacental passage of maternal anti-AChR antibodies. Symptoms include feeding and respiratory difficulties, generalized weakness, and less commonly, ptosis. They resolve within a few weeks.

Immunosuppressive treatment should be maintained during pregnancy to ensure good control of the mother's myasthenia and to reduce the likelihood of neonatal weakness.

Much more rarely, the infant is born with arthrogryposis multiplex congenita, secondary to profound intrauterine weakness and lack of movement. This relates to maternal antibodies which target the fetal form of the acetylcholine receptor (see above—Neuromuscular transmission) and in some cases the mother herself has been asymptomatic.

Future research

This may provide a better understanding of the immune processes involved, and thus lead to the development of selective treatments that avoid generalized immune suppression or other unwanted effects of the currently available drugs.

Lambert–Eaton myasthenic syndrome (LEMS)

This is a presynaptic disorder, characterized by limb-girdle weakness and symptoms of autonomic dysfunction, which is often associated with small-cell lung cancer. Delayed diagnosis is common. Symptomatic and immunosuppressant therapies are available.

Epidemiology

Some 60 per cent of patients have cancer-associated LEMS, caused by small-cell lung cancer and the peak presentation is in the fourth to sixth decades. The other 40 per cent have non-cancer-associated LEMS and may present from childhood onwards. It is estimated that 3 per cent of patients with small-cell lung cancer develop LEMS, but that the diagnosis is frequently not made. The weakness is often attributed to non-specific cachectic effects and the disorder is not either suspected or investigated. LEMS may predate the appearance of the cancer by as much as 5 years.

Pathogenesis

Both forms are associated with IgG class antibodies, which reduce the number of functional presynaptic P/Q-type voltage-gated calcium channels by cross-linking adjacent channels. This causes reduced calcium influx and therefore reduced quantal release of acetylcholine. As in myasthenia, patients with LEMS have an increased incidence of other forms of autoimmune disease, including a rare association with acquired myasthenia gravis.

Small-cell lung cancers express voltage-gated calcium channels and it is proposed that the tumour triggers an antibody response to those channels, the antibodies then cross-react with the calcium channels at the neuromuscular junction, causing LEMS.

Clinical features

Most patients present with an abnormality of gait and complain that their legs feel heavy or weak. Symptomatic upper limb weakness tends to present later. Autonomic dysfunction is common, but infrequently volunteered, and includes dryness of the mouth and constipation. In males, impotence may predate limb weakness. Compared with myasthenia gravis, ocular symptoms are rarely severe or particularly troublesome, and bulbar weakness is rare.

On examination, mild ptosis and diplopia may be evident. The abnormality of gait is often more striking than demonstrable weakness when testing on the examination couch. Partly this is because of the phenomenon of postexertional potentiation. Physiologically, with sustained effort there is mobilization of nerve calcium stores and consequently increased quantal release of acetylcholine. Clinically, this augmentation is apparent in two ways. First, strength increases after a few seconds of maximal effort. Second, the tendon reflexes, which are reduced or absent, increase or appear following 10 to 15 s of maximal contraction of the relevant muscle. Sensory testing is normal.

Diagnosis

Single-fibre electromyography, as in myasthenia gravis, shows increased jitter and blocking, and repetitive nerve stimulation studies show decrement at certain frequencies. However, the characteristic neurophysiological finding, which reflects the clinical observations made above, is of a small-amplitude compound muscle action potential which shows potentiation, sometimes enormous, 15 s after voluntary maximal contraction. Diagnosis is confirmed by demonstrating the presence of antivoltage-gated calcium channel antibodies, which are detectable in 95 per cent of cases.

Treatment

Pyridostigmine may offer some symptomatic benefit, but 3,4-diaminopyridine is more effective and the drug of choice (but is only available from specialist centres). 3,4-Diaminopyridine blocks the voltage-gated potassium channels (see Fig. 1), thereby prolonging the duration of the nerve action potential and allows a greater influx of calcium. The maximum dose of 3,4-diaminopyridine is 100 mg daily.

When an associated cancer is unlikely (young patients, non-smokers, more than 5 years since onset and no cancer apparent), treatment with alternate-day prednisolone (up to 1.5 mg/kg body weight per dose) and azathioprine (2.5 mg/kg body weight per day), as in myasthenia gravis, can be highly effective.

In a smoker in whom a cancer is not identified at presentation, it is prudent to repeat chest imaging (CT or MRI) yearly for 5 years.

In cancer-associated LEMS, removal of the tumour often leads to symptomatic improvement. Although there is some reluctance to use immunosuppression in patients with known cancer, alternate-day prednisolone may be used if there has been an inadequate symptomatic response to 3,4-diaminopyridine.

Plasma exchange and intravenous immunoglobulin both give short-term benefit and can be used in cancer-associated and non-cancer-associated LEMS.

Prognosis

In cancer-associated LEMS the prognosis is largely determined by the tumour. In non-cancer-associated LEMS many patients can be rendered symptom free, but some prove very resistant to treatment.

Congenital myasthenic syndromes

This is a rare group of conditions with an overall prevalence in the order of 1 in 200 000 population. They are genetically determined (usually autosomal recessive—so a history of consanguinity is common), non-autoimmune disorders. Major clinical features include onset in infancy, fatiguable weakness, a decremental response to repetitive nerve stimulation, and absence of anti-AChR antibodies. A significant exception to this generalization is the classic slow-channel syndrome, which may present in infancy or adult life, and is inherited as an autosomal dominant trait. The syndromes may be classified on the basis of the site of the defect of neuromuscular transmission, but this is not always certain. A revised classification is likely to evolve as the molecular basis of each is identified. Diagnosis depends upon electrophysiological tests, morphological studies of the end-plate region in muscle biopsy specimens, and increasingly on identification of the specific genetic defect.

Presynaptic disorders

These are the least well characterized of the myasthenic disorders. They include disorders of acetylcholine resynthesis or packaging (previously known as familial infantile myasthenia, now called congenital myasthenic syndrome with episodic apnoea), and a recently described condition with paucity of synaptic vesicles with reduced quantal release. Symptoms respond to anticholinesterase drugs. The episodic apnoea syndrome has recently been shown to be caused by choline acetyltranasferase mutations.

End-plate acetylcholinesterase deficiency

Fatiguable weakness is usually evident from birth. A single nerve stimulus may give rise to a repetitive compound muscle action potential response. The molecular basis is a mutation within the ColQ polypeptide gene. ColQ anchors acetylcholinesterase to the basal lamina. In the absence of the enzyme the acetylcholine receptors have a prolonged exposure to acetylcholine. Anticholinesterase drugs, not surprisingly, are ineffective. No specific treatments are available.

Postsynaptic disorders

These disorders are associated with mutations in the genes that encode the acetylcholine receptor subunits. They may affect the number of receptors or the kinetic properties of the central ion channel.

The most common in the United Kingdom is acetylcholine receptor deficiency, which is most frequently caused by mutations in the ε-subunit gene. Presentation is at birth or within the first few years of life. There is generalized weakness, delayed motor milestones, feeding difficulties, and extraocular muscle involvement. There is a good response to anticholinesterase drugs and 3,4-diaminopyridine.

The low-affinity, fast-channel syndrome is phenotypically similar to acetylcholine receptor deficiency and may be associated with α-, δ-, or ε-subunit mutations. The mechanism is altered kinetics of the receptor ion channel.

The slow-channel syndrome is also a kinetic disorder, associated with mutations in different subunits and in different domains within those subunits. It is an autosomal dominant disorder with variable penetrance that may not become symptomatic until adult life or may remain subclinical. It tends to be progressive and characteristically produces weakness of periscapular muscles and of finger extensors. As in end-plate acetylcholinesterase deficiency, electromyography may show a repetitive response to a single nerve stimulus. Anticholinesterase drugs are unhelpful, but quinidine may be beneficial.

Neuromyotonia

This term describes a condition in which peripheral nerve overactivity leads to spontaneous muscle activity. It is thus quite different from classic myotonia, which relates to an abnormality of muscle fibre membrane activity. Neuromyotonia may be seen in association with a variety of inherited disorders (notably neuropathies and spinal muscular atrophy), but the commonest form is acquired. The acquired form may be idiopathic, but recognized associations include tumour (thymoma—sometimes also in association with myasthenia gravis; bronchial carcinoma) and acquired demyelinating polyneuropathies. Most acquired cases are autoimmune in origin and relate to the presence of antibodies directed against voltage-gated potassium channels in the peripheral nerve (Fig. 1), for which an assay is now available. As noted above, activation of these channels is an important factor in nerve repolarization—the symptoms of neuromyotonia can be understood in terms of prolonged depolarization and excessive release of acetylcholine.

The main clinical features are muscle stiffness, cramps, and twitching (myokymia), which may be localized or generalized. Voluntary muscle contraction may precipitate or exacerbate the abnormal activity. The myokymia persists during sleep and general anaesthesia. Additional symptoms include peripheral paraesthesias and excess sweating, and rarely, mood change, disturbed sleep, and hallucinations.

Apart from the muscle twitching (which may be confused with the fasciculation of denervation), physical examination may be normal. Mild weakness may be evident, proximally or distally. In long-standing cases, muscle hypertrophy (simply a form of work hypertrophy) may be present. Tendon reflexes may be reduced.

Electromyography shows highly characteristic, and diagnostic, doublet, triplet, or multiplet motor unit discharges, or periods of continuous motor unit discharge, with a high (up to 300 Hz) intraburst frequency. Fibrillation and fasciculation potentials may also be seen. Further confirmation of the diagnosis comes from antivoltage-gated potassium channel antibody assay, which is positive in about 50 per cent of cases using the currently available assay. Chest imaging should be considered to exclude thymoma and bronchial carcinoma.

Most patients gain symptomatic relief from carbamazepine, phenytoin, or lamotrigine. If the benefit is insufficient, immunosuppression with prednisolone and azathioprine is often helpful. Intractable cases may respond to plasma exchange and intravenous immunoglobulin.

Further reading

The neuromuscular junction and neuromuscular transmission

Vincent A (2001). The neuromuscular junction and neuromuscular transmission. In: Karpati G, Hilton-Jones D, Griggs R, eds. *Disorders of voluntary muscle.* Cambridge University Press, Cambridge.

Myasthenia gravis

Aarli JA (1999). Late-onset myasthenia gravis: a changing scene. *Archives of Neurology* **56**, 25–7.

Gajdos P *et al.* and the Myasthenia Gravis Clinical Study Group (1997). Clinical trial of plasma exchange and high-dose intravenous immunoglobulin in myasthenia gravis. *Annals of Neurology* **41**, 789–96.

Newsom-Davis J, Besson D (In press). Myasthenia gravis and myasthenic syndromes: autoimmune and genetic disorders. In: Karpati G, Hilton-Jones D, Griggs R, eds. *Disorders of voluntary muscle.* Cambridge University Press.

Lambert–Eaton syndrome

Elrington GM *et al.* (1991). Neurological paraneoplastic syndromes in patients with small cell lung cancer: a prospective survey of 150 patients. *Journal of Neurology, Neurosurgery and Psychiatry* **54**, 764–67.

Maddison P *et al.* (1999). Favourable prognosis in Lambert–Eaton myasthenic syndrome and small-cell lung carcinoma. *Lancet* **353**, 117–18.

Motomura M *et al.* (1995). An improved diagnostic assay for Lambert–Eaton myasthenic syndrome. *Journal of Neurology, Neurosurgery and Psychiatry* **58**, 85–7.

Motomura M *et al.* (1997). Incidence of serum anti-P/Q-type and anti-N-type calcium channel autoantibodies in the Lambert–Eaton myasthenic syndrome. *Journal of the Neurological Sciences* **47**, 35–42.

Congenital myasthenic syndromes

Beeson D *et al.* (1993). Primary structure of the human muscle acetylcholine receptor: cDNA cloning of the gamma and epsilon subunits. *European Journal of Biochemistry* **215**, 229–38.

Beeson D, Palace J, Vincent A (1997).Congenital myasthenic syndromes. *Current Opinion in Neurology* **10**, 402–7.

Engel AG, Ohno K, Sine S (1999). Congenital myasthenic syndromes. *Archives of Neurology* **56**, 163–7.

Neuromyotonia

Hart IK *et al.* (1997). Autoantibodies detected to expressed K^+ channels are implicated in neuromyotonia. *Annals of Neurology* **41**, 238–46.

Newsom-Davis J (1997). Autoimmune neuromyotonia (Isaacs' syndrome): an antibody-mediated potassium channelopathy. *Annals of the New York Academy of Sciences* **835**, 111–19.

24.18 Paraneoplastic syndromes

Jerome B. Posner

Introduction

The term paraneoplastic syndrome refers to disorders of an organ or tissue caused by cancer but occurring at a site distant from the tumour or its metastases. Organs or tissues commonly involved include the skin (for example paraneoplastic pemphigus), the endocrine system (for example paraneoplastic hypercalcaemia or paraneoplastic Cushing's syndrome), and the central and peripheral nervous system. The nervous system can be damaged directly or the damage may be indirect, such as when paraneoplastic hypercalcaemia or paraneoplastic Cushing's syndrome causes secondary nervous system dysfunction. Table 1 lists paraneoplastic syndromes involving the central and peripheral nervous system. Only the direct paraneoplastic syndromes are discussed here. More extensive reviews of paraneoplastic syndromes and other effects of systemic cancer on the nervous system can be found in the further reading section.

Incidence

Neurological examination of patients with cancer often reveals mild abnormalities such as proximal leg weakness or diminished Achilles reflexes. Most of these mild, usually subclinical, abnormalities result from metabolic or nutritional disturbances associated with advanced cancer. These disorders are not usually classified as paraneoplastic syndromes. In fact, most paraneoplastic syndromes occur in patients not known to have cancer at the time the neurological symptoms develop. Furthermore, most paraneoplastic syndromes are significantly disabling. If one limits oneself to 'true paraneoplastic syndromes' as indicated in Table 1, the disorders are rare. In one series of almost 1500 patients, only 3 had paraneoplastic cerebellar degeneration, and none had subacute sensory neuronopathy. With the exception of the Lambert–Eaton myasthenic syndrome (**LEMS**), a disorder that affects about 3 per cent of patients with small-cell lung cancer, paraneoplastic syndromes probably affect fewer than 1 per cent of patients with cancer.

Table 1 Examples of paraneoplastic syndromes affecting the nervous system

Example(s)	Area most affected
Limbic encephalitis (dementia)	Cerebral hemisphere(s)
Cerebellar Purkinje cell degeneration	Cerebellum
Opsoclonus/myoclonus	Brainstem
Carcinoma-associated retinopathy	Retina
Necrotizing myelopathy	Spinal cord
Stiff person syndrome	Spinal cord
Sensory neuronopathy	Dorsal root ganglia
Sensory/sensorimotor neuropathy	Peripheral nerve
Autonomic neuropathy	Peripheral nerve
Lambert–Eaton myasthenic syndrome	Neuromuscular junction
Dermatomyositis	Muscle
Encephalomyelitis	Diffuse

Despite their low incidence, paraneoplastic syndromes are important for several reasons.

1. They usually develop before the cancer has been identified and so their presence may lead to the detection of small and potentially curable cancers.
2. Certain paraneoplastic syndromes characterized by specific autoantibodies suggest a specific cancer site.
3. The paraneoplastic syndrome is often more disabling than the cancer and may, in some instances, be the cause of death.
4. A paraneoplastic syndrome or an antibody associated with a paraneoplastic syndrome (see below) may predict an indolent course for the cancer.
5. The presence of specific antibodies in the serum of patients with a paraneoplastic syndrome identifies the neurological disorder as paraneoplastic and, as indicated above, sometimes strongly suggests the location of the underlying tumour.
6. Paraneoplastic antibodies identify proteins normally restricted to neurones that are of importance in the development and maintenance of neurones.

Pathogenesis

Current evidence suggests that paraneoplastic syndromes affecting the nervous system result from an autoimmune reaction to the tumour: protein antigens that are normally restricted to the nervous system are expressed in some cancers. The immune system recognizes the antigen in the cancer as foreign and some patients mount an immune response. The immune response has the dual effect of retarding the growth of the tumour but damaging those portions of the nervous system that express the antigen. A few of these so-called paraneoplastic antigens are normally expressed not only in the nervous system but also in the testis which, like the nervous system, is an immunologically privileged site. The best evidence for an immune-mediated mechanism comes from studies of the LEMS. Voltage-gated calcium channel proteins are found in all small-cell lung cancers. Some patients develop antibodies against these proteins. The antibodies react with voltage-gated calcium channels found in the presynaptic neuromuscular junction to prevent calcium from entering the junction, which in turn prevents the release of acetylcholine. The decreased release of acetylcholine causes the weakness that characterizes the syndrome. If one removes the antibody from the patient by plasma exchange, the patient's symptoms improve. If one injects experimental animals with the antibody from the patient, the syndrome is reproduced.

Evidence of immune-mediated mechanisms in most other paraneoplastic syndromes is less firm. However, several lines of evidence suggest that immune-mediated mechanisms are also pathogenetic in syndromes involving the central nervous system.

1. In some but not all patients with a paraneoplastic syndrome, the serum and cerebrospinal fluid contain high titres of autoantibodies that react

with both tumour and those portions of the nervous system damaged by the paraneoplastic syndrome.

2. The titre of the antibody relative to total IgG is higher in cerebrospinal fluid than in serum.
3. In some patients, T-cell infiltrates of limited T-cell receptor families are found in the tumour and the nervous system.
4. One report describes intracellular IgG in the brain of patients who die of a paraneoplastic syndrome.

Several different autoantibodies have been found in the serum of patients with different paraneoplastic syndromes. The antibodies often identify patients with a specific clinical syndrome and with a specific underlying tumour (Table 2). For example, the anti-Yo antibody, which reacts with Purkinje cells of the cerebellum and some ovarian and breast cancers, is almost always associated with the syndrome of paraneoplastic cerebellar degeneration and with breast, ovarian, or other gynaecological cancers. In a few patients, the antibody and the paraneoplastic syndrome have been associated with other cancers, including cancers in men. Conversely, most patients with paraneoplastic cerebellar degeneration associated with non-gynaecological cancers either demonstrate other antibodies that react with Purkinje cells or do not have antibodies identifiable by current techniques. For example, some patients with paraneoplastic cerebellar degeneration express the anti-Hu antibody, an antibody usually associated with small-cell lung cancer and paraneoplastic encephalomyelitis or sensory neuronopathy.

Some autoantibodies are associated with specific tumours but widely varying paraneoplastic syndromes. For example, the anti-Hu antibody is almost always associated with small-cell lung cancer (occasionally neuroblastoma, prostate cancer, or mesenchymal chondrosarcoma), but may be associated with several different clinical syndromes usually encompassed by the term encephalomyelitis. The clinical abnormalities include limbic encephalitis (see below), paraneoplastic cerebellar degeneration, brainstem encephalitis, sensory neuronopathy, and autonomic failure. Some or all of these clinical abnormalities may be found in the same patient.

In some patients with paraneoplastic syndromes no antibodies are found. A good example is opsoclonus/myoclonus associated with neuroblastoma in children. Most observers believe that this paraneoplastic disorder is immune-mediated, particularly because it responds to ACTH. The failure to find an antibody does not mean that one is not present, only that current techniques cannot identify it. Another good example is LEMS. Standard histochemical and immunoblotting techniques cannot identify an antibody; only by the special techniques of electron microscopic histochemistry or immune precipitation can the P/Q type calcium channel antibodies be identified. These findings give some hope that by using better techniques, antibodies may be found in some currently antibody-negative paraneoplastic syndromes.

Diagnosis

Certain clinical clues suggest to the physician that a patient with a neurological disorder may be suffering from a paraneoplastic syndrome. These are summarized in the following paragraphs.

Most paraneoplastic syndromes evolve subacutely. The disorder usually becomes apparent to the patient within a few days and often within several weeks has reached its peak. A few patients develop symptoms overnight. Occasional patients have a more protracted course, slowly evolving over several months. However, disorders that evolve slowly over many months to years are unlikely to be paraneoplastic.

Most paraneoplastic syndromes stabilize after weeks to months. As indicated above, symptoms usually progress rapidly but the progression usually ceases within several months.

The neurological disorders are usually severe. Most patients have substantial disability by the time they first consult a physician. Mild or waxing and waning neurological disorders are usually not paraneoplastic. For example, the patient with paraneoplastic cerebellar degeneration is usually unable to walk, unable to write, and sometimes because of the oscillopsia associated with nystagmus, unable to read or watch television. Many patients cannot sit unsupported.

The neurological findings are often characteristic. Those disorders are listed in Table 1. A subacutely developing pancerebellar disorder, the rapid development of opsoclonus (see below), or the development of LEMS strongly suggests cancer as the underlying cause. However, none of the syndromes, even the most characteristic, is invariably associated with cancer. Thus, only about two-thirds of patients with LEMS have cancer and only about 15 per cent of patients with myasthenia gravis have a tumour (almost

Table 2 Antineuronal antibody associated paraneoplastic disorders

Antibody	Neuronal reactivity	Protein antigens	Cloned genes	Tumour	Paraneoplastic symptoms
Anti-Hu	Nucleus>cytoplasm (all neurones)	35-40 Kd	HuD, HuC,Nel-N1	SCLC, neuroblastoma, sarcoma, prostate	PEM, PSN, PCD, autonomic dysfunction
Anti-Yo	Cytoplasm Purkinje cells	34, 36 Kd	CDR34, CDR62	Ovary, breast, lung	PCD
Anti-Ri	Nucleus>cytoplasm (CNS neurones)	55, 80 Kd	Nova	Breast, gynaecological cancer, lung, bladder	Ataxia/opsoclonus
Anti-Tr	Cytoplasm Purkinje cells	?	–	Hodgkin's disease	PCD
Anti-VGCC	Presynaptic neuromuscular junction	VGCC 64 Kd	P/Q type MysB	VGCC, SCLC	LEMS
Anti-Retinal	Photoreceptor, ganglion cells	23. 65, 145, 205 Kd	Recoverin	SCLC, melanoma, gynaecological cancer	CAR, MAR
Anti-Amphiphysin	Presynaptic	128Kd	Amphiphysin	Breast, SCLC	Stiff-person syndrome, PEM
Anti-CRMP5 (Anti-CV2)	Oligodendrocytes, neurones, cytoplasm	66 Kd	CRMP5 (POP66)	SCLC, thymoma	PEM, PCD, chorea, sensory neuropathy
Anti-PCA2	Purkinje cytoplasm and other neurones	280 Kd		SCLD	PEM, PCD, LEMS, others
Anti-Ma1	Neurones (subnucleus)	40 Kd	Ma1	Lung, others	Brainstem, PCD
Anti-Ma2	Neurones (subnucleus)	41.5 Kd	Ma2	Testis	Limbic brainstem encephalitis
ANNA 3	Nuclei, Purkinje cells	170 Kd		Lung cancer	Sensory neuropathy, PEM

CAR, cancer associated retinopathy; MAR, melanoma associated retinopathy; PEM, paraneoplastic encephalomyelitis; PSN, paraneoplastic sensory neuronopathy; PCD, paraneoplastic cerebellar degeneration; VGCC, voltage-gated calcium channel; SCLC, small-cell lung cancer.

always thymoma). Probably about half of patients with subacute cerebellar degeneration have cancer.

Paraneoplastic syndromes involving the central nervous system are often accompanied by cerebrospinal fluid pleocytosis, elevated protein, increased IgG, and oligoclonal bands. The spinal fluid findings are more likely to be abnormal early in the course of disease and revert to more normal values later on. In particular, the pleocytosis, rarely more than 30 to 40 cells, may be gone within a few weeks of the onset of disease. The immunoglobulin abnormalities usually persist.

Paraneoplastic syndromes often affect one particular portion of the nervous system with additional subtle or minor findings suggesting dysfunction in other areas. For example, paraneoplastic cerebellar degeneration selectively affects Purkinje cells of the cerebellum, causing pancerebellar neurological symptoms. Some patients will also be found to be mildly demented and demonstrate extensor plantar reflexes or sensory changes. These widespread changes have led to the term encephalomyelitis when the central nervous system is involved and neuromyopathy when the peripheral nerves and muscles are involved.

The physician encounters the patient with a paraneoplastic syndrome in one of two settings. In the first, the patient is known to have or have had cancer and then develops a neurological disorder. The cancer may be under active treatment, may have recurred after a remission, or may be assumed to have been cured in the remote past. Because paraneoplastic syndromes are the least common of the neurological complications of systemic cancer (Table 3), the physician must rule out all of the other causes before considering the disorder to be paraneoplastic. Unless a paraneoplastic antibody is found in the serum, the diagnosis is one of exclusion.

In the second setting, the patient is not known to have cancer. The physician must consider if the clinical findings fit a paraneoplastic syndrome (Table 1) and order the appropriate antibody studies (Table 2). Although the presence of a paraneoplastic antibody usually establishes the diagnosis, its absence does not. If an antibody is present and the search for an underlying cancer is negative, the physician is obligated to follow the patient carefully, searching periodically for a cancer.

Treatment

Some paraneoplastic syndromes, such as LEMS, respond to immunosuppression or to treatment of the underlying cancer (Table 4). Some syndromes, such as opsoclonus/myoclonus, may remit spontaneously, but for most paraneoplastic syndromes, treatment is unrewarding and most patients remain with severe neurological disability even if the cancer is cured. Most treatment has involved immunosuppression, particularly for those syndromes associated with autoantibodies. It is possible that the rapid onset of the syndromes does not allow sufficient time for accurate early diagnosis and for treatment to begin before irreversible neural damage has occurred. With earlier diagnosis, therapy may be more successful.

Table 3 Neurological complications of cancer

Metastases
Brain
Spinal cord
Leptomeninges
Cranial and/or peripheral nerves
Non-metastatic effects of cancer
Metabolic disorders:
Organ failure
Endocrinopathies
Nutritional problems
Tumour secretions of ectopic substances
Vascular disorders:
Hypocoagulability (haemorrhage)
Hypercoagulability (infarction)
Infections
Side-effects of therapy:
Surgery
Irradiation
Chemotherapy
'Remote effects' or paraneoplastic syndromes

Specific syndromes

Brain and cranial nerves (Table 5)

Paraneoplastic cerebellar degeneration

The disorder may complicate any malignant tumour but is most common with lung cancer (especially small-cell), gynaecological neoplasms, and Hodgkin's disease. Males and females are both affected and the age incidence reflects the age distribution of the cancer. Neurological manifestations precede detection of the associated tumour in over one-half of patients, rarely by up to 4 years. Alternatively, paraneoplastic cerebellar degeneration may develop after diagnosis of the neoplasm. In some instances, the tumour is not found until autopsy. Typically, the disorder begins as gait ataxia that over a few days to months progresses to severe truncal and appendicular ataxia with dysarthria and often nystagmus. The nystagmus is frequently downbeating. Vertigo with or without nausea and vomiting is common and many patients complain of diplopia. The cerebellar signs are bilateral but may be asymmetrical. A more rapid onset within a few hours or days or a slower progression sometimes occurs. The cerebellar deficit usually stabilizes but, by then, the patient is often incapacitated. Spontaneous improvement sometimes occurs, particularly when associated with Hodgkin's disease.

The cerebrospinal fluid may be normal, but early in the illness usually shows a mild pleocytosis. Oligoclonal bands may be present. Cytological examination of the cerebrospinal fluid and contrast-enhanced MRI of the neuraxis rule out leptomeningeal metastases. MR scans typically are normal early, but later show signs of progressive cerebellar atrophy with prominent cerebellar folia and a dilated fourth ventricle.

The pathological hallmark of paraneoplastic cerebellar degeneration is loss of Purkinje cells, affecting all parts of the cerebellum. Less striking changes in the cerebellar cortex may include thinning of the molecular layer with microglial proliferation and astrocytic gliosis, proliferation of Bergmann astrocytes, and slight thinning of the granular layer with decreased numbers of granule cells.

When typical, the clinical picture of paraneoplastic cerebellar degeneration is almost pathognomonic. When atypical, the disorder must be distinguished from a cerebellar tumour (primary or metastatic) and from leptomeningeal metastases (by MRI and cerebrospinal fluid examination, respectively), from late-onset, non-paraneoplastic cerebellar degenerative disorders, cerebellar haemorrhage and infarction, abscess, prion diseases, cerebellar ataxia related to 5-fluorouracil or high-dose cytarabine, and metabolic disorders, especially alcoholic cerebellar degeneration. In alcoholic cerebellar degeneration, the ataxia predominantly involves the lower extremities; dysarthria and nystagmus are unusual.

There have been occasional reports of a partial or near-complete remission of paraneoplastic cerebellar degeneration following treatment of the primary tumour. The presence of ocular flutter or opsoclonus indicates a better chance of improvement, but this may be a different paraneoplastic syndrome (see below). Only rarely is immunosuppression beneficial and most patients do not respond. It is possible that if begun early in the illness, before Purkinje cells are irreversibly damaged, plasmapheresis and immunosuppressive drugs might have a beneficial effect. Symptomatic improvement in the ataxia occurs in a few patients using clonazepam in doses varying from 0.5 to 1.5 mg daily. Buspirone may also give modest relief.

Table 4 Treatment of paraneoplastic neurological syndromes

Syndrome	Treatment
Paraneoplastic syndromes that usually respond to treatment:	
Lambert–Eaton myasthenic syndrome (LEMS)	Tumour therapy, plasma exchange, intravenous immunoglobulin, 3,4 diaminopyridine
Myasthenia gravis	Tumour therapy, plasma exchange, intravenous immunoglobulin, immunosuppressants
Dermatomyositis	Steroids, immunosuppressants, intravenous immunoglobulin
Opsoclonus/myoclonus (children)	Steroids, ACTH, tumour therapy
Carcinoid myopathy	Tumour therapy, cyproheptadine
Neuropathy (osteosclerotic myeloma)	Tumour therapy, radiation
Paraneoplastic syndromes that may respond to treatment:	
Vasculitis (nerve/muscle)	Steroids
Opsoclonus/myoclonus (adults)	Steroids, tumour therapy, protein A column, clonazepam, diazepam, baclofen
Paraneoplastic cerebellar degeneration (Hodgkin's disease)	Tumour therapy
Opsoclonus/ataxia (anti-Ri)	Steroids, cyclophosphamide
Guillain–Barré (Hodgkin's disease)	Tumour therapy, plasma exchange, intravenous immunoglobulin
Stiff person syndrome	Tumour therapy, steroids, diazepam, baclofen, intravenous immunoglobulin
Neuromyotonia	Plasma exchange
Paraneoplastic syndromes that usually do not respond to treatment:	
Paraneoplastic cerebellar degeneration:	
Small-cell lung cancer (irrespective of anti-Hu)	
Anti-Yo antibodies (cancer of ovary, breast)	
Paraneoplastic encephalomyelitis/sensory neuronopathy:	
Limbic encephalopathy (steroids)	
Cerebellar degeneration	
Brainstem encephalopathy	
Myelopathy	
Sensory neuronopathy	
Autonomic dysfunction (central or peripheral)	
Cancer-associated retinopathy	
Paraneoplastic syndromes that may improve spontaneously:	
Acute motor neuronopathy and lymphoma	
Paraneoplastic cerebellar degeneration associated with Hodgkin's disease	
Acute polyradiculopathy associated with Hodgkin's disease	
Limbic encephalopathy	
Opsoclonus/myoclonus (children or adults)	

Opsoclonus/myoclonus

Opsoclonus, a disorder of eye movements consisting of almost continuous arrhythmic, multidirectional, involuntary, high-amplitude conjugate saccades that are often accompanied by synchronous blinking of the lids, is a paraneoplastic syndrome complicating neuroblastoma in children and a variety of tumours in adults. Opsoclonus may be an isolated neurological sign, but is often accompanied by myoclonus of the trunk, limbs, head, diaphragm, larynx, pharynx, and palate, and ataxia. When opsoclonus is a paraneoplastic syndrome of adults it may be accompanied by paraneoplastic cerebellar degeneration. Opsoclonus/myoclonus is also associated with viral infections, postinfectious encephalitis, trauma, intracranial tumours, hydrocephalus, thalamic haemorrhage, and toxic encephalopathies from thallium or lithium, amitriptyline overdose, and diabetic hyperosmolar coma. Opsoclonus occurs in about 2 per cent of children with neuroblastomas. Neurological symptoms precede identification of the neuroblastoma at least 50 per cent of the time and the tumour often is not obvious on examination; thus, recognition of the neurological syndrome is an important clue to the presence of a neuroblastoma. When a neuroblastoma is associated with opsoclonus/myoclonus, there is a higher than expected incidence of intrathoracic tumours and of tumours with a benign histology. The prognosis of the neuroblastoma is better if opsoclonus/myoclonus is associated than when there is no neurological complication, an observation not explained by earlier diagnosis when neurological symptoms are present. The neurological disorder responds to ACTH and to intravenous immunoglobulin but not to prednisone. However, most patients suffer residual neurological damage, usually cognitive.

Table 5 Paraneoplastic syndromes affecting brain and cranial nerves

Subacute cerebellar degeneration
Opsoclonus/myoclonus
Limbic encephalitis and other dementias
Brainstem encephalitis
Optic neuritis
Retinal degeneration

Opsoclonus/myoclonus is less common in adults. Nevertheless, about 20 per cent of adult patients reported with opsoclonus/myoclonus have an underlying cancer. The neurological symptoms usually precede diagnosis of the tumour and commonly progress over several weeks, although more rapid or slower progression may be observed. Opsoclonus often is associated with truncal ataxia, dysarthria, myoclonus, vertigo, and encephalopathy. The cerebrospinal fluid may show a mild pleocytosis and a mildly elevated protein. The MRI is usually normal, but brainstem abnormalities have been reported.

Neuropathological findings have been variable. In some patients there are no identifiable abnormalities. In others, the changes resembled those of paraneoplastic cerebellar degeneration with a loss of Purkinje cells, inflammatory infiltrates in the brainstem, Bergmann gliosis, and loss of cells from the granular layer of the cerebellum.

The prognosis for recovery or partial remission of the neurological disorder is better for paraneoplastic opsoclonus/myoclonus than it is for paraneoplastic cerebellar degeneration. Improvement may follow treatment of the underlying tumour, and spontaneous partial remissions occur. Remissions have been reported to follow treatment of the tumour or immunosuppressive treatment including immunoadsorptive therapy using a protein A column.

Limbic encephalitis

Limbic encephalitis may occur as an isolated finding or as a more extensive encephalomyelitis. The neurological symptoms often precede diagnosis of the tumour by up to 2 years; sometimes the cancer is not detected until autopsy. Symptoms usually progress over several weeks but the course may be more insidious. Anxiety and depression are common early symptoms, but the most striking feature is a severe impairment of recent memory. Other manifestations include agitation, confusion, hallucinations, partial or generalized seizures, and hypersomnia. Progressive dementia usually occurs, but occasionally there may be a spontaneous remission. The cerebrospinal fluid commonly shows a pleocytosis and an elevated protein concentration. MR scans are usually normal but medial temporal abnormalities have been reported.

Inflammatory pathological changes affect the grey matter of the hippocampus, cingulate gyrus, pyriform cortex, orbital surfaces of the frontal lobes, insula, and the amygdaloid nuclei.

No treatment has proved uniformly beneficial although spontaneous remissions have been reported and some patients have improved after treatment of the underlying tumour.

Brainstem encephalitis

Paraneoplastic brainstem encephalitis is often associated with clinical and pathological evidence of encephalomyelitis elsewhere within the central and peripheral nervous systems, but may occur as the dominant or an isolated clinical finding. It is commonly associated with small-cell lung cancer, but an identical clinicopathological syndrome may be seen in the absence of a malignancy.

The clinical features vary according to the brainstem structures involved in the pathological process. Common manifestations include vertigo, ataxia, nystagmus, vomiting, bulbar palsy, oculomotor disorders, and corticospinal tract dysfunction. Less common clinical features include deafness, myoclonus of the branchial musculature, hypoventilation, and movement disorders including chorea or Parkinson's syndrome.

Neurological symptoms may develop before or after discovery of the malignancy. The pathological changes are identical to those observed in other forms of paraneoplastic encephalomyelitis.

Visual loss

Paraneoplastic syndromes can affect retinal photoreceptors, either rods or cones or both. They can cause a retinal vasculitis or optic neuropathy. Paraneoplastic retinal degeneration, also called cancer-associated retinopathy, usually occurs in association with small-cell cancer of the lung, melanoma, and gynaecological tumours. Typically, the visual symptoms include episodic visual obscurations, night blindness, light-induced glare, photosensitivity, and impaired colour vision. Visual symptoms usually precede the diagnosis of cancer. The symptoms progress to painless visual loss. They may begin unilaterally but usually become bilateral. Visual testing demonstrates peripheral and ring scotomas and loss of acuity. Funduscopic examination may reveal arteriolar narrowing and abnormal mottling of the retinal pigment epithelium. The electroretinogram is abnormal. Cerebrospinal fluid is typically normal, although elevated immunoglobulin levels have been reported. Inflammatory cells are sometimes seen in the vitreous by slit-lamp examination.

Pathologically, a loss of photoreceptors and ganglion cells with inflammatory infiltrates and macrophages is usually noted. The other parts of the optic pathway are preserved, although a loss of myelin and lymphocytic infiltration of the optic nerve may occur.

Treatment of cancer-associated retinopathy is usually unsuccessful although a recent report describes improvement in some patients with the use of intravenous immunoglobulin.

Table 6 Paraneoplastic syndromes affecting spinal cord and dorsal root ganglia

Necrotizing myelopathy
Subacute motor neuronopathy
Motor neurone disease
Myelitis
Sensory neuronopathy

Spinal cord and dorsal root ganglia (Table 6)

Necrotizing myelopathy

This is an extremely rare remote effect of cancer. The initial symptoms of muscle weakness and sensory loss in the arms and legs may be asymmetrical, but eventually signs become bilateral and symmetrical. Back or radicular pain may precede other neurological signs. Cerebrospinal fluid abnormalities may include an elevated level of protein and a mild pleocytosis. Swelling of the spinal cord may be apparent on MRI. Typically, the neurological deficit progresses rapidly over days or a few weeks, ultimately leading to respiratory failure and death. There is no effective treatment.

Pathologically, there is widespread necrosis of the spinal cord, often most marked in the thoracic segments. The necrosis involves all components of the spinal cord with white matter usually more affected than grey matter.

Motor neurone disease (amyotrophic lateral sclerosis)

Paraneoplastic syndromes include: (i) amyotrophic lateral sclerosis with both upper and lower motor neurone dysfunction; (ii) progressive muscular atrophy, a pure lower motor neurone syndrome that is sometimes reversible and also associated with lymphoproliferative disorders; and (iii) primary lateral sclerosis, a pure upper motor neurone syndrome associated with solid tumours as well as lymphoproliferative disorders. The clinical and pathological characteristics differ little from non-paraneoplastic motor neurone disease save for the fact that the paraneoplastic disorders are often more rapid in onset and evolution, sometimes reverse spontaneously, and, at autopsy, may be more inflammatory than non-paraneoplastic disorders.

Myelitis

Paraneoplastic myelitis is usually a part of the encephalomyelitis syndrome with inflammatory lesions elsewhere in the brain and dorsal root ganglia as well as the spinal cord. The clinical picture is characterized by patchy wasting and weakness of muscles, sometimes combined with fasciculations. The upper extremities are often more severely affected than the legs, reflecting predominant involvement of the cervical spinal cord. There may be striking weakness of neck and intercostal muscles, resulting in respiratory failure. Sensory symptoms may be present. Autonomic dysfunction results from involvement of autonomic neurones.

Sensory neuronopathy

In contrast to the common axonal or demyelinating sensory neuropathies, paraneoplastic sensory neuronopathy where the dorsal root ganglion is the site of pathology is a rare syndrome. At least two-thirds of the patients have small-cell lung cancer. Symptoms typically begin before the cancer is identified, with dysaesthetic pain and numbness in the distal extremities or occasionally in the arm(s), face, or trunk. The symptoms may be asymmetrical at onset but progress over days to several weeks to involve the limbs, trunk, and sometimes the face, causing a severe sensory ataxia. All sensory modalities are affected, distinguishing this disorder from cisplatin neuropathy, in which pin and temperature sensation are spared. Deep tendon reflexes are lost but motor function is preserved. The cerebrospinal fluid is typically inflammatory.

Table 7 Paraneoplastic syndromes affecting peripheral nerves

Subacute or chronic sensorimotor peripheral neuropathy
Acute polyradiculoneuropathy (Guillain–Barré syndrome)
Mononeuritis multiplex and microvasculitis of peripheral nerve
Brachial neuritis
Autonomic neuropathy
Peripheral neuropathy associated with myeloma

Early pathological changes are limited mostly to the dorsal root ganglia, in which both a loss of neurones and the presence of lymphocytic inflammatory infiltrates are noted. About 50 per cent of patients with paraneoplastic sensory neuronopathy have pathological changes that may be clinically inapparent in other regions of the nervous system.

In most patients, treating the underlying tumour or removal of the autoantibody by plasmapheresis or immunosuppressive therapy does not alter the course of the neurological disease, although there are isolated reports of responses to immunotherapy. Occasional patients have a mild and indolent neuropathy.

Peripheral nerves (Table 7)

Sensory and sensorimotor neuropathy

Peripheral neuropathies, particularly mild distal sensorimotor neuropathies, are quite common in patients with cancer. In one study of lung cancer the incidence was 16 per cent. The incidence is even higher if one defines the disorder by electrical evidence in clinically asymptomatic patients. However, many patients may have suffered from the metabolic or nutritional ravages of late cancer and would not be considered by the definitions here to have true paraneoplastic syndromes.

Some patients not known to have cancer, and who are not evidently systemically ill, present to the neurologist with a peripheral neuropathy which may be quite severe and disabling. It is estimated that in those patients whose initial evaluations do not reveal an obvious cause (such as vitamin deficiency, amyloidosis, diabetes), about 10 per cent will eventually prove to have cancer as the underlying reason for the peripheral neuropathy. Therefore, one should seriously consider a cancer diagnosis in such patients. Paraneoplastic peripheral neuropathy may take several clinical and pathological forms. The most common is the distal, symmetrical, subacutely developing, sensory neuropathy which may be either axonal or demyelinating. A relatively pure sensory neuropathy, a mononeuritis multiplex due to microvasculitis, and acute polyradiculopathy, a focal neuropathy such as brachial neuritis, or an autonomic neuropathy may also be paraneoplastic. Most of these neuropathies are not associated with autoantibodies and the diagnosis is often one of exclusion.

Neuromuscular junction and muscle (Table 8)

Paraneoplastic disorders of the neuromuscular junction include the Lambert–Eaton myasthenic syndrome and myasthenia gravis. These disorders have a common pathogenetic mechanism—they are caused by antibodies against ion channels and, whether paraneoplastic or not, they respond to immunological treatment. Another ion channel disorder included in this section is neuromyotonia, which is not confined to the neuromuscular junction. Finally, because of its similarity to neuromyotonia, the stiff person syndrome is also included in this section.

Table 8 Paraneoplastic syndromes affecting neuromuscular junction and muscle

Lambert–Eaton myasthenic syndrome
Myasthenia gravis
Dermatomyositis, polymyositis, acute necrotizing myopathy
Neuromyotonia and stiff person syndrome

Lambert–Eaton myasthenic syndrome (LEMS)

LEMS results from a reduced release of acetylcholine at presynaptic nerve terminals. The same P/Q-type voltage-gated calcium channels are found in small-cell lung cancers. Interestingly, the richest source of P/Q-type voltage-gated calcium channels is the cerebellum, perhaps explaining the occasional relationship of paraneoplastic cerebellar degeneration and LEMS.

LEMS can be treated either by immune suppression or by treatment of the underlying cancer when present. Patients with small-cell lung cancer associated with LEMS have a better prognosis than patients with small-cell lung cancer who do not develop a paraneoplastic disorder.

Myasthenia gravis

Myasthenia gravis occurs in 30 per cent of patients with thymomas, and approximately 15 per cent of patients with myasthenia gravis are found to have a thymoma.

Polymyositis and dermatomyositis

Only a minority of patients suffering from these disorders have an underlying malignancy as the cause; elderly patients are more likely to have an underlying malignancy. Dermatomyositis with typical cutaneous changes is more likely than polymyositis to be paraneoplastic. Females and males are affected in approximately equal numbers. Symptoms of the muscle weakness generally precede identification of the cancer. The tumour may be at any site, but breast, lung, ovarian, and gastric malignancies are the most common. Hodgkin's disease and prostate and colon cancer are also reported offenders.

Corticosteroids, cyclosporine, and other immunosuppressants have been used successfully. Other reports suggest that high-dose intravenous immunoglobulin is useful in patients unresponsive to other forms of immunosuppression.

Neuromyotonia and stiff person syndrome

Muscle cramps are a common complication of cancer, sometimes related to electrolyte imbalance or induced by chemotherapy. A much rarer but clinically significant paraneoplastic disorder is acquired neuromyotonia. The disorder is characterized by muscle stiffness, cramps, and obviously rippling and twitching muscles, sometimes leading to sustained abnormal postures. Relaxation after voluntary contraction is delayed. Symptoms persist during sleep but are abolished by curare. Sudden prolonged bursts of high-frequency, involuntary, repetitive muscle action potentials are seen on electromyography.

The muscle spasms and rigidity are sometimes precipitated by activity, forcing patients to become sedentary. The disorder arises from peripheral nerves and is sometimes a part of the encephalomyelitis syndrome. The disorder is usually non-paraneoplastic, but may be associated with cancer including thymomas and small-cell lung cancer. Antibodies against voltage-gated potassium channels are often positive. Plasma exchange improves the patient's condition. Some patients respond to anticonvulsants. Injection of IgG from affected patients into experimental animals can reproduce the syndrome.

The stiff person syndrome may superficially resemble neuromyotonia, but has a central origin. The disorder is clinically characterized by stiffness and rigidity with episodic spasms of axial muscles. A variant of the syndrome affects the limbs. Painful reflex spasms can occur in response to tactile stimuli or startle. Muscle action potentials are normal on electromyography but the activity is continuous and excessive and increased by voluntary activity. The disorder is not usually associated with cancer, but in some patients the underlying syndrome is paraneoplastic.

Further reading

Dalmau JO, Gultekin HS, Posner JB (1999). Paraneoplastic neurologic syndromes: Pathogenesis and physiopathology. *Brain Pathology* **9**, 275–84. [Part of a comprehensive symposium of paraneoplastic syndromes in that issue of *Brain Pathology*.]

Darnell RB (1996). Onconeural antigens and the paraneoplastic neurologic disorders: At the intersection of cancer, immunity, and the brain. *Proceedings of the National Academy of Sciences of the United States of America* **93**, 4529–36. [An excellent summary of the biology of paraneoplastic syndromes.]

Das A, Hochberg FH, McNelis S (1999). A review of the therapy of paraneoplastic neurologic syndromes. *Journal of Neuro-oncology* **41**, 181–94. [A review of current treatments.]

Griswold W, Drlicek M (1999). Paraneoplastic neuropathy. *Current Opinion in Neurology* **12**, 617–25. [A summary of peripheral neuropathy associated with cancer.]

Posner JB (1995). *Neurologic Complications of Cancer.* FA Davis, Philadelphia. [A comprehensive review of metastatic and non-metastatic neurological complications of cancer.]

24.19 Diseases of the peripheral nerves

P. K. Thomas

Pathophysiological considerations

The peripheral nerves consist of bundles (fascicles) of unmyelinated and myelinated axons that have their cell bodies in the anterior horns of the spinal cord, dorsal root ganglia, or autonomic ganglia. The fascicles are surrounded by a lamellated cellular sheath, the perineurium, which provides a diffusion barrier that separates the intrafascicular or endoneurial compartment from the extracellular tissues. Peripheral nerve trunks usually consist of several fascicles bound together by the mainly collagenous epineurial connective tissue. The nutrient vessels connect with a longitudinal anastomotic network of arterioles and venules in the epineurium. This in turn communicates through perforating vessels with a longitudinal intrafascicular capillary anastomotic network. This anastomotic system is extremely efficient: experimentally it is very difficult to produce ischaemia of nerve trunks by ligation of nutrient vessels. The occurrence of an ischaemic neuropathy, therefore, implies widespread vascular insufficiency. A blood–nerve barrier, comparable to the blood–brain barrier, exists in peripheral nerves (except in the sensory and autonomic ganglia). This, in conjunction with the diffusion barrier provided by the perineurium, probably regulates the composition of the endoneurial connective tissue fluid and thus the ionic environment of the nerve fibres.

All nerve fibres, whether myelinated or unmyelinated, are closely related to satellite cells, the cells of Schwann. There is evidence that they may provide metabolic support for the axons, which often extend for very considerable distances from their perikarya. In myelinated fibres the myelin segments are derived by the spiralling of Schwann cell surface membrane around the axons. The axon is exposed at the nodes of Ranvier, which represent the gaps between adjacent myelin segments. Conduction in unmyelinated axons takes place by the spread of a continuous wave of depolarization, the action potential, that migrates along the axolemma. In myelinated fibres, because of the high electrical resistance of the lipid in the myelin lamellae, the generation of the action potential is restricted to the region of the nodes of Ranvier. Conduction is therefore saltatory, jumping from one node to the next by local currents that traverse the axon and the extracellular tissue fluid. By this means, conduction velocity is increased from about 1 m/s in unmyelinated axons to 60 to 70 m/s in the largest myelinated fibres in human nerves.

The majority of the synthetic mechanisms in neurones are sited in the cell bodies. Synthesized materials are then transported down the axons to the termination of the fibres by an active transport system. This involves a fast system with a rate of about 400 mm/day, and a slow system, in which the structural proteins travel at 1 to 2 mm/day. The system is bidirectional: apart from the two anterograde fluxes, there is a retrograde system transporting materials, including neurotrophic factors, back from the periphery to the cell body. The retrograde system may be involved in the regulation of protein synthesis in the cell body and probably carries the signal for chromatolysis which ensues on transection.

Disorders of peripheral nerve function can be categorized in terms of the site of the primary disturbance. Conditions that lead to the death of the neurone as a whole, with the loss of the cell body and the axon, are categorized as neuronopathies. Conditions that have a selective effect on axons are termed axonopathies. A selective effect on axonal conduction is seen in poisoning with tetrodotoxin, which blocks the sodium channels at the nodes. Axonopathies may be focal or generalized. Focal axonopathies occur as a result of insults such as trauma or ischaemia. Axonal interruption leads to wallerian-type degeneration below the site of the injury. Recovery has to take place by axonal regeneration which is a slow process: the rate of axonal regeneration is about 1 to 2 mm/day.

Generalized axonopathies often lead to a selective degeneration of the distal portion of the fibres which then extends proximally. The axons are said to 'die back' towards the cell bodies. This pattern is seen in many toxic neuropathies and neuropathies due to nutritional deficiency. It has been suggested that in these conditions the axonal breakdown may result either from interference with enzymes involved in glycolysis which provide the metabolic energy for axonal transport mechanisms, or from cofactor deficiency or inactivation. As the enzymes are synthesized in the cell bodies and then transported down the axons, the further the distance from the cell body the greater will be the likelihood of the occurrence of metabolic insufficiency. This probably accounts for the distal distribution of many such neuropathies, as longer axons will be more vulnerable. Recovery again has to take place by axonal regeneration. In many distal axonopathies that involve the peripheral nervous system, not only does the degeneration affect the distal parts of the motor and sensory axons in the periphery, but the terminal parts of the centrally directed axons derived from the dorsal root ganglion cells also degenerate. Thus degeneration may be found in the rostral portions of the posterior columns. This process has been referred to as central–peripheral distal axonopathy. Neuropathy from iminodipropionitrile blocks the slow axonal transport system and leads to large swellings in the proximal parts of the axons that contain aggregations of neurofilaments (proximal axonopathy).

Other neuropathies primarily affect the myelin, either directly, or through an interference with Schwann cell function. The consequence is a selective demyelination with relative preservation of axonal integrity. This may be restricted to the region of the nodes of Ranvier (paranodal demyelination) or involve whole internodal segments (segmental demyelination) with consequent conduction block. The selective myelin damage may occur, for example, as the result of a cell-mediated attack on myelin by sensitized mononuclear cells, which is the likely explanation of the Guillain–Barré syndrome. Another instance is in diphtheritic neuropathy where the demyelination is considered to be secondary to an interference with Schwann cell protein metabolism. Local compression by a tourniquet also gives rise to selective damage to myelin through mechanical effects, although more severe pressure also causes axonal interruption. In diffuse demyelinating neuropathies, the distribution of the clinical effects, as for distal axonopathies, is often maximal peripherally. Presumably, this is a statistical effect: the longer the nerve fibre, the more likely it is to develop a region of demyelinating conduction block.

Recovery after paranodal or segmental demyelination occurs by remyelination. Initially, the newly formed myelin is thin, which results in an abnormally slow conduction velocity. Such reductions in conduction velocity may be focal, for example in relation to localized myelin damage in entrapment neuropathies, or widespread as in the Guillain–Barré syndrome or the inherited demyelinating neuropathies. In the latter, motor nerve conduction velocity is sometimes reduced to 10 m/s or less.

Finally, in other neuropathies the nerve fibres may be secondarily damaged by processes that primarily affect the connective tissues of nerve or the vasa nervorum. Usually a combination of demyelination and axonal loss occurs.

Clinical categories of neuropathy

Mononeuropathy, multifocal neuropathy, and polyneuropathy

Peripheral neuropathies may be divided into two broad categories depending upon the distribution of the involvement. The first category comprises lesions of isolated peripheral nerves or nerve roots termed mononeuropathy or multiple isolated lesions termed multifocal neuropathy (multiple mononeuropathy or 'mononeuritis multiplex'). The lesions in a widespread multifocal neuropathy may summate to produce a symmetrical disturbance, but the history or a careful examination may indicate the involvement of individual nerves. Isolated or multiple isolated peripheral nerve lesions arise from conditions that produce localized damage, such as mechanical injury, nerve entrapment, thermal, electrical, or radiation injury, vascular causes, granulomatous, neoplastic, or other infiltrations, and nerve tumours.

Secondly, there may be a diffuse and bilaterally symmetrical disturbance of function which can be designated polyneuropathy. When such a process affects the spinal roots, or affects the roots and the peripheral nerve trunks, the terms polyradiculopathy and polyradiculoneuropathy are sometimes employed. In general terms, polyneuropathies result from causes that act diffusely on the peripheral nervous system, such as metabolic disturbances, toxic agents, deficiency states, and certain instances of immune reaction. Isolated nerve lesions may sometimes be superimposed upon a symmetrical polyneuropathy, as a consequence, for example, of pressure lesions in a patient confined to bed. In certain polyneuropathies, there is an abnormal susceptibility to pressure lesions.

Symptomatology

Weakness or paralysis may be due either to conduction block in the motor nerve fibres or to axonal degeneration. Conduction block is related to demyelination with preservation of axonal continuity (neurapraxia). Recovery may occur by remyelination and may be rapid and complete. This can be the situation in localized nerve lesions, for example 'Saturday night' paralysis of the radial nerve, or in more widespread polyneuropathies, such as in acute inflammatory demyelinating polyneuropathy (Guillain–Barré syndrome). If axonal interruption takes place, axonal degeneration occurs below the site of interruption. The muscle weakness is accompanied by denervation atrophy and electromyographic signs of denervation. In a reversible process, recovery has to take place by axonal regeneration which is often slow and incomplete. An important recovery mechanism in conditions in which muscles become partially denervated is reinnervation of denervated muscle fibres by collateral sprouting from the remaining intact axons.

In generalized symmetrical polyneuropathies, the muscle weakness and wasting are commonly peripheral in distribution with an onset in the lower limbs. This results in bilateral footdroop and a 'steppage' gait in which an affected individual lifts his feet to an abnormal extent to avoid catching his toes against the ground. Involvement of the upper limbs begins with weakness and wasting of the small hand muscles and usually weakness of the finger and wrist extensors before the forearm flexor muscles are affected. At times, a symmetrical involvement of the proximal musculature in the limbs occurs in polyneuropathies, for example in the Guillain–Barré syndrome or porphyric neuropathy. Fasciculation due to spontaneous contraction of isolated motor units is most often a feature of anterior horn cell disease but may be encountered in peripheral neuropathies, as may muscle cramps. Postural tremor, mainly affecting the upper limbs and resembling essential tremor, may be seen in patients with chronic demyelinating polyneuropathies with slow conduction velocity. This 'neuropathic tremor' is most often encountered in type I hereditary motor and sensory neuropathy, chronic inflammatory demyelinating polyneuropathy, and IgM paraproteinaemic neuropathy. A rare manifestation of peripheral neuropathy is the occurrence of continuous repetitive discharges in motor nerve fibres leading to generalized muscular rigidity or 'neuromyotonia' (Isaacs' syndrome, continuous motor unit activity syndrome).

Loss of the tendon reflexes is a frequent accompaniment of a peripheral neuropathy, and usually first affects the ankle jerks. In assessing the clinical findings, it is important to remember that the ankle jerks may be lost in later life, probably as a result of senile changes in the peripheral nerves.

Sensory symptoms and sensory loss in symmetrical polyneuropathies are usually distal in distribution, giving rise to the 'glove and stocking' pattern of involvement. Only rarely is a proximal pattern encountered. The sensory loss may affect all modalities or be restricted to certain forms of sensation. If the loss is restricted, two broad patterns are discernible. In the first, the impairment predominantly affects the sense of joint position and vibration and touch–pressure sensibility, corresponding to a predominant loss of function in the larger myelinated nerve fibres. Sensory ataxia is the salient manifestation in 'large fibre' sensory neuropathies. Loss of postural sensibility may lead to sensory ataxia in the limbs and to 'pseudoathetosis', that is, involuntary movements, most often of the fingers and hands, that occur, for example, when a patient holds their arms outstretched with their eyes closed. In the second pattern of selective sensory loss, pain and temperature sensibility are predominantly affected, often associated with loss of autonomic function, corresponding to a predominant loss of small myelinated and unmyelinated axons. 'Trophic changes' and pain may complicate such small fibre neuropathies. The most important factor in their genesis is the loss of the protective effect of pain sensation with the consequent development of persistent ulceration or more extensive tissue loss, most commonly in the feet, and neuropathic joint degeneration.

Paraesthesiae are a frequent feature in peripheral neuropathy. These are usually of a tingling nature ('pins and needles'), but, especially in 'small fibre' neuropathies, may involve thermal sensations, most often with a burning quality. The paraesthesiae may be aggravated by touching or stroking the skin. Stimuli that are normally not painful may acquire an unpleasant quality (allodynia) and painful stimuli may give rise to an excessive or hyperpathic response, in which the stimulus, for example a pinprick, is abnormally intense. With repeated stimulation at the same site, the pain that is felt may spread widely and reach an intolerable intensity. An unusual symptom encountered most often in uraemic neuropathy is that of 'restless legs' (Ekbom's syndrome). Affected individuals experience sensations in the feet and legs that they find difficult to describe but which are temporarily relieved by movement of the feet and legs. 'Ekbom's syndrome' may also occur in the absence of any detectable disease process.

Spontaneous pains of an aching or lancinating character may complicate a number of generalized polyneuropathies. Severe paroxysms of lancinating pain occur in trigeminal neuralgia, but here the responsible lesion may well lie within the central nervous system. Causalgia constitutes a particularly troublesome painful syndrome, most often following gunshot wounds injuring the median nerve, the lower trunk of the brachial plexus, or the tibial nerve. It is a severe persistent pain, often with a burning quality that is characteristically aggravated by emotional factors. Sympathectomy relieves a high proportion of such cases.

Disturbances of autonomic function are occasionally the salient abnormality in a peripheral neuropathy, as in the Riley–Day syndrome, or they may accompany other manifestations, and can be observed both with localized peripheral nerve lesions and in generalized neuropathies.

Diagnosis and investigation

The history and physical examination frequently indicate that the disturbance has affected the peripheral nerves. If confirmation is required, this may usually be obtained by nerve conduction studies. Conduction may be examined in motor and sensory nerve fibres, and can give evidence of both localized and generalized neuropathies. Severely reduced conduction velocity may occur as a result of segmental demyelination or because of conduction in regenerating axons of small calibre after axonal degeneration.

Examination of the cerebrospinal fluid is not commonly of value in the diagnosis of peripheral neuropathies, although the substantially elevated protein content that often occurs in the Guillain–Barré syndrome may be helpful, as may inflammatory changes in some neuropathies.

Nerve biopsy is rarely required in establishing the existence of a peripheral neuropathy, but may be of diagnostic value in establishing the cause of the neuropathy, particularly in conditions that affect the vasa nervorum or neural connective tissues, in some 'storage' disorders and in inflammatory demyelinating neuropathies.

Individual nerves

Phrenic nerve (C2–C4)

This nerve innervates the diaphragm. When the diaphragm is totally paralysed, the normal protrusion of the upper abdomen during inspiration is lost, or is replaced by retraction (paradoxical movement). Radiographically, paralysis may be detected by unilateral or bilateral elevation of the diaphragm in a chest radiograph and its failure to descend on inspiration. The phrenic nerve may be involved in its course through the neck or thorax by wounds or tumours such as bronchial carcinoma, and it is sometimes affected in idiopathic brachial plexus neuropathy (neuralgic amyotrophy).

Nerve to serratus anterior (C5–C7)

The serratus anterior acts as a fixator of the scapula, holding the scapula against the chest wall when forward pressure is exerted by the arm. It is involved in forward movement of the shoulder as in a rapier thrust and in elevation of the arm, when it rotates the scapula. When serratus anterior is paralysed in isolation, the position of the scapula is normal at rest but if the extended arm is pushed forwards against resistance, 'winging' of the scapula becomes evident. The vertebral border, particularly in its lower portion, stands away from the chest wall. The nerve to serratus anterior may be involved in penetrating wounds, but usually in association with damage to the brachial plexus. It may be injured by forcible depression of the shoulder. Serratus anterior weakness is a common component of idiopathic brachial plexus neuropathy (neuralgic amyotrophy) and it is not infrequently encountered as an isolated and unexplained lesion.

Brachial plexus

The brachial plexus may be affected by penetrating wounds of the neck, in fractures and dislocations of the shoulder and clavicle, as a result of traction on the arm, by pressure from an aneurysm or a cervical rib, and by neoplastic involvement.

Traction lesions

Traction on the arm may result in damage to the plexus itself or may lead to avulsion of the spinal roots from the cord. If the roots are avulsed, sensory nerve action potentials will be preserved if recorded from affected fingers despite total anaesthesia, and the histamine flare response will be preserved in anaesthetized skin. This follows from the fact that the nerve fibres are interrupted proximal to the dorsal root ganglia and therefore the peripheral sensory axons do not degenerate.

In severe traction lesions, commonly encountered in current medical practice as a result of motorcycle or aircraft accidents, the whole of the plexus may be damaged. With forcible downward displacement of the shoulder, as when someone is thrown forwards and the shoulder strikes against an obstacle, only the upper part of the plexus, involving the contribution from the fifth and sixth cervical nerve roots, may be damaged. This may also be encountered as a birth injury from traction on the head, or on the trunk in a breech presentation (Erb's palsy), and rarely in anaesthetized patients during operation or in individuals carrying heavy rucksacks. Selective injury to the lower part of the plexus involving the contributions from the eighth cervical and first thoracic nerve roots occurs as a result of traction with the arm extended, as when an individual falls from a height and tries to save himself by hanging on to a ledge. It may also occur as a birth injury following traction with the arm extended (Klumpke's paralysis), but is less common than upper plexus damage.

Selective damage to the upper portion of the plexus (C5 and C6 roots or upper trunk) results in paralysis of deltoid, biceps, brachialis, brachioradialis, and sometimes supraspinatus, infraspinatus, and subscapularis. If the roots are avulsed from the cord, the rhomboids, serratus anterior, levator scapulae, and the scalene muscles will be affected. The arm hangs at the side, internally rotated at the shoulder, with the elbow extended and the forearm pronated in the 'waiter's tip' position. Abduction at the shoulder and flexion at the elbow are not possible. The biceps and brachioradialis jerks are lost. Sensory loss affects the lateral aspect of the shoulder and upper arm and the radial border of the forearm. Selective paralysis of the lower brachial plexus (C8, T1) results in paralysis of all the intrinsic hand muscles and a consequent claw-hand deformity, weakness of the medial finger and wrist flexors, and sensory loss along the medial border of the forearm and hand and over the medial two fingers. Cervical sympathetic paralysis, giving rise to Horner's syndrome, is frequently associated.

When the spinal roots are avulsed from the cord, regeneration is impossible and intractable spontaneous pain may be a highly troublesome sequel. Where the injury is distal to the dorsal root ganglia, lesions of the upper portion of the brachial plexus recover more satisfactorily than lower plexus lesions. The value of surgical repair is still a controversial issue. In the Erb's form of birth injury, weakness of abduction at the shoulder and flexion at the elbow often persist, although there may be little residual sensory loss. Full recovery takes place in about a third of the cases. It is less likely to occur with lower plexus injuries or if the whole plexus is involved. Early recognition and the application of measures to reduce the risk of joint contractures are important. Surgical treatment is of limited value.

Thoracic outlet syndromes

The contribution of the eighth cervical and first thoracic roots to the brachial plexus may be damaged by angulation over an abnormal rib or, more usually, a fibrous band arising from the seventh cervical vertebra and attached to the first rib. Although local structures such as the tendon of scalenus anterior may be involved in the production of symptoms, the isolation of a separate 'scalenus anterior syndrome' or of 'costoclavicular compression' is not justified. The subclavian artery may be affected by cervical ribs giving rise to aneurysmal dilatation and vascular symptoms such as Raynaud's syndrome and embolic phenomena, but the simultaneous occurrence of both neural and vascular phenomena is rare.

Damage to the lower part of the brachial plexus leads to weakness and wasting of the small hand muscles, and of the medial forearm wrist and finger flexors. Occasionally, there is selective wasting of the thenar pad in the hand, mimicking to some extent the appearances of the carpal tunnel syndrome. Numbness, pain, and paraesthesiae occur along the inner border of the forearm and hand, extending into the medial two fingers. The pain tends to be provoked by carrying heavy articles with the hand on the affected side. Horner's syndrome may be a feature. Nerve conduction studies are helpful when there are difficulties in distinguishing a cervical rib syndrome from a lesion of the ulnar or median nerves on clinical grounds.

Surgical removal of the rib or fibrous band often leads to abolition of the pain and paraesthesiae, but recovery of power in the small hand muscles is usually disappointing.

Neoplastic involvement

Tumours may arise locally in the brachial plexus, such as neurofibromata in von Recklinghausen's disease (type I neurofibromatosis) or a solitary neurinoma, or the plexus may be invaded by tumours arising in other structures. In the latter case the commonest situation is involvement of the lower part of the plexus by an apical carcinoma of the lung (Pancoast's syndrome), which gives rise to wasting and weakness of the small hand muscles and of the medial forearm wrist and finger flexors, pain and sensory loss affecting the medial border of the forearm and hand, and cervical sympathetic paralysis. Other tumours that may invade the brachial plexus include carcinoma of the breast and malignant lymphomas affecting the lymph glands in the root of the neck.

Neuralgic amyotrophy

This condition was not clearly differentiated from the other painful paralytic disorders of the shoulder and upper arm, such as root compression from disc prolapse, until the Second World War. It has been described in a variety of terms, including 'idiopathic brachial plexus neuropathy' and 'paralytic brachial neuritis'. It may follow immunizing procedures, in particular the administration of antitetanus serum or operations, or occur without recognizable antecedent event. It can occur on a genetic basis as an autosomal dominant disorder, hereditary neuralgic amyotrophy (HNA), with variable penetrance. This has been mapped to chromosome 17p.

The disorder develops acutely with intense pain in the shoulder region which may take some weeks before it subsides completely although generally it ceases after a few days. Paralysis of the muscles of the shoulder girdle becomes evident within a day or two of the onset of the pain, sometimes also of the arms or of the diaphragm. It may be unilateral or bilateral and may be associated with sensory loss. More distal upper limb muscles may at times be affected, as may the phrenic nerve, and, occasionally, the recurrent laryngeal nerve. The cerebrospinal fluid is consistently normal. The affected muscles show electromyographic evidence of denervation. Recovery is usually ultimately satisfactory. Not all cases recover fully and recurrences may occur. A comparable disorder can affect the lumbosacral plexus (idiopathic lumbosacral plexus neuritis).

The pattern of muscle involvement and sensory disturbances suggests that the neuralgic myotrophy affects the brachial plexus in a patchy manner. An immune reaction is assumed but not established. The condition takes the same course whether or not it follows an immunizing procedure. Corticosteroids do not influence either the initial pain or the ultimate outcome.

Post-irradiation brachial plexus neuropathy

Brachial plexus damage may occur as a sequel to radiotherapy for breast carcinoma or tumours in the neck. The onset of symptoms is usually several years after treatment, but may be within months. It can be difficult to distinguish from tumour recurrence but is less likely to be painful. Magnetic resonance imaging may be helpful in diagnosis.

Radial nerve (C5–C8)

The long course of the radial nerve and its position in relation to the humerus make this nerve unusually susceptible to external compression. It is a continuation of the posterior cord of the brachial plexus. In the upper arm it supplies triceps and anconeus and the skin on the back of the arm just above the elbow through the posterior cutaneous nerve of the arm. The lateral aspect of the lower part of the upper arm is supplied by the lower lateral brachial cutaneous branch and the dorsal aspect of the forearm by the posterior cutaneous nerve of the forearm. Muscular branches of the radial nerve innervate brachioradialis and extensor carpi radialis longus and brevis. The superficial branch of the nerve is its continuation. It descends along the radial border of the forearm and supplies the skin over the dorsum of the hand and the thumb, index, and middle fingers. The deep branch posterior interosseus nerve winds around the lateral aspect of the radius, passes through supinator, which it supplies, and innervates extensor digitorum, extensor digiti minimi, extensor carpi ulnaris, and often extensor carpi radialis brevis, abductor pollicis longus, extensor pollicis longus and brevis, and extensor indicis.

The nerve may be injured in wounds of the axilla so that the paralysis includes triceps, resulting in loss of extension at the elbow. The most frequent type of injury is compression of the nerve in the middle third of the arm against the humerus. This is encountered as 'Saturday night paralysis' in which an individual falls asleep when intoxicated with their upper arm over the arm of a chair. Triceps is spared, but brachioradialis, supinator, and all the forearm extensor muscles are paralysed. Sensory impairment is limited to the dorsum of the hand. Commonly the lesion consists of a localized conduction block (neurapraxia) so that muscle wasting does not occur and a muscle response can be obtained on electrical stimulation of the nerve below the level of the lesion. Recovery is complete within a matter of weeks. A cock-up wrist splint may be helpful while recovery is awaited. At times, there is some associated axonal degeneration so that electromyographic evidence of denervation is detectable and full recovery is correspondingly delayed.

Many muscles not supplied by the radial nerve work at a disadvantage when the wrist and finger extensors are paralysed. These defects must not be mistaken for signs of injury to other nerves. Owing to the flexed position of the wrist, gripping is impaired, but if the power of the wrist and finger flexors is tested with the wrist extended, it can be shown to be normal. The action of the interossei in abducting and adducting the fingers is also feeble when the wrist is flexed, but full power is demonstrable if these muscles are tested with the hand resting flat on a table.

A lesion of the posterior interosseus nerve gives rise to weakness confined to abduction and extension of the thumb and extension of the index finger. Supinator is spared, together with brachioradialis and the radial wrist extensors, and there is no sensory loss. The nerve may be compressed under the arcade of Frohse or during its transit through supinator.

Axillary nerve (C5, C6)

This is a branch of the posterior cord of the brachial plexus. It supplies deltoid and teres minor and the skin over deltoid through the upper lateral brachial cutaneous nerve. It may be damaged in injuries to the shoulder and the chief symptom is an almost complete inability to raise the arm at the shoulder. In the past, it was sometimes injured by pressure from a crutch ('crutch palsy').

Musculocutaneous nerve (C5, C6)

This nerve is rarely damaged alone, but may be involved in injuries to the brachial plexus. It supplies coracobrachialis, biceps, and brachialis and the skin over the lateral aspect of the forearm through the lateral cutaneous nerve of the forearm. Flexion at the elbow is still possible by brachioradialis, but is weak, and sensation may be impaired along the radial border of the forearm.

Median nerve (C6–C8, T_1)

The median nerve arises from the medial and lateral cords of the brachial plexus and descends with the brachial artery through the upper arm, entering the forearm deep to the bicipital aponeurosis. It has no muscular branches above the elbow. It supplies all the muscles in the anterior aspect of the forearm except flexor carpi ulnaris and the medial half of flexor digitorum profundus. The main trunk of the nerve supplies pronator teres, flexor carpi radialis, palmaris longus, and flexor digitorum superficialis. Through the anterior interosseus branch, it also supplies the lateral aspect of flexor digitorum profundus, flexor pollicis longus, and pronator quadratus. The main trunk passes deep to the flexor retinaculum of the wrist and its recurrent muscular branch supplies abductor pollicis brevis, opponens pollicis, and contributes to the innervation of flexor pollicis brevis. It also supplies the lateral two lumbrical muscles and the skin of the lateral aspect of the palm and the lateral three and a half digits over their palmar aspects and terminal parts of their dorsal aspects.

Lesions in the forearm

The median nerve may be injured in the region of the elbow or compressed at the level of the pronator teres muscle. Entrapment neuropathies in the upper forearm, however, are uncommon. Occasionally the anterior interosseus branch is involved in isolation.

Complete lesions of the median nerve at the elbow give rise to paralysis of pronator teres, the radial flexor of the wrist, the long finger flexors except the ulnar half of the deep flexor, most of the muscles of the thenar eminence, and the two radial lumbricals. In brief, there is an inability to flex the index finger and the distal phalanx of the thumb, flexion of the middle finger is weak, and opposition of the thumb is defective. The appearance of the hand has been described as simian; it shows ulnar deviation, the index and middle fingers are more extended than normal, and the thumb lies in the same plane as the fingers.

In more detail, pronation is incomplete and defective. The patient attempts to overcome this by rotating the whole limb at the shoulder. Paralysis of the wrist flexors is evident when attempts are made to flex against resistance. The tendon of flexor carpi ulnaris stands out alone and the hand goes into ulnar deviation. Flexion of the fingers is good in the ulnar two fingers, although weaker than normal. The index finger cannot be flexed, and the middle finger only incompletely. Flexion at the metacarpophalangeal joints is possible in all fingers, including the index, and flexion at these joints with extension at the interphalangeal joints is accomplished by the interossei and lumbricals. If the proximal phalanx of the thumb is immobilized, it will be found that flexion of the terminal phalanx is abolished because of paralysis of flexor pollicis longus. Paralysis of the thenar muscles gives rise to defective abduction and opposition of the thumb. By means of the adductor, the thumb can be drawn into the palm, but as the radial fingers cannot be flexed or the thumb opposed, it is impossible to place the tip of the thumb on the fingers.

Sensory loss is evident over the lateral three and a half digits and the lateral aspect of the palm, although individual variations occur. There is almost complete anaesthesia over the two terminal phalanges of the index and middle fingers. This degree of sensory loss, combined with the motor deficit, renders the thumb and index fingers almost useless and makes paralysis of the median the most serious single nerve lesion in the upper limb.

Vasomotor and trophic changes often ensue. The skin in the distribution of the median nerve tends to become reddened, dry, and atrophic. The pulp of the affected fingers becomes atrophic and ulceration occasionally develops in the tip of the index finger. The nails may become white and atrophic.

After a total transection of the nerve in the region of the elbow, even with a satisfactory surgical repair, recovery is slow and rarely complete, particularly with respect to the innervation of the hand.

With partial lesions of the median nerve in the arm or forearm, causalgia may be a troublesome consequence. This most often follows gunshot wounds. The pain develops at any time from a few hours to 45 days after the injury. The pain is severe and unremitting, frequently of a burning or smarting quality. Upon this may be superimposed severe paroxysms of pain provoked by touching or jarring the limb or by emotional factors. Vasomotor and sudomotor changes may be associated. The skin usually becomes dry and scaly, but excessive sweating may be a feature. The patient adopts a protective attitude towards the limb, so that fixation of the joints of the fingers and wrist may develop, together with atrophic changes in the skin and subcutaneous tissue. About 80 per cent of cases of true causalgia are relieved by sympathectomy. Untreated, the pain gradually subsides over months or years.

Lesions at the wrist

The superficial situation of the median nerve at the wrist renders it liable to injury in lacerations sustained by falling against a window with the hand outstretched or in suicidal attempts. It may also be damaged as an occupational hazard by individuals who exert repeated pressure on the butt of the hand.

Much the most common lesion at this site is the carpal tunnel syndrome, in which the median nerve is compressed as it passes deep to the flexor retinaculum. The usual presentation is with acroparaesthesiae. These consist of numbness, tingling, and burning sensations felt in the hand and fingers, the pain sometimes radiating up the forearm as far as the elbow or even as high as the shoulder or root of the neck. The paraesthesiae are sometimes restricted to the radial fingers, but may affect all the digits as some fibres from the median nerve are distributed to the fifth finger through a communication with the ulnar nerve in the palm. The attacks of pain and paraesthesiae are most common at night and often wake the patient from sleep. They are then relieved by shaking the hand. The hand tends to feel numb and useless on waking in the morning but recovers after it has been used for some minutes. The symptoms may recur during the day following use, or at times if the patient sits with the hands immobile. Such symptoms of acroparaesthesiae may persist for many years without the appearance of symptoms of median nerve damage. In other patients, weakness of the thenar muscles develops, particularly of abduction of the thumb, and is associated with atrophy of the lateral aspect of the thenar eminence (Fig. 1). Sensory loss may appear over the tips of the median innervated fingers. Occasionally patients present with symptoms of median nerve deficit in the hand without attacks of acroparaesthesiae having occurred, or motor and sensory signs may be discovered incidentally in the absence of symptoms, particularly in older individuals.

The symptoms are usually characteristic. If confirmation is required in atypical cases, this can generally be obtained by nerve conduction studies. In patients who are experiencing frequent attacks of acroparaesthesiae, the symptoms may be reproduced by inflating a sphygmomanometer cuff around the arm above arterial pressure for 2 min. At times percussion over the carpal tunnel may elicit a Tinel's sign, or symptoms may be provoked by hyperextension of the wrist or sustained flexion (Phalen's sign).

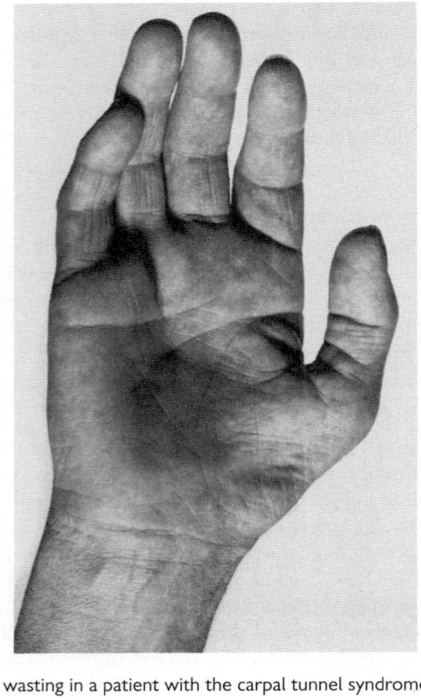

Fig. 1 Thenar wasting in a patient with the carpal tunnel syndrome.

The majority of cases occur in middle-aged and often obese housewives. In younger women it is commonly associated with excessive use of the hands, and it may develop in males after unaccustomed use of the hands, such as in house painting or fly fishing. In these instances, tenosynovitis of the flexor tendons is responsible. It may also be caused by tuberculous tenosynovitis at the wrist or involvement of the wrist joint in rheumatoid arthritis. It may develop as a consequence of osteoarthritis of the carpus, perhaps related to an old fracture. Other predisposing causes are pregnancy, myxoedema, acromegaly, and infiltration of the flexor retinaculum in primary and hereditary amyloidosis.

In cases in which muscle weakness and wasting, or sensory loss, are present when the patient is first seen, treatment should be decompression of the nerve by section of the flexor retinaculum. In patients with acroparaesthesiae alone and in which the cause is probably tenosynovitis at the wrist, reduction in the amount of activity engaged in with the hands may be sufficient to allow the symptoms to subside. Injection of the carpal tunnel with a long-acting corticosteroid preparation may give temporary relief. Splinting of the wrist to reduce movement during the day may also be useful. If the symptoms persist despite conservative measures, decompression is then advisable.

The majority of patients with acroparaesthesiae are relieved by decompression. In patients with sensory impairment and cutaneous hyperaesthesia, such symptoms may persist for prolonged periods despite decompression. If denervation of the thenar muscles has been present for a long time, full recovery may not occur.

Ulnar nerve (C7, C8, T1)

This nerve arises from the medial cord of the plexus, usually with a contribution from the lateral cord. It descends in the medial side of the upper arm, passes around the elbow in the ulnar groove, and enters the forearm under an aponeurotic band between the humeral and ulnar heads of flexor carpi ulnaris. It then runs superficial to flexor digitorum profundus to the wrist and enters the hand between the pisiform bone and the hook of the hamate, superficial to the flexor retinaculum. After penetrating the hypothenar muscles, its deep branch crosses the palm and ends in flexor pollicis brevis.

In the upper arm, branches arise that supply flexor carpi ulnaris and the medial part of flexor digitorum profundus. In the forearm, the dorsal branch arises that winds around the ulna and supplies the skin over the dorsal aspect of the hand and the medial one and a half fingers. In the hand, a superficial branch supplies palmaris brevis and the skin over the medial aspect of the palm and the medial one and half fingers. The deep branch, after supplying the hypothenar muscles, innervates the interossei, the third and fourth lumbricals, adductor pollicis, and part of flexor pollicis brevis.

Lesions at the elbow

Total paralysis from lesions at this level, including the branches to flexor carpi ulnaris and flexor digitorum profundus, gives rise to wasting along the medial side of the forearm flexor mass. There is weakness of flexion of the fourth and fifth fingers. If the proximal portions of these fingers are held immobilized, flexion of the terminal phalanges is not possible. When the hand is flexed to the ulnar side against resistance, the tendon of flexor carpi ulnaris is not palpable. Paralysis of the hypothenar muscles abolishes abduction of the fifth finger. Paralysis of the interossei and the medial two lumbricals gives rise to the 'claw hand' deformity (Fig. 2). The action of these muscles is to flex the fingers at the metacarpophalangeal joints with the fingers extended at the interphalangeal joints. In the claw hand, the posture of the fingers is opposite to this, namely, extension of the metacarpophalangeal joints with flexion at the interphalangeal joints. Although all the interossei are paralysed, the defect is seen mainly in the ulnar fingers since the radial lumbricals supplied by the median nerve are still active. The long extensors of the fingers, being unopposed, overextend the proximal joints, and the flexor digitorum superficialis flexes the proximal interphalangeal joints.

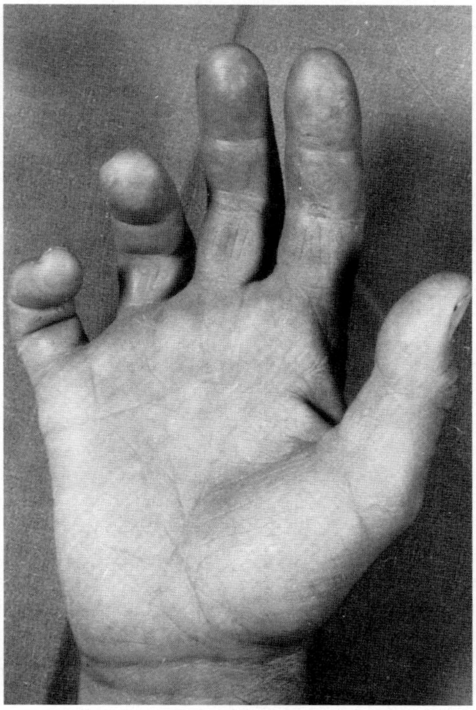

Fig. 2 'Claw hand' deformity in a patient with an ulnar nerve lesion.

In the hand, there is wasting of the hypothenar muscles, of the interossei, and of the medial part of the thenar eminence. Movements of abduction and adduction of the fingers are weak, as is adduction to the extended thumb against the palm. Sensory loss affects the dorsal and palmar aspects of the medial side of the hand and the medial one and a half fingers.

The ulnar nerve may be damaged by dislocations or fracture dislocations at the elbow and is sometimes compressed in individuals who habitually lean on their elbows. Entrapment may occur in the cubital tunnel as the nerve underlies the aponeurotic band between the two heads of the flexor carpi ulnaris. This is most likely to occur in those performing heavy manual work or if there is an excessive carrying angle at the elbow, as may occur following a previous malunited supracondylar fracture of the humerus ('tardy ulnar palsy'). The medial wall of the cubital tunnel is formed by the elbow joint; osteoarthritis of the elbow can lead to osteophytic encroachment on the tunnel and compression of the ulnar nerve. In the cubital tunnel syndrome, the ulnar nerve is often palpably enlarged in the ulnar groove and for a short distance proximally. Ulnar nerve lesions are not infrequent in leprosy. Here the enlargement of the nerve tends to be maximal at a little distance above the elbow.

When it is suspected that the nerve has been subjected to repeated compression at the elbow, surgical transposition to the front of the medial epicondyle should be considered. If the nerve is compressed in the cubital tunnel, decompression by slitting the aponeurosis may suffice.

Lesions at the wrist or in the hand

Damage to the nerve at the wrist will spare the dorsal branch, so that cutaneous sensation over the dorsum of the hand and fingers is spared. A lesion just proximal to the wrist will give rise to sensory impairment on the palmar aspect of the hand and fingers alone, and weakness of all the ulnar-innervated intrinsic hand muscles. A slightly more distal lesion spares the superficial branch of the nerve and therefore produces no sensory deficit. Finally, damage to the deep palmar branch spares the hypothenar muscles, but causes weakness of the other ulnar-innervated small hand muscles. Lesions at the wrist or in the hand are usually the result of compression by ganglia or by repeated occupational trauma. Damage to the deep palmar branch, for example, may be caused by firm pressure in the palm from a screwdriver or drill. If occupational pressure is the cause, recovery follows cessation of the precipitating cause. Should improvement fail to occur after an appropriate interval, surgical exploration to establish whether a ganglion is present is merited.

It is not always easy on clinical grounds to decide whether the lesion is at the elbow or the wrist. Compression of the nerve in the cubital tunnel, for example, may spare the branches to the flexor carpi ulnaris and flexor digitorum profundus. In these circumstances, nerve conduction studies may be helpful, as they may in distinguishing between lesions of the ulnar nerve and damage to the eighth cervical and first thoracic spinal roots.

Lumbosacral plexus

Lesions of the lumbosacral plexus are not common. The plexus may be involved in pelvic malignancy, such as from carcinoma of the uterine cervix, bladder, prostate, or rectum, or be the site of a local neural tumour. It may be compressed by a haematoma in patients receiving anticoagulant therapy or suffering from haemophilia, or be involved in fractures of the pelvis. The lumbosacral cord may be compressed against the rim of the pelvis by the fetal head during parturition, with consequent weakness of the anterior tibial and peroneal muscles, and sensory impairment in the distribution of the fourth and fifth lumbar dermatomes. The superior gluteal nerve may also be affected. Recovery is initially good but may not be complete. The plexus may be affected in diabetic amyotrophy. Rare instances of idiopathic lumbosacral plexus neuropathy are encountered, comparable to the corresponding disorder that affects the brachial plexus.

Femoral nerve (L2–L4)

This nerve arises from the lumbar plexus, crosses the iliac fossa between the psoas and iliacus muscles, and enters the thigh deep to the middle of the inguinal ligament. In the iliac fossa it supplies the iliacus, and in the thigh, pectineus, sartorius, and quadriceps femoris, and anterior cutaneous branches to the front of the thigh. The continuation of the femoral nerve is the saphenous which supplies the skin over the medial aspect of the lower leg as far as the medial malleolus.

Damage to the femoral nerve causes weakness of knee extension, wasting of quadriceps, loss of the knee jerk, and sensory impairment over the front of the thigh and in the distribution of the saphenous nerve. With a proximal lesion, there may also be weakness of hip flexion from paralysis of iliacus.

The femoral nerve may be injured in fractures of the pelvis or femur, in dislocations of the hip, and at times during operations on the hip. It may be involved by psoas abscesses, tumours, or implicated in wounds of the thigh. It is commonly involved in large psoas muscle haematomas in haemophiliacs (see Section 22) and in diabetic amyotrophy. Owing to the rapid dispersion of the branches in the thigh, partial lesions are common from wounds at this site. The nerve to quadriceps is most often injured. The resulting paralysis causes considerable difficulty in walking as the knee cannot be locked in extension and gives way, especially when descending stairs. The saphenous nerve is sometimes damaged in operations for the treatment of varicose veins.

Obturator nerve (L2–L4)

The nerve emerges from the lateral border of psoas, crosses the lateral wall of the pelvis, and enters the thigh through the obturator foramen where it supplies gracilis, adductor longus and brevis, adductor magnus, obturator externus, and sometimes also pectineus, and the skin over the lower medial aspect of the thigh.

Damage to the obturator nerve results in weakness of adduction and internal rotation at the hip, pain in the groin, and sensory impairment on the medial part of the thigh. The nerve may be involved in neoplastic infiltration in the pelvis and can be damaged by the fetal head or by forceps during parturition.

Lateral cutaneous nerve of the thigh (L2, L3)

This nerve arises from the lumbar plexus, passes obliquely across iliacus and enters the thigh under the lateral part of the inguinal ligament. It supplies the skin over the anterolateral aspect of the thigh.

Meralgia paraesthetica is an entrapment neuropathy resulting from compression of this nerve as it passes under the inguinal ligament. It is more common in men, who are often obese, and may be unilateral or bilateral. The symptoms consist of numbness in the territory of the nerve combined with tingling or burning paraesthesiae provoked by prolonged standing, or following excessive walking. Weight loss may be helpful, and in many instances the condition subsides spontaneously. Decompression of the nerve is rarely necessary.

Sciatic nerve (L4, L5, S1–S3)

The sciatic nerve enters the thigh through the sciatic notch. It is composed of the tibial and peroneal divisions which are usually bound together within a common sheath, the tibial division lying medially. It descends through the posterior aspect of the thigh, initially deep to gluteus maximus, and supplies semitendinosus, semimembranosus, and the long head of biceps through its peroneal division. It separates into the tibial and common peroneal nerves in the lower thigh, which supply all the muscles below the knee, and both nerves contribute to the formation of the sural nerve.

Total interruption of the sciatic nerve gives rise to foot drop. Walking is possible, but the patient cannot stand on the toes or the heel of the affected foot and the ankle is unstable. All movement below the knee is paralysed. If the injury is in the upper thigh, flexion of the knee is also weak. The skin is completely anaesthetized over the entire foot except for the medial border which is supplied by the saphenous nerve. Pressure sores may develop. The anaesthesia extends upwards on the posterolateral aspect of the calf in its lower two-thirds. The sense of joint position is abolished in the foot and toes. Beyond this area of complete anaesthesia, there is a wide zone in which sensibility may be diminished. Sweating is absent on the sole and dorsum of the foot, but is preserved on the medial side. The ankle jerk is lost but the knee jerk is retained.

The sciatic nerve may be involved in pelvic tumours and can be injured by fractures of the pelvis or femur or during hip replacement operations. After the radial and ulnar, it is implicated in gunshot wounds more frequently than any other nerve. Partial injury of the tibial division may be followed by causalgia. Incomplete lesions of the nerve may be caused by pressure of the nerve against the hard edge of a chair in individuals who fall asleep while intoxicated. Similar lesions may occur in diabetic subjects, in whom the peripheral nerves are more susceptible to pressure neuropathy.

The syndrome of root pain and sciatica is considered in Chapter 24.3.11.

Tibial nerve (L4, L5, S1–S3)

After separating from the peroneal division of the sciatic nerve in the lower thigh, this nerve passes through the popliteal fossa and enters the calf deep to gastrocnemius through the fibrous arch of soleus. It descends through the calf to the medial side of the ankle, passes beneath the flexor retinaculum, and divides into the medial and lateral plantar nerves. It supplies popliteus, all the muscles of the calf, and, through the plantar nerves, the small muscles of the sole of the foot and sensation to the sole.

When the nerve is interrupted, the patient is unable to plantarflex or invert the foot, to flex the toes, or to stand on the ball of the foot. Paralysis of the interossei leads to a claw-like deformity of the toes. Sensation is lost over the sole. Causalgia may arise after partial lesions. Injury to the distal portion of the nerve by a penetrating injury or deep wound of the calf gives rise to paralysis of the intrinsic muscles of the foot but spares the muscles acting at the ankle. Sensation is lost on the sole of the foot and this may be accompanied by pain. If the injury is distal to the origin of the branches to flexor hallucis longus and flexor digitorum longus, the lesion may escape detection since paralysis of the small foot muscles and sensory loss over the sole may be overlooked.

The tibial nerve is occasionally compressed under the flexor retinaculum (tarsal tunnel syndrome), usually precipitated by osteoarthritis or post-traumatic deformities at the ankle or by tenosynovitis. Burning pain and tingling paraesthesiae occur in the sole, usually following prolonged standing or walking. The condition is generally unilateral. Careful examination may demonstrate wasting of the intrinsic muscles in the medial aspect of the foot, and sensory impairment over the sole. Nerve conduction studies may be helpful diagnostically. Treatment is by surgical section of the flexor retinaculum.

Painful neuromas sometimes develop on the digital branches of the plantar nerves. These give rise to the syndrome of Morton's metatarsalgia in which pain occurs in the anterior part of the foot on standing. A localized area of tenderness is detectable on palpation. The condition is relieved by excision of the neuroma.

Common peroneal nerve (L4, L5, S1, S2)

After separating from the tibial division of the sciatic nerve in the lower part of the thigh, this nerve descends through the popliteal fossa, winds around the neck of the fibula, and divides into its superficial and deep branches. The superficial peroneal nerve passes down in front of the fibula, supplies peroneus longus and brevis, and emerges in the lower leg, supplying the skin on the lateral aspect of the lower leg. It crosses the extensor retinaculum and supplies the skin on the dorsum of the foot and the second to the fifth toes. The deep peroneal branch continues to wind around the fibula, pierces the anterior intermuscular septum, and descends on the anterior interosseous membrane. It innervates tibialis anterior, extensor digitorum longus, extensor hallucis longus, and peroneus tertius. It passes deep to the extensor retinaculum after which it supplies the extensor digitorum brevis and the skin of the adjacent sides of the first and second toes.

Damage to the common peroneal nerve is more frequent than injury to its two branches because of its vulnerable superficial position at the neck of the fibula. It gives rise to foot drop with paralysis of dorsiflexion and eversion at the ankle and of toe extension. Cutaneous sensation is impaired over the lateral aspect of the lower leg and ankle and on the dorsum of the foot.

The common peroneal nerve may be compressed at the neck of the fibula by habitual sitting with the legs crossed, prolonged squatting, pressure during sleep or while anaesthetized, and various other events. It can be damaged by traction caused by fractures of the tibia and fibula and is sometimes damaged by ischaemia in the anterior tibial compartment syndrome. Paralysis caused by external pressure frequently gives rise to a local conduction block (neurapraxia) with satisfactory recovery within a few weeks. If electromyography indicates that nerve degeneration has taken place a foot drop support should be provided while axonal regeneration is awaited.

Sural nerve (L5, S1–S2)

This arises from the sciatic nerve and descends to the back of the calf, winds around to the lateral side of the ankle, and reaches the lateral border of the foot. It supplies the skin in this distribution. Sensory impairment occasionally results from pressure on the nerve as it lies in a superficial situation in the back of the calf.

Generalized neuropathies

Neuropathies related to metabolic and endocrine disorders

Diabetes mellitus

A significant degree of peripheral neuropathy develops in about 15 per cent of patients with diabetes, although a substantially greater number either have minor symptoms without signs, or evidence of a subclinical neuropathy either on clinical examination or on the basis of abnormalities of nerve conduction. In general, the neuropathies that appear can be divided into symmetrical sensory and autonomic polyneuropathies on the one hand, and isolated peripheral nerve lesions or multifocal neuropathies on the other. Mixed syndromes are common.

The commonest form is a symmetrical sensory polyneuropathy, giving rise to numbness and tingling paraesthesiae in the toes and feet and less often in the fingers. Aching or lancinating pains in the feet and legs, particularly at night, may be a troublesome feature. Examination reveals loss of vibration sense in the feet, depression of the ankle jerks, and distal cutaneous sensory impairment. Neuropathic plantar ulcers and occasionally Charcot joints are an important complication. Loss of pain sense results in perforating ulcers on the feet and neuropathic joint degeneration, particularly in the toes and in the tarsal joints; impaired postural sense may give rise to an ataxic gait. An acute painful diabetic neuropathy also occurs that predominantly affects the lower limbs. The onset is often associated with poor diabetic control and precipitate weight loss ('diabetic neuropathic cachexia').

Autonomic neuropathy frequently accompanies the sensory neuropathy and may be the salient manifestation. It rarely occurs in isolation. Pupillary disturbances usually take the form of a reduced response to light. Gustatory facial sweating provoked by the smell and taste of food can be troublesome. Anhidrosis may occur distally in the limbs; if it is extensive and also affects the trunk, heat intolerance may result. Symptoms referable to the alimentary tract include dysphagia from oesophageal involvement, episodes of vomiting related to gastric atony, and episodic nocturnal diarrhoea, often alternating with periods of constipation. Those related to the genitourinary system include impotence, retrograde ejaculation, and bladder atony with difficulty in voiding and urinary retention with overflow. Vascular denervation sometimes results in orthostatic hypotension, and cardiac denervation may be demonstrable by an elevated resting heart rate and the absence of beat-to-beat variation with respiration. The risk of diabetic polyneuropathy is reduced by strict glycaemic control.

Isolated nerve lesions tend to occur more commonly in elderly diabetic subjects. At times they develop insidiously, at others they have an abrupt onset with pain. Of the cranial nerves, the nerves to the external ocular muscles, particularly the third and sixth, and also the facial nerve, are the most often affected. In contradistinction to the effects of compression of the third nerve by a carotid aneurysm, the pupillary innervation is often spared. In the limbs, the lesions tend to occur at the common sites of compression or entrapment. It seems likely that the nerves of diabetics exhibit an excessive vulnerability to damage from pressure.

Diabetic amyotrophy, or proximal diabetic neuropathy, represents a particular example of a multifocal neuropathy that develops usually in elderly obese diabetics. It consists of an asymmetric proximal motor syndrome that affects the anterior thigh muscles and hip flexors, and sometimes also the anterolateral muscles of the lower leg. Less commonly it is symmetric. Its onset may be acute or insidious and is often accompanied by pain, particularly at night. There is generally little or no associated sensory loss. The knee jerks are usually depressed or absent. Inflammatory lesions including vasculitis have recently been demonstrated in peripheral nerves in proximal diabetic neuropathy, leading to trials of immunomodulatory therapy.

The causation of diabetic neuropathy is uncertain. It tends to occur more often in poorly controlled diabetics, but the correlation is not close. It may occur for the first time on initiation of treatment with insulin, or be the presenting symptom in maturity onset diabetes. There is evidence to suggest that diabetic microangiopathy is important in the genesis of isolated nerve lesions. Metabolic factors are probably more important in the origin of the symmetric polyneuropathies, but their nature is uncertain. An increased concentration of sorbitol in nerves secondary to hyperglycaemia may be involved in causing nerve fibre dysfunction.

Focal peripheral nerve lesions and diabetic amyotrophy, if of acute onset, often recover adequately, as does acute painful diabetic neuropathy when satisfactory glycaemic control is achieved. Symmetric sensory and autonomic neuropathy, once established, recovers less satisfactorily, even with good diabetic control. Correcting the hyperglycaemia by continuous subcutaneous insulin infusion or pancreatic transplantation will stabilize the neuropathy. Trials of aldose reductase inhibitors to reduce sorbitol accumulation have, so far, not given clear evidence of improvement in neuropathy.

Care of the feet is vitally important in diabetic sensory neuropathy, to prevent the development of chronic ulceration. Pain may sometimes be helped by carbamazepine, tricyclic antidepressants, phenothiazines, or mexiletine. Hypotension can be improved by raising the head of the bed at night or by support bandages to the legs; more severe cases may require treatment with fludrocortisone. Gastroparesis may respond to metoclopramide, domperidone, or erythromycin; persistent vomiting may necessitate a Roux-en-Y gastroenterostomy. Diabetic diarrhoea can be helped by low-dosage tetracycline or diphenoxylate, loperamide, or codeine phosphate. Diabetic cystopathy can be managed in the earlier stages by regular voiding and cholinergic treatment with bethanechol. Urinary tract infections should be treated promptly. Bladder neck resection can be useful in carefully selected cases. Penile papaverine injections can be employed for erectile impotence, and sildenafil (Viagra) may be helpful in early cases. Silicone implants should be avoided because of the risk of infection.

Amyloidosis

The various forms of amyloid disease are described in Section 11.12. The peripheral nerves may be involved in primary amyloidosis due to a benign plasma cell dyscrasia and in amyloidosis related to myeloma (light chain amyloidosis). There are also several dominantly inherited forms of amyloid neuropathy, the most important of which are due to mutations in the gene for transthyretin (*TTR*), including the Portuguese type (see later). Isolated lesions may occur from the infiltration of amyloid into nerves or from compression of the median nerve in the carpal tunnel because of deposits in the flexor retinaculum. More strikingly, a generalized neuropathy may develop. It begins with selective loss of pain and temperature sensation in the feet and later in the hands. Motor involvement, loss of tendon reflexes, and impairment of other sensory modalities occur later. Autonomic involvement is an early feature, causing impotence, orthostatic hypotension, bladder atony, and disturbances of alimentary function. Amyloid deposits are present in the peripheral nerve trunks, which may be enlarged, and in the dorsal root and sympathetic ganglia.

No treatment influences the progress of the neuropathy apart from liver transplantation in neuropathy due to *TTR* mutations (see Section 11). The use of stem cell transplantation is being explored in amyloidosis related to malignant plasma cell dyscrasias. The spontaneous pains are sometimes improved by carbamazepine or tricyclic antidepressant drugs. Care must be taken to prevent damage to the anaesthetic feet, lower legs, and hands. Autonomic symptoms may require treatment as described for diabetic neuropathy.

Carpal tunnel syndrome is frequent in patients on long-term haemodialysis related to deposition of amyloid in the flexor retinaculum derived from retained β_2-microglobulin.

Uraemia

Uraemic neuropathy did not become a clinical problem until the advent of treatment of endstage renal failure by haemodialysis. It occurs in patients with severe chronic renal failure. It was most often seen in patients under treatment with periodic haemodialysis but is now much less frequently a problem. The symptoms are usually predominantly sensory, with numbness and tingling paraesthesiae in the feet. 'Restless legs' (Ekbom's syndrome) are often a conspicuous feature (see Section 24.22). A distal motor neuropathy may be associated and occasional cases are purely motor. The condition is improved by increased haemodialysis and more effectively by renal transplantation. A retained metabolite is assumed to be the cause, but this has not so far been identified.

Myxoedema

Compression of the median nerve in the carpal tunnel in myxoedema has already been discussed. Rarely a generalized mixed motor and sensory neuropathy develops. This improves on treatment of the hypothyroidism.

The slow contraction and relaxation observed in the tendon reflexes is not due to a disturbance of peripheral nerve function, but to an alteration in the contractile mechanism of the muscle fibres.

Acromegaly (see Section 12)

The occurrence of the carpal tunnel syndrome in acromegaly has also been mentioned. A rare manifestation of this condition is a sensorimotor polyneuropathy in which the peripheral nerves are thickened because of an overgrowth of the neural connective tissues. A similar neuropathy is occasionally observed in pituitary gigantism.

Critical illness polyneuropathy

A generalized polyneuropathy involving widespread axonal degeneration may be encountered in patients in intensive care units with sepsis and multiple organ failure. The neuropathy is discovered when attempts are made to wean them from the ventilator. The precise cause of this condition which has been termed critical illness polyneuropathy is unknown. Slow recovery occurs.

Other metabolic disorders

It has been claimed that a generalized peripheral neuropathy may be caused either by acute or chronic hepatic failure, but this is probably uncommon. A mild painful sensory neuropathy is occasionally encountered in primary biliary cirrhosis, sometimes related to xanthomatous deposits in the cutaneous nerve trunks. A motor neuropathy is a rare sequel to severe recurrent hypoglycaemia.

Toxic neuropathies

Industrial, environmental, and pharmaceutical substances

Acrylamide

This substance is widely employed industrially. The monomer is neurotoxic and causes peripheral neuropathy with mixed motor and sensory features. Ataxia is prominent and is possibly the result of concomitant cerebellar damage. Distal axonal degeneration occurs and slow recovery takes place on cessation of exposure.

Arsenic

Arsenical poisoning is occasionally seen as a result of accidental or homicidal ingestion of insecticides containing arsenic, or from indigenous medicines in India. Gastrointestinal symptoms develop after acute ingestion, followed by a mixed sensory and motor neuropathy after 1 to 3 weeks. Desquamation of the skin of the feet and hands takes place after about 6 weeks and white lines (Mees' lines) appear in the nails. With ingestion of smaller quantities on a chronic basis, gastrointestinal symptoms are less obtrusive and a slowly progressive neuropathy makes its appearance. The skin may become generally pigmented or show focal 'raindrop' pigmentation, and hyperkeratosis of the palms of the hands and soles of the feet may appear.

Slow recovery in the neuropathy occurs with removal from exposure. Chelating agents are of value in treating the non-neurological complications, but it is uncertain whether they are effective for the neuropathy.

Lead

Lead neuropathy is now a rare occurrence in Britain, although it was encountered as a consequence of the contamination of drinking water by lead pipes in old buildings. Subclinical neuropathy may be detectable in lead workers. It remains a hazard in certain parts of the world from the use of lead glazes in pottery. Lead neuropathy is predominantly motor, typically giving rise to wrist and foot drop. The 'lead colic' that may occur is probably a manifestation of autonomic involvement. Other features of lead poisoning that may be associated include a sideroblastic anaemia and a 'lead line' on carious teeth. The neuropathy improves on cessation of lead intake; the utility of treatment with BAL (dimercaprol), edetate, or penicillamine is uncertain.

Mercury

Exposure to inorganic mercury salts and to organic mercurial compounds may lead to neurological damage, as in 'Minamata disease' which was related to consumption of fish contaminated by organic mercury. Dementia, cortical blindness, and ataxia occur, together with sensory changes in the limbs attributed to a sensory neuropathy, although how far these have a peripheral origin is uncertain. Historically, a peripheral neuropathy was an important component of 'pink disease' which was caused by the administration of mercury-containing purgatives.

Thallium

This is present in certain pesticides and rodent poisons and was formerly used as a depilatory agent. Accidental or homicidal poisoning is occasionally encountered. Abdominal pain and diarrhoea are followed after 2 or 5 days by the development of a mixed motor and sensory neuropathy which is often painful. Evidence of central nervous system damage may be present with behaviour disorder, optic neuropathy, and choreiform movements. Alopecia develops later, after about 2 or 3 weeks, and renal damage may be produced. Diethyldithiocarbamate, which binds thallium, has been employed in treatment.

Triorthocresyl phosphate

This substance is used industrially as a high-temperature lubricant. Outbreaks of a sensorimotor neuropathy, often accompanied by evidence of damage to the central nervous system, occur periodically, usually as a consequence of the contamination of cooking ingredients or utensils. The original description was in relation to illegal liquor distillation (ginger jake paralysis) in the United States during the prohibition era. In more recent years, a large outbreak occurred in Morocco from the use of contaminated cooking oil. Recovery is slow and often incomplete.

Other industrial substances

Carbon disulphide, used in the manufacture of rayon, occasionally gives rise to a mild sensory neuropathy. Neuropathy may occur as a result of industrial exposure to the organic solvents *n*-hexane and methyl-*n*-butyl ketone. The former is also encountered as a consequence of solvent abuse; *n*-hexane, which has an intoxicant action, has been used as a solvent in certain glues. Other industrial agents causing neuropathy are ethylene oxide and methyl bromide. Trichlorethylene (or an impurity) has caused trigeminal neuropathy.

Iatrogenic

Cisplatin

This platinum derivative (*cis*-diaminedichloroplatinum) is used in the treatment of malignancy, including carcinoma of the ovary. A predominantly sensory neuropathy that recovers poorly may develop after the administration of several courses. Ototoxicity is more frequent, causing high-tone deafness and tinnitus.

Isoniazid

A mixed motor and sensory neuropathy may be produced by isoniazid and is more likely to occur in individuals who acetylate the drug slowly. The neuropathy is related to an interference with pyridoxine metabolism. Axonal degeneration occurs in the peripheral nerves. The neuropathy recovers slowly on cessation of administration of the drug and may be prevented by giving pyridoxine, which does not interfere with the antituberculous action of the isoniazid.

Nitrofurantoin

Excessively high blood levels of this preparation, as may occur in patients with reduced renal function, can cause a mixed motor and sensory neuropathy.

Vincristine

A neuropathy will occur in all subjects if sufficient amounts of this cytotoxic agent are administered. Mild sensory symptoms and the loss of tendon reflexes may have to be accepted if a satisfactory therapeutic effect of the drug is to be achieved. If the neuropathy advances, bilateral weakness of the extensors of the wrist and fingers develops, followed by more widespread weakness. The neuropathy improves satisfactorily if the drug is withdrawn or if the dosage is reduced.

Other substances

Less important drugs that may give rise to neuropathy are adriamycin, amiodarone, dapsone, disulfiram, gold, metronidazole, misonidazole, nitrous oxide (with a myelopathy), suramin, and zimeldine. A mild sensory neuropathy may develop after prolonged administration of phenytoin, and neuropathy was one of the complications produced by thalidomide. Pyridoxine, if taken in large doses, as 'megavitamin therapy', causes a sensory neuropathy.

Deficiency neuropathies

Beri beri neuropathy (see also Section 10)

This disorder is predominantly encountered in populations subsisting on diets composed largely of polished rice, but a similar neuropathy may be observed in other malnourished communities. Thiamine deficiency is probably involved, but a deficiency of other vitamins of the B group may also be implicated. A distal motor and sensory neuropathy develops which is frequently accompanied by spontaneous aching pain in the extremities, cutaneous hyperaesthesia, and tenderness of the soles of the feet and calves. Involvement of the recurrent laryngeal nerves may lead to hoarseness of the voice. The neuropathy may be associated with a cardiomyopathy ('wet beri beri'). Thiamine deficiency is established by the finding of reduced activity of erythrocyte transketolase. This enzyme requires thiamine as a cofactor.

Distal axonal degeneration occurs in the peripheral nerves and slow recovery ensues with vitamin replacement.

Strachan's syndrome

Strachan's syndrome, originally described in Jamaica but also observed in other parts of the world under conditions of nutritional deprivation, is characterized by the combination of a painful sensory neuropathy with amblyopia and at times deafness, in association with an orogenital dermatitis. It is assumed to be due to B vitamin deficiency, but the precise deficit has not been identified. It improves with B vitamin supplementation.

Alcoholic neuropathy

This always occurs on a background of nutritional deficiency. The dietary intake of the alcoholic is high in carbohydrates and low in vitamins. Moreover, alcoholics are known to have a reduced capacity to absorb thiamine. A direct toxic effect of alcohol on peripheral nerves may also be involved. The clinical features of alcoholic neuropathy are similar to those of beri beri. Other deficiency states may coexist, such as the Wernicke–Korsakoff syndrome. Improvement may take place with vitamin replacement and reduced alcohol intake, but it is beset with the usual difficulties met in treating alcoholic patients.

Pyridoxine deficiency

Attention has already been drawn to the fact that isoniazid neuropathy is related to an interference with pyridoxine metabolism. Pyridoxine deficiency may contribute to the neuropathy that occurs in nutritional deficiency states, and possibly accounts for the mild neuropathy of pellagra.

Pantothenic acid deficiency

Experimental deficiency of pantothenic acid in human volunteers is known to give rise to a sensory neuropathy, and the administration of pantothenic acid has been reported to alleviate the 'burning feet' syndrome which sometimes develops in deficiency states.

Vitamin B_{12} deficiency

Vitamin B_{12} deficiency, from whatever cause, may be responsible for the development of a distal sensory neuropathy, with 'glove and stocking' sensory loss and paraesthesiae, and areflexia, either in isolation or in association with a myelopathy or other central nervous system manifestations. Haematological changes are not always present. The peripheral neuropathy improves more satisfactorily with treatment than the central disturbances. This condition is considered in detail in Chapter 24.3.9.

A peripheral neuropathy is one component of Nigerian ataxic neuropathy, in which the other features are posterior column degeneration, sensorineural deafness, and optic atrophy. It has been suggested that an interference with vitamin B_{12} metabolism by cyanide derived from cassava in the diet, combined with nutritional deficiency, may be responsible.

Chronic severe vitamin E deficiency has recently been established as a cause for peripheral neuropathy in combination with a spinocerebellar degeneration. This may occur in abetalipoproteinaemia, and isolated vitamin E deficiency, both of autosomal recessive inheritance, and in congenital biliary atresia, cystic fibrosis, and occasional adults with chronic intestinal malabsorption.

Inflammatory and post-infective neuropathies

Leprous neuropathy

Peripheral nerve involvement in leprosy is considered in Chapter 7.11.24.

Guillain–Barré syndrome (acute idiopathic inflammatory polyneuropathy)

Guillain–Barré syndrome is characterized by a polyneuropathy that develops over the course of a few days up to maximum of 4 weeks. Cases that progress for up to 8 weeks (subacute Guillain–Barré syndrome) are probably distinct. An identifiable infection may precede the onset of the neuropathy by 1 to 3 weeks. This is commonly an upper respiratory tract infection or an infection with an enterovirus, Epstein–Barr virus, or mycoplasma. More recently *Campylobacter jejuni* has been recognized as an important cause, as has human immunodeficiency virus (**HIV**) infection. Other cases may follow surgical operations. In approximately 40 per cent of cases no antecedent event is identifiable.

The neuropathy may be ushered in by severe lumbar or interscapular pain. Motor involvement usually predominates over sensory loss and may be of a proximal, distal, or generalized distribution, and in severe cases affects the respiratory musculature. Distal paraesthesiae in the limbs are common and, if sensory loss occurs, it tends to affect tactile, vibratory, and postural sensibility. The cranial nerves may be affected, in particular the facial nerves, but bulbar involvement also occurs sometimes. A complete 'locked-in' state may develop. Autonomic disturbances may be associated, including bladder atony, ileus, hypertension (possibly the result of denervation of the carotid sinus), and orthostatic hypotension. Associated central nervous system involvement is occasionally encountered, particularly after infectious mononucleosis, and such cases are sometimes excluded from the Guillain–Barré syndrome as such. Papilloedema sometimes develops, possibly related to impaired resorption of cerebrospinal fluid because of the elevated protein content. Further variants are a combination of an external ophthalmoplegia, ataxia, and tendon areflexia (Miller Fisher syndrome), as possibly are instances of acute sensory neuropathy or pandysautonomia.

Nerve conduction studies reveal evidence of demyelination in most cases, but at times the findings indicate an axonopathy ('axonal' Guillain–Barré syndrome), as is seen in the acute motor axonal neuropathy or motor and sensory axonal neuropathy that occurs as an annual epidemic in children in northern China. Cerebrospinal fluid protein is usually raised, often to a substantial degree, but it may be normal, particularly in the early stages. The cell content is usually normal, but there may be a mild lymphocytic pleocytosis; this is more likely to occur in cases related to HIV infection or infectious mononucleosis. The Miller Fisher syndrome is frequently associated with circulating anti-GQ1b antibodies. Histologically, the abnormalities are maximal in the spinal roots but also occur diffusely throughout the peripheral nerves. In the demyelinating form, focal perivascular accumulations of inflammatory cells are associated with segmental demyelination of the nerve fibres and relative preservation of axonal continuity. Recovery occurs by remyelination. The disease probably represents a cell-mediated hypersensitivity reaction in which myelin is stripped off the axons by mononuclear cells. Whether antibody-mediated demyelination is also involved is not yet established. Severe axonal loss may be a 'bystander effect' or represent direct axonal damage in cases of axonal Guillain–Barré syndrome.

Most cases of Guillain–Barré syndrome recover satisfactorily within weeks or months. Severely affected patients, particularly those that require assisted respiration and in whom extensive axonal degeneration occurs, recover slowly and often show residual muscle weakness. Occasional patients have recurrences, which are sometimes multiple.

Although widely employed in the past, controlled trials of treatment with corticosteroids have shown no beneficial effects. Plasma exchange and high-dose intravenous human immunoglobulin have both been shown to improve the rate of recovery if given before the nadir of the disease. Because of significant morbidity, particularly with plasma exchange, and cost, these forms of treatment are best reserved for more severe cases. Severely affected patients may require extensive support in an intensive care unit because of respiratory failure and autonomic dysfunction.

Chronic inflammatory demyelinating polyneuropathy

Instances of peripheral neuropathy occur that resemble Guillain–Barré syndrome in that the neurological involvement is predominantly motor and the cerebrospinal fluid protein level is elevated, but which pursue either a chronic relapsing or chronic progressive course. They are also associated with widespread demyelination in the spinal roots and peripheral nerves and with inflammatory infiltrates. Nerve conduction velocity is usually markedly reduced and conduction block may be evident. Cases with a purely sensory ataxic neuropathy also occur, as do others with localized involvement, most often of the brachial plexus. Both the generalized and focal cases may respond to treatment with corticosteroids, plasma exchange, or high-dose intravenous human immunoglobulin. Cytotoxic drugs may be required in refractory cases. The response is less satisfactory in the chronic progressive cases.

Patients have recently been identified with a chronic multifocal motor neuropathy with persistent conduction block associated with GM1 ganglioside antibodies. They probably represent a variant of chronic inflammatory demyelinating polyneuropathy. They may respond to immunosuppressive therapy or plasma exchange.

Lyme borreliosis

Lyme borreliosis is a multisystem disease caused by a tick-borne spirochaete *Borrelia burgdorferi* (see Chapter 7.11.30). The peripheral nervous system is frequently affected both during the phase of early disseminated infection and during the late stage. Cranial neuropathies or an acute or subacute radiculoneuritis characterize involvement in the early stages, and a mild, predominantly distal, neuropathy characterizes the late stage. Nerve biopsies show perivasculitis and nerve fibre degeneration, but spirochaetes are not identifiable. Laboratory diagnosis is based on the detection of specific antibodies to *B. burgdorferi* but seronegative cases occur, as may false positive reactions. Treatment, which is with doxycycline and amoxicillin, may therefore have to be given on clinical suspicion of the disease.

Human immunodeficiency virus infection (see Chapter 24.14.4)

A variety of neuropathies may be related to HIV-1 infection, particular types tending to occur in different phases of the disease. Characteristically, Guillain–Barré syndrome or chronic inflammatory demyelinating polyneuropathy occur at the time of seroconversion, when the patient is otherwise well, and a multifocal vasculitic neuropathy occurs in the early symptomatic stage. A distal, often predominantly sensory and painful neuropathy occurs mainly in the later AIDS phase, and an aggressive lumbosacral polyradiculoneuropathy from cytomegalovirus infection is encountered in advanced cases. Neuropathy may also occur in patients with human T-cell leukaemia virus (HTLV-I) infection. The treatment of HIV infection is discussed in Chapter 7.10.21.

Sarcoid neuropathy

Sarcoidosis (see Section 17) may give rise to a multifocal neuropathy with a particular tendency to involve the facial nerves, or to a generalized neuropathy. The neuropathy may be restricted to the cranial nerves (polyneuritis cranialis). Evidence of involvement of other systems is not always present and sarcoid tissue may or may not be detectable on biopsy.

Diphtheritic neuropathy

The neuropathy of diphtheria (Chapter 7.11.1) is caused by the exotoxin which produces segmental demyelination by interfering with Schwann cell function, probably by affecting protein synthesis. The nerves are not invaded by the bacteria.

Palatal weakness tends to develop after 2 to 3 weeks following pharyngeal diphtheria, and local muscle paralysis after a similar interval following cutaneous diphtheria. Paralysis of accommodation and sometimes of the external ocular muscles appears after an interval of 4 to 5 weeks. A generalized predominantly motor neuropathy of distal distribution may develop after 5 to 7 weeks. In severe cases the respiratory muscles are affected, but if death occurs it is usually as a result of an associated myocarditis.

Neuropathy in autoimmune connective tissue disorders

Peripheral nerve involvement may be encountered in a wide range of the 'collagen-vascular' disorders. Polyarteritis nodosa characteristically gives rise to a multifocal neuropathy, often with considerable pain. Wegener's granulomatosis may similarly be associated with a florid neuropathy and, in both instances, the peripheral nerve damage is related to necrotizing angiitis of the vasa nervorum. Such changes may also occur in rheumatoid arthritis in association with a florid multifocal neuropathy; at other times, a less aggressive neuropathy is observed, either in the form of a distal sensory neuropathy or one restricted to the digital nerves. Entrapment neuropathies also occur in rheumatoid arthritis, for example median nerve compression in the carpal tunnel, related to inflammatory changes in articular synovial tissues or tendon sheaths.

An ataxic sensory neuropathy related to a sensory ganglionitis can complicate the Sjögren sicca syndrome. A clinical constellation that combines a distal sensory neuropathy with a trigeminal sensory neuropathy, and myotonic pupils with the sicca syndrome is particularly characteristic. A multifocal neuropathy can also be seen in patients with Sjögren's syndrome.

The neuropathy of polyarteritis nodosa or rheumatoid arthritis may respond to corticosteroids or cyclophosphamide. The neuropathy of Sjögren's sicca syndrome is largely refractory to treatment.

Neoplastic and paraneoplastic neuropathy

Peripheral neuropathy may develop as a non-metastatic complication of carcinoma, most often bronchial or gastric, or lymphoreticular proliferative disorders. The precise mechanism of production of the neuropathy is uncertain. The neuropathy may antedate the discovery of the carcinoma by as much as 2 or 3 years. In relation to carcinoma of the bronchus, the neuropathy may be purely sensory, either subacute or chronic, often with troublesome distal dysaesthesiae, or mixed sensory and motor. The sensory neuropathy is associated with circulating antineuronal Purkinje cell and anti-Hu antibodies. Guillain–Barré syndrome may be encountered in Hodgkin's disease and in chronic lymphocytic leukaemia, and a subacute, mainly motor neuropathy in relation to lymphoma. Non-metastatic carcinomatous neuropathies may regress following removal of the underlying tumour, or may remain unaffected.

Direct invasion of cranial nerves or spinal roots may occur in cases of malignant infiltration of the meninges and of the cervical and lumbosacral plexuses from local malignancies. Infiltration of peripheral nerve trunks is seen most commonly from malignant lymphomas.

Paraproteinaemic neuropathy

A sensory or sensorimotor polyneuropathy related to benign monoclonal paraproteins (monoclonal gammopathies of undetermined significance) has emerged in recent years as an important cause of late onset neuropathy. The neuropathy is usually demyelinating, and in some with features similar or identical to chronic inflammatory demyelinating polyneuropathy. A postural upper limb tremor is often a prominent feature. The paraprotein is most commonly immunoglobulin M, less frequently immunoglobulins G or A. The immunoglobulin M paraproteins can be demonstrated on surviving myelin sheaths in nerve biopsies, where they are probably acting as demyelinating antibodies. Neuropathies associated with immunoglobulin G or A paraproteins may respond to corticosteroids, intravenous immunoglobulin, plasma exchange or immunosuppressive drugs; the response in immunoglobulin M paraproteinaemic neuropathy is disappointing. Although a distal sensorimotor and often painful axonal neuropathy may be associated with myeloma, a demyelinating neuropathy accompanied by a dermatoendocrine syndrome may be encountered, referred to as the Crow–Fukase or POEMS syndrome (**P**olyneuropathy, **O**rganomegaly, o**E**dema, **M** protein, **S**kin changes). A mixed sensorimotor neuropathy occurs which may be associated with papilloedema. The skin changes consist of excessive pigmentation and hypertrichosis. Peripheral oedema develops. Partial syndromes may occur in which all features of the syndrome are not present. The disorder is most often related to osteosclerotic myeloma.

Multifocal, predominantly lower limb, neuropathy may be caused by single or mixed cryoglobulins in myeloma, lymphoma, systemic lupus erythematosus, rheumatoid arthritis, or Waldenström's macroglobulinaemia. They may be the result of vasculitis produced by the deposition of immune complexes in the walls of the vasa nervorum, or to intravascular precipitation of cryoglobulin. These neuropathies occasionally respond to treatment either with immunosuppressive or cytotoxic drugs, or to repeated plasma exchange.

Genetic neuropathies

Porphyria (see also Section 11)

A predominantly motor neuropathy may complicate acute attacks in the autosomal dominant disorders of acute intermittent and variegate porphyria and hereditary coproporphyria, and in the recessively inherited δ-aminolaevulinic acid dehydratase deficiency. It tends to affect the proximal muscles to a greater extent. There may be associated sensory loss which, although sometimes distal in distribution, can affect the trunk and the proximal portions of the limbs. The tendon reflexes are lost, with occasional paradoxical sparing of the ankle jerks. Accompanying autonomic features include abdominal pain and vomiting, tachycardia and hypertension; mental confusion, psychotic behaviour, and epilepsy.

The explanation of the neurological damage has not been established. Axonal degeneration occurs in the peripheral nerves so that recovery is slow and often incomplete.

Attacks may be provoked by a variety of drugs, including barbiturates, sulphonamides, and the contraceptive pill, and by alcohol, probably by enzyme induction in the liver (see Section 14).

Treatment with oral or intravenous glucose, or by infusions of laevulose or haematin, has been shown to reduce the urinary excretion of porphyrin precursors, but a beneficial effect on the neurological disturbances has not been established.

Familial amyloid polyneuropathy

A number of inherited amyloid neuropathies have been recognized, the commonest being those related to point mutations in the gene for transthyretin, formerly known as prealbumin, which is on chromosome 18. The commonest is the Portuguese type where there is a substitution of valine for methionine in the transthyretin molecule. The neuropathy begins with the involvement of small nerve fibres, leading to a distal loss of pain and temperature sensation and autonomic failure. Spontaneous pain is often a feature and a mutilating acropathy frequently develops. The onset is commonly in the fourth or fifth decades and the disorder is slowly progressive, leading to death within about 10 years. Transthyretin is produced mainly in the liver and liver transplantation may halt the progression of the disease. In other types of hereditary amyloid neuropathy with differing clinical features, the amyloid is derived from a variant apolipoprotein A1 (Iowa form) or plasma gelsolin (Finnish form).

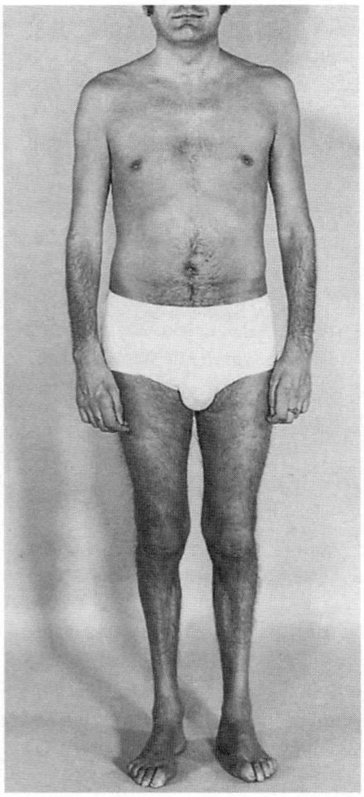

Fig. 3 Patient with type I hereditary motor and sensory neuropathy (Charcot–Marie–Tooth disease) showing symmetrical distal lower limb muscle wasting.

Hereditary motor and sensory neuropathy types I and II and X-linked (Charcot–Marie–Tooth disease, peroneal muscular atrophy); hereditary neuropathy with liability to pressure palsies

Hereditary motor and sensory neuropathies type I and II (or Charcot–Marie–Tooth 1, Charcot–Marie–Tooth 2) usually present during childhood or adolescence with difficulty in walking or because of foot deformity. The deformity is most commonly pes cavus associated with clawing of the toes and sometimes with an equinovarus position of the foot. Muscle weakness tends to affect the lower leg muscles and may give rise to bilateral foot drop with a 'steppage' gait. The muscle wasting is often restricted to below the knees, producing a 'stork leg' appearance (Fig. 3). Weakness and wasting of the small hand muscles may appear later. The tendon reflexes become depressed or lost, and there is a variable degree of distal sensory loss. This is the Charcot–Marie–Tooth phenotype. Progress of the disease is slow and cases with little disability or which are asymptomatic are common.

In the commoner type I families, there is a diffuse demyelinating neuropathy. The onset is most frequently in the first decade. Foot deformity and scoliosis occur more often than in the type II disease. Sensory loss and ataxia tend to be greater and generalized tendon areflexia is usual. Weakness in the hands appears earlier. The peripheral nerves may be thickened. Cases with ataxia and upper limb tremor are sometimes referred to as the Roussy–Lévy syndrome. The onset in the type II form, which is an axonal neuropathy, is most often in the second decade but it may be delayed until middle or even late adult life. Inheritance in both types I and II hereditary motor and sensory neuropathy is usually autosomal dominant. The disorder in type I hereditary motor and sensory neuropathy is most often caused by a segmental duplication on chromosome 17p11.2 (hereditary motor and sensory neuropathy HMSN Ia) which includes the gene for peripheral myelin protein 22 (*PMP22*). Other cases are related to mutations in the gene for myelin protein zero (hereditary motor and sensory neuropathy Ib). X-linked hereditary motor and sensory neuropathy is due to mutations in the gene for connexin 32. The clinical features resemble hereditary motor and sensory neuropathy I but female carriers are asymptomatic or only mildly affected. Several separate loci have so far been identified for hereditary motor and sensory neuropathy II but the gene products are not known.

Nerve conduction velocity is severely reduced in type I cases, moderately reduced in the X-linked form, and either normal or only slightly reduced in type II.

Affected individuals may be helped by the use of orthotic appliances and sometimes by surgical correction of foot deformity or tendon transfer.

Hereditary neuropathy with liability to pressure palsies is an autosomal dominant disorder in which affected individuals develop recurrent focal peripheral nerve or brachial plexus lesions produced by compression or stretch injury. It has been shown usually to be due to a segmental deletion on chromosome 17p11.2, i.e. it is the reciprocal of hereditary motor and sensory neuropathy Ia. Nerve fibres show focal regions of myelin thickening (tomacula).

Hereditary motor and sensory neuropathy type III (Dejerine–Sottas disease and congenital hypomyelination)

The Dejerine–Sottas phenotype consists of a severe slowly progressive mixed motor and sensory polyneuropathy with an onset in childhood. There is hypomyelination and extensive demyelination in the peripheral nerves, and there may be accompanying hypertrophic changes (concentric Schwann cell proliferation). Striking enlargement of the peripheral nerve trunks may be evident. These cases are most often due to de novo *PMP22* or P zero (*P0*) mutations. Some cases result from mutations in the early growth response gene 2 (*EGR2*). A severe congenital hypomyelination neuropathy can also result from *P0* or *EGR2* mutations.

Refsum's disease

This is a rare disorder inherited as an autosomal recessive trait that gives rise to a mixed motor and sensory polyneuropathy accompanied by a variety of other clinical features, including ataxia, anosmia, pigmentary retinal degeneration, pupillary abnormalities, deafness, cardiomyopathy, and ichthyosis. The presentation is usually during adolescence or early adult life and the course may be steadily progressive or relapsing. The peripheral nerves become thickened and display hypertrophic changes. Nerve conduction velocity is usually severely reduced.

The disorder is due to an inability to metabolize phytanic acid, a long-chain fatty acid, which accumulates in the blood and tissues. Phytanic acid is largely of dietary origin, and clinical improvement may be achieved with diets low in phytanic acid. Plasma exchange is effective for acute episodes of deterioration.

Hereditary sensory and autonomic neuropathies

Predominantly sensory neuropathies may occur with either an autosomal dominant or recessive inheritance. The symptoms in the latter instance are usually present from birth; in the former they generally develop during the second or third decades. In both, the sensory loss often leads to a mutilating acropathy, with neuropathic joint degeneration and chronic cutaneous ulceration, particularly of the feet (Fig. 4). Autonomic features are dominant in the recessive disorder of familial dysautonomia (Riley–Day syndrome). A further rare recessive neuropathy combines congenital insensitivity to pain and anhidrosis. Most cases of 'congenital insensitivity to pain' are probably examples of small-fibre neuropathies.

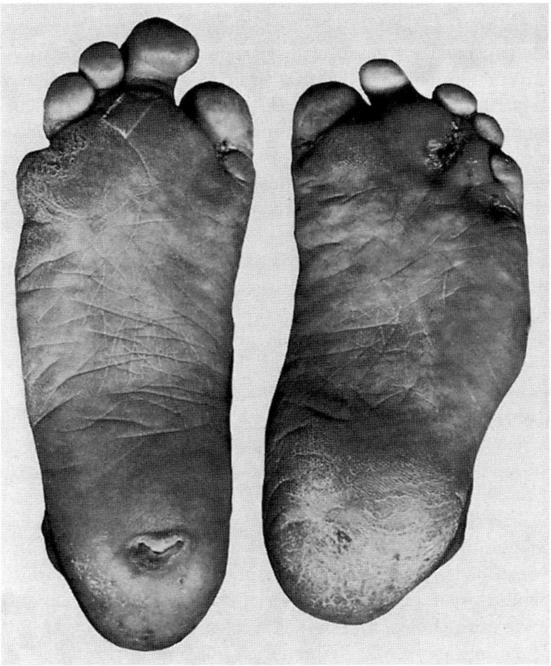

Fig. 4 Chronic foot ulceration and deformity in a case of hereditary sensory neuropathy.

Familial dysautonomia

Otherwise known as the Riley–Day syndrome, this recessively inherited disorder is encountered most often in Jewish populations. There is an aplasia of peripheral autonomic neurones that leads to a variety of symptoms, including absence of tears, unexplained pyrexia, cutaneous blotching, and episodic sweating attacks. These symptoms are present at birth and are accompanied by congenital insensitivity to pain related to an associated sensory neuropathy. In early infancy there is usually difficulty in feeding because of poor sucking, and repeated episodes of aspiration pneumonia. Later, stunted growth and often kyphoscoliosis become evident. The disorder has been mapped to chromosome 9.

Other hereditary neuropathies (see also Section 11)

Peripheral nerve involvement occurs in metachromatic and globoid cell leucodystrophy, adrenomyeloneuropathy, Fabry's disease, hereditary high-density lipoprotein deficiency (Tangier disease), hereditary abetalipoproteinaemia, and cholestanolosis. Giant axonal neuropathy is a rare autosomal recessive disorder with an onset in childhood, characterized by segmental axonal enlargements containing accumulations of neurofilaments. Affected children usually have abnormally curly hair and may have enlarged tangerine-coloured tonsils.

Cryptogenic neuropathy

Despite extensive investigation, the cause of a substantial number of peripheral neuropathies remains unknown. This applies in particular to examples of chronic progressive axonopathies, some of which may be instances of late onset type II hereditary motor and sensory neuropathy. A careful family history in such cases may reveal evidence of undetected neuropathy in relatives. Prolonged follow-up in other cases may disclose underlying malignancy.

Further reading

Asbury AK, Thomas PK (1995). *Peripheral nerve disorders. A practical approach*, 2nd edn. Butterworths, London.

Birch R, Bonney C, Wynn Parry CB (1998). *Surgical disorders of the peripheral nerves.* Churchill Livingstone, Edinburgh.

Dawson DM, Hallett M, Millender LH (1990). *Entrapment neuropathies*, 2nd edn. Little, Brown, Boston.

Dyck PJ, Thomas PK (1999). *Diabetic neuropathy*, 2nd edn. WB Saunders, Philadelphia.

Dyck PJ *et al.* (1993). *Peripheral neuropathy*, 3rd edn. WB Saunders, Philadelphia.

Harding AE (1995). From the syndrome of Charcot, Marie and Tooth to disorders of peripheral myelin proteins. *Brain* **118**, 809–18.

Hughes RAC (1990). *Guillain–Barré syndrome.* Springer, London.

Kimura J (1980). *Electrodiagnosis of diseases of nerve and muscle. Principles and practice*, 2nd edn. FA Davis, Philadelphia.

Stewart JD (2000). *Focal peripheral neuropathies*, 3rd edn. Lippincott, Williams and Wilkins, Philadelphia.

24.20 Neurological complications of systemic autoimmune and inflammatory diseases

Neil Scolding

Introduction

The range and breadth of diseases of the nervous system caused by immunological, infective, or inflammatory disturbances is very large. It includes 'primary' or idiopathic neuroimmune disorders, which may affect any part of the neuraxis (for example multiple sclerosis and Guillain–Barré syndrome) and which are very familiar to neurologists. However, 'secondary' disorders, where the neurological disturbance reflects involvement of the nervous system in a systemic inflammatory disease, are often no less common than idiopathic immune disorders, but most neurologists are rather less familiar and possibly less comfortable with them.

Systemic lupus erythematosus

Systemic lupus erythematosus, like many autoimmune diseases, occurs more in women than men—perhaps 20 times more commonly. Black people are more commonly affected than white. The neurologist should not (but usually does) omit direct enquiry and focused systemic examination to exclude fever and general malaise, skin changes—classically, the malar butterfly rash and/or photosensitivity—and large and small joint arthritis. Glomerulonephritis, pleurisy and pneumonitis, pericarditis and (so-called) Libmann–Sachs endocarditis, and haematological disorders—anaemia, thrombocytopenia, leucocytopenia, and the generation of circulating anticoagulants—also occur. Other laboratory abnormalities include the presence of a variety of autoantibodies, including antinuclear antibodies and anti-native DNA antibodies. The diagnosis—particularly for research and therapeutic trial purposes—is now commonly based on the widely accepted revised diagnostic criteria suggested by the American College of Rheumatology. The presence of any four (or more) of the listed features, 'serially or simultaneously, during any interval of observation' are sufficient for the diagnosis, with an estimated specificity and sensitivity of 96 per cent.

Neurological complications

Neurological involvement in systemic lupus erythematosus is seen in perhaps 50 per cent of cases; neurological presentation, in perhaps 3 per cent of cases. Central nervous system disease is much more frequent than neuromuscular involvement, and is a poor prognostic sign, reducing the overall survival figures, and representing the third commonest cause of death (after renal involvement and iatrogenic causes).

An enormous variety of central nervous system disease complications can occur, reflecting two broad pathogenetic mechanisms—thromboembolic (triggered either by changes in endothelial surfaces or by coagulation disturbances, including lupus anticoagulant activity) and more direct autoimmune events affecting the target tissue—neurones or glia—in which soluble and cellular mediators are implicated.

Headache (including that associated with dural sinus thrombosis), acute or subacute encephalopathy, fits, myelitis, strokes and movement disorders (especially chorea), ataxia and brainstem abnormalities, and cranial and peripheral neuropathies are all seen in the context of systemic lupus erythematosus. Psychiatric and cognitive disturbances have also long been associated with lupus.

Stroke, the lupus anticoagulant, and the primary phospholipid syndrome

The thrombotic tendency in patients with systemic lupus erythematosus and lupus anticoagulant manifests itself principally in the form of stroke and recurrent spontaneous abortion. Intra-abdominal and deep venous thrombosis, and peripheral arterial thrombosis are also seen. Thrombocytopenia is a key additional feature. Importantly, Hughes also showed that a similar clinical picture was associated with the presence of anticardiolipin antibodies (ACA) and/or lupus anticoagulant in patients without serological or clinical evidence of lupus, and introduced the term 'antiphospholipid syndrome'.

ACAs represent an independent risk factor for stroke. Central nervous system thrombosis in patients with primary or secondary antiphospholipid syndrome takes the form of completed arterial stroke, repeated transient ischaemic attacks, multi-infarct dementia, and cerebral venous sinus thrombosis. Vascular visual problems, including amaurosis fugax and ischaemic retinopathy, also occur. Chorea too is associated with antiphospholipid antibodies; the putative link with migraine may be factitious.

A severe acute ischaemic encephalopathy is also described, with confusion, obtundation, and a hyperreflexic quadriparesis (usually asymmetrical), with or without systemic disturbances (dermatological and renal). Cerebrospinal fluid examination may show only a raised protein; a fatal outcome is common. The disorder may represent a focal variant of the recently described 'catastrophic antiphospholipid syndrome', in which there is severe multi-organ failure and a mortality of the order of 60 per cent.

There are both clinical and pathological similarities between microangiopathic complications of lupus and the syndrome of thrombotic thrombocytopenic purpura. In this latter uncommon disorder, multi-organ involvement is also seen, with hepatic and renal disease, and fever, together with thrombocytopenia and an associated purpuric rash and other haemorrhagic complications. Neurologically, an encephalopathy occurs, often with fits, with or without focal deficits. Pathologically, there are widespread microangiopathic changes in the brain and systemically. Plasma exchange is commonly recommended.

Diagnosis of central nervous system lupus

Cerebrospinal fluid examination may reveal a raised protein level and a neutrophil or lymphocyte pleocytosis. It is clearly vital in such cases to exclude infectious complications of immune suppressants or steroids, now a major cause of death in patients with lupus. Serological tests are discussed elsewhere. MRI changes are common, though neither invariable nor specific. Cerebrospinal fluid oligoclonal band analysis is positive in up to 50 per cent of patients with central nervous system lupus and, interestingly, these changes can resolve with successful immunotherapy. A skin biopsy can be extremely helpful in suspected lupus (see Chapter 18.10.2).

The management of neuropsychiatric lupus

Symptomatic therapies are important in patients with encephalopathies, epilepsy, and/or psychiatric ailments. Disease-modifying therapeutic efforts fall into two categories depending on the presumed underlying mechanisms: (i) stroke prevention in cerebral ischaemia, particularly that associated with ACA, probably best achieved with moderate- to high-dose warfarin, and (ii) immunotherapy of 'other' central nervous system complications. Here, intravenous methyl prednisolone followed by oral steroids is the mainstay of treatment. Cyclophosphamide may be given for severe or steroid-resistant disease, with azathioprine to maintain remission and spare steroids. Plasmapheresis synchronized with cyclophosphamide, and intravenous immunoglobulin, may prove useful.

Rheumatoid arthritis

An inflammatory peripheral neuropathy occurs in approximately 30 per cent of seropositive rheumatoid cases. A relatively benign mononeuritis is typical, but a more severe and aggressive axonal polyneuropathy or mononeuritis multiplex may be seen when rheumatoid arthritis is accompanied by a vasculitis. More common than either are entrapment neuropathies of conventional distribution, precipitated by synovial swelling. Pannus formation and cervical spine subluxation with resulting cord compression represent the commonest cause of central nervous system involvement. More rarely, rheumatoid vasculitis, or deposition of rheumatoid nodules, may involve the central nervous system; the former warrants treatment with cyclophosphamide and steroids.

Sjögren's syndrome

Sjögren's syndrome characteristically comprises a triad of: (i) keratoconjunctivitis sicca, and (ii) xerostomia, occurring in approximately 50 per cent of cases (iii) in the context of another connective tissue, usually rheumatoid arthritis. Speckled antinuclear antibodies of the anti-Ro (SS-A) or anti-La (SS-B) type are present in up to 75 to 80 per cent of patients. Conventionally, the principal neurological manifestations have been held to be peripheral, with descriptions of both a mainly sensory neuropathy and of myositis. Trigeminal sensory neuropathy is also classically described.

More recently, attention has been drawn to various central nervous system complications of the disorder, with seizures, focal stroke-like or brainstem neurological deficits, and encephalopathy with or without an aseptic meningitis, often with raised cerebrospinal fluid pressure, protein, and white cell count, together with oligoclonal immunoglobulin bands. Psychiatric abnormalities may occur; spinal cord involvement may take the form of an acute transverse myelitis, a chronic myelopathy, or intraspinal haemorrhage. Occasionally, the features resemble those of multiple sclerosis (optic neuropathy is particularly associated) although most such patients have additional features of peripheral neuropathy or myositis.

Steroids may be insufficient for the treatment of patients with central nervous system complications of Sjögren's syndrome; more powerful immunosuppressants are probably more useful, although, as is so often the case, their value is yet to be proved objectively.

Systemic sclerosis

Systemic sclerosis results from the excessive deposition of collagen in the skin and other affected tissues. The cutaneous manifestation, scleroderma, may exist in isolation, but in multisystem disease, it is accompanied by Raynaud's phenomenon, calcinosis and atrophy of subcutaneous tissues, telangiectasia, and oesophageal strictures. Neurological complications are not common. Peripheral nervous system disease predominates, particularly painful trigeminal neuropathy; myopathy with an elevated creatine phosphokinase also occurs. A myelopathy may be associated. No treatment is of proven benefit.

Mixed connective tissue disease

In this disorder, features of scleroderma, polymyositis, and systemic lupus erythematosus coincide, and high levels of antibodies directed against extractable nuclear antigens—ribonucleoproteins—are found. Rheumatoid factor is also often present. In common with both systemic sclerosis and Sjögren's syndrome, trigeminal neuralgia and/or sensory neuropathy are described.

Seronegative arthritides

Ankylosing spondylitis

Neurological disease in the setting of ankylosing spondylitis usually reflects advanced bony disease; a cauda equina syndrome is well reported, unexplained, and difficult to treat.

Reiter's disease

The clinical triad of seronegative arthropathy, non-specific urethritis, and conjunctivitis, usually following venereal or dysenteric infection, constitutes Reiter's syndrome. As many as 25 per cent of patients are reported to have neurological features. Peripherally, radiculitis and polyneuritis occur; central nervous system disorders include aseptic meningoencephalitis, seizures, and psychiatric disturbances, particularly paranoid psychosis. Cranial neuropathies, pyramidal signs, and myelopathy are also reported. A recent report suggests that cyclosporin may be of value in severe Reiter's disease.

Psoriasis

Included as the third seronegative arthropathy, the neurology of psoriasis is not extensive. Cord compression from cervical psoriatic spondylosis is described, but reports of a complicating polyneuritis have not been substantiated.

Vasculitis

The vasculitides are a heterogeneous group of disorders which share certain pathological features, particularly intramural inflammation and necrotic changes within the walls of blood vessels. Their classification is complex, with subdivisions into: (i) idiopathic vasculitic disorders, for example giant cell arteritis and Wegener's granulomatosis; (ii) vasculitis secondary to collagen diseases, malignancy, viral infection, and so on; and (iii) vasculitis according to pathological features, largely vessel size (see Section 18.10). Nervous system involvement can occur in any of the systemic vasculitides. Additionally, isolated vasculitis of the central or peripheral nervous system is recognized, where little or no inflammation is apparent outside the nervous system—primary central (or peripheral) nervous system angiitis. In both primary and secondary vasculitis of the nervous system, neurological features arise from inflammation and necrosis of the vasculature, principally through infarction.

The clinical features of vasculitis of the nervous system

The picture of peripheral nerve vasculitis is relatively straightforward: a mixed sensory and motor neuropathy, usually rapidly progressive, and often painful. About 50 per cent of patients present with mononeuritis multiplex, the remainder with a more diffuse asymmetrical polyneuropathy or a distal symmetric neuropathy.

Central nervous system disease is infinitely more varied; focal or multifocal infarction, or diffuse ischaemia, affecting any part of the brain, explaining the protean manifestations, wide variation in disease activity, course, and severity, and the absence of a pathognomic or even a typical clinical picture. Thus, in primary and secondary intracranial vasculitis, the following are seen: headache, focal and generalized seizures, stroke-like episodes causing hemispheric or brainstem deficits, acute and subacute encephalopathies, progressive cognitive changes, behavioural disturbances, chorea, myoclonus and other movement disorders, and optic and other cranial neuropathies. The course is commonly acute or subacute, but monophasic, chronic progressive, and spontaneously relapsing–remitting presentations all occur. Despite this range, three broad clinical categories of presentation may be delineated: (i) phenotypically resembling atypical multiple sclerosis ('MS-plus'), with a relapsing–remitting course, and features such as optic neuropathy and brainstem episodes accompanied by other features less common in multiple sclerosis—seizures, severe and persisting headaches, encephalopathic episodes, or hemispheric stroke-like episodes; (ii) acute or subacute encephalopathy, with headache with an acute confusional state, progressing to drowsiness and coma; and (iii) intracranial mass lesion—with headache, drowsiness, focal signs, and (often) raised intracranial pressure. This grouping carries neither pathological nor therapeutic implications, but may help improve recognition of the condition. Systemic features, such as fever and night sweats, livedo reticulares, or oligoarthropathy, may be present (although often only revealed on direct enquiry) even in so-called isolated central nervous system vasculitis.

Diagnosis and management

The diagnosis of cerebral vasculitis involves the exclusion of alternative possibilities (Table 1), the confirmation of intracranial vasculitis, and pursuit of the causes of vasculitis.

Confirming cerebral vasculitis

No single simple investigation is universally useful in confirming cerebral vasculitis. Serological markers, including antineutrophil cytoplasmic antibodies (**ANCA**), are important. Spinal fluid examination is, like the erythrocyte sedimentation test, often abnormal, but lacks specificity, with changes in cell count and/or protein in 65 to 80 per cent of cases; oligoclonal immunoglobulin bands may be present. Magnetic resonance imaging may disclose ischaemic areas, periventricular white matter lesions, haemorrhagic lesions, and parenchymal or meningeal enhancing areas, but lacks both specificity and sensitivity. Contrast angiography may show segmental (often multifocal) narrowing and areas of localized dilatation or beading, often with areas of occlusion, rarely also with aneurysms. Again, these changes are not specific, and angiography carries a false-negative rate of perhaps 50 per cent, and a risk of 10 per cent for transient neurological deficit, and 1 per cent for permanent deficit. Nuclear imaging of labelled leucocytes and examination of the ocular vasculature may be useful.

Table 1 Some disorders which may mimic cerebral vasculitis

Other vasculopathies:	Infections:
Susac's syndrome	Lyme disease
Homocysteinuria	AIDS
Ehlers–Danlos syndrome	Endocarditis
Radiation vasculopathy	Whipple's disease
Köhlmeyer–Degos disease	Viral encephalitis
Fibromuscular dysplasia	Legionella/mycoplasma pneumonia
Fabry's disease	Tumours and malignancy:
Moyamoya disease	Atrial myxoma
Amyloid angiopathy	Multifocal glioma
CADASIL	Cerebral lymphoma
Marfan's syndrome	Paraneoplastic disease
Pseudoxanthoma elasticum	Multiple cholesterol emboli
Viral or fungal vasculitis	Thrombotic thrombocytopenic purpura
Other immune/inflammatory diseases:	Cerebral sinus thrombosis
Sarcoidosis	Mitochondrial disease
Lupus and antiphospholipid disease	
Behçet's syndrome	
Multiple sclerosis/ADEM	
Thyroid encephalopathy	

CADASIL, cerebral autosomal dominant arteriopathy with subcortical infarcts and leukoencephalopathy; ADEM, acute disseminated encephalomyelitis.

Histopathological confirmation, taking a biopsy of an abnormal area of brain where possible, or 'blind' biopsy, incorporating meninges and non-dominant temporal white and grey matter, is important. Biopsy may reveal an underlying process not otherwise suspected with profound therapeutic implications, such as infective or neoplastic (principally lymphomatous) vasculopathies, but is not a trivial procedure, carrying a risk of serious morbidity estimated at 0.5 to 2 per cent—although immune-suppressant treatment may have a higher morbidity than biopsy, emphasizing the rationale behind this procedure.

Once a vasculitic process has been confirmed, the specific defining characteristics of the primary and secondary vasculitides must be painstakingly sought.

Neurological vasculitis complicating systemic vasculitides

Wegener's granulomatosis predominantly affects the upper and lower respiratory tracts—the nose (often with destructive cartilaginous change causing saddle nose deformity), sinuses, larynx, trachea, and lungs. Ocular involvement may occur; renal disease is usual. cANCA is positive, with proteinase-3 specificity, and the biopsy is characteristic, with granulomatous vasculitis. Microscopic polyangiitis is a multisystem small-vessel vasculitis which can involve almost any organ, or may rarely be confined to a single organ. Renal involvement is almost invariable. The diagnosis usually rests upon a combination of renal biopsy and ANCA serology (commonly pANCA). Classic polyarteritis nodosa is now recognized as an unusual disorder which may have some overlap and coexist with microscopic polyangiitis, but often occurs alone. Medium-sized vessels are affected in polyarteritis nodosa, and the kidneys are again commonly involved; renal angiography may reveal microaneurysms. pANCA testing is also often positive in Churg–Strauss syndrome, a multisystem disease characterized pathologically by a granulomatous necrotizing vasculitis, and clinically by prominent asthma with an eosinophilia. Small-vessel vasculitis commonly affects postcapillary venules. The skin is most commonly involved, usually with purpura or urticaria; the common presence of an allergic precipitant has led historically to the term hypersensitivity vasculitis often being used synonymously in this context; cutaneous leucocytoclastic vasculitis is the currently preferred epithet.

In all these disorders, peripheral nervous system involvement, with mononeuritis multiplex, is considerably more common than central nervous system disease, ranging from up to 70 per cent in patients with classic polyarteritis nodosa and microscopic polyangiitis, to around 30 per cent in patients with Wegener's disease. Central nervous system disease can, however, also occur. Direct effects of the granulomatous process—either by contiguous invasive spread or from remote metastatic granulomas—represent a mode of neurological involvement unique to Wegener's disease.

Neurological vasculitis complicating non-vasculitic systemic disorders

Although the clinical picture of cerebral vasculitis may closely be mimicked by systemic lupus erythematosus, a non-inflammatory vasculopathy is far more commonly responsible, but rare instances of vasculitis are described. In contrast, seropositive rheumatoid disease is a well-recognized precipitant of vasculitic mononeuritis multiplex and of central nervous system vasculitis. There are rare reports of central nervous system vasculitis in the context of systemic sclerosis, Sjögren's syndrome, and mixed connective tissue disease. The clinical features of cryoglobulinaemia represent the combined consequences of hyperviscosity and of immune complex deposition-triggered vasculitis, particularly in mixed cryoglobulinaemia, when associated with hepatitis C infection. Skin disease, with purpura progressing to necrotic ulceration, and renal and joint involvement are common. However, the diagnosis will only be made if blood is collected into a plain tube, immediately placed in water in a vacuum flask at 37°C, taken to the laboratory, and tested immediately. Peripheral neuropathy occurs in a quarter of patients with essential cryoglobulinaemia; central nervous system involvement is rare. Peripheral nerve disease, and/or histologically and angiographically evident vasculitis of the central nervous system, usually in the context of granulomatous meningitis, may occur in sarcoidosis.

Drug-induced vasculitis

The issue of vasculitis and drugs is complex. The most compelling evidence of a direct association relates to amphetamines, with clinical and histological evidence of multisystem necrotizing vasculitis. The majority of strokes occurring with cocaine abuse are associated with arterial spasm, platelet aggregation, severe abrupt hypertension, or migrainous phenomena, not vasculitis, although histologically proven cerebral vasculitis does occur.

Infections

At least three mechanisms may underlie microbe-related vascular damage—direct invasion, immune complex formation and deposition, and (in part related to the second) secondary cryoglobulinaemia. Although the association of hepatitis C infection with cryoglobulinaemia and small-vessel vasculitis has been stressed above, other infections, including hepatitis B, Epstein–Barr virus, cytomegalovirus, Lyme disease, syphilis, malaria, and coccidiomycosis have also been linked to mixed cryoglobulinaemia.

Primary invasion of the vascular wall by the infectious agent is, however, the commonest precipitant of infection-associated vasculitis. *Histoplasma*, *Coccidioides*, and *Aspergillus* spp. are among the fungal causes of this picture, usually confined to immune-suppressed patients—although this includes diabetes mellitus. In HIV infection, cytomegalovirus and *Toxoplasma* may precipitate vasculitis, and syphilitic cerebral vasculitis has re-emerged in the context of HIV. More general bacterial causes of meningeal or cerebral infection—mycobacteria, pneumococci, and *Haemophilus influenzae*—may also trigger intracranial vasculitis.

Herpes zoster can precipitate cerebral vasculitis in approximately 0.5 per cent of cases, usually causing a monophasic illness, with hemiparesis contralateral to the eye disease. However, more generalized necrotizing and granulomatous vasculitis can also occur.

Malignancy, lymphomatoid granulomatosis, and malignant angioendothelioma

Leucocytoclastic vasculitis (often dermatological) may occur in association with a variety of cancers as a paraneoplastic phenomenon. Central nervous system disease in the context of Hodgkin's disease with a pathological picture indistinguishable from conventional isolated central nervous system angiitis is reported. Lymphomatoid granulomatosis is a lymphomatous disorder centred on the vascular wall, with destructive change and secondary inflammatory infiltration lending the appearance of true vasculitis; the infiltrating neoplastic cell is of T-lymphocyte derivation. Cutaneous and pulmonary involvement are common, with nodular cavitating lung infiltrates, and neurological manifestations occur in 25 to 30 per cent of cases; they are the presenting feature in approximately 20 per cent. Neoplastic or malignant angioendotheliosis is also a rare, nosologically separate disorder, wherein the neoplastic process is intravascular (within the lumen) and the lymphomatous cells are B-cell derived and characteristically do not invade the vascular wall. The neurological features of each disorder are similar, largely representing those of cerebral vasculitic disease; in malignant angioendotheliomatosis, lung involvement is not the rule; characteristic skin manifestations occur.

Treatment of cerebral vasculitis

Prospective controlled randomized trials remain conspicuous by their absence, but retrospective analyses support the use of cyclophosphamide with steroids in vasculitis. In proven cerebral vasculitis—as in lupus—a 3- to 4-month induction regime might comprise high-dose intravenous then oral steroids, with oral or pulsed intravenous cyclophosphamide; this is followed by a maintenance regime of alternate-day steroids with azathioprine. In resistant disease, methotrexate (10 to 25 mg once weekly; again, with steroids) or intravenous immunoglobulin may be useful.

Two eponymous primary disorders may involve the central nervous system. Cogan's syndrome is an unusual disorder, mostly affecting young adults, characterized by recurrent episodes of interstitial keratitis and/or scleritis with vestibuloauditory symptoms, which may be complicated by central or peripheral nervous system or systemic vasculitis. In Eale's disease, an isolated retinal vasculitis occurs, causing visual loss; again, neurological complications are well described.

Giant cell arteritis

Giant cell arteritis, the most common large-vessel vasculitis, rarely affects individuals under 55 years of age. It affects women twice as commonly as men, with an overall prevalence of 100/10 000. Generally it presents with uni- or bilateral scalp pain, often severe, with exquisite tenderness. Additional symptoms include jaw claudication and polymyalgia rheumatica, with stiffness and aching of the shoulder girdle, worse in the mornings, and occasionally general malaise. The affected temporal artery (-ies) may be thickened and cord-like, often non-pulsatile, and tender. A raised erythrocyte sedimentation rate, often accompanied by a normochromic normocytic anaemia, must be followed by temporal artery biopsy—a specimen of several centimetres in length is recommended to help avoid false-negative results, which may occur because of the focal or multifocal nature of the disorder.

Histopathological examination of the vessel reveals changes of vasculitis, with an inflammatory infiltrate comprising mononuclear and giant cells; the latter phagocytose the elastic laminae, causing characteristic fragmentation. Immunoglobulin and complement deposits are apparent in lesions, but activated T cells predominate in the inflammatory infiltrate, suggesting cell-mediated immune damage. Vasculitic changes may still be apparent in biopsies taken 14 days or more after the commencement of steroids.

Neurological complications

Blindness occurs in approximately one-sixth of treated patients with temporal arteritis, as a consequence of anterior ischaemic optic neuropathy following vasculitic involvement of the posterior ciliary arteries and/or the ophthalmic artery, from which they are derived. A typical picture comprises (locally) painless loss of acuity, commonly severe, often with an altitudinal field defect. The fundal appearances may be normal, although swelling (usually mild) may be seen. Intracranial involvement is much less common; vertebral artery involvement is typical.

Treatment

Oral steroids should be used immediately there is serious suspicion of the disease, and in high doses (60 to 80 mg a day) in view of the risk of permanent blindness. The dose is generally reduced slowly (5 mg decrements weekly) after 4 to 7 days to a maintenance dose of perhaps 10 mg daily; thereafter, some would suggest continuing for 12 to 24 months before closely monitored phased withdrawal. Such a duration of steroid therapy, particularly in this elderly population, should direct attention to the treatable or preventable long-term consequences of corticosteroids, particularly osteoporosis, diabetes, cataract, and peptic ulceration.

Behçet's disease

Behçet's disease is a chronic relapsing multisystem inflammatory disorder whose clinical manifestations vary. The classic triad of recurrent uveitis with oral and genital aphthous ulceration remains clinically useful, although formal diagnostic criteria have now been proposed and generally adopted. Recurrent oral ulceration (at least three times in one 12-month period) is an absolute criterion; any two of (i) recurrent genital ulceration, (ii) uveitis (anterior or posterior) or retinal vasculitis, (iii) skin lesions, including erythema nodosum, or acneform nodules, pseudofolliculitis, or papulopustular lesions, or (iv) a positive pathergy test (read at 24 to 48 h) are also required to confirm the diagnosis.

Approximately one-third of patients develop neurological involvement, although this includes the very common occurrence of benign headache. Cerebral venous sinus thrombosis is one of the more specific serious complications; others include sterile meningoencephalitis, encephalopathy, brainstem syndromes, cranial neuropathies, and cortical sensory and motor deficits. Psychiatric and progressive cognitive manifestations are reported. Investigation may reveal an active cerebrospinal fluid, and oligoclonal IgA and IgM bands—but apparently not IgG—may be present. Evoked potentials may be diagnostically useful. MRI abnormalities are non-specific.

Treatment of Behçet's disease

Recent retrospective studies indicate an improved survival in patients with Behçet's disease of the central nervous system treated with steroids and immunosuppressants. The place of thalidomide in steroid-unresponsive Behçet's disease is currently under review; chlorambucil is often advocated. Monitoring treatment is difficult—neither the erythrocyte sedimentation rate nor C-reactive protein levels are useful; MRI might have such a role.

Sarcoidosis

Sarcoidosis is a multisystem granulomatous disease of unknown aetiology commonly affecting the lungs and, in approximately 5 per cent of patients, the nervous system. Optic and other cranial neuropathies (especially involving the facial nerve), often due to meningeal infiltration, and brainstem and spinal cord disease are the commoner manifestations. Cognitive and neuropsychiatric abnormalities are reported. Peripheral nerve and muscle involvement is also well described.

The diagnosis can be difficult. Serum and cerebrospinal fluid ACE levels may be elevated; the cerebrospinal fluid may reveal more general abnormalities of protein or cell count and oligoclonal bands may be present. Whole-body gallium scanning remains a useful indicator of systemic disease. Cranial MRI may show multiple white matter lesions or meningeal enhancement. The diagnosis is confirmed where possible by biopsy, either of cerebral or meningeal tissue, or of lung or conjunctiva where appropriate.

The mainstay of medical treatment in neurosarcoidosis is corticosteroids, although response rates as low as 29 per cent have been reported. Methotrexate, azathioprine, hydroxychloroquine, and cyclophosphamide have been used in steroid-resistant cases.

Organ-specific autoimmune disease

Ulcerative colitis and Crohn's disease

While differences in the frequency and type of, for example, dermatological or articular complications may occur between ulcerative colitis and Crohn's disease, the neurological complications, seen in around 5 per cent of patients, are similar. Three types of central nervous system disease have been associated: cerebrovascular accidents, mostly precipitated by the hypercoagulable state, and including venous or arterial thromboembolism, cerebral sinus venous thrombosis, and (more rarely and less explicably) vasculitis; epileptic seizures, focal and generalized, and not always in connection with dehydration or sepsis; and, in some reports, a slowly progressive myelopathy.

Peripheral neuropathy is seen in 0.5 to 1.0 per cent of cases and an acute Guillain–Barré syndrome is the commonest phenotype. Lastly, myopathy, sometimes of metabolic origin but mostly inflammatory, is also reported.

Table 2 Neurological features of Whipple's disease (in approximate order of frequency)

Cognitive changes, dementia, and/or psychiatric disease
Supranuclear gaze palsy
Pyramidal signs
Hypothalamic features—somnolence, polydipsia, increased appetite, hypogonadism
Myoclonus
Oculomasticatory myorythmia
Cranial neuropathies.
Fits
Eye disease—keratitis, uveitis, papilloedema, ptosis
Ataxia

Whipple's disease

Whipple's disease is an uncommon multisystem disorder characterized by arthropathy, respiratory symptoms, anaemia, fever, erythema nodosum, and severe wasting in addition to steatorrhoea and abdominal distension, caused by *Tropheryma whippelii*. Approximately 10 per cent of patients have neurological involvement; 5 per cent present in this way. A wide variety of features is seen (Table 2).

Diagnosis and management

Up to 20 per cent of cases of cerebral Whipple's disease occur in the absence of gastrointestinal or indeed other systemic symptoms. CT and MR scanning may be normal, although the latter can also reveal non-specific abnormalities—multiple high-signal intensity areas on T_2-weighted images, or more striking enhanced mass lesions warranting biopsy. Similarly, the cerebrospinal fluid may be normal, or show an elevated protein and/or raised cell count; widely varying ratios of monocytes and polymorphonucleocytes are reported. One-third of cerebrospinal fluid samples may reveal pathognomic periodic acid–Schiff-stained bacilli; repeat spinal fluid examination increases this yield. Approximately 30 per cent of cases have a non-informative small bowel biopsy, although electron microscopy increases the sensitivity. Lymph node biopsy can also be useful. Polymerase chain reaction analysis of blood, lymph node, spinal fluid, small bowel tissue, or brain is increasingly used.

Whipple's disease usually responds to tetracyclines, penicillin, or more commonly nowadays, co-trimoxazole. Prompt treatment is vital in patients with neurological disease, which may (if untreated) run a profoundly aggressive and, not unusually, rapidly fatal course. Successful reversal of neurological deficits, including cognitive impairment, may follow antibiotic treatment.

Coeliac disease

Coeliac disease (non-tropical sprue) is an immunologically mediated disorder resulting from intolerance to dietary gluten; it causes weight loss with steatorrhoea and/or diarrhoea, and malabsorption. In common with other enteropathies, neurological sequelae of a predictable nature may complicate coeliac disease as a direct consequence of malabsorption. Central nervous system complications apparently unrelated to deficiency states may also occur in perhaps 10 per cent of patients. Rarely, vasculitis is responsible, but the cause of the most commonly described and distinctive central nervous system association, a progressive cerebellar or spinocerebellar degeneration, with eye movement disorders, myoclonus, and occasionally epilepsy, remains unresolved.

Major psychiatric complications and dementia are well described as a significant cause of morbidity, and have been studied in detail.

Thyroid disease

Hyperthyroidism and myxoedema both carry neurological complications generally considered direct consequences of abnormal thyroxine levels—anxiety, tremor, and occasionally chorea in thyrotoxicosis; and lethargy, myopathy, and dementia in hypothyroidism (see Chapter 12.4). By contrast, Grave's ophthalmoplegia and Hashimoto's encephalopathy are both thought to be immunologically driven.

In dysthyroid eye disease, the orbit and extraocular muscles are oedematous and infiltrated with inflammatory cells and glycosaminoglycans, resulting in proptosis and a restrictive ophthalmopathy. Up-gaze limitation is the commonest presenting sign. Vision is occasionally threatened by a complicating infiltrative or compressive optic neuropathy. Circulating thyroid-stimulating hormone (TSH) receptor-stimulating antibodies cross-reactive with orbital fibroblasts are found. Steroid treatment and radiotherapy are equally effective.

Hashimoto's encephalopathy exhibits a female:male ratio of up to 9:1. Most cases are clinically and biochemically euthyroid at presentation, and two modes of presentation occur. The relapsing–remitting variety causes stroke-like episodes, with or without mild cognitive impairment, focal or generalized seizures, and episodes of encephalopathy. The second group present with a more diffuse progressive disease, with dementia, psychotic features, seizures, and occasionally myoclonus, tremor, and/or ataxia; focal neurological deficits are uncommon.

Imaging by CT or even MR is often normal, as is angiography, though isotope brain scanning may show patchy uptake. Spinal fluid examination may reveal a raised protein level but typically a normal cell count. Very high titres of antithyroid antibodies are found, usually antimicrosomal. Most patients respond well to steroid treatment; some have received further immunosuppressive therapy, such as cyclophosphamide or azathioprine.

Stiff man syndrome

Stiffness on examination of muscles occurs in an enormous number of disorders (Table 3). In the great majority, a clinical diagnosis can be made from the nature of the stiffness, the context, and the associated neurological and general clinical findings. Muscle stiffness as a primary disorder is much less common. It occurs in three major conditions – tetanus and neuromyotonia and the stiff man syndrome. Neuromyotonia has a peripheral origin in the distal axon and neuromuscular junction, while the stiff man syndrome is a CNS disease.

Table 3 Causes and differential diagnosis of stiff muscles

Disorders in which stiffness is the principal manifestation
Stiff man syndrome
Neuromyotonia
Progressive encephalomyelitis with rigidity
Schwarz-Jampel syndrome
Tetanus
Strychnine poisoning
Disorders in which other signs may predominate
Pyramidal disorders
Extrapyramidal disease
Neuroleptic malignant syndrome
Malignant hyperthermia (during anaesthesia)

Stiff man (or person) syndrome is an uncommon disorder, relatively recently recognized and generally now agreed to be of autoimmune origin. It appears to be a disorder unique among CNS diseases – a primary, non-malignant immune-mediated process caused by antibodies directed against a specific subpopulation of (spinal) neurones. It may be associated with diabetes mellitus, or with systemic autoimmune diseases, particularly lupus, and rarely is seen as an apparent paraneoplastic disorder, but in the majority of cases it occurs in isolation.

Clinical features

It presents with adult onset slowness, aching discomfort and stiffness of muscles, mainly but not exclusively, axial, and with painful muscle cramps, progressing slowly over months and years. Spasms, often noise-, startle-, or action-induced, may be very severe – tendon and muscle rupture may occur. Walking may become clumsy and unsteady. There is no disturbance of sphincter function. Examination reveals normal power and tendon reflexes, downgoing plantar responses, and no abnormalities either of sensation or (barring spasms) coordination. However, axial and abdominal wall rigidity is apparent, and there may be proximal limb muscle stiffness, agonists and antagonists acting simultaneously. An hysterical origin for the symptoms is often wrongly assumed. Asymmetrical contraction of the paraspinal muscles causes a characteristic lordotic and often scoliotic posture.

Investigations

Brain and spinal cord imaging is normal. The spinal fluid is usually normal, but for the common finding of oligoclonal immunoglobulin bands. Electrophysiological muscle examination reveals continuous muscle activity despite invitation to relax, with normal motor unit morphology. ('The patient was unable to relax during the examination' should raise suspicion.) Importantly, voluntary contraction of antagonists fails to inhibit the activity in the muscle under examination. Abnormal activity – and likewise spasms – does not persist during sleep; its central origin is confirmed by its disappearance following pharmacological peripheral nerve block or spinal or general anaesthesia, in contrast to the abnormal activity demonstrable in neuromyotonic syndromes.

Pathogenesis and detection of specific antibodies

The syndrome is thought to result from an imbalance between excitatory (catecholaminergic) and descending inhibitory (γ-amino butyric acid or GABA-ergic) influences on spinal motor neurones. Antibodies directed against glutamic acid decarboxylase (GAD), the enzyme responsible for producing GABA from glutamic acid, which therefore react with GABA-ergic neurones (and with pancreatic islet β-cells) are present in 60 per cent of patients. A clonal B cell response against GAD is apparent within the CSF, partly accounting for the oligoclonal immunoglobulin bands.

In patients with cancer and stiff man syndrome, antineuronal antibodies of a different specificity to a synaptic vesicle-associated protein amphiphysin, may be found. Additionally, in the more serious stiff or progressive encephalomyelitis with rigidity (**PEWR**), with stiffness accompanied by cranial neuropathies, myoclonus, ataxia, diminished tendon jerks, and (especially) extensor plantar responses, MRI brain stem and spinal cord changes occur, and the CSF shows a pleomorphic leucocytosis. The course is substantially more aggressive, with death in 3 to 10 years. GAD antibodies may be found, but in PEWR seen in the context of cancer, antibodies against amphiphysin can also be present.

Treatment

Benzodiazepines (particularly), tizanidine, and also baclofen and occasionally sodium valproate are used therapeutically. More experimental treatments have included intrathecal baclofen and paraspinal botulinum toxin.

There is now Class 1b evidence for the value of intravenous immunoglobulin.

Further reading

Adams M *et al.* (1987). Whipple's disease confined to the central nervous system. *Annals of Neurology* **21**, 104–8.

Adelman DC, Saltiel E, Klinenberg JR (1986). The neuropsychiatric manifestations of systemic lupus erythematosus: an overview. *Seminars in Arthritis and Rheumatism* **15**, 185–99.

Akman-Demir G, Serdaroglu P, Tasci B (1999). Clinical patterns of neurological involvement in Behçet's disease: evaluation of 200 patients. The Neuro-Behçet Study Group. *Brain* **122**, 71–82.

Alexander EL (1986). Central nervous system (CNS) manifestations of primary Sjögren's syndrome: an overview. *Scandinavian Journal of Rheumatology Supplement* **61**, 161–5.

Andonopoulos AP *et al.* (1990). The spectrum of neurological involvement in Sjögren's syndrome. *British Journal of Rheumatology* **29**, 21–3.

Averbuch Heller L, Steiner I, Abramsky O (1992). Neurologic manifestations of progressive systemic sclerosis. *Archives of Neurology* **49**, 1292–5.

Bathon JM, Moreland LW, DiBartolomeo AG (1989). Inflammatory central nervous system involvement in rheumatoid arthritis. *Seminars in Arthritis and Rheumatism* **18**, 258–66.

Bennett RM, Bong DM, Spargo BH (1978). Neuropsychiatric problems in mixed connective tissue disease. *American Journal of Medicine* **65**, 955–62.

Brain L, Jellinek EH, Ball K (1966). Hashimoto's disease and encephalopathy. *Lancet* **ii**, 512–14.

Caselli RJ, Hunder GG (1994). Neurologic complications of giant cell (temporal) arteritis. *Seminars in Neurology* **14**, 349–53.

Cerinic MM *et al.* (1996). The nervous system in systemic sclerosis (scleroderma). Clinical features and pathogenetic mechanisms. *Rheumatic Diseases Clinics of North America* **22**, 879–92.

Cooke WT, Smith WT (1966). Neurological disorders associated with adult coeliac disease. *Brain* **89**, 683–722.

Dalakas MC, Li M, Fujii M, Jacobowitz DM (2001). Stiff person syndrome: quantification, specificity, and intrathecal synthesis of GAD65 antibodies. *Neurology* **57**, 780–4.

Dalakas MC, *et al.* (2001).High-dose intravenous immune globulin for stiff-person syndrome. *New England Journal of Medicine* **345**, 1870–6.

Dresner SC, Kennerdell JS (1985). Dysthyroid orbitopathy. *Neurology* **35**, 1628–34.

Dropcho EJ (1996). Antiamphiphysin antibodies with small-cell lung carcinoma and paraneoplastic encephalomyelitis. *Annals of Neurology* **39**, 659–67.

Dyck PJ *et al.* (1987). Nonsystemic vasculitic neuropathy. *Brain* **110**, 843–54.

Eldor A (1998). Thrombotic thrombocytopenic purpura: diagnosis, pathogenesis and modern therapy. *Baillière's Clinical Haematology* **11**, 475–95.

Ellis SG, Verity MA (1979). Central nervous system involvement in systemic lupus erythematosus: a review of neuropathologic findings in 57 cases, 1955–1977. *Seminars in Arthritis and Rheumatism* **8**, 212–21.

Elsehety A, Bertorini TE (1997). Neurologic and neuropsychiatric complications of Crohn's disease. *Southern Medical Journal* **90**, 606–10.

Giang DW (1994). Central nervous system vasculitis secondary to infections, toxins, and neoplasms. *Seminars in Neurology* **14**, 313–19.

Good AE (1974). Reiter's disease: a review with special attention to cardiovascular and neurologic sequelae. *Seminars in Arthritis and Rheumatism* **3**, 253–86.

Hankey G (1991). Isolated angiitis/angiopathy of the CNS. Prospective diagnostic and therapeutic experience. *Cerebrovascular Disease* **1**, 2–15.

Jain R *et al.* (1994). Systemic lupus erythematosus complicated by thrombotic microangiopathy. *Seminars in Arthritis and Rheumatism* **24**, 173–82.

Johnson RT, Richardson EP (1968). The neurological manifestations of systemic lupus erythematosus. *Medicine (Baltimore)* **47**, 337–69.

Leonard TJ *et al.* (1984). Graves' disease presenting with bilateral acute painful proptosis, ptosis, ophthalmoplegia, and visual loss. *Lancet* **2**, 431–3.

Levine SR, Brey RL (1996). Neurological aspects of antiphospholipid antibody syndrome. *Lupus* **5**, 347–53.

Louis ED *et al.* (1996). Diagnostic guidelines in central nervous system Whipple's disease. *Annals of Neurology* **40**, 561–8.

Matthews WB (1968). The neurological complications of ankylosing spondylitis. *Journal of the Neurological Sciences* **6**, 561–73.

Moersch FP, Woltman HW (1956). Progressive fluctuating muscular rigidity and spasm ("stiff man syndrome"): report of a case and observations in 13 other cases. *Mayo Clinic Proceedings* **31,** 421–7.

Moore PM (1994). Vasculitis of the central nervous system. *Seminars in Neurology* **14**, 307–12.

Moore PM, Lisak RP (1995). Systemic lupus erythematosus: immunopathogenesis of neurologic dysfunction. *Springer Seminars in Immunopathology* **17**, 43–60.

Neuwelt CM *et al.* (1995). Role of intravenous cyclophosphamide in the treatment of severe neuropsychiatric systemic lupus erythematosus. *American Journal of Medicine* **98**, 32–41.

Nishino H *et al.* (1993). Neurological involvement in Wegener's granulomatosis: an analysis of 324 consecutive patients at the Mayo Clinic. *Annals of Neurology* **33**, 4–9.

Oksanen V (1986). Neurosarcoidosis: clinical presentations and course in 50 patients. *Acta Neurologica Scandinavica* **73**, 283–90.

Pincelli C *et al.* (1994). Psoriasis and the nervous system. *Acta Dermato-venereologica Supplementum (Stockholm)* **186**, 60–1.

Puechal X *et al.* (1995). Peripheral neuropathy with necrotizing vasculitis in rheumatoid arthritis. A clinicopathologic and prognostic study of 32 patients. *Arthritis and Rheumatism* **38**, 1618–29.

Scolding NJ (1999). Cerebral vasculitis. In: Scolding NJ, ed. *Immunological and inflammatory diseases of the central nervous system*, pp 210–58. Butterworth-Heinemann, Oxford.

Scolding NJ (1999). Neurological complications of rheumatological and connective tissue disorders. In: Scolding NJ, ed. *Immunological and inflammatory diseases of the central nervous system*, pp 147–80. Butterworth-Heinemann, Oxford.

Scolding NJ (1999). Organ-specific autoimmune and inflammatory disease and the CNS. In: Scolding NJ, ed. *Immunological and inflammatory diseases of the central nervous system*, pp 181–92. Butterworth-Heinemann, Oxford.

Scolding NJ, ed (1999). *Immunological and inflammatory diseases of the central nervous system*, pp. 138–46. Butterworth–Heinemann, Oxford.

Scolding NJ *et al.* (1997). The syndrome of cerebral vasculitis: recognition, diagnosis and management. *Quarterly Journal of Medicine* **90**, 61–73.

Solimena M, DeCamilli P (1991). Autoimmunity to glutamate decarboxylase (GAD) in stiff man syndrome and insulin-dependent diabetes. *Trends in Neurosciences* **14**, 452–57.

Stern BJ *et al.* (1985). Sarcoidosis and its neurological manifestations. *Archives of Neurology* **42**, 909–17.

Zajicek JP (1999). Sarcoidosis and the nervous system. In: Scolding NJ, ed. *Immunological and inflammatory diseases of the central nervous system*, pp 193–209. Butterworth-Heinemann, Oxford.

24.21 Developmental abnormalities of the central nervous system

C. M. Verity, H. Firth, and C. ffrench-Constant*

Normal development of the human central nervous system (CNS)

The human CNS, like that of all vertebrates, develops from a two-dimensional sheet of cells into a complex three-dimensional structure. Within the CNS individual neurones establish precise connections over long distances. The resulting neural networks control and support behaviours ranging from simple reflex activities to the most complex functions of the brain. Given this complexity, it is not surprising that a range of abnormalities results from failures in distinct stages of development. This chapter describes normal development of the human CNS and uses it as a framework to discuss disorders of each phase as well as those that result from multiple disturbances of these complex processes. We have included only structural abnormalities of the CNS that are present at birth and have not reviewed the numerous metabolic and degenerative disorders that can affect the infant brain.

Induction

This is a process by which one group of cells acts upon another group so that the second group differentiates or in some way alters its behaviour. Following the development of the three cell layers of the early embryo (ectoderm, mesoderm, and endoderm), signals from the underlying mesoderm (the 'inducer') instruct a region of the ectoderm (the 'induced tissue') to adopt a neural fate.

Neural tube formation

The neural ectoderm folds to form a tube which separates from the ectoderm and runs most of the length of the embryo. Closure starts at a level corresponding to the future hindbrain/spinal cord junction and then proceeds both towards the head (rostrally) and the tail (caudally). The most caudal part of the neural tube is formed by the thickening of the neural plate and the subsequent formation of a cavity (rather than a tube as is seen rostrally).

Regionalization and specification

Once the neural tube has developed, specification of different regions and individual cells within these regions occurs. This patterning occurs in both the rostrocaudal and dorsoventral axis. The three basic regions of the CNS (forebrain, midbrain, and hindbrain) develop at the rostral end of the tube, with the spinal cord more caudally. Within the developing cord the specification of the different populations of neural precursors (neural crest, sensory neurones, interneurones, glial cells, and motor neurones) is observed in progressively more ventral locations. This process reflects the interaction between genes whose expression defines individual territories or cell types, and diffusible signalling molecules secreted by adjacent areas of the embryo.

Some of the genes and signalling molecules involved in these processes were originally identified by genetic studies in the fruit fly *Drosophila melanogaster*, and appear to be very highly conserved throughout evolution. Of particular importance are a family of genes, called homeotic genes, most of which contain a conserved sequence called a homeobox encoding a protein motif called a homeodomain. This motif binds DNA sequences involved in the regulation of expression of other genes important in development, and so can regulate cell differentiation. For example, homeotic genes have been shown in *Drosophila* to define the identity of individual segments of the fly's body, so that homeotic mutations alter segment identity. The same basic mechanism patterns the vertebrate CNS. In addition, two of the key extracellular signalling molecules, encoded by the genes *wingless* and *sonic hedgehog* (*shh*), were first identified in *Drosophila*.

An example of how these genes and signalling molecules interact is provided by the process of ventral induction. This is illustrated by the specification of motor neurones and glial cells in the spinal cord. Initially the cells of the tube have no axis. The notocord, a transient structure ventral to the neural tube, then produces *shh* protein. This induces the ventralization of the adjacent tube and the expression of two homeobox-containing genes (*PAX6* and *NKX2.2*) in this region. These genes in turn allow motor neurones to develop in the ventral tube, but this requires further exposure to *shh*. Because it is produced in ventral sites, the *shh* molecule is present in a gradient from ventral to dorsal, and this provides further patterning information. Motor neurone specification occurs at a higher concentration of *shh* than that required for the specification of the glial precursor cells. As a consequence, motor neurones develop correctly in a location ventral to the glial cells.

Proliferation and migration

Following the establishment of the basic plan of the CNS, the most dorsal cells of the tube (the neural crest) migrate away to form much of the peripheral nervous system. At the same time, cell proliferation and migration within the tube leads to thickening of the wall and the movement of the many different cell types to their correct locations. The developing forebrain cortex provides a good example. An area called the germinal matrix adjacent to the lumen of the neural tube (which will become the ventricular system) contains populations of neural stem cells that divide to generate committed precursor cells of the different cell lineages of the CNS—neurones and the two glial cell types, oligodendrocytes and astrocytes. These precursor cells then migrate to their final locations. Many of the neurones migrate along specialized cells called radial glial cells, whose processes span the entire thickness of the developing cortex, before leaving the glial fibre to join a specific cortical layer. The time at which the precursor cells are generated defines which type of neurone they will become, and the cortex is built in an 'inside-out' pattern with each neuronal type then migrating beyond its predecessors before leaving the radial fibre. In this way, the six layers of the cortex each containing different neuronal populations are established. Abnormalities of migration in mice and humans

* We are very grateful to Dr Nagui Antoun (Addenbrooke's Hospital, Cambridge), Dr Fred Pickworth (Norfolk and Norwich Hospital), and Mr Paul Chamberlain (John Radcliffe Hospital, Oxford) for the images shown in this chapter and for advice on their interpretation.

have been linked to specific genetic mutations. For example mice with abnormalities in an extracellular matrix molecule called reelin or in its receptors show aberrant patterns of cortical lamination and cerebellar development.

Connection and selection

Once each cell type is specified and in an appropriate location, axon outgrowth and the formation of synapses occurs. These connections are made both locally and over considerable distances, as for example in the contralateral connections made by axons running in the corpus callosum (a fibre tract crossing from one side of the brain to the other). The mechanisms by which the vast number of connections are made are complex and incompletely understood. There are both attractive and repulsive cues that guide growth cones within the CNS. Examples are the netrins, that are attractive to most outgrowing axons and are produced by the ventral floor plate of the spinal cord before axons grow into it, and the semaphorins that can repel growth cones. In addition there is evidence that recognition molecules such as cadherins and ephrins can regulate cell–cell adhesion and intracellular signalling and allow axons to select precise targets once they have arrived in the appropriate location. In many cases such signalling and recognition molecules exist as large families of related molecules, a diversity that may underlie the development of such complex connections. Finally, cells that fail to establish the correct connections undergo programmed cell death (apoptosis) as a result of a failure to obtain factors produced by the target cells that are required for survival. In this way, errors in pathfinding or cell production can be corrected at a later stage. At the same time, neurones establish close interactions with glial cells that either form the myelin sheaths essential for rapid impulse conduction (oligodendrocytes) or regulate the extracellular environment of the neurone and so play a homeostatic role essential for correct function (astrocytes).

Although developmental abnormalities can occur at any stage of gestation, some developmental events such as neural tube formation and specification occur in the first month after conception. This is important from a clinical standpoint, as developmental abnormalities resulting from environmental factors can occur before pregnancy is confirmed. Dietary folic acid supplements can reduce the risk of neural tube defects but need to be taken from the very earliest stages of pregnancy and should be started before conception.

Structural abnormalities resulting from disturbances of normal CNS development

Disorders of neural tube formation

Introduction

The neural tube usually fuses completely between 18 and 26 days after ovulation. Failure of closure leads to malformations that include anencephaly, encephalocele, spina bifida, and spina bifida occulta. These neural tube defects are aetiologically related and if one member of a family is affected there is an increased risk in the relatives for all types of neural tube defect. They are malformations of the neuroectoderm which are associated to a variable extent with abnormalities of the surrounding mesodermal structures. The term dysraphism is used when there is continuity between the posterior neuroectoderm and cutaneous ectoderm.

Epidemiology

The prevalence of neural tube defects varies according to geography and race, although they are among the most common congenital abnormalities in most countries. High rates (more than 8 per 1000 births) have been reported in Northern Ireland, Egypt, India, and China. There are worldwide reports of decreasing prevalence rates. In England there was a peak in 1954 to 1955 followed by a substantial decline which started in the early 1970s. The epidemiological evidence suggests that this decrease was not entirely due to prenatal screening, and it also preceded the widespread use of periconceptual vitamin supplemention, so some of the decrease remains unexplained. By 1994 the prevalence of neural tube defects in England and Wales was just under 0.8 per 1000 total births. In the United Kingdom anencephaly and spina bifida are of approximately equal prevalence and together make up 95 per cent of all neural tube defects.

Aetiology

Genetic factors

Most neural tube defects are a complex interaction between several genes and environmental factors. Major genes have been identified in the mouse that may mutate and cause neural tube defects, but their relevance to human defects is still not clear. More is being discovered about the identity of modifier genes. For instance mutations in the methylene tetrahydrofolate reductase gene are associated with elevated blood homocysteine levels in pregnant women and and increased risk of neural tube defects. However, the relative risks are low (about twofold) and mutation analysis is not used in routine clinical practice. Neural tube defects occur in many different syndromes and many chromosome disorders, but if a neural tube defect is the only anomaly, karyotyping is not indicated.

Environmental factors

Periconceptual multiple vitamin supplements containing folic acid have been shown to reduce the incidence of neural tube defects. In England it is currently recommended that, to prevent a first occurrence of neural tube defect, women who are planning pregnancy should take 400 μg of folic acid daily before conception and during the first 12 weeks of pregnancy. To prevent recurrence of neural tube defect the dose should be 4 to 5 mg per day.

Some drugs taken during pregnancy may increase the risk of neural tube defects in the fetus. These include sodium valproate and folic acid antagonists such as trimethoprim, triamterene, carbamazepine, phenytoin, phenobarbitone, and primidone.

Prenatal diagnosis

α-Fetoprotein levels in maternal serum

The fetal liver is the main source of α-fetoprotein (AFP), which leaks through open neural tube defects into the amniotic fluid and then into the maternal blood. This abnormal increase in maternal serum α-fetoprotein is best detected at 16 to 18 weeks of pregnancy. Maternal serum screening does not detect closed defects (those covered by skin) and is less sensitive in women taking the antiepileptic drug sodium valproate.

Ultrasonography

This is recommended for all at-risk women—those with positive serum α-fetoprotein screening, those who have had one or more affected child, and those taking drugs associated with neural tube defects in the fetus. Anencephaly can be detected by ultrasound from the 12th week of gestation and spina bifida from 16 to 20 weeks (Fig. 1(a and b)). However, even the best ultrasonographers may occasionally miss spina bifida, particularly in the L5–S2 region.

Amniocentesis

This has been largely superseded by detailed ultrasound imaging. When adequate ultrasound images cannot be obtained, amniocentesis with measurement of of α-fetoprotein and assay of neuronal acetylcholinesterase provides an alternative method of prenatal diagnosis.

Cranial dysraphism

Anencephaly

This is a lethal defect that results from failure of fusion of the rostral folds of the neural tube between days 18 to 25 of embryonic development. The cranial vault is absent and an angiomatous membranous mass lies on the floor of the cranium. The eyes are protruberant because of shallow orbits and there is variable involvement of the spinal cord. Before the advent of prenatal diagnosis by ultrasound most anencephalic babies were born in the last 3 months of gestation; now an increasing number of such pregnancies are terminated. In liveborn anencephalic babies the initial neurological examination may be surprisingly normal if brainstem structures are reasonably intact and seizures may be seen despite the absence of cerebral hemispheres. However, the infants usually die in hours or days.

Cephaloceles

A cephalocele is a herniation of cranial contents through a skull defect. There are several subtypes: a cranial meningocele contains only meninges, an encephalocele contains brain tissue, and a ventriculocele contains part of the ventricle within the herniated portion of brain. Cephaloceles are less common than anencephaly or spina bifida, occurring in 1 to 3 per 10 000 live births. They are associated with other brain abnormalities such as agenesis of the corpus callosum or abnormal gyration. They may be part of a recognized syndrome, so it is important to look for abnormalities in other parts of the body. Sometimes neurosurgery is indicated.

Posterior cephaloceles This is the commonest group in Western countries and the majority are occipital encephaloceles. They are of variable size and may be above or below the tentorium. The latter are often associated with severe cerebellar defects, such as the Chiari III malformation (see under posterior fossa abnormalities). The prognosis depends on the size of the encephalocele, the site, and the associated abnormalities, such as hydrocephalus. Visual impairment may result from involvement of the occipital lobes. There may be motor and intellectual impairment and seizures.

Anterior cephaloceles These are more common in some parts of Asia. Frontoethmoidal cephaloceles may protrude into the nose, the ethmoid, or the orbit. They often include olfactory tissue and frontal lobe tissue and can present with nasal blockage or cerebrospinal fluid leakage. Sphenoidal cephaloceles can cause pharyngeal obstruction and recurrent meningitis and may be associated with abnormalities in the secretion of somatotrophin, gonadatrophin, or antidiuretic hormone.

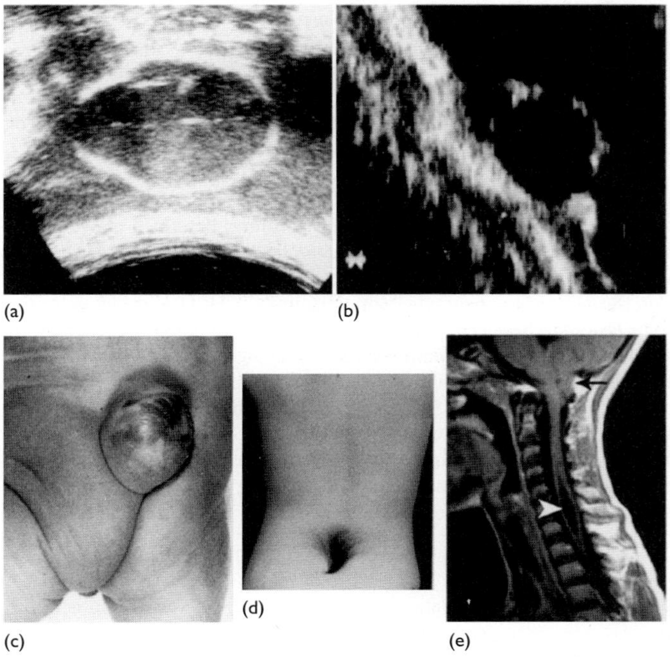

Fig. 1 (a) Prenatal ultrasound of a child with a neural tube defect, showing the 'lemon sign' resulting from the change in shape of the back of the skull (on the left-hand side in the image) which is associated with the Chiari II malformation described in the text. (b) Prenatal ultrasound of a child with a neural tube defect, showing a cystic lumbar meningomyelocele in the caudal neural tube. (c) Lumbar meningomyelocele. Photograph of a newborn infant. (d) Chiari I malformation and syringomyelia in an asymptomatic girl aged 11 years. Photograph of tuft of hair seen over the lumbar region at birth. The associated CNS malformations are shown in scan (e). (e) Chiari I malformation and syringomyelia. T_1-weighted sagittal MRI shows there is herniation of the cerebellar tonsils through the foramen magnum (arrow) and a syrinx of the lower cervical spinal cord (C5–C7) (arrow head). The associated tuft of lumbar hair is shown in photograph (d).

Spinal dysraphism

Spina bifida

This can be divided into spina bifida occulta, which consists of failure of closure of the vertebral arches without an external lesion, and spina bifida cystica in which there is a cystic lesion on the back. The lesion may be either a meningocele without neural tissue or a myelomeningocele in which the spinal cord is a component of the cyst wall.

The term rachischisis is used for the most severe defect, which is a widely patent dorsal opening of the spine, often associated with anencephaly.

Myelomeningocele

The spinal defect This is the abnormality found in 80 to 90 per cent of children with spina bifida cystica. It is lumbosacral in about 80 per cent of cases and consists of a sac covered with a thin membrane which may leak cerebrospinal fluid (Fig. 1(c)). Neurological abnormalities depend on the level of the lesion, which is best judged clinically by determining the upper limit of sensory loss. There is usually a mixture of upper and lower motor neurone signs depending on the level. Whatever the level of the lesion, there is disturbance of bladder and bowel sphincters and also bladder detrusor dysfunction. The sensory level correlates with the severity of abnormalities in the urinary tract and is also related to long-term disability. Higher lesions of the cord are associated with bladder outlet obstruction, dilatation of the upper urinary tract, and chronic pyelonephritis.

Hydrocephalus This complicates most cases of lumbosacral meningomyelocele. Ultrasound studies show hydrocephalus in about 90 per cent of cases at birth, even though the head circumference is normal. Usually it is associated with the Chiari II malformation (see below), although it may be due to aqueduct stenosis or have no clear structural cause. If there is evidence of progressive ventricular dilatation (often detected with ultrasound) or signs of increasing intracranial pressure, insertion of a ventriculoperitoneal shunt is usually necessary.

Chiari II malformation This is present in about 70 per cent of cases of meningomyelocele. It is the most common of the four types of Arnold–Chiari malformation. It consists of downward protrusion of the medulla below the foramen magnum to overlap the spinal cord. The medulla is kinked and the cerebellar vermis indented by the posterior lip of the foramen magnum. The fourth ventricle is elongated and the midbrain distorted, which can cause early or late problems. These include palsies resulting from involvement of the lower cranial nerves and central apnoea (which may be misdiagnosed as epilepsy in older children).

Almost all cases of Chiari II malformation are associated with meningomyelocele. In contrast the other types of Arnold–Chiari malformations (I, III, and IV) are not associated with spina bifida and are dealt with in the section on posterior fossa abnormalities.

Management Treatment of infants with meningomyeloceles became possible with the development of ventriculoatrial and ventriculoperitoneal shunts. In the early 1960s it was argued that closure of the defect within 24 h of birth reduced mortality and morbidity by avoiding infection and reducing trauma to the exposed neural tissue. The early active management of all cases was questioned by Lorber who proposed that surgery should be selective. He reported four adverse criteria that he thought were contraindications to treatment: a high level of paraplegia, clinically evident hydrocephalus at birth, lumbar kyphosis, and the presence of other major malformations. However, using these criteria the outcome was uncertain; many infants survived even though they did not have closure of the defect within 24 h, and some children with a supposedly good prognosis were left with major disabilities after surgery. Selective surgical management is therefore not universally practised and this remains a controversial area.

Now the emphasis has moved towards prevention. It is recommended that women planning to conceive supplement their diet with folic acid, which reduces the risk of neural tube defects. Screening of maternal serum for α-fetoprotein is possible and prenatal diagnosis by ultrasound and amniocentesis is available. This is discussed above in the section on neural tube defects.

Meningocele

Here there is protrusion of the meninges outside the spinal canal: the sac does not contain any neural tissue. Meningoceles account for about 5 per cent of cases of spina bifida cystica. There is no associated hydrocephalus and the neurological examination is usually normal. They must be distinguished from meningomyeloceles because the prognosis is so different.

Occult spinal dysraphism

The term spina bifida occulta is often applied to a defect of the posterior arch of one or more lumbar or sacral vertebrae (usually L5 and S1). It is found incidentally by radiography in 25 per cent of children admitted to hospital and may be regarded as a normal variant. However, it must not be assumed that spina bifida occulta is always benign. If examination of the skin over the spine reveals a naevus, hairy patch (Fig. 1(d)), dimple, sinus, or subcutaneous mass, further evaluation is necessary. Even if there are no associated abnormalities of sphincter or limb control on MRI of the spinal cord is indicated. A spinal cord malformation may cause an asymmetrical lower motor neurone weakness with wasting, deformity, and diminished reflexes in the lower limb. Alternatively there may be a progressive gait disturbance with spasticity. Either presentation may be associated with disturbed bladder control. Several different abnormalities may be found.

Dorsal dermal sinuses may connect the skin surface to the dura or to an intradural dermoid cyst. They are most commonly found in the occipital and lumbosacral regions. An open sinus tract can cause recurrent meningitis so ideally they should be explored and excised before infections occur. Lipomyelomeningoceles present as a bulge in the lumbosacral region, usually lateral to the midline. They consist of a lipoma or lipofibroma attached to a low lying abnormal spinal cord and are often associated with a meningocele. Diastematomyelia is the presence of a sagittal cleft which divides the spinal cord into two halves, each surrounded by its own pia mater. A bony or cartilaginous spur may transfix the cord, fixing it in a low position as the child grows. The cleft is usually in the low thoracic or lumbar region, but cervical clefts have been reported. In 75 per cent of cases of diastematomyelia an overlying midline skin abnormality is present and plain radiographs show abnormalities in most cases—these include abnormal segmentation of vertebrae, spina bifida, and scoliosis.

Treatment of occult spinal dysraphism

If an abnormality involving the cord or nerve roots is found, there is often a good case for neurosurgical intervention. The aim is to free the spinal cord from its abnormal attachments to allow for growth and prevent further damage. Early intervention may prevent worsening motor deficits and urological complications, but the indications for intervention are controversial.

Other developmental abnormalities of the spinal cord

Syringomyelia

This is a tubular cavitation of the spinal cord as opposed to hydromyelia which is dilatation of the central canal of the cord—a distinction that may be difficult to make clinically. Syringomyelia is often associated with the Chiari I malformation and hydrocephalus (Fig. 1(e)). It tends to be in the cervical region but may involve the whole cord. It rarely becomes symptomatic in children. Treatment is controversial. Shunting of the abnormal cavity is sometimes performed and posterior fossa exploration may be undertaken if there is a Chiari I malformation.

Sacral agenesis

This is strongly associated with maternal diabetes mellitus. Absence of the sacrum and coccyx is usually associated with abnormalities of the lumbosacral cord. There may be arthrogryposis at birth (defined as a fixed deformity of one or more joints). A flaccid neurogenic bladder causes incontinence and there are sensory and motor deficits in the legs.

Disorders of regionalization

Failure of normal development of the most anterior portion of the neural tube (the mediobasal prosencephalon) and associated structures due to disturbances in the process of ventral induction described above may result in various abnormalities of the brain and face. The most severe CNS abnormality is holoprosencephaly in which there is failure of the prosencephalon to separate into two cerebral hemispheres. The mildest is olfactory aplasia without other cerebral malformations. The severity of the associated facial abnormalities tends to parallel those in the brain. In the most severe facial abnormality there is anophthalmia and absence of the nose. However there may be just mild hypotelorism (closely set eyes), a single central incisor tooth, or the face may be normal.

Holoprosencephaly (prosencephaly)

This occurs with a frequency of approximately 1 in 14 000 births. There is failure of formation of the two cerebral hemispheres resulting in abnormalities of varying severity. The causes may be chromosomal, multifactorial, or monogenic and there may be associated facial and midline malformations.

Aetiology

This is time specific and stimulus non-specific. There is a very short vulnerable period, because ventral induction probably occurs prior to 23 days, just before the elaboration of the optic vesicles (24 days), which explains its relative rarity (6 per 10 000 live births in one study). Environmental factors may be important: it is at least 20 times more common in the infants of mothers with diabetes than in the general population.

Genetic factors are also important. At least 12 genetic loci and several holoprosencephaly (*HPE*) genes have been identified in humans. Some of these genes can be linked to signalling pathways described above in the section on CNS development. One (*HPE3* on chromosome 7q36) is the *sonic hedgehog* gene encoding a secreted protein required for ventral induction throughout the neuraxis. Mutations in PATCHED-1, the receptor for *sonic hedgehog*, have been found in individuals with holoprosencephaly. In addition *ZIC2*, present on chromosome 13q32 and encoding a human homologue of the *drosophila odd-paired* gene is implicated in *wingless* signalling. Two other genes, *SIX3* and *TGIF*, both encode homeodomain proteins of undefined function. A number of chromosomal abnormalities have also been recognized in association with holoprosencephaly. These include trisomy and other abnormalities of chromosome 13, partial deletion of the short arm of chromosome 18, ring chromosome 18, and partial trisomy of chromosome 7.

Clinical features

In alobar holoprosencephaly the completely undivided forebrain is in the shape of a horseshoe surrounding a single cavity. The thalami are fused but the brainstem and cerebellum are well developed. The associated facial abnormalities are severe—there may be anophthalmia or cyclopia in which there is a single orbit. In holoprosencephaly with median cleft lip there is marked hypotelorism. In semilobar holoprosencephaly the brain is divided into two hemispheres posteriorly but anteriorly the two hemispheres are fused (Fig. 2). In lobar holoprosencephaly there is almost complete separation of the hemispheres and the face may be normal. The head is usually microcephalic unless there is associated hydrocephalus.

The most severely affected infants die in the neonatal period. Less severely affected patients may live for months or years. The survivors often develop infantile spasms or other seizures. Some patients with significant structural abnormalities may survive to adulthood but usually there are

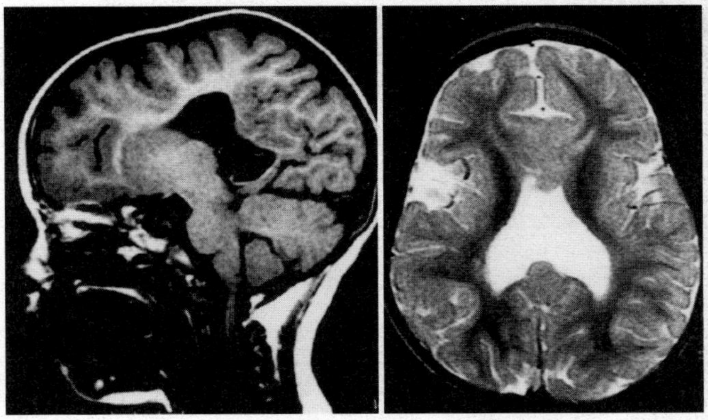

(a) (b)

Fig. 2 (a) Semilobar holoprosencephaly in a girl aged 2 years imaged with T_1-weighted sagittal MRI. This midline view shows absence of the corpus callosum and fusion of the frontal lobes. (b) Semilobar holoprosencephaly in the same patient using T_2-weighted axial MRI. There is fusion of the frontal lobes of both cerebral hemispheres and a common central ventricle.

severe learning difficulties. Associated anomalies include congenital heart disease, scalp defects, and polydactly. Holoprosencephaly may be part of syndromes such as the Meckel–Gruber syndrome and the Aicardi syndrome.

Genetic counselling

Families have been described in which there is dominant inheritance of minor features and one or more children with holoprosencephaly. It is therefore important to look for minor signs in both parents of an affected child. These include orbital hypotelorism, median cleft lip, flat nose with or without a single nostril, anosmia, and a single central incisor.

Prenatal diagnosis can be made by ultrasound from the 16th week of pregnancy and holoprosencephaly accounts for a proportion of the cases of hydrocephalus diagnosed antenatally. Orbital hypotelorism is a reliable diagnostic feature for antenatal diagnosis by ultrasound.

Disorders of cortical development

Modern brain imaging, in particular MRI, has resulted in the identification of many previously unrecognized developmental abnormalities of the cerebral cortex. Following the classification used by Aicardi this section is divided into disorders of proliferation, migration, and cortical organization.

Disorders of proliferation and differentiation

Microcephaly

This is an abnormally small head, which is disproportionately small in relation to the rest of the body. A child is microcephalic when the head circumference is below the normal range (less than the 0.4th centile), defined by head growth charts appropriate for sex and race. Some children with microcephaly are neurologically normal.

Genetic causes of microcephaly There is a genetically determined type of microcephaly in which the inheritance is usually autosomal recessive with at least three loci currently identified, but may be autosomal dominant or X linked. Characteristically there is marked microcephaly but the neurological problems are relatively mild. They consist of fine motor incoordination and hyperkinetic behaviour with moderate learning difficulties and seizures. However, it is more usual to find that patients with microcephaly have more significant abnormalities of the nervous system such as pyramidal tract signs and profound learning difficulties. Microcephaly is a feature of more than 450 syndromes listed in the Oxford Dysmorphology Database, so it is a challenge to differentiate genetic from other causes.

Non-genetic causes of microcephaly Ionizing radiation in the first two trimesters of the pregnancy, intrauterine infections, drugs and other chemicals, circulatory disturbance, and perinatal hypoxic–ischaemic events can all cause microcephaly. Poor dietary control in mothers with phenylketonuria is also an important cause of microcephaly, as the fetal brain is very sensitive to the toxic effects of phenylalanine. Sometimes serial head circumference measurements are necessary to make the diagnosis. When there is a significant perinatal insult to the brain the head circumference may be normal at birth with subsequent failure of growth in the first few months of life. However, the first head circumference measurement at birth may be misleading because of skull moulding during delivery.

It is important to perform a skull radiograph to look for evidence of early closure of all the cranial sutures (total craniosynostosis). In some types of genetic microcephaly the head size falls off as late as 32 to 34 weeks of gestation or even after birth. Prenatal diagnosis by ultrasound may be difficult.

Megalencephaly

The term macrocephaly is used when the head circumference is above the normal range for the age, sex, and race of the child. This may result from abnormalities outside the brain parenchyme such as hydrocephalus, arachnoid cysts, congenital abnormalities of the cerebral veins, fluid collections over the surface of the brain, or abnormalities of the skull. Cranial imaging is necessary to make the diagnosis. This discussion deals only with megalencephaly, which is increased size of the brain itself.

Many normal individuals have large heads. When assessing a child with a large head it is important to exclude a developmental or neurological abnormality. A large head may be part of a specific disorder, for example one of the neurocutaneous syndromes, or an overgrowth disorder such as Sotos syndrome. Large heads can run in normal families ('familial megalencephaly') and it is important to check the head circumference of the parents. However, there are kindreds in which some of the family members with large heads have learning problems.

Sometimes megalencephaly is associated with significant learning difficulties, autism, neurological abnormalities, and seizures, and this combination of features can have a genetic basis. The brains may have bulky gyri and usually all parts of the cerebrum are diffusely enlarged, with normal-sized or mildly enlarged ventricles. Occasionally particular parts of the brain such as the cerebellum are disproportionately large. No consistent microscopical alterations are reported in the cortex, but minor anomalies such as small heterotopias may be found. The pathogenesis of this type of megalencephaly is not clear: it may be caused by overproduction of CNS cells, possibly combined with failure of apoptosis.

Hemimegalencephaly or unilateral megalencephaly may involve all parts of the brain on the same side or there may be enlargement of one hemisphere only. In the affected hemisphere there are broadened and coarse gyri and sometimes areas of polymicrogyria. The microscopic abnormalities vary. There may be disorganized masses of grey matter without laminar organization or nodular heterotopias of grey matter: giant neurones may be found.

The neurological problems associated with hemimegalencephaly can be severe. Sometimes there are intractable seizures, which may start in infancy, associated with marked developmental delay and sometimes with hemiparesis. There may be overgrowth of one side of the face or of one side of the whole body. Some infants may present with prenatal or perinatal onset of seizures and die early. Others may develop seizures later which may be refractory to drug treatment, and they may be candidates for hemispherectomy.

Disorders of migration

Migration defects occur when neurones of the subependymal matrix zone lining the ventricular cavity (the ventricular zone) fail to reach their intended destination in the cerebral cortex. This results in either major or minor disturbances of development which may be focal or diffuse. If neurones fail to leave the ventricular zone entirely, periventricular heterotopias result. If neurones leave the ventricular zone but then fail to complete their migration in the cortex, this causes lissencephaly. If, however, only a subpopulation of neurones are affected and the others complete their migration normally, then this results in nodular or band heterotopias. Migration disorders are found as part of recognized syndromes and there are also acquired types resulting from intrauterine infections, circulatory disturbances, and toxins (alcohol or phenytoin for example).

Agyria–pachygyria (lissencephaly)

This is a group of disorders of varying severity. There may be complete absence of gyri, in which case the terms agyria or lissencephaly (greek: 'smooth brain') are used. Pachygyria describes a reduced number of broadened and flat gyri with less folding of the cortex than normal. There may be varying degrees of agyria–pachygyria in the same brain.

Type I lissencephaly

Here the brain is small with only the primary and sometimes a few secondary gyri. The cortex is thick with the white matter forming a thin rim along the ventricles (Fig. 3(a)). In the brainstem the olivary nuclei are ectopic and the pyramids are hypoplastic or absent. In the cerebellum the dentate nuclei are abnormally convoluted. There may be associated agenesis of the corpus callosum. Infants with type I lissencephaly may be divided into the majority who have no dysmorphic features ('isolated lissencephaly sequence') and those with the dysmorphic features of the Miller–Dieker syndrome.

The Miller–Dieker syndrome Characteristically in this syndrome there is postnatal growth deficiency and occasional microcephaly. The dysmorphic features include a tall narrow forehead, a depressed nasal bridge, anteverted nares, midfacial hypoplasia, a prominent upper lip with a thin vermilion border, retrognathism, and hypervascularization of the retina. Hypotonia and seizures are associated. MRI and CT scans show lissencephaly together with a midline focus of calcification in the callosal remnant in about 40 per cent of cases (this is rarely seen in the isolated lissencephaly sequence). About 50 to 70 per cent of cases have a deletion of 17p13.3 by light microscopy and almost all the remainder have a submicroscopic deletion demonstrable by fluorescent *in situ* hybridization of chromosomes using gene probes. This region includes the *LIS1* gene, mutations in which are associated with isolated lissencephaly and which is also required for correct neuronal migration in mice. It has been suggested, therefore, that deletions of the *LIS1* gene cause the lissencephaly seen in the Miller–Dieker syndrome and that the facial dysmorphism is caused by loss of adjacent genes.

Isolated lissencephaly sequence This is a heterogeneous group. Many have a deletion of, or mutations within, the *LIS1* gene. Mutations in a second gene, *doublecortin* (*DCX*) have also been shown to cause lissencephaly.

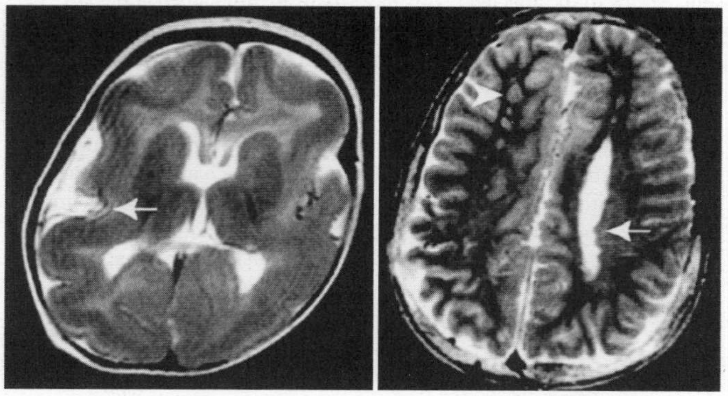

(a) (b)

Fig. 3 (a) Lissencephaly type I in a girl aged 5 months who is visually and socially unresponsive, displays poor feeding, and increased tone. The T_2-weighted axial MRI shows a smooth cerebral cortex with absence of normal gyri and sulci. On the right a vertically orientated shallow sylvian fissure is seen (arrow). (b) Nodular heterotopias in a boy aged 13 years. The T_2-weighted axial image shows the nodular heterotopias are subependymal (arrow) and subcortical (arrow head).

DCX is on the X chromosome, explaining why inheritance of isolated lissencephaly sequence in some cases is X linked. While affected males in these families show the full isolated lissencephaly sequence phenotype, carrier females can show band heterotopia in which a subset of neurones fail to complete migration and form bilateral symmetrical ribbons of grey matter in the centrum semiovale. This is thought to reflect X inactivation of the normal *DCX* gene in these neurones, while those that inactivate the mutation-containing X chromosome migrate normally. In addition to *LIS1* and *DCX*, mutations in the human gene encoding *reelin* (RELN) have recently been described in lissencephaly associated with cerebellar hypoplasia. As described above, *reelin* gene mutations are found in some naturally-occurring mouse mutants with abnormal neuronal migration, and so this provides a direct link between the animal and human studies. Possible non-genetic causes include intrauterine cytomegalovirus infection and early placental insufficiency. Clinically there is severe mental retardation and diplegia together with partial seizures and infantile spasms.

Diagnosis of type I lissencephaly The diagnosis of type I lissencephaly is made by CT or MRI, which show a thick cortical plate with no or few sulci separated from the white matter by an undulating border. The differential diagnosis includes peroxisomal disorders such as Zellweger syndrome, but these have their own specific features. Some cases are due to cytomegalovirus infection and there may be associated periventricular calcification. Prenatal diagnosis is not possible by ultrasound before 24 weeks as tertiary sulci do not appear before then.

Genetic counselling In the Miller–Dieker syndrome, if a deletion is found in the *LIS1* gene and the parental chromosomes are normal, the recurrence risk is less than 1 per cent. In the isolated lissencephaly sequence, if chromosome and DNA studies are negative and the other differential diagnoses are excluded, the empirical recurrence risk is 5 to 7 per cent.

Type II lissencephaly or Walker–Warburg syndrome

This is also called 'cobblestone lissencephaly' and is a completely different malformation from type I lissencephaly. The smooth cortex has a granular surface and is covered with meninges that are thickened due to mesenchymal proliferation. The cerebellum is small with an absent vermis and the pyramidal tracts are usually absent. Hydrocephalus is present in 75 per cent of cases. Microscopically there is complete disorganization of the cortex which consists of neurones separated by bundles of gliomesenchymal tissue continuous with the meninges. More deeply there is a thin layer of white matter lying above islands of heterotopic grey matter. These abnormalities probably result from overmigration of neuroglial precursors through a disrupted pial–glial limiting membrane.

Clinical features The clinical features include both nervous system and muscle abnormalities. The infants are very abnormal at birth. The eyes show retinal dysplasia, microphthalmia, and anomalies of the anterior segment. There may be hydrocephalus or sometimes microcephaly. Usually there is an elevated creatine kinase and necrosis of fibres in all muscles, similar to that seen in severe muscular dystrophy.

Diagnosis The diagnosis of type II lissencephaly is confirmed by MRI or CT scan, which show that the cortex is thinner than in type I lissencephaly and there are characteristic trabeculae penetrating the cortex from the white matter with the appearance of a double cortical layer due to the subcortical heterotopic islands. There is agenesis of the cerebellar vermis and often a posterior encephalocele or large posterior fontanelle.

Differential diagnosis There are a group of conditions involving muscle, eye, and brain that all follow recessive inheritance. It seems likely that the cerebro-ocular–muscle syndrome (COMS) is identical to the Walker–Warburg syndrome for which the gene locus is not yet identified. Fukuyama-type muscular dystrophy is associated with severe mental retardation. It is relatively common in Japan and is due to mutations in the Fukutin gene at 9q31–33. Muscle–eye–brain disease is found in Finland. The eye and brain abnormalities are less severe and the gene locus is on 1p32–34.

Non-lissencephalic cortical dysgenesis

Polymicrogyria (microgyria) is the most important type of abnormality in this section, although the aetiology remains poorly understood. Sometimes the surface of the cortex is relatively smooth resembling pachygyria because the small gyri pile upon each other to form a thickened cortex. The histology of polymicrogyria varies. In unlayered microgyria there is a single cell layer between the white matter and the molecular layer. In classic four-layered microgyria the cortex consists of a molecular layer, an upper dense layer, a layer of low cellular density containing myelinated fibres, and a deep cellular layer. It is suggested that the developmental disturbance occurs near the fifth month of pregnancy. Case reports of polymicrogyria in the infant brain after maternal trauma or asphyxiation during the pregnancy suggest that the abnormality may sometimes be due to failure of cerebral perfusion with resulting hypoxia.

The clinical manifestations of polymicrogyria depend on the location and extent of the abnormalities. Small patches may be found incidentally in the absence of symptoms, but there may be involvement of the whole cortex, or areas of polymicrogyria may border porencephalic cysts in patients with neurological disabilities. There is a bilateral perisylvian syndrome (or anterior operculum syndrome) in which bilateral opercular abnormalities are seen on MRI, some of which have the appearance of polymicrogyria. These patients have a pseudobulbar palsy with dysarthria, and loss of voluntary control of the face and tongue leading to drooling and difficulty feeding. Familial occurrence has been reported on several occasions.

Heterotopias

Periventricular heterotopias are abnormal collections of neurones in the subependymal region. They may be part of a complex malformation syndrome such as the Aicardi syndrome. They may be isolated and clinically silent or associated with seizures. A gene responsible for periventricular heterotopia, the *filamin 1* (FLN1) gene, has been identified on the X chromosome. Filamin protein reorganizes the cytoskeleton, consistent with a role in cell migration. Families with periventricular heterotopia have been described in which females are affected while affected males appear to die before or soon after birth. It is likely that the heterotopias present in affected females result from X inactivation of the normal *FLN1* gene in those cells, while those cells inactivating the abnormal *FLN1* gene migrate normally. Males have only one X chromosome and so all cells will fail to migrate—a lethal phenotype in these families. However, in other families some surviving males with periventricular heterotopias have now been shown to have *FLN1* mutations.

Subcortical heterotopias can be divided into two groups. Nodular heterotopias of grey matter are found in association with other migration disorders and may be the cause of partial seizures (Fig. 3(b)). Subcortical laminar heterotopias are also known as band heterotopias or 'double cortex' and may be inherited as an X-linked trait, as discussed above. Patients with subcortical heterotopias often have seizures, which may be focal or generalized, and they may also have intellectual problems although some do develop normally.

Disorders of cortical organization

There is increasing interest in developmental abnormalities within the cerebral cortex that are relatively subtle compared with those described above, as they may represent important causes of epilepsy and developmental delay. It is likely that this group of disorders will become increasingly well recognized as imaging and other investigative techniques improve.

Cortical microdysgenesis

In 1971 Taylor and colleagues described localized cortical abnormalities in the brains of 10 patients with intractible epilepsy. The lesions could only be seen microscopically and consisted of an excess of large abnormal cells scattered throughout the cortical layers. The abnormal neurones were restricted to sharply delineated areas of cortex and also formed foci in the depths of sulci.

Experiments have been performed in rats using microelectrodes to freeze small areas of cortex, leading to microgyri at these sites. They show that focal cortical abnormalities are associated not only with alterations in the membrane properties and synaptic connections of the neurones directly involved, but also with much more widespread abnormalities of neuronal circuits. Thus there may be more global effects on cerebral function than expected from the size of the lesion.

Microscopic abnormalities of cortical arrangement have been described in the brains of patients with epilepsy or learning difficulties. They include persistence of the subpial layer, aggregates of large neurones in the plexiform zone, a fragmented appearance of the superficial neuronal layers, excess ectopic cells in the cortex, and excess numbers of cells in the molecular layer. Such abnormalities can be found in normal individuals. These abnormalities may cause cortical excitability in generalized epilepsy and localized temporal lobe cortical dysgenesis might lead to dyslexia. Cortical dysgenesis has been reported in autism, schizophrenia, and fetal alcohol syndrome. The extent to which these findings explain abnormal brain function is an area of active research.

Focal cortical dysplasia

It is now known that cortical dysplasias are an important cause of early-onset seizures that may be focal or generalized (Fig. 4(a–c)). Patients with refractory epilepsy should therefore have the best possible imaging, even if they have generalized seizures. Resection of cortical dysplasias may improve seizure control, but this is a challenging field because the preoperative assessment must take into account the widespread anatomical and functional abnormalities associated with cortical dysplasias.

Combined and overlapping cerebral malformations

There is overlap between the different malformations even though they are often described as distinct entities. This is not surprising—the teratogenic periods are so closely spaced that overlaps are likely if there is an environmental cause. Also, in genetically determined syndromes, more than one developmental process may be affected giving predictable combinations of cerebral malformations.

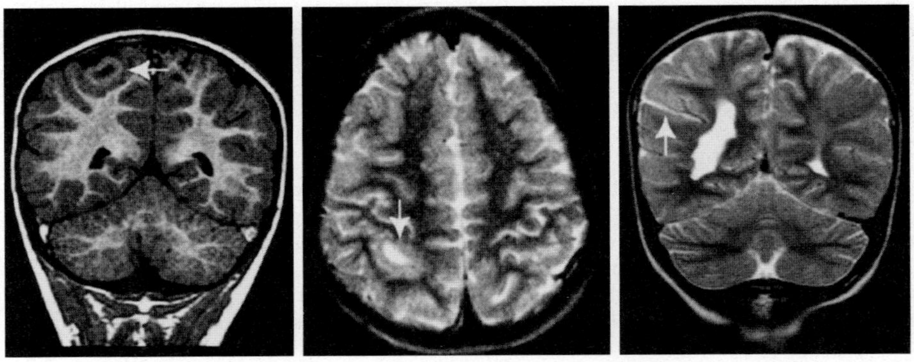

(a) (b) (c)

Fig. 4 (a) Cortical dysplasia in a boy aged 4 years. Focal seizures started at 1 year of age and consisted of a giggle, flexion of the left arm, and a vacant stare. T_1-weighted coronal MRI shows cortical dysplasia in the right parietal region (arrow). (b) The same patient. On T_2-weighted axial MRI, the cortical dysplasia is marked with an arrow. (c) Cortical dysplasia in a boy aged 3 years. Seizures commenced at 9 months of age and consisted of daytime absences and nocturnal generalized tonic–clonic seizures. A T_2-weighted coronal MRI shows an abnormal fissure in the cortex on the right (arrow). The right lateral ventricle is abnormal in size and shape.

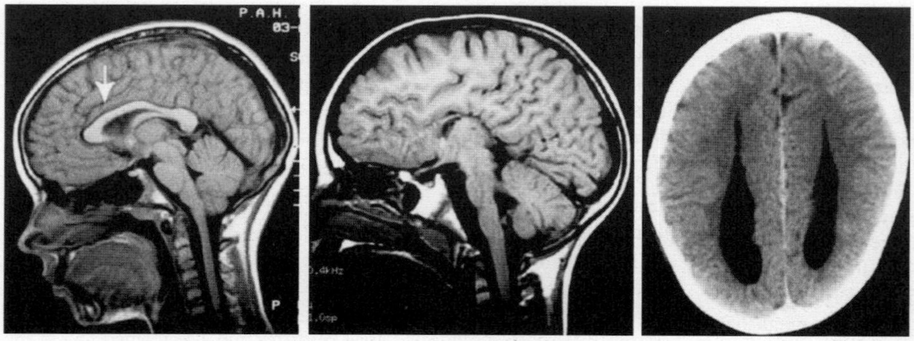

(a) (b) (c)

Fig. 5 (a) Normal brain in a girl aged 2 years. A T_1-weighted sagittal MRI shows normal corpus callosum and cingulate gyrus (arrow). (b) Agenesis of the corpus callosum in a girl aged 6 years who has microcephaly and moderate learning difficulties. A T_1-weighted sagittal MRI shows absence of the corpus callosum and of the cingulate gyrus, which normally runs parallel to the corpus callosum. (c) Agenesis of the corpus callosum in the same girl as (b). Axial CT shows typical appearance of parallel lateral cerebral ventricles, with divergence of the anterior horns of the ventricles and colpocephaly (dilated posterior part of the lateral ventricles).

Agenesis of the corpus callosum

The true prevalence of this abnormality is not accurately known because it can be present without any symptoms. Estimated prevalence has varied from 0.05 to 70 per 10 000 in the general population, increasing to 230 per 10 000 in children with developmental disabilities.

Embryology

The corpus callosum forms within the commissural plate, a thickening of the lamina terminalis which is the frontal boundary of the neural tube. At 11 to 12 weeks the first fibres cross the midline to form the corpus callosum, which displaces the fornix and extends back in the occipital direction to assume the adult form by 18 to 20 weeks. There are two types of 'true' callosal agenesis. These are: (i) defects in which axons are unable to cross the midline and become large aberrant longitudinal fibre bundles, called Probst bundles, along the medial walls of the cerebral hemispheres; and (ii) defects in which the commissural axons or their parent cell bodies fail to form in the cerebral cortex. The former is probably the most common type, the latter is seen in the Walker–Warburg syndrome and other types of lissencephaly. There are also two secondary types: (i) absence associated with major malformations of the embryonic forebrain, such as holoprosencephaly; and (ii) degeneration or atrophy, as is seen in some syndromes in which the corpus callosum is thinned but not shortened.

Pathology

Agenesis of the corpus callosum may be complete or partial. Either the anterior or the posterior part may be missing. When there is complete absence there is no cingulate gyrus. There is associated enlargement of the occipital horns of the lateral ventricles, known as colpocephaly. Other associated abnormalities include cysts dorsal to the third ventricle, heterotopias, gyral abnormalities, cephaloceles, lipomas of the corpus callosum, eye abnormalities, and hydrocephalus.

Aetiology

Isolated callosal agenesis may be inherited as an autosomal recessive, autosomal dominant, or X-linked recessive trait, but none of these loci have been mapped and non-syndromic genetic transmission is rare. It has been associated with several chromosomal rearrangements. These include trisomy 18, trisomy 13, and many deletions and duplications. Also it has been reported in more than 20 autosomal and many X-linked malformation syndromes. Callosal agenesis is part of the fetal alcohol syndrome and is seen in metabolic disorders including glutaric aciduria type 2, peroxisomal disorders, pyruvate dehydrogenase deficiency, and non-ketotic hyperglycinaemia.

Clinical findings

Non-syndromic forms are the most common. When agenesis of the corpus callosum is the only lesion there may be no symptoms, although tests of perception and language may demonstrate disturbances of integration of hemispheric function. However, even if there is no clearly defined syndrome, some patients have mental retardation, seizures, or cerebral palsy. Sometimes there is macrocephaly, which may be due to cysts lying dorsal to the third ventricle or to hydrocephalus.

Diagnosis

This depends on brain imaging (Fig. 5(a–c)). The abnormalities that can be found are widely spaced parallel lateral ventricles, colpocephaly (enlarged posterior horns of the lateral ventricles), upward displacement of the third ventricle, absent callosal tissue, or midline dorsal cyst. Prenatal ultrasound allows diagnosis from the 20th week of gestation. After birth, MRI is best because it gives sagittal views of the corpus callosum. The scan should be carefully reviewed for other midline anomalies (such as agenesis of the septum pellucidum) or generalized defects (such as lissencephaly).

The eyes should be examined to look for optic nerve hypoplasia (as seen in septo-optic dysplasia) or choroidal lacunae (as seen in the Aicardi syndrome). In neonates with seizures or other significant neurological problems the cerebrospinal fluid should be taken to measure glycine (raised in non-ketotic hyperglycinaemia) and lactate (raised in mitochondrial encephalomyelopathy). A karyotype should be performed and urine sent to measure amino and organic acids. If there is evidence of septo-optic dysplasia (see below), pituitary function should be checked.

Genetic counselling

This depends on the specific diagnosis. When callosal agenesis is discovered on antenatal scan the prognosis is difficult to assess because the isolated lesion can be associated with normal development. A decision to terminate the pregnancy may depend on the demonstration of associated abnormalities.

Porencephaly

The term porencephaly is often used indiscriminately for all large cavities in the brains of infants. Friede recommends using the term only for circumscribed hemispheric necrosis that occurs *in utero* before the adult features of the hemisphere are fully developed (Fig. 6(b)). The developmental origin of such lesions is shown by their smooth walls and from disturbances in the development of the adjoining cortex. These disturbances may take the form of polymicrogyria or of local distortion of the gyral pattern. In contrast, areas of damage resulting from insults in the terminal phase of the pregnancy or in postnatal life have irregular shaggy walls and do not alter the gyral environment except by atrophy or scarring.

Schizencephaly

This term is used to describe clefts which traverse the full thickness of the hemisphere, connecting the ventricle to the subarachnoid space. They are described as type I or 'fused-lip' when the walls of the cleft are opposed, and type II or 'open-lip' when cerebrospinal fluid separates the walls (Fig. 6(d)). Some authors think that the clefts are usually the result of destruction of brain tissue and the term porencephaly should be used for them all. However, there is now evidence that some of them are genetic—familial and sporadic cases have been recognized in association with mutations in the homeobox gene *EMX2*. This is one of the vertebrate homeobox genes expressed in the extended regions of the developing rostral brain of mouse

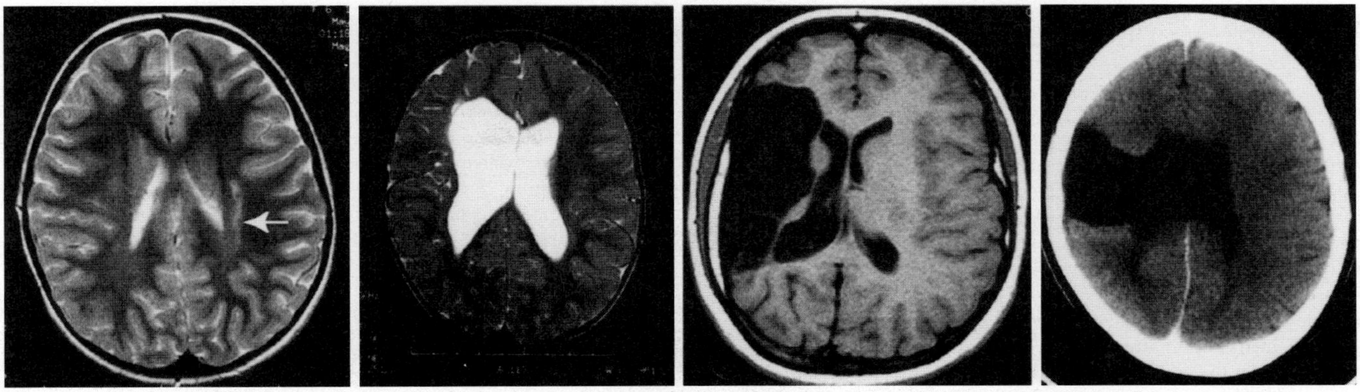

Fig. 6 (a) Cerebral palsy: spastic diplegia. Probable periventricular leucomalacia in a girl aged 6 years. There was threatened premature labour at 29 and 32 weeks, but she was born at term with no perinatal problems. She walked late with a diplegic gait. T_2-weighted axial MRI shows abnormal signal change lateral to the body of the left lateral ventricle and posterolateral to the posterior horn of the left lateral ventricle (arrow). This a characteristic distribution of periventricular leucomalacia, but such scan appearances should be interpreted with caution because there are other causes of white matter abnormalities in children (e.g. the leucodystrophies). (b) Cerebral palsy: left hemiplegia. Porencephalic cyst in a boy aged 18 months. He was delivered by forceps at 38 weeks with no resuscitation, but nasogastric feeding for several days after birth. At 10 months of age he was not moving the left arm normally. T_2-weighted axial MRI shows there is dilatation of the anterior horn of the right lateral ventricle with loss of overlying cerebral cortex and a small periventricular cyst adjacent to the anterior horn of the right lateral ventricle. These abnormalities may result from periventricular leucomalacia. Such loss of tissue due to *in utero* damage of the developing brain is called a porencephalic cyst. (c) Cerebral palsy: left hemiplegia. Tissue loss in middle cerebral artery territory in a young woman aged 17 years. There were no perinatal problems; reduced movement of left arm from 6 months of age; nocturnal generalized tonic–clonic seizures from 4 years of age; normal intelligence; abnormal posture of left hand; and shortening of the left leg. T_1-weighted axial MRI shows there is a loculated cystic lesion in the distribution of the supply of the middle cerebral artery. Also *ex vacuo* enlargement of the right lateral ventricle and small ipsilateral left hemicranium. (d) Open-lipped schizencephaly in a 49-year-old female. An axial CT scan shows there is a wide cleft joining the right lateral ventricle to the subarachnoid space.

embryos that are thought to play a role in patterning the forebrain. The clefts are frequently bilateral and symmetrical, the most severe form being large bilateral defects. Even when unilateral, they are often combined with cortical dysplasia of the opposite hemisphere.

Clinical features

These are variable, depending on the site and size of the lesion. Epilepsy is common and sometimes the only problem is isolated partial seizures.

There may be hemiplegia, quadriplegia, and learning difficulties of variable degree. If there is bilateral involvement of both opercular regions, there may be facial apraxia and speech difficulties. The diagnosis is best made by MRI.

Hydranencephaly

In this condition the cerebral hemispheres are mostly replaced by fluid-filled sacs. The defect typically corresponds to the territory of the anterior and middle cerebral arteries, although the major cranial arteries do not usually show evidence of obstruction. Preservation of the temporal lobes and the tentorial parts of the occipital lobes is common. The extent of preservation of the basal ganglia varies. The cause of hydranencephaly is not clear in many cases. It has been described after intoxication of pregnant women with gas at about the 25th week of gestation. It can result from intrauterine infections and has been described in association with a proliferative vasculopathy.

Affected infants may be born after a normal pregnancy and be surprisingly normal on neurological examination for the first few weeks of life. Gradually the infants become hypertonic and irritable. They may develop infantile spasms, which is surprising because of the almost complete lack of cerebral hemispheres. The head may enlarge because of associated hydrocephalus. The diagnosis can be made by transillumination of the skull, which lights up like a lantern in a darkened room. Similar appearances can be caused by hydrocephalus with a very thin cortical mantle, so MRI is indicated to confirm the diagnosis. Infants with hydranencephaly often die in a few months, but they may survive for several years and may need a ventriculoperitoneal cerebrospinal fluid shunt if there is progressive hydrocephalus.

Septo-optic dysplasia

This is the association of optic nerve hypoplasia with absence of the septum pellucidum. Disturbances of the hypothalamopituitary axis may occur. The most severely affected patients are blind and have severe learning difficulties. The optic discs have a characteristic double contour: the true disc at the centre is small and there is a peripheral ring about the size of a normal optic nerve head. It important to search for evidence of endocrine disturbances when these abnormal discs are identified—deficiences of growth hormone, corticotrophin, luteinizing hormone, and follicle-stimulating hormone have been described, together with hypoglycaemia and diabetes insipidus. Most cases are sporadic, but a homozygous mutation in the homeobox gene *HESX1* has been identified in familial septo-optic dysplasia. Also some sporadic cases of the more common mild forms of pituitary hypoplasia are associated with heterozygous mutations of the *HESX1* gene.

Malformations of posterior fossa structures

These malformations are now identified more accurately using prenatal ultrasound and MRI, which is superior to CT scanning for showing posterior fossa structures.

Cerebellar and brainstem development

Embrology

At the end of the fourth week of gestation the neural tube divides into the three primary brain vesicles—the prosencephalon, the mesencephalon, and the rhombencephalon. The last further subdivides into the metencephalon and the myelencephalon. The cerebellar hemispheres (neocerebellum) are derived primarily from the metencephalon, while the vermis (palaeocerebellum) is derived from the mesencephalon.

Experiments in animals demonstrate that a critical area for vertebrate cerebellar development occurs at the junction of the mesencephalon and the metencephalon in the region of the isthmus. An early abnormality in the isthmus that affects the mesencephalic contribution to midline cerebellar structures could contribute to the pathogenesis of syndromes that involve agenesis or hypoplasia of the cerebellar vermis, such as Joubert syndrome.

Aplasia and hypoplasia of the cerebellum

This is a heterogeneous group of conditions that affect cerebellar development in various ways—total cerebellar aplasia is exceptional and unilateral hypoplasia occurs. Neocerebellar aplasia (Fig. 7(a)) is characterized by a small vermis and extreme smallness or absence of the cerebellar hemispheres except for persistent flocculi. There may be associated anomalies in the brainstem such as dysplasia of the inferior olivary nucleus and other brainstem nuclei.

Some cases are associated with genetic syndromes, many of which are poorly defined. Recent attention has been drawn to a group of disorders classified under the broad headings of pontocerebellar hypoplasia or olivopontocerebellar atrophy. Pontocerebellar hypoplasia is found in carbohydrate-deficient glycoprotein syndrome type 1 and cerebromuscular dystrophies (Walker-Warburg syndrome, Fukuyama syndrome, and muscle-eye-brain diseases—see above). There are at least two types of autosomal recessive pontocerebellar hypoplasias (type I and type II). MRI demonstrates cerebellar hypoplasia together with a hypoplastic ventral pons. It has been speculated that some of these cases are due to mutations of *engrailed* genes which are essential for the development of the segmental precursors of the pons and cerebellum in the mouse brain.

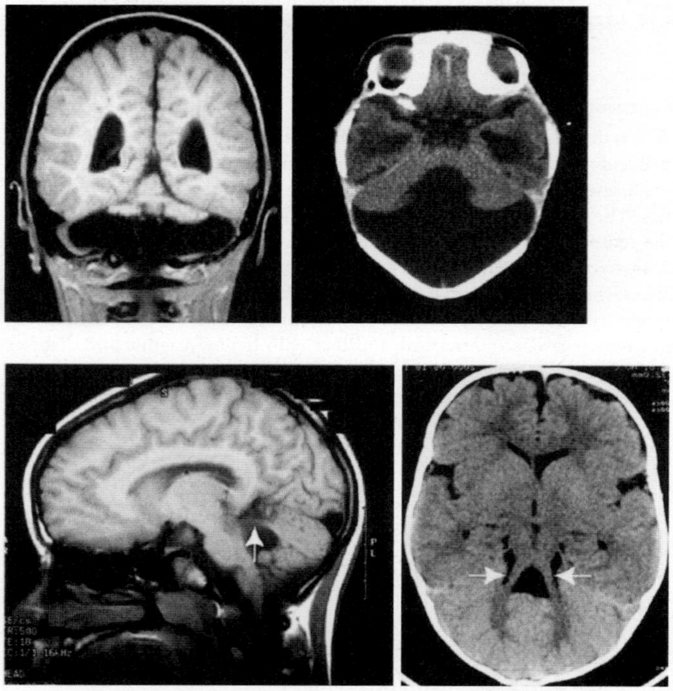

Fig. 7 (a) Cerebellar hypoplasia in a boy aged 5 years, who was born preterm at 26 weeks of gestation, with no neurological problems apart from absence seizures of unknown cause. T_1-weighted coronal MRI shows almost complete absence of the cerebellar hemispheres and hypoplasia of the cerebellar vermis. (b) Dandy–Walker malformation in a 1-year-old girl. Axial CT scan shows absence of the roof of the fourth ventricle. A large cyst is continuous with the fourth ventricle and fills the posterior fossa. (c) Joubert syndrome in a girl aged 10 years. T_1-weighted sagittal MRI shows the superior cerebellar peduncles run horizontally (arrow) and the cerebellar vermis is absent. (d) Joubert syndrome in a girl aged 9 months who is hypotonic and visually unresponsive, with 'wandering' nystagmus. Axial CT shows the superior cerebellar peduncles (arrows) run horizontally and stand out because of the absence of the vermis ('molar tooth sign'). The prominent fourth ventricle has a typical shape (sometimes looking like a 'bat wing').

The Chiari malformations

There are four types. The Chiari II malformation is usually associated with a meningomyelocele and is dealt with in the section on neural tube defects. In the Chiari I malformation there is downward displacement of the lower cerebellum, including the tonsils. It rarely cause symptoms in childhood but may be associated with hydrocephalus and syringomyelia. The Chiari III malformation consists of downward displacement of the cerebellum into a posterior encephalocele and the Chiari IV malformation is a form of cerebellar hypoplasia.

Abnormalities of the vermis

Dandy–Walker malformation and Dandy–Walker variant

Two main complexes have been described. The Dandy–Walker malformation (Fig. 7(b)) consists of the following triad: (i) complete or partial agenesis of the vermis, (ii) cystic dilatation of the fourth ventricle, and (iii) enlarged posterior fossa with upward displacement of lateral sinuses, tentorium, and torcula. A Dandy–Walker variant has been recognized more recently and consists of variable dysplasia of the vermis without enlargement of the posterior fossa. There is an association between Dandy–Walker malformations and chromosomal abnormalities including trisomies 13 and 18. Dandy–Walker malformation is listed as a feature of 80 syndromes in the London Dysmorphology Database.

Prenatal ultrasound studies show that the majority of fetuses with both complexes have other anomalies. The commonest CNS anomaly was ventriculomegaly and the commonest non-CNS anomalies were structural heart defects. Other associated CNS abnormalities include holoprosencephaly, agenesis of the corpus callosum, occipital encephaloceles, and abnormal migration of the inferior olive.

Clinical features The outcome of fetuses with both Dandy–Walker malformation and Dandy–Walker variant ranges from severe mental and physical handicap to normal development. In general the outcome is worst if there are associated abnormalities and best for isolated Dandy–Walker variant. Intrauterine deaths occur and some infants do not survive the neonatal period, the poor early outcome being related to the extra-CNS abnormalities. However, the abnormality is often recognized only when the infant is investigated for the signs of hydrocephalus, which may not become apparent until late in the first year of life. Sometimes there is a bulging occiput which alerts suspicion. Another presentation may be later in life with learning difficulties. Cerebellar signs tend not to be prominent, but cranial nerve palsies, nystagmus, and truncal ataxia have been described.

Diagnosis The cerebellar vermis starts to form in the ninth week of gestation, beginning superiorly so that fusion of the two cerebellar hemispheres is completed when the inferior part of the vermis is formed at 15 weeks. However, in a small proportion of infants this happens later, so that conclusive prenatal ultrasound diagnosis cannot be made until 18 weeks. When the diagnosis is made there should be an exhaustive screen for associated structural and chromosomal anomalies because these determine the prognosis. Radiological diagnosis is relatively straightforward for the Dandy–Walker malformation. Dandy–Walker variant may be difficult to distinguish from a prominent cisterna magna or a retrocerebellar arachnoid cyst. Sagittal MRI can then help to differentiate whether the vermis is partly absent or alternatively is fully present but displaced.

Genetic counselling If a chromosomal anomaly is identified or a syndrome diagnosis is made, appropriate counselling is given. If there are no associated abnormalities and the chromosomes are normal, the recurrence risk is 1 to 5 per cent.

Joubert syndrome

This rare autosomal recessive disorder is characterized by brainstem and cerebellar malformations. The disease is genetically heterogeneous, and one locus has been mapped to chromosome 9q.

Neuropathology The neuropathological features include absence or hypoplasia of the posteroinferior part of the cerebellar vermis. In some cases enlargement of the fourth ventricle and the cisterna magna has been reported. Microscopically, heterotopias have been seen in the cerebellar hemispheres with fragmentation of the dentate nuclei. Brainstem abnormalities include absence of the pyramidal decussation, abnormal inferior olivary nuclei, and subtle dysplasias in the nuclei of the solitary and descending trigeminal tracts and of the dorsal columns.

Clinical features The common abnormalities are marked hypotonia (particularly in the neonatal period and infancy), poor balance (walking occurs in 50 per cent of cases and is late—at approximately 4 years), and variable cognitive problems (some affected children are unable to talk but others develop language, read, and write). Typically CT or MRI shows the 'molar tooth' sign in the axial plane, which consists of: (i) a deeper than normal posterior interpeduncular fossa, (ii) prominent or thickened superior cerebellar peduncles, and (iii) vermian hypoplasia or dysplasia. MRI in the coronal and axial plane shows clefting of the vermis; in the sagittal plane it shows an abnormally shaped and rostrally placed fourth ventricle (Fig. 7(c and d).

The associated abnormalities are dysmorphic facial features (high rounded eyebrows, broad nasal bridge, epicanthus, anteverted nostrils, triangular-shaped open mouth with irregular tongue protrusion, low-set coarse ears), episodic hyperpnoea and/or apnoea in up to 75 per cent of patients (most marked in the neonatal period), eye abnormalities (retinal dysplasia, colobomata, nystagmus, strabismus, ptosis, and oculomotor apraxia), and microcystic renal disease.

Neurological syndromes resulting from disturbances of brain development

The cerebral palsies

Introduction

The cerebral palsies are defined as a heterogeneous collection of non-progressive disorders of movement and posture due to defects or lesions of the immature brain.

It can be seen that this is a broad definition, but it does need to be used carefully. It is not satisfactory to label a child with neurological problems as suffering from 'cerebral palsy' and go no further. It is important to determine the type and distribution of the abnormality of motor control. In addition to motor deficits, patients with cerebral palsy may suffer with other neurological problems, such as learning difficulties, epilepsy, and hearing or visual loss. It is important to evaluate these, although they are not present in all cases.

Although the underlying causes of the cerebral palsy syndromes are by definition not progressive, the symptoms and signs of cerebral palsy do change with age. For instance some children who are destined to have major problems with spasticity are initially very hypotonic. In some cases it can be difficult to be sure whether or not a child with suspected cerebral palsy has a progressive underlying disorder. It may be necessary to allow the passage of time and children may be 3 or 4 years old before the diagnosis of cerebral palsy can be made with confidence.

Classification

Patients may be classified according to the type of motor abnormality as follows: spastic, dyskinetic (dystonic or athetoid), ataxic, or hypotonic. The clinical picture is rarely clear-cut and individuals may exhibit complex mixtures of motor disability.

Patients are subclassified according to the distribution of motor abnormality—in diplegia the legs are involved more than the arms, in quadriplegia all four limbs are involved, and in hemiplegia just one side of the body is involved.

In practice there is considerable interobserver disagreement when classifying patients with cerebral palsy. However, it is important to use a classification system for research and management because different types of cerebral palsy tend to have distinct causes, different associated deficits, and different prognoses.

Epidemiology

There is a relative shortage of data from developing countries, so the statistics quoted here are for developed countries. Although the risk of cerebral palsy is higher for preterm infants, most children with cerebral palsy are born at term. Overall cerebral palsy rates are therefore determined mainly by the numbers of term infants born with cerebral palsy.

Overall cerebral palsy rates since the mid-1950s have remained remarkably constant at about 2 to 2.5 per 1000 live births, although there have been some fluctuations with time. In 1970 the rate fell to 1.5 in Sweden, Western Australia, and Mersey (United Kingdom), rising again in the 1980s.

Cerebral palsy rates stratified by birth weight show marked changes with time. Most population-based registers have shown increases in rates in infants of very low birth weight (less than 1500 g) since the 1970s. For instance, in Mersey in the early 1970s the rate in infants of very low birth weight fluctuated around 10 per 1000 live births. In the late 1970s the rate increased sharply to about 50 per 1000 live births, presumably because more children of very low birth weight were surviving with neurological deficits. This increase was seen for all cerebral palsy types. However, to put the increasing cerebral palsy rates in survivors of very low birth weight in perspective, during this time an increasing proportion of patients were also surviving unimpaired. Another important point is that very low birth weight survivors with cerebral palsy are only a small proportion of the total number of children with cerebral palsy and therefore have very little effect on overall cerebral palsy rates.

Relative rates of the different types of cerebral palsy vary according to the series. In the Western Australian Cerebral Palsy Register 1980–1992 cohort the proportions of cases of congenital (as opposed to postneonatal) cerebral palsy were as follows: spastic hemiplegia 33.6 per cent, spastic diplegia 29.7 per cent, spastic quadriplegia 18.1 per cent, ataxic 7.6 per cent, dyskinetic 10.0 per cent, and hypotonic 0.9 per cent.

Aetiology

Although it has been thought that cerebral palsy results primarily from 'birth asphyxia', recent studies suggest that abnormal events around the time of birth play only a limited role. Genetic causes are clearly important as there can be a significant recurrence risk to future children, particularly in populations where consanguineous marriage is relatively common. Families have been reported in which spastic diplegia and quadriplegia (often with associated mental retardation) appear to be inherited in autosomal recessive, autosomal dominant, or X-linked recessive patterns. It is said that the highest risk of recurrence is in the category of children with ataxic cerebral palsy: both autosomal dominant and autosomal recessive inheritance have been reported. However, there are many conditions which cause ataxia in children. It is therefore important to search for an underlying cause before giving genetic advice, rather than to 'lump' this group and give an overall recurrence risk.

Other possible causes before conception or in early pregnancy

Maternal iodine deficiency in early pregnancy may cause endemic cretinism (which causes spastic diplegia and deafness): this is the most important cause of cerebral palsy worldwide. Abnormal thyroid function in pregnancy may play a role in developed countries. Exposure to toxins during pregnancy may cause cerebral palsy—recognized examples are methylmercury, alcohol, and carbon monoxide poisoning. Viral infections which are vertically transmitted before the third trimester often result in cerebral malformations—those best known are toxoplasmosis, rubella, and cytomegalovirus. Finally, there are some fetal malformation syndromes that include brain abnormalities and cause cerebral palsy.

The role of very preterm birth

The rate of cerebral palsy among neonatal survivors born before 33 weeks is up to 30 times higher than among those born at term. This may be because of increased survival of very preterm infants whose brains are already damaged or because preterm infants are vulnerable to cerebral damage after birth. It seems likely that there is a combination of these mechanisms. Cerebral ultrasound scans performed in newborn babies have shown that the strongest predictor of cerebral palsy in these infants is periventricular leucomalacia. This term is used for abnormal echolucency, often associated with cystic change, which is found particularly in the white matter dorsolateral to the lateral ventricles (Fig. 6(a)). It is difficult to time the onset of the pathological processes that lead to the appearance of these lesions. At present there is evidence that many different factors result in preterm birth and it is not known how they contribute to cerebral palsy.

The role of intrauterine growth restriction

Babies born small for their gestational age are at increased risk of cerebral palsy and the risk increases with the degree of birth weight deficit. The underlying mechanism is not clear and the majority of small-for-dates infants do not have cerebral palsy.

The role of multiple births

The prevalence of cerebral palsy is much higher in twins than in singletons, particularly in those who survive after the other twin has died *in utero* and in monochorionic twins. The risk rises with the number of fetuses carried. Causes include low birth weight, congenital anomalies, cord entanglement, and abnormal vascular connections.

The role of birth asphyxia

In the 1970s it was expected that more intensive monitoring of the fetus during labour, coupled with earlier obstetric intervention, would improve neonatal outcome. The major effects of electronic monitoring of the heart rate during labour have been an increase in caesarean section rates and a reduced rate of neonatal seizures, however it has had no impact on the rates of cerebral palsy. The proportion of cerebral palsy cases associated with intrapartum events has been estimated by several epidemiological studies to be only about 10 per cent. However, there may be some cases caused by intrapartum events that are preventable.

In 1999 a consensus statement for the International Cerebral Palsy Task Force outlined a template for defining a causal relationship between acute intrapartum events and cerebral palsy. The statement emphasized the difficulty of retrospectively identifying the antenatal causes of cerebral palsy in the individual case and the non-specific nature of the clinical signs that lead to the suspicion of fetal hypoxia in labour. It proposed that the terms 'fetal distress' and 'birth asphyxia' should be replaced by the term 'non-reassuring fetal status' and suggested eight criteria for defining an acute intrapartum hypoxic event. The hope is that more general use of these criteria will reduce the number of cases of cerebral palsy that are wrongly attributed to an acute event during labour.

Cerebral palsy acquired after the neonatal period

Cerebral palsy registers in Sweden, Mersey, and Western Australia report rates varying from about 1 to 6 per 10 000 live births. Causes include CNS infections, accidental and non-accidental head injuries, cerebrovascular accidents, and hypoxia (suffocation, near drowning).

Brain imaging in children with cerebral palsy

The pathological processes that cause cerebral palsy have been investigated using ultrasonography, MRI, and CT scanning. One study found that about a quarter of children with a hemiplegia had normal CT scans, whilst an MRI study of a heterogeneous group of children with cerebral palsy found abnormalities in 93 per cent of the patients.

The studies have in many cases been performed years after birth on heterogeneous groups of children with cerebral palsy attending specialized clinics. The commonest lesion in preterm infants is periventricular leucomalacia, which is necrosis of periventricular white matter in the watershed regions dorsal and lateral to the lateral ventricle (Fig. 6(a)). This is said to be characteristic of damage in the early third trimester. In term infants there are a number of different findings, which are said to occur only in infants born at or near term. These are infarcts in the arterial border zones in the parasagittal regions leading to cortical and subcortical injury, bilateral lesions of the basal ganglia and the thalamus, areas of subcortical leucomalacia, and multicystic leucomalacia (replacement of the brain tissue by fluid-filled cysts). Periventricular leucomalacia and localized gyral abnormalities are also seen in infants born at term.

Children with hemiplegias are sometimes found to have periventricular leucomalacia, porencephalic cysts (Fig. 6(b)), or cortical/subcortical lesions in the middle cerebral artery territory distribution (Fig. 6(c)). The lesions tend to be unilateral, but bilateral lesions are seen. Rarely they may have schizencephaly (Fig. 6(d)), focal pachygyria, or focal heterotopia.

Although brain scans in children with cerebral palsy are performed a long time after the insult, the nature of the lesions allows some assessment of the timing of cerebral damage. Like the epidemiological studies the brain imaging studies suggest that perinatal brain injury occurs in a relatively small proportion of cases.

Life expectancy

Different studies have followed patients with cerebral palsy for 10 years or more and have yielded similar findings. The survival rates have been about 90 per cent when all the types of cerebral palsy are considered together. The prognosis is best for those with hemiplegia and worst for those with quadriplegia. A population-based study in Canada found that 30-year survival rates were: hemiplegia 96 per cent, diplegia 95 per cent, and quadriplegia 83 per cent. The factors associated with reduced survival rates are severe mental retardation, lack of basic functional skills (mobility, independent feeding), and epilepsy.

Hydrocephalus

This results from expansion of the ventricles secondary to a block in the normal flow pathway of cerebrospinal fluid. Cerebrospinal fluid is produced by the choroid plexus in the lateral ventricles, from where it flows through the foramen of Munro into the third ventricle and then the fourth ventricle via the aqueduct of Sylvius. It leaves the ventricular system via small openings in the roof of the fourth ventricle, the foramina of Magendie and Luschka. From here the fluid flows in the subarachnoid space before being reabsorbed into the blood supply via arachnoid villae.

Two major forms of hydrocephalus are recognized. In communicating hydrocephalus the ventricular pathways are clear and a failure of reabsorption (following, for example, bleeding into the subarachnoid space) results in increased cerebrospinal fluid volume. In obstructive or non-communicating hydrocephalus the blockage occurs at one of the ventricular levels, with expansion of the ventricular system above the block (Fig. 8). The major clinical sign that results is increasing head circumference following the ventricular enlargement, and this allows the distinction from cases in which increased ventricular size reflects cerebral atrophy. Mental retardation can result from both the damage associated with ventricular expansion and other abnormalities associated with the underlying cause of the problem.

Sometimes hydrocephalus is genetically determined; stenosis of the aqueduct between the third and fourth ventricle can result from mutations in the cell adhesion molecule L1-CAM. Hydrocephalus then occurs in association with hypoplasia of the corpus callosum, mental retardation, spastic paraplegia, and adducted thumbs. This X-linked syndrome has been given the extremely unfortunate acronym CRASH syndrome and mutations in *L1-CAM* are found in as many as 75 per cent of cases with a family history and 15 per cent of apparently isolated cases. The developmental abnormalities of the cerebellum in both the Dandy–Walker syndrome and the Arnold–Chiari malformation (see above) may also be associated with obstructive hydrocephalus. While treatment via a ventriculoperitoneal

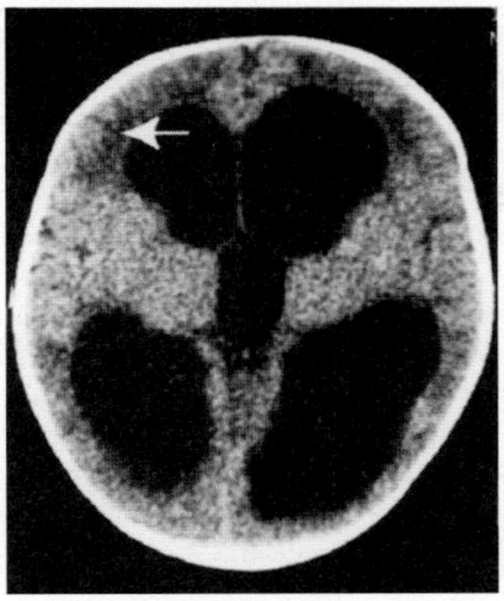

Fig. 8 Aqueduct stenosis in a boy aged 1 month with a bulging anterior fontanelle and increasing head circumference. Axial CT shows a gross dilatation of the third and lateral ventricles (the fourth ventricle is not shown, but was normal in size). Note the periventricular low density due to transependymal exudation of cerebrospinal fluid under pressure (arrow).

shunt can relieve the obstruction, the other abnormalities associated with these developmental problems remain.

Effects of alcohol on the developing nervous system

Worldwide, alcohol is one of the commonest causes of learning difficulty and neurobehavioural disturbance in young children. The incidence of fetal alcohol sydrome depends on geographical location. An international survey in 1997 found that in the United States the incidence per 1000 live births in Seattle was 2.8 and in Cleveland was 4.6. The combined rate of fetal alcohol sydrome and alcohol-related neurodevelopmental disorder in Seattle was estimated at nearly 1 per cent of all live births. The reduced brain mass and neurobehavioural disturbances associated with fetal alcohol syndrome may be related to the recent observation in rats that ethanol can trigger widespread apoptotic neurodegeneration.

Regular and binge drinking can both cause fetal alcohol syndrome and alcohol-related neurodevelopmental disorder. Unlike many other teratogens, alcohol has harmful effects throughout pregnancy. There is a significant risk of fetal alcohol syndrome associated with high-dose exposure (estimated blood alcohol concentrations of 150 mg per decilitre or more, at least weekly for several weeks in the first trimester).

In addition to microcephaly, structural anomalies of the brain such as partial or complete agenesis of the corpus callosum or cerebellar hypoplasia may occur. Children with fetal alcohol syndrome may have impaired fine motor skills, sensorineural deafness, poor hand–eye co-ordination and a poor tandem gait. A complex pattern of behavioural and cognitive abnormalities is observed following exposure to teratogenic levels of alcohol in pregnancy. These include learning difficulties, poor impulse control, problems with social perception, deficits in higher level receptive and expressive language, poor capacity for abstraction, and difficulties with memory, attention, and judgement.

Congenital infections

Cytomegalovirus, herpes simplex, parvovirus, rubella, syphilis, toxoplasmosis, and varicella are all recognized as teratogens. Primary infection rather than reinfection of the mother during pregnancy is more likely to result in congenital infection. The risk of congenital infection and the outcome of such infection is crucially dependent on the stage of pregnancy. This brief account focuses on the effects of congenital infection on the developing nervous system.

Congenital infection should be considered in the differential diagnosis of microcephaly. Intracranial calcification identified on a cranial ultrasound or CT scan during the investigation of developmental delay or seizures should arouse suspicion of congenital infection, especially cytomegalovirus or toxoplasmosis (calcification is not picked up well by MRI). Detailed ophthalmological assessment may reveal clues such as chorioretinitis or cataract that may help in the retrospective diagnosis of congenital infection. Chorioretinitis (pigmentary retinopathy) is characteristic of intrauterine infection by cytomegalovirus or toxoplasmosis. Audiometry is important since sensorineural deafness is a common sequel to congenital infection with cytomegalovirus, rubella, and toxoplasmosis.

The risk of maternal–fetal transmission with primary cytomegalovirus infection is as high as 40 per cent, however fewer than 10 per cent of infants with intrauterine infection are symptomatic at birth. Of those who are symptomatic as neonates, approximately 90 per cent have some of the characteristic features including microcephaly, periventricular calcification, chorioretinitis, optic atrophy, and sensorineural deafness. Of the 90 per cent of infants who are asymptomatic at birth, approximately 15 per cent have sequelae including sensorineural deafness and/or developmental delay.

Intrauterine infection with herpes simplex virus is rare. Congenitally affected infants may have microcephaly, chorioretinits, and microphthalmos. Neonatal infection acquired at the time of delivery, which may occur with primary infection of the mother with herpes simplex virus in the third trimester, is a commoner cause of neurodisability than congenital infection. Neonatal infection may cause meningitis and encephalitis with resulting neurological damage. The risks of perinatally acquired infection may be reduced by appropriate obstetric intervention (such as delivery by caesarian section for women with active genital lesions resulting from herpes simplex virus) and by treatment of affected neonates with acyclovir.

The classic triad of defects associated with congenital rubella syndrome is sensorineural deafness, congenital heart disease, and eye abnormalities (retinopathy, cataracts, microphthalmos, and congenital glaucoma). Microcephaly and developmental delay may also occur. The spectrum of defects in an individual child is determined by the stage of pregnancy at which intrauterine infection occurs. The risk of congenital infection is more than 90 per cent below 10 weeks and falls to zero beyond 18 weeks.

The risk of intrauterine infection with toxoplasmosis increases with the stage of pregnancy at which the mother acquires her primary infection; however the sequelae of intrauterine infection diminish with advancing gestation. Congenital toxoplasmosis syndrome includes hydrocephalus, intracranial calcification, microcephaly, seizures, and developmental delay. There may also be sensorineural deafness and chorioretinitis with visual impairment.

Congenital varicella syndrome follows primary maternal varicella occurring at 1 to 20 weeks of gestation, but the risk of sequelae is small at around 2 per cent. Cataracts and chorioretinitis may occur together with hypoplasia of the optic disc. Microcephaly and porencephaly have been described.

Clinical approach to diagnosis and genetic counselling

Assessing the nervous system in children

History

General

The importance of the history cannot be overemphasized. Children may give a history themselves, but usually the parents or carers are an essential source of information and this may be amplified by teachers, therapists, and other health professionals.

Past history

The pregnancy details are important. Significant events in the first trimester may be a threatened miscarriage, hyperemesis, or a viral infection—the mother may have been taking medication. Later there may have been unsatisfactory fetal growth (perhaps poor head growth assessed by ultrasound) or reduced fetal movements. The perinatal history is relevant, including weeks of gestation at the time of delivery, details of labour and delivery, birth weight, and head circumference. In the neonatal period the infant may have required treatment for early hypoglycaemia, seizures, or breathing or feeding difficulties. A developmental history is essential—particular areas of concern in infants are lack of social response, absence of a social smile, poor fixing and following of the eyes, and lack of symmetrical organized limb movements. Later a characteristic pattern of delayed development may emerge—for instance global delay is found in the most severe brain abnormalities or there may be mainly motor delay in the milder forms of cerebral palsy.

Family and social history

Information should be obtained about first-degree and more distant relatives. Considerable effort may be needed to obtain relevant facts—some families conceal or do not know about relatives with severe disability, perhaps because they are in instituitions. It is important to know about consanguinity, also about epilepsy, motor disorders, and severe or mild learning disabilities. Social factors are important in determining the environment in which the child grows up and they also determine the quality of care available for a child with significant disability.

Examination

Observation of spontaneous activity is essential. The form of this depends on the degree of disability, but if the child is able to play this should be encouraged. It may be helpful to use toys, bricks, beads for threading, paper, and crayons. The quality and symmetry of spontaneous movements should be noted and also any abnormal movements. It is best to assess muscle power by watching the child run, jump, and climb stairs. Fine motor function can be assessed whilst the child is drawing or threading beads.

Developmental assessment may be formally undertaken in infants using one of the standardized schedules, such as the Bailey Scales of Infant Development or the Denver Developmental Screening Test. Later the Wechsler Preschool and Primary Scale of Intelligence (WPPSI) and the Wechsler Intelligence Scale for Children (Revised) (WISC-R) may be used. The latter assessments are usually undertaken by a clinical or educational psychologist.

The conventional examination of the nervous system may be difficult in infants or young children. The examiner may need to adapt the order of events or even come back later—a useful assessment cannot be made if an infant is deeply asleep or upset and crying. Examination of the cranial nerves should be made as much like play as possible by using a toy to observe eye movements and by encouraging the child to smile, whistle, close the jaw tight, stick out the tongue, and so on.

Dysmorphic features are particularly relevant in the context of a suspected abnormality of the nervous system. There may be birth marks (capillary haemangiomata of the face in Sturge–Weber syndrome or midline skin abnormalities such as hairy patches or dimples over the spine in cord abnormalities). Other important skin abnormalities may not be very obvious at birth but become so in infancy or early childhood. Examples are the pale ash-leaf patches, shagreen patches, and angiofibromas of the face ('adenoma sebaceum') that are found in tuberous sclerosis or the café-au-lait patches found in neurofibromatosis type I.

A full eye examination is essential. In babies it may be necessary to dilate the eyes and come back to perform fundoscopy whilst the child is feeding (and therefore quiet!). Indirect ophthalmoscopy by an experienced ophthalmologist is probably best for older children. There may be hypo- or hypertelorism which may be associated with midline defects of the brain (for example hypotelorism in holoprosencephaly and hypertelorism in agenesis of the corpus callosum), so the interpupillary distance and the distance between the inner canthi should be measured and checked on standard charts. There may be abnormalities of the iris (such as colobomata in trisomy 13, the CHARGE association, and other syndromes that involve the nervous system; Lisch nodules in neurofibromatosis type I; or Kayser–Fleischer rings in Wilson's disease). Pale hypoplastic optic nerve heads are seen in septo-optic dysplasia and other congenital and acquired conditions. Significant retinal abnormalities include the chorioretinitis seen in congenital toxoplasmosis or cytomegalovirus infections and the retinal 'lacunae' seen in Aicardi syndrome.

Growth should be assessed by measuring weight, length (height), and head circumference and plotting them on standard charts. In particular the head circumference should be related to the age of the child and to the other measurements (see sections on microcephaly and megalencephaly above). Changes with time may be significant—for instance, after a severe perinatal insult, the head circumference may initially be in the normal range and then fall progressively further below the expected centile line in the first few months of life, which can be important in dating the insult to the brain. Babies may be upset by having their heads measured, so this is best left to the end of the examination.

Investigations

The cornerstone of investigations in children or adults with suspected disorders of CNS development is MRI to investigate brain structure. It is important to discuss the investigation with a neuroradiologist as special imaging sequences not normally performed may be required to visualize relevant abnormalities, for example subependymal nodules in tuberose sclerosis. Infants and young children may require sedation or anaesthesia for the procedure. CT scanning does not provide the resolution of CNS structure obtained with MRI, but may be valuable if intracerebral calcification is suspected (as in tuberous sclerosis or cytomegalovirus infection).

Further investigations will depend on the specific diagnosis in question. Metabolic disorders can cause structural abnormalities in the developing CNS, and routine investigations that may be appropriate include plasma and urine amino acids, together with urine organic acids. In addition, further specific investigations may be indicated, for example in suspected Zellweger's syndrome which is associated with pachygyria and which is caused by abnormalities of very long chain fatty acid metabolism. Mutation analysis of specific genes may confirm a clinical diagnosis. Fluorescent *in situ* hybridization studies of chromosome regions using labelled probes that will bind (hybridize) to specific gene sequences may detect microdeletion syndromes such as Miller–Dieker by revealing an absence of fluorescent labelling on one of the pair of chromosomes.

These investigations may then allow diagnosis and accurate assessment of risks for other family members following extended family testing. Molecular genetic techniques are improving very rapidly and new tests will become available. It is therefore valuable to take blood in order to extract and store DNA or establish a lymphoblastoid cell line if no precise diagnosis can be reached, especially if life expectancy is short. Immediately after death it may be appropriate to obtain a muscle or liver biopsy to help establish a diagnosis. Also skin may be obtained to establish a fibroblast culture. Later other tissues can be frozen if a full postmortem examination is performed. The ability to perform new tests many years after the death of the index case may be extremely valuable to other family members concerned about risks to their own offspring.

Risk assessment, prenatal diagnosis, and genetic counselling

When families request genetic advice regarding a developmental disorder of the nervous system they usually have four questions in mind: what is it?, why did it happen?, will it happen again?, and what can be done to reduce the chance of it happening again, or to detect it if it does? If it is possible to make a specific diagnosis, these questions can often be answered with some accuracy.

Risk assessment

An important component of risk assessment is the construction of a three-generation family tree, with detailed enquiry and if necessary examination and investigation of close relatives for subtle expression of a disorder, or evidence of carrier status. Sometimes the diagnosis will immediately identify the recurrence risk. For example Zellweger syndrome always follows an autosomal recessive pattern of inheritance (hence there is a 1 in 4 risk of recurrence in future pregnancies). For many of the developmental anomalies discussed in this chapter, the causes are heterogeneous with a variety of different mechanisms resulting in similar clinical endpoints.

The assessment of holoprosencephaly provides an example of the steps involved in risk assessment. It may occur in an individual with a chromosomal anomaly such as trisomy 13, or a variety of subtle chromosome deletions such as del (18p), del (7q). It may also follow an autosomal dominant pattern of inheritance with incomplete penetrance and variable expression (mutations in the *sonic hedgehog* gene in some families), or be a feature of a recognizable syndrome such as Smith–Lemli–Opitz, which follows an autosomal recessive pattern of inheritance. Assessing the risk for a particular family depends upon careful integration of the clinical picture in the affected individual with information from the family tree and the results of investigations.

If it is not possible to identify the precise aetiology, and common causes have been excluded as far as possible by appropriate investigation, it is usually possible to offer an empirical recurrence risk after examination of the parents. For example, in a family where the child has holoprosencephaly with no additional features suggestive of a syndromic cause and who has normal chromosomes, the next step is a careful examination of both parents to look for the subtle features of autosomal dominant holoprosencephaly (such as single central incisor, hypotelorism). They should also both have a cranial MRI. If these assessments are normal, then the empirical recurrence risk is 5 to 6 per cent.

Prenatal diagnosis

Prenatal diagnosis and termination of affected pregnancies is only one of a range of reproductive options open to parents at increased risk of having children with neurodevelopmental abnormalities, but for many couples it is the option of choice. Other options include embarking on a further pregnancy and accepting the risk of recurrence, or electing against any further pregnancies and perhaps considering adoption. For the majority of developmental disorders of the nervous system, preimplantation genetic diagnosis is not yet feasible. For a condition following mendelian inheritance the option of donor gametes could be discussed. For a condition with a strong environmental component it is imperative that measures are taken to minimize the risk of exposure in a future pregnancy. For neural tube defects, periconceptual supplementation with high-dose folate has been shown to reduce the risk of recurrence in future pregnancies (see above).

When a specific diagnosis has been made and a chromosomal anomaly, genetic mutation, or biochemical defect has been identified, it is usually possible to offer prenatal diagnosis by chorionic villus sampling at 11 weeks of gestation in a future pregnancy. If this is not the case, detailed ultrasound scanning may be helpful in some instances; for example, neural tube defects where anencephaly can be clearly visualized by 13 to 14 weeks of gestation, and spina bifida by 18 to 20 weeks. For other conditions such as isolated lissencephaly, no features are likely to be visible on an ultrasound scan before 24 weeks of gestation, and for isolated microcephaly often not until 32 to 34 weeks of gestation or later. The limitations of detailed ultrasound scanning in these circumstances will need to be discussed frankly with the parents.

Genetic counselling

Providing accurate genetic advice about developmental anomalies of the nervous system is a challenging task. Referral for specialist advice is strongly recommended.

Further reading

Aicardi J (1998). *Diseases of the nervous system in childhood*, 2nd edn. Mac Keith Press, London.

Baraitser M. (1997). *The genetics of neurological disorders*, 3rd edn. *Oxford Monographs on Medical Genetics 34.* Oxford University Press, Oxford.

Bock G, Marsh J, eds (1994). *Neural tube defects. Ciba Foundation Symposium 181.* John Wiley, Chichester.

Faerber EN, ed. (1995). *CNS magnetic resonance imaging in infants and children. Clinics in Developmental Medicine No. 134.* Mac Keith Press, London.

Friede RL (1989). *Developmental neuropathology*, 2nd (revised and expanded) edn. Springer-Verlag, Berlin.

Gleeson JG, Walsh CA (2000). Neuronal migration disorders: from genetic diseases to developmental mechanisms. *Trends in Neuroscience* **23**, 352–9.

Govaert P, de Vries LS (1997). *An atlas of neonatal brain sonography. Clinics in Developmental Medicine No. 141–2.* Mac Keith Press, London.

Maclennan A, for the International Cerebral Palsy Task Force (1999). A template for defining a causal relationship between acute intrapartum events and cerebral palsy: international consensus statement. *British Medical Journal* **319**, 1054–9.

Miller G, Clark GD, eds (1998). *The cerebral palsies. Causes, consequences, and management.* Butterworth-Heinemann, Boston.

Milunsky A, ed. (1998). *Genetic disorders and the fetus. Diagnosis, prevention and treatment*, 4th edn. Johns Hopkins University Press, Baltimore.

Norman MG *et al.* eds (1995). *Congenital abnormalities of the brain. Pathologic, embryologic, clinical, radiologic and genetic aspects.* Oxford University Press, New York.

Pless IB, ed (1994). *The epidemiology of childhood disorders.* Oxford University Press, New York.

Stanley F, Blair E, Alberman E. (2000). *Cerebral palsies: epidemiology and causal pathways. Clinics in Developmental Medicine No.151.* Mac Keith Press, London.

Swaiman KF, Ashwal S, eds (1999). *Paediatric neurology. Principles and practice*, 3rd edn. Mosby, St Louis.

Wallis D, Muenke M (2000). Mutations in holoprosencephaly. *Human Mutation* **16**, 99–108.

24.22 Disorders of muscle

24.22.1 Introduction: structure and function

M. Hanna

Basic anatomy of skeletal muscle

We possess more than 150 voluntary (skeletal) muscles most of which are attached to the skeleton at both ends through tendons. Complex voluntary movements of the body are achieved by integrated activity of different skeletal muscle groups. To the naked eye a transverse section of any skeletal muscle reveals small units known as muscle fascicles. Each skeletal muscle fascicle is composed of many basic structural units known as muscle fibres (Fig. 1). Muscle fibres are cylindrical structures that may be several centimetres long and 50 to 100 μm in diameter. A muscle fibre is a highly specialized cell. Like any other cell it has a membrane (the sarcolemma), it contains cytoplasm (the sarcoplasm), and it has an endoplasmic reticulum (the sarcoplasmic reticulum) as well as other subcellular organelles such as mitochondria. However, unlike cells from many other tissues, muscle cells are multinucleate. Typically the nuclei are positioned at the edges of the muscle fibre. The sarcolemma of muscle fibres possesses specialized regions known as motor endplates. These endplate regions are the points at which the axon innervating a muscle fibre forms synapses. Release of acetylcholine from the presynaptic region transmits the axonal action potential to the muscle fibre membrane by binding to postsynaptic acetylcholine receptors located in the sarcolemma at the endplate. The sarcolemma is differentially permeable to ions. This allows different concentrations of ions to be maintained inside and outside the membrane and this is critical in maintaining the resting membrane potential. A chain of important structural proteins maintain the integrity of the sarcolemma by linking intracellular muscle fibre cytoskeletal proteins to the extracellular matrix. These structural proteins include dystrophin (located in a subsarcolemmal distribution), the dystrophin-associated glycoprotein complex (a trans-sarcolemmal protein complex), and laminin (located extracellularly). These important proteins may be dysfunctional in certain forms of genetic muscle diseases (see Chapter 24.22.2).

After staining, or if suitably illuminated, muscle fibres are seen to have regular cross-striations that extend right across the inside of the fibre, dividing it up into sarcomeres (Fig. 1). The parts of the cross-striations are identified by letters. The light I band is divided by the dark Z line and the dark A band has the lighter H zone in its centre. The region between two adjacent Z lines is called a sarcomere. The cross-striations are due to the presence of the principal contracile filamentous proteins, actin and myosin, in the sacroplasm. These filamentous proteins are arranged in rod-like structures known as myofibrils. A single myofibril contains many protein filaments. In life, myofibrils are transparent on routine light microscopy, but if viewed with a polarizing microscope, a typical pattern of cross-striations can be seen within individual myofibrils. The correct understanding of the basic microscopic anatomy of this pattern of cross-striations was critical to the discovery of the sliding filament theory of skeletal muscle contraction.

The sliding filament theory of skeletal muscle contraction

The protein filaments contained within myofibrils are of two types; the thin filaments are composed of actin, tropomyosin, and troponin and the thick

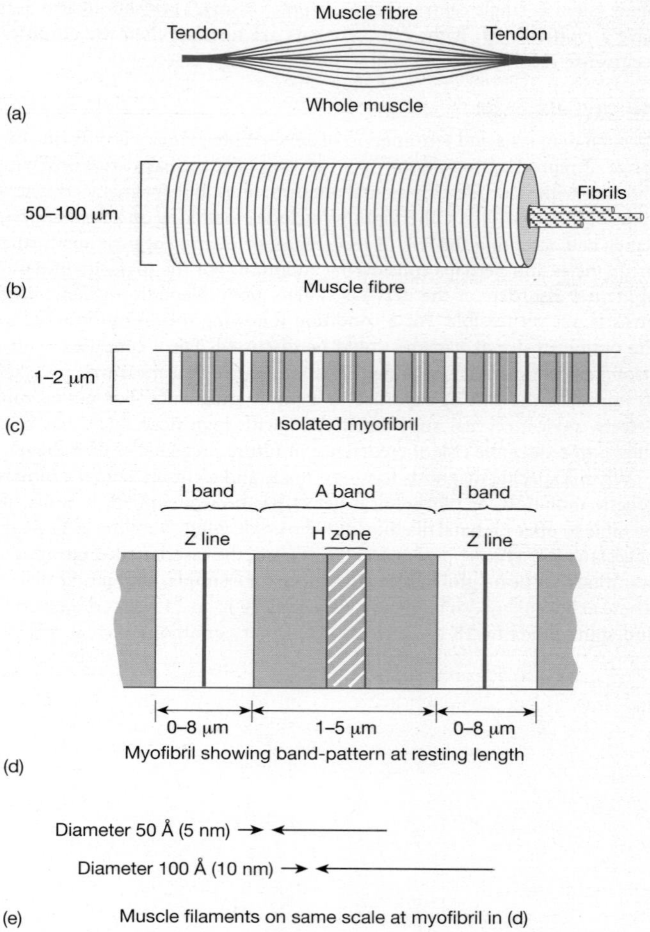

Fig. 1 The dimensions and arrangement of the contractile components in a muscle. The whole muscle (a) is made up of fibres (b) which contain cross-striated myofibrils (c, d). These are constructed of two types of protein filaments (e), put together as shown in Fig. 2

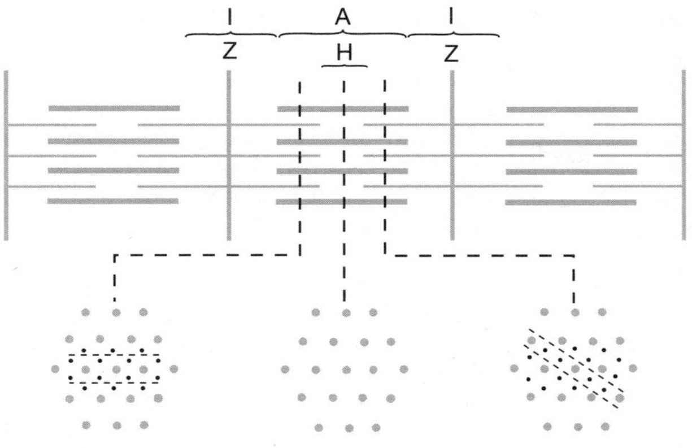

Fig. 2 Diagram illustrating the arrangement of the different kinds of protein filament (thick filaments: myosin; thin filaments: actin) in a myofibril. At the top are three sarcomeres drawn as they would appear in longitudinal section. Below are transverse sections through the H zone and other parts of the A band where the thick and thin filaments interdigitate. The plane of section determines whether, in electron micrographs, there seem to be one or two thin (actin) filaments between two thick (myosin) ones. (Reproduced from Huxley and Hanson, 1960, with permission.)

filaments are composed of myosin (Fig. 2). The thick filaments are approximately twice the diameter of the thin filaments.

The thick filaments are lined up to form the A bands, whereas the array of thin filaments forms the less dense I bands. The lighter H bands in the centre of the A bands are the regions where, when the muscle is relaxed, the thin filaments do not overlap the thick filaments. The Z lines transect the myofibrils and connect to the thin filaments. If a transverse section through the A band is examined under the electron microscope, each thick filament is found to be surrounded by six thin filaments in a regular hexagonal array (Fig. 2). The myosin molecules have large globular heads at their C-terminal portions (Fig. 3). The heads contain an actin-binding site that hydrolyses ATP. During muscle contraction, cross-linkages occur between the heads of the myosin molecules and the actin molecules (Fig. 3).

The thin filaments are composed of two chains of actin that form a long double helix. Tropomyosin molecules are long filaments located in the groove between the two chains of actin. Troponin molecules are small globular units located at intervals along the tropomyosin molecules. Troponin has three components: troponin T, responsible for binding to tropomyosin; troponin I, which inhibits the interaction of actin and myosin; and troponin C, which contains the binding sites for the Ca^{2+} ions that initiate contraction (Fig. 3).

The process by which shortening of the contractile elements of muscle is brought about is sliding of the thin filaments over the thick filaments. The width of the A band is constant, whereas the Z lines move closer together when the muscle contracts and further apart when it is stretched. The sliding during muscle contraction is produced by breaking and reforming of the cross-linkages between actin and myosin. The immediate source of energy for contraction is hydrolysis of ATP localized to the myosin head.

Neural activation of muscle fibres—the motor unit

The motor unit is the final common pathway for all voluntary muscle activity. The motor unit is composed of an anterior horn cell (located within the spinal cord), its peripheral axon, the axon terminal branches, the associated neuromuscular junctions, and the muscle fibres innervated. The muscle fibres of a single motor unit are spatially dispersed throughout a muscle and only a few fibres innervated by the same anterior horn cell are contiguous. The number of motor units varies greatly between muscles, from approximately 1000 in leg muscles to 100 in intrinsic hand muscles. The number of muscle fibres per motor unit also varies greatly. Motor units also differ in physiological and biochemical characteristics. Two main types of motor units are recognized, each composed of a single muscle fibre type. Type 1 muscle fibres contain many mitochondria and are slightly smaller than type 2 muscle fibres as they contain myofibrils, which are more slender. Type 1 fibres contain a high concentration of oxidative enzymes and more fat. Type 2 fibres are larger, contain fewer mitochondria, but have a higher concentration of glycogen and enzymes involved in anaerobic metabolism such as myophosphorylase. All skeletal muscles contain a mixture of both fibre types, typically in a chequerboard pattern when stained appropriately (with the myofibrillar ATPase reaction) and visualized under light microscopy (Fig. 4). Type 1 fibres are also known as slow fibres since they contract and relax slowly and are abundant in muscles concerned mainly with maintaining posture. In contrast, type 2 fibres contract and relax quickly and are also known as twitch fibres. Type 2 fibres can be further subdivided into type 2a and 2b based on their intensity of staining with myofibrillar ATPase reaction at different pHs (Table 1).

Normally muscle fibres do not contract in isolation, rather the muscle fibres which comprise the motor unit contract together in response to depolarization of an anterior horn cell. Such depolarization is transmitted along the axon until it invades the nerve terminal. This results in opening of voltage-gated calcium channels located in the presynaptic membrane. Calcium enters the nerve terminal down an electrochemical gradient. The resulting increase in presynaptic calcium concentration promotes fusion of acetylcholine-containing vesicles normally present in the nerve terminal with the presynaptic membrane. Quanta of acetylcholine are released into the synaptic cleft and diffuse to the postsynaptic membrane to bind to and

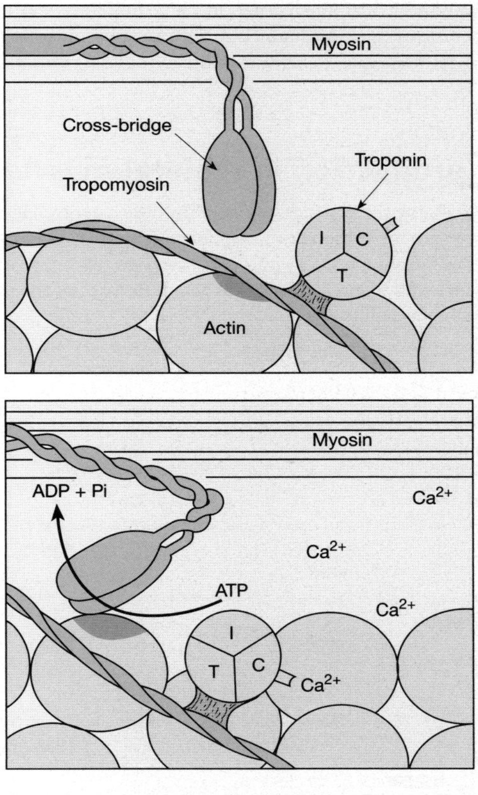

Fig. 3 Initiation of muscle contraction by Ca^{2+} ions. The cross-bridges (heads of myosin molecules) attach to binding sites on actin (striped areas) and swivel when tropomyosin is displaced laterally by binding of Ca^{2+} ions to troponin C. (Modified from Katz AM, 1975, Congestive heart failure. *New England Journal of Medicine* **293**, 1184.)

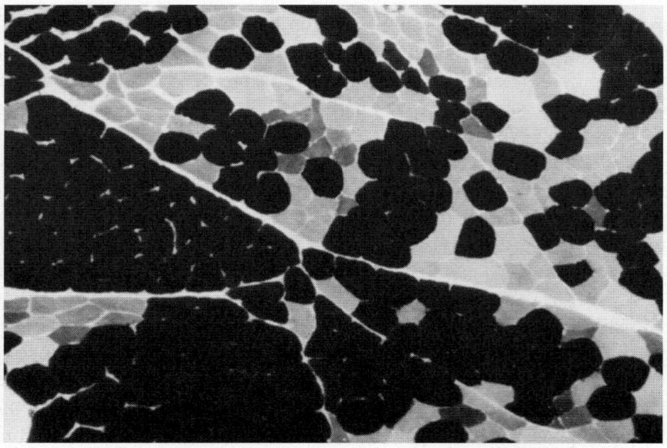

Fig. 4 A transverse section of human skeletal muscle obtained by biopsy from a patient with spinal muscular atrophy stained for the myofibrillar ATPase reaction after preincubation at pH 4.6. There is extensive evidence of fibre type grouping, particularly of the type 1 fibres, resulting from reinnervation. Magnification ×150. (Kindly supplied by Dr Margaret Johnson.)

activate acetylcholine receptors. Acetycholine binding causes opening of its receptor channel allowing cations to enter the muscle fibre in the endplate region. This cation flux depolarizes the postsynaptic membrane resulting in a mini-endplate potential. The summation of endplate potentials results in the excitation of the postsynaptic membrane, which is then conducted along the muscle fibre membrane. The excitation is transmitted into the muscle fibre by invaginations of the sarcolemma known as the T-tubule system. Activation of calcium channels in the T-tubule system membrane results in opening of calcium channels in the sarcoplasmic reticulum. Calcium is then released into the muscle fibre cytoplasm, initiating muscle contraction.

Energy production in skeletal muscle

Resting skeletal muscle requires remarkably little energy. However, the requirement for energy production may increase dramatically in response to exercise, since energy is required for muscle contraction. Adenosine triphosphate (ATP) is the main source of energy in muscle. ATP is required for shortening of the contractile filaments and also for the active reuptake of calcium into the sarcoplasmic reticulum after each muscle contraction. Maintenance of electrochemical gradients across the sarcolemma also requires ATP. Resynthesis of ATP from ADP is essential for normal muscle function. The two main energy-producing pathways in muscle are glycolysis in the sarcoplasm and oxidative phosphorylation in the mitochondria. Resynthesis of ATP from ADP is also aided by phosphocreatine and the creatine kinase reaction. Creatine kinase catalyses the transfer of high-energy phosphate from phosphocreatine to ADP in circumstances in which ATP demand may outstrip ATP production, for example at the very beginning of exercise before oxidative phosphorylation or glycolysis is activated. Glycolysis is the main pathway of ATP synthesis in anaerobic conditions and results in the generation of lactate. Oxidative phosphorylation is the major ATP-generating pathway in aerobic conditions. The main fuel sources in skeletal muscle are glucose, glycogen, and fatty acids. In anaerobic conditions, glycogen is the main energy source. In aerobic exercise, glycogen and glucose are utilized initially, but after approximately 30 min, fatty acids are the main energy source. In resting aerobic muscle, fatty acids provide the principal source of fuel. Several muscle diseases are recognized in which energy metabolism is impaired and are known as the metabolic myopathies.

Table 1 Histochemical and physiological characteristics of the three major types of muscle fibre

	Fibre type		
	1	2A	2B
Enzyme reactions			
NADH–tetrazolium reductase and SDH	+++	++	+
Myofibrillar ATPase:			
pH 9.4	+	+++	+++
pH 4.6	+++	–	+++
pH 4.3	+++	–	–
Phosphorylase	+	+++	+++
Physiological properties			
Twitch speeds	Slow	Fast	Fast
Fatigue resistance	+++	++	+
Nomenclature			
Peter *et al.* (1972)	Slow twitch Oxidative	Fast twitch Oxidative–glycolytic	Fast twitch Glycolytic
Burle *et al.* (1971)	S (slow contracting)	FR (fast contracting, fatigue resistant)	FF (fast contracting, fast fatigue)

From Walton and Mastaglia (1980).

Diseases of human skeletal muscle—overview

Human muscle diseases may be conveniently divided into those which are genetically determined and those which are acquired (Table 2).

The clinical history in muscle diseases

Although a muscle biopsy is usually needed to determine the exact type of muscle disease, the clinical history and examination are usually sufficient to determine whether a muscle disease is present or absent. Since many muscle diseases are genetically determined, it is particularly important to consider the family history. A careful drug history is also essential.

Although many diseases may affect skeletal muscle (Table 2), there are three main symptoms with which patients may present: muscular pain, muscular weakness, and fatiguability. A further important but less common symptom is darkening of the urine (pigmenturia) due to release of myoglobin from damaged muscle. This occurs particularly in the metabolic myopathies. Unless pigmenturia has been dramatic, patients may not volunteer this symptom. Muscle pain is a common symptom, but in only about one-third of patients presenting with this symptom will an underlying muscle disease be identified. In those without a definable muscle disease, many are considered to have a psychogenic cause for their muscle pain, although some may have as yet undefined disorders of muscle metabolism. Sometimes it can be difficult for the patient and the physician to distinguish between pain originating in muscle and pain originating in

Table 2 A simple classification of human muscle diseases

Genetically determined muscle diseases
Muscular dystrophies, such as Duchenne/Becker
Congenital myopathies, such as nemaline
Muscle ion channel disorders, such as hyper-/hypokalaemic periodic paralysis
Metabolic myopathies, such as McArdle's disease (myophosphorylase deficiency) and mitchondrial myopathies
Acquired muscle diseases
Inflammatory muscle diseases, such as polymyositis/dermatomyositis
Degenerative muscle diseases, such as inclusion body myositis
Endocrine muscle diseases, such as hyper-/hypothyroid myopathies
Toxic and drug-induced muscle diseases, due to alcohol/corticosteroids

joints or bones. Certain rheumatological diseases may result in joint pain as well as muscle pain. For example, systemic lupus erythematosus may cause arthritis and polymyositis. Muscle pains may take the form of cramps, which are involuntary contractions of muscle groups. Simple muscle cramps are not uncommon in the elderly and frequently occur at night. There is usually no underlying muscle disease but drugs such as diuretics (which induce hypokalaemia) may be implicated. In younger patients, muscle cramps may be the presenting feature of a metabolic muscle disease such as McArdle's disease. Muscle pain brought on by exertion is a particular feature of the metabolic muscle diseases. Muscle contractures may also be a source of muscle pain in patients with metabolic myopathies. Patients experience a pain similar to a cramp, but unlike a cramp, electromyography reveals that a contracture is electrically silent.

Muscle weakness is a common feature of muscle diseases and the distribution of weakness in most is in the proximal limb muscles. Patients may complain of difficulty performing tasks which involve lifting their arms up to or above their head, such as brushing hair. Proximal lower limb muscle weakness causes difficulties getting out of low chairs and in climbing stairs. Muscle diseases often affect the limb musculature symmetrically—although there are important exceptions to this. For example, one of the common autosomal dominant muscular dystrophies, fascioscapulohumeral muscular dystrophy, often affects the limb muscles in an asymmetrical fashion. Some muscle diseases may affect the facial musculature as well as that of the limb. Symptoms may include difficulty in whistling, in closing the eyes, or in articulating. Respiratory muscle disease may cause breathlessness. It is important to determine the natural history of muscle weakness. In most genetically determined muscle diseases, weakness progresses slowly over years; occasionally the patient may experience attacks of weakness separated by periods when they seem to have normal strength, as in the periodic paralyses. The muscle weakness in the inflammatory muscle diseases usually develops more rapidly.

Fatiguability is defined as an increase in weakness with exercise. Patients may describe that they can start a particular physical activity but the longer they continue the weaker they become. They may also complain that they become weaker as the day goes on. Myaesthenia gravis, a disorder of neuromuscular transmission, is the principal cause of fatiguability. In patients with myaesthenia gravis, fatiguability can usually be demonstrated at the bedside. Patients with metabolic muscle diseases may also experience fatiguability.

The physical examination in muscle disease

The examination may be broadly divided into two aspects. First, an examination is made to establish whether there are any clues to the cause of the muscle disease. In this context, the general physical examination is very important. Particular attention is paid to eliciting signs which might indicate an underlying endocrine or rheumatological disorder. For example, signs of hyper-/hypothyroidism, Cushing's syndrome, or of rheumatological disorders such as systemic lupus erythematosus. Inspection of the skin may reveal the appearances of dermatomyositis. The second part of the examination involves examining the muscular system to determine the extent and severity of the condition; this may in addition give further clues to the aetiology. The muscles are inspected for any atrophy or hypertrophy (as occurs in some muscular dystrophies) or for any spontaneous activity of the muscle fibres (such as fasciculation, which might indicate an anterior horn cell disorder). The muscles should be palpated for any tenderness or swelling, which may occur in inflammatory muscle diseases. Myotonia is a delayed relaxation of muscle after contraction. This may be observed by asking the patient to clench their fist and then to open it rapidly. A patient with myotonia is unable to open the clenched fist rapidly due to an inability to relax the contracted muscles quickly. Myotonia may also be evident on percussion of muscle. The examination of muscle power is carried out systematically starting with the cranial musculature before proceeding to the arms and legs. The degree of weakness is assessed with reference to the Medical Research Council grading scale (0 to 5). The distribution of weakness is also noted, since different muscle diseases have characteristic patterns of weakness. Bedside assessment of respiratory muscles including the diaphragm is also important, although detailed assessment of these muscles requires formal spirometry. Finally, the tendon reflexes are elicited. These are generally preserved in acquired muscle diseases, except when there is advanced weakness; however, they may be lost relatively early in the course of dystrophies.

Investigating the patient with muscle disease

Investigations are generally only instituted when the history and examination have provided clear evidence that the patient has symptoms and/or signs of muscle disease. The investigations are aimed primarily at determining the exact type of muscle disease as it is essential to establish whether the patient has a treatable muscle disease, such as an inflammatory myopathy. Many investigations of increasing complexity and invasiveness are available.

Simple blood tests allow an assessment of the endocrine and nutritional status of the patient (such as thyroid function, the consumption of excess alcohol, or the presence of vitamin D deficiency). Measurement of the blood creatine kinase is important as this can be an indicator of the degree of muscle fibre damage or necrosis. The creatine kinase is generally elevated in the inflammatory muscle diseases and in many of the muscular dystrophies.

Increasingly, DNA-based testing is available from simple blood samples. This can be particularly helpful and in some situations may obviate the need for further more-invasive tests, such as a muscle biopsy. For example, if analysis of the dystrophin gene on the X chromosome identifies a pathogenic mutation known to associate with Duchenne muscular dystrophy, the diagnosis is confirmed. It is likely that there will be greater availability of DNA-based tests for genetic muscle disease in the future and this will become an increasingly important aid to diagnosis.

The diagnosis of metabolic muscle diseases may be achieved by specific dynamic tests. For example, McArdle's disease can be diagnosed using the ischaemic lactate test, and mitochondrial disease may be suspected on the basis of subanaerobic exercise tests (both these tests are described in the relevant section).

Detailed nerve conduction studies and electromyography are useful in determining whether a patient has a neuropathy, a defect in neuromuscular junction transmission, or a myopathy. Electromyography is useful in characterizing any spontaneous activity of muscle, such as fasciculations or myotonia. Although electromyography is generally useful in confirming the presence of a myopathy, it is less useful in determining the cause.

Muscle biopsy allows a detailed analysis of the internal architecture of muscle and is an extremely valuable and safe investigation in carefully selected patients. Using a range of histochemical stains, histochemical enzyme reactions, and immunological techniques on frozen muscle biopsy sections, much information of diagnostic use can be obtained. Different muscle diseases often reveal characteristic patterns of abnormalities, which are usually identified by light microscopic techniques. Using basic histochemical stains the features of different muscular dystrophies are generally similar; the most common features being marked variations in fibre diameter, internal nuclei, fibre splitting, fibre necrosis and regeneration, and increase in connective tissue. However, a more precise diagnosis of the type of muscular dystrophy can now be obtained by immunostaining techniques. Antibodies which are raised against specific membrane proteins allow quantitative analysis. For example, staining using antibodies directed against dystophin reveals no or very little dystrophin in cases of Duchenne muscular dystrophy (Fig. 5). Prominent inflammatory infiltrates are typically seen in muscle sections from patients with inflammatory myopathies. Figures 5, 6, and 7 show the muscle biopsy features of some of the metabolic myopathies. In some cases the changes seen on the biopsy clearly indicate a myopathic process, but it is not possible to be more specific in the absence of typical immunological, inflammatory, or metabolic changes.

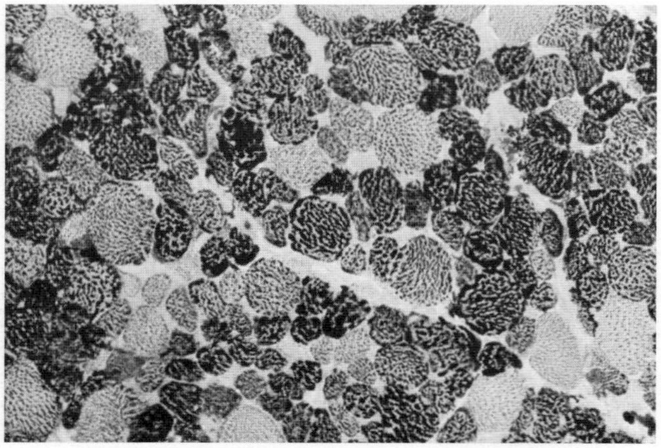

Fig. 5 A transverse section of human skeletal muscle obtained from a patient with carnitine deficiency and stained with Sudan black B. The massive accumulation of neutral fat, especially with the type 1 fibres, is evident. Magnification ×196.

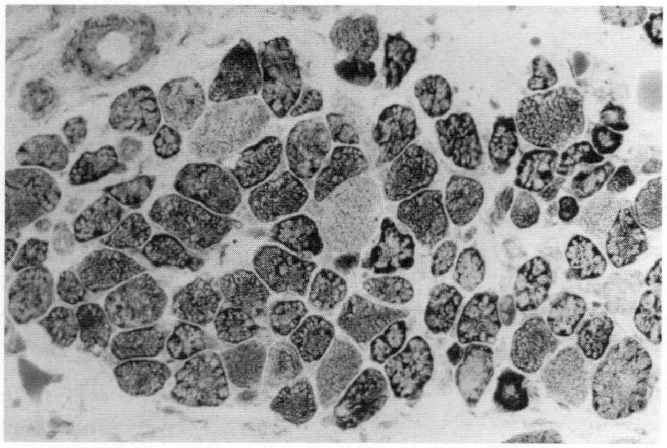

Fig. 6 A transverse section of skeletal muscle obtained from a patient with mitrochondrial myopathy, stained for the MADH-TR reaction. The type 1 fibres are darkly stained and show the typical reticulated appearance of so-called 'ragged-red fibres' with massive mitochondria, particularly in many fibres just deep to the sarcolemma. Magnification ×384. (Kindly supplied by Dr Margaret Johnson.)

Further reading

Huxley HE, Hanson J (1960). In: Bourne GH, ed. *The structure and function of muscle*, Vol.1. Academic Press, New York.

Walton JN, Mastaglia FL (1980). The molecular basis of muscle disease. In: Thompson RHS, Davison AN, eds. *The molecular basis of neuropathology.* Edward Arnold, London.

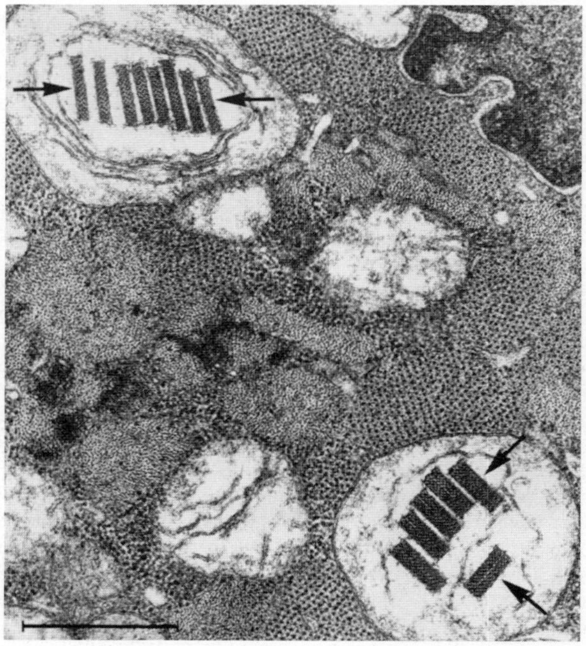

Fig. 7 A transverse section of a biopsy specimen obtained from one quadriceps muscle in a patient with mitrochondrial myopathy showing arrays of paracrystalline inclusions in the damaged mitochondria. Bar = 1 μm. (Kindly supplied by Dr Michael Cullen.)

24.22.2 Muscular dystrophy

K. Bushby

Introduction

Muscular dystrophy is not a single disease. Many different types of muscular dystrophy can be recognized: all are primary, genetically determined disorders of muscle and all cause muscle weakness, which is usually progressive. The various types of muscular dystrophy share several characteristic findings on muscle biopsy, most notably a variation of fibre size, evidence of muscle fibre necrosis, and usually replacement of muscle tissue by fat and fibrous tissue. These pathological findings are often but not always accompanied by elevation of the serum creatine kinase. While the key clinical sign in muscular dystrophy is muscle weakness, the distribution of that weakness and the association with other features such as wasting, hypertrophy, and joint contractures are the defining features which are most helpful in making a clinical diagnosis, together with age at presentation and rate of progression. Unusual manifestations of muscular dystrophy are muscle pain, rhabdomyolysis, and myoglobinuria. Complications may include cardiac and respiratory failure or anaesthetic problems. These complications may be specific to particular types of muscular dystrophy. Taken in conjunction with the clinical findings in any patient, precise diagnostic tests (either through DNA analysis or protein analysis of a muscle biopsy sample) are available for a growing number of these disorders, as knowledge of the underlying mechanism of disease for each of these entities has increased. Confirmation of the type of muscular dystrophy in any individual patient is critical to the provision of appropriate

Box 1 Basis of the classification of muscular dystrophies

- Clinical description.
- Genetics (autosomal dominant/recessive/X-linked).
- Underlying gene/protein defect.
- Localization or function of the protein involved.

management, prognostic advice, and genetic counselling. No form of muscular dystrophy is currently curable, although various experimental therapeutic procedures are under investigation.

Classification of the muscular dystrophies

Various classifications of the muscular dystrophies have been proposed, reflecting historical advances in the understanding of this group of diseases (Box 1). The current basis for classification combines an appreciation of the clinical features with the ability to determine the molecular basis for the disease. Therefore the eponymous names (for example Duchenne muscular dystrophy) still in common usage reflect the detailed clinical descriptions provided by early clinicians: other disease names reflect the recognized pattern of muscle involvement in a particular condition (for example facioscapulohumeral muscular dystrophy). Disease designations based on the genetic or protein defect in a particular disorder (for example dystrophinopathy) are becoming more widely used, reflecting the fact that some disorders previously believed to be clinically distinct actually represent different manifestations of lesions at the same locus. Genetic analysis has also revealed an unsuspected level of heterogeneity with different genetic causes for disorders which show superficial clinical similarities. This can be seen most strikingly within the 'limb girdle' group of muscular dystrophies.

The pathophysiology of the muscular dystrophies

Biochemical and physiological experiments failed to shed any light on the mechanisms by which muscular dystrophy could arise, and it has only been since the cloning of the *dystrophin* gene in 1987 that progress has been made. It is now quite clear that proteins involved in several different functions within the muscle cell can, when altered or absent, cause muscle damage and account for the pathological and clinical features of a muscular dystrophy. Some of these proteins are components of the membrane of the muscle fibre which may have a structural or signalling role, others are components of the nuclear envelope or are muscle-specific enzymes (see Fig. 1).

General points on the diagnosis of muscular dystrophy

Box 2 summarizes some of the major considerations in arriving at the correct diagnosis of a muscular dystrophy. History taking at the time of presentation (Box 3) may be particularly informative. The clinical history may be pathognomonic. Detailed diagnostic information is given in the following text relating to specific diseases. The main tools for specific diagnosis in muscular dystrophy are the use of antibodies for the immunolabelling of muscle biopsy sections and/or the application of specific DNA-based genetic analysis.

General points on the management of the muscular dystrophies

Despite the fact that no cures for muscular dystrophy are established, there are many issues for management which may be important or specific to the various types. However, there is as yet little systematic or comprehensive clinical research into management and randomized trials of management regimes are few and far between. It is nonetheless appropriate that where possible, patients with a diagnosis or a suspected diagnosis of muscular dystrophy should be referred to a specialist clinic. The multidisciplinary approach of these clinics ensures that patients have access to the full range of diagnostic facilities, are able to obtain specialized physiotherapy advice, and can obtain accurate genetic counselling where this is required. Access to patient support organizations and their staff is also of paramount importance. The diagnosis of any kind of muscular dystrophy, in that it inevitably implies a progressive and incurable disease, possibly with implications for children or other relatives, is a considerable burden and one which needs to be recognized and supported.

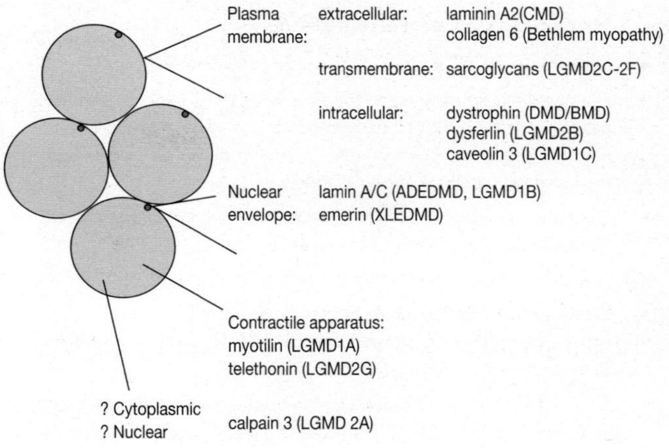

Fig. 1 Schematic diagram to show localization within the muscle fibre (where known) of the proteins known to be involved in producing a dystrophic phenotype. In particular, groups of proteins localizing to the plasma membrane or nuclear envelope have been implicated in a number of different types of muscular dystrophy.

Box 2 Diagnosis of muscular dystrophy

- History (especially motor milestones, age at onset, physical prowess as a child).
- Age of patient (congenital/childhood/teenage/adult presentation).
- Pattern of muscle involvement on examination (predominantly proximal/distal, upper limb/lower limb, symmetrical/asymmetrical).
- Pattern of associated features on examination (contractures, muscle wasting, hypertrophy).
- Level of serum creatine kinase in active disease (massive elevation in dystrophinopathy, sarcoglycanopathy, dysferlinopathy, calpainopathy, congenital muscular dystrophy (some); moderate elevation in facioscapulohumeral muscular dystrophy, Emery Dreifuss muscular dystrophy, congenital muscular dystrophy (some); normal to mild elevation in autosomal dominant limb girdle muscular dystrophy, facioscapulohumeral muscular dystrophy (some)).
- Electromyography (to exclude neurogenic causes of weakness, especially if serum creatine kinase is not markedly elevated).
- Muscle imaging (ultrasound scans can confirm muscle involvement, but to confirm pattern of muscle involvement need MRI/CT).
- Muscle biopsy, histology, and storage of frozen biopsy material for further analysis.
- Specialized analysis of muscle biopsy (immunocytochemistry, immunoblotting, electron microscopy).
- DNA analysis.

Box 3 History taking in muscle disease

- Question in detail about early motor development.
- Eliciting what actually were the first symptoms experienced by a patient may be difficult but is important in highlighting the initial pattern of muscle involvement—lower limb versus upper limb/ proximal versus distal musculature.
- Asking 'when were you at your fastest' may be informative in determining age of peak motor performance.
- Ask about performance at school sports.
- Particularly useful indicators in that respect are the ability to climb ropes (upper girdle weakness), muscle pain on running, a tendency to spend all the time in goal at football(!).
- Do not assume that difficulty climbing stairs always indicates proximal muscle weakness—it may reflect an inability to push up on the toes.
- Ask specifically about the ability to stand on tiptoe/stand on heels. The need to wear heels on shoes at all times may indicate Achilles tendon contractures.
- Patients who had early Achilles tendon contractures may have had them operated on before being referred for diagnosis. Ask about this.

The congenital muscular dystrophies

The congenital muscular dystrophies (**CMD**) are defined by their very early childhood onset. They comprise a number of disorders with different molecular pathological bases for the diseases.

Presentation

1. Neonatal presentation:
   - hypotonia, which may be prenatal
   - feeding problems (usually mild)
   - joint contractures, especially knees, hips, and ankles (see Fig. 2).
2. Early childhood presentation:
   - delayed motor milestones
   - failure to thrive
   - repeated respiratory infections.
3. Later childhood presentation (rare):
   - mainly proximal muscle symptoms
   - history of delayed motor milestones
   - rigid spine, contractures of ankles, hips, and knees.

Differential diagnosis

In the neonatal and early childhood presentation the main clinical diagnostic confusion (after excluding central causes of hypotonia) – may be with spinal muscular atrophy (check *SMN/NAIP* genes), congenital myotonic dystrophy (facial weakness is usually more pronounced and diagnosis can be excluded on genetic testing), and congenital myopathy (may be distinguished on muscle biopsy). In all of these conditions, serum creatine kinase is either normal or much lower than seen in many congenital muscular dystrophies.

With later childhood presentation the differential diagnosis is as above, plus Duchenne muscular dystrophy (though calf hypertrophy is usually more pronounced and serum creatine kinase is typically higher—biopsy will exclude the diagnosis) or childhood presentation of a limb girdle type of muscular dystrophy.

Classification

There are several recognized forms of congenital muscular dystrophy, and as there is considerable heterogeneity in the group which remains, many more different entities are ultimately likely to be distinguished at the genetic level. The first level of subdivision is on the basis of whether clinically there is a 'pure' muscle phenotype, or whether there is also prominent involvement of the central nervous system and eyes. In the types of congenital muscular dystrophy with a 'pure' muscle phenotype clinically, the next major subdivision is based on the presence or absence of a muscle protein merosin or laminin A2. Examination of collagen VI labelling in the muscle fibre may also be informative (see Table 1).

Establishing the diagnosis

Serum creatine kinase may in some kinds of congenital muscular dystrophy be normal, but is typically elevated at least twofold, and up to 20-fold or more in the laminin A2 deficient group. Muscle biopsy shows dystrophic changes and examination of LAMA2 or collagen VI in muscle or skin is used to distingush cases with normal and abnormal or absent protein. Secondary changes in laminin A2 probably reflect the involvement of a number of different primary mutations. Mutations in the gene *FKRP* are responsible for some of these cases. Magnetic resonance imaging of the brain is a useful adjunct to diagnosis as it will confirm the presence of white matter changes always present after 6 months of age in primary LAMA2

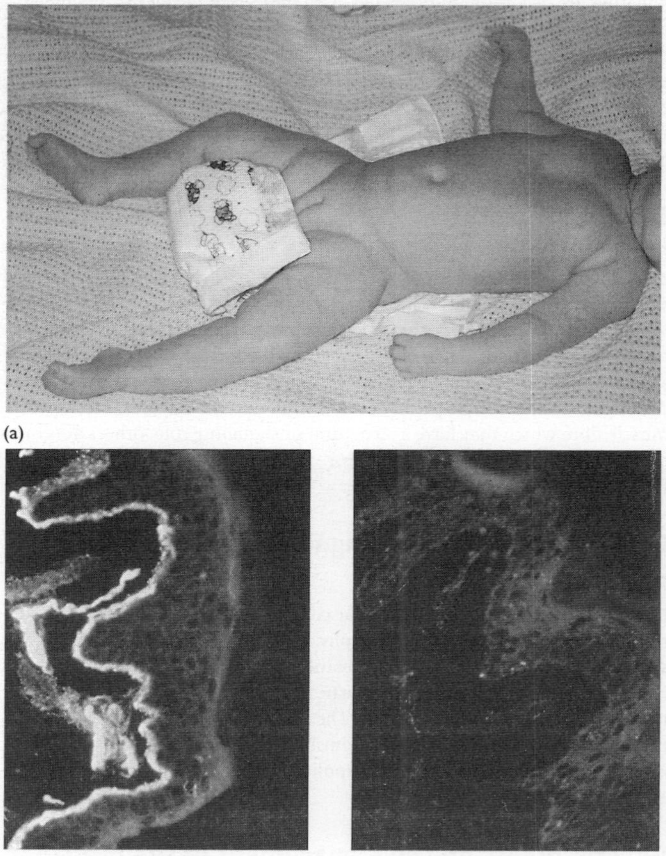

(a) (b) (c)

Fig. 2 (a) Typical clinical picture of a baby presenting with merosin negative muscular dystrophy. Note the hypotonic posture, and mild contractures of the hips, knees, and ankles. (b), (c) Immunofluorescence picture of skin biopsy labelled with an antibody to laminin A2 (merosin) showing normal and absent labelling patterns. This investigation can be carried out on a variety of tissues including skin, muscle, or placenta.

deficiency, and the characteristic brain malformations in the other types of congenital muscular dystrophy (see Table 1).

Prognosis and management

The muscle weakness in congenital muscular dystrophy may be relatively static, but the complications of that weakness can be severe, and vary according to the precise diagnosis. The degree of muscle weakness is quite variable. In primary laminin A2 deficient congenital muscular dystrophy, the severity of the disease correlates roughly with the abundance of laminin A2 in the muscle, with children completely lacking laminin A2 rarely achieving independent ambulation. Others may learn to walk independently but this is usually much later than usual, and these children may later lose this ability. Joint contractures and scoliosis are major complications of the disease and cause much additional disability, requiring careful management by physiotherapy, standing regimes, splinting, bracing, and surgery where appropriate. Feeding problems may be intractable and lead to chronic malnutrition unless treated by nasogastric or gastrostomy feeding. Malnutrition may contribute to susceptibility to chest infections, which is also heightened by weakness of the respiratory muscles. These children are at risk of respiratory failure and their follow-up should include monitoring for this complication which can be effectively managed by the provision of non-invasive home nocturnal ventilation. Cardiac failure is reported in some children, mainly in the group lacking laminin A2.

The overall prognosis depends on the type of congenital muscular dystrophy. Children with the most severe forms are at risk of dying in early childhood. If they survive this period, with appropriate management of feeding problems, respiratory, and cardiac complications, survival into adult life is the norm. In the 'pure' forms of congenital muscular dystrophy

Table 1 The congenital muscular dystrophies

	Pure CMD (normal LAMA2)	Pure CMD (primary loss of LAMA2)	Pure CMD (secondary loss of LAMA2)	Fukuyama muscular dystrophy	Muscle–eye–brain disease	Walker–Warburg syndrome
CNS involvement (radiological)	Usually normal	White matter radiolucency (seen after 6 months of age) essential to distinguish primary and secondary LAMA2 deficiency	May be present in some types	Poly-microgyria	Pachygyria, cobblestone cortex, cerebral atrophy, small cerebellar vermis and brainstem	Type II lissencephaly, may be ventricular dilatation and encephalocele
CNS involvement (clinical)	Usually normal	About 30% have epilepsy. IQ normal	May be present in some types	IQ usually reduced	IQ reduced	IQ severely reduced
Ocular involvement	Normal	May have restricted eye movements	Probably normal	Myopia	Myopia, retinal degeneration, cataracts	Anterior chamber abnormalities, corneal opacities, micro-ophthalmia
Epidemiology	Many different entities: individual frequencies unknown	About 1/3 of CMD seen in USA and Europe have absent *LAMA2*	Many different entities: individual frequencies unknown	Common in Japan, rarely reported elsewhere	Common in Finland, rarely reported elsewhere	Seen worldwide. Rare, prevalence unknown
Diagnostic investigations	Collagen VI is abnormal in Ullrich's CMD. *SEPN1* mutations are described in a form of CMD with rigid spine syndrome (RSMD1)	LAMA2 examination in muscle, skin, or placenta (for prenatal diagnosis)	*LAMA2* reduced in muscle or skin. A subgroup of these patients have *FKRP* mutations	Analysis of *fukutin* gene (predominant insertion mutation seen in Japan)	Linkage to chromosome 1 has been described. No specific diagnostic tests to date	No known molecular basis to date
Notes	A highly variable group, undoubtedly comprising a number of different entities. One cause of this phenotype is mutations in the *collagen 6* genes, causing Ullrich''s congenital muscular dystrophy, and another is *SEPN1* mutations, causing rigid spine syndrome	Primary loss of *LAMA2* invariably accompanied by the typical CNS changes. Secondary loss of *LAMA2* is not.	This is a highly variable group and the molecular basis for the different sybtypes is not yet fully understood	A broad clinical spectrum seen in association with FCMD: some children achieve independent walking, but all are severely handicapped	Molecular genetic testing may sort out some of the diagnostic overlaps between these different groups	Most severe end of the CMD spectrum, CNS abnormalities typically dominate. Survival rare beyond age 2

Abbreviations: CMD, congenital muscular dystrophy; LAMA2, laminin A2; CNS, central nervous system; FCMD, Fukuyama congenital muscular dystrophy.

the intellect is normal, and these children should be encouraged to pursue the best possible education, with appropriate support for their physical difficulties. Fukuyama congenital muscular dystrophy (FCMD), muscle–eye–brain disease (MEBD), and Walker–Warburg syndrome (WWS) may be dominated by intellectual and visual handicap. General management issues remain the same; however, on the whole all of these groups carry a much poorer prognosis (see Table 1).

Genetic counselling

All these disorders are autosomal recessive in inheritance. As the molecular basis for these disorders becomes better established, specific prenatal and carrier testing will become more widely referable in this group of conditions.

Dystrophin deficiency

This group, including two of the most common forms of muscular dystrophy, Duchenne and Becker muscular dystrophy, involve the same gene and protein. These are X-linked diseases, caused by mutations, most of which are deletions, in the *dystrophin* gene.

Presentation

Duchenne muscular dystrophy

- All patients are symptomatic within the first 3 years of life though the mean age at diagnosis is 4 years 10 months.
- Motor milestones are often delayed (half of cases are not walking by 18 months).
- Speech is also frequently delayed.
- Patient is unable to run—there is a pronounced waddling gait on attempting to rush.
- Patient is unable to jump with both feet together or to hop—there is no spring in the step.
- 'Climbs up legs' on rising from the floor—Gower's manoeuvre.
- Rarely presents with anaesthetic complications.

Becker muscular dystrophy

- The mean age at onset of Becker muscular dystrophy is 11 years, though the range of age at presentation is extremely wide and the diagnosis may be made at any age.
- A proportion will have had delayed motor milestones (this may correlate as much with reduction in IQ as with major motor problems at that age).
- Many describe being unable to keep up with peers at school.
- Difficulty with high steps, climbing hills.
- Muscle pains after exercise are a common complaint especially in teenagers (rarely myoglobinuria).

Manifesting carriers of Duchenne muscular dystrophy/Becker muscular dystrophy

A highly variable group, who may occasionally be as severely affected as those with Duchenne muscular dystrophy or as mildly or more mildly than those with Becker muscular dystrophy.

Dystrophin-associated cardiomyopathy

Symptoms and signs of hypertrophy progressing to dilated cardiomyopathy in the absence of major muscle symptoms. Some patients have elevated serum creatine kinase.

Establishing the diagnosis

The clinical presentation of Duchenne muscular dystrophy is very characteristic. Hypertrophy of the calf muscles is almost universal (see Fig. 3), sometimes accompanied by muscle hypertrophy elsewhere, most frequently involving deltoid, parts of the quadriceps, the tongue, and masseters. Wasting of the pectoral and scapular muscles leads to hypotonia around the shoulders detected as the child 'slipping through the hands' on being lifted. In the lower limbs, quadriceps power is weaker than that of the hamstrings. Formal examination of a small child may be difficult, and the main clinical tool is observation of walking, attempting to run, jump, and climb stairs, and to rise from the floor. It is imperative to give the child space to attempt to run, as this will bring out the lack of spring in the step and the lack of fluidity of the attempted running.

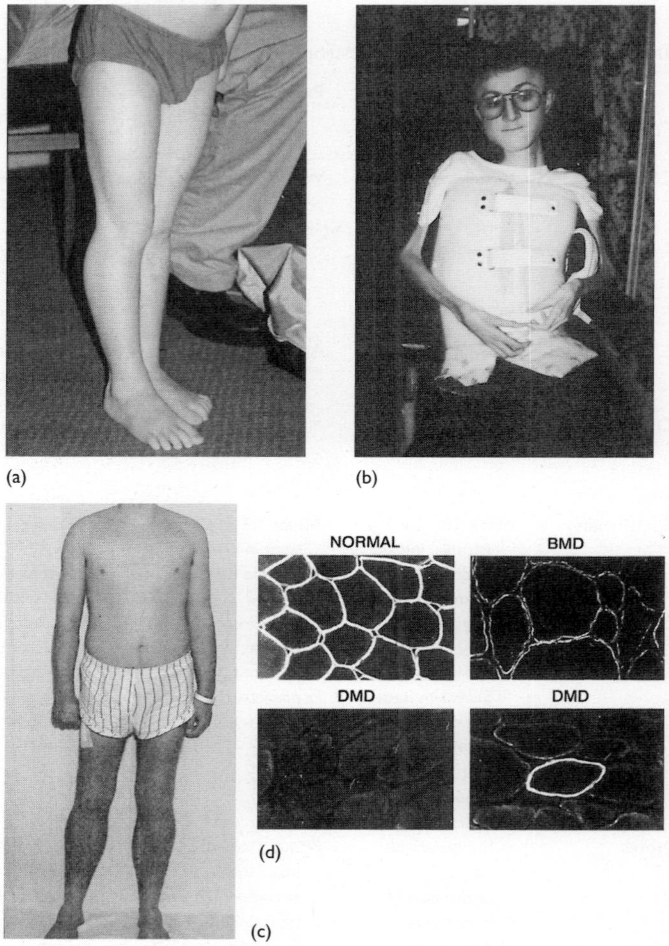

Fig. 3 (a) Child with Duchenne muscular dystrophy at presentation, showing the marked calf and quadriceps hypertrophy and tendency to rise onto the toes. (b) Teenage boy in the later stages of the disease, showing the complications of marked immobility, scoliosis, and muscle wasting. This young man has now been maintained on home nocturnal ventilation successfully for more than 7 years. (c) Clinical pattern at presentation in a young man with Becker muscular dystrophy. Note hypertrophic muscles in calves and quadriceps and mild wasting around the shoulder girdle. (d) Immunocytochemical analysis of dystrophin in normal muscle, Becker muscular dystrophy muscle, and Duchenne muscular dystrophy muscle. In normal muscle, dystrophin labels evenly around the periphery of the muscle fibres. This labelling is typically patchy and reduced in Becker muscular dystrophy, and is either completely or nearly completely absent in Duchenne muscular dystrophy.

Becker muscular dystrophy has been described as a 'slow motion version of Duchenne muscular dystrophy' in that the pattern of muscle involvement in these two allelic disorders is essentially identical (see Fig. 3), but progresses at a much slower rate in Becker muscular dystrophy. Patients with Becker muscular dystrophy may be quite strong on formal muscle examination, but tend to show subtle signs of proximal muscle weakness on climbing stairs or running. They frequently have hypertrophy involving the same muscle groups as seen in Duchenne muscular dystrophy. Some patients have pes cavus.

Serum creatine kinase is always massively elevated, even to more than 200 × normal, but levels of serum creatine kinase do not distinguish the severity of the disease. Muscle biopsy and electromyography are non-specifically dystrophic. Molecular confirmation of the diagnosis is essential to assist in defining prognosis and to provide appropriate genetic counselling. Genetic analysis readily confirms the diagnosis in the 60 to 80 per cent of patients in whom a deletion of the *dystrophin* gene is present: in all patients the diagnosis can be established by the finding of absent or reduced dystrophin in the muscle biopsy (see Fig. 3). This analysis also allows the distinction of dystrophinopathy from the rarer (in most populations) limb girdle types of muscular dystrophy.

Prognosis

Within the 'dystrophinopathy' group the prognosis is highly variable. By definition, those patients with Duchenne muscular dystrophy lose the ability to walk by the age of 12. The development of scoliosis, respiratory failure, and cardiomyopathy (see Box 4) during the teenage years can all be managed so that survival into or beyond the late 20s is becoming more common. Patients with Becker muscular dystrophy are ambulant beyond 16 years of age, and may remain able to walk independently into their fifth decade or longer. These patients are susceptible to cardiac failure at any age from the teens onward and should be monitored for this complication on a regular basis (see Box 4). Respiratory failure is a late complication in Becker muscular dystrophy and correlates with very late stage disease. Lifespan in Becker muscular dystrophy may be normal, or reduced in more severe disease. An 'intermediate' group is also recognized who lose ambulation between 12 and 16: their overall prognosis is also intermediate between Duchenne muscular dystrophy and Becker muscular dystrophy. Around 8 per cent of carriers of Duchenne muscular dystrophy or Becker muscular dystrophy may develop some signs of the disease: rarely this is in a full blown form comparable to the disease in the boys. In practise, there is a continuum of severity with the highest incidence in the Duchenne muscular dystrophy group (birth incidence 1 in 3500 male live births). As lifespan is so much longer in the Becker muscular dystrophy group, however, the prevalence of the two conditions is roughly similar (about 24 per million population in northeast England).

Over the whole group, there is a correlation between dystrophin abundance (as measured in a muscle biopsy sample) and severity: children with completely absent dystrophin tend to be confined to a wheelchair slightly earlier than children whose biopsies contain low levels of dystrophin. Patients with Becker muscular dystrophy have much higher levels of dystrophin (Fig. 3). These dystrophin levels also correlate in most cases with the type of mutation found in the *dystrophin* gene—in Duchenne muscular dystrophy most deletions are out of frame, not supporting the production of dystrophin, while Becker muscular dystrophy patients typically have in-frame deletions, allowing the production of a reduced amount of dystrophin of a slightly smaller size.

While these correlations are useful in a general sense, they are not absolutely predictive of outcome in an individual case, and must always be taken in the context of the clinical features of the patient. They can be useful though in giving the best possible guide to prognosis, especially in those patients with Becker muscular dystrophy who present early or who are identified by neonatal screening or the incidental finding of a high serum creatine kinase level.

Box 4 Practice point: cardiac involvement in dystrophinopathy

- All patients with dystrophinopathy are at risk of developing cardiomyopathy which progresses with age. It is frequently asymptomatic, and needs to be sought through full cardiac assessment including echocardiography, as treatment with antifailure medication may improve function and prognosis.
- Cardiac transplantation has been used successfully in patients with Becker muscular dystrophy and manifesting carriers of dystrophinopathy.
- Cardiac compromise is the major determinant of operative risk in boys with Duchenne muscular dystrophy, and all should have a full cardiac assessment in advance of any surgery at any age.

Management

Duchenne muscular dystrophy—the early stages

Proper management of a child with Duchenne muscular dystrophy starts with awareness of the possibility of the diagnosis in any boy who is not walking by the age of 18 months or whose mobility is poor compared with his peers. The current mean age at diagnosis of nearly 5 years reflects a typical but unacceptable delay of at least 2 years since the onset of disease is noticed by the parents. The principal impetus to early diagnosis at present is the ability to offer parents the option of prenatal diagnosis in subsequent pregnancies. When specific treatments become available, there will also be a need to implement such treatments before the disease is too advanced.

Once the diagnosis has been considered, measurement of the serum creatine kinase will confirm the suspicion and ideally a referral into a specialist unit should be made at this stage. The specialist unit should have rapid-track access to DNA diagnostic and muscle biopsy facilities to confirm the diagnosis as quickly as possible. Duchenne muscular dystrophy is a devastating diagnosis, and should be given to the family following guidelines for the best practice for disclosure of bad news—the parents should be seen together wherever possible in complete privacy, they should have time to sit and ask questions, and have access to experienced staff for support and further information. Access to support groups and the relevant national charity is also appropriate. Supporting information should also be passed immediately to the general practitioner, health visitor, and school who may never have looked after a child with this type of condition before.

Since Duchenne muscular dystrophy is an X-linked condition, early access to genetic counselling is also vital shortly after diagnosis (see Box 5).

In the early stages of the disease it is advisable for the child to be introduced to a community physiotherapist for advice on stretching, which at this stage can usually concentrate on the ankles and hips, with the emphasis on the maintenance of symmetry. Boys frequently develop a toe-walking gait which is partially compensatory for their proximal muscle weakness—walking splints or ankle–foot orthoses are therefore not appropriate at this stage and any early Achilles tendon contractures are better managed through passive stretching and night-time below-knee splints. At the point at which walking becomes impossible independently, the child can often be rehabilitated in long leg callipers or knee–ankle–foot orthoses. Lengthening of the Achilles tendon is often necessary to allow the child to do well with knee–ankle–foot orthoses. The length of time children walk in knee–ankle–foot orthoses varies from child to child—residual muscle strength is probably the best predictor of how long a child will use them for mobility, but motivation on the part of the child's family and school is also a key factor.

Despite a consensus that use of corticosteroids does prolong ambulation for up to a couple of years, various questions about side-effects and long-term complications remain and thus corticosteroids are not universally used. Where steroids are considered, intermittent treatment probably offers the best balance between efficacy and side-effects.

Duchenne muscular dystrophy—after mobility is lost

Inevitably there comes a point in Duchenne muscular dystrophy where even the ability to stand supported in knee–ankle–foot orthoses is lost and the child is confined permanently to a wheelchair. The provision of an electric chair with indoor and outdoor access is critical to the best possible maintenance of independence. Seating in the chair should also be carefully addressed to promote an upright and symmetrical posture. Scoliosis is an almost universal complication of Duchenne muscular dystrophy and close liaison with the orthopaedic department is necessary to co-ordinate management which in the long term is likely to include spinal surgery. Physiotherapy priorities shift towards postural support, the prevention and containment of contractures, and respiratory maintenance. Measurements of forced vital capacity carried out regularly provide an indication of the trend of respiratory function—forced vital capacity usually plateaus soon after confinement to a wheelchair and thereafter falls. The timing of surgery for scoliosis therefore needs to take this variable into account, though cardiomyopathy is probably an even greater risk factor in the timing of surgery (see Box 4).

As forced vital capacity falls further, boys are at serious risk of chest infections and ultimately nocturnal respiratory failure. Symptoms of this respiratory failure may be extremely insidious and totally missed unless explicitly sought (see Box 6). Routine overnight pulse oximetry (which can readily be carried out at home provided the equipment is available) can show a trend of deteriorating overnight oxygenation and, together with the monitoring of symptoms, highlight the time at which elective nocturnal respiratory support, ideally initially at least through non-invasive means, should be provided. Such respiratory support abolishes symptoms, reduces the tendency to chest infections, and undoubtedly improves lifespan.

In the late stages of Duchenne muscular dystrophy, nutrition may be of concern. Loss of weight occurs in most boys as the disease progresses, and issues of diet and the possibility of supplemental nutrition need to be addressed.

The actual cause and timing of death in Duchenne muscular dystrophy is hard to predict. Some patients will die of a particularly severe chest infection. In others cardiomyopathy may be difficult to control or a cardiac arrhythmia may arise. Early onset of cardiomyopathy is a poor prognostic sign. Talking about death to these patients and their parents, helping them to prepare and also addressing their fears and uncertainties is another important but easily neglected aspect of management.

Education

On average, children with Duchenne muscular dystrophy have an IQ around one standard deviation below the normal mean; often a striking verbal-performance deficit is also observed. Schooling should offer the best possible environment for learning, including full attention to information technology equipment, while supporting the very real physical needs of the child. Families and areas vary as to whether this will be best provided through mainstream or special schooling. With a good education and medical support, boys with Duchenne muscular dystrophy and the appropriate intellectual potential can go on to higher education, and where possible, should be encouraged to do so.

Becker muscular dystrophy

Management issues in Becker muscular dystrophy tend to cover the same broad areas as Duchenne muscular dystrophy, but with the deterioration in muscle function over a much longer timescale. Certain complications, such as scoliosis, are very unusual. Other complications, such as cramping

Box 5 Genetic counselling in dystrophinopathy is an essential part of the management of any family where a diagnosis of dystrophinopathy has been made because the potential implications go far beyond the index case

- These are X-linked diseases.
- The new mutation rate in the dystrophin gene is high.
- Most cases of Duchenne muscular dystrophy are born now in families with no prior history of the disease.
- None the less, even in these families, other female relatives (through the maternal line) are at risk of being carriers.
- The essential piece of information is the delineation of the dystrophin mutation in the affected child (easy to find in the 60 per cent in whom the mutation is a deletion, harder and much more specialized if it is not).
- In the presence of a known mutation, female relatives can be offered testing directly to see if they are carriers or not.
- They may choose to have prenatal diagnosis on the basis of that testing.
- Even if mothers of boys with Duchenne muscular dystrophy can be shown not to be somatic carriers of the mutation in their son, they still may have a proportion of egg cells containing the mutation (a situation known as 'germline mosaicism'). They therefore remain at a 10 to 20 per cent risk of having another affected child in a future pregnancy.
- Boys with Duchenne muscular dystrophy do not often have children, but men with Becker muscular dystrophy often do (overall fitness reduced to around 2/3). All of their daughters are obligate carriers of Becker muscular dystrophy, but none of their sons are at risk.

Box 6 Respiratory failure in neuromuscular disease is a complication which needs to be specifically sought

- It may be the result of intercostal muscle or diaphragmatic weakness or a combination of the two. The presence of a scoliosis or other spinal deformity may be an additional factor.
- Nocturnal problems tend to dominate.
- Frank symptoms of morning CO_2 retention may be seen (poor colour, morning sickness, headaches, confusion) but these are late symptoms and the problem should be detected by investigation or careful history taking before this stage.
- Increasing frequency of chest infections may indicate incipient respiratory failure.
- Subtle signs include loss of appetite and weight loss, loss of energy and enthusiasm.
- Poor sleep, increasing wakefulness at night, inability to lie flat may also be seen together with a tendency to fall asleep during the day.
- Difficulties swallowing and difficulty completing sentences may also be seen.
- In many muscle diseases, the main risk of respiratory failure is when the patient is no longer able to walk independently and weakness is pronounced (for example Duchenne muscular dystrophy, Becker muscular dystrophy, congenital muscular dystrophy, facioscapulohumeral muscular dystrophy, limb girdle muscular dystrophy, etc.).
- In other muscle diseases, respiratory failure may be an earlier feature and present while the patient is still ambulant (for example multicore and other congenital myopathies, some forms of congenital muscular dystrophy).

muscle pains after exercise, which can be a particular problem in the teenage years, are more common. Despite the fact that Becker muscular dystrophy is much milder than Duchenne muscular dystrophy it can represent a considerable and insurmountable disability for the person who has it, and problems with adjustment, poor self-esteem, and poor body image are all fairly common in this group. No hard data exist to define completely any intellectual problems in Becker muscular dystrophy, but on average it is likely that this group has a general reduction in IQ, though probably not to the extent seen in Duchenne muscular dystrophy. Cardiac complications may occur at any age in Becker muscular dystrophy (see Box 4): respiratory complications tend to be a feature of the late stages of the disease.

Facioscapulohumeral muscular dystrophy

Facioscapulohumeral muscular dystrophy is an example of a muscular dystrophy named for the most characteristic pattern of muscle involvement observed (that of involvement of the facial, scapular, and humeral muscles predominantly). However, other muscle groups usually become involved with time and may even be involved at onset.

Presentation

- Age at presentation is variable. Most affected individuals manifest some symptoms by their teens or twenties. Occasionally symptoms may be very minor, even late in adult life.
- Symptoms may, unusually for a muscular dystrophy, be very markedly asymmetrical.
- Early symptoms typically include facial weakness (inability to bury eyelashes or puff cheeks; this often goes unnoticed), shoulder girdle weakness manifesting as problems in reaching high shelves, changing lightbulbs, or climbing ropes, and foot drop.

An infantile form of facioscapulohumeral muscular dystrophy is recognized with early childhood onset, extremely marked facial weakness and progressive weakness of both the shoulder and pelvic girdle musculature. Lumbar lordosis may be profound. Hearing loss and retinal telangiectasia may be seen in any patient with facioscapulohumeral muscular dystrophy but are particularly associated with this most severe form of the disease.

Differential diagnosis

The clinical pattern of facioscapulohumeral muscular dystrophy can be very distinctive, and the asymmetry of muscle involvement is a major clue. However, facial weakness may be very variable, and if it is absent or subtle, confusion can arise with forms of limb girdle muscular dystrophy.

Diagnostic investigations

Serum creatine kinase may be normal or mildly elevated. Muscle biopsy and electromyography (EMG) provide supportive evidence for a muscular dystrophy; some inflammatory features are sometimes also seen in the biopsy. Most cases (if not all) of facioscapulohumeral muscular dystrophy are linked to chromosome 4q35. Although the nature of the gene responsible for facioscapulohumeral muscular dystrophy is not yet known, a DNA-based test is available which can confirm the diagnosis in 95 per cent of cases. This test involves the demonstration of a DNA deletion which is consistently associated with the disease. It is likely that this deletion alters the expression of an unknown gene close to the telomere of chromosome 4q (position effect variegation).

Prognosis and management

Infantile facioscapulohumeral muscular dystrophy is a progressive disease which leads to early confinement to a wheelchair and the development of such complications as scoliosis and respiratory failure. This condition is most frequently seen as a result of a new dominant mutation in cases with no family history, and these children often have particularly large DNA deletions on chromosome 4. The development of a lumbar lordosis, seen also in later onset facioscapulohumeral muscular dystrophy, together with secondary hip flexion contractures, can be very disabling. Bracing may be partially successful at controlling the lordosis, but at the expense of some loss of mobility.

More typically, facioscapulohumeral muscular dystrophy is a slowly progressive disease. As the disease progresses it can involve the proximal as well as the distal lower limb muscles. Around 20 per cent of patients with facioscapulohumeral muscular dystrophy will become unable to walk independently, most over the age of 40. Involvement of the proximal lower limbs before the age of 20 years is a poor prognostic sign, indicating an increased likelihood of needing to use a wheelchair. Some patients describe progression as being stepwise in nature, with periods of faster deterioration alternating with phases of plateauing of their symptoms. Footdrop is a common complaint, which can be helped by the provision of daytime ankle–foot orthoses. A significant proportion of patients with facioscapulohumeral muscular dystrophy complain of painful muscles, for which no cause can be found, and for which pain relief may be difficult. Some patients find swimming or a small dose of antidepressants useful for this symptom. More severely affected patients with facioscapulohumeral muscular dystrophy may develop respiratory failure or swallowing problems and these complications should be sought. Cardiomyopathy is rarely reported.

Genetic counselling

Facioscapulohumeral muscular dystrophy is an autosomal dominant disease and as such an affected person has a 50 per cent chance of transmission to his or her offspring, regardless of sex. Use of the new DNA diagnostic techniques have shown that up to 30 per cent of cases of facioscapulohumeral muscular dystrophy may represent new dominant mutations. Germline mosaicism is also common. Genetic analysis has also shown a higher proportion of asymptomatic gene carriers than expected, with females overrepresented in this group. The availability of a relatively straightforward genetic test in this disorder has opened up the possibility of presymptomatic and prenatal testing, which were previously impossible. However, despite an overall correlation between the size of the deletion found and the severity of the symptoms, the DNA test is not useful in predicting the severity of the disease—people in individual families with apparently the same sized deletion may have a very variable experience of the disease (see Fig. 4).

Emery Dreifuss muscular dystrophy

Emery Dreifuss muscular dystrophy has a highly characteristic phenotype. X-linked recessive, autosomal dominant, and autosomal recessive forms are recognized, and the genes involved in these conditions both encode proteins which are components of the nuclear envelope (see Fig. 5). The gene involved in X-linked Emery Dreifuss muscular dystrophy is *emerin*, and the gene involved in autosomal dominant and autosomal recessive Emery Dreifuss muscular dystrophy is *lamin A/C*.

Presentation

- Patients may present at any age, most typically in the early teens, though symptoms may be present much earlier than that.
- Contractures of the ankles and elbows and rigidity of the spine often predate any clear weakness.
- Consequently, these patients have frequently had Achilles tendon release before the diagnosis is suspected.
- Weakness and wasting are typically humeroperoneal in distribution.

A key part of these conditions, which may rarely be present at presentation, is cardiac involvement, most typically arrhythmias (see below). An alternative phenotype (limb girdle muscular dystrophy 1B, see Box 7 and Fig. 5) exists in combination with mutations in the same gene as autosomal dominant Emery Dreifuss muscular dystrophy (*lamin A/C*). These patients may present with purely cardiac disease, or with a more proximal 'limb girdle muscular dystrophy' presentation, without prominent contractures. *Lamin A/C* mutations are also described in patients with partial lipodystrophy without prominent muscle weakness.

Confirming the diagnosis

Serum creatine kinase is typically mildly elevated in Emery Dreifuss muscular dystrophy. Muscle biopsy shows non-specific histological features: in X-linked Emery Dreifuss muscular dystrophy, emerin is absent in muscle and skin. Detection of mutation in the *emerin* gene is necessary to offer genetic counselling to female relatives at risk of being carriers.

The involvement of *lamin A/C* (the gene responsible for autosomal dominant Emery Dreifuss muscular dystrophy) cannot be determined by antibody analysis in muscle, but requires the demonstration of a *lamin A/C* mutation. A secondary deficiency of laminin β-1 may be seen in muscle from some patients with autosomal dominant Emery Dreifuss muscular dystrophy, but is not specific to this condition. Many *lamin A/C* mutations arise *de novo*, and germline mosaicism is common.

Differential diagnosis

Other muscular dystrophies may present with contractures as an important component (Fig. 5). Some forms of congenital muscular dystrophy may be associated with contractures and a rigid spine. Bethlem myopathy may present congenitally (often with torticollis) or in early childhood: here finger flexion contractures, elicited especially on wrist extension, are more prominent and cardiac involvement is not associated. Bethlem myopathy is itself genetically heterogeneous, involving mutations in any of the genes for collagen 6A1, 6A2, and 6A3. Like autosomal dominant Emery Dreifuss muscular dystrophy, some cases of Bethlem myopathy show a secondary reduction in laminin β-1 staining in muscle biopsy: the significance of this is uncertain.

In some cases, calpainopathy (limb girdle muscular dystrophy 2A) may be associated with contractures of the ankles, elbows, fingers, and paraspinal muscles. However, the associated weakness here is predominantly proximal and of a characteristic distribution (see below). These patients have typically a higher creatine kinase, absent calpain 3 on biopsy and *CAPN3* mutations.

Prognosis and management

The prognosis in Emery Dreifuss muscular dystrophy relates almost directly to the ability to manage the life-threatening arrhythmias to which every patient with either the X-linked or dominant form is susceptible. Severe arrhythmias are inevitable by the third decade. All patients with this diagnosis should therefore be under regular cardiological review, and cardiac pacing once a rhythm disturbance is detected may be life-saving. However, in autosomal dominant Emery Dreifuss muscular dystrophy the risk of cardiomyopathy remains and may be less amenable to routine treatment.

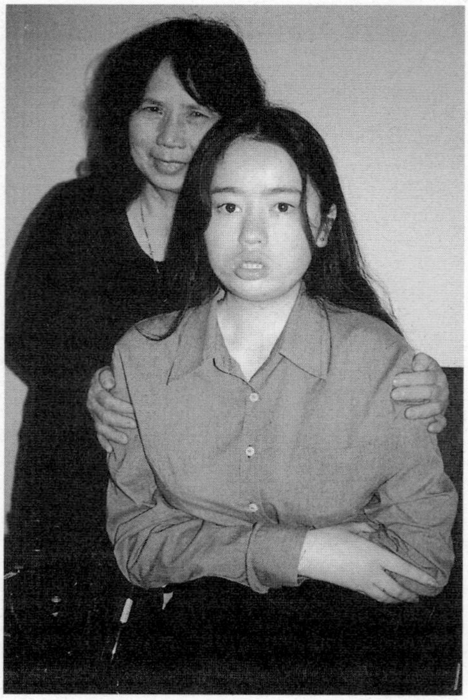

Fig. 4 Mother and daughter with facioscapulohumeral muscular dystrophy. The mother is extremely mildly affected and has minimal symptoms. By contrast the daughter was affected from early childhood and has been wheelchair dependent outside from her early teens. Note the daughter's expressionless face and her posture—she is leaning forwards due to a combination of her marked lumbar lordosis, a major feature of the condition, and hip flexion contractures.

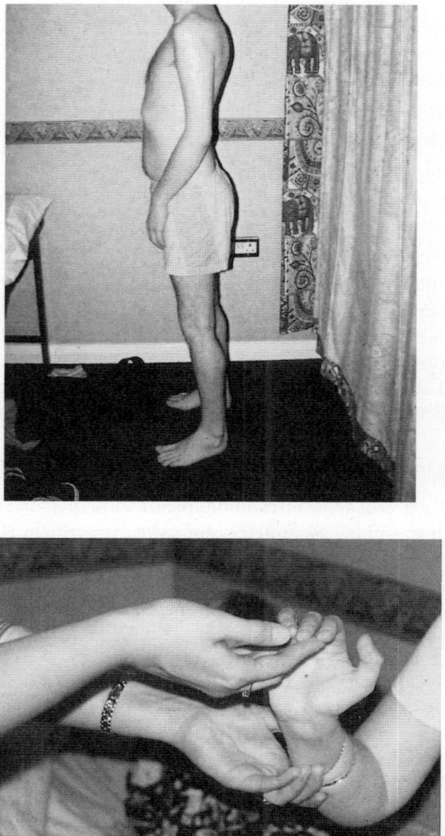

(a)

(b)

Fig. 5 Muscular dystrophy phenotypes characterized by prominent contractures. (a) This patient has autosomal dominant Emery Dreifuss muscular dystrophy, with a proven mutation in his *lamin A/C* gene. The elbow and Achilles tendon contractures seen here, combined with his markedly rigid spine, are very similar to the pattern of contractures and weakness seen in the X-linked form of the disease. (b) Bethlem myopathy in a woman with marked contractures of the elbows, ankles, and spine. In addition she has finger flexion contractures, demonstrated here by attempting to straighten the fingers with the wrist extended.

Box 7 Autosomal dominant Emery Dreifuss muscular dystrophy and limb girdle muscular dystrophy 1B—the 'laminopathies'

- These disorders are caused by mutations in the lamin A/C gene. Lamin A/C, like emerin, is a component of the nuclear envelope.
- The phenotype is variable, depending on the presence or not of contractures as a major component of the phenotype.
- Where contractures are present, these typically involve the elbows, Achilles tendons, and spine. In these patients, there is often a humeroperoneal pattern of muscle weakness as in X-linked Emery Dreifuss muscular dystrophy.
- Where contractures are less of a feature, patients typically present with proximal muscle weakness.
- In both groups, cardiac involvement is the most important complication. Arrythmias may lead to sudden death and should be sought and treated appropriately.
- A phenotype with exclusively cardiac involvement has also been described.
- New mutations and germline mosaicism is common in this group.

Management of the contractures in Emery Dreifuss muscular dystrophy is the other main issue, and will involve close liaison with a physiotherapist. Operative treatment of contractures, especially at the Achilles tendons, is commonly performed, but while such surgery does work in the short term, contractures often recur. With increasing age, however, contractures often stabilize. Muscle weakness may worsen but progression is usually very slow.

The limb girdle muscular dystrophies

The broad definition of limb girdle muscular dystrophy comes from the classification of Walton and Nattrass in 1954 when the term was suggested to describe those patients with weakness of the proximal musculature who did not fulfil the criteria for the X-linked muscular dystrophies or for facioscapuluhumeral muscular dystrophy. The term has always encompassed a heterogeneous group of disorders: now that many of them can be distinguished at the gene or protein level it is no longer sufficient to use it without qualification as to the specific type of disease (see Tables 2 and 3). The type of limb girdle muscular dystrophy may be suggested by the precise pattern of muscle involvement, with confirmation from a combination of genetic and protein analysis. The ability to provide a precise diagnosis in limb girdle muscular dystrophy has greatly improved the prognostic and genetic information which can be given to these patients.

The approach to diagnosis in limb girdle muscular dystrophy

Could it be dominant disease?

Autosomal dominant limb girdle muscular dystrophy represents only around 10 per cent of the total limb girdle muscular dystrophy population, and limb girdle muscular dystrophies 1A, 1C, 1D, and 1E have been very rarely reported (see Table 2). In families with a dominant history the most likely diagnoses are facioscapulohumeral muscular dystrophy (exclude facioscapulohumeral muscular dystrophy on DNA analysis especially if there is any suspicion of facial weakness), limb girdle muscular dystrophy 1B (allelic with autosomal dominant Emery Dreifuss muscular dystrophy—see Box 7), and Bethlem myopathy. New mutations are common, however, so that if the clinical features are suggestive of one of these disorders, then the diagnosis should be pursued even in the absence of a family history. Features which should raise the suspicion of dominant disease are less marked elevation of creatine kinase (typically normal to fives times normal in dominant disease and much higher than this in active recessive disease) or the presence of early and prominent contractures.

What is the age and nature of the presentation?

Variability in the age of presentation and of rate of progression is usual in the various autosomal recessive types of limb girdle muscular dystrophy. However, some broad conclusions can be helpful (Fig. 6). Childhood presentation is most common in sarcoglycanopathy, which may superficially resemble dystrophinopathy, with frequent calf (and other muscle) hypertrophy. Adult onset cases are less frequent and are essentially 'Becker like' in presentation. However, whatever the age at presentation, in sarcoglycanopathy, quadriceps is almost always stronger than the hamstrings. This is the reverse of the pattern seen in dystrophin deficiency. Calpainopathy may

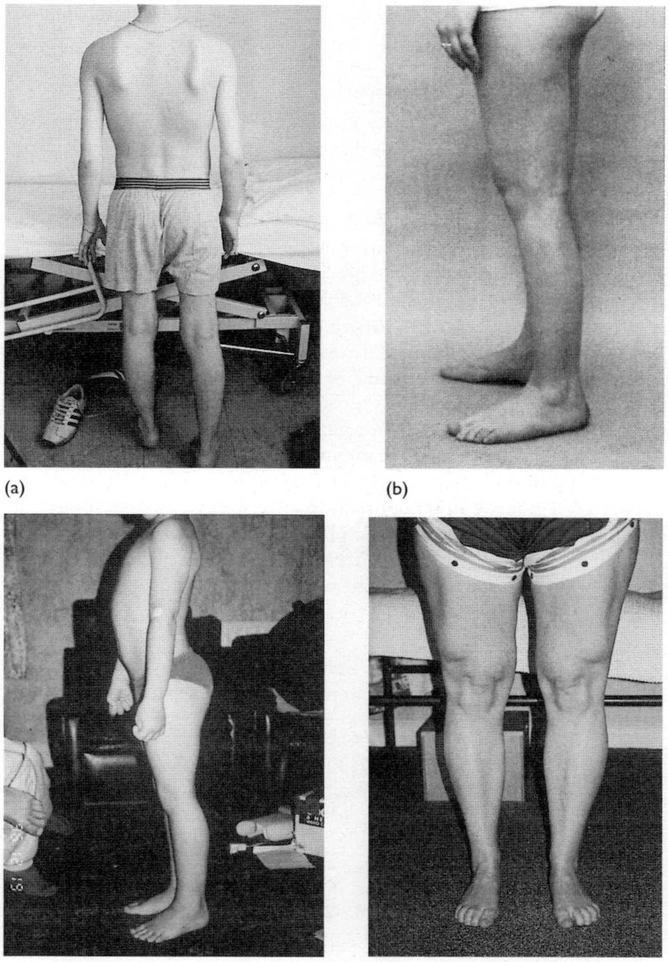

(a) (b) (c) (d)

Fig. 6 Typical clinical pictures of patients with different types of autosomal recessive limb girdle muscular dystrophy. (a) Calpainopathy or limb girdle muscular dystrophy 2A; note the predominantly atrophic pattern of muscle involvement and Achilles tendon contractures. The stance is often wide-based due to the imbalance of the hip abductors and adductors. (b) Dysferlin deficiency or limb girdle muscular dystrophy 2B. Note the wasting of the posterior calf muscles and flat-footed stance. (c) Child with γ sarcoglycanopathy or limb girdle muscular dystrophy 2C. Note the lordotic posture and scapular winging, both of which may be more marked at presentation in sarcoglycanopathy than in dystrophin deficiency. (d) Adult with γ sarcoglycanopathy, to illustrate the variability in severity of sarcoglycan deficiencies and the muscular hypertrophy which may be as marked or more marked than in dystrophin deficiency.

present with early childhood symptoms, especially contractures of the Achilles tendons, but onset is most commonly between 8 and 15 years of age. Dysferlinopathy typically presents in the late teens or early twenties, and early features may include proximal weakness or distal involvement (usually manifesting as difficulty standing on tiptoe).

Which investigations should be performed?

Serum creatine kinase is greatly elevated in all forms of autosomal recessive limb girdle muscular dystrophy, but may be only marginally elevated or within the normal range in autosomal dominant limb girdle muscular dystrophy. EMG confirms a primary myopathic process and standard analysis of the muscle biopsy shows dystrophic changes (which especially in dysferlinopathy can be accompanied by evidence of inflammation). Specialized investigations are always necessary to attempt to determine the type of limb girdle muscular dystrophy, and require a muscle biopsy as the starting point for immunologically based diagnosis (see Fig. 7), taken in conjunction with the clinical features.

Scheme for specialized investigations

Do the clinical features or family history suggest a specific disorder (see Boxes 8, 9, and 10)? If so look for that first.

The sarcoglycanopathies

Dystrophin staining may be mildly abnormal in these patients reflecting the close and interdependent relationship between the proteins of the dystrophin associated complex; but the predominant abnormality on immunolabelling or immunoblotting will be the absence or reduction of one or more of the sarcoglycans. The pattern of reduction of these proteins may give a clue as to the primary gene involvement. In γ sarcoglycanopathy, there may be preservation of some or all of the other sarcoglycans, with specific loss of γ sarcoglycan. α Sarcoglycanopathy may similarly present with a selective reduction, or with more widespread loss or reduction in labelling for all members of the complex. In δ and β sarcoglycanopathy there is typically loss of the whole sarcoglycan complex. Determining the primary protein involved is important to direct genetic analysis. Detection of the mutation is necessary to offer prenatal diagnosis and specific genetic counselling, but as there are few recurrent mutations in the *sarcoglycan* genes the search for mutations can be very time-consuming: hence the need to obtain the best possible information from immunolabelling before embarking on detection of mutations.

Calpainopathy

Here the sarcoglycans are normal, as is dystrophin. Currently available antibodies to calpain 3 do not work on tissue sections but need to be used on immunoblotting. Detection of reduced or absent calpain on immunoblotting (Fig. 7) indicates the need to search for *calpain 3* mutations, which are highly variable, generally non-recurrent, and which may involve any part of the large (24 exons) gene. However, a secondary reduction in calpain 3 may also be seen in some cases of dysferlin deficiency. Hence the need to use all antibodies in combination to ensure that the primary problem can be identified correctly and the appropriate gene searched for mutations.

Dysferlinopathy

Here all other proteins with the possible exception of calpain 3 are within the normal range and deficiency of dysferlin can be demonstrated on tissue sections or immunoblotting. Decreased or absent dysferlin in muscle is an indication to proceed to mutation detection. The *dysferlin* gene is very large

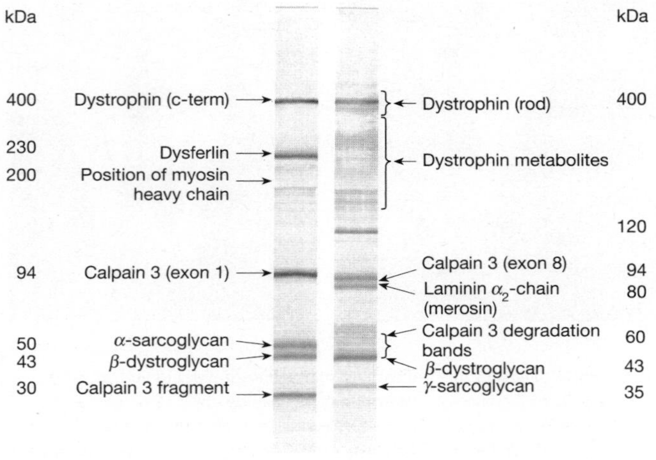

Fig. 7 Multiplex Western blotting as an approach to diagnosis in limb girdle muscular dystrophy. Two strips of a Western blot of control human skeletal muscle protein extracts immunostained with a mixture of antibodies to the proteins indicated. Absence or reduced intensity of a particular species compared with the other proteins labelled in the same lane can indicate which gene and protein is implicated in that patient's disease. (By courtesy of Dr L. V. B. Anderson, University of Newcastle upon Tyne.)

Box 8 Clinical features of sarcoglycanopathies

- Most frequently present in childhood, but may present at any age. Intrafamilial variability is common.
- These conditions are most closely related clinically to dystrophinopathy which will be the major differential diagnosis and have a similar spectrum of severity.
- Typically motor milestones are less delayed than in dystrophinopathy.
- Muscle hypertrophy is common.
- Intelligence is not affected.
- Cardiomyopathy is an important complication, though not universal, and should be sought through careful surveillance.
- Respiratory failure is an important late complication.
- Scoliosis is seen in the most severely affected individuals.
- Prognosis overall is typically better than dystrophinopathy presenting at a similar age.

Box 9 Clinical features of calpainopathy

- This is the most common form of limb girdle muscular dystrophy in most populations.
- May present at any age but typically 8 to 15 years.
- Highly selective muscle involvement: posterior thigh weakness, and wasting; scapular winging common at onset.
- Muscle hypertrophy rare—tends to be predominantly atrophic pattern.
- Preservation of hip abductor muscles even at late stages contributes to characteristic wide-based stance.
- Most have Achilles tendon contractures: a subgroup presents with much more prominent contractures in an Emery Dreifuss muscular dystrophy-like pattern.
- Progression is variable but never as fast as Duchenne muscular dystrophy.
- Cardiac involvement is not common but respiratory impairment may be seen in late stages.
- Prognosis in all but the most severe and early onset cases is good.

Box 10 Dysferlinopathy: clinical features

- Presentation most commonly in late teens or early twenties.
- Patients often report good muscle prowess before onset of disease. Serum creatine kinase may not be massively elevated in presymptomatic cases.
- Occasional patients present with unilateral calf swelling which may be tender and lead to the clinical diagnosis of myositis.
- Primary muscle involvement is always in the lower limbs, with absence of upper girdle involvement at onset.
- Lower limb involvement may be of proximal muscles or distal muscles. The distal muscles involved first are typically posterior (leading to difficulty standing on tiptoe as an early feature) but may be anterior.
- Progression is typically slow and life expectancy is not reduced. This is the usually mildest type of limg girdle muscular dystrophy.
- Cardiomyopathy is not reported and respiratory involvement is usually mild and at a very late stage only.
- This phenotype is genetically heterogeneous, with another locus for Miyoshi myopathy on chromosome 10.
- The main differential diagnosis, especially in patients presenting with distal weakness, may be an alternative form of distal myopathy. Typically here the creatine kinase is not so high.

(55 exons), and as with the other forms of limb girdle muscular dystrophy, mutations are highly variable.

Laminopathy

Some (but by no means all) patients with *lamin A/C* mutations have a secondary reduction of the muscle protein laminin β-1 on immunolabelling of tissue sections. The confirmation of the diagnosis is by demonstration of a *lamin A/C* mutation.

Other forms of limb girdle muscular dystrophy

Limb girdle muscular dystrophy 2G and 2H appear relatively restricted in their geographical distribution. Limb girdle muscular dystrophy 2I is seen worldwide and is due to mutations in *FKRP*. This type of locus can be associated with cardiomyopathy.

Management

Once the diagnosis is secure, management should include monitoring and treatment for the specific complications of the various subtypes. If a clear diagnosis is not possible (for example where appropriate samples are not available or where the diagnosis cannot be reached even after exhaustive investigation) the management should as a minimum include physiotherapy and regular cardiac and respiratory surveillance.

Oculopharyngeal muscular dystrophy

Oculopharyngeal muscular dystrophy is unusual in that it has an exceptionally late presentation.

Presentation

- Presentation is typically in the sixth decade.
- It commonly presents with ptosis, dysphagia to solids, and dysphonia which may be as severe as in myotonic dystrophy.
- Other features include ophthalmoparesis, facial weakness, and proximal muscle weakness.

Diagnosis

The muscle biopsy in oculopharyngeal muscular dystrophy typically shows the presence of rimmed vacuoles and intranuclear inclusions. DNA analysis confirms the presence of an expanded guanine–cytosine–guanine repeat in the *poly(A) binding protein 2* gene.

Prognosis and management

Ptosis can be managed surgically, but frequently recurs. Dysphagia may respond, at least partially, to surgical intervention with myotomy of the cricopharyngeal muscle and other annular muscle fibres. Potentially life-threatening complications may include aspiration pneumonia and regurgitation. Progression of the limb muscle weakness is highly variable.

Genetic counselling

Oculopharyngeal muscular dystrophy is an autosomal dominant disorder. Genetic analysis offers the potential for presymptomatic testing if this is specifically sought.

Prospects for specific treatment in muscular dystrophy

Drug treatments have a limited place in the treatment of muscular dystrophy at present. Despite many small-scale studies reporting the beneficial use of steroids in prolonging ambulation in Duchenne muscular dystrophy and possibly the sarcoglycanopathies as well, these treatments are not universally applied due to reservations about side-effects and the true cost–benefit equation for this intervention. Steroids do not appear to be beneficial in facioscapulohumeral muscular dystrophy: β agonists are currently under trial in this condition after some fairly positive findings in a pilot study.

Treatments to modify the underlying disease are not yet available for clinical application. Gene transfer experiments in animal models have proved the general feasibility of this approach to these genetic diseases, at least on a small scale. Modification of mutations, either by drugs or other means, is an area of research, as is the concept of upregulating the production of ancillary proteins.

Supportive treatment for patients and their families remains the mainstay of treatment at present, and this is likely to be the case for the current generation of patients at least. This treatment is ideally provided through a specialized multidisciplinary team, bringing together with the 'myologist' the skills of medical and associated colleagues from physiotherapy, occupational therapy, genetics, cardiology, respiratory medicine, and orthopaedics.

Further reading

Bushby K, Anderson LVB, eds (2000). *Molecular methods in medicine: the muscular dystrophies.* Humana Press, New York. [A practical guide to DNA and protein based diagnosis in many types of muscular dystrophy.]

Emery AEH, ed (1998). *Neuromuscular disorders: clinical and molecular genetics.* Wiley, Chichester. [A 'state of the art' review of the level of knowledge about a variety of neuromuscular disorders in 1998.]

Emery AEH, ed. (2001). *The muscular dystrophies.* Oxford University Press. [Authoritative reviews of the different types of muscular dystrophy.]

Karpati G, Hilton-Jones D, Griggs RC, eds (2001). *Disorders of voluntary muscle*, 7th edn. Cambridge University Press, Cambridge, UK. [The book contains sections on basic physiology and anatomy of muscle as well as approaches to clinical diagnosis and management.]

With the rate of change in the last few years in the information we have available about genetically determined diseases, the most up to date reviews of the subject may be found on the Internet rather than in traditional textbooks. Online Mendelian Inheritance in Man (http://www3.ncbi.nlm.nih.gov) provides a good starting point for up to date information on a range of subjects. The Leiden muscular dystrophy database (http://www.dmd.nl) offers specific information on the muscular dystrophies.

Table 2 Dominant types of limb-girdle muscular dystrophy and related disorders

	Type of muscular dystrophy (gene symbol)					
	LGMD 1A	**LGMD 1B**	**ADEDMD**	**LGMD 1C (*CAV3*)**	**LGMD 1D (*FDC-CDM*)**	**LGMD 1E**
Distribution	Single large USA family	Described in Dutch families	French, British, other families	Two reports	One large family (> 25 affected)	Two families
Status of diagnosis	Linkage to 5q gene mutations *myotilin* gene mutations	Overlapping candidate region to ADEDMD (*lamin A/C*)	Mutations identified in *lamin A/C* gene	Mutations reported in caveolin 3 gene (*CAV3*) on 3p25. Mutations hetero-zygous in three families, homozygous in one	3cM locus on 6q22	Linkage to 9cM region on 7q
Age at onset	Adult	4–38 years	Childhood, adult	?Childhood	Males, late 2nd decade. Females about 10 years later	Young adults
Mode of presentation	Usually upper LG: may be more distally or in LL. Distal LG rarely involved	Proximal LL musculature.May be painful muscles, mild elbow contractures. UL muscles less involved. CT data show selective muscle involvement: rectus femoris and gracilis spared	Criteria for ADEDMD include early contractures AT, elbows and spine, humero-peroneal muscle weakness. Presentation may be with cardiac symptoms alone	Proximal muscle weakness, calf hypertrophy	Proximal muscle weakness. Dilated cardiomyopathy and conduction disturbance also common	Skeletal muscle and/or cardiac disease
Early development	Normal	Normal	May present with early contractures	N/K	N/K	Late
Rate of progression	Slow, none WCB	Progression of skeletal muscle weakness usually slow	Variable	N/K	N/K	Slow M > F, rarely WCB
Hypertrophy	None	No	May see hypertrophy of EDL muscle in foot	Calf hypertrophy reported in two pedigrees	Calf hypertrophy can be seen	No
Contractures	May be AT contractures	May be mild elbow contractures. Rigid spine not seen	Contractures very prominent in ADEDMD presentation	N/K	N/K	No
Cardiac status	Normal	AV conduction disturbance, age related: 100% penetrant by age 45. Infrequent dilated cardio-myopathy	AV conduction defect, may be dominant or only feature in some family members	N/K	AV conduction disturbance	Normal
Other features	Nasal quality to voice in 50%. Anticipation has been reported	Mild facial weakness in a minority	N/K	N/K	Males more severely affected for both cardiac and skeletal muscle disease	Some patients had dysphagia
Creatine kinase	Not more than 3–4 × ULN	N to 6× normal	N/K	N/K	Normal to 4× N	1.5 to 3× normal
Biopsy	N/K	Non-specific	N/K	N/K	Dystrophin	Myopathic or dystrophic

Abbreviations: LGMD, limb girdle muscular dystrophy; LG, limb girdle; ADEDMD, autosomal dominant Emery Dreifuss muscular dystrophy; AT, Achilles tendons; WCB, wheelchair bound; N/K, not known; ULN, upper limit of known; N, normal; LL, lower limbs; UL, upper limbs; AV, atrioventricular; EDL,

Table 3 Recessive types of limb-girdle muscular dystrophy

	Type of muscular dystrophy (gene symbol)					
	Calpainopathy (LGMD 2A) (*CAPN3*)	**Dysferlinopathy (LGMD 2B/MM) (*DYSF*)**	**Sarcoglycanopathies (LGMD 2C–2F) (*SGCA, SGCB, SGCC, SGCD*)**	**LGMD 2G**	**LGMD 2H**	**LGMD 2I**
Distribution	Worldwide, some isolates (e.g. Reunion, Amish, Basque)	Worldwide. Founder effect in Libyan Jewish population. ?Others	Worldwide. Regional differences in different types	Brazil	Manitoba Hutterites	Worldwide
Status of diagnosis	Protein, mutations	Protein, mutations	Protein, mutations (may not be readily found in all patients)	Protein, mutations	Linkage to 9q31–33	Mutations in *FKRP*
Protein	Calpain 3 deficiency detectable by monoclonal antibody on blots	Dysferlin deficiency detectable on sections and blots	• Dystrophin may be mildly abnormal • γ and α: may see selective reduction • β and δ: mostly see depletion of all	Telethonin deficiency on sections and blots	Not yet	Secondary reduction in laminin A2 or laminin β1 in some muscle biopsies
Mutations	Widely distributed, few recurrent. All types of mutation seen, large deletions rare. Changes may be non-pathogenic. Except in homozygotes, difficult to correlate mutation type with rate of progression	Widely distributed, few so far recurrent	• α R77C seen in 42% of chromosomes • γ two predominant mutations, N. African and gypsy. Otherwise mutations very heterogeneous • Missense mutations mainly in extracellular domain	Few yet described	Not yet	Common mutation (C826A) responsible for many cases
Age at onset	Typically 8–15, may be from early childhood or adulthood	Most present around 20 (± 5 years). Onset not in first decade	α most variable—may be from childhood to adulthood. γ, β, δ tend to be more severe. Majority of all types will present in first decade	Childhood	8–27 years, usually mid 20s	Congenital form may be very severe: ranges to very mild disease in LGMD group
Mode of presentation and selective muscle involvement	Highly selective pattern of muscle involvement wasting post. compartment of thighs, scapular winging. Sparing of hip abductors. Relative involvement of muscle groups important	Variable. May be: • lower limbs first • proximal alone, mixed proximal/distal alone • distal presentation most commonly posterior, may be anterior	Weakness, toe walking, muscle pains/cramps are typical presentations. Main muscles—shoulder girdle involvement more prominent than DMD, scapular involvement, hamstrings more than quadriceps, lordosis, foot drop in some before loss of mobility	May be distal involvement at presentation with foot drop. Other patients with proximal disease	Proximal involvement, may present with back pain, fatigue, waddling gait	Proximal muscle weakness
Early development	Motor milestones normal; physical prowess in childhood may be less good than peers	Normal—good athletic prowess	Motor milestones less delayed than DMD, even if later very severe	N/K	Unremarkable	Normal in LGMD cases

Table 3 Continued

	Type of muscular dystrophy (gene symbol)					
	Calpainopathy (LGMD 2A) (*CAPN3*)	**Dysferlinopathy (LGMD 2B/MM) (*DYSF*)**	**Sarcoglycanopathies (LGMD 2C–2F) (*SGCA, SGCB, SGCC, SGCD*)**	**LGMD 2G**	**LGMD 2H**	**LGMD 2I**
Rate of progression	May not be linear—can see rapid change with no gender effect. Otherwise gradual with time. Age at death probably typically in 60s	Usually slow—some more rapidly progressive Cases have similar age at onset	Variability main feature: • poor correlation between age at onset/ progression • rate of progression very variable • may be great intrafamilial variation, even with sibs	Noticeable late teens/early twenties	Slow	Variable, usually mild
Age of confinement to wheelchair	20–30+	Typically beyond 30s. Seems to be normal lifespan	Earliest 9 years. Variability in mild cases very marked. Occasional asymptomatic cases in adult life (esp. α). Typically even most severe cases live to 30s	4 WCB 31–39	3 WCB in 40s	In mild cases 40+
Atrophy	Posterior compartment of thighs, latissimus dorsi	Typically distal LL, biceps—may be very selective. Atrophy of proximal deltoid, hypertrophy of distal	Anterior and posterior thighs, shoulder girdle	Widespread	Proximal wasting in some	Proximal
Hypertrophy	Occasionally see calf hypertrophy	Very rare—a few cases have transient calf hypertrophy at presentation which may be painful	Common in calves, also elsewhere. May be macroglossia	Additional potentially linked family had calf hypertrophy	Not obvious	Common in calf muscles
Contractures	AT contractures common. Occasionally more widespread	No	AT contractures, lordosis, hip flexion contractures (may be problem in rehab.). Scoliosis less common than DMD even when WCB	No	No	Not common in LGMD forms
Facial involvement	Mild facial weakness unusual. Also macroglossia very occasionally seen	No facial weakness	No facial weakness, may see macroglossia. In later stages typical transverse smile	N/K	Facial weakness (previously described in this group) not seen	Mild facial weakness common
Cardiac status	Normal	Normal	α usually not present (one Dutch patient). β, γ, δ may be important	Normal	Normal	Cardiomyopathy significant complication
Respiratory status	Respiratory impairment may be significant in some	Normal	Common, may be at later stage than DMD	N/K	Normal	Some cases require nocturnal ventilation
Intellectual function	Normal	Normal	Normal	N/K	Normal	Normal
Creatine kinase	10–100× normal	May be low or mildly raised in young presymptomatic cases, rising to huge elevation by early teens. Very high in active phase of disease, falling with age	10–100× normal	At least 7.5× normal	250–4280 (lowest in advanced disease)	10–100 × normal
Biopsy	Dystrophic	Dystrophic plus inflammation, may be perivascular or more widespread	Dystrophic	Rimmed vacuoles in some biopsies	Dystrophic changes	Dystrophic

Table 3 Continued

	Type of muscular dystrophy (gene symbol)					
	Calpainopathy (LGMD 2A) (*CAPN3*)	Dysferlinopathy (LGMD 2B/MM) (*DYSF*)	Sarcoglycanopathies (LGMD 2C–2F) (*SGCA, SGCB, SGCC, SGCD*)	LGMD 2G	LGMD 2H	LGMD 2I
Other	Muscle imaging confirms highly selective pattern of muscle involvement	Muscle imaging may reveal asymptomatic proximal changes in distal onset and vice versa. Phenotypes may vary with same mutation and between sibs	Genotype–phenotype correlations: α-null tend to be more severe; β truncating very severe, huge variation with missense. Majority in γ are truncating mutations. δ mutations so far are rare	N/K	N/K	Allelic with a form of congenital muscular dystrophy
Note	Finnish anterior tibial MD homozygotes may show reduction of calpain on blots	May have been misdiagnosed as polymyositis or distal myopathy	Main differential diagnosis is with dystrophinopathy. Occasional cases may resemble calpainopathy. No clinical guidelines to distinguish subgroups, though very mild disease most likely to be α	N/K	N/K	N/K

Abbreviations: LGMD, limb girdle muscular dystrophy; DMD, Duchenne muscular dystrophy; WCB, wheelchair bound; N/K, not known; LL, lower limbs; AT, Achilles tendon.

24.22.3 Myotonia

David Hilton-Jones

Introduction

The term myotonia, and related terms such as paramyotonia and neuromyotonia, cause much confusion. Various diseases accompanied by myotonia have different molecular origins and many associated symptoms and signs. Myotonia can be considered as a symptom, as a physical sign, or as a neurophysiological phenomenon, but understanding is perhaps best served by discussing these in reverse order.

The basic neurophysiological finding is of repetitive muscle-fibre action potentials following a stimulus, which may be voluntary contraction or muscle percussion. The repetitive electrical activity causes muscle contraction, and thus myotonia is characterized by delayed muscle-fibre relaxation following such a stimulus. Electromyography demonstrates the repetitive firing. Characteristically, the discharge gradually declines in amplitude and frequency, producing the so-called 'dive-bomber' sound in the monitoring loudspeaker.

As a physical sign, myotonia is demonstrated either as delayed muscle relaxation following voluntary contraction (for example grip myotonia, Fig. 1), or as persistent muscle dimpling following percussion (percussion myotonia, Fig. 2).

As a symptom, complaints relating to myotonia differ between patients with myotonic dystrophy, which is by far the most common cause of myotonia, and those with myotonia congenita. In myotonic dystrophy, even when grip myotonia is readily evident on examination, the patient may offer no symptoms. They are more likely to complain of hand weakness than of myotonia. When the myotonia is symptomatic, the patient complains of difficulty releasing objects after a tight grip. This is sometimes striking. One patient first noted grip myotonia in early adult life, when he was appointed as a teacher at a school—as his future headmaster shook his hand to congratulate him, he was embarrassingly unable to release his grip. In myotonic dystrophy, bulbar symptoms relating to myotonia are quite common—patients complain of their tongue or jaw 'locking' when speaking or swallowing and tongue myotonia on percussion may be demonstrated.

By contrast, in myotonia congenita weakness is absent and the myotonia, which is generalized, is problematic, particularly in the lower limbs. Patients complain of stiffness which is most evident on trying to initiate movement after rest. Thus, the patient who has been sitting in the waiting room rises and walks with profound leg stiffness, somewhat reminiscent of spasticity, into the consulting room. A classic presentation is the soldier on the parade ground—after a prolonged period 'standing to attention', the order to march results in his falling due to leg muscle stiffness. One such patient also demonstrated marked grip myotonia—on an unfortunate occasion he alighted from a bus but, unable to release his grip from the handrail before the bus departed, was dragged along the road.

In most disorders, myotonia lessens with repeated activity of the muscle. Thus, the sign becomes less striking with repeated percussion of the thenar eminence or attempts to demonstrate grip myotonia. As a symptom, for example, the leg stiffness in myotonia congenita lessens as the patient continues to walk. In paramyotonia the reverse is seen, with myotonia increasing with activity—so-called paradoxical myotonia. Some, but by no means all, patients complain that their myotonia is worse in the cold. This is again a particular characteristic of paramyotonia.

Classification of myotonic disorders

As with many other inherited neuromuscular disorders, nomenclature and classification are currently in a state of flux as molecular mechanisms are being unravelled. For clinical purposes a useful distinction is between those multisystem disorders in which weakness is a significant feature, and which are therefore referred to as dystrophies, and the non-dystrophic myotonias (Table 1).

The nomenclature for the gene loci of myotonic dystrophies has been revised recently. Classic myotonic dystrophy was previously called dystrophia myotonica, which gave rise to the abbreviation DM. It shows no genetic heterogeneity, all cases being associated with a trinucleotide repeat expansion in the 3′ untranslated region of a novel protein kinase gene on chromosome 19q. This locus is referred to as DM1. Many cases of proximal myotonic myopathy, a recently described disorder, are linked to chromosome 3q, and that locus is designated DM2. However, some cases of proximal myotonic myopathy do not link to DM2. As yet, other loci have not been identified, but as they are they will be designated DM3, DM4, and so on.

The most common non-dystrophic myotonias are the autosomal dominant and recessive forms of myotonia congenita, both of which are caused by mutations of the skeletal muscle chloride channel (*CLC-1*) gene. Different mutations of the skeletal muscle sodium channel gene (*SCN4A*) give

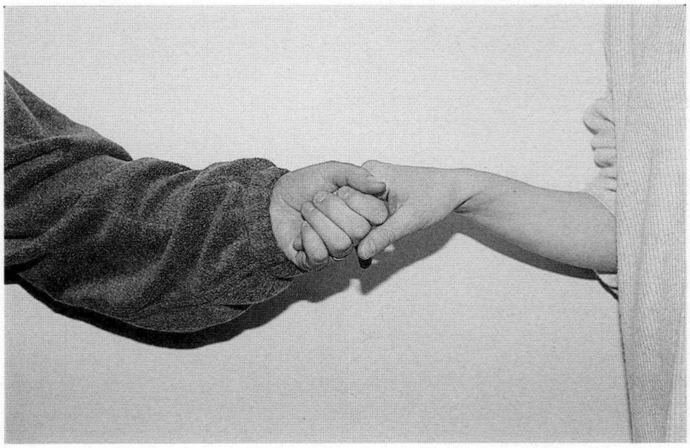

(a)

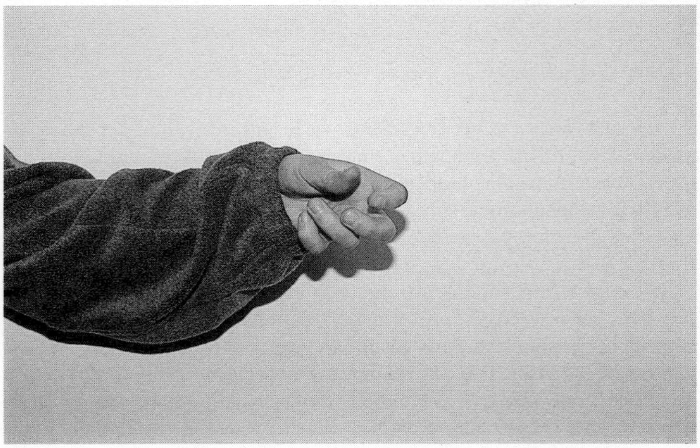

(b)

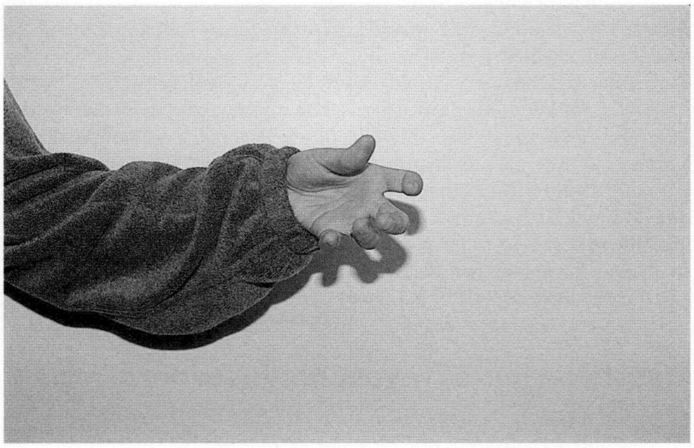

(b)

Fig. 1 Grip myotonia. The patient was asked to grip the examiner's fingers tightly for 3 s, and then to release the grip as rapidly as possible. The following two photographs were taken at 3-s intervals.

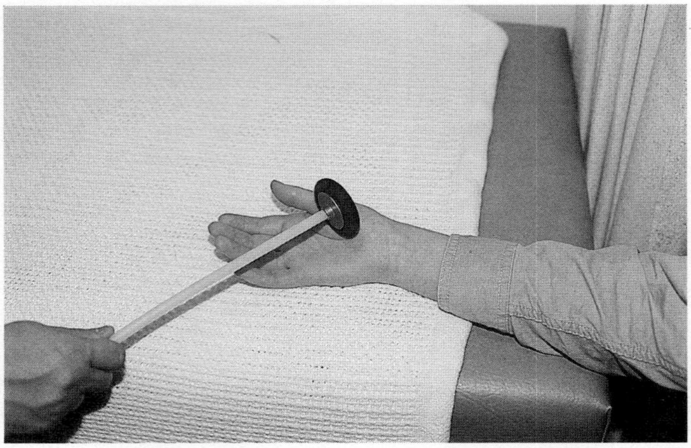

(a)

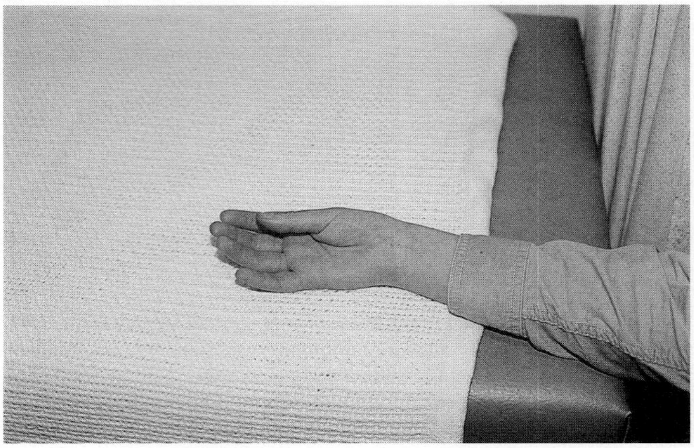

(b)

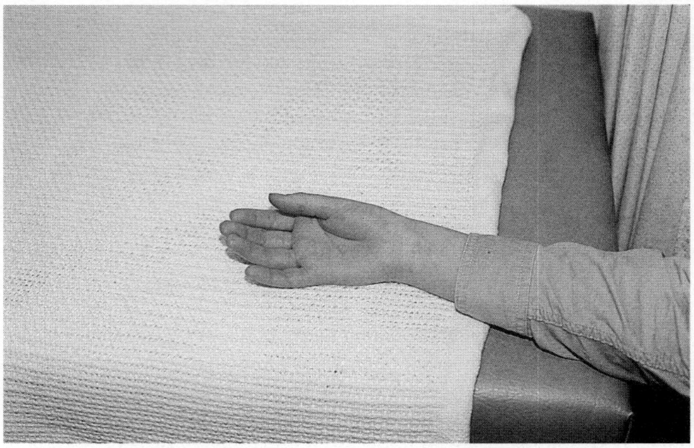

(b)

Fig. 2 Percussion myotonia. Following a sharp tap, the thenar eminence muscles contract and then relax slowly (subsequent photographs taken at 3-s intervals).

Table 1 The classification of myotonic disorders

Myotonic dystrophies(multisystem myotonic myopathies)	Non-dystrophic myotonias
Myotonic dystrophy (Chromosome 19q, DM1)	Chloride channelopathies—myotonia congenita (Chromosome 7q)
Proximal myotonic myopathy (Chromosome 3q, DM2, and other loci)	Sodium channelopathies—paramyotonia congenita (Chromosome 17q)
	Schwartz–Jampel syndrome—chondrodystrophic myotonia (Chromosome 1p and other loci)

rise to hyperkalaemic periodic paralysis and related disorders, including paramyotonia congenita. These chloride and sodium channelopathies, together with the calcium channel disorders causing hypokalaemic periodic paralysis, are discussed further in Chapter 24.22.5.

Schwartz–Jampel syndrome is a very rare recessive disorder of infantile onset, characterized by skeletal abnormalities, abnormal facial appearance, and abnormal muscle electrical activity. Electromyography may show typical myotonia as well as periods of continuous electrical activity which are probably neural in origin. It is genetically heterogeneous. Some cases are linked to chromosome 1p. One patient with a clinical diagnosis of Schwartz–Jampel syndrome was subsequently found to have a sodium channel mutation.

Myotonic dystrophy

Myotonic dystrophy is the most frequent cause of myotonia and indeed is also the most prevalent muscular dystrophy in adults. It is a multisystem disorder that has very important (but sometimes rather neglected) manifestations other than skeletal muscle dysfunction, involving cardiac conduction tissues, smooth muscle, eyes, and the central nervous system. Clinical severity ranges from death *in utero* to a condition so mild that it may be asymptomatic and without abnormal physical signs in old age. The molecular basis is now known (an expansion of an unstable trinucleotide repeat in a gene coding for a novel protein kinase), but it is not yet clear how this leads to the various manifestations of the disease. Myotonic dystrophy provides a dramatic example of the phenomenon of 'anticipation', by which succeeding generations may be much more severely affected than their predecessors, and this correlates with the size of the genetic expansion.

Epidemiology

The disease is seen worldwide, with a particularly high frequency in French Canadians in Quebec (originating from a single immigrant couple). Incidence and prevalence figures are unreliable, and probably mostly underestimates, because of the difficulty in ascertaining asymptomatic individuals. A generally accepted prevalence value is 5/100 000 population.

Pathogenesis

The molecular basis is the expansion of a trinucleotide (cytosine–thymine–guanine, **CTG**) repeat sequence in the 3′ untranslated region of the myotonic dystrophy protein kinase (*DMPK*) gene on chromosome 19q. The function of this novel putative serine–threonine protein kinase is unknown. In the normal population the size of the repeat is in the range CTG_{5-37}, with a trimodal distribution of 5, 11 to 17, and 19 to 37 repeats. Expansions in the range CTG_{37-49} are believed to represent premutations. Individuals with myotonic dystrophy have repeats in the range $CTG_{50-5000}$ and, as noted below, there is a correlation between the size of the repeat and clinical severity, and an inverse correlation between repeat size and age of onset.

A fundamental concept is that the expanded gene is unstable. It is mitotically unstable, and so the size of the gene increases with age. There is somatic mosaicism, so that the expansion is not the same size in different tissues. Diagnostic studies are based on measurement of the expansion size in blood lymphocyte DNA.

More important is intergenerational CTG-repeat instability, which explains why the disease tends to increase in severity in subsequent generations. The gender of the parent of origin is important. In most transmissions the allele size increases. However, there appears to be a threshold limit for sperm, and males never transmit the very large expansions associated with congenital myotonic dystrophy (see below), which only occurs when the mother is the gene carrier. There is some evidence of meiotic drive, which leads to preferred transmission of the abnormal expanded allele.

It remains uncertain as to how the basic molecular abnormality causes the various manifestations of the disease. One theory is that the expansion affects the expression of other genes in the DM locus apart from *DMPK*, such as the DM locus-associated homeodomain protein (*DMAHP*) gene. Another theory is that nuclear accumulation of RNA transcripts from the expanded *DMPK* gene affects processing of other mRNAs, thus having a knock-on effect on the translation of many proteins.

Clinical features

From the above it is apparent that there is a continuous distribution of expanded allele size, and that there is a relationship between allele size and disease severity, and between allele size and age of onset. While accepting that some patients will fall between these categories, for practical clinical purposes myotonic dystrophy can be considered to give rise to three main patterns of disease:

- congenital
- classic or early adult onset
- late onset, asymptomatic, or oligosymptomatic.

Because it is the best known, and illustrates the multifarious manifestations of myotonic dystrophy, the classic form will be discussed first.

Classic form

Onset is in adolescence or early adult life. The principal manifestations are summarized in Table 2. A number of rarer or clinically less important associations are also recognized. These include reduced fertility, testicular atrophy, insulin resistance (but rarely overt diabetes), retinopathy, eye movement disorder, peripheral neuropathy, disturbed tests of endocrine

Table 2 Main clinical features of classic myotonic dystrophy

System	Manifestations
Neuromuscular	Weakness Myotonia
Ocular	Cataract
Central nervous system	Excessive daytime sleepiness Low IQ Sensorineural deafness
Cardiovascular	Heart block Dysrhythmias Sudden death
Respiratory	Recurrent infections Sleep apnoea
Hair	Premature balding
Gastrointestinal	Dysphagia Irritable bowel syndrome Pseudo-obstruction

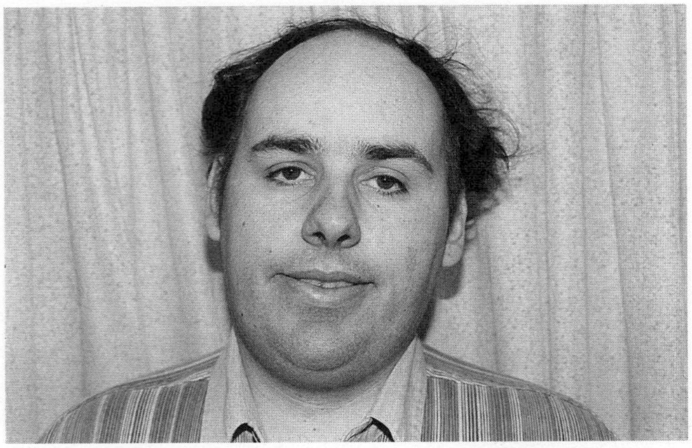

Fig. 3 Adult-onset myotonic dystrophy. Typical facial features (see text).

function, hypotension, pilomatrixomas, and reduced levels of immunoglobulins and complement.

Skeletal- and smooth muscle

The features of myotonia have already been discussed. The distribution of muscle weakness is highly characteristic. Wasting and weakness of the facial muscles, combined with premature male-pattern balding, gives rise to the typical facial appearance of the condition (Fig. 3). The temporalis muscle is atrophic, giving a sunken appearance over the temples. There is ptosis. Eye closure is weak and in severe cases the sclera may remain visible. The jaw tends to hang down. Neck flexion is weak and in some, but not all patients, there is evident atrophy of the sternomastoid muscles. In the limbs, and in marked contrast to most other myopathic disorders, the weakness is predominantly distal. In the upper limbs there is weakness and wasting of the small hand muscles and of the long wrist and finger flexor and extensor muscles in the forearm. There is often profound weakness of grip and the patient complains of difficulty with tasks such as wringing-out a cloth and removing the lid from a bottle. A simple hand-held dynamometer reveals the extent of the weakness—whereas a normal female would easily exceed 35 kg, patients of either sex may manage only 1 or 2 kg. In the lower limbs there is weakness of ankle dorsiflexion, presenting as tripping easily and foot drop. As the disease advances, weakness becomes evident more proximally, but the marked distal predilection remains throughout.

Bulbar muscle weakness presents with dysarthria and dysphagia. Smooth muscle involvement contributes towards the dysphagia. Symptoms akin to those of irritable bowel syndrome are frequent. Constipation is common, pseudo-obstruction rare. There may be evidence of incoordinate uterine contraction in labour.

Ocular

Cataracts develop at an early age. The initial manifestation is multicoloured opacities in the subcapsular regions, readily seen on slit-lamp examination. Identification of cataracts used to be important in screening asymptomatic family members for the disease, but that has now been replaced by DNA testing. In practice, the cataracts are managed as any other cataracts, being operated on when vision is significantly impaired. Early-onset cataracts should always raise the suspicion of myotonic dystrophy.

Central nervous system

Central nervous system disease is expressed in two main ways. As a group, patients with myotonic dystrophy have a lower IQ than average, but many mildly affected patients have intelligence within the normal range. They are often perceived as apathetic or lacking self-motivation. There is some neuropsychological evidence of specific defects of frontal lobe functioning. The second principal feature is excessive daytime sleepiness which affects over three-quarters of patients, some profoundly. This appears to be a central phenomenon and is only rarely attributable to obstructive sleep apnoea/nocturnal sleep disturbance.

Cardiovascular

Cardiovascular dysfunction is arguably the most important extramuscular manifestation of myotonic dystrophy and is probably responsible for most of the not infrequently reported cases of sudden unexpected death. The most commonly recognized pattern is of progressive conduction disturbance. Thus, in very early cases the ECG is normal. Subsequently, the P–R interval gradually lengthens until first-degree block is present. Later features include bundle branch and complete heart block. Tachyarhythmias also occur, most frequently atrial flutter or fibrillation. Symptoms include palpitation, dizzy spells, and fainting. Prolonged ECG monitoring and sometimes intracardiac electrophysiological studies are indicated if such symptoms are reported, or the standard ECG shows significant change. All patients should have an ECG annually, and be advised to report any cardiac symptoms immediately. Rhythm disturbances precipitated by anaesthesia or surgery are common, as are respiratory problems. For these reasons, patients should carry a medical alert bracelet/medallion and, for elective admissions for surgery, be reminded to inform the anaesthetist of their diagnosis. The latter is particularly important for asymptomatic individuals diagnosed on the basis of DNA studies following family screening, as they may not consider themselves to be at risk—they are. Although there is some correlation between cardiac involvement and overall severity of the myotonic dystrophy, it is not absolute and individuals with minimal muscle involvement may have significant ECG changes.

Heart muscle disease, as opposed to disordered cardiac conducting tissues, is not clinically significant and routine echocardiography is not required.

Respiratory

Recurrent chest infections are common and relate to respiratory muscle weakness and the tendency to aspirate. In advanced disease, death is often secondary to pneumonia. Respiratory insufficiency may become apparent following anaesthesia, with difficulty in weaning from the ventilator. Chronic hypoventilation and hypercapnia may cause excessive daytime sleepiness, but in practice is much less common than the presumed central mechanism already mentioned. However, it must be considered and excluded (for example by overnight oximetry and blood gas measurements) if felt to be a possibility. Particular warning features would include a history of disturbed night-time sleep, snoring, waking with headaches, and the development of secondary polycythaemia.

Congenital myotonic dystrophy

By simple definition, this form of myotonic dystrophy is evident at birth, but in reality the spectrum of early-onset myotonic dystrophy is much wider. The exclusive (with only very rare exceptions) maternal transmission of congenital myotonic dystrophy has already been discussed. Many fetuses carrying large expansions are aborted spontaneously in early pregnancy and there is a high rate of fetal wastage. Because of the unstable nature of the CTG-repeat and the associated phenomenon of anticipation, it is not uncommon for the mother to be unaware of her own diagnosis at the time of birth. In that situation, the diagnosis in the infant is not always immediately apparent, as there are no entirely specific clinical features. In other infants the disorder is not evident at birth and thus is not strictly congenital, but symptoms become apparent within the first few years of life.

There is often a history of polyhydramnios and poor fetal movement in the pregnancy. The child is born hypotonic ('floppy') and talipes is present in about one-half. Respiratory and feeding difficulties may necessitate assisted ventilation or an oxygen tent, and feeding by nasogastric tube. Some die in the neonatal period from respiratory complications, but somewhat surprisingly, there are few further deaths in the survivors until the late teens and early adult life. There is generalized weakness, including the face—the jaw hangs open and the mouth has a characteristic tented or

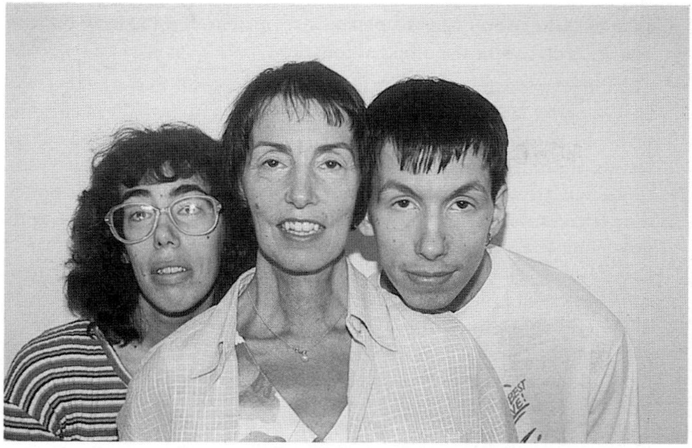

Fig. 4 Myotonic dystrophy. The affected mother's two children have the congenital form of the disease.

carp-like (as in fish) appearance. Myotonia is not evident clinically and even electromyographically may not appear for several years.

In those who survive, hypotonia resolves and motor function improves over the following few years, but during adolescence the features of the classic adult form of the disease appear (Fig. 4).

Mental retardation is invariable and may be severe. Most require special-needs schooling. Bowel involvement is common with faecal soiling and irregular bowel habit. Curiously, cataracts are relatively uncommon.

The overall prognosis is poor. Some 25 per cent die in the first 18 months of life, most in the neonatal period. One-half survive into the mid-30s, death most commonly resulting from respiratory involvement, but with a proportion of sudden deaths almost certainly due to cardiac conduction defects. Few achieve an independent adult life.

Late-onset form

This form is associated with a small CTG-repeat expansion. It is typically asymptomatic or oligosymptomatic and is diagnosed during family studies or by an alert ophthalmologist when the patient presents with cataracts. Skeletal muscle disease may be absent, or confined to mild myotonia and weakness confined to the hands. Balding may be a feature. It is not uncommon to see the parents of a patient with the classic adult form of the disease and not be able to identify the transmitting parent on clinical examination.

Importantly, even patients with such minimal symptoms may occasionally develop significant cardiac conduction problems and they should have annual electrocardiograms.

Management

The essential management issues in myotonic dystrophy are:

- genetic counselling
- annual ECG
- anaesthetic risks
- physical therapies
- cataract surgery.

A particular concern relates to the genetic phenomenon of anticipation and the potential for an asymptomatic mother, ignorant of the diagnosis, to give birth to a congenitally affected child. When the diagnosis of myotonic dystrophy is established in a family member it is imperative that at-risk relatives are offered screening. Prenatal diagnosis, by chorionic villous sampling, can then be offered.

Annual ECG should be performed in all patients. They and their medical attendants must be aware of the cardiorespiratory complications associated with anaesthesia. They should be encouraged to wear an appropriate medical alert bracelet or medallion. A few patients require nocturnal positive-pressure ventilation by face mask, but most excessive daytime sleepiness is not related to respiratory insufficiency. Recurrent chest infections are common. Annual influenza vaccination should be advised. Pneumococcal vaccination is also given but is of uncertain value.

Physiotherapy and occupational and speech therapy all have a role, as does the use of orthotic devices (for example for foot drop). Bowel problems in the congenital form require specific advice and counselling.

Cataract surgery is required when vision is significantly impaired.

Proximal myotonic myopathy

In the last few years a number of families have been described with an autosomal dominant multisystem disorder similar to myotonic dystrophy, but who do not have the chromosome 19 CTG expansion. Many, but not all, show linkage to chromosome 3q. In some countries (such as Germany) these conditions seem to be almost as common as myotonic dystrophy, but in others (such as the United Kingdom) they appear to be rare. Some issues concerning classification were discussed earlier.

Various names and abbreviations have been given to these conditions, including proximal myotonic myopathy, proximal myotonic dystrophy and DM2.

Despite the superficial similarities to myotonic dystrophy, there are also differences. Onset is usually in adult life. Myotonia tends to be more symptomatic than in myotonic dystrophy and patients complain of stiffness and muscle pain. Unlike myotonic dystrophy, the weakness tends to be more marked proximally, and may show significant fluctuation from day to day. Cataracts may be indistinguishable from those seen in myotonic dystrophy. Cardiac conduction problems appear to be less common. Male hypogonadism and deafness occur. There is considerable clinical variability even between families linked to the same chromosome 3q locus, indicating allelic heterogeneity.

Further reading

Myotonic dystrophy

Brook JD *et al.* (1992). Molecular basis of myotonic dystrophy: expansion of a trinucleotide (CTG) repeat in the 3' end of a transcript encoding a protein kinase family member. *Cell* **68**, 799–808.

Harper P (2001). *Myotonic dystrophy*, 3rd edn. WB Saunders, London.

Koch MC *et al.* (1991). Genetic risks for children of women with myotonic dystrophy. *American Journal of Human Genetics* **48**, 1084–91.

Lazarus A *et al.* (1999). Relationships among electrophysiological findings and cardiac status, heart function, and extent of DNA mutation in myotonic dystrophy. *Circulation* **99**, 1041–6.

Reardon W *et al.* (1993). The natural history of congenital myotonic dystrophy: mortality and long term clinical aspects. *Archives of Disease in Childhood* **68**, 177–81.

Proximal myotonic myopathy

Moxley RT (1996). Proximal myotonic myopathy: mini-review of a recently delineated clinical disorder. *Neuromuscular Disorders* **6**, 87–93.

Ranum LPW *et al.* (1998). Genetic mapping of a second myotonic dystrophy locus. *Nature Genetics* **19**, 196–8.

Udd B *et al.* (1997). Proximal myotonic dystrophy—a family with autosomal dominant muscular dystrophy, cataracts, hearing loss and hypogonadism: heterogeneity of proximal myotonic syndromes? *Neuromuscular Disorders* **7**, 217–28.

Wieser T *et al.* (2000). A family with PROMM not linked to the recently mapped PROMM locus DM2. *Neuromuscular Disorders* **10**, 141–3.

24.22.4 Metabolic and endocrine disorders

David Hilton-Jones and Richard Edwards

Introduction

This section deals with disorders of voluntary muscle that arise either as the result of a disturbance of muscle metabolism, or disordered ion flux. In many cases precise mechanisms have yet to be defined.

The term 'metabolic myopathy' is applied to those disorders in which there is a primary defect, usually an enzyme deficiency, in the biochemical pathways associated with energy generation (ATP synthesis). This group includes the mitochondrial disorders, which are some of the most common causes of primary metabolic myopathy seen in clinical practice.

Endocrine myopathies and nutritional and toxic myopathies, including those that are drug-induced, can be considered as secondary (acquired) metabolic myopathies.

Defects in genes coding for subunits of the skeletal-muscle sodium and calcium channels underlie primary hyperkalaemic and hypokalaemic periodic paralysis, respectively. Both autosomal dominant and autosomal recessive myotonia congenita are caused by mutation in the skeletal-muscle chloride channel. Mutations affecting two skeletal-muscle calcium channels, the dihydropyridine (**DHP**) and ryanodine (**RYR1**) receptors, are associated with malignant hyperthermia (**MH**). The congenital myopathy central core disease is allelic to MH and is associated with *RYR1* mutations.

The cardinal symptoms of myopathy are weakness, fatigue, and/or pain; altered excitability may also occur. It is important that the physician appreciates several points:

- There are non-specific effects, such as loss of muscle, that may be far more important as a cause of weakness than the energetic consequences of the biochemical defect. Visual inspection and circumference measurements tend to underestimate the extent of wasting, which may be better documented by quantitative scanning methods (magnetic resonance imaging (**MRI**) or computed tomography (**CT**)).
- Not all the biochemical abnormalities cause symptoms. Clinical expression of the underlying defect depends on the habitual demands on the muscle for movement and weight-lifting.
- A patient with a metabolic myopathy may have common, non-myopathic, musculoskeletal complaints which have no relation to the inherited or acquired defect.
- Muscle symptoms may have no physiological connection with the underlying defect and may be consequences of somatization or other psychological process.
- The practical assessment of metabolic myopathy should include consideration of the WHO ICIDH-2 (2000) classification of the functioning and disability criteria of impairment, activities, and participation (revised from the International Classification of Impairments, Disabilities, and Handicaps (**ICIDH**) of WHO 1980). In this generic consideration, the relationship between antigravity muscle strength and the body weight to be carried is crucial: performance may be improved as much or more by weight reduction as by therapeutic attempts to reverse the myopathy, providing that calorie restriction does not aggravate the metabolic defect—for example, in the case of carnitine palmitoyl transferase deficiency, where carbohydrate starvation may exacerbate the energy supply problem of the underlying enzyme defect.
- An objective assessment of a response to treatment requires the measurement of individual muscle strength and/or timing of the performance of tasks relevant to the patient's symptoms and the everyday life demands placed on the diseased muscles.
- Metabolic myopathies are unusual or rare conditions that are very variable in presentation. They are not easy to discuss in the light of current, evidence-based healthcare philosophies, which are largely based on the results of randomized controlled trials (**RCTs**) of therapeutic interventions. The treatments of the metabolic myopathies tend to fall under the general rubric of 'orphan drugs' and 'orphan diseases', since, as with other rare diseases, a commercial return on the investment in research and development to deliver effective treatments is unlikely. Furthermore, in view of their rarity, there is little or no chance of formal treatment evaluation by RCTs. These conditions are therefore still to be evaluated by thoughtful clinical research employing the most relevant modern biochemical and physiological approaches.
- The patient with a metabolic myopathy is a person, and therefore far more important and complex to understand and help than the underlying metabolic diagnosis, difficult though that may be. It is essential to the humane and effective management of such a patient to see the individual as coping in a personal and social sense despite the metabolic impairment. The aim is to determine what is likely to best improve the patient's overall quality of life. Here, as with other disabilities, the constructive analysis and recommendations of the World Health Organization are useful as a basis for working with the patient to determine an individual management plan. (Table 1).

Primary metabolic myopathies

The principal energy currency of living cells is adenosine triphosphate (**ATP**). Whereas in most organs the rate of ATP utilization is fairly constant, in voluntary muscle the change from rest to strenuous activity may increase the demand on ATP generation several thousand-fold. If that demand is not met, contractile failure (that is to say, fatigue or weakness) will develop and may be accompanied by the destruction of muscle fibres. In many of the primary metabolic myopathies it is often assumed that exercise-induced symptoms relate to a failure of ATP generation, and although this is probably not always correct, it is a useful generalization. Whilst exercise-induced symptoms are often a striking feature of this type of metabolic myopathy, they are not always present. Some patients develop a chronic progressive myopathy.

Table 1 Key features of disability evaluation and management in metabolic myopathy

Body	Person	Society
Impairment	*Activities* (limitations)	*Participation* (restriction)
Metabolism/ function/structure		
Severity, localization, duration	Difficulties, duration, assistance needed	Extent, facilitators, environmental demands of barriers
Harmful consequences, e.g. myoglobinuria, falls	Physical and mental adaptive responses	Positive or negative psychosocial factors
Treatment options—modification of chemistry by diet or drugs?	Counselling for exercise-behaviour modification; avoidance of excessive weight gain; mechanical solutions, e.g. wheelchair/bicycle	Better popular understanding of side-effects of prescription drugs and alcohol; positive attitudes to assisting those with locomotor disability, improved access

[a] Developed from WHO 2000.

The main fuels providing energy for ATP generation in skeletal muscle are glycogen, fatty acids, and glucose (Fig. 1). Their relative contributions depend upon the state of nutrition and, more importantly, the level and duration of exercise. A gross oversimplification of these pathways aids understanding of the clinical features of the different forms of metabolic myopathy.

At rest, the main fuel source is circulating free fatty acids, with a lesser contribution from circulating glucose. Small amounts of ATP may be generated directly from glycolysis, but the production of the energy-rich electron carriers (reduced nicotinamide adenine dinucleotide (NADH) and reduced flavin adenine dinucleotide ($FADH_2$)) from fatty acid β-oxidation, and the Krebs' cycle are more important. Transfer of electrons to molecular oxygen through the electron transport chain of the mitochondria releases energy for the generation of ATP (oxidative phosphorylation)

The increased demand on ATP generation during early strenuous exercise cannot be met by oxidative pathways. The resting blood flow provides an inadequate delivery of oxygen and substrate, and compression of blood vessels by the contracting muscle exacerbates the problem. ATP is therefore generated by the breakdown of muscle-fibre stores of glycogen (anaerobic glycolysis). The relative lack of oxygen leads to increasing levels of NADH and pyruvate. NADH accumulation would inhibit glycolysis, and thus ATP generation, and is avoided by the reduction of pyruvate to lactate, explaining the lactic acidosis seen in disorders of oxidative metabolism.

Adaptive processes occur as exercise continues; muscle blood flow increases, the respiratory rate rises, and free fatty acids are mobilized from adipose stores. Glycogen stores in muscle become depleted and circulating free fatty acids become the main energy source, with a very small contribution from circulating glucose.

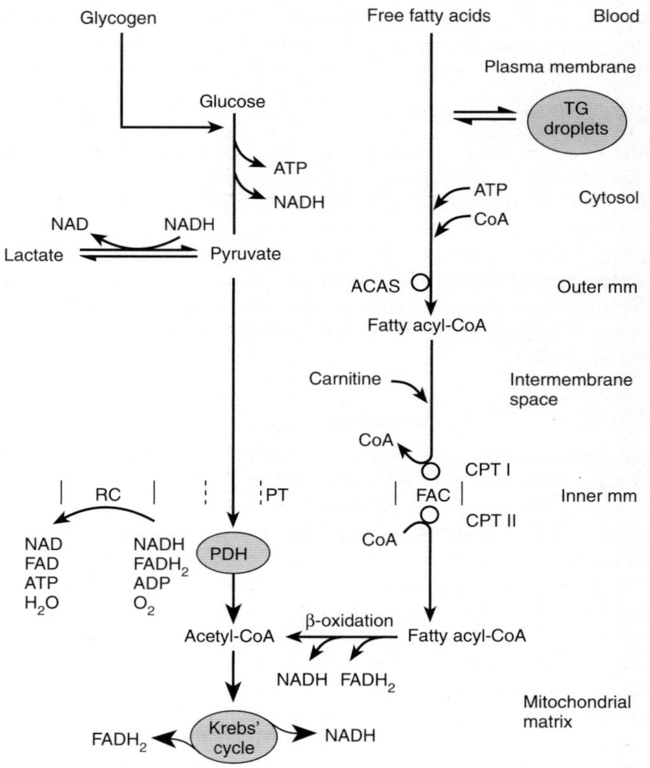

Fig. 1 Major pathways associated with energy production in skeletal muscle. ACAS, acyl-CoA synthetase; ADP, adenosine diphosphate; ATP, adenosine triphosphate; CoA, coenzyme A; CPT, carnitine palmityl transferase; FAC, fatty acyl-carnitine; FAD, flavin adenine dinucleotide; $FADH_2$, reduced FAD; mm, mitochondrial membrane; NAD, nicotinamide adenine dinucleotide; NADH, reduced NAD; PDH, pyruvate dehydrogenase complex; PT, pyruvate translocase; RC, respiratory chain; TG, triglyceride.

Certain deductions can be made from the above that are largely borne out in clinical practice. Disorders of glycogen and glucose metabolism are typically asymptomatic at rest, but produce symptoms early in exercise when anaerobic glycolysis is important for energy supply. If low levels of exercise can be sustained, symptoms can improve as fatty acid oxidation increases ('second wind' phenomenon in McArdle's disease). Disorders of fatty acid metabolism, insufficient to cause symptoms at rest, are likely to be exposed by sustained exercise and fasting. The central role of oxidative phosphorylation explains why disorders of the respiratory chain may be symptomatic at rest. The clinical presentation will also depend upon whether the enzyme defect is restricted to skeletal muscle or is more generalized, thereby causing dysfunction of other tissues and organs. Systemic features may dominate in disorders of β-oxidation and in mitochondrial disorders but are absent in McArdle's disease because the defective enzyme is muscle-specific.

Disorders of glycogen and glucose metabolism (see also Section 11.3)

Several of the glycogenoses show significant skeletal-muscle involvement. The major pathways of metabolism, and the enzymes associated with these disorders, are shown in Fig. 2. They are autosomal recessive disorders, except for the X-linked recessive, phosphoglycerate kinase deficiency. In most of these disorders the serum creatine kinase is elevated at rest, and massively so after exercise-induced muscle damage.

Acid maltase deficiency (type II glycogenosis)

Acid maltase is a lysosomal enzyme not directly involved in energetic pathways, and exercise-induced symptoms are absent. In the infantile form (Pompe's disease) there is widespread organomegaly as well as skeletal-muscle involvement, and death occurs by the age of 2 years due to cardiac or respiratory failure. The adult form is of considerable importance and has probably been underdiagnosed. The most obvious feature is a slowly progressive, painless, proximal myopathy. Diaphragmatic involvement is an important characteristic, and many of these patients first present with respiratory failure. Nocturnal assisted ventilation alleviates sleep-disordered breathing and may prolong survival for many years. Muscle biopsy showing glycogen-containing vacuoles is usually suggestive; but the definitive diagnosis is established by enzyme assay in muscle, fibroblasts, or leucocytes, or by demonstrating glycogen granules by Periodic acid–Schiff (**PAS**) staining in lymphocytes on a peripheral blood film.

There is an intermediate juvenile form, with limited survival.

Myophosphorylase deficiency (type V glycogenosis—McArdle's disease)

The onset of symptoms is usually during childhood, and the cardinal features are pain, weakness, and stiffness of muscles early in exercise, relieved by rest. Strenuous exercise, such as helping to push a car or lift heavy furniture, may induce painful, electrically silent, muscle contractures. Muscle fibre breakdown is reflected in myalgia and myoglobinuria (dark red/black urine), which, if severe, may cause renal failure. Muscle breakdown is accompanied by a large release of creatine kinase (**CK**) into the blood, and a failure to see such a rise in serum CK levels should cast doubt on a diagnosis of myoglobinuria. Conversely, if renal failure is present then no myoglobinuria may be seen and the only evidence of rhabdomyolysis is the raised CK level. However, symptoms may ease ('second wind' phenomenon) if low levels of activity are maintained, as circulating free fatty acids and glucose become available as alternative fuels.

Progressive proximal weakness frequently develops and is sometimes the mode of presentation in late-onset cases.

Failure of lactate generation (accompanied by increased blood ammonia and hypoxanthine concentrations) during ischaemic forearm exercise is consistent with the diagnosis. However, this is not specific since it also occurs in other glycogenolysis disorders, and may be seen to some extent in acquired conditions such as alcoholic myopathy or hypothyroidism. Also, the test may give a misleading ('false-negative') result if the myophosphorylase deficiency is only partial. The definitive diagnosis is established by histochemical demonstration of the absence of phosphorylase staining (or by enzyme assay) on muscle biopsy, or by genetic studies of the coding and expression of muscle phosphorylase.

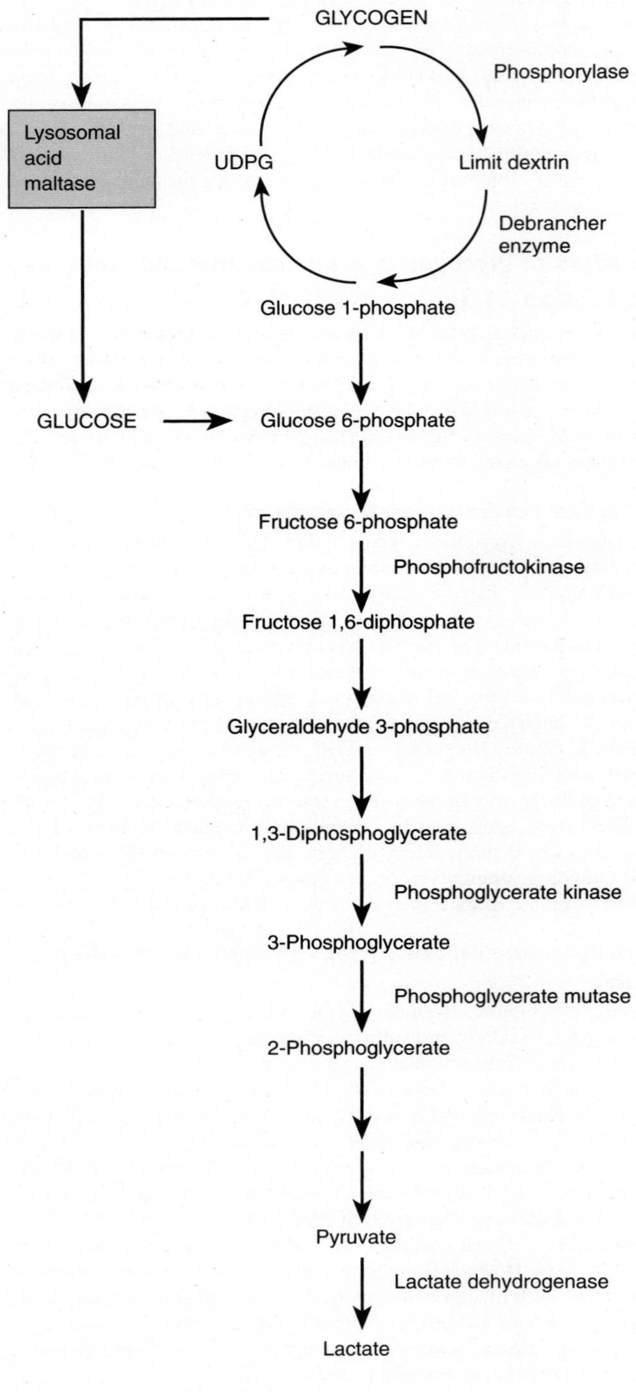

Fig. 2 Pathways of glycogenolysis and glycolysis. Enzymes known to be associated with particular clinical syndromes are shown.

Debrancher enzyme deficiency (type III glycogenosis—Cori–Forbes disease)

In infancy and childhood the main features of this disorder are hepatomegaly, hypoglycaemia, and failure to thrive. During adolescence muscle symptoms become more prominent. A small group of patients first present during adult life with muscle symptoms, but may give a history of a protuberant abdomen in childhood. Both exercise intolerance and a slowly progressive proximal myopathy are present.

It has recently been recognized that most patients develop a potentially fatal cardiomyopathy.

The ischaemic forearm test shows impaired lactate generation, muscle biopsy shows glycogen accumulation, and the administration of glucagon fails to produce a hyperglycaemic response. Enzyme assay can be performed on muscle, liver, erythrocytes, and leucocytes.

Phosphofructokinase deficiency (type VII glycogenosis—Tarui's disease)

The clinical picture is very similar to that of myophosphorylase deficiency, but a phosphofructokinase (**PFK**) deficiency in erythrocytes leads to the additional features of haemolytic anaemia and gout. Unlike patients with myophosphorylase deficiency, ingested glucose does not improve exercise tolerance in those with PFK deficiency because of the position of PFK in the sequence of enzymes in the glycolytic pathway (Fig. 2). Diagnosis is established by enzyme assay in muscle.

Defects of distal glycolysis

Deficiencies of phosphoglycerate kinase, phosphoglycerate mutase, and lactate dehydrogenase have been described recently. All three are associated with exercise intolerance and myoglobinuria. It is possible that other defects of glycolysis, causing similar symptoms, remain to be discovered.

Treatment

There is, as yet, no specific treatment for any of the disorders described above. Attempts at dietary manipulation have generally proved unsuccessful. Patients must be aware of the risk to renal function from myoglobinuria, and try to avoid intense exercise. There is evidence, in patients with muscle pain due to McArdle's disease and other metabolic myopathies, that maintaining a reasonable level of aerobic fitness is beneficial, by sustaining sufficient activity of muscle mitochondria to provide energy from oxidative phosphorylation to adapt for the deficiencies in energy availability from glycogenolysis.

Disorders of lipid metabolism

Unlike glycolysis, lipid metabolism is entirely dependent upon oxidative processes. Moreover, there is a close relationship between the disorders described below and defects of the mitochondrial respiratory chain; for example, lipid accumulation in muscle is a common histological feature in respiratory chain disorders.

Free fatty acids, mainly from the blood but also from triglyceride droplets stored within muscle fibres, are a major fuel at rest and during sustained exercise (see Fig. 1). They are converted to fatty acyl-coenzyme A (**CoA**) at the outer mitochondrial membrane which, within the mitochondrial matrix, can undergo β-oxidation. A transport system involving carnitine and the enzyme system carnitine palmityl transferase (**CPT**) is required to enable fatty acyl-CoA to cross the inner mitochondrial membrane. Defects involving carnitine, CPT, and β-oxidation are recognized.

Carnitine deficiency

Muscle carnitine deficiency, causing fluctuating weakness and lipid storage (intracellularly in myocytes), and systemic carnitine deficiency causing weakness and recurrent, often fatal, Reye-like episodes, have been described. It has become apparent that in most cases of so-called systemic carnitine deficiency, and perhaps even in some purely myopathic cases, the carnitine deficiency is secondary to another metabolic disorder: most commonly defects of β-oxidation or of the mitochondrial respiratory chain.

Defects of β-oxidation

Many enzyme deficiencies have been described, but clinical features are limited. They may present during the neonatal period with hypotonia, hypoglycaemia, cardiomyopathy, failure to thrive, and early death. Such defects may be a cause of some cases of sudden infant death syndrome. Later-onset cases develop Reye-like crises, muscle weakness, and cardiomyopathy. Secondary carnitine deficiency is common. A high carbohydrate and low fat diet may help.

Carnitine palmitoyl transferase deficiency

This rare disorder shows a male predominance. Symptoms are precipitated by sustained exercise (for example, a route march) or prolonged fasting, and consist of muscle pain followed by myoglobinuria, which may cause renal failure. The diagnosis may be suggested by showing impaired ketone body production during fasting, but is proven by enzyme assay in skeletal muscle. A high carbohydrate, low fat diet may reduce the number of attacks.

Myoadenylate deaminase deficiency

Deficiency of myoadenylate deaminase has been suggested as a cause of exercise-induced myalgia, weakness, and cramps but its exact status remains controversial. It is almost certainly an unusual cause of significant myalgia. It has been described as an incidental finding in muscle needle biopsies taken from normal volunteers to study muscle chemistry in sports science research. The enzyme catalyses the reaction adenosine monophosphate (**AMP**) → inosine monophosphate (**IMP**) + ammonia (NH3). Theoretically, this reaction may aid ATP production by removing AMP and increasing flux through the adenylate kinase reaction 2ADP→ ATP + AMP. The diagnosis is established from the absence of a rise in the plasma ammonia level during forearm exercise testing and from the histochemical demonstration of absent enzyme activity.

Endocrine myopathies

Although weakness is a common symptom in many endocrine disorders, the mechanisms are generally poorly understood. However, the myopathy responds to treatment of the underlying hormonal disorder, and extensive investigation of the myopathic component is rarely required. The commonest pattern is limb-girdle weakness.

Thyroid disorders (see also Chapter 12.4)

Thyrotoxicosis

Typically, weakness develops shortly after the onset of other thyrotoxic symptoms, and 80 per cent of patients have demonstrable weakness at presentation. The shoulder-girdle muscles tend to be involved before the pelvic musculature. Muscle atrophy is usually slight. Asymmetrical and distal weakness, myalgia, cramps, and fasciculations are rare findings.

The serum creatine kinase level is usually normal, but electromyography shows features consistent with muscle disease. The myopathy responds to treatment of the thyrotoxicosis.

Thyrotoxic periodic paralysis

Most cases have been reported in individuals from the Orient, with a strong male predominance. Clinical features closely mimic those of familial hypokalaemic periodic paralysis. The weakness is disproportionate to any muscle wasting. The onset of paralytic attacks usually follows the development of hyperthyroid symptoms but the attacks cease when the patient is rendered euthyroid.

Thyroid ophthalmopathy (Graves' ophthalmoplegia)

The classic features of this condition include eyelid lag, retraction, and swelling, as well as progressive swelling of the extraocular muscles and orbital soft tissues leading to proptosis and diplopia and, in severe cases, corneal ulceration, papilloedema, and optic atrophy. An extremely important but often missed variant is the patient who presents with minimal diplopia only.

In mild cases, MRI or CT imaging is useful for detecting extraocular muscle swelling. Simple tests of thyroid function may be normal. Estimation of antithyroglobulin and antimicrosomal antibodies, and the performance of a thyrotrophin-releasing hormone (**TRH**) stimulation test may be required. Thyroid-stimulating immunoglobulins are present in most patients.

If thyrotoxic, the patient should be rendered euthyroid. Lid retraction may respond to topical 10 per cent guanethidine. Persisting major eye problems may require high-dose prednisolone, plasma exchange, or orbital decompression. Tarsorrhaphy protects the cornea.

Thyroid disease and myasthenia

Patients with myasthenia gravis have an increased incidence of thyroid disease, including hyperthyroidism, hypothyroidism, Hashimoto's thyroiditis, and increased antibodies to thyroglobulin or microsomal fractions. Thyroid disease may pre-date or follow the onset of myasthenia and must be considered as a cause of deterioration in an otherwise stable patient with myasthenia. Some 5 per cent of patients with myasthenia will develop thyroid disease, but only about 0.1 per cent of thyrotoxic patients develop myasthenia.

Hypothyroidism

Although hypothyroid myopathy may be asymptomatic, mild weakness is probably present in most patients. Muscle biopsy characteristically shows evidence of type II (fast twitch, glycolytic, high intrinsic force) muscle fibre atrophy with type I fibre dominance. Even in the absence of weakness the serum creatine kinase level is often markedly raised. Slow relaxation of the tendon jerks may be present in isolation. Muscle pain and cramps are common. In children, the combination of hypothyroidism, weakness, and muscle hypertrophy is referred to as the Kocher–Debré–Semelaigne syndrome. In adults, Hoffman's syndrome describes the combination of hypothyroidism, weakness, muscle hypertrophy, cramps, and myoedema (the formation of a localized ridge of muscle following direct percussion). They probably represent variants of the same disorder.

All hypothyroid myopathic symptoms respond to thyroxine replacement.

Pituitary–adrenal axis disorders

Clinically, the most important of these is iatrogenic steroid myopathy, discussed below under 'Glucocorticoid excess'.

Acromegaly

Proximal weakness, pelvic more than shoulder girdle, is present in about one-half of patients. Common complaints include tiredness, weakness, and myalgia; muscle wasting is slight. Serum creatine kinase levels are normal or slightly raised. Normalizing growth-hormone levels improves the myopathy, but recovery may be incomplete.

Hypopituitarism

Growth-hormone deficiency in childhood impairs muscle and skeletal development proportionately; weakness is not usually a feature. In adults, panhypopituitarism causes generalized weakness and fatigue, which usually responds to thyroxine and cortisone-replacement therapy. Replacement of growth hormone in growth hormone-deficient adults has been associated with varying degrees of improvement in the strength of wasted muscles.

Glucocorticoid excess

ACTH excess, from a functioning pituitary adenoma or from ectopic production, is usually associated with high glucocorticoid levels, producing pituitary or ectopic Cushing's syndrome. Weakness is common and thought to relate to glucocorticoid excess. Weakness may occur in Nelson's syndrome, in which there is a high level of ACTH but no glucocorticoid excess.

The myopathy associated with Cushing's syndrome is probably related to glucocorticoid excess, and the clinical features are essentially the same as those of iatrogenic steroid myopathy. The 9α-fluorinated steroids, including dexamethasone, triamcinolone, and betamethasone, appear to have the greatest myopathic potential. Topical steroids can cause myopathy.

The most common picture is of a slowly progressive limb-girdle wasting and weakness, pelvic more than shoulder girdle, often accompanied by myalgia. The drug-induced form may have a more acute onset. Myopathy without other features of glucocorticoid excess is unusual. The serum creatine kinase level is usually normal and muscle biopsy shows non-specific type II fibre atrophy.

Steroid withdrawal is followed by recovery over several months. If steroid therapy for the primary disorder has to be continued then a non-fluorinated compound such as prednisolone should be used, preferably on an alternate-day basis. Successful treatment of Cushing's syndrome leads to recovery.

Conn's syndrome

Weakness is present in about 75 per cent of patients and is due to the associated hypokalaemia. Secondary hypokalaemic periodic paralysis may occur.

Addison's disease

Weakness, fatigue, and myalgia occur in up to one-half of patients. Rare myopathic presentations include progressive flexion contractures and secondary hyperkalaemic periodic paralysis.

The serum creatine kinase level is normal or slightly increased. Glucocorticoid replacement therapy is curative.

Disorders of calcium, vitamin D, and parathyroid hormone metabolism (see also Chapter 12.6)

There are complex interactions between vitamin D metabolism, calcium and phosphate homeostasis, and parathyroid hormone activity. Myopathy occurs in several clinical situations, but the precise pathophysiological mechanisms are unclear.

Osteomalacia

Weakness is the presenting symptom in one-third of patients, affecting predominantly the pelvic girdle musculature. Bone pain is prominent. The serum creatine kinase level is usually normal. Muscle biopsy may show type II fibre atrophy, sometimes severe.

The pain responds fairly rapidly to vitamin D treatment, but the weakness recovers more slowly and may be incomplete.

Primary hyperparathyroidism

Myalgia, stiffness, and complaints of fatigue are common, but overt weakness is rare. Symptoms resolve when the underlying parathyroid adenoma is removed and serum calcium levels fall.

Renal osteodystrophy

Endstage renal failure is frequently accompanied by a predominantly pelvic girdle myopathy, sometimes with buttock and thigh pain. Symptoms respond to dialysis, transplantation, or vitamin D treatment.

Dialysis osteodystrophy

Some patients undergoing dialysis develop a severe myopathy with bone pain, fractures, and vitamin D resistance. It probably relates to aluminium toxicity. Fatigue and muscle weakness are common. Objective muscle testing is needed to distinguish true changes in muscle function from the non-specific causes of fatigue and ill health seen in patients on dialysis.

Ischaemic myopathy

Rarely, a painful ischaemic myopathy with arterial narrowing due to calcium deposition complicates renal failure. Skin ulceration and bowel infarction may also occur.

Nutritional and toxic myopathies

Whilst malnutrition causes muscle wasting, specific myopathic effects of nutritional deficiencies are uncommon, a notable exception being vitamin D deficiency, discussed above. Myopathies due to ingested toxins are relatively more common than the inherited metabolic myopathies and include those due to alcohol, and therapeutic-drug excess or idiosyncrasy.

Alcoholic myopathies

Chronic alcoholics may develop subacute or slowly progressive, proximal muscle weakness with mild-to-moderate wasting, and with muscle-biopsy evidence of type II fibre atrophy, mainly affecting the lower limbs. Occasionally the wasting is more generalized, since alcoholism may be associated with neurogenic muscle atrophy secondary to concomitant thiamin deficiency and more generalized malnutrition. It is thus still debated whether the so-called chronic alcoholic myopathy is purely myopathic, neuropathic, or both, and whether the cause is a direct toxic effect of alcohol or a secondary phenomenon, perhaps relating to malnutrition. Abstinence may lead to some degree of recovery.

Much more dramatic is acute alcoholic myopathy ('alcoholic rhabdomyolysis'), which usually occurs during or shortly following a binge. There may be widespread cramps, pain, and weakness. However, the most striking feature is the development of extremely painful muscle swelling, which may be localized or generalized. Myoglobinuria presents a threat to renal function, and hyperkalaemia may be present in severe cases. The serum creatine kinase is elevated and muscle biopsy shows acute necrosis. Recovery, which may be incomplete, occurs over several weeks.

Vitamin E deficiency

Vitamin E deficiency probably causes a myopathy, but interpretation is confused by the presence of additional neurological problems including neuropathy and ataxia.

Drug-induced myopathies

Drug-induced neuromuscular disorders are common, under-recognized and under-reported. Numerous drugs have been implicated, several mechanisms are responsible (Table 2), and some drugs can affect both muscle and peripheral nerves (for example, vincristine, D-penicillamine, and perhexiline).

Skeletal-muscle channelopathies

The term 'channelopathy' has come into common usage since the last edition of this textbook. Ion channels may be ligand-gated or voltage-gated. In the field of muscle diseases, the most important ligand-gated channel is the skeletal-muscle nicotinic acetylcholine receptor, at the neuromuscular junction. Antibody-mediated destruction underlies acquired myasthenia gravis, whereas inherited mutations of genes coding for the subunits of the receptor are the basis of several forms of congenital myasthenic syndrome. Acquired neuromyotonia and Lambert–Eaton myasthenic syndrome are caused by antibody-mediated damage to the voltage-gated potassium and calcium channels, respectively, of the terminal axon, and are discussed, together with myasthenia gravis and the myasthenic syndromes, in Chapter 24.17.

The following section is concerned with inherited disorders of skeletal-muscle voltage-gated sodium, calcium, and chloride channels. In passing, it should be noted that channelopathies are not confined to muscle, and note was made above of two neuronal channelopathies. Other disorders caused by an inherited channel defect include certain forms of epilepsy (nocturnal frontal lobe epilepsy, benign neonatal convulsions), episodic ataxia, hemiplegic migraine, deafness, night-blindness, cardiac long-QT syndromes, and nephrolithiasis.

Periodic paralyses

Marked hypokalaemia and hyperkalaemia from whatever cause may produce weakness or paralysis (secondary periodic paralysis). The primary periodic paralyses are familial, dominantly inherited disorders characterized by recurrent attacks of paralysis. These have previously been subdivided into hyperkalaemic, hypokalaemic, and normokalaemic forms on the basis of changes in the serum potassium level during attacks. Recent evidence has shown that the primary abnormality in the hyperkalaemic and normokalaemic forms is a mutation affecting the adult skeletal-muscle sodium channel, whereas the hypokalaemic form is caused by a mutation affecting the skeletal-muscle calcium channel.

Hypokalaemic periodic paralysis

Attacks usually start during the second decade of life and then vary in frequency from daily to years between episodes. Weakness may be present on waking or develop during the day, typically in response to a heavy carbohydrate meal or during rest after strenuous exercise. The weakness involves the legs more than the arms, proximal muscles more than distal, and it may be asymmetrical. Bulbar and respiratory muscle weakness is rare. Attacks last from hours to several days. The tendon reflexes may be depressed or lost during an attack. Permanent and progressive proximal weakness often develops by middle age. The serum potassium level typically falls during an attack, but not necessarily outside the normal range.

Table 2 Drug-induced myopathies

Focal damage/fibrosis	Intramuscular – opiates – antibiotics – paraldehyde
Necrosis	Heroin Clofibrate ε-aminocaproic acid
Myoglobinuria/rhabdomyolysis	Heroin Methadone Amphetamines Barbiturates Diazepam Isoniazid Carbenoxolone Phenformin Amphotericin B
Inflammatory myopathy	Procainamide D-Penicillamine
Hypokalaemic weakness	Diuretics Carbenoxolone Liquorice Purgatives
Subacute or painless proximal myopathy	Corticosteroids Chloroquine β-Blockers
Myasthenia	D-penicillamine Aminoglycosides
Malignant hyperthermia	Suxamethonium Cyclopropane Halothane Enflurane Ketamine

The disorder is caused by a mutation in the *CACNA1S* gene (on chromosome 1) encoding the dihydropyridine receptor (**DHPR**) component of the skeletal-muscle calcium channel. The DHPR is located within the transverse tubular system, and acts as a voltage-sensor for the ryanodine receptor (RYR1) component of the calcium channel, which is located in the sarcoplasmic reticulum and is responsible for triggering calcium release and thus muscle contraction. Different mutations in the same gene, and mutations in the *RYR1* gene, are associated with malignant hyperthermia (see below).

Acetazolamide is the treatment of choice to prevent attacks. Acute attacks respond to oral potassium, given as an unsweetened aqueous solution.

Apparently-identical attacks may occur in association with thyrotoxicosis and resolve when the patient is rendered euthyroid.

Hyperkalaemic periodic paralysis

Attacks tend to start at an earlier age than in the hypokalaemic form, and do not last as long. Precipitants include cold, fasting, rest after exercise, pregnancy, alcohol intake, and potassium loading. Readily utilized carbohydrate sources, such as a sweet drink, may abort an attack. A progressive proximal myopathy may also develop. Myotonia is present in some patients (see below). The serum potassium level may rise during an attack, but the change is often slight.

The underlying abnormality is a mutation within the *SCNA4* gene (on chromosome 17) encoding the α-subunit of the skeletal-muscle sodium channel.

Mild attacks respond to carbohydrate ingestion. Kaliuretic diuretics usually prevent attacks.

Paramyotonia congenita

Paramyotonia congenita describes a dominantly inherited condition characterized by cold-induced weakness and muscle stiffness (paramyotonia), and which is sometimes accompanied by periodic paralysis. The relationship between this disorder and primary hyperkalaemic periodic paralysis had been much debated, but recent evidence has shown that hyperkalaemic periodic paralysis, hyperkalaemic periodic paralysis with myotonia, paramyotonia congenita, and paramyotonia congenita with periodic paralysis are allelic disorders involving the *SCNA4* gene (on chromosome 17) encoding the α-subunit of the skeletal-muscle sodium channel.

Myotonia congenita

Autosomal dominant (Thomsen's disease) and recessive (Becker-type) forms of this condition are recognized, with the recessive type being much commoner. Onset tends to be earlier in the dominant form but both usually become apparent in childhood. There is muscle stiffness, worse after rest and exacerbated by cold; minimal or no weakness, readily demonstrable percussion myotonia; and muscle hypertrophy, which tends to be more marked in the recessive form.

Both the recessive and dominant forms are caused by mutations in the *CLCN1* gene (on chromosome 7) encoding the skeletal-muscle chloride channel.

Malignant hyperthermia (MH)

The main features of this autosomal dominant disorder are a rapidly rising body temperature and generalized muscular rigidity during anaesthesia. Additional features include skin mottling, cyanosis, tachypnoea, tachycardia, cardiac dysrhythmias, and autonomic instability. Attacks in susceptible individuals may be triggered by suxamethonium and anaesthetic agents (halothane, cyclopropane, enflurane, ketamine). A similar, but probably different, disorder may be associated with heavy exercise in very hot conditions (for example, recruits undergoing route marches on mountains during a hot summer).

Attacks are life-threatening. Treatment consists of withdrawing the offending agent and providing general supportive measures and intravenous dantrolene (2 mg/kg body weight).

Disturbed calcium homeostasis underlies the attacks, with excessive calcium-ion influx into the sarcoplasmic reticulum. The disorder is genetically heterogeneous. In many families the underlying abnormality affects the skeletal-muscle calcium channel with either a mutation in the ryanodine receptor (*RYR1*) gene (on chromosome 19), or in the *CACNA1S* gene (on chromosome 1). *RYR1* mutations may also cause central core disease (**CCD**)—CCD and MH are allelic disorders and may occur together in the same individual or independently. Other *CACNA1S* gene mutations cause hypokalaemic periodic paralysis.

Screening for MH susceptibility involves muscle biopsy and *in vitro* testing for a reduced contractile threshold to halothane and caffeine. False-positive results are common but false-negative results appear to be very rare. It is hoped that specific molecular biological tests will become available. A significant practical problem is the management of family members who fear they may be at risk. As with those patients who have suffered hyperpyrexia under anaesthesia (even in whom repeated exposure has not led to a consistent re-occurrence), it is advisable for those individuals of proven or suspected risk to wear at all times some form of bracelet or locket giving details of the risk, in case they are casualties in an emergency such as a road accident.

Myoglobinuria

This important symptom and sign must be differentiated from haematuria and haemoglobinuria. Red cells are visible on microscopy in the former but not in the latter. In all three conditions, the haemoperoxidase stick test is positive.

Myoglobin is a protein that acts as an oxygen store within skeletal-muscle fibres. Myoglobinuria causes a dark-brown/red discoloration of the urine, the main concern being that the protein can cause renal tubular necrosis and thus renal failure. Numerous disorders are known to be associated with myoglobinuria (Table 3). In the metabolic disorders, the presumed mechanism is failure of substrate utilization or supply when energy demands increase during exercise or starvation. In other disorders, there is disruption of the plasma membrane. Apparently idiopathic cases are probably due to an unidentified metabolic defect or infection.

Table 3 Causes of myoglobinuria

Metabolic	Glycogenoses Carnitine palmitoyl transferase deficiency Severe electrolyte disturbance
Excessive activity/ temperature	Marathon running Military training Status epilepticus Malignant hyperthermia Neuroleptic malignant syndrome
Drugs and toxins	Several drugs (see Table 1) Venoms and animal toxins
Infection	Viral Toxic shock Clostridial infection/gangrene
Ischaemia and trauma	Crush Coma Any cause of severe ischaemia Compartment syndrome Electric shock
Inflammatory myopathies	Dermatomyositis Polymyositis

Rhabdomyolysis is considered further in Section 28.

Further reading

General

Brooke MH (1986). *A clinician's view of neuromuscular diseases*, 2nd edn. Williams and Wilkins, Baltimore.

Engel AG, Franzini-Armstrong C, eds (1994). *Myology*, 2nd edn. McGraw-Hill, New York.

Karpati G, Hilton-Jones D, Griggs R, eds (2001). *Disorders of voluntary muscle*, 7th edn. Cambridge University Press.

Lane RJM, ed. (1996). *Handbook of muscle disease.* Marcel Dekker, New York.

Scheinberg IH, Walshe JM, eds (1986). *Orphan diseases and orphan drugs.* Fulbright Papers 3. Manchester University Press.

WHO (1980). *International classification of impairments, disabilities, and handicaps.* World Health Organization, Geneva.

WHO (2000). *International classification of functioning and disability ICIDH-2.* http://www3.who.int/icf/icftemplate

Metabolic myopathies

Angelini C (1990). Defects of fatty-acid oxidation in muscle. *Ballière's Clinical Endocrinology and Metabolism* **4**, 561–82.

Barsy T, Hers H-G (1990). Normal metabolism and disorders of carbohydrate metabolism. *Ballière's Clinical Endocrinology and Metabolism* **4**, 499–522.

Bartram C, *et al.* (1994). McArdle's disease: a rare frameshift mutation in exon 1 of the muscle glycogen phosphorylase gene. *Biochimica et Biophysica Acta* **1226**, 341–3.

Hilton-Jones D, *et al.*, eds (1995). *Metabolic myopathies.* WB Saunders, London.

Layzer RB (1990). Muscle metabolism during fatigue and work. *Ballière's Clinical Endocrinology and Metabolism* **4**, 441–59.

Wagenmakers AJM, Coakley JH, Edwards RHT (1988). The metabolic consequences of reduced habitual activities in patients with muscle pain and disease. *Ergonomics* **31**, 1519–27.

Endocrine myopathies

Fells P (1991). Thyroid-associated eye disease: clinical management. *Lancet* **338**, 29–32.

Ruff RL, Weissmann J (1988). Endocrine myopathies. *Neurologic Clinics* **6**, 575–92.

Weetman AP (1991). Thyroid-associated eye disease: pathophysiology. *Lancet* **338**, 25–8.

Nutritional and toxic myopathies

Argov Z, Mastaglia FL (1994). Drug-induced neuromuscular disorders in man. In: Walton JN, Karpati G, Hilton-Jones D, eds. *Disorders of voluntary muscle*, 6th edn, pp 989–1029. Churchill Livingstone, Edinburgh.

Channelopathies

Ebers GC, *et al.* (1991). Paramyotonia congenita and hyperkalemic periodic paralysis are linked to the adult muscle sodium channel gene. *Annals of Neurology* **30**, 810–16.

Fontaine B, *et al.* (1990). Hyperkalemic periodic paralysis and the adult muscle sodium channel a-subunit gene. *Science* **250,** 1000–2.

Fontaine B, *et al.* (1991). Different gene loci for hyperkalemic and hypokalemic periodic paralysis. *Neuromuscular Disorders* **1**, 235–8.

Greenberg DA (1997). Calcium channels in neurological disease. *Annals of Neurology* **42**, 275–82.

Gronert GA (1980). Malignant hyperthermia. *Anesthesiology* **53,** 395–423.

Koch MC, *et al.* (1992). The skeletal muscle chloride channel in dominant and recessive human myotonia. *Science* **257,** 797–800.

Lehmann-Horn F, Jurkat-Rott K (1999). Voltage-gated ion channels and hereditary disease. *Physiological Reviews* **79**, 1317–72.

MacLennan DH, *et al.* (1990). Ryanodine receptor gene is a candidate for predisposition to malignant hyperthermia. *Nature* **343,** 559–61.

Myoglobinuria

Penn, AS (1986). Myoglobinuria. In: Engel AG, Banker BQ, eds. *Myology*, pp 1785–805. McGraw-Hill, New York.

24.22.5 Mitochondrial encephalomyopathies

P. F. Chinnery and D. M. Turnbull

Introduction

Mitochondria are ubiquitous intracellular organelles that are involved in many different metabolic pathways. Disorders of intermediary metabolism (such as fatty acid β-oxidation or tricarboxylic acid cycle defects) involve mitochondrial enzymes, but the term 'mitochondrial encephalomyopathy' usually means a disease which is due to an abnormality of the final common pathway of energy metabolism—the mitochondrial respiratory chain. The respiratory chain is essential for aerobic metabolism, and respiratory chain defects characteristically affect tissues and organs that are heavily dependent upon oxidative metabolism (such as the central nervous system, the eye, skeletal muscle, myocardium, and endocrine organs).

Recent studies have demonstrated the central role of the mitochondrion in the pathophysiology of well-established diseases such as Friedreich's ataxia and Wilson's disease, but these are not primarily disorders of the mitochondrial respiratory chain and are not considered here.

Biochemistry and genetics of the respiratory chain

The intermediary metabolism of carbohydrates, amino acids, and fatty acids generates the reduced cofactors NADH, NADPH, and $FADH_2$. These cofactors transfer electrons to the mitochondrial respiratory chain. As the electrons are passed through complexes I to IV of the respiratory chain along the inner mitochondrial membrane, protons are pumped out of the mitochondrial matrix into the intermembrane space. This creates an electrochemical gradient that is harnessed by complex V (ATP synthase) to generate ATP from ADP. Each respiratory chain complex contains many polypeptide subunits, some of which are coded by genes within the nucleus and some of which are encoded by the mitochondrial genome. Although all of the polypeptides encoded in mitochondrial DNA (**mtDNA**) have been known for over a decade, many nuclear genes involved in mitochondrial biogenesis have yet to be characterized.

The mitochondrial genome encodes seven complex I subunits (NADH-ubiquinone oxidoreductase), one of the complex III subunits (ubiquinol-cytochrome *c* oxidoreductase), three of the complex IV (cytochrome *c* oxidase, or **COX**) subunits, and the ATPase 6 and ATPase 8 subunits of complex V. Interspaced between the protein-encoding genes are two ribosomal RNA genes (12S and 16S rRNA), and 22 transfer RNA genes that provide the necessary RNA components for the mitochondrial translation machinery. The remaining polypeptides, including all of the complex II subunits, are synthesized from nuclear gene transcripts within the cytosol. These are subsequently imported into the mitochondria through the inner and outer membrane translocation complexes. There are many additional proteins that are essential for the normal assembly and function of the mitochondrial respiratory chain. As a result, mitochondrial respiratory chain disorders can be due to mutations affecting both nuclear and mitochondrial genes.

The classification and investigation of mitochondrial respiratory chain disorders has been revolutionized by the recent advances in our understanding of the underlying genetic defects. By the year 2000, over 70 different point mutations and over 100 different deletions of mtDNA had been associated with a wide variety of different diseases. One factor that contributes to the frequency of mitochondrial mutations is the absence in mitochondrial DNA polymerase of the 'proof-reading' property of nuclear DNA polymerase where exonuclease activity greatly enhances the fidelity of replication. Very recently a number of nuclear genetic defects have been identified in some patients with respiratory chain defects (Table 1).

Basic mitochondrial genetics

There are two main differences between nuclear DNA and mtDNA that are important for the expression and transmission of mitochondrial genetic disease, as follows.

Heteroplasmy and the threshold effect

Each mammalian cell contains over 1000 copies of the small (16.5 kb) mitochondrial genome; there are on average 5 to 15 mtDNA molecules in each organelle. Individuals with mtDNA disease often harbour a mixture of

Table 1 Genetic basis of mitochondrial encephalomyopathies

Nuclear DNA defects

Nuclear genetic disorders of the mitochondrial respiratory chain:
- Leigh syndrome (complex I deficiency—mutations in AQDQ subunit on Chr 5)
- Optic atrophy and ataxia (complex II deficiency—mutations in Fp subunit of SDH on Chr 3)
- Leigh syndrome (complex IV deficiency—mutations in *SURF I* gene on Chr 9q1)

Nuclear genetic disorders associated with multiple mtDNA deletions:
- Autosomal dominant external ophthalmoplegia (mutations in *POLG*, *TWINKLE*, and *ANT1*)
- Mitochondrial neurogastrointestinal encephalomyopathy (thymidine phosphorylase deficiency—mutations in thymidine phosphorylase gene on Chr 22q13.32-qter)

Mitochondrial DNA defects

Rearrangements (deletions and duplications):
- Chronic progressive external ophthalmoplegia
- Kearns–Sayre syndrome
- Diabetes and deafness

Point mutations:*
- Protein-encoding genes
  - Leber's hereditary optic neuropathy (G11778A, T14484C, G3460A)
  - Neurogenic weakness with ataxia and retinitis pigmentosa/Leigh syndrome (T8993G/C)
- tRNA genes
  - MELAS (A3243G, T3271C, A3251G)
  - MERRF (A8344G, T8356C)
  - Chronic progressive external ophthalmoplegia (A3243G, T4274C)
  - Myopathy (T14709C, A12320G)
  - Cardiomyopathy (A3243G, A4269G)
  - Diabetes and deafness (A3243G, C12258A)
  - Encephalomyopathy (G1606A, T10010C)
- rRNA genes
  - Non-syndromic sensorineural deafness (A7445G)
  - Aminoglycoside-induced non-syndromic deafness (A1555G)

* mtDNA nucleotide positions refer to the L-chain.

mutated and wild-type (normal) mtDNA—a situation known as heteroplasmy. Single cells only express a respiratory chain defect when the proportion of mutated mtDNA exceeds a critical threshold. Different organs, and even adjacent cells within the same organ, may contain different amounts of mutated mtDNA. This variability, coupled with tissue-specific differences in the threshold and the varied dependence of different organs on oxidative metabolism, explains in part why certain tissues are preferentially affected in patients with mtDNA disease. In general, postmitotic (non-dividing) tissues such as neurones, skeletal and cardiac muscle, and endocrine organs harbour much higher levels of mutated mtDNA and are often clinically involved. In contrast, rapidly dividing tissues such as the bone marrow are only rarely clinically affected (one example is Pearson's syndrome—see below).

Maternal inheritance and the transmission of heteroplasmy

After fertilization of the oocyte, sperm mtDNA is actively degraded. As a consequence, mtDNA is transmitted exclusively down the maternal line. This means that affected males with mtDNA disease cannot transmit the genetic defect. Deleted molecules are rarely, if ever, transmitted from clinically affected females to their offspring. By contrast, a female harbouring a heteroplasmic mtDNA point mutation, or mtDNA duplications, may transmit a variable amount of mutated mtDNA to her children. Early during development of the female germ line, the number of mtDNA molecules within each oocyte is reduced before being subsequently amplified to reach a final number of around 100 000 in each mature oocyte. This restriction and amplification (also called the mitochondrial 'genetic bottleneck') contributes to the variability between individual oocytes, and the different levels of mutant mtDNA seen in the offspring of a single female.

Clinical presentation of respiratory chain disorders

Mitochondrial encephalomyopathies are highly variable both clinically and at the genetic level. The same clinical syndrome can be caused by different genetic defects (which may be within nuclear or mitochondrial genes), but the same genetic defect may present in a variety of different ways. In general, adults who present with mitochondrial disease are often found to have a defect of mtDNA. Children often present with different clinical features and are more likely to have a nuclear genetic defect. It is often possible to identify well-defined clinical syndromes, but many patients present with a collection of clinical features that are highly suggestive of respiratory chain disease but do not fit into a discrete clinical category.

Defined clinical syndromes (Table 2)

Large-scale deletions can cause chronic progressive external ophthalmoplegia and bilateral ptosis. Some of these patients have minimal disability and may have limited skeletal muscle involvement. In contrast, similar deletions may also cause chronic progressive external ophthalmoplegia with bilateral sensorineural deafness, cerebellar ataxia, pigmentary retinopathy, diabetes mellitus, and cardiac conduction defects leading to complete heart block. When this begins in teenage years and is associated with a raised cerebrospinal fluid protein, it is called the Kearns–Sayre syndrome, which is a progressive neurological disorder associated with severe disability. Hypoparathyroidism and hypothyroidism are well-recognized features of Kearns–Sayre syndrome. The vast majority of cases of chronic progressive external ophthalmoplegia and Kearns–Sayre syndrome are sporadic. These two syndromes are the extremes of a spectrum of disease and many individuals lie somewhere between the pure extraocular muscle and severe central neurological phenotypes.

Table 2 Clinical syndromes

Disorder	Primary features	Additional features
Chronic progressive external ophthalmoplegia	External ophthalmoplegia and bilateral ptosis	Mild proximal myopathy
Kearns–Sayre syndrome	Progressive external ophthalmoplegia onset before age 20 with pigmentary retinopathy Plus one of the following: cerebrospinal fluid protein greater than 1 g/l, cerebellar ataxia, or heart block	Bilateral deafness Myopathy Dysphagia Diabetes mellitus Hypoparathyroidism Dementia
Pearson's syndome	Sideroblastic anaemia of childhood Pancytopenia Exocrine pancreatic failure	Renal tubular defects
Mitochondrial encephalomyopathy with lactic acidosis and stroke-like episodes (MELAS)	Stroke-like episodes before age 40 years Seizures and/or dementia Ragged-red fibres and/or lactic acidosis	Diabetes mellitus Cardiomyopathy (hypertrophic leading to dilated) Bilateral deafness Pigmentary retinopathy Cerebellar ataxia
Myoclonic epilepsy with ragged-red fibres (MERRF)	Myoclonus Seizures Cerebellar ataxia Myopathy	Dementia Optic atrophy Bilateral deafness Peripheral neuropathy Spasticity Multiple lipomas
Leber's hereditary optic neuropathy	Subacute bilateral visual failure Males:females approximately 4:1 Median age of onset 24 years	Dystonia Cardiac pre-excitation syndromes
Leigh syndrome	Subacute relapsing encephalopathy with cerebellar and brainstem signs	Basal ganglia lucencies
Infantile myopathy and lactic acidosis (fatal and non-fatal forms)	Hypotonia in the first year of life Feeding and respiratory difficulties	Fatal form may be associated with a cardiomyopathy and/or the Toni–Fanconi–Debre syndrome

Pearson's syndrome of exocrine pancreatic failure, sideroblastic anaemia, and marrow panhypoplasia is usually due to a mtDNA deletion. Pearson's syndrome usually presents in infancy and a number of individuals who have survived into later childhood subsequently developed the Kearns–Sayre phenotype.

Pathogenic point mutations of mtDNA are more common than rearrangements. This is partly because mtDNA deletions cause sporadic disease, whereas many mtDNA point mutations are transmitted down the maternal line. The A3243G mutation in the leucine (UUR) tRNA gene was first described in a patient with mitochondrial encephalomyopathy with lactic acidosis and stroke-like episodes (MELAS). Different families harbouring the same genetic defect may have different phenotypes. For example, some families harbouring A3243G have predominantly diabetes and deafness, some families have chronic progressive external ophthalmoplegia, and some present with a cardiomyopathy. It is currently not known why this is the case but it is likely that additional nuclear genetic factors play an important role in modifying the expression of the primary mtDNA defect. This single mutation is important since it has been estimated that between 0.5 and 1.5 per cent of cases of diabetes mellitus in the general population are associated with the A3243G mutation.

Patients may present with myoclonic epilepsy, ataxia, optic atrophy, and have ragged-red fibres in skeletal muscle (MERRF) and this may also be due to a point mutation of mtDNA (for example A8344G).

mtDNA mutations are the major cause of visual loss in young adult males. About half of all males who harbour one of three point mutations of mtDNA (G11778A, T14484C, G3460A) develop bilateral sequential visual loss in the second or third decade—a disorder known as Leber's hereditary optic neuropathy (LHON). The majority of individuals with these mutations are homoplasmic—harbouring only mutated mtDNA. It is not clear why the disease only affects approximately half of the males and 10 per cent of females who inherit the primary mtDNA defect. Environmental factors, such as alcohol and tobacco, partly explain the variable penetrance of this disorder; however, additional, as yet unknown, nuclear genetic factors may also be important.

Leigh syndrome (subacute necrotizing encephalomyopathy) is a relapsing encephalopathy with prominent cerebellar and brainstem signs that usually presents in childhood and is associated with characteristic neuroimaging abnormalities involving the basal ganglia. Leigh syndrome can be due to an X-linked pyruvate dehydrogenase deficiency or a defect of the mitochondrial respiratory chain. Complex I deficiency or COX deficiency are common findings in Leigh syndrome. In these patients it may be possible to identify recessive mutations in nuclear complex I genes, or genes involved in the assembly of the respiratory chain complexes (for example *SURF 1*). Point mutations at position 8993 in the ATPase 6 gene of mtDNA may cause neurogenic weakness with ataxia and retinitis pigmentosa. These particular mutations are also associated with some forms of childhood Leigh syndrome.

COX deficiency may also present in childhood with an infantile myopathy and a severe lactic acidosis, which may also be associated with a cardiomyopathy and the Toni–Fanconi–Debre syndrome. Despite maximal supportive intervention, this is usually a fatal disorder and a severe depletion of mtDNA occurs in a proportion of these cases. It is important to recognize that isolated myopathy and lactic acidosis may be self-limiting, often with a significant improvement by 1 year of age and complete resolution by the age of 3 years.

Non-specific clinical presentations

Although the foregoing diseases and numerous other syndromes may strongly suggest a mitochondrial aetiology (Fig. 1 and Table 2), many patients do not present with a characteristic phenotype. Children may present in the neonatal period with a metabolic encephalopathy and systemic lactic acidosis, often associated with hepatic and cardiac failure. This may be associated with a depletion in the total amount of mtDNA within affected tissues. Although this syndrome may be fatal, in some it is a self-limiting disorder. Childhood presentations may be even less specific, with neonatal hypotonia, feeding and respiratory difficulties, and failure to thrive. A respiratory chain defect should be considered in any patient who has a disease with multiple organ involvement, particularly if there are central neurological features (such as seizures and dementia), a myopathy, cardiomyopathy, and endocrine abnormalities such as diabetes mellitus (Fig. 1). Bilateral sensorineural deafness and ocular features (retinopathy, optic atrophy, ptosis, and ophthalmoparesis) are common. Renal tubular defects, gastrointestinal hypomotility, cervical lipomatosis, and psychiatric features are also well described in patients with respiratory chain disease.

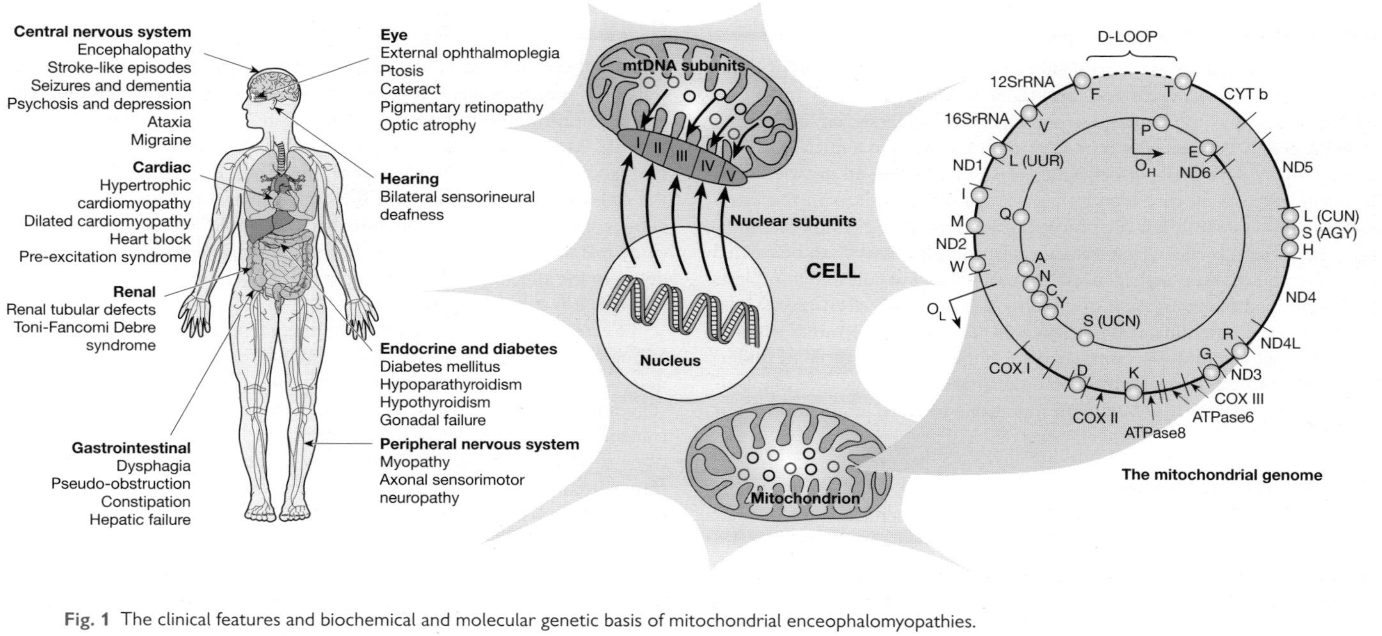

Fig. 1 The clinical features and biochemical and molecular genetic basis of mitochondrial enceophalomyopathies.

Investigation of respiratory chain disease

The investigation of patients with a suspected mitochondrial encephalomyopathy involves the careful assimilation of clinical and laboratory data. In a significant proportion of cases (such as Leber's hereditary optic neuropathy), it is possible to identify a specific clinical syndrome with a clear maternal family history. Under these circumstances it is appropriate to carry out a molecular genetic test on a blood sample. In many situations, particularly in sporadic cases, this is not appropriate because the clinical features overlap with those of many other disorders. Even if the patient has a mitochondrial disorder, numerous different genetic defects may be responsible, some of which will not be detectable by analysis of blood samples.

Investigations fall into two main groups: clinical investigations used to characterize the pattern and nature of the different organs involved, and specific investigations to identify the biochemical or genetic abnormality.

General clinical investigations

It is essential to search for the more common features of respiratory chain disease. This includes cardiac assessment (ECG and echocardiography) and endocrine assessment (oral glucose tolerance test, thyroid function tests, alkaline phosphatase, fasting calcium, and parathyroid hormone levels). The organic and amino acids in urine may be abnormal even in the absence of overt tubular disease. Measuring blood and cerebrospinal fluid lactate levels is more helpful in the investigation of children than adults. These measurements must be interpreted with caution because there are many causes of blood and cerebrospinal fluid lactic acidosis, including fever, sepsis, dehydration, seizures, and stroke. The cerebrospinal fluid protein may be elevated. The serum creatine kinase level may be raised but is often normal. Neurophysiological studies may identify a myopathy or neuropathy. Electroencephalography may reveal diffuse slow-wave activity consistent with a subacute encephalopathy, or evidence of seizure activity. Cerebral imaging may be abnormal, showing lesions of the basal ganglia, high signal in the white matter on MRI, or generalized cerebral atrophy.

Specific investigations

A skeletal muscle biopsy is invaluable in the investigation of respiratory chain disease. Histochemical and biochemical investigations, in conjunction with the clinical assessment, often indicate where the underlying genetic abnormality must lie.

Histochemistry and biochemistry

Histochemical analysis may reveal subsarcolemmal accumulation of mitochondria (so-called 'ragged-red' fibres), or COX deficiency. A mosaic of COX-positive and COX-negative muscle fibres suggests an underlying mtDNA defect. Patients who have COX deficiency due to a nuclear genetic defect usually have a global deficiency of COX affecting all muscle fibres. Electron microscopy may identify paracrystalline inclusions in the intermembrane space, but these are non-specific and may be seen in other non-mitochondrial disorders. Respiratory chain complex assays can be carried out on various tissues. Skeletal muscle is preferable, but cultured fibroblasts are useful in the investigation of childhood mitochondrial disease. Measurement of the individual respiratory chain complexes determines whether an individual has multiple complex defects that would suggest an underlying mtDNA defect, involving either a tRNA gene or a large deletion. Isolated complex defects may be due to mutations in either mitochondrial or nuclear genes.

Molecular genetic investigations

Under certain circumstances, the clinical and biochemical features may point towards a specific genetic defect, and it may be possible to detect this abnormality in a blood sample. Children presenting with Leigh syndrome and who have an isolated deficiency of one of the respiratory chain subunits may have a point mutation within the nuclear-encoded respiratory chain subunit or assembly genes. These have been identified by direct sequencing of the appropriate exons.

For some mtDNA defects (particularly mtDNA deletions) the abnormality is not detectable in a DNA sample extracted from blood, and the analysis of DNA extracted from muscle is essential to establish the diagnosis. The first stage is to look for mtDNA rearrangements or mtDNA depletion by Southern blot analysis and long-range polymerase chain reaction (**PCR**). This is followed by PCR or restriction fragment length polymorphism analysis for common point mutations. Many patients with mitochondrial disease have a previously unrecognized mtDNA defect and it is necessary to sequence directly the mitochondrial genome. Interpretation of the sequence data can be extremely difficult. mtDNA is highly polymorphic and any two normal individuals may differ by up to 60 base pairs. In the strictest sense, a mutation can only be considered to be pathogenic if it has arisen independently several times in the population, it is not seen in controls, and it is associated with a potential disease mechanism. These stringent criteria depend upon a good knowledge of polymorphic sites in the background population. If a novel base change is heteroplasmic, this suggests that it is of relatively recent onset. Family, tissue segregation, and single cell studies may show that higher levels of the mutation are associated with mitochondrial dysfunction and disease, which strongly suggests that the mutation is causing the disease.

Management

There is currently no definitive treatment for patients with mitochondrial disease. Management is aimed at minimizing disability, preventing complications, and genetic counselling.

Supportive care and surveillance

Many patients with mitochondrial disorders require follow-up over many decades. An integrated approach is essential involving the primary physician, other specialist physicians (ophthalmology, diabetes, and cardiology), specialist nurses, physiotherapists, and speech therapists. Vigilant clinical monitoring over many years can prevent the development of complications, such as those secondary to cardiac and endocrine involvement. Specific procedures may be indicated at various stages of disease. These include cardiac pacing, ptosis correction, cataract surgery, and percutaneous gastrostomy.

Genetic counselling

The detailed investigation of patients with respiratory chain disease usually leads to a specific molecular genetic diagnosis, particularly in adults. This has profound implications on the counselling given to patients and their families. Most children with respiratory chain disease are compound heterozygotes with recessive nuclear gene mutations. If it is possible to identify the causative mutations in both the offspring and parents, then this will allow confident genetic counselling for the whole family. If, as in many cases, it is not possible to identify the underlying gene defect, or the genetic defect in the affected child cannot be traced back to the parents, then counselling is less straightforward.

If a causative mtDNA defect is identified, then the implications for counselling are distinctly different. Males cannot transmit pathogenic mtDNA defects. Patients who carry mtDNA deletions rarely have a family history suggestive of mtDNA disease, and there is no significant risk that they will transmit the mtDNA defect to any offspring. There are a few rare exceptions to this rule where the propensity to develop mtDNA deletions is transmitted as an autosomal dominant or autosomal recessive trait. By contrast, women harbouring pathogenic mtDNA point mutations may transmit the genetic defect to their offspring. The mitochondrial genetic 'bottleneck' leads to a variation in the proportion of mutated mtDNA that is transmitted to any offspring (see above). It is therefore possible for a female to have mildly affected as well as severely affected children. The risk of having affected offspring varies from mutation to mutation, and although there does appear to be a relationship between the level of mutated mtDNA in the mother and the risk of affected offspring, there are insufficient data from prospective studies to allow accurate risk prediction.

Prognosis

In general the prognosis depends upon the extent of central neurological involvement. Patients with Leber's hereditary optic neuropathy rarely have significant central neurological features and have a normal lifespan. The prospect for visual recovery varies. After the initial nadir, individuals harbouring the G11778A mutation are the least likely to regain functional vision, whilst those harbouring the T14484C mutation are the most likely to regain their sight.

Children presenting with an encephalopathy have a poor prognosis. Although residual neurological deficits are common after repeated childhood encephalopathic episodes, the disease may enter a more stable 'chronic' phase during teenage years and adulthood. A similar course may be seen in adults presenting with a relapsing encephalopathy. In contrast, a large proportion of adults with mtDNA defects and chronic progressive external ophthalmoplegia have very mild disease that may remain limited to the extraocular muscles for many decades. For certain mutations, there also appears to be a relationship between the proportion of mutated mtDNA in skeletal muscle and the severity of the disease. Although the proportion of mutated mtDNA in muscle may give some guide to prognosis, there is insufficient information available to allow accurate prognostic counselling based upon these determinations. A significant proportion of patients have distinct phenotypes associated with unique genetic defects and the prognosis must be guarded in these families.

Pharmacological treatments and novel approaches under development

Standard doses of vitamin C and K, thiamine, riboflavin, and ubiquinone (coenzyme Q10) may be of some benefit. These treatments have no significant side-effects and are relatively cheap, but their efficacy is largely based upon anecdotal reports. Novel treatments are, however, under development. Dichloracetate can be used to reduce lactic acid levels but may cause an irreversible toxic neuropathy. The efficacy of dichloracetate is currently being assessed in clinical trials. Exercise is important for patients with mtDNA disease, and isometric muscle contraction may lead to an improvement in muscle strength. Drug-induced muscle necrosis followed by proliferation of myoblasts may also be important for the treatment of mitochondrial myopathy and ptosis, but this approach is only at the experimental stage. Finally, several centres are investigating methods for correcting the underlying mtDNA defect by gene therapy.

Further reading

Anderson S *et al.* (1981). Sequence and organization of the human mitochondrial genome. *Nature* **290**, 457–65.

Andrews RM *et al.* (1999). Reanalysis and revision of the Cambridge Reference Sequence. *Nature Genetics* **23**, 147. [Benchmark reference sequences for normal human mtDNA.]

Chinnery PF *et al.* (1998). MELAS and MERRF: the relationship between maternal mutation load and the frequency of clinically affected offspring. *Brain* **121**, 1889–94. [First paper to show a relationship between maternal mutation load and the outcome of pregnancy.]

Chinnery PF *et al.* (1999). Clinical mitochondrial genetics. *Journal of Medical Genetics* **36**, 425–36. [A detailed description of the clinical aspects of mitochondrial disease.]

Dahl H-HM (1998). Getting to the nucleus of mitochondrial disorders: identification of respiratory chain-enzyme genes causing Leigh syndrome. *American Journal of Human Genetics* **63**, 1594–7. [A review of the nuclear genes causing Leigh syndrome.]

DiMauro S, Schon EA (1998). Nuclear power and mitochondrial disease. *Nature Genetics* **19**, 214–5. [An excellent introduction to nuclear genes and diseases involving mitochondria, including Wilson's disease, Friedreich's ataxia, and hereditary spastic paraparesis.]

Harding AE *et al.* (1995). Pedigree analysis in Leber hereditary optic neuropathy families with a pathogenic mtDNA mutation. *American Journal of Human Genetics* **57**, 77–86. [Important paper summarizing the risks of blindness for the most common mutations causing Leber hereditary optic neuropathy.]

Howell N *et al.* (1998). Mitochondrial DNA mutations that cause optic atrophy: how do we know? *American Journal of Human Genetics* **62**, 196–202. [A succinct discussion of the molecular genetics and disease mechanisms in Leber hereditary optic neuropathy.]

Jackson MJ *et al.* (1995). Presentation and clinical investigation of mitochondrial respiratory chain disease. *Brain* **118**, 339–57. [Clinical features and investigation of a large series of adults with mitochondrial disease.]

Larsson N-G, Clayton DA (1995). Molecular genetic aspects of human mitochondrial disorders. *Annual Review of Genetics* **29**, 151–78. [A review of basic mitochondrial genetics.]

Lightowlers RN *et al.* (1997). Mammalian mitochondrial genetics: heredity, heteroplasmy and disease. *Trends in Genetics* **13**, 450–5. [A discussion of the basic principles of mitochondrial genetics.]

Poulton J, Macaulay V, Marchington DR (1998). Mitochondrial genetics '98: Is the bottleneck cracked? *American Journal of Human Genetics* **62**, 752–7. [A contemporary review of the approaches to the inheritance of heteroplasmic mtDNA defects.]

Smeitink J, van den Heuvel L (1999). Human miotochondrial complex I in health and disease. *American Journal of Human Genetics* **64**, 1505–10. [Comprehensive review of nuclear complex I genes and human disease.]

Taylor RW *et al.* (1997). Treatment of mitochondrial disease. *Journal of Bioenergetics and Biomembranes* **29**, 195–205. [A discussion of current therapy and novel treatment approaches under development.]

Wallace DC (1999). Mitochondrial diseases in mouse and man. *Science* **283**, 1482–8. [A review of recent scientific developments and mouse models for mitochondrial disease.]

24.22.6 Tropical pyomyositis (tropical myositis)

D. A. Warrell

Definition

The term 'tropical pyomyositis' should be restricted to primary muscle abscesses arising within skeletal muscles. This condition must be distinguished from abscesses extending into muscle either from subcutaneous sites following infection through the skin, or from osteomyelitis or suppuration originating in tissues other than muscle.

Geographical occurrence

Tropical myositis has been reported from most parts of tropical Africa, Malaysia, Thailand, India, Indonesia, Oceania, Central and South America, and the Caribbean. It is common in many tropical countries, accounting for 4 per cent of admissions to a hospital in Uganda and for 2.2 per cent of all surgical admissions to a hospital in eastern Ecuador. In temperate climates, pyomyositis was extremely rare, but is becoming more common in patients immunosuppressed due to the human immunodeficiency virus (**HIV**), lymphomas, chemotherapy of malignant diseases, asplenia, Felty's syndrome, and other conditions.

Aetiology

Staphylococcus aureus is the organism most commonly cultured from the abscesses. *Streptococcus pyogenes* (usually group A) is responsible for a few cases, but tropical pyomyositis must be distinguished from streptococcal necrotizing myositis (also known as peracute streptococcal pyomyositis or spontaneous streptococcal gangrenous myositis) which is more fulminant and diffuse and has a very high mortality. Other isolates have included *S. pneumoniae, Haemophilus influenzae, Escherichia coli, Pseudomonas* species, and anaerobes. In Thailand, most cases of pyomyositis are caused by *Burkholderia pseudomallei.* The strikingly different incidence of pyomyositis in tropical and temperate countries has not been explained. In Africa and South America, the condition appears to be relatively more common in indigenous peoples. A history of preceding trauma to the affected muscle is obtained from more than 20 per cent of patients in most series. It has been suggested that, by analogy with osteomyelitis, a muscle haematoma provides a nidus for blood-borne infection. A number of predisposing causes has been suggested: preceding viral infection (for example, an arbovirus), general debilitation, and nematode infections—particularly toxocariasis, *Lagochilascaris minor*, and filariasis. None has been supported by convincing evidence, but sickle-cell disease may be a genuine predisposing cause in a minority of cases. Most of the abscesses associated with helminth infections should not be termed 'pyomyositis' as they are inter- rather than intramuscular. For example, *Dracunculus medinensis* can give rise to deep intermuscular abscesses secondarily infected with *Staphylococcus aureus.*

Pathology

The abscesses may be large, are usually loculated, and are situated within skeletal muscles beneath the deep fascia. Histologically, there is focal muscle necrosis with an infiltration of mononuclear cells and inflammatory oedema.

Clinical features

Tropical pyomyositis can occur at any age but its highest incidence is in the second decade. It is commoner in males. The earliest symptom is pain and tenderness of the affected muscle. Any of the skeletal muscles may be involved, but those of the trunk and lower limbs are the most commonly affected. Usually there is a single localized abscess, but multiple abscesses in distantly separated muscles can occur. At an early stage, an ill-defined tender and thickened area may be palpable in the muscle. Later, a localized, very tender, and hot swelling is palpable. There may be redness and oedema of the overlying skin, but the skin is not primarily involved. The swelling is usually non-fluctuant and there is no local lymphadenopathy. Symptoms and signs usually develop over a few days. Peripheral leucocytosis is not invariable. Eosinophilia is frequently described but is usually common in the populations most affected by tropical pyomyositis. In spite of considerable muscle destruction at the site of the abscess, serum concentrations of muscle enzymes may not be elevated, but in some cases there is myoglobinaemia, myoglobinuria, and acute renal failure. Complications are uncommon, but consist of spread of infection from the affected muscle to other structures such as joints resulting in septic arthritis, to the pleural cavity resulting in empyema, or by haematogenous spread to the heart valves. Mortality in inpatients is said to be less than 1.5 per cent.

Diagnosis

The differential diagnosis is from pus tracking from abscesses in other organs and tissues, muscle haematomas, torn muscles, certain highly vascular or necrotic tumours of connective tissue or muscle (such as rhabdomyosarcoma), and the inflammatory and allergic swellings resulting from the migration of helminths such as *Loa loa* and *Gnathostoma, Paragonimus*, and sparganum spp. *Staphylococcus aureus* is usually cultured from the pus, but blood cultures are positive in less than 5 per cent of cases. Ultrasound, computed tomography (**CT**), and especially magnetic resonance imaging (**MRI**) scans are useful for localizing abscesses and guiding needles for diagnostic and therapeutic aspiration.

Treatment

Full surgical exploration, debridement, and drainage are essential. Because the abscesses are usually loculated, needle aspiration is inadequate. Parenteral treatment with a β-lactamase-resistant penicillin (flucloxacillin) should be started immediately, but if group A *Streptococcus* is cultured, benzyl penicillin or clindamycin are the drugs of choice.

Further reading

Chiedozi LC (1979). Pyomyositis: review of 205 cases in 112 patients. *American Journal of Surgery* **137**, 255–9.

Gibson RK, Rosenthal SJ, Lukert BP (1984). Pyomyositis: increasing recognition in temperate climates. *American Journal of Medicine* **77**, 768–72.

Hossain A, *et al.* (2000). Nontropical pyomyositis: analysis of eight patients in an urban center. *American Surgeon* **66**, 1064–6.

Levin MJ, Gardner P, Waldvogel FA (1971). 'Tropical' pyomyositis. An unusual infection due to *Staphylococcus aureus. New England Journal of Medicine* **284**, 196–8.

Marcus RT, Foster WD (1968). Observations on the clinical features, aetiology and geographical distribution of pyomyositis in East Africa. *East African Medical Journal* **45**, 167–76.

Norrgren H, *et al.* (1997). Increased prevalence of HIV-2 infection in hospitalized patients with severe bacterial diseases in Guinea-Bissau. *Scandinavian Journal of Infectious Diseases* **29**, 453–9.

Smith PG, *et al.* (1978). The epidemiology of tropical myositis in the Mengo districts of Uganda. *Transactions of the Royal Society of Tropical Medicine and Hygiene* **72**, 46–53.

Soler R, *et al.* (2000). Magnetic resonance imaging of pyomyositis in 43 cases. *European Journal of Radiology* **35**, 59–64.

Vassilopoulos D, *et al.* (1997). Musculoskeletal infections in patients with human immuno-deficiency virus infection. *Medicine (Baltimore)* **76**, 284–94.

25

The eye in general medicine

25 The eye in general medicine

Peggy Frith

The significance of disorders of the eye in general medicine

Because the eye may be involved in so many diseases, it is essential that clinicians are familiar with ocular manifestations, learn how to examine the eye, and in particular, are proficient with the ophthalmoscope. Ocular findings may point to the diagnosis of a particular systemic disorder and in some cases an eye complication may need urgent and specific treatment.

Red eye

The pattern of redness suggests a possible diagnosis and other features help to confirm this, as shown in Table 1. The slit lamp shows specific features found in some types of conjunctivitis, the staining pattern of corneal lesions, cells diagnostic of uveitis within the eye chambers, and raised eye pressure of glaucoma. Iritis is described with ankylosing spondylitis, and scleritis with rheumatoid arthritis.

Dry eye

Lack of tears may have a systemic cause, particularly if there is also dryness of the mouth—sicca syndrome. Sicca with an identifiable systemic association is known as Sjögren's syndrome (as with rheumatoid arthritis, systemic sclerosis, mixed connective tissue disease), graft-versus-host disease, or sarcoidosis. The eyes feel gritty and are red or sticky (see rheumatoid arthritis below). Artificial tear drops can help, but severely dry eyes are a miserable problem which can be very difficult to manage.

Loss of vision

A clear history of the visual loss is important. Visual acuity should be measured in each eye, using glasses or a pinhole to correct for any error of focus. Major impairment of vision in one eye gives an asymmetrical pupil response to a bright light. There is a limited number of important causes within the retina or optic nerve (see Table 2).

The Ophthalmoscope

The optic nerve head is usually visible through an undilated pupil, but it is impossible to assess the retina reliably without using a mydriatic. Short-acting drops, such as tropicamide 1 per cent, work within 15 min and last about 2 h, with no risk of causing acute glaucoma. The pupil should not be dilated if the patient has a suspected subarachnoid haemorrhage, coma, or recent head injury. The central fovea is seen if the patient looks directly into the light, and in patients with diabetes the area temporal to the fovea should also be examined. A clouded view suggests opacity in the lens or vitreous, best seen by adjusting focus on to the pupil margin to give a red reflection against which opacities stand out as black shadows, especially if the pupil is dilated. The peripheral retina, for example in sickle-cell retinopathy, is best seen with the indirect ophthalmoscope.

Superficial flame-shaped haemorrhages, though not unique to hypertension, demand measurement of blood pressure. Deeper dot and blot haemorrhages temporal to the macula suggest diabetes, vein occlusion if unilateral or localized, or a haematological disorder if bilateral. Subhyaloid haemorrhage, confined in front of the retina and behind the vitreous, forms a dense focus which may sediment into a characteristic flat-topped shape, typical of bleeding from new vessels—as in diabetes or after retinal vascular occlusion—or secondary to a bleeding diathesis or trauma, including non-accidental injury. Most haemorrhages are asymptomatic and will resolve, but vision falls if the fovea is involved or if blood leaks into the vitreous itself, causing floaters.

Shiny hard exudates consist of protein and lipid; if in circles (circinate), focal vascular leakage may be associated with diabetes, whereas a star around the fovea forms with resolving retinal oedema, as in treated hypertension or papilloedema. Commonly confused with exudates are retinal drusen, which are more uniform and discrete, usually scattered around the retina or congregated close to the fovea. Cotton wool spots are fluffy pale patches indicating swollen nerve fibre axons at sites of microvascular closure. They are always significant (see Table 3). Retinal infiltrates look like cotton wool spots but consist of cells spilled into the vitreous. These are visible with the slit lamp, as in active toxoplasmosis, cytomegalovirus retinitis, sarcoidosis, Behçet's syndrome, or ocular lymphoma. Discrete punched-out scars suggest healed foci of inflammation of the retina and underlying choroid, of which the most common cause is toxoplasmosis.

Fluorescein angiography

This can define the type and severity of retinal vascular disorders. The dye, injected intravenously, demonstrates patterns of perfusion both in the retina and underlying choroidal circulation, outlines abnormalities of the vessels such as microaneurysms, and identifies sites of leakage indicating damage to retinal vessels or the formation of new vessels. Angiography is valuable diagnostically and indicates where laser treatment is needed. Anaphylactic reactions and even fatalities have been reported, so patients must be carefully selected.

Visual fields

The visual fields should be examined in patients with visual loss. Even large defects may go unnoticed. A unilateral central or altitudinal (top or bottom of field) defect suggests an anterior lesion, in retina or optic nerve; a bitemporal defect implicates the optic chiasm; and a homonymous defect the visual path posterior to the chiasm. With bilateral occipital infarction, visual loss may be difficult to define and pupil reactions are normal. A CT scan may be advisable. If there is unaccountably poor vision in one eye, a defect of focus or an amblyopic (lazy) eye resulting from a squint or refractive error in childhood may be responsible: the first should improve with a pinhole device but the second will not.

Eye changes in diabetes (Plates 1–5)

Retinopathy, the most common serious eye complication in diabetes, is the principal reason for blind registration of younger adults from industrial countries. Annual retinal screening is essential, as early treatment can prevent blindness and patients with sight-threatening changes are often asymptomatic.

Older patients especially may have cataract, glaucoma, retinal vein occlusion, and occasionally ischaemic optic neuropathy. Diabetic eye disease is discussed fully in Chapter 12.11.1.

Table 1 Findings in the red eye

Cause	Features	Possible systemic associations
Conjunctivitis	• Redness of conjunctiva, both eye and inside lid • Sticky discharge • Discomfort rather than pain or photophobia • Follicles may be visible	Bacterial or viral infection Sicca
Episcleritis	• Redness of eye only, may be sectorial • Not sticky • Discomfort rather than pain • Common • Not serious and no threat to sight	Systemic inflammatory in a minority
Scleritis	• Redness as episcleritis, may be intense and bluish • Pain which may be intense • Uncommon • Serious disorder with threat to sight • Systemic problem often present	Rheumatoid arthritis Wegener's granulomatosis
Iritis (anterior uveitis)	• Redness mostly around the cornea, may be bluish • Pain and photophobia usual • Corneal precipitates may be visible • Pupil small and may festoon on dilating	Sarcoidosis Ankylosing spondylitis Behçet's syndrome Some infections
Corneal lesion (keratitis)	• Redness often sectorial and adjacent to lesion • Pain photophobia and watering usual • Fluorescein staining will highlight	Herpes virus infection Vasculitis Cogan's syndrome (rare)
Acute glaucoma	• Redness of the entire eye, often bluish • Pain may be intense and vomiting common • Cornea steamy • Eye feels cricket-ball hard • Pupil dilated, oval, and fixed	Dilating drops (rare with tropicamide 1 per cent alone)

Table 2 Some causes of a relative afferent pupil defect

Central retinal artery occlusion (occasionally vein)
Ischaemic optic neuropathy, as in giant cell arteritis
Optic neuritis
Extensive retinal detachment
Advanced unilateral glaucoma
Optic nerve compression

The eye in hypertension

In the hypertensive patient retinal changes will help determine if treatment is necessary, if it is adequate, or if it is needed urgently. Description of individual features is preferable to grading. Unless the pupil is dilated, it is easy to miss or to underestimate retinal changes. A bright halogen bulb and a green or 'red-free' filter helps accentuate vessels and haemorrhages. Haemorrhages or cotton wool spots, indicating acute changes, are most likely to be seen temporal and nasal to the optic nerve head, around the major vessels. Blurring of the margins of the optic nerve head, indicating disc oedema, must be excluded.

Long-standing hypertension and ageing produce similar changes. Arterioles are narrowed, irregular, or tortuous and the wall may be thickened, showing an increase in reflected light described as copper or silver wiring. There may be nipping at the arteriovenous crossings so that the underlying vein appears to be constricted. Long-standing changes often persist with treatment of hypertension but may be reversed in younger patients.

Classification of hypertensive retinopathy

Perhaps the best known grading of hypertensive retinopathy is the Keith–Wagner classification:

Grade 1, mild narrowing or sclerosis of retinal arteries;

Grade 2, moderate to marked narrowing or sclerosis with light reflex and arteriovenous crossing changes;

Grade 3, in addition, haemorrhages or cotton wool spots; and

Grade 4, in addition, swelling of the optic nerve head (papilloedema).

Grades 3 and 4 indicate severe, accelerated, or 'malignant' retinopathy, but disc swelling is no longer regarded as a reliable feature in assessing urgency for treatment—the prognosis is similar for grades 3 and 4.

Blood pressure high enough to damage the renal and cerebral circulation is best recognized by inspecting retinal vessels, even in the absence of visual symptoms. Diastolic pressure likely to be associated with severe retinal changes is usually 110 mmHg or higher at some stage. Proteinuria is almost invariable.

Acute, severe retinal changes indicate either leakage or closure of smaller vessels. Flame haemorrhages are seen particularly around the vessel trunks above and below the macula, temporal to the optic disc (Plate 6). These indicate leakage of blood from fine superficial capillary branches supplying the nerve fibre layer. Bleeding deeper in the retina forms blot-like haemorrhages which, if widespread or in a wedge shape from an arteriovenous crossing, indicate occlusion of the central or a branch retinal vein. Haemorrhages resolve with treatment of hypertension. Only foveal haemorrhage causes visual impairment.

Table 3 Some causes of cotton wool spots

Diabetes
Accelerated hypertension
Retinal vein occlusion (sometimes)
Microemboli or hyperviscosity
Acute pancreatitis
Vasculitis
HIV retinopathy
Migraine attack

Cotton wool spots indicate closure of capillaries supplying the nerve fibres. Microinfarcts cause stasis of axoplasmic flow and intra-axonal contents accumulate, distending and opacifying the fibres and producing the pale fluffy appearance. Spots gradually resolve with treatment. In the absence of hypertension, an inflammatory vasculitis such as systemic lupus erythematosus should be suspected.

Hypertensive damage causes disruption of endothelial tight junctions in retinal vessels so that fluid, protein, and lipid leak into the extracellular spaces within the retina. These are removed by macrophages and processed into shiny hard exudates which may persist for many months. Hard exudates imply leakage for more than a matter of days. They are common in resolving hypertensive retinopathy, forming a characteristic star around the fovea. In hypertension, exudate rarely forms in the ring-shaped circinate pattern typical of diabetes.

Papilloedema implies hypertensive damage to the disc capillaries or cerebral oedema with raised intracranial pressure, attributable to hypertension. Sudden reduction of blood pressure may cause acute, sometimes irreversible, loss of vision also with a risk of stroke.

Histopathology

In the early phases of severe retinopathy there is disruption of endothelial cells or tight junctions followed by vessel wall damage leading to occlusion, sometimes with fibrinoid necrosis or frank thrombosis.

Non-retinal eye changes in hypertension

Occasional patients with severe hypertension, especially those with eclampsia or renal failure, may suffer pronounced visual loss secondary to occlusive changes in the vessels supplying the optic nerve head or in the choroid underlying the retina itself. The tissues become swollen and pale and the retina may even become detached by fluid. Rarely, patients with secondary hypertension may have eye manifestations of genetic disorders such as neurofibromatosis type 1, von Hippel-Lindau, or Sipple's syndrome (see below).

Ocular vascular occlusion

Retinal vascular occlusion is a common cause of blindness, especially in elderly patients. This can be a valuable warning of vascular disease elsewhere, particularly affecting the cerebral circulation.

Retinal artery occlusion

Occlusions of central retinal arteries or their branches, are almost always embolic, arising in the carotid system in the neck, or intracranially, or in the heart. Usually, they start abruptly with permanent loss of function once the retina has infarcted. Central artery occlusion results in profound loss of vision. Branch occlusion causes a visual field defect that often has a horizontal (altitudinal) edge which the patient may be able to define. Recovery of vision is unlikely but prognosis for the other eye is good, especially if an underlying cause can be corrected (Table 4).

Amaurosis fugax

Transient retinal ischaemia causes brief episodes of blindness limited to one eye (amaurosis fugax), usually lasting for a few seconds, some for up to a few minutes, rarely longer. Loss of vision may be total or partial, affecting the upper or lower half of the field like a blind moving up or down. Recovery is usually complete. Most attacks are painless and associated symptoms rare. There may be a history of cerebral transient ischaemic attacks on other occasions. Emboli have been seen passing through the retinal circulation during an attack, moving from central to branch arterioles where they may disperse or become permanently trapped.

Table 4 Associations with retinal artery occlusion

Vascular embolic	Atheroma of carotid bifurcation, carotid siphon, or aortic arch
	Paradoxical embolus (rare)
Cardiac	Thrombus from left atrium or ventricle; atrial fibrillation, myocardial infarct, cardiomyopathy
	Myxoma (rare)
	Mitral valve prolapse (mechanism not known)
	Aortic or mitral valve degeneration or prosthesis
	Endocarditis
Vasculitis	Polyarteritis, systemic lupus erythematosus, syphilis
	Giant cell arteritis (in a minority)
	Takayasu aortitis
Sickle-cell disease	

Clinical findings

Initially, the infarcted retina swells and becomes opaque leaving a 'cherry' red spot at the fovea where the intact underlying choroidal circulation shows through. The territory of an occluded branch artery may become whitened for several days or a few weeks (Plate 7), then subside to leave thinned retina and narrowed, often sheathed, vessels. The optic nerve head may atrophy over ensuing months as the nerve fibres die. If much of the retina is infarcted, there is a defect in the afferent pupil response which persists when other signs have subsided. Emboli may be visible at any stage, in the central or branch vessels, often at a bifurcation. Most emboli are small, glistening white or yellow pieces of cholesterol from atheromatous plaque. Larger, round, solid white emboli, which usually lodge proximally within or near the disc in the larger vessels, may have come from a calcified heart valve, whereas fibrin and platelet emboli from thrombosed plaque or cardiac thrombus may look dark or grey.

Associated findings include an ipsilateral carotid bruit, heart murmur, or dysrhythmia (particularly atrial fibrillation), absent pulses or bruits at other sites, and hypertension.

Investigation and management

No treatment is worthwhile acutely, apart from firm ocular massage which might dislodge an unstable central embolus. Fluorescein angiography is necessary only if the clinical picture is not typical. Risk factors are assessed by measuring blood pressure, full blood count, blood sugar, lipids, and renal function. Even in the absence of a bruit, carotid Doppler ultrasonography is useful for detecting atheromatous plaque at the bifurcation, with a view to carotid surgery.

Management involves reducing risk factors such as smoking, hypertension, obesity, or other abnormalities. Patients unsuitable for surgery are given long-term aspirin.

Retinal vein occlusion

Retinal venous occlusion usually occurs *in situ*. Risk factors include age, hypertension, diabetes, haematological disorders, and glaucoma (Table 5). Symptoms develop less abruptly than with arterial occlusion. Commonly

Table 5 Associations with retinal vein occlusion

Hypertension	
Diabetes	
Smoking	
Hyperlipidaemia	
Haematological	Raised cell or platelet count, hyperviscosity such as myeloma
Glaucoma	
Clotting tendency	Antiphospholipid syndrome, deficiency of protein S, C, or antithrombin III, Leiden mutation
Vasculitis	Sarcoidosis, Behçet's syndrome

the patient wakes with blurred vision. With a central vein occlusion, haemorrhages are scattered throughout the fundus, the characteristic 'blood-storm' pattern (Plate 8), often with cotton wool spots. Less complete block causes sparse scattered haemorrhages, but foveal oedema may impair vision. Branch vein occlusion, usually at an arteriovenous crossing, causes a wedge-shaped sector of haemorrhage in the area of drainage, its apex towards the optic disc. Vision may improve, depending on the state of the fovea, and the outlook for the opposite eye is good if risk factors are minimized. If the retina is ischaemic, the risk of retinal new vessel formation may be prevented by laser treatment. Acute signs of occlusion may persist for many weeks or months. Curly collateral vessels may develop at the disc or peripheral retina.

Investigation and management

Blood pressure, blood sugar, full blood count, and erythrocyte sedimentation rate should be measured. Ocular pressure is checked as glaucoma is a treatable risk factor. Plasma protein electrophoresis, viscosity, and blood coagulation (including antiphospholipid antibodies or lupus anticoagulant) are tested in younger patients, particularly if the changes are recurrent, bilateral, or associated with thrombosis elsewhere. Other possibilities include sarcoidosis or Behçet's syndrome, particularly if the patient describes floaters or the slit lamp shows inflammatory cells within the eye. Risk factors such as blood pressure, smoking, and obesity must be addressed. The benefit of long-term aspirin in patients with venous occlusion is unproven.

Chronic ocular ischaemia

Eye ischaemia is associated with arterial disease anywhere from the aortic arch to the ophthalmic artery. The eye is often painful and red with impaired vision. On slit lamp examination, intraocular pressure is low and there are dilated vessels on the iris with protein flare in the anterior chamber. Cataract may obscure dilated and tortuous retinal vessels, often with scattered haemorrhages. New vessels may form. In younger patients this syndrome may suggest congenital or acquired proximal arterial occlusion, particularly Takayasu's arteritis. In older patients, surgical relief of stenosis may save and even improve vision.

Occlusion of vessels supplying the optic nerve

Giant cell arteritis is associated with occlusion of ciliary (rather than the central retinal branches of the ophthalmic artery) causing acute ischaemia of the optic nerve (see below). Some patients have non-inflammatory occlusion from atheroma. Rarely, acute optic nerve ischaemia, sometimes bilateral, is associated with catastrophic postpartum or gastrointestinal haemorrhage; prognosis for recovery of vision is poor.

The eye in systemic inflammatory diseases

Sarcoidosis

External eye

Asymptomatic sarcoid granulomas may occur in the eyelids or conjunctiva. They are solid, raised, of variable size, often clustered, and characteristically yellowish in colour. Biopsies may be made of them at slit lamp examination. 'Blind' biopsy of normal-looking conjunctiva is not fruitful. Dry eye is common causing grittiness, reduced Schirmer's test, fluorescein staining of the cornea, perhaps with enlarged lacrimal glands.

Uveitis

Iritis (anterior uveitis) is common. It is usually bilateral and recurrent; sometimes severe and damaging. Acutely, the eye is red, painful, and photophobic. Large, greasy precipitates, said to resemble mutton fat, are seen on the internal surface of the cornea by slit lamp. Granulomas may be visible; Busacca's (in the iris), Koeppe's (at the pupil margin). Repeated attacks of iritis cause cataract, glaucoma, or particularly if there is also hypercalcaemia, calcified corneal band keratopathy.

Posterior uveitis causes cells to appear in the vitreous, noticed by the patient as floaters. These may obscure the view of the fundus and may aggregate into characteristic strands or 'snowballs'. Granulomas in retina or choroid are visible as pale foci behind a haze of cells. Vision may be further impaired by fluid leaking from inflamed retinal vessels and collecting around the fovea. Inflamed retinal branch veins look dilated, irregular, later sheathed, and may be surrounded by inflammatory cells; fluorescein angiography shows a segmental pattern of leakage. Occlusive retinal phlebitis of branch veins, causing focal retinal haemorrhages, strongly suggests sarcoidosis. Differential diagnoses are Behçet's syndrome or 'idiopathic' retinal vasculitis without systemic features.

Sarcoid can also cause an optic neuropathy. Sarcoid granulomas behind the eye may cause exophthalmos or cranial nerve palsy.

Corticosteroids are given topically for anterior and systemically for posterior lesions.

Behçet's syndrome (see also Chapter 18.10.5)

Uveitis (iritis and retinal vasculitis) is a defining feature of Behçet's syndrome. Recurrent attacks progressively damage the eye with risk of blindness. In Japan and Turkey, Behçet's syndrome is the commonest cause of uveitis. The incidence in northern Japan is about 1 per 10 000 population, of whom roughly 75 per cent have ocular inflammation at some stage. Untreated, blindness results in 50 per cent of eyes within 5 years of the first ocular attack. Males with the HLA B5 haplotype, particularly the BW51 subtype, are at highest risk of eye disease.

Ocular inflammation is usually bilateral, sometimes with a gap of many years between involvement of each eye. Iritis is typically acute with pain, redness, and photophobia. Hypopyon is characteristic but not unique to Behçet's syndrome (Plate 9). Attacks may settle spontaneously, but the eye may be damaged so short intensive courses of corticosteroid drops and mydriatics are recommended.

Retinal vasculitis particularly involves capillaries and branch veins. Inflammatory cells spill into the vitreous giving rise to floaters. Inflamed vessels leak, causing foveal oedema and an increase in visual impairment with distortion of central vision and risk of permanent foveal damage. Occlusion of inflamed branch veins causes haemorrhages and cotton wool spots (Plate 10). Vision is permanently affected if occlusion involves the fovea. Fluorescein angiography indicates severity of leakage and closure. With recurrent attacks, the retina gradually dies, vessels become sheathed, and the optic nerve head atrophies. Neovascularization may cause vitreous haemorrhage. Acute retinal infiltration with polymorphonuclear leucocytes causes white fluffy patches which indicate active inflammation, strongly suggestive of Behçet's syndrome.

Management is difficult. No regime of immunosuppression tolerable in the long term will prevent all inflammation. Systemic corticosteroids limit acute damage. Longer-term agents such as azathiaprine, clorambucil, colchicine, or cyclosporin A seem to be helpful but their impact on blindness is uncertain.

In a patient dying of cerebral involvement 10 years after the onset of treated eye disease there were collections of T_4 lymphocytes within and around walls of retinal vessels. Many cells were positive for interleukin 2, and HLA DR-positive cells were found in eye tissue, despite heavy immunosuppression.

Giant cell arteritis

Ischaemic, irretrievable visual loss is a feared complication. On systemic corticosteroid treatment the risk of visual loss and blindness falls, provided initial doses are adequate. Patients presenting with visual loss are at high risk of further loss in that eye or of rapid involvement of the second eye; they should be started on high doses until the symptoms, erythrocyte sedimentation rate, and C-reactive protein are controlled. This usually takes days rather than weeks. In patients presenting with bilateral involvement, intravenous methylprednisolone is justified. Temporal artery biopsy is valuable and helps to confirm the diagnosis and the need for continued treatment in patients with visual loss.

Vision may be lost overnight or during the daytime. Patients may have experienced episodes of transient visual loss in the preceding weeks or days. Initially loss may be partial involving either the top or bottom half of the visual field, but often becomes total. The optic nerve head is characteristically pale and swollen (Plate 11). The afferent pupil response is usually decreased compared with the normal eye. Occlusion of the central retinal artery, producing a pale retina and cherry-red foveal spot, is uncommon.

Takayasu's arteritis

This is an inflammatory disorder involving large arteries which can cause an aortic arch syndrome with raised erythrocyte sedimentation rate and C-reactive protein, typically in younger patients. There may be amaurosis fugax or retinal vascular changes of chronic ocular ischaemia, sometimes with anastomoses at the optic nerve head, or scleritis or iritis.

Wegener's granulomatosis

Episcleritis is very common in the active stages and many patients notice that their eyes become red when the disease flares. Occasionally there is a more severe painful scleritis involving the cornea with the risk of corneal thinning and even perforation. Acutely the eye is red and the slit lamp may reveal infiltrates of inflammatory cells in the peripheral cornea. Scleritis and sight-threatening sclerokeratitis respond poorly to topical treatment and require systemic immunosuppression. A pulsed intravenous regime may be needed for initial control.

In patients with 'limited' Wegener's granulomatosis of the upper airway, the orbit may be involved, usually secondarily to disease in the adjacent sinuses but sometimes in isolation. Retro-orbital granuloma produces proptosis, usually painful, and may involve cranial nerves including the optic nerve, with an acute threat to vision (Plate 12). Some patients have a positive antineutrophil cytoplasmic antibody (ANCA) test, although the titres may be low. Many respond to immunosuppression, but high doses may be required for local control.

Polyarteritis nodosa

Inflammation of the eye coat, similar to Wegener's granulomatosis, may produce episcleritis, scleritis, or keratitis. Complications may be severe, requiring systemic immunosuppression. The retinal vessels may be involved, with or without hypertensive changes, and branch arteriolar closure is characteristic. Uveitis is not a feature.

Relapsing polychondritis

This systemic inflammatory disorder involving cartilage is associated with inflammation of the eye coat, similar to rheumatoid arthritis. Half the patients will have eye features at some stage. Episcleritis and scleritis are most common, sometimes with severe corneal features similar to Wegener's granulomatosis and polyarteritis nodosa. Uveitis, retinitis, Sjögren's syndrome, and ischaemic optic neuropathy also occur.

Systemic lupus erythematosus

Episcleritis may occur with exacerbations in systemic lupus activity; the more serious scleritis is uncommon. Retinal vascular occlusions—particularly venous but sometimes branch arterial—may be linked with the antiphospholipid syndrome. Retinopathy with cotton wool spots is associated with active vasculitis, anaemia, and perhaps, moderate hypertension. Ischaemic optic neuropathy with acute irretrievable loss of vision is unusual. Some patients, particularly those with mixed connective tissue disease, have Sjögren's syndrome. Uveitis is not a feature of systemic lupus. Cutaneous lupus may involve the eyelids with oedema and the lid margins may develop scarring inflammatory plaques.

Dermatomyositis

Purple coloration of the eyelids and oedema of the lids and conjunctiva are typical findings. Less common is retinal ischaemia with microinfarcts.

Kawasaki's disease

Bilateral conjunctivitis without discharge is a cardinal feature of Kawasaki's syndrome, characteristically found in young children. Other features are fever, rash, lymphadenopathy, and changes in the other mucosa and nails. Cells may be found in the anterior chamber (mild iritis) and cornea (keratitis) using the slit lamp. The eyes do not need specific treatment.

Multiple sclerosis

Uveitis can occur in multiple sclerosis. Low-grade subtle changes, such as sheathing of the peripheral retinal veins with inflammatory cells within the vitreous, are common in patients with optic neuritis. Fluorescein angiography reveals inflammation and leakage of the retinal veins even though the retina itself does not usually contain myelin. Association of ocular and neurological features also occurs in sarcoidosis and Behçet's syndrome, but in these conditions eye inflammation is usually more pronounced.

Vogt–Koyanagi–Harada syndrome

This curious and uncommon clinical syndrome comprises deafness or meningoencephalitis with cerebrospinal fluid lymphocytosis in the acute stages and bilateral pan uveitis, almost exclusively in patients of Asian origin. There are HLA associations. Inflammatory cells collect within the retinal pigment epithelium and may cause fluid detachment of the retina or deeper layers, associated with decreased vision. There is a response to systemic corticosteroids, with relapses if the dose is reduced. In the chronic phase of the disease there is depigmentation of skin, hair, or eyelashes (poliosis).

Cogan's syndrome

In young adults, especially males, eye inflammation may be associated with deafness or vestibular dysfunction and proximal aortitis or inflammation of medium-sized arteries. Keratitis with patchy cell infiltration in the corneal stroma may lead to corneal vascularization, as in syphilitic keratitis. Some patients have anterior uveitis, scleritis, inflammation of the eye coat, or retinitis. The disorder responds to systemic corticosteroid, which may prevent total deafness if given early enough.

Inflammatory bowel disease

About 10 per cent of patients with Crohn's disease have episcleritis, scleritis, or iritis. Corneal or retinal inflammation is uncommon. Episodes of episcleritis may be associated with exacerbation of the bowel disorder. Eye problems are less common in ulcerative colitis.

Pancreatitis

Ischaemic retinopathy and acute visual loss may occur. There is retinal oedema with cotton wool spots. Fluorescein angiography shows closure of branch retinal arterioles and capillaries, with patches of retinal non-perfusion.

Whipple's disease

This rare disorder is suggested by the association of a malabsorbing enteropathy with arthritis, ocular inflammation, or particular neurological features. There are retinal haemorrhages, diffuse retinal and choroidal vasculitis with cells in the vitreous, or keratitis. Central nervous system features include cranial nerve palsies, papilloedema, and brainstem involvement. The diagnosis is confirmed by small bowel biopsy (see Chapter 14.9.6).

Rheumatoid arthritis

The commonest problem is keratoconjunctivitis sicca, apparently due to autoimmune damage to lacrimal tissue with lymphocytic infiltration and destructive fibrosis. The eyes are uncomfortable, gritty, and often sticky due to low-grade lid infection and poor flushing of the eye surface. Signs include reduced Schirmer's test and staining of the conjunctiva with fluorescein where epithelial cells are shed, particularly of the surface exposed between the eyelids. Symptoms may respond to topical tear substitutes containing methylcellulose: most common is hypromellose. In some patients filaments of adherent mucus may disperse with topical acetyl cysteine treatment (Ilube). Severe dry eye is best managed by a specialist who will watch for complications, particularly corneal ulceration. Other systemic conditions associated with Sjögren's syndrome include systemic sclerosis, mixed connective tissue disease, lupus erythematosus, and sarcoidosis.

Episcleritis is common and may indicate an exacerbation of systemic activity. It rarely needs treatment, but may respond to oral non-steroidal anti-inflammatory agents.

Scleritis, usually found in patients with active vasculitis, is more serious. The eye is usually painful, red, and boggy. The inflammatory process may spread from the posterior eye into the internal eye or to the orbit. Any patient with rheumatism and a painful eye should be referred for specialist assessment, even if the eye is white. Scleritis is an ischaemic vasculitic process involving the vessels which supply the sclera. It responds best to systemic immunosuppression with corticosteroids, sometimes with a cytotoxic agent. Pulsed intravenous treatment may be needed to control the acute attack. Untreated scleritis may cause scleral thinning (Plate 13), corneal ulceration, and perforation of the eyeball. Patients are rarely suitable for corneal grafting.

Ankylosing spondylitis

Ankylosing spondylitis is the most common association with iritis in young patients, particularly men, who should be asked about pain and stiffness of the spine or sacroiliac joints. Radiographs of lumbar spine or sacroiliac joints, or HLA B27 haplotype may be positive. One-third of patients with ankylosing spondylitis will develop eye features at some stage.

The eye is painful, aching, photophobic, and red. The slit lamp shows the cells diagnostic of iritis floating in the anterior chamber and sedimented on the back surface of the cornea as keratic precipitates (Plate 14). Posterior synechias may form, often with the iris constricted: a mydriatic may break these adhesions. This treatment should be continued until inflammation has settled so that the pupil remains large and the iris mobile. Inflammatory cells usually clear quite rapidly with 1 to 2 weeks of topical corticosteroids. Patients with ankylosing spondylitis should be warned that recurrent iritis should be treated early and effectively; there is a 50 per cent chance of recurrence.

Reiter's syndrome

Arthritis, urethritis, cervicitis, or colitis together suggests Reiter's syndrome, especially in HLA B27-positive patients. A self-limiting sterile conjunctivitis is common in the early stages, causing a red sticky eye. Later, iritis may be the dominant recurrent feature. Features and management are similar to ankylosing spondylitis. Other differential diagnoses of arthritis with iritis include sarcoidosis, Behçet's syndrome, psoriasis, and gonorrhoea, with intestinal involvement, inflammatory bowel disease, or Whipple's disease. Sometimes, posterior uveitis, scleritis, or keratitis develop.

Juvenile chronic arthritis

Children most at risk have chronic, seronegative, pauciarticular disease, perhaps involving only one digit or an ankle, especially younger girls positive for antinuclear antibody. The picture is usually one of a low-grade recurrent iritis over several months or years. There may be no symptoms or redness of the eye in the early stages; slit lamp examination is essential. Cells appear in the anterior chamber when inflammation is active. Untreated inflammation can damage the cornea, lens, and aqueous drainage causing band keratopathy, cataract, glaucoma, and risk of blindness. Topical treatment may prevent secondary problems, but some patients will lose useful vision in both eyes. Other causes of iritis in children include sarcoidosis, ankylosing spondylitis, toxocariasis, leukaemia, and retinoblastoma.

Ocular features of blood disorders

Retinal changes are common in haematological disorders even if vision is normal. Bilateral changes result from anaemia, hyperviscosity, and haemostatic abnormalities. The signs are easily missed unless the pupils are dilated.

Hypoxia or hyperviscosity cause retinal vein enlargement, scattered retinal haemorrhages, and cotton wool spots: 'slow flow' or 'stasis' retinopathy. If blood pressure and blood sugar are normal, bilateral retinal haemorrhages suggest a blood disorder. Full blood count, erythrocyte sedimentation rate, and plasma protein electrophoresis should be checked. Roth spots, haemorrhages with a white centre, occur in leukaemia and hyperviscosity. Blood may leak in front of the retina to form a dense, rounded, often boat-shaped, subhyaloid blotch; leakage into the vitreous will cause floaters or clouding of vision.

Leukaemias

Although retinopathy is common in acute and chronic leukaemias, visual symptoms are unusual. The retinal haemorrhages are non-specific, though Roth spots represent focal collections of white cells (Plate 15). If the white cell count is very high, frank infiltration of the retina or optic nerve head causes pale fluffy areas. Leukaemic cells may spill into the vitreous. Chronic leukaemias may cause a slow-flow picture from chronic retinal hypoxia. Retinopathy may improve with chemotherapy. In acute lymphoblastic leukaemia, collections of cells may form a mass retro-orbitally (causing proptosis), or on the iris masquerading as iritis. Ocular infiltrations may respond to radiotherapy. Associated infections (such as orbital mucormycosis), chemotherapy, or radiotherapy may affect the eye. Bone marrow transplantation is associated with cataract and dry eye whilst graft-versus-host disease may cause conjunctival scarring and severe dry eye.

Lymphomas

Lymphoma may occur around or inside one or both eyes, in isolation, in disseminated disease, or in relapse; usually non-Hodgkin, low-grade, B-cell lymphomas. Externally, they form firm swellings in the eyelid or conjunctiva, resembling smoked salmon. In the orbit lymphomas may cause neuro-ophthalmic signs. T-cell tumours may infiltrate the internal eye, particularly iris or choroid. The rare ocular reticulum cell sarcoma ('histiocytic' lymphoma), can masquerade as uveitis, but with a pale mass in the choroid or retina visible through a cloudy vitreous. The monoclonal cells may spread from or to the brain, often the frontal or temporal lobes, so repeated cranial scanning is necessary. Immunocytochemistry of cells obtained by vitreous biopsy is diagnostic. Ocular lymphomas usually respond to local radiotherapy.

Bleeding tendencies

Pronounced or repeated subconjunctival haemorrhage, hyphaema, or vitreous haemorrhage suggests a bleeding diathesis. Bleeding may be spontaneous or follow minor trauma or eye surgery. In haemophilia, bleeding around or inside the orbit may compress the optic or other cranial nerves.

Clotting tendencies

Thrombophilias, including factor V Leiden, protein S, protein C, or antithrombin III deficiencies, are associated with retinal vascular occlusion, especially in the veins. Closure of choroidal vessels affects vision if fluid exudes to detach the retina; this pattern suggests thrombotic thrombocytopenic purpura or disseminated intravascular coagulation. Retinal venous or arterial occlusions occur in systemic lupus erythematosus with lupus anticoagulant or antiphospholipid antibodies. The optic nerve head may be involved, causing amaurosis fugax or ischaemic optic neuropathy. A full clotting screen is indicated in patients with retinal vein thrombosis if another site is involved, episodes are multiple, or there is a family history of juvenile thrombosis at any site.

Sickling disorders

Minor eye features are common in the sickling haemoglobinopathies and may assist diagnosis. Major eye features occur in less than half the patients. They are more common with haemoglobin SC and sickle-cell thalassaemia (**SThal**) than in haemoglobin S homozygotes (**SS**). Unilateral blindness is uncommon, even in SC patients; bilateral blindness is rare. As early treatment improves prognosis, screening the retina of high-risk patients is important. The risk of acute painful or chronic painless glaucoma is increased. Orbital infarction or pneumococcal ophthalmitis are rare. Patients may suffer a stroke affecting the visual field.

Conjunctival signs are more marked in haemoglobin SS than SC. Small conjunctival vessels develop linear, saccular, or comma-shaped dilatations, more prominent in children and after topical phenylephrine drops.

Bleeding into the retina causes a round 'salmon patch'. After resolution over several weeks, haemosiderin is left as iridescent spots in the superficial retina. Deeper haemorrhages damage the underlying retinal pigment layer leaving a permanent black 'sunburst' scar. Bleeds are usually asymptomatic and do not threaten vision.

Sickling in terminal branches of retinal arterioles produces signs in about half the patients. Their prevalence is related to age as most new vessels form between the ages of 10 and 25 years, rarely after 40. In SC patients blindness usually occurs between the ages of 20 and 30 years. Severe retinal ischaemia with new vessel formation is twice as common in haemoglobin SC and SThal as in SS. The risk of sight-threatening vitreous haemorrhage is related to the number and size of new vessels.

After their pupils are dilated, patients must be screened using the indirect ophthalmoscope or an accessory lens at the slit lamp. The earliest sign of peripheral ischaemia is closure of arterioles in the superior temporal sector (stage I) with a paler background and narrow white vessels. If these areas extend and become confluent, anastomotic loops form (stage II), then tufts of new vessels (stage III). As the tufts grow forwards into the vitreous they often look like coral 'seafans'. Fluorescein angiography reveals profusely leaking new vessels whose size can be assessed before or after treatment. Many new vessel tufts will autoinfarct from sickling in the feeder arteriole; they will not then bleed but others may form, so the patient must still be observed.

There are no symptoms until vitreous haemorrhage occurs (stage IV). Small haemorrhages produce a sudden shower of many small floaters, like 'midges'. Large haemorrhages cause sudden marked cloudiness with reduced red reflex. If the retina is distorted or detached (stage V) there may be flashes of light and a visual field defect. Some patients lose central vision, gradually with macular ischaemia or suddenly with foveal haemorrhage or central retinal artery occlusion. Retinal vein occlusion is not associated with sickling.

Screening and treatment

Annual retinal screening is recommended for patients aged 20 to 30 years, especially for SC and SThal diseases. New vessels should be reassessed every few months. If they do not autoinfarct and their size increases or vitreous haemorrhage occurs, laser treatment should cause regression and reduce the risk of early blindness.

Infectious diseases and the eye

Organisms on the surface of the eye can be identified from swabs. Those inside the eye are identified from their pattern of involvement; it is rarely necessary to aspirate material from inside the eye. Treatment for superficial eye infections is by topical antimicrobial drops or ointments, whereas internal infections demand systemic therapy; the choice is partly dictated by penetration into the eye cavities. Rarely, drugs are injected directly into the vitreous to supplement systemic treatment in achieving high intraocular levels.

Bacterial infections

The commonest bacterial eye infection is conjunctivitis caused by *Staphylococcus aureus*, *Haemophilus* spp., or the pneumococcus. Topical chloramphenicol is effective as drops (hourly for the first 24 h then three times daily for several days) with ointment at night. Cellulitis is usually caused by the same organisms; *Haemophilus* is common in children; systemic amoxycillin is the regimen of choice. Retro-orbital spread is an ophthalmic emergency requiring admission to hospital for investigation. If the patient is systemically ill or has orbital signs (proptosis, double vision, or loss of vision), intravenous treatment is warranted.

Metastatic endophthalmitis results when bloodborne bacteria seed to the internal eye (Plate 16). The commonest sources are meningeal, urinary, and endocardial; the most likely organisms are staphylococci, *Neisseria* spp., or streptococci. *Bacillus cereus* and fungi (see below) may complicate intravenous drug abuse and unusual opportunistic organisms must also be considered in immunosuppressed patients. There is visual impairment with pain. Cells and debris within the eye chambers blur the ophthalmoscopic view, though a pale chorioretinal focus of infection may be visible. Blood, urine, and cerebrospinal fluid cultures are necessary. Tapping of the internal eye for vitreous microscopy and culture is justified in some cases. In infective endocarditis, retinal haemorrhages and microembolic infarcts are common, classically in the form of Roth spots.

Tuberculosis can cause indolent granulomatous uveitis, either of the iris or choroid. The eye is frequently involved in leprosy with a risk of blindness; specific iritis and cataracts occur in the lepromatous form. Corneal scarring complicates facial palsy and/or reduced corneal sensation.

In syphilis, uveitis or neuroretinitis occur in the secondary stage and optic neuropathy or Argyll Robertson pupils in the tertiary stage. Congenital syphilis is associated with interstitial keratitis and a salt-and-pepper retinopathy. *Leptospira icterohaemorrhagiae* commonly causes an early conjunctivitis with subconjunctival haemorrhages and a late uveitis. Late Lyme disease may cause ocular inflammation.

The gonococcus causes a marked purulent conjunctivitis in the newborn baby or in those sexually exposed. Tularaemia is associated with a severe granulomatous conjunctivitis with local lymph node enlargement. Botulism causes paralysis of the ocular muscles, sometimes with autonomic signs, with diphtheria as a differential diagnosis. Brucellosis can cause optic neuritis or uveitis—consider this especially in slaughterhouse or farm workers. Actinomycetes can infect the tear canaliculi. Rarely, *Nocardia* spp. can infect the internal eye with a focal chorioretinitis.

Chlamydial eye infection (see also Chapter 7.11.40)

Trachoma is the most common cause of chronic conjunctivitis and worldwide a preventable cause of blindness. At least 600 million people are infected, and about 6 million blinded. *Chlamydia trachomatis* serotypes A to C cause a chronic conjunctivitis with follicles which look like pale grains of rice in the conjunctiva. Scarring of the lids associated with inturning of eyelashes may accelerate corneal scarring. The diagnosis is confirmed by seeing inclusions in conjunctival scrapes or by culturing the organism from swabs. World Health Organization recommendations for control are topical tetracycline ointment twice daily for 7 days six times a year, or six doses of oral doxycycline at 5 mg/kg given monthly.

The genital serotypes of chlamydia cause acute conjunctivitis. The eye is red and sticky, and lymphoid follicles are found in the conjunctiva lining the eyelids. Infection is persistent, responding only partially to topical chloramphenicol. Systemic tetracycline (or erythromycin) with topical tetracycline is effective.

Viral infections and the eye

Adenovirus conjunctivitis is the most common viral infection. It is usually caused by highly contagious, potentially epidemic types 3, 4, 7, 8, or 19. The eye is acutely red and uncomfortable with scanty discharge. Lymphoid follicles may be visible in the conjunctiva lining the eyelids and the preauricular node may be enlarged. Symptoms may continue for some weeks, but recovery is usually uneventful and treatment rarely necessary. The most important differential diagnosis is chlamydial infection, in which eye discharge is more profuse.

In systemically ill patients with fever, rash, and red eyes, measles, meningococcal, or disseminated gonococcal infection may be implicated and in some parts of the world, relapsing fevers (borreliosis) or rickettsoses. Conjunctivitis with marked local lymphadenopathy (oculoglandular syndrome) may be attributable to adenovirus, chlamydia, mumps, or other rarer causes.

Primary herpes simplex can cause conjunctivitis. Secondary herpes infection is associated with recurrent attacks of dendritic corneal ulceration which can result in corneal scarring and poor vision, especially if treated with topical corticosteroid. Herpes zoster can cause corneal ulceration, iritis, glaucoma, and delayed cranial nerve palsies including optic neuropathy. Patients with ophthalmic shingles should be referred for slit lamp examination if there is red eye or visual impairment. All herpes viruses can cause retinal infection, particularly in the immunosuppressed patient; simplex and zoster can cause potentially blinding necrotizing retinitis, which progresses rapidly and may respond poorly to systemic antiviral therapy.

Cytomegalovirus causes progressive retinitis with characteristic haemorrhages and patchy retinal necrosis (see below). In transplant recipients, cytomegalovirus infection may respond to reduction of immunosuppression.

Measles may cause a scarring corneal inflammation, an important cause of blindness in undernourished children. Inflammation of the internal eye is less common. Neuro-ophthalmic associations occur in subacute sclerosing panencephalitis. Congenital rubella and varicella are associated with cataract and retinopathy in infancy. Iritis is characteristic of mumps. Molluscum contagiosum, cowpox, and orf can cause lid infection.

Fungal infections

Indolent fungal keratitis is associated with contact lens wear, diabetes, exposure to inoculation in the garden or field, and intravenous opiate abuse. Metastatic endophthalmitis is usually caused by *Candida albicans* in association with immunosuppression, irradiation, intravenous drug use/abuse, and poorly controlled diabetes. Small, dense, white 'snowballs' are seen in the vitreous with white foci of infection visible in the choroid and overlying retina (Plate 17). Retinal haemorrhage is uncommon. Diagnosis can be confirmed by vitreous biopsy which provides the opportunity to inject antifungals into the eye. The differential diagnosis of a white focus with hazy vitreous full of cells includes purulent endophthalmitis, toxoplasmosis, intraocular lymphoma, sarcoid, or tuberculosis.

Peri- and retro-orbital infection is characteristic of invasive mucormycosis in the same groups at risk of candida, especially debilitated patients receiving treatment for haemtological malignancies and in severe diabetic ketoacidosis. The infection spreads rapidly, often involving the vascular supply and producing tissue necrosis, particularly blackening of the hard palate. Medical treatment is combined with surgical debridement.

In endemic areas such as the Mississippi basin, *Histoplasma capsulatum* produces a multifocal scarring chorioretinitis described as 'histo spots'.

Rickettsial infection

There are petechial haemorrhages of the bulbar conjunctiva with marked redness. Retinal haemorrhages also occur.

Protozoal infections

Toxoplasma gondii causes congenital infection of the retina and underlying choroid, if the mother acquired a primary infection in pregnancy. This is especially common in France and Brazil. The primary scarring focus in the eye may involve the macula or optic nerve head resulting in congenitally poor vision. More commonly, an asymptomatic scar reactivates later in life, releasing cells into the vitreous (Plate 18). An inactive scar may be visible in the other eye. Patients presents with visual blurring, often describing 'floaters'. Presumptive diagnosis is based on clinical findings and positive blood serology. Acute attacks are best treated promptly by an ophthalmologist with several weeks of combined systemic clindamycin or co-trimoxazole and corticosteroid. Some infants have associated cerebral toxoplasmosis.

Retinal haemorrhages are commonly found in patients with cerebral malaria (see Chapter 7.13.2). Retinal toxicity has not been reported with standard use of antimalarials, but has been reported with chloroquine abuse.

Ulcers and nodules of cutaneous leishmaniasis may be seen on the eyelids in endemic areas. Retinal haemorrhages are common in kala-azar, particularly when there is associated anaemia.

Keratosis may occur in African trypanosomiasis (Chapter 7.13.10). In Latin America, oedema of the eyelids, lacrimal gland, and local lymph nodes (Romaña's sign) develops in the weeks following a periocular bite by a reduviid ('kissing') bug transmitting *Trypanosoma cruzi*, the causatial agent of Chagas disease (Chapter 7.13.11).

Acanthamoeba can cause an indolent and potentially blinding keratitis in contact lens wearers or after corneal abrasion.

Pneumocystis choroiditis is discussed in Chapters 7.10.21 and 7.12.6.

Helminth infections

Onchocerciasis ('river blindness') (see Chapter 7.14.1) is a common cause of blindness, particularly in Africa. Microfilarias lodge particularly in the choroid causing insidiously progressive destructive and scarring chorioretinitis. Lymphatic filariasis rarely affects the eye.

Nematode worms of *Toxocara canis* (see Chapter 7.14.7) form a visible mass beneath the retina with uveitis and sometimes whitening of the pupil. The differential diagnosis is a tumour such as retinoblastoma.

Some adult worms invade the eye surface. *Loa loa* (see Chapter 7.14.1) may be felt by the patient and be visible to an observer beneath the bulbar conjunctiva; it may be removed surgically. In Japan, the fly-transmitted 'oriental eye worm' *Thelazia* occurs in the conjunctival sac. In South-East Asia, *Gnathostoma* infects the eyelids or internal eye where the larvas may be visible with the slit lamp.

When pork is eaten, trichinosis (*Trichinella spiralis* infection) affects extraocular muscles, causing pain, periorbital oedema, proptosis, and defective eye movements. There may be internal eye involvement.

Sparganosis (see Chapter 7.15.4) can cause conjunctivitis, swelling, itching, proptosis, and blindness.

The larval form of cysticercosis may be visible inside the eye in either chamber, looking like a motile pearl or toxocara-like mass. Posterior uveitis and retinitis may occur. Orbital involvement is rare. Orbital cysts, perhaps calcified, may occur in patients with hydatid disease.

In schistosomatasis an urticarial conjunctivitis is associated with egg deposition, but the interior of the eye is rarely involved.

Myiasis can involve the eye and orbit (ophthalmomyiasis externa) (Chapter 7.17).

Human immunodeficiency virus infection and AIDS (see also Chapter 7.10.21)

Eye signs are common, particularly in the later stages of AIDS. The retina and optic nerve head are most commonly involved. In patients with coexisting central nervous system infection, eye features may prove an important clue. Definitive diagnosis in life is possible only by retinal biopsy, which is rarely if ever justified. The cellular response within the eye is much scantier than usual. Opportunistic pathogens tend to be facultative intracellular parasites. Cytomegalovirus retinitis is the most common problem in patients with AIDS in the United Kingdom and United States, but is rarely seen in patients with haemophilia or in Africa where non-specific retinopathy and herpes zoster ophthalmicus are more common.

Retinal microvascular disease is common. Cotton wool spots (Plate 19) are commonly seen in relatively early HIV infection with haemorrhages, Roth spots, and microaneurysms. There may be closure and sheathing of the peripheral retinal venous branches and occasional microvascular closure around the fovea producing visual loss; this retinal pattern is common in patients in Africa, particularly children.

Cytomegalovirus retinitis

This was the most common ocular complication in sexually acquired HIV infection in the United Kingdom and United States, affecting about one in three of such patients in the later stages of AIDS when the CD4 T-cell count fell below 100. The incidence has fallen and the prognosis improved strikingly since the introduction of highly active antiretroviral therapy (**HAART**) (see Chapter 7.10.21).

The typical appearance is of patchy areas of pale crumbled-looking retina with associated scattered haemorrhages (sometimes said to look like pizza), most commonly around branch vessels (Plate 20). These are areas of cytomegalovirus replication with oedematous and necrotic retina and some cells, mostly neutrophils and macrophages, although the cell response within the eye cavity is usually scanty. The patches spread contiguously from their borders and, untreated, may enlarge over the course of several weeks. Retinal death results eventually in blindness. Before HAART, the average life expectancy of patients with AIDS in conjunction with cytomegalovirus retinitis was about 9 months.

Differential diagnoses of these appearances include branch retinal vein occlusion, toxoplasmosis, early acute retinal necrosis, candida, or cryptococcus. Definitive diagnosis is difficult. Culture and serology discourage a diagnosis only if they are repeatedly negative.

Adequate doses of virustatic (cidofovir, ganciclovir, or foscarnet) damp down the infection. The lesions become atrophic with resolution of the pale and haemorrhagic features and arrest of spread. Ganciclovir treatment is initiated with 2 weeks of twice daily intravenous doses of 5 mg/kg. The dose is reduced if there is renal impairment. The daily maintenance dose is 5 mg/kg intravenously or 3 g orally. The most important complication is bone marrow suppression. To avoid toxicity, ganciclovir may be given by direct injection into the eye (vitreous), but this is rarely justified as the treatment must be repeated perhaps weekly and the infection is usually bilateral and elsewhere in the body. If the CD4 cell count remains low, breakthrough of retinitis is common and is treated by repeating the induction course of ganciclovir, or by switching to foscarnet or cidofovir.

Spread of retinitis will occur if treatment is interrupted and will often smoulder on during the treatment course; breakthroughs after several weeks are treated by increasing the dose or changing to another agent. Ophthalmic supervision is important as it is more accurate to assess the lesions by indirect ophthalmoscopy, preferably with serial retinal photographs to document progression at the edges of lesions.

In patients with cytomegalovirus retinits, the low CD4 cell count must be improved with HAART and once the count is securely above 100/μl, maintenance therapy for cytomegalovirus may usually be suspended.

Other infections

Especially in non-industrial countries, HIV infection is a common cause of herpes zoster ophthalmicus. Retinal infection with herpes zoster or simplex may also cause rapidly spreading retinal death, as acute retinal necrosis (**ARN**) with pale oedematous areas lacking the crumbled texture and haemorrhages characteristic of cytomegalovirus retinitis. Often there is involvement of the optic nerve with optic neuritis and sometimes there may be encephalitis. Vision can be lost bilaterally, within days if untreated. Intravenous acyclovir may halt spread within the retina.

Syphilis in HIV infection may cause iritis or optic neuritis, often bilateral. There may be retinitis with a vitreous cell reaction, abnormal cerebrospinal fluid, or other signs of central nervous system involvement. Non-specific treponemal serology may be negative, so specific tests must be done. Eye complications are treated with benzathine penicillin, using a regime suitable for central nervous system infection.

Toxoplasmal choroidoretinitis in HIV-infected patients may show a fluffy focal retinal lesion with cells in both chambers. These signs may explain accompanying optic neuritis or encephalitis. Treatment is with clindamycin, without corticosteroids.

Pneumocystis pneumoniae may occasionally cause a multifocal choroidoretinitis with multiple, pale, rounded patches visible beneath the retina, and cryptococcus an acute optic neuropathy associated with meningitis.

Disorders of the thyroid and parathyroid

Eye signs result either from imbalance of thyroid hormones or from an immunological disorder of both the thyroid (Graves' disease) and retro-orbital tissues; the most common cause of proptosis/exophthalmos, referred to as 'Graves' ophthalmopathy' or 'ophthalmic Graves' disease'.

Cosmetic problems and eye discomfort are common, but a threat to vision may be an acute emergency. Evolution of eye signs is often independent of current thyroid status; the patient may be euthyroid, hyperthyroid, or hypothyroid, and correction of hormone imbalance may not affect eye features. Commonly, orbital disease appears in patients who have become hypothyroid after treatment for hyperthyroidism.

Orbital disorders result from infiltration of orbital tissues by T cells, stimulated by autoantibodies which cross-react with adipocytes. Initially, fibroblasts are stimulated to produce mucinous material and oedema within muscle or fat; later this leads to fibrosis and atrophy.

Werner's classification is as follows.

Class 0, signs and symptoms both absent;

Class 1, signs without symptoms;

Class 2, both symptoms and signs of soft tissue involvement;

Class 3, proptosis indicating orbital involvement;

Class 4, eye muscle involvement with double vision;

Class 5, secondary corneal involvement; and

Class 6, optic nerve involvement with loss of vision.

The eyelids may be swollen in both hyper- and hypothyroidism, especially on waking. In hyperthyroidism, upper lid retraction reveals white sclera above the upper cornea and there is lid lag. Raised orbital pressure causes congestion and redness of the eye, particularly over the visible tendon insertions of the lateral rectus muscles and conjunctival swelling (chemosis) (Plate 21). Diplopia is common; it is usually vertical, worse on waking and looking upwards.

Proptosis causes white sclera to appear, often asymmetrically, below the lower corneal margin. This can be measured from the bony rim of the orbit using an exophthalmometer, which gives a useful impression of progression. Thyroid function and autoantibody tests may be normal in patients with typical eye disease. Scans, especially coronal MRI views, can show enlargement of ocular muscles. Severe protrusion with upper lid retraction exposes the cornea to damage; corneal abrasion, ulceration, and perforation can develop rapidly and so patients with a protruding eye, impaired blinking, pain, or fluorescein staining of the cornea are an ophthalmic emergency.

Orbital pressure may be highest in patients without much proptosis as protrusion has a decompressing effect. Optic nerve compression causes visual blurring, perhaps with a central scotoma, loss of colour definition, or relative afferent pupillary defect. The optic nerve head may be swollen. Scanning shows enlarged extraocular muscles. Urgent management is necessary.

Cosmetic orbital surgery is rarely justified, but upper lid surgery is sometimes worthwhile. Discomfort is difficult to treat; simple artificial tears may be tried. Immunosuppression seems justified for active inflammation. Initially, diplopia is best managed with a plastic Fresnel prism stuck on to a spectacle lens. Stable diplopia may need a permanent spectacle prism, surgery, or botulinum toxin injection. Corneal exposure demands lateral tarsorrhaphy or temporarily taping the lids or single lid suture under local anaesthesia.

Optic nerve compression needs urgent orbital decompression; medically, using high-dose systemic corticosteroid; surgically, by removing bone from the orbital walls, or by orbital radiotherapy in severe cases.

Another cause of a congested protuberant eye is an orbital mass, usually unilateral. Few conditions mimic thyroid eye disease in having bilateral if asymmetrical signs. Upper lid signs are particularly helpful in suggesting this diagnosis. Orbital pseudotumour or myositis is characteristically more painful and a caroticocavernous arteriovenous fistula may cause a frontotemporal bruit. The conditions are differentiated neuroradiologically.

Parathyroid disorders

Hyperparathyroidism producing hypercalcaemia may cause calcium deposition (band keratopathy), a lacy opacity spreading horizontally from the margins inwards. The eyes may be red and feel gritty.

In hypoparathyroidism and pseudohypoparathyroidism, hypocalcaemia causes lens opacities. Small white or coloured crystals beneath the lens capsule may not impair vision. Papilloedema from intracranial hypertension is rare and reversible by correcting hypocalcaemia.

Multiple endocrine neoplasia syndrome

In type IIb of this rare autosomal dominant condition, prominent corneal nerves are easily detected by slit lamp. Conjunctival neuromas or thickened eyelids may occur.

The eye in diagnosis of inherited conditions (Table 6)

Marfan's syndrome (see Chapter 19.1)

Most patients have reduced vision, commonly due to myopia and astigmatism which may be inferred from their spectacle lenses. Slit lamp reveals lens dislocation upwards (Plate 22). The iris trembles with eye movement (iridodonesis), because it is poorly supported by an abnormally mobile lens. The dislocated lenses are best retained. Careful correction of focus can improve vision dramatically in early childhood, preventing permanent amblyopia. Differential diagnoses of dislocated lenses are isolated ectopia lentis (without other marfanoid features) and homocystinuria (with marfanoid habitus).

Neurofibromatosis type 1 (see Chapter 24.6.1)

Most patients have raised, yellowish/brown, multiple, Lisch nodules of the iris visible by slit lamp which must be distinguished from common, simple, flat iris freckles. Corneal, retinal, or orbital neurofibromas/schwannomas may be found. There is an increased incidence of glaucoma. Screening and management of intracranial tumours associated with neurofibromatosis

Table 6 Eye findings in some inherited disorders

Eyelid	
Epicanthus	Turner's syndrome (XO), trisomy 18 (Edward's syndrome), Down's syndrome, deletions 13q, 18, 4p, 5p
Ptosis	Kearns–Sayre disease, myotonic dystrophy, Turner's syndrome (XO), 13q deletion
Conjunctiva	
Telangiectasia	Osler–Weber–Rendu syndrome, Louis–Bar syndrome, Sturge–Weber syndrome, Fabry's disease, fucosidosis
Pingueculas	Gaucher's disease
Cornea	
Kayser-Fleischer ring	Wilson's disease
Cornea verticillata	Fabry's disease
Corneal crystals	Cystinosis
Corneal clouding	Mucolipidoses, mucopolysaccharidoses, Lowe's syndrome, X-linked ichthyosis, tyrosinaemia, Tangier disease, trisomy 18
Thickened corneal nerves	Multiple endocrine neoplasia type IIb
Keratoconus	Down's syndrome
Iris	
Iris tremor (iridodonesis)	Marfan's syndrome
Lisch nodule	Neurofibromatosis type 1
Iris transillumination	Albinism
Aniridia (absent iris)	Wilm's tumour/11p deletion
Coloboma (cat eye)	Trisomy 22
Brushfield spots	Down's syndrome
Lens	
Lens dislocation	Marfan's syndrome, homocystinuria, ectopia lentis
Lenticonus	Alport's syndrome
Cataract, infantile	Galactosaemia, galactokinase deficiency, Down's syndrome, Lowe's syndrome
Cataract, childhood	Skeletal, chromosomal, and dermatological syndromes
Cataract, adult	Myotonic dystrophy, Wilson's disease, neurofibromatosis type 2, Fabry's disease, mannosidosis
Retina	
Retinal angioma	von Hippel–Lindau disease, Sturge–Weber syndrome
Retinal phacoma	Tuberous sclerosis, neurofibromatosis type 1
Angioid streaks	Pseudoxanthoma elasticum
Retinal dysplasia	Norrie's disease, incontinentia pigmenti
Macular abnormality	Batten's disease, Farber's disease, Gaucher's disease
Macular cherry red spot	Sialidosis, Niemann–Pick disease, Tay–Sachs disease
Pigmentary retinopathy	Usher's disease, mitochondrial myopathy (some), Refsum's disease, Kearns–Sayre disease, abetalipoproteinaemia, Hurler's syndrome, Laurence–Moon–Biedl syndrome
Pigmented patches	Gardner's syndrome
Gyrate atrophy	Hyperornithinaemia
Retinoblastoma	13q deletion
Vascular anomaly	Fucosidosis
Crystals	Cystinosis, oxalosis, Alport's syndrome
Sclera	
Blue sclera	Osteogenesis imperfecta
Thinned sclera	Ehlers–Danlos syndrome
Pigmented sclera	Alkaptonuria
Glaucoma	Neurofibromatosis type 1, Sturge–Weber syndrome

type 1, including optic nerve or chiasmal gliomas, is controversial. Neurofibromatosis type 2 is associated with posterior subcapsular cataracts.

von Hippel–Lindau disease

Retinal angiomas may be the presenting and sole features. They are usually bilateral and multiple in the mid-peripheral retina, so indirect ophthalmoscopy is advised. They start as a very small lesion no bigger than a microaneurysm which enlarge, later developing dilated, tortuous feeder and draining retinal vessels. Early peripheral angiomas may be destroyed by laser, preferably before they bleed or cause retinal detachment. Juxtapapillary angiomas at the optic nerve head may affect vision early in their development and are difficult to treat (Plate 23). Prolonged eye follow-up is needed.

The eye in diagnosis of inherited premalignant conditions

Gardner's syndrome is deep retinal pigmentation with polyposis coli; the dark retinal patches, multiple and usually bilateral, are best seen by indirect ophthalmoscopy. Absence of the iris (aniridia) is associated with renal Wilm's tumour, especially if there is a chromosome 11p deletion. Retinoblastoma, when associated with deletion of chromosome 13q, is inheritable as a dominant trait with high penetrance, together with other tumours such as osteosarcomas. In multiple endocrine neoplasia syndrome type IIB, associated especially with thyroid malignancy, there are enlarged corneal nerves and other ocular abnormalities (see above). von Hippel–Lindau disease is also associated with malignant renal tumours.

Ocular drug toxicity

Few drugs require ophthalmic screening but visual loss can result from poisoning.

Antimalarials

The risks of chloroquine are discussed in Chapter 7.13.2. Patients may develop a dose-dependent retinal toxicity of the 'bull's eye' type with permanent reduction in central vision (Plate 24).

Hydroxychloroquine (Plaquenil) carries a lower risk of retinal damage. Monitoring is recommended only in patients taking more than the standard dose of up to 400 mg daily.

Ethambutol (see Chapter 7.11.22)

Toxicity, rare at doses of 15 mg/kg or less, is usually related to total dose, and is therefore least likely in the first 6 months of treatment. However, idiosyncratic toxicity in the first few weeks has been reported. Patients with symptoms of optic neuropathy should stop taking the drug immediately and should be warned to report any change in visual clarity or colour vision. Visual acuity, colour vision (100 Hue test),and optic disc appearance are monitored 3-monthly during treatment. Previous optic nerve damage or renal failure increase the risk. The early changes usually recover if the drug is stopped.

Corticosteroids

Lens opacities, typically posterior subcapsular, producing light scatter and glare, are visible by slit lamp or the ophthalmoscope set to catch the red reflex in focus, particularly if the pupil is dilated. Surgery may be necessary.

Eye signs in poisonings (see Chapter 8.2)

Quinine poisoning can blind by damaging the retina and optic nerve head. Ethyl alcohol (antifreeze) damages the optic nerve. Cyanide in raw cassava can blind.

Organophosphate pesticides and other anticholinesterases constrict the pupil by parasympathetic stimulation. Vision is not affected. Opiates also constrict the pupil. Atropine-like compounds, including nightshade berries, dilate the pupils ('gardeners's mydriasis') (see Chapter 8.3).

The external eye is vulnerable to ammonia, alkalis (including lime, cement, and plaster), acids, and some riot control agents. Primary treatment is prolonged irrigation for up to 20 min, using tap water (or even milk if necessary), followed by specialist referral.

Blindness worldwide

The World Health Organization defines blindness as binocular vision of Snellen 6/60 or less. More than 45 million people are estimated to be blind worldwide; perhaps two-thirds of these have visual impairment that prevents self-sufficiency.

Trauma

Physical or chemical eye injuries are a common cause of visual loss where prevention and treatment are poor. Emergency eye surgery and antibiotics can save vision.

Cataract

There is no known method of preventing cataract, which remains the most common cause of blindness in populations with limited surgical services. As the lens ages, its protein structure changes and the lens opacifies. Malnutrition, dehydration, diabetes, and perhaps sunlight accelerate lens ageing. In some populations, primitive surgical 'couching' or dislodging of the lens within the eye makes matters worse. Implanting artificial lenses is impracticable in many countries and, even if surgery is successful, correction by spectacles needed afterwards is often unsatisfactory. In poorer countries attention is focused on organizing the training and deployment of mobile surgical teams to carry out as many effective operations as possible.

Glaucoma

Nerve fibres within the rim of the optic nerve head are damaged by relatively high intraocular pressure and impaired blood supply. The central cup of the nerve head enlarges and visual field is irretrievably lost long before central acuity is affected, so the early stages are usually asymptomatic and painless. Even in wealthy populations, screening for early glaucoma is difficult and some patients progress to blindness despite all efforts. Those most at risk have a first-degree relative with glaucoma.

Age-related macular degeneration

The central retina around the fovea has an extraordinarily high metabolic turnover. In some patients, the efficiency of recycling metabolic products fails, abnormal material is deposited in the retina, and tissue integrity breaks down. Drusen may form around the fovea. They do not impair vision themselves but may herald formation of aberrant vessels which grow into the fovea from the choroid beneath, and may leak and may leak or bleed to form a scar with an irregular 'disciform' shape. This permanently damages the fovea. The patient loses detailed central vision, although peripheral vision allows them to navigate independently. Only a few patients at an early stage are ever likely to benefit from laser coagulation.

Diabetic retinopathy

This remains an important cause of blindness in younger patients. Major problems are organization of effective screening programmes and deployment of laser treatment. Over 50 per cent of blindness is preventable if laser treatment is given early enough.

Trachoma

Blindness occurs in populations who have poor eye hygiene and repeated fly-borne infection. Vaccination is not feasible. The only effective means of control is intermittent topical or systemic tetracycline treatment. Surgery for established scarring is less effective on a mass scale.

Vitamin A deficiency (xerophthalmia)

This most commonly affects young children and may destroy the whole eye. Lack of vitamin A causes conjunctival and corneal dryness and keratinization (xerosis) with Bitot's spots. The cornea softens (keratomalacia), ulcerates, and may perforate and become infected, resulting in endophthalmitis. Vitamin A is found in many green leafy vegetables and palm oil. Measles keratitis increases the risk of corneal scarring in malnourished children.

Onchocerciasis (river blindness)

This is estimated to cause blindness in 1 million people. Recently the disease has been largely controlled, thanks to vector control and the widespread use of ivermectin.

Further reading

Easty DL, Sparrow JM, eds (1999). *Oxford textbook of ophthalmology.* Oxford University Press. [For reference purposes.]

Fraunfelder FT, ed. (2000). *Drug-induced ocular side effects and drug interactions.* Lea & Febiger. [A compendium, regularly updated.]

Frith PA, ed. (2001). *The eye in clincal practice,* 2nd edn. Blackwell Scientific Publications. [A basic practical exposition for non-specialist clinicians.]

Nussenblatt RB, Palestine AG (1995). *Uveitis, fundamentals and clinical practice,* 2nd edn. Year Book Medical Publishers Inc. [For clinical aspects and conundrums.]

Taylor D, ed. (1997). *Paediatric ophthalmology,* 2nd edn. Blackwell Scientific Publications. [For comprehensive clinical coverage.]

26

Psychiatry and drug related problems

26.1 General introduction

Michael Sharpe

Modern psychiatric medicine represents a substantial body of knowledge and skills, much of which is of potential value to the physician. It is therefore unfortunate that psychiatry and medicine have become so divorced from one another. Based on the questionable intellectual foundations of mind–body dualism, this separation has shaped research, planning, and services. In recent years, the split seems to have widened as medicine has focused increasingly on the basic biology of disease and psychiatric services have tended to make psychoses such as schizophrenia their central concern. Despite this, there is much evidence to show that physicians are faced every day with diagnostic and management problems for which the larger body of psychiatric knowledge and skills are relevant. Indeed, it could be argued that much of the criticism of clinical medicine in recent years reflects a lack of attention to the non-biological aspects of patient's illnesses. Examples include failures to establish therapeutic relationships with patients, to properly manage distress, and to effectively understand and manage complaints that are medically unexplained.

Psychiatric knowledge of relevance to medicine includes a practically useful, if imperfect, classification system, with an increasingly sophisticated psychological and neurobiological underpinning, and a range of pharmacological and psychological treatments, each with a substantial evidence base. Skills of relevance to the physician include the ability to assess the patient's mental as well as physical state, the detection of symptoms of depressive and anxiety disorders, and the eliciting of the patient's own understanding of their illness. These factors can be of substantial importance in the patient's management. Attitudes are also important, it being no secret that some physicians are dismissive toward patients who are perceived as 'psychiatric'. The acceptance of patients' concerns, even if apparently illogical, the tolerance of difficult behaviours, and a degree of reflectiveness in moderating one's own response; all are valuable in all medical settings.

Although physicians do a great deal of 'psychiatry' themselves, specialist help is not infrequently required, but psychiatric and psychological services can be problematic for the hospital physician to access because of the separation of psychiatric and medical services. In recent years, however, there has been a slow but steady growth of general hospital-based psychiatry and psychology services dedicated to the needs of medical patients, often termed 'liaison psychiatry' or 'health psychology', respectively. Such services offer improved integration of medical and psychiatric practice.

The sections that follow hopefully provide a practical and accessible summary of those aspects of assessment and management conventionally deemed 'psychiatric', but which are in fact central to the practice of medicine: They include:

- guidance on taking a psychiatric history from a medical patient in a way that is manageable within a medical setting;
- information about relevant psychiatric diagnoses, including organic mental disorder, depression and anxiety, reactions to stress, somatoform disorders and eating disorders, as well as basic coverage of the less commonly encountered but important psychiatric diagnosis of bipolar disorder, schizophrenia, and obsessive–compulsive disorder;
- practical advice on the management of depression and anxiety when it coexists with disease, somatic symptoms that are unexplained by disease, deliberate self-harm, and on how to cope with acute behavioural emergencies;
- a substantial section on the highly prevalent and clinically significant problem of alcohol and substance misuse.

Some might regard this section as an 'add on' that is of questionable relevance to the practising physician. Rather, it is better considered as a more detailed look at some aspects of medicine that are of relevance to the management of many of the medical conditions described in this book. It therefore forms part of an integrated approach to illness in which biological, psychological, and social strands of patient assessment and management run in parallel.

For the interested reader who wishes to find out more about psychiatry in general or liaison psychiatry in particular standard texts are listed below.

Further reading

Gelder M *et al.* (1996). *Oxford textbook of psychiatry*, 3rd edn. Oxford University Press, Oxford.

Royal Colleges of Physicians and Royal College of Psychiatrists (1995). *The psychological care of medical patients; recognition of need and service provision.* Royal College of Physicians, London.

Rundell JR, Wise MG, (1996). *Textbook of consultation–liaison psychiatry.* American Psychiatric Press, Washington DC.

Sharpe M (1998). Psychiatry in relation to other areas of medicine. In: Johnstone JC, Freeman CPL, Zealley AK, eds. *Companion to psychiatric studies*, 6th edn, pp 785–806. Churchill Livingstone, Edinburgh.

26.2 Taking a psychiatric history from a medical patient

Eleanor Feldman

Listen to the patient, he is telling you what is wrong
William Osler

This chapter covers issues that physicians and surgeons need to know about concerning psychiatric history-taking in general hospital patients. It would not be appropriate for a non-psychiatrist to attempt to take a full psychiatric history, involving as it does at least one hour's discussion covering relationships in the family of origin and a detailed biography to establish premorbid personality and aetiological factors, plus further discussion with at least one other informant. However, all patients should be screened for the most common problems: cognitive dysfunction, mood disorder, anxiety states, and alcohol and substance misuse. The assessment of cognitive dysfunction is predominantly a matter of mental state examination rather than taking a history and is covered in Chapter 26.4 and Chapter 30.2. Substance misuse is covered in some detail in Section 26.7. Chapter 26.5.2 covers how to assess a patient following attempted suicide, and the diagnostic features of patients with eating disorders are discussed in Chapter 26.5.5.

It is not necessary to screen routinely for psychotic symptoms as functional psychosis rarely presents for the first time in general hospital cases. If hallucinations and delusions do emerge during an inpatient's stay, then the most likely cause is an acute organic brain syndrome, and careful testing of orientation in time and observation for fluctuations in conscious level will usually confirm delirium. If in doubt, psychiatric advice should be sought.

Screening questions in routine assessment

Depression and anxiety

Significant proportions of general hospital patients will have diagnosable mental health problems. (Tables 1 and 2) Frequently these will impinge on the physical health and well being of the patient. Stress affects the immune response; depression and anxiety are often comorbid with physical illness, either preceding it, or arising largely as a result of it; depressed and anxious people frequently have increased worry about physical health and experience minor physical symptoms as severe and intolerable. Antidepressants may help.

Table 1 Prevalence of psychiatric disorder in 453 medical inpatients

Psychiatric disorder	Men (%)	Women (%)
Anxiety/depression	12 (4–6)*	16 (8–10)*
Alcohol problems	18	4
Dementia and delirium (patients over 70 years only)	23	38

*Expected figures in the general population.

Screening for depression and anxiety need not take much time in itself (Box 1). However, if the patient gives positive answers it is helpful for these to be explored in more depth when time allows and in a private interview room. Patients will be aware when you are under pressure or in a rush, and this will inhibit them from telling you important things and you from wanting to hear about them. Therefore, indicating that you think something is important and will come back to them when you can set aside more time is very helpful and reassuring to the patient.

Questions about mood disorder are best construed as part of an enquiry into general health and the 'person as a whole', and most patients are pleased to discover that their physician takes an interest in their general well being. Starting with a non-directive enquiry about sleep **before** coming into hospital (most patients have sleep disturbance **in** hospital) is a natural way to link physical and emotional health: difficulty sleeping is a common denominator in stress, anxiety, and depression and a description of a disturbed sleep pattern may also assist you in distinguishing endogenous depression characterized by early morning wakening and diurnal mood variation. The reasons for any sleep disturbance, whatever they may be, are important in general health and will often reveal what troubles and worries a patient. Again ask this non-directively; do not be tempted to offer the patient a multiple choice of explanations. By open questioning, you will guide the patient into revealing what difficulties they are facing and most will find it a relief to tell you. At this stage, it is best to listen empathically and let the patient tell you their story. It may seem to you that you are doing nothing, but the patient gains great relief by being heard and understood, and you are gaining their trust and eliciting valuable information.

The rare patient who objects to a sensitive enquiry intended to be helpful will have a reason to be defensive, and a history from the family practitioner or another informant will usually explain all. If you find the patient defensive and there always seem to be reasons why there is no-one else you can talk to, so that you cannot even confirm the patient's identity, then this is characteristic of those with factitious disorder using a false identity.

It is also advisable to screen for a past history of mental disorder, either when screening for the patient's past medical history, or if you have already elicited current mental health problems. Use the vernacular language of the

Table 2 Prevalence of anxiety/depression in medical outpatients according to final medical diagnosis

	Definite organic pathology (*n* = 91)	Recognized syndromes (e.g. irritable bowel syndrome, fibromyalgia) (*n* = 42)	No organic diagnosis (*n* = 58)
Anxiety/depression (%)	12	43	33

culture of that patient; for example, in my own culture it would be: 'Have you ever had any troubles with your nerves or had to see a doctor about your nerves?'. Positive answers should then be explored non-directively by saying something like: 'Tell me more about that'. Hence, there need be only a few screening questions to lead effectively into a discussion of most mood disorders, worries, and stress. As important as the questions themselves will be, the way in which they are asked, the time available for discussion, and the physician's own willingness to listen and take note, are equally—if not more—important.

The importance of the alcohol use history

Insomnia and mood and anxiety disorders may be associated with heavy alcohol use. This alone may depress mood and give rise to early morning wakening, appetite changes, and weight loss. For this reason, a diagnosis of depressive illness cannot be made until the patient has been through alcohol withdrawal and been dry for a few weeks. If the alcohol problem is missed, incorrect advice and treatment will be given.

Patients are often defensive and evasive when they have an alcohol problem and persistent probing is needed to elicit the precise amount. Questions need to be asked as a routine and in a non-judgemental friendly way (Box 2). It is important to know the average intake in terms of units, rather than a vague qualitative response such as 'social drinking' or 'moderate drinking'. The CAGE questions may also be asked as a routine in anyone who drinks excessively (also in Box 2).

Box 1 Screening and probing questions for mood and anxiety disorder

Screening for current problems

- How have you been sleeping (before you came into hospital)?

Probing: sleep, worry, and mood

If not sleeping well, ask about the pattern of, and perceived reason for, sleep disturbance:

- Is it difficulty getting off to sleep?—If Yes: how long before you fall asleep?
- Are you woken intermittently? Why? (may be due to physical symptoms)—Do you get back to sleep easily?
- Do you wake early and find you can't get back to sleep?—If Yes: how early?

If they have good nights and bad nights:

- What proportion are good or bad; is it 50:50 or better or worse than that?

If sleeping badly:

- Why do you think you are sleeping badly? (This is a natural opportunity for patients to reveal what is worrying them)
- Are you kept awake with worries going round and round your mind?

At this point you will find out what is bothering the patient—after they have confided this in you, it is then empathic to ask:

- How have you been feeling in your spirits?

If a patient reveals problems, it is appropriate now to ask about their previous mental health.

Screening for past mental health problems:-

- Have you ever had trouble with your nerves?
- Ever seen a doctor about your nerves?
- Ever taken tablets for your nerves or to help you sleep?

Box 2 Screening for alcohol problems

Routine questions

On an average week, how much alcohol do you drink?

What do you like to have (spirits, wine, beer, etc.)?

How many measures/glasses/pints?

How often do you drink that much?

Did you used to drink much more than that?

If so, when and how much?

CAGE questions:

Do you feel you should **C**ut down on your drinking?

Does anyone **A**nnoy you or get on your nerves by telling you to cut down your drinking?

Do you feel bad or **G**uilty about your drinking?

Do you have a drink first thing in the morning to steady your nerves or get rid of a hangover (**E**ye-opener)?

A positive answer to one or more questions is indicative of problems

Recognizing and dealing with somatized anxiety and depression

Stress, anxiety, and depression can also be the main reasons for physical symptoms (Table 3). When patients experience the unpleasant physical symptoms that arise from their bodily reactions to emotional states, it is natural for them to complain of these to their medical attendants rather than present their primary complaint as an emotional disorder, which they will often regard as secondary to their physical symptoms, or make no connection at all. This is the common phenomenon known as somatization.

Table 3 Some common physical symptoms of anxiety/depression

Common physical symptoms of anxiety
Dry mouth
Difficulty swallowing, lump in throat, choking
Chest discomfort: pain or tightness
Breathing difficulty, feeling of smothering—can't catch breath
Heart pounding, missing beats, beating faster
Fear of dying/heart attack/collapse in an attack
Sweating, e.g. palms of hands
Trembling or shaking of hands or limbs/legs wobbly or 'like jelly'
Hot or cold sweats, flushes
Butterflies in stomach, abdominal discomfort, nausea
Vomiting
Diarrhoea
Light-headedness, dizziness, feeling faint
Tingling or numbness in hands, feet, or around mouth (secondary to hyperventilation)
Urinary frequency
Headache
Any musculoskeletal pain (especially back, neck, shoulders) including tenderness
Sleep disturbance (getting off to sleep and broken sleep and/or bad dreams)
Common physical symptoms of depression
Symptoms of anxiety as above (depression and anxiety often coexist)
Tiredness, can be extreme lethargy
Physically slowed up
Pain
Loss of appetite
Weight loss
Loss of libido
Poor sleep with early morning wakening

Misinterpretation by patients and their doctors of the symptoms of chronic tension, as well as sympathetic hyperarousal and hyperventilation in panic disorder, may lead to inappropriate extensive searches for organic abnormalities and provide no relief from suffering for the patient. Indeed, the patient's suffering increases as they are left with continuing uncertainty as to the cause of very distressing symptoms, and they become sensitive to the increasing scepticism and exasperation displayed by their doctors. In a study at a cardiac clinic in London, 50 to 60 per cent of patients had normal cardiac function on investigation, and many of these were experiencing the palpitations, dyspnoea, and chest discomfort of anxiety; 21 per cent showed evidence of hyperventilation. The common physical effects of hyperarousal and hyperventilation affect most organ systems and parts of the body from head (ache) to toe (tingling) (see Table 3), and so these patients find their way into every specialist clinic in the hospital.

If you have patients with such unexplained physical symptoms, then the most acceptable way of exploring the possibility of these syndromes is to enquire systematically about all the common symptoms listed in Table 3. Patients often have a few more symptoms that are not on the list and are usually not bothered by all. Once organic causes have been excluded, the diagnosis of panic disorder can be made on the history of physical symptoms alone, and an explanation can be given to the patient in terms of the physiological effects of adrenaline plus overbreathing. It is particularly important that the physician makes it clear that the symptoms are genuine, and that the tests only show that nothing is wrong because we do not use tests for the transient physiological changes accounting for the symptoms.

Treatments for panic disorder include low doses of antidepressants and cognitive–behavioural therapy, and give very good results. The majority of patients will accept psychiatric referral if it is made clear: that you **do** believe their symptoms are real (which they are); you are **not** saying that they are mad, or making it up, or it is all in their minds; and that there **is** a treatment that is effective and not addictive or harmful. It helps if you know the psychiatrist and know what the patient is likely to experience. Left untreated these patients may become severely disabled and continue to undergo expensive and unnecessary medical investigation.

Recognizing depression in someone with good reasons to be unhappy

To be ill and in discomfort is generally to be unhappy, and the more serious the illness, the greater the pain, the greater the loss and the tragedy, so much more the misery. Worry about health and fears for the future are to be expected. How can a doctor tell when an ill person's unhappiness amounts to a depressive illness requiring specific intervention, and when is it an appropriate adjustment reaction to grievous circumstance? Some of the cardinal diagnostic features of depressive illness much emphasized in general psychiatric practice are of little use in these circumstances, so that in patients with physical reasons for poor appetite and weight loss, and sleep disturbed by pain or other physical symptoms, we must look for other indicators of mood disorder. Endicott has thus suggested modifications to the diagnostic criteria for depression (see Box 3).

The emphasis is placed on the predominantly negative thinking style that is pervasive. A depressed person cannot be cheered up when nice things happen, will not be interested in things he/she used to enjoy, will be excessively pessimistic, and have an exaggerated sense of guilt and worthlessness.

Box 3 Endicott's criteria for depression in the medically ill

Presence of five out of these nine symptoms for at least 2 weeks:

1. *Fearful or depressed appearance*
2. Social withdrawal or decreased talkativeness
3. Psychomotor retardation or agitation
4. Depressed mood, subjective or observed
5. Marked diminished interest or pleasure in most of the activities, most of the day
6. *Brooding self-pity or pessimism*
7. Feelings of worthlessness or excessive or inappropriate guilt
8. Recurrent thoughts of death or suicide
9. *Mood is non-reactive to environmental events*

Symptoms in italics replace DSM-III-R* symptoms as follows:

weight change

sleep disturbance

fatigue or energy loss

diminished ability to think, concentrate; indecisiveness

**Diagnostic and statistical manual of mental disorder, third edition, revised* (1987).

Final comment

It is important to screen for mental health problems: they are common in general medical patients and failure to recognize and deal with them will often interfere with the management of the physical health of the patient. Moreover, depression itself can kill, and if by screening you identify depression, you should ask about hopelessness and suicidal ideation. How to do this sensitively is covered in Chapter 26.5.2.

Further reading

American Psychiatric Association (1987). *Diagnostic and statistical manual of mental disorder, third edition, revised.* APA, Washington, DC.

Bass C, *et al.* (1988). Panic anxiety and hyperventilation in patients with chest pain, *Quarterly Journal of Medicine* **69**, 949–59.

Endicott J (1994). Measurement of depression in out-patients with cancer. *Cancer* **53**, 2243–8.

Feldman E, *et al.* (1987). Psychiatric disorder in medical in-patients. *Quarterly Journal of Medicine* **63**, 405–12.

Mayfield DG, Johnstone RGM (1980). Screening techniques and prevalence estimation in alcoholism. In: Fann WE, *et al.*, eds. *Phenomenology and treatment of alcoholism*, pp.33–44. Spectrum, New York.

Van Hemert AM, *et al.* (1993). Psychiatric disorders in relation to medical illness among patients of a general medical outpatient clinic. *Psychological Medicine* **23**, 167–73.

26.3 Neuropsychiatric disorders

Laurence John Reed, Tom Stevens, and Michael D. Kopelman

Introduction

'Neuropsychiatry' is concerned with disorders of affect, cognition, and behaviour that arise from overt disorder in cerebral function, or from indirect effects of extracerebral disease. The term has largely replaced the earlier expression 'organic psychiatry', which originated in the classification of mental disorders as either 'organic' or 'functional' on the basis of the presence or absence of pathological changes in the brain. The latter distinction has become increasingly ambiguous as a result of the development of new methods for detecting abnormal brain pathology and pathophysiology in so-called 'functional' disorders such as depression and schizophrenia. Indeed, the most recent version of the *Diagnostic and statistical manual of mental disorders, fourth edition* (DSM-IV, American Psychiatric Association) states, 'the term organic mental disorder is no longer used in DSM-IV because it incorrectly implies that 'non-organic' mental disorders do not have a biological basis'. Nevertheless, a creative conflict has always pertained between neurological and psychological theories of behaviour and, in the absence of satisfactory alternatives, these terms have retained a place in clinical practice. In part, this serves to demarcate the uneasy and shifting boundary between disorders predominantly diagnosed and managed by physicians and psychiatrists, respectively.

This chapter is divided into two parts. First, we provide a consideration of practical issues related to the assessment, investigation, and management of patients manifesting cognitive and behavioural change. Second, we discuss specific cerebral and extracerebral disorders that commonly involve or are accompanied by cognitive or behavioural change. This bipartite organization is intended to help in the identification of possible diagnoses causing particular behavioural features, and also to alert clinicians to the likely neuropsychiatric sequelae of specific medical disorders.

Assessment, investigation, and management of patients with cognitive and behavioural change

The assessment and classification of mental and behavioural disorders is a frequent source of misunderstanding and confusion for clinicians, the process being undermined by the absence of robust clinical and laboratory markers for these conditions. Moreover, the clinical terminology used to describe certain symptoms and signs (such as 'confusion') is often unsatisfactory and unreliable. Although the major systems of classification are broadly similar, they continue to use different terminology: for instance, the World Health Organization's *International classification of diseases, tenth edition* (ICD-10) retains the term 'organic disorders', whereas DSM-IV uses the broad grouping 'delirium, dementia, amnesic and other cognitive disorders'. In addition, some of the operational diagnoses may have little validity in assisting the clinician to determine the appropriate investigation and treatment, for example the ICD-10 'unspecified organic personality and behavioural disorders due to brain disease, damage and dysfunction'. Nevertheless, there is consensus on the essential clinical features of these disorders, and in this section we shall describe their assessment on the basis of a number of core features underpinning the differential diagnosis.

Differential diagnoses

Acute versus chronic disorder

The differentiation of acute and chronic cognitive disorder essentially determines the boundary between delirium and dementia. This distinction should be apparent from the history and mode of presentation, although difficulties may arise where a clear history is lacking due to disturbed communication or the absence of an adequate informant. However, they can usually be distinguished on the basis of the characteristic clinical features described below. Essentially, a conspicuous impairment of attention is typical of an acute disorder, together with a fluctuating course and prominent perceptual disturbance. However, the 'acute on chronic' disorder, where there is a delirium superimposed on a chronic cognitive disorder, should not be overlooked.

Cognitive versus psychiatric disorder

This distinction between a cognitive and a psychiatric disorder is not always easy. It is important to recognize that an apparent cognitive abnormality may be seen in psychiatric disorders such as schizophrenia and depression. In depression, impairment of memory and concentration together with somatic complaints may lead to a misleading impression of dementia, so-called 'pseudodementia' or 'reversible dementia'. Likewise, the distinction between acute psychotic disorders and delirium can be difficult where both conditions show behavioural disturbance and disturbed communication. The risks associated with the wrongful categorization of delirium as psychosis are high: delirium is a medical emergency with high morbidity and mortality, and it is potentially reversible. Likewise, the attribution of a psychiatric disorder as delirium or dementia bears costs in terms of performing unnecessary investigations and pursuing the wrong therapy in an inappropriate setting, thereby compounding any illness behaviour.

Specific versus generalized cognitive impairment

If cognitive impairment is identified, it needs to be determined whether this is generalized to many cognitive functions or affects a specific function such as memory, planning, perception, language, or attention. Identification of a specific impairment, such as the amnesic syndrome, offers important clues as to the aetiology and management and is more likely to result from a focal brain lesion (as opposed to an extracerebral disorder).

Reversible versus irreversible

The range of causes of any cognitive impairment needs to be fully assessed. In particular, it is essential that those conditions that can be reversed or arrested should be specifically considered, for example human immunodeficiency virus (HIV) infection and cerebral neoplasms. It is equally important that any treatable psychiatric disorder is identified.

Table 1 Causes of acute behavioural change

- Delirium
- Alcohol and substance misuse
- Psychosis
- Personality disorder
- Acute stress reaction
- Adjustment disorder
- Depression
- Dissociative disorder
- Malingering

Acute cognitive and behavioural change

Assessment

A wide range of disorders may cause acute emotional and behavioural disturbance (Table 1). One of the most problematic aspects of assessment is the distinction between an acute psychotic episode and delirium. The clinical features of delirium (also known as 'acute organic brain syndrome' or 'acute confusional state') and of the 'functional' psychoses typical of schizophrenia or affective disorder share a number of characteristics. First, both involve a pervasive disruption of thought, cognition, communication, and behaviour in the patient, hence presenting particular difficulties in assessment. Second, both conditions may involve abnormalities of perception in the form of hallucinations or illusions; abnormalities of belief, in the form of delusions or overvalued ideas; psychomotor abnormalities, including hypo- or hyperactivity; disturbance of the sleep–wake cycle; and emotional disturbance encompassing the range from depression to irritability and euphoria. These similarities cause practical difficulties in diagnostic differentiation, and they also hint that an absolute distinction between 'functional' psychosis and 'medical' delirium is probably untenable.

Delirium

A thorough history of the antecedents and onset of any behavioural and mental disturbance, as well as details of any past medical or psychiatric contact, will yield important clues as to the likelihood of an organic aetiology to behavioural change. The unco-operative or mute patient presents a particular challenge as important historical details may not be forthcoming, such as head injury, substance misuse, foreign travel, diabetes, or other medical disorders. Furthermore, accurately eliciting a mental and cognitive state is problematic, and it is in this group that a history from an informant, ward staff, or relatives is especially important. The diagnosis of delirium should be suspected where the history of behavioural disturbance is of recent onset, fluctuating, and there is evidence of deterioration at night. Difficulty in communicating with a patient is frequently the first indication of an underlying delirium.

The elderly and general hospital inpatients are particularly vulnerable to delirium. Any change of environment such as a recent admission to residential care or pre-existing cognitive impairment will heighten this vulnerability. Visual and hearing impairments are also more frequently observed in this group. Amongst inpatients the problem is compounded by inadequate information, impersonal environments, and confusing exposure to a myriad of different professionals. It is common for the diagnosis to be missed where there is no overt agitation or antisocial behaviour.

Behavioural changes seen with delirium include irritability, repetitive purposeless movements, and disorganization or difficulty performing routine tasks such as undressing. It is important to recognize that patients may be both overactive and noisy or inactive and slow.

The predominant clinical feature of delirium has been described as 'clouding of consciousness' or 'clouding of the sensorium'. These terms lack consensus definitions or clarity in practice, but have traditionally been used to describe a combination of orientation, attention, and memory deficits. Consequently, deficits of attention are stressed in diagnostic criteria, which in the delirious patient may range from distractibility and inability to follow complicated conversations, through an almost complete inability to register information or to concentrate, progressing in the extreme case to diminished consciousness and coma. Furthermore, such attentional difficulties tend to have a sudden onset and to fluctuate over time. Thinking tends to be muddled and speech may show considerable perseveration. The illusions and hallucinations associated with delirium tend to include a strong visual component, although auditory hallucinations and misperceptions are common. Delusions are usually simple, persecutory in nature, fluctuating, and transient.

It should be noted that if delirium and cognitive impairment are simply assessed by orientation in time, place, and person, then 'mild' or 'early' delirium may be missed, and it is therefore important to use additional tests of concentration and memory. All patients should be screened with a small battery of bedside cognitive tests that include specific tests of concentration such as serial subtractions and an assessment of memory for recent events and new information. The Mini-Mental State Examination (**MMSE**), supplemented with a few additional memory tests, is often used.

Psychiatric disorder

The characteristic clinical features of psychiatric disorders are covered in Chapter 26.5.6. Here we will discuss the features of acute behavioural disturbance that are suggestive of a psychotic illness or other psychiatric disorder. This issue is especially important in the emergency medical setting where such patients may be perceived as 'time-wasting' and 'not medical', and their medical needs may be crucially neglected.

A past history of psychiatric contact or treatment should be sought in all those with behavioural disturbance, as this is an indicator of putative psychiatric causation. In those with an underlying psychiatric disorder there is usually a background of insidious behavioural disturbance or personality change, and this will often become apparent from any informant. Delusions in psychotic disorders tend to be complex, bizarre, and consistently held, but this may not be so in early cases. Visual hallucinations are rare in psychosis. Marked attentional and memory deficits are not typical of psychosis, although more subtle attentional problems and a range of other cognitive deficits may be present. Distractibility as a consequence of internal experiences may give the impression of confusion and attentional impairment, although careful cognitive assessment will usually indicate preserved function.

Delirium in those with psychiatric disorder

The diagnosis of delirium is particularly difficult in those with a history of severe psychiatric disorder and/or learning disability. Difficulty in communicating with and examining such patients, who may have baseline cognitive impairment, means that delirium is particularly likely to be overlooked. Patients with severe mental illness will often attend for emergency consultations where the initial impression is of deterioration in their mental state, often coupled with a recent history of failing to comply with prescribed treatment or a disengagement from services provided. It should always be remembered that there is a high rate of undiagnosed physical illnesses in this population, and their risk of delirium is also raised because of serious side-effects from psychotropic medication, including neuroleptic malignant syndrome and lithium toxicity that can result in a deteriorating mental state. In addition, other aspects of these patients' behaviour place them at risk of physical illness, such as coexisting substance and alcohol dependency.

Investigation

It is necessary to exclude the wide range of medical conditions (Table 2) that may lead to delirium. A history of alcohol and/or illicit substance misuse may offer important indicators of aetiology. Although not always easy, a thorough physical examination with particular attention to neurological examination is essential in the assessment of all patients with acute disturbance. In addition, a routine screen—including blood count, electrolytes,

Table 2 Causes of delirium

• Infection	Pneumonia, urinary tract infection, septicaemia, any other infection e.g. HIV, malaria, encephalitis etc
• Vitamin deficiencies	Thiamine, nicotinic acid and vitamin B_{12} deficiency
• Epileptic	Complex partial seizures, postictal states, petit mal epilepsy
• Metabolic	Hypoxia, hypercapnia, electrolyte and acid–base disturbances, liver disease, uraemia, hypothermia, hyperthermia, and porphyria
• Endocrine	Hypoglycaemia, hypo- and hyperthyroidism, addisonian crisis, hypo- and hyperparathyroidism, hypopituitarism
• Trauma	Head injury, acute post-traumatic psychosis
• Vascular	Cerebrovascular accident, subarachnoid haemorrhage, hypertensive encephalopathy
• Toxic	Alcohol and drug withdrawal and intoxication, carbon monoxide poisoning
• Iatrogenic	Drug toxicity—anticonvulsants

liver and thyroid function, and C-reactive protein (**CRP**)/erythrocyte sedimentation rate (**ESR**)—is required, as this might indicate delirium where the diagnosis is in doubt. Infection is implicated in around one-third of hospital inpatients who are delirious, and a mid-stream urine sample (**MSU**) and chest radiograph are usually warranted in addition to routine blood testing in these patients. Relevant history and findings on physical examination usually guide more specific investigation. Encephalitis and intracerebral haemorrhage sometimes present with acute disturbance and cognitive impairment with no additional abnormalities in the history and clinical examination. An urgent computed tomography (**CT**) head scan or magnetic resonance imaging (**MRI**) is indicated where the immediate cause of acute cognitive impairment is not apparent or there are focal neurological signs. Appropriate tests for infectious diseases such as malaria, trypanosomiasis, typhoid fever, and typhus will also need to be considered when there is a history of foreign travel. An electroencephalogram with evidence of progressive cortical slowing may suggest a delirium and the need for a more extensive investigation where the diagnosis is in doubt.

Management

The management of delirium essentially consists of treating the underlying cause. Containment of any behavioural disturbance should involve general measures in the first instance, rather than psychotropic drug treatment, although sedation is necessary in some cases. Careful and repeated explanation of the diagnosis, investigations, and treatment to the patient and relatives is important. The patient should be nursed in a bright, simple room with minimal changes in staff and good lighting at night to reduce perceptual disturbance. Drugs, especially psychoactive and anticholinergic agents that may exacerbate confusion, should be reduced to a minimum. Where sedation is required then a regular oral antipsychotic such as haloperidol or chlorpromazine can be administered, although the clinician should be alert to the powerful antidopaminergic side-effects of these drugs. (See Chapter 26.4 for further discussion of these issues.)

Behavioural disturbance in patients with alcohol and substance misuse

This group of patients often present considerable demands on clinicians due to the wide range of associated physical morbidity that follows from substance and alcohol misuse. Approximately one-quarter of all male medical admissions have been found to have a current or previous alcohol problem. Such individuals commonly attend accident and emergency departments in a state of withdrawal or intoxication that engender negative attitudes from clinical staff. Often there is an expectation that the behavioural disturbance is due to intoxication or a withdrawal syndrome, without adequate assessment of any other physical pathology. Alternatively, such patients may attempt to minimize their alcohol and drug history so that the contribution of these to their complaints may not be immediately apparent.

Table 3 Causes of behavioural disturbance associated with a history of alcohol dependency

- Alcohol intoxication
- Alcohol withdrawal
- Alcoholic blackouts
- Delirium tremens
- Wernicke's encephalopathy
- Head injury
- Intracranial haemorrhage
- Pneumonia
- Tuberculosis
- Hepatic encephalopathy
- Epilepsy
- Hypoglycaemia
- Hypomagnesaemia
- Withdrawal and other alcohol-related seizures
- Alcoholic hallucinosis.

Patients with a history of excessive alcohol consumption are vulnerable to a large number of complications that may precipitate a delirium (see Table 3) and care is needed to assess all of these possibilities. The onset of hallucinations may be mistakenly labelled as a consequence of delirium tremens without consideration of other 'organic' or 'functional' disorders.

Delirium tremens carries a mortality risk of approximately 5 per cent and, furthermore, there is the danger that a withdrawal or intoxication syndrome may mask the emergence of other complications of alcohol and substance misuse. A history of recent blackouts or seizures should alert the physician to the possibility of hypoglycaemia or epilepsy. A careful assessment of the mental state is needed to differentiate 'functional' disorders, such as alcoholic hallucinosis, from schizophrenia as treatment of a mental disorder may be overlooked. Physical examination should include a careful assessment for signs of cirrhosis or acute hepatic encephalopathy. Investigation is essential to distinguish underlying conditions such as hepatic encephalopathy and hypoglycaemia from delirium tremens and should include full blood count, liver function tests, electrolyte and γ-glutamyl transferase (**GGT**) measurements, glucose estimation, chest radiographs, and a CT or MRI scan of the brain where there is a suspicion of head trauma contributing to the disturbance. In particular, Wernicke's encephalopathy should be considered since it may be seen in up to 3 per cent of all admissions for alcohol complications. (See Chapters 26.7.1, 26.7.2, and 26.7.3 for further discussion of these issues.)

Chronic and subacute cognitive and behavioural disturbance

Assessment

In the assessment of patients with a more insidious onset of cognitive or psychiatric disturbance there can again be uncertainty as to the relative aetiological roles of organic or psychiatric factors. This may lead to unnecessary investigations at both considerable expense and discomfort to the patient, with attention diverted from appropriate management. Moreover, failure to consider a treatable cerebral disorder such as a space-occupying lesion may lead to avoidable and irreversible brain damage. Table 4 outlines a list of cognitive and psychiatric disorders that may exhibit evidence of cognitive impairment. The diagnostic uncertainty pertaining to

Table 4 Disorders presenting with chronic/subacute cognitive and behavioural disturbance

Cognitive
• Dementia
• Frontal lobe syndrome
• Amnesic disorder
Psychiatric
• Depression
• Schizophrenia
• Dissociative disorder

the assessment of chronic cognitive impairment is highlighted by the somewhat misleading term 'pseudodementia' used to denote a psychological aetiology.

The diagnostic challenges in this group of patients are exemplified by the complex differentiation between dementia and depression or 'depressive pseudodementia', where there are changes in behaviour, mood, intellectual functioning, and cognitive performance. Differentiation is complicated by the fact that depressed mood is a frequent prodrome (and possibly even a risk factor) for an emerging dementia such as Alzheimer's. Furthermore, depression is a common complication or consequence of Alzheimer's and other dementias. It is therefore essential in the clinical setting that the relative contributions of psychiatric and pathological factors in any given case are considered, and that assessment includes a thorough physical, neurological, and psychiatric examination.

Dementia

Dementia is a syndrome involving a pervasive impairment of higher cortical functions and resulting from widespread brain pathology. The aetiology and characteristic clinical features of dementia are described in detail in Chapters 24.13.8 and 30.2, summarized in Table 5, and the most important causes are shown in Table 6. In the investigation of dementia it is essential to identify or exclude reversible causes: this should therefore include a complete blood count, electrolyte and metabolic screen, thyroid screen, vitamin B_{12} and folate levels, syphilis serology, urinalysis, chest radiography, and electrocardiography, and head CT or MRI scan. These investigations are sufficient to diagnose most treatable dementias. Any uncertainty about the extent of cognitive impairment necessitates formal neuropsychological assessment using instruments such as the Weschler Adult Intelligence Scale (**WAIS**-R or WAIS-111), as well as standard memory and executive tests.

The presence of a family history of early-onset cognitive impairment may indicate the need for genetic screening for Alzheimer's and Huntington's disease after appropriate counselling. Other potential evaluations include MRI, electroencephalography, cerebrospinal fluid examination, and possibly cerebral blood flow and metabolism measures (single-photon emission computed tomography (**SPECT**) and positron-emission tomography (**PET**)). Brain biopsy can be of additional assistance in diagnosing the cause of the dementia when justified by the clinical setting. For example, any suggestion of Creutzfeldt–Jakob disease would make an electroencephalogram (**EEG**) essential, and focal neurological signs would indicate the need for neuroimaging to exclude a space-occupying lesion. A known history of HIV infection would warrant a lumbar puncture. Evidence of extrapyramidal disturbance should alert the clinician to the possibility of Wilson's disease, necessitating serum copper and caeruloplasmin level investigation and slit-lamp examination for Kayser–Fleischer rings. These issues are discussed more completely in Chapter 24.13.8.

Table 5 Clinical features of dementia

• Behaviour	Disorganized, inappropriate, and distractible behaviour. Lack of interest and initiative. Personality change, antisocial behaviour, sleep disturbance, incontinence. Self-neglect
• Mood	Anxiety, agitation, irritability, and depression. Lability of mood
• Thinking and perception	Delusions, illusions, and hallucinations
• Cognition	Disorientation, anterograde and retrograde amnesia, impairment in comprehension and language. Aphasia, apraxia, and agnosia
• Insight	Impaired

Table 6 Causes of dementia

• Degenerative	Alzheimer's, vascular dementia, Pick's disease, Creutzfeldt–Jakob disease, Parkinson's disease, multiple sclerosis, normal-pressure hydrocephalus
• Infection	Neurosyphilis, Whipple's disease, HIV
• Metabolic	Renal dialysis (aluminium toxicity), liver failure, metachromatic leucodystrophy.
• Endocrine	Hypothyroidism
• Vitamin deficiency	Vitamin B12 and folate deficiency, pellagra
• Space-occupying	Subdural haemorrhage, tumour
• Traumatic	Punch-drunk syndrome
• Genetic	Wilson's disease, Huntington's chorea
• Autoimmune	Systemic lupus erythromatosus (**SLE**)
• Anoxia	Respiratory failure, cardiac arrest, carbon monoxide poisoning
• Toxic	Alcohol dementia, heavy metal poisoning (lead, arsenic, mercury, and thallium)

New cases of psychotic disorder

Missing an underlying 'organic' diagnosis remains a continuing concern of clinicians responsible for the assessment and treatment of new cases of an apparent psychosis. Clinical experience and numerous case reports attest to the wide range of disorders that may emerge following the initial diagnosis of a 'functional' psychosis. One follow-up study of a sample of patients with first-episode schizophrenia found that 15 out of 268 cases studied had 'organic' disorders that appeared relevant to the mental state: 13 patients out of these 15 had salient features in the medical history or neurological signs that could have alerted the clinician to the underlying disorder, the two exceptions both having a diagnosis of neurosyphilis. HIV is increasingly prevalent in this population and one recent cohort identified a known diagnosis of HIV in 4 per cent, with many subjects not tested. An assessment of risk factors for HIV is therefore required in all new cases of psychotic disorder. Overall, the literature suggests that the risks of missing organic illness are low, provided that a thorough clinical assessment is performed.

Some debate remains over the degree of investigation appropriate for the onset of psychosis. Certainly patients with cognitive impairment, abnormal neurological signs, atypical illnesses not responding to treatment, or other indications from the history, warrant further investigation. Where appropriate, this should include neuroimaging, electroencephalography, syphilis serology, and other investigations indicated by the clinical picture. Increasingly, neuroimaging provides important information relevant to the management of a particular case, although in the absence of specific indications the identification of treatable neurological disease is low.

Focal cognitive disorders

A variety of neuropsychiatric syndromes may arise from regional cerebral impairments of diverse cause in the absence of generalized cognitive impairment.

Clinical features

Amnesic disorders

The essential clinical feature of an amnesic disorder is a profound impairment in new learning relative to any generalized cognitive impairment. The impairment in recent memory is usually associated with disorientation in time and the patient is unable to retain information for more than a few seconds. A common cause of the amnesic syndrome is the Wernicke–Korsakoff syndrome resulting from thiamine deficiency in association with chronic alcoholism or, occasionally, malnutrition or malabsorption. The Wernicke phase of this disorder is characterized by confusion, nystagmus, abducent and conjugate gaze palsies (ophthalmoplegia), and ataxia. These features are commonly accompanied by peripheral neuropathy. Prompt treatment with thiamine replacement is vital in order to avert a chronic and disabling amnesic disorder (the Korsakoff syndrome).

The neuropathology of amnesic disorders usually involves lesions within the limbic system, including the thalamus and posterior hypothalamus, medial temporal lobes, and mamillary bodies. The crucial pathology in Korsakoff's syndrome is thought to involve neuronal loss, gliosis, and microhaemorrhages that produce disruption of mammilothalamic circuits. Pathology elsewhere in the paraventricular and periaqueductal grey matter, the frontal lobes, and in white matter pathways traversing the diencephalons, are common accompanying features. Amnesia can also be seen in herpes simplex encephalitis, carbon monoxide poisoning, other causes of cerebral anoxia, thalamic infarction, subarachnoid haemorrhage, head injury, deep midline space-occupying lesions, or tuberculous meningitis.

Frontal lobe syndromes

Particular neuropsychiatric interest is attached to the consequences of damage to the anterior regions of the brain. These are frequently neurologically 'silent', but they can also result in remarkable alterations in behaviour and personality, with preservation of cognitive functions such as memory and intelligence. Thus, psychiatric manifestations may be the only signs of frontal brain disease, and psychiatric disturbance may be an impediment to medical management. Two clinical pictures that frequently coexist are recognized. The first is characterized by a loss of initiative, indifference, lack of motivation, with impoverished speech and communication to the extreme of mutism. The second is characterized by disinhibition, impulsivity (occasionally with aggression), lack of ability to sustain attention and concentration, and loss of sensitivity to social cues: in general, such patients are excessively talkative and they may confabulate spontaneously. Both such syndromes have been subsumed under the term 'dysexecutive syndrome' (also known as 'strategy application disorder'), which attempts a unitary cognitive psychological perspective on the condition. Interesting parallels have been drawn between the clinical frontal lobe syndrome and the features of neurological conditions such as Parkinson's disease and psychiatric disorders such as the negative syndrome in schizophrenia: in both these examples it is thought that impaired dopaminergic neurotransmission in prefrontal brain regions gives rise to the particular symptomatology.

Temporal lobe syndromes

A variety of syndromes, depending upon the particular area affected, are recognized following temporal lobe damage. Personality disturbance may be seen, although usually with neurological impairments. A particular variant of this is the Kluver–Bucy syndrome following bilateral lesions to the medial and lateral temporal lobes: this results in irresistible impulses to touch objects and place them in the mouth, combined with a lack of initiative, placidity, and visual agnosia. Dominant lobe lesions may produce aphasia, 'surface' dyslexia, and/or dysgraphia, frequently accompanied by neurological impairments on the contralateral side. Non-dominant lesions may particularly affect facial, spatial, or autobiographical memory, or may appear to be cognitively 'silent'. There is a recognized association between temporal lobe lesions, particularly those giving rise to epileptic activity, and psychosis, which may bear striking similarities with that seen in schizophrenia or affective disorder. Last, severe bilateral medial temporal lobe damage usually gives rise to a profound amnesic syndrome, with an almost complete loss of the ability to learn new material (anterograde amnesia) and a variable degree of retrograde loss of memory, whilst pathology in the left inferior temporal gyrus can produce severe deficits in semantic memory.

Parietal lobe syndromes

Parietal lobe lesions are associated with two particular sets of higher cognitive impairments: first, loss of visuospatial abilities, resulting in apraxias and spatial disorientation including left–right disorientation; second, loss of higher sensory perception, resulting in astereognosis and body image disturbance, which may be of such severity that there is a denial of disability, anosognosia, and visuospatial neglect. There may also be involvement of the occipital lobe, which can produce additional homonymous field defects, occasionally associated with visual hallucinations.

Diencephalic syndromes

Lesions to the deep midline structures of the thalamus, hypothalamus, and brainstem are associated with an amnesic syndrome, particularly exemplified by the Wernicke–Korsakoff syndrome. Deep midline tumours can produce a similar picture. More posterior brainstem lesions are associated with hypersomnia and placidity, which may be insidious: this was memorably described in a patient with 'akinetic mutism' due to a juxtapituitary meningioma.

Investigation of focal cognitive disorders

Cognitive assessment

Neuropsychological tests require the patient's co-operation and may fail to discriminate reliably between a cognitive and psychiatric disorder. However, they may furnish important indications of localized cerebral dysfunction and assist the clinician in monitoring the progress of any cognitive impairment. A wide range of tests is available to evaluate the pattern of disability, and these may also contribute important information to assist rehabilitation.

Brain imaging

The most useful range of investigations in suspected neuropsychiatric disorders comprise brain imaging techniques, the technology and application of which has expanded greatly in recent years. The most widely available, computed tomography (CT), is able to visualize most cerebral lesions, but should nowadays be reserved for the investigation of acute progressive cerebral damage such as stroke or subarachnoid haemorrhage, where time is of the essence and management decisions must be made rapidly. In more insidious, less acute contexts, the brain imaging of choice is magnetic resonance imaging (MRI), which allows both a higher spatial resolution with fine anatomical detail and a choice of endogenous/exogenous tissue-contrast modalities, producing greater diagnostic yield. MRI is more sensitive than CT in identifying small vascular lesions or demyelination, but less sensitive in detecting calcified lesions. Sequential assessments of cerebral atrophy and quantitative approaches can facilitate the accurate assessment of disease progression.

The EEG is frequently employed in the investigation of neuropsychiatric disorder as it is both widely available and a sensitive, if relatively non-specific, indicator of cerebral dysfunction. Focal abnormalities are characteristic of epilepsy that may, in turn, reflect vascular change. Diffuse slowing (that is to say, a shift to lower frequency ranges) is a sensitive indicator of brain dysfunction arising from metabolic and degenerative processes that correlates with the degree of cognitive impairment, although with relatively little specificity. Characteristic EEG changes are associated with Huntington's disease (pronounced flattening of traces), sporadic Creutzfeldt–Jakob disease (repetitive and triphasic spike discharges), and in association with specific drugs. Medial temporal slowing can be suggestive of early Alzheimer dementia.

The imaging of cerebral metabolism, blood flow, and receptor density, using techniques such as SPECT and PET, provide an alternative perspective on cerebral dysfunction. These are proving increasingly valuable in neuropsychiatry, although more for research than clinical purposes.

The past decade has seen an enormous expansion in functional brain imaging that allows assessment of brain regional engagement during cognitive processing. Changes in regional cerebral blood flow using PET, or in regional haemoglobin oxygenation status using blood oxygenation level-dependent (**BOLD**) functional MRI (**fMRI**), can be measured during cognitive performance. Such dynamic assessments remain essentially research techniques, allowing measurement of regional brain function and functional connectivity between linked brain areas. However, they may well offer clinical value in diagnosis and disease stratification in the future.

Neuropsychiatric causes of psychiatric disorders

Neuropsychiatric causes of psychiatric disorder are shown in Table 7.

'Organic mood disorder'

A variety of medical conditions are associated with prominent affective disorder, including anxiety, elation, and depressive symptoms. In many of these there appears to be a direct relationship between the presence of brain disease and depression, and the latter does not just seem to reflect the disabling social consequences of chronic disease, although the 'psychological reaction' to the disablement may still be an important contributory factor. In this connection, the severity of the depression is poorly correlated with the 'objective' disability or the prognosis of the disorder, and some disorders, such as multiple sclerosis, can be associated with either euphoria or depression or mood swings between the two extremes.

'Organic personality disorder'

'Organic personality disorder' is an unhappy term employed in ICD-10 to denote acute or (more typically) insidious changes in personality, defined as a significant alteration in the habitual disposition and behaviour of a patient from their premorbid state. The syndrome is increasingly well recognized, although often in retrospect. Most prominently affected is the degree of emotional expression and levels of activity, in the absence of pronounced cognitive alterations, except where 'higher level' functions such as planning complex actions or anticipation of social and emotional consequences are affected. Causes comprise intracerebral insults and consequent damage, most commonly to the frontal, temporal, or subcortical regions, or a range of rare degenerative conditions (Table 8).

Table 7 Neuropsychiatric causes of psychiatric disorders

• Intracranial disorder	Cerebrovascular stroke, head injury, Parkinson's disease, multiple sclerosis, brain tumour, epilepsy, Huntington's disease, postencephalitic
• Endocrine disorder	Hypothyroidism, hyperthyroidism, hyperparathyroidism, hypopituitarism, Addison's disease, Cushing's disease, hypoglycaemia, diabetes mellitus
• Systemic disorder	Hepatic failure, renal failure, pernicious anaemia, rheumatoid arthritis, systemic lupus erythematosus, malignant neoplasia, viral infection (particularly infectious mononucleosis, influenza)
• Pharmacological causes	Corticosteroids, oestrogens (e.g. hormone replacement therapy), oral contraceptives, L-DOPA, clonidine, methylphenidate, withdrawal from stimulant agents, e.g. amphetamines

Table 8 Causes of organic personality disorder

Intracerebral insult	Cerebrovascular stroke, head injury, tumour (frequently frontal/sphenoidal meningioma), abscess, encephalitis (frequently herpes encephalitis, which has a recognized tropism for frontotemporal brain regions), subdural haematoma(chronic)
Neurodegenerative conditions	Huntington's disease, Wilson's disease (hepatolenticular degeneration), Pick's disease, Creutzfeldt–Jakob disease, subcortical dementias

Specific conditions giving rise to acute, subacute, or insidious cognitive and behavioural change

This section attempts to address two aspects of psychiatric problems associated with medical conditions: (1) to prompt the recognition and exploration of psychiatric abnormality in 'high-risk' conditions where such associations are well recognized; and (2) to encourage appropriate medical examination and investigation in the presence of outwardly psychiatric abnormality.

Psychological or psychiatric disorder may become manifest as an adjustment reaction to medical disability, malaise, and handicap, and this can affect not only the patient, but also family members, who often bear the practical burden of care. Psychological disorder may also result from a specific compromise of cerebral function, either directly or systemically mediated. For example, postoperative psychiatric disturbance is common and usually the result of infective, metabolic, or drug-induced delirium. However, the simple circumstances of operation may lead to the precipitation of disorientation in the presence of an insidious dementia, or a withdrawal syndrome in an alcohol-dependent individual. Furthermore, the emotional reaction in response to life-threatening and life-altering circumstances may be profound following major surgery. These factors interact, and the ultimate expression of mental disturbance depends upon a particular patient's premorbid disposition and social circumstances, as well as specific illness factors. Nevertheless, the recognition and specific ascertainment of the presence of mental disturbance in certain conditions has profound diagnostic and prognostic importance.

Neurological disorders

Cerebrovascular disorders

The psychiatric complications associated with stroke have illustrated the relevance of a neuropsychiatric perspective. Early studies recognized distinct emotional reactions associated with cerebral damage. These included the catastrophic reaction (often extreme or disproportionate emotional outburst to small demands); the indifference reaction (associated with fatuous mood, indifference to failures, and unilateral neglect and anosognosia); and pathological laughter/crying (also known rather pejoratively as emotional incontinence, where emotional displays occur seemingly spontaneously or to trivial provocation). More recent and carefully controlled studies have revealed that, contrary to expectation, the mood consequences of stroke are disproportionate to the objective disability and show a consistent relationship with the location of the lesion, with anterior lesions being strongly associated with depression.

Cerebral tumours

Cerebral tumours are frequently associated with psychiatric disability, ranging from 'understandable' reactions to the diagnosis to frank syndromes resulting from impaired brain function. Minor psychological disturbance including anxiety, depression, and occasionally hysterical symptoms may be seen before the medical diagnosis is made, and specific signs of cerebral

Table 9 Neuropsychiatric consequences of head injury

Delirium
Focal cognitive disorder (frontal lobe syndrome, amnestic disorder)
Global cognitive disorder
Subdural haematoma
Post-traumatic epilepsy
Delusional syndrome and hallucinosis
Affective syndrome
Post-traumatic disorder
Anxiety disorder
Personality change
Conversion disorders
Postconcussional syndrome
Alcohol misuse

pathology need to be excluded in this group of patients. The regional syndromes outlined above are notable in cases of primary or secondary cerebral tumours, in particular when the tumour is rapidly progressive or where multiple brain regions are involved with metastases. The most common adult-onset primary tumour is the ostensibly 'benign' meningioma, which is notoriously slow growing (estimates of growth indicate that tumours at diagnosis have often been present for some 10 to 15 years), and thus cerebral function is only slowly compromised. Coupled with their propensity for a frontal location, in which there may be few frank neurological signs, this can lead to tragic cases of progressive personality deterioration being overlooked. More dramatic impairments of cerebral function are particularly associated with rapidly progressive tumours in which raised intracranial pressure, irritative epileptic phenomena, and an overall distortion in brain structure may combine to produce delirium and dementia. There can be remote effects of malignant disease on cerebral function: hypercalcaemia may present with an acute confusional state or with other psychological/psychiatric manifestations, and some forms of lung carcinoma (in particular) secrete growth factor/endocrine hormones that result in neurodegenerative changes and a dementia-like picture. Last, both episodic and prolonged confusional states have been reported in malignant disease in the absence of a clear metabolic disturbance or focal brain involvement, for example in diffuse leptomeningeal disease.

Head injury

The most prominent group suffering head injury are young men who have sustained a motor vehicle injury. Recent neuropsychiatric interest in the condition stems from recognition that the problems suffered involve impairment in personality, affect, and social/occupational function more prominently than the objective dysfunction would suggest should be the case. The wide range of neuropsychiatric sequelae recognized after head injury are outlined in Table 9. The most disabling and distressing problems for both patients and carers are the emotional and behavioural effects and, in particular, the personality change.

Impairment of consciousness is characteristic after all but the most mild head injuries and features of delirium are often seen after severe injuries. The period of post-traumatic amnesia (**PTA**), representing the time that elapses between the moment of injury and the restoration of memory for everyday events, is an important predictor of outcome. This is correlated with personality change as well as intellectual impairment and neurological disorder. By contrast, memory loss for the events of the trauma itself appears to protect against the development of post-traumatic stress disorder.

Cognitive impairment following head injury is usually more apparent after a PTA exceeding 24 h, and testing reveals that performance and nonverbal intelligence are more vulnerable to the effects of trauma than verbal and vocabulary-based intelligence. Penetrating and localized injuries tend to result in more focal cognitive deficits dependent on the site of injury. Dysexecutive syndrome and short-term memory impairment are commonly seen.

Personality change is particularly common after severe head injury and frontal lobe damage and includes irritability, impatience, apathy, and lability of mood. There is an inability to learn from experience, with poor judgement and lack of initiative. Aggression and sexual disinhibition may necessitate high levels of subsequent care. Delusional disorders are frequently observed in the early stages of recovery and may reflect the persistence of disordered cognition; mood and anxiety disorders are also often seen. Premorbid alcohol misuse may have predisposed to the trauma and alcohol tolerance can decline markedly after severe injury. Problems with heavy drinking are not uncommon in this group, which may reflect poor insight and drinking in response to stressful circumstances. Caution is needed to exclude chronic subdural haematoma and post-traumatic epilepsy before ascribing emotional and behavioural change to a psychiatric diagnosis.

Complex rehabilitation strategies are often needed to manage this group of patients and novel pharmacological management are being assessed.

Epilepsy

In assessing epilepsy it is important to establish the extent of underlying cerebral damage giving rise to the epileptic discharge, as well as the nature and severity of any cognitive impairment. While compatible with normal intelligence, epilepsy is more common in patients with a learning disability, and is related to its severity, presumably as both epilepsy and a learning difficulty arise from underlying cerebral dysfunction. Thus the capacity of individuals to manage their epilepsy is highly variable and poses an important problem for management. Furthermore, there is a relationship between emotional state and definite epileptic seizures, indicating an interesting brain–mind relationship.

The neuropsychiatric consequences of epilepsy are best considered in terms of peri-ictal and interictal disorders, which are outlined in Table 10. Further information is available in Chapter 24.13.3.

Intracranial infections

Subacute encephalopathies

A well-recognized manifestation of acute cerebral infection is dramatic behavioural disturbance, which may involve violence and delirium—this forms a relatively common diagnostic problem, with particular value placed on a correct diagnosis. Of note are, first, that the groups relatively predisposed to the development of encephalitis are alcohol and drug misusers, where attitudes of medical staff may exert a pejorative effect; second, that the disordered behaviour may be sufficiently extreme to render medical examination and management difficult. While not rigorously studied, herpes simplex encephalitis is particularly implicated in such presentations, perhaps as the most common encephalitis and also because of tropism of

Table 10 Neuropsychiatric complications of epilepsy

Ictal and peri-ictal disorders	
Prodromal states	Tension, irritability, and depression may be seen
Complex partial seizures	Automatisms, distortions of perception, hallucinations, déjà vu, unusual disturbances of memory, thinking. Sudden changes in affect
Interictal disorders	
Cognitive impairment	This usually reflects underlying brain damage, and developmental consequences of repeated seizures and treatment with anticonvulsants
Personality	Probably only related to severe epilepsy where there is underlying brain damage
Schizophrenia-like psychosis	Associated with temporal lobe epilepsy
Depression	Suicide is four times more frequent in epileptics: those with adverse social factors and temporal lobe epilepsy are particularly at risk

the virus to frontal and temporal regions. Damage in these areas can lead to impairment of behaviour and language, and occasionally to acute psychotic features such as auditory hallucinations. Other forms of encephalitis can also produce striking behavioural change.

Neurosyphilis

In historical terms syphilitic infection is considered an archetype for neuropsychiatric disorder. It was formerly called the 'great mimic' in that a large variety of presentations were recognized, including frank neurological features, insidious cognitive deterioration, affective disturbance (particularly grandiose mania), and personality coarsening. Whilst its incidence is low, particular groups such as immigrants and those with coexistent HIV infection are at increased risk. More recently, partially treated neurosyphilis means that atypical presentations have become the norm. Although neurological features, such as the Argyll–Robertson pupil, may raise suspicions, these are rare; in practice, possible exposure needs to be elicited and routine laboratory testing carried out on a regular basis.

HIV and AIDS

Human immunodeficiency virus and the acquired immunodeficiency syndrome (**AIDS**) now form the most common infection 'cluster' associated with prominent psychiatric features. Primarily, the most common reactions are to the psychological impact of the diagnosis and its prognosis, which can result in profound depression or anxiety states and needs careful management. It is now recognized that HIV has a direct tropism for neuronal tissue and may result in a frank encephalopathy, producing progressive cognitive impairment in a so-called AIDS–dementia complex. The encephalopathy is also associated with features of mania. Gathering evidence suggests that this may be reversible using antiretroviral combination therapy.

New-variant Creutzfeldt–Jakob disease

New-variant Creutzfeldt–Jakob disease (**nvCJD**) commonly presents with neuropsychiatric problems, particularly with subtle memory disturbances (which may result from the disproportionate tropism of prions for the thalamus and diencephalon), intermittent delirium with violent outbursts, auditory hallucinations, and mutism. It is rapidly progressive, and while thalamic involvement can be recognized at an early stage on neuroimaging, the diagnosis can only be confirmed by brain biopsy with immunostaining for prion precursor protein. Less invasive tonsillar biopsy methods, which require specialist referral, have also been developed for diagnosis.

Neurodegenerative conditions

Multiple sclerosis and demyelinating disorders

A strong association with cognitive impairment (between 40 and 60 per cent) and mood disorder is recognized in multiple sclerosis. The cognitive deficits seem to subtend from disturbed 'frontal' or executive function, as does depressed mood, and both show little relationship with motor disability or with demonstrable lesion load.

Parkinson's disease and movement disorders

There are four particular aspects of neuropsychiatric disturbance relevant to the consideration of idiopathic and atypical parkinsonian syndromes, including multisystem atrophy:

1. A prodromal period without frank movement disorder is well recognized and may be typified by depression, personality change, and sensory changes, reflecting the onset of nigrostriatal degeneration. This must proceed to about 80 per cent loss before the development of motor signs relatively late in the disease process.
2. Dopaminergic replacement therapy, whether with cholinergic antagonists, dopamine agonists, or L-levodopa (**l-DOPA**), is associated with a substantial incidence of psychosis and delirium.
3. There is a strong association between Parkinson's disease and depression, with estimates of prevalence in community samples of about 7.5 per cent for major depressive disorder and 45 per cent for mild depressive symptoms. This association is widely divergent from objective disability, and probably reflects a prominent dopaminergic influence on mood and motivation.
4. A substantial proportion of sufferers develop 'diffuse' (extranigrostriatal) Lewy-body disease leading to focal and general cognitive deficits and dementia.

Particular mention should be made here of iatrogenic movement disorder attendant upon antipsychotic medication. All currently available antipsychotic agents have dopamine D2-antagonist activity and provoke parkinsonism, dyskinesias, and dystonia, although newer agents, in particular clozapine, have a lower propensity for this effect. Tardive dyskinesias and provoked parkinsonian syndromes do not necessarily remit on cessation of the antipsychotic agent.

Mental retardation

Although beyond the immediate scope of this chapter, the diverse conditions that give rise to learning disorders have been the subject of intense recent interest. In particular, their strong associations with attention-deficit hyperactivity disorder (**ADHD**), fetal alcohol syndrome, and autism have underscored a probable neuropsychiatric basis. From a neurodevelopmental perspective, attention deficit in children is strongly linked to conduct disorder and may have diverse consequences in adulthood, providing an archetype for the understanding of personality disorder, traditionally not viewed in neuropsychiatric terms. (See Chapter 24.21 for further discussion of some of these issues.)

Another relevant area of interest is the concept of behavioural phenotypes, where consistent behavioural abnormalities are associated with distinct genotypic abnormalities. For example, the frequently occurring chromosomal disorders of Down's syndrome, Turner's syndrome, and Klinefelter's syndrome have distinct and consistent neuropsychiatric aspects, albeit of variable degree. In Turner's syndrome, while overall IQ is variable, distinct difficulties in visuospatial function give rise to large verbal-performance IQ deficits.

Extracerebral disorders

Endocrine disorder

Endocrine disorder has an important influence on mental function and characteristic associations with neuropsychiatric disorder are found. The use of 'routine' blood tests of endocrine function has resulted in the earlier detection of problems, such that florid states are rarely seen. The focus of clinical interest in this area is upon 'preclinical' endocrine dysfunction, the complications arising from the disorder, and their treatment.

Diabetes mellitus

The neuropsychiatric aspects of diabetes mellitus, both insulin-dependent (**IDDM**) and non-insulin dependent (**NIDDM**) forms, may be considered in four areas:

1. The syndrome itself and the constraints of optimal management have a considerable impact on the lives of sufferers. The disorder is stigmatizing, especially in the young, and has significant associated morbidity and increased mortality, both factors that confer the risk of impaired psychological development, personality difficulties, and affective disorder. There is clear evidence of a relationship between 'stress', emotional disturbance, and impaired glycaemic control, although whether this is directly or indirectly (through neglect of diet and treatment) mediated is unclear.
2. Hypoglycaemic episodes are associated with frank behavioural disturbance and automatisms, as described below.
3. A series of studies have identified significant intellectual impairments in a subset of sufferers of diabetes, an attribute particularly associated

with an earlier age of onset, and the frequency and severity of hypoglycaemic episodes. While this strongly suggests that episodic hypoglycaemia results in brain damage in this subgroup, the so-called 'hypoglycaemic encephalopathy', an alternative possibility is that these patients are less able to manage their diabetes. This is of particular importance for those suffering 'brittle' diabetes, whose dietary and insulin requirements prove unpredictable, and who manage only poor glycaemic control; also for those suffering hypoglycaemia-unawareness, where incipient hypoglycaemia fails to trigger counter-regulatory neuroendocrine responses, thereby resulting in unpredictable hypoglycaemic episodes.

4. Later complications of diabetes, particularly if the diabetes is suboptimally controlled, include cerebral atherosclerosis and an increased risk of stroke, focal neuropsychological syndromes, and multi-infarct dementia.

Thyroid disorder

It is rare for classical presentations of thyroid disease to be missed in clinical practice, but interesting to note that surveys reveal that more than 5 per cent of attendees at psychiatric consultations have an abnormality in thyroid function. While not all of this group would benefit from treatment for thyroid disease, it underscores the insidious nature of thyroid dysfunction, and the rule should be to exclude this whenever suspicions are aroused. In particular, hypothyroidism may commonly manifest as apathy, depression, memory impairment, and dementia, with prominent cognitive slowing. If recognized and treated early, the condition may be reversible, although in long-lasting cases of hypothyroidism it is rarely so. Neonatal hypothyroidism or 'cretinism' is now rare as a result of routine screening, but again this indicates the importance of adequate thyroid function for cerebral development. Occasionally, adult hypothyroidism may be associated with psychosis (most commonly a delirium with prominent agitation), famously termed 'myxoedema madness'.

Hyperthyroidism is almost ubiquitously associated with a subjective feeling of tension, irritability, and high arousal. Initially this may be confused with anxiety, but in more severe cases behaviour can be frankly disturbed, although the individual concerned generally retains insight. Hypomania has been reported, as has a paradoxical apathetic state—both are rare. Thyroid 'crises' with delirium are occasionally seen following radioiodine treatment.

It should be noted that both hypo- and hyperthyroidism are common consequences of lithium treatment of bipolar affective disorder. This introduces the possibility of confusing a thyroid disorder with the recurrence of affective disorder, although it should be effectively excluded by the routine monitoring of lithium treatment.

Cushing's syndrome

The excess endogenous corticosteroid production in Cushing's syndrome appears to give rise to apathy and depression, with irritability and occasionally frank behavioural disturbance. The depression is often marked and may progress to stupor. Interestingly, exogenous steroids can give rise not only to anxiety and irritability, but also to hypomania and euphoria, which are rarely seen in Cushing's syndrome itself.

Phaeochromocytoma

The episodic release of adrenergic hormones from phaeochromocytoma classically gives rise to dizziness, tremulousness, palpitations, and the subjective feeling of intense fear, leading to confusion with anxiety and panic attacks. The diagnostic feature is the elevation of blood pressure during an attack, and if such attacks are reported, routine testing for adrenergic metabolites should be conducted. Attacks are occasionally of sufficient intensity to lead to confusion and delirium.

Pituitary disorder

Panhypopituitarism with consequent adrenal failure produces a characteristic neuropsychiatric picture with apathy, fatigue, weight loss, inability to attend and concentrate, and memory impairment. The disorder may therefore be confused with chronic fatigue, depression, or even dementia. The weight loss has been confused with anorexia nervosa, although neither appetite disturbance nor distorted body image is usually found with panhypopituitarism. Acromegaly can also result in a rather characteristic apathy and lack of concern, with occasional depression and irritability, perhaps reflecting a degree of global hypopituitrism.

There are two other particular neuropsychiatric issues that arise in consideration of a pituitary disorder. First, cerebral irradiation of pituitary tumours may give rise to collateral damage to adjacent brain structures, and there are reports of memory impairment, perhaps reflecting diencephalic and/or hippocampal damage. Second, endocrine replacement therapy following pituitary ablation may be suboptimal; indeed, replacement of sex steroids is occasionally omitted because of their propensity to release sexual drive, which may be inappropriate.

Gonadal dysfunction

Considerable attention has been devoted to the influence of the menopause and the consequent fall in oestrogen and progesterone on the development of depressive disorders in women. However, given the association with changing social role, this is a complex area. The consensus is that a lack of these hormones does play a significant part in the development of minor depressive disorders, which are significantly ameliorated by hormone replacement therapy. As a corollary, recent studies of testosterone deficiency in men have identified an association with depression, anxiety, irritability, insomnia, weakness, fatigue, diminished libido, impotence, and poor memory. Given the significant confound with ageing, this remains a controversial area.

Further reading

Amiel SA (1997). Hypoglycaemia in diabetes mellitus—protecting the brain. *Diabetologia* **40**(Suppl. 2), S62–8.

Baddeley AD (1986). *Working memory.* Clarendon Press, Oxford.

Bain BK (1998). CT scans of first-break psychotic patients in good general health. *Psychiatric Services* **49**, 234–5.

Deary IJ, Frier BM (1996). Severe hypoglycaemia and cognitive impairment in diabetes. *British Medical Journal* **313**, 767–8.

D'Ercole A, *et al.* (1991). Diagnosis of physical illness in psychiatric patients using axis III and a standardised medical history. *Hospital and Community Psychiatry* **42**, 395–400.

Folstein MF, Folstein SE, McHugh PR (1975). 'Mini mental state'. A practical method for grading the cognitive state of patients for the clinician *Journal of Psychiatric Research* **12**, 189–98.

Frackowiak RSJ, *et al.* (1997). *Human brain function.* Academic Press, London.

Guinan EM, *et al.* (1998). Cognitive effects of pituitary tumors and their treatments: two case studies and our investigation of 90 patients. *Journal of Neurology, Neurosurgery, and Psychiatry* **65**, 870–6.

Harper C (1983). The incidence of Wernicke's encephalopathy in Australia—a neuropathological study of 131 cases. *Journal of Neurology, Neurosurgery and Psychiatry* **46**, 593–8.

Hebb DO (1945). Man's frontal lobe: a critical review. *Archives of Neurology and Psychiatry* **54**, 10–24.

Hodges JR (1994). *Cognitive assessment for clinicians.* Oxford Medical Publications, Oxford.

Jacobson R, Kopelman M (1998). *Organic psychiatric disorders.* In: Wilkinson G, Stein G, eds. *College seminars in adult psychiatry.* Gaskell, London.

Johnstone EC, Macmillan F, Crow TJ (1987). The occurrence of organic disease of possible or probable aetiological significance in a population of 268 cases of first episode schizophrenia. *Psychological Medicine* **17**, 371–9.

Kopelman MD (1994). Structured psychiatric interview. *British Journal of Hospital Medicine* **52**, 93–8 and see **52**, 277–81.

Kopelman MD (1995). The Korsakoff syndrome. *British Journal of Psychiatry* **166**, 154–73.

Lewis S, Higgins N (1996). *Brain imaging in psychiatry.* Blackwell Science, Oxford.

Lishman WA (1997). *Organic psychiatry, the psychological consequences of cerebral disorder,* 3rd edn. Blackwell Scientific Publications, Oxford.

Mendez MF, Cummings JL, Benson DF (1986). Depression in epilepsy. *Archives of Neurology* **43**, 766–70.

Raskind MA (1998). The clinical interface of depression and dementia. *Journal of Clinical Psychiatry* **59**(Suppl. 10), 9–12. [Review; 22 refs]

Ron MA, Feinstein A (1992). Multiple sclerosis and the mind. *Journal of Neurology, Neurosurgery, and Psychiatry* **55**, 1–3.

Rutter M., Taylor E, Hersov L (1994). *Child and adolescent psychiatry: modern approaches.* Blackwell Science, Oxford.

Sacks O (1995). *An anthropologist on Mars.* Picador, London.

Silver JM, Yudofsky SC, Hales RE (1994). Neuropsychiatry of traumatic brain injury. American Psychiatric Press, Washington DC.

Sternbach H (1998). Age-associated testosterone decline in men: clinical issues for psychiatry. *American Journal of Psychiatry* **155**, 1310–18.

Susser E *et al.* (1997). HIV infection among young adults with psychotic disorders. *American Journal of Psychiatry* **154**, 864–6.

Tandberg E, *et al.* (1996). The occurrence of depression in Parkinson's disease. A community-based study. *Archives of Neurology* **53**, 175–9.

Taylor D, Lewis S (1993). Delirium. *Journal of Neurology, Neurosurgery, and Psychiatry* **56**, 742–51.

Toone BJ, Garralda MF, Ron MA (1982). The psychoses of epilepsy and the functional psychoses: a clinical and phenomenological comparison. *British Journal of Psychiatry* **141**, 256–61.

World Health Organization (1992). The ICD-10 classification of mental and behavioural disorders. WHO, Geneva.

Zeidler M *et al.* (1997). New variant Creutzfeldt–Jakob disease: psychiatric features. *Lancet* **350**, 908–10.

26.4 Acute behavioural emergencies

Eleanor Feldman

This chapter covers the assessment and management of patients with acute behavioural disturbance in the general hospital.

Compromised cerebral function can lead to acute behavioural problems in any unit in a general hospital, but behavioural emergencies are most frequently encountered in accident and emergency departments and on wards to which deliberate self-harm patients have been admitted. The physician needs to be able to evaluate the causes of disturbance, understand how to calm the situation before resorting to sedation, know what emergency medication may safely be used if required, and have a confident understanding of his own, and other hospital staff's, legal rights and duties under local jurisdiction. Whilst all hospitals should have specialist help available from a psychiatrist, in many circumstances a physician will be the first doctor on the scene and may need to take immediate action to prevent harm.

Evaluating the causes of disturbance

A priority is to discover whether or not the patient is severely physically ill with compromised cerebral function and suffering from delirium. 'Delirium' is a term often used interchangeably with such phrases as 'toxic confusional state', 'acute confusional state', and 'acute organic brain syndrome'. It accounts for the majority of acute behavioural disturbances arising in patients in a general hospital who have no previous history of mental or behavioural disorder. Delirium in a young adult may signal severe life-threatening illness, but most patients will be elderly, many with a degree of dementia on to which the delirium is superimposed.

Delirium is a reversible organic mental syndrome with an acute or subacute onset, typically fluctuating in severity and often worse at night. Patients will have disturbed attention and concentration and no clear memory of events once they recover. They may be somnolent and have decreased psychomotor activity, or have the opposite with agitation and aggression. Mood changes occur, as do delusions (usually fleeting) and hallucinations, with the latter being in any sensory modality, commonly visual. Clinical features present in delirium are listed in Table 1.

Where mood disorder, delusions, and hallucinations are prominent, the patient's history and cognitive function are particularly helpful in distinguishing delirium from acute functional psychoses such as schizophrenia, mania, or psychotic depression. The most sensitive indicator of generalized cognitive dysfunction is disorientation in time, which may be subtle (see Table 1). The underlying cause of the delirium must be found and treated, but in the meantime any behavioural disturbance needs to be managed. Table 2 lists the causes of delirium.

It is worth noting that a patient who appears disorientated in person but shows no sign of other cognitive impairment is not delirious, but may be in a dissociative state or possibly be presenting with a factitious disorder.

How to calm the situation before resorting to sedation

Whatever the cause of a behavioural disturbance, there are general principles in the management of all such patients.

Staff behaviour

Disorientated and psychotic patients are often in a state of nightmarish terror, whilst patients disinhibited by drugs or alcohol are less in control of their aggressive tendencies. In all cases, staff need to remain calm and polite in their dealings with patients, as anxiety and hostility on the part of staff will only serve to escalate fear and aggression in the patient. Speech should be gentle, calm, and soft spoken, but also clear, confident, and honest. The patient should be treated with normal respect and staff should not forget to introduce themselves and explain what is happening at every point. The same few staff should have contact with a disorientated patient and, for inpatients, catering staff and cleaners should be kept away. Disorientated patients need to be reminded repeatedly where they are and what is happening. Non-verbal communication should mirror this calm and gentle approach. Touching the patient without permission or getting too close may be misinterpreted as an attack. An unpredictable patient should never be seen without support staff being present in the background and within earshot. Furthermore, the patient should not be backed into a corner of the room, and staff should remain close to the door. No attempts to control

Table 1 Clinical features of delirium

History	
Onset	Acute, often at night
Course	Fluctuating, with lucid intervals; typically worse at night
Duration	Brief, from hours to weeks if untreated
Sleep–wake cycle	Always disrupted
Cognitive function	
Awareness	Reduced
Alertness	Abnormally low or high
Attention	Impaired, causing distractibility; fluctuates over the course of the day
Orientation	Impairment for time is the most sensitive indicator, and may be subtle, e.g. correct day and date, but mistaking morning for afternoon. Impairment for place indicates more severe impairment. Impairment for person only is compatible with most severe generalized cognitive dysfunction
Memory	Always impaired. After recovery there is little or no memory for recent events during the period of disturbance
Other features of mental state	
Speech	Incoherent, hesitant, slow, or rapid
Mood	Mood changes may be prominent and take any form; irritability is common
Thinking	Disorganized and delusional, delusions tend to fluctuate and not be fixed
Perceptions	Illusions and hallucinations, commonly visual

Table 2 Causes of delirium

1.	Intoxication by drugs and poisons A wide range of drugs, including tricyclic antidepressants, anticholinergics, hypnotic sedatives, antiparkinsonian agents, anticonvulsants, digoxin, etc. Alcohol, illicit drugs, inhaled solvents Industrial poisons
2.	Withdrawal syndromes, especially of alcohol and hypnotic sedatives
3.	Infections, systemic or intracranial (meningitis, encephalitis)
4.	Metabolic encephalopathies Acid–base or electrolyte imbalance Hypoglycaemia Hypoxia, hypercapnia Hepatic or renal failure Wernicke's encephalopathy and other vitamin B deficiencies Endocrine disorders, for example Cushing's disease, Addison's disease Porphyria
5.	Multifocal and diffuse brain disease Anoxia, fat embolism Vasculitis Cerebrovascular disease Raised intracranial pressure, hydrocephalus
6.	Head trauma
7.	Epilepsy, including postictal states and non-convulsive status
8.	Focal brain lesions, particularly to the brainstem or right hemisphere

and restrain the patient should be made unless staff are trained in these techniques.

Facilities in an accident and emergency department

Accident and emergency (**A&E**) departments need an interview room designed for use with behaviourally disturbed patients. The room should be situated within sight and hearing of A&E staff, not isolated in an inaccessible part of the department, nor at the end of a corridor. It should be well lit, in a good state of decoration in quiet calming colours. No furniture or fittings should be usable as weapons. In the interests of safety the room should have more than one outwardly opening door and an observation window so that the occupants can be seen from outside. There should be an easily accessible 'panic button' with connection to the staff area nearby.

Facilities on an inpatient unit

Acutely disturbed inpatients are best managed in a well-lit, single-bedded room: delirious patients are more prone to visual misperceptions in the shadows of half light. The room should be sparsely furnished with no objects that can be used as weapons. The door should have an observational glass panel. If the room is not on the ground floor, the window in the room should be made safe, with reinforced glass and a means of preventing the window from being fully opened. The room should be fitted with an appropriate alarm system.

What emergency medication may be safely used if required?

It may be necessary to sedate a patient when all other efforts to calm them and make the situation safe have failed. The reality is that there is usually much less capacity to contain behavioural disturbance in a general hospital than would be the case on a psychiatric unit: there are usually no specialist psychiatric nurses available, ward layout is not designed for patients with disturbed behaviour, and other ill patients in the vicinity may be placed at risk. If non-drug calming measures fail, early intervention is desirable to bring disturbed behaviour under control as soon as possible. None the less, the decision to restrain and sedate a patient is not to be undertaken lightly. Whilst this experience may not be recalled by someone with delirium, it is very traumatic for a fully orientated and aware person, and this includes someone with psychosis. That person could develop post-traumatic stress disorder, and the experience may seriously compromise their future cooperation with the required medical and psychiatric treatment. The intervention must be carried out with kindness and as gently as possible. The general principles whereby medication can be used as safely as possible are summarized in Table 3.

Recommended drugs

Major tranquillizers

There are three major tranquillizers in common usage in emergencies: chlorpromazine, haloperidol, and droperidol. These are generally safe and effective for rapid tranquillization. All lower the seizure threshold and should be avoided in patients at risk of seizures, including those in alcohol withdrawal. They are also to be avoided in patients with pre-existing parkinsonism and they have proved dangerous in dementia with Lewy bodies. Hypotension is the most common of the potentially serious side-effects and is most frequent with chlorpromazine. Extrapyramidal side-effects are also relatively frequent, making the use of an antiparkinsonian drug such as procyclidine advisable prophylactically, especially in patients with organic brain syndromes. Acute dystonic reactions may be confused with the severe neck stiffness of meningitis or a spastic posture, thereby adding to diagnostic difficulty in organic brain syndromes of unknown cause. For a patient in spinal traction a dystonic reaction would be very dangerous. The most hazardous complication overall is cardiorespiratory arrest: the true incidence of this is unknown, but it is less of a risk with haloperidol than with chlorpromazine.

Haloperidol has been widely studied with regard to its rapidity of action: intramuscular injection brings about a quicker improvement than oral administration, with significant improvement within 30 min at minimum, although 1 to 2 h is more usual. The usual intramuscular dose is 5 to 10 mg, repeated every 60 min, to a maximum dose over 24 h of around 18 mg. Doses in the elderly should be much lower: Jacoby recommends a single small dose of no more than 2 mg oral haloperidol, with effect assessed after an hour, and in general no more than 6 to 9 mg given orally over 24 h. The

Table 3 Using sedation in cases of behavioural emergencies: Do's and Don'ts

Do:
- Offer oral medication as a syrup before resorting to the parenteral route
- Use drugs that are well absorbed intramuscularly
- Use dose titration with repeated smaller doses in cases where the cause of the disturbance is unknown
- Carefully record the patient's mental state and time and dose of drugs used
- Observe patients carefully following rapid tranquillization
- Record a treatment plan in the notes for continuation of medication, and review this regularly
- Use antiparkinsonian drugs with neuroleptics to prevent dystonic reactions
- Use reduced doses for the elderly

Don't:
- Sedate patients with head injuries: observation of conscious level is an indicator of clinical state
- Use major tranquillizers where seizures are a risk, e.g. known epilepsy, alcohol withdrawal
- Give drugs intravenously
- Use a depot medication for rapid tranquillization
- Use drugs with parkinsonian side-effects if parkinsonism present

patient should be assessed between doses, rather than given a regular regimen, since individual response is unpredictable and doses need careful titration to avoid oversedation and severe extrapyramidal effects.

Chlorpromazine is the least rapidly effective of the two commonly used major tranquillizers and carries the greatest risk of cardiovascular side-effects; it need not be used where haloperidol is available. If it is all that is available, then a dose of 50 to 100 mg chlorpromazine would be appropriate for a first dose to assess the patient's response. The oral route should always be offered first, but where this fails, the intramuscular route is generally preferred over the intravenous on grounds of safety and ease of access. A reasonable general assumption is about a 2:1 oral:parenteral equivalent dose.

In summary, haloperidol is the most rapidly effective major tranquillizer by the safe and convenient intramuscular route. Small doses of haloperidol should be preferred in the elderly.

Minor tranquillizers

The benzodiazepines are sedative drugs with low toxicity. The principal adverse effect is respiratory depression, and prolonged use results in tolerance and dependence. They raise the seizure threshold and may be used as anticonvulsants, so are helpful in cases where there is a risk of seizures and in other conditions where major tranquillizers are contraindicated. Flumazenil allows rapid reversal of respiratory depression. Its short half-life (1 h) means repeated administration may be necessary. There have been concerns about paradoxical disinhibition and release of aggression with benzodiazepines, but these have been overstated in the past and at less than 1 per cent are no greater than placebo.

In general, intramuscular lorazepam appears as effective as a sedative as intramuscular haloperidol, even in mania, and has fewer adverse effects. In a small study in patients with mania the peak reduction in agitation occurred 60 to 120 min after oral administration, but 45 to 75 min after intramuscular and 5 to 10 min after intravenous injection. It appeared more effective than haloperidol during the first 2 h if patients were already receiving antipsychotic drugs: 10 patients who received lorazepam on one occasion and haloperidol on another spent less time in seclusion after lorazepam medication. Doses reported in studies have ranged from 2 to 10 mg every 1 to 2 h. The maximum single dose reported is 40 mg and maximum daily doses from about 20 to 40 mg. No serious adverse effects have been reported with lorazepam use over 1 to 2 weeks. Ataxia has occurred above 10 mg/day, with nausea and confusion at the highest doses. When given by intramuscular injection lorazepam should be diluted with an equal volume of water or saline for injection.

Diazepam is poorly and erratically absorbed after intramuscular injection, making it less suitable for emergency sedation than lorazepam. It has a long half-life and accumulation is likely with repeated doses. Intravenous diazepam is effective in calming behavioural disturbance within 15 min, the diazemuls preparation causing less venous inflammation.

It is often useful to combine an antipsychotic with a benzodiazepine for the most effective safe sedation. The most studied combination has been parenteral haloperidol with lorazepam. It has been claimed that this reduces the total dose of antipsychotic required, but there are case reports where an intravenous combination of these drugs has caused cardiorespiratory arrest. In an open trial the combination of haloperidol and lorazepam given intramuscularly was effective more rapidly than either drug alone, occurring within 30 min in most patients, compared to nearing 60 min for most receiving a single drug.

The management of different syndromes

Psychosis

If a non-organic psychotic illness such as schizophrenia, mania, or psychotic depression is suspected, a psychiatrist should be contacted as soon as possible. Where disturbance is extreme and the patient represents a risk to themselves or others the recommended drug is haloperidol 5 to 10 mg orally or intramuscularly. Further doses can be given hourly according to response. Lorazepam 2 to 4 mg orally or intramuscularly can be added to treat patients who are extremely disturbed. The benzodiazepine antagonist, flumazenil, should be available in case of respiratory depression. Evidence from the notes of known psychiatric patients may suggest that higher doses may be required. The elderly should be treated with half the normal adult doses. Acute dystonic reactions to major tranquillizers respond to procyclidine 5 mg intramuscularly or orally.

Alcohol and drug states

Patients with alcohol withdrawal and disturbed behaviour should be treated acutely with diazepam 10 mg orally or lorazepam 2 mg intramuscularly. They should then be placed on an alcohol withdrawal regime including thiamine to prevent Wernicke's encephalopathy.

Patients suffering from acute drug or alcohol intoxication or drug withdrawal (but **not** alcohol withdrawal) should be treated with haloperidol 5 mg orally or intramuscularly, and continuing disturbance should be treated as for psychosis.

Care following tranquillization

Patients should not be left unattended in the hours following rapid tranquillization. Observations should be recorded every 15 min for 1 hour on a form detailing the following information:

1. Conscious level:
   (a) awake and active,
   (b) awake and calm,
   (c) asleep but rousable,
   (d) asleep and unrousable.
2. Respiratory rate, blood pressure, and oxygen saturation in patients in conscious levels 1(c) and 1(d)—arterial gases should be measured if oxygen saturation is less than 92 per cent.
3. Blood pressure should always be measured if antipsychotic drugs have been given.
4. Reassessment at 1 h to look for evidence of dystonia.

When the acute situation has been calmed, a decision should be made as to whether parenteral or oral medication should be used to keep things under control, also regarding the need for specialist advice. There should be further consideration of the overall treatment plan and levels of nursing and medical observation. There should be a daily reassessment of mental state, and specialist advice should be sought if the patient remains disturbed after 3 days.

Drug interactions

Pharmaceutical formularies contain further information on drug interactions and these should be consulted for patients taking other drugs including alcohol, antiepileptic drugs, levodopa, and lithium.

Legal rights and duties under local jurisdiction

Unlike clinical matters, legal issues are limited by state and national boundaries. Most states and countries will have statute laws covering the treatment of mental disorder in situations of non-consent, but these laws may not allow treatment for coexisting medical disorders where the treatment of the latter is not a recognized treatment of the mental disorder. Clinicians require an understanding of local statute law and common law covering circumstances where patients have a diminished capacity to give meaningful consent to medical intervention in their best interests. This aspect of clinicians' training has often been neglected and the law in this area may be confusing for clinicians who must apply it in an emergency situation. Whilst psychiatrists may have a good understanding of statute law in relation to the treatment of mental disorder, they may not be so conversant with the legal issues surrounding non-consent for the treatment of physical illness. Hospital managers can assist their staff by drawing up guidance in conjunction with their legal advisors, the professions concerned, and any standing body or commission involved in the monitoring and regulation of statutory powers relevant to these circumstances. The author has discussed the legal situation in England and Wales in detail elsewhere (Feldman, in press).

Further reading

Anonymous (1991). Management of behavioural emergencies. *Drugs and Therapeutics Bulletin* **29**, 62–4.

Feldman EJ (2000). The use of the Mental Health Act and common law in mentally disordered general hospital patients. In: Ledingham JGG, Warrell D, eds. *Concise Oxford textbook of medicine*, pp.1443–6. Oxford University Press, Oxford.

Friedman T (2000). Medical management of acute behavioural disturbance in the general hospital. In: Peveler R, Feldman E, Friedman T, eds. *Liaison psychiatry: planning services for specialist settings*, pp.51–60. Gaskell, London.

Hodges JR (1994). *Cognitive assessment for clinicians.* Oxford Medical Publications, Oxford.

Jacoby R (1998). Drugs causing confusion and drugs to treat confusion. *Prescribers' Journal* **38**, 242–8.

Storer D (2000). Liaison psychiatry services in the accident and emergency department. In: Peveler R, Feldman E, Friedman T, eds. *Liaison psychiatry: planning services for specialist settings*, pp.14–26. Gaskell, London.

26.5 Psychiatric disorders as they concern the physician

26.5.1 Grief, stress, and post-traumatic stress disorder

Jenny Yiend and Tim Dalgleish

Grief

Introduction

Grief could be described as a natural response to an objectively significant loss, most commonly the death of a loved one, although whether the boundaries defining a 'significant loss' should be stretched further (and if so, how far) remains controversial. It involves primarily psychological reactions, although it may also lead to social and physical responses. 'Normal grief', which requires no clinical intervention, can be distinguished from 'pathological grief', also variously called 'atypical, traumatic, neurotic, morbid, complicated, or unresolved grief'. However, it should be stated clearly at the outset that the concept of an abnormal form of grief is not represented in current official diagnostic manuals, and as such is not an established clinical condition. Indeed, the lack of consensus over terminology in the literature illustrates the urgent need for quality research to establish clear and universally accepted diagnostic criteria. Despite this confusion, many professionals now recognize some form of abnormal grief response as an appropriate target for active intervention, the key features being: (1) an excessive intensity of the grief reaction (inappropriate within the culture); and (2) of an unusually prolonged duration.

Epidemiology

Considering the ubiquity of bereavement, the consequences of grief are of global importance. Incidence rates for pathological grief are not available; estimates of prevalence vary from 14 to 34 per cent, based primarily on samples drawn from the United States and Europe. In geographical areas prone to natural disasters and places engaged in active military conflict these rates will obviously rise significantly in line with death rates, and in such cases particular attention should be paid to the concurrent trauma that will have accompanied the loss (see under Stress, below).

Mortality

Much evidence shows that the bereaved in general (irrespective of whether a pathological response develops) are at greater risk of dying themselves than would be expected given mortality rates in the population at large. Mortality is elevated by a factor of two to three, applying not only to spousal loss, but also to parental, sibling, and child loss. These findings have proven robust across cultures and generations. The point of highest risk is the weeks and months immediately following the loss, although the data suggest it remains elevated for several years. This evidence should alert the clinician to pay particular attention to all forms of presenting grief, whether normal or pathological.

Within a bereaved population additional factors moderate this mortality risk, although it remains elevated for all subgroups. Thus, the younger bereaved are at a higher relative risk of death themselves than the older, as are widowers compared to widows (although remarriage selectively reduces the risk in widowers). The cause of bereavement is also important, mortality risk being particularly elevated for bereavements involving suicide, accidents, liver cirrhosis, and heart disease.

Hard evidence concerning the underlying reason for reduced longevity following bereavement is scarce, but factors both directly and indirectly related to the loss may be involved. For example, psychological consequences such as the loss of the will to live might directly lead to increased suicides and carelessness. Indirectly, the change in lifestyle necessitated by bereavement may lead to the adoption of health-impairing behaviours (neglect of diet, exercise, general well being) or may create psychological stress, which in turn could have serious negative consequences for health (see 'Stress' below).

Psychiatric comorbidity

Acute bereavement is associated with an increased risk for a range of psychiatric disorders, including major depression, panic disorder, generalized anxiety disorder (**GAD**), and post-traumatic stress disorder (**PTSD**). Any of these may occur comorbidly with pathological grief, when between 17 and 31 per cent will also meet criteria for major depression, 13 per cent panic disorder, 39 per cent GAD, and 9 per cent PTSD. However, these figures should be treated with caution since the criteria for 'pathological' and the timing and consistency of assessment can greatly affect the results. What is clear though, is that the rate of comorbidity following bereavement is significant, with estimates suggesting more than half of the bereaved suffer from two disorders. Hence, having diagnosed one disorder in the bereaved patient (be it psychiatric or pathological grief), the clinician should be particularly alert to the possible presence of additional, complicating disorders. It is unclear whether this comorbidity is best conceived as the presence of one disorder predisposing the patient to additional pathology, or simply the presence of two coexisting disorders whose symptoms may or may not aggravate each other. Whichever, it is essential that both domains of symptoms are separately monitored and, to the extent that it differs, treatment for both disorders is given.

Clinical features

Normal grief

The literature on normal grief reveals that we have yet to achieve a precise characterization of the process and a clear demarcation of its boundaries. Many theorists propose that there are distinct 'stages' of grief, and while opinions vary about the precise number and nature of stages, it is common to consider at least three. These are:

- an initial period of shock, including emotional numbing and disbelief. This stage may last from hours to weeks.
- a subsequent phase of acute mourning, involving an acknowledgement of the death together with intense emotional states that typically engulf

the individual in periodic 'waves' of feeling. Somatic discomfort, social withdrawal, and preoccupation with thoughts of the deceased may accompany this. There may also be 'identification' with the deceased, in which the individual adopts characteristic behaviours, mannerisms or habits of the loved one, and may even experience physical symptoms associated with the cause of death ('grief facsimile symptoms'). This phase may last for several months.

- a period of restoration of normal function during which the characteristics of acute mourning are gradually replaced by feeling able to continue with life. A shift in focus occurs away from the deceased and towards the future. While memories and a sense of loss may remain, there is recognition of having grieved and a will to move on.

More recent theories have placed less emphasis on chronological stages, preferring instead to consider particular domains or clusters of symptoms that may fluctuate in intensity throughout the period of grieving. Table 1 summarizes some of these symptoms of grief.

Pathological grief

As stated earlier, the concept of 'abnormal' grief superseding what might be construed as normal and therefore requiring medical intervention, is not currently an officially acknowledged pathology. However, many workers are calling for a set of universally accepted diagnostic criteria to be developed, and in the meantime Jacobs has proposed a preliminary set that should prove helpful to the practising clinician. These represent a consensus opinion drawn up at a recent conference of experts, and as such incorporate a variety of perspectives on grief and its manifestations. They are formulated in the American Psychiatric Association's *Diagnostic and statistical manual of mental disorders* (**DSM**) style and are reproduced in Table 2.

Several features are worth noting.

- First, diagnosis requires the actual death of a significant other, thereby excluding any other forms of loss (physical separation, loss of non-human objects: animals, body parts, material possessions). This remains controversial.
- Second, observable psychological distress in response to the death is essential, although it may be delayed. Thus a total non-response (the absence of any observable or reported signs of grief), which may be of concern to the practising clinician, would not warrant a positive diagnosis. In such cases the best approach may be close monitoring of the patient over time, together with probing for signs of intrusive thoughts or behaviours relating to the deceased, despite emotional numbing.
- Third, criterion B represents symptoms of particular severity. They fall into four broad categories: avoidance and numbing (1, 3, 4, 5); disorganized behaviour or experience (2, 6, 7, 9); identification symptoms (10); and anger (11). The recommendation is that at least four of these should be present for a positive diagnosis, in addition to the core response of distressing preoccupation listed under A.
- Fourth, criteria D and C are central to distinguishing normal from pathological grief. They embody the notion, described earlier and consistent throughout DSM-IV, that there must be significant impairment of functioning together with an abnormally long duration of symptoms. The latter is set, somewhat arbitrarily, at 2 months.

The core domains for positive diagnosis can therefore be summarized as severity, duration, and functioning.

Differential diagnosis

Bereavement and comorbid psychiatric disorder

DSM-IV criteria for the diagnosis of major depression include specific guidelines for the circumstances of bereavement. In effect, this acknowledges that depressive-like symptoms will be fairly ubiquitous following bereavement and criteria are therefore more stringent. Specifically, either a 2-month (rather than a 2-week) duration of symptoms is required, or alternatively the presence of particular symptoms such as marked functional impairment, psychotic symptoms, or suicidal ideation is necessary.

Table 1 Symptoms of normal grief

Psychological					Social	Physical
Emotional	**Cognitive**	**Behavioural**	**Perceptual**	**Pathological**		
Longing, yearning for deceased	Disbelief, shock	Searching, seeking out things and places associated with the deceased	Hallucinations	Despair	Social withdrawal and isolation	Sighing
Numbness	Preoccupying thoughts of the deceased	Aimlessness	Illusions	Arousal	Social inhibition	Crying
Sadness, nostalgia	Loss of interest, meaning	Avoidance	Dreams, nightmares	Anxiety, panic	Loss of compassion for others	Insomnia
Anger	Intrusive, unpleasant images	Identification behaviours (mimicking habits of the deceased)		Anorexia-like symptoms	Problems functioning at work	Fatigue, lethargy, apathy
Irritability	Mental disorganization (trouble concentrating, making decisions)	Coping strategies		Suicidal ideation		Vague somatic symptoms
Guilt	Acceptance and remembering	New commitments				
Loneliness						

Table 2 Proposed criteria for traumatic grief*

Criterion A:
1. Person has experienced the death of a significant other.
2. The response involves intrusive, distressing preoccupation with the deceased person (e.g. yearning, longing, or searching).

Criterion B:
In response to the death the following symptoms are marked and persistent:
1. Frequent efforts to avoid reminders of the deceased (e.g., thoughts, feelings, activities, people, places).
2. Purposelessness or feelings of futility about the future.
3. Subjective sense of numbness, detachment, or absence of emotional responsiveness.
4. Feeling stunned, dazed, or shocked.
5. Difficulty acknowledging the death (e.g. disbelief).
6. Feeling that life is empty or meaningless.
7. Difficulty imagining a fulfilling life without the deceased.
8. Feeling that part of oneself has died.
9. Shattered world view (e.g. lost sense of security, trust, or control).
10. Assumes symptoms or harmful behaviours of, or related to, the deceased person.
11. Excessive irritability, bitterness, or anger related to the death.

Criterion C:
The duration of disturbance (symptoms listed) is at least 2 months.

Criterion D:
The disturbance causes clinically significant impairment in social, occupational, or other important areas of functioning.

* The authors are grateful to Brunner/Mazel, a member of the Taylor & Francis Group, for permission to reproduce this Table.

Although no specific guidelines for other comorbid psychiatric disorders are given, the clinician would be well advised to apply similar principles of increased severity or extended duration before making a positive diagnosis.

Pathological grief and comorbid psychiatric disorder

Pathological grief, by the working definition given above, occurs exclusively in the circumstances of the death of a significant other. While this objective criterion helpfully restricts diagnosis, it remains necessary to distinguish between this and other possible psychiatric disorders that may follow bereavement.

- *Major depressive episode*—is distinguished by a pervasive and general depressed mood disturbance, in contrast to the episodic pangs of grief focused around the absence of the deceased. Other characteristic symptoms of pathological grief are absent (e.g. Criterion B: 1, 4, 5, 7, 8, 9, 10, 11)
- *Panic disorder and GAD*—are distinguished primarily by the absence of characteristic symptoms of pathological grief, and in the former by the presence of acute episodes of severe anxiety or panic attacks.
- *PTSD*—this is perhaps the most problematic differential diagnosis. Could pathological grief be construed as a specific example of PTSD? Only further research will resolve this question. For the present, we suggest that the following features be considered: pathological grief, in contrast to PTSD, does not require exposure to an objectively traumatic event (although this may occur in cases of violent death). In pathological grief, symptoms of avoidance and hyperarousal are less prominent than in PTSD. Symptoms of pathological grief are centred on the deceased person (pining, searching for them, sensitivity for signs of them in the environment), whereas those of PTSD centre around the traumatic event itself (re-experiencing the trauma, intrusive thoughts about the trauma, general hypervigilance). Finally, where both disorders are suspected, it is advisable to focus treatment initially on PTSD.

Treatment

Normal grief will resolve spontaneously over time. Treatment options for pathological grief fall into the categories of pharmacology, psychotherapies, cognitive/behavioural therapies, and self-help strategies. In common with other psychological disorders, maximum benefit may often be obtained by the prudent combination of drugs with psychological treatments. In practice, individual circumstances and the local availability of treatments will inevitably impose restrictions.

Pharmacology

The few studies available looking specifically at drug treatments following bereavement suggest that both tricyclic antidepressants and selective serotonin-reuptake inhibitors (**SSRIs**) may provide effective relief of symptoms. The tricyclics appear to be more confined in their effects, influencing primarily depressive symptoms, whereas the SSRIs may have a broader action, additionally counteracting symptoms reflecting trauma, such as avoidance and emotional numbing. SSRIs have the additional advantage of more tolerable side-effects, as well as being safer in overdose. Individual circumstances, side-effect profiles, and any known personal or family history of response to treatment can act as a guide in the selection of therapy.

Psychotherapies

Psychodynamic forms of psychotherapy tend to be favoured nowadays over those of a psychoanalytical persuasion. The former centre around the developing relationship between therapist and client, and focus on ongoing changes in the presenting psychological processes observed in the client. Current opinion suggests that this form of psychotherapy may yield more effective results within a shorter time frame than psychoanalytical techniques, which tend to focus more on a re-evaluation of personal history as the means to personal change.

Psychotherapies that have been used specifically to treat the bereaved include crisis intervention and brief dynamic psychotherapy. One study of crisis intervention psychotherapy, given immediately after the loss, lasted for several months and involved reviewing aspects of the lost relationship within the context of the psychodynamic relationship. A significant reduction in symptoms was noted. By contrast, in a study of a psychodynamic therapy starting several months after the loss, only a marginal symptom improvement was found.

Cognitive/behavioural therapies

Cognitive–behaviour therapy (**CBT**) is a popular form of treatment for many psychological disorders. It combines behavioural techniques, such as relaxation and exposure, with cognitive restructuring in which the patient is encouraged to identify and alter maladaptive styles of thinking that are thought to maintain ongoing psychological distress. While there is no data specifically considering the efficacy of this treatment for bereavement, it is likely to confer similar benefits to those noted elsewhere. In relation to separation anxiety disorder, which could be considered as a childhood analogue of pathological grief, a 60 per cent recovery to normal functioning has been reported, sustained over a follow-up year.

Exclusively behavioural techniques have also been used. These involve exposure to feared or avoided stimuli in order to produce habituation, and may also incorporate relaxation techniques to aid this process. Guided mourning and trauma desensitization are two such treatments. Both appear to selectively reduce somatic and avoidance symptoms, having less of an effect on depressive symptoms and preoccupations with the deceased.

Self-help

Self help groups should not be overlooked as a possible supplement to treatment, either to aid transition following successful treatment, or in a preventive capacity. Some evidence suggests that, with appropriately trained group leaders, benefits conferred may be equivalent to some of the more formal treatments discussed above.

Finally, the reader is referred to an excellent text by Jacobs, an expert in the area, which outlines one possible practical approach to treatment endorsed by the author (see p 81 therein), as well as a diagnosis/treatment algorithm (see p 76 therein).

Prognosis

Pathological grief responses may be chronic and unremitting without medical intervention, and a prolonged course of 2 years or more is likely where symptoms persist beyond the first year. In the case of normal grief, most of the acute symptoms of mourning may be expected to dissipate within several months to a year, but some level of emotional involvement may persist indefinitely. Those at higher risk of a pathological grief response may include the young, women, those who suffer multiple losses, and those who have suffered childhood loss. The risk is increased following sudden, unexpected, violent, or suicidal death. An ambivalent or insecure relationship to the deceased ('attachment disturbance') also increases risk, as do personality traits such as neuroticism, dependency, and schizoid personality. Finally, transient features displayed in an individual, such as the inability to accept an imminent death, or severe distress during a terminal illness, increase that individual's risk for pathological grief.

Prevention

Primary measures fall largely in the domain of social policy, such as gun control, safe driving practice, or healthy living styles. These can directly reduce deaths due to unnatural causes. However, the clinician may also play a role by moderating the impact of death, particularly when it is sudden or unexpected. This would include allowing ample time to be spent with a dying or indeed a deceased patient in a quiet and supportive atmosphere, which can enable associated others to more effectively assimilate their loss.

Secondary prevention might include screening bereaved populations at high risk. At the level of the individual this would involve ascertaining the risk profile of a recently bereaved patient and, where this is high, maintaining contact, monitoring progress, and providing early intervention where appropriate.

Tertiary prevention, to moderate the extent of disability, can be implemented by considering appropriate medium- to long-term treatments. Patients may well present late in the course of pathological grief, prompted only by severe functional impairment or social pressure. Although early intervention is preferable, an appropriate selection from the treatment options discussed above is still likely to confer some benefit.

Areas of controversy needing further research

Perhaps the major controversy of concern to clinicians is whether the concept of 'pathological grief' warrants a distinct diagnostic category, or whether it is best subsumed under existing pathologies such as PTSD or major depression. The high comorbidities and the question of the differential diagnosis support the latter view; factor analysis of symptom clusters, their differential response to drugs, and the distinct risk profiles support the former. However, the question of labelling becomes clinically unimportant, to the extent that the treatment for these pathologies overlaps.

Other controversies are:

- the model of distinct 'stages of grief', which some advocate more than others;
- the extent to which the absence of grief might be considered pathological;
- the duration of normal grief, which some argue is indefinite;
- the nature of the grief object, which some restrict to the death of an intimate, while others extend far more broadly to include non-death and non-human loss.

The following issues also warrant investigation:

- cultural differences in the expression and experience of grief;
- the factors responsible for the relationship between bereavement and increased health and mortality risks.

Stress and post-traumatic stress disorder

Introduction

Stress often refers to an external object, event, or situation that causes physical and psychological effects on an individual as a result of increased levels of arousal. These effects are usually experienced as unpleasant and undesirable, although there is a close correspondence with the excitement that occurs when a positive, desirable interpretation is adopted, for example during dangerous sports. The term 'stress' is perhaps more appropriately used to refer to the subjective experience of these effects, and the agent causing them is more accurately termed 'the stressor'.

Societal and lifestyle changes in developed nations, as well as media coverage, have given prominence to the role of stressors and their adverse effects, although in practice these are prevalent universally. While a moderate degree of stress can be helpful to enhance performance, chronic stress is indeed associated with negative outcomes. Stress can be a risk factor for various physical health problems, most notably coronary heart disease, infectious diseases, immune function, and cancer. In addition 'background stress' (the presence of low-level chronic stressors) is known to potentiate an individual's negative response to acute stressors, and thus can be considered a vulnerability factor for negative outcome. Within psychiatry the effect of stressors has been extensively studied. They are known to raise the probability of relapse and, more controversially, are believed to play a part in triggering the onset of some disorders. Examples include schizophrenia, where interventions developed to reduce the levels of interpersonal stress within families ('expressed emotion') have proved effective. Similarly, in major depression much research has been conducted on the role of 'life events' (for example, death of a spouse, loss of a job, going on holiday).

For the non-psychiatric patient the adverse effects of stressors can usually be addressed through lifestyle changes such as increased exercise, improved diet, relaxation techniques, reduction of working hours, and delegation of responsibilities. All these measures require an adjustment of personal priorities, which some may be unwilling to do. Where stress arises from unavoidable personal circumstances (for example, care-giving, financial or relationship problems), the role of the clinician includes referral to appropriate support services to enable the stressors to be addressed at their source.

An additional option, provided within the DSM-IV system, is a diagnosis of adjustment disorder. This may be appropriate where a discrete, identifiable stressor exists and causes either significant impairment in functioning, or distress beyond that which would normally be expected given the nature of the stress. However, this disorder (by definition) is time-limited by and closely coupled to the external stressor itself, although it may be classed as chronic where the stressor or its consequences persist indefinitely. Specifically, symptoms must commence within 3 months of the onset of the stressor and cease within 6 months of its termination. It is also of note that bereavement is specifically excluded as a qualifying stressor. Nevertheless, where these criteria are fulfilled and other psychiatric diagnoses have been excluded, the clinician may wish to offer appropriate psychological interventions as described below.

We will use the term 'trauma' where extreme stress occurs in response to an acute, intense episode brought about by a specific, objectively identifiable, external event. A trauma (defined under Clinical features, below) may be distinguished from a stressor primarily in terms of the objective intensity and severity of the experience or incident. It is now recognized that a proportion of people exposed to such a trauma go on to develop a clinical pathology, post-traumatic stress disorder (PTSD). PTSD, the subject of the rest of this section, was first introduced into the diagnostic nomenclature in 1980 with the publication of DSM-III, and it subsequently appeared in the World Health Organization's *International classification of disease* (**ICD**) system in 1992.

Epidemiology

Traumatic events are common, estimates suggesting that most Americans will experience at least 1 trauma over a lifetime. The lifetime prevalence of PTSD in the general population is between 1 and 14 per cent according to DSM-IV, with a recent review suggesting this level is higher in women (10 to 12 per cent) than men (5 per cent). Estimates of lifetime prevalence among trauma victims vary widely according to the criteria and populations sampled, but somewhere between 3 and 58 per cent of people who experience a trauma will go on to develop PTSD at some time in their lives, although more recent reviews put the figure as high as 60 to 80 per cent. Clearly geographical factors will influence these figures, leading to significant increases in areas prone to natural disasters or human conflict. In common with most psychiatric disorders there appears to be high comorbidity in PTSD, with 80 per cent of sufferers meeting the criteria for at least one other psychiatric disorder.

Clinical features

The primary, essential feature for a positive diagnosis of PTSD is the prior experience of an objectively traumatic event. DSM-IV distinguishes two components: first, the nature of the event itself, which should involve an 'actual or perceived threat to life or physical integrity'—typical events including active combat, rape or other assault, natural disasters, and serious accidents. Witnessing such events is also included within the concept of 'experiencing'. Second, individuals should have an extreme emotional response to the event, which DSM-IV describes as intense fear, helplessness, or horror.

A pathological reaction to such a trauma is characterized by symptoms that fall into three clinically observed domains: re-experiencing, avoidance/numbing, and hyperarousal. Avoidance and numbing may be better considered separately, although DSM-IV does not do so. Typical examples of these symptoms are as follows.

- *Re-experiencing*—including nightmares, flashbacks, intrusive thoughts, and images relating to the trauma. Such symptoms have often been considered to be the hallmark of PTSD.
- *Avoidance*—typically anything that could remind the individual of or be associated with the trauma is avoided. This can include people, places, activities, and conversations.
- *Numbing*—emotional responsiveness is generally reduced. This may include an inability to experience certain feelings and feelings of detachment or other dissociative symptoms (e.g. depersonalization, dissociative amnesia, derealization).
- *Hyperarousal*—this includes insomnia, anger, irritability, hypervigilance, problems with concentration, exaggerated startle.

DSM-IV requires at least one symptom of re-experiencing, three of avoidance/numbing, and two of hyperarousal to be present for a positive diagnosis. It also currently specifies three subtypes of PTSD—acute, chronic (where symptoms have lasted under or over 3 months, respectively), and delayed onset (where 6 months or more has elapsed after the stressor before the emergence of symptoms).

Finally, DSM-IV introduced a new, related diagnostic category—acute stress disorder (ASD)—which essentially is an acute form of PTSD. The symptoms are identical, but the diagnosis can be made as early as 2 days' post-trauma, thereby encouraging earlier intervention. Persistence of symptoms beyond 1 month results in the diagnosis reverting to PTSD. For ASD three of five dissociative/numbing symptoms are required, reflecting the belief that these are predictive of longer term psychopathology. Although the diagnosis remains controversial, it does provide the clinician with a clear indication for early intervention in certain cases.

Differential diagnosis

Normal reactions to trauma

As with grief, the key features that distinguish PTSD from non-pathological reactions to trauma are intensity, duration, and functioning. The intensity of the pathological reaction is captured by the nature of the symptoms themselves, with the presence of numbing symptoms thought to be the most effective distinguisher of victims with PTSD from those without. In addition, symptoms must have been present for at least 1 month and must be causing clinically significant distress or impairment in functioning.

Other psychiatric conditions

Subsets of the features of PTSD often overlap with other psychiatric conditions, but distinguishing characteristics are usually present. First, in PTSD there is an instigating traumatic event, which is not required for any of the other anxiety disorders. Second, the symptoms of nightmares and flashbacks are specific for PTSD and do not characterize other anxiety disorders. Third, emotional numbing, which occurs in the place of the normally expected emotional reactions, is strongly and uniquely characteristic to PTSD.

PTSD, considered to be an anxiety disorder, shares several anxiety-related symptoms, particularly from the hyperarousal cluster. Hypervigilance, sleep disturbance, irritability, and concentration problems are all common to GAD. Similarly, fear and avoidance are common to the phobias. Intrusive thoughts may also occur in obsessive–compulsive disorder (**OCD**), major depression, and GAD. Conversely, PTSD sufferers may exhibit compulsive behaviours of the type associated with OCD, such as repetitive cleansing procedures, or continual checking of locks and security devices, perhaps following rape or other kinds of assault. Although rates of comorbidity are indeed high (see above), dual diagnoses should only be made where the full criteria for both disorders are met.

Treatment

Crisis intervention

This approach, also called 'psychological debriefing', aims to treat all survivors of a trauma in the hope of reducing subsequent pathology. It takes place in a single session, within days of the incident, most forms of treatment being given individually or in small groups. Typically, there are several structured phases including each individual sharing their own general perspective ('recreating the event'), their thoughts at the time, the worst aspect of the event, and their reactions to it. There is usually also a teaching element, covering common reactions to trauma and how to deal with them.

Without doubt participants subjectively feel this type of intervention to be helpful and valuable. However, the research findings on its efficacy are mixed: a recent review revealed that there have been few randomized controlled trials, but that these show little observable benefit, some even reporting a negative outcome. One current view holds that benefits are greater if the treatment is delayed for a week or so, until the initial shock subsides. Unless and until future empirical data supports their worth, clinicians should be cautious about the use of indiscriminatory immediate intervention. The treatment options discussed below are suitable for individuals who go on to develop PTSD following trauma.

Pharmacology

The main difficulty regarding drug treatment is the current dearth of clinical trials, hence what follows cannot be more than tentative advice, based primarily on clinical experience.

Antiadrenergic agents

Agents such as β-blockers are effective in the short term in reducing symptoms of hyperarousal and re-experiencing. Patients respond quickly, although tolerance is likely to develop. They are perhaps most appropriate for those whose individual prognosis is good, or where immediate symptom relief is required, before pursuing other treatment options.

Antidepressants

Most antidepressants provide at least some symptom relief, but the benefits are generally considered to be modest for classes such as tricyclics and monoamine oxidase inhibitors (**MAOIs**), and issues of side-effect profiles and overdose safety mean that SSRIs tend to be preferred. Recent data suggests that SSRIs may be effective in reducing symptoms from all symptom domains, and therefore they are currently the preferred option for the long-term drug treatment of PTSD. Two additional points are worth noting. First, uncertainty persists about the speed of action of these drugs, with estimates for the onset of beneficial effects varying between 2 weeks and 1 month. Patients should therefore be prepared for some delay. Second, some SSRI side-effects, such as arousal and insomnia, although usually short-lived, will be particularly difficult for the patient with PTSD to tolerate.

Psychological treatments

Many different types of psychological therapy have been used to treat patients with PTSD, most appearing to impart some benefit in terms of symptom relief and improved psychological and social functioning, but longer term benefits remain unclear. Similarly, the potential for additional gains to be made by combining psychological treatments with each other or with drugs remains largely unexplored. Some of the commoner therapies are given below.

Cognitive–behavioural therapies

These are the psychological treatments of first choice for patients with PTSD because most are relatively brief and have a well-established efficacy, both from clinical experience and empirical research. Treatments are similar to those used for other anxiety disorders, such as specific phobia, but they focus specifically on trauma-related material. Therapies may differ in the particular components included, but generally they fall into one of two groups, exposure treatments or anxiety management.

Exposure treatments Exposure treatments involve repeated exposure to trauma-related material on the basis that this will reduce undesirable responses, either through simple habituation or as a result of concurrent cognitive reprocessing. Treatments vary in the type of exposure used. Imaginal techniques involve the patient reliving (describing verbally, writing down, or role playing) the trauma within the treatment room. *In vivo* exposure involves confronting, in real-life but safe situations, places or objects that provide reminders of the trauma. Other variables include the length of exposure (brief or prolonged) and the level of arousal induced (high or low). Prolonged imaginal exposure is currently the favoured technique of many therapists for the treatment of PTSD because of its relative efficacy and time-efficiency.

Some forms of exposure treatment, for example systematic desensitization, adopt a hierarchical approach in which exposure is graded in difficulty, starting with least feared stimuli and progressing in tandem with patient improvement. Relaxation procedures may also be employed: these are known to be unnecessary for treatment efficacy, but may help to encourage patient participation in an initially unpleasant procedure.

Exposure techniques are time-efficient and easy for patients to learn. Good quality, consistent data supports their efficacy. However, as noted, compliance may be a genuine problem, particularly in those with prominent avoidance symptoms.

Anxiety management Anxiety management training aims to teach patients to control and cope with their symptoms, rather than focusing on elimination or cure. Stress inoculation training is one such technique that has been commonly used for PTSD. Treatment usually involves components of both education and skills training. The latter may include deep relaxation, quick relaxation, breathing control, thought stopping, and role play. Anxiety management programmes are more complex to administer and more intellectually demanding for patients than other treatment options. However, they are likely to be particularly appropriate for PTSD patients with symptoms of chronic, general arousal. In addition, they may be indicated at later stages, for example where maximal benefit has been achieved from other treatment options and the patient is left with residual symptoms.

Psychotherapies

Both psychodynamic and psychoanalytical techniques (see 'Grief' above) have been used to treat PTSD. Such therapies tend to vary enormously in nature, encompassing individual and group approaches and lasting anywhere from a few sessions to over a year. The available data reveals improvements following treatment, but methodological flaws preclude any clear conclusions. Where alternatives exist, it may well be advisable to pursue these options first.

Hypnotherapy

Hypnosis has reportedly been used with some success. However, there is a lack of sound published data to confirm this, although one controlled study suggests that hypnosis is effective and may be particularly suitable for reducing intrusive symptoms (re-experiencing cluster).

*Eye-movement desensitization and reprocessing (**EMDR**)*

This is a controversial treatment, largely because of the surprising claims made by its originator, the lack of rigorous scientific testing to confirm its supposed efficacy, and the lack of any obvious theoretical basis or justification for its beneficial effects. Treatment involves focusing on a disturbing trauma-related thought or image, while visually tracking a movement, for example the therapist's finger. The primary components are therefore production of saccadic eye movements and exposure. Until methodologically sound data is available, clinicians are advised to consider this technique with caution.

Prognosis

The evidence suggests that most treatments are effective in reducing symptoms and improving quality of life, but it seems that the magnitude of these benefits is limited. Many sufferers retain some symptoms despite having received optimal treatment. Although little data exists on the efficacy of combining treatment options (for example, drugs alongside psychological techniques), it may be appropriate to consider this in resistant cases. In addition, where residual symptoms persist, it may be appropriate to shift goals towards rehabilitation and the successful management of symptoms.

What factors influence the chance of recovery following exposure to trauma? Known risk factors for the development of PTSD include the following: the severity of (including proximity to) the trauma; bereavement as a result of the trauma; presence of a pre- or comorbid psychiatric disorder; certain personality traits, for example neuroticism; and the absence of adequate social and psychological support. All appear to be predictors of poor outcome. Recent reviews suggest that neither age nor ethnic group interacts with pathological response to trauma and that PTSD-symptom expression is similar across age groups and cultures.

Areas of controversy needing further research

Controversial issues largely overlap with those requiring further research in this relatively newly recognized area. Particular attention should be paid to:

- SSRIs as a drug treatment of first choice;
- combined treatment approaches;
- crisis intervention as an immediate, unselective, post-trauma intervention;
- the eye-movement desensitization and reprocessing technique;
- long-term outcomes;
- the new diagnostic category, acute stress disorder;
- postconcussional disorder—a category provided for further study (Appendix B, DSM-IV). Symptoms occur following a closed head injury with concussion and include cognitive (specifically, attention

and memory), emotional (anxiety, depression, irritability), and physical (sleep problems, fatigue, headache) problems.

Further reading

American Psychiatric Association (1994). *Diagnostic and statistical manual of mental disorders*, 4th ed. APA, Washington DC.

Breslau N, *et al.* (1998). Trauma and post-traumatic stress disorder in the community. *Archives of General Psychiatry* **55**, 626–32.

Brom D, Kleber RJ, Defres PB (1989). Brief psychotherapy for posttraumatic stress disorders. *Journal of Consulting and Clinical Psychology* **57**, 607–12.

Bryant RA, Harvey AG (1997). Acute stress disorder: a critical review of diagnostic issues. *Clinical Psychology Review*, **17**, 757–73.

Davis LL, *et al.* (1997). Post-traumatic stress disorder and serotonin: new directions for research and treatment. *Journal of Psychiatry and Neuroscience* **22**, 318–26.

Foa EB, Rothbaum BO (1998). *Treating the trauma of rape: cognitive behavioral therapy for PTSD.* Guilford Press, New York.

Friedman MJ (1998). Current and future drug treatment for posttraumatic stress disorder. *Psychiatric Annals* **28**, 461–8.

Frueh BC, Brady KL, deArellano MA (1998). Racial differences in combat related PTSD: empirical findings and conceptual issues. *Clinical Psychology Review* **18**, 287–305.

Greenwood DC, *et al.* (1996). Coronary heart disease: a review of the role of psychosocial stress and social support. *Journal of Public Health Medicine*, **18**, 221–31.

Gump BB, Matthews KA (1999). Do background stressors influence reactivity to and recovery from acute stressors? *Journal of Applied Social Psychology* **29**, 469–94.

Irwin M, Pike J (1993). Bereavement, depressive symptoms and immune function. In: Stroebe MS, Stroebe W, Hansson RO, eds. *Handbook of bereavement: theory, research, and intervention*, pp 160–71. Cambridge University Press, Cambridge.

Jacobs S (1999). *Traumatic grief: diagnosis, treatment and prevention.* Brunner Mazel, Philadelphia.

Kim K, Jacobs S (1993). Neuroendocrine changes following bereavement. In: Stroebe MS, Stroebe W, Hansson RO, eds. *Handbook of bereavement: theory, research, and intervention*, pp 143–59. Cambridge University Press, Cambridge.

Kleber RJ, Brom D (1987). Psychotherapy and pathological grief: a controlled outcome study. Israeli *Journal of Psychiatry and Related Sciences* **24**, 99–109.

Marmar CR, *et al.* (1988). A controlled trial of brief psychotherapy and mutual help group treatment of conjugal bereavement. *American Journal of Psychiatry* **145**, 203–9.

Marshall RD, Spitzer R, Liebowitz MR (1999). Review and critique of the new DSM-IV diagnosis of acute stress disorder. *American Journal of Psychiatry* **156**, 1677–85.

Mawson D, *et al.* (1981). Guided mourning for morbid grief: A controlled study. *British Journal of Psychiatry* **138**, 185–93.

Prigerson HG, *et al.* (1995). The inventory of complicated grief: a scale to measure symptoms of maladaptive loss. *Psychiatry Research* **59**, 65–79.

Prigerson HG, *et al.* (1997). Traumatic grief as a risk factor for mental and physical morbidity. *American Journal of Psychiatry* **154**, 617–23.

Raphael B (1977). Preventive intervention with the recently bereaved. *Archives of General Psychiatry* **34**, 1450–4.

Shalev AY, Bonne O, Eth S (1996). Treatment of posttraumatic stress disorder: a review. *Psychosomatic Medicine* **58**, 165–82.

Shapiro F (1989). Eye movement desensitization: a new treatment for PTSD. *Journal of Behavior Therapy and Experimental Psychiatry* **3**, 211–17.

Shapiro F (1995). *Eye movement desensitization and reprocessing: basic principles, protocols and procedures.* Guilford Press, New York.

Simon RI (1999). Chronic posttraumatic stress disorder: a review and checklist of factors influencing prognosis. *Harvard Review of Psychiatry* **6**, 304–12.

Solomon SD (1997). Psychosocial treatment of posttraumatic stress disorder. *In Session-Psychotherapy in Practice* **3**, 27–41.

Solomon SD, Davidson JRT (1997). Trauma: prevalence, impairment, service use and cost. *Journal of Clinical Psychiatry* **58**(Suppl. 9), 5–11.

Stroebe MS, Stroebe W, Hansson RO, eds (1993). *Handbook of bereavement: theory, research, and intervention.* Cambridge University Press, Cambridge.

Weintraub D, Ruskin PE (1999). Posttraumatic stress disorder in the elderly: a review. *Harvard Review of Psychiatry* **7**, 144–52.

World Health Organization (1992). The ICD-10 classification of mental and behavioural disorders: clinical descriptions and diagnostic guidelines. WHO, Geneva.

26.5.2 The patient who has attempted suicide

Keith Hawton

Introduction

The term 'attempted suicide' is usually applied to all acts of deliberate self-harm, in other words deliberate self-poisoning or self-injury. In many ways this is a misleading term since the primary motivation for, or aim of, deliberate self-harm is often not death but some other purpose, such as communication of distress, blotting out an unbearable state of mind, or trying to change the behaviour of other people. Such 'non-suicidal' aims, however, often involve the use of the suicidal message to enhance the impact of such intentions. Because of this and the popularity of the term 'attempted suicide' among physicians, this terminology will be used throughout this chapter.

Attempted suicide is a major and increasing healthcare problem in most developed, and some developing, countries. In the United Kingdom, for example, there are approximately 170 000 general hospital presentations for self-poisoning or self-injury each year. Attempts occur in older children, but the behaviour becomes more common in adolescence, increasing rapidly in frequency in females from the age of 12 years, with peak rates in the late teens and early twenties. The increase with age occurs more slowly in males, rates peaking in the mid- to late twenties. In recent years there has been an increase in attempts by young males, which parallels the trend for completed suicide.

The vast majority of hospital-referred attempts involve self-poisoning. In the United Kingdom the substances most frequently involved are non-opiate analgesics, particularly paracetamol and paracetamol-containing compounds, and psychotropic agents, especially antidepressants and minor tranquillizers. Most self-injuries involve patients cutting themselves.

A wide variety of patient characteristics and problems can lead to attempted suicide. These include psychiatric disorders (especially depression, substance abuse, and anxiety disorders), personality difficulties, and poor coping resources. The more common life difficulties experienced by patients include interpersonal problems and broken relationships (especially in the young), employment difficulties, legal problems, and alcohol and drug misuse.

An important feature of attempted suicide is that it is often repeated, with at least 12 to 25 per cent of people repeating the act within a year. In the United Kingdom between 1 and 2 per cent die by suicide within a year and 3 to 5 per cent within 8 to 10 years. In settings where the patient population tends to be older the risk of suicide within a year of an attempt may be as high as 6 to 10 per cent.

This chapter focuses on the management of those who attempt suicide in the general hospital. It is imperative that patients should not only receive adequate physical care but that their psychiatric and psychosocial problems and needs are assessed.

Arrival of patients at the general hospital

In addition to the immediate assessment of the medical consequences of self-poisoning or self-injury, accident and emergency department staff should be capable of conducting a brief assessment of a patient's psychiatric status and risk. In particular, they need to determine whether a patient has a serious psychiatric disorder (for example, psychosis or severe depression) and/or is actively suicidal such that urgent attention by the psychiatric service is required. Dangerous tablets or other potential methods of self-harm should be removed.

Staff should be aware that a large number of patients leave hospital accident and emergency departments before a psychiatric assessment can be conducted. Such patients often have substance abuse disorders and a history of previous attempts, and may show behavioural disturbance in the department. Many have features associated with suicide risk, and tend to present to hospital with further repeat attempts more often than patients who are assessed in the accident and emergency department. These facts highlight the need for accident and emergency staff to have basic skills in assessment, and for them to be able to readily obtain urgent psychiatric assessment when they judge it to be necessary. Where a patient is thought to be at serious risk but wanting to leave hospital, medical staff can, in the United Kingdom at least, restrain the patient under common law until a psychiatric opinion can be obtained and, if necessary, a Mental Health Act order completed.

Medical care

Management of the medical complications of suicide attempts is dealt with in Chapter 26.6.1, but an obvious difficulty for physicians can arise with those patients who have attempted suicide and refuse potentially life-saving treatment for the physical consequences of their acts. The dilemma is whether to instigate such treatment against a patient's will. This problem most often presents in those who have poisoned themselves, such as with large overdoses of paracetamol, in which early treatment can prevent the development of potentially fatal liver damage.

In the United Kingdom the issue primarily comes down to one of mental capacity. To show that patients have the capacity to refuse treatment, they:

(1) must be able to understand and retain information on the treatment proposed, its indications, and its main benefits, as well as possible risks and the consequences of non-treatment;

(2) must be shown to believe that information; and

(3) must be capable of weighing up the information in order to arrive at a conclusion.

If a clinician instigates treatment against a patient's wishes in spite of the patient appearing to have capacity, then the clinician is at risk of being accused of battery. Where the patient is judged as lacking capacity, essential treatment can either be instigated: (1) directly by a physician, or (2) after the patient has been placed on a Mental Health Order because of the degree of mental illness, in which case the treatment for the physical condition is given because the overdose is judged to be the result of mental illness.

In situations of dire emergency most clinicians would instigate essential treatment to save the patient's life and then try to sort out the legal issues afterwards. Such understandable action is unlikely to lead to successful litigation if the clinician acted in a way that he/she judged at the time to be in the patient's best interest.

Psychiatric assessment

Psychiatric assessment should not usually take place until a patient has recovered from any acute medical effects of an attempt. Clearly, more urgent assessment is indicated if the patient is severely disturbed or regarded as being at acute risk. In some centres, general medical and nursing staff may have to carry out these assessments, either because this is local policy or because of inadequacy of the local psychiatric service. General hospital staff should in any case be familiar with how to conduct an assessment so that they can do this at times of emergency.

Table 1 Factors that should be covered in the assessment of patients having attempted suicide

- Life events that preceded the attempt
- Motives for the act, including suicidal intent and other reasons
- Problems faced by the patient
- Psychiatric disorder
- Personality traits and disorder
- Alcohol and drug misuse
- Family and personal history
- Current circumstances, such as:
  - social (e.g. extent of social relationships)
  - domestic (e.g. living alone or with others)
  - occupation (e.g. whether employed)
- Psychiatric history, including previous suicide attempts
- Risk of a further attempt
- Risk of suicide
- Coping resources and supports

A semi-structured assessment procedure is recommended. The main factors that should be covered are listed in Table 1. A useful way of assessing the events and the patient's problems that preceded the act, the nature of the attempt, possible motivation, and suicidal intent, is to obtain a very detailed account of the few days leading up to the act. Whenever possible the patient's account should be supplemented by enquiry of other informants such as a partner, relatives, and friends. Information should also be sought from professionals and others involved in the patient's care, including the general practitioner.

Suicidal intent and other motives

Suicidal intent (that is to say, the extent to which the patient wished to die at the time of the attempt) can usefully be assessed by examining the circumstances of the act and the explanation given by the patient and by the relatives or friends. Circumstances suggesting high suicidal intent include:

- act carried out in isolation;
- act timed so that intervention unlikely;
- precautions taken to avoid discovery;
- preparations made in anticipation of death (e.g. making will, organizing insurance);
- preparations made for the act (e.g. purchasing means, saving up tablets);
- communicating intent to others beforehand;
- extensive premeditation;
- leaving a note;
- not alerting potential helpers after the act.

It is also important to take account of what the patient and others say about the purpose of the act. Approximately one-third of patients will say that they definitely wanted to die, although in some cases the circumstances of the act will suggest otherwise. There is a small but important group of patients who will claim they did not wish to die when the circumstances strongly suggest high suicidal intent—such patients may be at increased risk of making a repeat attempt, which has a high chance of being fatal. A useful questionnaire which can assist in the assessment of suicidal intent is the Beck Suicidal Intent Scale.

It is extremely important to recognize that the apparent physical danger of an overdose is a poor and potentially misleading measure of the extent to which a patient may have wanted to die. Many patients are ignorant of the relative dangers of substances taken in overdose, although increasing attention to suicidal behaviour by the media may be changing this. Thus a small overdose of a benzodiazepine hypnotic or even an antibiotic may represent a serious attempt at suicide for some patients, whereas a large overdose of a highly dangerous analgesic might be taken with low intent by others. People in the medical and allied professions represent an exception, and usually the danger of their acts is a good measure of intent. Very dangerous self-injuries are often associated with high suicidal intent, but this is not always so.

Assessment of the motives for deliberate self-poisoning and self-injury should be based on the precedents, circumstances of the act, the patient's account, that of other informants, and deduction by the clinician. Motivational reasons that frequently underly this behaviour include:

- to die;
- to escape from unbearable anguish;
- to get relief;
- to change the behaviour of others;
- to escape from a situation;
- to show desperation to others;
- to get back at other people/make them feel guilty;
- to get help.

Risk of a repeated attempt and of suicide

Estimation of the risk of repetition and of suicide following attempted suicide, both short-term and long-term, is a very important part of the assessment. Factors associated with an increased risk of a repeat include:

- previous attempt(s);
- personality disorder;
- alcohol or drug abuse;
- previous psychiatric treatment;
- unemployment;
- lower social class;
- criminal record;
- history of violence;
- age between 25 and 54 years;
- single, divorced, or separated.

Factors associated with an increased risk of suicide in this population include:

- older age;
- male gender;
- unemployed or retired;
- separated, divorced, or widowed;
- living alone;
- poor physical health;
- psychiatric disorder (particularly depression, alcoholism, schizophrenia, and 'sociopathic' personality disorder);
- high suicidal intent in current episode;
- violent method involved in current attempt (e.g. attempted hanging, jumping);
- leaving a suicide note;
- previous attempt(s).

It is essential, however, to recognize that such predictive measures are notoriously imprecise. For repetition, this is because the predictive factors are relatively crude and, whilst those patients who show the risk factors have a high risk of repeating, a substantial proportion of repeaters, possibly more than half, do not demonstrate many risk factors.

Coping resources and supports

Assessment of coping resources and supports should be based on past behaviour under stress and the patient's account of whom they can turn to for support. It is particularly important to assess whether the patient has specific difficulties in problem-solving as these can be an important target for psychosocial therapy. The best evidence for such difficulties will be a description of the methods used to solve problems in the past. It is always important to determine whether current problem-solving is impaired by depression or other psychiatric disorders.

Care after attempted suicide

Patients who have attempted suicide are frequently ambivalent about accepting help, or even frankly dismissive of it. However, this may be understandable in the context of acts that often represent attempts at interpersonal communication or have other functions unconnected with help-seeking. Furthermore, many patients come from socioeconomic backgrounds in which help-seeking for emotional problems is rarely considered. Therefore clinicians may have to work hard in some cases to explain to patients how treatment might be of benefit. These factors also mean that a brief intervention, such as problem-solving, is likely to be more acceptable to a sizeable proportion of patients than more lengthy therapeutic approaches.

The assessment procedure can itself be highly therapeutic. Patients may be provided with their first opportunity to discuss their difficulties with a clinician. Joint interviews with family members can help highlight issues that need addressing and assist with communication problems.

Some patients thought to be at high risk of suicide refuse psychiatric treatment when this is judged to be essential. Management comes down to a judgement of whether the patient is suffering, or likely to be suffering, from a mental illness that necessitates hospital assessment and/or treatment. In most countries, if a patient thought to be at serious risk and/or mentally ill has presented to a general hospital following attempted suicide but is refusing to stay for a psychiatric assessment, accident and emergency department staff would be judged to be acting reasonably if they restrained the patient under 'common law' until a psychiatric opinion could be obtained.

Currently, there is inadequate evidence for the efficacy of treatments for patients who have attempted suicide, at least with regard to the prevention of repetition of attempts. This is partly to do with methodological flaws in the design of studies, and also because most studies have included too few patients. In one trial, repetition of attempts was reduced in multiple repeaters who received the depot neuroleptic flupentixol, compared with patients who received a placebo. Intensive and prolonged psychological therapy has been associated with promising results in female patients with a history of multiple acts of self-harm and borderline personality disorder. There are also promising results for brief problem-solving therapy.

Clinical services for patients who have attempted suicide

At one time the assessment of patients who attempted suicide was regarded as primarily the responsibility of psychiatrists. Increases in the clinical responsibilities of non-medical clinical staff and findings from research have resulted in a major change in the pattern of services in many places. In the United Kingdom it has been demonstrated that nurses, social workers, and other clinicians can assess these patients reliably, make effective aftercare arrangements, and provide effective therapy. This has resulted in official guidelines that reflect these findings.

It is imperative that staff of whatever discipline who are involved in this work have reasonable background experience and skills in the management of patients with emotional and psychiatric disorders, and that they be properly trained in the assessment and treatment of patients who have attempted suicide. They must also have support from senior psychiatrists, especially for patients with severe psychiatric disorders and where compulsory admission to hospital may be required. They must also be highly motivated and have good support systems in place, because working with such patients can be extremely demanding.

The functioning of a service for patients who have attempted suicide but do not require physical treatment in specialized settings (for example, in an intensive care unit) can be improved if they are admitted to one short-stay medical ward, rather than to a large number of wards. The attitudes of general medical and nursing staff to these patients can be negative, especially towards patients whose acts they perceive as having a low suicidal intent. Clinical experience shows that attitudes are far more favourable when admission to a single ward is possible. General medical and nursing staff in such wards acquire experience in managing these patients, and also develop closer working relationships with members of the service for attempted suicide.

The development of high-quality general hospital services for patients who attempt suicide should be a major element in any national or local suicide-prevention strategy.

Specific subgroups of patients

Alcohol and drug abusers

Many patients who attempt suicide have problems related to alcohol and drug abuse, and these factors, especially alcohol abuse, increase the risk of both repetition and eventual suicide. All attempters should be screened for substance abuse. Recognition of such problems in the general hospital may provide a special opportunity for treatment, which may be an important factor in preventing further suicidal behaviour as well as reducing physical and social harm.

Children and very young adolescents

Very young patients are usually admitted to a paediatric ward where this is available in the general hospital. It is advisable that all very young attempters be admitted to hospital rather than be dealt with in the accident and emergency department, since they require particularly careful and often prolonged assessment, including interviews with their families and the possible involvement of community statutory services (for example, social services).

The elderly

Attempted suicide in the elderly, while less common than in younger people, very often involves high suicidal intent. Routine admission to a medical bed is therefore also recommended for this group. Close links should be established with the local psychogeriatric service (if one exists) so that clinicians from the service can provide assessment and make arrangements for their aftercare.

Further reading

Bancroft J, *et al.* (1979). The reasons people give for taking overdoses: a further inquiry. *British Journal of Medical Psychology* **52**, 353–65.

Beck AT, Beck R, Kovacs M (1975). Classification of suicidal behaviors: I. Quantifying intent and medical lethality. *American Journal of Psychiatry* **132**, 285–7.

Crawford MJ, Wessely S (1998). Does initial management affect the rate of repetition of deliberate self harm? Cohort study. *British Medical Journal* **317**, 985.

Department of Health and Social Security (1984). *The management of deliberate self-harm.* HN **84**, 25. Department of Health and Social Security, London.

Eddleston K, Resvi Sheriff MH, Hawton K (1998). Deliberate self-harm in Sri Lanka—an overlooked tragedy in the developing world. *British Medical Journal* **317**, 133–5.

Hassan TB, *et al.* (1999). Managing patients with deliberate self harm who refuse treatment in the accident and emergency department. *British Medical Journal* **319**, 107–9.

Hawton K, Catalan J (1987). *Attempted suicide: a practical guide to its nature and management*, 2nd edn. Oxford University Press, Oxford.

Hawton K, van Heerinogen K (2000). *The international handbook of suicide and attempted suicide.* Wiley, Chichester.

Hawton K, *et al.* (1998). Deliberate self-harm: a systematic review of the efficacy of psychosocial and pharmacological treatments in preventing repetition. *British Medical Journal* **317,** 441–7.

Nordentoft M, *et al.* (1993). High mortality by natural and unnatural causes: a 10 year follow up study of patients admitted to a poisoning treatment centre after suicide attempts. *British Medical Journal* **306**, 1637–41.

Royal College of Psychiatrists (1994). *The general hospital management of adult deliberate self-harm*, Council Report CR32. Royal College of Psychiatrists, London.

Royal College of Psychiatrists (1998). *Managing deliberate self-harm in young people*, Council Report CR63. Royal College of Psychiatrists, London.

26.5.3 Medically unexplained symptoms in patients attending medical clinics

Christopher Bass and Michael Sharpe

Historical background

Throughout history, patients have presented with subjective somatic complaints that their doctors could not explain in terms of objectively identifiable disease. Medical advances have improved the precision with which disease can be identified, but has not solved the problem. Many complaints remain unexplained and continue to present a challenge to doctors.

The proposed explanations for medically unexplained symptoms have changed over the last 300 years; early ideas located their cause in a disturbance of a bodily organ, often the uterus. Attention then focused on the peripheral nervous system, later the central nervous system, and more recently the cause has been assumed to be in the patient's mental functioning. These changing aetiological theories have been reflected in the varied terms used for such complaints: the organ theory gave rise to hysterical and hypochondriacal; the nervous system theory to nervous, functional nervous illness, and neurasthenic; and the mental theory to psychological, psychogenic, and somatization.

Changes in theory led to changing approaches to management. Early treatments were focused on the organ believed to be giving rise to the symptoms. Consequently manipulations of, and even removal of, the female reproductive organs was practised. When the proposed explanation shifted to the peripheral nervous system the preferred treatments became tonics, electrical stimulation, and other means to regenerate nervous energy. As interest shifted to the central nervous system, hypnosis became a favoured treatment and was used by famous physicians such as Charcot. By the end of the nineteenth century many physicians came to consider hypnosis unnecessary and explanation and advice to be sufficient. It was only in the twentieth century that, with the rise in popularity of psychoanalysis, medically unexplained symptoms began to be seen as a 'mental' problem requiring psychiatric treatment. Much subsequent thinking has emphasized psychological and psychiatric theories and treatments.

At the beginning of the twenty-first century many doctors continue to regard medically unexplained symptoms as psychological in origin because there is no abnormality on standard investigation. However, it has become increasingly obvious that patients dislike the psychological approach, which they see as dismissive and stigmatizing. As a result of these conflicting views patients often seem to be left in a 'no man's land' between a psychiatric conceptualization, which they reject, and a biomedical approach that they see as rejecting them. Recent developments in neuroscience have suggested that many unexplained symptoms do have a basis in the functioning of the nervous system, as hypothesized more than 100 years ago. An approach that recognizes this, whilst also drawing on evidence-based psychological and psychiatric treatment, appears to be the most productive.

Introduction

Definition and terminology

Various terms have been used to describe symptoms that are unexplained by identifiable disease processes. These include:

- *Medically unexplained*—A simple operational term, but with the potential disadvantage of suggesting that psychophysiological explanations are not 'medical'.
- *Functional*—Originally meaning a disturbance of bodily function rather then structure, it is unfortunately used pejoratively to mean 'all in the mind'.
- *Somatization*—A widely used term implying a psychological problem expressed somatically. It should arguably be restricted to cases where the somatic symptoms are plausibly understood as an expression of identifiable emotional disorder.
- *Conversion*—Used specifically to refer to loss of function such as weakness of a limb. Implies (as does somatization) that the symptoms are due to a 'conversion' of psychological problems, usually without good evidence.
- *Somatoform*—A diagnostic category in the psychiatric classifications. Intended to be atheoretical but obviously linked to the idea of somatization.

In conclusion, there is no entirely satisfactory term: the best term scientifically is probably 'medically unexplained', or perhaps 'unexplained by identifiable disease', but many textbooks and computer databases use the term 'somatoform'.

Symptoms

Almost any symptoms can be medically unexplained. Common examples include:

- pain (including back pain, chest pain, abdominal pain, and headache);
- fatigue;
- dizziness;
- 'fits', funny turns, and feelings of weakness.

Syndromes

Unexplained symptoms have been grouped into various 'functional' syndromes. Each medical specialty has at least one (Table 1): for rheumatologists, prominent muscle pain and tenderness is fibromyalgia; for gastroenterologists, abdominal pain with altered bowel habit is irritable bowel syndrome; and for infectious-disease specialists, chronic fatigue and myalgia is a postviral or chronic fatigue syndrome.

It has been argued that these syndromes do not necessarily reflect separate conditions, but merely reflect the tendency of specialists to focus only on those symptoms most pertinent to their specialty. The research literature offers support for this hypothesis by revealing substantial overlap between syndromes in their constituent symptoms, proposed aetiological factors, and response to treatment.

Table 1 Functional somatic syndrome by speciality

Gastroenterology	Irritable bowel syndrome, non-ulcer dyspepsia
Gynaecology	Premenstrual syndrome, chronic pelvic pain
Rheumatology	Fibromyalgia
Cardiology	Atypical or non-cardiac chest pain
Respiratory medicine	Hyperventilation syndrome
Infectious diseases	(Chronic postviral) fatigue syndrome
Neurology	Tension headache, non-epileptic attacks
Dentistry	Temporomandibular joint dysfunction, atypical facial pain
Ear, nose, and throat	Globus syndrome
Allergy	Multiple chemical sensitivity

The significance of medically unexplained symptoms and syndromes

Medically unexplained somatic complaints are a common and important but relatively neglected medical problem, constituting a major part of the work of most doctors. Whilst sometimes regarded as merely 'worried well', patients with medically unexplained complaints often suffer disability and distress at least as severe as that of those whose symptoms are explained by disease. Their doctors often find them difficult to help. They are also expensive to the healthcare system because they attend multiple specialist services and receive extensive, but unproductive, investigation and treatment. Many not surprisingly turn to unconventional treatments that are of unproven effectiveness. Some are financially exploited. This situation is clearly unsatisfactory.

Aetiology

The precise aetiology of many medically unexplained symptoms is unknown, but there is evidence that biological, psychological, and social factors all play a role. The degree to which each of these contributes probably varies from case to case. Rather than seeking a single factor, it is helpful to consider multiple factors and to distinguish between those that predispose to the development of medically unexplained symptoms, those that precipitate them, and those that act to perpetuate them. Table 2 provides a summary of possible aetiological factors, perpetuating factors being especially important since they are targets for treatment. For example, a person may be predisposed by virtue of genetics or childhood experience to develop irritable bowel syndrome. This may have been precipitated by a combination of infection and psychological stress. The factors that perpetuate it may include neurophysiological mechanisms, fear of gastrointestinal disease, social stress, chronic anxiety, and iatrogenic factors such as overinvestigation.

Epidemiology and classification

Epidemiology

Medically unexplained somatic symptoms are extremely common in the general population in all countries, some of whom will visit doctors, usually because of concern about the cause or because of severe discomfort and disability.

- *Primary care*—Medically unexplained symptoms are the principal reason for 25 to 50 per cent of all consultations in primary care. A minority are referred for a specialist opinion.

Table 2 The aetiology of medically unexplained symptoms

	Predisposing	Precipitating	Perpetuating
Biological	Genetic	Acute illness/injury	Neurophysiological and other mechanisms
Psychological	Childhood abuse	Stresses	Concern and beliefs about symptoms Anxiety or depression Abnormal illness behaviour
Social	Childhood illness 'models'	Life events	Iatrogenesis and lack of effective treatment Financial and other gain from being ill Behaviour of family and others

- *Hospital outpatient care*—At specialist outpatient clinics between one-quarter and one-third of new patients have symptoms that remain unexplained by disease. A small number of such patients are admitted to hospital.
- *Hospital inpatient care*—The proportion of medical inpatients with unexplained complaints is lower than amongst outpatients, but these patients can be particularly costly to the service. One Scandinavian study found that a relatively small number of patients with recurrent multiple medically unexplained symptoms (referred to as somatization disorder as described below) were consuming a significant proportion of the country's hospital inpatient budget.

Classification

There are, rather confusingly, parallel medical and psychiatric classification schemes for medically unexplained complaints. The former emphasizes the type of symptom and lists functional syndromes by organ system as in Table 1; the latter emphasizes the number of symptoms and associated psychological factors, with the main categories as listed in Table 3. The implication of these parallel classifications is that most patients will qualify for both a medical and a psychiatric diagnosis. Both may be useful in guiding management and prognostication, hence a combined medical/psychiatric diagnosis such 'irritable bowel syndrome/anxiety disorder' is probably more useful than either alone.

An alternative multidimensional classification system that combines both the medical and psychiatric approach has been suggested and may have additional clinical value. An example is shown in Table 4.

Pathogenesis and pathophysiology

Although the physiological mechanisms of symptom production are not fully understood in many cases, some physiological abnormalities and putative mechanisms have been identified, for example the effect of overbreathing in causing non-cardiac chest pain. These physiological mechanisms interact with psychological and social factors to perpetuate the illness. Hence, overbreathing gives rise to chest pain and paraesthesias, which is interpreted by the patient as a cardiac problem, leading to anxiety and the seeking of medical care. Medical investigation increases the anxiety, leading to further hyperventilation, and so on. Some suggested physiological mechanisms are listed in Table 5.

General clinical features

Pointers to a patient having medically unexplained complaints may be apparent before the initial consultation. The referral letter and medical notes may reveal frequent attendance at medical services, numerous negative (and often repeated) investigations, and a previous history of unsuccessful surgery.

At the consultation multiple symptoms are suggestive. However, the only way of confidently diagnosing complaints as medically unexplained is when the appropriate history, examination, and investigation reveal one or more somatic symptoms that remain unexplained by disease. It should be remembered that patients often have both symptoms that are explained by disease and others that are unexplained. An example is the frequent co-occurrence of epilepsy and non-epileptic attacks. Several general points are worth noting:

- Many (but not all) unexplained medical complaints are simply somatic symptoms of depression or anxiety.
- Most medically unexplained complaints reflect genuine suffering. The deliberate manufacturing of complaints with the intent to mislead is uncommon in ordinary medical practice. However, some degree of exaggeration and even frank deception in order to obtain financial gain is not uncommonly encountered in medicolegal practice.
- Although management may be based on general principles, psychiatric diagnosis may indicate additional specific and evidence-based treatment strategies.

Differential diagnosis

The main medical differential diagnosis is from symptoms due to disease. Difficulties are likely to involve unusual presentations of common diseases and rare diseases. Missed disease is always a concern, but once a patient has been carefully assessed the emergence of a 'missed' disease is the exception rather than the rule.

Management

The general principles of management are outlined in Table 6.

Table 3 The main psychiatric categories of medically unexplained symptoms

• Predominantly worry about disease	—*hypochondriasis*
• Predominant concern about symptoms	—*somatization*
(a) Somatic presentation of	—*depression and anxiety*
(b) A small number of symptoms	—*simple somatoform disorders*
(c) Chronic multiple symptoms	—*somatization disorder (Briquet's syndrome)*
• Loss of function	—*conversion disorder*
• Dislike of body parts	—*body dysmorphic disorder*
• Other unusual presentations	
• Deliberate deception	—*factitious disorder and malingering (including Munchausen's syndrome)*

Table 4 A multidimensional classificatory scheme of medically unexplained symptoms

- Duration of illness
- Number of symptoms
- Degree of disability
- Severity of depression/anxiety
- Strength of patients fears/beliefs

Patient assessment

When assessing the patient the main tasks are to:

- Understand the nature of the presenting symptoms. For example, what does the patient mean by their complaint of fatigue? Is it lack of energy (non-specific), sleepiness (suggesting a sleep problem), or lack of motivation (suggesting depression)?
- Find out what other symptoms the patient has. It is worth asking for an exhaustive list: the more symptoms, the more likely it is that they will be medically unexplained.
- Ask the patient what they think or fear is wrong with them. This can reveal the reason they are worried about the symptoms (for example, 'it could be cancer') and allow appropriately targeted education and reassurance to be given.
- Seek evidence of 'stress'. Life stresses may be a contributory factor. Furthermore, most patients find 'stress' to be a more acceptable explanation than psychiatric diagnoses such as depression or anxiety.
- Systematically seek evidence of depression and anxiety. This is often best done toward the end of the consultation so that the patient does not feel they are being dismissed as 'just psychiatric'. A useful approach is to empathize with the understandable distress resulting from the symptoms, thereby avoiding antagonizing the patient by giving the impression that the doctor believes that the cause of the symptoms is psychological.
- Physically examine the patient. This may reveal unsuspected signs of disease and also helps to convince the patient that they have been taken seriously and properly assessed.
- Perform appropriate investigations. It should be noted that misdiagnosis is relatively uncommon, and a balance needs to be struck between the risk of missing disease and the potential iatrogenic harm resulting from excessive investigation.

Table 5 Examples of possible physiological mechanisms for medically unexplained physical symptoms that are supported by evidence

Non-cardiac chest pain	Chest wall pain from overbreathing
Localized chronic pain	Neuronal plasticity
Fibromyalgia	Changed CNS pain sensitivity
Chronic fatigue	Neuroendocrine changes
Irritable bowel	Changed neuronal control of bowel motility

Table 6 Principles of general management of medically unexplained symptoms

- Exclude disease, but avoid unnecessary investigation or referral
- Seek specific treatable psychiatric syndromes
- Demonstrate to the patient that you believe their complaints
- Take a full and sympathetic history
- Establish a collaborative relationship
- Give the patient a positive explanation, including but not overemphasizing psychological factors
- Encourage a return to normal functioning

Giving reassurance explanation and advice

As well as being reassured that there is no evidence they have an unpleasant disease, patients benefit from being given a positive and credible explanation for their symptoms and practical advice on what to do next.

Reassurance

Giving appropriate reassurance is an important part of the medical consultation. This is most effective if based on the patient's actual concerns, so it is important to ask them what they are worried about before reassuring them. Many patients report that having a physical examination is particularly reassuring. A detailed explanation of what the tests that they have had do and don't show can also help. Clearly, it may be unwise to state categorically that the patient has no disease. However, it can be explained that it is not possible to do this, whilst emphasizing as unambiguously as possible that the probability they have the disease they fear is very low. Beware of the patient who repeatedly asks for reassurance about the same issue—they may have hypochondriasis (see below).

Explanation

Patients also need a positive explanation for their symptoms. It is nearly always unhelpful to explain that the symptoms are 'just psychological' or 'all in the mind'. Such statements are likely to reduce confidence in the doctor and may paradoxically increase the patient's concern about missed disease. It is also potentially harmful to suggest that the patient has a disease when they do not, or to collude with their idea that they do so. This may lead to inappropriate coping behaviour, for example obtaining a wheelchair rather than seeking rehabilitation. Rather, it is useful to describe a plausible physiological mechanism for the symptom that emphasizes the link with psychosocial factors and helps the patient to see their symptoms as reversible. For example, it can be explained that in irritable bowel syndrome psychological stress results in increased activation of the autonomic nervous system, leading to constriction of smooth muscle in the gut wall, which in turn causes pain. The symptoms may therefore be perpetuated by a vicious circle in which pain leads to anxiety, and anxiety leads to further pain. It can then be explained (perhaps using a diagram) that this mechanism is reversible by targeting these perpetuating factors. It is helpful to offer an optimistic prognosis, but an unrealistically precise prediction ('you will be better next week') is unwise as it is likely to lead to loss of faith in the doctor if not fulfilled.

Advice

A positive plan of action that specifies both what the patient can change and what the doctor can do is helpful. The patient can be advised how to overcome probable perpetuating factors, for example by resolving stress causing social problems or by practising relaxation. The doctor can offer to review progress, to prescribe (for instance, an 'antidepressant' drugs) and if appropriate to refer, for example, to physiotherapy or psychology. Action by the doctor gives the patient a sense that they are being taken seriously and not (as they may have experienced before) being dismissed. Writing to the patient as well as to the general practitioner to summarize the conclusions of the medical assessment and the proposed plan reinforces messages that may otherwise be easily forgotten.

'Antidepressant' drugs

Antidepressant drugs are most useful when the patient is depressed, but they can also be tried when he or she is not. A specific explanation of why they are being prescribed is needed if they are to be acceptable to the patient. Depending on the circumstances, one of the following two approaches is suggested. The first is to explain that the term 'antidepressant' is a misnomer: in fact the drugs are broad-spectrum 'nervous tonics' of proven value for sleep and pain as well as for depression. The second is to be explicit that they are being prescribed for depression, but emphasize that depression is understandable given the somatic symptoms the patient is suffering. Both these explanations minimize blame and stigma.

A systematic review of antidepressants for medically unexplained symptoms found them to be moderately effective overall. The odds ratio (**OR**) for improvement with antidepressant treatment compared with placebo was 3.4, with the size of effect similar across the different functional syndromes. However, there was a high dropout rate from treatment, emphasizing the need for careful explanation and follow-up to ensure adherence.

Psychological therapies

Explanation, reassurance, and advice are important psychological therapies. Where insufficient they can be reinforced by a formal psychological treatment. The most widely used are behavioural or cognitive–behavioural treatment (**CBT**), although other psychological treatments may have a role. CBT aims to help the patient to improve by examining their way of thinking about and coping with their symptoms. The treatment works by changing potentially illness-perpetuating beliefs and coping behaviours.

A systematic review of CBT for medically unexplained symptoms found that it was significantly superior to non-specific treatment in 70 per cent of trials. Individual behavioural components of CBT, such as graded exercise, have also been studied and are of value, but are probably less effective. Overall research supports the use of specialist CBT and other behavioural therapies in the management of patients with medically unexplained symptoms.

Referral for psychological or psychiatric management

The decision to refer will be based on the physician's assessment of the patient and an appraisal of the available services. Ideally, all medical clinics would have dedicated specialist psychiatric or psychology services: this is rarely the case in practice. It is wise to find out who is willing and interested in receiving referrals in the immediate locality. If the options are few, however, the healthcare team may wish to make the case for the provision of better services.

Reasons to refer include:

- very severe disability;
- suspected somatization disorder;
- specific service available, e.g. for chronic pain or chronic fatigue syndrome (**CFS**);
- patient remains distressed despite explanation and reassurance;
- suicide risk.

When explaining the referral to the patient it is wise to:

- Emphasize the reality of the patient's symptoms.
- Be positive about the service you are referring to.
- Do not prematurely imply you think the origin of their complaint is psychological.

A patient is more likely to attend for a referral if you have said: 'I see you have real and troublesome symptoms. I am pleased to tell you that they do not indicate a disease but am sorry to say that I do not have a simple cure I can prescribe. However, I can recommend and refer you to a specialist service for your problem', than if you have said: 'there is clearly nothing wrong with you; it must all be in your mind. There is nothing to do now but to refer you to the shrinks.'

What happens in practice?

In practice the ideal management described above is inconsistently applied and iatrogenic psychological and physical damage is probably common. The specific evidence-based treatments of antidepressants and CBT are rarely offered and frequently refused by patients. We could do better.

Prognosis

The prognosis for those patients whose symptoms are sufficiently severe and persistent for them to be referred to a specialist service is often poor. It is not uncommon for persistent symptoms and disability to persist for years, especially if untreated The prognosis is best for those patients who were well before the onset of the complaint and whose symptoms are expressions of uncomplicated depressive and anxiety disorders. It is worst for those patients with long-standing multiple symptoms.

Prevention

We do not know enough about the aetiology of medically unexplained complaints to implement primary prevention. Parenting behaviour and social factors such as the stigma associated with psychiatric illness and the nature of benefit and litigation systems appear to play a role.

Secondary prevention is important, as effective early management probably reduces the risk of chronicity, whereas poor explanation and over-investigation probably perpetuates it.

Tertiary prevention is the effective management of chronic somatization and requires a proactive management plan as described above.

Quality of life and psychological aspects

Patients with medically unexplained symptoms may have considerable functional impairment and a markedly reduced quality of life. Two disorders in particular, fibromyalgia and chronic fatigue syndrome, are associated with marked functional impairment and can have important consequences on a person's ability to work. Some patients may become involved in medicolegal claims, especially if the symptoms were temporally related to an accident or injury.

Areas of uncertainty and controversy

Many aspects of medically unexplained somatic complaints are controversial. Perhaps the most controversial issue is whether they are best regarded as a psychiatric/psychological or as a medical problem. This issue has been particularly prominent in controversy over chronic fatigue syndrome/ myalgic encephalomyelitis (**ME**).

Any clinician who sees patients with medically unexplained symptoms (and most do) is likely to agree that they are difficult to manage effectively. Furthermore, the core of this problem is frequently a clash between the physician and the patient in how the illness is viewed. A consideration of the changes in medical fashion for explaining such symptoms over the last few hundred years should encourage humility. Further study that integrates psychosocial and physiological perspectives is required, both to improve our understanding and to help us to explain these problems effectively to our patients.

Common syndromes

This section will cover specific aspects of the main psychiatric categories of medically unexplained symptoms listed in Table 3.

Predominant worry about disease—hypochondriasis

The central feature of hypochondriasis is a persistent preoccupation with the possibility that one has a serious and progressive physical disease. These fears have persisted despite the fact that repeated investigations and examinations have identified no adequate physical cause, and appropriate reassurance that there is no physical disease has been given.

Example

The patient is a young woman. Her urgent referral is faxed by her general practitioner (**GP**). She has attended the general practice clinic daily for the last 2 weeks. Her history is of headache. On enquiry her main concern is that she has developed a brain tumour. The background history reveals that her father died of a brain tumour 2 years ago; he was told it was only a 'tension headache' by the GP. Examination is normal but she is very anxious indeed and repeatedly asks for a brain scan and for your reassurance that she doesn't have a tumour.

Management and prognosis

Assessment should elicit the patient's specific fears. A useful question is: 'what is your worst fear?' The patient's catastrophic fear leads understandably to their behaviour and anxiety. For example, a patient with headache who thinks, 'I have a brain tumour' will be anxious and seek urgent medical attention. That is to say the somatic symptoms (headache) leads to thoughts (brain tumour) that in turn lead to anxiety and to certain behaviours (visiting doctors). It also causes muscular tension that leads to further pain and so on. Eliciting this causal sequence from the patient, and describing it to them, perhaps with a diagram, aids explanation. Reassurance that they do not have a tumour is appropriate. However, repeated reassurance can worsen concern about disease and should be avoided. Depressive disorder should be treated. CBT can be effective. Many acute cases resolve, but the condition can become chronic.

Somatic presentation of depression and anxiety

One of the commonest causes of medically unexplained somatic complaints is undiagnosed depression. Because depression is (erroneously) thought of as a purely 'mental illness', it is readily forgotten that it has somatic symptoms. These include:

- fatigue;
- increased pain complaints;
- loss of weight and appetite;
- loss of libido;
- in severe forms there may be negative ruminations on health that in rare cases can be delusional.

Another very common cause of unexplained symptoms is anxiety in a generalized form (generalized anxiety disorder) or episodic severe form (panic disorder). Somatic symptoms of anxiety include:

- fatigue;
- dizziness;
- paraesthesias;
- chest pain and palpitations;
- shortness of breath (especially 'getting enough breath in').

Example

A 50-year-old man presents to the Accident and Emergency department with chest pain and fatigue. Investigations are negative. Only after admission to hospital does a junior doctor examine the patient's mental state and find a persistent low mood, loss of interest, and negative thinking, with episodic anxiety associated with overbreathing and many somatic symptoms. The diagnosis is panic disorder and depressive disorder.

Management and prognosis

Treatment is by reassurance, explanation, and treating the depression and anxiety. This can be achieved by prescribing an antidepressant agent combined with explanation and active follow-up to ensure adherence. In some cases psychological treatment may also be required. The prognosis for recovery within 6 months is good, although there is a risk of relapse. Patients should continue to take the antidepressant drug for at least 6 months to prevent early relapse.

Simple somatoform disorders

This presentation refers to the patient with a single or small number of somatic complaints that do not appear to be simply expressions of depression or anxiety. This diagnosis includes undifferentiated somatoform disorder and somatoform pain disorder. The most common type of clinical problem in this group is the patient with chronic persistent pain in one site, for example chronic back pain or chronic headache. The physical symptoms may have commenced after a trivial injury or accident, but the subsequent disability is usually out of proportion to the organic findings. A medicolegal case may be pending, which often makes management more difficult.

Example

A middle-aged man presents with widespread pain. He believes that his symptoms are a result of occupational exposure to printing ink. He is medically retired. There is a history of depression some 12 months ago, but no evidence of current depressive or anxiety disorder. Examination is normal. The patient walks with a stick and seems concerned to demonstrate to you how ill he is.

Management and prognosis

Explanation and symptomatic treatment including cognitive–behavioural therapy is appropriate. Antidepressants may be tried on an empirical basis. The prognosis for chronic complaints is fairly poor, although improvement often occurs over many months. Physical rehabilitation may be useful.

Somatization disorder (Briquet's syndrome)—patients with chronic multiple complaints

'Somatization disorder', or Briquet's syndrome, is a term used to describe patients—mostly women—who have a lifelong history of multiple recurrent somatic complaints, which usually include conversion symptoms. If looked for, such patients are relatively easy to identify. Although the patient's current presenting complaint may be of only one or two symptoms, for example chest pain or shortness of breath, scrutiny of the past medical notes reveals numerous outpatient visits to different clinics with symptoms such as abdominal pain and bloating, diffuse muscular pains and tenderness, and chronic lassitude over previous years. A history of childhood abuse is common.

Example

The patient is a middle-aged woman, referred to as a 'heart sink' patient by the GP. She presents with dizziness, bloating of her stomach, and generalized weakness. She has three volumes of medical notes documenting presentations with a range of symptoms including pain in a number of sites, irritable bowel symptoms, menstrual problems, and transient loss of sight. She has had many investigations, a hysterectomy and three laparotomies, and she is taking many medications including oral opiates. However, review of her notes does not reveal any convincing evidence of any proven disease and examination reveals only a number of operation scars.

Management and prognosis

If possible, it is sensible to review the case notes before the patient arrives in the clinic. It is worth asking why the patient has been referred now: the GP may have become frustrated or angry, or helpless in the face of repeated complaints, or unable to cope with or contain the patient's distress. Management requires a reduction in the patient's and their general practitioner's expectation of medical 'cure', and a shift toward the development of coping strategies. Further investigation should be strictly limited to that which is clearly indicated, but may be difficult to avoid. Practical management strategies are listed in Table 7.

Depression is common in such patients, may give rise to some of the symptoms, and should be treated. Long-term follow-up by a hospital doctor, general practitioner, psychiatrist or a combination of these is desirable.

Table 7 Management of patients with chronic persistent symptoms

- Try to be **proactive** rather than **reactive**. Arrange to see the patient at regular, fixed intervals, rather than allowing him/her to dictate the timing and frequency of the visits.
- During the appointment aim to **broaden the agenda** with the patient. This involves establishing a **problem list** and allowing the patient to discuss relevant psychosocial problems.
- **Reduce** or taper unnecessary drugs.
- Whenever possible, try to **minimize** the contact the patients have with other specialists or practitioners. This will reduce **iatrogenic harm** and make **containment** easier if only one or two practitioners are involved.
- Try to co-opt a relative as a **therapeutic ally** to implement your management goal.
- Reduce your **expectation of cure**: instead aim for **containment** and **damage limitation**.
- Encourage the patient (and yourself) to think in terms of **coping and not curing**.

A realistic aim is for limited improvement and prevention of iatrogenic harm. The condition is very likely to persist.

Conversion disorder

The presentation is loss of function of a body part, most often a limb, or abnormal body movements. This is not thought to be produced intentionally, as with factitious disorder and malingering, but rather 'subconsciously'. In reality this distinction is difficult. Persistence of the symptom even when the patient believes they are unobserved helps to differentiate intentional and non-intentional symptom production. Other oft-quoted signs such as 'belle indifference' are unreliable. In acute cases the symptoms may have arisen in the context of severe interpersonal stress or conflict. The patient may have experienced a family member with similar symptoms.

Example

A young woman is referred for unexplained weakness of her left side. She reports being unable to move her left arm and leg following a bang on the head. Enquiry reveals that she was sexually assaulted the week before her symptoms began. She has no explanation for the symptoms and seems unconcerned about them. On examination her left arm and leg appear weak, with a 'collapsing' pattern of weakness, but there are no abnormalities of reflexes. A magnetic resonance imaging (**MRI**) brain scan is normal.

Management and prognosis

For the acute case an early return to function should be encouraged. Physiotherapy may be useful. Depression should be sought and treated if present. The patient should also be offered an opportunity to talk about stressors. In chronic cases treatment is more difficult and may best be achieved via referral to a physical rehabilitation service. In chronic cases there may be long-term invalidism with dependence on state benefits.

Body dysmorphic disorder—requests for surgery to a body part in the absence of a conspicuous abnormality or deformity

Patients who are dissatisfied with some aspect of their bodily appearance or shape may find their way into the clinics of physicians and surgeons. Some of these patients are preoccupied with an imagined defect in appearance, such as a large nose. Others have more substantial concerns, such as disliking a limb sufficiently to desire its amputation. Even in the presence of a physical abnormality, the person's concern appears to be markedly excessive.

Example

A 30-year-old woman complains about the shape of her nose and blames this for many failures in her life. She requests plastic surgery.

Management and prognosis

In the absence of a conspicuous physical abnormality or deformity, it is usually prudent to seek a psychiatric opinion. There is some evidence for the effectiveness of CBT. Surgery sometimes helps, but should only be carried out after careful consideration.

Other unusual presentations

Atypical eating disorders

Some patients who attend with symptoms of abdominal pain after food, vomiting, anorexia, or constipation may have a covert eating disorder. Judicious enquiry about weight loss, amenorrhoea, and laxative use may help to establish the correct diagnosis, which may have been present for many years. See Chapter 26.5.5 for further discussion.

Chronic constipation that has not responded to conventional treatment

Patients may report constipation for two or three decades that has proved unresponsive to appropriate treatment. There is often no identifiable organic cause, and some are referred to surgeons for colectomy. All such patients require a thorough psychiatric assessment before major decisions about treatment are implemented. Biofeedback has been shown to benefit some patients, but resources for this treatment are scarce.

Loin-pain haematuria syndrome

This is a rare syndrome that is poorly understood. Patients may abuse opiate analgesics, and a proportion is thought to simulate their pain. It is unwise to carry out renal autotransplantation, because the pain can recur on the opposite side of the body.

Factitious disorders

Patients with factitious disorder deliberately feign or simulate illness, which is in contrast to the disorders described above. The term 'factitious disorder' is preferable to the eponym Munchausen's syndrome, because this stereotype is often misleading—Munchausen's syndrome generally being applied to wandering, untreatable, male sociopaths. Over three-quarters of patients with factitious disorders are women, over half of whom work in medically related occupations. They often report a large number of childhood illnesses and operations. High rates of substance abuse, mood disorder, and personality disorder have been reported. Some patients exploit genuine disease (usually chronic) to create dramatic medical emergencies.

Example

A young man is repeatedly admitted with breakdown of an abdominal surgical wound. He is observed rubbing dirt into the wound. When confronted with this he discharges himself immediately.

Management and prognosis

A supportive confrontation is required. This means presenting the patient with the evidence that they have been manufacturing symptoms, together with the acknowledgement that they have an emotional problem and an offer of psychological help. Ideally, the physician and psychiatrist do this jointly. There is some evidence that psychological support following hospital discharge may be associated with an improved outcome. Patients with more stable social networks have a better prognosis than wanderers.

Malingering

Malingering is the deliberate simulation or exaggeration of physical or psychiatric symptoms for obvious and understandable gain, for example monetary compensation, disabled status, and avoidance of criminal prosecution or conscription. Doctors are often reluctant to diagnose malingering lest it adversely affect the individual's healthcare, occupation, or legal case. However, it does occur, especially in medicolegal contexts. Common examples include malingered cognitive deficit and postinjury back/neck pain in patients seeking compensation or disability payment. The initial physical injury may be established, but the length and severity of symptoms, disability, and distress are disproportionate. There is probably a continuum from minor embellishment of symptoms to frank malingering.

Example

A 30-year-old man is seen in order to produce a legal report for the purpose of claiming compensation. He reports severe back pain following a car accident 2 years ago and is in a wheelchair. There are no neurological signs and no muscle wasting. He is later seen lifting his wheelchair into the boot of his car.

Management and prognosis

Assessment of suspected malingering requires the methodical use of all sources of information. It may only be possible to make the diagnosis positively when covert surveillance reveals behaviour clearly at odds with the reported disability. If management is required it is by confrontation, although it is more common that the identification of malingering ends the behaviour (and the legal case).

Further reading

Barsky AJ, Borus JF (1999). Functional somatic symptoms. *Annals of Internal Medicine* **130**, 910–21.

Barsky AJ (1998). A comprehensive approach to the chronically somatizing patient. *Journal of Psychosomatic Research* **45**, 301–6.

Bass C, Gill D (2000). Factitious disorders and malingering. In: Gelder M, *et al*., eds. *New Oxford textbook of psychiatry* pp. 1126–32. Oxford University Press, Oxford.

Bowman ES (1998). Pseudoseizures. *Psychiatric Clinics of North America* **21**, 649–57.

Carson AJ, *et al.* (2000). Do medically unexplained symptoms matter? A prospective cohort study of 300 new referrals to neurology outpatient clinics. *Journal of Neurology, Neurosurgery and Psychiatry* **68**, 207–10.

Creed F, Mayou RA, Hopkins A (1992). *Medical symptoms not explained by organic disease.* The Royal College of Psychiatrists and the Royal College of Physicians of London, London.

Chambers J, Bass C, Mayou R (1999). Non-cardiac chest pain: assessment and management. *Heart* **82**, 656–7.

Drossman DA (1995). Diagnosing and treating patients with refractory functional gastrointestinal disorders. *Annals of Internal Medicine* **123**, 688–97.

Fink P, *et al.* (1999). Somatization in primary care. Prevalence, health care utilization, and general practitioner recognition. *Psychosomatics* **40**, 330–8.

Kroenke K, Swindle R (2000). Cognitive–behavioral therapy for somatization and symptom syndromes: a literature synthesis. *Psychotherapy and Psychosomatics* **69**, 205–15.

Mayou RA, Bass C, Sharpe M (1995). *Treatment of functional somatic symptoms.* Oxford University Press, Oxford.

O'Malley PG, *et al.* (1999). Antidepressant therapy for unexplained symptoms and CNS syndromes. *Journal of Family Practice* **48**, 980–90.

Sharpe M (1998). Doctor's diagnoses and patient's perceptions; lessons from the chronic fatigue syndrome. *General Hospital Psychiatry* **20**, 335–8.

Sharpe M, Bass C (1992). Pathophysiological mechanisms in somatization. *International Review of Psychiatry* **4**, 81–97.

Smith RC (1991). Somatization disorder: defining its role in clinical medicine. *Journal of General and Internal Medicine* **6**, 168–75.

Wessely S, Nimnuan C, Sharpe M (1999). Functional somatic syndromes: one or many?. *Lancet* **354**, 36–9.

26.5.4 Anxiety and depression

L. Chwastiak and W. Katon

Introduction

Depression and anxiety are more commonly seen in primary care than any other condition except hypertension. Over half of all patients with mental health disorders are cared for solely by a primary care provider, and many seek help from their physician because they attribute symptoms of depression and anxiety to a physical problem. Physicians fail to make an accurate diagnosis in at least 50 per cent of those with depressive or anxiety disorders. This failure occurs because of time limitations, lack of knowledge, focus on presenting physical symptoms, fear of opening 'Pandora's box', and the stigma associated with psychiatric illness. As a result, only about half of those patients with major depression receive the dose and duration of treatment with antidepressants that meets United States Agency for Health Care Policy and Research (**AHCPR**) guidelines. Fewer than half of patients with anxiety disorders in primary care are treated with specific medications or psychotherapy.

Early recognition of depressive and anxiety disorders is important because they can be treated effectively, often in primary care. The detection and treatment of anxiety and depression can prevent patient discomfort and unnecessary expensive diagnostic investigations, which are often ordered to investigate unexplained physical symptoms. More serious complications may also be prevented, such as the progression of psychiatric illness, loss of employment and impairment of social roles, decreased adherence to medical treatment, and suicide.

Epidemiology

Depression and anxiety are very common and frequently follow a chronic course. The National Comorbidity Survey (**NCS**) found, through a structured psychiatric interview, that almost 50 per cent of community respondents in the United States had at least one lifetime DSM-III-R (*Diagnostic and statistical manual of mental disorders, third edition, revised*) psychiatric disorder. Major depression was the most common disorder with a lifetime prevalence of 17.3 per cent and a 12-month prevalence rate of 10.3 per cent. The point prevalence of depression in Western industrialized nations is from 2.3 to 3.2 per cent for men and 4.5 to 9.3 per cent for women; lifetime risk is 7 to 12 per cent for men and 20 to 25 per cent women. The reasons for gender differences are poorly understood, but are thought to include endocrine, biological, and sociocultural factors: women have been found to have experience higher rates of childhood (especially sexual) abuse.

The prevalence rates of depression are higher for medical patients than for the general population: 6 to 10 per cent of primary care patients; and 10 to 14 per cent medical inpatients meet the criteria for major depression. In patients with at least two chronic physical illnesses, the 12-month prevalence rate of major depression was 12.5 per cent. Major depression is commonly associated with cardiovascular disease (prevalence rate of 25 per cent), cancer (20 to 45 per cent), cerebrovascular accidents (26 to 34 per cent), chronic pain (33 to 35 per cent), and Parkinson's disease (40 per cent). Depression and panic disorder are also common in 'medically unexplained' syndromes (Table 1, and see Chapter 26.5.3).

Some 16 per cent of people experience an anxiety disorder sometime during their lifetime. These disorders are commoner in women, with a 12-month prevalence of panic disorder in community samples of 3.2 per cent in women and 1.3 per cent in men, and a lifetime prevalence of 5 per cent and 2 per cent, respectively. Infrequent panic attacks occur in up to one-third of individuals. Only 26 per cent of patients with panic disorder present to a mental health setting: one-third present to an emergency room, and over a third to their primary physician.

Table 1 Prevalence of depression and panic disorder

	Prevalence (%)	
	Panic disorder	Major depression
Community	1–3	3–5
Primary care	7	6–10
Medical inpatients	2–3	10–14
High utilizers of primary care	22	25
Chest pain and negative angiography	33–43	40
Irritable bowel syndrome	29	35
Unexplained dizziness	13	12
Headaches	5–15	9–25
Chronic fatigue	11–30	30–50

About 80 per cent of psychiatric disorders are comorbid disorders: almost half the cases of depression and anxiety occur in the same patients at the same time. About 25 per cent of patients with major depression, dysthymia, and anxiety disorders also have a history of substance abuse.

Costs

Worldwide, depression is the leading cause of years lived with disability. In the United States in 1990, the estimated total annual cost of major depression was $44 billion, and for anxiety disorders it was $42.3 billion, of which $23 billion was attributed to non-psychiatric medical costs, reflecting the high degree of medically unexplained symptoms these patients experience. Patients with anxiety and depression make more emergency visits, primary care visits, and more telephone calls to their physicians, have more medical tests and evaluations, take more medications, and are more likely to be admitted to hospital for a medical disorder than patients who do not have these disorders. As many as 50 per cent of 'high utilizers' of medical care services have a current depressive or anxiety disorder. Even after controlling for age and pre-existing medical comorbidity, patients with depression receive two to four times as much non-psychiatric medical care as patients without depression, and those with panic disorder use three times as many services as other primary care patients.

In patients with chronic medical illness, depressive and anxiety disorders are associated with an amplification of physical symptoms, additional functional impairment, and a decreased ability to adhere to medication and important lifestyle changes (exercise and diet). Depression reduces the effectiveness of rehabilitation in older patients with stroke, Parkinson's disease, heart disease, fractures, and pulmonary disease. Effective treatment of major depression reduces physical symptoms and functional impairment in patients with chronic medical illness.

The indirect costs of depression and anxiety include mortality, absenteeism from work, and adverse effects on family roles. In the WHO study in primary care, depression was associated with 6.1 disability days per month—as much or more than eight chronic illnesses, including coronary artery disease and arthritis. Anxiety disorders usually strike people at the beginning of their working lives, and may last for many years. Some studies reported that over half of those with panic disorder were not working, and others were forced to take lower-paying or part-time jobs near their homes. The lost economic productivity is easier to quantify than the other indirect costs: lost earning time of family or friends bringing patients to treatment, decreased efficiency at work, the toll on families, the future costs to society of children reared by an unemployed or housebound parent. The role functioning of patients with panic disorder is substantially lower than that of patients with chronic medical illnesses, but higher than that of depressed patients.

Pathophysiology

Depressive and anxiety disorders are complex syndromes that are diagnosed based on clinical criteria. No clear anatomical, physiological, or biochemical explanation has been found. Pathophysiological hypotheses for these disorders involve endocrine characteristics, abnormalities in levels of particular neurotransmitters, and neuroanatomical changes.

Data support an underlying genetic component for major depression, panic disorder, generalized anxiety disorder, and obsessive–compulsive disorder. There are significantly higher rates of depression and panic disorder in first-degree relatives of patients with these disorders. Twin studies have shown a higher rate of concordance for monozygotic compared to dizygotic twins in patients with panic disorder and major depression.

Mood disorders are associated with heterogeneous dysregulation of the biogenic amines, noradrenaline (norepinephrine) and serotonin being the two neurotransmitters most implicated. In animal models, long-term treatment with virtually all antidepressants is associated with a decrease in the sensitivity of postsynaptic β-adrenergic and type-2 serotonin receptors. Anxiety disorders are associated with abnormalities of the same neurotransmitters as well as in receptors of the neurotransmitter γ-aminobutyric acid (GABA), an inhibitory neurotransmitter found mainly in the cerebral cortex.

A variety of neuroendocrine abnormalities have been reported in patients with mood disorders, but it is unclear whether these are the cause of the mood disorder, or reflect an underlying brain disorder. Among the more consistent observations in patients with major depression is dysfunction of the hypothalamic–pituitary–adrenal (**HPA**) axis, presenting as elevation of basal cortisol, dexamethasone-mediated negative feedback resistance, increased cerebrospinal fluid levels of corticotropin-releasing factor (**CRF**), and an ACTH response to challenge with exogenous CRF. These features appear to be markers of state rather than trait: they usually normalize after successful treatment.

There is evidence suggesting that panic disorder is associated with specific biological abnormalities in the central nervous system. Stimulation of the locus coeruleus in the pons increases anxiety, and selective serotonin-reuptake inhibitors (**SSRIs**), tricyclic antidepressants, monoamine oxidase inhibitors (**MAOIs**), and benzodiazepines all decrease the firing rates of neurones in this area.

Diagnosis and clinical manifestations

Patients with depression or anxiety initially present with physical complaints 50 to 70 per cent of the time. They often complain of vague symptoms or report multiple somatic symptoms in a variety of anatomical locations, or experience greater dysfunction than can be attributed to their known medical disorders. Patients with panic disorder often selectively focus on the somatic components of anxiety, such as chest pain or palpitations, attributing their increased anxiety and tension to the frightening nature of somatic symptoms.

When depression or anxiety are suspected, simple screening questions may be helpful: 'Are you feeling sad, blue, or depressed?' 'Have you lost interest and pleasure in most things you usually enjoy?' 'Do you have sudden episodes or attacks where your heart beats fast, your chest is tight, it feels hard to breathe and you feel shaky?' The physician should enquire about the patient's explanatory model for his or her symptoms: 'Why do you think you get these symptoms?'

History is the single best diagnostic tool. The physician should elicit the patient's concerns and fears, current life situation, family and other support systems, and concurrent medical problems. A family history of psychiatric problems (depression, anxiety, substance use disorders) should also be obtained. Screening questions about a childhood or adult history of physical or sexual abuse or domestic violence are important and can be woven into the usual questions about family medical history. Adverse childhood and adult traumatic experiences are associated with an increased risk of

Table 2 DSM-IV criteria for major depressive episode

Five (or more) of the following symptoms, present most of the time for the past 2 weeks; at least one of the symptoms is either depressed mood or loss of interest or pleasure:

- Depressed mood
- Loss of interest or pleasure in activities
- Weight loss or gain (change of more than 5 per cent of body weight in a month)
- Sleep disorder (insomnia or hypersomnia)
- Psychomotor agitation or retardation
- Fatigue or loss of energy
- Feelings of worthlessness, or excessive or inappropriate guilt
- Diminished ability to concentrate or make decisions
- Recurrent thoughts of death or suicidal ideation, plan or attempt

anxiety and affective disorders in adulthood. Over half of the depressed women in one primary care study reported experiencing physical abuse as adults.

The physician should explain carefully that anxiety and depression reflect a biological predisposition that is provoked during a period of life stress, but major depression is not the uniform outcome of any stressful event. Risk factors that predispose patients to anxiety or depression include a personal or family history of depression or substance abuse, serious medical illness, lack of social support, or a history of early childhood trauma or neglect. Risk factors that can precipitate an acute episode or perpetuate the disorder include poor physical health, divorce, poor interpersonal relationships, illness or death in a family member, low socioeconomic status, or a stressful work situation.

Major depressive episodes last at least 2 weeks and are characterized by at least five of nine criteria, including at least one of the two primary criteria of depressed mood and loss of interest or pleasure in nearly all activities (Table 2). There are two to three times as many people with 'minor' depressive symptoms that fall short of major depression criteria: these have a higher rate of spontaneous recovery.

Physical symptoms are predictive of a good response to treatment: patients with middle insomnia (awakening between 0200 and 0400 h) or a diurnal variation in mood are more likely to respond to antidepressant medications.

Several dimensions of depression severity should be assessed: the frequency and chronicity of depressive symptoms, the impact of depression on the patient's ability to function, the potential for suicide, and the presence of psychotic or manic symptoms. Dysthymic disorder is characterized by a chronically depressed mood that occurs most of the day, more days than not, for at least 2 years. Dysthymic disorder is associated with many of features of major depression, but differs in its onset, duration, persistence, and severity of symptoms. Dysthymia is associated with impaired functioning and may not remit spontaneously.

Patients with anxiety have cognitive, affective, and somatic symptoms. The key feature distinguishing panic disorder from other anxiety disorders is the episodic nature of the attacks. Panic attacks are characterized by the sudden onset of intense apprehension, fear or terror, and by the abrupt development of at least four of the symptoms listed in Table 3, reaching a peak within 10 min. Panic disorder is diagnosed when attacks are recurrent, produce persistent fear, or become significantly disruptive to the patient's life.

Laboratory studies

An adequate diagnostic work-up for anxiety or depression may include a complete blood screen, urinalysis, and routine laboratory tests of renal and liver function. Selected patients should receive an electrocardiogram or chest radiograph. Thyroid function studies are recommended in perimenopausal or postmenopausal women. Given the sizeable differential diagnosis for a patient presenting with anxiety or depression, the extent of work-up must be tailored for each case.

Suicide

The risk of suicide should be evaluated in all patients with depressive and anxiety disorders. The risk of suicide attempts and suicidal ideation more than doubles in depressed patients with comorbid anxiety or physical illness. Other risk factors for suicide include gender (elderly White males are at highest risk), alcoholism, severe medical illness, psychosis, and lack of social support. The topic of suicidal ideation can be approached gradually with a non-specific question such as, 'Do you ever feel so discouraged that life does not seem worth living?'

Asking about suicide will not increase a patient's risk. Enquiries about suicide can reassure the patient and enable the physician and patient together to make a plan to prevent suicide, including deciding together whether emergency psychiatric consultation or hospitalization is necessary. Physicians should consider using a 'no harm contract': meaning that patients are simply asked to contract with the physician in writing that they will contact the physician if they think that they are losing control of a suicidal impulse. Although data on the effectiveness of this technique are not available, it seems sensible and is standard clinical practice in many centres.

For further discussion of these issues see Chapter 26.5.2.

Treatment

Whilst depression and anxiety are usually recurrent or chronic disorders, their clinical course can be markedly improved with timely, evidence-based treatments. Many patients can be treated successfully by primary care or general physicians. A meta-analysis of 28 randomized controlled trials found an overall efficacy rate of 54 to 65 per cent for the treatment of

Table 3 DSM-IV criteria for panic disorder

Both 1 and 2:

1. *Recurrent unexpected panic attacks: discrete period of intense fear or discomfort, in which four (or more) of the following symptoms develop abruptly and reach a peak within 10 min:*

Palpitations	Dizziness
Sweating	Derealization or depersonalization
Trembling or shaking	Fear of losing control or going crazy
Shortness of breath or choking	Fear of dying
Chest pain	Chills or hot flushes
Nausea or abdominal distress	

2. *At least one of the attacks has been followed by 1 month (or more) of one (or more) of the following:*
   Persistent concern about having additional attacks
   Worry about the implications of the attack or its consequences
   A significant change in behaviour related to the attacks

depression in the primary care setting, which is comparable to the response of patients seen by psychiatrists.

Physicians need to educate patients about the nature of depression or anxiety and how symptoms can be managed. They should explore background problems, define treatment goals, and dispel negative perceptions (for example, that antidepressant therapy is addictive). Patients should be reassured that they are not 'crazy', nor are their symptoms a manifestation of their own failure or shortcomings. There are several important educational points to cover. Depression and anxiety are quite common and are associated with important physiological changes. With proper treatment, these disorders almost always improve or remit; but relapses and recurrences can occur, so follow-up is essential. Physicians should enquire about the patient's concerns regarding a diagnosis of depression or anxiety, and also their worries about medical disorders. Raising the possibility of referral to a psychiatrist or other mental health professional early may make it easier to accept later.

Patients should be educated about the types of available treatments. Identifying the patient's desires and goals for treatment can provide a focus for the management of problems that can otherwise seem to be poorly defined and overwhelming. This can also increase patients' sense of participation in their care. Successful disease management programmes developed for asthma and diabetes that have emphasized educating patients to be partners in their medical care have resulted in significant improvements in adherence to treatment and in outcomes. Similar approaches appear to be successful in managing those with depression and panic disorder.

Pharmacotherapy

The decision to prescribe antidepressant therapy should be based on the number of symptoms, the level of dysfunction, and previous episodes of depression or anxiety. Before initiating antidepressant therapy, the physician should educate the patient regarding potential side-effects, the need to take medication regularly, and the usual time period and course to recovery.

The different classes of antidepressant drugs show virtually equivalent efficacy in the treatment of outpatients with major depressive disorder. The consensus on the pharmacotherapy of panic disorder also described equivalent efficacy of tricyclic antidepressants (**TCAs**), SSRIs, MAOIs, and high-potency benzodiazepines. For other forms of anxiety (social phobia and post-traumatic stress disorder), there is more evidence of the efficacy of SSRIs and MAOIs compared to TCAs.

The choice of medication should therefore be made on issues other than efficacy, such as side-effects, cost, adherence, and physician familiarity and comfort with prescribing particular agents. Primary care providers should become familiar with one or two medications with minimal side-effects from each of the major classes of antidepressants: TCAs, heterocyclics, and SSRIs. In each case the aim is to optimize treatment benefit and lower risk. Factors to be considered include the possibility of side-effects, history of response or a failure to respond, possible drug interactions, the presence of other psychiatric or medical conditions, familial response to a specific agent, and patient age.

The SSRIs have become the first-line treatment for major depression, dysthymia, and panic disorder, primarily because their improved side-effect profiles are associated with improved adherence to treatment. In the primary care setting, patients are significantly more likely to discontinue TCAs than SSRIs, those started on an SSRI being 7.5 times more likely to have a duration and an average dose of medication consistent with treatment guideline recommendations. The initial prescription of fluoxetine results in fewer side-effects, a lower rate of medication switching, and no difference in clinical outcomes, quality of life outcomes, or overall treatment costs when compared to TCAs. Although SSRIs are more expensive, total treatment costs per depressive episode are similar for patients treated with SSRI or TCA medication.

Randomized controlled trials have failed to show efficacy for antidepressant medication in patients with minor depression, largely because the placebo response rate was so high. Watchful waiting is appropriate for these patients, although the physician should recognize that they are at a higher risk of developing a major depressive episode.

Classes of medications

For a discussion of the pharmacology, side-effects, and interactions of tricyclic antidepressants, SSRIs, MAOIs, and other agents used in the treatment of anxiety and depression, see Section 26.6.1.

Selective serotonin-reuptake inhibitors (SSRIs)

The advent of the SSRIs (fluoxetine, paroxetine, sertraline, fluvoxamine, citalopram) and the newer atypical antidepressants (amfebutanone (buproprion), nefazodone, and venlafaxine) has significantly increased the number of patients receiving pharmacological treatment for depression and anxiety in a primary care setting. These new agents have fewer adverse side-effects and are safer for treating elderly patients and those with comorbid medical illnesses. SSRIs are also much safer than the tricyclic antidepressants if taken in overdose. They do not cause postural hypotension or cardiac conduction delay.

These agents have the advantage that the starting dose may also be an effective treating dose. This is most clearly the case for fluoxetine (20 mg), but may also be true for paroxetine (20 mg), sertraline (50 mg), and citalopram (20 mg). The frail elderly and those with liver disease require smaller starting doses (generally one-half of the recommended starting dose). Fluoxetine has the longest half-life (24–27 h) and a long-acting active metabolite (half-life of 7 days). This medication can be taken every other day, and the doses can eventually be given once or twice weekly to allow for smooth tapering when the drug is being withdrawn. The other SSRIs have half-lives of about 24 h and have no active metabolites with longer half-lives. This allows once-daily dosing and rapid washout. Amfebutanone (buproprion), venlafaxine, and nefazodone have shorter half-lives (14 h), so must be given at least twice a day; sustained release forms of amfebutanone and venlafaxine can be taken once daily.

Table 4 describes common side-effects of these medications: those such as anxiety, insomnia, nausea, headache, and agitation occur in fewer than 20 per cent of patients. When they do occur, they are usually mild and may respond to a reduction in the dose of medication. Sexual dysfunction (decreased libido and anorgasmia) may occur in up to one-third of patients treated with SSRIs; the addition of amfebutanone (buproprion) (75 to 150 mg a day in divided doses) or buspirone (20–40 mg) may alleviate these sexual side-effects. Strategies for the management of other common side-effects are listed in Table 5.

Patients with anxiety disorders are especially sensitive to the SSRI side-effects of jitteriness, restlessness, agitation, and insomnia. Low doses should be prescribed initially (5–10 mg paroxetine; 12.5–25 mg of sertraline; 25 mg fluvoxamine; 5 mg fluoxetine) for approximately 1 week, then gradually increasing to full therapeutic doses. To completely alleviate panic attacks in most cases requires: 20 to 50 mg paroxetine, citalopram, or fluoxetine; 50 to 200 mg of sertraline; and 100 to 300 mg of fluvoxamine. Similar schedules and dosages are used to treat patients with social phobia, post-traumatic stress disorder, and generalized anxiety disorder.

The SSRIs (but not amfebutanone (buproprion)) have all been shown to inhibit the cytochrome P-450 system in the liver, thus potentially leading to drug interactions (see Chapter 26.6.1). Amfebutanone is an effective antidepressant that may be especially useful because it does not cause the sexual side-effects common to the SSRIs, but it has been associated with a 1.5 per cent increase in prevalence of seizures compared to other antidepressants. The medication should not be given to individuals at risk for seizures (those with a history of seizures or head injury), and should never be administered in a single dose greater than 150 mg. Patients with a history of bulimia also have an increased risk of seizures on amfebutanone, and should not be prescribed this medication. The starting dose of 75 mg

Table 4 Side-effects of medications used to treat depression and anxiety

	Sedation, fatigue	Anti-cholinergic	Dizziness	Insomnia; agitation	Headache	Weight gain	GI	Anorgasmia
TCA								
Amitriptyline	3+	3+	3+	0	0	2+	1+	1+
Desipramine	1+	1+	1+	1+	0	2+	1+	1+
Doxepin	3+	3+	3+	0	0	2+	1+	1+
Imipramine	2+	3+	3+	1+	0	2+	1+	1+
Nortriptyline	2+	2+	1+	0	0	2+	0	1+
Protriptyline	1+	3+	1+	1+	0	2+	1+	1+
Heterocyclics								
Trazodone	3+	0	2+	0	0	2+	0	0
SSRIs								
Fluoxetine	0	0	0	2+	1+	0	1+	2+
Sertraline	1+	0	0	1+	0	0	2+	2+
Paroxetine	1+	1+	0	1+	0	0	0	2+
Fluvoxamine	0	0	0	1+	0	1+	2+	2+
Citalopram	1+	0	0	1+	0	0	0	1+
Aminoketone								
Amfebutanone (buproprion)	0	0	0	1+	0	0	0	1+
Venlafaxine	0	0	0	1+	0	0	2+	1+
Nefazodone	1+	0	0	1+	0	0	0	0
Mirtazapine	2+	0	0	0	0	1+	0	0

GI, gastrointestinal; TCA, tricyclic antidepressant; SSRIs, selective serotonin-reuptake inhibitors.

twice per day should be increased every week to achieve a therapeutic level of between 300 and 450 mg/day.

Tricyclic antidepressants

The heterocyclic medications include the tricyclic antidepressants and several other agents that are similar in structure, including maprotiline, amoxapine, and trazodone. These medications are similar in their side-effects and dosing strategies (see Chapter 26.6.1).

Low starting doses are required, with a gradual increase to a therapeutic level. For treating depression, generalized anxiety disorder, or panic disorder, physicians should begin at 10 to 25 of imipramine, gradually increasing the dose by 10 to 25 mg every 4 or 5 days. The ultimate dosage is variable, with some patient responding at a low dosage (50–100 mg), and others needing up to 300 mg.

Plasma levels can be measured, but these function primarily as crude indicators of whether or not the patient is taking the medication. Clinicians should treat the patient, and not the blood level, since many with high or low blood levels may do very well clinically. Nortriptyline is an exception, as it has a therapeutic window (50–150 ng/ml): levels below or above this are less likely to lead to remission of depression.

Table 5 Managing the side-effects of pharmacotherapy

Insomnia	Move dose to early part of the day Add trazodone 50–100 mg at bedtime or nortriptyline 25–50 mg at bedtime Switch to paroxetine or fluvoxamine
Nausea or diarrhoea	Take medication with food Reduce dose for 4–7 days, then reintroduce higher dose Add H_2 blocker Switch to nortriptyline
Sedation	Move dose to bedtime Switch to fluoxetine or sertraline
Anorgasmia	Add amfebutanone (buproprion) 75 mg once or twice per day Weekend drug holidays (not fluoxetine) Switch to nefazodone

Other agents

For the small subgroup of patients with anxiety disorders who do not tolerate SSRIs or TCAs, high-potency benzodiazepines may be an effective second-line treatment. Alprazolam, lorazepam, and clonazepam have all been shown to be more effective than placebo for the treatment of panic disorder. Patients can be started at 0.25 mg clonazepam three times per day, with a gradual increase by 0.25 mg every 2 to 3 days until the attacks stop. Symptoms of generalized anxiety disorder can be alleviated in most cases with a clonazepam dose between 0.25 to 0.5 mg twice daily and 1 mg two or three times daily, or lorazepam 0.5 to 1 mg three times daily. These agents are best used in conjunction with an SSRI or TCA at the beginning of treatment. After 6 to 8 weeks, when the antidepressant begins to have its optimal effects in treating anxiety symptoms, the benzodiazepine can usually be tapered with a 10 per cent dose reduction per week.

Buspirone is an azapirone with affinity for 5-HT1A and dopamine receptors that has been approved for the treatment of patients with generalized anxiety disorder. It is non-sedating, and there are no withdrawal symptoms with abrupt discontinuation. There are also no synergistic effects with alcohol. Buspirone is typically effective at doses of 30 to 60 mg, divided two or three times daily. Common side-effects include dizziness, nausea, headache, and nervousness. These can be reduced by using lower starting doses of 5 mg two or three times daily and advancing as tolerated.

Beta-adrenergic blockers may be useful for treating performance anxiety. Propranolol is used at doses of 10 to 80 mg per day (ideally taken 2 h before the anticipated exposure). Atenolol at 30 to 100 mg may be preferred since it has fewer CNS side-effects (exacerbating depression).

MAOIs are potentially the most effective class of medication for panic or certain types of depression. However, their regular use in primary care or by general physicians is precluded by the lack of familiarity with these agents, and the potential for hypertensive crisis that can ensue from not following a low-tyramine diet or taking an over-the-counter stimulant medication (like pseudoephedrine).

St John's Wort Clinicians need to ask patients in a routine and non-judgemental manner about their use of alternative treatments, and should know enough about the more common ones to assess for deleterious effects or interactions. St John's wort has been widely used in Europe. A recent meta-analysis found it to be more effective than placebo and of similar effectiveness to low-dose TCAs in the short-term treatment of mild depression.

However, a recent study comparing treatment with an SSRI versus St John's wort found that St John's wort was less effective in treating major depression. Gastrointestinal effects, including nausea, pain, loss of appetite, and diarrhoea occurred at a rate of 0.55 per cent in a German study of 3250 patients taking 300 mg three times a day. It may cause a sunburn-like reaction, mucosal inflammation, pruritis, and can lead to significant depression of the blood level of ciclosporin in organ transplant recipients, even leading to rejection.

Special issues in pregnancy

Mild postpartum 'blues' occur in 30 to 75 per cent of women immediately after delivery. Symptoms include labile mood, tearfulness, irritability, anxiety, and sleep and appetite disturbances lasting 4 to 10 days. If physical symptoms and depressed mood persist for 2 weeks, patients should be evaluated for postpartum major depression, which is relatively common, having a prevalence rate of approximately 10 per cent. Symptoms usually begin during the third trimester. A history of depression, limited social support, marital conflict, and ambivalence about the pregnancy increase the risk of depression during pregnancy and in the postpartum period.

Pharmacotherapy for depression during pregnancy requires an assessment of the risks and benefits of treatment for both mother and fetus. The risks of not treating depression may include suicide, poor maternal and fetal nutrition, an obstetric complication, and the continuation of depression into the postpartum period, with effects on mother and child bonding. Psychotherapy can be helpful in resolving interpersonal and psychosocial conflicts without exposing the mother or fetus to medications. Although psychotherapy is the first-line treatment for mild to moderate depression during pregnancy or after the birth of a child, antidepressant treatment may be warranted in severe major depression.

SSRIs are considered the first-line pharmacotherapy for depression during pregnancy. The Fluoxetine Pregnancy Database, based on 1103 prospectively reported pregnancies, reported rates of fetal malformation and spontaneous abortion similar to rates in pregnancies not exposed to fluoxetine. A prospective, controlled multicentre study to assess fetal safety and risks of the SSRIs (fluvoxamine, paroxetine, and sertraline) found that exposure to SSRIs was not associated with an increased risk for major malformations or higher rates of miscarriage, stillbirth, or prematurity. There do not appear to be adverse effects on global intelligence quotient, or language or behavioural development in preschool children exposed *in utero* to either tricyclic antidepressants or fluoxetine.

Data regarding the excretion of antidepressants in breast milk are limited. The American Academy of Pediatrics Committee on Drugs concluded: 'antidepressants are drugs whose effect on nursing infants is unknown but may be of concern'. Several studies have shown only small amounts of SSRIs in breast milk and infant serum samples. Children have been followed through their enrolment in kindergarten with no evidence of negative effects on global intelligence, language, or behaviour.

Monitoring

Regular visits are essential for patients with depression and anxiety. Brief visits every 2 weeks are usually indicated during the first 6 weeks of treatment to evaluate the dosage and side-effects of medications, and any changes in the patient's condition. With appropriate counselling beforehand and a regular discussion of side-effects, patients are more likely to adhere to a full medication trial, and this can also be encouraged by telephone monitoring. The physician should record the main symptoms that the patient presents at the beginning of treatment, and review these at each follow-up visit. After they have been on a therapeutic dose of medication for 4 weeks, the treatment response should be evaluated. Simply asking the patient to note the degree of progress on a scale of 1 to 5 can be helpful in assessing either an improvement or worsening of the target symptoms. Empirically validated, self-rating scales, such as the Patient Health Questionnaire, administered at initial diagnosis and at follow-up, can be useful in assessing treatment response. A 25 per cent or greater reduction in baseline symptoms constitutes a reasonable basis for extending the initial treatment. If there has been no response or only a partial response in symptoms, the dose of the medication should be increased to the upper therapeutic range.

Some two-thirds of patients with major depression respond to an antidepressant within 3 weeks after reaching a therapeutic plasma level. This success rate can be increased to 90 per cent by switching initial non-responders to another class of antidepressant, or by augmentation strategies using additional medication or psychotherapy. However, if a patient fails to improve adequately with first-line therapy, the diagnosis and the treatment plan must be reassessed. There may be unrecognized comorbid anxiety or substance abuse, and treatment failure is commonly due to inadequate dosing or lack of adherence to medication.

Once the patient is stabilized on a medication (usually 6–12 weeks), monthly visits are important for support. If chronic prophylactic treatment is necessary, visits every 3 months are usually appropriate. Consensus statements recommend a treatment period of between 6 and 9 months for a major depressive episode. Pharmacotherapy should be discontinued slowly over a period of 7 to 21 days. If tapered too quickly, almost all antidepressants (except fluoxetine) can produce withdrawal syndromes that include sleep disturbance, mood changes, anxiety, sensory disturbance, malaise, muscle aches, vertigo, sweating, fatigue, and gastrointestinal upset.

Patients who have remitted during the acute phase of pharmacotherapy for anxiety and depressive disorders remain at substantial risk of relapse during the subsequent 12 months: 37.1 per cent of depressed primary care patients experience further depressive symptoms during this time. There are three main risk factors are associated with relapse: (1) persistence of subthreshold depressive symptoms 7 months after the initiation of antidepressant therapy; (2) history of three or more previous episodes of major depression; and (3) chronic mood symptoms for more than 2 years. Patients with two of these risk factors are approximately three times more likely to relapse than those without. Between 50 and 60 per cent of patients who have had a single major depressive episode will have a second one; 70 per cent of those who have two episodes will have a third; and 90 per cent of those who have had three episodes will have a fourth. For patients with three or more depressive episodes or dysthymia and major depression, the AHCPR guidelines recommend treatment for 2 years or more.

The optimal duration of treatment for anxiety disorders has not been as well established by controlled studies. Treatment is recommended for 6 to 9 months after the first episode. Maintenance therapy should be considered for those with either a chronic history since adolescence, or three or more recurrences. Panic disorder is a recurrent or chronic disease in the majority of cases. In a review of 16 studies, most patients had improvement in symptoms with treatment, but few experienced complete resolution. As panic disorder progresses, attacks become more frequent, and are preceded by anticipatory anxiety. Patients may begin to associate environmental events with anxiety, leading to avoidance behaviour. The disorder may culminate in agoraphobia: being afraid to leave the house because of the association with panic attacks.

Electroconvulsive therapy (ECT)

ECT is still the most effective treatment available for the treatment of depression: it can be life-saving in some cases, and in the frail elderly it may be safer than antidepressants. Some reversible short-term memory loss is a common side-effect, but this reverts to normal in almost all cases. Patients with recurrent depression who receive effective ECT treatment should be treated with prophylactic medication or maintenance ECT once the acute course of the treatment has finished.

Psychotherapy

Randomized controlled trials support the efficacy of psychosocial interventions provided to ambulatory medical patients with psychiatric disorders. Problem-solving skills and other behavioural techniques, most of which can be provided as simple self-help materials, are part of the psychosocial support that general physicians can provide in a disease management programme for depressive or anxiety disorders. As in all chronic illnesses, lifestyle changes should be reinforced: good sleep habits, adequate exercise, and minimization of caffeine and alcohol intake.

There are three short-term psychotherapies used to specifically target the symptoms of major depression: cognitive–behavioural therapy (**CBT**), interpersonal psychotherapy (**IPT**), and problem-solving therapy (**PST**). CBT is directed at the negative and distorted thinking patterns and subsequent maladaptive behaviours that often accompany depressive episodes. IPT helps the patient learn to manage the current interpersonal relationship difficulties that are sometimes related to the development and maintenance of depressive symptoms. PST helps activate patients to break down global problems to smaller units that they can begin to attempt to solve.

Patients with major depression treated with CBT and IPT experience as much relief from symptoms by 16 weeks and those with PST by 11 weeks as those taking medication alone. Given these findings, physicians need not rely as heavily on drug treatments as they typically have, and should consider psychosocial interventions if the patient prefers them and they are available.

In a meta-analysis of studies on panic disorder, psychological coping strategies involving relaxation training, cognitive restructuring, and exposure worked comparably with both antidepressant and benzodiazepine medications. The combined somatic exposure and cognitive therapy used by Barlow and Clark helps patients confront and alter maladaptive cognitions (for example, thoughts of a heart attack or stroke when experiencing a rapid heartbeat). A meta-analysis of the treatment of generalized anxiety disorder concluded that CBT is more efficacious than control treatments and at least equal in efficacy to anxiolytics.

Specialty referral

Referral to a psychiatrist should be considered when the physician is confused about the primary diagnosis, as in distinguishing an anxiety disorder from depression with anxiety or substance abuse disorder. Referrals should also be made when adequate treatment does not lead to an improvement in symptoms within 10 to 12 weeks, or several medication trials have failed. Patients with suicidal behaviour require specialty care (see Chapter 26.5.2).

Other disorders

Generalized anxiety disorder is characterized by constant, non-episodic anxiety that affects the patient for more than 6 months and interferes with normal function. In community samples, lifetime prevalence rates are 5.1 per cent. Medical problems such as hyperthyroidism should be ruled out as the cause of the symptoms of motor tension and autonomic hyperactivity. This disorder can be treated effectively with SSRIs, TCAs, buspirone, and benzodiazepines; the first three classes should be tried first, given their lower potential for habituation and dependence.

Post-traumatic stress disorder (**PTSD**) is a syndrome that can occur after a person experiences trauma outside the range of normal human experience (accidents, abuse, rape, and natural disasters). The lifetime prevalence in the general population is between 1 and 9 per cent. The most frequent traumas in civilian cases involve adult domestic violence and childhood abuse. Symptoms include flashbacks, nightmares, and/or severe distress (or numbness) to stimuli that concretely or symbolically resemble the event—or to many stimuli (generalization), hypervigilance, or other persisting signs and symptoms of autonomic arousal, and secondary depression. Cases of PTSD are occasionally seen in primary care or by general physicians, with these patients often having a combination of symptoms of PTSD, panic, major depression, and an increased risk of alcohol and drug abuse. The alcohol and drugs are often taken to try to blunt excessive anxiety symptoms. Treatment of PTSD usually includes medication and psychotherapy, recent trials showed SSRIs to be more effective than placebo.

Specific phobias are characterized by episodic anxiety in response to a specific precipitant: intense excessive fear makes patients avoid the situation. Examples of stimuli for simple phobias are airplanes, heights, and insects, although most patients with simple phobias do not seek care for the condition. Social phobia is the fear of humiliation or failure in public situations (such as public speaking, meeting strangers, and eating in restaurants), and many with this condition also have major depression (58.3 per cent of cases of social phobia), or other anxiety disorders in (panic disorder, 27.8 per cent; generalized anxiety disorder, 30.6 per cent). Since social phobia is often present from childhood or adolescence, patients often consider the marked social anxiety and avoidance as part of their personality. Recent studies have shown that SSRIs are more effective than placebo in the treatment of social phobia; effective cognitive–behavioural techniques have also been developed. Propranolol (10–80 mg) may be useful for treating non-generalized social phobia that occurs in one situation, such as public speaking.

Obsessive–compulsive disorder (**OCD**) is characterized by regular intrusive thoughts or obsessions about aggression, sex, religion, theft, or loss—or other covering mental rituals such as counting objects or letters. Patients may also have persistent rituals or compulsions that are so frequent or complex that they interfere with normal function. They experience these obsessions and compulsions as intrusive, silly, and upsetting. Most patients with OCD have experienced major depressive episodes. Pharmacological treatment is indicated: although clomipramine had been the first-line treatment for many years, recent randomized controlled trials have shown SSRIs to be as effective. Treatment with SSRIs should continue for at least 10 weeks before it is considered ineffective. Randomized trials have shown behavioural treatments to be effective; these focus on exposure to feared activities and prevention of compulsive responses.

Conclusions

The healthcare problems of depression and anxiety are as common, and as treatable, as asthma and hypertension. If a patient does not improve with initial management, he or she should be referred to a mental health specialist. Routine follow-up is essential: these disorders follow a relapsing and remitting course in 70 to 80 per cent of patients, and become chronic disorders in up to 20 per cent. Lifelong monitoring of symptoms with the patient and his or her family is required.

Further reading

Ballenger JC, *et al.* (1998). Consensus statement on panic disorder from the International Consensus Group on Depression and Anxiety. *Journal of Clinical Psychiatry* **59**(Suppl. 8), 47–54.

Ballenger JC, *et al.* (1999). Consensus statement on the primary care management of depression from the International Consensus Group on Depression and Anxiety. *Journal of Clinical Psychiatry* **60**(Suppl. 7), 54–61.

Brown C, Schulberg HC (1995). The efficacy of psychosocial treatments in primary care: a review of randomized clinical trials. *General Hospital Psychiatry* **17**, 414–24.

Clinical Practice Guideline Number 5 (1993). Treatment of major depression. *Depression in primary care*, Vol. 2, AHCPR publication 93–0551. US Dept Health Human Services, Agency for Health Care Policy and Research, Rockville MD.

Clum G, Surls R (1993). A meta-analysis of treatments for panic disorder. *Journal of Consulting and Clinical Psychology* **61**, 317–26.

Edlund MJ (1990). The economics of anxiety. *Psychiatry in Medicine* **8**(2), 15–26.

Katerndahl DA, Realini JP (1995). Where do panic attack sufferers seek care? *Journal of Family Practice* **40**, 237–43.

Katon W, *et al.* (1990). Distressed high utilizers of medical care: DSM-III diagnoses and treatment needs. *General Hospital Psychiatry* **12**, 355–62.

Katon W, *et al.* (1992). Adequacy and duration of antidepressant treatment in primary care. *Medical Care* **30**, 67–76.

Kessler RC, *et al.* (1994). Lifetime and 12-month prevalence of DSM-IIIR psychiatric disorders in the United States: results of the National Comorbidity Survey. *Archives of General Psychiatry* **51**, 8–19.

Kim HL, *et al.* St. John's wort for depression: a meta-analysis of well-defined clinical trials. *Journal of Nervous and Mental Disease* **187**(9), 532–8.

Kulin NA, *et al.* (1998). Pregnancy outcome following maternal use of new selective serotonin reuptake inhibitors: a prospective controlled multi-center study. *Journal of the American Medical Association* **279**, 609–10.

Lin EH, *et al.* (1998). Relapse of depression in primary care: rate and clinical predictors. *Archives of Family Medicine* **7**, 443–9.

Mynors-Wallis LM, *et al.* (1995). Randomized controlled trial comparing problem solving treatment with amitriptyline and placebo for major depression in primary care. *British Medical Journal* **310**, 441–5.

Ormel J, *et al.* (1994). Common mental disorders and disability across cultures: results from the WHO Collaborative Study on Psychological Problems in General Health Care. *Journal of the American Medical Association* **272**, 1741–8.

Roy-Byrne P, *et al.* (1998). Pharmacotherapy of panic disorder: proposed guidelines for the family physician. *Journal of the American Board of Family Practice* **11**(4), 282–90.

Schulberg HC, Katon W (1998). Treating major depression in primary care practice: an update of Agency for Health Care Policy and Research Practice Guidelines. *Archives of General Psychiatry* **55**(12), 1121–7.

Simon GE, vonKorff M, Barlow W (1995). Health care costs of primary care patients with recognized depression. *Archives of General Psychiatry* **52**, 850–6.

Spitzer RL, *et al.* (1995). Health-related quality of life in primary care patients with mental disorders: results from the PRIME-MD 1000 study. *Journal of the American Medical Association* **274**, 1511–17.

Stein MB, *et al.* (1999). Social phobia in the primary care medical setting. *Journal of Family Practice* **48**(7), 514–19.

Wells KB, *et al.* (1989). The functioning and well-being of depressed patients: results from the Medical Outcomes Study. *Journal of the American Medical Association* **262**, 914–19.

26.5.5 Eating disorders

Christopher G. Fairburn

Introduction

The term 'eating disorder' refers to a persistent and severe disturbance of eating habits which results in impaired physical health or psychosocial functioning. The disturbance should not be secondary to any general medical disorder or to any other psychiatric condition. Anorexia nervosa and bulimia nervosa are the best characterized of the eating disorders. Anorexia nervosa has been recognized for many years, with physicians in the 19th century providing particularly good accounts of the disorder. By contrast, bulimia nervosa was first described in 1979. Anorexia nervosa and bulimia nervosa are closely related, in that they have many features in common and some patients move from one disorder to the other. Other eating disorders are encountered, most of which appear to be variants of anorexia nervosa or bulimia nervosa. These disorders are classified as 'atypical eating disorders'.

Eating disorders should not be confused with obesity—a general medical condition in which there is excess body fat (see Chapter 10.5). Eating disorders may coexist with obesity, although in practice most people with an eating disorder have a normal or low body weight.

Anorexia nervosa and bulimia nervosa

Definition of anorexia nervosa

To make a diagnosis of anorexia nervosa, three features need to be present:

1. *A characteristic set of attitudes to shape and weight in which self-worth is judged largely, or even exclusively, in terms of shape and weight*—Whereas most people evaluate themselves on the basis of their perceived performance in a variety of domains (such as their relationships, work, sport, artistic ability, etc.), in anorexia nervosa shape and weight dominate self-evaluation. This overevaluation of shape and weight may be regarded as the core psychopathology of the disorder since most other features appear to be secondary to it.
2. *The active maintenance of an unduly low body weight*—This is the principal behavioural expression of the extreme concerns about shape and weight. For diagnostic purposes, an 'unduly low body weight' may be defined as a weight at least 15 per cent below that expected for the person's age, height, and sex, or as a body mass index below 17.5.
3. *Amenorrhoea* (in postmenarchal females who are not taking an oral contraceptive)—Although required for official diagnostic purposes, the symptom of amenorrhoea has little discriminatory value. A clinical diagnosis of anorexia nervosa may be made in its absence.

Definition of bulimia nervosa

Bulimia nervosa also has three necessary diagnostic features:

1. *The same core psychopathology as that seen in anorexia nervosa, with self-worth being judged in terms of shape and weight.*
2. *Repeated episodes of uncontrolled overeating*—These bulimic episodes (commonly referred to as 'binges') involve the consumption of unusually large amounts of food, given the circumstances, and a sense of loss of control at the time. It is this latter feature that distinguishes binge-eating from simple overeating.
3. *The regular practice of extreme weight-control behaviour*—People with bulimia nervosa diet intensely, they may overexercise, and many engage in self-induced vomiting and the misuse of laxatives or diuretics. This behaviour is an expression of their extreme concerns about shape and weight, although it is further encouraged by the episodes of loss of control over eating.

It should be noted that there is no weight criterion for bulimia nervosa. In practice, body weight is generally unremarkable. This is because the overeating and weight-control behaviour tend to cancel each other out. There are some patients with anorexia nervosa who have binges like those seen in patients with bulimia nervosa, and who could therefore be eligible for both diagnoses. In practice, both diagnoses are not given: instead, the convention is that the diagnosis of anorexia nervosa takes precedence over that of bulimia nervosa.

Epidemiology

Anorexia nervosa is largely confined to females aged between 10 and 30 years and to Western societies. Estimates of the incidence of the disorder range from 0.10 to 8.2 per l00 000 population per annum, the higher figure being likely to be the more accurate. Estimates of its prevalence amongst adolescent girls, the group most at risk, range from 0.2 per cent to 0.8 per cent. The disorder is uncommon among men with about 10 per cent of patients being male. The social class distribution seems to be uneven with an over-representation of cases from upper socioeconomic groups, but the extent to which this is a result of referral bias is not known. It has been suggested that the disorder has become more common over recent decades, but other explanations for the apparent increase cannot be ruled out. These include alterations in diagnostic practice, better detection, increased help-seeking, and changes in the demographic structure of the population. Irrespective of whether the incidence has increased, anorexia nervosa is a major cause for concern. The disorder has one of the highest mortality rates of any psychiatric illness and it can be extremely difficult to treat.

Bulimia nervosa affects a slightly older age group than anorexia nervosa, with most cases being in their twenties. It also appears to have a broader social class distribution. The disorder is considerably more common than anorexia nervosa, the prevalence rate among young women (15 to 40 years) being between 1 per cent and 2 per cent, most of whom are not in treatment. Whilst there are no satisfactory data on the incidence of bulimia nervosa, it seems that the disorder has become much more common since the early 1970s. From being viewed as an unusual variant of anorexia nervosa, bulimia nervosa is now the most common eating disorder seen in clinical practice. It rarely occurs among men and, like anorexia nervosa, it appears to be largely confined to Western societies.

General clinical features

Anorexia nervosa

In anorexia nervosa the overevaluation of shape and weight results in a pursuit of weight loss and thinness. To the extent that this is successful, the disorder is 'egosyntonic'; that is, it is not viewed by the person as a problem—indeed, it has been noted that patients view it more as an achievement than as an affliction. As a consequence, there is little motivation to change or seek help.

The low weight is primarily the result of the strict and self-imposed restriction of food intake. Typically, the range of foods eaten is limited with those foods viewed as fattening being avoided. Except in long-standing cases, appetite persists and for this reason the term 'anorexia' is misleading. Restlessness and frequent intense exercising are common, and contribute to the low weight. Self-induced vomiting and the misuse of laxative and diuretics are practised by a subgroup, and some have occasional binges.

Driving the disturbed eating habits is the so-called 'body image disturbance'. This has several aspects. There is the core psychopathology, already mentioned, in which self-worth is judged largely in terms of shape and weight. In addition, there is sometimes a perceptual component involving overestimation of body size. This may be a consequence of the patients' frequent checking of their own body, and in some this becomes so distressing that it is abandoned, although the concerns about shape and weight persist. In almost every case there is preoccupation with thoughts about food, eating, shape, and weight, which may be expressed as an avid interest in cooking, nutrition, fitness, and health.

Depression, anxiety, irritability, lability of mood, and obsessional features are all common concomitants of anorexia nervosa. Typically, they get worse as weight is lost and improve with weight regain. Outside interests also decline and there may be marked social withdrawal. Suicidal thoughts may be present and the risk of suicide should always be kept in mind when assessing patients.

Bulimia nervosa

The clinical features of bulimia nervosa are similar to those of anorexia nervosa. There is the same over-evaluation of shape and weight, and this also leads to body checking and extreme methods of weight control. The main differences lie in the frequent bulimic episodes and the fact that body weight is generally unremarkable. The other important difference is that, as a consequence of the loss of control over eating, the disorder is 'egodystonic'; that is, it is viewed by the patient as a problem. This makes treatment much easier.

The binges involve the consumption of sizeable amounts on food (typically over 2000 kcal per episode) and they are a source of distress and shame. Typically, they are kept secret. In most cases, they are followed by self-induced vomiting or the taking of laxatives or diuretics, although there is a subgroup of patients who do not 'purge'. Between the binges, food intake is severely restricted. Depressive and anxiety symptoms are prominent in bulimia nervosa, more so than in anorexia nervosa, and some patients have problems with alcohol or drug misuse.

Physical and laboratory features

The physical abnormalities seen in anorexia nervosa have been the subject of much interest. They used to be viewed as evidence of a primary pituitary or hypothalamic disorder, but it is now thought that they are secondary to the disturbed eating habits and the patient's state of starvation. The physical abnormalities encountered in bulimia nervosa resemble those seen in anorexia nervosa except that they are less severe.

Symptoms and signs in anorexia nervosa

Many patients with anorexia nervosa have no physical complaints. However, systematic enquiry often reveals a heightened sensitivity to the cold and a variety of gastrointestinal symptoms such as constipation, fullness after eating, bloatedness, and vague abdominal pains. Other symptoms include restlessness, low sexual appetite, and poor sleep with early morning wakening. In females who are not taking an oral contraceptive, amenorrhoea is, by definition, present. Occasional patients complain of infertility.

On examination, the degree of emaciation may be striking. Growth may be stunted in those with a prepubertal onset and there may be failure of breast development. Unlike patients with hypopituitarism, axillary and pubic hair are preserved and there is no breast atrophy. A fine downy hair (lanugo) is commonly present on the back, arms, and side of the face. Typically, the skin is dry and the hands and feet are cold. There may be hypothermia. Blood pressure and pulse are low and some patients have dependent oedema.

Abnormalities on investigation in anorexia nervosa

Endocrine abnormalities

Many of the abnormalities encountered have been reproduced in studies of the physiological effects of dieting and starvation, and are reversed by the restoration of healthy eating habits and a normal weight. Luteinizing hormone-releasing hormone (**LHRH**) secretion is impaired and, as a result, levels of luteinizing hormone (**LH**), follicle-stimulating hormone (**FSH**), and oestradiol are low. There is an immature pattern of LH release. The LH response to LHRH is reduced, but the FSH response is normal or exaggerated.

Hypothalamic disturbance is also evident in a delayed thyroid-stimulating hormone (**TSH**) response to thyrotropin-releasing hormone (**TRH**). In addition, there is reduced peripheral conversion of thyroxine (T4) to triiodothyronine (T3), and an increased conversion of T4 to inactive reverse T3. These changes are seen in other chronic illnesses. T4 levels are in the low-normal range, whereas T3 levels are depressed. Clinical evidence of hypothyroidism includes sensitivity to cold, constipation, dry skin, and bradycardia.

Plasma cortisol levels are raised and the normal diurnal variation is lost. These changes are due in part to the increased half-life of cortisol seen in starvation, and in part to a relative increase in cortisol production. Growth-hormone levels are also increased, another secondary effect of starvation. Prolactin secretion is normal. Leptin levels are low.

Haematological changes

A normocytic normochromic anaemia is found in a minority of patients and is sometimes attributable to a low intake of iron or folate. Mild neutropenia is common. The erythrocyte sedimentation rate (**ESR**) is generally low.

Other metabolic abnormalities

Hypercholesterolaemia is frequently present. The mechanism is not understood. Increased serum beta-carotene may also be found and reflects increased dietary intake. Life-threatening hypoglycaemia very occasionally occurs, but may not present typically due to impaired sympathetic response. Dehydration is not uncommon, and electrolyte disturbance is found in those who vomit frequently or misuse large quantities of laxatives or diuretics.

Other abnormalities

Brain imaging studies have revealed enlargement of the cortical sulci and cisternes and dilatation of the ventricles. This appears to be reversible and has been termed 'pseudoatrophy'.

There is delayed gastric emptying and a prolonged gastrointestinal transit time. This may account for the common complaints of fullness after eating, bloatedness, and constipation. Acute gastric dilatation is a rare complication which can be provoked by episodes of extreme overeating or attempts at refeeding that are too vigorous.

In more long-standing cases bone mineral density is reduced, probably as a result of oestrogen deficiency and low weight. There is a heightened risk of fractures, particularly of the lumbar vertebrae. The bone loss appears to reverse with weight regain and the resumption of regular menstruation.

Symptoms and signs in bulimia nervosa

There are few physical complaints in bulimia nervosa. Those most commonly encountered are irregular or absent menstruation, weakness and lethargy, vague abdominal pains, and toothache. On examination, appearance is usually unremarkable. Salivary gland enlargement may be present: typically, this involves the parotids and gives the patient's face a slightly rounded appearance. Sometimes it is associated with a raised serum amylase level, the increase being in the salivary isoenzyme. The underlying pathophysiology is not understood. In those who vomit there may be calluses on the dorsum of the dominant hand (Russell's sign) due to the fingers being used to stimulate the gag reflex. Also, there may be significant erosion of the dental enamel particularly on the lingual surface of the upper front teeth. A minority of patients, particularly those who take large quantities of laxatives or diuretics, have intermittent peripheral or facial oedema.

Abnormalities on investigation in bulimia nervosa

Of most importance is the electrolyte disturbance which is encountered in about half of those who vomit or take laxatives or diuretics. Metabolic alkalosis, hypochloraemia, and hypokalaemia are the most common abnormalities and may account for the weakness and tiredness (and in rare instances hypokalaemic paralysis) experienced by some patients. The overall picture may resemble Bartter's syndrome. Severe electrolyte disturbance is occasionally encountered, particularly low potassium levels, but even when it is long-standing there may be surprisingly few accompanying symptoms. Despite concern about possible cardiac arrhythmias, nephrogenic diabetes insipidus, and the suggestion that chronic hypokalaemia may induce changes in the renal proximal tubular cells, aggressive treatment of this type of chronic electrolyte disturbance is rarely appropriate: instead, it should be monitored while treatment is focused on the eating disorder itself.

Endocrine abnormalities are also encountered in bulimia nervosa. They resemble those seen in anorexia nervosa, but are not as severe. They are thought to be secondary to the strict dieting and are probably reversible, given that the menstrual disturbance responds to the correction of the eating disorder.

Aetiology

It is generally accepted that anorexia nervosa and bulimia nervosa are the result of a complex interplay of physiological, psychological, and social processes. These have different influences at different stages in the development and subsequent course of the disorder. The understanding of the exact nature of these processes is limited, although there is increasing convergence between the findings of biological and psychosocial studies.

Development of anorexia nervosa and bulimia nervosa

Anorexia nervosa generally starts in mid-adolescence with a period of voluntary dietary restriction that proceeds to get out of control. Whereas everyday adolescent dieting is neither persistent nor extreme, in anorexia nervosa it becomes unremitting and intense. As a result body weight falls and a state of semi-starvation eventually develops. Concerns about shape and weight may pre-date the onset of the dieting or develop as weight is lost.

Bulimia nervosa starts in a similar way, although the age of onset is typically some years later. There is dietary restriction and it too leads to weight loss (sufficient to result in a period of anorexia nervosa in about 25 per cent of cases), but instead of dietary control being maintained, it becomes punctuated by episodes of binge-eating. This breakdown in control generally occurs within 2 years of onset. At first the episodes of overeating may be both modest in size and intermittent, but gradually they become larger and more frequent. As a result, the lost weight is regained and body weight returns to about the level at which the dieting first began. By this point the disorder tends to be self-perpetuating. At some stage in this sequence of events self-induced vomiting or laxative misuse may be adopted to compensate for the episodes of overeating. In practice they have the opposite effect, because these patients' belief in their effectiveness at preventing energy absorption undermines their attempts to control their eating.

Risk factors and processes

Epidemiological studies have implicated a variety of risk factors in the development of anorexia nervosa. These may be divided into four classes:

1. Being female, adolescent, and living in a Western society. These individuals are under social pressure to diet.
2. Being exposed to a microenvironment that further encourages dieting. This includes being brought up in a family in which there is intense interest in shape, weight, or eating, sometimes as a result of one or more family members having a frank eating disorder. Social or occupational pressures to diet are another example.
3. Being exposed to factors that increase the risk of psychiatric disturbance in general and depression in particular. These include a family history of psychiatric disorder, especially depression, and exposure to adverse childhood experiences such as parenting deficits and sexual and physical abuse.
4. The presence of the psychological traits of perfectionism, inflexibility, and low self-esteem.

A similar set of risk factors has been implicated in bulimia nervosa, although it seems that there is more exposure to social factors that encourage dieting. For example, there are strikingly raised rates of parental and childhood obesity (antedating the eating disorder), both of which are likely to sensitize individuals to their appearance and weight, and thereby make them prone to diet. The risk factors for psychiatric disturbance are also prominent, whereas the traits of perfectionism and inflexibility are less pronounced. One additional class of risk factor is parental substance abuse. How this might operate is not clear, although it does seem that those who develop bulimia nervosa are prone to mood fluctuations and that some may learn to modulate them by consuming large quantities of food, alcohol, or psychoactive drugs.

An important question is why people with bulimia nervosa have repeated episodes of loss of control over eating, whereas those with anorexia nervosa do not. Several factors appear to be relevant. First, the traits of perfectionism and inflexibility are less prominent, which may result in the person being less able to maintain strict self-control. Second, the mood fluctuations may interfere with dietary restraint. Third, the vulnerability to obesity, and perhaps therefore overeating, may also be relevant.

Genetic factors and neurobiological mechanisms

Family-genetic studies have demonstrated that eating disorders run in families, with familial aggregation being particularly evident in anorexia nervosa. The relative extent of genetic and environmental contributions is unclear: the findings of the few twin studies have been inconsistent and there have been no adoption studies.

The nature of any inherited vulnerability is not known. The liability appears not to be shared with that for other psychiatric disorders. However, there is some evidence of shared familial transmission between the various eating disorders, and between anorexia nervosa and 'obsessive–compulsive personality disorder', a personality construct that overlaps with certain of the traits mentioned earlier. Thus anorexia nervosa and obsessive–compulsive personality disorder may be common phenotypic expressions of a similar genotype. Clearly there may also be genetically determined abnormalities in the regulation of weight and eating habits.

Attempts to identify susceptibility genes have focused on those implicated in serotonin (5-hydroxytryptamine, **5-HT**) neurotransmission. This transmitter is of particular interest for a number of reasons: (1) it is known to have an important role in the control of both eating and mood; (2) there is some evidence of trait-related abnormalities in brain 5-HT function in both anorexia nervosa and bulimia nervosa; and (3) it has been found that dieting influences brain 5-HT function in women. There is some evidence, albeit inconsistent, that anorexia nervosa is associated with a polymorphism of the 5-HT_{2A} receptor.

Maintaining factors and processes

Several processes maintain the dietary restriction that is central to anorexia nervosa. One is the potent and strongly reinforcing sense of self-control that these people get from restricting their eating. Another is the resulting weight loss, given the overevaluation of shape and weight. A third is the effect on others of refusing to eat, which can be of special significance when there are dysfunctional relationships. A fourth is secondary to certain aspects of the starvation state. For example, the social withdrawal and preoccupation with food and eating both narrow the focus of the person's interests, and the delayed gastric emptying produces feelings of fullness even after eating modest amounts of food.

In bulimia nervosa similar maintaining processes operate. For example, the periods of successful dietary control are strongly reinforcing, as is the initial weight loss. However, there are also important differences. First, since the disorder is usually kept secret, there may be no reinforcing effects on others. Second, since body weight is generally unremarkable, starvation-related mechanisms are less relevant. Third, the repeated binges, while being aversive and a stimulus to change, strongly encourage further dieting as they undermine the sense of being in control and magnify fears of weight gain.

Treatment

Patients with eating disorders vary in the severity of their presenting symptoms and in their response to treatment. Some have a brief period of disturbance which spontaneously remits and does not recur; in others treatment is needed, but there is full and lasting recovery; while in others the disorder persists and may prove intractable.

The treatment of bulimia nervosa has been the subject of numerous randomized controlled trials. The most effective treatment is a specific form of cognitive–behaviour therapy. This is a psychological treatment which directly addresses both the disturbed eating habits and the abnormal attitudes to shape and weight. It involves about 20 sessions over 5 months and generally results in substantial improvement, with about half the patients making a complete and lasting recovery. Antidepressant drugs are the only pharmacological treatment to have shown promise. They result in a decline in the frequency of binge-eating and associated compensatory behaviour, and an improvement in mood, but their effect is not as great as that obtained with cognitive–behaviour therapy and, more importantly, it is often not maintained. Some patients respond to simple and brief forms of cognitive–behaviour therapy. These may be implemented in primary care. Indeed, a 'stepped care' management strategy has been advocated in which a simple treatment (such as cognitive–behavioural self-help) is used first, with more intensive and specialized treatments (such as full cognitive–behaviour therapy) being reserved for those who do not respond.

There has been relatively little research on the treatment of anorexia nervosa. This is for a number of reasons, including the low prevalence of the disorder and the fact that treatment may take a year or more. Another barrier to research and, indeed treatment, is the egosyntonic character of the disorder.

In principle, there are three aspects to the management of anorexia nervosa. The first is persuading patients that they need help, and maintaining their motivation thereafter, which is crucial given their reluctance to change. The second is weight restoration. The third is addressing the patient's overevaluation of shape and weight, eating habits, and general psychosocial functioning.

Weight restoration is needed to reverse the effects of starvation and of itself usually leads to substantial improvement in the patient's physical and psychological state. Weight restoration may be achieved on an outpatient, day-patient, or inpatient basis. Indications for hospital admission include risk of suicide, adverse home circumstances, and failure of outpatient treatment. Physical indications include a body mass index below 13.5, rapid weight loss, and the presence of medical complications such as marked oedema, severe electrolyte disturbance, hypoglycaemia, or significant intercurrent infection. Under such circumstances admission should be to a general medical ward or a psychiatric unit with good access to general medical help. Weight restoration may be achieved in either setting, but it is a great advantage if the staff are experienced in the management of patients with anorexia nervosa, and in a psychiatric unit it is generally easier to arrange the other aspects of treatment. Inpatient care should always be regarded as a preliminary to outpatient treatment.

There is no single way of addressing overevaluation of shape and weight, eating habits, and general psychosocial functioning. Leading approaches include various forms of family therapy, primarily for younger patients, and adaptations of cognitive–behaviour therapy. Training is needed to deliver these treatments, and they are best conducted on an outpatient basis.

Drug treatment has almost no role, although occasionally it is appropriate to use drugs to stimulate the resumption of regular menstruation, so long as body weight has reached a reasonable level and the patient is eating healthily.

Prognosis

Whilst at least half of those with anorexia nervosa recover in terms of their weight and menstrual function, sensitivity about shape and weight often persists and eating habits may remain disturbed. Up to one-quarter develop bulimia nervosa. The standardized mortality ratio is significantly raised, deaths being either a direct result of medical complications or due to suicide. The outcome in males appears to be similar to that in females. Few consistent predictors of outcome have been identified, exceptions being a long history and late onset, both of which are associated with a worse prognosis.

The outcome in bulimia nervosa is also varied, although it is substantially improved by cognitive–behaviour therapy. The mortality rate does not appear to be raised. No consistent predictors of outcome have been identified. Both anorexia nervosa and bulimia nervosa 'breed true', in that they do not seem to evolve into any other disorder.

Prevention

Programmes for the primary and secondary prevention of anorexia nervosa and bulimia nervosa have been developed, but none has been satisfactorily evaluated. The primary prevention programmes tend to focus on schoolgirls, the group most at risk. However, two specific difficulties have been encountered: first, there is a danger of magnifying concerns about shape and weight rather than reducing them; and second, there is potential for conflict between the content of these programmes and those directed at the prevention of obesity.

Pregnancy and childrearing

This topic has come to the fore with the emergence of bulimia nervosa, since pregnancy does not often occur in the course of anorexia nervosa. It is now clear that eating disorders can have untoward effects. They generally improve during pregnancy, but the amount of weight gained may be abnormally low or high. The effects on the fetus have yet to be established, although there have been reports of intrauterine growth retardation and low birth weight. Childrearing is impaired in some cases with adverse effects on the child's feeding and growth.

Atypical eating disorders

More than one-third of those who present for the treatment of an eating disorder do not meet the diagnostic criteria for anorexia nervosa or bulimia nervosa. Such patients have an 'atypical eating disorder', the equivalent North American term being an 'eating disorder not otherwise specified'. These eating disorders have received little attention. Many are similar in form to anorexia nervosa or bulimia nervosa and respond similarly to treatment.

Binge-eating disorder

The one atypical eating disorder to have been delineated is termed 'binge-eating disorder'. It is characterized by recurrent binge-eating in the absence of the extreme weight-control behaviour seen in anorexia nervosa and bulimia nervosa. The binge-eating occurs against the background of a general tendency to overeat. It seems to be more an habitual response to negative mood states than an intermittent breakdown of dietary restraint as occurs in bulimia nervosa. Not surprisingly, many of these patients are overweight or obese.

Little is known about the distribution of binge-eating disorder. It appears to affect an older age group than anorexia nervosa and bulimia nervosa, and cases among men are not uncommon. About 10 per cent of those attending obesity clinics have the disorder. The treatment that shows most promise is conventional behavioural weight control. As in bulimia nervosa, cognitive–behavioural self-help programmes help a subgroup of cases. The value of drug treatment is unclear.

Further reading

Andersen AE, Bowers W, Evans K (1997). Inpatient treatment of anorexia nervosa. In: Garner DM, Garfinkel PE, eds. *Handbook of treatment for eating disorders*, pp 327–53. Guilford Press, New York.

Fairburn CG, Marcus MD, Wilson GT (1993). Cognitive-behavioral therapy for binge eating and bulimia nervosa: a comprehensive treatment manual. In: Fairburn CG, Wilson GT, eds. *Binge eating: nature, assessment and treatment*, pp 361–404. Guilford Press, New York.

Fairburn CG, Brownell KD (2002). *Eating disorders and obesity: a comprehensive handbook*, 2nd edn. Guilford Press, New York.

Garner DM, Garfinkel PE (1997). *Handbook of treatment for eating disorders*. Guilford Press, New York.

Lilenfeld LR, Kaye WH (1998). Genetic studies of anorexia and bulimia nervosa. In: Hoek HW, Treasure JL, Katzman MA, eds. *Neurobiology in the treatment of eating disorders*, pp 169–94. Wiley, Chichester.

Mitchell JE, Pomeroy C, Adson DE (1997). Managing medical complications. In: Garner DM, Garfinkel PE, eds. *Handbook of treatment for eating disorders*, pp 383–93. Guilford Press, New York.

Russell GFM, Treasure J, Eisler I (1998). Mothers with anorexia nervosa who underfeed their children: their recognition and management. *Psychological Medicine* **28**, 93–108.

Wilson GT, Fairburn CG (2002). Treatments for eating disorders. In: Nathan PE, Gorman JM, eds. *A guide to treatments that work* 2nd edn. Oxford University Press, New York.

26.5.6 Schizophrenia, bipolar disorder, obsessive–compulsive disorder, and personality disorder

S. Lawrie

Recent research, using reliable diagnostic criteria based on clinical features since diagnostic laboratory tests are not available, has established that all of these conditions have both biomedical and psychosocial components. The *Diagnostic and statistical manual of mental disorders, 4th edition* (**DSM-IV**) has been most rigorously developed and is used here.

Schizophrenia

Schizophrenia and bipolar disorder are psychoses, that is to say they include phenomena that qualitatively differ from everyday experience. Schizophrenia is characterized by delusions, hallucinations, disorganized speech/behaviour, and negative symptoms.

Onset is in early adulthood (median age 25 years). The sex incidence is equal, but women tend to be affected later than men. The incidence is only 15 in 100 000 of the population per year, but the prevalence is about 5 in 1000 due to chronicity, and the lifetime risk is 1 per cent.

Aetiology

Genetic factors account for 80 per cent of the liability to schizophrenia, but no major genes have been identified. Having an affected relative increases the risk 5 to 50 times, depending on the relationship. Other risk factors include obstetric complications, developmental problems, and cannabis use, but these only double the risk. Stressful life events can be precipitants, but only in those otherwise predisposed.

There are subtle abnormalities of brain structure and function (particularly of the temporal and frontal lobes) in both chronic and first episode cases. Developmental changes in brain structure (for example, synaptic pruning) and function (for example, dopamine sensitivity) are thought to disrupt frontotemporal integration and bring on symptoms, but direct evidence is lacking.

Clinical features

Hallucinations and delusions are 'positive symptoms', that is, abnormal by their presence. Hallucinations are perceptions in the absence of stimuli. They are usually auditory 'voices' speaking the patients' thoughts or commenting on their actions. Hallucinations in other senses can occur but suggest a neurological disorder. Delusions are unshakeable false beliefs. Persecutory ('paranoid') delusions are common but occur in all psychoses. Delusions of passivity (actions or feelings 'made' by external forces) and other bizarre beliefs are more specific. The other positive symptom is 'thought disorder'—an illogical sequence of thoughts (as revealed in speech).

'Negative symptoms' are features that are abnormal by their absence. Common symptoms include a loss of emotion ('flat affect'), apathy, self-neglect, and social withdrawal. These may be prodromal, but are more common in chronic patients, and can be confused with depression or parkinsonism.

Differential diagnosis

Prodromal symptoms can be similar to depression. Delusions of passivity can be confused with obsessional ideas, but the latter are recognized as one's own. Drug intoxication can cause positive symptoms, but also disorientation. Neurological causes, for example temporal lobe epilepsy or brain tumours, are rare. The distinction of schizophrenia from bipolar disorder is based on whether psychotic or affective features predominate. Rarely, if both are present equally, a diagnosis of schizoaffective disorder is appropriate.

Management

Acute positive symptoms generally respond well to any antipsychotic drug (Table 1). These work by dopamine-receptor blockade. The main adverse effects are sedation, weight gain, and extrapyramidal syndromes (acute dystonia, akathisia, parkinsonism, tardive dyskinesia). These are best avoided by minimizing dosage, but dystonias and parkinsonism respond to anticholinergics. Medication should be continued for at least 2 years to reduce relapse rates.

Patients often refuse medication, due to adverse effects or lack of insight. Some are suitable for depot medication (intramuscular injections of esterified antipsychotics, see Table 1). The new 'atypical' antipsychotics have fewer adverse effects, but this is primarily because they are prescribed in relatively low doses. It is claimed that they are effective in those with negative and treatment-resistant positive symptoms, but clozapine is the only proven such treatment. Clozapine is the definitive atypical antipsychotic, with relatively high serotonin:dopamine-receptor blockade, but carries a considerable risk of neutropenia and agranulocytosis. These treatments are not contraindicated in pregnancy, as they confer only a small increased risk of teratogenicity and an untreated psychosis is more dangerous.

There are few effective non-drug treatments. Cognitive therapy may reduce symptoms and improve drug compliance. Illness education reduces relapse rates, as does teaching social skills, but these may primarily work by improving drug compliance.

Primary prevention is not a realistic prospect until better understanding of the pathogenesis of schizophrenia allows early detection. There is, however, some evidence that earlier treatment with antipsychotics may be associated with a better prognosis.

Prognosis

The prognosis is generally poor. About 25 per cent of patients will only have one or two episodes, but most will suffer chronic symptoms, numerous relapses, unemployment, and social isolation. Most patients smoke heavily, and many abuse alcohol/drugs, resulting in a high premature mortality rate. Suicide is all too common, at 10 to 15 per cent over a lifetime.

Table 1 Commonly used antipsychotic drugs

Type/name of drug	Optimal dose*	Main side-effects
Phenothiazines		
Chlorpromazine	400–600 mg daily	Sedation
Thioridazine	400–600 mg daily	Anticholinergic
Trifluoperazine	20–30 mg daily	Extrapyramidal
Butyrophenones		
Haloperidol	8–12 mg daily	Extrapyramidal
Benzamides		
Sulpiride	800–1200 mg daily	Minimal
Pimozide	8–10 mg daily	Minimal
Depot injections		
Flupentixol decanoate	40 mg every 2 weeks	Extrapyramidal
Fluphenazine decanoate	25 mg every 2 weeks	Extrapyramidal
Haloperidol decanoate	100 mg monthly	Extrapyramidal
New drugs		
Risperidone	6 mg daily	Weight gain
Olanzapine	15 mg daily	Weight gain
Atypicals		
Clozapine	200–300 mg daily	Hypersalivation

* This dose of chlorpromazine is established from meta-analyses. Others are calculated as chlorpromazine equivalents, but these are uncertain for depot, new, and atypical drugs.

Bipolar disorder (BPD)

The key features of bipolar disorder ('manic depression') are episodic increases or decreases in mood, thoughts, and activity, lasting at least 1 week. The prevalence, incidence, and lifetime risk of BPD are similar to schizophrenia (at 0.5 per cent, 0.01 per cent, and 1 per cent, respectively) and the sex incidence is also equal, but the mean age at onset is 21 years in both sexes in BPD.

Aetiology

The risk factors for BPD are similar to those for schizophrenia. Genetic influences are equally strong, but other associations are weaker in BPD. There may be specific abnormalities in monoamine metabolism and neuroendocrine function in BPD, for example a first 'high' may be precipitated by antidepressants, stimulants, steroids, or childbirth.

Clinical features

If 'hypomanic', such patients feel 'high', report rapid thoughts, have limitless energy, require little sleep, and are 'disinhibited', that is they are overfamiliar and take risks. They speak quickly ('pressure of speech') and jump between topics ('flight of ideas'), but with logical connections between thoughts. If psychotic ('manic'), their delusions and hallucinations are usually 'mood congruent', for example 'grandiose delusions' of special abilities.

If depressed, their mood is low, activities are not enjoyed ('anhedonia'), interests are diminished, energy is low, sleep is disturbed, appetite is reduced, and weight may fall. Patients typically think they are worthless, the future is hopeless, and they may be suicidal. Severe 'melancholic' depression is accompanied by early morning wakening, 'diurnal mood variation' (feeling worst in the morning), and 'psychomotor retardation' (head down, expressionless face, little spontaneous activity). Any psychotic symptoms are again mood-congruent, for example delusions of sin or guilt, 'voices' criticizing the patient.

Occasionally, one encounters 'mixed states', where patients have some features of (hypo)mania and depression simultaneously.

Differential diagnosis

Some one-third of patients will have several depressive episodes before their first 'high'. With no previous history, especially if old, (hypo)mania may rarely be attributable to thyroid disease or dementia. In established cases, the main differential is schizophrenia as individual symptoms can be similar (e.g. low mood and flat affect, thought disorder, and flight of ideas) but the key is that BPD is an episodic disturbance of mood.

Management

The treatment of depression is discussed elsewhere. 'High' patients may reject treatment, but most will later report feeling out of control and gratitude for being treated. (Hypo)mania generally responds well to antipsychotic drugs (see Table 1). Lithium is also effective, particularly with high serum levels (of about 1.0 mmol/l). Carbamazepine and sodium valproate are alternative 'mood stabilizers', with fewer adverse effects, but may be less effective. Valproate is the best treatment in 'rapid cycling disorder' (four or more illness episodes annually). Acute mixed episodes are probably best treated with mood stabilizers alone.

Prophylaxis is required if patients have two or more episodes in 5 years. Lithium (maintained at 0.5–1.0 mmol/l) is the treatment of choice as it reduces both (hypo)manic and depressive relapses, and may reduce suicide rates. Common adverse effects are dose-related and include diarrhoea, tremor, thirst, polyuria, and weight gain. Long-term effects can include hypothyroidism and renal impairment. Lithium is excreted in competition with sodium, so thiazide diuretics, non-steroidal agents, and dehydration can precipitate toxicity. Sudden vomiting, coarse tremor, sedation, or dysarthria require urgent medical treatment to avoid seizures, renal failure, and death.

Lithium is contraindicated in pregnancy and breast feeding, as it increases the rate of Fallot's tetralogy 10- to 20-fold and can cause neonatal toxicity. Carbamazepine and sodium valproate are associated with spina bifida. Best practice is therefore to use antipsychotics for symptom control until after delivery. Mood stabilizers should then be reinstituted, and bottle feeding commended, as relapse is very common postnatally.

Early diagnosis and self-medication can minimize relapses in established cases, but primary prevention is not presently possible.

Prognosis

Acute episodes generally respond to treatment, but 10 per cent of patients will be ill for a year and 50 per cent of (hypo)manic patients immediately become depressed. Recurrence is the norm, and becomes more frequent with age. Many patients have chronic symptoms between episodes, such that only 25 per cent of patients fully recover. Employment and social difficulties are common. Before treatment was possible, the annual mortality from cardiovascular collapse or suicide was 10 per cent. This is now the lifetime rate of suicide.

Obsessive compulsive disorder (OCD)

OCD is characterized by recurrent, unwanted thoughts that are recognized as one's own and/or repeated acts ('rituals') to relieve tension. Originally viewed as a neurosis, DSM-IV does not use this ambiguous term and classifies OCD as an anxiety state. OCD is common, with a prevalence of 1 per cent and lifetime risk of 2 to 3 per cent. The peak prevalence is in the fourth decade, with an earlier onset and slight excess in women.

Aetiology

OCD runs in families but twin studies are inconclusive. Obsessional personality is a risk factor, as are other personality disorders, childhood conduct disorder, and Tourette's syndrome. OCD can arise after lesions of the frontal lobes and basal ganglia; regions also implicated by studies of brain structure and function in patients. Follow-up functional imaging has found recovery is associated with normalized metabolism in these areas of the brain. Effective drugs all inhibit serotonin (5-hydroxytryptamine, **5-HT**) reuptake, and neurochemical evidence also suggests postsynaptic serotoninergic hypersensitivity and/or low synaptic 5-HT concentrations.

Clinical features

Patients are commonly ill for years before they come to medical attention. Obsessions are thoughts that are recurrent, resisted, and unwanted, but regarded as one's own. The thought may be a fear of contamination, excessive doubt, a somatic concern, a desire for precision, or an aggressive or sexual impulse. Usually, several obsessions coexist. Obsessional slowness and precision are more common in men.

Compulsions are obsessional acts, based on these thoughts and usually performed as a means to reduce anxiety, that are not in themselves pleasurable. Checking, cleaning, and counting are the most common acts. Most are performed in private as they are recognized as senseless.

Differential diagnosis

Rituals and superstitions are common in childhood, but are only pathological if they cause distress. Distinguishing OCD from depression/anxiety can be difficult, as secondary depression is frequent in OCD, and thoughts in depression and anxiety can have an obsessional quality. Obsessions can also be similar to phobias, but obsessives actually seek out anxiety-provoking stimuli whereas phobics avoid them.

Management

Both drugs and psychotherapy are effective in OCD. The tricyclic antidepressant clomipramine and the 'selective' serotonin-reuptake inhibitors (**SSRIs**) work, but high doses may be required. Clomipramine is probably most effective, particularly in treating patients with comorbid depression, but has unpleasant adverse effects (sedation, weight gain, anticholinergic). Maintaining drug treatment for 1 year reduces relapse rates.

The most effective psychotherapeutic techniques are behavioural. 'Exposure' to anxiety-provoking stimuli (with or without therapist 'modelling') and 'response prevention' (avoiding rituals by persuasion, monitoring, or adopting alternative behaviours) should also involve family members. This is more effective against compulsions than obsessions. Recent trials suggest that the combination of antidepressants and exposure may be best of all.

Prognosis

Response to treatment may take months and symptoms tend to recur if drugs are stopped. About 10 per cent of cases progressively deteriorate, particularly men with an early-onset OCD. Suicide was regarded as rare in OCD but recent studies challenge this view.

Personality disorder (PD)

PD is commonly seen as distinct from psychiatric 'illness' and untreatable. It is ironic that many PDs were originally described because they had links to particular psychiatric disorders, and that recent research has rediscovered these and found possible treatments.

PD is defined as culturally abnormal experience or behaviour, with onset in early adulthood, that is pervasive and inflexible, leading to distress or impairment. Only a brief description of subtypes (Table 2) and specific points is possible here.

Aetiology

Paranoid and borderline traits are clearly heritable, and schizotypy is genetically and biologically linked to schizophrenia. Paranoid and antisocial PDs are more common in men; borderline, histrionic, and dependent PDs in women. Childhood adversity is a general risk factor but specific effects are difficult to identify. Child sexual abuse, for example, may be linked to self-harm and substance abuse rather than any particular PD. Psychopaths have mild frontal lobe deficits—and similar head trauma related changes in personality have been described.

Clinical features

Many patients meet more than one set of PD criteria. Some borderline patients report auditory and visual hallucinations. Dysthymia (formerly depressive PD) and cyclothymia (also formerly a PD) are now seen as mild depression and bipolar disorder, respectively. Paranoid, schizotypal, obsessional, and avoidant PDs may be similarly reclassified in the future.

Differential diagnosis

The main differential is with the associated psychiatric disorder and other PDs. As a rule, the eccentric cluster can present similarly to schizophrenia, the emotional cluster-like bipolar disorder, and the anxious cluster with anxiety states. Borderline PD can cause diagnostic difficulties with both schizophrenia and BPD.

Management

Clinical management has conservative aims, but pressure is being put on psychiatrists to do more. Few treatments have been evaluated for PD *per se*.

Cognitive therapy may generally reduce the frequency of deliberate self-harm. Dysthymia responds to antidepressants; paranoid, schizotypal, and borderline patients may benefit from antipsychotic drugs; and obsessional PD may respond to SSRIs.

Prognosis

Recurrent deliberate self-harm and eventual suicide is common. Patients with PDs who develop other psychiatric disorders also have a poor prognosis for that disorder.

Concluding remarks

Psychiatric disorders are common, involuntary, distressing, and disabling. Like most medical disorders, they are caused by biological, psychological, and social factors. They can be successfully treated, but are often chronic and associated with social rejection. Stigmatization remains a big problem, not least from doctors.

Further reading

Abramowitz JS (1997). Effectiveness of psychological and pharmacological treatments for obsessive–compulsive disorder: a quantitative review. *Journal of Consulting and Clinical Psychology* **65**, 44–52. [As recommended in the Cochrane Library]

Altshuler L, *et al.* (1996). Pharmacologic management of psychiatric illness during pregnancy: dilemmas and guidelines. *American Journal of Psychiatry* **153,** 592–606. [High quality systematic review]

American Psychiatric Association (1994). *The diagnostic and statistical manual of mental disorders,* 4th edition. APA, Washington DC. [Diagnostic criteria for all psychiatric disorders, with background information]

Cannon M, Jones P (1996). Epidemiology of schizophrenia. *Journal of Neurology, Neurosurgery and Psychiatry* **61,** 604–13. [Comprehensive review of the epidemiology of schizophrenia]

Daly I (1997). Mania. *Lancet* **349,** 1157–60. [Accessible review of bipolar disorder]

Frith C (1995). Schizophrenia: functional imaging and cognitive abnormalities. *Lancet* **346,** 615–20. [One of a generally excellent series of reviews about schizophrenia]

Haslam DRS, *et al.* (1997). The treatment of bipolar disorder: review of the literature, guidelines and options. *Canadian Journal of Psychiatry* **42,** Suppl. 2. [Best available synthesis of the literature on the treatment of bipolar disorder, although Cochrane reviews are in progress]

Hawton K, *et al.* (1999). Deliberate self-harm: the efficacy of psychosocial and pharmacological interventions. In: *The Cochrane Library,* Issue 3. Update software, Oxford. [Systematic review and meta-analysis of treatments for self-harm, including five personality disorder trials]

Johnson JG, *et al.* (1999). Childhood maltreatment increases risk for personality disorders during early adulthood. *Archives of General Psychiatry* **56,** 600–6. [Community-based longitudinal study of the antecedents of personality disorder]

Johnstone EC, Freeman CPL, Zealley AK, eds (1998). *Companion to psychiatric studies,* 6th edn. Churchill Livingstone, Edinburgh. [Detailed and well-referenced textbook of psychiatry]

McIntosh A, Lawrie SM (2001). Schizophrenia. In: *Clinical evidence* pp. 695–716. British Medical Journal, London. [Regularly updated summary of efficacious treatments for schizophrenia, including summaries of relevant Cochrane reviews]

Table 2 Personality disorders

Type	Prevalence*	Essential features	Associated disorders	Possible treatments
Eccentric				
Paranoid	2% generally 5% outpatients 20% inpatients	Suspicious; distrustful	Paranoid psychoses; depression	Antipsychotics
Schizoid	3% generally	Social detachment; emotional restriction	Brief psychotic episodes; depression	None known
Schizotypal	3% generally	Strange ideas or experiences; social discomfort	Schizophrenia; depression	Antipsychotics
Emotional				
Histrionic	2–3% generally 10–15% patients	Attention-seeking; overemotional; seductive	Somatization disorder; conversion; depression	None known
Antisocial (psychopathic)	3% generally 50% prisoners	Callous disregard for others	Substance abuse; depression	None known
Narcissistic	1% generally 10% patients	Grandiose; need for admiration; lack of empathy	Depression; anorexia; substance abuse	None known
Borderline	2% generally 10% outpatients 20% inpatients	Unstable moods and relationships; impulsive	Depression; anorexia; substance abuse	Antipsychotics; cognitive therapy
Anxious				
Obsessive– compulsive	1% generally 5% patients	Perfectionistic; controlled	Obsessive– compulsive disorder	Selective serotonin-reuptake inhibitors
Dependent	30% patients	Clinging; submissive; need for care	Depression; anxiety	None known
Avoidant	1% generally 10% outpatients	Social inhibition; fear of criticism; timid	Anxiety states	Psychotherapy

* Refers to prevalence in psychiatric settings.

26.6 Psychiatric treatments

26.6.1 Psychopharmacology in medical practice

P. J. Cowen

Introduction

Psychotropic drugs are widely used in medical practice so that most clinicians are likely to have under their care a number of patients receiving treatment with psychoactive medication (Table 1). Practitioners therefore need to have an understanding of the uses and side-effects of psychotropic drugs, particularly of the way in which such medication can interact with drugs used to treat other medical disorders.

The majority of psychotropic drugs are prescribed for the treatment of depressive and anxiety disorders. This reflects the frequency of these conditions in both primary care and general hospital settings; accordingly, drug treatment for anxiety and depression will often be instituted both by general practitioners and hospital clinicians. Similarly, while the principal use of antipsychotic drugs is in the treatment of schizophrenia, such agents are also frequently used in general hospitals in the management of organic psychoses. Finally, while treatment with mood-stabilizing drugs, such as lithium, will generally be initiated by psychiatrists, patients receiving long-term therapy may well require treatment for coexisting medical disorders, because of which a knowledge of the effects of lithium on different body systems and its liability to produce adverse drug interactions will be required.

Drug overdose

The effects of deliberate or accidental overdose of psychotropic drugs will also involve physicians (see Chapters 8.1 and 26.5.2). Related to this is the general point that when prescribing psychotropic drugs, particularly for depressed patients, the risk of overdose should always be considered. If such a risk is present the practitioner should: (1) ensure that medication is dispensed in small amounts; (2) consider asking a close relative to supervise the medication; (3) use a relatively non-toxic drug, if possible.

Pharmacokinetic factors

Most psychotropic drugs are highly lipophilic and well absorbed from the gastrointestinal tract. They are metabolized by the liver to water-soluble derivatives which are eliminated by the kidney, hence their half-life will be prolonged in patients with hepatic or renal impairment and in the elderly. Where psychotropic medication is added to another drug treatment the possibility of drug interaction must be considered. For example, selective serotonin-reuptake inhibitors are potent inhibitors of hepatic cytochrome P-450 enzymes and can thereby increase plasma levels of coadministered drugs such as warfarin.

Withdrawal of psychotropic medication

Psychotropic and many other classes of drugs produce neuroadaptive changes during their repeated administration. Readjustment has to occur when drug treatment is stopped, and this may appear clinically as a withdrawal or abstinence syndrome. Characteristic abstinence syndromes have been described for the antidepressants and anxiolytics, while the sudden

Table 1 Classification of clinical psychotropic drugs

Name	Examples of classes	Indications
Antipsychotic	Phenothiazines Butyrophenones Substituted benzamides	Acute treatment of schizophrenia and mania, prophylaxis of schizophrenia
Antidepressant	Tricyclic antidepressants Monoamine oxidase inhibitors Selective serotonin-reuptake inhibitors	Major depression (acute treatment and prophylaxis), anxiety disorders, obsessive–compulsive disorder (5-HT-uptake blockers)
Mood stabilizer	Lithium Carbamazepine Valproate	Acute treatment of mania, prophylaxis of recurrent mood disorder
Anxiolytic	Benzodiazepines Azapirones (buspirone)	Generalized anxiety disorder
Hypnotic	Benzodiazepines Cyclopyrrolones (zopiclone) Imidazopyridines (zolpidem)	Insomnia

discontinuation of lithium can provoke a 'rebound' mania, hence it is prudent to withdraw psychotropic drugs slowly whenever possible. It is clearly also important to be able to distinguish withdrawal syndromes from relapse of the disorder being treated.

Compliance and concordance with treatment

In psychotropic drug prescribing, compliance is an even greater problem than in general therapeutics. Psychoactive drugs frequently have unpleasant side-effects and, while side-effects are experienced early in treatment, several days may elapse before a therapeutic response is evident. In addition, patients may not see the need for treatment or believe that it can help them. Careful explanation accompanied by written instructions can help to ensure that necessary medication is taken.

It is increasingly recognized that the successful and safe use of medication requires a collaborative relationship between patient and doctor. The term 'concordance' may therefore be preferred to 'compliance', which carries the implicit assumption that the patient's job is to obey instructions. It is therefore important to acquire an understanding of the patient's attitude to his or her illness as well its treatment. For example, discussion that helps patients to weigh the advantages and disadvantages of drug treatment ('compliance therapy') has been shown to benefit those with schizophrenia.

Antidepressant drugs

All currently employed antidepressant drugs, through one mechanism or another, increase the activity of serotoninergic (5-hydroxytryptamine, **5-HT**) and/or noradrenergic neurones in the CNS. The pharmacological actions of both noradrenaline (norepinephrine) and 5-HT in the synapse are terminated by specific reuptake pumps that draw these neurotransmitters back into the presynaptic nerve ending. Most antidepressants potentiate the action of 5-HT and noradrenaline by blocking this reuptake process.

Tricyclic antidepressants

Pharmacology

Tricyclic antidepressants inhibit the neuronal uptake of noradrenaline (norepinephrine) and 5-HT. They have numerous other pharmacological properties, but these are thought to contribute to their adverse effect profile rather than their therapeutic activity. However, some of these adverse effects, for example, sedation, can prove beneficial in certain circumstances.

Principal drugs

These are amitriptyline, clomipramine, desmethylimipramine, dothiepin, doxepin, imipramine, lofepramine, and nortriptyline.

Indications and use

Tricyclic antidepressants are still the most widely prescribed drug treatment for the management of depressive illness, but their use, particularly in less severe depressive states, is waning in favour of newer compounds that are better tolerated (see below). However, none of the newer antidepressants is more efficacious than the tricyclics and their therapeutic activity in severely ill patients is not as well established. For this reason, unless there are specific contraindications, tricyclic antidepressants should be preferred in depressed inpatients or in those with marked melancholic features.

Depressed patients with prominent sleep disturbance and anxiety should be treated with a sedating antidepressant such as amitriptyline; for other patients, less sedating compounds such as lofepramine or nortriptyline can be used. To obtain tolerance to side-effects, it is usual to begin treatment at a low dose, for example 25 to 50 mg of amitriptyline at night, and to increase the amount over about 2 to 3 weeks to the usual therapeutic dose, which ranges between 75 and 200 mg daily for amitriptyline and imipramine. Tricyclic antidepressants have long half-lives and a single daily dose taken at night is usually appropriate. Patients should be warned about side-effects because this helps to ensure compliance in the early stages of treatment. They should also be advised that a clear therapeutic response may not appear for up to 2 to 4 weeks.

If treatment is successful, it is usual to continue the antidepressant for 4 to 6 months at the original dose if tolerance allows (so called 'continuation therapy'). This reduces the risk of early relapse by about half. Some patients with recurrent depressive illness require long-term prophylactic treatment with antidepressant drugs. This should be considered in those who have had more than two episodes of depression in the previous 5 years, particularly if the episodes have been severe in terms of symptomatology and impact on work and social functioning.

Side-effects

As well as inhibiting the uptake of noradrenaline (norepinephrine) and 5-HT, tricyclic antidepressants possess antagonist properties at a variety of neurotransmitter receptors, including muscarinic cholinergic receptors, α_1-adrenoceptors, and H_1-histamine receptors. These receptor-antagonist effects account for much of the adverse effect profile of these agents, particularly their anticholinergic properties (Table 2). Tricyclics also possess membrane-stabilizing effects that underlie their most serious side-effect of cardiotoxicity, which can be particularly problematic in tricyclic overdose, where ingestion of less than 1 g can sometimes prove fatal. Lofepramine, however, is relatively safe in overdose. Tricyclics should be used with caution in patients with cardiovascular disease. They also lower the seizure threshold and can thereby aggravate pre-existing epilepsy or sometimes cause seizures *de novo*.

Drug interactions

Tricyclic antidepressants antagonize the hypotensive effects of α_2-adrenoceptor agonists such as clonidine, but can be safely combined with thiazides and angiotensin-converting enzyme (**ACE**) inhibitors. The ability of tricyclics to block noradrenaline (norepinephrine) reuptake can lead to hypertension with systemically administered noradrenaline and adrenaline (epinephrine). Tricyclics should not be used in conjunction with antiarrhythmic drugs, particularly amiodarone. Plasma levels of tricyclics can be increased by numerous other drugs including cimetidine, sodium valproate, calcium-channel blockers, and selective serotonin-reuptake inhibitors (**SSRIs**).

Newer antidepressants

Principal drugs

These can be classified as follows:

- *selective 5-HT reuptake inhibitors (SSRIs)*: citalopram, fluoxetine, fluvoxamine, paroxetine, sertraline;

Table 2 Some adverse effects of tricyclic antidepressants

Pharmacological action	Adverse effects
Muscarinic-receptor blockade (anticholinergic)	Dry mouth, tachycardia, blurred vision, glaucoma, constipation, urinary retention, sexual dysfunction, cognitive impairment
α_1-Adrenoceptor blockade	Drowsiness, postural hypotension, sexual dysfunction, cognitive impairment
Histamine H_1-receptor blockade	Drowsiness, weight gain
Membrane-stabilizing properties	Cardiac conduction defects, cardiac arrhythmias, epileptic seizures
Other	Rash, oedema, leucopenia, elevated liver enzymes

- *selective noradrenaline (norepinephrine)-reuptake inhibitors:* reboxetine;
- *selective noradrenaline- and serotonin-reuptake inhibitors:* venlafaxine;
- *monoamine-receptor antagonists*: mirtazapine, nefazodone, and trazodone.

Pharmacology

The actions of SSRIs are essentially confined to inhibition of 5-HT reuptake. Their use is associated with a sustained increase in brain 5-HT neurotransmission. By contrast, reboxetine inhibits only the reuptake of noradrenaline (norepinephrine). Venlafaxine is a potent blocker of 5-HT reuptake and at higher doses blocks the reuptake of noradrenaline as well. Nefazodone and trazodone have weak 5-HT-and noradrenaline-reuptake inhibiting properties. They also act as antagonists at 5-HT_2 receptors, and trazodone is a potent α_1-adrenoceptor antagonist. Mirtazapine is also a 5-HT_2-receptor antagonist, but in addition blocks inhibitory presynaptic α_2-adrenoceptors, resulting in an increased release of noradrenaline

All these compounds lack the cardiotoxicity and the anticholinergic effects of conventional tricyclic antidepressants. They are therefore safer in overdose and, in general, somewhat better tolerated. In the broad range of depressed subjects they have equal efficacy to tricyclics but, as noted above, it is not clear if this extends to the most severely ill patients.

Indications for use

The newer antidepressants should be used to treat patients in whom the use of tricyclic antidepressants is contraindicated because of their anticholinergic and cardiotoxic effects. In addition, some patients unable to tolerate a clinically effective dose of a tricyclic agent may find that one of the newer drugs causes fewer side-effects. The lack of sedation associated with SSRIs, reboxetine, venlafaxine, and nefazodone can be beneficial in outpatients striving to carry out their usual activities. Unlike tricyclic antidepressants, many of the newer drugs do not stimulate appetite and may therefore be appropriate in patients in whom weight gain would be undesirable. Finally, in patients where the risk of overdose cannot be minimized, the newer drugs may be preferred because of their lower acute toxicity.

Side-effects

The main adverse effects of the newer antidepressants are shown in Table 3. The major distinction between compounds is whether or not they are sedating. The sedating antidepressants have the advantage of improving sleep at an early stage but may impair cognitive function, while the reverse is true for SSRIs, venlafaxine, and reboxetine. Like tricyclic antidepressants, the newer compounds appear to lower seizure threshold to some extent, though this effect may be less with trazodone and SSRIs. SSRIs may increase the risk of upper gastrointestinal bleeding, particularly if given in conjunction with non-steroidal anti-inflammatory drugs (**NSAIDs**).

Drug interactions

SSRIs, with the exception of citalopram, slow the metabolism of numerous other drugs including warfarin, theophylline, anticonvulsants, antipsychotics, and tricyclic antidepressants. Dangerous interactions, characterized by 5-HT neurotoxicity, have been reported between SSRIs, venlafaxine, and monoamine oxidase inhibitors (**MAOIs**). This may be particularly problematic with fluoxetine, whose active metabolite norfluoxetine has a half-life of 7 to 10 days. At least 5 weeks should therefore elapse between stopping fluoxetine and prescribing a monoamine oxidase inhibitor. SSRIs may also produce 5-HT toxicity in combination with lithium. Trazodone and mirtazapine may increase the sedative effects of other centrally acting drugs. Nefazodone can raise plasma levels of terfenadine, causing a risk of cardiac arrhythmias. Nefazodone also elevates plasma levels of carbamazepine and digoxin. Reboxetine should not be given with other agents that might potentiate noradrenaline (norepinephrine) function (such as MAOIs) or increase blood pressure (such as ergot derivatives).

Monoamine oxidase inhibitors

Pharmacology

Monoamine oxidase inhibitors (MAOIs) block the enzyme monoamine oxidase, which deaminates the neurotransmitters, 5-HT, noradrenaline (norepinephrine), and dopamine. Monoamine oxidase exists in two forms, known as type A (which deaminates noradrenaline and 5-HT) and type B (which preferentially deaminates dopamine and tyramine). Conventional MAOIs irreversibly deactivate both type A and type B monoamine oxidase. This has two main consequences of importance for MAOI use: (1) there is a potential for serious food and drug interactions; and (2) the consequent drug and food restrictions need to be continued for 2 weeks after cessation of MAOI treatment so that new monoamine oxidase can be synthesized.

Recently a new MAOI, moclobemide, has been introduced. This differs from conventional MAOIs in that its inhibition of monoamine oxidase is reversible, and it selectively inhibits type A monoamine oxidase only. This leads to an increase in brain noradrenaline and 5-HT levels, but other amines such as tyramine are little affected. These factors make moclobemide much less likely than the older monoamine oxidase inhibitors to produce adverse food and drug interactions, giving it a significant safety advantage. However, while moclobemide has been shown to be effective in the treatment of moderately depressed outpatients, studies have not thus far demonstrated its efficacy in the patient groups for whom conventional MAOI treatment is currently reserved (see below).

Table 3 New antidepressants

Drug	Mechanism	Adverse effects
SSRIs	5-HT-reuptake blockade	Nausea, insomnia, headache, anxiety, rash, sweating, sexual dysfunction, low sodium state, extrapyramidal movement disorders (rare), seizure (rare)
Venlafaxine	5-HT- and noradrenaline (norepinephrine)-reuptake blockade	Nausea, headache, insomnia, sweating, anxiety, hypertension (high doses), sexual dysfunction
Reboxetine	Noradrenaline-reuptake blockade	Dry mouth, sweating, constipation, insomnia
Trazodone	5-HT_2-receptor antagonism α_1-Adrenoceptor blockade	Sedation, dizziness, nausea, postural hypotension, priapism (rare), cardiac arrhythmias (rare)
Nefazodone	5-HT_2-receptor antagonist	Headache, fatigue, dizziness, dry mouth, nausea, somnolence
Mirtazapine	$5\text{-HT}_2/\ \alpha_2$-receptor agonist	Sedation, weight gain, abnormal liver function tests, reversible agranulocytosis (rare)

Principal drugs

These are isocarboxazid, phenelzine, tranylcypromine, and moclobemide.

Indications and use

Conventional MAOIs are rarely used as a first choice of antidepressant, except where a patient is known to have responded to them in the past. They are usually reserved for subjects who have failed to respond to tricyclic antidepressants, newer antidepressants, or electroconvulsive therapy, where a very useful antidepressant effect can often be achieved.

Phenelzine and tranylcypromine are the two most commonly prescribed MAOIs. The usual therapeutic dose for phenelzine is between 30 and 90 mg daily. As with tricyclic antidepressants, patients should be informed about side-effects and advised that a therapeutic response from monoamine oxidase inhibitors may not be apparent for 3 to 4 weeks. Once a response is obtained, it is usually necessary to continue treatment for several months.

Side-effects

Monoamine oxidase inhibitors may cause the following side-effects:

- *central nervous system*: dizziness, muscular twitching, insomnia, confusion, mania;
- *cardiovascular:* tachycardia, postural hypotension, hypertension;
- *other:* dry mouth, blurred vision, impotence, peripheral oedema, hepatocellular damage, leucopenia.

Food and drug interactions

The major hazard of conventional MAOI treatment is through interaction with indirect sympathomimetics, that is, agents that release noradrenaline from nerve endings. The usual source of the interaction is tyramine in certain foodstuffs, especially cheese and meat extracts. Tyramine is usually metabolized by monoamine oxidase in the gut wall and liver, but in patients taking MAOIs large amounts may enter the systemic circulation, resulting in hypertension and even cerebrovascular accidents. Similar adverse effects have been reported when sympathomimetic drugs, such as amphetamines or ephedrine, are administered to patients taking monoamine oxidase inhibitors. Ephedrine or its derivatives are frequently present in cold cures: patients must therefore be warned against self-medication without seeking advice.

Hypertensive episodes resulting from the interaction of sympathomimetic drugs and monoamine oxidase inhibitors are best treated with an α_1-adrenoceptor antagonist. If one is unavailable, intramuscular chlorpromazine is an alternative.

MAOIs also produce important interactions with other commonly used drugs, including opiates, insulin, and oral hypoglycaemic agents. Except in special circumstances, combination with tricyclic antidepressants is best avoided. Combination with clomipramine, SSRIs, and venlafaxine can cause a 5-HT neurotoxicity syndrome and is contraindicated.

From the foregoing it will be apparent that conventional monoamine oxidase inhibitors should only be prescribed to patients capable of adhering to the necessary dietary restrictions. Written instructions listing prohibited foods should be provided. No additional medication should be given until the possibility of an adverse drug interaction has been excluded.

Moclobemide

Moclobemide is well tolerated, although insomnia and nausea may occur. Unlike conventional monoamine oxidase inhibitors, moclobemide does not cause significant interaction with tyramine, and adverse drug interactions also seem to be less likely. However, caution is recommended when prescribing with opiates, and combined use with SSRIs and sympathomimetic agents should be avoided. Because of the reversible nature of moclobemide's interaction with monoamine oxidase and its short half-life (about 3 h), normal monoamine oxidase activity is restored within a day of stopping treatment.

Mood-stabilizing drugs

Lithium

Pharmacology

Lithium salts have inhibitory effects on receptor-transduction systems, particularly second messengers such as cyclic-AMP and phosphoinositol. Lithium also produces marked increases in some aspects of brain 5-HT function.

Indications and use

The main uses of lithium are:

- prophylaxis of recurrent affective disorders, especially manic depressive illness;
- acute treatment of mania;
- augmentation of antidepressant medication in patients with resistant depression.

The excretion of lithium from the body is critically dependent on the kidney. Since there is little margin between the therapeutic plasma levels of lithium (0.5 to 0.8 mmol/l) and those causing toxicity (>1.2 mmol/l), the introduction of lithium therapy should be preceded by clinical and laboratory assessment of renal function. Renal function tests should include urinalysis and estimations of plasma creatinine and electrolyte levels, with measurement of creatinine clearance if there is any suggestion of impaired renal function.

Patients should initially be treated with 200 to 400 mg daily of lithium carbonate, usually as a single dose at night. Slow-release preparations of lithium are available, but their pharmacokinetics *in vivo* are very similar to those of the standard preparation. Dosage should be adjusted every 5 to 7 days on the basis of plasma lithium determinations obtained approximately 12 h after the last dose. For prophylaxis of recurrent mood disorders, plasma levels of 0.5 to 0.8 mmol/l are usually satisfactory; but some patients—particularly those with an acute manic episode—may require higher levels (0.8 to 1.0 mmol/l). Most patients achieve adequate plasma levels with lithium carbonate dosages of between 600 and 1200 mg daily, and following this their lithium requirement is generally stable.

In the absence of clinical indications it is usually sufficient to check lithium levels every 2 to 3 months and repeat renal function tests every 6 months. Lithium can also cause hypothyroidism, so thyroid function tests should be performed prior to treatment and at 6-monthly intervals thereafter. If necessary, lithium can be combined with thyroxine replacement therapy. Sudden withdrawal of lithium in bipolar patients can cause an acute rebound mania and should be avoided if at all possible.

Side-effects

Many patients suffer from a fine tremor and nausea; diarrhoea may occur, especially at the start of treatment (Table 4). Some degree of thirst and polyuria is common, and a few patients develop nephrogenic diabetes insipidus, probably caused by lithium blocking the effect of ADH on the renal tubule. Most patients taking lithium have a demonstrable impairment of tubular concentrating ability, although this is rarely of clinical significance. Glomerular function is not usually affected by lithium, but glomerular damage and interstitial fibrosis have been reported following lithium toxicity. There are reports that long-term lithium treatment can occasionally cause long-term renal impairment. However, this risk is low provided the plasma concentrations of lithium are kept within the therapeutic range and episodes of toxicity are avoided.

Up to 80 per cent of the lithium filtered by the renal glomerulus is reabsorbed by the proximal tubule. Conditions such as diarrhoea and excessive

Table 4 Some adverse effects and interactions of lithium

Central nervous system	Drowsiness, lethargy, headache, memory impairment, fine tremor
Cardiovascular system	Conduction defects (rare)
Gastrointestinal system	Nausea, vomiting, diarrhoea
Genitourinary system	Polydipsia, polyuria, nephrogenic diabetes insipidus
Endocrine system	Hypothyroidism (T4 ↓ TSH ↑), hyperglycaemia, hyperparathyroidism
Other	Leuoccharacteristics, skin rash, weight gain
Drug interaction (lithium level ↑)	Diuretics, NSAIDs, metronidazole, spectinomycin, ACE inhibitors
Signs of toxicity (plasma level: >1.2 mmol/l)	Nausea, vomiting, coarse tremor, drowsiness, dysarthria, seizures, coma, renal failure, cardiovascular collapse

T4, thyroxine; TSH, thyroid-stimulating hormone; NSAIDs, non-steroidal anti-inflammatory drugs; ACE, angiotensin-converting enzyme.

sweating, which induce renal sodium retention, also result in increased lithium reabsorption by the kidney and elevated plasma lithium levels.

Drug interactions

Thiazide diuretics, through their effect on sodium excretion, increase lithium reabsorption and can produce lithium toxicity unless the dose of lithium is reduced and plasma concentrations carefully monitored. It is said that loop and potassium-sparing diuretics are less likely to alter lithium clearance, but it is prudent to monitor lithium levels carefully when using these drugs. Plasma lithium levels may also be increased by concomitant administration of NSAIDs, and a similar effect may be produced by metronidazole. Lithium levels may be increased by ACE inhibitors and lowered by theophylline. While the effects of lithium on cardiac conduction are usually considered benign, the effects of cardiac glycosides on conduction may be potentiated. Lithium can cause neurotoxicity (at normal plasma levels) with calcium-channel blockers and carbamazepine. Finally, lithium may increase the liability of antipsychotic drugs to cause extrapyramidal movement disorders.

Lithium toxicity

Acute lithium toxicity usually appears at plasma levels above 1.2 mmol/l. Early signs are coarse tremor, drowsiness, and dysarthria. Higher plasma concentrations (>2.0 mmol/l) can lead to seizures, coma, and death. Since lithium toxicity is potentially fatal, any suspicion of intoxication should lead to the immediate withdrawal of lithium treatment and close monitoring of serum lithium and plasma electrolyte and creatinine concentrations. Severely ill patients with high serum lithium levels may require dialysis.

Carbamazepine

Pharmacology

Like certain other anticonvulsant drugs, carbamazepine blocks neuronal sodium channels. The relationship of this effect to its therapeutic actions in affective disorder is uncertain. Similarly to lithium, carbamazepine facilitates some aspects of brain 5-HT neurotransmission.

Indications and use

Carbamazepine is effective in the acute treatment of mania and in the prophylaxis of bipolar affective disorder. It is used in patients who have difficulty tolerating or fail to respond to lithium therapy, when it may be given in combination with lithium.

The dose range of carbamazepine employed to treat patients with affective illness is similar to that used in the treatment of seizure disorders. Initial treatment should be with 100 mg of carbamazepine twice daily, with the dose increased according to tolerance over the next 2 to 4 weeks. The effective dose range in the treatment of bipolar disorder is generally between 600 and 1200 mg daily, although some patients require higher doses. Plasma level monitoring may be used to help avoid toxicity.

Side-effects

Dizziness, drowsiness, and nausea are common early in treatment, particularly with rapid dose titration, but tolerance to these effects usually develops. Persistent ataxia and diplopia may indicate plasma carbamazepine levels in the toxic range. A moderate degree of leucopenia is often seen during carbamazepine treatment and agranulocytosis can occasionally develop, such that it is prudent to monitor the white cell count as well as the carbamazepine level during treatment. Skin rashes are also quite common. Other rarer adverse effects include hyponatraemia and liver cell damage. Circulating thyroid hormone level may be lowered by carbamazepine treatment, but thyroid-stimulating hormone (**TSH**) levels generally remain in the normal range and clinical hypothyroidism is unusual. Carbamazepine can impair cardiac conduction and should be used with caution in patients with cardiovascular disease.

Drug interactions

Carbamazepine increases the metabolism of a number of other drugs, including tricyclic antidepressants, haloperidol, oral contraceptive agents, warfarin, and other anticonvulsants. A similar mechanism may underlie the decline in the plasma carbamazepine level sometimes seen during continued treatment. The carbamazepine level may be increased by erythromycin and by some calcium-channel blockers, such as diltiazem and verapamil. Reversible neurotoxicity has been reported when carbamazepine is combined with lithium.

Sodium valproate

Pharmacology

Valproate is a simple branch-chain fatty acid with a mode of action that is unclear, although there is some evidence that it can slow the breakdown of the inhibitory neurotransmitter γ-aminobutyric acid (**GABA**). This action could account for its anticonvulsant properties, but whether it also underlies the psychotropic effects is unclear.

Indications and use

Like carbamazepine, sodium valproate was first introduced as an anticonvulsant. Recent studies have shown that it is clearly effective in the management of acute mania: the drug is licensed for this purpose in the United States, but not in the United Kingdom. In the United States, valproate is widely used in the longer term prophylaxis of bipolar disorder, but there is little evidence for this indication from randomized trials.

Valproate can be started at a dose of 400 to 600 mg daily, which may be increased once or twice weekly to between 1 and 2 g daily. Plasma levels of valproate do not correlate well with either its anticonvulsant or mood-stabilizing effects, but it has been suggested that efficacy in the treatment of mood disorders is usually apparent when plasma levels are above 50 μg/ml.

Side-effects

Common side-effects of valproate include gastrointestinal disturbances, tremor, sedation, weight gain, and transient hair loss. Serious side-effects are rare, but fatal hepatic toxicity has been reported, as has acute pancreatitis. Valproate may also cause thrombocytopenia and inhibit platelet aggregation, and increases in plasma ammonia have been reported.

Drug interactions

Valproate potentiates the effects of central sedatives. It has been reported to increase the side-effects of other anticonvulsants (without necessarily improving anticonvulsant control). It may increase plasma levels of phenytoin and tricyclic antidepressants.

Antipsychotic drugs

Conventional (typical) and atypical agents

Pharmacology

Antipsychotic drugs, also known as major tranquillizers or neuroleptics, are a group of agents of varied structure that are used to treat schizophrenia and other psychoses. Conventional or typical antipsychotic agents have in common the ability to block dopamine receptors in the central nervous system, and it is likely that their antipsychotic effect is caused by blockade of dopamine D2 receptors in mesolimbic and mesocortical brain regions.

Atypical antipsychotic drugs have been developed more recently. These have a varied pharmacology, but a much lower likelihood than conventional agents of producing extrapyramidal side-effects at therapeutic doses. Some are highly selective dopamine D_2-receptor antagonists with selectivity for mesolimbic dopamine receptors, for example sulpiride and amisulpiride. Others (for example, risperidone, olanzapine, and quetiapine) have high affinities for the 5-HT_2 receptor that exceed their affinities for the D_2 receptor. Finally, clozapine is also a potent 5-HT_2-receptor antagonist but a weak D_2-receptor antagonist, which accounts for its particularly low risk of inducing extrapyramidal movement disorders.

Principal drugs

These are the:

- *conventional (typical) antipsychotic drugs*: chlorpromazine, haloperidol, flupentixol, fluphenazine, loxapine, pimozide, thioridazine, and trifluoperazine;
- *atypical antipsychotic drugs*: amisulpiride, olanzapine, quetiapine, risperidone, sulpiride.

Indications and use

Antipsychotic drugs are used mainly in the management of schizophrenia. They are also used to treat mania and are sometimes given to depressed patients who have psychotic symptoms or who are particularly agitated. Antipsychotic drugs are also used in the management of disturbed behaviour arising from other causes (for example, confusional states), but their use as non-specific tranquillizing agents should (if possible) be limited to short-term use because of potentially serious side-effects.

In the treatment of acute confusional states, haloperidol, in doses of 1.0 to 5.0 mg is often helpful. This can be administered either orally or parenterally, with the dose repeated after an hour if the patient remains disturbed. Cardiovascular and respiratory side-effects are unlikely with this drug, but acute dystonias can occur and should be treated appropriately (Table 5). Antipsychotic drugs such as risperidone are used for the treatment of confused elderly patients. It is worth noting that some groups of demented patients (particularly those with Lewy-body type dementia) may suffer severe extrapyramidal effects from comparatively low doses of antipsychotic drugs.

The treatment of patients with schizophrenia or mania with antipsychotic drugs requires careful monitoring and persistence because the full therapeutic response may be delayed for some weeks. Furthermore, the dose of antipsychotic drug required may vary considerably from patient to patient, and also within the same patient at different stages of the illness. Lower doses of conventional antipsychotic drugs are now employed for the treatment of these disorders, since positron-emission tomography (**PET**) imaging studies have revealed that an adequate blockade of dopamine D_2 receptors can be obtained with oral doses of 5 to 10 mg of haloperidol daily or 200 to 400 mg of chlorpromazine. Higher doses of these agents can produce sedation and behavioural calming, but at the expense of movement disorders and decreased compliance subsequently.

If a patient has responded to an antipsychotic drug it is usual to continue the medication for a number of months into remission. Frequently it is necessary to administer medication on a long-term basis to prevent relapse, in which case the use of long-acting intramuscular preparations will improve compliance. The decanoates of fluphenazine, flupentixol, and haloperidol are most commonly used.

Atypical antipsychotic drugs should be used when patients experience extrapyramidal movement disorders on low doses of typical agents. In addition, clozapine can be effective in up to 50 per cent of patients with schizophrenia whose symptoms have not responded to typical antipsychotic drugs. It is effective in the treatment of both positive and negative symptoms of schizophrenia; the latter often showing a poor response to typical agents. Whether the other atypical agents are effective in treatment-resistant patients is not yet fully clear. Clinical impression is that some patients can indeed show a useful response, but the frequency of a positive outcome may be less than with clozapine.

Table 5 Extrapyramidal disorders and antipsychotic drugs

Disorder	Description	Treatments employed
Dystonic reaction	Involuntary muscle contraction, especially face and jaw, occulogyric crisis	1. Benzatropine (1–2 mg IM or IV) 2. Diazepam (10 mg IV)
Akathisia	Sense of subjective motor restlessness, continual pacing	1. Reduce dose of antipsychotic drug 2. Benzatropine (1–6mg daily) 3. Propranolol (40–120mg daily) 4. Diazepam (10–30mg daily)
Parkinsonism	Rigidity, bradykinesia, tremor	1. Reduce dose of neuroleptic 2. Benzatropine (1–6 mg daily)
Tardive dyskinesia (late onset)	Choreoathetoid movements, especially tongue, lips, and jaw	1. Withdraw antipsychotic drug 2. Vitamin E 3. Atypical antipsychotic drug
Neuroleptic malignant syndrome (rare)	Fever, muscular rigidity, coma, death	1. Discontinue neuroleptic 2. Intensive care support 3. Bromocriptine 4. Dantrolene

IM, intramuscular; IV, intravenous.

Table 6 Atypical antipsychotics

Drug	EPS[1]	Prolactin	Weight gain	Adverse effects
Amisulpiride	+	↑	+	Insomnia, agitation, nausea, constipation, Q–T prolongation (rare)
Sulpiride	+	↑	+	Insomnia, agitation, abnormal liver function tests
Clozapine	0	0	+++	Agranulocytosis—white cell monitoring mandatory, myocarditis and myopathy (rare), fatigue, drowsiness, dry mouth, sweating, tachycardia, postural hypotension, nausea, constipation, ileus, urinary retention
Olanzapine	+/0	0	+++	Somnolence, dizziness, oedema, hypotension, dry mouth, constipation
Quetiapine	0	0	++	Somnolence, dizziness, postural hypotension, dry mouth, abnormal liver function tests, Q–T prolongation (transient)
Risperidone	+	↑	++	Insomnia, agitation, anxiety, headache, impaired concentration, nausea, abdominal pain

[1]EPS, extrapyramidal symptoms.
0, not present; +, sometimes; ++, often; +++, can be excessive.

Side-effects

Movement disorders

Through their blockade of brain dopamine receptors, typical antipsychotic drugs produce a variety of extrapyramidal movement disorders that can mimic signs of basal ganglia disease (Table 5). Many patients exhibit symptoms of parkinsonism very similar to those of the idiopathic disorder, although tremor is less prominent. A side-effect that appears early in treatment is acute dystonia, which can present with abnormal postures or dramatic muscular spasms involving the face and limbs. Laryngeal spasm with respiratory distress can also occur. A history of recent antipsychotic drug use can help avoid misdiagnoses (it is not unusual, for example, for such reactions to be viewed as 'hysterical'). Another movement disorder that patients find very distressing is akathisia, which is a state of motor restlessness, often with agitation and dysphoria. Distinguishing this reaction from symptoms arising from the underlying psychiatric disorder may not be easy.

All these movement disorders may be treated by a reduction in dosage of the antipsychotic drug or by the introduction of anticholinergic medication such as benzatropine. However, anticholinergic drugs should not be prescribed routinely with antipsychotic medication because of the risk of misuse for their euphoriant effects.

Later in treatment, tardive dyskinesia may develop. This consists of involuntary repetitive movements, usually involving the tongue and lips, though other parts of the body may be involved. The condition may be associated with a supersensitivity of postsynaptic dopamine receptors in the basal ganglia. Unfortunately, this disorder cannot be treated easily, and anticholinergic medication may make it worse. If possible, the antipsychotic drug should be stopped, but this decision is often difficult because of the risk of relapse of the psychiatric disorder.

Atypical antipsychotic drugs are much less likely to cause movement disorders. Risperidone, however, is a potent D_2-receptor antagonist as well as a 5-HT_2-receptor antagonist and can produce some movement disorders at the upper end of its dose range (above 4 to 6 mg daily). Whether atypical antipsychotic drugs are generally less likely to cause tardive dyskinesia is not yet clear. The risk does appear to be less with clozapine, olanzapine, and risperidone.

Neuroleptic malignant syndrome

A rare but potentially very serious reaction to antipsychotic drugs is the neuroleptic malignant syndrome (Table 5). This is characterized by fever, rigidity, and altered consciousness, together with tachycardia and labile blood pressure. Laboratory investigations usually reveal a leucocytosis together with markedly raised levels of creatinine phosphokinase. Antipsychotic drug treatment should be withdrawn immediately if the neuroleptic malignant syndrome is suspected. Management in an intensive care facility may be needed to deal with cardiovascular, respiratory, and renal complications. Treatment with a dopamine-receptor agonist, such as bromocriptine, and the antispasticity agent dantrolene may be beneficial.

Other side-effects of antipsychotic drugs

Antipsychotic drugs, especially chlorpromazine and thioridazine, can produce a variety of side-effects due to blockade of muscarinic receptors and α-adrenoceptors (Table 2). Other side-effects include:

- *endocrine*: elevated prolactin levels, amenorrhoea, and galactorrhoea;
- *skin*: rashes, pigmentation, and photosensitivity (especially phenothiazines);
- *other*: precipitation of seizures, hypothermia (especially chlorpromazine), cardiac arrhythmias (pimozide), weight gain, cholestatic hepatitis, leucopenia, and retinitis pigmentosa (thioridazine in doses >800 mg daily).

The most common side-effects of atypical antipsychotic drugs are shown in Table 6.

Drug interactions

Antipsychotic drugs potentiate the effects of other central sedatives. They may delay the hepatic metabolism of tricyclic antidepressants and antiepileptic drugs, leading to increased plasma levels of these agents. The hypotensive properties of chlorpromazine and thioridazine may enhance the effects of antihypertensive drugs. Antipsychotic drugs, particularly pimozide and thioridazine, can increase the Q–T interval and should not be given with other drugs likely to potentiate this effect, such as antiarrhythmics, astemizole, terfenadine, cisapride, and tricyclic antidepressants. There are also reports of an increased risk of cardiac arrhythmias when pimozide has been combined with clarithromycin and erthyromycin. Clozapine should not be given with any agent likely to potentiate its depressant effect on the white cell count such as carbamazepine, cotrimoxazole, and penicillamine. SSRIs slow the hepatic metabolism and increase blood levels of several antipsychotic drugs, including haloperidol, risperidone, and clozapine.

Antianxiety agents

Benzodiazepines

Pharmacology

Benzodiazepines enhance the action of the neurotransmitter γ-aminobutyric acid (GABA) in the central nervous system by binding to a specific benzodiazepine receptor located in a complex with a GABA receptor and a chloride-ion channel. The pharmacological effects of benzodiazepines are attributed to the facilitation of GABA neurotransmission.

Principal drugs

These are alprazolam, chlordiazepoxide, diazepam, flurazepam, lorazepam, lormetazepam, nitrazepam, and temazepam.

Indications and use

The prescription of benzodiazepines is now decreasing following concern about their liability to produce dependence. Alternative therapies are available for most anxiety-related disorders, and it is recommended that the drug treatment of anxiety and insomnia should be limited to a few weeks' duration. The major indication for the use of benzodiazepines is to help patients in a crisis, when generalized anxiety and insomnia are causing functional impairment and reducing their ability to cope. Patients should be advised that the drug treatment will be of short duration to help them manage their immediate difficulties.

All benzodiazepines have hypnotic and anxiolytic properties. The major distinction of clinical importance is their length of action. Derivatives with short half-lives, such as temazepam, are suitable hypnotics because of their relative lack of a hangover effect. Other benzodiazepines, for example diazepam, have long half-lives and are metabolized to active compounds. These may be used for the treatment of anxiety, either in the form of regular dosing, or on the now preferred 'as required' basis with an agreed maximum daily dose.

Side-effects and interactions

Benzodiazepines have a low acute toxicity. Their adverse effects are extensions of their clinical effects and include the following: drowsiness, psychomotor impairment, dizziness, ataxia, and paradoxical aggression (rare). Benzodiazepines potentiate the effects of other centrally acting sedatives, particularly alcohol. The effects of benzodiazepines are potentiated by cimetidine.

Patients who have taken clinical doses of a benzodiazepine for more than a few months may show a withdrawal syndrome when the medication is stopped. In many respects this syndrome resembles an anxiety state, but perceptual disturbances and acute dysphoria may also occur. It is thus apparent that benzodiazepines can cause physical dependence, and, although the withdrawal syndrome is less severe than that seen following the cessation of barbiturates, patients frequently find it extremely difficult to stop their medication. A gradual reduction is usually best. Generally, withdrawal from a long-acting benzodiazepine is easier than from a short-acting preparation, and if patients taking short-acting benzodiazepines have difficulty withdrawing, then a switch to a long-acting preparation may be helpful.

Other drugs that increase brain GABA function

Zopiclone, zolpidem, and zaleplon

Zopiclone is a cyclopyrrolone derivative marketed for the treatment of insomnia. It binds to a site close to the benzodiazepine receptor and thereby facilitates brain GABA function. By contrast to the benzodiazepines, which reduce the amount of slow-wave (deep) sleep at night, zopiclone has little effect on sleep architecture and is relatively free from a daytime 'hangover' effect. It is claimed to be less likely than benzodiazepine hypnotics to produce tolerance and withdrawal effects, but cases have been reported. The most common adverse effects of zopiclone include bitter taste, nausea, dry mouth, irritability, and headache.

Zolpidem is an imidazopyridine derivative, which also binds to a site close to the benzodiazepine receptor. It has a very short duration of action and, like zopiclone, has little effect on sleep architecture or daytime performance. Its possible adverse effects include nausea, dizziness, headaches, and diarrhoea. Zoleplon is a pyrazolopyrimidine derivative with pharmacological properties similar to zopiclone and zolpidem. However, its half-life is only about an hour which means that it can be used to re-induce sleep after nocturnal waking.

Clomethiazole

Clomethiazole also binds at the GABA-receptor complex, but its clinical effects resemble those of barbiturates rather more than those of the benzodiazepines. It can cause serious respiratory depression in overdose, particularly in combination with alcohol. Because of its short half-life (4 to 5 h), clomethiazole is also used as a hypnotic in the elderly, where dependence has not been reported.

Drugs altering monoamine function

Buspirone

Buspirone is a 5-HT_{1A}-receptor agonist structurally unrelated to benzodiazepines. It is effective in the treatment of generalized anxiety disorder (less so in patients previously exposed to benzodiazepines) but has a slow onset of action (1 to 3 weeks). Unlike benzodiazepines, buspirone does not cause significant sedation or cognitive impairment and appears unlikely to cause dependence. It does not have hypnotic properties. Side-effects include nervousness, dizziness, and headache.

Other drugs

Tricyclic antidepressants and SSRIs are effective in the management of patients with a range of anxiety disorders, including generalized anxiety. They are generally preferred to benzodiazepines for the treatment of agoraphobia with and without panic attacks. SSRIs are also effective in the treatment of obsessive–compulsive disorder and social phobia, but tricyclics (with the exception of clomipramine) are not.

Further reading

Cowen PJ (1997). Pharmacotherapy for anxiety disorders: drugs available. *Advances in Psychiatric Treatment* **3**, 66–71.

Ferrier IN, Tyrer SP, Bell AJ (1999). Lithium therapy. *Recent Topics from Advances in Psychiatric Treatment* **2**, 76–83.

Nutt D, Bell C (1997). Practical pharmacotherapy for anxiety. *Advances in Psychiatric Treatment* **3**, 79–85.

Porter R, Ferrier N, Ashton H (1999). Anticonvulsants as mood stabilisers. *Advances in Psychiatric Treatment* **5**, 96–103.

Richelson E (1999). Receptor pharmacology of neuroleptics: relation to clinical effects. *Journal of Clinical Psychiatry* **60**(Suppl. 10), 5–14.

Spigset O, Martensson B (1999). Drug treatment of depression. *British Medical Journal* **318**, 1188–91.

Stahl SM (2000). *Essential psychopharmacology*, 2nd edn. Cambridge University Press, Cambridge.

Stahl SM (1999). Selecting an atypical antipsychotic by combining clinical experience with guidelines from clinical trials. *Journal of Clinical Psychiatry* **60**(Suppl. 10), 31–41.

26.6.2 Psychological treatment in medical practice

Michael Sharpe and Simon Wessely

What is psychological treatment?

Psychological treatments in medicine come in two main forms. First are formal psychological interventions, which usually have particular labels and content, such as counselling or behaviour therapy, and which are rarely delivered by physicians. Second, and arguably more important, is the doctor–patient interaction itself. This can also be regarded as a psychological treatment; an intervention that has an important and unavoidable psychological impact, whether for good or ill.

Psychological treatment and the medical consultation

The psychotherapeutic importance of the medical encounter was perhaps best acknowledged and described at a time when physicians had less to offer in terms of biological therapies, and consequently placed more emphasis on what they could achieve by talking with the patient. Hence, one less-welcome consequence of the increasing specialization and dependence on technology in modern medicine has been a relative neglect of the psychological aspects of the encounter, most particularly in hospital medicine. Despite the power of modern drug and surgical therapies, there remains a great and possible increasing need for the psychotherapeutically helpful medical consultation. This is especially the case when there is diagnostic uncertainty and when the patient is distressed.

Psychotherapeutic consultations (doing good)

The key ingredients of the psychologically helpful consultation are those described by Jerome Frank as factors common to all psychological treatments, including:

- establishing a good, confiding, and collaborative relationship with the patient;
- giving an explanation to the person of what is wrong with them;
- offering a clearly described plan of action;
- giving a positive message.

Medical encounters are often suboptimal in these general, but important, non-specific factors. The nature of the encounter and its context may not provide an opportunity for the patient to confide in the doctor. The doctor may convey verbally or non-verbally that he does not wish to hear the patient's story or concerns. A positive explanation for the person's symptoms is often lacking and there may be no clear plan of action.

Simple steps can be taken to remedy these shortcomings. It is desirable that attention be paid to the physical arrangements for the consultation. The days when patients were first told that they have cancer on an open ward round may be gone, but many consultations offer scant privacy and opportunity for the patient to ask questions. Some consultations will take time. Whilst to some extent others such as nurses can supplement the doctor's role, it is important that time and privacy are recognized and insisted on as essential therapeutic tools. Taking an interest in the patient's symptoms (even those that are not of diagnostic value) and their fears about these (even if they appear illogical) is essential. Unless this is done the patient may feel they have not been listened to and ignore subsequent advice. It is hard to give effective reassurance if one does not know what the patient fears: time spent on such matters is not therefore a distraction from the diagnostic process, but critical to the overall aim of helping the patient to feel better.

A clear explanation and plan of action is important. All too often patients complain that doctors told them what they didn't have, but not what they did have. This usually happens when the patient's symptoms are not adequately explained by identifiable disease (see Chapter 26.5.3), but even when a clear explanation cannot be given, a positive plan of action usually can. There is evidence that a positive approach has a beneficial effect on outcome.

The provision of hope and an expectation of improvement has long been an ingredient of the doctor–patient relationship. This should not be false hope, for example if the patient has a terminal condition the message should not be a false message that the condition can be cured, but rather that their symptoms will be managed and the doctor will provide ongoing help for them.

Psychological iatrogenesis (doing harm)

Iatrogenesis is not only the result of prescribing the wrong drug or doing the wrong operation: what doctors say to patients can also have powerful negative effects. These include:

- *Dismissive messages*: for example, telling a patient with medically unexplained symptoms 'there is nothing wrong with you—it's "all in the mind", you are imagining it'. This is not only likely to damage your relationship with the patient, but may also send him or her into the arms of less scrupulous practitioners.
- *Excessively optimistic predictions*: for example, telling a patient who has not yet been adequately assessed 'I'm sure it's nothing serious'. This may lead to the patient losing faith in the doctor who made the predictions (and to legal redress) if it turns out to be incorrect.
- *Excessively negative predictions*: for example, telling a person with possible multiple sclerosis 'its probably best if you come to terms with the idea of a wheelchair'. This is likely to lead to the patient becoming unnecessarily distressed.
- *Ill-considered or unhelpful explanation for the illness*: for example, telling the person who is depressed that it's 'probably a virus'. This can set them off on the wrong track for how they should cope and what treatment they should seek.
- *Poorly thought out or ill-informed advice*: for example, telling a patient with indigestion to avoid all foods that are associated with the symptoms. For some patients this can fuel excessive dietary restriction. An elegant demonstration of this type of problem was found in a study of schoolchildren whose parents were told (sometimes incorrectly) that their children had abnormal hearts and should avoid exertion: at follow-up the children with normal hearts were as disabled as those with heart disease.

Specific psychological treatments

Specific psychological treatments may be broadly divided into simple counselling interventions, more intense but short-term psychotherapeutic interventions such as cognitive–behavioural therapy, and longer-term treatments such as long-term psychotherapy. These have a potentially important role in medical practice in improving quality of life and adherence to recommended treatments, and there is some evidence that they may even improve survival. Certainly there is empirical support for better integration of psychological therapies into standard medical care.

Counselling

Simple counselling may have a role in helping people express distress and talk through acute problems, for instance adjustment to a worrying diagnosis such as that of cancer. Whereas the provision of reassurance and emotional support is clearly important, whether or not this qualifies as a specific 'treatment' or needs to be given by a mental health professional is doubtful. Rather it should be regarded as a generic skill to be possessed by all health workers.

Short-term specific psychological therapies

Short- and medium-term specific therapies such as cognitive–behavioural therapy and interpersonal therapy are of documented effectiveness. Both are as effective as antidepressant medication in the treatment of depression. Cognitive–behavioural therapy is also of value in the treatment of patients with anxiety and panic disorders and has a specific role in those with unexplained somatic symptoms (see Chapter 26.5.3). It has been shown in randomized trials to be of benefit in patients with chronic unexplained pain, chronic fatigue syndrome, hypochondriasis, irritable bowel syndrome, non-cardiac chest pain, and other poorly understood conditions.

Cognitive–behavioural therapy is based on a collaborative relationship. The cognitive aspects refer to the patient being helped to re-evaluate and optimize their understanding of their illness. The behavioural part involves some form of target setting, activity scheduling and trying out new ways of coping. Interpersonal therapy is similar, but focuses on the person's relationships and social roles, rather than on their thoughts and behaviours.

Long-term psychotherapy

For persons with problems not amenable to brief therapy, such as ongoing difficulty in adjusting to disease and/or personality problems, there is a case for longer term psychological therapy, but the availability of such therapy is very limited.

Making a referral for specialist psychological treatment

The first requirement for making a referral for specialist psychological treatment is to ensure that there is a service available and to find out what types of referrals are accepted. The second is to make sure that the patient understands why they have been referred and to establish that they are likely to attend.

Services

Psychological treatment services will ideally be located in organizational and geographical proximity to the medical consultation. In reality they often are not. It is therefore desirable for the physician to familiarize themselves with what is available, how long the patient will have to wait, and how they will be received before the need to make a referral arises.

Making the referral

It is often helpful to discuss the referral with the service to ensure it is appropriate. For example, the psychological problems may appear obvious to the physician but regarded as untreatable personality characteristics by the service being referred to. If medical investigation or treatment is ongoing it will help if uncertainties are made explicit in the referral letter and new findings communicated as they arise.

Explanation to the patient

The first and perhaps most important aspect of explaining such a referral to the patient is to make is clear to them that you are not implying that their illness is 'all in the mind', but rather that there is a psychological aspect that deserves attention. The second is to convey a positive attitude towards psychotherapy as being a sensible approach with a realistic chance of helping them. It helps if you have some knowledge of what they can expect. Finally, it can be important, if appropriate, to indicate that you will see the patient after the psychological treatment, meaning that you do not simply regard this as a way of disposing of them.

Summary

There has been an unfortunate separation of biomedical and psychosocial aspects of patient management in our medical system. This is maintained by a number of factors, including geographical separation of services and the short time available for medical consultations. None the less, all medical interactions have an inescapable psychological component and the potential to help or harm the patient. There are basic aspects of a consultation that will maximize the opportunity of doing good; there are other ways of handling consultations that may do harm and should be avoided.

Specific psychological treatments have an important role, especially for those who are distressed in relation to a medical condition, and for those who have unexplained physical symptoms. Whilst there is a general supportive role for counselling, most of the evidence of effectiveness is in support of short- and medium-termed structured psychological treatment such as cognitive–behavioural therapy. A small number of patients, such as those with long-standing problems adjusting to an illness or personality problems, might benefit from longer term psychotherapy, although the evidence for the effectiveness of this is limited.

Further reading

Andrews G (1996). Talk that works: the rise of cognitive behaviour therapy. *British Medical Journal* **313**, 1501–2.

Clark DM, Fairburn CG (1997). *Science and practice of cognitive behaviour therapy.* Oxford University Press, Oxford.

Frank JD (1967). *Persuasion and healing.* Johns Hopkins Press, Baltimore, MD.

Guthrie E (1996). Emotional disorder in chronic illness: psychotherapeutic interventions. *British Journal of Psychiatry* **168**, 265–73.

Kroenke K, Swindle R (2000). Cognitive–behavioral therapy for somatization and symptom syndromes: a literature synthesis. *Psychotherapy and Psychosomatics* **69**, 205–15.

Price JR (2000). Managing physical symptoms: the clinical assessment as treatment. *Journal of Psychosomatic Research* **48**, 1–10.

Spiegel D (1999). Healing words: emotional expression and disease outcome. *Journal of the American Medical Association* **281**, 1328–9.

Thomas KB (1987). General practice consultations: is there any point being positive? *British Medical Journal* **294**, 1200–2.

26.7 Alcohol and drug related problems

26.7.1 Alcohol and drug dependence

Mary E. McCaul and Gary S. Wand

Diagnosis

In the 1970s, Edwards and Gross first characterized the alcohol-dependence syndrome. Today, this syndrome is the basis of alcohol- and other drug-dependence criteria for both major diagnostic systems: the *World Health Organization international classification of diseases, tenth revision* (**ICD-10**) and the *American Psychiatric Association diagnostic and statistical manual of mental disorders, fourth edition* (**DSM-IV**). For a diagnosis of dependence, both systems require a clustering of at least three of the following symptoms during a 12-month period:

(1) tolerance (i.e. increasing amounts of drug needed to achieve the desired effect);

(2) characteristic physiological withdrawal;

(3) difficulties in controlling onset, termination, or amount of substance use;

(4) neglect of important social, occupational, or recreational activities because of substance use;

(5) increased time required to obtain, use, or recover from substance use; and

(6) continued use despite persistent negative physical or psychological consequences.

In DSM-IV, dependence is subtyped for the presence/absence of physiological withdrawal and tolerance, and recovery status is characterized for duration (early versus sustained remission) and symptom status (partial versus full remission). International studies have found remarkable consistency in the dependence syndrome across diverse geographical and cultural settings, suggesting that fundamental biological processes underpin the disorder.

By contrast, cross-cultural reliability has not been established for the less severe diagnoses of harmful use (ICD-10) and substance abuse (DSM-IV), defined by the negative consequences of alcohol and drug use. This may stem from the greater subjectivity of defining 'harm' within a particular social and cultural context, compared to the more physically based dependence symptoms of withdrawal and tolerance. Similarly, specific levels of hazardous alcohol consumption have not been defined: acceptable amounts vary across cultures, time, and individuals as a function of health, pregnancy, age, and gender.

It is sometimes difficult to disentangle the signs and symptoms of substance abuse and dependence from other common psychiatric and medical conditions. Given their prevalence, alcohol and other drug use should be explored carefully with every patient; there are few socioeconomic, racial/ethnic, or educational predictors of who may experience these problems. Patients should be queried for substance use versus abstention, recent, lifetime, and heaviest use patterns, and finally any problems associated with use. Particular attention should be given to those who report family members with alcohol or drug problems. Additionally, certain behaviours often suggest hazardous levels of substance use; these include cigarette smoking, missing work, neglecting family responsibilities, poor nutrition and hygiene, and high rates of injury and accidents.

This chapter focuses on the harmful use of alcohol, stimulants, and opioids because of their prevalence and severe medical and psychosocial consequences. Although of importance, marijuana, nicotine, sedative, hallucinogen, and inhalant use will not be covered (some of these are discussed in Chapter 26.7.3, and for review, see APA 1994).

Epidemiology of alcohol and drug use, abuse, and dependence

There is considerable cultural variation in alcohol- and drug-use patterns and definitions of harmful or pathological levels of consumption. In North America and Europe the use of alcohol is widespread: in a recent multinational study, approximately one-quarter of primary healthcare patients reported at least one alcohol-related problem in the last year. The North American and European lifetime prevalence of alcohol dependence is approximately 9 per cent (range: 5.5 per cent in The Netherlands to 14.3 per cent in the United States) and the prevalence of drug dependence is about 4 per cent (range: 0.7 per cent in Mexico to 7.5 per cent in the United States). Alcohol-related problems account for approximately 4 per cent of the total burden of disease and injury in the world.

In comparison to alcohol use, the prevalence of drug use in Europe and North America is considerably lower, with approximately one-third of persons reporting lifetime drug use. Globally, the use of substances other than alcohol is generally considered socially aberrant, and rates of use remain low. In the United States there was a large increase in the prevalence of cocaine use during the 1970s and 1980s, and currently about 10 per cent of people report lifetime cocaine use: 2 per cent report use in the past year and 1 per cent report current use. In the United States less than 1 per cent of the population reports heroin use in the past year. Use of most illicit drugs peaks in young adults and then declines with age.

Aetiology of alcohol and drug dependence

Many people have tried alcohol or drugs, but only a subset develop dependence, with an interplay of genetic, psychological, and environmental factors increasing dependence vulnerability. A family history of alcohol or drug dependence remains one of the strongest predictors of risk, with heritability estimates for alcohol dependence ranging from 45 to 65 per cent for men and women. Genetic factors associated with an increased risk for alcohol dependence may include inborn abnormalities in dopamine, opioid, and serotonin neurotransmitter systems.

Drugs of abuse influence several different brain neurotransmitter systems, many of these primary responses leading to secondary effects involving dopamine. For example, morphine and heroin first bind to opioid receptors, which then increase the activity of midbrain mesolimbic dopamine neurones that send projections to interconnected forebrain structures such as the prefrontal cortex and striatum. The nucleus accumbens, a region at the base of the striatum, is the key zone that mediates the rewarding effects of drugs such as amphetamine and cocaine, which act directly by increasing dopamine levels at this site, as does ethanol ingestion. Opioid antagonists block ethanol-induced release of nucleus accumbens dopamine, implicating opioidergic activity as an intermediary between ethanol exposure and dopamine release. Genetic, as well as psychological and environmental effects, on this key mesolimbic system may contribute to individual differences in dependence vulnerability.

Psychological factors also appear to increase a person's vulnerability for alcohol or drug dependence. A recent international study found strong associations between anxiety and mood disorders and substance-use disorders, despite large differences in their prevalence across study sites. Anxiety disorders were very likely to pre-date the onset of the substance-use disorders, suggesting aetiological significance. By contrast, mood disorders did not indicate as strong a temporal relationship. In a recent United States household survey, over three-quarters of alcohol-dependent persons were diagnosed with at least one additional psychiatric disorder, with anxiety disorders having the highest prevalence, 61 per cent of women and 36 per cent of men meeting lifetime diagnostic criteria. Some types of people are at increased risk for alcoholism as a result of antisocial tendencies and high excitement-seeking behaviours. Antisocial personality disorder increases the risk of alcohol dependence approximately fourfold for men and over fivefold for women. Cross-cultural consistency in patterns of comorbidity suggests that, while cultural factors may influence the availability and type of substance exposure, the associations between psychopathology as risk factors and the sequelae of substance disorders are probably independent of particular cultural norms and standards.

Finally, environmental and social processes—including marital discord, parental hostility, poor parental monitoring, and high parental tolerance of adolescent drinking—influence a person's vulnerability for alcohol and drug dependence.

Laboratory diagnosis of alcohol- and drug-use disorders

A diagnosis of alcohol or drug dependence is not based primarily on laboratory findings, but rather on the behavioural manifestations of uncontrolled substance use. None the less, laboratory assessments can be useful for confirming recent alcohol or drug use, supporting other evidence of regular use, and providing information about alcohol- and drug-related physical problems. For patients enrolled in treatment, periodic testing can be used to monitor their progress and encourage accurate verbal reports of recent use.

To confirm recent use, measurements are made of current alcohol or drug concentrations in blood, urine, or other body fluids. Blood alcohol levels are measured in milligrams of alcohol per decilitre of blood and can be readily obtained from breath or blood samples. Impairment from alcohol is common above 50 mg/dl and climbs steeply as the blood alcohol level reaches 100 mg/dl and higher: a very elevated value without significant impairment indicates high alcohol tolerance resulting from chronic, heavy drinking. Urine or blood toxicology screens are commonly effective in detecting most illicit drugs for up to 72 h following use.

Most markers (including liver enzymes—aspartate aminotransferase (**AST**), alanine aminotransferase (**ALT**), gamma-glutamyl transferase (**GGT**)—and estimation of macrocytosis, mean cell volume (**MCV**)) have not provided sufficient sensitivity and specificity for use in widespread screening for alcohol problems. Various non-alcohol-related diseases produce similar changes in these markers to those produced by excessive alcohol use. Recent findings indicate that an increase in carbohydrate-deficient transferrin (**CDT**) levels is highly specific for heavy alcohol use (>50 g ethanol/day for at least 1 week), although its usefulness in women or for screening heterogeneous populations of drinkers may be limited.

Alcohol pathology, treatment, and pregnancy complications

Alcohol-related pathology

Age-adjusted morbidity and mortality rates increase as a function of the amount and duration of alcohol consumption, and these rates are increased two- to threefold among chronic, heavy drinkers. Alcohol consumption affects virtually every major organ system. The primary causes of excess mortality include liver disease, severe respiratory infections, cancer of the upper respiratory and digestive systems, cardiovascular disease, suicides, and violence.

Gastrointestinal system

Heavy alcohol use is associated with acute abdominal pain, nausea, and vomiting. With regular, heavy alcohol use, a variety of medical complications involving the gastrointestinal tract and related organ systems can develop. Oesophageal disorders include oesophagitis, oesophageal varices, and oesophageal mucosal tears with bleeding. Common upper gastrointestinal symptoms are gastritis, duodenitis, and ulcer disease. Some of these effects result from direct mucosal irritation by alcohol.

Liver

Because the liver receives portal blood directly from the intestines and is the primary site of alcohol metabolism, liver damage is one of the most common health consequences of chronic, heavy drinking. Two main types of alcohol-related liver injury are inflammation (alcoholic hepatitis) and progressive scarring (fibrosis or cirrhosis), the mechanisms of the toxic effects being shown in Table 1. Despite multiple pathways for alcohol-induced hepatic injury, only some chronic, heavy drinkers experience serious liver damage. Vulnerability to liver injury may result from genetic variations in the enzymes that metabolize alcohol (ADH and **ALDH** (aldehyde dehydrogenase)) and in cytochrome P4502E1 activity. Women experience higher rates of hepatic injury at lower cumulative alcohol levels than men.

Table 1 Mechanisms for alcohol's toxic effects on liver

- Peroxidation of liver cells, resulting from the interaction of free radicals and superoxide anions produced during the metabolism of alcohol with proteins, lipids, and DNA
- Increased hypoxia and associated damage, secondary to increased production of vasoconstrictors by Kupffer cells and endothelial cells in liver sinusoids
- Reduced production of protective eicosanoids (such as prostaglandins) and increased production of toxic eicosanoids (such as thromboxane B_2)
- Accumulation of acetaldehyde (the first oxidative metabolite of alcohol) in the liver, thereby increasing the risk of free-radical production, acetaldehyde–protein adduct formation, and acetaldehyde-induced impairment of protein secretion. Acetaldehyde–protein adducts stimulate collagen production, leading to fibrosis and cirrhosis
- Increased production of cytokines, including tumour necrosis factor-α (**TNF-α**) and transforming growth factor-β (**TGF-β**), associated with Kupffer-cell stimulation

This been attributed to a toxic interaction of female sex hormones and alcohol-metabolizing enzymes, also to lower levels of gastric ADH in women compared to men, resulting in reduced first-pass metabolism in the stomach and higher blood alcohol levels following equivalent alcohol doses. Hepatic injury is also facilitated by nutritional factors, including depletion of antioxidant vitamins and glutathione and a diet high in polyunsaturated fats or iron. Finally, other medical conditions including infection with hepatitis B and C viruses are known to increase the risk of liver damage in alcoholics. These issues are discussed in more detail in Section 14.20.

Cardiovascular

In healthy individuals, moderate alcohol use reduces mortality from atherosclerotic cardiovascular disease, due in part to alcohol's effects of decreasing low-density lipoprotein (**LDL**) and increasing high-density lipoprotein (HDL) cholesterol. By contrast, heavy drinking is associated with an increased risk for cardiac arrhythmias, cardiomyopathy, and sudden cardiac death. Heavy alcohol consumption is also associated with systolic and diastolic hypertension, significantly increasing the risk of stroke by 250 to 450 per cent. In those with established arrhythmias, hypertension, or hyperlipoproteinaemia, even moderate alcohol use may aggravate symptoms.

Pulmonary

At high doses, alcohol decreases respiratory rate, airflow, and oxygen transport, hence increasing pulmonary disease symptoms in affected patients. Alcohol also reduces key pulmonary defences against infection, including: mucociliary clearance; macrophage mobilization, killing, and clearance; and phospholipid metabolism. These actions directly contribute to the increased rates of pulmonary infections (e.g. pneumococcal and Gram-negative pneumonias) in chronic, heavy drinkers.

Neurological

Chronic, heavy alcohol consumption causes structural changes in the brain, particularly in the cerebellum, limbic system, diencephalon, and cerebral cortex. Enlargement of the ventricles and widening of the fissures and sulci over the cerebral hemispheres suggest cortical atrophy. Severely dependent patients may experience a significantly decreased blood flow in the frontal, cortical, and periventricular regions of the cerebral cortex.

A variety of cognitive deficits have been associated with regular, heavy alcohol use, including slowed information-processing, poor attention, difficulties with abstraction, solving problems, and learning new information, and reduced visuospatial abilities. Chronic irreversible damage includes ataxia and gait disturbances, polyneuropathy, dementia, and the Wernicke–Korsakoff syndrome. These are discussed further in Chapter 24.15.

Endocrine

Endocrine abnormalities result from the direct toxic effects of chronic, heavy alcohol use and indirect effects associated with alcohol-related liver disease and malnutrition. Chronic alcohol exposure is particularly damaging to the gonadal axis, resulting in impaired sex hormone production. Male alcoholics often develop gynaecomastia, impotence, and testicular atrophy. Alcohol-dependent women often develop menstrual abnormalities. Both sexes have a higher incidence of osteoporosis resulting in part from reduced sex hormone levels.

Chronic, heavy alcohol use is also associated with activation of the hypothalamic–pituitary–adrenal axis (**HPA**), especially during acute alcohol withdrawal. Some alcoholics develop clinical and biochemical features of Cushing's syndrome or 'the psuedo-Cushing syndrome'. By contrast, HPA responsiveness is temporarily dampened following alcohol withdrawal. As alcohol-dependent individuals cycle through periods of intoxication and withdrawal, the HPA cycles through hyper- and hypoactivity. This alcohol-induced cyclical pattern of corticotropin-releasing factor (**CRF**) and cortisol secretion may induce various pathological states, for instance episodes of sustained hypercortisolism may exacerbate osteoporosis, diabetes mellitus, and hypertension, as well as impairing growth, reproductive ability, and immune function. Further, hypercortisolism accompanying alcohol withdrawal increases excitatory amino acid levels within the central nervous system, resulting in neurotoxicity and worsening withdrawal symptoms such as seizures.

Table 2 Other alcohol-related endocrine abnormalities

Pituitary–gonadal axis:
Decreased LH and FSH
Decreased testosterone and oestrogen
Impotence, gynaecomastia, testicular atrophy and infertility in men
Menstrual abnormalities and infertility in women
Pituitary–adrenal axis:
Hypercortisolism
Altered glucocorticoid negative feedback
Bones:
Osteoporosis
Carbohydrate metabolism:
Glucose intolerance
Alcoholic hypoglycaemia
Alcoholic ketoacidosis
Lactic acidosis
Lipid abnormalities:
Hypertriglyceridaemia
Electrolyte abnormalities:
Low calcium and magnesium
Sodium retention

LH, luteinizing hormone; FSH, follicle-stimulating hormone.

Other alcohol-related endocrine abnormalities are shown in Table 2.

Cancers

Heavy alcohol consumption significantly increases the risk of oesophageal cancers through the local actions of alcohol-metabolizing enzymes on oesophageal cells, and by the increased production of cytochrome P4502E1 in the oesophageal mucosa. This risk is considerably increased by smoking, which has a strikingly high prevalence in heavy drinkers. Other cancers increased by chronic heavy alcohol use include breast, thyroid, skin, laryngeal, and nasopharyngeal. Compromised immune function associated with heavy drinking may contribute to these elevated cancer rates.

Injury

Accidental injuries are a major cause of increased morbidity and mortality among chronic, heavy drinkers. Alcohol use has been implicated in 15 to 63 per cent of fall fatalities, 33 to 61 per cent of burn fatalities, and 44 per cent of fatal traffic accidents. In a study of emergency-room patients admitted for blunt or penetrating trauma, almost half had a positive blood alcohol level (as do half of all those who die from unintentional injuries).

Treatment of alcohol disorders

Inpatient settings have traditionally been used for the early phases of treatment, particularly acute detoxification and short-term residential programmes. Outpatient settings have provided longer term, abstinence-maintenance treatment. With growing concern over the cost-effectiveness of services, outpatient utilization has increased across all treatment phases.

Alcohol-withdrawal management

Alcohol withdrawal is potentially life-threatening. However, fewer than 10 per cent of alcohol-dependent patients are at risk for severe withdrawal symptoms, which: appear within the first 24 h after drinking cessation; intensify; and then decrease over 2 to 3 days. Symptoms generally result from disinhibition of the γ-aminobutyrate (**GABAergic**) system and the resulting overactivation of the autonomic nervous system. Primary symptoms include tremor, sweating, headache, restlessness, anxiety, nausea, vomiting, disorientation, hallucinations, and seizures. The level of alcohol consumption typically determines symptom severity, but comorbid medical conditions can exacerbate the problem and complicate its management.

Repeated, unmedicated withdrawal episodes may increase the risk of future alcohol withdrawal seizures (kindling), and hence withdrawal management using benzodiazepines is recommended for most patients. Symptom-driven protocols that base medication frequency and dosage on regular withdrawal severity assessments are increasingly preferred over traditional fixed-dose regimens. These decrease the total amount and duration of medication and withdrawal-symptom severity. For most patients, alcohol withdrawal can be successfully treated on an outpatient basis. (See Chapter 26.7.3 for further discussion.)

Pharmacotherapy for alcohol dependence

There is considerable interest in developing medications to use in conjunction with psychosocial therapies to improve treatment retention and reduce relapse. Until recently, the only pharmacotherapy for alcoholism was disulfiram (Antabuse), an alcohol-sensitizing medication that produces flushing, nausea, vomiting, increased blood pressure, and heart rate when combined with alcohol. However, there is limited empirical support for the effectiveness of disulfiram because of poor patient acceptance and compliance.

As described above, various neurotransmitter systems contribute to alcohol reward, tolerance, and dependence, so providing an empirical basis for the development of pharmacotherapies to treat alcohol craving or reduce alcohol reward or intoxication. If persistent and intrusive thoughts about drinking (in other words, craving) and within-treatment 'slips' could be effectively treated, this would improve patients' retention in psychosocial services and decrease their risk of relapse. In clinical trials, opioid receptor antagonists (such as naltrexone) have decreased craving and alcohol consumption, whilst improving objective markers of drinking such as liver function test results. Of particular interest, placebo-treated subjects who drank were far more likely to progress to persistent heavy drinking than naltrexone-treated subjects who drank. Acamprosate, an *N*-methyl-D-aspartate (**NMDA**)-receptor antagonist, also increases abstinence and improves treatment retention; it is widely marketed in Europe and is currently under a Food and Drug Administration (**FDA**) review for alcoholism treatment in the United States.

Alcohol-dependent patients with a concurrent psychiatric disorder are at an increased risk of substance-abuse treatment non-compliance, relapse, psychosocial and interpersonal problems, greater severity of psychiatric symptoms, and suicide attempt and completion. The psychiatric disorder often requires treatment concurrently with the substance-use disorder and may not improve simply as a result of reduced alcohol and drug use (for example, serotonergic medications may be effective in reducing drinking in alcohol-dependent patients with concurrent major depression, possibly secondary to improvements in mood and overall psychosocial functioning). A newer non-benzodiazepine anxiolytic, buspirone, has also been found to increase substance-abuse treatment participation and duration, and improve outcomes on measures of anxiety, depression, and global psychopathology compared to placebo treatment.

Psychosocial treatments

Most substance-abuse patients are treated in outpatient rather than inpatient facilities (that is, detoxification, residential rehabilitation, therapeutic communities). Outpatient programmes typically offer assessment and diagnosis, individual and group therapy, and referral for other needed services. Recently, outpatient services have increasingly introduced focused, empirically validated treatment interventions, such as cognitive–behavioural skills training programmes, relapse-prevention groups, and marital and family therapy. Family involvement in treatment and patient participation in community-based, self-help programmes such as Alcoholics Anonymous (**AA**) can improve long-term, post-treatment outcomes.

Alcohol-related pregnancy complications

Although many women reduce unhealthy behaviours, including alcohol and drug use and cigarette smoking during pregnancy, approximately one in five women in the United States reports drinking alcohol while pregnant. Among pregnant drinkers, 8 per cent drink on 6 or more days during the month, and 30 per cent consume three or more drinks per drinking day, hence alcohol use remains high during pregnancy despite well-documented and publicized maternal and fetal risks. Because no safe alcohol limits have been established during pregnancy, women are targeted for early intervention at lower alcohol-use levels during pregnancy.

At its most extreme, alcohol consumption during pregnancy can result in the fetal alcohol syndrome, characterized by facial dysmorphology, growth retardation, and CNS disorders, which is the most common preventable cause of mental retardation. Other more common fetal effects have been labelled 'alcohol-related birth defects', and include: reductions in weight, height, and head circumference; decreased cognitive abilities and school achievement; and, possibly, an increased risk of behavioural problems such as attention deficits and impulsiveness. The current global estimated incidence of fetal alcohol syndrome is approximately 1 in 1000 live births in the general obstetric population and 4.3 per 100 births among heavy drinkers.

Pathology, treatment, and pregnancy complications of stimulant drugs

Stimulant-related pathology

Stimulants including amphetamines and cocaine work primarily on three CNS neurotransmitters, norepinephrine (noradrenaline), serotonin, and dopamine. They acutely increase norepinephrine neuronal activity by increasing presynaptic synthesis and blocking reuptake from the synaptic cleft. Effects of which include hypertension, tachycardia, dilated pupils, diaphoresis, vasoconstriction, and tremor. Norepinephrine levels in brain decrease in the longer term, leading to depression, confusion, restlessness, suicidal ideation, and irritability. Stimulants also acutely diminish CNS serotonin activity, contributing to insomnia. Effects on dopamine transmission, particularly in ventral tegmental/corticomesolimbic regions, are thought to mediate the high potential of stimulants for abuse. Acutely, dopamine transmission is increased, but chronic cocaine use depletes central dopamine levels, such that short-term euphoria, increased energy, and alertness is followed by depression and subsequent drug administration.

Drug-related pathology often results from the method of administration or lifestyle issues (for example, prostitution) rather than direct drug toxicity. Chronic intranasal administration increases rhinitis, maxillary sinusitis and necrosis, and perforation of the nasal septum. Smoked cocaine increases pulmonary complications including pneumonitis, obliterative bronchiolitis, asthma, and pulmonary haemorrhage. Finally, intravenous administration increases the risk of infectious diseases, including human immunodeficiency virus (**HIV**) infection, endocarditis, hepatitis, and sepsis, as well as abscesses and cellulitis at the injection site.

Cocaine use is associated with a number of other serious medical problems, particularly cardiovascular complications, including cardiac arrhythmias, myocardial infarction, myocarditis, cardiomyopathy, endocarditis, and aortic dissection. Myocarditis was present in approximately 20 per cent of regular cocaine users in one autopsy study.

A serious neurological complication of cocaine use and a leading cause of cocaine-associated deaths is seizures. The seizure threshold decreases with repeated cocaine use and associated kindling. Additionally, acute cocaine use increases the risk of stroke secondary to focal artery vasospasm, thrombosis, and elevated blood pressure. Chronic use can result in significant hypoperfusion in the frontal, periventricular, and temporoparietal areas, changes that have been linked to deficits in attention, concentration, learning, visual and verbal memory, and visuomotor integration.

Stimulant use can lead to significant psychiatric symptoms, both acutely and chronically. Acute symptoms include grandiosity, impulsiveness, and aggression. Common complications of chronic use include panic attacks, paranoia, depression, delirium, and hypersomnia.

Medical problems are more frequent among female than male drug abusers. Common complaints include infections, anaemia, sexually transmitted diseases (particularly gonorrhoea, trichomonas, and chlamydia), hepatitis, urinary tract infections, and gynaecological problems. Substance-abusing women are at an increased risk of developing a variety of reproductive dysfunctions compared with other women, including amenorrhoea, anovulation, luteal-phase dysfunction, ovarian atrophy, spontaneous abortion, and early menopause.

Treatment of stimulant-use disorders

Withdrawal management

Stimulant withdrawal is characterized by primarily psychological rather than physical symptoms. The acute 'crash' following discontinuation of intense cocaine use is notable for depression, agitation, cocaine craving, and hypersomnia. Prolonged withdrawal symptoms include anhedonia, anergia, and cocaine craving.

Pharmacotherapy

There has been little progress in identifying effective pharmacological treatments for stimulant dependence and, as a result, psychosocial treatments remain the mainstay of care. Because chronic cocaine use depletes brain dopamine levels, pharmacotherapeutic research has focused predominantly on dopamine agonists. Antidepressants have also been explored for the treatment of dysphoric symptoms accompanying cocaine cessation.

Psychosocial treatments

Retention for longer rather than shorter periods in outpatient treatment is associated with improved long-term, postdischarge outcomes across alcohol, cocaine, and opiate treatments. For cocaine-dependent patients receiving outpatient psychosocial treatments, retention in care for 90 days or longer is associated with a reduced risk of cocaine relapse. Abstinence-focused treatments appear most effective for promoting long-term recovery.

Stimulant-related pregnancy complications

Approximately 2 per cent of pregnant women in the United States report illicit drug use. Across a variety of drug classes, drug-abusing women experience a clinically significant increase in obstetric complications compared with non-drug-using women. Maternal cocaine abuse is associated with intrauterine growth retardation, decreased birth weight, length and head circumference, anaemia, increased risk of intrauterine or perinatal infections (hepatitis, sexually transmitted diseases (**STDs**) and HIV), and cardiac abnormalities. Maternal complications specifically associated with cocaine use include reduced maternal weight gain, precipitous delivery, placental abruption, preterm labour and delivery, and spontaneous abortion. Drug-using women generally participate in fewer prenatal services than non-drug-using women, compromising the delivery of adequate prenatal care for these more complicated pregnancies. Maternal drug use also adversely affects infant health, the most obvious neonatal complication associated with maternal stimulant abuse being drug withdrawal, including tremors, irritability, high-pitched and excessive crying, poor feeding, and abnormal sleep patterns. The overall morbidity for drug-exposed neonates is over twice that of non-drug-exposed neonates.

Pathology, treatment, and pregnancy complications of opioid drugs

Opioid-related pathology

As described above for stimulants, the pathology associated with regular heroin use often results from the method of drug administration or lifestyle issues. Approximately one-quarter of heroin-dependent individuals die from homicide, suicide, accidents, and infectious disease within 10 to 20 years of initiating regular use.

Infections including abscesses, cellulitis, endocarditis, and septicaemia are common among opioid users: many stem from intravenous drug administration, the use of unsterile injection equipment, and contaminated drugs.

Infection with the hepatitis C virus, associated with an increased mortality rate, is a growing concern among intravenous drug users. In the United States, as many as two-thirds of patients seeking drug treatment are positive for hepatitis C; hepatitis B is also fairly common. Both contribute to the liver dysfunction frequently observed in these patients.

More than 30 per cent of adult and 50 per cent of paediatric **AIDS** (acquired immunodeficiency syndrome) cases in the United States are directly or indirectly associated with intravenous drug use, and in both the United States and Europe over one-third of drug-treatment patients are infected with HIV. As a result, more-aggressive, harm-reduction strategies are recommended by some to reduce the spread of HIV, and needle-exchange programmes in which drug-dependent persons can exchange used for new injection equipment are increasing. Other sexually transmitted diseases including syphilis, gonorrhoea, trichomonas, and chlamydia also are common, especially among female drug users.

Tuberculosis (**TB**) emerged in the 1990s as a significant concern among intravenous drug users, with its rising prevalence attributed to increased susceptibility to TB infection among HIV-positive, immunocompromised drug users, and the emergence of antibiotic-resistant strains of the tubercle bacillus.

Treatment of opioid-use disorders

Withdrawal management

Opioids produce a very characteristic withdrawal syndrome, although the speed of onset and duration vary as a function of the half-life of the particular drug. Heroin or morphine withdrawal begins 8 to 12 h following the last dose and subsides over 5 to 7 days. Methadone withdrawal begins 12 to 16 h after the last dose, peaks in approximately 3 days, and can persist for 3 weeks or longer. Typical symptoms include: gastrointestinal distress such as cramping, diarrhoea, nausea, vomiting; arthralgias or myalgias; increased respiratory rate; lacrimation; yawning; rhinorrhoea; piloerection; anxiety, restlessness and irritability; tachycardia and hypertension.

Clonidine, marketed for the treatment of hypertension, is widely used for opioid-withdrawal management and is mainly effective for alleviating milder withdrawal symptoms and anxiety-related complaints. However, because of the high morbidity and mortality associated with heroin use, opioid-substitution therapy is the treatment of choice in the United States and Europe, and generally recommended for opioid-dependent people who have failed in prior drug-free treatments. Opioid-substitution therapy replaces the use of illicit, short-acting, injected, impure drugs with longer and orally active medications of known potency and purity. Outcomes include withdrawal symptom suppression, reduced drug craving, blockade of the euphoric effects of heroin or other opioid administration, and patient engagement in rehabilitative services. Individual and group counselling and urine testing for illicit drugs are part of routine care in most programmes. HIV/AIDS has heightened the importance of treatment approaches focused on reducing or eliminating injection drug use as opposed to achieving drug-free status. Methadone is commonly used for short- and long-term management of heroin and other opioid withdrawal. Buprenorphine, a mixed agonist and antagonist drug, may offer particular advantages for opioid-withdrawal management, although it does not have current United States approval. The details of pharmacotherapeutic management are discussed in Chapter 26.7.3.

Because of the breadth of psychosocial problems associated with chronic opioid use, individual and group counselling sessions are standard treatment components. Patients evidence their greatest improvements in comprehensive care programmes that integrate medical, psychiatric, family, legal, and social services.

Opioid-related pregnancy complications

Complications associated with regular heroin use include spontaneous abortion, amnionitis, chorioamnionitis, intrauterine growth retardation, placental insufficiency, postpartum haemorrhage, pre-eclampsia, premature labour, premature rupture of membranes, eclampsia, toxaemia, and placental abruption. Symptoms of neonatal drug withdrawal are very similar to those of adults, and include CNS hyperirritability, loose stools and other gastrointestinal dysfunction, nasal stuffiness, yawning, sneezing, increased lacrimation, and fever. As described above for stimulants, there is a high frequency of other fetal/neonatal complications, including suboptimal APGAR scores, low birth weight, prematurity, and an increased risk of intrauterine or perinatal infections.

Maternal and infant morbidity and mortality are significantly improved among women receiving opioid-replacement treatment, a major benefit for the fetus being the prevention of repeated, medically unsupervised withdrawal episodes. Maintenance has also been shown to improve the frequency of prenatal care, decrease illicit drug use, improve nutritional status, and decrease risky lifestyles. Infants of methadone-maintained mothers need to be closely monitored and, in most cases, treated for opiate withdrawal, typically using paregoric. Symptom onset is often delayed and duration may be unusually prolonged because of reduced metabolic clearance.

Prevention and early intervention

Given the high prevalence of alcohol and drug disorders, all physicians treat patients with these problems. It is estimated that as many as 20 per cent of primary care patients and 25 to 40 per cent of inpatients are alcohol-dependent or problem drinkers. Physicians should routinely enquire about drinking and other drug use (prescribed and illicit), and facilitate the referral and management of patients with these problems. Most alcohol-related health consequences are experienced not by those who are alcohol-dependent, but by the much larger group of hazardous drinkers whose problems are at an early or relatively mild stage. Brief advice on setting safe drinking limits can have a significant and sustained impact on drinking levels in this at-risk population. These interventions begin with a focused assessment of alcohol and drug use and related problems, followed by a brief, highly directive interaction in which the health professional provides personalized feedback based on the assessment findings (for instance, elevated liver function test results or other medical problems, absenteeism or lateness at work, marital distress). Finally, the provider offers specific drinking-reduction strategies, such as goal-setting for 'sensible' drinking and assigning relevant reading materials. Brief interventions reduce overall alcohol use, binge-drinking episodes, and hospital admissions and are easily conducted in various healthcare settings, including that of primary care. (For further discussion see Chapter 26.7.2.)

Areas of uncertainty/controversy

Controlled alcohol use versus abstinence

Controlled drinking as a therapeutic goal for alcoholism treatment remains controversial, particularly in the United States. Less than one-quarter of surveyed treatment programmes in the United States found controlled drinking acceptable, compared with approximately three-quarters of surveyed United Kingdom programmes. Even the United States and United Kingdom programmes that endorsed controlled drinking recommended it as a therapeutic goal for fewer than 25 per cent of patients based on their dependence severity, drinking history duration, psychological dependence, family history of alcoholism, prior treatment outcomes, and current health damage. Although controlled drinking may offer a harm-reduction option in a subset of treatment-resistant patients, abstinence generally produces the most positive long-term outcomes for patients in treatment.

Pharmacotherapy versus drug-free treatment

Pharmacotherapy for abstinence maintenance continues to be controversial. In part, this may stem from treatment providers' concerns about cross-addiction, but it also reflects the current paucity of medication options for alcoholism treatment. It is very likely that in the next decade new and more effective pharmacotherapies will be identified, and physicians will need to encourage the appropriate use of these medications by their patients since it is unlikely that the momentum for change will come from within specialty alcoholism-treatment facilities.

Smoking cessation as a concurrent treatment goal

While smoking rates have declined in the general population, estimates of smoking prevalence among alcohol- and drug-dependent persons have generally been stable and in the range of 75 per cent to 90 per cent. Indeed, smoking can now be considered as a risk marker of heavy alcohol and drug use, particularly among pregnant women. Historically, treatment professionals have discouraged a concurrent cessation of nicotine and other substance use. However, patients in treatment for alcoholism who decrease or eliminate cigarette use have comparable or slightly improved rates of alcohol abstinence compared with patients who continue smoking. Thus, smoking cessation concurrent with or in close proximity to substance-abuse treatment may decrease the risk of post-treatment relapse. This is a critical area for future research and intervention, given the excessive morbidity and mortality associated with nicotine dependence among alcohol and other drug abusers.

Further reading

American Psychiatric Association (1994). *Diagnostic and statistical manual of mental disorders, 4th edition*. American Psychiatric Association, Washington, DC.

Fleming MF, *et al.* (1997). Brief physician advice for problem alcohol drinkers. A randomized controlled trial in community-based primary care practices. *Journal of the American Medical Association* **277**, 1039–45.

Gianoulakis C (1996). Implications of endogenous opioids and dopamine in alcoholism: human and basic science studies. *Alcohol and Alcoholism Supplement* **1**, 33–42.

Lieber CS (2000). Alcoholic liver disease: new insights in pathogenesis lead to new treatment. *Journal of Hepatology* **32**(Suppl.), 113–28.

Ling W, Rawson RA, Compton MA (1994). Substitution pharmacotherapies for opioid addiction: from methadone to LAAM and buprenorphine. *Journal of Psychoactive Drugs* **26**, 119–28.

Mayo-Smith MF (1997). Pharmacological management of alcohol withdrawal. *Journal of the American Medical Association* **278**, 144–51.

Merikangas KR, *et al.* (1998). Comorbidity of substance use disorders with mood and anxiety disorders: results of the International Consortium in Psychiatric Epidemiology. *Addictive Behaviors* **23**, 893–907.

Reich T, *et al.* (1999). Genetic studies of alcoholism and substance dependence. *American Journal of Human Genetics* **65**, 599–605.

Swift RM (1999). Drug therapy for alcohol dependence. *New England Journal of Medicine* **340**, 1482–90.

Wagner CL, *et al.* (1998). The impact of prenatal drug exposure on the neonate. *Obstetric and Gynecology Clinics of North America* **25**, 169–94.

Wand GS, Froehlich JC (1991). Alterations in hypothalamo-hypophysial function by ethanol. In: Muller E, MacLeod R, eds. *Neuroendocrine perspectives*, Vol. 9, pp 45–126. Springer-Verlag, New York.

26.7.2 Brief interventions against excessive alcohol consumption

Nick Heather and Eileen Kaner

Introduction

Harm caused by excessive drinking extends far beyond 'alcoholism' or severe alcohol dependence. Alcohol-related problems can be of many different kinds—medical, interpersonal, social, psychological, financial, vocational, legal—and can be associated with various patterns of drinking. For example, problems related to acute alcohol intoxication, such as accidents, violence, and public disorder offences, need not involve high levels of regular consumption or dependence. Even in the area of medical harm, research has shown that patients who develop chronic liver disease are usually only mildly dependent on alcohol, probably because those who escape florid symptoms of dependence are able to sustain a consistent pattern of heavy drinking over many years. When those at risk of harm are added to those who have already incurred it, the number of individuals whose lives may be adversely affected by their drinking becomes very large.

Among specialists in the treatment and prevention of alcohol problems, there is now a consensus that a prior focus on the alcoholism concept had distracted attention from the full range of alcohol problems that occur. This is not to imply, of course, that patients suffering from severe alcohol dependence should be ignored, only that the scope of treatment and preventive efforts should be broadened in an attempt to reduce the aggregate of alcohol-related harm in our society. Brief interventions in medical practice have a crucial role to play in this strategy.

Definitions

Excessive alcohol consumption

'Excessive alcohol consumption' is a term that includes both 'hazardous' and 'harmful' drinking. In the *International classification of diseases* (10th revision), the hazardous use of a psychoactive substance is defined as: 'An occasional, repeated or persistent pattern of use...which carries with it a high risk of causing future damage to the medical or mental health of the user but which has not yet resulted in significant medical or psychological ill effects'. Harmful use is defined as: 'A pattern of use which is already causing damage to health. The damage may be physical or mental'.

Hazardous and harmful alcohol consumption can also be defined by drinking limits recommended by medical authorities in various countries. In the United Kingdom, a joint working group of the Royal Colleges of Physicians, Psychiatrists, and General Practitioners in 1995 defined low risk (or 'sensible') consumption as up to 21 units/week for men and 14 units/week for women, increasing risk (here hazardous) as 22 to 50 units/week for men and 15 to 35 units/week for women, and high risk (here harmful) consumption as above 50 units/week for men and above 35 units/week for women (one unit = 8 g ethyl alcohol). Subsequently, a United Kingdom government report on sensible drinking effectively increased the drinking limits, by advising the public that men could drink up to 4 units/day and women up to 3 units/day. These revised recommendations have been severely criticized and medical practitioners are best advised to continue using the previous limits.

Brief interventions

As delivered by non-alcohol specialists, brief interventions refer to a collection of methods incorporated into routine practice aimed at helping patients who drink excessively to reduce their consumption to low-risk levels. These interventions are often called 'opportunistic' because they typically take advantage of opportunities that arise when people present to a medical facility for reasons unconnected with a possible alcohol problem. Brief interventions are normally restricted to individuals with only low levels of alcohol dependence or alcohol-related problems, those more seriously impaired usually being referred to specialist services. However, this is not always the case, and some doctors feel able to offer intensive treatment to more serious cases, often with advice or help from specialists in the form of shared-care arrangements. Although normally directed at a reduced drinking goal, there is no reason why brief interventions should not be targeted at total abstinence in appropriate circumstances or if the patient prefers it. However, for patients with relatively low levels of dependence and problems, insistence on abstinence is almost always a disincentive to a change in behaviour.

Prevalence

The latest United Kingdom General Household Survey in 1996 showed that 27.5 per cent of adult (over 16 years of age) males and 13 per cent of adult females reported drinking over the limits recommended by the Royal Colleges. Among young (16–24 years of age) men and women, the figures rose to 35 per cent and 21 per cent, respectively. There are reasons for believing that even these figures may be underestimates, but they nevertheless reveal the enormous extent of excessive drinking in the general population of the United Kingdom.

Patients with alcohol problems consult their general practitioners nearly twice as often as the average, their most common problems being gastrointestinal, psychiatric, and accidents. Some 40 harmful drinkers and a further 100 hazardous drinkers would be expected in every 2000 patients in primary care, but it is likely that the primary care physician will be unaware of the problem in more than half of these. In surgical and general medical wards, estimates range up to 30 per cent of all male admissions and 15 per cent of female admissions. Again, few of these patients will be identified as excessive drinkers. It is also well established that excessive drinkers are over-represented among patients of accident and emergency services.

Aims and targets of brief interventions

Opportunistic identification and brief intervention for excessive drinking are often justified as a means of early intercession and secondary prevention of alcohol problems. The attempt is made to help the patient reduce consumption or abstain before seriously adverse consequences arise, and before alcohol dependence and problems have reached levels that make intensive treatment difficult. However, as noted above, brief interventions can also be seen as making an important contribution to the public health approach in reducing alcohol-related harm at the population level. As public health measures, there is no incompatibility between the widespread implementation of brief interventions in medical practice and the adoption of fiscal, legislative, and other alcohol-control policies. These two strategies can be seen as mutually reinforcing and as acting synergistically to reduce and prevent alcohol-related harm.

Brief interventions in the sense defined here should be clearly distinguished from briefer forms of treatment given by specialist alcohol or addiction agencies. Among a number of differences, brief treatment by specialists typically takes longer to deliver than the kind of interventions we are considering here. Various types of brief intervention will be described below, but here it may be noted that they range in length from a few minutes of structured advice, up to perhaps five sessions of counselling spread over 6 months. Doctors, nurses, and other healthcare professionals (for example, specially employed counsellors) can be involved in the delivery of brief interventions.

Effectiveness of brief interventions

There is now abundant evidence that brief interventions delivered in medical settings are effective in leading to reduced alcohol consumption. Randomized controlled trials in general practice demonstrating the effectiveness of such interventions have been carried out in the United Kingdom, the United States, Canada, and Australia, and other trials are currently underway in several non-English-speaking countries. These studies indicate that intervention reduces drinking by an average of about 25 per cent. The best estimate of the proportion of patients who show a good outcome is 15 per cent among men and somewhat less among women, although it is possible than many women will respond simply by having their attention drawn to their drinking in an assessment (that is to say, without a specific intervention). Studies conducted in the 'real-world' conditions of general practice show somewhat less benefit than in those carried out under optimal research conditions, but nevertheless they support the effectiveness of brief interventions. Research in general hospital wards has been less extensive, and evidence for their effectiveness is less impressive, although still positive. Studies of the effectiveness of interventions in accident and emergency departments are just beginning.

It may be that some doctors will find the success rates described above unacceptably low. They may recall many patients who have been advised to cut down, but who have ignored this advice. However, given that up to 80 per cent of the population consult a healthcare professional at least once a year, brief interventions—if widely implemented—would undoubtedly represent a powerful means of reducing excessive drinking in the population at large. From the clinical perspective, patients who do not respond at first may do so on subsequent occasions, and even if advice seems to be ignored, it may well influence an evolving process of behaviour change. The disjunction in aims between the public health approach, which regards even very low success rates as beneficial, and the clinical perspective of most medical practitioners, in which the welfare of the individual patient is paramount, must be recognized, but the widespread and consistent implementation of brief interventions can serve both causes.

Practical approach to brief interventions

Identifying excessive drinkers

Screening is the process of identifying patients whose alcohol consumption places them at increased risk of psychological or physical complications and who might benefit from early detection and brief intervention. There are a number of laboratory indicators of excessive alcohol consumption, such as mean corpuscular volume (**MCV**), γ-glutamyl transferase (**GGT**), and blood alcohol concentration (**BAC**). However, in medical practice, standardized questionnaires have been found to have a greater sensitivity and specificity than laboratory indicators; they are also far less intrusive and more acceptable to patients.

Although there are a number of standardized questionnaires, most were developed to detect a severe level of alcohol dependence (in other words, 'alcoholism'). The Alcohol Use Disorders Identification Test (**AUDIT**) is the only standardized instrument designed specifically to detect hazardous and harmful drinking in both primary and secondary healthcare settings. AUDIT is a 10-item questionnaire that includes items on drinking frequency and intensity (binge drinking), together with experience of alcohol-related problems and dependence (see Fig. 1). At a score of 8 out of a possible 40, the ability of AUDIT to detect genuine excessive drinkers (sensitivity) and to exclude false cases (specificity) is 92 per cent and 93 per cent, respectively.

Management of excessive drinkers

Patients who are drinking at hazardous levels (AUDIT 8–12 for men and 7–12 for women) should be offered brief intervention. Excessive drinkers who show prima facie evidence of significant alcohol dependence (AUDIT 13+ for women and 15+ for men) should normally receive a fuller assessment of their dependence and alcohol-related problems, including the impact of their drinking on their social functioning. Unless skills and resources exist to assess and treat these patients at the generalist level, they should be offered referral to a specialist alcohol or addiction treatment agency.

Types of brief intervention

The most basic form of brief intervention is simple advice to cut down, delivered in a persuasive but non-judgemental fashion and with clear guidance on consumption targets. This advice should, as far as possible, be personalized by taking into account the particular circumstances of the individual patient, their level of consumption in relation to population norms for their sex, and an appeal to any specific alcohol-related difficulties they may recognize as applying to them, including social and psychological as well as medical problems.

Advice can be supported by the offer of self-help material, and a follow-up appointment to check on their progress in cutting down will also be helpful. Successive feedback of GGT readings or other laboratory markers of alcohol consumption can be a powerful motivator. All this can be accomplished in a 5 to 10 min consultation, and specially developed brief intervention packages are available to assist this task. One such package is the Drink-Less Programme, which was developed for a WHO Collaborative Project on brief interventions in primary healthcare. It has been adapted for use in the United Kingdom, with separate versions for doctors and nurses, and is available at a small cost to cover production expenses from the Department of Primary Health Care, University of Newcastle upon Tyne.

Some doctors may prefer to spend more than 5 to 10 min on intervention, or may have the assistance of nursing or other colleagues with the time and expertise to devote to intervention. In either case, the opportunity arises to engage the patient more thoroughly in the change process. One possibility here is to use a condensed form of a type of treatment that is frequently offered in specialist alcohol treatment centres, known as cognitive–behavioural therapy. In this approach, the attempt is made to identify the types of stress and 'high-risk situations' that lead to excessive drinking in the individual case, and then train the patient in ways of coping with these stressors or situations without heavy drinking. Attention is also paid to modifying cognitive factors (for example, unhelpful beliefs about alcohol, subconscious positive expectations about its effects, lack of confidence in the ability to alter drinking behaviour) that may impede the patient's attempts to change. This form of intervention could be implemented in one session of, say, 40 min, but would probably be more effective if delivered over a series of three to five meetings over several months.

Condensed cognitive–behavioural therapy is most suitable for patients who clearly recognize that damage to their lives is being caused by alcohol and who are ready to try to change their drinking. With patients who refuse to recognize the possibility of harm and who are firmly set against change, probably nothing much can be done except to offer educational material and ask them to return if they change their minds. Between these two extremes, however, there is a large group of patients who will be fluctuating in their concern about their drinking, will be experiencing conflict about the advantages and disadvantages of heavy drinking, and will be ambivalent about attempting to cut down or abstain. For these patients, the approach that should be used is known as 'brief motivational interviewing'. This is based on the fact that ambivalence about changing behaviour is a common feature in healthcare consultations. Although some patients will respond immediately to the delivery of health advice, others will be less ready to change their drinking behaviour and direct persuasion may cause such patients to become defensive. The most effective way of helping ambivalent patients to change is to explore their conflict and encourage them to express their own reasons for concern and arguments for change. It must be emphasized that both condensed cognitive–behavioural therapy and brief motivational interviewing should not be attempted without proper training.

Implementing brief interventions

In a survey of general practitioners (**GPs**; primary care physicians) carried out in the English Midlands during 1995 to 1996, it was found that the levels of detection and intervention for excessive drinking were low. As in studies of junior hospital doctors, it appeared that the GPs did not routinely enquire about alcohol, and that any enquiries were mainly restricted to new patient registrations or those with obvious physical symptoms. Compared with earlier surveys, there was an increase in numbers of GPs

Dear Patient,

As part of my service I am examining lifestyle issues likely to affect the health of my patients. This information is important because it will assist me in giving the best treatment and highest possible standard of care. To help me do this, I would like you to complete this questionnaire in the waiting room before your appointment. When you have finished, please bring it along to your consultation. I will explain the results to you during your consultation with me. Your answers to these questions will be treated in strict confidence. No details of your name are on the carbon copy.

What is your name? ....

What is your age? ....

What is your sex? (please tick) ☐Male ☐Female

Current occupation ....

Level of education (please tick)

OFFICE USE ONLY
ADVISED ☐ → or → **BOOKLET** ☐ / **CARD** ☐

Primary school ☐ Some secondary/high school ☐ Completed secondary/high school ☐ Technical or trade certificate ☐ University, CAE, tertiary education ☐

One Standard Drink is

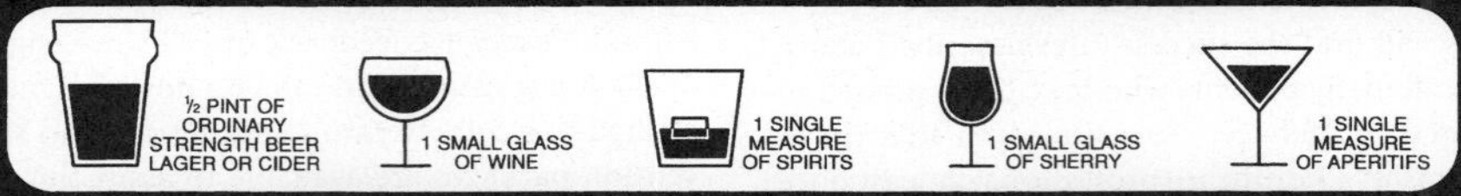

½ PINT OF ORDINARY STRENGTH BEER LAGER OR CIDER
1 SMALL GLASS OF WINE
1 SINGLE MEASURE OF SPIRITS
1 SMALL GLASS OF SHERRY
1 SINGLE MEASURE OF APERITIFS

Please tick the box next to your answer

1. How often do you have a drink containing alcohol?
   Never ☐ (0) Monthly or less ☐ (1) 2 to 4 times a month ☐ (2) 2 to 3 times a week ☐ (3) 4 or more times a week ☐ (4)
2. How many standard drinks containing alcohol do you have on a typical day when you are drinking? (see above diagram)
   1 or 2 ☐ (0) 3 or 4 ☐ (1) 5 or 6 ☐ (2) 7 to 9 ☐ (3) 10 or more ☐ (4)
3. How often do you have 6 or more standard drinks on one occasion? (see above diagram)
   Never ☐ (0) Less than monthly ☐ (1) Monthly ☐ (2) Weekly ☐ (3) Daily or almost daily ☐ (4)
4. How often during the last year have you found that you were not able to stop drinking once you had started?
   Never ☐ (0) Less than monthly ☐ (1) Monthly ☐ (2) Weekly ☐ (3) Daily or almost daily ☐ (4)
5. How often during the last year have you failed to do what was normally expected from you because of your drinking?
   Never ☐ (0) Less than monthly ☐ (1) Monthly ☐ (2) Weekly ☐ (3) Daily or almost daily ☐ (4)
6. How often during the last year have you needed an alcoholic drink in the morning to get yourself going after a heavy drinking session?
   Never ☐ (0) Less than monthly ☐ (1) Monthly ☐ (2) Weekly ☐ (3) Daily or almost daily ☐ (4)
7. How often during the last year have you had a feeling of guilt or remorse after drinking?
   Never ☐ (0) Less than monthly ☐ (1) Monthly ☐ (2) Weekly ☐ (3) Daily or almost daily ☐ (4)
8. How often during the last year have you been unable to remember what happened the night before because you had been drinking?
   Never ☐ (0) Less than monthly ☐ (1) Monthly ☐ (2) Weekly ☐ (3) Daily or almost daily ☐ (4)
9. Have you or someone else been injured as a result of your drinking?
   No ☐ (0) Yes, but not in the last year ☐ (2) Yes during the last year ☐ (4)
10. Has a relative or friend, doctor or other health worker been concerned about your drinking or suggested you cut down?
    No ☐ (0) Yes, but not in the last year ☐ (2) Yes during the last year ☐ (4)

Thank you

The numbers in parentheses refer to the points scored for each answer, the sum of the 10 questions being the patient's overall score. (max = 40)
The points allocated to each answer are not displayed on the form that the patient completes.

Fig. 1 The audit questionnaire.

who felt that working with alcohol issues was a legitimate part of medical practice, but fewer doctors saw themselves as being effective in this work. The main barriers to implementing brief interventions were stated as insufficient time and training and lack of help from government policy; the main incentives related to the availability of appropriate support services and the proven effectiveness of brief interventions.

As this chapter has shown, there is very good evidence for the effectiveness of brief interventions and it is clearly necessary to disseminate this information more widely. With regard to other barriers and incentives, strenuous efforts are now being made to persuade policy-makers and decision-makers at national, regional, and district levels to create the conditions that are needed to support the widespread implementation in routine medical practice of brief interventions against excessive alcohol consumption.

Further reading

Anderson P (1996). *Alcohol and primary health care.* WHO Regional Publications, European Series No. 64. World Health Organization, Copenhagen. [A comprehensive and authoritative guide to alcohol issues encountered in primary healthcare]

Faculty of Public Health Medicine/Royal College of Physicians (1991). *Alcohol and the public health: the prevention of harm related to the use of alcohol.* Macmillan, London. [An excellent coverage of the wider context of alcohol-related harm]

Heather N (1995). Brief intervention strategies. In: Hester RK, Miller WR, eds. *Handbook of alcoholism treatment approaches: effective alternatives*, 2nd edn, pp. 105–22. Allyn and Bacon, Needham Heights. [A review of brief intervention approaches and the evidence of their effectiveness]

Heather N, Robertson I (1998). *Problem drinking*, 3rd edn. Oxford University Press, Oxford. [An introduction to the broad changes in theory, research, and practice in the alcohol field over the last 20–30 years]

Israel Y, *et al.* (1996). Screening for problem drinking and counseling by the primary care physician–nurse team. *Alcoholism: Clinical and Experimental Research* **20**, 1443–50. [One of the best trials of brief interventions yet published, paying particular attention to issues of acceptability to physicians, nurses, and patients]

Kaner E, *et al.* (1999). Intervention for excessive alcohol consumption in primary health care: attitudes and practices of English general practitioners. *Alcohol and Alcoholism* **34**, 559–66.

Rollnick S, Kinnersley P, Stott N (1993). Methods of helping patients with behaviour change. *British Medical Journal* **307**, 188–90. [A key article on the motivational interviewing approach in medical settings]

Rollnick S, Mason P, Butler C (1999). *Health behaviour change: a guide for practitioners.* Churchill Livingstone, Edinburgh. [A recent and highly recommended guide to the negotiation of behaviour change, including drinking, in healthcare settings]

Royal Colleges of Physicians, Psychiatrists and General Practitioners (1995). *Alcohol and the heart in perspective: sensible limits reaffirmed.* Report of a joint working party. Royal College of Physicians, London.

Sanchez-Craig M (1990). A brief didactic treatment for alcohol and drug-related problems. *British Journal of Addiction* **85**, 169–77. [A guide to condensed cognitive–behavioural therapy for alcohol and other drug problems]

Saunders JB, *et al.* (1993). Development of the Alcohol Use Disorders Identification Test (AUDIT): WHO Collaborative Project on early detection of person with harmful alcohol consumption—II. *Addiction* **88**, 791–804.

Wallace PG, Cutler S, Haines A (1988). Randomised controlled trial of general practitioner intervention in patients with excessive alcohol consumption. *British Medical Journal* **297**, 663–8. [The first and still widely quoted trial showing a clear benefit of brief interventions in general practice]

26.7.3 Problems of alcohol and drug users in the hospital

Carol Ann Huff

Introduction

Alcohol and drug use are two of the most common problems facing physicians and nurses caring for patients in a general medical or surgical unit. It is estimated that up to 25 per cent of adult inpatients have a problem with alcohol or drug use. The implications of this are significant, and many studies have shown that those who abuse alcohol and/or drugs have higher rates of healthcare utilization, more complications, and longer hospital stays. Unfortunately, many of these problems go undetected or are not detected until the patient is in active withdrawal, which complicates their care. When an alcohol or drug use problem is not identified, both physicians and patients miss an important opportunity for counselling and effective early interventions.

There are many reasons why a diagnosis of alcohol or drug abuse may be missed. These include failure on the part of physicians to obtain a complete history of alcohol and drug use, including the quantity and pattern of use of both illicit and prescription medications as well as any personal or family history of substance abuse. Patients contribute to missed diagnoses through denial and minimization of their use of alcohol and drugs, in many cases because they fear social, occupational, legal, and insurance repercussions that may result from the identification of a drug or alcohol problem. These concerns are not unfounded and cannot be fully overcome, but they can be minimized by asking open-ended questions in a non-judgemental and supportive manner.

Central to the success of efforts to deal with those who abuse alcohol or drugs are educational programmes on the nature of addiction and its successful treatment. This in turn leads to the development of a supportive environment, which affords excellent patient care, minimizes ward disruptions, and encourages patients to seek assistance for alcohol or drug-related problems in conjunction with their other medical needs.

Epidemiology

Alcohol and drug use are common problems affecting people of all religions, socioeconomic classes, and geographical areas. Epidemiological studies estimate the lifetime prevalence of alcohol abuse at approximately 13 per cent and problem drug use at 6 per cent. Men are twice as likely as women to develop a drug or alcohol problem. Around 30 per cent of patients with mental illness have a concomitant substance abuse disorder, ranging from approximately 25 per cent in those with anxiety disorders to 50 per cent in those with schizophrenia. Similarly, half of the patients who abuse alcohol or drugs also have a mental illness. Polysubstance use is common and is seen in more than 75 per cent of patients seeking treatment for substance abuse.

It is estimated that more than 50 per cent of accidents and traumas are related to alcohol and or drug use. Many medical illnesses are directly or indirectly related to such use. These include gastrointestinal disorders (for example, bleeding, cirrhosis, and pancreatitis), infectious diseases (for example, pneumonia, human immunodeficiency virus (**HIV**) infection, and hepatitis) and cardiac problems (for example, ischaemia, infarction, and arrhythmias). Patients presenting with these and other medical problems are often the ones in whom a diagnosis of alcohol or drug dependence is not suspected and thus missed entirely, or only made when the patient is in withdrawal.

Clinical features and treatment of intoxications

Alcohol

The clinical picture of alcohol intoxication depends on the rate of ingestion, metabolism, and tolerance of an individual to alcohol's effects. Although legal intoxication is a blood alcohol level of 100 mg/dl, behavioural, psychomotor, and cognitive changes can be seen at levels as low as 20 to 30 mg/dl in those without tolerance. Euphoria occurs at 25 to 50 mg/dl, incoordination at 50 to 100 mg/dl, ataxia at 100 to 200 mg/dl, stupor at 200 to 400 mg/dl, and coma at 400 to 500 mg/dl. Some people become somnolent after modest alcohol ingestion, do not experience euphoria, and therefore rarely abuse alcohol.

The neurological signs of intoxication include slurred speech, impaired coordination, nystagmus, and gait disturbance. Signs of increased sympathetic activity including tachycardia, hypertension, mydriasis, and skin flushing often accompany these changes. Whilst patients may present with what appears to be mere alcohol intoxication, physicians must also be aware of the potential for superimposed problems requiring acute care including hypoglycaemia, subdural haematoma, systemic infections (including aspiration pneumonia), and other ingestions (including methanol, antifreeze, and sedatives).

Alcoholic coma is a medical emergency with a mortality rate approaching 5 per cent. Management requires prompt recognition, careful clinical examination, and an expeditious history, usually from a friend, of the amount and rate of alcohol ingested, as well as any other drugs or medications. If the patient is stuporous or has excessive secretions, he or she should be intubated immediately to provide airway protection and ventilatory support. Once the patient's cardiopulmonary status is stabilized, full investigation—including arterial blood gases, serum chemistries, toxicology screens, and imaging studies—can be undertaken to look for complicating factors when clinically appropriate. Patients may require close monitoring in an intensive care unit with respiratory, cardiovascular, and haemodynamic support and, in some cases, haemodialysis.

Opiates

An opiate overdose can be a life-threatening emergency and requires prompt recognition and institution of therapy. The characteristic signs include varying degrees of clouded consciousness (ranging from somnolence to obtundation), pinpoint pupils, and marked respiratory depression. Aside from protection of the airway, administration of oxygen, and provision of respiratory support as required, treatment involves the administration of an opiate antagonist, usually naloxone. If intravenous access is not available, then this should be administered intramuscularly. The starting dose is 0.2 to 0.4 mg and the onset of action is rapid, typically seen within 2 to 3 min of intravenous administration or 15 min after intramuscular administration. If no response is seen, the dose may be increased. Patients typically respond to doses of less than 2 mg of naloxone, and if the maximum dose of 10 mg is given and the patient has not responded it is unlikely that an opiate overdose is the cause of the problem. The half-life of naloxone is about 90 min, hence re-dosing may be needed, particularly if the overdose is due to a long-acting agent, such as methadone. Pulmonary oedema is often associated with the severe respiratory distress and may improve with restoration of the respiratory drive, but may also require positive-pressure ventilation to fully alleviate it.

Withdrawal syndromes

The clinical features and treatment of withdrawal syndromes are summarized in Table 1.

Alcohol

Clinical features of alcohol withdrawal

Chronic exposure to alcohol leads to upregulation of neural mechanisms within the central nervous system to counteract the depressant effects of alcohol. When the amount of alcohol ingested is diminished or abruptly stopped, these adaptive mechanisms are left unopposed and a hyperexcitable state ensues. This hyperexcitable state can lead to a range of symptoms, from tremulousness and disordered perceptions to seizures and frank delirium, also known as delirium tremens. This spectrum of findings is known collectively as the alcohol withdrawal syndrome.

The first signs of withdrawal begin 6 to 8 h after the alcohol-dependent person's last drink. Tremor is the earliest, most common, and most easily recognized sign. It is coarse, generalized, rapid, and intensified by motor activity and stress. It may be severe enough to interfere with basic motor activities. At this stage, patients are often irritable and complain of nausea and vomiting. In the absence of resumed alcohol consumption or treatment, many go on to develop signs of sympathetic overactivity including diaphoresis, tachycardia, mild hypertension, facial flushing, and increased body temperature. These symptoms peak in intensity between 48 and 72 h and gradually subside by day 4 to 5 unless alcohol consumption is resumed. Anxiety, insomnia, and mild autonomic dysfunction may persist for up to 6 months after alcohol cessation and can predispose some patients to early relapse.

Table 1 Patterns of withdrawal and treatment

Drug options		Onset	Duration	Signs and symptoms	Treatment
Alcohol		6–8 h	4–5 days	Tremor, autonomic instability, seizures, delirium	Benzodiazepines
Opiates					
•	heroin	6–8 h	5–7 days	Nausea, vomiting, diarrhoea, myalgias, bone pain, rhinorrhoea, irritability, intense craving	Opiate replacement Clonidine NSAIDs Dicyclomine Loperamide Lomotil
•	methadone	22–24 h	14–21 days		
Cocaine		30–60 min	72–100 h	Dysphoria, anxiety, insomnia, depression, intense craving	Supportive care; rarely, benzodiazepines
Benzodiazepines					
•	alprazolam	6–12 h	Variable	Irritability, tremor, insomnia, orthostatic hypotension, delirium, seizures	Benzodiazepine substitution, phenobarbitol
•	diazepam	24–48 h	Variable		

Some 25 per cent of patients with tremor and autonomic instability develop perceptual disturbances. These include hyperacusis, vivid nightmares, and, in some cases, auditory hallucinations which peak in intensity 24 to 36 h after alcohol intake is stopped. The auditory hallucinations can last for several weeks and are termed 'alcoholic hallucinosis'. This condition can be distinguished from schizophrenia by its temporal association to alcohol cessation and its lack of recurrence unless drinking is resumed.

Generalized tonic–clonic seizures occur in up to one-third of patients with chronic alcohol dependence when their alcohol ingestion is stopped. The seizures are usually isolated and begin within the first 12 to 24 h of stopping, occasionally they occur in groups of three or four within a 6-hour period. Alcohol withdrawal accounts for 15 per cent of all seizures, and alcoholics who have seizures during one episode of withdrawal are likely to have them during subsequent episodes of withdrawal. The seizures are self-limited and do not require treatment beyond that given to the patient for alcohol withdrawal, unless another cause is found. Only rarely do alcohol withdrawal seizures progress to status epilepticus.

Delirium tremens is the most severe form of alcohol withdrawal and is seen in about 5 per cent of alcoholics. It is characterized by a state of agitated arousal, global confusion, and disorientation. Patients are delusional, have vivid hallucinations, and insomnia. They exhibit signs of sympathetic hyperactivity: fever, tachycardia, mydriasis, and diaphoresis. The onset is 2 to 4 days after alcohol cessation and may be the first sign of withdrawal in a previously unrecognized alcoholic. Patients are terrified, combative, and often destructive. An episode of delirium tremens may last from 24 to 72 h and often ends as abruptly as it starts. Relapses occur and may continue for days to weeks, often with intervening periods of lucidity. Aggressive treatment with benzodiazepines is essential to calm the patient, control his or her behaviour, and ensure that they do not harm themselves or others.

Treatment of alcohol withdrawal

There are three main aspects to the treatment of alcohol withdrawal. First, one must perform a thorough, yet expeditious, evaluation to look for coexisting medical illnesses. This can usually be accomplished through a careful history, physical examination, and selected laboratory studies. Second, one must ensure adequate nutrition. Patients who abuse alcohol often consume most of their daily calories in the form of alcoholic beverages, which contain carbohydrates but are devoid of minerals, protein, and vitamins. As such, most alcoholics are deficient in folic acid, thiamine, pyridoxine, and nicotinic acid and need to have these vitamins replaced. The most important is thiamine and the patient should be given 100 mg a day for 5 to 7 days. The first dose should be given intravenously or intramuscularly to ensure absorption, and later be changed to an oral preparation. In addition to thiamine, patients should be given a multivitamin and folic acid preparation daily for at least 1 week. Thiamine should be given prior to or concurrent with the administration of dextrose-containing fluids, as glucose increases the need for thiamine and may precipitate or worsen a Wernicke's encephalopathy if given to patients who are thiamine-deficient.

The third aspect of treatment is to replace the central nervous system depressant effect of alcohol with a pharmacological agent that can be tapered over 3 to 5 days. There are several drugs that can be used, but benzodiazepines have the highest margin of safety and are therefore preferred. Diazepam and chlordiazepoxide are the most commonly used, in part because of their longer half-lives. Lorazepam or oxazepam are preferred in patients with hepatic dysfunction, as they do not require hepatic metabolism.

Patients with only a slight tremor or minimal autonomic hyperactivity do not require pharmacotherapy. If additional symptoms are present or patients are in moderate to severe distress, a benzodiazepine should be given. The goal of treatment is to keep the patient sleepy, but easily rousable. Each patient's requirements will therefore differ depending on their tolerance, sex, age, and concomitant medical problems. As a general rule, the average male can be managed with diazepam 10 mg four times a day for the first 1 to 2 days, followed by 10 mg twice daily for 2 days, and 10 mg once a day for 2 days. If chlordiazepoxide is used, the average dose is 25 to 50 mg four times a day for 2 days, followed by 20 mg a day for 2 days, then 5 mg a day for 2 days. An individual patient's requirements may differ and can best be determined by frequently monitoring vital signs, symptoms, and mental status. In women, the starting doses are usually reduced by 20 per cent. The goal of early recognition and treatment is to prevent the development of delirium tremens.

Delirium tremens is a medical emergency and should raise suspicion as to the presence of an intercurrent illness, such as pancreatitis, pneumonia, hepatic failure, or a subdural haematoma. It requires an expeditious assessment, followed by the rapid administration of intravenous benzodiazepines. Between 5 and 10 mg of diazepam may be given every 5 to 15 min until the patient is calm. Maintenance therapy is needed every 1 to 4 h after this, and may exceed 200 mg a day for a period of 3 to 5 days. The goal of treatment is to calm the patient without oversedation until the symptoms have passed. Although this syndrome is being increasingly recognized and treated, it still has a reported mortality rate of 1 to 5 per cent, which is usually due to an intercurrent illness.

Carbamazepine is effective in treating mild to moderate alcohol withdrawal, but data are limited on its efficacy in preventing seizures and delirium tremens, and its use is limited by side-effects in up to 10 per cent of patients. Although commonly used in emergency settings, there is a paucity of data to support the use of phenytoin in treating alcohol or drug-withdrawal seizures and thus, if started, it should not be continued beyond 5 to 7 days unless an underlying seizure disorder is identified. Antipsychotic drugs have no role in the treatment of mild withdrawal. They are sometimes used as adjuncts in the treatment of delirium tremens, although caution must be exercised as they can lower the seizure threshold.

Opiates

Clinical features of opiate withdrawal

The onset and duration of withdrawal depends on which opiate the patient is dependent upon. Opiates with short half-lives have a more rapid onset and shorter duration of symptoms than opiates with longer half-lives. Withdrawal from morphine or heroin usually begins 6 to 8 h after the last dose in a tolerant person and lasts 5 to 7 days. Methadone has a half-life of 22 to 24 h and withdrawal begins more slowly and lasts much longer. **LAAM** (L-α-acetylmethadol) has the longest half-life and thus, the longest withdrawal syndrome in the absence of opiate replacement.

Although uncomfortable, opiate withdrawal is not life-threatening. The symptoms are the opposite of the acute effects of the drugs. They include fatigue, anxiety, irritability, and insomnia. Patients complain of abdominal cramping, nausea, vomiting, and diarrhoea. They frequently yawn, experience rhinorrhoea, excess lacrimation, and increased bronchial secretions. Sweating is common, may be profuse, and is often associated with piloerection. Patients complain of bone pain and myalgias and say that they feel as though they have influenza. These symptoms are accompanied by intense craving for opiates. The physical signs of opiate withdrawal include mydriasis and mild elevations in blood pressure, body temperature, and respiratory rate.

Treatment of opiate withdrawal

Many patients with opiate dependence will have attempted self-detoxification without significant success. As such, when these patients are admitted to the hospital, it is best to treat their withdrawal symptoms pharmacologically. This not only alleviates their discomfort, but also improves the ability of the entire healthcare team to treat their presenting problems and to assess their willingness to seek treatment for their substance abuse. Several approaches can be used, including the use of opiate replacement therapy or through the use of non-opiate medications to treat the symptoms of withdrawal.

Opiate withdrawal is most effectively treated by the administration of opiates. This can be accomplished by giving a long-acting opiate such as methadone, or by using an opiate with agonist and antagonist properties, such as buprenorphine. When methadone is used, the principle is to give enough methadone on the first day to alleviate the patient's symptoms and then to decrease the dose by 10 to 20 per cent per day over the next 5 to 10 days. Estimating the amount of methadone that an individual patient needs is difficult, and it is generally best to give a test dose of 10 to 20 mg and monitor the patient's response over the next 1 to 2 h. This ensures that the patient is not overmedicated and also that the symptoms are improving. If not, an additional dose or doses may be given then or 12 h later if symptoms recur. Although there are no special licensing requirements for the use of methadone in hospital patients in the United States, its use in the outpatient treatment of opiate dependence is restricted to licensed facilities. As such, when therapy needs to be continued beyond the length of hospital stay, either for detoxification or maintenance, the patient must be referred to a licensed treatment facility. This makes its use in treating medically ill inpatients challenging, particularly as the length of hospital stays continues to decline.

An alternative approach is to use buprenorphine, an opioid with partial μ-agonist/antagonist properties. As such, it treats the symptoms of opiate withdrawal, and blocks the effects of additional opioid stimulation in a dose-dependent manner. It has poor bioavailability and therefore must be given sublingually or parenterally. Its advantages include less physical dependence, a lower risk of overdose, and a less intense withdrawal syndrome. Its half-life is approximately 3 h. The initial dose is usually 0.3 to 0.6 mg intramuscularly or 2 to 4 mg sublingually, repeated at 6 to 8 h intervals and tapered over 4 to 5 days.

The symptoms of opiate withdrawal can also be managed with non-opiate medications. The α2-agonists, such as clonidine, decrease the sympathetic nervous system overactivity in patients with opiate withdrawal. They decrease the patient's nausea, vomiting, abdominal cramping, and diarrhoea, but do little to alleviate myalgias, back pain, and craving for opiates. Most patients respond to oral doses of clonidine 0.1 to 0.3 mg given every 6 to 8 h for the first 24 to 48 h, followed by a taper over the next 3 to 5 days. Dose-limiting side-effects are orthostatic hypotension and somnolence. Clonidine neither shortens the duration of withdrawal nor prevents relapse.

Symptomatic treatment of abdominal cramps and diarrhoea can be achieved with Lomotil® (diphenoxylate and atropine) or loperamide and dicyclomine. Both diphenoxylate and loperamide are opioids with low addictive potential as they are poorly absorbed from the gastrointestinal tract. Myalgias and bone pain may be treated with non-steroidal anti-inflammatory drugs (**NSAIDs**) such as ibuprofen or naproxen, and rhinorrhoea can be managed with nasal decongestants such as pseudoephedrine. Insomnia should be managed expectantly: the routine use of sedatives is discouraged as they have no specific effect on opiate withdrawal and can also be misused.

Cocaine

Withdrawal from cocaine leads to intense neuropsychological symptoms, including dysphoria and intense cravings for more cocaine. Despite these symptoms, which are often severe, cocaine withdrawal is not life-threatening and has no associated physiological instability. Patients with a long history of cocaine use or recent bingeing may also complain of depression, anxiety, anhedonia, and profound fatigue. Nevertheless, patients can usually be managed with reassurance and supportive care, but may require psychiatric assistance if they are suicidal. On rare occasions, a brief course of benzodiazepine therapy (less than 24 h) may be needed if cravings and anxiety are of an intensity to jeopardize the team's ability to care for the patient.

Sedative/hypnotics

Clinical features of sedative/hypnotic withdrawal

The development of a sedative withdrawal syndrome varies in onset and severity based on the half-life of the drug involved, the degree of dependence, and the duration of daily use. Benzodiazepines are the most commonly prescribed sedatives, and although safer than barbiturate and non-barbiturate hypnotics, they still have the potential for abuse and the development of dependence. Benzodiazepine dependence can occur in as little as a month if higher than usual doses are taken on a daily basis, or after several months when standard doses are used. Withdrawal can therefore be seen in a wide range of patients when these drugs are stopped, including those who are unaware of their physical dependence.

The signs and symptoms of sedative withdrawal are variable and do not always follow a specific sequence in their development. Mild irritability, tremor, diaphoresis, and sleep disturbances are common. Physical findings can include orthostatic hypotension, tachycardia, fever, seizures, and delirium. With long-acting preparations, such as diazepam, the onset of symptoms may be delayed for 24 to 48 h after the drug is discontinued and does not peak in intensity until 5 to 7 days later. Symptoms may appear sooner when a shorter acting agent such as alprazolam is involved. A previously unappreciated sedative dependence may first be recognized 2 to 3 days into a patient's hospital stay, when some or all of the above symptoms and signs appear. Thus, it is important to consider benzodiazepine dependence in patients who are symptomatic, even if a history of benzodiazepine use has not been previously elicited.

Treatment of sedative/hypnotic withdrawal

Treatment of sedative/hypnotic withdrawal requires close medical attention, with monitoring for seizures. Detoxification is best accomplished with sedative substitution and gradual tapering in a controlled setting. As with opiate dependence, it is usually best to substitute an agent with a longer half-life, such as diazepam, clonazepam, or phenobarbital for the sedative of abuse. Each patient's level of dependence needs to be determined by giving a test dose and monitoring the patient's response, rather than relying on the patient's historical reports. Tolerance to the subjective effects of sedatives develops quickly; while tolerance to sedation remains low, unexpected central nervous system depression may occur if too large a dose is given. In the absence of sedation or intoxication, it is likely that the patient's tolerance is higher and indicates that a larger dose will be needed. Once the patient's requirements are determined, the dose is divided and can be gradually reduced over 14 to 21 days. This time course may require extension in patients with severe symptoms or a history of withdrawal seizures.

Pain management in patients with substance abuse disorders

Adequate pain management is an integral component of the successful care of all patients who require admission to hospital. This is particularly true for patients with a concomitant alcohol or drug use problem as they are more likely to sustain traumatic injuries and have a higher rate of medical and surgical illnesses. As pain is primarily subjective, physicians and nurses must rely on the patient's assessment of the adequacy of analgesia. Physical signs such as tachycardia, diaphoresis, and hypertension that are associated with acute pain are neither sensitive nor specific, and thus cannot be relied upon in assessing the adequacy of treatment. This is further complicated in patients with problems of dependence, as these findings may also be signs of withdrawal. The complex behavioural and psychological phenomena associated with addiction can alter the patient's perception of pain, and some studies suggest that patients with alcohol or drug-dependence may have a lower tolerance for pain.

Managing pain in this population can therefore be difficult even for experienced clinicians. Yet, by using a systematic approach, one can make a good assessment of the problem and provide the best chance for a successful outcome, diminishing the chances of developing an adversarial relationship between the patient and the medical staff.

The six steps to consider are listed in Table 2.

1. The first and most important step is to identify the source of the patient's pain and direct primary therapy towards it. Examples of this

Table 2 Acute pain management in a patient with alcohol or drug dependence

1.	Identify aetiology of the acute pain syndrome and direct therapy to the underlying cause
2.	Identify whether the patient has an active or remote history of alcohol/drug abuse, in particular opiates, and whether the patient is receiving methadone maintenance therapy
3.	Institute opiate analgesics for pain control: (a) select an opiate with agonist properties (b) determine dose, dosing interval, and route of administration
4.	Consider non-opioid analgesics: (a) NSAIDs (b) nerve blocks, regional anaesthesia
5.	Anticipate, recognize, and intervene in aberrant behaviour
6.	Utilize a multidisciplinary approach with consultation of appropriate services early: (a) substance abuse (b) psychiatry (c) pain (if available)

include antibiotics and debridement for an abscess and realignment of a broken bone.

2. The next step is to determine whether the patient has a history of active or remote substance abuse. This helps in determining the dose and frequency of analgesia, as those with a history of active opiate use or who are in methadone maintenance programmes are likely to be tolerant to opiates. Physicians should pay close attention to symptoms of anxiety and depression which can not only influence one's perception of pain, but may require concomitant intervention.
3. The third step involves selecting the appropriate opioid analgesic based on a clear understanding of the pharmacology of the agent selected and the person in whom it is to be used. Patients with tolerance will need higher doses at more frequent intervals to achieve the same analgesic effect as those who are not tolerant. Using opiates with both agonist and antagonist properties is generally not a good way to manage acute pain in dependent patients, as these drugs have lower analgesic potential due to difficulty in overcoming their antagonist activity. While patient-controlled analgesia is very useful in the non-addicted patient, its use in those with drug dependence is usually discouraged because of concerns about the 'high' that patients can receive from intravenous bolusing of opiates.
4. The fourth step involves the addition of non-opioid analgesics, including NSAIDs such as ibuprofen, or ketorolac if parenteral administration is needed. These medications can be effective, usually as adjuncts to opiates, in the treatment of acute pain. They are most helpful in cases where dose-limiting toxicities of opiates have been reached without optimal analgesia. Regional nerve blocks should also be considered in the appropriate clinical setting.
5. The fifth step is the recognition and prevention of aberrant behaviour. Patients with an active drug or alcohol problem can frequently have difficulty with limit-setting and, despite optimal medical care and pain management, may continue to seek drugs, either in the form of prescribed medications or through illicit use during their hospital stay. Patients may tamper with intravenous catheters and infusion devices, may attempt to crush oral medications for intravenous administration, or may surreptitiously use illicit drugs or alcohol. These behaviours are unacceptable and clear limits must be set. This is often best accomplished by discussing with the patient what is acceptable behaviour and which behaviours will not be tolerated. Utilization of behaviour contracts, limitation of visitors, and supervised medication administration have all been employed with some success in individual situations.
6. The last step includes early consultation with substance abuse and psychiatric services to assess the patient's readiness for treatment, to encourage change, and to allow for appropriate referrals to aftercare treatment. In using a multidisciplinary approach to the patient's care, the medical and substance use issues can be addressed simultaneously. This is beneficial both to patients and healthcare providers, and is essential when behavioural management becomes an issue.

Summary

Alcohol and drug dependence are common among patients admitted to a general medical or surgical unit. These problems are frequently missed or may not be detected until a patient exhibits physical or psychological signs of withdrawal. As awareness of the problem increases and physicians become more comfortable recognizing and treating them, these problems will differ little from other medical conditions that are commonly encountered in the hospital and clinic settings.

Further reading

Cheskin LJ, Fudala PJ, Johnson RE (1994). A controlled comparison of buprenorphine and clonidine for acute detoxification from opioids. *Drug and Alcohol Dependence* **36**, 115–21. [Demonstrated that buprenorphine and clonidine have similar efficacy in opiate withdrawal, but buprenorphine has fewer side-effects.]

Gossop M (1988). Clonidine and the treatment of the opiate withdrawal syndrome. *Drug and Alcohol Dependence* **21**, 253–9. [Nice review.]

Jaffe JH (1990). Drug addiction and abuse. In: Gilman AG, *et al*, eds. *Goodman and Gilman's the pharmacological basis of therapeutics*, 8th edn, pp 522–73. Pergamon Press, New York.

Lader M, Morton S (1991). Benzodiazepine problems. *British Journal of Addiction* **86**, 823–8.

Mayo-Smith MF for The American Society of Addiction Medicine Working Group on Pharmacological Management of Alcohol Withdrawal (1997). Pharmacological management of alcohol withdrawal. *Journal of the American Medical Association* **278**, 144–51. [A meta-analysis providing evidence-based guidelines.]

Moore RD, *et al.* (1989). Prevalence, detection and treatment of alcoholism in hospitalized patients. *Journal of the American Medical Association* **261**, 403–7. [Demonstrated underdiagnosis of alcohol abuse in hospital patients.]

Portenoy RK, Payne R (1997). Acute and chronic pain. In: Lowinson JH, *et al.*, eds. *Substance abuse: a comprehensive textbook*, pp 563–89. Williams and Wilkins, Baltimore, MD.

Regier DA, *et al.* (1990). Comorbidity of mental disorders with alcohol and other drug abuse: results from the epidemiologic catchment area (ECA) study. *Journal of the American Medical Association* **264**, 2511–18. [Population-based study estimating the lifetime prevalence of alcohol and drug disorders in patients with comorbid psychiatric illness.]

Samet JH, Stein MD, O'Connor PG (1997). Alcohol and other substance abuse. *Medical Clinics of North America* **81**, 831–1075. [Concise review of many aspects of alcohol and drug abuse.]

Smith DE, Wesson DR (1999). Benzodiazepines and other sedative-hypnotics. In: Galanter M, Kleber HD, eds. *Textbook of substance abuse treatment*, pp 239–50. American Psychiatric Press, Washington DC. [Comprehensive review.]

US Department of Health and Human Services (1999). *Results of the 1998 National Household Survey on Drug Abuse.* National Institute on Drug Abuse, Rockville, MD. [National survey of the prevalence of alcohol and drug use.]

27

Forensic medicine and the practising doctor

27 Forensic medicine and the practising doctor

Anthony Busuttil

Introduction

The interface and borders between the law and the medical profession are becoming increasingly wider and more far-reaching, and a doctor has to keep in mind his or her legal responsibilities and duties from the very first day of their practice. Sound ethical principles should form the backbone of professional clinical practice, ensuring competence and integrity of the medical practitioner. The doctor–patient relationship is a partnership based on mutual trust, respect, and confidence with the fundamental rights of every patient being adhered to always and respected fully. These patient rights are succinctly enshrined in the *Declaration of Lisbon* agreed to in September 1981 by the 34th Assembly of the World Medical Association (Box 1).

In addition to dealing with natural illnesses, the services of the medical practitioner, whether in primary care or in hospital practice, are often called upon when injuries and other forms of abuse have taken place, also when death has occurred, particularly if death was sudden and unexpected. As a direct consequence of this, the doctor may acquire information that suggests a suspicious and potentially criminal event. In such instances the doctor's duty of care and bond of confidentiality to the patient must be carefully balanced against his duties as a citizen of a country in which homicide cannot go undetected and crime cannot be condoned.

The courts

It is to be recalled at all times that the system in the courts in Britain, in contrast to other parts of Europe, is very firmly based on the so-called adversarial system, with the sole exception of the HM Coroners' Courts at which an inquisitorial system is in place. In the adversarial system within the criminal courts, the object of the forensic exercise is for those acting for the prosecution on behalf of the State (Her Majesty in England, Wales, and Northern Ireland and the Lord Advocate—or Procurator Fiscal—in Scotland) to prove that the charges laid against the person in the dock (the 'plaintiff' in England and the 'accused' in Scotland) can be proved 'beyond reasonable doubt'. The charges are drafted in terms of alleged contraventions of the Statutes of Criminal Law or of 'common law'. This is a universal system of unwritten law, applied commonly and universally throughout the land, which employs a set of principles, tenets, and maxims that can provide answers to legal problems and can be applied by the judiciary in deciding on cases. Over the years common law has been interpreted and re-moulded by the decisions of one generation of judges after another; these are written down and can be alluded to and quoted in decisions and judgments made by other judges. As a hierarchy of courts developed, thereby enabling an appeal against a decision reached in a lower court to a more senior court, decisions taken by higher courts became binding on lower courts—the concept of 'precedent'. The courts do this by adducing evidence taken under oath or affirmation from witnesses in open court. This enables in minor (summary) cases, the judge, or in serious cases (indictable or solemn cases), the members of the jury (15 in Scotland, 12 in the rest of the United Kingdom) to come to decision. If the verdict is one of 'guilty', the judge will sentence the accused according to tariffs—fines, custodial sentences, community work, etc.—laid down in Statute. The object of the defence is to attempt to cast doubt and demolish the evidence that is being given: they do so through their own witnesses, of which the accused may be one, and by cross-examination of the prosecution witnesses.

The medical practitioner in active employment is usually exempt from jury service but may have to give evidence to fact either as an 'ordinary' witness, like any other citizen, or as a 'professional' witness, by divulging to the court information which he or she has gathered in their professional capacity, for example about injuries, physical or mental illness of the persons in the dock, or other witnesses who have suffered injury. In matters of a scientific and medical nature, when the courts wish to be informed and have explained to them matters which do not fall within the ambit of common knowledge and common sense, persons of a sufficient experience and expertise in the particular subject who can suitably assist may be called as witnesses. By giving information about these matters to the court in this capacity the witness is referred to as an 'expert' (*ex*: from; *peritia*: specialized skill). They are not there to come to a decision on behalf of the court, but solely to assist to the best of their capacity with information, and if required, also to give opinions based on their professional experience and expertise. Details of their qualifications and specialization would be brought to the attention of the courts at the commencement of the expert evidence.

In HM Coroners' courts, whose sole limit is the investigation of death, the questions are asked of all the witnesses by the Coroner, who has to come to a decision at the end of the public 'inquest' as to the identity of the person who has died, when and where they died, and how they came about

Box 1 Declaration of Lisbon

Recognising that there may be practical, ethical and legal difficulties, a physician should always act according to his/her conscience and always in the best interest of the patient. The following Declaration represents some of the principal rights that the medical profession seeks to provide to patients. Whenever legislation or governmental action denies these rights of the patient, physicians should seek by appropriate means to assure and restore them

a. The patient has the right to choose his physician freely.

b. The patient has the right to be cared for by a physician who is free to make clinical and ethical judgements without outside interference.

c. The patient has the right to accept or refuse treatment after receiving adequate information.

d. The patient has the right to expect that his physician will respect the confidential nature of his medical and personal details.

e. The patient has the right to die with dignity.

f. The patient has the right to receive or decline spiritual and moral comfort, including the help of a minister of an appropriate religion.

their death. There is no such office in Scotland, where death investigations are carried out in private by the Procurator Fiscal. There are no public inquests except for deaths in custody and in the course of work as a consequence of the employment; in all other cases the Lord Advocate decides whether 'in the public interest' a 'Fatal Accident Inquiry' is required.

In civil cases one party—persons, or company, or corporate body—sues another party, and the arbiter in almost all such cases is a judge or judges. Both sides can call witnesses, including expert witnesses, to give evidence, and all witnesses can be cross-examined. The only remedy in the civil courts is a pecuniary one, namely the award of monetary damages. The case requires to be proven 'on the balance of probabilities'.

Duties at a death

Death can be said to have occurred in the body of a person when there is either:

- an irreversible cessation of all function of the brain; or
- an irreversible cessation of the circulation of blood.

In this country there is no statutory definition of death as exists elsewhere, for example in the United States or in New South Wales, Australia. There is also no statutory requirement that the diagnosis of the fact of death is invariably made by a doctor; it is however customary that all diagnoses of death are confirmed by a medical practitioner.

When a doctor is called to a person thought to be have died, six principal responsibilities have to be considered (Fig. 1):

1. To confirm the **fact of death** and **document** this at the time.
2. To exclude on medical grounds, where possible, any **suspicions of foul play or negligence** in relation to the death.
3. To identify whether there is a **requirement to report the death** to the appropriate authorities who have a statutory (Her Majesty's Coroners in England, Wales, and Northern Ireland) and/or 'common law' (Procurators Fiscal in Scotland) duty to investigate deaths.
4. To issue a **medical certificate of the causes of death** (commonly referred to as the **Death certificate**) when in a position to do so.
5. If **unable to issue** a Death certificate, to **refer the death to the legal authorities**.
6. If appropriate, and if the medical practitioner is suitably qualified, to issue **other certification** which may be required in relation to the death and the disposal of the decedent.

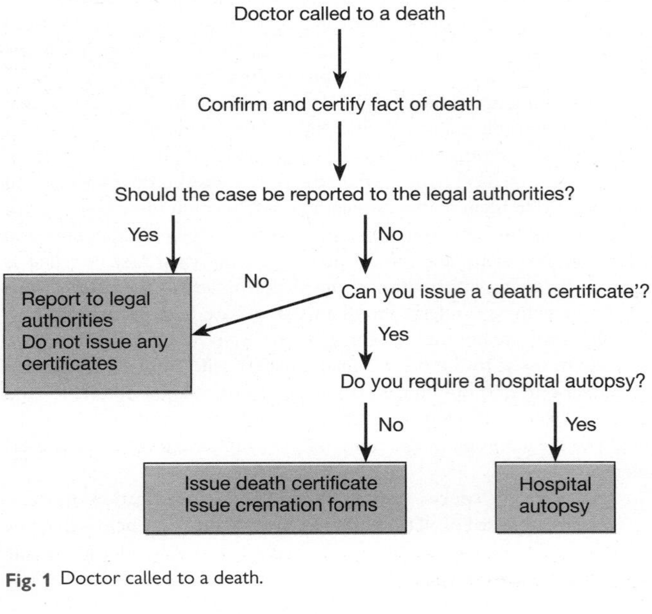

Fig. 1 Doctor called to a death.

Confirming and documenting death

In the recently deceased it is essential that a formal clinical examination is carried out to ensure that the pumping action of the heart and breathing have both ceased. This should be done by auscultation over the chest for a timed period of about 2 min. It is also useful to feel the tension in the eyes, which decreases quite promptly after death (due to a lack of blood pressure) and to look into the pupils, which assume a mid-position: the corneal and light reflexes disappear. If the cornea is still transparent and moist (usually until about 10 min after death if the eyelids were closed) and if in any doubt, it may be useful to examine the eye with an ophthalmoscope: the blood in the retinal veins breaks up into segments within 10 s of clinical death in the majority of instances, a phenomenon variously referred to a 'railroading' or 'cattle-trucking'. In all deaths, there is also blanching of all retinal vessels if the eyeball is pressed with a finger.

In the presence of severe mutilation and burning, or if the body is showing obvious features of decomposition, these tests are obviously superfluous and to carry them out would not be sensible.

Great care must be taken in situations in which vital functions and general metabolism may have been decreased to such an extreme as to simulate death. For a doctor to be caught out in such situations is not only a major embarrassment but may lead to civil action for damages and disciplinary procedures for erroneous certification. Such 'apparent death' or 'suspended animation' can take place in instances where there has been:

- an overdose of CNS depressant drugs
- hypothermia from exposure or medical complaints
- (electrocution)
- (drowning)
- (psychiatric catatonic states).

When in any doubt, particularly when such conditions are present in combination, and particularly in the young, it is always wise to attempt full resuscitation (or 're-animation' as it is referred to in Europe) (see Chapter 16.3).

In all situations when death has been medically confirmed, this must be fully documented on the case notes with the entry timed, dated, and signed. This should be done at the time or as soon afterwards as is reasonable, and the entry should list the clinical tests carried out.

Brain death

The diagnosis of brain death (or 'brainstem death') in patients in an apnoeic coma should be done accurately and positively, even in the presence of a beating heart and machine-maintained respiration, by an appropriately qualified and suitably experienced—at least 5 years' registration—medical practitioner. Tests have to be carried by two doctors and on two occasions several hours apart. Details are discussed in Chapter 16.6.3. In brief:

- Any potentially reversible condition that has led to cerebral depression must be positively excluded. The coma must not be due to CNS depressant drugs, neuromuscular blocking agents (muscle relaxants), hypothermia, or metabolic abnormalities, particularly hypoglycaemia, renal or hepatic failure.

Once all these conditions have been excluded, the simple tests used to confirm that brain death has occurred are that:

- both pupils should be fixed, though not necessarily equal and rounded, and do not react to light;
- no response occurs to corneal stimulation with cotton wool;
- no response is found to the presence of the endotracheal tube or any cough response to suction applied to the tracheal lumen;
- no eye movements occur when 20 ml of ice-cold water are injected into the external auditory meati, having previously established clear access to the ear drums;

- no motor cranial nerve responses are elicited to painful stimuli, e.g. ear-lobe pinching, supraorbital pressure;
- there is no spontaneous breathing with the onset of hypercapnia by disconnecting the respiratory for a sufficiently lengthy period to allow the $Paco_2$ to build up.

If brain death is thus diagnosed, the time when this has been definitively established can be taken as the 'time of death', and not the time that the respiratory support is withdrawn. Any subsequent harvesting of organs will therefore be carried out on a cadaver in whom artificial respiratory and other support has been retained.

The time of death

The actual time of death will always precede the time that 'life is pronounced extinct', and the duration of this period—often referred to as the 'postmortem interval'—is frequently unknown and unknowable. Forensic pathologists are often involved in making estimates of this period by utilizing such phenomena as cooling of the body after death, the onset and distribution of rigor mortis, etc. This is an area fraught with problems and inaccuracies, and one that the non-forensically qualified medical practitioner should best refrain from venturing into and giving any professional opinions on. In those instances where the estimation of the postmortem interval is of specific importance, this matter should be referred to those who are forensically qualified.

Excluding foul play

Doctors, similarly with all other professional persons, have an overriding duty to the 'society' in which they practise, that allows breaches of medical confidentiality when it comes to ensuring that crime is prevented, fully investigated, and detected. Thus, if a medical practitioner suspects or has good reason to believe that a particular death was due to a criminal or negligent act, it is his or her unalienable public duty to ensure that this incident is reported to the police, and that no certification is completed, no matter how obvious the cause of death may be. If the doctor has acted in 'good faith' in such instances, even if their suspicions are eventually found to be unfounded on due investigation, they do not lay themselves open to civil litigation by informing about the death.

No matter the age of the decedent, but particularly so in the elderly and in children, other considerations should not obscure or side-track the doctor from accepting the possibility that death was due to a criminal or negligent act. In this respect, it may be of some importance, as part of the diagnosis of the fact of death, to look carefully for petechial facial haemorrhages in all decedents, particularly around the eyes, behind the ears, on the labial mucosa, and specifically in the conjunctivae. In the absence of known coagulation problems, their presence on the face should always be taken seriously, especially in babies, and if found should always raise the possibility of death being due to a mechanical form of asphyxia, suggesting the possibility of another party's involvement in the death.

Reporting deaths to the legal authorities

Certain categories of deaths are always reportable to the legal authorities. These include all violent deaths, deaths from all types of accidents, including medical mishaps—no matter how long before the death this accident took place, deaths from suicide and suspected suicide, deaths in legal custody and in secure mental institutions, deaths in fires and explosions, from suspected poisoning, from industrial diseases, and from other diseases which by law are notifiable—these include tuberculosis and hepatitis (but not HIV-related deaths). Deaths in which a medical, surgical, or therapeutic mishap may have contributed to or caused the death of the patient always have to be reported.

If the cause of death is not known and yet there is no other reason why the death should be reported, that death is an uncertified death and thus has to be reported. In such instances this notification should precede any attempts to secure an autopsy.

Death certification

This is a privilege accorded to doctors as a consequence of fulfilling the criteria for their registration with the General Medical Council, and thus any misuse or abuse of this principle would render the doctor liable to a disciplinary procedure. The death certificate is an important statutory document and also a very important public health record: it should be filled in carefully and with all due consideration.

The certifier of the Causes of Death does so to 'the best of my knowledge and belief' and records both the immediate causes of death (Part I), these to be placed in a sequence with the initial line (a) being the condition which chronologically resulted from the condition in the second line (b) and so on. Other conditions that have contributed to the death or accelerated it should be listed in Part II of the certificate.

The mode of dying, for example cardiac arrest, cardiac failure, coma, are inappropriate terms to use in this context, except if they are qualified by the underlying causative pathological condition, such as ischaemic heart disease. Terms such as 'senility' and 'old age' should strictly refer to decedents above the age of 80 years, and then only when there was no further recent superimposed pathology. 'Natural causes' is not acceptable. However, it is accepted that in certain instances the determination of the cause of death would have to await laboratory studies, for example overdose deaths, and in such instances a death certificate indicating this may be acceptable.

Reporting to the legal authorities

The bereaved are understandably often in a very distressed state, and great care and sensitivity should be exercised in ensuring that their grief is not made more acute. Any delays in certification would compound such grief, yet the doctor should not feel pressurized, and every effort should be made to follow the rules and regulations strictly. Religious observances and rites, and other social considerations and conventions may also be brought to bear on the doctor. Although the family of the deceased should be heard out with deference and respect, the certifying doctor should not compromise his or her position in any way. If the doctor cannot certify the death or is bound to report it for any other reason, then the case should be referred further.

Consent to a hospital autopsy and to the retention of organs or tissues therefrom can only be sought if the cause of death is known and all other legal requirements have been abided by. This consent should be given in writing by the next-of-kin on the forms designated for this purpose.

Other certification

In the United Kingdom the disposal of the deceased's body by cremation is covered by Statute and Statutory Regulations. For human remains to be disposed of by cremation a series of forms have to be endorsed by medical practitioners. Form B can be signed by any registered doctor and gives details of the death and its causes; form C, a confirmatory certificate, can only be signed by a doctor who has been fully registered for 5 years. Both doctors need to have inspected the body after death, have conferred, and the second doctor needs to have spoken to some other person who had treated, nursed, or been otherwise directly involved in the patient's last illness. The duty of the 'Medical Referee to the Crematorium' is to scrutinize these certificates and the application for cremation (Form A), and if fully satisfied authorize the cremation to proceed. In cases reported to the legal authorities the Coroner or Procurator Fiscal signs the forms that should otherwise have been signed by the two medical practitioners. In all instances, permanent pacemakers and radioactive implants have to be removed prior to cremation.

If the body has to be transported abroad or to other parts of Great Britain, there may be a requirement of further certificates to enable this to take place. These include certificates from the legal authorities enabling the movement of the body outwith their jurisdiction and confirming they require no further access to it, a 'freedom from infection' certificate and often an 'embalming certificate'.

Particular causes of death

Deaths resulting from and in the course of medical care

No matter how vigilant and caring medical and surgical treatment may be, occasional deaths will occur in the course of treatment as a direct consequence of the treatment. This may due to an allergic or idiosyncratic response to medication, and much more rarely through error, such as giving an excessive dose of a drug, or from accidents (for example, intra-arterial versus intravenous injection) and mishaps (for example, internal bleeding after a liver biopsy). For this reason, deaths that occur during operation or in the early postoperative period, deaths during investigative procedures, in the course of the administration of a general or local anaesthetic, or in the progress of clinical trials, invariably become the subject of a legal investigation.

Such deaths in the course of medical care raise the spectre of litigation and claims of medical negligence. There should be absolute transparency in divulging all the facts about such deaths, which should always be investigated by a pathologist who is completely independent of the hospital or other establishment in which the death has occurred, and who has some previous experience in such investigations. The investigating pathologist requires access to all the medical notes of the deceased patient, full statements from the doctors and nursing staff involved, detailing their involvement (disconcertingly, often acquired by the police), a thorough examination of any equipment used, access to batches of drugs used and blood samples collected **premortem**. Such investigations will invariably require the assistance and participation of a number of 'experts' in other fields.

Sudden infant deaths

The careful investigation of death in infancy and childhood has led to major successful prophylactic campaigns; perhaps if unexpected adult deaths were to be looked at as carefully, similar preventive measures could be implemented. These deaths have also led to the production of universally acceptable protocols for postmortem examination that involve photography, radiology, microbiology, virology, immunology, genetics, etc. If this approach were to be emulated in other death investigations, the end-product therefrom would be much enhanced.

As infectious diseases no longer take a major toll in infancy in most developed countries, and as serious congenital conditions are no longer as prevalent, the most important cause of the sudden death of infants after the first month of life and within the first year is the 'sudden infant death syndrome' (**SIDS**, sometimes referred to as 'cot death' or 'crib death'). The original definition, still applicable, is of 'sudden death of any young child that is unexpected by the history, and in which a thorough post mortem examination fails to demonstrate an adequate cause of death'. Most pathologists would also wish to have a thorough inspection of the scene of the death to exclude potentially noxious environmental agents, for instance carbon monoxide exposure.

The diagnosis of SIDS is therefore only made by carefully and meticulously excluding any other causes, and is a morbid anatomical diagnosis rather than a clinical one; an autopsy is therefore a *sine qua non* to reach this diagnosis. It is especially important to exclude congenital metabolic abnormalities such as medium-chain acyl coenzyme A dehydrogenase (**MCAD**) deficiencies by appropriate testing (plasma/blood spot acylcarnitine profiles in MCAD deficiencies) and thus alert the family to possible further recurrences. Trauma and poisoning by alcohol, or with other sedative or anxiolytic preparations, also have to be excluded specifically on appropriate autopsy samples; the 'Münchhausen syndrome by proxy', first described by Meadow in 1977, is another condition to be aware of.

The incidence of SIDS has decreased dramatically in many industrialized countries as a result of major public health educational campaigns advising parents about the risk factors and means of prevention. Overheating of the child is one such risk factor. Parents are instructed to prevent this by removing the child's headgear when indoors, and by ensuring that the sleeping child does not wear excessive clothing or has too many bedclothes, by preventing the ambient bedroom temperature from being too high, and by seeking medical advice when the child appears feverish. The dangers of cigarette smoking close to the baby have also been emphasized as an important risk factor for this and other childhood complaints. The 'back-to-sleep' campaign, that is ensuring that the child is placed in the prone sleeping position, is based on another epidemiologically established important risk factor. Paradoxically, immunization of the child for common childhood illnesses, once thought related to SIDS, has been shown to be protective and is thus further encouraged in this connection.

The actual pathogenetic cause of SIDS is still uncertain in the majority of instances: hypoxia, cardiac arrhythmias, hypoglycaemia, loss of vascular tone, reflex apnoea, and heat shock have all been proposed, as well as the 'superantigen' effects of bacterial toxins. Other important aspects of the epidemiology of this condition is the seasonal incidence, the familial recurrence, the increased incidence in boys, and the increased association with certain ethnic groups, such as Native Americans and Australian Aborigines, and its absence in others, for example immigrant families from the Indian Subcontinent. The pathognomonic feature of SIDS, which is yet to be explained, is the finding of diffuse, internal petechial haemorrhages overlying the thymus and beneath the pleura and the pericardium.

Sudden unexpected nocturnal deaths in adults

The syndrome of sudden unexpected nocturnal deaths (**SUND**) occurs in young adults and adolescents, mainly in immigrant workers from SE Asia employed in Singapore and Saudi Arabia, and in refugees from the Far East. These decedents are usually employed in manual jobs in the building or the gardening trades, and have been residing in their adoptive country for several months. They are almost exclusively males who smoke or who are passively exposed to smoke in their environment, and who have a recent history of a mild upper respiratory tract infection; petechiae may also be found internally. These deaths mostly occur during sleep and at night.

Various theories have been put forward, including vitamin B and other nutritional deficiencies, familial cardiac arrhythmias, brainstem epilepsy, *Pfeifferinella mallei* infection, stress and homesickness, bacterial toxin production from nasopharyngeal colonization by *Staphylococcus aureus,* but no specific and recurring cause has been identified.

It is also the case that a full autopsy, with comprehensive toxicological and histological investigations, in the occasional sporadic death of an adolescent native of this country fails to yield a cause of death. Such deaths have been labelled as 'deaths from SUND' in Great Britain. However, it must be kept strictly in mind that this diagnosis is also one of exclusion, and should be used sparingly and appositely.

Survivors of violence

Sexual assaults

Over the last few decades the police have appropriately received positive and favourable publicity regarding the manner in which they deal with the survivors of alleged sexual abuse, and investigate their formal complaints. This has enabled more of those who have been abused in this manner to come forward and report the abuse suffered. In spite of this, however, it is not infrequent that the first disclosure of such abuse, particularly abuse which had occurred some time previously—on occasions, several years earlier—is initially made to a doctor in the course of a confidential consultation, perhaps on a totally unrelated matter. The medical practitioner is thus placed in a situation in which they are party to highly confidential and sensitive information relating to a potentially very serious crime, whose investigation requires careful and specialized investigation. This requires the careful interviewing of the survivor of this crime, the description of general and genital injuries, the meticulous collection of trace evidence, and of course the presentation of all this expertly in the criminal courts.

In this situation—as in many other similarly problematic circumstances—the doctor has to determine for himself whether or not, in the eyes of the law, the person disclosing abuse has full competence to take decisions. In Scotland and the rest of the United Kingdom, the legal age above which legally valid consent to medical treatment can be given is 16 years. If the patient is competent in terms of age and of mental and physical faculties, then in all such instances the doctor must firmly put to them the option of immediately involving the police. The police are much more knowledgeable about the process of investigation of allegations of sexual abuse and better equipped for the purpose than any medical practitioner is likely to be. If after due consideration the patient does not wish to inform the police for any or no reason, then patient confidentiality must be maintained.

All efforts should be made to ensure that any problems related to possible sexual abuse are adequately dealt with, including any worries that the patient may have about the possibilities of an unwanted pregnancy, sexually transmitted diseases including HIV infection, and the physical and mental trauma sustained. If the police are brought into the picture, the patient may still require some further support.

In Scotland, below the age of 16 years, the consent by a minor is only competent if in the view of the particular medical practitioner that patient fully understands the implications of the treatment being offered, and this consent can be extended to consent to medical procedures. Elsewhere, medical decisions of all types are also governed by the child's understanding of the proposed line of action or procedure—referred to as '*Gillick*-competence' in the United Kingdom. If the consent to involve the police is not forthcoming from a minor, then the doctor has to decide whether in the interest of the particular young patient, this decision should be overruled, and perhaps whether those with parental responsibility for the child are to become involved at this stage. This decision-taking tightrope has to be negotiated very carefully, with the best interests of the patient always paramount and with the medical practitioner acting 'in good faith'. Advice from more senior colleagues, from forensic medical practitioners, and from the medical defence unions is often invaluable in such instances.

In the case of young children who are 'not-legally competent', appropriate multidisciplinary guidelines have been put together by every health authority and health board. In these a close co-operation between the health services, the police, the education department, and the social work department forms the basis of the investigation and further management of these cases. These guidelines should be adhered to strictly.

If the police are not involved it may be very difficult to collect evidence that would stand up in a court of law. If the doctor is inexperienced in such examinations then their competence and expertise will be called into serious question by the courts in any eventual adversarial criminal court case; a gynaecological or surgical colleague may have to be involved. For instance, the taking of swabs for seminal fluid analysis may fall short in terms of the unbroken continuity of the chain of evidence and the exclusion of cross-contamination that the courts would always require. These difficulties should be brought specifically to the attention of any patient who is reluctant to involve the police.

Another way to ensure that any physical evidence of injury to the genital area is recorded permanently at the time of the medical examination is to utilize videocolposcopy, as is now almost invariably performed in examinations of this type in prepubertal children to avoid problems with second examinations and nuances of varying interpretations.

It is a fact of life that a very significant number of prosecutions initiated in sexual assaults fail to produce a conviction. By the very nature of this crime, these incidents are usually perpetrated in private with no eye-witnesses to the event. It often boils down to the oral evidence given in court by the two parties, and to which of the two, tested by cross-examination, the members of the jury are prepared to accept.

The medical notes

On the principle that contemporaneous recording will always provide good evidence in court, and in many cases that will be the best evidence, it is essential that all members of staff keep regularly annotated and thorough medical notes that are adequate, comprehensive, and comprehensible. Conciseness is not an issue at all in these instances: the notes made may be telegrammatic, provided that they convey all that has transpired on that occasion in terms of how the patient was dealt with and managed.

It is important to record dates and timings, to ensure that each page bears the name of the patient (or a 'sticker' bearing their details).

In those patients who allege assault, or have been otherwise injured, the manner and method of presentation, as well as the triage procedures all have to be documented in full. It may be said that some of these issues are normally attended to by other clerical staff; however, it does no harm when urgency and the vagaries of practice has put the system out of kilter, and indeed sometimes saves the day, for the doctor to record such important details, or at least ensure that they have been properly recorded.

The narrative given of the presenting complaint should be carefully recorded at the time, and what is even more important, it is essential to document who gave the initial information that has found its way on to the notes. If it is the ambulance crew or the accompanying relative or police officer from which you obtained this information, indicate so, as this renders it second-hand or 'hearsay information' in a forensic context. If the patient has given you specific details about how their injuries were acquired, transcribe these into text. In cases that may end up in court it is important not to attempt to précis, filter, or alter the information as originally given, perhaps in an attempt to make it sound more plausible and coherent: it should be documented as it was imparted to the doctor at the time.

Always indicate the findings on clinical examination. State what you did and when, and the investigations that were carried out by you (for example, blood pressure, peritoneal lavage), or asked for, either at the accident and emergency department itself (such as breath testing for alcohol, urinalysis for blood), and/or elsewhere (such as blood gases, serum electrolytes). It is also important to ensure that when the reports of such tests are available that these are also quoted in the notes, even if this information has been given to you over the telephone.

If radiographs have been ordered, make sure that in addition to your own viewing thereof and a recording of the diagnosis made by you on your personal 'reading' of them at the time, that the films are also subsequently reported on by the radiology department. These reports will serve as confirmation of your diagnosis and should always find their way into the patient's notes. For instance, it is of little assistance if you believe that there was a fracture of the maxilla or of the nasal bones, both clinically and on radiography, but this has not been confirmed anywhere in the notes in an 'official' radiological report.

If there has been a referral to other units (for example, neurosurgery, maxillofacial surgery, or burns units), this must also be recorded, preferably with a copy of the letter of referral. Consultations with other colleagues, for instance the physicians on call, the otorhinolaryngological specialist registrar, should be fully documented for any future reference.

Describing wounds

It is absolutely essential that wounds in injured persons are carefully described in the medical notes. This holds true whether the presentation is in hospital or in primary care. Domestic violence is on the increase, and the setting up of primary care-manned units in the community is becoming more frequent. It is not a valid excuse to claim that because the doctor to whom the patient presented initially was not an accident and emergency doctor, there was no obligation on them to record appropriate details. (See Box 2.)

A wound in the medicolegal sense is any traumatically induced abnormality, and this ranges from erythema to abrasion to cuts through the skin or mucous membranes to any internal injury.

Box 2 Wounds

In a systematic way:

For each wound:

1. Define the wound.
2. Locate the wound in relation to fixed anatomical points.
3. Measure the wound (with its edges in apposition).
4. Describe its edges, its immediate surroundings, and its floor.
5. Describe the wound in terms of its orientation or pattern.
6. State whether recent or old.
7. Discuss its severity, either individually or collectively.
8. Record the baseline general physiological parameters of the patient, e.g. pulse rate, blood pressure, respiratory rate, Glasgow Coma Scale.
9. Consider sketching the wound freehand or on a line diagram.
10. Consider photographing the wound.

For each external 'wound', describe its shape (vertical, transverse, lozenge-shaped), and its exact location—the latter by reference to standard fixed anatomical sites (for example, suprasternal notch, the prominence of the seventh cervical vertebra), and not variable ones such as the nipple or the umbilicus.

The wound should be measured with some degree of accuracy, and if the wound happens to be oriented in any particular manner, this should also be recorded; similarly document any collar of abrasion and bruising around it, and any pattern in the wound itself.

In forensic practice, trivial wounds that may not require any active treatment may be as important as those that are more serious. Abrasions in the form of fingernail scratches may be as important as any full-thickness lacerations that may be coexistent on the same patient. Therefore try to refer to all wounds in your description.

Be careful to define each wound appropriately. By definition, a laceration indicates a wound with very irregular (and perhaps bruised) edges, and the presence of bridging of incompletely damaged tissue in its base. Furthermore, a laceration, again by definition, is also a wound caused by a blunt-force injury—that is to say a force that has stretched the skin excessively, and more usually over a bony point or surface, causing the elasticity of the epidermis and dermis or of a mucosal surface (such as the lip, the vagina, or anus) to be so exceeded that, as a consequence, there is splitting and tearing apart of the skin or mucosa at the site of application of the force.

A sharp and pointed object will produce an incision or an incised wound with clean-cut straight undamaged edges. However, it is often impossible to indicate what specific weapon did cause the injury; for example, a sharp shard of glass, a kitchen knife, and the sharp edge of a tin can all produce incised wounds which look identical, even to someone with plenty of experience in wound interpretation. In the case of lacerations and bruises the difficulty may be even more pronounced. All that one would be able to say with any degree of accuracy is that among other objects that could have produced the wound, its appearances are consistent with having been produced by the particular weapon that is being suggested.

If there is a penetrating stab wound, it is essential to record the length of the wound track after it has been probed or explored, also to what depth the wound has extended, and, if this has been identified, which direction the track leads away from the skin. If the wound has penetrated beyond the skin, it would be important to denote which layers have been breached.

Although it may prove impossible to record individually all the wounds sustained, the use of simple line-drawings with the inclusion thereon of brief comments may be very effective.

Also recall that fractures, dislocations, and internal injuries fall under the category of wounds in this context. Any foreign bodies which have been retrieved from wounds, no matter how banal they may look (for example, grit, glass), may have very important evidential value and should never be discarded.

Wounding in the legal context

The legal practitioner, when looking through descriptions of wounds, often has different priorities and different questions from medics in their mind. Occasionally, these may not be immediately apparent or deemed relevant by the medic, but these queries may be expressed in writing or in court. Samples of such questions include: 'How much force was required to produce the wound under review?'; 'Could the particular wound have been inflicted accidentally, or as part of a self-defence type of response by the patient to an assault on him?'; 'Was the wound inflicted by a right-handed or left-handed assailant?'; 'Were all the wounds inflicted in the course of one assault?'

It is the counsel of perfection only to answer such questions if one feels experienced and fully competent to so do. An off-the-cuff remark on such matters that cannot be substantiated on robust cross-examination may cost dearly in lost face, and perhaps even in reputation, in the witness box.

It is important to be very circumspect about the ageing of wounds; inter-individual variation is such that one can only provide general answers to questions on this matter. If a wound is showing healing as demonstrated by scabbing, then it will be about 2 days old, and one which is scarred almost a week old, but statements must be as general as that. Ageing of bruises is particularly fraught, in that the colour change that can be seen as the haemoglobin that has extravasated into tissues is changed to bilirubin and biliverdin, depends on a number of variable local and systemic factors.

Of specific importance to the criminal justice system are also such matters as the severity of the wound in question, and whether a particular wound could be considered as being life-threatening. On the basis of the 'soil and seed' concept, severity should be assessed by the damage produced by the trauma, the amount of blood lost, the degree of surgical shock present; also on the amount of days lost from work, the age of the patient, associated medical conditions that decrease the rate of healing, the ease with which it could be dealt with medically, etc. Indeed, any answers to questions about severity should always be predicated by a series of reasons indicating why the opinion given is being proffered. In doing so it may be useful to distinguish between whether or not the particular wound is 'serious' and 'life-threatening', or whether wounds in that specific anatomical location (for example, neck, anterior chest wall) in general terms are serious and life-threatening. For example, a penetrating stab wound of the chest may not have actually produced a pneumothorax, but had it been slightly deeper or its track slightly more medial or more lateral it could have: thus within these caveats, the wound can be considered as serious and potentially life-threatening. The fact that a particular injury can be salvaged with relative ease in a hospital does not necessarily detract from its degree of severity. Any inevitable or avoidable delay in seeking or obtaining medical help, any intervening wound infection, etc., should also be listed to enable a more balanced assessment of wound severity.

The after-effects of the wounding are also of importance. Any scarring left behind by the wounding, which may be considered as cosmetically disfiguring, even if surgical in origin, can increase the 'legal' severity of the wound, and similarly any residual pain and stiffness of an injured joint.

Photographs of injury

Photographs of wounds may be extremely useful if in due course the case comes to a court hearing: pictures taken prior to stapling or suturing may clearly convey to a jury more poignantly the degree and variety of injury sustained. This may require close co-operation with the police, and above all the 'informed' consent of the patient, if at the time they are in a state in which they are legally capable (*capax*) to give this. If the patient is unconscious and the case is very likely to have been the result of criminal violence, there should be close co-operation with the police. If the management of the patient will not suffer adversely, any reasonable requests for photography made by the police should be considered—even if only a Polaroid—

and if at all possible acquiesced to. In all such instances there must always be a careful and considered balance between one's professional obligation as a medical practitioner to provide optimal care and confidentiality for the patient, and one's duty as a citizen of a country in which violence cannot be condoned and for which its perpetrators are brought to justice in the course of a fair trial.

Photographs of wounds after they have been debrided and sutured may not be as useful as photographic documentation prior to such treatment, but they are better than nothing. Patterned injuries which may have to be matched to other weapons (for example, footwear imprints, imprints from blows) may need to be photographed in black and white, in colour, and under different light sources (such as ultraviolet light). If photography cannot be used for any reason, then consider sketching the wound freehand or use anatomical outline drawings to indicate the location and appearances: this will also economize on text.

Human bites

On occasions, human bites may be the presenting injuries. In these instances photography may be essential, and furthermore, valuable information can be gained from appropriately thorough and specialized examination. There may be enough material on the skin to secure a DNA profile of the perpetrator, and an odontological opinion may be able to produce a dental chart of the offending jaws for matching purposes. This cannot be done without the involvement of the police at an early stage, and, as always, the patient's own informed consent would be required.

Intoxication

Alcohol tends to feature prominently in persons who have been assaulted or accidentally injured, and it may be useful for the purposes of the courts to document the degree of intoxication observed in the victims or in the perpetrators. Although 'alcohol' can often be smelled on the breath, it must be remembered that it is not ethanol that is being picked up, but congeners such as esters and other organic compounds that have been consumed together with the alcohol. As with alcohol, these are excreted for a lengthy period after drinking has stopped.

Alcohol is absorbed from the upper gastrointestinal tract, mostly the duodenum, and disseminated uniformly and in an unimpeded fashion throughout all body compartments that contain water. Hence, the amount of water in the body, which relates to body weight and to gender, will influence the eventual concentration and therefore the effects of the alcohol consumed. Typically, the consumption of 1 pint (568 ml) of ordinary beer or a double public-house measure (about 55 ml) of spirits (40 per cent (v/v)—alcohol concentration) will result in a blood alcohol (ethanol) concentration of 30 mg of alcohol per 100 ml of blood, or 13 μg of alcohol per 100 ml of breath. The corresponding legally prescribed limits for driving in Britain are 80 mg for blood and 35 μg for breath.

One should only carry out a formal blood alcohol estimation if this has potential therapeutic indication, and then only with the knowledge and consent of the patient. Alcohol is a CNS depressant and the effects of alcohol intoxication can be elicited by tests of neuromuscular coordination and of higher central functions, including the Glasgow Coma Scale. The eyes will also show evidence of sustained lateral nystagmus and the pupils will be dilated.

In those who may be under the influence of 'controlled substances', with or without additional alcohol intoxication, a full neurological examination should be carried out and recorded. However, it is often unhelpful and profligate to carry out urinary or blood tests for the presence of drugs.

Access to information

The same rules of medical confidentiality apply wherever the patient is seen. Relay of information to others has to be carefully controlled. The police frequently seek information, either acutely and/or after the patient has been discharged. It is therefore important that some basic rules are laid down, enabling the police to know what information will and what will not be divulged to them, without the patient first having been approached and their formal consent obtained.

In terms of statute in the United Kingdom, the police have every right to ask for full details of those persons whom they believe have been driving a 'mechanically propelled vehicle' which has been involved in a collision, and who have been admitted to hospital. Similarly, in relation to acts of terrorism, the police have a right to obtain information. In other instances it is a question of whether, in terms of their inquiries, information should be divulged to police officers who are seeking it. The admission of a person who is likely to die (or as they would put it, 'a condition that is likely to prove fatal'), whether this is the result of an accident or a criminal assault, is cause enough to bring information to the attention of the police.

If the patient or their legal representative requests a copy of the medical notes, this legitimate request cannot be refused unless it can be shown—if need be to the scrutiny of a Crown Court judge (or a Sheriff, in Scotland)—that disclosure of the notes may disclose the identify of a third party or be detrimental to the physical and/or mental heath of that particular patient. Barring this, such records should be handed over: staff in local hospital medical records' departments are trained to deal with such requests appropriately.

The forensic use of molecular biological techniques—DNA profiling evidence

DNA-based evidence has revolutionized forensic practice over the last few years. Based on the principles that all cells of an organism are derived from one fertilized ovum, and that mitotic division of cells is uniform and precise, all cells inside an organism that contain a nucleus retain an identical DNA content. Thus, DNA from hair, buccal cells, semen, and white blood cells derived from the same individual is identical, and it is possible to determine the exact origin of a particular cell or group of cells if their DNA can be matched to that of some other cells of the same origin. Furthermore, as half of a cell's DNA has originated from each of the parents, it is also possible to derive the genetic origin of a particular cell by comparison of its DNA content with that of its parents.

Variable number of tandem-repeat loci

Groups of DNA loci that are used extensively in forensic analysis are those counting variable numbers of tandem repeats (**VNTR**). These are not genes, since they do produce any known product, and those used in forensic analysis have no known biological role. They are thus less likely to be influenced by natural selection, which can lead to different frequencies in different populations. A typical VNTR region contains 500 to 10 000 base pairs, containing many tandemly repeated units, each 15 to 35 base pairs in length. The exact number of repeats, and hence the length of the VNTR, varies from one allele to another, and different alleles may be identified by their relative lengths. VNTRs have a very high mutation rate, leading to changes in their length, with an individual mutation usually resulting in a change in length by only one or a few repeating units. This leads to a very large number of alleles, often 100 or more, no one of which is common, although only 15 to 25 can be distinguished practically. This means that the number of possible pairs of alleles forming the genotype at a locus is considerable, and given that testing of several different such loci can be combined, the total number of genotypes becomes enormous. For example, for n alleles there are n homozygous genotypes and $n(n-1)/2$ heterozygous ones, in other words: if $n = 20$, there are a total of 210 genotypes, and if four loci are examined with 20 alleles each, then 210^4 or about 2 billion genotypes are possible (assuming that all four alleles are inherited independently).

The main uses of the DNA profiling method in forensic cases are:

1. The identification of crime suspects from trace evidence left behind at the scene, e.g. a specimen of blood from the deceased is found to match stains on the clothing, etc. of the accused person.
2. The elimination of crime suspects in crimes where there has been deposition of body fluids, e.g. the DNA profile of the seminal sample taken from the vagina of the victim does not match that obtained from the white cells of the peripheral blood of the alleged perpetrator of the rape.
3. Paternity testing, when it is necessary to establish which one of two or more males is the actual biological father of a particular child, e.g. in incest or rape cases. Fetal tissue is also suitable for such testing (and is often used).
4. Identification of an unknown person or of unknown mutilated human remains, by comparing material taken at postmortem examination with material, such as hair or blood, which is authenticated as belonging to a particular person during life. This has been extended to buried remains, e.g. the Romanovs, Mengele.
5. Mass disasters—this technique assists with the identification of individuals provided a premortem sample is available for comparison, and has the ability to match together different and separated parts of the same body.
6. Mass screening ('a genetic man-hunt') of a well-circumscribed population from which the murderer or rapist is known to have originated. This was the first use of DNA profiling in a criminal context in the United Kingdom.
7. DNA databases—allowing crimes committed by the same perpetrator in which body fluids have been deposited at the site of the crime to be associated, i.e. serial crimes and previous offenders to be linked with a specific 'new' crime, or resolution of historical unsolved cases.
8. Disputed maternity, e.g. in cases of infanticide and child destruction, when it requires to be proven that a particular child is indeed the offspring of a particular woman.
9. Settlement of immigration problems in relation to the admission into a country of blood relatives rather than 'friends'.

In the civil courts, DNA profiling has also been proving useful in such cases as:

(1) divorce (associated with alleged adultery);
(2) disputed paternity (and more rarely maternity): in settling estates after death;
(3) in immigration disputes (when a country only allows entry of certain closely related relatives, born outside that country, of newly established residents);
(4) in disputed pedigrees of animals and origins of biological material.

The forensic applications of DNA profiling are not universally available, and therefore these tests are yet to completely replace and supplant conventional blood grouping methods involving the ABO and isoenzyme (for example, **PGM** (phosphoglucomutase)), systems. In some countries such as the United Kingdom and Switzerland this has already taken place.

The important limitation of DNA profiling is the amount of DNA-containing material available for carrying out the appropriate testing. This is particularly the case when dealing with peripheral blood: only the leucocytes within it that can be of assistance, meaning that a substantial quantity of these cells must be available.

Polymerase chain reaction techniques

In 1987 the polymerase chain reaction (**PCR**) technique was introduced, enabling the rapid and specific, *in vitro*, enzymatic amplification of DNA fragments. This laboratory synthesis utilizes a heat-stable enzyme, DNA polymerase (formerly obtained from a thermophilic bacterium found in hot natural springs and called '*Thermus aquaticus*'—thus '*Taq* polymerase'). The other essential reagents are primers, which are small complementary fragments of single-stranded DNA, also produced artificially. With the correct reaction conditions, a pair of primers can be made to attach themselves to single complementary strands of DNA, and in the presence of an excess of bases in the solution, marshal the formation of replicas of the original DNA fragments. Repeated reaction cycles can be conducted until sufficient quantities of the product are formed to enable standard DNA profiling techniques to be carried out.

The PCR technique is so sensitive that even a very small amount of tissue, such as a single hair root, a single buccal cell, or a single spermatozoon, may be sufficient to produce a DNA profile that is adequate for matching purposes. It can also amplify denatured DNA, and even material from paraffin-embedded histology blocks and formaldehyde-fixed tissue is suitable for replication.

Very strict control of laboratory technique is required in conducting PCR procedures as any minute amount of DNA present in the sample will be replicated. Controls are of the essence in demonstrating the absence of contamination. Protective clothing is necessary when evidence is being collected at scenes of crime, as is careful attention to detail in terms of the collection of material for DNA analytical procedures.

HLA-DQα

A further development is related to one of the genes that controls transplant rejection, *DQA*, coding for a protein HLA-DQα that shows substantial variation in its base sequence from one individual to another. The most variable fragment of this gene may be readily amplified by PCR to distinguish eight different alleles, of which six are used in forensic practice, and thus 21 different combinations of two alleles—6 homozygous and 15 heterozygous. In practice, a reverse blot is used, with the nylon membrane containing preattached probes specific for the individual alleles, making a quick, reliable, and very useful preliminary test if one is required. On average the DQα profile of a person is identical with that of about 7 per cent of the population.

Mitochondrial DNA

Mitochondrial DNA contains a segment called the control region, which is highly variable and has the following additional properties:

1. This DNA can survive in extensively decomposed tissues.
2. It can be successfully amplified, even from the most unpromising tissues such as bones.
3. It is strictly maternally inherited.

Analysis of mitochondrial DNA has been used most frequently in looking at historical cases, and in instances where nuclear DNA is in short supply or where it has been denatured by, for example, contact with soil and the bacteria therein.

Other advances

Microsatellites or short tandem-repeat loci (STRL)

Microsatellites are much shorter than the minisatellites (VNTRs) and comprise 2- to 4-base pair repeats only. They are very common, are distributed widely throughout the genome, and can be amplified singly or together by PCR. Individual specificity can be achieved by typing several loci sequentially. The method can be used with severely decomposed and burnt bodies, using the DNA from a portion of spared voluntary muscle or red bone marrow.

Amplitype polymarker (PM) DNA

This method analyses several loci simultaneously: **LDLR** (low-density lipoprotein receptor), **GYPA** (glycophorin A, the MN blood groups), **HBGG** (haemoglobin gammaglobulin), D7S8 (an anonymous genetic marker on chromosome 7), and **GC** (group-specific component). Each has two to three alleles per locus.

Minisatellite repeat mapping or digital typing

This analyses for length variation and detects sequence differences within the base sequences repeated in VNRTs.

DNA identikit

In the future it may be possible to describe physical (for example, blue eyes, red hair) or other characteristics of a subject from their DNA sequence, thereby obtaining hints as to their actual identity.

Estimation of the population frequency of a DNA pattern

DNA 'exclusions' are easy to interpret: if technical artefacts can be excluded, a non-match is definitive proof that two samples have come from two different sources. However, 'DNA inclusions' cannot be interpreted without knowledge of how often a match might be expected to occur in the general population at random. In simple terms, if two DNA profiles match then there are two logical possibilities: first, that the DNA profile at the scene, on clothing, etc. is actually that of the suspect; and second, that it comes from someone else who has the same profile as the suspect. The commoner the particular DNA profile, the greater is the likelihood that it could come from someone other than the suspect; by contrast, if the suspect's profile happens to be a rare one, then the chances of this are much less likely. Thus the frequency of a particular profile in a particular population must be known to enable this comparison.

The statistical analysis of profiling data has caused problems to the courts: judiciary, jurors, and lawyers alike. Population frequencies of various profiles have been established, a standard method being to count occurrences in a random sample of the appropriate population and then to use classical statistical formulas to place upper and lower confidence limits on the estimate. Because estimates used in forensic science should avoid placing undue weight on incriminating evidence, an upper confidence limit of the frequency should be used in court, which is appropriate in the forensic context because any loss of power can be offset by studying additional loci.

The product rule should be used to estimate the frequency of a particular DNA profile frequency. If the race of the particular individual is known, the database for that particular race should be used; if not, calculations for all prevalent racial groups should be used. The probability that two randomly chosen individuals have a particular phenotype is the square of its frequency in the population. The probability that two randomly chosen persons have the same unspecified genotype is the sum of the squares of the frequencies of all the genotypes. If there are n loci, and the sum of the squares of the genotype frequencies at locus 1 is $p1$, then the exclusion power is (1 minus ($p1$, $p2......pn$)).

Population frequencies that are quoted for DNA purposes are not based on actual counting but on theoretical models based on principles of population genetics. Each matching allele is assumed to provide statistically independent evidence, and the frequencies of the individual alleles are multiplied together to calculate a frequency of the complete DNA pattern. Although a databank might contain only 500 persons or less, multiplying the frequencies of enough separate events might result in an estimation frequency of their all occurring in the same person of $1{:}10^9$. However, the scientific validity of this multiplication rule depends on whether the events are actually statistically independent. In organizing databanks it is essential that ethnic groups are considered separately, and in the United Kingdom databanks for Caucasian, Afro–Caribbeans, Indians, Pakistanis, Chinese, etc. have yet to be established.

Further reading

Aitken CGG (1995). *Statistics and the evaluation of evidence for forensic scientists.* Wiley, Chichester.

Balarajan R, Reileigh VS, Botting B (1989). Sudden infant death syndrome and post neonatal mortality in immigrants in England and Wales. *British Medical Journal* **298**, 716–20.

Balding DJ, Donnelly P (1994). How convincing is DNA evidence? *Nature* **368**, 285–6.

Beckwith JB (1970). Discussion of terminology and definition of the Sudden Infant Death Syndrome. In: Bergman AB, Beckwith JB, Ray GC, eds. *Proceedings of the Second International Conference on the Causes of Sudden Death in Infancy,* pp 14–22. University of Washington Press, Seattle, WA.

Blackwell CC (1999). Sudden infant death syndrome. *FEMS Immunology and Medical Microbiology* **25**(1–2), Special issue.

Blackwell CC, *et al.* (1994). SUND among Thai immigrants in Singapore: the possible role of toxigenic bacteria. *International Journal of Legal Medicine* **106**, 205–8.

Budowle B, *et al.* (1995). Validation and population studies of the loci LDRL, GYPA, HBGG, D7S8 and Gc (PM loci), and the HLD-DQα using a multiplex amplification and typing procedure. *Journal of Forensic Science* **40**, 45–54.

Busuttil A (1993). Domestic violence. In: Mason JK, ed. *The pathology of trauma,* 2nd edn, Chapter 10, pp. 121–37. Hodder and Stoughton, London.

Comey CT, *et al.* (1993). PCR amplification and typing of HLA-DQ α gene in forensic samples. *Journal of Forensic Science* **38**, 239–49.

Evett IW, *et al.* (1996). Establishing the robustness of short-tandem-repeat statistics for forensic applications. *American Journal of Human Genetics* **58**, 398–407.

Hazelwood RR, Burgess AW, eds (1995). *Practical aspects of rape investigation.* CRC Press, Boca Raton, FL.

Jeffreys AJ, *et al.* (1991). Minisatellite repeat coding as a digital approach to DNA typing. *Nature* **354**, 204–9.

Karlsson T, Ormastad K, Rajs J (1988). Patterns in sharp force fatalities—a comprehensive forensic medical study. *Journal of Forensic Science* **33**, 448–61.

Kevorkian J (1961). The *fundus oculi* as a '*post mortem* clock'. *Journal of Forensic Science* **6**, 261–8.

Knight B, ed. (1995). *The estimation of the time since death in the early post-mortem period.* Edward Arnold, London.

Lander S, Budowle B (1994). DNA fingerprinting laid to rest. *Nature* **371**, 735–8.

Langlois NEI, Gresham GA (1991). The ageing of bruises: a review and study of colour changes with time. *Forensic Science International,* **50**, 227–38.

Millroy CM, Rutty GN (1997). If a wound is 'neatly incised' it is not a laceration? *British Medical Journal* **315**, 1312.

Morris JA, Haran D, Smith A (1987). Hypotheses: common bacterial toxins as a possible cause of the sudden infant death syndrome. *Medical Hypotheses* **22**, 211–22.

Ormstad K, *et al.* (1986). Patterns in sharp force fatalities—a comprehensive medical study. *Journal of Forensic Science* **31**, 529–42.

Pallis C (1983). *The ABC of brain stem death.* British Medical Journal, London.

Rao VG, Wetli CV (1988). The pathological significance of conjunctival petechiae. *American Journal of Forensic Medicine and Pathology* **9**, 32–4.

Raza NW, *et al.* (1999). Exposure to cigarette smoke, a major risk factor for SIDS: effects of cigarette smoke on inflammatory responses to viral infection and bacterial toxins. *FEMS Immunology and Medical Microbiology* **25**, 145–54.

Royal College of Physicians and the Royal College of Pathologists (1982). Medical aspects of death certification. A Joint Report of the Royal College of Physicians and the Royal College of Pathologists. *Journal of the Royal College of Physicians, London* **16**, 205–18.

Tomlin PJ (1967). 'Railroading' in retinal vessels. *British Medical Journal* **3**, 722–3.

Valdes-Dapena M (1992). A pathologist's perspective on the sudden infant death syndrome. *Pathology Annual* **27**, 133–64.

Webb E, *et al.* (1999). A comparison of fatal with non-fatal injuries in Edinburgh. *Forensic Science International* **99**, 179–87.

Weir BS (1993). DNA fingerprinting report. *Science,* **260**, 473.

Weir BS, Hill WG (1993). Population genetics of DNA profiles. *Journal of Forensic Science* **33**, 219–26.

Wilson MR, *et al.* (1993). Guidelines for the use of mitochondrial DNA sequencing in forensic science. *Crime Laboratory Digest* **20**, 69–77.

Winton R (1982). The Declaration of Lisbon. *Medical Journal of Australia* **1**, 101–4.

Wroblewski B, Ellis M (1970). Eye changes after death. *British Journal of Surgery* **56**, 69–72.

28

Sports and exercise medicine

28 Sports and exercise medicine

R. Wolman

Introduction

Traditionally, sports medicine has concentrated on injuries that occur during exercise, and therefore has come under the umbrella of orthopaedic surgery. However, with the pursuit of sporting excellence a range of different exercise-related medical disorders are now recognized. These are associated with intense levels of training and may have a detrimental effect on long-term health, as may drugs (and nutrients) that are frequently taken to enhance training and performance. Physicians are therefore increasingly being confronted with medical problems related to sport. This section will cover some of the medical disorders that occur with sport and physical training. It will also address the use of drugs and some of the common overuse injuries that occur with sport.

Developments in exercise physiology over the last 30 years have led to improved training regimes for athletes. A spin-off from this has been the recognition of the benefits of exercise in health promotion and disease management. Exercise prescription now forms an important part of some treatment programmes, with evidence for its use in the management of a range of disorders, including heart disease, diabetes, obesity, hypertension, osteoporosis, arthritis, back pain, chronic fatigue syndrome, and depression. These will be covered in other sections.

Female athlete triad

History

Amenorrhoea in athletes was first recognized in the late 1970s. Prior to this it was unusual for women to train sufficiently hard to develop this syndrome. Since 1980 there has been a growth in the popularity of aerobic sports and in the number of endurance competitions for women, whose first Olympic marathon was in 1984 and first 10 000 metres was in 1988. The other important factor has been the fashion for thinness, which really began in the 1970s. These two changes in female behaviour are the main factors responsible for the development of this syndrome.

In the early 1980s it was thought that training intensity was the main underlying aetiological factor, but studies in the late 1980s indicate that a high proportion of these athletes also have disordered eating habits. It was also thought that the bone density of amenorrhoeic athletes would be normal, as the high levels of exercise would compensate for the low levels of oestrogen. However, studies from 1984 onwards have shown that amenorrhoeic athletes have low bone density. This female athlete triad therefore consists of disordered eating, amenorrhoea, and osteoporosis.

Incidence and aetiology

The female athlete triad is associated with endurance sports. The incidence of amenorrhoea varies in different sports and is a reflection of the requirements for that particular activity, in terms of training intensity, calorie restriction, and age group (Fig. 1).

Training intensity can be difficult to quantify in certain sports, but in runners it is relatively easy as the number of miles run per week provides an accurate estimate. Some work has shown that the incidence of amenorrhoea increases as weekly training mileage increases, with an incidence of about 50 per cent in those running more than 80 miles per week.

Disordered eating is commonly seen in female athletes and may occur in over 60 per cent of competitors in sports such as gymnastics. In many cases this is the result of constant pressure from coaches, and sometimes parents, to maintain a prescribed body weight and appearance. In some of these cases the eventual outcome may be an overt eating disorder and anorexia nervosa. The two most relevant nutritional deficiencies are of calories and calcium.

The importance of calorie restriction is seen in rowers, where the incidence of amenorrhoea is significantly higher amongst lightweights (who have to be below 59 kg in order to compete) than their heavyweight counterparts. Both groups have similar training regimes, but the lightweights frequently consume restricted diets in order to 'make the weight' for competition. Furthermore, nutritional studies on runners show that those with amenorrhoea have a lower daily calorie intake than their eumenorrhoeic counterparts.

Age is also important, with athletes in their late teens being more vulnerable to menstrual irregularity than those in their twenties. In activities such as gymnastics and ballet, where there are many teenage performers, there is a high incidence of amenorrhoea, both primary and secondary.

Pathophysiology

Endurance training is associated with menstrual dysfunction. At relatively low levels of training a shortened luteal phase may occur, which can be associated with reduced progesterone levels and anovulatory cycles. These abnormalities become more frequent as training intensity increases and

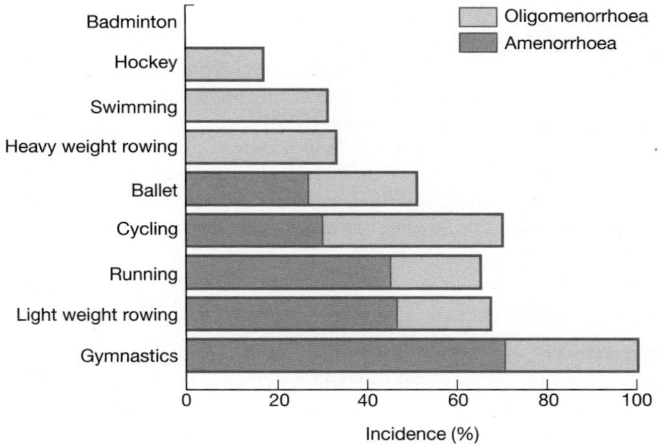

Fig. 1 The incidence of amenorrhoea amongst élite athletes in different sports. (Data taken from Wolman RL, Harries MG (1989). *Clinical Sports Medicine* **1**, 95–100, with permission.)

eventually cycles may become irregular (oligomenorrhoea) or absent (amenorrhoea). In those sports where training starts before puberty there is often a delay in the menarche. Typically this is seen in gymnasts and ballerinas where, on average, the menarche is delayed by 1 year. However, primary amenorrhoea may result, and in some cases the athlete may be in their twenties before menstruation begins.

There are many similarities between the female athlete triad and anorexia nervosa, and many believe that these are part of the same spectrum of ill health. The psychological profiling of patients with both disorders is very similar. Furthermore, in both there is disordered eating, energy imbalance, and low body weight. The aetiology of the amenorrhoea is also similar, with slowing of the gonadotrophin-releasing hormone (**GnRH**) pulse generator in terms of both amplitude and frequency, leading to a reversible hypogonadotrophic hypogonadism with severe impairment of oestrogen production, which seems to be a reversion to the prepubertal pattern of gonadotrophin release.

Over the last 15 years or so, attention has been directed towards exploring the factors responsible for the suppression of the GnRH pulse generator. There are several hypotheses, including endorphin release, central 'stress', and energy deprivation, in each of which hormones are released that may influence hypothalamic function, including cortisol, insulin-like growth-factor binding protein-1 (**IGFBP-1**) and leptin (aside from endorphin). The inhibitory action of opioids on the GnRH pulse generator is now well established. However, although endorphin levels increase with acute aerobic training (which may account for the so-called 'runners high'), there is much less evidence that they remain elevated with regular exercise, hence endorphin release alone is unlikely to account for the gonadal suppression seen in athletes.

Serum cortisol levels are elevated in amenorrhoeic athletes compared to their eumenorrhoeic counterparts. This represents central 'stress' and occurs as a result of the central activation of corticotrophin-releasing hormone (**CRH**). CRH increases GnRH sensitivity to opioid inhibition, and therefore in combination with endorphin release provides a possible mechanism for amenorrhoea. The raised cortisol level may also adversely affect bone density (see below).

An alternative hypothesis is that amenorrhoea occurs as a result of energy deprivation (Fig. 2). Several independent studies have demonstrated that the energy (calorie) intake of amenorrhoeic athletes is significantly lower than their eumenorrhoeic counterparts, even when matched for exercise intensity. This produces a relative energy imbalance, that is to say a low-energy intake in the diet compared to a high-energy output in the form of exercise, which results in weight loss. Amenorrhoeic athletes, like those with anorexia nervosa, have a low body mass index (usually below 18) and low body fat (usually below 17 per cent). Furthermore, they have a lower resting metabolic rate and reduced levels of insulin, insulin-like growth factor-1 (**IGF-1**), and tri-iodothyronine. These changes are seen in situations of energy deprivation, but it is uncertain whether any of these three hormones act as a metabolic signal influencing the release of GnRH.

Two other possible candidates are IGFBP-1 and leptin. The level of IGFBP-1 is directly suppressed by insulin, and in amenorrhoeic athletes this is elevated. Serum leptin levels are related to body fat and are reduced in anorexia nervosa and probably in the female athlete triad. Further work is needed to determine whether either of these hormones have a direct effect on the GnRH pulse generator.

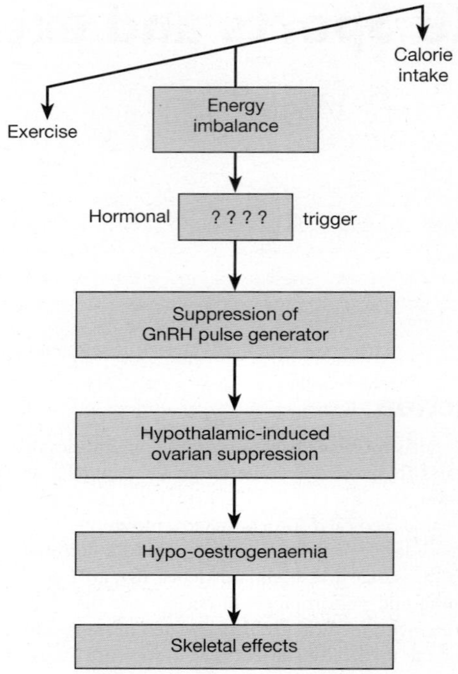

Fig. 2 Energy deprivation hypothesis for the female athlete triad.

Skeletal effects

Bone density

The bone density of amenorrhoeic athletes is reduced. This is seen most obviously in the spine where there is a high proportion of trabecular bone, but other sites such as the proximal femur and wrist may also be affected. The fall in bone density is predominantly due to low oestrogen levels, but other factors may be important since bone density does not always improve when oestrogen replacement is given (see below). Levels of IGF-1, which has important anabolic effects on the skeleton, are reduced, whilst those of cortisol, which has a catabolic action, are elevated in the female athlete triad: either of these hormonal changes could enhance the fall in bone density.

The type of exercise undertaken modifies the fall in bone density. For example, amenorrhoeic rowers have a higher spinal bone density than amenorrhoeic runners, presumably due to intense exercise involving the trunk. Amenorrhoeic gymnasts have higher spinal and femoral neck bone density than amenorrhoeic runners, probably due to weight training and jumping activity involved in gymnastic training.

With short episodes of amenorrhoea (6 to 12 months) the fall in bone density is reversible once normal menstruation is restored. With longer episodes, however, the changes may become irreversible and bone density remains persistently low. Occasionally the bone loss is severe, leading to bone densities similar to those seen in postmenopausal women, and in this subgroup there is a significant risk of osteoporotic fracture. More commonly, bone density reduction is less extreme and the risk is of premature osteoporosis (10 to 15 years early).

Other skeletal effects

Stress fractures occur more frequently in amenorrhoeic athletes, which may be related to low bone density. Stress injuries to bone commonly occur in athletes: these are usually repaired, preventing the development of a full stress fracture. The repair mechanism may be less effective in those with amenorrhoea who have low levels of oestrogen and IGF-1, both of which are important in maintaining skeletal integrity.

Athletes with delayed menarche and primary amenorrhoea may have delayed skeletal maturation, including delayed epiphyseal closure that may increase the risk of epiphyseal injury.

Investigation and management

It is important to exclude other causes of amenorrhoea. This will include taking an accurate history to establish a relationship between training and menstrual abnormalities. Investigations should aim to exclude other causes of amenorrhoea (see Chapters 12.2 and 12.8.1) and the serum tri-iodothyronine level should be measured, which is likely to be low in the female

Table 1 Investigation of the female athlete triad

• Exclude other causes of amenorrhoea
• Serum tri-iodothyronine measurement
• Nutritional assessment for energy and calcium
• Bone mineral density

athlete triad. A nutritional screen is helpful to assess calorie and calcium intake, and bone density should be measured (Table 1).

Once the diagnosis is established the most effective treatment is to re-establish natural menstruation (Table 2). This can be achieved with a combination of reducing training intensity (with the help of the coach) and increasing calorie intake (with the aid of a dietitian). It is very important to educate the athlete about both the short- and long-term risks of remaining amenorrhoeic, otherwise many athletes will not accept this type of intervention. Psychological intervention may be necessary in those athletes where an eating disorder is apparent (see Chapter 26.5.5).

In those athletes who remain amenorrhoeic despite attempts at adjusting their training and diet, oestrogen replacement (either the oral contraceptive or hormone-replacement therapy) should be given. Unfortunately some athletes may have difficulty tolerating this. Furthermore, anecdotal experience suggests that this is not always effective, probably for the reasons given above. Calcium supplements should be considered, especially in those with low intakes, and vitamin D supplements may also be helpful. Experience with bisphosphonates and raloxifene in this age group is too limited to offer clear advice.

Progress should be monitored with bone densitometry. In those who remain amenorrhoeic either the progressive fall in bone density or recurrent injuries will eventually force them to make lifestyle adjustments in terms of training and nutrition. By then it may be too late, hence emphasis needs to be placed on education and counselling at an early stage.

Overtraining syndrome

Introduction

This condition and its associated symptoms are well recognized in the athletic population, but the pathophysiology is poorly understood. It tends to occur in athletes doing high-intensity endurance training and is rarely seen in those who partake in strength and power sports. The most common presentation is with underperformance, for example a worsening of the times for the athletes' favoured events. Often the initial response is to assume that the training is inadequate and therefore to increase the intensity even more. This will perpetuate the problem, eventually forcing the athlete to seek medical advice.

Aetiology

Athletes must train hard to improve their performance. This can lead to transient fatigue and underperformance, hence intensive training should be followed by a period of relative rest to allow regeneration and recovery. This cyclical method of training is called 'periodization' and produces adaptation, allowing progressive increases in training intensity and performance. During the period of intense training, known as 'overreaching', it is common for the athlete to complain of muscle soreness, fatigue, and stress-related symptoms. As part of the stress response serum cortisol may rise, whilst testosterone may decrease, and creatine phosphokinase may be elevated as a reflection of transient muscle damage. These clinical and biochemical features should recover during the rest period. Overreaching is a necessary part of training if the athlete's performance is going to improve.

Table 2 Treatment of the female athlete triad

• Decrease amount of exercise—with the help of the coach
• Increase energy intake—with the help of a dietitian
• Consider psychological intervention
• Oestrogen replacement—HRT or oral contraceptive
• Calcium and vitamin D
• ?Bisphosphonates
• ?Raloxifene

In some situations the athlete may not allow sufficient time for rest in between periods of heavy training. This leads to under-recovery and prevents full adaptation to increased training loads. This may occur when there is a rapid increase in training intensity, with very prolonged training, and at times of stressful competition. It may also occur when the athlete is exposed to other stresses, including intercurrent infection, travel across several time zones, or other unrelated psychoemotional stresses. In the adolescent athlete it may be seen during a rapid growth spurt. This combination of stresses may lead to underperformance, which will usually respond to a rest period of 2 weeks, but if the athlete fails to recognize the early signs the symptoms become more severe and may require a more prolonged rest period to achieve full recovery.

Pathophysiology

Over the last 15 years or so there have been many studies investigating the pathophysiology of the overtraining syndrome, and these have generated several hypotheses. Unfortunately studies are not always directly comparable because they use different definitions for the syndrome and may perform their evaluations at different stages in its evolution.

Neuroendocrinological features

There are effects on the hypothalamic–pituitary–adrenal axis. In some overtrained athletes there is a rise in salivary cortisol levels and a low testosterone:cortisol ratio. This reflects a rise in free-cortisol levels, which correlates with the depressed mood state seen in some athletes. There is a decreased pituitary ACTH response to insulin-induced hypoglycaemia, and reduced adrenal responsiveness to ACTH. The latter effect leads to a compensatory elevation of ACTH in the early stages of the overtraining syndrome, but in an advanced stage both ACTH release and the cortisol response may be reduced. There is also evidence of sympathetic involvement, with increased resting noradrenaline (norepinephrine) levels associated with decreased nocturnal excretion.

Central fatigue and the branched-chain amino acids

Prolonged endurance exercise leads to a depletion of glycogen stores in muscles and the liver, at which point muscle requires alternative sources of energy. Mobilization of fatty acids provide this, producing increased levels in plasma, where they are bound to albumin. The branched-chain amino acids (valine, leucine, and isoleucine) are another alternative fuel for muscle, with an increased rate of oxidation during exercise. In plasma, fatty acids compete with tryptophan for binding to albumin, hence an increase of bound fatty acids leads to an increase in plasma levels of free tryptophan. Tryptophan and the branched-chain amino acids pass the blood–brain barrier in competition for the same amino acid carrier, an increase in free plasma tryptophan and a decrease in branched-chain amino acids favouring the entry of free tryptophan into the brain. Tryptophan is converted to the neurotransmitter 5-hydroxytryptamine (5-HT, serotonin) in the brain, which plays a role in the induction of sleep and fatigue and has an inhibitory effect on the hypothalamus. This hypothesis might therefore explain some of the effects that are seen in the overtraining syndrome, but human overtraining studies, including interventions with glycogen and with branched-chain amino acids, have so far been inconclusive.

Glutamine and the immune system

The relationship between exercise and the immune system remains controversial. The leucocytosis of exercise is well recognized, and there is also evidence of impaired neutrophil function following intensive exercise, which may explain why upper respiratory tract infections are probably more common following a marathon. They also seem to be more frequent

Table 3 Symptoms of overtraining

- Underperformance
- Loss of appetite
- Depression and anxiety
- Sleep disturbance
- Fatigue
- Upper respiratory tract infections
- Raised, resting heart rate

in the overtraining syndrome, although it is uncertain whether this is cause or effect.

Glutamine metabolism provides one possible explanation for the relationship between immune function and exercise. Glutamine is a free amino acid that is utilized at high rates by rapidly dividing cells such as leucocytes, and therefore considered important for normal immune function. Plasma levels fall with intensive exercise, possibly due to the increased glutamine requirement for gluconeogenesis and increased uptake by the liver, gut, and kidney. There is evidence that glutamine supplements may reduce the risk of infection in endurance athletes and also that plasma glutamine levels can act as a marker of the overtraining syndrome, but more research is needed in this area.

Clinical features

The overtraining syndrome is characterized by performance deterioration refractory to normal regeneration strategies. Variable combinations of symptoms are seen in association with this (Table 3). The athlete will commonly complain of fatigue and heaviness in the muscles, which they tend to ignore in the early stages. Sleep disturbance is common with difficulty getting off to sleep, early waking, and feeling unrefreshed on waking. They may complain of depression, anxiety, and irritability, with loss of appetite and of libido. There may also be a history of upper respiratory tract infections.

The resting heart rate may be elevated, but this gradually returns to normal (usually very low in an élite endurance athlete) as recovery occurs. Physiological testing may show an increased heart rate response to exercise, a reduced maximum oxygen consumption (V_{O_2}**max**), and an impaired heart rate recovery following exercise. Maximum power output may also be reduced.

Blood tests show non-specific changes consistent with heavy training such as dilutional anaemia and raised muscle enzymes (in some cases the creatine phosphokinase level may be increased several thousand times). There may be evidence of a recent viral illness such as a positive Paul Bunnell test. It is also important to recognize that underperformance may be secondary to an underlying medical disorder such as anaemia, diabetes, or thyroid disease: these secondary causes are rare, but should always be considered.

Management

Prevention

As our understanding of this syndrome improves it may be possible to prevent it from occurring. This is not possible at present, because although it is related to prolonged intensive exercise, the ability to withstand the stress of training varies significantly between different athletes. Furthermore, there is currently no screening test that can reliably predict the onset of the syndrome. Resting heart rate can provide a guide: this is consistently low (within a couple of beats) in the healthy endurance athlete, but with overreaching and overtraining this may increase significantly (by 5–10 beats/min) and only returns to the previous low level when recovery occurs. Psychological assessment can also provide a guide, with the **POMS** (Profile of Mood State) questionnaire proving to be useful in this respect.

It is important to incorporate rest days into any training regime. Racehorses can develop a syndrome similar in many respects to the human overtraining syndrome, and in one study where they were given an alternate-day regime of hard training day/easy training day the frequency of the equine equivalent of the overtraining syndrome decreased and performance improved. There have now been several human studies where rest days have been incorporated into the training regime (for example, four heavy training days, two light training days, and one rest day per week): these seem to be associated with a reduction in the frequency of the syndrome.

It is also important to ensure that dietary intake is sufficient at times of intensive training, especially in terms of carbohydrate and hydration. It is surprising how many athletes are unaware of the nutritional components of diet and have an intake that is inadequate for the intensity of their training.

Treatment of the established syndrome

As many of the symptoms of this syndrome are non-specific, it is important to exclude other causes of underperformance and fatigue, including infection, thyroid disease, diabetes, and anaemia. In most cases tests for these disorders will be negative.

The treatment of the established syndrome requires rest to allow regeneration and recovery. Most athletes will only accept absolute rest for a few days, hence it is important to follow this up with a period of relative rest, that is allowing very low intensity training. The exercise can then be slowly progressed, but it may take up to 12 weeks to achieve full recovery. Many athletes are pleasantly surprised about how well they have maintained their performance despite 12 weeks of light training.

In addition to relative rest, it is important to adopt a holistic approach to treatment. This includes assessing other coexistent stresses and making use of relaxation techniques. Nutrition is important and further advice on this should be offered as appropriate. Athletes should monitor their progress by measuring their resting heart rate, which will decrease as recovery occurs.

Medical complications in sport

Although injuries are the dominant feature of sports medicine, there are several well-recognized medical disorders that occur as a result of sport and physical activity. Some are associated with acute bouts of exercise and others with more prolonged periods of training. The female athlete triad is discussed above, and sudden cardiac death and exercise-induced asthma are dealt with elsewhere.

Delayed-onset muscle soreness, rhabdomyolysis, and heat stroke

Strenuous exercise can produce transient damage to the muscle. Delayed-onset muscle soreness can occur several hours after a bout of unaccustomed, intensive eccentric exercise, reaching a peak between 1 and 3 days. It is associated with objective muscle weakness, which can last for up to 10 days. There are increased serum levels of creatine kinase and myoglobin, with muscle oedema and structural change revealed on magnetic resonance imaging (**MRI**) (*T*2-weighted sequences) and muscle biopsy, respectively. These findings are most obvious after 2 to 3 days. The structural damage fully repairs and the symptoms and laboratory abnormalities resolve by 10 days. This phenomenon is commonly seen following marathon running, when creatine kinase levels may rise to over 2000 IU/l (Fig. 3).

There is less muscle damage when a bout of similar intensive eccentric exercise is repeated. This is known as the 'repeated bout effect' and is probably due to a series of adaptations taking place at neural, connective tissue, and cellular levels. These changes make the muscle more resistant to damage with further bouts of intensive exercise.

It is rare for large amounts of myoglobin to be released from muscle during exercise ('exertional rhabdomyolysis'), but when it does occur it can be life-threatening by causing acute renal failure, often with severe hyperkalaemia (see Chapter 20.4). This is associated with intensive eccentric exercise, dehydration, and hyperthermia and forms part of the syndrome of heat stroke.

There is high heat production with exercise: 75 per cent of the energy expended is converted to heat during running. Heat dissipation therefore becomes extremely important, with evaporation through sweating being the most important mechanism, and anything that impairs sweat evaporation will put the athlete at risk of hyperthermia and heat stroke. This can occur in extreme environmental conditions such as high temperature and high humidity, and is more likely when the athlete is dehydrated. A poorly prepared athlete lacking fitness, who is inadequately acclimatized to the heat, has had a recent illness (for example, a cold or gastroenteritis), or wears excessive clothing is more at risk. Nowadays heat stroke is more commonly seen in fun runs than in marathons, when there are often a large number of poorly prepared participants. Furthermore, it can occur when the environmental conditions are not particularly extreme, suggesting that heat production during exercise is the most important factor.

The pathophysiology, clinical features, and management of heat stroke is dealt with elsewhere (Chapter 8.5.1). As patients with heat stroke require immediate treatment, on-site resuscitation facilities should be available at competitions and fun runs. Management includes the use of intravenous therapy and increasing heat loss through evaporation (the patient should be put in the shade and then wetted with lukewarm water and fanned). It is

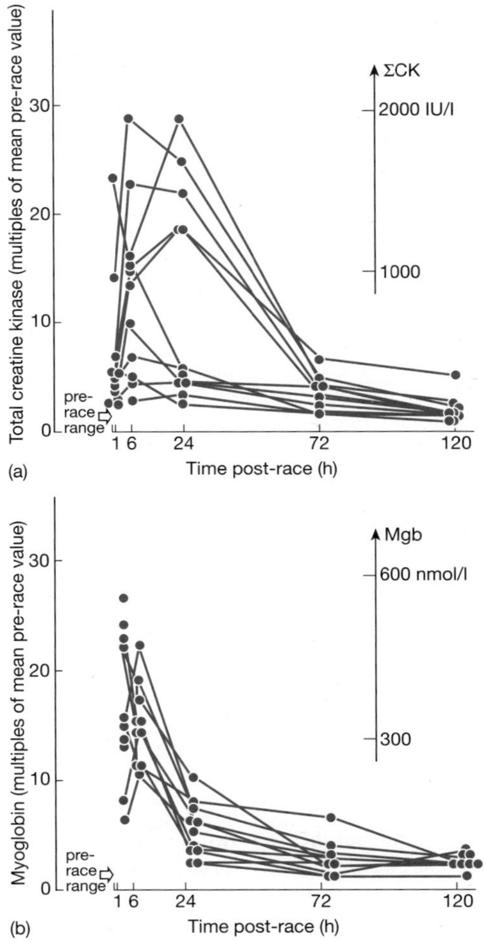

Fig. 3 Changes in (a) serum total creatine kinase (CK) and (b) plasma myoglobin in young men who had completed a marathon (running times: mean, 194 min; range, 163–280 min). (Taken from Young, *et al.* (1984). *European Journal of Clinical Investigation* **14**, 2, 58, with permission.)

Table 4 Recommendations to minimize the risk of developing exertional heat stroke

• Organized competitions and events should avoid the hottest time of the year and the hottest part of the day.
• Training and fitness will improve thermoregulation during exercise, and therefore participants should be given advice about how to prepare for an event.
• A minimum of 7–10 days' acclimatization to the heat should take place prior to the event.
• The athlete should be adequately hydrated prior to the event, and there should be opportunities to rehydrate during the event.
• Participants should avoid competitions and events when they are unwell, e.g. with an upper respiratory tract infection or gastroenteritis.

possible to minimize the risk of developing exertional heat stroke by paying attention to certain recommendations (Table 4).

Exercise-induced gastrointestinal symptoms

Up to 50 per cent of long-distance runners will complain of gastrointestinal (**GI**) symptoms. These include reflux/heartburn, intestinal cramps, the urge to defecate, and diarrhoea, which may be bloody. The lower GI symptoms are probably due to reduced blood flow (splanchnic blood flow decreases by up to 80 per cent with intensive endurance activity) and possibly mechanical (jarring) stress on the gut (as symptoms are more common in runners than cyclists). The relative gut ischaemia may lead to the release of several GI hormones, including secretin, glucagon, and vasoactive intestinal polypeptide: the latter can remain elevated for up to 2 h after the termination of exercise. These hormones will increase secretion into the gut while also reducing absorption, effects that are enhanced by dehydration.

Exercise-induced GI symptoms can usually be controlled with appropriate advice and tend to decrease with adequate training. Adaptive changes occur with gradual increases in training volume and intensity, such that there may be an improvement in blood flow through the splanchnic circulation. It is also important for athletes to be adequately hydrated both before and during exercise: they should therefore take account of the ambient temperature and humidity and adapt their fluid intake accordingly. Hypertonic drinks should be avoided as they will tend to increase the risk of dehydration.

Exercise-related anaemia

Haemoglobin concentrations in highly trained endurance athletes are often at the lower end of the normal range or even just below it. In most cases this reflects a dilutional state where, although red cell mass increases with exercise, there is a proportionally greater increase in plasma volume. A true runners' anaemia may be caused by faecal blood loss (see above), also from intravascular haemolysis caused by high foot-impact forces ('march haemoglobinuria'). A similar traumatic haemoglobinuria also occurs in congadrum players due to high impact on the hands.

Fitness to exercise

Sudden death in sport

Although it often attracts headlines in the press, sudden death in sport is very rare. The frequency of sudden death varies from about 0.5 per 100 000 to 6 per 100 000 per year, depending on the age group being assessed, the level of underlying fitness, and the intensity of activity. Fatal arrhythmia seems to be the most common mechanism of death (Table 5). Atherosclerotic coronary artery disease is the most common cause in those over

Table 5 Cardiac causes of sudden death

- Coronary artery disease
- Hypertrophic cardiomyopathy
- Myocarditis
- Coronary artery anomalies
- Aortic rupture (Marfan's syndrome)
- Aortic valve stenosis
- Right ventricular dysplasia
- Conduction defects

40 years of age: in younger athletes underlying causes include cardiomyopathy, valvular heart disease, and Marfan's syndrome.

Myocarditis (see Chapter 15.8.1) is another possible cause of sudden death in sport. This is usually viral in origin, in particular cocksackie B virus, but a series of sudden death cases amongst Swedish orienteers was found to be associated with *Chlamydia pneumoniae* myocarditis. Cardiac concussion is a rare cause of sudden death, thought to be due to a dysrhythmia resulting from a non-penetrating precordial blow from a projectile, such as a cricket ball or an ice hockey puck.

Screening

Although it is accepted that people with certain cardiac risk factors, such as those with hypertrophic cardiomyopathy or aortic stenosis, should avoid competitive sports, there is limited value in cardiac screening of athletes. This is because of the rarity of these abnormalities, the rarity of sudden death, and the cost of screening. It is estimated that 200 000 athletes would have to be screened to find one at-risk case. There is also limited predictive accuracy of some of the cardiac investigations. This is the case with electrocardiography (**ECG**), where it may be difficult to distinguish the physiological changes of the athletes' heart with the pathological changes seen with hypertrophic cardiomyopathy. Further cardiac investigation should probably be restricted to those with a history of cardiac and/or exercise-related symptoms, a relevant family history, or abnormalities found on cardiac auscultation.

Prevention of sudden death in sport

Athletes with confirmed myocarditis should be withdrawn from competitive sports for at least 6 months, while those with more general viral illness should abstain from sport until they have recovered.

Sudden death is most likely to occur in high-intensity competitive sports (for instance, squash), and in this situation the athlete should be offered a basic medical assessment (personal and family history and physical examination) prior to competition. The need for a medical assessment is less important in those participating in recreational sports. Although acute bouts of exercise increase the risk of cardiac death, this transient increase in risk is outweighed by the cardiac benefits of habitual exercise. The importance of graded increases in exercise intensity, allowing cardiac and musculoskeletal adaptations to occur, should be stressed.

Overuse injuries

Overuse injuries are the most common type of injury seen in a sports medicine clinic. It is usually relatively straightforward to make the diagnosis from the history and examination. However, it is equally important to determine the aetiological factors responsible for the injury to prevent a recurrence. These can be divided into training methods, equipment, and biomechanical factors (see Table 6).

Injuries can occur when the training is increased too quickly, when there is an inadequate warm-up or cool-down period, and when there is inadequate flexibility training to complement the overall programme. Injuries can also occur when the athlete suddenly changes from one surface or gradient to another. Equipment factors are also important, which is especially the case for footwear in weight-bearing sport, where it is vital that the shoes provide adequate support for the sport being undertaken and are not overly worn out. In racket sports the size, weight, and string tension of the racket are important factors that may influence the risk of injury.

It is important to consider biomechanical factors in athletes as the repetitive nature of their activities (for example, running action, tennis serve, or cricket bowling) may magnify any minor malalignment. It is therefore necessary to assess for various factors, including leg-length difference, wide pelvis, pelvic tilt, femoral neck anteversion, and tibia varum. The shape of the foot on standing should also be considered, as both overpronated and rigid, high-arched feet can cause problems. Variations in anatomy of the bones may also increase the risk of injury, such as the hooked acromium and rotator cuff impingement in throwers and the os trigonum and posterior ankle impingement in dancers and footballers.

The type of injury will depend on the age of the athlete as this determines the weakest point in the musculoskeletal chain. In the growing adolescent the point of attachment of the tendon to bone is vulnerable, and injuries such as Osgood–Schlatter's disease at the tibial tubercle and Severs disease at the calcaneus are commonly seen. In the young adult tendinitis and injuries at the musculotendinous junction are particularly common, while in the elderly athlete degenerative injuries of the tendon and joint are seen.

Stress (or fatigue) fractures occur as a result of bone overload. They occur when training is increased too quickly, as in rapid preparation for a marathon, or when there are biomechanical factors that increase the stress load on bone, for example rigid, high-arched feet. They also occur more commonly in amenorrhoeic athletes than in their eumenorrhoeic counterparts. Clinically the athlete usually has point tenderness. A bone scan or MRI will allow an accurate diagnosis to be made, although the plain radiograph may be negative.

Drugs and ergogenic aids in sport

Introduction

The use of drugs and nutritional supplements in competitive sports is widespread. The main reason for this is to enhance performance, but supplements are also taken to improve general health and to increase resistance to infection. In theory, this would reduce the risk of developing coincidental medical problems and hence minimize interruptions to training. The scientific evidence for many of these substances is flimsy, but athletes are often prepared to try them on the basis of the anecdotal experience of fellow athletes, advice from their coach, or even from suppliers at the local gym. Furthermore, surveys suggest that athletes are willing to take substances for short-term performance enhancement, even if it puts their long-term health at risk. The banning of some substances has had an effect on some athletes, but others continue to take them and are prepared go to extremes to avoid detection.

With most performance-enhancing drugs there is a large interindividual response, but the cause for this is not fully understood. Studies on most drugs and nutritional supplements have therefore been unable to demonstrate consistent efficacy. There is a large potential placebo effect, which may obscure any pharmacological action. Large randomized controlled trials would be helpful, but these are virtually impossible to do because most athletes would be unwilling to accept a placebo. Furthermore, if there is any possibility of the drug enhancing performance it is likely already to have been banned by the sports governing body. Studies on the non-athletic population, who exercise at much lower levels, may not be representative of the effects seen in athletes. Moreover, athletes often take a variety of substances in extremely large doses, which makes it difficult to compare the results with the lower doses given in the general population in terms of efficacy and (especially) safety.

Anabolic agents

Anabolic–androgenic steroids

Testosterone, first synthesized in the 1930s, has both anabolic and androgenic effects. Since then several synthetic derivatives have been produced in an attempt to provide a steroid with predominant anabolic actions. The first recorded use of anabolic–androgenic steroids (**AAS**) was during the Second World War when they were given to German troops to increase their aggressiveness. In 1952 the Russian weightlifting team was suspected of taking them when they won three gold medals at the Helsinki Olympic Games. This increased the interest in these drugs, and by 1958 a United States pharmaceutical company had developed AAS. The dangers gradually became apparent, but it was not until 1975 that the International Olympic Committee banned their use.

AAS enhance muscle strength and power but have no effect on aerobic performance. They are also thought to have psychological effects and can promote aggressiveness, which in its most extreme form may lead to 'roid rage'. Athletes may also experience euphoria and reduced fatigue while taking AAS, a combination of effects that may allow them to train harder and for longer.

Although AAS will increase muscle strength in non-exercising people, the greatest increases in strength occur when AAS are taken in conjunction with resistance exercise (Fig. 4). The reason for this may be that physiological stress occurs with intense resistance exercise and leads to increased levels of glucocorticoids, thereby producing a catabolic state with a negative nitrogen balance that anabolic steroids can reverse.

Human growth hormone

The physiological effects of human growth hormone (**HGH**) include nitrogen retention, increased protein synthesis and tissue growth, and an increase in fat-free mass. Recombinant HGH was first produced in 1984 and (although expensive) its use by athletes has since increased.

The anabolic effects of HGH make it potentially valuable as an ergogenic aid for athletes participating in power sports. Furthermore, as it is not detected by most drug-test screenings performed by sports governing bodies, it is an attractive option when compared to anabolic steroids. However,

Table 6 Common overuse injuries seen in sport

Injury	Site	Sport	Aetiology	Treatment
Plantar fasciitis	Undersurface of the foot	Running	Overpronation	NSAID, physiotherapy orthotic, splint
Achilles tendinitis	Posterior ankle	Running	Overpronation, high arches, footwear	Physiotherapy, NSAID, orthotics
Severs	Posterior ankle	Running	Early adolescence	Relative rest
Os trigonum	Posterior ankle	Dance, football	Repetitive plantar flexion	Excision
Flexor hallucis longus tendinitis	Medial ankle	Dance	Poor turnout, overpronation	Rest, physiotherapy
Compartment syndrome	Shin, calf	Running, walking, dance	Increased training intensity	Rest, physiotherapy surgery
Patellofemoral joint syndrome	Anterior knee	Running, dance, cycling, swimming —breaststroke	Overpronation, wide q angle, femoral neck anteversion	Physiotherapy, orthotic, biomechanical correction
Osgood–Schlatter	Anterior knee—tibial tubercle	Running, jumping	Adolescence	Rest, physiotherapy
Patellar tendinitis	Anterior knee	Jumping sports	Increased training intensity	Physiotherapy
Iliotibial band friction syndrome	Lateral knee	Running	Tight ITB, overpronation	Physiotherapy, ITB stretches
Trochanteric bursitis	Lateral hip	Running, dance	Tight ITB, wide pelvis	Physiotherapy, ITB stretches, steroid injection
Iliopsoas bursitis	Anterior hip	Dance	Poor trunk stability	Physiotherapy, steroid injection
Spondylolysis	Low back	Dance, tennis, gymnastics, cricket bowling	Increased lumbar lordosis, spinal hyperextension	Rest, physiotherapy, ?surgery
Subacromial impingement	Shoulder	Throwing sports, tennis, swimming	Hooked acromium, instability, poor scapula control	Physiotherapy, steroid injection, surgery

ITB, iliotibial band.

so far there has been only limited research to determine its effectiveness in increasing muscle strength and power.

β_2-Agonists

This group of drugs was initially banned by the sporting bodies because of their stimulant action. However, in the last few years they have gained interest as muscle strengthening agents when taken orally. During the 1992 Barcelona Olympics, two American power athletes were found to have taken clenbuterol.

Animal studies show that clenbuterol can produce muscle hypertrophy. Studies of β_2-agonists in healthy men, in patients following lower limb surgery, and those with spinal cord injury, all showed gains in muscle strength following an exercise programme when compared to a placebo group. However, there is very little data on their effect in highly trained athletes. Although they act as bronchodilators, there is no evidence that they can improve aerobic fitness in non-asthmatics.

Creatine

Creatine was first recognized as an ergogenic aid in the early 1990s and was used by athletes in the 1992 Barcelona Olympics. It is an amino acid present in meat, normal daily intake being less than 1 g. The highest concentration of creatine is in skeletal muscle, in particular in type-II muscle fibres, where most is in the form of creatine phosphate, providing a source of energy and assisting in the restoration of ATP following exercise. Creatine phosphate may also assist in buffering when the pH falls due to lactic acid accumulation during exercise.

Supplements are usually taken in high dosage for a limited period (for example, 25 g for 6 days), following which muscle concentrations of free creatine and creatine phosphate remain elevated for several weeks. It is generally pointless to take high-dose supplementation beyond this period as the majority of muscle creatine uptake occurs during the first few days, but some athletes take a maintenance dose of 2 g/day.

Following this regime many athletes report that they are able to increase their training loads, and studies suggest that supplementation does improve high-intensity performance, especially when repeated exercise bouts are carried out (for example, repetitive sprinting and cycling). The ergogenic effects also extend to strength and power events such as weight-lifting. No effect is seen in predominantly aerobic events.

Overall, there is only limited information on the effects of creatine supplementation, but these are consistent with the role of creatine phosphate in enhancing the restoration of ATP. The increase in muscle strength possibly occurs by allowing greater training intensity, leading to an enhanced training response. Within a few days of taking creatine there is a weight gain of between 2 and 5 kg: a large proportion of which can be accounted for by an increase in intracellular fluid volume (it is well known that urine volume decreases during the period of supplementation), but there may also be an increase in fat-free mass.

There are theoretical concerns regarding the side-effects of using large doses of creatine for prolonged periods. These include adverse effects on the kidney, although, so far, there have been no confirmed reports of this. There are also anecdotal reports of increases in muscle cramps and concerns regarding the impact of weight gain, especially in athletes competing in weight-category sports (for example, boxing and wrestling). In these sports the athlete often has to lose weight rapidly to 'make the weight' for competition, and if they have gained extra weight with the use of creatine they may have to severely dehydrate to achieve such weight reduction.

As supplementation with creatine seems capable of enhancing performance there are ethical issues regarding its use. Some feel it should be banned, others argue against this on the basis that it is a component of a normal meat diet and is therefore no different to taking carbohydrate supplements.

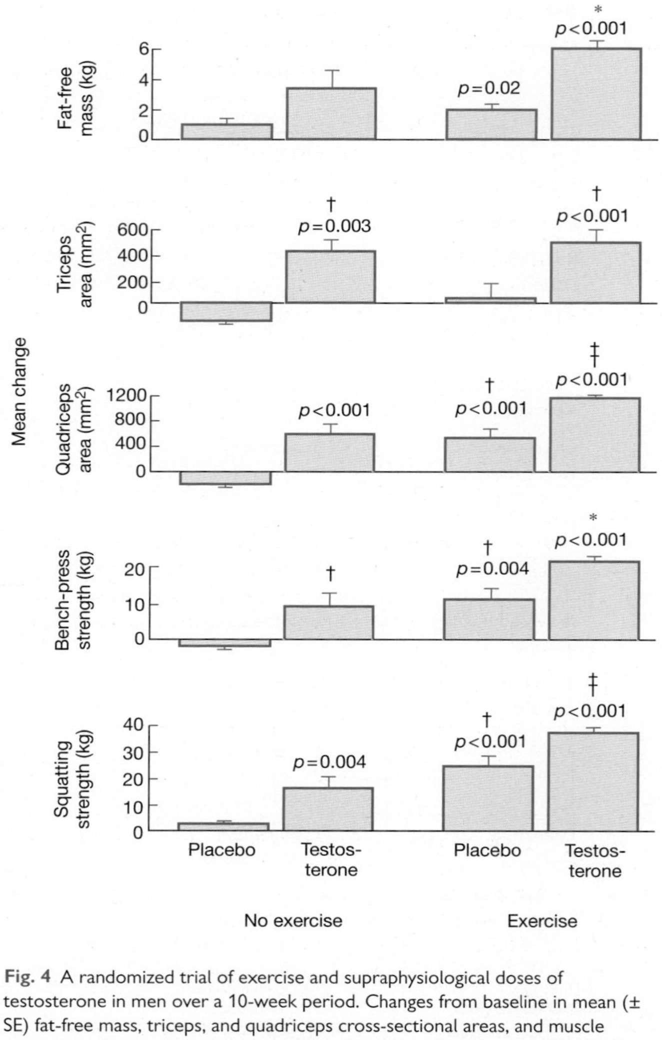

Fig. 4 A randomized trial of exercise and supraphysiological doses of testosterone in men over a 10-week period. Changes from baseline in mean (± SE) fat-free mass, triceps, and quadriceps cross-sectional areas, and muscle strength in the bench-press and squatting exercises. Note the greatest effect is obtained with a combination of exercise and testosterone.

Stimulants

Amphetamines, ephedrine, and cocaine

These stimulate the central and sympathetic nervous systems. As sympathomimetic agents they increase heart rate, blood pressure, metabolic rate, and plasma levels of free fatty acids. These actions could theoretically enhance aerobic performance, but not without risk. There were at least two amphetamine-related deaths in cyclists in the early years of their use (one in the Rome Olympic Games in 1960 and the other in the 1968 Tour de France) and there have also been several deaths in athletes associated with the use of both ephedrine and cocaine.

Research on the use of amphetamines suggests that they have little direct physiological effect during exercise but that they can mask pain and fatigue during activity. This may allow athletes to exercise closer to their limit, which may produce a positive effect, especially on endurance performance. However, this could also have a detrimental effect on health by inhibiting the athlete's awareness of early warning signs (for example, injury or dehydration). The same may apply to ephedrine and cocaine. Ephedrine is also used by athletes to reduce fat and increase fat-free mass, but there is little evidence for this effect. Cocaine can produce euphoria and also lead to addiction, which has caused great concern regarding its use amongst athletes.

Caffeine

Caffeine, which is chemically related to the theophyllines, is metabolized in the liver to produce dimethylxanthine. When used prior to prolonged exercise (in a dose of 3–6 mg/kg body weight, 1 h before exercise) it can delay fatigue and enhance endurance performance, although there is significant individual variation. Although caffeine is known to have effects on the central nervous system, adipose tissue, and skeletal muscle, the mechanism by which it reduces fatiguability is unclear. It has several unwanted effects, including insomnia, headache, and gastrointestinal irritation, but its diuretic effect is of particular concern, especially in athletes competing in hot climates.

The International Olympic Committee considers caffeine to be a performance-enhancing drug. However, it would be impossible to have an outright ban on a substance that is present in so many foods and drinks, hence an athlete found to have a urine concentration of more than 12 mg/l is deemed to be guilty of a doping offence. This has its limitations as some athletes can obtain a performance-enhancing effect at urine concentrations well below this level.

Other agents

β-Blockers

By reducing heart rate this group of drugs reduces aerobic capacity and therefore decreases endurance. However, they are effective in skill sports, with studies confirming that shooters improve their performance when taking β-blockers. These drugs probably exert their effect by reducing hand tremor and heart rate: top-class shooters tend to shoot between one heartbeat and the next, and therefore a reduction in heart rate is helpful. They have also been shown to be effective in treating stage fright in musicians.

Diuretics

Athletes use diuretics when they need to lose weight rapidly. This occurs in sports such as boxing, judo, and light-weight rowing when the individual needs to make a particular weight classification for competition. Diuretics are very effective in producing short-term weight loss, in the order of 4 per cent over 24 h. However, this can lead to dehydration and electrolyte disturbance, both of which can affect performance. Frequently the athlete will have up to 20 h between the weigh-in and competition: this gives sufficient time to replace the fluid loss, but is insufficient to re-establish normal electrolyte balance, which can lead to medical complications during competition, including renal failure, severe hyperkalaemia, and rhabdomyolysis.

Erythropoietin and blood doping

A modest increase in red cell mass of up to 5 per cent occurs with adaptation to endurance training. This can take several months. However, some athletes artificially increase their red cell mass either by infusing previously stored red cells or by the use of erythropoietin. Infusing red cells has probably been used since the early 1970s in sports such as distance running, cycling, and cross-country skiing. In 1984 the United States men's cycling team confessed to using it during the Olympics, and won gold medals. Erythropoietin has probably been used by athletes since the late 1980s and may well have been responsible for a number of deaths seen in cyclists in the last 12 years.

Although homologous transfusions are used by athletes, autologous transfusion is probably more common. During this process several units of blood are removed from the athlete and then stored for several weeks, while the blood count is naturally restored to normal. The red cells are then reinfused, thereby increasing the red cell count, which will be sustained for a few weeks. The alternative method of increasing red cell mass is to administer erythropoietin, when the red cell count rises gradually over several weeks and remains elevated as long as the treatment continues.

Physiological studies confirm improved exercise performance with the use of these techniques to increase the blood count. Maximal aerobic power, submaximal endurance, and race performance have all been shown to improve. Blood doping may also provide a thermoregulatory advantage for those exercising in the heat, and some benefit for those exercising at altitude.

Medical risks include those associated with transfusions. Even autologous infusions can cause problems through clerical errors and mishandling of the stored blood product. Risks also occur in association with the high haematocrit, with blood viscosity rising exponentially as the haematocrit increases above 30 per cent thus leading to an increased risk of thromboembolic events. There have now been numerous deaths related to the use of blood doping by athletes.

Although blood doping is banned by all the main sports governing bodies there is no reliable test for detecting either autologous red cell infusion or erythropoietin administration. It is therefore difficult to prove that an athlete has used this technique and to provide a consistent deterrent.

Bicarbonate

A metabolic acidosis occurs with anaerobic exercise and is thought to be responsible for the progressive fatigue that occurs. By inducing a metabolic alkalosis prior to exercise, it may be possible to delay the onset of fatigue and improve exercise performance. Several studies have been undertaken to assess the effect of pre-exercise bicarbonate ingestion on performance. There are conflicting results from these studies, some showing a benefit, others not. The reason for these differences is probably due to variations in the duration and intensity of exercise, the dosage of bicarbonate, and the length of time between taking bicarbonate and the onset of exercise. Bicarbonate is most likely to have an effect with exercise of only a few minutes duration, when given 2 to 3 h before exercise, and at a dose of about 0.3 g of sodium bicarbonate per kg body weight. Side-effects of this ingestion include vomiting and diarrhoea, which may limit the potential benefits. Bicarbonate is not banned by the sports governing bodies.

Further reading

Bhasin S, *et al.* (1996). The effects of supraphysiologic doses of testosterone on muscle size and strength in normal men. *New England Journal of Medicine* **335**, 1–7. [Comprehensive review]

Brouns F, Beckers E (1993). Is the gut an athletic organ? Digestion, absorption and exercise. *Sports Medicine* 15(4): 242–257. [Comprehensive review]

Budgett R (1998). Fatigue and underperformance in athletes: the overtraining syndrome. *British Journal of Sports Medicine* **32**, 107–10. [Comprehensive clinical review]

Budgett R, *et al.* (2000). Redefining the overtraining syndrome as the unexplained underperformance syndrome. *British Journal of Sports Medicine* **34**, 67–8. [Summary of current thinking]

Clarkson PM, Thompson HS (1997). Drugs and sport. Research findings and limitations. *Sports Medicine* **24**, 366–84. [Comprehensive review]

Foster C, Lehmann M (1997). Training/overtraining: the first Ulm symposium. *Medicine and Science in Sports and Exercise* **30**, 1137–78. [Comprehensive scientific review]

Futterman LG, Myerburg R (1998). Sudden death in athletes. *Sports Medicine* **26**, 335–50. [Comprehensive review]

Huston TP, *et al.* (1985). The athlete heart syndrome. *New England Journal of Medicine* **313**, 24–30. [Comprehensive review, especially of ECG changes in athletes]

Jenkins PJ, Grossman A (1993). The control of the gonadotrophin-releasing hormone pulse generator in relation to opioid and nutritional cues. *Human Reproduction* **8**, 154–61. [Comprehensive review]

Loucks AB, *et al.* (1992). The reproductive system and exercise in women. *Medicine and Science in Sports and Exercise* **24**, S288–S293. [Comprehensive review]

Maron BJ (1986). Structural features of the athletes' heart as defined by echocardiography. *Journal of the American College of Cardiology* **7**, 190–203. [Comprehensive review of echo changes in athletes]

Maughan RJ (1999). Nutritional ergogenic aids and exercise performance. *Nutrition Research Reviews* **12**, 255–80. [Comprehensive review]

McHugh MP, *et al.* (1999). Exercise-induced muscle damage and potential mechanisms for the repeated bout effect. *Sports Medicine* **27**, 157–70. [Comprehensive review]

Mittleman MA, *et al.* (1993). Triggering myocardial infarction by heavy physical exertion. *New England Journal of Medicine* **329**, 1677–83). [Important trial demonstrating the risk of myocardial infarction with unaccustomed physical activity]

Neely FG (1998). Biomechanical risk factors for exercise-related lower limb injuries. *Sports Medicine* **26**, 395–413. [Comprehensive review]

Otis CL, *et al.* (1997). American College of Sports Medicine position stand. The female athlete triad. *Medicine and Science in Sport and Exercise* **29**, i–ix. [Comprehensive review]

Renstrom PAFH (1999). An introduction to chronic overuse injuries. In: Harries MG, *et al.*, eds. *Oxford textbook of sports medicine*, pp 633–48. Oxford University Press. [Comprehensive review]

Robinson TL, *et al.* (1995). Gymnasts exhibit higher bone mass than runners despite similar prevalence of amenorrhoea and oligomenorrhoea. *Journal of Bone and Mineral Research* **10**, 26–35. [Important trial showing difference between gymnasts and runners]

Sawka MN, *et al.* (1996). American College of Sports Medicine position stand. The use of blood doping as an ergogenic aid. *Medicine and Science in Sport and Exercise* **28**, i–viii. [Comprehensive review]

Walsh NP, *et al.* (1998). Glutamine, exercise and immune function. *Sports Medicine* **26**, 177–91. [Comprehensive review of the role of glutamine]

Wolman RL, *et al.* (1990). Menstrual status and exercise are important determinants of spinal trabecular bone density in female athletes. *British Medical Journal* **301**, 516–18. [Important trial showing difference between rowers and runners]

Zanker CL, Swaine IL (1998). The relationship between serum oestradiol concentration and energy balance in young women distance runners. *International Journal of Sports Medicine* **19**, 104–8. [Important trial demonstrating the effects of energy imbalance in athletes]

29

Adolescent medicine

29 Adolescent medicine

R. Viner

Introduction

Young people between 10 and 20 years of age comprise 12 to 15 per cent of the population in most developed countries, and are increasingly recognized as a distinct patient group requiring a special approach. Few diseases are unique to adolescence, but adolescents have a distinct epidemiology of disease and present a constellation of symptoms and problems not found in children or adults. Special communication skills are needed to take an accurate history and elicit clinical signs in young people. The effective treatment of illness in adolescence requires adept management of compliance, consent, and confidentiality, and relationships between the young person and their family.

The most serious health problems affecting young people are primary care issues, including teenage pregnancy, drug misuse, mental health problems, and violence. However, young people with acute or chronic medical conditions present management challenges to physicians—challenges that are mounting with the increasing incidence of chronic illness in adolescence.

What is adolescence?

Strictly speaking, adolescence is the period between childhood and adulthood. Theoretical definitions abound; Freud saw adolescence as the period of recapitulation of the childhood Oedipal complex, while Erickson claimed that the struggle between Identity and Role Confusion typified adolescence. The World Health Organization defines adolescence as between 10 and 20 years of age. However, chronological definitions take little account of the timing of the developmental changes at the heart of the concept of adolescence.

Some have suggested that adolescence is merely a socially constructed rite of passage. These claims ignore the biological changes of puberty and psychological developments driven by increasing maturation of the central nervous system. The most useful definition is that adolescence is a period of biopsychosocial maturation leading to functionally independent adult life.

Adolescent development

All clinical interactions with adolescents must be seen against a developmental background. The timing and tempo of the events of biological, psychological, and social development each proceed independently, although they are deeply intertwined (Table 1).

Biological changes

The biological changes of adolescence are puberty, the pubertal growth spurt, and accompanying maturational changes in other organ systems. These include maturation of enzyme systems (such as cytochrome P-450), accretion of peak bone mass, and the development of sexually dimorphic adult patterns in blood lipids, haemoglobin, and red cell indices. It is important for physicians to be able to identify the pubertal stage in adolescents, particularly in chronic illness. The defining event of puberty in girls is the menarche. The biological changes of adolescence are universal to all races, as are psychological changes driven by increasing brain myelination. However, most psychological and social development is culture-specific, varying with the social and cultural norms of childhood and adult roles in society.

Psychological development

Before adolescence, children think concretely, understanding only the immediate and short-term consequences of actions or events. Ideas and concepts can be manipulated only by using concrete representations. From the age of 12 years onwards, thought patterns begin to become formal operational or abstract, with the ability to manipulate ideas rather than things, imagine the future, and conceive multiple outcomes of actions. These capacities are important for the development of a settled personal and sexual identity.

Social development

The essential social tasks of adolescence are developing a sense of personal identity, moving from dependence to relative independence, and developing mature relationships with peers. Rather than achieving 'independence' from the family; adolescence involves renegotiating family relationships from a position of increasing adult equality. These challenges will exist across all cultures; however, the point at which successful completion is expected varies greatly.

Why is medicine different when dealing with adolescents?

Clinical medicine with adolescents is different because adolescents have special patterns of disease and special needs in the management of illness. Few diseases, aside from disorders of puberty, are specific to adolescence. However, the causes of mortality and morbidity in adolescents are distinct from both children and adults. Environmental and social causes of mortality (for example, accidents and suicide) account for a larger proportion of total adolescent mortality than at any other age (Fig. 1). Young people are one of the only groups in which overall mortality rates have fallen little during the past 40 years.

Common paediatric or adult diseases present with different patterns during adolescence. Type I diabetes has its peak age of incidence around 12 to 14 years. Puberty accelerates the progression of diabetic complications and the metabolic control of diabetes is poorer during adolescence than at any other age, due both to the growth-hormone excess of puberty and the psychosocial challenges of chronic illness management. Cancer during adolescence is remarkable for its combination of 'late' presentations of paediatric cancers, 'age-specific' cancers of adolescence (for example, bone tumours), and early-onset 'adult-type' carcinomas.

Medical challenges of adolescent development

The real challenges of medicine in adolescents come from the reciprocal impacts of adolescent development on disease management and quality of life. This is especially true in chronic conditions (Table 2) that may retard adolescent development, producing pubertal and growth delay, delayed social independence, poor body and sexual self-image, and educational and vocational failure. Physicians and paediatricians must monitor growth and pubertal development in chronic illness, until well into the early twenties.

Being chronically ill, having a visible disability, or being required to adhere to difficult treatment regimens is specially difficult during adolescence. Alienation from the peer group and absence from school cause social isolation, failure of socialization, and educational underachievement. The importance of helping young people with chronic illness or disability to develop independent adult living and vocational skills has been shown in longitudinal follow-up studies.

Conversely, developmental issues affect the management of illness. Poor adherence (compliance) and poor disease management are almost 'the rule' in adolescence. Immature abilities to imagine future consequences make the prevention of long-term complications of illness a poor motivator for compliance. Medical advice may be rejected as part of growing independence from parents, particularly in chronic paediatric illnesses where medical staff have become medical 'parents'. Adherence and disease control are also put at risk by the developmental need to explore possible modes of future behaviour, no matter how dangerous (derogatively referred to as 'adolescent risk-taking'). Risky behaviour such as smoking, alcohol, and recreational drug use are as common in adolescents with chronic illness or disability as in the general population.

The management of ill-health in adolescence

Most doctors have adolescent patients, but few are experienced or skilled in dealing with such patients. American studies suggest that only around one-third of physicians and paediatricians enjoy working with adolescents, and that another third have very little interest in caring for them. The effective clinical management of any disease in an adolescent requires a non-judgemental communication style, a knowledge of adolescent development, an awareness of consent and confidentiality issues, and an ethnographic approach that aims at understanding the health beliefs and situations in which the young person manages their disease.

Communication with young people

Neither the standard paediatric consultation (doctor communicates with parents) nor the standard adult consultation (doctor communications solely with patient) is appropriate for adolescents. It is best to see young people together with their parents, and also by themselves. While time consuming, this is essential for obtaining an accurate history, understanding their motivations and goals, and for getting accurate information about risky behaviour.

Table 1 Biopsychosocial development during adolescence

	Biological	Psychological	Social
Early adolescence	Early puberty *Girls*: Breast bud and pubic hair development (Tanner stage II) Initiation of growth spurt *Boys*: Testicular enlargement Beginning of genital growth (stage II)	Thinking remains concrete, but with development of early moral concepts Progression of sexual identity development: • development of sexual orientation—possibly by experimentation • possible homosexual peer interest • reassessment and restructuring of body image in the face of rapid growth	Realization of differences from parents Beginning of strong peer identification Early exploratory behaviour(smoking, violence)
Mid adolescence	*Girls*: Mid to late puberty (stage IV–V) and completion of growth Menarche (stage IV event) Development of female body shape with fat deposition *Boys*: Mid puberty (stages III and IV) Spermarche and nocturnal emissions Voice breaking Initiation of growth spurt (stage III–IV)	Emergence of abstract thinking, although ability to imagine future applies to others rather than self (self seen as 'bullet-proof') Growing verbal abilities; adaptation to increasing educational demands Conventional morality(identification of law with morality) Development of fervently held ideology (religious/political)	Establishment of emotional separation from parents Strong peer group identification Increased risky behaviour(smoking, alcohol, drugs, sexual exploration) Heterosexual peer interests develop Early vocational plans Development of an educational trajectory; early notions of vocational future
Late adolescence	*Boys*: Completion of pubertal development (stage V) Continued androgenic effects on muscle bulk and body hair	Complex abstract thinking Postconventional morality(ability to differentiate law from morality) Increased impulse control Further completion of personal identity Further development or rejection of ideology and religion—often fervently	Further separation from parents and development of social autonomy Development of intimate relationships—initially within peer group, then separation of couples from peer group Development of vocational capability, potential or real financial independence

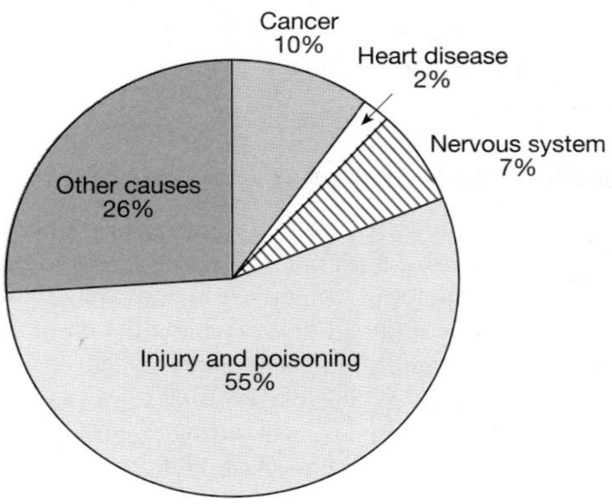

Fig. 1 Causes of death for 15- to 19-year-olds in the United Kingdom, 1997 (*Mortality statistics*, The Stationery Office. DH2, No. 23).

Frameworks have been developed for best practice with young people, the best known being **HEADSS** which reminds clinicians to cover the important domains of: home life; education; activities (friendships, social relationships, exercise); drugs; sexuality (intimate relationships, risky behaviour); and suicide (depression and self-harming). But having a framework is not enough; the key skills required for effective communication with young people are an understanding of adolescent development, empathy, respect and a non-judgemental attitude, understanding the link between physical and emotional well being, and provision of a physically and emotionally safe environment in which a clinical interaction can take place.

Table 3 summarizes these points.

Confidentiality and consent issues

Adolescents require from clinicians confidentiality, respect, and clinical excellence. Services that are not considered to be confidential are less likely to be used by young people. Confidentiality (including keeping confidentiality from parents) should be assured to young people, unless they are found to be at risk from suicide, sexual abuse, or they reveal plans to harm others.

Adolescents can fall into a no-man's land between parental rights over minors and adult rights. In most countries, including the United Kingdom, adolescents are now deemed to have adult rights to consent to treatment if they are legally competent, regardless of their parents' wishes. The legal criteria for competence differ between countries, but usually require the ability to give informed consent and understand the benefits and risks of treatment or non-treatment. In the United Kingdom, competence is presumed over the age of 18 years, while adolescents between 16 and 18 years can consent to treatment but cannot refuse life-saving treatment. Under 16 years of age, adolescents are presumed incompetent unless they demonstrate otherwise.

Adherence issues

There is little evidence that young people with chronic diseases are any less compliant to medical regimens than adults. Many struggle with the responsibility of organizing difficult regimens; others manipulate their regimen as part of their conflict with parents; and many adhere to a regimen of their own choosing—but one that may have little relationship to that prescribed. Practical measures to improve adherence to medical regimens are outlined in Table 4. The most important aspect is to 'decriminalize' non-adherence by recognizing that some non-adherence is universal, and to work with the adolescent to tailor the regimen to meet their health goals.

Transition

Adolescents with continuing health problems will require transfer from paediatric to adult services. Much more than just a clinic transfer, transition requires a change from the family-centred developmentally focused paediatric approach (which infantilizes the adolescent) to an adult medical culture that acknowledges patient autonomy and reproduction and employment issues but neglects growth, development, and family concerns.

Traditional methods of transfer of care by referral letter can lead to adolescents settling poorly into the new service or even dropping out of medical supervision altogether. This period is particularly dangerous for those diseases where adult services or skills are poorly developed, such as in 'paediatric' metabolic diseases or congenital heart disease. All paediatric specialist clinics should have transition policies and guidelines, especially where many adolescents are transferring. Preparation for transition should begin in early adolescence, and young people should only move to adult care when they have the necessary experience to survive independently in the adult service.

Table 2 Reciprocal effects of chronic illness or disability and adolescent development

Effects of chronic illness or disability on development	Effects of developmental issues on chronic illness or disability
Biological Delayed puberty Short stature Reduced bone mass accretion	*Biological* Increased caloric requirement for growth may impair response to diseases Pubertal hormones may affect the disease (e.g. growth hormone impairs metabolic control in diabetes)
Psychological Infantilization Adoption of the role of being a sick person Egocentricity persists into late adolescence Impaired development of sense of sexual or attractive self	*Poor adherence and poor disease control* due to: • poorly developed abstract thinking and planning(reduced ability to plan and prepare using abstract concepts) • difficulty in imagining the future; self-concept as being 'bullet-proof' • rejection of medical professionals as part of separation from parents • exploratory (risk-taking) behaviour
Social Reduced independence at a time of when independence is normally developing Failure of peer relationships then intimate (couple) relationships Social isolation Educational failure and then vocational failure; failure of development of independent living ability	*Associated health risk behaviours* Chaotic eating habits may result in poor nutrition Smoking, alcohol, and drug use often in excess of normal population rates Sexual risk-taking, possibly from realization of limited lifespan

Table 3 Practical points for clinical interactions with young people

1. Assure confidentiality—both in the clinical interaction and in the clinical/hospital set-up.
2. See young people by themselves as well as with their parents.
3. Be empathic, respectful, and non-judgemental.
4. Be yourself; don't be an adolescent and don't use hip jargon; don't be their friend. Maintain appropriate boundaries
5. Provide an emotionally and physically safe environment. A gender balance among staff is important, particularly where physical examinations are undertaken.
6. Ensure you take a full psychosocial history, including HEADSS (home life, education, activities, drugs, sexuality, suicide, and depression).
7. Use immediate motivators not future motivators to change behaviour. Remember that growth and puberty are excellent motivators for improved disease control in young people with chronic illness.

Drug, alcohol, sex, and health promotion

By 15 years of age, around 24 per cent of adolescents in Britain are regular smokers, 38 per cent will be regular alcohol consumers, and around 25 per cent are sexually active. Young people with chronic illness have similar rates of risk, although few physicians (especially paediatricians) address smoking, alcohol, or sex issues with young people with chronic conditions. Healthy behaviour begun in adolescence continues into adult life, and health promotion during early adolescence can discourage smoking, drug use, and unsafe sexual behaviour. Over 70 per cent of adolescents visit a doctor every year; each clinical interaction should provide an opportunity for health promotion.

Table 4 Practical measures to improve adherence in adolescents

'Decriminalize' non-compliance. Ask: 'Most (young) people have trouble taking medications. How many days a week do you manage to take them all?'
Involve the adolescent as much as possible in planning the regimen, choosing the drugs (if there is an alternative), and deciding on dose-timing. Young people are more likely to adhere to programmes for which they feel responsible.
Search for motivating factors that will help the young person continue with treatment. Issues about growth, weight, and appearance are often useful in chronic illness.
Make a contract with the young person in which each side agrees to fulfil certain conditions.
Provide written instructions (in adolescent-friendly language) about the treatment regimen.
Focus the regimen on the least chaotic time in the adolescent's daily life. This is usually in the morning and before leaving for school.
For complex regimens, don't assume adherence is the same for each drug. Adolescents may faithfully adhere to some and never take others because of beliefs about the drug or side-effects. Discuss compliance and explore beliefs and knowledge about each medication separately.
Find ways to involve the family without increasing parent–adolescent conflict about independence, e.g. assign the parents 'check-points' every 2–3 days but forbid constant nagging (which usually reduces compliance!).
Don't assume that non-adherence results from ignorance or that education will improve compliance.

(Taken with permission from Viner *et al.* 2000.)

Psychological issues of illness in adolescence

Epidemiological studies show that up to 20 per cent of adolescents may suffer mental health problems, most not being serious and frequently presenting with physical symptoms. Conversely, many young people with chronic medical conditions suffer adverse psychological sequelae, particularly depression and anxiety and adjustment disorders. During the developmental changes of adolescence, the psyche and soma are inextricably interrelated. Assessment and management of the reciprocal psychosocial impacts of adolescence and chronic illness (see Table 2) are a central part of medicine for adolescents. Severe or chronic illness in adolescence should be managed by multidisciplinary teams, including mental health, social, and youth workers and teachers as well as doctors and nurses.

Conclusions

Adolescent medicine demands that special attention be paid to communication, compliance, and risk behaviour, as the person develops. Greater skill in dealing with young people is required in all areas of the medical profession. These skills can be learned; evidence from randomized trials suggests that training in techniques for communicating with young people is effective and is valued by doctors and young people alike.

Further reading

Kramer T, Garralda ME (1998). Psychiatric disorders in adolescents in primary care. *British Journal of Psychiatry* **173**, 508–13.

British Medical Association (2001). *Consent, rights and choices in health care for children and young people.* BMJ, London.

Kyngas HA, Kroll T, Duffy ME (2000). Compliance in adolescents with chronic diseases: a review. *Journal of Adolescent Health* **26**, 379–88.

Goldenring JM, Cohen E (1988). Getting into adolescent heads. *Contemporary Pediatrics* **July**, 75–90.

Leffert N, Petersen AC (1995). Patterns of development during adolescence. In: Rutter M, Smith DJ, eds. *Psychosocial disorders in young people*, pp 67–103. Wiley, London.

MacKenzie RG (1990). Approach to the adolescent in the clinical setting. *Medical Clinics of North America* **74**, 1085–95.

Sanci LA, *et al.* (2000). Evaluation of the effectiveness of an educational intervention for general practitioners in adolescent health care: randomised controlled trial. *British Medical Journal* **320**, 224–30.

Viner RM (1999). Transition from paediatric to adult care. Bridging the gaps or passing the buck? *Archives of Disease in Childhood* **81**, 271–5.

Viner RM, *et al.* (2000). *Improving adherence to treatment in adolescents with chronic conditions: a practical evidence-based approach.* Society for Adolescent Medicine, San Diego, CA.

White PD (1999). Transition to adulthood. *Current Opinion in Rheumatology* **11**, 408–11.

Zirinsky L (1993). The psychological impact of illness in adolescence. In: Brook CDG, ed. *The practice of medicine in adolescence*, pp 25–34. Edward Arnold, London.

30

Geratology

30.1 Medicine in old age

John Grimley Evans

Few, if any, diseases occur only in old age. The speciality of geriatric medicine is defined less in terms of the diseases it treats than in the range of responsibility it accepts. This responsibility embraces preventative care, health promotion, and diagnosis and treatment of acute illness followed by rehabilitation and resettlement of patients in the community. Some diseases are so much more common in later life that geriatricians will necessarily have more experience in managing them than will some other physicians. However, the great majority of what is to be found in a textbook of medicine will apply to older as well as to younger adults. Indeed it is an ethical duty of doctors to assume, in the absence of evidence to the contrary, that treatments that are effective for younger adults are at least as effective for those who are older.

Some aspects of medical practice need to take account of common age-associated changes in physiology. This chapter will briefly review some of these areas, but it begins with an outline of the background to medicine in later life provided by the universal processes of human ageing.

Ageing

Table 1 summarizes the sources of differences between young and old people. True ageing comprises those processes whereby differences arise because older people change from what they were when younger. However, not all differences between young and old people are due to ageing:

1. Selective survival leads to very old people showing genetic, sociobehavioural, and psychological differences from younger members of the same ethnic groups. Not surprisingly, differences include a lower prevalence of genes, social factors, and lifestyles associated with the risk of fatal diseases. Psychological variables with survival value include higher intelligence, better education, and a will for self-determination.

2. Cohort effects are prominent as causes of differences between young and old in changing societies. Apart from the effects of poverty and poor nutrition in early life, people born 70 years ago were raised and educated in a society very different from that of young people today. In longitudinal studies, where people are tested against their own former selves, declines in mental abilities appear less dramatic and later than in cross-sectional comparisons with younger individuals. Unfortunately most popular notions of the effects of ageing are based on uncritical acceptance of the findings of cross-sectional studies. Differences between young and old in psychological function partly reflect changes in educational emphasis, for example on computer skills rather than irregular Latin verbs. Also relevant, however, are changes in the cultural valuation of matters such as verbal abilities and good manners over the decades. Older people in England speak more slowly than the young not because they are slower witted but because 70 years ago it would have been considered ill-bred to talk as fast as is the custom nowadays. Another problem with cross-sectional studies is that they distort the pattern of ageing by blurring differences between individuals. Many individuals show preservation of mental function until the last year of life when abilities decline rapidly in what is sometimes termed the 'terminal drop'. With age the proportion of individuals who are in this phase will increase, so lowering the average performance of age groups. The true ageing pattern of a relatively constant level of performance followed by abrupt decline is therefore obscured by an appearance of continuous progressive decay.

3. Differential challenge. Since ageing is characterized by loss of adaptability it can only be accurately assessed by presenting individuals of different ages with similar challenges. In practice, society is organized so that older people may be faced with more severe challenges than are the young, and their poorer outcomes may then be attributed to ageing rather than inequity. This is particularly important in assessing the benefits potentially available to older people from medical interventions. There is abundant evidence from the United Kingdom and the United States that older people are on average provided with poorer quality health care than are younger adults. In the United States this is well documented for cancer treatment and in the United Kingdom for treatment of heart disease. In both countries the problem seems to arise from ageist prejudice among health workers at a local level in that its effects vary from district to district and hospital to hospital. Although less readily documented, there can be little doubt that ageism is as rife in primary as in secondary care. American studies have shown that primary care physicians spend less time with older patients than with younger ones even though the problems of the former are the more numerous, serious, and complex.

Table 1 Sources of differences between younger and older people

True ageing	Primary	Intrinsic Extrinsic
	Secondary	Species level Individual level
Non-ageing	Selective survival Cohort effects Differential challenge	

True ageing

Ageing, in the sense of senescence, is a progressive loss of adaptability of an individual organism as time passes. As we grow older the homoeostatic mechanisms on which survival depends become on average less sensitive, slower, less accurate, and less well sustained. Sooner or later we encounter a challenge from the internal or external environment to which we can no longer mount an effective response and we die. An increase in the risk of death with age is therefore the biological hallmark of senescence. In the human species death rates, which are high in the early years of life, fall to a nadir around the age of 12 to 13 at which point ageing first becomes manifest as rates turn upwards and continue through late adolescent perturbations due to violent and accidental deaths, to mount continuously and broadly exponentially throughout adult life (Fig. 1). The lowest point on

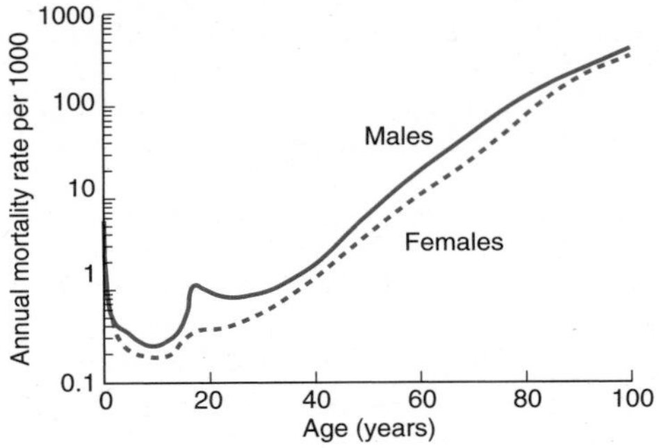

Fig. 1 Sex- and age-specific total mortality rates. England and Wales 1988.

the age-specific mortality curve which marks the onset of manifest senescence has been constant in England and Wales for over 100 years. It presumably therefore represents the point of maximum biological fitness. This is, in fact, to be expected since evolutionary pressure will lead to maximum fitness at the time of onset of reproductive capacity.

As individuals, we age at different rates and with different patterns. Although average performance on measures of physical and psychological function may decline with age, interindividual variance increases and there will be many people in their eighties or beyond performing within a range normal for young adults. It is important to assess older people as individuals when making judgements about their function and capacity to benefit from medical interventions and not to assume that they are all average members of their age group.

Primary ageing

Primary ageing is the product of interactions between intrinsic, genetically determined, factors and extrinsic factors in lifestyle and environment. Some interactions are specific. A high dietary sodium intake will cause hypertension in genetically predisposed individuals, and excess dietary calories will lead to obesity and type 2 diabetes with its associated problems in people carrying the so-called 'thrifty genes' that allowed our intermittently starving ancestors to survive periods of famine by laying down body fat during the good times. Other interactions have more general effects: for example lack of exercise hastens the ageing of bone, muscle, and the cardiovascular system. Cigarette smoking impairs lung function, has anti-oestrogenic effects, brings forward the age of the menopause, and reduces bone density in addition to causing a variety of cancers.

Extrinsic factors in ageing are identified by epidemiological studies of people ageing under different conditions and by interventional studies of the effects of lifestyle or environmental modification. Epidemiological studies can be difficult to interpret because of clustering of lifestyle factors. Thus women who are health conscious enough to take hormone replacement therapy are more likely to be non-smokers, take regular exercise, have regular health checkups, and watch their weight and blood pressure. Statistical methods aimed, for example, at detecting a specific effect of hormone therapy on cardiovascular disease by 'adjusting' for the other factors are unreliable for ineluctable statistical reasons. Only a randomized placebo-controlled trial could settle this particular issue, but randomized trials of lifestyle modifications are rarely practicable.

The strongest evidence that extrinsic factors must be important comes from changes over time in the pattern of ageing. There have been dramatic improvements in the incidence of coronary heart disease and in some cancers over recent years. Conversely, there has in several countries been an increase in the age-specific incidence of fractures of the proximal femur. Overall, however, over the last 20 years older people in the United States have been living longer and also enjoying a falling prevalence of chronic disability. The presumption is that this is because of the adoption of healthier lifestyles including the use of preventative measures such as control of blood pressure, together with the rational and timely deployment of health interventions which reduce disability, such as hip replacement and coronary surgery. We have no idea whether similar changes are occurring in the United Kingdom or elsewhere, but the American evidence tells us that it could be made to happen.

Intrinsic ageing is due to cumulative damage to cells and their components which comes about because the body's systems of damage control are less than 100 per cent efficient. Damage control comprises processes of prevention, detection, repair, and replacement. Damage occurs from a variety of sources including heat, radiation, glycation (non-enzymatic cross-linking by sugar molecules of proteins, nuclear and mitochondrial DNA, and other biological polymers), and from free oxygen radicals generated in particular by mitochondrial metabolism.

Damage control is expensive in terms of energy. Although it might be biologically feasible to attain 100 per cent accuracy in damage control, organisms which achieved potential immortality in this way would still die from accident, predation, disease, famine, or warfare. They would therefore be at an evolutionary disadvantage in competition with organisms that devoted somewhat less of their resources to retarding ageing but were thereby able to maintain a higher average reproduction rate. Evolutionary pressure towards a longer lifespan will arise as environments become safer, when a slower reproduction rate can be more than compensated for by ensuring greater survival of offspring by strategies such as choice of breeding season or parental care. None the less, for any species in a specific ecological niche, investment of resources in damage control to retard ageing and prolong lifespan will always be at a level less than is necessary to abolish ageing. Thus, although maximum lifespan has increased enormously over the history of our species, we have not completely eliminated the accumulation of damage that manifests as ageing.

The fact that our lifespan has increased so rapidly, however, suggests that a fairly small number of genes may have an important effect. For the reasoning outlined above these genes are likely to be relevant to processes of damage control. Systematic comparisons of the genomes of centenarians with younger people are under way in the hope of identifying 'longevity assurance genes' whose mechanisms of action might be manipulable. Meanwhile, experimental attempts to slow intrinsic ageing are aimed at reducing the sources of damage, particularly from free oxygen radicals. Interventions under investigation include increasing the levels of free radical scavengers in cells, and reducing the production of radicals by limiting food intake and inessential mitochondrial metabolism.

Secondary ageing

Secondary ageing refers to adaptations to primary ageing changes. At the species level the female menopause is thought to be an adaptation to the age-associated increase in risk of maternal and infant death with age. In terms of getting genes into succeeding generations a woman in middle age will do better to give up increasingly dangerous and ineffective efforts to produce children containing 50 per cent of her genes and instead to devote her energies to the survival of her grandchildren each containing 25 per cent of her genes. At the individual level secondary ageing is most obvious in psychological adaptations to age-associated changes in memory and physical capabilities. Adaptations to changes in memory may range from minor obsessive traits to an old person's refusal to go shopping for fear they might get lost. The first is not obsessive–compulsive disorder and the second is not agoraphobia. Doctors need to be aware in a general way of the possibility of secondary ageing in order to resist unthinking attempts to 'normalize' some physiological parameter or aspect of behaviour where the deviation from the normal is in fact adaptive.

Sex differences in ageing

As Fig. 1 shows, death rates in females are lower than in males at all ages. In Westernized societies women outlive men by 5 to 6 years on average. Epidemiological evidence suggests that in the United Kingdom nearly four of these extra years are due to intrinsic differences between the sexes while the remining difference has developed during the twentieth century due to extrinsic effects. There is a paradox in that although women outlive men they are much more likely to become disabled and dependent in old age. As discussed below, the physical basis for this probably lies largely with sex differences in muscle bulk rather than particular disease entities. However, the impact of disability on an elderly woman is increased by the likelihood that she married a man older than herself and so has outlived her husband (and all too often his occupational pension) by more than the average sex difference in lifespan. It has also to be admitted that a woman is more likely to be capable of looking after a disabled husband than man is of caring for disabled wife. The sum of these biological, environmental, and social factors emerges in dependency rates in later life. Although one man in seven who reaches the age of 65 in the United States can expect to spend a year or more in a nursing home before death, the proportion for women is one in three.

Age-associated changes of medical significance

Anatomical and physiological changes associated with ageing are described in almost every body system. Most start to become apparent in early or middle adult life but their magnitude and practical significance vary considerably.

The cardiovascular system

Interpretation of changes in cardiovascular function in old age is made difficult by the age-associated increase in prevalence of ischaemic heart disease. The principal anatomical alterations in the cardiovascular system include an increase in the amount of fibrous tissue in the skeleton of the heart and in the myocardium and valves and an accumulation of lipofuscin in the myocardial fibres. This last change has no evident functional significance. There is also an increase in amyloid material in the aged heart, but again this does not usually appear to have clinical significance. There is a decrease in the elasticity of the aorta and its main branches, accompanied by an increase in the diameter and length.

There is a minor decline in resting heart rate and maximum heart rate on exercise. These changes probably relate to a decrease in the number of pacemaker cells in the sinoatrial node and to alterations in their reactivity to sympathetic and parasympathetic stimuli. Cardiac output at rest does not fall with age, but maximum exercise-induced cardiac output falls to a variable extent. Mean arterial venous oxygen differences are unaltered. Since the older heart in exercise shows a smaller increase in cardiac rate than is seen in younger patients, the increased cardiac output is achieved by a relatively greater increase in stroke volume than in younger adults. The older heart is essentially more dependent than the young on the Frank–Starling mechanism for increasing output.

Owing to diminished compliance due to heart wall hypertrophy and crosslinking of proteins, the older heart takes longer to fill during diastole then does the young heart. The older patient is therefore relatively intolerant of tachycardia since at very fast rates stroke volume and cardiac output will decline. In addition, the low compliance of the ventricular wall leads to an increase in the relative importance of atrial output to diastolic filling.

Management of heart disease in older people

For various, though less than cogent, reasons older people tend to be omitted from randomized controlled trials, but it has to be assumed for ethical reasons that treatments shown to be effective for younger patients will be at least as effective for the old. In some instances benefits will be greater in later life because of the increase in background risk of morbidity or mortality. This is documented in the use of thrombolytic treatment for acute myocardial infarction and for the benefits of β-blockers after infarction. A recent study (The Heart Outcomes Prevention Evaluation Study) of the benefit of the angiotensin-converting enzyme inhibitor ramipril in secondary prevention of cardiovascular events in high-risk patients showed benefits at least as great in patients aged over 65 as in those younger.

While lack of evidence relating specifically to relevant age groups should not prevent older people from receiving treatment, care is needed with treatments for which an age-associated increase in the risk of undesirable side-effects may be expected. For example, anticoagulation in atrial fibrillation may need more careful and frequent supervision for an older person than for a younger one. The benefit of β-blockade in improving survival in chronic heart failure has so far only been demonstrated for patients aged up to 80, and since the likelihood of ill-effects of β-blockade increases with age, treatment of older patients should be introduced with low doses and increased slowly ('start low, go slow').

Blood pressure

Ordinary vascular pressures are unchanged (except for a slight rise on exercise) as is pulmonary blood volume. Mean systemic arterial pressure rises in most, but not all, populations, and presumably represents a response of susceptible individuals to environmental factors such as excessive salt intake and perhaps sociocultural stress. In populations in which blood pressure rises, systolic arterial pressure increases more than diastolic, probably as an expression of reduced elasticity of the large arteries. As ageing progresses, diastolic pressure rises to a peak and then falls. The combination of these processes leads to the increasing prevalence in old age of isolated systolic hypertension. This is a risk factor for cardiovascular disease and especially for stroke. Trials show that up to at least the age of 85 reduction of systolic pressure reduces the risk of stroke. Indeed this is another area in which, in terms of numbers needed to treat, reduction of blood pressure in older patients is more effective than at younger ages.

Trials of the treatment of high blood pressure in older people have used conventional drugs, and the assumption has been that it is the fall in blood pressure that matters and the drug used is less important. In terms of average effectiveness β-blockers tend to become less effective as hypotensive agents with age while calcium channel blockers become more effective. Concerns expressed over the long-term safety of calcium channel blockers are not convincing. Conventional treatment is of stepped-care type in which drugs are added in sequence if the response is inadequate. Recent studies in younger patients have emphasized individual variability in responsiveness to different classes of antihypertensive drug such as angiotensin-converting enzyme inhibitors, diuretics, β-blockers, and calcium channel blockers. The varying efficacy probably reflects differences in the underlying mechanisms of the hypertension in individual patients. Instead of launching immediately into stepped care, therefore, a formal trial of different classes of drugs should first be undertaken in the hope of finding a suitable monotherapy. These findings need to be verified in older people, but the idea is intuitively attractive.

An important consideration in managing hypertension at older ages is impairment of the responses of blood pressure to postural change. Baroreceptor responses are often blunted in later life, possibly as a result of sclerotic changes in the carotid sinus, and there may in addition be failure of central and perhaps peripheral vasoconstrictor responses to falling blood pressure. Older people are more susceptible to the risk of hypovolaemia. Postprandial hypotension is also common in older populations and may be a constraint on management of hypertension. When assessing older people taking medication that may affect blood pressure, lying and standing pressures should be used routinely. The role of ambulatory blood pressure monitoring in the management of treatment remains to be defined, but can be helpful in identifying episodes of unexpectedly low pressure that are missed in the clinic.

Atrial fibrillation

As noted earlier, loss of cardiac wall compliance with age increases the importance of the atrial phase of diastolic ventricular filling. Not surprisingly, therefore, the onset of atrial fibrillation, particularly if it is associated with a high ventricular rate, often has serious consequences for an older patient. Intermittent atrial fibrillation is also one of the recognized causes of recurrent syncope at later ages. Rate control is often a matter of clinical urgency for an older patient following the onset of atrial fibrillation, and electrical conversion may be required. Unless some definable precipitant such as myocardial infarction or thyrotoxicosis is present the likelihood of subsequent recurrence and permanence of atrial fibrillation rises with age. Longer-term management needs to take this into account.

Large trials have now established that in the absence of contraindications, patients aged 60 and over with atrial fibrillation should receive long-term anticoagulant therapy in order to reduce their three- to fivefold increased risk of stroke. Patients with associated valvular disease or a dilated left atrium are at even higher risk of stroke. Even in the absence of overt stroke, computed tomography scanning has shown that older patients in atrial fibrillation have a higher prevalence of 'silent' cerebral infarcts; anticoagulant therapy may therefore reduce the subsequent incidence of multi-infarct dementia.

Oral anticoagulants have more powerful pharmacodynamic effects in later life and the higher risk of complications calls for more intensive medical supervision of an old person taking anticoagulation than of a younger one. The target international normalized ratio of 2 to 2.5 is appropriate and it is prudent to reduce pre-existing high blood pressure. Where anticoagulants are thought to carry unacceptable risks, owing for example to poor compliance, intermittent high alcohol intake, or frequent falls, antiplatelet therapy should be considered. Published trials relate mostly to aspirin, and newer drugs such as clopidogrel require further evaluation in older patients.

In young patients, paroxysmal atrial fibrillation does not seem to be associated with an enhanced risk of stroke. The situation is less clear for patients aged over 60, some of whom will develop intermittent atrial fibrillation as they progress towards chronic established atrial fibrillation. There is epidemiological evidence that the risk of stroke may be greatest during this phase. Geriatricians will therefore normally anticoagulate an elderly person with intermittent fibrillation.

Respiratory system

The interpretation of changes in respiratory function with age is complicated by a high prevalence of cigarette smoking in many populations. Total lung volume does not alter but vital capacity falls and residual volume increases with age so that over the age of about 60 the critical closing volume exceeds the functional residual volume. Ventilatory capacity falls with age at a slower rate in non-smokers than in smokers. Ventilation-perfusion inequality increases slightly, probably mainly as a result of increasing inequality of ventilation. These changes in lung function reflect a decrease in elasticity of the lungs and of respiratory muscular strength but the overall consequences are minimal in terms of their effect on the blood gases. Closure of small airways during resting breathing can produce crepitations at the lung basis posteriorly in older patients. As an isolated finding these should not be overinterpreted as a sign of left ventricular failure. These same changes can also lead to areas of atelectasis in ill older patients or following surgery. Physiotherapy for older patients after surgery should therefore concentrate on expanding the lung bases rather than clearing sputum.

The principles of management of respiratory disease do not vary with the age of the patient. Diagnostic probabilities may need to be adjusted for age and for cohort effects. Cough due to left ventricular failure or to oesophageal reflux disease may become more common, and older people are more likely to have experienced past industrial exposures, for example to asbestos and coal dust.

Renal function and fluid and electrolyte balance

Old people are particularly susceptible to disorders of fluid and electrolyte balance. This is due in part to age-associated changes in physiology and partly to a higher incidence of challenges to homoeostasis from disease and drugs.

Renal function

Age-related changes in renal function are well documented. The glomerular filtration rate falls as do tubular reabsorptive and secretory capacities. Typically, these changes exceed the decline in lean body mass so that serum urea and creatinine concentrations rise slightly. Several formulae have been devised to try to estimate the glomerular filtration rate from serum creatinine taking age, weight, and sex into account. Various forms of the Cockroft–Gault equation are available as a means of estimating creatinine clearance from serum creatinine and body weight. This formula is only approximate and can mislead in extreme old age and in the presence of obesity where calculation based on ideal body weight or lean mass body weight may be more accurate. Where accuracy is important, such formulae are no substitute for formal creatinine clearance based on a 24-h urine collection.

The response to an acid load is impaired and the maximum rate of secretion of hydrogen ions falls. Changes in blood pH in response to an acid load are therefore greater in magnitude and longer in duration than in younger people. Response to antidiuretic hormone is reduced and water conservation less efficient.

Thirst

A delayed response to fluid deprivation due to impaired thirst mechanisms in old age may compound the effect of delayed renal responses to changes in fluid status. The sensation of thirst is decreased in later life. In an experimental study of 24 h of fluid deprivation younger volunteers felt thirsty while older volunteers did not. When given access to water the older volunteers drank less than the young. Similar differences between young and old were found following infusions of hypertonic saline in which the younger volunteers were able to adjust serum osmolality by water ingestion more accurately than the old. It is not clear, however, to what extent the changed physiology is due to insensitivity of the osmoreceptors and baroreceptors rather than to a deficit in the opioid-mediated drinking drive.

The decline in thirst sensitivity with age is one reason why older people are at enhanced risk of dehydration. This effect may be exaggerated if an old person voluntarily restricts fluid intake in the hope of controlling urinary urgency or incontinence, or to avoid having to call for nursing assistance when in hospital.

Conversely some elderly people, often hypertensive women, show an enhanced thirst response to diuretics (particularly amiloride) with increased water intake and hyponatraemia.

Other age-associated changes

Average renin and aldosterone levels diminish with age with consequent impairment of sodium conservation. Renal concentrating ability is also reduced, which is partly due to a decrease in medullary hypertonicity and partly to impaired renal responsiveness to vasopressin which may result in excessive water losses. The ability of older patients to cope with volume expansion is also impaired and older individuals take longer to excrete a sodium load. There is also a possibility that vasopressin secretion may be impaired.

Secretion of atrial natriuretic peptide in response to hypervolaemia may be reduced in older people and the responsiveness of the kidney to atrial natriuretic peptide may also be reduced.

Implications for clinical care

Assessment of fluid status is an essential component of the evaluation of an elderly patient who is unwell. Sometimes a degree of fluid deprivation will have preceded the illness because some older patients deliberately minimize their fluid intake with the hope of reducing problems of urinary urgency and incontinence. During an illness the most sensitive assessment of fluid balance is by daily weighings, but every attempt should be made to maintain accurate fluid balance charts as well. Infections, commonly pneumonia or urinary tract infections, are frequent causes of dehydration. This is in part due to loss due to fever, which may be overlooked if body temperature is not measured with especial care and after a patient has recovered from travelling in a cold ambulance to hospital. Older people are also more susceptible than the young to the effects of high environmental temperature.

Many old people are on long-term diuretic treatment which can exacerbate the effects of illness as well as causing problems in their own right. In addition to hypovolaemia and postural hypotension, hyponatraemia and disorders of potassium balance can be caused by diuretic therapy. Diuretics may precipitate hyperuricaemia and gout in older patients and destabilize diabetes. The significance of the lipid-raising effect of diuretics on lipid levels in old age is less clear. As noted above, some older people, especially women with hypertension, seem particularly susceptible to diuretics and overcompensate for diuresis with excess water intake so leading to hyponatraemia.

As far as possible dehydration should be corrected by oral intake. Intravenous therapy provides for more rapid and accurate correction but care must be taken over the rapidity of correction of hypo- or hypernatraemia. Subcutaneous fluid replacement is now established as an option where intravenous access is difficult or fluid correction is less than urgent. The infusion needle can be placed subcutaneously in the abdominal wall, the axilla, or the subclavicular area, but for a confused patient between the shoulder blades can be a less troublesome site. Hyaluronidase, 1500 iu, can be given as a bolus through the cannula if the infusion runs too slowly but is expensive, does not improve comfort, and is not usually necessary with an older patient. The infusion site should be changed every 24 or 48 h. Normal saline is well-tolerated by this route, and 5 per cent dextrose can also be given safely at doses up to 1 ml/min (1.5 litres per day). If necessary, potassium chloride up to 40 mmol can be added to each litre of solution, but this may increase complication rates due to local inflammation and secondary infection of the infusion site. Colloid and hyperosmolar solutions should not be given subcutaneously.

Urinary incontinence

This socially disabling condition affects approximately 2 per cent of middle-aged men and 12 per cent of middle-aged women and increases with age to a prevalence of around 8 per cent in men and 16 per cent in women over the age of 75 years. A number of classifications of urinary incontinence have been proposed and Table 2 presents a common version. The patient with acutely developing incontinence due to illness or injury should be reassured and every effort should be made to ensure that it does not continue into a chronic form. As with all problems of older people, possible iatrogenic causes must be reviewed, including rapidly acting diuretics and sedative drugs. Excessive urine output due to hyperglycaemia or hypercalcaemia may present with urinary incontinence, but nocturnal urinary frequency and incontinence due to unrecognized heart failure is much more common. Faecal impaction is another common remediable cause of urinary incontinence in hospitalized older people.

Many patients with dementia become incontinent, but incontinence should never be attributed solely to dementia unless the latter is severe and until all treatable causes have been excluded. Functional incontinence due to the inability of an old person to reach a toilet in time is unnecessarily prevalent, particularly in hospitals where old people with mobility problems may have their beds too far from the toilet or where nurses cannot or do not answer bells promptly.

Table 2 Forms of urinary incontinence

Acute	
Transitory due to illness, delirium, epilepsy, etc.	
Established	
Infection	may be the consequence rather than the cause of incontinence. Treatment should not be continued if incontinence persists after the urine is sterile
Functional	difficulty in getting to a toilet
Stress	loss of urine on coughing or straining
Urge	often due to precipitate bladder contractions
Overflow	secondary to obstruction of bladder outflow. Diagnosis may need postvoiding ultrasound. May be due to constipation
Fistulous	for example, fistula between bladder and vagina
Disinhibitory	occurs in frontal brain damage and dementia
Behavioural	a form of social manipulation (rare)

Overflow incontinence when the bladder is only able to overcome an outlet obstruction at high volumes is common in men with prostate difficulties. It is diagnosable by postvoiding ultrasound examination and often requires surgical intervention. Where that is not feasible, or if a patient declines surgery, medical approaches including α-adrenergic blockers (given with care on account of the risk of hypotension) may be helpful. Where there is prostate enlargement there is some evidence for benefit from finasteride which inhibits 5α-reductase, which metabolizes testosterone to the more potent dihydrotestosterone. This can lead over a period of some months to a reduction in prostatic size and improvement in urinary flow rates and obstructive symptoms. There are some antiandrogenic side-effects including impotence and decreased libido, and the drug has to be handled with care by women of child-bearing potential, a fact which may be relevant to carers or nurses involved in dispensing the drug.

Urge incontinence is usually due to instability of the detrusor muscle of the bladder and may also arise through irritation of the bladder by infected urine when it responds to appropriate antibiotic therapy. After identifying the sensitivities of the infecting organism, antibiotic treatment is given and urine culture repeated. If the incontinence is not improved despite eradication of the infection antibiotics should not be continued. Studies have shown no benefit from treatment of asymptomatic urinary infections in older patients. The contractions of an unstable bladder may be inhibited by anticholinergic drugs but these must be used with care as they may induce glaucoma and constipation. Lipid-soluble anticholinergic drugs may also cross the blood–brain barrier and cause delirium. The drugs most commonly in use on account of claims of some degree of specificity for bladder receptors are oxybutynin and tolterodine.

The certain diagnosis of unstable bladder and associated urethral dysfunction requires invasive investigation including cystometry. In practice most cases of urinary incontinence in older patients can be dealt with empirically, and invasive investigations should be reserved for the more intractable cases. It is useful for medical and nursing teams providing care for older people in the community and residential settings or hospitals to agree on a general plan for approaching problems of incontinence. Figure 2 outlines an example of such an approach. In many instances urinary incontinence may be a problem only at night. A single dose of imipramine in the evening may be of benefit, partly through its anticholinergic effects. Setting an alarm to wake the patient to empty his or her bladder prophylactically may also be of benefit. For some patients a small dose of a rapidly acting diuretic in the afternoon followed by restriction of fluids until bedtime will enable the cardiovascular system to reabsorb fluid pooled during the day in the lower limbs without an inconvenient increase in urinary output. The use of dDAVP or other analogues of vasopressin at bedtime in order to produce an antidiuresis during the night has been reported but it carries a high risk of fluid overload and hyponatraemia in older patients.

Long-term catheterization may need to be considered in intractable situations. This is an invasive procedure with a risk of complications and should be undertaken only after the agreement of the patient. Some older patients will choose catheterization in preference to incontinence pads. Catheters should be inserted and changed under strict asepsis and with consideration of antibiotic cover for patients with cardiac valvular disease or joint prostheses. The urine of an older patient with an indwelling catheter will almost inevitably become infected. Although treatment of symptomatic infection must be considered, and the risk of ascending pyelonephritis and haemosepsis kept in mind, repeated courses of antibiotics can lead to colonization with highly resistant organisms. This is particularly undesirable in institutional care. Although a somewhat old-fashioned approach, manipulation of urinary pH by potassium citrate can help and urinary antiseptics such as hexamine hippurate can also be effective. The last should not be given with alkalinizing agents, and although theoretically less effective where an indwelling catheter prevents bladder filling it can be helpful. It should be avoided in renal failure.

Where possible, leg bags should replace the undignified bag-on-a-stand with which so many hospitals unnecessarily advertise their older patients' disability. Problems of backflow when the patient's bladder is lower than the bag when sitting usually indicate a need for a more suitable chair than for putting the bag on the floor.

For older men who are incontinent only at night a condom-type appliance with drainage bag may be helpful, although leakage and discomfort are common complications. No reliable analogous device has yet been produced for women.

A wide range of incontinence pads and holders is available. Specialist incontinence nurses are available in many hospitals and primary care districts who can advise on the most suitable treatment for individual patients. Charities concerned with disabled people are also a valuable source of expert advice.

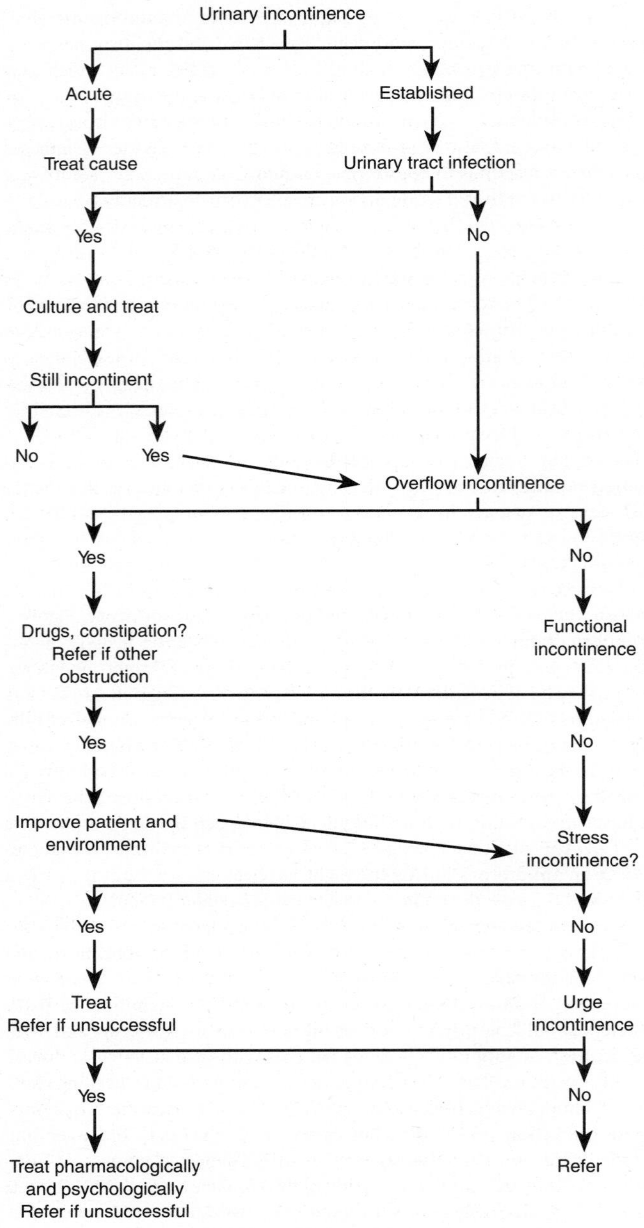

Fig. 2 Illustrative algorithm for management of urinary incontinence in elderly patients 'Refer' indicates referral to specialist urologist or gynaecologist.

The gastrointestinal system

Gastric atrophy becomes increasingly common as age advances but many older people retain full capacity for hydrogen ion secretion. Minor atrophic changes in the mucosa of the small bowel are described but there is no significant change in the absorption of nutrients that are absorbed by passive diffusion. Bacterial overgrowth syndrome may occur in an older patient with an anatomically normal bowel, and needs to be included in the differential diagnosis of diarrhoea, partially intermittent diarrhoea, and malabsorption. The increased risk with age is thought to reflect gastric hypoacidity and reduced motility of the small bowel. Reduced motility of the large bowel is also common and may be associated with diverticular disease or overuse of purgatives.

There is an age-associated reduction in hepatic mass and blood flow, with some consequent changes in first-pass metabolism of drugs and gastrointestinal hormones, but no significant changes in hepatic function as measured by conventional tests.

Gastrointestinal disease

Older people are liable to the full range of gastrointestinal disorders. Even coeliac disease may present for the first time in old age. Gastrointestinal haemorrhage is common and frequently associated with the ingestion of non-steroidal anti-inflammatory drugs. Management of an older patient is along conventional lines but age-associated loss of adaptability should be compensated for by an increased readiness to institute invasive monitoring and to intervene endoscopically or operate sooner rather than later in deteriorating situations. Uncertainty among junior hospital medical staff can be reduced by locally agreed guidelines for management of what is a common but dangerous emergency. Guidelines will only be effective if adhered to by surgeons as well as physicians.

Constipation is a common complaint among older people, but before initiating treatment it may be helpful to ensure that a patient's expectations of bowel function are reasonable. The implications of a recent change of bowel habit must also not be missed. Where chronic constipation is a problem, a daily intake of 10 to 20 g of dietary fibre should be aimed at, with if necessary a stool softening agent such as lactulose. Doses of stimulant laxatives such as senna may be necessary but should be avoided as much as possible.

Faecal incontinence

Recurrent faecal incontinence, with our without associated urinary incontinence, affects about 1 per cent of people aged over 65. Faecal and double incontinence are associated with a range of anorectal and neurological disorders including dementia. In later life, however, the commonest cause is rectal or sigmoid overloading due to constipation (faecal impaction). In middle-aged women a pelvic neuropathy, sometimes possibly a consequence of childbirth, is encountered as a risk of faecal incontinence and may be improved by surgical intervention. Any form of acute or chronic diarrhoea will also lead to incontinence in a proportion of cases. Faecal impaction most commonly occurs in the rectum and can be readily diagnosed by rectal examination. 'High' impaction can occur at the recto-sigmoid junction and above and may need to be diagnosed by a plain abdominal radiograph. High impaction must always raise the possibility of obstruction by a carcinoma or inflammatory stricture due to diverticulitis. Treatment of impaction requires enemas and suppositories, rarely manual evacuation, and then a regular regime of a stool softening medication such as lactulose.

In some cases where faecal incontinence is an intractable problem it can be ameliorated by giving constipating medicine such as loperamide with bowel lavage once a week. This is not an easy regime to establish but can be of help for an old person who wishes to remain in his or her home or to ease nursing problems in residential care.

The locomotor system

Muscle mass, strength, and power

Significant and progressive alterations in average body composition appear in the fifth decade of life. There is a decline in lean body mass with a corresponding fall in oxygen consumption largely attributable to a decline in muscle mass. This is also associated with a decline in muscle strength and power. (As in physics, strength is conceptualized as maximum force and power as the maximum rate of doing work.) The consequences of this trend are more prominent in women who, on average, start adult life with less muscle tissue than men. The age-associated decline is such that by the age of 80 the great majority of women in economically advanced societies are unable to rise from a chair without using their arms to help. This is probably the chief reason why disability levels are so much higher in old women than old men. Improvement in muscular power can be achieved even in the very old by appropriate exercise regimes, which should be considered as part of the rehabilitation programme of an older person who has had to be off his or her feet for more than a day or two.

Bone and joints

Fractures: osteoporosis

The major changes with age in the bony skeleton, which include a steep increase in the prevalence of osteoporosis after middle age, are discussed in Section 19. Loss of bone tissue with age occurs in all humans but appears to vary in severity with place, time, and race. The most important manifestation of the decline in bone mass is a reduction in the mechanical strength of bone and an increase in the tendency to fracture. Although many fractures increase in risk with age and the rising prevalence of osteoporosis, the three 'classical' osteoporotic fractures are those of the vertebrae, the distal forearm, and the proximal femur. Vertebral fractures start to appear at the time of menopause in women and increase in prevalence thereafter. The great majority of limb bone fractures in old age are caused by simple falls. The epidemiological pattern of fractures is partly determined by the causes of falls, the speed of protective responses, and the presence or absence of 'passive' protective factors such as floor coverings, clothing, muscle, or subcutaneous fat. Women are more likely than men to fall and there is an exponential increase in the risk of falling from about the age of 60. It is therefore not surprising that there is a similarly exponential increase in the risk of proximal femoral fracture with a much higher risk in women over the same age range. However, distal forearm fractures which show a steep increase around the age of menopause do not continue to increase in incidence through old age. This probably indicates that the older the person is the less likely he or she is in a fall to throw out an arm in time as a protective response.

Fractures: osteomalacia

Osteomalacia is now rare as a cause of falls and fractures in old age, but it may need to be considered in an older person who has been housebound, has a low dietary vitamin D intake, and takes drugs such as antiepileptics that induce hepatic enzymes that destroy vitamin D derivatives. Age-associated changes in the ability to synthesize vitamin D in the skin and to absorb calcium from the gut are coupled with a reduction in the renal 1α-hydroxylase activity that metabolizes vitamin D into its highly active 1,25-dihydroxy vitamin form. Relative vitamin D deficiency may play a part in the genesis of osteoporosis. There is a growing literature suggesting that minor degrees of vitamin D deficiency during the winter in temperate latitudes may lead to compensatory increases in parathyroid hormone secretion and negative bone balance. This can be prevented by a daily intake of 400 to 600 iu of vitamin D from October to April.

Arthritis

The reasons for the virtual universal occurrence of osteoarthritic changes in many joints in later life are uncertain but may include the mechanical effects of time-related wear and tear, age-associated changes in the metabolism of joint cartilage,and subchondral bone, or a disease process unrelated to age. The epidemiology of knee osteoarthritis suggests that wear and tear from occupation injury and obesity is important. Obesity seems both to predispose to arthritis of the knee and to be a factor in making the arthritis painful. Weight loss is therefore an important therapeutic approach. In contrast, osteoarthritis of the hip seems often to be a long-term consequence of minor (or major) forms of congenital dysplasia of the hip and the effects of occupation and obesity are much less clear. There is evidence of a genetic predisposition to the syndrome of generalized osteoarthritis.

Falls

Falls and the fear of falls are important causes of morbidity among older people. Community surveys indicate that a quarter of people aged 65 to 69 fall at least once in the course of a year and this annual prevalence doubles by the age of 80. Women are more liable to falls than men. This may partly reflect greater activity but is also related to lower muscular strength. Falls are a cause of direct and potentially fatal injuries such as fractures and head injury. Old people who are unable to get themselves up again may suffer the additional problems arising from a 'long lie'. These include hypothermia, pressure sores, and rhabdomyolysis. The last can in severe cases lead to acute renal failure and serum muscle enzymes should be checked in old people presenting to medical care after a fall with long lie. Significant haemorrhage following falls is an increasing problem as more older people are being prescribed anticoagulants for atrial fibrillation. A history of falls is a relevant issue in deciding whether an older person should be established on anticoagulants.

Falling, especially if associated with inability to rise again, is an extremely unpleasant experience for most older people and fear of further falls can lead to a form of 'postfall syndrome' in which the patient becomes morbidly afraid of falls, progressively more immobile (which may increase the risk falls as much as decreasing it), and socially isolated. Old people with this condition may seek premature institutional care or may be pressurized into care by worried family or neighbours. Falls by old people that come to medical attention need therefore to be taken seriously and possible preventive interventions sought. There have also been some studies of primary prevention at a community level but the cost-effectiveness of these approaches has not yet been established.

Causes of falls

Some general age-associated changes contribute to the rise in risk of falls. The syndrome of non-rotatory dizziness, which is common in later life and epidemiologically associated with an enhanced risk of falls, probably represents a temporary failure of the brain to achieve a coherent integration of positional data from eyes, inner ear, and proprioceptors. Proprioceptive information is reduced by increased variance in neural conduction time from peripheral tissues, and by damage to receptors in joint capsules by arthritis in the neck and elsewhere. The older patient therefore becomes increasingly dependent on vision for spatial orientation. Poor lighting levels or a visually confusing environment, as experienced on a moving escalator for example, can be particularly hazardous.

A large number of more specific risk factors for falls have been identified. These are typically classified as intrinsic to the patient and extrinsic in the environment, but as with all such dichotomies interactions are important. Interpretation in terms of causality can be uncertain because of confounding factors. In observational studies sedative and antidepressant drugs emerge as commonly associated with an increased risk of falls. Long-acting benzodiazepines and antidepressants are probably directly associated with an increased risk, but a link between diuretic therapy and falls found in some studies is probably more often mediated by the cardiovascular disease for which the drugs have been prescribed.

Some falls are no more than a misfortune that afflicts all of us by chance. An older person who falls only once or twice in a year will commonly be found to have no specific remediable cause. Old people who fall more than twice in a 12-month period should be investigated further. Extrinsic causes in the home should be identified, and the help of a skilled occupational therapist may be needed. Inadequate lighting, slippery floors, inadequate

Table 3 Some medical causes of falls

Cardiovascular
Hypotension (postural, exertional, postprandial, drug-induced, induced by bed rest)
Cardiac arrhythmia
Syncope (micturition, cough, defaecation, carotid sinus sensitivity)
Neuromuscular
Epilepsy
Transient ischaemic attacks
Menière's disease
Parkinsonism and multisystem disorders
Myopathy
Neuropathy or myelopathy
Unstable knee due to quadriceps weakness
Visual field defect or inattention
Dementia
Intermittent delirium (drugs, alcohol, hypoglycaemia)

handholds, sloppy footwear, and loose rugs are common hazards. Where falls are not readily explicable in terms of an identifiable environmental hazard medical appraisal is needed. Table 3 lists some of the commoner medical causes of falls. Patients who find themselves on the floor with no memory of falling may have been unconscious at least momentarily and this suggests cardiac dysrhythmia, syncope, or epilepsy. Such a history may not be obtained consistently from patients subsequently shown to suffer from syncope, however, and this possibility has to be borne in mind for any older patient suffering repeated falls. Full investigation requires tilt-table and carotid sinus massage testing. The mechanism of syncope may be predominantly cardioinhibitory in which case a demand pacemaker can be of benefit. Syncope that is mediated by systemic hypotension is less amenable to treatment.

Ambulatory electrocardiographic monitoring is a commonly requested investigation for older patients suffering falls or intermittent lapses of consciousness. Findings can be difficult to interpret in the absence of symptomatic events during recording because the prevalence of intermittent cardiographic abnormalities is high in later life. None the less, intermittent arrhythmias or significant pauses may be identified that justify a trial of therapy if compatible with the clinical history.

Where no remediable causes of falls can be established thought needs to be given to tertiary prevention of the consequences of further falls. A physiotherapist should train the older person in getting up after a fall or in moving across the floor to an alarm or telephone to summon help. An alarm system may need to be installed in the patient's home provided he or she can be trained to use it. Otherwise, some system of regular surveillance by statutory services, volunteers, or good neighbours may be more useful. The risks of further falls need to be discussed fully with the patient and with concerned relatives. The right of an old person to continue to live in his or her own home, even where that carries some risk, may need to be defined for relatives pressing for institutionalization to relieve their anxieties rather than the patient's.

The endocrine system

Historically, there have been many attempts to explain ageing as a consequence of sequential endocrine failure, in the hope that suitable replacement therapy might halt or reverse the process. Apart from the obvious changes in ovarian function with the menopause, there are minor declines in circulating thyroid hormone levels, a reduction in the rate of secretion of insulin in response to raised blood sugar levels, and a decline in tissue sensitivity to insulin. The release of antidiuretic hormone in response to osmotic loads increases, perhaps in association with reduced renal responsiveness and changes in the sensitivity of blood volume receptors. There is little evidence of any abnormality of parathyroid, adrenal, or pituitary function as a universal feature of old age. The response of the adrenals and of adrenocorticotrophin secretion to stress is essentially unaltered. Indeed, following injury ACTH secretion is more prolonged in older patients than younger but the significance of this is unclear.

There is a gradual age-associated decline in average testosterone levels in ageing men. There is no abrupt change corresponding to the female menopause, nor, on evolutionary grounds, would one expect there to be. Testosterone implants are available in the private medical sector in some countries but there is at present no scientific justification for the claimed benefits of 'normalizing' testosterone at young adult levels. Some older men have been found to have very low levels of growth hormone and in uncontrolled experiments show increases in muscle bulk and strength when replacement therapy is provided. Functional benefits have yet to be demonstrated, and side-effects from growth hormone can be severe.

Blood levels of dehydroepiandrosterone, a weak androgen, are high in fetal life, decline after birth, and then rise again from puberty into early adult life. There follows a steep decline with age and there have been reports of improvements in function and wellbeing in later life from supplements. Again, larger and better trials are needed.

Diabetes mellitus

The clinical presentation of diabetes in old age may differ from that of younger patients. Many patients are diagnosed as a result of routine testing during a medical or surgical illness and some because of the development of disorders associated with diabetes such as peripheral vascular disease or cataract. Relatively few present because of classical symptoms such as weight loss and polyuria but a small proportion present with life-threatening metabolic decompensation in a hyperosmolar state.

There is now sufficient evidence to justify trying to control hyperglycaemia. Dietary treatment and oral hypoglycaemic agents are firstline treatment but insulin should not be withheld if it is necessary for control of hyperglycaemia. Shorter-acting oral hyperglycaemic drugs such as gliclazide are preferred and longer-acting drugs such as chlorpropramide and glibenclamide should not be used for older patients.

Diabetes mellitus interacts with other risk factors for cardiovascular disease. Diabetic patients of any age should be persuaded to give up smoking. Control of blood pressure is very important, with evidence to support the use of angiotensin-converting enzyme inhibitors in preference to other classes of drugs. Hypercholesterolaemia should be reduced.

The specific complications of diabetes occur more frequently in older than in younger patients. The majority of patients blind from diabetes are aged over 60 and the prognosis of diabetic retinopathy in old age is less favourable than at younger ages. Photocoagulation remains effective, and the results of cataract extraction are excellent except when retinopathy is contributing to the visual impairment.

Foot care is an important aspect of the management of diabetes and it is important to bear in mind that peripheral neuropathy and vascular disease may render the elderly diabetic patient particularly prone to pressure sores of the heels if confined to bed for any length of time.

Hypothyroidism

Most cases of hypothyroidism in old age are of autoimmune origin, although previous thyroid surgery and radio-iodine therapy account for a proportion. Classical clinical signs such as cold intolerance, hair loss, and coarsening of the skin are less common as presentations in old age than an insidious decline in health and mobility with psychiatric manifestations, particularly depression. Hypothyroid coma, sometimes associated with severe headache and fits, and hypothermia are less common but important presentations. The most physical signs are a change in voice and delayed relaxation in tendon reflexes, often most easily recognized in the arm reflexes of an older patient.

The principle of 'start low, go slow' in prescribing for older people is important when starting thyroid replacement therapy, particularly if myocardial ischaemia is known to be present. A problem in management may be failure to comply with treatment and the responsible doctor must ensure that lifelong treatment is in fact lifelong. It may be necessary to enlist the aid of a relative, neighbour, or visiting nurse in ensuring compliance.

Hyperthyroidism

Hyperthyroidism is less common in old age than hypothyroidism but is even more likely to present in an 'atypical' manner. Weight loss, anorexia, gastrointestinal, and cardiovascular symptoms predominate. Cardiac failure, often associated with atrial fibrillation resistant to digitalis, is a common cardiac presentation. Eye signs and goitre are less common in elderly patients, and apathy or depression, rather than tremor and agitation, may be prominent.

Treatment is begun with carbimazole followed when thyroid function is returned to normal by radio-iodine. Thyroid replacement therapy is often required later either because of an ablative dose of radio-iodine or because of subsequent decline in thyroid function. Careful follow-up is therefore necessary.

The nervous system

Age changes in the nervous system are among the most important because of their significance in the psychology and psychiatry of ageing and in the production of disorders of movement. Numbers of neurones in some parts of the nervous system, for example the motor neurones of the spinal cord, the Purkinje cells of the cerebellum, the cells of the substantia nigra, and parts of the neocortex, fall with age. There are no changes in other parts, for example in several brainstem nuclei. Anatomical abnormalities of the neurones that remain are also described including the accumulation of lipofuscin and the loss of dendrites and dendritic spines in cortical neurones. The anatomical basis of alterations in cortical function may thus be due both to a reduction in the number of neurones and in the connections between them. There is a reduction in peripheral nerve conduction velocities, both motor and sensory, differing in different nerves and reflecting a fallout of fibres of all sizes. There is also an increase in the variance of nerve conduction velocities which probably contributes to the inaccurate transmission of information and may impair the cognitive function of the brain as a parallel computer. The increase in nerve conduction variance may explain the frequent bilateral loss of ankle tendon reflexes above the age of 60. Loss of vibration sense in the feet and ankles may be another manifestation of the same process. Although commonly of no clinical significance, such findings need to be interpreted with care as it is important not to overlook a peripheral neuropathy, due for example to vitamin B_{12} deficiency.

Temperature control

Central autonomic nuclei, for example the intermediolateral cells in the spinal cord and first- and second-order autonomic neurones outside the central nervous system, show a fall in cell numbers with age. Associated changes in autonomic function include alterations in the control of heart rate (see above) and abnormalities of temperature regulation. Older people are more susceptible to hypothermia and to heat stroke. The threshold for appreciation of skin temperature changes may increase by as much as tenfold over the age range. This contributes to older people's inability to recognize temperature change and to respond appropriately. There is reduced cutaneous vasoconstriction in response to cold and impaired vasodilatation and sweating in response to increase in body temperature. Reduction in sweating is due in part to a reduction in the number of sweat glands. Failure of shivering is common and makes hypothermia more likely, while coexisting undernutrition, even of brief duration, reduces hepatic thermogenesis.

Hypothermia

In many countries, especially the United Kingdom, there is an excess of deaths during winter. This is mostly due to influenza and to cardiovascular disease and the contribution from hypothermia is very small. None the less the diagnosis is important as it can easily be missed in its early stages and carries a high fatality. Most elderly patients with hypothermia present after a period of 2 or 3 days of cold weather, but it is entirely possible for hypothermia to develop in hospital in midsummer at United Kingdom latitudes especially if disease or drugs play a part. The fall in central temperature occurs over 24 to 48 h and its principal manifestations are progressive ataxia and slowing of cerebration continuing to stupor and finally coma. On clinical examination, the skin on unexposed surfaces such as the axilla, chest, and abdomen feels cold to the touch. There may be oedema of the face and eyelids resembling that of myxoedema but due to redistribution of fluid between the intra- and extracellular compartments and resolving with correction of hypothermia. The pulse is slow unless severe physical illness has raised it towards normal, and the blood pressure is difficult to record or is low. Tendon reflexes are normal unless there is associated hypothyroidism. The diagnosis is made by recording the rectal or other form of core temperature, and this should be done without delay on all occasions when an oral temperature is recorded at 35 °C or less. The electrocardiogram may show characteristic bradycardia and J waves (Fig. 3), but in severe hypothermia there is often atrial fibrillation with a slow ventricular response.

Hypothermia in elderly patients carries a high fatality. Although patients with hypothermia due to drugs commonly recover, those with severe physical illness as a cause usually die. Management is rendered difficult by the absence of comparative trials. There is no rational basis for the use of steroids, and intravenous fluids are dangerous because they may produce pulmonary oedema. Intravenous glucose is not metabolized and insulin is ineffective in the hypothermic state. In some younger patients, particularly those suffering acute accidental hypothermia, there may be benefits from rapid warming, but in older patients slow rewarming is the usual practice. A rise in body temperature, optimally 0.5 °C/h, is obtained by exposing the patient to a relatively high ambient temperature of 30 °C. Improvement is shown by an increase in rectal temperature and pulse rate, maintained blood pressure, and improvement in level of consciousness.

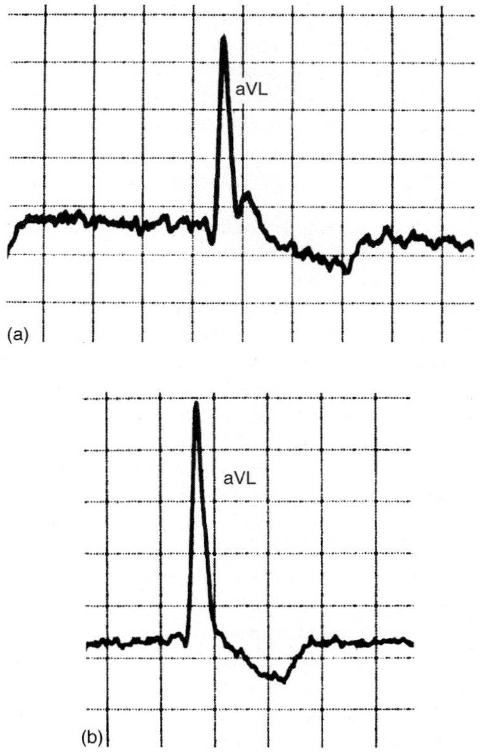

Fig. 3 An Osborne (J) wave seen in the electrocardiogram of a patient during hypothermia (a) and after recovery (b). The characteristic deflection lies between the QRS complex and the beginning of the ST segment. The pathophysiology of the J wave is uncertain.

An elderly patient who has recovered from hypothermia should be regarded as at risk for further episodes, and relatives and social agencies should be alerted. The long-term prognosis is better in patients who have survived an episode of hypothermia due to identifiable causes.

Hyperthermia

An increase in mortality on continuing care wards and among elderly people living at home has been recognized during heat waves. It is not known how many of the extra deaths are due specifically to hyperthermia, in the sense of rise in body temperature, rather than to dehydration or general stress. As with hypothermia part of the problem seems to be the failure of the older person to recognize that a problem is developing and for many a cool environment is not easily available. Adequate fluid intake should be recommended and tepid bathing may be the only available way of preventing a rise in body temperature.

Vision

Age-associated changes in the eye and ear are well documented. Decrease in elasticity of the lens begins early in life but only becomes symptomatic in the fifth decade when presbyopic hypermetropia results from failure of accommodation due to changes in the lens itself and in its capsule and suspensory ligaments. Cataracts increase in prevalence with age but vary in frequency between racial groups and with factors such as diabetes and family history. The media of the eye become less translucent with age and there is more scattering of light. Older people therefore have lower contrast sensitivity than the young and need more light and sharper contrast in reading material and in important environmental cues such as marker strips along the edges of steps. At a practical level, use of the inverse square law in placing lights nearer to what they are required to illuminate may be preferable to simply increasing their wattage. The eye media also become yellow with age so that the older eye is less sensitive to blue, a problem that can on occasion lead to mistakes in medication as the older patient fails to register which tablet is 'the blue one'. The public environment, including buildings such as hospitals, is often unnecessarily difficult for older people to use because of failure by architects to understand the visual problems of an ageing population.

Driving

Vision is an important determinant of fitness to drive a car. The loss of the right to drive can interfere seriously with an older person's quality of life as well as having a profound symbolic impact as a sign of disability and social marginalization. The common notion that older drivers are dangerous is exaggerated. In terms of preventing fatal road accidents the most effective intervention would be to refuse licences to males aged under the age of 25. Accident rates are very high for drivers, especially men, in early adult life where high-speed accidents with high injury and fatality rates are characteristic. Rates then fall into middle age but begin to rise again after the age of 70. At later ages, however, accidents tend to occur at low speeds with correspondingly low death and injury rates, and typically involve side collisions at road intersections. One reason for this may be a diminution in the size of the functional visual field with age. There is laboratory evidence that the functional visual field can be enlarged by training but the practical impact is not yet convincing. As with so many other aspects of modern life, road design could be improved to make travel safer and pleasanter for the increasing numbers of older drivers in society.

In addition to vision, a range of attributes including cognitive function and physical ability in manipulating controls, contribute to a person's ability to drive safely. In the absence of gross abnormalities, an older person's driving ability can only be assessed in a road test. Clinical examination and computer simulation are not adequate substitutes.

Specialized testing may also lead to useful advice about modifications to an old person's car that will enhance safety.

Hearing

A degree of high-tone deafness (presbyacusis) is probably universal in humans. It reflects several mechanisms and although it is partly an intrinsic true age change, there is little doubt of the importance of prolonged exposure to industrial and other environmental noise. Loss of high-tone hearing with the associated difficulty in following one voice against a background of others is socially and occupationally disabling. Minor degrees of deafness also have a more subtle effect on cognitive performance. Normal language has a high degree of informational redundancy, so that in conversation the hearer has often already understood and is preparing an answer before the speaker has concluded. Hearers who have to concentrate on listening to complete sentences in order to be sure they have understood are at a disadvantage in terms of processing and reacting to what is being said. This is all too often interpreted as cognitive impairment, and in confrontational situations, such as legal proceedings, can be exploited by unscrupulous interlocutors.

Psychiatric disorders in later life

Physicians should be aware that there is always a psychological element to physical disease. At one extreme physical symptoms and even signs can be a manifestation of a somatization syndrome. At the other extreme there will inevitably be a psychological reaction to physical illness. This may include a panic reaction, but more commonly fear and anxiety manifest in different ways ranging from denial of symptoms to morbid preoccupation with them. It is part of a physician's duty to recognize the psychological dimension to a patient's illness and to respond to it appropriately. All this is true at any age but requires particular thought with older patients for whom the possibility of death is a constant presence and disability a constant dread. These problems may be compounded with a degree of cognitive impairment, background depression, and an increased susceptibility to delirium. For practical reasons the physician will need to deal directly with a broad range of such problems but should be ready to invoke the aid of psychogeriatrician colleagues in situations that are less than straightforward.

Delirium

Delirium, one form of acute confusional state, can affect an acutely ill patient of any age but becomes more common in later life. Any toxic febrile condition can precipitate delirium as can primary insult to the brain such as stroke, meningitis, encephalitis, or subarachnoid haemorrhage. The mechanisms of delirium remain obscure but there is suggestive evidence that in toxic states it may involve the leakage across the blood–brain barrier of neuroactive compounds, normally not present in the bloodstream or normally excluded from passage into the brain. In some instances the patient may be quiet, drowsy, and withdrawn, perhaps quietly muttering, but more commonly a delirious older patient is agitated, restless, noisy, paranoid, and sometimes aggressive. The diagnosis must be suspected in old person who shows an abrupt deterioration in cognitive function or an abrupt change in personality. In toxic conditions such as urinary infection, haemosepsis, or pneumonia the delirium may appear before any other signs of infection such as fever or leucocytosis.

The central element of management is to diagnose and treat the underlying cause and in some instances this may call for the 'blind' institution of antibiotic therapy while cultures of blood and urine are awaited. Although an agitated depression can be made more manageable by sedative drugs such as haloperidol these bring with them a risk of secondary complications and as far as possible doses should be kept to a minimum and the patient's disturbed behaviour handled by skilled nursing. This will be facilitated by an attempt to understand what the patient is experiencing as the cause for his or her behaviour. In a delirious state consciousness is clouded and experience may have a dreamlike quality with all that means in a sense of ill-understood dread and powerlessness to escape or defend oneself. Memory is impaired so that although careful explanation to the patient of who people are and what is happening is an important part of care it may need to be repeated at frequent intervals. Attention is disrupted so that the patient may not be listening when spoken to or may focus on some unimportant feature of the environment which may take on particular and often menacing significance. This is often coupled with misinterpretation of what is seen or heard so that a smoke alarm in the ceiling becomes a Martian death ray machine, or a pop song on a distant television set becomes the howling of a fellow prisoner in a torture chamber. In some instances, characteristically where alcohol or certain drugs have played a part in the delirium, visual hallucinations may occur which are often of a frightening or threatening kind.

Where possible a delirious patient should be nursed in a quiet room with good lighting and preferably in the company of a well-known friend or family member. Extraneous noise should be avoided as far as possible and constant reassurance and explanation provided. It is reassuring to delirious old people if doctors are dressed and behave like doctors, and nurses like nurses of more gracious times. Being addressed in old age by some over-familiar ambiguous stranger using one's forename can be alarming. All forms of physical restraint are terrifying and should not be used.

Patients with pre-existing brain disease such as dementia are more prone than average to delirium but one of the differential diagnoses of delirium is of the acute panic and alarm of a demented person removed from their familiar environment. It is important to recognize this syndrome of 'decompensated dementia' in an older patient since if they are not returned as quickly as possible to their familiar environment their cognitive hold on reality may become permanently disrupted. The accident and emergency unit of a busy general hospital is a common setting for this problem.

Dementia

Dementia is distressingly common in later life with a prevalence of approximately 5 per cent over the age of 65. In its fully developed form it is conceptualized as an acquired global impairment of cognitive function. At earlier stages it is diagnosed on the basis of progressive impairment in two or more areas of cognition (memory, language, visuospatial and perceptual ability, thinking and problem-solving, personality) sufficient to interfere with work, social function, or relationships, in the absence of delirium or major 'non-organic' psychiatric disorders such as depression (section XXX). In the earlier stages, diagnosis may require formal neuropsychological testing. At present the diagnosis is essentially clinical, although functional neuroimaging is showing promise as a diagnostic aid.

The commonest cause of dementia in old age is Alzheimer's disease with cardiovascular causes second. Normal pressure hydrocephalus, classically associated with the triad of urinary incontinence, apraxia of gait, and mild cognitive impairment, is always sought for even though operative ventricular shunting often confers no benefit. Dementia with cortical Lewy bodies is being increasingly recognized. Although commonly described as a subacute disorder it is likely that more chronic forms will become increasingly recognized. Mood disorders, particularly depression, are common in the early stages and visual hallucinations are an early and persistent feature. Parkinsonian symptoms and signs are commonly present but are rarely severe. The importance of recognizing the disease lies in the particular sensitivity of sufferers to the ill-effects of phenothiazine drugs, which should be avoided.

Unfortunately there is little in the way of specific treatment for dementia. Patients with vascular dementia are commonly prescribed aspirin, although there is little evidence at present to support this practice. Patients in atrial fibrillation with stepwise progressive dementia suggestive of cerebral emboli will normally be offered anticoagulation, although careful supervision of dosage and monitoring of the international normalized ratio may be required. The memory defect of Alzheimer's disease is associated with a deficiency of acetylcholine in the brain and drugs which inhibit cholinesterase in the brain are now becoming available. The first of these, tacrine, had too severe a side-effect profile to be clinically useful but its successors, donepezil, galantamine, and rivastigmine, are proving more acceptable. Both drugs bring about a small improvement in cognitive function but, as to be expected, do not retard the continuous decline in function associated with the underlying dementing process. There is evidence that some patients with clinically diagnosed Alzheimer's disease do not respond to these drugs and it is important that if they are tried some formal measurement of cognitive function be applied at baseline and then a decision taken at a 6-week review as to whether the drug should be continued. If cognitive function has declined further the drug is not worthwhile. If there is been improvement or maintenance of function further review should take place at 12 weeks. Side-effects of these drugs are to be expected due to their cholinergic properties and include nausea, stomach cramps, and diarrhoea.

Depression

Depression is probably no more common in old age than at any other time of life but its effects can be more prominent and disabling. The present generation of older people are often unwilling to acknowledge that they may have a mental illness so that the clinical presentation and treatment may be complicated by denial and somatization. The classical features of depression may be present but more subtle manifestations such as a change of personality or behaviour, self-neglect, and asocial behaviour may be the presenting feature. Late-onset alcoholism or other forms of drug abuse, usually of sleeping tablets or pain killers, may also be symptoms. It is also important to recognize depression complicating physical disease; for example, rehabilitation of a stroke patient is often interrupted by the understandable onset of a depressive illness. As a physical sign avoidance of eye contact by an older patient can be very significant even if other aspects of demeanour are not typical of depression. Treatment is along conventional lines and old people respond as well as young to antidepressants. Doses should start low and be increased with care, particularly with drugs such as the tricyclics which because of their anticholinergic properties may induce delirium. The risk of suicide increases steeply with age and is particularly high in older men. Where a suicide is thought to be a high risk urgent psychogeriatric help should be sought and in such circumstances, or in the case of an old person whose health is compromised by withdrawal and refusal to eat, electroconvulsive therapy may be life saving.

Paraphrenia

Although for a long time thought to be a form of late-onset schizophrenia, this syndrome is now suspected more often to have its basis in organic brain damage. It is usually readily recognized as a primary psychiatric illness but may occasionally present to the physician, sometimes in a patient brought up to an accident and emergency unit because of abnormal behaviour. Chronic undernutrition due to delusional ideas about food being poisoned or unsafe is one of the causes for the geriatric syndrome of 'failure to thrive'. In contrast with earlier-onset schizophrenia, personality is usually well preserved and although the patient may have alarming delusions they rarely become dangerously aggressive. The typical patient is an elderly solitary female, somewhat deaf with prominent semistructured auditory hallucinations. Ideas of being subjected to influence from outside, extraterrestrial aliens, or merely the television set are common and auditory noises attributed to the neighbours may lead to friction. The physician should not necessarily leap to the conclusion that a patient's description of strange noises is necessarily delusional. The old lady diagnosed as paraphrenic before the family of illegal immigrants living in her roof space was discovered is a possibly apocryphal but cautionary tale. Patients with paraphrenia require skilled psychogeriatric care, but can often be supported in their own homes if visiting psychiatric nurses or social workers can establish adequate rapport.

Unusual personalities

Old people display the same range of personalities as seen at any other age, from the delightfully eccentric to the perfectly odious. A syndrome of self-neglect, commonly, though unhelpfully, called the Diogenes syndrome, is well recognized. Characteristically this affects an old person living alone with a good work record and rather rigid personality, who for obscure reasons accumulates enormous piles of rubbish through a pathological inability to throw anything away. Such a patient may come to medical attention through the consequences of self-neglect, but sometimes as a victim of burglary and violence as a consequence of their being assumed by local villains to be the archetypal rich old miser. Complaints from neighbours about rat infestations, fire risks, or odours may also precipitate medical attention.

Other forms of personality disorder may resurface in old age, perhaps when protective spouses die or families and other carers reach the limit of their tolerance. Placement problems can arise since aggressive, abusive, or even merely 'difficult' behaviour can be hard to accommodate where some form of collective living is required.

Clinical pharmacology and the older patient

In epidemiological studies, the incidence of adverse effects of drugs increases with age. It has been suggested that at least 10 per cent of hospital admissions of older people in the United Kingdom are due in whole or part to adverse reactions to drugs. Higher incidences have been reported from general practice. Conventionally, adverse drug reactions are categorized into the idiosyncratic, usually due to host factors such as allergy or genetic susceptibility, and the dose-related, which are undesirably intense effects of the drug's pharmacological actions. In some instances adverse drug reactions are related to both dose and duration of exposure; the adverse effects of long-term high-dose steroids in older people being an example. Most adverse drug reactions affecting older people are dose-related or dose and duration-related. The chief reason for this is that more older people than younger take medications and are also more likely to be taking multiple medications with the risk of interactions. Although patients suffering from cognitive or visual impairment are at risk of making mistakes with their medications, there is no evidence that older people are any worse than younger ones at following treatment advice. Unnecessarily complex drug regimens may cause problems in compliance, and care in prescribing is an important aspect of good-quality medical care for older people. There are some age-associated changes in pharmacokinetics and, probably, pharmacodynamics that increase the risk of adverse drug reactions.

Bioavailability

In general there is no significant change with age in intestinal absorption of drugs that are absorbed, as most are, by passive diffusion. Absorption of substances such as iron, thiamine, calcium, and vitamin B_{12} which undergo active transport across the intestinal mucosa may be lower in older people. Loss of gastric acidity and bacterial overgrowth in the small intestine increase in prevalence with age and may affect drug absorption. The absorption of levodopa increases with age, probably because of reduced dopa decarboxylase activity in the gastric mucosa.

Hepatic metabolism

First-pass metabolism in the liver has an important effect on the bioavailability of drugs. The size of the liver declines with age, as does the density of its blood supply. For drugs such as propanolol and morphine that undergo significant first-pass metabolism, a higher proportion of drug absorbed from the intestine will reach the systemic circulation. Hepatic drug metabolism has been classified into phase 1 (oxidation–reduction) reactions mediated by the mixed-function oxidase system and phase 2 (conjugation) reactions. The clearance of some drugs (chlordiazepoxide and diazepam) metabolized by phase 1 reactions is retarded with age, but conjugation reactions seem unimpaired. Phase 2 reactions are, however, a potential site for important interactions between drugs that share common pathways of elimination. As with all age-associated phenomena, these are generalizations based on averages derived from groups of people of different ages. They reflect in part the increasing prevalence with age of 'frail' people with multiple disease and acquired impairments, and may not apply to individuals who are fit and healthy.

Body composition

Average body composition changes with age. Even though total body weight may not alter, muscle mass and total body water fall, while fat increases. These changes affect volumes of distribution of drugs and also have consequences for drug binding and retention. Water-soluble drugs such as digoxin, gentamicin, theophylline, and cimetidine have reduced volumes of distribution in older patients. Although, in acute single-dose studies, these drugs may produce higher serum levels in older than in younger patients, higher levels will lead to more rapid excretion. There is therefore no consistent effect in steady state conditions. Lipid-soluble drugs such as hypnotics and anaesthetics, diazepam and thiopental for example, have increased volumes of distribution contributing to prolonged serum half-lives in older people.

Renal function

Particular care is required in prescribing drugs that undergo renal elimination. As noted earlier, most individuals show an age-associated decline in glomerular filtration, which may be intensified by illness or medications, and which can retard the elimination of drugs, such as digoxin, that are largely excreted renally. Drugs eliminated by renal tubular secretion, such as penicillins and aminoglycosides, are also affected by the age-associated decline in renal mass and loss of nephrons.

Blood–brain barrier

The blood–brain barrier comprises the mechanical barrier provided by the endothelial cells of the cerebral vasculature with their characteristic tight (non-porous) junctions, and the metabolic barriers provided by the glial cells. It is not clear whether there is any general age-associated change in the efficiency of the blood–brain barrier. An increased susceptibility of older people to the adverse effects of benzodiazepines is well documented, but it is not known whether this is a pharmacodynamic effect at receptor level or where such drugs enter the brain in higher concentration in later life. Clinically, patients with cerebrovascular disease often seem more susceptible than average to drugs acting on the central nervous system, and this should be borne in mind when prescribing, but again it is not known whether this represents increased permeability of the blood–brain barrier or a pharmacodynamic effect.

Protein binding

There is a very small reduction in serum albumin concentration in healthy elderly people which has no clinical significance. The much greater reduction in albumin levels in many elderly people in hospital is due to the effects of disease and subnutrition and is a predictor of poor prognosis. Low serum albumin levels might in theory increase the proportion of unbound and metabolically active drugs that are normally highly protein bound. Interactions due to one drug displacing another from protein binding sites is also an enhanced theoretical possibility. Bound drugs that might be affected are particularly warfarin, tolbutamide, and phenytoin, and common displacing drugs are aspirin and sulphonamides. Other things being equal, any effect should be transient as the unbound drug is also more rapidly eliminated, but with older patients it is wise to be alert to any avoidable possibility of harm.

Pharmacodynamic effects

Age-associated increases in the effects (including adverse effects) of some drugs are not readily explicable in terms of gross pharmacokinetic changes, and pharmacodynamic effects at receptor level have been proposed. Such effects may contribute to the increased susceptibility of older people to benzodiazepines and warfarin, and to the age-associated reduction in sensitivity of β_1 receptors to adrenergic β-blockers. The susceptibility of older people to gastric complications of non-steroidal anti-inflammatory drugs may also have a pharmacodynamic element.

Preventing adverse drug effects

The possibility of an adverse drug reaction needs to be included in every differential diagnosis considered for an older patient. It is important to seek information about over-the-counter and self-prescribed preparations (perhaps 'borrowed' from a spouse or neighbour) as well as prescribed drugs. The use of over-the-counter drugs by older people varies between countries and social classes but is generally increasing. Table 4 lists some of the commoner adverse drug reactions seen in clinical practice. In addition to the effects listed in Table 4, older people often feel non-specifically unwell when taking drugs, especially antibiotics. Another frequent problem arises from oesophageal dysmotility, which is common in later life and can cause temporary delay in the clearance of tablets or capsules from the lower oesophagus into the stomach. This can cause local oesophagitis, which may be misinterpreted as ischaemic heart disease or an indicator of gastro-oesophageal reflux. Although well recognized as an adverse effect of alendronate, virtually any drug can cause the problem, and antibiotic capsules are among the most common. The remedy is for the patient to take tablets or capsules while standing and to wash them down well with a glass of water. Some older patients find that following tablets or capsules with a small piece of bread will stimulate enough oesophageal peristalsis to clear the drugs into the stomach.

Of the drugs causing adverse effects listed in Table 4, diuretics are probably the commonest offenders because they tend to be over-prescribed in general practice, usually for minor stasis oedema in older women. In terms of severity and permanence of damage, steroid-induced osteoporosis is one of the most serious complications of drug therapy for older people. If there is a possibility of steroid therapy becoming prolonged, as when prescribed for polymyalgia rheumatica or giant-cell arteritis, treatment to prevent osteoporosis should be initiated from the time of first prescription. For older patients this will normally consist of oral supplements of vitamin D and calcium with a bisphosphonate.

Table 5 outlines the principles of safer prescribing for older patients. Most of these are self-evident. In choosing a drug for an older patient a common problem, already alluded to, is that all too often there is no evidence on effectiveness specific to older people. Other things being equal, one is wise to choose a class of drug for which there is relevant evidence rather than extrapolate from data on younger patients. In general, with drugs with powerful and potentially dangerous effects, shorter-acting forms are preferable to longer, even though this may complicate dosage regimens. Thus, with oral hypoglycaemic drugs, tolbutamide or gliclazide should be prescribed in preference to chlorpropamide or glibenclamide. Benzodiazepines are best avoided entirely for older patients, but if essential for sleep disturbance only shorter-acting forms should be used and only for short periods. In a range of studies, longer-acting benzodiazepines have been consistently associated with falls. Although allegedly short acting, temazepam has longer effects on psychological function than its plasma half-life would suggest and is best regarded as a longer-acting drug.

Table 4 Common adverse drug reactions affecting older people

Drug group.	Common effects
ACE inhibitors	Renal failure
Diuretics	Hypokalaemia, hyponatraemia, hypotension, hypovolaemia, hyperglycaemia, gout, urinary retention
Benzodiazepines	Drowsiness, confusion, falls
Digoxin	Anorexia, nausea, confusion, cardiotoxicity
NSAIDs	Gastropathy, gastric ulcer, gastrointestinal haemorrhage, fluid retention, renal impairment, hypertension
Opiates	Drowsiness, confusion
Anticholinergics	Dry mouth, constipation, urinary retention, delirium, glaucoma
Levodopa	Delirium, hallucinations, dyskinesias
Antidepressants	Delirium, anticholinergic effects, falls
β-blockers*	Weariness, weakness, reduced exercise reserve, confusion
Aminoglycosides	Renal and auditory impairment
Tranquillizers	Dyskinesias, hypotension, oversedation
Hypoglycaemics	Neuroglycopenia
Antihypertensives	Postural hypotension
Steroids	Osteoporosis

ACE inhibitors, angiotensin-converting enzyme inhibitors; NSAIDs, non-steroidal anti-inflammatory drugs.

*Adverse reactions may be caused by eye-drops.

Table 5 Principles of good prescribing for older patients

1. Check
Is the diagnosis clear?
Is treatment really necessary?
What other diseases does the patient have?
Does the patient have renal or hepatic impairment?
Does the patient have cognitive impairment?
What other drugs is the patient taking?
Is there any history of adverse drug effects?

2. Choice of drug
Is there relevant evidence of effectiveness?
Short- rather than long-acting
Distinctive colour and shape
Simple dosage regime

3. Dosage
Adjustment needed for renal or other problems?
If in doubt 'start low, go slow'

4. Surveillance
What adverse effects should be watched for?
Who should do the watching?
When should dosage be reviewed?
When can the drug be stopped?

Various prescribing practices are aimed at helping patients to avoid mistakes in medication. If possible drugs should be chosen to minimize the number of different times a day that they have to be taken. Combinations of four and three times a day regimes can be particularly troublesome if followed religiously. Patients should be helped by knowing what each of the medications they are taking is intended to do. Although there is little direct evidence in support, it is common geriatric practice to try to offer older patients drugs with distinctive shapes and colours rather than a collection of anonymous white tablets. Such a policy has to be consistent across repeat prescriptions and may call for specific rather than generic prescribing with attendant increases in costs. Patients discharged from specialist geriatric or psychogeriatric departments are often given cards with specimens of each prescribed tablet attached with transparent tape against a description of its purpose and dosage schedule. This can be helpful provided that general practitioners and pharmacists continue to provide the same brands of drug. A more reliable approach is to make use of one of the various forms of box or packet in which tablets can be sorted, by pharmacist or carer, into separate compartments labelled by day and time. These can be helpful to patients and also to carers who need to check whether drugs have been taken or not.

Arrangements should be made for regular and frequent review of medications given to older people, not least because dosage adjustments are often required with longer-term therapy. Even more important, no drug should be prescribed without thought to when it should be stopped, and unintended continuation of treatments is one source of unnecessary morbidity in old people. Pill counts are helpful in detecting inadvertent non-compliance with therapy. Surveillance of drug therapy for older patients is also important if adverse effects are to be detected promptly. It may be constructive to involve carers in the surveillance process. While it is clearly wise practice to warn patients and carers about possible adverse effects,

Table 6 Characteristics of illness in later life

Multiple pathology
Non-specific or cryptic presentation
Rapid deterioration if untreated
High incidence of complications
Need often for active rehabilitation after recovery
Social and housing needs common

comprehensive warnings of the type included in packet inserts can frighten people into not taking the drug at all.

General approaches to medical care for older people

Conditions such as stroke, cancer, heart disease, and dementia increase in incidence and prevalence with age, but old people do not suffer from any diseases that never afflict younger adults. It is in the treatment of the patient rather than of the disease that medical care for older people has to provide particular emphasis and sensitivity. Central is the loss of adaptability characteristic of age. Older patients may have little physiological reserve to cope with even minor shortcomings in care. Loss of adaptability may need to be compensated for in the design of medical services. More frequent checking of the international normalized ratio of older patients taking anticoagulants, and readier deployment of invasive monitoring for older patients after trauma or at risk of cardiovascular instability are examples.

Table 6 sets out some of the characteristics of illness in later life of which health workers must be aware and to which health services should be ready to respond. All of these characteristics are directly or indirectly aspects of the loss of adaptability that is the fundamental property of ageing. The first four underlie a need for rapid access to high-quality diagnostic and treatment facilities when an older person falls ill. Because of the frequent conjunction of multiple diseases with non-specific presentation, older people often need more investigations than do younger patients to establish an accurate diagnosis. An elderly patient with pneumonia may present with delirium or falls before any localizing signs appear in the chest. In infections, fever may appear late and may be missed if core temperature is not accurately measured or the patient is not given time to recover from a cold ambulance drive. Visceral pain from the peritoneum in acute appendicitis or intestinal perforation, or from the heart in myocardial infarction, may be reduced or absent in older patients. The slowness of the aged body in mounting its defences can lead to rapid deterioration unless an accurate diagnosis is made and correct treatment instituted urgently.

Reduced adaptability in old age also leads to a high incidence of secondary complications both of disease and treatment with consequent need for careful surveillance by medical and nursing staff. Good-quality medical and nursing care depends on scrupulous attention to detail, since even the smallest error of judgement or lack of observation may have serious consequences for the patient. A typical example lies with the development of pressure sores. A young person can usually lie immobile for 4 h without suffering serious pressure sores. An older person can develop sores in half that time. Pressure sores are most likely to develop if a patient is lying on a hard surface; particular hazards include time spent lying on a hospital trolley in a casualty department or on an operating table while junior orthopaedic surgeons spend an age doing their first hip replacement. High-quality care for an older population puts demands on the managers as well as the practitioners in health services.

Specialist geriatric care

The last two items in Table 6 underlie the need for specialist geriatric rehabilitation teams to be closely linked to the working of acute medical and surgical services. Most older patients, approximately 70 per cent of those referred to British hospitals as medical emergencies, have fairly straightforward illnesses such as pneumonia, myocardial infarction, or deep venous thrombosis. Treatment can be along normal lines, and patients discharged directly back home. The average length of stay will need to be longer than for younger patients because older people need longer to recover full function after a debilitating illness, and they are more likely to be living alone with no one to support them during convalescence. A proportion of older people admitted to medical wards, typically 10 to 15 per cent, have complex illnesses and functional problems that call for the multiprofessional approach of a specialist geriatric service if best outcomes are to be attained. Such patients need to be identified early on in their illness, and the ideal way of ensuring this is for physicians with special responsibility for older people to be part of the clinical team on acute medical wards. This approach ensures that the majority of older people, whose chief need is unimpeded access to the skills of other specialties, are not disadvantaged as they may be if admitted initially to a purely geriatrics service.

The approach to an elderly patient

Table 7 outlines the four stages that should structure the approach to elderly patients, especially those with complex problems.

Assessment

Assessment may require contributions from all members of the core geriatric team—doctor, nurse, occupational therapist, physiotherapist, and social worker. In addition to dealing with technical matters, this stage should also be seen by the team as an opportunity for 'getting to know' the patient as an individual and for building mutual trust and friendship. Functional assessment is best documented in terms of performance as measured using standard scales agreed both among the geriatric team and with the relevant social services of community teams who will care for the patient after discharge. A wide range of scales is available, but one of the commonest in use for activities of daily living is the Barthel scale (Fig. 4). This is robust and reliable if the rules of administration are agreed and followed. It is useful as an indicator of needs for help but is primarily applicable to patients with moderate to severe disabilities. At higher levels of performance, scales for assessment of instrumental activities of daily living such as ability to use the telephone or travel on public transport may be more relevant.

Assessment of mental function usually calls for a global performance scale and may also require assessment of mood. The abbreviated mental test score (Table 8) is widely used in British hospitals and is easily applied but was developed for use in geriatric and psychogeriatric inpatient units; a patient scoring at the significantly low score of 7 out of 10 is quite severely impaired. Milder degrees of impairment are better detected by the Folstein mini-mental status examination. Neither the mental test score nor the mini-mental status examination is a diagnostic instrument, and reduced

Table 7 The four-stage 'geriatric process'

1. Assessment
Health (diagnoses, prognosis)
Function (physical, mental)
Resources (culture, education, social, economic)
2. Agree objectives of care
What does the patient want?
What is feasible?
3. Specify the management plan
To close the ecological gap between what the patient can do and what his or her environment requires:
therapeutics—improve the patient
prosthetics—reduce the demands of the environment
4. Regular review
Is progress as expected?
Does the plan need changing?

BARTHEL Index of Activities of Daily Living

Name:
Address:

Hospital No: D of B:

Aim to record what the patient actually DOES do in daily life, not what he/she can do.
The score reflects the degree of INDEPENDENCE from help provided by another person:
– if supervision is required, the patient is NOT independent,
– if aids and devices are used but no help is required, the patient IS independent.

Use the best available evidence, asking the patient or relatives, carers, nurses and therapists, and using common sense. Observing the patient is helpful, but direct testing is NOT necessary.
Middle categories imply that the patient supplies over 50% of the effort.
Ask about abilities before admission or acute illness, and enter in the column marked "Estimate of previous score".

BOWELS:
2 continent (for preceding week).
1 occasional accident (once a week or less).
0 any worse grade of incontinence (or needs enemas for continence).

BLADDER:
2 continent (for preceding week), or able to manage any device (eg. catheter and bag) without help.
1 occasional accident (once a day or less), or catheterized and needs help with device.
0 any worse grade of incontinence.

FEEDING, food placed within reach by others:
2 able to cut up food, spread butter etc. without help.
1 needs some help cutting or spreading.
0 needs to be fed.

GROOMING:
1 independent washing face, combing hair, shaving, & cleaning teeth (when implements are provided).
0 needs help.

DRESSING:
2 independent putting on all clothes, incl. fastening buttons, zips etc. (Clothes may be adapted)
1 needs some help, but can do at least half.
0 needs more help than this.

TRANSFER, bed to chair and back:
3 needs no help
2 needs minor help, verbal or physical: can transfer with one person easily, or needs supervision.
1 needs major help; two people or one strong/trained person, but can sit unaided.
0 cannot sit; needs skilled lift by two people (or hoist).

TOILET USE:
2 able to get on and off toilet or commode, undress & dress sufficiently, & wipe self without physical or verbal help.
1 needs some help, can wipe self and do some of the rest with *minimal help* only.
0 needs some help with this.

MOBILITY around house or ward, indoors:
3 may use aid (stick or frame etc. *but not wheelchair*).
2 needs help of one person, verbal or physical, including help standing up.
1 independent in wheelchair, incl. able to negotiate doors & corners unaided.
0 needs more help than this.

STAIRS:
2 independent up and down, and can carry any necessary walking aid
1 needs help, verbal or physical or help carrying aid.
0 unable.

BATHING
1 able to get in and out of the bath or shower, wash self without help (may use any aids)
0 unable.

Estimate of previous score ↓	DATE of ASSESSMENT →				
	BOWELS: 2 continent 1 occ. accident ≤ 1/wk 0 incontinent				
	BLADDER: 2 continent 1 occ. accident ≤ 1/day 0 incontinent				
	FEEDING 2 independent 1 needs some help 0 dependent				
	GROOMING face/hair/teeth/shave 1 independent 0 needs help.				
	DRESSING 2 independent 1 can do half 0 dependent				
	TRANSFER 3 independent 2 minor help 1 major help (can sit) 0 unable				
	TOILET USE 2 independent 1 needs some help 0 dependent				
	MOBILITY 3 independent 2 walks with one 1 wheelchair indep. 0 unable				
	STAIRS 2 independent 1 needs help 0 unable				
	BATHING 1 independent 0 dependent				
	TOTAL SCORE				

Fig. 4 The Barthel activities of daily living scale with instructions for administration. (Formatted by courtesy of Dr S. J. Winner.)

Table 8 The abbreviated mental test score

1.	Age: must be correct
2.	Time: correct to nearest hour without looking at watch or clock
3.	'42 West Street': give this or similar address, ask for it to be repeated to ensure that it has been heard correctly. Ask for it at the end of the test
4.	Month: exact
5.	Year: exact, except in January or February when previous year is acceptable
6.	Name of place: if not in hospital ask for type of place or area of town
7.	Date of birth: exact
8.	Start of the Second World War: exact year
9.	Name of present monarch
10.	Count backwards from 20 to 1: prompt if necessary, 20, 19, 18..., but no further prompts. Patients can hesitate and self-correct but no other errors are allowed
	Score: 8–10 probably normal, 7 probably abnormal, 0–6 abnormal. Change in score of 3 or more is probably significant

Formatted by Dr S.J. Winner.

scores may reflect any cause of impaired cognitive function including dementia, depression, or delirium. If depression is suspected, a screening questionnaire such as the geriatric depression scale may be helpful but should not be regarded as an adequate substitute for a skilled and sensitive clinical assessment.

Understanding a patient's cultural and educational background is an important stage in ensuring good communication and information needs. Protection of patients' autonomy is imperative but forcing patients to make worrying decisions they do not understand is to mistake the form for the substance. The most important resource available to an older patient is often his or her family who must be appropriately involved in planning care. 'Appropriately' implies taking their needs and priorities into account but not letting them over-ride those of the patient.

Setting the objectives of care

The second stage of setting objectives of care is essentially a dialogue and negotiation between the doctor who knows what could effectively be done, and the patient who decides what should be done. This should be an essential stage of care for any patient but is often omitted with younger patients for whom it is usually assumed, not always appropriately, that prolongation of life is the only objective to be considered. Older people may have other priorities; they may value dignity and independence more than life. If alone in the world they may have the privilege of being able to please themselves without having to worry about the effects their decision may have on others. It is at this stage of care that issues of quality of life are most important. Standard questionnaires are of limited worth because they assume that everyone shares the same system of values. In identifying what a person enjoys in life, and the effects that different treatment options may have on a particular patient's quality of life, more individualized methods are required. Psychometrically based questionnaires responsive to the value systems of individual patients are under development, and interactive computer programs can help with specific issues such as choice of treatment of prostatic hypertrophy, but for older patients with complex problems it has yet to be shown that anything is more reliable than compassionate human interchange. Once objectives have been agreed they need to be specified clearly in the notes and, subject to the patient's agreement, explained to relevant family members and future carers.

The management plan

Formulating a management plan calls for appropriate and timely treatment for any relevant acute diseases together with rehabilitation of the patient for resettlement in the future abode of choice, usually his or her own home. In order to achieve this the management plan must provide for bridging any 'ecological gap' between what patients can do and what their homes are going to demand. The gap is closed by improving the patient through therapeutic interventions and reducing the demands of the environment by prosthetic interventions. Therapeutic interventions often involve the whole geriatrics team. A hemiplegic stroke patient, for example, might be helped by the doctor improving exercise tolerance through tighter management of heart failure, the physiotherapist improving walking, the occupational therapist teaching him or her how to dress, the nurse devising the best programme for the diuretic therapy and ensuring proper nutrition, and the social worker steadying morale and sense of security about future support in the community. At the same time that the therapeutic programme is under way plans should be going forward for any prosthetic changes to the patient's home that are likely to be needed. These may include aids and adaptations such as extra banisters on stairs, grab rails in the bathroom, a raised toilet seat, fitting an alarm, as well as providing for personal help for shopping, bathing, supervision of medication, or other needs. In difficult situations rehousing, or, in the worst case, the ultimate prosthetic environment of institutional care might have to be arranged. It is important that the therapeutic and prosthetic programmes are managed in step since it can be extremely demoralizing for a patient who is physically and psychologically ready to go home to have to wait because aids and services are not yet in place.

Home visits with the patient prior to discharge can be very helpful both in identifying what prosthetic input is necessary and also in reassuring an apprehensive patient and possibly anxious relatives that a return home is feasible. The team must pay careful attention to the needs of relatives and others involved in the patient's care. Those who will make a personal contribution may need to spend time in the rehabilitation ward under the tutelage of nurses or therapists learning any necessary skills in helping the patient both physically and psychologically. An important element in this may be to prevent carers from being too helpful, as that can lead later to the patient becoming unnecessarily dependent. A less welcome aspect of the rehabilitation team's dealing with relatives is in relation to objections, often from those who will be contributing least to a patient's later care, that attempts at return into the community are impractical and 'she would be much better off in a nursing home'. This situation is often more complex than it seems in that it may reflect family tensions arising from half a century of unspoken animosities. The problem may also arise because relatives think that responsibility for the success or failure of the discharge will fall upon them, or feel guilty that they will not be able to contribute, or fear criticism for not doing so. The first step in negotiations is therefore always to try to find out what social and psychological crosscurrents are running—an activity in which all members of the team need to acquire skill, although the social worker is the most specifically trained. Discussion with a primary care physician who has known the patient and family for years can often prove illuminating. Tact and avoidance of confrontation are called for, followed sometimes by delicate diplomacy in negotiating between differing factions in a patient's family. It may surprise some to learn that this aspect of the work of specialist geriatrics departments, far from being seen as an impediment to rational medicine, is actually a source of great professional satisfaction when done well.

A follow-up visit 10 days or so after discharge is also helpful, both to make sure that all is well and for the rehabilitation team to savour the satisfaction of seeing their patient happily back in his or her natural habitat or to learn from any insufficiencies.

Regular review of a patient's progress is usually formalized in a weekly multiprofessional meeting. The meeting is chaired by the clinically responsible doctor, but decisions are collective and must be formally recorded in the patient's notes. In addition to a general review of progress towards treatment goals, an important task for the meeting is to recognize when progress is not as had been expected. This may mean that the original plan was inappropriate, either in setting unrealistic goals or in specifying a less than optimum treatment programme. More often the problem arises because some new factor has intervened to interrupt the patient's progress. This may range from medical problems such as a depressive illness (a particularly common sequela in stroke), a drug side-effect, or urinary tract infection, to psychosocial factors such as discouragement from something a visitor has said, or some adverse change in the ward environment. The new factor should be dealt with or the management plan or treatment goals modified as appropriate. Relevant family members and carers, as well as the patient, should be informed if significant changes to aims and means of rehabilitation are made.

The future

Populations are ageing throughout the world and for more than a decade the majority of the world's population of people aged over 65 have been living in developing rather than developed countries. The older patient is now the norm, and the practice of medicine and the design of services must continue to adapt. The demand for medical care will rise as the numbers of older people increase and new medical technologies become increasingly appropriate for frailer patients. These changes must be planned for, but in so far as they represent the fact that more people are living longer and more actively, they should be welcomed as one aspect of the progress of civilization. Emphasis in health care needs to shift from the prolongation of life at all costs to the prevention and cure of disability. This needs to apply at all ages. Age-based rationing of health care is not compatible with the democratic ideal, nor would it make economic sense as it would merely substitute the long-term costs of disablement for the short-term price of treatment. But in association with the development of rational heath care systems there needs to be a public health strategy for the lifelong primary prevention of disability. Because of the age-associated loss of adaptability, the later in life a potentially disabling disease strikes the more likely the patient is to die from it rather than linger on in disability. Postponement of disease is prevention of disability. Our collective aim is to spend a long time living and a short time dying.

Further reading

Browne JP *et al.* (1994) Individual quality of life in the healthy elderly. *Quality of Life Research* **3**, 235–44.

Dickerson JEC *et al.* (1999). Optimisation of antihypertensive treatment by crossover rotation of four major classes. *The Lancet* **353**, 2008–13.

Fiatarone MA *et al.* (1994). Exercise training and nutritional supplementation for physical frailty in very elderly people. *New England Journal of Medicine* **330**, 1769–75.

Grimley Evans J *et al.*,eds (2000). *The Oxford textbook of geriatric medicine*, 2nd edn. Oxford University Press, Oxford.

Holliday R (1995). *Understanding ageing.* Cambridge University Press, Cambridge.

Manton KG, Gu X (2001). Changes in the prevalence of chronic disability in the United States black and nonblack population above age 65 from 1982 to 1999. *Proceedings of the National Academy of Sciences of the USA* **98**, 6354–9.

Phillips PA *et al.* (1984). Reduced thirst after water deprivation in healthy elderly men. *New England Journal of Medicine* **311**, 753–9.

Salim A *et al.* (1998). Subcutaneous hydration in the elderly. In: Armand MJ *et al*, eds. *Hydration and aging.* pp. 201–8. Springer Publishing Company, New York.

The Heart Outcomes Prevention Evaluation Study Investigators (2000). Effects of an angiotensin-converting-enzyme inhibitor, ramipril, on cardiovascular events in high-risk patients. *New England Journal of Medicine* **342**, 145–53.

30.2 Mental disorders of old age

Robin Jacoby

Mental disorders of old age are of the greatest importance because:

- demographic trends in **all** countries are leading to a marked increase in the number of elderly persons, especially the very old;
- this age group is particularly prone to debilitating mental illness;
- presentations of mental illness in the elderly may differ from those at younger ages and go unrecognized;
- the pattern of morbidity differs; the elderly suffering more from organic disorder—delirium and dementia;
- mental and physical illness often occur together, the one sometimes masking the other.

Elderly inpatients on non-psychiatric wards show high rates of mental disorder of various sorts. Community rates are also high. For instance, the prevalence of dementia is about 7 per cent over 65 years of age, but approaches 20 per cent in those over 80. For major depressive illness defined by ICD-10 or DSM-IV the prevalence is no more than 3 per cent, but for pervasive depressive symptoms, which most psychiatrists would consider in need of treatment, it is around 12 per cent. There are no valid data for the prevalence of very-late-onset schizophrenia-like psychosis. The closure of large mental institutions in most developed countries has resulted in a greatly increased number of elderly patients in the community suffering from chronic schizophrenia that began much earlier in their lives.

Assessment

Factors to be considered are:

- the setting in which the patient is examined;
- the patient's ability to provide information.

Assessment in the patient's own home gives invaluable clues about premorbid adjustment, activities of daily living, and even causes of an abnormal mental state—for example, a waste bin full of empty whisky bottles. Patients in general hospital wards should be assessed in a side-room if possible. Many elderly patients are unable to give a history. It is therefore essential to find reliable informants, even if this means disturbing neighbours or making long-distance telephone calls. Doctors visiting patients outside hospital should carry equipment for physical examination. A low-reading thermometer, sphygmomanometer, and sugar-detection urine sticks may also prove invaluable at home in detecting the cause of mental disturbance.

Examination of the mental state of an elderly person is essentially the same as for any adult, but with differences of emphasis. More attention is paid to the level of consciousness, particularly subtle fluctuations throughout 24 h. For patients with suspected dementia a full cognitive examination is undertaken, frequently in several brief sessions because patients become easily fatigued and unable to co-operate. Tired or inattentive patients may fail a test that they might otherwise have been able to perform satisfactorily. Systematic evaluation of all higher cerebral functions, such as memory, praxis, and language, is essential. On general hospital wards or home visits the routine administration of standardized questionnaires is of value as an alerting mechanism, but not a substitute for full evaluation. The Mini-Mental State Examination (**MMSE**) is the preferred questionnaire because it assesses a range of higher cerebral functions, not just memory and orientation.

Because the capacity to live independently is frequently compromised in elderly people and becomes the crucial determinant of social outcome, it is essential to assess the patient's ability to perform activities of daily living (**ADL**)—dressing, feeding, toilet care, and so on. Impairment in ADL may reveal dyspraxia or agnosia undisclosed by formal clinical tests. The informant's account is important, as patients' assessments of their own abilities may be misleading.

Delirium

The clinical features of delirium are described elsewhere. The elderly are particularly susceptible because:

- They more commonly suffer from the physical disorders that cause delirium: hypoxia, infections, toxicity (especially from drugs), and metabolic and CNS disorders.
- Many have a decreased cerebral reserve because of incipient or overt dementia.

An underlying physical cause for delirium must therefore be sought assiduously, as it is generally more important to treat this than the mental symptoms. Physical illnesses causing delirium can be relatively minor: for example, a urinary tract infection, especially in patients with dementia. Because the elderly generally suffer high physical morbidity they tend to receive more prescribed medication. Single or multiple drugs, as well as drug withdrawal effects, are potent causes of delirium. Management is essentially that of the underlying cause and psychotropic drugs should be avoided whenever possible. However, short-term treatment of mental symptoms and behavioural disturbance with a small dose of a neuroleptic drug is sometimes unavoidable to allow medical treatment to proceed unhindered.

Dementia

The importance of dementia lies not only in the suffering it causes to patients but also in the demands it makes upon family caregivers and the medical and social services. The clinical features of the dementia syndrome are described in Chapter 24.13.8. Global impairment is required for diagnosis, and memory loss alone, of which elderly people invariably complain, is **not** a sufficient criterion. Accurate diagnosis is required because:

- treatable or arrestable causes may be discovered;
- management can be planned and implemented;

- caregivers are helped by a clearer understanding of the process affecting the patient and its likely course;
- knowledge of the underlying conditions is accrued and advanced.
- treatment with a central cholinesterase inhibitor may be indicated.

Rational management requires an appreciation of the practical implications of cognitive impairment: for example, ensuring nutrition in a patient with dyspraxic inability to feed herself. However, the non-cognitive, behavioural, and psychiatric disturbances in dementia are the manifestations which cause most problems to caregivers and often require management by specialist services. Patients should be maintained at home for as long as possible, both for humane reasons and because they will have lost the capacity to adapt easily to a new environment. This is best achieved through a continuing partnership between clinicians, family caregivers, and local statutory and voluntary social services. Such interagency co-operation and discussion facilitates access to community services, which include those brought to the patient—meals, nursing, bathing, house cleaning—and day care away from home. Intercurrent illness should be treated along with other medical problems, such as incontinence, which is due more commonly to urinary tract infections and faecal impaction, respectively, than to the underlying disease processes of dementia. Attention must be given to principal caregivers (most frequently spouses or adult daughters, but sometimes unrelated neighbours), who show high levels of psychiatric morbidity themselves due to their burden of care.

Affective illness

Depression

Depressive illness in the elderly differs only in emphasis from that in earlier life, varying from mild dysthymia to major psychosis with high risk of suicide. Psychosocial factors are as important, but genetic loading is usually lower in patients with late-onset depression. Cerebral organic change is more common in late-onset cases.

Psychomotor retardation is frequent, as in younger patients, but anxiety and agitation are also characteristic. Delusions of guilt and unworthiness are typical, but hypochondriacal or nihilistic beliefs also often occur. Histrionic or other bizarre behaviour, which is out of premorbid character, is also seen. Some patients with severe depression perform badly on cognitive tests, so called 'depressive pseudodementia', which may lead to a wrong diagnosis of organic dementia,. Hypochondriacal delusions together with anorexic weight loss can be mistaken for physical illness, such as cancer. Some patients may even deny low mood ('masked depression'), but the presence of other typical affective manifestations and a favourable response to antidepressant treatment reveal the correct diagnosis. The clinician should not avoid treating depression in patients, such as those with severe physical illnesses, simply because they appear to have a valid reason to be unhappy.

The elderly are vulnerable to the unwanted effects of psychotropic drugs but respond well to standard antidepressants. Selective serotonin-reuptake inhibitors (**SSRIs**) are usually preferred as first-choice drugs because of their safety and fewer side-effects. However, tricyclics, such as amitriptyline and imipramine, are highly effective, especially in major depression, if care is taken to observe the general principle of small initial doses increasing slowly to lower therapeutic doses than are given to younger patients. The elderly also respond well to electroconvulsive therapy (**ECT**), regarded by many as the treatment of choice for deluded and/or suicidal patients. Extreme age, dementia, and physical infirmity are **not** contraindications to electroconvulsive therapy. After recovery from an episode of major depression, antidepressant treatment should be continued for at least 2 years, and probably indefinitely.

Mania/hypomania

Manic illness, which accounts for about 5 per cent of psychogeriatric admissions, is usually less florid than in younger patients. Mixed manic and depressive pictures have been described as typical, but are probably not more common in old age than before. Cerebral organic disease is found in a high proportion of cases. Diagnosis is sometimes difficult to make because patients may present with a rather non-specific psychosis, or one mimicking delirium. The clinician should therefore enquire about a previous history of affective illness. Secondary mania, defined as a first onset in close temporal relationship with a physical illness or drug treatment in patients with no previous history of affective disorder, is also seen. Patients respond well to treatment with neuroleptics and lithium carbonate in the acute phase. Lithium is also widely used to prevent relapse. Here, frequent monitoring of renal and thyroid function is essential, and the serum lithium level should be maintained at the lower end of the therapeutic range, that is to say around 0.6 mmol/l.

Paranoid disorders

Paranoid ideas, usually but not invariably of persecution, are common in dementia and affective disorder. In dementia they tend to be transient, variable, and unsystematized. In affective disorder they are usually mood-congruent, for example persecution deserved because of guilt. Persecutory ideas are also seen in paranoid personalities and acute paranoid reactions, but very-late-onset schizophrenia-like psychosis* is the main paranoid syndrome of old age, equivalent to, but distinct from, paranoid schizophrenia of earlier adult life. The following aetiological factors have been consistently reported:

- a high female to male ratio (up to 7:l);
- a family history of schizophrenia intermediate between the general population and younger schizophrenic patients;
- social isolation and poor premorbid interpersonal relationships;
- low marriage and fecundity rates compared with age-matched peers;
- long-standing deafness.

The clinical picture is sometimes indistinguishable from early-onset paranoid schizophrenia, but the patient usually presents with a few simple delusions and associated auditory hallucinations. For example, she may complain of hearing the neighbours plotting against her, or impugning her sexual virtue. Medication with atypical antipsychotic drugs, such as risperidone or olanzapine, to minimize the risk of extrapyramidal side-effects, is the treatment of choice. However, neuroleptics rarely extinguish delusional beliefs that become 'encapsulated', meaning set aside or compartmentalized and not permitted to intrude into so many aspects of mental and daily life, as happens during the acute phase of illness. Adherence to treatment is often poor but can be improved with the help of a community psychiatric nurse.

Neurotic, personality, and other disorders

These are too complex to discuss briefly and the reader is referred to specialist texts. However, some general principles can be stated. It is essential to differentiate lifelong neurosis from neurotic symptoms of first onset in old age because the latter, predominantly anxiety and phobia, are most likely to indicate an underlying depressive illness. Elderly patients with lifelong neurosis have frequently adapted to their disability in spite of continued

* Recent international agreement states that cases with onset between 40 and 59 years of age should be termed 'late-onset schizophrenia'; whereas cases from 60 years onwards should be called 'very-late-onset schizophrenia-like psychosis'.

suffering. Mild and moderate lifelong personality deviations are common, but severe disorders are occasionally encountered, such as the senile squalor (Diogenes) syndrome, which can require compulsory removal from home under mental or public health legislation. Illicit drug taking is rare among the present generation of elderly, but the abuse of prescribed drugs, notably benzodiazepines, is common. Alcohol abuse is increasingly recognized as a cause of mental and social disability in elderly people.

Further reading

Folstein MF, Folstein SE, McHugh PR (1975). 'Mini Mental State'. A practical method for grading the cognitive state of patients for the clinician. *Journal of Psychiatric Research* **12**, 189–98.

Jacoby R, Oppenheimer C, eds (2002). *Psychiatry in the elderly*, 3rd edn. Oxford University Press, Oxford.

31

Palliative care

31 Palliative care

Robert Twycross and Mary Miller

In Western countries, about 25 per cent of the population die of cancer. Even more die of progressive non-malignant disease. In this chapter the focus is on symptom management in patients with far-advanced cancer.

Palliative care is far more than symptom relief. It addresses physical, psychological, social, and spiritual aspects of suffering, thereby helping patients to come to terms with their impending death as constructively as they can while living as actively and creatively as possible. Palliative care also provides a parallel support system to help families cope during the patient's illness and in bereavement; it is best provided by a multiprofessional team.

General principles of symptom management ('EEMMA')

The principles underlying management are:

- *evaluation*: diagnosis of each symptom before treatment;
- *explanation*: explanation to the patient before treatment;
- *management*: individualized treatment;
- *monitoring*: continuing review of the impact of treatment;
- *attention to detail*: no unwarranted assumptions.

Evaluation is based on probability and pattern recognition. For example, hiccup in advanced cancer is mostly associated with gastric stasis or distension, and the most common cause of pruritus is dry skin. Symptoms are not always caused by the disease itself but by treatment, debility, or a concurrent second disorder. Some symptoms are caused by multiple factors. **Explanation** by the doctor of the cause(s) of a symptom does much to reduce its psychological impact on the sufferer.

Management falls into three categories:

- correct the correctable
- non-drug measures
- drugs.

By adopting a multimodality approach, although the underlying disease cannot be cured, it is generally possible to obtain significant, and sometimes complete, relief.

Drugs for a persistent symptom should be prescribed regularly on a prophylactic basis. The use of drugs 'as needed' instead of regularly is the cause of much needless distress. Although many symptoms respond to a combination of non-drug and drug measures, often the main part of the management of symptoms such as anorexia, weakness, and fatigue is helping the patient (and family) accept the irreversible physical limitations of terminal disease.

Patients vary, and it is not always possible to predict the optimum dose of opioids, laxatives, and psychotropic drugs. Adverse effects may also jeopardize patient compliance. **Monitoring** is crucial, with adjustments made as necessary.

Attention to detail is important at every stage of symptom management. It is equally important in relation to the non-physical aspects of care—all symptoms are exacerbated by anxiety and fear.

Pain

At diagnosis, between 20 and 50 per cent of patients with cancer have pain. Prevalence varies according to the primary site of the cancer and metastatic spread. In advanced cancer, 75 per cent of patients have pain and two-thirds of these have multiple pains.

Evaluation

Each pain described by the patient should be recorded on a body chart with a comment about the probable cause (Fig. 1). In addition, pain may be classified as:

- nociceptive, i.e. pain caused by physical and/or chemical stimulation of free nerve endings;
- neuropathic, i.e. pain caused by compression or injury to the peripheral or central nervous systems.

Nerve compression pain, like nociceptive pain, is aching in character. On the other hand, nerve injury pain tends to be superficial and burning, and associated with allodynia (light touch caused pain). There may also be

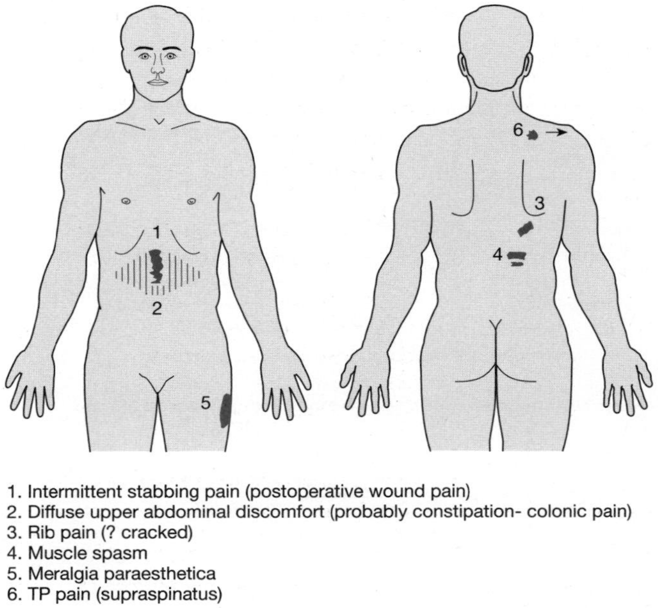

Fig. 1 Pain chart of a 63-year-old woman with cancer of the pancreas, 10 days postoperatively. TP, myofascial trigger point.

spontaneous stabbing pain with or without an underlying aching component. Peripheral neuropathic pain is neurodermatomal in distribution, not local to the lesion, and there may be associated numbness.

A history of analgesic use is part of the evaluation. Not all pains respond equally to analgesics, and information about the benefits of specific medication (or lack of it) may help to identify the underlying mechanism. A detailed pain history coupled with physical examination is generally sufficient to guide management. Further radiological investigations are necessary in only a minority of patients.

Management

Although analgesics are the mainstay of management, it is important not to overlook correctable causes of pain or ignore other treatment modalities (Box 1). Analgesics can be divided into three classes: non-opioid (antipyretic), opioid, and adjuvant. Their use is governed by the following maxims:

- *By the mouth*—the oral route is the preferred route, including for morphine and other strong opioids.
- *By the clock*—analgesics should be given regularly and prophylactically for persistent pain; 'as needed' medication is irrational and inhumane.
- *By the ladder*—use the 3-step analgesic ladder (Fig. 2).
- *Individualized treatment*—analgesic combinations and doses should be determined individually for each patient.
- *Use adjuvant medication*—meaning adjuvant analgesics, antidotes for adverse effects (e.g. laxatives, antiemetics), and psychotropic medication.

Non-opioids

The non-opioid (antipyretic) analgesics comprise paracetamol/acetaminophen and the non-steroidal anti-inflammatory drugs (**NSAIDs**). Paracetamol can be taken by two-thirds of patients who are hypersensitive to aspirin. NSAIDs and paracetamol can be used together with an additive effect. The main drawback with paracetamol is the frequency of administration, generally every 4 to 6 h.

Box 1 Pain management in cancer

Modification of the pathological process
Radiation therapy
Hormone therapy
Chemotherapy
Surgery

Analgesics
Non-opioid (antipyretic)
Opioid
Adjuvant
- corticosteroids
- antidepressants
- antiepileptics
- muscle relaxants
- antispasmodics

Non-drug methods

Physical
- massage
- heat
- transcutaneous electrical nerve stimulation (TENS)

Psychological

Relaxation
Cognitive–behavioural therapy
Psychodynamic therapy

Interruption of pain pathways
Local anaesthesia
- lidocaine (lignocaine)
- bupivacaine

Neurolysis
- chemical (e.g. alcohol, phenol)
- cold (cryotherapy)
- heat (thermocoagulation)

Neurosurgery
- cervical cordotomy

Modification of way of life and environment
Avoid pain-precipitating activities
Immobilization of the painful part
- cervical collar
- surgical corset
- slings
- orthopaedic surgery

Walking aid
Wheelchair
Hoist

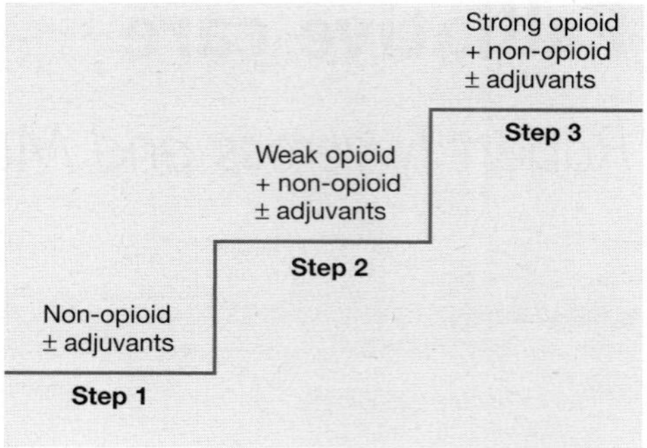

Fig. 2 The World Health Organization analgesic ladder for cancer pain management.

NSAIDs inhibit cyclo-oxygenase (**COX**), an important enzyme in the arachidonic acid cascade which results in the production of tissue and inflammatory prostaglandins. COX exists in two forms; COX-1 is present in all normal tissues, whereas COX-2 is more limited in its distribution but massively induced by inflammation (Fig. 3). Recently introduced COX-1 sparing NSAIDs and specific COX-2 inhibitors cause less gastric toxicity than most dual COX inhibitors.

NSAIDs are of particular benefit for pains associated with inflammation, for example soft tissue infiltration and bone metastases. NSAIDs differ in their effect on platelet function. In patients undergoing chemotherapy or with thrombocytopenia from another cause, it is best to use an NSAID which has no effect on platelet function (Table 1).

Weak opioids

There is little to choose between codeine, dextropropoxyphene, and dihydrocodeine in terms of efficacy. Pentazocine is not recommended; it acts for only 2 to 3 h and often causes psychotomimetic effects (hallucinations, feelings of unreality, dysphoria). Generally, a weak opioid should be added to a non-opioid, not substituted for one. If a weak opioid is inadequate

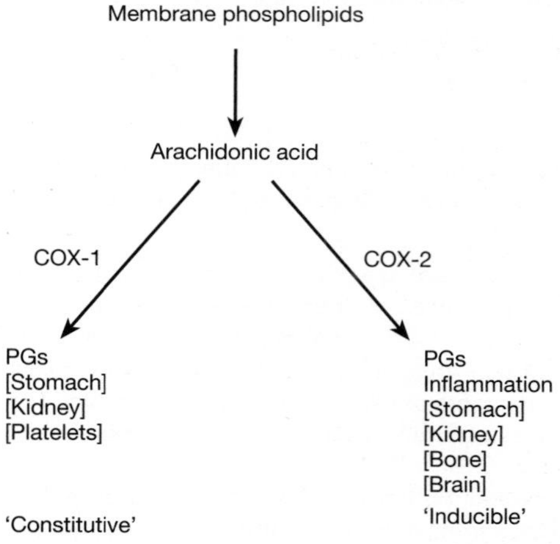

Fig. 3 The different effects of COX-1 and COX-2.

when given regularly in an optimal dose, change to morphine (or an alternative strong opioid); do not switch from a weak opioid to a weak opioid.

Tramadol forms a bridge between the classic weak and the classic strong opioids. By injection, it is one-tenth as potent as morphine. By mouth, it is about one-fifth as potent as morphine because of its high oral bioavailability. Tramadol has a dual mechanism of action, partly via opioid receptors and partly by blocking the presynaptic reuptake of 5-hydroxytryptamine (5-HT, serotonin) and noradrenaline (norepinephrine), similar to a tricyclic antidepressant. Tramadol causes less constipation than codeine and morphine.

Strong opioids

The use of strong opioids is dictated by therapeutic need, not by brevity of prognosis.

Morphine is the strong opioid of choice for treating cancer pain (Box 2), and is generally given with an NSAID (and/or paracetamol). Morphine is available as tablets (for example, 10 mg, 20 mg) or in a solution (for example, 2 mg and 20 mg in 1 ml). Modified-release preparations are mostly administered twice a day, some once a day.

Morphine rarely causes respiratory depression in patients with pain because pain is a physiological antagonist to the central depressant effects of morphine. However, morphine is potentially dangerous in renal failure. Its main metabolites are morphine-3-glucuronide (**M3G**) and morphine-6-glucuronide (**M6G**). Both cumulate in renal failure but, whereas M3G is inactive, M6G is more potent than morphine. In this circumstance, there is danger of sedation and respiratory depression if the dose is not closely monitored and, if necessary, reduced both in quantity and frequency.

Psychological dependence (addiction) does not occur when morphine is used appropriately as an analgesic. Physical dependence—a phenomenon seen with many psychoactive drugs when taken for prolonged periods (months rather than weeks)—does not prevent a step-by-step reduction in the dose of morphine if the pain ameliorates, for example as a result of radiotherapy or a nerve block. Tolerance to morphine is not a practical problem.

Other modes of administration are necessary at times (Fig. 4). Transdermal fentanyl patches, available in several sizes (25, 50, 75, 100μg/h over 3 days), are an alternative option for patients on a stable dose of morphine, and for those with a tablet phobia or dysphagia. Patients who have not been taking morphine should always start on the lowest dose. Fentanyl is less constipating than morphine. However, acquisition costs are much higher.

Injections are indicated when there is:

- persistent nausea and vomiting;
- severe dysphagia (alternatively use transdermal fentanyl);
- extreme weakness;
- a diminished level of consciousness.

In the United Kingdom, diamorphine hydrochloride (diacetylmorphine) is used when injections are necessary. It is more soluble than morphine salts and large amounts can be given in small volumes. By injection, diamorphine is twice as potent as morphine. Because of rapid deacetylation, however, diamorphine by mouth is essentially a prodrug for morphine and is only marginally more potent than morphine.

There are several opioid receptor subtypes (μ, κ, δ). Opioids differ in their receptor-site affinity, intrinsic activity, and concomitant non-opioid effects. These differences can be capitalized on in patients who are intolerant of morphine (mainly a μ-receptor agonist) by converting, for example, to methadone (μ-receptor agonist with non-opioid properties) or oxycodone (μ-, κ-receptor agonist).

When switching from another strong opioid to oral morphine (or vice versa), the initial dose depends on the relative potency of the two drugs (Table 2). The main reason for changing from morphine to another opioid is intolerance of morphine, for example marked dysphoria, sedation, and/or persistent hallucinations. Pethidine is not recommended for cancer pain—it acts for only 2 to 3 h.

Adjuvant analgesics

Adjuvant analgesics are miscellaneous drugs that relieve pain in specific circumstances. The main ones are corticosteroids, antidepressants, antiepileptics, muscle relaxants, and antispasmodics.

Corticosteroids

Corticosteroids are particularly useful for pain associated with nerve root or nerve trunk compression, and with spinal cord compression. Dexamethasone, 4 to 8 mg once a day, is prescribed for the former and 12 to 20 mg (sometimes more) for cord compression together with radiotherapy.

Antidepressants and antiepileptics

Nerve injury pains often do not respond well to non-opioids and opioids because of central (dorsal horn) sensitization. Additional measures are commonly necessary to obtain satisfactory relief. These aim to:

- dampen the hyperexcitability of damaged peripheral nerves;
- inhibit the glutamate excitatory system in the dorsal horn;
- enhance the γ-aminobutyric acid (**GABA**) inhibitory system in the dorsal horn (Fig. 5).

For example, amitriptyline 25 to 75 mg at night (an antidepressant) and sodium valproate 400–1000 mg at night (an antiepileptic) can be used either singly or together. These should generally be given in addition to morphine and a non-opioid analgesic if the nerve injury pain is associated with an infiltrating cancer, but they may well be effective alone in 'pure' nerve injury pain (for example, chronic postsurgical incision pain, postherpetic neuralgia).

Table 1 NSAIDs and platelet function

Drug	Effect on platelets	Comment
Dual COX inhibitors		
Aspirin	+	*Irreversible* platelet dysfunction as a result of acetylation of platelet COX-1
Non-acetylated salicylates (e.g.choline magnesium trisalicylate, diflunisal, salsalate)	–	No effect at recommended doses
Classical NSAIDs *except diclofenac*, e.g. ibuprofen, flurbiprofen, ketorolac, naproxen	+	Reversible platelet dysfunction
Diclofenac	–	Although diclofenac *in vitro* is a potent reversible inhibitor of platelet aggregation, typical oral doses *in vivo* do not affect platelet function
COX-1 sparing NSAIDs		
Nimesulide, celecoxib, meloxicam	–	
Specific COX-2 inhibitors		
Rofecoxib	–	

Box 2 Starting patients on oral morphine

Morphine is indicated in patients with pain that does not respond to the optimized combined use of a non-opioids and a weak opioid.

The starting dose of morphine is calculated to give a greater analgesic effect than the medication already in use:

- If the patient was previously receiving a weak opioid, give 10 mg every 4 h or modified-release 20–30 mg every l2 h.
- If changing from another strong opioid, a much higher dose of morphine may be needed (Table 2).
- If the patient is frail and elderly, a lower dose (e.g. 5 mg every 4 h) helps to reduce initial drowsiness, confusion, and unsteadiness.
- Because of cumulation of an active metabolite, a lower and/or less frequent regular dose may be preferable in renal failure, e.g. 5–10 mg every 6 h.

If the patient takes two or more 'as needed' doses in 24 h, the regular dose should be increased by 30 to 50 per cent every 2 to 3 days.

Upward titration of the dose of morphine stops when the pain is relieved or intolerable undesirable effects supervene. In the latter case, it is generally necessary to consider alternative measures. The aim is to have the patient free of pain and mentally alert.

Modified-release morphine may not be absorbed satisfactorily in patients troubled by frequent vomiting or those with diarrhoea or an ileostomy. M/r morphine should be used with caution if there is evidence of renal failure.

Scheme 1: ordinary (normal-release) morphine tablets or solution

- morphine given 4-hourly regularly 'by the clock' with 'as needed' doses of equal amounts up to 1-hourly;
- after 1–2 days, adjust the dose upwards if the patient still has pain or is using two or more 'as needed' doses per day;
- continue with 4-hourly doses regularly with 'as needed' doses of equal amounts up to 1-hourly;
- increase the regular dose by 30 to 50 per cent every 2 to 3 days until there is adequate relief throughout each 4-h period;
- *a double dose at bedtime obviates the need to wake the patient for a 4-hourly dose during the night.*

Scheme 2: ordinary (normal-release) morphine and modified-release morphine

- begin as for Scheme 1;
- when the 4-hourly dose is stable, replace with modified-release morphine every l2 h, or once daily if a 24 h preparation is prescribed
- each l2-hourly dose will be *three times* the previous 4-hourly dose; a once-daily dose will be *six times* the previous 4-hourly dose, rounded to a convenient number of tablets;
- continue to provide ordinary morphine solution or tablets for 'as needed' use. Give the equivalent of a 4-hourly dose, i.e. 1/6 of the total daily dose.

Scheme 3: modified-release morphine and ordinary (normal-release) morphine

- starting dose generally modified-release morphine 20-30 mg 12-hourly or 40–60 mg once daily;
- use ordinary morphine tablets or solution for 'as needed' medication; give about 1/6 of the total daily dose;
- increase the dose of modified-release morphine by 30 to 50 per cent every 2–3 days until there is adequate relief around the clock.

Box 2 *Continued*

Supply an antiemetic in case the patient becomes nauseated, e.g. haloperidol 1.5 mg to be taken immediately and then regularly at bedtime.

Prescribe laxatives, e.g. co-danthrusate or senna ± docusate; adjust the dose as necessary.

Suppositories and enemas continue to be necessary in about one-third of patients.

Constipation may be more difficult to manage than the pain.

Warn all patients about the possibility of initial drowsiness.

If swallowing is difficult or there is persistent vomiting, morphine may be given per rectum by

suppository; the dose is the same as by mouth. Alternatively give half the oral dose by injection,

or one-third as diamorphine, preferably by subcutaneous infusion.

For outpatients, write out the drug regimen in detail with times, names of drugs and amount to

be taken. Arrange for follow-up.

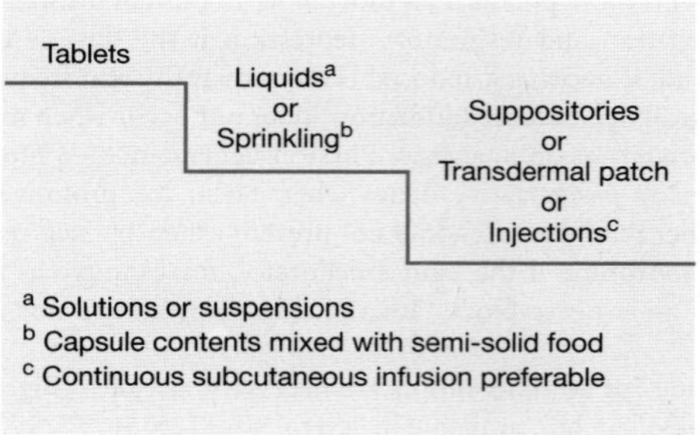

Fig. 4 The different effects of COX-1 and COX-2.

Table 2 Approximate analgesic equivalence to oral morphine

Analgesic	Potency ratio with morphine[1]	Duration of action (hours)[2]
Codeine Dihydrocodeine Dextropropoxyphene[3]	1/10	3–6
Pethidine	1/8	2–4
Tramadol	1/5[4]	4–6
Oxycodone	1.5–2[4]	5–6
Methadone	5–10[5]	8–12
Hydromorphone	7.5	4–5
Buprenorphine (sublingual)	60	6–8
Fentanyl (transdermal)	100–150	72

[1]Multiply dose of opioid by its potency ratio to determine the equivalent dose of morphine sulphate.

[2]Dependent in part on the severity of pain and on dose; often longer lasting in the very elderly and those with renal dysfunction.

[3]Multiple doses; single doses less potent.

[4]Tramadol and oxycodone are both relatively more potent by mouth because of high bioavailability; parenteral potency ratios with morphine are 1/10 and 3/4, respectively.

[5]Methadone: a single 5 mg dose is equivalent to morphine 7.5 mg. However, its long plasma half-life and broad-spectrum of action result in a much higher than expected potency ratio when given repeatedly.

Gabapentin is the only antiepileptic drug that is specifically licensed in the United Kingdom for the relief of neuropathic pain. The effective dose varies between 100 and 1200 mg given three times a day. Like many drugs acting on the central nervous system, gabapentin can cause drowsiness; most patients with cancer cannot tolerate more 600 mg three times a day.

With nerve injury pain which does not respond to such measures, it may be necessary to supplement or replace the antidepressant and antiepileptic with a glutamate (**NMDA**, *N*-methyl-D-aspartate) receptor-channel blocker, for example methadone and ketamine. A few patients (<1 per cent) require spinal analgesia (for example, morphine plus bupivacaine, with or without clonidine) or a neurolytic procedure to obtain adequate relief. Some patients derive benefit from other non-drug measures, for instance transcutaneous electrical nerve stimulation (**TENS**).

Antispasmodics and muscle relaxants

Muscle spasm pain (cramp) secondary to underlying bone pain and/or skeletal deformity is common in cancer patients. Myofascial trigger-point pains also occur. For these the correct approach is not more analgesics but explanation, physical therapy (massage and local heat), diazepam, and relaxation therapy. Trigger points can be injected with a local anaesthetic and a corticosteroid, for example bupivacaine 0.5 per cent and depot methylprednisolone.

Antispasmodics such as hyoscine butylbromide and glycopyrronium (given by subcutaneous infusion) are necessary in some patients with inoperable endstage intestinal obstruction.

Nausea and vomiting

Nausea and vomiting occurs in about half of the patients with advanced cancer. Intestinal obstruction, gastric stasis, drugs, and biochemical abnormalities are responsible in about 80 per cent of cases. It is often the sequence of events (plus an appropriate level of suspicion) that points to the likely cause.

In **acute** bowel obstruction there is typically a single discrete lesion, whereas in **chronic** obstruction (persistent or remittent) there may well be several sites of partial obstruction in both small and large bowels. Retroperitoneal disease may cause visceral neuropathy and functional obstruction. In consequence, the quartet of symptoms and signs that point to a diagnosis of acute intestinal obstruction (abdominal distension, pain, vomiting, and constipation) is often not so obvious in patients with advanced cancer and chronic obstruction. For example, distension may be minimal because of multiple intra-abdominal malignant adhesions. Bowel sounds vary from absent to overactive with borborygmi; tinkling bowel sounds are unusual. Some patients have diarrhoea rather than constipation.

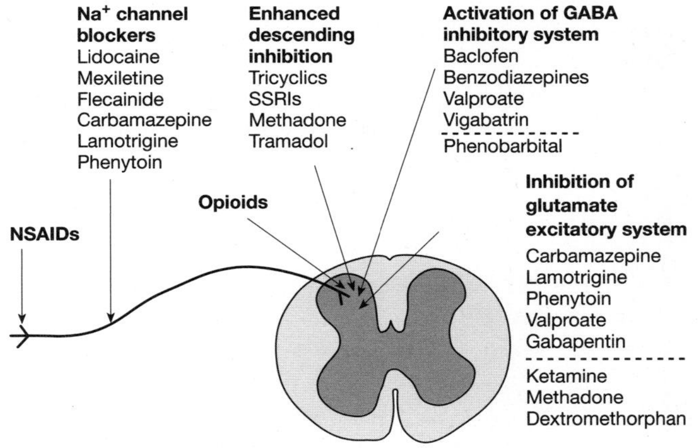

Fig. 5 Impact of analgesics and adjuvant analgesics on peripheral nerves and the dorsal horn of the spinal cord. Drugs below the dotted lines are channel blockers; the rest are receptor ligands.

Box 3 Clinical features of gastric stasis

Some or all of the following symptoms may occur:
- early satiety
- postprandial fullness
- epigastric bloating
- epigastric discomfort
- heartburn
- belching
- hiccup
- nausea
- retching
- vomiting

On examination there may be:
- epigastric distension
- a succussion splash

The absence of these features does not rule out symptomatic gastric stasis.

If associated with autonomic neuropathy, there is often evidence of other autonomic abnormalities,

e.g. orthostatic hypotension without a compensatory tachycardia.
- bowel sounds are generally normal but may be decreased if the stasis is opioid-induced

The use of metoclopramide (a prokinetic drug) often leads to improvement and the resolution of the succussion splash.

A degree of gastric stasis is present in many patients with advanced cancer. Diagnosis depends on a high level of clinical suspicion and pattern recognition (Box 3). There are several causes of gastric stasis and multiple factors may be responsible:

- dysmotility dyspepsia (often long-standing);
- drugs, e.g. opioids, antimuscarinics;
- cancer of the head of the pancreas (disrupts duodenal transit);
- retroperitoneal disease leading to neural dysfunction;
- spinal cord compression;
- paraneoplastic autonomic neuropathy;
- diabetic autonomic neuropathy.

Management

Correct the correctable

Medication may need to be modified, ascites drained, and hypercalcaemia corrected (unless coincidental in a moribund patient). Surgery for bowel obstruction should be considered if all the following criteria are all fulfilled:

- an easily reversible cause seems likely, e.g. postoperative adhesions or a single discrete neoplastic obstruction;
- the patient's general condition is good, i.e. does not have widely disseminated disease and has been independent and active; and
- the patient is willing to undergo surgery.

Surgical intervention for bowel obstruction is contraindicated in each of the following circumstances:

- previous laparotomy findings preclude the prospect of a successful intervention;
- diffuse intra-abdominal carcinomatosis as evidenced by diffuse palpable intra-abdominal tumours;
- massive ascites that reaccumulates rapidly after paracentesis.

Non-drug measures

Make sure that the patient is not assailed by food smells from the kitchen. Offer only small helpings of food. Possibly try an acupressure band on one or both wrists.

Drugs

The initial choice generally lies between four drugs: metoclopramide, haloperidol, hyoscine butylbromide, and cyclizine (Box 4). Second-line drugs may need to be added or substituted in some patients.

A systematic approach for inoperable bowel obstruction is shown in Fig. 6. For those with severe colic or who are not passing flatus, prokinetic drugs are contraindicated and step 1 is omitted. Bulk-forming, osmotic, and stimulant laxatives should be stopped, but patients may well benefit from a faecal softener, for example docusate 100 to 200 mg once to twice a day. Octreotide, a somatostatin analogue, has intestinal antisecretory properties and is occasionally indicated. It is much more expensive than hyoscine butylbromide but has no antimuscarinic effects. A venting gastrostomy is rarely necessary for symptom relief in patients with advanced cancer and bowel obstruction.

Patients who are inoperable and are managed by drug therapy should be allowed to drink and eat small amounts of their favourite beverages and food. Some patients find that they can manage food best in the morning. Antimuscarinic drugs and diminished fluid intake often result in a dry mouth. This is generally relieved by conscientious mouth care. A few millitres of fluid every 30 min, possibly given as a small ice cube, is often helpful.

Constipation

Constipation (difficulty in defaecation) is common in advanced cancer. Diminished food and fibre intake, lack of exercise, and drugs are common causal factors.

Evaluation

Many patients who are constipated do not need a rectal examination (by definition, an assault which must be justifiable). On the other hand, a rectal examination is essential in patients with faecal leakage or diarrhoea to confirm or exclude faecal impaction.

In non-obese patients, firm faeces are often palpable in the left iliac fossa and left side of the abdomen. Faeces may also be palpable in the transverse colon, and occasionally in the ascending colon as well, together with caecal distension and tenderness. Bowel sounds are variable. Sometimes it is not clear whether the problem is severe constipation, chronic intestinal obstruction, or both. Although plain radiographs confirm the presence of retained faeces, they cannot reliably differentiate between the two conditions. Pattern recognition and probability may enable a presumptive diagnosis to be made, but sometimes only the passage of time and the response (or lack of response) to treatment confirm whether it is just constipation or obstruction.

Management

Laxatives are the mainstay of treatment for patients with a limited physical capacity and reduced intake of food and fibre. For patients not taking an opioid, start with senna or bisacodyl tablets, adding a faecal softener (for example, docusate) if necessary. Alternatively, a combination preparation (for example, codanthramer, codanthrusate) can be substituted (Box 5). Some patients do better with lactulose but may require 30 ml twice daily or more. Opioids cause constipation by decreasing propulsive activity and increasing non-propulsive activity in both the small and large bowel; peristalsis is impeded and absorption of fluid and electrolytes is facilitated. So-called stimulant laxatives act principally by reducing intestinal ring contractions, thereby facilitating propulsive activity.

About one-third of patients receiving morphine continue to need rectal measures (suppositories, enemas, digital evacuation) either regularly or intermittently. Danthron-containing laxatives are inadvisable in patients with faecal leakage or incontinence because danthron can cause a contact skin burn. Because of concern that it may be carcinogenic, danthron-containing laxatives are now only licensed for use in terminally ill patients.

Box 4 Guidelines for the management of nausea and vomiting in palliative care

1. After clinical evaluation, document the most likely cause(s) of the nausea and vomiting in the patient's case notes.
2. Ask the patient to record their symptoms and response to treatment.
3. Treat correctable causes/exacerbating factors, e.g. drugs, constipation, severe pain, infection, cough, hypercalcaemia. *Correction of hypercalcaemia may not be appropriate in a dying patient.*

Anxiety exacerbates nausea and vomiting from any cause and may need specific treatment, pharmacological and/or psychological.

4. Prescribe the most appropriate first-line antiemetic for the most likely main cause: immediately, regularly, and 'as needed'. Give subcutaneously if continuous nausea or frequent vomiting, preferably by subcutaneous infusion.

First-line antiemetics:

Prokinetic antiemetic

For gastritis, gastric stasis, functional bowel obstruction:

- metoclopramide 10 mg immediately by mouth, and then four times a day; or 10 mg immediately subcutaneously, and 40–100 mg/24 h as a subcutaneous infusion, and 10 mg 'as needed' up to four times daily.

Antiemetic acting principally in chemoreceptor trigger zone (area postrema)

For most chemical causes of vomiting, e.g. morphine, hypercalcaemia, renal failure:

- haloperidol 1.5–3 mg immediately by mouth, and at bedtime; or 2.5–5 mg immediately subcutaneously, and 2.5–10 mg/24 h by subcutaneous infusion and 2.5–5 mg 'as needed' up to four times daily.

Metoclopramide also acts here.

Antispasmodic and antisecretory antiemetic

If bowel colic and/or need to reduce gastrointestinal secretions:

- hyoscine butylbromide 20 mg immediately subcutaneously, and 80–160 mg/24 h by subcutaneous infusion, and 20 mg 'as needed' up to every lR.

Antiemetic acting principally in the vomiting centre

For organic bowel obstruction, raised intracranial pressure, motion sickness:

- cyclizine 50 mg immediately by mouth, and two or three times per day; or 50 mg immediately subcutaneously, and 100–150 mg/24 h by subcutaneous infusion, and 50 mg 'as needed' up to four times daily.

5. Review the dose of antiemetic every 24 h, taking note of 'as needed' use and the patient's diary.
6. If there is little or no benefit, despite optimizing the dose, have you got the cause right?
    - if no, change to an alternative first-line antiemetic and optimize
    - if yes, provided the first-line antiemetic has been optimized *add* or *substitute* the second-line antiemetic
    - for patients with obstructive vomiting, follow the steps in Fig. 6.

Box 4 *Contunued*

Second-line drugs for nausea and vomiting

Broad-spectrum antiemetic

If first-line antiemetics (in appropriate combination, dose, and route) are inadequate:

- *levomepromazine (methotrimeprazine) 6–12.5 mg by mouth or subcutaneously immediately, at bedtime, and* 'as needed' up to four times daily.

Corticosteroids

Adjuvant antiemetic

- *dexamethasone 8–16 mg immediately by mouth or subcutaneously, and once daily; consider reducing the dose after 7 days.*

5-HT3-receptor antagonist

Use when there is a massive release of 5-HT (serotonin) from enterochromaffin cells or platelets, e.g. chemotherapy, abdominal radiation, bowel obstruction, renal failure:

- tropisetron 5 mg *immediately by mouth or subcutaneously, and once daily.*

7. Some patients with nausea and vomiting need more than one antiemetic.
8. *Do not prescribe a prokinetic and an antimuscarinic drug concurrently because the latter blocks the cholinergic final common pathway through which prokinetics act.*
9. Except in organic bowel obstruction consider converting to the oral route after 72 h of good control with injections.
10. Continue antiemetics indefinitely unless the cause is self-limiting.

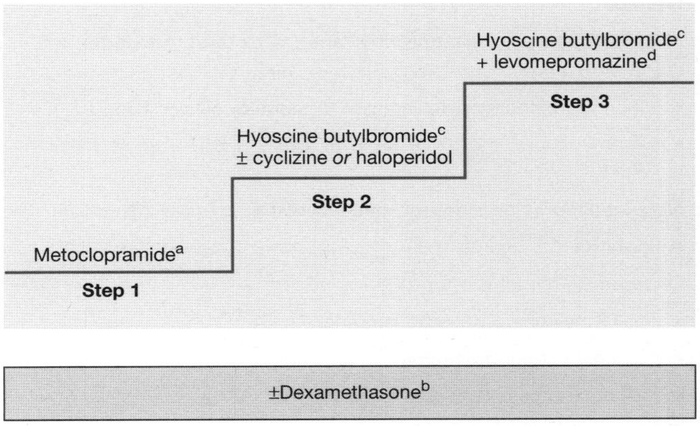

[a] If obstruction complete or severe colic, *omit step 1.*
[b] The place of corticosteroids in inoperable bowel obstructions is controversial; consider a trial of dexamethasone 8–16 mg once daily for 7 days.
[c] If not available, use glycopyrronium 600–1200 μg/24 h instead.
[d] If levomepromazine is too sedative, revert to step 2 but give both cyclizine and haloperidol.

Fig. 6 Antiemetics for endstage bowel obstruction. These are normally given by subcutaneous injection/infusion. (a) If the obstruction complete or there is severe colic, start at step 2. (b) The role of corticosteroids in bowel obstruction is controversial; consider a trial of dexamethasone 8–16 mg once a day for 5 days. (c) If not available, use glycopyrronium 600–1200 μg/24 h instead. (d) If levomepromazine is too sedative, revert to step 2 and add haloperidol.

Dyspnoea

Dyspnoea is an unpleasant subjective awareness of difficulty in breathing. Objective signs generally include tachypnoea (an increased rate of respiration) and sometimes hyperpnoea (an increased depth of respiration). Dyspnoea becomes more common as death approaches; overall it is experienced by about 70 per cent of patients with advanced cancer.

Evaluation

In most patients with advanced cancer, dyspnoea is caused by several factors, for example chronic obstructive pulmonary disease, progressive intrathoracic malignant disease, anaemia of chronic disease, weakness (Box 6). The history and examination are often sufficient to determine the main causes.

Management

Non-drug measures

The key to successful management at the end of life is at an earlier stage, when dyspnoea on exertion first becomes a symptom. Acknowledgement of and discussion about the terror associated with acute episodes of breathlessness, for instance when climbing stairs, is very important. Referral to a

Box 5 Management of opioid-induced constipation

- Ask about the patient's past (premorbid) and present bowel habit and use of laxatives; record date of last bowel action.
- Do a rectal examination if faecal impaction is suspected or if the patient reports diarrhoea or faecal incontinence (to exclude impaction with overflow).
- For inpatients, keep a daily record of bowel actions.
- Encourage fluids generally, and fruit juice and fruit specifically.
- When an opioid is first prescribed, prescribe co-danthrusate[a] (one capsule at bedtime) prophylactically; although occasionally appropriate to optimize a patient's existing bowel regimen, rather than change automatically to co-danthrusate.
- If already constipated, prescribe co-danthrusate (two capsules at bedtime).
- Adjust the dose every few days according to results, up to three capsules three times a day.
- If the patient prefers a liquid preparation, use co-danthrusate suspension; 5 ml is equivalent to one capsule.
- If more than 3 days since the last bowel action, 'uncork' with suppositories, e.g. bisacodyl 10 mg and glycerol 4 g.
- If suppositories are ineffective, administer a high phosphate enema; possibly repeat the next day.
- If the maximum dose of co-danthrusate is ineffective, switch to an osmotic laxative, e.g. lactulose 20–30 ml twice daily or macrogol 3350 1 to 3 sachets daily ± a reduced dose of co-danthrusate.
- If co-danthrusate causes abdominal cramps, divide the total daily dose into smaller more frequent doses, e.g. change from co-danthrusate two capsules twice daily to one capsule four times daily or change to lactulose or macrogol 3350.
- An osmotic laxative may be preferable to co-danthrusate in patients with a history of colic with other colonic stimulants.

[a] In the USA, use Peri-Colace (casanthranol 30 mg + docusate sodium 100 mg) capsules instead.

Box 6 Causes of breathlessness in advanced cancer

Caused by cancer	Related to cancer and/or debility
Pleural effusion(s)	Anaemia
Obstruction of main bronchus	Atelectasis
Replacement of lung by cancer	Pulmonary embolism
Lymphangitis carcinomatosa	Pneumonia
Mediastinal obstruction	Empyema
Pericardial effusion	Weakness
Massive ascites	
Abdominal distension	**Concurrent causes**
Cachexia–anorexia syndrome	Chronic obstructive pulmonary disease (COPD)
Caused by treatment	Asthma
Pneumonectomy	Heart failure
Radiation-induced fibrosis	Acidosis
Chemotherapy	
bleomycin	
doxorubicin	

physiotherapist for breathing advice and relaxation techniques is important.

Correct the correctable

Specific treatment should be given for specific causes, for example: bronchodilators for reversible airways obstruction; diuretics for cardiac failure; aspiration and pleuradesis for pleural effusion; and radiotherapy or stenting for superior vena caval obstruction.

Drugs

When the patient is close to death, breathlessness may be present at rest as well as on exertion, or become apparent on minimal activity. Often the patient is bedbound, more because of breathlessness than weakness. In this situation, an opioid (to slow the respiratory rate towards normal), an anxiolytic, and oxygen therapy may all be helpful (Box 7).

Anorexia

Anorexia (diminished or absent appetite) is normal in advanced cancer.

Evaluation

Anorexia may be primary (cachexia–anorexia syndrome) or secondary. Secondary anorexia may be caused by:

- medication which causes dyspepsia or nausea, e.g. NSAIDs, opioids, antibiotics, selective serotonin-reuptake inhibitors (**SSRIs**);
- nausea;
- pain;
- altered taste;
- difficulty feeding because of weakness, dysphagia, or a sore mouth;
- fatigue;
- psychological distress, e.g. fear, anxiety, depression.

Patients are generally more tolerant of anorexia than their families, for whom it is a source of great concern. Many patients state that their carers try too hard to encourage eating, resulting in conflict. Eating is an important social interaction and anorexia may be interpreted by the family as giving in to the cancer. Explanation should be given about the cause(s) of anorexia and the limitations of treatment.

Management

Correct the correctable

Review the current medication for a possible cause; treat pain, nausea, and sore mouth. Obtain dietary advice to minimize the impact of an altered sense of taste.

Non-drug measures

'A little of what you fancy when you fancy' is good advice. Frequent snacks high in calories and low in bulk are preferable to traditional meals.

Drugs

If anorexia appears to be mainly due to early satiety, a prokinetic agent should be tried, for example metoclopramide 10 mg four times daily by mouth.

Prednisolone (15 to 20 mg once a day) or dexamethasone (2 to 4 mg once daily) help about 50 per cent of patients. To avoid cumulative adverse effects, a corticosteroid should be discontinued if there is no benefit after a week or, if effective, reduced to a maintenance dose. Patients and families should be forewarned that the benefit often lasts for only a few weeks.

Medroxyprogesterone acetate (400 mg once daily up to 500 mg twice daily) or megestrol acetate (160 mg once daily up to 800 mg once daily) often lead to weight gain after 3 to 4 weeks, particularly in patients with breast cancer, as a result of an increase in both fat and body water. The effect may last for months. Progestogens are much more expensive than corticosteroids.

Box 7 Relief of breathlessness at rest in a dying patient

Bronchodilators

The use of bronchodilators should be reviewed and tested clinically for efficacy; it may be necessary to use a spacer to ensure adequate inhalation from an inhaler, or to convert to a nebulizer. Benefit is not always correlated with improvement in peak flow.

Opioids

Morphine reduces respiratory drive and can be used to ease the sensation of dyspnoea:

- if on morphine for pain, increase the dose by 50 per cent;
- if not on oral morphine, 5–6 mg every 4 h is a good starting dose.

Nebulized morphine is not recommended; it is no better than saline.

Anxiolytics

Diazepam by mouth is a good choice:

- 5–10 mg immediately and bedtime;
- 2–5 mg in the very elderly;

reduce dose after several days if drowsy.

Use midazolam subcutaneously for patients who find tablets difficult to take:

- 2.5–5 mg immediately and 'as needed';
- 10–20 mg/24 h by subcutaneous infusion.

Oxygen

Oxygen 4 L/min, preferably via nasal prongs, should be tried to see if benefit gained either continuously or before and during activity (e.g. moving from bed to commode or chair). The benefit of oxygen is not dependent on correction of hypoxaemia; a trial of therapy is the only way to determine benefit, not improvement in blood gases.

Cachexia

Cachexia (marked weight loss and muscle wasting) occurs in up to 80 per cent of patients with advanced cancer. Muscle wasting results in weakness and fatigue. The incidence is highest in cancers of the gastrointestinal tract and lung.

Evaluation

Cachexia is caused by several interrelated metabolic disturbances (Box 8). Concurrent exacerbating factors may be reversible and should be considered.

Management

Correct the correctable

As for anorexia (see above).

Non-drug measures

Avoid routine weighing. Explain that 'forced feeding' cannot correct primary cachexia. Some patients benefit psychologically from powdered or liquid nutritional supplements, and a few gain weight. Dietary advice is important if there are changes in taste sensation.

Drugs

As for anorexia. In most patients the effect is small or non-existent. Management is often best focused on acceptance and adaptation.

Dehydration

As the dying patient becomes weaker, intake of both food and fluid becomes less. Decreased fluid intake may be caused by dysphagia, nausea, anorexia, lack of energy and interest, and a reduced level of consciousness, either singly or in combination. There is a big difference between acute and chronic dehydration. Whereas the former is accompanied by intense thirst, this is not the case in dying patients when there is a slow progressive reduction in fluid intake. Conscientious mouth care (cleaning and moistening) is generally all that is called for. As a general rule, intravenous fluids should not be administered if the decreased intake is best interpreted as part of the process of dying. Guidelines from the British Medical Association support this approach.

Confusion

An acute confusional state (delirium) eventually occurs in most dying patients. This typically manifests as disorientation, bewilderment, and drowsiness, often compounded by a spectrum of cognitive disturbances such as poor concentration, impairment of short-term memory, misinterpretation, paranoid ideas, hallucinations, rambling incoherent speech, agitation, and noisy aggressive behaviour.

Box 8 Causes of cachexia in advanced cancer

Paraneoplastic	Concurrent
Cytokines produced by host cells and tumour (e.g. TNF, IL-6, IL-3[a])	Anorexia → deficient food intake
Abnormal host metabolism of protein, carbohydrate, and fat	Vomiting
Increased metabolic rate → increased energy expenditure	Diarrhoea
Nitrogen trap by the tumour	Malabsorption
	Bowel obstruction
	Debilitating effect of surgery, radiotherapy, chemotherapy
	Ulceration } excessive loss of body protein
	Haemorrhage } excessive loss of body protein

aTNF, tumour necrosis factor; IL, interleukin.

Box 9 Common causes of acute confusion in the dying

Cancer	Drugs
paraneoplastic effect	sedative
cerebral involvement	psychostimulant
Infection	antiparkinsonian
Dehydration	Drug withdrawal
Change of environment	psychotropics
Unfamiliar excessive stimuli	alcohol
too hot	nicotine
too cold	Biochemical derangement
wet bed	hypercalcaemia
crumbs in bed	hyponatraemia
creases in sheets	hypoglycaemia
pain	hyperglycaemia
constipation	Cerebral anoxia
retention of urine	anaemia
pruritus	cardiac failure
Anxiety	Organ failure
Depression	hepatic
Fatigue	renal

Evaluation

Multiple factors may contribute to confusion (Box 9). Biochemical investigations are generally contraindicated in patients close to death. It is important not to overlook urinary retention and faecal impaction.

Management

Correct the correctable

The patient's drug regimen should be reviewed and a reduction in psychoactive drugs considered, for example amitriptyline 75 mg once a day reduced to 25 mg once a day. Occasionally nicotine or alcohol withdrawal may be the main cause (see below). Pneumonia often precipitates confusion. Treating pneumonia with antibiotics is generally inappropriate in a debilitated, bedbound, dying patient.

Non-drug measures

The presence of a close relative or friend is generally helpful. Visual cues (day, date, soft light, and photographs) and auditory cues (favourite music) may help (Box 10).

Drugs

If the patient is agitated, haloperidol should be given, for example 1.5 to 5 mg by mouth or 2.5 to 5 mg subcutaneously. Diazepam or midazolam should be added if the patient remains agitated after 5 to 10 mg of haloperidol (Box 10). If nicotine or alcohol withdrawal is suspected and the patient is unable to smoke or drink, specific treatment should be considered—for instance, transdermal nicotine patches, or a benzodiazepine with or without thiamine for delirium tremens.

Terminal anguish

Terminal anguish is a tormented state of mind that relates to long-standing unresolved emotional problems and/or interpersonal conflicts, or to long-hidden unhappy memories often with a guilty content. These problems have festered in the mind but have never been brought into the open. The possibility of such an outcome highlights the need to make every effort to deal with psychological 'skeletons in the cupboard' before the patient becomes too weak to be able to address them. A few patients, however, resist every attempt to explore what has been suppressed.

Terminal anguish is managed in the same way as an agitated confusional state, for instance by combining an antipsychotic and a benzodiazepine.

Large doses may be required and sometimes the more sedative levomepromazine (methotrimeprazine) is preferable to haloperidol. A dose of 50 to 100 mg per 24 h is often very sedative, but this (or more) is what may be necessary to ensure calm. On rare occasions, it may be necessary to use subcutaneous phenobarbital (Box 10).

Death rattle

Evaluation

The inability to clear secretions from the oropharynx and trachea results in noisy (rattling) breathing as the secretions oscillate with respiration. When a death rattle develops the patient is almost always unconscious and untroubled by the secretions. It helps the family to appreciate this, but some families still find it distressing.

Box 10 Treatment of acute confusion

Non-drug measures

Explanation to patient, family, nurses.

Stress that patient is not going mad.

Stress that almost always there are lucid intervals.

Continue to treat patient as a sane, sensible person.

Be aware that illusions, hallucinations, and nightmares may reflect unresolved fears and anxiety.

Drugs

Use drugs only if symptoms are marked, persistent, and cause distress to the patient and/or family. Review sooner rather than later if a sedative drug is prescribed in case it exacerbates symptoms.

Specific

Dose reduction of present psychotropic medication?

If hypoxic or cyanosed, give oxygen.

If cerebral tumour, give dexamethasone 8–16 mg once daily. *Correction of cerebral oedema may not be appropriate in a dying patient.*

If nicotine withdrawal, give nicotine either as a nasal spray or transdermal patch.

General

Haloperidol 1.5–5 mg by mouth or subcutaneously, particularly if hallucinations and paranoid ideas.

Diazepam 5–10 mg by mouth or midazolam 5–10 mg subcutaneously if still restless after two doses of haloperidol (or give concurrently if there is myoclonus):

- initial dose depends on previous medication, weight, age, and severity of symptoms;
- subsequent doses depend on initial response;
- daily- or twice-daily maintenance doses are generally adequate;
- sometimes more frequent administration is necessary.

In extreme situations, it may be necessary to deeply sedate a dying agitated patient, e.g.:

- levomepromazine 25–50 mg immediately and 50–200 mg/24 h subcutaneously;
- phenobarbital 100–200 mg immediately and 800–1600 mg/24 h subcutaneously.

Management

Non-drug measures

Placing the unconscious patient in the recovery (semi-prone) position aids the drainage of secretions from the mouth. Suctioning is generally contraindicated; it can distress a patient who is otherwise settled.

Drugs

Because antimuscarinic drugs do not dry up secretions already present, it is important to act at the first sign of rattling. Hyoscine hydrobromide (0.4 to 0.6 mg immediately subcutaneously and 1.2 mg by subcutaneous infusion over 24 h) or hyoscine butylbromide (Buscopan; 20 mg subcutaneous at once and 20 to 40 mg by infusion over 24 h) are both widely used. Glycopyrronium may be used instead, for example, 0.2 mg immediately subcutaneously and 0.6 mg by infusion over 24 h). Such measures are successful in about 50 to 60 per cent of patients. Intravenous diuretics are of benefit if there is concomitant left ventricular failure, which is unusual.

Ethical considerations

The cardinal principles that underpin clinical practice, including palliative care, are:

- respect for patient autonomy (patient choice);
- beneficence (do good);
- non-maleficence (minimize harm);
- justice (fair use of available resources).

These four principles need to be applied against the background of respect for life and an acceptance of the ultimate inevitability of death. Thus, in practice, three dichotomies need to be held in balance:

- the potential benefits of treatment versus the potential risks and burdens;
- striving to preserve life but, when the burdens of life-sustaining treatments outweigh the potential benefits, then withdrawing or withholding such treatments and providing comfort in dying;
- individual needs versus the needs of society.

Principle of double effect

The principle of double effect states that:

> A single act having two possible foreseen effects, one good and one harmful, is not always morally prohibited if the harmful effect is not intended.

This is a universal principle without which the practice of medicine would be impossible. It follows inevitably from the fact that all treatment has an inherent risk. However, discussions of the principle of double effect are often limited to the use of morphine or similar drug to relieve pain in terminally ill patients. This gives the false impression that the use of morphine in this circumstance is a high-risk strategy. When correctly used morphine (and other strong opioids) are very safe drugs, safer than NSAIDs, which are widely prescribed with relative impunity. The use of both classes of analgesic is justified on the basis that the benefits of pain relief far outweigh the risk of serious adverse effects. Indeed, clinical experience suggests that those whose pain is relieved live longer than would have been the case if they had continued to be exhausted and demoralized by severe unremitting pain.

However, the intended aim of treatment must be the relief of suffering and not the patient's death. Although a greater risk is acceptable in more extreme circumstances, it remains axiomatic that effective measures that carry less risk to life should normally be used. Thus, in an extreme situation, although it may occasionally be necessary (and acceptable) to render a patient unconscious, it remains unacceptable (and unnecessary) to cause death deliberately. Deliberate hastening of death by intentionally giving an overdose of one or more drugs (euthanasia) is illegal in almost all countries. Palliative care and euthanasia are essentially mutually exclusive philosophies.

Appropriate treatment

A doctor is not obliged legally or ethically to preserve life 'at all costs'. Priorities change when a patient is clearly dying. There is no obligation to employ treatments if their use can best be described as prolonging the process of dying. A doctor has neither duty nor right to prescribe a lingering death. In palliative care, the primary aim of treatment is not to prolong life but to make the life that remains as comfortable and as meaningful as possible. Part of the art of medicine is to decide when to allow death to occur without further medical impediment.

However, it is not a question of to treat or not to treat but what is the most appropriate treatment given the patient's biological prospects and his personal and social circumstances? Appropriate treatment for an acutely ill patient may be inappropriate in the dying (Fig. 7). Nasogastric tubes, intravenous infusions, antibiotics, cardiac resuscitation, and artificial respiration are all primarily support measures for use in acute or acute-on-chronic illnesses to assist a patient through the initial crisis towards recovery of health. The use of these measures in patients who are irreversibly close to death is generally inappropriate (and therefore bad practice) because the burdens of such treatments exceed their potential benefits.

Although the possibility of unexpected improvement or recovery should not be totally ignored, there are many occasions when it is appropriate to 'give death a chance'. Interest in hydration and nutrition often becomes minimal as death draws near. The patient's disinterest or positive disinclination is part of the process of letting go.

At the end

Although eventually you may feel powerless in the face of approaching death, patients are generally more realistic. They know you cannot perform a miracle and time is limited. Despite possibly having nothing new to offer, it is important for the doctor to:

- continue to visit;
- quietly indicate that, 'The important thing now is to keep you comfortable';
- simplify medication;
- arrange for medication to be given sublingually, rectally, or by continuous subcutaneous infusion when the patient cannot swallow;
- continue to inform the family of the changing situation;
- control agitation, even if it results in sedation;
- listen to the nurses.

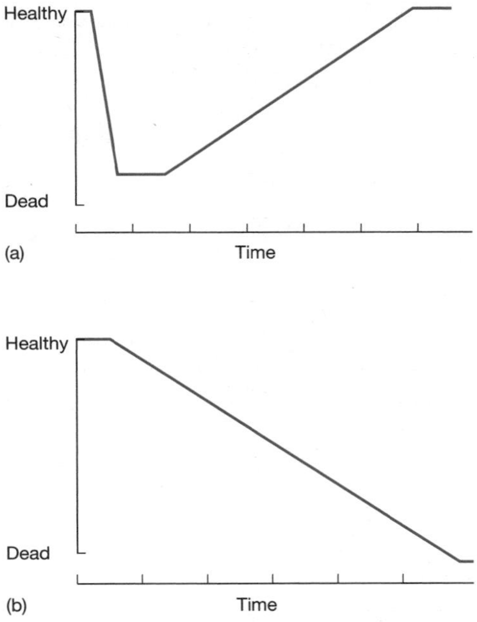

Fig. 7 (a) A graphical representation of acute illness. Biological prospects are generally good. Acute resuscitative measures are important and enable the patient to survive the initial crisis. Recovery is aided by the natural forces of healing; rehabilitation is completed by the patient on his own, without continued medical support. (b) A graphical representation of terminal illness. Biological prospects progressively worsen. Acute and terminal illnesses are therefore distinct pathophysiological entities. Therapeutic interventions that can best be described as prolonging the distress of dying are essentially futile and inappropriate.

Further reading

BMA Report (1999). *Withholding and withdrawing life-prolonging medical treatment.* BMA, London.

Doyle D, Hanks GWC, MacDonald N, eds (1997). *Oxford textbook of palliative medicine*, 2nd edn. Oxford Medical Publications, Oxford.

National Council for Hospice and Specialist Palliative Care Services (1997). Artificial hydration (AH) for people who are terminally ill. *European Journal of Palliative Care* **4,** 124.

Sindrup SH, Jensen TS (1999). Efficacy of pharmacological treatments of neuropathic pain: an update and effect related to mechanism of drug action. *Pain* **83,** 389–400.

Twycross R. (1999). *Introducing palliative care*, 3rd edn. Radcliffe Medical Press, Oxford.

Twycross R, Wilcock A, Charlesworth S, Dickman A (2002). *Palliative care formulary*, 2nd edn. Radcliffe Medical Press, Oxford.

32

Reference intervals for biochemical data

32 Reference intervals for biochemical data

P. A. H. Holloway and A. M. Giles

Classification of laboratory results

Intervals are presented in the following format;

for individual tests see general text:

Everyday tests and enzymes Table 1

Blood gases Table 2

Paediatric reference ranges Table 3

Hormones Table 4

Tumour markers Table 5

Vitamins and related tests Table 6

Lipids and lipoproteins Table 7

Proteins and immunoproteins Table 8

Trace elements and metals Table 9

Urinary values Table 10

Faecal values Table 11

Cerebrospinal fluid Table 12

Functional tests Table 13

Therapeutic drugs Table 14

Common drug toxicology Table 15

Introduction

The precise quantitation of a substance in easily accessible body fluids is an integral part of the clinical assessment of patients. The results are used in screening for disease as well as in diagnosis and for monitoring the response to therapy in established disease. Much diagnostic weight rests on single determinations and patterns of biochemical tests. To this end it is important to consider biological variations between healthy individuals, inherent variations in laboratory methods, and the errors of sampling and hospital practice which can influence every determination. The first (and the last) are the provinces of the physician ordering the test. The second is the concern of the laboratory which provides quality control and the reference intervals for the test.

An important growth area in diagnostic pathology is emerging in the field of 'point-of-care' testing (**POCT**), particularly in the critical care environment. Whilst technology has advanced to enable rapid analytical turnaround times in POCT—usually far less than 10 min from sample withdrawal to result—with consequent hastening to clinical decision-making, the laboratory responsibility for interpretation and overseeing test results is partially devolved to the nurse or doctor at the bedside. In this context there is greater need for an understanding of the appropriate reference intervals as well as of any limitations on the analytical precision when compared to central laboratory methods.

'Normal range' and 'abnormal' results

Clinical diagnostic decisions may depend equally upon finding a 'normal' or 'abnormal' result for any test requested. The physician should be clear as to the meaning of these terms. An important task of the clinical biochemist is therefore to provide relevant sets of reliable reference data. For any individual the ideal reference value for an analyte should be that obtained when that individual is healthy. However, in practice, laboratory test results are interpreted by comparison to traditional, but often inadequately, defined reference intervals (formerly termed 'normal' ranges). The wide belief that biological data assume a gaussian distribution is inappropriate. Most biological data are not symmetrically distributed and require statistical tools that assume other kinds of distribution or are independent of distribution form. Ideally, each laboratory should establish sets of reference intervals derived from a local reference population.

Reference interval

In the past many texts quoted a 'reference range' defined as the mean ± 2 standard deviations from the mean of results obtained from the reference population. This is, however, not now the commonest method applied to clinical biochemistry tests. Many of the 'intervals' quoted in clinical practice are in fact derived from a skew-distribution, which is calculated from the geometric mean to include 95 per cent of values obtained from what is considered to be a 'healthy' population (95 per cent confidence intervals). The merits of a diagnostic test are determined by the relationship between the data for healthy and unhealthy populations, and an example of a relatively poor test is given in Fig. 1. By whatever criteria it is obtained, the reference interval is compounded of both physiological variation and the irreducible error. More elaborate statistical handling of human biochemical data is available for individual tests, but is not generally required in making a diagnosis. By way of warning, however, it will readily be appreciated that if this criterion of health (that is, the biochemical results within 95 per cent limits for the given value), is applied to multiple tests in any individual, then with a battery of say 12 tests only 50 per cent of 'normal' individuals will be found to be 'healthy'. An important example of the limitations of strict referral to the 'reference interval' is highlighted by plasma total cholesterol measurements within certain populations, where established reference intervals may be considered to contain a considerable proportion of individuals with 'undesirable' or 'unhealthy' values. In such situations it may be appropriate to define an 'ideal' or 'optimum' range for that parameter. Other difficulties arise from situations where the reference interval has not been constructed from a population of matched ethnic mix.

In conclusion, the use of the following tables of reference intervals for biochemical tests must therefore include an appreciation of the limitations in reference intervals of analytical variation and differences between methods of analysis, as well as sex, age, posture, diet, and other biological variables, as well as sampling, that contribute to such an operation. The physician should constantly bear in mind the need to see individual results

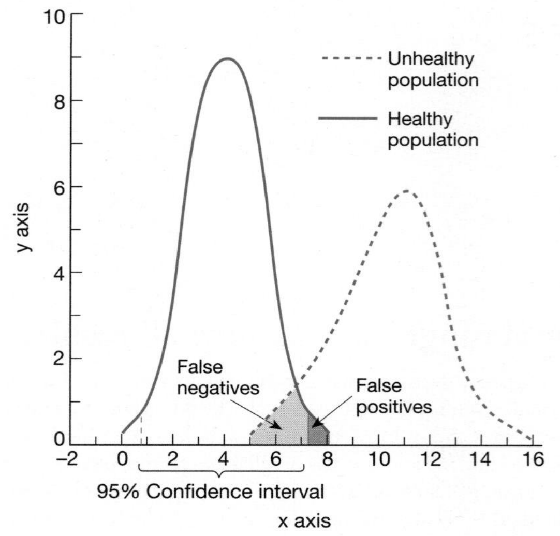

Fig. 1 Theoretical distributions of an analyte in healthy (symmetrical) and unhealthy (negatively skewed) populations.

of laboratory tests in their clinical context, and not to hesitate in questioning an unexpected or unlikely result.

The reference intervals given here are predominantly those established for laboratory investigations available at the John Radcliffe Hospital in Oxford, in the United Kingdom. Throughout the tables intervals are given in SI and conventional units, together wherever possible with the factor for converting from SI to conventional. Where appropriate, specific, specimen collection details are given, although it should be recognized that with varied methodologies for most assays it is not possible to make these prescriptive.

Table 1 Everyday tests (adult)

Determination	Sample⊥	SI units		Conversion factor (SI to conventional)	Conventional units	
Alcohol						
legal limit (UK)	B or P	<17.4	mmol/l	× 4.6	<80	mg/dl
Albumin	P	35–50	g/l	× 0.1	3.5–5.0	g/dl
in pregnancy	P	25–38	g/l	× 0.1	2.5–3.8	g/dl
Ammonia	B	<40	µmol/l	× 1.4	<56	µg/dl
α-Amylase	P	25–180	somogyi units/dl	× 1.83	46–330	U/l
Anion gap $(Na^+ + K^+) - (HCO_3^- + Cl^-)$*	P	12–16	mmol/l	× 1	12–16	mEq/l
Bilirubin	P	3–17	µmol/l	× 0.058	0.2–1.0	mg/dl
Bicarbonate*	P	22–28	mmol/l	× 1	22–28	mEq/l
Calcium						
ionized	P	1.0–1.25	mmol/l	× 4.0	4.0–5.0	mg/dl
total	P	2.12–2.65	mmol/l	× 4.0	8.5–10.6	mg/dl
total in pregnancy	P	1.95–2.35	mmol/l	× 4.0	7.8–9.4	mg/dl
Chloride	P	95–105	mmol/l	× 1	95–105	mEq/l
Cholesterol+	P	3.9–7.8	mmol/l	× 38.6	150–300	mg/dl
Copper	P	12–26	µmol/l	× 6.37	76–165	mg/dl
Creatinine	P	70-150	µmol/l	× 0.011	0.7–1.7	mg/dl
in pregnancy	P	24–68	µmol/l	× 0.011	0.27–0.76	mg/dl
Digoxin•						
children	P	2.0–3.0	nmol/l	× 0.78	1.6–2.3	ng/ml
adults	P	1.0–2.0	nmol/l	× 0.78	0.8–1.6	ng/ml
Glucose (fasting)	P	3.0–5.0	mmol/l	× 18	54–90	mg/dl
Glycated haemoglobin (HbA1C)	B	5–8%		× 1	5–8%	
Iron						
M	S	14–31	µmol/l	× 5.59	78–174	µg/dl
F	S	11–30	µmol/l	× 5.59	62–168	µg/dl
Total iron-binding capacity (TIBC)	S	45–75	µmol/l	× 5.59	250–420	µg/dl
Lactate						
venous	B	0.5–2.2	mmol/l	× 9.0	4.5–19.8	mg/dl
arterial	B	0.5–1.6	mmol/l	× 9.0	4.5–14.4	mg/dl

Table 1 continued

Determination	Sample⊥	SI units		Conversion factor (SI to conventional)	Conventional units	
Magnesium	P	0.75–1.05	mmol/l	× 2.0	1.5–2.1	mEq/l
Osmolality	P	278–305	mosm/kg	× 1	278–305	mosm/kg
Phosphate (inorganic)	P	0.8–1.45	mmol/l	× 3.1	2.48–4.5	mg/dl
Potassium¶	P	3.5–5.0	mmol/l	× 1	3.5–5.0	mEq/l
Protein (total)	P	60–80	g/l	× 0.1	6.0–8.0	g/dl
Sodium	P	135–145	mmol/l	× 1	135–145	mEq/l
Troponin T°	P	<0.1	ng/ml	× 1	<0.1	ng/ml
Troponin I†	P	<0.2	ng/ml	× 1	<0.2	ng/ml
Urea	P	2.5–6.7	mmol/l	× 2.8	7.8–18.7	mg/dl
in pregnancy	P	2.0–4.2	mmol/l	× 2.8	5.6–11.0	mg/dl
Urea nitrogen (BUN)	P	1.16–3.12	mmol/l	× 2.8	7.0–18.7	mg/dl
Uric acid						
M	P	M 210–480	μmol/l	× 0.169	3.5–8.1	mg/dl
F	P	F 150–390	μmol/l	× 0.169	2.5–6.5	mg/dl
in pregnancy	P	100–270	μmol/l	× 16.9	1.7–4.5	mg/dl
Zinc	P	6–25	μmol/l	× 6.54	39–163	μg/dl

* See Table 2.
⊥ B, whole blood; S, serum; P, plasma; U, urine; M, male; F, female.
\+ Current distribution in the United Kingdom. Desirable upper limit 5.2 mmol/l (200 mg/100 ml).
Requires collection under anaerobic conditions (as for blood gases).
Avoid use of tourniquet.
• 6 hours post-dose.
Collection tube must contain inhibitor of glycolysis (e.g. fluoride and oxalate).
¶ Avoid delayed separation and conditions inducing haemolysis (e.g. heat extremes, agitation).
° To exclude myocardial infarction 12–24 h from onset of chest pain.
† Same use as Troponin T. Method: DPC Immulite. Typical 12-h postinfarct value >30 ng/ml.

Diagnostic enzymes

Enzyme		**Sample**	**Reference intervals**	
Acid phosphatase				
total		S	1–5	U/l
prostatic		S	0–1	U/l
Alkaline phosphatase*	Adult	P	80–250	U/l
Alanine-transaminase (ALT (SGPT))		P	5–35	U/l
α-Amylase		P	25–180	somogyi units/dl
Angiotensin-converting enzyme (ACE)		S	21–54	U/l
Aspartate-transaminase (AST (SGOT))		P	15–42	U/l
Creatine kinase (CK)	M	P	24–195	U/l
	F	P	24–170	U/l
Creatine kinase MB (CKMB)∞				
activity			<25	U/l
	±		<6	% total CK
mass			<5	ng/ml
Gamma-glutamyl transferase (GGT)*	M	P	11–51	U/l
	F	P	7–35	U/l
Lactate dehydrogenase (LDH)				
total		P	240–525	U/l
Pseudocholinesterase		P	2.25–6.9	kU/l

Cholinesterase	*Phenotype*	*Percentage inhibition with:* *Fluoride*	*Dibucaine*
Normal homozygote	$Ch_1^UCh_1^U$	40–50	82–88
Abnormal homozygote	$Ch_1^DCh_1^D$	70–81	14–30
	$Ch_1^FCh_1^F$	30–35	60–73
Abnormal heterozygote	$Ch_1^UCh_1^D$	44–60	60–68
	$Ch_1^UCh_1^F$	37–41	70–79
	$Ch_1^DCh_1^F$	47–52	59–63

SGPT, serum glutamate pyruvate transaminase; SGOT, serum glutamate oxaloacetate transaminase; MB, myocardial bound; other abbreviations as Table 1.
* Adult values. See Table 3 for intervals in paediatrics.
∞ To exclude myocardial infarction 8–48 h from onset of chest pain.
General comment: Enzyme reference intervals are assay-dependent. Check with local laboratory.

Table 2 Blood gases

	SI units	Conversion factor (SI to conventional)		Conventional units	
Anion gap $(Na^+ + K^+) - (HCO_3^- + Cl^-)$	12–16	mmol/l	× 1	12–16	mEq/l
Arterial CO_2 ($Paco_2$)	4.7–6.0	kPa	× 7.52	35–45	mmHg
Mixed venous CO_2 ($Pvco_2$)	5.5–6.8	kPa	× 7.52	41–51	mmHg
Arterial oxygen (Pao_2)	12.0–14.5	kPa	× 7.52	90–109	mmHg
Mixed venous oxygen (Pvo_2)	4.0–6.0	kPa	× 7.52	30–45	mmHg
Newborn arterial oxygen	5.3–8.0	kPa	× 7.52	40–60	mm Hg
H^+ ion activity	36–44	nmol/l	× 1	36–44	nmol/l
Arterial pH	7.35–7.45	pH units		7.35–7.45	pH units
Bicarbonate					
arterial—whole blood	19–24	mmol/l	× 1	19–24	mmol/l
venous—plasma	22–28	mmol/l	× 1	22–28	mmol/l
cord blood	14–22	mmol/l	× 1	14–22	mmol/l
Base excess	± 2	mmol/l	× 1	± 2	mEq/l
Carboxyhaemoglobin:					
non-smoker				<2%	
smoker				3–15%	
toxic at:				>15%	
coma at:				>50%	
Strong ion difference (SID) apparent: $(Na^+ + K^+ + Ca(i)^{2+} + Mg(i)^{2+}) - (lactate^- + Cl^-)$	40–42	mmol/l	× 1	40–42	mmol/l

(i) = ionized.

Table 3(a) Paediatric reference intervals (for immunoglobulins see Table 3(b))

	Sample	SI units		Conversion factor (SI to conventional)	Conventional units	
Alkaline phosphatase (*p*-nitrophenylphosphate method at 37 °C)						
<1 year	P	30–250	IU/l	× 1	30–250	IU/l
1–14 years		150–570	IU/l	× 1	150–570	IU/l
>14 years		80–250	IU/l	× 1	80–250	IU/l
Ammonia♥						
newborn	P	64–107	µmol/l	× 1.4	90–150	µg/dl
0–2 weeks		56–92	µmol/l	× 1.4	79–129	µg/dl
>1 month		21–50	µmol/l	× 1.4	29–70	µg/dl
Aspartate transaminase						
1–3 years	P	20–60	IU/l	× 1	20–60	IU/l
4–6 years		15–50	IU/l	× 1	15–50	IU/l
Bicarbonate						
infants	P	18–22	mmol/l	× 1	18–22	mEq/l
older children		20–26	mmol/l	× 1	20–26	mEq/l
Bilirubin						
first week of life	P	100–200	µmol/l (total)	× 0.058	6–11.6	mg/dl
after first week of life		2–14	µmol/l (total)	× 0.058	0.11–0.8	mg/dl
and throughout childhood		0–0.4	µmol/l (direct)	× 0.058	0–0.02	mg/dl
Calcium						
1–3 weeks	P	1.9–2.85	mmol/l	× 4.0	7.6–11.4	mg/dl
3 weeks and above		2.12–2.65	mmol/l	× 4.0	8.5–10.6	mg/dl
β-Carotene♣						
<1 year (upper limit falls with age up to 3½ years)	S	1.3–6.3	µmol/l	× 53	69–334	µg/dl
3½ years onwards		1.9–2.8	µmol/l	× 53	101–148	µg/dl

Table 3(a) continued

	Sample	SI units		Conversion factor (SI to conventional)	Conventional units	
Creatinine*						
cord blood	P	57–100	μmol/l	× 0.011	0.6–1.10	mg/dl
2 weeks–6 years		33–61	μmol/l	× 0.011	0.37–0.67	mg/dl
6 years–10 years		39–70	μmol/l	× 0.011	0.44–0.77	mg/dl
>12 years		49–81	μmol/l	× 0.011	0.54–0.82	mg/dl
Creatinine clearance						
3–13 years	U and P	94–142	ml/min per 1.73 m^2			
Creatine kinase (CK) (method: CK Boehringer at 37 °C)						
neonates	P	75–400	U/l	× 1	75–400	U/l
infants 3–12 months		10–145	U/l	× 1	10–145	U/l
children 1–15 years		15–130	U/l	× 1	15–130	U/l
Gamma-glutamyl transferase (GGT)						
0–1 month	P	12–271	U/l	× 1	12–271	U/l
1–2 months		9–159	U/l	× 1	9–159	U/l
2–4 months		7–98	U/l	× 1	7–98	U/l
4–7 months		5–45	U/l	× 1	5–45	U/l
7–12 months		4–27	U/l	× 1	4–27	U/l
1–15 years		3–30	U/l	× 1	3–30	U/l
Glucose (fasting)						
cord	S	2.5–5.3	mmol/l	× 18.0	45–95	mg/dl
premature/low birth weight		1.1–3.3	mmol/l	× 18.0	20–60	mg/dl
neonate		1.67–3.3	mmol/l	× 18.0	30–60	mg/dl
1 day		2.2–3.3	mmol/l	× 18.0	40–60	mg/dl
1–7 days		2.8–4.6	mmol/l	× 18.0	50–83	mg/dl
>7 days		3.3–5.5	mmol/l	× 18.0	60–100	mg/dl
Homovanillic acid (HVA): urine						
Upper limits of normal in children:						
0–1 years	U	25	mmol/mol creat	× 1.6	40	μg/mg creat
1–3 years		17	mmol/mol creat	× 1.6	27	μg/mg creat
3–5 years		16	mmol/mol creat	× 1.6	26	μg/mg creat
5–8 years		14	mmol/mol creat	× 1.6	23	μg/mg creat
8–11 years		11.1	mmol/mol creat	× 1.6	18	μg/mg creat
>11 years		7		× 1.6	11	μg/mg creat
Immunoreactive trypsin (upper limit	B	<70	μg/l			
of normal)	S	<130	μg/l			
Total protein						
1st month	P	51	g/l (mean)			
1st year		61	g/l (mean)			
children:						
1–6 years		61–78	g/l			
7–16 years		66–82	g/l			
Lactate	P—venous	0.5–2.2	mmol/l	× 9	4.5–19.8	mg/dl
	P—arterial	0.5–1.6	mmol/l	× 9	4.5–14.4	mg/dl
	B	0.5–1.7	mmol/l	× 9	4.5–15.3	mg/dl
	CSF	<2.8	mmol/l	× 9	<25.2	mg/dl
Metadrenaline: urine						
Upper limits of normal in children: total metadrenaline (metadrenaline + normetadrenaline)						
0–1 years	U	2.8	mmol/mol creat	× 1.74	4.5	μg/mg creat
1–2		3.0	mmol/mol creat	× 1.74	5.2	μg/mg creat
2–5		1.8	mmol/mol creat	× 1.74	3.1	μg/mg creat
5–10		1.6	mmol/mol creat	× 1.74	2.8	μg/mg creat

Table 3(a) continued

	Sample	SI units		Conversion factor (SI to conventional)	Conventional units	
10–15		1.0	mmol/mol creat	× 1.74	1.7	μg/mg creat
15–18		0.5	mmol/mol creat	× 1.74	0.9	μg/mg creat
Phosphate (inorganic)·						
newborn	P	1.20–2.78	mmol/l	× 3.1	3.7–8.6	mg/dl
young children		1.29–1.78	mmol/l	× 3.1	4.0–5.5	mg/dl
girls 15 years		0.9–1.38	mmol/l	× 3.1	2.8–4.3	mg/dl
boys 17 years		0.83–1.49	mmol/l	× 3.1	2.6–4.6	mg/dl
(over the age of 7 years there is a steady fall to reach adult levels at 15–17 years)						
Potassium¶						
newborn	P	up to 6.6	mmol/l	× 1	up to 6.6	mmol/l
>1 month–6 years		4.1–5.6	mmol/l	× 1	4.1–5.6	mmol/l
boys 7–16 years		3.3–4.7	mmol/l	× 1	3.3–4.7	mmol/l
girls 7–16 years		3.4–4.5	mmol/l	× 1	3.4–4.5	mmol/l
Sweat sodium♠		10–40	mmol/l	×1.0	10–40	mEq/l
Sweat chloride♠		0–50	mmol/l	×1.0	0–50	mEq/l
Thyroid-stimulating hormone (TSH) (outside neonatal period)	S	0.5–5.0	mU/l	×1.0	0.5–5.0	μU/ml
Uric acid						
childhood (will rise until adulthood—further during puberty in boys but not in girls)	P	0.06–0.24	mmol/l	× 16.8	1.0–4.0	mg/dl
boys 16 years		0.23–0.46	mmol/l	× 16.8	3.8–7.7	mg/dl
girls 16 years		0.19–0.36	mmol/l	× 16.8	3.2–6.0	mg/dl
Vanillylmandelic acid (VMA): urine						
Upper limits of normal in children:						
0–1 years	U	13.9	mmol/mol creat	× 1.76	24.5	μg/mg creat
1–3		11	mmol/mol creat	× 1.76	19.4	μg/mg creat
3–5		10.5	mmol/mol creat	× 1.76	18.5	μg/mg creat
5–8		10	mmol/mol creat	× 1.76	17.6	μg/mg creat
8–11		7.5	mmol/mol creat	× 1.76	13.2	μg/mg creat
>11		7	mmol/mol creat	× 1.76	12.3	μg/mg creat

* Values depend also on gestational age.

Typical definition of hypoglycaemia: low birth wt, <1.5 mmol/l × 18.0 <27 mg/dl; normal wt, 0–3 days, <1.7 mmol/l × 18.0 <31 mg/dl; >3 days, <2.2 mmol/l × 18.0 <40 mg/dl (SI units, conversion factor, Conventional units, respectively).

** Values from *Handbook of clinical immunochemistry*, 5th edn 1996. PRU Publications, Sheffield.

Collection tube must contain inhibitor of glycolysis (e.g. fluoride and oxalate).

Collection must be into bottles containing acid.

· Affected by diet—particularly milk feed.

¶ Avoid delayed separation and conditions inducing haemolysis (e.g. heat extremes, agitation).

♣ Avoid exposure to light.

♥ Requires extra care in cleaning collection site and particularly avoidance of contamination with urine.

♠ Requires extra care in cleaning collection site with deionized water.

Creat, creatinine; other abbreviations as Table 1.

Table 3(b) Serum immunoglobulins

		IgG (g/l)	IgA (g/l)	IgM (g/l)
Cord		5.2–18.0	0.00–0.02	0.02–0.2
Weeks	0–2	5.0–17.0	0.01–0.08	0.05–0.2
	2–6	3.9–13.0	0.02–0.15	0.08–0.4
	6–12	2.1–7.7	0.05–0.4	0.15–0.7
Months	3–6	2.4–8.8	0.1–0.5	0.20–1.0
	6–9	3.0–9.0	0.15–0.7	0.40–1.6
	9–12	3.0–10.9	0.20–0.7	0.60–2.1
Years	1–2	3.1–13.8	0.3–1.2	0.50–2.2
	2–3	3.7–15.8	0.3–1.3	0.50–2.2
	3–6	4.9–16.1	0.4–2.0	0.50–2.0
	6–9	5.4–16.1	0.5–2.4	0.50–1.8
	9–12	5.4–16.1	0.8–2.8	0.50–1.9
	12–15	5.4–16.1	0.8–2.8	0.50–1.9

Table 4 Hormones

	Sample	SI units		Conversion factor (SI to conventional)	Conventional units	
Adrenaline (epinephrine)⊗*f*	P	0.03–1.31	nmol/l	× 183	5.5–240	pg/ml
Adrenaline	U	<100	nmol/24 h	× 0.183	<18.3	μg/24 h
ACTH⊗*f*	P	3.3–15.4	pmol/l	× 4.55	15–70	ng/l
Aldosterone						
recumbent	P	100–450	pmol/l	× 0.03	3–14	ng/dl
midday		2-fold increase of recumbent level				
Aldosterone	U	10–50	nmol/24 h	× 0.36	4–18	mg/24 h
Angiotensin II	P	5–35	pmol/l	× 1.0	5.5–35.0	pg/ml
Antidiuretic hormone (ADH)	P	0.9–4.6	pmol/l	× 1.0	0.9–4.6	ng/l
Calcitonin						
M	P	<100	nmol/l	× 1.0	<100	ng/l
F		<30	nmol/l	× 1.0	<30	ng/l
Catecholamines	U	<2.6	μmol/24 h	× 169	<440	μg/24 h
Cortisol⊗						
00.00 h	P	80–280	nmol/l	× 0.036	3–10	μg/dl
09.00 h		280–700	nmol/l	× 0.036	10–25	μg/dl
free	U	<280	mmol/24 h	× 0.036	<10	μg/dl
Follicle-stimulating hormone (FSH)						
follicular phase	P/S	0.5–5.0	U/l	× 1.0	0.5–5.0	mIU/ml
ovulatory peak		8–15	U/l	× 1.0	8–15	mIU/ml
luteal phase		2–8	U/l	× 1.0	2–8	mIU/ml
postmenopause		>30	U/l	× 1.0	>30	mIU/ml
male		0.5–5.0	U/l	× 1.0	0.5–5.0	mIU/ml
Gastrin∅						
M (+F >60 y)	P	<50	pmol/l	× 2.0	<100	ng/l
F (16–60 y)		<38	pmol/l	× 2.0	<76	ng/l
Glucagon∅	P	<50	pmol/l	× 0.35	<17.5	ng/dl
Growth hormone⊗	P	<20	mU/l	× 1.0	<20	μU/ml
Homovanillinic acid (HVA)	U	<43	μmol/24 h	× 0.18	<8	μg/24 h
Human chorionic gonadotrophin	S	<5	U/l	× 1.0	<5	U/ml
Insulin (fasting)	P	<15	mU/l	× 1.0	<15	μU/ml
Insulin C-peptide (fasting)*f*	P	<0.4 (undetectable in hypoglycaemia)	nmol/l	× 3.0	<1.2	
Insulin-like growth factor-1 (IGF-1)	P	0.52–3.4	kU/l	× 1.0	0.52–3.4	U/ml

Table 4 continued

	Sample	SI units		Conversion factor (SI to conventional)	Conventional units	
Luteinizing hormone						
premenopausal	P/S	6–13	U/l	× 1.0	6–13	mIU/ml
follicular phase		3–12	U/l	× 1.0	3–12	mIU/ml
ovulatory peak		20–80	U/l	× 1.0	20–80	mIU/ml
luteal phase		3–16	U/l	× 1.0	3–16	mIU/ml
postmenopause		>30	U/l	× 1.0	>30	mIU/ml
male		3–8	U/l	× 1.0	3–8	mIU/ml
Metadrenaline	U	<2	μmol/24 h	× 0.195	<0.39	mg/24 h
(adults)	U (24 h)	0.03–0.69	mmol/mol creat	× 1.74	0.05–1.20	μg/mg creat
3-Methoxytyramine (adults)	U	<2	μmol/24 h	× 0.165	<0.33	mg/24 h
Neurotensin	P	<100	pmol/l	× 1.67	<167	ng/l
Noradrenaline⊗*f*	P	0.47–4.14	mmol/l	× 169	79–700	ng/ml
Normetadrenaline	U	<3	μmol/24 h	× 0.183	<0.55	ng/24 h
17-β-Oestradiol	P					
follicular phase		75–260	pmol/l	× 0.27	20–70	pg/ml
mid-cycle		370–1470	pmol/l	× 0.27	100–400	pg/ml
luteal phase		180–1100	pmol/l	× 0.27	50–300	pg/ml
male		<220	pmol/l	× 0.27	<60	pg/ml
Parathormone (PTH) (intact)*f*	P	0.9–5.4	pmol/l	× 4.0	3.6–22	mg/dl
Pancreatic polypeptide (PP)∅	P	<200	pmol/l	× 4.1	<820	ng/l
Progesterone						
M	P	<5	nmol/l	× 0.314	<1.6	ng/ml
postovulation		15–77	nmol/l	× 0.314	4.7–24	ng/ml
follicular		<3	nmol/l	× 0.314	<1	ng/ml
17-Hydroxyprogesterone (newborn)	P	7–16	nmol/l	× 33.0	230–530	ng/dl
Prolactin⊗						
M	P	<450	U/l	× 1.0	<450	mIU/ml
F		<600	U/l	× 1.0	<600	mIU/ml
Renin activity						
recumbent	P	1.1–2.7	pmol/ml per h	× 4.4	4.8–11.9	μg/dl per h
erect after 30 min (depends on diuretics, salt intake, etc.)		3.0–4.3	pmol/ml per h	× 4.4	13.2–19	μg/dl per h
Sex-hormone binding protein (SHBG)						
M	S	17–52	nmol/l	× 0.027	0.5–1.4	μg/dl
F		35–104	nmol/l	× 0.027	1–3	μg/dl
Somatostatin∅	P	30–166	pmol/l	× 0.163	5–27	ng/dl
Testosterone						
M	P/S	9–42	nmol/l	× 0.29	2.6–12.1	ng/ml
F		1–2.5	nmol/l	× 0.29	0.3–0.7	ng/ml
Thyroid-stimulating hormone	P	0.5–5.5	mU/l	× 1.0	0.5–5.5	mIU/ml
Thyroid-binding globulin	P	13–28	mg/l	× 1.0	13–28	mg/l
Tri-iodothyronine (T3)	P	1.0–3.0	nmol/l	× 65.0	65–195	ng/dl
Free T3 (FT3)	P	3.3–8.2	pmol/l	× 65.0	214–533	pg/dl
Thyroxine (T4)	P	70–140	nmol/l	× 0.076	5.3–10.6	μg/dl
Free T4 (FT4)	P	9–25	pmol/l	× 0.068	0.6–1.7	ng/dl
Vanillylmandelic acid (VMA)	U	<35	μmol/24 h	× 0.20	<7	μg/24 h
Vasoactive intestinal polypeptide (VIP)∅	P	<30	pmol/l	× 3.33	<100	ng/l

Values vary with dietary sodium and plasma renin activity.
⊗Should be collected under maximal resting conditions.
Collection must be into bottles containing acid.
∅Collected into heparinized tubes containing protease inhibitor (e.g. Trasylol).
*f*Requires rapid separation and freezing.
Creat, creatinine; y, years of age; other abbreviations as Table 1.

Table 5 Tumour markers

	Sample	Reference intervals	
Alpha-fetoprotein (AFP)	S	<10	kU/l
Carcinoembryonic antigen (CEA)	S	<10	μg/l
Neurone-specific enolase (NSE)	S	<12	μg/l
Prostatic-specific antigen (PSA)	S	<4	μg/l
Human chorionic gonadotrophin (HCG)	S	<5	IU/l
Ca125	S	<35	U/ml
Ca19–9	S	<33	U/ml

Table 6 Vitamins and related tests

Vitamins	Sample	SI units		Conversion factor (SI to conventional)	Conventional units	
Vitamin A (retinol)						
M	S	1.06–3.35	μmol/l	× 28.6	30–96	μg/dl
F		0.84–2.95	μmol/l	× 28.6	24–84	μg/dl
β-Carotene*						
M	S	0.01–6.52	μmol/l	× 53.7	0.5–350	μg/dl
F		0.019–2.93	μmol/l	× 53.7	1.02–158	μg/dl
Vitamin B						
Thiamine (B_1)	P	>40	nmol/l	× 0.025	>1	μg/dl
as rbc thiamine diphosphate	B				320–550	ng/g Hb
as rbc transketolase		<1.3	TPP α effect			
Riboflavin (B_2)	S	100–630	nmol/l	× 0.038	4–24	μg/dl
as rbc glutathione reductase	B	<70	% activation			
Pyridoxine (B_6)	P (EDTA)	20–120	nmol/l	× 0.247	5–30	ng/ml
as rbc aspartate transaminase	B	<150	% activation			
Vitamin B_{12}	S	138–780	nmol/l	× 1.36	187–1060	ng/l
Folate	S	12–33	μmol/l	× 0.442	5.3–14.6	μg/l
	B (rbc)	500–1300	μmol/l	× 0.442	221–575	μg/l
Vitamin D metabolites						
25-(OH)D	S	17–125	nmol/l	× 0.4	7–50	μg/l
1,25-$(OH)_2D_3$		50–120	pmol/l	× 0.4	20–48	pg/ml
Vitamin E (α-tocopherol)	S	11.5–35	μmol/l	× 0.43	5–15	μg/ml

rbc, Red blood cells; TPP, thiamine pyrophosphate; EDTA, ethylene diamine tetraacetic acid; other abbreviations as Table 1.

*See paediatric table.

Upper limit reduced by ~50 per cent in winter.

Check with local laboratory for ideal collection conditions.

Table 7 Lipids and lipoproteins

	Sample	SI units		Conversion factor (SI to conventional)	Conventional units	
Cholesterol*	P	3.9–7.8	mmol/l	× 38.7	150–300	mg/dl
ideal upper limit		5.2	mmol/l	× 38.7	200	mg/dl
acceptable upper limit		6.5	mmol/l	× 38.7	250	mg/dl
Triglyceride (fasting)	P	0.55–1.90	mmol/l	× 88.4	48.6–168	mg/dl
Non-esterified (free) fatty acids (NEFA)						
M	S	0.19–0.78	mmol/l	× 26.7	5.1–20.9	mg/dl
F		0.06–0.9	mmol/l	× 26.7	1.6–24	mg/dl
Lipoproteins (as cholesterol)						
LDL	S	1.55–4.4	mmol/l	× 38.7	60–170	mg/dl
ideal upper limit		3.4	mmol/l	× 38.7	130	mg/dl
acceptable upper limit		4.2	mmol/l	× 38.7	160	mg/dl
HDL	S	0.8–2.0	mmol/l	× 38.7	30–77	mg/dl
ideal M	S	>0.9	mmol/l	× 38.7	>35	mg/dl
ideal F		>1.2	mmol/l	× 38.7	>46	mg/dl
Total cho/HDL						
ideal	S	<5	ratio			

LDL, low-density lipoproteins; HDL, high-density lipoproteins; cho, cholesterol; other abbreviations as Table 1.

*Values increase with age.

Table 8 Proteins and immunoproteins

	Sample	Reference intervals	
Albumin	P	35–50	g/l
α_1-Antitrypsin	S	107–209	mg/l
Complement			
C3		65–190	mg/dl
C4		15–50	mg/dl
Caeruloplasmin	S	16–60	mg/dl
C1 esterase inhibitor	S	15–35	mg/dl
C-reactive protein (CRP)	S	<10	mg/l
CSF IgG:albumin ratio		<22	%
Ferritin	S	14–200	μg/l
Fibrinogen	P	2–4	g/l
D-Dimer	S	<500	μg/l
Haptoglobins	S	0.6–2.6	g/l
Immunoglobulins*			
IgG	S	6.0–13.0	g/l
IgA		0.8–3.0	g/l
IgM		0.4–2.5	g/l
IgE[F]		<120	kU/l
Mast-cell tryptase[A]	P[J]/S	2–14	μg/l
Methylhistamine[v]	U	10–25	ng/μmol creat.
β_2-Microglobulin	S	<3	mg/l
	U	4–370	μg/l or 30–370 μg/24 h
Thyroid microsomal antibodies			
M	S		<1/400
F (<44 years)	S	<1/400	
F (>44 years)	S	<1/6400	
Total protein	P	60–80	g/l
	U	<140	g/l
β_1-Transferrin	S	1.2–2.0	g/l
Viscosity	S	1.4–1.9	(ratio to water)

Abbreviations as Table 1.

*See Table 3.

[F]IgE specific to different antigens can be measured by radioallergosorbent test (RAST).

[J]EDTA plasma.

[A]For anaphylaxis sample within 1 h and 3 h and 24 h after reaction. Systemic anaphylaxis >40 μg/l. If 14–40 + raised urine methylhistamine = local IgE-mediated reaction. If 14–40 + normal urine methylhistamine anaphylactoid.

[v]Random urine taken ~3 h after ?anaphylactic reaction and repeat >24 h later for baseline.

Table 9 Trace elements and metals

	Sample	SI units		Conversion factor (SI to conventional)	Conventional units	
Aluminium[θ]	S	<0.4	μmol/l	× 27	<10	μg/l
toxic		>7.4	μmol/l	× 27	>200	μg/l
	Dialysis fluid	<1.1	μmol/l	× 27	<30	μg/l
Arsenic	B (EDTA)	0.03–0.83	μmol/l	× 7.5	0.2–6.2	μg/dl
Bromide						mmol/l
unexposed	S	≤0.15	mmol/l	× 75	<11	mg/l
toxic		>20	mmol/l	× 75	>1500	mg/l
Cadmium						
non-smokers	B	<27	nmol/l	× 0.11	<3	μg/l
smokers	B	<54	nmol/l	× 0.11	<6	μg/l
	U	<10	nmol/mmol creat	× 1.0	<10	μg/g creat
Chromium	S	<10	nmol/l	× 0.025	<0.25	μg/l
	U	<5	nmol/24 h	× 0.05	<0.25	μg/24 h
Cobalt	S	1.7–6.8	nmol/l	× 0.06	0.1–0.4	μg/l
	U	<17.0	nmol/l	× 0.06	<1	μg/l

Table 9 continued

	Sample	SI units		Conversion factor (SI to conventional)	Conventional units	
Copper						
0–6 months	P	3.1–11.0	μmol/l	× 6.54	20–72	μg/dl
6 years		14–30	μmol/l	× 6.54	92–196	μg/dl
12 years		12.6–25	μmol/l	× 6.54	82–164	μg/dl
adult M		11–22	μmol/l	× 6.54	72–144	μg/dl
adult F		13–24	μmol/l	× 6.54	85–157	μg/dl
pregnancy–term		18.5–47	μmol/l	× 6.54	121–307	μg/dl
	U[∀]	0.47–0.55	μmol/l	× 6.54	3.1–3.6	μg/l
Gold (therapeutic)	S	2.5–10.2	μmol/l	× 0.2	0.5–2.0	mg/l
Iron						
M	S	12–30	μmol/l	× 5.5	66–165	μg/dl
F	S	9–30	μmol/l	× 5.5	50–165	μg/dl
Lead						
environmental exposure						
children	B	<0.5	μmol/l	× 20.5	<10	μg/dl
adults	B	<1.4	μmol/l	× 20.5	<30	μg/l
severe overexposure	B	≥3.4	μmol/l	× 20.5	≥70	μg/l
Manganese	B	73–210	nmol/l	× 0.057	4–12	μg/l
	S	9–24	nmol/l	× 0.057	0.5–1.3	μg/l
	U	2–27	nmol/l	× 0.057	0.1–1.5	μg/l
Mercury	B	<20	nmol/l	× 0.2	<4	μg/l
	U[∀]	<50	nmol/24 h	× 0.2	<10	μg/24 h
	EMU	<5	nmol/mmol creat	× 2.0	<10	μg/g creat
Selenium	U	<3.8	μmol/24 h	× 7.9	<30	mg/g creat
children	P[θ]	0.44–1.43	μmol/l	× 79	35–113	μg/l
adults	P[θ]	0.89–1.65	μmol/l	× 79	70–130	μg/l
Silver	B	<2.8	nmol/l	× 0.107	<0.3	μg/l
Thallium	B	<5	nmol/l	× 0.2	<1	μg/l
	U	<5	nmol/l	× 0.2	<1	μg/l
Zinc	S	11–24	μmol/l	× 0.065	0.7–1.6	mg/l
	U	4.5–9	μmol/24 h	× 0.065	0.3–0.6	mg/24 h

EMU, early-morning urine sample; creat, creatinine; other abbreviations as Table 1.
[θ]Usually requires special collection tube provided by laboratory and rapid separation.
[∀]24-h collection into bottle previously washed with nitric acid.
Check with local laboratory for ideal collection conditions.

Table 10 Urinary values

	SI units		Conversion factor (SI to conventional)	Conventional units	
Aldosterone	10–50	nmol/24 h	× 0.36	4–18	μg/24 h
Albumin	<80	mg/24 h	× 1.0	<80	mg/24 h
α-Aminolaevulinic acid♣	9.9–53.4	μmol/24 h	× 0.13	1.3–7	mg/24 h
Amylase					
secretion rate	1–17	somogyi U/h	× 1.0	1–17	somogyi U/h
clearance	0.01–0.04	of creatinine clearance value			
Arginine	1.3–6.5	μmol/mol creat	× 1.49	1.9–9.7	mg/g creat
Ascorbic acid	34–68	μmol/l	× 0.179	6–12	mg/l
Calcium	2.5–7.5	mmol/24 h	× 40	100–300	mg/24 h
Catecholamines	<2.6	μmol/24 h	× 169	<440	μg/24 h
Chloride	110–250	mmol/24 h	× 1.0	110–250	mEq/24 h
Copper[∀]	0.47–0.55	μmol/l	× 6.54	3.1–3.6	μg/l
Cortisol	60–1500	nmol/l	× 0.036	2–54	μg/dl
	<280	nmol/24 h	× 0.036	<10	μg/24 h
Creatinine*					
male	9.0–17.0	mmol/24 h	× 0.11	1.0–1.9	g/24 h
female	7.5–12.5	mmol/24 h	× 0.11	0.8–1.4	g/24 h
pregnancy	8.0–13.5	mmol/24 h	× 0.11	0.9–1.5	g/24 h
Cystine	4.7–42	μmol/mmol creat	× 2.0	9–84	mg/g creat
	83–830	μmol/24 h	× 0.12	10–100	mg/24 h

Table 10 Continued

	SI units		Conversion factor (SI to conventional)	Conventional units	
Glucose	0.06–0.84	mmol/l	× 18.0	1.1–15.1	mg/dl
Homovanillic acid (HVA)—adults	<43	μmol/24 h	× 0.18	<8	μg/24 h
Hydroxyindole-acetic acid (5-HIAA)	16–73	μmol/24 h	× 0.19	3–14	mg/24 h
Hydroxymethyl-mandelic acid (HMMA)	16–48	μmol/24 h	× 0.2	3.2–9.6	mg/24 h
Iron	<1.8	μmol/24 h	× 0.56	<1.0	mg/24 h
Lead	<0.4	μmol/l	× 200	<80	μg/l
Lysine	15–53	μmol/mmol creat	× 1.28	19–68	mg/g creat
Methylhistamine	10–25	ng/μmol creat.			
β_2-Microglobulin[α]	4–370	μg/l			
Magnesium	3.3–4.9	mmol/24 h	× 24.5	80–120	mg/24 h
Ornithine	4–17	μmol/mmol creat	× 1.1	4.5–19	mg/g creat
Osmolality|	350–1000	mosm/kg			
Oxalate	<450	μmol/24 h	× 0.09	<40	mg/24 h
Phosphate (inorganic)	15–50	mmol/24 h	× 0.03	0.5–1.5	g/24 h
Porphyrins♣					
coproporphyrin	50–350	nmol/24 h	× 0.67	34–234	μg/24 h
porphobilinogen	0.9–8.8	μmol/24 h	× 0.20	0.18–1.8	mg/24 h
uroporphyrin	0–49	nmol/24 h	× 0.83	0–41	μg/24 h
Potassium	20–60	mmol/l	× 1.0	20–60	mEq/l
	40–120	mmol/24 h	× 1.0	40–120	mEq/24 h
Protein	<120	mg/24 h			
Pregnancy	<300	mg/24 h			
Sodium	50–125	mmol/l	× 1.0	50–125	mEq/24 h
	100–250	mmol/24 h	× 1.0	100–250	mEq/24 h
Urea	250–500	mmol/24 h	× 0.06	15–30	g/24 h
Uric acid*	<5.0	mmol/24 h	× 0.167	<0.84	g/24 h
pregnancy (except late)	<7.0	mmol/24 h	× 0.167	<1.17	g/24 h
Urobilinogen	<6.7	μmol/24 h	× 0.59	<4	mg/24 h
Vanillylmandelic acid (VMA)	<35	μmol/24 h	× 0.20	<7	μg/24 h
Zinc	2.1–11.0	μmol/24 h	× 65.5	137–720	μg/24 h

*Partially influenced by diet.
|Range of young adults, declines with age—see text.
♣Avoid exposure to light.
[α]Must be kept alkaline.
Collection must be into bottles containing acid.
[γ]24-h collection into bottle previously washed with nitric acid.
Check with local laboratory for ideal collection conditions

Table 11 Faecal values

	SI units		Conversion factor (SI to conventional)	Conventional units	
Fat (on normal diet)	<7	g/24 h	× 1.0	<7	g/24 h
Nitrogen	70–140	mmol/24 h	× 0.014	1–2	g/24 h
Urobilinogen	67–473	μmol/24 h	× 0.59	40–280	mg/24 h
Coproporphyrin♣	<0.46	nmol/g dry weight	× 0.654	<0.30	μg/g dry weight
Protoporphyrin♣	<2.67	μmol/24 h	× 561	<1500	μg/24 h
Protoporphyrin♣	≤0.11	nmol/kg dry weight	× 561	≤60	μg/g dry weight
Total porphyrin♣					
(ether soluble)	10–200	nmol/g dry weight			
(ether insoluble)	0–24	nmol/g dry weight			

♣Avoid exposure to light.

Table 12 Cerebrospinal fluid

	SI units		Conversion factor (SI to conventional)	Conventional units	
Glucose	3.3–4.4	mmol/24 h	× 18.0	59–79	mg/dl
Protein	0.15–0.40	g/l	× 1.0	0.15–0.40	g/l
Chloride	122–128	mmol/l	× 1.0	122–128	mEq/l
Lactate	<2.8	mmol/l	× 9.0	<25.2	mg/dl
Xanthochromia[c]	Bilirubin ± haemoglobin not detected by spectrophotometry				

Collection tube must contain inhibitor of glycolysis (e.g. fluoride and oxalate).

[c]To exclude subarachnoid haemorrhage. Specimen (first tap only) collected ≥6 h postonset of symptoms, centrifuged, and separated immediately.

Table 13 Functional tests

Fat absorption	100-g fat load: an increase of 1.0 mmol/l (90 mg/dl) either 2 or 4 h after load from the fasting level (esterified fatty acids). Significantly abnormal if increase is <0.55 mmol/l (50 mg/dl)		
Xylose absorption	25-g dose xylose: normal urine excretion should be greater than 4 g/5-h period. Children only: normal plasma xylose >1.6 mmol/l, 1 h after 25 g (or 1 g/kg) xylose		
Creatinine clearance	Normal: 90–120 ml/min		
	Calculation:	[urine creatinine (mmol/l) × vol. (ml/min)]/[plasma creatinine (mmol/l)]	
Renal functional capacity (GFR)	Male	age 20	105–270 ml/min per 1.73 m^2
		age 50	95–138 ml/min per 1.73 m^2
		age 70	70–110 ml/min per 1.73 m^2
	Female	age 20	104–158 ml/min per 1.73 m^2
		age 50	90–130 ml/min per 1.73 m^2
		age 70	74–114 ml/min per 1.73 m^2
Maximum concentrating ability 800/1200 mosm/kg			
Minimum urinary pH 5.3 (after acid load)			
Tubular phosphate reabsorption (TRP)	Urine collection 08.00–12.00 h + plasma (fasting)		
	Calculation:	TRP = 1 – (phosphate clearance/creatinine clearance) = 1– [(UP × PCre)/(UC × PPhos)] × 100	
		Adults† <80%	
Maximum tubular phosphate reabsorption (TM phos/GFR)	Calculated from nomogram* using TRP (decimal) and plasma phosphate		
		TM phos/GFR: adults,† 0.8–1.35 mmol/l (2.5–4.2 mg/dl)	
Ischaemic lactate test	Fasting lactate:		0.5–1.5 mmol/l (4.5–13.5 mg/dl)
	Immediate postexercise:		approximately 5 mmol/l (45 mg/dl)
	25 minutes postexercise:		return to normal
	Type V glycogen storage disease:		no response to exercise
Adrenal			
Dexamethasone suppression of adrenal cortex	(1)	Overnight dexamethasone suppression—dose 2 mg at 24.00 hours Plasma cortisol at 09.00 h <200 nmol/l	
	(2)	High dose: 2 mg dexamethasone every 6 h	
	NB:	Pituitary-dependent Cushing's disease: plasma and urine often gives values below 50% of basal level. Other aetiologies result in values above 50%	
Short Synacthen® (tetracosactide)	Dose—0.25 mg IM:		plasma cortisol >580 nmol/l or increase of >250 nmol/l

Table 13 continued

Depot Synacthen® (tetracosactide + zinc)	Dose—1 mg IM:	Normal cortisol >900 nmol/l at 4–6 h: ACTH-deficient patients may only reach this value at 24 h or even after further injections. Addison's disease results in <10% increment over basal at any of these times, even after further injections
Response to insulin hypoglycaemia (plasma glucose <2.2 mmol/l) plasma cortisol >600 nmol/l or 2× basal		
Growth hormone	(1) Fasting:	<20 mU/l
	(2) Glucose suppression (75 g):	60 min, 90 min, 120 min: <5 mU/l
	(3) Insulin hypoglycaemia:	peak >20 mU/l
Glucose and insulin	Overnight fasting:	glucose 3.0–5.0 mmol/l (54–90 mg/dl)
	Overnight fasting:	plasma insulin 2–13 mU/ml (mean 5 mU/ml)
	If fasting:	plasma glucose >7.0 mmol/l (126 mg/dl); whole blood >6.1 mmol/l (110 mg/dl); diagnosis of diabetes certain and GTT unnecessary
	If random:	plasma glucose >11.1 mmol/l (200 mg/dl) diagnosis of diabetes certain
‡Criteria for diabetes in 75-g oral GTT	Fasting plasma glucose:	>7.0 mmol/l (126 mg/dl)
	120-min plasma glucose:	>11.1 mmol/l (200 mg/dl)
	NB: GTT results rise with age; after the age of 50 years, samples taken after glucose loading rise by approximately 0.55 mmol/l per decade	
Hypoglycaemia	If plasma glucose <2 mmol/l, plasma insulin should not exceed 1.5 mU/ml	
Glucagon stimulation test (alternative to insulin hypoglycaemic-stress test for pituitary function)	Overnight fast: test requires clinical supervision Baseline blood for glucose, growth hormone (GH), and cortisol Glucagon 1 mg subcutaneous (adjust for excesses in body wt) Bloods at 30-min intervals for glucose, growth hormone, and cortisol Normal response is rise of GH to >20 mU/l (usually 120–180 min postdose) and peak cortisol should exceed 550 nmol/l (19.8 μg/dl)	

GFR, glomerular filtration rate; UP, urine phosphate; UC, urine creatinine; PCre, plasma creatinine; PPhos, plasma phosphate; GTT, glucose tolerance text; IM, intramuscular.

*From Walton and Bijvoet (1975). *Lancet* Aug 16, 309–10.

†Paediatric intervals are given in Kruse, Kracht, and Göpfert (1982). *Archives of Disease in Childhood* **57**, 217–23.

‡WHO (1999). *WHO definition, diagnosis and classification of diabetes mellitus and its complications.* WHO, Geneva.

Table 14 Therapeutic drugs

	Sample	SI units		Conversion factor (SI to conventional)	Conventional units	
Amikacin						
trough	S	≤17	μmol/l	× 0.59	≤10	μg/ml
peak		34–51	μmol/l	× 0.59	20–30	μg/ml
Amitryptiline	S	360–720	nmol/l	× 0.28	100–200	μg/l
toxic		>1800	nmol/l	× 0.28	>500	μg/l
Carbamazepine	P	34–51	μmol/l	× 0.235	8.0–12.0	μg/ml
Clonazepam						
fluoride/oxalate		79–248	nmol/l	× 0.317	25–85	μg/l
		(NB based on pre-dose sample)				
Digoxin						
children	P	2.0–3.0	nmol/l	× 0.76	1.6–2.3	ng/ml
adults		1.0–2.0	nmol/l	× 0.76	0.8–1.6	ng/ml
		(NB therapeutic-range sample taken at least 6 h after dose)				
Ethosuximide	P	280–710	μmol/l	× 0.14	40.0–100	μg/ml
Gentamicin						
trough	S	≤4	μmol/l	× 0.48	≤2	μg/ml
peak		10–22	μmol/l	× 0.48	5–11	μg/ml
Lithium						
therapeutic	S	0.5–1.5	mmol/l	× 1.0	0.5–1.5	mEq/l
toxic		>2.0	mmol/l	× 1.0	>2.0	mEq/l
Netilmicin						
trough	S	≤6	μmol/l	× 0.48	≤3	μg/ml
peak		10–22	μmol/l	× 0.48	5–11	μg/ml
Primidone	P	23–55	μmol/l	× 0.22	5–12	μg/ml
Phenobarbital	P	65–172	μmol/l	× 0.23	15–40	μg/ml
Phenytoin	P	40–80	μmol/l	× 0.24	10–20	μg/ml
Quinidine	S	6–15	μmol/l	× 0.33	2–5	μg/ml
Quinine	S	31–46	μmol/l	× 0.32	10–15	μg/ml
Sodium valproate	P	0.3–0.7	μmol/l	× 144	43.0–101	μg/ml
Theophylline						
adult	P	55–110	μmol/l	× 0.18	10–20	μg/ml
paediatric		27–55	μmol/l	× 0.18	5–10	μg/ml
Vancomycin						
trough	S	3–7	μmol/l	× 1.44	4–10	μg/ml
peak		12–18	μmol/l	× 1.44	17–26	μg/ml

Abbreviations as Table 1.

Samples should be taken pre-dose, usually at least 6 h post-dose.

Check with local laboratory for ideal collection conditions.

Table 15 Common drug toxicology

	Sample	SI units		Conversion factor (SI to conventional)	Conventional units	
Amphetamine	P	>1500	nmol/l	× 0.135	>200	μg/l
Cocaine	P	>3300	nmol	× 0.303	>1000	μg/l
Methadone	P	>6.5	μmol/l	× 310	>2000	μg/l
Paracetamol* (acetaminophen) (risk of liver damage)	P	>1.3	mmol/l	× 151	>200	mg/l
Quinidine	P	>18	μmol/l	× 0.32	>6	μg/ml
Salicylate (therapeutic limit)	P	<2.5	mmol/l	× 138	<350	mg/l

Abbreviations as Table 1.

* Sample taken 4-h post-overdose.

33
Emergency medicine

33 Emergency medicine

J. D. Firth, C. A. Eynon, D. A. Warrell, and T. M. Cox

1 Heart and circulation

1.1 Cardiac arrest

See Chapter 16.3 in main text

Clinical features	**History** (1) Sudden collapse
	Examination (1) Patient unresponsive (2) Airway, breathing—no respiration or agonal breathing (3) Circulation—pulse not palpable
Immediate management	See Figs 1 and 2

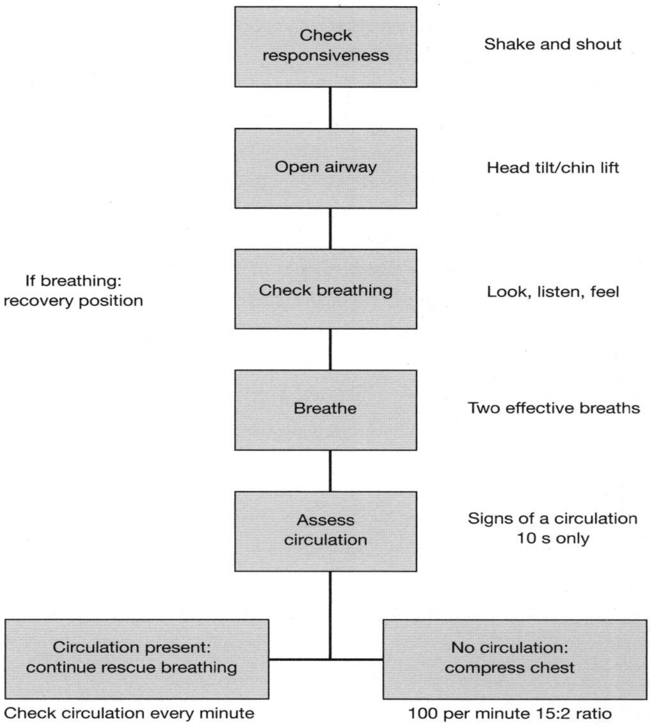

Fig. 1 European Resuscitation Council guidelines for adult basic life support.

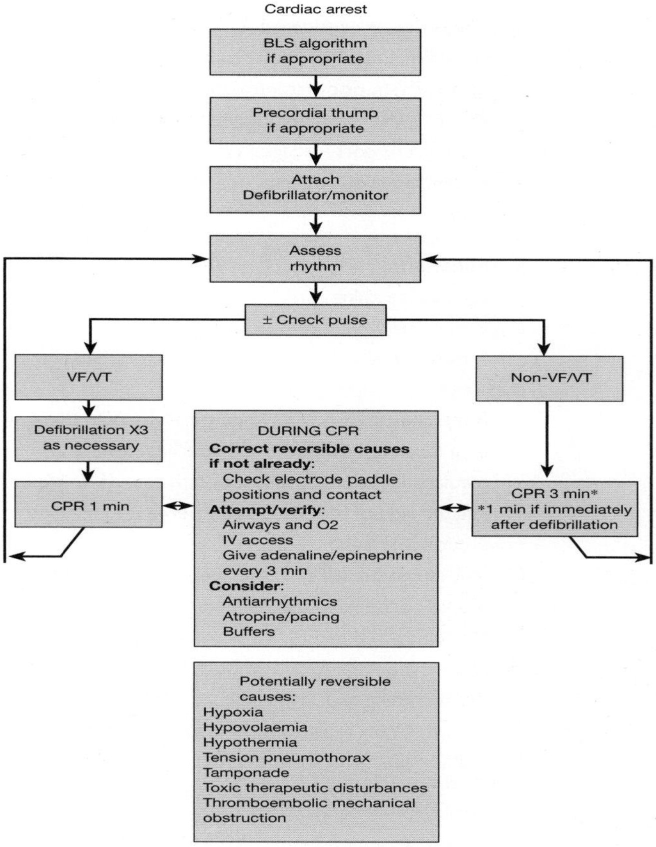

Fig. 2 European Resuscitation Council guidelines for advanced life support.

1.2 Cardiorespiratory collapse: the patient *in extremis*

See Chapter 16.1 in main text

Clinical features

History

A patient who is *in extremis* is unlikely to be able to give a lucid history and may die during (unwise) interrogation, but the following clues may be elicited and be very useful diagnostically:

(1) Chest pain—suggests myocardial infarction or other cardiorespiratory catastrophe
(2) Chest and back pain—dissection of thoracic aorta must be seriously considered
(3) Abdominal pain—suggests ruptured abdominal aortic aneurysm or other intra-abdominal emergency
(4) Recent surgery—pulmonary embolism likely
(5) High fever/rigors—suggests infective cause
(6) Recent travel to relevant area—malaria until proven otherwise

Examination

Airway and breathing
(1) Is the airway patent?
(2) Is the patient making a respiratory effort, and is the chest expanding with it?
(3) Is the chest expanding symmetrically? Could there be a tension pneumothorax? (trachea deviated, mediastinum shifted, absent breath sounds on hyperinflated side of the chest, see Emergency Medicine section 2.3)
(4) Widespread crackles in the chest—suggests pulmonary oedema in this context (see Emergency Medicine, section 1.8).
(5) Does the patient look as though they could keep this breathing up for the next 10 min?—If not, the patient is very likely to need respiratory support. Call for assistance from the ICU immediately

Circulation
(1) Do the peripheries feel cold or warm?—if warm, sepsis is likely
(2) Pulse rate and rhythm—if rate <60/min or >120/min, consider whether arrhythmia is primary cause of hypotension
(3) Blood pressure
- Is there a postural drop if the patient is moved from lying to being propped up? If so, indicates intravascular volume depletion in this context.
- Does BP fall substantially on inspiration? If so, indicates large intrathoracic pressure swings with breathing (likely in upper airway obstruction or asthma) or cardiac tamponade

(4) What is the JVP?
- If low, indicates intravascular volume depletion or dilated circulation
- If high, suggests primary cardiorespiratory problem

General
(1) Rash—purpura suggests meningococcal or other septicaemia
(2) Temperature—high fever suggests infection
(3) Loss of left radial pulse, or BP lower in left arm than right arm, indicates aortic dissection
(4) Abdominal tenderness/peritonism—suggests ruptured abdominal aortic aneurysm or other intra-abdominal emergency

See Table 1 for further information

Immediate management

Airway and breathing
(1) Ensure airway is clear: consider oropharyngeal airway
(2) Keep oxygen saturation >92 per cent (monitor using pulse oximetery), giving high flow oxygen (10 l/min) by face mask with reservoir bag if needed
(3) If tension pneumothorax, decompress immediately (see Emergency Medicine, Section 10.4.3.1).
(4) Give intravenous naloxone (0.8–2.0 mg repeated at intervals of 2–3 min to a maximum of 10 mg) if there is any suspicion that patient has received opioids
(5) Consider elective intubation and ventilation

Circulation
Obtain IV access using a safe technique (see Emergency Medicine, section 10.1)
Also: begin resuscitation according to volume status as indicated in Table 2
(1) Insert urinary catheter and monitor fluid input/output hourly in any patient with cardiorespiratory collapse.
(2) Give broad spectrum antimicrobial cover to any patient with unexplained cardiorespiratory collapse, e.g. cefotaxime 1 g intravenously twice daily, as dictated by clinical suspicion of likely pathogen (see Emergency Medicine, section 7.7)

Key investigations

See Table 1

Further management

Determined by underlying condition.

Table 1 Examination and investigation of the patient with cardiorespiratory collapse

Diagnosis		Key finding on examination	Key initial investigation	Definitive investigations
Cardiovascular	Myocardial infarction	No specific findings likely	ECG	ECG, cardiac enzymes
	Arrhythmia	Pulse rate and rhythm	ECG	ECG
	Aortic dissection	Absence or reduction in one or more peripheral pulse, especially left radial. Blood pressure lower in left arm than right	CXR showing widened mediastinum	Imaging of aorta, usually by CT scan or trans-oesophageal echocardiography
	Cardiac tamponade	Raised JVP. Pulsus paradoxus (pulse becomes impalpable on inspiration in extreme cases)	CXR may show globular heart. ECG may show low voltage complexes or electrical alternans	Echocardiography
Cardiorespiratory	Pulmonary embolus	Raised JVP. Right ventricular heave. Loud P2. Right ventricular gallop rhythm Signs of DVT in leg	ECG may show features of acute right heart strain	Ventilation/perfusion scan. Imaging of pulmonary vessels by CT scan or pulmonary angiography
	Pulmonary oedema	Gallop rhythm, crackles	CXR	Usually cardiac—ECG, echocardiography
Respiratory	Tension pneumothorax	Tracheal deviation. Hyperexpansion of one side of chest. Mediastinal shift. Absent breath sounds on one side of chest	CXR – but should be treated on basis of clinical diagnosis (see text)	CXR – but should be treated on basis of clinical diagnosis (see text)
	Pneumonia	May have high fever Signs of consolidation or pleurisy	CXR	CXR, blood culture, serological tests
	Asthma	Wheezes, but beware of silent chest	Response to treatment (β-agonist), but CXR excludes pneumothorax and other respiratory diagnoses	Peak flow measurements before and after β-agonist
	Exacerbation of COPD	Features of COPD	A clinical diagnosis, but CXR excludes other respiratory diagnoses	See Chapter 17.6
Abdominal	Gastrointestinal haemorrhage	Usually obvious, but don't forget rectal examination for blood/ melaena in the patient with unexplained hypotension	A clinical diagnosis	Endoscopy
	Perforated viscus	Peritonism	Erect chest radiograph to look for free air under diaphragm	CT scan or laparotomy, depending on clinical situation
	Pancreatitis	Peritonism Bruising in flanks	Serum amylase	Imaging of pancreas, usually by CT scan
	Ruptured abdominal aortic aneurysm	Peritonism Palpable aneurysm Bruising in flanks	A clinical diagnosis.	CT scan or laparotomy, depending on clinical situation
Sepsis		May have high fever. May have warm peripheries and bounding pulse, but could be cold and shut down. No specific findings likely, but look for rash or localized infection, e.g. abscess. Malaria if relevant travel history	A clinical diagnosis	Blood culture
Metabolic	Many possible causes, e.g. renal failure, hepatic failure, profound acidosis, but collectively these are rare causes of presentation with cardiorespiratory collapse	May have evidence of organ failure, or of drug overdose. May have no specific findings	Electrolytes, renal and liver function tests. Blood gases.	As indicated following initial tests

Table 1 Continued

Diagnosis	Key finding on examination	Key initial investigation	Definitive investigations
Anaphylaxis	Facial, tongue and throat swelling. Stridor. Wheeze. Urticarial rash. Skin erythema or extreme pallor	A clinical diagnosis	Serum mast cell tryptase. Specific IgE for suspect allergens. See Chapter 16.4 for further discussion

Notes

(1) Primarily neurological disorders may compromise the airway or ventilation, but rarely cause cardiovascular collapse. If a patient with cardiovascular collapse has a severely depressed conscious level (GCS <8) or focal neurological signs, then the assumption—until proven otherwise—should be that the neurological impairment is secondary to the cardiovascular collapse and not the cause of it.

(2) See other sections in this Emergency Medicine chapter for further details of conditions listed in this Table.

Table 2 Immediate clinical response to determination of volume status in the patient with cardiorespiratory collapse

Main problem	Key clinical signs	Immediate management
Hypotension	Peripheries cool and shut down Postural hypotension Low jugular venous pressure Lungs clear	Intravenous fluid (0.9% saline or plasma expander) given rapidly (0.5 litre boluses) until there is clear evidence that physical signs are being restored to normal, then slow rate infusion
Breathing difficulty	High jugular venous pressure Gallop rhythm Basal crepitations	Do not give fluid Sit up Consider intravenous loop diuretic and/or venodilator Consider need for ventilation
Hypotension and breathing difficulty	Peripheries cool and shut down High jugular venous pressure May be gallop rhythm Basal crepitations	Will almost certainly need urgent ventilation Call for help from ICU/anaesthetist before the patient suffers cardiorespiratory arrest Trial of fluid infusion may be appropriate: give 200 ml of plasma expander, keeping patient under continuous observation and terminating infusion immediately in the event of clinical deterioration

Notes

(1) All patients should be given high flow oxygen.

(2) Vigorous attempts should be made to diagnose and treat the underlying condition concurrent with efforts to resuscitate.

(3) Is resuscitation being effective in restoring organ perfusion? Do not forget the value of the urinary catheter: if the patient is passing urine, then their kidneys are being perfused effectively.

(4) If the patient remains hypotensive despite 'optimization' of intravascular volume then consideration can be given to the use of inotropes and vasoactive agents: see Chapter 16.2 for further discussion.

1.3 Acute myocardial infarction (AMI)

See Chapters 15.4.2.3 and 15.4.2.4 in main text

Clinical features

History

(1) Ischaemic chest pain
(2) Cardiorespiratory collapse
(3) May be non-specific or silent, especially in the elderly or in diabetics

Examination

May be normal, but look for
(1) 'Pump failure'—cool peripheries, hypotension
(2) Pulmonary oedema—see Emergency Medicine, section 1.8.
(3) Cardiac—gallop rhythm, murmurs

Immediate management

If cardiorespiratory collapse, as described in Emergency Medicine, section 1.2

Otherwise

(1) Give high flow oxygen by facemask.
(2) Give aspirin 300 mg p.o. immediately, chewed or dispersed in water (if not given before admission to hospital)
(3) Give adequate analgaesia, e.g. (i) diamorphine by slow intravenous injection at 1 mg/min, usual maximum initial dose is 5 mg, but may be repeated if necessary, or (ii) morphine by slow intravenous injection at 2 mg/min, usual maximum initial dose is 10 mg, but may be repeated if necessary. Both to be accompanied by appropriate antiemetic, e.g. metoclopramide 10 mg IV over 1–2 min, or cyclizine 50 mg IV over 1–2 min (caution in severe heart failure)
(4) If appropriate, give thrombolysis as soon as possible (Tables 3 and 4)
(5) If appropriate, consider percutaneous intervention (Table 5)

Key investigations

To establish the diagnosis

(1) ECG—looking for ST segment elevation and/or (presumed or proven) new bundle branch block

(2) Cardiac biochemical markers (troponins, CK-MB)

Other important tests

(1) Assess risk factors for ischaemic heart disease, e.g. cholesterol

(2) As indicated by clinical examination, e.g. chest radiograph to look for pulmonary oedema; echocardiography to assess LV function or cause of pansystolic murmur (?mitral valve dysfunction, ?ventricular septal defect)

Further management

Consider

(1) β-Blockade
- Early—if no contraindication (e.g. hypotension, heart failure, heart block) give, e.g. atenolol 5 mg IV over 5 min, repeated after 10–15 min
- Long term—if no contraindication continue oral β-blockade for at least 2–3 years.

(2) Angiotensin converting enzyme inhibition
- Early—start within 24 h in patients who are normotensive and continue for at least 5–6 weeks
- Long term—recommended for any patient with left ventricular dysfunction

(3) Long term aspirin (75–150 mg/day)

(4) Long term statin (lipid lowering agent) will benefit most if not all patients after AMI

Note

(1) Treat complications, e.g. venodilator or diuretic for pulmonary oedema. Severe heart failure/shock may require ventilation, inotropes +/– intra-aortic balloon pump

(2) Diabetic patients will benefit from intensive insulin therapy during admission with AMI and afterwards

(3) For all patients: give advice regarding lifestyle issues before and after discharge from hospital—smoking, diet, exercise—also regarding resumption of normal activities. Consider referral to cardiac rehabilitation services

(4) Consider need for specialist cardiological opinion and/or investigation by cardiac stress test (e.g. treadmill exercise tolerance test) and/or coronary angiography

Table 3 Thrombolysis in acute myocardial infarction (AMI)

Indications

Must satisfy three criteria:
(1) Typical chest pain at rest for >20 min
(2) ST elevation in two contiguous leads (> or = 1 mm inferiorly, > or = 2 mm anteriorly), or (presumed or proven) new bundle branch block
(3) Within 12 h of onset, but consider at 12–24 h if continuing pain

Contraindications

Absolute contraindications
(1) Bleeding—active internal bleeding; proven active peptic ulcer
(2) Brain—cerebrovascular accident within the past 6 months (or at any time if haemorrhagic stroke); known intracranial neoplasm or aneurysm
(3) Suspected aortic dissection
(4) Uncontrolled hypertension—SBP >180 mmHg or DBP >110 mmHg after pain relief and nitrates
(5). Pregnancy

Relative contraindications
(1) Recent (<6 weeks) major trauma/surgery/injury or traumatic resuscitation (>10 min or sufficient to fracture rib)
(2) Symptoms suggesting active peptic ulceration
(3) Defective haemostasis
(4) Lactation/peripartum
(5) Severe liver disease/oesophageal varices
(6) Severe renal disease
(7) Bacterial endocarditis
(8) Acute pancreatitis
(9) On warfarin with INR outside therapeutic range

Note that the following are not contraindications:
(1) Proliferative diabetic retinopathy
(2) Previous cardiopulmonary resuscitation, unless this is prolonged (>10 min) or associated with obvious trauma
(3) Therapeutic anticoagulation

Examples of agents

(1) Streptokinase 1 500 000 units by IV infusion over 60 min
(2) Recombinant tissue-type plasminogen activator, e.g.

Alteplase™
- Accelerated regimen (within 6 h of AMI): 15 mg by IV injection, followed by IV infusion of 50 mg over 30 min, then 35 mg over 60 min (lower doses in patients <65 kg)
- Standard regimen (6–12 h from AMI): 10 mg by IV injection, followed by IV infusion of 50 mg over 60 min, then 40 mg over 120 min (lower doses in patients <65 kg)

Tenecteplase™
- 30–50 mg (6000–10 000 units, depending on body weight) by intravenous injection over 10 s

Reteplase™
- 10 units intravenously over not more than 2 min, followed 30 min later by another 10 units intravenously over not more than 2 min

Notes

(1) Use of rt-PA is preferred if anterior AMI presenting within 6 h of onset; cardiogenic shock (SBP <80 mmHg); streptokinase given more than 5 days previously; streptokinase allergy. In some health care systems use of rt-PA is restricted to younger patients because of cost considerations.

(2) Most treatment regimen use 24 h of intravenous heparin as adjunctive therapy when recombinant tissue-type plasminogen activator is used (consult product literature).

(3) Problems during streptokinase infusion: see Table 4.

Table 4 Problems during streptokinase infusion

Problem	Immediate action	Further action
Common		
Hypotension (SBP<90 mmHg)	Stop infusion until blood pressure recovers	Recommence infusion more slowly (to complete over 2 h) OR switch to rt-PA regimen (see Table 3)
Rigors	Stop infusion until rigor settles	Recommence infusion more slowly (to complete over 2 h) OR switch to rt-PA regimen (see Table 3)
Ventricular fibrillation	Cardiovert	Continue infusion at usual rate
Uncommon		
Allergic reaction	Stop infusion Give hydrocortisone 100 mg IV and chlorpheniramine 10 mg IV	Recommence infusion more slowly if possible (to complete over 2 h) OR switch to rt-PA regimen (see Table 3)
Haemorrhage (major)	Stop infusion	Consider fresh frozen plasma/cryoprecipitate
Stroke	Stop infusion	Urgent CT head

Table 5 Indications for percutaneous intervention in acute myocardial infarction

Primary percutaneous intervention is an alternative to thrombolysis when it can be performed:
(1) within 60–90 min of admission
(2) by individuals skilled in the procedure (>75 cases per annum)
(3) in a high volume centre (>200 cases per annum)
(American College Cardiology/American Heart Association guidelines)

Primary percutaneous intervention is specifically indicated when there is:
(1) Contraindication to thrombolysis
(2) Haemodynamic compromise
And should be considered as
(3) Salvage procedure after failed thrombolytic therapy

1.4 Unstable angina or non-ST segment elevation myocardial infarction (non-Q-wave myocardial infarction)

See Chapters 15.4.2.3 and 15.4.2.4 in main text

Clinical features

History
(1) Ischaemic chest pain at rest or on minimal exertion
(2) Chest tightness/breathlessness

Examination
Usually no specific signs, but may be
(1) 'Pump failure'—cool peripheries, hypotension
(2) Pulmonary oedema—breathing difficulty, pulmonary crackles (see Emergency Medicine, section 1.8)
(3) Cardiac—gallop rhythm, murmurs

Immediate management

(1) Give high flow oxygen by facemask.
(2) Give aspirin 300 mg orally immediately, chewed or dispersed in water (if not given before admission to hospital)
(3) Give thienopyridine, e.g. clopidogrel 300 mg orally (then 75 mg daily)
(4) Give nitrate, e.g. (1) sublingual glyceryl trinitrate (GTN), 0.3–1 mg repeated as required; (2) buccal GTN, up to 5 mg, with tablet placed between upper lip and gum and left to dissolve; (3) intravenous infusion of isosorbide dinitrate at initial dose of 2 mg/h (increasing as necessary to maximum of 20 mg/h to relieve pain and as limited by hypotension)
(5) If pain not relieved by nitrate give adequate analgaesia, e.g. (1) diamorphine by slow intravenous injection at 1 mg/min (usual maximum initial dose is 5 mg, but may be repeated if necessary), or (2) morphine by slow intravenous injection at 2 mg/min (usual maximum initial dose is 10 mg, but may be repeated if necessary). Both to be accompanied by appropriate antiemetic, e.g. metoclopramide 10 mg IV over 1–2 min, or cyclizine 50 mg IV over 1–2 min (caution in severe heart failure)
(6) Give low molecular weight heparin, e.g. enoxaparin 1 mg/kg (100 units/kg) every 12 h, or dalteparin 120 units/kg every 12 h (maximum 10 000 units twice daily), unless contraindicated
(7) Give intravenous or oral β-blocker (see Emergency Medicine section 1.3) unless contraindicated
(8) Consider heart-rate-lowering calcium antagonist (e.g. diltiazem or verapamil) if β-blocker is contraindicated in patient without left ventricular dysfunction
(9) Consider glycoprotein IIb/IIIa inhibitor in high risk groups, e.g. those with ST segment depression and/or troponin positive, or those receiving urgent percutaneous intervention for unstable angina or non-ST segment elevation AMI. Agents tested in large scale randomized trials include abciximab, eptifibatide, and tirofiban
(10) Consider percutaneous intervention (Table 5)

Key investigations

To establish the diagnosis
(1) ECG—looking for transient ST segment shift with pain; T wave changes are less specific and ECG may be normal
(2) Cardiac biochemical markers (troponins, CK-MB)

Other important tests
As for acute myocardial infarction (see Emergency Medicine section 1.3)

Further management

(1) Angiotensin converting enzyme inhibition—recommended for any patient with left ventricular dysfunction
(2) Long-term aspirin (75–150 mg/day).
(3) Long-term statin (lipid lowering agent) will benefit most patients with ischaemic heart disease
Consider:
(4) Clopidogrel 75 mg/day

Note

(1) For all patients: give advice regarding lifestyle issues before and after discharge from hospital—smoking, diet, exercise—also regarding resumption of normal activities. Consider referral to cardiac rehabilitation services

(2) Consider need for specialist cardiological opinion and/or investigation by cardiac stress test (e.g. treadmill exercise tolerance test) and/or coronary angiography

1.5 Dissection of the thoracic aorta

See Chapter 15.14.1 in main text

Clinical features

History

(1) Chest pain, particularly if of sudden onset, tearing in quality, and radiating to the back

(2) Collapse

Examination

(1) Patient will usually look very unwell: cool peripherally, hypotensive

(2) Look for loss/reduction of one or more peripheral pulses: most likely is compromise of the left subclavian artery. Check left radial pulse in comparison with right; measure blood pressure in both arms; any deficit on the left strongly supports the diagnosis of aortic dissection. Examine also for reduction of carotid or femoral pulse(s)

(3) Evidence of focal ischaemia, eg. focal neurological deficit ('stroke')

(4) Could the patient have Marfan's syndrome? (risk factor)

Immediate management

If cardiorespiratory collapse, as described in Emergency Medicine, section 1.2

(1) The key to correct management is a high index of clinical suspicion that aortic dissection might be the diagnosis. Most patients with chest pain and circulatory collapse have acute myocardial infarction, the management for which (thrombolysis) could clearly be fatal in the patient with aortic dissection

(2) Give high flow oxygen by facemask

(3) Give adequate analgaesia, e.g. (i) diamorphine by slow intravenous injection at 1mg/min (usual maximum initial dose is 5mg, but may be repeated if necessary) or (ii) morphine by slow intravenous injection at 2 mg/min (usual maximum initial dose is 10 mg, but may be repeated if necessary). Both to be accompanied by appropriate antiemetic, e.g. metoclopramide 10 mg IV over 1–2 min, or cyclizine 50 mg IV over 1–2 min (caution in severe heart failure)

Key investigations

To establish the diagnosis

(1) CT angiography of chest

(2) Transoesophageal echocardiography

Other important tests

(1) Chest radiograph—look for widened mediastinum

(2) ECG—may have features of acute myocardial infarction (usually inferior) if dissection has compromised a coronary artery (usually right coronary artery)

(3) Cardiac biochemical markers—to exclude acute myocardial infarction

(4) Full blood count, clotting screen, electrolytes, renal and liver function tests—may give a lead to an underlying medical condition and will establish baseline

(5) Group and save/crossmatch blood.

Further management

(1) Reduce blood pressure using agents that will not cause tachycardia or increase the rate of cardiac ejection, e.g. titrate IV labetolol (initial dose 1 mg/min) or esmolol (50–200 μg/kg/min) to achieve SBP <110 mmHg. If blood pressure remains too high, add intravenous infusion of sodium nitroprusside (0.5–8 μg/kg/min) after β-blockade established (pulse <60 /min)

(2) Obtain opinion from cardiothoracic surgeon: immediate surgical repair will usually be the best management for patients with dissection of the ascending aorta (Stanford Type A) who are in reasonable condition

1.6 Bradycardia

See Chapters 15.2.3 and 15.6 in main text

Clinical features

History

(1) Syncope or presyncope

(2) Fatigue/breathing difficulty

(3) Drugs (especially β-blockers)

Examination

The most important immediate issue is to decide whether or not the circulation is compromised: is the patient cool peripherally? What are the rate, rhythm, and blood pressure? Is there pulmonary oedema (see Emergency Medicine, section 1.8)?

If seen in the presence of bradycardia, note rate and

(1) Abnormal rhythm, e.g. dropped beats in second degree AV block

(2) Other cardiovascular abnormality, e.g. cannon waves in JVP in third degree (complete) AV block

(3) Temperature (hypothermia—see Emergency Medicine, section 9.4)

Immediate management

Obtain ECG

If the patient is haemodynamically compromised

(1) Give atropine, 0.3–1.0 mg IV, repeated as necessary
(2) Consider isoprenaline, 0.5–10 μg/min by IV infusion
(3) Consider temporary pacing (see Emergency Medicine, section 10.3)
(4) Consider glucagon 50–150 μg/kg intravenously in 5 per cent glucose in cases of β-blocker overdose, with precautions to protect the airway in case of vomiting (NB unlicensed indication and dose)

Key investigations

To establish the diagnosis

12-lead ECG

Other important tests

(1) Electrolytes (particularly potassium)
(2) Cardiac biochemical markers (depending on context)
(3) Chest radiograph—look at heart size and for evidence of pulmonary oedema
(4) 24 h ECG monitor (if symptoms intermittent and 12-lead ECG not diagnostic)
(5) Echocardiography (if clinical suspicion that heart is structurally abnormal)

Further management

Dependent on diagnosis. If not reversible likely to require permanent pacing

1.7 Tachycardia

See Chapters 15.2.3 and 15.6 in main text

Clinical features

History

(1) Syncope or presyncope
(2) Palpitations
(3) Fatigue/breathing difficulty
(4) Chest pain

Examination

The most important immediate issue is to decide whether or not the circulation is compromised: is the patient cool peripherally? What are the rate, rhythm and blood pressure? Is there pulmonary oedema (see Emergency Medicine, section 1.8)?

Physical examination is unlikely to aid diagnosis of the particular type of tachycardia, excepting for the presence of an irregularly irregular rhythm in atrial fibrillation. However, note the following:

(1) Jugular venous pulse—absence of 'a' waves in AF; rapid flutter waves in atrial flutter; cannon waves in ventricular tachycardia
(2) First heart sound—variable intensity in AF
(3) A dilated heart increases the chance that tachycardia is ventricular in origin

Immediate management

Obtain ECG

If cardiorespiratory collapse, as described in Emergency Medicine, section 1.2

FOR ARRHYTHMIAS THAT ARE POORLY TOLERATED, SYNCHRONISED DC SHOCK (UNDER GENERAL ANAESTHESIA OR DEEP SEDATION) USUALLY PROVIDES RAPID RELIEF.

Management otherwise depends upon clinical context and type of tachycardia

Key investigations

To establish the diagnosis

(1) 12-lead ECG (see Table 6)

Other important tests

(1) Electrolytes (particularly potassium)
(2) Cardiac biochemical markers (depending on context)
(3) Chest radiograph—look at heart size and for evidence of pulmonary oedema
(4) 24 h ECG monitor (if symptoms intermittent and 12-lead ECG not diagnostic)
(5) Echocardiography (if clinical suspicion that heart is structurally abnormal)
(6) Thyroid function tests (in atrial fibrillation)

Further management

Uncertain of the diagnosis of a broad complex tachycardia? See Table 7

With severe haemodynamic compromise

Atrial fibrillation/flutter

- DC cardioversion, or
- Amiodarone, 5 mg/kg over 20–120 min followed by 1200 mg/24hrs until sinus rhythm restored (into central venous catheter), or
- Sotalol, 1.5 mg/kg intravenously over 30 min.

Atrioventricular nodal re-entry (AVNRT) and atrioventricular re-entry tachycardias (AVRT) (supraventricular tachycardias, SVTs)

- Adenosine, 3 mg intravenously given over 2 s, if necessary followed by 6 mg after 1–2 min, and then by 12 mg after a further 1–2 min (note—contraindicated in those with asthma, and patients taking dipyridamole are very sensitive, requiring reduced initial dose of 0.5–1 mg)
- Verapamil, 5–10 mg by slow intravenous injection over 2–3 min is an alternative in patients with asthma, but NOT in those who might have ventricular tachycardia, or in those who are receiving β-blockers

Ventricular tachycardia

- DC cardioversion (see Emergency Medicine, section 1.1)

Without severe haemodynamic compromise

Atrial fibrillation/flutter

Duration <48 h or trans-oesophageal echocardiography shows no intracardiac thrombus

- Consider prompt chemical or synchronised DC cardioversion.
- Flecainide (Class 1C) 2 mg/kg intravenously over 30 min if there is no evidence of ischaemic heart disease or left ventricular dysfunction
- Amiodarone or sotalol (Class III) can be used to restore sinus rhythm and maintain it
- Digoxin is useful for rate control only but will not restore sinus rhythm. If digoxin is ineffective in controlling ventricular rate, and cardioversion is unsuccessful or inappropriate, consider adding verapamil or β-blocker

Duration >48 h or thrombus on trans-oesophageal echocardiography

- Anticoagulate for 4–6 weeks before synchronised DC cardioversion

Note

- Atrial fibrillation arising in the context of intercurrent illness is usually best managed by treatment of the underlying medical condition and with digoxin (plus or minus verapamil or β-blocker) to control ventricular rate. The patient is likely to return to sinus rhythm when the underlying condition has resolved

Atrioventricular nodal re-entry (AVNRT) and atrioventricular re-entry (AVRT) tachycardias (supraventricular tachycardias, SVTs)

- Vagal stimulation by respiratory manoeuvres (Valsalva), prompt squatting, or pressure over one carotid sinus (but not the latter in those with recent ischaemia, digitalis toxicity, or in the elderly)
- Adenosine if vagal stimulation fails
- Other options include verapamil, β-blocker, flecainide, sotalol, or amiodarone

Ventricular tachycardia

- Consider synchronized DC cardioversion.
- Lignocaine (lidocaine) 50–100 mg as intravenous bolus over a few min followed immediately by infusion of 4 mg/min for 30 min, 2 mg/min for 2 h and then 1 mg/min up to 24 hr.
- Other antiarrhythmics that can be used include amiodarone, sotalol, procainamide and disopyramide—but seek expert help.

Torsade de pointes

This form of ventricular tachycardia requires particular treatment

- Give magnesium sulphate, 8 mmol of magnesium over 10–15 min, repeated once if necessary
- If torsade is associated with bradycardia and pauses, consider isoprenaline infusion or overdrive atrial/ventricular pacing to increase heart rate

Table 6 ECG criteria to distinguish VT from SVT with aberrant conduction

Feature favouring diagnosis of VT	Notes	
Atrioventricular (AV) dissociation	The most reliable criterion for VT	
Capture/fusion beats	Both occur rarely but their presence usually secures the diagnosis of VT	
Wide QRS complex	QRS width (s)	Predictive value for VT (%)
	<0.12	14
	0.12–0.14	43
	>0.14	100
Concordance across chest leads	QRS complexes all positive or all negative is reliable pointer to VT	
Extreme left axis deviation and/or a definite axis shift compared with previous ECGs	Strong indicator of VT	

Table 7 A practical clinical approach to broad-complex tachycardia

Clinical	Note	Working diagnosis
History	Myocardial infarction, ischaemic heart disease, or congestive heart failure present	VT
ECG	Features in Table 6 present	VT
Effect of adenosine (given as described in Emergency Medicine, section 1.7)	Inconclusive	VT
	Reversion of tachycardia	Atrioventricular nodal re-entry (AVNRT) or atrioventricular re-entry (AVRT) tachycardias (supraventricular tachycardias, SVTs). May also reveal (but unlikely to revert) atrial flutter or fibrillation

Notes

(1) Wrongly diagnosing an SVT is potentially disastrous, whereas manoeuvres to treat VT are unlikely to compromise the patient with SVT.

(2) History—patients with VT can have paroxysmal self-terminating episodes that are indistinguishable from those reported by patients with SVT.

(3) Examination—the haemodynamic state of the patient CANNOT be used to differentiate between VT and SVT: patients with VT can be haemodynamically stable, and those with haemodynamic compromise can have SVT.

1.8 Pulmonary oedema

See Chapter 15.15.2.2 in main text

Clinical features

History

(1) Breathing difficulty
(2) Orthopnoea, paroxysmal nocturnal dyspnoea
(3) Palpitations
(4) Chest pain
(5) Ankle oedema
(6) Of any cardiac disorder

Examination

(1) How unwell is the patient? If very ill, see Emergency Medicine, section 1.2
(2) Respiratory rate, cyanosis, peripheral circulation (cold, clammy), pulse rate and rhythm (?arrhythmia, see sections 1.6 and 1.7), blood pressure, JVP (likely to be elevated), apex beat (displaced in congestive cardiac failure), heart sounds (gallop rhythm, murmurs), crackles and/or wheezes in chest, peripheral oedema (suggests biventricular failure in this context)

Immediate management

If cardiorespiratory collapse, as described in Emergency Medicine, section 1.2

(1) Sit the patient up
(2) Give high flow oxygen via reservoir bag to achieve Pao_2 >92%
(3) Give frusemide 40–80 mg intravenously

If not improving rapidly

(4) Give either
- Diamorphine by slow intravenous injection at 1 mg/min (usual maximum initial dose is 5mg, but may be repeated if necessary), or
- Morphine by slow intravenous injection at 2 mg/min (usual maximum initial dose is 10 mg, but may be repeated if necessary)
- Both to be accompanied by appropriate antiemetic, e.g. metoclopramide 10 mg IV over 1–2 min (not cyclizine in severe heart failure)

(5) Unload with intravenous nitrate, e.g. isosorbide dinitrate 2–20 mg/h
(6) Consider elective ventilation: non-invasive or after endotracheal intubation

Key investigations

To establish the diagnosis

Chest radiograph

Other important tests

(1) ECG—look for arrhythmia or acute myocardial infarction
(2) Cardiac biochemical markers

Further management

Depending on clinical context

(1) Acute myocardial infarction—see Emergency Medicine, section 1.3
(2) Arrhythmia—see Emergency Medicine, sections 1.6 and 1.7
(3) Acute mechanical cause—e.g. aortic incompetence, mitral regurgitation, ventricular septal defect—may require surgical intervention

1.9 Deep venous thrombosis and pulmonary embolus

See Chapter 15.15.3.1 in main text

Clinical features

History

Deep venous thrombosis

(1) Calf/leg pain
(2) Calf/leg swelling
(3) Features to suggest PE

Pulmonary embolus

(1) Shortness of breath, developing over hours, days, or (sometimes) weeks
(2) Pleuritic chest pain, haemoptysis (lung infarction, peripheral emboli)
(3) Circulatory collapse (massive PE)
(4) Features to suggest DVT

Deep venous thrombosis and pulmonary embolus
Risk factors—immobilization, recent surgery, previous episodes, malignancy, travel, family history etc.

Examination

Deep venous thrombosis

(1) Calf/leg swelling—measure circumference 10 cm below tibial tuberosity: difference between sides of >1cm likely to be significant
(2) Calf tenderness; palpable cord; positive Homan's sign
(3) Dilated superficial veins; leg feels warmer than the other
(4) Check for signs of PE
(5) Consider alternative diagnoses—especially Baker's cyst, cellulitis, haematoma in muscle

Pulmonary embolus

(1) May be no abnormal signs
(2) Tachypnoea (70% of cases), crackles (50%), tachycardia (30%), pleural rub (<10%)
(3) Circulatory collapse with cool peripheries, hypotension, and cyanosis. Look particularly for signs of right heart strain: elevated JVP, parasternal heave, S3 over right ventricle, loud P2
(4) Check for signs of DVT
(5) Consider alternative diagnoses—especially pneumonia, musculoskeletal pain

Note

(1) Low grade fever is common in both DVT and PE

(2) In cases of DVT or PE—perform rectal/pelvic examination (before discharge from hospital)

Immediate management

If cardiorespiratory collapse, as described in Emergency Medicine, section 1.2

If index of clinical suspicion for PE is high, start IV standard (unfractionated) heparin pending the results of investigation

Key investigations

To establish the diagnosis

Tests commonly used to demonstrate the presence of thrombus/embolus are as follows:

- DVT—venous ultrasonography, contrast venography
- PE—lung ventilation/perfusion (VQ) scan, CT pulmonary angiogram, or pulmonary angiogram

Many patients referred for medical opinion have a low probability of having DVT or PE and not all require imaging to exclude DVT or PE. Follow management algorithms as follows:

- DVT—see Table 8
- PE—see Table 9

Other important tests

Pulmonary embolus

(1) ECG—commonest abnormality is sinus tachycardia and/or non-specific ST segment or T wave abnormalities. Look for signs of right heart strain, e.g. T wave inversion in V1/V2, S1Q3T3, axis shift

(2) Chest radiograph—look for atelectasis or pulmonary parenchymal abnormality, also pleural effusion. May be normal

(3) Arterial blood gases—look for hypoxia; but normoxia does not exclude PE

Deep venous thrombosis and pulmonary embolus

(1) Full blood count, electrolytes, renal and liver function tests—may give a lead to an underlying medical condition and will establish baseline

(2) At a later stage a thrombophilia screen may be appropriate, also investigations dictated by clinical findings or investigations detailed above

Further management

(1) Anticoagulation with standard (unfractionated) heparin (Table 10) *or* low molecular weight heparin (e.g. Tinzaparin 175 units anti-Factor Xa IU/kg subcutaneous o.d.) *until* oral anticoagulation (usually with warfarin, Table 11) is established

(2) In cases with circulatory collapse consider thrombolysis, e.g.

- Streptokinase by intravenous infusion of 250 000 units over 30 min, then 100 000 units/h for 12–72 h, OR
- Alteplase 10 mg by intravenous infusion over 1–2 min, followed by 90 mg over 2 h (maximum 1.5 mg/kg in patients of <65kg)

Notes

(1) No monitoring of low molecular weight heparin treatment is required

(2) Methods of reversing anticoagulation are shown in Table 12

Table 8 Pre-test clinical probability scoring system and care pathway for the patient with suspected deep venous thrombosis

Pre-test probability score

Criteria	Score
Active cancer	+1
Paralysis, plaster cast	+1
Bed rest >3 days, surgery within 4 weeks	+1
Tenderness along veins	+1
Entire leg swollen	+1
Calf swollen >3 cm	+1
Pitting oedema	+1
Collateral veins	+1
Alternative diagnosis likely	–2

Pre-test probability

Low	0
Moderate	1 or 2
High	3 or more

Management algorithm

Pre-test probability score	**Action**	**Result**	**Further action**
0 or 1	Perform D-dimer	Negative	No further investigation
		Positive	Perform ultrasonography
2 or more	Do not perform D-dimer		
	Perform ultrasonography	Negative	Withhold treatment and repeat ultrasonography in 10–14 days. If serial ultrasonography is negative, pulmonary embolism rarely occurs
		Positive	Diagnosis of venous thrombosis established

Notes

(1) Pre-test probability score from Wells *et al.* (1997). *Lancet* **350**, 1795–8.

(2) This management algorithm is typical of many used, but further prospective evaluation is warranted.

(3) If the physician's judgement is that deep venous thrombosis is very likely in a particular case, then they should proceed to investigations directed at detecting thrombus in leg veins whatever the scoring algorithm would suggest. If the result of ultrasonography is negative, and repeat ultrasonography in 10 to 14 days is also negative, pulmonary embolism rarely occurs.

(4) All patients who are discharged with 'deep venous thrombosis excluded' should be given written information describing how they can be reassessed if symptoms worsen or fail to settle over the next few days.

Table 9 Pre-test clinical probability scoring system and care pathway for the patient with suspected pulmonary embolism

Pre-test probability score

Criteria	Score
Clinical signs and symptoms of deep venous thrombosis (minimum of leg swelling and pain with palpation of deep vein region)	+3
No alternative diagnosis	+3
Heart rate >100/min	+1.5
Bed rest >3 days, surgery within 4 weeks	+1.5
Previous DVT or PE	+1.5
Haemoptysis	+1
Malignancy	+1

Pre-test probability

Low (approximately 2–4% chance of PE)	0 or 1
Moderate (approximately 20% chance of PE)	2 to 6
High (approximately 60% chance of PE)	More than 6

Table 9 Continued

Management algorithm

Pre-test probability score	Action	Result	Further action
O or 1	Perform D-dimer	Negative	No further investigation
		Positive	Perform ventilation-perfusion lung scanning (see notes)
2 or more	Do not perform D-dimer		
	Perform ventilation-perfusion lung scanning	Normal scan	No further investigation—PE is excluded
		Low/intermediate probability	Scan is non-diagnostic—perform further investigation (see notes)
		High probability	Diagnosis of PE established

Notes

(1) Pre-test probability score from Wells *et al.* (2000). *Thrombosis and Haemostasis* **83**, 416–20.

(2) This management algorithm is typical of many used, but further prospective evaluation is warranted. If ventilation-perfusion lung scanning gives a low or intermediate probability result it should be regarded as non-diagnostic and further action determined by the pre-test probability as follows. (a) If the pre-test probability is low (score 0 or 1), then perform bilateral venous ultrasonography—if this is negative, pulmonary embolism can be considered excluded without further testing. With a low probability clinical assessment, serial leg tests are unnecessary. (b) If the pre-test probability is high (score 2 or more), and the patient has adequate cardiopulmonary reserve, then serial ultrasonography of the leg veins over 10–14 days may be performed. If serial ultrasonography is negative, pulmonary embolism rarely occurs. If cardiopulmonary reserve is inadequate, proceed to a definitive diagnostic test for pulmonary embolism (pulmonary angiography or perhaps spiral computed tomography).

(3) If the physician's judgement is that pulmonary embolism is very likely in a particular case, then they should proceed to investigations directed at detecting pulmonary embolism, whatever the scoring algorithm would suggest.

(4) All patients who are discharged with 'pulmonary embolism excluded' should be given written information describing how they can be reassessed if symptoms worsen or fail to settle over the next few days.

Table 10 A schedule for infusion of standard (unfractionated) heparin to obtain APTT ratio 1.5–2.5

(1) Measure APTT at start of therapy and at least daily thereafter
(2) Give IV loading dose of 5000 units by bolus injection, followed by
(3) IV infusion of heparin 500 units/ml (dilute 25 000 units heparin to 50 ml total volume with 0.9% saline) at the following rate:

Bodyweight (kg)	Initial rate (ml/h)
50	1.8
60	2.2
70	2.5
80	2.9
90	3.2
100	3.6
120	4.4

(4) Check APTT 6–12 h after start of treatment and then at least once daily, adjusting the infusion rate according to the APTT as follows:

APTT ratio	Continue infusion at
>7.0	Stop for 30 min and then reduce by 1.0 ml/h (check APTT 4 h later)
5.1–7.0	Reduce by 1.0 ml/h (check APTT 4 h later)
4.1–5.0	Reduce by 0.6 ml/h (check APTT 4 h later)
3.1–4.0	Reduce by 0.2 ml/h
2.6–3.0	Reduce by 0.1 ml/h
1.5–2.5	No change
1.2–1.4	Increase by 0.4 ml/h
<1.2	Increase by 0.8 ml/h (check APTT 4 h later)

Protocol in use in Addenbrooke's Hospital, Cambridge (by courtesy of Dr T. Baglin).

Table 11 A schedule for anticoagulation with warfarin designed to achieve an INR of 2.0–3.0

Day 1 INR	Day 1 Warfarin	Day 2 INR	Day 2 Warfarin	Day 3 INR	Day 3 Warfarin	Day 4 INR	Day 4 Warfarin
<1.4	10	<1.8	10	<2.0	10	<1.4	>8
		1.8	1	2.0–2.1	5	1.4	8
		>1.8	0.5	2.2–2.3	4.5	1.5	7.5
				2.4–2.5	4	1.6–1.7	7
				2.6–2.7	3.5	1.8	6.5
				2.8–2.9	3	1.9	6
				3.0–3.1	2.5	2.0–2.1	5.5
				3.2–3.3	2	2.2–2.3	5
				3.4	1.5	2.4–2.6	4.5
				3.5	1	2.7–3.0	4
				3.6–4.0	0.5	3.1–3.5	3.5
				>4.0	0	3.6–4.0	3
						4.1–4.5	Miss next day's dose, then 2 mg
						>4.5	Miss out 2 days' doses, then 1 mg

(1) INR measured from sample taken at 08.00–11.00 hours; (2) warfarin dose (in mg) given at 17.00–19.00 hours; (3) protocol in use in Addenbrooke's Hospital, Cambridge (by courtesy of Dr T. Baglin).

Table 12 Reversal of anticoagulation

Anticoagulant	Method	Notes
Standard (unfractionated) heparin	(1) Stop heparin (2) Give protamine by slow IV injection: 1 mg neutralizes 100 units of heparin if given within 15 min of heparin. Give less if a longer time has elapsed because heparin is rapidly excreted. Maximum dose of protamine is 50 mg	(1) There is no point in giving FFP or other clotting concentrates: they do not contain heparin-neutralizing activity (2) Excess protamine is anticoagulant
Low molecular weight heparin	(1) Stop heparin (2) Administer protamine by slow IV injection, maximum 50 mg. This is less effective at neutralizing the effect of LMW heparin than it is for standard heparin. There is no good evidence on which to base dosage	(1) There is no point in giving FFP or other clotting concentrates: they do not contain heparin-neutralizing activity (2) Excess protamine is anticoagulant
Warfarin	Immediate reversal (e.g. patient bleeding with high INR) (1) Stop warfarin (2) Vitamin K 1 mg IV (3) Fresh frozen plasma, 2–4 units, IV (4) Re-check INR Controlled reversal (e.g. high INR but patient not bleeding) (1) INR <8. Stop warfarin. Re-check INR in 3 days (2) INR >8. Stop warfarin. Give vitamin K 5–10 mg p.o. INR re-checked in 24 h should show a fall	(1) In extremis give up to 5 mg of vitamin K IV (2) Large volumes of FFP (up to 2 litres) can be required to effect complete reversal of warfarin (3) The role of factor concentrates (II, VII, IX, X) is being evaluated Continue warfarin in lower dose (if indicated) when INR back in therapeutic range.

1.10 Cardiac tamponade

See Chapter 15.9 in main text

Clinical features

History

(1) There are no specific features to indicate this condition
(2) Can follow acute myocardial infarction, aortic dissection, cardiac trauma (including iatrogenic with cardiac catheterization)
(3) There may be evidence of a condition that can cause pericardial effusion, e.g. tuberculosis, cancer, advanced renal failure

Examination

The key to making this rare but very important (because treatable) diagnosis is to consider it in any patient with unexplained cardiorespiratory collapse. Look for:

Signs of tamponade

(1) Grossly elevated JVP that rises (if its top can be seen) on inspiration (Kussmaul's sign)
(2) Pulsus paradoxus—meaning an exaggerated fall in systolic blood pressure on inspiration (normal <10 mmHg), but a rapid screening test for severe cases is to ask 'does the radial pulse disappear on inspiration'?

Evidence of a (large) pericardial effusion, although these will NOT be present unless there is a pre-existing effusion

(3) Increased area of cardiac dullness
(4) Quiet heart sounds

Immediate management

If the patient is *in extremis* proceed as in Emergency Medicine, section 1.2

As soon as the diagnosis of cardiac tamponade is established, perform or arrange for immediate/urgent pericardial aspiration (see Emergency Medicine, section 10.2.3)

Give colloid, e.g. gelofusin 500 ml by rapid intravenous infusion, to support blood pressure

Key investigations

To establish the diagnosis

(1) Echocardiography.
- The most sensitive test for the presence of pericardial fluid.
- Diastolic collapse of right ventricle or right atrium and a striking increase in the amplitude of septal motion with respiration indicate severe circulatory embarrassment

(2) Cytology and culture of pericardial fluid

Other important tests

(1) Chest radiograph—look for globular heart (almost invariably with clear lung fields)

(2) ECG—look for low voltage QRS complexes and electrical alternans (in large pericardial effusion) and for evidence of acute myocardial infarction

Further management

As determined by underlying condition

1.11 Accelerated ('malignant') hypertension

See Chapter 15.16.3 in main text

Clinical features

History

(1) Headache
(2) Blurring of vision
(3) Drowsiness
(4) Epileptic fits

Examination

(1) Blood pressure—will usually be grossly elevated with diastolic pressure >130 mmHg, but note that accelerated hypertension can occur at lower pressures than this and the diagnosis is established not by a particular elevation of blood pressure but by signs of fibrinoid necrosis

(2) Ocular fundi
- Grade III retinopathy: flame-shaped superficial haemorrhages, 'dot and blot' haemorrhages, cotton wool spots (retinal microinfarcts), hard exudates
- Grade IV retinopathy: as Grade III + papilloedema

(Note that there is no difference in management or prognosis of patients with Grade III or Grade IV disease)

(3) Urine—stix testing shows proteinuria and haematuria, microscopy may show red blood cell casts

Also look for signs of

(4) Pulmonary oedema—see Emergency Medicine, section 1.8

(5) Aortic dissection—see Emergency Medicine, section 1.5

(6) Scleroderma—scleroderma renal crisis

Immediate management

In an uncomplicated case:

(1) Admit to hospital
(2) Bed rest
(3) No smoking (causes an acute rise in blood pressure)
(4) Aim to lower diastolic pressure into range 100–105 mmHg over 2–3 days using:
- Atenolol 25–50 mg orally, or
- Nifedipine 10–20 mg of modified release preparation orally (tablets, not sublingual)
- Further dosing determined by response
- Maximum initial fall in blood pressure should not exceed 25% of presenting value

In a complicated case (aortic dissection, epileptic fitting, acute pulmonary oedema, oral medication not possible) use intravenous infusion of:
- Labetolol, initial bolus of 20 mg, then at 20 mg/h, increased as necessary every 30 min to maximum of 120 mg/h, or
- Sodium nitroprusside at initial dose of 0.25–0.5 μg/kg/min, increasing up to 8 μg/kg/min

Key investigations

To establish the diagnosis

Accelerated hypertension is a clinical diagnosis

Other important tests

(1) ECG—looking for evidence of left ventricular hypertrophy and acute myocardial ischaemia

(2) Chest radiograph—looking for heart size, pulmonary oedema, and (if chest/back pain) for aortic dissection

(3) Electrolytes and renal function—if serum creatinine >250 μmol/l renal function is likely to deteriorate further (at least in the short term)

(4) 'Autoimmune/vasculitic' serology—ANCA, ANA etc.—for evidence of multisystem disorder that can present with accelerated phase hypertension and which (if present) will require specific treatment

(5) CT angiography of chest if aortic dissection suspected

Further management

When acute emergency is controlled, all patients that have suffered from accelerated phase hypertension require thorough investigation for secondary causes of hypertension

1.12 Anaphylactic shock

See Chapter 16.4 in main text

Clinical features

History

(1) Facial, tongue or throat swelling
(2) Stridor or wheeze
(3) Sudden collapse
(4) Premonitory aura—apprehension, light-headedness, dizziness, tingling or itching of skin
(5) Exposure to preciptant

Examination

(1) Cyanosis
(2) Hypotension
(3) Facial, tongue, or throat swelling
(4) Stridor or wheeze
(5) Urticaria, angio-oedema, skin erythema, or extreme pallor

Immediate management

(1) High flow oxygen (10 l/min) by face mask with reservoir bag to keep $Pa\text{O}_2$ >92%.
(2) Adrenaline (epinephrine)
- Give 0.3–0.5 ml of 1:1000 (0.3–0.5 mg) intramuscularly, repeated every 5–10 min as needed

If this is ineffective, or if the patient is about to die
- Give 1–4 mg (1–4 ml) of 1:1000 adrenaline nebulized with oxygen, and
- Make up 1:100 000 preparation of adrenaline by drawing up 1ml of 1:1000 adrenaline (total of 1 mg) in 20 ml syringe, adding 9 ml of 0.9% saline to give total volume of 10 ml. Discard all but 2 ml (leaving 200 μg of adrenaline in the syringe), and then draw up further saline to a total volume of 20 ml, giving a final concentration of 10 μg/ml. Give 0.75–1.5 mg/kg of 1:100 000 adrenaline IV at 10–20 μg/min (1–2 ml/min) initially, repeated as necessary

(3) Colloid—give 10–20 ml/kg as rapid intravenous infusion if patient is hypotensive

Second line therapy, after cardiorespiratory stability has been achieved:

(4) Give H1-blocker, eg. chlorpheniramine 10–20 mg IV, repeated up to 40 mg in 24 h (change to oral when patient tolerates)
(5) Give H_2-blocker, e.g. ranitidine 50 mg IV three times daily (change to oral when patient tolerates)
(6) Give hydrocortisone 5 mg/kg IV, then 2.5 mg/kg IV four times daily (change to oral prednisolone 40 mg daily when patient tolerates)
(7) Give salbutamol 5 mg (repeated as necessary) via oxygen-driven nebulizer if bronchospasm is a persistent problem

Key investigations

To establish the diagnosis

(1) Anaphylaxis is a clinical diagnosis
(2) Mast cell tryptase

Other important tests

(1) ECG, chest radiograph, electrolytes, renal function, arterial blood gases (depending on context)

Further management

(1) Determination of allergen (if any)
(2) Advice regarding avoidance
(3) Medic Alert bracelet
(4) Instruction regarding self-injection of adrenaline and supply of appropriate medication, e.g. EpiPen™

2 Respiratory

2.1 Acute on chronic respiratory failure

See Chapters 17.6 and 17.7 in main text

Clinical features

History

(1) Chronic respiratory condition—usually chronic obstructive pulmonary disease
(2) Recent increase in breathlessness
(3) Evidence of infection—fever, sweats, increased sputum production, increased sputum purulence
(4) 'Cor pulmonale'—worsening ankle oedema

Examination

(1) Cyanosis
(2) Respiratory rate
(3) Temperature
(4) Evidence of carbon dioxide retention—drowsiness, asterixis, metabolic flap
(5) Chest signs—of chronic respiratory condition, of infection, and exclude pneumothorax
(6) Signs of cor pulmonale—elevated JVP, right ventricular heave, right ventricular gallop, loud P2, congested liver, ascites, peripheral oedema
(7) Check PEFR if patient is able to use PEF recorder
(8) Check pulse oximetry.

Is the patient getting exhausted? Remember that a 'normal' respiratory rate in the patient who looks very tired may mean that they are close to death.

Immediate management

The patient who is extremely ill

If the patient is *in extremis*, proceed as in Emergency Medicine, section 1.2, with the exception that a high concentration of inspired oxygen should NOT be given to patients who are KNOWN to have acute on chronic respiratory failure. If the patient is known to have chronic respiratory failure:

(1) Give controlled oxygen (24–28% or 1–2 l/min by nasal prongs)
(2) Initiate other aspects of management listed below
(3) Check arterial blood gases, adjusting inspired oxygen concentration if allowed by clinical response, $Pa{O_2}$, $Pa{CO_2}$, and pH (pH, not hypoxia, is the most important factor related to survival in patients with acute on chronic respiratory failure)
(4) Consider need for urgent intubation and ventilation if matters do not improve rapidly

Note

If it is UNCERTAIN whether or not a patient has acute on chronic respiratory failure, then high concentration oxygen should be given to all patients who are extremely ill. All such patients require continued close monitoring of their clinical state and arterial blood gases, allowing (amongst other things) detection of the few who will have acute on chronic respiratory failure and lose their respiratory drive in response to high concentration oxygen

The patient who is moderately unwell

(1) Give 24% oxygen, increasing concentration to 28% (or 1 to 2 l/min by nasal prongs) depending on the results of subsequent blood gas analysis
(2) Give nebulized β_2-agonist, e.g. salbutamol 2.5–5 mg, terbutaline 5–10 mg, using air as the driving gas, repeated as required
(3) Give nebulized anticholinergic, e.g. ipatropium bromide 500 μg (can be combined with β_2-agonist), repeated as required
(4) Give diuretic, e.g. frusemide 40–80 mg IV, if evidence of fluid overload
(5) Give corticosteroid, e.g. hydrocortisone 100 mg IV twice daily or prednisolone 30 mg orally once daily
(6) Give antibiotic that will cover likely respiratory pathogens if two of the following symptoms are present—increased breathlessness, increased sputum volume, or increased sputum purulence, e.g. amoxycillin 250 mg orally three times daily or (if allergic to penicillin) clarithromycin 250–500 mg orally twice daily (intravenously if oral administration not possible)
(7) Consider aminophylline, loading dose (in patient not previously treated with theophylline) of 5 mg/kg given intravenously over 20 min, then an infusion of 0.5 mg/kg/h aiming for serum concentration in the range 10–20 mg/l
(8) Consider need for non-invasive positive pressure ventilation if patient does not improve.

Note—use intravenous fluids to correct and prevent dehydration

Key investigations

To establish the diagnosis

(1) Chest radiograph—looking for focal consolidation and to exclude pneumothorax
(2) Sputum culture

To determine severity and monitor response to treatment

(3) Arterial blood gases
(4) Serial measurements of peak flow

Other important tests

(1) Full blood count
(2) Electrolytes, renal and liver function
(3) ECG

Further management

(1) Optimization of treatment for chronic pulmonary condition, usually chronic obstructive pulmonary disease
(2) Emphasize need to stop smoking

2.2 Tension pneumothorax

See Chapters 16.2 and 17.12 in main text

Clinical features

History

(1) Collapse with extreme difficulty in breathing

Examination

(1) Patient looks as though they are about to die
(2) Gasping respiratory effort
(3) Cyanosis
(4) Chest looks asymmetrical, being prominent on side of tension
(5) Tracheal deviation, away from side of tension
(6) Mediastinal shift, away from side of tension, most reliably detected by percussion of cardiac dullness
(7) Chest is silent on side of tension, the only breath sounds being heard in the opposite axilla

Immediate management

Insert needle to decompress chest, see Emergency Medicine, section 10.4.3

Key investigations

To establish the diagnosis

(1) Tension pneumothorax is a clinical diagnosis to be treated immediately without delay for investigation

Note

(1) The signs of tension pneumothorax are not subtle, but you will not make the diagnosis unless you consider it and seek the presence of the signs listed above
(2) If a patient appears to be dying and you think that they might have a tension pneumothorax, then—after calling for help and initiating resuscitation (see Emergency Medicine, section 1.1)—there is nothing to be lost (and potentially much to be gained) from an attempt at chest decompression

Other important tests

Chest radiograph will confirm diagnosis of pneumothorax after decompression

Further management

Insertion of chest drain (see Emergency Medicine, section 10.4.3.3) after tension has been relieved

2.3 Upper airway obstruction

See Chapter 17.8.1 in main text

Clinical features

History

(1) Extreme difficulty in breathing
(2) Coughing /choking
(3) Noisy breathing
(4) Difficult/unable to speak
(5) 'Something stuck'

Examination

(1) Extreme but ineffective respiratory effort
(2) Cyanosis
(3) Drooling (cannot swallow saliva)
(4) Stridor

Immediate management

(1) Heimlich manoeuvre if the patient has inhaled a foreign body
- Patient sitting or standing—rescuer stands or kneels behind patient, encircling the patient's waist with their arms, placing one fist just above the navel (well below xiphoid process) and using their other hand to press the fist into the patient's abdomen with a quick upward thrust. Repeat as necessary
- Patient lying—place patient on their back. Rescuer kneels astride patient and puts the palm of one hand between the navel and xiphisternum, places their other hand on top of this, and pushes upwards and inwards

(2) If Heimlich manoeuvre is inappropriate or has failed
- If there is time and you have the expertise—spray the pharynx with local anaesthetic (e.g. 5% cocaine and adrenaline) and examine the pharynx and upper airway by indirect laryngoscopy to establish the cause of obstruction and allow (if possible) its removal (with finger sweep under direct vision or long handled forceps) or passage of an endotracheal tube
- If there is time and you are not experienced in upper airway management—call immediately for help from anaesthetic or ENT colleagues

Key investigations

To establish the diagnosis

(1) Upper airway obstruction is a clinical diagnosis

Other important tests

As dictated by cause of obstruction

Further management

As dictated by cause of obstruction
See Emergency Medicine, section 10.4.2.3

2.4 Asthma

See Chapter 17.4.4 in main text

Clinical features

History

(1) Worsening asthma
(2) Increasing difficulty breathing
(3) Decrease in exercise tolerance
(4) Increasing wheeze
(5) Chest tightness
(6) Cough
(7) Difficulty in speaking
(8) Fall in self-monitored peak flow
(9) Failure to obtain improvement with use of regular β_2-agonist

Precipitating factor

(1) Exposure to known precipitant, eg. exercise, cold air, dusty environment

(2) Respiratory infection, e.g. upper respiratory tract infection

Examination

Moderate uncontrolled acute asthma

(1) Breathlessness

(2) Wheeze

(3) Chest tightness

(4) Peak flow 50–70% of predicted or personal best

Acute severe attack

(1) Cannot complete sentences in one breath

(2) Increased respiratory rate: >25 breaths/min

(3) Use of accessory muscles of respiration

(4) Tachycardia: >110/min

(5) Peak flow <50% of predicted or personal best

Life-threatening asthma

(1) Exhaustion or poor respiratory effort

(2) Inability to speak.

(3) Altered level of consciousness.

(4) Cyanosis

(5) Silent chest.

(6) Hypotension or bradycardia

(7) Peak flow <33% of predicted or personal best (or unrecordable)

Note

(1) A 'normal' respiratory rate is consistent with the patient being near to death if they are exhausted

(2) Always check carefully for signs of pneumothorax

(3) Always check pulse oximetry

(4) Asking the patient to count out loud as far as they can on a single breath provides a rapid, quantitative, and repeatable measure of respiratory function

Immediate management

If cardiorespiratory collapse, as described in Emergency Medicine, section 1.2

Moderate uncontrolled acute asthma

(1) β_2-Agonist via spacer and mask or nebulizer (see below)

(2) Oral prednisolone 30 mg once daily

(3) Inhaled steroids—commence or increase dose

Acute severe attack

(1) Oxygen, high flow with reservoir bag if needed, to achieve $P\text{aO}_2$ >92%

(2) Salbutamol 5 mg or terbutaline 10 mg via oxygen-driven nebulizer, repeated up to every 15–30 min as needed, and then 4 hourly

(3) Steroids—hydrocortisone 200 mg intravenously four times daily or prednisolone 30–60 mg orally once daily

Life-threatening attack or patient failing to improve

(4) Add ipatropium 0.5 mg to nebulized β_2-agonist

(5) Give aminophylline, loading dose (in patient not previously treated with theophylline) of 5 mg/kg given intravenously over 20 min, then an infusion of 0.5 mg/kg/h aiming for serum concentration in the range 10–20 mg/l. Omit loading dose if patient already taking oral theophylline

Consider intravenous salbutamol (3–20 μg/min) or terbutaline (1.5–5 μg/min) infusion

Note

(1) IF THE PATIENT IS DETERIORATING, CALL FOR HELP FROM THE INTENSIVE CARE UNIT SOONER RATHER THAN LATER—ELECTIVE INTUBATION AND VENTILATION IS BETTER THAN THAT DONE AFTER CARDIORESPIRATORY ARREST (SEE CHAPTER 16.1)

(2) Use intravenous fluids to correct and prevent dehydration

Key investigations

To establish the diagnosis

Acute asthma is a clinical diagnosis

Other important tests

(1) Chest radiograph—exclude pneumothorax

(2) Arterial blood gases—markers for life-threatening asthma being:

- Normal or high $P\text{aCO}_2$ (>5 kPa)
- Low pH
- Severe hypoxia ($P\text{aO}_2$ <8 kPa) in spite of high flow oxygen treatment

(3) Electrolytes, renal and liver function, full blood count

Further management

(1) Optimization of long-term asthma management

(2) Education regarding how to recognize severe attacks and how to respond when they develop

2.5 Pneumonia

See Chapter 17.5.2.1 in main text

Clinical features

History

(1) Breathing difficulty

(2) 'flu-like prodrome

(3) High fever, sweats, rigors

(4) Pleuritic chest pain

(5) Sputum production (but note that this is not expected in atypical pneumonia)

(6) Travel

(7) Pet birds

Examination

(1) Fever

(2) Respiratory—cyanosis, respiratory rate, focal lung signs (consolidation, pleural rub, pleural effusion)

(3) Circulation—peripheral perfusion (hot or cold), pulse, blood pressure
(4) Look at the sputum (if any)
(5) Always check pulse oximetry

British Thoracic Society definition of severe pneumonia states that one or more of the following must be present in a patient with clinical and/or radiological signs of pneumonia:
(1) Respiratory rate >30/min
(2) Systolic blood pressure <90 mmHg
(3) Pa_{O_2} <8 kPa (breathing room air)
(4) Multilobar involvement on chest radiograph
(5) Blood urea >7 mmol/l

Immediate management

If cardiorespiratory collapse, as described in Emergency Medicine, section 1.2
(1) Oxygen, high flow with reservoir bag if needed, to achieve Pa_{O_2} >92%
(2) Appropriate antimicrobial agent

British Thoracic Society guidelines for treatment of community-acquired pneumonia

- Mild/moderate pneumonia
  Oral therapy with extended spectrum penicillin (eg. amoxicillin 250–500 mg three times daily) alone or with a macrolide (eg. clarithromycin 250–500 mg twice daily). Omit the penicillin in patients with penicillin allergy
- Severe pneumonia
  Intravenous therapy with a second- or third-generation cephalosporin (e.g. cefotaxime 1g twice daily) plus a macrolide (e.g. erythromycin 500 mg four times daily)
- Suspected legionnaire's disease
  High-dose intravenous erythromycin (1g four times daily) plus consider adding oral rifampicin (0.6–1.2 g daily in two to four divided doses)

In areas/countries where there is serious concern that *S. pneumoniae* may be resistant to penicillin and other agents

- Mild/moderate pneumonia
  Second- or third-generation cephalosporin (e.g. cefotaxime 1g intravenously twice daily) plus macrolide (e.g. erythromycin 500 mg orally or intravenously four times daily), OR fluoroquinolone (e.g. levofloxacin 500 mg orally or intravenously once or twice daily) alone
- Severe pneumonia
  Second/third-generation cephalosporin (e.g. cefotaxime 1 g intravenously twice daily) plus macrolide (e.g. erythromycin 500 mg intravenously four times daily), OR second-/third-generation cephalosporin (e.g. cefotaxime 1g intravenously twice daily) plus fluoroquinolone (e.g. levofloxacin 500 mg intravenously twice daily)

Note
(1) If staphylococcal pneumonia is suspected, add flucloxacillin 1g intravenously four times daily
(2) See Chapters 17.5.2.2 and 17.5.2.3 for discussion of antimicrobial treatment of patients with hospital-acquired pneumonia or pneumonia in the immunocompromised
(3) Intravenous fluids to maintain adequate hydration

Key investigations

To establish the diagnosis
(1) Chest radiograph—looking for focal consolidation (lobar pneumonia) or more widespread interstitial shadowing.
(2) Blood culture.
(3) Sputum culture.
(4) Blood sample for serological testing.

To establish severity
Arterial blood gases—if patient is very ill or pulse oximetry shows Pa_{O_2} <92%

Other important tests
Full blood count, electrolytes, renal and liver function

Further management

Follow up chest radiograph to ensure complete resolution

3 Gastrointestinal and hepatological

3.1 Upper gastrointestinal haemorrhage

See Chapter 14.3.2 in main text

Clinical features

History

(1) Haematemesis or 'coffee-ground' vomiting
(2) Melaena
(3) Presyncope
(4) Indigestion or reflux or medication for these symptoms
(5) Retching before haematemesis (consider Mallory Weiss tear)
(6) Previous upper gastrointestinal investigation or surgery
(7) To suggest recent development of anaemia
(8) Drugs that predispose to upper gastrointestinal haemorrhage—aspirin, non-steroidal anti-inflammatory agents, anticoagulants
(9) Risk factors for, or presence of, chronic liver disease (consider varices)
(10) Anorexia and weight loss (consider malignancy)

Examination

(1) State of circulation—temperature of peripheries, pulse rate, blood pressure, jugular venous pressure
(2) Mucous membranes—chronic anaemia
(3) Evidence of chronic liver disease—jaundice and other manifestations (consider varices)
(4) Evidence of portal hypertension—especially splenomegally (consider varices)
(5) Lymphadenopathy—especially in left supraclavicular fossa (consider malignancy)
(6) Abdomen—for epigastic mass (consider malignancy)
(7) Rectal examination—for blood/melaena

Notes

(1) The most reliable signs of intravascular volume depletion are postural hypotension (sitting versus lying) and a low jugular venous pressure
(2) Clinical assessment of severity, see Table 13

Immediate management

If cardiorespiratory collapse, as described in Emergency Medicine, section 1.2

(1) Establish intravenous access with one or more large-bore peripheral venous cannulae (look in the antecubital fossae in the patient who is shut down). If you cannot do this, then insert femoral venous catheter (see Emergency Medicine, section 10.1.3). DO NOT ATTEMPT TO INSERT AN INTERNAL JUGULAR OR SUBCLAVIAN VENOUS CATHETER INTO A PATIENT WHO OBVIOUSLY HAS SEVERE INTRAVASCULAR VOLUME DEPLETION (see Chapter 16.1 for discussion).
(2) If clinical evidence of intravascular volume depletion, give 1000 ml of intravenous fluid (colloid, e.g Gelofusin™, or 0.9% saline) as fast as possible. Repeat clinical examination. If the patient still has intravascular volume depletion, give further 500 ml of fluid as fast as possible. Repeat cycle until arterial pressure and jugular venous pressure restored towards normal, then slow down rate of infusion. Use blood instead of colloid/saline as soon as it is available
(3) Cross-match blood for transfusion
(4) Consider need for urgent upper gastrointestinal endoscopy
(5) If oesophageal varices—see Table 14

Also

(1) Keep oxygen saturation >92% (monitor using pulse oximetery), giving high flow oxygen (10 l/min) by face mask with reservoir bag if needed
(2) Insert urinary catheter and monitor fluid input/output hourly in any patient with substantial gastrointestinal haemorrhage—a satisfactory urine output is the best gauge of adequate resuscitation
(3) Correct any coagulopathy—see Emergency Medicine, section 1.9, Table 3 (iatrogenic overanticoagulation) and section 9.1 (disseminated coagulation)
(4) Nurse to avoid aspiration, and do not insert nasogastric tube, which makes this more likely

Key investigations

To establish the diagnosis (and also potentially therapeutic)

(1) Upper gastrointestinal endoscopy
- Within 24 h of admission in anyone with a substantial gastrointestinal bleed
- Urgently if oesophageal varices are suspected or the patient is actively bleeding

See Table 13 for assessment of risk of rebleeding and mortality after endoscopy

Other important tests

(1) Full blood count—but remember that the initial haemoglobin concentration is a poor estimate of the volume of acute blood loss
(2) Electrolytes, renal and liver function tests
(3) Coagulation screen
(4) To pursue possibility and causes of chronic liver disease (if clinically indicated)

Further management

(1) Inform surgical colleagues of all cases of substantial gastrointestinal haemorrhage immediately
(2) Dependent on cause of haemorrhage, e.g.
- Acid suppression for ulcer healing—high dose intravenous proton pump inhibitor, e.g. omeprazole 80 mg bolus followed by 8 mg/h
- Eradication of *H. pylori*

Table 13 Risk of rebleeding and mortality following upper gastrointestinal haemorrhage (Rockall score)

Clinical parameters				
Score	0	1	2	3
Age (years)	<60	60–79	80+	
Shock	SBP >100 mmHg Pulse <100/min	SBP >100 mmHg Pulse >100/min	SBP <100 mmHg	
Comorbidity	None	Other	Cardiac failure Ischaemic heart disease	Renal failure Liver failure
Total clinical score	0	2	4	6
Mortality (%)	0.2	5	24	49

Endoscopic parameters				
Score	0	1	2	3
Diagnosis	No lesion seen Mallory Weiss	Other diagnosis	Malignancy	
Major stigmata of recent haemorrhage	None		Blood in upper gastrointestinal tract Adherent clot Visible vessel	

Total clinical and endoscopic score	0	2	4	6	8+
Mortality (%)	0	0.2	5	17	41
Re-bleeding (%)	5	5	14	32	41

SBP, systolic blood pressure

Table 14 Management of bleeding from oesophageal varices

Resuscitation	**As described above in Emergency Medicine, 3.1**
Coagulopathy	Correct if present • Give vitamin K, 1 mg IV • Maintain platelet count >25 × 10⁹ /l • Give 2 units of fresh frozen plasma for every 4 units of blood or packed cells
Pharmacological measures to reduce haemorrhage	Consider • Vasopressin, 20 units intravenously over 15 min, followed by 20 U/h IV • Terlipressin, 2–4 mg intravenous bolus, followed by 1–2 mg IV every 4–6 h as needed for up to 72 h • Octreotide 50 μg intravenous bolus, followed by 50μg/h IV for 5 days Note • Nitrates are often given (sublingually, as transdermal patch, or intravenously) concurrently with vasopressin to reduce side-effects
Urgent endoscopy	Banding or sclerotherapy can stop bleeding, hence immediate liaison with specialist gastroenterological/hepatological services is essential in cases of suspected variceal haemorrhage
Sengstaken-Blakemore tube	Consider if • Haemorrhage is torrential • Other factors prevent safe emergency endoscopy

3.2 Lower gastrointestinal haemorrhage

See Chapter 14.3.2 in main text

Clinical features

History

(1) Haemorrhoids
(2) Abdominal pain—if long-standing and intermittent may suggest diverticular disease, if severe may indicate mesenteric ischaemia
(3) Previous lower gastrointestinal investigation or surgery
(4) To suggest recent development of anaemia
(5) Anorexia, weight loss, recent alteration in bowel habit (consider malignancy)
(6) Drugs that predispose to gastrointestinal haemorrhage—aspirin, non-steroidal anti-inflammatory agents, anticoagulants
(7) Risk factors for, or presence of, chronic liver disease (consider rectal varices)
(8) Family history—colonic polyps/neoplasia, hereditary haemorrhagic telangiectasia

Examination

(1) State of circulation—temperature of peripheries, pulse rate, blood pressure, jugular venous pressure
(2) Mucous membranes—chronic anaemia
(3) Jaundice—suggests malignancy or chronic liver disease
(4) Lymphadenopathy—suggests malignancy
(5) Abdomen—for localized tendeness, peritonism or palpable mass
(6) Rectal examination—for piles and blood
(7) Peripheral vasculature—generalized disease increases likelihood of mesenteric ischaemia
(8) Telangiectasiae on skin or mucosae

Notes

The most reliable signs of intravascular volume depletion are postural hypotension (sitting versus lying) and a low jugular venous pressure

Immediate management

If cardiorespiratory collapse, as described in Emergency Medicine, section 1.2

(1) Establish intravenous access—as Emergency Medicine, section 3.1
(2) If clinical evidence of intravascular volume depletion, resuscitate as described in Emergency Medicine, section 3.1
(3) Cross-match blood for transfusion

Also

(4) Keep oxygen saturation >92% (monitor using pulse oximetery), giving high flow oxygen (10 l/min) by face mask with reservoir bag if needed
(5) Insert urinary catheter and monitor fluid input/output hourly in any patient with substantial gastrointestinal haemorrhage—a satisfactory urine output is the best guage of adequate resuscitation
(6) Correct any coagulopathy—see Emergency Medicine, Section 1.9, Table 3 (iatrogenic overanticoagulation) and Section 9.1 (disseminated intravascular coagulation)

Key investigations

To establish the diagnosis

In all patients

(1) Proctoscopy and rigid sigmoidoscopy

As required:

(2) Colonoscopy
(3) Mesenteric angiography

Other important tests

(1) Full blood count
(2) Electrolytes, renal and liver function tests, coagulation screen, inflammatory markers
(3) To pursue possibility and causes of chronic liver disease (if clinically indicated)

Further management

(1) Inform surgical colleagues of all cases of substantial gastrointestinal haemorrhage immediately
(2) Dependent on cause of haemorrhage

3.3 Acute colitis

See Chapters 14.11 and 14.17 in main text

Clinical features

History

(1) Bowel motions—frequency and type (blood, mucus, pus)
(2) Abdominal pain
(3) Rapidity of onset
(4) Systemic features—fever, malaise, anorexia
(5) Previous episodes/known colitic disease
(6) Recent diet (contaminated or infected food)
(7) Have close contacts also been ill?
(8) Recent antibiotic treatment (consider *C. difficile*)
(9) Use of non-steroidal anti-inflammatory agents
(10) Associated vomiting
(11) Travel
(12) Risk factors for HIV (in some cases)

Examination

(1) State of circulation—temperature of peripheries, pulse rate, blood pressure, jugular venous pressure
(2) Signs of toxicity—fever
(3) Mucous membranes—chronic anaemia, ulceration, Candida
(4) Abdomen—for distension, localized tenderness, peritonism or palpable mass, or altered bowel sounds (absent, reduced)
(5) Rectal and perineal examination—for fistulae and nature of stool (blood, pus)
(6) Peripheral vasculature—generalized disease increases likelihood of ischaemic colitis
(7) Peripheral oedema—suggests hypoproteinaemia and chronic disease in this context

Notes

The most reliable signs of intravascular volume depletion are postural hypotension (sitting versus lying) and a low jugular venous pressure

Immediate management

If cardiorespiratory collapse, as described in Emergency Medicine, section 1.2

(1) Fluid and potassium resuscitation as necessary—see Emergency Medicine, sections 3.1 and 5.5.
(2) Most cases of acute colitis do not require antimicrobial therapy and settle with rehydration and time, the results of stool culture and rectal biopsy (which should be available in 24–48 h) being used to guide further treatment decisions. However, patients who are very ill with marked systemic symptoms and bloody diarrhoea (indicating probable colitis) should be given antimicrobial therapy pending culture results. Treat empirically with, e.g. ciprofloxacin (500–750 mg orally twice daily, or 200–400 mg intravenously twice daily) and metronidazole (400 mg orally three times daily or 500 mg intravenously three times daily).
(3) Also, in cases of known colitis (and to be considered in those with new and undiagnosed presentations of colitis), give steroids to those who are very ill, e.g. hydrocortisone 100 mg intravenously every 6 h or prednisolone 60 mg orally once daily

Note the features of a severe acute attack of ulcerative colitis (Table 15)

Key investigations

To establish the diagnosis

In all patients

(1) Abdominal radiograph—to assess extent of inflammation and to exclude toxic megacolon (required before proctoscopy/sigmoidoscopy), and erect chest radiograph—looking for air under diaphragm (perforation)
(2) Flexible or rigid sigmoidoscopy and rectal biopsy
(3) Stool—microscopy, culture and testing for *C. difficile* toxin

(4) Blood cultures

Other important tests

(1) Full blood count
(2) Group and save or crossmatch blood
(3) Electrolytes, renal and liver function tests, inflammatory markers, coagulation screen

Further management

(1) Inform surgical colleagues of all cases of acute colitis, urgently if radiography shows perforation or toxic dilatation
(2) Nurse in side room (if possible) until infective cause excluded
(3) Further management dependent on cause of colitis
(4) Note that suspected or proven food poisoning and typhoid are notifiable diseases in the UK

Table 15 Features that indicate a severe acute attack of ulcerative colitis

Bowels	Open 9–12 times in the first 24 h
Pulse	>100 /min
Fever	>38°C
Albumin	<30 g/l
CRP	>45 mg/dl
Abdominal radiograph	Toxic megacolon Mucosal islands Dilated small bowel

3.4 Acute hepatic failure

See Chapter 14.21.3 in main text

Clinical features

Definitions

(1) Acute hepatic failure is hepatocellular jaundice, hypertransaminasaemia, and prolongation of the prothrombin time associated with an acute liver disease
(2) Fulminant hepatic failure is acute liver failure with hepatic encephalopathy, most definitions specifying that this must occur within a particular time (variable) from the onset of clinical evidence of liver disease (usually jaundice)

History

(1) Jaundice—not always present in fulminant hepatic failure
(2) Confusion/drowsiness—note timing of onset of mental changes in relation to jaundice
(3) Relevant to cause of acute liver failure, e.g. paracetamol overdose, full drug history (prescribed and non-prescribed), risk factors for viral hepatitis
(4) Is there a background of chronic liver disease?—alcohol, risk factors for viral hepatitis
(5) Autoimmune conditions (associated with autoimmune chronic active hepatitis)
(6) Family history (Wilson's is a rare cause of fulminant hepatic failure)

Examination

(1) State of circulation—vital signs are normal in the early stages. Tachycardia and hypotension occur later. Hypertension and bradycardia are very late and sinister signs of cerebral oedema
(2) Jaundice
(3) Liver—usually tender, but normal size or only slightly enlarged in acute hepatic failure. If hepatomegaly consider hepatic venous obstruction (Budd Chiari), malignant infiltration, chronic liver disease
(4) Ascites—if substantial consider Budd Chiari
(5) Encephalopathy
  - Grade 1—mild confusion, irritability, decreased attention
  - Grade 2—drowsiness, lethargy, inappropriate behaviour
  - Grade 3—somnolent but rousable, disorientated
  - Grade 4—coma
(6) Signs of chronic liver disease

Notes

Focal neurological signs are not expected in acute hepatic failure. If present they suggest a focal cerebral lesion, most likely haemorrhage in this context

Immediate management

If cardiorespiratory collapse, as described in Emergency Medicine, section 1.2

Acute hepatic failure

(1) Oxygen, high flow with reservoir bag if needed, to achieve Pa_{O_2} >92% (monitor with pulse oximetry)
(2) Treat/prevent hypovolaemia—give 4.5% serum albumin intravenously to keep CVP at +10 cm of water
(3) Treat/prevent hypoglycaemia—give 50% glucose intravenously (central line) at 5–10 ml/h (monitor BM stix regularly)
(4) *N*-Acetyl cysteine by intravenous infusion
  - Paracetamol overdose
    150 mg/kg in 200 ml 5% dextrose over 15 min, then 50 mg/kg in 500 ml 5% dextrose over 4 h, then 100 mg/kg in 1000 ml 5% dextrose over 16 h
  - Other diagnosis
    150 mg/kg in 1000 ml 5% dextrose over 24 h
(5) Give prophylactic broad spectrum antibiotic, eg. cefotaxime 1 g intravenously twice daily
(6) Give prophylaxis against gastrointestinal stress ulceration, e.g. ranitidine (150 mg orally twice daily, 50 mg intravenously three times daily)

Hepatic encephalopathy

To prevent or treat

(1) Removal or correction of precipitating factors
  - Drugs—stop all if possible, particularly sedatives/

hypnotics and diuretics
- Fluid and electrolyte balance—maintain carefully. Avoid/treat dehydration, hypoglycaemia, hypokalaemia, hypophosphataemia

(2) Minimize absorption of nitrogenous substances

The following treatments may or may not be given
- Give enemas ($MgSO_4$ or phosphate) to encourage bowel emptying
- Give disaccharide laxative, e.g. lactulose 30–50 ml three times daily, dosage then adjusted to produce 2–3 soft stools daily
- Give broad spectrum poorly-absorbed antibiotic, e.g. neomycin 1 g four times daily by mouth

(3) If Grade 3 or 4 encephalopathy, also
- Intubate and ventilate
- Give parenteral feeding

Notes

(1) Hyponatraemia is common and due to water excess rather than sodium deficiency. It should be treated with fluid restriction and not by infusion of saline

(2) If there is a history of chronic high alcohol intake or malnourishment, give thiamine intravenously BEFORE giving glucose to avoid risk of precipitating Wernicke's encephalopathy, e.g. PabrinexTM intravenous high potency injection, 10 ml (2 ampoules) over 10 min (repeated three times daily)

(3) Insert urinary catheter and monitor fluid input/output hourly in any patient with acute hepatic failure

(4) Cerebral oedema
- Avoidance—Avoid overfilling with intravenous fluids
- Treatment—Nurse in quiet room with trunk and head elevated at 40°; consider transfer to facility where intracranial pressure can be monitored; consider mannitol 1 g/kg as intravenous bolus of 20% solution (if plasma osmolality <315 mosmol/kg and the patient is not oliguric), repeated 4 hourly (0.5 g/kg) if previous infusion induced a diuresis

Key investigations

To establish the presence of acute liver failure

(1) Liver blood tests—bilirubin, transaminases (ALT, AST, gGT)

(2) Prothrombin time/coagulation screen

To establish the cause of liver disease

If no history of paracetamol overdose

(1) Hepatitis B core IgM, hepatitis A IgM, liver autoantibodies, immunoglobulins

(2) Abdominal ultrasound and Doppler of hepatic veins—looking for size/echogenicity of liver, splenomegaly, signs of Budd Chiari

(3) If <40 years: serum copper and caeruloplasmin; ophthalmic examination for Kayser-Fleischer rings (Wilson's disease)

Note

(1) Tap ascites if present—microscopy, culture, and sensitivity. Culture/swab blood, urine, nasal, high vagina

(2) Do not correct coagulopathy unless the patient is bleeding: the prothrombin time is an important prognostic indicator

(3) Where the prothrombin time (in s) is greater than the time after a paracetamol overdose (in h), there is a substantial risk of developing acute liver failure

Other important tests

(1) Full blood count

(2) Glucose, renal function tests, amylase

(3) Arterial blood gases

Further management

(1) Discuss all cases of acute hepatic failure with a specialist (transplant) centre (see Table 16): urgent orthotopic liver transplantation may be required and appropriate

(2) Dependent on cause of hepatic failure

Table 16 Guidelines for referral to a specialist (transplant) centre in case of paracetamol overdose

Parameter	Day 2 (24–48 h)	Day 3 (48–72 h)	Day 4 (72–96 h)
Arterial pH	<7.3	<7.3	–
INR	>3	>4.5	Any rise
Encephalopathy	Present	Present	Present
Creatinine	>200 μmol/l	>200 μmol/l	>250 μmol/l
Hypoglycaemia	Present	Present	Present

3.5 The acute abdomen

See Chapter 14.3.1 in main text

Clinical features

History

(1) Abdominal pain—duration, constant or colicky, where is it worst (point with one finger), radiation

(2) Gastrointestinal symptoms—anorexia, nausea, vomiting, diarrhoea, constipation (precisely when were the bowels last open), blood in vomit or stool

(3) Urinary symptoms—frequency, pain on micturition, haematuria

(4) Gynaecological symptoms—last menstrual period, vaginal discharge

(5) To suggest sepsis—sweats, fevers, rigors

(6) History of gastrointestinal problems—indigestion, peptic ulceration, gallstones, pancreatitis

(7) History of atheromatous vascular disease—ischaemic heart disease, cerebrovascular disease, peripheral vascular disease (increase the likelihood

of bowel ischaemia or of abdominal aortic aneurysm, also relevant to surgical risk)

Examination

(1) State of circulation—temperature of peripheries, pulse rate, blood pressure, jugular venous pressure
(2) Signs of toxicity—fever
(3) Foetor
(4) Abdomen
- Inspection—distension, movement on respiration
- Palpation—tenderness, guarding, rigidity, rebound tenderness, palpable mass
- Auscultation—bowel sounds
- Check all hernial orifices and abdominal aorta

(5) Rectal examination—for tenderness and nature of stool, blood in stool
(6) Vaginal examination—tenderness, pelvic mass
(7) Test urine for blood

Immediate management

If cardiorespiratory collapse, as described in Emergency Medicine, section 1.2

(1) Establish intravenous access—as Emergency Medicine, section 3.1
(2) If clinical evidence of intravascular volume depletion, resuscitate as described in Emergency Medicine, section 3.1
(3) Immediate liaison with surgical colleagues
(4) Provide effective analgaesia e.g.
- Non-steroidal anti-inflammatory agent: e.g. diclofenac 75 mg intramuscularly, repeated after 30 min if necessary
- Opioid: e.g. morphine 5 mg subcutaneously plus 5 mg intramuscularly, repeated if necessary and accompanied by appropriate antiemetic, e.g. metoclopramide 10 mg IV over 1–2 min, or cyclizine 50 mg IV over 1–2 min

(5) Nasogastric tube
(6) Urinary catheter

Key investigations

To establish the diagnosis

(1) Abdominal radiograph—is there intestinal obstruction?
(2) Erect chest radiograph—is there gas under the diaphragm indicating intestinal perforation?
(3) Serum amylase—a substantial increase suggests pancreatitis
(4) Abdominal ultrasound—?free fluid/swollen appendix/ovarian cyst
(5) Abdominal CT scan

Note

Patients with generalized peritonitis require an urgent LAPAROTOMY provided that pancreatitis has been excluded. DO NOT DELAY. If the patient requires resuscitation, then make arrangements for theatre whilst initiating resuscitation and continue to resuscitate in the anaesthetic room. Do not wait 'until the patient is a bit better' before involving anaesthetic and surgical colleagues

Other important tests

(1) Full blood count
(2) Group and save or crossmatch blood
(3) Electrolytes, renal and liver function tests
(4) Coagulation screen

Further management

Dependent on the cause of the acute abdomen

Note

(1) Adhesive small bowel obstruction may resolve with conservative management
(2) Remember rare 'medical' causes of abdominal pain, e.g. pneumonia, shingles, drugs (digoxin), diabetes, sickle cell crisis, porphyria, familial mediterranean fever ... remember also that these are rare: if in doubt, diagnose a common condition

4 Renal

4.1 Acute renal failure

See Chapter 20.4 in main text

Clinical features

History

(1) There are no specific features to suggest acute renal failure: presentation is dominated by the precipitating condition
(2) Previous renal or urinary tract disease
(3) Drugs, prescribed and non-prescribed
(4) Evidence of multisystem disease
(5) ALWAYS seek the results of previous tests of renal function

Examination

(1) State of circulation—temperature of peripheries, pulse rate, blood pressure, jugular venous pressure
(2) Evidence of infection—fever, localizing signs
(3) Breathing—evidence of pulmonary oedema or acidosis (Kussmaul)
(4) Abdominal—is the bladder palpable? (obstruction)
(5) Rectal—is there pelvic malignancy? (obstruction)
(6) General—signs indicating multisystem disorder: rash, joints, eyes, nose. Are muscles swollen/tender? (rhabdomyolysis)

Note

The most reliable signs of intravascular volume depletion are postural hypotension (sitting versus lying) and a low jugular venous pressure

Immediate management

If cardiorespiratory collapse, as described in Emergency Medicine, section 1.2

Treatment of life-threatening complications
(1) Hyperkalaemia—see Emergency Medicine, section 5.4
(2) Pulmonary oedema—see Emergency Medicine, section 1.8
(3) Severe acidosis, causing circulatory compromise
(4) 'Gross uraemia', causing encephalopathy or bleeding

Aside from immediate life-saving medical treatments, patients with these features will need urgent renal replacement therapy (preferably by haemodialysis or haemofiltration, as dictated by clinical context) unless their renal function can be restored rapidly

Optimization of intravascular volume—many patients presenting with acute renal failure will be volume deplete
(1) Establish intravenous access—as Emergency Medicine, section 3.1
(2) If clinical evidence of intravascular volume depletion, resuscitate as described in Emergency Medicine, section 3.1

Oxygen, high flow with reservoir bag if needed, to achieve PaO_2 >92%

Make diagnosis of cause of renal failure
(1) Is it acute or chronic?—previous biochemical measurements; renal size on ultrasonography (small kidneys indicate chronic disease)
(2) Is it due to urinary obstruction?—history of problems with urinary flow, urinary stones etc.; dilated pelvicalyceal system on ultrasonography (but beware of obstruction without dilatation)
(3) Is it due to renal inflammation?—dipstick proteinuria and haematuria; urinary red cell casts
(4) Is it due to prerenal failure/acute tubular necrosis?—clinical context; evidence of circulatory compromise/intrvascular volume depletion

Note

(1) Stop all drugs that can be haemodynamically deleterious to renal function unless there is a very pressing indication for them, e.g. non-steroidal anti-inflammatory agents, angiotensin converting enzyme inhibitors, angiotensin II receptor blockers; also stop all nephrotoxic agents (e.g. aminoglycosides) and substitute non-toxic alternative
(2) Insert urinary catheter and monitor fluid input/output hourly in any patient with acute renal failure—remove after 24 h if the patient is anuric/oliguric

Key investigations

To establish the diagnosis

Renal function tests—acute renal failure is usually diagnosed clinically on the basis of rapid rise in serum creatinine

Other important tests

(1) ECG—looking for manifestations of hyperkalaemia
(2) Electrolytes—especially potassium
(3) Full blood count, coagulation screen, liver function tests
(4) Creatine kinase (rhabdomyolysis)
(5) Blood and other cultures—if clinically indicated
(6) Autoimmune/vasculitic screen (anti-GBM, ANCA, ANA, immunoglobulins, cryoglobulins)—if clinically indicated
(7) Ultrasonography of urinary tract—to determine renal size and look for evidence of obstruction
(8) Chest radiograph—looking for pulmonary oedema or (less likely) evidence of lung haemorrhage in pulmonary-renal syndrome
(9) Arterial blood gases—quantitate acidosis

Further management

Dependent on the cause of acute renal failure

Note

(1) When intravascular volume has been restored to normal (JVP clearly visible/CVP in normal range; no postural drop in blood pressure), fluid input should

then be given in equal volume to measured output of urine and other fluids, plus an allowance (500–1000 ml/day) for insensible losses. The prescription of fluid should be refined on the basis of (at least) twice daily clinical examination and daily measurement of the patient's weight

(2) Precise diagnosis of the cause of acute renal failure due to renal inflammation (glomerulonephritis, tubulointerstitial nephritis, vasculitis) will probably require renal biopsy

(3) If imaging suggests urinary obstruction, then this requires urgent relief, e.g. by urethral catheterization, suprapubic catheterization or percutaneous antegrade nephrostomy as appropriate

4.2 Rhabdomyolysis

See Chapter 20.5 in main text

Clinical features

Rhabdomyolysis is the breakdown of muscle fibres, when leakage of potentially toxic cellular contents into the circulation can lead to hypovolaemia, acidosis, hyperkalaemia, acute renal failure, and disseminated intravascular coagulation.

History

Muscular symptoms

(1) Pain, tenderness—focal or generalized
(2) May be none

Related to cause

(1) Focal muscle damage
- Obvious—e.g. crush injury, high-voltage electrical injury
- Not so obvious—e.g. ischaemic injury following arterial embolus to limb; pressure damage following prolonged immobilization (commonly coma)

(2) Generalized muscle damage
- Excessive muscular activity
  - Severe exercise—e.g. marathon running
  - Epileptic fitting—prolonged (see Emergency Medicine, section 6.5)
  - Status asthmaticus
  - Severe dystonia
  - Acute psychosis
- Infections
  - Septicaemia—see Emergency Medicine, section 7.7
  - Viral myositis—e.g. influenza
- Toxins
  - Prescribed drugs—e.g. HMG CoA reductase inhibitors
  - Substance abuse—e.g. alcohol, barbiturates, opioids, methanol, ethylene glycol (antifreeze), cocaine, amphetamine, ecstacy (MDMA), LSD (lysergic acid diethylamide)
  - Other—e.g. snake bite, spider (black widow), bee sting (multiple), carbon monoxide, toluene, hemlock (quail that have eaten hemlock)
- Heatstroke (see Emergency Medicine, section 9.3)
- Malignant hyperpyrexia (see Emergency Medicine, section 9.3)
- Neuroleptic malignant syndrome (see Emergency Medicine, section 9.3)
- Myopathies
  - Consider particularly if rhabdomyolysis occurs without clear precipitant
  - Metabolic—ask for history of intermittent muscular fatigue/pain, e.g. McCardle's syndrome
  - Inflammatory—e.g. polymyositis
- Metabolic /endocrine
  - Hypothyroidism
  - Electrolyte disturbance—e.g. hypokalaemia
  - Diabetic ketoacidosis

Examination

General

(1) Vital signs—temperature, pulse rate, blood pressure, respiratory rate
(2) Full physical examination

For cause of rhabdomyolysis

(1) Muscles
- Are any swollen or tender?
- Is there a compartment syndrome?

(2) Ischaemia
- Are legs and arms all well perfused?
- Can you feel all peripheral pulses?

(3) Pressure damage
- Look especially at the back of the head, spine, pelvis and heels—pressure sores indicate likelihood of pressure damage to muscles

(4) Systemic condition
- Rash—septicaemia (common), dermatomyositis (very rare)
- Slow relaxing tendon jerks (hypothyroidism)

Immediate management

As for acute renal failure: see Emergency Medicine, section 4.1

To prevent rhabdomyolysis from leading to renal failure

(1) Restore intravascular volume rapidly: see Emergency Medicine, section 3.1

(2) Monitor
- Urine output—urethral catheter
- Urinary pH—dipstick

(3) Fluid

Encourage brisk diuresis (urine output >150 ml/h) of alkaline urine (myoglobin more soluble at elevated pH)—when intravascular volume has been restored give:
- 0.9% sodium chloride/5% dextrose (alternating

bags), or 0.45% sodium chloride and 2.5% dextrose (same bag), at 200 ml/h—adjust rate to achieve urine output of approx 200 ml/h
- 1.25% sodium bicarbonate (=150 mmol/l each of sodium and bicarbonate) at 25 ml/h—adjust rate to achieve urinary pH>7

(4) Mannitol / diuretic
If urine output remains low give:
- Mannitol—1 g/kg as 20% solution intravenously over 30–60 min
and/or
- Diuretic—e.g. frusemide 40 mg (push) –500 mg (over 2 h) intravenously

Note

(1) If urine output remains low, then infusion of fluid as described here will inevitably lead to overload—FLUID INFUSION MUST BE REDUCED OR STOPPED BEFORE PULMONARY OEDEMA DEVELOPS. Then proceed as for acute renal failure (see Emergency Medicine, section 4.1)

(2) There is no randomized controlled trial proof of the efficacy of a regimen comprising high volume fluid infusion/alkalinization/mannitol such as that described here, but use of this (or similar) treatment produces outcomes far superior to historical controls

(3) Do not correct hypocalcaemia with calcium (risk of inducing / worsening metastatic calcification)

Key investigations

To establish the diagnosis

(1) Urine
- Dipstick test positive for blood, but microscopy shows no red blood cells

(2) Blood
- Creatine kinase—grossly elevated in severe cases (>10,000 IU/l)

Other important tests

(1) ECG
- Look for features of hyperkalaemia (see Emergency Medicine, section 5.4)

(2) Blood
- Electrolytes
  Hyperkalaemia—POTENTIALLY LIFE THREATENING. May develop rapidly. See Emergency Medicine, section 5.4
  Hypocalcaemia, hyperphosphataemia, hyperuricaemia
- Renal function
- Liver function tests—elevated transaminases from muscle (also LDH)
- Coagulate on screen—risk of disseminated intravascular coagulation

(3) As dictated by clinical suspicion, e.g.
- Blood cultures
- Thyroid function tests
- Muscle biopsy

Further management

(1) Dependent on the cause of rhabdomyolysis

(2) Compartment syndrome—measure compartment pressure. Consider fasciotomy if elevated

5 Metabolic and endocrine

5.1 Hypoglycaemia

See Section 12.11 in main text

Clinical features

History

(1) Coma
(2) Epileptic fitting
(3) Confusion and/or delirium
(4) Focal neurological signs (including hemiplegia, uncommon)

The patient may not be able to give any useful history: obtain as much information as possible from others in attendance (relatives, friends, ambulance crew, bystanders etc.). Ask in particular regarding:

(1) Diabetes mellitus
(2) Patient self-medication, and access to insulin/oral hypoglycaemic agents
(3) Previous episodes
(4) Alcohol and food consumption
(5) Other medical conditions

Examination

Immediate priorities

(1) Airway, breathing, circulation
(2) Glasgow Coma Score
(3) Bedside stick test for blood glucose

Other features

(4) Typically very pale and shut down peripherally with a cold sweat
(5) Evidence that the patient is diabetic: search for Medic Alert bracelet/necklace, medication (insulin, oral hypoglycaemic agents), documentation (glucose monitoring, outpatient clinics), sites of insulin injection
(6) Evidence of chronic liver disease or endocrine disorder

Immediate management

If cardiorespiratory collapse, as described in Emergency Medicine, section 1.2

Give glucose after establishing hypoglycaemia by bedside stick test, as follows:

- Patient alert and co-operative: give glucose 10–20 g by mouth (2 teaspoons sugar, or 3 sugar lumps, or one 23 g oral ampoule of Hypostop™ gel)
- If impaired consciousness and not protecting airway: give glucose 50% solution, 50 ml intravenously (note that the solution is viscous and irritant if extravasated, hence give through large bore needle/cannula into large vein)
- If impaired consciousness, not protecting airway and intravenous access not possible: give glucagon 1 unit (= 1 mg) intramuscularly

Repeat blood sugar measurement 10 min later: repeat glucose if still hypoglycaemic

Note

Hypoglycaemic symptoms are unusual if the plasma glucose is >2.5 mmol/l, but the threshold varies from person to person; hence it is appropriate to administer one dose of glucose intravenously (50% solution, 50 ml) to any patient with impaired consciousness whose plasma glucose is <3.0 mmol/l

Key investigations

To establish the diagnosis

Blood glucose—take sample through cannula BEFORE giving intravenous glucose

Other important tests

Hypoglycaemia in a known diabetic is unlikely to require further investigation. However, if the situation is not clear-cut, then a serum sample should be taken BEFORE intravenous glucose (or intramuscular glucagon) is given for serum insulin and C-peptide levels—to determine whether hypoglycaemia is due to endogenous or exogenous insulin

The following investigations may also be appropriate

- Electrolytes, renal and liver function tests
- Blood and other cultures—if clinical suspicion of sepsis
- Tests for endocrine disease—adrenocortical insufficiency, hypothyroidism, hypopituitarism
- Salicylate level—if possibility of overdose
- Chest radiograph—?aspiration in any patient who has been unconscious

Further management

Dependent on the cause of hypoglycaemia

Note

(1) Hypoglycaemia may recur—patients who have been given intravenous glucose and recovered from hypoglycaemia should be observed for at least 12 h, longer if they have taken long acting insulin/oral hypoglycaemic agents
(2) Education—most cases of hypoglycaemia occur in known diabetics and can be avoided by the patient checking their blood glucose and responding appropriately in the event of warning signals

5.2 Diabetic ketoacidosis

See Section 12.11 in main text

Clinical features

History

(1) Polyuria and polydipsia
(2) Drowsiness
(3) To suggest precipitating condition—often infection, but can be any acute illness
(4) Monitoring and treatment of diabetes (in known diabetics)—in particular recent details of blood glucose measurements and medication with insulin or oral hypoglycaemic agents

Examination

(1) State of circulation/dehydration—temperature of peripheries, skin turgor, pulse rate, blood pressure, tongue and mucous membranes, eyes, jugular venous pressure
(2) Breathing—in particular for indication of acidosis (Kussmaul) and for smell of ketones
(3) Glasgow Coma Score.
(4) Evidence of infection—fever, localizing signs, including careful examination of the feet and skin for ulceration/sepsis

Note

(1) The most reliable signs of intravascular volume depletion are postural hypotension (sitting versus lying) and a low jugular venous pressure
(2) Examine carefully for evidence of complications of diabetes, but not in the immediate emergency setting

Immediate management

If cardiorespiratory collapse, as described in Emergency Medicine, section 1.2

(1) Restoration of intravascular volume/hydration—patients will typically have a total body fluid deficit of 3–6 litres
  - Establish intravenous access—as Emergency Medicine, section 3.1
  - Give 1 litre of colloid as fast as possible (if hypotensive and shut down peripherally, if not, then omit this and proceed directly to give saline)
  - 0.9% saline, 1 litre over 30 min, then
  - 0.9% saline, 1 litre over 1 h, with potassium (see below), then
  - 0.9% saline, 1 litre over 2 h, with potassium (see below), then
  - 0.9% saline, 1 litre every 4–6 h until rehydrated, with potassium (see below)
  - When blood glucose <15 mmol/l, switch from saline to 5% dextrose infusion until eating normally (do NOT simply allow the glucose concentration to keep falling into the normal range, reducing the insulin infusion rate to low levels according to the sliding scale. The patient continues to require insulin in dosage sufficient to allow them to metabolize ketones effectively)

(2) Correction of electrolyte imbalance—all patients will have a very substantial deficit in body potassium, even though serum potassium concentration will usually be elevated at presentation. Replace potassium as follows, monitoring the serum concentration every few hours:

Serum potassium (mmol/l)	Potassium (mmol) added to each litre of fluid replacement
<3	40
<4	30
<5	20

(3) Correction of hyperglycaemia
Give insulin (actrapid 50 units mixed in 50 ml of 0.9 per cent saline) intravenously according to a sliding scale as follows:

Blood glucose, measured hourly (mmol/l; reagent stick	Insulin rate (units/h)
<4	0.5
4–7	1
7.1–11	2
11.1–15	3
15.1–19	4
19.1–24	5
>24	6

(4) Correction of acidosis
Acidosis will correct with restoration of circulating volume and administration of insulin; hence most cases do NOT require administration of bicarbonate. However, consider giving sodium bicarbonate (1.26% solution, 500 ml by intravenous infusion over 1 h) in cases where there is profound acidosis (e.g. arterial pH<7.0) that is thought to be causing circulatory compromise

Also

(1) Empty the stomach with nasogastic tube—gastroparesis/acute gastric dilatation is a particular risk in diabetic ketoacidosis, with a high risk of vomiting and aspiration, which can be fatal
(2) Give prophylaxis against venous thromboembolism (high risk) with low molecular weight heparin, e.g. enoxaparin 40 mg by subcutaneous injection once daily

And

Treat any precipitating condition vigorously. Note that surgical attention may be required, in particular when there is foot sepsis

Note

(1) Hyperosmolar non-ketotic diabetic coma (HONK)
  - Typically occurs in elderly patients with non-insulin dependent diabetes mellitus (NIDDM)
  - Glucose usually >40 mmol/l

- Not ketoacidotic (by definition)
- Look for plasma osmolality >350 mosmol/kg, calculated as 2 × (Na+K) + Urea + Glucose (all measured in mmol/l)
- Give colloid and 0.9% saline as for diabetic ketoacidosis, but switch to 0.45% saline when intravascular volume deficit is replaced (no postural hypotension, JVP clearly visible) if serum sodium remains >150 mmol/l
- Insulin requirements are typically low: hence use a reduced dose of insulin on the sliding scale to avoid hypoglycaemia

Key investigations

To establish the diagnosis

(1) Blood glucose
(2) Reagent stick test of urine for ketones

Other important tests

(1) Serum electrolytes
(2) Arterial blood gases
(3) Full blood count, renal and liver function tests
(4) 'Infection screen'—chest radiograph, urine and blood culture, swab any potentially infected site
(5) ECG (may have silent infarct)

Further management

Education—most cases of diabetic ketoacidosis occur in known diabetics and can be avoided. The key issue to emphasize is that illness increases insulin requirements, hence diabetics who are ill:

(1) Still need to take insulin, even if they are not eating
(2) Should check their blood glucose regularly (up to every 2 h or so)
(3) Should give themselves frequent appropriate doses of short-acting insulin if their blood glucose starts to rise
(4) Should have access to a phone number that they can call for advice if they run into problems

5.3 Metabolic acidosis

See Section 11.11 in main text

Clinical features

History

In the Emergency Medicine context presents non-specifically with

(1) Altered conscious level
(2) Circulatory collapse
(3) Hyperventilation.

Key points to establish

(4) In what circumstances was the patient found?
(5) History of diabetes mellitus
(6) History of chronic renal failure
(7) Overdose—most commonly salicylates
(8) Consumption of poison—e.g. ethylene glycol, methanol, antifreeze

Note

Medical conditions that can cause profound metabolic acidosis (with normal anion gap, see below) include:

(1) Severe diarrhoeal illness
(2) Renal tubular acidosis

Examination

(1) State of circulation—temperature of peripheries, pulse rate, blood pressure, jugular venous pressure
(2) Breathing—in particular for indication of acidosis (Kussmaul) and for smell of ketones
(3) Glasgow Coma Score

Immediate management

If cardiorespiratory collapse, as described in Emergency Medicine, section 1.2

Restoration of intravascular volume

(1) Establish intravenous access—as Emergency Medicine, section 3.1
(2) If clinical evidence of intravascular volume depletion, resuscitate as described in Emergency Medicine, section 3.1

Oxygen, high flow with reservoir bag if needed, to achieve $Pa\text{O}_2$ >92%

Should bicarbonate be given? This is a contentious issue: if acidosis is severe (pH<7.0) and there is circulatory compromise, give intravenous sodium bicarbonate (e.g. 1.26% solution, 500 ml by intravenous infusion over 1 h; or an equivalent amount of bicarbonate as a more concentrated solution if the patient is fluid overloaded), then assess clinical response and repeat estimation of arterial blood gases.

Note

Correction of metabolic acidosis requires careful attention to serum potassium concentration: profound hypokalaemia can occur if this is neglected

Key investigations

To establish the diagnosis

(1) Arterial blood gases—show metabolic acidosis (by definition)
(2) Plasma glucose and reagent stick test for urinary ketones—to exclude diabetic ketoacidosis (see Emergency Medicine, section 5.2)
(3) Plasma salicylate concentration—to exclude overdose
(4) Renal function tests—to exclude uraemic acidosis
(5) Plasma potassium—acidosis may be associated with hypokalaemia or hyperkalaemia, but with profound deficit in total body potassium in both situations. Close monitoring required
(6) Blood lactate concentration—many types of severe illness are associated with lactic acidosis, especially overwhelming sepsis
(7) Plasma bicarbonate concentration
(8) Calculate the anion gap: are there unusual anions in the blood? The blood 'anion gap', calculated as (Na^+

$+ K^+) - (Cl^- + HCO_3^-)$, usually equals 10–18 mmol/l. If there is acidosis with a high anion gap, then there must be an unmeasured substance in the blood, in which case discuss measurement of specific toxins with a clinical biochemist

Other important tests

(1) Full blood count, electrolytes, liver function tests
(2) Blood paracetamol level (rarely causes profound acidosis, but combined overdoses are common)
(3) Chest radiograph—consider aspiration in any patient with a depressed conscious level
(4) Abdominal radiograph—in cases of unexplained normal anion gap acidosis: renal tubular acidosis may be associated with nephrocalcinosis

Further management Dependent on the cause of metabolic acidosis

5.4 Hyperkalaemia

See Chapters 20.2.2 and 20.4 in main text

Clinical features

History

(1) Hyperkalaemia does not produce specific symptoms. Patients may sometimes develop 'odd feelings' in their muscles, but these are rarely dramatic
(2) Cardiac arrest
(3) Context—almost always occurs in the context of acute or chronic renal failure

Examination

(1) Hyperkalaemia does not produce specific signs
(2) Cardiac arrhythmia

Immediate management

If there are ECG changes that are more severe than tenting of the T waves:

(1) Give 10 ml of 10% calcium gluconate by slow intravenous injection, repeated as necessary until ECG shows clear evidence of returning towards normal

If ECG changes are not severe, or after giving calcium gluconate:

(2) Give 10–20 units of soluble insulin in 50 ml of 50% dextrose intravenously over 20 min, and/or
(3) Give nebulized β_2-agonist, e.g salbutamol 10 mg

These treatments will lower serum potassium concentration by 1–2 mmol/l over 20–30 min and buy a few hours of time, but hyperkalaemia will recur unless the cause can be treated rapidly, hence consider:

(4) Referral to nephrological services for renal replacement therapy

Note

(5) Intravenous infusion of sodium bicarbonate 50–100 mmol (approx. 300–600 ml of 1.26% solution or approx. 50–100 ml of 8.4% solution) can usefully be employed to treat hyperkalaemia in the setting of severe acidosis. In other cases it has no advantage over insulin/dextrose or β_2-agonist and has the disadvantages of not only requiring a substantial sodium/fluid load (a problem in those who are already overloaded), but also that concentrated solutions are chemically irritant and hence must be administered through central venous lines

Key investigations

To establish the diagnosis

(1) ECG—the following changes occur progressively as the plasma potassium concentration rises
- Tenting of T waves
- PR interval lengthens and P wave diminishes before disappearing
- QRS complex widens
- 'Sine wave' pattern

(2) Serum potassium concentration >5.5 mmol/l

Other important tests

(1) Renal function tests
(2) To determine cause of acute renal failure—if clinical context is appropriate

Further management

(1) Ion exchange resins, eg. calcium resonium™ 15 g in water three of four times daily by mouth (with concurrent prescription of a laxative), or 30 g in methylcellulose solution given as an enema, retained for 9 h and then removed by irrigation—these can be helpful in patients with persistent (but not life-threatening) hyperkalaemia who would not otherwise require renal replacement therapy. Note, however, that ion exchange resins take at least 4 h to have any effect and are NOT an emergency treatment for hyperkalaemia
(2) Stop all drugs that might exacerbate hyperkalaemia unless there is a very pressing need for them and no alternative is available, e.g. potassium supplements, potassium-sparing diuretics, angiotensin converting enzyme inhibitors, angiotensin II receptor antagonists, trimethoprim, heparin
(3) Dependent on the cause of hyperkalaemia

5.5 Hypokalaemia

See Chapter 20.2.2 in main text

Clinical features

History

(1) In almost all cases of hypokalaemia there are no symptoms (or only non-specific symptoms) attributable to the low plasma potassium concentration
(2) Cardiac arrhythmia (rare)
(3) Muscular paralysis (very rare)
(4) Relevant to cause of hypokalaemia

Examination

(1) Hypokalaemia does not produce specific signs
(2) Cardiac arrhythmia
(3) Muscular paralysis (very rare)

Immediate management

Emergency treatment is rarely required.

If life-threatening cardiac arrhythmia or muscular paralysis

- Give 40 mmol of potassium intravenously via volumetric pump over 1 h, then repeat measurement of serum potassium concentration and adjust rate of potassium infusion as appropriate

If thyrotoxic periodic paralysis

- Give propanolol 3 mg/kg orally

Key investigations

To establish the diagnosis

(1) Defined by serum potassium concentration <3.5 mmol/l, severe <3.0 mmol/l

Other important tests

(1) ECG – looking for flattening of the T wave, depression of the ST segment, and the development of a prominent U wave, also for arrhythmia
(2) To determine cause of hypokalaemia

Further management

Dependent on the cause of hypokalaemia

5.6 Hyponatraemia

See Chapter 20.2.1 in main text

Clinical features

History

(1) Does not produce specific symptoms
(2) Altered consciousness, epileptic fitting
(3) Relevant to cause of hyponatraemia

Examination

(1) Glasgow Coma Score
(2) Fluid status
- Intravascular volume depletion—low JVP, postural hypotension
- Clinically normal volume status
- Volume expansion—peripheral oedema

Immediate management

Chronic asymptomatic hyponatraemia

Do NOT aim to correct rapidly:

(1) If intravascular volume depletion—give 0.9% saline intravenously until intravascular volume restored, then restrict water intake
(2) If euvolaemic or hypervolaemic—restrict fluid intake to 1000 ml/day. Provide swabs to moisten the mouth and give the fluid allowance as ice cubes in aliquots throughout the day

Acute symptomatic hyponatraemia

Infuse saline intravenously, with the aim of:

- Effecting initial correction of serum sodium concentration at a rate of 1 mmol/l/h
- Reducing the rate of correction/stopping infusion of saline as soon as the patient's neurological condition begins to improve, or when serum sodium is elevated into the range 120–125mmol/l. DO NOT ATTEMPT RAPID CORRECTION OF SODIUM CONCENTRATION INTO THE NORMAL RANGE (probably increases risk of inducing central pontine myelinolysis)

Saline concentration	Rate of infusion (ml/h)
0.9%	3.3 × body weight (kg)
1.8%	1.7 × body weight (kg)
3.0%	1 × body weight (kg)

Monitor the serum sodium concentration regularly and adjust infusion as required

Note

If glucocorticoid deficiency is possible, then give steroid replacement immediately, e.g. hydrocortisone 100mg intravenously 6 hourly, until the diagnosis is excluded

Key investigations

To establish the diagnosis

(1) Defined by serum sodium concentration <130 mmol/l

Other important tests

(1) Plasma and urinary osmolality
(2) Urinary sodium concentration

Further management

Dependent on the cause of hyponatraemia

5.7 Hypercalcaemia

See Chapter 12.6 in main text

Clinical features

History

(1) Does not produce specific symptoms
(2) Acute hypercalcaemia—general malaise, anorexia, thirst, polyuria, constipation. In severe cases vomiting, confusion, coma
(3) Chronic hypercalcaemia—urinary stones, abdominal pain, mental disturbance
(4) Relevant to cause of hypercalcaemia

Examination

(1) Acute hypercalcaemia does not produce specific signs
(2) Fluid status
- Intravascular volume depletion—postural hypotension, low JVP
- Dehydration—reduced skin turgor, dry mucous membranes

(3) Evidence of malignancy

Immediate management

If cardiorespiratory collapse, as described in Emergency Medicine, section 1.2.

(1) Restoration of intravascular volume (if necessary)—as described in Emergency Medicine, section 3.1
(2) Saline diuresis—give 0.9% saline intravenously at a

rate of 1 l/6 h until calcium restored towards normal, assuming adequate urinary output (monitor carefully, and examine the patient regularly for signs of fluid overload). Give loop diuretic, e.g. frusemide 40–80 mg orally or intravenously twice daily, if urine output slow to increase

When diuresis initiated:

(3) Bisphosphonate, e.g. disodium pamidronate, 15–60 mg by intravenous infusion at a rate of 1 mg/min, repeated as necessary to give up to a total of 90 mg over 2–4 days

Also:

(4) Glucocorticoids, e.g. prednisolone 40–60 mg daily, if hypercalcaemia is due to sarcoidosis, vitamin D toxicity, or haematological malignancy

Note

If glucocorticoid deficiency is possible, then give steroid replacement immediately, e.g. hydrocortisone 100mg intravenously 6 hourly, until the diagnosis is excluded

Key investigations

To establish the diagnosis

(1) Defined by serum calcium concentration >2.6 mmol/l, acute symptomatic cases usually >3.0 mmol/l.

Other important tests

(1) Full blood count, electrolytes, renal and liver function tests

(2) Serum PTH, immunoglobulins. Protein electrophoresis of serum and urine

(3) Chest radiograph

(4) Directed by clinical suspicion of malignancy

Further management

Dependent on the cause of hypercalcaemia

5.8 Addisonian crisis

See Chapter 12.7.1 in main text

Clinical features

History

(1) Cardiovascular collapse

(2) Context of non-specific symptoms compatible with glucocorticoid deficiency: tiredness, weakness, dizziness, anorexia, weight loss, gastrointestinal disturbance. May have salt craving

(3) Related to cause: personal or family history of autoimmune/endocrine disease, steroid usage (and cessation), tuberculosis, recent flank pain (?adrenal haemorrhage/infarction)

(4) May occur in context of septicaemia

Examination

(1) State of circulation—temperature of peripheries, pulse rate, blood pressure, jugular venous pressure

(2) Hyperpigmentation—palmar creases, scars and buccal mucosae

(3) Loss of axillary and pubic hair in women

(4) Vitiligo

Immediate management

If cardiorespiratory collapse, as described in Emergency Medicine, section 1.2.

(1) Restoration of intravascular volume—give 0.9% saline intravenously as described in Emergency Medicine, section 3.1

(2) Steroid, e.g. hydrocortisone 100 mg intravenously (give immediately, then every 6 h)

Key investigations

To establish the diagnosis

(1) Serum cortisol and ACTH—taken at the time of venous cannulation for resuscitation

(2) Short synacthen test—performed later

Other important tests

(1) Electrolytes, glucose, renal function tests, calcium, full blood count

(2) Autoantibodies (adrenal, thyroid, intrinsic factor)

(3) Thyroid function

(4) Plasma renin activity—to assess mineralocorticoid status (high renin in primary adrenal insufficiency; not high in secondary adrenal insufficiency, where mineralocorticoid reserve is normal)

(5) Chest radiograph—small heart, ?evidence of TB.

(6) Adrenal CT scanning (where not available, abdominal radiograph—when adrenal calcification suggests TB)

Further management

(1) Long-term steroid replacement therapy: usually hydrocortisone (30 mg/day in divided doses), also fludrocortisone (50–150 μg/day) if mineralocorticoid deficient

(2) Education—patients need to know that they will require increased steroid dosage at times of intercurrent illness. All patients must carry a steroid card. Medic Alert bracelet

5.9 Thyrotoxic crisis

See Chapter 12.4 in main text

Clinical features

History

(1) Usually known thyroid disease

(2) Compatible with thyrotoxicosis: weight loss, palpitations, heat intolerance, sweating, diarrhoea, tremor, agitation/anxiety/irritability

(3) Precipitant of thyrotoxic crisis: infection, trauma, withdrawal of antithyroid drug therapy, radio-iodine treatment, iodinated contrast dyes, thyroid surgery, childbirth

(4) Personal or family history of autoimmune/endocrine disease

Examination

(1) Hyperpyrexia
(2) Profuse sweating
(3) Extreme restlessness, confusion, psychosis, eventually progressing to coma
(4) Cardiac arrhythmia—particularly fast atrial fibrillation. Eventually cardiorespiratory collapse
(5) Signs of thyroid disorder—goitre, eye signs of Graves' disease

Immediate management

THYROTOXIC CRISIS IS A POTENTIALLY FATAL DISORDER THAT REQUIRES IMMEDIATE TREATMENT ON THE BASIS OF CLINICAL SUSPICION

If cardiorespiratory collapse, as described in Emergency Medicine, section 1.2.
Restoration of intravascular volume—as described in Emergency Medicine, section 3.1
Oxygen, high flow with reservoir bag if needed, to achieve $Pa{O_2}$ >92%
Give

(1) Antithyroid drug: propylthiouracil is better than carbimazole in thyrotoxic crisis
   - Propylthiouracil 600 mg orally or via NG tube given immediately, then 250 mg every 6 h (may also be given rectally if severe vomiting prevents oral/NG route), or
   - Carbimazole 20 mg orally or via NG tube given immediately, then 20 mg every 6 h
(2) Iodide, starting 1–4 h after the antithyroid drug
   - Aqueous iodine oral solution, e.g. Lugol's (iodine 5%, potassium iodide 10% in purified water) 5 drops orally or via NG tube every 6 h
(3) Hydrocortisone, 200 mg intravenously, then 100 mg every 8 h
(4) Propanolol, 1 mg by intravenous injection over 1 min, repeated if necessary every 2 min to maximum of 5 mg, then 40–80 mg orally every 6 h
(5) Active cooling—cooling blankets, antipyretics (use paracetamol, not aspirin, which displaces thyroid hormone from thyroid-binding globulin)

Consider

(6) Digoxin for atrial fibrillation—may need larger dose than usual
(7) Diuretics for pulmonary oedema

Also

(8) Specific treatment of precipitating event (if possible)

Key investigations

To establish the diagnosis

Thyroid function tests—these confirm the diagnosis of hyperthyroidism, but note that the diagnosis of thyrotoxic crisis is made on clinical grounds. The severity of disturbance of the thyroid function tests does not correlate with the clinical picture

Other important tests

(1) Full blood count, electrolytes, renal and liver function tests, calcium
(2) Autoantibodies (adrenal, thyroid, intrinsic factor)
(3) ECG—arrhythmia, especially atrial fibrillation
(4) Chest radiograph—pulmonary oedema, infection

Further management

Dependent on the cause of thyrotoxicosis

5.10 Pituitary apoplexy

See Chapter 12.2 in main text

Clinical features

History

Most commonly

(1) Sudden onset retro-orbital headache
(2) Visual field defect

Sometimes

(3) Nausea and vomiting
(4) Meningism
(5) Altered conscious level
(6) Diplopia

Also

(6) Compatible with hypopituitarism or hyperprolactinaemia: lethargy, reduced libido, oligomenorrhoea/amenorrhoea, impotence, galactorrhoea

Examination

(1) Glasgow Coma Score
(2) Vision—acuity and fields
(3) Eye movements—looking for ophthalmoplegia
(4) Signs of underlying pituitary disease, e.g. acromegaly, are rarely present

Immediate management

If cardiorespiratory collapse, as described in Emergency Medicine, section 1.2.
Oxygen, high flow with reservoir bag if needed, to achieve $Pa{O_2}$ >92%
On clinical suspicion of diagnosis

(1) Take blood for serum cortisol assay to establish baseline retrospectively
(2) Take blood for urgent prolactin assay
(3) Assume anterior pituitary dysfunction and give
   - Corticosteroid, e.g. hydrocortisone 100 mg intravenously (immediately, then every 6 h)

Key investigations

To establish the diagnosis

MRI (or CT) scan of pituitary fossa—looking for haemorrhage into pituitary adenoma or other tumour

Other important tests

(1) Electrolytes, glucose, renal function, calcium, full blood count, coagulation screen
(2) Anterior pituitary function—baseline tests: cortisol, thyroid function tests, prolactin, LH, FSH, oestrogen/testosterone

Further management

All cases require

(1) Full endocrine evaluation
(2) Management dependent on hormonal deficiencies and the cause of pituitary apoplexy

Prolactin <1500 mU/l

(1) If vision is severly affected—urgent surgical decompression
(2) If vision is not severely affected—consider surgical decompression within one week (improves visual and endocrine outcomes)

Prolactin >1500 mU/l (suggests prolactinoma)

(1) A conservative (non-surgical) approach may be adopted if there is no progressive visual or neurological deficit and prolactin levels are very high, suggesting a prolactinoma
(2) Start immediate treatment with dopamine agonist drug such as bromocriptine or cabergoline

5.11 Acute porphyria

See Chapter 11.5 in main text

Clinical features

History

Intermittent episodes of:

(1) Acute abdominal pain, vomiting and constipation
(2) Severe proximal limb and/or back pain
(3) Seizures, coma
(4) Psychiatric disturbance

Notes

(5) Family history—nearly all the acute porphyrias are dominantly inherited, but many carriers are latent
(6) Rash—in variegate and hereditary coproporphyria (which can cause acute neurovisceral attacks) but NOT in acute intermittent porphyria
(7) Precipitant—alcohol, sex steroids, drugs (see Table 17), anaesthetic agents, starvation

Examination

(1) Cardiovascular—looking for sinus tachycardia, hypertension
(2) Abdominal—may have signs indistinguishable from those of the acute 'surgical' abdomen, but tenderness is usually lacking
(3) Neurological—Glasgow Coma Score (if appropriate); look for sensorimotor neuropathy, respiratory muscle weakness

Immediate management

If cardiorespiratory collapse, as described in Emergency Medicine, section 1.2.

If coma, as described in Emergency Medicine, section 6.1

Oxygen, high flow with reservoir bag if needed, to achieve $Pa{O_2}$ >92%

(1) Stop all known precipitant drugs, especially any that have recently been prescribed. Consult Table 17 before prescribing ANY agent
(2) Give 5% dextrose intravenously, 1 litre every 8 h (except if hyponatraemic, when give reduced volume of more concentrated dextrose solution). Start high carbohydrate diet when patient able to eat
(3) Give haem arginate, 3 mg/kg once daily for 4 days (maximum 250 mg daily) by intravenous infusion in 0.9% saline over at least 30 min

Notes

(1) Supplies of haem arginate can be obtained from Orphan Europe Ltd., 32 Bell Street, Henley-on-Thames, Oxon RG9 2BH. Tel 44(0)1491–414333. e-mail: info.uk@orphan-europe.com. Also from the on-call pharmacist at the University College of Wales, Cardiff ([029] 2074 7747); St James' University Hospital, Leeds ([0113] 243 3144 or [0113] 283 7010); St Thomas' Hospital, London ([020] 7928 9292)
(2) Seizures pose difficulties since many anticonvulsants precipitate or worsen porphyric attacks: temazepam, lorazepam, and midazolam are probably safe
(3) Distress may be helped by chlorpromazine. Morphine and pethidine (safe) may be required
(4) Propanolol is useful for controlling hypertension and extreme tachycardia

Key investigations

To establish the diagnosis

(1) Detection of porphyrin precursors in fresh urine (which may rarely become red/purple/brown on standing)

Other important tests

(1) Electrolytes—may cause profound hyponatraemia. Monitor serum sodium daily in the acute phase
(2) Full blood count, renal and liver function tests, calcium
(3) ECG

Further investigation to exclude serious abdominal or neurological disease will be determined by clinical presentation, especially if excretion of haem precursors is normal, e.g.

(4) Amylase/chest and abdominal radiograph/CT abdomen/senior surgical opinion
(5) CT brain/lumbar puncture

Note

In a patient with known porphyria, the absence of excess porphobilinogen (PBG) or δ-aminolaevulinic acid (ALA) in the urine renders acute porphyria an unlikely cause of the current illness

Further management

(1) Seek expert advice to establish diagnosis and investigate family
(2) Medic Alert bracelet important as warning to health care personnel in the future

Table 17 Drugs unsafe for use in acute porphyrias

Drug groups (please check **FIRST**)	
Amphetamines	Diuretics[6]
Anabolic steroids	Ergot derivatives[7]
Antidepressants[1]	Gold salts
Antihistamines[2]	Hormone replacement therapy[5]
Barbiturates[3]	Menopausal steroids5
Benzodiazepines[4]	Progestogens[5]
Cephalosporins	Sulphonamides[8]
Contraceptives, steroid[5]	Sulphonylureas[9]
Individual drugs (please check groups above FIRST)	
Alcohol	Lidocaine (lignocaine)[14]
Aluminium-containing antacids[10]	Lisinopril
Aminoglutethimide	Loxapine
Amiodarone	Mebeverine
Azapropazone	Mefenamic acid
Baclofen	Meprobamate
Bromocriptine	Methotrexate
Busulfan	Methyldopa
Captopril	Metoclopramide[15]
Carbamazepine	Metyrapone
Carisoprodol	Miconazole
Chloral hydrate[11]	Mifepristone
Chlorambucil	Minoxidil[15]
Chloramphenicol	Nalidixic acid
Chloroform[12]	Nifedipine
Ciclosporin	Nitrofurantoin
Clonidine	Orphenadrine
Cocaine	Oxybutynin
Colistin	Oxycodone
Cyclophosphamide	Oxymetazoline
Cycloserine	Oxytetracycline
Danazol	Pentazocine[13]
Dapsone	Pentoxifylline (oxpentifylline)
Dexfenfluramine	Phenoxybenzamine
Dextropropoxyphene[13]	Phenylbutazone
Diclofenac	Phenytoin
Doxycycline	Piroxicam
Econazole	Prilocaine
Enflurane	Probenecid
Erythromycin	Pyrazinamide
Etamsylate	Ranitidine
Ethionamide	Rifabutin[16]
Ethosuximide	Rifampicin[16]
Etomidate	Simvastatin
Fenfluramine	Sulfinpyrazone
Flucloxacillin	Sulpiride
Flupentixol	Tamoxifen
Griseofulvin	Theophylline[17]
Halothane	Thioridazine
Hydralazine	Tinidazole
Hyoscine	Triclofos[11]
Isometheptene mucate	Trimethoprim
Isoniazid	Valproate[4]
Ketoconazole	Verapamil
Ketorolac	Zuclopenthixol

Quite modest changes in chemical structure can lead to changes in porphyrinogenicity but where possible general statements have been made about groups of drugs; these should be checked first.

[1] Includes tricyclic (and related) and MAOIs; fluoxetine thought to be safe.

[2] Cetirizine, chlorphenamine, cyclizine, diphenhydramine, doxylamine, ketotifen, loratadine, and alimemazine (trimeprazine) thought to be safe.

[3] Includes methohexital, primidone, and thiopental.

[4] Status epilepticus has been treated successfully with intravenous diazepam; temazepam is thought to be safe; where essential, seizure prophylaxis has been undertaken with clonazepam or valproate. Clobazam, lorazepam, and midazolam probably safe.

Table 17 Continued

[5] Progestogens are more porphyrinogenic than oestrogens; oestrogens may be safe at least in replacement doses. Progestogens should be avoided whenever possible by all women susceptible to acute porphyria; however, where non-hormonal contraception is inappropriate, progestogens may be used with extreme caution if the potential benefit outweighs risk. The risk of an acute attack is greatest in women who have had a previous attack or are aged under 30 years. Long-acting progestogen preparations should never be used in those at risk of acute porphyria.

[6] Acetazolamide, amiloride, bumetanide, cyclopenthiazide and triamterene have been used.

[7] Includes ergometrine (oxytocin probably safe), lisuride and pergolide.

[8] Includes co-trimoxazole and sulfasalazine.

[9] Glipizide is thought to be safe.

[10] Absorption limited but magnesium-containing antacids preferable.

[11] Although evidence of hazard is uncertain, manufacturer advises avoid.

[12] Small amounts in medicines probably safe.

[13] Buprenorphine, codeine, diamorphine, dihydrocodeine, fentanyl, morphine, and pethidine are thought to be safe.

[14] Bupivacaine is thought to be safe; lidocaine (lignocaine) and prilocaine may be used with caution.

[15] May be used with caution if safer alternative not available.

[16] Rifamycins have been used in a few patients without evidence of harm—use with caution if safer alternative not available.

[17] Includes aminophylline.

Reproduced from *British National Formulary* (March 2002), 43 with addition of lisinopril to list of unsafe drugs.

6 Neurological

6.1 Coma

See Chapter 24.13.1 in main text

Clinical features

History

Coma is defined as a Glasgow Coma Score (GCS) <8, hence the patient will not be able to give any useful history. Obtain as much information as possible from others in attendance (relatives, friends, ambulance crew, bystanders etc.). Ask in particular regarding:

(1) The circumstances in which the patient was found
(2) Alcohol consumption
(3) Diabetes mellitus
(4) Epilepsy
(5) Drugs of abuse, in particular opioids
(6) Head injury
(7) Regular medications
(8) Past medical history

Examination

Initial survey

(1) Airway, breathing, circulation
(2) Reagent stick test for blood glucose (?hypoglycaemia)
(3) Check for small pupils and slow respiratory rate (?opioid overdose)
(4) Check temperature (?hypothermia)
(5) Look for Medic Alert bracelet or necklace
(6) Check Glasgow Coma Score (see Table 18)

Further examination

(1) State of circulation—temperature of peripheries, pulse rate, blood pressure, JVP
(2) Respiratory—look for evidence of aspiration
(3) Neurological
    - Focal/lateralizing signs—a structural lesion is likely if these are present
    - Meningism
    - Movements (can be subtle)—status epilepticus
(4) Tongue biting or incontinence of urine—suggest (but do not prove) epilepsy
(5) Back of head and neck—for bruising or bleeding to suggest head injury
(6) Ears and nose—for bleeding or CSF leak to suggest basal skull fracture
(7) Search pockets etc. for clues—e.g. anticonvulsant tablets

Immediate management

If cardiorespiratory collapse, as described in Emergency Medicine, section 1.2

Nurse in recovery position (when injury to neck excluded).

Oxygen, high flow with reservoir bag if needed, to achieve Pa_{O_2} >92%. Consider oropharyngeal airway

Patients with a GCS <8 are likely to need endotracheal intubation to protect and maintain their airway if they do not respond to glucose or naloxone. This is obligatory if they need to be moved from an area where they can be given intensive nursing care to one where they cannot, e.g. to CT scanner

Establish intravenous access

(1) If hypoglycaemic—give 50 ml of 50% glucose (dextrose monohydrate) intravenously. IF IN DOUBT, TREAT
(2) If possibility of opioid overdose—give naloxone 0.8–2 mg intravenously, repeated at intervals of 2–3 min to a maximum of 10 mg. IF IN DOUBT, TREAT
(3) If hypothermic—start rewarming

Key investigations

To establish the diagnosis

(1) Glucose.
(2) CT brain—if diagnosis not clinically apparent and patient not improving rapidly. Look for:
    - Extradural, subdural, subarachnoid, or intracerebral haemorrhage
    - Signs of raised intracranial pressure
    - Focal ischaemia (may not be visible on early scan)
(3) Blood film for malaria—if relevant travel history

Other important tests

(1) Electrolytes, renal and liver function tests, calcium, full blood count
(2) ECG—note that 'ischaemic' changes can occur in subarachnoid haemorrhage
(3) Chest radiograph—?aspiration pneumonia
(4) Arterial blood gases—if diagnosis not clear, or if Pa_{O_2} <92% on air
(5) Sepsis screen (selected cases)
(6) Lumbar puncture (selected cases)
(7) EEG (selected cases, ?non-convulsive status)

Further management

Dependent on the cause of coma.

Table 18 Glasgow Coma Scale

Eye opening	Score	Verbal	Score	Motor (best response in any limb)	Score
Spontaneously	4	Orientated	5	Obeys commands	6
To speech	3	Confused conversation	4	Localizes to pain	5
To pain	2	Words	3	Withdraws to pain	4
None	1	Sounds	2	Flexor (decorticate) response to pain	3
		None	1	Extensor (decerebrate) response to pain	2
				None	1

The Glasgow Coma Score is obtained by adding the best eye, verbal and motor responses together: minimum = 3, maximum = 15, coma = 8 or less, significant deterioration = fall by 2 points or more.

Painful stimulation: rub knuckles on sternum, squeeze pencil or biro against nail bed. Do not use methods that might lead to bleeding or bruising, which includes supraorbital pressure.

6.2 Acute confusional state

See Chapter 24.8 and Section 30 in main text

Clinical features

History

Is the patient confused?:

(1) Establish that the patient is not dysphasic rather than confused

(2) Abbreviated Mental Test (AMT) score—a score of 6 or less is likely to indicate impaired cognition
- Age
- Time (to nearest hour)
- What year is it?
- Name of institution
- Recognition of two persons (can the patient identify your job and that of a nurse?)
- Date of birth (day and month)
- Year of First World War
- Name of present monarch
- Count backwards from 20 to 1

(3) The patient who is confused cannot (by definition) give an accurate and reliable account of themselves

Obtain as much information as possible from others in attendance (relatives, friends, ambulance crew, bystanders etc). Ask in particular regarding:

(1) The situation in which the patient was found

(2) Any recent change in health, in particular:
- Symptoms to suggest infection
- Medications—especially any recent change

(3) Previous cognitive function

(4) Alcohol consumption (consider intoxication, withdrawal, Wernicke's encephalopathy)

(5) Drugs of abuse (if relevant)

(6) Regular medications

(7) Past medical history

(8) Social circumstances

Examination

(1) General appearance—well-presented clothing and cleanliness indicates an acute problem or an assiduous carer.

(2) Nutritional state—reflects previous weeks/months

(3) Hydration state—reflects previous 48 h

(4) Full physical examination—look in particular for:
- Temperature—pyrexia or hypothermia
- Pulse rate, blood pressure, JVP—hypotension from any cause can lead to confusion
- Evidence of sepsis—in particular chest, urine, cellulitis
- Neurological—focal signs (indicating a focal neurological lesion, most commonly stroke), head injury, Wernicke's encephalopathy
- Evidence of organ failure—cardiac, respiratory, hepatic, renal
- Urinary retention or faecal impaction
- Hip or pelvic fracture.

Immediate management

If cardiorespiratory collapse, as described in Emergency Medicine, section 1.2.

Oxygen, high flow with reservoir bag if needed, to achieve $Pa{O_2}$ >92%

If hypoglycaemic—give 50 ml of 50% glucose (dextrose monohydrate) intravenously. IF IN DOUBT, TREAT

(1) Fluids—encourage oral intake, but if intravenous fluids are required, then insert venous cannula into flat site and bandage carefully

(2) Treat any obvious precipitating condition—if none apparent then consider initiating antibiotic treatment for, e.g. urinary infection, on a 'best guess' basis (e.g. ciprofloxacin 500 mg orally twice daily, but note local hospital policy)

(3) Anticipate and avoid problems:
- Do not exacerbate confusion—nurse in lit room (darkness makes confusion worse), expose to limited number of staff (many people 'popping in' increase confusion), enlist assistance from relatives/carers/friends (a sensible person that the patient knows can be enormously helpful)
- Pressure areas—appropriate mattress
- Urine—try to avoid catheterization if possible (will make any infection harder to clear), but need to strike a difficult balance with concern for skin/pressure areas
- Bowels—suppositories, laxative, enema as required
- Venous thromboembolism—low molecular weight heparin, e.g. enoxaparin 20 mg subcutaneously once daily

(4) Sedation—try to avoid if possible, but if necessary

use risperidone 0.5 mg orally twice daily (increased in steps of 0.5 mg twice daily to 1–2 mg twice daily) or haloperidol 0.5–2 mg orally/intramuscularly two to three times daily. (Dosage of both drugs appropriate for the elderly—higher doses likely to be required for younger patients)

Key investigations

To establish the diagnosis

These will be guided by any clinical leads, but as non-specific presentation is common, the following are advisable in almost all patients:

(1) Reagent stick test for blood glucose.
(2) Full blood count, electrolytes, renal and liver function tests, calcium, phosphate, cardiac enzymes, glucose, thyroid function, inflammatory marker (CRP or ESR)
(3) Oxygen saturation—check arterial blood gas if Pa_{O_2} <92%. on air
(4) Sepsis screen—urine dipstick test, urine and blood culture
(5) Chest radiograph
(6) ECG

Other important tests

Guided by clinical findings or results of screening investigations, e.g. new focal neurological signs—imaging of brain by CT scan or MRI

Further management

Dependent on the cause of confusion

6.3 Acute stroke

See Chapter 24.13.7 in main text

Clinical features

History

May be difficult to obtain, particularly if the patient has dysphasia. If this is the case, get as much information as possible from others in attendance (relatives, friends, ambulance crew, bystanders etc.)

(1) Focal neurological deficit—usually of sudden onset
(2) Previous episodes—stroke, transient ischaemic attack, amaurosis fugax
(3) Risk factors
(4) Other medical conditions
(5) Medications
(6) Normal level of functioning—do they need help with activities of daily living?
(7) Social circumstances

Examination

(1) Airway, breathing, circulation
(2) Neurological
   - Glasgow Coma Score
   - Nature of focal deficit (see Table 19)
(3) Cardiovascular—pulse rate and rhythm (?atrial fibrillation), blood pressure, carotid bruits, cardiac murmurs, absent peripheral pulses

Immediate management

If cardiorespiratory collapse, as described in Emergency Medicine, section 1.2.

(1) Nurse in recovery position if impairment of consciousness
(2) Oxygen, high flow with reservoir bag if needed, to achieve Pa_{O_2} >92%. Consider oropharyngeal airway
(3) Establish intravenous access
(4) Reagent stick test for blood glucose: if hypoglycaemic—give 50 ml of 50% glucose (dextrose monohydrate) intravenously. IF IN DOUBT, TREAT

Notes

(1) Urgent neurosurgical assessment is required for patients with large cerebellar infarcts or haemorrhages or hydrocephalus, and for some cases with cerebral haemorrhage
(2) There is no proven benefit for drugs in the limitation of neural damage, including corticosteroids, nimodipine, plasma volume expanders, barbiturates. or glutamate receptor antagonists. Patients treated rapidly (?within 3 h of stroke) may benefit from thrombolysis, but this should only be given in centres that use the treatment routinely, and preferably in the context of controlled trials

Key investigations

To establish the diagnosis

CT or MRI brain—also to distinguish between infarction and haemorrhage

Other important tests

(1) Full blood count, electrolytes, renal and liver function tests, calcium, inflammatory markers (CRP or ESR), coagulation screen
(2) ECG—look for arrhythmia or signs of recent myocardial infarction
(3) Chest radiograph—?aspiration pneumonia
(4) Echocardiography; ultrasound/Doppler examination of carotid arteries—in selected cases

Further management

Short term

(1) Nursing and physiotherapy—protect pressure areas, attention to bladder and bowels, prevent contractures, aid recovery of function, psychological support
(2) Hydration/nutrition—If swallowing impaired, stop oral feeding and start intravenous fluids
(3) Blood pressure—this is commonly elevated immediately after a stroke, cerebral autoregulation is impaired, and aggressive attempts to reduce it are likely to cause more harm than good. If BP >220/130 then many physicians would treat, e.g. using modified release nifedipine 10 mg orally, but some would only do so if there was evidence that the hypertension were causing acute organ damage

(4) Venous thromboembolism—high risk: use compression stockings
(5) Antiplatelet therapy—usually aspirin 300 mg once daily – should be started to prevent recurrence as soon as haemorrhage has been excluded
(6) Blood glucose—use intravenous sliding scale of insulin (see Emergency Medicine, section 5.2) to obtain good control in diabetics

Medium/long term
(1) Rehabilitation and social support as required
(2) Control of vascular risk factors—hypertension, hyperlipidaemia, cessation of cigarette smoking
(3) Consider imaging of the carotid arteries in all patients who have made a reasonable recovery from a carotid territory stroke: endarterectomy may be indicated

Table 19 A practical classification of stroke (the Oxfordshire community stroke subclassification system)

Total anterior circulation syndrome (TACS)	Large cortical stroke in middle cerebral artery, or middle and anterior cerebral artery territories	New higher cerebral dysfunction (e.g. dysphasia, dyscalculia, visuospatial disorder) + Homonymous visual field defect + Ipsilateral motor and/or sensory deficit involving two out of three of face, arm, or leg
Partial anterior circulation syndrome (PACS)	Cortical stroke in middle or anterior cerebral artery territories	Two out of three components of TACS Or New higher cerebral dysfunction alone Or Motor/sensory deficit more restricted than those classified as LACS (e.g. monoparesis)
Lacunar syndrome (LACS)	Subcortical stroke due to small vessel disease	Pure motor stroke Or Pure sensory stroke Or Sensorimotor stroke Or Ataxic hemiparesis Or Dysarthria and clumsy hand Note that evidence of higher cortical involvement or disturbance of consciousness excludes a lacunar syndrome

Table 19 Continued

Posterior circulation syndrome (PCS)	Ipsilateral cranial nerve palsy with contralateral motor/sensory deficit Or Bilateral motor and/or sensory deficit Or Disorder of conjugate eye movement Or Cerebellar dysfunction without ipsilateral pyramidal involvement (which would be an ataxic hemiparesis and classified as LACS) Or Isolated homonymous visual field defect

6.4 Subarachnoid haemorrhage

See Chapter 24.13.7 in main text

Clinical features

History
(1) Presentation is very variable: typically severe headache ('worst ever') of sudden onset, but can vary from minor symptoms to collapse/coma or sudden death
(2) Previous episodes; recent unusual headache
(3) Risk factors—hypertension, cigarette smoking, alcohol (binge drinking), adult polycystic kidney disease, connective tissue disorders (some)

Examination
(1) Airway, breathing, circulation
(2) Glasgow Coma Score
(3) Focal neurological signs—in particular:
- Third nerve palsy—posterior communicating artery aneurysm
- Sixth nerve palsy—posterior fossa aneurysm, but usually a false localizing sign
- Bilateral leg weakness—anterior communicating artery aneurysm
- Dysphasia/hemiparesis—middle cerebral artery aneurysm

(4) Neck rigidity
(5) Retinal haemorrhages
(6) Cardiovascular—arrhythmia, hypertension

Immediate management

If cardiorespiratory collapse, as described in Emergency Medicine, section 1.2.
(1) Nurse in recovery position if impairment of consciousness.
(2) Oxygen, high flow with reservoir bag if needed, to achieve $Pa{O_2}$ >92%. Consider oropharyngeal airway
(3) Establish intravenous access and resuscitate if volume depleted or dehydrated
(4) Bed rest for all patients

(5) Nimodipine 60 mg orally every 4 h, started within 4 days of subarachnoid haemorrhage and continued for 21 days, should be given to all patients with subarachnoid haemorrhage who are not hypotensive (systolic BP <110 mmHg). This is to prevent ischaemic neurological deficit
(6) Keep arterial pressure <160/100 mmHg (using conventional agents)

Key investigations

To establish the diagnosis

(1) CT brain, without contrast, taking thin cuts through the base
(2) Lumbar puncture—perform not earlier than 12 h after the ictus if CT normal: look for xanthochromia after centrifugation of CSF

Other important tests

(1) Electrolytes, renal and liver function tests, full blood count, coagulation screen
(2) ECG—note that 'ischaemic' changes can occur in subarachnoid haemorrhage
(3) Chest radiograph—?aspiration pneumonia

Further management

Depends on the patient's clinical condition: if

- GCS = 12 or more, or
- GCS <12 with space occupying intracranial haemorrhage or hydrocephalus

Then surgery should be considered in patients with proven intracranial aneurysms: hence discuss with neurosurgical colleagues with a view to arranging four-vessel angiography (CT angiograms may be done first, and sometimes instead)

6.5 Status epilepticus

See Chapter 24.13.3 in main text

Clinical features

Definition

Continuous seizures or serial (two or more) discrete seizures between which there is incomplete recovery of consciousness

History

(1) Loss of consciousness, usually with obvious fitting
The patient will not be able to give any useful history. Obtain as much information as possible from others in attendance (relatives, friends, ambulance crew, bystanders etc.). Ask in particular regarding:
(2) The circumstances in which the patient was found
(3) Past history of epilepsy
(4) Alcohol consumption
(5) Any possible drug abuse
(6) Diabetes mellitus
(7) Regular medications
(8) Any other medical history

Examination

Initial survey

(1) Airway, breathing, circulation
(2) Signs of injury—especially of tongue, which can compromise breathing
(3) Respiratory—?aspiration
(4) Glasgow Coma Score
(5) Medic Alert bracelet/necklace

Further examination

(1) Vital signs—temperature, pulse rate, blood pressure
(2) Neurological
    - Pupil size and reactions
    - Other brainstem signs
    - Symmetry of tone and reflexes in the limbs
    - Neck stiffness
    - Note that focal signs may indicate focal pathology, but can be seen as a post-ictal phenomenon (i.e. Todd's paresis)
(3) Search pockets etc. for clues—e.g. anticonvulsant tablets

Immediate management

If cardiorespiratory collapse, as described in Emergency Medicine, section 1.2.

(1) Place in recovery position (if possible)
(2) Oxygen, high flow with reservoir bag if needed, to achieve Pa_{O_2} >92%. Consider oropharyngeal airway, but do not try to insert one against resistance i.e. when the patient is actually fitting
(3) Establish intravenous access.
(4) Reagent stick test for blood glucose—if hypoglycaemic: give 50 ml of 50% glucose (dextrose monohydrate) intravenously. IF IN DOUBT (GLUCOSE <3 mmol/l), TREAT
(5) Anticonvulsant—first line
    - Lorazepam 0.1 mg/kg intravenously at 2 mg/min. THE FIRST LINE TREATMENT OF CHOICE
    - Diazepam 10–20 mg intravenously at a rate of 5 mg/min. This may be repeated after 30–60 min if necessary, and can be followed by infusion (add 10–40 mg of diazepam to 100 ml of 5% dextrose to make a solution containing 0.1- 0.4 mg/ml) at a rate of e.g. 5 mg/h, adjusted according to clinical response, but with maximum dose of 3 mg/kg body weight over 24 h
(6) Anticonvulsant—second line. If seizure activity still continues, consider
    - Fosphenytoin, 15 mg phenytoin-equivalent (PE)/kg body weight (fosphenytoin 1.5 mg = phenytoin 1 mg) by intravenous infusion at a rate of 100–150 mg PE/min, followed by 4–5 mg PE/kg daily in 1–2 divided doses. Dose adjusted according to clinical response and trough plasma phenytoin levels. THE SECOND LINE TREATMENT OF CHOICE

- Phenytoin, 15 mg/kg body weight by intravenous infusion at a rate not exceeding 50 mg/min, followed by 100 mg every 6–8 h. Dose adjusted according to clinical response and trough plasma-phenytoin levels

(7) Anticonvulsant—Third line treatments. If seizure activity still continues, consider
- Phenobarbital (phenobarbitone), 20 mg/kg by intravenous infusion at a rate of not more than 50–75 mg/min, maximum dose 1000 mg. Note that this treatment may lead to respiratory depression. THE THIRD LINE TREATMENT OF CHOICE
- Paraldehyde, 5–10 ml by deep intramuscular injection (not more than 5 ml at any one site), or 10–20 ml administered by enema as a 10% solution in physiological saline or mixed with an equal volume of olive oil. Note that this treatment is only to be used if other treatments listed above are not available

(8) Anaesthesia. If seizure activity still continues after first, second and third line treatments (or earlier if required to achieve adequate airway protection/ventilation):
- Call anaesthetist and arrange ICU admission for anaesthesia with thiopental or propofol. Ventilate with EEG monitoring until clinical and EEG epileptic activity ceases

Key investigations

To establish the diagnosis

Status epilepticus is a clinical diagnosis, although EEG is used to diagnose the very rare condition of non-convulsive status in a patient with unexplained coma

Other important tests

(1) A reagent stick test for blood glucose should be performed in all patients.

The intensity of further investigation depends on the context: the patient that is known to have epilepsy who has frequent prolonged seizures does not require extensive investigation after each and every one. In other cases:

(2) Glucose, electrolytes, renal and liver function tests, calcium, creatine kinase, anticonvulsant level (if appropriate)

And consider:

(3) Arterial blood gases.
(4) Chest radiograph—?aspiration
(5) ECG
(6) Sepsis screen
(7) Toxicology screen
(8) CT or MRI brain
(9) Lumbar puncture—only after imaging to exclude raised intracranial pressure or intracerebral mass

Further management

Dependent on the cause of status epilepticus

6.6 Spinal cord compression

See Chapters 24.13.16 and 24.13.17 in main text

Clinical features

History

Cord compression

(1) Leg weakness—developing over hours or days
(2) Sensory symptoms—in particular, is there a sensory level, which can be suspended?
(3) Bladder disturbance

Cause of cord compression

(1) Back pain
(2) Intervertebral discs—any previous problem?
(3) Malignancy—any known previous, or any features to suggest this diagnosis, e.g. anorexia, malaise, weight loss
(4) Infection—sweats, fevers, rigors. Tuberculosis. Risk factors for osteomyelitis or abscess, e.g. previous septicaemia (particularly staphylococcal), intravenous drug abuse, haemodialysis

Examination

Cord compression

(1) Motor—look for increased tone, weakness, and hyperreflexia below the site of the lesion. Do the plantars go up or down?
(2) Sensory—is there a sensory level, which can be suspended? In particular, check for sensory loss in the saddle area, which would suggest a cauda equina lesion
(3) Bladder—is this palpable?

Cause of cord compression

(1) General examination for signs of malignancy—e.g. cachexia, clubbing, lymphadenopathy, pallor, jaundice, chest/abdominal examination, pelvic mass
(2) Suggestion of infective cause—temperature

Immediate management

(1) Nurse on pressure-relieving mattress
(2) Relieve urinary retention with urethral catheter (if appropriate)
(3) EMERGENCY IMAGING AND CONSULTATION WITH NEUROSURGICAL COLLEAGUES
(4) Specific treatments depending on precise diagnosis
- Disc protrusion—surgical decompression
- Metastasis—high dose steroids (e.g. methylprednisolone) and radiotherapy
- Abscess—surgical decompression/drainage; antimicrobials. For an immunocompetent patient with a pyogenic abscess give intravenous antimicrobials as follows: third-generation cephalosporin, e.g. cefotaxime 1–2 g 12 hourly PLUS flucloxacillin 1–2 g 6 hourly PLUS metronidazole 500mg 8 hourly. Modify regimen when microbiological

results are available.
- Spinal cord tumours (rare)—neurosurgical intervention may be appropriate

Note

Acute spinal cord injury—give methylprednisolone 30 mg/kg as intravenous bolus over 1 h, followed by 4.0 mg/kg/h for 23 h

Key investigations

To establish the diagnosis

MRI spine, performed as an emergency (if this is not available, discuss best available imaging modality with radiological colleagues, e.g. CT scan, myelography)

Other important tests

(1) Full blood count, electrolytes, renal and liver function tests, calcium, inflammatory markers, coagulation screen, immunglobulins, and protein electrophoresis
(2) Urinary Bence Jones protein
(3) Chest radiograph

Other tests as dictated by clinical suspicion, e.g. blood cultures, lymph node biopsy

Further management

Dependent on the cause of spinal cord compression

6.7 Acute inflammatory polyneuritis (Guillain Barré)

See Chapter 24.19 in main text

Clinical features

History

(1) Sensory symptoms—begin distally and ascend symmetrically
(2) Motor—weakness, usually ascending (but can sometimes be proximal), symmetrical. Muscle pain is common (particularly lower back or interscapular)
(3) Legs usually worst affected, but can sometimes be arms
(4) Progression usually occurs over days (no longer than 4 weeks, by definition) but can sometimes be more rapid
(5) Patients often have upper respiratory tract or diarrhoeal illness (especially *Campylobacter jejuni*) in the few weeks prior to onset

Examination

(1) Motor—reduced tone; lower motor neurone weakness, distal > proximal; areflexia. May have facial involvement and ophthalmoplegia (Miller Fisher syndrome)
(2) Sensory—glove and stocking sensory disturbance, often mild
(3) Respiratory—RESPIRATORY FAILURE DUE TO MUSCLE WEAKNESS IS AN AVOIDABLE CAUSE OF DEATH: check forced vital capacity and monitor frequently
(4) Autonomic—look for variable pulse rate, variable arterial pressure, intestinal ileus, urinary retention

Immediate management

(1) Respiratory
- CONSIDER ELECTIVE ASSISTED VENTILATION SOONER RATHER THAN LATER IF THE PATIENT IS TIRING
- Note that tracheal suction can trigger hypotension or bradycardia in the presence of autonomic dysfunction

(2) Cardiac
- Monitor ECG
- Arrhythmias can be fatal—treat as appropriate
- Use antihypertensive drugs with extreme caution (if at all) in the face of autonomic dysfunction

(3) Fluids
- If gag reflex impaired—stop oral feeding and start intravenous fluids
- Will need to consider PEG feeding as an early option

(4) Nursing and physiotherapy
- Keep chest clear
- Protect pressure areas
- Attention to bladder and bowels
- Prevent contractures: move all joints through their full range of movement daily
- Aid recovery of function
- Psychological support: emphasize that most cases recover well

(5) Pain—give non-steroidal anti-inflammatory agents as required. Consider amitriptyline, carbamazepine, gabapentin
(6) Compression stockings and low molecular weight heparin (e.g. enoxaparin 40 mg subcutaneously once daily)—to reduce the risk of venous thromboembolism
(7) Intravenous immunoglobulin, 0.4 g/kg body weight/day, for 5 days—give to all patients, excepting those with very mild disease

Key investigations

To establish the diagnosis

Acute inflammatory polyneuritis (Guillain Barré syndrome) is primarily a clinical diagnosis: investigation may confirm it, but initial management is dictated by clinical suspicion

(1) Nerve conduction studies—the earliest abnormality is impersistence or absence of F waves. Peripheral demyelination starts proximally in the nerve roots, hence distal conduction velocities and motor latencies are often normal early in the illness, even when there is profound weakness
(2) Lumbar puncture—look for elevated protein (but not cells)
(3) Anti GQ1b antibodies—present in all cases that are

associated with ophthalmoplegia

Other important tests

Relevant to cause

(1) Stool culture and serology for *Campylobacter jejuni*

(2) Serology for atypical pneumonias

(3) CSF analysis for viral infection

Need to exclude

Acute intermittent porphyria—see Emergency Medicine, section 5.11

General

(1) Full blood count, electrolytes, renal and liver function tests, plasma calcium, magnesium and phosphate concentrations

(2) ECG

(3) Chest radiograph

Further management

Dependent on the nature of any residual disability. Significant weakness remains in about 10% of cases, especially those with the axonal form

6.8 Myasthenia gravis

See Chapter 24.22.2 in main text

Clinical features

History

Myasthenic crisis

(1) Breathing difficulty due to muscular weakness in a patient with known myasthenia.

Presentation of myasthenia

(2) Droopy eyelid(s)/double vision

(3) Difficulty chewing, swallowing, talking (nasal speech), holding the head up

(4) Limb weakness

(5) Symptoms less severe in the morning, getting worse as the day goes on

(6) Exacerbation by intercurrent illness, pregnancy, menses, and by some drugs

Examination

Myasthenic crisis

(1) Exhaustion

(2) Ineffective respiratory effort

(3) Inability to clear airway secretions

(4) Cyanosis

(5) Low vital capacity

Also

(6) Check for focal lung signs

Myasthenia

Muscular weakness that becomes worse with repetitive effort (fatiguability)

Immediate management

Respiratory failure caused by muscular weakness in a patient with myasthenia can be due to a myasthenic crisis (attributable to the disease itself) or rarely to an overdose of anticholinesterases (cholinergic crisis). These cannot reliably be distinguished on clinical grounds, hence safe management consists of:

(1) Airway, breathing, circulation

(2) Intubate and ventilate

(3) Stop all anticholinesterases.

IF there is specialist expertise, AND in conjunction with someone skilled in intubation, then edrophonium chloride, 2 mg by intravenous injection, can be used to discriminate between underdosage and overdosage of cholinergic drugs

Key investigations

To establish the diagnosis

Myasthenic crisis is a clinical diagnosis

Of myasthenia gravis

(1) Edrophonium chloride (Tensilon) test: after pretreatment with atropine (0.6 mg intravenously), give edrophonium 2 mg intravenously and look for transient improvement in e.g. ptosis, diplopia, dysarthria. If no improvement after 1–2 min give edrophonium 8 mg intravenously and watch for effect. Note that this test has limited sensitivity and specificity

(2) Serum acetylcholine receptor antibodies—highly specific, being present in 85% of patients with generalized myasthenia

(3) Electromyography: look for increased jitter, also decremental response to repetitive nerve stimulation—this test has good sensitivity and specificity

Other important tests

In myasthenic crisis

(1) Arterial blood gases

(2) Chest radiograph

(3) Electrolytes, renal and liver function tests, calcium, phosphate, full blood count

(4) Sepsis screen (if appropriate)

Further management

In myasthenic crisis consider the following:

(1) Plasma exchange—e.g. 50 ml/kg body weight/day for 4 or 5 days

(2) Intravenous immunoglobulin—e.g. 0.4 g/kg body weight/day, for 5 days

Long-term treatment of myasthenia. Consider:

(1) Immunosuppression—usually prednisolone (starting at a low dose of e.g. 10 mg on alternate days) and azathioprine (2.5 mg/kg body weight/day)

(2) Anticholinesterase, e.g. pyridostigmine bromide 30–120 mg at suitable intervals throughout the day (total daily dose 0.3–1.2 g). Together with antimuscarinic agent if needed

(3) Thymectomy

6.9 Acute Wernicke's encephalopathy

See Chapters 26.3 and 26.7.3 in main text

Clinical features

History

(1) Alcoholism—usually, but also other states of nutritional deficiency and protracted vomiting
(2) Difficulty standing/walking
(3) Confusion

The patient will almost certainly not be able to give a reliable history: corroborate as much information as possible from other sources (relatives, friends, general practitioner etc.)

Examination

Related to Wernicke's encephalopathy, the classic triad of:

(1) Ophthalmoplegia
- Horizontal and vertical nystagmus
- Weakness/paralysis of lateral rectus muscles
- Weakness/paralysis of conjugate gaze

(2) Ataxia—predominantly affecting stance and gait, often without clear-cut intention tremor
(3) Confusion, confabulation

Related to clinical context:

(1) Cardiovascular—look for evidence of intravascular volume depletion and/or dehydration
(2) Consider other complications of alcoholism
- Acute alcohol withdrawal
- Acute liver failure
- Chronic liver disease and its complications

(3) Consider other causes of an acute confusional state—see Emergency Medicine, section 6.2
(4) Nutritional status

Immediate management

Thiamine—give parenteral thiamine immediately, usually in combination with other vitamins B and C, e.g. Pabrinex™ I/V high potency, 2–3 pairs of ampoules intravenously over 10 min every 8 h (each pair of ampoules contains ascorbic acid 500 mg, anhydrous glucose 1 g, nicotinamide 160 mg, pyridoxine hydrochloride 50 mg, riboflavin 4 mg, and thiamine hydrochloride 250 mg in a total of 10 ml). Note—facilities for treating anaphylaxis should be available

Key investigations

To establish the diagnosis

(1) Wernicke's encephalopathy is a clinical diagnosis
(2) Red cell transketolase—a reduced level confirms thiamine deficiency

To exclude other conditions

CT scan brain—should be done in all cases because of the high incidence of structural lesions, e.g. subdural haematoma, in this group of patients

Other important tests

Depending of clinical context, consider as for acute confusional state—see Emergency Medicine, section 6.2

Further management

(1) After 3–5 days, switch from intravenous to oral vitamin replacement, e.g. thiamine 50 mg once daily + vitamin B tablets, Compound, Strong, 1–2 tablets three times daily + vitamin C 100 mg once daily
(2) If alcohol withdrawal—see Emergency Medicine, section 8.2
(3) Other aspects: as for acute confusional state—see Emergency Medicine, section 6.2—except avoid antipsychotics which lower seizure threshold
(4) Long term—measures to help alcoholism

7 Infectious disease

7.1 Malaria

See Chapter 7.13.2 in main text

Clinical features

Clinical features

Falciparum malaria is the life-threatening form and the immediate concern in patients presenting to medical services in malarious areas, or who have travelled to such areas

Transmitted to man by the bite of an infected *Anopheles* mosquito. The interval between bite and first symptom is usually 7–14 days. Most patients with imported falciparum malaria present within 3 months of return from the malarious area, but a few present up to 1 year or more later

History

(1) Risk of exposure to malaria—anyone who has travelled to a malarious area and presents to medical attention with a febrile illness has malaria until proved otherwise

Symptoms of malaria

(2) Early—malaise, headache, backache, myalgia, anorexia, low grade fever.

(3) Later—dizziness, nausea, vomiting, abdominal discomfort, diarrhoea, rigors and drenching sweats.

Symptoms of cerebral malaria

(4) Gradual decline in conscious level over several hours

(5) Generalised epileptic convulsion without post-ictal recovery of consciousness (present in 50 per cent of adult cases).

Note

'Classical' tertian (48 h) or subtertian (36 h) periodicity of fever spikes is rarely seen in falciparum malaria

Examination

(1) Vital signs—temperature, pulse rate, blood pressure, respiratory rate. A high fever (rising to >39°C) is typical, which can be of any periodicity

(2) General—anaemia, jaundice

(3) Abdominal—ook for moderate tender enlargement of liver and/or spleen

(4) Neurological—look for signs of cerebral malaria
- Glasgow Coma Score—reduced (by definition in cerebral malaria)
- Focal signs—note presence of dysconjugate gaze, brisk tendon reflexes, ankle clonus, extensor plantar responses and absent abdominal reflexes; and of decorticate or decerebrate posturing in severe cases
- Fundi—retinal haemorrhages are common (exudates and papilloedema also occur)

Notes

(1) The following are NOT found in malaria
- Lymphadenopathy
- Rash—excepting herpes simplex 'cold sores' in some cases
- Focal signs

(2) Signs of hypoglycaemia may be misinterpreted as merely being manifestations of cerebral malaria

Immediate management

If cardiorespiratory collapse, as described in Emergency Medicine, section 1.2

Oxygen, high flow with reservoir bag if needed, to achieve Pa_{O_2} >92%

If clinical evidence of intravascular volume depletion, establish intravenous access and resuscitate as described in Emergency Medicine, section 3.1

If hypoglycaemic—give 50 ml of 50% glucose (dextrose monohydrate) intravenously, followed by infusion of 10% glucose at sufficient rate to maintain blood glucose concentration >3 mmol/l. IF IN DOUBT, TREAT

Antimalarial drugs for falciparum malaria (adult dosages)

Assume chloroquine-resistance

Patients who can swallow and retain tablets

Use ONE of the following regimen

(1) Mefloquine
- By mouth: 15–25 mg/kg of mefloquine base (maximum 1500 mg), divided into two doses 6–8 h apart

(2) Proguanil with atovaquone ('Malarone')
- By mouth: 4 tablets (each containing 100 mg proguanil and 250 mg atovaquone) once daily for 3 days

(3) Artemether with lumefantrine ('Riamet')
- By mouth: 4 tablets (each containing 20 mg artemether and 120 mg lumefantrine) twice daily for 3 days

(4) Quinine—*the treatment of choice in many countries*
- By mouth: 600 mg of quinine salt every 8 h for 7 days
- Afterwards: when the 7 day course is completed, give tetracycline 250 mg four times daily for 7 days or doxycyline 100 mg daily for 7 days

(5) Fansidar™ (each tablet containing pyrimethamine 25 mg and sulfadoxine 500 mg)
- 3 tablets as single dose.

Patients with severe malaria or who cannot swallow and retain tablets

Use ONE of the following regimen:

(1) Quinine—*the treatment of choice in many countries*
- By intravenous infusion: loading dose of 20 mg/kg dihydrochloride salt (maximum 1400 mg) diluted in 10 ml/kg isotonic fluid and given over 4 h, then

after 8 h give maintenance dose of 10 mg/kg (maximum 700 mg) over 4 h, repeated following further 8 h gaps until patient can swallow tablets to complete 7 day course
- By intravenous infusion in the intensive care unit: loading dose of 7 mg/kg dihydrochloride salt by infusion pump over 30 min, followed immediately by 10 mg/kg (maintenance dose) over 4 h, repeated after 8 h gaps as above.
- By intramuscular injection (if intravenous infusion not possible): loading dose of 20 mg/kg of dihydrochloride salt diluted to 60 mg/ml, by deep intramuscular injection (half dose into each anterior thigh) with strict sterile precautions, then 10 mg/kg every 8–12 h until patient can take oral medication
- Afterwards: when the 7 day course is completed, give tetracycline 250 mg four times daily for 7 days or doxycycline 100 mg daily for 7 days

(2) Quinidine—replaces quinine for parenteral treatment of malaria in the USA
- By intravenous infusion: loading dose of 15 mg/kg of quinidine base given over 4 h, then 7.5 mg/kg given over 4 h three times daily until the patient can swallow and take quinine. Followed by tetracycline or doxycycline as above

(3) Artesunate
- By intravenous 'push': loading dose of 2.4 mg/kg followed by 1.2 mg/kg at 12 and 24 h, then 1.2 mg/kg daily for 6 days

(4) Artemether
- By intramuscular injection: loading dose of 3.2 mg/kg on the first day (in one or two doses), followed by 1.6 mg/kg/day for 6 days

Other measures

(1) High fever—control by fanning, tepid sponging, cooling blankets, antipyretics (e.g. paracetamol 15 mg/kg in tablets, or powder washed down an NG tube, or as suppositories)
(2) Anaemia—transfuse with whole blood or packed cells if haematocrit falls to <20% or if there is severe bleeding
(3) Urine output—insert urinary catheter to monitor closely
(4) Cerebral malaria—appropriate nursing care for the unconscious patient. Control convulsions (see Emergency Medicine, section 6.5). Consider elective intubation and ventilation if airway in danger of compromise
(5) Hyperparasitaemia—consider exchange transfusion or haemophoresis in non-immune patients who are severely ill, who have deteriorated on conventional treatment, and who have parasitaemia >10%

Key investigations

To establish the diagnosis

Depends on the detection of parasitaemia (stop antimalarial chemoprophylaxis)
(1) Repeated examination of thick and thin blood films (8–12 hourly for 72 h) by an experienced microscopist
(2) Antibody detection technique, e.g. dipstick antigen-capture assay

Note

If patient remains unwell and no other diagnosis can be made, then consider therapeutic trial even if early smears are negative

Other important tests

(1) Reagent stick test for blood glucose—?hypoglycaemia
(2) Full blood count—anaemia with evidence of haemolysis is usual. Neutrophilia is common, but white cell count can be normal or low
(3) Electrolytes, renal and liver function, glucose, coagulation screen—mild hyponatraemia is common
(4) Arterial blood gases
(5) Blood culture—to exclude secondary bacterial septicaemia in those with an obvious focus of such infection and in patients who are very unwell or have a raised blood white cell count
(6) Depending on clinical context (mainly to exclude differential diagnoses)—CT brain, lumbar puncture, chest radiograph

Further management

Emphasize need for avoidance and prophylaxis with any future travel to malarious areas

7.2 Meningitis

See Chapters 7.11.3, 7.11.5, 7.11.12, and 24.14.1 in main text

Clinical features

Clinical features

Acute bacterial meningitis has a mortality of 70–100% if untreated and is the immediate concern in patients presenting to medical services

History

General symptoms
(1) Early—malaise, headache, fever, vomiting, diarrhoea
(2) Later—increasingly severe headache, photophobia, drowsiness
(3) Very late—coma, convulsions

Localizing (if meningitis secondary to infection elsewhere)
(4) Respiratory—pneumococcal disease (pneumonia)
(5) Ear—*H. influenzae* (otitis media)

Also
(6) Contact with a case of meningitis
(7) Previous history of meningitis
(8) History of immunodeficiency

(9) Pregnancy—increased risk of Listeria
(10) Travel history—particularly meningococcal disease

Examination

(1) Vital signs—temperature, pulse rate, blood pressure, respiratory rate
(2) General
- Skin: petechiae/purpura—characteristic of meningococcal disease, but not specific
- Conjunctivae/palate: petechiae—characteristic of meningococcal disease, but not specific
- Posture—patients with severe meningism often lie with the back and neck in hyperextension

(3) Neurological
- Meningism—neck stiffness. Kernig's sign (with the leg flexed at the hip, an attempt by the clinician to passively extend the knee is resisted by hamstring spasm)
- Ocular fundi—papilloedema indicates raised intracranial pressure, but absence of papilloedema does not exclude this
- Cranial nerve lesions—most commonly VIth (false localizing sign)

(4) Other—in secondary meningitis there may be signs of primary focus, e.g. pneumonia, otitis media, CSF shunts/reservoirs

Immediate management

If cardiorespiratory collapse, as described in Emergency Medicine, section 1.2
Oxygen, high flow with reservoir bag if needed, to achieve $P\text{aO}_2$ >92%
If clinical evidence of intravascular volume depletion, establish intravenous access and resuscitate as described in Emergency Medicine, section 3.1

Antimicrobial chemotherapy (empirical treatment, adult dosages)

Spontaneous meningitis

Drug	Dose	Route	Frequency	Duration*
Cefotaxime	2 g	IV	4 hourly	2 weeks
Or				
Ceftriaxone	2 g	IV	12 hourly	2 weeks
If high prevalence of penicillin-resistent pneumococci, then add				
Vancomycin	1 g	IV	12 hourly	2 weeks
If underlying immunosuppression, pregnancy or age >65 years, then add				
Ampicillin	2 g	IV	4-6 hourly	3 weeks

Post-traumatic meningitis

Community acquired

Treat as for spontaneous meningitis

Nosocomial

Drug	Dose	Route	Frequency	Duration*
Probability of *Pseudomonas* spp. high				
Ceftazidine	2 g	IV	8 hourly	3 weeks
Or				
Meropenem	2 g	IV	8 hourly	3 weeks
Probability of *Pseudomonas* spp. low				
Cefotaxime	2 g	IV	4 hourly	3 weeks
Or				
Ceftriaxone	2 g	IV	12 hourly	3 weeks

Shunt-associated meningitis

Insidious onset

Drug	Dose	Route	Frequency	Duration*
Vancomycin	1 g	IV	12 hourly	2 weeks
PLUS				
Vancomycin	5–10 g	IT	48–72 hourly	2 weeks

Acute onset

Treat as for nosocomial post-traumatic meningitis

Notes

* Antimicrobial therapy can be refined as soon as organism is isolated, otherwise patients with suspected bacterial meningitis should receive treatment with the regimen indicated.
Doses of antimicrobials to be adjusted in renal failure (especially vancomycin)
IV, intravenous; IT, intrathecal.

Key investigations

To establish the diagnosis

(1) Epidemiological data (any current epidemics)
(2) Lumbar puncture to obtain specimen of CSF—looking in bacterial meningitis for:

General appearance
- Cloudy or purulent, but can be clear

Microscopy
- White cell count—usually raised (although can rarely be normal, i.e. <6 lymphocytes/μl) with neutrophils accounting for >80% of cells, but can have a lymphocytic pleocytosis in early bacterial meningitis or with *L monocytogenes*
- Gram stain—shows organisms in 50–80% of cases

Biochemical testing
- Glucose—usually reduced (<40% that of a parallel serum sample)
- Protein—usually elevated (>0.45 g/l)

Microbiological culture
Bacterial antigen detection for common pathogens
PCR for meningococcal disease

Notes

(1) Give antibiotics immediately—before referral to hospital, and if in hospital before lumbar puncture—in cases of suspected meningococcal meningitis/septicaemia

(2) Lumbar puncture should not be performed if there are
- Symptoms or signs to suggest raised intracranial pressure, namely
  - Drowsiness/coma
  - Focal neurological signs
  - Loss of retinal vein pulsation/papilloedema
  - Bradycardia/hypertension
- Local skin sepsis at the sight of puncture
- Clinical suspicion of spinal cord compression
- Bleeding diathesis

(3) If symptoms or signs suggest raised intracranial pressure—arrange for CT brain to exclude space occupying lesion or cerebral oedema

Other important tests

For specific diagnosis

(1) Blood culture
(2) Throat swab—for viral and bacteriological culture
(3) Skin lesion—disrupt with needle and make contact slide for Gram stain.
(4) Blood sample—in EDTA (as full blood count) for bacterial PCR

Other

(1) Full blood count
(2) Electrolytes, renal and liver function, glucose, clotting screen
(3) Arterial blood gases (severe cases)
(4) Chest radiography—?pneumonia (pneumococcal disease), ?aspiration (if impaired conscious level)
(5) CT/MRI brain—may demonstrate skull fractures or parameningeal septic foci

Further management

(1) Meningitis is a notifiable disease
(2) If meningococcal meningitis
- Household and other intimate contacts—give prophylaxis (e.g. rifampicin 600 mg orally twice daily for 2 days, or ciprofloxacin 750 mg orally as single dose) and immunize if serogroup C or A
- Staff—prophylaxis is not required unless mouth to mouth resuscitation given

7.3 Encephalitis

See Chapters 7.10.2, 7.10.12, 7.10.6.1, and 24.14.2 in main text

Clinical features

Clinical features

Encephalitis is an acute inflammation of the brain and/or spinal cord (encephalomyelitis) presenting as alteration of consciousness, convulsions and/or focal neurological signs. It is usually caused by an acute viral infection of the central nervous system (typically Herpes simplex, Japanese encephalitis, or an arthropod-borne virus), or it complicates a systemic viral infection such as measles (post-infectious encephalomyelitis) or vaccination (post-vaccinal encephalomyelitis). Case fatality is extremely variable but may exceed 40% when there is no antiviral therapy (e.g. Japanese encephalitis), and there is a high incidence of permanent neurological sequelae

History

General symptoms (after incubation period of a few days to 2 weeks)

(1) Early—fever, headache, neck stiffness, vomiting
(2) Later—psychiatric symptoms, altered consciousness, convulsions

Localizing symptoms

(3) Altered behaviour, hallucinations, temporal lobe seizures—Herpes simplex encephalitis
(4) Rashes—preceding illness (e.g. measles, varicella, post-infectious encephalomyelitis); concurrent (e.g. West Nile virus encephalitis)

Also

(5) Recent vaccination (vaccinia, nervous tissue rabies vaccine)
(6) Current seasonal epidemic (arthropod-borne encephalitides)
(7) Travel history—to endemic area (e.g. Central Europe/Scandinavia—tick-borne encephalitis)

Examination

(1) Vital signs—temperature, pulse rate, blood pressure, respiratory rate, Glasgow Coma Scale
(2) General
- Skin: rashes—West Nile virus, enteroviruses etc.
- Mucous membranes: cold sores (Herpes simplex encephalitis)

(3) Neurological
- Meningism
- Ocular fundi—papilloedema indicates raised intracranial pressure, but absence of papilloedema does not exclude this
- Cranial nerve lesions—most commonly VI (false localizing sign)

(4) Other—in post-infectious encephalomyelitis there may be signs of the preceding illness, e.g measles, varicella, mumps etc.

Immediate management

If cardiorespiratory collapse, as described in Emergency Medicine, Section 1.2

If convulsing, as described in Emergency Medicine, Section 6.5

Oxygen, high flow with reservoir bag if needed, to achieve Pa_{O_2} >92%

(1) Antiviral treatment
- Aciclovir—where it is affordable, treatment with

aciclovir should be started immediately in all undiagnosed cases in which viral encephalitis is included in the differential diagnosis. Specifically, aciclovir is recommended for Herpes simplex, Herpes simiae (B), Herpes zoster, and Epstein-Barr virus encephalitides: dose 10 mg/kg every 8 h by intravenous infusion (reduced in renal impairment)

- Ribavirin (tribavirin)—for the rare encephalitides associated with RNA virus infections (e,g, Lassa fever, Argentine haemorrhagic fever, Hanta virus, Crimean-Congo haemorrhagic feverm and Rift Valley Fever) ribavirin (tribavirin) has been recommended: 2 g loading dose by intravenous infusion, then 1 g every 6 h for 4 days, then 0.5 g 8 hourly for 6 days

(2) Other measures
- Corticosteroids—sometimes used for post-vaccinal encephalomyelitis (controversial)
- Reduction of severe intracranial hypertension—intravenous mannitol or mechanical hyperventilation

Key investigations

To establish the diagnosis

(1) Epidemiological data (any current epidemics)
(2) Lumbar puncture to obtain specimen of CSF—looking in viral encephalitis for:

Microscopy
- White cell count—usually raised (but normal in 10–15% of patients with Herpes simplex encephalitis at first examination), with lymphocytes and other mononuclear cells predominant except in early infections
- Gram stain to exclude bacterial meningoencephalitis

Biochemical testing
- Glucose—usually normal or increased, but low levels have been reported
- Protein—usually elevated into range 0.5–1.5 g/l

Virology
- PCR
- Specific viral IgM (microcapture technique)
- Viral isolation—e.g. mumps, enteroviruses, lymphocytic choriomeningitis virus

(3) Other samples
- Skin lesions—immunofluorescence (Herpes zoster) and electron microscopy (Herpesviruses)
- Nasopharyngeal aspirate—measles
- Stool—enteroviruses
- Serology (acute/convalescent titres)—mumps, Coxsackie viruses, arthropod-borne viruses

Other important tests

(1) Full blood count
(2) Arterial blood gases (severe cases)
(3) CT/MRI—may demonstrate focal lesions (e.g. Herpes simplex encephalitis) or cerebral oedema

Note

The diagnosis of viral encephalitis should not be made too hastily as the differential diagnosis is broad and other treatable causes (e.g. cerebral malaria, bacterial or fungal meningoencephalitides) may be ignored

7.4 Tetanus

See Chapter 7.11.20 in main text

Clinical features

Tetanus, caused by toxins of *Clostridium tetani* in contaminated wounds, remains common in some developing countries but is preventable by vaccination. It is now rare in developed countries but, because it is decreasingly familiar, is less likely to be diagnosed. The case fatality ranges from 20–60%, although in expert hands this may be reduced to 6%, even in severe cases

History

(1) Recent wound, especially penetrating, contaminated or with necrosis, is identified in 75–85% of cases

Also

(2) Problems in head, neck, mouth—trismus due to a painful local condition is an important differential diagnosis
(3) Drugs—a dystonic drug reaction is an important differential diagnosis

Symptoms of tetanus

After an incubation period of usually 6–10 days (less than 15 days in 90% of cases):
- Non-specific—malaise, fever, sweating, and headache
- Suggestive—muscle stiffness (especially of the jaws), spasms, and dysphagia.

Examination

Features of tetanus

(1) Muscles
- Trismus, risus sardonicus, neck retraction
- Rigidity of erector spinae and abdominal muscles (board-like rigidity)
- Opisthotonos
- Tonic contractions/spasms of the stiff muscles
- Spasms of respiratory muscles and larynx threaten to cause asphyxia
- Local tetanus may involve only muscles in the region of the wound, e.g. cephalic tetanus

(2) Autonomic nervous system
- Fluctuating heart rate, blood pressure, and temperature with sweating and hypersalivation

Clinical grading is of prognostic significance:
- I (mild)—trismus and generalized stiffness without respiratory embarrassment or spasms

- II (moderate)—marked rigidity, brief spasms, mild respiratory embarrassment, and dysphagia
- III and IV—frequent prolonged spasms, respiratory embarrassment with apnoeic spells, severe dysphagia. and cardiovascular abnormalities

Also

- Features of alternative diagnosis, e.g. local cause of trismus

Note

(1) Incubation period less than 4 days and period of onset (trismus to first spasm) less than 48 h are associated with high mortality

(2) In developed countries, patients are often elderly (missed childhood vaccination)

Immediate management

If cardiorespiratory collapse, as described in Emergency Medicine, Section 1.2

If convulsing, as described in Emergency Medicine, Section 6.5

Oxygen, high flow with reservoir bag if needed, to achieve $Pa\text{O}_2$ >92%

(1) If apnoeic/asphyxiating/hypoxaemic—emergency tracheostomy, assisted ventilation with oxygen. See Emergency Medicine, section 10.4.2

(2) Tetanus immune globulin

In all cases—give before manipulating the wound:

- EITHER equine tetanus immune globulin 10 000 units intravenously (beware of anaphylaxis, see Emergency Medicine, section 1.12)
- OR (preferably, if available) human tetanus immune globulin 5000 units intravenously

(3) The wound

Antibiotics to sterilize

- EITHER—Metronidazole 500 mg, orally (if possible) or intravenously, three times a day for 10 days
- OR—Benzyl penicillin 2 megaunits intravenously four times a day for 8 days

Thorough surgical débridement of the wound after tetanus immune globulin has been given

(4) Other measures

- Sedatives/muscle relaxants
- Diazepam 5–20 mg three times a day by mouth (mild cases) or by continuous intravenous infusion (moderate-severe cases)
- Tracheostomy (moderate and severe cases)
- Neuromuscular blockade (pancuronium/vecuronium) and mechanical ventilation (severe cases)

Further management (severe cases in the intensive care unit)

(1) Ventilatory support

(2) Control of autonomic nervous system disturbances

- Hypertension—cautious use of low dose short-acting β-blockers
- Brady/tachyarrhythmias—treat only if causing significant haemodynamic disturbance, see Emergency Medicine, Section 1.7

(3) Prevention of deep vein thrombosis—low molecular weight heparin

Note

Avoid use of excessive doses of diazepam

Key investigations

THE DIAGNOSIS OF TETANUS IS ENTIRELY CLINICAL

(1) Wound swab—but failure to culture *Clostridium tetani* from the wound does NOT exclude the diagnosis of tetanus

(2) Lumbar puncture—the cerebrospinal fluid is normal

Note

The differential diagnosis includes the many local causes of trismus, dystonic reactions to drugs, tetany, strychnine poisoning, meningitis, and rabies (cephalic tetanus)

Further management

Infection does not confer immunity: give full course of active immunization (tetanus toxoid) after recovery

7.5 Rabies

See Chapter 7.11.9 in main text

Clinical features

Clinical features

Rabies is a zoonotic viral infection of the central nervous system, endemic in domestic dogs and cats, wild carnivores, bats etc., in most parts of the world. It is transmitted to humans by bites of rabid mammals, usually dogs. The case fatality of rabies encephalomyelitis is virtually 100%, but the disease is preventable by modern post-exposure treatment started soon after the bite

History

(1) Animal contact

- History of dog (or other mammal) bite (but may be distant or forgotten, especially with insectivorous bat bites in USA) or a lick by a mammal on broken skin
- Travel history to rabies endemic area
- Post-exposure treatment—see Emergency Medicine, section 7.6

(2) Incubation period

- Usually between 20 and 90 days (extreme range 4 days to 19 years)

(3) Prodromal symptoms

- Non-specific—fever, chills, malaise, weakness, tiredness, headache
- Suggestive—itching, pain, or paraesthesiae at the site of the healed bite wound

(4) A few days later

- Furious rabies—difficulty swallowing (especially

water), causing spasms of breathing and great anxiety (with or without pain in the throat)
- Extreme susceptibility to draughts, causing similar spasms
- Bizarre behaviour
- Periods of extreme excitement, hallucinations, terror, aggression with lucid intervals

(5) After several more days
- Lapse into coma and convulsions
- Sudden death during a hydrophobic spasm
- Paralytic rabies—ascending weakness with sensory symptoms often starting in the bitten limb; sphincter problems; dysphagia, drooling, and respiratory weakness

Examination

(1) Wound
- Evidence of healed bite

(2) Neurological
- Clinical examination may be normal
- Excitable behaviour interspersed with lucid intervals
- Furious rabies—violent, jerky spasms of inspiratory muscles associated with evident terror provoked by attempts to drink or exposure to a draught of air
- Paralytic rabies—ascending flaccid paralysis with fasciculations, sensory loss, sphincter dysfunction
- Weakness of muscles of deglutition and respiration
- Excitable behaviour interspersed with lucid intervals

(3) Autonomic nervous system
- Signs of overactivity—hypersalivation, sweating, labile pulse rate and blood pressure

Immediate management

Although life can be prolonged by invasive, intensive care (tracheostomy, paralysis, mechanical ventilation, cardiac monitoring etc.), the chances of a successful outcome are so low that there is a strong case for palliative care to relieve pain and anxiety

Key investigations

To establish the diagnosis during life

(1) Skin punch biopsy (hairy area, e.g. nape of neck)
- Detection of virus by direct fluorescent antibody in nerves surrounding hair follicles

(2) Saliva
- Virus may be isolated

(3) Blood
- Rabies-neutralizing antibody titre—elevated in unvaccinated patient (but may be negative for 7 days after clinical illness has begun)

(4) CSF analysis
- May be normal, but protein usually elevated, and may have elevated white blood cell count
- Rapid PCR (experimental)
- Virus may be isolated
- Rabies-neutralizing antibody titre—elevated in unvaccinated patient (but may be negative for 7 days after clinical illness has begun)

(5) Other important tests
- Given the appalling outcome of rabies it is important to pursue the possible differential diagnosis of a rapidly progressing encephalitis (see Emergency Medicine, section 7.3) if there is ANY doubt about the diagnosis

To establish the diagnosis in the biting animal (dog etc.)—brain smear with detection of virus by direct fluorescent antibody or viral isolation. Euthanizing the biting dog and examining its brain immediately is now recommended, rather than observing it for onset of rabid symptoms over a 10-day period

Further management

Attempt to identify/capture/examine (by veterinarian)/test the animal responsible for the bite

7.6 Animal bites/stings

See Chapters 7.11.9 and 8.2 in main text

Clinical features

A very wide range of animals may inflict bites and stings. Serious consequences may result from trauma, envenoming, allergy or infection

History

(1) Timing
- The event is usually painful and memorable and so precisely timed by the victim.

(2) Immediate symptoms—distress associated with a terrifying event and attributable to trauma, envenoming or allergy
- Trauma
  - Pain, bleeding, dysfunction (depending on site and severity of injury)
- Envenoming
  - Snake bite
    Local—pain, swelling, persistent bleeding, bruising, blistering, painful enlargement of draining lymph nodes
    Systemic—syncope/collapse (may be early and transient), spontaneous systemic bleeding (gums, nose etc.), vomiting, progressive weakness starting with ptosis, blurred vision, inability to open mouth, swallow, speak etc., generalized muscle aches and tenderness, passage of black urine (rhabdomyolysis)
  - Scorpion sting
    Local—very severe pain, mild swelling
    Systemic—vomiting, sweating, faintness, difficulty with breathing, muscle spasms
  - Spider bites
    Local—pain, sweating and gooseflesh (neuro-

toxic) or progressive skin changes (red, white, and blue sign; necrotic)
Systemic—vomiting, faintness, colic and muscle spasms
- Jellyfish stings
  Local—severe pain, blistering, contact rash
  Systemic—collapse, vomiting
- Fish stings
  Local—very severe pain
  Systemic—rarely collapse

- Allergy
  - Hymenoptera stings (bees, wasps, hornets, yellowjackets, ants)
    Local—pain, swelling (may be negligible)
    Systemic—early syncope and collapse, raised, itchy rash, swelling of mouth, lips, tongue, and gums, chest tightness, wheezing, asthma attack, abdominal colic, vomiting, diarrhoea (all of these may develop within a few minutes of the sting)

(3) Delayed symptoms—attributable to infection
Earliest onset at about 12 h (*Pasteurella multocida*)
Local—pain, swelling, redness, heat, purulent discharge
Systemic—sometimes severe generalized symptoms (sepsis)

Examination

(1) Vital signs
Temperature, pulse rate, blood pressure, respiratory rate, Glasgow Coma Scale

(2) Trauma
Injuries to soft tissues, joints, tendons, bones (crush fractures), body cavities (e.g. haemothorax), evisceration, dead tissue, foreign material in the wound (broken teeth, claws, earth etc.). May be severe/life-threatening

Note that effects of trauma may be associated with envenoming and/or allergy and/or infection (e.g. marine coral cuts, stingray, and sea urchin injuries)

(3) Envenoming—see History

(4) Allergy—features of anaphylaxis (Emergency Medicine, section 1.12)

(5) Infection
Local—pain, swelling, redness, heat, purulent discharge
Systemic—sepsis syndrome (see Emergency Medicine, section 7.7)

Note

(1) Human bites
- May be of medicolegal significance: document carefully, also any other evidence of injury (sketch and photograph)
- High risk of infection with group A β-haemolytic streptococci, *Staph. aureus* (40% of wounds), *Haemophilus, Klebsiella, Eikenella corrodens*, and anaerobes
- May be self-inflicted—typically lips, buccal cavity, fingers, clenched-fist injuries of knuckles

(2) Dog, cat/other mammal bites
- Associated with high risk of infection with a wide range of pathogens, notably *Pasteurella multocida, Capnoctyophaga canimorsus, Staph. aureus, Clostridium tetani*, and other anaerobic bacteria, rabies virus etc.

Immediate management

First-aid

(1) Trauma
Control pain and bleeding, contain wound with bandaging, give plasma expander if available, transport to medical care

(2) Envenoming
Snake bite
- Immobilize the patient, especially the bitten limb
- Avoid harmful remedies
- Transport the patient to medical care
- Neurotoxic bites only—pressure immobilization and splinting with a long crepe bandage
- Venom ophthalmia (spitting cobras and rinkhals)—irrigate affected eye with liberal quantities of bland fluid (e.g. water, milk) and apply 1% epinephrine drops for pain (if available)

Note
- Tourniquets, incisions, suction, electric shock, cryotherapy, snake stones etc. should NEVER be used

(3) Other bites and stings
- Fish stings—immerse stung part in uncomfortably-hot but not scalding water (maximum 45°C)
- Scorpion stings and other painful bites and stings—local 1% lignocaine with digital block or strong systemic analgesia (if available)
- Jellyfish stings
  Box jellyfish (North Australia, Indo-Pacific)—wash area with dilute acetic acid/vinegar
  Atlantic jellyfish—apply a slurry of baking powder
- Bee stings—remove the sting as quickly as possible
- Tick bites—apply surgical spirit to the animal and prise out the mouth parts with forceps

Hospital management

If anaphylaxis, as described in Emergency Medicine, section 1.12

If cardiorespiratory collapse, as described in Emergency

Medicine, section 1.2

Oxygen, high flow with reservoir bag if needed, to achieve Pa_{O_2} >92%

If clinical evidence of intravascular volume depletion, establish intravenous access and resuscitate as described in Emergency Medicine, section 3.1

(1) Trauma
- Explore wound under anaesthesia, débriding and removing foreign material.
- Treat specific injuries to vital structures
- Delayed primary suture.

(2) Envenoming

Antivenom treatment

In cases of envenoming by snakes, fish, scorpions, spiders, box jellyfish, and ticks, administer antivenom intravenously (provided that an appropriate specific antivenom is available) if any of the following are present:
- Paralysis (ptosis etc)
- Spontaneous systemic bleeding (gums, GI tract etc)
- Incoagulable blood
- Shock, ECG abnormalities
- Black urine (myoglobinuria, haemoglobinuria)
- Severe/rapidly progressive local envenoming

Beware of antivenom reactions (anaphylactic or serum): treat/prevent as follows:
- Treatment with adrenaline (1/1000, 0.3–0.5 ml intramuscularly = 0.3–0.5 mg dose, repeated as necessary) plus anti-H_1 (e.g. chlorpheniramine 10–20 mg IV) plus corticosteroid (e.g. hydrocortisone 5 mg/kg IV) at the first sign of a reaction is preferred to routine prophylaxis EXCEPT in atopic subjects with severe asthma and those who have suffered previous reactions to antivenom. See Emergency Medicine, section 1.12

Key investigations

Trauma
- Appropriate radiological imaging to define extent of the injury

Snake bites
- Simple 20 min whole blood clotting test or rapid coagulation screen
- Stick test urine for blood: positive may indicate red blood cells (?disseminated intravascular coagulation) or myoglobin (rhabdomyolysis)
- Australia only—rapid EIA venom detection kit, using swab from the bite wound
- Tensely-swollen limbs—measure intracompartmental pressure as guide to fasciotomy

Other important tests
- Depending on clinical context/severity—ECG, full blood count, electrolytes, renal and liver function tests, muscle enzymes (creatine kinase), arterial blood gases, chest radiograph

Further management

Trauma (bites by large animals)

(1) Definitive wound closure with skin grafts etc.

(2) Infection risk
- Bacterial

  Prophylactic antibiotics for severe/multiple wounds or wounds of the fingers or in response to cultures:

  Amoxicillin/clavulanic acid—(expressed as) amoxicillin 250 mg three times daily by mouth (prophylaxis, mild case) to 1 g three times daily intravenously (treatment, severe case)

  OR

  Second/third generation cephalosporin, e.g. cefotaxime 1–2g 6 hourly intravenously
- Tetanus

  Give tetanus toxoid or, if unimmunized, consider tetanus immunoglobulin
- Rabies

  Consider possibility of rabies exposure and (if appropriate) give **rabies post-exposure treatment**
  - Thorough wound cleaning—scrub under running tap with soap and water; irrigate with plain water
  - Apply virucidal agent such as 40–50% alcohol or 1% iodine
  - Avoid suturing.
  - Vaccination:
    - Start active vaccination using tissue culture vaccine: dividing one dose (0.5–1 ml) between 8 sites intradermally produces the most rapid antibody response) PLUS
    - Start passive immunization: give equine rabies immunoglobulin, 40 units/kg body weight, OR—preferably if available—human rabies immunoglobulin, 20 units/kg body weight, infiltrate around the wound, with the residue given intramuscularly distant from the site of rabies vaccination

Envenoming

(1) Nursing
- Avoid elevation of the bitten limb

(2) Surgery
- Débridement of necrotic tissue with immediate split skin grafting
- Avoid hasty and unjustified fasciotomy (especially if the blood is still incoagulable).

(3) Myoglobinuric renal failure—try to prevent by correcting hypovolaemia and acidosis and encouraging diuresis (see Emergency Medicine, section 4.2)

7.7 Septic shock

See Chapters 4.4 and 7.5 in main text

Clinical features

Clinical features

Septic shock is a condition associated with severe infection in which there is hypotension (systolic blood pressure <90 mmHg) unresponsive to fluids or requiring vasoactive drugs for its correction. The causative septicaemia may be with Gram-positive or Gram-negative bacteria, yeasts, viruses, or protozoa. Failure of one or more organ systems is common

History

(1) Systemic features
- Early—malaise, lethargy, nausea, vomiting, fever, sweating, shivering/rigors
- Later—restless, anxious, confused, agitated.
- May develop rapidly (minutes—hours), e.g. meningococcaemia, or gradually

(2) Localized features
- Related to causative infection—e.g pneumonia, urinary tract infection, infected intravascular catheter, meningitis, after large bowel surgery etc.

(3) Risk factors
- Complication of surgery, instrumentation, burns, or other trauma.
- Complication of preceding illness, e.g 'flu predisposing to staphylococcal pneumonia
- Travel history—could the patient have malaria? (see Emergency Medicine, section 7.1)

Examination

(1) Vital signs
- Temperature—fever or hypothermia
- Tachycardia
- Tachypnoea
- Hypotension
- Peripheries warm (vasodilated) or cold and cyanosed (vasoconstricted)
- Glasgow Coma Score

(2) Evidence of the causative infection
- Complete physical examination to look for focus of infection. Do not forget to examine the back and perineum/rectum (localized abscess).

(3) Evidence of organ failure
- Respiratory—central cyanosis (check pulse oximetry), crackles. Risk of adult respiratory distress syndrome (ARDS)
- Renal – low urine output. Risk of prerenal renal failure or acute tubular necrosis
- Liver—jaundice
- Neurological—confusion
- Haematological—abnormal bleeding/gangrene of extremities

Notes

(1) Look for evidence of predisposition to infection—elderly, immunosuppressed, asplenic, malignant disease, artificial heart valve, prosthetic material etc.

(2) Streptococcal toxic shock syndrome—erythematous rash, local severe pain and swelling (necrotizing fasciitis/myositis)

(3) Staphylococcal toxic shock syndrome—diarrhoea, myalgia, rash (desquamating), often associated with menstruation/tampon use

Immediate management

If cardiorespiratory collapse, as described in Emergency Medicine, section 1.2

Oxygen, high flow with reservoir bag if needed, to achieve $Pa{O_2}$ >92%

If clinical evidence of intravascular volume depletion, establish intravenous access and resuscitate as described in Emergency Medicine, section 3.1

(1) Fluid/circulatory
- 500 ml crystalloid IV every 30 min until central venous pressure is 8–12 mmHg
- If mean arterial pressure <65 mmHg—give vasopressors
- If mean arterial pressure >90 mmHg—give vasodilators
- Central venous oxygen saturation <70% (measured in blood from pulmonary artery or central venous catheter)—transfuse packed red cells to increase haematocrit to at least 30% and give dobutamine initial dose 2.5 μg/kg/min intravenously, increasing until central venous oxygen saturation is 70% or higher

(2) Respiratory
- Consider early intubation and mechanical ventilation

(3) Antibiotics

Give broad-spectrum, empirical treatment

Community-acquired septicaemia:
- Aminoglycoside (e.g. gentamicin 5 mg/kg intravenously once daily, assuming normal renal function) + broad-spectrum penicillin (e.g. amoxicillin, 500 mg 8 hourly to 1 g 6 hourly, intravenously)
  OR
- Broad-spectrum cephalosporin (e.g. cefotaxime, 1 g 12 hourly to 2 g 6 hourly, intravenously)

Hospital-acquired septicaemia:
- Aminoglycoside (e.g. gentamicin 5 mg/kg intravenously once daily, assuming normal renal function) + broad-spectrum anti-Pseudomonal penicillin (e.g. Tazosin® 2.25–4.5 g [= Piperacillin 2–4 g + tazobactam 250–500 mg] 6 hourly intravenously)
  OR
- Ceftazidime, 1 g 12 hourly to 2 g 8 hourly, intravenously
  OR

- Meropenem 500 mg–1 g 12 hourly intravenously
  OR
- Imipenem with cilastatin, 500 mg–1 g (of imipenem) 6 hourly intravenously

Pseudomonas infection suspected:
- Aminoglycoside (e.g. gentamicin 5 mg/kg intravenously once daily, assuming normal renal function) + broad-spectrum anti-Pseudomonal penicillin (e.g. Tazosin® 2.25–4.5 g [= Piperacillin 2–4 g + tazobactam 250–500 mg] 6 hourly intravenously)

Gram positive infection suspected:
- Add flucloxacillin 1–2g 12 hourly intravenously
  OR
- Vancomycin 1g 12 hourly intravenously (assuming normal renal function)

Anaerobic infection suspected:
- Add metronidazole 500 mg 8 hourly intravenously

Meningococcaemia
- Benzylpenicillin 2.4 g 4 hourly intravenously
  OR
- Cefotaxime 2 g 6 hourly intravenously

Streptococcal toxic shock syndrome
- Benzylpenicillin 1.2–2.4 g 6 hourly intravenously, or Cefotaxime 2 g 6 hourly intravenously
  PLUS
- Clindamycin 600–1200 mg 6 hourly intravenously

Note

(1) Aminoglycosides, vancomycin—dosage dependent on renal function; always monitor levels

(2) Other aspects
- For patients with shock, acidosis, oliguria, or hypoxaemia with evidence of end organ dysfunction—consider recombinant human activated protein C
- Supportive treatment for specific organ failure—mechanical ventilation, renal replacement therapy (haemofiltration, haemodialysis)
- Surgical—e.g. urgent fasciotomy and débridement for streptococcal necrotizing fasciitis/myositis
- Strict normalization of blood glucose between 4.4 and 6.1 mmol/l using intravenous infusion of Actrapid insulin on sliding scale

Key investigations

To establish the source of infection

(1) Blood culture

(2) Other cultures as determined by clinical signs or imaging, e.g. needle aspiration of fluid collections

Other

(3) Full blood count—leucocytosis or leucopenia

(4) Electrolytes, renal and liver function tests, glucose, clotting screen, muscle enzymes (creatine kinase, ? rhabdomyolysis)

(5) Arterial blood gases—pH, $p\text{O}_2$, $p\text{CO}_2$, base excess

8 Psychiatry

8.1 Acute alcohol withdrawal

See Chapters 26.3 and 26.7.3 in main text

Clinical features

History

Related to alcohol withdrawal

(1) Agitation and anxiety
(2) Tremor
(3) Sweating
(4) Insomnia
(5) Nausea and vomiting
(6) Hallucinations—tactile, visual, auditory
(7) Grand mal seizures.

Also

(8) Drinking history—how much alcohol does the patient usually drink? Have they recently been drinking particularly heavily, or have they stopped?

Examination

Related to alcohol withdrawal:

(1) Agitation and anxiety
(2) Confusion
(3) Tremor
(4) Sweating
(5) Tachycardia and hypertension

Related to clinical context:

(6) Cardiovascular—look for evidence of intravascular volume depletion and/or dehydration
(7) Consider other complications of alcoholism
  - Wernicke's encephalopathy:
    - Ophthalmoplegia
      - Horizontal and vertical nystagmus
      - Weakness/paralysis of lateral rectus muscles
      - Weakness/paralysis of conjugate gaze
    - Ataxia—predominantly affecting stance and gait, often without clear-cut intention tremor
  - Acute liver failure
  - Chronic liver disease and its complications
(8) Consider other causes of an acute confusional state – see Emergency Medicine, section 6.2
(9) Nutritional status

Immediate management

(1) Sedation
  - Patient can take oral medication—reducing schedule of chlordiazepoxide, e.g. 30 mg four times daily (day 1); 20 mg three times daily and 30 mg at night (day 2); 10 mg three times daily and 20 mg at night (day 3); 5 mg three times daily and 10 mg at night (day 4); 5 mg in the morning and 10 mg at night (day 5); 5 mg at night (day 6), then stop
  - Patient cannot take oral medication—clomethiazole (chlormethiazole), 0.8% solution, initially 2.5–7.5 ml/min (20–60 mg/min) until light sleep is induced from which the patient can easily be roused, with the rate of infusion then reduced to the lowest possible to maintain this state. Note—careful monitoring for respiratory depression is required: resuscitation facilities must be available. Switch to oral sedation when possible

(2) Thiamine—give parenteral thiamine immediately, usually in combination with other vitamins B and C as Pabrinex™ I/V high potency, 2–3 pairs of ampoules intravenously over 10 min every 8 h (each pair of ampoules contains ascorbic acid 500 mg, anhydrous glucose 1 g, nicotinamide 160 mg, pyridoxine hydrochloride 50 mg, riboflavin 4 mg and thiamine hydrochloride 250 mg in a total of 10 ml). Note—facilities for treating anaphylaxis should be available

Then

(3) Glucose—treat/prevent hypoglycaemia.
  - DO NOT GIVE GLUCOSE BEFORE THIAMINE—DANGER OF PRECIPITATING WERNICKE'S ENCEPHALOPATHY
  - If hypoglycaemic—give 50 ml of 50% glucose (dextrose monohydrate) intravenously. IF IN DOUBT, TREAT
  - If not hypoglycaemic—start 5% dextrose infusion at 50 ml/h to prevent hypoglycaemia (if hyponatraemic used reduced volume of more concentrated dextrose solution)

Key investigations

To establish the diagnosis

Acute alcohol withdrawal is a clinical diagnosis

Other Important tests

Depending of clinical context, consider as for acute confusional state—see Emergency Medicine, section 6.2

Further management

(1) After 2 days, switch from intravenous to oral vitamin replacement, e.g. thiamine 50 mg once daily + Vitamin B tablets, Compound, Strong, 1–2 tablets three times daily + Vitamin C 100 mg once daily
(2) Other aspects: as for acute confusional state—see Emergency Medicine, section 6.2—except avoid antipsychotics which lower seizure threshold
(3) Long term—measures to help alcoholism

8.2 Drug overdosage

See Chapters 8.1 in main text

Clinical features

History

The overdose

(1) Nature, time and quantity of drug ingested
(2) Circumstantial evidence
(3) Concurrent alcohol consumption

Also

(4) Assessment of intent
(5) Past medical history, medications and allergies
(6) Past psychiatric history

Note

Be cautious in accepting the patient's account at face value. Assume that overdoses of multiple drugs are likely

Examination

Initial survey

(1) Airway, breathing, circulation

(2) Reagent stick test for blood glucose (?hypoglycaemia)

(3) Check for small pupils and slow respiratory rate (?opioid overdose)

(4) Check temperature (?hypothermia)

(5) Check Glasgow Coma Score (see Table 18)

Further examination

(6) Look for features indicated in Table 20.

Immediate management

If cardiorespiratory collapse, as described in Emergency Medicine, section 1.2

Nurse in recovery position if Glasgow Coma Score impaired

Oxygen, high flow with reservoir bag if needed, to achieve Pa_{O_2} >92%.

Consider oropharyngeal airway or cuffed endotracheal tube depending on level of consciousness

ECG monitor—but do not treat arrhythmias unless these are associated with profound hypotension

Establish intravenous access

(1) If hypoglycaemic—give 50 ml of 50% glucose (dextrose monohydrate) intravenously. IF IN DOUBT, TREAT

(2) If possibility of opioid overdose—give naloxone 0.8–2 mg intravenously, repeated at intervals of 2–3 min to a maximum of 10 mg. IF IN DOUBT, TREAT

(3) If hypothermic—start rewarming

Prevention of drug absorption—see Table 21

Specific antidote (if available)—see Table 22

If in doubt—discuss management with a Poisons Centre: the following single number for the UK National Poisons Information Service directs the caller to the relevant local centre: 0870 600 6266

Key investigations

To establish the diagnosis

(1) Serum drug levels, e.g. paracetamol, salicylates, iron, theophylline, lithium

(2) Save serum sample for measurement of other toxins after discussion with clinical chemist, e.g. paraquat

Note

Record time of blood sampling accurately on specimen tube and in notes

Other Important tests

(1) Electrolytes, glucose, renal, liver and bone function tests, full blood count, clotting screen

(2) ECG

Consider

(3) Arterial blood gases

(4) Carboxyhaemoglobin level

(5) Chest radiograph—look for evidence of aspiration or pulmonary oedema

(6) Abdominal radiograph

See Table 23

Further management

(1) Dependent on the nature of overdose taken

(2) As dictated by psychiatric condition (if any)

Table 20 Clinical features of drug overdose

Clinical feature	Drug to consider
Vital signs	
Hypothermia	Alcohol Phenothiazines
Hyperthermia	Amphetamines Sympathomimetics, including cocaine Monoamine oxidase inhibitors Salicylates Ecstasy
General appearance	
Sweating	Salicylates
Venepuncture marks	Drug abuse
Cardiovascular	
Cardiac arrhythmia	Tricyclics Amphetamines Potassium Theophylline Digoxin β-Blockers
Hypertension and tachycardia	Amphetamines Sympathomimetics
Hypotension	Sedatives Narcotics Hypnotics Iron Tricyclics Alcohol
Respiratory	
Hyperventilation	Salicylates
Hypoventilation	Opioids Sedatives Hypnotics
Gastrointestinal	
Oral ulceration	Strong acids or alkalis
Haematemesis	Iron Salicylates
Eyes	
Pinpoint pupils	Opioids

Table 20 Continued

Dilated pupils	Anticholinergics Tricyclics Cocaine
Neurological	
Drowsiness (depressed GCS)	Alcohol Sedatives Opioids Hypnotics Salicylates Tricyclics
Confusion	Alcohol
Ataxia	Tricyclics
Excitability	Antihistamines Salbutamol Solvents
Dystonia	Metoclopramide Haloperidol Phenothiazines

Table 21 Prevention of absorption of drugs taken in overdose

Indications	Contraindications	Notes
Gastric lavage		
• Within 2 h of ingestion of life-threatening amount of toxic substance • May be extended up to 6 h after drugs that delay gastric emptying (e.g. salicylates, opioid analgaesics, anticholinergic drugs)	• Inability to maintain the airway (unless intubated with cuffed endotracheal tube) • Ingestion of corrosives or organic solvents	• Save lavage sample for analysis
Ipecacuanha		
• No indication (for use in adults)		• No evidence of reduced drug absorption in poisoned patients
Activated charcoal		
• Within 2 h of ingestion of life-threatening amount of toxic substance • Consider repeat doses for some toxins, e.g. slow-release preparations, carbamazepine, dapsone, digoxin, paraquat, phenobarbitone, quinine, amanita phalloides (death cap mushroom)	• Drugs that are not bound to charcoal, e.g. iron salts, lithium, ethanol, methanol, ethylene glycol, cyanide salts, acids/alkalis, organic solvents, mercury, lead, fluorides, potassium salts	• Standard adult dose is 50 g • Can be given after gastric lavage

Table 22 Antidotes used in drug overdose

Overdose	Antidote
Benzodiazepines	Flumazenil 0.2 mg IV over 15 s, then 0.1 mg at 60-s intervals (maximum total dose 1–2 mg). If drowsiness recurs after arousal, consider IV infusion at 0.1–0.4 mg/h
β-Adrenoceptor blockers (if severe hypotension)	Atropine 0.6–3.0 mg IV *If no response to atropine* Glucagon 50–150 μg/kg IV in 1 min, then 1–5 mg/h by IV infusion
Digoxin	Digoxin-specific Fab antibodies, IV over 30 min. Dose determined in relation to patient's body weight and serum digoxin concentration (or 380–760 mg if potentially life-threatening toxicity and serum digoxin concentration not known)
Iron salts	Desferrioxamine mesilate 15 mg/kg/h IV (max 80 mg/kg over 24 h)
Opioids	Naloxone 0.8–2.0 mg IV/IM, repeated at intervals of 2–3 min to maximum 10 mg. If drowsiness recurs after arousal, consider IV infusion (2 mg in 500 ml 0.9% saline, rate adjusted according to response)
Paracetamol	Methionine 2.5 g orally, followed by 2.5 g 4 hourly (×3 further doses), OR *N*-acetylcysteine 150 mg/kg IV in 15 min, then 50 mg/kg over 4 h, then 100 mg/kg over 16 h (in 5% dextrose)
Phenothiazines (dystonia)	Benzatropine mesilate 1–2 mg IV/IM or procyclidine 5–10 mg IV/IM
Warfarin	Vitamin K_1 (phytomenadione) 5 mg slow IV

All dosages are for adults.

Table 23 Laboratory data in drug overdose

Abnormality	Drug to consider
Hypokalaemia	Sympathomimetic drugs Diuretics
Hyperkalaemia	Cardiac glycosides (e.g. digoxin) β-Blockers Potassium salts
Hypoglycaemia	Insulin Oral hypoglycaemic agents Ethanol Salicylates
Metabolic acidosis	Methanol Ethylene glycol Salicylates Tricyclics Carbon monoxide Cyanide
Carboxyhaemoglobin	Carbon monoxide Smoke
Chest radiograph—pulmonary oedema	Opioids Salicylates Inhalation of toxins (ammonia, chlorine, oxides of nitrogen)
Abdominal radiograph—radio-opacities	Button batteries Iron Sustained release potassium tablets

9 Other conditions

9.1 Disseminated intravascular coagulation

See Chapters 22.5.5 and 22.5.6 in main text

Clinical features

Disseminated intravascular coagulation (DIC) is a systemic disorder in which haemorrhage (main problem in 90% of cases) and thrombosis can occur at the same time. It involves the generation of intravascular fibrin and the consumption of procoagulants and platelets. May be acute or chronic (only acute discussed here)

History

Presence of DIC

(1) Bleeding
- Skin—extensive superficial bruising; oozing from venepuncture/intramuscular injection sites, around indwelling catheters/tubes
- Mucosa—mouth, nose, gastrointestinal tract, (lungs), (renal tract)
- Internal—brain, other organs

(2) Thrombosis
- Microthrombotic lesions
- Skin—often on fingers/toes
- Internal organs—dysfunction of brain, kidneys, lungs

Related to cause of DIC

(1) Sepsis—bacterial, viral, fungal, parasitic (malaria)
(2) Major trauma—including burns, surgery
(3) Toxins—e.g. venoms (see Emergency Medicine, section 7.6)
(4) Obstetric—placental abruption, eclampsia, amniotic fluid embolism
(5) Cancer—metastatic carcinoma of stomach, colon, pancreas, breast, lung; mucin-secreting adenocarcinomas; leukaemia (especially acute promyelocytic leukaemia)
(6) Blood transfusion—incompatible, massive
(7) Liver disease—acute hepatic failure
(8) Others—heatstroke (see Emergency Medicine, section 9.3), prosthetic devices (e.g. shunts, ventricular assist devices)
(9) Idiopathic—purpura fulminans

Examination

(1) Vital signs
(2) Evidence of bleeding or thrombosis
(3) Related to possible cause (see above)

Immediate management

If cardiorespiratory collapse, as described in Emergency Medicine, section 1.2

(1) Underlying cause
Treat aggressively
Give broad-spectrum antimicrobials to cover sepsis if diagnosis not clear (see Emergency Medicine, section 7.7)

(2) When diagnosis of DIC established by laboratory testing, give (as appropriate)
- Fresh-frozen plasma—to keep prothrombin time and activated partial thromboplastin time below a value 1.5 times the upper limit of control values
- Cryoprecipitate/fibrinogen concentrates—to keep fibrinogen levels >1g/l
- Platelets—to keep platelets >50×109/l
- Blood (packed red blood cells)—to keep haematocrit >0.30

Note

(1) If the patient continues to bleed/clot 4–6 h after initiation of treatment of underlying cause and the supportive measures described above, then—ONLY WITH EXPERT HAEMATOLOGICAL ADVICE—consider:
- Antithrombin III, 100 U/kg intravenously over 3 h (loading dose), then continuous infusion of 100 U/kg/24h. Used in moderate/severe DIC when levels of antithrombin III are very low
- Heparin, 20 000–30 000 units/24h, by continuous intravenous infusion—to inhibit further thrombogenesis. Used when thrombosis is the main clinical problem

(2) Possibility of adrenal infarction (Waterhouse-Friederichson)—give steroid (e.g. hydrocortisone 50–100mg 6hourly intravenously) if circulatory compromise

Key investigations

To establish the diagnosis

There is no single diagnostic test for DIC: look for the following

(1) Appropriate clinical context
(2) Platelet count—decreased
(3) Prothrombin time and activated partial thromboplastin time—both increased
(4) Fibrinogen/fibrin degradation products (FDPs) and/or D-dimer—both present/elevated

Other haematological features that may be present include

(1) Antithrombin III level—reduced: useful test for diagnosis and therapeutic monitoring
(2) Fibrinogen—reduced
(3) Fibrinopeptide A—breakdown product of fibrinogen, elevated
(4) Thrombin time—prolonged
(5) Blood film—may show red cell fragmentation/microangiopathic haemolytic anaemia

Other Important tests

Dependent on clinical context

Further management
Dependent on clinical context

9.2 Sickle cell crises

See Chapters 22.4.7 in main text

Clinical features

History

There are several clinical conditions

(1) Pain crisis—severe pain in limbs, hips, back, chest or abdomen
(2) Chest/lung syndrome—breathlessness, pleuritic chest pain
(3) Brain/neurological syndrome—epileptic fits, transient ischaemic attacks, strokes

And less commonly in adults

(4) Aplastic crisis—presents with breathlessness and fatigue. Usually seen in children. Associated with parvovirus infection
(5) Sequestration crisis—presents with profound anaemia. Usually seen in babies and young children when the spleen and/or liver enlarge rapidly due to trapping of red blood cells. Hepatic sequestration can occur in adults
(6) Priapism

Also

(7) Previous sickle cell crises.
(8) Precipitating factors—extremes of heat and cold, infections/fever (often upper respiratory tract, 'flu), heavy exercise, emotional stress, any situation producing hypoxia
(9) Family history—patterns of crises may follow through generations

Note

(1) The patient or their relatives/friends generally know that they have sickle cell disease and are often knowledgeable about the condition
(2) The pain is
- Genuine
- Excruciating
- Varies in character and location

Examination

(1) Airway, breathing, circulation
(2) Glasgow Coma Scale
(3) Vital signs—pulse rate, blood pressure, respiratory rate, temperature

Note particularly

(4) General examination—pallor
(5) Chest—local tenderness and signs of infection.
(6) Bones—tenderness
(7) Liver or spleen—look for enlargement due to hepatosplenic sequestration (particularly in children, uncommon in adults)
(8) Priapism.
(9) Infection—fever may be the only sign

Remember that there may be no localizing signs

Immediate management

If cardiorespiratory collapse, as described in Emergency Medicine, section 1.2

(1) Oxygen, high flow with reservoir bag if needed, to achieve $Pa{O_2}$ >92%. Monitor with pulse oximeter.
(2) Fluid—establish intravenous access (may be difficult, asking patient's advice on best site is often helpful) and give 1 litre of 0.9% saline rapidly, then repeat 4–6 hourly for duration of crisis (assuming satisfactory urine output)
(3) Analgaesia
- Intravenous e.g. (1) diamorphine by slow intravenous injection at 1 mg/min, usual maximum initial dose is 5 mg, but may be repeated if necessary, or (2) morphine by slow intravenous injection at 2 mg/min, usual maximum initial dose is 10 mg, but may be repeated if necessary. Both to be accompanied by appropriate antiemetic, e.g. metoclopramide 10 mg IV over 1–2 min, or cyclizine 50 mg IV over 1–2 min
- Intramuscular/subcutaneous—if it is not possible to establish intravenous access, then give diamorphine (0.05 mg/kg) or morphine (0.1 mg/kg) subcutaneously, repeated after 1 h if necessary

(4) Warmth—wrap in warm blankets if the patient feels cold
(5) Antibiotics—e.g. amoxicillin 500 mg intravenously every 8 h + benzypenicillin 1.2 g intravenously every 6 h
(6) Prophylaxis against venous thromboembolism—give low molecular weight heparin, e.g. enoxaparin 20 mg subcutaneously once daily

Key investigations

To establish the diagnosis

Sickle cell crisis is a clinical diagnosis

Other Important tests

(1) Full blood count, reticulocytes, group and save
(2) Electrolytes, renal and liver function, glucose
(3) Cultures—blood, sputum, urine, throat swab
(4) Arterial blood gases
(5) Chest radiograph—may show widespread patchy infiltrate that is difficult to distinguish from infection
(6) HbS level (percentage of total Hb)—if exchange transfusion considered
(7) Abdominal radiograph, serum amylase (abdominal syndrome)
(8) Serology to detect acute parvovirus B19 infection (aplastic crisis)

Notes

Other investigations as dictated by clinical context, e.g. CT scan brain if focal neurological signs

Do not order plain radiographs of all sites of pain

Further management

Seek expert advice

Chest syndrome with hypoxia, neurological symptoms or priapism (also seek urological advice) are all indications for exchange transfusion to reduce the HbS to <30% of total Hb

Consider hydroxyurea to reduce frequency of crises

9.3 Heat stroke

See Chapters 8.5.1 and 26.6.1 in main text

Clinical features

Hyperthermia is a failure of thermal homeostasis that allows the core temperature to rise above 40°C. It can result from exposure to environmental heat with/without prolonged physical exercise (especially if heat dissipating mechanisms are impaired) and/or from increased metabolic heat production. Heat stroke is hyperthermia with severe central nervous system abnormalities such as delirium, convulsions, or coma. Its case fatality ranges from 17–70%

History

Predisposing factors

(1) Exposure to high ambient temperature ± high humidity (e.g. in a heatwave)
(2) Prolonged strenuous physical exercise at any ambient temperature, especially if insulation from clothing is excessive and the patient is unacclimatized
(3) Drugs
  - Neuroleptic malignant syndrome—psychiatriac/recreational dopaminergic drugs, e.g. phenothiazines, thioxanthene, butyrophenones, amphetamines
  - Malignant hyperpyrexia—occurs in people with a rare genetic predisposition (autosomal dominant) when exposed to various inhaled or local anaesthetic agents
(4) Previous history of heat intolerance

Symptoms

Heat exhaustion

(1) General—irritability, weakness, lethargy, fatigue, dizziness, headache, muscle cramps/myalgias
(2) Gastrointestinal—nausea, vomiting, diarrhoea
(3) Respiratory – hyperventilation/tachypnoea

Heatstroke

Any or all of the symptoms of heat exhaustion, plus

(4) CNS dysfunction—impaired judgement, abnormal behaviour, disorientation, hallucinations, confusion, convulsions, loss of consciousness

Examination

(1) Vital signs—core (rectal) temperature 40° or more (by definition), hypotension, tachycardia, tachypnoea
(2) Related to temperature control mechanisms
  - Sweating—present (>50% cases)or absent (<50%). Hot dry skin is a late finding
  - Piloerection
(3) General—weakness, dehydration, bleeding (disseminated intravascular coagulation)
(4) Neurological—impaired consciousness (Glasgow Coma Scale), seizures, opisthotonus, decerebrate rigidity, cerebellar dysfunction, oculogyric crises, fixed dilated pupils
(5) Signs of predisposing condition—e.g. obesity, skin disease, thyrotoxicosis

Note

Muscular rigidity is a feature of neuroleptic malignant syndrome and malignant hyperpyrexia but not of heat-stroke

Immediate management

If cardiorespiratory collapse, as described in Emergency Medicine, section 1.2

Oxygen, high flow with reservoir bag if needed, to achieve $Pa{O_2}$ >92%

If clinical evidence of intravascular volume depletion, establish intravenous access and resuscitate using isotonic saline as described in Emergency Medicine, section 3.1

(1) Cooling
  Should be done rapidly
  Remove to shade or cooler place
  Remove clothes
  - External methods
    Tepid spongeing and fanning; ice packs to neck, axillae, groin; cover with wet sheet—as available
    Hypothermia bed/blanket
    Immersion in cold water with vigorous massage—effective at lowering body temperature but associated with more complications than evaporative cooling and not generally recommended
  - Internal methods
    Ice water gastric lavage, ice water rectal lavage, ice water intraperitoneal lavage, mechanical ventilation with cooled gases, cardiac bypass—anecdotal success reported for these treatments
(2) Monitor urine output—consider urethral catheter
(3) Correct fluid, electrolyte and acid-base abnormalities (see below)
(4) Malignant hyperpyrexia and neuroleptic malignant syndrome
  - Stop drug/anaesthetic
  - Treat muscle spasms/rigidity—give dantrolene sodium by rapid intravenous injection, 1 mg/kg repeated as required to a cumulative maximum of 10 mg/kg

Notes

(1) In the field—stop exertion at the first sign of heat exhaustion, remove excess clothing, move into shade, encourage oral fluids
(2) Do not give salicylates—which do not reduce body temperature and may exacerbate coagulopathy
(3) Do not give paracetamol (acetaminophen)—which does not reduce body temperature and may worsen hepatic damage

Key investigations

Heat stroke is a clinical diagnosis

Important tests

(1) Electrolytes and renal function—risk of hypokalaemia, hyponatraemia, hypocalcaemia, hypomagnesaemia, hypophosphataemia, impaired renal function (hyperkalaemia if renal failure and rhabdomyolysis)
(2) Glucose—may have hyperglycaemia; also risk of hypoglycaemia
(3) Full blood count—high haematocrit indicates haemoconcentration
(4) Liver blood tests—elevated transaminases almost always found in heatstroke and indicate hepatotoxicity and/or muscle damage
(5) Muscle enzymes—elevated creatine kinase indicates muscle damage (rhabdomyolysis)
(6) Albumin/serum proteins—elevated values indicate haemoconcentration
(7) Coagulation tests—evidence of DIC (see Emergency Medicine, sectioin 9.1)
(8) Amylase—?pancreatitis
(9) ECG, troponin—evidence of myocardial damage
(10) Arterial blood gases—?lactic acidosis

Other tests that may be indicated include

(1) Chest radiograph—?aspiration
(2) CT scan head—?alternative cause of CNS dysfunction

Further management

(1) Monitor results of active cooling
 - Beware of seizures (see Emergency Medicine, section 6.5)
 - Beware of cardiac arrhythmias—only treat if causing significant haemodynamic compromise (see Emergency Medicine, section 1.7)

(2) Supportive care as appropriate
Respiratory failure—consider intubation and mechanical ventilation
Circulatory failure—treat hypotension with volume repletion and, if necessary, vasopressor drugs
Renal failure—in case of rhabdomyolysis, prevent renal damage by correcting acidosis and hypovolaemia and promoting diuresis (see Emergency Medicine, section 4.2)
Sodium depletion (hyponatraemia, muscle cramps)—sodium repletion with isotonic saline

Note

After recovery—advice to prevent recurrence

9.4 Hypothermia

See Chapters 8.5.2 in main text

Clinical features

History

Two distinct contexts
(1) Cold exposure, in patient of any age
(2) Multifactorial cause, often in the elderly patient
 - Immobility/falls
 - Cognitive impairment
 - Alcohol
 - Vasodilating drugs
 - Autonomic dysfunction, eg. diabetes mellitus
 - Poor socio-economic conditions

Note

Elderly patients with hypothermia have often been found on the floor at home following a fall

Examination

Initial survey
(1) Airway, breathing, circulation
(2) Reagent stick test for blood glucose (?hypoglycaemia)
(3) Check for small pupils and slow respiratory rate (?opioid overdose)
(4) Temperature—using a low-range rectal thermometer: <35°C (by definition).
(5) Check Glasgow Coma Score (see Table 18)

Futher examination

(1) General appearance—cold, pale mottled skin (whereabouts on the body, if anywhere, does the skin feel warmer?). At 32–35°C, shivering; at <32°C, muscular rigidity
(2) Cardiovascular—bradycardia and hypotension
(3) Respiratory—look for evidence of aspiration, pneumonia or pulmonary oedema
(4) Neurological
 - May range from mild inco-ordination to confusion, lethargy, and coma. Pupils may be dilated and non-reactive
 - Focal/lateralizing signs may indicate stroke that has precipitated hypothermia

(5) Endocrine—could the patient be hypothyroid?

Immediate management

Depends on the clinical context

If cardiorespiratory collapse, as described in Emergency Medicine, section 1.2

Treat for hypoglycaemia and/or opioid overdose if appropriate

The patient with hypothermia of gradual onset (usually elderly, usually multifactorial cause)

(1) Re-warm—slowly in warm room covered with a blanket or 'Bair hugger' (do not use foil blankets which retard re-warming)
(2) Oxygen—give oxygen as necessary to keep Pa_{O_2} >92%
(3) Fluids—establish intravenous access. Note risk of pulmonary oedema, hence do not infuse fluid rapidly. If hypotensive, infuse 1 litre 0.9% saline over 2 h, checking for lung crackles and/or worsening gas exchange as this progresses. Repeat or slow rate of infusion as determined by clinical response
(4) ECG monitoring—risk of ventricular tachycardia/fibrillation
(5) Antibiotics—as appropriate for pulmonary infection, which is common in this context, e.g. cefotaxime 1 g 12 hourly intravenously

The patient with cold exposure or severe hypothermia (<30°C) or with hypothermia of any cause complicated by life threatening arrhythmia

Re-warm—rapidly, using both:

(1) Active external re-warming—apply heat to body surface, e.g. hot water bottles/warmed IV bags (not too hot, must be comfortably bearable against your own skin) in groins and axillae, warmed blankets, radiant heaters
(2) Active core re-warming
    - Non-invasive—give warmed (42–46°C) humidified oxygen and warmed (43°C) intravenous fluids
    - Invasive—gastric, colonic, bladder, and peritoneal lavage with warmed (43°C) 0.9% saline solutions

Notes

(1) Patients with hypothermia are best managed in an ICU setting: they may require treatment of arrhythmia and/or ventilatory support
(2) Arrhythmias
    - Avoid use of catecholamines (arrhythmogenic)
    - Only treat if life-threatening (ventricular fibrillation or asystole)—For VF, attempt defibrillation up to three times, but not more until core temperature >30°C. The drug of choice is probably bretylium 5–10 mg/kg intravenously over 15–30 min, repeated after 1–2 h to total dose of 30 mg/kg. Magnesium sulphate (8 mmol of magnesium) given intravenously over 10–15 min (repeated once if necessary) has also been reported to be effective. Lignocaine (lidocaine) is not effective in hypothermic VF, and the International Liaison Committee on Resuscitation guidelines suggest avoiding this drug, also epinephrine and procainamide, because of the risk of accumulation to toxic levels
(3) Diagnosis of death—this can be difficult. Patients with severe hypothermia can appear clinically dead. Resuscitative efforts must continue until the core temperature is 30–33°C, i.e. THE PATIENT IS NOT DEAD UNTIL THEY ARE WARM AND DEAD

Key investigations

To establish the diagnosis

Hypothermia is defined as a core temperature <35°C

Other important tests

(1) Full blood count, electrolytes, glucose, renal and liver function tests—note that severe hyperkalaemia is common in profound hypothermia. Serum potassium must be monitored closely during rewarming, even if initially normal
(2) Calcium (low), amylase (high)—in pancreatitis, an important complication of hypothermia
(3) Thyroid function tests—?hypothyroid
(4) Arterial blood gases—to look for hypoxia and/or acidosis
(5) ECG—look for sinus bradycardia, J wave ('junctional' wave—a broad slurred deflection that is superimposed on the distal limb of the QRS complex), prolonged QT interval. Note that the muscular tremor of shivering can lead to artefact on the ECG, which should not be confused with ventricular fibrillation
(6) Chest radiograph—look for aspiration, pneumonia, pulmonary oedema

Further management

Dependent on the cause of hypothermia. Prevention of recurrence is likely to require socio-economic intervention in the elderly, e.g. provision of heating, increased supervision

10 Practical procedures

10.1 Central vein cannulation, arterial cannulation and invasive monitoring

10.1.1 Femoral vein cannulation

The optimum position is with the patient supine, but their head and torso can be propped up to an angle of 15 to 30° if this is more comfortable. The key landmark is the femoral pulse, which should be palpated one finger-breadth below the crease of the groin. The femoral vein lies one finger-breadth medial to the femoral artery (the mnemonic NAVY, Nerve Artery Vein Y-fronts, can be useful in remembering the anatomy). The needle should therefore enter the skin one finger-breadth medial to the femoral artery and one finger-breadth below the groin crease (Fig. 1). It should be advanced in the line of the leg, angled rostrally at about 60° to the skin, and with its bevel pointing forwards. When the vein is punctured the guidewire should pass directly up the femoral vein and into the inferior vena cava.

10.1.2 Internal jugular vein cannulation

10.1.2.1—The low lateral approach

The patient is supine with the head turned away from the side of the puncture. A towel may be placed under both shoulders to extend the neck. After preparation of the skin and drapes, and insertion of local anaesthetic, the bed is tilted to a 25° head down position. The needle is inserted just lateral to the posterior border of the clavicular head of the sternocleidomastoid muscle, about one finger-breadth above the clavicle, with its bevel pointing caudally. It is then advanced parallel to the line of the clavicle and just behind the sternocleidomastoid muscle. The internal jugular vein, which lies superficially at this point, is cannulated close to its junction with the subclavian vein (Fig. 2(a)). As soon as the vein is entered the needle is angulated caudally to ease cannulation, the guidewire passing directly into the innominate vein. The risk of complications was lower with this technique than for any other method of central venous cannulation used in one series of over 5400 cases (see Chapter 16.1).

10.1.2.2—The axial approach

The patient is positioned as described for the low lateral approach to the internal jugular vein (Fig. 2(b)). The needle is inserted in the centre of the triangle defined by the sternal and clavicular heads of the sternocleidomastoid muscle and the clavicle itself. It should be angulated caudally, at about 60° to the skin, and in a line pointing towards the ipsilateral anterior superior iliac spine.

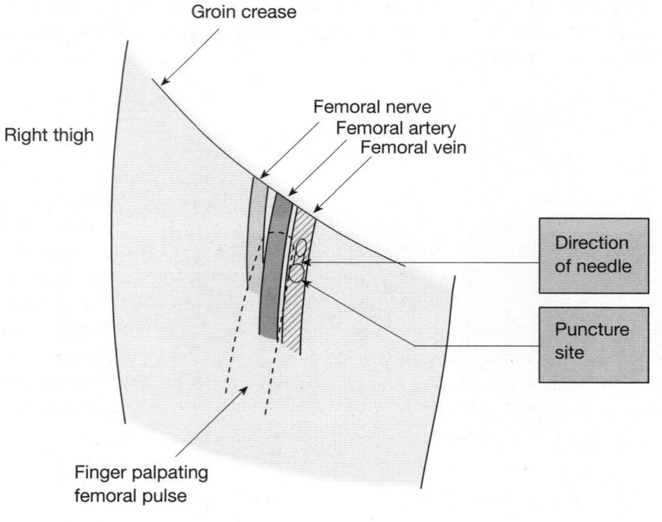

Fig. 1 The approach to the femoral vein.

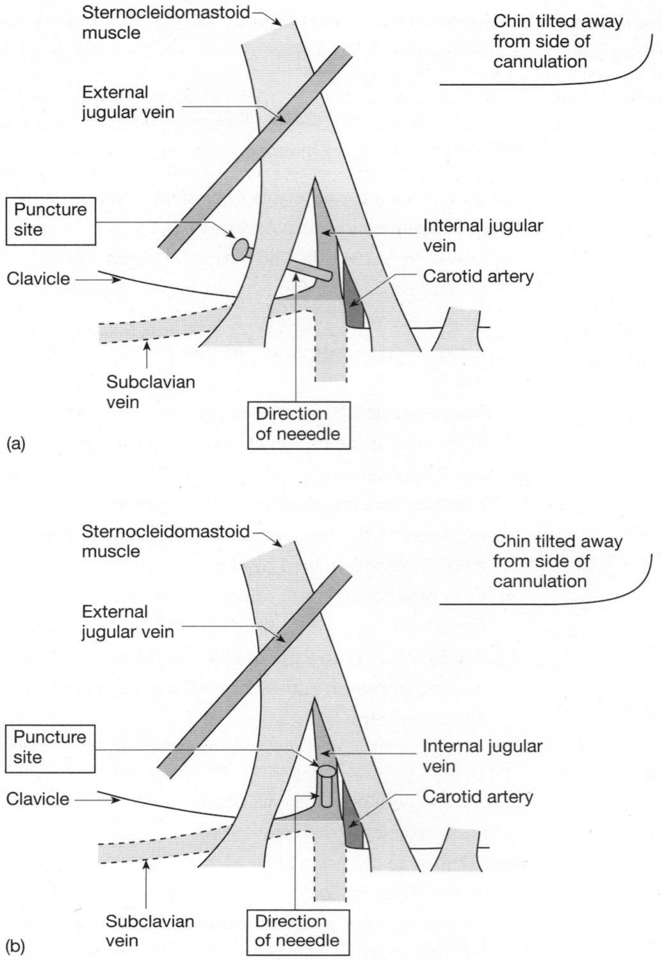

Fig. 2 (a)The low lateral approach to the internal jugular vein. (b)The axial approach to the internal jugular vein.

10.1.3 Subclavian vein cannulation

10.1.3.1—The infraclavicular approach (Fig. 3(a))

The patient is positioned as described for the low lateral approach to the internal jugular vein, excepting that instead of a towel being placed under both shoulders it should be positioned under the spine, allowing the shoulders to retract to reduce the risk of pneumothorax. The needle enters the skin below the mid-point of the lower border of the clavicle and is advanced under the clavicle towards the upper edge of the junction of the clavicle with the manubrium.

10.1.3.2—The supraclavicular approach (Fig. 3(b))

The patient is positioned as described for the infraclavicular approach to the subclavian vein. The needle is inserted into the angle between the superior border of the clavicle and the posterior border of the clavicular head of sternocleidomastoid and advanced caudally, medially and ventrally.

10.1.4 Pulmonary artery flotation catheter

Central venous cannulation should be performed as described above (sections 10.1.2 and 10.1.3) and a pulmonary artery (PA) catheter introducer inserted. Ensure that the balloon at the end of the PA catheter inflates completely and uniformly, and then slowly advance the catheter whilst watching the pressure trace on the monitor. The balloon should be inflated when the catheter is advanced and deflated whenever the catheter is withdrawn. Pressure traces corresponding to the right atrium, the right ventricle and the pulmonary artery should be seen (Fig. 4). As a rough guide, the waveform should change for every 10 cm that the catheter is advanced. Inflation of the balloon when the catheter is in a medium sized pulmonary artery allows it to 'wedge' and occlude distal flow. To obtain valid readings, the catheter tip should reside in a region of the lung where pulmonary venous pressure exceeds alveolar pressure. The pressure recorded at the tip of the catheter (pulmonary capillary wedge pressure, PCWP) provides indirect measurement of the left atrial pressure, which reflects left ventricular end-diastolic pressure if the chamber is not diseased. Values for cardiac output and mixed-venous blood chemistries may also be directly measured. A number of variables such as systemic vascular resistance and left ventricular stroke work may be derived from values measured with a PA catheter.

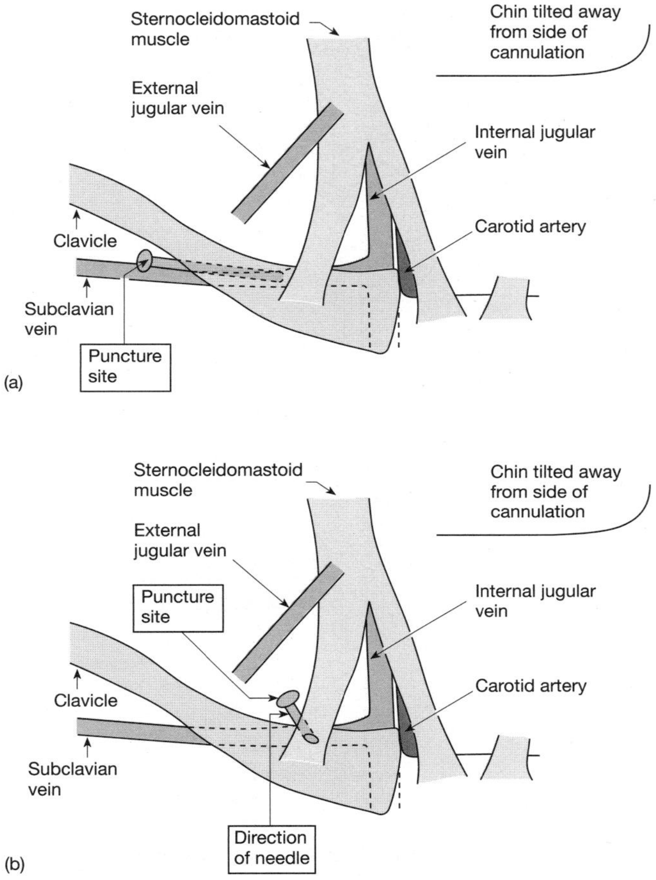

Fig. 3 (a)The infraclavicular approach to the subclavian vein. (b)The supraclavicular approach to the subclavian vein.

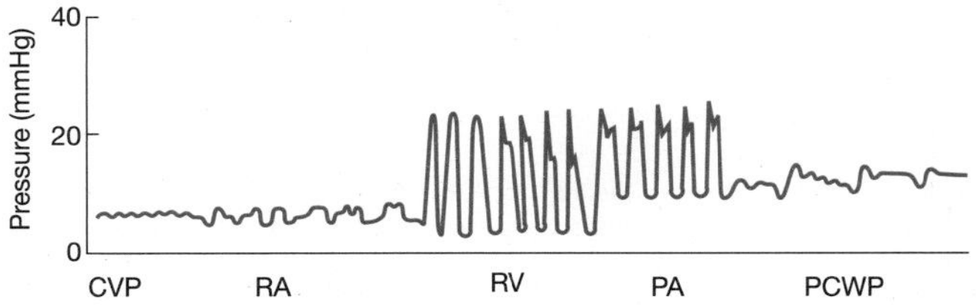

Fig. 4 Pressure tracings obtained on insertion of a pulmonary artery flotation catheter. CVP, central venous pressure, RA, right atrium, RV, right ventricle, PA, pulmonary artery, PCWP, pulmonary capillary wedge pressure.

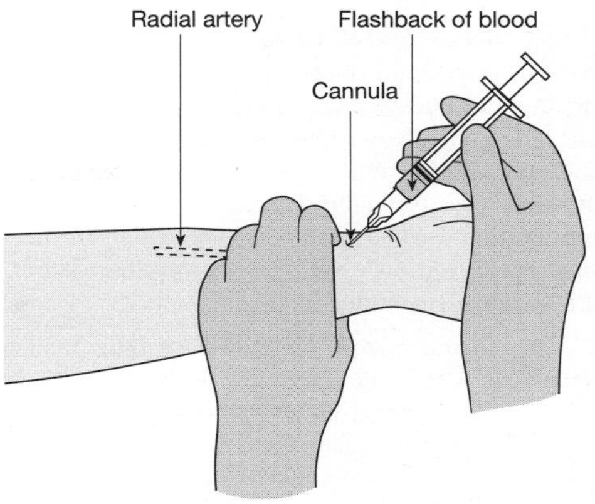

Fig. 5 Puncture of the radial artery.

10.1.5 Arterial puncture/cannulation

Before attempting to puncture or cannulate the radial artery, check the patency of the ulnar artery by applying pressure to the radial artery and asking the patient to clench their fist firmly. On relaxing the fist, the hand should pink up within 10 s (Allen test).

A 25G needle (orange) is perfectly adequate to obtain an arterial blood gas (ABG) sample from a radial artery. 18G (green) or 23G (blue) is needed for a femoral sample. Use either a preheparinized ABG syringe or draw up 1 ml of 1000 u/ml heparin into a syringe and then completely expel the heparin.

Lay the index and middle fingers of your non-dominant hand along the line of the artery as a guide (Fig. 5). For radial and brachial samples, hold the syringe at 45 to 60° to the skin and slowly advance in the line of the artery. For femoral samples, hold the syringe at 90° to the skin. A flash of blood into the syringe indicates successful puncture. Some syringes will fill to a predetermined volume, others require aspiration of 1 to 2 ml.

After successful arterial puncture, press on the site for 3 min (5 if anticoagulated) to prevent haematoma formation.

Arterial cannulation may be performed either with a cannula over a needle (similar to a venflon) or with a Seldinger technique. After preparation of the skin and insertion of local anaesthetic, the method of arterial puncture should be as described above, with the exception that for all arterial cannulations the needle should be inserted at 45° to the artery. Once arterial puncture has been confirmed, the cannula should be advanced over the needle, or the guidewire passed directly into the artery and the cannula then advanced over the guidewire.

10.2 Cardiac procedures

10.2.1 DC cardioversion

Synchronized cardioversion is the treatment of choice for symptomatic tachyarrhythmias. Conscious patients must be anaesthetized or sedated. Suitable monitoring and facilities for dealing with cardiac arrest should be available. Modern defibrillators incorporate a switch that allows the shock to be synchronised with the R wave of the ECG to reduce the risk of inducing ventricular fibrillation. Gel pads should be applied to the chest wall and cardioversion carried out in the same manner as for defibrillation. The energy required depends on the underlying rhythm. Synchronization means that there may be a delay between pressing the defibrillator buttons and the discharge of the shock when the next R wave occurs.

10.2.2 Cardiac pacing (temporary)

Indications for emergency/acute temporary cardiac pacing are shown in Table 24.

10.2.2.1 External (transcutaneous) pacing

10.2.2.1.1 Percussion pacing Percussion pacing can be used as a temporising measure in some patients with profound bradycardia causing clinical cardiac arrest. It is particularly useful for ventricular standstill where P waves are visible on the ECG. A series of gentle blows should be applied to the lower left sternal edge using the closed fist. Using trial and error, a site can sometimes be found which results in stimulation of the ventricular myocardium. If percussion does not produce a cardiac output, orthodox pacing or CPR should be instituted immediately.

10.2.2.1.2 Transcutaneous pacing Most modern transcutaneous pacing systems are integrated with an ECG monitor/defibrillator. Pacemaker electrodes should be placed in either an anterior-posterior position or in the conventional anterior-lateral configuration. The pacemaker should be set to demand pacing to prevent a stimulus from falling on the T wave following a sponteaneous heart beat, with the rate set at 60 to 90/min for adults. The pacemaker current should be set at the lowest setting and gradually increased to obtain capture of the myocardium and a palpable pulse. The current required to obtain capture is generally in the range 50 to 100 mA and will produce painful contraction of the patient's skeletal muscle. Conscious patients will require analgesia and/or sedation. If capture of the myocardium does not occur, alternative electrode placement should be tried.

Transcutaneous pacing is only a temporizing measure and arrangements should be made for urgent transvenous pacing.

10.2.2.2 Transvenous pacing (ventricular)

Temporary transvenous pacing can be achieved after cannulation of any central vein, but is most easily performed via the right internal jugular, right subclavian or right femoral vein, which can be cannulated as described in sections 10.1.1, 10.1.2 and 10.1.3.

The conventional Seldinger technique of guidewire and dilators is used to allow placement of a sheath (preferably haemostatic) of sufficient size to accept passage of the pacing wire in the vein that has been cannulated. The pacing wire is passed down the sheath and advanced towards the heart, the aim being to maneouvre it under fluoroscopic guidance into a position where its tip is at the apex of the right ventricule, angulated slightly downwards. Key aspects of the technique are shown in Fig. 6. Common problems and their solutions are described in Table 25.

After positioning the pacing wire, set the pacemaker to a rate of 70/min, or 10/min above the patient's ventricular rate, and to deliver a pulse of 3 V (or as directed by the manufacturer). A correctly positioned electrode should 'capture', such that each pacing spike is followed by a ventricular complex on the ECG. Establish the voltage threshold by gradually turning down the amplitude of the voltage delivered until capture is lost, which will usually be in the range 0.7 to1.0 V. To allow a safety margin, it is then appropriate in most circumstances to set the pacemaker to deliver a voltage of at least twice the threshold. Sensing can be checked only if there is spontaneous ventricular activity: this is best done by setting the pacemaker rate to between10 and 20/min below the spontaneous ventricular rate and looking on the ECG monitor and the pulse generator for evidence of pacing inhibition. Sensitivity is usually set to to its maximum. Common problems and their solutions are described in Table 26.

When the pacing wire is positioned appropriately and pacing is established, carefully remove the introducer sheath (in most cases), secure the wire with a strong suture (usually 2/0 silk), loop it once or twice on the skin, and then dress with a clear adhesive dressing.

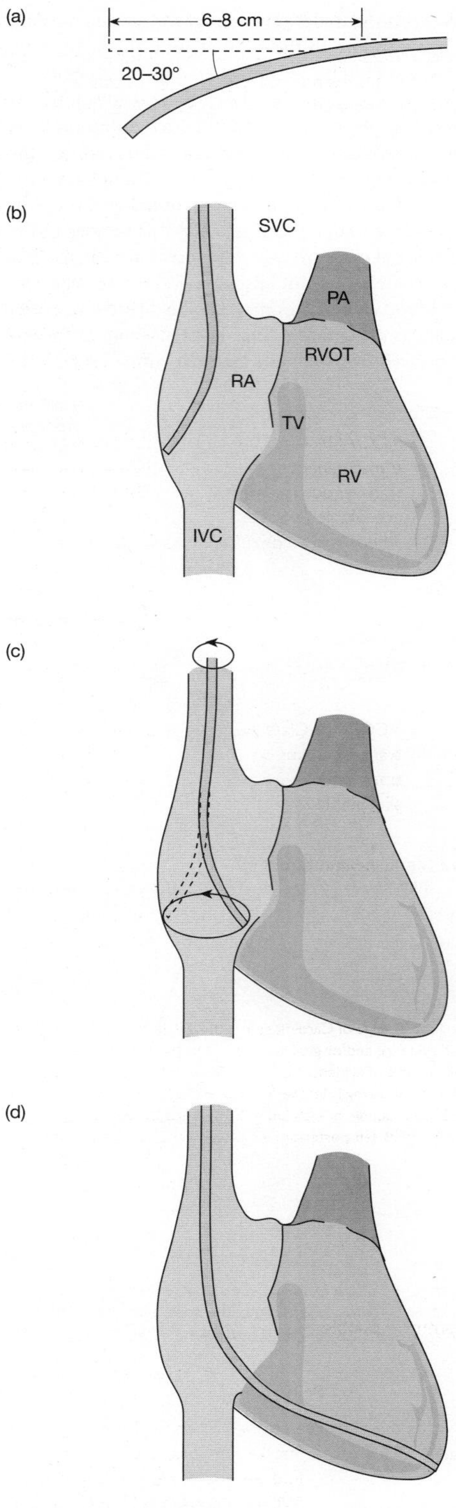

Fig. 6 Correct positioning of the electrode is helped if there is a 20 to 30° curve at the tip of the pacing wire. Mould the electrode to this shape using your fingers: it may need to be bent or straightened depending on its packaging. (a). Advance the wire until it lies vertically in the right atrium. It will usually assume a position where its tip points towards the free wall on the right side (b). Rotate the wire between your index finger and thumb until it points towards the patient's left (c). When it has done so, advance the wire steadily: it should pass through the tricuspid valve and along the floor of the right ventricle to the apex (d). SVC, superior vena cava; RA, right atrium; IVC, inferior vena cava; TV, tricuspid valve; RV, right ventricle; RVOT, right ventricular outflow tract.

Table 24 Indications for emergency/acute temporary cardiac pacing

Acute myocardial infarction	ACC/AHA Class I—transvenous pacing required	• Symptomatic bradycardia (sinus bradycardia with hypotension and type I second degree AV block with hypotension not responding to atropine) • Bilateral bundle branch block (alternating BBB or RBBB with alternating LAHB/LPHB) • New or indeterminate age bifascicular block with first degree AV block • Mobitz type II second degree AV block
	ACC/AHA Class IIa—transcutaneous or transvenous pacing acceptable (except where indicated)	• RBBB with LAHB or LPHB (new or indeterminate) • RBBB with first degree AV block • LBBB (new or indeterminate) • Recurrent sinus pauses (>3 s) not responsive to atropine • Incessant VT, for atrial or ventricular overdrive pacing (transvenous pacing required)
	ACC/AHA Class IIb—transcutaneous or transvenous pacing acceptable	• Bifascicular block of indeterminate age • New or indeterminate age RBBB
Bradycardia not associated with myocardial infarction	Transvenous pacing	• Asystole • Second or third degree AV block with haemodynamic disturbance or syncope at rest • Ventricular tachyarrhythmia secondary to bradycardia

ACC/AHA, American College of Cardiology/American Heart Association. Class I, conditions for which there is evidence and/or general agreement that pacing is beneficial, useful and effective. Class IIa, weight of evidence/opinion in favour of usefulness/efficacy of pacing. Class IIb, usefulness/efficacy of pacing is less well established by evidence/opinion. BBB, bundle branch block. LBBB, left bundle branch block. RBBB, right bundle branch block. LAHB, left anterior hemiblock. LPHB, left posterior hemiblock. AV, atrioventricular block. VT, ventricular tachycardia.

Table 25 Common problems in temporary transvenous ventricular pacing.

Problem	Possible solution
Wire will not cross the tricuspid valve	Feed the wire into the right atrium until it 'catches' and forms a large loop. It may pass into the IVC (if approaching from above) or SVC (if approaching from below), in which case it will need to be pulled back and then pushed forward until it does catch. When a large loop has been formed, rotate the wire until its tip flips through into the ventricle
Intubation of the coronary sinus	The wire appears to be in the right ventricle, but (sometimes) will not capture the ventricle at an acceptable output. On fluoroscopy the electrode tip is directed upwards and towards the left shoulder (and on a lateral chest radiograph is directed posteriorly rather than anteriorly). If satisfactory pacing cannot be obtained, then the pacing wire must be withdrawn into the right atrium and further attempts made to advance it across the tricuspid valve
Wire is in the right ventricle, but it is difficult to get it positioned at the apex	Pass the tip of the wire into the right ventricular outflow tract, then gently withdraw it whilst rotating between index finger and thumb. When the tip is angulated downwards, advance towards the apex of the ventricle Note that it can be difficult to get a good position at the apex if the pacing wire is too bent to start off with, hence the injunction to mould the tip with the fingers to obtain an angulation of 20–30° at the beginning of the procedure

Table 26 Failure to pace

Problem	Causes	Solution
No spikes seen and no output	Battery/generator failure Loose connections Oversensing	Replace battery/generator Check and tighten Reduce sensitivity or go to fixed rate pacing
Spikes seen, but no capture	Loose connections Exit block (high threshold)	Check and tighten Increase output. Check position of pacing wire (by fluoroscopy or plain radiograph). Consider re-positioning of electrode

Further reading

Fitzpatrick A, Sutton R (1992). A guide to temporary pacing. *British Medical Journal* **304**, 365–9.

Gammage MD (2000). Electrophysiology: temporary cardiac pacing. *Heart* **83**, 715–20.

10.2.3 Pericardiocentesis

Cardiac tamponade is the indication for pericardiocentesis as an emergency. Unless the patient is *in extremis* the procedure should, whenever possible, be performed with echocardiographic guidance by an operator experienced in the technique, as follows:

(1) Two-dimensional echocardiography is used to assess the size, distribution and haemodynamic effect of the effusion.

(2) The ideal entry site for pericardiocentesis is the point on the skin where the effusion is closest to the transducer and the fluid accumulation is maximal. The distance from the skin to the pericardial space is estimated, with the needle trajectory defined by the angulation of the hand-held transducer. A straight path that best avoids vital structures (also the internal mammary artery, which lies 3 to 5 cm lateral to the sternal margin) is chosen.

(3) After preparation of the skin and insertion of local anaesthetic, a 16 to 18 gauge polytef-sheathed (or similar) needle attached to a saline-filled syringe is advanced in the predetermined trajectory, with continued

gentle aspiration as it moves forward. On entering the pericardial fluid, the needle is advanced approximately 2 mm further, when the sheath is advanced over the needle and the steel core withdrawn.

(4) The position of the sheath in the pericardial space can be confirmed by injecting 5 ml of agitated saline through it, whilst observing the pericardial space with 2D-echocardiography (optional).

(5) Intrapericardial pressure can be directly measured with a manometer (optional); pericardial fluid can be sent for diagnostic tests (optional).

(6) A guidewire is advanced through the polytef sheath, which is removed over the guidewire. A small stab incision of the skin is made at the entry site, following which dilators are used to allow the insertion of a larger sheath (6–8 F) through which a pigtail angiocatheter can be introduced. After the pigtail catheter has been inserted the introducer sheath is removed, leaving only the smooth-walled pigtail catheter in the pericardial space. (Note that this technique is preferred to that of introducing the pigtail catheter directly over the guidewire because the catheter tip can occasionally pull the guidewire out of the pericardial sac, particularly if this is sclerotic.)

(7) Pericardial fluid is drained completely by syringe suction and the pericardial catheter is secured to the chest wall by suture and appropriate dressing.

(8) If left on continuous drainage, pericardial catheters become plugged. It is therefore better to perform intermittent aspiration, every 4 to 6 h or as clinically indicated, leaving the catheter flushed with saline in between times. It can be removed when drainage has been reduced to less than 25 to 30 ml/day and follow-up echocardiography shows no significant residual effusion (sooner if the catheter is causing problems).

If the patient is *in extremis* and/or echocardiography (with appropriate expertise) is not available, then a 'blind' subxiphoid approach is most often used:

(1) Sit the patient up at an angle of 45°.

(2) Insert the needle 3 cm below the xiphisternum at an angle of 30 to 45° to the skin and advance, applying gentle suction all the time (as above), in a line towards the patient's left shoulder.

(3) If the needle touches the heart, it will usually provoke ectopic beats. Some authorities recommend that the aspiration needle is attached to the 'V' lead terminal of an ECG cable (using insulated wire with a clip on each end, or simply with sticky tape) to allow continuous monitoring. If the needle touches the heart, then the character of the ECG changes, most particularly with the appearance of gross ST-segment elevation if the needle touches the right or left ventricle.

(4) When fluid is obtained, proceed as described above.

Further reading

Tsang TS, Freeman WK, Sinak LJ, Seward JB (1998). Echocardiographically guided pericardiocentesis: evolution and state-of-the-art technique. *Mayo Clinic Proceedings* **73**, 647–52.

10.3 Arterial blood gases (Table 27)

Table 27 Parameters that may be measured or derived by blood gas machines

Normal range	Notes
pO_2	
>10.6 kPa (80 mmHg), when breathing air	(1) Can only be interpreted if the inspired oxygen concentration is known (2) Hypoxia defined as po_2 <8 kPa when patient breathing air. (3) If patient is breathing with supplemental oxygen, a 'hypoxaemia score' can be calculated as:
	Hypoxaemia score = po_2 (mmHg)/Fio_2
	If a patient was breathing air and had a po_2 at the lower limit of the normal range, then their hypoxaemia score would equal 10.6 × 7.6/0.21, or about 380. If they had a po_2 of 8 kPa, then their hypoxaemia score would be 8 × 7.6/0.21, or about 290
	In assessing a patient breathing supplemental oxygen a value of <300 is usually taken as indicating significant compromise (Note: 1 kPa = 7.6 mmHg)
pCO_2	
4.7–6.0 kPa (35–45 mmHg)	(1) po_2 < 8 kPa with pco_2 < 6.5 kPa = type 1 respiratory failure. (2) po_2 < 8 kPa with pco_2 > 6.5 kPa = type 2 respiratory failure (3) Low pco_2 indicates hyperventilation, which may be primary or secondary, the latter being indicated by a base excess more negative than −2 (see below) (4) High pco_2 indicates hypoventilation, which may be primary or secondary, the latter being indicated by a base excess more positive than +2 (see below)
pH	
7.37–7.43	(1) pH < 7.35 defines acidosis (2) pH > 7.45 defines alkalosis
H^+	
37–43 nmol/l	(1) H^+ >45 nmol/l defines acidosis (2) H^+ <35 nmol/l defines alkalosis
HCO_3^-	
19–24 mmol/l	(1) Measurement of arterial or venous (normal range 22–28 mmol/l in plasma) bicarbonate concentration is often helpful in analysis of patients with acid-base disturbance 2. Changes in bicarbonate concentration occur slowly (over many hours or days), hence evidence of compensatory change, e.g. high bicarbonate concentration in the patient with elevated pco_2, indicates that the respiratory abnormality is chronic

Table 27 Continued

Base excess	
+2 to −2 mmol/l	Are measured abnormalities of pH or pco_2 due to metabolic or respiratory processes?
	Many blood gas machines display a value for the base excess (or deficit), which is a value derived from primary (directly measured) data using an algorithm, the principles of which are as follows:
	(1) Predict the pH that would arise in normal blood in the presence of the pco_2 actually measured: if the pco_2 is high, then the predicted pH is low, and vice versa (2) Calculate the amount of acid or base that would have to be added to the blood to change the predicted pH to the pH measured. This is the base deficit/excess and an estimate of the degree of 'metabolic' as opposed to 'respiratory' disturbance. A base excess more negative than −2 indicates metabolic acidosis; a value more positive than +2 indicates metabolic alkalosis

10.4 Airway and respiratory procedures

10.4.1 Mechanical support of ventilation

10.4.1.1 Continuous positive airways pressure

Continual positive airway pressure (CPAP) exerts a dilating force on the upper airway (hence its use in obstructive sleep apnoea), and also recruits collapsed alveoli and increases functional residual capacity. This improves lung compliance, reducing the work of breathing, which is a benefit in a range of clinical circumstances.

CPAP can be used for patients with acute or acute on chronic hypoxaemia who are not exhausted or in ventilatory failure (meaning elevated pco_2), e.g. acute pulmonary oedema, postoperative atalectasis, pneumonia. It is not appropriate and is contraindicated for patients who are too obtunded to cooperate, who are unable to protect their airway, who have haemodynamic instability or life-threatening arrhythmias, life-threatening hypoxaemia, or exhaustion.

CPAP is applied via a tight fitting face or nose mask, the usual range for pressure being 2.5 to 10 cmH_2O. Once applied, patient comfort, respiratory rate and arterial blood gases should be monitored. Some patients are unable to tolerate the face mask: gastric distension, vomiting, aspiration, eye irritation, conjunctivitis, and facial-skin necrosis are other complications.

10.4.1.2 Non-invasive positive pressure ventilation

Masks that are used for CPAP can also be used to provide non-invasive positive pressure ventilation (NIPPV, often more simply referred to as NIV). The difference between the two treatments is that in CPAP a constant pressure is applied to the airway, but no airflow occurs in the absence of respiratory muscle activity. By contrast, in NIV a pulse of positive pressure is applied to assist respiration, the usual arrangement being that this is triggered by a sensor that detects a fall in pressure in the facial mask when the patient initiates a breath. If a positive pressure is also applied in the expiratory phase (EPAP) in addition to the pulse delivered to support inspiration, then then this is known as bilevel pressure support (BIPAP).

Contraindications for and complications of NIV are the same as those for CPAP.

10.4.1.3 Invasive ventilation

Invasive ventilation may be applied via a tracheal tube or tracheostomy. Ventilation can be adjusted by altering the minute volume (respiratory rate × tidal volume). Oxygenation is adjusted by altering inspired oxygen concentration and positive end-expiratory pressure (PEEP, which acts in a similar manner to CPAP by recruiting collapsed alveoli and reducing the work of breathing). Most ventilators for adults are volume generators that deliver a fixed tidal volume regardless of changes in lung mechanics. If the lungs become stiffer, then inflation pressure will increase to deliver the same tidal volume.

The change from inspiration to expiration is usually time cycled; that from expiration to inspiration is usually either time cycled or triggered by the patient if they are breathing spontaneously. The following values can be used as a guide when initially setting up a ventilator for an adult:

- Tidal volume should be 10–15 ml/kg
- Respiratory rate 10–12/min
- Ratio of inspiratory to expiratory time (I:E ratio) set at 1:2, but for patients with chronic obstructive pulmonary disease or asthma, a smaller I:E ratio is often used (e.g. 1:3) to prevent gas trapping and hyperinflation.
- Concentration of inspired oxygen depends on the clinical context: the patient with normal lungs who requires respiratory support because of respiratory muscle weakness does not need a high $F\text{io}_2$ (start with say 28 per cent), whereas the patient with severe problems with gas exchange, eg. bilateral pneumonia or acute respiratory distress syndrome, will require a high $F\text{io}_2$ (start with say 60–80 per cent).

Once ventilation is established, the various parameters should be adjusted (and others added, e.g. CPAP) according to the patient's clinical condition and the results of repeated measurement of arterial blood gases.

10.4.2 Management of the airway

10.4.2.1 Endotracheal intubation

Endotracheal intubation remains the gold standard for airway management as it provides a method of oxygenating and ventilating the patient, whilst securing the airway from vomitus and secretions.

Intubation should be preceded by ventilation with high concentration oxygen. The neck should be slightly flexed and the head extended (an assistant holding the neck in a neutral position if trauma to the cervical spine is suspected). The mouth should be inspected for loose teeth or dentures, which should be removed, as should any secretions or vomitus (by suction). A trained assistant should apply cricoid pressure to prevent passive regurgitation.

The laryngoscope should be introduced over the right side of the tongue, moving the tongue to the left. The tip of the blade should be positioned in the valecula (between the epiglottis and the base of the tongue) and lifted upwards and away from the operator to expose the vocal cords (Fig. 7(a)). The endotracheal tube should be introduced so that the cuff is positioned just beyond the cords (Fig. 7(b)).

After successful intubation, the patient should be ventilated with high concentration oxygen, the endotracheal tube secured and the tube cuff inflated. Positioning of the endotracheal tube should be confirmed by listening over the apices and the bases of the lungs, and over the stomach. If available, an end-tidal carbon dioxide monitor should be attached to the endotracheal tube.

10.4.2.2 Laryngeal mask airway

The laryngeal mask airway (LMA) is used widely in routine anaesthetic practice and is increasingly used for immediate airway management in cardiac arrest. Pulmonary aspiration associated with the use of a LMA is uncommon provided high inflation pressures are avoided.

The patient should be supine with the neck slightly flexed and the head extended (an assistant holding the neck in a neutral position if trauma to the cervical spine is suspected). The LMA should be held like a pen, and introduced into the mouth with the distal aperture facing towards the patient's feet. The tip should be applied to the palate and advanced until it reaches the posterior pharynx. The LMA is then pressed backwards and downwards until the resistance of the hypopharynx is felt (Fig. 8), when the cuff of the LMA should be inflated. If insertion is satisfactory, the end of the LMA will rise slightly. Positioning of the LMA should be confirmed by listening over the apices and the bases of the lungs, and over the stomach. If available, an end-tidal carbon dioxide monitor should be attached.

10.4.2.3 Cricothyroidotomy

10.4.2.3.1 Needle cricothyroidotomy Insertion of a needle or a cannula (typically a large bore intravenous cannula) through the cricothyroid membrane is a useful emergency technique that allows short-term provision of oxygen until a definitive airway can be placed. The cannula should be connected to high flow oxygen with either a Y connector or a side hole cut into the tubing between the cannula and the oxygen supply (Fig. 9). Intermittent insufflation can be achieved by closing the Y connector or side hole with a thumb for one second and then releasing it for three seconds. Inadequate exhalation leads to accumulation of carbon dioxide, hence this technique of ventilation can only be used for 30 to 45 minutes.

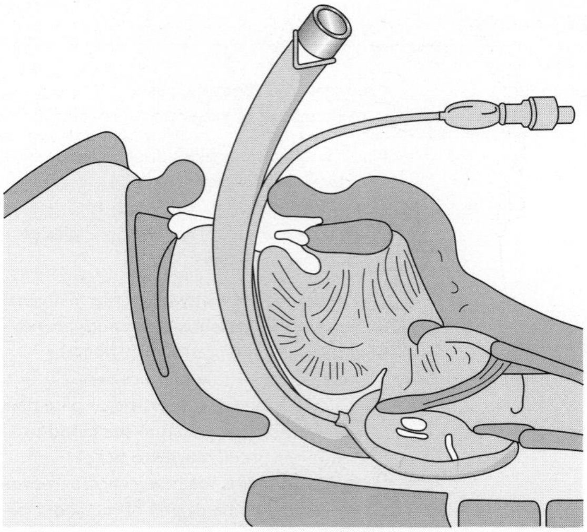

Fig. 8 Laryngeal mask airway inserted into the hypopharynx. The inflated cuff surrounds and isolates the entrance to the larynx.

10.4.2.3.2 Surgical cricothyroidotomy The skin over the cricothyroid membrane should be cleaned and local anaesthetic inserted (in patients who are conscious). A horizontal skin incision is made and extended through the cricothyroid membrane (Fig. 10). A curved haemostat (forceps) is then used to dilate the opening and a small, cuffed endotracheal tube or tracheostomy tube inserted. The position of the tube should be confirmed by auscultation of the lungs and over the stomach, and the tube then secured.

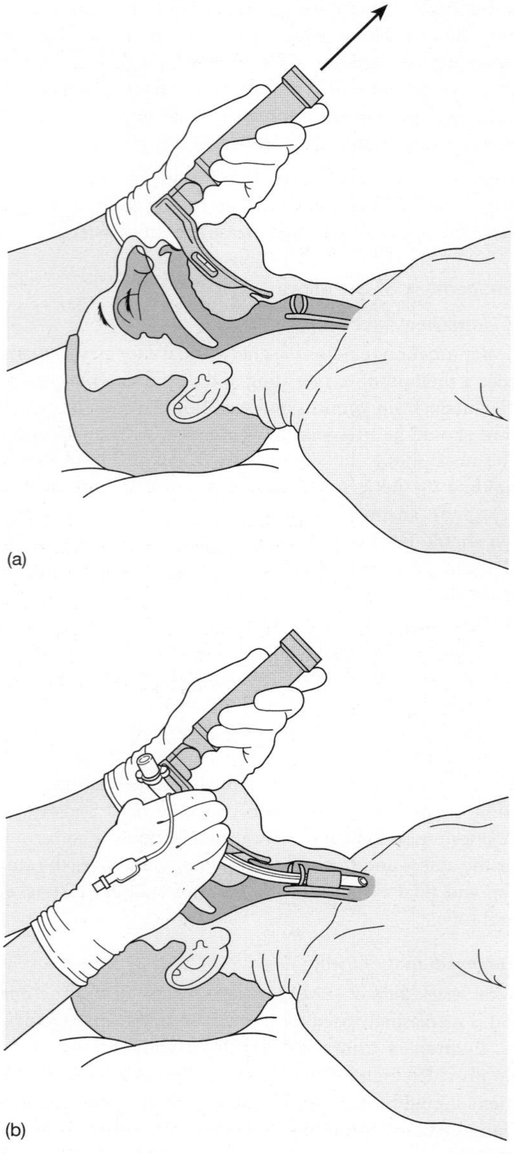

Fig. 7 (a) Position of the laryngoscope before insertion of the endotracheal tube. (b) Placement of the endotracheal tube.

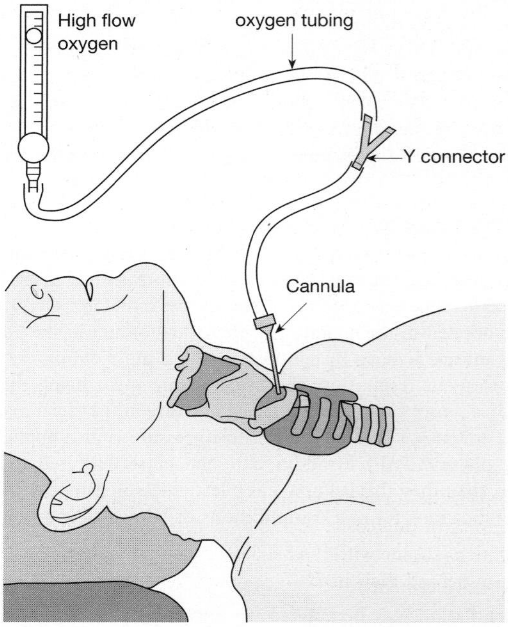

Fig. 9 Oxygenation via a cannula through the cricothyroid membrane.

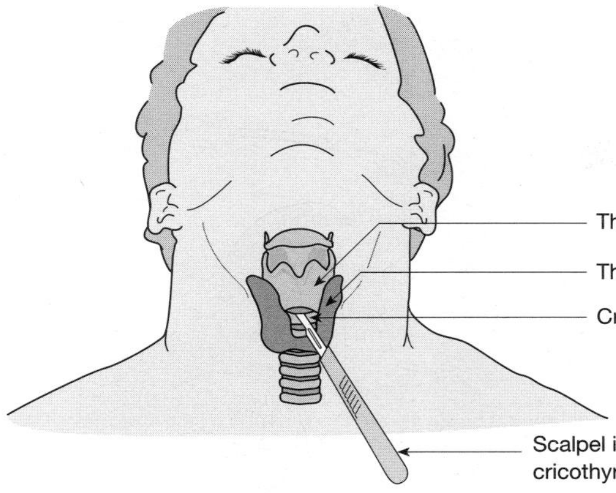

Fig. 10 Technique of surgical cricothyroidotomy.

10.4.3 Percutaneous procedures on the chest

10.4.3.1 Chest decompression

The rapidly deteriorating patient with clinical signs of a tension pneumothorax requires immediate needle decompression of the chest. The second intercostal space on the side of the tension pneumothorax should be identified, and an over the needle cannula or any hollow needle should be inserted in the midclavicular line, directing it just superior to the rib into the intercostal space. Listen for a sudden escape of air when the needle enters the pleural cavity. The cannula should be secured and arrangements made for an intercostal drain to be inserted as soon as the tension pneumothorax has been decompressed.

10.4.3.2 Chest aspiration

Chest aspiration may be considered for any symptomatic spontaneous pneumothorax, irrespective of its size. The advantages over intercostal tube drainage are that, if successful, needle aspiration means a shorter hospital stay, less pain, and less scarring.

The British Thoracic Society guidelines recommend an anterior approach using the second intercostal space in the midclavicular line. Other authors recommend a posterior approach, with the patient in a sitting position with the arms gripping the knees, and using the secone, third, or fourth intercostal space medial to the scapula.

The skin should be prepared and local anesthetic infiltrated down to the pleura. A 16 G cannula is inserted perpendicular to the skin and just over the superior border of the rib. The cannula is then connected to a three-way tap, the second port of which is connected to a 50 ml syringe, and the third to a length of tubing that runs to open under the surface a container of sterile water (Fig. 11). Aspiration should be continued until either resistance is felt or the patient coughs excessively.

The success (or otherwise) of aspiration can be determined by repeat chest radiography. The procedure may be repeated if not successful or if the pneumothorax recurs. Success is less likely for older patients and in those with chronic lung disease or recurrent pneumothorax, also after aspiration of more than 2.5 litres.

10.4.3.3 Chest drain

Always confirm the correct side for chest tube insertion. The usual site is the fourth to sixth intercostal space anterior to the midaxillary line. Position the patient supine with the head of the bed slightly elevated and the patient's arm behind their head. Clean and drape the area for tube insertion.

Infiltrate local anaesthetic down to the parietal pleura (10–20 ml of 1 per cent lignocaine). Make a 2 to 3 cm transverse incision at the site and blunt dissect through the subcutaneous tissues, just over the superior surface of the rib. Puncture the parietal pleura with the end of the dissection forceps and insert a gloved finger into the incision to ensure that the pleural space has been entered.

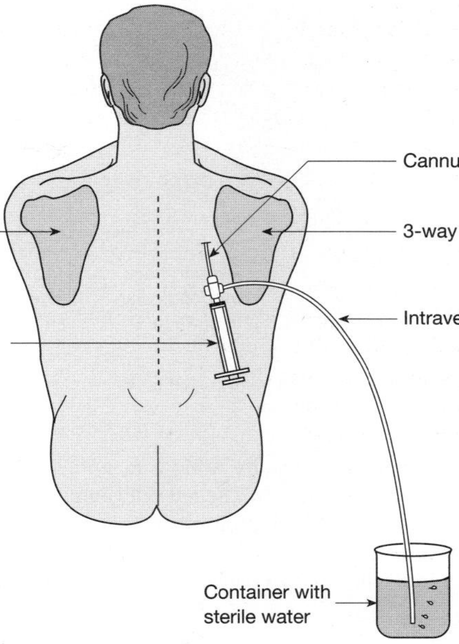

Fig. 11 Chest aspiration (posterior approach).

Remove the trocar from the intercostal drain and slide the drain over your finger into the pleural cavity, when 'fogging' of the tube should be seen. Connect the end of the intercostal tube to an underwater-seal apparatus and confirm correct placement by ensuring that the fluid level is swinging with respiration.

Insert two 3/0 monfilament sutures at 90° to the line of the skin incision, one on either side of the chest drain, but do not tie them. They will be used to close the skin when the chest drain is removed (and are much better than a purse string suture, which produces an unsightly scar, for this purpose). Suture the tube in place with a separate 1/0 or 2/0 silk suture, tied around it as many times as its length allows. If the skin incision is gaping on either side of the drain, close this with one or more 3/0 sutures. Place a gauze dressing around the site and secure with strong tape, wrapping some of this around the tube to secure it firmly.

Obtain a chest radiograph to confirm satisfactory placement and effect of the chest drain.

10.5 Lumbar puncture

Ensure that there are no contraindications to lumbar puncture (LP), namely raised intracranial pressure, bleeding tendency, local sepsis, posterior fossa or spinal cord mass lesion.

The patient should be positioned on the bed (Fig. 12(a)) with their knees drawn up towards the chest to open the space between the spinous processes and with their spine parallel to the bed. Prepare and drape the skin and locate the puncture site (L3/L4 or L4/L5).

Anaesthetize the skin and subcutaneous tissues using 5 to 10 ml of 1 per cent lignocaine. Insert the LP needle at 90° to the skin. Advance slowly, aiming between two spinous processes (Fig. 12(b)). As the needle enters the dural space, there is a slight loss of resistance. Remove the stylet and ensure that CSF drips freely from the needle. If it does not, insert the stylet and advance the needle a few millimetres then check again.

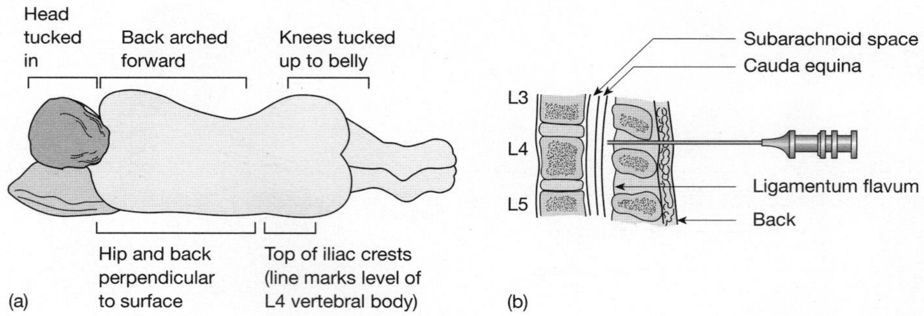

Fig. 12 (a) The patient should lie curled up to increase the spave between the vertebrae. (b) The needle should be slowly advanced until it penetrates the ligamentum flavum.

Check the opening CSF pressure using a manometer (normally 6–15 cmH_2O) then collect CSF samples. The red cell count in consecutive samples can sometimes help to distinguish subarachnoid haemorrhage from a bloody tap, but this is not always reliable and the sample should also be examined for xanthochromia (oxyhaemoglobin and bilirubin) when subarachnoid haemorrhage is possible. Always send blood samples for glucose and protein estimation at the same time, the CSF glucose concentration normally being 60 to 80 per cent of the blood level.

The patient should be asked to remain lying flat for 2 to 4 h to reduce the severity of post-LP headache.

Index

Note: Numbers 1., 2. and 3. preceding the page numbers denote the volume. Numbers in italic refer to tables and/or illustrations separate from the text.